Appendices From CVT XIII on website

Appendix III   AAFCO Dog and Cat Food Nutrient Profiles

The following tables are provided for reference purposes only. Although these data may be useful when interpreting clinical laboratory samples, some of the methods referenced in the footnotes have been supplanted by newer techniques. Thus the reader must use care when extrapolating between methodologies. In some cases, the studies cited have not been repeated with new analyzers, so although the general trends are still relevant, the exact values may vary considerably due to differences in instrumentation. The clinician should always consult the reference standards provided by the laboratory or the analyzer manufacturer when interpreting results of laboratory tests. Additionally all laboratory results should be viewed in the context of the specific patient and recent or current treatments.

Appendix IV   Hematology—Coulter S Plus IV with Manual Differential Counts

Appendix V   Hematology—Technicon H-1 Hematology Analyzer

Appendix VI   Système International (SI) Units in Hematology

Appendix VII   Hematology—Manual or Semiautomated Methods

Appendix VIII   Canine Hematology (Means) at Different Ages—Manual or Semiautomated Methods

Appendix IX   Canine Hematology (Means and Ranges) with Different Ages and Genders—Manual or Semiautomated Methods

Appendix X   Canine Hematology at Different Ages

Appendix XI   Effects of Pregnancy and Lactation on Canine Hematology (Means)

Appendix XII   Relative Distribution of Cell Types in Canine Bone Marrow

Appendix XIII   Feline Hematology (Means and Ranges) with Different Ages and Genders—Manual or Semiautomated Methods

Appendix XIV   Feline Hematology (Means) at Different Ages

Appendix XV   Effects of Pregnancy and Lactation on Feline Hematology (Means)

Appendix XVI   Relative Distribution of Cell Types in Feline Bone Marrow

Appendix XVII   Clinical Chemistry—Hitachi 911

Appendix XVIII   Clinical Chemistry—Selected Manual Procedures

Appendix XIX   Système International (SI) Units in Clinical Chemistry

Appendix XX   Serum Protein Fractions

Appendix XXI   Serum Iron and Iron-Binding Capacities in Iron-Deficient and Normal Dogs

Appendix XXII   Serum Immunoglobulin Concentrations of Normal Beagle Dogs at Various Ages

Appendix XXIII   Acid-Base and Blood Gases

Appendix XXIV   Coagulation Screening Tests

Appendix XXV   Specific Coagulation Tests

Appendix XXVI   Quantitative Tests of Gastrointestinal Function

Appendix XXVII   Tests of the Endocrine System

Appendix XXVIII Système International (SI) Units for Hormone Assays

Appendix XXIX   Urinary and Renal Function Tests

Appendix XXX   Bronchoalveolar Lavage Fluid Cell Populations

Appendix XXXI   Cerebrospinal Fluid (CSF)

Appendix XXXII   Cerebrospinal Fluid Biochemical Analytes in Histologically Normal Cats

Appendix XXXIII Characteristics of Body Cavity Fluids in Healthy Dogs and Cats

Appendix XXXIV   Cytologic Findings in Normal and Abnormal Canine Synovial Fluids

Appendix XXXV   Canine Semen

Appendix XXXVI   Canine Prostatic Fluid (Third Fraction)

Appendix XXXVII Electrocardiography

D1710823

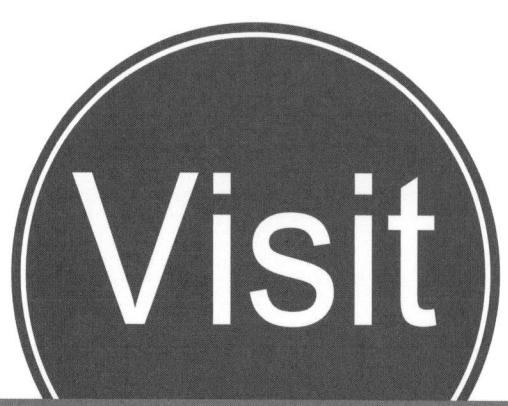
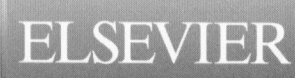

KIRK'S

CURRENT
VETERINARY
THERAPY
XV

KIRK'S
CURRENT VETERINARY THERAPY XV

Editors

**John D. Bonagura, DVM, MS, DACVIM
(Cardiology, Internal Medicine)**
Professor
Department of Veterinary Clinical Sciences
College of Veterinary Medicine
The Ohio State University
Head, Cardiology and Interventional Medicine Service
The Ohio State University Veterinary Medical Center
Columbus, Ohio

**David C. Twedt, DVM, DACVIM
(Internal Medicine)**
Professor
Department of Clinical Sciences
College of Veterinary Medicine and Biomedical Sciences
Colorado State University
Fort Collins, Colorado

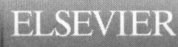

ELSEVIER
SAUNDERS

3251 Riverport Lane
St. Louis, Missouri 63043

Notice

Knowledge and best practice in this field are constantly changing. As new research and
experience broaden our knowledge, changes in practice, treatment and drug therapy may
become necessary or appropriate. Readers are advised to check the most current
information provided (i) on procedures featured or (ii) by the manufacturer of each
product to be administered, to verify the recommended dose or formula, the method and
duration of administration, and contraindications. It is the responsibility of the
practitioner, relying on their own experience and knowledge of the patient, to make
diagnoses, to determine dosages and the best treatment for each individual patient, and to
take all appropriate safety precautions. To the fullest extent of the law, neither the
Publisher nor the Editor assumes any liability for any injury and/or damage to persons or
property arising out of or related to any use of the material contained in this book.

The Publisher

A Note about Drug Dosages

Some chapters include dosage recommendations that may differ from information contained
in the drug formulary found in Appendix I: *Table of Common Drugs: Approximate Dosages*,
beginning on page 1307. We acknowledge the expertise of our individual chapter authors
and want to share their individual preferences with you. We have taken great care to ensure
the accuracy of all dosages provided throughout *Kirk's Current Veterinary Therapy XV*.

Vice President and Publisher: Linda Duncan
Content Strategy Director: Penny Rudolph
Content Manager: Shelly Stringer
Publishing Services Manager: Catherine Jackson
Senior Project Manager: David Stein
Design Direction: Paula Catalano

Printed in the United States

Last digit is the print number: 9 8 7 6 5 4 3 2 1

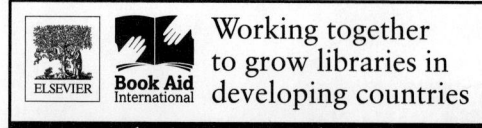

Working together
to grow libraries in
developing countries

www.elsevier.com • www.bookaid.org

Consulting Editors

Section I: Critical Care
Elisa M. Mazzaferro, MS, DVM, PhD, DACVECC
Staff Criticalist
Cornell University Veterinary Specialists
Stamford, Connecticut
Hyperthermia and Heat-Induced Illness

Section II: Toxicologic Diseases
Michael J. Murphy, DVM, JD, PhD
Professor Emeritus
University of Minnesota
Stillwater, Minnesota
Rodenticide Toxicoses
Nephrotoxicants
Small Animal Poisoning: Additional Considerations Related to Legal Claims
Sources of Help for Toxicosis
Treatment of Animal Toxicoses: Regulatory Points to Consider

Section III: Endocrine and Metabolic Diseases
Ellen N. Behrend, VMD, PhD, DACVIM
Jozey Griffin Professor
Clinical Sciences
Auburn University
Auburn, Alabama
Occult Hyperadrenocorticism: Is It Real?
Interpretation of Endocrine Diagnostic Test Results for Adrenal and Thyroid Disease

Robert J. Kemppainen, DVM, PhD
Professor
Anatomy, Physiology and Pharmacology
Auburn University College of Veterinary Medicine
Auburn, Alabama
Interpretation of Endocrine Diagnostic Test Results for Adrenal and Thyroid Disease

Section IV: Oncology and Hematology
Douglas H. Thamm, VMD, DACVIM (Oncology)
Associate Professor and Barbara Cox Anthony Chair in Oncology
Department of Clinical Sciences
College of Veterinary Medicine
Colorado State University
Fort Collins, Colorado
Talking to Clients about Cancer
Anticancer Drugs: New Drugs

Christine S. Olver, DVM, PhD, DACVP
Associate Professor
Clinical Pathology Section
Colorado State University
Fort Collins, Colorado
Lymphocytosis in Dogs and Cats
Bone Marrow Dyscrasias

Section V: Dermatologic and Otic Diseases
Andrew Hillier, BVSc, MACVSc, DACVD
Former Professor and Head of Dermatology and Otology
Veterinary Clinical Sciences
The Ohio State University
Columbus, Ohio
Senior Veterinary Specialist (Dermatology), Zoetis
Cyclosporine Use in Dermatology
Flea Control in Flea Allergy Dermatitis
Treatment of Superficial Bacterial Folliculitis

Lynette K. Cole, DVM, MS, DACVD
Associate Professor
Department of Veterinary Clinical Sciences
College of Veterinary Medicine
The Ohio State University
Columbus, Ohio
Principles of Therapy for Otitis
Systemic Antimicrobials for Otitis

Section VI: Gastrointestinal Diseases
David C. Twedt, DVM, DACVIM (Internal Medicine)
Professor
Department of Clinical Sciences
College of Veterinary Medicine and Biomedical Sciences
Colorado State University
Fort Collins, Colorado
Copper Chelator Therapy
Idiopathic Vacuolar Hepatopathy
Feline Cholangitis
Evaluation of Elevated Serum Alkaline Phosphatase in Dogs
Hepatic Support Therapy

Kenneth W. Simpson, BVM&S, MRCVS, PhD, DACVIM, DECVIM
Professor of Small Animal Medicine
Clinical Sciences
Cornell University
Ithaca, New York
Cobalamin Deficiency in Cats
Canine Colitis
Feline Cholangitis

Section VII: Respiratory Diseases
Lynelle R. Johnson, DVM, MS, PhD, DACVIM (SAIM)
Associate Professor
Medicine & Epidemiology
University of California—Davis
Davis, California
Rhinitis in Cats
Chronic Bronchial Disorders in Dogs

Section VIII: Cardiovascular Diseases
John D. Bonagura, DVM, MS, DACVIM (Cardiology, Internal Medicine)
Professor
Department of Veterinary Clinical Sciences
College of Veterinary Medicine
The Ohio State University
Head, Cardiology and Interventional Medicine Service
The Ohio State University Veterinary Medical Center
Columbus, Ohio
Congenital Heart Disease
Drugs for Treatment of Heart Failure in Dogs
Management of Heart Failure in Dogs
Ventricular Septal Defect

Brian A. Scansen, DVM, MS, DACVIM
Assistant Professor of Cardiology and Interventional Medicine
Veterinary Clinical Sciences
The Ohio State University
Columbus, Ohio
Tracheal Collapse
Congenital Heart Disease

Section IX: Urinary Diseases
India F. Lane, DVM, MS, EdD
Assistant Vice President
Office of Academic Affairs and Student Success
The University of Tennessee
Knoxville, Tennessee
Professor and Internist
Department of Small Animal Clinical Sciences
College of Veterinary Medicine
The University of Tennessee
Knoxville, Tennessee

Section X: Reproductive Diseases
Michelle Anne Kutzler, DVM, PhD, DACT
Banfield Professor of Companion Animal Industries
Animal and Rangeland Sciences
Oregon State University
Corvallis, Oregon
Postpartum Disorders in Companion Animals
Early Age Neutering in Dogs and Cats
Acquired Nonneoplastic Disorders of the Male External Genitalia

Section XI: Neurologic Diseases
Curtis W. Dewey, BS, DVM, MS
Associate Professor
Clinical Sciences
College of Veterinary Medicine
Cornell University
Ithaca, New York
Intracranial Arachnoid Cysts in Dogs
New Maintenance Anticonvulsant Therapies for Dogs and Cats
Peripheral and Central Vestibular Disorders in Dogs and Cats
Craniocervical Junction Abnormalities in Dogs

Section XII: Ophthalmologic Diseases
Anne J. Gemensky Metzler, DVM, MS, DACVO
Professor-Clinical Comparative Ophthalmology
Veterinary Clinical Sciences
College of Veterinary Medicine
The Ohio State University
Columbus, Ohio
Evaluation of Blindness

Amber Labelle, DVM, MS, DACVO
Assistant Professor
Veterinary Clinical Medicine
University of Illinois Urbana—Champaign
Urbana, Illinois
Corneal Ulcers
Canine Ocular Neoplasia
Feline Ocular Neoplasia

Section XIII: Infectious Diseases
Michael R. Lappin, DVM, PhD, DACVIM (SA Internal Medicine)
The Kenneth W. Smith Professor
Department of Clinical Sciences
Colorado State University
Fort Collins, Colorado
Protozoal Gastrointestinal Disease
Infectious Agent Differentials for Medical Problems
Infectious Causes of Polyarthritis in Dogs
Update on Vaccine-Associated Adverse Effects in Cats
Toxoplasmosis
Feline Infectious Peritonitis Virus Infections

Appendix I: Table of Common Drugs: Approximate Dosages
Mark G. Papich, DVM, MS
Professor of Clinical Pharmacology
College of Veterinary Medicine
North Carolina State University
Raleigh, North Carolina
Veterinary Teaching Hospital
College of Veterinary Medicine
North Carolina State University
Raleigh, North Carolina
Respiratory Drug Therapy
Appendix I: Table of Common Drugs: Approximate Dosages

Contributors

Jonathan A. Abbott, DVM, DACVIM (Cardiology)
Associate Professor of Cardiology
Small Animal Clinical Sciences
Virginia-Maryland Regional College of
    Veterinary Medicine
Virginia Tech
Blacksburg, Virginia
Associate Professor
Basic Sciences
Virginia Tech Carilion School of
    Medicine and Research Institute
Roanoke, Virginia
Subaortic Stenosis

Mark J. Acierno, MBA, DVM
Associate Professor
Veterinary Clinical Science
The Louisiana State University
Baton Rouge, Louisiana
Continuous Renal Replacement Therapy

Larry G. Adams, DVM, PhD, DACVIM (SAIM)
Professor
Small Animal Internal Medicine
Department of Veterinary Clinical
    Sciences
Purdue University
West Lafayette, Indiana
Laser Lithotripsy for Uroliths

Christopher A. Adin, DVM, DACVS
Associate Professor
Veterinary Clinical Sciences
The Ohio State University
Columbus, Ohio
*Mechanical Occluder Devices for Urinary
    Incontinence*

Darcy B. Adin, DVM
Associate Cardiologist
Cardiology
MedVet
Medical and Cancer Center for Pets
Worthington, Ohio
Tricuspid Valve Dysplasia

Hasan Albasan, DVM, MS, PhD
Minnesota Urolith Center
Veterinary Medicine
University of Minnesota
St. Paul, Minnesota
Canine Urate Urolithiasis
Laser Lithotripsy for Uroliths

Kelly E. Allen, MS, PhD
Department of Veterinary Pathobiology
Center for Veterinary Health Sciences
Oklahoma State University
Stillwater, Oklahoma
Hepatozoon americanum Infections

Karin Allenspach, Dr.Med.Vet., ECVIM-CA, FVH, PhD, FHEA
Doctor
Veterinary Clinical Sciences
Royal Veterinary College
London, Hertfordshire, Great Britain
Inflammatory Bowel Disease

Colleen M. Almgren, DVM, PhD
Staff Veterinarian
Clinical Toxicology
Pet Poison Helpline/SafetyCall
    International
Bloomington, Minnesota
Toxin Exposures in Small Animals

John D. Anastasio, DVM, DACVECC
Associate Veterinarian
Veterinary Emergency and Referral
    Center
Norwalk, Connecticut
Crystalloid Fluid Therapy

P. Jane Armstrong, DVM, MS, MBA
Professor
Small Animal Internal Medicine
Veterinary Clinical Sciences Department
University of Minnesota
St. Paul, Minnesota
Feline Hepatic Lipidosis
Feline Cholangitis

Clarke E. Atkins, DVM
Jane Lewis Seaks Distinguished Professor
    of Companion Animal Medicine
Department of Clinical Sciences
North Carolina State University
Raleigh, North Carolina
Feline Heartworm Disease

Anne Avery, VMD, PhD
Associate Professor, Director Clinical
    Immunology
Microbiology, Immunology and
    Pathology
Colorado State University
Fort Collins, Colorado
Lymphocytosis in Dogs and Cats

Sandra M. Axiak-Bechtel, DVM, DACVIM
Assistant Professor
College of Veterinary Medicine
University of Missouri
Columbia, Missouri
Pulmonary Neoplasia

Todd W. Axlund, DVM, MS, ACVIM (Neurology)
Metropolitan Veterinary Referral Group
Akron, Ohio
Treatment of Intracranial Tumors

Nicholas J. Bacon, MA, VetMB, DECVS, DACVS, MRCVS
Clinical Assistant Professor of Surgical
    Oncology
Small Animal Clinical Sciences
University of Florida College of
    Veterinary Medicine
Gainesville, Florida
Tumor Biopsy and Specimen Submission

Cindy Bahr
Hospital Administrator
Warner Center Pet Clinic
Woodland Hills, California
Neutriceutical Formulator
Complete Vites LLC
Calabasas, California
Pregnancy Diagnosis in Companion Animals

Dennis B. Bailey, DVM, DACVIM (Oncology)
Staff Oncologist
Oradell Animal Hospital
Paramus, New Jersey
*Treatment of Adverse Effects from Cancer
    Therapy*

Claudia J. Baldwin, DVM, MS
Associate Professor
Veterinary Clinical Sciences
Faculty
Center for Food Security and Public
    Health
Iowa State University
Ames, Iowa
Pregnancy Loss in the Bitch and Queen

Lora R. Ballweber, MS, DVM, DACVM (Parasitology)
Professor
Microbiology, Immunology and
    Pathology
Section Head, Parasitology
Veterinary Diagnostic Laboratory
College of Veterinary Medicine and
    Biomedical Sciences
Colorado State University
Fort Collins, Colorado
Appendix II: Treatment of Parasites

Tania Ann Banks, BVSc, FACVSc (Small Animal Surgery), GC (HEd)
Lecturer and Consultant Surgeon
Small Animal Surgery
The University of Queensland
St. Lucia and Gatton Campuses
Queensland, Australia
Soft Tissue Sarcomas

A. Catherine Barr, PhD
President Elect, AAVLD
Diplomate American Board of Toxicology
Quality Assurance & Safety Manager
Texas A&M Veterinary Medical
    Diagnostic Laboratory
Amarillo, Texas
*Top Ten Toxic and Nontoxic Household
    Plants*

**Vanessa R. Barrs, BVSc(hons),
    MVetClinStud, FANZCVSc (Feline
    Medicine)**
Associate Professor
Small Animal Medicine
Faculty of Veterinary Science
The University of Sydney
Sydney, New South Wales, Australia
Rhinitis in Cats

**Joseph W. Bartges, DVM, PhD,
    DACVIM, DACVN**
Professor of Medicine and Nutrition
Department of Small Animal Clinical
    Sciences
The Acree Endowed Chair of Small
    Animal Research
Department of Small Animal Clinical
    Sciences
Internist and Nutritionist
Small Animal Hospital
Veterinary Medical Center
The University of Tennessee
Knoxville, Tennessee
*Minilaparotomy-Assisted Cystoscopy for
    Urocystoliths*
Top Ten Urinary Consult Questions

Karin M. Beale, DVM, DACVD
Dermatologist
Gulf Coast Veterinary Specialists
Houston, Texas
Feline Demodicosis

Adrienne Bentley, DVM, DACVS
Staff Surgeon
Veterinary Medical and Surgical Group
Ventura, California
Drainage Techniques for the Septic Abdomen

Allyson Berent, DVM, DACVIM
Director of Interventional Endoscopy
Interventional Radiology/Interventional
    Endoscopy
The Animal Medical Center
New York, New York
Interventional Strategies for Urinary Disease

**Alexa M.E. Bersenas, DVM, MS,
    DACVECC**
Associate Professor
Clinical Studies
Ontario Veterinary College
University of Guelph
Guelph, Ontario, Canada
Antacid Therapy

**Nick Bexfield, BVETMED, DSAM,
    DECVIM-CA, MRCVS**
Department of Veterinary Medicine
University of Cambridge
Cambridge, United Kingdom
*Ascites and Hepatic Encephalopathy
    Therapy for Liver Disease*

Adam J. Birkenheuer
Associate Professor
Department of Clinical Sciences
College of Veterinary Medicine
North Carolina State University
Raleigh, North Carolina
Thrombocytopenia
Treatment of Canine Babesiosis

Karyn Bischoff, DVM, MS, DABVT
Assistant Professor
Population Medicine and Diagnostic
    Sciences
Diagnostic Toxicologist
New York State Animal Health Diagnostic
    Center
Cornell University
Ithaca, New York
Automotive Toxins
Aflatoxicosis in Dogs

Dana R. Bleifer, DVM
Owner
Warner Center Pet Clinic
Woodland Hills, California
Pregnancy Diagnosis in Companion Animals

**Manuel Boller, Dr.med.vet., MTR,
    DACVECC**
Senior Lecturer Emergency and Critical
    Care
Faculty of Veterinary Science
University of Melbourne
Melbourne, Victoria, Australia
Cardiopulmonary Resuscitation

**Michele Borgarelli, DVM, PhD,
    DECVIM-CA**
Associate Professor
Small Animal Clinical Sciences
Virginia-Maryland College of Veterinary
    Medicine
Virginia Tech
Blacksburg, Virginia
Pulmonary Hypertension

Shay Bracha, DVM
Assistant Professor Oncology
Department of Clinical Sciences
Assistant Professor
Department of Clinical
    Sciences-Oncology
College of Veterinary Medicine
Oregon State University
Corvallis, Oregon
Reproductive Oncology

**Allison Bradley, DVM, DACVIM
    (SAIM)**
Department of Clinical Sciences
College of Veterinary Medicine and
    Biomedical Sciences
Colorado State University
Fort Collins, Colorado
Copper Chelator Therapy

**Benjamin M. Brainard, VMD,
    DACVA, DACVECC**
Associate Professor of Emergency and
    Critical Care
Critical Care
Small Animal Medicine and Surgery
College of Veterinary Medicine
University of Georgia
Athens, Georgia
Thromboelastography

**Janice M. Bright, BSN, MS, DVM,
    DACVIM (Cardiology)**
Professor of Cardiology
Department of Clinical Science
Cardiologist
Veterinary Teaching Hospital
Colorado State University
Fort Collins, Colorado
Cardioversion

Susan J. Bright-Ponte, DVM
Office of Surveillance and Compliance
FDA Center for Veterinary Medicine
Rockville, Maryland
*Reporting Adverse Events to the Food and
    Drug Administration—Center for
    Veterinary Medicine*
*Treatment of Animal Toxicoses: Regulatory
    Points to Consider*

Marjorie B. Brooks, DVM, DACVIM
Director
Comparative Coagulation Laboratory
Population Medicine and Diagnostic
    Sciences
Cornell University
Ithaca, New York
*von Willebrand Disease and Hereditary
    Coagulation Factor Deficiencies*

**Michael R. Broome, DVM, MS,
    DABVP**
Advanced Veterinary Medical Imaging
Tustin, California
Radioiodine for Feline Hyperthyroidism

Scott A. Brown, VMD, PhD, DACVIM
Josiah Meigs Distinguished Teaching
    Professor
Department of Physiology and
    Pharmacology
Edward Gunst Professor of Small Animal
    Studies
Department of Small Animal Medicine
    and Surgery
College of Veterinary Medicine
University of Georgia
Athens, Georgia
*Use of Nonsteroidal Antiinflammatory
    Drugs in Kidney Disease*

Ahna G. Brutlag, DVM, MS, DAPT
Assistant Director of Veterinary Services
Pet Poison Helpline and SafetyCall
 International
Minneapolis, Minnesota
Antidepressants and Anxiolytics

**C.A. Tony Buffington, DVM, PhD,
 DACVN**
Professor
Veterinary Clinical Sciences
The Ohio State University
Columbus, Ohio
*Multimodal Environmental Enrichment for
 Domestic Cats*

**Barret J. Bulmer, DVM, MS,
 DACVIM-Cardiology**
Staff Veterinarian
Cummings School of Veterinary
 Medicine
Tufts University
Grafton, Massachusetts
Tufts Veterinary Emergency Treatment
 and Specialties
Cardiology
Walpole, Massachusetts
Mitral Valve Dysplasia

**Amanda K. Burrows, BVMS,
 MANZVSC, FANZVSC (Veterinary
 Dermatology)**
Adjunct Lecturer
Department of Veterinary and
 Biomedical Science
Director
Animal Dermatology Clinic—Perth
Director
Dermatology
Perth Veterinary Specialists
Perth, Western Australia, Australia
Actinic Dermatoses and Sun Protection
Avermectins in Dermatology

Kevin Byrne, DVM, MS
Chief of Staff
Allergy Ear and Skin Care for Animals
 LLC
Bensalem, Pennsylvania
Superficial Necrolytic Dermatitis

Julie K. Byron, DVM, MS, DACVIM
Associate Professor—Clinical
Veterinary Clinical Science
The Ohio State University
Columbus, Ohio
*Urinary Incontinence: Treatment with
 Injectable Bulking Agents*

Amanda Callens, BS, LVMT
Department of Small Animal Clinical
 Sciences
College of Veterinary Medicine
The University of Tennessee
Knoxville, Tennessee
*Minilaparotomy-Assisted Cystoscopy for
 Urocystoliths*
Top Ten Urinary Consult Questions

Clay A. Calvert, DVM
Professor Emeritus
Small Animal Medicine and Surgery
College of Veterinary Medicine
University of Georgia
Athens, Georgia
Syncope

Starr Cameron, BVetMed
Resident, Neurology/Neurosurgery
Department of Clinical Sciences
Cornell University Hospital for Animals
Ithaca, New York
*Peripheral and Central Vestibular Disorders
 in Dogs and Cats*

Nigel Campbell, BVetMed, PhD
Clinical Assistant Professor
College of Veterinary Medicine
North Carolina State University
Raleigh, North Carolina
Analgesia of the Critical Patient

**Elizabeth A. Carsten, DVM, DACVIM
 (SAIM)**
Manager
US Internal Medicine Consulting
IDEXX Laboratories, Inc.
Tucson, Arizona
Esophagitis

Sharon A. Center, BS, DVM, DACVIM
Professor, Internal Medicine
Clinical Sciences
College of Veterinary Medicine
Cornell University
Ithaca, New York
Acute Liver Failure

**Rosario Cerundolo, DVM, Cert. VD,
 DECVD, MRCVS**
Consultant in Dermatology
Dick White Referrals
Six Mile Bottom
Suffolk, United Kingdom
Alopecia X

**Daniel L. Chan, DVM, DACVECC,
 DACVN, FHEA, MRCV**
Senior Lecturer in Emergency and
 Critical Care
Veterinary Clinical Sciences
The Royal Veterinary College
University of London
North Mymms, Hertfordshire, United
 Kingdom
Nutrition in Critical Care

**Dennis J. Chew, DVM, DACVIM
 (Internal Medicine)**
Professor Emeritus
Veterinary Clinical Sciences
College of Veterinary Medicine
The Ohio State University
Columbus, Ohio
Feline Idiopathic Hypercalcemia
Treatment of Hypoparathyroidism
*Urinary Incontinence: Treatment with
 Injectable Bulking Agents*

**David B. Church, BVSc, PhD,
 MACVSc, MRCVS, ILTM**
Professor of Small Animal Studies
Department of Clinical Sciences and
 Services
The Royal Veterinary College
University of London
London, United Kingdom
Feline Hypersomatotropism and Acromegaly

**Cécile Clercx, DVM, PhD,
 DECVIM-CA (Internal Medicine)**
Professor of Clinical Sciences of
 Companion Animals and Equine
University of Liège
Faculty of Veterinary Medicine
Liège, Belgium
Eosinophilic Pulmonary Diseases

**Craig A. Clifford, DVM, MS,
 DACVIM (Oncology)**
Medical Oncologist
Director of Clinical Research
Oncology
Hope Veterinary Specialists
Malvern, Pennsylvania
Canine Hemangiosarcoma

**Joan R. Coates, DVM, MS, DACVIM
 (Neurology)**
Professor
Service Leader—Neurology and
 Neurosurgery Service
Department Veterinary Medicine and
 Surgery
College of Veterinary Medicine
University of Missouri
Columbia, Missouri
Canine Degenerative Myelopathy

Richard E. Cober, DV, MS
Clinical Instructor
Cardiology and Interventional Medicine
Veterinary Clinical Sciences
Veterinary Medical Center
The Ohio State University
Columbus, Ohio
Chesapeake Veterinary Cardiology
 Associates
Maryland and Virginia
Congenital Heart Disease

Patrick W. Concannon, PhD
Director Emeritus
Laboratory for Comparative
 Reproduction
Biomedical Sciences
Cornell University
College of Veterinary Medicine
Ithaca, New York
President
International Veterinary Information
 Service
Ithaca, New York
Estrus Suppression in the Bitch

Edward S. Cooper, VMD, MS, DACVECC
Associate Professor—Clinical, Small
  Animal Emergency and Critical Care
Veterinary Clinical Sciences
Head of Service—Small Animal
  Emergency and Critical Care
Veterinary Medical Center
The Ohio State University
Columbus, Ohio
Catecholamines in the Critical Care Patient

**Johanna C. Cooper, DVM, DACVIM
  (SAIM)**
Tufts Veterinary Emergency Treatment &
  Specialties
Walpole, Massachusetts
Diagnostic Approach to Hepatobiliary Disease

**Rhian Cope, BVSc, BSc (Hon 1),
  PhD, DABT, ERT, MRCVS**
Senior Advisor
Hazardous Substances
Environmental Risk Management
  Authority
Wellington, New Zealand
*Pesticides: New Vertebrate Toxic Agents for
  Pest Species*

**Brendan M. Corcoran, MVB, PhD,
  DPharm, MRCVS**
Professor
Veterinary Clinical Studies
Royal (Dick) School of Veterinary Studies
  and Roslin Institute
The University of Edinburgh
Edinburgh, Scotland, United Kingdom
Interstitial Lung Diseases

**Étienne Côté, DVM, DACVIM
  (Cardiology, Small Animal
  Internal Medicine)**
Associate Professor
Department of Companion Animals
Atlantic Veterinary College
University of Prince Edward Island
Charlottetown, Prince Edward Island,
  Canada
Feline Cardiac Arrhythmias

Nancy B. Cottrill, DVM, MS, DACVO
Staff Ophthalmologist
Massachusetts Veterinary Referral
  Hospital
Woburn, Massachusetts
*Anisocoria and Abnormalities of the
  Pupillary Light Reflex: The Neuro-
  ophthalmic Examination*

**Jamie M. Burkitt Creedon, DVM,
  DACVECC**
Head of the Emergency and Critical Care
  Service
Red Bank Veterinary Hospital of Cherry
  Hill
Cherry Hill, New Jersey
Critical Consultations
Allentown, New Jersey
*Critical Illness–Related Corticosteroid
  Insufficiency*

**Cheryl L. Cullen, DVM, MVetSc,
  DACVO**
CullenWebb Animal Neurology &
  Ophthalmology Centre
Riverview, New Brunswick, Canada
Feline Corneal Disease

William T.N. Culp
Assistant Professor
Department of Surgical and Radiological
  Sciences
University of California—Davis
Davis, California
Interventional Oncology

**Suzanne M. Cunningham, DVM,
  DACVIM (Cardiology)**
Assistant Professor of Cardiology
Clinical Sciences
Tufts Cummings School of Veterinary
  Medicine
North Grafton, Massachusetts
Chronic Valvular Heart Disease in Dogs

**James T. Custis III, DVM, MS,
  DACVR (RO)**
Assistant Professor
Veterinary Radiation Oncology
Environmental and Radiological Health
  Sciences
James L. Voss Veterinary Teaching
  Hospital and the Animal Cancer
  Center
Colorado State University
Fort Collins, Colorado
*Advances in Radiation Therapy for Nasal
  Tumors*

**Ronaldo Casimiro da Costa, DVM,
  MSc, PhD, DACVIM-Neurology**
Assistant Professor and Service Head
Neurology and Neurosurgery
Veterinary Clinical Sciences
The Ohio State University
Columbus, Ohio
*Diagnosis and Treatment of Cervical
  Spondylomyelopathy*

Autumn P. Davidson, DVM, MS
Clinical Professor
Medicine and Epidemiology
University of California—Davis
Davis, California
Staff Internist
Internal Medicine
Pet Care Veterinary Hospital
Santa Rosa, California
Dystocia Management
Canine Brucellosis

Douglas J. DeBoer, DVM
Professor of Dermatology
Department of Medical Sciences
University of Wisconsin
Madison, Wisconsin
Allergen-Specific Immunotherapy
Treatment of Dermatophytosis

**Linda J. DeBowes, DVM, MS, DAVDC,
  DACVIM (Small Animal)**
Shoreline Veterinary Dental Clinic
Seattle, Washington
Feline Caudal Stomatitis

**Joao Felipe de Brito Galvao, MV, MS,
  DACVIM (SAIM)**
Internal Medicine Specialist and Medical
  Director
Internal Medicine and Nuclear Medicine
VCA Arboretum View Animal Hospital
Downers Grove, Illinois
Feline Idiopathic Hypercalcemia
Treatment of Hypoparathyroidism

**Louis-Philippe de Lorimier, DVM,
  DACVIM (Oncology)**
Staff Medical Oncologist
Medical Oncology
Hôpital Vétérinaire Rive-Sud
Brossard, Québec, Canada
Canine Hemangiosarcoma

**Helio Autran de Morais, DVM, PhD,
  ACVIM (SAIM & Cardiology)**
Director
Lois Bates Acheson Veterinary Teaching
  Hospital
Oregon State University
Corvallis, Oregon
Acid-Base Disorders

**Robert C. DeNovo, DVM, DACVIM
  (SAIM)**
Professor
Internal Medicine
Associate Dean for Administration and
  Clinical Programs
Department of Small Animal Clinical
  Sciences
College of Veterinary Medicine
The University of Tennessee
Knoxville, Tennessee
Canine Megaesophagus

**Stephen P. DiBartola, DVM, DACVIM
  (Internal Medicine)**
Professor of Medicine
Veterinary Clinical Sciences
College of Veterinary Medicine
The Ohio State University
Columbus, Ohio
Acid-Base Disorders

**Pedro Paulo Vissotto de Paiva
  Diniz, DVM, PhD**
Assistant Professor of Small Animal
  Internal Medicine
College of Veterinary Medicine
Western University of Health Sciences
Pomona, California
Canine Bartonellosis

David C. Dorman, DVM, PhD
Professor of Toxicology
Department of Molecular Biomedical
    Sciences
College of Veterinary Medicine
North Carolina State University
Raleigh, North Carolina
Over-the-Counter Drug Toxicosis

**Steven Dow, DVM, PhD, DACVIM
    (SAIM)**
Professor
Department of Clinical Sciences
Internist
Veterinary Teaching Hospital
Colorado State University
Fort Collins, Colorado
*Management of Immune-Mediated
    Hemolytic Anemia in Dogs*
Cancer Immunotherapy
Immunotherapy for Infectious Diseases

**Patricia M. Dowling, DVM, MSc,
    DACVIM (LAIM), DACVCP**
Professor
Veterinary Clinical Pharmacology
Veterinary Biomedical Sciences
Western College of Veterinary Medicine
Saskatoon, Saskatchewan, Canada
Rational Empiric Antimicrobial Therapy

**Kenneth J. Drobatz, DVM, MSCE,
    DACVIM, DACVECC**
Professor and Chief,
Section of Critical Care
Department of Clinical Studies
Director, Emergency Service
Critical Care
Mathew J. Ryan Veterinary Hospital of
    the University of Pennsylvania
University of Pennsylvania
Philadelphia, Pennsylvania
Oxygen Therapy

**Eric K. Dunayer, MS, VMD, DABT,
    DABVT**
Associate Professor
Veterinary Clinical Sciences
School of Veterinary Medicine
St. Matthew's University
Grand Cayman, Cayman Islands
*Human Foods with Pet Toxicoses: Alcohol to
    Xylitol*

**Janice A. Dye, DVM, MS, PhD,
    DACVIM (SA-IM)**
Principal Investigator
Environmental Public Health Division
National Health and Environmental
    Effects
Research Laboratory, ORD
US Environmental Protection Agency
Research Triangle Park, North Carolina
*Respiratory Toxicants of Interest to Pet
    Owners*

David A. Dzanis, DVM, PhD, DACVN
Regulatory Discretion, Inc.
Santa Clarita, California
*Nutrition in the Bitch and Queen During
    Pregnancy and Lactation*

Susan M. Eddlestone, DVM, DACVIM
Associate Professor
Veterinary Clinical Sciences
School of Veterinary Medicine
The Louisiana State University
Baton Rouge, Louisiana
*Canine and Feline Monocytotropic
    Ehrlichiosis*

**Nicole P. Ehrhart, VMS, MS, DACVS,
    ACVS Founding Fellow Surgical
    Oncology**
Professor, Surgical Oncology
Department of Clinical Sciences
Colorado State University
Fort Collins, Colorado
James Voss Veterinary Teaching Hospital
Osteosarcoma

Bruce E. Eilts, DVM, MS DACT
Associate Professor
School of Veterinary and Biomedical
    Sciences
James Cook University
Townsville, Queensland, Australia
Professor Emeritus
Department of Veterinary Clinical
    Sciences
School of Veterinary Medicine
The Louisiana State University
Baton Rouge, Louisiana
Medical Termination of Pregnancy

**Jonathan Elliott, MA, VetMB, PhD,
    Cert SAC, DECVPT, MRCVS**
Professor of Veterinary Clinical
    Pharmacology and Vice Principal for
    Research
Veterinary Basic Sciences
Royal Veterinary College
University of London
London, England
*Chronic Kidney Disease: International Renal
    Interest Society Staging and Management*

**Gary C.W. England, BVetMed, PhD,
    DVetMed, DVR, DVRep, DECAR,
    DACT, FHEA, FRCVS**
Department of Veterinary Surgery
School of Veterinary Medicine and
    Science
University of Nottingham
Sutton Bonington, Loughborough,
    United Kingdom
Breeding Management of the Bitch

**Amara H. Estrada, DVM, DACVIM
    (Cardiology)**
Associate Professor and Associate Chair
Small Animal Clinical Sciences
University of Florida
Gainesville, Florida
Dilated Cardiomyopathy in Dogs
Pulmonic Stenosis

Cristian Falzone, DVM, DECVN
Department of Neurology
Small Animal Diagnostics
Zugliano (VI), Italy
Department of Neurology
Malpensa Veterinary Clinic
Samarate (VA), Italy
Metabolic Brain Disorders

Timothy M. Fan, DVM, PhD
Associate Professor
Veterinary Clinical Medicine
University of Illinois at
    Urbana—Champaign
Urbana, Illinois
Osteosarcoma

**James P. Farese, DVM, DACVS (ACVS
    Founding Fellow of Surgical
    Oncology)**
Staff Surgeon
VCA Animal Care Center of Sonoma
    County
Rohnert Park, California
Surgical Oncology Principles

Claude Favrot, DVM
Prof. Dr.
Head of the Dermatology Service
Clinic for Small Animal Internal
    Medicine
Vetsuisse Faculty
University of Zurich
Zurich, Switzerland
*Diagnostic Criteria for Canine Atopic
    Dermatitis*

**Anne Fawcett, BA (Hons), BVSc(Vet)
    (Hons), BVSc(Hons), MVetStud
    CMAVA**
Lecturer
Faculty of Veterinary Science
University of Sydney
Sydney, New South Wales, Australia
Associate
Sydney Animal Hospitals Inner West
Sydney, New South Wales, Australia
*Nontuberculous Cutaneous Granulomas in
    Dogs and Cats (Canine Leproid
    Granuloma and Feline Leprosy
    Syndrome)*

Edward C. Feldman, DVM
Professor of Small Animal Internal
  Medicine
Department of Medicine & Epidemiology
University of California—Davis
Davis, California
*Hypercalcemia and Primary
  Hyperparathyroidism in Dogs*
*Large Pituitary Tumors in Dogs with
  Pituitary-Dependent
  Hyperadrenocorticism*

**Alberto L. Fernandez Mojica, DVM,
  DACVECC**
Associate Professor
Small Animal Medicine and Surgery
Assistant Medical Director
Veterinary Teaching Hospital
Small Animal Medicine and Surgery
School of Veterinary Medicine
St. Georges University
St. Georges, Grenada, West Indies
Intravenous Lipid Emulsion Therapy

**Jeanne E. Ficociello, VMD, MS,
  DACVIM**
Small Animal Internal Medicine
VCA South Shore Animal Hospital
South Weymouth, Massachusetts
Neospora caninum

Hille Fieten, DVM, MSc
Clinical Sciences of Companion Animals
Faculty of Veterinary Medicine
Universiteit Utrecht
Utrecht, The Netherlands
Copper-Associated Hepatitis

Julie R. Fischer, DVM, DACVIM
Staff Internist
Veterinary Specialty Hospital of San
  Diego
Internal Medicine
San Diego, California
*Persistent Escherichia coli Urinary Tract
  Infection*

Randall B. Fitch, DVM, MS, DACVS
Ladera Ranch, California
Evaluation of Canine Orthopedic Trauma

**Derek Flaherty, BVMS, DVA,
  DECVAA, MRCA, MRCVS**
Professor of Veterinary Anaesthesia and
  Analgesia
School of Veterinary Medicine
University of Glasgow
Glasgow, Scotland, United Kingdom
Anesthesia for the Critical Care Patient

**Daniel J. Fletcher, PhD, DVM,
  DACVECC**
Assistant Professor
Emergency and Critical Care
Clinical Sciences
College of Veterinary Medicine
Cornell University
Ithaca, New York
Crystalloid Fluid Therapy
Cardiopulmonary Resuscitation
*Treatment of Cluster Seizures and Status
  Epilepticus*

**Andrea Flory, DVM, DACVIM
  (Oncology)**
Medical Oncologist
Veterinary Specialty Hospital
San Diego, California
*Chemotherapeutic Drug Handling and
  Safety*

Marnin A. Forman, DVM, DACVIM
Head of Department
Staff Internist
Internal Medicine
Cornell University Veterinary Specialists
Stamford, Connecticut
Feline Exocrine Pancreatic Disorders

**Lisa J. Forrest, VMD, DACVR
  (Radiology, Radiation Oncology)**
Professor
Surgical Sciences
Professor
Carbone Cancer Center
University of Wisconsin—Madison
Madison, Wisconsin
Nasal Tumors

**Susan F. Foster, BVSc, MVetClinStud,
  FANZCVS**
Adjunct Senior Lecturer in Small Animal
  Medicine
Department of Veterinary Clinical
  Sciences
Murdoch University
Murdoch, Western Australia, Australia
Small Animal Medical Consultant
Vetnostics
Sydney, Australia
Nasopharyngeal Disorders

**Philip R. Fox, DVM, MSc, BSc,
  DACVIM/ECVIM-CA (Cardiology),
  DACVECC**
Head of Cardiology
The Animal Medical Center
New York, New York
Director
Caspary Institute of the Animal Medical
  Center
New York, New York
*Arrhythmogenic Right Ventricular
  Cardiomyopathy in Cats*

Linda A. Frank, MS, DVM, DACVD
Professor of Dermatology
Department of Small Animal Clinical
  Sciences
College of Veterinary Medicine
The University of Tennessee
Knoxville, Tennessee
Staphylococci Causing Pyoderma

Lisa M. Freeman, DVM, PhD, DACVN
Professor
Department of Clinical Sciences
Tufts Cummings School of Veterinary
  Medicine
North Grafton, Massachusetts
Nutritional Management of Heart Disease

Valérie Freiche, DVM
Vet Clinic
Internal Medicine
Alliance
Bordeaux, France
*Brachycephalic Airway Obstruction
  Syndrome*

Cecilia Friberg, DVM, DACVD
Owner, Veterinary Dermatologist
Animal Dermatology Center of Chicago,
  P.C.
Chicago, Illinois
Ototoxicity

Janet A.M. Fyfe, PhD
Senior Scientist
Mycobacterium Reference Laboratory
Victorian Infectious Diseases Reference
  Laboratory
North Melbourne, Victoria, Australia
Deputy Head
WHO Collaborating Centre for
  Mycobacterium Ulcerans
(Western Pacific Region)
North Melbourne, Victoria, Australia
*Nontuberculous Cutaneous Granulomas in
  Dogs and Cats (Canine Leproid
  Granuloma and Feline Leprosy
  Syndrome)*

Sara Galac, DVM, PhD
Assistant Professor
Department of Clinical Sciences of
  Companion Animals
Faculty of Veterinary Medicine
Universiteit Utrecht
Utrecht, The Netherlands
*Ectopic ACTH Syndrome and Food-
  Dependent Hypercortisolism in Dogs*

Leana V. Galdjian, DVM
Veterinarian
Rose City Veterinary Hospital
Pasadena, California
Veterinarian
Warner Center Pet Clinic
Woodland Hills, California
Pregnancy Diagnosis in Companion Animals

Tam Garland, DVM, PhD, DABVT
Toxicology Section Head
Texas A&M Veterinary Medical
 Diagnostic Laboratory
College Station, Texas
Aflatoxicosis in Dogs

Laurent S. Garosi, DVM, MRCVS, DECVN, RCVS-Recognized Specialist in Veterinary Neurology
Head of Neurology/Neurosurgery Service
 Head
Neurology and Neurosurgery
Davies Veterinary Specialists
Higham Gobion, England
Vascular Disease of the Central Nervous System

Laura D. Garrett, DVM, DACVIM (Oncology)
Clinical Associate Professor
Veterinary Clinical Medicine
University of Illinois
Urbana, Illinois
Plasma Cell Neoplasms

Anthony T. Gary, DVM, DACVIM
Owner/Veterinarian
Arkansas Veterinary Internal Medicine
Little Rock, Arkansas
Evaluation of Elevated Serum Alkaline Phosphatase in Dogs

Frédéric P. Gaschen, Dr.med.vet., Dr.habil.
M.L. Martin Professor
Veterinary Clinical Sciences
School of Veterinary Medicine
The Louisiana State University
Baton Rouge, Louisiana
Gastric and Intestinal Motility Disorders

Rudayna Ghubash, DVM, DACVD
Veterinarian
Animal Dermatology Clinic
Marina del Rey, California
Feline Viral Skin Disease

Urs Giger, PD Dr.med.vet., MS, FVH, DACVIM (Small Animal Internal Medicine), DECVIM-CA (Internal Medicine), DECVCP (Clinical Pathology)
Charlotte Newton Sheppard Professor
Section of Medical Genetics, School of
 Veterinary Medicine, and Division of
 Hematology
Senior Faculty Clinician
Ryan Veterinary Hospital
Director of Metabolic Genetics and
 Deubler Testing Laboratory (PennGen)
Section of Medical Genetics
University of Pennsylvania
Philadelphia, Pennsylvania
Professor of Internal Medicine
Department of Small Animal Medicine
VetSuisse
University of Zurich
Zurich, Switzerland
Blood Typing and Crossmatching to Ensure Blood Compatibility

Margi Gilmour, DVM
Associate Professor
Veterinary Clinical Sciences
Oklahoma State University
Stillwater, Oklahoma
Canine Nonulcerative Corneal Disease

Juliet R. Gionfriddo, DVM, MS, DACVO
Professor
Clinical Sciences
Colorado State University
Fort Collins, Colorado
Ocular Emergencies

Elizabeth A. Giuliano, DVM, MS, DACVO
Associate Professor
Veterinary Medicine and Surgery
University of Missouri
Columbia, Missouri
Tear Film Disorders in Dogs

Richard E. Goldstein, DVM, DACVIM (Small Animal Internal Medicine), DECVIM-CA
Chief Medical Officer
The Animal Medical Center
New York, New York
Infectious Causes of Polyarthritis in Dogs

Rebecca E. Gompf, DVM, MS
Associate Professor of Cardiology
Department of Small Animal Clinical
 Sciences
College of Veterinary Medicine
The University of Tennessee
Knoxville, Tennessee
Ventricular Septal Defect

Jody L. Gookin, DVM, PhD
Associate Professor
Department of Clinical Sciences
North Carolina State University
Raleigh, North Carolina
Protozoal Gastrointestinal Disease

Sonya G. Gordon, DVM, DVSc, DACVIM (Cardiology)
Department of Small Animal Clinical
 Science
College of Veterinary Medicine and
 Biomedical Science
Texas A&M University
College Station, Texas
Canine Heartworm Disease
Patent Ductus Arteriosus

Carlos M. Gradil, DVM, MS, PhD, DACT
Ext. Associate Professor
Veterinary and Animal Sciences
University of Massachusetts
Amherst, Massachusetts
Adjunct Associate Professor, Clinical
 Sciences
Tufts University
North Grafton, Massachusetts
Ovarian Remnant Syndrome in Small Animals

Gregory F. Grauer, DVM, MS, DACVIM
Professor and Jarvis Chair of Medicine
Department of Clinical Sciences
Kansas State University
Manhattan, Kansas
Staff Internist
Veterinary Medical Teaching Hospital
Kansas State University
Manhattan, Kansas
Proteinuria/Albuminuria: Implications for Management

Deborah S. Greco, DVM, PhD, DACVIM
Senior Research Scientist
Nestle Purina PetCare
St. Louis, Missouri
Complicated Diabetes Mellitus
Alternatives to Insulin Therapy for Diabetes Mellitus in Cats

Craig E. Greene, DVM, MS, DACVIM
Emeritus Professor
Department of Small Animal Medicine
 and Surgery
College of Veterinary Medicine
University of Georgia
Athens, Georgia
Pet-Associated Illness

Clare R. Gregory, DVM, DACVS
Professor Emeritus
Surgical and Radiological Sciences
School of Veterinary Medicine
University of California—Davis
Davis, California
Staff Surgeon
PetCare Animal Hospital
Santa Rosa, California
Immunosuppressive Agents

Joel D. Griffies, DVM DACVD
Animal Dermatology Clinic
Marietta, Georgia
Topical Immunomodulators

Carol B. Grindem, DVM, PhD, DACVP
Professor of Clinical Pathology
Department of Population Health and
Pathobiology
North Carolina State University
Raleigh, North Carolina
Thrombocytopenia

Amy M. Grooters, DVM, DACVIM
Professor, Companion Animal Medicine
Veterinary Clinical Sciences
The Louisiana State University
Baton Rouge, Louisiana
Systemic Antifungal Therapy
Pythiosis and Lagenidiosis

Julien Guillaumin, Doct. Vet. DACVECC
Assistant Professor—Clinical
Veterinary Clinical Sciences
Veterinary Medical Center
The Ohio State University
Columbus, Ohio
Ventilator Therapy for the Critical Patient

Lynn F. Guptill, DVM, PhD, DACVIM (SAIM)
Associate Professor
Veterinary Clinical Sciences
Purdue University
West Lafayette, Indiana
Feline Bartonellosis

Amanda Guth, DVM, PhD
Research Scientist
Animal Cancer Center
Clinical Sciences
Colorado State University
Fort Collins, Colorado
Cancer Immunotherapy

Sharon M. Gwaltney-Brant, DVM, PhD, DABVT, DABT
Adjunct Instructor
Department of Comparative Biosciences
University of Illinois College of
Veterinary Medicine
Urbana, Illinois
Toxicology Consultant
Veterinary Information Network
Davis, California
Drugs Used to Treat Toxicoses
Lead Toxicosis in Small Animals

Timothy B. Hackett, DVM, MS
Professor
Emergency and Critical Care Medicine
Clinical Sciences
Colorado State University
Fort Collins, Colorado
Stabilization of the Patient with Respiratory Distress
Transfusion Medicine: Best Practices

Susan G. Hackner, BVSc, MRCVS, DACVIM, DACVECC
Chief Medical Officer & Chief Operating
Officer
Cornell University
Veterinary Specialists
Stamford, Connecticut
Pulmonary Thromboembolism

Kevin A. Hahn, DVM, PhD, ACVIM (Oncology)
Chief Medical Officer
Science & Technology
Hill's Pet Nutrition, Inc.
Topeka, Kansas
Drug Update: Masitinib
Pulmonary Neoplasia

Annick Hamaide, DVM, PhD, DECVS
Associate Professor
Department of Clinical Sciences
(Companion Animals)
School of Veterinary Medicine
University of Liege
Liege, Belgium
*Medical Management of Urinary
Incontinence and Retention Disorders*

Ralph E. Hamor, DVM, MS, DACVO
Clinical Professor
Veterinary Clinical Medicine
University of Illinois at
Urbana-Champaign
Urbana, Illinois
Orbital Disease

Rita M. Hanel, DVM, DACVIM, DACVECC
Assistant Professor of Emergency and
Critical Care
Department of Clinical Sciences
College of Veterinary Medicine
North Carolina State University
Raleigh, North Carolina
Pneumonia

Bernie Hansen, DVM, MS, DACVECC, DACVIM (Internal Medicine)
Associate Professor
Department of Clinical Sciences
North Carolina State University
Raleigh, North Carolina
Pneumonia

William R. Hare Jr., DVM, MS, PhD, DABVT, DABT
Veterinary Medical Officer—Retired
Animal and Natural Resources Institute
USDA-ARS
Beltsville, Maryland
Urban Legends of Toxicology: Facts and Fiction

Katrin Hartmann, Dr.vet.med., Dr. habil., DECVIM-CA
Professor
Center of Clinical Veterinary Sciences
Clinic of Small Animal Medicine
Munich, Germany
Management of Feline Retrovirus-Infected Cats

Andrea M. Harvey, BVSc, DSAM (Feline), DECVIM-CA, MRCVS
Feline Specialist
Small Animal Specialist Hospital
Sydney, New South Wales, Australia
Australian Representative
International Society of Feline Medicine
Feline Primary Hyperaldosteronism

Elizabeth A. Hausner, DVM, DABT, DABVT
Center for Drug Evaluation and Research
United States Food and Drug
Administration
Silver Spring, Maryland
Herbal Hazards

Eleanor C. Hawkins, DVM
Professor, Internal Medicine
Department of Clinical Sciences
North Carolina State University College
of Veterinary Medicine
Raleigh, North Carolina
Respiratory Drug Therapy

Silke Hecht, Dr.Med.Vet., DACVR, DECVDI
Associate Professor Radiology
Department of Small Animal Clinical
Sciences
College of Veterinary Medicine
The University of Tennessee
Knoxville, Tennessee
*Applications of Ultrasound in Diagnosis and
Management of Urinary Disease*

Romy M. Heilmann, Dr.Med.Vet
Veterinary Resident Instructor
Small Animal Internal Medicine/
  Graduate (PhD) Student
Gastrointestinal Laboratory
Department of Small Animal Clinical
  Sciences
College of Veterinary Medicine and
  Biomedical Sciences
Texas A&M University
College Station, Texas
Laboratory Testing for the Exocrine Pancreas

Carolyn J. Henry, DVM, MS
Professor of Oncology
Veterinary Medicine and Surgery
Interim Associate Director of Research
Internal Medicine
Hematology/Oncology Division
Ellis Fischel Cancer Center
Faculty Facilitator of One Health/One
  Medicine
Office of the Provost
Mizzou Advantage Program
College of Veterinary Medicine
University of Missouri
Columbia, Missouri
Mammary Cancer

Meghan E. Herron, DVM, DACVB
Clinical Assistant Professor
Veterinary Clinical Sciences
The Ohio State University
Columbus, Ohio
Drugs for Behavior-Related Dermatoses

**Steve L. Hill, DVM, MS, DACVIM
  (SAIM)**
Clinical Associate Faculty
Veterinary Medicine
Western University of Health Sciences
College of Veterinary Medicine
Pomona, California
Staff Internist, Partner, Hospital
  Co-Owner
Internal Medicine
Veterinary Specialty Hospital of San
  Diego
San Diego, California
President
Comparative Gastroenterology Society
  (CGS)
Feline Hepatic Lipidosis

**Armando E. Hoet, DVM, PhD,
  DACVPM**
Director, Veterinary Public Health
  Program
Veterinary Preventive Medicine
  Department
College of Veterinary Medicine
The Ohio State University
Columbus, Ohio
*Disinfection of Environments Contaminated
  by Staphylococcal Pathogens*

**Daniel F. Hogan, DVM,
  DACVIM-Cardiology**
Associate Professor and Chief,
  Comparative Cardiovascular Medicine
  and Interventional Cardiology
Veterinary Clinical Sciences
College of Veterinary Medicine
Purdue University
West Lafayette, Indiana
Arterial Thromboembolism

**Steven R. Hollingsworth, DVM,
  DACVO**
Associate Professor of Clinical
  Ophthalmology
Department of Surgical and Radiological
  Sciences
School of Veterinary Medicine
University of California—Davis
Davis, California
Diseases of the Eyelids and Periocular Skin

**Fiona K. Hollinshead, BVSC (Hons),
  PhD, MACVS, DACT**
Adjunct Senior Lecturer
Veterinary Science
The University of Sydney
Sydney, New South Wales, Australia
Matamata Veterinary Services
Matamata, New Zealand
Endoscopic Transcervical Insemination

David Holt, BVSc, DACVS
Professor of Surgery
Department of Clinical Studies
School of Veterinary Medicine
University of Pennsylvania
Philadelphia, Pennsylvania
Drainage Techniques for the Septic Abdomen
Pleural Effusion

Heidi A. Hottinger, DVM, DACVS
Soft Tissue Surgeon & Practice Partner
Surgery, Orthopedics & Neurology
Gulf Coast Veterinary Specialists
Houston, Texas
Canine Biliary Mucocele

Geraldine Briony Hunt, DVM
Professor of Small Animal Soft Tissue
  Surgery
Veterinary Surgical & Radiological
  Sciences
University of California—Davis
Davis, California
Nasopharyngeal Disorders

Kate Hurley, DVM, MPVM
Director, Koret Shelter Medicine Program
Center for Companion Animal Health
University of California—Davis
Davis, California
Feline Upper Respiratory Tract Infection

**Toshiroh Iwasaki, DVM, PhD,
  DAICVD**
Professor
Veterinary Internal Medicine
Tokyo University of Agriculture &
  Technology
Fuchu, Tokyo, Japan
Interferons

**Hilary A. Jackson, BVM&S, DVD,
  DACVD, MRCVS**
Dermatology Referral Service
Honorary Teacher
University of Glasgow Veterinary School
Glasgow, Scotland, United Kingdom
*Elimination Diets for Cutaneous Adverse
  Food Reactions: Principles in Therapy*

**Karl E. Jandrey, DVM, MAS,
  DACVECC**
Assistant Professor of Small Animal
  Emergency & Critical Care
Veterinary Surgical & Radiological
  Sciences
University of California—Davis
Davis, California
William R. Pritchard Veterinary Medical
  Teaching Hospital
Davis, California
Thromboelastography

**Albert E. Jergens, DVM, PhD,
  DACVIM**
Professor
Veterinary Clinical Sciences
Iowa State University
Ames, Iowa
*Current Veterinary Therapy: Antibiotic
  Responsive Enteropathy*

Beth M. Johnson, DVM, DACVIM
Clinical Assistant Professor of Medicine
Department of Small Animal Clinical
  Sciences
College of Veterinary Medicine
The University of Tennessee
Knoxville, Tennessee
Canine Megaesophagus

**Eileen McGoey Johnson, BS, DVM,
  MS, PhD**
Associate Professor
Department of Veterinary Pathobiology
Oklahoma State University
Stillwater, Oklahoma
Hepatozoon americanum Infections

Valerie Johnson, DVM, DACVECC
T32 Fellowship Grant Trainee
Microbiology, Immunology, and
  Pathology
Veterinary Teaching Hospital
Colorado State University
Fort Collins, Colorado
*Management of Immune-Mediated
  Hemolytic Anemia in Dogs*

Andrea N. Johnston, DVM, DACVIM
Clinical Instructor
Clinical Sciences
College of Veterinary Medicine
Cornell University
Ithaca, New York
Portal Vein Hypoplasia (Microvascular Dysplasia)

Debra A. Kamstock, DVM, PhD, DACVP
Chief Pathologist and Director
KamPath Diagnostics & Investigation
Fort Collins, Colorado
Faculty Affiliate
College of Veterinary Medicine and Biomedical Sciences
Colorado State University
Fort Collins, Colorado
Tumor Biopsy and Specimen Submission

Shinichi Kanazono, DVM
Veterinary Medicine and Surgery
College of Veterinary Medicine
University of Missouri
Columbia, Missouri
Canine Degenerative Myelopathy

Margo Karriker, PharmD, FSVHP
Clinical Pharmacist
University of California Veterinary Medical Center—San Diego
San Diego, California
University of California—Davis
Davis, California
Chemotherapeutic Drug Handling and Safety

Aarti Kathrani, BVetMed (Hons), PhD, MRCVS
Resident
Small Animal Internal Medicine
Clinical Sciences
Cornell University
Ithaca, New York
Inflammatory Bowel Disease

Linda K. Kauffman, BS, DVM
Clinician
Veterinary Clinical Sciences
Iowa State University
Ames, Iowa
Pregnancy Loss in the Bitch and Queen

Bruce W. Keene, DVM, MSc, DACVIM (Cardiology)
Professor
Department of Clinical Sciences
North Carolina State University
Raleigh, North Carolina
Drugs for Treatment of Heart Failure in Dogs
Management of Heart Failure in Dogs

Charlotte B. Keller, Dr.Med.Vet., DACVO, DECVO
West Coast Veterinary Eye Specialists
New Westminster, British Columbia, Canada
Epiphora

Robert Allen Kennis, DVM, MS, DACVD
Associate Professor
Department of Clinical Sciences
Auburn University
Auburn, Alabama
Bilaterally Symmetric Alopecia in Dogs
Occult Hyperadrenocorticism: Is It Real?
Flea Control in Flea Allergy Dermatitis

Michael S. Kent, DVM, MAS, DACVIM (Medical Oncology), DACVR (Radiation Oncology)
Associate Professor
Surgical and Radiological Sciences
School of Veterinary Medicine
University of California—Davis
Davis, California
Oral Tumors

Marie E. Kerl, DVM, MPH, DACVIM (SAIM), DACVECC
Associate Teaching Professor
Veterinary Medicine and Surgery
University of Missouri
Columbia, Missouri
Recognition and Prevention of Hospital-Acquired Acute Kidney Injury

Peter P. Kintzer, DVM, DACVIM
Medical Affairs Manager
IDEXX Laboratories
Westbrook, Maine
Canine Hypoadrenocorticism
Differential Diagnosis of Hyperkalemia and Hyponatremia in Dogs and Cats

Rebecca Kirby, DVM, DACVIM, DACVECC
Animal Emergency Center
Glendale, Wisconsin
Colloid Fluid Therapy
Disseminated Intravascular Coagulation

Claudia A. Kirk, DVM, PhD, DACVN, DACVIM (SAIM)
Professor and Head
Department of Small Animal Clinical Sciences
College of Veterinary Medicine
The University of Tennessee
Knoxville, Tennessee
Obesity

Deborah W. Knapp, DVM
Dolores L. McCall Professor of Comparative Oncology
Veterinary Clinical Sciences
Purdue University
West Lafayette, Indiana
Urinary Bladder Cancer

Hans S. Kooistra, DVM, PhD, DECVIM-CA
Department of Clinical Sciences of Companion Animals
Faculty of Veterinary Medicine
Universiteit Utrecht
Utrecht, The Netherlands
Ectopic ACTH Syndrome and Food-Dependent Hypercortisolism in Dogs

Peter Hendrik Kook, Dr.Med.Vet., DACVIM, DECVIM
Department for Small Animals
Clinic for Small Animal Internal Medicine
University of Zurich
Zurich, Switzerland
Gastroesophageal Reflux

Bruce G. Kornreich, DVM, PhD, DACVIM (Cardiology)
Associate Director for Education and Outreach
Cornell Feline Health Center
Cardiologist
Department of Clinical Sciences
College of Veterinary Medicine
Cornell University
Ithaca, New York
Bradyarrhythmias

Marc S. Kraus, DVM, DACVIM (Cardiology, Internal Medicine)
Senior Lecturer
Department of Clinical Sciences
College of Veterinary Medicine
Cornell University
Ithaca, New York
Syncope

Annemarie T. Kristensen, DVM, PhD, DACVIM-SA, DECVIM-CA (Oncology)
Professor, Section Head
Internal Medicine and Clinical Pathology
Department of Veterinary Clinical and Animal Sciences
Faculty of Health and Medical Sciences
University of Copenhagen
Copenhagen, Denmark
Hypercoagulable States

Ned F. Kuehn, DVM, MS, DACVIM (SAIM)
Chief of Internal Medicine
Michigan Veterinary Specialists
Southfield, Michigan
Rhinitis in Dogs

Kate S. KuKanich, DVM, PhD, DACVIM (Internal Medicine)
Assistant Professor
Department of Clinical Sciences
Kansas State University
Manhattan, Kansas
Surveillance for Asymptomatic and Hospital-Acquired Urinary Tract Infection

Kenneth W. Kwochka, DVM, DACVD
Veterinary Manager
Health and Wellness
Bayer HealthCare Animal Health
Shawnee Mission, Kansas
Topical Therapy for Infectious Diseases

Mary Anna Labato, DVM, DACVIM (SAIM)
Clinical Professor
Clinical Sciences
Cummings School of Veterinary Medicine
Tufts University
North Grafton, Massachusetts
Medical Management of Nephroliths and Ureteroliths
Calcium Oxalate Urolithiasis

Susan E. Lana, DVM, MS, DACVIM (Oncology)
Associate Professor
Clinical Sciences
Colorado State University
Fort Collins, Colorado
Lymphocytosis in Dogs and Cats

Cathy E. Langston, DVM, DACVIM (SAIM)
Staff Veterinarian
Nephrology, Urology, and Dialysis
Animal Medical Center
New York, New York
Recognition and Prevention of Hospital-Acquired Acute Kidney Injury

Susan M. LaRue, DVM, PhD, DACVS, DACVR (Radiation Oncology)
Professor
Environmental and Radiological Health Sciences
James L. Voss Veterinary Teaching Hospital and the Animal Cancer Center
Colorado State University
Fort Collins, Colorado
Advances in Radiation Therapy for Nasal Tumors

James A. Lavely, DVM, DACVIM Neurology
Neurology and Neurosurgery
VCA Animal Care Center
Rohnert Park, California
Priapism in Dogs

Eric C. Ledbetter, DVM, DACVO
Robert Hovey Udall Assistant Professor of Ophthalmology
Clinical Sciences
College of Veterinary Medicine
Cornell University
Ithaca, New York
Canine Conjunctivitis

Justine A. Lee, DVM, DACVECC, DABT
Associate Director of Veterinary Services
Pet Poison Helpline, a Division of SafetyCall International
Minneapolis, Minnesota
Intravenous Lipid Emulsion Therapy

Michael S. Leib, DVM, MS
C.R. Roberts Professor
Small Animal Clinical Sciences
Virginia-Maryland Regional College of Veterinary Medicine
Virginia Tech
Blacksburg, Virginia
Gastric Helicobacter spp. and Chronic Vomiting in Dogs

Jonathan M. Levine, DVM, DACVIM (Neurology)
Assistant Professor
Neurology/Neurosurgery
Small Animal Clinical Sciences
Texas A&M University
College Station, Texas
Canine Intervertebral Disk Herniation

Christine C. Lim, DVM, DACVO
Assistant Clinical Professor
Department of Veterinary Clinical Sciences
College of Veterinary Medicine
University of Minnesota
St. Paul, Minnesota
Tear Film Disorders of Cats

Julius M. Liptak, BVSc, MVetClinStud, FACVSc, DACVS, DECVS
Adjunct Professor
University of Guelph
Guelph, Ontario, Canada
Adjunct Professor
St. Matthews University
Grand Cayman, Cayman Islands
Specialist Small Animal Surgeon
Alta Vista Animal Hospital
Ottawa, Ontario, Canada
Soft Tissue Sarcomas

Susan E. Little, DVM, PhD, DACVM (Parasitology)
Regents Professor and Chair
Veterinary Pathobiology
Center for Veterinary Health Sciences
Oklahoma State University
Stillwater, Oklahoma
Hepatozoon americanum Infections

Meryl P. Littman, VMD, DACVIM
Professor of Medicine
Clinical Studies
School of Veterinary Medicine
University of Pennsylvania
Philadelphia, Pennsylvania
Borreliosis

Remo Lobetti, BVSc, MMeVet (Med), PhD, DECVIM
Doctor
Bryanston Veterinary Hospital
Bryanston, South Africa
Pneumocystosis

Dawn Logas, DVM, DACVD
Owner/Staff Dermatologist
Veterinary Dermatology Center
Maitland, Florida
Ear-Flushing Techniques

Cheryl A. London, DVM, PhD, ACVIM (Oncology)
Associate Professor
College of Veterinary Biosciences
The Ohio State University
Columbus, Ohio
Drug Update: Toceranib

Catherine A. Loughin, DVM, DACVS, DACCT
Staff Surgeon
Department of Surgery
Long Island Veterinary Specialists
Plainview, New York
Craniocervical Junction Abnormalities in Dogs
Diagnosis and Treatment of Degenerative Lumbosacral Stenosis

Virginia Luis Fuentes, MA, VetMB, PhD, CertVR, DVC, MRCVS, DACVIM, DECVIM-CA (Cardiology)
Professor of Veterinary Cardiology
Department of Veterinary Clinical Sciences and Services
The Royal Veterinary College
Hatfield, Hertfordshire, United Kingdom
Feline Myocardial Disease

Jody P. Lulich
Professor
Co-Director
Minnesota Urolith Center
University of Minnesota
St. Paul, Minnesota
Canine Urate Urolithiasis
Laser Lithotripsy for Uroliths

Katharine F. Lunn, BVMs, MS, PhD, MRCVS, DACVIM
Associate Professor
Clinical Sciences
North Carolina State University
Raleigh, North Carolina
Leptospirosis

John M. MacDonald, MEd, DVM, DACVD
Professor of Dermatology
Small Animal Hospital
Department of Clinical Sciences
Auburn University
Auburn, Alabama
Acral Lick Dermatitis

Kristin A. MacDonald, DVM, PhD, DACVIM (Cardiology)
Veterinary Cardiologist
VCA—Animal Care Center of Sonoma County
Rohnert Park, California
Infective Endocarditis

Catriona M. MacPhail, DVM, PhD
Associate Professor
Department of Clinical Sciences
College of Veterinary Medicine and Biomedical Sciences
Colorado State University
Fort Collins, Colorado
Laryngeal Diseases

Dennis W. Macy, DVM, MS
Professor Emeritus
Clinical Sciences
College of Veterinary Medicine and Biomedical Sciences
Colorado State University
Fort Collins, Colorado
Chief of Medical Oncology
Department of Oncology
Desert Veterinary Specialist
Palm Desert, California
Owner Cancer Care Specialist
West Flamingo Animal Hospital
Las Vegas, Nevada
Update on Vaccine-Associated Adverse Effects in Cats

David J. Maggs, BVSc, DACVO
Professor
Department of Surgical and Radiological Sciences
University of California—Davis
Davis, California
Pearls of the Ophthalmic Examination

Herbert W. Maisenbacher III, VMD, DACVIM (Cardiology)
Clinical Assistant Professor
Small Animal Clinical Sciences
College of Veterinary Medicine
University of Florida
Gainesville, Florida
Dilated Cardiomyopathy in Dogs
Pulmonic Stenosis

Giovanni Majolino, DVM
Specialist in Small Animal Diseases
Reproduction
Clinic Majolino-Ranieri
Collecchio (Parma), Italy
Aspermia/Oligospermia Caused by Retrograde Ejaculation in Dogs

Richard Malik, DVSc, DipVetAn, MVetClinStud, PhD, FASM, FACVSc
Adjunct Professor
School of Animal & Veterinary Sciences
Charles Sturt University
Wagga Wagga, New South Wales, Australia
Senior Staff Specialist
Double Bay Veterinary Clinic
Sydney, New South Wales, Australia
Valentine Charlton Veterinary Specialist
Centre for Veterinary Education
University of Sydney
Sydney, New South Wales, Australia
Nontuberculous Cutaneous Granulomas in Dogs and Cats (Canine Leproid Granuloma and Feline Leprosy Syndrome)

Alison C. Manchester, BS
Veterinary Student Research Assistant
College of Veterinary Medicine
Cornell University
Ithaca, New York
Canine Colitis

Dominic J. Marino, DVM, DACVS, DACCT, CCRP
Long Island Veterinary Specialists
Plainview, New York
Craniocervical Junction Abnormalities in Dogs

Jessica E. Markovich, DVM, DACVIM
Department of Clinical Sciences
Tufts Cummings School of Veterinary Medicine
North Grafton, Massachusetts
Internal Medicine and Clinical Nutrition
VCA Emergency Animal Hospital & Referral Center
San Diego, California
Medical Management of Nephroliths and Ureteroliths

Stanley L. Marks, BVSc, PhD, DACVIM (Internal Medicine, Oncology), DACVN
Professor
Department of Medicine and Epidemiology
School of Veterinary Medicine
University of California—Davis
Davis, California
Oropharyngeal Dysphagia

Rosanna Marsella, DVM, DACVD
Professor
Small Animal Clinical Sciences
University of Florida
Gainesville, Florida
Pentoxifylline

Julie M. Martin, DVM, MS, DACVIM (Cardiology)
Veterinary Referral Center of Colorado
Rocky Mountain Veterinary Cardiology
Englewood, Colorado
Cardioversion

Linda G. Martin, DVM, MS, DACVECC
Associate Professor
Critical Care Medicine
Department of Veterinary Clinical Sciences
Washington State University
Pullman, Washington
Approach to Critical Illness–Related Corticosteroid Insufficiency
Approach to Hypomagnesemia and Hypokalemia

Karol A. Mathews, DVM, DVSc, DACVECC
Professor Emerita
Clinical Studies
Ontario Veterinary College
University of Guelph
Guelph, Ontario, Canada
Gastric Dilation-Volvulus

Elizabeth A. Mauldin, DVM, DACVP, DACVD
Associate Professor of Dermatopathology, CE
Department of Pathobiology
School of Veterinary Medicine
University of Pennsylvania
Philadelphia, Pennsylvania
Primary Cornification Disorders in Dogs

Glenna E. Mauldin, DVM, MS
Western Veterinary Cancer Centre
Western Veterinary Specialist and Emergency Centre
Calgary, Alberta, Canada
Nutritional Support of the Cancer Patient

Dianne I. Mawby, DVM, MVSc, DACVIM
Clinical Associate Professor
Department of Small Animal Clinical Sciences
College of Veterinary Medicine
The University of Tennessee
Knoxville, Tennessee
Top Ten Urinary Consult Questions

Robert J. McCarthy, DVM, MS, DACVS
Clinical Associate Professor
Veterinary Clinical Sciences
Tufts Cummings School of Veterinary Medicine
North Grafton, Massachusetts
Tufts Foster Hospital
Cummings School of Veterinary Medicine
North Grafton, Massachusetts
Owner
Veterinary Surgery of Central Massachusetts
Grafton, Massachusetts
Emergency Management of Open Fractures
Ovarian Remnant Syndrome in Small Animals

Mary A. McLoughlin, DVM, MS, DACVS
Associate Professor
Veterinary Clinical Sciences
Small Animal Surgery
College of Veterinary Medicine
Veterinary Medical Center
The Ohio State University
Columbus, Ohio
Urinary Incontinence: Treatment with Injectable Bulking Agents

Erick A. Mears, DVM, DACVIM
Medical Director
BluePearl Veterinary Partners
Specialty & Emergency Medicine for Pets
Tampa, Florida
Canine Megaesophagus

Karelle A. Meleo, DVM, ACVIM, ACVR
Chief Oncologist
Animal Cancer Specialists
Seattle, Washington
Treatment of Insulinoma in Dogs, Cats, and Ferrets

Colleen L. Mendelsohn, DVM, DACVD
Animal Dermatology Clinic
Tustin, California
Topical Antimicrobials for Otitis

Stacy D. Meola, DVM, MS
ECC Resident
Emergency
Wheat Ridge Veterinary Specialists
Wheat Ridge, Colorado
Emergency Wound Management and Vacuum-Assisted Wound Closure

Kathryn M. Meurs, DVM, PhD
Professor
Department of Clinical Sciences
College of Veterinary Medicine
North Carolina State University
Raleigh, North Carolina
Arrhythmogenic Right Ventricular Cardiomyopathy

Vicki N. Meyers-Wallen, VMD, PhD, DACT
Associate Professor
Baker Institute for Animal Health
Cornell University
Ithaca, New York
Inherited Disorders of the Reproductive Tract in Dogs and Cats

Matthew W. Miller, DVM, MS, DACVIM (Cardiology)
Professor of Cardiology
Small Animal Veterinary Clinical Sciences
Senior Research Scientist
Texas A&M Institute for Preclinical Studies
Charter Fellow
Michael E. DeBakey Institute
Texas A&M University
College Station, Texas
Canine Heartworm Disease
Patent Ductus Arteriosus

Darryl L. Millis, MS, DVM, DACVS, CCRP
Associate Professor of Orthopedic Surgery
Department of Small Animal Clinical Sciences
College of Veterinary Medicine
The University of Tennessee
Knoxville, Tennessee
Physical Therapy and Rehabilitation of Neurologic Patients

Leah Ann Mitchell, PhD
Research Scientist
Department of Clinical Sciences
Colorado State University
Fort Collins, Colorado
Cancer Immunotherapy

N. Sydney Moïse, DVM, MS
Professor of Medicine (Cardiology)
Clinical Sciences
College of Veterinary Medicine
Cornell University
Ithaca, New York
Bradyarrhythmias
Supraventricular Tachyarrhythmias in Dogs

Eric Monnet, DVM, PhD, DACVS, DECVS
Professor
Clinical Sciences
Colorado State University
Fort Collins, Colorado
Laryngeal Diseases

William E. Monroe, DVM, MS, DACVIM (SAIM)
Professor, Small Animal Clinical Sciences
Department of Small Animal Clinical Sciences
Virginia-Maryland Regional College of Veterinary Medicine
Virginia Tech
Blacksburg, Virginia
Canine Diabetes Mellitus

Hernán J. Montilla, DVM.
Assistant Professor
Clinical Science
Clinical Instructor
Theriogenology
Veterinary Teaching Hospital
Oregon State University
Corvallis, Oregon
Methods for Diagnosing Diseases of the Female Reproductive Tract

Erin Mooney, BVSc, DACVECC
Clinical Tutor
Department of Emergency and Critical Care
University of Melbourne
Werribee, Victoria, Australia
Pneumothorax

Antony S. Moore, BVSc, MVSc, DACVIM (Oncology)
Co-Director
Veterinary Oncology Consultants
Wauchope, New South Wales, Australia
Consultant
Animal Referral Hospital
Homebush, New South Wales, Australia
Malignant Effusions

George E. Moore, DVM, MS, PhD, DACVIM (SAIM), DACVPM (Epi)
Professor
School of Veterinary Medicine
Comparative Pathobiology
Purdue University
West Lafayette, Indiana
Vaccine-Associated Adverse Effects in Dogs

Adam Mordecai, DVM, MS, DACVIM
Veterinary Medical Referral Service
Veterinary Specialty Center
Buffalo Grove, Illinois
Rational Use of Glucocorticoids in Infectious Disease

Karen A. Moriello, DVM, DACVD
Professor of Dermatology
American College of Veterinary Dermatology
Department of Medical Sciences
University of Wisconsin—Madison
Madison, Wisconsin
Treatment of Dermatophytosis
Dermatophytosis: Investigating an Outbreak in a Multicat Environment

Daniel O. Morris, DVM, MPH
Associate Professor of Dermatology
Clinical Studies
School of Veterinary Medicine
University of Pennsylvania
Philadelphia, Pennsylvania
Malassezia Infections

Ralf S. Mueller, Dr.Med.Vet., Dr.habil., DACVD, Fellow ANZCVSc, DECVD
Professor of Veterinary Dermatology
Center of Clinical Veterinary Medicine
Chief of Dermatology and Allergy
Center of Clinical Veterinary Medicine
Ludwig Maximilian University Munich
Munich, Germany
Canine Demodicosis

Suzanne Murphy, BVM&S, MSc (Clin Onc), DECVIM-CA (Onc), MRCVS
Head of Hospital
Centre for Small Animal Studies
Animal Health Studies
Lanwades Park, Kentford, Suffolk, United Kingdom
Thyroid Tumors

Russell Muse, DVM, DACVD
Animal Dermatology Clinic
Tustin, California
Diseases of the Anal Sac

Anthony J. Mutsaers, DVM, PhD, DACVIM (Oncology)
Assistant Professor
Department of Clinical Studies
Department of Biomedical Sciences
Ontario Veterinary College
University of Guelph
Guelph, Ontario, Canada
Metronomic Chemotherapy

Kathern E. Myrna, MS, DVM, DACVO
Assistant Professor
Small Animal Medicine and Surgery
University of Georgia
Athens, Georgia
Feline Retinopathies

Masahiko Nagata, DVM, PhD, DAICVD
Director
Dermatology Service
Animal Specialist Center
Chofu,Tokyo, Japan
Canine Papillomaviruses

Larry A. Nagode, DVM, MS, PhD
Emeritus Associate Professor
Veterinary Biosciences
The Ohio State University
Columbus, Ohio
Treatment of Hypoparathyroidism

Jill Narak, DVM, MS, DACVIM (Neurology)
Assistant Professor, Neurology & Neurosurgery
Department of Small Animal Clinical Sciences
College of Veterinary Medicine
The University of Tennessee
Knoxville, Tennessee
Treatment of Intracranial Tumors

Jennifer A. Neel, DVM, DACVP (Clinical)
Assistant Professor in Veterinary Clinical Pathology
Department of Population Health and Pathobiology
College of Veterinary Medicine
North Carolina State University
Raleigh, North Carolina
Thrombocytopenia

Reto Neiger, Dr.med.vet., PhD, DECVIM-CA, DACVIM
Professor for Small Animal Internal Medicine
Justus-Liebig-Universtat-Giessen
Small Animal Clinic
Giessen, Germany
Canine Hyperadrenocorticism Therapy
Gastric Ulceration

O. Lynne Nelson, DVM, MS, DACVIM
Associate Professor
Veterinary Clinical Sciences
Washington State University
Pullman, Washington
Pericardial Effusion

Richard W. Nelson, DVM, DACVIM (Small Animal)
Professor
Department of Medicine and Epidemiology
School of Veterinary Medicine
University of California—Davis
Davis, California
Insulin Resistance

Sandra Newbury, DVM
Koret Shelter Medicine Program
School of Veterinary Medicine
University of California—Davis
Davis, California
Adjunct Assistant Professor
Department of Pathobiology
University of Wisconsin
Madison, Wisconsin
Dermatophytosis: Investigating an Outbreak in a Multicat Environment

Sandra M. Nguyen, BVSc (Hons I) DACVIM (Oncology)
Animal Referral Hospital
Sydney, Australia
Canine Ocular Neoplasia
Feline Ocular Neoplasia

Rhett Nichols, DVM, ACVIM
The Animal Endocrine Clinic
New York City, New York
Internal Medicine Consultant
Antech Diagnostics
Irvine, California
Clinical Use of the Vasopressin Analog Desmopressin for the Diagnosis and Treatment of Diabetes Insipidus

Stijn J.M. Niessen, DVM, PhD, DECVIM, PGCVetEd, FHEA, MRCVS
Lecturer, Internal Medicine
Veterinary Clinical Sciences
The Royal Veterinary College
North Mymms, Hertfordshire, United Kingdom
Research Associate
Diabetes Research Group
Medical School Newcastle
Newcastle-Upon-Tyne, Tyne and Wear, United Kingdom
Feline Hypersomatotropism and Acromegaly

Benjamin G. Nolan, DVM, PhD, DACVIM (SAIM)
Staff Internist
Internal Medicine
Veterinary Specialty Center
Middleton, Wisconsin
Calcium Oxalate Urolithiasis

Roberto E. Novo, DVM, MS, DACVS
Veterinary Surgeon
Columbia River Veterinary Specialists
Vancouver, Washington
Surgical Repair of Vaginal Anomalies in the Bitch

Tim Nuttall, BSc, BVSc, CertVD, PhD, CBiol, MSB, MRCVS
The Royal (Dick) School of Veterinary Studies
The University of Edinburgh
Easter Bush Veterinary Centre
Roslin, United Kingdom
Topical and Systemic Glucocorticoids for Otitis

Frederick W. Oehme, DVM, Dr. Med. Vet, PhD
Professor Emeritus
Diagnostic Medicine/Pathobiology
Kansas State University
Manhattan, Kansas
Urban Legends of Toxicology: Facts and Fiction

Thierry Olivry, Dr Vet, PhD, DACVD, DECVD
Professor of Immunodermatology
Department of Clinical Sciences
College of Veterinary Medicine
North Carolina State University
Raleigh, North Carolina
Treatment Guidelines for Canine Atopic Dermatitis

Carl A. Osborne, DVM, PhD, DACVIM
Veterinary Clinical Sciences Department
College of Veterinary Medicine
University of Minnesota
St. Paul, Minnesota
Canine Urate Urolithiasis

Catherine A. Outerbridge, DVM, MVSc
Associate Professor of Clinical Dermatology
Department of Veterinary Medicine and Epidemiology
William Pritchard Veterinary Medical Teaching Hospital
Dermatology Service
University of California—Davis
Davis, California
Diseases of the Eyelids and Periocular Skin

Mark A. Oyama, DVM, DACVIM (Cardiology)
Professor
Department of Clinical Studies
University of Pennsylvania
Philadelphia, Pennsylvania
Ventricular Arrhythmias in Dogs
Bradyarrhythmias and Cardiac Pacing

Philip Padrid, DVM
Associate Professor of Medicine
Department of Molecular Medicine
University of Chicago
Chicago, Illinois
Associate Professor of Small Animal Medicine
The Ohio State University
Columbus, Ohio
Regional Medical Director
VCA/Antech
Los Angeles, California
Chronic Bronchitis and Asthma in Cats

Lee E. Palmer, DVM
Resident, Emergency and Critical Care
Small Animal Clinical Sciences
Auburn University
Small Animal Teaching Hospital
Auburn, Alabama
Approach to Hypomagnesemia and Hypokalemia

Lee Anne Myers Palmer, VMD
Office of Surveillance and Compliance
FDA Center for Veterinary Medicine
Rockville, Maryland
Reporting Adverse Events to the Food and Drug Administration—Center for Veterinary Medicine

David L. Panciera, DVM, MS
Anne Hunter Professor of Small Animal Medicine
Department of Small Animal Clinical Sciences
Virginia-Maryland Regional College of Veterinary Medicine
Virginia Tech
Blacksburg, Virginia
Complications and Concurrent Conditions Associated with Hypothyroidism in Dogs

Romain Pariaut, DVM, DACVIM (Cardiology), DECVIM-CA (Cardiology)
Assistant Professor of Cardiology
Veterinary Clinical Sciences
Louisiana State University
Baton Rouge, Louisiana
Supraventricular Tachyarrhythmias in Dogs

Edward E. (Ned) Patterson, DVM, PhD, DAVIM
Associate Professor
Veterinary Clinical Sciences
Veterinary Medical Center
University of Minnesota
St. Paul, Minnesota
Methods and Availability of Tests for Hereditary Disorders of Dogs and Cats

Dominique Peeters, DVM, DECVIM-CA
Associate Professor
Companion Animals Clinical Sciences
University of Liège
Liège, Belgium
Eosinophilic Pulmonary Diseases

Simon M. Petersen-Jones, DVetMed, PhD, DVOphthal, DECVO, MRCVS
Myers-Dunlap Endowed Chair in Canine Health
Department of Small Animal Clinical Sciences
Michigan State University
East Lansing, Michigan
Canine Retinopathies

Mark E. Peterson, DVM, DACVIM
Director
Department of Endocrinology and Nuclear Medicine
Animal Endocrine Clinic
New York, New York
Canine Hypoadrenocorticism
Clinical Use of the Vasopressin Analog Desmopressin for the Diagnosis and Treatment of Diabetes Insipidus
Differential Diagnosis of Hyperkalemia and Hyponatremia in Dogs and Cats
Hyperadrenocorticism in Ferrets
Radioiodine for Feline Hyperthyroidism
Treatment of Insulinoma in Dogs, Cats, and Ferrets

Michael E. Peterson, DVM, MS
Staff Veterinarian
Reid Veterinary Hospital
Albany, Oregon
Reproductive Toxicology and Teratogens

Brenda Phillips, DVM, ACVIM (Oncology)
Medical Oncologist
Veterinary Specialty Hospital of San Diego
San Diego, California
Chemotherapeutic Drug Handling and Safety

Fred S. Pike, DVM, DACVS
Clinical Associate Faculty
Western University of Health Sciences
College of Veterinary Medicine
Pomona, California
Staff Surgeon and Associate Medical Director
Veterinary Specialty Hospital of San Diego
San Diego, California
Extrahepatic Biliary Tract Disease

Lauren Riester Pinchbeck, DVM, MS, DACVD
Veterinary Dermatologist and Partner
Northeast Veterinary Dermatology Specialists
Shelton, Connecticut
New Haven, Connecticut
Hopewell Junction, New York
Norwalk, Connecticut
Yonkers, New York
White Plains, New York
Systemic Glucocorticoids in Dermatology

Simon R. Platt, BVM-S, MRCVS, DECVN, DACVIM (Neurology)
Associate Professor Neurology and Neurosurgery
Small Animal Medicine and Surgery
College of Veterinary Medicine
University of Georgia
Athens, Georgia
Vascular Disease of the Central Nervous System

Michael Podell, MSc, DVM, DACVIM (Neurology)
Owner
Chicago Veterinary Neurology and Neurosurgery Group
Chicago, Illinois
Ototoxicity

Cyrill Poncet, DVM, DECVS
Head
Department of Soft Tissue Surgery
Fregis Hospital
Arcueil, Paris, France
Brachycephalic Airway Obstruction Syndrome

Robert H. Poppenga, DVM, PhD, DABVT
Professor of Diagnostic Veterinary Toxicology
California Animal Health and Food Safety Laboratory
School of Veterinary Medicine
University of California—Davis
Davis, California
Herbal Hazards

Cynthia C. Powell, DVM, MS, DACVO
Professor, Veterinary Ophthalmology
Clinical Sciences
Colorado State University
Fort Collins, Colorado
Feline Uveitis

Pascal Prélaud, DV, DECVD
Clinique Veterinaire Advetia
Paris, France
Treatment Guidelines for Canine Atopic Dermatitis

Barrak M. Pressler, DVM, PhD, DACVIM
Assistant Professor of Internal Medicine
Veterinary Clinical Sciences
The Ohio State University
Columbus, Ohio
Glomerular Disease and Nephrotic Syndrome

Jessica M. Quimby, DVM, PhD, DACVIM (Internal Medicine)
Clinical Instructor
Clinical Sciences
Colorado State University
Fort Collins, Colorado
Immunotherapy for Infectious Diseases

Ian K. Ramsey, BVSc, PhD, DSAM, DECVIM-CA, MRCVS
Professor of Small Animal Medicine
School of Veterinary Medicine
University of Glasgow
Glasgow, Scotland, United Kingdom
Canine Hyperadrenocorticism Therapy

Jacquie S. Rand, BVSc, DVSc, MACVS, DACVIM
Professor of Companion Animal Health
Centre for Companion Animal Health, School of Veterinary Science
University of Queensland
St. Lucia, Queensland, Australia
Feline Diabetes Mellitus

Amy J. Rankin, DVM, MS, DACVO
Assistant Professor Ophthalmology
Clinical Sciences
Kansas State University
Manhattan, Kansas
Feline Glaucoma

Kent R. Refsal, DVM, PhD
Professor, Endocrine Section
Diagnostic Center for Population and Animal Health
Michigan State University
Lansing, Michigan
Feline Primary Hyperaldosteronism

Claudia E. Reusch, Dr. med.vet., DECVIM-CA
Professor
Clinic for Small Animal Internal Medicine
Vetsuisse Faculty
University of Zurich
Zurich, Switzerland
Diabetic Monitoring

Caryn A. Reynolds, DVM, DACVIM (Cardiology)
Assistant Professor
Department of Veterinary Clinical Sciences
Louisiana State University
Baton Rouge, Louisiana
Ventricular Arrhythmias in Dogs

Keith P. Richter, DVM
Hospital Director and Staff Internist
Internal Medicine Department
Veterinary Specialty Hospital of San Diego
San Diego, California
Feline Gastrointestinal Lymphoma
Extrahepatic Biliary Tract Disease

Jyothi V. Robertson, DVM
Shelter Medicine Consultant
Koret Shelter Medicine Program
School of Veterinary Medicine
University of California—Davis
Davis, California
Owner-Principal Consultant
JVR Shelter Strategies
Belmont, California
Feline Upper Respiratory Tract Infection

Kenita S. Rogers, DVM, MS
Associate Dean for Professional Programs & Biomedical Sciences
College of Veterinary Medicine
Professor of Oncology
Small Animal Clinical Sciences
Texas A&M University
College Station, Texas
Collection of Specimens for Cytology

Stefano Romagnoli, DVM, MS, PhD, DECAR (European College of Animal Reproduction)
Professor
Clinical Veterinary Reproduction
University of Padova
Legnaro, Italy
Aspermia/Oligospermia Caused by Retrograde Ejaculation in Dogs

Wayne S. Rosenkrantz, DVM, ACVD
Owner/Partner
Animal Dermatology Clinic
Tustin, California
Topical Therapy for Pruritus
House Dust Mites and Their Control
Pyotraumatic Dermatitis ("Hot Spots")

Karen L. Rosenthal, DVM, MS
Dean and Professor of Exotic Animal Medicine
School of Veterinary Medicine
St. Matthew's University
Grand Cayman, Cayman Islands
Hyperadrenocorticism in Ferrets

Linda Ross, DVM, MS, DACVIM (SAIM)
Associate Professor
Clinical Sciences
Tufts Cummings School of Veterinary Medicine
North Grafton, Massachusetts
Medical Management of Acute Kidney Injury

Edmund J. Rosser Jr., DVM, DACVD
Professor and Head of Dermatology
Small Animal Clinical Sciences
College of Veterinary Medicine
Michigan State University
East Lansing, Michigan
Therapy for Sebaceous Adenitis

Jan Rothuizen, DVM, PhD, DECVIM-CA
Clinical Sciences of Companion Animals
Faculty of Veterinary Medicine
Universiteit Utrecht
Utrecht, The Netherlands
Copper-Associated Hepatitis

Philip Roudebush, DVM, DACVIM
Adjunct Professor
Department of Clinical Studies
College of Veterinary Medicine
Kansas State University
Manhattan, Kansas
Flatulence

Elizabeth A. Rozanski, DVM, DACVECC, DACVIM (SAIM)
Associate Professor
Clinical Sciences
Tufts Cummings School of Veterinary Medicine
North Grafton, Massachusetts
Crystalloid Fluid Therapy
Pneumothorax

Craig G. Ruaux, BVSc (Hons), PhD, MANZCVSc, DACVIM (SAIM)
Assistant Professor
Small Animal Internal Medicine
Veterinary Clinical Sciences
Oregon State University
Corvallis, Oregon
Treatment of Canine Pancreatitis

Elke Rudloff, DVM, DACVECC
Director of Education
Animal Emergency Center and Specialty
    Services
Glendale, Wisconsin
President
Veterinary Emergency Critical Care
    Society
Colloid Fluid Therapy
Disseminated Intravascular Coagulation

**Wilson K. Rumbeiha, BVM, PhD,
    DABVT, DABT**
Professor of Veterinary Toxicology
Veterinary Diagnostics and Production
    Animal Medicine
College of Veterinary Medicine
Iowa State University
Ames, Iowa
Parasiticide Toxicoses: Avermectins
Nephrotoxicants

John E. Rush, DVM, MS
Professor
Clinical Sciences
Tufts Cummings School of Veterinary
    Medicine
North Grafton, Massachusetts
Pacing in the ICU Setting
Chronic Valvular Heart Disease in Dogs

Marco Russo, DVM, PhD, MRCVS
Senior Lecturer in Obstetrics and
    Diagnostic Reproductive Imaging
Department of Veterinary Medicine and
    Animal Sciences
University of Naples "Federico II"
Naples, Italy
Special Lecturer in Veterinary Diagnostic
    Imaging and Reproduction
The School of Veterinary Medicine and
    Science
The University of Nottingham Sutton
    Bonington Campus
Sutton Bonington
Leicestershire, England
Breeding Management of the Bitch

**Roberto A. Santilli, DVM, PhD,
    DECVIM-CA (Cardiology)**
Chief
Cardiology Division
Clinica Veterinaria Malpensa
Samarate, Varese, Italy
Supraventricular Tachyarrhythmias in Dogs

Kari Santoro-Beer, BS, DVM
Resident
Emergency and Critical Care
Department of Clinical Studies
Matthew J. Ryan Veterinary Hospital
University of Pennsylvania
Philadelphia, Pennsylvania
Shock

John S. Sapienza, DVM, DACVO
Department Chief and Head
Ophthalmology
Long Island Veterinary Specialists
Plainview, New York
Canine Glaucoma

**Ashley B. Saunders, DVM, DACVIM
    (Cardiology)**
Assistant Professor
Department of Small Animal Clinical
    Sciences
Texas A&M University
College Station, Texas
Patent Ductus Arteriosus

**Jimmy H. Saunders, DVM, PhD,
    DECVDI**
Professor, Doctor
Department of Veterinary Medical
    Imaging and Small Animal
    Orthopaedics
Ghent University
Merelbeke, Belgium
Imaging in Diagnosis of Endocrine Disorders

Patricia A. Schenck, DVM, PhD
Section Chief
Endocrine Diagnostic Section
Diagnostic Center for Population and
    Animal Health
Michigan State University
Lansing, Michigan
Assistant Professor
Pathobiology and Diagnostic
    Investigation
Michigan State University
Lansing, Michigan
Feline Idiopathic Hypercalcemia
Treatment of Hypoparathyroidism

**Karsten Eckhard Schober, DVM,
    PhD, DECVIM (CA)**
Associate Professor
Veterinary Clinical Sciences Department
College of Veterinary Medicine
The Ohio State University
Columbus, Ohio
Feline Myocardial Disease
Myocarditis

**J. Catharine R. Scott-Moncrieff, MA,
    Vet MB, MS**
Professor
Veterinary Clinical Sciences
Purdue University
West Lafayette, Indiana
Canine Hypothyroidism
*Nutritional Management of Feline
    Hyperthyroidism*

Davis M. Seelig, DVM, PhD
Assistant Professor
Department of Veterinary Clinical
    Sciences
University of Minnesota
St. Paul, Minnesota
Plasma Cell Neoplasms

Bernard Séguin, DVM, MS, DACVS
Associate Professor
Animal Cancer Center
Colorado State University
Fort Collins, Colorado
Oral Tumors

**Rance K. Sellon, DVM, PhD,
    DACVIM (Small Animal Internal
    Medicine; Oncology)**
Associate Professor
Veterinary Clinical Sciences
Washington State University
Pullman, Washington
*Rational Use of Glucocorticoids in Infectious
    Disease*

**G. Diane Shelton, DVM, PhD,
    DACVIM (Internal Medicine)**
Professor
Department of Pathology
School of Medicine
University of California—San Diego
La Jolla, California
Oropharyngeal Dysphagia
*Treatment of Autoimmune Myasthenia
    Gravis*
Treatment of Myopathies and Neuropathies

Robert G. Sherding, DVM, DACVIM
Professor Emeritus
Department of Veterinary Clinical
    Sciences
College of Veterinary Medicine
The Ohio State University
Columbus, Ohio
Respiratory Parasites

Traci A. Shreyer, MA
Applied Animal Behaviorist-Program
    Specialist
Veterinary Clinical Sciences and
    Veterinary Preventive Medicine
College of Veterinary Medicine
The Ohio State University
Columbus, Ohio
*Multimodal Environmental Enrichment for
    Domestic Cats*

**Deborah C. Silverstein, DVM,
    DACVECC**
Assistant Professor of Critical Care
Clinical Studies
University of Pennsylvania Ryan
    Veterinary Hospital
Philadelphia, Pennsylvania
Adjunct Professor
Pharmacology
Temple School of Pharmacy
Philadelphia, Pennsylvania
Shock

Kaitkanoke Sirinarumitr
Associate Professor
Department of Companion Animal
  Clinical Sciences
Faculty of Veterinary Medicine
Head of Small Animal Reproduction
  Clinic
Vice Director
Kasetsart University Teaching Hospital
Kasetsart University
Bangkhaen, Bangkok, Thailand
*Benign Prostatic Hypertrophy and Prostatitis
  in Dogs*

**D. David Sisson, DVM,
  DACVIM-Cardiology**
Professor of Cardiovascular Medicine
Department of Clinical Sciences
Oregon State University
Corvallis, Oregon
Bradyarrhythmias and Cardiac Pacing

**Annette N. Smith, DVM, MS,
  DACVIM (Oncology & SAIM)**
Associate Professor
Clinical Sciences
Auburn University
Auburn, Alabama
Treatment of Intracranial Tumors

Frances O. Smith, DVM, PhD, DACT
Owner
Smith Veterinary Hospital, Inc.
Burnsville, Minnesota
President
Orthopedic Foundation for Animals, Inc.
Columbia, Missouri
Pyometra

**Patricia J. Smith, MS, DVM, PhD,
  DACVO**
Animal Eye Care
Fremont, California
Canine Retinal Detachment

Ian Brett Spiegel, VMD, MHS, DACVD
Chief of Dermatology and Allergy
Veterinary Specialty and Emergency
  Center
Levittown, Pennsylvania
Chief of Dermatology and Allergy
Animergy
Raritan, New Jersey
Chief of Dermatology and Allergy
Jersey Shore Veterinary Emergency
  Service
Lakewood, New Jersey
Cutaneous Adverse Drug Reactions

**Jörg M. Steiner, Dr.Med.Vet., PhD,
  DACVIM, DECVIM-CA, AGAF**
Professor and Director
Gastrointestinal Laboratory
Department of Small Animal Clinical
  Sciences
Texas A&M University
College Station, Texas
Laboratory Testing for the Exocrine Pancreas

Janice C. Steinschneider, MA, JD
Supervisory Regulatory Counsel
Center for Veterinary Medicine
Office of Surveillance & Compliance
Food and Drug Administration
Rockville, Maryland
*Treatment of Animal Toxicoses: Regulatory
  Points to Consider*

Rebecca L. Stepien, DVM, MS
Clinical Professor—Cardiology
Department of Clinical Sciences
School of Veterinary Medicine
Staff Cardiologist
Chief of Staff
Small Animal Services
University of Wisconsin
Madison, Wisconsin
Systemic Hypertension

**Rachel Sternberg, DVM, DACVIM
  (Oncology)**
Medical Oncologist
VCA Arboretum View Animal Hospital
Downers Grove, Illinois
Plasma Cell Neoplasms

Rachel A. Strohmeyer, DVM, MS
Kingston, Washington
*Infectious Diseases Associated with Raw
  Meat Diets*

Beverly K. Sturges, DVM, DACVIM
Radiological & Surgical Sciences
University of California—Davis
Davis, California
*Diagnosis and Treatment of Atlantoaxial
  Subluxation*

**Jan S. Suchodolski, MedVet,
  DrMedVet, PhD**
Clinical Assistant Professor
Small Animal Clinical Sciences
Associate Director
Gastrointestinal Laboratory
College of Veterinary Medicine
Texas A&M University
College Station, Texas
Probiotic Therapy

**Lauren Sullivan, DVM, MS,
  DACVECC**
Assistant Professor
Clinical Sciences
Colorado State University
Fort Collins, Colorado
*Stabilization of the Patient with Respiratory
  Distress*
*Critical Illness–Related Corticosteroid
  Insufficiency*
Transfusion Medicine: Best Practices

Patricia A. Sura, MS. DVM, DACVS
Staff Surgeon
BluePearl Veterinary Partners
Louisville, Kentucky
*Minilaparotomy-Assisted Cystoscopy for
  Urocystoliths*

**Jane E. Sykes, BVSc(Hons), PhD,
  DACVIM**
Professor
Medicine & Epidemiology
University of California—Davis
Davis, California
*Canine Infectious Respiratory Disease
  Complex*
Systemic Antifungal Therapy

**Harriet M. Syme, BSc, BVM, PhD,
  DACVIM, DECVIM, MRCVS**
Senior Lecturer in Small Animal Internal
  Medicine
Department of Veterinary Clinical
  Sciences
The Royal Veterinary College
North Mymms, Hatfield, Hertfordshire,
  United Kingdom
Feline Hyperthyroidism and Renal Function

Joseph Taboada, DVM, DACVIM
Professor
Small Animal Internal Medicine
Associate Dean
Student and Academic Affairs
School of Veterinary Medicine
Louisiana State University
Baton Rouge, Louisiana
Systemic Antifungal Therapy

Lauren R. Talarico, DVM
Neurology/Neurosurgery Resident
Department of Clinical Sciences
Cornell University
Ithaca, New York
*Treatment of Noninfectious Inflammatory
  Diseases of the Central Nervous System*

**Patricia Ann Talcott, MS, DVM,
  PhD, DABVT**
Professor, Director of Admissions
Department of Integrative Physiology
  and Neuroscience
Toxicology Section Head
Washington Animal Disease Diagnostic
  Laboratory
College of Veterinary Medicine
Washington State University
Pullman, Washington
Insecticide Toxicoses

**Séverine Tasker, BSc, BVSc, PhD,
  DSAM, DECVIM-CA, PGCertHE,
  MRCVS**
Senior Lecturer in Small Animal
  Medicine
School of Veterinary Sciences
University of Bristol
Bristol, North Somerset, United Kingdom
*Canine and Feline Hemotropic
  Mycoplasmosis*

John H. Tegzes, MA, VMD, DABVT
Professor, Toxicology
Director, Year 1 Curriculum
College of Veterinary Medicine
Western University of Health Sciences
Pomona, California
Lawn and Garden Product Safety

Vincent J. Thawley, VMD
Resident in Emergency & Critical Care
Clinical Studies
Matthew J. Ryan Veterinary Hospital
University of Pennsylvania
Philadelphia, Pennsylvania
Oxygen Therapy

Alan P. Théon, Dr Med Vet, MS, PhD, DACR-RO
Professor
Radiology and Surgery
School of Veterinary Medicine
Oncology Service Chief
Veterinary Medical Teaching Hospital
University of California—Davis
Davis, California
Large Pituitary Tumors in Dogs with Pituitary-Dependent Hyperadrenocorticism

Emily K. Thomas, BA, VetMB
Emergency and Critical Care Resident
Matthew J. Ryan Veterinary Hospital
University of Pennsylvania
Philadelphia, Pennsylvania
Acute Respiratory Distress Syndrome

Randall C. Thomas, DVM, DACVD
Veterinary Dermatologist
Southeast Veterinary Dermatology & Ear Clinic
Mt. Pleasant, South Carolina
Treatment of Ectoparasitoses

William B. Thomas, DVM, MS, DACVIM (Neurology)
Associate Professor, Neurology and Neurosurgery
Department of Small Animal Clinical Sciences
College of Veterinary Medicine
The University of Tennessee
Knoxville, Tennessee
Congenital Hydrocephalus

Justin D. Thomason, DVM, DACVIM (Internal Medicine)
Assistant Professor of Cardiology
Department of Clinical Sciences
Veterinary Health Center
Kansas State University
Manhattan, Kansas
Syncope

Elizabeth J. Thomovsky, DVM
Clinical Assistant Professor
Veterinary Clinical Sciences
Purdue University
West Lafayette, Indiana
Drug Incompatibilities and Drug-Drug Interactions in the ICU Patient

Karen M. Tobias, DVM, MS, DACVS
Professor, Small Animal Surgery
Department of Small Animal Clinical Sciences
College of Veterinary Medicine
The University of Tennessee
Knoxville, Tennessee
Portosystemic Shunts

Lauren A. Trepanier, DVM, PhD, DACVIM, DACVCP
Professor and Director of Clinician Scientist Training
Department of Medical Sciences
University of Wisconsin—Madison
Madison, Wisconsin
Medical Treatment of Feline Hyperthyroidism
Drug-Associated Liver Disease

Gregory C. Troy, DVM, MS, DACVIM
Professor
Dr. and Mrs. Dorsey Mahin Endowed Professor
Department of Small Animal Clinical Sciences
Virginia-Maryland Regional College of Veterinary Medicine
Virginia Tech
Blacksburg, Virginia
American Leishmaniasis

Michelle M. Turek, DVM, DACVIM (Oncology), DACVR (Radiation Oncology)
Assistant Professor
Radiation Oncology
Veterinary Anatomy and Radiology
College of Veterinary Medicine
University of Georgia
Athens, Georgia
Perineal Tumors

Shelly L. Vaden, DVM, PhD, DACVIM
Professor, Internal Medicine
Department of Clinical Sciences
College of Veterinary Medicine
North Carolina State University
Raleigh, North Carolina
Glomerular Disease and Nephrotic Syndrome

David M. Vail, DVM, DACVIM (Oncology)
Professor of Oncology
Barbara A. Suran Chair in Comparative Oncology
School of Veterinary Medicine
University of Wisconsin
Madison, Wisconsin
Rescue Therapy for Canine Lymphoma
Anticancer Drugs: New Drugs

Alexandra van der Woerdt, DVM, MS, DACVO, DECVO
Staff Ophthalmologist
The Animal Medical Center
New York, New York
Canine Uveitis

Linda M. Vap, DVM, DACVP
Instructor
Microbiology, Immunology and Pathology
Colorado State University
Fort Collins, Colorado
Quality Control for the In-Clinic Laboratory

Julia K. Veir, DVM, PhD, DACVIM (SAIM)
Assistant Professor
Clinical Sciences
Colorado State University
Fort Collins, Colorado
Canine Parvoviral Enteritis

Carlo Vitale, DVM, ACVD
VCA—San Francisco Veterinary Specialists
San Francisco, California
Methicillin-Resistant Staphylococcal Infections

Katrina R. Viviano, DVM, PhD, DACVIM (Internal Medicine)
Clinical Assistant Professor
Department of Medical Sciences
University of Wisconsin
Madison, Wisconsin
Drug Incompatibilities and Drug-Drug Interactions in the ICU Patient

Petra A. Volmer, DVM, MS, DABVT, DABT
Manager of Pharmacovigilance
Ceva Animal Health
Lenexa, Kansas
Human Drugs of Abuse and Central Nervous System Stimulants

Lori S. Waddell, DVM, DACVECC
Adjunct Assistant Professor
Critical Care
Clinical Studies
School of Veterinary Medicine
University of Pennsylvania
Philadelphia, Pennsylvania
Acute Respiratory Distress Syndrome
Pleural Effusion

Andrea Wang, MA, DVM, DACVIM
Small Animal Internal Medicine Resident
Veterinary Teaching Hospital
University of Georgia
Athens, Georgia
Pet-Associated Illness

Wendy A. Ware, DVM, MS, DACVIM (Cardiology)
Professor
Departments of Veterinary Clinical Sciences and Biomedical Sciences
Staff Cardiologist
Lloyd Veterinary Medical Center
Iowa State University
Ames, Iowa
Pericardial Effusion

Erin N. Warren, DVM, MS
Small Animal Intern
Department of Small Animal Clinical
    Sciences
College of Veterinary Medicine
The University of Tennessee
Knoxville, Tennessee
Treatment of Intracranial Tumors

A.D.J. Watson, BVSc, PhD
Department of Veterinary Clinical
    Sciences
The University of Sydney
Glebe, New South Wales, Australia
*Chronic Kidney Disease: International Renal
    Interest Society Staging and Management*

**Penny J. Watson, MA, VetMD,
    CertVR, DSAM, DECVIM, MRCVS**
Senior Lecturer in Small Animal
    Medicine
Department of Veterinary Medicine
University of Cambridge
Cambridge, United Kingdom
Chronic Hepatitis Therapy

Craig B. Webb, PhD, DVM
Associate Professor
Clinical Sciences
Colorado State University
Fort Collins, Colorado
Probiotic Therapy

**Cynthia R.L. Webster, DVM,
    DACVIM (Internal Medicine)**
Professor
Clinical Science
Tufts Cummings School of Veterinary
    Medicine
Grafton, Massachusetts
*Diagnostic Approach to Hepatobiliary
    Disease*
*Portal Vein Hypoplasia (Microvascular
    Dysplasia)*

Glade Weiser, DVM, DACVP
Professor, Special Appointment
Department of Microbiology,
    Immunology & Pathology
Colorado State University
Fort Collins, Colorado
Quality Control for the In-Clinic Laboratory

Douglas J. Weiss, DVM, PhD, DACVP
Emeritus Professor
Department of Veterinary and
    Biomedical Sciences
University of Minnesota
St. Paul, Minnesota
Nonregenerative Anemias

Chick Weisse, VMD, DACVS
Director of Interventional Radiology
Staff Surgeon
Interventional Radiology/Surgery
Animal Medical Center
New York, New York
Interventional Oncology
Tracheal Collapse
Interventional Strategies for Urinary Disease

**Sharon L. Welch, DABVT, DABT,
    DVM**
Veterinarian, Toxicologist
Pet Poison Helpline
Bloomington, Minnesota
Toxin Exposures in Small Animals

**Elias Westermarck, DVM, PhD,
    DECVIM**
Professor Emeritus of Medicine
Department of Equine and Small Animal
    Medicine
University of Helsinki
Helsinki, Finland
Tylosin-Responsive Diarrhea

Jason Wheeler, DVM, MS, DACVS
Small Animal Surgeon
Virginia Veterinary Specialists
Charlottesville, Virginia
*Emergency Wound Management and
    Vacuum-Assisted Wound Closure*

Richard Wheeler, DVM, DACT
Small Animal Reproduction
Veterinary Teaching Hospital
College of Veterinary Medicine and
    Biomedical Sciences
Colorado State University
Fort Collins, Colorado
Vulvar Discharge

Maria Wiberg, DVM, PhD
Clinical Teacher
Department of Equine and Small Animal
    Medicine
Faculty of Veterinary Medicine
University of Helsinki
Helsinki, Finland
Exocrine Pancreatic Insufficiency in Dogs

K. Tomo Wiggans, DVM
Resident, Comparative Ophthalmology
Department of Surgical and Radiological
    Sciences
University of California—Davis
Davis, California
Ocular Emergencies

Bo Wiinberg, DVM, PhD
Head of Translational Haemophilia
    Pharmacology
Biopharmaceuticals Research Unit
Novo Nordisk A/S
Maaloev, Denmark
Hypercoagulable States

David A. Wilkie, DVM, MS, ACVO
Professor
Veterinary Clinical Sciences
The Ohio State University
Columbus, Ohio
Disorders of the Lens

**Michael D. Willard, DVM, MS,
    DACVIM**
Professor
Department of Small Animal Clinical
    Sciences
Texas A&M University
College Station, Texas
Esophagitis

**Marion S. Wilson, BVMS, MVSc,
    MRCVS**
Director
TCI Ltd
Feilding, New Zealand
Endoscopic Transcervical Insemination

Tina Wismer, DVM, DABVT, DABT
Medical Director
ASPCA Animal Poison Control Center
Urbana, Illinois
*ASPCA Animal Poison Control Center Toxin
    Exposures for Pets*

Angela Lusby Witzel, DVM, PhD
Assistant Clinical Professor
Department of Small Animal Clinical
    Sciences
College of Veterinary Medicine
The University of Tennessee
Knoxville, Tennessee
Obesity

**J. Paul Woods, DVM, MS, DACVIM
    (Internal Medicine, Oncology)
    CVMA Certificate of
    Specialization in Small Animal
    Internal Medicine**
Professor
Department of Clinical Studies
Small Animal Medicine & Oncology
Ontario Veterinary College Health
    Sciences Centre
University of Guelph
Guelph, Ontario, Canada
Small Animal Medicine
Thames Valley Veterinary Services
The Lawson Research Institute
London, Ontario, Canada
Feline Cytauxzoonosis

Paul A. Worhunsky, DVM
Veterinary Resident
Clinical Sciences
College of Veterinary Medicine
Cornell University
Ithaca, New York
Sage Centers for Veterinary Speciality
    and Emergency Care
Campbell, California
Cobalamin Deficiency in Cats

Panagiotis G. Xenoulis, DVM, Dr.Med.Vet., PhD
Gastrointestinal Laboratory
Department of Small Animal Clinical Sciences
Texas A&M University
College Station, Texas
Approach to Canine Hyperlipidemia

Vicky K. Yang, DVM, PhD
Cardiology Resident
Tufts Cummings School of Veterinary Medicine
North Grafton, Massachusetts
Pacing in the ICU Setting

Debra L. Zoran, DVM, PhD, DACVIM-SAIM
Associate Professor and Chief of Medicine
Small Animal Clinical Sciences
Texas A&M University
College Station, Texas
Diet and Diabetes
Protein-Losing Enteropathies

To my Dad, Peter J. Bonagura, with admiration and gratitude.

JDB

To my wife Liz and my son Ryan for their love and support
and to all the animals that make the veterinary profession so worthwhile.

DCT

Preface

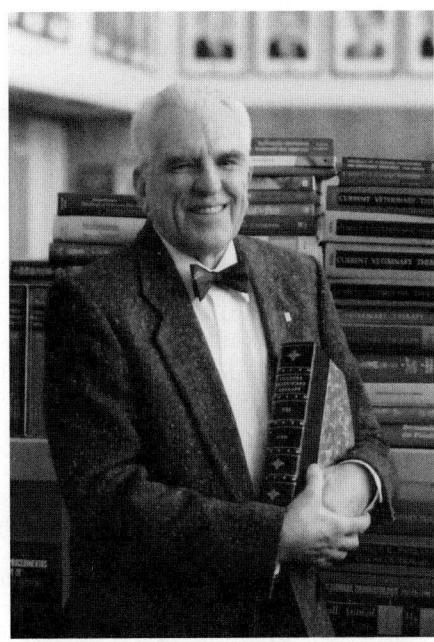

(Photograph provided by Cornell University.)
Robert W. Kirk, DVM, 1922-2011

This 15th volume of *Current Veterinary Therapy* continues the tradition of presenting practicing veterinarians and students with concise chapters focused on the treatment of medical disorders of dogs and cats. This is the first volume to be published since the passing of Dr. Robert W. Kirk, who founded and edited new editions of this series for nearly three decades. Bob Kirk was a giant in the profession, a man with a remarkable impact on veterinary education and clinical practice. In introducing *Current Veterinary Therapy XV*, I believe it is appropriate to both remember Dr. Kirk and to consider his intent for creating this book. Therefore this preface will be a bit more personal than usual, as I try to express my admiration for Dr. Kirk and the importance of this clinician-educator to our profession. To that end I will quote Dr. Donald F. Smith, Dean Emeritus of the College of Veterinary Medicine at Cornell University, who has written about Bob's legacy, and also will include some excerpts from the Preface of Dr. Kirk's first edition of *Current Veterinary Therapy* (published as *CVT 1964-1965* [i.e., before the Roman numerals were added]).

Dr. Smith wrote in his tribute:

A 1946 graduate of Cornell, Dr. Kirk was one of the most accomplished clinical veterinarians, authors and educators of the 20th century. His knowledge of general small animal medicine was established through several years in private practice, then honed in his three decades of advanced medical practice, including dermatology, at Cornell University. When he retired in 1985, he was one of the most decorated and widely-known small animal veterinarians in the world. Among his many accomplishments was his famous book, Current Veterinary Therapy, *which he edited by himself through its first ten editions. This series of books has sold more than a quarter of a million copies and has been translated into many languages. As a student, I studied from the fourth edition that my friends and I simply knew as Kirk.*

A native of Stamford, Connecticut, Dr. Kirk came to Cornell in 1943 intent on becoming a large animal veterinarian. The

draw of pet medicine intrigued him, though, and he worked in mixed practices as well as the ASPCA in New York City after graduation. Kirk was recruited in 1952 to ....(help) usher in a new age of pet health care at Cornell. He insisted on the highest quality of medicine but always with a view to practicality and service. Dr. Kirk had an enormous impact on the development of small animal medicine. He was a founding member of the American College of Veterinary Internal Medicine, and also the specialty of veterinary dermatology. His students and residents populated some of the most important university hospitals and private practices in the country.

I never had the opportunity to practice alongside Dr. Kirk—he was a faculty member at Cornell, while I have spent most of my career at Ohio State. Nevertheless, his influence on me as a student, trainee, and faculty member was significant. As Dr. Smith remarked, "Dr. Kirk was both professor and practitioner," and Bob's ability to teach, publish, and demonstrate practical skills in the clinical arena represented the characteristics I greatly admired in him and in my other mentors. My association with Bob Kirk was actually longer than he ever realized! I spent much of the summer between my second and third years of veterinary school "with Dr. Kirk," highlighting each chapter in *CVT IV* (the orange one, for those who know the editions by their colors). I studied Volume V (the yellow cover) and the gigantic sixth volume (with that slightly unnatural green cover) during my residencies. Bob later told me that volume six kept breaking its binding, so he needed to limit the page count in future editions; I still struggle with that issue. As a young faculty member I was asked to write a chapter for *CVT VII* and can recall how honored I felt. I served as the consulting editor for cardiology for the next three editions and associate editor for *CVT X*, learning from a distance how Bob managed his textbook. Then one day as we sat on a picnic bench at a New England VMA meeting, Dr. Kirk (and his wife Helen) asked me to assume editorship of *CVT*. During this conversation, Bob discussed in some detail his vision for future editions of the textbook. This opportunity—to edit what at the time was the best known veterinary textbook—evoked feelings of personal satisfaction but also of daunting obligation to not mess it all up. I have never quite shaken those emotions.

Dr. Kirk indicated the purpose of *Current Veterinary Therapy* in the preface to his first edition, namely "to provide the small animal clinician with easily accessible information on the latest accepted methods of treating medical conditions in a pet practice." Since assuming editorial duties, I have tried to maintain his focus while adapting the textbook to the remarkable medical advances our profession has witnessed over the past four decades. To control the book size, I have limited the *CVT* to medical disorders of dogs and cats; when surgical treatments are indicated, the reader is referred to other available sources. Diagnosis is not the focus of *CVT*, although our authors usually provide basic information regarding diagnostic studies, and a few chapters focus entirely on establishing a correct diagnosis. As Dr. Kirk wrote in the first edition, "the text assumes that a secure diagnosis has been obtained"; achieving that accurate diagnosis is as important today as it was 50 years ago when he wrote his first volume.

The organization of the 15th edition of *Kirk's Current Veterinary Therapy* will be familiar to long-time users. Sections are devoted to multisystem specialties of critical care medicine, endocrine and metabolic disorders, hematology and oncology, infectious diseases, and toxicology. Sections that focus on specific organ systems detail cardiovascular, dermatologic and otic, gastrointestinal, neurologic, ophthalmologic, respiratory, reproductive, and urinary system diseases. There are a total of 365 chapters, with 279 chapters in the textbook and 86 chapters on the companion website and in all electronic versions of *CVT XV*. Some of the appendices have been moved to the website to gain page space, but the often-copied Table of Common Drugs: Approximate Dosages is still found in both electronic and print versions of the book. When navigating *CVT*, most readers find the Table of Contents, which is divided into individual sections, and the Index to be their best guide. The chapters also have been extensively cross referenced.

We continue our policy of integrating this new volume with the "still current" chapters from Volume XIV of *Current Veterinary Therapy*. These chapters have been updated by the authors and are reprinted because of their clinical importance. Others have been updated and appear on the companion website. *CVT XV* is available for today's veterinary students and practitioners both as a print book and as an e-book accessible on any mobile device (eReader, tablet, or laptop). I firmly believe that the student or first-time reader of "Kirk" who holds only this current volume will find the information so useful as to forgive the occasional omission of a topic, or be convinced to go online when that subject is covered only in the electronic version of the book. Owing to the large number of potential chapters, we have elected not to reprint some chapters in which new information is minimal or where we simply could not allocate the page space.

The organization and overall editing of this new volume has been shared with Dr. David Twedt, Professor of Clinical Sciences at Colorado State University. I first met Dave when he tried to train me during my internship at the Animal Medical Center in New York, and from that point on I have admired his intellect, common sense, clinical acumen, sense of humor, and kindness. David is an internist and gastroenterologist of extraordinary skill and experience, as evidenced by his publications, his world travel as an invited lecturer, and his recent receipt of the ACVIM Distinguished Service Award. This is a capstone award bestowed on one individual annually and marks a distinguished career of service to veterinary internal medicine; Dr. Twedt is a most deserving recipient. *CVT* is so much better with David's input and I am thankful for his collaboration and friendship.

Dr. Kirk knew that the quality of the textbook depended mainly on the recruitment of authors with expertise and clinical experience, and we have been fortunate to enlist over 300 outstanding clinicians and clinical scientists to help with *CVT XV*. As with Dr. Kirk's first *CVT* volume, we have asked our contributors to provide what the "author regards as the best treatment at present," accepting that some will be "traditional," whereas others are "just emerging" and will require more definition. We practice in an era in which clinical trial evidence is considered the standard; however, definitive trial data are often lacking due to a variety of factors (including insufficient research funding and insufficient numbers of clinical scientists in veterinary schools). We ask our authors to inform us about evidence-based treatments, but also ask them to explain how they manage their own patients in practical terms, even in the absence of definitive studies. Our contributors have done a tremendous job of summarizing available therapies within the confines of relatively

short chapters, and both Dr. Twedt and I are highly appreciative of their efforts.

These chapter submissions have been guided and reviewed by our Consulting Editors, with one or two experts overseeing each of the 13 textbook sections. Collectively, these clinical specialists have evaluated each chapter in *CVT*, offering their perspective and providing oversight for content accuracy and currency. We are truly grateful to each of these outstanding clinicians for their guidance, editorial input, and time.

Ultimately, our readers—practicing veterinarians and veterinary students studying clinical science—decide the fate of a textbook. Too many books become ornaments on shelves (or now pretty pictures on digital devices). We certainly hope that readers will find the volumes of *CVT* useful to their practices. No single textbook can cover the vast subject of veterinary medicine, and thus we have maintained our niche, focusing (as Dr. Kirk directed) on medical therapies of canine and feline diseases. There are a large number of textbooks addressing diagnosis and other volumes detailing subspecialty medicine and surgery. It is our hope that *CVT* will find a useful place between these other resources and be a first choice when managing patients in your clinical practice.

Extraordinary efforts have been made to ensure accuracy in treatment recommendations, especially in the dosing of drugs (as so many are used in an extralabel manner). We are very interested in hearing from readers about things they like about *CVT*, as well as suggestions for improvement. Should a potential error be encountered, I would be indebted to any reader willing to take the time to notify me or the publisher of their concern.

I would like to close by reiterating that Dr. Kirk was a role model as an academic clinician. He practiced, contributed to scientific discovery, and disseminated what he learned himself and from others through his teaching and writings. He recognized talent in others and collaborated with many outstanding clinicians and scientists during his career. Although he was a pioneer of our profession in so many ways, to me he was foremost a clinician-educator and mentor. In this regard, I would like to briefly acknowledge and thank three other veterinarians who have greatly influenced my career. Dr. Robert Hamlin has taught me cardiology continuously, with brilliance, imagination, and enthusiasm for over 40 years. His helpfulness and impact on educating veterinary students and future cardiologists around the world cannot be overestimated. Bob inspired me to an academic career, and I will forever be thankful for his example. Dr. William Kay was still a practicing neurologist when he taught and mentored me during my internship at the Animal Medical Center (and later during my professional career). Bill taught me how to approach all sorts of difficult, complicated, and challenging situations in a forthright manner. I am indebted to him for these lessons. Dr. Stephen Ettinger was a great friend to Bob Kirk, and he stands as another giant of our profession. His textbooks, *Canine Cardiology* and *Textbook of Veterinary Internal Medicine*, were highly influential to me as a clinician and author. I have learned even more by talking to Steve and observing his intellect, innovation, passion, and persistence. Along with Dr. Kirk, these mentors have offered me guidance, support, and opportunities throughout my career; without their help and friendship, someone else would likely be writing this preface.

Acknowledgments

In addition to our contributors, David and I would like to thank everyone at Elsevier who worked so hard to bring this new edition to publication. Shelly Stringer, Content Manager, was our daily go-to person. Shelly patiently listened to all of my excuses, managed thousands of details, and kept us moving toward the target with grace and helpfulness. David Stein, Senior Production Manager at Elsevier, was superb while wearing multiple hats as senior copy editor and production leader. He carried the book through edited manuscript and page proofs while fixing hundreds of my errors with aplomb. Whitney Noble was often working behind the scenes in various aspects of organization, communication, website structure, and textbook production. I've no doubt she performed many other essential tasks, but largely under the radar of the authors and editors. Once again the overall supervision and guidance of *CVT* was managed most capably by Content Strategy Director Penny Rudolph. Penny knew when we needed her insight and direction and otherwise supported us throughout the creation of this new volume. Special thanks are extended to Dr. Debra Primovic, a practicing veterinarian, for indexing yet another volume of *CVT* with care and clinical perspective. Dr. Twedt and I would like to thank each of these individuals, along with others at Elsevier who worked to bring *Current Veterinary Therapy XV* to publication.

John D. Bonagura, DVM
Columbus, Ohio

Contents

Section I: Critical Care

1 Crystalloid Fluid Therapy, 2
   John D. Anastasio, Daniel J. Fletcher, and Elizabeth A. Rozanski
2 Colloid Fluid Therapy, 8
   Elke Rudloff and Rebecca Kirby
3 Catecholamines in the Critical Care Patient, 14
   Edward S. Cooper
4 Shock, 18
   Kari Santoro-Beer and Deborah C. Silverstein
5 Cardiopulmonary Resuscitation, 26
   Daniel J. Fletcher and Manuel Boller
6 Drug Incompatibilities and Drug-Drug Interactions in the ICU Patient, 32
   Katrina R. Viviano and Elizabeth J. Thomovsky
7 Nutrition in Critical Care, 38
   Daniel L. Chan
8 Stabilization of the Patient with Respiratory Distress, 44
   Timothy B. Hackett and Lauren Sullivan
9 Acute Respiratory Distress Syndrome, 48
   Emily K. Thomas and Lori S. Waddell
10 Oxygen Therapy, 52
   Vincent J. Thawley and Kenneth J. Drobatz
11 Ventilator Therapy for the Critical Patient, 55
   Julien Guillaumin
12 Analgesia of the Critical Patient, 59
   Nigel Campbell
13 Anesthesia for the Critical Care Patient, 63
   Derek Flaherty
14 Hyperthermia and Heat-Induced Illness, 70
   Elisa M. Mazzaferro
15 Thromboelastography, 74
   Karl E. Jandrey and Benjamin M. Brainard
16 Critical Illness–Related Corticosteroid Insufficiency, 78
   Lauren Sullivan and Jamie M. Burkitt Creedon
17 Evaluation of Canine Orthopedic Trauma, 80
   Randall B. Fitch
18 Emergency Management of Open Fractures, 83
   Robert J. McCarthy
19 Emergency Wound Management and Vacuum-Assisted Wound Closure, 87
   Stacy D. Meola and Jason Wheeler
Web Chapter 1 Acid-Base Disorders, e1
   Helio Autran de Morais and Stephen P. DiBartola
Web Chapter 2 Drainage Techniques for the Septic Abdomen, e9
   Adrienne Bentley and David Holt
Web Chapter 3 Gastric Dilation-Volvulus, e13
   Karol A. Mathews
Web Chapter 4 Pacing in the ICU Setting, e21
   John E. Rush and Vicky K. Yang

Section II: Toxicologic Diseases

20 ASPCA Animal Poison Control Center Toxin Exposures for Pets, 92
   Tina Wismer
21 Toxin Exposures in Small Animals, 93
   Colleen M. Almgren and Sharon L. Welch
22 Urban Legends of Toxicology: Facts and Fiction, 97
   Frederick W. Oehme and William R. Hare Jr.

23 Drugs Used to Treat Toxicoses, 101
   Sharon M. Gwaltney-Brant
24 Intravenous Lipid Emulsion Therapy, 106
   Justine A. Lee and Alberto L. Fernandez Mojica
25 Human Drugs of Abuse and Central Nervous System Stimulants, 109
   Petra A. Volmer
26 Antidepressants and Anxiolytics, 112
   Ahna G. Brutlag
27 Over-the-Counter Drug Toxicosis, 115
   David C. Dorman
28 Top Ten Toxic and Nontoxic Household Plants, 121
   A. Catherine Barr
29 Herbal Hazards, 122
   Elizabeth A. Hausner and Robert H. Poppenga
30 Lawn and Garden Product Safety, 130
   John H. Tegzes
31 Rodenticide Toxicoses, 133
   Michael J. Murphy
32 Insecticide Toxicoses, 135
   Patricia Ann Talcott
33 Pesticides: New Vertebrate Toxic Agents for Pest Species, 142
   Rhian Cope
34 Parasiticide Toxicoses: Avermectins, 145
   Wilson K. Rumbeiha
35 Human Foods with Pet Toxicoses: Alcohol to Xylitol, 147
   Eric K. Dunayer
36 Automotive Toxins, 151
   Karyn Bischoff
37 Lead Toxicosis in Small Animals, 156
   Sharon M. Gwaltney-Brant
38 Aflatoxicosis in Dogs, 159
   Karyn Bischoff and Tam Garland
Web Chapter 5 Nephrotoxicants, e29
   Wilson K. Rumbeiha and Michael J. Murphy
Web Chapter 6 Reporting Adverse Events to the Food and Drug Administration—Center for Veterinary Medicine, e35
   Susan J. Bright-Ponte and Lee Anne Myers Palmer
Web Chapter 7 Respiratory Toxicants of Interest to Pet Owners, e43
   Janice A. Dye
Web Chapter 8 Small Animal Poisoning: Additional Considerations Related to Legal Claims, e49
   Michael J. Murphy
Web Chapter 9 Sources of Help for Toxicosis, e53
   Michael J. Murphy
Web Chapter 10 Treatment of Animal Toxicoses: Regulatory Points to Consider, e54
   Michael J. Murphy, Susan J. Bright-Ponte, and Janice C. Steinschneider

Section III: Endocrine and Metabolic Diseases

39 Bilaterally Symmetric Alopecia in Dogs, 164
   Robert Allen Kennis
40 Imaging in Diagnosis of Endocrine Disorders, 167
   Jimmy H. Saunders

41   Approach to Critical Illness–Related Corticosteroid Insufficiency, 174
     Linda G. Martin
42   Canine Hypothyroidism, 178
     J. Catharine R. Scott-Moncrieff
43   Feline Hyperthyroidism and Renal Function, 185
     Harriet M. Syme
44   Canine Diabetes Mellitus, 189
     William E. Monroe
45   Diabetic Monitoring, 193
     Claudia E. Reusch
46   Diet and Diabetes, 199
     Debra L. Zoran
47   Insulin Resistance, 205
     Richard W. Nelson
48   Feline Diabetes Mellitus, 208
     Jacquie S. Rand
49   Feline Hypersomatotropism and Acromegaly, 216
     Stijn J.M. Niessen and David B. Church
50   Occult Hyperadrenocorticism: Is It Real? 221
     Ellen N. Behrend and Robert Allen Kennis
51   Canine Hyperadrenocorticism Therapy, 225
     Ian K. Ramsey and Reto Neiger
52   Ectopic ACTH Syndrome and Food-Dependent Hypercortisolism in Dogs, 230
     Sara Galac and Hans S. Kooistra
53   Canine Hypoadrenocorticism, 233
     Peter P. Kintzer and Mark E. Peterson
54   Feline Primary Hyperaldosteronism, 238
     Kent R. Refsal and Andrea M. Harvey
55   Feline Idiopathic Hypercalcemia, 242
     Joao Felipe de Brito Galvao, Dennis J. Chew, and Patricia A. Schenck
56   Approach to Hypomagnesemia and Hypokalemia, 248
     Lee E. Palmer and Linda G. Martin
57   Obesity, 254
     Angela Lusby Witzel and Claudia A. Kirk
58   Approach to Canine Hyperlipidemia, 261
     Panagiotis G. Xenoulis
Web Chapter 11   Hypercalcemia and Primary Hyperparathyroidism in Dogs, e69
     Edward C. Feldman
Web Chapter 12   Clinical Use of the Vasopressin Analog Desmopressin for the Diagnosis and Treatment of Diabetes Insipidus, e73
     Rhett Nichols and Mark E. Peterson
Web Chapter 13   Complicated Diabetes Mellitus, e76
     Deborah S. Greco
Web Chapter 14   Complications and Concurrent Conditions Associated with Hypothyroidism in Dogs, e84
     David L. Panciera
Web Chapter 15   Large Pituitary Tumors in Dogs with Pituitary-Dependent Hyperadrenocorticism, e88
     Alan P. Théon and Edward C. Feldman
Web Chapter 16   Differential Diagnosis of Hyperkalemia and Hyponatremia in Dogs and Cats, e92
     Peter P. Kintzer and Mark E. Peterson
Web Chapter 17   Hyperadrenocorticism in Ferrets, e94
     Karen L. Rosenthal and Mark E. Peterson
Web Chapter 18   Interpretation of Endocrine Diagnostic Test Results for Adrenal and Thyroid Disease, e97
     Robert J. Kemppainen and Ellen N. Behrend
Web Chapter 19   Medical Treatment of Feline Hyperthyroidism, e102
     Lauren A. Trepanier
Web Chapter 20   Nutritional Management of Feline Hyperthyroidism, e107
     J. Catharine R. Scott-Moncrieff
Web Chapter 21   Radioiodine for Feline Hyperthyroidism, e112
     Mark E. Peterson and Michael R. Broome
Web Chapter 22   Treatment of Hypoparathyroidism, e122
     Joao Felipe de Brito Galvao, Dennis J. Chew, Larry A. Nagode, and Patricia A. Schenck
Web Chapter 23   Treatment of Insulinoma in Dogs, Cats, and Ferrets, e130
     Karelle A. Meleo and Mark E. Peterson
Web Chapter 24   Alternatives to Insulin Therapy for Diabetes Mellitus in Cats, e135
     Deborah S. Greco

Section IV: Oncology and Hematology

59   Immunosuppressive Agents, 268
     Clare R. Gregory
60   Management of Immune-Mediated Hemolytic Anemia in Dogs, 275
     Valerie Johnson and Steven Dow
61   Thrombocytopenia, 280
     Jennifer A. Neel, Adam J. Birkenheuer, and Carol B. Grindem
62   von Willebrand Disease and Hereditary Coagulation Factor Deficiencies, 286
     Marjorie B. Brooks
63   Disseminated Intravascular Coagulation, 292
     Elke Rudloff and Rebecca Kirby
64   Hypercoagulable States, 297
     Bo Wiinberg and Annemarie T. Kristensen
65   Lymphocytosis in Dogs and Cats, 301
     Susan E. Lana, Christine S. Olver, and Anne Avery
66   Quality Control for the In-Clinic Laboratory, 306
     Glade Weiser and Linda M. Vap
67   Transfusion Medicine: Best Practices, 309
     Lauren Sullivan and Timothy B. Hackett
68   Bone Marrow Dyscrasias, 314
     Christine S. Olver
69   Talking to Clients about Cancer, 318
     Douglas H. Thamm
70   Tumor Biopsy and Specimen Submission, 322
     Debra A. Kamstock and Nicholas J. Bacon
71   Chemotherapeutic Drug Handling and Safety, 326
     Andrea Flory, Brenda Phillips, and Margo Karriker
72   Treatment of Adverse Effects from Cancer Therapy, 330
     Dennis B. Bailey
73   Cancer Immunotherapy, 334
     Leah Ann Mitchell, Amanda Guth, and Steven Dow
74   Advances in Radiation Therapy for Nasal Tumors, 338
     James T. Custis III and Susan M. LaRue
75   Malignant Effusions, 341
     Antony S. Moore
76   Interventional Oncology, 345
     William T.N. Culp and Chick Weisse
77   Nutritional Support of the Cancer Patient, 349
     Glenna E. Mauldin
78   Metronomic Chemotherapy, 354
     Anthony J. Mutsaers
79   Drug Update: Toceranib, 358
     Cheryl A. London
80   Drug Update: Masitinib, 360
     Kevin A. Hahn
81   Oral Tumors, 362
     Michael S. Kent and Bernard Séguin
82   Perineal Tumors, 366
     Michelle M. Turek
83   Urinary Bladder Cancer, 370
     Deborah W. Knapp

84 Mammary Cancer, 375
Carolyn J. Henry

85 Rescue Therapy for Canine Lymphoma, 381
David M. Vail

86 Plasma Cell Neoplasms, 384
Rachel Sternberg, Davis M. Seelig, and Laura D. Garrett

87 Osteosarcoma, 388
Nicole P. Ehrhart and Timothy M. Fan

88 Canine Hemangiosarcoma, 392
Craig A. Clifford and Louis-Philippe de Lorimier

89 Thyroid Tumors, 397
Suzanne Murphy

Web Chapter 25 Anticancer Drugs: New Drugs, e139
Douglas H. Thamm and David M. Vail

Web Chaptre 26 Blood Typing and Crossmatching to Ensure Blood Compatibility, e143
Urs Giger

Web Chapter 27 Soft Tissue Sarcomas, e148
Tania Ann Banks and Julius M. Liptak

Web Chapter 28 Collection of Specimens for Cytology, e153
Kenita S. Rogers

Web Chapter 29 Nasal Tumors, e157
Lisa J. Forrest

Web Chapter 30 Nonregenerative Anemias, e160
Douglas J. Weiss

Web Chapter 31 Pulmonary Neoplasia, e165
Kevin A. Hahn and Sandra M. Axiak-Bechtel

Web Chapter 32 Surgical Oncology Principles, e168
James P. Farese

Section V: Dermatologic and Otic Diseases

90 Diagnostic Criteria for Canine Atopic Dermatitis, 403
Claude Favrot

91 Treatment Guidelines for Canine Atopic Dermatitis, 405
Thierry Olivry and Pascal Prélaud

92 Cyclosporine Use in Dermatology, 407
Andrew Hillier

93 Allergen-Specific Immunotherapy, 411
Douglas J. DeBoer

94 Systemic Glucocorticoids in Dermatology, 414
Lauren Riester Pinchbeck

95 Topical Therapy for Pruritus, 419
Wayne S. Rosenkrantz

96 Elimination Diets for Cutaneous Adverse Food Reactions: Principles in Therapy, 422
Hilary A. Jackson

97 Flea Control in Flea Allergy Dermatitis, 424
Robert Allen Kennis and Andrew Hillier

98 Treatment of Ectoparasitoses, 428
Randall C. Thomas

99 Canine Demodicosis, 432
Ralf S. Mueller

100 Staphylococci Causing Pyoderma, 435
Linda A. Frank

101 Treatment of Superficial Bacterial Folliculitis, 437
Andrew Hillier

102 Topical Therapy for Infectious Diseases, 439
Kenneth W. Kwochka

103 Methicillin-Resistant Staphylococcal Infections, 443
Carlo Vitale

104 Nontuberculous Cutaneous Granulomas in Dogs and Cats (Canine Leproid Granuloma and Feline Leprosy Syndrome), 445
Anne Fawcett, Janet A.M. Fyfe, and Richard Malik

105 Treatment of Dermatophytosis, 449
Karen A. Moriello and Douglas J. DeBoer

106 Dermatophytosis: Investigating an Outbreak in a Multicat Environment, 452
Sandra Newbury and Karen A. Moriello

107 Disinfection of Environments Contaminated by Staphylococcal Pathogens, 455
Armando E. Hoet

108 Principles of Therapy for Otitis, 458
Lynette K. Cole

109 Topical and Systemic Glucocorticoids for Otitis, 459
Tim Nuttall

110 Topical Antimicrobials for Otitis, 462
Colleen L. Mendelsohn

111 Systemic Antimicrobials for Otitis, 466
Lynette K. Cole

112 Ototoxicity, 468
Michael Podell and Cecilia Friberg

113 Ear-Flushing Techniques, 471
Dawn Logas

114 Primary Cornification Disorders in Dogs, 475
Elizabeth A. Mauldin

115 Alopecia X, 477
Rosario Cerundolo

116 Actinic Dermatoses and Sun Protection, 480
Amanda K. Burrows

117 Drugs for Behavior-Related Dermatoses, 482
Meghan E. Herron

118 Superficial Necrolytic Dermatitis, 485
Kevin Byrne

119 Cutaneous Adverse Drug Reactions, 487
Ian Brett Spiegel

Web Chapter 33 Acral Lick Dermatitis, e172
John M. MacDonald

Web Chapter 34 Avermectins in Dermatology, e178
Amanda K. Burrows

Web Chapter 35 Canine Papillomaviruses, e184
Masahiko Nagata

Web Chapter 36 Diseases of the Anal Sac, e187
Russell Muse

Web Chapter 37 Feline Demodicosis, e191
Karin M. Beale

Web Chapter 38 Feline Viral Skin Disease, e194
Rudayna Ghubash

Web Chapter 39 House Dust Mites and Their Control, e197
Wayne S. Rosenkrantz

Web Chapter 40 Interferons, e200
Toshiroh Iwasaki

Web Chapter 41 Pentoxifylline, e202
Rosanna Marsella

Web Chapter 42 Pyotraumatic Dermatitis ("Hot Spots"), e206
Wayne S. Rosenkrantz

Web Chapter 43 Therapy for Sebaceous Adenitis, e209
Edmund J. Rosser Jr.

Web Chapter 44 *Malassezia* Infections, e212
Daniel O. Morris

Web Chapter 45 Topical Immunomodulators, e216
Joel D. Griffies

Section VI: Gastrointestinal Diseases

120 Feline Caudal Stomatitis, 492
Linda J. DeBowes

121 Oropharyngeal Dysphagia, 495
Stanley L. Marks

122 Gastroesophageal Reflux, 501
Peter Hendrik Kook

123 Antacid Therapy, 505
Alexa M.E. Bersenas

124 Gastric *Helicobacter* spp. and Chronic Vomiting in Dogs, 508
Michael S. Leib

125 Gastric and Intestinal Motility Disorders, 513
Frédéric P. Gaschen

126 Current Veterinary Therapy: Antibiotic Responsive Enteropathy, 518
Albert E. Jergens

127 Cobalamin Deficiency in Cats, 522
Kenneth W. Simpson and Paul A. Worhunsky

128 Probiotic Therapy, 525
Craig B. Webb and Jan S. Suchodolski

129 Protozoal Gastrointestinal Disease, 528
Jody L. Gookin and Michael R. Lappin

130 Canine Parvoviral Enteritis, 533
Julia K. Veir

131 Inflammatory Bowel Disease, 536
Karin Allenspach and Aarti Kathrani

132 Protein-Losing Enteropathies, 540
Debra L. Zoran

133 Feline Gastrointestinal Lymphoma, 545
Keith P. Richter

134 Canine Colitis, 550
Kenneth W. Simpson and Alison C. Manchester

135 Laboratory Testing for the Exocrine Pancreas, 554
Romy M. Heilmann and Jörg M. Steiner

136 Exocrine Pancreatic Insufficiency in Dogs, 558
Maria Wiberg

137 Treatment of Canine Pancreatitis, 561
Craig G. Ruaux

138 Feline Exocrine Pancreatic Disorders, 565
Marnin A. Forman

139 Diagnostic Approach to Hepatobiliary Disease, 569
Cynthia R.L. Webster and Johanna C. Cooper

140 Drug-Associated Liver Disease, 575
Lauren A. Trepanier

141 Acute Liver Failure, 580
Sharon A. Center

142 Chronic Hepatitis Therapy, 583
Penny J. Watson

143 Copper Chelator Therapy, 588
Allison Bradley and David C. Twedt

144 Ascites and Hepatic Encephalopathy Therapy for Liver Disease, 591
Nick Bexfield

145 Portosystemic Shunts, 594
Karen M. Tobias

146 Portal Vein Hypoplasia (Microvascular Dysplasia), 599
Andrea N. Johnston and Cynthia R.L. Webster

147 Extrahepatic Biliary Tract Disease, 602
Keith P. Richter and Fred S. Pike

148 Idiopathic Vacuolar Hepatopathy, 606
David C. Twedt

149 Feline Hepatic Lipidosis, 608
Steve L. Hill and P. Jane Armstrong

150 Feline Cholangitis, 614
David C. Twedt, P. Jane Armstrong, and Kenneth W. Simpson

Web Chapter 46 Canine Biliary Mucocele, e221
Heidi A. Hottinger

Web Chapter 47 Canine Megaesophagus, e224
Beth M. Johnson, Robert C. DeNovo, and Erick A. Mears

Web Chapter 48 Copper-Associated Hepatitis, e231
Hille Fieten and Jan Rothuizen

Web Chapter 49 Esophagitis, e237
Michael D. Willard and Elizabeth A. Carsten

Web Chapter 50 Evaluation of Elevated Serum Alkaline Phosphatase in Dogs, e242
Anthony T. Gary and David C. Twedt

Web Chapter 51 Flatulence, e247
Philip Roudebush

Web Chapter 52 Gastric Ulceration, e251
Reto Neiger

Web Chapter 53 Hepatic Support Therapy, e255
David C. Twedt

Web Chapter 54 Oropharyngeal Dysphagia, e259
G. Diane Shelton

Web Chapter 55 Tylosin-Responsive Diarrhea, e262
Elias Westermarck

Section VII: Respiratory Diseases

151 Respiratory Drug Therapy, 622
Eleanor C. Hawkins and Mark G. Papich

152 Feline Upper Respiratory Tract Infection, 629
Jyothi V. Robertson and Kate Hurley

153 Canine Infectious Respiratory Disease Complex, 632
Jane E. Sykes

154 Rhinitis in Dogs, 635
Ned F. Kuehn

155 Rhinitis in Cats, 644
Lynelle R. Johnson and Vanessa R. Barrs

156 Brachycephalic Airway Obstruction Syndrome, 649
Cyrill Poncet and Valérie Freiche

157 Nasopharyngeal Disorders, 653
Susan F. Foster and Geraldine Briony Hunt

158 Laryngeal Diseases, 659
Catriona M. MacPhail and Eric Monnet

159 Tracheal Collapse, 663
Brian A. Scansen and Chick Weisse

160 Chronic Bronchial Disorders in Dogs, 669
Lynelle R. Johnson

161 Chronic Bronchitis and Asthma in Cats, 673
Philip Padrid

162 Pneumonia, 681
Rita M. Hanel and Bernie Hansen

163 Eosinophilic Pulmonary Diseases, 688
Cécile Clercx and Dominique Peeters

164 Pleural Effusion, 691
David Holt and Lori S. Waddell

165 Pneumothorax, 700
Elizabeth A. Rozanski and Erin Mooney

166 Pulmonary Thromboembolism, 705
Susan G. Hackner

167 Pulmonary Hypertension, 711
Michele Borgarelli

Web Chapter 56 Interstitial Lung Diseases, e266
Brendan M. Corcoran

Web Chapter 57 Respiratory Parasites, e269
Robert G. Sherding

Section VIII: Cardiovascular Diseases

168 Nutritional Management of Heart Disease, 720
Lisa M. Freeman

169 Systemic Hypertension, 726
Rebecca L. Stepien

170 Bradyarrhythmias, 731
Bruce G. Kornreich and N. Sydney Moïse

171 Supraventricular Tachyarrhythmias in Dogs, 737
Romain Pariaut, Roberto A. Santilli, and N. Sydney Moïse

172 Ventricular Arrhythmias in Dogs, 745
Mark A. Oyama and Caryn A. Reynolds

173 Feline Cardiac Arrhythmias, 748
Étienne Côté

174 Congenital Heart Disease, 756
Brian A. Scansen, Richard E. Cober, and John D. Bonagura

175 Drugs for Treatment of Heart Failure in Dogs, 762
John D. Bonagura and Bruce W. Keene

176 Management of Heart Failure in Dogs, 772
Bruce W. Keene and John D. Bonagura

177 Chronic Valvular Heart Disease in Dogs, 784
John E. Rush and Suzanne M. Cunningham

178 Dilated Cardiomyopathy in Dogs, 795
Amara H. Estrada and Herbert W. Maisenbacher III

179 Arrhythmogenic Right Ventricular Cardiomyopathy, 801
Kathryn M. Meurs

180 Feline Myocardial Disease, 804
Virginia Luis Fuentes and Karsten Eckhard Schober

181 Arterial Thromboembolism, 811
Daniel F. Hogan

182 Pericardial Effusion, 816
O. Lynne Nelson and Wendy A. Ware

183 Feline Heartworm Disease, 824
Clarke E. Atkins

184 Canine Heartworm Disease, 831
Matthew W. Miller and Sonya G. Gordon

Web Chapter 58 Arrhythmogenic Right Ventricular Cardiomyopathy in Cats, e277
Philip R. Fox

Web Chapter 59 Bradyarrhythmias and Cardiac Pacing, e281
Mark A. Oyama and D. David Sisson

Web Chapter 60 Cardioversion, e286
Janice M. Bright and Julie M. Martin

Web Chapter 61 Infective Endocarditis, e291
Kristin A. MacDonald

Web Chapter 62 Mitral Valve Dysplasia, e299
Barret J. Bulmer

Web Chapter 63 Myocarditis, e303
Karsten Eckhard Schober

Web Chapter 64 Patent Ductus Arteriosus, e309
Matthew W. Miller, Sonya G. Gordon, and Ashley B. Saunders

Web Chapter 65 Pulmonic Stenosis, e314
Amara H. Estrada and Herbert W. Maisenbacher III

Web Chapter 66 Subaortic Stenosis, e319
Jonathan A. Abbott

Web Chapter 67 Syncope, e324
Marc S. Kraus, Justin D. Thomason, and Clay A. Calvert

Web Chapter 68 Tricuspid Valve Dysplasia, e332
Darcy B. Adin

Web Chapter 69 Ventricular Septal Defect, e335
Rebecca E. Gompf and John D. Bonagura

Section IX: Urinary Diseases

185 Applications of Ultrasound in Diagnosis and Management of Urinary Disease, 840
Silke Hecht

186 Recognition and Prevention of Hospital-Acquired Acute Kidney Injury, 845
Marie E. Kerl and Cathy E. Langston

187 Proteinuria/Albuminuria: Implications for Management, 849
Gregory F. Grauer

188 Glomerular Disease and Nephrotic Syndrome, 853
Shelly L. Vaden and Barrak M. Pressler

189 Chronic Kidney Disease: International Renal Interest Society Staging and Management, 857
Jonathan Elliott and A.D.J. Watson

190 Use of Nonsteroidal Antiinflammatory Drugs in Kidney Disease, 863
Scott A. Brown

191 Medical Management of Acute Kidney Injury, 868
Linda Ross

192 Continuous Renal Replacement Therapy, 871
Mark J. Acierno

193 Surveillance for Asymptomatic and Hospital-Acquired Urinary Tract Infection, 876
Kate S. KuKanich

194 Persistent *Escherichia coli* Urinary Tract Infection, 880
Julie R. Fischer

195 Interventional Strategies for Urinary Disease, 884
Allyson Berent and Chick Weisse

196 Medical Management of Nephroliths and Ureteroliths, 892
Jessica E. Markovich and Mary Anna Labato

197 Calcium Oxalate Urolithiasis, 897
Benjamin G. Nolan and Mary Anna Labato

198 Canine Urate Urolithiasis, 901
Jody P. Lulich, Carl A. Osborne, and Hasan Albasan

199 Minilaparotomy-Assisted Cystoscopy for Urocystoliths, 905
Joseph W. Bartges, Patricia A. Sura, and Amanda Callens

200 Multimodal Environmental Enrichment for Domestic Cats, 909
Traci A. Shreyer and C.A. Tony Buffington

201 Medical Management of Urinary Incontinence and Retention Disorders, 915
Annick Hamaide

202 Mechanical Occluder Devices for Urinary Incontinence, 919
Christopher A. Adin

203 Top Ten Urinary Consult Questions, 923
Dianne I. Mawby, Amanda Callens, and Joseph W. Bartges

Web Chapter 70 Laser Lithotripsy for Uroliths, e340
Jody P. Lulich, Larry G. Adams, and Hasan Albasan

Web Chapter 71 Urinary Incontinence: Treatment with Injectable Bulking Agents, e345
Julie K. Byron, Dennis J. Chew, and Mary A. McLoughlin

Section X: Reproductive Diseases

204 Breeding Management of the Bitch, 930
Gary C.W. England and Marco Russo

205 Methods for Diagnosing Diseases of the Female Reproductive Tract, 936
Hernán J. Montilla

206 Endoscopic Transcervical Insemination, 940
Marion S. Wilson and Fiona K. Hollinshead

207 Pregnancy Diagnosis in Companion Animals, 944
Dana R. Bleifer, Leana V. Galdjian, and Cindy Bahr

208 Dystocia Management, 948
Autumn P. Davidson

209 Postpartum Disorders in Companion Animals, 957
Michelle Anne Kutzler

210 Nutrition in the Bitch and Queen During Pregnancy and Lactation, 961
David A. Dzanis

211 Pyometra, 967
Frances O. Smith

212 Vulvar Discharge, 969
Richard Wheeler

213 Surgical Repair of Vaginal Anomalies in the Bitch, 974
     Roberto E. Novo
214 Early Age Neutering in Dogs and Cats, 982
     Michelle Anne Kutzler
215 Estrus Suppression in the Bitch, 984
     Patrick W. Concannon
216 Medical Termination of Pregnancy, 989
     Bruce E. Eilts
217 Inherited Disorders of the Reproductive Tract in Dogs and Cats, 993
     Vicki N. Meyers-Wallen
218 Ovarian Remnant Syndrome in Small Animals, 1000
     Carlos M. Gradil and Robert J. McCarthy
219 Pregnancy Loss in the Bitch and Queen, 1003
     Linda K. Kauffman and Claudia J. Baldwin
220 Benign Prostatic Hypertrophy and Prostatitis in Dogs, 1012
     Kaitkanoke Sirinarumitr
221 Methods and Availability of Tests for Hereditary Disorders of Dogs and Cats, 1015
     Edward E. (Ned) Patterson
222 Reproductive Oncology, 1022
     Shay Bracha
223 Reproductive Toxicology and Teratogens, 1026
     Michael E. Peterson
224 Acquired Nonneoplastic Disorders of the Male External Genitalia, 1029
     Michelle Anne Kutzler
Web Chapter 72   Aspermia/Oligospermia Caused by Retrograde Ejaculation in Dogs, e350
     Stefano Romagnoli and Giovanni Majolino
Web Chapter 73   Priapism in Dogs, e354
     James A. Lavely

Section XI: Neurologic Diseases

225 Congenital Hydrocephalus, 1034
     William B. Thomas
226 Intracranial Arachnoid Cysts in Dogs, 1038
     Curtis W. Dewey
227 Treatment of Intracranial Tumors, 1039
     Erin N. Warren, Jill Narak, Todd W. Axlund, and Annette N. Smith
228 Metabolic Brain Disorders, 1047
     Cristian Falzone
229 New Maintenance Anticonvulsant Therapies for Dogs and Cats, 1054
     Curtis W. Dewey
230 Treatment of Cluster Seizures and Status Epilepticus, 1058
     Daniel J. Fletcher
231 Treatment of Noninfectious Inflammatory Diseases of the Central Nervous System, 1063
     Lauren R. Talarico
232 Peripheral and Central Vestibular Disorders in Dogs and Cats, 1066
     Starr Cameron and Curtis W. Dewey
233 Canine Intervertebral Disk Herniation, 1070
     Jonathan M. Levine
234 Canine Degenerative Myelopathy, 1075
     Joan R. Coates and Shinichi Kanazono
235 Diagnosis and Treatment of Atlantoaxial Subluxation, 1082
     Beverly K. Sturges
236 Diagnosis and Treatment of Cervical Spondylomyelopathy, 1090
     Ronaldo Casimiro da Costa
237 Craniocervical Junction Abnormalities in Dogs, 1098
     Curtis W. Dewey, Dominic J. Marino, and Catherine A. Loughin
238 Diagnosis and Treatment of Degenerative Lumbosacral Stenosis, 1105
     Catherine A. Loughin
239 Treatment of Autoimmune Myasthenia Gravis, 1109
     G. Diane Shelton
240 Treatment of Myopathies and Neuropathies, 1113
     G. Diane Shelton
241 Vascular Disease of the Central Nervous System, 1119
     Laurent S. Garosi and Simon R. Platt
Web Chapter 74   Physical Therapy and Rehabilitation of Neurologic Patients, e357
     Darryl L. Millis

Section XII: Ophthalmologic Diseases

242 Pearls of the Ophthalmic Examination, 1128
     David J. Maggs
243 Evaluation of Blindness, 1134
     Anne J. Gemensky Metzler
244 Canine Conjunctivitis, 1138
     Eric C. Ledbetter
245 Tear Film Disorders in Dogs, 1143
     Elizabeth A. Giuliano
246 Corneal Ulcers, 1148
     Amber Labelle
247 Canine Nonulcerative Corneal Disease, 1152
     Margi Gilmour
248 Feline Corneal Disease, 1156
     Cheryl L. Cullen
249 Canine Uveitis, 1162
     Alexandra van der Woerdt
250 Feline Uveitis, 1166
     Cynthia C. Powell
251 Canine Glaucoma, 1170
     John S. Sapienza
252 Feline Glaucoma, 1177
     Amy J. Rankin
253 Disorders of the Lens, 1181
     David A. Wilkie
254 Canine Retinopathies, 1188
     Simon M. Petersen-Jones
255 Feline Retinopathies, 1193
     Kathern E. Myrna
256 Orbital Disease, 1197
     Ralph E. Hamor
257 Canine Ocular Neoplasia, 1201
     Sandra M. Nguyen and Amber Labelle
258 Feline Ocular Neoplasia, 1207
     Sandra M. Nguyen and Amber Labelle
Web Chapter 75   Diseases of the Eyelids and Periocular Skin, e363
     Catherine A. Outerbridge and Steven R. Hollingsworth
Web Chapter 76   Canine Retinal Detachment, e370
     Patricia J. Smith
Web Chapter 77   Epiphora, e374
     Charlotte B. Keller
Web Chapter 78   Ocular Emergencies, e377
     K. Tomo Wiggans and Juliet R. Gionfriddo
Web Chapter 79   Tear Film Disorders of Cats, e384
     Christine C. Lim
Web Chapter 80   Anisocoria and Abnormalities of the Pupillary Light Reflex: The Neuro-ophthalmic Examination, e388
     Nancy B. Cottrill

Section XIII: Infectious Diseases

259 Infectious Agent Differentials for Medical
     Problems, 1212
     Michael R. Lappin
260 Rational Empiric Antimicrobial Therapy, 1219
     Patricia M. Dowling
261 Infectious Causes of Polyarthritis in Dogs, 1224
     Richard E. Goldstein and Michael R. Lappin
262 Immunotherapy for Infectious Diseases, 1229
     Steven Dow and Jessica M. Quimby
263 Systemic Antifungal Therapy, 1234
     Jane E. Sykes, Amy M. Grooters, and Joseph Taboada
264 Infectious Diseases Associated with Raw
     Meat Diets, 1239
     Rachel A. Strohmeyer
265 Pet-Associated Illness, 1244
     Andrea Wang and Craig E. Greene
266 Vaccine-Associated Adverse Effects in Dogs, 1249
     George E. Moore
267 Update on Vaccine-Associated Adverse
     Effects in Cats, 1252
     Dennis W. Macy and Michael R. Lappin
268 Treatment of Canine Babesiosis, 1257
     Adam J. Birkenheuer
269 Canine Bartonellosis, 1261
     Pedro Paulo Vissotto de Paiva Diniz
270 Feline Bartonellosis, 1267
     Lynn F. Guptill
271 Borreliosis, 1271
     Meryl P. Littman
272 Management of Feline Retrovirus-Infected Cats, 1275
     Katrin Hartmann
273 *Hepatozoon americanum* Infections, 1283
     Kelly E. Allen, Eileen McGoey Johnson, and Susan E. Little
274 Leptospirosis, 1286
     Katharine F. Lunn
275 *Neospora caninum*, 1290
     Jeanne E. Ficociello
276 Canine and Feline Monocytotropic Ehrlichiosis, 1292
     Susan M. Eddlestone
277 Toxoplasmosis, 1295
     Michael R. Lappin
278 Rational Use of Glucocorticoids in
     Infectious Disease, 1299
     Adam Mordecai and Rance K. Sellon
279 Feline Infectious Peritonitis Virus Infections, 1303
     Michael R. Lappin
Web Chapter 81   American Leishmaniasis, e396
     Gregory C. Troy
Web Chapter 82   Canine and Feline Hemotropic
     Mycoplasmosis, e398
     Séverine Tasker
Web Chapter 83   Canine Brucellosis, e402
     Autumn P. Davidson
Web Chapter 84   Feline Cytauxzoonosis, e405
     J. Paul Woods
Web Chapter 85   Pneumocystosis, e409
     Remo Lobetti
Web Chapter 86   Pythiosis and Lagenidiosis, e412
     Amy M. Grooters

Appendix I   Table of Common Drugs: Approximate
     Dosages, 1307
     Mark G. Papich

Appendix II   Treatment of Parasites, 1335
     Lora R. Ballweber

Index, 1339

SECTION I

Critical Care

Chapter 1: Crystalloid Fluid Therapy 2
Chapter 2: Colloid Fluid Therapy 8
Chapter 3: Catecholamines in the Critical Care Patient 14
Chapter 4: Shock 18
Chapter 5: Cardiopulmonary Resuscitation 26
Chapter 6: Drug Incompatibilities and Drug-Drug Interactions in the ICU Patient 32
Chapter 7: Nutrition in Critical Care 38
Chapter 8: Stabilization of the Patient with Respiratory Distress 44
Chapter 9: Acute Respiratory Distress Syndrome 48
Chapter 10: Oxygen Therapy 52
Chapter 11: Ventilator Therapy for the Critical Patient 55
Chapter 12: Analgesia of the Critical Patient 59
Chapter 13: Anesthesia for the Critical Care Patient 63
Chapter 14: Hyperthermia and Heat-Induced Illness 70
Chapter 15: Thromboelastography 74
Chapter 16: Critical Illness–Related Corticosteroid Insufficiency 78
Chapter 17: Evaluation of Canine Orthopedic Trauma 80
Chapter 18: Emergency Management of Open Fractures 83
Chapter 19: Emergency Wound Management and Vacuum-Assisted Wound Closure 87

The following web chapters can be found on the companion website at www.currentveterinarytherapy.com

Web Chapter 1: Acid-Base Disorders
Web Chapter 2: Drainage Techniques for the Septic Abdomen
Web Chapter 3: Gastric Dilation-Volvulus
Web Chapter 4: Pacing in the ICU Setting

CHAPTER 1
Crystalloid Fluid Therapy

JOHN D. ANASTASIO, *Malvern, Pennsylvania*
DANIEL J. FLETCHER, *Ithaca, New York*
ELIZABETH A. ROZANSKI, *North Grafton, Massachusetts*

Crystalloids are water-based solutions containing electrolyte and nonelectrolyte solutes and are capable of entering all body compartments. They are the most common fluid type used therapeutically in veterinary medicine.

The major goals of crystalloid fluid therapy are restoration of intravascular volume (in shock), replacement of interstitial fluid deficits (in dehydration), and provision of maintenance fluid needs for dogs or cats at risk of dehydration. Fluid therapy is not warranted in cases in which heart failure cannot be excluded, as in the hypothermic tachypneic cat, and it should be used with caution if anuria is a possibility. The route of fluid administration is determined based on the goals of fluid therapy and the likelihood that these goals may be reasonably met with the planned therapeutic approach. The authors assume that most practitioners employ fluid therapy on a regular basis, and thus the purpose of this chapter is to highlight some controversial and emerging aspects of fluid therapy.

Types of Crystalloid Fluids

Crystalloids are classified as isotonic, hypotonic, or hypertonic in relation to plasma osmolality. Isotonic crystalloids are by far the most commonly used fluid type in veterinary medicine (Table 1-1). Also known as replacement fluids, isotonic crystalloids are used to replace fluid deficits that may have developed from excessive loss. The electrolyte composition of isotonic fluid is typically similar to that of plasma. These solutions may also be classified as acidifying (e.g., normal saline) or buffering (e.g., lactated Ringer's solution [LRS], Normosol-R, Plasma-Lyte 148) solutions. Buffering solutions are considered balanced due to an electrolyte composition that is roughly equal to plasma. Normal saline is not a balanced solution and is acidifying due to a relatively high concentration of chloride and a lack of buffer, both of which decrease plasma bicarbonate.

The clinical relevance of isotonic fluid choice is perhaps less important than commonly believed, although it is reasonable to closely evaluate the electrolyte composition of the fluid choice in relation to the patient's needs. For example, 0.9% saline might be preferred in cases of head trauma, hypercalcemia, or metabolic alkalosis caused by gastrointestinal (GI) obstruction.

Some believe that LRS administration to patients with hepatic dysfunction is contraindicated. A recent study in healthy dogs found that LRS given at a rate of 180 ml/kg/hr resulted in a significant increase in plasma lactate concentration within 10 minutes of infusion. However, the clinical significance of this finding is uncertain, especially considering the extreme fluid rates needed to raise the plasma lactate. Additionally, the impact of lactate-containing solutions has never been investigated in patients with liver disease. In the absence of fulminant low-output hepatic failure, the benefits of using LRS for treatment of hypovolemia and metabolic acidosis likely outweigh the risks. Alternatively, balanced isotonic crystalloids with acetate or gluconate may be considered. However, these molecules also require hepatic metabolism to bicarbonate (albeit less than LRS) to exert their buffering effects.

Hypotonic crystalloids have a lower tonicity relative to plasma and contain additional free water. These solutions may be termed *maintenance fluids*. Hypotonic fluids are primarily used when volume replacement is adequate but ongoing fluid therapy is deemed necessary, such as for a dog recovering from maxillary fracture that is not yet eating. When fluid therapy is needed in the patient with cardiac failure, hypotonic solutions also may be preferable.

Hypertonic crystalloids (e.g., 7.5% saline) can be used for short-term, rapid resuscitation and intravascular volume expansion, as well as for treatment of head trauma. These solutions pull water from the interstitium down the concentration gradient into the intravascular space. They are preferred in euhydrated but hypovolemic patients. These fluids cause interstitial and intracellular dehydration and therefore must be followed by administration of isotonic crystalloids. The addition of electrolytes and dextrose may increase the tonicity of isotonic fluids to a hyperosmolar range (see Table 1-1). Hypertonic crystalloids are not intended for long-term use.

Fluid Management of Hypovolemic Shock

Hypovolemic shock can occur in dogs and cats in association with trauma, massive gastrointestinal hemorrhage, spontaneous hemoperitoneum (e.g., ruptured splenic mass), untreated gastrointestinal disease (e.g., parvovirus infection), gastric dilation-volvulus (GDV), diabetic ketoacidosis, and renal failure. Fluid administration is a mainstay of shock management.

The term *shock dose of fluids* has been popularized in emergency and critical care medicine. Twenty years ago it was commonly recommended to give a specific dose of fluids to animals in shock (generally 90 ml/kg in dogs and

TABLE 1-1

Composition of Commonly Used Fluids*

Fluid	Glucose (g/L)	Na⁺ (mEq/L)	Cl⁻ (mEq/L)	K⁺ (mEq/L)	Ca²⁺ (mEq/L)	Mg²⁺ (mEq/L)	Buffer (mEq/L)	Osmolarity (mOsm/L)	Cal/L	pH
5% Dextrose	50	0	0	0	0	0	0	252	170	4.0
10% Dextrose	100	0	0	0	0	0	0	505	340	4.0
2.5% Dextrose in 0.45% NaCl	25	77	77	0	0	0	0	280	85	4.5
5% Dextrose in 0.45% NaCl	50	77	77	0	0	0	0	406	170	4.0
5% Dextrose in 0.9% NaCl	50	154	154	0	0	0	0	560	170	4.0
0.45% NaCl	0	77	77	0	0	0	0	154	0	5.0
0.9% NaCl	0	154	154	0	0	0	0	308	0	5.0
3% NaCl	0	513	513	0	0	0	0	1026	0	5.0
7.5% NaCl	0	1283	1283	0	0	0	0	2567	0	5.0
23.4% NaCl	0	4004	4004	0	0	0	0	8008	0	5.0
Ringer's lactated solution	0	130	109	4	3	0	28 (L)	272	9	6.5
2.5% Dextrose in Ringer's lactated solution	25	130	109	4	3	0	28 (L)	398	94	5.0
5% Dextrose in Ringer's lactated solution	50	130	109	4	3	0	28 (L)	524	179	5.0
2.5% Dextrose in half-strength Ringer's lactated solution	25	65.5	55	2	1.5	0	14 (L)	263	89	5.0
Normosol M in 5% dextrose	50	40	40	13	0	3	16 (A)	364	175	5.5
Normosol R	0	140	98	5	0	3	27 (A) 23 (G)	294	18	6.4
Plasma-Lyte A	0	140	98	5	0	3	27 (A) 23 (G)	294	17	7.4
Plasma-Lyte 148	0	140	98	5	0	3	27 (A) 23 (G)	294	17	5.5
Plasma-Lyte 56 in 5% dextrose	50	40	40	13	0	3	16 (A)	363	170	5.5
Procalamine	0	35	41	24.5	3	0	47 (A)	735	0	8.8
20% Mannitol	0	0	0	0	0	0	0	1099	0	
7.5% NaHCO₃	0	893	0	0	0	0	893 (B)	1786	0	
8.4% NaHCO₃	0	1000	0	0	0	0	1000 (B)	2000	0	
10% CaCl₂	0	0	2720	0	1360	0	0	4080	0	
14.9% KCl	0	0	2000	2000	0	0	0	4000	0	
50% Dextrose	500	0	0	0	0	0	0	2780	1700	4.2

L, Lactate; *A*, acetate; *G*, gluconate; *B*, bicarbonate; *Cal*, calorie.
*Please see text for more explanation.

60 ml/kg in cats). The volume was set to replace an entire blood volume with crystalloids administered over a period of 1 hour or less. Similarly, administration of shock volumes of fluids was considered the norm in human patients until publication of the landmark study investigating immediate versus delayed fluid resuscitation for hypotensive patients (Bickell et al, 1994). The results of that study challenged the idea that if some fluids are good, more must be better. Multiple experimental studies and clinical trials in people have subsequently demonstrated that excessive crystalloid or synthetic colloid fluid therapy is associated with dilutional coagulopathy, decreased wound healing, increased risk of sepsis, and acute lung injury leading to acute respiratory distress syndrome (ALI/ARDS). Current resuscitation efforts in massively traumatized humans have focused on treatment with blood and blood products. It is unlikely that most veterinary hospitals have a blood bank with sufficient resources to resuscitate all dogs and cats with blood, but this may become a therapeutic possibility in the future.

So what do these studies mean for the clinician treating a patient in hypovolemic shock? Intravascular fluid support is clearly indicated to restore or maintain circulating blood volume. However, the dose of fluid should not be a specific volume but rather a quantity titrated to *restore perfusion parameters* such as heart rate, mucous membrane color, and peripheral pulse quality to normal values. Blood pressure (BP) is maintained in most cases of shock owing to compensatory mechanisms. Normal BP does not exclude hypovolemia and should be interpreted with caution in patients with other signs of shock. Lactate is a useful surrogate marker of inadequate tissue perfusion, with increased lactate (>2.5 mmol/L) associated most commonly with hypoperfusion. It should be recognized that blood lactate may increase with patient struggling, with excessive muscle activity, in association with metabolic alternations (e.g., neoplasia), and with some medications, most notably prednisone (Boysen et al, 2009).

A reasonable starting point for fluid administration is 15 to 20 ml/kg of crystalloids over 10 to 15 minutes with reassessment of patient parameters, especially those of perfusion. Additionally, attention should be directed to the underlying cause of the hypovolemic shock so that the cause can be treated directly through surgical or other medical therapy. If a patient is not responding rapidly to initial fluid therapy, urgent response is needed to reverse shock. It helps to know the average response time for a specific disease and to understand other comorbidities that may accompany the specific injury. For example, if stabilization is not occurring, major differentials include ongoing bleeding into the abdomen, thorax, or fracture site (femur/pelvis) or possibly pneumothorax.

Other useful monitoring parameters include heart rate, respiratory rate, pulse quality, lactate, packed cell volume, total solids, urine production, and attitude. Goals for fluid therapy in shock are restoration of circulating plasma volume to reverse oxygen debt and normalization of the above parameters. Fluid therapy may be tapered over several hours if the resuscitation goals have been met and the patient remains stable.

Fluids should be given as a bolus in the patient with evidence of intravascular volume depletion, as suggested by tachycardia, dull mentation, pale mucous membranes, or hypotension. If vomiting and diarrhea are associated with extreme hemoconcentration, such as a packed cell volume of greater than 60% in non-greyhound dogs (or > 70% in greyhounds), a fluid bolus also may be used to decrease blood viscosity and improve hemodynamics. A fluid bolus is not needed in a pet that is simply dehydrated.

Hypotensive or Low-Volume Resuscitation

Extrapolating from medicine, limited-volume resuscitation (also know as low-volume or hypotensive resuscitation) has gained some momentum in veterinary medicine. The goal of low-volume resuscitation is administration of fluid volumes sufficient to achieve a mean arterial BP of 60 to 80 mm Hg, ensuring adequate tissue and organ perfusion while preventing clot disruption. This method, used for people with uncontrolled cavitary hemorrhage requiring surgical stabilization, aims to have patients in the operating room within an hour of first response to minimize the time that they are hypotensive. Short transitions from the emergency room to the operating room can be difficult to attain in the veterinary setting. Although surgical intervention is usually unnecessary for traumatic hemoabdomen, other causes of hemoabdomen, such as ruptured neoplasia, are likely to require surgery. In this latter setting, low-volume resuscitation may be beneficial for the patient earmarked for surgery. However, this approach requires careful patient monitoring so that prolonged hypotension and the complications of poor tissue perfusion and organ dysfunction are avoided.

Occasionally, there is confusion between low-volume resuscitation and resuscitation with hypertonic saline (HTS) and colloids. One popular method is to mix 43 ml of hetastarch with 17 ml of 23.4% hypertonic saline in a 60-ml syringe and then dose this at 4 to 5 ml/kg over 10 to 15 minutes. Although HTS and colloids represent a smaller volume of fluid than an equivalent dose of crystalloids and may be infused more rapidly than an isotonic crystalloid, the approaches are not interchangeable. Use of HTS and colloid results in a higher plasma volume than administered due to an interstitial fluid shift to the vascular space.

In one small unpublished study of nontraumatic hemoabdomen, dogs randomized to hypertonic saline and hetastarch showed a more rapid time to stabilization than did dogs randomized to crystalloids; however, no differences were noted in either outcome or transfusion needs.*

Fluids for Rehydration

Isotonic crystalloids are commonly used for rehydration and may be administered subcutaneously (SC [or SQ]) or intravenously (IV). Fluid therapy for rehydration is typically based on the formula

---

*Tara Hammond, DVM, DACVECC, personal communication.

TABLE **1-2**

Historical and Physical Examination Findings Relative to Estimated Dehydration

% Dehydration	Historical Findings	Physical Examination Findings
<5%	Excessive fluid loss	Appears normal
5-6%	Excessive fluid loss	Slightly dry mucous membranes, early loss of skin elasticity (skin tent)
7-8%	Excessive fluid loss Quiet/lethargy	Dry mucous membranes, increased skin tent, possible prolonged CRT
8-10%	Excessive fluid loss Quiet/lethargy	Dry mucous membranes, decreased skin tent, mild tachycardia with exertion
10-12%	Excessive fluid loss Weak	Dry mucous membranes, decreased skin tent, tachycardia, sunken eyes
>12%	Collapsed, long-standing or severe fluid losses	Hypovolemic shock; other findings are typically present but due to severity of signs may not be appreciated

$$\frac{\text{Maintenance needs} + \text{percent dehydration} + \text{ongoing losses}}{24 \text{ Hours}} = \text{Volume to be infused}$$

Maintenance fluid is usually calculated at 40 to 60 ml/kg/ day, with calculations ideally based on *lean body weight*. Smaller animals tend to need more fluids per day, while larger animals require a smaller amount on a non-linear per kilogram basis. Dehydration percentage can be calculated many ways, most commonly based on a combination of historical and physical examination findings (Table 1-2). Clinical signs of dehydration include tacky or dry mucous membranes, increased skin turgor, eyes sunken within orbits, and weight loss. Moisture of mucous membranes and skin turgor, however, are at best crude estimates of dehydration. Patients who pant excessively may have dry mucous membranes, and young or obese patients with dehydration may be assessed as having normal skin turgor due to a large amount of SC water or fat. Conversely, older euhydrated patients may be assessed as dehydrated due to a lack of SC fat and elastin. Ongoing fluid losses should be estimated and reassessed over the first 12 to 24 hours of fluid therapy.

As an example, a 20-kg dog with severe vomiting and diarrhea is estimated to be 10% dehydrated; one approach to fluid therapy might be:

1. Calculate maintenance fluids: 60 ml/kg/day × 20 kg = 1200 ml/day.
2. Calculate dehydration fluids: 20 kg × 0.1 × 1000 = 2000 ml (percentage dehydration may be converted to a decimal, and the result multiplied by 1000 to determine ml).
3. Estimate ongoing losses: This is harder to do, but one might guess 250 ml. The sum of 1200 + 2000 + 250 = 3450 ml or approximately 144 ml/hr infused over 24 hours to rehydrate the patient. For this example fluid rate would likely be rounded to 150 ml/hr. Some clinicians prefer to rehydrate over 12 hours and then decrease fluid rates based on the patient's response. Acute changes in body weight also can be used to judge fluid loss, with 1 gm roughly equal to 1 ml of fluid.

Fluids are sometimes dosed in "multiples of maintenance" such as twice maintenance fluids. Twice maintenance fluids is basically the same as maintenance fluids plus 5% dehydration deficits; thus this may be used if preferred or if easier for calculation purposes. However, an animal with polyuria/polydipsia (PU/PD) may have higher than average maintenance needs, and this method may underestimate the patient's actual needs. Conversely, some disorders can make a patient intolerant of an otherwise reasonable volume of crystalloid. This is more likely when there is enhanced potential for sodium and water retention as can occur with advanced cardiac disease, hyperthyroidism, hypoproteinemia, and moderate-to-severe anemia.

No matter which formula is used to calculate fluid rates, the patient should be evaluated at regular intervals. Parameters to reassess include the physical examination findings, urine production, heart rate, attitude, and body weight. Jugular venous pressure is an often-overlooked estimate of volume status, especially in cats. Onset of tachypnea also may indicate circulatory overload. The patient should be evaluated for evidence of overhydration or ongoing dehydration. Additionally, patients should be observed for improvement in the clinical signs that caused the dehydration, such as vomiting or polyuria. Daily weights and in-house laboratory testing such as packed cell volumes and total solids are also helpful, as is following serum electrolytes and acid-base status. Fluid rates should be assessed and altered as needed, at least twice a day, and the fluid therapy discontinued as soon as the patient is recovered. In patients with ongoing renal disease or in situations in which it is unclear if the patient can drink enough to maintain hydration, it helps to taper fluids over 24 to 48 hours. In animals with resolved disorders, such as acute gastroenteritis, fluid therapy may be abruptly stopped.

Fluid Therapy in Special Cases

Crystalloid therapy is one of the most important treatments available to critically ill veterinary patients. Certain diseases require specific considerations, and fluid plans should be tailored to meet individual needs. Some important examples follow.

Polyuria/Polydipsia

Fluid therapy in conditions of PU/PD can be challenging. As illness progresses, the animal may be drinking large amounts (>50 ml/kg/day) of fluids; after dehydration develops, the patient needs much higher than anticipated fluid volume replacements in order to achieve rehydration. It helps to recall the common diseases that usually result in loss of urine concentrating ability, including renal diseases, hyperthyroidism, hypercalcemia, hypoadrenocorticism, hepatic shunts, and diabetes insipidus. Also, other common conditions can result in dilute urine including unregulated or poorly regulated diabetes mellitus and hyperadrenocorticism, as well as exogenous glucocorticoid therapy, phenobarbital therapy, and treatment with diuretics. It is especially difficult to know the prerenal contribution to azotemia in a dehydrated patient who has been receiving furosemide. Additionally, postobstructive diuresis, as follows urethral obstruction, may create large volumes of dilute urine.

Dogs that pant or vocalize excessively may also have increased fluid needs, a finding that may be underappreciated. Some of these patients lose so much free water with panting and vocalizing that hypernatremia may develop.

Pulmonary Contusion

Patients with pulmonary contusions (as well as some other parenchymal injuries such as noncardiogenic pulmonary edema) have altered vascular permeability and increased lung water at the site of the contusion. Fluid therapy, especially colloids, can extravasate and exacerbate the functional lung injury, worsening ventilation (V)/perfusion (Q) mismatch and gas exchange. However, many traumatized animals are also hypovolemic and require some IV fluids to restore circulating intravascular volume and support arterial BP. This leads to a dilemma: deciding to volume resuscitate these patients with pulmonary lesions versus fluid-restricting to prevent worsening of the lung injury. Guidelines advanced by some criticalists are to err on the conservative side for crystalloid fluid resuscitation (e.g., 10 to 25 ml/kg as a bolus) and to avoid colloids. Additionally, pneumothorax commonly accompanies lung contusion, so if the patient is showing respiratory compromise, further diagnostic imaging or diagnostic thoracocentesis is recommended.

Head Trauma

Patients with head trauma commonly present in hypovolemic shock; to maintain cerebral perfusion and reduce cerebral ischemia, fluid therapy should be implemented to restore and maintain normal mean arterial BP (80 to 100 mm Hg). To prevent fluid therapy from contributing to cerebral edema, patients without electrolyte disturbances should be administered 0.9% saline. Water is able to freely cross the blood-brain barrier (BBB), but sodium is not. Because it has the highest sodium concentration of the isotonic crystalloids, 0.9% saline is least likely to contribute to cerebral edema.

Additionally, some euhydrated patients with hypotension due to hypovolemia and clinical signs of increased intracranial pressure (altered mentation, cranial nerve deficits, abnormal postures) can be treated with 7% hypertonic saline (2 to 4 ml/kg over 15 to 20 minutes). The high osmolarity of this solution draws water across the BBB as well as from the interstitium, reducing cerebral edema. This solution also has beneficial rheologic effects, increases cardiac contractility, and reduces edema and dysfunction of the BBB. As described earlier, a mixture of 23.4% hypertonic saline and a synthetic colloid will have similar effects, with the added benefit of prolonged volume expansion compared with administration of a crystalloid alone (see Chapter 2).

Cardiopulmonary Arrest

Administration of IV fluids in euvolemic or hypervolemic patients with cardiopulmonary arrest (CPA) does not increase cardiac output and, due to the resulting increase in venous pressure, commonly reduces tissue blood flow and perfusion. Coronary artery perfusion pressure is defined as the diastolic aortic pressure minus right atrial pressure; thus increasing right atrial pressure will decrease coronary artery perfusion pressure. However, administration of IV fluids during cardiopulmonary resuscitation (CPR) is reasonable in patients with documented or suspected hypovolemia, although it is wise to use conservative doses of isotonic crystalloids (20 ml/kg over 15 to 20 minutes) during CPR. In the postarrest period, hemodynamic optimization targeted at restoring adequate oxygen delivery and tissue perfusion is essential. Crystalloid fluid therapy helps restore intravascular volume and compensate for the peripheral vasodilation that commonly occurs due to acidemia (from respiratory and metabolic acidosis), hypoxic endothelial damage, and ischemia-reperfusion injury. Ideally, intravascular volume status should be assessed objectively in these patients using central venous pressure with a target of 6 to 10 cm H_2O. In patients without central lines, indirect measures such as extent of jugular vein filling, oral mucous membrane color, and capillary refill time may be helpful. Due to the high incidence of postarrest cerebral edema, 0.9% saline (or 7% hypertonic saline in euhydrated patients) is preferred. For further information on goal-directed postarrest care, see Chapter 5.

Potassium Supplementation

Potassium supplementation to crystalloids is warranted in hypokalemic therapy and in patients at risk for potassium depletion. Risk factors for hypokalemia include anorexia, PU/PD, diuretic therapy, hypomagnesemia, metabolic alkalosis, insulin therapy, β-agonist toxicity, and catecholamine therapy. Some clinicians routinely use a sliding scale (Table 1-3) to help determine the amount of potassium to add to the fluids. Animals with marked potassium deficits can be PU/PD patients (e.g., diabetic patients or patients with chronic renal failure) and require larger volumes of crystalloids for maintenance or they can be dehydrated cardiac patients receiving diuretic therapy necessitating fluid rates that are more conservative. Potassium supplementation rates should be adjusted accordingly in these individuals. The reported maximum

TABLE **1-3**

Sliding Scale for Addition of Potassium to IV Fluids (Originally Proposed by Dr. Richard Scott)*

Serum Potassium (mEq/L)	Milliequivalents of KCl to Add to 1 L Fluids	Maximal Fluid Infusion Rate (ml/kg/hr)
<2.0	80	6
2.1-2.5	60	8
2.6-3.0	40	12
3.1-3.5	30	18
3.6-5.0	20	25

*See text for more details and for other options for rate of potassium supplementation. Do not exceed 0.5 mEq/kg/hr. Use central line for concentrations > 60 mEq/L of potassium to decrease the likelihood of phlebitis.

potassium that should be administered to non-oliguric patients is 0.5 mEq/kg/hr (0.5 mmol/kg/hr), although some patients with severe polyuria and cellular potassium depletion (e.g., diabetic ketoacidosis) may require higher rates in rare instances. High concentrations (>60 mEq/L) of potassium in fluids irritate the peripheral vessels and should ideally be given through a central catheter.

Two examples may be instructive. In the first an elderly 4-kg cat has chronic renal failure, anorexia, and serum potassium of 2.7 mmol/L. He is approximately 10% dehydrated, and his fluid replacement needs are calculated to be 28 ml/hr owing to his degree of dehydration and pre-existing PU/PD. If we chose to correct his potassium deficits at one half the maximal allowable supplementation rate (see above), the dose would be 1 mEq KCl per hr, with a total volume infusion of 30 ml/hr. This supplementation would represent the addition of 35 mEq of KCl per liter of isotonic crystalloid. In the second example, a cat of identical age and body weight is diagnosed with congestive heart failure due to hypertrophic cardiomyopathy. He was treated aggressively with furosemide, is currently out of heart failure, but is slightly dehydrated and persistently anorexic, with a serum potassium of 2.8 mEq/L. If a conservative crystalloid fluid rate of 5 ml/hr is selected and again supplemented with potassium at one half the maximal allowable infusion rate, a concentration of 200 mEq of KCl per liter of crystalloid would be required. This concentration would be irritating to the vessels, and thus ideally a central line might be used. Alternatively, it may be preferable to decrease the added potassium to 60 mEq/L (or less) and supplement potassium orally.

Route of Fluid Administration

Fluids may be administered SC, intraosseously (IO),* or IV. Older textbooks describe intraperitoneal fluid therapy, but this route is rarely used. The route of fluid reflects the goals of fluid therapy and the preferences of both the clinician and the client. IV fluid therapy is the standard for hospitalized patients and in urgent situations. Some solutions, such as hypertonic solutions or those supplemented with high concentrations of potassium, only should be administered IV. However, SC fluids may be more practical in some situations and the following comments pertain to this route of administration.

SC fluids are warranted in smaller animals that are dehydrated or at risk of dehydration (e.g., patients with chronic renal failure). For hospitalized pets or those treated as outpatients, SC fluids can be administered and then permitted to absorb slowly. The rate of fluid absorption depends on the volume administered, the patient's hydration status, and the perfusion to the SC space. Some elderly cats take a long time to absorb fluids, and fluids may migrate to gravity-dependent areas such as the limbs. Most clients can be taught to administer SC fluids at home, and this treatment is often well tolerated. For some clients, long-term SC fluid therapy is most easily accomplished with the placement of a SC port,* which prevents the need to "stick" the patient. In most cases, the standard needle, dripset, and fluid bag are preferred. Overall, complications from SC fluids are uncommon. However, potential complications include failure to absorb fluids adequately and SC pooling. Rarely, injection site infections or abscesses have been observed, most frequently in the immunocompromised patient (e.g., a puppy with parvoviral enteritis). Only *isotonic* fluids should be given SC; 20 mEq/L KCl may be added, but no other additives. Hypotonic and hypertonic fluids should never be administered SC.

Dosage for SC fluids depends on patient size, underlying renal function, the size of the SC, and the degree of dehydration. The single most important determinate of fluid dosing in dehydration is the presence or absence of a PU/PD condition (see earlier). A cat with chronic renal failure may benefit from 150 to 250 ml/cat per day for months, whereas a cat with moderate GI upset may be adequately rehydrated with a single dose of 100 ml.

References and Suggested Reading

Bickell WH et al: Immediate versus delayed fluid resuscitation for hypotensive patients with penetrating torso injuries, *N Engl J Med* 331(17):1105-1109, 1994.

Boysen SR et al: Effects of prednisone on blood lactate concentrations in healthy dogs, *J Vet Intern Med* 23(5):1123-1125, 2009.

DiBartola SP, Bateman S: Introduction to fluid therapy. In *Fluid, electrolyte, and acid-base disorders in small animal practice*, ed 4, St Louis, 2012, WB Saunders.

Drobatz KJ, Cole SG: The influence of crystalloid type on acid-base and electrolyte status of cats with urethral obstruction, *Vet Emerg Crit Care* 18:355-361, 2008.

Hammond TN, Holm JL: Limited fluid volume resuscitation, *Compend Contin Educ Vet* 31(7):309-321, 2009.

Pachtinger GE, Drobatz K: Assessment and treatment of hypovolemic states, *Vet Clin North Am Small Anim Pract* 38(3):629-643, 2008.

*EX-IO, Vidacare, San Antonio, TX.

*GIF tube, PractiVet, Phoenix, AZ.

CHAPTER 2
Colloid Fluid Therapy

ELKE RUDLOFF, *Glendale, Wisconsin*
REBECCA KIRBY, *Glendale, Wisconsin*

Severe intravascular volume depletion associated with conditions such as hemorrhage, trauma, systemic inflammatory response syndrome (SIRS) diseases, and various metabolic diseases ultimately results in poor tissue perfusion, tissue hypoxia, and cellular energy depletion. As a consequence, vascular tone can be lost and capillary permeability can be increased, leading to maldistribution of fluid between fluid compartments. Timely and appropriate intravascular fluid resuscitation becomes the mainstay of treatment to restore perfusion and oxygen delivery.

The goals of resuscitation and maintenance fluid therapy in the critically ill animal are to restore and maintain perfusion and hydration without causing volume overload and complications caused by pulmonary, peripheral, or brain edema. By using colloid fluids in conjunction with crystalloid fluids (see Chapter 1), goal-driven resuscitation (also known as end-point resuscitation) can be achieved more rapidly and with less fluid volume compared with crystalloid fluids alone. Maintaining an effective circulating volume can be challenging when there is vascular leakage, vasodilation, excessive vasoconstriction, inadequate cardiac function, hypoalbuminemia, or ongoing fluid loss. Whether a fluid administered intravenously remains in the intravascular compartment or moves into the interstitial or intracellular spaces depends on the dynamic forces that affect fluid movement between body fluid compartments.

Fluid Dynamics

The body fluids are distributed between three major compartments: intracellular, intravascular, and interstitial. The cellular membrane defines the intracellular space and is freely permeable only to water. Most ions must enter the cell by specific mechanisms such as channels, solvent drag, carriers, or pumps. Intracellular ions help retain water within the cell by osmosis. The intravascular space is contained within a vascular semipermeable "membrane" composed of a single thin glycocalyx surface lining the endothelium. Fluid and nutrient exchange between the blood and the tissues occur primarily at the level of the capillary membrane. Larger molecules such as the plasma proteins (albumin, fibrinogen, and globulins) are too large to freely cross this semipermeable membrane.

The modified Starling-Landis equation defines the forces that control the rate of the flow of fluid between the capillary and interstitium as:

$$V = k\,[(HP_c - HP_i) - \sigma\,(COP_c - COP_{gc})] - Q$$

where V = filtered volume, k = filtration coefficient, HP = hydrostatic pressure, c = capillary, i = interstitial fluid, gc = subendothelial glycocalyx, σ = membrane pore size, COP = colloid osmotic pressure, and Q = lymph flow.

The main components that control intravascular fluid volume include intravascular colloid osmotic pressure (COP) and hydrostatic pressure (HP) (Figure 2-1). Eighty percent of the COP is produced by albumin, which is the most abundant extracellular protein. The pressure generated by albumin is augmented by its negative charge, which attracts cations (e.g., sodium) and water around its core structure. This unique dynamic is termed the *Gibbs-Donnan effect*. Vascular permeability to ion species, ionic concentration gradients, and electrochemical charges influence the movement of ions such as sodium, potassium, and chloride. Capillary membrane pore size and the filtration coefficient control the ease with which larger molecules such as albumin leave the intravascular space. Pore size varies from tissue to tissue (e.g., continuous capillaries in the brain and fenestrated capillaries in the liver). The filtration coefficient is variable and partly dependent on the amount of albumin in the intravascular space and within the interendothelial cleft.

The dynamics of normal fluid movement across the capillary membrane can change with certain diseases. Fluid moves from the intravascular to the interstitial or third-space compartment under certain conditions (Figure 2-2 and Table 2-1). Plasma COP can increase with water loss (hemoconcentration), remain the same when there is acute hemorrhage, or decrease with protein loss. In addition to capillary dynamics, the composition of intravenously administered fluids determines how these fluids are distributed across fluid compartments.

Basic Colloid Fluid Pharmacology

The two major categories of intravenous fluids are crystalloids (see Chapter 1) and colloids. A crystalloid fluid is a water-based solution with small molecules permeable to the capillary membrane. A colloid fluid is a crystalloid-based solution that contains large molecules that do not easily cross normal capillary membranes. When large volumes are needed for intravascular fluid resuscitation, crystalloids alone may fail to provide effective intravascular volume support without causing interstitial volume overload and edema.

Ultimately the selection of a colloid or a combination of a colloid with a crystalloid for intravenous

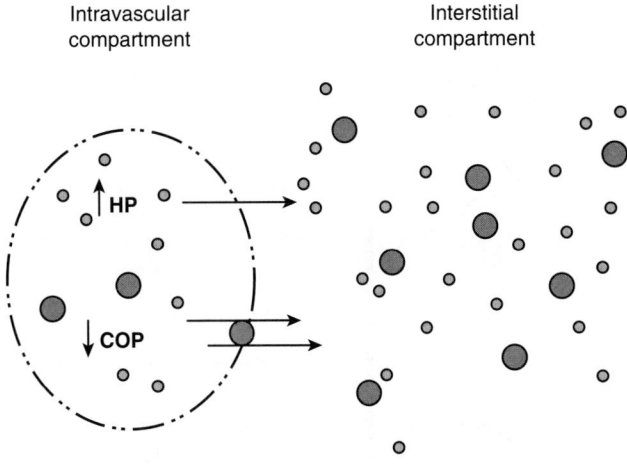

Figure 2-1 The main components of the Starling-Landis equation that affect intravascular water content include intravascular hydrostatic pressure (HP) and colloid osmotic pressure (COP). The intravascular HP is a result of intravascular volume, cardiac output (CO), and systemic vascular resistance (SVR). Under normal conditions the HP favors the movement of fluid from the vessel into the interstitium. The COP is the force that opposes intravascular HP, supporting intravascular water retention. The COP is generated by the presence of large molecules (primarily proteins) that do not readily pass the capillary membrane and create an osmotic effect.

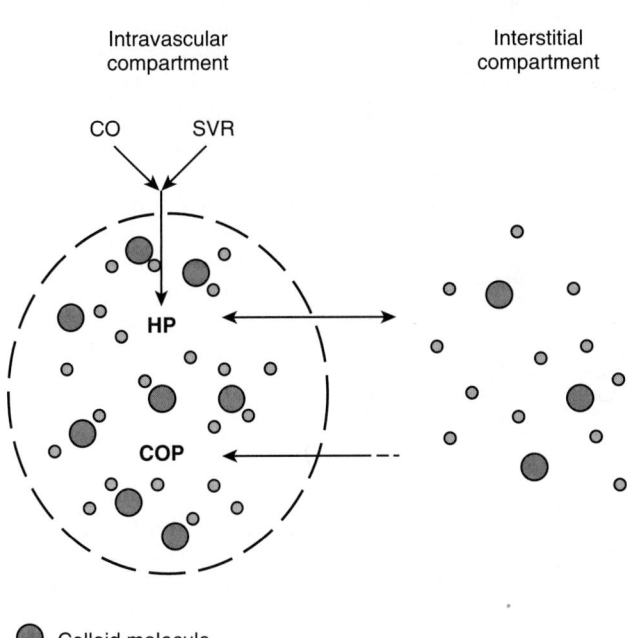

Figure 2-2 Fluid can pass out of the intravascular space under several conditions listed in Table 2-1: increased intravascular hydrostatic pressure (HP), increased capillary permeability, decreased filtration coefficient, and decreased intravascular colloid osmotic pressure (COP). These conditions lead to the consequences of peripheral edema and hypovolemia.

TABLE 2-1

Examples of Conditions That Result in Movement of Fluid Out of the Intravascular Space

Condition	Example
Plasma to interstitial HP gradient increases over the COP gradient	Hypertension Fluid overload
Capillary membrane pore size becomes larger	SIRS-associated diseases • Pancreatitis • Peritonitis • Sepsis • Severe gastroenteritis • Burns • Multitrauma • Vasculitis
The filtration coefficient changes	Burns Hypoalbuminemia Hypervolemia
Intravascular COP falls below interstitial COP	Hypoalbuminemia • SIRS disease • Liver dysfunction • Protein-losing nephropathy/enteropathy

COP, Colloid osmotic pressure; *HP,* hydrostatic pressure; *SIRS,* systemic inflammatory response syndrome.

resuscitation and maintenance is based on the pharmacology of the fluid and the disorder that requires treatment. Each colloid solution is unique, and knowledge of the composition and pharmacology of the fluid is needed to make an appropriate colloid selection for an individual patient's needs (Table 2-2). Differences in macromolecular structure and weight dictate the colloid osmotic effect, method of excretion, and half-life of the colloid solution. The larger the number of small molecules per unit volume of the colloid, the greater will be the initial colloid osmotic effect and plasma volume expansion. When the number of large molecules per unit volume of colloid is high, the colloid is retained longer within the vascular space.

Solutions that contain naturally produced proteins such as albumin (whole blood, plasma products, and concentrated human and canine albumin solutions) or hemoglobin (hemoglobin-based oxygen carriers [HBOCs]) are referred to as natural colloids. Solutions that contain synthetically derived colloid particles such as hydroxyethyl starches (HESs) (hetastarch and tetrastarch) are referred to as synthetic colloids.

Large-volume fluid resuscitation decreases the concentration of coagulation proteins in the plasma and can cause a dilutional coagulopathy. Synthetic colloids are not a substitute for blood products when albumin, hemoglobin, antithrombin, or coagulation proteins are needed. At the present time, albumin products and HESs are the most readily available and commonly used colloids in the United States. Although HBOCs are not available for clinical use at this time, they are being

TABLE 2-2

Characteristics of Colloid Fluids

Colloid	Osmolarity (mOsm/L)	pH	Na+ (mEq/L)	Cl− (mEq/L)	K+ (mEq/L)	Mg2+ (mEq/L)	Ca2+ (mEq/L)	Dextrose (g/L)	Buffer	COP (mm Hg)	Miscellaneous
Natural											
Whole blood	300	Variable	140	100	4	0	0	0-4	None	20	
Frozen plasma	300	Variable	140	110	4	0	0	0-4	None	20	
25% Human albumin			0	0	0	0	0	0	None	200	
Lyophilized canine albumin			0	0	0	0	0	0	None		
Oxyglobin	300	7.8	150	118	4	0	0	0	Lactate	40	
Synthetic											
6% Hetastarch 600/0.7 (Hespan)	310	5.5	154	154	0	0	0	0	None	32	C2:C6 = 4-5:1
6% Hetastarch 670/0.75 (Hextend)	307	5.9	143	124	3	0.9	5	0.99	Lactate	31	C2:C6 = 4:1
6% Tetrastarch 130/0.4 (VetStarch)	308	4-6.5	154	154	0	0	0	0	None	36	C2:C6 = 9:1
10% Pentastarch 260/0.45 (Pentaspan)	326	5.0	154	154	0	0	0	0	None	66	C2:C6 = 4.5:1

COP, Colloid osmotic pressure.

continuously evaluated in experimental studies and are expected to be reintroduced in the near future.

Albumin

Albumin, the most abundant colloid molecule in plasma, can be administered through plasma transfusions, canine lyophilized albumin, or concentrated (25%) human albumin. Allogeneic blood products contain approximately 2.5% albumin. The size of the albumin molecule is constant, and the higher the concentration of albumin, the greater the colloid osmotic effect per milliliter of solution. Plasma transfusions have an albumin concentration equal to that of plasma and may not increase intravascular COP significantly when administered as the sole colloid solution. Availability of plasma in an unfrozen form (i.e., liquid plasma) reduces the time to administration; refrigerated liquid plasma is also advocated by some for use during resuscitation of coagulopathic animals.

Because of its high concentration of albumin and high COP (200 mm Hg), 25% human albumin has the greatest capability for increasing plasma COP. When capillary permeability is normal, 25% albumin can be an effective colloid for rapid intravascular volume expansion. It also can be used to minimize interstitial edema in animals with hypoalbuminemia caused by inadequate albumin production or renal and gastrointestinal albumin loss. However, when increased capillary permeability allows plasma albumin to pass into the interstitium, the initial intravascular COP benefits of albumin infusion are temporary and increased interstitial COP and edema may result.

Human albumin has physiochemical properties that differ from canine and feline albumin, and complications appear to occur at a higher rate (about 20%) with human albumin administration in dogs than with allogeneic transfusions. This risk is reduced when the solution is diluted to a 5% concentration with 0.9% saline and administered over 10 to 24 hours. Acute and delayed immune-mediated reactions have been reported after the administration of human albumin, allogeneic plasma, and blood, requiring vigilant monitoring for allergic reactions when any of these colloids are used. Accordingly, these colloids are administered slowly for the first hour, with careful monitoring for adverse reactions, before increasing to standard recommended rates of infusion.

A 5-g lyophilized canine albumin (www.ABRInt.net) recently has been developed for use as a replacement colloid in the treatment of hypoalbuminemia in dogs. It is stored in a dehydrated powder form and reconstituted with isotonic saline to a desired concentration. Information on its clinical use is limited to albumin replacement in dogs with hypoalbuminemia and septic peritonitis, but not for volume replacement.

Hemoglobin-Based Oxygen Carrier Solutions

The hemoglobin contained in HBOC solutions binds with oxygen, transporting it to the tissues. Because of their small size, HBOC molecules sometimes can pass through the microcirculation more effectively than red blood cells. Their colloidal properties, oxygen-carrying capacity, and low antigenicity may make HBOC solutions an ideal fluid for animals with severe anemia, hypotension, or hypovolemia.

Oxyglobin (Dechra) is a stroma-free, ultrapure bovine-origin polymerized hemoglobin solution approved by the Food and Drug Administration for therapeutic use in dogs with anemia. Oxygen is bound to hemoglobin by a chloride-dependent process, facilitating its release at the capillary. In addition to acting as a temporary oxygen-carrying substitute for red blood cells, the product maintains osmotic pressure and exerts a vasoconstricting effect that can reduce the volume required for resuscitation. It can be stored at room temperature with a 3-year shelf life if unopened, making it more readily available and transportable than whole blood; has universal compatibility; and is unlikely to transmit hematogenous diseases. Oxyglobin is excreted in the urine and bile. Limitations include a short half-life (40 hours) once administered, interferences with enzyme-based chemistry analyses, and requirements for red blood cell replacement if significant anemia is present. Side effects occur most commonly in euvolemic patients and include pulmonary edema, vomiting and diarrhea, and hypertension. These can be minimized by slow administration of small quantities, titrated to effect.

Hydroxyethyl Starch

HES, the parent name of a synthetic polymer of glucose (98% amylopectin), is made from a waxy species of plant starch (either maize or sorghum). It is a highly branched polysaccharide that closely resembles glycogen and is formed by the reaction between ethylene oxide and amylopectin in the presence of an alkaline catalyst. The molecular weight and molar substitution can be adjusted by replacing hydroxyl groups with hydroxyethyl groups at the C2, C3, and C6 positions on the glucose molecule. The greater the substitution on position C2 in relation to C6 (the C2:C6 ratio), the slower the degradation of the molecule by amylase. Renal function has been shown to decline after infusion of hetastarch with molar substitutions greater than 0.62 in human patients undergoing surgery and receiving 10% (hyperoncotic) solutions. This adverse effect has not been identified in animals. Renal effects of lower molar substitutions and 6% solutions are currently under evaluation.

The number-averaged molecular weight (M_n) is the arithmetic mean of the molecular weights of the polymers in solution. Weight-averaged molecular weight (M_w) is the sum of the number of molecules at each M_n divided by the total of all molecules. This weight is generally larger when larger polymers are present in a solution.

The classification of different HES products includes the ratio of the M_w and the degree of substitution. There are three HES products clinically available in the United States at this time: hetastarch (0.7-degree substitution), pentastarch (0.5-degree substitution), and tetrastarch (0.4-degree substitution). Hetastarch can be purchased in 0.9% saline (Hespan; M_w of 450 kD) or in lactated Ringer's solution (LRS) (Hextend; M_w of 670 kD). The electrolyte and buffer compositions of Hextend may reduce the incidence of hyperchloremic acidosis. Hextend also contains 0.45 mmol/L of magnesium and 99 mg/dl (0.99%) of dextrose. A tetrastarch, VetStarch (M_w of 130 kD), is new to the U.S. veterinary market; this solution's higher C2:C6 ratio (9:1) increases its half-life compared with the hetastarch solutions. Pentaspan is a 10% pentastarch solution (M_w of 200 kD) that has a lower average molecular weight than hetastarch.

Although HES can adversely affect von Willebrand's factor, factor VIII, and platelet function, as well as reduce fibrin polymerization, clinical evidence of bleeding has not been reported in animals receiving 6% HES 450/0.7 (Hespan) at doses up to 20 ml/kg/day. The use of 6% hetastarch in LRS (Hextend) may be associated with fewer coagulation abnormalities when compared with 6% hetastarch in saline (Hespan) because it contains calcium, which can become depleted in coagulopathic states. Because of a lower M_w and degree of substitution, the use of 6% HES 130/0.4 is associated with few coagulation abnormalities, and doses up to 50 ml/kg have been recommended.

A differential charge may exist between administered HES molecules and the capillary pore, blocking the passage of HES molecules into the interstitium. This property is independent of molecular size. HESs may also down-regulate and decrease expression of endothelial surface adhesion molecules, which has been reported to decrease cytokine release, inflammation, endothelial injury, and leukocyte migration into the interstitium. HESs have been shown to reverse changes in microvascular permeability caused by oxygen-free radicals during reperfusion injury. This may explain why HES molecules remain in the vascular space in the septic patient when albumin does not (Marx et al, 2002).

Smaller HES molecules are filtered through the glomerulus and excreted in the urine, excreted through the bile, or passed into the interstitium and ingested by macrophages. Larger molecules are degraded by α-amylase into smaller HES molecules. Ongoing studies will better define the safety of various HES solutions on renal function. The authors have observed signs of nausea, occasional vomiting, and hypotension with rapid infusion of hetastarch in cats. Slow administration of small-volume increments has eliminated these side effects in cats.

Clinical Use

Goals for colloid administration include increasing intravascular volume and improving systemic blood flow while maintaining intravascular COP. Selection of a specific colloid or colloids is based on individual traits of the product and the disease under treatment (Tables 2-2 and 2-3). In hypercoagulable animals, the hetastarch solutions may be more useful, whereas in hypocoagulable animals, the tetrastarches may be more suitable for volume expansion. Because at least 75% of the volume of isotonic crystalloid administered into the intravascular fluid compartment translocates into the interstitial fluid compartment within 45 minutes, there is an increased risk for formation of interstitial edema in clinical settings of moderate to severe hypovolemia or systemic inflammation (see Figure 2-2). The 6% HES solutions are effective for expanding intravascular volume while minimizing interstitial edema. The 10% HES solutions are considered hyperoncotic and can increase intravascular volume by 175%.

When there is a coexistent coagulopathy, VetStarch may be the colloid of choice for acute volume replacement. If large volumes of HES are required to restore perfusion, plasma or whole blood transfusions may be

TABLE 2-3

Colloid Choices and Resuscitation Goals Used Based on Hypovolemic Condition in Dogs*

Condition	Resuscitation Colloid	Resuscitation Goal
Hypovolemic and/or traumatic shock	6% HES Oxyglobin	MAP 60-80 mm Hg HR normal CVP 8-10 cm H$_2$O
Trauma or edema in the brain or lungs	6% HES Oxyglobin	MAP 60 mm Hg[†] HR <140 beats/min CVP 5-8 cm H$_2$O
Hypovolemic shock with hemorrhage	Oxyglobin Whole blood pRBC + 6% HES	MAP 60 mm Hg[†] HR <140 beats/min CVP 5-8 cm H$_2$O
Hypovolemic heart failure in a critically hypotensive animal	6% HES	MAP 60 mm Hg[†] HR <180 beats/min
Hypovolemia in the chronically hypoalbuminemic animal	6% HES	MAP 60-80 mm Hg HR normal CVP 8-10 cm H$_2$O

HES, Hydroxyethyl starch; HR, heart rate; MAP, mean arterial pressure; pRBC, packed red blood cell transfusion; CVP, central venous pressure.
*Colloid fluids are always used in conjunction with crystalloid fluids and appropriate analgesia.
†Systolic arterial pressure >90 mm Hg.

required to supplement coagulation proteins and restore clotting times. Oxyglobin is selected when there is a need to improve tissue oxygenation associated with maldistribution of blood flow or anemia. Blood component transfusions are an option when anemia or coagulopathies exist.

Based on the disease process and resuscitation needs, a single colloid or a combination of colloids is selected to obtain the desired benefits. Colloids are typically administered in combination with isotonic crystalloids. When more than one type of colloid is needed, the colloids are usually administered *consecutively* rather than simultaneously. Dogs can tolerate rapid intravenous infusion of 6% HES for immediate intravascular resuscitation. In the cat all forms of colloid are administered more slowly (over 5 to 15 minutes).

The volume of fluids to administer for resuscitation is directed toward achieving desired clinical end-points of heart rate, blood pressure, central venous pressure, pulses, and capillary refill time. This method is described as early goal-directed therapy in humans and end-point or goal-oriented resuscitation in animals. The objective is to infuse the least amount of fluids necessary to achieve and maintain end-point perfusion parameters for the condition being treated. These perfusion parameters for most clinical conditions will be those measured in normal animals. When the patient is at risk for heart failure, hemorrhage, or brain or lung edema, low-normal end points (e.g., low-normal blood pressure and near-normal heart rates) are selected to avoid exacerbation of hemorrhage or edema.

When low-normal resuscitation end points are the goal, replacement isotonic crystalloids are administered initially (10 to 15 ml/kg) with 6% HES (3- to 5-ml/kg increments) titrated to effect (up to 20 ml/kg). When normal end points are desired, larger volumes of replacement isotonic crystalloids can be administered initially (20 to 40 ml/kg) with 6% HES at larger volumes (10 to 15 ml/kg) titrated as needed (up to 30 ml/kg).

Hypothermia, hypotension, and bradycardia are typical clinical findings in the cat in hypovolemic shock. Hypothermia perpetuates hypotension and must be rapidly corrected as part of the resuscitation plan to prevent fluid overload. Initially replacement isotonic crystalloids are administered (10 to 15 ml/kg), and 6% HES (3 to 5 ml/kg) titrated to reach a systolic indirect peripheral blood pressure higher than 40 mm Hg. Maintenance crystalloids and colloids are given at this time while aggressive external warming is provided to bring the rectal temperature above 98° F (within 30 minutes). It is common for the arterial blood pressure and heart rate to reach desired end points after warming is achieved without the administration of additional resuscitation fluids. However, additional crystalloid and colloid doses can be administered if blood pressure remains suboptimal despite warming, assuming the underlying disorder is volume related and not the result of cardiogenic shock (in which case therapy should be focused on improving cardiac pump function, typically with dobutamine or dopamine).

Bolus infusions of colloids are titrated in succession, and clinical parameters are assessed in between boluses until end-point parameters are achieved. When large volumes are required to reach resuscitation end points, coagulation parameters are closely monitored and coagulation factors replaced as needed. Once the resuscitation goal has been achieved, a continuous-rate infusion (CRI) of 6% HES (20 to 30 ml/kg/day) or Oxyglobin (cat: 10 ml/kg/day; dog: 30 ml/kg/day) can be used to maintain the intravascular COP until the capillary integrity is restored and recovery is eminent. Crystalloids are administered simultaneously to restore and maintain hydration and replacement of ongoing losses.

When end-point parameters have not been reached despite adequate fluid replacement, causes of nonresponsive shock should be ruled out and vasoactive agents considered. Oxyglobin has a vasoconstricting effect and can be used in situations resulting in persistent vasodilation. When Oxyglobin is used in the dog for its vasoconstricting properties, 5 ml/kg incremental infusions are given to reach desired end points (to a total of 30 ml/kg). In hypotensive cats, 1- to 3-ml incremental infusions of Oxyglobin can be administered slowly to effect (up to 10 ml/kg) with little risk of acute volume overload and pulmonary edema. An Oxyglobin CRI (10 ml/kg/day in the cat and 30 ml/kg/day in the dog) is then initiated to maintain the blood pressure along with crystalloids for maintenance of hydration and ongoing losses.

When a critical animal does not require aggressive intravascular volume resuscitation but may benefit from intravascular colloid support, 20 ml/kg 6% HES can be administered over 2 to 4 hours by CRI. When there is normal capillary permeability and albumin replacement is desired, 25% human albumin (diluted to a 5% solution, 2 ml/kg/hr over 10 to 12 hours) or lyophilized canine albumin (diluted to a 5% or 16% solution, 800 mg/kg over 6 hours) can be selected and infused as a CRI to reach desired albumin levels. Plasma is administered when there is need for albumin, coagulation factors, or antithrombin. The dose of plasma is variable, with an end-point goal of maintaining or improving albumin, coagulation factor, and antithrombin concentrations. The rate of plasma infusion is calculated to maximize volume infusion without causing fluid overload.

Perfusion and hydration parameters are closely monitored during and after colloid infusion. Early clinical signs of fluid intolerance include serous nasal discharge, chemosis, tachypnea, dull lung sounds (pleural effusion), "moist" lung sounds or crackles (pulmonary edema), gelatinous subcutaneous swelling (peripheral edema), and jugular venous distention. Signs of allergic reaction include facial swelling, urticaria, abrupt hypotension, tachycardia, nausea, vomiting, fever, and hyperemia. Monitoring for acute allergic reaction and anaphylaxis is more important in patients receiving transfusions and concentrated albumin.

References and Suggested Reading

Ballinger WF II, Solanke TF, Thompson WL: Effect of hydroxyethyl starch upon survival of dogs subjected to hemorrhagic shock, *Surg Gynecol Obstet* 122:33, 1966.

Barron M, Wilkes M, Navickis R: A systemic review of the comparative safety of colloids, *Arch Surg* 139:552, 2004.

Bonagura JD, Twedt D, editors: *Kirk's current veterinary therapy XIV (small animal practice)*, Philadelphia, 2009, Saunders, p 61.

Gold MS et al: Comparison of hetastarch to albumin for perioperative bleeding in patients undergoing abdominal aortic aneurysm repair: a prospective, randomized study, *Ann Surg* 211:482, 1990.

Haak C, Rudloff E, Kirby R: Comparison of Hb-200 and 6% hetastarch 450/0.7 during initial fluid resuscitation of 20 dogs with gastric dilatation-volvulus, *J Vet Emerg Crit Care* 22:201-210, 2012.

Kirby R, Rudloff E: Crystalloid and colloid fluid therapy. In Ettinger S, Feldman E: *Textbook of veterinary internal medicine*, ed 6, St Louis, 2005, Saunders, p 412.

Marx G et al: Hydroxyethyl starch and modified fluid gelatine maintain plasma volume in a porcine model of septic shock with capillary leakage, *Intensive Care Med* 28:629, 2002.

Marx G et al: Resuscitation from septic shock with capillary leakage: hydroxyethyl starch (130 kD), but not Ringer's solution maintains plasma volume and systemic oxygenation, *Shock* 21:336, 2004.

Mathews K, Barry M: The use of 25% human serum albumin: outcome and efficacy in raising serum albumin and systemic blood pressure in critically ill dogs and cats, *J Vet Emerg Crit Care* 15(2):110, 2005.

Molnar Z et al: Fluid resuscitation with colloids of different molecular weight in septic shock, *Intensive Care Med* 30:1356, 2004.

Muir W, Wellman M: Hemoglobin solutions and tissue oxygenation, *J Vet Intern Med* 17:127, 2003.

Prittie J: Optimal end points of resuscitation and early goal-directed therapy, *J Vet Emerg Crit Care* 16:329, 2006.

Tian J et al: Hydroxyethyl starch (130 kD) inhibits Toll-like receptor 4 signaling pathways in rat lungs challenged with lipopolysaccharide, *Anesth Analg* 113:112, 2011.

Trow A et al: Evaluation of the use of human albumin in critically ill dogs: 73 cases (2003-2006), *Am Vet Med Assoc* 233:607-612, 2008.

Viganó F et al: Administration of 5% human serum albumin in critically ill small animal patients with hypoalbuminemia: 418 dogs and 170 cats (1994-2008), *J Vet Emerg Crit Care* 20:237, 2010.

Wehausen C, Kirby R, Rudloff E: Evaluation of the effects of bovine hemoglobin glutamer-200 on systolic arterial blood pressure in hypotensive cats: 44 cases (1997-2008), *J Am Vet Med Assoc* 238:909, 2011.

Zikria BA et al: Macromolecules reduce abnormal microvascular permeability in rat limb ischemia-reperfusion injury, *Crit Care Med* 17:1306, 1989.

CHAPTER 3

Catecholamines in the Critical Care Patient

EDWARD S. COOPER, *Columbus, Ohio*

Catecholamines are the primary effectors of the sympathetic nervous system (SNS) and play a major role in cardiovascular homeostasis in normal and pathophysiologic stress. Physiologic sympathetic outflow, which is maintained through a basal level of stimulation from the vasomotor center and adrenal secretion of catecholamines, sustains appropriate heart rate, vascular tone, and blood pressure. Endogenous catecholamines include norepinephrine (NE) and dopamine (DA), both primarily released by sympathetic nerve fibers, and epinephrine (EPI), primarily released by the adrenal gland. A number of stimuli, including pain, fear, hypoxemia, anemia, and hypotension, can increase the release of these sympathetic mediators and subsequent activation of adrenergic receptors. The resulting "fight or flight" response is characterized by tachycardia, increased cardiac output, and elevation of blood pressure.

The actions of catecholamines are largely determined by the location and type of receptor activated. These receptors are classified as presynaptic or postsynaptic.

Presynaptic receptors have a regulatory effect on the amount of NE released from the nerve terminal, increasing or decreasing it depending on the receptor type. Postsynaptic receptors are subdivided into synaptic/junctional (having the most significant role in tissue activation) and extrajunctional (only stimulated with massive catecholamine release). A number of different receptor types (and subtypes) have been elucidated and include α-adrenergic (α_1, α_2), β-adrenergic (β_{1-3}), and dopaminergic (DA1, DA2). Each receptor type has a relative distribution within certain tissues, a varying affinity for the adrenergic neurotransmitters, and specific physiologic effects when activated.

Catecholamines exert their effects by binding with a receptor and then triggering intracellular signaling pathways. Although these effects are complicated and modulated by vagal input, circulating hormones, and locally produced mediators, some general points deserve emphasis. Vascular postsynaptic α_1 and α_2 receptors increase intracellular calcium levels, leading to vasoconstriction.

TABLE **3-1**

Receptor Activities of Catecholamine/Vasoactive Drugs

Drug	α_1	α_2	β_1	β_2	DA1	DA2	V_1
Epinephrine	++++	+++	+++	++	–	–	–
Dopamine							
0.5-3 µg/kg/min	–	–	+	+	++++	++++	–
3-10 µg/kg/min	+	(+)	++	+	++	++	–
10-20 µg/kg/min	+++	(+)	+	(+)	+	+	–
Norepinephrine	++++	++	++	–	–	–	–
Dobutamine	–	–	++++	++	–	–	–
Vasopressin	–	–	–	–	–	–	++++

Presynaptic α_2 receptors diminish the release of NE and promote down-regulation of sympathetic outflow, with resultant vasodilation and diminished cardiac output. β Receptors modify cyclic adenosine monophosphate (cAMP) levels, which alter cytosolic calcium levels depending on the tissue location. Postsynaptic β_1 receptors, which are largely located on myocardial cells, increase intracellular (cytosolic) calcium, leading to increased contractility (inotropy) along with enhanced reuptake of calcium in diastole that speeds myocardial relaxation (lusitropy). In specialized tissues such as the sinoatrial (SA) and atrioventricular (AV) nodes the postsynaptic β_1 receptors both enhance calcium entry and stimulate funny current to increase heart rate (chronotropy) and speed of conduction across the SA and AV nodes. Myocardial β_2 activation has mostly similar effects, although these receptors are extrajunctional and require significant stimulation. β_2 receptors located in bronchial and vascular tissues promote vascular smooth muscle relaxation, which results in bronchodilation and vasodilation. For tissues with multiple types of adrenergic receptors, the net effect of activation depends on receptor prevalence and affinity for catecholamine stimulation.

Specific Catecholamines

Given the varied effects and tissue beds that are subject to sympathetic stimulation, there is significant potential for therapeutic manipulation through administration of exogenous catecholamines. In critical care patients these medications are primarily used to augment catecholamine effects on the cardiovascular system, especially when the endogenous response might be insufficient or become exhausted. Determining which catecholamine to use is largely based on its relative receptor activities (Table 3-1), the clinical scenario in which intervention is needed (Table 3-2), and the potential for adverse effects.

Epinephrine

EPI is nonselective in its receptor activation and has effects on all α and β receptors. The α effects primarily cause vasoconstriction, although the net impact on

TABLE **3-2**

Commonly Used Catecholamine/Vasoactive Drugs

Drug	Indications	Dose Range
Epinephrine	CPR	0.01 mg/kg IV
	Anaphylaxis, asthmatic crisis	0.01-0.02 mg/kg
Dopamine	Decreased CO, myocardial failure	3-10 µg/kg/min CRI
	Vasodilatory shock	10-20 µg/kg/min CRI
Norepinephrine	Vasodilatory shock	0.1-1.0 µg/kg/min CRI
Dobutamine	Decreased CO, myocardial failure	2-20 µg/kg/min CRI (dog)
		1-5 µg/kg/min CRI (cat)
Vasopressin	CPR	0.8 U/kg
	Vasodilatory shock	0.01-0.04 units per dog per min

CPR, Cardiopulmonary resuscitation; *CO,* cardiac output.

peripheral resistance is partially offset by β_2-induced vasodilation. The β effects promote an increase in cardiac output as well as bronchodilation. Given this combination of activities, EPI is primarily used in the treatment of patients with cardiopulmonary arrest, anaphylaxis, or severe asthmatic crisis. Potential adverse effects include excessive vasoconstriction, especially to the splanchnic circulation; increased myocardial oxygen demand; arrhythmias; tachycardia; hyperglycemia; and hypokalemia.

The primary beneficial effect of EPI in cardiopulmonary resuscitation (CPR) is α-induced vasoconstriction (and resultant increase in diastolic pressure) rather than any direct cardiac effects from β stimulation. Coronary circulation is an essential component of successful resuscitation, and diastolic pressure is a major determinant for coronary perfusion pressure. In addition, EPI has beneficial effects on cerebral perfusion and oxygen delivery. Despite these potential benefits, available evidence shows no clear survival benefit with administration of EPI in

CPR (Neumar et al, 2010). However, EPI remains the drug of choice in CPR because it has been shown to improve rates of return of spontaneous circulation (ROSC).

Ideal dosing has been a subject of some debate. Although it has increased α_1 stimulation, "high-dose" EPI (0.1 mg/kg) has not proved any more effective in achieving ROSC than "low-dose" EPI (0.01 mg/kg) in most clinical circumstances of arrest. Also, with "low-dose" EPI some of the adverse effects of EPI are avoided in the postresuscitation period, especially if repeated doses are needed, and this "low-dose" approach currently is recommended in CPR (Neumar et al, 2010). One must be mindful of the concentration of epinephrine used (1:1000 vs 1:10,000). For "low-dose" EPI, standard dosing with 1:10,000 is 0.1 ml/kg (or 1 ml/10 kg). If only 1:1000 is available, it should be diluted 1:10 in sterile water and then administered as above. This can be repeated every 3 to 5 minutes (after each one to two cycles of compressions) until ROSC or cessation of CPR. When administered via the endotracheal route if intravenous (IV) access is unavailable, doses administered during CPR should be doubled.

Another potential application of EPI is in the treatment of anaphylaxis/anaphylactic shock. The combination of vasoconstriction and bronchodilation makes EPI, along with IV fluids and oxygen therapy, ideally suited to help reverse the major life-threatening aspects of anaphylaxis. In addition, EPI serves to decrease production and release of mediators involved in the pathogenesis of anaphylaxis. Although there is some evidence of improved outcomes with a constant rate infusion (CRI) of EPI (Mink et al, 2004), bolus dosing of 0.01 to 0.02 mg/kg IV (potentially repeated after 15 to 20 minutes) is still currently recommended. EPI also may be beneficial as a bronchodilator for cats in asthmatic crisis, dosed at 0.01 to 0.02 mg/kg IV or subcutaneously (SC).

Dopamine

DA exerts its varied effects on α and β_1 receptors both directly and indirectly (by promoting release of NE) and also stimulates dopaminergic receptors. Its receptor activities (and thereby its effects) are highly dose dependent, and a short plasma half-life (~2 min) requires that it be used as a CRI. At very low doses (0.5 to 3 µg/kg/min) DA receptors are potentially activated, promoting renal, coronary, and splanchnic vasodilation. At intermediate doses (3 to 10 µg/kg/min) DA effects diminish and β effects predominate, with increases in heart rate and contractility. At higher doses (10 to 20 µg/kg/min) α-adrenergic activities predominate, with a net effect of vasoconstriction and increased peripheral resistance. However, there can be significant variation and overlap of these effects from patient to patient and these dosing ranges only serve as a guideline. Typical indications for DA include inotropic support in myocardial dysfunction/failure and pressor support in vasodilatory shock. Potential adverse effects include excessive vasoconstriction, tachycardia, and arrhythmias.

DA can be used in the β activity range for patients with impaired myocardial contractility or forward flow, especially if cardiogenic shock is suspected. In addition to positive inotropic effects, β_2 activation can promote peripheral vasodilation and decrease afterload, further supporting forward flow. Caution must be exercised at higher doses because triggering α effects could promote vasoconstriction and impair cardiac output by increasing afterload.

DA also can be used as a pressor in the treatment of hypotension caused by vasodilation, such as that associated with sepsis or anesthesia. For this purpose high doses are needed to stimulate α receptors. Patients should have close electrocardiograph (ECG) and (ideally direct arterial) blood pressure monitoring to most effectively titrate therapy. Given the short half-life of DA, adjusting doses every 10 to 20 minutes to reach target pressures is reasonable.

It was previously believed that low-dose infusion of DA was beneficial in the treatment of oliguric renal failure by promoting renal blood flow and glomerular filtration rate (GFR). However, human clinical trials have failed to show any clear benefit, and DA is no longer recommended for this purpose (Hollenberg, 2011).

Norepinephrine

NE activates α and β_1 receptors, with virtually no β_2 stimulation. The net effect is marked vasoconstriction with no offsetting vasodilation from β_2, along with some positive inotropic and chronotropic effects. NE-induced tachycardia is offset by reflex vagal stimulation triggered by a rise in blood pressure. Its primary application is in vasodilatory (septic) shock that is refractory to volume expansion. NE must be administered as a CRI with dose ranges from 0.1 to 1.0 µg/kg/min, titrated to desired blood pressure. Similar to DA, the short half-life of NE allows for rapid achievement of steady state and dose adjustment every 10 to 20 minutes. Given the potent vasoconstrictive effects, ideally NE should be administered through a central venous catheter. Potential adverse effects include excessive vasoconstriction and tissue ischemia, arrhythmias, and increased myocardial oxygen demand.

Dobutamine

Dobutamine (DO) is a fairly selective β_1 agonist, although there are dose-dependent α_1 and β_2 activities. The net effect is an increase in contractility, a possible decrease in ventricular filling pressures, and minimal impact on peripheral vascular tone, depending on the infusion rate. At higher doses, DO can also have some positive chronotropic effects that can serve to further increase cardiac output. These effects make DO ideally suited to the treatment of cardiogenic shock, secondary myocardial dysfunction and impaired contractility, such as that seen with dilated cardiomyopathy. Increased cardiac output, and potential for improved tissue perfusion, may also confer benefit in noncardiogenic causes of shock (e.g., hemorrhagic or vasodilatory), especially if the patient has not been responsive to intravascular volume loading. DO has an extremely short half-life (~2 min) and so rapidly achieves onset of action and steady state as a CRI. Dose ranges for dogs and cats are 2 to 20 µg/kg/min and 1 to 5 µg/kg/min, respectively. Infusions are started at the low end of the dose range and titrated every 10 to 20 minutes until desired effect or maximum dosing is reached. Potential adverse effects include increased myocardial oxygen demand, tachycardia, and arrhythmias (especially at higher doses).

Vasopressin

Although vasopressin (VP) is not a catecholamine, it deserves some consideration as a vasoactive agent in the context of this discussion. VP released by the pituitary gland in response to increased plasma osmolarity or to hypovolemia promotes vasoconstriction directly through activation of V_1 receptors. It also potentiates the effects of catecholamines and inhibits endothelial nitric oxide production. It has been demonstrated that endogenous VP levels, while increased initially, can become depleted in certain disease states such as sepsis and hemorrhagic shock (Scroggin and Quandt, 2009). The effects of VP, unlike those of catecholamines, are not diminished by severe acidemia. Given these attributes, VP is primarily used in critically ill patients to increase systemic blood pressure and improve coronary perfusion. One potential indication is CPR with recommended dosing of 0.8 U/kg, which can be repeated in 3- to 5-minute intervals. Another potential application is refractory vasodilatory (septic) shock, after volume resuscitation and other pressor therapies have failed to raise blood pressure. Clear dosing recommendations have not been established but published ranges include 0.5 to 5.0 mU/kg/min (Silverstein et al, 2007) or 10 to 40 mU/min (Scroggin and Quandt, 2009). Potential adverse effects of VP include severe peripheral and splanchnic vasoconstriction with associated diminished cardiac output and ischemic injury.

Cardiopulmonary Resuscitation

As previously stated, EPI has long been the drug of choice during CPR. However, EPI can have significant adverse effects, especially in the postresuscitative period. Other catecholamines (NE, phenylephrine) have been studied in comparison to EPI but failed to show benefit. In experimental models VP has resulted in improved neurological outcomes and rates of ROSC, but human clinical trials have largely demonstrated effects equivalent to those of EPI.

Current American Heart Association advanced life support guidelines suggest that these drugs are equally effective and that VP can replace the first or second dose of EPI (Neumar et al, 2010). A randomized, blinded clinical trial in dogs with naturally occurring cardiac arrest also has demonstrated similar outcomes with VP and EPI (Buckley, 2011). It is therefore reasonable to consider alternating administration of these agents (e.g., EPI, VP, EPI) during CPR.

Septic Shock

Catecholamine therapy seems intuitive in septic shock to curtail excessive vasodilation, especially if hypotension is refractory to fluid resuscitation. Numerous studies have attempted to determine the optimal pressor to use in human patients. Based on the available evidence, the 2008 Surviving Sepsis Campaign guidelines suggest that either DA or NE can be used as first-line medications (Dellinger et al, 2008). However, more recent studies comparing DA and NE found an equivalent impact on 28-day survival but fewer side effects (tachycardia and arrhythmias) associated with NE (De Backer, 2012).

VP also has been investigated extensively in the treatment of septic shock. A large-scale human clinical trial demonstrated that VP had outcomes equivalent to NE and actually demonstrated superiority in patients with less severe septic shock (Russell et al, 2008). VP has been shown to decrease catecholamine requirements. Given the available information, it is reasonable to consider DA or NE as a first-line agent, with consideration of VP for additional pressor support. For patients with evidence of decreased cardiac output and/or myocardial dysfunction, provision of a positive inotrope (such as DA or DO), potentially in conjunction with pressor therapy, may also be of benefit.

References and Suggested Reading

Buckley GJ, Rozanski EA, Rush JE: Randomized, blinded comparison of epinephrine and vasopressin for treatment of naturally occurring cardiopulmonary arrest in dogs, *J Vet Intern Med* 25:1334-1340, 2011.

De Backer D et al: Dopamine versus norepinephrine in the treatment of septic shock: a meta-analysis, *Crit Care Med* 40(3):725-730, 2012.

Dellinger RP et al: Surviving Sepsis Campaign: International guidelines for management of severe sepsis and septic shock: 2008, *Crit Care Med* 36:296-327, 2008.

Hollenberg S: Vasoactive drugs in circulatory shock, *Respir Crit Care Med* 183:847-855, 2011.

Long KM, Kirby R: An update on cardiovascular adrenergic receptor physiology and potential pharmacological applications in veterinary critical care, *J Vet Emerg Crit Care* 18:2-25, 2008.

Mink SN et al: Constant infusion of epinephrine, but not bolus treatment, improves haemodynamic recovery in anaphylactic shock in dogs, *Clin Exp Allergy* 34(11):1776-1783, 2004.

Neumar RW et al: Part 8: Advanced cardiac life support, *Circulation* 122:S729-S767, 2010.

Russell JA et al: Vasopressin versus norepinephrine infusion in patients with septic shock, *N Engl J Med* 358:877-887, 2008.

Scroggin RD, Quandt J: The use of vasopressin for treating vasodilatory shock and cardiopulmonary arrest, *J Vet Emerg Crit Care* 19(2):145-157, 2009.

Silverstein DC et al: Vasopressin therapy in dogs with dopamine-resistant hypotension and vasodilatory shock, *J Vet Emerg Crit Care* 17(4):399-408, 2007.

CHAPTER 4

Shock

KARI SANTORO-BEER, *Philadelphia, Pennsylvania*
DEBORAH C. SILVERSTEIN, *Philadelphia, Pennsylvania*

Shock is a state of severe hemodynamic and metabolic derangements. It is characterized by poor tissue perfusion from low or unevenly distributed blood flow that leads to a critical decrease in oxygen delivery (DO_2) in relation to oxygen consumption (VO_2) (Figure 4-1) or inadequate cellular energy production. If the shock state is not promptly recognized and treated, neurohormonal compensatory mechanisms will lead to stimulation of the renin-angiotensin-aldosterone system, as well as baroreceptor- and chemoreceptor-mediated release of catecholamines and subsequent production of counterregulatory hormones (glucagon, adrenocorticotropic hormone [ACTH], and cortisol). These changes will increase cardiovascular tone, activate a variety of biochemical mediators, and stimulate inflammatory responses that contribute to the shock syndrome. This progression can cause or exacerbate uneven microcirculatory flow, poor tissue perfusion, tissue hypoxia, altered cellular metabolism, cellular death, and vital organ dysfunction or failure.

Box 4-1 lists the different types of shock, but this classification can be overly simplistic. Critically ill patients are subject to complex etiologic and pathophysiologic events and therefore may suffer from more than one type of shock simultaneously. The rationale for the functional classification of shock is the presumption that each underlying illness identified can be associated with a specific pathophysiologic process and rapid, appropriate therapy can be administered.

Clinical Presentation

Depending on the type and clinical phase of shock, the patient's clinical signs will vary. Dogs in compensatory shock demonstrate mild-to-moderate mental depression, increased heart rate, increased respiratory rate, peripheral vasoconstriction with cold extremities as well as pale mucous membranes, and a shortened capillary refill time with normal blood pressure. As compensatory mechanisms fail, patients may develop severe mental depression, prolonged capillary refill time, increased heart rate, poor pulse quality, and decreased arterial blood pressure.

Dogs with sepsis or a systemic inflammatory response syndrome (SIRS) can show clinical signs of hyperdynamic or hypodynamic shock. The initial hyperdynamic phase of sepsis is characterized by tachycardia, fever, bounding peripheral pulse quality, and hyperemic mucous membranes secondary to peripheral vasodilation. If septic shock or SIRS progresses unchecked, a decreased cardiac output and signs of hypoperfusion may ensue as a result of cytokine effects on the myocardium or myocardial ischemia. Clinical alterations may then include tachycardia, pale (and possibly icteric) mucous membranes with a prolonged capillary refill time, hypothermia, poor pulse quality, and dull mentation. Hypodynamic septic shock is the decompensatory stage of sepsis and without intervention results in organ damage and death. Finally, the gastrointestinal (GI) tract is considered the shock organ in dogs and often leads to ileus, diarrhea, hematochezia, or melena.

In cats the hyperdynamic phase of shock is rarely recognized. Also, in contrast to dogs, cats with shock have unpredictable changes in heart rate; they may exhibit tachycardia or bradycardia. In general, cats typically present with pale mucous membranes (and possibly icterus), weak pulses, cool extremities, hypothermia, and generalized weakness or collapse. In cats the lungs seem to be the organ most vulnerable to damage during shock or sepsis, and signs of respiratory dysfunction are common (Schutzer et al, 1993; Brady et al, 2000; Costello et al, 2004).

Patient Monitoring

General Diagnostics

Basic diagnostic tests, including venous or arterial blood gases, a complete blood cell count, blood chemistry panel, coagulation panel, blood typing, and urinalysis, should be completed for all patients in shock to assess the extent of organ injury and identify the cause of the shock state. Thoracic and abdominal radiographs, abdominal ultrasound, and echocardiography may be indicated once the patient is stabilized. Thoracic imaging can help distinguish cardiogenic from other forms of shock.

Monitoring Perfusion and Oxygen Delivery

The magnitude of oxygen deficit is a key predictor in determining outcome in patients with shock. Therefore optimizing tissue perfusion and DO_2 are goals of effective therapy, and thorough monitoring is necessary to achieve this objective. An optimally perfused patient maintains the following characteristics: central venous pressure between 5 and 10 cm H_2O (2 to 5 cm H_2O in cats); urine production of at least 1 ml/kg/hr; a mean arterial pressure (MAP) between 70 and 120 mm Hg and diastolic pressure above 40 mm Hg; normal body temperature, heart rate, heart rhythm, and respiratory rate; and moist, pink mucous membranes with a capillary refill time of less than 2 seconds. Monitoring these parameters creates the baseline for patient assessment. Additional monitoring

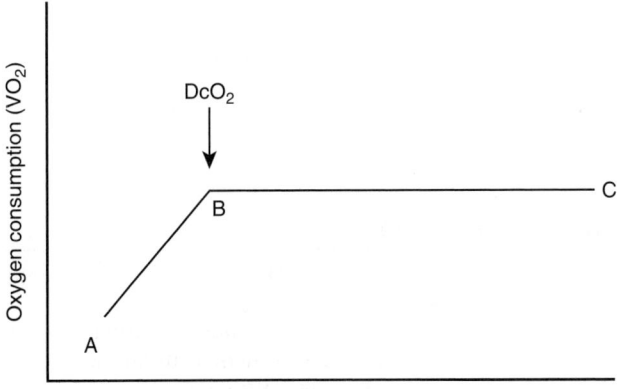

Figure 4-1 The relationship between oxygen delivery and oxygen consumption. In region B-C, the oxygen consumption remains constant as oxygen delivery is increased. The oxygen supply is in excess of consumption and VO_2 is termed supply-independent. During shock, as metabolic demand (VO_2) increases or DO_2 diminishes (C-B), OER rises to maintain aerobic metabolism so that consumption can remain independent of delivery. However, at point B, called critical DO_2 (DcO_2), the maximum OER is reached. This is believed to be 60% to 70%, and beyond this point any further increase in VO_2 or decline in DO_2 must lead to tissue hypoxia. (Data from Mellema M: Cardiac output, wedge pressure and oxygen delivery, *Vet Clin North Am Small Anim Pract* 31(6):1175, 2001.)

BOX 4-1

Functional Classifications and Examples of Shock

Hypovolemic: A Decrease in Circulating Blood Volume
- Hemorrhage
- Severe dehydration
- Trauma

Cardiogenic: A Decrease in Forward Flow from the Heart
- Congestive heart failure
- Cardiac arrhythmia
- Cardiac tamponade
- Drug overdose (e.g., anesthetics, β-blockers, calcium channel blockers)

Distributive: A Loss of Systemic Vascular Resistance
- Sepsis
- Obstruction (heartworm disease, saddle thrombosis)
- Anaphylaxis

Metabolic: Deranged Cellular Metabolic Machinery
- Hypoglycemia
- Cyanide toxicity
- Mitochondrial dysfunction
- Cytopathic hypoxia of sepsis

Hypoxemic: A Decrease in Oxygen Content in Arterial Blood
- Anemia
- Severe pulmonary disease
- Carbon monoxide toxicity
- Methemoglobinemia

elements that may prove beneficial include measurements of blood lactate, indices of systemic oxygenation transport, and mixed venous oxygen saturation.

Blood Lactate Levels

Critically ill patients with inadequate tissue perfusion, DO_2, or oxygen uptake often develop a hyperlactatemia and acidemia that reflect the severity of tissue hypoxia. Human patients with lactic acidosis are at greater risk of developing multiple organ failure and demonstrate a higher mortality rate (Nguyen et al, 2004). High blood lactate levels may also help to predict mortality in dogs (Boag and Hughes, 2005; de Papp et al, 1999; Nel et al, 2004; Lagutchik et al, 1998). The normal lactate level in adult dogs and cats is reported to be less than 2.5 mmol/L; lactate concentrations greater than 7 mmol/L are considered severely elevated (Boag et al, 2005). However, normal neonatal and pediatric patients may have higher lactate concentrations (McMichael et al, 2005). In addition, sample collection and handling techniques can affect lactate concentration (Hughes et al, 1999). Serial lactate measurements can be taken during the resuscitation period to gauge response to treatment and evaluate the resuscitation end points; the trends in lactate concentrations are a better predictor of outcome than are single measurements in both human and veterinary patients (Husain et al, 2003; Zacher et al, 2010; Green et al, 2011; Conti-Patara et al, 2012). The ability of the body to correct an elevated lactate concentration is directly correlated to survival.

Cardiac Output Monitoring and Indices of Oxygen Transport

The most direct way to assess the progress of resuscitation in shock patients is to measure indices of systemic oxygen transport. Measurement and monitoring of these values requires right-sided cardiac catheterization, which is performed using a specialized pulmonary artery catheter (PAC), also termed *Swan-Ganz catheter* or *balloon-directed thermodilution catheter*. When connected to appropriate electronic monitoring systems, the PAC allows access for the measurement of central venous and pulmonary arterial pressure, mixed venous blood gases (PvO_2 and SvO_2), pulmonary capillary wedge pressure (PCWP), and cardiac output. With these data additional information regarding the function of the circulatory and respiratory systems can be derived (i.e., stroke volume, end-diastolic volume numbers, systemic vascular resistance index, pulmonary vascular resistance index, arterial oxygen content, mixed venous oxygen content, DO_2 index, VO_2 index, and oxygen extraction ratio). The cardiac output is most commonly determined using thermodilution methods, although other techniques are available, including noninvasive Doppler-based methods.

A PAC can provide the clinician with useful information to assess and monitor the cardiovascular and pulmonary function of shock patients. It may also help the clinician evaluate the response to therapeutic interventions and allow titration of fluid therapy, vasopressors, and inotropic agents. Cardiac output and systemic DO_2 should be optimized by intravascular volume loading until the PCWP approaches 18 to 20 mm Hg. A higher

PCWP (>18 to 20 mm Hg) promotes the formation of pulmonary edema, further impairing oxygenation and overall oxygen transport. Higher cardiac index (CI), DO_2, and VO_2 measurements have been linked with improved survival in critically ill human patients. Finally, the use of a PAC does not necessarily translate into reduced mortality in the critically ill shock patient; it is an invasive monitoring technique that is not without risk.

Although much information can be obtained from it, the PAC has a number of limitations. The accuracy of its measurements relies on catheter placement, calibration of transducers, coexisting cardiac or pericardial disease, and interpretation of waveforms and measurements or calculations. Thus PAC placement should be performed by experienced individuals, and interpretation of the data should be systematic. In veterinary practice today, PAC catheters and monitoring systems are largely confined to academic centers and to specialty referral practices. In humans the most common complications that occur during or after PAC insertion include arrhythmias, pulmonary injuries, thromboembolism, and sepsis.

Mixed Venous Oxygen Saturation and Central Venous Oxygen Saturation

Mixed venous oxygen saturation (SvO_2) can be used to assess changes in the global tissue oxygenation (oxygen supply-to-demand). If VO_2 is constant, SvO_2 is determined by cardiac output, hemoglobin concentration, and systemic arterial oxygen tension. The SvO_2 decreases if DO_2 is reduced by low cardiac output, hypoxia, or severe anemia, or if the VO_2 is increased (as with fever). SvO_2 is increased in hyperdynamic stages of sepsis and cytotoxic tissue hypoxia (e.g., cyanide poisoning). A reduction in SvO_2 may be an early sign that the patient's clinical condition is deteriorating. Also, SvO_2 may be a surrogate for measuring the CI during resuscitative efforts.

Ideally SvO_2 is measured in a blood sample derived from a PAC because this represents a true mixed venous oxygen sample. However, in cases in which the insertion of a PAC is not possible or desirable, SvO_2 can be determined within the central circulation using a central venous catheter in the cranial vena cava. SvO_2 is then termed *central venous oxygen saturation ($ScvO_2$)*. In critically ill patients with circulatory failure of any origin, $ScvO_2$ values generally are higher than SvO_2, but the two measurements closely parallel one another. Therefore the presence of a low $ScvO_2$ likely indicates an even lower SvO_2. The difference between the two values is usually about 5% and can be explained by blood flow redistribution and differences in VO_2 across the hepatosplanchnic, coronary, and cerebral circulations during shock states. The potential value of this monitoring was shown in a study comparing two algorithms for early goal-directed therapy in human patients with severe sepsis and septic shock (Rivers et al, 2001). In this study maintenance of a continuously measured $ScvO_2$ above 70% (in addition to maintaining central venous pressure above 8 to 12 mm Hg, MAP above 65 mm Hg, and urine output above 0.5 ml/kg/hr) resulted in a 15% absolute reduction in mortality compared with the same treatment without $ScvO_2$ monitoring (see Early Goal-Directed Therapy section later in the chapter for further details). $ScvO_2$ measurement in small animals has not gained widespread use, but clinical research in critically ill and septic dogs suggests that it may prove useful as a diagnostic, prognostic, and monitoring tool in the future (Conti-Patara et al, 2012; Hayes et al, 2011).

Therapy of Shock

Optimal therapy of the shock state involves careful patient monitoring, as discussed in the previous section, and specific treatments that include oxygen and various forms of fluid therapy tailored to the clinical situation. Additional treatment often involves vasopressors, inotropic agents, antimicrobials, gastrointestinal protectants, and nutritional support.

Oxygen

If the animal is not breathing or displays signs of impending respiratory fatigue, immediate intubation and positive-pressure ventilation should be instituted. If the animal is breathing spontaneously, oxygen is administered (see Chapters 10 and 11). This can involve flow-by methods (50 to 150 ml/kg/min) such as simply holding the oxygen tubing to the nose or administering oxygen into a mask, hood, or bag. Nasal or nasopharyngeal catheter(s) are effective methods of oxygen administration (using rates of 50 to 100 ml/kg/min per catheter). Once the vital signs are obtained, vascular access is established and fluid administration is initiated if indicated. Preliminary diagnostics and appropriate treatment should be rapidly initiated to maximize DO_2 to the tissues and prevent irreversible shock.

Fluid Therapy

Vascular Access

The first and most important therapeutic goal for non-cardiogenic shock is to restore the effective circulatory volume. Appropriate vascular access is essential for rapid administration of large volumes of fluid. Poiseuille's law of flow states that resistance to flow through a catheter is directly proportional to the length of the catheter and inversely related to the fourth power of the radius. Thus large-bore, short intravenous catheters should be placed in a central or peripheral vein for resuscitation. For cats and small dogs 18- or 20-gauge catheters should be used; for larger dogs multiple venous catheters (14- to 18-gauge) should be placed. Faster intravenous fluid administration can be further facilitated by applying pressure around the fluid bag with a commercial pressure device or a blood pressure cuff.

Crystalloids

Isotonic crystalloids remain the cornerstone of treatment for noncardiogenic shock. Examples include 0.9% saline, lactated Ringer's solution, Normosol-R, and Plasma-Lyte A. A shock dose of isotonic crystalloid solution is approximately one blood volume (i.e., 90 ml/kg in the dog and 50 ml/kg in the cat). The fluid administered rapidly distributes into the extracellular fluid compartment so that only approximately 25% of the delivered volume remains in the intravascular space by 30 minutes after infusion (Silverstein et al, 2005). Although theoretically this increase in interstitial fluid volume might predispose to interstitial edema and deranged oxygen transfer to the cells, this has not been proven in human clinical trials. However, it is important that excessive fluid volumes are not administered to prevent volume overload. The general recommendation is that one third to one half of the shock dose be administered as quickly as possible, followed by additional boluses as indicated by clinical parameters and repeated physical examination. In patients that are bleeding it may even be advantageous to perform "hypotensive resuscitation" (to a MAP of approximately 60 mm Hg) until the hemorrhage is controlled since aggressive fluid therapy in this setting can worsen bleeding and outcome. For animals with coexisting head trauma, the isotonic crystalloid of choice is 0.9% saline since it contains the highest concentration of sodium and is least likely to contribute to cerebral edema (see Chapter 1).

Hypertonic Solutions
Hypertonic (7% to 7.5%) saline administration causes a transient osmotic shift of water from the extravascular to the intravascular compartment. It is administered in small volumes (3 to 5 ml/kg) intravenously (IV) over 5 to 10 minutes. In addition to the fluid compartment shift caused by hypertonic saline, there is evidence that it may also help reduce endothelial swelling, increase cardiac contractility, cause mild peripheral vasodilation, and decrease intracranial pressure. Because of the osmotic diuresis and rapid redistribution of the sodium cations that ensue following the administration of hypertonic saline, the intravascular volume expansion is transient (<30 minutes) and additional fluid therapy must be used (Silverstein et al, 2005). Hypertonic saline may be administered in conjunction with synthetic colloids.

Synthetic Colloids
Colloids are large molecules (molecular weight >20,000 daltons) that do not readily sieve across the vascular membrane (see Chapter 2). The colloidal particles in the most commonly used synthetic colloids (e.g., hydroxyethyl starch) are suspended in 0.9% saline or a lactated electrolyte solution. The synthetic colloid solutions are hyperoncotic to the normal animal and therefore pull fluid into the vascular space and help to retain it there in animals with normal vascular permeability. They cause an increase in blood volume that is greater than that of the infused volume and help to retain this fluid in the intravascular space in animals with normal capillary permeability. Hetastarch solutions (e.g., Hextend or Hespan) are 6% solutions with particles ranging from 10,000 to 1,000,000 daltons in molecular weight, a weight-average molecular weight of 450,000 daltons, a number-average molecular weight of 69,000 daltons, and a colloid osmotic pressure of approximately 34 mm Hg *in vitro*. The recommended dose of synthetic colloids for the treatment of shock is up to 20 ml/kg in the dog and up to 10 ml/kg in the cat (note that rapid administration of hydroxyethyl starch in the cat has been reported to cause vomiting).

Excessive volumes can lead to volume overload, coagulopathies, and hemodilution. At volumes greater than 40 ml/kg/day, an increase in incisional bleeding has been reported with hetastarch solutions, which may be due to increased blood pressure and microcirculatory flow as well as dilutional and direct effects of hetastarch on coagulation. Hetastarch affects von Willebrand's factor, platelet function, and factor VIII function. Clinical evidence of bleeding has not been reported in animals receiving doses up to 20 ml/kg/day. VetStarch, a 6% tetrastarch solution in 0.9% saline that was recently approved for veterinary use (also known as Voluven in human medicine), contains particles ranging from 110,000 to 150,000 daltons, a weight-average molecular weight of 130,000 daltons, and a COP of 40 mm Hg *in vitro* (unpublished data). Because of its lower weight-average molecular weight and low molar substitution, VetStarch is purportedly less likely to cause adverse renal and coagulation side effects and may provide a safer alternative for short-term oncotic support. The magnitude and duration of its effects in small animal patients require further investigation.

Synthetic colloid solutions are appropriately used for shock therapy in acutely hypoproteinemic animals (total protein less than 3.5 g/dl) with a decreased colloid osmotic pressure. They can also be used with isotonic or hypertonic crystalloids to maintain adequate plasma volume expansion with lower interstitial fluid volume expansion and to expand the intravascular space with smaller volumes over a shorter time period. Despite multiple clinical studies in humans, there is no definitive documentation that colloids are superior to crystalloids for resuscitation, and the price of colloids is significantly greater than that of crystalloids. Total protein readings via refractometer are not valid in animals receiving synthetic colloid therapy; daily measurements of colloid osmotic pressure are recommended, with a goal of 16 to 18 mm Hg.

Hypertonic Saline Plus Synthetic Colloid Solutions
To prolong the effect of the resuscitation fluids, a hypertonic saline/synthetic colloid mixture can be administered for the treatment of shock. A 1:2.5 ratio of 23.4% NaCl with hetastarch makes an approximately 7.5% saline mixture (17 ml of 23.4% NaCl and 43 ml of hydroxyethyl starch). It should be administered in small volumes (3 to 5 ml/kg) over 5 to 10 minutes.

Blood Component Therapy
The need for blood products during resuscitation depends on the patient's disease process. Most fluid-responsive shock patients tolerate acute hemodilution to a hematocrit of less than 20%. In animals with acute blood loss that are unresponsive to fluid therapy alone, the hematocrit should be maintained above 25% to maximize oxygen-carrying capacity. Excessive increases in hematocrit should be avoided since this will increase blood viscosity. Most animals can tolerate an acute loss of 10% to 15% of blood volume without requiring a blood transfusion. Acute hemorrhage exceeding 20% of the blood volume often requires transfusion therapy in addition to the initial fluid resuscitation discussed previously. In

animals with acute blood loss requiring transfusion therapy, fresh whole blood or packed red blood cells and fresh frozen plasma should be used in an attempt to stabilize clinical signs of shock, maintain the hematocrit above 25%, and promote clotting times within the normal range (see Chapter 2).

Packed red blood cells and fresh frozen plasma are administered at a dose of 10 to 15 ml/kg, and fresh whole blood at a dose of 20 to 25 ml/kg. Refrigerator-stored plasma or frozen plasma that is more than 1 year old no longer contains labile coagulation factors (V, VIII, and von Willebrand's). Platelets are only present in fresh whole blood, platelet-rich plasma, or plasma concentrate, and use of these products is indicated in animals with thrombocytopenia- or thrombocytopathia-induced bleeding disorders or with massive hemorrhage. Cryopreserved, lyophilized platelets are also available for dogs and offer the benefits of immediate availability and long-term storage, but early research suggests decreased *in vivo* recovery and survival compared with platelet concentrate (Callan, Appleman, and Sachais, 2009). However, animals with life-threatening bleeding due to thrombocytopenia or thrombocytopathia will likely benefit, at least in the short term, from the administration of any platelet-containing transfusion product.

Plasma products are most commonly used in animals with profound blood loss, a coagulopathy, or severe hypoalbuminemia. The ability of these products to increase colloid osmotic pressure is limited compared with the hyperoncotic synthetic colloids, although blood products do supply a small amount of albumin. Cryoprecipitate may be administered to bleeding dogs with fibrinogen, fibronectin, factor VIII, or von Willebrand's factor deficiencies. Blood products generally should be administered over at least 1 to 2 hours to monitor for a transfusion reaction and avoid volume overload, but it may be necessary to bolus these products in life-threatening situations. A blood type should be determined in all animals, especially cats, before transfusions are given. Cross-matching also helps to decrease the incidence of transfusion reactions. Hemoglobin-based oxygen carrier (HBOC) solutions may be useful in cases of anemia to increase oxygen delivery to the tissues. Due to the small size of free hemoglobin, HBOCs also may increase perfusion to constricted or partially thrombosed capillary beds. Although HBOCs have these theoretical benefits and a long shelf life, they are not widely used due to inconsistent supply, undesirable side effects, and lack of clear benefit over other products.

Human Serum Albumin Solution

Animals with severe hypoalbuminemia (<1.5 g/dl) may benefit from treatment with 25% human albumin. Albumin is crucial in the transport of drugs, hormones, chemicals, toxins, and enzymes. Preliminary studies in dogs show that human albumin administration in dogs increases circulating albumin concentrations, total solids, colloid osmotic pressure, and blood pressure. Potential risks are similar to those for any blood transfusion (i.e., fever, vomiting, increased respiratory effort) in addition to the potential for increasing clotting times. Both healthy normoalbuminemic and critically ill dogs

with hypoalbuminemia developed anti–human albumin antibodies following infusion. Albumin-induced anaphylaxis and delayed hypersensitivity reactions have been described when concentrated human albumin was administered rapidly to healthy normoalbuminemic dogs, but only anecdotal reports have described a similar phenomenon when concentrated human albumin was administered to critically ill patients. This highlights the importance of careful case selection and monitoring during and after administration (Mathews and Barry, 2005; Trow et al, 2008; Francis et al, 2007). Due to antigenicity, repeated dosing is not recommended. Canine serum albumin is now commercially available in the United States, but more study is needed regarding its efficacy.

Vasopressors and Positive Inotropes

Shock patients that remain hypotensive despite intravascular volume resuscitation often require vasopressor therapy with or without inotropic support. Since both cardiac output and systemic vascular resistance affect DO_2 to the tissues, therapy for hypotensive patients includes maximizing cardiac function with fluid therapy and adding inotropic drugs or modifying vascular tone with vasopressor agents when necessary. Commonly used vasopressors include catecholamines (epinephrine, norepinephrine, and dopamine) and the sympathomimetic drug phenylephrine and vasopressin (see Chapter 3).

Different sympathomimetics cause various changes in the cardiovascular system, depending on the specific receptor stimulation caused by the drug. Conventionally, adrenergic receptor location and function involve the α_1 and β_2 receptors located on the vascular smooth muscle cells that lead to vasoconstriction and vasodilation, respectively, whereas β_1 receptors in the myocardium primarily modulate inotropic and chronotropic activity. In addition, there are dopaminergic-1 receptors in the renal, coronary, and mesenteric microvasculature that mediate vasodilation and dopaminergic-2 receptors in the synaptic nerve terminals that inhibit the release of norepinephrine.

Dopamine has various potential actions on adrenergic and dopaminergic receptors. Primarily dopaminergic effects are seen at low intravenous dosages (1 to 5 μg/kg/min); mainly β-adrenergic effects are seen at moderate dosages (5 to 10 μg/kg/min); mixed α- and β-adrenergic effects are present at high dosages (10 to 15 μg/kg/min); and primarily α-adrenergic effects are seen at very high dosages (15 to 20 μg/kg/min). The actual dose-response relationship is unpredictable in a given patient because it depends on individual variability in enzymatic dopamine inactivation, receptor down-regulation, and the degree of autonomic derangement. Dopamine can be used as a single-agent therapy to provide both inotropic and pressor support in animals with vasodilation and decreased cardiac contractility. In comparison to other pressor drugs, dopamine is a less potent inotrope than epinephrine or dobutamine and less vasoconstricting than norepinephrine. The cardiovascular effects of dopamine may dissipate after several days of therapy, perhaps because of receptor down-regulation and/or induction of increased postsynaptic norepinephrine release. Despite the beneficial effects of dopamine on cardiac output and blood pressure, it may have deleterious effects on renal, mesenteric, and skeletal blood flow.

Norepinephrine has mixed α- and β-adrenergic receptor agonist effects with preferential α-receptor activity. Therefore the effects on heart rate and contractility are less potent, and norepinephrine is commonly used as a pressor agent in animals with normal or increased cardiac output states. Canine septic shock models have demonstrated that the effects of norepinephrine on cardiac function are diminished compared with those of nonseptic controls. In septic patients with cardiac insufficiency and vasodilation, it may be desirable to use norepinephrine in conjunction with dobutamine (a potent β-agonist) to prevent the deleterious effects of increasing afterload in the face of a diseased heart. Renal blood flow may improve in animals with septic shock so long as arterial blood pressure is normalized. Conversely, norepinephrine administration to dogs with hypovolemic shock induces deleterious renal vasoconstriction. Norepinephrine has also been shown to improve urine output and creatinine clearance when added to dopamine or dobutamine in human patients with septic shock. Enhanced splanchnic DO_2 and increases in gastric mucosal pH are evident in humans who receive norepinephrine therapy for the treatment of hypotensive septic shock. The vasopressor dosage of norepinephrine in humans (and extrapolated to dogs) is 0.1 to 1.0 µg/kg/min IV.

Epinephrine is a potent pressor with mixed α- and β-agonist activity. Although epinephrine is thought to have more potent β-agonist effects than norepinephrine, individual response is quite variable in patients with systemic inflammatory diseases and hypotension. Epinephrine may significantly impair splanchnic blood flow compared with norepinephrine and dobutamine (in combination). This is most likely because of the strong α-adrenergic activity of epinephrine with subsequent vasoconstriction in regional vascular beds, although epinephrine also activates vasodilatory β-receptors. The vasopressor dosage of intravenous epinephrine is 0.01 to 0.1 µg/kg/min and for primarily β-agonist effects 0.005 to 0.02 µg/kg/min. Epinephrine is rarely used as a sole first-line vasopressor agent because of its potential side effects, but it may be necessary in critically ill animals. Epinephrine also inhibits mast cell and basophil degranulation and therefore is the drug of choice in patients suffering from anaphylactic shock. It is also commonly used for the treatment of cardiac arrest.

Phenylephrine is a pure α-agonist drug that causes profound vasoconstriction. It has been shown to cause an increase in cardiac output and blood pressure, presumably as a result of increased venous return to the heart and activation of α_1 receptors in the myocardium. Typically phenylephrine is used in patients that are unresponsive to other sympathomimetics, although it can be used as a sole first-line agent in vasodilated, hypotensive animals. Since phenylephrine has no β-agonist activity, it is the least arrhythmogenic of the sympathomimetic pressor drugs and therefore is desirable in animals that develop tachyarrhythmias in response to other pressor agents. The intravenous dosage range is 0.5 to 3 µg/kg/min.

Dobutamine is a β-agonist with weaker, dose-dependent α-effects. It increases cardiac output, DO_2, and VO_2 without causing vasoconstriction at lower doses. Therefore it is useful in animals with shock caused by cardiac insufficiency. Dobutamine may worsen or precipitate tachyarrhythmias and may precipitate seizure activity in cats. The intravenous dosage range is 1 to 5 µg/kg/min in cats and 2.5 to 20 µg/kg/min in dogs.

Vasopressin is a nonadrenergic vasopressor agent. It has both direct and indirect effects on the vascular smooth muscle via the V_1 receptors and induces vasoconstriction in most vascular beds. In vitro vasopressin is a more potent vasoconstrictor than phenylephrine or norepinephrine. At low doses this drug causes vasodilation in renal, pulmonary, mesenteric, and cerebral vasculature in an attempt to maintain perfusion to these vital organs. Low flow states secondary to hypovolemia or septic shock are associated with a biphasic response in endogenous serum vasopressin levels. There is an early increase in the release of vasopressin from the neurohypophysis in response to hypoxia, hypotension, or acidosis, which leads to high levels of serum vasopressin. This plays a role in the stabilization of arterial pressure and organ perfusion in the initial stages of shock. There appears to be a subsequent decrease in circulating vasopressin levels, most likely a result of a depletion of hypothalamic stores. Therefore the use of vasopressin in animals in the later stages of shock, especially those that exhibit vasodilation and are refractory to catecholamine therapy, may be beneficial. The drug also enhances sensitivity to catecholamines and therefore may allow the dose of concurrent catecholamine therapy to be lowered. Experimental studies in dogs have demonstrated an increase in blood pressure and cardiac output with minimal side effects. A clinical case series using vasopressin at 0.01 to 0.04 units per dog per min found an increase in blood pressure following vasopressin therapy as well. This drug will require further investigation but may be considered in animals with catecholamine-resistant vasodilatory shock.

Antimicrobial Therapy

Early antimicrobial therapy is crucial in shock patients with proven or suspected sepsis. Studies have shown that time from triage to administration of appropriate antimicrobial therapy is a primary determinant of mortality in human patients with severe sepsis and septic shock (Gaieski et al, 2010). If possible, properly collected cultures of blood, urine, respiratory secretions (collected by endotracheal wash, transtracheal wash, or bronchoscopy), and other available body fluids (i.e., pleural, peritoneal, or cerebrospinal fluid) should be sampled carefully before antimicrobial therapy is begun. Broad-spectrum antibiotic therapy should be initiated pending culture and sensitivity results. Empiric antibiotic choices should be effective against gram-positive and gram-negative organisms and anaerobes. Initial combinations might include ampicillin (22 mg/kg IV q6-8h) and enrofloxacin (15 mg/kg IV q24h in dogs, 5 mg/kg IV q24h in cats); ampicillin and amikacin (15 mg/kg IV q24h); cefazolin (22 mg/kg IV q8h) and amikacin, ampicillin, and cefotaxime (25 to 50 mg/kg IV q6h); or clindamycin

(10 mg/kg IV q8-12h) and enrofloxacin. Single agents such as ticarcillin/clavulanic acid (50 mg/kg IV q6h), cefoxitin (15 to 30 mg/kg IV q4-6h), or imipenem (5 to 10 mg/kg IV q6-8h, if bacterial resistance is suspected) could be used initially as well.

Gastrointestinal Protection

Stress-related mucosal disease (SRMD) and subsequent upper GI bleeding are frequently seen in critically ill humans and may also occur in dogs and cats. Clinical signs of hematemesis, hematochezia, or melena should alert the clinician to potentially serious GI hemorrhage. Hypoperfusion of the upper GI mucosa during shock, excessive gastric acid secretion, and impaired mucosal defense mechanisms (mucus secretion, production of growth factors) contribute to the development of SRMD. Furthermore, in human patients other factors are thought to increase the risk of stress-related GI hemorrhage including prolonged mechanical ventilation, extensive burns, hepatic failure, renal failure, coagulopathy, head injuries, multiple trauma, high-dose corticosteroids, nonsteroidal antiinflammatory drug use, and absence of enteral nutrition. In veterinary patients the incidence of SRMD and clinically significant bleeding is unknown; therefore no guidelines are available for their management.

The initial strategy in critically ill dogs and cats should be to ensure adequate GI perfusion and use early enteral nutrition. High-risk patients should receive pharmacologic prophylaxis for stress-related GI hemorrhage. Based on the currently available evidence in human medicine, it appears that proton pump inhibitors (PPIs) are superior to histamine-2 receptor antagonists (H_2RAs), which are superior to sucralfate in the prevention of SRMD in adult critical-care patients. Drugs available include oral omeprazole 0.7 to 1 mg/kg, or esomeprazole sodium IV (0.5 mg/kg), pantoprazole 0.5 mg/kg PO q24h or 0.7 to 1 mg/kg IV q24h, famotidine (H_2RA) 0.5 to 1 mg/kg IV q12-24h, ranitidine (H_2RA) 0.5 to 4 mg/kg IV q8-12h, and sucralfate (protectant) 0.25 1 g/25 kg PO q6-8h. Recent evidence suggests that ranitidine and famotidine may not adequately decrease acid production in dogs at clinically recommended doses (Bersenas et al, 2005; Cook et al, 1999; Tolbert et al, 2011).

Nutrition

Following initial stabilization of the shock patient, nutritional status should be addressed (see Chapter 7). Adequate nutrition is critical in patients with secondary hypermetabolic states such as sepsis. The enteral route (orally or via nasoesophageal, esophagostomy, gastrostomy, or jejunostomy tube) is preferable if the animal is normotensive, not vomiting, and alert. Parenteral nutrition should be administered if the enteral route is not feasible or contraindicated. If the blood glucose falls below 60 g/dl, 0.5 to 1 ml/kg of 50% dextrose should be diluted 1:1 with sterile water and administered IV over 1 to 2 minutes. The fluids should also be supplemented with dextrose as needed (2.5% to 7.5%). Hyperglycemia should be avoided since it has been associated with an increased likelihood of infection and a poorer prognosis.

Novel Therapeutic Strategies

Early Goal-Directed Therapy

For many years it has been recognized that critically ill patients in shock benefit from rapid normalization of abnormal physiologic functions. Many therapeutic strategies have been studied, including reestablishing normal or even supranormal hemodynamic indices' values to improve patient outcome. Although supranormal resuscitation has not proven beneficial, early goal-directed therapy has shown promise (Kern and Shoemaker, 2002).

Early goal-directed therapy is performed using a series of predefined resuscitation end points to help clinicians resuscitate shock patients as soon as the syndrome is recognized. The aim of these specific end points is to adjust cardiac preload, contractility, and afterload to balance systemic DO_2 with demand. Recently the effect of early goal-directed therapy was evaluated in a prospective, randomized clinical trial that included humans who presented to an emergency room with severe sepsis, septic shock, or sepsis syndrome (Rivers et al, 2001). During the first 6 hours of resuscitation from sepsis-induced hypoperfusion, patients treated with early goal-directed therapy received, in a sequential fashion, fluid resuscitation, vasopressors or dilator agents, red-cell transfusions, and inotropic medications to achieve target levels of central venous pressure (8 to 12 mm Hg), MAP (65 to 90 mm Hg), urine output (as least 0.5 ml/kg of body weight), and $ScvO_2$ (at least 70%). The other group of patients was treated following a standard therapy at their clinician's discretion. Ultimately patients resuscitated following the early goal-directed therapy plan had higher survival rates. In dogs and cats, initiating a similar early goal-directed therapy strategy immediately after recognition of a shock syndrome might be beneficial. Recent research examining the use of goal-directed therapy in dogs with sepsis appears promising, and the use of "resuscitation bundles" will likely prove beneficial in future studies (Conti-Patara et al, 2012).

Relative Adrenal Insufficiency and Use of Steroids

Adrenal insufficiency of critical illness is a well-recognized clinical entity in humans, especially those suffering from sepsis (Cooper and Stewart, 2003). These patients have an increased morbidity and mortality, and early studies supported the use of physiologic doses of steroids to improve outcome. More recently, however, studies have shown that although steroids might reverse shock more quickly, there is no difference in mortality between groups and there may be higher rates of superinfection in patients given steroids (Sprung et al, 2008). Adrenal insufficiency may be secondary to both a decrease in glucocorticoid synthesis (i.e., adrenal insufficiency) and peripheral resistance to glucocorticoids. The diagnosis of the dysfunction relies on assessment of plasma cortisol (+/- aldosterone) before and after exogenous corticotropin administration (ACTH stimulation test). A relative adrenal insufficiency may lead to refractory hypotension in shock patients or those with critical illness since steroids normally suppress endogenous vasodilators such as the kallikrein-kinin system, prostacyclin, and nitric oxide. Glucocorticoids also modify the renin-angiotensin-aldosterone system and up-regulate angiotensin II receptors in the vasculature. Although administration of glucocorticoids may suppress aldosterone secretion secondary to ACTH deficiency, this has not been well-demonstrated in dogs (Corrigan et al, 2010). The use of physiologic doses of steroids in people with refractory hypotension has been well studied (Annane et al, 2004). Critically ill, hypotensive animals may also benefit from physiologic doses of corticosteroids, but further research is required to confirm this (Martin et al, 2008) (see Chapter 16). There is controversy regarding the definition of an "adequate" response, the dose of ACTH that should be administered, and the constituents of "replacement" therapy.

In specific situations critically ill patients might benefit from glucocorticoid supplementation. Etomidate, which blocks the synthesis of cortisol by reversible inhibition of 11β-hydroxylase, has an inhibitory effect on adrenal function in critically ill patients and has been associated with an increase in intensive care unit mortality. Patients receiving treatment with corticosteroids for chronic autoimmune or inflammatory diseases and those receiving replacement therapy for hypoadrenocorticism should receive at least physiologic doses of prednisone or dexamethasone during severe illness.

References and Suggested Reading

Annane D et al: Corticosteroids for treating severe sepsis and septic shock, *Cochrane Database Syst Rev* 1 CD002243, 2004.

Bersenas AM et al: Effects of ranitidine, famotidine, pantoprazole, and omeprazole on intragastric pH in dogs, *Am J Vet Res* 66(3):425, 2005.

Boag A, Hughes D: Assessment and treatment of perfusion abnormalities in the emergency patient, *Vet Clin North Am Small Anim Pract* 35(2):319, 2005.

Brady CA et al: Severe sepsis in cats: 29 cases (1986-1998), *J Am Vet Med Assoc* 217(4):531, 2000.

Callan MB, Appleman EH, Sachais BS: Canine platelet transfusions, *J Vet Emerg Crit Care* 19(5):401-415, 2009.

Conti-Patara A et al: Changes in tissue perfusion parameters in dogs with severe sepsis/septic shock in response to goal-directed hemodynamic optimization at admission to ICU and the relation to outcome, *J Vet Emerg Crit Care* 22(4):409, 2012.

Cook D et al: Risk factors for clinically important upper gastrointestinal bleeding in patients requiring mechanical ventilation, *Crit Care Med* 27(12):2812, 1999.

Cooper MS, Stewart PM: Corticosteroid insufficiency in acutely ill patients, *N Engl J Med* 348:727, 2003.

Corrigan AM et al: Effect of glucocorticoid administration on serum aldosterone concentration in clinically normal dogs, *Am J Vet Res* 71(6):649, 2010.

Costello MF et al: Underlying cause, pathophysiologic abnormalities, and response to treatment in cats with septic peritonitis: 51 cases (1990-2001), *J Am Vet Med Assoc* 225(6):897, 2004.

de Papp E et al: Plasma lactate concentration as a predictor of gastric necrosis and survival among dogs with gastric-volvulus: 102 cases (1995-1998), *J Am Vet Med Assoc* 215(1):49, 1999.

Francis AH et al: Adverse reactions suggestive of type III hypersensitivity in six healthy dogs given human albumin, *J Am Vet Med Assoc* 230:873, 2007.

Gaieski DF et al: Impact of time to antibiotics on survival in patients with severe sepsis or septic shock in whom early goal-directed therapy was initiated in the emergency department, *Crit Care Med* 38(4):1045, 2010.

Green TI et al: Evaluation of initial plasma lactate values as a predictor of gastric necrosis and initial and subsequent plasma lactate values as a predictor of survival in dogs with gastric diltation-volvulus: 84 dogs (2003-2007), *J Vet Emerg Crit Care* 21(1):36-44, 2011.

Hayes GM et al: Low central venous oxygen saturation is associated with increased mortality in critically ill dogs, *J Small Anim Prac* 52(8):433, 2011.

Hughes D et al: Effect of sampling site, repeated sampling, pH and Pco_2, on plasma lactate concentration in healthy dogs, *Am J Vet Res* 60(4):521, 1999.

Husain FA et al: Serum lactate and base deficit as predictors of mortality and morbidity, *Am J Surg* 185(5):485, 2003.

Kern JW, Shoemaker WC: Meta-analysis of hemodynamic optimization in high-risk patients, *Crit Care Med* 30(8):1686, 2002.

Lagutchik MS et al: Increased lactate concentrations in ill and injured dogs, *J Vet Emerg Crit Care* 8(2):117, 1998.

Martin LG et al: Pituitary-adrenal function in dogs with acute critical illness, *J Am Vet Med Assoc* 233:87, 2008.

Mathews KA, Barry M: The use of 25% human serum albumin: outcome and efficacy in raising serum albumin and systemic blood pressure in critically ill dogs and cats, *J Vet Emerg Crit Care* 15(2):110, 2005.

McMichael MA et al: Serial plasma lactate concentration in 68 puppies aged 4 to 80 days, *J Vet Emerg Crit Care* 15(1):17, 2005.

Nel M et al: Prognostic value of blood lactate, blood glucose and hematocrit in canine babesiosis, *J Vet Intern Med* 18(4):471, 2004.

Nguyen HB et al: Early lactate clearance is associated with improved outcome in severe sepsis and septic shock, *Crit Care Med* 32(8):1637, 2004.

Rivers E et al: Early goal directed therapy in the treatment of severe sepsis and septic shock, *N Engl J Med* 345:1368, 2001.

Schutzer KM et al: Lung protein leakage in feline septic shock, *Am Rev Respir Dis* 147:1380, 1993.

Silverstein DC et al: Assessment of changes in blood volume in response to resuscitative fluid administration in dog, *J Vet Emerg Crit Care* 15(3):185, 2005.

Sprung CL et al: Hydrocortisone therapy for patients with septic shock, *N Engl J Med* 358:111, 2008.

Tolbert K et al: Efficacy of oral famotidine and 2 omeprazole formulations for the control of intragastric pH in dogs, *J Vet Intern Med* 25:47, 2011.

Trow AV et al: Evaluation of human albumin in critically ill dogs: 73 cases (2003-2006), *J Am Vet Med Assoc* 233(4):607, 2008.

Zacher LA et al: Association between outcome and changes in plasma lactate concentration during presurgical treatment in dogs with gastric dilatation-volvulus: 64 cases (2002-2008), *J Am Vet Med Assoc* 236(8):892, 2010.

CHAPTER 5
Cardiopulmonary Resuscitation

DANIEL J. FLETCHER, *Ithaca, New York*
MANUEL BOLLER, *Melbourne, Victoria, Australia*

Veterinary protocols for cardiopulmonary resuscitation (CPR) have been largely adapted from those promoted by the American Heart Association for humans. The Reassessment Campaign on Veterinary Resuscitation (RECOVER) recently completed a systematic review of the literature relevant to veterinary CPR and developed the first evidence-based, consensus CPR guidelines for small animals (Fletcher et al, 2012). The clinical questions examined during the evidence evaluation process were partitioned into five domains: (1) Preparedness, (2) Basic Life Support (BLS), (3) Advanced Life Support (ALS), (4) Monitoring, and (5) Post–Cardiac Arrest Care.

Preparedness

Delays in initiation of CPR for patients with cardiopulmonary arrest (CPA) consistently result in poor outcomes. It is therefore crucial that veterinary practices are well-prepared for early recognition of CPA and immediate initiation of high-quality resuscitation. CPR training that includes both didactic components and opportunities to practice psychomotor skills is recommended for all veterinary personnel who may be called on to assist in a crisis. Refresher training and drills at minimum 6-month intervals have been shown to improve performance, and structured assessment and feedback after training maximizes the effectiveness of that training. A fully stocked crash cart that is routinely audited for content should be available in an easily accessible central location. Cognitive aids such as CPR algorithm charts and emergency drug dosing charts improve adherence to guidelines and individual performance during CPR. After every CPR attempt, a debriefing session during which team performance is discussed and critically evaluated can identify misconceptions and improve future team performance.

Diagnosis of Cardiopulmonary Arrest

CPA is an important differential diagnosis for any acutely unresponsive patient. It is a clinical diagnosis based on the presence of unconsciousness, lack of breathing, and absence of a palpable pulse. Regardless of the clinician's index of suspicion for CPA in an individual patient, a rapid assessment focused on ruling out CPA should be undertaken immediately when an animal is unresponsive. A standardized approach based on evaluation of airway, breathing, and circulation (ABC) quickly identifies CPA and allows immediate intervention should the diagnosis be made. Because the benefits of starting CPR

immediately in a patient with CPA far outweigh the risks of performing CPR on an unresponsive patient not in CPA, the clinician should not delay starting CPR in any patient in which there is a suspicion of CPA.

Thorough *airway* evaluation is crucial in acutely presenting unresponsive patients. Airway obstruction prevents effective ventilation and delivery of oxygen to the tissues, and failure to identify obstruction likely leads to unsuccessful resuscitation. The airway should be visually inspected by opening the mouth, pulling out the tongue, and examining the oral cavity, pharynx, laryngeal area, and arytenoids. Digital palpation from the oral cavity back to the laryngeal area may reveal foreign objects, masses, or swellings causing airway obstruction. If direct visualization and digital palpation are obstructed by conformation or swollen tissues, a laryngoscope should be used if available. If fluid is preventing visualization, swab the mouth out or use suction to clear the area. If the patient is roused by manipulation of the airway, use caution to avoid being bitten.

When evaluating an unresponsive patient, assessment of *breathing* and particularly the rapid identification of apnea (respiratory arrest) are of primary concern. If there are no obvious chest excursions on initial visual inspection, breathing can be further assessed by lightly touching the chest and feeling for chest movements, auscultation of the chest for lung sounds, or placing cotton or a slide in front of the nares and looking for movement or fogging, respectively.

Rapid assessment of the *circulation* via palpation of the femoral or dorsal metatarsal pulses, palpation for an apex heartbeat, or cardiac auscultation should be undertaken; however, if CPA cannot be definitively ruled out, CPR should be initiated immediately rather than performing further diagnostic assessment of the circulation. This is important because (1) several studies in human medicine have shown that pulse palpation is an insensitive test for diagnosis of CPA, which also may be the case in dogs and cats, and (2) a large body of literature indicates that even small delays in initiating CPR in pulseless patients reduce the likelihood of successful resuscitation. Therefore the ABC assessment described above should take no more than 10 to 15 seconds to complete.

Basic Life Support

BLS is the crucial first step in CPR and should be initiated immediately following diagnosis of CPA using the circulation, airway, breathing (CAB) concept. BLS includes delivery of chest compressions, establishment of an airway, and positive pressure ventilation. Circulation should be addressed first because ventilation is ineffective if there is no cardiac output, and evidence suggests a worsening outcome the longer chest compressions are delayed.

Circulation: Chest Compressions

Patients with CPA have no forward blood flow out of the heart and no delivery of oxygen to the tissues. Immediate consequences are the exhaustion of cellular energy stores, cell depolarization, and thus loss of organ function. If persisting for more than a few minutes, this results in increasing severity of ischemic organ injury and sets the stage for escalating reperfusion injury on reinstitution of tissue blood flow. The initial goal of chest compressions is therefore to provide (1) pulmonary blood flow for oxygen upload and carbon dioxide (CO_2) elimination and (2) tissue perfusion for oxygen delivery to restore cellular metabolic activity. Experimental evidence suggests that even well-executed external chest compressions produce only approximately 30% of normal cardiac output, so great care must be taken to perform compressions with proper technique. Chest compressions should be started as soon as possible after diagnosis or suspicion of CPA. Delay in the start of high-quality chest compressions reduces the likelihood of return of spontaneous circulation (ROSC).

Chest compressions should be delivered with the dog or cat in *lateral* recumbency (with a few exceptions noted below). The recommended compression depth is one third to one half the width of the chest. Regardless of species or size, the chest compression rate should be 100 to 120 per minute. Use of aids to ensure correct compression rate, such as a metronome or a song with the correct tempo (e.g., "Staying Alive") is recommended. Leaning or residual compression of the chest between compressions must be avoided to allow full elastic recoil. Chest compressions should be delivered without interruption in cycles of 2 minutes, and a new compressor should take over after each cycle to attenuate the effect of rescuer fatigue. Any interruption in compressions should be as short as possible because it takes approximately 60 seconds of continuous chest compressions before coronary perfusion pressure (CPP) reaches its maximum. CPP in turn is a critical determinate of myocardial blood flow and the likelihood of ROSC.

The physiology of blood flow generation is fundamentally different during CPR compared with spontaneous circulation. Two distinct theories have been advanced to explain how chest compressions lead to systemic blood flow. The *cardiac pump theory* is based on the concept that the left and right ventricles are directly compressed, increasing the pressure in the ventricles, opening the pulmonic and aortic valves, and providing blood flow to the lungs and the tissues, respectively. Recoil of the chest between compressions due to the elastic properties of the rib cage creates negative pressure within the chest, thereby improving filling of the ventricles before the next compression. The *thoracic pump theory* is based on the concept that external chest compressions raise overall intrathoracic pressure, which forces blood from intrathoracic vessels into the systemic circulation, with the heart acting as a passive conduit.

Given the chest wall stiffness in medium and large dogs, blood flow generated by the thoracic pump mechanism likely predominates in these patients. Therefore it is recommended that the chest be compressed over the highest point on the lateral thoracic wall with the patient in lateral recumbency. In contrast, in very keel- or deep-chested dogs (e.g., Doberman pinschers, sight hounds) it is reasonable to do chest compressions directly over the heart as the cardiac pump mechanism likely predominates in dogs with this conformation. In markedly barrel-chested dogs (e.g., English bulldogs), compressions over the sternum with the patient in dorsal recumbency may be more effective in eliciting the thoracic pump mechanism than lateral chest compressions. In these and other large dogs with low chest compliance, considerable compression force is necessary for CPR to be effective. The compressor should maintain locked elbows with one hand on top of the other, and the shoulders should be directly above the hands. This allows compressions to be done using the core muscles rather than the biceps and triceps, reducing fatigue and maintaining optimal compression force. If the patient is on a table and the elbows cannot be locked, a stool should be used or the patient should be placed on the floor to allow correct technique.

Most cats and small dogs tend to have higher thoracic compliance and narrower chests than larger dogs, making the cardiac pump mechanism achievable in these patients; therefore chest compressions should be done directly over the heart. Compressions may be performed using the same two-handed technique as described above for large dogs or may be done using a single-handed technique in which the compressing hand is wrapped around the sternum and compressions are achieved from both sides of the chest by squeezing. Circumferential compressions of the chest using both hands also may be considered.

Airway and Breathing: Ventilation

If an endotracheal (ET) tube and laryngoscope are available, the patient should be intubated as soon as possible. Both dogs and cats can be intubated in lateral recumbency, so chest compressions should continue during ET tube placement. If an ET tube is not readily available, mouth-to-snout ventilation provides improved oxygenation and CO_2 removal. The patient's mouth should be held closed firmly with one hand. The neck is extended to align the snout with the spine, opening the airway as completely as possible. The rescuer makes a seal over the patient's nares with his/her mouth and blows firmly into the nares to inflate the lungs. The chest should be visually inspected during the procedure and the breath continued until a normal chest excursion is accomplished. An inspiratory time of approximately 1 second should be targeted.

In nonintubated patients ventilated using the mouth to snout technique, ventilation *cannot* be performed simultaneously with chest compressions because air will flow into the esophagus and stomach rather than into the lungs when the lungs are compressed during chest compressions. Therefore 30 chest compressions should be delivered, immediately followed by two breaths. Alternating compressions and ventilations should be continued for 2-minute cycles, and the rescuers rotated every cycle to prevent fatigue. In contrast, chest compressions and ventilations should be performed *simultaneously* in intubated patients because the inflated cuff of the ET tube allows alveolar ventilation during a chest compression; interruptions in chest compressions are thereby minimized. Intubated patients should be ventilated at a rate of 10 breaths per minute with an inspiratory time of approximately 1 second. If a respirometer is available, a tidal volume of approximately 10 ml/kg should be targeted. This low-minute ventilation is adequate during CPR since pulmonary blood flow is reduced in comparison with an animal with spontaneous circulation. Care should be taken not to hyperventilate the patient because low arterial CO_2 tension leads to cerebral vasoconstriction, decreasing cerebral perfusion and delivery of oxygen to the brain.

Advanced Life Support

Once BLS procedures have been implemented, the CPR team should initiate ALS, which includes monitoring, drug therapy, electrical defibrillation, and open chest CPR. Drug therapy is preferably administered by the intravenous or intraosseous route. Therefore placement of a peripheral or central intravenous catheter or an intraosseous needle is recommended but should not interfere with continuation of BLS (i.e., chest compression and ventilation).

Monitoring

Many commonly employed monitoring devices are of limited use during CPR due to their susceptibility to motion artifact and the low likelihood that sufficient perfusion is present to allow accurate readings. Low-yield monitoring devices include pulse oximeter and indirect blood pressure monitors, including Doppler and oscillometric devices. The two most useful monitoring devices during CPR are the electrocardiogram (ECG) and end-tidal CO_2 (ETCO$_2$) monitor.

Electrocardiogram
Although the ECG is highly susceptible to motion artifact and is of limited use during ongoing chest compressions, an accurate rhythm diagnosis is essential to guide drug and defibrillation therapy. The goal of ECG monitoring during CPR is to diagnose which of the three most common arrest rhythms are present (Figure 5-1): asystole; pulseless electrical activity (PEA), also known as electrical-mechanical dissociation (EMD); or ventricular fibrillation (VF). The ECG should be quickly evaluated while compressors are being rotated between 2-minute cycles of CPR, the rhythm diagnosis should be called out to the group by the team leader, and differing opinions on the diagnosis should be solicited during training. Discussion about the rhythm diagnosis should not prevent rapid resumption of chest compressions.

End-Tidal Carbon Dioxide
$ETCO_2$ data can be used in multiple ways during CPR and is highly resistant to motion artifact regardless of the technology employed (i.e., side stream or mainstream). If available, $ETCO_2$ monitoring is recommended in dogs and cats during CPR. In conjunction with direct visualization of the arytenoids during intubation, thoracic auscultation, and observation of chest excursions when providing positive pressure breaths with a resuscitator bag, the presence of measureable CO_2 by $ETCO_2$ monitoring is supportive of correct placement of the ET tube. Because $ETCO_2$ is proportional to pulmonary blood flow, it can also be used as a measure of chest compression efficacy. However, the relationship between $ETCO_2$ and pulmonary blood flow is also confounded by ventilation, with higher ventilation rates or tidal volumes leading to a decrease in $ETCO_2$. A constant quality of ventilation is therefore crucial for the use of $ETCO_2$ as a metric of quality of chest compressions. Upon ROSC, $ETCO_2$ dramatically increases due to the rapid increase in circulation and therefore is a valuable early indicator of ROSC during CPR.

Drug Therapy

Depending on the arrest rhythm, vasopressors, parasympatholytics, and/or antiarrhythmics may be indicated in dogs and cats with CPA. In addition, in some cases reversal agents, intravenous fluids, and alkalinizing drugs may be indicated. Strict adherence to evidence-based CPR algorithms is recommended to increase the quality of CPR, the likelihood of ROSC, and the chance of survival to hospital discharge.

Vasopressors
Regardless of the arrest rhythm vasopressors are recommended to increase peripheral vasoconstriction. Because a limited cardiac output of only 30% of normal is achieved during optimal external chest compressions, shunting of blood away from the periphery and toward the core (e.g., heart, lungs, brain) is essential to maintain perfusion to these vital organs. Epinephrine is a catecholamine that causes peripheral vasoconstriction via stimulation of α_1 receptors. It is a nonspecific catecholamine that also acts on β_1 and β_2 receptors, but the α_1 effects have been proved the most beneficial during CPR. Initially low doses (0.01 mg/kg IV/IO every other cycle of CPR) are recommended, but after prolonged CPR, a higher dose (0.1 mg/kg IV/IO every other cycle of CPR) may be considered. Epinephrine also may be administered via ET tube (0.02 mg/kg low dose; 0.2 mg/kg high dose) by feeding a long catheter through the ET tube and diluting the epinephrine 1:1 with sterile isotonic saline.

Vasopressin is an alternative vasopressor that exerts its vasoconstrictive effects via activation of peripheral V_1 receptors. It may be used interchangeably with epinephrine during CPR at a dose of 0.8 U/kg IV/IO every other cycle of CPR. Potential benefits of vasopressin include continued efficacy in acidic environments in which α_1 receptors may become unresponsive to epinephrine and lack of cardiac β_1 effects (positive inotropy and positive chronotropy), which may otherwise cause increased myocardial oxygen consumption and worsened myocardial ischemia upon ROSC. Vasopressin also can be administered via ET tube by feeding a long catheter through the

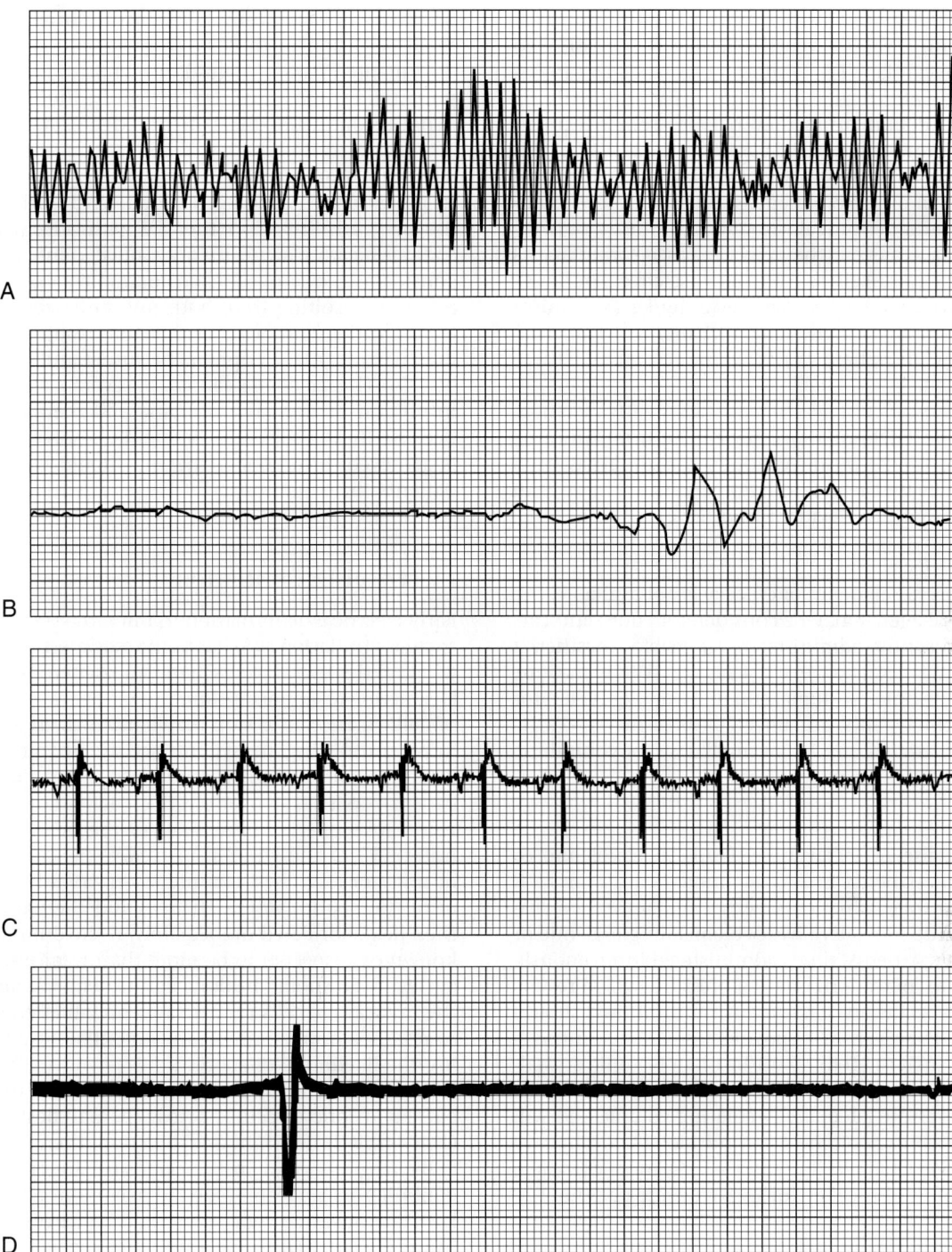

Figure 5-1 The most common arrest rhythms in dogs and cats. **A,** Ventricular fibrillation. **B,** Asystole. **C** and **D,** Pulseless electrical activity (PEA), also known as electrical-mechanical dissociation (EMD). Note that the ECG waveform in PEA is highly variable and can be indistinguishable from a perfusing rhythm; however, in all cases PEA is associated with lack of a palpable pulse. Paper speed 25 mm/sec.

ET tube and diluting the vasopressin 1:1 with sterile isotonic saline.

Anticholinergics
Atropine is an anticholinergic, parasympatholytic drug that has been extensively studied in CPR. Although only a few studies have shown a beneficial effect, there is limited evidence of a detrimental effect, and atropine at a dose of 0.04 mg/kg IV/IO may be considered during CPR in dogs and cats and is reasonable in all dogs and cats with asystole or PEA associated with increased vagal tone. Atropine also may be administered via ET tube (0.08 mg/kg) by feeding a long catheter through the ET tube and diluting the atropine 1:1 with sterile isotonic saline.

Antiarrhythmics

Although nonperfusing ventricular fibrillation or ventricular tachycardia (VF/VT) should be treated as early as possible with electrical defibrillation, patients with VF refractory to defibrillation may benefit from treatment with amiodarone at a dose of 2.5 to 5 mg/kg IV/IO. This drug has been associated with anaphylactic reactions and hypotension in dogs, so patients should be closely monitored for signs of peripheral vasodilation, wheals, or hives once ROSC is achieved (the newly released formulations for IV may be less likely to cause adverse effects in dogs). Treatment with diphenhydramine (2 mg/kg IM) and/or antiinflammatory corticosteroids (0.1 mg/kg dexamethasone sodium phosphate IV) is warranted should these signs be noted.

If amiodarone is not available, patients with VF refractory to electrical defibrillation may benefit from lidocaine 2 mg/kg slow IV/IO push. Although this drug has been shown to increase the defibrillation threshold in dogs in one study, benefit was evident in others.

Reversal Agents

Although specific evidence of efficacy is not available, the use of reversal agents may be considered in dogs and cats that were recently administered reversible anesthetic/analgesic drugs. Naloxone (0.04 mg/kg IV/IO) may be used to reverse opioids, flumazenil (0.01 mg/kg IV/IO) for benzodiazepines, and atipamezole (0.14 mg/kg IV/IO for large dogs to 0.32 mg/kg for small dogs) or yohimbine (0.1 mg/kg IV/IO) for α_2 agonists.

Intravenous Fluids

The routine use of intravenous fluids in euvolemic or hypervolemic patients is not recommended during CPR but is reasonable in patients with documented or suspected absolute or relative hypovolemia. In euvolemic or hypervolemic patients, fluids administered intravenously serve solely to increase right atrial pressure, which results in decreased perfusion of the brain and heart and should be avoided. However, in hypovolemic patients, intravenous fluids, such as 10 to 30 ml/kg of an isotonic crystalloid solution depending on the degree of hypovolemia, will help to restore adequate circulating volume and will increase the efficacy of chest compressions and improve perfusion. (See Chapters 1, 2, and 4 for a more complete discussion of fluid therapy for hypovolemic patients.)

Corticosteroids

The routine use of high-dose corticosteroids during CPR in dogs and cats is not recommended. Although one retrospective study showed an association between administration of corticosteroids and increased rate of ROSC in dogs and cats, the type and dose of steroids administered were highly variable and the study design did not allow determination of a cause-and-effect relationship (Hofmeister et al, 2009). Other studies have shown no benefit or harm from the use of steroids during CPR. Non-CPR studies have demonstrated that single high doses of corticosteroids in dogs frequently lead to gastrointestinal ulceration and bleeding, which could also cause other ill effects such as bacterial translocation. In addition, corticosteroids suppress the immune system and reduce prostaglandin production in the kidney, a primary mechanism employed by the kidney to maintain renal perfusion in the face of hypotension. Because the documented risks of high-dose steroids far outweigh the potential benefit shown in one study, the use of steroids is not recommended in patients with CPA.

Alkalinization Therapy

In patients with prolonged CPA of greater than 10 to 15 minutes, alkalinization therapy with administration of sodium bicarbonate (1 mEq/kg, once, diluted IV) may be considered. Prolonged CPA commonly leads to severe acidemia resulting from both metabolic acidosis, due to lactate and uremic acids, and venous respiratory acidosis, due to inadequate peripheral perfusion and accumulation of CO_2. This acidemia can cause severe vasodilation and inhibition of normal enzymatic and metabolic activity. Because these issues may be rapidly resolved once ROSC is achieved, bicarbonate therapy should be reserved for patients with prolonged CPA and with documented severe acidemia (pH < 7.0).

Electrical Defibrillation

Early electrical defibrillation in human patients with ventricular fibrillation (VF) has been associated with increased ROSC and survival to discharge in numerous studies and is superior to antiarrhythmic medical therapy. The goal of defibrillation is to stop the ventricular myocardial cells from contracting dyssynchronously by simultaneously driving them all into a refractory period, allowing the pacemakers to take over electrical activation and coordinated subsequent contractions of the heart. If the duration of VF is known or suspected to be of duration of 4 minutes or less, chest compressions should be continued until the defibrillator is charged and the patient should then be defibrillated immediately. If the duration of VF is known or suspected to be more than 4 minutes, one full cycle of CPR should be done before defibrillating to allow the myocardial cells to generate enough energy substrate to restore a normal membrane potential, thereby increasing the likelihood of success.

Defibrillators may be either monophasic (delivering a current in one direction across the paddles) or biphasic (delivering a current in one direction, then reversing and delivering a current in the opposite direction). Biphasic defibrillators are recommended over monophasic defibrillators because a lower current (and hence less myocardial injury) is required to successfully defibrillate the patient. For monophasic defibrillators, an initial dose of 4 to 6 J/kg should be used, whereas biphasic defibrillation should start at 2 to 4 J/kg. The second dose may be increased by 50%, but subsequent doses should not be further increased. Operators should be intimately familiar with equipment operations and safety precautions pertinent to defibrillation.

After defibrillation, chest compressions should be resumed immediately and a full 2-minute cycle of CPR administered before reassessing the ECG and determining if the patient is still in VF and should be defibrillated again. Brief assessment of the ECG immediately after defibrillation to determine if a perfusing rhythm has resulted is reasonable, but should minimally delay resumption of chest compressions.

Open Chest CPR

Direct cardiac massage during open chest CPR generates superior cardiac output compared with closed chest CPR but is more invasive, is more expensive, and requires surgical closure and more intensive care if ROSC is achieved. Indications for open chest CPR include pleural space disease, pericardial disease, flail chest, or other significant thoracic wall defects. Direct cardiac massage also should be done in patients undergoing thoracic or abdominal surgery that develop CPA under anesthesia during the surgery. In the case of abdominal surgery, an incision can be made in the diaphragm and cardiac massage performed from an abdominal approach. Finally, in very large, obese, or broad-chested dogs, closed chest CPR is unlikely to be effective, and open chest CPR should be initiated as soon as possible provided the owner has consented.

Post–Cardiac Arrest Care

Patient outcome is determined by the events that led to CPA and the duration of the cardiac arrest but also by the processes unfolding during and after reperfusion. Two thirds of human cardiac arrest victims that achieve ROSC die during the postresuscitation phase. In veterinary medicine, only 16% of dogs and cats initially successfully resuscitated were found to survive to hospital discharge in one study (Hofmeister et al, 2009).

Abnormalities that the clinician is confronted with in dogs and cats in the postresuscitation phase result from a combination of anoxic brain injury, postischemic myocardial dysfunction, the systemic response to ischemia and reperfusion, and the persistent precipitating pathology (e.g., underlying disease processes). Consequently, the clinical abnormalities in these post–cardiac arrest cases are highly variable and therapy should be aimed at alleviating the clinical signs resulting from these abnormalities.

Early hemodynamic optimization, similar to algorithms described for severe sepsis and septic shock (see Chapter 4), has proved effective in human cardiac arrest survivors and should be considered in hemodynamically unstable small animals after cardiac arrest. Central venous oxygen saturation of at least 70% or normalization of lactate levels should be used as global perfusion metrics and end points for resuscitation. Central venous pressure monitoring is also a useful guide for fluid therapy because left ventricular dysfunction may increase the risk for hydrostatic pulmonary edema, while the ischemia-reperfusion injury increases the tendency toward permeability pulmonary edema. Cerebral autoregulation of blood flow may be impaired and adequate cerebral blood flow may depend on a sufficiently high cerebral perfusion pressure, in turn demanding a mean arterial pressure of 80 mm Hg or higher.

The efficacy of mild therapeutic hypothermia (core temperature of 32° to 34°C [89.6° to 93.2°F]) for 12 to 24 hours after ROSC has been shown to improve neurological outcome after cardiac arrest in humans and other species, including dogs, that remain comatose 1 to 2 hours after resuscitation. Whether therapeutic hypothermia is a feasible strategy for veterinary patients that remain comatose after cardiac arrest remains to be shown, but rapid active rewarming is probably detrimental, and the development of hyperthermia is certainly harmful. It is therefore important to monitor the body temperature after cardiac arrest. Active rewarming should be avoided and passive rewarming should not be allowed to occur faster than 0.5°C per hour. Patients should also be carefully monitored for seizures and treated aggressively with diazepam (0.5 mg/kg IV/IO) if they occur.

Short-term mechanical ventilation to ensure optimal arterial oxygen tension (80 to 100 mm Hg) and CO_2 levels (35 to 40 mm Hg) and to prevent respiratory arrest in the comatose post–cardiac arrest patient is optimal if available but is not required for patients that are ventilating sufficiently. In all cases, adequacy of ventilation should be monitored using $ETCO_2$ or arterial blood gas analysis. Ample experimental evidence substantiates the detrimental effects of oxidative injury after ischemia-reperfusion, particularly when reperfusion occurs under hyperoxic conditions. Titration of oxygen to achieve normoxemia (e.g., targeting a SpO_2 level of 94% to 96%) is a reasonable strategy to reduce oxidative injury while maintaining adequate tissue oxygenation. Additional supportive patient care is determined by the patients' underlying disease processes and by concomitant organ dysfunctions such as ileus and renal failure.

Prognosis

There are limited data in the veterinary literature regarding prognosis for patients receiving CPR after CPA. Although overall survival rates have been reported to be quite low, the underlying cause of the arrest may contribute significantly. Patients that experience CPA as a consequence of severe, untreatable, or progressive chronic diseases are less likely to experience good outcomes. However, perianesthetic CPA carries a better prognosis for survival to discharge (as high as 47% in one recent retrospective veterinary study), and aggressive, prolonged CPR attempts in these cases are reasonable. Adherence to these evidence-based CPR guidelines may help improve the likelihood of survival in these cases.

References and Suggested Reading

Berg RA et al: Part 5: Adult basic life support: 2010 American Heart Association Guidelines for Cardiopulmonary Resuscitation and Emergency Cardiovascular Care, *Circulation* 122(18 Suppl 3):S685-S705, 2010.

Fletcher DJ et al: Part 7: Clinical guidelines: RECOVER initiative for evidence and consensus based guidelines for cardiopulmonary resuscitation in dogs and cats, *J Vet Emerg Crit Care* 22(Suppl 1):S102-S131, 2012.

Hofmeister EH et al: Prognostic indicators for dogs and cats with cardiopulmonary arrest treated by cardiopulmonary cerebral resuscitation at a university teaching hospital, *J Am Vet Med Assoc* 235(1):50-57, 2009.

Neumar RW et al: Part 8: Adult advanced cardiovascular life support: 2010 American Heart Association Guidelines for Cardiopulmonary Resuscitation and Emergency Cardiovascular Care, *Circulation* 122(18 Suppl 3):S729-S767, 2010.

Neumar RW et al: Post-cardiac arrest syndrome: epidemiology, pathophysiology, treatment, and prognostication, *Circulation* 118(23):2452-2483, 2008.

CHAPTER 6

Drug Incompatibilities and Drug-Drug Interactions in the ICU Patient

KATRINA R. VIVIANO, *Madison, Wisconsin*
ELIZABETH J. THOMOVSKY, *West Lafayette, Indiana*

Patients in a veterinary intensive care unit (ICU) suffer from a variety of diseases and are treated with many drugs. An adverse drug event (ADE) typically results from increased drug plasma concentrations and leads to toxicity or to subtherapeutic drug plasma concentrations and therapeutic failure. In addition to drug interactions associated with well-known pharmacologic effects, such as the additive effects of a β-blocker with a calcium channel blocker, pathophysiologic changes in critically ill patients impact the disposition (i.e., absorption, distribution, metabolism, and excretion) of drugs, placing the critically ill patient at increased risk for ADEs. Those treating ICU patients should be mindful of interactions between disease and drug management.

Adverse Drug Events

An ADE is broadly defined in human medicine as "any noxious, unintended, and undesired effect of a drug, which occurs at doses used in humans for prophylaxis, diagnosis, or therapy... [This excludes] therapeutic failures, intentional or accidental poisoning or drug abuse, and adverse effects due to errors in administration or compliance" (Bowman, Carlstedt, and Black, 1994). These ADEs can be dose-dependent (predictable) or dose-independent (unpredictable) and are relatively common in human ICUs, reported at approximately 29.7 per 100 ICU admissions (WHO, 2000). There are no data available about the incidence of ADEs in veterinary ICU patients.

Drug administration is a key part in the treatment and management of ICU patients. The clinician can minimize ADEs and maximize medication efficacy by considering both the pharmacologic properties of the drugs being administered and patient characteristics that can modify drug effects. Factors that contribute to ADEs can be divided into two categories: drug-related factors and patient-related factors. Drug-related factors refer to the basic physical and chemical incompatibilities that exist when certain drugs are combined. These most commonly occur when drugs are given in succession through an intravenous catheter or fluid delivery line and can be anticipated (Table 6-1). A less appreciated drug-related factor that can contribute to ADEs is the formulation.

For example, long-acting drug formulations such as methylprednisolone acetate, triamcinolone acetonide, and cefovecin can persist in the body for weeks, eliminating the option of drug withdrawal if side effects develop. In addition, long-acting glucocorticoids do not allow a controlled dose taper and long-acting antibiotics increase the risk of developing antimicrobial resistance.

More difficult to predict are those patient-related factors that predispose to ADEs. ICU patient populations at increased risk for ADEs include those that are dehydrated or have decreased total body water, receiving multiple concurrent medications (polypharmacy), or that have altered organ function (Table 6-2). In addition, the very young and elderly patient populations are at increased risk for ADEs. A number of examples can be cited and are the main focus of this chapter.

Most drugs are metabolized by the liver and excreted by the kidneys, and therefore dysfunction of these organs may limit excretory capacity of drugs. Similarly, whenever there is decreased drug delivery (e.g., with decreased perfusion, severe dehydration, or massive vasodilation), the kidneys and liver cannot effectively remove drugs from the body. Drugs also must be distributed from the blood to various organs to exert their effects. Disorders such as severe dehydration, vasodilation, and cardiac disease may alter blood flow, affecting drug distribution. The distribution of lipophilic drugs to tissues also is altered in older patients owing to a greater proportion of body fat when compared with younger animals. Finally, protein binding affects drug distribution such that liver failure, systemic inflammation, or protein loss can alter drug distribution throughout the body.

Liver Disease

Alterations in drug clearance, drug extraction, and drug biotransformation and metabolism are major concerns in cases of liver disease. Clearance depends largely on hepatic blood flow and protein binding. Key drug (phase I and phase II) metabolizing enzymes housed in the liver are essential to convert lipophilic drugs to more soluble metabolites needed for excretion in the urine or the bile. To reduce the risk of toxicity, drugs metabolized

TABLE 6-1

Physical and Chemical Drug Incompatibilities of IV-Administered Drugs

Drug	Interaction	Recommendation
Aminoglycosides	Inactivated by penicillins (high concentrations)	Do not infuse drugs at the same time in same syringe or IV line. Flush IV lines between administration of penicillins and aminoglycosides
Amphotericin B	Drug precipitation if diluted with most solutions	Only dilute with 5% dextrose or sterile water
Antacids Dairy products	Decreased oral absorption of fluoroquinolones, tetracyclines, and digoxin due to drug chelation with divalent and trivalent cations (Ca^{2+}, Mg^{2+}, Al^{3+})	Avoid antacids or dairy products in patients treated with oral fluoroquinolones, tetracyclines, or digoxin or give drugs intravenously
Blood or pRBC	Many solutions result in RBC damage	Only dilute with 0.9% saline
Calcium gluconate	Many drugs: cephalothin, amphotericin B, fluoroquinolones, dobutamine, metoclopramide, methylprednisolone, calcium channel blockers (diltiazem, amlodipine, verapamil), and citrated blood or plasma	Do not use calcium gluconate in same IV line or syringe with these drugs
Heparin	Many drugs: aminoglycosides (gentamicin, amikacin), β-lactam antibiotics, benzodiazepines, and morphine	Flush IV line with saline before and after the administration of heparin. The use of nonheparinized saline to flush IV lines is preferred to heparinized saline.
Lactated Ringer's solution (LRS)	Citrated blood products (microthrombi formation associated with citrate's chelation of calcium) Fluoroquinolones (drug precipitation)	Use alternative fluid therapy that does not contain calcium (e.g., 0.9% saline, Plasma-Lyte, Normosol) Do not infuse fluoroquinolones into IV line filled with LRS
Pentobarbital	Penicillin: inactivation and drug precipitation	Do not mix in same syringe or IV line
Regular insulin	Adsorbs to surface of polymeric IV lines	Saturate the internal surface of polymeric IV lines by initially running the insulin solution through line before beginning patient infusion
Sodium bicarbonate	Many drugs: LRS, vitamin C, dobutamine HCl, dopamine HCl, epinephrine HCl, metoclopramide, vitamin C	Flush IV line with saline before administration of sodium bicarbonate. Do not administer in IV line if patient receiving LRS
Sucralfate	Decreased oral absorption of fluoroquinolones, tetracyclines, and digoxin due to chelation with aluminum	Administer oral fluoroquinolones, tetracyclines, and digoxin 2 hours before sucralfate administration or use IV administration.
Vitamin B complex	Penicillin: inactivation and drug precipitation	Do not mix in same syringe or IV line
Vitamin B₁ (thiamine HCl)	Unstable in alkaline solutions	Do not mix with alkalinizing solutions, carbonates, or citrates

pRBC, Packed red blood cells.

exclusively by the liver should have dosages reduced when hepatic failure is evident. For example, dose reductions should be considered for metronidazole, chloramphenicol (dog), phenobarbital, and benzodiazepines in the setting of liver failure, accepting that there are no specific algorithms available in veterinary patients to estimate the degree of dose reduction. For most other drugs, unless fulminant liver failure is present it is difficult to accurately predict the need for dosage adjustments associated with liver disease. Drugs whose liver metabolism is limited by hepatic blood flow (i.e., lidocaine, propranolol, midazolam, and opioids) may have increased plasma drug concentration in patients with altered hepatic blood flow associated with impaired cardiovascular function or hypotension. Additionally, the use of these drugs in patients with chronic liver disease or with portosystemic

shunting may increase the risk of side effects or systemic toxicity.

The major phase I metabolic machinery of the liver is the cytochrome P450 (CYP 450) enzyme system. Drugs can either inhibit or induce CYP 450 enzymes and result in clinically significant drug-drug interactions if coadministered. Additionally, cholestasis can sometimes decrease the activity of CYP 450 enzymes in the liver. Table 6-3 summarizes some of these potentially significant drug interactions based on CYP 450 enzyme inhibition or induction.

Other drug interactions closely associated with CYP 450 metabolism involve drugs that are inhibitors or substrates of P-glycoprotein, or both. P-glycoprotein is the most well-characterized drug transporter in veterinary medicine. Inhibitors of P-glycoprotein include

TABLE 6-2

Drug Interactions and Suggested Therapeutic Adjustments in Commonly Used Drugs in Critically Ill Patients

Drug	Comorbidity	Rationale	Therapeutic Adjustments
Aminoglycosides	Kidney failure	Elimination by glomerular filtration Nephrotoxicity—drug accumulates in the epithelial cells of the proximal renal tubule	Interval adjustment*
	Sepsis, systemic inflammation	Water-soluble antibiotic Distributes to areas of edema, lowering plasma drug concentrations	Dose based on accurate current body weight
Atenolol	Kidney failure	~50% excreted unchanged in the urine	Use with caution in patients with kidney dysfunction; consider conservative dosing or dose reduction†
Benzodiazepines	Liver failure	Metabolized in liver → increased plasma drug concentrations	Dose reduction
Cephalosporins (e.g., cephalothin, cefazolin)	Kidney failure	Excreted unchanged by the kidneys → serum half-life prolonged in patients with impaired kidney function	Dose reduction‡
Chloramphenicol	Liver failure	Dogs: Eliminated primarily by hepatic metabolism (glucuronidation)	Dose reduction‡
	Kidney failure	Cats: Excrete > 25% unchanged in the urine	Dose reduction‡
Digoxin	Cardiac failure	Significant distribution to skeletal muscle	Dose based on lean body weight and use TDM
	Hypokalemia	Increases the risk of digoxin toxicity (less K⁺ available to competitively bind to Na⁺/K⁺ ATPase of myocytes)	Correct hypokalemia
Dopamine	Metoclopramide	Metoclopramide acts as a dopamine antagonist → potential to decrease the efficacy of dopamine	Clinical significance unknown
Enalapril	Kidney failure	Half-life increased in patients with impaired kidney function	Dose reduction†
Fluoroquinolones	Kidney failure Sepsis, systemic inflammation	~20%-50% excreted unchanged in the urine Lipid-soluble antibiotic	Interval adjustment* Dose on lean body weight
Furosemide	Kidney failure KBr	Serum half-life prolonged Inhibits renal tubular reabsorption of bromide, increasing excretion	Dose reduction† Increase KBr dosage to achieve therapeutic conc.—recommend TDM
H₂ blockers	Kidney failure	~33% excreted unchanged in the urine	Dose reduction†
Lidocaine	Reduced hepatic blood flow	Rapidly metabolized by the liver to active metabolites, reduced hepatic blood flow, decreased clearance	Dose reduction
	Cardiac disease Hypokalemia	Elimination half-life prolonged Reduces drug efficacy	Dose reduction Correct hypokalemia
Metoclopramide	Kidney failure	~25% excreted unchanged in the urine	Dose reduction‡
Metronidazole	Liver failure	Lipophilic antibiotic requires significant liver metabolism	Dose reduction: suggested dose = 7.5 mg/kg twice daily
Midazolam	Reduced hepatic blood flow	Liver metabolism is blood flow limited	Dose reduction
	Hypoalbuminemia	High protein binding (~97%)	Caution when used concurrently with other highly protein-bound drugs (e.g., sulfonamides, NSAIDs) Risk of increased plasma concentrations and prolonged duration of action
Mirtazapine	Kidney disease	Delayed clearance	Interval reduction§
	Tramadol, MAOIs (e.g., selegiline, amitraz)	Increase CNS concentrations of serotonin and noradrenergic neurotransmission	Increase risk of serotonin syndrome‖

TABLE 6-2

Drug Interactions and Suggested Therapeutic Adjustments in Commonly Used Drugs in Critically Ill Patients—cont'd

Drug	Comorbidity	Rationale	Therapeutic Adjustments
NSAIDs	Kidney disease	COX inhibition: loss of prostaglandin-mediated autoregulation of renal hemodynamics	DO NOT USE (high potential for renal toxicity)
	Hypoalbuminemia	High protein binding (~ 99%)	Caution when used concurrently with other highly protein-bound drugs (e.g., sulfonamides, benzodiazepines) Risk of increased plasma concentrations and prolonged duration of action
	Glucocorticoids	Phosphodiesterase A$_2$ inhibition: significant risk of GI ulceration and perforation	The concurrent use of glucocorticoids and NSAIDs is CONTRAINDICATED
Omeprazole	Clopidogrel	CYP 2C19 inhibition → reduced bioactivation of clopidogrel	Reduced efficacy of clopidogrel Use pantoprazole
Opioids	Reduced hepatic blood flow	Elimination by hepatic metabolism	Dose reduction
Penicillins	Kidney failure	Eliminated primarily through the kidneys (tubular secretion)	Dose reduction[‡]
Phenobarbital	Liver failure	Primary liver metabolism	Dose reduction–TDM recommended
Propranolol	Reduced hepatic blood flow	Metabolism primarily by the liver	Dose reduction
Sulfonamides	Kidney failure	Primarily renal excretion	Dose reduction[‡]
Tetracyclines (other than doxycycline)	Kidney failure	Eliminated unchanged by glomerular filtration Prolonged elimination half-life and drug accumulation in patients with impaired kidney function	Dose reduction[‡]

COX, Cyclooxygenase; CYP, cytochrome P450; GI, gastrointestinal; KBr, potassium bromide; MAOIs, monoamine oxidase inhibitors; NSAIDs, nonsteroidal antiinflammatory drugs; TDM, therapeutic drug monitoring.
*Consider interval adjustment for concentration-dependent antibiotics:
New interval = Standard interval × [1 ÷ (Normal serum creatinine / Patient's serum creatinine)]
[†]New dose = Standard dose × (Normal serum creatinine / Patient's serum creatinine).
[‡]Consider dose adjustment for time-dependent antibiotics: New dose = Standard dose × (Normal serum creatinine / Patient's serum creatinine).
[§]Mirtazapine 1.88 mg/cat every 48 hours is recommended dose in cats with chronic kidney disease (Quimby et al, 2011).
[‖]Clinical signs consistent with serotonin syndrome include agitation, tachycardia, hyperthermia, mydriasis, muscle twitching, vomiting, or diarrhea.

TABLE 6-3

Potential Drug-Drug Interactions Based on CYP 450 Substrate Drug Inhibition or Induction

Drug	CYP 450 Induction/Inhibition	CYP 450 Substrates	Drug Interaction
Cimetidine	CYP 2E1, 2C9 inhibition	Theophylline	Prolonged elimination half-life and decreased clearance
Chloramphenicol	CYP 2B11 inhibition	Phenobarbital Propofol	Prolonged elimination half-life
Fluoroquinolones Enrofloxacin Marbofloxacin	CYP 1A2 inhibition	Theophylline	Increased plasma concentrations (inhibition of clearance)
Ketoconazole	CYP 3A12 inhibition	Cyclosporine Midazolam	Increased plasma concentrations Prolonged elimination half-life
Phenobarbital	CYP 3A12 induction CYP not identified	Digoxin Propranolol	Decreased elimination half-life Decreased bioavailability and elimination half-life

ketoconazole, diltiazem, lidocaine, and cyclosporine (also a P-glycoprotein substrate). The coadministration of a P-glycoprotein substrate with an inhibitor may result in a clinically significant drug interaction. For example, ketoconazole increases the oral absorption of cyclosporine via its inhibition of P-glycoprotein, although CYP 3A inhibition also contributes to this drug interaction.

In addition to drug clearance and enzyme inhibition, another concern with hepatic failure is hypoalbuminemia. Albumin is the most common site in plasma for drug binding. Patients with hypoalbuminemia have an increase in the fraction of unbound drug, often leading to a higher concentration of pharmacologically active free drug. The clinical impact of hypoalbuminemia may be most relevant for highly protein-bound drugs (i.e., drugs with > 90% protein binding) that have a narrow therapeutic range. In these cases, low albumin levels lead to more pharmacologically active free drug at standard dosing, increasing the risk of toxicity. Examples of common drugs with high protein binding include nonsteroidal antiinflammatory drugs (NSAIDs) and benzodiazepines (see Table 6-2).

Kidney Disease

The kidneys are involved in clearance of many water-soluble (hydrophilic) drugs. Drug clearance is compromised either due to decreased drug delivery to the kidneys (as with massive vasodilation, decreased perfusion, or severe dehydration) or if intrinsic renal disease is present.

In human patients the standard recommendation is that dosage adjustments for drugs primarily eliminated by the kidney should occur when 67% of renal function (i.e., when urine concentrating ability) is lost. Creatinine clearance is the best guide for drug dosage adjustments because functional tubular secretion and creatinine clearance decrease at parallel rates. For drugs excreted in the urine, the elimination half-life remains stable until the creatinine clearance is reduced by 30% to 40%.

Unfortunately, creatinine clearance is not readily available in dogs and cats; therefore the patient's serum creatinine may be used to estimate creatinine clearance and thus aid in proportionally adjusting the dosages of those drugs primarily excreted by the kidneys. However, this approach has limitations because the relationship between serum creatinine and creatinine clearance is linear only up to a serum creatinine of about 4 mg/dl. Therefore clinically monitoring the patient's response following dosage adjustment remains important. Table 6-2 outlines drugs in which dosage adjustments are recommended for patients with kidney disease. Due to the potential for direct renal toxicity, nephrotoxic drugs (e.g., NSAIDs) should be completely avoided in patients with kidney disease.

Serum creatinine can be used to reduce the dose or to adjust the dosing interval. Drugs commonly adjusted by dose are those with relatively high safety margins that require a minimum drug concentration during the dosing interval. Examples include time-dependent antibiotics such as penicillins and cephalosporins, anticonvulsants, and cardiac drugs. The new drug dose is calculated using the following equation:

$$\text{New dose} = \text{Standard dose} \times \frac{\text{Normal serum creatinine}}{\text{Patient's serum creatinine}}$$

Interval adjustment is most appropriate for drugs that remain effective at low concentrations or have a long elimination half-life. These include the concentration-dependent antibiotics with postantibiotic effects such as aminoglycosides and fluoroquinolones, as well as glucocorticoids. The new dosing interval is calculated using the following equation:

$$\text{New interval} = \text{Standard interval} \times \left(1 \div \frac{\text{Normal serum creatinine}}{\text{Patient's serum creatinine}}\right)$$

Uremic patients are also at increased risk for drug toxicities due to altered tissue receptors, changes in protein binding, or electrolyte abnormalities. For example, acidic drugs such as NSAIDs, penicillins, furosemide, and anticonvulsants have decreased protein binding, increased concentration of free active drug, and increased clearance in uremic patients. Basic drugs such as diazepam, propranolol, and prazosin have increased protein binding, decreased concentrations of free drug, and decreased clearance in uremic patients. The clinical significance of altered protein binding of acidic and basic drugs is difficult to predict based on the compensatory changes in drug clearance in association with the increase or decrease in free drug available for metabolism and elimination. Dosage adjustments should be made on an individual basis.

Cardiovascular Disease

The most common form of cardiac disease seen in the ICU setting is cardiac failure, primarily due to left-sided congestive heart failure (CHF). In CHF there is an increase in total body water as well as a decrease in the effective perfusion of tissues. Together these alter the distribution of drugs to common sites such as skeletal muscle or reduce the delivery to sites of drug clearance such as the liver and kidney. For example, clearance of drugs dependent on hepatic blood flow (lidocaine, propranolol, calcium channel blockers, and opioids) may be reduced, resulting in accumulation or toxicity. Similarly impaired renal perfusion can lead to toxicosis of drugs requiring renal elimination such as digoxin and potentially atenolol. Dosage adjustments should therefore be considered in CHF patients for drugs that have significant distribution to skeletal muscle as well as for those cleared by the liver or kidney. For example, digoxin has significant distribution to skeletal muscle and therefore should be dosed on lean body weight (see Table 6-2).

Diuretics such as furosemide alter the amount of total body water, which further impacts drug distribution while potentially increasing the clearance of some drugs by the kidneys, provided renal perfusion is not markedly diminished from volume contraction. Furosemide also significantly alters serum potassium and magnesium concentrations, and these electrolyte disturbances can alter the action of some drugs. For example, hypokalemia increases the risk of digoxin toxicity and decreases the efficacy of lidocaine (see Table 6-2).

Other cardiovascular conditions seen in the ICU are of concern. The patient with either a tachyarrhythmia or bradyarrhythmia may experience reductions of cardiac output and blood delivery of drugs to the kidney and liver. Systemic hypertension can impair cardiac output and more importantly cause end-organ damage to the kidneys.

Gastrointestinal Disease

Patients are often treated for gastrointestinal (GI) disease in the ICU. Typically, the GI tract manifests disease as inflammation, bleeding, or alterations in motility. GI disease can be the primary condition or secondary to another disease (e.g., GI bleeding associated with sloughing of the gut lining due to hypoperfusion). Changes in motility can be transient (e.g., as with anesthetic-related events), secondary to the effects of other medications, or a result of the patient's primary disease.

GI drug absorption is a function of GI pH, motility, epithelial permeability, surface area, and blood flow. In the critically ill patient, changes in GI motility and blood flow can influence the rate and extent of absorption of orally administered drugs. This can cause prolonged time for oral drug absorption and delay the drug's onset of action. In addition, opioid administration negatively impacts GI motility. In the critically ill patient intravenous drugs are often indicated to remove any questions about compromised oral absorption or peripheral hypoperfusion. Once the patient is stabilized hemodynamically and has resumed eating, oral, subcutaneous, or intramuscular drug administration can be reintroduced. Table 6-2 lists some of the common therapies used in patients with GI disease and associated with clinically significant drug-drug interactions. Additional clinically significant drug interactions associated with GI therapies involve drugs that modify gastric pH (especially cimetidine), sucralfate, and NSAIDs.

Drugs that raise gastric pH such as the H₂ blockers and proton pump inhibitors may impact the oral absorption of some drugs, as well as exert other effects on drug metabolism. Cimetidine is a particularly notable H₂ blocker with CYP 450 inhibition, which alters the disposition of substrate drugs such as theophylline, cyclosporine, and verapamil, leading to drug-drug interactions (see Table 6-3). Among other H₂ blockers, famotidine and ranitidine do not inhibit CYP 450 and therefore are preferred in small animal patients when H₂ blockers are used to treat gastric ulceration. However, these drugs—as well as the proton pump inhibitors related to omeprazole (Prilosec)—increase gastric pH, enhancing absorption of drugs that are weak bases and impairing absorption of drugs that are weak acids. For example, some of the drugs used in critically ill patients that are weak acids include aspirin, diazepam, furosemide, ketoconazole, and itraconazole (Reynolds, 1990). To optimize oral absorption of these drugs, H₂ blockers or proton pump inhibitors should be discontinued. Alternatively in cases of GI disease, the clinician can choose drugs whose oral absorption is not altered by gastric pH (e.g., fluconazole).

Other drugs used to manage GI ulceration include aluminum-containing antacids and sucralfate. These drugs prevent the oral absorption of drugs that can chelate with aluminum including fluoroquinolones, tetracyclines, and digoxin. If sucralfate is indicated in a patient concurrently treated with oral fluoroquinolones, tetracyclines, or digoxin, the recommendation is to administer the other drugs 2 hours prior to the administration of sucralfate to optimize drug absorption.

NSAIDs inhibit cyclooxygenase (COX-1 and/or COX-2) and glucocorticoids inhibit phospholipase A₂. The net effect of each drug class is to decrease prostaglandin production and lead to clinically significant GI ulceration and bleeding. The concurrent administration of NSAIDs and glucocorticoids is contraindicated due to the high risk of GI ulceration and perforation.

Sepsis/Infection/Systemic Inflammation

Septic patients suffer from complex and multifactorial disease processes (see Chapter 4). However, in cases of significant inflammation (whether idiopathic or resulting from generalized or localized infection) most patients develop some degree of vasodilation and injury to vascular endothelium. In both situations, blood flow to the liver and kidneys is decreased and this can impair drug elimination. Other organs are often ineffectively perfused, which can lead to reduced efficacy in organs targeted by specific drugs. Significant inflammation leads to reduced albumin production by the liver, often causing dramatic reductions in albumin levels (see Table 6-2).

Drug dosage adjustments are recommended in septic patients with third-spacing or peripheral edema. Lipid-soluble drugs such as fluoroquinolones should be dosed based on lean body weight. Water-soluble drugs like aminoglycosides will distribute to areas of edema and decrease drug plasma concentrations; they are best dosed using an accurate current body weight. In addition, drugs with a narrow therapeutic window that carry a high risk of toxicity should be dosed on lean body weight. However, although dehydration or volume contraction can increase the plasma concentration of drugs, drug dosage adjustments are NOT recommended in critical patients that are volume contracted; instead therapy should focus on fluid resuscitation prior to administration of drugs.

Neurologic Disease

Many ICU patients are hospitalized for treatment of neurologic disease. The most common diseases include seizures, inflammatory brain disease, brain tumors, head trauma, and disorders increasing intracranial pressure (ICP). In the majority of situations, aside from traumatically induced increased ICP, these patients are systemically normal. Therefore the concerns of treatment largely relate to the effects of the medications themselves or their interactions with other drugs. For example, phenobarbital accelerates the elimination half-life of drugs like digoxin, propranolol, and phenobarbital through CYP 450 induction. Furosemide increases bromide excretion, effectively decreasing potassium bromide plasma levels.

References and Suggested Reading

Bowman L, Carlstedt BC, Black CD: Incidence of adverse drug reactions in adult medical inpatients, *Can J Hosp Pharm* 47:209-216, 1994.

Close SL: Clopidogrel pharmacogenetics: metabolism and drug interactions, *Drug Metabol Drug Interact* 26:45-51, 2011.

Ogilvie BW et al: The proton pump inhibitor, omeprazole, but not lansoprazole or pantoprazole, is a metabolism-dependent inhibitor of CYP2C19: implications for coadministration with clopidogrel, *Drug Metab Dispos* 39(11):2020-2033, 2011.

Quimby JM et al: Studies on the pharmacokinetics and pharmacodynamics of mirtazapine in healthy young cats, *J Vet Pharmacol Ther* 34:388-396, 2011.

Quimby JM et al: The pharmacokinetics of mirtazapine in cats with chronic kidney disease and in age-matched control cats, *J Vet Intern Med* 25:985-989, 2011.

Reynolds JC: The clinical importance of drug interactions with antiulcer therapy, *J Clin Gastroenterol* 12:S54-S63, 1990.

WHO Collaborating Centre for International Drug Monitoring: Safety monitoring of medicinal products: guidelines for setting up and running a pharmacovigilance centre, London, UK, 2000, Uppsala Monitoring Centre, *EQUUS*.

CHAPTER 7

Nutrition in Critical Care

DANIEL L. CHAN, *Hertfordshire, United Kingdom*

Critical illness in animals induces unique metabolic changes that put them at high risk for malnutrition and its deleterious effects. The rationale for providing nutritional support in critical illness is based on a number of pathophysiologic factors. In diseased states the inflammatory response triggers alterations in cytokine and hormone concentrations and shifts metabolism toward a catabolic state. In the absence of adequate food intake, the predominant energy source for the host is derived from accelerated proteolysis. Thus the animal may preserve fat deposits in the face of loss of lean muscle tissue. Consequences of malnutrition include negative effects on wound healing, immune function, strength (both skeletal and respiratory), and ultimately the overall prognosis. An important point with regard to nutritional support of hospitalized patients is that the immediate goal is not to achieve "weight gain," per se, which mostly likely reflects shift in water balance, but rather to minimize further loss of lean body mass. Reversal of malnutrition hinges on resolution of the primary underlying disease. Provision of nutritional support is aimed at restoring nutrient deficiencies and providing key substrates for healing and repair.

Patient Selection

As with any intervention in critically ill animals, nutritional support carries some risk of complications. This risk likely increases with the severity of the disease, and the clinician must therefore consider many factors in deciding when to institute nutritional support. Of utmost importance is the patient's cardiovascular status, which must be stable before initiation of any nutritional support.

Processes such as gastrointestinal motility, digestion, and nutrient assimilation are altered when perfusion is reduced. Feeding under such circumstances is likely to result in complications. Other issues that should be addressed before nutritional support begins include patient hydration, electrolyte imbalances, and abnormalities in acid-base status.

In animals that have been stabilized, careful consideration must be given to the appropriate time to initiate nutritional support. A previously held notion that nutritional support is unnecessary until 10 days of inadequate nutrition have elapsed is outdated. Commencing nutritional support within 3 days of hospitalization (sometimes as early as within the first 12 hours), even before determining the diagnosis of the underlying disease, is a more appropriate goal in most cases; however, other factors should also be considered as discussed in the next section.

Nutritional Assessment

Indicators of malnutrition in animals that have been proposed include unintentional weight loss (typically greater than 10% of body weight), poor hair coat quality, muscle wasting, signs of inadequate wound healing, and hypoalbuminemia. However, these abnormalities are not specific to malnutrition and often occur as late complications of a variety of systemic diseases. A greater emphasis is placed on evaluating overall body condition rather than simply noting body weight. Body condition scores (BCSs) have been shown to be reproducible, reliable, and clinically useful in nutritional assessment. Fluid shifts may significantly impact body weight, but BCSs are not affected by fluid shifts and therefore are helpful in assessing critically ill animals. More recently, lean muscle loss has also been evaluated in cats and this may become a component of nutritional assessment in small animals (Michel et al, 2011).

In light of the limitations to assessing nutritional status, it is crucial to identify early risk factors that may predispose patients to malnutrition such as anorexia of greater than 5-days' duration, serious underlying disease (e.g., severe trauma, sepsis, peritonitis, acute pancreatitis), and large protein losses (e.g., protracted diarrhea, draining wounds, burns). Nutritional assessment also identifies factors that can impact the nutritional plan such as specific electrolyte abnormalities; hyperglycemia, hypertriglyceridemia, or hyperammonemia; or comorbid illnesses such as renal, cardiac, or hepatic disease, including various forms of neoplasia. In the presence of such abnormalities the nutritional plan should be adjusted accordingly to limit acute exacerbations of any preexisting condition.

Finally, since many of the techniques required for implementation of nutritional support (e.g., placement of most feeding tubes, intravenous catheters for parenteral nutrition) necessitate sedation or anesthesia, the patient must be properly evaluated and stabilized first. When the patient is deemed too unstable for general anesthesia, temporary measures of nutritional support that do not require anesthesia (e.g., nasoesophageal tube placement, placement of peripheral catheters for parenteral nutrition) should be considered.

Nutritional Plan

Nutrition should be provided as soon as it is feasible, with careful consideration of the most appropriate route of nutritional support. Providing nutrition via a functional digestive system is the preferred route of feeding, and particular care should be taken to evaluate if the patient can tolerate enteral feedings. Even if the patient can only tolerate small amounts of enteral nutrition, this route of feeding should be pursued and supplemented or augmented with parenteral nutrition (PN) as necessary to meet the patient's nutritional needs. However, if an animal demonstrates complete enteral feeding intolerance, some form of PN should be provided. Implementation of the devised nutritional plan also should be gradual, with the goal of reaching target level of nutrient delivery within 48 to 72 hours. Adjustments to the nutritional plan are made on the basis of frequent reassessment and the development of any complications.

Calculating Nutritional Requirements

Based on indirect calorimetry studies in dogs, there has been a recent trend toward formulating nutritional support simply to meet resting energy requirements (RERs) rather than more generous illness energy requirements (IERs). For many years clinicians used to multiply the RER by an illness factor between 1.1 and 2 to account for purported increases in metabolism associated with different disease states. However, now less emphasis is being placed on these extrapolated factors, and the current recommendation is to use more conservative

energy estimates (i.e., start with the animal's RER) to avoid overfeeding and its associated complications. Examples of complications resulting from overfeeding include gastrointestinal intolerance, hepatic dysfunction, and increased carbon dioxide production. Although several formulas are proposed to calculate the RER, a widely used allometric formula can be applied to both dogs and cats of all weights. The formula most commonly used by the author is:

$$RER = 70 \times (\text{current body weight in kilograms})^{0.75}$$

Alternatively, for animals weighing between 3 and 25 kg, the following may be used:

$$RER = (30 \times \text{current body weight in kilograms}) + 70$$

Hospitalized dogs should be supported with 4 to 6 g of protein per 100 kcal (15% to 25% of total energy requirements), whereas cats are usually supported with 6 g or more of protein per 100 kcal (25% to 35% of total energy requirements). In most cases estimation of protein requirements is based on clinical judgment and recognition that in certain disease states (e.g., peritonitis, draining wounds) protein requirements are markedly increased.

Parenteral Nutritional Support

PN, formerly referred to as total PN (TPN) or partial PN (PPN), is the intravenous delivery of nutrients (e.g., dextrose, amino acids, lipid emulsion, vitamins, minerals, electrolytes) to patients. This can be achieved via a central vein (central PN [CPN]) or a peripheral vein (peripheral PN [PPN]). Factors that influence how PN should be administered include feasibility of central venous access and the osmolarity of the PN solution, with the recommendation to use the central route when the osmolarity of solution exceeds 850 mOsm/L.

Crystalline amino acid solutions are an essential component of PN. The importance of supplying amino acids relates to the maintenance of positive nitrogen balance and repletion of lean body tissue, which may be vital in the recovery of critically ill patients. Supplementation of amino acids may support protein synthesis and spare tissue proteins from being catabolized via gluconeogenesis. The most commonly used amino acid solutions (e.g., Travasol, Aminosyn II) contain most of the essential amino acids for dogs and cats, with the exception of taurine. However, because PN is typically not used beyond 10 days, the lack of taurine does not become a problem in most circumstances. Amino acid solutions are available in different concentrations from 4% to 15%, but the most commonly used concentration is 8.5%. Amino acid solutions are also available with and without electrolytes.

Lipid emulsions are the calorically dense component of PN and a source of essential fatty acids. Lipid emulsions are isotonic and available in 10% to 30% solutions (e.g., Intralipid, Liposyn III). These commercially available lipid emulsions are made primarily of soybean and safflower oil and provide predominantly long-chain polyunsaturated fatty acids, including linoleic, oleic, palmitic, and stearic acids. The emulsified fat particles are comparable in size to chylomicrons and are removed from the circulation via the action of peripheral lipoprotein lipase. Side effects attributed to lipid emulsions include liver dysfunction and immune suppression. Newer lipid emulsions with fewer side effects have been developed, and one such product composed of soybean oil, medium chain triglycerides, olive oil, and fish oil (i.e., SMOF lipid) is available in Europe and may become more widely distributed in the future (Goulet et al, 2010). There is a persistent misconception regarding the use of lipids in cases of pancreatitis. Although hypertriglyceridemia may be a risk factor for pancreatitis, infusions of lipids have not been shown to increase pancreatic secretion or worsen pancreatitis and therefore are considered safe. However, the one exception is in cases in which serum triglyceride concentrations are severely increased, indicating a clear failure of triglyceride clearance. Although specific data regarding the maximal safe level of lipid administration in veterinary patients are not available, it would seem prudent to maintain normal serum triglyceride concentrations in patients receiving PN. Another concern surrounding the use of lipids in PN is their purported immunosuppressive effects via impairment of the reticuloendothelial system, particularly in PN solutions containing a high percentage of lipids. Despite *in vitro* evidence supporting the notion that lipid infusions can also suppress neutrophil and lymphocyte function, studies have not yet correlated lipid use and increased rates of infectious complications.

Electrolytes, vitamins, and trace elements also may be added to the PN formulation. Depending on the hospital and the individual patient, electrolytes can be added to the admixture, included as part of the amino acid solution, or left out altogether and managed separately. Because B vitamins are water soluble, they are more likely to become deficient in patients with high-volume diuresis (e.g., renal failure, diabetes mellitus), and supplementation could be considered. Since most animals receive PN for only a short duration, fat-soluble vitamins usually are not limiting; therefore supplementation is not typically required. The exception is in obviously malnourished animals in which supplementation may be necessary. Trace elements serve as cofactors in a variety of enzyme systems and can become deficient in malnourished patients as well. In people receiving PN, zinc, copper, manganese, and chromium are routinely added to the PN admixture. These are sometimes added to PN admixtures for malnourished animals, but their compatibility with the solution must be verified.

The addition of other parenteral medications to the PN admixture is possible; however, their compatibility also must be verified. Drugs that are known to be compatible and sometimes added to PN include heparin, insulin, potassium chloride, and metoclopramide. Although the addition of insulin to PN is often necessary in people, the hyperglycemia seen in veterinary patients with PN usually does not require insulin administration, except for patients with known diabetes mellitus.

Parenteral Nutrition Compounding

Based on the nutritional assessment and plan, PN can be formulated according to the worksheets found in Boxes 7-1 and 7-2. For CPN (see Box 7-1) the first step is the calculation of the patient's RER. Protein requirements (grams of protein required per day) are then calculated, taking into consideration factors such as excessive protein losses or severe hepatic or renal disease. The energy provided from amino acids is accounted for in the energy calculations and subtracted from the daily RER to estimate the total nonprotein calories required. Some protocols do not account for the energy provided by amino acids in the calculations, which may lead to overfeeding in critically ill animals. The nonprotein calories are usually provided as a 50:50 mixture of lipids and dextrose; however, this ratio can be adjusted in cases of persistent hyperglycemia or hypertriglyceridemia (e.g., a higher proportion of calories would be given from lipids in an animal with hyperglycemia). The calories provided from each component (amino acids, lipids, and dextrose) are then divided by their respective caloric density, and the exact amounts of each component are added to the PN bags in an aseptic fashion. The amount of CPN delivered often provides less than the patient's daily fluid requirement. Additional fluids can either be added to the PN bag at the time of compounding or be provided as a separate infusion.

For formulation of PPN, Box 7-2 provides a step-by-step protocol in which patients of various sizes can receive 70% of their RER and approximately meet their daily maintenance fluid requirement. In very small animals (≤3 kg), the amount of PPN will exceed the maintenance fluid requirement and increase the risk for fluid overload; thus adjustments may need to be made. Also, in animals requiring conservative fluid administration (e.g., congestive heart failure), these calculations for PPN may provide more fluid than would be safe. This formulation has been designed so that the proportion of each PN component depends on the weight of the patient, such that a smaller animal (between 3 and 5 kg) receives proportionally more calories from lipids compared with a large dog (>30 kg) that receives more calories in the form of carbohydrates. This allows the resulting formulation to approximate the patient's daily fluid requirement.

Ideally, compounding of PN should be done aseptically under a laminar flow hood using a semiautomated, closed-system PN compounder (e.g., Automix compounder). If the appropriate facilities and equipment are not available, it may be preferable to have a local human hospital, compounding pharmacy, or human home health care company compound PN solutions using the formulations listed in Boxes 7-1 and 7-2. Alternatively, commercial ready-to-use preparations of glucose or glycerol and amino acids suitable for (peripheral or central) intravenous administration are available (e.g., ProcalAmine). Although ready-to-use preparations are convenient, they provide only 30% to 50% of caloric requirements when administered at maintenance fluid rates and as a result should only be used for interim nutritional support or to supplement low-dose enteral feedings.

Parenteral Nutrition Administration

The high osmolarity of CPN solutions (often > 1200 mOsm/L) requires its administration through a

BOX **7-1**

Worksheet for Calculating a Central Parenteral Nutrition Formulation

1. Resting energy requirement (RER)

$$70 \times (\text{current body weight in kg})^{0.75} = \text{kcal/day}$$

or for animals 3-25 kg, can also use:

$$30 \times (\text{current body weight in kg}) + 70 = \text{kcal/day} \quad \text{RER} = \rule{2cm}{0.4pt} \text{kcal/day}$$

2. Protein requirements	Canine	Feline
Standard	5 g/100 kcal	6-7 g/100 kcal
Decreased requirements (hepatic/renal failure)	3 g/100 kcal	3-4 g/100 kcal
Increased requirements (protein-losing conditions)	6-7 g/100 kcal	6-7 g/100 kcal

$(\text{RER} \div 100) \times \rule{2cm}{0.4pt}$ g/100 kcal = $\rule{2cm}{0.4pt}$ g of protein required per day (protein req)

3. Volumes of nutrient solutions required each day
a. 8.5% amino acid solution = 0.085 g of protein per milliliter
$\rule{2cm}{0.4pt}$ g of protein per day required ÷ 0.085 g/ml = $\rule{2cm}{0.4pt}$ ml of amino acids per day
b. Nonprotein calories:
The calories supplied by protein (4 kcal/g) are subtracted from the RER to get total nonprotein calories needed:
$\rule{2cm}{0.4pt}$ g of protein required per day × 4 kcal/g = $\rule{2cm}{0.4pt}$ kcal provided by protein
RER − kcal provided by protein = $\rule{2cm}{0.4pt}$ nonprotein kcal needed per day
c. Nonprotein calories are usually provided as a 50:50 mixture of lipid and dextrose. However, if the patient has a preexisting condition (e.g., diabetes, hypertriglyceridemia), this ratio may need to be adjusted.

*20% lipid solution = 2 kcal/ml
To supply 50% of nonprotein kcal
$\rule{2cm}{0.4pt}$ lipid kcal required ÷ 2 kcal/ml = $\rule{2cm}{0.4pt}$ ml of lipid
*50% dextrose solution = 1.7 kcal/ml
To supply 50% of nonprotein kcal
$\rule{2cm}{0.4pt}$ dextrose kcal required ÷ 1.7 kcal/ml = $\rule{2cm}{0.4pt}$ ml of dextrose
4. Total daily requirements
$\rule{2cm}{0.4pt}$ ml of 8.5% amino acid solution
$\rule{2cm}{0.4pt}$ ml of 20% lipid solution
$\rule{2cm}{0.4pt}$ ml of 50% dextrose solution
$\rule{2cm}{0.4pt}$ ml total volume of total parenteral nutrition solution
5. Administration rate
Day 1: $\rule{2cm}{0.4pt}$ ml/hr
Day 2: $\rule{2cm}{0.4pt}$ ml/hr
Day 3: $\rule{2cm}{0.4pt}$ ml/hr

*Be sure to adjust the patient's other fluids accordingly!

central venous (jugular) catheter, whereas PPN solutions can be administered through either a jugular catheter or catheters placed in peripheral veins. The concern with high osmolarity is that it may increase the incidence of thrombophlebitis, although this has not been well characterized in veterinary patients. The administration of any PN requires a dedicated catheter used solely for PN administration that is placed using aseptic technique. In most cases this requires placement of additional catheters because PN should not be administered through existing catheters that were placed for reasons other than PN. Long catheters composed of silicone, polyurethane, or tetrafluoroethylene are recommended for use with any type of PN to reduce the risk of thrombophlebitis. Multilumen catheters are often recommended for CPN because they can remain in place for long periods and separate ports can also be used for blood sampling and administration of additional fluids

and intravenous medications without the need for separate catheters placed at other sites. Injections into the PN catheter infusion port or administration lines should be strictly prohibited.

Because of the various metabolic derangements associated with critical illness, PN should be instituted gradually over 48 hours. Administration of PN is typically initiated at 50% of the RER on the first day and increased to the targeted amount by the second day. In most cases PPN can be started without gradual increase. It is also important to adjust the rates of other fluids being concurrently administered. For both forms of PN, the animal's catheter and infusion lines must be handled aseptically at all times to reduce the risk of PN-related infections.

PN should be administered as continuous-rate infusions over 24 hours via fluid infusion pumps. Inadvertent delivery of massive amounts of PN can result if administration is not regulated properly. Once a bag of PN is set

BOX 7-2

Worksheet for Calculating a Peripheral Parenteral Nutrition Formulation

1. Resting energy requirement (RER)

$$70 \times (\text{current body weight in kg})^{0.75} = \text{kcal/day}$$

or for animals 3-25 kg, can also use:

$$30 \times (\text{current body weight in kg}) + 70 = \text{kcal/day RER} = \underline{\hspace{2cm}} \text{kcal/day}$$

2. Partial energy requirement (PER)
Plan to supply 70% of the animal's RER with peripheral parenteral nutrition (PPN):

$$\text{PER} = \text{RER} \times 0.70 = \underline{\hspace{2cm}} \text{kcal/day}$$

3. Nutrient composition
(NOTE: For animals ≤3 kg, the formulation will provide a fluid rate higher than maintenance fluid requirements. Be sure that the animal can tolerate this volume of fluids)
a. Cats and dogs 3-5 kg:
PER × 0.20 = _____ kcal/day from carbohydrate
PER × 0.20 = _____ kcal/day from protein
PER × 0.60 = _____ kcal/day from lipid
b. Cats and dogs 6-10 kg:
PER × 0.25 = _____ kcal/day from carbohydrate
PER × 0.25 = _____ kcal/day from protein
PER × 0.50 = _____ kcal/day from lipid
c. Dogs 11-30 kg:
PER × 0.33 = _____ kcal/day from carbohydrate
PER × 0.33 = _____ kcal/day from protein
PER × 0.33 = _____ kcal/day from lipid
d. Dogs >30 kg:
PER × 0.50 = _____ kcal/day from carbohydrate
PER × 0.25 = _____ kcal/day from protein
PER × 0.25 = _____ kcal/day from lipid
4. Volumes of nutrient solutions required each day
a. 5% dextrose solution = 0.17 kcal/ml
_____ kcal from carbohydrate ÷ 0.17 kcal/ml = _____ ml of dextrose per day
b. 8.5% amino acid solution = 0.085 g/ml = 0.34 kcal/ml
_____ kcal from protein ÷ 0.34 kcal/ml = _____ ml of amino acids per day
c. 20% lipid solution = 2 kcal/ml
_____ kcal from lipid ÷ 2 kcal/ml = _____ ml of lipid per day
5. Total daily requirements
_____ ml of 5% dextrose solution
_____ ml of 8.5% amino acid solution
_____ ml of 20% lipid solution
_____ ml of total volume of PPN solution
6. Administration rate
This formulation provides an approximate maintenance fluid rate.
_____ ml/hour of PPN solution

Be sure to adjust the patient's other fluids accordingly!

up for administration, it is not disconnected from the patient even for walks or diagnostic procedures—the drip regulator is decreased to a slow drip and accompanies the patient throughout the hospital. Administration of PN through a 1.2-micron in-line filter (e.g., 1.2-micron downstream filter) is also recommended and is attached at the time of setup. This setup process is performed daily with each new bag of PN. Each bag should only hold 1 day's worth of PN, and the accompanying fluid administration sets and in-line filter are changed at the same time using aseptic technique. PN should be discontinued when the animal resumes consuming an adequate amount of calories of at least 50% of RER. CPN should be discontinued gradually over a 6- to 12-hour period, but PPN can be discontinued without weaning.

Enteral Nutritional Support

In critically ill animals with a functional gastrointestinal tract, feeding tubes are the standard mode of nutritional support. As discussed previously, a key decision is determining whether the patient can undergo general anesthesia for placement of feeding tubes. In animals with surgical disease requiring laparotomy, placement of gastrostomy or jejunostomy feeding tubes should receive particular consideration. Feeding tubes commonly used in critically ill animals are nasoesophageal, esophagostomy, gastrostomy, and jejunostomy. Newer techniques available in some institutions include fluoroscopy-guided jejunal tubes. The decision to choose one tube over another is based on the anticipated duration of nutritional support (e.g., days versus months), the need to circumvent certain segments of the gastrointestinal tract (e.g., oropharyngeal injury, esophagitis, pancreatitis), clinician experience, and suitability of patient to withstand anesthesia (very critical animals may only tolerate placement of nasoesophageal feeding tubes). Another consideration for choosing the most appropriate tube is the expectation of how well the animal will tolerate enteral feedings. Nasoesophageal and esophagostomy feeding tubes may not be ideal in animals that have persistent vomiting or regurgitation and that are also mostly recumbent. In these animals, gastrostomy or jejunal tubes may be preferable.

Monitoring for Complications

Because the development of complications in critically ill animals can have serious consequences, close monitoring is an important aspect of nutritional support. With implementation of enteral nutrition, possible complications include vomiting, diarrhea, fluid overload, electrolyte imbalances, feeding tube malfunction, and infectious complications associated with the feeding tube insertion site. Metabolic complications are more common with PN and include the development of hyperglycemia, lipemia, azotemia, hyperammonemia, and electrolyte abnormalities.

Rarely nutritional support can be associated with severe abnormalities that are sometimes referred to as the refeeding syndrome. Strategies to reduce risk of complications include observing aseptic techniques when placing feeding tubes and intravenous catheters, using conservative estimates of energy requirements (i.e., RER), and careful patient monitoring. Parameters that should be monitored during nutritional support include body temperature; respiratory rate and effort; signs of fluid overload (e.g., chemosis, tachypnea, pulmonary crackles, increased body weight); and serum concentrations of glucose, triglycerides, electrolytes, blood urea nitrogen, and creatinine. Detection of any abnormality should prompt full reassessment.

Pharmacologic Agents in Nutritional Support

Since critically ill animals are often anorexic, there is the temptation to use appetite stimulants to increase food intake. Unfortunately appetite stimulants are generally unreliable and seldom result in adequate food intake in critically ill animals. Pharmacologic stimulation of appetite is often short-lived and only delays true nutritional support. This author does not believe that appetite stimulants have a place in the management of hospitalized animals when more effective measures of nutritional support such as placement of feeding tubes are more appropriate. Appetite stimulants may be considered in recovering animals once they are home in their own environment, since ideally the primary reason for loss of appetite should be reversed by time of hospital discharge.

Future Directions in Critical Care Nutrition

The current state of veterinary critical care nutrition revolves around proper recognition of animals in need of nutritional support and implementation of strategies to best provide nutritional therapies. Important areas that need further evaluation in critically ill animals include the optimal composition and caloric target of nutritional support and strategies to minimize complications and optimize outcome. Recent findings implicating development of hyperglycemia with poor outcome in critically ill humans have led to more vigilant monitoring and stricter control of blood glucose, with obvious implications for nutritional support. Evidence of a similar relationship in dogs and cats is mounting, and ongoing studies are focusing on the possible consequences of hyperglycemia. Until further studies suggest otherwise, efforts to reduce the incidence of hyperglycemia in critically ill animals, especially those receiving nutritional support, should be strongly pursued.

Other exciting areas of clinical nutrition in critically ill humans include the use of special nutrients that possess immunomodulatory properties such as glutamine, arginine, and n-3 fatty acids. In specific populations these agents used singly or in combination have demonstrated promising results, even in severely affected people. However, results have not been consistent, and ongoing trials continue to evaluate their efficacy. To date there is limited information on the use of these nutrients to specifically modulate disease in clinically affected animals. Future studies should focus on whether manipulation of such nutrients offer any benefit in animals.

References and Suggested Reading

Brunetto MA et al: Effects of nutritional support on hospital outcome in dogs and cats, *J Vet Emerg Crit Care* 20:224, 2010.

Buffington T, Holloway C, Abood A: Nutritional assessment. In Buffington T, Holloway C, Abood S, editors: *Manual of veterinary dietetics*, St Louis, 2004, Saunders, p 1.

Chan DL: Nutritional requirements of the critically ill patient, *Clin Tech Small Anim Pract* 19:1, 2004.

Freeman LM, Chan DL: Total parenteral nutrition. In DiBartola SP, editor: *Fluid, electrolyte, and acid-base disorders in small animal practice*, ed 3, St Louis, 2006, Saunders, p 584.

Goulet O et al: A new intravenous fat emulsion containing soybean oil, medium-chain triglycerides, olive oil, and fish oil: a single-center, double-blind randomized study on efficacy and safety in pediatric patients receiving home parenteral nutrition, *J Parenter Enteral Nutr* 34:485, 2010.

Michel KE et al: Correlation of a feline muscle mass score with body composition determined by dual-energy x-ray absorptiometry, *Br J Nutr* 106:S57, 2011.

Novak F et al: Glutamine supplementation in serious illness: a systematic review of the evidence, *Crit Care Med* 30:2022, 2002.

Pyle SC, Marks SL, Kass PH: Evaluation of complications and prognostic factors associated with administration of total parenteral nutrition in cats: 75 cases (1994-2001), *J Am Vet Med Assoc* 255:242, 2004.

Torre DM, deLaforcade AM, Chan DL: Incidence and significance of hyperglycemia in critically ill dogs, *J Vet Intern Med* 21:971, 2007.

Van den Berghe G et al: Intensive insulin therapy in critically ill patients, *N Engl J Med* 345:1359, 2001.

Walton RS, Wingfield WE, Ogilvie GK: Energy expenditure in 104 postoperative and traumatically injured dogs with indirect calorimetry, *J Vet Emerg Crit Care* 6:71, 1998.

CHAPTER 8

Stabilization of the Patient with Respiratory Distress

TIMOTHY B. HACKETT, *Fort Collins, Colorado*
LAUREN SULLIVAN, *Fort Collins, Colorado*

Respiratory distress in small animals presents a therapeutic dilemma. By the time owners identify a problem, their animal may be so severely compromised that diagnostic testing and treatment could stress the pet to the point of respiratory and cardiac arrest. Thus diagnostic testing may be delayed or restricted to avoid placing the patient at further risk. In these circumstances, the clinician must quickly develop a rational list of differential diagnoses and treatments, while providing basic supportive care. Initial steps toward stabilization of the respiratory system, such as oxygen supplementation, thoracocentesis, and possibly airway control via endotracheal intubation or temporary tracheotomy, may be necessary before proceeding with diagnostics. This chapter reviews the pathophysiologic mechanisms behind respiratory distress and provides guidance on anatomic localization of the disease, recommendations for initial stabilization, and appropriate sequencing of diagnostic tests.

Pathophysiology of Respiratory Distress

Work of breathing, or the effort required for effective pulmonary gas exchange, depends mainly on two forces within the respiratory system: (1) airway resistance, which opposes airflow during inspiration and expiration and (2) elastic recoil, which is the tendency for the lungs to collapse following inspiration. In animals with respiratory tract pathology, additional energy and effort may be required to overcome these forces. The clinician who is faced with managing respiratory distress requires greater understanding of airway resistance and elastic recoil, as well as their contributions to overall work of breathing.

Airway resistance is the pressure difference between the alveoli and the mouth divided by flow rate. Airway caliber is critical in determining resistance. If the radius of the airway is halved, resistance increases sixteenfold; in comparison, doubling airway length only increases resistance by a factor of two. Therefore small changes in airway caliber can lead to noticeable clinical signs. The major site of airway resistance in healthy animals is the medium-sized bronchi. Airway resistance is determined by lung volume, bronchial smooth muscle tone, and dynamic airway compression. At reduced lung volumes, radial traction supporting the bronchi is lost and airway caliber is reduced. Similarly, bronchial muscle contraction narrows airways and increases resistance. Bronchoconstriction is mediated by reflex stimulation of irritant receptors in the upper airways or increased parasympathetic activity. Dynamic airway collapse is seen with forceful respiration. Sudden changes in intrathoracic pressure can affect the diameter of large airways. Intrathoracic and extrathoracic airway collapse, airway foreign bodies, and mass lesions also result in increased airway resistance.

The resting lung volume is a balance between the elastic properties of the lung (favoring alveolar collapse) and the elastic properties of the chest wall (favoring alveolar expansion). This resting lung volume, understood as the volume of air remaining in the lungs at the end of a normal breath, is called the functional residual capacity (FRC). At the normal FRC, the lung is very compliant. Compliance or stiffness is the change in lung volume for any given applied pressure. In a healthy state with compliant lungs, small changes in intrapleural pressure cause a large change in lung volume, subsequently drawing fresh air into the respiratory tract. A pressure-volume curve of the lung shows the change in the work of breathing at normal and reduced lung volumes (Figure 8-1). Most common pulmonary parenchymal diseases (e.g., pulmonary edema, pneumonia) increase FRC, flatten the pressure-volume curve, and decrease compliance. Significant pleural space disease resulting in lung collapse (e.g., pneumothorax, diaphragmatic hernia) produces similar changes in lung compliance and FRC.

Respiratory Failure

Impaired respiration occurs secondary to inadequate ventilation or inadequate gas exchange. If sufficiently severe, this impairment can progress to respiratory failure, a life-threatening situation that often necessitates aggressive intervention. *Failure of ventilation* is the inability to move fresh air into the pulmonary alveoli, resulting in high blood carbon dioxide levels (hypercarbia) and low blood oxygen levels (hypoxemia). *Failure of gas exchange* occurs at the level of the blood-air barrier, resulting in hypoxemia with or without hypercarbia. In cases of impaired gas exchange, the hypoxemic patient initially hyperventilates in an effort to improve oxygenation. This results in low blood carbon dioxide levels and a respiratory alkalosis. With progression of disease and onset of respiratory

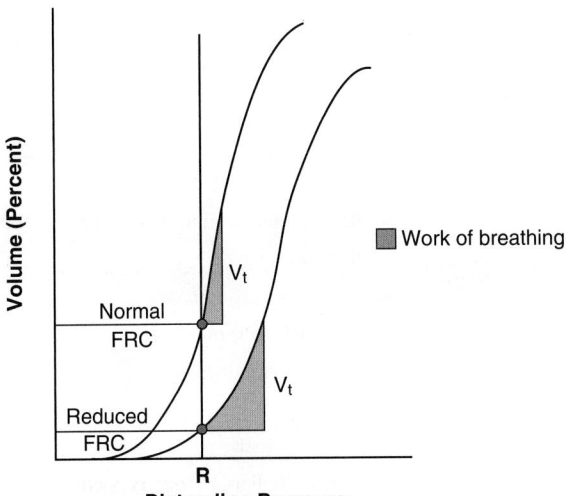

Figure 8-1 Pulmonary compliance equals the slope of the pressure volume curve at the functional residual capacity (FRC) or resting volume of the lung. The x-axis, *R*, is the pressure required to move a volume of air (shown in the y-axis). With a reduced FRC, a greater distending pressure is required to move an equal tidal volume. This requires more work and therefore more energy. *V*ₜ, Tidal volume.

failure, effective exchange of both oxygen and carbon dioxide is lost, resulting in hypoxemia and hypercarbia. Appropriate differentiation of the type of respiratory failure is critical when moving forward with proper medical intervention. Close observation of respiratory pattern and physical examination findings are especially helpful in determining the likely cause and appropriate therapeutic interventions (Table 8-1).

Physical Examination

Due to the fragile nature of most animals in respiratory distress, physical restraint for close examination, radiography, or intravenous catheterization may need to wait until the patient is less anxious and breathing more comfortably. In such cases, determination of the problem underlying respiratory distress often can be accomplished with observation alone. There are several key observations that optimize the information gained and help the clinician tailor treatment to the most likely underlying disease.

One of the more common descriptors used by clinicians when observing an animal in respiratory distress is the term *dyspneic*. Dyspnea is frequently used in veterinary medicine to designate animals with difficult or labored breathing, whereas in human medicine the term describes the sensation of an unpleasant sensory experience. In human medicine not all dyspneic patients have increased respiratory efforts, nor do all patients with labored breathing have the sensation of dyspnea. Dyspnea can be subjective and difficult to assess in nonverbal patients, thus making identification of these sensations particularly challenging in veterinary medicine.

The sensation of air hunger is often stressful. The results of this stress are a more rapid breathing pattern

and increased levels of circulating catecholamines, which only further increase the animal's oxygen requirements. Clinical signs associated with the underlying disease are frequently exacerbated when these patients increase their respiratory rate or effort. For example, disorders characterized by dynamic airway narrowing (e.g., laryngeal paralysis, tracheal collapse, bronchitis) become more severe when airflow velocity increases due to reduced pressure within the airway lumen. This further compromises the airway cross-sectional area and illustrates how increasing oxygen demand, coupled with impaired respiratory function, can have additive consequences. This is one reason why sedatives/tranquilizers that reduce this stress response can help the dyspneic animal breathe more efficiently and why these drugs are often imperative to successful management of respiratory distress (Table 8-2). Identification and treatment of dyspnea are important first steps before moving on to the physical examination.

When in distress, animals adopt a respiratory pattern to minimize their work of breathing. Characterization of the breathing pattern can be helpful in anatomic localization of the disease. Specific points to evaluate include the phase of respiration affected and the overall breathing pattern (see Table 8-1). The first step is to determine if the increased work of breathing is occurring on inspiration, expiration, or both. Increased work of breathing on inspiration often localizes the problem to the upper airways (e.g., laryngeal paralysis, extrathoracic tracheal collapse), whereas increased work of breathing on expiration indicates intrathoracic or lower airway disease (e.g., intrathoracic tracheal collapse, bronchitis). Increased work of breathing on both inspiration and expiration suggests a fixed lesion within the airway (e.g., airway foreign bodies, intraluminal masses, external compression of the airway).

Following anatomic localization of the respiratory pathology, further characterization of the respiratory pattern can help narrow down the differential diagnoses (see Table 8-1). Animals with airway obstruction generally breathe slower and deeper to minimize the resistance to airflow. Loud respiratory noise may be evident without a stethoscope. A rapid, shallow respiratory pattern, also known as a restrictive pattern, is observed in animals with pulmonary parenchymal disease (e.g., pneumonia, pulmonary edema) and in some animals with pleural space diseases. A third breathing pattern, known as an inverse or asynchronous pattern, might also be evident with pleural space disease. This pattern is characterized by paradoxical movement of the chest wall on inspiration (the thorax collapses in) and on expiration (the thorax expands out), which is the reverse of normal chest wall movement.

Upper airway and thoracic auscultation can be highly beneficial in the initial evaluation and can be accomplished without stressing the patient. An obvious heart murmur or gallop sound may indicate congestive heart failure. In many cases of airway obstruction, noise that is loudest over the obstruction can be heard during slow breathing. Wheezing with prolonged expiration suggests either bronchial narrowing (bronchitis or asthma) or obstruction/collapse of a principal bronchus. When

TABLE 8-1

Common Causes of Respiratory Distress in Dogs and Cats

Problem	Phase Affected/Respiratory Pattern	Emergency Treatment
Upper Airway Obstruction		
Laryngeal paralysis	Inspiratory/Obstructive	O_2, sedation, antiinflammatory, +/– tracheostomy
Extrathoracic tracheal collapse	Inspiratory/Obstructive	O_2, sedation, antitussive
Airway mass lesion	Fixed/Obstructive	O_2, sedation, +/– tracheostomy
Airway foreign body	Fixed/Obstructive	O_2, sedation, Heimlich maneuver
Laryngeal stenosis	Fixed/Obstructive	O_2, sedation, +/– tracheostomy
Lower Airway Obstruction		
Intrathoracic tracheal collapse	Expiratory/Obstructive	O_2, sedation, antitussive
Bronchitis	Expiratory/Obstructive	O_2, sedation, antiinflammatory, bronchodilator
Airway mass lesion	Fixed/Obstructive	O_2, sedation
Airway foreign body	Fixed/Obstructive	O_2, sedation, Heimlich maneuver
Pulmonary Parenchymal Disease		
Pneumonia	Inspiratory/Restrictive	O_2, IV fluids, antibiotic, physical therapy
Cardiogenic pulmonary edema	Inspiratory/Restrictive	O_2, sedation, fluid restriction/diuretics
Noncardiogenic pulmonary edema	Inspiratory/Restrictive	O_2, sedation
Pulmonary hemorrhage	Inspiratory/Restrictive	O_2, sedation, FFP
Pulmonary neoplasia	Inspiratory/Restrictive	O_2, sedation
Pleural Space Disease		
Chylothorax	Inspiratory/Restrictive/Inverse	O_2, thoracocentesis
Pneumothorax	Inspiratory/Restrictive/Inverse	O_2, thoracocentesis
Pyothorax	Inspiratory/Restrictive/Inverse	O_2, thoracocentesis
Pleural hemorrhage	Inspiratory/Restrictive/Inverse	O_2, FFP, thoracocentesis
Diaphragmatic hernia	Inspiratory/Restrictive/Inverse	O_2, sedation, surgical correction
Pulmonary Thromboembolism	Hyperventilation	O_2, sedation, thrombolytic, anticoagulation

Phase affected describes either inspiratory or expiratory dyspnea, with increased effort and time devoted to that phase of respiration. Fixed obstructive pattern will have increased effort during both phases of respiration. Obstructive pattern is generally deeper with a loud stridor. Restrictive pattern breathing is rapid and shallow.

O_2, Oxygen supplemented by face mask, blow-by, nasal cannula, oxygen cage, oxygen tent, or positive pressure ventilation. FFP, fresh frozen plasma. Physical therapy consists of nebulization and coupage to loosen airway secretions.

attempting to differentiate pleural space disease from parenchymal diseases particular attention should be directed to identification of a pleural fluid line (muffled breath sounds ventrally) or pulmonary crackles (indicating diffuse small airway or lung parenchymal disease). Unfortunately, an absence of crackles does not exclude the presence of pulmonary parenchymal disease.

Initial interventions (e.g., oxygen supplementation, minimization of stress and sedation) are often performed concurrently with observation and brief thoracic auscultation. Once these steps are complete, a more thorough physical examination is warranted. This should include close monitoring of vital signs, assessment of cardiovascular status, and a thorough thoracic auscultation if not already done. Following the physical examination, additional interventions may be required (e.g., thoracocentesis, temporary tracheotomy) or definitive diagnostics can be performed.

Diagnostics

Radiography

Radiography is typically indicated for animals presenting with respiratory signs because radiographic changes or patterns can help further determine the cause of the distress. As indicated earlier, radiography should be delayed until the patient is more stable. Thoracic and cervical radiographs can be used to diagnose collapsing trachea, tracheal or laryngeal foreign bodies, and mass lesions. It is possible to assess airway dynamics by taking inspiratory and expiratory views of the trachea or with fluoroscopy (or bronchoscopy).

Thoracic radiographs are indicated for suspected lower airway disease, with careful attention paid to classic radiographic patterns of the pulmonary parenchyma. Bronchial patterns develop as the peribronchiolar tissues

TABLE 8-2

Drugs Used to Calm Dyspneic Dogs and Cats

Drug	Initial Dose and Route	Notes
Butorphanol tartrate*	0.2-0.4 mg/kg IM or IV	Respiratory distress/anxiety in cats
Acepromazine*	0.01-0.02 mg/kg IV	Respiratory distress/anxiety in dogs
Methadone	Dogs: 0.1-0.5 mg/kg IV, or 0.5-2 mg/kg SC or IM Cats: 0.05-0.1 mg/kg IV, or 0.2-0.6 mg/kg IM or SC	Additional sedation in dogs and cats
Propofol	2-4 mg/kg IV, to effect	Slowly titrated to gain airway control
Morphine	Dogs: 0.2-0.5 mg/kg IV, IM, or SC Cats: 0.1 mg/kg IV, IM, or SC (can increase to 0.2 mg/kg if necessary)	Relax splanchnic vasculature in cases of pulmonary edema. In addition to those listed above

*Can be used in combination (if there are no contraindications).

become inflamed, often consistent with lower airway disease (e.g., asthma, chronic bronchitis). Interstitial patterns develop with thickening of the fibrous structures of the lung, as seen with pulmonary neoplasia or fungal infections. Alveolar patterns, characterized radiographically by air bronchograms, are caused by fluid accumulation in the alveoli. These may be secondary to cardiogenic or noncardiogenic pulmonary edema, pneumonia, or hemorrhage. Radiographic distribution of the alveolar pattern can help further distinguish the cause of disease. A cranioventral opacity, most commonly observed in the right middle lung lobe, usually indicates aspiration pneumonia. A dorsocaudal distribution is seen with many causes of noncardiogenic edema (e.g., airway obstruction, electrocution, post-ictal, with near-drowning). A perihilar alveolar pattern, observed around the base of the heart, can be seen with cardiogenic edema. In addition, these cases often have signs of left atrial enlargement and pulmonary venous congestion. Any condition affecting the pleural space (e.g., fluid accumulation, pneumothorax, diaphragmatic hernia) should also be identified with a radiograph. Radiographic signs consistent with pleural space disease include visualization of widened pleural fissures, retraction of lung lobe margins, blunting of the costophrenic angle on the ventrodorsal view, and the silhouette sign with the heart and the diaphragm.

Ultrasonography

The use of ultrasound in the emergency setting has significantly increased in recent years. There is a clear trade-off between obtaining immediate results and the quality of the examination that can be performed based on both patient and operator (experience) factors. When used in a focused manner, a "fast" thoracic ultrasound examination can be helpful. Importantly, appropriate equipment (including transducer frequencies) must be available, the examiner should have sufficient training in ultrasound imaging techniques, and the clinician must learn to interpret the obtained images correctly. In the patient with respiratory distress, ultrasound imaging is especially useful for identifying pleural effusion and pericardial effusions, assessing left atrial size (for left-sided congestive heart failure), and identifying a gas/fluid interface consistent with lung parenchymal disease.

Complete blood counts may be useful for distinguishing inflammatory diseases from stress. Coagulation testing is indicated in patients with pleural space or parenchymal bleeding and assists in identification of acquired coagulopathies requiring clotting factor and vitamin K replacement therapy. Serum biochemical profiles aid in evaluating organ function, documenting concurrent diseases, and evaluating serum albumin concentrations. Arterial blood gas samples, although sometimes difficult to obtain in small and critical patients, are useful for assessing ventilation, oxygenation, and acid-base status. A high partial pressure of carbon dioxide indicates hypoventilation, whereas a low value confirms hyperventilation. Partial pressure of oxygen and oxygen saturation of arterial blood inform the clinician about efficacy of gas exchange and assist in determining the magnitude of the respiratory dysfunction.

Recently several tests have been identified that may help distinguish cardiac from primary respiratory causes of respiratory distress. The cardiac troponin I (cTnI) and serum N-terminal pro-B-type natriuretic peptide (NT-proBNP) can be elevated in patients with cardiac disease and may help determine the primary disease process in these patients. Importantly, the specific cut-off values for the natriuretic peptides differ between test type (BNP versus NT-proBNP), between patient type (dog versus cat), and depending on whether disease is isolated or concurrent (heart disease only, respiratory disease only, or both). The sensitivity, specificity, and practical application of these tests are still under investigation but may hold some future promise in point-of-care testing.

Treatment Plan

Once the cause of respiratory distress is localized to a region of the airway, lung, or pleural space, specific diagnostics and definitive therapy can be initiated. Light sedation and supplemental oxygen often are required to manage the case before more definitive therapy is directed. Providing an oxygen source via an induction chamber, oxygen cage, nasal cannula, face mask, or semiclosed Elizabethan collar can quickly raise the inspired oxygen concentration and improve clinical signs. In patients with high airway obstructions, supplemental oxygen can be delivered through a large needle placed directly into the trachea or via a temporary tracheotomy.

Patients with pronounced expiratory dyspnea and expiratory wheezes likely have bronchial inflammation, narrowing, or collapse. Regardless of cause or species affected, the emergency plan includes supplemental oxygen, inhaled bronchodilator (see Chapter 161), and a

The cause of lung parenchymal disease should be identified because it is likely to dictate treatment. Patients with pneumonia are usually systemically ill. Fever, dehydration, leukocytosis with an inflammatory left shift, and inflammatory airway cytology are all signs of pulmonary infection. In addition to supplemental oxygen, these patients should receive intravenous fluids, antibiotics, and physical therapy to encourage loosening and clearance of the infectious material. A mitral murmur, lung crackles, and serous-to-pink-tinged acellular airway fluid may indicate pulmonary edema, requiring diuretic therapy (see Chapter 176). Blood in the airway is seen with trauma and acquired coagulopathies such as rodenticide intoxication and, if severe enough, may require transfusion of clotting factors and/or red blood cells (see Chapter 31).

With pleural fluid accumulation, fluid cytology and radiographs are often necessary to distinguish the cause (see Chapter 164). Thoracocentesis is a valuable therapeutic and diagnostic tool when approaching pleural space disease. If pleural accumulation of air or fluid is rapid or if the fluid is viscous and inflammatory, a thoracostomy tube can facilitate drainage and allow repeated evacuation of the pleural space.

Respiratory distress in dogs and cats can be challenging. Definitive diagnostic investigation may not be possible at the time of presentation, but critical observation and focused physical examination help rank differential diagnoses of respiratory distress. The clinician should have a thorough understanding of the manifestations of multiple differentials of respiratory distress based on the pattern of breathing and be able to quickly identify appropriate treatments. A rational emergency diagnostic and treatment plan is based on understanding of respiratory function and alterations associated with specific diseases.

References and Suggested Reading

Lee JA, Drobatz KJ: Respiratory distress and cyanosis in dogs. In King LG, editor: *Textbook of respiratory disease in dogs and cats*, St Louis, 2004, Saunders, pp 1-12.

Mandell DC: Respiratory distress in cats. In King LG, editor: *Textbook of respiratory disease in dogs and cats*, St Louis, 2004, pp 12-17.

Mellema MS: The neurophysiology of dyspnea, *J Vet Emerg Crit Care* 18(6):561-571, 2008.

Oyama MA, et al: Assessment of serum N-terminal pro-B-type natriuretic peptide concentration for differentiation of congestive heart failure from primary respiratory tract disease as the cause of respiratory signs in dogs, *J Am Vet Med Assoc* 235(11):1319-1325, 2009.

Payne EE, et al: Assessment of a point-of-care cardiac troponin I test to differentiate cardiac from noncardiac causes of respiratory distress in dogs, *J Vet Emerg Crit Care* 21(3):217-225, 2011.

West JB: Pulmonary pathophysiology: the essentials, ed 8, Philadelphia, 2012, Lippincott Williams & Wilkins.

CHAPTER 9

Acute Respiratory Distress Syndrome

EMILY K. THOMAS, *Philadelphia, Pennsylvania*
LORI S. WADDELL, *Philadelphia, Pennsylvania*

Acute respiratory distress syndrome (ARDS) is a severe inflammatory disorder of the lungs that can result in life-threatening respiratory failure in dogs and cats. It can be caused by a wide range of precipitating conditions, all of which lead to lung inflammation, alveolar capillary leakage, and protein-rich pulmonary edema. Acute lung injury (ALI) is a milder form of inflammatory injury to the lungs that also can progress to ARDS.

Risk Factors

ARDS has many potential causes. It may result either from direct pulmonary insult or from a generalized inflammatory response such as systemic inflammatory response syndrome (SIRS) or sepsis. Box 9-1 lists many of the risk factors proposed in dogs, but this list is not exhaustive. Sepsis of either pulmonary or nonpulmonary origin is the most common predisposing cause of ARDS identified in dogs. Risk factors have not been characterized in cats, but the few available reports suggest similar underlying etiologies. A single patient may have multiple precipitating causes.

Pathophysiology

The pathogenesis of ARDS is similar regardless of the underlying etiology and is characterized by an overwhelming inflammatory process that leads to epithelial

Risk Factors for the Development of ARDS in Dogs

Direct Lung Injury
Common Causes
Microbial pneumonia
Aspiration pneumonia
Pulmonary contusions

Less Common Causes
Smoke inhalation
Near-drowning
Lung lobe torsion
Noncardiogenic pulmonary edema

Indirect Lung Injury
Common Causes
Sepsis/SIRS
Shock
Severe trauma

Less Common Causes
Pancreatitis
Systemic infection
Multiple transfusions
Drugs and toxins
Organ torsion

Differential Diagnoses

Cardiogenic pulmonary edema
Volume overload
Pulmonary thromboembolism
Bacterial pneumonia
Atelectasis
Pulmonary hemorrhage
Neoplasia

damage in the lung. Macrophages, neutrophils, and pro-inflammatory cytokines such as tumor necrosis factor and interleukin-1β interact to cause alveolar and vascular epithelial injury.

Three overlapping phases of inflammation are typically described. The *exudative phase* begins as a diffuse vascular leak syndrome, with infiltration of erythrocytes and inflammatory cells and effusion of protein-rich fluid into the alveoli; progressive pulmonary edema and hemorrhage result. Activation of inflammatory cells causes release of harmful mediators that contribute to ongoing lung injury. Synthesis of surfactant is impaired, with consequent alveolar collapse. Hyaline membranes (organized proteinaceous debris) form within the alveoli.

In the *proliferative phase* that follows, a proliferation of type II pneumocytes and fibroblasts occurs in an attempt to repair damaged tissue. This leads to interstitial fibrosis. Lastly, the *fibrotic phase* is characterized by collagen deposition and the development of varying degrees of fibrosis before eventual resolution.

Historical Findings and Clinical Features

The hallmark sign of ARDS is an acute history of severe respiratory distress. It is most commonly seen in intensive care unit patients with other underlying diseases but may affect any animal with a predisposing risk factor. The earliest signs, tachypnea and increased respiratory effort, rapidly progress to severe respiratory distress. Signs may develop within hours or up to 4 days after an inciting event.

Clinical examination usually reveals severe respiratory distress with cyanosis. Dogs may expectorate a pink,

foamy fluid from the lungs. In the early stages harsh airway or loud bronchial sounds are heard on thoracic auscultation, but these rapidly progress to crackles. If the animal is intubated, sanguineous fluid may drain from the endotracheal tube. Tachycardia is common secondary to severe hypoxemia, with poor oxygen delivery to the tissues. Evidence of other underlying or systemic disease may be found.

Diagnosis

In small animal veterinary medicine four criteria are required to diagnose ARDS (Wilkins et al, 2007). Respiratory distress should be *acute in onset* (< 72 hours), with one or more *known risk factors* present (see Box 9-1). Evidence of *inefficient gas exchange* is required, together with evidence of *pulmonary capillary leak* without increased pulmonary capillary pressure. Evidence of *pulmonary inflammation* is an optional fifth criterion. Other differential diagnoses should be considered if the above criteria are not met in a patient (Box 9-2).

Inefficient Gas Exchange

Severe hypoxemia in arterial blood gas results provides evidence of inefficient gas exchange. Hypoxemia is further defined as a $PaO_2:FiO_2$ ratio of 200 or lower (ARDS) or 300 or lower (ALI) or as an increased alveolar-arterial gradient (normal value < 15 mm Hg while breathing room air). For accurate calculation, a known FiO_2 is required (such as room air, oxygen cage, or mechanical ventilation). During mechanical ventilation, positive end-expiratory pressure (PEEP) or continuous positive airway pressure (CPAP) may reduce hypoxemia and affect results. The extent of hypoxemia is often sufficient to increase respiratory drive, resulting in hyperventilation and hypocarbia. However, if end-stage lung disease or respiratory muscle fatigue occurs, hypercarbia may be seen.

Pulmonary Capillary Leak

Thoracic radiographs show characteristic diffuse, bilateral, pulmonary alveolar infiltrates (Figure 9-1), providing evidence of pulmonary capillary leak. Infiltrates affect more than one quadrant and may be asymmetrical or patchy. The ventral lung lobes may be the most severely affected. The heart and blood vessels should also be evaluated. Cardiomegaly, left atrial enlargement,

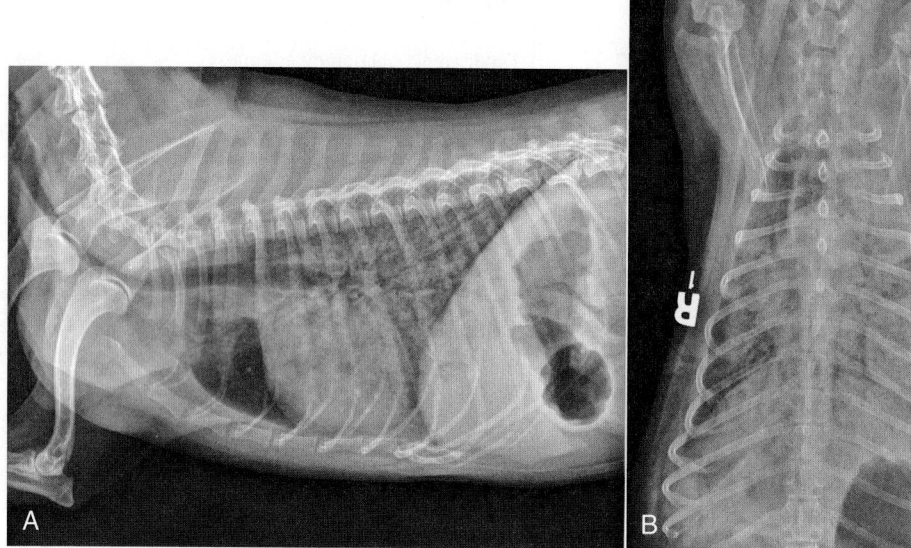

Figure 9-1 Left lateral **(A)** and dorsoventral **(B)** radiographs showing diffuse, pulmonary alveolar infiltrates in an 11-year-old dog presenting with acute respiratory distress after anesthesia for a dental procedure. The cardiac silhouette is only partially visible but is normal in size, with normal pulmonary vasculature.

distended pulmonary vessels, or concurrent pleural effusion may suggest increased pulmonary capillary pressure secondary to congestive heart failure or fluid overload, rather than ARDS. If this is suspected, echocardiography is indicated to rule out cardiogenic pulmonary edema or volume overload. Pulmonary capillary leak with normal cardiac function may also be seen with noncardiogenic pulmonary edema related to seizures or acute upper airway obstruction. The pathogenesis is not fully understood, but mechanical disruption of the capillary endothelium from acute overload of the pulmonary circulation secondary to massive sympathetic stimulation and systemic vasoconstriction may contribute to the leak. Typically, this type of edema resolves over 24 to 48 hours with treatment, although in severe cases it can progress to ARDS. Radiographs commonly show asymmetric infiltrates with predominantly right-sided or caudodorsal quadrant involvement.

A central venous catheter may be placed for both diagnostic and management purposes. Elevation of the central venous pressure (CVP), as well as visible jugular venous distention prior to catheter placement, may suggest congestive heart failure or fluid overload. Until recently, pulmonary arterial catheters were frequently used in humans to assess pulmonary capillary wedge pressure and left heart function (see Chapter 4). However, placement is invasive, and their use was not shown to improve outcome. Less invasive methods of assessment (such as echocardiography) are recommended in veterinary patients.

Additional Diagnostics

Typical abnormalities in the complete blood count (CBC) include leukopenia due to sequestration of white blood cells in the periphery and in the lungs and thrombocytopenia due to platelet sequestration or consumption. Changes in the serum biochemical profile (SBP) are often nonspecific, but hypoalbuminemia is common due to underlying disease and exudative protein loss into the pulmonary edema fluid. Prolonged coagulation times and elevated fibrin degradation products or D-dimers may indicate a consumptive coagulopathy.

Cytologic evaluation and culture of bronchoalveolar lavage or transtracheal wash samples provide useful additional diagnostic information—if the animal is stable enough to perform these diagnostics. Neutrophilia of the lavage sample fulfills the optional fifth diagnostic criterion for evidence of pulmonary inflammation. Culture results will guide antibiotic therapy.

Therapeutics

The first priority of treatment is to address the underlying cause of SIRS or primary lung injury, if possible, so that the source of ongoing injury is removed. Other than this, supportive care is the mainstay of treatment, and specific treatments for ARDS are still lacking despite ongoing research. However, improvements in supportive care have significantly reduced mortality in humans over the last decade.

Respiratory Support

Animals with mild ALI may respond to oxygen supplementation alone (see Chapter 10) and may appear more comfortable following sedation with butorphanol (0.1 to 0.4 mg/kg IV, IM). However, ARDS patients usually require positive pressure ventilation (PPV) to achieve adequate gas exchange (see Chapter 11). PPV with PEEP recruits alveoli and increases functional residual capacity, allowing ventilation at lower FiO_2 and preventing cyclical alveolar reopening and stretching with each breath. FiO_2 should be 0.6 or lower to prevent oxygen toxicity. A strategy of protective lung ventilation should be employed, with tidal volumes as low as possible (ideally 6 to 8 ml/kg) in order to prevent overdistention of normal alveoli, shear stress, and progression of lung injury. Excessively high airway pressures (> 30 cm H_2O) may cause further lung injury and should be avoided.

Fluid Therapy

Fluid administration should be carefully evaluated to prevent fluid overload and worsening of pulmonary dysfunction. Measurement of CVP may aid in targeting fluid therapy. If volume overload is present, judicious administration of diuretics such as furosemide is indicated, with close monitoring of renal function. Colloidal support (fresh frozen plasma, synthetic colloids, or 25% human albumin solutions) is required for hypoproteinemic patients.

Pharmacotherapy

Many treatments have shown promising results in experimental animal models, including corticosteroids, nitric oxide, exogenous surfactant, β_2 agonists, and a variety of cyclooxygenase, thromboxane, and leukotriene inhibitors. However, none have been shown to have an effect on morbidity or mortality in human clinical trials. Therapies currently under investigation include mesenchymal stem cell therapy and inflammatory modulation using immunonutrition.

Drugs used in veterinary patients with ARDS are limited to antibiotics (if appropriate for underlying disease) and supportive measures (diuretics, fluid therapy, anesthesia if PPV is required) as outlined above. A constant rate infusion of low-dose furosemide (0.1 mg/kg hour) has proved beneficial at decreasing lung water and peak airway pressure in dogs with experimentally induced ARDS. Low-dose corticosteroids may be considered in patients with severe, early (< 72 hours) ARDS, but their use has not been substantiated by scientific data.

Patient Monitoring

Patients require intensive care monitoring, with frequent arterial blood gas analysis, pulse oximetry, arterial blood pressure, urine output, temperature, electrocardiogram, thoracic radiographs, CBC, serum biochemical analyses, and coagulation monitoring. Patients are at high risk for aspiration pneumonia, and appropriate nursing care with careful use of analgesics and sedation should be provided.

Prognosis

Humans with ARDS have an expected survival rate of 40% to 60% and often require mechanical ventilation for 4 to 6 weeks. Death may be caused by respiratory failure or by progressive multiple organ dysfunction and failure. Mortality in dogs and cats is even higher, and a grave prognosis must be given.

References and Suggested Reading

DeClue AE, Cohn LA: Acute respiratory distress syndrome in dogs and cats: a review of clinical findings and pathophysiology, *J Vet Emerg Crit Care* 17(4):340-347, 2007.

Dushianthan A et al: Acute respiratory distress syndrome and acute lung injury, *Postgrad Med J* 2011; Jun 4 (Epub ahead of print).

Wilkins PA et al: Acute lung injury and acute respiratory distress syndromes in veterinary medicine: consensus definitions: The Dorothy Russell Havemeyer Working Group on ALI and ARDS in Veterinary Medicine, *J Vet Emerg Crit Care* 17(4):333-339, 2007.

Parent C et al: Clinical and clinicopathologic findings in dogs with acute respiratory distress syndrome: 19 cases (1985-1993), *J Am Vet Med Assoc* 208(9):1419-1427, 1996.

Parent C et al: Respiratory function and treatment in dogs with acute respiratory distress syndrome: 19 cases (1985-1993), *J Am Vet Med Assoc* 208(9):1428-1433, 1996.

CHAPTER 10
Oxygen Therapy

VINCENT J. THAWLEY, *Philadelphia, Pennsylvania*
KENNETH J. DROBATZ, *Philadelphia, Pennsylvania*

Inadequate oxygen delivery to the tissues is commonly encountered in critically ill patients and results in a shift to anaerobic metabolism to support cellular functions. Cellular energy production declines and lactic acid accumulates, which may exacerbate tissue injury and can lead to organ dysfunction or even death. Ensuring adequate tissue oxygenation is a principal goal in the critical care setting. This chapter explores the major determinants of tissue oxygen delivery as well as several methods that may be employed in an effort to improve blood oxygen content.

Indications for Oxygen Therapy

Oxygen therapy is indicated in situations in which there is inadequate oxygen delivery to the tissues (hypoxia). Oxygen delivery depends on cardiac output, hemoglobin concentration, oxygen saturation of hemoglobin, and the amount of oxygen dissolved in plasma. It can be compromised by a number of pathophysiologic conditions including hypoxemia (poorly oxygenated arterial blood); decreased blood flow from cardiovascular shock, congestive heart failure, or vascular obstruction; anemia; or decreased hemoglobin affinity for oxygen such as in carbon monoxide intoxication or methemoglobinemia.

Clinical signs of hypoxemia include tachypnea, orthopnea, and open-mouth breathing. Patients may appear anxious and stand with their head and neck extended and elbows abducted. Severely hypoxemic patients may be syncopal, obtunded, or comatose. Cyanosis is an insensitive marker for hypoxemia because it is only detected when the arterial partial pressure of oxygen is less than 50 mm Hg and there is greater than 5 g/dl of desaturated hemoglobin. Furthermore, cyanosis is not apparent in patients with severe anemia or mucous membranes that are pale due to hypoperfusion.

There are five principal causes of hypoxemia. *Low inspired partial pressure of oxygen*, which may occur in intubated patients breathing an oxygen-poor gas mixture, patients rebreathing dead space gas, or patients living at a high altitude, can result in poorly oxygenated arterial blood. *Hypoventilation* occurs most frequently as a result of airway obstruction, neuromuscular disease, pleural space disease, or pain or in conditions that result in dysfunction of the chest wall or diaphragm. *Impaired diffusion* of oxygen across the alveolar-capillary membrane is an uncommon cause of hypoxemia. Diseases that result in pneumocyte proliferation or accumulation of cellular infiltrates or interstitial fibrin deposits may lead to thickening of the alveolar membrane and diffusion barrier.

The most common cause of hypoxemia seen clinically is *ventilation/perfusion (V/Q) mismatch*, which occurs when pulmonary blood passes by poorly ventilated alveoli. V/Q mismatch is seen with pneumonia, pulmonary edema, hemorrhage, pulmonary thromboembolism, neoplasia, and acute respiratory distress syndrome (ARDS). *Right-to-left vascular shunt* represents an extreme case of V/Q mismatch and may be seen in cases of lung lobe collapse or in some congenital cardiac defects. This is the only cause of hypoxemia that does not respond to oxygen supplementation.

Measuring blood oxygenation can be accomplished via either pulse oximetry or arterial blood gas analysis. Pulse oximetry estimates the percent oxygen saturation of hemoglobin (SpO_2), whereas arterial blood gas analysis measures the amount of dissolved oxygen in plasma (PaO_2). The relationship between SpO_2 and PaO_2 is demonstrated by the oxygen-hemoglobin dissociation curve. A shift in the curve to the right indicates improved oxygen delivery to the tissues, with a decrease in pH or an increase in temperature or in concentration of 2,3-diphosphoglycerate. An increase in pH or a decrease in temperature or in concentration of 2,3-diphosphoglycerate shifts the curve to the left, indicating an increased binding affinity of hemoglobin for oxygen.

A PaO_2 less than 80 mm Hg or SpO_2 less than 93% indicates hypoxemia, and oxygen supplementation is warranted. When pulse oximetry and arterial blood gas analysis are unavailable, the decision to supplement oxygen should be based on physical examination findings that suggest hypoxemia or decreased tissue oxygen delivery. However, not all patients with clinical signs referable to the respiratory system are hypoxemic. For example, tachypnea may be noted with anxiety, pain, increased temperature, or metabolic acidosis. If there is any doubt, supplemental oxygen should be provided.

Techniques for Oxygen Supplementation

There are several methods available to provide supplemental oxygen, including flow-by, face mask, nasal or nasopharyngeal catheter, tracheal catheter, oxygen cage, and mechanical ventilation. The method selected depends on the severity of hypoxemia, the desired fraction of inspired oxygen (FiO_2), the expected duration of therapy, equipment availability, patient compliance, and underlying disease process(es). Sedation is often administered to patients with respiratory distress and in some situations may facilitate the delivery of supplemental oxygen.

52

Flow-By Oxygen

Flow-by oxygen, administered by holding the oxygen hose a few centimeters from the nose or mouth if the patient is panting, is a quick and easy method to provide short-term supplemental oxygen. Flow-by also may be useful in determining whether a patient is responsive to oxygen therapy before initiating long-term treatment. An FiO_2 of 30% to 40% may be achieved by using oxygen flow rates of 2 to 5 L/min. Constant nursing attention is required because many patients turn away from the oxygen source. This method is also somewhat wasteful because a significant amount of oxygen may bypass the patient.

Face Mask

Face masks are another option for short-term oxygen supplementation that can be set up quickly with minimal equipment. An FiO_2 of 50% to 60% is possible with a well-fitted mask and a flow rate of 8 to 12 L/min. Poorly fitting masks should be avoided because they may limit the amount of oxygen delivered and create dead space that increases the work of breathing. Some patients may struggle during placement of a face mask, increasing tissue oxygen consumption and exacerbating hypoxemia; nasal catheterization or the use of an oxygen cage is suggested in these patients. Long-term use of a face mask is generally only possible in sedated or moribund patients.

Nasal Catheter

Nasal catheters are useful for providing long-term oxygen supplementation and can be placed with ease in most patients. Advantages of nasal catheters include rapidity of placement and the ability to provide an FiO_2 up to 90% while maintaining free access to the patient. Major disadvantages include the inability to accurately monitor delivered FiO_2 and patient intolerance that may result in attempts to remove the catheter.

To place a nasal catheter, first instill topical anesthetic (2% lidocaine or proparacaine) into the naris. A soft red rubber catheter (size 5 to 10 French) is premeasured from the naris to the medial canthus of the eye and marked at the level of the naris. Nasopharyngeal catheters can be placed by measuring from the naris to the ramus of the mandible. The tip of the catheter is lubricated and placed into the ventromedial aspect of the naris and then advanced quickly but gently to the premeasured length. Suture, staples, or tissue adhesive is used to secure the catheter to the face as close to the naris as possible and more proximally (ventral to the ear or on the forehead). Care should be exercised to avoid entrapment of the patient's whiskers when securing the tube.

Nasal prongs designed for humans may be used in place of a nasal catheter in patients that are not very mobile. Prongs are cut shorter as needed to fit snugly into the nares; they can be secured in place by tightening the tubing behind the head. Nasal prongs are easily dislodged but may be useful in sedated, very ill, or brachycephalic patients.

The oxygen flow rate selected depends on the size of the patient, but, in general, flow rates of 50 to 100 ml/kg/min can provide an FiO_2 of 30% to 50%. If a higher FiO_2 is desired, placement of bilateral catheters is recommended because flow rates exceeding 100 ml/kg/min may be uncomfortable for the patient and can injure the nasal mucosa. Humidification is suggested as oxygen bypasses the nasal passages and may dry and injure the respiratory mucosa. This can be accomplished by using a commercial in-line bubble humidifier or by bubbling the oxygen through an intravenous fluid bottle filled with sterile water.

Complications of nasal oxygen administration include nasal mucosal jet lesions, sneezing, nasal discharge, epistaxis, and gastric dilation. If local irritation is observed, the catheter should be removed and replaced in the opposite naris. A new catheter should be placed in the opposite naris every 48 hours to limit nasal mucosal injury.

Tracheal Catheter

Tracheal catheters are useful in patients that will not tolerate a nasal catheter or for patients with anatomic abnormalities or pathology that precludes placement of a nasal catheter. Although mucosal injury is less likely to occur than with a nasal catheter, tracheal catheters are more technically challenging to place, are more invasive, and often do not remain in place if the patient is mobile.

Tracheal catheters can be placed by percutaneously inserting a large-gauge through-the-needle catheter into the trachea between two rings caudal to the larynx. The catheter is advanced to just above the carina at the level of the fifth rib. The needle is then withdrawn from the skin and secured in place. Alternatively, a red rubber catheter or argyle feeding tube may be used in place of a through-the-needle catheter. In this case, following appropriate local anesthesia and sedation, a small incision is made on the ventral cervical midline approximately four tracheal rings caudal to the larynx. A combination of sharp and blunt dissection is used to expose the trachea by laterally retracting the sternothyroid and sternohyoid muscles. A transverse incision is made through the annular ligament between two tracheal rings, and hemostatic forceps are used to guide the tube into the tracheal lumen.

Humidified oxygen with flow rates similar to those for nasal catheters is used. Major complications include tracheal jet injury, tracheitis, and kinking at the insertion site. Displacement of the catheter can lead to subcutaneous oxygen insufflation and subcutaneous emphysema, which may result in pneumomediastinum or pneumothorax.

Oxygen Cage

Oxygen cages are sealed compartments that allow for accurate control of FiO_2, ambient temperature, humidity, and carbon dioxide (CO_2) elimination. Both commercial and custom-built cages are available but the ability to provide an FiO_2 greater than 40% is limited except in the more expensive models. Most oxygen cages have a

Plexiglas front to allow direct visualization of the patient at all times, as well as a conduit for monitoring leads and fluid lines that prevents oxygen from leaking out of the cage. Ambient temperature should be set at 22°C (70°F) with a relative humidity of 40% to 50%, although this may be adjusted as needed for hypothermic or hyperthermic patients.

The major advantage of the oxygen cage is that it is a noninvasive method of supplementing oxygen in patients that may not tolerate more invasive measures. In addition, the relatively quiet environment may be beneficial for anxious dyspneic patients. Frequently monitoring the patient's temperature is essential because hyperthermia may develop, especially in large-breed dogs. For these patients, oxygen via nasal catheter is suggested.

Disadvantages of oxygen cages include the equipment expense, oxygen waste, and isolation of the patient from the clinician. Within moments of the cage being opened, the FiO_2 drops to room air level, which may cause clinical deterioration in the patient. Physical examination, pulse oximetry, and blood gas analysis with the door open do not accurately reflect the condition of the patient inside the cage.

Mechanical Ventilation

Mechanical ventilation is recommended in patients with ventilatory failure or severe pulmonary pathology resulting in persistent hypoxemia despite supplemental oxygen (see Chapter 11). Other indications for mechanical ventilation include impending respiratory fatigue, intracranial hypertension, and postresuscitation from cardiopulmonary arrest. Patients requiring high FiO_2 for a prolonged period are at risk for pulmonary oxygen toxicity and may benefit from mechanical ventilation because the use of positive end-expiratory pressure (PEEP) may allow for a reduction in FiO_2.

Hyperbaric Oxygen Therapy

Hyperbaric oxygen therapy (HBOT) involves exposing the patient to 100% O_2 at supraatmospheric pressures, significantly increasing PaO_2 and promoting oxygen diffusion to the tissues. HBOT accelerates tissue healing, stimulates leukocyte and macrophage function, and has some antimicrobial effects. Although uncommonly used, applications of HBOT include skin flaps and grafts, poorly healing wounds, clostridial infections, and carbon monoxide toxicity. Complications that may arise with HBOT include pneumothorax, tympanic membrane rupture, oxygen-induced seizures, and pulmonary oxygen toxicity.

Complications Associated with Oxygen Therapy

Oxygen therapy is commonly used in hospitalized patients; however, the potential for toxicity has been long recognized. Oxygen toxicity is thought to result from excessive production of reactive oxygen radicals that cause degradation of intracellular sulfhydryl groups and cellular membranes. Pulmonary endothelial permeability increases and protein-rich fluid accumulates in the interstitium and alveoli, leading to severe pulmonary dysfunction.

Other complications include absorption atelectasis, peripheral arterial vasoconstriction, pulmonary vasodilation, and decreased erythropoiesis. In chronically hypercapnic patients, central chemoreceptors become less sensitive to the effects of CO_2 and hypoxia becomes the major impetus for breathing. Oxygen therapy in these patients may decrease the respiratory drive or worsen V/Q mismatch due to release of hypoxic pulmonary vasoconstriction allowing blood flow to poorly ventilated alveoli.

Weaning From Oxygen Therapy

Weaning should be attempted only after the underlying cause of hypoxia has been identified and addressed. There is no standard time over which weaning occurs; rather, weaning ideally takes place slowly while observing the patient's response because abrupt discontinuation of oxygen therapy can lead to rapid deterioration. Oxygen therapy should be reinstituted if the patient shows signs of respiratory distress at any point during weaning. Monitoring pulse oximetry or arterial blood gases during weaning may help determine whether continued therapy is indicated.

References and Suggested Reading

Court M: Respiratory support of the critically ill small animal patient. In Murtaugh RJ, Kaplan PM, editors: *Veterinary emergency and critical care medicine*, St Louis, 1992, Mosby, pp 575-580.

Drobatz KJ, Hackner S, Powell S: Oxygen supplementation. In Bonagura J, Kirk R, editors: *Kirk's current veterinary therapy XII: small animal practice*, Philadelphia, 1995, WB Saunders, pp 175-179.

Dunphy ED et al: Comparison of unilateral versus bilateral nasal catheters for oxygen administration in dogs, *J Vet Emerg Crit Care* 12:245-251, 2002.

Edwards ML: Hyperbaric oxygen therapy. Part 2: application in disease, *J Vet Emerg Crit Care* 20:289-297, 2010.

Jenkinson S: Oxygen toxicity, *New Horiz* 1:504-511, 1993.

Tseng LW, Drobatz KJ: Oxygen supplementation and humidification. In King L, editor: *Textbook of respiratory disease in dogs and cats*, St Louis, 2004, Saunders, pp 205-213.

CHAPTER 11

Ventilator Therapy for the Critical Patient

JULIEN GUILLAUMIN, *Columbus, Ohio*

In humans, modern mechanical ventilation (MV) took off during the Copenhagen poliomyelitis epidemic of 1952. Survival rates in the 1960s were 30% to 40% but dramatically improved to almost 90% in the early 1980s. MV in veterinary medicine is lagging behind its human counterpart, with less than 250 dogs and 100 cats reported in the clinical literature.

Indications

The indications for MV in veterinary medicine include (1) ventilatory failure characterized by hypercarbia, with a cutoff of $PaCO_2$ greater than 60 mm Hg or $PvCO_2$ greater than 65 mm Hg; (2) hypoxemic failure, with objective cutoffs including a PaO_2 lower than 60 mm Hg or pulse oximetry lower than 90% despite oxygen therapy ($FiO_2 \geq 60\%$); and (3) increased work of breathing with a risk of respiratory arrest. This last criterion is a subjective assessment of a patient showing evidence of respiratory fatigue or substantial distress, even if the blood gas values are still acceptable. Under these circumstances, delayed intervention is unethical and medically inappropriate.

Prognosis

There are only three large retrospective studies of MV in veterinary medicine (Table 11-1). Another set of four studies researched specific populations of canine patients (see Table 11-1). The prognosis for survival to discharge varies greatly depending on the primary disease process. Survival to discharge is reported to be up to 86% for animals with toxicoses, who are usually younger patients with reversible causes and no pulmonary parenchymal disease; 40% for those with pulmonary contusions; and 11% for post–cardiopulmonary resuscitation (CPR) patients (Hopper, 2007). The overall prognosis ranges from 21% to 71% in dogs and from 15% to 42% in cats (see Table 11-1).

Placing a Patient on the Mechanical Ventilator

Selection of drugs for anesthetic induction and sedation depends on the clinician's preference and the patient's status (see Chapter 13). Some unconscious patients may not require drugs, but most will not tolerate MV without sedation. Various options are available. Most clinicians use a combination of benzodiazepine and an opioid and then add propofol, barbiturates, ketamine, or dexmedetomidine as needed. For the benzodiazepines, midazolam is preferred over diazepam because diazepam binds to plastic syringes and infusion lines, can precipitate with other drugs, and is less available. Fentanyl is usually the opioid of choice, at "anesthetic doses" of 6 to 20 µg/kg/hr. Propofol is generally a safe anesthetic but its use generates some concerns, notably involving volume, cost, hyperlipidemia, and bacterial contamination because of the soy-based carrier. Long-term propofol use in cats is discouraged because it can cause Heinz body anemia. Pentobarbital was most widely used (65% to 80%) in veterinary medicine in the 1990s but has become obsolete. Although induction and plane of anesthesia are smooth on barbiturates, tremors and seizures can potentially occur at the time of weaning. Ketamine has some cardiovascular sparing effects and requires small volumes when administered as a constant-rate infusion. Dexmedetomidine has cardiovascular side effects including bradycardia, hypotension, and vasoconstriction but can be used at "microdoses" to enhance analgesia and sedation and to decrease the opioid and propofol requirement in some patients.

Paralytics such as nondepolarizing neuromuscular blocking agents (NMBAs) are controversial in human medicine. NMBAs should only be used as a last resort and the clinician should first attempt to troubleshoot both the machine and the patient when patient-ventilator dyssynchrony (PVD) occurs.

Choosing the Correct Settings of the Mechanical Ventilator

A mechanical ventilator moves gas (a mixture of oxygen and medical air) in and out of the lungs. All modern mechanical ventilators follow the equation of motion that links machine characteristics that can be manipulated and patient characteristics that depend on the primary disease and can change over time:

$$Pressure = Volume/Compliance + Resistance \times Flow$$

The clinician enters variables into the machine to program the breath that will be delivered. With a pressure-controlled breath, the machine delivers a breath up to a specific airway pressure. With a volume-controlled breath (technically flow-controlled), the machine delivers a certain volume in a given inspiratory time by controlling

TABLE 11-1

Available Retrospective Studies or Case Series of Mechanical Ventilation in Small Animal Clinical Patients

First Author–University–Reference	Timeframe	Population	Median (Range) Duration of MV (Hours)	Survival to Discharge (%)
King–U Penn–*J Am Vet Med Assoc* 204(7):1045-1052, 1994.	1990-1992	7 cats and 34 dogs with MV > 2 hours	28 (2-137)	38 (dogs); 42 (cats)
Campbell–U Penn–*J Am Vet Med Assoc* 217(10):1505-1509, 2000.	1994-1998	10 dogs with thoracic trauma	32 (8-77)	33
Beal–U Penn–*J Am Vet Med Assoc* 218(10):1598-1602, 2001.	1991-1999	14 dogs with cervical spinal disorders	108 (10-312)	71
Lee–U Penn–*J Am Vet Med Assoc* 226(6):924-931, 2005.	1993-2002	53 cats with any MV	11 (1-176)	15
Hopper–UC Davis–*J Am Vet Med Assoc* 230(1):64-75, 2007.	1990-2001	124 dogs and 24 cats with MV > 24 hours	48 (24-356)	29 (dogs); 21 (cats)
Hoareau–U Penn–*J Vet Emerg Crit Care* 21(3):226-235, 2011.	1990-2008	15 dogs with brachycephalic syndrome	15 (2-240)	27
Rutter–Tufts Cummings U–*J Vet Emerg Crit Care* 21(5):531-541, 2011.	2003-2009	14 dogs with LMN disease	109 (5-261)	21

MV, Mechanical ventilation; *LMN,* lower motor neuron.

the flow of gas. Also, the clinician may choose to provide positive end-expiratory pressure (PEEP), in which the baseline pressure at the end of expiration remains supra-atmospheric. This helps to prevent alveolar collapse and recruit alveolar units.

The ventilator can generate different types of breath. In mandatory breaths, the ventilator determines either the delivery and/or the end of inspiration. Spontaneous breaths are initiated and terminated by the patient. Mandatory breath can be assisted, with the patient triggering the breath that is then delivered and terminated by the machine, or controlled, with the system triggering, delivering, and terminating the breath. This is called assist/control (A/C) or continuous mandatory ventilation (CMV).

The ventilator can *support* a spontaneous breath by adding some positive pressure to "support" its tidal volume. With synchronized intermittent mandatory ventilation (SIMV), both spontaneous and mandatory breaths can be delivered in a synchronized manner, with the machine triggering, delivering, and cycling the breath if the patient does not. Newer modes, such as airway pressure release ventilation (APRV), are more frequently used for humans than for animals.

When MV is initiated, the goal is to achieve the least aggressive settings to maintain adequate oxygenation (PaO_2 80 to 100 mm Hg) and ventilation ($PaCO_2$ 35 to 45 mm Hg). The general guidelines for initial settings in animals are:

- Mode A/C (or CMV) to provide maximum ventilatory support until the patient is stabilized. Some clinicians initially use "hybrid" modes such as SIMV.
- Peak airway pressure of 15 to 25 cm H_2O.
- Tidal volume of 10 ± 2 ml/kg, although in severe hypoxemic failure ("protective lung strategy"), tidal volumes are aimed for smaller than normal volumes (4 to 6 ml/kg).
- Respiratory rate of 20 breaths per minute.
- Inspiratory time of 1 sec, giving an inspiratory:expiratory ratio of 1:2.
- PEEP 2 to 5 cm H_2O, although higher levels of PEEP can recruit and prevent derecruitment of alveolar units ("open lung strategy").

Inspiratory pressure, respiratory rate, and PEEP can be manipulated to maintain acceptable oxygenation and ventilation. Peak inspiratory pressures up to 40 to 60 cm H_2O and PEEP up to 20 cm H_2O have been used to stabilize patients in severe respiratory failure.

Patient Care

Long-term ventilation can be associated with several nursing care complications, including decubitus ulcers, peripheral edema, corneal ulceration, and oral ranula. These complications occur in at least 5% to 10% of MV veterinary patients. Well-padded tables, regular repositioning, and passive range of motion should be performed every 4 to 6 hours. Ocular ulcer prevention should be done by regular application of artificial tears. Oral care is an important part of the nursing of the MV patient. Canine patients on MV appear prone to ranula development and tongue swelling. Oral care with saline, diluted chlorhexidine solution, a commercial oral rinse, and/or protection with glycerin-soaked gauze is important.

Providing early nutrition is essential for the ventilated patient. Ventilated patients can be fed enterally or parenterally. The combination of central parenteral nutrition

---

BOX **11-1**

Tracheostomy Tube Care

- Clean stoma q12h (please ask primary clinician about tracheostomy tube dressing).
1. Gather supplies and wash hands.
2. If necessary, remove old dressing, being careful to keep tracheostomy tube in place.
3. Inspect the site around the tracheostomy stoma for signs of skin breakdown, infection, or irritation.
4. Using an antiseptic solution (e.g., chlorhexidine), clean and prep the skin around the stoma as for a surgical procedure.
5. Using a cotton swab with a rolling motion, clean the skin area around the stoma and under the flange of the tube. Dried mucus and secretions can be removed by gently wiping with gauze soaked in saline. Wipe gently away from the opening.
6. Pat dry with a clean dry swab or pad.
7. If necessary, place clean tracheostomy dressing or a 4" × 4" gauze sponge folded in half under the flange.
8. Change tracheostomy ties as necessary if soiled.
- Change and clean inner cannula (if applicable) q8h, or more frequently as needed if inner cannula becomes obstructed.
1. Gather supplies and wash hands.
2. Fill the removable basin with diluted 0.05% chlorhexidine.
3. Glove, with nonsterile vinyl gloves, and gently remove old inner cannula. Discard gloves.
4. Glove, using sterile gloves.
5. Grab new inner cannula from the sterile pack or the removable basin. Rinse the inner cannula thoroughly with sterile water.
6. Dry the inner cannula using a sterile gauze sponge.
7. Insert new sterile disposable inner cannula into tube.
8. While still wearing sterile gloves, clean old inner cannula by gently removing encrustations and mucus using a sterile trach brush or sterile pipe cleaners.
9. Place the old, but now clean, inner cannula in the removable basin.
- Nebulization q4-8h.
- Change artificial nose every 5-7 days or if grossly soiled.
- Suction PRN: Please ask primary clinician about saline instillation.
- DO NOT routinely change tracheostomy tube. Follow protocol as needed.
1. Gather supplies and wash hands.
2. Glove with sterile gloves.

3. Remove the tracheostomy tube from the package and remove the inner cannula (if applicable) using aseptic technique.
4. Thread the outer cannula with neck tapes.
5. Test inflate the cuff and deflate it (if applicable).
6. Place the obturator into the outer cannula.
7. Lubricate the tip of the tube and the obturator with water-soluble lubricant to ease insertion.
8. When the new tube is fully ready for insertion, cut the tapes on the old tube.
9. Grasp the old tube by the neck flange and remove it in a downward motion.
10. When the old tube is out, immediately insert the new tube using gentle inward pressure and stay sutures.
11. IMMEDIATELY remove the obturator, inflate the cuff (if applicable).
12. Have an assistant wearing examination gloves secure the neck tapes with a square knot with enough space between the neck and the tie to allow one finger space.

Patient Care with a Cuffed Tracheostomy Tube
- If patient is spontaneously breathing, please DO NOT inflate the cuff.
- If patient is ventilated, check cuff pressure q12-24h (goal is 15-20 mm Hg).

Troubleshooting
If tracheostomy tube falls out:
- DON'T PANIC.
- Assess patient's breathing, as most of the patients will still breathe through normal airways or stoma.
- You may use stay sutures to help keep the stoma open if necessary.
- Ask for help.
- Be ready to insert a new tube or proceed to an orotracheal intubation: sedation or anesthesia drugs, adequate material, oxygen source, and so forth.
If acute dyspnea:
- Provide oxygen +/– sedation.
- Check patency of tracheostomy tube with chest auscultation and/or feeling from air moving out of the tube.
- If patency of tracheostomy tube is lost, the options are:
  - Change inner cannula if applicable.
  - Suction tube.
  - Change tube.

Adapted from The Ohio State University—Intensive Care Unit, Standard Operating Procedures Book.

and enteral nutrition can provide the patient's full caloric requirement and promote enterocyte health (see Chapter 7). Enteral nutrition may also decrease the risk of bacterial translocation. When enteral feeding is instituted, residual gastric contents should be monitored and a promotility agent added.

Tracheal intubation should be done using a sterile endotracheal (ET) tube and aseptic technique. A low-pressure, high-volume, cuffed polyvinyl chloride ET tube is the most commonly used tube in veterinary medicine. Less rigid silicone ET tubes are also available. Rubber ET tubes are not recommended. The ET tube should be suctioned and changed whenever necessary.

With a tracheostomy, MV patients often can tolerate the machine with mild sedation, eliminating the need for anesthesia. Tracheostomy also avoids complications associated with the ET tube including ranula and macroglossia. The reported tracheostomy rate in veterinary medicine is 20% to 30%, a number similar to that for human patients, but is increased to 70% for patients in ventilatory failure. A high incidence of complications is reported in cats with tracheostomy, so appropriate warning and proper care are warranted (Box 11-1).

MV patients have open airways with a continuous flow of dry gas, so the inspired air needs to be humidified to prevent desiccation of the respiratory mucosa using inline humidifier systems or "artificial noses," such as a heat and moisture exchanger or a hygroscopic condenser humidifier.

Ventilator patients are usually severely physiologically compromised and require intensive monitoring. Central catheters can be placed to monitor central venous pressure and for sampling. Arterial lines (femoral or dorsopedal) are the preferred method to measure blood pressure and can be used for blood sample collection. Urinary catheters are often placed to facilitate nursing care and quantify urine output. Other monitoring includes cardiac output, fluid balance (i.e., *ins and outs*, body weight), and ventilator waveform display (i.e., flow-time, pressure-time, volume-time, pressure-volume, and flow-volume). The ventilator waveforms help to identify PVD or changes in pulmonary compliance.

Ventilated patients have an abnormal fluid homeostasis. In one study, healthy mixed-breed dogs that were ventilated for 24 hours receiving 5 ml/kg/hr of fluids had a decrease in urine output and an increase in urine specific gravity and showed edema with no significant changes in serum sodium concentration or cardiac index. Urine output improved following administration of low-dose furosemide. Polyuria and resolution of edema occurred following weaning from MV. This scenario is very common in clinical patients, with edema reported in up to 40% in veterinary studies. Several theories may account for the fluid-retaining state observed in MV patients. The syndrome of inappropriate antidiuretic hormone (SIADH) secretion is a well-reported consequence of MV in both humans and experimental canine studies and is also reported with use of opioids, especially fentanyl, in dogs. Use of positive pressure ventilation and (high) PEEP may also decrease venous return and cardiac output, which in turn can stimulate the release of ADH and aldosterone.

Complications of Mechanical Ventilation

Ventilator-induced lung injury (VILI) is a global term that includes barotrauma, volutrauma, atelectrauma, and biotrauma. Barotrauma is a misnamed process that involves formation of extraalveolar air in the form of pneumothorax or subcutaneous emphysema. Pneumothorax is reported in up to 15% of human patients and up to 30% of veterinary patients with MV. Gradients between the intraalveolar and extraalveolar pressures cause air to dissect along vascular sheaths and accumulate in the extraalveolar space. There is poor correlation between leak of air from the lungs and peak airway pressure. It has been postulated that *"there is no pressure above which you will always cause a pneumothorax and there is no pressure below which you will never cause a pneumothorax."*

Volutrauma is a complication of MV caused by stretch-induced trauma to the alveoli that increases epithelial and endothelial permeability. Atelectrauma results from cyclic opening and closing of alveoli that creates lung inflammation. In addition, the production of inflammatory mediators can cause direct local lung injury as well as worsening systemic inflammation in a process called biotrauma.

Oxygen toxicity describes the damage due to free radical and reactive oxygen species formation. Propagation of oxygen-derived free radical species can lead to DNA damage, lipid peroxidation, cell membrane disruption, and inactivation of sulfhydryl-containing proteins. In the lung, oxygen causes an inflammatory syndrome resembling acute respiratory distress syndrome (ARDS) with an exudative and proliferative phase (see Chapter 9). In the brain, oxygen toxicity is associated with blindness and/or seizures. Oxygen toxicity to the brain and lungs appears to be related to PaO_2 rather than alveolar oxygen or FiO_2.

Wide individual and species sensitivity to oxygen are reported, but the current dogma is that oxygen toxicity can occur when FiO_2 is 100% oxygen for more than 24 hours in humans, dogs, and cats. Clinically, FiO_2 should be lowered to 60% or less as soon as possible.

Ventilator-associated pneumonia (VAP) is a common complication of MV, and affects 10% to 50% of MV patients. Early onset VAP can be defined by the presence of two or more of the following: purulent respiratory secretions, increase or decrease in temperature, increase or decrease in white blood cell count, and worsening gas exchange within 48 hours of MV initiation. Risk factors for development of VAP include trauma, tracheostomy, duration of MV, multiple invasive lines, enteral feeding, and blood transfusion. The Centers for Disease Control and Prevention published guidelines for VAP prevention in human patients. Recommendations such as staff education, avoiding routine change of ventilator circuits, hand decontamination, use of gloves, and oral hygiene are guidelines that can be implemented in veterinary medicine. Oral and gastric decontamination with antibiotics, systemic antibiotic prophylaxis, or gastroprotectants is not recommended currently as it is unclear if it decreases the incidence of VAP in humans.

Weaning a Patient From Mechanical Ventilation

The objective for every MV patient is to be weaned off the ventilator. As the primary disease process is successfully treated or heals, the clinician should require the patient to breathe on its own with a decreased magnitude of ventilator support. Weaning should be attempted if there is evidence for improvement of the underlying cause for respiratory failure, there is adequate oxygenation (e.g., PaO_2/FiO_2 ratio above 200 to 300 on a PEEP less than 4 cm H_2O), hemodynamic stability, and spontaneous breath taken by the patient.

Weaning methods depend on the patient, the disease process, the clinician, and the ventilator itself. In general, sedation is decreased to achieve increased spontaneous breathing, to assess the ability of the patient to generate adequate tidal volume, and to maintain oxygenation without signs of ventilator fatigue with lowered FiO_2 or PEEP. Ventilator settings are modified to decrease the amount of pressure support or mandatory breath. The patient is then disconnected from the machine but usually remains intubated and is provided with supplemental oxygen. Following extubation, the patient is placed on other forms of supplemental oxygen until there is a complete resolution of its hypoxemia and the patient is able to sustain appropriate oxygenation on room air before being discharged from the hospital.

References and Suggested Reading

Corona TM, Aumann M: Ventilator waveform interpretation in mechanically ventilated small animals, *J Vet Emerg Crit Care* 21(5):496-514, 2011.

Ethier MR et al: Evaluation of the efficacy and safety for use of two sedation and analgesia protocols to facilitate assisted ventilation of healthy dogs, *Am J Vet Res* 69(10):1351-1359, 2008.

Fisk BA, Moores LK: Sedation, analgesia, and neuromuscular blockage. In MacIntyre NR, Brandson RD, editors: *Mechanical ventilation*, ed 2, St Louis, 2009, Saunders Elsevier, pp 235-251.

Haskins SC, King, LG: Positive pressure ventilation. In King LG, editor: *Textbook of respiratory disease in dogs and cats*, St Louis, 2004, Saunders Elsevier, pp 217-229.

MacIntyre NR et al: Evidence-based guidelines for weaning and discontinuing ventilatory support: a collective task force facilitated by the American College of Chest Physicians; the American Association for Respiratory Care; and the American College of Critical Care Medicine, *Chest* 120(6 Suppl):375S-95S, 2001.

Stapleton RD, Steingert KP: Ventilator-induced lung injury. In MacIntyre NR, Brandson, RD, editors: *Mechanical ventilation*, ed 2, St Louis, 2009, Saunders Elsevier, pp 206-212.

Wunsch H et al: Use of intravenous infusion sedation among mechanically ventilated patients in the United States, *Crit Care Med* 37(12):3031-3039, 2009.

CHAPTER 12

Analgesia of the Critical Patient

NIGEL CAMPBELL, *Raleigh, North Carolina*

Clinical pain is seen with trauma or surgery and often accompanies acute illness. This acute pain can contribute to the postinjury stress response and increase overall morbidity and mortality. If the initial pain response is not well controlled, adaptive responses occur in the pain pathways that lead to peripheral and central sensitization and hyperalgesia ("wind-up"). To get the best results, analgesia should be preemptive and multimodal whenever possible. To ensure that analgesia is adequate, frequent reassessment of patient comfort should be performed. This chapter reviews a number of drug therapies used for preventing and treating pain in dogs and cats. In addition, routes of administration and delivery of analgesic drugs are considered.

Opioids

Opioids, the primary drugs for treating pain in the critical patient, also provide mild to moderate sedation, depending on the agent. The most commonly used opioids are the pure mu agonists (morphine, hydromorphone, oxymorphone, and fentanyl) and the partial mu agonist, buprenorphine. Butorphanol, a kappa agonist and a mu antagonist, provides less analgesia but more sedation. Fentanyl, a potent analgesic, has a very short half-life and therefore should be administered as a constant rate infusion (CRI) or a transdermal patch.

Methadone is a mu-receptor agonist that also inhibits N-methyl-D-aspartate (NMDA) receptors. It has similar duration and action to morphine but produces less sedation and vomiting. Intramuscular injection can be painful in cats.

Tramadol is a weak mu-receptor agonist that also inhibits neuronal reuptake of norepinephrine and serotonin. There are reports of adequate analgesia being provided by oral tramadol (Lamont et al, 2008). Because of the risk of serotonin syndrome, tramadol should not be used in patients receiving monoamine oxidase inhibitors. Side effects can include sedation or dysphoria, especially in cats.

Buprenorphine is increasingly used in clinical practice. In addition to parenteral administration, it can be administered via the oral transmucosal route (OTM). This route has been demonstrated to provide analgesia in the cat at 0.02 mg/kg (Robertson et al, 2005). However, in the dog this dose has lower bioavailability and seems to provide little analgesia. A higher OTM dose (0.12 mg/kg) has greater bioavailability, and in a study of dogs undergoing ovariohysterectomy (OVH) it appeared to be an alternative for postoperative pain management when given immediately before anesthetic induction (Ko et al, 2011). However, drug cost and the volume that must be administered (in bigger dogs) may be concerns. Buprenorphine SR is an injectable, sustained-released (polymer) formulation that is designed to release buprenorphine over a 72-hour period; in cats undergoing OVH this appeared to have an efficacy and adverse effect profile comparable to twice-daily OTM administration of buprenorphine (Catbagan et al, 2011). There have been anecdotal reports of some dogs exhibiting dysphoria and anorexia when buprenorphine SR is used at higher doses.

Potential Adverse Effects of Opioids

Critical patients often have altered drug metabolism. Therefore the respiratory depressant effects and dysphoria or excitement seen with higher doses of opioids in healthy patients may be observed with normal or even lower doses in critically ill animals. Opioids can be reversed readily with the use of naloxone; however, buprenorphine is harder to reverse due to its higher affinity for the mu receptor.

Morphine can cause histamine release and lead to the development of hypotension and therefore is given intramuscularly (IM) or subcutaneously (SC) or is diluted for very slow intravenous (IV) administration. Bradycardia can occur with opioid use but is usually of little clinical significance and can be easily treated with atropine or glycopyrrolate. Mu agonists can cause nausea and vomiting even after a single dose and can contribute to a decrease in gut motility or ileus with more chronic exposure.

Of the opioids, hydromorphone and methadone are the most likely to cause panting in dogs. This can lead to potential problems with gas exchange and difficulties when monitoring respiratory rate in dyspneic patients. Therefore these two opioids are best avoided in patients with respiratory compromise or hypoxemia. Additionally, perioperative use of hydromorphone has been associated with the development of postanesthetic hyperthermia, which can be severe (40 to 42°C [104 to 108°F]), in cats. If hyperthermia occurs, cooling measures should be used; if the patient's temperature does not drop, reversal agents such as naloxone should be administered. Careful monitoring of body temperature and respiratory rate in patients receiving opioids, especially cats, is recommended.

Nonsteroidal Antiinflammatory Drugs

Nonsteroidal antiinflammatory drugs (NSAIDs) work by inhibiting cyclooxygenase (COX) and preventing the production of prostaglandins (PGs), which decreases inflammation to provide analgesia. NSAIDs have a longer onset of action (45 to 60 minutes) compared with opioids and most provide analgesia for an extended period (12 to 24 hours). When used in combination with opioids, NSAIDs can have a synergistic effect and provide improved analgesia compared with use of either drug class alone.

Side effects of NSAIDs include gastrointestinal ulceration, renal damage, and a decrease in platelet function. Accordingly, obvious contraindications to NSAIDs include gastrointestinal ulceration or bleeding, platelet dysfunction, renal dysfunction, and concurrent corticosteroid use. Furthermore, hypotension, intravascular volume depletion (from vomiting, diarrhea, hemorrhage, or other fluid losses), and congestive heart failure can also constitute relative or absolute contraindications because these disorders can compromise function of the kidneys and gastrointestinal tract. Thus NSAIDs are most safely used in normovolemic, hemodynamically stable patients. However, carprofen did not cause clinically relevant adverse effects in dogs anesthetized for fracture repair, even when it was administered before surgery or given to patients with trauma-induced alterations in renal function or hemostasis (Bergmann et al, 2005).

Numerous NSAIDs are available in veterinary medicine. Those most commonly used in dogs include carprofen, deracoxib, firocoxib, and meloxicam. Only carprofen and meloxicam are available in an injectable form, so these tend to be used more in hospitalized patients that cannot tolerate oral administration of drugs. Commonly used NSAIDs in the cat are carprofen, ketoprofen, and meloxicam. NSAIDs must be used with caution in this species as cats have a low capacity for hepatic glucuronidation, which can lead to accumulation. Because of this, cat doses should never be extrapolated from those used in dogs.

α₂-Adrenergic Agonists

α_2-Adrenergic agonists produce sedation and analgesia. Other effects include peripheral vasoconstriction with reflex bradycardia followed by centrally mediated vasodilation, respiratory depression, diuresis, and muscle relaxation. Due to the profound cardiovascular changes that occur with α_2-adrenergic agonists (e.g., up to a 50% decrease in cardiac output), they should be limited to patients that are normovolemic and with stable cardiovascular status. Atropine or glycopyrrolate should not be administered concurrently with α_2-adrenergic agonists because coadministration can lead to the development of hypertension and cardiac arrhythmias.

Dexmedetomidine is now the most commonly used α_2-adrenergic agonist in small animal medicine, having replaced medetomidine. Dexmedetomidine is the pharmacologically active enantiomer found in the racemic preparation of medetomidine. Dexmedetomidine can be given IV or IM or used as a CRI. α_2-Adrenergic agonists can be easily reversed with atipamezole administered IM. The IV administration of atipamezole for reversal should be avoided because its use can lead to hyperexcitability or aggression.

Other Drugs

N-Methyl-D-Aspartate Antagonists

Ketamine is an NMDA antagonist that can be used as an adjunct to other analgesia methods to help prevent central sensitization and hyperalgesia. It is usually used as a CRI after a loading dose IV but can also be effective in the short term when given as a single dose. The dosages used are subanesthetic, so sedation generally does not occur.

Amantadine is an antiviral agent that is also an NMDA antagonist. It has been beneficial in the treatment of chronic pain from osteoarthritis when used orally in conjunction with NSAIDs (Lascelles et al, 2008), but further research is required to see if it has a role in the treatment of acute pain.

Gabapentin

Gabapentin is an anticonvulsant drug that is helpful in the treatment of chronic neuropathic pain. It modulates voltage-gated calcium channels. Gabapentin is frequently recommended as part of chronic pain management in veterinary patients despite very few studies of its use. Perioperative administration of gabapentin in dogs undergoing forelimb amputation produced no significant difference in pain scores compared with administration of a placebo (Wagner et al, 2010). Further research is warranted to see if gabapentin is helpful in the management of acute pain.

Routes of Administration

Drugs used to control pain are delivered by a variety of parenteral routes (including IM, IV, and SC) or through oral administration. Some drugs are most effectively administered by an IV CRI in the critical care setting. Additionally anesthetics can be administered locally, by epidural delivery, and via transdermal delivery systems.

Constant Rate Infusions

CRIs offer the best means of achieving analgesia in the critical patient because they provide a consistent level of pain control that can be increased or decreased (within defined limits of dose) to suit the needs of the patient. Fentanyl is probably the most commonly used drug administered by CRI. Side effects of fentanyl can include nausea, bradycardia, and dysphoria as well as respiratory depression (at higher doses). A loading dose is given followed by the CRI. Ketamine can be used as a CRI to help prevent central sensitization and wind-up. Lidocaine CRIs have been shown to provide analgesia, but the exact mechanism has yet to be elucidated. A lidocaine CRI should NOT be used in cats because systemic toxicity is very likely due to a reduced ability to metabolize lidocaine. Neither ketamine nor lidocaine CRIs should be the sole method of analgesia; rather, they should be used in combination with a CRI of an opioid such as fentanyl or morphine.

Local Anesthesia

Local anesthetic drugs work by blocking sodium channels to prevent nerve conduction and are one of the best ways to provide analgesia and prevent wind-up. The most commonly used drugs are lidocaine, which has a rapid onset of action (within 5 minutes) and lasts for 1 to 2 hours, and bupivacaine, which has a longer onset of effect (20 to 30 minutes) but a much longer duration of action (4 to 6 hours). Local infiltration, nerve blocks, splash blocks, and other local anesthetic protocols only last as long as

the duration of the drug chosen. Additionally, some knowledge and training are required to effectively administer nerve blocks (Lemke and Dawson, 2000).

To achieve a longer effect, wound or soaker catheters can be used. These are fenestrated catheters placed into a surgical or wound site before closure or near a nerve(s) that innervate the affected area. These catheters allow for a continuous nerve block or local wound infiltration. Soaker catheters have been shown to be an effective, viable means of providing local analgesia in postoperative veterinary patients (Hansen, 2008).

Care must be taken when using local anesthetics, especially through a wound catheter, not to exceed the recommended safe dose, particularly in cats, a species especially sensitive to the toxic effects of local anesthetic drugs (Table 12-1). Signs of toxicity typically begin as nausea, progressing to hyperexcitability, tremors, seizures, and then cardiovascular collapse. Vomiting may be observed, especially in dogs.

Epidural Analgesia

Epidural administration of drugs is an excellent way to provide analgesia to the caudal half of the body, including the abdomen. Preservative-free morphine (morphine PF) is used most commonly; having low lipid solubility, this drug remains in the epidural space longer than other opioids, with effects lasting 12 to 24 hours (Valverde, 2008). Buprenorphine has also been used effectively in the epidural space. Local anesthetic drugs can also be used in epidural analgesia but may lead to motor paralysis. Bupivacaine is usually administered, instead of lidocaine, because of its longer duration of action (2 to 4 hours).

Side effects of epidurals can include vomiting, urinary retention, pruritus, and delayed regrowth of fur at the clipped site. The failure rate for epidurals is 20% to 30%. Epidural catheters allow more long-term analgesia but require strict asepsis and can be technically difficult to place. Radiographic verification is recommended after placement of epidural catheters. Contraindications for use of an epidural include hypotension, sepsis, coagulopathy, and skin infection at the site. Further information on epidurals and epidural catheters can be found in the references (Valverde, 2008).

Transdermal Analgesia

Fentanyl patches can be used to provide long-term analgesia, but both onset of action and duration of effect can vary considerably. Uptake depends on many factors, including dermal blood flow, presence of fur, obesity, hypothermia, hypovolemia, and proximity to an external heat source. Because of this variation in uptake, animals must be closely monitored for either underdosing or overdosing. It takes 12 to 24 hours after application of the patch for steady-state plasma fentanyl concentrations to be achieved. For this reason, the patch needs to be placed the night before the infliction of surgical pain or alternate drugs must be administered to provide systemic analgesia until the fentanyl patch takes effect. The patch lasts approximately 72 hours in the dog and up to 5 days in the cat. These patches must be appropriately applied to

TABLE 12-1

Dosages of Analgesic Drugs

Drug	Dog	Cat
Opioids		
Buprenorphine	0.01-0.03 mg/kg IV, IM q6-8h; 0.12 mg/kg OTM	0.01-0.02 mg/kg IV, IM, SC, OTM q6-8h
Buprenorphine SR	0.12-0.27 mg/kg SC	0.12 mg/kg SC
Butorphanol	0.2-0.4 mg/kg IV, IM q1-4h	0.2-0.8 mg/kg IV or SC q2-6h
Fentanyl	3-5 µg/kg IV (lasts 5-20 min)	
Fentanyl CRI	2-3 µg/kg LD IV, then 2-6 µg/kg/hr (6-30 µg/kg/hr intra-op)	
Fentanyl-Transdermal	2-4 µg/kg/hr	
Hydromorphone	0.22 mg/kg IV, IM, SC q4-6h	0.1-0.2 mg/kg IV, IM, SC q4-6h
Hydromorphone CRI	0.05-0.1 mg/kg/hr	0.01-0.05 mg/kg/hr
Methadone	0.1-0.5 mg/kg IV q4h; 0.2-1.0 mg/kg IM q4h	0.1-0.5 mg/kg IV q4-6h; 0.2-0.6 mg/kg IM q4-6h
Morphine	0.5-1.0 mg/kg IM, SC q4-6h; epidural: 0.1 mg/kg PF	0.1 mg/kg IM; epidural: 0.1 mg/kg PF
Morphine CRI	0.15-0.5 mg/kg LD SLOWLY IV, then 0.1-0.2 mg/kg/hr	0.2 mg/kg LD slowly IV, then 0.05-0.1 mg/kg/hr
Naloxone	0.01-0.04 mg/kg IV, IM	
Oxymorphone	0.03-0.1 mg/kg IV, IM, SC q4h	0.01-0.05 mg/kg IV q4h; 0.01-0.1 IM, SC q4h
Tramadol	3-10 mg/kg PO q8-12h	3-5 mg/kg PO q12h
NSAIDs		
Carprofen	4.4 mg/kg SC once; 4.4 mg/kg q24h or 2.2 mg/kg PO q12-24h PRN	2-4 mg/kg IV or SC once only
Deracoxib	1-2 mg/kg PO q24h Post-op pain: 3-4 mg/kg PO q24h for up to 7 days	
Firocoxib	5 mg/kg PO q24h Post-op pain: 5 mg/kg PO q24h for up to 3 days	
Ketoprofen	1-2 mg/kg IV, IM, or SC once; 1 mg/kg PO q24h up to 5 days	2 mg/kg SC q24h for up to 3 days; 1 mg/kg PO q24h for up to 5 days
Meloxicam	0.1-0.2 mg/kg IV or SC once; 0.1 mg/kg PO q24h PRN	0.2-0.3 mg/kg SC once only; 0.2 mg/kg SC followed by 0.05 mg/kg PO q24h for up to 4 days; 0.1 mg/kg PO on day 1, then 0.05 mg/kg PO q24h
α₂-Agonists		
Atipamezole	0.05-0.2 mg/kg IM	
Dexmedetomidine	1-5 µg/kg IV; 1-20 µg/kg IM	1-5 µg/kg IV; 1-10 µg/kg IM
Dexmedetomidine CRI	0.5-2.5 µg/kg/hr	
Other Drugs		
Amantadine	3-5 mg/kg PO q24h	
Bupivacaine	Up to 2 mg/kg for nerve blocks; 0.5 mg/kg for epidurals	Up to 1 mg/kg for nerve blocks; 0.5 mg/kg for epidurals
Bupivacaine (wound catheters)	Up to 2 mg/kg q6h	Up to 1 mg/kg q6-8h
Gabapentin	5-40 mg/kg PO q12h	5-20 mg/kg PO q12h
Ketamine	Analgesia without sedation: 0.1-1 mg/kg IV or IM	
Ketamine CRI	0.5 mg/kg IV LD, then 2 µg/kg/min (10 µg/kg/min intra-op)	
Lidocaine	Up to 4 mg/kg for nerve blocks	Up to 2 mg/kg for nerve blocks
Lidocaine CRI	1-2 mg/kg LD IV then 30-50 µg/kg/min	NOT IN CATS
Lidocaine: Transdermal (10 × 14–cm patch)	1.4-2.3 kg (body weight) = ⅛ to ¼ patch; 2.7-4.5 kg = ½ patch; 5-9.1 kg = 1 patch; 9.5-18 kg = 2 patches; 18.6-27.3 kg = 2.5 to 3 patches; 27.7-45.5 kg = 3 to 4 patches	

IV, Intravenous; *IM,* intramuscular; *LD,* loading dose; *OTM,* oral transmucosal route; *PF,* preservative-free; *PO,* orally; *PRN,* as needed; *SC,* subcutaneous.

prevent ingestion, which might be fatal (and if therapy is continued in the home setting, parents must be advised about potential toxicity to children should a patch be ingested).

Lidocaine is also available in a 5% patch and has been shown to provide local analgesia when placed after surgery. The patches can be cut to shape and are usually placed on either side of the incision. No systemic toxic effects have been seen in the dog or cat, but local skin irritation can occur (Weil et al, 2007).

References and Suggested Reading

Bergmann HM, Nolte IJ, Kramer S: Effects of preoperative administration of carprofen on renal function and hemostasis in dogs undergoing surgery for fracture repair, *Am J Vet Res* 66:1356-1363, 2005.

Catbagan DL et al: Comparison of the efficacy and adverse effects of sustained-release buprenorphine hydrochloride following subcutaneous administration and buprenorphine hydrochloride following oral transmucosal administration in cats undergoing ovariohysterectomy, *Am J Vet Res* 72:461-466, 2011.

Ko JC et al: Efficacy of oral transmucosal and intravenous administration of buprenorphine before surgery for postoperative analgesia in dogs undergoing ovariohysterectomy, *J Am Vet Med Assoc* 238:318-328, 2011.

Gaynor JS, Muir WM: *Handbook of veterinary pain management,* ed 2, St Louis, 2009, Mosby Elsevier.

Hansen B: Analgesia for the critically ill dog or cat: an update, *Vet Clin North Am Small Anim Pract* 38:1353-1363, 2008.

Lamont LA: Adjunctive analgesic therapy in veterinary medicine, *Vet Clin North Am Small Anim Pract* 38:1187-1203, 2008.

Lascelles BD et al: Amantadine in a multimodal analgesic regimen for alleviation of refractory osteoarthritis pain in dogs, *J Vet Intern Med* 22:53-59, 2008.

Lemke KA, Dawson SD: Local and regional anesthesia, *Vet Clin North Am Small Anim Pract* 30:839-857, 2000.

Quandt J, Lee JA: Analgesia and constant rate infusions. In Silverstein DC, Hopper K, editors: *Small animal critical care medicine,* St Louis, 2009, Saunders Elsevier, pp 710-716.

Robertson SA et al: PK-PD modeling of buprenorphine in cats: intravenous and oral transmucosal administration, *J Vet Pharmacol Ther* 28:453-460, 2005.

Valverde A: Epidural analgesia and anesthesia in dogs and cats, *Vet Clin North Am Small Anim Pract* 38:1205-1230, 2008.

Wagner AE et al: Clinical evaluation of perioperative administration of gabapentin as an adjunct for postoperative analgesia in dogs undergoing amputation of a forelimb, *J Am Vet Med Assoc* 236:751-756, 2010.

Weil A, Ko J, Inoue T: The use of lidocaine patches, *Compend Contin Educ Vet* 29:208-210, 2007.

CHAPTER 13

Anesthesia for the Critical Care Patient

DEREK FLAHERTY, *Glasgow, Scotland*

Critically ill animals may require chemical restraint for a variety of procedures, ranging from minor interventions such as diagnostic imaging to major surgery. Although a clinician may be tempted to avoid anesthesia due to its inherent risks and instead perform complete procedures under sedation alone, deep sedation is likely to be a greater risk to the animal than "full" general anesthesia. Patients under deep sedation may be unable to maintain and protect their airway, may be breathing room air, and are rarely closely monitored during sedation. However, with general anesthesia the animal usually has an endotracheal tube in place, is receiving supplemental oxygen, and usually has one person dedicated to monitoring and maintaining physiologic function. This is not to say that sedative techniques should be avoided in critically ill animals, merely

that they should only be used in situations in which the procedure can be performed under "light" sedation (often combined with local anesthesia) using drugs that are minimally depressant to the cardiovascular (CV) and respiratory systems. If these caveats cannot be met, general anesthesia is usually preferable. In all critical care patients undergoing any form of chemical restraint, secure intravenous access always should be available, and oxygen should be supplemented at every opportunity.

It is impossible to be prescriptive in terms of the anesthetic requirements of every critically ill animal, but, in general, this type of patient usually presents primarily with underlying dysfunction of the cardiovascular system, the respiratory system, or the central nervous system, although there is often multiorgan pathology.

Anesthesia for Patients with Cardiovascular Dysfunction

CV dysfunction may be related to volume depletion, vascular dysfunction, heart rhythm disturbances, advanced heart disease, or overt congestive heart failure. Appropriately categorizing CV risk and dysfunction is an important aspect of sedation and anesthesia of these patients. Special consideration should be directed to the preanesthetic period, induction of anesthesia, and maintenance.

Specific Patient Groups

The main forms of CV dysfunction encountered in critical care patients relate to hypovolemia or to cardiac arrhythmias. Additionally, some older dogs are affected by advanced valvular heart disease or chronic heart failure. In cats cardiomyopathies (sometime occult) are relatively common.

Hypovolemic Patients

Hypovolemia may be present as a result of dehydration (e.g., protracted vomiting with intestinal obstruction) or blood loss. Virtually all sedative and anesthetic agents cause a degree of CV depression, so the use of these drugs in patients with depleted circulatory volume can result in a severe drop in arterial blood pressure (BP). Consequently, restoration of the circulating blood volume should be undertaken prior to any form of chemical restraint, although there may be an argument for "delayed resuscitation" in those animals with internal hemorrhage (see Chapter 1).

Even following adequate volume resuscitation in hypovolemic patients, it is wise to provide chemical restraint by choosing agents with the least CV-depressant effects and using the lowest doses possible, usually through coinduction and balanced anesthetic techniques (see sections on "Induction of Anesthesia" and "Maintenance of Anesthesia").

Patients with Cardiac Arrhythmias

Cardiac arrhythmias are common in critical care patients. Although these may result from underlying cardiac disease, a number of extracardiac factors also may be responsible (e.g., hypoxemia, hypercapnia, electrolyte disorders). Regardless of etiology, the aim should be to restore normal cardiac rhythm before induction of anesthesia through treatment of underlying pathology, correction of exacerbating factors (e.g., hypokalemia), and judicious use (when necessary) of appropriate antiarrhythmic drugs (see Chapters 171 and 172). However, even with these measures, restoration of normal sinus rhythm may not always be possible, and consideration needs to be given to selection of an anesthetic technique that will not further exacerbate the arrhythmia.

The main aims in critically ill patients with preexisting cardiac arrhythmias are to avoid agents that are proarrhythmic (e.g., α_2-adrenergic agonists, thiopental, halothane) and use balanced anesthetic techniques to minimize the dose of any one agent. Hypoxemia, hypercapnia, and hypotension should be avoided in these animals because they may significantly exacerbate any preexisting arrhythmia. Thus consideration should be paid to preoxygenation prior to induction of anesthesia, oxygen supplementation during the procedure (even if the procedure is performed solely under sedation), and possibly the use of intermittent positive pressure ventilation to avoid excessive hypercapnia, accepting that controlled ventilation may carry detrimental CV side effects (see the section on "Intermittent Positive Pressure Ventilation" later). Drugs that may be required to manage acute exacerbations of the arrhythmia (such as lidocaine) or extremes of heart rate (atropine or glycopyrrolate; esmolol or propranolol) should be readily available. Not only should these drugs be close at hand, but the appropriate volume to be administered calculated in advance. The electrocardiogram should be monitored before, during, and after the anesthetic periods.

Premedication/Sedation of Patients with CV Dysfunction

A significant proportion of critical care cases with CV dysfunction may not require sedative premedication, particularly those that are severely hypovolemic. In general, patients with any degree of hypovolemia should not be given acepromazine because it causes vasodilation and will drop BP. The α_2-adrenergic agonists (xylazine, medetomidine, dexmedetomidine) also should be avoided because they profoundly decrease cardiac output by affecting afterload and heart rate. In contrast, both opioids and benzodiazepines are relatively cardiostable and are extremely useful when dealing with high-risk CV cases.

Although paradoxical excitement can occur when benzodiazepines alone are administered to healthy animals, this is much less likely when used in depressed, critically ill patients. Combining these drugs with an opioid also improves the degree of sedation and limits the likelihood of excitation. The two benzodiazepines commonly used in small animals are diazepam and midazolam. Diazepam is best administered intravenously because it is poorly absorbed and relatively painful when given intramuscularly; midazolam is preferable if the intramuscular route is to be used. Although the latter is significantly more expensive than diazepam, it can be mixed in the same syringe with opioid drugs; this cannot be done with diazepam because precipitation may occur.

A variety of opioids (see Chapter 12) may be used in combination with the benzodiazepines, and the choice depends to a large extent on the procedure that the animal is undergoing. If there is preexisting moderate to severe pain, or if such pain is anticipated following the procedure, a full mu-agonist such as oxymorphone, hydromorphone, morphine, or methadone would be most appropriate because these can be titrated to the degree of pain. Partial agonists such as butorphanol or buprenorphine may be suitable alternatives but are less efficacious analgesics and should be limited to mild to moderate pain only. The full opioid agonists can also be antagonized (most commonly by naloxone) if the situation suddenly deteriorates, although this is uncommon if excessive doses are avoided. Table 13-1 lists suggested doses for each agent.

TABLE **13-1**

Opioids Commonly Used for Sedation/Premedication of Critically Ill Animals with CV Disease

Drug	Suggested Dose and Administration Route	Approximate Duration	Comments
Morphine	0.1-1.0 mg/kg, SC, IM, or IV	4-6 hr (dog) 6-8 hr (cat)	Morphine may cause emesis and should be avoided when this is contraindicated (e.g., esophageal foreign body; raised intracranial pressure; penetrating eye injury). Morphine may cause histamine release, particularly when given IV; thus, if the IV route is used, the drug should be diluted and administered slowly over approximately 10 min. Doses at the lower end of the scale should be used in cats to avoid excitation.
Meperidine (pethidine)	3.5-5 mg/kg IM (dog) 5-10 mg/kg SC or IM (cat)	1-1.5 hr	Meperidine is contraindicated by the IV route because it may cause massive histamine release/cardiac arrest. Does not tend to achieve therapeutic analgesic levels in dogs when given SC, but may do so in cats if given at higher doses.
Methadone	0.1-1.0 mg/kg SC, IM, or IV	4-6 hr	Much less likely to cause vomiting than morphine. Antagonist at the NMDA receptor so may help block/reverse central sensitization.
Hydromorphone	0.05-0.1 mg/kg SC, IM, or IV	~4 hr	May cause vomiting, so contraindicated in similar situations to morphine (see above). May cause hyperthermia in cats.
Buprenorphine	0.01-0.02 mg/kg SC, IM, or IV	~6 hr	Partial opioid agonist. Duration of analgesia variable, with some studies suggesting up to 12 hr.
Butorphanol	0.2-0.8 mg/kg SC, IM, or IV	? 1-1.5 hr	Partial opioid agonist/agonist-antagonist. Analgesic efficacy extremely variable. Duration of action probably shorter than generally accepted.

IM, Intramuscularly; *IV,* intravenously; *NMDA,* n-Methyl-D-Aspartic Acid; *SC,* subcutaneously.

There is huge variability between individual patients in terms of dose requirements and analgesic response, and the doses/durations in Table 13-1 are intended only as a general guide.

Induction of Anesthesia

Most of the commonly used induction agents (thiopental, propofol, alfaxalone) can cause hypotension even in healthy patients, and in critical animals this can be profound. For this reason, these agents are not recommended by themselves for anesthetic induction in patients with limited CV reserve. Although combinations of ketamine/diazepam are considered relatively "cardiac-safe" in healthy animals (in that cardiac output and arterial BP are usually well maintained), the high preexisting (often maximal) sympathetic tone evident in most critically ill patients means that the animal may not be able to compensate for the direct negative inotropic effects of ketamine in the same manner as healthy animals; as a result, BP may fall to a similar extent to that of the previously discussed induction agents.

Etomidate is a nonbarbiturate sedative-hypnotic drug often used as an intravenous induction drug in human patients with CV disease because it has minimal effects on cardiac output and arterial BP. Although not licensed for veterinary use, it has been extensively used in dogs and cats with significant preexisting arrhythmias, cardiac pathology, or ongoing hypovolemia. This drug must be used with attention to potential adverse effects. Due to the high osmolarity of the solution, etomidate can cause pain on injection and thrombophlebitis. As a result, it is probably best administered into a free-flowing intravenous fluid line so it is suitably diluted before it enters the patient's vein; this is probably more important in cats due to the small vein size. Etomidate can also cause myoclonus (twitching) at induction, as well as excitement and muscle movements during anesthetic recovery; this is much more common if the drug has not been preceded by a benzodiazepine or a potent opioid such as fentanyl. Additionally, etomidate causes suppression of cortisol production, so should only be administered as a single intravenous induction dose or acute hypoadrenocorticism may be observed. Some anesthesiologists recommend administering physiologic doses of glucocorticoids on the day that a patient receives etomidate.

With all the aforementioned anesthetic induction agents, it is essential to minimize the dose used when administered to patients with unstable CV status. This can be achieved using a coinduction technique, which implies the use of one or more additional drugs alongside the main hypnotic agent. The coinduction drug(s) used should be capable of reducing the dose of hypnotic required to produce unconsciousness, while at the same time having minimal CV-depressant effects of their own. The most common coinduction agents used are the potent, short-acting opioids, such as fentanyl and alfentanil, and the benzodiazepines, diazepam and midazolam.

For coinduction, one of these opioids or benzodiazepines (or a combination) is administered intravenously immediately before the chosen hypnotic agent, resulting in a reduced dose requirement for the latter and reduced CV depression.

As an alternative, and particularly for those animals with severe CV compromise in which even a small dose of hypnotic drug may not be tolerated, a combination benzodiazepine/opioid induction protocol can be very useful. Because both groups of drugs are relatively cardiostable, they can be given in fairly high doses to achieve induction of anesthesia. The most common technique utilizes a combination of fentanyl and diazepam: a dose of 10 μg/kg fentanyl and a dose of 0.5 mg/kg diazepam are drawn up into separate syringes. After a 3- to 5-minute period of preoxygenation by facemask, half the fentanyl (5 μg/kg) is administered intravenously, followed by half of the diazepam (0.25 mg/kg). Adequate time must be allowed for the drugs to reach peak effect, since this technique results in slower induction than traditional intravenous induction techniques. In addition, the appearance of animals following benzodiazepine/opioid induction is different to that following "classical" anesthetic induction; these patients may occasionally remain in sternal recumbency and often appear quite awake, with centrally positioned glazed eyes. However, even in this state many still tolerate intubation of the trachea. If anesthesia is inadequate for endotracheal intubation, further increments of the two drugs are delivered until unconsciousness is achieved. On occasion, particularly if the animal was not significantly depressed prior to induction of anesthesia, inadequate hypnosis may not be achieved after the full doses of diazepam and fentanyl have been administered; unconsciousness can then be produced with an intravenous hypnotic such as propofol or alfaxalone, but only very small doses of these agents are required due to the anesthetic sparing effects of both fentanyl and diazepam. High doses of fentanyl can result in bradycardia; this can usually be avoided if the drug is given very slowly over several minutes, but it is wise to have an antimuscarinic (atropine or glycopyrrolate) drawn up and ready to administer, if necessary. Alternatively, some authorities recommend *pretreatment* with an antimuscarinic if a benzodiazepine/opioid induction technique is to be used, although this may in itself lead to some CV instability due to the likely transient tachycardia.

Maintenance of Anesthesia

All the volatile anesthetic agents cause CV depression, either by direct effects on myocardial contractility (halothane) or by vasodilation (isoflurane, sevoflurane), and these effects are dose-dependent, so it is important to use as low a vaporizer setting as possible. Nitrous oxide, on the other hand, has minimal effects on CV function and allows a reduction in the concentration of volatile agent required to maintain anesthesia. Consequently, inclusion of nitrous oxide (if available) generally allows better preservation of cardiac output and arterial BP. Similarly, potent *short-acting* opioids given by intermittent intravenous bolus injection (fentanyl) or by constant rate infusion (fentanyl, alfentanil, remifentanil) are also extremely useful in reducing the requirement for volatile anesthetics and promoting a relatively stable CV status during anesthesia; this is commonly referred to as a balanced anesthetic technique (although, more correctly, this term only applies if neuromuscular blocking drugs are also used). While exerting minimal direct effects on contractility and arterial BP, these short-acting opioids can reduce cardiac output by causing profound bradycardia and less frequently ventricular asystole. These adverse effects are more common when opioids are given by intravenous bolus injection, and especially if high doses are used.

These complications, although seemingly more common with alfentanil and remifentanil, can occur with all three drugs and can be avoided in several ways:

- Avoid giving intravenous boluses, and only use constant rate infusions (CRIs), bearing in mind that it takes time for a CRI to achieve stable therapeutic blood levels if not preceded by a bolus dose.
- Preadminister atropine or glycopyrrolate immediately before these drugs (more important prior to alfentanil or remifentanil boluses than fentanyl, and probably unnecessary if only using them by CRI).
- Most importantly, when using IV bolus techniques, slowly titrate the dose to the pulse rate during several minutes of administration.

The downside to the relative cardiostability of the short-acting opioids relates to marked respiratory depression, so intermittent positive pressure ventilation is likely to be required (see the section on "Intermittent Positive Pressure Ventilation" later). Appropriate doses for the short-acting opioids during maintenance of anesthesia are given in Table 13-2. When these agents are not available, longer-acting agents, such as oxymorphone, morphine, or methadone, should be considered.

Regional local anesthesia (e.g., epidural analgesia) should also be considered to minimize the requirement for anesthetic maintenance agents, as well as to maximize postoperative pain relief. These techniques are well described in the literature (see References and Suggested Reading) and generally require some training before they are mastered.

Neuromuscular blocking drugs ("muscle relaxants") may also be used in critically ill patients to minimize anesthetic requirements. Because these drugs have neither hypnotic nor analgesic activities, care should be paid at all times to maintenance of unconsciousness. These agents should not be used by those unfamiliar with them.

Finally when dealing with patients with compromised CV systems, attention should be paid to support of *oxygenation*, since these patients are likely to suffer severe detrimental effects from even short periods of hypoxemia. This principle is applicable from preinduction through recovery because respiratory depressant effects of the anesthetic agents are likely to persist even after completion of the procedure.

Intermittent Positive Pressure Ventilation

As described earlier, critically ill animals often receive potent short-acting opioid drugs as part of their

TABLE **13-2**

Doses of Short-Acting Opioids Used During Maintenance of Anesthesia*

Drug	IV Bolus Dose	IV CRI Dose	Potential Side Effects
Fentanyl	2-5 µg/kg (lasts ~ 20 min after single bolus dose)	0.1-0.7 µg/kg/min (dog) 0.1-0.5 µg/kg/min (cat)	Respiratory depression/apnea. Bradycardia.
Alfentanil	5-10 µg/kg (only lasts ~5 min after single bolus dose, so not commonly used in this manner during maintenance of anesthesia)	1-2 µg/kg/min	Respiratory depression/apnea. Bradycardia. Potential asystole if bolus dose not preceded by atropine or glycopyrrolate.
Remifentanil	Not recommended as a bolus	0.1-0.5 µg/kg/min	Respiratory depression/apnea. Bradycardia. Potential asystole if bolus dose not preceded by atropine or glycopyrrolate.

*Note: none of these are licensed for animal use.

anesthesia. This may result in significant respiratory depression with the consequent need for controlled ventilation (intermittent positive pressure ventilation [IPPV]), especially when higher opioid doses are used. IPPV also may be required during general anesthesia for other reasons such as preexisting respiratory impairment or during thoracotomy. In addition, the commonest acid-base disturbance encountered in ill animals is metabolic acidosis; the body's normal response to this is a respiratory compensation with increased ventilation to lower carbon dioxide levels. However, because virtually all anesthetic agents depress ventilation, respiratory compensation may be inadequate or so depressed that a combined metabolic *and* respiratory acidosis develops. In these cases pH declines dramatically and severe acidemia may develop.

Thus it may be prudent to consider IPPV when anesthetizing animals with preexisting metabolic acidosis and to hyperventilate them to maintain carbon dioxide at lower-than-normal levels to compensate for the metabolic acidosis. Among its adverse effects, IPPV tends to impair venous return, which reduces cardiac output and arterial BP. Many patients with moderate-to-severe metabolic acidosis are already hypotensive; thus institution of IPPV may actually worsen the degree of CV compromise. This creates a dilemma: allowing spontaneous ventilation in animals with metabolic acidosis may cause a further drop in pH with potential for worsening CV function, whereas institution of IPPV may help normalize pH but also depresses CV function. There is no "right answer" in this situation and judgment is required. If IPPV is used in any high-risk patient, inflation pressures should be kept as low as possible to minimize the depression of CV function.

Sodium Bicarbonate

Intravenous sodium bicarbonate may be indicated in patients with moderate-to-severe metabolic acidosis. However, its use is somewhat controversial because administration is not without potential side effects. Although metabolic acidosis itself may undoubtedly lead to detrimental metabolic and negative inotropic consequences, the adverse effects of sodium bicarbonate therapy may outweigh the benefits. Sodium bicarbonate combines with hydrogen ions in the body to produce carbonic acid, which rapidly dissociates into water and carbon dioxide. If ventilatory function is impaired, carbon dioxide can accumulate, leading to respiratory acidosis. Thus sodium bicarbonate therapy should only be considered when there is already adequate respiratory compensation. If carbon dioxide is higher than expected, the animal is unlikely to be able to eliminate the additional carbon dioxide produced by the administration of sodium bicarbonate. Even in animals with normal ventilation, the production of carbon dioxide following sodium bicarbonate administration can lead to a paradoxical cerebrospinal fluid (CSF) acidosis, since sodium bicarbonate cannot cross the blood-brain barrier (due to its ionization) but carbon dioxide can readily diffuse across. Animals receiving IPPV during sodium bicarbonate administration may require an increase in tidal volume or respiratory rate to eliminate the additional carbon dioxide being generated. Other possible side effects of sodium bicarbonate administration include an overshoot metabolic alkalosis, hypernatremia, hypokalemia, and hypocalcemia, as well as a leftward shift of the oxyhemoglobin dissociation curve, which limits oxygen delivery to tissues. Although alternative alkalinizing solutions are available (e.g., tromethamine [THAM]), they are less commonly used than sodium bicarbonate.

Due to the potential adverse effects described previously, there are no generally accepted guidelines for sodium bicarbonate administration. The cause of the acidosis should be established first, the most common in the majority of veterinary patients being lactic acidosis associated with hypovolemia. Thus attempts at restoration of circulating volume should be undertaken as a first-line measure. Although this may not completely eliminate the acidosis, it is often sufficient to correct it to a milder level (pH >7.2) in which sodium bicarbonate may not be required. When it is determined that ventilation is adequate and metabolic acidosis severe, sodium bicarbonate is probably indicated. Dosage is based on blood-gas analysis and calculated as:

$$0.3 \times \text{body weight (kg)} \times \text{base deficit (mmol/L)}$$
$$= \text{mmol of } HCO_3^- \text{ required.}$$

Sodium bicarbonate is available in a variety of concentrations, but the 8.4% solution is most convenient since 1 ml of this concentration contains 1 mmol (mEq) of HCO_3^-. Initially, approximately one half of the total volume calculated is infused over 20 to 30 minutes, and a repeat blood-gas analysis is then performed to avoid overcorrection. The aim of sodium bicarbonate therapy is not necessarily to restore the pH to within the normal range but to increase it to a level where it is less likely to be detrimental to the patient.

Anesthesia for Patients with Respiratory Dysfunction

Critical care animals with respiratory impairment can be broadly subdivided into those suffering from pleural space disorders (e.g., pneumothorax), those with parenchymal disease such as pneumonia, and those with major airway obstruction. The most important point when dealing with these patients is to attempt to improve or stabilize respiratory function as much as possible prior to general anesthesia. In some cases, such as an obstructed airway due to laryngeal paralysis, anesthesia is required to correct the problem and allow intubation. In most cases of pneumothorax or pleural effusion thoracocentesis should be done first. Optimally this would proceed with oxygen supplementation and local anesthesia; however, some patients require sedation or anesthesia. Unless thoracocentesis can be performed under mild sedation and a local anesthetic block, it may be safer to administer general anesthesia because moderate-marked sedation may worsen respiratory function without the clinician having any control over ventilation.

In terms of anesthesia, the general rule with the majority of respiratory disorders is to go from minimal interference to maximal support. This implies that in most cases premedication should either be withheld altogether or should be light. Thus drug choice is not particularly critical, but doses should be kept low. It is usually best to avoid potentially emetic drugs (e.g., xylazine, morphine, hydromorphone) in animals with respiratory compromise. Likewise, choice of induction agent is probably not important, but it should be given as a rapid bolus rather than titrated to effect, to achieve endotracheal intubation as quickly as possible. From this point, ventilation can be supported if necessary by IPPV. One additional point: preoxygenate all critically ill animals with respiratory impairment for 3 to 5 minutes prior to administration of the induction agent.

A number of agents are suitable for anesthetic maintenance in these animals, although those providing a more rapid recovery (e.g., sevoflurane) may offer benefits. The tendency of nitrous oxide to expand gas-filled spaces would contraindicate its use during anesthetic maintenance in animals with closed pneumothorax; it should also be used with caution in other forms of respiratory disease unless adequacy of oxygenation can be confirmed by pulse oximetry or arterial blood-gas analysis. Regardless of the maintenance agent used, anesthetic-induced respiratory depression may persist for

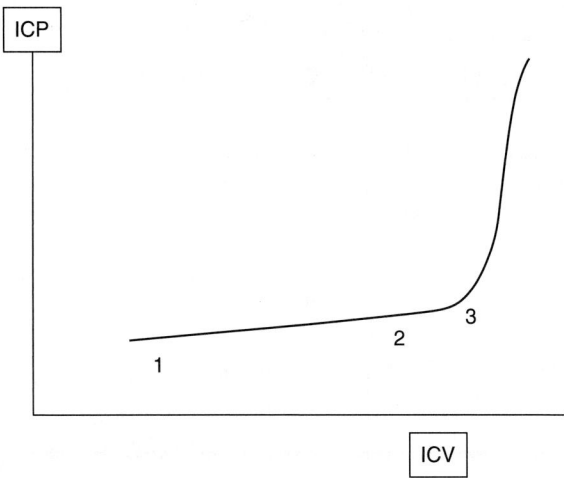

Figure 13-1 Intracranial elastance curve.

some time in recovery, so supplemental oxygen should be provided during this period.

Anesthesia for Patients with Intracranial Pathology

Administration of anesthesia for patients with intracranial pathology is not for the faint-hearted. A thorough understanding of the physiology underlying cerebral blood flow (CBF) and intracranial pressure (ICP) and the influence of sedative and anesthetic agents on these parameters is a prerequisite for successful anesthetic outcome.

A few basic principles can be enumerated. The cranial vault is a rigid structure containing brain tissue, blood, and CSF. An increase in the volume of any one of these three components necessitates a reduction in volume of one of the others or an increase in ICP will ensue. As intracranial volume (ICV) increases, rises in ICP are initially prevented in normal patients by a process of isobaric spatial compensation. This entails initial redistribution of CSF from the cranial vault to the spinal compartment; once this reserve is exhausted, venous blood is redistributed away from the cranial vault. When these two mechanisms have been expended, however, continuing increases in ICV will result in ICP increasing sharply (Figure 13-1).

If the animal is sitting at point 1 on the intracranial elastance curve (see Figure 13-1) and there is an increase in ICV for some reason (for instance, an increase in blood flow to the brain), there is likely to be movement of the graph to the right toward point 2. However, the compensatory effects previously described prevent an increase in ICP. If, on the other hand, the animal starts at point 2 on the graph, any small increase in ICV can lead to a dramatic increase in ICP. Unfortunately, it is not possible to determine at what point on the curve a patient lies, and one should therefore assume that any small increase in ICV will increase ICP. Precautions are taken to prevent this (see later).

Cerebral function depends on adequate cerebral perfusion pressure (CPP), which is defined as the difference

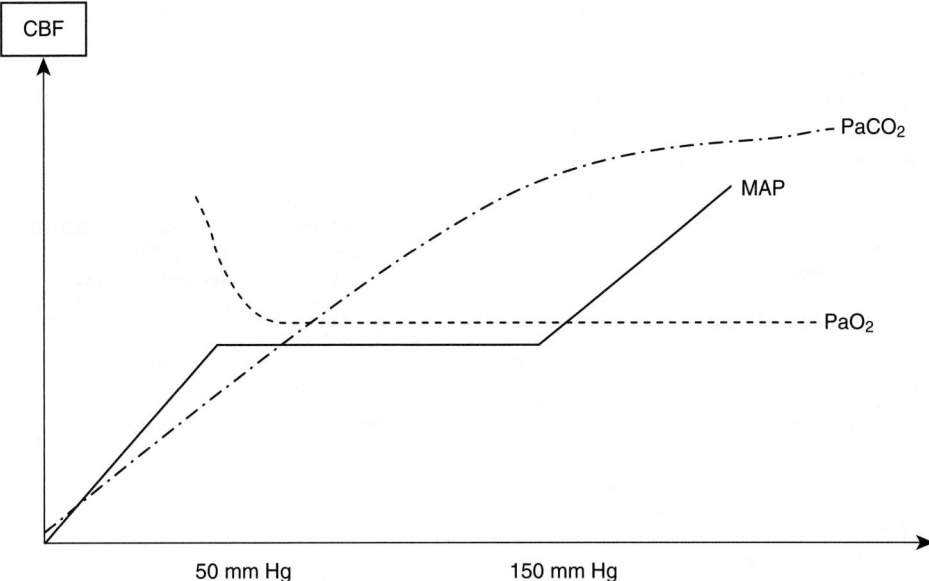

Figure 13-2 Effect of mean arterial blood pressure (MAP), PaO_2, and $PaCO_2$ on cerebral blood flow (CBF).

between mean arterial pressure (MAP) and ICP or central venous pressure (CVP), whichever is greater:

$$CPP = MAP - ICP$$

If ICP increases for any reason, cerebral perfusion can be maintained only if MAP rises. Marked elevations in MAP may occur in some patients, and these can trigger a baroreceptor response, resulting in a subsequent bradycardia. This is the so-called Cushing's response, and should be suspected in any head trauma patient with bradycardia. When a Cushing's response is suspected, arterial BP should be measured and there should be an attempt to lower ICP, usually by administering mannitol (0.25 to 1 g/kg intravenously over 20 minutes). Use of antimuscarinics to treat the bradycardia in these animals is contraindicated because this may lead to marked hypertension, which may in turn result in brain herniation.

The brain normally compensates for variations in arterial BP through autoregulation; thus CBF is usually maintained at a constant level between MAPs of approximately 50 to 150 mm Hg. Hypotension and hypertension lead to a decrease or increase in CBF, respectively (Figure 13-2).

Alterations in $PaCO_2$ have profound effects on CBF, with a directly proportionate relationship between $PaCO_2$ levels of 20 to 80 mm Hg (see Figure 13-2). Thus, as CO_2 levels increase, CBF also increases, and this may lead to elevations in ICP if compensatory mechanisms are already maximal (see Figure 13-1). This has important implications for control of ventilation during anesthesia in animals with intracranial disease. Within the normal physiologic range, changes in PaO_2 have minimal effects on CBF (see Figure 13-2). However, hypoxemia ($PaO_2 <$ 60 mm Hg) dramatically increases CBF.

General anesthesia can increase CBF and ICP through a variety of mechanisms. A number of the drugs commonly used for premedication, induction, and maintenance of anesthesia have effects on the cerebral vasculature. Sedative premedication may not be required in cases with intracranial pathology because consciousness may already be depressed. However, if required, opioids may provide mild sedation without significant effects on ICP. Morphine and hydromorphone should be avoided, however, due to the potential for vomiting, which can lead to an acute, dramatic elevation of ICP. In addition, acepromazine should also be avoided as it induces vasodilation, which increases CBF. If additional sedation is required after opioid administration, low doses (1 to 2 µg/kg) of medetomidine or dexmedetomidine appear to have minimal effects on ICP in experimental studies.

Most induction agents are compatible with cranial pathology, with the exception of ketamine, which increases cerebral metabolic rate and CBF. To this author's knowledge, no studies have assessed the effects on alfaxalone on CBF or ICP.

Patients should be preoxygenated for 3 to 5 minutes by facemask prior to induction of anesthesia to avoid potential hypoxemia, with consequent increase in CBF. Similarly, endotracheal intubation induces a hypertensive response that can be avoided by ensuring that anesthesia is not excessively light prior to intubation and by administering either a short-acting potent opioid (fentanyl, alfentanil) or a bolus of lidocaine (dogs only), intravenously, just before attempted intubation.

Both isoflurane and sevoflurane are suitable for maintenance of anesthesia in these patients, provided excessive depth is avoided, with several human studies suggesting that sevoflurane may result in improved outcome. Propofol CRI appears to be a suitable alternative maintenance technique in dogs.

Since all anesthetics depress ventilation, the resultant increase in $PaCO_2$ can lead to vasodilation, which increases CBF (see Figure 13-2), and potentially ICP. For this reason, IPPV should be undertaken, with the aim of maintaining $PaCO_2$ at approximately 35 to 40 mm Hg in dogs and 30 to 35 mm Hg in cats.

Finally, care should be taken with maintenance fluid provision in patients with intracranial pathology. Lactated Ringer's solution (Hartmann's solution) is slightly hypotonic and may promote cerebral edema; 0.9% saline is generally a better choice. Excessive administration rates also should be avoided.

References and Suggested Reading

Kushner LI: Guidelines for anesthesia in critically ill feline patients. In Drobatz KJ, Costello MF, editors: *Feline emergency and critical care medicine*, Iowa, 2010, Wiley-Blackwell, pp 39-52.

Kushner LI: Pain management in critically ill feline patients guidelines. In Drobatz KJ, Costello MF, editors: *Feline emergency and critical care medicine*, Iowa, 2010, Wiley-Blackwell, pp 63-76.

Leece E: Neurological disease. In Seymour C, Duke-Novakovski T, editors: *BSAVA manual of canine and feline anaesthesia and analgesia*, ed 2, Gloucester, 2007, British Small Animal Veterinary Association, pp 284-295.

Lemke KA: Pain management II: local and regional anaesthetic techniques. In Seymour C, Duke-Novakovski T, editors: *BSAVA manual of canine and feline anaesthesia and analgesia*. ed 2, Gloucester, 2007, British Small Animal Veterinary Association, pp 104-114.

CHAPTER 14
Hyperthermia and Heat-Induced Illness

ELISA M. MAZZAFERRO, *Stamford, Connecticut*

Hyperthermia, defined as a severe elevation body temperature from 40.5° to 43°C (104.9° to 109.4°F), can occur with exposure to elevated ambient temperatures and high ambient humidity, after strenuous activity, or as a normal physiologic process in response to endogenous or exogenous pyrogens. A fever differs from hyperthermia in that with a fever, or pyrogenic hyperthermia, the thermoregulatory center set point in the hypothalamus is elevated in response to infection and inflammation. Nonpyrogenic hyperthermia is abnormal and is secondary to an inability to dissipate heat. Animals that exercise or are allowed to work or exert themselves under conditions of high environmental temperatures can develop hyperthermia in as little as 30 minutes unless adequate access to shade, water, and rest period is available.

Pathophysiology

Core body temperature is controlled by a thermoregulatory center that is located in the hypothalamus. Heat balance occurs through the actions of heat-gaining and heat-dissipating mechanisms. Heat gain occurs through oxidative metabolic processes after eating, exercise or increased metabolic activity, and elevated environmental temperature. Heat-dissipating mechanisms mitigate heat gain and include changes in behavior such as

seeking a cooler location, peripheral vasodilation, and evaporative cooling in the form of respiratory heat exchange, radiation, and convection. When environmental temperature increases and approaches body temperature, evaporative heat loss becomes important to maintain normothermia. Domestic animals such as dogs and cats that largely lack sweat glands depend primarily on the dissipation of heat in the form of evaporative cooling from the respiratory system during panting. Panting is an adaptive mechanism to help dissipate heat and prevent hyperthermia. As body temperature increases, the thermoregulatory center in the hypothalamus is activated, senses a change in temperature, and sends a relay of signals to the panting center. The animal responds by panting, increasing both dead space ventilation and evaporative cooling mechanisms in an attempt to dissipate heat. Evaporative cooling occurs as air comes in contact with the mucous membranes of the upper airways. Evaporative cooling mechanisms are not efficient if high ambient humidity is present, and the body's core temperature continues to rise. Early, an increase in dead space ventilation occurs, with little effect on carbon dioxide elimination. As hyperthermia progresses, however, metabolic alkalosis can occur. With prolonged hyperthermia, the body's normal adaptive mechanisms no longer compensate, and cerebrospinal fluid hypocapnia and alkalosis, factors that normally decrease panting, are no longer effective, and panting continues.

Convection is a second method of cooling by which heat is passively transferred from an overheated animal to a cooler surface. Peripheral vasodilation increases blood flow to the skin and periphery and helps to dissipate heat by convective mechanisms. Peripheral vasodilation causes a state of relative hypovolemia, and in order to maintain adequate blood pressure, splanchnic vessels constrict to maintain adequate circulating volume. Catecholamines are released, causing an increase in heart rate and cardiac output. Early in hyperthermia, there is an increase in cardiac output and decrease in peripheral vascular resistance. However, as hyperthermia progresses, blood pressure and cardiac output decrease when the body can no longer compensate. Perfusion to vital organs decreases and can result in widespread organ damage if left untreated.

Widespread thermal injury occurs to neuronal tissue, cardiac myocytes, hepatocytes, renal parenchymal and tubular cells, and the gastrointestinal tract. The combined effects of decreased organ perfusion, enzyme dysfunction, and uncoupling of oxidative phosphorylation are a decrease in aerobic glycolysis and an increase in tissue oxygen debt, both of which contribute to increased lactate production and lactic acidosis. Lactic acidosis can occur within 3 to 4 hours of initial heat-induced injury.

Direct thermal injury to renal tubular and parenchymal cells, decreased renal blood flow, and hypotension cause hypoxic damage to the tubular epithelium and cell death. As hyperthermia progresses, renal vessel thrombosis can occur with disseminated intravascular coagulation (DIC). Consistent findings in patients affected with severe hyperthermia are renal tubular casts and glycosuria on urinalysis in the presence of normoglycemia. Rhabdomyolysis can also be associated with severe myoglobinuria and pigment-associated damage to the renal tubular epithelium.

The gastrointestinal tract is a key factor in multiorgan failure associated with hyperthermia. Decreased mesenteric and gastrointestinal perfusion and thermal injury to enterocytes often result in a disruption of the gastrointestinal mucosal barrier, with subsequent bacterial translocation. Bacteremia and elevation of circulating bacterial endotoxin can lead to sepsis, systemic inflammatory response syndrome (SIRS), and multiorgan failure. Patients with severe hyperthermia can present with hematemesis and severe hematochezia, and often slough the lining of their gastrointestinal tract.

Thermal damage to the liver can result in decreased hepatic function, with elevations of hepatocellular enzyme activities and increased alanine transaminase (ALT), aspartate transaminase (AST), and total bilirubin. Necropsy findings in one retrospective study of 42 dogs with hyperthermia found centrilobular necrosis, widespread tissue congestion, hemorrhagic diathesis, and pulmonary infarction. Persistent hypoglycemia in affected patients may be associated with hepatocellular dysfunction and glycogen depletion. Decreased hepatic macrophage function and portal hypotension can also predispose the patient to sepsis, with associated bacteremia and SIRS.

Virchow's triad (vascular endothelial injury, venous stasis, and a hypercoagulable state) develops during hyperthermia and heat-induced illness. Widespread endothelial damage with exposure of subendothelial collagen and tissue factor cause systemic platelet activation, consumption of clotting factors, and activation of the fibrinolytic pathway. Sluggish blood flow during periods of hypotension, decreased production of clotting factors, and loss of natural anticoagulants such as antithrombin from the gastrointestinal tract combine to predispose the patient to DIC. Massive global thrombosis associated with DIC can result in multiorgan dysfunction syndrome (MODS) and death.

Finally, hyperthermia can cause direct damage to neurons, neuronal death, and cerebral edema. Thrombosis or intracranial hemorrhage can also occur with DIC. Damage to the hypothalamic thermoregulatory center, localized intraparenchymal bleeding, infarction, and cellular necrosis can all lead to seizures. Altered levels of consciousness are among the most common clinical signs of heat-induced illness. As hyperthermia progresses, severe central nervous system depression, seizures, coma, and death may occur. The potential for reversal of cerebral edema is related to the duration of the neurons to heat exposure. Severe abnormalities in mentation are associated with a negative outcome in animals with hyperthermia. In one retrospective study of dogs, the only presenting clinical sign that was negatively associated with outcome was if the animal was comatose on presentation. A less favorable outcome was also associated with the development of stupor, coma, or seizures within 45 minutes of presentation.

Risk Factors

A number of factors can increase the risk of heat stroke, including high ambient humidity, upper airway obstruction, laryngeal paralysis, brachiocephalic airway syndrome, collapsing trachea, obesity, and a previous history of hyperthermia or heat-induced illness. A lack of shade and no allowance for a cooldown period after exercise can predispose an animal for the development of exertional heatstroke or exertional hyperthermia. Any animal that works or exercises in a hot humid climate without acclimation must be allowed time to rest in a cool, shady place with plenty of water every 30 minutes.

Differential Diagnoses

Differential diagnoses in patients with rectal temperatures greater than 40.5°C (104.9°F) include a number of infectious and immune-mediated inflammatory diseases, such as those of the central nervous system (e.g., meningitis and encephalitis). Hypothalamic mass lesions affecting the thermoregulatory center are another cause, although rare. Other potential differential diagnoses include malignant hyperthermia (particularly in Labrador retrievers) and unwitnessed seizure activity. Toxins such as metaldehyde, strychnine, and neurogenic mycotoxins can also cause seizures and muscle tremors that can lead to hyperthermia. Opiates, especially hydromorphone, can result in profound hyperthermia, especially in cats.

In an animal with no other signs of infection or systemic inflammation, heatstroke or hyperthermia must be considered on the list of differential diagnoses. This issue is important when considering treatment, as pyrogenic hyperthermia (fever) is a normal physiologic process in response to any number of endogenous or exogenous pyrogens. This occurs as the body attempts to kill the offending organism or mount an immunologic response. Nonpyrogenic hyperthermia results from an inability to adequately dissipate heat. Therefore antipyretic agents (such as nonsteroidal antiinflammatory drugs [NSAIDs]) are not only ineffective in reducing body temperature in animals with heat-induced illness, but are also contraindicated due to their potentially adverse side effects of reducing gastrointestinal and renal perfusion; they also contribute to gastrointestinal ulceration and renal failure.

Clinical Signs

Patients that present with heat-induced illness or hyperthermia often have a history of excessive panting, collapse, vomiting, ataxia, hypersalivation, seizures, or diarrhea. Other clinical signs can include lethargy, muscle fasciculations or tremors, altered level of consciousness, seizure, hematuria, cyanosis, epistaxis, swollen tongue, head tremors, vocalization, stridor, and dilated pupils. Changes in mentation, oliguria, vomiting, hematemesis, diarrhea, respiratory distress, icterus, and petechial hemorrhages can occur almost immediately after heat-induced illness or within 3 to 5 days after the inciting event. All animals that have sustained heatstroke and hyperthermia should be watched carefully during this period.

Laboratory Changes

Animals with hyperthermia should have serial complete blood counts (CBCs), biochemical analyses, coagulation tests (prothrombin test [PT], activated partial thromboplastin time [aPTT]), arterial blood gas, venous lactate, and urinalyses performed. Prerenal and renal azotemia may be present, with elevations in serum blood urea nitrogen (BUN) and creatinine secondary to renal tubular necrosis. Higher mortality has been reported when serum creatinine is greater than 1.5 mg/dl in dogs with heat-induced illness. Hepatocellular injury and hepatic thrombosis can cause elevation in serum ALT, AST, alkaline phosphatase, and total bilirubin. The presence of hypocholesterolemia, hypoalbuminemia, and hypoproteinemia has been associated with a less favorable outcome. Additionally, serum total bilirubin and creatinine were found to be higher in nonsurvivors than survivors. Elevations in creatine kinase (CK) and AST can occur secondary to rhabdomyolysis. Blood glucose may be decreased, but this is an inconsistent finding. A higher mortality rate has been observed in heatstroke patients whose blood glucose remained low despite aggressive supplementation or was less than 47 mg/dl.

Packed cell volume and total solids may be increased secondary to hypovolemia and dehydration, with subsequent hemoconcentration. Elevations in peripheral nucleated red blood cells have been associated with increased morbidity and mortality in dogs with heat-induced illness. Thrombocytopenia, prolonged PT and aPTT, and elevated fibrin degradation products (FDPs) may be observed in the presence of DIC. Thrombocytopenia is one of the most common clinicopathologic abnormalities observed in animals with heat-induced illness; however, in one study there was no significant difference in platelet counts of survivors versus nonsurvivors. Thrombocytopenia may not become apparent for several days after the initial insult, so serial CBCs should be performed over time in the most critical animals. The presence of coagulation abnormalities may or may not be associated with an increased risk of mortality. In one study, a calculated discomfort index, but not environmental temperature, was significantly associated with the development of DIC. Arterial blood gas analyses can be variable, with a respiratory alkalosis and metabolic acidosis and a mixed acid-base disturbance. The need for administration of sodium bicarbonate is a negative prognostic indicator. Urinalysis may reveal the presence of renal tubular casts or glucosuria, both indicators of renal tubular epithelial damage. Myoglobinuria secondary to rhabdomyolysis also can contribute to severe acute renal tubular necrosis.

Treatment

Management of hyperthermia and heat-induced illness involves first treating the hyperthermia, along with providing cardiovascular support, and then treating any complications associated with the hyperthermia. These complications often occur simultaneously and may be evident in a critical patient at the time of presentation. Other problems may be recognized and require treatment during the course of hospitalization and recovery. Cornerstones of therapy include restoring effective cooling measures, restoring circulating intravascular blood volume, improving glomerular filtration and renal blood flow, stabilizing electrolyte balance, and providing broad-spectrum antibiotics to minimize complications of bacterial translocation and sepsis. Rapid early recognition of hyperthermia and instituting early cooling measures are extremely important and can be performed by the first responders before the patient presents to the hospital. First, the animal should be moved to a cool area in the shade or indoors, away from direct sunlight. Next, the animal should be sprayed or covered with cool, but not cold, water. Cool packs can be placed in the axillary and inguinal regions. Air conditioning or cool fans also can help to dissipate heat and improve convective cooling mechanisms. The patient must be cooled to 39.4° C (103° F) within 30 to 60 minutes of initial presentation, but overcooling should be avoided. Immersion in ice baths or cold water is absolutely contraindicated because cold water immersion causes peripheral vasoconstriction and prevents vasodilation, one of the primary methods of cooling. Vasoconstriction results in further elevation of core body temperature and thus should be avoided at all costs. In one retrospective study, animals that were cooled prior to presentation by their owners had a more favorable prognosis and decreased risk of mortality than animals that were not cooled at the time of initial injury. A more recent study, however, found that cooling before time of presentation did not significantly affect outcome.

The thermoregulatory center cannot function properly in animals with heat-induced illness, so overcooling can be associated with poor prognosis. Cooling the patient to lower than 39.4°C (103°F) causes a rapid drop in core temperature, and shivering can occur, which increases metabolic rate and further increases core body temperature. In one study, patients who were presented with hypothermia were more likely to die. Massaging the skin can increase peripheral circulation, improve peripheral blood flow, and improve heat dissipation. Other methods of cooling that have been described but that offer no real advantage or improvement to clinical outcome include administration of cool intravenous fluids, gastric lavage, cold-water enemas, and cool peritoneal lavage. Placing alcohol on the footpads has been described, but can further complicate overcooling, and is not recommended. Time is of the essence, and the first responder should get the animal to a veterinary facility as soon as possible. Animals that present to the veterinarian within 90 minutes of the inciting event have a more favorable prognosis than animals that are presented later.

Intravenous fluids should be administered judiciously during the early stages of hyperthermia and heat-induced illness. Initially, fluid loss is not severe unless third-spacing of fluid and loss from the gastrointestinal tract occur. Oversupplementation of crystalloids during this time can potentially increase the chance of or worsen cerebral edema and cause pulmonary fluid overload. Fluids should be tailored to each patient's individual needs and can be administered based on central venous pressure, acid-base and electrolyte status, blood pressure, thoracic auscultation, and colloid oncotic pressure.

A balanced electrolyte fluid such as Normosol-R, Plasma-Lyte A, or lactated Ringer's solution can be given as determined by calculated dehydration deficits. If a free water deficit is present, as evidenced by hypernatremia, the clinician should calculate the free water deficit and replace it slowly over a period of 24 hours to prevent further cerebral edema. Experimental evidence has also suggested that hydroxyethyl starch may be superior to saline alone for resuscitating animals with hyperthermia.

Oxygen should be administered in animals with signs of upper airway obstruction. If laryngeal paralysis is present, sedative and anxiolytic agents such as acepromazine should be considered. In severe cases of upper airway obstruction and laryngeal edema, antiinflammatory doses of glucocorticoids can also be administered to decrease airway edema. General anesthesia and airway intubation should be considered in the most severely affected animals. Empiric glucocorticoids in patients without signs of airway obstruction are contraindicated because they can further impair renal perfusion and predispose to gastrointestinal ulceration.

Broad-spectrum antibiotics such as a second-generation cephalosporin (Cefoxitin 30 mg/kg IV q8h), ampicillin (22 mg/kg IV q6-8h) with enrofloxacin (10 mg/kg IV q24h), and sometimes metronidazole (10 mg/kg IV q8h) should be administered to decrease bacteremia. Nephrotoxic antibiotics should not be administered because compromised renal function is a serious concern in patients with hyperthermia.

Antipyretic agents such as dipyrone, flunixin meglumine, carprofen, and etodolac are *contraindicated* for a number of reasons. First, the actions of such drugs are ineffective at decreasing temperature in an animal with a deranged hypothalamic thermoregulatory center. Their use may be justified in animals with pyrogenic hyperthermia but not in animals with heat-induced illness. Second, antiprostaglandins can potentially worsen hypothermia if present. Finally, in high doses antiprostaglandin drugs have been shown to decrease renal perfusion and can predispose the patient to gastrointestinal ulceration.

Serious complications of hyperthermia include oliguria, ventricular arrhythmias, and seizures, and the need to treat any of these has been associated with a poorer outcome in some published studies. Urine output should be quantitated and calculated to observe if oliguric or anuric renal failure is present. After volume resuscitation, urine output should be 1 to 2 ml/kg/hr. If urine output is less, a constant rate infusion of dopamine at 3 to 5 μg/kg/min can be started to increase renal perfusion and urine output. Ventricular arrhythmias should be monitored by electrocardiograph (ECG) and treated when necessary. The presence of ventricular rhythm disturbances and the need for antiarrhythmic therapy in the form of lidocaine (see Chapter 172) may be associated with a less favorable outcome in the hyperthermic patient. Finally, seizures should be controlled with diazepam (see Chapter 230).

Prognosis

Severe hyperthermia can result in widespread organ failure and must be recognized and treated promptly. In most cases, prognosis is guarded to grave, depending on the presence of underlying diseases and complications. Mortality rates are directly associated with the duration and intensity of hyperthermia. In one study, mortality rate was 50%. Obesity, renal failure, and DIC all increase the risk of death associated with hyperthermia. Permanent renal, hepatic, and cerebral damage can occur, including permanent changes in the hypothalamic thermoregulatory center that can predispose the patient to further hyperthermic episodes. In most cases, the clinician must give a guarded prognosis. If death is going to occur, it usually happens within the first 24 hours of the incident. If an animal survives past 48 hours of hospitalization, the outcome is generally favorable. Animals who present with coma or hypothermia after a hyperthermic event generally have a very grave prognosis, even with extremely aggressive therapy.

References and Suggested Reading

Aroch I et al: Peripheral nucleated red blood cells as a prognostic indicator in heatstroke in dogs, *J Vet Intern Med* 23:544-551, 2009.

Bouchama A, Knochel JP: Heat stroke, *N Engl J Med* 346:1978, 2002.

Bruchim Y et al: Heat stroke in dogs: a retrospective study of 54 cases (1999-2004) and analysis of risk factors for death, *J Vet Intern Med* 20:38, 2006.

Bruchim Y et al: Pathological findings in dogs with fatal heat-stroke, *J Comp Pathol* 140(2-3):97-104, 2009.

Diehl KA et al: Alterations in hemostasis associated with hyper-thermia in canine model, *Am J Hematol* 64:262, 2000.

Drobatz KJ, Macintire DK: Heat-induced illness in dogs: 42 cases (1976-1993), *J Am Vet Med Assoc* 209(11):1894, 1996.

Flournoy SW, Wohl JS, Macintire DK: Heatstroke in dogs: patho-physiology and predisposing factors, *Comp Cont Educ Pract Vet* 25:410-418, 2003.

Flournoy SW, Wohl JS, Macintire DK: Heatstroke in dogs: clinical signs, treatment, prognosis and prevention, *Comp Cont Educ Pract Vet* 25:422-431, 2003.

Haskins SC: Thermoregulation, hypothermia, hyperthermia. In Ettinger S, editor: *Textbook of veterinary internal medicine*, ed 4, Philadelphia, 1995, WB Saunders.

Holloway SA: Heatstroke in dogs, *Comp Cont Educ Pract Vet* 14(12):1598, 1992.

Johnson SI, McMichael M, White G: Heatstroke in small animal medicine: a clinical practice review, *J Vet Emerg Crit Care* 16(2):112-119, 2006.

Liu CC et al: Hydroxyethyl starch produces attenuation of circu-latory shock and cerebral ischemia during heat stroke, *Shock* 22(3):288, 2004.

Reiniker A, Mann FM: Understanding and treating heat stroke, *Vet Med* May:344-355, 2002.

CHAPTER 15
Thromboelastography

KARL E. JANDREY, *Davis, California*
BENJAMIN M. BRAINARD, *Athens, Georgia*

Viscoelastic point-of-care coagulation instruments have become more popular owing to their unique ability to detect both hypocoagulability and hyper-coagulability using a whole blood sample. Viscoelastic analyzers measure changes in the viscosity or elasticity of a blood sample as it turns from liquid to a fibrin clot during coagulation. The use of whole blood is ideal to re-create the physiology of coagulation *ex vivo* because it summates the contribution of each individual compo-nent (e.g., platelets, red blood cells, plasma factors) to hemostasis. The testing duration is generally short and the blood sample volumes required are relatively small. The most common viscoelastic coagulation machines used in veterinary medicine include the Thrombelasto-graph (TEG, Haemonetics [formerly Haemoscope]), Sono-clot, and rotational thrombelastometer (ROTEM). This chapter emphasizes some important technical aspects of thromboelastography, outlines principles of interpreta-tion including some complicating factors, and highlights the potential value of this technology for monitoring coagulation disorders in veterinary patients.

Thromboelastography

The principle behind thromboelastography is the mea-surement of the viscoelastic characteristics of clotting blood. Clot formation occurs in a rotating plastic cylindri-cal cuvette (the cup) with a stationary suspended piston (the pin) that is lowered into the center of the cuvette.

The cup rotates through an angle of 4°45' with a 10-second cycle period. The pin is attached to a thin metal torsion wire. As clot formation progresses, the fibrin that is gener-ated physically links the pin to the cup. As this connec-tion strengthens, the rotation of the cup is transmitted to the pin and this torque is translated into the TEG tracing by the torsion wire. The graphic tracing is dis-played in real time via the computer interface and pro-prietary software.

The thromboelastograph generates a qualitative tracing, as well as quantitative values to describe the clot (Figure 15-1). The R-time is the time in minutes from when that blood is placed in the TEG until initial fibrin formation. Reaction time generally reflects coagulation factor levels but does not always correlate with prothrom-bin time (PT) and activated partial thromboplastin time (aPTT). The K-time measures in minutes the time it takes from initiation of clotting for a TEG tracing to reach a predetermined level (20 mm) of clot strength. The α-angle measures in degrees the rate of fibrin buildup and cross-linking as a function of amplitude and time. Both K-time and α-angle are affected by the availability of fibrinogen, factor XIII, and to a lesser degree platelets. The maximum amplitude (MA, measured in mm), the widest part of the TEG tracing, is a direct result of fibrin produc-tion and platelet function and represents the final clot strength. Another measure of clot firmness is the elastic shear modulus (G, in dynes/second/cm^2) and is calculated from the MA using the equation:

$$G = 5000 \times MA/(100 - MA)$$

In addition to clot production, the TEG also demonstrates fibrinolysis; the percent decrease in the amplitude of the tracing 30 and 60 minutes following the MA is indicated as the lysis parameters (CL 30 and LY 30 and CL 60 and LY 60, respectively, measured in %). Lysis parameters are a measure of clot stability. Table 15-1 lists normal values for TEG parameters that have been reported in the literature.

TEG Operation

There are no standard protocols for veterinary TEG; in general, samples are run as recalcified citrated samples

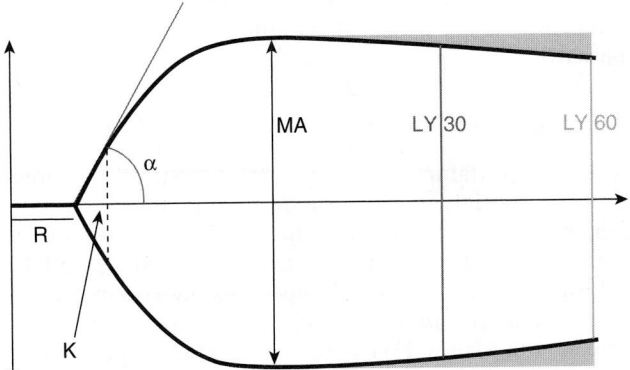

Figure 15-1 A generalized TEG tracing showing the most commonly reported values and how they relate to the tracing. *R,* R-time or reaction time, the time to the formation of the first fibrin strands; *K,* K-time, the time from the R-time until the tracing reaches 20 mm in width; *Angle,* α-angle, a measure of the rate of clot formation; *MA,* maximum amplitude, the widest part of the tracing, corresponding to the final clot strength; *LY 30* and *LY 60,* the ratio of the amplitude at 30 and 60 minutes following the generation of MA to the MA; these parameters represent the speed of clot dissolution or fibrinolysis.

(typically 3.2% sodium citrate at a 1:9 v/v ratio), at 37° C, and after a 30-minute rest period at room temperature. Vibration, shock, mixing, and rapid shifts in temperature during the rest period should be avoided. Although some laboratories use only recalcification with calcium chloride before starting the assay, this method depends on contact activation (intrinsic pathway) and may result in a prolonged assay time, especially in horses. This method is also associated with operator variability. The use of very dilute (1:50,000) or moderately dilute (1:3400) tissue factor (TF; Innovin, Siemens Healthcare) has been described in many species and decreases interoperator variability. Haemonetics provides prefilled vials containing a liquid kaolin solution, which strongly activates coagulation via the intrinsic pathway. Kaolin activation also decreases variability and has been described in small animal species. A recent publication that studied various activators (native, TF, and kaolin) for TEG analysis of cat blood showed that the activators are not interchangeable due to large coefficients of variation between activators.

Because of variability between users and institutions, each institution should develop a specific protocol, decide on a specific reference interval, and identify a limited number of operators to maximize useful information from the assay. Protocols should specify guidelines for sample collection, a standard sample rest period following blood sampling, and a standard temperature for both the rest period and the TEG analysis. For research studies, a single operator is preferable, and duplicate testing should be considered if possible. If limiting the number of operators is not feasible, an activator such as TF or kaolin should be used.

TEG Interpretation

In general, animals may be considered hypercoagulable if they have all or some of the following TEG characteristics: a faster time to the start of clot formation (a shorter R-time), a steeper α-angle (corresponding to more rapid clot formation), and a greater MA than the reference

TABLE **15-1**

Survey of Reference Intervals or Experimental Ranges Generated for TEG in Dogs and Cats Using Various Activation Methods*

Species, Activation Method	R-time (min)	K-time (min)	α-Angle (deg)	Maximum Amplitude (MA, mm)	n	Reference
Dog, recalcification	2.1-11.0	1.2-4.6	39-74	44.5-61.7	120 (reference interval)	Pittman 2010
Dog, kaolin	1.8-8.6	1.3-5.7	36.9-74.6	42.9-67.9	56 (reference interval)	Bauer 2009
Dog, tissue factor (1:50000)	2.8-8.7	2.3-7.7	27.5-58.7	39.0-59.0	18 (range)	Wiinberg 2005
Cat, recalcification	3.3-19.8	1.9-6.6	32.5-64.6	38.3-60.7	15 (range)	Marschner 2010
Cat, kaolin	2.4-9.5	1.2-3.9	45.5-73.5	46.8-66.1	15 (range)	Marschner 2010
Cat, tissue factor (1:50,000)	3.2-12.5	1.9-5.8	34.1-64.3	40.3-62.8	15 (range)	Marschner 2010

*All samples rested at room temperature for 30 minutes prior to initiation of the test, with the exception of the canine kaolin–activated samples, which rested for 1 hour.

range. Some animals may display all these characteristics and some only an increased α-angle and MA. In human studies, the only parameter that has been correlated to an increased risk of thrombosis is an MA larger than the reference range. An association between TEG parameters and outcome measures has yet to be established in veterinary medicine. Animals with hypocoagulable states typically display a prolonged R-time if they have a decrease in coagulation factors. If animals are hypocoagulable due to thrombocytopenia, the R-time remains normal (because it is determined by plasma proteins), but the α-angle and MA will be significantly decreased. In coagulopathic patients with low fibrinogen due to conditions such as disseminated intravascular coagulopathies (DIC), the α-angle and MA will also be narrow compared with reference ranges.

Clinical Utility

The use of the TEG in veterinary medicine has grown rapidly since the initial report in 2000, in which hypercoagulability was described in puppies with parvoviral enteritis. Hypercoagulability in this population was characterized by increased MA and was correlated to other laboratory measures such as decreased antithrombin and increased fibrinogen concentration. Four of nine puppies in this group had clinical evidence of catheter-associated phlebitis or venous thrombosis.

One study used TF-activated TEG to describe both hypercoagulability and hypocoagulability in dogs with various types of metastatic neoplasia. TF-activated TEG has also been used to illustrate hypercoagulability and hypocoagulability in dogs with DIC. Dogs with a hypocoagulable TEG are more likely to have clinical bleeding. When TEG was compared against standard tests of coagulation in dogs admitted to an intensive care unit (ICU), positive associations were found between MA and α-angle and fibrinogen and platelet count, as well as between PT, aPTT, and R-time.

Recent reports have addressed the usefulness or application of the TEG to the understanding of many disease states across species. These diseases include protein-losing nephropathies and enteropathies (where tendencies toward hypercoagulability were identified), hyperadrenocorticism (where affected dogs did not have TEG parameters different from a control group), and immune-mediated hemolytic anemia (where affected dogs also displayed hypercoagulability). Kaolin-activated TEG was used to evaluate coagulation in cats with hypertrophic cardiomyopathy (HCM) and indicated that, although individual cats may be hypercoagulable, there is significant overlap in values between healthy cats and those with HCM.

Important Aspects of TEG Interpretation

The TEG tracing is significantly affected by hematocrit (Hct). As Hct drops, the tracing appears progressively hypercoagulable, with both a steeper angle and a larger MA. It is unclear if this is an *in vitro* phenomenon due to an altered ratio of plasma to cells or if it represents actual *in vivo* hypercoagulability. Platelet count is also important. Patients with thrombocytopenia less than 50 to

75×10^3 platelets/μL generate a hypocoagulable tracing. The TEG tracing (specifically MA) is also directly correlated to the patient's fibrinogen concentration.

Ongoing research in the veterinary TEG community is directed toward evaluating the effects of variable rest periods, test temperatures, and venipuncture techniques. With longer rest periods (greater than 60 minutes), the tracing appears progressively hypercoagulable. Resting the sample for 30 minutes at room temperature or at 37° C has no effect on the tracing (the TEG warms the blood to 37° C over 2.5 minutes, and the sample is greater than 30° C within 30 seconds). TEG reference intervals generated at 37° C and at 39° C appear similar. The quality of both venipuncture and the postsampling handling of blood is also important; as with any samples for coagulation testing, blood for the TEG should be obtained with minimal stasis or trauma. Overall, consistency of technique is the most important aspect of generating TEG tracings that are interpretable and comparable between patients.

Modifications to Thromboelastography

Samples contaminated with unfractionated or low-molecular-weight heparin or from patients treated with heparins may display significant TEG abnormalities. Unfractionated heparin concentrations as low as 0.1 U/ml result in excessively prolonged R-times and may complicate data interpretation. For this reason, Haemonetics also manufactures TEG cups that contain a proprietary dose of heparinase. These cups are run in the same fashion as those without additives, but the heparinase inactivates any heparin present in the sample; theoretically this results in a tracing that shows the underlying coagulation status of the patient. This is an attractive technique not only for quality control of samples obtained via an indwelling catheter, but also because it may allow monitoring of the underlying coagulation state of animals that are receiving therapeutic doses of heparins. The only downside is that there is a specific dose of heparinase in each cup, and depending on the amount of heparin in the sample, complete inactivation may not occur. The heparinase cups may also be useful for generating a therapeutic monitoring protocol for patients receiving low-molecular-weight heparin.

The whole blood TEG tracing may also be modified by the addition of inhibitory substances. In humans, the *in vitro* addition of cytochalasin D and abciximab results in a significant decrease in MA and α-angle. In dogs, *in vitro* cytochalasin D is effective and results in a decreased MA and α-angle, but abciximab does not affect the tracing.

TEG performed on citrated whole blood is not sensitive to platelet inhibition from commonly used drugs such as clopidogrel or aspirin; however, TEG PlateletMapping offers a way to work around this problem. Instead of a citrated sample, heparinized blood is obtained. The heparin prevents *de novo* thrombin formation and allows the TEG to be used as a modified platelet aggregometer. In order to create the tracing, Haemonetics provides an activator consisting of a mixture of reptilase (to convert fibrinogen to fibrin, in the absence of thrombin) and activated factor XIII (to cross-link the fibrin). The addition of this activator (activator F) and a platelet agonist such as adenosine diphosphate (ADP) or arachidonic acid (AA) allows platelet activation and subsequent integration of platelets and fibrin into a clot that is demonstrable on the machine. Activator F used alone induces an MA resulting from fibrin(ogen) already present in the sample. AA or ADP combined with activator F generates an MA resulting from platelet activation and subsequent fibrin binding induced by the agonists. The percentage difference between the MA of these various measures is calculated to show the reduction in platelet function as a result of antiplatelet medications. This assay is sensitive to clopidogrel treatment in dogs and presumably would work for aspirin as well. To the authors' knowledge, it has not been evaluated in cats, and the reptilase activator limits its use in horses. Inhibiting platelet function in the PlateletMapping assay, as a concept, may allow better differentiation in hypercoagulable animals if the coagulation changes arise from the platelet component or the plasma protein component, but further work is necessary to standardize this assay.

The TEG as a Tool for Therapeutic Monitoring

As noted earlier, the TEG is very sensitive to heparin, and even subtherapeutic levels result in significantly prolonged assay times and may not generate a tracing. This may be partially avoided through the use of an activator such as TF, but even this may not be able to distinguish high concentrations of heparin. A recent *in vitro* study evaluating the use of heparinase cups and low-dose (1:50,000) TF activation identified different doses of dalteparin in canine whole blood, and the author (BMB) has used high-dose (1:3400) TF and normal cups to evaluate dogs receiving both unfractionated and low-molecular-weight heparin.

In both dogs with hemophilia and those with factor VII deficiency the TEG demonstrated hypocoagulability. The TEG can presumably be used to monitor dogs that have other factor deficiencies as they are addressed therapeutically, although the value of a TEG analysis versus standard coagulation testing (e.g., PT, aPTT) in this context is debatable. *In vitro* studies in children have also demonstrated the sensitivity of the TEG in monitoring the reversal of tissue plasminogen activator (t-PA)–induced fibrinolysis by ε-aminocaproic acid (EACA); the TEG may be useful for this purpose in companion animals treated with EACA.

A TEG analysis can give information about global hemostasis that is difficult to obtain using other currently available methodologies. Although the machine has a strong theoretic place in clinical veterinary medicine, standardization of protocols and clear correlations with other assessments of coagulation are necessary before the TEG becomes an instrument for everyday clinical evaluation of hemostasis in veterinary species.

References and Suggested Reading

Bauer N, Eralp O, Moritz A: Establishment of reference intervals for kaolin-activated thromboelastography in dogs including an assessment of the effects of sex and anticoagulant use, *J Vet Diagn Invest* 21(5):641-648, 2009.

Donahue SM, Otto CM: Thromboelastography: a tool for measuring hypercoagulability, hypocoagulability, and fibrinolysis, *J Vet Emerg Crit Care* 15(1):9-16, 2005.

Ganter MT, Hofer CK: Coagulation monitoring: current techniques and clinical use of viscoelastic point-of-care coagulation devices, *Anesth Analg* 106(5):1366-1375, 2008.

Kol A, Borjesson DL: Application of thrombelastography/thromboelastometry to veterinary medicine, *Vet Clin Pathol* 39(4):405-416, 2010.

Marschner CB et al: Thromboelastography results on citrated whole blood from clinically healthy cats depend on modes of activation, *Acta Vet Scand* 52:38, 2010.

Pittman JR, Koenig A, Brainard BM: The effect of unfractionated heparin on thrombelastographic analysis in healthy dogs, *J Vet Emerg Crit Care* 20(2):216-223, 2010.

Wiinberg B et al: Validation of human recombinant tissue factor-activated thromboelastography on citrated whole blood from clinically healthy dogs, *Vet Clin Pathol* 34(4):389-393, 2005.

CHAPTER 16

Critical Illness–Related Corticosteroid Insufficiency

LAUREN SULLIVAN, *Fort Collins, Colorado*
JAMIE M. BURKITT CREEDON, *Cherry Hill, New Jersey*

Cortisol is a key hormone in the maintenance of homeostasis in both health and disease. It contributes to several important physiologic processes including immunologic, cardiovascular, and inflammatory modulation. The adrenal glands depend on an intact hypothalamic-pituitary-adrenal (HPA) axis for continuous and appropriate amounts of cortisol production. The adrenal glands must continually synthesize cortisol to meet cellular needs, with very little cortisol actually stored in the glands themselves.

Impairment or dysfunction of the HPA axis is identified in approximately 40% of critically ill humans, depending on the underlying disease, and is most frequently observed in patients with severe sepsis, septic shock, trauma, or hemorrhagic shock. A similar incidence has been recently documented in critically ill dogs. Dysfunction of the HPA axis results in a relative, not necessarily absolute, decrease in cortisol production. This endocrine dysfunction was initially thought to result from insufficient cortisol production by the adrenal glands, and thus it was initially called *relative adrenal insufficiency* (RAI). Further elucidation of this disease has led clinicians to understand that dysfunction may occur anywhere along the HPA axis, and therefore *critical illness–related corticosteroid insufficiency* (CIRCI) is now the preferred term. The end result, insufficient production of cortisol to meet physiologic needs during severe illness, contributes significantly to morbidity and mortality within the critical care setting. An easily recognizable sign of critical illness–related HPA axis dysfunction is hypotension that is refractory to fluid resuscitation and vasopressor therapy.

Pathophysiology

Although exact mechanisms require further investigation, CIRCI is a result of several aberrations evident during critical illness. Primary adrenal dysfunction may be due to hemorrhage or microvascular thrombi within the adrenal glands or due to drugs that suppress steroidogenesis. Secondary adrenal dysfunction occurs higher in the HPA axis, at the level of the hypothalamus or anterior pituitary gland. Inflammatory cytokines may cause suppression at the level of these structures, decreasing production of corticotropin-releasing hormone (CRH) or adrenocorticotropic hormone (ACTH). Finally, increased cortisol clearance, alterations in cortisol transport, or decreased cortisol receptor affinity may also contribute to the development of CIRCI. A glucocorticoid deficiency is the final result of these mechanisms, but mineralocorticoid activity does not appear to be affected and usually remains intact.

There may also be a genetic contribution to the development of CIRCI in dogs. P-glycoprotein plays a role in regulation of the HPA axis, and this axis may be suppressed in dogs with multidrug resistance protein 1 (MDR1) mutations. A study of healthy collies found that dogs with the MDR1 mutation had significantly lower basal plasma cortisol concentrations, as well as lower cortisol concentrations after ACTH stimulation. Some practitioners anecdotally report that herding breeds appear to have worse outcomes in response to stress; increased risk of HPA axis dysfunction and CIRCI may possibly explain this observation. Although this suggests that HPA axis testing is prudent in certain breeds of critically ill dogs, CIRCI may occur in any breed and warrants further investigation in any critically ill dog or cat that demonstrates clinical signs compatible with CIRCI.

Diagnosis

CIRCI should be considered as a differential diagnosis in any critically ill animal that remains hypotensive despite adequate fluid resuscitation and vasopressor support. Other nonspecific signs may include fever, gastrointestinal upset, weakness, and depression, although it is difficult to clarify if these are signs of CIRCI or of the systemic inflammation that led to the CIRCI. The gold standard for definitively diagnosing CIRCI remains debatable in human and veterinary medicine. A basal cortisol should never be the sole diagnostic test used because these levels can often be normal or elevated. An ACTH stimulation test, along with appropriate clinical suspicion, is the current recommendation for identification of animals with CIRCI.

In dogs, 0.5 µg/kg (low dose) to 250 µg/dog (standard dose) of cosyntropin can be administered IV, with serum cortisol concentration measured just prior to cosyntropin administration ("pre-ACTH") and serum cortisol concentration measured 1 hour after cosyntropin administration ("post-ACTH"). A Δ-cortisol can then be determined by subtracting the pre-ACTH cortisol from the post-ACTH cortisol. A similar protocol can be used in cats by injecting 125 µg/cat IM, then calculating Δ-cortisol from measured pre-ACTH and 1-hour post-ACTH cortisol samples. According to a recent review article about CIRCI in small animals, CIRCI can be highly suspected in critically ill dogs if one of the following criteria is met: (1) normal or elevated basal cortisol, ACTH-stimulated cortisol is less than the normal reference range; (2) normal or elevated basal cortisol, ACTH-stimulated cortisol that is greater than baseline by less than 5%; (3) a Δ-cortisol of 3 µg/dl or less; or (4) improvement in cardiovascular status following glucocorticoid supplementation (e.g., improvement in arterial blood pressure, weaning from vasopressors). Criteria for diagnosing critically ill cats with CIRCI are still undetermined.

There is still much controversy concerning the use of the ACTH stimulation test when diagnosing CIRCI in humans and animals; however, most clinical veterinary research has used this test to identify HPA axis dysfunction. There are several recognized limitations to the ACTH stimulation test when diagnosing CIRCI. This test only evaluates the ability of the adrenal glands to make cortisol, but does not evaluate the integrity of the entire HPA axis. It also does not evaluate the cortisol responsiveness of peripheral glucocorticoid receptors. Additionally, normal cortisol reference ranges for critically ill dogs and cats have not been established. Also, total cortisol measures both the fraction of cortisol that is protein bound and the fraction that is freely circulating. Only freely circulating cortisol is biologically active. Thus concentrations of free cortisol may be altered in critical illness even when the total cortisol is normal, a discrepancy the ACTH stimulation test does not address. Finally, recent studies in humans suggest that there may be little or no correlation between ACTH stimulation test results and hypotension's responsiveness to low doses of hydrocortisone in septic shock. Because of these limitations to the ACTH stimulation test, the appropriate method(s) for diagnosing CIRCI in human and veterinary medicine will likely change after additional investigation.

Veterinary Evidence

Several clinical studies that evaluated the presence of CIRCI in critically ill animals have been published. One prospective cohort study (Martin et al, 2011) observed 31 dogs with a variety of acute critical illnesses including sepsis, severe injuries, and gastric dilation-volvulus (GDV). Of these 31 dogs, 55% demonstrated at least one biochemical abnormality suggestive of HPA axis dysfunction (defined as an ACTH-stimulated cortisol less than the reference range, a plasma endogenous ACTH concentration less than the reference range, or no response to an ACTH stimulation test). In this study, dogs with a Δ-cortisol of 3 µg/dl or less were 5.7 times more likely to require vasopressor therapy. A second study (Burkitt et al, 2007) evaluated 33 septic dogs and identified CIRCI in 48% of the population. These authors also found that dogs with a Δ-cortisol of 3 µg/dl or less were at higher risk for developing systemic hypotension and were also 4.1 times more likely to die.

In one case report (Durkan et al, 2007) a critically ill cat recovering from polytrauma developed CIRCI, defined as an inadequate response to ACTH stimulation and a Δ-cortisol of 3.2 µg/dl. One study of 19 septic cats (Costello et al, 2006) reported that the septic cats had a decreased cortisol response to ACTH compared with normal cats, but made no specific recommendation for diagnosis in the species. Ongoing work in septic cats to determine the appropriate identification of CIRCI will hopefully provide some future guidelines for this species.

Treatment and Prognosis

Hydrocortisone (0.5 mg/kg IV QID, or 0.08 mg/kg/hr as a constant rate infusion) is considered the glucocorticoid of choice when treating CIRCI because it is structurally identical to endogenous cortisol in dogs and has a relatively short duration of HPA axis suppression. The dose of hydrocortisone used is considered *low dose*, with the intent of improving cardiovascular stability without predisposing to further complications (e.g., new infections, superinfections). Hydrocortisone is considered to be one fourth as potent as prednisone, allowing extrapolations to be made if hydrocortisone is unavailable for treatment. Clinical markers for successful hydrocortisone therapy include improvement in blood pressure or other cardiovascular parameters and successful weaning from vasopressor therapy.

Hydrocortisone therapy can be weaned (approximately 25% per day) once the animal's condition has stabilized and the underlying disease is resolving. An ACTH stimulation test should be repeated following discontinuation of exogenous glucocorticoids to ensure that CIRCI is no longer present. The endocrine dysfunction observed with CIRCI is typically transient and recoverable, meaning animals should not require glucocorticoid supplementation long term. Prognosis is largely based on the severity of the underlying disease, but the presence of CIRCI typically indicates significant illness that requires intensive care and owner commitment.

References and Suggested Reading

Burkitt JM et al: Relative adrenal insufficiency in dogs with sepsis, *J Vet Intern Med* 21:226-231, 2007.

Costello MF et al: Adrenal insufficiency in feline sepsis. In Proceedings: ACVECC Postgraduate Course 2006: *Sepsis in veterinary medicine*, p. 41. 2006.

Durkan SD et al: Suspected relative adrenal insufficiency in a critically ill cat, *J Vet Emerg Crit Care* 17(2):197-201, 2007.

Guma N, Brewer W: Relative adrenal insufficiency in the critical care setting, *Compend Contin Educ Small Anim* 30(12):E1-E9, 2008.

Martin LG et al: Pituitary-adrenal function in dogs with acute critical illness, *J Am Vet Med Assoc* 233(1):87-95, 2008.

Martin LG: Critical illness–related corticosteroid insufficiency in small animals, *Vet Clin Small Anim* 41:767-782, 2011.

Peyton JL, Burkitt JM: Critical illness–related corticosteroid insufficiency in a dog with septic shock, *J Vet Emerg Crit Care* 19(3):262-268, 2009.

CHAPTER 17

Evaluation of Canine Orthopedic Trauma

RANDALL B. FITCH, *Ladera Ranch, California*

Clinical evaluation of the trauma patient for orthopedic injury is multifaceted. Although outward injuries such as fractures may be apparent, an awareness of more insidious threats is also of critical importance. Cardiovascular stability and the identification of associated injuries should be prominent considerations inasmuch as mortality rates for trauma patients are reported at 7% to 12.5% (from spontaneous death or euthanasia). Additionally, between 39% and 60% of small animals that present with fractures have recognizable thoracic trauma. This chapter emphasizes the diagnostic approach to the dog with orthopedic trauma (see Chapter 18).

Recognition and stabilization of life-threatening conditions may delay a thorough orthopedic evaluation. Also, key components of a typical orthopedic evaluation such as gait assessment can be especially challenging and may require support with a sling or harness. Other barriers to a complete examination include bandages and splints that may have been placed due to lacerations, abrasions, or fractures. Therefore completion of a thorough orthopedic examination may need to be performed over time.

Historical information helps clarify the cause of injury and expected associated injuries. For example, patients with gunshot wounds have a higher incidence of additional penetrating injuries to the abdomen or thorax, whereas patients who suffer vehicular trauma have a high incidence of pelvic trauma. These incidence and risk factors impact the diagnostic workup and treatment performed. Preexisting conditions should not be overlooked because they may become especially relevant following trauma and are often forgotten in the excitement of patient stabilization.

Orthopedic Examination

Although a complete gait and mobility workup may not be feasible immediately following trauma, standing weight-bearing assessment remains an important tool for appraising a patient's neurologic and orthopedic functions. The position of the limbs with the patient in a standing position allows the clinician to assess muscle strength, girth, and tone and search for any neurologic injury such as radial nerve injury or brachial plexus trauma. If functional changes are noted in the limb, further neurologic evaluation should be pursued including spinal reflexes and sensation.

Additional assessment involves lifting each limb to determine the amount of weight placement, proprioception, and weight balance between limbs. Further neurologic evaluation is indicated if weakness or conscious proprioceptive deficits are found. Limbs should be compared for differences in symmetry. The vertebral column should be examined for any derangement. Weight distribution, posture, weight bearing, and limb positioning should be assessed from multiple perspectives (from both sides, front, and back). Many orthopedic injuries have characteristic postural changes easily recognized in a standing position (as with coxofemoral luxation). A systematic approach or checklist is likely to improve efficiency and accuracy of diagnosis. The standing examination provides the most direct and specific assessment of weight bearing, symmetry, and function.

Palpation

Starting with the cervical spine, one can manipulate and palpate the osseous and muscular structures to detect discomfort. The clinician should flex and extend the neck through full range of motion, including lateral, dorsal, and ventral flexion. The spine should be palpated throughout its extent. In addition to the spine, pelvis, forelimbs, and hind limbs should be assessed carefully and systematically to include palpation of bone, ligament, and muscles and evaluation of nervous system function.

Examination of the Forelimbs

Palpation of the forelimbs should include palpation of each scapula for normality and symmetry. The spine of the scapula serves as an excellent barometer for assessing forelimb muscle atrophy, an indicator of preexisting forelimb lameness. It is useful to compare both muscular tone and development especially near osseous landmarks such as the spine, acromion process, and the greater tubercle of the humerus.

The examiner should flex and extend all forelimb joints, including the shoulder, elbow, and carpus and each phalange. The latter also should be assessed carefully for swelling. Each forelimb joint should be evaluated for stability, displacement, or increased joint laxity. Shoulder luxations often demonstrate displacement, but subluxations are more subtle and require stress maneuvers to reveal instability. Elbow luxations are predominantly displaced laterally, with observable and palpable displacement of the radial head. Injuries to the carpus commonly produce hyperextension of the joint, which often requires stressed-view radiographs to document fully.

Limb fractures (of the humerus, radius, or ulna) often produce mechanical instability and displacement. Mechanical integrity of many of the long bones can be assessed through torsional stress. This is done by stabilizing the proximal aspect and rotating the distal aspect of the bone. The distal joint can be used as a lever when the limb is in flexion. For example, humeral integrity is evaluated by palpating the greater tubercle, which stabilizes the proximal humerus. By rotating the elbow to 90 degrees the antebrachium is used as a lever to apply controlled torsional stress to the humeral shaft. Rotation of the distal aspect of the humerus should produce proportional torsional rotation at the greater tubercle.

Palpation of osseous structures is performed not only to detect displacement but also to identify discomfort (osteodynia) caused by bone contusion, "greenstick" fracture, or nontraumatic preexisting disorders such as neoplasia or panosteitis.

Shoulder
While assessing shoulder range of motion, the clinician should stabilize the scapula. To test shoulder integrity the acromion process is stabilized while the joint is placed in extension. Assessment for medial shoulder stability is complex due to contributions of the collateral ligaments and the additional support of regional muscles. Sedation is advantageous, with the patient in lateral recumbency. With the scapula stabilized and the shoulder in extension, valgus stress is applied on the limb by lifting the limb upward (in abduction) to determine medial stability. Normal glenohumeral abduction angles are less than 30 degrees and using the opposite shoulder for comparison is helpful. Assessment of lateral collateral stability is more difficult due to interference of the thorax and is done with varus stress applied. The shoulder range of motion, degrees of varus and valgus freedom, and rotation movement should be compared with the contralateral limb. Many shoulder joints pop or click without significance, but any translation of the humeral head in relationship to the acromion process is abnormal.

Radius, Ulna, and Elbow
The radius and ulna are palpated from distal to proximal, and torsional stress is applied to assess stability. Injuries to the elbow are common. Flexion and extension of the elbow allow not only range of motion assessment, but also access to the anconeus, olecranon, and caudal joint structures. In full elbow flexion the carpus should almost touch the shoulder. With the elbow in extension and flexed at 90 degrees, integrity of the collateral ligaments is checked by applying medial and lateral force to the radius and ulna. Lateral condylar fractures are common. In these fractures, pain and displacement can be detected with digital pressure applied across the condyles.

Carpus
Carpal range of motion should be identified, as should any discomfort related to movement. Maximum extension of the carpus should be about 180 to 190 degrees,

with flexion of 45 degrees (the digit pads should rest against the forearm when flexed). Hyperextension injuries of the carpus result in excessive extension and pain. In some cases, the patient must be sedated to evaluate the degree of hyperextension or identify injuries to the collateral ligaments. Stressed-view radiographs are required in addition to standard views whenever stability is in question.

Examination of the Pelvis and Rear Limbs

Following evaluation of the forelimbs, the orthopedic evaluation is systematically continued caudally across the thoracic, lumbar, and sacral spine until the pelvis is reached. Pelvic fractures and luxations are common presentations in trauma patients. Side-by-side comparison of pelvic symmetry is an effective aid for detecting pelvic injury. Side-by-side comparison of gluteal muscles and pelvic bony prominences (specifically the iliac crests, tuber ischi, and greater trochanters) can detect injuries to the pelvis. Integrity of the hemipelvis, sacroiliac, or coxofemoral joints can be assessed through palpation of these landmarks. Additional evaluation in lateral recumbency helps confirm injury by allowing more detailed orthopedic examination. Lateral recumbency also facilitates neurologic evaluation of the limb including evaluation of spinal reflexes (femoral and sciatic nerves), sensation, the perineum (anal tone and reflexes), the rectum, and the tail.

Further evaluation of the pelvic limb begins with palpation of the femur and thigh muscles to determine if there is swelling, sensitivity to deep palpation, palpable instability, or crepitation. Many fractures of the femur or tibia can be discovered through specific palpation using proximal and distal osseous landmarks and applying torsional stress as previously described.

Palpation of the distal limb is more easily performed with the patient in lateral recumbency. This provides better visual access to the medial surface of the lower limb for detection of lacerations, punctures, and abrasions. The rear limbs should be examined as previously discussed for the forelimb.

Metatarsus
The metatarsus is examined by placing stress in both mediolateral and dorsoplantar directions. Minor laxity is expected across the tarsometatarsal joints. Luxation, fractures, and swelling in the metatarsal region, including the calcaneus, are often detectable with palpation. With the metatarsal joint in flexion or extension, regional fractures, instability of the collateral ligaments and styloid process, and joint effusion may be evident. If joint flexion and extension are limited, periarticular osteophytes and joint degeneration may be present. Palpation of the calcaneal tendon at its point of insertion in the tibia may reveal pain, swelling, or displacement.

Stifle Joints
Stifle joints are common sites of injury, and therefore the clinician should concentrate on palpation of the stifles for abnormalities. Swelling, capsular fibrosis, and

osteoarthritis are palpable during both standing and recumbent examinations and may obscure the normal anatomic features such as the patellar ligament. Preexisting stifle injuries are often exacerbated in trauma patients and may require further treatment. With the patient in lateral recumbency, injury to the cruciate and collateral ligaments may be identified as well as abnormalities of the quadriceps mechanism including the patella, the patellar tendon, and the tibial crest. Patellar stability can be assessed using torsional stress to displace the patella. This is done by extending the stifle, internally rotating the foot, and applying digital pressure to the patella medially. Externally rotating the foot, while simultaneously applying lateral stress, can be used to test for lateral patellar laxity. Valgus and varus force can be applied to the stifle to evaluate the integrity of the collateral ligaments. The medial collateral ligament is typically tighter compared with the lateral collateral ligament, which has mild rotational laxity.

Evaluation for a cranial or caudal drawer sign is used to test the integrity of the cranial and caudal cruciate ligaments. Muscle tension, regional swelling, and coexisting injuries can make this evaluation more challenging and it may require reexamination. Drawer evaluation should be performed through a range of joint angles from flexion to extension to detect partial tears. Reduced drawer motion is often noted in patients with chronic cruciate ligament injuries due to the secondary periarticular fibrosis that restricts stifle motion. Drawer motion is not only an indicator of cranial cruciate ligament instability, but also evident with a torn caudal cruciate ligament (which is commonly traumatic). Fractures of the distal femur can also be confused with stifle joint injuries.

Femur and Coxofemoral Joint

Integrity of the femur is tested with torsional stress by first identifying the greater trochanter with the stifle flexed (90 degrees) and then rotating the distal femur using the lower limb like a lever. Normally the limb should move as one unit, with the corresponding rotation noted proximally and distally. Muscles and tendons overlying the femur also should be palpated.

Injuries of the hip region are common and include coxofemoral (sub)luxations, femoral neck fractures, and acetabular fractures. Hip joint motion and comfort can be evaluated by flexing and extending the hip with a hand placed over the greater trochanter. During hip extension, the femur in a normal hip should extend caudally to a position almost parallel to the pelvis and without inducing pain. Degenerative joint disease is a common preexisting condition that limits range of motion and may induce pain and predispose to coxofemoral luxation. The integrity of the proximal femur and acetabulum can be evaluated by placing digital pressure on the greater trochanter and then placing the hip through a range of motion including torsional rotation of the femur. Crepitus is abnormal and may indicate proximal femoral neck or acetabular fractures. Capital physeal fractures produce palpable displacement of the proximal femur similar to a coxofemoral luxation. Acetabular fractures commonly produce medial displacement of the proximal femur that is detectable with digital pressure placed on the greater trochanter. Further evaluation of the femoral neck may require "frog legged" radiographic views with the hind limbs abducted as well as standard lateral and extended ventrodorsal views of the pelvis.

Coxofemoral luxation can result in displacement in any direction, with craniodorsal being most common. Patients with craniodorsal displaced hip luxation exhibit lameness and external rotation of the affected limb. The greater trochanter in these patients is caudomedially displaced with shortening of the affected limb length when compared with the contralateral limb on physical examination. In the normal hip, thumb placement between the greater trochanter and ischiatic tuberosity is displaced with external rotation of the limb. In the presence of a coxofemoral luxation, the thumb is not displaced with external rotation as the femoral head is not engaged into the acetabulum, allowing the femur to slide cranially. In patients with ventrally displaced coxofemoral luxation, the affected limb is comparatively longer when compared with the contralateral limb due to its ventral displacement. In addition, the limb is adducted and internally rotated.

As indicated earlier, evaluation of the pelvis relies heavily on assessment of osseous landmarks including the iliac wings, ischiatic tuberosity, and greater trochanter. The pubic region is more assessable in lateral recumbency. Injuries to the pubis include contusions, gravity-dependent bruising, pubic fractures, prepubic tendon ruptures, and abdominal trauma.

Other Issues

In patients with orthopedic trauma, additional evaluation should include assessment of neurologic status and vascular integrity. Vascular compromise is indicated by changes in limb color, temperature, and pulse quality. Thoracic trauma, abdominal trauma including body wall herniation (e.g., prepubic tendon injury associated with pelvic trauma), and head trauma also can be present in the patient with multiple trauma. For these reasons, a complete orthopedic evaluation may not be achievable until cardiovascular and respiratory stability are achieved.

Open Fractures

Open fractures are special situations in which the wound requires immediate attention (clipping, bacterial culture, lavage, and dressing) and the fracture requires immobilization. They occur in association with a skin wound and are subdivided based on severity, contamination, and exposure of underlying bone. Shear injuries are severe open fractures in which the overlying soft tissues have been sheared away, typically due to abrasion from the road with minimal tissue available for closure. In shear injuries the joint and bone are typically exposed and require delayed closure and stabilization with bandaging over several weeks. Ultimately, the success rate even for these shear injuries is high, approaching 91% to 98% with appropriate treatment. However, initial case management is intensive and often requires daily bandage changes. In many cases referral to a specialist is the best approach once the patient is stable.

Definitive stabilization is commonly performed following many days to weeks of wound care. Daily wet-to-dry bandage changes combined with surgical débridement are used to achieve a clean, healthy wound before surgical stabilization with implants can occur (see Chapter 19). For more details on management see Chapter 18.

References and Suggested Reading

Beardsley SL, Schrader SC: Treatment of dogs with wounds of the limbs caused by shearing forces: 98 cases (1975-1993), *J Am Vet Med Assoc* 207(8):1071-1075, 1995.

Breshears L et al: Radiographic evaluation of ilial fracture fixation in the dog (69 cases), *Vet Comp Orthop Traumat* 15:64-72, 2004.

Crowe DT: Assessment and management of the severely polytraumatized small animal patient, *J Vet Emerg Crit Care* 16(4):264-275, 2006.

Kolata RJ, Kraut NH, Johnston DE: Patterns of trauma in urban dogs and cats: a study of 1000 cases, *J Am Vet Med Assoc* 164(5):499-502, 1974.

Kuntz CA et al: Sacral fractures in dogs: a review of 32 cases, *J Am Anim Hosp Assoc* 31:142-148, 1995.

Pavletic MM, Trout NJ: Bullet, bite and burn wounds in dogs and cats, *Vet Clin North Am Small Anim Pract* 36:873-893, 2006.

Roush JK: Management of fractures in small animals, *Vet Clin North Am Small Anim Pract* 35:1137-1154, 2005.

Shamir MH et al: Dog bite wounds in dogs and cats: a retrospective study of 196 cases, *J Vet Med* 49:107-112, 2002.

Sigrist NE, Doherr MG, Spreng DE: Clinical findings and diagnostic value of post-traumatic thoracic radiographs in dogs and cats with blunt trauma, *J Vet Emerg Crit Care* 14(4):259-268, 2004.

Simpson SA, Syring R, Otto CM: Severe blunt trauma in dogs: 235 cases (1997-2003), *J Vet Emerg Crit Care* 19(6):588-602, 2009.

Streeter EM et al: Evaluation of vehicular trauma in dogs: 239 cases (January-December 2001), *J Am Vet Med Assoc* 235(4):405-408, 2009.

CHAPTER 18

Emergency Management of Open Fractures

ROBERT J. MCCARTHY, *North Grafton, Massachusetts*

Open fractures, defined as those in which fractured bone has been exposed to the external environment, represent between 5% and 10% of all fracture cases seen in small animal practice. Any open fracture must be considered contaminated and a source of potential infection. These fractures require immediate intervention and should be treated as surgical emergencies.

Open fractures constitute a wide spectrum of injury severity and related consequences, and various classification systems have been developed based on factors such as wounding mechanism, hard and soft tissue damage, location, degree of contamination, and fracture configuration. Perhaps the most useful classification scheme was described by Gustilo, and is based primarily on the degree of soft tissue injury. In this system three different types of open fracture are possible (Table 18-1). Type I open fractures are associated with the lowest energy trauma, have a wound less than 1 cm long, and are generally clean. Type 2 open fractures have a wound greater than 1 cm long but no extensive soft tissue damage, flaps, or

avulsions. Type III open fractures have been divided into three subtypes based on worsening prognosis. Type IIIA fractures have adequate soft tissue coverage despite potentially extensive soft tissue laceration or flaps. In type IIIB fractures there is extensive soft tissue loss with periosteal stripping and bone exposure, often associated with massive contamination. Type IIIC fractures have concomitant arterial injury. Any fracture associated with high-energy trauma is classified as a type III injury, *regardless* of wound size.

As with most classification systems, the Gustilo system has limitations. Many fractures do not fit perfectly into a single category. Furthermore, classification is only useful if it helps guide clinical management or determine prognosis. Although multiple studies have been published in human patients, this information is not readily available for dogs and cats. In reality there is a continuum of open fracture from simple to complex, with multiple variables determining recommended treatment protocol and prognosis.

TABLE 18-1

Classification of Open Fractures

Classification	Description
Type I	Wound < 1 cm in size and clean
Type II	Wound > 1 cm in size without extensive soft tissue damage, flaps, or avulsions
Type IIIA	Adequate soft tissue coverage of a fracture despite potentially extensive soft tissue laceration or flaps
Type IIIB	Extensive soft tissue injury loss with periosteal stripping and bone exposure Usually associated with massive contamination
Type IIIC	Open fracture associated with arterial injury

Any open fracture caused by high-energy trauma is classified as type III.

BOX 18-1

Treatment Protocol for Management of Patients with Open Fracture

1. Evaluate patient status and treat life-threatening injuries
2. Control hemorrhage
3. Place sterile dressing and bandage during patient stabilization
4. Assess vascular and neurologic status of limb
5. Obtain preliminary deep wound culture
6. Start antibiotic therapy
7. Manage pain
8. Obtain radiographs
9. Perform definitive surgical débridement and fracture fixation within 6-8 hours if possible

Initial Assessment and Emergency Management

Treatment of an open fracture should be started at home. Owners are instructed to minimize all limb manipulation and to cover the wound and exposed bone with a sterile dressing if possible. A clean cloth or diaper is an appropriate alternative if bandage materials are not available. Owners should be warned that injured animals may bite, and they should consider placing a muzzle if necessary. Compression is usually sufficient to control hemorrhage during transport to the hospital.

Initial veterinary management is directed toward evaluation and treatment of other potentially life-threatening injuries and pain management, unless the wound is inadequately covered or is hemorrhaging profusely (Box 18-1). In this situation a sterile dressing and pressure wrap should be applied. Ligation of actively bleeding vessels is occasionally required. Protruding bone should not be forced back into the wound at this time since this allows additional contamination of the fracture site.

Evaluation of the stabilized patient begins with a thorough case history. Owners are questioned regarding the cause of the injury and the environment in which the injury occurred. Whether the animal was "run into" or "run over" is significant because in the latter situation a substantial crushing component is more likely. The environment where the injury occurred may help determine potential wound contaminants and dictate the choice of future antibiotic therapy.

Initial wound evaluation should be directed toward a careful assessment of the neurologic and vascular status of the limb because these findings may alter treatment options. Simple diagnostic tests include clipping a toenail short to check for active bleeding, evaluation of extremity pulses distal to the wound by palpation or by Doppler flow detection, limb temperature assessment, and patient recognition of extremity sensation. Although the degree of wound contamination and apparent soft and bony tissue trauma should be determined, limb manipulation must be minimized and wound probing avoided because these procedures increase contamination, cause vascular damage, and result in pain. Potential problems associated with small puncture wounds should not be underestimated because debris may be under the skin, deep in the wound and medullary cavity. Preliminary deep wound cultures should be obtained at the time of initial wound evaluation. In humans 50% to 70% of open fractures produce positive results when cultured at presentation, and in 66% of cases the bacteria cultured at presentation are the same as those later isolated from infected wounds. After the wound is assessed and cultured, radiographs are obtained and a more functional immobilization dressing is applied. The purpose of this bandage is to prevent additional contamination, preserve vasculature, and decrease pain. Most organisms that are recovered from the wound after the development of an orthopedic infection can be traced to the hospital; thus early protection of the wound is critical. Sterile dressings should be used in all cases and strict asepsis maintained. A splint is generally applied to support open fractures below the elbow or stifle, whereas a spica-type bandage is required to immobilize fractures more proximal on the limb. Fractures proximal to the elbow or stifle are frequently difficult to immobilize properly, and in many cases it may be preferable simply to cover the wound and confine the animal to a small cage.

Antibiotics are always indicated for animals with open fractures because all wounds are contaminated and wounds that occurred longer than 6 to 8 hours before definitive surgical débridement and lavage are infected. In humans antibiotics administered within 3 hours of injury significantly decrease the rate of future wound infection. Risk of infection may be greater in animals with open fractures because of decreased host defense mechanisms caused by stress or because of vascular compromise. Choice of antibiotic is based on the cause of injury, nature of the wound, likely bacterial contaminants, and knowledge of commonly isolated bacteria from patients with osteomyelitis. *Staphylococcus* spp. cause between 50% and 60% of bone infections in dogs, and many of these infections are monomicrobial. In general, concerns about penetration of antibiotics into bone interstitial fluid are unfounded.

First-generation cephalosporins such as cefazolin (Kefzol, 20 mg/kg q8h) are often the initial drugs of choice because they are broad spectrum, can be given intravenously, are usually effective against β-lactamase–producing *Staphylococcus* spp., and are relatively inexpensive. If contamination with a gram-negative organism is expected, a fluoroquinolone antibiotic such as enrofloxacin (Baytril, 5 to 10 mg/kg SC q24h) or a penicillin-derivative such as imipenem (Primaxin, 5 to 10 mg/kg IV q6-8h) may be added. Anaerobic infections are more common than previously thought, and clindamycin (Antirobe, 5 to 10 mg/kg PO q12h) or metronidazole (Flagyl, 25 to 40 mg/kg PO q12h) should be considered in addition to first-generation cephalosporins in animals with severely necrotic, avascular wounds. The initial choice of antibiotic is altered when culture and sensitivity test results become available. In type I and II open fractures that are not infected, antibiotic use can be discontinued immediately after fracture repair. In any type III open fracture or in type I or II open fractures that are infected, more prolonged use is indicated. In general, antibiotic therapy is continued for about 1 month in these cases. Antibiotics can be discontinued at that time if there is no clinical or radiographic evidence of infection.

Recognition of pain is difficult in dogs and cats because even animals with severe pain may show no overt clinical signs. Open fractures are associated with extensive pain and anxiety in humans, and a similar situation is expected in animals. Pain should be treated with narcotic analgesics (see Chapter 12). Buprenorphine (Buprenex, 0.01 to 0.02 mg/kg IV or IM q6-8h), hydromorphone (Dilaudid, 0.05 to 0.2 mg/kg IV, IM, or SC q2-6h), methadone (Methadone hydrochloride, 0.1 to 0.3 mg/kg IV, IM, or SC q2-6h), and fentanyl (Sublimaze, 2 to 10 µg/kg/hr constant rate infusion [CRI] for dogs; 1 to 3 µg/kg/hr for cats CRI) all provide good analgesia, although fentanyl may be best for severe pain. A dermal fentanyl patch may be an adjunct for providing longer-term analgesia but should not be used in animals with poor peripheral perfusion because absorption will be unreliable. Fentanyl patches should also not contact heating pads because absorption may be increased to a level causing toxicity.

Surgical Débridement

Patients with open fractures frequently require long hospitalization, multiple surgical procedures, and expensive medications; thus, before initiating definitive wound management and fracture repair, owners should be informed of the potential prognosis and cost. It is essential that the veterinarian communicate treatment options and prognosis in a manner that allows clients to understand the situation and then make rational, realistic decisions for themselves and their pets. An estimate in writing of the anticipated expense and treatment should be provided. Limb amputation may be a necessary alternative in some cases. Definitive surgical débridement of the open fracture wound should be performed as soon as safely possible, preferably within 6 to 8 hours after injury. This period is considered the *golden period* in which the wound is contaminated but bacteria have not had the opportunity to multiply and spread through adjacent tissues. If the patient is not yet stable enough for

anesthesia, initial débridement can be attempted with a local anesthetic or a regional anesthesia technique such as an epidural. Neuroleptanalgesia also can be considered.

Surgical preparation and removal of gross debris may be performed in the surgical preparation area, but definitive débridement is performed in the operating room. Most orthopedic infections originate from hospital organisms; thus strict aseptic technique is important. Sterile water-soluble gel can be placed in the wound to avoid contamination with hair while clipping. A water-impermeable barrier is placed between the limb and the rest of the body and surgery table during débridement to prevent wicking of contaminated fluids from the environment into the operative field.

The goal of surgical débridement is to convert a contaminated wound to a clean one. All foreign material and contaminated or dead tissue are removed, but undermining wound edges and extensive soft tissue dissection are avoided. Sharp dissection technique is preferred. Dependable features for predicting viability of muscle are ability to bleed, consistency, and contractility. Although commonly used, color is actually a relatively poor criterion because it depends greatly on the available light. If viability is questionable, it is better to leave tissue in place and remove it if necessary during a second procedure. As a guideline for débriding bone, if the bone has no soft-tissue attachment and is not critical for reconstruction of the fracture, it is excised. Bone that has no soft-tissue attachment but is critical for fracture reconstruction should be saved. Any bone that has good soft-tissue attachment is saved in the fracture site.

Wounds are irrigated with liters of isotonic saline. Tap water has been used for wound irrigation but is not recommended because its hypotonicity may potentiate cellular damage. There is no evidence for incorporation of antibiotics, antiseptics, or reducing agents into lavage fluids in dogs and cats. In fact, each of these additives probably delays wound healing by inhibiting cellular proliferation. Various irrigation devices have been recommended, including professionally manufactured pulsating irrigation delivery systems, 35-ml syringes with 18-gauge needles, saline bottles with needle holes drilled in the cap, bulb syringes, and spray bottles. The target pressure for wound lavage is 6 to 8 psi, and this pressure is reproducibly accomplished by flushing with fluid from a 1-liter bag pressurized to 300 mm Hg with a cuff. Fluid is administered through a drip set attached to a 16- to 22-gauge needle. Too great a pressure with any method is generally indicated by the production of fluid bubbles in the local areolar tissue. Bullets retrieved from gunshot fracture wounds should be saved because of the potential for future litigation. A deep wound culture is obtained at the end rather than the beginning of surgery because this has been shown to correlate better with later infection.

Fracture Repair

Fracture fixation is performed as soon as safely possible, preferably during the initial wound débridement. If immediate fixation is planned, the operative field, the equipment, and the surgeon's gown and gloves should all be changed after the wound débridement. Rigid stabilization of the fracture increases patient comfort, improves blood supply to the tissues, facilitates wound healing, and promotes resistance to infection.

A number of techniques can be used for fracture repair. In general, after surgical débridement type I open fractures can be treated in the same manner as a closed fracture. Higher-grade open fractures require special consideration when planning repair. External coaptation with splints and casts is rarely appropriate since wound care is difficult and stabilization is generally inadequate. Use of intramedullary pins is avoided if possible because they impede medullary circulation, may spread bacteria through the medullary cavity, and when used alone do not provide rigid stabilization. Bone screw and plate fixation can be used, but placement of a large metallic foreign body at the fracture site is a disadvantage. Implants potentiate bacterial proliferation because the surfaces become covered with glycolipid, which allows *Staphylococcus* spp. and other gram-positive organisms to adhere. The extensive open surgical approach required for bone plating also further compromises vascularity. Despite these limitations, rigid fixation with a bone plate and screws is generally acceptable and usually results in uncomplicated healing.

External skeletal fixation is often the technique of choice because fixation pins can be placed away from damaged tissue and rigid stabilization is possible. External skeletal fixation is economical, is readily available, and does not require specialized equipment. The wound can be visualized and treated as needed. The Ilizarov ring external skeletal fixator may be particularly useful in these patients because very small fixation pins under tension are used.

Autogenous cancellous bone grafts are indicated in many open fractures, since cortical defects are common and these fractures may heal slowly because of vascular and soft-tissue damage. Transplanted cancellous bone facilitates bone healing by means of osteoconductive, osteoinductive, and osteogenic properties. Cancellous bone grafts rarely become infected, and when they do they undergo harmless liquefactive necrosis. The graft should be collected with a separate set of equipment and gloves to avoid contamination of the graft site. Alternately a combination of cancellous allograft and demineralized bone matrix providing osteoconductive and osteoinductive properties can be obtained commercially (Osteo-Allograft Mix). In severely avascular wounds bone grafting should be delayed 1 to 2 weeks to allow sufficient proliferation of granulation tissue to provide vascular support for the graft. If delayed grafting is performed, the incision should be through previously undamaged tissue if possible. Although cortical allografts have been used successfully in open fractures, they are not recommended because the risk of sequestration and resorption is high. Autogenous vascular bone grafts transplanted by microsurgery may prove beneficial in the future.

Wound Closure

Wound closure can be performed if débridement results in a surgically clean wound with adequate vascularity that can be closed without tension. Dead space drainage should be accomplished with aseptically placed closed suction drains. In general, more severe type II and all type III open fractures should be handled as open wounds with delayed primary or secondary closure. If there is any doubt, it is always better to leave the wound open.

References and Suggested Reading

Egger EL: Emergency treatment of musculoskeletal trauma. In Bright RM, editor: *Surgical emergencies*, New York, 1986, Churchill Livingstone, p 175.

Grant GR, Olds RB: Treatment of open fractures. In Slatter D, editor: *Textbook of small animal surgery*, Philadelphia, 2003, Saunders, p 1793.

Gustilo RB, Anderson JT: Prevention of infection in the treatment of 1,025 open fractures of long bones: retrospective and prospective analyses, *J Bone Joint Surg* 58:453-458, 1976.

Piermattei DL, Flo GL, DeCamp CE: Open fractures. In Piermattei DL, Flo GL, DeCamp CE, editors: *Small animal orthopedics and fracture repair*, Philadelphia, 2006, Saunders, p 145.

Seligson DS, Henry SL: Treatment of compound fractures, *Am J Surg* 161:696-701, 1991.

CHAPTER 19

Emergency Wound Management and Vacuum-Assisted Wound Closure

STACY D. MEOLA, *Wheat Ridge, Colorado*
JASON WHEELER, *Charlottesville, Virginia*

A variety of wounds are seen during emergency practice. Many wounds in small animal practice are traumatic in origin, such as lacerations, bite wounds, open fractures, degloving injuries, and those resulting from automobile accidents and penetrating/projectile objects. Additionally, envenomations, burns, and surgical dehiscence are commonly encountered. The mechanism of injury, the time from injury, and the level of wound contamination are all crucial management factors. Patient characteristics including age, obesity, nutritional status, serum albumin, and concurrent diseases such as hyperadrenocorticism, diabetes mellitus, and neoplasia also affect wound healing.

The so-called golden period is the time from injury to development of infection with 10^5 organisms/gram of tissue. This time period, which on average lasts 6 hours, provides the best opportunities for wound management and closure.

Wound healing begins immediately after injury and occurs in four phases. The first phase, the inflammatory phase, lasts up to 5 days and begins with hemostasis and the release of cytokines and inflammatory mediators to initiate migration of neutrophils toward the wound. The second phase is débridement of the wound by neutrophils and monocytes that mature to macrophages. Macrophages and neutrophils clean the wound bed of debris, bacteria, foreign material, and necrotic tissue. Débridement lasts for 3 to 5 days and sets up the wound bed for repair. The repair phase usually begins 3 to 5 days after the initial injury and lasts up to several weeks. During the repair phase angiogenesis, fibroplasia, and collagen synthesis set up the meshwork for epithelialization of the wound. The final phase, maturation of the wound, may last for years as connective tissue and collagen fibers remodel to increase wound strength.

Initial Assessment and Treatment

Severe wounds are commonly seen in association with multiple traumatic injuries. The wounds are often impressive and can distract the clinician from more life-threatening concurrent injuries. While the patient's life-threatening injuries are addressed, the wound should be covered or bandaged for basic stabilization and to prevent further contamination by nosocomial organisms.

The wound can be evaluated, cleaned, and definitively managed at a later time.

Initial Patient Management

The patient's cardiovascular status should be fully stabilized with fluid therapy (see Chapters 1 and 2) and analgesic drugs such as pure mu opioid agonists administered (see Chapter 12) prior to addressing the wound. The wound should be covered with a sterile towel or sterile lubricating gel to prevent fur from contaminating the wound during clipping. The wound should be clipped with wide margins of 3 to 5 cm to allow for bandages or closure and to fully assess the wound's margins.

Once the wound has been adequately clipped of fur it should be flushed to reduce contamination and facilitate evaluation. A 1-L fluid bag placed into a pressure cuff inflated to 300 mm Hg, attached to a 16-gauge needle provides ideal pressure of 7 to 8 psi with which to flush the wound without causing further tissue damage and bacterial contamination (Gall and Monnet, 2010).

Wound Evaluation and Flushing

Wounds should be fully evaluated before establishing a plan for repair. Extremities with wounds should be checked for distal pulses and sensation. Wounds with skin flaps should be evaluated for adequate blood supply, recalling that most arteries flow from rostral to caudal and proximal to distal. Accordingly, inverted V-shaped skin flaps with the narrow tip rostral or proximal may not heal properly. Crushing injuries, including bite wounds, may have an area of devitalized tissue beneath the wound surface and a compromised vascular supply that is inapparent initially. On average, tissue takes 24 to 72 hours to "declare itself." Unfortunately, it is often very difficult to predict which tissues will become necrotic. Finally, wounds should be evaluated for joint or bone involvement or for penetration into cavities such as the thorax and abdomen.

Prior to closure and after flushing, the wound should be cultured to ensure appropriate antibiotic coverage. Radiographs should be taken of any extremity wound or if communication with the pleural or peritoneal spaces is suspected. A contrast fistulagram study of the wound tract can be performed using an ionic (diluted 1:1 with saline) or nonionic contrast agent to determine the extent of the wound or penetration into the thorax or abdomen.

Wound Closure

There are four categories of wound closure: primary closure, delayed primary closure, secondary closure, and second-intention healing. Primary closure occurs within 24 hours of injury. Delayed primary closure occurs within 3 to 5 days of injury but before the development of granulation tissue. Secondary closure commences once granulation tissue is present, approximately 5 days after the injury. Second-intention healing occurs when the wound is left open to heal from the inside out; this takes much longer than primary or delayed primary closure.

Vacuum-Assisted Wound Closure

Primary closure of a wound may not be possible for a number of reasons including loss of tissue, wound size, location of the injury, severe contamination, or concern for further devitalization of the wound edges. A variety of wound bandages are available for these situations. Commonly used débriding wound bandages include wet-to-dry, dry-to-dry, sugar or honey, and vacuum-assisted wound closure (VAC) bandages. This last type of bandage is discussed in more detail in the next section.

Clinical Advantages of VAC Bandages

VAC wound closure bandage therapy has been adapted successfully from the treatment of acute and chronic non-healing wounds in humans. Early swine models (Morykwas et al, 1997) showed a 63% increase in granulation tissue with continuous suction and a 103% increase with intermittent suction over standard wet-to-dry bandages. In this study, bacterial clearance of the wounds occurred at day 4 with the VAC bandage, whereas greater than 10^6 organisms/gram were isolated at day 7 in controls. When VAC bandages were applied to humans with chronic non-healing wounds, closure and a favorable outcome occurred in 171 of 175 patients (Agenta and Morykwas, 1997).

VAC bandages are indicated in large contaminated wounds, burns, chronic open wounds, surgically dehisced wounds, and skin flaps and grafts, as well as to improve mesh graft survival. They can also be used in the treatment of septic peritonitis, but discussion of this is beyond the scope of this textbook (see Web Chapter 2). VAC bandages apply subatmospheric pressure to the tissue bed, decreasing interstitial fluid, tissue edema, and bacterial contamination. At the same time increases are observed in vascular supply, granulation tissue formation, epithelial cell migration, and cell mitosis. Recently the reduction of bacterial load with VAC therapy has been questioned; however, bacteria cultured from wounds in recent studies did not appear to hinder the formation of healthy granulation tissue. Despite higher aerobic bacterial load in wounds treated with VAC therapy, granulation tissue developed sooner (3 days) compared with wounds treated with standard dressings (Demaria et al, 2011). None of the wounds demonstrated signs of clinical

infection, which supports the theory that healthy granulation tissue does not develop in infected wounds and is a marker of wound health.

Suction can be applied to the wound in a continuous or intermittent fashion. The advantage of continuous suction is that it requires less specialized equipment and is less painful. The advantage of intermittent suction is increased wound healing. Intermittent suctioning is cycled as 5 minutes on and 2 minutes off. The ideal suction pressure that increases blood flow to a wound is −125 mm Hg. To reduce seroma formation in surgically closed wounds, suction pressure is −50 mm Hg.

Application

VAC bandage kits are commercially available (KCI Animal Health, San Antonio, TX); however, less expensive bandages can be made from routine supplies in a veterinary hospital (Box 19-1). Patients should be fully anesthetized for the initial placement of a VAC bandage. The wound should be clipped with wide margins and flushed. All grossly necrotic tissue should be débrided.

Key steps in VAC bandage application include the following:

1. Sterile open cell foam is cut to conform to, then packed into, the wound (Figure 19-1, A); multiple pieces of foam can be used as long as they are touching or overlapping (Figure 19-1, B).
2. The egress tubing is fenestrated for additional openings and is tunneled into the foam or placed between two layers of foam; this tubing never should be placed on the wound itself.
3. The egress tube is sutured into place using a finger-trap suture pattern.
4. The foam is stapled to the edges of the wound to keep the foam in place.
5. A thin rim of stoma paste is applied approximately 2 cm from the entire circumference of the wound and the egress tube (Figure 19-1, C).
6. The foam and wound edges are sprayed with an adhesive.
7. The suction tubing is connected to the egress tubing and suction is applied before the application of the adhesive dressing to allow the foam to contract the

BOX 19-1

VAC Supplies

1. Open cell polyurethane foam (pore size 400-600 μm)
2. Red rubber tubing
3. Skin staples
4. Suture
5. Adhesive spray
6. Stoma paste
7. Occlusive dressing (such as Ioban)
8. Suction tubing
9. Suction canister
10. Suction pump or wall suction

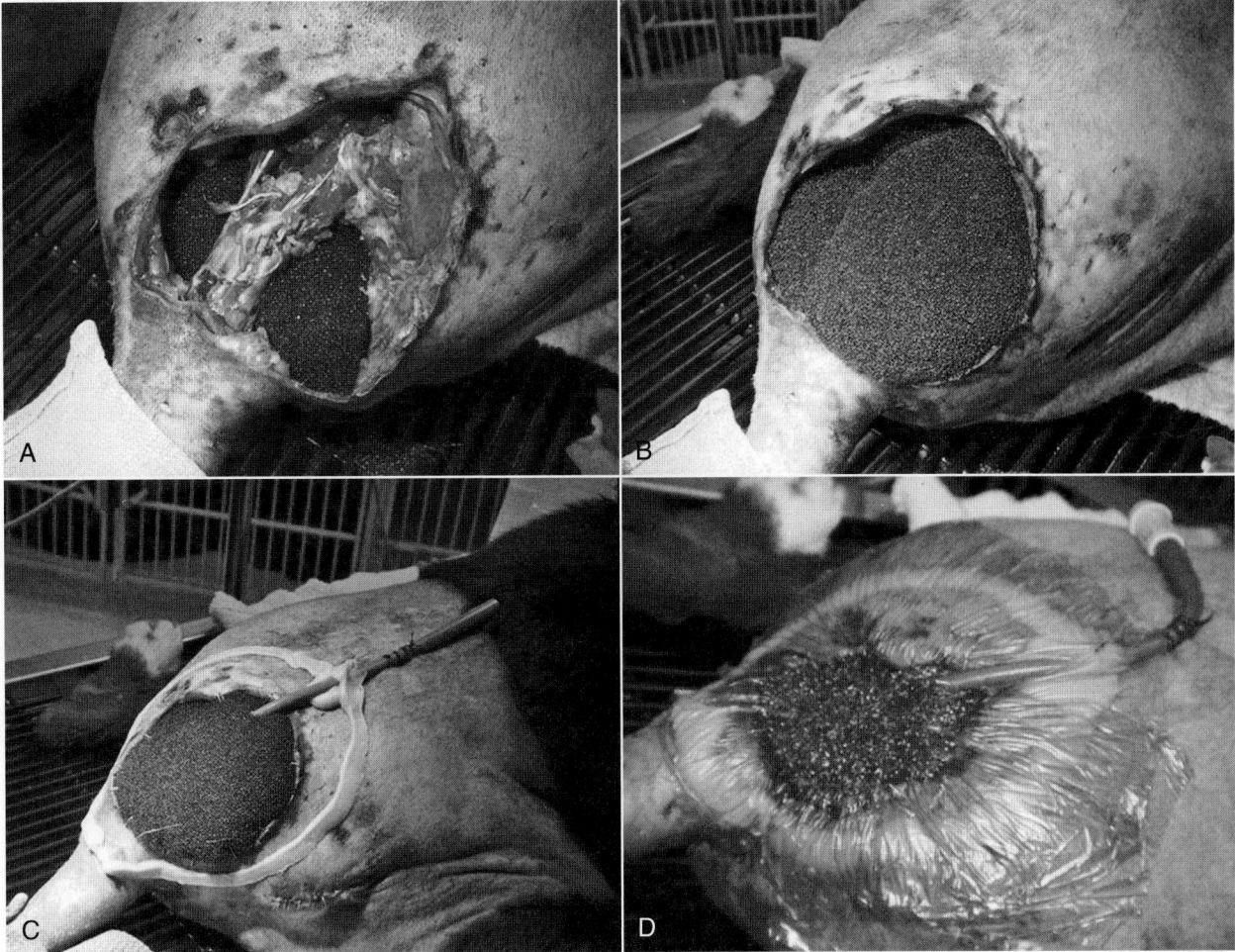

Figure 19-1 Application of a VAC bandage. **A,** The sterile open cell foam is packed into the wound. **B,** Additional pieces of foam are added to fill the wound bed. **C,** The egress tubing is placed between the foam layers and secured. The foam is stapled to the wound edges and stoma paste is applied around the wound edges and the egress tube. **D,** The adhesive dressing is placed over the foam and suction is applied, giving the raisin appearance.

wound as the adhesive dressing adheres to the skin edges.

8. Sufficient suction has been applied when the foam is shriveled and looks like a "raisin" (Figure 19-1, *D*).

If the wound is on an extremity, the VAC bandage can be covered lightly with a soft padded bandage to protect the adhesive dressing. A small window should be cut in the bandage to allow an area to view the VAC bandage to ensure suction is still applied.

VAC bandages should be changed every 2 to 3 days. A VAC bandage left on for longer than 5 days can cause growth of granulation tissue into the foam, requiring surgical extraction of the foam from the wound. VAC bandages may be changed under general anesthesia or heavy sedation. It is common in the authors' practice to attempt primary closure after 3 days of VAC therapy; however, this is largely case dependent.

Managing and Troubleshooting VAC Bandages

VAC bandages require 24-hour hospitalization and monitoring by a trained staff. If suction is lost for long periods,

the wound becomes macerated and granulation tissue growth stops. The VAC bandage should be checked hourly for the raisin appearance. The suction tubing can be clamped with a large Carmalt forceps and disconnected to allow for walking the patient or administering other treatments that require disconnection from the suction apparatus.

The most common sites of bandage leakage are at the egress tubing, at skin folds, in regions of high motion, and in tears to the adhesive film. Most leaks can be repaired by reapplying a second adhesive film on top of the first film and reapplying stoma paste around the egress tubing.

Cautions and Contraindications

VAC bandages never should be placed on a distal extremity in a 360-degree fashion with the digits or the distal paw exposed. This type of VAC bandage placement will function as a tourniquet. If a wound is present on an extremity and is not small enough to place within a localized, noncircumferential VAC bandage, the distal extremity including the digits should be covered in foam and incorporated into the bandage. The VAC bandage will not harm the intact or uninjured tissue distal to the wound.

VAC bandages are contraindicated in a number of situations including: (1) dirty wounds that have not been débrided, (2) wounds that are actively bleeding or complicated by a coagulopathy, (3) wounds with untreated osteomyelitis, or (4) wounds contaminated with neoplastic cells. VAC bandages should not be placed over large blood vessels where the foam could erode through the vessel and lead to rapid exsanguination.

Complications

Few complications occur when VAC bandages are applied correctly. Pain is the most commonly reported complication, but is decreased with the use of continuous suction. Analgesia in the form of nonsteroidal antiinflammatory drugs (NSAIDs) or opioids is administered as needed for concurrent injuries or for the VAC therapy itself. The most common complication observed by the authors is mild local dermatitis at the site of the stoma paste. If the paste is allowed to fall off with time, less irritation occurs. Adhesion of the foam to the wound bed can be decreased by ensuring proper intervals between bandage changes. Mild bleeding is also possible. Two cases of toxic shock have been reported in humans; however, to the authors' knowledge no cases have been reported in veterinary patients.

References and Suggested Reading

Argenta LC, Morykwas MJ: Vacuum-assisted closure: a new method for wound control and treatment: clinical experience, *Ann Plast Surg* 38(6):563-577, 1997.

Demaria M et al: Effects of negative pressure wound therapy on healing open wounds in dogs, *Vet Surg* 40(6):658-669, 2011.

Gall TT, Monnet E: Evaluation of fluid pressures of common wound-flushing techniques, *Am J Vet Res* 71(11):1384-1386, 2010.

Kirkby KA et al: Vacuum-assisted wound closure: application and mechanism of action, *Compend Contin Educ Vet* 31(12):E1-E7, 2009.

Kirkby KA et al: Vacuum-assisted wound closure: clinical applications, *Compend Contin Educ Vet* 32(3):E1-E7, 2010.

Morykwas MJ et al: Vacuum-assisted closure: a new method for wound control and treatment: animal studies and basic foundation, *Ann Plast Surg* 38(6):553-562, 1997.

SECTION II

Toxicologic Diseases

Chapter 20:   ASPCA Animal Poison Control Center
              Toxin Exposures for Pets   92
Chapter 21:   Toxin Exposures in Small Animals   93
Chapter 22:   Urban Legends of Toxicology: Facts and Fiction   97
Chapter 23:   Drugs Used to Treat Toxicoses   101
Chapter 24:   Intravenous Lipid Emulsion Therapy   106
Chapter 25:   Human Drugs of Abuse and Central
              Nervous System Stimulants   109
Chapter 26:   Antidepressants and Anxiolytics   112
Chapter 27:   Over-the-Counter Drug Toxicosis   115
Chapter 28:   Top Ten Toxic and Nontoxic
              Household Plants   121
Chapter 29:   Herbal Hazards   122
Chapter 30:   Lawn and Garden Product Safety   130
Chapter 31:   Rodenticide Toxicoses   133
Chapter 32:   Insecticide Toxicoses   135
Chapter 33:   Pesticides: New Vertebrate
              Toxic Agents for Pest Species   142
Chapter 34:   Parasiticide Toxicoses: Avermectins   145
Chapter 35:   Human Foods with Pet Toxicoses:
              Alcohol to Xylitol   147
Chapter 36:   Automotive Toxins   151
Chapter 37:   Lead Toxicosis in Small Animals   156
Chapter 38:   Aflatoxicosis in Dogs   159

**The following web chapters can be found on the companion website at
www.currentveterinarytherapy.com**

Web Chapter 5:   Nephrotoxicants
Web Chapter 6:   Reporting Adverse Events to the Food and Drug
                  Administration–Center for Veterinary Medicine
Web Chapter 7:   Respiratory Toxicants of Interest to Pet Owners
Web Chapter 8:   Small Animal Poisoning: Additional Considerations
                  Related to Legal Claims
Web Chapter 9:   Sources of Help for Toxicosis
Web Chapter 10:   Treatment of Animal Toxicoses: Regulatory Points
                  to Consider

CHAPTER 20

ASPCA Animal Poison Control Center Toxin Exposures for Pets

TINA WISMER, *Urbana, Illinois*

"Common things happen commonly" is a good adage for veterinary toxicology. Knowing which toxicoses happen most frequently can help when formulating a list of differential diagnoses. The Animal Poison Control Center (APCC) of the American Society for Prevention of Cruelty to Animals (ASPCA) began as the Illinois Animal Poison Information Center (IAPIC) in November 1978 at the University of Illinois. When it first started the center averaged one call per day and dealt mostly with large animal–related inquiries (48% ruminants, swine, horses, and poultry). By 1981 it received up to six calls a day, with 63% being small animal–related inquiries (dogs 49%, cats 14%).

During 2010 there were approximately 167,000 cases opened concerning possible animal poisoning. It should be noted that these data reflect exposure and not confirmed toxicosis. Domestic dogs made up the majority of exposures with 84.9%, followed by cats with 13.2%, birds and small mammals (ferrets, lagomorphs, and rodents) with 0.7%, and livestock (horses and cows) with only 0.5%. These changing demographics may reflect the fact that animals living in a house have more opportunities for exposure to various substances than livestock, which live in a more controlled environment. It also reflects the urbanization of North America, with more pets living inside as family members. Most calls are initiated by the owner (75.9%), but 18.5% stem from veterinary personnel.

The majority of dog and cat poisonings are accidental, with ingestion of dropped pills the most common scenario. Oral exposures to toxins make up 85.6% of all inquiries. Dermal exposures are next with 6.2%, followed by a combination of dermal/oral with 3.6%. Although exposures are steady throughout the year, the summer months always show an increase in calls (Figure 20-1). This may be due to pets having increased access to the outdoors and its associated toxins (plants, herbicides, insecticides), pets having increased exposure to flea and tick treatments, or children being at home on vacation and possibly not being as vigilant with keeping substances out of a pet's reach. The 2 weeks around Christmas have a 10% increased call volume, mostly related to chocolate, a popular gift given during a hectic season in which pets may not be as carefully monitored. October, with Halloween, also has an increased call volume related to pets ingesting candy and chocolate.

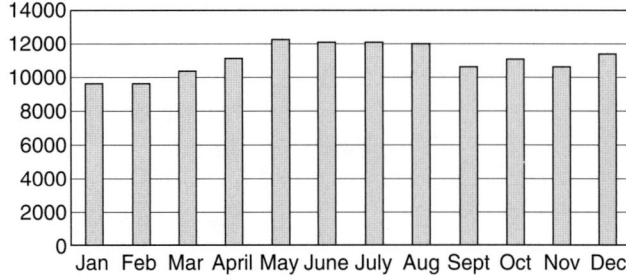

Figure 20-1 Monthly distribution of cases at the ASPCA APCC.

TABLE 20-1

Dog and Cat Exposures to the Most Common Categories of Substances (2010)

Poison	Dog	Cat	Total	Percentage
Human prescription pharmaceuticals	7983	884	8867	16.8
Toxic foods	7790	185	7975	15.1
Insecticides	7209	3514	10723	20.4
Rodenticides	5307	218	5525	10.5
Veterinary pharmaceuticals	5022	442	5464	10.4
Human OTC pharmaceuticals	4959	300	5259	10.0
Plants	2143	1107	3250	6.2
Household*	1700	80	1780	3.4
Herbicide	1173	106	1279	2.4
Miscellaneous	697	136	833	1.6
Cleaning products	510	114	624	1.2
Lawn, garden	417	15	432	0.8
Automotive	261	45	306	0.6
Foreign body	184	8	192	0.4
Bite, sting, envenomation	134	19	153	0.3
Totals	45489	7173	52662	

OTC, Over-the-counter.
*Household toxins include items such as fire starter logs, mothballs, glues, paints, batteries, and coins.

The previous information offers some epidemiologic bias including:

1. The APCC's telephone number has been publicized primarily among veterinarians but is also available to people with Internet access.
2. Calls are more likely when clinical signs develop than when no signs are apparent.
3. Calls from owners are more likely after exposure to a substance that has received media attention (see Chapter 22).
4. Once veterinarians have become familiar with the clinical signs and treatment of a toxicosis, they are less likely to call about that agent again.

Despite these inherent biases, the pattern of species involvement and substance exposure trends has been quite consistent for years (Table 20-1).

Dogs are most commonly exposed to human prescription pharmaceuticals. They ingest dropped pills or may chew up vials of medication. Cats are overrepresented in the insecticide category when compared with other poison categories. For example, many calls were initiated by owners who had applied non–feline-approved flea products to their cats. Other calls related to cats drooling after the application of an insecticide (a spot-on or spray product). People may be more likely to call about their indoor-only cats, and therefore cats are likely to be underrepresented in the outdoor toxin categories, such as automotive products, lawn and garden chemicals, and herbicides.

The frequency of poison exposures depends on the animal's activity level and sensitivity. An agent's availability and prevalence of use are also important factors. Most households contain ibuprofen or acetaminophen, agents at the center of a large percentage of the calls to the APCC involving over-the-counter medications. Pharmaceuticals, plants, and other compounds that are widely available are more likely to cause clinical poisonings; again, "common things happen commonly."

CHAPTER 21

Toxin Exposures in Small Animals

COLLEEN M. ALMGREN, *Bloomington, Minnesota*
SHARON L. WELCH, *Bloomington, Minnesota*

Pet Poison Helpline (PPH), a division of SafetyCall International, has been providing fee-for-service animal toxicology and poison information since 2004. The help line is available to animal owners, veterinarians, veterinary students, veterinary technicians, pesticide control officers, and others 24 hours a day, 7 days a week, 365 days a year on a fee-per-case basis. The help line is staffed by board-certified veterinary toxicologists (Diplomate of the American Board of Veterinary Toxicology [DABVT], Diplomate of the American Board of Toxicology [DABT]), veterinarians, and certified veterinary technicians. A variety of board-certified veterinary specialists and allied health professionals including pharmacists, physicians, zoologists, and others with advanced training are available 24/7 for consultation.

Call volumes for animal toxicology cases have increased steadily over the past several years (Figure 21-1). Whether this represents an actual increase in exposures, an increase in awareness and use of available animal toxicology services, or both is unclear. The call distribution represents a sample of the type of animal toxicology questions posed to small animal practitioners. The source of these calls, species affected, age of animals, and toxin and foreign body types are briefly summarized.

Call Source

During the 12-month period beginning July 1, 2010 and ending June 30, 2011, PPH received over 30,000 animal toxicology calls. About 60% of calls originated from pet owners and 30% from veterinarians, veterinary hospitals, or clinics. The remaining calls came from myriad sources including zoological gardens, farms, ranches, pesticide control offices, restaurants, and pet stores.

Species Affected

Dog exposures accounted for 90% of the calls, with cat exposures accounting for 9%. The remaining 1% involved primarily caged birds, ferrets, rabbits, small rodents, sugar gliders, other pocket pets, potbellied pigs, goats, chickens, horses, fish, turtles, and a rare primate.

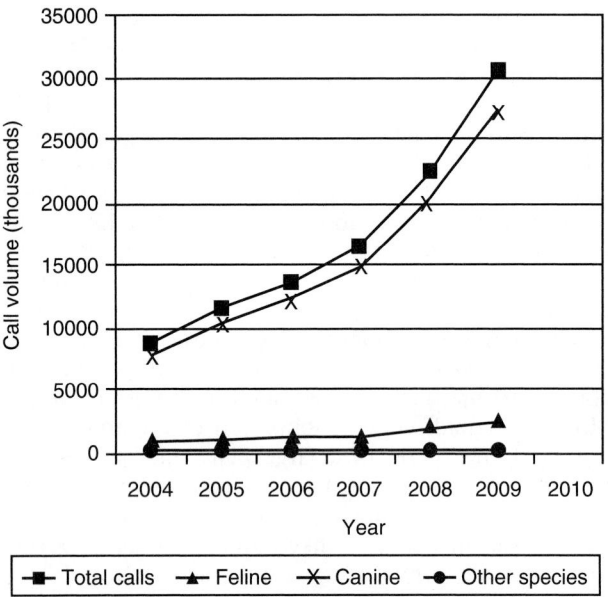

Figure 21-1 Total call volume 2004-2011.

TABLE 21-1

Category of Deaths

Category	Number of Deaths
House and garden	
Insecticide	2
Metaldehyde	1
Rodenticide	2
Ethylene glycol	1
Caffeine	2
Human drugs (prescription and over-the-counter)	11
Household products	1
Xylitol	1
Other	10

The majority of canine exposures were attributed to the following breeds: 7014 calls pertaining to mixed breeds, followed in decreasing order by the Labrador retriever (2673), golden retriever (1065), Chihuahua (793), Yorkshire terrier (771), cocker spaniel (629), beagle (625), and boxer (614). Cats were split between domestic short-hair, domestic longhair, and mixed breed or unknown.

Thirty-one deaths were reported during the 12-month period from July 1, 2010 to June 30, 2011 (Table 21-1). This number may be falsely low because some cases had unknown or undocumented outcomes. Twenty-four dogs, three cats, two guinea pigs, and one sugar glider died or were humanely euthanized. The most common cause of death in all species was from ingestion of human medications, followed by rodenticides; pesticides or other products used around the house and garden to eliminate insects, rodents, or weeds; and unknown toxins. Ten of the recorded deaths were due to unrelated causes (e.g.,

underlying disease conditions and neoplasia including hemangiosarcoma).

Age

Most of the calls involved younger animals. Of canine-related calls, 76% concerned dogs 5 years old and younger, with 21.9% concerning dogs 6 to 12 years old. Very few calls (2.1%) involved dogs in the 13- to 19-year age range. Of cat-related calls, 67.8% involved cats in the 0- to 5-year age range and 24.6% in the 6- to 12-year age range; 7.6% of the calls involved cats 13 years and older. No age-related data were retrieved for the other species.

Call Types

For the purpose of investigating the specific toxin/foreign body responsible for the call, calls were divided into nine general categories (Table 21-2) Subdivisions were used in each category as needed to further classify information.

Plants and Mushrooms

Almost all calls involving *plants and mushrooms* (1513) originated from the caller's home. When corrected for increasing monthly volume, the number of calls per month was relatively steady across the calendar year. Two small spikes occurred: one in December when the number of poinsettia calls increased and one in April associated with an increase in Easter lily calls. Other common plant calls included oxalate-containing plants, azalea, sago palm, marijuana, cyclamen, and all varieties of lilies. More than 60% of the plant ingestions involved symptomatic cats and were primarily associated with some form of lily or oxalate-containing plant. Sago palm and marijuana exposures were limited to the dog population.

Human Drugs and Herbal Supplements

Over 4000 *human drugs and herbal supplements* were identified as potential toxins. This number does not reflect the actual call volume because multidrug ingestions occurred with some frequency and were generally associated with the most serious and life-threatening ingestions. Within this category human prescription drugs constituted about 60% of calls, while exposure to over-the-counter (OTC) drugs and nutraceuticals constituted about 40% of the calls.

Oral products accounted for almost all of the *human prescription drug exposures*, with very few calls involving ingestion of topical agents, patches, suppositories, lollipops, and inhaled or injectable substances. Within the human prescription drug division, antidepressant drugs, antianxiety drugs, newer sleep-inducing drugs, drugs for attention-deficit disorder, and cholesterol-lowering drugs were overrepresented. Despite the large number of calls generated by these drugs, few serious outcomes occurred. Two of the drug-related canine deaths were from ingestion of topical 5-fluorouracil products. Baclofen and other prescription pain medications were responsible for many of the extremely symptomatic canine patients.

TABLE 21-2

Classifications of Call Type

Call Type	Yearly Call Volume
Human drugs and nutraceuticals	>12,000
Pesticides	
Rodenticides	1715
Fertilizers and plant foods	524
Insecticides	380
Herbicides	215
Metaldehyde	30
Plants	1408
Mushrooms	105
Mycotoxins	14
Food	
Chocolate	1924
Xylitol	846
Vitis sp. (grapes, raisins, currants)	374
Allium sp. (onion, garlic, chives)	154
Coffee	102
Tea	85
Alcoholic beverages	59
Macadamia nuts	45
Bread/bread dough	29
Household products	
Cleaners, disinfectants, bleach	840
Paint, stain, varnish	294
Soap	185
Batteries	125
Pool and spa chemicals	67
Air fresheners, potpourri	58
Deodorant	47
Other (primarily automotive)	
Ethylene glycol	54
Brake fluid	20
Transmission fluid	8
Veterinary drugs	>2400

OTC drugs and nutraceuticals showed a slightly different picture, with about 10% of the ingestions involving topical medications and ophthalmic solutions. Within this category, pain medications such as acetaminophen (APAP), aspirin, ibuprofen, and naproxen were the drugs most commonly ingested, followed by cough and cold products, multivitamins, herbal supplements, and calcium-containing supplements. With the exception of the pain medications and imidazoline decongestants (naphazoline, oxymetazoline, tetrahydrozoline, xylometazoline), clinical signs in this group were generally mild and self-limiting. Two feline drug-related deaths occurred from APAP overdose.

Foreign Bodies

Surprisingly, silica gel packets made up over 50% of the calls falling into the *foreign body* category. Labrador and golden retrievers accounted for the majority of victims in this category. Other common foreign body ingestions included batteries of all types, plastic, fireplace starter logs, pens, pencils, coins, glues, heat wraps, hand/foot warmers, ice packs, and dryer sheets. Some of the more interesting items ingested included taxidermy specimens, 40 starfish, fiberglass insulation, drywall, part of a home foundation, light bulbs, and glass.

Household Products

Exposures involving *household products* were equally split between dogs and cats. The exposures were divided into those involving laundry products, general cleaning products, toilet products, carpet-cleaning or carpet-freshening products, and essential oils. When further analyzed, cat exposures occurred most often in the laundry and bathroom area, whereas dog ingestions occurred throughout the home and involved primarily carpet-freshening agents and general cleaning products. Clinical signs in this category for all species were usually mild and self-limiting. Essential oils were more likely to cause significant clinical signs than other agents in this category.

Food-Related Products

Of the 3618 *food-related calls*, over half involved dogs ingesting some form of chocolate. This was consistent for every month. Other food products included nuts (almonds, macadamia nuts, and hazelnuts), onions, grapes and raisins, and xylitol-containing products (gums, mints, cough drops, and other sugar-free items). When corrected for increasing call volume, a distinct increase occurred in December and again in late March and early April. Butter, gravy, meat products, eggnog, and alcohol ingestions all increased in December, presumably because of increased availability and decreased surveillance. The number of chocolate and candy ingestions increased around Easter, Halloween, Christmas, and to a lesser extent Valentine's Day, again presumably because of the greater availability.

House, Lawn, and Garden Products

Almost 2900 calls involved exposures to *house, lawn, and garden products* (i.e., products meant to eliminate insects and other pests or rodents, herbicides, fertilizers). Pyrethrin-based insecticides accounted for over 80% of the insecticide calls, followed by avermectin or ivermectin, hydramethylnon, imidacloprid, and boric acid. Outcomes in this group varied from no clinical signs to severe, with cats having the most severe symptoms (especially when exposed to permethrin-based products formulated for dogs). Moderate to severe clinical signs (tremors, seizures) were also noted in some dogs ingesting granular bifenthrin products. Calls regarding a carbamate, organophosphate, or arsenic compound occurred much less frequently, but the outcome was generally much more critical. Deaths in the insecticide group were from exposure to either a concentrated product or very large amounts of a more dilute product. A genuine seasonal occurrence occurred with these calls, with the incidence highest in summer and lowest in winter.

Most of the *rodenticide* calls concerning ingestion of long-acting anticoagulant agents involved dogs. Call numbers varied little from month to month. Most calls originated from the caller's home and were managed with no clinical signs. Calls originating from a health care facility were often associated with more severe clinical signs and required prolonged care and treatment. Brodifacoum and bromadiolone ingestions occurred with the most regularity. The remainder of the rodenticide calls included difethialone, diphacinone, and bromethalin. Several calls involved some form of sticky board exposure and typically involved cats or small dogs. The distribution of rodenticide calls is expected to change dramatically in the near future due to new regulations restricting the use of long-acting anticoagulant rodenticides. Bromethalin exposures are expected to become much more prevalent.

Household *herbicide and fertilizer* calls were almost always of low toxicity and involved a taste, touch, or lick of a product or ingestion of treated grass. Rarely did any clinical effects develop, and signs that occurred involved primarily vomiting and mild gastrointestinal irritation. There was a distinct seasonal occurrence to these calls, with the lowest call volume in December and January and the highest in early spring and summer.

Metaldehyde

Metaldehyde, although technically a pesticide, was counted separately because calls related to this product were almost always associated with a moderate-to-severe clinical outcome. This product is used for controlling snails, slugs, and other gastropods. In addition to the inherent toxicity, the product is often placed and forgotten until dug up and ingested by a curious dog. One documented canine death was attributed to metaldehyde.

Veterinary Products

Dogs and cats were equally represented in calls involving *veterinary products*. Topical flea and tick products, including pyrethrin-based products, showed a seasonal occurrence, whereas nonsteroidal antiinflammatory drug ingestion was steady from month to month. Clinical signs and outcomes were worse with pyrethrin-based flea products, especially in cats. Other calls, primarily those involving dogs, concerned heartworm medication, prescription animal drugs, anthelmintics, and nutraceuticals. Clinical effects for almost all these categories were mild and self-limiting with the exception of avermectins including ivermectin.

Others

The remaining calls were lumped into the *other* category. Within this group, *automotive products* were the most prevalent, with more than 82 exposures in the 12-month period. Of these, 54 were known exposures to ethylene glycol, which was responsible for one reported feline death. Fortunately no reported canine deaths occurred.

Personal care products such as shampoo, soap, nail polish remover, deodorant, and other items accounted for numerous calls but were all of low toxicity and generally resulted in few clinical effects. Oddly, animal and insect bites or stings occurred year-round, with two to three calls occurring each month. The outcome was generally good, and clinical signs were mild to moderate.

Although dog exposures made up the vast majority of calls, clinical effects were usually mild, and the outcome was excellent. Despite the smaller number of calls, cats seemed to have a more difficult time with ingestions, often exhibiting significant clinical signs. This may be because of their relatively smaller body size or differences in metabolic pathways.

Summary

In summary, PPH handled over 30,000 calls from July 1, 2010 to June 30, 2011, with 31 reported and documented deaths. The majority of calls originated from the caller's home, and the animals involved generally had no-to-few clinical signs and were treated at home with no referral to a veterinary facility. About 90% of the calls involved young dogs, followed by cats and a variety of other species. The most commonly reported exposures were to human pharmaceuticals and OTC drugs/nutraceuticals, followed by rodenticides, pesticides, and other agents used in the lawn and garden.

References and Suggested Reading

Barton J, Oehme FW: The incidence and characteristics of animal poisonings seen at Kansas State University from 1975-1980, *Vet Hum Toxicol* 23(2):101, 1981.

Buck WB: A poison control center for animals: liability and standard of care, *J Am Vet Med Assoc* 302(8):1118, 1993.

Forrester MB, Stanley SK: Patterns of animal poisonings reported to the Texas Poison Center Network: 1998-2002, *J Am Vet Med Assoc* 46(2):96, 2004.

Haliburton JC, Buck WB: Animal poison control center: summary of telephone inquiries during first three years of service, *J Am Vet Med Assoc* 182(5):514, 1983.

Hornfeldt CS, Murphy MJ: Poisonings in animals: a 1990 report of the American Association of Poison Control Centers, *Vet Hum Toxicol* 34(3):248, 1992.

Hornfeldt CS, Jacobs MR: A poison information service for small animals offered by a regional poison center, *Vet Hum Toxicol* 33(4):339, 1991.

Hornfeldt CS, Borys DJ: Review of veterinary cases received by the Hennepin Poison Center in 1984, *Vet Hum Toxicol* 27(6):525, 1985.

Klaassen CD, editor: *Casarett and Doull's toxicology: the basic science of poisons*, ed 7, New York, 2008, McGraw-Hill Professional.

Osweiler GD et al: *Blackwell's five-minute veterinary consult clinical companion, small animal toxicology*, Ames, IA, 2011, Wiley-Blackwell.

Peterson ME, Talcott PA: *Small animal toxicology*, ed 2, St Louis, 2006, Elsevier Saunders.

Plumlee KH: *Clinical veterinary toxicology*, St Louis, 2004, Mosby.

CHAPTER 22

Urban Legends of Toxicology: Facts and Fiction

FREDERICK W. OEHME, *Manhattan, Kansas*
WILLIAM R. HARE JR., *Beltsville, Maryland*

Tens of thousands of potentially toxic exposures are reported to U.S. animal poison control centers annually. Most of these exposures are not life threatening, and many do not cause harm. Understanding the realistic significance of these exposures depends on knowledge of the animal species, the actual toxicity of the chemical to which the animal was exposed, and the circumstances surrounding the exposure.

All substances must be considered potentially toxic; however, whether clinical toxicity occurs is often simply a matter of whether a dose delivered to the animal is high enough to cause toxicosis. Considerations in formulating a toxicologic risk assessment include (1) the toxic substance and its chemical and physiologic characteristics such as concentration and formulation, (2) characteristics of the animal involved such as species, size, age, sex, and physiologic condition, and (3) the exposure characteristics, which include the route and duration of exposure. Ingestion is by far the most common route of exposure. Therefore, given the numerous chemical and biologic variables involved in any exposure instance, it is unsurprising that not all exposures to toxic substances result in clinical toxicosis. The role of the clinician is to review the specific circumstances surrounding an exposure and offer appropriate judgment and recommendations. Favorable outcomes depend on prompt veterinary intervention following any potentially harmful exposure.

Brand name products often change ingredients through the years, which often alters the hazard. Products with similar names and intended mimicry in names can cause confusion when determining an assessment of relative risk. Therefore it is always important to read the label, determine the ingredients, and be certain that an actual exposure did occur. It is also critical to examine the patient.

All too frequently, however, individuals with emotional concerns and limited chemical and medical knowledge become vocal in news and electronic media—for example, the Internet—in declaring toxic problems inappropriately. These are often blanket statements incriminating products or situations as being the absolute cause of animal illnesses or death. Once these statements become ingrained in the media and are circulated widely, they become *urban legends*. Such urban legends may be repeatedly presented to veterinary practitioners as inquiries, concerns, or even *facts*.

The truth is that almost all urban legends are exaggerations of potentially risky situations or misinterpretations of related information that are erroneously applied to everyday events or behaviors. It then becomes the responsibility of veterinarians to apply their knowledge and people skills to clarify these concerns and hopefully place the urban legend in its appropriate category.

The following are a selected number of statements concerning potentially toxic exposure situations that have commonly been reported to veterinarians. In some cases the concerns may be valid, whereas in others evidence of significant risk simply does not exist. Many urban legends are rumors spread through Internet communications. It almost goes without stating to be careful of Internet misinformation. As much as we all appreciate information, to quote former President Ronald Reagan, "Information is good information only if it can be verified."

Consider how you would respond to the following statements. Are they true, false, or possible? Remember that often it is the combination of variables that ultimately affects the outcome of every chemical exposure!

Home Care and Cleaning Products

- **Ingestion of any small desiccant sachet "Fresh-Packet" is harmless to dogs and cats.**

  False: These products serve as a desiccant, as the name implies, to control spoilage due to accumulation of moisture and/or oxidation. They may contain silicates (Na_2SiO_3), activated carbon (charcoal), iron compounds (FeN_3O_9), or other desiccants. In addition, sometimes the silicate products contain a color indicator ($CoCl_2$) that turns pink when hydrated. Each of these ingredients may irritate the gastric mucosa; the iron-containing packets and color indicator–containing packets can be toxic to dogs and cats.

- **Ingestion of Swiffer WetJets kills dogs by liver failure.**

  False: This product contains water (80% to 90%), propylene glycol (1% to 4%), isopropyl alcohol (1% to 4%), and preservatives (0.1%). Propylene glycol is much less toxic than ethylene glycol found in antifreeze, and this concentration of propylene glycol taken orally should not present a hazard. If there is a problem following ingestion, most likely a foreign body has been introduced or it is the result of a preexisting condition.

- **Ultra Clorox contains lye and therefore is potentially dangerous for your dog.**

  False: Both ultra Clorox and regular Clorox bleach formulations contain 5.25% aqueous sodium hypochlorite but not sodium hydroxide (i.e., lye). However, sodium hypochlorite is still corrosive and may cause harm from eye or skin contact, ingestion, or inhalation. It is often used as a good premise disinfectant, but it is best to keep it away from pets.

- **Pot-scrubbing sponges contain dangerous amounts of Agent Orange (2,4-D + 2,4,5-T).**

  False: Packages of these commercially available sponges are moist inside because a liquid antimicrobial is included to ensure that no fungal growth develops. The antimicrobial agent is a nontoxic disinfectant and even has some perfume added. Now hands will smell nice after "doing pots and pans." However, if the sponges become grease filled and are ingested, they could lead to gastrointestinal obstruction. It is best to properly dispose of these products following their use.

- **Febreze, the odor elimination product, is dangerous for household pets.**

  False: Zinc chloride, present in the pre-1998 formulation, was removed, and now the product is sold as a pump spray rather than as an aerosol that could have been an inhalation hazard to some birds in confined spaces. Febreze contains water, alcohol, a corn-derived odor eliminator, and fragrance. Toxicity is not expected with routine use, even with exaggerated exposure.

- **Resolve spot and stain carpet cleaner is lethal when ingested by dogs and cats.**

  False: This product contains soap, sodium bicarbonate, alcohols 1.5% (ethanol, 2-propanol, and carbinol), glycols 1% (propylene glycol and methyl ether), citrus/pine scent, and water. It is not a lethal formulation. It can cause temporary minor eye irritation and mild gastrointestinal upset if ingested. It is best to keep all household products out of a pet's reach.

Foods

- **Macadamia nuts produce muscle weakness in dogs.**

  True: Weakness, depression, and vomiting usually occur 6 or more hours after ingestion of about 1 nut per kilogram of body weight, or more. Weakness and depression gradually improve after 24 hours in dogs without significant preexisting medical conditions.

- **Ingestion of grapes and raisins may result in acute renal failure in dogs.**

  True: Vomiting, polydipsia, and lethargy can occur 5 to 6 hours after ingestion, followed by anorexia, anuria, tremors, and diarrhea. One to two grapes per kilogram of body weight has been reported as sufficient to induce adverse clinical signs in some dogs. Significant ingestion warrants prompt decontamination (emesis), followed by oral dosing with activated charcoal. In addition, aggressive fluid therapy within 48 hours may prevent acute renal failure from developing. Interestingly, this syndrome

has not been reported in cats, and many dogs ingesting grapes or raisins do not develop clinical signs of toxicosis.

- **Ingestion of sugarless candy/gum containing xylitol is poisonous to dogs.**

  True: Weakness, ataxia, and total collapse may occur 30 to 60 minutes following ingestion of significant amounts of sugarless candy, gum, or breath-mints. Xylitol promotes insulin release by the pancreas, which results in profound hypoglycemia. Absorption is rapid, and activated charcoal is not efficacious in most instances. Acute hypoglycemia is best treated with intravenous dextrose—an initial bolus followed by continuous intravenous drip, with blood glucose concentrations being monitored over the next 12 to 24 hours (see Web Chapter 24).

- **Tea is a good poisoning antidote for cats and dogs.**

  False: Tea contains 300 to 1200 mg/oz of caffeine, whereas semisweet chocolate contains 22 to 138 mg/oz, making tea on average 5 to 10 times more toxic than chocolate. Tea does have other beneficial actions, but for cats and dogs the bad effects from the high caffeine usually outweigh potential good effects.

- **Ingestion of chocolate can poison cats and dogs.**

  True: Chocolates contain the methylxanthines caffeine and theobromine, which can be toxic. Unsweetened baking chocolate contains the most methylxanthines (40 and 390 mg/oz for caffeine and theobromine, respectively), and white chocolate has the least (0.8 and 0.2 mg/oz, respectively). The higher the cocoa content of the chocolate, the higher the methylxanthine risk per ounce of chocolate. Hyperactivity, polydipsia, vomiting, diuresis, diarrhea, restlessness, tachycardia, cardiac arrhythmia, and seizures usually occur in a progressive fashion beginning shortly after significant ingestions. Treatment should be directed at decontamination, control of anxiety and seizures, and the support of renal elimination through fluid diuresis.

- **Ingestion by dogs of cocoa beans, coca hulls, cola, coffee, and tea leaves may require emergency treatment.**

  True: All contain variable but potentially toxic concentrations of methylxanthines (caffeine, theobromine, and theophylline). Depending on the dose ingested, acute vomiting, excitement, cardiac irregularities, tremors, and seizures may result. Treatment includes early digestive tract evacuation plus activated charcoal/cathartics, diazepam for seizures, and lidocaine or atropine for life-threatening cardiac effects.

- **Onions and garlic can be bad for dogs.**

  True: Although *bad* is a relative term, too much acute exposure—or to a lesser extent, chronic, low-level dietary exposure—to onion or garlic may produce depression, rapid heart and respiratory rates, and pale mucous membranes. The anemia results from free radicals that cause Heinz bodies to form, damage to red blood cells, hemolysis, and methemoglobinemia. Effects persist for several days after exposure stops. Vitamin C and/or administration of other antioxidants may have therapeutic benefits. Cooked onions and garlic are much less of a hazard than the raw food.

- **Ingestion of Greenies treats is enjoyable but not risk free for cats and dogs.**

  True: Greenies are hard, green, molded bone-shaped treats that contain wheat gluten, glycerin, cellulose, and other additives that are both enjoyable and nutritious for pets. Greenies are intended to be chewed before ingestion to help prevent oral odors, tartar buildup, and gingivitis. Unfortunately pets occasionally swallow large pieces of these hard treats rather than chewing them into smaller pieces. Ingestion of large pieces of Greenies has the potential of creating an esophageal or intestinal obstruction and fails to accomplish the intended use.

Plants and Herbs

- **Herbal products can harm cats and dogs.**

  True: When left open and available, potpourri, garden herbs, cooking powders, perfumes, and various odorants and similar scent products are attractive to cats. The essential oils in such materials are irritants, which cause damage to sensitive respiratory cells, skin epithelium, and mucous membranes in general. Some herbal supplements may also contain steroids, benzodiazepines, heavy metals, analgesics, nonsteroidal antiinflammatory drugs, caffeine, atropine, and other constituents that are hazardous to pets that ingest or have contact with them.

- **Ingestion of Easter lilies (*Lilium longiflorum*) is highly poisonous to cats.**

  True: Vomiting, hypersalivation, depression, and anorexia usually occur within 1 to 2 hours after ingestion, followed by anuria and severe renal failure 2 to 4 days later. All parts of the plant should be considered poisonous, and almost all species of *Lilium* should be considered toxic. Dogs only appear to be affected with gastrointestinal upset. The sooner treatment is begun, the better the prognosis.

- **Ingestion of poinsettia flowers or leaves can make cats and dogs sick.**

  True: *Native* poinsettia (*Euphorbia pulcherrima*) belongs to the large *Euphorbia* genus of flowering plants. This genus may contain a milk-like sap that contains diterpenoid esters. These compounds can act as irritants. On the other hand, cats or dogs chewing or ingesting the cultivated *ornamental* poinsettia flower or leaves rarely exhibit more than mild gastrointestinal upset or simply drool from the plant's taste. Serious consequences are rarely seen. Treatment usually consists of washing away the sap with a drink of water or milk.

Other Ingestions

- **Ingestion of pennies and other coins is hazardous to household pets.**

  True: U.S. pennies minted since 1982 are copper coated, weigh 2.5 g, and contain 97.5% zinc. Although the adverse clinical signs of zinc poisoning, characterized by severe gastroenteritis and marked intravascular hemolysis, may be delayed following the ingestion of pennies, significant lodging of pennies in the acid media of the stomach increases the risk of zinc poisoning. Coins of other value do not contain zinc but can cause foreign body GI trauma.

- **Centipedes, if eaten by pets, can cause harm to the ingesting animal.**

  True: All species of the order Scolopendromorpha (i.e., centipedes having 21 or 23 pairs of legs) are venomous and can inflict harm by their bites or because they have been ingested. These centipedes have a stinging apparatus connected to their first pair of legs. Little is known of their venom; however, endopeptidase, cardiotoxin (toxin-S), serotonin, histamine, lipids, and various polysaccharides have been identified. No fatalities have been reported, but ingestion can produce vomiting, anxiety, and an irregular heartbeat or may simply induce a mild digestive upset.

- **Ingestion of caterpillars and butterflies by cats and dogs can be harmful.**

  True: Several types of hair, setae, or bristles cover the bodies of butterflies, moths, and their caterpillars. These hairs are irritants and sometimes are associated with venomous glands. No less than 200 varieties of these insects are known to be poisonous. Harm may result as a dermatologic syndrome, an ophthalmic injury, or respiratory and digestive syndromes. Mild gastrointestinal upset appears to be the most common hazard.

- **Parenteral administration of penicillin G procaine can cause spinal cord damage.**

  False: Penicillin G procaine (procaine penicillin G) is an equimolar salt of procaine and penicillin G in sterile solution. Penicillin G is one of the safest parenteral antimicrobial drugs available for use in animals. It has been used successfully for more than 50 years. However, there are always exceptions. A significant amount of penicillin G procaine injected directly into the spinal cord or even injected epidurally could cause spinal cord damage. Likewise, use of penicillin in animals known to be hypersensitive to penicillin is problematic. Use is contraindicated in guinea pigs and chinchillas, as well as in certain species of birds, snakes, turtles, and lizards.

- **Vitamins A and D have toxic potential for most animals.**

  True: Excessive amounts of vitamin A promote bone lesions with potential development of exostoses, which in turn may cause pressure on spinal nerves, resulting in paresis or other nerve deficits. Excessive amounts of vitamin D lead to hypercalcemia and calcium deposition of soft tissues, resulting in gastrointestinal, cardiopulmonary, and renal pathophysiology.

- **Ingestion of lipstick by cats or dogs results in lead poisoning.**

  False: The formulation of lipstick and other cosmetics is closely regulated and does not include lead as a constituent. However, many of the paints used in arts and crafts still contain potentially dangerous levels of heavy metals (including lead, barium, cadmium, and mercury). Red, yellow, orange, green, violet, vermillion, white, and black paints may contain toxic heavy-metal pigments and may also be potentially carcinogenic.

- **DEET mosquito repellent products are safe for use on cats and dogs.**

    False: All DEET (N,N-diethyl-meta-toluamide)– containing mosquito repellent products are potentially toxic to cats and dogs. Hypersalivation, vomiting, anxiety, tremors, ataxia, and seizures may occur within 6 hours following excessive exposure. Animals need to be decontaminated (dermal washing, oral-activated charcoal), their hydration monitored, and supportive therapy initiated as soon as possible following exposure. There is no antidote.

- **Ingestion of environmental mosquito larvicides containing *Bacillus thuringiensis israelensis (BTI)* is deadly to cats and dogs.**

    False: All mosquito prevention products containing BTI for use around the home (e.g., floating donuts, granules, liquids, briquettes) are generally safe. They may potentially cause gastrointestinal upset 3 to 6 hours following ingestion, and on rare occasions ingestion of floating donuts could result in formation of a gastrointestinal obstruction. However, they do help eliminate mosquito pests.

- **Human drugs tend to be less toxic to dogs and cats and therefore accidental ingestion is not usually a problem.**

    False: Human medications have a much narrower margin of safety in animals and any accidental ingestion should therefore be regarded as potentially toxic. Among the most hazardous are pain relief medications and antidepressants. However, all human medications should be regarded as hazardous to animals, unless prescribed by a veterinarian.

- **Anything and everything can be potentially toxic for a companion animal.**

    True: DOSE ALONE CAN MAKE ALL THE DIFFERENCE!

As may be seen from the previous examples of urban legends taken from various Internet sites, some have selected validity, some are clearly erroneous, and others are half-truths and depend on the circumstances of exposure. Veterinarians called on to respond to clients' concerns about such electronic postings or related neighborhood rumors must use their knowledge, experience, and common sense to provide appropriate, realistic, and professional clarifying information.

In some instances questions about the real toxicologic facts may develop, and other professional resources may be researched. Colleagues certified by the American Board of Veterinary Toxicologists (www.abvt.org) are widely available and can be contacted at nearby universities or animal poison centers. Clarification of related chemical details and the expertise of veterinary toxicologists are usually no more than a telephone call or computer keyboard click away; once the networking has been initiated, keep the phone number or online address in a readily available and visible place. Misconceived or erroneous urban legends fade away slowly!

References and Suggested Reading

Gupta RC: *Veterinary toxicology: basic and clinical principles*, New York, 2007, Academic Press.
Material Safety Data Sheets (MSDS): For commercial products MSDSs are available from manufacturers off their websites.
Peterson ME, Talcott PA: *Small animal toxicology*, ed 2, St Louis, 2006, Elsevier.
Plumlee KH: *Clinical veterinary toxicology*, St Louis, 2004, Mosby.

CHAPTER 23

Drugs Used to Treat Toxicoses

SHARON M. GWALTNEY-BRANT, *Mahomet, Illinois*

Paracelsus, who some consider the "Father of Toxicology," declared in the sixteenth century, "All substances are poisons; there is none which is not a poison. The right dose differentiates a poison from a remedy." Given the large number of potential poisons (toxicants) in the world and the wide variety of clinical effects these toxicants have on biological systems, it is not surprising that a vast range of compounds have been used in attempting to treat the effects of these toxicants on the body.

Antidotes

In the broadest definition, any compound that is used to counteract the effects of a toxicant is an *antidote*. The compound can interfere with the absorption, distribution, metabolism, or elimination of a toxicant; reduce or eliminate the adverse effects of that toxicant; or perform any combination of these biological effects. As our understanding of the mechanisms of action of various compounds increases, so does our ability to choose the most appropriate drugs to counter the adverse effects of toxicoses. This knowledge puts to rest the legend of the "universal antidote," that mythical compound that can counter the effects of any poison. Table 23-1 lists drugs commonly used in the management of toxicoses.

Mechanisms of Action

Antidotes are frequently classified into two groups based on their mechanisms of action: chemical antidotes and pharmacologic antidotes. *Chemical antidotes,* which interact directly with a toxicant to alter the toxicant's action in the body, include metal chelators, antibodies, and agents causing pharmacologic compartmentalization, as well as some other drugs. Metal chelators bind to metal ions, forming complexes that prevent the metal from reaching its target tissue and enhancing elimination of the chelate-metal complex. Immunologic products include intact immunoglobulins, such as IgG, and isolated F(ab') fragments, such as digoxin-specific F(ab') fragments, antivenoms, and antivenins. These drugs also bind target compounds, which prevents or reduces toxicant action and enhances excretion. Chemical chelators also may act as *sinks* by forming pharmacologic compartments that sequester toxicants, thereby reducing their ability to react with target tissues. Cholestyramine and intravenous lipid emulsions are examples of drugs thought to act in this fashion.

Pharmacologic antidotes neutralize or antagonize the effects of toxicants. Some such as fomepizole block metabolic enzymes and thereby reduce the formation of toxic metabolites; others such as naloxone act as receptor antagonists; and still others such as methocarbamol counter the effects of the toxicant.

Clinical Use of Antidotes

Although antidotes can be valuable assets in the management of toxicoses, there can be challenges when attempting to use them in veterinary practice. Some antidotes can be difficult to obtain; for example, botulinum antitoxin is only available through the Centers for Disease Control and Prevention and a few researchers. Others may be too expensive for some animal owners; for example, F(ab') crotalid antivenin costs more than $1,000.

Furthermore, not all antidotes are innocuous; injudicious use of excessive or inappropriate antidotes may result in clinical consequences that are more serious than those caused by the original toxicant. For example, methylene blue is an oxidation-reduction agent that has been used to treat methemoglobinemia; however, its precise dosing is required to prevent worsening of methemoglobinemia, especially in cats.

Approach to Patient Management

The veterinary clinician faced with a case of potential poisoning must carefully evaluate the patient and manage the clinical signs that are present in a systematic manner (i.e., *"treat the patient, not the poison"*). Because we lack specific chemical or pharmacologic antidotes for many toxicants, veterinarians are frequently forced to rely on "symptomatic and supportive" care when dealing with patients with toxicoses. The good news is that in many cases, successful outcomes can be attained by using good clinical judgment.

Initial Assessment

Patients should be assessed on presentation for any immediate life-threatening signs that need to be addressed. An efficient but thorough physical examination should be completed and vital signs carefully recorded. Specific tests, such as fluorescein staining for corneal ulcers, electrocardiography to identify heart rhythm disturbances, and thoracic radiography for pulmonary injury or a risk of aspiration, and routine

TABLE **23-1**

Drugs Used in Toxicology*

Drug	Indication
Acepromazine	Sedation for agitation caused by psychotropic drugs (e.g., amphetamines, phenylpropanolamine, pseudoephedrine)
N-acetylcysteine (Mucomyst, Acetadote)	Management of acetaminophen toxicosis Hepatoprotectant
Activated charcoal	Adsorption of ingested toxicants (poor adsorption of many metals and minerals, small molecules [e.g., alcohols]) Multidose protocols: monitor for hypernatremia
Aluminum hydroxide	Antacid; use for ingestion of corrosives or ulcerogenic drugs (e.g., NSAIDs)
Anti-digoxin Fab fragments, ovine origin (Digibind, DigiFab)	Management of cardiac glycoside toxicosis (drugs, plants, toads) in which life-threatening arrhythmias have not resolved with symptomatic therapy or serum potassium levels > 5 mmol/L
Antitoxin, botulinum, equine origin	Management of clinical signs of botulism
Antitoxin, tetanus, equine origin	Management of clinical signs of tetanus
Antivenin Crotalidae polyvalent, equine origin Polyvalent, immune Fab, ovine origin (Cro Fab)	Management of North American crotalid envenomation (rattlesnake, copperhead, water moccasin)
Antivenin *Micrurus* (Wyeth)	Management of North American elapid envenomation (coral snake)
Antivenin *Latrodectus* (Merck)	Management of envenomation by black widow spider
Antivenom, *Centruroides* immune F(ab')$_2$, equine origin (Anascorp)	Treatment of clinical signs of North American scorpion envenomation
Apomorphine	Induction of emesis; may not be effective in cats because they have few dopaminergic receptors in their CNS emetic center
Ascorbic acid	Antioxidant Urinary acidifier
Atipamezole hydrochloride (Antisedan)	Reversal of bradycardia, hypotension, and sedation from α-agonists (e.g., amitraz, xylazine, imidazole decongestants)
Atropine	Test dose for suspected organophosphorus (OP) or carbamate toxicosis Management of bradycardia or excessive bronchial secretions from OP or carbamate toxicosis Treatment of bradycardia from cardiac depressant drugs (e.g., digoxin)
Bicarbonate, sodium	Management of acidosis (e.g., ethylene glycol)
Blood, whole	Replacement therapy for anemia (e.g., anticoagulant rodenticides)
Buprenorphine	Management of pain
Calcitonin, salmon	Treatment of hypercalcemia (e.g., vitamin D or analogs)
Calcium EDTA	Heavy metal chelator (lead)
Calcium gluconate, calcium chloride	Management of fluoride or calcium channel blocker toxicosis Management of hypocalcemia
Cholestyramine resin polystyrene	Ion-binding resin; may help remove agents that undergo extensive enterohepatic recirculation Hepatotoxic mushroom ingestion
Chlorpromazine	Antiemetic Sedation for agitation caused by psychotropic drugs (e.g., amphetamines, pseudoephedrine)
Cyproheptadine	Assist in management of serotonin syndrome and serotonergic effects of psychotropic drugs (e.g., SSRI)
Dantrolene	Management of *Latrodectus* (black widow spider) bites; management of malignant hyperthermia from hops
Dapsone	Management of dermal necrosis from *Loxosceles* (recluse spider) bites
Deferoxamine mesylate (Desferal, Novartis)	Heavy metal chelator (iron)
Dextrose	Treatment of hypoglycemia due to xylitol, α-lipoic acid, or antidiabetic drug (e.g., sulfonylurea) toxicosis

TABLE 23-1

Drugs Used in Toxicology*—cont'd

Drug	Indication
Diazepam	Sedation for CNS stimulation or seizures; use with caution with sympathomimetic (e.g., amphetamine) intoxication because paradoxical excitation may occur
Dimercaprol (BAL)	Heavy metal chelator (arsenic, lead, mercury)
Diphenhydramine	Management of acute allergic reactions; antiemetic
Epinephrine	Systemic treatment of acute anaphylaxis
Esmolol	Management of ventricular arrhythmias; ultra–short acting β-blocker
Ethanol	Prevent formation of toxic metabolites in ethylene glycol toxicosis
Etidronate	Treatment of hypercalcemia (e.g., vitamin D or analogs)
Flumazenil	Benzodiazepine antagonist used to aid in severe benzodiazepine overdose
Fomepizole (Antizol-Vet)	Prevent formation of toxic metabolites in ethylene glycol toxicosis
Furosemide	Diuretic for use in management of pulmonary edema secondary to inhaled toxicants Enhance calcium excretion in hypercalcemia (e.g., cholecalciferol toxicosis)
Glucagon	Manage hypotension (e.g., β-adrenergic blocker, calcium channel blocker, tricyclic antidepressant toxicosis); manage hypoglycemia (e.g., antidiabetic drug toxicosis)
H₂-blockers (cimetidine, famotidine, nizatidine, ranitidine)	Reduce gastric acid production Prevention and healing of gastrointestinal ulcers (e.g., NSAIDs)
Hemoglobin glutamer-200, bovine (Oxyglobin)	Replacement therapy for anemia (e.g., anticoagulant rodenticides); does NOT provide clotting factors Improved perfusion of tissues with pressure hypoperfusion (e.g., snakebite swelling)
Hydroxocobalamin (Cyanokit)	Management of cyanide toxicosis
Hydrogen peroxide USP, 3%	Induction of emesis; CAUTION: overuse can result in esophagitis or gastritis
Intravenous lipid solution, intravenous fat emulsion (20%; Liposyn, Intralipid)	Management of intoxication by highly lipid-soluble compounds (e.g., avermectins, baclofen, calcium channel blockers); emerging modality that some consider experimental; should be reserved for severe cases that are poorly responsive to other therapy
Kaolin-pectin	Demulcent and putative adsorbent; CAUTION: many formulations now contain salicylates
Lactulose	Laxative and reduces blood ammonia levels Management of liver insufficiency (e.g., *Cycas* toxicosis)
Leucovorin calcium	Management of folate antagonist (methotrexate, trimetrexate) overdoses
Lidocaine	Management of ventricular arrhythmias
Magnesium hydroxide	Antacid; use for ingestion of corrosives or ulcerogenic drugs (e.g., NSAIDs)
Magnesium sulfate	Cathartic
Mannitol	Management of oliguric renal failure Treatment of cerebral edema
Maropitant (Cerenia)	Antiemetic
Methocarbamol	Management of muscle tremors, rigidity, convulsive activity (e.g., permethrin toxicosis, metaldehyde toxicosis)
Methylene blue	Treatment of methemoglobinemia; use with extreme caution, especially in cats (many clinicians no longer recommend); DO NOT USE new methylene blue from staining kits
Metoprolol	Management of tachycardia
Milk	Diluent May reduce pain from exposure to insoluble calcium oxalate–containing plants
Misoprostol (Cytotec)	Synthetic prostaglandin; prevention and healing of gastrointestinal ulcers (e.g., NSAIDs)
Naloxone	Opiate antagonist; management of opioid toxicosis
Neostigmine, physostigmine, pyridostigmine	Management of toxicosis from non-depolarizing neuromuscular blocking agents, botulism, atropine, coral snake envenomation, and anticholinergics
Nitroprusside	Treatment of hypertension
Norepinephrine	Treatment of hypotension

Continued

TABLE 23-1

Drugs Used in Toxicology*—cont'd

Drug	Indication
Ondansetron (Zofran)	Antiemetic
Pamidronate (Aredia)	Treatment of hypercalcemia (e.g., vitamin D or analogs)
D-Penicillamine	Heavy metal chelator (arsenic, copper, lead)
Pentobarbital	Management of seizures
Phenobarbital	Management of seizures
Plasma, frozen plasma, fresh frozen	Management of coagulopathy from anticoagulant rodenticides; provide clotting factors
Pralidoxime chloride (Protopam)	Treatment of nicotinic signs of OP insecticide intoxication
Prednisone	Adjunct therapy in hypercalcemia (e.g., cholecalciferol)
Propofol	Management of seizures
Propranolol	Management of tachycardia or other cardiac arrhythmias; management of hypokalemia in albuterol toxicosis
Protamine sulfate	Management of heparin overdoses
Proton pump inhibitors (e.g., omeprazole, lansoprazole, pantoprazole)	Reduce gastric acid production Prevention and healing of gastrointestinal ulcers (e.g., NSAIDs)
Prussian blue	Management of thallium toxicosis
Pyridoxine (vitamin B_6)	Management of seizures from penicillamine, *Gyromitra* mushroom, isoniazid, and hydrazines; adjunct therapy for ethylene glycol toxicosis
SAMe	Hepatoprotectant
Silymarin	Hepatoprotectant
Sodium sulfate	Cathartic
Sorbitol	Cathartic
Succimer (Chemet, Lundbeck)	Heavy metal chelator (arsenic, lead, mercury)
Sucralfate	Management and prevention of esophageal (slurries) and gastrointestinal ulceration
Trientine (Syprine)	Heavy metal chelator (copper)
Vitamin K_1 (phytonadione)	Treatment of anticoagulant rodenticide coagulopathy
Xylazine	Emetic, especially for cats
Yohimbine	Reversal of bradycardia, hypotension, and sedation from α-agonists (e.g., amitraz, xylazine, imidazole decongestants)

*See Appendix for dosages.
CNS, Central nervous system; *EDTA,* ethylenediaminetetraacetic acid; *NSAIDs,* nonsteroidal antiinflammatory drugs; *SAMe,* s-adenosyl methionine; *SSRI,* selective serotonin reuptake inhibitor; *USP,* United States Pharmacopeia.

clinical laboratory tests should be performed as clinically indicated.

Initial Treatments

Critical problems require immediate management. *Seizures and convulsions* generally respond well to standard anticonvulsants such as barbiturates and benzodiazepines; general anesthetics should be considered in refractory cases. Life-threatening *cardiac arrhythmias* or *respiratory issues* should be managed with appropriate antiarrhythmic medications (see Chapters 171 and 172), oxygen (see Chapter 10), and other drugs as needed (see Chapter 8). Severe *hemorrhage* or *anemia* may require blood transfusion (see Chapter 67) and *oxygen supplementation.* *Severe hyperthermia* (see Chapter 14), *electrolyte abnormalities, hypoglycemia* or *hyperglycemia,* and other metabolic derangements should be managed as needed (see Section I). Supportive care could include control of non–life-threatening signs, such as vomiting, maintenance of hydration, thermoregulation, and pain management (see Chapter 12).

Decontamination

Decontamination of clinically stable patients may be considered depending on the time frame of the exposure, the toxicant involved, and the potential for adverse effects from the decontamination procedure. Decontamination most commonly applies to surface exposures and to oral ingestions of potential toxicants. Grooming behavior can extend a topical exposure to a systemic exposure. Surface exposures are usually treated by irrigation of the skin, hair, or eyes with copious volumes of water, along with washing using a mild detergent. Care must be directed to effects on body temperature, especially in depressed or sedated animals. In cases of ocular contact, the cornea and eyelids should be gently irrigated with eyewash or sterile saline.

When a toxic substance is ingested consideration should be given to inducing emesis, administration of activated charcoal, and administration of a cathartic. However, as discussed in other chapters in this section, these treatments should not be administered to every animal or for every toxicant.

Emetics include (1) xylazine (0.44 mg/kg IM for cats; 1.1 mg/kg IM for dogs; note: xylazine can be reversed with yohimbine); (2) apomorphine in dogs (0.25 mg/kg of the crushed tablet in the conjunctival sac; rinse the conjunctival sac after vomiting; note: apomorphine can be reversed with naloxone); and (3) hydrogen peroxide (3%) in dogs (1 to 2 ml/kg PO to a maximum of 45 ml). Emesis should not be induced if the animal has been vomiting or if toxicant exposure has occurred over 3 hours before admission to the hospital. Moreover, it is not recommended to induce vomiting when a corrosive chemical has been ingested, if the animal cannot gag, or when there is evidence of preexistent or developing esophageal, cardiac, respiratory, or central nervous system disease. Marked sedation or loss of consciousness is a contraindication for emetics.

Activated charcoal (1 to 4 g/kg) may be beneficial as a nonspecific adsorbent for specific toxicoses (see Chapters 26 and 27). Activated charcoal will adsorb many larger molecules such as many pharmaceutical products, pesticides, and plant toxins. However, it is not indicated for ingestion of caustic (alkaline) chemicals, petroleum distillates, or small molecules such as alcohols, some mineral acids, or ionized metals or minerals (e.g., sodium, lithium). Administration can proceed by the oral route (in conscious animals that can swallow) or by orogastric tubing in dogs or nasogastric tubing in cats (the commonly used route in most emergency practices). In conscious animals, if emesis has been induced, administration of activated charcoal should be delayed for about 30 minutes to minimize the risk of spontaneous vomiting of charcoal or aspiration. If the patient is anesthetized or comatose, a cuffed endotracheal tube should be inserted to protect the airway. Re-dosing at one half of the original dose can be considered at 4- to 8-hour intervals for toxicants that undergo enterohepatic recirculation including phenobarbital, methylxanthines (chocolate), theophylline, marijuana, ivermectin (see Chapter 34), and nonsteroidal antiinflammatory drugs (see Chapter 27), among others. Potential risks include aspiration of activated charcoal, peritonitis if there is gastrointestinal ulceration or perforation, discoloration of the alimentary mucosa thereby complicating endoscopic evaluation, and hypernatremia due to fluid shifts following multidose activated charcoal regimens.

A *cathartic* reduces the time a toxicant is exposed to the gastrointestinal tract. These may be administered with the first dose of activated charcoal; in multidose activated charcoal regimens, cathartics are generally given with every third charcoal dose. Cathartics include sorbitol and magnesium or sodium sulfate salts. These may be incorporated into some commercial activated charcoal products or administered separately. The dosage of magnesium sulfate is approximately 5 to 20 g per dog and 2 to 4 g per cat. Magnesium sulfate is not administered in patients with kidney failure.

Specific Treatments

Table 23-1 list some of the specific drug treatments used when managing pets with toxicosis. Clinicians are advised to check dosages carefully and to appreciate differences between canine and feline dosing (see Appendix). Some of the specific uses of these drugs are described in greater detail in other chapters within this section.

References and Suggested Reading

American Board of Veterinary Toxicology: Review of veterinary antidotes. Available at: http://www.abvt.org/public/docs/reviewofveterinaryantidotes.pdf. Accessed Dec 1, 2011.

Bright SJ, Post LO: *Veterinary antidotes and availability: an update,* Center for Veterinary Medicine, US Food and Drug Administration. Available at: http://www.abvt.org/public/docs/antidoteupdate08.pdf, 2008. Accessed Dec 1, 2011.

Gwaltney-Brant SM, Rumbeiha WR: Newer antidotal therapies, *Vet Clin North Am Small Anim Pract* 32:323-339, 2002.

CHAPTER 24

Intravenous Lipid Emulsion Therapy

JUSTINE A. LEE, *Minneapolis, Minnesota*
ALBERTO L. FERNANDEZ MOJICA, *St. Georges, West Indies, Grenada*

Intravenous lipid emulsion (ILE), also known as intravenous fat emulsion (IFE), has been used in human and veterinary medicine as a part of total parenteral nutrition (TPN) or partial parenteral nutrition (PPN) for the past several decades. It also has been used as a vehicle for drug delivery for emulsions, such as propofol. More recently, ILE has been recommended as a potential antidote for lipophilic drug toxicosis.

In the 1970s and 1980s, studies that evaluated the effects of ILE on the pharmacokinetics of chlorpromazine and cyclosporine in rabbits and phenytoin in rats demonstrated potential support for use of ILE in certain drug toxicities. Almost 2 decades later, Weinberg and colleagues reintroduced the potential beneficial effects of ILE in the treatment of the fat-soluble, local anesthetic bupivacaine toxicosis. Since then, several animal studies and human and animal case reports have reported successful use of ILE. Toxicoses that are reportedly responsive to ILE treatment include bupivacaine, lidocaine, clomipramine, verapamil, bupropion, mepivacaine, ropivacaine, haloperidol, quetiapine, doxepin, carvedilol, carbamazepine, flecainide, hydroxychloroquine, amlodipine, propranolol, calcium channel blockers (e.g., diltiazem), and macrocyclic lactones (e.g., moxidectin, ivermectin). However, success with ILE has been variable, ranging from no improvement to complete resolution of clinical signs. That said, ILE is considered a potential antidote in cases of lipid-soluble toxicities in which cardiopulmonary arrest (CPA) and standard resuscitation have failed to result in return of spontaneous circulation (ROSC). Currently, no prospective, randomized studies are available in human or veterinary medicine regarding the use of ILE because it is currently reserved for catastrophic toxicities and severe clinical signs.

In veterinary medicine, recent publications describe the use of ILE for macrocyclic lactones, lidocaine, pyrethrins, and calcium channel blocker toxicoses (Crandell et al, 2009; O'Brien et al, 2010; Clarke et al, 2011; Brückner et al, 2012; Maton et al, 2013). A state-of-the-art review was recently published introducing the first recommendations on the use of ILE in veterinary medicine (Fernandez et al, 2011). Pet Poison Helpline, an animal poison control center based in Minneapolis, has experienced anecdotal success with the use of ILE for certain additional medications with a narrow margin of safety (e.g., baclofen, cholecalciferol, β-blockers).

Mechanism of Action

The precise mechanism of action through which ILE increases the rate of recovery and augments conventional resuscitation efforts in various cases of lipophilic drug toxicosis is currently unknown. It is possible that the potential antidotal effects of ILE vary with the lipophilicity of the toxic agent or that more than one mechanism of action is operative. Current theories regarding ILE's mechanism of action are:

- Providing myocytes with energy substrates, thereby augmenting cardiac performance.
- Restoring myocardial function by increasing intracellular calcium concentration.
- Acting as a lipid sink by sequestration of lipophilic compounds into the newly created intravascular lipid compartment (a lipid or pharmacologic sink). With this lipid sink hypothesis, compartmentalization of the drug into the lipid phase results in a decreased free drug concentration available to tissues.
- Increasing the overall fatty acid pool, which overcomes inhibition of mitochondrial fatty acid metabolism (e.g., bupivacaine toxicosis).

Currently, the most supported hypotheses are that ILE improves cardiac performance and provides a lipid sink effect in the vascular compartment.

Current Published Human Research Information and Data

The vast majority of ILE publications in human medicine stem from case reports. Initial human case reports related to the use of ILE as a treatment in local anesthesia-related CPA that was unresponsive to cardiopulmonary resuscitation (CPR). In 2006, the first case study was published involving a patient who developed seizures and cardiac arrest shortly after receiving a nerve block with a mixture of bupivacaine and mepivacaine (Rosenblatt et al, 2006). After 20 minutes of unsuccessful CPR and advanced cardiac life support (ACLS), 100 ml of a 20% ILE was administered (1.2 ml/kg IV bolus), followed by an additional constant rate infusion (CRI) (0.5 ml/kg/min, IV, over 2 hours). Sinus rhythm and ROSC occurred shortly after administration of the ILE bolus. The patient recovered uneventfully. Similar reports have since been published demonstrating an amelioration or reversal of the adverse effects of bupivacaine, mepivacaine, and ropivacaine with ILE. However, ILE has not proven to be consistently effective in all cases of lipophilic drug toxicosis, presumably related to the lipid solubility of the toxin in question.

Current Published Veterinary Information

Experimental studies: In contrast to the available human data, most of the animal publications are in the form of experimental studies. One of the first investigations performed in 1974 evaluated *in vivo* and *ex vivo* rabbit models of chlorpromazine toxicosis. In the *in vivo* arm of the study, all control rabbits dosed with 30 mg/kg IV chlorpromazine died, whereas all control rabbits in the ILE pretreatment group lived. The study also reported significantly decreased free chlorpromazine after the addition of ILE to rabbit blood. A similar study evaluating coadministration of 20% ILE on the pharmacokinetics of cyclosporine in rabbits reported decreased total body clearance and volume of distribution of cyclosporine with ILE administration.

In 1998, Weinberg and colleagues evaluated the effects of pretreatment with ILE in a rodent model of bupivacaine-induced asystole and reported a 48% increase in median lethal dose (LD_{50}) in the ILE-treated group. Several years later, this author evaluated the effect of saline fluid versus ILE in the treatment of bupivacaine-induced cardiotoxicity in 12 dogs in which all animals in the saline control group failed to develop ROSC and died, whereas all the ILE-treated patients survived. Additional details of these and related studies can be found in the review of Jamaty et al.

Case Reports

The first clinical case using 20% ILE in veterinary medicine was described by Crandell et al in a 16-week-old Jack Russell terrier with moxidectin toxicosis. In this case, 2 ml/kg of ILE (IV, bolus) was administered, followed by 4 ml/kg/hr (0.07 ml/kg/min, IV) for 4 hours. ILE treatment began 10 hours after moxidectin exposure, and then was repeated approximately 25 hours after exposure (0.25 ml/kg/min, IV, for 30 minutes). Several subsequent cases reported ILE use.

In 2010, O'Brien et al reported on ILE-treated lidocaine toxicosis. A 5-year-old cat received a SC injection of about 20 mg/kg of lidocaine for surgical closure of a wound in the left hind limb. Less than 5 minutes after administration, severe lethargy and respiratory distress were noticed. Marked cardiovascular, respiratory, and neurologic abnormalities were seen on arrival to the emergency room approximately 25 minutes later. Initial therapy consisted of oxygen support, crystalloid fluid resuscitation, and a 20% ILE bolus administered at 1.5 ml/kg [0.68 ml/lb]) over a 30-minute period. Shortly after initiation of ILE administration, the cat was more responsive to stimuli and was able to hold its head up. Significant neurologic improvement was noticed by the end of the lipid infusion. The cat survived to discharge with no adverse effects reported. In this case it is likely that the toxic effects of

lidocaine may have improved without the use of ILE; however, its use appeared to reduce the duration of clinical signs and minimize the overall morbidity associated with this toxicosis.

Later, Clarke et al reported the use of ILE in a Border collie that developed ivermectin toxicosis after ingesting 6 mg/kg of equine ivermectin paste. Treatment with a 20% ILE bolus administered at 1.5 ml/kg over 10 minutes, followed by a CRI of 0.25 ml/kg/min for 60 minutes was performed. This was the first clinical study to demonstrate the lipid sink hypotheses based on serial ivermectin serum levels.

Since then, numerous case reports have been published demonstrating the use of ILE in dogs and cats (Brückner and Schwedes, 2012), some with successful resolution of clinical signs and some demonstrating lack of efficacy (Wright et al, 2011).

When to Use ILE

ILE therapy is generally considered relatively safe. Nevertheless, in human medicine ILE is reserved for severe toxicosis and life-threatening clinical signs when conventional therapies have failed. This differs from veterinary medicine, in which ILE is generally initiated earlier in the course of treatment. In veterinary medicine, ILE is warranted for toxicities associated with lipid-soluble compounds in which a high morbidity has been reported, the patient is symptomatic, and traditional therapies have failed or are cost-prohibitive.

Dosing of ILE

Initial human dosing guidelines for ILE administration stem from two main sources: a publication entitled *Guidelines for the Management of Severe Local Anesthetic Toxicity* by the Association of Anaesthetists of Great Britain and Ireland (AAGBI) and publications authored by Dr. Guy Weinberg, who created a website (www.lipidrescue.org) in which the use of ILE is well described. Following the publication of these guidelines, there was an increase in both the availability of and the willingness to use ILE in hospitals for humans, particularly in areas in which local anesthetic drugs were administered. These dosing recommendations were based on experimental animal studies and human case reports.

Currently in veterinary medicine, the dosing of ILE is extrapolated from human data and the use of ILE is considered extralabel. The current human guidelines for the use of ILE recommend that infusion with ILE should only be attempted when standard resuscitation protocols have failed to establish adequate ROSC and that CPR should continue during ILE administration. Dosage recommendations for 20% ILE are 1.5 ml/kg (IV, bolus over 1 minute), followed by a CRI of 0.25 ml/kg/min (IV, for 30 to 60 minutes). The bolus dose can be repeated twice in 5-minute intervals if CPA persists. If progressive hypotension is noticed, the CRI rate of administration can then be further increased to 0.5 ml/kg/min (IV). A total limit of 8 to 12 ml/kg/day has been suggested.

Fernandez et al recommended the following dosage in veterinary medicine based on extrapolation from human dosing and the dose used for TPN and PPN administration in veterinary medicine: administration of an initial 20% ILE bolus in the range between 1.5 ml/kg and 4 ml/kg (between 0.3 g/kg and 0.8 g/kg, IV, over 1 minute), followed by a CRI of 0.25 ml/kg/min (0.05 g/kg/min, IV, over 30 to 60 minutes) as a generally conservative start in dogs. In patients that are nonresponsive after this traditional dosing, additional individual bolus aliquots can be given slowly at up to 7 ml/kg (1.4 g/kg, IV). The authors recommended intermittent bolusing at 1.5 ml/kg q4-6h for 24 hours with anecdotal success. In addition, follow-up CRI doses of 0.5 ml/hr (0.1 g/kg/hr) can be continued until clinical signs improve (not to exceed 24 hours) or until serum is lipemic. That said, there have been no safety studies evaluating the use of ILE in the clinically poisoned veterinary patient, and careful monitoring and risk assessment is imperative.

Fat Overload Syndrome

Rare complications exist with ILE therapy. Delayed or subacute reactions to ILE are commonly referred to as *fat overload syndrome* (FOS). Reactions are often the result of accidental administration of excessive volumes or rates that overwhelms the endogenous lipid clearance mechanisms. FOS is characterized by hyperlipidemia, hepatomegaly, icterus, splenomegaly, thrombocytopenia, increased clotting times, hemolysis, and variable end-organ dysfunction. In humans, long-chain triglyceride emulsions administered at rates above 0.11 g/kg/hr (ILE 20% = 0.55 ml/kg/hr) can be associated with adverse effects. The syndrome can also occur when ILE is administered to patients with decreased plasma clearance of lipids. This complication appears to be reported in the literature more often with the use of soybean oil-based emulsions than with other formulations. However, this could be because these types of emulsions are more frequently used for parenteral nutrition.

Management of FOS consists of both discontinuation of ILE administration and supportive care. Resolution of clinical signs is expected after the ILE is metabolized, but permanent organ damage has been reported. Plasma exchange has been recommended for cases of FOS that failed to respond to conservative therapy.

Heparin, which elicits significant effects in lipid metabolism, has been clinically used to prevent adverse events from ILE administration. Although heparin can potentially minimize hyperlipidemia, its routine use with ILE therapy is not currently recommended. By enhancing the release of lipoprotein lipase (LPL) and hepatic lipase, heparin may reduce the lipid compartment in the blood and, potentially, the beneficial properties of ILE when used for the treatment of a lipid-soluble toxicant. Until further studies evaluate the underlying mechanisms of action of how ILE therapy works and is influenced by LPL, heparin should be reserved only for those patients at risk to develop FOS or other adverse events. If heparin administration is considered for the treatment of FOS, it should ideally be used as a CRI to have continued effects on LPL levels.

Controversies of ILE

If an effective therapy or antidote is already well established in the field of veterinary toxicology, its continued use is recommended over ILE due to the unknown effects of ILE administration. Keep in mind that certain therapeutics (e.g., anticonvulsants) may be made ineffective with the administration of ILE; hence supportive therapy is always warranted prior to experimental use of ILE. However, if the patient has undergone cardiovascular collapse secondary to toxicosis or demonstrates significant clinical signs of toxicosis (e.g., from baclofen, ivermectin, or moxidectin), ILE should be considered. As administration of ILE increases the free fatty acid concentration, it may have negative inotropic effects and induce cardiac arrhythmias in the hypoxic myocardium. Therefore appropriate medical management, volume resuscitation, and adequate oxygenation are imperative as the first-line defense in the treatment of the critically ill patient with a lipophilic compound intoxication prior to any consideration of the use of ILE.

The administration of ILE for the treatment of local anesthetic or other lipophilic drug toxicosis in veterinary medicine is still in its infancy and the potential is currently unknown. The judicious use of this new potential antidote should be considered based on the lipophilic nature of the drug. The higher the affinity of a drug for lipids and the higher the volume of distribution, the more suitable it is to be potentially reversed by administration of ILE. An animal poison control helpline should ideally be consulted prior to administration of ILE to ensure appropriate use and fat-solubility for the toxicant.

References and Suggested Reading

Association of Anaesthetists of Great Britain and Ireland. Available at: http://update.anaesthesiologists.org/wp-content/uploads/2009/12/Management-of-local-anaesthetic-toxicity.pdf Accessed November 25, 2012.

Brückner M, Schwedes CS: Successful treatment of permethrin toxicosis in two cats with an intravenous lipid administration, *Tierärztl Prax* 40:129-134, 2012.

Clarke DL et al: Use of intravenous lipid emulsion to treat ivermectin toxicosis in a Border collie, *J Am Vet Med Assoc* 239:(10):1328-1333, 2011.

Crandell DE, Weinberg GL: Moxidectin toxicosis in a puppy successfully treated with intravenous lipids, *J Vet Emerg Crit Care* 19(2):181-186, 2009.

Fernandez AL et al: The use of intravenous lipid emulsion as an antidote in veterinary toxicology, *J Vet Emerg Crit Care* 21(4):309-320, 2011.

Jamaty C et al: Lipid emulsions in the treatment of acute poisoning: a systematic review of human and animal studies, *Clin Toxicol* 48:1-27, 2010.

Kollef MH et al: The fat overload syndrome: successful treatment with plasma exchange, *Ann Intern Med* 112(7):545-546, 1990.

Krieglstein J, Meffert A, Niemeyer DH: Influence of emulsified fat on chlorpromazine availability in rabbit blood, *Experientia* 30(8):924-926, 1974.

LipidRescue: Resuscitation for cardiac toxicity. Available at: http://lipidrescue.org. Accessed November 10, 2011.

Maton BL et al: The use of high-dose insulin therapy and intravenous lipid emulsion to treat severe, refractory diltiazem toxicosis in a dog, *J Vet Emerg Crit Care* 23(3):321-327, 2013.

O'Brien TQ et al: Infusion of a lipid emulsion to treat lidocaine intoxication in a cat, *J Am Vet Med Assoc* 237:1455-1458, 2010.

Rosenblatt MA et al: Successful use of a 20% lipid emulsion to resuscitate a patient after a presumed bupivacaine-related cardiac arrest, *Anesthesiology* 105(1):217-218, 2006.

Turner-Lawrence DE, Kerns W II: Intravenous fat emulsion: a potential novel antidote, *J Med Toxicol* 4(2):109-114, 2008.

Weinberg GL et al: Pretreatment or resuscitation with a lipid infusion shifts the dose-response to bupivacaine-induced asystole in rats, *Anesthesiology* 88:1071-1075, 1998.

Weinberg G et al: Lipid emulsion infusion rescues dogs from bupivacaine-induced cardiac toxicity, *Reg Anesth Pain Med* 28:198-202, 2003.

Weinberg G: Lipid infusion resuscitation for local anesthetic toxicity, *Anesthesiology* 105:7-8, 2006.

Wright HM et al: Intravenous fat emulsion for treatment for ivermectin toxicosis in three dogs homozygous for the ABCB1-1Δ gene mutation, *J Vet Emerg Crit Care* 21(6):666-672, 2011.

CHAPTER 25

Human Drugs of Abuse and Central Nervous System Stimulants

PETRA A. VOLMER, *Champaign, Illinois*

Animal exposures to human *drugs of abuse* occur periodically in veterinary medicine. In many cases the owners are reluctant to admit that the animal was exposed until it is in severe distress. Often illicit drugs are contaminated with other compounds that may possess pharmacologic activity, causing unique combinations of clinical signs. Diagnosis of a toxicosis is often based on characteristic clinical signs and history of exposure. Over-the-counter drug-testing kits are available at most pharmacies. These kits are designed for rapid determination of drug presence in urine and, although designed for in-home human use, may provide important diagnostic information in the veterinary clinical setting. Some kits may test for as many as 12 drugs. Although these kits are often useful clinically, further confirmation may be needed in medicolegal circumstances.

Amphetamines

Amphetamines are a class of compounds that includes a number of prescription and illicit products, all derivatives of the parent compound amphetamine. Most animal exposures are a result of the accidental ingestion of human prescription products used for the treatment of obesity, narcolepsy, and attention-deficit hyperactivity disorder. Examples include dextroamphetamine (Dexedrine), methylphenidate (Ritalin, Concerta), pemoline (Cylert), phentermine (Fastin), and the combination of dextroamphetamine and amphetamine (Adderall). Exposure to unlawful amphetamine compounds can also occur. Street names for amphetamines can include *speed,*

uppers, dex or dexies, and *bennies.* Methamphetamine production is on the rise in clandestine laboratories in many areas of the United States. Street names for methamphetamine can include *ice* and *glass* for the clear, translucent crystals and *crystal, crank,* and *meth* for the white or yellow powder form. Designer amphetamines include 4-methylaminorex *(ice, U4EUh),* methcathinone *(cat),* 3,4-methylenedioxy-N-methylamphetamine (MDMA [*ecstasy, XTC, Adam, MDA*]), and 3,4-methylenedioxy-N-ethylamphetamine (MDEA [*Eve*]) (Volmer, 2006; Llera and Volmer, 2006).

The amphetamines as a class are well absorbed orally, with peak plasma levels occurring by 1 to 3 hours; thus clinical signs can develop rapidly. Some pharmaceutical products are extended-release preparations, with the result of prolonging absorption and delaying the onset of signs. Amphetamine and its metabolites are excreted in the urine in a pH-dependent manner, so that a lower pH enhances excretion (Baggot and Davis, 1972). Amphetamines have a stimulant effect on the cerebral cortex through release of catecholamines, acting as a dopamine excitatory receptor agonist and enhancing release of serotonin. Toxic dosages of amphetamine products are low: the oral median lethal dosage for amphetamine sulfate in the dog is 20 to 27 mg/kg; for methamphetamine hydrochloride it is 9 to 11 mg/kg (Zalis et al, 1965). Signs in field cases can be seen at dosages much lower than experimental lethal dosages.

Exposed animals exhibit signs associated with stimulation. Behavioral effects can include initial restlessness, pacing, panting, and an inability to sit still. These signs can progress to pronounced hyperactivity, hypersalivation, vocalization, tachypnea, tachycardia, tremors, hyperthermia, seizures, and potentially death. In some cases animals may exhibit depression, weakness, and bradycardia.

Diagnosis is based on clinical signs and history of exposure. Amphetamines can be detected in urine. Over-the-counter drug-testing kits may be of use in diagnosing an exposure in the acute clinical setting.

Animals should be stabilized and then decontaminated. Animals with known ingestions of amphetamine products less than 30 minutes prior can undergo induction of emesis followed by administration of activated charcoal and a cathartic. Animals already exhibiting signs of stimulation such as restlessness or worse should not be induced to vomit because of the risk of aspiration. Similarly, if the product is rapidly absorbed with the possible rapid onset of signs, emesis is not recommended. For those cases gastric lavage followed by the instillation of activated charcoal and a cathartic is a safer approach. Sustained-release medications may require repeated doses of activated charcoal.

Excitability, tremors, seizures, and other stimulant signs associated with amphetamine intoxication can be treated with acepromazine (0.5 to 1 mg/kg slowly intravenously [IV]; allow 15 minutes for onset of action; repeat as needed and monitor arterial blood pressure) or chlorpromazine (10 to 18 mg/kg IV repeated as needed with blood pressure monitoring). Phenothiazine tranquilizers have been shown to have a protective effect when used to treat amphetamine toxicoses (Catravas et al, 1977). Diazepam is not recommended because it can exacerbate the stimulatory signs in some animals. Phenobarbital, pentobarbital, and propofol (dosed carefully "to effect") may also be used to treat or mitigate severe central nervous system (CNS) signs. In addition, cyproheptadine, a serotonin antagonist, may help reduce the CNS signs. It has been used successfully to dampen the excessive stimulation from overexposure to antidepressant medications designed to increase serotonin in nerve synapses. Cyproheptadine is dosed at 1.1 mg/kg rectally in dogs.

Tachyarrhythmias should be treated with a β-blocker such as propranolol, esmolol, atenolol, or metoprolol. Hyperthermia should be corrected using a water mist and fans. Animals should be monitored to prevent subsequent hypothermia and housed in a dark, quiet environment to avoid external stimulation.

Intravenous fluids act to protect the kidneys and enhance elimination. Tremendous muscle stimulation can result in rhabdomyolysis and subsequent myoglobinuria, as well as a metabolic acidosis. Urinary acidification can promote elimination of amphetamines but must not be undertaken if the animal has compromised renal function or if acidosis is already present.

Cocaine

There are two main forms of cocaine: the hydrochloride salt and the pure cocaine alkaloid or *freebase*. The hydrochloride salt is a powder that readily dissolves in water and is usually self-administered by humans either intravenously or intranasally. Some street names for cocaine powder include *coke, girl, gold or star dust, snow, blow, nose candy,* and *white lady*. Freebase is the conversion of the hydrochloride salt form to the pure cocaine alkaloid. The pure alkaloid thus created exists in a flake, crystal, or rock form that vaporizes when heated, making a popping or cracking sound (i.e., *crack, rock,* or *flake*). Freebase is usually smoked but is sometimes taken orally (Volmer, 2006).

Cocaine is rapidly and well absorbed from all mucosal surfaces. Inflamed or irritated surfaces may promote absorption. Cocaine is rapidly and extensively metabolized in the liver and excreted in the urine. Cocaine is a strong CNS stimulant. It acts to block the reuptake of serotonin and norepinephrine and has the ability to block cardiac sodium channels (Parker et al, 1999).

The overall effect of cocaine intoxication is one of stimulation. Animals initially become restless and hyperactive. Signs can progress rapidly to tremors, tachycardia, hypotension, prolongation of QRS intervals, tachypnea, and seizures.

Diagnosis is usually based on clinical signs and history of exposure. Over-the-counter drug-testing kits may be helpful in diagnosing a cocaine toxicosis.

Treatment is aimed at stabilizing the patient, followed by decontamination. Because clinical signs can develop rapidly, increasing the risk of aspiration, caution should be used if inducing emesis. A safer approach may be to perform gastric lavage with administration of activated charcoal and a cathartic. Tremors and seizures can be controlled with diazepam, chlorpromazine, or a barbiturate. Pretreatment with chlorpromazine effectively antagonized the effects of cocaine in experimentally dosed dogs (Catravas and Waters, 1981). Administration of sodium bicarbonate decreases the likelihood of development of ventricular arrhythmias, shortens the prolonged QRS complex duration, counteracts the reduction in mean arterial blood pressure, and reverses cocaine-induced sodium channel blockade (Llera and Volmer, 2006). Severe tachyarrhythmias can be treated with a β-blocker such as propranolol or esmolol. Intravenous fluids should be administered to maintain renal blood flow and promote excretion. Acid-base and electrolyte status should be monitored and corrected. Hyperthermia can be severe in cocaine intoxications. Correction of body temperature can be achieved with evaporative cooling measures such as misting the animal with cool water and placing the patient in front of a fan until normal body temperature is reached. Alternatively the patient can be immersed in a tepid water bath while monitoring body temperature.

Marijuana

Tetrahydrocannabinol (THC), the major active cannabinoid in marijuana, can be found in all parts of the marijuana plant. Street names include *pot, Mary Jane, MJ, weed, grass, puff,* and *hemp*. Hashish is the dried resin from flower tops and can contain up to 10% THC. Hashish oil can contain up to 20% THC. Sinsemilla is seedless marijuana (Volmer, 2006).

THC is highly lipophilic, is highly protein bound, has a large volume of distribution, and undergoes enterohepatic recirculation. All these characteristics result in slow elimination from the body (Otten, 2002). Only 10% to 15% of THC or its metabolites are excreted in the urine, with the remainder through the feces via the bile. Marijuana has a wide margin of safety, with a minimum oral lethal dose in the dog of greater than 3 g/kg. However, clinical signs can occur at 1000 times less than this dose (Thompson et al, 1973).

Onset of clinical signs can occur within 30 to 60 minutes and can include depression, disorientation, lethargy, ataxia, bradycardia, vomiting, tremor, mydriasis, hypothermia, and urine dribbling. Analysis for THC can be performed on stomach contents and urine.

Treatment is primarily symptomatic and supportive. The cannabinoids have a wide margin of safety, and toxicoses are rarely fatal. If the animal is not exhibiting any clinical signs and no other contraindications exist, emesis should be induced. Because enterohepatic recirculation may prolong the residence time of the cannabinoids in the body, repeated doses of activated charcoal are recommended. Body temperature should be monitored for hypothermia and corrected. In most cases recovery should occur within 24 to 72 hours.

Opioids

Opium, the dried milky exudate of the poppy plant, contains 24 alkaloids, including morphine, codeine, and thebaine. The opioids are synthetic compounds that bind to the opioid receptor and are classed as agonists, partial agonists, or antagonists. They differ in their specificity and efficacy at different types of receptors. Four major opioid receptors have been identified, with most of the clinically useful opioids binding to mu receptors. Naloxone is a pure competitive antagonist with no agonist activity and has a high affinity for the mu receptor (Volmer, 2006).

Most animal exposures involve ingestion of pharmaceutical preparations. Some common opioids include codeine, fentanyl, hydrocodone, hydromorphone, levorphanol, loperamide, meperidine, methadone, and oxycodone. The opioids are well absorbed from the gastrointestinal tract and rapidly metabolized in the liver. Morphine is glucuronidated, and the glucuronide is then excreted by the kidney. Clinical signs can include vomiting, defecation, salivation, lethargy and depression, and ataxia. In severe cases respiratory depression, constipation, hypothermia, coma, seizures, and pulmonary edema are possible.

Emesis is recommended for recent ingestions in animals that are not exhibiting clinical signs. Pylorospasm produced by the opioid may cause much of the drug to remain in the stomach; thus gastric lavage, activated charcoal, and a cathartic may be effective even several hours after ingestion. Respiratory depression is the most common cause of death with opioid overexposure and should be treated by establishment of a patent airway, assisted ventilation, and oxygen. Naloxone (0.01 to 0.02 mg/kg IV, intramuscularly, or subcutaneously) reverses respiratory depression but does not restore full consciousness. Naloxone may need to be repeated as clinical signs indicate.

Barbiturates

Members of barbiturates are all derivatives of barbituric acid. The barbiturates are used therapeutically as sedatives and anticonvulsants. Animal exposures can result from iatrogenic overdose, ingestion of illicit preparations, accidental administration of euthanasia solutions, and ingestion of euthanized carcasses. Illicit products are known as *downers, reds, Christmas trees,* and *dolls* (Volmer, 2006).

The barbiturates are well absorbed orally or following intramuscular injection. Lipid solubility of the drug determines the distribution of the barbiturate in the body and the duration of effect. The barbiturates are metabolized in the liver by hepatic microsomal enzymes and excreted in the urine. Acutely the barbiturates may interfere with metabolism of other drugs by binding to hepatic P-450 enzymes, preventing their action on other compounds. Chronic exposure to barbiturates acts to increase microsomal enzyme activity (enzyme induction), thus enhancing the biotransformation of both exogenous and some endogenous substances. Approximately 25% of phenobarbital is excreted unchanged in the urine. It can be ion trapped in the urine by urinary alkalinization, increasing excretion fivefold to tenfold (Haddad and Winchester, 1998). The efficacy of ion trapping for other barbiturates is not as distinct.

Barbiturates activate γ-aminobutyric acid A receptors and inhibit excitatory glutamate receptors. Clinical signs can include depression, ataxia, incoordination, weakness, disorientation, recumbency, coma, hypothermia, tachycardia or bradycardia, and death. Barbiturates can be detected in stomach contents, blood, urine, liver, and feces.

For recent ingestions in animals exhibiting no other clinical signs, emesis followed by repeated dosages of activated charcoal and a cathartic is recommended. Activated charcoal acts as a *sink*, encouraging the barbiturate to diffuse back into the intestine from the circulation, even for compounds administered parenterally (Plumb, 2005). Gastric lavage followed by activated charcoal and a cathartic is a safer alternative for animals exhibiting clinical signs (and risking aspiration from induction of emesis). Death is usually the result of respiratory depression; therefore intubation, administration of oxygen, and assisted ventilation may be required. Body temperature should be monitored and corrected. Ventricular fibrillation and cardiac arrest can result from some barbiturates and be exacerbated by profound hypothermia (Haddad and Winchester, 1998). Supportive care, including intravenous fluids, is recommended. Forced alkaline diuresis may facilitate the excretion of some barbiturates, especially phenobarbital.

References and Suggested Reading

Baggot JD, Davis LE: Pharmacokinetic study of amphetamine elimination in dogs and swine, *Biochem Pharmacol* 21:1967, 1972.

Catravas JD et al: The effects of haloperidol, chlorpromazine and propranolol on acute amphetamine poisoning in the conscious dog, *J Pharmacol Exp Ther* 202:230, 1977.

Catravas JD, Waters IW: Acute cocaine intoxication in the conscious dog: studies on the mechanism of lethality, *J Pharmacol Exp Ther* 217:350, 1981.

Haddad LM, Winchester JF: Barbiturates. In Haddad LM, Shannon MW, Winchester JF, editors: *Clinical management of poisoning and drug overdose*, ed 3, Philadelphia, 1998, Saunders, p 521.

Llera RM, Volmer PA: Hazards faced by police dogs used for drug detection, *J Am Vet Med Assoc* 228:1028, 2006.

Otten EJ: Marijuana. In Goldfrank LR, et al, editors: *Toxicologic emergencies*, ed 7, New York, 2002, McGraw-Hill, p 1055.

Parker RB et al: Comparative effects of sodium bicarbonate and sodium chloride on reversing cocaine-induced changes in the electrocardiogram, *J Cardiovasc Pharmacol* 34:864, 1999.

Plumb DC: Phenobarbital. In Plumb DC, editor: *Plumb's veterinary drug handbook*, ed 5, Ames, IA, 2005, Blackwell Publishing, p 620.

Thompson GR et al: Comparison of acute oral toxicity of cannabinoids in rats, dogs, and monkeys, *Toxicol Appl Pharmacol* 25:363, 1973.

Volmer PA: Recreational drugs. In Peterson M, Talcott P, editors: *Small animal toxicology*, ed 2, Philadelphia, 2006, Saunders, p 273.

Zalis EG et al: Acute lethality of the amphetamines in dogs and its antagonism by curare, *Proc Soc Exp Biol Med* 118:557, 1965.

CHAPTER 26

Antidepressants and Anxiolytics

AHNA G. BRUTLAG, *Minneapolis, Minnesota*

Prescription antidepressants and anxiolytic drugs routinely rank among the most commonly prescribed agents in the United States. Additionally, they are commonly used in veterinary medicine for a variety of behavioral disorders including separation anxiety, storm phobias, inappropriate urine marking, stereotypic behaviors, and psychogenic alopecia (see Chapter 117). Although mild adverse effects may be noted at therapeutic doses, severe toxicosis and death may result following overdose, especially if these drugs are ingested with other drugs with serotonergic properties (such as monoamine oxidase inhibitors or 5-hydroxytryptophan). Because of their frequent use, the palatability of some flavored veterinary formulations, and the potential for severe intoxication, unintentional overdoses of antidepressants rank among the most commonly reported cases to Pet Poison Helpline.

Antidepressants and anxiolytics encompass several drug classes, the most common of which include selective serotonin reuptake inhibitors (SSRIs), serotonin and norepinephrine reuptake inhibitors (SNRIs), tricyclic antidepressants (TCAs), benzodiazepines (BZDs), and nonbenzodiazepine (non-BZD) hypnotic agents. The pharmacologic and pharmacokinetic properties of these different classes vary greatly and account for a wide range of toxicities and mechanisms of action. Although some drugs, such as many SSRIs or TCAs, may cause severe intoxication in smaller dosages, others, such as BZDs, have a wider margin of safety and are less likely to

result in severe toxicosis or death. Thus obtaining the exact name of the medication ingested by the pet is crucial to determine a proper course of treatment and guide prognosis. Due to the wide variability in clinical signs and treatments available for these drugs, along with the potential for severe intoxication, consultation with an animal poison control center is recommended (see Chapters 20 and Web Chapter 9).

Considerations for Decontamination

Appropriate decontamination procedures are paramount to successful treatment for most poisonings. Because many antidepressants and anxiolytics are rapidly absorbed, resulting in central nervous system (CNS) depression within 15 to 30 minutes of ingestion, decontamination must be judicious. For agents discussed in this chapter, the induction of emesis at home is not always advisable due to the increased risk of aspiration secondary to CNS depression. Additionally, emesis should never be induced in a symptomatic animal. Often, decontamination is most safely performed in a veterinary setting. Therefore educating receptionists, technicians, and other "front-line" agents about contraindications to emesis induction is imperative.

In cases of very recent ingestion (less than 5 minutes), the induction of emesis may be attempted at home in dogs (not cats) by administering fresh hydrogen peroxide, 3% (1 to 5 ml/kg, PO). Pet Poison Helpline typically recommends administering 1 ml/kg as the first dosage. If the dog has not vomited within 5 to 10 minutes and remains asymptomatic, a second dosage of 2 ml/kg may be administered. Offering a small amount of food prior to the administration of hydrogen peroxide may increase its effectiveness. Unfortunately, there are currently no safe and effective at-home emetic agents for cats. Products such as table salt, mustard, and syrup of ipecac are no longer recommended in any veterinary species.

If emesis cannot be safely induced in the dog at home, apomorphine (0.03 to 0.04 mg/kg) should be administered IV, IM, or by placing the tablet directly into the subconjunctival sac. If subconjunctival apomorphine is used, the subconjunctival sac must be flushed thoroughly after emesis or protracted vomiting may occur. Apomorphine use in cats is not recommended due to poor efficacy and the potential for CNS stimulation. Instead, xylazine (0.44 mg/kg, IM) may be administered. Reversal with yohimbine (0.1 mg/kg, IM, SC, or slowly IV) or atipamezole (Antisedan, 25 to 50 µg/kg, IM or IV) should be performed if severe CNS and/or respiratory depression develop from this treatment.

If the patient is symptomatic, the induction of emesis is contraindicated, but gastric lavage may still be effective provided the ingestion was recent (<60 minutes), a large number of pills were ingested and are likely located within the stomach, or the ingested drug results in delayed gastric emptying (e.g., TCAs).

Activated charcoal (1 to 5 g/kg, PO) with a cathartic such as sorbitol also may be administered in effort to adsorb the toxicants. In order to reduce the risk of aspiration, administration via an orogastric tube is advised in any symptomatic patient. Magnesium-based cathartics are not typically recommended due to the risk that ileus may result with subsequent hypermagnesemia (e.g., in cases of TCA ingestion). If the ingested toxicant undergoes enterohepatic recirculation (e.g., TCAs) or is a sustained-release formulation, administration of activated charcoal up to 6 hours after ingestion may still be beneficial. Additionally, multiple doses of activated charcoal (1 to 2 g/kg without a cathartic q4-6h for 24 hours) may be administered.

Selective Serotonin Reuptake Inhibitors and Others

SSRIs block the reuptake of serotonin in the presynaptic membrane, which results in an increased concentration of serotonin in the CNS. Common SSRIs include fluoxetine (Prozac in human medicine, Reconcile in veterinary medicine), citalopram (Celexa), escitalopram (Lexapro), paroxetine (Paxil), and sertraline (Zoloft), many of which are highly protein bound and all of which undergo hepatic metabolism.

The range of toxicity varies depending on the drug and species. Cats are typically more sensitive to these agents, necessitating lower therapeutic doses and exhibiting lower ranges of toxicity. Animals with seizure disorders, cardiovascular disease, or hepatic impairment may be at greater risk for toxicosis. Small overdoses of SSRIs typically cause sedation or agitation, hypersalivation, vomiting, and mydriasis. Larger overdoses may result in tremors,

seizures, nystagmus, dysphoria, vocalization, aggressive behavior, ataxia, and bradycardia. As the degree of overdose increases, so does the risk for the development of serotonin toxicity (also called serotonin syndrome), a toxidrome characterized by central nervous, autonomic, and neurobehavioral signs such as muscle rigidity, increased reflexes, tremors, hyperthermia, hypertension, and transient blindness.

Treatment of SSRI overdoses is largely supportive and symptomatic; no specific antidote is available. Appropriate decontamination is recommended (see previous section). Cyproheptadine (dogs [1.1 mg/kg] and cats, [2 to 4 mg total dose] q4-6h, PO or rectally), a serotonin antagonist, is useful in reducing the severity of signs, especially vocalization and dysphoria. Agitation may be treated with acepromazine (0.05 to 0.2 mg/kg, IV, IM, or SC PRN) or chlorpromazine (0.5 to 1 mg/kg, IV or IM PRN). Due to the risk for sedation and hypotension from phenothiazines, one should start at the low end of the dosage range and increase the dose as needed. Some animals may require larger doses than are listed here. For seizures in the absence of serotonin toxicity, benzodiazepines (e.g., diazepam, 0.25 to 0.5 mg/kg, IV PRN) are effective. In cases of serotonin toxicity, benzodiazepines may exacerbate neurologic signs; therefore barbiturates (e.g., phenobarbital 3 to 5 mg/kg repeated every 20 minutes for 2 to 3 doses, IV) are recommended. Additional treatments include methocarbamol for tremors (55 to 220 mg/kg, IV slowly and to effect) and IV fluids (balanced crystalloids, 1.5 to 2.5 times maintenance) for thermal cooling and to maintain hydration and adequate tissue perfusion. β-Blockers (e.g., propranolol 0.02 to 0.06 mg/kg, slowly IV) can be considered for tachycardia and hypertension if these problems are not corrected following sedation.

Clinical signs of overdose with other antidepressants such as duloxetine (Cymbalta), a SNRI, and venlafaxine (Effexor), a bicyclic antidepressant, are similar to those associated with an SSRI overdose. Because of their mechanism of action, these agents have an added element of increased presynaptic concentrations of norepinephrine and/or dopamine. This may lead to sympathomimetic signs (e.g., mydriasis, tachycardia, hyperthermia, hypertension). Treatment is similar to SSRI overdoses but more focus on sedation may be needed. Extremely high doses of chlorpromazine (10 to 18 mg/kg, IV) or acepromazine may be required.

Benzodiazepines and Non-Benzodiazepine Hypnotics

BZDs are commonly used as antianxiety agents, anticonvulsants, muscle relaxants, and sedatives/hypnotics. Non-BZD hypnotics are typically used as sleep aids. Although the two groups have different pharmacologic profiles, both exert their effects through the inhibitory neurotransmitter γ-aminobutyric acid (GABA) and have similar clinical effects and treatment regimens. Common BZDs used off-label in veterinary medicine include alprazolam (Xanax), diazepam (Valium), lorazepam (Ativan), midazolam (Versed), and zolazepam found in combination with tiletamine, a dissociative agent (Telazol).

Other BZDs frequently used in human medicine include clonazepam (Klonopin), oxazepam (Serax), and temazepam (Restoril). Common non-BZD hyptnotics or sleep aids include zolpidem (Ambien), eszopiclone (Lunesta), and zaleplon (Sonata).

Both families of drugs have a relatively wide margin of safety and fatalities are uncommon following a one-time overdose. Chronic use of oral BZDs in cats, however, can result in fulminant hepatic failure and is not recommended. Following ingestion, clinical signs may develop rapidly (within 30 to 60 minutes) and commonly include CNS depression, ataxia, and/or aggression. Rare signs include hypotension, hypothermia, coma, or seizures. Paradoxically, approximately 50% of animals ingesting these agents display neurologic stimulation and excitement.

Treatment of acute ingestions consists of appropriate decontamination (see previous section), supportive care, and, if necessary, the reversal agent/antidote flumazenil (Romazicon). The need for treatment is based on the degree of overdose and the severity of signs. In symptomatic animals, body temperature and blood pressure should be monitored and treated accordingly with warming measures and intravenous crystalloids or colloids to maintain adequate tissue perfusion. In cases of paradoxical stimulation, benzodiazepines should not be used because they may exacerbate the clinical signs. Instead, acepromazine (0.05 to 0.2 mg/kg, IV or IM PRN) or medetomidine (1 to 10 µg/kg, IV, IM, or SC PRN) are recommended. The reversal agent flumazenil (0.01 mg/kg, IV to effect PRN) is the antidote for benzodiazepine overdoses but is recommended only in cases with severe CNS or respiratory depression. It reverses the sedative and muscle relaxant effects within about 5 minutes and, due to the short half-life, should be repeatedly given as needed.

Tricylic Antidepressants

TCAs are structurally similar to phenothiazines and act on numerous receptors by inhibiting the neuronal reuptake of norepinephrine, serotonin, and dopamine in the CNS. They also have an affinity for muscarinic and histamine (H_1)-receptors and can cause a sodium and potassium channel blockade to varying degrees. The most common TCAs used in veterinary medicine include amitriptyline and clomipramine (Clomicalm).

In general, TCAs have a very narrow margin of safety with mild adverse effects possible at therapeutic dosages and serious effects possible following minor (2 to 3×) overdoses. Thus any overdose should be considered serious. Unlike the other drug families discussed in this chapter, TCAs may lead to profound cardiac toxicosis in addition to neurologic signs. Following ingestion, clinical signs may develop within the first few hours and may include severe CNS depression and seizures along with anticholinergic signs such as mydriasis, tachycardia, urinary retention, and a slowed gastrointestinal (GI) transit time. Due to the inhibition of fast sodium channels in the cardiac ventricles, slowed depolarization may lead to bradycardia, hypotension, and arrhythmias. Cardiovascular collapse is often the cause of death in domestic animals following overdose.

Treatment of acute ingestions consists of appropriate decontamination (see previous section) and aggressive supportive care; no specific antidote is available. Laboratory values, especially venous blood gas analysis, electrolytes, and blood glucose, should be monitored closely. If hypoglycemia occurs, supplement dextrose at 2.5% to 5% in intravenous fluids. Continuous electrocardiographic (ECG) monitoring is recommended to identify arrhythmias, widening QRS complexes, prolonged PR or Q-T intervals, and flattened or altered T waves. Administer IV crystalloids at 1.5 to 2.5 times maintenance to correct hypotension and maintain perfusion. Cyproheptadine may be helpful (see the section on SSRIs). If seizures occur, rule out hypoglycemia and, if needed, treat with diazepam (0.25 to 0.5 mg/kg, IV PRN) or barbiturates (e.g., phenobarbital 3 to 5 mg/kg, IV PRN). Phenothiazines should not be administered because these may exacerbate the clinical signs. The duration of signs is highly variable (hours to days) and animals should be hospitalized until asymptomatic.

References and Suggested Reading

Gwaltney-Brant SM, Albretsen JC, Khan SA: 5-Hydroxytryptophan toxicosis in dogs: 21 cases (1989-1999), *J Am Vet Med Assoc* 216(12):1937-1940, 2000.

Isbister GK, Buckley NA: The pathophysiology of serotonin toxicity in animals and humans: implications for diagnosis and treatment, *Clin Neuropharmacol* 28(5):205-214, 2005.

Lancaster AR et al: Sleep aid toxicosis in dogs: 317 cases (2004-2010), *J Vet Emerg Crit Care* 21(6):658-665, 2011.

Quandt J: Benzodiazepines. In Osweiler GD et al, editors: *Blackwell's five-minute veterinary consult, clinical companion: small animal toxicology*, Ames, IA, 2011, Blackwell Publishing Ltd, pp 148-154.

Sioris KM: Selective serotonin reuptake inhibitors (SSRIs). In Osweiler GD et al, editors: *Blackwell's five-minute veterinary consult, clinical companion: small animal toxicology*, Ames, IA, 2011, Blackwell Publishing Ltd, pp 195-201.

Wismer TA: Antidepressant drug overdoses in dogs, *Vet Med* July:520-525, 2000.

CHAPTER 27

Over-the-Counter Drug Toxicosis

DAVID C. DORMAN, *Raleigh, North Carolina*

According to the U.S. Food and Drug Administration (FDA) there are over 300,000 over-the-counter (OTC) drug products. These drugs represent approximately 60% of all medications purchased in the United States. The general public may assume that OTC products are safe because they do not require a prescription, thus leading to more frequent administration errors. Exposure to prescription and OTC drugs remains a significant concern for small animal owners and veterinarians. According to the Animal Poison Control Center (APCC) of the American Society for Prevention of Cruelty to Animals (ASPCA), exposure to human medications accounted for nearly 25% of all calls made to that Center in 2010. The APCC also reports that the OTC drugs ibuprofen, naproxen, and other nonsteroidal antiinflammatory drugs (NSAIDs), as well as acetaminophen and pseudoephedrine were among the 10 most frequent causes of drug-related exposure. Exposure to OTC drugs may occur from the administration of these drugs by an owner or veterinarian or through accidental ingestions in the home. Most OTC drug exposures result from ingestion, and the observed clinical signs often represent an exaggeration of the pharmacologic effects of the drug.

The formulation examples described in this chapter should not be considered comprehensive, but rather should serve to highlight some of the OTC products available. Formulations of these and other OTC products may change over time. Therefore it is critical that veterinarians clearly identify the full product name and the current formulation of the OTC in question. Certain OTC products can contain multiple active ingredients. For example, some products used to treat cold and flu-like symptoms contain combinations of aspirin, ibuprofen, acetaminophen, caffeine, diphenhydramine, and other agents. Coexposure to multiple drug formulations can dramatically complicate the management of the exposed animal. This chapter considers several of the newer OTC drugs in the marketplace and provides updates on the management of other more frequently encountered OTC drugs.

General Treatment and Diagnostic Considerations

Unless otherwise noted, the following general management recommendations can be applied to animals exposed to the OTC drugs discussed in this chapter. Initial treatment is focused on stabilizing vital signs, decreasing exposure dose through gastrointestinal decontamination

and other methods, and providing symptomatic treatment. In general, induction of emesis and other means of gastrointestinal decontamination is most effective when performed within 2 hours of ingestion. Many OTC drug formulations have been designed for rapid gastrointestinal absorption and systemic delivery, resulting in a shortening of this therapeutic window. Activated charcoal (1 to 2 g/kg, PO, SID or BID to TID) combined with an osmotic or saline cathartic (e.g., sodium sulfate at 250 mg/kg PO, SID) is generally the preferred method of gastric decontamination following ingestion of a potentially toxic dose of an OTC drug. Gastric lavage, followed by activated charcoal, is indicated after massive ingestion. Certain OTC drugs undergo extensive enterohepatic recirculation; therefore repeated doses of activated charcoal are indicated. Occasionally OTC tablets or capsules form concretions in the gastrointestinal tract. Consequently adsorbents, cathartics, and lavage procedures may be of value even several hours after exposure.

So-called intralipid therapy has also been increasingly used in the initial management of animals exposed to certain toxicants. This therapy was first applied clinically to people to reverse the cardiotoxicity associated with bupivicaine and other local anesthetic agents. More recently, intralipids have been used by veterinarians to reverse central nervous system (CNS) signs and cardiac arrhythmias associated with lipophilic drug overdoses such as ivermectin, permethrin, and baclofen (Fernandez et al, 2011; Gwaltney-Brant and Meadows, 2012; Kaplan and Whelan, 2012). The pharmacologic basis for how intralipid therapy works remains the subject of debate. Intralipids may form a lipid sink for lipophilic drugs, resulting in reduced tissue distribution of the drug and enhanced drug clearance. The lipids may also serve as an energy source that stabilizes tissue metabolism. Administration of a bolus in the range of between 1.5 and 4 ml/kg (0.3 to 0.8 g/kg IV over 1 min), followed by a continuous rate infusion (CRI) of 0.25 ml/kg/min (0.05 g/kg/min IV over 30 to 60 min), has been suggested for dogs (Fernandez et al, 2011). At this time the use of intralipid therapy in the management of OTC drugs can not be broadly advocated but may be warranted with cardiotoxic or neurotoxic drugs or OTC drugs that are highly lipophilic. Support of vital functions is a principle of therapy. Airway control with assisted ventilation and supplemental oxygen may be required. Seizures should be treated with standard anticonvulsants such as diazepam (2.5 to 5 mg/kg IV). Intravenous fluids, inotropic agents such as dopamine (2.5 to 10 µg/kg/min) or dobutamine (5 to 20 µg/kg/min), and electrolytes should be given to control hypotension and hemorrhage, maintain renal function, and correct electrolyte imbalances. In general, the highly protein-bound OTC drugs are not amenable to enhanced elimination by forced diuresis. Additional therapeutic considerations also are provided for individual drugs discussed in this chapter. It is important to remember that clinical signs associated with OTC exposure can emerge at different times; therefore repeated reevaluation of the animal and appropriate modifications of the treatment approach are always in order.

A definitive diagnosis for toxicoses resulting from the OTC drugs described in this chapter generally relies on a known history of exposure, development of compatible clinical signs, and confirmation of drug residues using appropriate analytic chemical methods. There may be a delay in obtaining analytic results, therefore veterinarians should not delay treatment for this confirmation.

Nonsteroidal Antiinflammatory Drugs

There has been an increase in the number of NSAIDs available in the U.S. market. Several NSAIDs (e.g., aspirin, ibuprofen, and naproxen) are available OTC. Other prescription NSAIDs include celecoxib, sulindac, piroxicam, indomethacin, etodolac, meloxicam, ketoprofen, nabumetone, and ketorolac tromethamine. Most NSAIDs act as nonselective inhibitors of the enzyme cyclooxygenase (COX), inhibiting both the cyclooxygenase-1 (COX-1) and cyclooxygenase-2 (COX-2) isoenzymes. COX catalyzes the formation of prostaglandins and thromboxane from arachidonic acid. Aspirin irreversibly inhibits COX, while the other commonly used NSAIDs (e.g., ibuprofen, naproxen) reversibly inhibit COX. Prostaglandins mediate a variety of normal physiologic functions including regulation of renal blood flow. Prostaglandins are also vasodilatory and cytoprotective in the gastrointestinal tract.

The inhibitory activity of NSAIDs on COX activity explains not only their beneficial antiinflammatory effects, but also in part accounts for their adverse effects on platelet, gastrointestinal, and renal function. For example, piroxicam and indomethacin exert their highest activity against COX-1 and demonstrate high gastrointestinal toxicity. In comparison, the selective COX-2 inhibitors (e.g., deracoxib, robenacoxib) have less inhibitory effects on blood clotting, have better gastrointestinal tolerability, and can be less nephrotoxic than NSAIDs, which are either nonselective or selective COX-1 inhibitors.

There are significant species differences in the elimination and biotransformation of NSAIDs, resulting in variable half-lives of elimination that can influence drug toxicity. For example, the elimination half-life of aspirin in cats approaches 40 hours, compared with 7.5 to 8 hours in dogs. The plasma elimination half-life of piroxicam has been reported as 37 to 40 hours in dogs, 12 to 13 hours in cats, and 30 to 86 hours in humans. Cats are thought to be more sensitive than dogs to some of the toxic effects of NSAIDs; however, there is insufficient information available to indicate whether this is a consistent finding for all NSAIDs. Two important protective determinants in NSAID-induced toxicity are high COX-2 selectivity and short blood half-life.

Toxicoses from NSAIDs can occur from either a single high-dose exposure or following repeated exposure to lower doses. In many cases even a small increase in the recommended therapeutic NSAID dose (e.g., a 25% to 100% dose increase) can lead to adverse effects. Common clinical signs observed with NSAID toxicosis include vomiting, CNS depression, anorexia, diarrhea, and ataxia. Dogs are particularly sensitive to the ulcerogenic effects of NSAIDs, especially when combined with corticosteroid use. The onset of gastrointestinal signs often occurs within the first 2 to 6 hours after ingestion, with the onset of gastrointestinal hemorrhage and ulceration occurring 12 hours to 4 days after ingestion. Severe gastric lesions may occur, however, with only minimal overt clinical signs. Lesions associated with NSAID gastroenteropathy include perforations, ulcers, and hemorrhages in the upper (stomach and duodenum) and, on occasion, lower (colon) gastrointestinal tract. Once ulceration has occurred, bleeding into the lumen of the gut may be exacerbated if blood clotting is inhibited. Blood loss, anemia, iron deficiency, and melena may be observed. Gastric erosions, ulcers, and evidence of hemorrhage may be detected by endoscopy. Recent studies have shown that dogs with NSAID-induced gastric lesions develop a marked elevation in plasma C-reactive protein (CRP), serum amyloid-A (SAA), haptoglobin, fibrinogen concentrations, and white blood cell counts. This rapid acute phase protein response occurs in concert with gastric mucosal injury and may be potentially useful together with rectal examination of fecal contents and gastroscopy in the diagnosis and monitoring of gastric injury.

Massive NSAID ingestion is also associated with renal failure characterized by oliguria and azotemia initially, followed by either an oliguric or anuric clinical course. The onset of renal failure often occurs within the first 12 hours after NSAID exposure but may be delayed 3 to 5 days. The liver is another target organ for certain NSAIDs (e.g., carprofen); however, it remains unknown whether this effect is idiosyncratic, dose related, or both. Other clinical effects that have been reported include decreased platelet aggregation leading to increased bleeding time, bone marrow depression, allergic reactions, and seizures.

Therapeutic considerations for NSAID toxicosis variably include gastrointestinal decontamination and, when needed, administration of crystalloid fluids (such as 0.45% saline and 2.5% dextrose, IV), whole blood, inotropic agents such as dopamine (2.5 µg/kg/min) or dobutamine (5 to 20 µg/kg/min), and electrolytes to control hypotension and hemorrhage, manage acute bleeding ulcers, maintain renal function, and correct electrolyte abnormalities. A variety of pharmacologic approaches have been used in humans to reduce the risk of NSAID-induced gastrointestinal toxicity. These approaches include the use of histamine (H_2)-receptor antagonists (ranitidine, famotidine, and cimetidine) and proton pump inhibitors (PPIs) (e.g., omeprazole). The effectiveness of these drugs following an acute massive dose NSAID exposure in veterinary medicine has not been fully evaluated, but they are often prescribed.

Sucralfate (0.5 to 1 g q8-12h PO [dog]; 0.25 g q8-12h PO [cat]), cimetidine (10 mg/kg q8h IM, IV, PO), ranitidine (2 mg/kg q8h IV, PO [dog]; 2.5 mg/kg q12h IV [cat] or 3.5 mg/kg q12h PO [cat]), and omeprazole (0.7 mg/kg q24h PO [dog]) have proved beneficial in the management of gastric ulcers. Misoprostol (2 to 5 µg/kg, PO, q8h, dog), a synthetic prostaglandin E_1 analog, prevents aspirin-induced gastric ulcers in dogs (Ward et al, 2003) but is generally less effective after an ulcer forms. Misoprostol also is associated with adverse side effects such as abdominal pain, vomiting, and diarrhea. Studies in humans suggest that PPIs (e.g., omeprazole) may be more effective in treating NSAID-related dyspepsia (indigestion) and also in healing gastric and duodenal ulcers in patients that continue to receive an NSAID. Metoclopramide (0.2 to 0.4 mg/kg q6-8h PO or SC) may be helpful in the control of vomiting. Mild gastrointestinal irritation may be treated symptomatically with nonabsorbable antacids such as magnesium or aluminum hydroxide. Bismuth subsalicylate antacid formulations are contraindicated. The NSAID should also be discontinued and other analgesic options considered if needed.

Specific NSAIDs

Ibuprofen
Ibuprofen is available OTC as 200 mg tablets and pediatric liquid preparations under a number of proprietary names (Advil, Medipren, Midol, Motrin IB, Nuprin, Pamprin IB). Prescription forms include capsules (200 to 800 mg), sustained-release capsules (100 and 200 mg), and 100 mg suppositories. Dogs ingesting single ibuprofen doses less than 100 mg/kg and cats ingesting less than 50 mg/kg generally remain asymptomatic. As with other NSAIDs, repeated doses of ibuprofen in dogs and cats increase the likelihood of clinical signs. Ibuprofen at 5 mg/kg q12h PO has been used to reduce pain and inflammation in dogs, but 8 mg/kg q24h PO for 30 days is likely to produce gastrointestinal irritation and hemorrhage. A single oral dose of ibuprofen above 125 mg/kg is associated with ulcers and erosions in the gastric antrum and pylorus. Acute doses greater than 250 to 300 mg/kg in either dogs or cats have resulted in clinical signs of acute renal failure in addition to gastrointestinal lesions.

Naproxen
Naproxen (e.g., Aleve) is available OTC as 200 mg tablets. Prescription forms (Anaprox and Naprosyn, Naprelan) include oral suspensions, capsules (250, 375, and 500 mg), delayed-release tablets (375 and 500 mg), and suppositories (500 mg). Naproxen is approximately 10 times more potent that aspirin as a COX inhibitor. In dogs, the drug has a half-life of 35 to 74 hours and naproxen probably undergoes extensive enterohepatic recirculation. Toxicosis in a dog given 5.6 mg/kg of naproxen for 7 days involved signs of anemia, melena, and renal and hepatic dysfunction.

Ketoprofen
Ketoprofen (Orudis KT, Actron) was previously available as 12.5 mg tablets; however, this OTC formulation has been withdrawn. Prescription forms include capsules (25 to 100 mg), sustained-release capsules (100 and 200 mg), and suppositories (100 mg). There are limited toxicology data available for ketoprofen in dogs and cats. As with many other NSAIDs, repeated doses increase the likelihood of development of clinical signs. Ketoprofen at 2 mg/kg PO for 4 days, followed by 1 mg/kg daily PO for up to 90 days, was associated with prolonged bleeding time (by day 7 of dosing) and gastric lesions at the end of the study.

Salicylates
The ingestion of aspirin (acetylsalicylic acid) and salicylate-containing products remains a significant risk to companion animals. As mentioned previously, aspirin irreversibly inhibits COX, especially the COX-1 isoform. Other features that distinguish aspirin from most other NSAIDs include more extensive hepatic metabolism (to salicylic acid), extensive phase II metabolic conjugation with glucuronic acid, and more widespread systemic delivery. The plasma half-life of elimination of salicylates is approximately 8 and 38 hours in dogs and cats, respectively.

Like the other NSAIDs, aspirin overdose can result in gastric irritation, gastric ulceration, oliguria and other renal effects, and seizures. Additional clinical signs have been attributed to respiratory alkalosis and secondary hyperpnea followed by metabolic acidosis. Gastric ulcers developed in beagles within 2 hours after oral administration of aspirin at 100 mg/kg (Cavanagh et al, 1998). This lesion was reduced by pretreatment with the H_2-receptor antagonists cimetidine and ranitidine. Aspirin-induced hepatitis has also been reported in cats. Treatment of salicylate toxicosis is similar to that used for other NSAIDs. In humans severe aspirin poisoning (acidemia, severe CNS depression, cerebral edema, cardiac or renal failure) is often associated with plasma salicylate concentrations in excess of 35 to 50 mg/dl. In these cases, alkaline diuresis, repeated doses of oral activated charcoal, hemodialysis, and other methods to enhance elimination should be attempted.

Many OTC products such as Pepto-Bismol contain salicylates. Some familiar products have undergone several iterations that could prove confusing to veterinarians and owners. For example, Kaopectate has undergone a series of changes from its original kaolin and pectin formulation (up to the 1980s), to attapulgite (a magnesium aluminum phyllosilicate) in the early 1990s, to one containing bismuth salicylate (at 17.5 or 35 mg/ml) since 2003. Certain preparations of other familiar OTC drugs can also contain salicylates. Maalox Total Stomach Relief contains bismuth subsalicylate at 35 mg/ml. In contrast, a related product, Maalox Advanced Maximum Strength Liquid, contains aluminum hydroxide (80 mg/ml), magnesium hydroxide (80 mg/ml), and simethicone (8 mg/ml).

Acetaminophen

Acetaminophen is a para-aminophenol derivative with antipyretic and analgesic activity, but minimal antiinflammatory effects. Unlike most NSAIDs, acetaminophen does not inhibit neutrophil activation, has little ulcerogenic potential, and has no effect on platelets or bleeding time. Acetaminophen may act by inhibiting COX or via interactions with the cannabinoid and serotonergic systems of the CNS.

The metabolism of acetaminophen, which plays a key role in its toxic effects, initially involves cytochrome P-450 metabolism of the parent drug to a more toxic intermediate. This intermediate can undergo conjugation (glucuronidation or sulfation), can be detoxified by conjugation with glutathione, or can react with tissue macromolecules, resulting in toxic effects. Toxicosis develops when the animal's ability to glucuronidate or sulfate the intermediate is overwhelmed and/or when tissue glutathione stores have become depleted. Cats are very sensitive to acetaminophen toxicosis because they are deficient in glucuronyl transferase and therefore have limited capacity to glucuronidate this drug.

Acetaminophen demonstrates dose-dependent adverse effects. As with the NSAIDs, poisoning can occur with repeated exposure at lower doses. In cats, toxicity can occur following exposure to 10 to 40 mg/kg. When used, the recommended therapeutic dose in dogs is 10 to 15 mg/kg PO TID, and signs of acute toxicity usually occur with doses in excess of 100 mg/kg. Adverse effects common to dogs and cats include CNS depression, vomiting, methemoglobinemia, tachycardia, hyperpnea, and weakness. Cats primarily develop methemoglobinemia within a few hours, followed by Heinz body formation. Clinical signs of methemoglobinemia have been reported in three of four dogs dosed at 200 mg/kg. Other clinical signs of acetaminophen toxicosis include icterus, vomiting, hypothermia, facial or paw edema (more common in cats), cyanosis, dyspnea, hepatic necrosis, and death. Liver damage (centrilobular necrosis) occurs most commonly in dogs and is often delayed, with signs and clinicopathologic changes appearing 24 or more hours after ingestion.

Treatment of acetaminophen toxicosis relies on timely gastrointestinal decontamination (within 1 to 2 hours), prevention or treatment of methemoglobinemia and hepatic damage, and additional supportive care. Activated charcoal administration may need to be repeated, especially with extremely high exposure doses, since acetaminophen undergoes enterohepatic recirculation. N-acetylcysteine has been a mainstay in the prevention of acetaminophen toxicosis. This sulfhydryl-containing drug augments the animal's ability to use glutathione to detoxify reactive acetaminophen metabolites. The loading dose of N-acetylcysteine is 140 mg/kg of a 5% solution IV or PO (diluted in 5% dextrose or sterile water), followed by 70 mg/kg PO QID for generally seven more treatments. Vomiting is a potential side effect of this drug. Administration of activated charcoal and oral N-acetylcysteine is generally separated by 1 hour because activated charcoal can decrease the bioavailability of N-acetylcysteine. Fluids and blood transfusions may be needed to manage dehydration, methemoglobinemia, Heinz body anemia, and hemolysis. Ascorbic acid (30 mg/kg, PO or injectable, BID-QID) is used to decrease methemoglobin levels. Cimetidine (5 to 10 mg/kg PO, IM, or IV), a cytochrome P-450 inhibitor, may help reduce formation of toxic metabolites and prevent liver damage; however, this therapy remains largely untested. Additional treatments may be required because certain OTC products also contain aspirin, caffeine, and other drugs.

Proton Pump Inhibitors

Another group of drugs that has emerged in the OTC market are the PPIs. The PPIs decrease gastric acid secretion through inhibition of the H^+/K^+ adenosine triphosphatase enzyme system at the surface of the gastric parietal cells involved in acid secretion. The PPIs are used to control and treat peptic ulcers, reflux esophagitis, and the Zollinger-Ellison syndrome in humans. Veterinary uses for these drugs include the treatment of gastric ulcers and other stomach acid–related disorders. For example, omeprazole has been used in dogs at 0.5 to 1.0 mg/kg PO SID for the control of gastric ulcers. Approved PPIs include omeprazole (Prilosec), lansoprazole (Prevacid), rabeprazole (Aciphex), pantoprazole (Protonix), and esomeprazole (Nexium). Omeprazole became the first PPI approved by the FDA for OTC sales in 2003.

Toxicity data for PPIs in animals are largely lacking. The lethal dose 50% (LD_{50}) of omeprazole in rodents is reportedly greater than 4 g/kg. Repeated high-dose exposure to omeprazole resulted in virtually complete inhibition of acid secretion in experimental animals, leading to hypergastrinemia. As a class, the PPIs are well tolerated in humans, with the most commonly reported side effects including headache, constipation, diarrhea, dizziness, and rash (Parikh and Howden, 2010). Anaphylactic and allergic reactions to PPI therapy have also been reported in humans. Other side effects with low incidence reported in humans include an increased risk for hip fractures and acute interstitial nephritis. Forrester (2007) reported on the experiences of the six poison control centers of the Texas Poison Center Network with PPI exposure between 1998 and 2004. Forrester found that most exposures were classified as having no effect, with almost all the rest classified as having minor effect. No cases were classified as involving major effects or death. The most frequently reported adverse clinical effects were gastrointestinal effects (nausea and abdominal pain), neurologic effects (drowsiness, dizziness, and headache), dermal effects, and cardiovascular defects. Based on this experience, management of the acutely exposed dog or cat would rely on gastrointestinal decontamination methods mentioned previously and supportive therapy as needed.

H_1-Antihistamines

The four major types of histamine receptors, H_1, H_2, H_3, and H_4, differ in their basal expression and functions. H_1-antihistamines act as inverse agonists (they have also been classified previously as H_1-receptor blockers or antagonists) that combine with and stabilize the inactive form of the H_1-receptor, shifting the equilibrium toward the inactive state (Simons, 2004). The H_1-antihistamines include ethanolamine, ethylenediamine, alkylamine, piperazine, piperidine, and phenothiazine subtypes. Clinically the first-generation H_1-antihistamines are sedating, whereas newer second-generation compounds are relatively nonsedating in humans. More than 40 H₁-antihistamines are available and these agents are among the most widely used of all OTC and prescription medications. Examples of antihistamines include diphenhydramine, chlorpheniramine, dimenhydrinate, and cyclizine. Antihistamines are common ingredients in cough and cold and allergy medications. Others (e.g., diphenhydramine) have been used to control motion sickness and as a sleep aid. OTC antihistamines include fexofenadine hydrochloride (Allegra). Both tablet (60 and 180 mg) and suspension forms (6 mg/ml) are available OTC. Some tablet formulations (Allegra D) also contain 120 or 240 mg of pseudoephedrine. Other OTC antihistamines include cetirizine hydrochloride (Zyrtec). Both tablet (10 mg) and liquid gel (10 mg) preparations are available OTC. Some tablet formulations (Zyrtec-D) contain 5 mg of cetirizine and 120 mg of pseudoephedrine. Loratadine is also available OTC and is sold as a liquid-filled capsule, a syrup, an immediate-acting and extended-release tablet, and a rapidly disintegrating tablet. Some tablet formulations (Claritin-D) contain 5 mg of loratadine and 120 mg of pseudoephedrine.

First-generation H₁-antihistamines have antimuscarinic and α-adrenergic blockade activity and may cause dose-related prolongation of the QT interval (Simons, 2004). Clinical signs are primarily limited to sedation, ataxia, vomiting, and diarrhea; however, CNS excitement or seizures also may be observed. Additionally, the anticholinergic effects of H₁ antagonists may result in other clinical signs including dry mucous membranes, tachycardia, urinary retention, and hyperthermia. Toxicity data for these agents in dogs are generally lacking. The acute oral LD₅₀ of clemastine is 175 mg/kg in the dog.

Symptomatic treatment should include steps to limit absorption such as an emetic and activated charcoal. Maintenance of hydration is important because these agents are primarily excreted in urine (Papich, 1990). Serious anticholinergic effects may be treated with physostigmine (0.02 mg/kg IV) and diazepam administered for seizures (Plumb, 2011).

H₂-Blockers

The H₂-blockers, famotidine, ranitidine, nizatidine, and cimetidine, inhibit gastric acid secretion and are also available on the OTC market. The incidence of adverse reactions to these agents is low in humans owing, in part, to the limited function of H₂-receptors in organs other than the stomach and poor CNS penetration. In dogs anesthetized with nitrous oxide and halothane, IV doses of cimetidine greater than 3 mg/kg resulted in decreased heart rate and blood pressure and left ventricular pressure, while cardiac output and coronary blood flow were only affected at doses of 30 mg/kg. In laboratory animals, high doses of cimetidine have resulted in tachycardia and respiratory failure. Cimetidine inhibits cytochrome P-450 activity, slows the metabolism of drugs that are substrates for cytochrome P-450, and prolongs the half-life and thus increases the serum levels of phenytoin, theophylline, diazepam, lidocaine, procainamide, phenobarbital, propranolol, and warfarin. The dosage of these drugs should

be adjusted and the patient should have increased therapeutic monitoring (Plumb, 2011). Hepatic blood flow is also reduced and this may decrease the clearance of flow-limited drugs such as propranolol and lidocaine. In addition, cimetidine-induced leukopenia and thrombocytopenia have been reported.

Famotidine is reported to be safer than cimetidine in dogs and is extensively used in clinical practice, although it may produce a negative inotropic effect or exacerbate cardiac arrhythmias (this is rarely observed). In humans, 40% to 45% of the dose is absorbed. Massive oral exposure of famotidine (>2 g/kg) may cause vomiting, restlessness, and hyperemia. Higher doses may depress cardiovascular function and lead to circulatory collapse.

Nizatidine is well absorbed (>90%) in humans PO. Overdose in humans is characterized by cholinergic signs including lacrimation, salivation, emesis, miosis, and diarrhea. The oral LD₅₀ of nizatidine in dogs is 2600 mg/kg. In acute toxicity studies, however, a single oral dose of 800 mg/kg was not lethal in dogs.

Ranitidine, unlike cimetidine, has apparently minimal effects on hepatic metabolism. In laboratory species doses over 200 mg/kg/day have been associated with muscular tremors, vomiting, and rapid respiration (Plumb, 2011).

Overdose with H₂-antagonists may be treated by limiting intestinal absorption and symptomatic therapy. If tachycardia and respiratory failure develop after cimetidine exposure, β-adrenergic blockers (a trial dose of esmolol to start) and ventilatory support are suggested. Cholinergic signs seen with nizatidine may be treated with atropine and supportive therapy.

Nicotine

Several OTC nicotine-based 2 or 4 mg polacrilex chewing gums and replacement transdermal patches are available in the United States as nicotine replacement therapy used in smoking cessation. Nicotine polacrilex is a resin complex of nicotine and polacrilin, which is a cation-exchange resin prepared from methacrylic acid and divinylbenzene. The gum may also contain sorbitol as a sweetener and buffering agents to enhance buccal absorption of nicotine. The rate of release of nicotine from the resin complex in chewing gum is variable and depends on the vigor and duration of chewing. Nicotine transdermal patches typically contain 8.3 to 114 mg of the free alkaloid. All patches have significant residues of nicotine (2 to 83 mg) even after 24 hours of application. Some patches consist of a drug reservoir containing nicotine in an ethylene-vinyl acetate copolymer matrix that delivers the drug via a rate-controlling polyethylene membrane. Other sources of nicotine include smokeless tobacco, cigarettes (these contain approximately 15 to 25 mg nicotine), cigars, and related products.

Nicotine is a cholinergic (nicotinic) receptor agonist that exhibits both stimulant (low-dose) and depressant (high-dose) effects in the peripheral nervous system and CNS. Nicotine's cardiovascular effects are usually dose dependent. Nicotine may increase circulating levels of cortisol and catecholamines. The drug is quite toxic (the minimal oral lethal dose in dogs and cats is approximately 10 mg/kg), and the toxic effects develop rapidly after ingestion. Nicotine-induced clinical effects may include muscle tremors, hypertension, tachycardia, tachypnea, vomiting, hypersalivation, CNS depression or excitation, mydriasis, ataxia, weakness, seizures, and death from respiratory paralysis.

Management of nicotine overdose generally involves gastric decontamination followed by symptomatic and supportive therapy. If vomiting has not occurred following an acute ingestion of nicotine, the stomach should be emptied immediately by inducing emesis or by gastric lavage. Activated charcoal and a saline cathartic should be given immediately following gastric emptying. Activated charcoal should be given every 6 to 8 hours following ingestion of transdermal patches because delayed nicotine release may occur. Vigorous intravenous fluid support and additional therapy should be instituted if hypotension or cardiovascular collapse occurs. Seizures should be treated with standard anticonvulsants such as diazepam. Atropine may be given for bradycardia, excessive bronchoconstriction, or diarrhea. Assisted pulmonary ventilation may be necessary for the management of respiratory paralysis.

Herbal Supplements

Accidental ingestion of herbal supplements by dogs and cats may result in toxicity. Herbal products are often heterogeneous, may produce multiple effects, and may affect multiple organ systems, including the nervous, cardiovascular, gastrointestinal, hepatic, renal, and hematologic systems (see Chapter 29).

References and Suggested Reading

Cavanagh RL, Buyniski JP, Schwartz SE: Prevention of aspirin-induced gastric mucosal injury by histamine H_2 receptor antagonists: a crossover endoscopic and intragastric pH study in the dog, *J Pharmacol Exp Ther* 243:1179-1184, 1987.

Fernandez AL et al: The use of intravenous lipid emulsion as an antidote in veterinary toxicology, *J Vet Emerg Crit Care* 21:309-320, 2011.

Fitzgerald KT, Bronstein AC, Flood AA: "Over-the-counter" drug toxicities in companion animals, *Clin Tech Small Anim Pract* 21:215-226, 2006.

Forrester MB: Pattern of proton pump inhibitor calls to Texas poison centers, 1998-2004, *J Toxicol Environ Health A* 70:705-714, 2007.

Gwaltney-Brant S, Meadows I: Use of intravenous lipid emulsions for treating certain poisoning cases in small animals, *Vet Clin North Am Small Anim Pract* 42:251-262, 2012.

Kaplan A, Whelan M: The use of IV lipid emulsion for lipophilic drug toxicities, *J Am Anim Hosp Assoc* 48:221-227, 2012.

Papich MG: Toxicoses from over-the-counter human drugs, *Vet Clin North Am Small Anim Pract* 20:431, 1990.

Parikh N, Howden CW: The safety of drugs used in acid-related disorders and functional gastrointestinal disorders, *Gastroenterol Clin North Am* 39:529-542, 2010.

Physicians' desk reference for nonprescription drugs, dietary supplements, and herbs 2011, ed 32, Montvale, NJ, 2011, Physicians' Desk Reference Inc.

Plumb DC: *Plumb's veterinary drug handbook*, ed 7, Hoboken, 2011, Wiley, John & Sons.

Poortinga EW, Hungerford LL: A case-control study of acute ibuprofen toxicity in dogs, *Prev Vet Med* 35:115-124, 1998.

Simons FE: Advances in H_1-antihistamines, *N Engl J Med* 351:2203-2217, 2004.

Ward DM et al: The effect of dosing interval on the efficacy of misoprostol in the prevention of aspirin-induced gastric injury, *J Vet Intern Med* 17:282-290, 2003.

CHAPTER 28

Top Ten Toxic and Nontoxic Household Plants

A. CATHERINE BARR, *College Station, Texas*

Dogs and cats often eat lawn grass and then vomit, but otherwise they are not considered sick. Similarly, there are other house and yard plants that if ingested may or may not cause a pet to vomit but do not typically induce serious adverse effects. Many veterinary practitioners handle calls about these plants and manage the situation by having the owner observe the animal at home. In most cases, if the pet is interested in eating at its next normal feeding time, follow-up medical care is not needed.

However, other common house and yard plants contain potentially toxic agents; if a pet eats any of these, it may require medical management and closer observation. This chapter lists the "top 10" nontoxic and toxic plants encountered by veterinary toxicologists in the United States with the hope that the information provided will be of practical use to the clinician or technical staff dealing with a concerned owner about a potential intoxication.

Nontoxic Plants

Using the popular "top 10" approach, Box 28-1 lists in alphabetical order (by common name) plants for which no reference to toxicity in dogs or cats has been found.

Toxic Plants

In contrast, a number of plants or plant groups are more likely to result in serious adverse effects if ingested by dogs and cats. The "top 10" toxic home and yard plants most frequently encountered by veterinary toxicologists across the United States are listed in Box 28-2. These are subdivided by the major form of clinical toxicosis.

There are very few true antidotes for plant intoxications. In the majority of cases, care consists mostly of decontamination and symptomatic/supportive measures. Management of some of these toxicoses is discussed elsewhere in this volume.

References and Suggested Reading

Barr AC: Household and garden plants. In Peterson ME, Talcott PA, editors: *Small animal toxicology*, ed 2, St Louis, 2006, Saunders, pp 345-410.

Milewski LM, Khan SA: An overview of potentially life-threatening poisonous plants in dogs and cats, *J Vet Emerg Crit Care* 16(1):25-33, 2006.

BOX 28-1

Top 10 Nontoxic Plants

African violets: *Ionantha saintpaulia* hyb.
Boston ferns: *Nephrolepis exaltata*
Camellias: *Camellia* spp./hyb.
Chrysanthemums: *Chrysanthemum* spp./hyb.
Geraniums: *Pelargonium* spp./hyb.
Grass, turf: Common lawn grasses (e.g., fescue, Bermuda, St. Augustine, Kentucky bluegrass)
Hibiscus, althea: *Hibiscus rosa-sinensis* hyb.
Orchids: *Cattleya, Bletia, Brassia, Cymbidium, Dendrobium, Laeliocattleya, Oncidium, Phalaenopsis* spp./hyb.
Roses: *Rosa* spp./hyb.
Sedums: *Sedum* spp./hyb.

BOX 28-2

Top 10 Toxic Plants

Oral Irritation
Araceae: Members of this family include *Alocasia* spp./hyb. (e.g., elephant ear), *Anthurium* spp./hyb. (e.g., flamingo flower), *Caladium* spp./hyb., *Dieffenbachia* spp./hyb. (e.g., dumb cane), *Philodendron* spp./hyb., *Zantedeschia* spp./hyb (e.g., calla lily), and many others

Cardiovascular Effects
Kalanchoe: *Kalanchoe* spp.
Rhododendron: *Azalea* spp./hyb, *Rhododendron* spp./hyb.
Oleander: *Nerium oleander*
Yew: *Taxus* spp.

Renal Effects
Lilies: *Lilium* spp./hyb., *Hemerocallis* spp./hyb.
Grapes/raisins: *Vitis* spp./hyb.

Severe Gastrointestinal/Hepatic Effects
Autumn crocus: *Colchicum autumnale*
Castor beans: *Ricinus communis*
Sago palms: *Cycas* spp./hyb.

CHAPTER 29
Herbal Hazards

ELIZABETH A. HAUSNER,* *Beltsville, Maryland*
ROBERT H. POPPENGA, *Davis, California*

Many people use herbal medicines and dietary supplements for their own health, and increasingly these products are administered for the health of their pets. The increasing popularity of herbals may be seen in the volume of sales. Despite economic difficulties, sales in 2010 increased by 3.3% over 2009, with receipts totaling about $5 billion (American Botanical Council). In addition to herbs sold in mass-market, chain, health food, and specialty stores, on-line sales of these products are substantial. The Internet has evolved into a powerful tool for offering information, misinformation, and access to a plethora of products from virtually every corner of the world. Accordingly, toxicities from plants not indigenous to this country can and should be considered in differential diagnoses of possible plant toxicosis.

Regulations

In 1994 Congress passed the Dietary Supplement and Health Education Act (DSHEA), creating a new category of substances termed *dietary supplements*. Dietary supplements include minerals, vitamins, amino acids, herbs, and any product sold as a dietary supplement before October 15, 1994. The Food and Drug Administration (FDA) Center for Veterinary Medicine interpreted the DSHEA as not applying to substances used in animals, leaving veterinary herbals and dietary supplements regulated as foods, food additives, or new animal drugs, depending on the ingredients and their intended use. DSHEA was followed by the Dietary Supplement and Nonprescription Drug Consumer Protection Act, effective December, 2007. This law requires collection of adverse event (AE) reports by manufacturers, distributors, and retailers, with reporting of serious AEs to the FDA. Dietary supplement labels are also required to provide information to facilitate reporting of AEs (Abdel-Rahman et al, 2011). Because there is an assumption of underreporting of AEs for prescription pharmaceuticals, it is reasonable to assume that underreporting of AEs for herbals will occur. Of course, nothing prevents a product intended for human use from being used in or on animals, and at this time there is scant information on AEs of dietary supplements in animals. Ultimately of equal or greater concern than intoxication from herbal remedies is the potential delay in seeking treatment for otherwise treatable diseases handled inappropriately with a supplement or herb.

Intoxication Scenarios

There are a number of scenarios in which animals may experience an adverse reaction to or toxicosis from an herbal preparation. It is worth noting that in several reports the incidence of animal intoxication from an herb, herbal preparation, or dietary supplement seems to parallel its popularity (Ooms, Khan, and Means, 2001; Gwaltney-Brant, Albretsen, and Khan, 2000). The following list provides situations in which toxicosis may occur:

1. The components of a supplement are correctly identified and the preparation contains a known toxicant. For example, the dried rootstocks of *Aconitum* spp. contain several constituents that are acutely cardiotoxic (Lin, Chan, and Deng, 2005). Pennyroyal oil containing the putative toxin pulegone was responsible for the death of a dog after dermal application to control fleas (Sudekum et al, 1992).
2. The intoxication may be chronic rather than acute as in the case of pyrrolizidine alkaloids, which are found in many plant species and when ingested over time cause severe liver disease (Prakash et al, 1999; Stedman, 2002).
3. Errors may be made when preparing a remedy. For example, human illness was caused when an anise seed preparation was contaminated with the highly toxic *Conium maculatum* (poison hemlock) seed (deSmet, 1991). An outbreak of renal interstitial fibrosis in women taking Chinese herbs for weight loss was attributed to the use of *Aristolochia fangchi* instead of *Stephania tetrandra* in imported powdered extracts (Vanherweghem, 1998).
4. Herbal preparations may unintentionally contain contaminants or intentionally contain chemical adulterants. Many Chinese herbal patent medicines contain drugs such as nonsteroidal antiinflammatory drugs (NSAIDs) or sedatives (Ko, 1998). Also, heavy metal and pesticide contamination has been reported (Ernst, 2002b; Saper et al, 2004; Harris et al 2011). Salmonellosis has been reported in humans taking rattlesnake capsules contaminated with *Salmonella arizonae* (Fleischman, Haake, and Lovett, 1989).
5. The active constituents in herbal preparations can interact with other concurrently administered drugs, resulting in adverse interactions. For example, buckthorn bark and berries taken chronically can increase the loss of potassium, thus potentiating the action of cardiac glycosides and antiarrhythmic agents (DerMarderosian, 2001). Potassium loss may

---

*The views and opinions expressed are those of the authors and do not represent the FDA.

be exacerbated by simultaneous use of thiazide diuretics, corticosteroids, and licorice root (DerMarderosian, 2001). In addition, active constituents in herbal preparations can induce liver-metabolizing enzymes, which can alter the metabolism and kinetics of coadministered conventional drugs. For example, eucalyptus oil induces liver enzyme activity (DerMarderosian, 2001). This scenario of adverse pharmacologic interactions may occur when the owner does not inform the veterinarian of the intentional use of herbal preparations.

6. Finally, pets may consume improperly stored remedies, resulting in ingestion of a large quantity of a product.

Active Herbal Constituents

There are many different ethnic traditions of herbal medicine use, with many plants having roles in these remedies. The following broad classes of active chemical constituents occur in plants: volatile oils, resins, alkaloids, polysaccharides, phenols, glycosides, and fixed oils (Hung, Lewin, and Howland, 1998). Volatile oils are odorous plant ingredients (e.g., catnip, garlic, citrus). Resins are complex chemical mixtures that can be strong gastrointestinal irritants. Alkaloids are a heterogeneous group of alkaline, organic, and nitrogenous compounds. Glycosides are sugar esters containing a sugar (glycol) and a nonsugar (aglycon). In some cases the glycosides are not toxic. However, hydrolysis of the glycosides after ingestion can release toxic aglycons. Fixed oils are esters of long-chain fatty acids and alcohols. Herbs containing fixed oils are often used as emollients, demulcents, and bases for other agents; in general these are the least toxic of the plant constituents.

There is a misperception that preparations from plants are inherently safe because they occur in nature compared with synthesized chemicals. However, many plant-derived chemicals are biologically active and therefore potentially toxic. Concentrated extracts of a number of herbs have proven to be toxic even if the entire plant may be used with relative safety. Although green tea is consumed by many people with apparent safety, an extract of green tea marketed in Europe caused a significant number of adverse hepatic events, including fulminant hepatitis. The extract was withdrawn from the market (Gloro et al, 2005).

Toxicity of Specific Herbs or Other Natural Products

Some of the most commonly encountered herbals are discussed in the following paragraphs; others are listed in Table 29-1.

Blue-Green Algae

Blue-green (BG) algae are single-celled organisms that have been promoted for their nutritional properties. Several BG algal species produce potent toxins. *Microcystis*

aeruginosa produces the hepatotoxic microcystins. *Anabaena flos-aquae* produce the neurotoxins anatoxin-a and anatoxin a$_s$. *Aphanizomenon flos-aquae* produce the neurotoxins saxitoxin and neosaxitoxin. Efforts are underway to better define the risks associated with ingestion of potentially toxigenic BG algae and to establish safe concentrations of total microcystins in marketed products. Spirulina has also been promoted as a nutritional supplement and is not considered a toxigenic BG algae genus. However, some products have been found to be contaminated with mercury. Microbial contamination could possibly be a concern if harvested algae grow in water contaminated with human or animal wastes.

Ephedra or Ma Huang

The dried young branches of ephedra (*Ephedra* spp.) have been used for their stimulating and vasoactive effects. In addition, ephedra has been used in several products promoted for weight loss. The plant constituents responsible for biologic activity are the sympathomimetic alkaloids ephedrine and pseudoephedrine. A case series involving intoxication of dogs following ingestion of a weight-loss product containing guarana (caffeine) and ma huang (ephedrine) has been reported (Ooms, Khan, and Means, 2001). Estimated doses of the respective plants associated with adverse effects were 4.4 to 296.2 mg/kg for guarana and 1.3 to 88.9 mg/kg for ma huang. Symptomatology included hyperactivity, tremors, seizures, behavioral changes, emesis, tachycardia, and hyperthermia. Ingestion was associated with mortality in 17% of the cases. North American species of ephedra (also called Mormon tea) have not been shown to contain the sympathomimetic alkaloids.

Citrus aurantium ("bitter orange" or "Seville orange") has appeared in many products labeled as "ephedrine-free" and is also combined with caffeine and/or guarana. The primary active components of *C. aurantium* are synephrine (structurally similar to epinephrine), octopamine (structurally similar to norepinephrine), and N-methyltyramine. The overall effect is that of stimulation (Fugh-Berman and Myers, 2004). Studies in humans have shown that bitter orange–containing preparations cause tachycardia and increases in systolic and diastolic pressure (Haller, Benowitz, and Jacob, 2005). Signs of intoxication are similar to those seen with ephedra.

Guarana

Guarana is the dried paste made from the crushed seeds of *Paullinia cupana* or *P. sorbilis,* a fast-growing shrub native to South America. The primary active component in the plant is caffeine, with concentrations that range from 3% to 5% compared with 1% to 2% for coffee beans. Currently the most common forms of guarana include syrups, extracts, and distillates used as flavoring agents and as a source of caffeine for the soft-drink industry. More recently it has been added to weight-loss formulations in combination with ephedra. Oral lethal doses of caffeine in dogs and cats range from 110 to 200 mg/kg of body weight and 80 to 150 mg/kg of body weight, respectively (Carson, 2001; also see Ephedra earlier in the

TABLE 29-1

Additional Herbs of Toxicologic Concern

Scientific Name	Common Names	Active Constituents	Target Organs
Acorus calamus	Acorus, calamus, sweet flag, sweet root, sweet cane, sweet cinnamon	β-Asarone (procarcinogen)	Liver: potent hepatocarcinogen
Aesculus hippocastanum	Horse chestnut, buckeye	Esculin, nicotine, quercetin, rutin, saponins, shikimic acid	Gastrointestinal, nervous
Arnica montana and *A. latifolia*	Arnica, wolf's bane, leopard's bane	Sesquiterpene lactones	Skin: dermatitis
Atropa belladonna	Belladonna, deadly nightshade	Atropine	Nervous: anticholinergic syndrome
Conium maculatum	Poison hemlock	Coniine, other similar alkaloids	Nervous: nicotine-like toxicosis
Convallaria majalis	Lily of the valley, mayflower, conval lily	Cardiac glycosides	Cardiovascular
Cytisus scoparius	Scotch broom, broom, broom tops	l-Sparteine	Nervous: nicotinic-like toxicosis
Datura stramonium	Jimsonweed, thorn apple	Atropine, scopolamine, hyoscyamine	Nervous: anticholinergic syndrome
Dipteryx odorata	Tonka, tonka bean	Coumarin	Hematologic: anticoagulant
Euonymus europaeus; E. atropurpureus	European spindle tree; wahoo, eastern burning bush	Cardiac glycosides	Cardiovascular
Eupatorium perfoliatum; E. purpureum	Boneset, thoroughwort; joe pye weed, gravel root, queen-of-the-meadow	Pyrrolizidine alkaloids	Liver
Heliotropium europaeum	Heliotrope	Pyrrolizidine alkaloids	Liver
Hyoscyamus niger	Henbane, fetid nightshade, poison tobacco, insane root, stinky nightshade	Hyoscyamine, hyoscine	Nervous: anticholinergic syndrome
Ipomoea purga	Jalap	Convolvulin	Gastrointestinal
Mandragora officinarum	Mandrake	Scopolamine, hyoscyamine	Nervous: anticholinergic syndrome
Podophyllum peltatum	Mayapple, mandrake	Podophyllin	Gastrointestinal: gastroenteritis
Sanguinaria canadensis	Bloodroot, red puccoon, red root	Berberine	Gastrointestinal
Solanum dulcamara, other *Solanum spp.*	Woody, bittersweet, climbing nightshade	Numerous glycoalkaloids including solanine and chaconine	Gastrointestinal, nervous, cardiovascular
Tussilago farfara	Coltsfoot	PA alkaloid, senkirkine	Liver
Vinca major and *V. minor*	Common periwinkle, periwinkle	Vincamine	Immune system

chapter for a discussion of a case series involving dogs ingesting a product containing guarana and ephedra; Ooms, Khan, and Means, 2001).

Kratom

Kratom usually refers to the leaves of *Mitragyna speciosa,* a plant indigenous to Southeast Asia. Kratom, or Krypton, has been used traditionally for pain, depression, and anxiety. There is some recent use for treating symptoms associated with opiate withdrawal. The leaves contain several active components including mitragynine and 7-hydroxymitragynine (Horie et al, 2005). While structurally similar to yohimbine, mitragynine acts as a mu opioid receptor partial agonist. The relatively minor component, indole alkaloid 7-hydroxymitragynine, is reported to be more potent than morphine. Kratom is a controlled substance in some countries, but not the United States (Babu et al, 2008). There are case reports in the literature describing adverse effects in humans but as yet little clinical information for animals (Kapp et al, 2011).

Noni Juice

Noni juice is derived from *Morinda citrifolia,* sometimes called "starvation fruit" due to a taste unappealing to humans. Traditionally, noni juice (also called Ba Ji'Tian, Indian Mulberry, or Wild Pine) has been used for a variety of conditions ranging from asthma to smallpox,

TABLE **29-2**

Salicylate-Containing Plants

Common Name	Latin Name	Salicylate Content
White willow	*Salix alba*	Variable
Sweet birch	*Betula lenta*	Variable
White birch	*Betula pendula*	Variable
Meadowsweet	*Filipendula ulmaria*	Variable

TABLE **29-3**

Salicylate-Containing Oils

Name	Salicylate Content
Wintergreen oil *(Gaultheria procumbens)*	98%
Hung Far Oil or Red Flower Oil	67%
Pak Far Oil or White Flower Oil	40%
Tiger Balm Liniment	28%
Kwan Loon Medicinal Oil	15%

Data from Davis JE: Are one or two dangerous? Methyl salicylate exposure in toddlers, *J Emerg Med* 32(1):63-69, 2007.

premenstrual syndrome, and leprosy but is not well studied for any of those. The herbal has a high potassium content that may predispose to interactions with potassium-sparing diuretics and certain antihypertensive medications. Xeronine and proxeronine are components mentioned in advertising, but at this time they have not been chemically identified or studied medically. Although there are several reports of hepatic damage in humans, there are insufficient data at this time to assess safety and efficacy in animals (Yue et al, 2011; Millonig et al, 2005; Stadlbauer et al, 2008).

Salicylate-Containing Preparations

Some of the available salicylate-containing plants and oils are listed in Tables 29-2 and 29-3, respectively.

Current indications for plant salicylate use include fever, rheumatism, and inflammatory conditions. The oils are readily absorbed through the skin. Both therapeutic and adverse effects occur through inhibition of prostaglandin synthesis. In addition, salicylates inhibit oxidative phosphorylation and Krebs cycle enzymes. Although salicylates are toxic to both dogs and cats, cats metabolize salicylates more slowly than other species and are therefore more likely to be overdosed. In cats acetylsalicylic (AS) acid is toxic at 80 to 120 mg/kg given orally for 10 to 12 days. In dogs AS at 50 mg/kg given orally twice a day is associated with emesis; higher doses can cause

depression, anorexia, diarrhea, bloody stool, melena, and metabolic acidosis. A dose of 100 to 300 mg/kg orally once daily for 1 to 4 weeks is associated with gastric ulceration; more prolonged dosing is potentially fatal (Osweiler, 1996).

Preparations for Diabetes Mellitus

A number of herbal agents are currently promoted for mitigating diabetes mellitus in humans and animals. One of these, *Gymnema sylvestre,* has been reported to decrease the taste of sugar in the mouth. This effect is reportedly due to glycosides called gymnemic acids. There are case reports of hepatic damage in humans from this supplement (Shiyovich et al, 2010).

Galega officinalis (goat's rue) was used in the Middle Ages to alleviate polyuria/polydipsia, a common manifestation of diabetes mellitus (and other conditions). Isolation and characterization of the active principle of *G. officinalis* led to the development of the prescription hypoglycemic agent metformin (Graham et al, 2011). *Galega* sp. has been associated with pulmonary edema in sheep (Keeler et al, 1986).

Stevia rebaudiana (sweet herb) is another putative treatment for diabetes mellitus. The diterpene glycosides, or steviol glycosides, provide the sweet taste associated with the plant (Kujur et al, 2010).

Lagerstroemia speciosa (Banaba leaf, Giant Crape-myrtle, Queen's Crape-myrtle), a deciduous tree found in India, Southeast Asia, and the Philippines, has a long history in ethnic medicine. There is evidence in both humans and animals to suggest a possible hypoglycemic effect (Ulbricht et al, 2007).

Momordica charantia (bitter melon, bitter squash, bitter gourd) is a vegetable grown in Asia, Africa, and the Caribbean. This plant is used in complementary and alternative medicine for treatment of diabetes mellitus, although a systematic review of the literature indicates insufficient data to evaluate *Momordica's* medical effects (Ooi et al, 2012).

At the present time there is insufficient information to assess either the safety or the efficacy of these supplements in companion animals. It should be noted that there are reports of herbal antidiabetic products adulterated with prescription pharmaceuticals (Ching et al, 2011).

Essential Oils

Essential oils are the volatile, organic constituents of fragrant plant matter and contribute to plant fragrance and taste. They are extracted from plant material by distillation or cold-pressing. A number of essential oils are not recommended for use (e.g., aromatherapy, dermal or oral use) because of their toxicity or potential for toxicity (Tisserand and Balacs, 1999). They are listed in Table 29-4. These oils have unknown or oral median lethal dose (LD$_{50}$) values in animals of 1 g/kg or less. Most toxicity information has been derived using laboratory rodents or mice. Such data should only be used as a rough guide since they cannot always be extrapolated to other species. *Essential Oil Safety: A Guide for Health Care Professionals* is

TABLE 29-4

Most Toxic Essential Oils

Oil	Genus/Species	Oral LD$_{50}$ (g/kg)	Toxic Component (%)
Boldo leaf	*Peumus boldus*	0.13	Ascaridole: 16
Wormseed	*Chenopodium ambrosioides*	0.25	Ascaridole: 60-80
Mustard	*Brassica nigra*	0.34	Allyl isothiocyanate: 99
Armoise	*Artemisia herba-alba*	0.37	Thujone: 35
Pennyroyal (Eur.)	*Mentha pulegium*	0.40	Pulegone: 55-95
Tansy	*Tanacetum vulgare*	0.73	Thujone: 66-81
Thuja	*Thuja occidentalis*	0.83	Thujone: 30-80
Calamus	*Acorus calamus* var angustatus	0.84	Asarone: 45-80
Wormwood	*Artemisia absinthium*	0.96	Thujone: 34-71
Bitter almond	*Prunus amygdalus* var amara	0.96	Prussic acid: 3
	Artemisia arborescens	Not established	Iso-thujone: 30-45
Buchu	*Agathosma betulina; A. crenulata*	Not established	Pulegone: 50
Horseradish	*Cochlearia armoracia*	Not established	Allyl isocyanate: 50
Lanyana	*Artemisia afra*	Not established	Thujone: 4-66
Pennyroyal (N. Am.)	*Hedeoma pulegioides*	Not established	Pulegone: 60-80
Western red cedar	*Thuja plicata*	Not established?	Thujone: 85

Data from Tisserand R, Balacs T: *Essential oil safety: a guide for health care professionals,* Edinburgh, UK, 1999, Churchill Livingstone.

an excellent reference for in-depth discussions of general and specific essential oil toxicity. The following essential oils are of particular concern.

Camphor

Camphor is an aromatic, volatile, terpene ketone derived from the wood of *Cinnamomum camphora* or synthesized from turpentine. Camphor oil is separated into four distinct fractions: white, brown, yellow, and blue camphor (Tisserand and Balacs, 1999). White camphor is the form used in aromatherapy and in over-the-counter (OTC) products (brown and yellow fractions contain the carcinogen safrole and are not normally available). OTC products vary in form and camphor content; external products contain 10% to 20% in semisolid forms or 1% to 10% in camphor spirits. It is used as a topical rubefacient and antipruritic agent. Camphor is rapidly absorbed from the skin and gastrointestinal tract, and toxic effects can occur within minutes of exposure. In humans signs of intoxication include emesis, abdominal distress, excitement, tremors, and seizures followed by central nervous system (CNS) depression characterized by apnea and coma. Fatalities have occurred in humans ingesting 1 to 2 g of camphor-containing products, although the adult human lethal dose has been reported to be 5 to 20 g (Tisserand and Balacs, 1999; Emery and Corban, 1999). A 1-tsp amount of camphorated oil (≈1 ml of camphor) was lethal to 16-month-old and 19-month-old children.

Citrus Oil

Citrus oil and citrus oil constituents such as D-limonene and linalool have been shown to have insecticidal activity. Although D-limonene has been used safely as an insecticide on dogs and cats, some citrus oil formulations or use of pure citrus oil may pose a poisoning hazard (Powers et al, 1988). Fatal adverse reactions have been reported in cats following the use of an "organic" citrus oil dip (Hooser, Beasley, and Everitt, 1986). Hypersalivation, muscle tremors, ataxia, lateral recumbency, coma, and death were noted experimentally in three cats following use of the dip according to label directions.

Melaleuca Oil

Melaleuca is derived from the leaves of the Australian tea tree *(Melaleuca alternifolia);* it is often referred to as tea tree oil. The oil contains terpenes, sesquiterpenes, and hydrocarbons. A variety of commercially available products contain the oil; shampoos and the pure oil have been sold for use on dogs, cats, ferrets, and horses. Tea tree oil toxicosis has been reported in dogs and cats (Villar et al, 1994; Bischoff and Guale, 1998). One case report describes the illness of three cats exposed dermally to pure melaleuca oil for flea control (Bischoff and Guale, 1998). Clinical signs in one or more of the cats included hypothermia, ataxia, dehydration, nervousness, trembling, and coma. There were moderate increases in serum alanine aminotransferase and aspartate aminotransferase concentrations. Two cats recovered within 48 hours following decontamination and supportive care. However, one cat died 3 days after exposure. The primary constituent of the oil, terpinen-4-ol, was detected in the urine of the cats. Another case involved the dermal application of 7 to 8 drops of oil along the backs of two dogs as a flea repellent (Kaluzienski, 2000). Within 12 hours one dog developed partial paralysis of the hind limbs, ataxia, and depression. The other dog only displayed depression. Decontamination (bathing) and symptomatic and supportive care resulted in rapid recovery within 24 hours.

Pennyroyal Oil

A volatile oil, pennyroyal oil is derived from *Mentha pulegium* and *Hedeoma* pulegioides. Pennyroyal oil has a long history of use as a flea repellent. There is one case report of pennyroyal oil toxicosis in the veterinary literature in which a dog was dermally exposed to pennyroyal oil at approximately 2 g/kg (Sudekum et al, 1992). Within 1 hour of application, the dog became listless, and within 2 hours it began vomiting. Thirty hours after exposure the dog exhibited diarrhea, hemoptysis, and epistaxis. Soon thereafter it developed seizures and died. Histopathologic examination of liver tissue showed massive hepatocellular necrosis.

Product Adulteration

There is a long history of Chinese patent medicines being adulterated with metals and conventional pharmaceuticals or containing natural toxins (Ko, 1998; Au et al, 2000; Ernst, 2002a; Dolan et al, 2003). Sedatives, stimulants, and NSAIDs are common pharmaceuticals added to patent medicines with no labeling to indicate their presence. Commonly found natural toxins in Chinese patent medicines include borneol (reduced camphor), aconite, toad secretions (*Bufo* spp., Ch'an Su), mylabris, scorpion-derived toxins, borax, *Acorus,* and strychnine (*Strychnos nux-vomica*) (Ko, 1998).

Chinese patent medicines often contain cinnabar (mercuric sulfide), realgar (arsenic sulfide), or litharge (lead oxide) as part of the traditional formula. Recently dietary supplements purchased largely from retail stores were tested for arsenic, cadmium, lead, and mercury (Dolan et al, 2003). Eighty-four of the 95 products tested contained botanicals as a major component of the formulation, while 11contained lead concentrations that would have exceeded recommended maximum levels in children and pregnant women had the products been used according to label directions.

Serious adverse health effects have been documented in humans using adulterated Chinese herbal medicines (Ernst, 2002a). There are no published cases in the veterinary literature, although we are aware of one case in which a small dog ingested a number of herbal tea "balls" that were prescribed to its owner for arthritis. The dog presented to a veterinary clinic in acute renal failure several days after the ingestion. Analysis of the formulation revealed low-level heavy metal contamination (mercury and lead) and large concentrations of caffeine and the NSAID indomethacin. The acute renal failure was most likely the result of NSAID-induced renal damage.

Drug-Herb Interactions

Drug-herb interactions refer to the possibility that an herbal constituent may alter the pharmacologic effects of a conventional drug given concurrently or vice versa. The result may be either enhanced or diminished drug or herb effects or the appearance of a new effect that is not anticipated from the use of the drug or herb alone. Possible interactions include those that alter the absorption, metabolism, distribution, and/or elimination of a drug or herbal constituent and result in an increase or decrease in the concentration of active agent at the site of action.

For example, herbs that contain dietary fiber, mucilage, or tannins might alter the absorption of another drug or herbal constituent. Herbs containing constituents that induce liver enzymes might be expected to affect drug metabolism and/or elimination (Blumenthal, 2000). Induction of liver metabolizing enzymes can increase the toxicity of drugs and other chemicals via increased production of reactive metabolites. The production of more toxic reactive metabolites is termed bioactivation (Zhou et al, 2004). Alternatively enhanced detoxification of drugs and other chemicals can decrease their toxicity or their therapeutic efficacy. Long-term use of herbs and other dietary supplements can induce enzymes associated with procarcinogen activation, thus increasing the risk of some cancers (Ryu and Chung, 2003; Zhou et al, 2004). The displacement of one drug from protein-binding sites by another agent increases the concentration of unbound drug available to target tissues. Pharmacodynamic interactions or interactions at receptor sites can be agonistic or antagonistic.

Diagnosis of Herbal Intoxication

Because of the nonspecific signs associated with most intoxications, the diagnosis of a causative agent is extremely difficult without a history of exposure or administration. Such information may not be forthcoming from clients since they may not equate use of an alternative therapy with conventional drug use and therefore may not reveal this information when queried about prior medication history. Also, clients may not volunteer such information because of embarrassment or belief that the veterinarian will not approve of the alternative therapy. Therefore it is important to specifically question clients regarding use of natural products, including herbs, supplements, and vitamins. An added complication is that, even with a history of exposure and a product package, the animal may have been exposed to adulterating or contaminating agents that are not listed on the package label.

Clinical laboratory tests (or postmortem findings) are rarely specific for intoxication from natural products; however, they do assist in determining affected organ systems and thus help formulate a differential list. It may be possible to detect specific herbal constituents in biologic specimens. For example, pulegone was detected in tissues from a dog intoxicated by pennyroyal oil (Sudekum et al, 1992). Currently however, analyses for organic natural products in tissues are not widely available, although analytic methods may improve as herbal use continues to increase.

Treatment of Herbal Intoxication

The adage "treat the patient and not the poison" is appropriate in most suspected poisonings caused by herbal preparations. Treatment consists of decontamination followed by general supportive care and is discussed elsewhere in this section (see Chapters 23 and 27). Indications and contraindications for decontamination procedures should be followed (Poppenga, 2004). Inducing emesis is contraindicated when there is high risk of aspiration (the patient is unconscious or there is neurologic depression) or the patient is having or is likely to have a seizure.

Generally dermal preparations can be removed by washing with a mild soap or detergent. Care should be exercised that the personnel performing this do not themselves become contaminated. Gloves, aprons, and good ventilation are necessary. It is also important to avoid hypothermia in the patient. Supportive care is based on the clinical signs exhibited by the patient. Body temperature, status of the major organ systems, hydration, acid-base balance, urine output, neurologic status, and cardiovascular function require regular monitoring and evaluation.

In rare cases an antidote might be available (e.g., digoxin-specific F(ab) fragments for cardiac glycosides). There are also specific considerations for several botanical agents. Intoxication with salicylates frequently results in acidosis. Urinary alkalinization using sodium bicarbonate may increase the elimination by trapping the ionized salicylate molecules in the urine. It is also important to protect the gastrointestinal tract against the ulcerogenic potential of the salicylates. Treatment may include a protectant such as sucralfate, a histamine H_2-receptor antagonist (cimetidine, ranitidine, or most often famotidine), a proton pump inhibitor (omeprazole), and potentially misoprostol (a PGE_1 analog).

In cases of poisoning from caffeine/guarana, ephedra, *Citrus aurantium,* and other materials causing CNS stimulation, the animal should be monitored for hyperthermia, dehydration, acidosis, cardiac arrhythmias, and seizures. Along with decontamination, fluid therapy increases urinary excretion and helps to correct electrolyte imbalances. Frequent premature ventricular complexes should be treated with lidocaine (without epinephrine). Tachyarrhythmias may require the use of a β-blocker. It must be remembered that β-blockers may also mask the early signs of shock or of hypoglycemia.

References and Suggested Reading

Abdel-Rahman A et al: The safety and regulation of natural products used as foods and food ingredients, *Toxicol Sci* 123(2): 333-348, 2011.

American Botanical Council: http//cmsherbalgram.org/press/2011/HerbalMarketReport2010.html. Last accessed November 11, 2011.

Au AM et al: Screening methods for drugs and heavy metals in Chinese patent medicines, *Bull Environ Contam Toxicol* 65:112, 2000.

Babu KM, McCurdy CR, Boyer EW: Opioid receptors and legal highs: *Salvia divinorum* and kratom, *Clin Toxicol* 46(2):146-152, 2008.

Bent S et al: The relative safety of ephedra compared to other herbal products, *Ann Intern Med* 138(6):468, 2003.

Birdsall TC: 5-Hydroxytryptophan: a clinically effective serotonin precursor, *Altern Med Rev* 3:271, 1998.

Bischoff K, Guale F: Australian tea tree *(Melaleuca alternifolia)* oil poisoning in three purebred cats, *J Vet Diagn Invest* 10:208, 1998.

Blumenthal M: Interactions between herbs and conventional drugs: introductory considerations, *Herbal Gram* 49:52, 2000.

Carson TL: Methylxanthines. In Peterson ME, Talcott PA, editors: *Small animal toxicology*, Philadelphia, 2001, Saunders, p 563.

Ching CK et al: Adulteration of herbal anti-diabetic products with undeclared pharmaceuticals: a case series in Hong Kong, *Br J Clin Pharmacol* Oct 28: 1365-2125, 2011.

Davis JE: Are one or two dangerous? Methyl salicylate exposure in toddlers, *J Emerg Med* 32(1):63-69, 2007.

DerMarderosian A, editor: *Review of natural products*, St Louis, 2001, Facts and Comparisons.

deSmet PAGM: Toxicological outlook on the quality assurance of herbal remedies. In De Smet PAGM et al, editors: *Adverse effects of herbal drugs 1*, Berlin, 1991, Springer-Verlag, p 1.

Dolan SP et al: Analysis of dietary supplements for arsenic, cadmium, mercury, and lead using inductively coupled plasma mass spectrometry, *J Agric Food Chem* 51:1307, 2003.

Emery DP, Corban JG: Camphor toxicity, *J Paediatr Child Health* 35:105, 1999.

Ernst E: Adulteration of Chinese herbal medicines with synthetic drugs: a systematic review, *J Intern Med* 252:107, 2002a.

Ernst E: Toxic heavy metals and undeclared drugs in Asian herbal medicines, *Trends Pharmacol Sci* 23(3):136, 2002b.

Fleischman S, Haake DA, Lovett MA: Salmonella arizona infections associated with ingestion of rattlesnake capsules, *Arch Intern Med* 149:705, 1989.

Fugh-Berman A, Ernst E: Herb-drug interactions: a review and assessment of report reliability, *J Clin Pharmacol* 52:587, 2001.

Fugh-Berman A, Myers A: *Citrus aurantium,* an ingredient of dietary supplements marketed for weight loss: current status of clinical and basic research, *Exp Biol Med* 229:698, 2004.

Gloro R et al: Fulminant hepatitis during self-medication with hydroalcoholic extract of green tea, *Eur J Gastroeterol Hepatol* 17:1135, 2005.

Graham GG et al: Clinical pharmacokinetics of metformin, *Clin Pharmacokinet* 50(2):81-98, 2011.

Grande GA, Dannewitz SR: Symptomatic sassafras oil ingestion, *Vet Hum Toxicol* 29:447, 1987.

Gwaltney-Brant SM, Albretsen JC, Khan SA: 5-Hydroxytryptophan toxicosis in dogs: 21 cases (1989-1999), *J Am Vet Med Assoc* 216:1937, 2000.

Haller CA et al: An evaluation of selected herbal reference texts and comparison to published reports of adverse herbal events, *Adverse Drug React Toxicol Rev* 21(3):143, 2002.

Haller CA, Benowitz NL, Jacob P III: Hemodynamic effects of ephedra-free weight-loss supplements in humans, *Am J Med* 118(9):998, 2005.

Harris ES et al: Heavy metal and pesticide content in commonly prescribed individual raw Chinese herbal medicines, *Sci Total Environ* 409(20):4297-4305, 2011.

Hooser SB, Beasley VR, Everitt JI: Effects of an insecticidal dip containing D-limonene in the cat, *J Am Vet Med Assoc* 189:905, 1986.

Horie S et al: Indole alkaloids of a Thai medicinal herb *Mitragyna speciosa* that has opioid agonistic effect in a guinea pig ileum, *Planta Med* 71(3):231-236, 2005.

Hung OL, Lewin NA, Howland MA: Herbal preparations. In Goldfrank LR et al, editors: *Goldfrank's toxicologic emergencies*, ed 6, Stamford, CT, 1998, Appelton and Lange, p 1221.

Kaluzienski M: Partial paralysis and altered behavior in dogs treated with Melaleuca oil, *J Toxicol Clin Toxicol* 38:518, 2000.

Kapp FG et al: Intra-hepatic cholestasis following abuse of powdered kratom *(Mitragyna speciosa)*, *J Med Toxicol* 7(3):227-231, 2011.

Keeler RF et al: Toxicosis from and possible adaptation to *Galega officinalis* in sheep and the relationship to *Verbesina encelioides* toxicosis, *Vet Hum Toxicol* 28(4):309-315, 1986.

Ko RJ: Herbal products information. In *Poisoning and toxicology compendium*, Cleveland, 1998, Lexi-Comp, p 834.

Kujur RS et al: Antidiabetic activity and phytochemical screening of crude extract of *Stevia rebaudiana* in alloxan-induced diabetic rats, *Pharmacognosy Res* 2(4):258-263, 2010.

Lazarou J, Pomeranz BH, Corey PN: Incidence of adverse drug reactions in hospitalized patients: a meta-analysis of prospective studies, *JAMA* 279 (15):1200, 1998.

Lin CC, Chan TYK, Deng JF: Clinical features and management of herb-induced aconitine poisoning, *Ann Emerg Med* 43:574, 2005.

Millonig G, Stadmann S, Vogel W: Herbal hepatotoxicity: acute hepatitis caused by a noni preparation *(morinda citrifolia)*, *Eur J Gastroenterol Hepatol* 17(4):445-447, 2005.

Ooi CP, Yassin Z, Hamid TA: *Momordica charantia* for type 2 diabetes mellitus, *Cochrane Database Syst Rev* Aug 15, 2012.

Ooms TG, Khan SA, Means C: Suspected caffeine and ephedrine toxicosis resulting from ingestion of an herbal supplement containing guarana and ma huang in dogs: 47 cases (1997-1999), *J Am Vet Med Assoc* 218:225, 2001.

Osweiler GD: Over-the-counter drugs and illicit drugs of abuse. In *The national veterinary medical series: toxicology*, Philadelphia, 1996, Williams & Wilkins, p 303.

Pirmohamed M et al: Adverse drug reactions as a cause of admission to hospital: prospective analysis of 18,820 patients, *Br Med J* 329:15, 2004.

Poppenga R: Treatment. In Plumlee KH, editor: *Clinical veterinary toxicology*, St. Louis, 2004, Mosby, p 13.

Powers KA et al: An evaluation of the acute toxicity of an insecticidal spray containing linalool, d-limonene, and piperonyl butoxide applied topically to domestic cats, *Vet Hum Toxicol* 30(3):206, 1988.

Prakash AS et al: Pyrrolizidine alkaloids in human diet, *Mutat Res* 443:53, 1999.

Ryu S, Chung W: Induction of the procarcinogen-activating CYP1A2 by a herbal dietary supplement in rats and humans, *Food Cosmet Toxicol* 41:861, 2003.

Saper RB et al: Heavy metal content of ayurvedic herbal medicine products, *JAMA* 292(23):2868, 2004.

Segelman AB et al: Sassafras and herb tea: potential health hazards, *JAMA* 236:477, 1976.

Shiyovich A, Sztarker I, Nesher L: Toxic hepatitis induced by *Gymnema sylvestre*, a natural remedy for type 2 diabetes mellitus, *Am J Med Sci* 340(6):514-517, 2010.

Stadlbauer V et al: Herbal does not at all mean innocuous: the sixth case of hepatotoxicity associated with *Morinda citrifolia* (noni), *Am J Gastroenterol* 103(9):2406-2407, 2008.

Stedman C: Herbal hepatotoxicity, *Semin Liver Dis* 22(2):195-206, 2002.

Sudekum M et al: Pennyroyal oil toxicosis in a dog, *J Am Vet Med Assoc* 200:817, 1992.

Tisserand R, Balacs T: *Essential oil safety: a guide for health care professionals*, Edinburgh, UK, 1999, Churchill Livingstone.

Ulbricht C et al: Banaba (*Lagerstroemia speciosa* L.): an evidence-based systematic review by the Natural Standard Research Collaboration, *J Herbal Pharmacotherapy* 7(1):99-113, 2007.

Vanherweghem LJ: Misuse of herbal remedies: the case of an outbreak of terminal renal failure in Belgium (Chinese herbs nephropathy), *J Altern Complement Med* 4:9, 1998.

Villar D et al: Toxicity of Melaleuca oil and related essential oils applied topically on dogs and cats, *Vet Hum Toxicol* 36:139, 1994.

Yang S, Dennehy CE, Tsourournis C: Characterizing adverse events reported to the California poison control system on herbal remedies and dietary supplements: a pilot study, *J Herb Pharmacother* 2(3):1, 2003.

Yue I et al: Acute hepatotoxicity after ingestion of *Morinda citrifolia* (noni juice) in a 14-year-old boy, *J Pediatr Gastroenterol Nutr* 52(2):222-224, 2011.

Zhou S et al: Herbal bioactivation: the good, the bad and the ugly, *Life Sci* 74:935, 2004.

CHAPTER 30

Lawn and Garden Product Safety

JOHN H. TEGZES, *Pomona, California*

Today's lawns and gardens are rife with products for making grass greener, controlling weeds and pests, and conserving water. These products can be classified by their intended use and include fertilizers, herbicides, mulches, and pesticides. They are often available in large volumes, stored in the garage, and applied throughout the year, making exposure to pets an everyday occurrence. Access can include pets eating concentrated product from bags and containers in storage areas and after application to lawns and gardens. Recent trends in lawn and garden care have created new dangers to pets including the increasing availability of products such as cocoa mulch. This chapter reviews some of the common fertilizers, herbicides, and mulches that are widely available, along with the clinical management of dogs and cats after exposure. Information on pesticides can be found in other chapters in this section.

Fertilizers

According to the Soil Science Society of America, fertilizers are defined as "any organic or inorganic material of natural or synthetic origin (other than liming materials) that is added to a soil to supply one or more plant nutrients essential to the growth of plants." Fertilizers include products that are granular or liquid and that contain either single ingredients or blends of plant nutrients. Plant nutrients can include nitrogen, phosphorus pentoxide (P_2O_5), water-soluble potash (K_2O), and secondary nutrients such as calcium, copper, iron, magnesium, and sulfur. Some fertilizers are acid-forming and decrease soil pH after application. Organic fertilizers include naturally occurring organic materials such as manure, guano, worm castings, and compost. Some commercial fertilizer products contain combinations of soil nutrients, herbicides, and insecticides.

The nutrient components of most fertilizers are unlikely to result in severe toxicity in dogs and cats. However, it is important to be aware of all ingredients in a particular product if ingestion occurs because treatment recommendations differ depending on the ingredients and their concentration. Regardless of the actual ingredients, fertilizers may cause vomiting and diarrhea if large amounts are ingested, a result of either irritant effects or bacterial contamination.

The main ingredients of nitrogen, phosphorus, and potash are of low toxicologic significance and do not pose the threat of severe toxicity. In a controlled study dogs that were exposed to urea-based fertilizer, herbicide, and insecticide mixtures via a stomach tube did not display clinical signs (Yeary, 1984). The volumes of mixtures given were extreme (10 ml/kg) and higher than those that could be eaten off grass after application. Based on these findings the ingestion of grass or walking or laying on lawns treated with fertilizers, alone or in combination with herbicides or insecticides, by dogs should not result in toxicologic effects requiring treatment.

Herbicides

There are more than 200 types of herbicides. Herbicides are used both in agriculture and on home gardens and yards to help eradicate weeds and unwanted plants. In general, herbicides are classified by their chemical class (Gupta, 2007). These chemical classes include phenoxy derivatives, urea and thiourea compounds, organic phosphorus/phosphonomethyl amino acids, triazines and triazoles, and others. Although most herbicides are generally not a high toxicologic risk for household pets, there are a few of which the small animal practitioner should be aware.

Organic Phosphorus/Phosphonomethyl Amino Acid Herbicides

Glyphosate, a broad-spectrum herbicide, is widely used by the general public on residential lawns and gardens. It has herbicidal activity against a vast range of annual and perennial weeds and is generally regarded as practically nontoxic to mammals and aquatic and avian species (Malik, Barry, and Kishore, 1989). Therefore it is unlikely that ingestions, even if directly from the container, will result in illness. Some dogs, however, experience vomiting, hypersalivation, and diarrhea after ingestion of glyphosate directly from the container. This is usually attributed to the inactive surfactant found in liquid formulations (Smith and Oehme, 1992). Dogs with protracted vomiting and/or diarrhea can be treated with antiemetics, antidiarrheals, and intravenous fluids, replacing electrolytes as needed based on serum electrolyte concentrations. These clinical effects usually resolve rapidly, and the prognosis is very good.

Phenoxy Acid Derivative Herbicides

The phenoxy acid derivatives are broad-spectrum herbicides used extensively for broad-leaf weed control. The chlorophenoxy herbicide 2,4-dichlorophenoxyacetic acid

(2,4-D) is commonly used around the home and in agriculture. Experimental data suggest that dogs are sensitive to toxicity, leading to gastrointestinal signs and myotonia when given doses of 175 or 220 mg/kg (Beasley, 1991). A case report involving an intact male weimaraner demonstrated clinical evidence of myotonia after an accidental (nonexperimental) exposure (Chen, Bagley, and Talcott, 2010). Toxicity after oral exposure leads initially to gastrointestinal signs of vomiting, diarrhea, and abdominal pain, although absence of these signs does not rule out exposure. Prolonged gastrointestinal signs may lead to fluid and electrolyte imbalances. Neurologic signs occur after high doses or chronic exposures and are characterized by myotonia. Sustained muscle contractions occur after stimulation because of a failure of the muscles to relax. Muscle stiffness, extensor rigidity, and a stiff-limbed gait are observed. Although reports of myotonia are rare following accidental ingestions of 2,4-D, treatment should still be undertaken, including decontamination with oral activated charcoal and supportive care, based on the clinical signs observed. Treatment with intravenous fluids helps to replace fluids and electrolytes lost due to gastrointestinal signs and may help to excrete the herbicide and its metabolites. Keeping the dog cage-rested while minimizing stimulation may help relieve signs of myotonia.

An association between lymphoma in dogs and the use of herbicides has been postulated. A case-control study in 1991 found an association between the use of 2,4-D on yards and the development of canine malignant lymphoma, with an odds ratio of 1.3 (Hayes et al, 1991). Additionally, the report documented a twofold increased risk of canine lymphoma in homes that used 2,4-D for 4 or more years. In 2001 another case-control study found an association between dogs living in an industrial area and the development of canine lymphoma. This same study also found an association between the use of chemicals by owners, specifically paints or solvents, and canine lymphoma (Gavazza et al, 2001). Additionally, a third case-control study reported in 2004 demonstrated an increased risk of transitional cell carcinoma of the urinary bladder in Scottish terriers associated with the use of phenoxy herbicides (Glickman et al, 2004). However, epidemiologic or observational studies such as those cited cannot demonstrate actual cause and effect. Moreover, depending on the study design, additional risk factors may or may not be included in the analysis. Nevertheless the development of neoplasias associated with chronic environmental exposure to phenoxy herbicides is a topic that will continue to be debated and investigated. Although these chronic environmental-type exposures do not require emergency veterinary care, clinicians need to be aware of them and educate owners of potential risks. At the least dog owners should be cautioned to limit access to lawns soon after herbicide applications if such applications cannot be avoided.

Similar to the debate about neoplasia in dogs, there has been speculation about an association between the use of herbicides, fertilizers, or plant pesticides and the development of hyperthyroidism in cats. One case-control study in 1988 found an association, but another case-control study in 2000 did not (Scarlett, Moise, and Rayl, 1988; Martin et al, 2000). Although a definitive connection requires further investigation, it may be prudent to inform owners that a risk may be present and have them limit cats from access to lawns soon after these applications.

Bipyridyl Derivative Herbicides

Paraquat is a bipyridyl herbicide with nonselective contact action. Paraquat use is very restricted but a few formulations are available. Instances of exposure in pets have occurred as a result of malicious poisoning; a series of alleged canine poisonings occurred in an urban dog park in 2003, providing clinical data regarding such exposures (Cope et al, 2004). Paraquat poisoning frequently leads to gastrointestinal signs of vomiting and anorexia soon after exposure. As time goes by, azotemia and progressive respiratory failure develop (Cope et al, 2004). Paraquat accumulates in the lungs, where it causes oxidative injury to type I and type II alveolar cells. As degeneration and sloughing of pneumocytes occur, the animal develops respiratory difficulty with poor exchange of respiratory gases. Often thoracic radiographs are normal in these cases, making ultimate diagnosis difficult unless the owner is aware of the paraquat exposure. In some patients, noncardiogenic pulmonary edema may be seen radiographically. Optimal therapy is uncertain and oxygen can accelerate further oxidative injury to pneumocytes. The dog should be maintained in a quiet environment with minimal stimulation on room air. Oxygen administration should be avoided, if possible. Unfortunately, most cases of paraquat poisoning are fatal, and treatment is supportive. Any animal with suspected ingestion of paraquat should be decontaminated as soon as possible after exposure with activated charcoal. After decontamination, any gastrointestinal signs can be treated with antiemetics and according to the specific signs the animal is exhibiting. Intravenous fluid administration is indicated to help maintain urine output and to protect the kidneys from accumulation and injury by paraquat. Most importantly, the animal should be kept calm and protected from unnecessary stimulation. The prognosis for most cases is poor.

Triazine and Triazole Herbicides

Atrazine is the major herbicide in this class. It has been studied extensively in laboratory animals, looking at both high-dose and low-dose chronic exposures and any association with disease. Generally, it is regarded as having low mammalian toxicity and is unlikely to cause illness in pets with normal household use (Gupta, 2007).

Mulches

Mulches are protective covers placed over soil in gardens to help retain moisture, reduce erosion, provide nutrients, and suppress weeds. Organic residue mulches are probably the most commonly used in households and include shredded bark and tree clippings, wood chips, sawdust, and other plant materials. Some mulches come mixed with animal manure to provide nutrients to soil. Compost is another effective mulch that also provides soil nutrients. These types of plant-based mulches generally are not a significant toxicologic risk but may pose risks associated with gastrointestinal foreign bodies and bacterial contamination.

Recently there has been increased use of cocoa mulch, which consists of shells of spent cacao beans used in chocolate production. Cocoa mulches are attractive to use around the home because of their dark brown color and chocolate aroma. However, some of these mulches can contain the methylxanthines theobromine and caffeine (Carson, 2006). Some dogs are attracted to cocoa mulch because of its smell, and ingestions in dogs are not uncommon. There is variability in the methylxanthine content in cocoa mulches, and not all ingestions result in significant toxicity. However, cocoa mulch ingestions should be treated as suspect methylxanthine toxicity. Clinical effects of toxicity can range from mild vomiting, restlessness, and diarrhea with low-dose ingestions to cardiac arrhythmias, muscular rigidity, hyperreflexia, ataxia, and terminal seizures with high-dose ingestions. Treatment includes decontamination with activated charcoal. Multiple doses of activated charcoal should be administered when prolonged or severe clinical signs are observed. Activated charcoal without a cathartic can be dosed at 1 to 2 g/kg PO every 3 to 6 hours for up to 3 days postexposure. Clinical signs should be treated based on the patient's presentation. Prolonged vomiting can be treated with antiemetics. Tachyarrhythmias are usually responsive to β-blockers such as esmolol, propranolol, or atenolol. Seizures can be treated initially with diazepam and barbiturates and progressed to constant-rate infusions of anesthetic drugs such as propofol for refractory seizure activity.

Treating the Poisoned Patient

Generally, the products reviewed in this chapter are of low toxicity; however, some dogs may be sensitive to certain products. It is prudent to follow these basic principles when treating a known or suspected toxicity. First, after the initial assessment of the patient, all dermal and oral exposures should be decontaminated by administering activated charcoal at 1 to 2 g/kg. If the product exposure was to the hair coat and/or skin, as much of the product as possible should be removed by either clipping the fur or brushing, followed by bathing with a gentle shampoo. Additionally, these patients should also receive oral activated charcoal because most animals self-groom and potentially will ingest the garden chemical that was in the hair coat.

Although some clinical signs can be anticipated after exposure to certain toxins, it is important to treat the patient and not the poison. As such, treatment plans need to be based on the clinical signs and assessment of the patient. Many garden products are irritants to the gastrointestinal tract, and vomiting may occur spontaneously after ingestion. Persistent vomiting can be treated with antiemetics. Cardiac arrhythmias should be treated on a case-by-case basis, paying attention to the overall hemodynamic stability of the patient. Most supraventricular tachyarrhythmias respond to β-blockers, most ventricular arrhythmias to lidocaine, and most bradyarrhythmias to atropine unless associated with shock (as in cats) or profound hypothermia. Neurologic and/or neuromuscular signs can include myotonia, rigidity and hyperreflexia, agitation and anxiety, tremors and seizures, and CNS depression. Depending on the clinical signs presented, some treatment options include the use of skeletal muscle relaxants such as methocarbamol. For agitation and seizures benzodiazepines or barbiturates are often useful. When these signs are severe or prolonged, constant rate infusions of drugs such as propofol are helpful. Fluid and electrolyte losses due to gastrointestinal signs can be replaced through the administration of intravenous fluids, while monitoring serum electrolytes helps to select the best type of fluid and additives.

References and Suggested Reading

Beasley VR et al: 2,4-D toxicosis I: a pilot study of 2,4-dichlorophenoxyacetic acid and dicamba-induced myotonia in experimental dogs, *Vet Human Toxicol* 33:435-440, 1991.

Carson TL: Methylxanthines. In Peterson ME, Talcott PA, editors: *Small animal toxicology*, ed 2, St Louis, 2006, Saunders, pp 845-852.

Chen AV, Bagley RS, Talcott PA: Confirmed 2,4-dichlorophenoxyacetic acid toxicosis in a dog, *J Am Anim Hosp Assoc* 46:43-47, 2010.

Cope RB et al: Fatal paraquat poisoning in seven Portland, Oregon dogs, *Vet Hum Toxicol* 46(5):258-264, 2004.

Gavazza A et al: Association between canine malignant lymphoma, living in industrial areas, and use of chemicals by dog owners, *J Vet Intern Med* 15:190-195, 2001.

Glickman LT et al: Herbicide exposure and the risk of transitional cell carcinoma of the urinary bladder in Scottish terriers, *J Am Vet Med Assoc* 224(8):1290-1297, 2004.

Gupta PK: Toxicity of herbicides. In Gupta RC, editor: *Veterinary toxicology*, New York, 2007, Elsevier, pp 567-586.

Hayes HM et al: Case-control study of canine malignant lymphoma: positive association with dog owner's use of 2,4-dichlorophenoxyacetic acid herbicides, *J Natl Cancer Inst* 83:1226-1231, 1991.

Malik J, Barry G, Kishore G: The herbicide glyphosate, *Biofactors* 2(1):17-25, 1989.

Martin KM et al: Evaluation of dietary and environmental risk factors for hyperthyroidism in cats, *J Am Vet Med Assoc* 217(6):853-856, 2000.

Scarlett JM, Moise NS, Rayl J: Feline hyperthyroidism: a descriptive and case-control study, *Prev Vet Med* 6:295-309, 1988.

Smith EA, Oehme FW: The biological activity of glyphosate to plants and animals: a literature review, *Vet Hum Toxicol* 34(6):531-543, 1992.

Soil Science Society of America Web site: Glossary of soil science terms. Available at: www.soils.org/publications/soils-glossary#. Accessed Oct 27, 2011.

Yeary R: Oral intubation of dogs with combinations of fertilizer, herbicide, and insecticide chemicals commonly used on lawns, *Am J Vet Res* 45(2):288-290, 1984.

CHAPTER 31

Rodenticide Toxicoses

MICHAEL J. MURPHY, *Stillwater, Minnesota*

Pesticides account for about 25% of toxin exposures in pets. Insecticides (see Chapter 32) and rodenticides represent the majority of these pesticide exposures. The rodenticides most frequently encountered by dogs and cats are anticoagulant rodenticides, cholecalciferol, strychnine, zinc phosphide, and bromethalin. Cholecalciferol is discussed in Web Chapter 5. The prevalence of rodenticide exposure in pets may change in upcoming years because the U.S. Environmental Protection Agency issued a direct final rule in 2008, with a final implementation date of June 2011 regarding residential rodenticide use. Briefly, rodenticides for residential use should be distributed in bait stations, and the second-generation anticoagulant rodenticides may no longer be directly available to residential users. The key aspects of toxicosis associated with anticoagulant rodenticides, bromethalin, strychnine, and zinc phosphide follow.

Anticoagulant Rodenticides

The anticoagulant rodenticides continue to be the pesticide most commonly inquired about by animal owners. These compounds (including warfarin, brodifacoum, bromadiolone, diphacenone, and chlorophacinone) represent a substantial proportion of actual toxicoses treated in veterinary and emergency clinics. All anticoagulant rodenticides act by inhibiting the recycling of vitamin K_1 from vitamin K_1 epoxide reductase. This inhibition leads to a reduction in the active forms of clotting factors II, VII, IX, and X in circulation, with factor VII and the extrinsic pathway affected initially. The reduction in the active forms of these factors leads to prolonged clotting times. Prolonged clotting time is most commonly measured by activated clotting time (ACT), one-stage prothrombin time (PT), activated partial thromboplastin time (APTT), or a combination of these tests in the clinic. Prolongation of these times to 15% to 25% above the upper end of the normal range is commonly interpreted as a coagulopathy. Toxic doses of anticoagulant rodenticides induce a coagulopathy. The coagulopathy is not always apparent on clinical presentation and typically is delayed for a number of days following ingestion. The so-called *second-generation* anticoagulant rodenticides have a much longer duration of action when compared to warfarin. The toxic dose and median lethal dose (LD_{50}) for various anticoagulant rodenticides in dogs and cats is quite variable. Data for specific compounds can be found in consultation with veterinary toxicologists (see www.abvt.org).

Anticoagulant rodenticide toxicosis should be considered in dogs or cats with dyspnea, exercise intolerance, coughing, or hemoptysis related to intrathoracic or intrapulmonary hemorrhage. Intrapulmonary hemorrhage occurs commonly in anticoagulant rodenticide toxicosis. Large pleural effusions and marked intrapulmonary bleeding (seen as a coarse, alveolar lung pattern) may be evident on thoracic radiography. Prolonged bleeding from venipuncture sites may be observed. Hematomas, hematemesis, melena, hemoptysis, hematuria, and pallor of mucous membranes are other relatively common clinical signs observed in animals with anticoagulant rodenticide toxicosis. Bleeding may occur in unusual locations such as the pericardial space or into the spinal cord. Of course, anticoagulant rodenticides represent just one cause of coagulopathies in dogs and cats, and other bleeding disorders must be considered.

Detection of the specific anticoagulant rodenticide in serum is the most definitive means of confirming exposure to an anticoagulant rodenticide in a live animal. Liver is the specimen of choice for a dead animal. This testing is now available in many veterinary diagnostic laboratories throughout the United States (see www.aavld.org).

Anticoagulant rodenticide–induced coagulopathies are commonly distinguished from other causes of coagulopathy in the clinic by a relatively rapid response to vitamin K_1 treatment. ACT, PT, and APTT are each dramatically shortened within 24 hours of initiating daily therapy with 2.5 to 5 mg/kg of vitamin K_1 administered orally or subcutaneously (but *not* intravenously or intramuscularly) with a small-gauge needle. Anaphylaxis can occur with parenteral administration of K_1 by any route. Failure to see an initial response may suggest that the coagulopathy is not caused by anticoagulant rodenticide exposure. *Oral* therapy is very effective; some clinicians divide the daily dose into two or three treatments and aim to enhance absorption of the vitamin by administration with a fatty meal, such as some canned dog foods.

In certain cases of recent ingestion (within 2 to 4 hours of presentation), general measures for treatment of toxicosis should be considered, including induction of emesis and administration of activated charcoal (see Chapter 23). Clotting tests are often normal in these cases, so they should be monitored for at least 3 days. Vitamin K_1 treatment should be administered if the clotting time is prolonged.

A severe coagulopathy may call for more than simple vitamin K_1 treatment, and the clinician must appreciate that effects of vitamin K_1 are not immediate. Animals with a packed cell volume less than 15 or those demonstrating complications of anemia may need fresh whole blood immediately. Furthermore, vitamin K_1 alone may be insufficient when results of coagulation tests show rapidly progressing prolongation in clotting times. In these cases, administration of fresh or frozen plasma may be needed to provide clotting factors. Blood product therapy may be required for 12 to 36 hours after initiating vitamin K_1 therapy to allow time for the synthesis of new functional clotting factors. Thoracocentesis may be needed if there is significant dyspnea related to bleeding within the pleural space. Rest, mild sedation, and oxygen are appropriate for intrapulmonary hemorrhage unless respiratory failure has developed, in which case short-term ventilation may be needed.

The dose and duration indicated for vitamin K_1 vary with the specific anticoagulant rodenticide responsible for the coagulopathy. Dosages of 1 to 2.5 mg/kg daily for 3 to 5 days were often effective in treating toxicoses caused by warfarin. Treatment of brodifacoum, diphacenone, and chlorophacinone often requires vitamin K_1 at 2.5 to 5 mg/kg daily for 2 to 4 weeks. Tests of clotting function can be useful guides for the duration of therapy. The bioavailability of vitamin K_1 is greatest when given orally; thus this route is preferred unless contraindicated because of vomiting. Vitamin K_1 may be given subcutaneously but should not be given intramuscularly or intravenously because of the increased risk of massive hemorrhage or anaphylaxis, respectively. Vitamin K_3 therapy is contraindicated because it is not effective and may induce oxidative damage to red cells.

Clients should be educated to remove all anticoagulant rodenticide bait from the pet's environment. Unfortunately, pets occasionally are reexposed to rodenticide bait following discharge from the clinic. The long-acting anticoagulant rodenticides may be present in the serum and liver of the pet for weeks following successful treatment and recovery. Accordingly some anticoagulant rodenticides may be detected by analytic chemistry techniques in animals with no demonstrable coagulopathy and consequently no toxicosis.

Bromethalin

Bromethalin is the active ingredient in rodenticide baits marked under the trade names Assault (Agrisel) and Terminator (Syngenta). The prevalence of bromethalin exposure may increase with the phase-out of second-generation anticoagulant rodenticides for residential consumer use. This compound acts by uncoupling oxidative phosphorylation and leads acutely to hyperexcitability followed by depression in the chronic phase of toxicosis. Muscle tremors, seizures, hind limb hyperreflexia, and death may be observed within approximately 10 hours after exposure to 5 mg/kg. Clinical signs can be progressive, with depression, recumbency, and coma preceding death. Clinical signs of toxicosis may persist for up to 12 days after exposure to 2.5 mg/kg of bromethalin.

With analysis of bait, stomach contents, or vomitus it is possible to confirm exposure to bromethalin in a veterinary patient. Analysis of tissues, including fat, may be used to confirm exposure at postmortem examination. Routine complete blood count, serum biochemistries, and urinalysis generally do not assist in the diagnosis of exposure to bromethalin.

No specific antidote exists. Aggressive charcoal therapy is aimed at reducing absorption and possible enterohepatic circulation of bromethalin. Mannitol and glucocorticoids have been used to reduce cerebral fluid pressure, but they may not reliably reverse clinical signs.

Strychnine

Strychnine distribution has been restricted in many areas of the United States. It has been replaced by zinc phosphide in many areas. Nevertheless, strychnine toxicosis is seen occasionally in clinical practice. Strychnine inhibits the postsynaptic buffering effects of glycine on sensory stimulation of motor neurons and interneurons. Consequently strychnine-poisoned animals appear apprehensive, tense, and stiff within minutes to hours of exposure. Rectal temperature may be increased from muscular hyperactivity. Clinical signs progress to tonic extensor rigidity, especially after sensory stimulation by light, sound, or touch. Animals often die in opisthotonos because of paralysis of respiratory muscles.

Urine samples obtained from a live animal and stomach contents retrieved from a dead animal are the samples of choice for analytic confirmation of exposure to strychnine. Other toxins can result in musculoskeletal stimulation, including mycotoxins, nicotine insecticides (see Chapter 32), and zinc phosphide (see next section). Tetanus and hypocalcemia are other considerations.

Therapy is centered on sedating the patient to prevent seizures. This allows time for strychnine metabolism. Pentobarbital (2 to 15 mg/kg IV for dogs), administered to effect, is the most often used sedative/anticonvulsant. Methocarbamol (55 to 220 mg/kg IV or PO) may be administered for muscle relaxation. One half of the dose can be given as a bolus, with the rest administered slowly to effect. Daily dose should not exceed 330 mg/kg. Although diazepam normally is the initial drug of choice for seizing animals, efficacy for strychnine-induced seizures is variable. Activated charcoal may be administered to reduce further absorption as long as precipitation of seizures is avoided. Stimulation should be avoided, and a quiet, darkened hospital kennel may be beneficial. The patient should be given good nursing care, with attention to clinical and vital signs, as well as rectal temperature. Other treatments may include intravenous fluids and urinary acidification (ammonium chloride) to assist with urinary excretion.

Zinc Phosphide

Zinc phosphide is used for rodent and mole control and marketed under an increasing number of trade names, including Bartlett Waxed Mouse-Bait, Burrow Oat Bait, Rodent Bait, Rodent Pellets, ZIP RTU Bait, ZP Rodent Bait, and ZP Tracking Powder. This compound has become more prevalent since it replaced strychnine in many areas of the United States.

Animals exposed to zinc phosphide have a rapid course of clinical signs. These can progress through anorexia, lethargy, dyspnea, vomiting (occasionally with hematemesis), ataxia, agitation, muscle tremors, weakness, recumbency, and death. Signs develop within minutes to hours of ingestion of a toxic dose of zinc phosphide. Detection of zinc phosphide in the vomitus of a live animal or stomach contents of a dead animal supports the animal's exposure to it. Unfortunately, this compound is volatile; freezing contents in air-tight receptacles may enhance the likelihood of detection in an analytic laboratory.

There is no specific antidote for zinc phosphide. Treatment is mainly supportive. Methods aimed at moving zinc phosphide from the stomach in known cases of ingestion, including emetics, can be used. Increasing gastric pH may be helpful by reducing phosgene liberation. Milk of magnesia has been used as a home remedy;

in the hospital gastric lavage with 5% sodium bicarbonate (take care to prevent bloat) may be used. Diazepam or pentobarbital may be needed for excessive musculoskeletal activity or seizures. In addition to intravenous fluid therapy, liver-supportive agents may be considered.

References and Suggested Reading

Murphy MJ: Rodenticides, *Vet Clin North Am Small Anim Pract* 32: 469, 2002.

CHAPTER **32**

Insecticide Toxicoses

PATRICIA ANN TALCOTT, *Pullman, Washington*

Insecticides used in the United States to which small animals have been exposed include the organophosphate and carbamate cholinesterase inhibitor insecticides, the pyrethrin and pyrethroid groups of insecticides, the triazapentadiene compound amitraz, botanical insecticides, and miscellaneous insecticides that do not fit in any of these aforementioned groups. Each of these groups is discussed in turn.

Organophosphate and Carbamate Insecticides

Organophosphate and carbamate insecticide poisonings are still one of the most commonly encountered toxicoses in small animals because of their widespread use on animals, around the house, and in agriculture (Hansen, 1995a,; Talcott, 2000). These insecticides may be used on animals intentionally or accidentally. Many exposures are accidental, caused by either inappropriate use by the applicator or accidental access to the product by the pet because of inappropriate storage or disposal. Many insecticide products are intended to be applied to the premises or other property, but some are components of pet products including shampoos, flea and tick collars, and insecticide dips.

These products are generally formulated with oily vehicles or solvents to increase contact time and enhance stability. Literally hundreds of formulations are marketed in the form of sprays, dips, shampoos, collars, foggers, or bombs. These marketed products are sometimes mixed with food items to intentionally or maliciously expose pets.

Hundreds of cholinesterase inhibitor insecticides are marketed in the United States. See Box 32-1 for a list of

some of the more commonly used chemicals. The toxicity of these chemicals varies widely. Unfortunately, there are few well-established toxic or lethal doses for dogs or cats reported in the literature. Dermal or oral exposures are commonly encountered by dogs or cats. The inhalation route of exposure is more common in humans. Most of the organophosphate and carbamate insecticides are rapidly metabolized by hepatic enzymes; then both the parent compound and its metabolites are rapidly eliminated in the urine. However, a few lipophilic compounds have longer half-lives, giving them a greater potential to cause central nervous system effects.

Both the organophosphate and carbamate insecticides inhibit acetylcholinesterase (AChE) and pseudocholinesterase enzymes to varying degrees. AChE is responsible for breaking down acetylcholine released at cholinergic sites. Thus animals poisoned with cholinesterase inhibitors often exhibit a mixture of clinical signs as a result of overstimulation of the nicotinic receptors of the somatic nervous system (skeletal muscle), sympathetic and parasympathetic preganglionic junctions, all parasympathetic postganglionic junctions (including a few sympathetic postganglionic junctions), and some neurons within the central nervous system.

The onset of clinical signs can vary between a few minutes to several hours, depending on the dose, the route of exposure, and the specific chemical involved. Commonly reported muscarinic signs include excessive salivation, anorexia, emesis, diarrhea, excessive lacrimation, miosis or mydriasis, dyspnea, excessive urination, and bradycardia or tachycardia. The mnemonics SLUD (i.e., salivation, lacrimation, urination, defecation) and DUMBBELS (i.e., diarrhea, urination, miosis, bronchospasm, bradycardia, emesis, lacrimation, salivation) are

BOX 32-1

Examples of Insecticides

Cholinesterase Inhibitors
Organophosphates
- Chlorpyrifos
- Coumaphos
- Cythioate
- Diazinon
- Dichlorvos
- Dimethoate
- Disulfoton
- Ethoprop
- Famphur
- Fenthion
- Malathion
- Mevinphos
- Parathion
- Phorate
- Phosmet
- Terbufos
- Tetrachlorvinphos

Carbamates
- Aldicarb
- Carbaryl
- Carbofuran
- Methiocarb
- Methomyl
- Oxamyl
- Propoxur

Pyrethrins, Pyrethroids
- Allethrin
- Bifenthrin
- Bioallethrin
- Cismethrin
- Cyfluthrin
- Cyhalothrin
- Cypermethrin
- Deltamethrin
- Esfenvalerate
- Fenfluthrin
- Fenvalerate
- Flumethrin
- Fluvalinate
- Permethrin
- Phenothrin
- Pyrethrin
- Pyrethrum
- Resmethrin
- Sumithrin
- Tetramethrin
- Tralomethrin

Triazapentadiene Compounds
- Amitraz

Botanicals
- d-Limonene
- Linalool
- Melaleuca oil
- Pennyroyal oil
- Rotenone

Miscellaneous
- Fipronil
- Imidacloprid
- Lufenuron
- Methoprene
- Methoxychlor
- Nitenpyram
- Pyriproxyfen
- DEET
- Avermectins

often used in the classroom as a device to remember these clinical signs. Prominent nicotinic signs include ataxia, weakness, and muscle twitching. In acute high-dose oral exposures, seizures can occur within 10 to 20 minutes. It is important to note that not all signs are seen in every poisoning case.

Death is generally the result of respiratory failure and tissue hypoxia caused by excessive respiratory secretions, bronchoconstriction, paralysis of the respiratory muscles, and direct depression of the respiratory center in the medulla. Cats appear to be particularly sensitive to chlorpyrifos; anorexia, muscle weakness, ataxia, and depression are the predominant features. Exposure to these more lipophilic compounds has been referred to as the intermediate syndrome; additional clinical features may include muscle tremors, abnormal mentation, and abnormal posturing with hyperesthesia.

A clinical diagnosis of organophosphate or carbamate poisoning relies heavily on observing compatible clinical signs and a history of known exposure. Inhibition of whole blood, plasma, serum, retinal, or brain cholinesterase activity (at least 25% to 50% of normal) suggests an exposure to these compounds and toxicosis if the clinical signs are compatible. Cholinesterase testing can still be performed after the administration of atropine and may still be useful several days after pesticide exposure. Lack of inhibition cannot rule out exposure to carbamate compounds because of the reversibility of their binding to the cholinesterase enzyme. In addition, because of the acuteness in onset of signs and possible death and the lack of some compounds to readily traverse the blood-brain barrier, brain cholinesterase may be normal in the acutely poisoned patient. Lower red blood cell counts may also lower true AChE activity; this is one reason to check the packed cell volume before running the assay. Therefore cholinesterase testing should be regarded as a screening tool, and false negatives and positives may occur. Tissue analysis for the organophosphate or carbamate insecticide is primarily reserved for confirming an exposure following a postmortem examination. Stomach and intestinal contents and samples from the liver, kidney, fat, and skin (in cases of suspect dermal exposures) should be collected, individually bagged and labeled, and kept frozen during shipment to a laboratory.

Changes observed on a complete blood count, serum chemistry panel, and urinalysis are typically very nonspecific and highly variable. Pancreatitis accompanied by significant elevations in amylase and lipase has been reported following exposures to certain organophosphate insecticides.

Treatment should be aimed at preventing further absorption through aggressive decontamination procedures and controlling the muscarinic and nicotinic clinical signs. Many dermal exposures lead to subsequent oral exposures, particularly in cats; thus multiple decontamination procedures may be needed. In the asymptomatic orally exposed patient, emetics such as 3% hydrogen peroxide or apomorphine are generally recommended. Three percent hydrogen peroxide is dosed at 1 ml/lb or 2.2 ml/kg PO, with a total dose not exceeding 10 ml in the cat or 50 ml in the dog, regardless of body weight (however, this volume has been routinely exceeded in dogs, and I have observed few serious complications). It can be used shortly after feeding a small amount of food. If emesis is contraindicated, a gastric lavage can be performed after inducing light anesthesia, followed by the placement of a cuffed endotracheal tube to prevent aspiration.

Induction of emesis and gastric lavage should always be followed with the use of activated charcoal and a cathartic. Administration of multiple activated charcoal doses may be warranted; care should be taken to reduce the subsequent cathartic doses and monitor the patient for the rare occurrence of hypernatremia or hypermagnesemia. A mild detergent bath and thorough rinsing are recommended in cases of dermal exposure. In the topically exposed patient, particularly in cats, exposure may be both dermal and oral because of excessive grooming. In these cases both dermal and oral decontamination procedures may be beneficial.

Atropine sulfate is used to control the muscarinic signs (e.g., miosis, salivation, diarrhea, bradycardia, bronchoconstriction). The usual dosage range is 0.20 to 0.50 mg/kg (one fourth IV, the remainder SC or IM; some individuals administer the entire dosage IV). The dosage selected should be just enough to provide adequate atropinization, and atropine may be repeated at half the initial dose if signs return. Hypersalivation is often the most useful clinical sign for monitoring atropine therapy. Oxygen therapy with or without artificial respiration may be required until the patient is breathing normally on its own.

Seizures, muscle tremors, or agitation can be controlled with intravenous diazepam, methocarbamol, or phenobarbital. Pralidoxime chloride ([2-PAM]; 10 to 20 mg/kg IM or SC BID or TID) can help reduce muscle tremors resulting from nicotinic receptor stimulation by an organophosphate. A clinical effect should be observed within the first 3 to 4 days, and treatment should be continued as long as improvement is observed. 2-PAM has its best effect if administered within 24 hours of exposure; however, some benefits may occur, particularly in cases involving large toxin exposures, if given within 36 to 48 hours. Rapid intravenous injection may cause tachycardia, muscle rigidity, transient neuromuscular blockage, and laryngospasm. The use of oximes in cases of carbamate poisonings is somewhat controversial (particularly since the carbamate binding is reversible); one should weigh the benefits and risks of its use in each case. It is impossible to tell based on clinical signs alone whether the exposure was caused by an organophosphate or a carbamate insecticide.

Diphenhydramine use is also controversial in the treatment of organophosphate and carbamate poisonings; I do not recommend it. One suggested dose of diphenhydramine in dogs is 2 to 4 mg/kg orally every 6 to 8 hours. However, there have been reports of excessive sedation or excitement and anorexia when used in dogs and cats.

Good supportive and nursing care, including intravenous fluid therapy, adequate nutritional management, and maintenance of normal body temperature and electrolyte balance, should also be considered in the acutely poisoned patient. Chlorpyrifos poisoning in cats requires special attention; these cats often show signs of ataxia, anorexia, depression, and muscle tremors for several days or weeks after initial exposure.

Pyrethrins/Pyrethroids

Pyrethrins are organic esters extracted with fat solvents from flower heads of the pyrethrum plant, *Chrysanthemum cinerariifolium*. Pyrethroids are their synthetic cohorts that vary in both structure and potency. Pyrethroids generally are more toxic to insects and mammals and persist longer in the environment than pyrethrins (Hansen, 1995b; Talcott, 2000). A number of commonly used pyrethrin and pyrethroid chemicals are listed in Box 32-1. Many of these pesticide formulations are registered for topical use on dogs and cats for flea and tick control. Other formulations are marketed for household use, and still others can be used in agriculture. These products can be purchased through many readily available outlets and packaged as sprays, dips, shampoos, and spot-on formulations. The percentages of active ingredient can range from less than 1% to as much as 65% or greater; therefore it is crucial to read the label thoroughly when using them.

There are hundreds of pyrethrin- and pyrethroid-containing formulations, sometimes combined in mixtures along with insect growth regulators, insect repellents, and various synergists. Piperonyl butoxide is a common additive to pyrethrin products. Although it possesses limited insecticidal activity, it acts as a synergist to extend the killing duration of the pyrethrin. The mode of synergistic activity is not conclusively known. Hypothesized mechanisms of the synergistic effect of piperonyl butoxide include (1) prolongation of the action of pyrethrins by preventing rapid oxidation; (2) formation of complexes with the pyrethrins that lead to higher insecticidal activity; and (3) delay of pyrethrin detoxification by the insect's tissue enzymes. A number of pyrethroid products also contain insect repellents.

N-octyl bicycloheptene dicarboximide, di-n-propyl isocinchomeronate, and butoxypolypropylene glycol are insect repellents often present in pyrethrin- and pyrethroid-containing products at concentrations ranging from 0.34% to 15%. Toxicity of these mixtures may be attributed solely to the pyrethrins and pyrethroids or be caused by the combined effects of the insecticides plus the additives, synergists, and solvents.

Pyrethrins work by stimulating the insect's central nervous system. This action results in muscular excitation, convulsions, and paralysis. When dissolved in thin oils, pyrethrins readily penetrate through the hard, chitinous covering of the insect, and their insecticidal action is rapid. Both pyrethrins and pyrethroids affect nervous tissue in mammals by reversibly prolonging sodium conductance, producing increased depolarizing afterpotentials that result in repetitive nerve firing. Their toxicity to mammals is low and, when used according to label instructions, should not induce deleterious effects in mammals. Toxicoses in mammals can be observed when these products are ingested or when there is overzealous heavy topical application, particularly in cats and small dogs. Many poisonings in clinical practice are the result of products labeled "for use in dogs only" being used on cats. There are also many anecdotal instances in which cats exhibited adverse effects following topical exposure to appropriately applied formulations. Clinical signs are normally observed within minutes to a few hours after exposure.

Clinical signs usually include excessive salivation (as a result of oral sensory stimulation), muscle tremors, depression, ataxia, anorexia, and vomiting. Less commonly reported adverse effects include weakness, dyspnea, diarrhea, hyperthermia or hypothermia, hyperesthesia (ear flicking, paw shaking; repeated contractions of the superficial cutaneous muscles), and recumbency. Occasionally one can see a topical allergic reaction characterized by urticaria, pruritus, and alopecia at the site of application. Death is rarely reported but can occur, typically following severe, uncontrollable seizure activity.

A clinical diagnosis of pyrethroid poisoning most heavily relies on obtaining a history of recent use and access to these products. The clinical signs closely mimic other poisonings (e.g., organophosphate and carbamate poisonings), and there are no specific clinicopathologic abnormalities routinely observed in affected animals. Laboratory methods for analyzing pyrethrin/pyrethroid residues are not routinely available but can be done to confirm exposure if necessary. Since clinical signs often mimic organophosphate or carbamate poisonings, assessing blood or brain cholinesterase is recommended to rule out these differentials. Cholinesterase activity is not inhibited in cases of pyrethrin/pyrethroid poisonings, whereas it may be in organophosphate or carbamate exposures and poisonings.

There is no specific antidote for pyrethrin/pyrethroid poisonings. Consequently treatment should be aimed at decontaminating the animal to prevent further absorption and addressing the clinical presentation. Bathing the animal in warm soapy water followed by a thorough rinsing is recommended for topical exposures. Long-haired dogs and cats may require multiple bathings-dryings-brushings or clipping to remove residues from the hair.

Oral ingestions can be treated with emetics, activated charcoal, and cathartics and more aggressively with light sedation and gastric lavage. Muscle tremors can usually be controlled with diazepam (0.5 to 1 mg/kg IV or to effect) or methocarbamol (55 to 220 mg/kg IV); it should be administered half rapidly, not to exceed 2 ml/min, and the rest to effect. Continuous monitoring of body temperature for hypothermia or hyperthermia is essential. Providing adequate hydration and electrolyte status is also important in achieving a positive outcome. The oral cavity can be rinsed to help control hypersalivation. The prognosis for the majority of pyrethrin/pyrethroid poisonings is excellent, with most animals recovering within 24 to 72 hours.

Amitraz

Amitraz is a formamidine pesticide that is present in some tick collars used on dogs. It is often present at a concentration of 9%. The collars are designed to kill ticks for 4 months. Toxicosis can occur in dogs that ingest a substantial portion of, or the entire, collar. The entire collar weighs 27.5 g, so each gram of collar contains approximately 90 mg of amitraz. However, the collar is a controlled-release device that releases amitraz in first-order kinetics over an effective period of more than 90 days. Therefore release is much higher when the collar is new than after it has been used for 4 months. Mitaban liquid concentrate contains 19.9% amitraz. It is used topically for the control and treatment of generalized demodicosis. Several different treatment protocols have been suggested, depending on the location and severity of the disease and the age of the affected animal. Amitraz is not recommended in lactating or pregnant animals or in animals that weigh less than 5 kg.

The lethal dose of amitraz is estimated to be about 100 mg/kg orally in dogs, although toxic doses as low as 10 to 20 mg/kg have been reported. Amitraz is well absorbed by the gastrointestinal tract. Clinical signs of toxicosis usually begin within 1 hour of ingestion, sometimes as early as 30 minutes.

Amitraz is a monoamine oxidase inhibitor, an α_2-adrenergic agonist, and an inhibitor of prostaglandin synthesis. Ocular exposure to this compound can lead to mild irritation. The clinical signs can be severe but often transient and rarely fatal. Most clinical signs are associated with the α_2-adrenergic properties of amitraz and include depression, sedation, ataxia, bradycardia, mydriasis, hypothermia, vomiting, polyuria, and gastrointestinal stasis or diarrhea. Other signs that have been reported include hyperthermia, gastric dilation, hypersalivation, dyspnea, anorexia, shock, tachycardia, urinary incontinence, disorientation, tremors, and coma (Duncan, 1993; Grossman, 1993; Hovda and McManus, 1993). Clinical laboratory data often reveal a hyperglycemia. Most signs, whether in mild exposures or excessive exposures followed by aggressive treatment, usually last no longer than 24 to 48 hours.

Treatment is aimed at decontamination to prevent further absorption and reversal of the adrenergic agonist effects. In the asymptomatic patient emesis should be induced with 3% hydrogen peroxide or apomorphine. Administering a non-oily laxative such as activated charcoal with a cathartic is recommended as long as no diarrhea is present. An enema to evacuate the colon may be administered 12 to 18 hours after ingestion if diarrhea has not occurred or the laxative does not produce the desired effect.

Abdominal radiography is recommended if a length of collar is the suspected source of the amitraz or if the depression/sedation is severe and prolonged. Retrieval of the collar or pieces of collar can be performed by endoscopy, gastrotomy, or enterotomy. Xylazine should be avoided because of the possibility of exacerbating hypotension. All surgical procedures and anesthesia protocols should be considered carefully because of the potential to exacerbate preexisting problems of gastric dilation or bradycardia. The probability of requiring these more invasive decontamination procedures is rare.

Since amitraz is not a cholinesterase inhibitor, atropine and 2-PAM are contraindicated in the treatment of amitraz poisoning. In moderately or severely affected patients who cannot be aroused, the α_2-antagonists, yohimbine or atipamezole, may be administered (Hsu, Lu, and Hembrough, 1986; Hugnet et al, 1996). Yohimbine is dosed at 0.1 mg/kg IV and since the duration of action is short (half-life = 1.5 to 2 hours), it may need to be repeated until the dog's clinical condition improves significantly. Atipamezole can be initiated at the conservative dose of 50 µg/kg IV. A typical dosage range for atipamezole, based on body surface area, is from 230 µg/kg to 100 µg/kg IV (for dogs ranging from 5 kg to 50 kg), or from 400 µg/kg to 140 µg/kg IM (for dogs ranging from 5 kg to 50 kg). This extralabel dosing can be further informed by consulting the Antisedan product insert for reversal of dexmedetomidine for that patient's specific *body surface area*. Both compounds should reverse amitraz-induced changes within 20 to 30 minutes. Body temperature should be monitored following yohimbine use to avoid hyperthermia. Fluid therapy (see Chapters 1 and 2) is also warranted in the bradycardic, dehydrated patient.

Botanical Oil Extracts

Various fragrant volatile oils that are currently marketed as having parasiticidal properties have been isolated from a number of plants. The most popular of these oils include d-limonene and linalool. These oils are sold as shampoos, sprays, and dips for flea and tick control on dogs and cats or for premise control. Some citrus oil extracts are also found in household cleaners. These oils are considered to be relatively nontoxic and are generally regarded as safe by the Food and Drug Administration. Both d-limonene and linalool are present in oils extracted from the skins of citrus fruits and are typically associated with poisonings in dogs and cats when used at excessive concentrations. Cats are more sensitive to developing clinical signs after exposures than dogs.

With normal use these compounds may cause temporary irritation to the eyes, skin, nose, throat, or respiratory tract. Adverse reactions to these compounds can occur following inhalation, dermal, or oral exposure. Clinical effects are often observed within 15 to 30 minutes after exposure. Typical signs after oral exposure include salivation, vomiting, diarrhea, and central nervous system depression. Other signs reported with higher exposures include muscle tremors, hypothermia, hypotension, ataxia, and mydriasis.

Ataxia, weakness, depression, and dermal irritation (e.g., scrotal, perianal) have been seen following topical applications. Seizures and death are rare and are presumed to be secondary to severe hypotension and hypothermia. There has been one report of erythema multiforme and disseminated intravascular coagulation in a dog following a dermal application of a d-limonene–containing dip (Rosenbaum and Kerlin, 1995). An acute necrotizing dermatitis and subsequent septicemia was reported in a 2-year-old cat following application of a d-limonene–containing insecticidal shampoo (Lee, Budgin, and Mauldin, 2002). Other signs reported included lethargy, inappetence, vocalization, and abnormal aggressive behavior.

Treatment is aimed at decontamination, with supportive care based on the clinical signs. Repeated bathing with warm, soapy water followed by thorough rinsing are recommended following topical applications. Gastric lavage with activated charcoal and a cathartic is recommended following oral ingestions. Body temperature and blood pressure should be monitored to prevent hypotension and hypothermia. Diazepam has been used to control the muscle tremors, and fluid therapy is generally recommended to prevent dehydration. Most affected animals recover within 24 hours.

Pennyroyal oil has long been used as a flea repellent and is sold as a shampoo, powder, or the pure oil itself. Pennyroyal is an herb consisting mainly of leaves from two different plants, *Mentha pulegium* and *Hedeoma pulegioides*. The oil is derived from the leaves and flowering tops of these plants. Pulegone constitutes approximately 85% of the pennyroyal oil and is metabolized to the toxic metabolite menthofuran by the liver. Toxicoses have been described in both animals and humans following dermal application and oral ingestion. Clinical signs are associated primarily with gastrointestinal upset, liver failure, and severe neurologic injury. Clinical signs include lethargy, vomiting, diarrhea, hemoptysis, epistaxis, dyspnea, miosis or mydriasis, seizures, and death (Anderson et al, 1996). Massive hepatic necrosis has been reported in the dog following topical application of the oil (Sudekum et al, 1992).

Pennyroyal oil ingestion is treated by decontaminating the stomach by gastric lavage and activated charcoal. Emesis is generally not suggested because of the rapid absorption of pennyroyal oil, the risk for developing aspiration pneumonia, and the potential for rapid onset of central nervous system depression. Repeated bathing with a mild detergent followed by thorough rinsings is recommended following topical applications. *N*-acetylcysteine has been suggested in cases in which there is a high risk of inducing a toxicosis, starting with a loading dose of 140 mg/kg and following with 70 mg/kg every 4 hours. *N*-acetylcysteine therapy should be beneficial within the first few hours of poisoning and should continue for at least 24 to 48 hours. The cytochrome P-450 inhibitor cimetidine has also been recommended in the treatment of this poisoning. Mice pretreated with cimetidine exhibited less liver disease associated with intraperitoneal pulegone administration than controls (Sztajnkrycer, 2003). Any additional therapy is supportive only and should be based on clinical signs; this may include the use of antiemetics and fluid therapy. Basic support for liver failure may include plasma transfusions, antibiotics, vitamin K$_1$, S-adenosylmethionine, vitamin E, and gastric protectants (sucralfate). A complete blood count, serum chemistry and coagulation profile, and urinalysis should be performed to monitor organ function.

Another essential oil, Melaleuca oil or tea tree oil, is obtained from the leaves of the Australian tea tree *(Melaleuca alternifolia)*. Melaleuca oil derivatives can be found in products used topically for skin infections, as insect repellents, as antipruritics, or as household cleaners. Melaleuca oil is known to contain as much as 60% terpenes; thus the clinical signs in poisoned patients strongly resemble those described for the essential oils d-limonene and linalool.

Toxicities with these products have been reported in cats, dogs, rats, and humans, after either oral ingestion or topical application. Most reports of poisoning in pets occur after misuse of high topical doses of the product. The lipophilic terpenes are readily and rapidly absorbed across the skin and mucosal lining of the gastrointestinal tract. Cats are thought to be more sensitive than dogs, and toxicities might be observed more frequently in this species because of their fastidious grooming habits.

The onset of clinical signs may occur within minutes to 8 hours after topical application. The time interval is highly dependent on dose and the extent of oral exposure following grooming behavior. The most common adverse signs include ataxia, incoordination, weakness, tremors, depression, hypothermia, and behavior abnormalities (Villar et al, 1994). Elevation in liver enzymes (alanine aminotransferase, aspartate aminotransferase) has been reported in cats following topical exposure (Bischoff and Guale, 1998).

Treatment is directed toward symptomatic and supportive care. Topical exposures warrant bathing with a mild detergent followed by a thorough rinsing. Long-haired pets may benefit from having their hair cut or trimmed. Activated charcoal and a cathartic can be administered in orally exposed pets. Monitoring basic life support measures and correcting any temperature, fluid, and electrolyte abnormalities may be indicated. Prognoses are generally favorable, and most affected animals recover over a 2- to 3-day interval.

Miscellaneous Insecticides (Methoprene, Lufenuron, Fipronil, Imidacloprid, Pyriproxyfen, Nitenpyram)

Many of the insecticides described in this section are used topically. When an adverse effect related to topical/oral exposure to these products is suspected, it is essential to read the label ingredients carefully. Many of the insecticides listed in the following paragraphs can occur as a single ingredient or in combination with other insecticides, mainly pyrethrins and pyrethroids. In addition, several adverse reactions reported such as salivation or skin irritation following dermal or oral exposures may be caused by the carriers present in the formulation. Typically these signs are mild and self-limiting.

Insect growth regulators are a relatively new category in the war against fleas and ticks. All act as analogs of juvenile growth hormones, thereby interrupting the normal growth patterns of the insect. Methoprene preferentially kills fleas and ticks in the larval stage by binding to and activating juvenile hormone receptors. It thereby prevents larvae from developing into adult fleas. Methoprene can be absorbed from the gastrointestinal tract, through the intact skin, or by inhalation. However, it is considered to be virtually nontoxic when ingested or inhaled and only slightly toxic after dermal absorption. Methoprene is not considered an eye or skin irritant.

Lufenuron, a benzoylphenyl urea, inhibits the synthesis, polymerization, and deposition of chitin in the eggs or exoskeleton of fleas. Lufenuron is highly lipophilic and readily accumulates in adipose tissue. Lufenuron has shown no synergistic or additive effects when combined with other insecticides. It has proven to be safe at recommended dosage regimens in puppies and kittens as young as 6 weeks of age, as well as in lactating dogs and cats and their offspring. Various studies in dogs and cats using up to 10 times the normal dosage have shown no serious health effects over an exposure period of 1 to 9 months. No adverse effects were seen in cats orally exposed to up to 17 times the recommended dosage. A mild decrease in food consumption was reported in puppies exposed from 8 weeks to 10 months of age to 18 to 30 times the recommended dosage. However, the majority of studies have shown no significant adverse effects on food consumption, body weight, hematology, clinical chemistries, and urinalyses following excessive exposures. Few effects on fertility and reproduction have been reported. Administration of lufenuron to breeding male and female dogs at 90 times the recommended dosage of 10 mg/kg resulted in a reduced pregnancy rate compared with controls. Pups born to treated females exhibited nasal discharge, pulmonary congestion, diarrhea, dehydration, and sluggishness. It appears that lufenuron concentrates in the milk at a 60:1 milk:blood concentration ratio (Ciba-Geigy Corporation).

Lufenuron, 90 mg/kg, was administered to breeding cats before mating and through gestation and lactation. Kittens born to these cats exhibited no adverse effects on health, growth, and survival (Ciba-Geigy Corporation, 1996; Shipstone and Mason, 1995). Plumb lists vomiting, lethargy, depression, urticaria, diarrhea, dyspnea, anorexia, and reddened skin as rare adverse effects (Plumb, 2005).

Fipronil is a phenylpyrazole flea and tick adulticide currently marketed as a spray and topical liquid that boasts a wide margin of safety. It can be used on dogs, cats, puppies, or kittens greater than 8 weeks old. No adverse effects were noted in studies in which dogs or cats were fed five times the maximum dose. Fipronil acts on the γ-aminobutyric acid–mediated chloride channels of invertebrates, thereby interrupting nervous transmission and leading to rapid death of the fleas and ticks. Mammals reportedly have receptors inside the chloride channel that are shaped differently than the invertebrate receptors, and fipronil is not thought to be able to bind these channels for a long period of time. Following dermal application, it is not considered systemically active and is thought to be sequestered in the pet's sebaceous glands. Mild skin irritation may occur following topical applications of these products.

Imidacloprid is another topically used adulticide that reportedly binds specifically to postsynaptic nicotinic acetylcholine receptors of insects and both kills adult fleas and exhibits some larvicidal action. Toxicity testing of imidacloprid has shown no adverse effects when used at five times the maximum dosage in dogs and cats. A few reports of alopecia and erythema have been observed following dermal application. Theoretically poisoning could occur by the oral route if the dosage or concentration were excessive. The most common complaint following ingestion is excessive salivation that is self-limiting. There is no specific antidote, and all treatment should be based on observed clinical problems. Topically exposed pets should be bathed and rinsed; orally exposed patients should be decontaminated by either emesis or lavage, followed by the use of activated charcoal and a cathartic.

Pyriproxyfen and nitenpyram are two of the relatively newer products that have entered the marketplace. Nitenpyram is a neonicotinoid derivative that binds and inhibits specific nicotinic acetylcholine receptors. It does not inhibit AChE activity. Pyriproxyfen is an insect growth regulator used topically to control insects. No significant adverse effects have been reported with either of these products.

References and Suggested Reading

Anderson IB: Pennyroyal toxicity: measurement of toxic metabolite levels in two cases and review of the literature, *Ann Intern Med* 124:726, 1996.

Bischoff K, Guale F: Australian tea tree (*Melaleuca alternifolia*) oil poisoning in three purebred cats, *J Vet Diagn Invest* 10:208, 1998.

Blagburn BL et al: Efficacy dosage titration of lufenuron against developmental stages of fleas in cats, *Am J Vet Res* 55:98, 1994.

Blagburn BL et al: Efficacy of lufenuron against developmental stages of fleas in dogs housed in simulated home environments, *Am J Vet Res* 56:464, 1995.

Blodgett DJ: Organophosphate and carbamate insecticides. In Peterson ME, Talcott PA, editors: *Small animal toxicology*, St Louis, 2006, Elsevier, p 941.

Campbell WR, Lynn RC: Tolerability of lufenuron (CGA-184699) in normal dogs and cats, *J Vet Intern Med* 3:2, 1992.

Ciba-Geigy Corporation: Program (lufenuron) for control of existing flea infestations, *Adv Pract Vet*, 1, 1996.

Ciba-Geigy Corporation: Summary of studies submitted as part of the new animal drug application, No 41-035, for lufenuron tablets, Ciba-Geigy Corp, Greensboro, NC, 800-637-0281.

Ciba-Geigy Corporation: Program (lufenuron): a radical breakthrough in flea control, Ciba Animal Health, Ciba-Geigy Animal Health, Greensboro, NC 27419.

Duncan KL: Treatment of amitraz toxicosis, *J Am Vet Med Assoc* 208(8):1115, 1993.

Fikes JD: Organophosphorus and carbamate insecticides, *Vet Clin North Am* 20(2):353, 1990.

Fikes JD: Feline chlorpyrifos toxicosis. In Bonagura JD, Kirk RW, editors: *Kirk's current veterinary therapy XI (small animal practice)*, Philadelphia, 1992, Saunders, p 188.

Grossman MR: Amitraz toxicosis associated with ingestion of an acaricide collar in a dog, *J Am Vet Med Assoc* 203(1):55, 1993.

Hansen SR: Management of adverse reactions to pyrethrin and pyrethroid insecticides. In Bonagura JD, Kirk RW, editors: *Kirk's current veterinary therapy XII (small animal practice)*, Philadelphia, 1995a, Saunders, p 242.

Hansen SR: Management of organophosphate and carbamate insecticide toxicoses. In Bonagura JD, Kirk RW, editors: *Kirk's current veterinary therapy XII (small animal practice)*, Philadelphia, 1995b, Saunders, p 245.

Hansen SR: Pyrethrins and pyrethroids. In Peterson ME, Talcott PA, editors: *Small animal toxicology*, St Louis, 2006, Elsevier, p 1002.

Hansen SR, Buck WB: Treatment of adverse reactions in cats to flea control products containing pyrethrin/pyrethroid insecticides, *Feline Pract* 20(5):25, 1992.

Hink WF et al: Evaluation of a single oral dose of lufenuron to control flea infestations in dogs, *Am J Vet Res* 55:822, 1995.

Hooser SB: d-Limonene, linalool, and crude citrus oil extracts, *Vet Clin North Am Small Anim Pract* 20(2):383, 1990.

Hovda LR, McManus AC: Yohimbine for treatment of amitraz poisoning in dogs, *Vet Hum Toxicol* 35(4):329, 1993.

Hsu WH, Lu ZX, Hembrough FB: Effect of amitraz on heart rate and aortic blood pressure in conscious dogs: influence of atropine, prazosin, tolazoline, and yohimbine, *Toxicol Appl Pharmacol* 84:418, 1986.

Hugnet C et al: Toxicity and kinetics of amitraz in dogs, *Am J Vet Res* 57(10):1506, 1996.

Kanzler K, editor: *Veterinary pharmaceuticals and biologicals*, 1995/1996, ed 9, Lenexa, KS, Veterinary Medicine Publishing, p 841.

Lee JA, Budgin JB, Mauldin EA: Acute narcotizing dermatitis and septicemia after application of a d-limonene–based insecticidal shampoo in a cat, *J Am Vet Med Assoc* 221(2):258, 2002.

Miller TA: Personal communication, Virbac, Inc, 3200 Meacham Blvd, Fort Worth, TX 76137.

Plumb DC: *Plumb's veterinary drug handbook*, ed 5, Ames, IA, 2005, Blackwell Publishing.

Rosenbaum MR, Kerlin RL: Erythema multiforme major and disseminated intravascular coagulation in a dog following application of a d-limonene–based insecticidal dip, *J Am Vet Med Assoc* 207(10):1315, 1995.

Shipstone MA, Mason KV: Review article: The use of insect development inhibitors as an oral medication for the control of the fleas *Ctenocephalides felis, C. canis* in the dog and cat, *Vet Dermatol* 6:131, 1995.

Sudekum M et al: Pennyroyal oil toxicosis in a dog, *J Am Vet Med Assoc* 200(6):817, 1992.

Sztajnkrycer MD: Mitigation of pennyroyal oil hepatotoxicity in the mouse, *Acad Emerg Med* 10(10):1024, 2003.

Talcott P: Toxicity of flea and tick products. In Bonagura JD, editor: *Kirk's current veterinary therapy XIII (small animal practice)*, Philadelphia, 2000, Saunders, pp 231, 233.

Valentine WM: Pyrethrin and pyrethroid insecticides, *Vet Clin North Am* 20(2):375, 1990.

Villar D et al: Toxicity of melaleuca oil and related essential oils applied topically on dogs and cats, *Vet Hum Toxicol* 36(2):139, 1994.

Whittem T: Pyrethrin and pyrethroid insecticide intoxication in cats, *Compendium* 17(4):489, 1995.

CHAPTER 33

Pesticides: New Vertebrate Toxic Agents for Pest Species

RHIAN COPE, *Lower Hutt, New Zealand*

Given that most indigenous animal life in New Zealand evolved for millions of years in the absence of terrestrial mammalian predators, the continued preservation of most endemic species is heavily contingent on effective suppression of introduced vertebrate predators with the use of vertebrate toxic agents.

In New Zealand the most common method for the control of feral cats and stoats is trapping, which is effective but labor intensive. Sodium fluoroacetate (1080) is also currently registered for feral cat control in the form of a fish/meat meal pellet for either bait stations or hand-laying, although it is not approved for stoat control. Notably, 1080 operations directed against brush tailed possums *(Trichosurus vulpecula),* rabbits *(Oryctolagus cuniculus),* and other mammalian pest species often serendipitously result in secondary poisoning of feral cats and stoats. However, 1080 is controversial because of genuine concern regarding secondary poisoning in nontarget domestic species, as well as the general public's concern over its use. Thus New Zealand has been placed in the position of seeking new toxicants and technologies for the control of vertebrate pest species.

New Zealand has recently approved a new vertebrate toxic agent for the control of feral cats *(Felis catus)* and stoats *(Mustela erminea):* para-aminopropiophenone (PAPP). The use of encapsulated sodium nitrite for the control of feral pigs *(Sus scrofa domesticus)* is currently in the final stages of regulatory approval. A third toxin, tutin, is currently under development. These toxins (toxicants) are the subjects of this chapter.

Para-Aminopropiophenone (PAPP)

PAPP was originally developed as a potential antidote for acute cyanide poisoning and for its radioprotective properties against X, gamma, and high-energy proton irradiation. PAPP is the most potent methemoglobin inducer of the para-aminoalkylphenones. It is capable of inducing clinically significant methemoglobinemia, oxidative hemolytic anemia, and Heinz body formation in a variety of vertebrate species including mustelids, cats, dogs, and rodents, as well as in various bird species.

In the United States, trials using PAPP for control of coyotes *(Canis latrans)* were conducted for the U.S. Fish and Wildlife Service. The coyote trials revealed problems with both formulation and regurgitation by dosed animals. Development of PAPP was not a priority after 1080 was registered for use in the Livestock Protection Collar. New Zealand PAPP formulations all contain an

antiemetic. This addition decreases the risk that vomiting of the bait will reduce the effectiveness of these formulations in targeted species. Unfortunately, the inclusion of an antiemetic potentially increases the hazard of PAPP baits ingested by nontarget species.

PAPP is readily metabolized, is not bioaccumulative, and does not accumulate in the environment. The risk of secondary toxicity to nontarget species is regarded as low. However, nontarget burrowing seabirds are considered to be at risk of inadvertent poisoning because of the current design of the bait stations.

Lethal Doses

PAPP has some selective toxicity for felids, mustelids, and canids. The lethal doses are: cats, 20 to 34 mg/kg; stoats, 37.1 to 94.8 mg/kg; ferrets *(Mustela furo),* 13 to 25 mg/kg; and dogs *(Canis familiaris),* 21.4 to 42.9 mg/kg. Birds and rodents are somewhat less susceptible, although there is some variability in the response of different bird species.

Methods of Use as a Vertebrate Toxic Agent

Veterinarians should understand how these agents are deployed and how most exposures occur. PAPP is available as a 410 g/kg paste mixed with meat to produce meat boli that contain about 22 mg PAPP/g. The boli are placed in bait stations. PAPP is designed to be a single-feed vertebrate toxic agent. However, prefeeding with mince for 2 weeks prior to laying the PAPP baits is recommended. Prepared mince baits should be used within 24 hours of preparation and remain toxic for several days.

A device in which a concentrated PAPP preparation is sprayed onto the ventrum of the animal and subsequently ingested via grooming is currently under development. This device is capable of dosing more than 100 animals without having to be reset or recharged.

Disposition

PAPP is rapidly and nearly completely absorbed after oral exposure. It is a protoxicant that undergoes metabolic activation *in vivo.* In rodents, the putative methemoglobin-producing metabolite is 4-(N-hydroxy) aminopropiophenone (PHAPP). However, there are species differences in metabolism. In rats PAPP is metabolized predominantly by N-acetylation. In dogs metabolism is predominantly by ring and aliphatic hydroxylation, with lower rates of N-hydroxylation occurring in male dogs; consequently bitches produce more methemoglobin for a given dose of PAPP than male dogs. In primates both N-acetylation and oxidation occur. Elimination kinetics after oral dosing follows a two-compartment model. The elimination of PAPP metabolites appears to be dependent on glucuronidation, implying that species with low glucuronidation capacity, such as cats, may have greater difficulty eliminating the compound.

Mode of Action

PAPP and its putative active metabolite PHAPP produce acute oxidative damage to the erythron, with resultant methemoglobinemia, Heinz body formation, and oxidative hemolysis. This results in decreased blood oxygen carrying capacity and tissue hypoxia. Frank methemoglobinemia is compounded by a concurrent left shift of the hemoglobin:oxygen dissociation curve, which further exacerbates tissue hypoxia. Peak methemoglobinemia occurs between 1 and 3 hours postingestion.

Clinical Signs

Clinical signs are consistent with rapid-onset, acute methemoglobinemia and oxidative hemolytic anemia. Cyanotic and/or muddy/brown mucous membranes combined with depression, exercise intolerance, elevated respiratory and heart rates, incoordination, tremor, hemorrhage from body orifices, and hemoglobinuria are likely clinical signs. Traditional pulse oximetry measurements are inaccurate and unreliable in patients with high methemoglobin fractions because methemoglobin absorbs light at wavelengths that also absorb deoxyhemoglobin and oxyhemoglobin. Thus methemoglobin interferes with the colorimetric testing that is used to obtain the percentage of oxyhemoglobin to deoxyhemoglobin. Traditional pulse oximetry of patients with low-level methemoglobinemia often reveals falsely low values for oxygen saturation and falsely high values in those with high-level methemoglobinemia. Pulse co-oximetry should be used if possible.

Laboratory and Necropsy Findings

Clinical pathology findings are typical of oxidative insult to the erythron: methemoglobinemia, sulfhemoglobinemia, elevated Heinz bodies, hemolysis (spherocytes, keratocytes or "bite" cells, "blister" cells, and irregularly contracted erythrocytes), hemoglobinemia, and hemoglobinuria. Surviving animals are likely to have elevated serum bilirubin. Gross and microscopic anatomic pathology findings are indicative of acute methemoglobinemia, acute oxidative hemolytic anemia, and general tissue hypoxia.

Treatment

Decontamination of the gastrointestinal tract is unlikely to be effective given the form of the baits, the rapid absorption of PAPP, and the likely interval between exposure and treatment. Supplemental oxygen is recommended. Methylene blue is the first-line antidote but should be used with caution if at all in cats (many consider this therapy contraindicated in this species). Methylene blue accelerates the enzymatic reduction of methemoglobin by NADPH-methemoglobin reductase to leukomethylene blue that, in turn, reduces methemoglobin. The initial dose is 1 to 2 mg/kg IV slowly over 5 minutes. Its effects should be seen in approximately 20 minutes to 1 hour. Patients may require repeated dosing, but high doses of methylene blue may actually induce a paradoxical methemoglobinemia, particularly in species that are prone to oxidative damage to erythrocytes (notably cats). Treatment failures may occur in patients with ongoing exposure, patients exposed to sulfhemoglobinemia, and individuals who have deficient NADPH-methemoglobin reductase enzymatic pathways.

Ascorbic acid is an alternative treatment for methemoglobinemia. Ascorbic acid produces the nonenzymatic reduction of methemoglobin. It is relatively slow acting compared with methylene blue. Treatment protocol is 30 mg/kg PO every 6 hours for six or seven doses.

The clinical effectiveness of N-acetylcysteine in PAPP poisoning has not been evaluated. It has been demonstrated to be of negligible benefit in human methemoglobinemias. However, it may be of some benefit in species with poor glucuronidation capacity (i.e., cats) because it may facilitate phase II sulfation by increasing the level of 3'-phosphoadenosine 5'-phosphosulfate in hepatocytes and thus the detoxification and excretion of the active PAPP metabolite. The concurrent use of N-acetylcysteine and methylene blue in cats should be avoided (particularly in male cats) because it causes severe depletion of blood glutathione levels and increases the elimination half-life of methemoglobin in this species. N-Acetylcysteine can be administered as a constant rate IV infusion (suggested dosage: 150 mg/kg IV over 1 hour, followed by 50 mg/kg over 4 hours, then 100 mg/kg over 16 hours). When administered orally the suggested loading dose is 140 mg/kg, followed in 4 hours by a maintenance dose of 70 mg/kg PO given every 4 hours). The drug has also been administered by inhalation and by the intratracheal route but it can be irritating. Dosing is commonly recommended to be continued for 72 hours; however, tailoring the duration of therapy to the patient's clinical situation is often desirable. Both oral and intravenous N-acetylcysteine treatments are usually well tolerated. In humans oral administration has commonly caused nausea and vomiting, and intravenous use has been associated with the development of anaphylactoid reactions. Generally these reactions are mild and self-limiting, but life-threatening anaphylactoid reactions and deaths have been reported. An alternative to N-acetylcysteine is S-adenosylmethionine (SAMe). SAMe may reduce methemoglobin formation in cats.

Whole blood transfusion or packed red cell transfusion is recommended provided that antidotal treatment has been instigated.

Prognosis

The prognosis for inadvertently poisoned domestic species is unknown at this time. It is likely to be guarded in cats and dependent on the interval between exposure and treatment.

Encapsulated Sodium Nitrite

Encapsulated sodium nitrite baits are currently in the final stages of regulatory approval in New Zealand for the control of brush tailed possums and feral pigs. The encapsulation of the sodium nitrite masks the bitter salty taste, thus improving palatability and consumption by the target species.

The baits contain 100 g/kg sodium nitrite and are hand-laid within bait stations. The bait stations are specifically designed to target feral pigs and to minimize nontarget species exposure.

Disposition and Mode of Action

Nitrites are generally rapidly absorbed from the gastrointestinal tract. Peak methemoglobin formation is typically within 1 to 2 hours following oral exposure. Nitrite is also rapidly excreted, largely by renal filtration, with an elimination half-life of about 30 minutes.

Nitrites act directly on the erythron to produce oxidative damage, methemoglobinemia, and nitrite-methemoglobinemia, as described above. Nitrites are also potent smooth muscle relaxants, which results in vasodilation, diminished vascular return, and hypotension. The net overall result of these effects is tissue hypoxia. Nitrite methemoglobin also reacts with endogenously generated hydrogen peroxide to form reactive intermediates, further exacerbating damage to the erythron.

The clinical signs, laboratory test results, and necropsy findings, as well as the treatment and prognosis, are identical to those described above for PAPP.

Tutin

Tutin is a potent convulsant sesquiterpene lactone toxin derived from the New Zealand tutu plant (Coriaria arborea) and other native Coriaria spp. In New Zealand tutin exposure has historically caused heavy losses among grazing livestock and is associated with outbreaks of toxic honey poisoning when bees feed on the honeydew exudate from the passion vine hopper (Scolypopa australis) that, in turn, has been feeding on the sap of tutu bushes. Within vine hoppers, tutin is metabolized to a second toxin, hyenanchin (8-hydroxytutin; or mellitoxin). Currently tutin is undergoing development as a potential vertebrate toxic agent in New Zealand.

Disposition and Mode of Action

Little is known about the disposition of tutin. It appears to be rapidly absorbed from the gastrointestinal tract. Tutin inhibits the action of neuronal glycine receptors at low concentrations and potentiates their activity at higher concentrations.

The resultant clinical signs in humans include vomiting, delirium, giddiness, increased excitability, stupor, coma, and violent epileptiform convulsions. In ruminants, clinical signs develop within 24 to 48 hours of ingestion and consist of drooling, nausea, excitement, convulsions, coma, and death. Cattle may become aggressive and bloated and may regurgitate. In sheep a "dummy" syndrome has been described in which poisoned animals stand still, are reluctant to move, and appear blind. Death usually occurs rapidly after exposure and often animals are just found dead.

The laboratory and necropsy findings of tutin toxicosis are nonspecific.

Treatment and Prognosis

Treatment of animals exposed to tutin is primarily symptomatic and supportive, with the goal of controlling the excitability and convulsions. Treatment with barbiturates is most commonly attempted.

The prognosis for tutin poisoning following plant ingestion in livestock is generally very guarded and relates to the level of consumption. Reports of successful treatment are rare. Although data are currently lacking on the proposed tutin-based vertebrate toxic agent(s), the likely higher concentration of the active agent in these formulations suggests a poor prognosis unless there is immediate treatment.

References and Suggested Reading

Bright JE, Marrs TC: A comparison of the methemoglobin-inducing activity of moderate oral doses of 4-dimethylaminophenol and p-aminopropiophenone, Toxicol Lett 13:81-86, 1982.

Bright JE, Marrs TC: The induction of methaemoglobin by p-aminophenones, Toxicol Lett 18:157-161, 1982.

Bright JE, Marrs TC: Kinetics of methaemoglobin production. (2). Kinetics of the cyanide antidote p-aminopropiophenone during oral administration, Hum Toxicol 5:303-307, 1986.

Bright JE et al: Sex differences in the production of methaemoglobinaemia by 4-aminopropiophenone, Xenobiotica 7:79-83, 1987.

Eason CT et al: Development of a new humane toxin for predator control in New Zealand, Integr Zool 5:31-36, 2010.

Fisher P, O'Connor CE, Morriss G: Oral toxicity of p-aminopropiophenone to brushtail possums (Trichosurus vulpecula), Dama wallabies (Macropus eugenii), and mallards (Anas platyrhynchos), J Wildl Dis 44:655-663, 2008.

Parton K, Bruere AN, Chambers JP: Tutu (Coriaria spp.). In Parton K, Bruere AN, Chambers JP, editors: Veterinary clinical toxicology, ed 3, Palmerston North, 2006, VetLearn, pp 343-345.

Savarie PJ et al: Comparative acute oral toxicity of para-aminopropiophenone (PAPP) in mammals and birds, Bull Environ Contam Toxicol 30:122-126, 1983.

Scawin JW, Swanston DW, Marrs TC: The acute oral and intravenous toxicity of p-aminopropiophenone (PAPP) to laboratory rodents, Toxicol Lett 23:359-365, 1984.

CHAPTER 34

Parasiticide Toxicoses: Avermectins

WILSON K. RUMBEIHA, *Ames, Iowa*

Avermectins are a group of parasiticidal drugs derived from soil *Streptomyces* microorganisms. Biochemically they belong to a group of compounds known as macrocyclic lactones and are related to milbemycins. These drugs are widely used for their parasiticidal properties. Representative drugs (and products) include ivermectin (Heartgard; Iverhart), selamectin (Revolution), doramectin (Dectomax), eprinomectin (Eprinex), moxidectin (Proheart; Advantage Multi), milbemycin (Interceptor), and abamectin. In general these drugs have a substantial margin of safety in dogs and cats and are very active against a wide range of parasites, including nematodes and arthropods. Practically they are highly effective at very low doses such as micrograms per kilogram of body weight. These drugs are not active against trematodes or cestodes. As such, they may be combined with other drugs that are active against trematodes and cestodes in some formulations. They are available for oral, topical, and parenteral formulations for use in different domesticated species and humans.

Toxicity of Avermectins and Milbemycins

Because of their wide safety margin, avermectins and milbemycins are used safely in the majority of dogs and cats. However, some specific breeds of dogs are more sensitive to this group of drugs (i.e., collies, Australian shepherds, Shetland sheepdogs, Old English sheepdogs, German shepherds, long-haired whippets, and silken windhounds). Recent findings have determined that these breeds express a mutation in the multidrug resistance *(MDR-1)* gene. This gene regulates the synthesis of P-glycoprotein, a 170-kDa transmembrane protein responsible for extruding drugs and other xenobiotics from the brain across the blood-brain barrier. A mutation in the *MDR-1* gene causes synthesis of a truncated P-glycoprotein molecule that is unable to perform this regulatory role. The result is that breeds of dogs with this mutation cannot efficiently extrude xenobiotics such as avermectins and milbemycins from the brain.. Studies have demonstrated higher concentrations of ivermectin in brain tissues of dogs with the mutated *MDR-1* gene than naïve control dogs that have normal-functioning P-glycoprotein.

Collies as a breed have the highest prevalence of the *MDR-1* mutation. Research from the United States, Europe, and Japan indicates that 75% of all collies carry this genetic mutation and explains why avermectin

toxicosis is more commonly observed in this breed. This statistic includes dogs that are either heterozygous carriers or homozygous for the mutant allele, making the animal sensitive. Note that collies not carrying this mutation (i.e., homozygous for the normal allele) have the same sensitivity to avermectin and milbemycin toxicity as other normal breeds of dogs.

It is worth noting that some mixed breeds of dogs carry a single recessive gene mutation, making them heterozygous carriers. These dogs have sensitivity to avermectins, which is between that of double recessive–sensitive mutants and naïve dogs with normal alleles.

Toxic Dose and Sources of Exposure

The monthly oral dose of ivermectin for prevention of heartworms in dogs and cats is 0.006 to 0.024 mg/kg (6 to 24 μg/kg of body weight), respectively. The median lethal dose (LD_{50}) of ivermectin in beagles is 80 mg/kg body weight. Most dogs with a normal *MDR-1* gene tolerate oral dosages as high as 2.5 mg/kg body weight before they start to exhibit clinical signs of poisoning to this drug. However, dogs with a double recessive *MDR-1* gene can only tolerate up to 0.1 mg/kg (100 μg/kg of body weight) of ivermectin. Sensitive collies tolerated doses of 28 to 35.5 μg/kg of body weight over a period of 1 year when administered oral chewable formulations of ivermectin. The highest observed nontoxic dose in cats is 1.3 mg/kg of body weight. However, toxicity in cats has been reported after as low as 0.3 mg/kg of body weight subcutaneously. Toxicosis to moxidectin was observed in a collie that received a dose 30 times higher than the recommended dose of 0.003 mg/kg of body weight. Toxicosis to milbemycin has been observed in collies at doses that are 10 times higher than the recommended therapeutic dose of 0.5 mg/kg orally. In one study collie sensitivity to milbemycin oxime at 10 mg/kg of body weight was judged to be clinically equivalent to that of ivermectin at 120 μg/kg of body weight. Selamectin is potentially toxic to sensitive collies at oral doses greater than 15 mg/kg of body weight. For the other avermectins, the minimum toxic doses in sensitive breeds of dogs are not well established.

Typically toxicosis to avermectins and milbemycins is observed in the more sensitive breeds of dogs when dosage errors occur at more than 5 to 10 times higher than recommended doses, depending on a specific drug; when dogs are accidentally given formulations for large animals; or when they eat a large number of drug tablets. Puppies and kittens are also very sensitive to both avermectins and abermectins and care should be taken to avoid iatrogenic intoxication.

Clinical Signs of Toxicosis

Following acute exposure, clinical signs are seen within a few hours. However, they may also become evident after several days of topical exposure. Typically clinical signs of avermectin and milbemycin toxicity are associated with depression of the central nervous system. Affected animals develop ataxia, weakness, and recumbency; if the dose is severe, respiratory failure and coma are evident. Some dogs exhibit signs of blindness, mydriasis, and muscle tremors; in some cases seizures have been reported. These clinical signs result from avermectins acting as agonists of the γ-aminobutyric acid (GABA) in the central nervous system. Other non-GABA–related effects include mydriasis, hypothermia, vomiting, salivation, and shallow breathing. Avermectin toxicosis is a protracted disease that may last *days or weeks*. Treatment should be directed with these time intervals in mind.

Diagnosis and Therapy of Toxicosis

Diagnosis of avermectin toxicosis consists of a history consistent with exposure to large quantities of one or more of these drugs, clinical signs consistent with avermectin intoxication, and chemical analysis of serum or blood plasma in live animals. In dead animals, adipose tissue, brain, and liver have been used for chemical analysis to confirm exposure to avermectins. However, there are no well-established concentrations of avermectins in these matrices that can be regarded as "diagnostic marker concentrations." Brain concentrations in excess of 100 ppb are supportive of ivermectin intoxication. History of excessive exposure and clinical signs consistent with avermectin toxicosis remain the two most important diagnostic criteria in live animals to date. In the United States there is a molecular genetics test for the presence of a mutant gene (available at the time of writing at Washington State University Veterinary Clinical Pharmacology Laboratory). This test, which uses cheek brush samples, is helpful in determining whether an individual dog is sensitive to avermectins and other drugs whose toxicokinetics are regulated by the *MDR-1* gene.

Therapy of avermectin toxicosis is symptomatic with no specific antidote. As such, prevention of absorption resulting from topical or oral exposure is key to successful therapy in cases of acute exposure. Animals exposed topically should be washed with mild dishwashing detergents and plenty of water. In cases of acute oral exposure, patients should be induced to vomit if exposure is within 1 to 2 hours. Apomorphine is recommended in dogs, and xylazine in cats as emetic drugs (see Chapter 23). Following emesis, activated charcoal can be given to bind the unexpelled drug. Avermectins are excreted largely unchanged through the feces. Activated charcoal also may be beneficial in binding these compounds that are normally excreted unmetabolized through bile and feces. Treatments with physostigmine, neostigmine, or picrotoxin have resulted in either temporary relief or mixed results.

Thus supportive care that includes fluid therapy, respiratory support, parenteral alimentation, and maintenance of normal body temperature is vital to a successful treatment outcome. Treatment of avermectin toxicosis is likely to be protracted since these drugs have prolonged half-lives in dogs of at least 2 days for ivermectin, 11 days for selamectin, and 19 days for moxidectin. The effective half-life is likely longer in *MDR-1* double recessive dogs, which are more likely to accumulate higher brain tissue concentrations.

References and Suggested Reading

Griffin J et al: Selamectin is a potent substrate and inhibitor of human canine P-glycoprotein, *J Vet Pharmacol Ther* 28:257, 2005.

Kawabata A et al: Canine MDR-1 gene mutation in Japan, *J Vet Med Sci* 67(11):1103, 2005.

Mealy KL: Ivermectin: macrolide antiparasitic agents. In Peterson ME, Talcott PA, editors: *Small animal toxicology*, Philadelphia, 2006, Saunders, p 785.

Mealy KL: Therapeutic implications of the MDR-1 gene, *J Vet Pharmacol Ther* 27:257, 2004.

Mealy KL, Bentjen SA, Waiting DK: Frequency of mutant MDR-1 allele associated with ivermectin sensitivity in a sample population of collies from northwestern United States, *Am J Vet Res* 63(4):479, 2002.

Nelson OL et al: Ivermectin toxicity in an Australian Shepherd dog with the MDR-1 mutation associated with ivermectin sensitivity in collies, *J Vet Intern Med* 17(3):354, 2003.

Paul AJ et al: Evaluating the safety of administering high doses of chewable ivermectin tablets to collies, *Vet Med* 86(6):623, 1991.

Pawde AM et al: Ivermectin toxicity in dogs, *Indian Ass Vet Res* 1(2):51, 1992.

Shoop WL, Mrozik H, Fisher MH: Structure and activity of avermectins and milbemycins in animal health, *Vet Parasitol* 59:139, 1995.

Tranquilli WJ, Paul AJ, Todd KS: Assessment of toxicosis induced by high-dose administration of milbemycin oxime in collies, *Am J Vet Res* 52 (7):1170, 1991.

CHAPTER 35

Human Foods with Pet Toxicoses: Alcohol to Xylitol

ERIC K. DUNAYER, *Grand Cayman, Cayman Islands*

Many foods commonly and safely eaten by people can have toxic effects in dogs and cats. Dogs, with their indiscriminate, food-driven behavior, are more likely than cats to ingest these foods. Often, the toxicant is an ingredient that neither the pet owner nor the veterinarian knows to be toxic.

Alcohol (Ethanol)

Ethanol, the type of alcohol found in beer, wine, and distilled spirits, is frequently ingested by dogs and occasionally ingested by cats. Dogs and cats may more readily consume alcoholic beverages if they contain sweet fruit juices or milk. Other products, such as mouthwashes and waterless hand sanitizers, may also contain ethanol. Because the growing yeast in rising bread produces ethanol and carbon dioxide, ingestion of raw bread dough can lead to both ethanol toxicosis and gastric distention.

Ethanol content greatly varies with the type of beverage: generally, it is 4% to 7% in beer, about 12% in wine, and from 40% to about 100% in distilled spirits. The reported proof of an alcoholic beverage is twice the percentage of ethanol (e.g., "80 proof" signifies 40% ethanol). In dogs, the minimum lethal ingested dose for ethanol is about 5500 mg/kg, but significant signs of toxicosis can develop with smaller exposures.

Following ethanol ingestion, onset of signs is rapid; initial signs appear within 15 to 30 minutes. Ataxia is usually observed first. Following ataxia, signs can rapidly progress to vomiting, central nervous system (CNS) depression, hypothermia, hypoglycemia, and coma. Ethanol is metabolized via alcohol dehydrogenase and aldehyde dehydrogenase. Both enzymes cause the release of numerous hydrogen ions, so significant metabolic acidosis can develop. Death is usually associated with CNS and respiratory depression, metabolic acidosis, and/or aspiration pneumonia.

Treatment is symptomatic and supportive. Emesis can be attempted but should not be used if signs have already appeared. Activated charcoal adsorbs small molecules, such as ethanol molecules, poorly and is not considered useful. Additionally, because of the high incidence of vomiting, its use can increase the risk of aspiration pneumonia. Intravenous fluids containing added dextrose and B vitamins should be started to correct any dehydration and hypoglycemia. Blood gases should be monitored, and significant acidosis should be corrected with sodium bicarbonate. If respiration is severely depressed, assisted ventilation through a cuffed endotracheal tube should be initiated (see Chapter 11). Yohimbine at 0.1 to 0.2 mg/kg IV has been reported to reverse some of the CNS depression. However, the effect is short-lived; the yohimbine may need to be repeated frequently. Dialysis (either hemodialysis or peritoneal dialysis) has been shown to rapidly clear ethanol and may be considered in the case of potentially lethal ingestions. Prognosis is good with small ingestions but can be guarded, especially in patients who are comatose or severely acidotic.

When a dog ingests yeasted bread dough, the warmth and low oxygen tension of the stomach environment augment the yeast's production of ethanol and carbon dioxide. In addition to ethanol toxicosis, expanding dough mass can lead to gastric distention with poor venous return and dyspnea secondary to diaphragmatic impingement. Therapy addresses both problems. In asymptomatic dogs, emesis can be attempted, but it often has little effect due to the weight and consistency of the dough mass. Gastric lavage with cold water can be used to chill or kill the yeast and reduce ethanol production. In severe cases, gastrotomy may be necessary to remove the dough mass.

Allium Plants Such as Onions and Garlic

Onions, garlic, scallions, and leeks belong to the genus *Allium*. The disulfides and thiosulfates in *Allium* spp. are metabolized to compounds that can cause oxidative damage to erythrocytes, with the resultant production of Heinz bodies and methemoglobinemia. Cats are particularly sensitive to the toxic effects of *Allium* spp. because feline hemoglobin contains many exposed sulfhydryl groups and because methemoglobin reductase is relatively inactive in cats. *Allium* spp. are toxic whether fresh, dried, or cooked and may be ingredients in other foods.

In dogs the minimum toxic dose of ingested onions is considered to be more than 0.5% body weight (>5 g/kg); garlic is more toxic than onions. Like cats, certain breeds of dogs such as the Japanese breeds (e.g., Akita, Shiba Inu) or those with hereditary red-blood-cell (RBC) enzyme deficiencies may be more sensitive to *Allium* spp. toxicosis. Because the damage to the RBCs is cumulative, the dose can be ingested over a period of days to weeks. Hours or days after ingestion, Heinz bodies appear, followed by hemolysis. The patient may show weakness (secondary to anemia), pale mucous membranes, and hemoglobinuria (often reported by the owner as bloody urine). With methemoglobinemia the mucous membranes, the blood, and possibly the urine become brownish due to methemoglobinuria from hemolyzed RBC. The patient may show variable degrees of dyspnea.

With recent ingestions, emesis may be useful; administration of activated charcoal should also be considered in significant ingestions. The dog or cat should be monitored for several days for the appearance of hemolysis or declining hematocrit. In severely anemic dogs or cats, RBC transfusions may be needed as support until increased hematopoieses replaces the lost RBCs. Patients with severe methemoglobinemia may need oxygen supplementation and blood transfusion. In cats, methylene blue is contraindicated as a treatment for methemoglobinemia. With control of signs, prognosis is generally good.

Hops

Hops, the female cones harvested from *Humulus* spp., are used in the brewing of beer and also are present in some herbal preparations. Canine exposure generally occurs when dogs ingest spent hops that have been discarded after being used for home production of beer. Canine ingestion of herbal products has also been associated with signs of toxicity. The toxic principle and doses are unknown.

Following ingestion, onset of signs is rapid; death can occur within 6 hours. The dogs develop malignant hyperthermia; body temperatures commonly exceed 42.2°C (108°F). Vomiting, tachypnea, and tachycardia are also common.

Prior to onset of signs, induction of emesis should be attempted. In symptomatic dogs, gastric lavage may be effective. Activated charcoal can be given; enemas may accelerate gastrointestinal passage. Intravenous fluids and thermoregulation should be instituted. Dantrolene, a peripheral muscle relaxant, has been used to treat malignant hyperthermia. Doses of either 2 to 3 mg/kg IV or 3.5 mg/kg PO q8-12h (canine dose) should be started immediately. Anecdotal reports have indicated that cyproheptadine at 1.1 mg/kg PO or rectally PRN may help control hyperthermia until dantrolene can be obtained. Prognosis is guarded, especially once hyperthermia has developed.

Macadamia Nuts

Macadamia nuts are harvested from *Macadamia integrifolia* or *M. tetraphylla* trees. They are consumed as nuts (sometimes chocolate-covered) or included in baked goods such as cookies. The toxic principle has not been identified. Dogs that ingest more than 2 g/kg of macadamia nuts may develop weakness and muscle tremors. Also, because the nuts are high in fat, pancreatitis is a possible sequela. Other nuts, such as almonds and walnuts, are not considered toxic in dogs.

After a dog ingests macadamia nuts, signs of toxicity usually develop within 12 hours. Vomiting is common. Weakness (especially in the hind limbs), tremors, and

TABLE 35-1

Approximate Methylxanthine Content of Various Products

Product	Caffeine (mg/oz for solids, mg/fl oz for fluids)	Theobromine (mg/oz)
Coffee beans	310-620	0
Coffee, brewed	13-25	0
Tea, dry	850-1130	0
Tea, brewed	5-15	0
White chocolate	0.85	0.25
Milk chocolate	6	58
Dark chocolate	20	130
Semisweet chocolate	22	138
Baker's chocolate	47	393
Cocoa powder	70	737

Note: For chocolates with a high percentage of cocoa (e.g., 70%), multiply the cocoa percentage by 400 mg/oz to obtain the methylxanthine content.

hyperthermia are frequently seen. Signs are generally mild and, in most cases, can be managed at home.

In cases of heavy ingestion of macadamia nuts, emesis and activated charcoal should be considered. Severe tremors can be controlled with methocarbamol (55 to 220 mg/kg slow IV PRN). Intravenous fluids may be useful in controlling hyperthermia. Prognosis is generally good.

Methylxanthines (Especially in Chocolate)

Methylxanthines—primarily caffeine and theobromine—are found in many foods, including coffee, tea, and chocolate. Methylxanthine content greatly varies by product (Table 35-1).

Chocolate comes in many forms, such as baker's chocolate, chocolate candy, and chocolate baked goods (e.g., cakes, cookies, brownies). Dogs are very attracted to chocolate foods that are high in sugar and fat. The Animal Poison Control Center of the American Society for Prevention of Cruelty to Animals (ASPCA) receives numerous reports of chocolate ingestion by dogs. The methylxanthine dose of chocolate should be calculated by combining the amounts of caffeine and theobromine in the product. However, in the case of chocolate baked goods or mixed-filled chocolates, estimating ingested doses of methylxanthine can be difficult.

In dogs, gastrointestinal upset can result from ingestion of even very small doses of methylxanthine but is most likely if the dose exceeds 20 mg/kg. Doses greater than 40 to 50 mg/kg can cause cardiac signs such as supraventricular or ventricular tachycardia; doses over 60 mg/kg can cause CNS signs such as tremors and seizures. The minimum lethal dose is 100 mg/kg.

After a dog ingests methylxanthine-containing agents, polydipsia is often the earliest sign. The dog may develop vomiting and diarrhea. Agitation can be seen at any dose.

If a dog ingests a large amount of chocolate, onset of cardiac and CNS signs may be delayed because ingesting a large amount of food can delay absorption.

Treatment of chocolate ingestion should include emesis and activated charcoal. Emesis can be induced up to 12 hours following ingestion because chocolate can remain in the stomach for a long time. Activated charcoal should be administered every 6 to 8 hours for as long as the dog is symptomatic. Theobromine has a long half-life in dogs due to enterohepatic recirculation, which can be interrupted by repeated doses of activated charcoal. Diuresis should be started to support cardiac output and to increase renal elimination. Resting tachycardias of greater than 160 to 180 bpm should be controlled with β-blockers such as propranolol (0.01 to 0.02 mg/kg q6h IV). Acepromazine (0.025 to 0.05 mg/kg IV PRN) can be used to control agitation, and diazepam (5 to 10 mg IV) can be used to manage seizures. Because methylxanthines can be absorbed though the urinary bladder wall, frequent walks or urinary catheters should be used to keep the bladder empty. Prognosis is good except in severe cases, especially when the owner delays seeking veterinary care.

Tremorgenic Mycotoxins in *Penicillium* Molds

Molds of the *Penicillium* spp. can produce the tremorgenic mycotoxins roquefortine or penitrem A. These molds can grow on spoiled foods such as dairy products, walnuts, spaghetti, and grains. They can also be found in compost heaps. Dogs can be exposed to the toxins if they get into trash that includes discarded food.

The toxins' precise mechanism of action is unknown. Onset of action can be rapid (within minutes to hours). In general, the more rapid the onset of signs, the more guarded the prognosis. Signs include vomiting and diarrhea, tachycardia, agitation, ataxia, muscle tremors, and seizures. Excessive muscle activity can cause lactic acidosis, rhabdomyolysis with leakage of myoglobin, myoglobinuric nephrosis, and severe hyperthermia with the development of disseminated intravascular coagulation (DIC).

In asymptomatic patients, emesis can be attempted. Gastric lavage may be useful if signs have already developed. Activated charcoal can limit toxin absorption, but care must be taken to avoid aspiration. Intravenous fluids should be started to provide cardiovascular support, treat hyperthermia, and protect the kidneys from myoglobinuric nephrosis. Acid-base abnormalities should be treated if significant. Tremors are best controlled by methocarbamol (55 to 220 mg/kg slow IV PRN). Seizures should be controlled with diazepam or barbiturates as needed. Prognosis is good unless the signs cannot be controlled or secondary complications such as DIC or acute renal failure develop.

Vitis Fruits (Grapes and Raisins)

In dogs, fruits of the *Vitis* spp. have been associated with development of acute renal failure secondary to acute proximal tubular necrosis. Anecdotal reports indicate that this association also may be identified in cats and ferrets. Toxicity has been noted in homegrown, store-bought, and organic *Vitis* spp. Grapes and raisins whose ingestion has resulted in confirmed toxicoses have been tested for the presence of pesticides, heavy metals, and nephrotoxic mycotoxins, but no causative agent of grape/raisin toxicosis has been identified.

Ingestion of more than 0.7 oz/kg of grapes or more than 0.11 oz/kg of raisins has been associated with signs of toxicosis, but lower doses also can be toxic. Some toxicologists think that cooked raisins, such as those found in raisin bread, are not toxic, but this hypothesis has not been confirmed. Many dogs do not develop signs of toxicosis after ingestion of grapes or raisins. This finding may indicate that the toxin is not always present or there may be undetermined factors in the dogs themselves that predispose to toxicity.

Following ingestion, vomiting is seen within 24 hours; among dogs that later develop renal failure, 100% vomit after exposure. Anorexia, lethargy, and weakness may also develop. Clinical pathology changes include increased creatinine, blood urea nitrogen (BUN), and phosphorus starting around 24 hours after ingestion; hypercalcemia may also occur. Urinary granular casts and glucosuria, both indicative of renal tubular damage, may be seen about 18 hours after ingestion. Oliguria and anuria may develop 48 to 72 hours after the ingestion.

Initial treatment should include emesis and multiple doses of activated charcoal. Enemas may expedite the movement of plant material through the gastrointestinal tract. Fluid diuresis at twice maintenance should be started as soon as possible and maintained for 48 hours. Baseline BUN, creatinine, phosphorus, and calcium should be obtained and monitored every 12 to 24 hours. If renal values are normal after 48 hours, fluids can be tapered off and the patient discharged. If acute renal failure develops, urine output should be monitored. Because grapes and raisins cause tubular epithelial necrosis but do not damage the basement membrane, there is the potential for repair of renal tubular injury, but it may be weeks or longer before normal renal function is restored. Dialysis can be used to support the patient until renal function recovers. Prognosis is good if the toxicosis is treated early (< 18 hours) but guarded once renal signs develop.

Xylitol (a Common Sweetener)

Xylitol is a sugar alcohol commonly used as a sweetener in chewing gums, mints, puddings, and baked goods. It can be purchased as a granulated powder for use in home baking or as a sweetener of foods such as beverages and cereals. Xylitol also is used as a sweetener in chewable vitamins, liquid medications, and oral-care products such as toothpastes and mouthwashes. At present, confirmed reports of xylitol toxicity are limited to dogs. (There have been unconfirmed reports of xylitol toxicity in ferrets.)

After a dog ingests xylitol, the pancreas releases a large amount of insulin, and there is rapid onset of hypoglycemia. The minimum toxic dose is about 75 to 100 mg/kg. However, determining ingested dose can be difficult; many products do not specify xylitol content. In many dogs, ingestion of xylitol has been associated with a transient increase in alanine aminotransferase (ALT); usually this increase is a few hundred U/L or less. Some dogs that have ingested more than 500 mg/kg of xylitol have developed severe, potentially fatal hepatic necrosis. However, it is unclear whether this reaction is dose-related or idiosyncratic.

Following ingestion of xylitol, signs can appear within 15 to 30 minutes. With respect to gum that contains xylitol, absorption of xylitol is variable so onset of signs can be delayed up to 12 hours. After a dog ingests xylitol, vomiting is frequently the first sign, followed by weakness, ataxia, collapse, and seizures. At presentation, dogs with xylitol toxicosis usually are profoundly hypoglycemic; however, sometimes they present collapsed but hyperglycemic, likely due to glucose rebound (Somogyi-like effect) from glycogen mobilization. Hypokalemia and hypophosphatemia associated with intracellular movement of the compounds are also common.

Dogs that develop hepatic necrosis from xylitol ingestion may not initially show signs of hypoglycemia and may not become symptomatic for 24 to 72 hours. These dogs often present with acute collapse secondary to hemorrhagic shock from internal bleeding. On presentation, they have severely elevated ALTs (often ranging from 1000 to more than 10,000 U/L), hyperbilirubinemia, mild-to-moderate elevation of alkaline phosphatase (ALP), and coagulopathy and/or DIC (prolonged prothrombin time [PT]/activated partial thromboplastin time [aPTT], thrombocytopenia, decreased fibrinogen, and/or increased D-dimers/fibrin degradation products [FDPs]). Additional findings include hypoglycemia secondary to the hepatic failure and either hypophosphatemia or hyperphosphatemia; the latter is associated with a poorer prognosis.

Emesis may be useful, depending on the type of xylitol product ingested. Gum can remain in the stomach for hours. Therefore, in the case of gum ingestion, delayed emesis may be considered. However, hypoglycemia, if present, should be corrected prior to emesis. Activated charcoal has not been effective in adsorbing xylitol and is not recommended. Blood glucose should be monitored hourly for the first 12 hours following exposure. If hypoglycemia develops, an intravenous bolus of dextrose (0.5 to 1 g/kg of 25%) should be given and followed with a constant rate infusion (CRI) of 5% dextrose in a balanced electrolyte solution. With large ingestions of xylitol, a dextrose solution infusion can be started preemptively. Hypokalemia, if severe (< 2.5 mmol/L), can be treated by intravenous supplementation.

Currently there is no consensus regarding the steps that should be taken to prevent severe hepatic necrosis because the cause has not been definitively determined. According to one theory, xylitol metabolism in the liver depletes ATP and leads to necrosis; therefore, in dogs that have ingested potentially hepatotoxic doses of xylitol, starting a dextrose infusion may increase the liver's ATP via glycolysis. According to a second theory, hepatic necrosis results from oxidative damage to the hepatocytes; thus, starting hepatic protectants such as N-acetylcysteine, S-adenosylmethionine (SAMe), or vitamins C and E may reduce oxidative damage. Neither treatment regimen has been proven effective.

If hepatic necrosis develops, treatment is supportive and symptomatic. Plasma transfusions can be used to provide clotting factors and control hemorrhage. Intravenous fluids with dextrose supplementation should be started.

The prognosis for dogs with simple hypoglycemia or mild ALT elevation is generally good. Dogs who develop fulminant hepatic necrosis have a guarded to poor prognosis; their mortality rate is high.

References and Suggested Reading

Dunayer EK: New findings on the effects of xylitol ingestion in dogs, *Vet Med* 101(12):791, 2006.

Duncan KL et al: Malignant hyperthermia-like reaction secondary to ingestion of hops in five dogs, *J Am Vet Med Assoc* 210(1):51, 1997.

Gwaltney-Brant S: Chocolate intoxication, *Vet Med* 96(2):108, 2001.

Hansen SR et al: Weakness, tremors, and depression associated with macadamia nuts in dogs, *Vet Hum Toxicol* 42(1):18, 2000.

Means C: Bread dough toxicosis in dogs, *J Vet Emerg Crit Care Soc* 13(1):39, 2003.

Simmons DM: Onion breath, *Vet Tech* 22(8):425, 2001.

CHAPTER 36

Automotive Toxins

KARYN BISCHOFF, *Ithaca, New York*

Various compounds used in vehicle maintenance and stored around the home have known toxic properties. An incomplete list of such chemicals includes ethylene glycol (EG), propylene glycol (PG), diethylene glycol (DEG), petroleum products, and methanol. EG is the most common component of antifreeze and unfortunately is the most common automotive product associated with poisoning in small animals. PG has been substituted for EG in antifreeze brands that are advertised as "safe" or "nontoxic," and although PG is not without adverse effects, it is much less toxic than EG.

Ethylene Glycol

EG, or 1,2-dihydroxyethane, is a colorless, sweet-tasting liquid with a density of 1.113, a high boiling point (197.2° C [326° F]), a low freezing point (−12.3° C [9.86° F]), and is miscible with water and alcohol. Less common sources of EG include deicer, hydraulic brake and transmission fluids, additives in motor oils, paints, inks, wood stains and polishes, photographic solutions, and industrial solvents.

EG is one of the most common causes of fatal poisoning in small animals, perhaps because it is readily available in most households, is toxic in low doses, and is palatable. Toxicosis is most common in the late autumn or early spring, when radiators have been drained and open containers may be available to pets. Dogs occasionally chew through closed containers. Denatonium benzoate, a bittering agent, has been added to antifreeze to make it less palatable. The states of Arizona, California, Georgia, Illinois, Maine, Maryland, Massachusetts, New Jersey, New Mexico, Oregon, Tennessee, Utah, Vermont, Virginia, Washington, and West Virginia require addition of bittering agents to commercial antifreeze at the time of this writing.

Toxicity and Toxicokinetics

The minimum lethal dose for EG in dogs is about 6.6 ml/kg. Cats are more sensitive, with a minimum lethal dose around 1.4 ml/kg. Dogs are more frequently affected than cats, although cats are likely to become intoxicated through grooming activity after dermal contamination. Intact animals are more frequently affected.

EG is absorbed rapidly from the gastrointestinal tract, particularly on an empty stomach. Peak plasma concentrations occur within 3 hours of ingestion. Metabolism begins within hours of ingestion and occurs predominantly in the liver, with minor renal and gastric metabolism. The metabolic pathway of EG is illustrated in Figure 36-1. The metabolism of EG to glycoaldehyde and then glycolic acid to glyoxylic acid are both rate-limiting steps. Oxalic acid is the most important final metabolite of EG. The plasma half-life of EG is approximately 3 hours, and elimination is almost complete within 24 hours. EG and its metabolites are eliminated in the urine.

Mechanism of Action

The severe clinical effects associated with EG ingestion are caused by metabolites. Acidosis is produced by such metabolic products as glycolic acid. Renal tubular damage is the most common cause of death in small animals poisoned with EG. Metabolites of EG are directly cytotoxic to renal tubular epithelium. Oxalic acid binds to calcium ions (Ca^{2+}) in the renal tubules (and in other tissues) to form calcium oxalate crystals, leading to hypocalcemia, obstruction of tubules, and renal epithelial damage. Renal blood flow can be compromised from acidosis.

Clinical Signs

EG toxicosis is described as having three sometimes overlapping stages, although early stages are often missed. The first stage, usually within 30 minutes of exposure, can last for 2 to 12 hours. Some animals vomit. Polyuria and polydipsia are described in dogs, and cats are frequently polyuric. Apparent "inebriation" presents as ataxia and hyporeflexia. Dogs often have a period of apparent recovery from this stage, but cats typically do not.

The second stage usually occurs 8 to 24 hours after exposure and is related to metabolic acidosis. Clinical signs include central nervous system (CNS) depression, changes in heart rate, hypothermia, muscle fasciculations, and sometimes coma. Cats often lose coordination in the pelvic limbs.

Animals that survive the first two stages enter the third stage, acute renal failure, which can begin from less than 1 to 3 days after EG ingestion. Animals progress through oliguria to anuria. Signs of uremia include oral ulcerations, salivation, vomiting, anorexia, and seizures. Palpation of cats often reveals large, painful kidneys.

Serum chemistries reveal an increased osmolal gap about an hour after EG ingestion, which usually declines within the first 18 hours. The anion gap increases in a few hours and can remain elevated for 48 hours. Hypocalcemia is reported due to calcium oxalate crystal formation. Phosphorus can be elevated early, as a result of the phosphate additives in antifreeze, and again as a consequence of renal failure. Other findings associated with

151

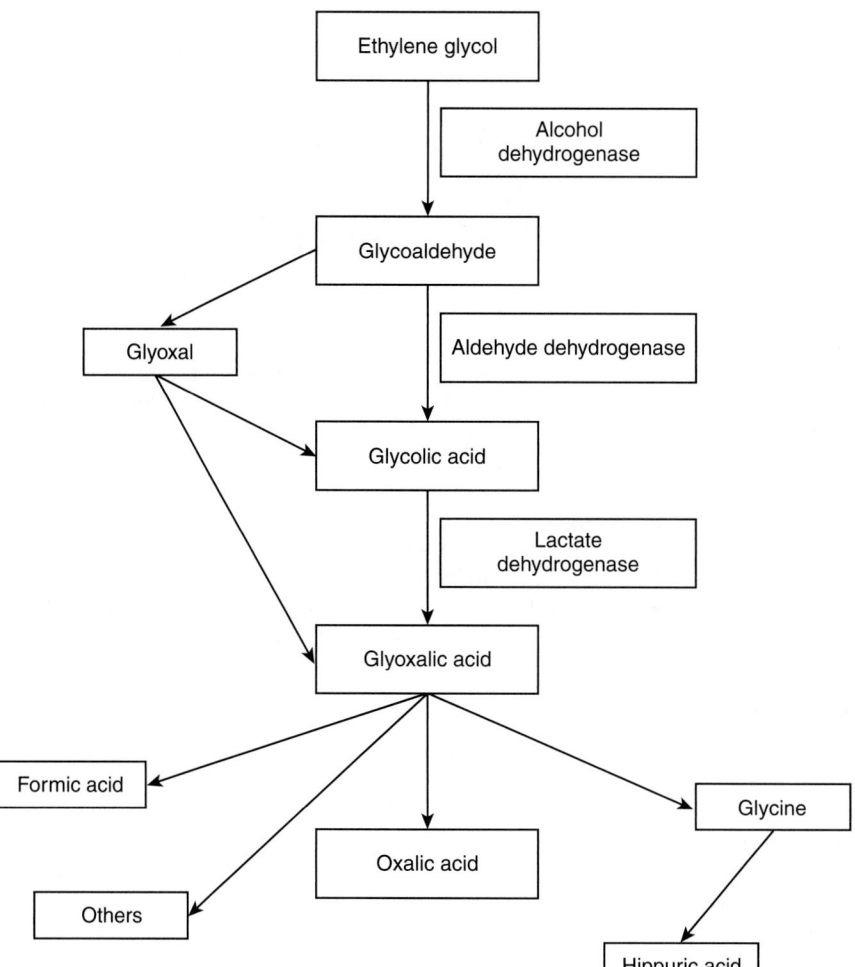

Figure 36-1 Hepatic metabolism of ethylene glycol.

renal failure include elevated serum urea nitrogen and creatinine, hyperkalemia, isosthenuria with low urine pH, hematuria, proteinuria, glycosuria, and granular and cellular casts. Calcium oxalate crystals are evident in urine within 8 hours of exposure, but are not a specific finding considering that crystalluria is identified in many healthy animals.

Diagnosis

Speed is of the essence in the diagnosis (and management) of EG toxicosis. The prognosis decreases precipitously the longer treatment is delayed. EG concentrations begin to decline within 6 hours of exposure and are often undetectable in blood or urine by the time the animal presents to the veterinarian, further complicating the diagnosis.

Various analytic tests have been used to confirm EG exposure. Commercial test kits are available, but some of these kits cross-react with PG, glycerol, sorbitol, ethanol, and other compounds that can be present in pet foods and pharmaceuticals; thus samples for testing should be collected before initiating treatment. Current test kits are able to detect EG at concentrations above 0.6 mg/dl, but due to rapid EG metabolism false-negative results can occur in samples collected more than 12 hours after

ingestion. Gas chromatography (GC) is frequently used to assay blood, urine, or kidney tissue for EG at diagnostic laboratories, although results are delayed by sample shipping and processing and false-negative results are still possible if the EG has been completely metabolized.

The findings of increased anionic and osmolal gaps along with the appropriate history and presentation are highly suggestive of EG toxicoses, but are not always seen. Calcium oxalate monohydrate crystals are commonly found in the urine. Fluorescent dye, which is sometimes added to antifreeze, is visible in the urine, in the vomitus, or around the oral cavity under Wood's lamp. However, other components of urine and some plastic containers also fluoresce.

The "halo effect," an ultrasound finding related to increased echogenicity of the renal cortex and medulla and decreased echogenicity at the corticomedullary junction and central medulla, is supportive (although not pathognomonic) for the diagnosis of EG toxicosis. This change occurs near the onset of anuria.

Postmortem findings are frequently used to confirm the diagnosis of EG toxicosis. Typical findings include gastric hemorrhage, pulmonary edema, and pale firm kidneys. Histologic changes include degeneration and necrosis of proximal convoluted tubular epithelium with intraluminal birefringent crystals. Chronicity is indicated by evidence of tubular regeneration, interstitial fibrosis, and glomerular atrophy and synechia. Oxalate crystals are sometimes found in other tissues, including the liver and CNS.

Management

The prognosis for EG toxicosis depends on the time of presentation. Animals treated early (stage 1) have an excellent prognosis, but the prognosis is poor for animals that present in renal failure (stage 3). Due to the rapid absorption of EG, gastrointestinal decontamination is unlikely to be beneficial.

Antidotes that act by inhibiting metabolism of EG by alcohol dehydrogenase include fomepizole and ethanol. Antidotal treatment should be started as early as possible for best effect but can still be attempted if the animal is presented to the clinician up to 32 hours postexposure.

Fomepizole
The preferred antidote is fomepizole (4-methylpyrazole). This product is used in dogs at an initial dose of 20 mg/kg IV, then 15 mg/kg IV at 12 and 24 hours, and then 5 mg/kg IV at 36 hours. Cats have recovered after being treated with the much higher doses of fomepizole of 125 mg/kg IV initially, then 31.25 mg/kg every 12 hours for three more doses. The dosing regimen can be extended if the dog or cat ingested a large amount of EG. Fomepizole causes less CNS depression than ethanol. Concurrent use of fomepizole and ethanol produces severe CNS depression due to ethanol toxicosis and is therefore *contraindicated*. The prognosis is good if fomepizole therapy is started within 8 to 12 hours of EG ingestion for dogs or within 3 hours for cats. Ethanol can be used if fomepizole is not immediately available. Fomepizole dosage must be adjusted if hemodialysis or peritoneal dialysis is used to treat renal failure.

Ethanol
Ethanol has been used for many years to treat EG toxicoses; however, ethanol enhances CNS depression and can cause respiratory depression. Animals remain stuporous during treatment, requiring close monitoring and supportive care. Ethanol is usually given IV to maintain blood concentrations of 50 to 100 mg/dl. A 5.5-ml/kg dose of 20% ethanol is given every 4 hours for the first five treatments and then every 6 hours for the next four treatments in dogs. Alternatively, dogs can be given a bolus dose of 1.3 ml of 30% ethanol followed by a constant rate infusion of 0.42 ml/kg/hr for 48 hours. Cats are given 5 ml/kg of 20% ethanol IV every 6 hours for five treatments and then every 8 hours for four treatments.

Monitoring
Patients should be monitored for hydration, urine production (which can be assessed via bladder catheterization), acid-base status, serum urea nitrogen, creatinine, electrolytes, and body temperature at least daily and treated symptomatically. Fluid therapy corrects dehydration and electrolyte imbalances and promotes diuresis: saline is used to establish urine flow in anuric patients, a slow infusion of bicarbonate solution is required to correct metabolic acidosis, and calcium gluconate is added to correct for hypocalcemia. Fluid therapy in patients with anuria may aggravate or cause pulmonary edema, and respiratory rate and depth must be monitored regularly. Tubular regeneration requires weeks or months, and urine concentrating ability can be lost indefinitely.

Propylene Glycol

PG, or 1,2-propanediol, has a density of 1.036 and is colorless, odorless, and almost flavorless. Like other antifreeze compounds, it has a high boiling point (189°C [372°F]) and a low freezing point (–60°C [140°F]) and is freely miscible with water and alcohol. PG is used commonly in recreational vehicles and as an alternative type of antifreeze to the more toxic EG. PG can be used as a deicer, a hydraulic fluid, an industrial solvent, a humectant, a plasticizer, and an ingredient in pharmaceuticals, cosmetics, and foods. PG is frequently kept in large barrels in veterinary clinics to treat ruminant ketosis. Although no longer used in cat food, PG is still classified as "Generally Recognized as Safe (GRAS)" by the U.S. Food and Drug Administration.

Toxicity, Toxicokinetics, and Mechanism of Action

PG is less toxic than other glycols. The median lethal doses (LD_{50}s) in laboratory animals are around 20 ml/kg. The LD_{50} in experimental dogs is 9 ml/kg. Dogs tolerate a diet containing up to 20% PG with minimal clinical effects; however, 5% to 6% PG in the diet causes increased Heinz body formation in kittens and cats. Cats given high doses of PG (approximately 40% of the diet) had mild neurologic signs, including ataxia and depression. Toxicosis has been reported in humans, horses, and cattle and experimentally produced in dogs, laboratory animals, goats, and chickens. The author has seen apparently malicious PG poisoning in a dog.

PG is absorbed rapidly from the gastrointestinal tract and lungs. About a third of the PG dose is excreted unchanged in the urine; the rest is metabolized mostly in the liver and kidneys. Lactic acid is a major metabolite. PG is conjugated to glucuronide in some species, but this metabolic pathway is inadequate in cats. Metabolites usually appear in the blood within 4 hours of exposure. PG is excreted completely within a day in dogs.

PG causes osmotic diuresis and a direct narcotic effect similar to ethanol, but at about one third the potency. The L-isomer of the lactic acid metabolite enters the citric acid cycle and is metabolized, but D-lactic acid is not readily metabolized and contributes to lactic acidosis. The mechanism of PG-mediated Heinz body formation in cats is not completely understood.

Clinical Signs and Diagnosis

Clinical signs in cats given high doses of PG include polyuria, polydipsia, and mild-to-moderate ataxia. Cats exposed to low dietary concentrations of PG, although asymptomatic, have increased numbers of Heinz bodies, reticulocytes, and low erythrocyte counts. Animals ingesting high dietary PG concentrations have increased blood D-lactic acid.

Osmotic diuresis occurs after oral or parenteral administration of a high dose of PG. Severe clinical signs of acute PG toxicosis are attributable to acidosis; hypotension, circulatory collapse, and respiratory arrest have been reported in cats. Pure PG is hyperosmolar and is likely to cause hemolysis if given intravenously. Postmortem lesions are nonspecific but can include a foul, garlic-like odor to gastrointestinal contents. Diagnosis is based on history and clinical signs. Serum, urine, tissues, or the suspected source of PG may be analyzed using GC.

Management

The prognosis for cats with chronic dietary exposure to PG is excellent. Heinz bodies resolve once the source of PG is removed. The prognosis for acute toxicosis is fair to guarded, depending on the clinical status of the animal. Decontamination using gastric lavage and activated charcoal is unlikely to be of benefit unless initiated within an hour of exposure due to rapid absorption of PG. Dehydration, acidosis, and hypoglycemia are treated routinely as needed. Antioxidants such as vitamins E and C and *N*-acetylcysteine do not show much benefit.

Diethylene Glycol

DEG has a specific gravity of 1.118 and is a colorless, nearly odorless, palatable liquid. It is an industrial solvent used in brake fluid, hydraulic fluid, lubricants, and canned cooking fuels. High mortality is reported in epidemic human poisonings.

Toxicity, Toxicokinetics, and Mechanism of Action

The LD_{50} of DEG in laboratory animals ranges from 3.6 to 11.6 ml/kg, making it more toxic than PG but less so than EG. DEG is rapidly absorbed through the gastrointestinal tract or damaged skin. Peak plasma concentrations occur within an hour or two. Similar to other glycols, DEG is metabolized primarily in the liver by alcohol and aldehyde dehydrogenases. DEG and metabolites are excreted in the urine, with nearly complete excretion within 36 hours. DEG produces a direct narcotic effect and renal damage, but oxalate crystals are not produced.

Clinical Signs and Diagnosis

Clinical signs of DEG toxicosis are similar in most species. CNS depression and vomiting are reported early but resolve and are followed by renal failure within a day or more. Cardiac abnormalities have been reported in some species. Serum chemistry findings include elevated urea nitrogen, creatinine, and potassium, as well as evidence of lactic acidosis.

Findings at necropsy usually include pale, swollen, mottled kidneys that bulge on cut surface. There is necrosis and degeneration of proximal convoluted tubular epithelium and tubular ectasia. Hepatic lipidosis and centrilobular necrosis have been reported. Hemorrhage involving the pericardium, adrenal medulla, lungs, and pleura has been reported in humans, and multifocal hemorrhage was observed by the author in one dog.

Diagnosis is based on a history of exposure, clinical signs, and lesions. Tissues or suspected source of DEG can be analyzed using GC, keeping in mind the rapidity of DEG elimination.

Management

Animals presenting soon after exposure have a fair-to-guarded prognosis, but once animals have evidence of renal failure, the prognosis is poor. Therapy includes symptomatic and antidotal treatments similar to those described earlier for EG toxicosis. The combination of dialysis and fomepizole treatment has been successfully used to treat human cases of DEG toxicosis. As with EG, the fomepizole dose must be adjusted when the patient is also undergoing dialysis.

Petroleum Compounds

Petroleum compounds include a wide variety of products with variable physical and chemical characteristics. Such compounds include fuels such as propane, gasoline, kerosene, and diesel; solvents such as paint thinner and degreasers; lubricants such as motor oil; and carriers for pesticides, paints, and drugs. Animals can ingest spilled hydrocarbons or drink from open containers. Material spilled on the skin causes dermatitis and can be ingested when the animal grooms. Animals are occasionally given petroleum products intentionally.

Toxicity, Toxicokinetics, and Mechanism of Action

Absorption occurs through the gastrointestinal tract, skin, and lungs. Low-molecular-weight compounds such as gasoline are better absorbed; high-molecular-weight compounds such as greases, mineral oils, and waxes are not well absorbed. Hydrocarbons are distributed to all major organs. Aliphatic hydrocarbons are oxidized in the liver to polar compounds that are more readily excreted. Respiratory excretion is important for volatile compounds, and highly volatile hydrocarbons can be excreted completely within 24 hours.

Highly volatile compounds are likely to be aspirated, and low-viscosity compounds have greater penetration into airways. Aspirated hydrocarbons dissolve lipids in cell membranes and cause degeneration and necrosis of the respiratory epithelium; secondary bacterial infections are common. Direct irritation of the skin and eyes is caused by the solvent effects of volatile hydrocarbons on cell membranes. Absorbed compounds interact with neuronal cell membranes to cause CNS depression.

Clinical Signs and Diagnosis

Early clinical signs of ingestion include increased salivation, head shaking, and pawing at the muzzle. Vomiting and colic are typically seen with more volatile compounds, and diarrhea with heavier compounds such as mineral oil. Aspiration is sometimes seen in the absence of apparent emesis. Signs of aspiration pneumonia include choking, coughing, gagging, dyspnea, and cyanosis. Signs of CNS involvement include ataxia, confusion, depression, narcosis, and coma. Tremors and convulsions have been reported in a few cases, as have cardiac arrhythmias and cardiovascular collapse.

Animals that die after hydrocarbon ingestion frequently have gross lesions typical of aspiration pneumonia, with oily material visible in small airways. Secondary bacterial pneumonia is evident in animals that die later. Centrilobular hepatic necrosis, myocardial necrosis, and renal tubular necrosis have been reported in animals surviving more than 24 hours. Dermatitis, characterized by alopecia with or without erythema, has been reported in cats and other species with dermal exposure to petroleum hydrocarbons.

Petroleum hydrocarbons float to the top of vomitus or stomach contents when mixed with warm water, and this is a rapid test for hydrocarbon exposure. If skimmed with a paper towel, these compounds evaporate quickly and have a characteristic odor that is often detectable on the breath or skin of the affected animal. Confirmation of exposure involves analysis of the gastrointestinal content or material on the skin, to be compared with suspected source material, via GC. Samples should be collected quickly and placed in glass containers or wrapped in foil, to avoid contact with plastic, and frozen until analysis can be performed.

Management

Early management involves identification of the compound involved. When possible, the owner should bring the container or label of the suspected source of exposure. Gastrointestinal detoxification must be pursued with great care. Emetics and instillation of oily cathartics are contraindicated because of the risk of aspiration. Gastric lavage of the sedated intubated animal and dosing with activated charcoal have been recommended.

Monitoring of the exposed animal should include auscultation and thoracic radiography to assess pulmonary status. Aspiration pneumonia is treated symptomatically with cage or stall rest, supplemental oxygen, and β_2-agonists if needed for bronchospasm. Corticosteroids increase the risk of bacterial infection and should not be used, but prophylactic antibiotics should be considered. Cardiac function should be monitored, and arrhythmia treated as needed.

The prognosis for animals that have ingested low-volatility compounds such as mineral oil or motor oil is good, assuming these products did not contain other toxicants such as pesticides or heavy metals. Management in this case involves cage rest and observation. Animals with no evidence of aspiration pneumonia 12 to 24 hours

after ingestion have a good prognosis. Uncomplicated aspiration pneumonia is usually resolved after 2 weeks, but the prognosis is poor if animals have extensive pulmonary lesions or present comatose.

If there is dermal contamination, especially with a viscous product like tar, vegetable oil is applied to the affected surface of the stabilized animal. This is followed by a mild detergent bath. Clipping of long or matted hair is useful, and animals should be kept warm.

Methanol

Methanol is used in automotive window washer fluids, gasoline antifreezes, canned cooking fuels, and various solvents. It is highly toxic to humans and other primates, causing formic acidosis, CNS disturbances, and retinal damage, with severe toxicosis resulting in death. Methanol is much less toxic to dogs and cats because they are able to efficiently metabolize formic acid using a folate-dependent enzyme system. Methanol is, in fact, less toxic in small animals than ethanol. Clinical signs of methanol toxicosis in dogs and cats are similar to those of inebriation with ethanol. Treatment is based on monitoring and symptomatic and supportive care. Treatment of veterinary patients other than primates with ethanol or fomepizole to inhibit alcohol dehydrogenase will intensify clinical signs and is discouraged.

References and Suggested Reading

Bischoff K: Diethylene glycol. In Peterson ME, Talcott PA, editors: *Small animal toxicology*, ed 2, St Louis, 2006a, Elsevier Saunders, p 693.

Bischoff K: Methanol. In Peterson ME, Talcott PA, editors: *Small animal toxicology*, ed 2, St Louis, 2006b, Elsevier Saunders, p 840.

Bischoff K: Propylene glycol. In Peterson ME, Talcott PA, editors: *Small animal toxicology*, ed 2, St Louis, 2006c, Elsevier Saunders, p 996.

Dalefield R: Propylene glycol. In Plumlee KH, editor: *Clinical veterinary toxicology*, St Louis, 2004a, Mosby, p 168.

Dalefield R: Ethylene glycol. In Plumlee K, editor: *Clinical veterinary toxicology*, St Louis, 2004b, Mosby, p 150.

Hill AS: Antioxidant prevention of Heinz body formation and oxidative injury in cats, *Am J Vet Res* 62:370, 2001.

Raisebeck MF, Dailey RN: Petroleum hydrocarbons. In Peterson ME, Talcott PA, editors: *Small animal toxicology*, ed 2, St Louis, 2006, Elsevier Saunders, p 986.

Tart KM, Powell LL: 4-Methylpyrazole as a treatment in naturally occurring ethylene glycol intoxication in cats, *J Vet Emerg Crit Care* 21: 268, 2011.

Thrall MA: Ethylene glycol. In Peterson ME, Talcott PA, editors: *Small animal toxicology*, ed 2, St Louis, 2006, Elsevier Saunders, p 986.

Thrall MA, Hamar DW: Alcohols and glycols. In Gupta RC, editor: *Veterinary toxicology basic and clinical principles*, ed 1, New York, 2007, Elsevier, p 605.

Valentine WM: Short-chain alcohols, *Vet Clin North Am Small Anim Pract* 20:515, 1990.

CHAPTER 37

Lead Toxicosis in Small Animals

SHARON M. GWALTNEY-BRANT, *Mahomet, Illinois*

Lead contamination of residential environments has decreased through removal of lead from residential paints, gasoline, and other household items. Accordingly, the incidence of lead poisoning in small animals has decreased over the last 30 years, and lead now accounts for less than 1% of reported accidental poisonings in pets. Nevertheless, lead intoxication in pets does occur, and the vagueness of clinical signs that frequently accompany lead poisoning can create diagnostic challenges.

Pathogenesis of Lead Toxicosis

Sources of Lead

Lead may be found in a wide variety of products, including paints, linoleum, caulking and putty compounds, solders, wire shielding, old metal tubing, certain weights (e.g., fishing sinkers, curtain weights), roofing felt, golf balls, ammunition, computer equipment, wine cork covers, pottery glazing, lead-containing toys, and lead arsenate pesticides. In addition, contaminated soil and water can be potential sources of lead. Exposure to organolead from various leaded petroleum products has decreased considerably following legislation restricting the use of leaded gasoline and oil in the United States.

The most common source of lead in cases of small animal poisoning is leaded paints from buildings erected before passage of the 1977 legislation requiring that residential paints contain no more than 0.06% (600 ppm) lead. In many cases older leaded paints have been painted over with unleaded paints, and it is estimated that 74% of privately owned homes built before 1980 still contain hazardous amounts of leaded paint. Renovation of these homes results in the generation of paint chips or dust that, if ingested by pets, can result in clinical lead intoxication. Cats may be at increased risk for toxicosis during these situations because of their grooming habits, which can result in significant ingestion of lead-containing particulates that collect in their fur.

Kinetics

The degree to which ingested lead is absorbed depends on variables such as the physical form of lead, particle size, and matrix association. In addition, patient variables that influence the degree of lead absorption from the gastrointestinal (GI) tract include age, diet, and preexisting disease. The acidic environment of the stomach favors ionization of the lead, which is then absorbed from the

duodenum. Lead shot embedded in soft tissues such as skeletal muscle is not appreciably absorbed and is not an important source of lead toxicosis. Conversely, lead shot that enters areas capable of active inflammation (e.g., joint cavities) may become solubilized by the enzymatic activity of the inflammatory reaction and could subsequently be absorbed.

Once absorbed, lead is carried primarily on the red blood cells, with less than 1% to 2% bound to albumin or free in the plasma. Unbound lead distributes widely through tissues, with the highest concentrations found in bone, teeth, liver, lung, kidney, brain, and spleen. Bone serves as a storage depot for lead, which substitutes for calcium in the bone matrix. During times of increased activity of bone remodeling such as fracture repair stored lead may be released from the bone, resulting in toxicosis. Lead crosses the blood-brain barrier and concentrates in the gray matter of the brain. This passage of lead into the brain occurs to a greater extent in young animals. Unbound lead crosses the placenta and is passed through the milk in lactating animals.

Most ingested lead is excreted in the feces unabsorbed. Lead in the blood passes through the glomerulus and accumulates in the renal tubular epithelium. During the natural process of sloughing of tubular epithelial cells, the lead is slowly eliminated from the body. Chelation therapy can greatly increase the rate of urinary excretion of lead by allowing the chelated lead to be passed in the urine without entering the tubular epithelium. Lead has a multiphasic half-life because of its distribution into depot areas such as bone and brain. In dogs intravenously administered lead, it has triphasic elimination half-lives of 12 days, 184 days, and 4,591 days.

Mechanism of Action

Lead has a wide variety of effects within the body, including interfering and competing with calcium ions, binding to cellular and enzymatic sulfhydryl groups, altering vitamin D metabolism, and inhibiting membrane-associated enzymes. Inactivation of the enzymes ferrochelatase and δ-aminolevulinic acid dehydratase causes impairment in heme synthesis, resulting in red blood cell abnormalities. Anemia can develop with chronic exposure to lead. GI signs in lead-intoxicated patients may be caused in part by alteration of smooth muscle contractility as a result of interference of lead on intracellular calcium-dependent mechanisms. Lead can disrupt the blood-brain barrier of immature animals by interfering

156

with normal endothelial cell function. Lead decreases cerebral blood flow and alters neuronal energy metabolism and neurotransmission within the central nervous system (CNS). Recently, the propensity of lead to induce oxidative damage through the production of reactive oxygen species has been the subject of much study. Lead-induced inhibition of endogenous antioxidant enzymes such as superoxide dismutase and catalase can lead to injury of cell macromolecules through a variety of oxidative pathways including lipid peroxidation of cellular membranes.

Lead Toxicity

Toxic dosages of lead reported for dogs range from 191 to 1,000 mg/kg, depending on the form of lead; 3 mg/kg/day caused vomiting and behavioral changes in cats. However, these dosages have little clinical relevance in most cases of lead toxicosis in small animals because the amount of lead ingested is rarely determined.

Young animals are at greater risk than mature animals because they absorb up to five times more lead following ingestion. Lead absorption is enhanced in animals deficient in calcium, zinc, iron, or vitamin D. Younger cats are thought to be at higher risk for development of lead-induced seizures.

Pathologic Findings

Few gross lesions have been described in dogs and cats with lead toxicosis. Necropsy may reveal the presence of lead objects, especially in the GI tract. Histopathologic findings may include degenerative changes within the white matter of the brain and spongiosis of the cerebrum. In dogs degenerative changes in the kidney and liver may be seen, occasionally associated with intranuclear inclusion bodies.

Clinical Signs and Diagnosis

The primary signs seen with lead intoxication in dogs and cats are related to GI upset. Anorexia, vomiting, diarrhea, weight loss, lethargy, and abdominal discomfort have been reported. In cats the most common signs are lethargy and anorexia. Neurologic signs may also occur but are less common than GI signs. Neurologic effects can include behavior changes, ataxia, tremors, seizures, and agitation. Less commonly polyuria, polydipsia, blindness, aggression, dementia, pica, vestibular signs, coma, and megaesophagus (cats) have been reported.

Laboratory and Radiographic Findings

In acute lead intoxication very few changes are expected in terms of clinical pathology. Anemia, basophilic stippling, and elevations in nucleated red blood cells (NRBCs) have been reported as indicative of lead toxicosis; however, these abnormalities are not consistently found and are not pathognomonic for lead toxicosis. Basophilic stippling and NRBCs (>40 NRBCs per 100 white blood cells) are more likely to occur in dogs than in cats with lead toxicosis.

Radiography may be helpful in identifying lead opacities within the GI tract. *Lead lines,* linear opacities in the epiphyses of long bones used to aid in diagnosis of lead toxicosis in humans, are not commonly found in domestic animals.

Diagnosis

The diagnosis of lead toxicosis can be difficult because the signs most commonly associated with this disease (anorexia, lethargy, vomiting) are nonspecific. Blood lead levels can be measured in a timely fashion and, when evaluated in light of compatible clinical signs, can be helpful in making a diagnosis. The widespread distribution of lead throughout the body can result in fluctuating blood levels, and the level of lead in the blood may not be indicative of the total body burden. Some animals may have fairly high blood lead levels without significant clinical signs, whereas other animals may have significant clinical signs with only moderately elevated blood lead levels. Most dogs and cats have background lead levels of 10 to 15 µg/dl (0.1 to 0.15 ppm); blood lead levels exceeding 30 to 35 µg/dl (0.3 to 0.35 ppm) along with appropriate clinical signs suggest lead toxicosis. Levels greater than 60 µg/dl are generally considered diagnostic for lead toxicosis.

Treatment and Prognosis of Lead Toxicosis

Management of lead toxicosis entails control of immediate clinical signs, removal of the immediate source of lead intoxication, chelation therapy, supportive care, and removal of other potential sources of lead from the environment. Seizures should be managed with anticonvulsants such as diazepam or barbiturates (see Chapter 230). Similarly, vomiting and diarrhea should be managed, and any fluid and electrolyte abnormalities should be corrected as needed (see Chapter 1).

Decontamination

GI decontamination must occur before chelation therapy because most chelators, with the exception of succimer, actually enhance the absorption of lead from the GI tract. Sulfate-containing cathartics (magnesium sulfate, sodium sulfate) may be administered to aid in emptying the GI tract and to precipitate the lead as lead sulfate, which is poorly absorbed. Large lead-containing objects (e.g., lead sinkers, lead weights) may require removal via endoscopy or gastrotomy/enterotomy if too large to pass using bulking cathartics. When cats are suspected of exposure through grooming, thorough bathing should be performed.

Chelation Therapy

Chelation therapy is intended to bind lead into a soluble complex that will be excreted via the urine. Because of the nephrotoxic nature of most chelators, as well as the lead chelate, it is imperative that renal function be assessed before and during chelation and that adequate hydration be maintained during chelation. Chelation of asymptomatic animals that have elevated blood lead levels is not recommended because the chelator may increase blood lead levels and precipitate clinical signs. In cases of asymptomatic animals with elevated blood lead levels, decontamination and removal from the source of lead will allow the animal to eliminate the lead at its own pace. Available chelators for lead include calcium disodium ethylenediaminetetraacetic acid (Ca-EDTA), British anti-Lewisite (BAL), penicillamine, and succimer (meso-2,3-dimercaptosuccinic acid).

Calcium EDTA

Ca-EDTA, the first chelator agent used for lead toxicosis, has an established track record in veterinary and human medicine. Sodium EDTA should *not* be used for chelation because it will bind serum calcium and cause hypocalcemia. Ca-EDTA is administered parenterally and may cause pain at the injection site. The dosage for dogs is 25 mg/kg q6h for 2 to 5 days (not to exceed 2 g per dog per day), with each dose divided every 8 hours, diluted to a final concentration of 10 mg of Ca-EDTA per milliliter of 5% dextrose and administered subcutaneously at different sites. Expect clinical improvement within 24 to 48 hours.

If further treatment is required after the first 5 days of therapy, a 5-day hiatus is recommended between treatments. Patients should be kept well hydrated during Ca-EDTA therapy. Side effects of Ca-EDTA therapy include lethargy, vomiting, diarrhea, and renal injury. Oral zinc supplementation may minimize the GI side effects.

British Anti-Lewisite (Dimercaprol)

BAL is occasionally used in combination with Ca-EDTA, especially when significant CNS signs are present. BAL increases both urinary and biliary excretion of lead. The dosage of BAL is 2 to 5 mg/kg intramuscularly every 4 hours for 2 days, then every 8 hours for 1 day, and then every 12 hours until recovery. BAL is contraindicated in animals with hepatic dysfunction, is nephrotoxic, and causes pain on injection. Other potential side effects include vomiting, hypertension, sulfur odor of breath, and seizures.

Penicillamine

Penicillamine is an oral medication that eliminates the need for painful injections of BAL and Ca-EDTA. It binds essential nutrients such as zinc, iron, and copper, and its chelates may be nephrotoxic. Reported dosage for dogs is 10 to 15 mg/kg q12h PO. Feline dosage is 125 mg per cat orally every 12 hours for 5 days. Adverse effects reported with penicillamine include vomiting, fever, lymphadenopathy, and blood dyscrasias. Long-term administration may result in deficiencies of some essential nutrients such as zinc and copper.

Succimer

An analog to BAL, succimer has several advantages over BAL, Ca-EDTA, and penicillamine. Succimer can be administered orally or, in vomiting animals, rectally. The dose is 10 mg/kg orally or rectally every 8 hours for 10 days. Succimer is much less likely to cause nephrotoxicity than the other three chelators, and it does not bind essential minerals such as copper, zinc, calcium, and iron.

Succimer does not enhance absorption of lead from the GI tract as do the other chelators, and it has been shown to decrease GI lead absorption in studies with rats. Succimer also has a lower incidence of GI side effects. It does impart a mercaptan odor to the breath, similar to BAL, which some clients may find objectionable.

Additional Therapy

Following chelation therapy, blood lead levels may show a rebound within 2 to 3 weeks as a result of redistribution of lead from bone and tissue stores. Provided that this rebound is not associated with significant clinical signs, further chelation is not indicated. However, it is prudent to have the animal's environment evaluated to be sure the rebound is not caused by reexposure to lead.

Supportive care involves providing adequate nutritional support since many animals with chronic lead toxicosis may be in a negative nutritional state because of chronic anorexia and vomiting. Hydration should be maintained, and force- or hand-feeding provided as needed. The use of antioxidants such as pyridoxine (vitamin B_6), thiamine (vitamin B_1), ascorbate (vitamin C), tocopherol (vitamin E), and N-acetylcysteine have been advocated by some to help minimize the oxidant effects of lead within the body, but controlled studies are lacking as to the efficacy of any of these treatment modalities. The animal's environment should be examined to identify and remove any additional sources of lead so that the animal does not become reexposed when reintroduced to its environment.

Prognosis

Provided that prompt and appropriate care is pursued, including removing the source of lead from the animal's environment, the prognosis for animals showing mild-to-moderate signs is favorable. Animals showing severe CNS signs or with repeated exposure to lead may merit a more guarded prognosis.

Public Health

The relative susceptibility of household pets to lead toxicoses makes them good sentinel animals for the potential for human exposure to lead. Veterinarians treating lead-intoxicated pets should ensure that pet owners are aware of the risk to family members, especially young children, from lead in the environment. Pet owners should be directed to their own health care professionals or public health officials for more information. Information on the risks of lead to human health can be found on the Environmental Protection Agency's website (www.epa.gov).

References and Suggested Reading

Casteel SW: Lead. In Peterson ME, Talcott PA, editors: *Small animal toxicology*, ed 2, St Louis, 2006, Elsevier Saunders, p 795.
Gwaltney-Brant SM: Lead. In Plumlee KH, editor: *Clinical veterinary toxicology*, St Louis, 2004, Mosby, p 204.

Gwaltney-Brant SM, Rumbeiha WK: Newer antidotal therapies, *Vet Clin Small Anim* 32:323, 2002.

Knight TE, Kent M, Junk JE: Succimer for treatment of lead toxicosis in two cats, *J Am Vet Med Assoc* 218:1946, 2001.

Knight TE, Kumar MSA: Lead toxicosis in cats—a review, *J Feline Med Surg* 5:249, 2003.

Thompson LJ: Lead. In Gupta RC, editor: *Veterinary toxicology: basic and clinical principles*, St Louis, 2007, Elsevier Academic Press, pp. 438-441.

CHAPTER 38

Aflatoxicosis in Dogs

KARYN BISCHOFF, *Ithaca, New York*

TAM GARLAND, *College Station, Texas*

Aflatoxicosis in dogs was first described as *hepatitis X* in 1952. The disease was experimentally reproduced in 1955 using contaminated feed and again in 1966 using purified aflatoxin B_1. Moldy corn poisoning of swine and turkey X disease were reported in the 1940s. Turkey X disease was linked to aflatoxin in 1961.

Aflatoxins are a group of related compounds produced as secondary metabolites of various fungi, including *Aspergillus parasiticus, A. flavus, A. nomius,* and some *Penicillium* spp. Aflatoxins are not produced by all strains of these fungi. The most common aflatoxins in grains are named, in part, for their fluorescent color: aflatoxins B_1 and B_2 fluoresce blue and aflatoxins G_1 and G_2 fluoresce green. Aflatoxin B_1 is the most common and most potent of the aflatoxins.

High-energy and high-protein agricultural crops are most often affected. Corn, peanuts, and cottonseed are frequently implicated; however, rice, wheat, oats, sweet potatoes, potatoes, barley, millet, sesame, sorghum, cacao beans, almonds, soy, coconut, safflower, sunflower, palm kernel, cassava, cowpeas, peas, and various spices have been affected. Ingestion of homemade pet foods, moldy garbage, and improperly stored dog foods also has been implicated in aflatoxicosis.

Mold can grow on crops in the field or during storage. Mycotoxin synthesis depends on factors such as temperature, humidity, drought stress, insect damage, and handling techniques.

Commercial grain is screened routinely for aflatoxins, but contamination of pet food has occasionally resulted from sampling errors. Uneven distribution of mold within a given lot of grain (by analogy, one moldy orange in a large bag of fruit or blue veins in a block of blue cheese) increases the risk of sampling error. A simple black light at 366 nm can be used to detect kojic acid, which fluoresces blue-green and is also produced by many aflatoxin-producing fungi, but its presence does not confirm the presence of aflatoxins, and its absence does not guarantee that aflatoxin is not present. More sensitive analyses that test directly for aflatoxins use enzyme-linked immunosorbent assays, high-performance liquid chromatography (HPLC), and liquid chromatography/mass spectrometry. Many pet food companies currently sample each lot of grain before use *and* sample postproduction batches of pet food for testing to minimize the problem of sampling error.

Toxicity

Dogs and cats are considered very sensitive to aflatoxin (Newbern and Butler, 1969). The oral median lethal dose (LD_{50}) for aflatoxins in dogs ranges from 0.5 to 1.8 mg/kg. It is difficult to determine the total dose of aflatoxin in field cases when detailed information on the amount ingested and period of exposure is not usually available. Exposure to dog food containing as low as 60 ppb of aflatoxin for 60 or more days has been implicated in aflatoxicosis.

The experimental oral LD_{50} for aflatoxin in cats is 0.55 mg/kg. There is anecdotal evidence of aflatoxicosis in cats known to have consumed contaminated dog food for approximately 3 months. The cats were lethargic and had vomiting and diarrhea. One of the affected cats died and had liver lesions compatible with aflatoxicosis.

Factors such as dose, genetic predisposition, and concurrent disease influence the course of aflatoxin poisoning. Generally, younger animals, particularly males, seem to be more susceptible. Aflatoxin-related deaths in pups sucking a clinically healthy dam have been reported. Pregnant and whelping bitches also appear to be more susceptible. Early castration decreases mortality in males of some species. Low dietary protein enhances hepatocyte damage, whereas nutritional antioxidants, vitamin A, and carotene decrease it.

Toxicokinetics

Aflatoxins are highly lipophilic and are absorbed rapidly and almost completely in the duodenum. Aflatoxins entering the portal circulation are highly protein bound. The unbound fraction is distributed to the tissues, with the highest concentration occurring in the liver.

The liver is the primary metabolic site for aflatoxins, although some metabolism occurs in the kidneys and small intestine. Phase I metabolism of aflatoxin B_1 by cytochrome P-450 enzymes produces aflatoxin M_1 and the reactive intermediate aflatoxin B_1 8,9-epoxide. During phase II metabolism aflatoxin B_1 8,9-epoxide is conjugated to glutathione in a reaction catalyzed by glutathione S-transferase.

Metabolites of aflatoxin are excreted in both urine and bile. Dogs excrete primarily aflatoxin M_1 in the urine. More than 90% of urinary excretion of metabolites occurs within 12 hours of dosing in dogs, and aflatoxin metabolites are no longer detectable by 48 hours. Conjugated aflatoxin is excreted predominantly in the bile. Approximately 1% of an oral dose of aflatoxin is excreted as aflatoxin M_1 in the milk in dairy cattle.

Mechanism of Action

Phase I metabolism of aflatoxin B_1 produces the highly reactive electrophile aflatoxin B_1 8,9-epoxide, which binds readily to cellular molecules, including nucleic acids, proteins, and subcellular organelles. Formation of deoxyribonucleic acid (DNA) adducts modifies the DNA template, altering the binding of DNA polymerase and thus affecting replication. Effects on ribosomal translocase inhibit protein production. These changes lead to necrosis of hepatocytes and other metabolically active cells such as renal tubular epithelium. Coagulopathy results from decreased prothrombin and fibrinogen production. Excretion of aflatoxin adducts is slow compared with the parent compound and other metabolites.

Aflatoxins are classified by the International Agency for Research on Cancer as class I human carcinogens. Hepatocellular carcinoma has been associated with chronic aflatoxin exposure and concurrent infection with hepatitis B virus. Aflatoxins are also known carcinogens in ferrets, ducks, trout, swine, sheep, and rats, but are **not** known to be carcinogenic in dogs or cats. Aflatoxin-induced neoplasia is rare in domestic animals in general, probably due to the limited life spans of most domestic species.

Clinical Signs

Although aflatoxicosis may be caused by prolonged exposure to contaminated food, the presentation in small animals is usually acute. Toxicosis has been reported in dogs after ingesting contaminated food for as long as 90 to 120 days before onset of clinical signs. The course of clinical aflatoxicosis is usually a few days but can be protracted for up to 2 weeks. Dogs can and do survive when the concentration is low or exposure is limited. Experimentally poisoned cats died of aflatoxicosis within a few days of onset of clinical signs, but in the anecdotal cases described above some affected cats survived.

The most commonly reported early clinical signs of aflatoxicosis in dogs include feed refusal or anorexia, weakness and obtundation, vomiting, and diarrhea. A few die unexpectedly without showing clinical signs. As the toxicosis progresses, dogs become icteric and can have bilirubinuria. Hepatic encephalopathy has been reported. Many dogs die from disseminated intravascular coagulation, evidence of which includes melena or frank blood in the feces, hematemesis, petechial hemorrhages, and epistaxis. Hemorrhage into the calvarium has been associated with seizures.

Diagnosis

Differential diagnoses for dogs in pet food–related cases of aflatoxicosis can include leptospirosis, parvovirus, anticoagulant rodenticide toxicosis, and a variety of hepatotoxic agents, including acetaminophen, cyanobacterial toxins, mushroom toxins, and cycad palms, as well as phosphine and iron.

Diagnosis of aflatoxicosis is often based on history, clinical signs, clinical pathology findings, and postmortem changes. Laboratory testing of dog food or other implicated material is helpful in confirming the diagnosis, but often all the contaminated food has been consumed by the time the animal becomes clinically affected. It is important to retain bar codes and lot numbers from containers of pet food when contamination is suspected because this information is critical for case tracking and in product recalls. Some laboratories test for aflatoxin M_1 in the urine, although urinary metabolites are no longer detectable 48 hours postexposure in dogs. Some laboratories have had success analyzing serum or liver for aflatoxin, but due to the low concentrations ingested and rapid metabolism and excretion, this too is of limited diagnostic use if negative.

Clinical Chemistry

Complete blood count, serum chemistry including bile acids, and urinalysis are recommended to support the diagnosis of aflatoxin poisoning and rule out other causes of liver failure. Total bilirubin is increased in aflatoxicosis. Alanine aminotransferase, alkaline phosphatase, and aspartate aminotransferase are frequently elevated, but the elevations do not correlate well with the magnitude of hepatic damage. Liver function tests have been used to support the diagnosis of aflatoxicosis, including decreased serum albumin, protein C, antithrombin II, and cholesterol, and increased prothrombin time.

Postmortem Findings

Diagnosis of aflatoxicosis is often made on necropsy. Common gross pathology findings include icterus; hepatomegaly, which could be mild; abdominal or pleural effusions; gastrointestinal hemorrhage; and multifocal petechia and ecchymosis.

The primary histologic changes of canine aflatoxicosis are associated with the liver, although necrosis of the proximal convoluted renal tubules has been reported. Liver lesions associated with acute aflatoxicosis include centrilobular necrosis, canalicular cholestasis, mild inflammation, and fatty degeneration of hepatocytes, which may contain one to many lipid vacuoles. Similarly, dogs with subacute toxicosis have hepatocytic fatty degeneration, canalicular cholestasis, and multifocal-to–locally extensive hepatic necrosis, often associated with neutrophilic inflammation and hepatocyte regeneration. However, as aflatoxicosis progresses, bridging portal fibrosis and bile duct proliferation become more prominent, and the central vein can be obscured by dilated sinusoids. Chronic aflatoxicosis is characterized by less fatty degeneration of hepatocytes and marked fibrosis and regeneration, disrupting the hepatic architecture. Lesions reported in cats are somewhat different. Experimentally affected cats had hepatomegaly with multifocal petechia. Hepatocytes contained mostly glycogen with minimal lipid. Bile duct hyperplasia was noted in cats that survived clinical aflatoxicosis for more than 72 hours.

Prognosis and Management

The prognosis for small animals with clinical aflatoxicosis is guarded, with a mortality rate of approximately two out of three affected dogs. Animals with severe clinical signs usually respond poorly to treatment. Early intervention, especially in preclinical exposed animals, greatly improves the chance of survival. Removal of contaminated food is key to survival. The food should be replaced with a high-quality protein diet.

As with most other conditions, patient assessment and stabilization are the first steps in management. Oral activated charcoal is appropriate to limit absorption in cases of recent high-dose exposure, as can occur when moldy garbage is ingested. Supportive care includes correcting hydration and electrolyte imbalances with intravenous fluids. B-vitamins and dextrose can be added to fluids. Vitamin K_1 therapy reportedly decreased clinical coagulopathy within 72 hours. Plasma transfusions have been used to improve clotting profiles in severely affected dogs. Gastroprotectants such as sucralfate and famotidine, and sometimes parenteral nutrition, are necessary in animals with severe gastroenteric signs. Vitamin E, a fat-soluble antioxidant, and liver protectants such as silymarin have been used clinically and experimentally. Silymarin is a mix of flavonolignans, such as silybin, from milk thistle (*Silybum marianum*). Silymarin decreased the hepatotoxic effects of dietary aflatoxin B_1 in experimental chickens. One proposed mechanism of action for silybin is decreasing the metabolism of aflatoxin B_1 to the epoxide form. *S*-adenosylmethionine (SAMe) has also been used

clinically as a hepatoprotectant in the treatment of aflatoxicosis. Sulfhydryl groups on SAMe are believed to bind aflatoxin B_1 8,9-epoxide. Although milk thistle and SAMe are considered liver supportive, combined therapy in patients with prolonged exposure to dietary aflatoxin could prevent aflatoxin adducts from being excreted.

N-acetylcysteine, given parenterally, has been used in severely intoxicated dogs. It is known to increase cytosolic and mitochondrial glutathione and may act directly as a free-radical scavenger. Experimentally *N*-acetylcysteine has been shown to enhance elimination of aflatoxin B_1 and prevent liver damage in poultry.

The antischistosomal drug oltipraz has been used to treat aflatoxicosis in humans and experimental animals. Oltipraz inhibits phase I enzymes, CYP1A2 in particular, that metabolize aflatoxin B_1 to the epoxide form. It also induces phase II enzymes, including glutathione S-transferase, to facilitate conjugation of aflatoxin B_1 8,9-epoxide. This drug protects against hepatocarcinogenesis in rats. Oltipraz has not been used in veterinary medicine to the authors' knowledge.

References and Suggested Reading

Bastianello SS et al: Pathological finding in a natural outbreak of aflatoxicosis in dogs, *Onderstepoort J Vet Res* 64:635, 1987.
Bingham AK et al: Identification and reduction of urinary aflatoxin metabolites in dogs, *Food Chem Toxicol* 42:1851, 2004.
Bruchim Y et al: Accidental fatal aflatoxicosis due to contaminated commercial diet in 50 dogs, *Res Vet Sci* 93(1):279-287, 2012.
Garland T, Reagor J: Chronic canine aflatoxin and management of an epidemic. In Panter KE, Wierenga TL, Pfister JA, editors: *Poisonous plants: global research and solutions*, Wallingford, Oxon, UK, 2007, CABI Publishing.
Meerdink GL: Mycotoxins. In Plumlee KH, editor: *Clinical veterinary toxicology*, St Louis, 2004, Mosby, p 231.
Newbern PM, Butler WH: Acute and chronic effects of aflatoxin on the liver of domestic and laboratory animals: a review, *Cancer Res* 29:236, 1969.
Stenske KA et al: Aflatoxicosis in dogs and dealing with suspected contaminated commercial foods, *J Am Vet Med Assoc* 228:1686, 2006.
Tedesco D et al: Efficacy of silymarin-phospholipid complex in reducing the toxicity of aflatoxin B 1 in broiler chickens, *Poult Sci* 83:1839, 2004.
Valdivia AG et al: Efficacy of N-acetylcysteine to reduce the effects of aflatoxin B 1 intoxication in broiler chickens, *Poult Sci* 80:727, 2001.
Wang JS et al: Protective alterations in phase 1 and 2 metabolism of aflatoxin B 1 by oltipraz in residents of Qidong, People's Republic of China, *J Natl Cancer Inst* 91:347, 1999.

SECTION III

Endocrine and Metabolic Diseases

Chapter 39:   Bilaterally Symmetric Alopecia in Dogs   164
Chapter 40:   Imaging in Diagnosis of Endocrine Disorders   167
Chapter 41:   Approach to Critical Illness–Related
               Corticosteroid Insufficiency   174
Chapter 42:   Canine Hypothyroidism   178
Chapter 43:   Feline Hyperthyroidism and Renal Function   185
Chapter 44:   Canine Diabetes Mellitus   189
Chapter 45:   Diabetic Monitoring   193
Chapter 46:   Diet and Diabetes   199
Chapter 47:   Insulin Resistance   205
Chapter 48:   Feline Diabetes Mellitus   208
Chapter 49:   Feline Hypersomatotropism and Acromegaly   216
Chapter 50:   Occult Hyperadrenocorticism: Is It Real?   221
Chapter 51:   Canine Hyperadrenocorticism Therapy   225
Chapter 52:   Ectopic ACTH Syndrome and Food-Dependent
               Hypercortisolism in Dogs   230
Chapter 53:   Canine Hypoadrenocorticism   233
Chapter 54:   Feline Primary Hyperaldosteronism   238
Chapter 55:   Feline Idiopathic Hypercalcemia   242
Chapter 56:   Approach to Hypomagnesemia and Hypokalemia   248
Chapter 57:   Obesity   254
Chapter 58:   Approach to Canine Hyperlipidemia   261

The following web chapters can be found on the companion website at www.currentveterinarytherapy.com

Web Chapter 11:   Hypercalcemia and Primary Hyperparathyroidism in Dogs
Web Chapter 12:   Clinical Use of the Vasopressin Analog Desmopressin for the
                   Diagnosis and Treatment of Diabetes Insipidus
Web Chapter 13:   Complicated Diabetes Mellitus
Web Chapter 14:   Complications and Concurrent Conditions Associated with
                   Hypothyroidism in Dogs
Web Chapter 15:   Large Pituitary Tumors in Dogs with Pituitary-Dependent
                   Hyperadrenocorticism
Web Chapter 16:   Differential Diagnosis of Hyperkalemia and Hyponatremia in Dogs
                   and Cats
Web Chapter 17:   Hyperadrenocorticism in Ferrets
Web Chapter 18:   Interpretation of Endocrine Diagnostic Test Results for Adrenal
                   and Thyroid Disease
Web Chapter 19:   Medical Treatment of Feline Hyperthyroidism
Web Chapter 20:   Nutritional Management of Feline Hyperthyroidism
Web Chapter 21:   Radioiodine for Feline Hyperthyroidism
Web Chapter 22:   Treatment of Hypoparathyroidism
Web Chapter 23:   Treatment of Insulinoma in Dogs, Cats, and Ferrets
Web Chapter 24:   Alternatives to Insulin Therapy for Diabetes Mellitus in Cats

CHAPTER 39

Bilaterally Symmetric Alopecia in Dogs

ROBERT ALLEN KENNIS, *Auburn, Alabama*

Endocrine diseases are among the many causes of symmetric alopecia in the dog. In certain situations the cutaneous manifestations of endocrine disease provide some of the most obvious clinical signs. However, the clinician must consider a number of common and uncommon disorders when approaching the dog with symmetric alopecia (Box 39-1). As with most dermatologic disorders, signalment, historical information, and physical findings are the starting points to a diagnosis, followed by performance of appropriate laboratory tests and the collection of a dermatologic minimum database. This chapter provides a concise and rational guide for achieving a diagnosis when confronted with a canine patient with bilaterally symmetric alopecia. More details about these specific conditions can be found in this section and in Section V of this textbook.

Pruritic Alopecia

By definition, alopecia means hair loss. It must be determined if the dog was pruritic and created the alopecia from trauma (e.g., biting, scratching, rubbing) or if the hair fell out spontaneously. Most endocrine and metabolic causes of alopecia are nonpruritic unless complicated by other lesions. For example, dogs with spontaneous hyperadrenocorticism may become pruritic if calcinosis cutis is present. Likewise, dogs with various metabolic disorders including hyperadrenocorticism may develop pruritus if secondary infection from bacteria or yeast occurs. The only pruritic endocrine disorder is hyperestrogenism. Pruritus in general is usually symmetric, and therefore trauma-induced alopecia may mimic metabolic causes of symmetric alopecia. Regardless of the cause, bilaterally symmetric alopecia is rarely identical on both sides. The presence of similar appearing lesions on both sides of the midline allows us to use this terminology.

The presence of pruritus leads to a list of differential diagnoses that include myriad allergic, parasitic, and infectious diseases. Historical evidence supports trauma-induced pruritus. A trichogram (sometimes referred to as a KOH prep) is an easy diagnostic procedure used to determine if the tips of the hairs are broken due to traumatic causes. Normal hairs should have a fine taper at the tip of the hairshaft, whereas broken hairs have blunted ends. Hairs are grasped at their base with hemostats or thumb forceps and removed with traction. They are then placed on a glass slide with a few drops of mineral oil or potassium hydroxide (KOH). Care should be taken to place the hairs in the same direction so that they can be examined from base to tip. The application of a cover slip aids in viewing. The hairs can be examined under the microscope using either 4× or 10× magnification objectives. Lowering the light condenser makes viewing easier by increasing the refractivity.

A KOH prep also can be used to identify other conditions. For example, in dermatophyte-infected hairs fungal spores (microconidia) may be visible. Affected hairs have a damaged cuticle, are asymmetric, and are usually much wider than normal hairs. The presence of macromelanosomes along with a damaged hair cuticle may assist in the diagnosis of color-dilution alopecia (Figure 39-1); however, the definitive diagnosis is based on clinical signs and histopathologic evaluation. Interestingly, large melanosomes may be seen in color-dilute breeds such as the weimaraner, but the cuticle is not damaged; therefore these breeds do not exhibit color-dilution alopecia (with rare exceptions).

If broken hairs are present due to pruritic causes, every effort should be made to identify and treat the underlying cause of the pruritus. Of note is the historical use of glucocorticoid medications because such treatment could potentially interfere with interpretation of prior and future laboratory results.

Clinical Evaluation

Historical information is important in all dermatologic cases. Questionnaire templates are available for clinical use in virtually every veterinary dermatologic textbook. These are an efficient way to collect the necessary data to help formulate a list of differential diagnoses. They also provide the client an opportunity to reflect on the history, which hopefully leads to a more accurate account of the clinical problem. The signalment alone may provide important data and should not be overlooked. Many endocrine skin disorders can be considered more likely based on the age of onset. Likewise, many breeds are overrepresented for certain endocrine causes of alopecia.

Atypical coloration, such as a "blue" or "fawn" Doberman pinscher, may predispose the dog to *color dilution alopecia* at a later age. Although the Doberman is one of the most common breeds associated with this disorder, the Chihuahua, chow-chow, and Yorkshire terrier have increased prevalence. Any dog that exhibits a dilution pattern may develop color dilution alopecia. As puppies, affected dogs have a normal hair coat (other than color) and they may develop alopecia as the adult hairs replace the puppy coat. It is impossible to predict the age of onset or severity of the alopecia in color-dilute situations.

Causes of Nonpruritic Canine Symmetric Alopecia

Hypothyroidism
Hyperadrenocorticism
Hypotestosteronism
Hyperestrogenism
Sertoli cell tumor–associated skin disease
Alopecia X
Color dilution alopecia
Cyclical flank alopecia
Anagen or telogen defluxion
Post-clipping alopecia
Traction alopecia
Follicular dysplasia
Acquired pattern alopecia

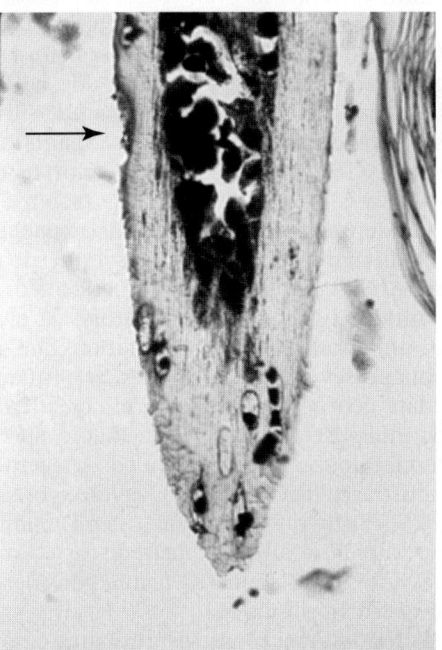

Figure 39-1 Photomicrogram of a hair. The base of the hair is at the bottom. Note the damaged cuticle *(arrow).* Macromelanosomes can be seen within the hair; the melanosomes are large and clumped compared with the normal appearance (being much smaller, punctate, and distinct from each other).

The sex status of the dog is also important when considering hyperestrogenism. Sertoli cell tumor is a testicular neoplasm more common in male dogs with retained testicles. Female dogs may develop postpartum hair defluxion. Lastly, traction alopecia may occur from the exuberant use of rubber bands or hair clips on some canine breeds; therefore the grooming and maintenance history is helpful in making this diagnosis.

A thorough investigation of all topical and systemic medications is required. Topical glucocorticoid medications can lead to local or systemic clinical signs such as skin atrophy, alopecia or follicular atrophy, changes in skin pigmentation, calcinosis cutis, and the development of secondary infections or demodicosis. Topical glucocorticoid medications have been responsible for inducing

some spectacular symmetric alopecias and should not be ignored when investigating the underlying cause of the problem. Topical steroids also can have a profound influence on serum biochemical test results, especially serum alkaline phosphatase. Other commonly used medications such as ketoconazole may not directly lead to the development of symmetric alopecia but may influence laboratory results.

Diagnostic Tests

Once pruritic causes of alopecia have been removed or ruled out, additional baseline information is needed. Several *deep skin scrapings* should be collected to search for Demodex mites. This is a mandatory diagnostic procedure for all alopecic dogs because Demodex mites may be associated with a roughly symmetric alopecia. Identification of the mites is easier if the light condenser is lowered, similar to the technique used for a trichogram discussed earlier. If mites are found, the possibility of an endocrinopathy as the true cause of the symmetric alopecia is still high. Hyperadrenocorticism, hypothyroidism, and the use of glucocorticoid medications are the most frequent underlying causes of generalized demodicosis in an adult dog. Conversely, adult-onset generalized demodicosis may be idiopathic in some cases.

Dermatophytosis may be associated with a symmetric alopecia. The presence of fungal spores may be identified with a trichogram. Dermatophytosis may be associated with endocrinopathies, with glucocorticoid administration, or with other medications exerting an immunosuppressive effect. A *fungal culture* (i.e., dermatophyte test media [DTM]) is inexpensive and easy to perform and should be included as a part of a minimum database for dogs presenting with alopecia regardless of the cause of the problem.

Direct impression samples collected for *cytologic evaluation* are a quick and easy procedure to identify bacterial or yeast organisms that may be contributing to the development of alopecia. A glass slide is pressed firmly against the skin surface or any moist surface lesion. If epidermal collarettes are present, the leading margin should be gently lifted using the side of the slide and the impression cytology collected from that site. The sample should be allowed to air dry before staining with a modified Wright's stain. The oil objective will be necessary to identify bacteria or yeast organisms.

Another option for sample collection is the *tape preparation,* especially when the lesions are dry and scaly or located in a difficult-to-sample site such as the interdigital regions. Clear acetate tape is pressed to the skin surface 2 to 3 times and placed sticky-side down onto a few drops of the third (purple) stain of the modified Wright's stain kit. The tape should be pressed firmly to the slide with paper towels to remove excess stain. The tape preparation can be evaluated at oil immersion without a cover slip.

Canine bacterial folliculitis is usually associated with focal or patchy-to-diffuse alopecia rather than bilaterally symmetric alopecia. Secondary infections may be a result of an underlying endocrinopathy. It is usually best to resolve any secondary infections with appropriate topical or parenteral medications before performing routine blood work or specific serum laboratory testing for endocrine diseases. Also, it is best to resolve these infections before biopsy samples are collected for histopathologic evaluation. Secondary infections may mask the underlying cause of the alopecia.

Skin Biopsy Samples

Submission of *skin biopsy samples* for histopathology is sometimes helpful in diagnosing the cause of canine symmetric alopecia. Because biopsy samples must be evaluated in light of available historical and serum biochemical results, all pertinent historical information also should be sent to the pathologist. Digital images of the alopecia and skin lesions also may be useful because many pathologists consult with clinical dermatologists to provide the best diagnostic service. Many causes of canine symmetric alopecia share similar histopathologic findings. Therefore it is essential to use the signalment, history, and laboratory and clinical findings to achieve a diagnosis. Occasionally histopathology alone is helpful in making a diagnosis. Cyclical flank alopecia, color dilution alopecia, and hyperadrenocorticism (if calcinosis cutis is present) can all be readily diagnosed with standard histopathology methods. However, alopecia X, hyperestrogenism, Sertoli cell tumor–associated skin disease, and hyperadrenocorticism (spontaneous or iatrogenic) are impossible to differentiate on histopathology without additional data. In short, endocrinopathies, acquired pattern alopecia, and post-clipping alopecia can be very difficult to sort out with histopathology alone.

Before the biopsy, the skin surface should not be surgically prepared. Long hairs may be clipped and gently brushed away from the collection site. A 6- to 8-mm Baker biopsy punch usually provides an adequate sample size. Samples should be taken from sites exhibiting early, middle, and late stages of the disease process (or mildly affected to severely affected regions). The location and description of each skin biopsy site should be noted and each sample placed in a separate container of formalin. This is especially important when attempting to differentiate endocrine causes of alopecia from acquired pattern alopecias (i.e. pattern baldness). Submitting a sample from a nonaffected area in this instance may be beneficial as a comparison to the other samples. It is imperative to submit samples in separate containers to avoid confusion about site of origin.

Laboratory Tests

Baseline laboratory data are usually needed to achieve a diagnosis for a dog presenting with bilaterally symmetric alopecia. A complete blood count (CBC), serum chemistry, and urinalysis provide the minimum data base. Abnormalities may provide clues that help direct selection of additional diagnostic procedures such as an adrenocorticotropic hormone (ACTH) stimulation test or low-dose dexamethasone suppression test when hyperadrenocorticism is suspected (see Chapters 42 and 51). In the diagnosis of hypothyroidism, a total thyroxine (T_4), free T_4, and thyroid-stimulating hormone (TSH) provide the minimum database. Some reference laboratories provide additional information such as autoantibodies. It is important to not rely on a single thyroid value (such as a T_4 or TSH) in making a definitive diagnosis. The data are best evaluated alongside the clinical signs. Even with values from quality reference laboratories, the diagnosis of hypothyroidism may be challenging (see Chapter 42 and Web Chapter 14). History, clinical findings, histopathology, and ruling out other causes of symmetric alopecia are important in achieving a diagnosis.

Because they can greatly affect the aforementioned tests, topical or parenteral glucocorticoid medications usually should not be used for 4 to 6 weeks prior to submitting laboratory tests. Milder topical glucocorticoids such as hydrocortisone are less likely to cause side effects. There are several potent topical steroids such as triamcinolone, betamethasone, and mometasone that increase the likelihood of developing iatrogenic Cushing's disease. The potency of the steroid and the duration of usage will be determining factors in evaluating the necessary withdrawal period, and it may be longer than 4 to 6 weeks. Clearly there are conditions to consider before suddenly stopping glucocorticoids, such as the dog with adrenal suppression that may need to be managed with physiologic doses of prednisone (see Chapter 53) and monitored closely with ACTH stimulation tests prior to complete withdrawal.

Some laboratories provide sex hormone panels to help sort out challenging cases of canine symmetric alopecia. A standard ACTH stimulation test is performed. Serum is then submitted chilled to the laboratory for evaluation. Both pre- and post-ACTH concentrations are provided for cortisol and several sex hormones. The interpretation of these data can be challenging and consultation with an endocrinologist or internal medicine specialist or with a dermatologist is recommended. A recent publication demonstrated elevations in 17-hydroxyprogesterone (17OHP) in healthy bitches during the normal reproductive cycle. Therefore all previously discussed diagnostic procedures should be evaluated before considering measurement of sex hormones.

In a related issue, a report of miniature poodles and Pomeranians with clinical signs of alopecia X indicated that these dogs had elevations of 17OHP post-ACTH stimulation. In these cases, trilostane therapy led to complete hair regrowth in all of the miniature poodles and 85% of the Pomeranians within a 4- to 8-week period (Cerundolo et al, 2004; see Chapter 115). However, trilostane may not improve the clinical signs associated with alopecia X in all dogs.

References and Suggested Reading

Bromel C et al: Serum 17α-hydroxyprogesterone concentrations during the reproductive cycle in healthy dogs and dogs with hyperadrenocorticism, *J Am Vet Med Assoc* 236(11):1208-1214, 2010.

Cerundolo R et al: Treatment of canine Alopecia X with trilostane, *Vet Dermatol* 15:285-293, 2004.

Behrend EN, Kennis RA: Atypical Cushing's syndrome in dogs: arguments for and against, *Vet Clin Small Anim* 40(2):285-296, 2010.

Kooistra HS, Galac S: Recent advances in the diagnosis of Cushing's syndrome in dogs, *Vet Clin Small Anim* 40(2):259-267, 2010.

CHAPTER 40

Imaging in Diagnosis of Endocrine Disorders

JIMMY H. SAUNDERS, *Merelbeke, Belgium*

Imaging Modalities in Endocrinology

Radiography has little value for imaging endocrine organs and is mainly used to detect lung metastases. Ultrasonography (US) is the most commonly used imaging modality for diagnosis of endocrine disorders because of its availability and relative low cost. Major endocrine organs such as the thyroid gland, parathyroid glands, and adrenal glands are superficially located, which makes them easily accessible with US using high-resolution transducers ($\geq$10 MHz). Additionally, US allows for fine-needle aspiration, tissue-core biopsy, or interventional procedures of endocrine organs to be performed in real-time. Two newer US techniques, which are still under clinical investigation, can help to improve the accuracy of gray-scale diagnostic US. Contrast-enhanced US involves intravenous injection of gas microbubbles as vascular contrast agents to improve the detection of perfusion and vascularity of both normal and abnormal organs. Changes in vascularity and blood flow are frequently seen secondary to pathology and are represented in time-intensity curves as alterations of the shape of the curve on contrast-enhanced US. The second method, elastography, is an US technique that evaluates the stiffness of tissues by measuring the displacement of ultrasound echoes before and after compression. Elastography thereby provides information about the mechanical properties of tissues and is currently used in people to differentiate malignant from benign lesions in thyroid tissue.

Computed tomography (CT) and magnetic resonance imaging (MRI) are very useful for evaluation of the extent, local invasiveness, and local or distant metastases of neoplastic processes. CT is the modality of choice for detection of lung metastases, whereas MRI provides excellent delineation of anatomic structures because of inherent high-contrast resolution and is the modality of choice for evaluation of presurgical tissue and vascular invasion. Both modalities allow visualization of intracranial structures and are particularly suited for imaging the pituitary gland. Dynamic CT contrast studies including targeted angiography or dual-phase CT are useful for examination of adrenal glands, pituitary gland, and pancreatic disorders.

The routine use of nuclear medicine in veterinary endocrinology is limited to thyroid scintigraphy. This modality is extremely useful to determine unilateral or bilateral lobe involvement, the status of the gland, the location of hyperfunctioning ectopic or accessory tissue, and distant metastases of thyroid tumors. Availability of scintigraphy is limited in veterinary medicine. Box 40-1 lists some useful imaging tips for evaluating endocrine disorders in dogs and cats.

Imaging the Thyroid Gland

The thyroid gland is composed of two separate lobes except in a few large-breed dogs in which an isthmus connects both lobes caudally. Thyroid lobes are oblong and span the dorsolateral aspect of the trachea, medial to the common carotid arteries, from the first to the eighth tracheal ring. The thyroid gland is supplied with arterial blood from a large cranial and a smaller caudal thyroid artery, both branches of the common carotid artery. The caudal thyroid artery is absent in cats. Venous drainage is via the cranial and caudal thyroid veins.

US is the primary modality for evaluation of the thyroid gland. The gland appears on US as a homogeneous, well-delineated, hyperechoic (compared with the surrounding musculature), fusiform structure. Measurements of the height (dorsoventral axis) of the thyroid gland and calculation of its volume using the formula of a rotation ellipse have the lowest variability and should be preferred in comparative and follow-up studies. On CT, the normal thyroid gland is homogeneous, ovoid or triangle-shaped, and hyperattenuating compared with the surrounding tissues (Table 40-1). The hyperattenuation is due to its natural high iodine content, which is an element with a high atomic number (53) compared with most other elements in the body (Figure 40-1, *A*). After intravenous injection of iodinated contrast medium, the gland shows usually diffuse enhancement. On MRI, the thyroid gland may appear heterogeneous, particularly on T2-weighted images, or homogeneous. On T1-weighted images, the thyroid gland is isointense to surrounding muscles in half of cases and shows intermediate signal intensity between fat and muscle in the other half. After contrast medium administration (gadolinium-based), the thyroid gland shows intensity between muscle and fat or is isointense to fat. On T2-weighted images, the thyroid gland shows intensity between muscle and fat. MRI is the best modality to evaluate local tissue invasion, detect cervical lymphadenopathy, and detect recurrent thyroid carcinoma after treatment.

Radionuclide iodine (^{123}I, ^{131}I) or pertechnetate (^{99m}TcO$_4$) is taken up by thyroid tissue and can be used for thyroid scintigraphy. In contrast to pertechnetate, iodine isotopes are incorporated in thyroglobulin (organification), enabling the determination of "true" uptake,

---

BOX 40-1

Imaging Tips for Evaluation of Endocrine Disorders

- Follow-up US studies of the thyroid gland should be performed by the same individual.
- Always perform radiography of the thorax or, even better, CT scan of the lungs in patients with a neoplastic process.
- Perform dynamic CT scans for examination of the adrenal glands, pituitary gland, and pancreas.
- Use vascular landmarks to find the adrenal glands on US.
- CT and MRI of the pituitary gland should be performed using thin slices (1 to 2 mm).
- The sensitivity of US for detection of metastasis within lymph nodes is greatly improved by use of contrast-enhanced US.

TABLE 40-1

Computed Tomography Attenuation Values of the Normal Thyroid Gland

Thyroid Gland	Canine	Feline
Precontrast attenuation (HU)	108	123
Postcontrast attenuation (HU)	169	169
Volume (mm³)	1150*	—

*Dog weighing 30 kg.

which could be more reflective of thyroid physiology. Despite this advantage of iodine, pertechnetate routinely is preferred because it is easily obtainable from an in-house molybdenum generator, is cheaper, and has a shorter half-life compared with iodine isotopes. On a normal scintigraphic study, the thyroid-to-salivary uptake ratio is less than 1. Injection of iodinated contrast medium on CT scan influences the results of nuclear imaging for 6 to 8 weeks. Gadolinium-based MRI contrast agents do not interfere with thyroid function and subsequent nuclear imaging.

Canine Thyroid Neoplasia

In dogs, thyroid neoplasia (mostly carcinomas, less commonly adenomas) is associated with a unilateral (66%) or bilateral (33%) mass caudal to the pharynx. Clinically detectable neoplasms usually are nonsecreting, resulting in euthyroidism throughout the course of the disease. In dogs with thyroid neoplasia, diagnostic imaging is used (1) to define the thyroid origin of the cervical mass, (2) to detect local or distant metastases, and (3) to evaluate local tissue invasion. Whatever imaging modality is used, it is sometimes difficult to document the thyroidal origin of the mass when its size severely disrupts the normal anatomy of the cervical area. Scintigraphy, CT, and to a lesser extent US may be indicated to determine whether large cervical masses arise from the thyroid gland or from other tissues. When the mass arises from tissues

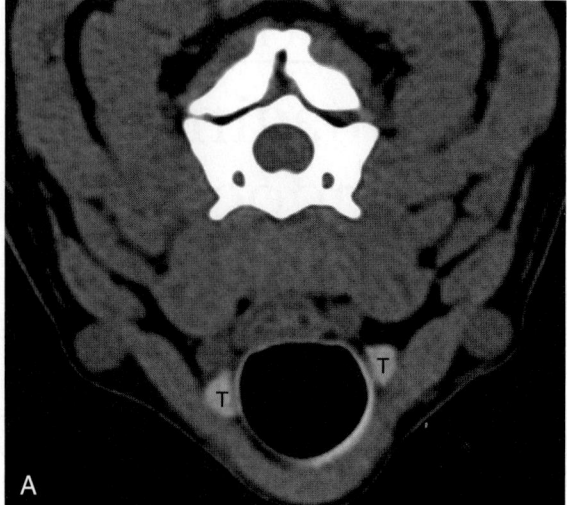

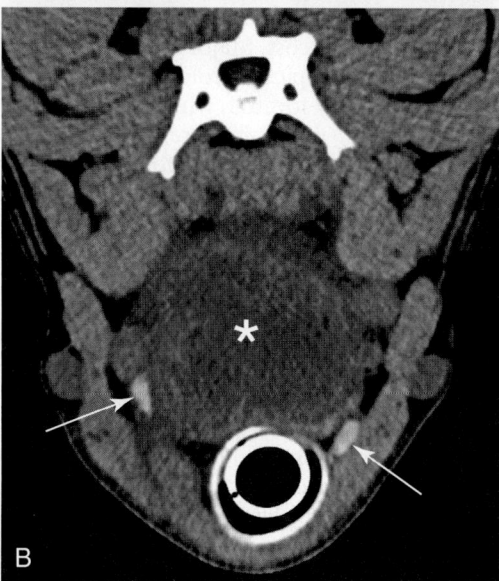

Figure 40-1 CT images of the thyroid gland. **A,** Precontrast CT scan of a normal adult dog shows the hyperattenuating thyroid glands *(T)*. **B,** Precontrast CT study of an adult dog with a large mass *(asterisk)* located dorsally to the trachea and extending from the caudal part of the pharynx to the level of the sixth cervical vertebra. Both thyroid glands *(arrows)* were entirely visible excluding a thyroid origin. An ectopic thyroid origin is also unlikely because of the dorsal location. The mass was a paraesophageal abscess. (Courtesy Olivier Taeymans, Tufts University.)

other than the thyroid, both thyroid lobes should be visible exhibiting a normal pattern (Figure 40-1, *B*). Additionally, US and CT can be used to guide a fine-needle aspiration or a core biopsy of a cervical mass.

With thyroid neoplasia, radiography may reveal a (sometimes mineralized) mass and possibly show displacement or compression of the trachea or the esophagus (mostly ventrally) or deformation of the larynx. Thyroid neoplasia appears as a large, heterogeneous mass involving most commonly the entire lobe or gland, with variable delineation, hypoechoic (US), isoattenuating to hypoattenuating (CT), or hyperintense (all routine MRI sequences); the mass sometimes may contain multiple cystic areas of necrosis or hemorrhage that alternate with areas of normal parenchyma, dense connective tissue, or mineralization. Thyroid carcinoma shows strong vascularization on power or color Doppler, contrast-enhanced US, and contrast-enhanced CT. CT is highly specific (100%) and MRI is highly sensitive (93%) in diagnosing thyroid carcinoma, whereas US has a moderate sensitivity (79%) and a poor specificity (33%). Main differential diagnosis is a carotid body tumor. On scintigraphy, thyroid tumors are of various sizes with irregular areas of pertechnetate uptake and usually heterogeneous distribution of radioactivity. Diffuse increased and decreased uptake patterns also have been described. If the tumor is secreting excessive amounts of thyroid hormones, moderate to extensive areas of increased, usually uniform, tracer uptake are detected, and the contralateral lobe exhibits suppressed uptake because of negative feedback onto the pituitary gland and resultant lack of thyroid-stimulating hormone (TSH) secretion. Unfortunately, increased uptake of radionuclide does not always correlate with increased production of thyroid hormones by the tumor. For instance, if the thyroid tumor destroys enough of the thyroid gland (≥75%) to cause subnormal thyroxine concentration, the pituitary gland increases its TSH release, and the remaining normal tissue is stimulated. The nonsecreting thyroid neoplasm shows decreased uptake, and the remaining normal tissue has increased uptake. Diagnostic imaging cannot reliably differentiate adenoma from carcinoma.

Distant pulmonary metastases from local invasion of the thyroid veins are common, and thoracic radiographs or lung CT scan should always be performed in cases of thyroid carcinoma. If a cranial mediastinal mass is present, neoplastic transformation of ectopic thyroid tissue should be considered. The second most common site of metastases is the retropharyngeal lymph nodes, which are best imaged on CT, MRI, and Doppler or contrast-enhanced US. Other sites of metastatic spread include abdominal organs (liver, kidneys, spleen, and adrenal glands), justifying standard abdominal US or CT to be performed, and also bone, bone marrow, brain, and spinal cord. Thyroid scintigraphy is a specific tool for identification of metastasis but is not considered sensitive. Scintigraphic visualization of metastases in the presence of an intact trapping mechanism in thyroid tumor cells indicates a high trapping ability of iodine in the tumor tissue, and this may be considered a predictive factor of radioiodine therapy effectiveness.

Even with the use of US, CT, or MRI, the detection of local tissue invasion by a thyroid carcinoma may be challenging. US is less sensitive than MRI and CT for detecting capsule disruption and local tissue invasion. US strongly depends on the skill of the operator and the quality of the US equipment, and it is limited for detection of retrotracheal and intrathoracic extension of the thyroid malignancy. The extension of tumor into adjacent soft tissues and vessels of the neck is the main purpose of CT and MRI in assessing patients with thyroid carcinoma, with MRI having the best contrast resolution. Posttreatment imaging should be performed at 3 to 6 months and include thoracic radiography and pertechnetate scintigraphy.

Canine Hypothyroidism

Hypothyroidism in adult dogs is almost always the result of a primary dysfunction of the thyroid gland resulting from an immune-mediated lymphocytic thyroiditis or idiopathic atrophy of the gland. With much practice and skill, US is a sensitive and quick test for the diagnosis of primary hypothyroidism. US features include decreased echogenicity, gland inhomogeneity, irregular capsule delineation, abnormal lobe shape, and decreased relative thyroid volume. These five parameters combined result in an overall sensitivity of 94.1% in hypothyroid dogs. A continuous decrease of thyroid volume is seen over time after treatment with levothyroxine, whereas the other features do not change significantly with time. Scintigraphy should show decreased or absent uptake of pertechnetate in primary hypothyroidism. However, the value of thyroid scintigraphy for detection of acquired primary hypothyroidism is controversial, and scintigraphic studies should be interpreted with caution.

In juvenile dogs, congenital primary hypothyroidism is only rarely diagnosed and can be the result of dysgenesis of the gland, dyshormonogenesis, or iodine deficiency. Radiography of the skeleton in patients with congenital hypothyroidism shows delayed closure of the sutures in the skull, delayed epiphyseal ossification, and epiphyseal dysgenesis (i.e., irregularly formed, fragmented, or stippled epiphyseal centers), mostly seen in the proximal tibia, humerus, femoral condyles, and vertebral bodies. The overall length of the long bones and vertebral bodies is reduced, and the skull is shortened and broad. Valgus limbs are common and result from retarded ossification of the carpal and tarsal bones. Thickening of the radial and ulnar cortices with increased medullary opacity and bowing of these bones also can be seen. Degenerative joint disease may develop at a later stage. Scintigraphy can be used to differentiate dysgenesis (minimal uptake) and dyshormonogenesis (normal or increased uptake).

Feline Hyperthyroidism

Hyperthyroidism is the most common endocrine disorder in cats; it is typically caused by functional thyroid adenomatous hyperplasia or hyperfunctioning adenoma. Thyroid lesions are bilateral in 70% of patients. Additionally, intrathoracic ectopic tissue has been reported in 8% to 25% of hyperthyroid cats (Figure 40-2). Ectopic thyroid tissue may be found everywhere between the base of the tongue and the base of the heart in a ventral location. On US, the thyroid glands of hyperthyroid cats initially appear increased in size, rounder, heterogeneous with hypoechoic or anechoic areas, and with an increased vascularity. Scintigraphy is characterized by increased radiopharmaceutical uptake in the area of the gland and allows assessment of bilateral versus unilateral disease, estimation of thyroid size or functional activity, identification of ectopic thyroid tissue, and potential detection of metastatic disease (see Figure 40-2). The mean thyroid-to-salivary ratio of abnormal lobes in hyperthyroid cats is 5.25 : 1 (range, 1.2 : 1 to 12.1 : 1). There is a good correlation between US and scintigraphy in differentiating

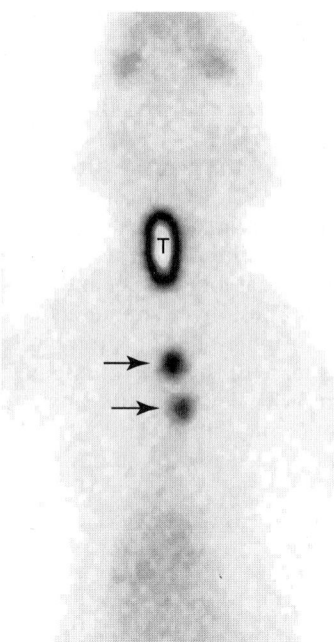

Figure 40-2 Scintigraphic image of a thyroid adenoma in an adult cat. Marked uptake is visible at the level of the left thyroid gland *(T)*. There are two areas of focal uptake at the entrance of the thorax corresponding to ectopic thyroid tissue *(arrows)*.

normal from abnormal thyroid lobes. Thyroid glands show decreased size, reduced rounding, reduced heterogeneity, and decreased vascularity 3 to 12 months after radioactive iodine treatment.

Imaging the Parathyroid Glands

US is a powerful tool for visualization of the normal parathyroid glands and for diagnosis of parathyroid tumors. The small (<2 mm in diameter and <3.3 mm in length) normal parathyroid glands are well-delineated structures that are anechoic to hypoechoic to the surrounding thyroid parenchyma. Parathyroid nodules greater than 4 mm in diameter are likely to be parathyroid adenomas or carcinomas.

Imaging the Adrenal Glands

Imaging of the adrenal glands is commonly performed to differentiate pituitary-dependent hyperadrenocorticism (PDH) from adrenal-dependent hyperadrenocorticism (ADH) in dogs based on morphologic criteria. Imaging also can be performed to help diagnose and evaluate neoplastic processes. However, abnormal hormonal secretion by the adrenal glands is not always accompanied by visible morphologic changes. Functional imaging modalities (single-photon emission computed tomography [SPECT], positron emission tomography [PET], functional MRI, contrast-enhanced US, contrast-enhanced CT) that allow differentiation of hyperfunctioning from nonfunctioning lesions are quickly emerging. This trend is reasonable because endocrinologic disorders should be approached dynamically in medical imaging as with hormonal testing.

The adrenal glands are small, paired abdominal glands located in the craniodorsal abdomen, medial to the ipsilateral kidney and adjacent to the aorta (left) and the caudal vena cava (right). These glands are composed of two morphologically and functionally different tissues: an outer cortex and an inner medulla. The cells of the adrenal cortex produce mainly cortisol and other glucocorticoids, whereas the chromaffin cells of the medulla produce catecholamines.

The US and CT approach and the appropriate MRI sequences needed for examination of the adrenal glands have been extensively described. The best landmarks for localization of the glands are vascular because both adrenal glands are cranial to the ipsilateral renal vessels and in the region of the celiac and cranial mesenteric arteries. In dogs, the normal glands are mainly linear in shape but have a variable degree of modification of their poles. This is especially evident in the cranial pole of the right gland, which tends to be consistently wider and of more variable shape. In cats, both glands are consistently oval to bilobed and contain mineralization in 30% of healthy cats. Adrenal glands are usually isoechoic to the cortex of the kidney and hypoechoic to surrounding fat. The cortex and the medulla can be frequently distinguished, with the cortex being hypoechoic and the medulla being hyperechoic. In other images, a hyperechoic rim is seen at the transition between cortex and medulla. Using MRI fast spin echo sequences, the adrenal glands may appear homogeneous and hypointense to surroundings or they may show a corticomedullary type of pattern with a hyperintense central area surrounded by a hypointense rim of tissue.

The visualization of both adrenal glands is mandatory during imaging examinations. Adrenal size is one of the imaging criteria used for differentiating normal glands from adrenal hyperplasia. A maximum diameter of 7.4 mm at the caudal pole offers a reasonable compromise to maximize sensitivity and specificity for both glands with regard to distinguishing normal from hyperplastic adrenal glands. More recent studies proposed the use of measurement values based on the dog's size or breed. A cutoff of 6.0 mm in small-breed dogs and 9.0 mm in large-breed dogs has been proposed in one study. In another study, upper thresholds for the left and right caudal height of the gland on a longitudinal slice of 7.9 mm and 9.45 mm (Labrador retriever) and 5.4 mm and 6.7 mm (Yorkshire terrier) have been suggested. It has still to be studied in which proportion the use of these more specific reference values may improve the sensitivity and specificity of US. The influence of stress and concurrent diseases on adrenal gland measurements has not been studied a great deal.

With the introduction of a radiolabeled microsphere methodology, which permitted independent measurement of blood flow into the two regions of the adrenal glands, it became apparent that the medulla and cortex in dogs regulate blood flow independently and that both regions receive levels of blood flow considerably greater than required for nutrient delivery. Abundant blood flow likely serves to speed entry of adrenal secretory products into the systemic circulation. Our preliminary experience with contrast-enhanced US has shown that normal adrenal glands give rise to diffuse, centrifugally intense, and homogeneous contrast enhancement because of the rich medullary capillary circulation. Abundant blood flow may also be linked to the high rate of adrenal involvement in metastatic cancer in dogs (21%) and cats (15%).

In most instances, "routine" evaluation of dogs with hyperadrenocorticism includes an abdominal US examination. US should be used as a test to help differentiate PDH from ADH and not as a screening test for Cushing's syndrome because of its low sensitivity and specificity for that diagnosis. US becomes more sensitive and specific when performed in association with biochemical studies. For instance, the sensitivity and specificity of adrenal US and endogenous adrenocorticotropic hormone determinations to identify the cause of hyperadrenocorticism were demonstrated to be 100% and 95%, respectively, for ADH when both indicate ADH. Measurements made on CT are of little value for directly determining the origin of hyperadrenocorticism. However, the use of an adrenal diameter ratio (maximal diameter ratio of the largest to the smallest adrenal glands) appears to distinguish PDH from ADH patients, with a ratio greater than 2.08 highly suggestive of ADH. A great advantage of CT and MRI is that they allow visualization of the pituitary gland and adrenal glands during the same examination.

Pituitary-Dependent Hyperadrenocorticism

The adrenal glands of dogs with PDH may have a plump appearance, are usually homogeneous and hypoechoic compared with the adjacent renal cortices, and are increased in size. Sometimes the glands show a heterogeneous parenchyma and focal areas of increased echogenicity. Contrast-enhanced US of the adrenal glands in untreated patients with PDH reveals a delayed appearance of the peak of enhancement in the cortex and medulla compared with normal control dogs. This delay might be related to the compression of the capillary network by the thickened cortex within the glands. High-dose trilostane treatment (60 mg daily for dogs weighing 5 to 20 kg or 120 mg daily for dogs weighing >20 kg) may induce an enlargement of the adrenal gland by more than 60% of its width or length. A more apparent distinction between the cortex and medulla also may be observed secondary to both a decrease in echogenicity of the hypoechoic outer zone and an increase in echogenicity in the hyperechoic center. After 1 year of treatment, the shape of the gland appears irregular, and the parenchyma becomes heterogeneous. It is the author's impression that these modifications are not as pronounced with lower dosages of trilostane.

Adrenal-Dependent Hyperadrenocorticism

Differentiating primary adrenocortical adenomas from carcinomas is difficult using morphologic imaging characteristics. Abdominal radiography may allow for visualization of an adrenal mass only if it is larger than 2 cm in diameter or calcified. On US and CT, carcinomas tend to be larger, rounder, irregularly outlined, and more invasive (into vessels or kidney) than adenomas (Figure 40-3). US has a sensitivity of 80% and a specificity of 90% for detection of a caval thrombus. Thrombi confined to the phrenicoabdominal vein are more likely to be missed on

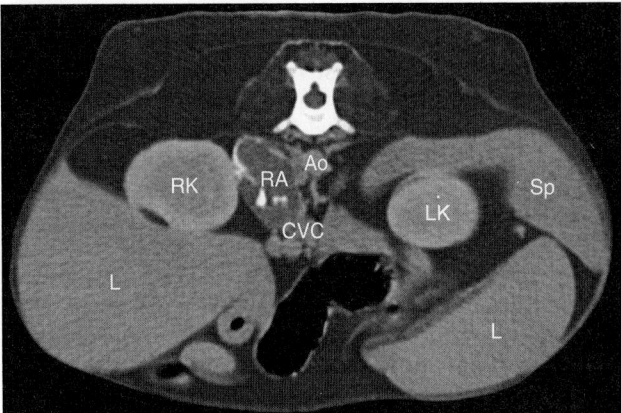

Figure 40-3 Transverse CT image of an adult dog with right adrenal carcinoma. The right adrenal gland *(RA)* is rounded, has heterogeneous density, and contains mineral densities at the periphery. Vascular compression, even invasion, is suspected. *Ao,* Aorta; *CVC,* caudal vena cava; *L,* liver; *LK,* left kidney; *RK,* right kidney; *Sp,* spleen.

both US and contrast-enhanced CT. For these reasons, detection of neoplastic involvement of adjacent structures is considered an important prognostic factor for surgical treatment.

The echogenicity or density of the mass, the presence of mineralization, or the finding of bilateral gland involvement cannot distinguish between adenoma and carcinoma. Bilateral adrenocortical tumors seem to be more common than previously assumed (up to 20% of all cases of ADH). If an adrenocortical tumor is unilateral and the contralateral gland is small (≤5 mm in width), a secreting adrenocortical tumor is highly suspected, but this finding is inconsistent.

Pheochromocytoma

On imaging, dogs with pheochromocytoma, a neuroendocrine tumor, may have normal adrenal glands (about 15%) or a mass lesion (about 85%) that may be unilateral or bilateral. Most US features of pheochromocytomas are similar to US features of adrenocortical tumors, but there are some important differences with pheochromocytoma: (1) calcification of the glands is rarely observed, (2) caval thrombi are more frequently observed, and (3) there is a direct correlation between size of the tumor and severity of clinical signs. MRI is a promising diagnostic modality for pheochromocytomas because it has the advantage of higher sensitivity for detection of hemorrhage and necrosis. Nuclear scintigraphy using radiolabeled metaiodobenzylguanidine has been used to localize adrenal, ectopic, and disseminated pheochromocytomas in dogs. p-[18F] Fluorobenzylguanidine is a norepinephrine analog that has been developed as a PET-imaging radiopharmaceutical for use in imaging tumors of neuroendocrine origin, including pheochromocytoma.

Other Adrenal Abnormalities

The benefit of imaging the adrenal glands in canine hypoadrenocorticism (Addison's disease) is quite limited. The adrenal glands in affected dogs can show a significant reduction in length and thickness on US, along with a change in shape. A left adrenal thickness of less than 3.2 mm is strongly suggestive of hypoadrenocorticism. However, imaging also can appear normal. In dogs with hypoadrenocorticism caused by adrenal necrosis after a brief treatment with trilostane, US initially demonstrates large hypoechoic adrenal cortices, which subsequently became small and heterogeneous.

Feline adrenal diseases are rare and mainly evaluated by US. Hyperadrenocorticism in cats shows similar imaging findings as in dogs. Feline hyperaldosteronism is most commonly caused by an adrenocortical tumor (44% carcinoma, 41% adenoma). Bilateral infiltration is not uncommon (22%) and rarely detected with US. Bilateral micronodular hyperplasia of the zona glomerulosa in cats is also reported in hyperaldosteronism and most likely is underdiagnosed because the adrenal gland may not show US abnormalities.

Incidentalomas ("incidental adrenal mass") are adrenal masses discovered during an imaging study performed for indications other than adrenal disease. Their frequency has dramatically increased since the advent of higher resolution imaging techniques. To manage the phenomenon, radiologists working in human medicine have proposed many algorithms. In veterinary medicine, decisions about the appropriate diagnostic workup for dogs with an adrenal incidentaloma should be based on clinical findings and the owner's willingness to have laboratory or imaging investigations performed. It may be helpful to consult with a specialist in endocrine disease.

Imaging the Pituitary Gland

The pituitary gland is located within the hypophyseal (sellar) fossa of the basisphenoid bone and consists of two embryologically distinct components: the neurohypophysis (centrally) and the adenohypophysis (peripherally). The normal pituitary gland is visible on both CT and MRI. Several protocols for dynamic CT and MRI examinations of the canine and feline pituitary gland have been described emphasizing the importance of obtaining thin slices (1 to 2 mm). On CT, mean precontrast attenuation values of the normal canine pituitary gland are approximately 50 HU in the central parts and 70 HU in peripheral parts. If a dynamic contrast CT scan is performed, earlier enhancement of the arterial phase of the centrally located neurohyphophysis ("pituitary flush") is observed first, followed by delayed enhancement of the adenohypophysis through the portal blood supply. The degree and timing of maximum enhancement vary with contrast medium dose, speed of injection, and patient factors. In dogs, maximum enhancements of the central and peripheral parts have been reported at 0 to 28 seconds and 14 to 70 seconds following peak enhancement of the maxillary artery. Maximum contrast enhancement occurs at 14 to 50 seconds from the onset of contrast medium injection in cats. On MRI, the neurohypophysis may be observed as a bright spot on precontrast T1-weighted images depending on the vasopressin concentration in the pars nervosa of the neurohypophysis.

CT and MRI are used for imaging the pituitary gland in dogs with suspected PDH or in cats with acromegaly;

both disorders are commonly due to a functional pituitary adenoma. Pituitary measurements may be used to differentiate adenoma from invasive adenoma (>1.9 cm in vertical height) combined with other criteria such as age. More commonly, normalization to a body index (brain area) is performed to evaluate the pituitary gland leading to the use of a height-to-brain ratio (P/B ratio = pituitary gland height in mm × 100/brain area in mm^2). This ratio is used on postcontrast images to distinguish normal (P/B ratio ≤0.31 mm^{-1}) from enlarged (P/B ratio >0.31 mm^{-1}) pituitary glands. A small or missing pituitary gland is observed in approximately 3% of dogs and is considered an incidental variant. However, care must be taken not to confuse an empty sella with a cystic malformation (Rathke's cleft) or cystic mass occupying the fossa. Pituitary cysts are not unusual in healthy dogs, particularly brachycephalic breeds, but they are also seen in dogs with congenital growth hormone deficiency (pituitary dwarfism).

Low-field MRI and dynamic CT provide comparable information regarding the diagnosis of pituitary adenoma in the diagnosis of PDH. Pituitary macroadenomas are characterized by suprasellar extension of a pituitary "mass" of variable size, homogeneity, and margination that may compress or invade the diencephalon. Macroadenomas are usually hyperintense on T2-weighted sequences and isointense on T1-weighted sequences (Figure 40-4, A and B). Most macroadenomas are enhanced after contrast administration (Figure 40-4, C). Because the normal pituitary naturally enhances after contrast administration, some contrast agent uptake in some adenomas may not be as great as for normal, surrounding tissues. Pituitary macroadenomas and rare adenocarcinomas share the same imaging features, although any osseous involvement or presence of metastases is consistent with carcinoma. Concurrent findings (e.g., hemorrhage, hydrocephalus, brain edema, mass effect) are similar to findings of other extraaxial brain tumors. A diagnosis of pituitary microadenoma is usually made by exclusion in dogs if no pituitary enlargement is identified on imaging. Both the pituitary flush on dynamic CT and the bright spot on precontrast T1-weighted MRI can identify an absent or displaced pituitary (neurohypophyseal) flush and indirectly suggest the presence of a microtumor. A normal CT study (conventional and dynamic) does not rule out PDH.

Imaging the Pancreas

Imaging the pancreas in patients with diabetes mellitus may provide useful information regarding the potential presence of an underlying pancreatitis that is usually of the chronic form and less likely of the acute form (Table 40-2). Acute pancreatitis causes a pancreatic mass effect or enlargement, changes in echogenicity (US) or density (CT), and lack of contrast enhancement on US and CT. Pancreatic enlargement also may be suspected on radiography when the duodenum is laterally displaced and the transverse colon is caudally displaced. Another feature can be peritonitis causing peritoneal effusion directly visible on US and CT and local inflammation of the mesentery, which appears hyperechoic on US

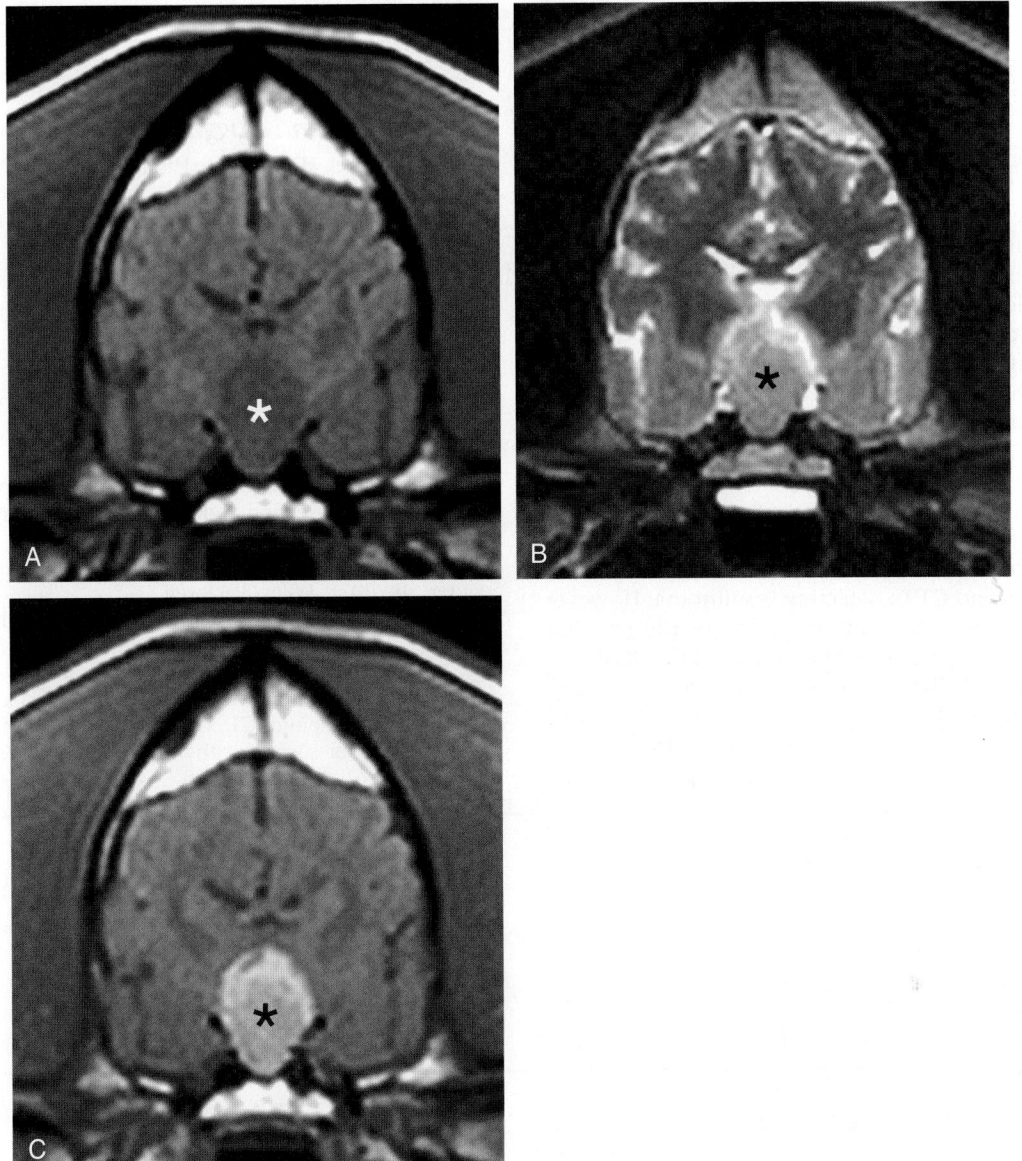

Figure 40-4 Transverse MRI of a pituitary macroadenoma *(asterisks)* in an adult dog. **A,** On T1-weighted image, the mass appears isointense (compared with surrounding musculature). **B,** On T2-weighted images, the mass is hyperintense. **C,** Postcontrast T1-weighted image shows moderate uptake of contrast agent.

and hazy or ill-defined on CT. Peritonitis secondary to pancreatitis is suspected radiographically when serosal detail is lost in the right cranial hemiabdomen and the descending duodenum is dilated and static. In severe cases, peripancreatic vasculature thrombosis is observed on CT. Pain on transducer pressure localized over the area of the pancreas is often a notable feature during US examination. Chronic pancreatitis can be associated with a reduced size of the pancreas, irregular widening of the pancreatic duct, the presence of intraparenchymal or extraparenchymal mineralization, and a mixed or mottled echogenicity (US) or density (CT) of the pancreatic parenchyma, best illustrated on postcontrast US and CT studies.

TABLE 40-2

Sensitivity of Imaging Modalities for Diagnosis of Pancreatic Disorders

Sensitivity	Acute Pancreatitis	Chronic Pancreatitis
Radiography	Low	Low
Ultrasonography	70% in dogs 10%-30% in cats	Low
Computed tomography	NR	Low

NR, Not reported.

Pancreatic Endocrine Neoplasia

Insulinoma is the most common canine pancreatic endocrine tumor; it is rare in cats. This tumor often metastasizes (liver, kidneys, regional lymph nodes) and is frequently accompanied by hypoglycemia and hyperinsulinemia. US can be used for the initial evaluation of dogs with hypoglycemia including detection of metastases. Insulinomas appear on US as solitary or multiple nodules or ill-defined areas of abnormal echogenicity, mainly smaller than 2.5 cm in diameter. Because of these features, the diagnosis of insulinomas using gray-scale US is challenging and often disappointing. It is the author's experience that contrast-enhanced US or dual-phase contrast CT greatly improves the detection of these tumors. Using these techniques, neuroendocrine tumors appear hypervascular showing a marked contrast-enhancing mass in the arterial phase and early decrease in enhancement in the portal phase contrary to the mildly contrast-enhancing pancreatic adenocarcinoma. SPECT appears as effective as US and CT in detecting insulinoma. However, intraoperative inspection and palpation of the pancreas remains more sensitive than the imaging modalities.

Gastrinoma (Zollinger-Ellison syndrome) is a rare gastrin-producing, non-β islet cell pancreatic tumor that results in gastric acid hypersecretion and gastrointestinal ulceration. US, CT, and somatostatin receptor scintigraphy are indicated to define the primary tumor and metastatic lesions.

References and Suggested Reading

Auriemma E et al: Computed tomography and low-field magnetic resonance imaging of the pituitary gland in dogs with pituitary-dependent hyperadrenocorticism: 11 cases (2001-2003), *J Am Vet Med Assoc* 235:409, 2009.

Barthez PY, Nyland TG, Feldman EC: Ultrasonography of the adrenal glands in the dog, cat, and ferret, *Vet Clin North Am Small Anim Pract* 28:869, 1998.

Harvey AM et al: Scintigraphic findings in 120 hyperthyroid cats, *J Feline Med Surg* 11:96, 2009.

Pey P et al: Contrast-enhanced ultrasonography of the normal canine adrenal gland, *Vet Radiol Ultrasound* 52:560, 2011.

Robben JH et al: Comparison of ultrasonography, computed tomography, and single-photon emission computed tomography for the detection and localization of canine insulinoma, *J Vet Intern Med* 19:15, 2005.

Schwarz T, Saunders J: *Veterinary computed tomography*, Chichester, UK, 2011, Wiley-Blackwell.

Taeymans O, Peremans K, Saunders JH: Thyroid imaging in the dog: current status and future directions, *J Vet Intern Med* 21:673, 2007.

Taeymans O, Penninck DG, Peters RM: Comparison between clinical, ultrasound, CT, MRI and pathology findings in dogs presented for suspected thyroid carcinoma, *Vet Radiol Ultrasound* 54:61, 2013.

CHAPTER 41

Approach to Critical Illness–Related Corticosteroid Insufficiency

LINDA G. MARTIN, *Pullman, Washington*

Critical illness–related corticosteroid insufficiency (CIRCI), previously known as relative adrenal insufficiency, is a topic of debate in both human and veterinary medicine. The clinical syndrome of CIRCI is controversial, but it has been reported in critically ill human patients with systemic inflammation associated with sepsis or septic shock, acute respiratory distress syndrome or acute lung injury, trauma, severe hepatic disease, and acute myocardial infarction, as well as following cardiopulmonary bypass. More recently, insufficient adrenal or pituitary function has been identified in dogs with sepsis or septic shock (Burkitt et al, 2007; Martin et al, 2008), trauma (Martin et al, 2008), gastric dilation-volvulus (Martin et al, 2008), and neoplasia (lymphoma and several types of nonhematopoietic tumors) (Boozer et al, 2005) and in cats with sepsis or septic shock (Costello et al, 2006), trauma (Durkan et al, 2007), and neoplasia (lymphoma) (Farrelly et al, 1999).

In contrast to patients with hypoadrenocorticism, patients with CIRCI usually have a normal or elevated basal serum cortisol concentration and a blunted cortisol response to an adrenocorticotropic hormone (ACTH) stimulation test. This syndrome is characterized by an inadequate production of cortisol in relation to an increased demand during periods of severe stress, such as critical illnesses. After recovery, hypothalamic-pituitary-adrenal (HPA) dysfunction resolves. The HPA dysfunction is transient and relative.

Pathophysiology and Causes

The pathogenesis of CIRCI in dogs and cats is unknown but it is most likely multifactorial, involving complex interactions between endocrine and immune systems. Possible mechanisms for the development of CIRCI in humans and animals include the following:

1. Proinflammatory cytokine-mediated inhibition of corticotropin-releasing hormone (CRH) and ACTH secretion resulting in decreased cortisol production
2. Proinflammatory cytokine-mediated corticosteroid receptor dysfunction and reduction in receptor numbers, whereby a reduction in the activity or number of receptors would reduce the ability of cells to respond appropriately to cortisol
3. Corticostatin-mediated (peptide produced by immune cells) ACTH receptor antagonism, resulting in impaired adrenocortical function via corticostatin competing with ACTH and binding to its receptor
4. Leptin-mediated (adipose-derived hormone) inhibition of HPA axis during stress or illness
5. Tissue resistance to the actions of cortisol, whereby several factors may be involved, including decreased cortisol access to tissues secondary to a reduction of circulating cortisol-binding globulin and increased cytokine-mediated conversion of cortisol (active) to cortisone (inactive)
6. Disruption of pituitary or adrenal gland function secondary to extensive tissue destruction by infection, infarction, hemorrhage, or thrombosis

The *ABCB1* gene mutation that results in lack of P-glycoprotein (Pgp) at the blood-brain barrier may also be a contributing factor in some dog breeds (e.g., collies, Shetland sheepdogs, Australian shepherds, Old English sheepdogs, English shepherds, German shepherds, long-haired whippets, silken windhounds). Pgp restricts the entry of cortisol into the brain, limiting cortisol's feedback inhibition of CRH and ACTH. In *ABCB1* mutant dogs, Pgp is not present, allowing greater concentrations of cortisol within the brain. There is greater feedback inhibition of the HPA axis and, ultimately, inhibition of sufficient cortisol secretion, potentially leading to the inability to respond appropriately to critical illness and stress.

Clinical Signs

Clinical signs of CIRCI can be vague and nonspecific, such as depression, weakness, fever, vomiting, diarrhea, and abdominal pain. In addition, clinical signs that are secondary to the underlying disease process responsible for CIRCI (e.g., septic shock, hepatic disease, trauma) can mask the clinical features of CIRCI. The most common clinical abnormality associated with CIRCI in critically ill human patients is hypotension refractory to fluid resuscitation, requiring vasopressor therapy. Hyponatremia and hyperkalemia, abnormalities consistent with aldosterone deficiency, are uncommon in humans with CIRCI and, to date, have not been reported in canine or feline critically ill patients with insufficient adrenal or pituitary function. Laboratory assessment of critically ill human patients with CIRCI may demonstrate eosinophilia or hypoglycemia or both, but these abnormalities are not consistently found in all humans with CIRCI. Eosinophilia and hypoglycemia have not been reported in critically ill veterinary patients with CIRCI.

Diagnosis

CIRCI should be considered as a differential diagnosis in all critically ill patients requiring vasopressor support. At the present time, there is no consensus regarding the identification of patients with CIRCI in human or veterinary medicine, and normal reference ranges do not exist for basal and ACTH-stimulated cortisol concentrations in critically ill dogs and cats.

Various tests have been recommended for diagnosing CIRCI, including random serum or plasma (total) basal cortisol concentration, serum free cortisol concentration, ACTH-stimulated cortisol concentration, delta cortisol concentration (the difference when subtracting basal from ACTH-stimulated cortisol concentration), the cortisol-to-endogenous ACTH ratio, and combinations of these methods. The optimal way to identify critically ill veterinary patients with CIRCI has yet to be determined.

Evaluation of adrenal function in veterinary patients typically involves administration of an ACTH stimulation test. The most commonly used protocol for ACTH stimulation testing in dogs involves intravenous administration of 5 µg/kg of cosyntropin, up to a maximum of 250 µg. In cats, intravenous administration of 125 µg/cat of cosyntropin is commonly used. Serum or plasma is obtained for cortisol analysis before and 60 minutes after ACTH administration for both dogs and cats. The standard doses of cosyntropin (5 µg/kg in dogs and 125 µg/cat) currently used are greater than the doses necessary to produce maximal adrenocortical stimulation in healthy small animals. Doses of 0.5 µg/kg in healthy dogs (Martin et al, 2007) and 5 µg/kg in healthy cats (DeClue et al, 2011) have been shown to induce maximal adrenocortical cortisol secretion. The use of higher doses is considered supraphysiologic and may hinder the identification of dogs and cats with CIRCI. Low-dose (0.5 µg/kg IV) ACTH stimulation testing has been compared with standard-dose (5 µg/kg IV) testing in critically ill dogs (Martin et al, 2010). Every critically ill dog that was identified to have insufficient adrenal function (i.e., ACTH-stimulated serum cortisol concentration below the reference range or <5% greater than the basal cortisol concentration) by the standard-dose ACTH stimulation test was also identified by the low-dose test. Additional dogs with adrenal insufficiency were identified by the low-dose ACTH stimulation test but not by the standard-dose test. ACTH administered at a dose of 0.5 µg/kg IV appears to be at least as accurate in determining adrenal function in critically ill dogs as the standard dose. The low-dose ACTH stimulation test may be a more sensitive diagnostic test in detecting patients with insufficient adrenal gland function than the standard-dose test.

Assays that measure cortisol concentration typically measure total hormone concentration (i.e., serum free or unbound cortisol plus a protein-bound fraction). However, the serum free cortisol fraction is thought to be responsible for the physiologic function of the hormone. Serum free cortisol concentrations may be a more precise predictor of adrenal gland function.

The relationship between free and total cortisol varies with serum protein concentration. In critically ill human patients, cortisol-binding globulin and albumin concentrations can decrease by approximately 50% because of catabolism at the inflammatory sites and inhibition of hepatic synthesis via cytokine induction. Serum total cortisol concentration may be falsely low in hypoproteinemic patients, resulting in overestimation of CIRCI. Serum free cortisol concentration is less likely to be altered in states of hypoproteinemia. Consequently, serum total cortisol concentrations may not accurately represent the biologic activity of serum free cortisol during critical illness. Several human studies suggest that serum free cortisol concentrations are a more accurate measure of circulating glucocorticoid activity than total cortisol concentrations. At this time, canine and feline studies are sparse, and the ability to measure serum free cortisol concentration is not widely available. However, serum free and total cortisol concentrations were compared in a group of 35 critically ill dogs having one of the following diseases: sepsis, severe trauma, or gastric dilation-volvulus (Martin et al, 2010). Fewer critically ill dogs with adrenal insufficiency (i.e., an ACTH-stimulated serum cortisol concentration below the reference range or <5% greater than the basal cortisol concentration) were identified by serum free cortisol concentration than by serum total cortisol concentration. However, basal and ACTH-stimulated serum total cortisol concentrations were not lower in hypoproteinemic dogs compared with normoproteinemic dogs. The significance of this finding is unknown, and further investigation is warranted in veterinary patients.

The delta cortisol concentration has been advocated as a method to identify critically ill patients with CIRCI in both human and veterinary medicine. A study in human patients with septic shock found that basal cortisol concentrations of 34 µg/dl (938 nmol/L) or less combined with delta cortisol concentrations of 9 µg/dl (250 nmol/L) or more in response to an IV 250 µg/person ACTH stimulation test were associated with a favorable prognosis. In addition, basal cortisol concentrations greater than 34 µg/dl combined with delta cortisol concentrations less than 9 µg/dl were associated with a poor prognosis. Because this protocol was successful in predicting outcome, a delta cortisol concentration less than 9 µg/dl is frequently used as the diagnostic criterion for CIRCI in critically ill human patients.

Veterinary studies have also assessed delta cortisol concentration as a criterion for diagnosing CIRCI in critically ill patients. One study found that septic dogs with delta cortisol concentrations of 3 µg/dl (83 nmol/L) or less after an IM 250 µg/dog ACTH stimulation test were more likely to have systemic hypotension and decreased survival (Burkitt et al, 2007). In addition, another study investigating acutely ill dogs (i.e., dogs with sepsis, severe trauma, or gastric dilation-volvulus) found that dogs with delta cortisol concentrations of 3 µg/dl or less after an IV 5 µg/kg ACTH stimulation test were more likely to require vasopressor therapy as part of their treatment plan (Martin et al, 2008). Sensitivity of delta cortisol concentrations of 3 µg/dl or less in the diagnosis of critically ill veterinary patients with CIRCI has yet to be determined.

A further confounding factor in interpreting pituitary-adrenal function tests of any kind is that parameters can change over time. Test results obtained on a single day may not reflect the findings on previous or future days. The relationship between abnormal parameters can also change over time. For example, dogs that died from parvoviral diarrhea had a lower delta cortisol concentration than dogs that survived on day 1 of hospitalization but not on day 3 (Schoeman and Herrtage, 2008).

Based on the current veterinary literature, three scenarios may indicate the presence of CIRCI in critically ill dogs (especially in the presence of refractory hypotension): (1) dogs with a normal or an elevated basal cortisol concentration and an ACTH-stimulated cortisol concentration less than the normal reference range, (2) dogs with a normal or an elevated basal cortisol concentration and an ACTH-stimulated cortisol concentration that is less than 5% greater than the basal cortisol concentration (flatline response), or (3) dogs with a delta cortisol concentration of 3 µg/dl or less (≤83 nmol/L). Based on a few clinical studies and case reports, CIRCI also appears to occur in cats. However, there is no consensus regarding the diagnostic criteria in cats at this time.

At the present time, it is recommended that ACTH stimulation testing not be used to identify human patients with septic shock who should receive supplemental corticosteroid therapy. This recommendation is based on the lack of compelling evidence demonstrating that a patient's response to ACTH administration predicts the benefit from corticosteroid therapy. Similarly, no studies in veterinary medicine have investigated the usefulness of ACTH stimulation (or other diagnostic) testing for identifying patients that would benefit from supplemental corticosteroid therapy. ACTH stimulation testing may still prove useful in veterinary patients if only to gain more information on the syndrome of CIRCI in animals and to help identify animals that should receive supplemental corticosteroid treatment. The results of ACTH stimulation testing also can be used to decide if corticosteroid therapy should be stopped or continued (see next section on Treatment).

Treatment

Critically ill human patients with CIRCI who are treated with supplemental doses of corticosteroids are more likely to be quickly weaned from vasopressor therapy and ventilatory support, and some treated groups are more likely to survive with CIRCI. However, the optimal dose and duration of treatment with glucocorticoids in human patients with CIRCI have yet to be determined. The dosages of glucocorticoids used to treat human patients with CIRCI are variously referred to as supplemental,

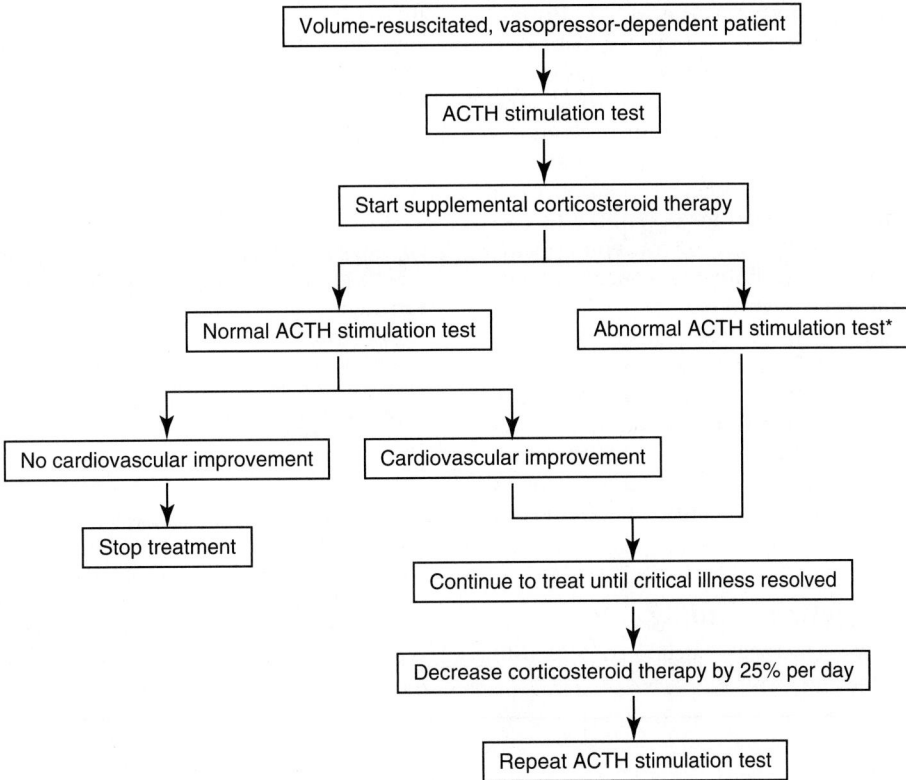

Figure 41-1 Treatment algorithm for the use of supplemental corticosteroids in veterinary patients with suspected CIRCI. *For CIRCI, abnormal ACTH stimulation test results are (1) normal or elevated basal cortisol concentration and ACTH-stimulated cortisol concentration less than the normal reference range, (2) normal or elevated basal cortisol concentration and ACTH-stimulated cortisol concentration less than 5% greater than the basal cortisol concentration (flatline response), or (3) delta cortisol concentration less than 3 µg/dl (<83 nmol/L).

physiologic, supraphysiologic, low dose, stress dose, or replacement.

Hydrocortisone appears to be the corticosteroid of choice to treat human patients with CIRCI. This choice is based on more recent studies (after 1997) that used longer courses of lower dose hydrocortisone and demonstrated improved shock reversal and survival rates. Earlier studies (before 1989) used predominantly short courses of high-dose dexamethasone, betamethasone, or methylprednisolone and reported increased mortality and higher secondary infection rates. Most human protocols have used hydrocortisone dosages of 200 to 300 mg IV per 24 hours for an average 70-kg person (2.9 to 4.3 mg/kg/24 hours IV). Typically, the total daily dose either is given as a constant rate infusion or is divided and given every 6 hours. Hydrocortisone is one fourth as potent as prednisone and one thirtieth as potent as dexamethasone. The equivalent dosages are prednisone 0.7 to 1 mg/kg/24 hours or dexamethasone 0.1 to 0.4 mg/kg/24 hours. The hydrocortisone dose currently recommended for CIRCI in human patients is supraphysiologic (the human physiologic dose of hydrocortisone is 0.2 to 0.4 mg/kg/24 hours), resulting in a serum cortisol concentration several times higher than achieved by ACTH stimulation.

Currently there are no guidelines for treatment of CIRCI in critically ill veterinary patients. However, it is reasonable to start volume-resuscitated, vasopressor-dependent critically ill animals on corticosteroid therapy

after performing an ACTH stimulation test. When the test results are available, treatment can be withdrawn in animals that responded normally to the ACTH stimulation test. Corticosteroids can be continued in patients that have (1) a normal or elevated basal cortisol concentration and an ACTH-stimulated cortisol concentration less than the normal reference range, (2) a normal or elevated basal cortisol concentration and an ACTH-stimulated cortisol concentration that is less than 5% greater than the basal cortisol concentration (flat line response), (3) a delta cortisol concentration 3 µg/dl or less (≤83 nmol/L), or (4) a clinically demonstrated significant improvement in cardiovascular status within 24 hours of starting corticosteroid therapy (Figure 41-1).

The appropriate dosage, duration, and type of corticosteroid therapy are unknown in veterinary patients with CIRCI. However, it is reasonable to give supplemental doses of corticosteroids at physiologic to supraphysiologic dosages: 1 to 4.3 mg/kg/24 hours IV of hydrocortisone (total daily dose can be divided into four equal doses and given every 6 hours or as a constant rate infusion), 0.25 to 1 mg/kg/24 hours IV of prednisone (total daily dose can be divided into two equal doses and given every 12 hours), or 0.04 to 0.4 mg/kg/24 hours IV of dexamethasone. Supplemental corticosteroid therapy should be started as soon as patients are observed to be poorly responsive to vasopressor therapy. If therapy is started before an ACTH stimulation test is done, dexamethasone should be used, and the ACTH stimulation test should be performed as soon as possible (within 4 hours). Prednisone and hydrocortisone cross-react on cortisol assays and falsely elevate the cortisol concentration; if a single dose of either corticosteroid is given, an ACTH stimulation test cannot be done for 12 hours. In the author's opinion, poor responsiveness to vasopressor therapy can be defined as the need for dopamine greater than 15 µg/kg/min or norepinephrine or epinephrine greater than 0.5 µg/kg/min to maintain a mean arterial blood pressure greater than 60 mm Hg.

Because HPA dysfunction in CIRCI is transient, lifelong therapy with corticosteroids is not thought to be required, and treatment is tapered after resolution of the critical illness. The corticosteroid dose can be tapered by 25% per day after resolution of the critical illness. An ACTH stimulation test should be repeated to confirm the return of normal adrenocortical function after discontinuation of corticosteroid supplementation.

References and Suggested Reading

Boozer AL et al: Pituitary-adrenal axis function in dogs with neoplasia, Vet Comp Oncol 3:194, 2005.
Burkitt JM et al: Relative adrenal insufficiency in dogs with sepsis, J Vet Intern Med 21:226, 2007.
Costello MF et al: Adrenal insufficiency in feline sepsis, Proceedings of the American College of Veterinary Emergency and Critical Care Postgraduate Course 2006, Sepsis in Veterinary Medicine, San Francisco, CA, 2006, p 41.
DeClue AE et al: Cortisol and aldosterone response to various doses of cosyntropin in healthy cats, J Am Vet Med Assoc 238:176, 2011.
Durkan S et al: Suspected relative adrenal insufficiency in a critically ill cat, J Vet Emerg Crit Care 17:197, 2007.
Farrelly J et al: Evaluation of pituitary-adrenal function in cats with lymphoma, Proceedings of the 19th Annual Veterinary Cancer Society Conference, Wood's Hole, MA, 1999, p 33.
Martin LG et al: Effect of low doses of cosyntropin on serum cortisol concentrations in clinically normal dogs, Am J Vet Res 68:555, 2007.
Martin LG et al: Pituitary-adrenal function in dogs with acute critical illness, J Am Vet Med Assoc 233:87, 2008.
Martin LG et al: Comparison of low-dose and standard-dose ACTH stimulation tests in critically ill dogs by assessment of serum total and free cortisol concentrations, J Vet Intern Med 24:685, 2010.
Schoeman JP, Herrtage ME: Adrenal function in critically ill puppies with parvoviral diarrhea, J Vet Intern Med 22:726, 2008.

CHAPTER 42
Canine Hypothyroidism

J. CATHARINE R. SCOTT-MONCRIEFF, *West Lafayette, Indiana*

Clinical signs of hypothyroidism result from decreased production of thyroxine (T_4) and triiodothyronine (T_3) by the thyroid gland. Acquired primary hypothyroidism is most common in dogs and usually is caused by either lymphocytic thyroiditis or idiopathic thyroid atrophy. Secondary hypothyroidism (deficiency of thyroid-stimulating hormone [TSH]) is less commonly recognized in dogs.

Cause

Approximately 50% of cases of primary hypothyroidism are caused by lymphocytic thyroiditis. Grossly, the thyroid gland may be normal or atrophic, whereas histologically there is multifocal or diffuse infiltration of the thyroid gland by lymphocytes, plasma cells, and macrophages. As thyroiditis progresses, the parenchyma is destroyed and replaced by fibrous connective tissue. Initially, thyroiditis may be subclinical, but progression to overt hypothyroidism can occur. Idiopathic thyroid atrophy, in which there is loss of thyroid parenchyma

and replacement by adipose and connective tissue, may represent end-stage thyroiditis rather than a separate disease process. Canine thyroiditis is believed to be immune mediated, and antithyroglobulin antibodies (ATAs) are a sensitive marker of thyroid inflammation. Approximately 50% of hypothyroid dogs have ATAs; however, the prevalence varies widely among breeds, which reflects a familial tendency for thyroiditis and resultant hypothyroidism.

Signalment

Any breed can develop hypothyroidism; however, some breeds, such as the golden retriever and the Doberman pinscher, have been reported to be at higher risk. Thyroiditis is clearly heritable in the beagle and the borzoi, and many other common breeds, such as the golden retriever, Great Dane, Irish setter, Doberman pinscher, and Old English sheepdog, have a high prevalence of ATAs. The rate of clinical progression of thyroiditis also varies among breeds. In beagles, the prevalence of thyroiditis can reach 40%, but if thyroiditis progresses to hypothyroidism, it occurs in middle age or later (Scott-Moncrieff et al, 2006). In other breeds, such as golden retrievers, thyroiditis appears to progress more rapidly, with some dogs diagnosed at 2 years of age. Middle-aged dogs generally are at increased risk of hypothyroidism. In one study, mean age at diagnosis was 7 years (range, 0.5 to 15 years).

Clinical Signs

Clinical features of hypothyroidism are insidious in onset, and hypothyroidism is commonly misdiagnosed because of nonspecific clinical signs affecting multiple body systems. Clinical signs attributable to decreased metabolic rate include lethargy, mental dullness, weight gain, unwillingness to exercise, and cold intolerance.

Dermatologic findings include dry scaly skin, changes in hair coat quality or color, symmetrical alopecia, seborrhea, and superficial pyoderma. Hyperkeratosis, hyperpigmentation, comedo formation, hypertrichosis, ceruminous otitis, poor wound healing, increased bruising, and myxedema also may occur. Alopecia is usually bilaterally symmetrical (see Chapter 39) and is first evident in areas of wear, whereas the head and extremities tend to be spared. The hair may be brittle and easily epilated, and loss of undercoat or primary guard hairs may result in a coarse appearance or a puppy-like hair coat. Fading of coat color may occur, and failure of hair regrowth after clipping is common. Hypothyroid dogs are also predisposed to recurrent bacterial infections of the skin.

Reproductive dysfunction has been attributed to hypothyroidism. There is little evidence for male reproductive dysfunction associated with hypothyroidism; however, bitches with radioactive iodine (^{131}I)–induced hypothyroidism have reduced fertility, prolongation of parturition, and higher periparturient mortality compared with euthyroid bitches (Panciera et al, 2007).

Both the peripheral nervous system and the central nervous system may be affected by hypothyroidism. Subclinical myopathy is well documented in hypothyroid dogs (Rossmeisl, 2010). Peripheral nerve dysfunction also has been described in association with hypothyroidism. Affected dogs have exercise intolerance, generalized weakness, ataxia, tetraparesis or paralysis, deficits of conscious proprioception, and decreased spinal reflexes. Some affected dogs have multifocal dysfunction of cranial nerves (facial, trigeminal, vestibulocochlear). Clinical signs resolve with levothyroxine sodium (L-thyroxine) supplementation. Rarely, central neurologic dysfunction (seizures, central vestibular dysfunction, disorientation, and mentation changes) is observed as a result of cerebral or cerebellar infarction, atherosclerosis, myxedema, coma, and blood viscosity changes secondary to hyperlipidemia. Overall, hypothyroidism is a rare cause of seizure disorders in dogs (Higgins et al, 2006). Although laryngeal paralysis and megaesophagus have been reported in association with hypothyroidism, treatment of hypothyroidism does not consistently result in resolution of clinical signs, and a causal relationship has not been established. Behavioral abnormalities that have been attributed to canine hypothyroidism include aggression and cognitive dysfunction; however, evidence for a causal association between behavioral problems and hypothyroidism is lacking.

Hypothyroidism can cause cardiovascular changes, such as sinus bradycardia, weak apex beat, low QRS voltage, and inverted T waves. Reduced left ventricular pump function has been documented in hypothyroidism and may exacerbate clinical signs in dogs with underlying cardiac disease. Although hypothyroidism is rarely the primary cause of myocardial failure in dogs, dilated cardiomyopathy and hypothyroidism may occur concurrently.

Congenital hypothyroidism results in mental retardation and stunted, disproportionate growth caused by epiphyseal dysgenesis and delayed skeletal maturation. Affected dogs are mentally dull and have large broad heads, short thick necks, short limbs, macroglossia, hypothermia, delayed dental eruption, ataxia, and abdominal distention. A palpable goiter may be present, depending on the cause of the congenital defect. Other clinical signs include gait abnormalities, stenotic ear canals, sealed eyelids, and constipation. Congenital hypothyroidism with goiter (CHG) caused by a nonsense mutation in the thyroid peroxidase gene has been recognized in toy fox terriers and rat terriers (Fyfe et al, 2003; Dodgson et al, 2012). A different missense mutation of the thyroid peroxidase gene causes CHG in Tenterfield terriers. Both defects are autosomal-recessive traits, and a deoxyribonucleic acid test that detects carriers of the defects is available through the laboratory of comparative medical genetics at Michigan State University.

Diagnosis

Hypothyroidism is clinically suspected based on evaluation of the signalment; history and physical examination; and results of a hemogram, biochemical panel, and urinalysis. Clinicopathologic changes that are commonly observed in dogs with hypothyroidism are normocytic, normochromic, nonregenerative anemia; fasting hypertriglyceridemia; and hypercholesterolemia.

Measurement of total T_4 concentration is a sensitive initial screening test for hypothyroidism. Additional tests that may aid in confirmation of the diagnosis include measurement of free T_4 and TSH concentration, provocative thyroid function testing, antibody tests for thyroiditis, and diagnostic imaging. In some equivocal cases, evaluation of response to thyroid hormone supplementation is necessary to confirm the diagnosis.

Basal Thyroid Hormone Concentrations

T_4 is the major secretory product of the thyroid gland, whereas most serum T_3 is derived from the extrathyroidal deiodination of T_4. Both T_3 and T_4 are highly protein bound to serum carrier proteins. Only unbound (free) hormone penetrates cell membranes, binds to receptors, and has biologic activity. Protein-bound hormone acts as a reservoir and buffer to maintain a steady concentration of free hormone in the plasma despite rapid alterations in release and metabolism of T_3 and T_4 and changes in

TABLE 42-1

Diagnostic Tests for Hypothyroidism in Dogs

	Sensitivity (%)	Specificity (%)	Accuracy (%)
Total T$_4$	89-100	75-82	85
Free T$_4$	80-98	93-94	95
TSH	63-87	82-93	80-84
TSH/T$_4$*	63-67	98-100	82-88
TSH/free T$_4$*	74	98	86

Data are compiled from three published studies of 100 hypothyroid dogs and 164 euthyroid dogs. Not all studies evaluated all diagnostic tests listed. T$_4$, Thyroxine; TSH, thyroid-stimulating hormone.
*A dog was considered to have hypothyroidism only if the T$_4$ or free T$_4$ was decreased and the TSH was increased.

TABLE 42-2

Canine Breeds with Unique Thyroid Hormone Reference Ranges

Breed	Total T$_4$ (↓ or N)	Free T$_4$ (↓ or N)	Total T$_3$ (↓ or N)	TSH (↑ or N)
Greyhound	↓	↓	Variable	N
Whippet	↓	N	—	N
Saluki	↓	↓	↓	↑
Sloughi	↓	↓ or ↑ (ED)	—	↑
Conditioned Alaskan sled dogs	↓	↓	↓	Variable

ED, Equilibrium dialysis; N, no change; T$_3$, triiodothyronine; T$_4$, thyroxine; TSH, thyroid-stimulating hormone; ↓, decreased; ↑, increased.

TABLE 42-3

Mean and Median Serum Total Thyroxine Concentrations of Samples Submitted to a Reference Laboratory for Dogs of Different Ages*

Age (years)	Mean T$_4$ (μg/dl)	Median T$_4$ (μg/dl)	No. Patients
0-2	1.94	1.9	1043
3-5	1.91	1.8	2773
6-8	1.83	1.6	6975
9-11	1.75	1.5	5064
12-14	1.67	1.4	4016
>14	1.46	1.2	736
All ages	1.78	1.5	20,607
Total T$_4$ reference range	1.0-4.0		

Data provided by IDEXX Laboratories, Inc., Westbrook, ME.
T$_4$, Thyroxine.
*Patients with age listed as zero were excluded.

plasma protein concentrations. Free T$_4$ is monodeiodinated within cells to T$_3$, which binds to receptors and induces the cellular effects of thyroid hormone. Basal thyroid hormone measurements used in the diagnosis of canine hypothyroidism are shown in Table 42-1.

Factors such as age, breed, drug therapy, and concurrent illness influence thyroid hormone concentrations without altering metabolically active free thyroid hormone concentrations. Not only do thyroid hormone concentrations in healthy dogs commonly fluctuate out of the reference range, but also numerous breeds have been identified as having thyroid hormone concentrations different than established laboratory reference ranges (Table 42-2). There is also a significant decline in thyroid hormone concentrations with age in dogs (Table 42-3), and many drugs have a marked influence on the thyroid axis (Table 42-4) (Daminet et al, 2003). Dogs treated with phenobarbital that have clinical signs of hypothyroidism are particularly challenging to evaluate for hypothyroidism because phenobarbital treatment causes both a decrease in thyroid hormone concentrations and sometimes an increase in TSH. Options include reevaluation after withdrawal of phenobarbital (and, if

necessary, transition to an alternative drug) or consideration of a therapeutic trial (see later).

In nonthyroidal illness, thyroid hormone concentrations tend to decrease, with the change being more severe with increasing severity of illness. Changes in hormone binding to serum carrier proteins (e.g., decreased protein concentration, reduced binding affinity, circulating inhibitors of binding), changes in peripheral hormone distribution and metabolism (e.g., reduced 5'-deiodinase activity), inhibition of TSH secretion, and inhibition of thyroid hormone synthesis all are proposed to contribute to this change. The magnitude of decrease depends on disease severity and is predictive of mortality. Thyroid hormone supplementation does not improve survival in euthyroid humans with decreased thyroid hormone concentrations or increase survival in euthyroid dogs with congestive heart failure (Tidholm et al, 2003). Medical conditions reported to decrease thyroid hormone concentrations in dogs include hyperadrenocorticism, diabetic ketoacidosis, hypoadrenocorticism, renal failure, hepatic disease, peripheral neuropathy, generalized megaesophagus, heart failure, neoplasia, critical illness or infection, and surgery or anesthesia. Estrus, pregnancy, obesity, and malnutrition also influence thyroid hormone concentrations. Interference by anti-T$_3$ and anti-T$_4$ antibodies can cause a spurious increase or decrease in the measured thyroid hormone concentration.

Total Thyroxine Concentration

Total T$_4$ concentration is the most commonly performed static thyroid hormone measurement and is a good initial screening test for canine hypothyroidism (see Table 42-1). Generally, a dog with a T$_4$ concentration well within the normal range may be assumed to have normal thyroid function; however, a basal T$_4$ concentration below the normal range is *not* diagnostic for hypothyroidism because many factors other than hypothyroidism may affect the basal T$_4$ concentration (see earlier discussion).

TABLE 42-4

Drugs That Have Been Shown to Influence Thyroid Function in Dogs

Drug	Total T$_4$ ($\downarrow$ or N)	Free T$_4$ ($\downarrow$ or N)	TSH ($\uparrow$ or N)	Clinical Signs of Hypothyroidism? (Yes/No)	Notes
Glucocorticoids	$\downarrow$	($\downarrow$ or N)	N	No	Effect dose and duration dependent
Phenobarbital	$\downarrow$	$\downarrow$	Slight $\uparrow$	No	TSH not increased outside reference range
Trimethoprim/ sulfonamides	$\downarrow$	$\downarrow$	$\uparrow$	Yes	Effect dose and duration dependent
Nonsteroidal antiinflammatory drugs					Effect varies depending on specific drug used
Aspirin	$\downarrow$	N	N	No	
Deracoxib	N	N	N	No	
Ketoprofen	N	N	N	No	
Meloxicam	N	N	N	No	
Carprofen	N	N	N	No	
TADs					Effect of other TAD drugs unknown in dog
Clomipramine	$\downarrow$	$\downarrow$	N	No	
Propranolol	N	N	N	No	
Potassium bromide	N	N	N	No	

Adapted from Daminet S, Ferguson DC: Influence of drugs on thyroid function in dogs, *J Vet Intern Med* 17:463, 2003.
N, No change; *TADs*, tricyclic antidepressants; *T$_4$*, thyroxine; *TSH*, thyroid-stimulating hormone; $\downarrow$, decreased; $\uparrow$, increased.

Free Thyroxine Concentration

Because only the unbound fraction of serum T$_4$ is biologically active, measurement of free T$_4$ should be more sensitive and specific for diagnosis of hypothyroidism than total T$_4$. Numerous different assays for measurement of free T$_4$ currently are used in dogs, and their diagnostic performance varies (Table 42-5) (Scott-Moncrieff et al, 2011). Although measurement of free T$_4$ concentration may be slightly more specific and sensitive for diagnosis of canine hypothyroidism than measurement of total T$_4$ depending on the assay used, concurrent illness, drug administration, and breed variability can still suppress free T$_4$ concentration. One additional advantage of free T$_4$ assays that use an equilibrium dialysis step is that the results are unaffected by antibody interference.

Total Triiodothyronine Concentration

In euthyroid dogs, T$_3$ concentration fluctuates in and out of the normal range even more than T$_4$ concentration; T$_3$ concentrations are less accurate in distinguishing euthyroid from hypothyroid dogs. Spurious T$_3$ measurements may also occur because of the presence of anti-T$_3$ antibodies.

Thyroid-Stimulating Hormone Concentration

Measurement of canine TSH concentration is helpful in dogs with a low total T$_4$ concentration because a low T$_4$ in conjunction with a high TSH is highly specific for the diagnosis of hypothyroidism (Table 42-6; also see Table 42-1). The main disadvantage of measuring TSH is the lack of sensitivity of this assay; approximately 30% of hypothyroid dogs have a TSH concentration within the

TABLE 42-5

Sensitivity, Sensitivity, and Accuracy of Four Assays for Free Thyroxine in Dogs

Assay	Sensitivity (%)	Specificity (%)	Accuracy (%)
Analog free T$_4$	80	97	89
MED IVD	92	90	91
MED AN	71	100	86
Two-step	96	90	93

The dog population included 56 dogs with clinical signs of hypothyroidism (31 euthyroid, 25 hypothyroid). Assays included the IMMULITE 2000 Veterinary Free T$_4$ (*Analog free T$_4$*), Direct Free T$_4$ by Equilibrium Dialysis (*MED IVD*), free T$_4$ by equilibrium dialysis (*MED AN*), and GammaCoat Free T$_4$ (*Two-step*) radioimmunoassay.
T$_4$, Thyroxine.

reference range. In dogs with ^{131}I-induced hypothyroidism, TSH concentrations decrease within a few months of onset of hypothyroidism and after 3 years are not significantly different from concentrations before thyroidectomy. This decrease in TSH concentrations occurs in conjunction with enlargement of the pituitary gland, hypersecretion of growth hormone, and hyposecretion of prolactin (transdifferentiation). Dogs with primary hypothyroidism also have hypersecretion of growth hormone and lack an increase in TSH after administration of thyrotropin-releasing hormone, suggesting that similar functional pituitary changes occur in spontaneous

TABLE 42-6

Interpretation of Basal Thyroid Hormone Concentrations*

	Normal T₄/Free T₄	Decreased or Borderline Normal T₄/Free T₄
Normal TSH	Normal dog Consider further thyroid testing only if strong clinical suspicion of hypothyroidism	Hypothyroid, normal variation, or concurrent illness Consider further diagnostic evaluation of thyroid function (e.g., thyroid autoantibodies, provocative testing) or therapeutic trial
Increased TSH	Early subclinical hypothyroidism or recovery from concurrent illness Consider reevaluation of thyroid function in 1-3 months; if strong clinical suspicion for hypothyroidism, evaluate for thyroiditis by measuring ATAs	Hypothyroid Lifelong therapy with L-thyroxine is indicated; use therapeutic monitoring to adjust dose

ATAs, Antithyroglobulin antibodies; *T₄*, thyroxine; *TSH*, thyroid-stimulating hormone.
*T₄, free T₄, TSH.

hypothyroidism. These findings may explain why some hypothyroid dogs have a TSH concentration within the reference range (Diaz-Espiñeira, 2008, 2009).

Thyroid-Stimulating Hormone Stimulation Test

The TSH stimulation test is a test of thyroid reserve. It is considered the "gold standard" test for assessment of thyroid function in dogs, but its use is limited by the expense of TSH. The protocol requires collection of a serum sample for measurement of T_4, intravenous administration of 75 to 150 µg of human recombinant TSH, and an additional blood sample for T_4 collected 6 hours later. The higher dose is recommended in dogs with concurrent disease and dogs receiving medications such as glucocorticoids or phenobarbital (Boretti et al, 2009). Hypothyroidism is confirmed by T_4 concentrations below the reference range for basal T_4 concentration before and after administration of TSH. Euthyroidism is confirmed by a T_4 concentration greater than 2.5 µg/dl after administration of TSH. Interpretation of intermediate results should take into consideration the clinical signs and severity of concurrent systemic disease.

Diagnostic Imaging

Ultrasonography may be useful in evaluation of dogs with suspected hypothyroidism (see Chapter 40). The thyroid gland in many hypothyroid dogs has a smaller volume and cross-sectional area compared with euthyroid dogs and tends to be less echogenic. Nuclear scintigraphy also has high discrimination for evaluation of dogs with suspected hypothyroidism; however, it is rarely performed in clinical practice (see Chapter 43).

Therapeutic Trial

Response to therapy is sometimes the most practical approach to confirming a diagnosis of hypothyroidism (Figure 42-1). After ruling out nonthyroidal illness, supplementation with L-thyroxine should be initiated at a dose of 20 µg/kg every 12 hours. If improvement is noted, therapy should be temporarily withdrawn. Recurrence of clinical signs is consistent with a diagnosis of hypothyroidism. If clinical signs do not recur, thyroid responsive disease, in which clinical signs improve secondary to the nonspecific effects of thyroid hormone, should be suspected. If there is no response to treatment after 2 to 3 months of appropriate therapy, and serum T_4 concentrations 4 to 6 hours after L-thyroxine administration are within the appropriate therapeutic range, therapy should be withdrawn and other diagnoses should be pursued.

Diagnosis of Thyroiditis

Antithyroglobulin Antibodies

ATAs are found in approximately 50% of hypothyroid dogs and are believed to be the result of leakage of thyroglobulin into circulation secondary to lymphocytic thyroiditis. A commercially available enzyme-linked immunosorbent assay for ATAs is a sensitive and specific indicator of thyroiditis, although false-positive results do occur. Because ATAs are more common in hypothyroid dogs than euthyroid dogs, their presence may be useful in evaluating the likelihood of thyroid dysfunction in dogs when other tests of thyroid function are equivocal. However, positive ATA titers can occur in euthyroid dogs.

The proportion of euthyroid dogs with ATAs that ultimately develop hypothyroidism is unknown. In one study, approximately 20% of euthyroid dogs with thyroiditis developed some evidence of thyroid dysfunction within 1 year based on either an increase in TSH or a decrease in T_4. A small percentage of dogs (15%) became ATA negative after 12 months. Possible causes for false-positive ATAs include nonspecific binding, recent vaccination, drug therapy, or viral infection.

Measurement of ATAs has been advocated for screening breeding stock with the aim of ultimately eliminating heritable forms of thyroiditis. The Orthopedic Foundation for Animals (OFA) maintains a thyroid registry and issues a breed database number to all dogs found to have normal thyroid function at 12 months of age (based on

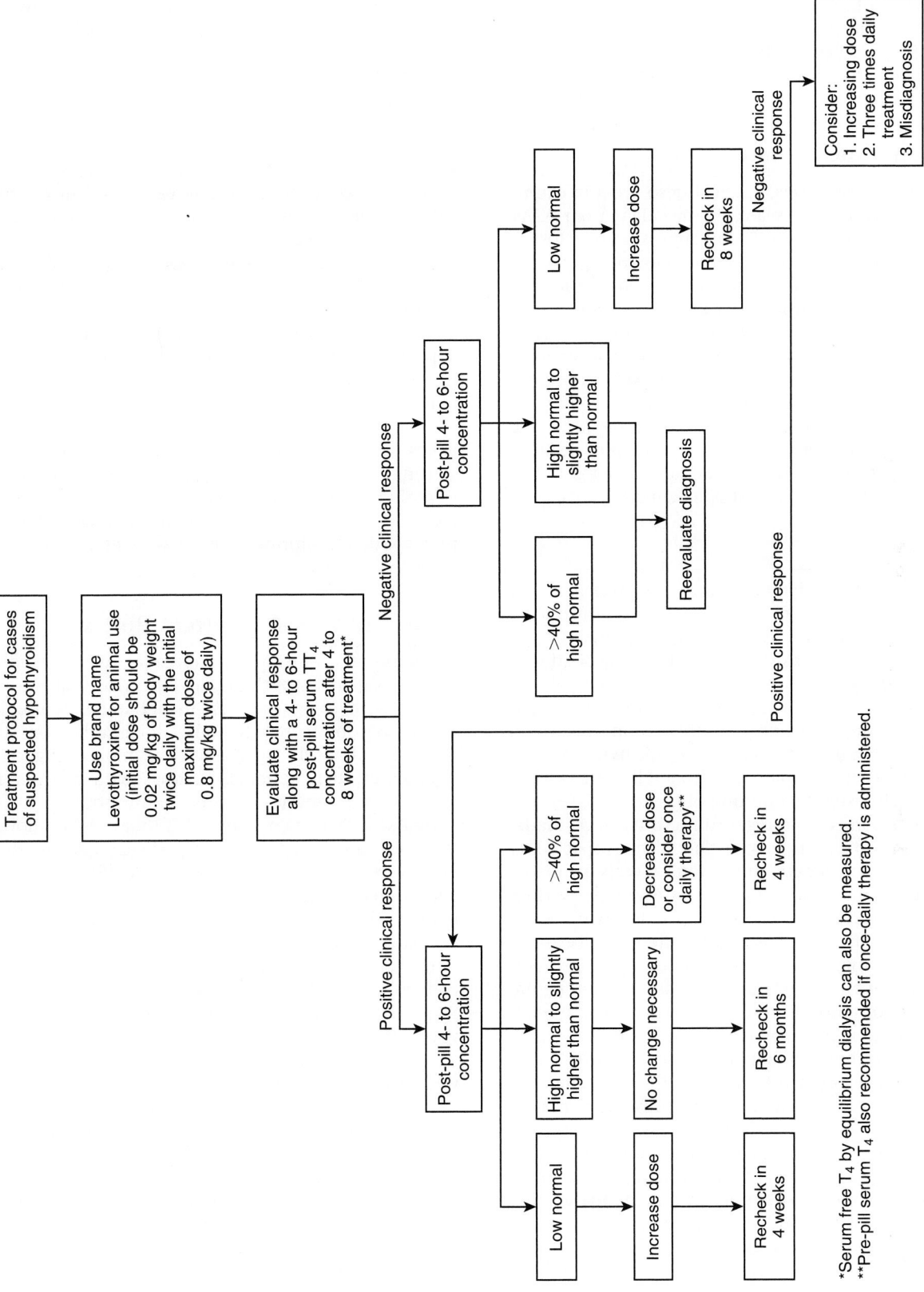

Figure 42-1 Algorithm outlining approach to treatment of canine hypothyroidism. (Modified from Scott-Moncrieff JCR, Guptill-Yoran L: Hypothyroidism. In Ettinger SJ, Feldman EC, editors: *Textbook of veterinary internal medicine: diseases of the dog and cat,* ed 6, St Louis, 2005, Elsevier.)

*Serum free T$_4$ by equilibrium dialysis can also be measured.
**Pre-pill serum T$_4$ also recommended if once-daily therapy is administered.

measurement of free T_4, TSH, and ATAs by an OFA-approved laboratory). Each dog also must be examined by a veterinarian. Because hypothyroidism usually develops after 1 year of age, it is recommended that reexamination and retesting occur at 2, 3, 4, 6, and 8 years of age.

Anti-T_3 and Anti-T_4 Antibodies

Antibodies directed against T_3 and T_4 also occur in canine thyroiditis, although they are less prevalent than ATAs. Anti-T_3 antibodies are identified in approximately 30% of hypothyroid dogs, and anti-T_4 antibodies are reported in 15% of hypothyroid dogs. Although some euthyroid dogs may be positive for anti-T_3 and anti-T_4 antibodies, the presence of antithyroid antibodies increases the likelihood of hypothyroidism in dogs with equivocal basal thyroid hormone concentrations. Antibodies directed against T_3 and T_4 may interfere with hormone assays; this usually leads to a spurious increase in the measured hormone concentration but can cause a spurious decrease in a few assays. Antithyroid antibodies do not interfere with response to L-thyroxine supplementation.

Treatment

Regardless of the underlying cause, the treatment of choice for hypothyroidism is L-thyroxine. Administration of L-thyroxine with food may decrease bioavailability, so it is important to be consistent about the time of administration of the medication in relation to feeding. Treatment with synthetic T_3 is not recommended because it has a shorter half-life, requires administration three times daily, and is more likely to cause iatrogenic hyperthyroidism. Treatment with T_3 may be indicated if there is inadequate gastrointestinal absorption of L-thyroxine because T_3 is better absorbed in the gastrointestinal tract. Inadequate absorption of L-thyroxine should be suspected in dogs in which therapeutic monitoring reveals an inadequate increase in thyroxine or decrease in TSH in dogs receiving higher than usual doses of L-thyroxine, especially in dogs with concurrent gastrointestinal disease. It is important to rule out nonthyroidal illness or the effects of drug therapy on the measured T_4 concentration before suspecting poor absorption of L-thyroxine because inadequate absorption is uncommon. The use of desiccated thyroid extract, thyroglobulin, or "natural" thyroid preparations is not recommended because the bioavailability and T_4-to-T_3 ratio of these compounds are variable, making consistent dosing difficult.

Twice-daily administration of T_4 at a dose of 0.02 mg/kg q12h PO is recommended initially. If clinical signs resolve and T_4 concentrations are within the therapeutic range after 4 to 8 weeks of therapy, the frequency of T_4 administration can be decreased to once daily. Because of individual variability in T_4 absorption and serum half-life, the dose should be adjusted based on the measured serum T_4 concentration 4 to 6 hours after dosing. Although considered uncommon, iatrogenic hyperthyroidism does occur, particularly in dogs inappropriately treated for hypothyroidism based solely on the results of a serum total T_4 concentration. Therapeutic monitoring minimizes the effect of any differences in potency and bioavailability between different brands of L-thyroxine and other factors that influence bioavailability such as time of feeding. For otherwise healthy adult dogs, T_4 concentration should be at the high end or slightly above the reference range 4 to 6 hours after dosing; however, therapy should be individualized based on clinical response, presence of concurrent illness, age, and concurrent drug administration. Concurrent measurement of serum TSH concentration may be helpful in interpretation of the T_4 concentration after administration of L-thyroxine (see subsequently).

Improvement in activity should be evident within the first 1 to 2 weeks of treatment; weight loss should be evident within 8 weeks. Achievement of a normal hair coat may take several months, and the coat may initially appear worse as telogen hairs are shed. Neurologic deficits improve rapidly after treatment, but complete resolution may take 8 to 12 weeks.

The plasma half-life of synthetic T_3 is 5 to 6 hours; it needs to be administered three times a day. The initial starting dose is 4.4 µg/kg q8h PO. Dogs treated for hypothyroidism with T_3 may be more susceptible to thyrotoxicosis and should be monitored carefully using therapeutic monitoring with measurement of T_3, T_4, and TSH.

Treatment with Concurrent Illness

The appropriate therapeutic range for hypothyroid dogs with concurrent nonthyroidal illness or that are being treated with drugs such as phenobarbital is unknown but is likely lower than the range for healthy dogs. Interpretation of results of therapeutic monitoring can be difficult in such patients. In dogs with a lower than ideal T_4 concentration after administration of oral L-thyroxine, a TSH concentration that persists above the reference range suggests inadequate supplementation or poor owner compliance; conversely, if TSH is suppressed and clinical signs have resolved, it is not necessary to increase the L-thyroxine dose to drive the T_4 concentration after L-thyroxine administration into the therapeutic range, especially in geriatric patients or patients with concurrent illness. Current assays for TSH are not sensitive enough to identify dogs that are oversupplemented with L-thyroxine.

Caution should be used when initiating treatment with thyroid hormone in certain disease states. Thyroid hormone supplementation increases myocardial oxygen demand and may cause cardiac decompensation in dogs with underlying heart disease. For this reason, the initial dose of L-thyroxine should be 25% to 50% of the usual starting dose. The dose may be increased incrementally based on the results of therapeutic monitoring and reevaluation of cardiac function. In dogs with concurrent hypoadrenocorticism, replacement of mineralocorticoid and glucocorticoid deficiency should be initiated before treatment with L-thyroxine because increased basal metabolic rate after supplementation may exacerbate electrolyte disturbances. Intravenous L-thyroxine at a dose of 4 to 5 µg/kg every 8 to 12 hours has been reported to be safe and effective for treatment of hypothyroid dogs with critical illness.

Treatment Failure

Incorrect diagnosis of hypothyroidism is the most common reason for treatment failure. Diseases such as hyperadrenocorticism, atopy, and flea hypersensitivity may have clinical signs similar to hypothyroidism and may be associated with decreased thyroid hormone concentrations. Many other disorders result in physiologically appropriate decreases in thyroid hormone concentrations. Other, less common reasons for a poor response to treatment include poor absorption of T_4 from the gastrointestinal tract or problems with owner compliance. These situations can be identified by therapeutic monitoring.

References and Suggested Reading

Boretti FS et al: Comparison of 2 doses of recombinant human thyrotropin for thyroid function testing in healthy and suspected hypothyroid dogs, *J Vet Intern Med* 23:856, 2009.

Daminet S et al: Influence of drugs on thyroid function in dogs, *J Vet Intern Med* 17:463, 2003.

Diaz-Espiñeira MM et al: Functional and morphological changes in the adenohypophysis of dogs with induced primary hypothyroidism: loss of TSH hypersecretion, hypersomatotropism, hypoprolactinemia, and pituitary enlargement with transdifferentiation, *Domest Anim Endocrinol* 35:98, 2008.

Diaz-Espiñeira MM et al: Adenohypophyseal function in dogs with primary hypothyroidism and non-thyroidal illness, *J Vet Intern Med* 23:100, 2009.

Fyfe JC et al: Congenital hypothyroidism with goiter in toy fox terriers, *J Vet Intern Med* 17:50, 2003.

Dodgson SE et al: Congenital hypothyroidism with goiter in Tenterfield terriers, *J Vet Intern Med* 26:1350, 2012.

Graham PA et al: Etiopathologic findings of canine hypothyroidism, *Vet Clin North Am Small Anim Pract* 37:617, 2007.

Higgins MA, Rossmeisl JH, Panciera DL: Hypothyroid associated central vestibular disease in 10 dogs: 1999-2005, *J Vet Intern Med* 20:1363, 2006.

Panciera DL et al: Effect of short-term hypothyroidism on reproduction in the bitch, *Theriogenology* 68:316, 2007.

Rossmeisl JH: Resistance of the peripheral nervous system to the effects of chronic canine hypothyroidism, *J Vet Intern Med* 24:875, 2010.

Scott-Moncrieff JC et al: Lack of association between repeated vaccination and thyroiditis in laboratory beagles, *J Vet Intern Med* 20:818, 2006.

Scott-Moncrieff JC et al: Accuracy of serum free thyroxine concentrations determined by a new veterinary chemiluminescent immunoassay in euthyroid and hypothyroid dogs [ECVIM Abstract EN-O-14], *J Vet Intern Med* 25:1493, 2011.

Shiel RE et al: Thyroid hormone concentrations in young healthy pretraining greyhounds, *Vet Rec* 161:616, 2007.

Shiel RE et al: Assessment of criteria used by veterinary practitioners to diagnose hypothyroidism in sighthounds and investigation of serum thyroid hormone concentrations in healthy Salukis, *J Am Vet Med Assoc* 236:302, 2010.

Tidholm A et al: Effect of thyroid hormone supplementation on survival of euthyroid dogs with congestive heart failure due to systolic myocardial dysfunction: a double-blind placebo controlled trial, *Res Vet Sci* 75:195, 2003.

CHAPTER 43

Feline Hyperthyroidism and Renal Function

HARRIET M. SYME, *Hertfordshire, Great Britain*

Physiology

Hyperthyroidism has numerous effects on both glomerular and renal tubular function. Thyroid hormones increase glomerular filtration rate (GFR) partly as a result of direct renal actions and partly secondary to cardiovascular and systemic hemodynamic effects that act to increase renal blood flow. When hyperthyroid patients are treated, GFR decreases and some cats become azotemic. Chronic kidney disease (CKD) is "unmasked" in some treated hyperthyroid cats; the renal disease is preexisting but is hidden by the increased GFR that accompanies the hyperthyroid state. Changes in GFR occur with all treatment modalities and should be considered the result of resolution of the hyperthyroid state and not a side effect of treatment.

The most significant hemodynamic effect of thyrotoxicosis is a profound decline in systemic vascular resistance secondary to dilation of resistance arterioles in the peripheral circulation. The decline occurs as a result of thyroid hormone–induced increases in tissue metabolism, release of locally acting vasodilators, and direct effects of the thyroid hormone triiodothyronine (T_3) on vascular smooth muscle. As a result of the decrease in systemic vascular resistance, effective arterial filling volume decreases, causing stimulation of the sympathetic and renin-angiotensin-aldosterone systems. Activation of this system stimulates renal sodium reabsorption, leading to an increase in plasma volume; this increases stroke volume and along with the increase in heart rate that occurs with hyperthyroidism enhances cardiac output. This renal tubular effect is augmented by impaired response of the renal tubules to natriuretic peptides associated with thyrotoxicosis. Taken together, these mechanisms explain how plasma volume increases and sodium excretion decreases in the hyperthyroid state despite increases in renal blood flow and GFR. The normal pressure-diuresis-natriuresis response of the kidneys is altered by direct and indirect actions of thyroid hormones. Tubular reabsorption of other electrolytes, including phosphorus, also is enhanced.

Epidemiology

In most published studies, about 10% of hyperthyroid cats are azotemic at the time of diagnosis. A further 15% to 49% of cats become azotemic in the first few months after starting treatment. The number of cats that develop azotemia depends on various factors but particularly on how well hyperthyroidism is controlled. If treatment results in a borderline hyperthyroid state, the change in GFR is not as great as for a patient that is well controlled; the cat may not become azotemic. However, adverse consequences of thyrotoxicosis may be persistent. Conversely, if a cat is rendered hypothyroid during treatment, the likelihood of developing azotemia is increased.

CKD is highly prevalent in geriatric cats. The prevalence of azotemia increases with age, and hyperthyroid cats tend to be elderly. Even so, it is unclear whether the very high prevalence of azotemic CKD in cats that are diagnosed and treated for hyperthyroidism can be explained simply by demographics. One commonly asked question that has yet to be resolved is whether the high prevalence of azotemic CKD in cats treated for hyperthyroidism is due to the fact that hyperthyroidism is damaging to the kidneys. The hyperthyroid state causes glomerular hyperfiltration, hyperphosphatemia, and proteinuria, all of which have been associated with progression of CKD in cats and other species. At the present time, direct evidence that the hyperthyroid state is injurious to the kidneys is lacking.

Diagnosis of Hyperthyroidism with Chronic Kidney Disease

Diagnosis of hyperthyroidism is usually straightforward; in a cat that shows compatible clinical signs, demonstration of elevated serum total thyroxine (T_4) concentration is all that is required. However, in patients with nonthyroidal illness, total T_4 concentration can be suppressed, often to within or below the laboratory reference range. This is a relatively common occurrence in cats with previously diagnosed azotemic CKD. In the author's clinics, hyperthyroidism is often suspected in cats with CKD many months before the diagnosis is confirmed by laboratory testing. Although these cats may exhibit classic signs of hyperthyroidism, the owner is unaware of any problem in many instances. The clinical suspicion arises when the cat is noted to lose weight while the serum

creatinine concentration is decreasing secondary to enhanced GFR. Together with palpation of a goiter, these changes, although often subtle, are highly suggestive of hyperthyroidism.

Numerous testing strategies are possible in this situation. One option is to wait and repeat total T_4 measurement in the hope that values will eventually be outside the reference range. An alternative option is to use a combination of diagnostic tests to confirm the diagnosis. A total T_4 measurement in the upper half of the laboratory reference range together with either an undetectable thyroid-stimulating hormone (TSH) concentration (<0.03 ng/ml using the canine Diagnostic Products Corporation [DPC] assay) or an increased free T_4 concentration is supportive of the diagnosis of hyperthyroidism, even though either of these tests (TSH, free T_4) when performed in isolation has relatively low specificity (i.e., results in many false-positive diagnoses). Other options include the use of provocative endocrine tests (i.e., T_3 suppression test or thyrotropin-releasing hormone stimulation test) or thyroid scintigraphy, but these tests have disadvantages including the need for specialist facilities, collection of multiple blood samples, tablet administration, and potential side effects.

Renal Function in Hyperthyroidism

In the hyperthyroid state GFR increases, causing decreases in serum or plasma concentrations of urea and creatinine. However, the changes in urea and creatinine that occur are not proportional to one another; the urea-to-creatinine ratio increases with hyperthyroidism, and it is common for hyperthyroid cats to have urea concentrations above the laboratory reference range. Elevated urea concentrations are found even in cats with good underlying renal function that do not go on to develop azotemia when treated. The reasons for the change in the urea-to-creatinine ratio are multifactorial. Urea may be relatively increased in the hyperthyroid state because of failure to fast the (polyphagic) patient before blood sampling and increased protein catabolism. Creatinine may also be relatively decreased, independent of the effects of GFR, because of a reduction in muscle mass.

Studies performed in hyperthyroid cats treated with radioactive iodine show that GFR decreases rapidly after establishment of euthyroidism with detectable changes in 1 week and that after 1 month little further change in GFR occurs. However, creatinine concentration takes longer to plateau after treatment, typically stabilizing after about 3 months. The urea concentration may increase slightly with treatment for hyperthyroidism, but this change is inconsistent.

Hyperthyroid cats may exhibit polydipsia and polyuria and consequently have relatively low urine specific gravity (USG). This finding was thought to be more common in cats with severe thyrotoxicosis, and the prevalence of these clinical signs is believed to have decreased in recent years as a result of earlier diagnosis. The cause of the polyuria and polydipsia is poorly understood. In experimental studies in rodents, hyperthyroidism was shown to inhibit the insertion of aquaporins, the channels through which water is absorbed in the renal distal tubules and collecting ducts, resulting in a form of nephrogenic diabetes insipidus. It also has been proposed that heat intolerance results in a psychogenic polydipsia in hyperthyroid animals. These effects are independent of any underlying renal dysfunction. Treatment of hyperthyroidism, despite the resulting decline in GFR, has very unpredictable effects on USG except in cats that become overtly azotemic.

Predicting Azotemia

At the present time there is no single test that can reliably predict renal function after treatment for hyperthyroidism. Predictive biomarkers that identify cats with CKD could be advantageous because they would allow management strategies, including closer monitoring of renal function, to be instituted before treatment. However, in view of the relatively good prognosis for cats that become azotemic when made euthyroid (see later), the importance of preemptive planning should not be overly stressed.

Direct estimation of GFR by measurement of plasma clearance of a substance (e.g., iohexol, inulin, creatinine) or by using nuclear medicine imaging techniques has been found to be predictive of the development of azotemia after treatment. However, these methods are impractical for routine clinical use. Additionally, estimates of GFR differ according to the methodology employed, so it is difficult to take suggested cut-points from one study and apply them in a different clinical setting.

In routine clinical practice, serum creatinine concentration is used as a marker of GFR, albeit a relatively insensitive one (given that in cats subjected to nephrectomy, at least seven eighths of the renal tissue has to be destroyed to induce azotemia). However, differences in creatinine concentration can reflect differences in GFR even when still within the laboratory reference range. In most studies in which it has been evaluated, cats with decreased creatinine concentrations (increased GFR) at baseline are less likely to develop azotemia when treated for hyperthyroidism. Despite this finding, creatinine is not a useful predictor in an individual cat. Although a statistical difference can be demonstrated in mean baseline creatinine concentrations between cats that develop azotemia and cats that do not, there is a great deal of overlap between the two groups.

It has been suggested that cats with concentrated urine (USG >1.035) are at a relatively low risk of developing azotemia after treatment for hyperthyroidism. However, this assertion has not been substantiated with data. USG is not independently associated with the development of azotemia in multivariable analyses.

Many other markers of renal function after treatment for hyperthyroidism have been evaluated, but none has been found to be consistently useful. Although hyperthyroid cats are frequently proteinuric (with more than half having urine protein-to-creatinine ratios >0.4), this variable also does not predict the development of azotemia with treatment.

Prognostic Significance of Azotemia

Almost all hyperthyroid cats are clinically improved when rendered euthyroid, including most that develop azotemia. Cats typically gain weight, other clinical signs associated with hyperthyroidism resolve, and owners are very pleased with their clinical condition. Unless renal function is systematically retested, the development of azotemia is likely to be undetected in many cats. In a recent study (Williams et al, 2010b) that compared the survival of cats that developed azotemia with cats that did not, no difference was found between the two groups (Figure 43-1, *A*). Results of that study suggest that the importance of the mild azotemia that commonly develops after treatment for hyperthyroidism may have been overemphasized previously. There is no rationale for undertreating hyperthyroidism to keep patients from becoming azotemic as has been suggested in the past.

The same study found that in cats that were inadvertently overtreated and made hypothyroid, the development of azotemia was of prognostic significance. The diagnosis of hypothyroidism was confirmed by documenting that the cats had a subnormal total T_4 concentration in combination with elevated TSH (>0.15 ng/ml using the DPC canine assay). Cats that were hypothyroid and azotemic had shorter survival times than cats that were hypothyroid and remained nonazotemic (Figure 43-1, *B*). The number of hypothyroid cats included in the study was small, so ideally these results should be replicated in a larger group before conclusions are drawn. In practical terms, such a study would be difficult because of the long follow-up periods required. What is unclear is why the survival of these cats was worse; the azotemia was relatively mild, and in the group of cats as a whole (i.e., euthyroid and hypothyroid combined) the survival of the azotemic cats was no worse than that of the cats that were nonazotemic. It is possible that although the clinical signs associated with hypothyroidism in cats are very subtle, hypothyroidism does contribute to patient morbidity, and in association with the azotemia it played a role in the patients' decline.

Although overall cats that develop azotemia with treatment of hyperthyroidism do very well, the same is not true of cats that are azotemic before treatment. Williams and colleagues (2010a) found that the survival time of cats that were azotemic (on the basis of plasma or serum creatinine concentration) before diagnosis and treatment was approximately 6 months (median survival, 178 days; range, 0 to 1505 days), which is considerably shorter than survival in cats that were not azotemic (median survival, 612 days; range, 0 to 2541 days).

Choice of Treatment Modality

It has been widely recommended that hyperthyroid cats be treated initially with drugs (methimazole or carbimazole) so that the effect of treatment can be reversed if necessary. This approach seems advisable in cats that are azotemic before they are treated for hyperthyroidism because survival times in these cats are known to be very poor, and a reversible treatment is warranted. Although clinical experience with the use of iodine-deficient diets

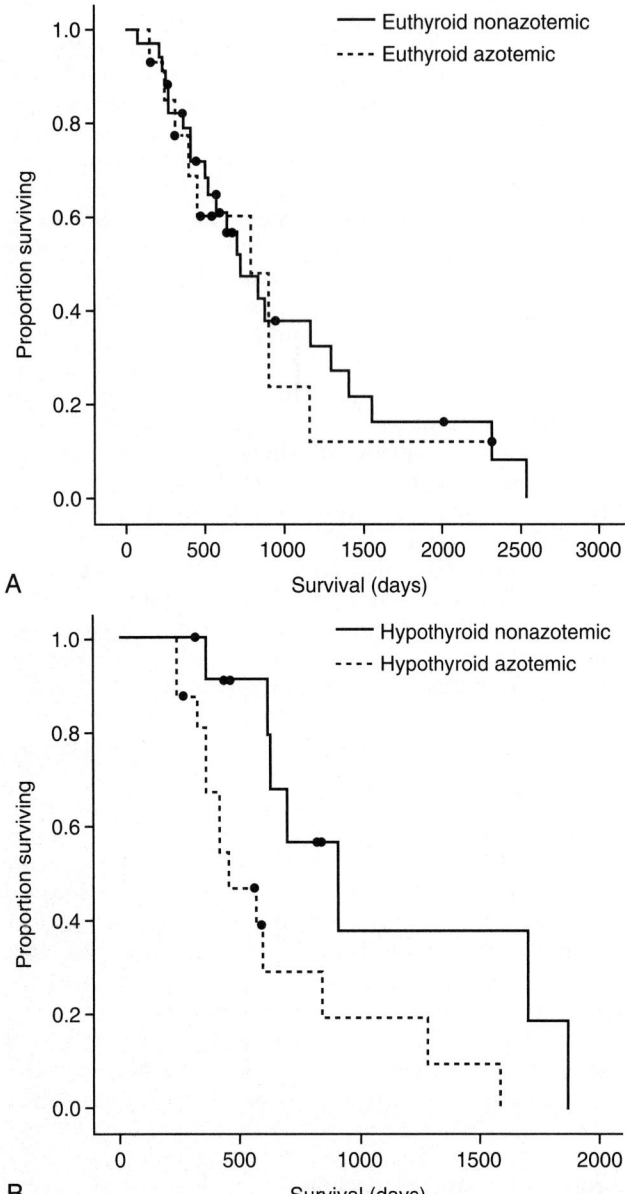

Figure 43-1 A, Kaplan-Meier survival curves of 47 cats treated for hyperthyroidism that were euthyroid after 6 months of treatment. Cats were grouped according to whether or not they were azotemic at the end of the 6-month follow-up period. *Circles* represent censored individuals. **B,** Kaplan-Meier survival curves of 28 cats treated for hyperthyroidism that were hypothyroid after 6 months of treatment. Cats were grouped according to whether or not they were azotemic at the end of the 6-month follow-up period. *Circles* represent censored individuals. (Data from Williams TL et al: Survival and the development of azotemia after treatment of hyperthyroid cats, *J Vet Intern Med* 24:863, 2010, with permission.)

(i.e., Hill's Y/D) is not yet widespread, this could also be a useful treatment in this setting (see Web Chapter 20). In most cats in which azotemia develops only after treatment, the recommendation to use only a reversible form of treatment initially may be overly cautious because many of these cats have long survival times, and the development of azotemia is not related to outcome except

in cats that become hypothyroid. However, a reversible form of treatment has been the author's usual practice unless the cat's owner is reluctant to attempt medical therapy. Medical or dietary treatment of cats before surgical thyroidectomy is generally advised to reduce the risks associated with general anesthesia. Reversible treatment may also be advised before radioactive iodine treatment, particularly if there are long waiting times for appointments, so the owner can be educated about the significance of azotemia if it develops with treatment.

In many situations medical treatment for hyperthyroidism before permanent therapy is inappropriate. First, if the cat cannot tolerate medical treatment with methimazole or carbimazole because of the development of serious side effects (e.g., facial excoriations, blood dyscrasias, hepatopathies), drug therapy must be permanently discontinued. A second situation is when the owner is unable or unwilling to medicate a cat with sufficient regularity to control the hyperthyroidism. In these situations, provided that the owner is aware that a proportion of cats develop azotemia with treatment for hyperthyroidism, the use of a definitive treatment modality (i.e., radioactive iodine or bilateral thyroidectomy) as first-line therapy is reasonable. In most patients the consequences of untreated or poorly controlled hyperthyroidism far outweigh the risks associated with definitive treatment.

In addition, development of azotemia with a reversible form of treatment should not preclude the definitive treatment of hyperthyroidism. Patients that have been treated with drugs or diet and have developed mild, stable renal azotemia may benefit from surgery or radioactive iodine therapy. However, if the patient is relatively poorly controlled with medical treatment (i.e., total T_4 concentration remains in the upper half of the laboratory reference range), the azotemia is likely to worsen if the patient is subsequently well controlled with surgery or radioactive iodine therapy.

One potential disadvantage of definitive methods of treatment for hyperthyroidism (radioactive iodine or bilateral thyroidectomy) is that a relatively large proportion of treated cats may develop hypothyroidism. Until recently, development of hypothyroidism after treatment was not considered to be of any great clinical significance, but the observation that hypothyroid azotemic cats have poorer survival than euthyroid or nonazotemic cats has altered this perception. Although hypothyroid cats do not typically become alopecic, they do exhibit other changes consistent with the diagnosis; they have lower heart rates and packed cell volumes, in addition to having higher creatinine concentrations. Decreased endogenous creatinine production has been demonstrated in hypothyroid dogs resulting in serum concentrations that are lower than would be predicted on the basis of GFR. It is unknown whether the same is true in cats, but if it is, the effects of hypothyroidism on renal function in the cat may be underestimated.

Treatment of Hypothyroidism

Azotemic, hypothyroid cats have been found to have shorter survival times than nonazotemic hypothyroid cats. However, it is uncertain if reversing hypothyroidism (by giving less methimazole or carbimazole or supplementing thyroxine after definitive therapy) would improve outcomes. Reversing the hypothyroid state would be expected to ameliorate the azotemia, if not resolve it entirely; whether this is beneficial has yet to be investigated. Probably most cats treated with radioactive iodine or bilateral thyroidectomy demonstrate, at least transiently, subnormal total T_4 concentrations. Hyperthyroidism causes suppression of pituitary TSH secretion, and recovery of pituitary thyrotrophs is likely to take several months in most instances. Differentiation between transient and permanent hypothyroidism is impossible (at least on the basis of endocrine testing) immediately after treatment for hyperthyroidism. Additionally, differentiating hypothyroidism from the effects of nonthyroidal illness (resulting in subnormal total T_4 concentrations) may be difficult. A protocol for TSH stimulation testing in cats is described, but the length of time needed following treatment to confirm that a patient has developed hypothyroidism is unknown. Observational data suggest that total T_4 concentrations generally return to normal or near-normal levels by 3 months after radioactive iodine treatment, so TSH stimulation testing after this time interval is probably reasonable.

References and Suggested Reading

Boag AK et al: Changes in the glomerular filtration rate of 27 cats with hyperthyroidism after treatment with radioactive iodine, *Vet Rec* 161:711, 2007.

Panciera DL, Lefebvre HP: Effect of experimental hypothyroidism on glomerular filtration rate and plasma creatinine concentration in dogs, *J Vet Intern Med* 23:1045, 2009.

Riensche MR, Graves TK, Schaeffer DJ: An investigation of predictors of renal insufficiency following treatment of hyperthyroidism in cats, *J Feline Med Surg* 10:160, 2008.

van Hoek I et al: Short- and long-term follow-up of glomerular and tubular renal markers of kidney function in hyperthyroid cats after treatment with radioiodine, *Domest Anim Endocrinol* 36:45, 2009.

van Hoek IM et al: Thyroid stimulation with recombinant human thyrotropin in healthy cats, cats with non-thyroidal illness and in cats with low serum thyroxin and azotaemia after treatment of hyperthyroidism, *J Feline Med Surg* 12:117, 2010.

Wakeling J et al: Diagnosis of hyperthyroidism in cats with mild chronic kidney disease, *J Small Anim Pract* 49:287, 2008.

Williams TL, Elliott J, Syme HM: Association of iatrogenic hypothyroidism with azotemia and reduced survival time in cats treated for hyperthyroidism, *J Vet Intern Med* 24:1086, 2010a.

Williams TL et al: Survival and the development of azotemia after treatment of hyperthyroid cats, *J Vet Intern Med* 24:863, 2010b.

CHAPTER 44
Canine Diabetes Mellitus

WILLIAM E. MONROE, *Blacksburg, Virginia*

Definition, Epidemiology, and Pathophysiology

Diabetes mellitus in dogs is a persistent defect of carbohydrate metabolism associated with an absolute deficiency of insulin in nearly all cases. Almost every affected dog requires administration of exogenous insulin for management of the disease. The underlying cause in dogs is poorly understood but is likely multifactorial, including genetic predisposition; infectious, toxic, or inflammatory damage to the pancreatic islets with progressive immune-mediated destruction; or predisposing conditions, such as natural or iatrogenic endocrine disorders, obesity, and hyperlipidemia that cause insulin resistance with subsequent β-cell exhaustion. The prevalence in North American teaching hospitals seems to have increased between 1970 (19 dogs per 10,000) and 1999 (64 dogs per 10,000) (Guptill et al, 2003). The prevalence in Europe is similar, although perhaps slightly variable depending on location. Females, neutered or intact, and neutered males are overrepresented, although female predisposition may be declining. The peak age of occurrence is 7 to 11 years, with 70% of patients older than 7 years at the time of diagnosis. Diabetes occurs rarely in dogs younger than 1 year of age.

Absolute insulin deficiency associated with canine diabetes mellitus is also associated with an increase in glucagon concentration. Together these changes lead to hyperglycemia, both from increased hepatic glucose production and from lack of peripheral use. When blood glucose concentration exceeds the renal threshold (180 to 220 mg/dl), osmotic diuresis occurs, leading to polyuria with secondary polydipsia. There is also fatty acid mobilization with consequent increased production of ketoacids by the liver because the peripheral tissues become energy starved. In addition, ketoacid production is increased because of the lack of the effects of insulin on lipoprotein lipase and hormone-sensitive lipase to facilitate the storage of fatty acids in adipocytes. As ketoacid production exceeds the quantity used for energy metabolism, acidemia occurs, and spillover of ketones into the urine contributes to polyuria. Without insulin, the ability of cells to use glucose is markedly diminished. Insulin deficiency reduces fatty acid deposition in adipocytes and decreases the incorporation of amino acids into protein. These metabolic abnormalities create a catabolic state with resultant weight loss despite adequate or excessive food consumption.

Diagnosis and Management Plan

The diagnosis of diabetes mellitus is based initially on a combination of clinical signs that generally include polyuria and polydipsia, weight loss despite a good appetite, and the demonstration of persistent hyperglycemia with glucosuria. Repeat blood and urine glucose testing to confirm the persistence of hyperglycemia is unnecessary if the clinical signs of polyuria, polydipsia, and polyphagia have been noted. Ketonuria may be present in 66% of dogs with uncomplicated diabetes mellitus. Increased serum alkaline phosphatase and alanine transaminase and hypertriglyceridemia are also common.

Once the diagnosis of diabetes mellitus has been established, it is important to determine if the dog has complicated diabetes (see Web Chapter 13). This determination is critical because diabetic ketoacidosis requires aggressive management in the hospital. Conversely, uncomplicated cases are better managed as outpatients. The major clinical criteria for determining if a dog requires aggressive management relate to clinical findings: Is the patient ill, anorexic, or vomiting, or, conversely, is the dog eating and drinking well and exhibiting a generally healthy attitude? Dogs that appear generally well and show a good appetite can be managed as uncomplicated diabetics even in the presence of ketonuria. Morbidity in these patients is rarely severe enough to require hospitalization and intensive care.

Before initiating therapy, it is important to discuss the effort and cost of management of a diabetic dog with the owner and identify comorbid conditions. Lifestyle or financial circumstances may prevent some owners from successfully managing a diabetic pet. Foremost, it is important that the clinician have a clear understanding of the owner's lifestyle and daily schedule so that a feasible treatment and monitoring protocol can be developed. Additionally, many older dogs manifest concurrent disease that can affect control of the diabetes or may influence the owner's decision to treat or not. A thorough medical evaluation should be conducted to identify concurrent diseases. In addition to the history and physical examination, recommended studies include a complete blood count, serum chemistries (including canine pancreatic lipase immunoreactivity), urinalysis, urine culture, thoracic radiographs, and abdominal ultrasonography or radiography.

Diet, Feeding Schedule, and Exercise

Diets that are high in fiber, low in simple sugars, and moderately restricted in fat and protein are generally recommended for diabetic dogs, although they may not provide an advantage over diets with moderate fiber and low carbohydrates (see Chapter 46). However, the most important aspect of diet for diabetic dogs is that it be a balanced diet that the dog will eat consistently.

If dogs receive insulin twice daily, it is recommended to feed two equal meals at the time of insulin administration. Some clinicians recommend that the dog be fed before injecting insulin and withholding the insulin injection anytime the dog does not eat its entire meal. Although this may work well for a dog that is a gluttonous eater, it is less effective for finicky eaters or dogs that eat small amounts throughout the day. The latter type of eaters may be given insulin routinely without having eaten their entire meal after it has been established that their eating pattern is consistent and glucose curves have confirmed hypoglycemia does not occur.

Even when insulin is given once daily, it is recommended that the dog be fed twice daily. The second meal should approximately coincide with the glucose nadir depending on when the owner can be home to feed. For patients that have a variable time to glucose nadir, the second meal of the day should be fed at a consistent time that approximates the average time of the nadir. Alternatively, the second meal should be presented 12 hours after the insulin injection. Feeding a larger portion of the daily diet around the time of the glucose nadir may lead to a glucose curve with less fluctuation. However, if Lente insulin given once daily provides adequate control, the glucose response can be improved in some cases by feeding the larger meal at the time of the insulin injection. Lente insulin contains 30% short-acting insulin (Semilente) and 70% long-acting insulin (Ultralente) and is absorbed in many dogs such that there are two peaks of insulin activity, with the earlier peak leading to the higher insulin concentration.

Exercise affects both the absorption of insulin and the metabolic use of glucose. Consequently, exercise levels should be kept constant with activity provided at the same times every day.

Insulin Therapy

As stated previously, virtually all diabetic dogs require insulin therapy. Both recombinant human insulin and porcine insulin have been advocated for canine diabetes. There is very little experience or published information about the use of synthetic insulin analogs in dogs (see later). The use of compounded insulin products is not recommended because of a lack of both consistency between batches and stringent control of the formulation.

The recommendation for insulin treatment in dogs involves administration of an insulin with intermediate duration of action twice daily. The only currently available intermediate-duration product is recombinant human neutral protamine Hagedorn (NPH) insulin (used extralabel for dogs). Porcine Lente insulin (Vetsulin) has been approved for use in dogs but cannot be sold in the United States at the present time because of concerns with stability and bacterial contamination associated with the manufacturing process. It is uncertain when or if the product will again be available in the United States.

There is some experience with this product because it has been and remains in use in Canada and many European countries under the brand name Caninsulin. Using Vetsulin, most dogs require injections every 12 hours for adequate control of blood glucose, with a median dose between 0.75 and 0.78 U/kg per injection (range, 0.28 to 1.4 U/kg) for dogs receiving insulin every 12 hours (Monroe et al, 2005). Using recombinant human NPH insulin, most dogs also appear to require two injections per day, with a median time to glucose nadir of 4 hours (range, 1 to ≥10 hours) and a range for duration of action 4 to 10 hours or longer. The median dose reported for well-controlled dogs is 0.63 U/kg every 12 hours (range, 0.4 to 0.97 U/kg) (Palm et al, 2009).

The long-acting protamine zinc insulin made with recombinant human insulin and approved for veterinary use in cats (ProZinc) may be useful for dogs for which intermediate-duration insulins provide too short of a duration of action (<8 hours) to provide adequate glycemic control when given twice daily.

Insulin glargine (e.g., Lantus, Aventis) is a human insulin analog in which the amino acid asparagine has been replaced by glycine within the α-chain and two arginine molecules have been added to the C-terminus of the β-chain. It is intended to be used as a long-acting, basal insulin in humans. There is little clinical information about the use of this product in dogs. It may be useful as a longer acting insulin in patients for which NPH or Lente insulins have too short a duration of action to provide adequate glycemic control with two daily injections. In a small number of dogs, insulin glargine was shown to be safe, providing good to moderate control in most of the patients with a median dose of 0.6 U/kg (range 0.11 to 1.07 U/kg) given every 12 hours. However, the time to glucose nadir was quite variable, and duration of action was not determined (Fracassi et al, 2012). Insulin detemir (Levemir) is a long-acting insulin that is used in humans as a basal insulin. The fatty acid myristic acid replaces threonine at position 30 on the β-chain, which causes strong binding between insulin detemir molecules and binding to albumin to prolong its metabolism. There is very little information about use of insulin detemir in dogs, but, similar to insulin glargine, it may be useful for dogs that need a long-acting product. An equivalent dose of detemir in dogs appears to be 25% of the dose of NPH insulin, and the duration of action may be too long to require dosing every 12 hours (Sako et al, 2011). Evidence-based information about the use of detemir or glargine in dogs is too sparse to make a clear recommendation for dosing frequency. It is very important to determine the duration of action and appropriate dose for each patient by performing glucose curves, which may need to be continued longer than 12 hours.

Determining Insulin Dose and Frequency of Administration

In dogs with uncomplicated diabetes, it is recommended to initiate treatment with an insulin product with intermediate duration of action, such as recombinant human NPH or porcine Lente, at a dose of 0.25 U/kg every 12 hours administered subcutaneously starting at a time in the morning that fits the client's schedule. Blood glucose is measured two or three times at 3-hour intervals during the first day to ensure that the dose is not so high as to create hypoglycemia. If the blood glucose decreases to less than 100 mg/dl at any time during the first day, the dose should be reduced by 25%, and blood glucose should again be monitored to ensure hypoglycemia does not develop before the dog is sent home. Because it can take several days for the dog to adjust to any change in insulin dose or product type, it is sent home to receive insulin injections for 5 to 7 days before the first recheck to monitor the response to the insulin. To prevent tissue irritation from injecting insulin at the same site while maintaining consistent absorption of insulin from each injection, it is recommended to alternate injections at approximately 1 to 2 inches on either side of the midline. The suggested level is over the thorax from just caudal to the scapulae to the last rib, alternating from side to side; this allows for injection sites with similar blood supply, skin thickness, and muscular activity.

Because each dog may react uniquely to any insulin product, the appropriate dose and number of injections per day must be determined by monitoring the blood glucose response to the product (see Chapter 45). A careful history should be taken and a thorough physical examination, including body weight, should be performed to determine if clinical signs have resolved or are resolving. In addition, one should perform a glucose curve at 5- to 7-day intervals until the appropriate protocol is determined, which often takes 4 to 6 weeks. Performing one or two blood glucose measurements after the morning injection to titrate the insulin dose is inadequate and often leads to poor glucose control and hypoglycemia. To provide adequate information, the glucose curve should be performed after feeding the same food and giving the same insulin product and dosage at the usual times on the morning of the test. Blood glucose is determined every 2 hours for 10 to 12 hours, beginning either just before the dog is fed and given insulin or within 1 hour of doing so, if possible, depending on the owner's schedule. Deciding to feed and give insulin to the dog at home before coming to the hospital depends on the following practical factors: (1) the time in the morning that the dog is usually fed and treated and (2) whether or not the dog is likely to eat normally in the hospital setting. It is best to keep feeding and insulin administration within 1 hour of the usual schedule while beginning the curve at a time that is practical for the owner and veterinarian.

Glucose concentration can be determined using a point-of-care analyzer or handheld glucose meter to reduce the amount of blood drawn and the associated trauma to the patient. Handheld glucose meters intended for use with human blood generally underestimate the serum or plasma glucose concentration by 10% to 15% compared with a reference laboratory. A relatively new meter (AlphaTRAK) intended for use in dogs and cats may be the most accurate for use with dog blood. The AlphaTRAK both overestimates and underestimates blood glucose concentration, but the degree of inaccuracy is small. However, when blood glucose is relatively low, it occasionally may overestimate the value, failing to identify hypoglycemia.

Based on the clinical response of the patient and the results of the blood glucose curves, the insulin dose is adjusted by 1 to 5 U per injection, depending on the size of the dog and blood glucose concentrations measured every 5 to 7 days. The dose is adjusted to obtain a blood glucose nadir concentration of 80 to 150 mg/dl and to attempt to maintain the blood glucose concentration less than 250 to 300 mg/dl. It is important to perform glucose curves to determine the duration of insulin activity, defined as the time after insulin injection when the blood glucose exceeds 250 mg/dl after a nadir of 80 to 150 mg/dl. To determine the duration of insulin activity accurately, the blood glucose nadir must decrease sufficiently (range, 80 to 150 mg/dl) so that glucose concentrations greater than 250 mg/dl can be considered as representing near-complete loss of the administered insulin effect. In addition, it is important that the blood glucose nadir concentration remain greater than 65 mg/dl; otherwise, counterregulatory hormonal responses may stimulate blood glucose concentrations to increase to more than 250 mg/dl prematurely, before the true duration of insulin activity has been exceeded. If the blood glucose concentration just before the next scheduled insulin injection is less than 150 mg/dl and the glucose nadir was appropriate, the dog should be fed without giving the next injection of insulin, and the glucose curve should be continued until the blood glucose exceeds 250 mg/dl to determine if the duration of activity of the insulin product is longer than 12 hours. If the blood glucose exceeds 250 mg/dl within 1 to 2 hours of feeding without giving insulin, the duration of insulin activity is likely very close to 12 hours. Some dogs do not have an increase in blood glucose for some time after the injected insulin has been completely metabolized unless they are fed to provide a glucose source. If the glucose increases after feeding without giving insulin as indicated, it is generally safe to continue giving the same dose of insulin every 12 hours.

If the duration of insulin activity is longer than 14 hours but shorter than 16 hours and an extended glucose curve or clinical signs indicate the blood glucose concentration becomes too low overnight, administering a dose of intermediate-duration insulin in the evening that is 25% to 50% lower than the morning dose provides safe and adequate control in most cases. If the duration of insulin activity is longer than 16 hours, the dog may be adequately controlled with one daily injection of the product.

If the duration of action of an intermediate-duration insulin that is given once daily is longer than 16 hours but the dog continues to have clinical signs of polyuria and polydipsia, particularly during the night, a different intermediate-acting preparation could be tried every 12 hours, or a longer acting product, such as protamine zinc insulin, insulin detemir, or insulin glargine, could be given once or twice daily. It cannot be overemphasized that when starting a diabetic dog on any insulin once or twice daily, the duration of the response to that product must be determined by means of an adequate glucose curve. There is great variation among dogs in the duration of action of insulin products; for example, an insulin that is considered of long duration may have an effect of less than 12 hours in certain dogs. Treating with once-daily insulin without adequate glucose monitoring often leads to hypoglycemia. This occurrence is explained by the tendency to continue to increase the daily insulin dose in response to continued polyuria and polydipsia when the actual problem is not an inadequate dose but an inadequate duration of activity.

Longer Term Monitoring of Insulin Therapy

Once the appropriate insulin preparation, dose, and dosing interval have been determined, it is appropriate to reevaluate the dog in 30 days. A history and physical examination should be conducted, and urine ketones, blood glucose curve, and perhaps fructosamine concentration should be measured. Thereafter, rechecks every 3 to 6 months are appropriate unless the dog develops problems, such as recurrence of polyuria or polydipsia, weight loss, signs of hypoglycemia, or another disease. The owner may be asked to check urine glucose and ketones periodically, but the dose of insulin should not be altered on the basis of urine glucose determinations alone. The presence of ketonuria or of consistently high urine glucose, particularly if checked in the afternoon, should prompt reevaluation by a veterinarian.

When an appropriate dose and schedule have been determined, it must remain consistent. The client must understand that, as with humans, the true insulin need is likely to vary from day to day, but the goal is to identify a dosage and schedule that prevent clinical signs on most days, without episodes of hypoglycemia. Realistic therapeutic goals are first to maintain the dog as an acceptable companion and pet and second to attempt to prevent formation of diabetic cataracts.

It has been well documented that fructosamine values in dogs that are well controlled can overlap with values in dogs that are poorly controlled, and glucose curve values can vary from day to day. It is important not to rely on just one parameter to determine adequacy of glucose control or to change the insulin dose. If the glucose curve values do not seem to coincide with the history and physical examination results, the glucose curve should be repeated at the hospital, by the owner at home, or using a continuous glucose monitoring device while the dog is in the home setting. Generally, the most reliable parameters for determining adequacy of glycemic control are demonstration of resolution of polyuria and polydipsia, normal appetite, and lack of clinical signs of hypoglycemia on clinical history and maintenance of body weight noted on physical examination.

Complications and Prognosis

Hypoglycemia is one of the most serious complications of insulin therapy in diabetic dogs. Owners should be educated about the clinical signs of hypoglycemia and should be instructed to feed a meal when signs of low blood glucose develop, assuming the dog is sufficiently aware to consume food safely. For dogs that are not fully conscious, the owner should be instructed to rub syrup or honey on the gingival mucosa in an attempt to revive the dog before calling a veterinarian.

Most dogs live for a few years with diabetes. The average survival is approximately 2 to 3 years, but survival likely depends on the age of onset, concurrent disease, ease of management, and owner commitment. Most dogs develop cataracts within 5 to 6 months of the diagnosis, and 80% develop cataracts by 16 months after diagnosis. In the future, a topical ophthalmic preparation containing an aldose reductase inhibitor, Kinostat, may be useful to reduce cataract development in diabetic dogs, but it is not currently commercially available in the United States.

References and Suggested Reading

Briggs C et al: Reliability of history and physical examination findings for assessing control of glycemia in dogs with diabetes mellitus: 53 cases (1995-1998), *J Am Vet Med Assoc* 217:48, 2000.

Fracassi F et al: Use of insulin glargine in dogs with diabetes mellitus, *Vet Rec* 170:52, 2012.

Gilor C, Graves TK: Synthetic insulin analogs and their use in dogs and cats, *Vet Clin North Am Small Anim Pract* 40:297, 2010.

Guptill L, Glickman L, Glickman N: Time trends and risk factors for diabetes mellitus in dogs: analysis of veterinary medical data base records (1970-1999), *Vet J* 165:240, 2003.

Kador PR et al: Topical KINOSTAT ameliorates the clinical development and progression of cataracts in dogs with diabetes mellitus, *Vet Ophthalmol* 13:363, 2010.

Monroe WE et al: Efficacy and safety of a purified porcine insulin zinc suspension for managing diabetes mellitus in dogs, *J Vet Intern Med* 19:675, 2005.

Mori A et al: Comparison of time-action profiles of insulin glargine and NPH insulin in normal and diabetic dogs, *Vet Res Commun* 32:563, 2008.

Palm CA et al: An investigation of the action of Neutral Protamine Hagedorn human analogue insulin in dogs with naturally occurring diabetes mellitus, *J Vet Intern Med* 23:50, 2009.

Rucinsky R et al: AAHA diabetes management guidelines. *J Am Anim Hosp Assoc* 46:215, 2010.

Sako T et al: Time-action profiles of insulin detemir in normal and diabetic dogs, *Res Vet Sci* 90:396, 2011.

CHAPTER 45

Diabetic Monitoring

CLAUDIA E. REUSCH, *Zurich, Switzerland*

The aim of therapy in diabetic pets is to eliminate the clinical signs of diabetes mellitus, prevent short-term complications (e.g., hypoglycemia, ketoacidosis), and enable a good quality of life. Most diabetic pets do well if blood glucose concentrations are kept at 5 to 15 mmol/L (90 to 270 mg/dl) throughout 24 hours. In diabetic cats, the possibility of achieving remission requires special attention. Remission may occur in 50% of cats, usually during the first 3 months of therapy. To increase the chance of remission, treatment should be started immediately after the diagnosis of diabetes is made, and one should aim for good glycemic control. Close supervision and frequent monitoring of blood glucose are critical. In cases where remission is overlooked, serious hypoglycemia may result.

Management of diabetic dogs and cats relies on the owner's observations of clinical signs and on periodic evaluation by a veterinarian. The latter includes assessment of the owner's observations, measurement of body weight, and determination of blood glucose and serum fructosamine concentrations. Previously, blood glucose measurements and generation of blood glucose curves (BGCs) were almost always performed in veterinary hospitals because most owners were unable to collect venous blood samples. Nowadays many owners of diabetic pets perform so-called home monitoring by measuring capillary blood glucose with a portable blood glucose meter (PBGM). Home monitoring of blood glucose has nearly completely displaced the measurement of urine glucose in the clientele in our practice.

Monitoring in the Hospital

Frequency of Reevaluations

After diagnosis of diabetes mellitus, the owner should be informed that it usually takes 2 to 3 months until stable glycemic control is achieved (see Chapters 44 and 48) and that lifelong regular reevaluations in the hospital are required. Initially, frequent reevaluations should be scheduled. With time, intervals between rechecks can be extended. In our hospital, reevaluations are suggested at 1 week, 3 weeks, 8 weeks, and 12 weeks after diagnosis and then at intervals of approximately every 4 months. More frequent reevaluations may be needed in cats in which it is difficult to regulate diabetes. In animals (usually cats) in which diabetic remission has been achieved, the owners should be informed about the possibility of a relapse. They should be advised to watch their pets with regard to recurrence of polyuria and polydipsia, polyphagia, and weight loss.

Serum Fructosamine

Fructosamine measurements are widely used as an indicator of glycemic control in diabetic dogs and cats. Measurement is done in serum using commercially available test kits adapted to autoanalysis. Storage at 25° C for 5 days does not cause a significant change in fructosamine concentrations, allowing shipping of serum samples. Because fructosamine is the product of an irreversible reaction between glucose and the amino groups of plasma proteins, it is assumed that its concentration reflects the mean blood glucose concentration of the preceding 1 to 2 weeks. Serum fructosamine concentration is not affected by short-term increases of blood glucose; therefore it is also a valuable tool to differentiate between diabetes and stress hyperglycemia in cats. If healthy cats are infused with glucose to maintain a marked hyperglycemia (30 mmol/L [540 mg/dl]), fructosamine concentrations exceed the upper limit of the reference range after 3 to 5 days; if an only moderate hyperglycemia (17 mmol/L [300 mg/dl]) is induced, fructosamine concentrations mostly fluctuate just below the upper limit of the reference range (Link and Rand, 2008).

Reference ranges for serum fructosamine concentration differ slightly among laboratories but usually are approximately 200 to 360 µmol/L. In most newly diagnosed diabetic dogs and cats, fructosamine levels are greater than 400 µmol/L, but they may reach 1500 µmol/L. Normal fructosamine levels may be seen in animals with a very short duration of diabetes mellitus. Fructosamine may also be normal in animals with certain concurrent diseases. Hypoproteinemia, hyperlipidemia, and azotemia in dogs and hypoproteinemia and uncontrolled hyperthyroidism in cats can decrease the fructosamine concentration. In these cases, fructosamine measurements should not be used for the diagnosis or the long-term management of diabetes mellitus.

In all other cases, it is helpful to measure fructosamine concentrations during routine reevaluations. The parameter is independent of stress and lack of food intake, which are both major influencing factors for blood glucose measurements in the hospital. Fructosamine concentrations increase when glycemic control worsens and decrease when glycemic control improves. Differences between two consecutive measurements have to exceed approximately 50 µmol/L to reflect a clinically significant difference in glycemic control.

Normoglycemia is not a general treatment goal in veterinary medicine, and even dogs and cats with well-controlled diabetes are slightly to moderately hyperglycemic throughout the day. Consequently, fructosamine usually does not become completely normal during therapy. In contrast, the finding of a normal fructosamine level (in particular, fructosamine levels in the lower half of the reference range) should raise concern for prolonged periods of hypoglycemia caused by insulin overdose. In cats in which fructosamine levels decrease into the normal range during therapy, the possibility of diabetic remission has to be considered. Fructosamine levels of 360 to 450 µmol/L usually suggest good control; levels of 450 and 550 µmol/L, moderate control; and levels greater than 600 µmol/L, poor metabolic control. In the last situation, fructosamine measurement does not help to identify the underlying problem. All reasons for poor regulation have to be considered, including insulin underdosage, too short duration of insulin effect, diseases causing insulin resistance, and the Somogyi phenomenon.

Over the years, we and others have sometimes seen discrepancies between fructosamine on the one hand and clinical signs and blood glucose concentration on the other hand. Although high fructosamine levels suggested poor control, the lack of clinical signs and glucose level within the desired range pointed to good control. The reason for the discrepancy remains ambiguous in most instances, but it is possible that there are individual differences with regard to the extent of protein glycation. In those cases, the assessment based on clinical signs should be given priority over assessment of fructosamine.

Diabetic ketoacidosis, dehydration, acidosis, and other unidentified factors may influence fructosamine concentrations. If a diabetic patient is hospitalized for any reason, fructosamine levels measured at the time of admission may differ considerably from the fructosamine concentration measured a few days later after successful therapy. It is advisable to repeat the measurement at the time of discharge and to use this level as a reference point for future measurements.

Fructosamine is a valuable adjunct parameter to monitor glycemic control. However, it should always be interpreted in conjunction with clinical signs and body weight.

Glycated Hemoglobin

Glycated hemoglobin has been measured in human medicine since the 1970s and is regarded as one of the cornerstones of assessment of glycemic control. Comparable to fructosamine, it is formed by nonenzymatic, irreversible attachment of glucose to an amino group of the globin part of the hemoglobin molecule. Although glycation kinetics are relatively complicated, it is commonly assumed that glycated hemoglobin reflects the average blood glucose concentration over the life span of the erythrocytes, which is 100 to 120 days in dogs and 70 days in cats. Glycated hemoglobin is rarely used as a long-term parameter in veterinary medicine at the present time. The main explanation for infrequent use pertains to the various assay techniques and the lack of standardization in veterinary medicine. Therefore results may not be comparable among laboratories. Glycated hemoglobin should be considered only if the assay has been validated for dogs and cats and assay-specific reference ranges have been established.

Blood Glucose Measurements and Blood Glucose Curves

Single blood glucose measurements are usually insufficient to assess glycemic control. Exceptions to this rule are dogs and cats with an unremarkable history and physical examination and a serum fructosamine of 360 to 450 µmol/L. In these cases, the finding of a blood glucose concentration of 10 to 15 mmol/L (180 to 270 mg/dl) around the time of insulin injection would support the assumption of good glycemic control and may render further blood glucose measurements unnecessary. In all other cases, there is a substantial risk of misinterpretation if only one glucose measurement is performed. Evaluation of a BGC is mandatory in the initial phases of diabetic regulation and in animals with persistence of clinical signs, ongoing weight loss, and fructosamine greater than 500 µmol/L. The BGC provides guidelines for making rational adjustments in insulin therapy.

We usually recommend that feeding and the insulin injection be done at home and that the animal be presented to the hospital as soon as possible thereafter. If technical difficulties are suspected, owners are asked to bring the animal to the hospital before the insulin administration and to perform the whole injection procedure under the supervision of a veterinarian or a technician. Blood samples are taken every 1 to 2 hours throughout the day until the next insulin injection whether the insulin is given in the hospital or not. To avoid multiple venipunctures, we collect capillary blood from the ear or the footpad using the same sampling technique and the same PBGM as the owners at home (see later).

BGCs enable the assessment of insulin efficacy, the glucose nadir, the time of peak insulin effect, the duration of the effect of insulin, and the degree of fluctuation in blood glucose. The most important parameters are insulin efficacy, glucose nadir, and duration of effect. Insulin efficacy is defined as the difference between the highest and the lowest glucose concentration and must be interpreted in the light of the highest blood glucose concentration and the insulin dosage. A relatively small difference (e.g., 2.8 mmol/L [50 mg/dl]) is acceptable in an animal in which the highest glucose concentration is less than 11 mmol/L (200 mg/dl); however, the same difference is unacceptable if the highest glucose level is greater than 17 mmol/L (300 mg/dl). Similarly, the same difference may indicate insulin efficacy in an animal receiving a small dosage of insulin (<0.25 to 0.5 U/kg) but may point to insulin resistance if the insulin dosage is high (>1.5 U/kg). Some newer insulins (e.g., insulin glargine) have been developed to provide a more constant level of insulin, which should render the difference between the highest and lowest glucose level relatively small (so-called peakless insulins). In some pets, this is definitely the case; in most, however, insulin glargine is not a peakless insulin, and efficacy may be evaluated as mentioned earlier. In cases in which glucose concentrations are constantly high, insulin underdosing, insulin resistance, technical problems with the insulin administration procedure, stress hyperglycemia in cats, and the counterregulatory phase of the Somogyi phenomenon have to be considered.

After insulin effectiveness is confirmed, the glucose nadir should be interpreted; this should ideally be 5.0 to 7.8 mmol/L (90 to 140 mg/dl). A lower nadir can be seen with insulin overdosage, excessive overlap of insulin action, lack of food intake, and strenuous exercise. It is also typically seen in diabetic cats in which the disease is progressing to remission. In cases in which overdosage is identified, the insulin dosage should be reduced by 10% to 50%. Excessive overlap of insulin action may require a change to an insulin with a shorter duration of action. If the nadir is greater than 7.8 to 9 mmol/L (140 to 160 mg/dl) despite insulin effectiveness, insulin underdosage, stress hyperglycemia, the counterregulatory phase of the Somogyi phenomenon, and technical problems of the owners have to be considered. If the animal is already being treated with a high insulin dosage, insulin resistance also may be possible. It is very important to identify the exact cause because treatment decisions differ and may be completely opposite of one another. For example, insulin underdosage is treated by increasing the insulin dosage by 10% to 25%, whereas the Somogyi phenomenon is treated by decreasing the dosage by approximately 50%.

Careful evaluation of the other parameters of glycemic control such as clinical signs and serum fructosamine is mandatory. In addition, it may be necessary to assess the owner's insulin administration technique. The counterregulatory phase of the Somogyi phenomenon may last 72 hours. Therefore several BGCs may be required to demonstrate a decrease of blood glucose to less than 3.5 mmol/L (60 mg/dl) followed by an increase in blood glucose to a concentration greater than 17 mmol/L (300 mg/dl) within a 12-hour period after insulin administration.

Duration of insulin effect is evaluated if the glucose nadir lies in the desired range of 5 to 7.8 mmol/L (90 to 140 mg/dl). The duration is defined as the time from insulin injection through the glucose nadir until the blood glucose exceeds 14 to 15 mmol/L (250 to 270 mg/dl). If the duration of insulin effect is less than 8 to 10 hours, animals usually show clinical signs of diabetes mellitus. In contrast, if the duration is longer than 14 hours, the risk of developing hypoglycemia secondary to overlapping insulin effect increases.

In some instances it is difficult to distinguish between too short duration of effect and the Somogyi phenomenon because BGCs may look alike. It is therefore important to reevaluate the patient soon (a few days to a week) after any treatment modification.

Problems Encountered with Monitoring Blood Glucose in the Hospital

Interpretation of BGCs generated in hospitalized animals may be difficult because of the potential influence of stress, abnormal housing conditions (e.g., lack of exercise), and decreased food intake on blood glucose concentrations. A study by Fleeman and Rand (2003) showed that there was a large day-to-day variability when BGCs were performed on consecutive days in diabetic dogs. In addition, BGCs are time-consuming and expensive; therefore they are often not performed as frequently as required. Many patients would benefit from more frequent blood glucose determinations. For example, adjustments of the insulin dosage on short notice are necessary in diabetic patients with infections (increased dosage) or at times of increased physical activity (mostly decreased dosage). Close monitoring of blood glucose is also indicated in diabetic patients that are treated for concomitant diseases such as hyperadrenocorticism or hypothyroidism that are known to cause insulin resistance. Similarly, intact bitches may require adjustments of the insulin dosage at the transition from one stage of the cycle to another. Because of the abolition of the resistance to insulin associated with these conditions, the required insulin dosage may have to be reduced drastically to prevent life-threatening hypoglycemia. It is difficult to manage these cases without frequent blood glucose determinations.

Monitoring at Home by the Owner

Frequency of Monitoring

Owners should assess their animals with regard to the clinical signs of diabetes mellitus on a daily basis. Body weight should be measured at least once a week. It is important that the owner be familiar with the clinical signs of the most important complications of diabetes mellitus (i.e., hypoglycemia, diabetic ketoacidosis). Measurement of blood glucose is also feasible for owners and may be recommended in many cases.

Home Monitoring of Blood Glucose

Problems with diabetic control in human patients are similar in principle to problems encountered in veterinary patients. Many of these issues have been largely eradicated since the late 1970s with the introduction of self-monitoring of blood glucose (SMBG) concentration. For SMBG, humans obtain a drop of capillary blood usually by pricking a fingertip with a lancing device. The drop is placed on a test strip, and the glucose concentration is measured using a PBGM. During the last 10 years, similar methods for monitoring blood glucose have been developed for dogs and cats and are now widely used. In Zurich, a lancing device creating a negative pressure (Microlet Vaculance) was used since the beginning of home monitoring, and the sampling technique had been called the "Vaculance method." This device is no longer available, and we replaced it with the Microlet 2 lancing device. However, many other devices are available, and the choice is a question of personal preference.

Capillary blood may be obtained from various sites. We prefer to sample from the inner aspect of the pinna. In cases in which this site is not feasible (e.g., blood drop too small, resistance of the pet), the metacarpal or metatarsal pads are used as alternative sites. In dogs, the buccal mucosa has been described as another site for capillary blood sampling; blood sampling by the so-called marginal ear vein technique is sometimes used in cats.

Since their introduction, the quality control of PBGMs has been a frequent topic of discussion in human medicine. Studies have shown that accuracy can vary greatly but generally tends to be poor for very low as well as for very high glucose concentrations. Factors with a possible effect on the results of glucose measurements include variation in hematocrit, altitude, environmental temperature and humidity, hypotension, hypoxia, and

triglyceride concentrations. It has become difficult to maintain an overview of the accuracy of all available PBGMs because new devices are frequently being developed by various companies; all of these new devices are claimed to be smaller in size, faster in action, and easier to handle than their predecessors.

Most PBGMs are made for use in humans; however, several companies are now marketing devices for veterinary use, claiming that they give more accurate results in dogs and cats than the counterparts made for humans. So far, independent studies have been published only for the AlphaTRAK. In both dogs and cats, glucose concentrations measured with the AlphaTRAK differed from glucose concentrations measured with the reference method. However, differences were considerably smaller than with other PBGMs (including the Ascensia Elite, which had been our preferred PBGM for many years) (Cohen et al, 2009; Zini et al, 2009). The differences between the AlphaTRAK readings and the reference method increase as blood glucose concentrations increase. In contrast to other PBGMs (which usually measure glucose concentration lower than the reference method), the AlphaTRAK may either underestimate or overestimate the true glucose concentrations. In rare instances, hypoglycemia may be overlooked. Besides better performance, additional advantages of the AlphaTRAK are the very small sample volume (0.3 μl) and the extended measurement range (1.1 to 41.7 mmol/L [20 to 750 mg/dl]).

Other "veterinary" PBGMs are already on the market, and many more are expected. It is very important that quality control studies are performed before these devices are used. However, measurements done with a PBGM deviate to a certain extent from the reference method. The American Diabetes Association recommends for "human" PBGMs that the error of the meter (i.e., difference from the reference method) should be less than 5%. This is a very ambitious goal and is frequently not reached. In veterinary medicine, analytic quality goals have not yet been established. For more than 10 years, we have used home monitoring of blood glucose (HM) in diabetic dogs and cats, and the results have been extremely positive. Most owners are very interested in measuring blood glucose in their pets, and about 70% have been capable and willing to perform HM on a long-term basis.

Several steps should precede the introduction of HM. The first step is a definitive diagnosis of diabetes mellitus. Additional tests to diagnose concurrent diseases may be indicated at this point. The owner receives detailed information about various aspects of diabetes mellitus and careful instruction on injection technique, and the concept of HM is mentioned for the first time. This consultation takes approximately 45 minutes. The second step consists of reevaluation of the patient after 1 week. Observations made by the owner are discussed, a clinical examination is performed, and fructosamine concentration and a 12-hour BGC are generated in the hospital. Treatment is adjusted if necessary. At the time of discharge, the importance of regular generation of BGCs during long-term monitoring of the disease is emphasized. In addition, the advantages of HM for owner and pet are discussed, and the owner is informed that this procedure can be started after the next reevaluation.

The third step follows approximately 3 weeks after the diagnosis has been made. The owner is given the opportunity to learn the technique of HM. A minimum of 30 minutes is required for teaching, which consists of repeated demonstrations of the use of the lancing device and the PBGM. The owner performs the technique several times on the pet. He or she is also taught how to calibrate the PBGM (if needed), how to check the meter's accuracy using the control strips, and how to record the blood glucose values on forms prepared by our clinic. HM is not started before the third week after a diagnosis of diabetes mellitus; this allows the owner time to become familiar with the disease and to gain experience with the injection of insulin. Introduction of HM is delayed to a later date if the owner does not seem ready for it.

When the owner is comfortable with the HM procedure, we request that a fasting blood glucose concentration be determined twice weekly and a BGC generated at least once monthly. The former serves to detect morning hypoglycemia, in which case the owner is instructed to call us. For determination of a BGC, the blood glucose is measured before the insulin injection (fasting) and every 2 hours thereafter. Because all our diabetic animals receive insulin twice daily, the BGC is performed over a 12-hour period. The owner sends the results of the BGC per fax or e-mail, and appropriate changes in treatment are discussed, if necessary, on the telephone. The assessment of the BGC generated at home follows the same rules as for the BGC generated in the hospital. Periodic reassessments of the entire procedure (capillary blood sampling, use of the PBGM, and correct reading of measurement) in the hospital are mandatory. For the first 2 months, the patient is reassessed at least once a month; after that time, the frequency of rechecks is reduced to approximately every 4 months.

It is important that owners performing HM have ready access to veterinary support, if required. Most of our clients call for advice one or more times, especially after the start of HM. Sometimes support via telephone is insufficient, and additional explanation or demonstration of the technique must be provided. By watching an owner perform the procedure, a veterinarian can identify and correct errors immediately. The most frequently encountered technical problem is failure to generate an adequate amount of blood. If repeated demonstration does not solve the problem, choosing an alternative sampling site (e.g., switching from pinna to footpad) may be helpful. Handling the PBGM usually is not a problem for owners, and most report that their pet tolerates blood collection well. The skin puncture does not seem to be painful, and the puncture sites are barely visible, even after numerous blood collections.

We (Casella et al, 2003, 2005) compared BGCs generated at home with BGCs generated in the hospital with regard to treatment decisions. In about 60% of cases, treatment decisions would have been the same; in about 40% of cases, treatment decisions would have been different. In the 40% in which treatment decisions would have differed, only 3% of dogs and 8% of cats would have had treatment decisions made that would have been contrary (e.g., increase versus decrease of insulin dosage); in the others, although the decisions would have been different, the clinical consequences would have been less. We also showed that there is a lot of variability if BGCs are performed at home on consecutive days (Alt et al, 2007). Single curves may not reflect the true glycemic situation regardless of whether they are generated in the hospital or at home. However, a major advantage of HM is that it enables frequent generation of BGCs, which may be of particular importance in animals that are difficult to regulate. More than one BGC can be performed at home before a decision is made concerning therapy. Performance of multiple curves at home is also beneficial for cats in which the degree of hyperglycemia attenuates and diabetic remission begins to show. In those cases, repetitive BGCs in short intervals are helpful to tailor insulin requirements and to avoid hypoglycemia.

Long-term compliance of pet owners is often good; many perform HM for several years. According to a retrospective survey in cat owners, only a few adjusted insulin dosages independently, and most of them called the hospital for advice. All cat owners believed that HM provides major advantages over in-hospital monitoring (Kley et al, 2004).

It has been argued that pet owners who are able to perform HM would visit the hospital less frequently. However, our observations over the last years do not support this argument. Frequency of in-hospital reevaluation does not differ among pets with or without HM.

HM is a valuable additional tool in the management of dogs and cats with diabetes mellitus. One of its major advantages is that blood glucose can be measured more frequently than when it has to be done in the hospital.

Monitoring of Urine Glucose

Until blood glucose measurement became possible, urine glucose testing was the main method of assessing glycemic control at home. Glucose is freely filtered at the glomerulus and actively resorbed by the proximal tubule. The resorption capacity for glucose is limited; when the blood glucose concentration exceeds the so-called renal threshold (approximately 10 mmol/L [180 mg/dl] in dogs and approximately 17 mmol/L [300 mg/dl] in cats), urine glucose excretion is thought to be roughly proportional to hyperglycemia. However, measurement of urine glucose may be misleading for several reasons, as follows:

1. The result does not reflect the actual blood glucose but is an average over the time of urine accumulation in the bladder.
2. A negative urine test does not differentiate between hypoglycemia, normoglycemia, or mild hyperglycemia.
3. Hydration status and urine concentration may affect the result.
4. In individual diabetic dogs and cats, the renal threshold may increase or decrease over time as is known to occur in humans; in those cases, severe hyperglycemia may exist without glucosuria, and glucosuria may occur with a normal BGC.

Very few clinical studies have been performed on the accuracy of urine glucose testing and its use for diabetic monitoring. A more recent study compared the Bayer

Urine Multistix (a frequently used test strip for urinalysis) with the Purina Glucotest in feline samples. The latter is a litter additive designed to monitor urine glucose concentrations of cats in their home environment. Both methods had high sensitivity and specificity for detection of glucose. However, with regard to estimations of severity of glucosuria, the Bayer Urine Multistix overestimated the glucose concentration in about 20% of samples. The Purina Glucotest inaccurately classified a similar percentage if evaluation was done immediately; however, the percentage decreased if the test was read 30 minutes or longer after exposure to urine. Underestimation of glucosuria occurred in 5.2% (Bayer Urine Multistix) and 1% (Purina Glucotest) of samples (Fletcher et al, 2011).

We usually do not adjust insulin dosages on urine glucose measurements, and we do not allow owners to do this. Owners who are unable to measure blood glucose but still want to monitor their pet may be advised to use urine glucose measurements in all urine samples voided throughout 1 day per week. Persistent glucosuria would suggest inadequate glycemic control and the need for thorough evaluation in the hospital. Persistently negative results may point to hypoglycemia (insulin overdosage, diabetic remission), and this also requires evaluation. In animals prone to developing diabetic ketoacidosis, we recommend that owners check the urine for ketone bodies on a regular basis (e.g., once to twice per week) to detect impending or actual ketoacidosis.

Continuous Glucose Monitoring

Continuous glucose monitoring systems (CGMS) were developed for humans almost 2 decades ago, and they have been introduced more recently into veterinary medicine. With this system, glucose concentration can be monitored without the need of continuous capillary blood sampling. The technology is designed to measure interstitial glucose instead of blood glucose. Interstitial fluid is easily accessible and has rapid equilibration with the blood; therefore interstitial and blood glucose concentrations have a good correlation.

Several CGMS are currently available. The first systems offered only retrospective analysis of the glucose concentrations after disconnecting the sensor and uploading the data, whereas the new generations measure and display the data immediately, allowing direct intervention (real-time = RT-CGMS). We started to use and to evaluate one system, the Guardian REAL-Time, a few years ago and consider it a highly valuable additional monitoring tool. The system uses a small electrode, which is inserted in the subcutaneous tissue and fixed with tape; the sensor is connected to a transmitter that is also fixed to the patient with tape and that sends data in a wireless fashion over a maximal distance of 3 m (10 feet) to a pager-sized monitor. Data are collected every 10 seconds, and a mean glucose value is computed every 5 minutes. The system still has some shortfalls at the present time: (1) It requires a 2-hour period for initialization during which no data are recorded; (2) it needs to be calibrated within 6 hours after initial calibration and then every 12 hours thereafter, which requires capillary blood sampling; and (3) the sensor, which is

quite expensive, can be used for only a few days. The monitor displays glucose concentrations from 2.2 to 22.4 mmol/L (40 to 400 mg/dl); concentrations outside this range are correctly recorded but need to be downloaded to be visualized. Based on currently available studies, CGMS provide clinically accurate estimates of blood glucose in diabetic dogs and cats. CGMS give much greater insight into glucose levels throughout the day and help to identify fluctuations, hypoglycemic episodes, and trends that may otherwise go unnoticed. CGMS are not a general replacement for other types of monitoring (e.g., glucose curve with a PBGM), but they may be helpful in difficult cases to regulate or in animals with diabetic ketoacidosis in which close monitoring is needed for several days. With some further improvements, CGMS also are likely to be used at home in the future.

References and Suggested Reading

Alt N et al: Day-to-day variability of blood glucose concentration curves generated at home in cats with diabetes mellitus, *J Am Vet Med Assoc* 230:1011, 2007.

Casella M et al: Home monitoring of blood glucose concentration by owners of diabetic dogs, *J Small Anim Pract* 44:298, 2003.

Casella M, Hässig M, Reusch CE: Home-monitoring of blood glucose in cats with diabetes mellitus: evaluation over a 4-month period, *J Feline Med Surg* 7:163, 2005.

Cohen TA et al: Evaluation of six portable glucose meters for measuring blood glucose concentration in dogs, *J Am Vet Med Assoc* 235:276, 2009.

Dietiker-Moretti S et al: Comparison of a continuous glucose monitoring system with a portable blood glucose meter to determine insulin dose in cats with diabetes mellitus, *J Vet Intern Med* 25:1084, 2011.

Fleeman LM, Rand JS: Evaluation of day-to-day variability of serial blood glucose concentration curves in diabetic dogs, *J Am Vet Med Assoc* 222:317, 2003.

Fletcher JM et al: Glucose detection and concentration estimation in feline urine samples with the Bayer Multistix and Purina Glucotest, *J Feline Med Surg* 13:705, 2011.

Graham PA, Mooney CT, Murray M: Serum fructosamine concentrations in hyperthyroid cats, *Res Vet Sci* 67:171, 1999.

Kley S, Casella M, Reusch CE: Evaluation of long-term home monitoring of blood glucose concentrations in cats with diabetes mellitus: 26 cases (1999-2002), *J Am Vet Med Assoc* 225:261, 2004.

Link KR, Rand JS: Changes in blood glucose concentration are associated with relatively rapid changes in circulating fructosamine concentrations in cats, *J Feline Med Surg* 10:583, 2008.

Moretti S et al: Evaluation of a novel real-time continuous glucose-monitoring system for use in cats, *J Vet Intern Med* 24:120, 2010.

Reineke EL et al: Accuracy of a continuous glucose monitoring system in dogs and cats with diabetic ketoacidosis, *J Vet Emerg Crit Care* 20:303, 2010.

Reusch C: Feline diabetes mellitus. In Ettinger SJ, Feldman EC, editors: *Textbook of veterinary internal medicine*, Vol 2, St Louis, 2010, Saunders, p 1796.

Reusch CE, Gerber B, Boretti FS: Serum fructosamine concentrations in dogs with hypothyroidism, *Vet Res Commun* 26:531, 2002.

Reusch CE, Haberer B: Evaluation of fructosamine in dogs and cats with hypo- or hyperproteinaemia, azotaemia, hyperlipidaemia and hyperbilirubinaemia, *Vet Rec* 148:370, 2001.

Reusch CE, Tomsa K: Serum fructosamine concentration in cats with overt hyperthyroidism, *J Am Vet Med Assoc* 215:1297, 1999.

Thompson MD et al: Comparison of glucose concentrations in blood samples obtained with a marginal ear vein nick technique versus from a peripheral vein in healthy cats and cats with diabetes mellitus, *J Am Vet Med Assoc* 221:389, 2002.

Wess G, Reusch C: Capillary blood sampling from the ear of dogs and cats and use of portable meters to measure glucose concentration, *J Small Anim Pract* 41:60, 2000.

Wiedmeyer CE, DeClue AE: Continuous glucose monitoring in dogs and cats, *J Vet Intern Med* 22:2, 2008.

Zeugswetter FK, Rebuzzi L, Karlovits S: Alternative sampling site for blood glucose testing in cats: giving the ears a rest, *J Feline Med Surg* 12:710, 2010.

Zini E et al: Evaluation of a new portable glucose meter designed for the use in cats, *Schweiz Arch Tierheilk* 151:448, 2009.

Zini E et al: Predictors of clinical remission in cats with diabetes mellitus, *J Vet Intern Med* 24:1314, 2010.

CHAPTER 46
Diet and Diabetes

DEBRA L. ZORAN, *College Station, Texas*

Diabetes mellitus in dogs and cats is a complex, multifactorial disease that develops secondary to a relative or absolute insulin deficiency or a dysfunctional response to insulin. The disease affecting dogs is primarily one of absolute insulin deficiency that occurs as a result of the complete loss of insulin production, most commonly caused by immune-mediated destruction of pancreatic β cells. The disease in cats is quite different and is similar to insulin-resistant (type 2) diabetes associated with chronic hyperglycemia, hyperinsulinemia, and obesity-induced insulin resistance that is seen in adult humans. Nevertheless, the end result in both forms of diabetes is persistent hyperglycemia and a relative or absolute lack of insulin that ultimately leads to abnormal lipid and protein metabolism that creates a catabolic state sometimes termed *starvation in the face of plenty*.

Insulin therapy is the mainstay of treatment for both diabetic dogs and cats (see Chapters 44 and 48), but because diabetes is a disease of disordered metabolism, nutritional therapy is a key component of the management of these patients. Although different mechanisms for development of diabetes exist for dogs and cats, concurrent pancreatitis or other conditions (e.g., obesity) may be important factors for both species that influence the nutritional plan. The general goals of dietary therapy in any diabetic dog or cat are broad based and include the following:

1. To achieve and maintain optimal body condition
2. To provide a nutritionally complete, balanced, and palatable food that is readily consumed (so that intake is predictable)
3. To provide nutritional support for any concurrent diseases requiring nutritional modification
4. To maintain consistency in the timing and type (e.g., ingredients and calories) of food to assist in achieving optimal glycemic control
5. To control the amount and types of dietary starch, because the primary determinant of postprandial glycemia is starch, present in the diet.

Although more studies (especially in cats) have been forthcoming in recent years, well-designed dietary studies in diabetic dogs and cats remain sparse, and dietary recommendations cannot be based solely on research. In addition, there are important differences between dogs and cats in dietary management strategies for this disease. This chapter reviews the most relevant aspects of nutritional management of diabetes, the major differences between dogs and cats, and the role of specific nutrients in the management of diabetes.

Dietary Management of Canine Diabetes Mellitus

Dogs with diabetes typically are presented for examination because of polyuria, polydipsia, polyphagia, or weight loss; many diabetic dogs have a thin body condition at the time of diagnosis. The goal of achieving optimal body condition in a diabetic dog requires a dietary strategy that not only assists in the control of postprandial glycemia but also allows the dog to regain its normal body weight (BW). Alternatively, some diabetic dogs are obese or have a normal body condition; in these dogs, the dietary strategy is still focused on achieving optimal body condition, but the type and amount of diet may differ from the diet for a dog that is very thin and needs to gain weight. No single dietary strategy works for all diabetic dogs; clinicians must tailor their dietary recommendations to fit the specific needs of the individual dog.

Dietary Fiber

For many years, diets containing increased amounts of dietary fiber have been recommended for dogs with diabetes because such diets may improve postprandial glycemia, presumably by delaying gastric emptying, slowing carbohydrate digestion and absorption, and altering gut hormones. No standards are set for what is considered to be high versus low fiber, just generally agreed-on ranges. Generally, high fiber is assumed to be greater than 15% dry matter (similar to many weight-loss diets); medium fiber, 5% to 15% dry matter; and low fiber, less than 5% dry matter. In addition, the term "dietary fiber" encompasses a wide variety of complex carbohydrates that have widely varying effects in the gastrointestinal (GI) tract. It is necessary to understand how dietary fiber is characterized and how these qualities affect glycemic control in diabetic dogs.

Dietary fiber is characterized by its degree of solubility, which also generally reflects both its degree of fermentability (i.e., how completely the intestinal bacteria can break it down) and its properties in water (e.g., intestinal juice). Highly soluble fibers, such as guar gum, have a great water-holding capacity and form a viscous gel-like solution in the lumen of the intestine. Conversely, insoluble fibers, such as cellulose, increase bulk and reduce intestinal transit time (i.e., increase speed of transit of ingesta through the small intestine), making nutrients (including starch) less available for digestion. In normal dogs fed diets high in soluble fibers, more rapid glucose absorption occurs because of increased intestinal glucose transport, glucagon-like peptide-1, and insulin secretion. However, it is unknown whether these same effects occur in diabetic dogs.

In studies comparing the effects of diets with soluble, insoluble, or mixed fiber in dogs with diabetes, there was no significant difference between the effects of diets on oral glucose tolerance testing; serum triglyceride levels; or the cholesterol content of high-density lipoproteins, low-density lipoproteins, or very-low-density lipoproteins. The only significant difference created by the diets was that total serum cholesterol concentrations were lower in dogs fed the diets containing mixed fiber.

Additional studies in diabetic dogs suggest that diets high in insoluble or mixed fiber may be associated with improved glycemic control. Insoluble-fiber diets appear to exert little physiologic effect on the canine GI tract compared with soluble-fiber diets and are not fermented by the bacterial flora; higher concentrations of these fibers may be added to diets with fewer side effects (e.g., diarrhea, flatulence). In other studies comparing a mixed-fiber diet with a lower fiber maintenance diet, diabetic dogs had significantly improved glycemic control when fed the mixed-fiber diet. However, regardless of the type or concentration of fiber added to the diet or the duration of time over which the diabetic dogs were monitored, there ultimately was no significant difference in the daily insulin requirement or fasting triglyceride levels.

Finally, there is a highly variable difference between dogs in their response to dietary fiber—in other words, there does not appear to be a uniform effect of fiber in all diabetics, and the effect of a type or amount of fiber in a diabetic dog is unpredictable. An investigation in diabetic dogs comparing a canned, high-fiber, moderate-starch diet with a diet that contained a moderate amount of fiber and starch found no significant difference between the diets in insulin requirements or glycemic response. The decision to use a diet with increased dietary fiber in the therapy of a diabetic dog should be based on individual circumstances because there is no clear indication that these diets are beneficial in all cases. For example, in dogs that may need to lose weight or dogs with poor glycemic control with a normal maintenance diet, diets containing increased insoluble or mixed fiber may be a reasonable choice. Alternatively, if the dog does not tolerate or refuses to eat a diet with increased amounts of fiber, the clinician should choose a maintenance or weight-loss diet containing lower fat and high complex carbohydrates. Table 46-1 lists different diets, both fiber-containing veterinary diets and non–fiber-containing diets, that may be considered for use in diabetic dogs (this is not an exhaustive list).

Dietary Carbohydrates, Fat, and Protein

The glycemic index classifies food based on its potential to increase blood glucose after absorption from the GI tract. To create diets that result in a lower, less prolonged postprandial blood glucose concentration, the glycemic index of the type of starch ingested can be considered when choosing a diet for a diabetic dog. In healthy dogs, the amount of starch in the diet is a major determinant of the glycemic index, no matter what type of dog food is tested. In one study of healthy dogs, rice-based diets resulted in significantly higher postprandial glucose levels, whereas sorghum-based diets (especially barley) resulted in the lowest glycemic response. However, predicting the glycemic index of food is based not only on the type of starch present in a diet but also on the matrix in which the carbohydrate is found, the type of processing the carbohydrate has undergone, and the total amount of carbohydrate consumed. Data about the responses of diabetic dogs to different diets and different types of carbohydrates are sparse, and it is difficult to make specific evidence-based recommendations for dogs with diabetes. However, because highly digestible diets designed for GI disease often contain rice-based carbohydrate sources, these diets may not be ideally suited for diabetic dogs.

Diabetic dogs also have abnormalities in lipid metabolism secondary to the lack of insulin production, including hypertriglyceridemia; hypercholesterolemia; and increases in lipoproteins, chylomicrons, and free fatty acids. In contrast to humans, who have increased risk of cardiovascular disease and stroke secondary to hypertriglyceridemia, the major consequence in dogs is the increased risk of pancreatitis, which complicates the management of diabetes and increases the risk for secondary complications and morbidity (see Chapters 58 and 137). In most diabetic dogs, the lipid values improve with

TABLE **46-1**

Selected Canine Diabetic Diet Comparisons of Prescription and Nonprescription Products*

Diet	Protein (% DM)	CHO Type	CHO (% DM)	Fat (% DM)	Fiber Type and Amount (% DM)	Calories (kcal/Cup or Can)
Hill's prescription diets w/d dry	19.2	Whole grain corn	50.8	8.7	Cellulose (16.4)	243
Hill's prescription diets w/d canned	17.9	Whole grain corn, cracked barley	52.6	12.7	Cellulose (12.4)	370
Hill's Science Diet adult light dry	24.3	Whole grain corn, soybean	49.6	8.8	Cellulose (12.4)	295
Hill's Science Diet adult light canned	19.5	Whole grain corn, soybean	56.8	8.6	Mixed 9.7	322
Purina veterinary diet DCO	25.3	Corn, pearled barley	47.8	12.41	Mixed 7.6	320
Purina veterinary diets OM (weight management) dry	31.0	Whole corn, soybean germ	44.2	7.2	Mixed 10.2	266
Purina veterinary diets OM (weight management) canned	48.0	Corn, gluten meal	16.7	14.6	Mixed 12.7	286
Purina Pro Plan weight management dry	30.5	Brewers rice, corn	40.7	10.2	Mixed 2.5	337
Royal Canin diabetic HF 18 dry	18.0	Rice, ground corn	49.8	7.0	Cellulose 12.6	273
Royal Canin Calorie Control CC High Fiber dry	22.5	Corn	36.3	8.0	Mixed 18.3	237

CHO, Carbohydrate; *DM,* dry matter.
*Based on current product guides.

the administration of insulin and feeding a diet containing lower fat and higher fiber content. Current recommendations by nutritionists suggest feeding a diet that contains less than 30% of metabolizable energy from fat; however, there are very few published data on the influence of dietary fat or the optimal level of fat in dogs with diabetes.

In humans with diabetes, supplementation with omega-3 fatty acids has been recommended to reduce serum lipid levels, blood pressure, and platelet aggregation—all benefits that are important to reduce the risk of stroke and cardiovascular disease. However, in some humans with diabetes, consumption of increased amounts of omega-3 fatty acids results in increased blood glucose concentrations and an overall reduction in glycemic control. The effects of omega-3 fatty acids have not been adequately evaluated in dogs with diabetes and it is unknown whether or not these same effects occur in dogs.

Finally, L-carnitine is a conditionally essential vitamin-like nutrient that has an essential role in fatty acid metabolism. Dog with poorly controlled diabetes are prone to ketogenesis, weight loss, and altered fat metabolism—all factors that can be attenuated by improved lipid metabolism that may occur with supplementation of L-carnitine. The amount of L-carnitine that is needed to achieve this effect in diabetic dogs is unclear, but in one report 50 ppm added to a canine diet improved lipid parameters in normal dogs. L-Carnitine supplementation is not routinely recommended for diabetics, but it could be considered in a patient with complications of lipid abnormalities (e.g., pancreatitis).

Protein catabolism occurs when insulin concentrations are low or ineffective. Catabolism of muscle proteins is a protective mechanism designed to supply substrate (amino acids) that can be used for gluconeogenesis. In diabetic dogs that are unregulated, not eating well, or being fed inadequate protein in the diet, muscle proteins are used. To prevent this loss of essential tissue, it is necessary that both an adequate quality and quantity of protein be supplied in the diet. In general, diets for diabetic dogs should contain a highly digestible (85% to 90%), high-quality protein (18% to 25% on a dry-matter basis) to reduce muscle catabolism. Such diets also provide adequate protein for maintenance and repair but do not appear to increase the risk of diabetic nephropathy.

Micronutrients

When a complete and balanced diet is fed in appropriate quantities for a dog's BW and condition, there is no need for additional vitamin and mineral supplementation in most diabetic dogs. However, in diabetic dogs that are not consuming a balanced diet (e.g., dogs consuming home-made or single-item diets) or that have uncontrolled diabetes, the risk of development of a micronutrient imbalance is increased.

The macrominerals most likely to be affected in diabetic dogs are potassium, magnesium, and phosphorus. In most dogs with adequate glycemic control that are consuming appropriate amounts of an adult maintenance food, either no macromineral imbalance occurs, or it self-corrects. Appropriate monitoring of electrolytes is an important aspect of clinical evaluation of any diabetic patient, but especially in any dog that has poorly controlled diabetes or is ill.

The importance of micronutrients in diabetics has been a topic of considerable interest in various species for many years. The most important micronutrients in diabetes are zinc, chromium, selenium, copper, and manganese. Of these nutrients, the essential role of zinc in the synthesis, storage, and secretion of insulin is clearly established; however, the exact mechanisms underlying altered zinc metabolism in diabetic dogs have not been identified; specific recommendations for supplementation are difficult. Excesses of zinc can be quite detrimental and can cause complications such as gastritis and gastric ulceration, copper deficiency, and hemolytic anemia. The same ambiguity exists for the use of chromium in diabetic dogs. Chromium is essential for normal carbohydrate and lipid metabolism, and supplementation in humans with diabetes improves insulin sensitivity and overall control; however, few studies have been performed in dogs with diabetes, and in one study no increase in glycemic control was observed.

The best approach in diabetic patients at the present time is to feed a complete and balanced diet that has micronutrients supplied according to the Association of American Feed Control Officials (AAFCO) recommendations for adult maintenance (see Appendix). If the dog is unwilling to eat this type of diet, a standard adult human vitamin-mineral supplement (1 tablet/dog/day) containing a United States Pharmacopeia (USP) label can be administered safely to help prevent development of a micronutrient deficiency. If a dog is unwilling to eat a commercially prepared, balanced diet, the best approach is to consult with or seek the guidance of a board-certified veterinary nutritionist to help develop and balance an appropriate diet that meets the long-term needs of the dog.

Food Type and Feeding Plans

As a general rule, most diabetic dogs, regardless of diet chosen, can be well managed with feeding a consistent diet at consistent times with concurrent administration of an appropriate amount of exogenous insulin. In addition, because there is no clear evidence that specific diets in diabetic dogs are essential to good glycemic control, the first rule of thumb is that the nutritional requirements of any concurrent disease in a diabetic dog should take precedence when choosing a diet. The next most important issue of diet selection is palatability to ensure that the dog consistently and predictably consumes the diet.

Both canned and dry foods are acceptable for diabetic dogs; however, because dry foods empty the slowest from the stomach, they have a greater effect in decreasing postprandial hyperglycemia than canned foods. Nevertheless, if the dog more consistently consumes a meal if it contains some canned food or if the dog needs the added water in its diet, canned foods are an acceptable diet for diabetics. Soft, moist foods should be avoided entirely because they contain large amounts of simple sugars (e.g., dextrose, fructose, sucrose, cane molasses)

TABLE 46-2

Calculating Calories

	Equations for Calculating Caloric Intake
Canine MER: Ideal BW	$125(BW_{kg})^{0.75}$ or $BW_{kg} \times 60\text{-}70$
Feline MER: Ideal BW	$50(BW_{kg})^{0.67}$ or $BW_{kg} \times 40\text{-}45$

BW, Body weight; *MER*, maintenance energy requirement.

that are highly digestible and result in a large increase in blood sugar. Generally, highly digestible foods (diets with >90% digestibility) designed for GI disease may result in greater postprandial hyperglycemia; they are likely not the best diets for diabetic dogs. Conversely, diets with less than 80% nutrient digestibility and low fat concentrations may not be sufficient to help a thin diabetic dog regain lost BW.

Finally, it is ideal to choose a diet that has a fixed formula (as opposed to an open formula) so that there are fewer variations in the diet formulation that can affect the individual response from batch to batch. Open-formula diets are diets found in a typical grocery store or pet specialty supply store, and their formulation changes with market prices. The glycemic index changes with the formulation over time, which may result in a variable insulin response.

Once the diet is chosen, the next most important aspect of dietary management is to impress on the owner the importance of feeding consistent amounts of food at consistent times. Giving treats can be accommodated, as long as the type (preferably low in fat and sugar) and the number of treats given are consistent every day. Ideally, diabetic dogs should be fed one half of their total daily energy requirement at a specified time in the morning at the time of insulin administration. The second half of the dog's energy requirements should be given at the evening meal, approximately 12 hours later, coinciding with the evening insulin administration.

Calculation of energy requirements for diabetic dogs should be based on maintenance energy needs of the dog's ideal BW (Table 46-2). However, if the dog fails to gain weight despite an appropriate amount of insulin and food, an increase in the energy density of the food or increased daily caloric intake will be required. A final key point for a successful dietary management strategy for diabetic dogs is simply to monitor the BW, body condition (muscle and fat mass), and glycemic control and adjust the diet as needed, but to maintain as much consistency as possible not only in the food type but also in the timing and amount.

Dietary Management of Feline Diabetes

As in diabetic dogs, dietary therapy is a very important aspect of successful management of diabetic cats. However, in contrast to dietary therapy of dogs for which multiple dietary strategies are available, dietary management of diabetic cats is aimed at improving metabolism, correcting obesity, and reversing persistent hyperglycemia by using high-protein, low-carbohydrate foods. There is strong and increasing evidence that a diet containing protein as the primary energy source and very low concentrations of carbohydrate is highly effective in achieving these goals in cats. In addition, because many diabetic cats are obese and have obesity-induced insulin resistance as part of their disease, high-protein diets are essential to preserving muscle mass, preventing hepatic lipidosis, and increasing metabolism to help promote fat burning. Although dietary therapy of feline diabetes has similar goals to that in dogs, the approach is specifically tailored to provide diets that more closely mimic their natural carnivorous diet.

Dietary therapy of feline diabetes has several major goals, as follows:

1. To correct or normalize BW—for most cats this means to achieve weight loss
2. To minimize hyperinsulinemia and hyperamylinemia that occurs secondary to persistent hyperglycemia resulting from obesity or other factors associated with insulin resistance
3. To use protein as the primary insulin secretagogue to stimulate endogenous insulin secretion by feeding a diet high in arginine (an amino acid found prominently in meat source proteins)
4. To provide a continuous source of gluconeogenic amino acids from meat source proteins to allow removal of all starches from the diet—reducing the degree and duration of postprandial hyperglycemia.

Obesity is a major medical problem in domestic cats. Most cats that live indoors with free access to food are either overweight (15% to 20% over ideal BW) or obese (>20% over ideal BW). Because obesity-induced insulin resistance is a major risk factor for development of diabetes mellitus, both from the perspective of prevention and from the perspective of treatment, weight loss is a key aspect of dietary therapy. To induce weight loss in cats, a dietary strategy must be include the following: (1) feeding a diet high in protein (>45% metabolizable energy) to decrease muscle mass loss and prevent lipid and energy metabolism derangements that occur during calorie restriction, (2) feeding a diet that is reduced in energy (both fat and carbohydrates) to stimulate fat mobilization, and (3) monitoring and adjusting the food consumption to BW and response to food reduction.

Lean muscle tissue is an essential element of basal metabolism and is necessary for normal insulin function. Many weight-loss diets are low calorie but not high enough in protein to preserve lean muscle tissue. In studies of cats comparing high-protein and moderate-protein diets during weight loss, cats consuming high-protein diets had greater success in achieving weight loss, lost fat mass while preserving lean tissue, and had a greater tendency to maintain stable weight after weight loss. Many diets may be acceptable for preservation of lean muscle tissue, but the goal should be to have fat less than 4 g/100 kcal, starch less than 5 g/100 kcal, and protein content greater than 10 g/100 kcal (in dry-matter terms it is equivalent to protein > 40% to 45%, depending

on the energy in the diet). Diets with this profile are easily obtained using canned food diets, and many options exist; however, extruded dry food diets require a minimum amount of carbohydrate in processing for the creation of the shape and texture. Dry foods often have larger amounts of carbohydrates or fat and can make calorie control or reduction of postprandial hyperglycemia difficult, if not impossible.

The other essential aspect of achieving weight loss is to control energy intake. In obese cats, meal feeding is required to be able to provide the specified calories needed to achieve restriction. Maintenance energy needs for indoor neutered cats that are of ideal BW are estimated to be 40 to 50 kcal/kg/day (or for the average 4- to 5-kg cat an intake of 160 to 200 kcal/day) (see Table 46-2). However, to achieve weight loss, the caloric intake must be restricted further, with a reduction in calories from this maintenance rate by 10% to 40%—which may mean intakes of 130 to 140 kcal/day for some cats. If the cat has been eating free choice food, the first step is to establish a meal feeding regimen with intake aimed at the ideal. Many canned diets have a high-protein, low-fat to moderate-fat, and low-carbohydrate profile and provide a way to control calories by volume; they are a good dietary choice for a feline weight-loss program. In addition, canned foods contain a large amount of water, which serves to dilute calories and still allow a larger portion size that helps increase satisfaction. In a comparison between a high-fiber food and a canned food with equal ingredients, cats fed the canned diets begged less and showed more signs of satiety than cats fed the dry high-fiber diets. Because caloric intake can be easily controlled, it is easier to create a high-protein and low-carbohydrate profile, and the increased water adds both moisture and volume to the meal, canned diets are a highly desirable option for cats needing to lose weight or to help manage diabetes. Table 46-3 lists the caloric differences among several high-protein, low-carbohydrate canned and dry diets and other diets that are fed to cats for weight loss.

In addition to weight loss, another major goal of a diet for diabetic cats is to control blood glucose levels and reduce hyperinsulinemia and associated hyperamylinemia, both of which are very important in preserving β-cell function. Previously, diets high in fiber and complex carbohydrates were recommended for dietary management of diabetic cats, similar to the approach in dogs. Although these diets may reduce postprandial hyperglycemia, it is not to the same degree as high-protein and low-carbohydrate diets, and they do not result in consistent weight loss without loss of muscle mass. In addition, they are not associated with a high percentage of cats reverting to a preclinical (non–insulin-requiring) diabetic state. Recent studies have shown that cats fed high-carbohydrate diets have a much longer postprandial hyperglycemia period (up to 8 to 10 hours), and this period is prolonged even further when the cat is obese (up to 18 hours) (Hewson-Hughes, 2011). This physiologic difference in carbohydrate handling creates an even greater strain on their pancreatic β cells under conditions of chronicity or inflammation. Thus, in contrast to dogs, the primary strategy in diabetic cats is to achieve clinical

TABLE 46-3

Selected Feline Diabetic Diet Comparisons of Prescription Products*

	Protein (% DM)	CHO (% DM)	Fat (% DM)	Calories (kcal/Cup or Can)
Hill's prescription diet m/d dry	51.1	15.1	21.8	495
Hill's prescription diet m/d canned	52.8	15.7	19.4	156
Purina veterinary diets DM dry	57.9	14.9	17.9	592
Purina veterinary diets DM canned	53.4	4.5	32.9	191
Royal Canin diabetic DS 44 dry	44.0	23.1	11.0	239

CHO, Carbohydrate; DM, dry matter.
*Based on product guides.

diabetic remission and normalize β-cell production, and the key dietary strategy in cats is reduction of postprandial blood glucose levels by feeding diets with extremely low levels of carbohydrate and replacing dietary carbohydrate with protein. In several more recent studies of newly diagnosed diabetics, cats placed on insulin and a high-protein and low-carbohydrate diet were four times more likely to achieve clinical remission; in cats that did not achieve remission, the amount of insulin required to control their diabetes was reduced by half.

In addition to the amount of carbohydrate, the type of carbohydrate in the diet appears to be important. For cats that consume only dry food diets and have some carbohydrate in their food, the source should be a complex carbohydrate with a low glycemic index (e.g., whole grains such as barley). However, studies in diabetic cats comparing these types of diets with complex carbohydrates with low-carbohydrate diets are lacking, and because cats do not require any carbohydrates in their diet and normally would eat very little in their natural diet, it seems reasonable to try to achieve that ideal.

Another major aspect of dietary therapy of feline diabetes—stimulation of insulin secretion—is also achieved by feeding a high-protein, low-carbohydrate diet because arginine is a potent insulin secretagogue. Even in cats with chronic, persistent hyperglycemia and resultant hyposecretion of insulin secondary to glucose stimulation, insulin secretion in response to arginine is normal to increased. Feline diets that are rich in animal source proteins contain abundant arginine, which contributes to endogenous insulin secretion in diabetic cats and subsequently may help lead to diabetic remission. In addition, the feeding of a high-protein, low-carbohydrate diet to diabetic cats ensures the presence of gluconeogenic amino acids for production of glucose for energy throughout the day; this is particularly important

for diabetic cats because of their ability to regain their own insulin secretory function at any time. A hypoglycemic crisis may be even more likely than in dogs, especially if cats are consuming high-carbohydrate diets that provide an immediate postprandial increase in blood glucose but do not provide a readily available energy source later in the day.

Finally, although cats prefer to eat small frequent meals (nibble or graze), it is very important that all diabetic cats are meal-fed so that the owner can observe the cat at the time of insulin administration and can be sure that the cat is eating appropriately at least twice daily. If the cat is prone to hypoglycemia or prefers small frequent meals, it is reasonable to divide the daily energy requirement into four separate feedings. This is easily done by using timed feeders, so the cat has the opportunity to eat multiple times per day while controlling intake but at the same time providing an energy source midday should the cat attain diabetic remission. Because diabetic remission is an important goal, especially in newly diagnosed obese or previously obese cats, frequent monitoring (both of weight loss and glycemic control) and access to small amounts of food is the best strategy. The specific techniques used to monitor successful control of blood glucose in diabetic cats are beyond the scope of this chapter but represent an essential aspect of diabetic management in cats (see Chapter 48). However, with appropriate use of diet in the management of feline diabetes, the goals of successful control, which include clinical remission of the diabetes, can be achieved.

References and Suggested Reading

Benner N et al: Use of a low-carbohydrate versus high-fiber diet in cats with diabetes mellitus, *J Vet Intern Med* 15:297, 2001.

Biourge VC: Feline diabetes mellitus: nutritional management, *Waltham Focus* 15:36, 2005.

Farrow HA, Rand JS, Sunvold GD: The effect of high-protein, high-fat, or high-carbohydrate diets on postprandial glycemia and insulin concentrations in normal cats, *J Vet Intern Med* 16:360, 2002.

Fleeman LM, Rand JS: Beyond insulin therapy: achieving optimal control in diabetic dogs, *Waltham Focus* 15:12, 2005.

Frank G et al: Use of a high-protein diet in the management of feline diabetes mellitus, *Vet Ther* 2:238, 2001.

Hewson-Hughes AK et al: The effect of dietary starch level on postprandial glucose and insulin concentrations in cats and dogs, *Br J Nutr* 12:51, 2011.

Kimmel SE et al: Effects of insoluble and soluble dietary fiber on glycemic control in dogs with naturally occurring insulin-dependent diabetes mellitus, *J Am Vet Med Assoc* 216:1076, 2000.

Marshall R, Rand JS: Insulin glargine and high-protein low carbohydrate diet are associated with high remission rates in newly diagnosed diabetic cats, *J Vet Intern Med* 18:401, 2004.

Mazzaferro EM et al: Treatment of feline diabetes mellitus using an alpha-glucosidase inhibitor and a low-carbohydrate diet, *J Feline Med Surg* 53:183, 2003.

Nelson RW et al: Effect of dietary insoluble fiber on control of glycemia in dogs with naturally occurring diabetes mellitus, *J Am Vet Med Assoc* 212:380, 1998.

Rand JS, Marshall R: Understanding feline diabetes mellitus: pathogenesis and management, *Waltham Focus* 15:5, 2005.

Remillard RL: Nutritional management of diabetic dogs, *Compend Contin Educ* 21:699, 1999.

CHAPTER 47

Insulin Resistance

RICHARD W. NELSON, *Davis, California*

Insulin resistance is defined as a condition in which a normal amount of insulin produces a subnormal biologic response. Insulin resistance may result from problems occurring before the interaction of insulin with its receptor (e.g., circulating insulin-binding antibodies), at the receptor (e.g., altered insulin receptor binding affinity or concentration), or at steps distal to the interaction of insulin and its receptor (e.g., block in insulin signal transduction). Postreceptor problems are difficult to differentiate clinically from receptor problems, and both often coexist. In dogs and cats, receptor and postreceptor abnormalities are usually attributable to obesity, inflammation such as pancreatitis or gingivitis, or a disorder causing excessive or deficient secretion of one or more insulin-antagonistic hormones, specifically glucagon, catecholamines, cortisol, and growth hormone. Clinically relevant problems caused by insulin resistance include development of diabetes mellitus, stimulation of ketogenesis and development of diabetic ketoacidosis (DKA), and interference with the effectiveness of exogenous insulin injections for treating diabetes mellitus.

Role in the Pathogenesis of Feline Diabetes and Diabetic Remission

Amylin is a polypeptide produced by pancreatic β cells in cats. It is stored in secretory granules that contain insulin and is cosecreted with insulin. Stimulants of insulin secretion stimulate the secretion of amylin. Chronic increased secretion of insulin and amylin, as occurs with obesity and other insulin-resistant states, results in aggregation and deposition of amylin in the pancreatic islets as amyloid. Amyloid fibrils cause apoptotic islet cell death. Deposition of islet amyloid and subsequent loss of β cells is progressive with persistent insulin-resistant states and ultimately results in diabetes mellitus. The severity of islet amyloidosis and loss of β cells determines, in part, a cat's need for insulin treatment to control hyperglycemia and the potential for diabetic remission once treatment is initiated. Total destruction of the islets results in insulin-dependent diabetes mellitus and the need for insulin treatment for the rest of a cat's life. Partial destruction of the islets may or may not result in clinically evident diabetes, insulin treatment may or may not be required to control hyperglycemia, and diabetic remission may or may not occur when treatment is initiated.

The presence, severity, and reversibility of insulin resistance is an important variable that influences the severity and progression of islet amyloidosis, treatment options at the time diabetes is diagnosed, and likelihood of diabetic remission in cats. Any chronic insulin-resistant disorder can have a deleterious impact on the population and function of β cells and play a role in the development of diabetes. Identification and correction of concurrent problems that cause insulin resistance is critical to the successful treatment of diabetes in cats (Box 47-1). Correction and subsequent avoidance of insulin resistance may result in diabetic remission in cats with partial loss of pancreatic β cells, and recurrence of insulin resistance may result in recurrence of symptomatic diabetes.

Role in Diabetic Ketoacidosis

Insulin is a powerful inhibitor of lipolysis and ketone production. A deficiency of insulin or the presence of insulin resistance, or both, promotes lipolysis, ketogenesis, and development of DKA. Virtually all dogs and cats with DKA have a relative or absolute deficiency of insulin and insulin resistance at the time DKA is diagnosed. Some diabetic dogs and cats develop ketoacidosis despite receiving daily injections of insulin, and circulating insulin concentrations may be increased. In these dogs and cats, insulin deficiency results from insulin resistance caused by an increase in insulin-antagonistic hormones, most notably glucagon, and the presence of concurrent disorders such as pancreatitis. Insulin dosages that were effective in controlling hyperglycemia become inadequate with development of insulin resistance and predispose a diabetic dog or cat to developing DKA. Almost all dogs and cats with DKA have some coexisting disorder, such as pancreatitis, infection, or hormonal excess or deficiency. Recognition and treatment of disorders that coexist with DKA are critical for successful management (see Box 47-1).

Role in Control of Hyperglycemia

Insulin resistance interferes with the actions of exogenously administered insulin, resulting in persistent hyperglycemia; glycosuria; clinical signs (polyuria, polydipsia, and weight loss); and development of complications of chronic diabetes, such as cataracts in dogs and peripheral neuropathy in cats. Persistent problems with diabetic regulation should raise suspicion for insulin resistance. However, other issues with the insulin treatment regimen should also be considered, such as an inadequate or excessive dosage of insulin and a short or prolonged duration of effect of the insulin preparation.

There is no insulin dosage that clearly defines insulin resistance. For most diabetic dogs and cats, control of hyperglycemia can usually be attained using a dosage of 1.0 U or less of an intermediate-acting or long-acting

BOX 47-1

Recognized Causes of Insulin Resistance in Diabetic Dogs and Cats

Conditions Typically Causing Severe Insulin Resistance	Conditions Typically Causing Mild or Fluctuating Insulin Resistance
Hyperadrenocorticism	Obesity
Acromegaly (cat)	Infections
Progesterone excess (diestrus in female dog)	Chronic pancreatitis
Diabetogenic drugs*	Chronic inflammation
	Disease of the oral cavity
	Renal insufficiency
	Liver insufficiency
	Cardiac insufficiency
	Hypothyroidism (dog)
	Hyperthyroidism (cat)
	Pancreatic exocrine insufficiency
	Hyperlipidemia
	Neoplasia
	Glucagonoma
	Pheochromocytoma
	Insulin autoantibodies

*Most notably glucocorticoids and progestins.

insulin preparation per kilogram of body weight given twice daily. Insulin resistance should be suspected if control of hyperglycemia is poor despite an insulin dosage greater than 1.5 U/kg, when excessive amounts of insulin (i.e., insulin dosage >1.5 U/kg) are necessary to maintain the blood glucose concentration less than 300 mg/dl, and when control of hyperglycemia is erratic and insulin requirements are constantly changing in an attempt to maintain control. Failure of the blood glucose concentration to decrease below 300 mg/dl is suggestive of, but not definitive for, the presence of insulin resistance. Failure of blood glucose concentration to decrease after insulin administration can also result from stress-induced hyperglycemia, induction of the Somogyi response, and other problems with insulin therapy. Similarly, a decrease in the blood glucose concentration to less than 300 mg/dl does not rule out insulin resistance because responsiveness to insulin may be present with disorders causing mild insulin resistance (e.g., obesity, chronic pancreatitis). Serum fructosamine concentrations are typically greater than 500 µmol/L in dogs and cats with insulin resistance and can exceed 700 µmol/L if resistance is severe. However, serum fructosamine concentrations can also be greater than 500 µmol/L with other problems involving the insulin treatment regimen.

The severity of insulin resistance depends in part on the underlying etiology. Insulin resistance may be mild and easily overcome by increasing the dosage of insulin or may be severe, causing persistent severe hyperglycemia regardless of the type and dosage of insulin administered. Some causes of insulin resistance are readily apparent at the time diabetes is diagnosed, such as obesity and the administration of insulin-antagonistic drugs (e.g.,

glucocorticoids). Other causes of insulin resistance are not readily apparent and require an extensive diagnostic evaluation to be identified. Generally, any concurrent inflammatory, infectious, hormonal, neoplastic, or organ system disorder can interfere with the effectiveness of insulin. The most common concurrent disorders interfering with insulin effectiveness in diabetic cats include diabetogenic drugs (e.g., glucocorticoids), severe obesity, chronic pancreatitis, kidney failure, hyperthyroidism, oral infections, acromegaly, and hyperadrenocorticism. The most common concurrent disorders interfering with insulin effectiveness in diabetic dogs include diabetogenic drugs (i.e., glucocorticoids), severe obesity, hyperadrenocorticism, diestrus, chronic pancreatitis, kidney failure, oral and urinary tract infections, hyperlipidemia, and insulin antibodies in dogs treated with beef insulin. Obtaining a complete history and performing a thorough physical examination is the most important step in identifying these concurrent disorders. If the history and physical examination fail to identify the underlying problem, a complete blood count, serum biochemical analysis, serum thyroxine concentration (cat), serum pancreatic lipase immunoreactivity (IDEXX Spec cPL), serum progesterone concentration (intact female dog), abdominal ultrasound, and urinalysis with bacterial culture should be considered to screen further for concurrent illness. Additional tests depend on the results of the initial screening tests.

Treatment and reversibility of insulin resistance depend on the etiology. Insulin resistance is reversible with treatable disorders (e.g., sodium levothyroxine treatment in a diabetic dog with concurrent hypothyroidism or ovariohysterectomy in an intact female diabetic dog in diestrus. In contrast, insulin resistance often persists with disorders that are difficult to treat, such as chronic recurring pancreatitis in diabetic dogs and cats or acromegaly in diabetic cats. In some situations, measures can be taken to prevent insulin resistance, such as avoidance of glucocorticoids in diabetic dogs and cats or performing an ovariohysterectomy at the time diabetes mellitus is diagnosed in an intact female dog.

Insulin Dosage Adjustments

In most diabetic dogs and cats, insulin resistance is not suspected until insulin dosages exceed 1.5 U/kg per injection and problems with hyperglycemia persist. Two common exceptions are obesity, which is readily recognizable, and treatment with insulin-antagonistic drugs, most notably glucocorticoids. Adjustments in the insulin dosage should always be considered at the time treatment of the insulin-resistant disorder is initiated. How much to decrease the insulin dosage is variable and depends in part on the severity of insulin resistance, the amount of insulin being administered, and the expected rapidity of improvement in insulin resistance after treatment of the disorder. For example, dogs with poorly controlled diabetes and newly diagnosed hypothyroidism have a rapid improvement in insulin resistance after initiating thyroid hormone treatment. Failure to decrease the insulin dosage may result in symptomatic hypoglycemia within days of starting thyroid hormone treatment. In contrast, correction of obesity and subsequent improvement in insulin resistance is a slow process associated with a gradual reduction in the insulin dosage over time as obesity improves. Avoiding hypoglycemia is the primary goal when adjusting the insulin dosage. I always err on the side of caution by not decreasing the insulin dosage too much rather than too little, recognizing that hyperglycemia is not life-threatening, but severe hypoglycemia can be. When in doubt, I decrease the insulin dosage to approximately 0.5 U/kg per injection for diabetic dogs and cats and rely on owner observations regarding the overall health of their pet and the presence of clinical signs suggestive of hypoglycemia. Home blood glucose monitoring and monitoring random urine samples for negative glycosuria may also be considered.

Glucocorticoids and Hyperadrenocorticism

Diabetic dogs and cats are often treated with glucocorticoids for treatment of concurrent disease (e.g., allergic skin disease). Glucocorticoids have the potential to cause severe insulin resistance, creating a tendency for large amounts of insulin to be administered in an attempt to control hyperglycemia. If glucocorticoids are required for treatment of a concurrent disease, the glucocorticoid dosage should be kept as low as possible and administered as infrequently as possible to minimize the severity of insulin resistance. Insulin dosage requirements are higher in the presence of insulin resistance to maintain some semblance of glycemic control. It is important to remember the interplay between dosage adjustments of glucocorticoids and the impact of the adjustment on severity of insulin resistance and insulin dosage requirements. Appropriate adjustments in the insulin dosage should be made whenever the glucocorticoid dosage is increased or decreased to minimize hyperglycemia or hypoglycemia, respectively.

Naturally occurring hyperadrenocorticism and diabetes mellitus are common concurrent diseases in dogs. For most dogs, glycemic control remains poor despite insulin therapy, and good glycemic control is generally not possible until the hyperadrenocorticism is controlled. The initial focus should be on treating the hyperadrenal state in a dog with poorly controlled diabetes and hyperadrenocorticism. Insulin treatment is indicated; however, aggressive efforts to control hyperglycemia should not be attempted. Rather, a conservative dosage (0.5 to 1.0 U/kg) of intermediate-acting insulin (i.e., NPH or Lente) should be administered twice a day to prevent ketoacidosis and severe hyperglycemia. Monitoring water consumption and frequency of urination is unreliable because both diseases cause polyuria and polydipsia, and polyuria and polydipsia may persist if poor control of hyperglycemia persists despite attaining control of hyperadrenocorticism. As control of hyperadrenocorticism is achieved, insulin resistance resolves, and tissue sensitivity to insulin improves. Home blood glucose monitoring and testing urine for the presence of glucose can be done by the owner to help prevent hypoglycemia and identify when insulin resistance is resolving. Any blood glucose concentration less than 150 mg/dl or urine sample found

to be negative for glucose should be followed by a 20% to 25% reduction in the insulin dosage and evaluation of control of the hyperadrenocorticism. Critical assessment of glycemic control and adjustments in insulin therapy should be initiated after hyperadrenocorticism is controlled.

Feline Acromegaly

Chronic excess secretion of growth hormone (GH) by a functional adenoma of the somatotropic cells of the pituitary pars distalis causes acromegaly in adult cats (see Chapter 49). Clinical manifestations of acromegaly result from the catabolic effects of GH and the anabolic effects of insulin-like growth factor-1 (IGF-1). GH-induced catabolic effects include insulin resistance, carbohydrate intolerance, hyperglycemia, and diabetes mellitus. Most cats are diabetic at the time acromegaly is diagnosed, and most have poorly controlled diabetes because of GH-mediated insulin resistance, which is usually severe. Cats typically have blood glucose concentrations that remain greater than 400 mg/dl regardless of the dosage or type of insulin being administered. Insulin dosages of 20 to 40 units per injection are common at the time acromegalic cats are referred to our hospital; these dosages have been attained in an effort to decrease the blood glucose concentration to less than 300 mg/dl. In my experience, control of hyperglycemia cannot be attained in most acromegalic cats. The goal of insulin treatment is to avoid severe hyperglycemia (blood glucose concentrations >600 mg/dl) and hypoglycemia, not to attain control of the diabetic state. I start with a long-acting insulin preparation at an initial dosage of 0.5 to 1.0 U/kg administered twice a day. I increase the insulin dosage based on the owner's perception of how the cat is doing as it relates to activity, grooming, and interactions with family members, not based on severity of polyuria, polydipsia, or polyphagia or persistent hyperglycemia or glycosuria. Severe hyperglycemia causes lethargy, obtundation, and the perception that the cat is "not feeling well." I consider increasing the insulin dosage if owners report these problems, especially if the blood glucose concentration is greater than 600 mg/dl. I am cautious when increasing the insulin dosage because of concerns for the development of severe life-threatening hypoglycemia that can occur unexpectedly in acromegalic cats, presumably as a result of sporadic reductions in GH secretion and subsequent improvement in insulin resistance. I rarely exceed 12 units of insulin per injection and then only because of owner concerns that their cat is "not feeling well" and only after measuring blood glucose concentrations to confirm the presence of severe hyperglycemia. Home blood glucose monitoring and testing urine for the presence of glucose by the owner should be encouraged to help prevent hypoglycemia and identify when insulin resistance has improved.

References and Suggested Reading

Appleton DJ et al: Insulin sensitivity decreases with obesity and lean cats with low insulin sensitivity are at greatest risk of glucose intolerance with weight gain, *J Feline Med Surg* 3:211, 2001.

Davison LJ et al: Anti-insulin antibodies in diabetic dogs before and after treatment with different insulin preparations, *J Vet Intern Med* 22:1317, 2008.

Durocher LL et al: Acid-base and hormonal abnormalities in dogs with naturally occurring diabetes mellitus, *J Am Vet Med Assoc* 232:1310, 2008.

Henson MS et al: Evaluation of plasma islet amyloid polypeptide and serum glucose and insulin concentrations in nondiabetic cats classified by body condition score and in cats with naturally occurring diabetes mellitus, *Am J Vet Res* 72:1052, 2011.

Hess RS et al: Concurrent disorders in dogs with diabetes mellitus: 221 cases (1993-1998), *J Am Vet Med Assoc* 217:1166, 2000.

Lowe AD et al: A pilot study comparing the diabetogenic effects of dexamethasone and prednisolone in cats, *J Am Animal Hosp Assoc* 45:215, 2009.

CHAPTER 48

Feline Diabetes Mellitus

JACQUIE S. RAND, *Queensland, Australia*

Diabetes mellitus is the second most common endocrinopathy in cats and affects approximately 1 in 50 to 1 in 400, depending on the population studied. Risk factors include advanced age, male sex, breed, obesity, physical inactivity, confinement indoors, and administration of glucocorticoids or progestins. Breeds reported at risk are Burmese in Australia, New Zealand, and the United Kingdom and Maine coon, domestic longhair, Russian blue, and Siamese in the United States.

Diagnosis of diabetes mellitus is based on the finding of persistently increased blood glucose concentration. In most cats, diabetes is usually not diagnosed until relatively late in the disease process when extensive β-cell function has been lost. The diagnosis is typically made when blood glucose concentration is above the renal threshold (i.e., >250 to 290 mg/dl [14 to 16 mmol/L]) and signs of polyuria, polydipsia, and weight loss are apparent. In contrast, in humans with type 2 diabetes, diagnosis is made earlier in the disease process. Because of this difference in diagnosis and extent of β-cell failure, most humans but only the minority of cats can be managed satisfactorily with oral hypoglycemic drugs.

At the present time, there is no consensus in the veterinary literature regarding the minimal blood glucose concentration in cats that should be classed as diabetic. Based on data in other species, blood glucose concentrations below the renal threshold but persistently greater than normal are likely associated with adverse effects, such as glucotoxic damage to β cells. Persistently mild hyperglycemia (e.g., >117 mg/dl fasted or >145 mg/dl unfasted to <180 mg/dl [>6.5 mmol/L fasted or >8.0 mmol/L unfasted to <10 mmol/L]) could be considered in cats to represent impaired fasting glucose, a state between normal and diabetic, which in human patients is considered to be prediabetic. Research is urgently required to define the cut-point between impaired fasting glucose and diabetes in cats; persistent blood glucose concentrations of 180 mg/dl (10 mmol/L) or greater likely indicate diabetes. In human patients with diabetes, 50% are undiagnosed, and there are more patients with prediabetes than diabetes. This is likely also the case in cats.

With the current availability of low-carbohydrate feline diets, research is needed to determine the most appropriate blood glucose concentration for institution of dietary management. Logically, if there are no contraindications such as azotemia, cats should be changed to a low-carbohydrate, high-protein diet whenever a persistently increased blood glucose concentration is present (e.g., >144 mg/dl [8 mmol/L] unfasted), and the diet is fed to achieve an ideal body weight. Cats should be monitored on a regular basis (e.g., every 3 to 6 months).

Pathogenesis of Diabetes in Cats

To manage diabetic cats effectively, an understanding of the pathogenesis and main features of feline diabetes is required. In developed countries, most owned cats with diabetes likely have type 2 diabetes, which is characterized by a relative lack of insulin secretion and insulin resistance. Insulin resistance reduces the glucose-lowering effect of a given amount of insulin. Diabetic cats are on average six times less sensitive to insulin than healthy cats, representing a similar magnitude of insulin resistance to that identified in humans with type 2 diabetes. Insulin resistance results from numerous mechanisms, and more than one mechanism is likely operating in most diabetic cats. A small percentage of cats have other specific types of diabetes resulting from β-cell destruction associated with pancreatitis and neoplasia or have marked insulin resistance from excess growth hormone or corticosteroids. In referral practice, cats with other specific types of diabetes account for a substantial proportion of diabetic cats; acromegaly (growth hormone–producing tumor) has been reported in 25% to 30% of diabetic cats, and pancreatic neoplasia was reported in necropsy specimens of 8% to 18% of diabetic cats at referral institutions in the United States. Pancreatitis is likely an underdiagnosed cause of diabetes, and anecdotal data indicate it might be a cause of diabetes in cats that achieve remission as well as cats that remain dependent on insulin throughout their life. Hyperthyroidism results in glucose intolerance and insulin hypersecretion, both of which are exacerbated in some cats after treatment of hyperthyroidism and might be the result of weight gain and resultant obesity.

Insulin Resistance

In humans, the most important causes of insulin resistance are genotype, obesity, and physical inactivity. These same factors are also the most likely causes of insulin resistance in cats. It is important to be aware of these predisposing factors so that they are appropriately managed. Obesity markedly decreases insulin sensitivity in cats. An increase in body weight from an ideal weight of 4 kg to 6 kg decreases insulin sensitivity by 50% in cats. Management of body condition is a vital part of therapy for prevention and management of feline diabetes as well as prevention of relapse in cats that have achieved diabetic remission. Physically inactive cats have been shown to be at risk of diabetes, and increasing physical activity improves insulin sensitivity in other species. One study in cats also found that active play for 10 minutes daily produced the same rate of weight loss as calorie restriction.

Genetic predisposition is likely a risk factor for insulin resistance and diabetes in cats. Lean cats with insulin sensitivity values below the median of the population were at three times greater risk of developing impaired glucose tolerance when they gained weight than cats with higher insulin sensitivity. Impaired glucose tolerance is the glycemic state between normal and diabetic. It is likely that these cats had underlying insulin resistance associated with genotype and that obesity would result in diabetes in some of these cats with time. Burmese cats are at increased risk of diabetes in Australia, New Zealand, and the United Kingdom and appear to have underlying insulin resistance.

High blood glucose concentration also contributes to insulin resistance. In dogs, it has been shown that this effect has a relatively short-term influence, with insulin resistance related more closely to glycemia over the previous 48 hours rather than over longer periods. This finding is relevant especially in the initial phases of treatment, and clinicians need to be aware that insulin sensitivity is increased with decreasing blood glucose concentration.

Drugs such as glucocorticoids and progestins produce insulin resistance and increase the risk of diabetes particularly when administered as long-acting preparations or given repeatedly. Glucocorticoids and progestins increase the risk of relapse in cats that have achieved diabetic remission.

Impaired Insulin Secretion

Insulin secretion is decreased in feline diabetes through many mechanisms, some of which are reversible. Loss of β cells in type 2 diabetes is thought to result from apoptosis triggered by factors associated with obesity and insulin resistance, including release of inflammatory adipokines. Loss of β cells also occurs as a result of islet amyloid deposition and intracellular formation of toxic amyloid fibrils. Reversible suppression of insulin secretion occurs when blood glucose or lipid concentrations are high. These conditions are called *glucotoxicity* and *lipotoxicity,* and both may act through similar intracellular mechanisms in the β cell. With time, chronic hyperglycemia irreversibly damages β cells, and they are permanently lost, which can lead to insulin-dependent diabetes.

Loss of β cells also occurs through pancreatitis, and approximately 50% of diabetic cats have histologic evidence of pancreatitis. In most cats, the severity of the lesion is not sufficient by itself to cause diabetes but potentially contributes to loss of β cells. However, pancreatitis is likely an underdiagnosed cause of diabetes in cats, and it is recommended that feline pancreatic lipase be measured in all newly diagnosed diabetic cats, especially cats with any signs that could be consistent with pancreatitis.

When insulin resistance is not involved, clinical signs of diabetes ensue once approximately 80% to 90% of β cells are lost. If insulin sensitivity is reduced, clinical signs of diabetes occur earlier with smaller loss of β cells. With obesity-induced insulin resistance, cats need 30% more insulin to maintain fasting glucose concentration than when they were lean, and so logically, they would develop diabetes earlier with less β-cell loss. Veterinarians need to impress on owners the importance of attaining an ideal body condition in their diabetic cats, cats at risk of diabetes, and cats in diabetic remission.

Diabetic Remission

Within days to months of beginning treatment with insulin, a proportion of diabetic cats are able to maintain euglycemia without therapy. This is called *diabetic remission.* The proportion of cats that achieve diabetic remission depends on how early tight glycemic control is instituted, the type of therapy, and the underlying cause of the diabetes. Cats require functioning β cells to attain remission. It is believed that reversal of glucotoxicity and lipotoxicity leads to diabetic remission. Therapies that provide the best glycemic control are likely to lead to the highest remission rates.

Factors shown to be associated with increased probability of remission include institution of rigorous glycemic control within 6 months of diagnosis (remission rate 84% compared with 34% after 6 months), use of a long-acting insulin (glargine or detemir), feeding a low-carbohydrate diet, and careful monitoring of blood glucose concentrations together with appropriate adjustment of insulin dosage. Recent treatment with corticosteroids was positively associated with remission in one study. Other factors associated with remission are mean blood glucose less than 290 mg/dl (16 mmol/L) within 3 weeks of initiation of treatment and older age of cat. Cats less likely to achieve remission have increased serum cholesterol concentration, evidence of plantigrade stance, and requirement of a higher maximum dosage of insulin to gain glycemic control (median dosage was 50% higher—0.66 U/kg versus 0.43 U/kg).

Cats in remission may relapse in weeks to months, and it is important that they are carefully monitored and managed in remission, ideally with weekly home blood glucose monitoring. With early reinstitution of insulin therapy, some cats can achieve remission again. Persistent mildly increased blood glucose concentrations, that is, impaired fasting glucose (145 to 180 mg/dl [8 to 10 mmol/L]); more severe glucose intolerance (first return to baseline glucose concentration at 5 hours after 1 g/kg glucose intravenously); obesity; and use of glucocorticoids or progestins likely increase the probability of relapse.

Management of Diabetes

The most important goals of therapy are to achieve diabetic remission in cats with newly diagnosed diabetes; resolve clinical signs; and avoid clinical hypoglycemia, which can be life-threatening. The best way to resolve clinical signs is to achieve diabetic remission. Treatments available for management of feline diabetes include dietary modification, insulin, and oral hypoglycemic drugs. The prevalence of diabetes is increasing as risk factors such as obesity and physical inactivity become more common. These risk factors also need to be addressed in management and prevention of diabetes. Maintaining ideal body weight and avoiding drugs such as corticosteroids and progestins are important for maintaining remission.

Diet

Diet is an important component of therapy, and a low-carbohydrate diet is vital for cats achieving diabetic remission because it decreases mean daily glucose concentration, an important contributor to recovery of β cells from glucose toxicity (see also Chapter 46). A high-carbohydrate diet (50% of energy from carbohydrate) can increase mean blood glucose concentrations 4 to 18 hours after eating by 20% to 25% and peak glucose concentrations by more than 30% compared with a moderate-carbohydrate diet (25% energy from carbohydrate); comparison with a low-carbohydrate diet is even more pronounced. Remission rates were significantly higher (68% versus 42%) in cats fed a low-carbohydrate diet (12% of energy from carbohydrate; 3.5 g/100 kcal ME) compared with cats fed a higher carbohydrate diet (26% of energy from carbohydrate; 7.6 g/100 kcal ME), despite similar protein content of the two diets. Cats eating an ultra-low-carbohydrate diet (5% of energy; 1.8 g/100 kcal ME) have even greater reduction in blood glucose concentration; however, no studies comparing remission rates in cats fed low-carbohydrate and ultra-low-carbohydrate diets have been published. Ultra-low-carbohydrate diets are often nearly all meat or fish, may

not be complete or balanced, and are high in phosphorus, which is of concern given the frequency of chronic kidney disease in diabetic cats.

Reducing carbohydrate content of the diet also decreases the demand on β cells to secrete insulin. Cats in diabetic remission likely have reduced β-cell mass. From the limited testing reported, most of these cats have impaired glucose tolerance, and about one third have impaired fasting glucose, meaning a glucose concentration above normal (117 mg/dl [6.5 mmol/L]) but less than diabetic (180 mg/dl [10 mmol/L]). It is vital that cats in remission be fed diets that minimize the amount of insulin required to be secreted to control postprandial glycemia. Feeding a low-carbohydrate diet once diabetic remission is achieved would likely prolong remission.

To achieve and maintain remission, it is important to attain an ideal body weight because of the negative impact of obesity on insulin sensitivity. Diet is also important for achieving weight loss. A minority of cats fed canned low-carbohydrate, high-protein diets self-restrict energy intake and lose weight spontaneously after their diet is changed. For most cats, energy intake needs to be restricted to achieve weight loss. Physical activity promotes weight loss and improves insulin sensitivity in other species, independent of body weight. Encouraging owners to engage in active play with their cat is likely beneficial.

Insulin Therapy

Insulin therapy is the mainstay of therapy in diabetic cats. Veterinary insulin preparations available for maintenance treatment of diabetic cats include porcine Lente insulin (40 U/ml; Caninsulin/Vetsulin) in Europe and Canada and human recombinant protamine zinc insulin (PZI) (40 U/ml; ProZinc) in North America. Human insulin preparations used for long-term maintenance of diabetic cats include neutral protamine Hagedorn (NPH), glargine, and detemir. Human Lente and Ultralente insulin preparations have been removed from the market in most countries. In Europe, veterinarians are legally required to use an insulin registered for veterinary use as the first line of therapy.

Choice of Insulin Type

In a trial of 24 cats, all 8 cats with newly diagnosed diabetes treated with glargine and an ultra-low-carbohydrate diet (5% of energy from carbohydrate; Nestle Purina DM canned) achieved remission compared with 3 of 8 treated with PZI and 2 of 8 treated with porcine Lente. These findings compare with 20% to 30% remission rates reported using other insulin preparations and a standard feline maintenance diet (typically 30% to 40% of energy from carbohydrate). One study reported 60% remission rates using PZI or Lente insulin and a low-carbohydrate diet. Trials using either glargine or detemir in cats previously treated with other insulins, predominantly Lente, achieved remission rates of 84% and 81% if cats were changed to intensive blood glucose monitoring and glargine or detemir therapy within 6 months of diagnosis of diabetes.

Glargine and detemir are long-acting insulins, and although their long duration of action is achieved by different modifications to the insulin molecule, they have similar clinical effects in cats. In cats with newly diagnosed diabetes, remission rates of greater than 80% to 90% often can be achieved using glargine or detemir combined with a low-carbohydrate or ultra-low-carbohydrate diet and frequent monitoring of blood glucose concentration and appropriate adjustment of insulin dosage. Lower remission rates occur in cats with long-term diabetes changed to glargine or detemir therapy. Diabetic remission is rare in cats that have been diabetic for more than 2 years.

Because of the huge advantage to the client and the cat in achieving diabetic remission, it is strongly recommended that the *first choice of insulin for diabetic cats be glargine or detemir.* If there is a legal requirement to use a veterinary insulin product first, PZI would be the first choice because it has a longer duration of action than Lente insulin. However, recombinant PZI is not yet licensed for veterinary use in Europe.

Lente and NPH insulins have too short a duration of action for optimal blood glucose control in cats. Using Lente or NPH insulin, even with an optimal dosage and the nadir glucose concentration in the normoglycemic range, most cats have a period of at least 2 to 4 hours before each insulin injection when there is no exogenous insulin action, and high blood glucose concentrations ensue, often 360 mg/dl (20 mmol/L) or greater. Because the blood glucose concentration is very high, administering a potent insulin such as Lente or NPH may result in a rapid decrease in blood glucose concentration. The hypothalamic neurons detect a decreasing blood glucose concentration and trigger counterregulatory mechanisms before hypoglycemia occurs. These neurons control their intracellular glucose concentration by limiting glucose uptake when plasma glucose concentration is high; with a rapidly decreasing blood glucose concentration, the neurons become hypoglycemic even at relatively high blood glucose concentration, and the resultant counter-regulatory mechanisms are often triggered when blood glucose concentration is still above the normal range. Cortisol, epinephrine, and glucagon are released, increasing blood glucose concentrations. The end result is further shortening of insulin action, which for some cats treated with Lente insulin is only about 3 hours. The counter-regulatory response also results in insulin resistance, and the following insulin injections may result in little appreciable glucose-lowering effect.

Recommendations for Using Glargine and Detemir

Glargine and detemir are long-acting insulins designed to provide basal insulin concentrations in humans with type 1 and 2 diabetes. Administration in humans is coupled with prandial administration of an ultra-short-acting insulin or oral hypoglycemic drug. In cats, because the postprandial period is so prolonged (12 to 24 hours) compared with humans, administration of an ultra-rapid-acting insulin at the time of eating is unlikely to be useful.

Glargine (Lantus) is produced by recombinant deoxy-ribonucleic acid (DNA) technology using *Escherichia coli.* The insulin molecule is modified by replacing asparagine at position 21 with glycine and by adding two arginine residues at the terminal portion of the B chain. It is supplied as a clear, colorless solution of monomeric insulin with a pH of 4.0. When injected into the subcutaneous tissues with a pH of 7.0, glargine forms hexamers, and microprecipitates deposit in the tissues. These microprecipitates slowly break down, releasing monomeric glargine into solution, which gives glargine its long duration of action. Because of this, the manufacturers state that glargine cannot be diluted or mixed with other insulin. Glargine is available only at a concentration of 100 U/ml, which makes accurate dosing a problem in cats, particularly when very low dosages are being administered close to remission. Some human patients dilute or mix glargine with other insulin. This causes glargine to precipitate and the solution to become cloudy, but it appears to retain some efficacy. Dilution is not recommended for feline patients except as a last resort, and dilution should occur just prior to injection.

Detemir (Levemir) is also produced by recombinant DNA technology but using yeast (*Saccharomyces cerevisiae*). The insulin molecule is modified via addition of an acylated fatty acid chain, which facilitates reversible binding to plasma proteins, particularly albumin, from where it is released slowly into plasma. It also self-associates at the injection site, which helps prolong its absorption and duration of action. Detemir can be diluted using the Insulin Diluting Medium supplied by the manufacturer or with sterile water or saline just prior to administration.

Glargine and detemir have been used successfully in cats with a starting dosage of 0.5 U/kg twice daily if blood glucose is 360 mg/dl (20 mmol/L) or greater, and 0.25 U/kg for lower blood glucose concentrations. The initial starting dosage should not exceed 3 U/cat twice daily. It is strongly recommended that glargine and detemir be administered twice daily in the first 4 months of therapy to maximize glycemic control and diabetic remission. Glargine administered once daily has been shown to be similar in effectiveness to Lente insulin twice daily.

The dosage generally should not be increased in the first week unless little or no glucose-lowering effect is evident after the third day. In many cats, the dosage needs to be reduced in the first 7 days. If the dosage is increased after the third day, it is important that intensive glucose monitoring be done. Increasing the dosage without monitoring can result in clinical hypoglycemia. It is recommended that close monitoring occur in the first 4 to 8 weeks of treatment with appropriate dosage adjustments because many cats achieve diabetic remission within this time. It is prudent to keep the cat in the hospital and check blood glucose concentration for the first 3 days after institution of treatment to check for evidence of hypoglycemia, or if the owner is capable, careful home monitoring of blood glucose concentration can be performed. If monitoring of blood glucose concentration is not possible, one can closely monitor urine glucose concentration and water drunk as indicators of glycemic control. If a marked decrease in water drunk occurs in the

BOX 48-1

Current Recommendations for Adjusting Dosage of Glargine, Detemir, and PZI in Diabetic Cats

Home blood glucose monitoring is highly recommended to provide additional data for insulin dosage adjustments. Blood glucose measurements are based on using a portable meter calibrated for feline blood or a serum chemistry analyzer. If using a meter calibrated for human blood, adjust glucose cut-points as required based on validation of the meter with a serum chemistry analyzer.

1. Starting Dosage
Begin with 1 U/cat if blood glucose less than 360 mg/dl (20 mmol/L) and 2 U/cat if 360 mg/dl (20 mmol/L) or greater.

2. Indications for Increasing Dosage
Assess response for 5 to 7 days after each dosage increase, before increasing dosage again; ideally, assess with daily home blood glucose monitoring, but if this is not possible, use clinical data such as water drunk, urine glucose monitoring, and presence or absence of clinical signs of hypoglycemia as a guide to response to therapy as well as weekly blood glucose curves generated during weekly veterinary checks.
- If preinsulin glucose concentration is 216 mg/dl (12 mmol/L) or greater, provided that nadir glucose is not less than 72 mg/dl (4 mmol/L), increase dosage by 0.25 to 1 U/injection, depending on the degree of hyperglycemia and if on a high (≥3 U/cat) or low dosage of insulin.
- If nadir (lowest) glucose concentration is 126 mg/dl (7 mmol/L) or greater, increase dosage by 0.25 to 1 U/injection, depending on the degree of hyperglycemia and if on a high (≥3 U/cat) or low dosage of insulin.
- After several weeks of therapy, aim for a nadir (lowest glucose) in the normal range (e.g., 72-126 mg/dl [4-7 mmol/L]).

3. Indications for Maintaining Same Dosage
- If pre-insulin glucose concentration is 180 to less than 216 mg/dl (10 to <12 mmol/L), maintain dosage.
- If nadir glucose concentration is 72 to 126 mg/dl (4 to 7 mmol/L), maintain dosage.

4. Indications for Decreasing Dosage
- If preinsulin glucose concentration is 180 mg/dl (10 mmol/L) or less, decrease dosage by 0.25 to 1 U/injection.
- If nadir glucose concentration is less than 54 mg/dl (3 mmol/L), decrease dosage by 0.5 to 1 U/injection.
- If severe clinical signs of hypoglycemia develop (e.g., seizures, coma), rub glucose syrup or honey into the gums and obtain veterinary attention immediately; administer 50% glucose intravenous bolus followed by 2.5% glucose infusion, then reduce dosage by 50% and check for remission.

- If mild clinical hypoglycemia develops (e.g., tremors, lethargy), this can often be managed by feeding the cat, preferably food containing a higher carbohydrate level, such as feline maintenance dry foods. However, it must be palatable enough to eat. Most weight-reducing and renal diets are high-carbohydrate diets, as are many grocery lines of dry food.
- For cats with unexpected biochemical hypoglycemia (i.e., no clinical signs) at the time of the next insulin injection, some owners find that they can manage the hypoglycemia by delaying the insulin injection until blood glucose increases to 180 mg/dl (10 mmol/L) and then giving the same dosage (the following scheduled dosage of insulin may need to be reduced or delayed), whereas others find it best to reduce the dosage once glucose increases to > 126 to 180 mg/dl (7 to 10 mmol/L), although this may result in subsequent hyperglycemia.
- For cats with a normal blood glucose, 60 to 126 mg/dl (3.5 to 7 mmol/L), at the time of the next insulin injection, initially test which of the alternative methods is best suited to the individual cat:
  1. Feed the cat and reduce the dosage by 0.25 to 0.5 IU depending on if the cat is on a low (<3 U/cat) or high dosage of insulin.
  2. Feed the cat, wait 1 to 2 hours, and when the glucose concentration increases to greater than 126 mg/dl (7 mmol/L), give the normal dosage. If the glucose concentration does not increase within 1 to 2 hours, reduce the dosage by 0.25 or 0.5 IU (as above).
  3. Split the dosage: feed the cat, and give one half to two thirds of the dosage immediately and give the remainder 1 to 2 hours later, when the glucose concentration has increased to greater than 126 mg/dl (7 mmol/L).
- If all these methods lead to increased blood glucose concentrations, give the full dosage if preinsulin blood glucose concentration is 72 to 126 mg/dl (4 to 7 mmol/L) and observe closely for signs of hypoglycemia. For most cats, the best results during the phase of increasing dosage or the maintenance phase generally occur when insulin dosage is as consistent as possible, giving the full normal dosage at the regular injection time.

5. Insulin Dosage Maintained or Decreased
The insulin dosage may be maintained or decreased depending on the water drunk, urine glucose, clinical signs, and length of time the cat has been treated with insulin.
- If nadir is 54 to 72 mg/dl (3 to 4 mmol/L), maintain or decrease dosage.

Updated recommendations can be found at www.uq.edu.au/vetschool/centrecah.
Modified with permission from Rand JS, Marshall RD: Diabetes mellitus in cats, *Vet Clin North Am Small Anim Pract* 35:211, 2005.

first week or urine glucose becomes negative, the cat should be rechecked because a lower insulin dosage is likely indicated. If no monitoring of blood glucose concentration, water drunk, or urine glucose concentration is possible, it is safer to begin with a dosage of 1 U/cat twice daily and increase the dosage weekly. Poor monitoring and inadequate tailoring of the dosage to control hyperglycemia delay or prevent diabetic remission. It

is recommended that cats be checked weekly by a veterinarian in the first 4 to 8 weeks after institution of therapy and the dosage be adjusted appropriately, even if the owner is performing frequent home monitoring of blood glucose concentration (Box 48-1).

Subcutaneous glargine can be used in combination with intramuscular glargine or regular insulin in treating ketoacidosis. Administered intramuscularly, glargine has a similar action to regular insulin. The recommended regimen is to administer 2 U glargine subcutaneously twice daily immediately and glargine or regular insulin intramuscularly at 1 U every 2 to 4 or more hours once fluid and electrolytes are being administered, aiming to keep glucose between 145 and 250 mg/dl (8 and 14 mmol/L). Intramuscular insulin is required until appetite returns or dehydration is resolved, which is 24 to 48 hours in most cats.

Occasionally, the dosage of glargine or detemir needs to be increased to 5 or 6 U/cat and rarely 10 U/cat or more twice daily over the first 1 to 2 months. In many of these cats, the dosage needs to be reduced when glycemic control is achieved. Careful monitoring is required to prevent hypoglycemia. In first accession practice, rarely is hyperadrenocorticism a cause for treatment failure; in contrast, acromegaly appears to be a common finding in cats with poorly controlled diabetes (see Chapter 49). When either condition is present, high dosages of insulin are often required, especially with acromegaly, which may require extreme dosages (>25 U/cat BID) to control blood glucose concentration. For cats on a high dosage of insulin (>5 U BID), screening for acromegaly should be done by measuring insulin-like growth factor-α; brain imaging may also be required (see Chapter 49).

In cats with signs of other specific types of diabetes in which the underlying disease is potentially reversible, such as hyperadrenocorticism, acromegaly, or pancreatitis, one should not delay insulin therapy and wait to determine if blood glucose normalizes after instituting specific therapy for the underlying condition that is contributing to insulin resistance or loss of β-cell function. If blood glucose concentrations are elevated (≥270 mg/dl [15 mmol/L]), insulin therapy should be instituted immediately to preserve β cells and not be delayed until after other specific therapy.

Determining if Diabetic Remission Is Present

Many cats achieve diabetic remission within 2 to 8 weeks. It is strongly recommended that insulin therapy not be withdrawn prematurely. Cats with almost normal β-cell function can tolerate 0.5 to 1 U once or twice daily and rarely develop clinical hypoglycemia. If insulin therapy is stopped prematurely and hyperglycemia recurs, it can take weeks or months to achieve the same level of glycemic control once insulin is reinstituted. It is recommended that insulin therapy continue for a minimum of 2 to 4 weeks after initiating treatment to facilitate β-cell recovery from glucotoxicity.

Insulin dosage should be decreased gradually based on dosing guidelines in Box 48-1. When preinsulin blood glucose concentration is less than 180 mg/dl (10 mmol/L) and total dosage is decreased to 0.5 U twice daily, the dosing frequency can be reduced to once daily. If after 1 to 2 weeks preinsulin blood glucose is still less than 180 mg/dl (10 mmol/L) and nadir glucose concentration is not above the normal range (72 to 126 mg/dl [4 to 7 mmol/L]), insulin therapy can be discontinued, and blood glucose concentration should be monitored during the day. If blood glucose increases to greater than 180 mg/dl (10 mmol/L) within 12 to 24 hours, insulin should be

immediately reinstituted at 1 U once or twice daily, and one should wait a minimum of 2 weeks before attempting withdrawal of insulin again. If blood glucose concentration is less than 180 mg/dl (10 mmol/L), one should continue to withhold insulin, checking blood glucose every 3 to 7 days for several weeks, and carefully monitor the cat for signs of hyperglycemia (increasing thirst and glycosuria). Owners should monitor glucose concentrations once a week, but if this is not possible, they should measure water drunk and monitor urine glucose concentration because increased thirst or glycosuria likely indicates relapse. If blood glucose is 180 mg/dl (10 mmol/L) or greater, insulin therapy should be reinstituted immediately. Some cats regain substantial β-cell function but require 0.5 to 1 U of insulin every 2 to 3 days to maintain normoglycemia.

Generally, blood glucose concentration following glargine or detemir administration does not change as quickly as with shorter acting insulins such as Lente; measuring blood glucose concentration every 4 hours is usually adequate. Critical time points to monitor are the blood glucose concentration just before each insulin injection (i.e., the preinsulin morning and evening glucose concentrations) when using glargine or detemir. For many cats treated with glargine or detemir, the evening blood glucose concentration is lower than the morning concentration and is often the nadir glucose concentration.

Occasionally, blood glucose concentration can change rapidly, especially during the night, and can increase from 54 mg/dl to 324 mg/dl (3 mmol/L to 18 mmol/L) in 2 hours. It is unclear whether this rapid increase in blood glucose is mediated by counterregulatory hormones (Somogyi phenomenon) or reflects marked hepatic gluconeogenesis associated with negligible insulin concentrations. A rapid increase in blood glucose is more common when glargine is given once daily. Cats with low normal glucose concentration when last monitored in the evening may have very high blood glucose concentrations the next morning. In some cats, decreasing the dosage of insulin decreases morning blood glucose concentration, suggesting that the morning hyperglycemia may be the result of a Somogyi response. The Somogyi phenomenon appears to be very rare in cats treated with glargine or detemir compared with shorter acting insulins such as Lente insulin. However, cats treated with glargine appear quite susceptible to stress-induced hyperglycemia associated with hospital monitoring of blood glucose. If marked hyperglycemia occurs in the hospital, it is critical that information be obtained on glycemic control at home before the hyperglycemia is attributed to treatment failure. Home monitoring of blood glucose concentration helps to clarify the level of glycemic control. If home monitoring of blood glucose concentration is not possible, owners should measure water drunk and urine glucose concentration.

Biochemical Hypoglycemia

Cats treated with glargine or detemir often have biochemical hypoglycemia without clinical signs of hypoglycemia. Humans treated with glargine have significantly lower frequency of clinical hypoglycemia compared with humans treated with NPH insulin. In cats, clinical hypoglycemia also appears to be less common with glargine or detemir than when Lente insulin is used. Biochemical hypoglycemia, with or without mild to moderate clinical signs, can usually be managed at home by feeding the cat, preferably a higher carbohydrate meal such as a dry maintenance feline diet. If a cat displays severe clinical signs such as seizures, glucose syrup or honey must be promptly rubbed into the gums, and veterinary attention should be sought immediately. Most cats showing signs of clinical hypoglycemia with glargine or detemir are in diabetic remission or achieve remission within a few weeks. If biochemical hypoglycemia without clinical signs is present at the time of an insulin injection, one should wait until blood glucose concentration is greater than 126 mg/dl (7 mmol/L) and then reduce the dosage by 0.25 to 0.5 U/cat depending on whether the insulin dosage is greater than or less than 3 U and the degree of hypoglycemia.

Monitoring Glycemic Control

Home blood glucose monitoring two to five times daily provides superior glycemic monitoring to weekly or less frequent glucose monitoring by the veterinarian. However, in the absence of daily home glucose monitoring, measurement of water drunk and urine glucose concentration are invaluable indicators of glycemic control. Diabetic cats with exemplary glycemic control drink volumes similar to nondiabetic cats (<10 ml/kg/24 hr if eating canned food and <60 ml/kg/24 hr with dry food). When using glargine or detemir, in contrast to Lente insulin, monitoring urine glucose concentration is less useful for detecting diabetic remission. This is because cats with well-controlled diabetes that still require glargine or detemir to control blood glucose concentrations have negative or trace urine glucose concentrations. However, urine glucose concentration is more useful for indicating a need for an increase in dosage when using glargine or detemir. Fractious cats can be stabilized solely using urine glucose concentrations and water drunk, although glycemic control is usually not as good as when combined with blood glucose monitoring; diabetic remission may be delayed or not achieved.

Daily home glucose monitoring, coupled with appropriate insulin dosage adjustments, facilitates early optimization of glycemic control and diabetic remission. Daily home glucose monitoring also allows immediate diagnosis of hypoglycemia when clinical signs are vague but suggestive of hypoglycemia. Clients still require frequent clinic visits during the initial stabilization phase to review the home log of blood glucose measurements and to adjust insulin dosage, but a serial glucose curve does not need to be obtained at the veterinary clinic. The confounding effects on blood glucose concentrations of stress and reduced food intake are avoided. Blood glucose should be measured at home before each insulin injection, and if possible, one to three more measurements should be obtained when the owners are home. Ideally, the cat should be monitored a minimum of two to three times daily (before each insulin injection and one other

time point) and once a week more intensely (e.g., five measurements) until remission is achieved or it is evident the cat will not achieve remission but glycemic control is excellent and insulin dose is stable. With newer portable glucose meters available, only a very small volume of blood (0.3 µL) is required, which can be readily sampled by owners from the ear or paw pad from most cats using a lancing device designed for use by pet owners or human diabetic patients.

Portable glucose meters are typically quite precise, but the accuracy is improved using a meter calibrated for feline blood, such as the AlphaTRAK. This increased accuracy is especially helpful for insulin dosage adjustments when blood glucose measurements are around the normal range. Meters calibrated for human use often measure 9 to 36 mg/dl (0.5 to 2 mmol/L) lower than the actual blood glucose concentration, which can make dosage adjustments problematic when the cat is close to achieving diabetic remission.

Storage of Glargine and Detemir

Although the manufacturers recommend discarding glargine and detemir within 4 weeks and 6 weeks, respectively, of opening, an open vial of insulin can usually be kept for up to 6 months if *refrigerated*. The manufacturer's recommendation is based on the risk of bacterial contamination with multiple-use vials. Vials that appear to have lost potency or develop any cloudy discoloration should be discarded immediately. The change may represent precipitation or bacterial contamination.

Oral Hypoglycemic Agents

Oral hypoglycemic drugs act by stimulating β cells to secrete insulin, by increasing insulin sensitivity, or by reducing glucose absorption from the gastrointestinal tract (see Web Chapter 24). Glipizide 2.5 to 7.5 mg/cat q12h is the most commonly used oral hypoglycemic drug in cats and acts by stimulating β cells. It should not be offered as a first line of therapy because of the poorer control of blood glucose concentration and the subsequently lower rate of diabetic remission (<20%) compared with insulin use. However, it can be lifesaving for cats when the owner would elect for euthanasia if insulin injections were the only available treatment. If the cat is easy to pill, glipizide may be used instead of insulin in cats that have insufficient β-cell function to achieve remission but require only minimal dosages of insulin to control hyperglycemia.

Acarbose inhibits brush-border α-glucosidase activity in the intestine and reduces postprandial blood glucose concentrations. Changing to an ultra-low-carbohydrate diet (<6% of energy) has a greater glucose-lowering effect than administering acarbose. However, cats that need a reduced-protein diet (moderate to high carbohydrate) for control of azotemia might benefit from the addition of acarbose at 12 to 25 mg/cat twice daily at the time of eating. Acarbose is minimally effective if the cat is eating multiple meals daily, which is typically the eating pattern of cats with chronic kidney disease by the time they require a restricted-protein diet. Acarbose is most effective when it is administered at the time of eating and the majority of food is consumed soon after it is offered, for example, the eating pattern commonly seen in obese cats that are fed restricted amounts of energy to lose weight. Acarbose should be administered twice daily, even if the cat is only fed once daily, because some food remains in the stomach for 12 to 24 hours when most of the food is consumed in one meal.

Summary

Management of diabetic cats is optimized by using glargine or detemir administered subcutaneously twice daily combined with a low-carbohydrate, high-protein, feline diabetes diet; careful monitoring of blood glucose concentration with appropriate insulin dosage adjustment; and obesity management. Using this protocol to keep maximum blood glucose concentration less than 200 mg/dl (11 mmol/L) can result in diabetic remission in approximately 90% of cats with newly diagnosed diabetes.

References and Suggested Reading

Bennett N et al: Comparison of a low carbohydrate–low fiber diet and a moderate carbohydrate–high fiber diet in the management of feline diabetes mellitus, *J Feline Med Surg* 8:73, 2006.

Elliott DA et al: Prevalence of pituitary tumors among diabetic cats with insulin resistance, *J Am Vet Med Assoc* 216:1765, 2000.

Feldman EC et al: Intensive 50-week evaluation of glipizide administration in 50 cats with previously untreated diabetes mellitus, *J Am Vet Med Assoc* 210:772, 1997.

Gilor C et al: Pharmacodynamics of insulin detemir and insulin glargine assessed by an isoglycemic clamp method in healthy cats, *J Vet Intern Med* 24:870, 2010.

Lepore M et al: Pharmacokinetics and pharmacodynamics of subcutaneous injection of long-acting human insulin analog glargine, NPH insulin, and ultralente human insulin and continuous subcutaneous infusion of insulin lispro, *Diabetes* 49:2142, 2000.

Link KRJ, Rand JS: Changes in blood glucose concentration are associated with relatively rapid changes in circulating fructosamine concentrations in cats, *J Feline Med Surg* 10:583, 2008.

Marshall RD et al: Intramuscular glargine with or without concurrent subcutaneous administration for treatment of feline diabetic ketoacidosis, *J Vet Emerg Crit Care* 23(3):286, 2013.

Marshall R, Rand JR, Morton JM: Treatment with glargine insulin improves glycemic control and results in a higher rate of non-insulin dependence than protamine zinc or lente insulins in newly-diagnosed diabetic cats, *J Feline Med Surg* 11:683, 2009.

Marshall RD, Rand JS, Morton JM: Glargine and protamine zinc insulin have a longer duration of action and result in lower mean daily glucose concentrations than lente insulin in healthy cats, *J Vet Pharmacol Ther* 31:205, 2008.

Marshall RD, Rand JS, Morton JM: Insulin glargine has a long duration of effect following administration either once daily or twice daily in divided doses in healthy cats, *J Feline Med Surg* 10:488, 2008.

Martin GJ, Rand JS: Control of diabetes mellitus in cats with porcine insulin zinc suspension, *Vet Rec* 161:88, 2007a.

Martin GJ, Rand JS: Comparisons of different measurements for monitoring diabetic cats treated with porcine insulin zinc suspension, *Vet Rec* 161:52, 2007b.

Nelson RW et al: Field safety and efficacy of protamine zinc recombinant human insulin for treatment of diabetes mellitus in cats, *J Vet Intern Med* 23:787, 2009.

Niessen SJM et al: Feline acromegaly: an underdiagnosed endocrinopathy? *J Vet Intern Med* 21:899, 2007.

Norsworthy G, Lynn R, Cole C: Preliminary study of protamine zinc recombinant insulin for the treatment of diabetes mellitus in cats, *Vet Ther* 10:24, 2009.

Roomp K, Rand J: Intensive blood glucose control is safe and effective in diabetic cats using home monitoring and treatment with glargine, *J Feline Med Surg* 11:668, 2009.

Roomp PK, Rand JS: Evaluation of detemir in diabetic cats managed with a protocol for intensive blood glucose control, *J Feline Med Surg* 14(8):566, 2012.

Slingerland LI et al: Indoor confinement and physical inactivity rather than the proportion of dry food are risk factors in the development of feline type 2 diabetes mellitus, *Vet J* 179:247, 2009.

Weaver KE et al: Use of glargine and lente insulins in cats with diabetes mellitus, *J Vet Intern Med* 20:234, 2006.

Websites

Selected articles and updated protocols are available at www.uq.edu.au/ccah.

CHAPTER 49
Feline Hypersomatotropism and Acromegaly

STIJN J.M. NIESSEN, *London, United Kingdom*
DAVID B. CHURCH, *London, United Kingdom*

The management of diabetes mellitus (DM) can be quite challenging in a significant percentage of cats. The inherently more autonomous nature of feline patients and the implications on compliance with optimal management might be partly to blame. An important additional consideration is the fact that we currently have a limited understanding of the etiopathogenesis of feline DM. What we do know is that to classify a cat as a typical type 2 diabetic automatically on documentation of persistent hyperglycemia and concurrent glucosuria is a tempting, yet inappropriate practice. Although feline DM used to be routinely attributed to pure insulin resistance phenomena, we now recognize that other processes can be concurrently or alternatively involved. β-Cell dysfunction is one such important process. Additionally, various other disorders outside the endocrine pancreas could play a crucial role in the etiology of the disease of a patient. At least in a subset of cases, understanding and recognizing the processes underlying feline DM affect the optimal management options.

Feline hypersomatotropism or acromegaly is recognized as an important alternative cause of feline DM largely as a result of two more recent prevalence studies (Niessen et al, 2007a; Berg et al, 2007). Hypersomatotropism refers to the pathologic overproduction and subsequent secretion of growth hormone (GH), which leads to the clinical syndrome of acromegaly. The excess GH, among other effects, causes a state of insulin resistance, which eventually results in DM. Most cats with GH hypersecretion are initially considered to have diabetes. The existence of individual nondiabetic acromegalic cases has been mentioned anecdotally, but the true prevalence of such cases is largely unknown. Because excess GH is diagnosed in a large proportion of cats that do not yet show the typical acromegalic phenotype, using the term *hypersomatotropism* instead of *acromegaly* might be more appropriate, although the terms are often used interchangeably.

Prevalence

GH induces the production of the peptide insulin-like growth factor-1 (IGF-1) (mainly by the liver and only in the presence of sufficient portal insulin concentrations). Serum IGF-1 concentrations are elevated in most acromegalic cats. The authors and colleagues performed a screening study among diabetic cats with variable glycemic control (from good to bad) (Niessen et al, 2007a); 59 of 184 (32%) assessed diabetic cats had IGF-1 concentrations strongly suggestive of acromegaly (>1000 ng/ml). Of these 59 cats, a subpopulation (n = 18) was more closely evaluated with intracranial contrast-enhanced computed tomography (CT) or magnetic resonance imaging (MRI) and serum GH measurement to establish conclusively the diagnosis of hypersomatotropism. The diagnosis was subsequently confirmed in 94% of these more carefully assessed cases, proving the original estimation of prevalence, made on the basis of increased IGF-1 concentrations only, to be close to the true prevalence in this diabetic cat population in the United Kingdom.

A retrospective North American study indicated that 26% of diabetic cats in the United States seemed to have acromegaly (Berg et al, 2007). Continued monitoring of diabetic cats in British first-line veterinary practices by the authors' research group has enabled assessment of more than 1200 serum samples of diabetic cats and has substantiated further a prevalence ratio of approximately 25%. This is very important information for any veterinary practitioner because a diagnosis of hypersomatotropism has a huge impact on prognosis and management of the diabetic cat in question (see section on Treatment and Prognosis later). The authors advocate routine screening of diabetic cats for the possible presence of hypersomatotropism, just as screening is done for urinary tract infections in diabetics, the presence of an adrenal tumor in cases with hyperadrenocorticism, or any underlying disease in cases with immune-mediated hemolytic anemia. However, the characteristics and dynamics of serum total IGF-1 concentration measurements as a screening tool should be taken into account (see subsequent section on Diagnosis).

Etiology

Traditionally, acromegaly in cats has been seen as a process caused by excess endogenous GH secretion caused by a pituitary adenoma (Figure 49-1). Until more recently, all reported cases that were subjected to postmortem examination, although bearing in mind the paucity of such reports, suggested this to be the case. A more systematic evaluation of pituitary histopathology in a larger number of patients is currently ongoing and indicates that a minority of cases lack the histopathologic features of a concrete acidophilic adenoma. Instead, acidophilic hyperplasia has been found in these cats (Figure 49-2), which phenotypically in terms of facial and other physical features were indistinguishable from other acromegalic cats (although a typical acromegalic phenotype is

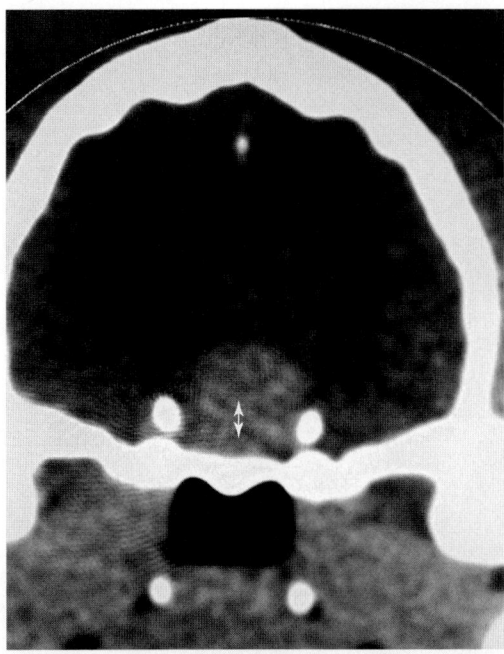

Figure 49-1 Transverse CT image of the brain of a cat with hypersomatotropism demonstrating the presence of a pituitary tumor *(double arrow)* at the level of the pituitary fossa.

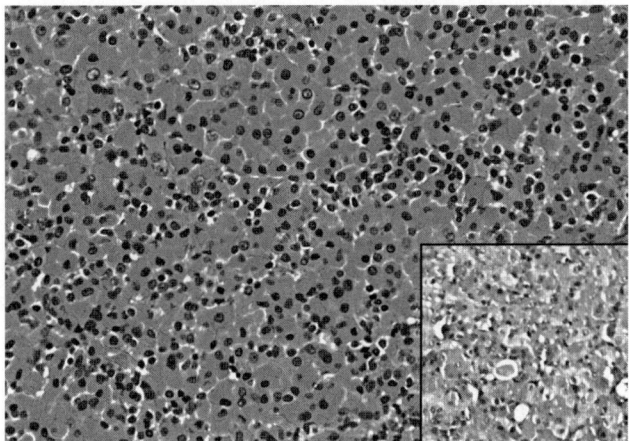

Figure 49-2 Microscopic image of the pituitary of a cat with hypersomatotropism demonstrating clear dominance of acidophils (red-staining cells that produce GH) instead of the expected mix of acidophils and basophils (deep blue–staining cells) in a healthy pituitary *(inset)*. (Hematoxylin and eosin staining, magnification ×400.)

not *persistently* present; see the section on Signalment and Presentation next). If there are at least two underlying etiologic mechanisms, questions arise over a possible interrelationship between them (e.g., hyperplasia becoming adenoma?). A comparison with current hypotheses on the etiology of feline hyperthyroidism is tempting in this regard. Given the fact that feline hyperthyroidism often affects both thyroid glands (albeit not always at the same time), it can be hypothesized that there is a suprathyroidal process driving the disease. Similarly, hypersomatotropism could be hypothesized to originate from the pituitary itself or to be driven by a suprahypophyseal process, possibly located in the hypothalamus.

TABLE 49-1	
Signalment Data and Insulin Requirements of 59 Acromegalic Cats	
Gender	47 male neutered, 6 female neutered, 5 intact males, 1 unknown
Breed	52 DSH, 3 domestic long hair, 4 unknown
Age (years)	Median, 11 (range, 6-17)
Body weight (kg)	Median, 5.8 (range, 3.5-9.2)
Insulin dose (total per injection)	Median 7 U BID (range, 1-35 U BID)

BID, Twice daily; *DSH,* domestic short hair.

Signalment and Presentation

Most reported feline acromegalic patients have been middle-aged to older male neutered domestic short hair cats with DM, although various breeds have been documented to be affected (Table 49-1). The presence of insulin-resistant DM has been shown to be a definite indicator for the presence of hypersomatotropism. Nevertheless, although in the authors' dedicated Acromegalic Cat Clinic insulin resistance is frequently a presenting sign, when routinely measuring IGF-1 in all diabetic cats, a significant number of acromegalic patients can be found that appear insulin sensitive at the time of the initial diagnosis. This finding may relate to "catching" these animals at an early time during their disease process, when hyperglycemia and insulin resistance–induced β-cell dysfunction and hyperglycemia-induced insulin resistance have not yet taken their toll. It is also known that hypersomatotropism-induced changes show a particularly gradual and slow onset. This might also be an explanation for the fact that a "typical" acromegalic phenotype is not consistently present. Previous failure to screen more subtle cases can explain our misconception about what an acromegalic cat should *always* look like. To illustrate the point of gradual onset, duration of clinical signs in the initial group of cats seen by the authors' research group ranged widely from 2 to 42 months with owners and attending clinicians often remaining unaware of any ongoing morphologic changes (Niessen et al, 2007a; Niessen, 2010). It seems tempting to draw comparisons to feline hyperthyroidism, where we currently rarely see the extreme hyperthyroid cat phenotype, possibly owing to increased preparedness to screen for this disease in elderly cats and increased awareness among clinicians and owners. Commonly encountered yet not consistently present clinical signs, assumed to be directly or indirectly caused by the excess of anabolic and catabolic GH and anabolic IGF-1, are denoted in Figure 49-3. The detected polyphagia might be extreme. Especially weight *gain* despite poor glycemic control should be a trigger to alert clinicians for the possible presence of acromegaly.

Cardiomyopathies (and resulting congestive heart failure), arthropathies, and nephropathies have been reported to ensue as part of the pathophysiology of acromegaly, presumably also being induced by excess GH and IGF-1 concentrations. However, because relatively few

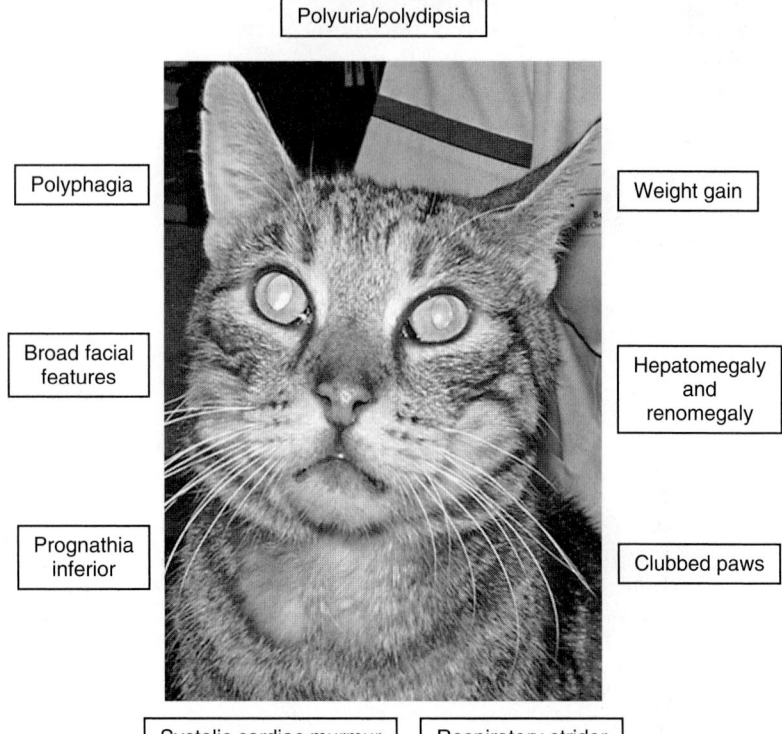

Figure 49-3 A cat with hypersomatotropism with advanced acromegalic features, including broad facial features and prognathia inferior (protrusion of the lower jaw). Boxes indicate common clinical signs associated with the syndrome. The presence of anisocoria is also noted. A large pituitary tumor was confirmed.

cases of feline acromegaly have been described so far, and most previous cases seem to have been at an advanced stage of acromegaly, this assumption warrants further investigation, especially in view of the high prevalence of concurrent disease, including cardiomyopathies, arthropathies and nephropathies, among nonacromegalic diabetic cats and nondiabetic geriatric cats in general. A comparison of routine clinical pathology parameters between acromegalic and nonacromegalic diabetic cats did not reveal a greater incidence of azotemia among acromegalic cats (Niessen, 2010). Pancreatic abnormalities, specifically hyperplasia, seem particularly prevalent in acromegalic cats based on postmortem examinations. "Snoring" or respiratory stridor has been noted by a large proportion of acromegalic cat owners and might relate to the increase in soft tissue in the oropharynx and soft palate induced by GH and IGF-1 causing a disturbed airflow. Finally, neurologic signs, including blindness, depression, anisocoria, and circling, rarely might occur as a consequence of a large pituitary adenoma exerting pressure on the surrounding central nervous system. The overall message should probably be that clinicians ought to remain open-minded about the signalment and presentation of acromegalic cats.

Diagnosis

Feline GH (serum or plasma), IGF-1 (serum), and intracranial imaging have been shown to be useful diagnostic studies. A suggested GH cutoff value of 10 ng/ml was shown to result in an acceptable specificity of 95% and sensitivity of 84% when using a recently developed feline GH assay (currently available only for research purposes at the Royal Veterinary College (RVC), London). Feline

GH also appeared relatively stable, allowing overnight transport of unseparated samples (Niessen et al, 2007b). However, measurement of feline GH or IGF-1 was shown to yield false-positive results in a few cases. Given the fact that GH shows considerable interspecies variation in structure, we can use only assays specifically validated for veterinary use. IGF-1 shows considerable species homology, with human IGF-1 radioimmunoassays having been shown to measure feline IGF-1 reliably. Nevertheless, in general and especially when it comes to determination of diagnostic cutoff concentrations (i.e., should one be suspicious of hypersomatotropism or not), it is recommended to use only IGF-1 assays that have been validated for use in (acromegalic) cats. The endocrine laboratory at Michigan State University in the United States and Cambridge Specialist Laboratories and the Royal Veterinary College in London in the United Kingdom offer IGF-1 assays.

Cases of acromegalic cats with a normal basal feline GH concentration have yet to be documented; however, false-negative IGF-1 results have been documented in a few cases. The duration of exogenous insulin administration could play a crucial role in false-negative IGF-1 results because hepatic IGF-1-production is induced via stimulation of insulin-dependent hepatic GH receptors. An insulin-deficient state can act as an inhibitor of IGF-1 production, resulting in low IGF-1 concentrations in diabetic patients before institution of exogenous insulin treatment or even during the first few weeks of treatment (Figure 49-4). When screening for the presence of acromegaly, these specific IGF-1 dynamics should be taken into account, and repeat IGF-1 determination should be considered 6 to 8 weeks into the treatment. Alternatively, if one wishes to determine IGF-1 only once, the latter

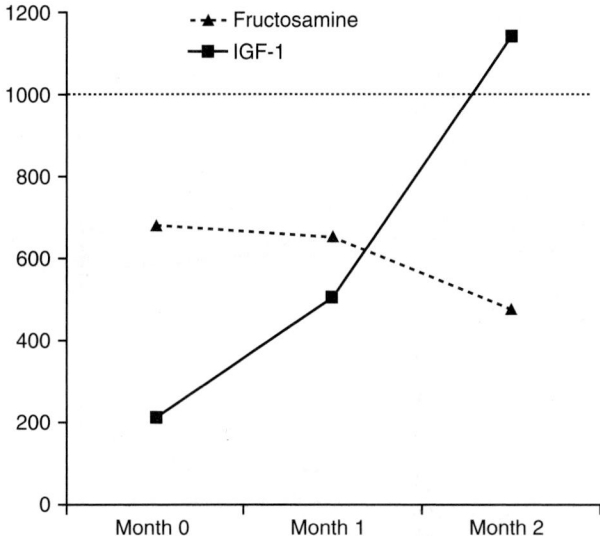

Figure 49-4 Serum IGF-1 in a cat with newly diagnosed diabetes at the time of diagnosis and after initiation of insulin therapy. IGF-1 concentration increases from a concentration not suggestive of hypersomatotropism to one at which it is likely *(above dotted line)* after 2 months of insulin therapy.

time point is recommended rather than at the time of diagnosis of DM.

Intracranial imaging (with contrast enhancement) seems useful in confirming the presence of hypersomatotropism, with MRI seemingly more sensitive than CT. However, cases with negative CT or MRI findings have been documented with the diagnosis eventually being confirmed on postmortem examination. When a structural pituitary abnormality is documented, it provides further circumstantial evidence for the presence of hypersomatotropism. However, it does not provide differentiation from a nonfunctional pituitary tumor or pituitary-dependent hyperadrenocorticism. More importantly, one could question the usefulness of intracranial imaging when a negative scan is obtained despite the presence of a documented hormonal imbalance (i.e., elevated feline GH or IGF-1 concentration in a diabetic patient). When imaging is negative, it seems more logical to have the ultimate premortem diagnosis of hypersomatotropism rely on hormonal assessment. Additionally, cases with subtle (microscopic) acidophilic hyperplasia or microadenoma instead of obvious (macroscopic) adenoma might be more likely to show negative intracranial imaging.

Finally, finding a mild elevation of IGF-1 (not in the acromegalic range) in a diabetic cat represents a dilemma. It is probably best followed up with a repeat measurement 1 or 2 months later because cases with a mild elevation secondary to either DM alone or genuine hypersomatotropism have been described. Nevertheless, a mild elevation in IGF-1 concentration in light of severe insulin resistance could justifiably trigger further diagnostic studies directed toward hypersomatotropism, particularly GH assessment (if available) and intracranial imaging, especially given the tremendous impact of the early diagnosis of the disease on prognosis and patient management.

Treatment and Prognosis

Broadly speaking, treatment options consist of treating the consequences of hypersomatotropism and treating the hypersomatotropism itself. When the disease is detected at an early stage, diabetic remission could result from effective treatment, and a *definitive* treatment option is often preferred. Medical, surgical, and radiation options are available.

Medical Treatment

Medical treatment options in cats have generally been aimed at inhibiting pituitary secretion of GH. Both somatostatins and dopamine agonists have natural affinity for pituitary receptors that facilitate such inhibition. However, administration of octreotide (short-acting somatostatin analog) and dopamine agonists (i.e., bromocriptine and selegiline) have not resulted in convincing clinical improvement of insulin sensitivity on dosing regimens employed so far. A trial with the long-acting somatostatin analog lanreotide also proved disappointing. For somatostatin analogs to work, the abnormal pituitary needs to express somatostatin receptors that are largely unaffected by mutations. Nevertheless, a decrease in plasma GH, adrenocorticotropic hormone, and cortisol concentrations has been documented in a small subset of acromegalic patients after intravenous injection of short-acting octreotide. At the present time, trials with longer acting synthetic somatostatin analogs targeting multiple somatostatin receptor types look the most promising of all attempted medical treatment options. A recent trial with the novel somatostatin analog Pasireotide conducted by the authors in eight affected cats resulted in a significant decrease in serum IGF-1 and insulin requirements in all cats, with two cats achieving diabetic remission (Personal communication, Dr. Stijn Niessen, 2013).

Surgical Treatment

Surgical treatment involves transsphenoidal hypophysectomy and is the main preferred treatment modality in humans. The successful application of hypophysectomy in acromegalic cats has been described, resulting in an immediate decrease in GH levels postoperatively and normalization of IGF-1 concentration as well as possible resolution of DM within weeks. Cryohypophysectomy constitutes another option, which has been reported to be successful in two cases. In the authors' clinic (RVC, London) hypophysectomy is also the preferred treatment option in cats. Availability of hypophysectomy is quite limited at the present time and, as is the case with human patients, success rates are closely correlated with the experience of the surgeon and the perioperative and postoperative management team.

Radiation Therapy

Radiation therapy is currently the most widely applied treatment modality and has been shown to reduce size and secretory capacity of the acidophilic adenoma successfully in most cases. Application of more refined protocols and Gamma Knife technology seems advantageous. More widespread availability of radiation facilities has aided its popularity as a treatment modality. Nevertheless, treatment is still relatively costly and often requires multiple fractions to be given under multiple general anesthetic episodes. The most important practical disadvantage is that clinical response, including the type of clinical response, is not guaranteed. Whether (and how much of) the hypersomatotropism resolves and whether (and how much of) the concurrent insulin resistance disappears remain unpredictable. Additionally, the time of onset (from weeks to >1 year after therapy) and duration are extremely variable. In contrast to outcome with hypophysectomy, IGF-1 and GH concentrations decrease, but they do not decrease to normal levels even in seemingly successfully treated animals (Figure 49-5). Nevertheless, diabetic stabilization as well as diabetic remission can occur in radiation-treated cats, although other negative sequelae of hypersomatotropism (e.g., cardiac, joint, and renal changes) might continue to develop. As soon as radiotherapy has started, owners and veterinarians should be alert for a sudden decrease in insulin resistance and the danger of an insulin overdose if it is missed. Home urine glucose or, even better, home blood glucose monitoring can provide a good safety mechanism during this time. Communication between veterinarian and owner should be optimal and regular in the period following radiation therapy.

Conservative Treatment

A more conservative approach ignores the underlying disease mechanism and focuses on the consequences of hypersomatotropism, specifically on gaining maximal control over DM. Eventually, most cats need high dosages of insulin or combinations of short-acting and long-acting insulin types to ensure an adequate quality of life for both pet and owner. Nevertheless, this approach can result in an adequate level of control in a minority of cases, although careful and continued assessment of quality of life is indicated. The use of more objective quality-of-life measurement tools designed for the diabetic pet might be useful in quantifying and monitoring the situation.

A long-term survival benefit has yet to be demonstrated with any treatment modality compared with treatment of DM alone, and documented survival times of acromegalic cats are currently lacking. Nevertheless, hypersomatotropism is a slowly progressive disease when left untreated, and the true gain might be in an increased quality of life when the underlying hypersomatotropism is targeted, and consequently better control of DM can be attained. Additionally, when treating hypersomatotropism in an early phase, before the onset of permanent β-cell damage and other possible pathology induced by GH and IGF-1, acromegaly-induced permanent DM possibly could be prevented.

Finally, these middle-aged to older patients might need additional treatment for comorbidities, which might or might not be related to hypersomatotropism. Arthropathies might require analgesia, and congestive heart failure

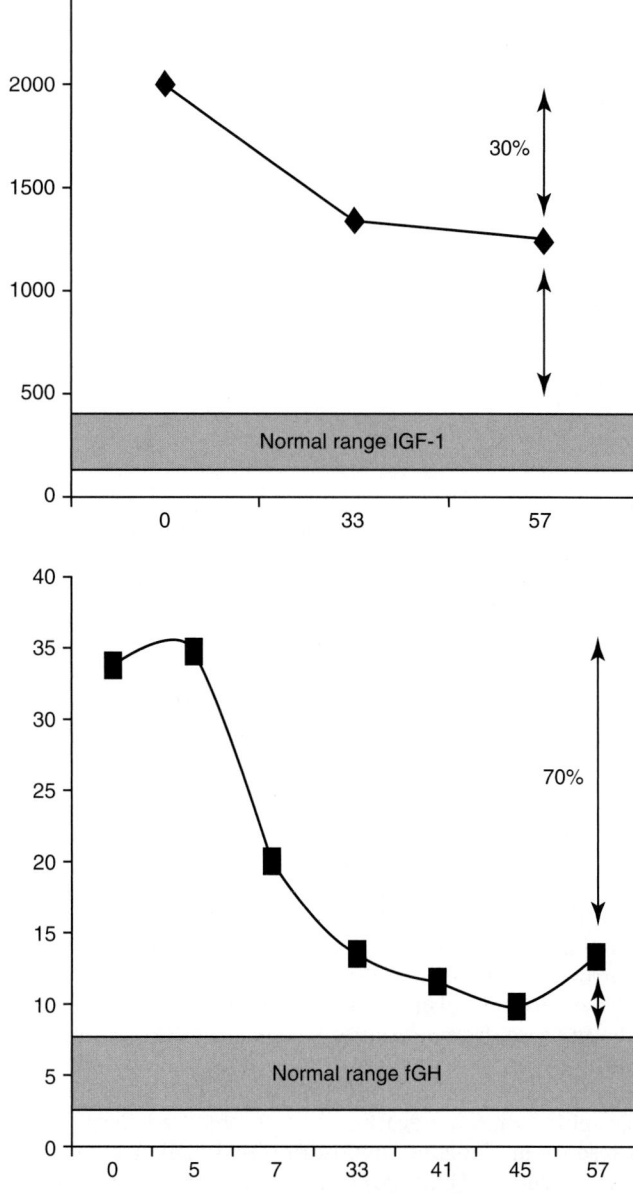

Figure 49-5 Graph displaying hormonal changes after radiotherapy of a cat with hypersomatotropism. *y-axis, top,* IGF-1 concentrations (ng/ml); *bottom,* feline GH concentrations (ng/ml). *x-axis, top and bottom,* weeks after radiation. Hormonal normalization is not achieved, although diabetic control improved. The percentage and *arrows* indicate the change in hormonal concentrations compared with original level and compared with reference interval.

might require treatment with angiotensin-converting enzyme inhibitors and diuretics. When using the latter two drugs, clinicians need to monitor carefully for electrolyte abnormalities, especially in view of concurrent aggravating osmotic diuresis caused by DM. Renal disease and hypertension require additional attention using standard recommended therapy.

References and Suggested Reading

Abraham LA et al: Treatment of an acromegalic cat with the dopamine agonist L-deprenyl, *Aust Vet J* 80:479, 2002.

Berg RI et al: Serum insulin-like growth factor-I concentration in cats with diabetes mellitus and acromegaly, *J Vet Intern Med* 2:892, 2007.

Dunning MD et al: Exogenous insulin treatment after hypofractionated radiotherapy in cats with diabetes mellitus and acromegaly, *J Vet Intern Med* 23:243, 2009.

Meij BP et al: Successful treatment of acromegaly in a diabetic cat with transsphenoidal hypophysectomy, *J Feline Med Surg* 12:406, 2010.

Niessen SJ: Feline acromegaly: an essential differential diagnosis for the difficult diabetic, *J Feline Med Surg* 12:15, 2010.

Niessen SJ et al: Feline acromegaly: an underdiagnosed endocrinopathy? *J Vet Intern Med* 21:899, 2007a.

Niessen SJ et al: Validation and application of an ovine radioimmunoassay for the diagnosis of feline acromegaly, *Vet Rec* 160:902, 2007b.

Peterson ME et al: Acromegaly in 14 cats, *J Vet Intern Med* 4:192, 1990.

Reusch CE et al: Measurements of growth hormone and insulin-like growth factor 1 in cats with diabetes mellitus, *Vet Rec* 158:195, 2006.

CHAPTER 50

Occult Hyperadrenocorticism: Is It Real?

ELLEN N. BEHREND, *Auburn, Alabama*
ROBERT ALLEN KENNIS, *Auburn, Alabama*

Because of the high incidence of hyperadrenocorticism (HAC) and the nonspecific clinical signs, older dogs are commonly screened for HAC with the low-dose dexamethasone suppression test (LDDST) or the standard adrenocorticotropic hormone (ACTH) stimulation test with measurement of serum cortisol before and after ACTH injection. Neither the LDDST nor ACTH stimulation test is perfect, however. For the LDDST and ACTH stimulation test, the sensitivity is approximately 95% and 80%, respectively, for diagnosing HAC. The specificity of the LDDST has been estimated to be 44% to 73%, whereas the specificity of the ACTH stimulation test is 59% to 86%. Because HAC occurs in older dogs, patients tested for HAC often have concurrent disease. At the least, if these dogs do not have HAC, they have a nonadrenal illness causing the clinical signs. Generally, the more severe the nonadrenal illness present, the more likely a false-positive test result for HAC is to occur.

Because of the imprecision of the tests, HAC can sometimes be a difficult diagnosis to make. Clinicians may be faced with situations in which their clinical impression is that patients have HAC, but the tests do not confirm the diagnosis, and no alternative diagnosis is identified. To explain such circumstances, much interest has focused more recently on a syndrome termed *occult HAC*. Dogs with occult HAC allegedly have clinical signs or routine laboratory abnormalities, or both, consistent with classic HAC but with normal LDDST and ACTH stimulation test results. Occult HAC is supposedly caused by diversion of the normal adrenocortical pathways for cortisol and aldosterone synthesis into overproduction of sex hormones instead. The syndrome is diagnosed by performance of an ACTH stimulation test with measurement of serum sex hormone concentrations before and after administration of ACTH.

However, it is the authors' opinion that conclusive evidence for the existence of occult HAC as a sex hormone–mediated condition is lacking. Here we evaluate the evidence both for and against the existence of occult HAC. In evaluating adrenal secretion of sex hormones and cortisol precursors, whether basal or ACTH-stimulated concentrations were measured in any study must be taken into account. For the diagnosis of standard HAC, determination of basal cortisol concentration is unreliable and never used by itself. No evidence exists that measurement of basal serum sex hormone concentrations are any more reliable for diagnosis of adrenal dysfunction. The following discussion focuses on ACTH-stimulated concentrations.

Adrenal Sex Hormone and Cortisol Precursor Secretion as a Cause of Bilaterally Symmetrical Alopecia

Evidence in Favor

Apart from the adrenal glands, sex hormones secreted from other sources can cause alopecia. A syndrome of castration-responsive alopecia has been recognized. Hyperestrogenism and hyperprogesteronism associated with Sertoli cell tumors, for example, can lead to bilaterally symmetrical alopecia.

The first report of clinical signs thought to be due to elevations in adrenal-derived sex hormone concentrations described bilaterally symmetrical alopecia and hyperpigmentation in seven Pomeranians (Schmeitzel and Lothrop, 1990). Classic HAC was ruled out on the basis of normal ACTH stimulation test and LDDST results. Progesterone, 17α-hydroxyprogesterone (17OHP), 11-deoxycortisol, dehydroepiandrosterone sulfate (DHEAS), testosterone, androstenedione, and estradiol were measured before and after administration of ACTH in 7 affected Pomeranians, 12 unaffected Pomeranians, and 19 non-Pomeranian control dogs. Only ACTH-stimulated 17OHP concentrations differed between affected and unaffected Pomeranians, but ACTH-stimulated progesterone and DHEAS concentrations were significantly higher in both affected and unaffected Pomeranians compared with controls. Given the constellation of abnormalities in affected and unaffected dogs, it was hypothesized the alopecia was due to a partial deficiency of 21-hydroxylase, an enzyme needed for cortisol synthesis. In humans with 21-hydroxylase deficiency, cortisol is not synthesized and its precursors, most notably 17OHP and androgens, accumulate. Because affected Pomeranians had normal cortisol concentrations, the enzyme deficiency was assumed to be partial. Family members of human patients with congenital adrenal hyperplasia have sex hormone elevations to a lesser magnitude and no clinical signs, explaining the findings (i.e., increased progesterone and DHEAS levels) in the unaffected Pomeranians (many of the affected and unaffected Pomeranians in the study were related). Subsequently, other dogs with alopecia X were reported to have ACTH-stimulated sex hormone concentrations above the reference range.

Evidence Against

Of six sex hormones assessed by Schmeitzel and Lothrop (1990) in the seven Pomeranians with alopecia X, only ACTH-stimulated serum 17OHP was significantly different between affected and unaffected dogs. However, when affected male and female dogs were assessed separately, the males did not have elevated serum 17OHP concentrations. In 276 dogs with alopecia X, only 73% had at least one basal or post-ACTH sex hormone concentration above the normal range (i.e., 27% had no elevations). Despite the preponderance of elevations in sex hormone concentrations, no consistent sex hormone abnormalities were identified. Of the ACTH-stimulated hormone concentrations, elevated progesterone was the most common abnormality, but it was found in only 36.2% of the patients. It was concluded that it is more appropriate to refer to alopecia X as "alopecia associated with follicular arrest rather than equating it with an adrenal hormone imbalance" (Frank et al, 2003).

Candidate genes in which mutations could cause the sex hormone abnormalities, including 21-hydroxylase and enzymes in the cortisol synthesis pathway, have been cloned. No mutations have been identified.

17α-Hydroxyprogesterone, Other Sex Hormones, and Cortisol Precursors as Causes of Occult Hyperadrenocorticism

Evidence in Favor

In a study of 24 dogs with clinical and routine laboratory findings suggestive of HAC, 11 dogs were assigned to group 1 that had typical HAC with elevated cortisol responses to ACTH. Of 13 dogs with normal ACTH response test results, 6 had positive LDDST results (group 2A), 4 had negative LDDST results (group 2B), and 3 had low plasma cortisol concentrations throughout testing so that the LDDST was uninterpretable (group 2C). Despite the variation in serum cortisol concentrations on the tests for standard HAC, all 23 dogs had elevated ACTH-stimulated 17OHP concentrations. It was concluded that ACTH-stimulated serum 17OHP concentration is elevated in dogs with classic and occult HAC, and measurement of serum 17OHP concentration is a marker of adrenal dysfunction (Ristic et al, 2002). Numerous other studies have since documented elevations in sex hormone concentrations in dogs with various forms of hypercortisolemia, either pituitary-dependent HAC (PDH) or HAC due to an adrenal tumor (AT).

In cases in which cortisol and sex hormones are both elevated, which hormones are causing clinical signs of HAC is difficult or impossible to determine. However, sporadic reports exist of dogs with sex hormone–secreting AT and low serum cortisol concentrations in which clinical signs of HAC were present, ostensibly secondary to the sex hormones.

Evidence Against

It is difficult to understand how sex hormones would cause clinical signs of HAC. The sex hormone mentioned most frequently as a cause of occult HAC is progesterone. However, because of the short half-life of progesterone, little is known about the effects of elevated serum concentrations. Chronic excesses in progesterone concentration are not unique. In estrus and diestrus, serum progesterone is elevated for 60 to 90 days and is higher than in dogs with HAC, but no clinical signs of HAC develop. In humans, clinically silent 17OHP-secreting AT occurs. Massive elevations in serum 17OHP occur with 21-hydroxylase deficiency in people, but clinically affected patients show signs either of aldosterone deficiency or androgen excess, not signs of HAC. Lastly, a "cryptic" syndrome of 21-hydroxylase deficiency exists in which affected people lack 21-hydroxylase and have hormonal abnormalities but no clinical signs. Similarly, in dogs with alopecia X, serum 17OHP concentrations can be quite elevated similar to what is seen with dogs with purported occult HAC; however, none of the classic systemic clinical signs, such as polyuria and polydipsia, polyphagia, pot belly, and panting, are reported.

Two mechanisms have been proposed for the ability of progesterone to cause signs of glucocorticoid excess. Synthetic progestins, compounds with progesterone-like actions, either may bind glucocorticoid receptors or may displace cortisol from its binding protein, elevating serum free cortisol concentrations. However, examination of Pomeranians with alopecia X refutes the likelihood of either mechanism occurring. If elevated serum 17OHP concentration, as seen in those dogs, is sufficient to cause clinical disease secondary to glucocorticoid actions of 17OHP, endogenous ACTH concentration should be suppressed because of negative feedback effects of glucocorticoids on the pituitary. For dogs with proven sex hormone–secreting tumors and signs of HAC despite hypocortisolemia, measured endogenous ACTH concentrations can be low. However, not all dogs with clinical signs supposedly caused by sex hormones have suppression of ACTH secretion. To the contrary, Pomeranians with elevated serum 17OHP concentrations had higher plasma ACTH concentrations than healthy dogs (Schmeitzel and Lothrop, 1990).

How AT could have a shift in hormone synthesis activity can be understood easily. Tumor cells are not normal and can undergo loss of differentiation, losing the ability to synthesize enzymes in the hormone synthesis pathways. In cases of pituitary-dependent occult HAC, how or why normal adrenocortical tissue should have altered steroid synthesis is unexplained.

The number of published cases of dogs with purported true occult HAC (i.e., presence of consistent clinical signs, ACTH stimulation test and LDDST both normal, and response to appropriate therapy) is quite small. In the initial study that attributed occult HAC to elevated 17OHP concentration, not all 24 dogs had occult HAC; 17 had standard ACTH stimulation test or LDDST results consistent with HAC and were not occult. Three dogs had normal ACTH stimulation test results and low plasma cortisol concentrations throughout the LDDST. These results are not unusual in dogs with AT. Only three dogs were diagnosed with PDH despite having both normal ACTH stimulation test and LDDST results (Ristic et al, 2002). In 64 dogs documented to have HAC, no dog was negative on both the ACTH stimulation test and the LDDST (Feldman, 1983). Of 57 dogs evaluated for HAC with cortisol measurements on an ACTH stimulation test and LDDST, 40 were diagnosed as having PDH, 12 as having AT, and 5 as possibly having occult HAC. The diagnosis of occult HAC was bolstered by a positive response to therapy in only 1 dog in the latter group, suggesting that only 1 of 57 dogs may have had occult HAC (Benitah et al, 2005).

Sex Hormone Panel Testing

Evidence in Favor

Measurement of serum sex hormone concentrations has been advocated as a means of diagnosing occult HAC. Use of a panel of hormones has been stated to increase sensitivity and specificity of the test over measurement of a single hormone alone. Elevations in concentrations of any hormone can be common, with estradiol elevations noted in approximately 40% of panels submitted to one reference laboratory.

Evidence Against

The specificity of sex hormone panel testing must be considered. It is reasonable to assume that dogs with nonadrenal illness (NAI) (e.g., a dog with diabetes mellitus) might not have the same ACTH response as healthy dogs because of adaptation of adrenocortical function to the stresses of chronic illness. Many stressed and sick dogs have increased cortisol concentrations and an exaggerated ACTH response but do not have HAC.

With regard to 17OHP, the specificity of the test may be only 70% (i.e., the chance of a false-positive result is 30%) (Chapman et al, 2003; Sieber-Ruckstuhl et al, 2008; Behrend et al, 2005; Monroe et al, 2012). In one study, serum cortisol, 17OHP, and corticosterone concentrations after ACTH stimulation were significantly correlated both in dogs with neoplasia and in dogs suspected to have HAC, suggesting that as adrenal function is increased either by adrenal disease or nonspecifically by NAI, production of all hormones increases proportionately (Behrend et al, 2005). When dogs suspected to have HAC but proven not to were compared to those that did have HAC, cortisol distinguished the two groups more clearly than did either 17α-hydroxypregnenolone or 17OHP (Chapman et al, 2003; Sieber-Ruckstuhl et al, 2008). The specificity of progesterone measurement in a single study was 55% (Monroe et al, 2012). In six dogs with either pheochromocytoma or a nonfunctional AT, concentrations of androstenedione, progesterone, 17OHP, testosterone, or estradiol were elevated in all (Hill et al, 2005). Dogs without adrenal disease clearly can have elevated sex hormone and cortisol concentrations, and sex hormones may be more likely to be falsely elevated by NAI compared with cortisol.

The ability of chronic NAI to affect sex hormone concentrations on an ACTH stimulation test has not received critical appraisal as has the effect on cortisol concentrations. The clinical significance of this test has not been determined.

Response to Treatment

Evidence in Favor

In dogs with either alopecia X or purported occult HAC, treatment with agents that affect pituitary or adrenal function has resulted in resolution of clinical signs. Melatonin is a neurohormone produced by the pineal gland that controls seasonal reproductive and hair growth cycles and that alters sex hormone concentrations in intact dogs. Melatonin was administered initially in 29 dogs with alopecia X, and 15 had partial hair regrowth at first reevaluation (Frank et al, 2004). In three Alaskan Malamutes with alopecia X, treatment with trilostane (3.0 to 3.6 mg/kg/day orally), a drug that inhibits adrenal hormone synthesis, resulted in complete hair regrowth within 6 months (Leone et al, 2005). Of 16 Pomeranians and 8 miniature poodles with alopecia X, 14 Pomeranians and all poodles had hair regrowth in response to trilostane; the mean dose that caused hair regrowth was 11.8 mg/kg/day (range, 5 to 23.5 mg/kg/day) in Pomeranians and 9 mg/kg/day (range, 6.1 to 15.0 mg/kg/day) in poodles (Cerundolo et al, 2004). (Note: The doses of trilostane are in general much higher than currently recommended.) In a study on occult HAC, nine dogs treated with trilostane or mitotane had clinical improvement. Decreased ACTH-stimulated cortisol or 17OHP concentrations were documented in four of the nine dogs (Ristic et al, 2002). Lastly, in one dog with clinical signs of HAC and normal post–ACTH stimulation cortisol and LDDST results but an elevated ACTH-stimulated 17OHP concentration, clinical signs resolved with mitotane therapy (Benitah et al, 2005).

Evidence Against

The response to mitotane, melatonin, or trilostane is not uniform or predictable. In 15 Pomeranians with alopecia X treated with melatonin (median, 1.3 mg/kg orally BID; range, 1.0 to 1.7 mg/kg orally BID) for 3 months, only 6 (40%) had mild to moderate hair regrowth (Frank et al, 2006). In the study evaluating 29 dogs with alopecia X that were treated with melatonin or mitotane, partial or complete hair regrowth was seen in only 62% overall. With mitotane, four of six dogs had partial to complete hair regrowth, and two had no hair regrowth (Frank et al, 2004). More importantly, serum sex hormone concentrations did not change significantly in response to treatment or correlate with whether a response was seen. Of the dogs with partial or complete hair regrowth, androstenedione, progesterone, and 17OHP were still elevated in 21%, 64%, and 36%, respectively. In 16 Pomeranians and 8 miniature poodles with alopecia X that responded to trilostane therapy, 17OHP concentrations were significantly elevated after therapy (Cerundolo et al, 2004). Similarly, two dogs with occult HAC treated with trilostane had clinical signs resolve despite 17OHP concentrations being higher with therapy (Ristic et al, 2002). Hair coat and other clinical signs improve despite further increases in concentrations of the sex hormones purportedly underlying the clinical signs.

Conclusion

Occult HAC caused by adrenal secretion of sex hormones has never been proven. There is evidence both in favor and against the theory. Using the research on alopecia X as an analogy for occult HAC and although elevations in sex hormone concentrations were widely documented in dogs with alopecia X, later research was unable to correlate elevations in any hormone with a clinical abnormality. The specificity of adrenal sex hormone panel testing needs to be carefully evaluated because evidence suggests that sex hormone concentrations may be commonly increased nonspecifically secondary to NAI. Furthermore, not all dogs with a diagnosis of occult HAC respond to therapy directed at minimizing adrenal hormone secretion. Sex hormones may be elevated even further by therapy, yet dogs may improve clinically.

References and Suggested Reading

Behrend EN et al: Serum 17-α-hydroxyprogesterone and corticosterone concentrations in dogs with non-adrenal neoplasia and dogs with suspected hyperadrenocorticism, *J Am Vet Med Assoc* 227:1762, 2005.

Benitah N et al: Evaluation of serum 17-hydroxyprogesterone concentration after administration of ACTH in dogs with hyperadrenocorticism, *J Am Vet Med Assoc* 227:1095, 2005.

Cerundolo R et al: Treatment of canine alopecia X with trilostane, *Vet Dermatol* 15:285, 2004.

Chapman PS et al: Evaluation of the basal and post-adrenocorticotrophic hormone serum concentrations of 17-hydroxyprogesterone for the diagnosis of hyperadrenocorticism in dogs, *Vet Rec* 153:771, 2003.

Feldman EC: Comparison of ACTH response and dexamethasone suppression as screening tests in canine hyperadrenocorticism, *J Am Vet Med Assoc* 182:506, 1983.

Frank LA et al: Retrospective evaluation of sex hormones and steroid hormone intermediates in dogs with alopecia, *Vet Dermatol* 14:91, 2003.

Frank LA, Donnell RL, Kania SA: Oestrogen receptor evaluation in Pomeranian dogs with hair cycle arrest (alopecia X) on melatonin supplementation, *Vet Dermatol* 17:252, 2006.

Frank LA, Hnilica KA, Oliver JW: Adrenal steroid hormone concentrations in dogs with hair cycle arrest (Alopecia X) before and during treatment with melatonin and mitotane, *Vet Dermatol* 15:278, 2004.

Hill KE et al: Secretion of sex hormones in dogs with adrenal dysfunction, *J Am Vet Med Assoc* 226:556, 2005.

Leone F et al: The use of trilostane for the treatment of Alopecia X in Alaskan malamutes, *J Am Anim Hosp Assoc* 41:336, 2005.

Monroe WE et al: Concentrations of noncortisol adrenal steroids in response to ACTH in dogs with adrenal-dependent hyperadrenocorticism, pituitary-dependent hyperadrenocorticism, and nonadrenal illness, *J Vet Int Med* 26:945, 2012.

Ristic JME et al: The use of 17-hydroxyprogesterone in the diagnosis of canine hyperadrenocorticism, *J Vet Intern Med* 16:433, 2002.

Schmeitzel LP, Lothrop CD: Hormonal abnormalities in Pomeranians with normal coat and in Pomeranians with growth hormone -responsive dermatosis, *J Am Vet Med Assoc* 197:1333, 1990.

Sieber-Ruckstuhl N et al: Evaluation of cortisol precursors for the diagnosis of pituitary-dependent hypercortisolism in dogs, *Vet Rec* 162:673, 2008.

CHAPTER 51

Canine Hyperadrenocorticism Therapy

IAN K. RAMSEY, *Glasgow, United Kingdom*
RETO NEIGER, *Giessen, Germany*

Hyperadrenocorticism, or Cushing's syndrome, results from a chronic excess of glucocorticoids and is one of the most common canine endocrinopathies. This chapter summarizes the current knowledge of the treatment of this syndrome, with attention focused on recent developments in the use of trilostane. For a detailed description of the more well-known aspects of this disease, readers should consult one of the standard textbooks.

Hyperadrenocorticism has two main spontaneous forms and may also be produced iatrogenically by the administration of steroids. The most common cause of hyperadrenocorticism is the overproduction of adrenocorticotropic hormone (ACTH) by a small, benign pituitary microadenoma (pituitary-dependent hyperadrenocorticism). A less common cause of hyperadrenocorticism, accounting for about 15% of cases, is the overproduction of cortisol by an adrenal tumor (adrenal-dependent hyperadrenocorticism).

It is useful, but not always essential, to distinguish between pituitary-dependent and adrenal-dependent hyperadrenocorticism. Differentiating between the two helps define the treatment that can be offered and provides information on the likely prognosis and progression of the condition. Interested readers should consult other texts for a full discussion of the various methods of achieving this distinction (e.g., low-dose dexamethasone suppression test, endogenous ACTH assay, abdominal ultrasonography).

Treatment of Pituitary-Dependent Hyperadrenocorticism

In general, all dogs with pituitary-dependent hyperadrenocorticism should be treated. However, cases identified fortuitously during routine health checks may not require immediate treatment. The risks of not treating hyperadrenocorticism, especially when more advanced, include the development of pancreatitis, diabetes mellitus, and calcium oxalate urolithiasis.

Treatment of pituitary-dependent hyperadrenocorticism may be associated with the unmasking of steroid-responsive diseases, including arthritis and atopic dermatitis. The sudden reduction in cortisol concentrations may result in rapid growth of a pituitary tumor, leading to neurologic signs such as ataxia, depression, apparent blindness, inappetence, aimless walking, seizures, and alteration in normal behavior patterns. Treatment may also be associated with a unilateral facial nerve paralysis; it is often unclear if this is a result of the disease or the treatment, but it is seen with both trilostane and mitotane therapy.

Owners of dogs with pituitary-dependent hyperadrenocorticism often request the "best" treatment. The response to this request is now more complicated than ever, and there are at least three effective treatments. No one regimen is perfect for all cases. Local laws and personal experience are important factors in determining the advice that is offered.

Surgical Options

Transsphenoidal hypophysectomy has been described for the treatment of pituitary tumors in dogs with pituitary-dependent hyperadrenocorticism. Only specialists working in suitable facilities should perform such surgery. The success rate in experienced hands is acceptable, but serious complications may occur.

Medical Options

Mitotane

Mitotane was once the mainstay of medical management of canine hyperadrenocorticism in many countries and is reviewed in detail elsewhere (Kintzer and Peterson, 1991). It is a cytotoxic agent that principally causes necrosis of the zona fasciculata and zona reticularis of the adrenal glands. It is slightly more efficacious than trilostane (see next section) but is reported to have a higher incidence of side effects (Kintzer and Peterson, 1991). Because it can be absorbed through the skin and is cytotoxic to humans, it should be handled carefully with gloves. Splitting tablets should be avoided when possible.

Mitotane is given initially as an induction course (50 mg/kg PO) administered once daily or divided twice daily, as required. Since it is a drug that has a narrow therapeutic index, stabilization in a hospital should be considered in some cases (e.g., dogs with concurrent diabetes) during the induction phase. The drug should be administered either in or immediately following a meal because this enhances its absorption. The induction course is monitored by carefully measuring the dog's water intake and observing its feeding behavior. Concomitant prednisone or prednisolone administration is generally not recommended. Mitotane can also be used at higher doses in a protocol designed to permanently destroy the adrenal gland. This protocol is no longer in widespread use, and interested readers are advised to consult relevant texts for further details.

Treatment is stopped when water consumption or the appetite starts to decrease. Once these end points are reached, if the animal is unusually listless, begins vomiting, or has diarrhea or 7 days of treatment have elapsed, an ACTH stimulation test is performed. A response signifying mild adrenal cortex suppression indicates satisfactory control. For most laboratories this means a post-ACTH cortisol less than 120 nmol/L (<4.3 μg/dl).

Most induction courses last 5 to 10 days. Almost all dogs with pituitary-dependent hyperadrenocorticism respond by day 14. Maintenance therapy (25 to 50 mg/kg PO every 7 days or divided into 2 or 3 smaller doses over the course of a week) is then given and checked by ACTH stimulation tests, initially every month and then every 3 months.

Many dogs relapse at some point and require adjustments to the dose of mitotane. If responses to ACTH stimulation tests suggest a failure of adrenal suppression (post-ACTH cortisol greater than 250 nmol/L [>9 μg/dl]) and clinical signs of hyperadrenocorticism, the dog should be treated with a 3-day reinduction course and the effects of this monitored with further ACTH stimulation tests at the end of the reinduction course. The maintenance dose should then be increased (usually best done by increases in frequency [e.g., from once every 7 days to once every 5 days]) and the ACTH stimulation test repeated in 1 month. When the clinical signs are minimal but the post-ACTH cortisol is greater than 250 nmol/L (>9 μg/dl), the dose frequency may be increased without a reinduction course.

Dogs that are treated with mitotane, particularly those that have been treated for several months, may develop acute signs of hypoadrenocorticism (e.g., severe depression, anorexia, vomiting, diarrhea). Intravenous fluids, glucocorticoids, and rest are usually effective. Mitotane administration should be discontinued until adrenal gland function has recovered, demonstrated by a post-ACTH cortisol concentration greater than 250 nmol/L (>9 μg/dl). The dose should then be decreased from the previous amount and/or frequency.

Occasionally there may be evidence of hyperkalemia and hyponatremia. If these occur, an ACTH stimulation test should be performed; post-ACTH cortisol would be expected to be less than 20 nmol/L (<0.7 μg/dl). Mineralocorticoids should be given if hyperkalemia has been documented and will likely be needed for the rest of the animal's life (see Chapter 53). Pancreatitis and hemorrhagic gastroenteritis are potential complications of the acute iatrogenic hypoadrenocorticism. Oral prednisolone (0.2 to 0.4 mg/kg PO every 24 hours) is given once the vomiting has subsided. Some dogs require this for life, but others may revert to their original state of hyperadrenocorticism.

Routine monitoring with ACTH stimulation tests is recommended; the frequency of monitoring largely depends on the clinical progression of the case. Some dogs receiving long-term prednisolone as a result of

mitotane-induced hypoadrenocorticism only require ACTH stimulation tests annually.

Some animals become intolerant of mitotane and show signs of gastrointestinal upset without a reduction in post-ACTH cortisol concentrations. These dogs should be treated by other means.

Trilostane

Trilostane is a synthetic steroid that competitively inhibits steroid synthesis by blocking 3β-hydroxysteroid dehydrogenase. The adrenal glands and in particular the synthesis of glucocorticoids are more susceptible to its action than are other steroid-producing tissues. The reasons for this are not known. Trilostane is now authorized in most European countries and in the United States for the treatment of pituitary-dependent and adrenal-dependent hyperadrenocorticism in dogs.

Trilostane has proven to be well tolerated by almost all dogs with pituitary-dependent hyperadrenocorticism in several published trials (totaling more than 120 dogs) summarized elsewhere (Ramsey, 2010). Few dogs develop signs of hypoadrenocorticism when treated with trilostane, although mild asymptomatic hyperkalemia is common. When hypoadrenocorticism does occur, dogs usually rapidly recover with appropriate therapy. The low prevalence of side effects compares favorably with those reported with mitotane.

Trilostane is safer for owners to handle when compared with mitotane. However, pregnant women are advised to wear gloves when handling the drug because it has been shown to cause abortion in monkeys given large doses.

Although few pharmacokinetic studies have been performed, trilostane is known to be short acting. The recommended starting dose is 2 to 5 mg/kg orally once daily, using the lower dosage range in small dogs. (Figure 51-1 is an algorithm of trilostane therapy.) Trilostane is better absorbed if given with food. It is effective in resolving the signs of pituitary-dependent hyperadrenocorticism in about 75% of cases (Neiger et al, 2002; Ruckstuhl, Nett, and Reusch, 2002). Polyuria, polydipsia, and polyphagia should dissipate within 4 weeks after starting trilostane. Skin changes should resolve within 4 months of starting treatment. All these improvements should be maintained as long as the dogs remain on adequate doses of trilostane.

The efficacy of the drug and the required dosages are assessed using ACTH stimulation tests carried out 7 to 14 days, 30 days, and 90 days after starting therapy. ACTH stimulation tests should be started 3 hours after dosing; however, it is probably acceptable to start as early as 2 hours after dosing and as late as 4 hours (such that the last sample is then taken at 5 hours). There are significant differences between the cortisol responses to ACTH if stimulation tests are performed at other times (Bell et al, 2006). Many dogs require a change in dose (increase or decrease), and much higher doses may be required in some cases.

Post-ACTH cortisol concentrations should be between 40 nmol/L (1.5 μg/dl) and 120 nmol/L (4.3 μg/dl). If the post-ACTH cortisol concentration is lower and there are clinical signs of hypoadrenocorticism, trilostane is

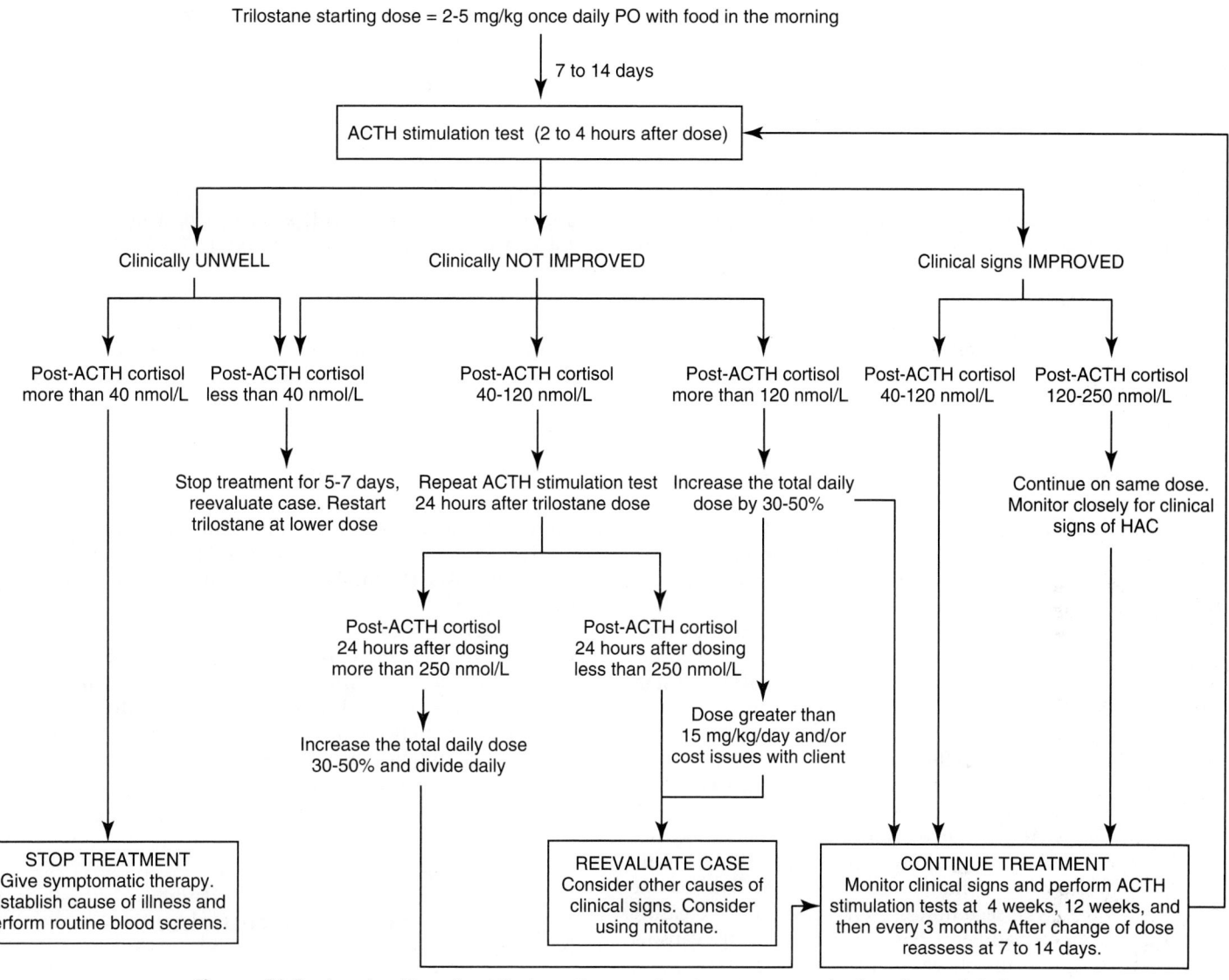

Figure 51-1 An algorithm for trilostane therapy showing steps to take based on clinical response.

stopped for 5 to 7 days and reintroduced at a lower dose. If clinical signs are not apparent (and cortisol concentrations are below 40 nmol/L), trilostane may be continued but the frequency of monitoring should be increased. If the post-ACTH cortisol concentration is higher, the dose of trilostane may need to be increased, depending on the resolution of clinical signs. However, if the post-ACTH cortisol concentration is between these two values and the patient appears not to be clinically well controlled, the trilostane may need to be given twice daily (and the total daily dose increased by approximately 50%). This can be investigated by performing an ACTH stimulation test 24 hours after the administration of trilostane. Post-ACTH cortisol concentrations greater than 250 nmol/L (9 µg/dl) 24 hours after the administration of trilostane in dogs with clinical signs of hyperadrenocorticism that are apparently adequately controlled with a post-ACTH cortisol between 40 and 120 nmol/L 3 to 5 hours after administration are an indication for twice-daily dosing. If an ACTH stimulation test is performed inadvertently at

times other than 2 to 6 hours after dosing, the post-ACTH cortisol concentration should be greater than 20 nmol/L (0.7 µg/dl) and less than 250 nmol/L (9 µg/dl).

Some earlier studies have recommended starting treatment with twice-daily dosing but a higher frequency of adverse effects were observed. However, later studies using lower starting doses demonstrated a lower rate of adverse events (equal to that achieved with once-daily dosing) and lower total daily doses when compared with other studies using once-daily dosing (Feldman, 2011). Whether the convenience of once-daily dosing is outweighed by the benefit of a lower total daily dose will be a client-dependent decision. The long-term effects of twice-daily dosing are unknown. Nevertheless, individual dogs may respond better to a twice-daily dosing regimen, and dogs treated once daily may require higher daily total drug. Diabetic dogs with concurrent hyperadrenocorticism should have trilostane and insulin given at the same frequency (usually this is twice daily), although detailed studies are lacking.

Once the clinical condition of the animal and the dose rate have been stabilized, the dog should be examined and an ACTH stimulation test performed every 3 months. Serum biochemistry (especially potassium measurement) can be performed periodically to check for hyperkalemia, but with increasing clinical experience this becomes less important. Many dogs relapse at some stage and require adjustments to the dosage of trilostane (generally increasing or decreasing by 30% to 50% of the previous dose). This may require individual compounding in some countries having only a limited range of capsule sizes.

Care should be exercised when using trilostane with aldosterone antagonists (such as spironolactone), and the effects of angiotensin-converting enzyme inhibitors may be potentiated. The drug should be used with greater caution in animals with preexisting renal or cardiac disease. No specific data on drug interactions exist, and these comments are purely precautionary. No unwanted drug interactions have been seen in dogs receiving trilostane and various nonsteroidal antiinflammatory drugs, antibiotics, insulin preparations, and levothyroxine. Trilostane should not be given when an animal is ill or having surgery because it reduces the stress response, which is important for such situations.

Minor side effects are sometimes seen, such as mild lethargy, decreased appetite, and slight electrolyte abnormalities. These may occur from 2 to 4 days after the start of the therapy and are often transient and respond to dose reduction.

Long-term adverse effects have not been documented, but adrenal glands increase in size in response to therapy, probably as a result of chronic overstimulation with endogenous ACTH. There is histopathologic evidence that, as well as adrenal hyperplasia, subclinical mild adrenal necrosis is common in treated dogs. This may be due to the hypersecretion of ACTH not only increasing the size of the adrenals but also paradoxically causing necrosis and hemorrhage of the adrenal glands. There have been no documented instances of adrenal tumors developing in trilostane-treated dogs.

Rarely adrenal necrosis may lead to more serious signs of vomiting, diarrhea, or lethargy due to hypoadrenocorticism. If this happens, trilostane should be stopped, and prednisolone given for 1 or 2 days. In some cases dogs will require glucocorticoid and mineralocorticoid supplementation for the rest of their lives. Some dogs may require very much lower doses of trilostane for the remainder of their lives (Reusch et al, 2007; Burkhardt et al, 2011).

The survival of dogs with pituitary-dependent hyperadrenocorticism treated with trilostane or mitotane has been compared (Barker et al, 2005). There was no significant difference between the 123 trilostane-treated dogs, surviving a median of 662 days (range 8 to 1971 days), and the 25 mitotane-treated dogs, surviving a median of 708 days (range 33 to 1339 days). A comparison of twice-daily trilostane with mitotane-induced adrenocorticolysis also did not demonstrate a significant difference.

Other Medical Treatments

Ketoconazole at high serum concentrations inhibits steroid synthesis and therefore exerts effects similar to those of trilostane. In those countries where trilostane and mitotane are unavailable, ketoconazole is indicated for the treatment of pituitary-dependent hyperadrenocorticism. Ketoconazole is hepatotoxic at high doses. The initial dose is 5 mg/kg q12h initially, then increase to 12 to 15 mg/kg q12h, based on laboratory results. An ACTH stimulation test is performed 1 week later. The same target range as for trilostane and mitotane is used, with a goal of post-ACTH cortisol concentrations between 20 and 120 nmol/L (0.7 to 4.3 µg/dl).

In the United States and some other countries, *selegiline* (L-deprenyl) is licensed for the treatment of pituitary-dependent hyperadrenocorticism. It is thought to increase dopamine concentrations in the brain and thereby decrease ACTH production. The dose is 1 mg/kg orally every 24 hours for 60 days, increasing to 2 mg/kg after this time if there is no response. If there is no response after a further month, alternative therapy should be considered. The current evidence indicates that there is minimal endocrinologic but some clinical improvement with selegiline therapy. Monitoring is based on subjective assessment; ACTH stimulation test results are not affected by selegiline.

Various other drugs have been suggested for the treatment of hyperadrenocorticism, including cabergoline, phosphatidylserine, retinoic acid, cyproheptadine, metyrapone, and aminoglutethimide. Some of these drugs have proven to be ineffectual; others have not been investigated. None are currently regarded as useful treatments for canine hyperadrenocorticism.

Treatment of Dogs with Pituitary-Dependent Hyperadrenocorticism and Neurologic Signs

Neurologic signs may develop during any stage of treatment; these usually indicate an expanding pituitary tumor. Magnetic resonance imaging and to a lesser extent computed tomography can diagnose such a tumor in dogs that have pituitary-dependent hyperadrenocorticism and neurologic signs. The presence of a large intracranial tumor should not be regarded as a poor prognostic sign per se, although the chance of intracranial hemorrhage (pituitary apoplexy) or the sudden expansion of the tumor following treatment is increased with larger tumors. The severity of the neurologic deficits associated with the pituitary tumor is the clinically most relevant prognostic indicator.

External beam radiotherapy has been used for pituitary tumors associated with pituitary-dependent hyperadrenocorticism. In general the neurologic signs improve more rapidly than the endocrinologic signs. There can be dramatic reduction in tumor size, but no long-term survival studies have been reported. With the availability of effective drugs to treat hypercortisolemia, radiotherapy should probably be considered only in cases of hyperadrenocorticism with neurologic signs. Treatment protocols vary among centers and need to be tailored to the individual patient.

Treatment of Adrenal-Dependent Hyperadrenocorticism

When treating adrenal-dependent hyperadrenocorticism, owners can opt for a high-risk surgical strategy with a potentially excellent but possibly disastrous outcome or a low-risk medical strategy with a more predictable but less positive outcome. Accurate imaging is essential in informing this decision. Good communication between veterinarians and their clients is essential when owners of dogs with hyperadrenocorticism are deciding which strategy is the most appropriate for them and their animal.

Surgical Options

Unilateral adrenalectomy is indicated for adrenal-dependent hyperadrenocorticism, but careful owner counseling is important since this form of hyperadrenocorticism may also be managed medically. The extent of any local invasion or metastatic spread should be investigated before surgery is performed.

Preoperative stabilization probably improves survival, but this has not been clearly demonstrated. Mitotane may be less useful than trilostane or ketoconazole in this respect because it may make the tumor more friable.

Medical Options

Mitotane

The cytotoxic properties of mitotane make it the logical choice for the long-term medical management of canine adrenal-dependent hyperadrenocorticism. Tumor regression has been demonstrated in some cases; however, most adrenal tumors are relatively resistant to the cytotoxic effects. This means that, when compared to dogs with pituitary-dependent hyperadrenocorticism, dogs with adrenal-dependent hyperadrenocorticism are more variable in their response to mitotane. They may respond very quickly to normal doses or they may require prolonged induction courses of mitotane at increased doses. Therefore careful patient monitoring is essential. Even if the response to an ACTH stimulation test was normal at the onset of treatment, the test can still be used to monitor mitotane therapy since the aim is to reduce the post-ACTH cortisol to less than 120 nmol/L (4.3 µg/ml). A starting dosage of 50 mg/kg orally every 24 hours or divided twice daily should be given. However, if there is no improvement in clinical signs or if the ACTH stimulation test results have not been suppressed after 10 days, the dosage can be increased to 75 mg/kg orally every 24 hours or divided twice daily.

Relapses are common during maintenance therapy. Furthermore, dogs may develop signs of mitotane toxicity (e.g., vomiting, anorexia, diarrhea) without control of cortisol production having been achieved.

Trilostane

Many dogs with adrenal-dependent hyperadrenocorticism have now been treated with trilostane. In the largest series, the survival of 22 dogs treated with trilostane was compared with that of 13 dogs treated with mitotane (Helm et al, 2011). Despite the fact that trilostane is not cytotoxic and thus has no effect on the growth of the tumor or metastases, there was no significant difference between the median survival time for animals treated with trilostane (353 days [range 4 to 1341]) when compared with the median survival time for animals treated with mitotane (102 days [range 33 to 982]).

Experience has shown that the same recommendations for treating dogs with pituitary-dependent hyperadrenocorticism with trilostane are valid for dogs with adrenal-dependent hyperadrenocorticism. Interestingly, the doses required to achieve clinical stabilization do not seem to increase significantly with time in dogs that do respond to the initial therapy.

References and Suggested Reading

Barker E et al: A comparison of the survival times of dogs treated for hyperadrenocorticism with trilostane or mitotane, *J Vet Intern Med* 19:810, 2005.

Bell R et al: Effects of once daily trilostane administration on cortisol concentrations and ACTH responsiveness in hyperadrenocorticoid dogs, *Vet Rec* 159:277, 2006.

Burkhardt WA et al: Adrenocorticotropic hormone, but not trilostane, causes severe adrenal hemorrhage, vacuolization, and apoptosis in rats, *Domest Anim Endocrinol* 40:155, 2011.

Feldman EC: Evaluation of twice-daily lower-dose trilostane treatment administered orally in dogs with naturally occurring hyperadrenocorticism, *J Am Vet Med Assoc* 238:1441, 2011.

Helm JR et al: A comparison of factors that influence survival in dogs treated with mitotane or trilostane with adrenal-dependent hyperadrenocorticism, *J Vet Intern Med* 25:251, 2011.

Kintzer PP, Peterson ME: Mitotane (o,p'-DDD) treatment of 200 dogs with pituitary-dependent hyperadrenocorticism, *J Vet Intern Med* 5:182, 1991.

Neiger R et al: Trilostane treatment of 78 dogs with pituitary-dependent hyperadrenocorticism, *Vet Rec* 150:799, 2002.

Ramsey I: Trilostane: a review, *Vet Clin North Am Small Anim Pract* 40:269, 2010.

Reusch CE et al: Histological evaluation of the adrenal glands of seven dogs with hyperadrenocorticism treated with trilostane, *Vet Rec* 160:219, 2007.

Ruckstuhl NS, Nett CS, Reusch CE: Results of clinical examinations, laboratory tests, and ultrasonography in dogs with pituitary-dependent hyperadrenocorticism treated with trilostane, *Am J Vet Res* 63:506, 2002.

CHAPTER 52

Ectopic ACTH Syndrome and Food-Dependent Hypercortisolism in Dogs

SARA GALAC, *Utrecht, The Netherlands*
HANS S. KOOISTRA, *Utrecht, The Netherlands*

Spontaneous hypercortisolism, or Cushing's syndrome, can be defined as the physical and biochemical changes that result from prolonged exposure to inappropriately high plasma concentrations of (free) cortisol, whatever its cause. In 80% to 85% of the spontaneous cases, hypercortisolism is adrenocorticotropic hormone (ACTH)-dependent, usually arising from hypersecretion of ACTH by a pituitary corticotroph adenoma. The remaining 15% to 20% of cases of spontaneous hypercortisolism are ACTH-independent and result from autonomous hypersecretion of glucocorticoids by an adrenocortical adenoma or adenocarcinoma. Recently, ectopic ACTH syndrome and food-dependent hypercortisolism have been described in dogs as well and should be added as differentials of spontaneous hypercortisolism.

Ectopic ACTH Syndrome

In about 5% to 10% of humans with Cushing's syndrome, the glucocorticoid excess is the result of ACTH secretion by a nonpituitary tumor. Ectopic ACTH secretion may be associated either with highly malignant tumors, small cell lung carcinoma being most common, or with a variety of less aggressive neuroendocrine tumors of bronchial, thymic, pancreatic, or gastrointestinal origin. Plasma ACTH concentrations and cortisol secretion rates can be extremely high in ectopic ACTH syndrome, and as a consequence the clinical manifestations can be very pronounced.

A typical finding is marked hypokalemia resulting from the severe cortisol excess exceeding the capacity of 11β-hydroxysteroid dehydrogenase type 2 (11β-HSD2). Normally, activation of the mineralocorticoid receptor by cortisol is prevented by the expression of 11β-HSD2 by the tissues that contain mineralocorticoid receptors. The 11β-HSD2 converts cortisol into cortisone that cannot activate mineralocorticoid receptors, thus protecting the mineralocorticoid receptor from activation by cortisol.

In ectopic ACTH syndrome, suppression of cortisol secretion is typically not seen on classic dynamic tests such as the high-dose dexamethasone suppression test (HDDST), underlining the autonomous character of ACTH secretion. Although the source of the ectopic ACTH release may be a very small tumor, modern diagnostic

imaging techniques in expert hands will succeed in locating it in the majority of cases (Newell-Price et al, 1998).

Ectopic ACTH syndrome has also been documented in dogs. The most convincing case report concerns an 8-year-old German shepherd (Galac et al, 2005). The dog was referred because of polyuria, polydipsia, polyphagia, and frequent panting. Physical examination revealed no abnormalities except an enlarged liver. Laboratory findings included an increase in plasma activity of alkaline phosphatase (111 U/L; reference range 15 to 69 U/L) and hypokalemia (3.4 mmol/L; reference range 3.6 to 4.8 mmol/L). Urine specific gravity was low (1.008). The basal urinary corticoid:creatinine ratios (UCCRs) on 2 consecutive days were 236 and 350×10^{-6} (reference range $< 10 \times 10^{-6}$) and as such compatible with hypercortisolism. After collection of the second urine sample, an oral HDDST was performed. The dog received 3 doses of 0.1 mg/kg body weight dexamethasone at 8-hour intervals and the third urine sample was collected on the following morning (i.e., 8 hours after the last dose of medication). The UCCR after dexamethasone administration (226×10^{-6}) was not suppressed more than 50% of the mean UCCR of the basal samples, leading to the diagnosis of nonsuppressible hypercortisolism (Galac et al, 2010). Plasma ACTH concentrations (159 and 188 ng/L; reference range 5 to 85 ng/L) were greatly elevated, pointing to dexamethasone-resistant pituitary-dependent hypercortisolism (PDH). Moreover, ultrasonography revealed equal enlargement of both adrenal glands. Because pituitary imaging did not reveal pituitary enlargement, a pituitary microadenoma was suspected. However, histologic examination of the pituitary tissue removed by transsphenoidal hypophysectomy revealed no adenoma. Immunohistochemical staining of the pituitary gland demonstrated normal growth hormone and α-melanocyte–stimulating hormone pattern, while ACTH immunopositive cells were identified only sporadically. Moreover, the clinical manifestations became exacerbated after surgery, including severe hypokalemia. Both the UCCR (1,518 and $2,176 \times 10^{-6}$) and the plasma ACTH concentration (281 ng/L) were further increased. In addition, there was no response of plasma concentrations of ACTH and cortisol to corticotropin-releasing hormone (CRH) administration, whereas in dogs with PDH plasma

230

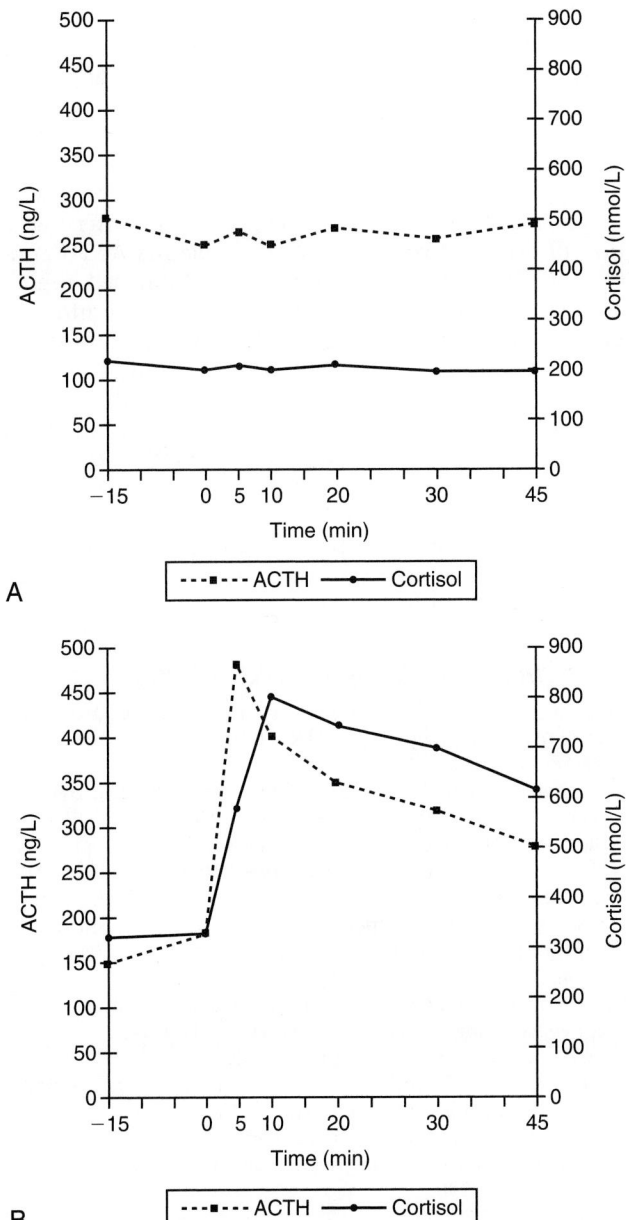

Figure 52-1 Plasma adrenocorticotropic hormone (ACTH) and cortisol concentrations before and after administration of corticotropin-releasing hormone (CRH; 1 μg/kg IV) at 0 min in an 8-year-old intact male German shepherd with ectopic ACTH secretion after complete hypophysectomy for initially presumed pituitary-dependent hypercortisolism **(A)** and in dogs with pituitary-dependent hypercortisolism **(B).** (Adapted from Meij BP, Mol JA, Bevers MM, Rijnberk A: Alterations in anterior pituitary function of dogs with pituitary-dependent hyperadrenocorticism, *J Endocrinol* 154:505-512, 1997.)

concentrations of ACTH and consequently cortisol increase within 5 and 10 minutes, respectively, after stimulation with CRH (Figure 52-1). Computed tomography of the abdomen revealed a tumor in the region of the pancreas. During laparotomy, a 5 mm nodule was located in the pancreas, together with an enlarged adjacent lymph node and nodular changes in the liver. Partial pancreatectomy, extirpation of the lymph node, and liver biopsy were performed, and histologic examination revealed a neuroendocrine tumor with metastases in the lymph node and liver. The second surgical intervention was not curative, probably because of additional metastatic tumor tissue that was not removed. Nevertheless, the dog did well for more than 2 years on treatment with trilostane (see Chapter 51).

Thus ectopic ACTH syndrome should be considered in cases of severe hypercortisolism with highly elevated plasma ACTH and cortisol concentrations that are not suppressible with high doses of dexamethasone, and in which diagnostic imaging does not reveal a pituitary tumor. In patients with ACTH-dependent hypercortisolism due to a pituitary corticotroph adenoma, administration of CRH (1 μg/kg body weight IV) usually results in a significant increase in plasma concentrations of ACTH and cortisol, whereas in patients with ectopic ACTH secretion CRH does not increase these plasma hormone concentrations.

The condition may not be extremely rare because there are two more individual case reports in which this diagnosis has been proposed. In another German shepherd a primary hepatic carcinoid was believed responsible for severe hypercortisolism with persistent hypokalemia (Churcher, 1999). In a dachshund with hypokalemia, an extrapituitary ACTH-producing microadenoma was considered as the cause, but a tumor was neither visualized by magnetic resonance imaging nor found on necropsy (Burgener et al, 2007).

Preferably, ectopic ACTH syndrome is treated by surgical removal of the tumor tissue. When the source of the ectopic ACTH secretion remains hidden or when surgical removal is not possible (e.g., due to the presence of metastases), medical treatment with drugs that eliminate the glucocorticoid excess should be initiated. Either trilostane, a competitive inhibitor of the 3β-hydroxysteroid dehydrogenase/isomerase system, or the adrenocorticolytic drug mitotane can be used to suppress adrenocortical cortisol hypersecretion.

Food-Dependent Glucocorticoid Excess

In addition to autonomous cortisol secretion by an adrenocortical tumor, ACTH-independent hypercortisolism may also result from expression of ectopic or hyperactive eutopic hormone receptors in the adrenal cortex. Ectopic receptors are not normally expressed (i.e., aberrant or inappropriate) in the adrenal cortex, while expression of eutopic receptors can be considered normal, but they can become hyperactive and as such abnormally functional. In humans, various adrenocortical membrane–bound receptors functionally coupled to steroidogenesis have been reported, including gastric-inhibitory polypeptide (GIP), catecholamine, vasopressin, serotonin, and luteinizing hormone (LH) receptors (Lacroix et al, 2001). Most of these receptors belong to the superfamily of G protein–coupled receptors that mimic the cellular events normally triggered by the ACTH receptor. Binding of the ligand to its receptor bypasses the physiologic negative feedback between the adrenal glands and the pituitary gland and leads to aberrant corticosteroidogenesis (Figure 52-2). Despite very low circulating ACTH

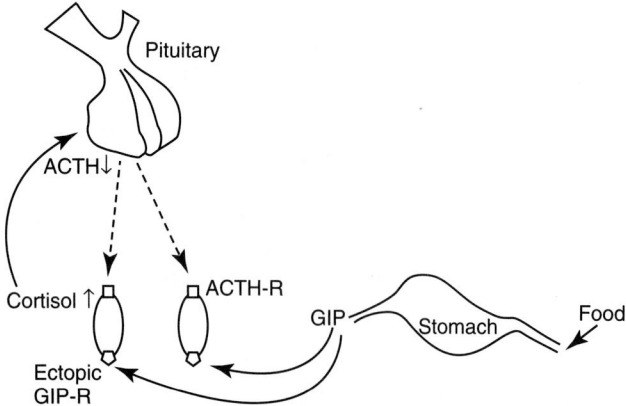

Figure 52-2 Mechanism of food-dependent hypercortisolism due to ectopic expression of the gastric-inhibitory polypeptide receptor (GIP-R). Food ingestion stimulates gastric-inhibitory polypeptide (GIP) secretion from the duodenum, which binds to ectopic adrenal GIP-Rs, leading to cortisol release. The negative feedback of cortisol on the hypothalamic-pituitary axis inhibits ACTH secretion.

concentrations, the adrenal glands are enlarged, and therefore this condition is also called primary macronodular adrenocortical hyperplasia.

Recently, food-dependent hypercortisolism, presumably due to ectopic adrenocortical expression of GIP receptors, was reported in a 6-year-old vizsla (Galac et al, 2008). In this dog with obvious clinical manifestations of hypercortisolism and slightly elevated UCCRs, the basal and CRH-stimulated plasma ACTH concentrations were suppressed, but diagnostic imaging did not reveal an adrenocortical tumor. Plasma cortisol concentration and UCCR increased more than 50% at about 2 and 3 hours after ingestion of a meal, respectively. Consistent with the diagnostic criteria for food-dependent hypercortisolism in humans, administration of octreotide (Sandostatin) at a dose of 3 µg/kg IM completely prevented the meal-induced hypercortisolemia.

Hypercortisolism due to the expression of aberrant adrenocortical hormone receptors should be suspected in dogs with clinical signs of hypercortisolism, suppressed basal plasma ACTH concentration, and bilateral adrenomegaly. Routine tests for hypercortisolism may be negative because hypercortisolemia only occurs after binding of the ligand to its receptor. A distinct increase in UCCR and/or plasma cortisol concentration after ingestion of a meal, low or undetectable plasma ACTH concentrations, and prevention of a meal-induced rise in plasma cortisol concentration by octreotide administration strongly suggest food-dependent hypercortisolism.

Hypercortisolism caused by the expression of aberrant adrenocortical hormone receptors is treated medically. In cases of food-dependent hypercortisolism, long-term octreotide therapy leads to down-regulation of somatostatin receptors on GIP-secreting intestinal cells and therefore becomes ineffective quite soon. Consequently, suppression of cortisol hypersecretion can be achieved by trilostane, or the adrenocorticolytic drug o,p'-DDD can also be used for this purpose.

References and Suggested Reading

Burgener IA et al: Empty sella syndrome, hyperadrenocorticism and megaoesophagus in a dachshund, *J Small Anim Pract* 48:584-587, 2007.

Churcher RK: Hepatic carcinoid, hypercortisolism and hypokalaemia in a dog, *Aust Vet J* 77:641-645, 1999.

Galac S et al: Hyperadrenocorticism in a dog due to ectopic secretion of adrenocorticotropic hormone, *Domest Anim Endocrinol* 28:338-348, 2005.

Galac S et al: ACTH-independent hyperadrenocorticism due to meal induced hypercortisolaemia in a dog, *Vet J* 177:141-143, 2008.

Galac S et al: Adrenals. In Rijnberk A, Kooistra HS, editors: *Clinical endocrinology of dogs and cats*, ed 2, Hannover, Germany, 2010, Schlütersche Verlag, pp 93-154.

Lacroix A et al: Ectopic and abnormal hormone receptors in adrenal Cushing's syndrome, *Endocr Rev* 22:75-110, 2001.

Newell-Price J et al: The diagnosis and differential diagnosis of Cushing's syndrome and pseudo-Cushing's states, *Endocr Rev* 19:647-672, 1998.

CHAPTER 53

Canine Hypoadrenocorticism

PETER P. KINTZER, *Westbrook, Maine*
MARK E. PETERSON, *New York, New York*

Spontaneous canine hypoadrenocorticism is a well-recognized but uncommon endocrine disorder. Hypoadrenocorticism is characterized by a deficiency of glucocorticoid and/or mineralocorticoid production by the adrenal cortices. Although mild destruction or atrophy of adrenocortical tissue can impair adrenocortical reserve, typically at least 90% of the adrenal cortex needs to be nonfunctional before clinical signs of hypoadrenocorticism are observed under nonstressful conditions.

Cause

Primary hypoadrenocorticism results from destruction or atrophy of the adrenal cortices and usually results in a deficiency of both glucocorticoid and mineralocorticoid secretion. Causes include idiopathic spontaneous (probably immune-mediated) primary hypoadrenocorticism (Addison's disease), iatrogenic disease resulting from mitotane or trilostane therapy, and very rarely adrenocortical destruction resulting from granulomatous disease, metastatic neoplasia, or hemorrhage.

A subset of dogs with primary hypoadrenocorticism have glucocorticoid deficiency, based on the findings of low basal and adrenocorticotropic hormone (ACTH)–stimulated serum cortisol values but normal serum sodium and potassium concentrations. This has been referred to as "atypical" hypoadrenocorticism. It has recently been reported that most dogs with "atypical" hypoadrenocorticism actually do not have measurable aldosterone levels (Mueller et al, 2007). In other words, most "atypical" cases do have aldosterone deficiency (as well as cortisol deficiency) and so are not so atypical after all. This has important implications as far as treatment recommendations are concerned. These dogs appear to maintain normal serum electrolyte concentrations by an alternative, aldosterone-independent, yet-to-be-defined mechanism. In most of these dogs electrolyte abnormalities eventually develop, but a few dogs do not develop serum electrolyte changes when followed for many months or years.

Secondary hypoadrenocorticism is caused by insufficient pituitary ACTH production and the resultant atrophy of the zona fasciculata of the adrenal cortices. The result is deficient glucocorticoid secretion; mineralocorticoid secretion is preserved. Causes include iatrogenic disease resulting from overly rapid discontinuation of long-term and/or high-dose glucocorticoid therapy, pituitary or hypothalamic lesions, or idiopathic isolated ACTH deficiency.

Diagnosis

Although most affected dogs present in young to middle age, naturally occurring hypoadrenocorticism has been reported in dogs ranging from 2 months to 14 years of age. A genetic predilection has been confirmed in standard poodles, leonbergers, and bearded collies and suggested in certain breeds such as Nova Scotia duck tolling retrievers, Portuguese water spaniels, Great Danes, rottweilers, and wheaten and West Highland white terriers. Female dogs are about twice as likely to develop naturally occurring hypoadrenocorticism as males.

The historical findings, clinical signs, and laboratory abnormalities associated with spontaneous hypoadrenocorticism are well described (Tables 53-1 and 53-2). The severity and duration of clinical signs vary greatly among cases, from the acute life-threatening addisonian crisis to the chronic intermittent or waxing and waning signs seen in some dogs with chronic hypoadrenocorticism. Many of the historical and clinical findings are nonspecific and also occur in many more common diseases, particularly gastrointestinal and renal disorders. No set of findings is pathognomonic for canine hypoadrenocorticism. A high index of suspicion is needed to recognize some cases, particularly those with normal serum electrolyte concentrations. Findings that should heighten this suspicion include a waxing/waning course, previous response to fluid or glucocorticoid therapy, and exacerbation of clinical signs in stressful situations.

The classic electrolyte abnormalities associated with spontaneous primary hypoadrenocorticism are hyperkalemia and hyponatremia and are seen in more than 80% of affected dogs. Prior treatment with fluids, steroids, or both may mask serum electrolyte changes. Therefore one should never exclude a diagnosis of primary hypoadrenocorticism in a dog suspected of having hypoadrenocorticism on a basis of normal serum electrolyte concentrations alone. Also, some dogs with secondary hypoadrenocorticism caused by isolated pituitary ACTH deficiency are hyponatremic with normal potassium concentrations. Although Addison's disease is often the first disorder thought of when these electrolyte abnormalities are found, the presence of hyperkalemia and hyponatremia cannot be relied on for the diagnosis of canine hypoadrenocorticism. Indeed these electrolyte abnormalities may be associated with a wide variety of diseases more common than hypoadrenocorticism, including gastrointestinal disorders, renal disease, effusive disorders, and acidosis (see Web Chapter 16).

TABLE 53-1

Clinical Findings in Dogs with Hypoadrenocorticism

Finding	Percent
Lethargy/depression	95
Anorexia	90
Vomiting	75
Weakness	75
Weight loss	50
Dehydration	45
Diarrhea	40
Waxing/waning course	40
Collapse	35
Previous response to therapy	35
Hypothermia	35
Slow capillary refill (perfusion) time	30
Shaking	25
Polydipsia/polyuria	25
Melena	20
Weak pulse	20
Bradycardia	18
Painful abdomen	8
Hair loss	5

TABLE 53-2

Laboratory Findings* in Canine Hypoadrenocorticism

Finding	Percent
Hyperkalemia	90
Hyponatremia	80
Na/K ratio <27	95
Hypochloremia	40
Hypercalcemia	30
Azotemia	85
Acidosis	40
Elevated ALT or AST	30
Hyperbilirubinemia	20
Hypoglycemia	15
Anemia	25
Eosinophilia	20
Lymphocytosis	10
Urine specific gravity <1.030	60

ALT, Alanine aminotransferase; *AST,* aspartate aminotransferase.
*Hypoalbuminemia and hypocholesterolemia are also sometimes observed.

Definitive diagnosis of hypoadrenocorticism requires demonstration of inadequate adrenal reserve. This is done by performing an ACTH stimulation test, considered the gold standard for diagnosis of hypoadrenocorticism. The preferred method is to determine serum cortisol concentrations before and 1 hour after the intravenous administration of 5 µg/kg of cosyntropin (Cortrosyn). Following reconstitution, the solution, when refrigerated, is stable for at least 4 weeks. Otherwise the remaining solution can be divided into aliquots and frozen.

If cosyntropin is not available, the ACTH stimulation test can also be performed by determining the serum cortisol concentration before and after the intramuscular injection of 2.2 U/kg of ACTH gel. ACTH gel (usually 40 U/ml) is available from several compounding pharmacies. The bioavailability and reproducibility of all these formulations have yet to be carefully evaluated. A study in dogs by Kemppainen, Behrend, and Busch (2005) using four compounded ACTH gels demonstrated increases in serum cortisol concentrations comparable to cosyntropin injection 1 hour after intramuscular injection of each of the four formulations but considerable variation at 2 hours after injection. The investigators recommended determining serum cortisol concentrations at both 1 and 2 hours post-ACTH administration when using a compounded ACTH gel. The determination of a third cortisol level would likely offset any presumed cost saving derived from using the compounded product. The potential for lot-to-lot variability in compounded ACTH gel formulations has not been evaluated. Therefore one should consider assessing the activity of each new vial by performing an ACTH stimulation test on a normal dog.

In normal dogs administration of a supraphysiologic dose of ACTH produces a rise in serum cortisol to values usually above 10 µg/dl (275 nmol/L). In contrast, dogs with hypoadrenocorticism have an absent or blunted response to ACTH administration. Basal and post-ACTH serum cortisol concentrations are less than 1 µg/dl (27 nmol/L) in over 75% of dogs and less than 2 µg/dl (55 nmol/L) in virtually all dogs with primary hypoadrenocorticism. Although the post-ACTH serum cortisol concentration may be as high as 2 to 3 µg/dl in a few dogs with secondary hypoadrenocorticism, the great majority of these dogs also have ACTH-stimulated cortisol concentrations of less than 2 µg/dl.

The ACTH stimulation test using intravenous cosyntropin can be performed during institution of initial treatment if dexamethasone is used for glucocorticoid replacement since dexamethasone does not interfere with the cortisol assay. If prednisone, prednisolone, methylprednisolone, or hydrocortisone has been administered, these treatments must be discontinued, and glucocorticoid supplementation changed to dexamethasone for at least 24 hours before ACTH stimulation testing. ACTH gel cannot be used in dehydrated or hypovolemic patients since impaired absorption may lead to inaccurate results. Alternatively, testing can be delayed until after the patient is stabilized.

A study in dogs compared an in-house cortisol assay (SNAP Cortisol) with a reference laboratory chemiluminescent assay; there was a very good correlation between the two assays. The in-house assay is particularly useful when a rapid determination of the presence of hypoadrenocorticism is desired, such as differentiating in an emergency patient between an addisonian crisis and a disease with a poorer prognosis such as acute renal failure.

Based on recent work (Lennon et al, 2007), a resting serum cortisol concentration above 2 μg/dl would make a diagnosis of hypoadrenocorticism very unlikely in a dog that had not recently received one or more doses of glucocorticoids. However, a low resting serum cortisol concentration is not diagnostic of hypoadrenocorticism and an ACTH stimulation test is necessary to confirm the diagnosis.

Secondary hypoadrenocorticism can be differentiated from atypical primary hypoadrenocorticism by measurement of a plasma ACTH level. Plasma ACTH is high (>500 pg/ml) with primary hypoadrenocorticism and undetectable-to-low with secondary hypoadrenocorticism. ACTH is labile; therefore the diagnostic laboratory performing the assay should be consulted for appropriate sample handling instructions. Plasma for ACTH determination must be collected before instituting therapy, especially glucocorticoid treatment. Even a relatively low dose of glucocorticoid may reduce previously high ACTH concentrations into the normal-to-low reference range; thus the results must be interpreted in conjunction with a careful drug history. To properly evaluate the endogenous ACTH test result, the dog ideally should not have received any form of steroid treatment in the preceding weeks. If plasma ACTH is measured in a dog that has received recent glucocorticoid treatment, a false-positive diagnosis of secondary hypoadrenocorticism may result.

Recently an alternate approach was proposed for assessing the pituitary-glucocorticoid axis in dogs by measuring basal cortisol and plasma ACTH concentrations and then calculating a cortisol-to-ACTH ratio (Javadi et al, 2006). Similarly the renin-angiotensin-aldosterone system was assessed by determining the basal plasma concentrations of aldosterone and plasma renin activity and then calculating an aldosterone-to-renin ratio.

Dogs with primary hypoadrenocorticism have low basal concentrations of cortisol with high plasma ACTH concentrations. In contrast, dogs with secondary hypoadrenocorticism have low plasma cortisol concentrations with low plasma ACTH concentrations. Therefore dogs with primary hypoadrenocorticism have much lower cortisol-to-ACTH ratios than do normal dogs or dogs with secondary hypoadrenocorticism, with little to no overlap in ratio values.

In states of aldosterone deficiency such as primary hypoadrenocorticism, the inability to retain sodium leads to hypovolemia, which subsequently stimulates renin release. Thus dogs with primary hypoadrenocorticism have low basal concentrations of aldosterone with high plasma renin activity. In secondary hypoadrenocorticism aldosterone secretion is not decreased; therefore plasma renin activity remains relatively normal. Accordingly, dogs with primary hypoadrenocorticism have much lower aldosterone-to-renin ratios than do normal dogs or dogs with secondary hypoadrenocorticism, again with little to no overlap in ratio values.

The advantage of using cortisol-to-ACTH and aldosterone-to-renin ratios is that such measurement of endogenous hormone variables in a single blood sample allows for the specific diagnosis of primary hypocortisolism and primary hypoaldosteronism. A dynamic stimulation test is not required. The use of these paired-hormone ratios generally allows for clear differentiation between primary and secondary hypoadrenocorticism; this dual assessment is particularly relevant when isolated hormone deficiency is suspected (i.e., isolated glucocorticoid deficiency or isolated mineralocorticoid deficiency).

Disadvantages of this approach to diagnosis include the considerable expense to measure plasma concentrations of cortisol, ACTH, aldosterone, and renin activity, as well as sample handling, including the absolute necessity of collecting blood for measurement of hormone and renin concentrations before any fluid or steroid treatment. Furthermore, it may be difficult to find a laboratory that can accurately measure plasma renin activity in dogs.

Treatment

The intensiveness of therapeutic intervention depends on the individual patient's condition. Acute hypoadrenocorticism (addisonian crisis) is a medical emergency requiring prompt treatment, whereas dogs with chronic hypoadrenocorticism generally do not need aggressive therapy, although many may benefit from hospitalization for parenteral fluids and glucocorticoids.

Acute Hypoadrenocorticism

If the clinical presentation is consistent with an addisonian crisis, treatment must be instituted immediately once blood is collected for a complete blood count, chemistry profile, and other indicated laboratory work and urine is obtained for urinalysis. Definitive diagnostic workup is done during the initial treatment and stabilization process. Goals of therapy are to restore plasma volume status, correct electrolyte and acid-base disturbances, improve vascular integrity, and provide an immediate source of rapid-acting glucocorticoid.

Of primary importance in therapy for acute hypoadrenocorticism is the rapid infusion of large volumes of intravenous fluids, preferably 0.9% saline, at an initial rate of 60 to 80 ml/kg/hr for 1 to 2 hours. This initial rate of infusion helps to address hypotension and hypovolemia. In addition, serum potassium concentration is reduced by dilution, increased renal perfusion, and thereby potassium excretion. A colloid also can be administered to address hypotension and hypovolemia, but this is rarely needed. The rate of saline infusion is then gradually reduced to a maintenance rate and eventually discontinued over a few days based on the dog's clinical response and laboratory parameters, including serial blood pressure, renal function, and electrolyte measurements. Urine output should be quantified to assess its adequacy and to help guide fluid therapy. If severe hyponatremia is present on initial evaluation, it should be corrected no faster than 10 to 12 mEq/dl per day over the first 48 hours of therapy. Overly rapid correction of hyponatremia can result in neurologic damage (myelinosis).

Also critically important to the therapy of acute hypoadrenocorticism is the intravenous administration of a rapid-acting glucocorticoid. Dexamethasone sodium phosphate (2 to 4 mg/kg) or prednisolone sodium succinate (15 to 20 mg/kg) is preferred; dexamethasone sodium phosphate must be used if the ACTH stimulation test is in progress. This initial dose of dexamethasone can be repeated in 2 to 6 hours if needed. Glucocorticoid supplementation is then gradually tapered to a maintenance dose of prednisone (0.1 to 0.2 mg/kg) over the next several days as dictated by clinical response. The maintenance dose of prednisone may not be reached until after the patient is at home. Parenteral supplementation is indicated until vomiting has ceased and oral intake has begun.

Hyperkalemia is often successfully corrected by parenteral fluid therapy alone. However, for severe hyperkalemia causing life-threatening myocardial toxicity manifested by significant arrhythmias (including atrial standstill, abnormal ST-T waves, and widening of the QRS complex), more aggressive therapy is necessary. Our preferred treatment is intravenous insulin and dextrose. Regular insulin (0.5 U/kg) is given intravenously. Glucose (2 to 3 g/U of insulin) is given half as an intravenous bolus and half in the intravenous fluids over the next 6 to 8 hours. These dogs must be closely monitored for hypoglycemia, with hourly blood glucose determinations. Dogs with hypoadrenocorticism are very sensitive to the glucose-lowering action of insulin; however, the administration of the rapid-acting glucocorticoid as described previously before or concurrent with insulin administration would be expected to counteract this tendency. Alternatively slow intravenous administration of 10% calcium chloride (0.1 ml/kg over 10 to 20 minutes) or $NaHCO_3$ (1 to 2 mEq/kg over 10 to 15 minutes) can be considered to treat hyperkalemic myocardial toxicity.

Hypoglycemia and metabolic acidosis may demand treatment in some cases. Dextrose (2.5% to 5%) is added to the intravenous fluids as needed. Symptomatic hypoglycemia is treated with a slow intravenous bolus of 0.5 to 1.5 ml/kg of 50% dextrose. Mild-to-moderate acidosis is usually corrected with parenteral fluid therapy. Severe metabolic acidosis (pH <7.1) is treated with sodium bicarbonate. The total dosage is calculated as follows:

Deficit in mEq
= (body weight in kilograms)(0.5)(base deficit)

One fourth of the calculated dosage is administered in the intravenous fluids over the next 6 to 8 hours, and then the acid-base status is reassessed. It is unusual for additional bicarbonate therapy to be needed.

No rapid-acting parenteral mineralocorticoid preparation is currently available for treatment of acute hypoadrenocorticism. This does not constitute a significant clinical problem because prompt aggressive treatment as described previously is sufficient to stabilize a dog suffering an addisonian crisis. Nonetheless we typically give a desoxycorticosterone pivalate (DOCP; Percorten-V) injection as soon as the diagnosis of primary hypoadrenocorticism is confirmed. Alternatively, fludrocortisone acetate (Florinef) can be used. Such mineralocorticoid supplementation is not harmful and may help correct serum electrolyte abnormalities.

Chronic Hypoadrenocorticism

Dogs with chronic hypoadrenocorticism present with clinical signs of varying severity and duration and do not require the aggressive therapy described previously for cases of acute hypoadrenocorticism. However, fluid therapy and parenteral glucocorticoid supplementation may be indicated in some cases, particularly if azotemia, dehydration, hypotension, or significant vomiting or diarrhea is present. In these dogs parenteral therapy is continued until these abnormalities have resolved and maintenance therapy can be instituted. Similarly, in dogs recovering from an addisonian crisis, maintenance therapy is instituted once the dog is stable and oral medication can be tolerated.

Dogs with naturally occurring primary hypoadrenocorticism that demonstrate the classic electrolyte abnormalities require both glucocorticoid and mineralocorticoid replacement therapy for life. Either DOCP or fludrocortisone can be used for chronic mineralocorticoid replacement. We typically institute treatment with DOCP given at 2.2 mg/kg subcutaneously or intramuscularly every 4 weeks. Side effects associated with DOCP therapy are rare. Most dogs are controlled with an injection every 4 weeks; a 3-week interval is uncommon and a 2-week interval is rare. After the first one or two injections of DOCP, electrolyte and creatinine levels are monitored at 2, 3, and 4 weeks following injection to determine the duration of action and help make dosage adjustments if necessary. Once stabilized, serum electrolyte and creatinine concentrations are checked every 3 to 6 months.

Although a DOCP dose of less than 2.2 mg/kg would be sufficient in some cases, a dose of 2.2 mg/kg is still recommended, at least for the initial treatment. Fewer than 5% of dogs require a DOCP dose greater than 2.2 mg/kg, and a starting dose of 2.2 mg/kg eliminates the need for the clinician to incrementally increase the DOCP dosage over the first several months of therapy, which can occur in dogs started on a lower initial DOCP dose. However, if financial constraints are a factor, one can attempt to gradually reduce the monthly dose of DOCP to the lowest effective dose based on close monitoring of serum electrolyte concentrations. Alternatively, the interval between DOCP injections can be incrementally lengthened (typically in 1-week intervals) as dictated by monitoring of serum electrolyte concentrations. Dogs with hypoadrenocorticism and congestive heart failure (such as some rottweilers with dilated cardiomyopathy) may require higher doses of furosemide the first 2 weeks following DOCP administration to prevent pulmonary edema (fludrocortisone represents an alternative treatment for this group).

Fludrocortisone acetate is given at an initial oral dosage of 0.01 to 0.02 mg/kg q24h, and the dosage is adjusted by 0.05 to 0.1 mg q24h as determined by serial serum electrolyte concentrations. After initiation of fludrocortisone therapy, serum electrolyte and creatinine levels should be monitored until stabilized within the normal range. Once this is achieved, the dogs should be reevaluated monthly for the first 3 to 6 months of therapy and then every 3 to 6 months thereafter. In many dogs in which fludrocortisone is used as a long-term mineralocorticoid replacement, the daily dose required to control the disorder gradually increases; this is most evident in the first 6 to 24 months of treatment. In most dogs the final fludrocortisone dosage needed is 0.02 to 0.03 mg/kg q24h. Very few dogs can be controlled on a dosage of 0.01 mg/kg q24h or less. Adverse effects (usually polyuria and polydipsia), development of a relative resistance to the effects of fludrocortisone, or financial considerations (especially when treating large- or giant-breed dogs) may necessitate a change to DOCP therapy in some dogs.

Many dogs with primary hypoadrenocorticism, particularly those receiving DOCP, require chronic glucocorticoid supplementation in addition to mineralocorticoid supplementation to prevent signs of glucocorticoid deficiency. In general, all dogs with primary hypoadrenocorticism are started on glucocorticoid replacement with prednisone or prednisolone (0.1 to 0.2 mg/kg/day) in conjunction with mineralocorticoid replacement (usually DOCP). If warranted because of the development of side effects, the glucocorticoid dosage can be tapered to alternate days and then discontinued if necessary to evaluate if glucocorticoids are needed as part of maintenance therapy. The fact that glucocorticoids can be discontinued without the recurrence of significant clinical signs in some dogs with hypoadrenocorticism is especially important in dogs that have developed signs of intolerance of glucocorticoid administration (e.g., polyuria/polydipsia) after treatment. In many of these dogs cessation of glucocorticoids reverses signs of iatrogenic hyperadrenocorticism, and mineralocorticoid replacement alone controls signs of hypoadrenocorticism. Nevertheless, additional glucocorticoid supplementation (2 to 10 times normal recommended replacement dosage) may be necessary during periods of stress such as illness, trauma, or surgery; therefore the owner should always have some glucocorticoid on hand and be informed of situations in which the dog might require glucocorticoid supplementation.

In those dogs with hypoadrenocorticism that maintain normal electrolytes ("atypical" hypoadrenocorticism), prednisone or prednisolone is given at a replacement dose of 0.1 to 0.2 mg/kg q24h. In addition we recommend that pre- and post-ACTH aldosterone concentrations (or the plasma ACTH concentration) be determined to differentiate primary from secondary hypoadrenocorticism. If aldosterone concentrations are low (or the plasma ACTH concentration high), DOCP is given at the standard dose. Given the recent findings that most dogs with "atypical" hypoadrenocorticism have subnormal aldosterone concentrations, if aldosterone (or ACTH) concentrations cannot be measured we recommend giving DOCP at

1 mg/kg monthly, monitoring electrolytes every 1 to 2 months and adjusting the DOCP dose as needed. If financial concerns prevent this, dogs with atypical primary hypoadrenocorticism can be started on glucocorticoid replacement therapy alone but must have serum electrolyte concentrations monitored every 1 to 2 months since most of these dogs will develop the typical electrolyte abnormalities after weeks to months and require mineralocorticoid supplementation as well.

Dogs with documented secondary hypoadrenocorticism (isolated pituitary ACTH deficiency) require only glucocorticoid replacement therapy. Oral administration of prednisone or prednisolone at a dosage of 0.1 to 0.2 mg/kg q24h usually suffices, except during periods of stress or illness when higher doses are necessary. If secondary hypoadrenocorticism has not been documented by the presence of undetectable-to-low plasma ACTH concentrations in hypoadrenal patients with normal serum electrolyte concentrations, one must continue to determine serum electrolyte concentrations on a regular (e.g., monthly) basis.

References and Suggested Reading

Church DB: Canine hypoadrenocorticism. In Mooney CT, Peterson ME, editors: *BSAVA manual of canine and feline endocrinology*, ed 3, Quedgeley, Gloucester, 2004, British Small Animal Veterinary Association, p 172.

Feldman EC, Nelson RW: Hypoadrenocorticism (Addison's disease). In Feldman EC, Nelson RW, editors: *Canine and feline endocrinology and reproduction*, ed 3, Philadelphia, 2004, Saunders, p 394.

Javadi S et al: Aldosterone-to-renin and cortisol-to-adrenocorticotropic hormone ratios in healthy dogs and dogs with primary hypoadrenocorticism, *J Vet Intern Med* 20:556, 2006.

Kemppainen RJ, Behrend EN, Busch KA: Use of compounded adrenocorticotropic hormone (ACTH) for adrenal function testing in dogs, *J Am Anim Hosp Assoc* 41:368, 2005.

Kintzer PP, Peterson ME: Diseases of the adrenal gland. In Birchard SJ, Sherding RG, editors: *Saunders manual of small animal practice*, ed 3, St Louis, 2006, Saunders, p 357.

Kintzer PP, Peterson ME: Treatment and long-term follow-up of 205 dogs with hypoadrenocorticism, *J Vet Intern Med* 11:43, 1997.

Lennon EM et al: Use of basal serum or plasma cortisol concentrations to rule out a diagnosis of hypoadrenocorticism in dogs: 123 cases (2000-2005), *J Am Vet Med Assoc* 231:413, 2007.

Mueller C et al: Investigation on the aldosterone concentration before and after ACTH application in 44 dogs with hypoadrenocorticism, *Kleintierpraxis* 52:216, 2007.

Peterson ME, Kintzer PP, Kass PH: Pretreatment clinical and laboratory findings in dogs with hypoadrenocorticism: 225 cases (1979-1993), *J Am Vet Med Assoc* 208:85, 1995.

CHAPTER 54

Feline Primary Hyperaldosteronism

KENT R. REFSAL, *Lansing, Michigan*
ANDREA M. HARVEY, *Sydney, Australia*

The term *primary hyperaldosteronism* (PHA) refers to the clinical consequences of mineralocorticoid excess arising from autonomous hyperfunction of the zona glomerulosa of the adrenal cortex. The first case of feline PHA related to an adrenocortical carcinoma was reported in 1983 (Eger, Robinson, and Huxtable, 1983). Since 1999, at least 40 additional affected cats have been described in individual case reports, case series, or book chapters. To date, the best-defined occurrences of PHA in cats are related to unilateral adrenocortical carcinoma or adenoma. Evidence for PHA related to idiopathic nodular hyperplasia of the zona glomerulosa was presented in a series of 11 cats with concomitant renal disease (Javadi et al, 2005). Increased awareness of the clinical manifestations has led to speculation that PHA may be the most common adrenocortical disorder in cats. This chapter summarizes the clinical features, diagnosis, and treatment of PHA in cats.

The Renin-Angiotensin-Aldosterone System: Regulation and Actions

The renin-angiotensin-aldosterone system (RAAS) acts to maintain extracellular fluid volume, circulatory pressure, and electrolyte homeostasis through integrated effects primarily on the vasculature and kidneys. Juxtaglomerular cells incorporated in afferent arterioles of renal glomeruli synthesize prorenin, of which some is converted to active renin and stored in secretory granules. Release of active renin from juxtaglomerular cells can be induced by different mechanisms. The predominant control of renin release is mediated through baroreceptors in the afferent arteriole, where a decrease in perfusion pressure stimulates renin release. In addition, cells of the macula densa in the distal convoluted tubule, in communication with juxtaglomerular cells, monitor sodium content in the glomerular filtrate. A decrease in sodium content stimulates renin secretion. Lastly, activity of sympathetic neurons communicating with cardiac baroreceptors stimulates renin release. In the circulation, renin cleaves angiotensinogen, a protein produced by the liver, into angiotensin I, which is in turn converted to angiotensin II by angiotensin-converting enzymes. Angiotensin II exerts potent biologic effects to mediate vasoconstriction, promote renal tubule reabsorption of sodium, and stimulate release of aldosterone from the zona glomerulosa of the adrenal cortex.

Aldosterone is synthesized from cholesterol through a series of steroid intermediates including progesterone, 11-deoxycorticosterone, and corticosterone in zona glomerulosa cells, mainly via stimulation by angiotensin II. Aldosterone secretion is also stimulated by a direct effect of hyperkalemia and, to a lesser extent, by adrenocorticotropic hormone (ACTH). Epithelial cells of renal tubules, salivary glands, and the colon are the classic mineralocorticoid-responsive tissues, where the effect of aldosterone is to promote reabsorption of sodium in exchange for loss of potassium and hydrogen ions.

In instances of reduced arterial blood volume, the RAAS can respond with sustained release of renin and aldosterone. Renin-stimulated aldosterone hypersecretion is referred to as secondary hyperaldosteronism, which usually occurs as a compensatory response to heart failure, gastrointestinal disease, water deprivation, or other causes of hypovolemia. Persistence of secondary hyperaldosteronism in an attempt to restore or maintain glomerular perfusion may contribute to the onset of hypokalemia or hypernatremia. In an experimental rat model, iatrogenic aldosterone excess promoted increased urinary loss of calcium and magnesium, with subsequent development of secondary hyperparathyroidism and reduced bone mineral content (Chhokar et al, 2005). Interestingly, cats with PHA and concomitant azotemia usually do not have hyperphosphatemia. It is possible that cats with PHA also have elevated parathyroid hormone levels, which would promote urinary excretion of phosphorus and allow serum phosphorus levels to remain normal (Graves, 2011).

Clinical Signs and Physical Examination Findings

Feline PHA is a disease of middle-aged to older cats. The reported age of onset ranges from 5 to 20 years, with a median age of 13 years for cats with adrenal neoplasia. The age for cases of adrenal hyperplasia appears similar, with reported ages ranging from 11 to 18 years. There appears to be no breed or sex predispositions. In 25 cats with PHA related to adrenal neoplasia, unilateral tumors were identified in 14 right and 9 left adrenal glands, with bilateral adrenal adenomas identified at postmortem examination in two cats.

The major clinical signs most commonly relate directly to increased aldosterone concentrations, which result in hypokalemia and arterial hypertension. PHA should be considered as a possible diagnosis in any cat presenting with arterial hypertension and/or hypokalemia, particularly if either appears to be refractory to treatment. The resulting presenting signs fall largely into two main groups:

- **Hypokalemic polymyopathy.** This is the most common reported presentation for cats with adrenal neoplasia. Cervical ventroflexion is the most frequently encountered sign of muscle weakness, but hind limb weakness and ataxia or, less commonly, limb stiffness, dysphagia, respiratory failure, and collapse may also occur. Signs of muscular weakness may be mild and episodic or insidious in onset, whereas in other cats these signs can be severe and acute in onset. Hypokalemic polymyopathy is reported to be a much less common presenting sign in cases of adrenal hyperplasia
- **Ocular signs of arterial hypertension.** These are a less common primary presentation in cats with adrenal neoplasia, but appear to be more common major presenting signs in cats with bilateral adrenal hyperplasia that tend to have more severe hypertension. Clinical signs may include intraocular hemorrhage or acute-onset blindness resulting from retinal detachment. This presentation is more likely in cats with systolic blood pressures above 200 mm Hg and can be the sole presenting sign. Subtle signs of hypertensive retinopathy evident on fundic examination (e.g., subretinal, intraretinal, and intravitreal hemorrhages, retinal edema) are more commonly observed.

Less common clinical findings in adrenal neoplasia cases include polyuria and polydipsia, polyphagia, and a systolic heart murmur. An adrenal mass may also be detected as an incidental finding on abdominal ultrasound examination or palpation in a normokalemic cat that may develop additional signs of hyperaldosteronism some time later (Renschler and Dean, 2009).

A different clinical presentation occurs less commonly in cats with excesses of other corticosteroids as well as aldosterone. There are published reports of cats with aldosterone-secreting adrenal tumors that have had concurrent hyperprogesteronism and the authors have also encountered similar cats (Brisco et al, 2009). In these cases signs of hyperprogesteronism/hyperadrenocorticism predominate, namely diabetes mellitus, polyuria, polydipsia, polyphagia, poor coat condition, seborrhea, thin fragile skin, and a potbellied appearance. Hypertension and persistent hypokalemia may be initially overlooked.

Because PHA affects older cats, concomitant nonadrenal illness may divert the clinician's attention from the possibility of hyperaldosteronism. For example, chronic kidney disease or hyperthyroidism may be assumed wrongly to be the cause of hypokalemia and/or hypertension. Left ventricular hypertrophy may also be present, resulting in typical clinical findings of cardiomyopathy such as a systolic heart murmur, tachycardia, gallop rhythm, or dysrhythmias. The changes could be believed to be secondary to hypertension and/or concurrent disease such as hyperthyroidism. However, the cardiac effects of elevated aldosterone are well recognized in humans, and it is therefore possible that cardiac disease could arise as a consequence of PHA. Consequently, the presence of left ventricular hypertrophy and the associated clinical findings should also prompt consideration of the presence of PHA. Congestive heart failure has been reported in one cat with concurrent PHA and hyperprogesteronism.

Laboratory Testing

Hematology and Chemistry Profile

There are no abnormalities on complete blood count (CBC) testing that are specific or characteristic for PHA in cats. Hypokalemia is a common finding with PHA, probably in part because the abnormality is viewed as a prerequisite for further investigation. However, hypokalemia has been less common or severe in cats with bilateral adrenal hyperplasia. Cats with PHA are typically not hypernatremic because of circulatory volume expansion related to sodium retention. In association with hypokalemia, varying elevations of creatine kinase activity are common. Evidence of metabolic alkalosis is often seen in response to aldosterone-mediated excretion of hydrogen ions. Approximately 50% of cats with PHA have elevations of serum urea and creatinine concentrations but usually without hyperphosphatemia (Djajadiningrat-Laanen, Galac, and Kooistra, 2011). Cats with PHA and azotemia at initial testing often exhibit progression of renal disease. Hyperglycemia or concurrent diabetes mellitus raises concern for an adrenal tumor producing excesses of progesterone and possibly other corticosteroids in addition to aldosterone.

Endocrine Testing

Interpretation of endocrine test results for diagnosis of PHA assesses evidence for an inappropriate mineralocorticoid excess accompanying hypertension and hypokalemia, especially if there has also been identification of an adrenal mass. The most readily available test is measurement of baseline aldosterone concentration in serum or plasma. To date, published reference intervals of baseline aldosterone in cats have an upper limit of approximately 550 pmol/L. Published baseline concentrations of aldosterone in cats with PHA related to adrenal neoplasia range from 800 to 45,000 pmol/L. To date, cats with PHA related to bilateral adrenal hyperplasia had baseline concentrations of aldosterone from within the reference range to a maximum of approximately 1000 pmol/L. Demonstration of an elevation of baseline aldosterone (especially > 1000 pmol) in a cat with hypertension, hypokalemia, and an adrenal mass provides excellent evidence to diagnose PHA. In cats with bilateral adrenal hyperplasia, evidence for autonomous, inappropriate production of aldosterone is based on suppressed plasma renin activity (PRA) and elevation of a calculated aldosterone-to-renin ratio (ARR). In the United States, no veterinary endocrine laboratory currently performs PRA assays. However, PRA assays available in human diagnostic laboratories are suitable for use in cats. Administration

TABLE 54-1

Baseline Concentrations of Progesterone, Corticosterone, and Cortisol in Feline Serum Submitted to a Diagnostic Laboratory for Measurement of Aldosterone

Aldosterone Result Category	<500 pmol/L Not Elevated	500-999 pmol/L Modest Increase	1000-3000 pmol/L Moderate Increase	>3000 pmol/L Very Elevated
Number of cats	25	24	23	34
Progesterone (nmol/L), ref in neutered cats < 5 nmol/L	1 (1-5) [4%]	1 (1-6) [13%]	2 (1-8) [17%]	7 (1-59) [59%]
Corticosterone (nmol/L), estimated ref <100 nmol/L	15 (9-110) [6%]	17 (9-117) [11%]	33 (11-213) [28%]	197 (9-1035) [72%]
Cortisol (nmol/L), ref 15-97 nmol/L	83 (4-245) [44%]	71 (11-276) [37%]	94 (15-264) [50%]	42 (4-291) [16%]

From Refsal KR, Mazaki-Tovi M: Baseline concentrations of progesterone, cortisol, and corticosterone in a laboratory survey of feline sera submitted for assay of aldosterone, Proceedings of the 19th ECVIM Companion Animals Congress, 2009, p 290 (abst).
Hormone concentrations are presented as median (range). The median age of cats in this survey was 13 years (range 1-19 years, with five cats younger than 7 years). When histories were included, hypokalemia and/or hypertension were the most frequent problems.
ref, Reference range, estimated for corticosterone. The percentage of samples above the reference range is shown as [%].

of spironolactone for symptomatic management of hypertension results in increases of baseline aldosterone concentrations in cats (MacDonald, Kittleson, and Kass, 2008). At present, the duration of spironolactone withdrawal necessary for reequilibration of endogenous mineralocorticoid function is not defined in cats. In human medicine, antihypertensive agents are discontinued for 2 weeks before diagnostic assessment of PHA is initiated.

As mentioned previously, some cats with PHA related to an adrenal carcinoma, diabetes mellitus, and dermatologic changes have had elevations of progesterone in addition to aldosterone (Briscoe et al, 2009). These cats had normal baseline concentrations of cortisol and blunted or normal increases of cortisol in response to ACTH stimulation. A laboratory survey of feline samples submitted for assay of basal aldosterone concentration suggests that elevations of progesterone and corticosterone of potential clinical significance are fairly common in samples in which aldosterone exceeds 3000 pmol/L (Refsal and Mazaki-Tovi, 2009; Table 54-1).

Diagnostic Imaging

Adrenal masses are rarely visible radiographically, but a mass seen on radiographs is more likely to be an adrenocortical carcinoma than adenoma. Pulmonary metastases can occur, albeit infrequently; therefore three-view thoracic radiographs to screen for metastases should be performed prior to consideration of surgery. Distant metastases may be missed if the size is below the detection limit of the technique. In one case, thoracic radiography failed to reveal pulmonary metastases 3 mm in diameter (Rijnberk et al, 2001).

Diagnostic imaging techniques such as ultrasonography, magnetic resonance imaging (MRI), and computed tomography (CT) are used to identify adrenal abnormalities and, in the case of neoplasia, to evaluate possible extension into the caudal vena cava and the presence of distant metastases. In cats with PHA in which adrenal

ultrasonography has been performed (n = 23), unilateral adrenal enlargement with evidence of an adrenal mass has been identified in all, ranging from 10 to 46 mm in diameter. The contralateral adrenal gland may appear normal in appearance or may be unidentifiable. A small or nondetectable contralateral adrenal gland would heighten concern for adrenal insufficiency following adrenalectomy, at least transiently. If the contralateral gland is not visualized, it cannot be assumed to be normal or small. Bilateral adrenal tumors have been reported with feline PHA that were not detected by ultrasound. In the reported cases of bilateral adrenal hyperplasia, ultrasonography and/or CT examination showed subtle abnormalities such as an increase in adrenal echogenicity or areas of calcification and thickening and/or rounding of one pole of one or both adrenal glands. However, the absence of visible adrenal changes may not rule out PHA related to bilateral adrenal hyperplasia.

Ultrasonography also should attempt to identify invasion of the caudal vena cava by the tumor or related thrombus and the presence of metastases to other organs. A close association between the tumor and the caudal vena cava is often evident, and imaging has not been useful in preoperative estimation of the likely ease of surgical removal of adrenal masses or likelihood for complications. While the presence of visible tumor in the caudal vena cava indicates that surgical removal may be difficult, the absence of visible tumor invasion by diagnostic imaging is no guarantee for an uncomplicated adrenalectomy. Even when there is a caval thrombus attached to an adrenal mass, successful removal with a good outcome is still possible (Rose et al, 2007).

CT and MRI are more commonly used in feline patients now, but further data are needed to define added enhancement for evaluation of PHA compared with ultrasound technology. One cat had a left adrenalectomy performed because ultrasonography and CT indicated asymmetrical thickening, but bilateral nodular hyperplasia of the zona glomerulosa was found at surgery. Two cats with bilateral adrenal hyperplasia had no visible adrenal changes on ultrasound or CT (Javadi et al, 2005).

Treatment and Prognosis

PHA Related to Adrenal Neoplasia

Adrenalectomy is a potentially curative treatment for unilateral adrenal neoplasia. However, adrenalectomy has been associated with high perioperative complications and mortality in cats with PHA, with a fatal outcome in 6 of 17 reported cases. The most common and severe complication was acute hemorrhage from the caudal vena cava. Other complications included acute renal failure, sepsis, suspected thromboembolism and arterial hypotension, and hypoglycemia. The risk for hemorrhage was not related to the type of neoplasia (adenoma versus carcinoma), presence of tumor extension, or hypertension as a presenting sign. The decision to undergo adrenalectomy should not be taken lightly, and owners must be fully informed of the unpredictable and potentially fatal complications.

Patients should be stabilized medically prior to surgery and meticulous preoperative planning is required. Initial treatment of PHA preoperatively is directed at controlling hypokalemia and/or hypertension. Potassium supplementation with gluconate salt at doses of 2 to 6 mmol PO q12h has been used, and intravenous potassium chloride may be required with more severe hypokalemia. Amlodipine besylate (0.625 to 1.25 mg per cat PO q24h) is the treatment of choice for hypertension. Hypertension is often alleviated but higher doses of amlodipine are sometimes required. Spironolactone, a competitive aldosterone receptor antagonist, is also recommended (2 to 4 mg/kg PO q24h), assisting in the control of both hypokalemia and hypertension. Severe facial dermatitis has been reported recently in Maine coon cats receiving spironolactone for management of hypertrophic cardiomyopathy (MacDonald, Kittleson, and Kass, 2008) but has not been reported in cats with PHA. Preoperative medical treatment may not normalize potassium levels but improvement of signs associated with myopathy usually is achieved.

Cats with concurrent hyperprogesteronism or hyperadrenocorticism pose additional surgical risks including wound dehiscence, sepsis, and thromboembolic disease but successful outcomes with adrenalectomy have been achieved. Effective medical management would also necessitate suppression of progestin and glucocorticoid production in addition to aldosterone antagonism from spironolactone. To date a protocol for such treatment has not been defined. One author (AH) has used trilostane in a cat with concurrent hyperaldosteronism and hyperprogesteronism. Treatment was only attempted for a short period when the clinical signs were very advanced and was not successful in suppressing progesterone concentration.

Some authors recommend additional dietary sodium supplementation during the first few weeks after unilateral adrenalectomy to avoid hyponatremia resulting from atrophy of the zona glomerulosa of the contralateral adrenal gland (Djajadiningrat-Laanen, Galac, and Kooistra, 2011). Although clinicians must be vigilant, complications of postoperative adrenal insufficiency (e.g., hypoadrenocorticism, hypoaldosteronism) have not been associated with excision of aldosterone-secreting tumors in cats.

The prognosis is good for cats with PHA that undergo adrenalectomy and survive the immediate perioperative and postoperative periods; eight of 17 adrenalectomized cats survived for at least 1 year, and two cats were alive 3.5 and 5 years postoperatively. To the authors' knowledge, there are no reports to date of successful surgical treatment of bilateral adrenal neoplasia associated with PHA. Bilateral adrenalectomy has been described for the treatment of pituitary-dependent hyperadrenocorticism and may be an option for PHA associated with bilateral neoplasia. Otherwise, long-term medical management as described previously would be advised.

Surgery is not always the treatment of choice for unilateral adrenal neoplasia. Other factors that are important to consider in the decision-making process include presence of any comorbid conditions, presence of distant metastasis, and financial limitations of the owner.

In cases where surgery is precluded for any of these reasons, medical management with combinations of potassium supplementation, amlodipine, and spironolactone can be continued long term. Reported survival times in four of five medically treated cats with PHA due to adrenal neoplasia ranged from 7 months to 984 days, with cats succumbing most commonly to chronic kidney disease or a thromboembolic episode. The survival time in one cat receiving medical treatment alone was limited to 50 days, attributed to noncompliance of the owners. In some cases, hypertension becomes refractory to medical management.

Bilateral Adrenal Hyperplasia

Currently, medical management with potassium supplementation, amlodipine besylate, and spironolactone, as described previously, is advised for long-term treatment of bilateral adrenal hyperplasia. The severity of hyperaldosteronism in these cats tends to be milder than in those with neoplasia, and normokalemia and normotension more likely may be sustained for long periods (Djajadiningrat-Laanen, Galac, and Kooistra, 2011). The long-term prognosis for PHA related to adrenal hyperplasia is less well documented to date.

Issues for the Future

In human medicine, unilateral adrenal adenoma (often <1 cm diameter) and bilateral adrenal hyperplasia account for more than 90% of PHA cases, and baseline aldosterone is usually normal or slightly elevated. Diagnosis of PHA involves identification of an elevated ARR as a screening test. A test designed to suppress normal mineralocorticoid function is then used as a confirmatory test (e.g., oral sodium loading, captopril suppression, or fludrocortisone suppression test). The debilitated condition or sizeable adrenal tumors described in many cats with PHA suggest an advanced stage of disease at initial diagnosis. As cats in less severe physical states are screened for PHA, there will be a need for mineralocorticoid function tests to provide optimal diagnostic confirmation of PHA. Administration of fludrocortisone acetate (0.05 mg/kg BID for 4 days) consistently suppressed urinary aldosterone-to-creatinine ratios in normal cats, showing the best current potential as a confirmatory test for feline PHA (Djajadiningrat-Laanen et al, 2008).

References and Suggested Reading

Briscoe K et al: Hyperaldosteronism and hyperprogesteronism in a cat, *J Fel Med Surg* 11:758-762, 2009.

Chhokar VS et al: Hyperparathyroidism and the calcium paradox of aldosteronism, *Circulation* 111:871-878, 2005.

Djajadiningrat-Laanen SC et al: Urinary aldosterone to creatinine ratio in cats before and after suppression with salt or fludrocortisone acetate, *J Vet Intern Med* 22:1283-1288, 2008.

Djajadiningrat-Laanen S, Galac S, Kooistra H: Primary hyperaldosteronism: expanding the diagnostic net, *J Fel Med Surg* 13:641-650, 2011.

Eger C, Robinson W, Huxtable C: Primary hyperaldosteronism (Conn's syndrome) in a cat; a case report and review of comparative aspects, *J Small Anim Pract* 24:293-307, 1983.

Graves TK: When normal is abnormal: keys to laboratory diagnosis of hidden endocrine disease, *Top Comp Anim Med* 26:45-51, 2011.

Javadi S et al: Primary hyperaldosteronism, a mediator of progressive renal disease of cats, *Domest Anim Endocrinol* 28:85-104, 2005.

MacDonald KA, Kittleson MD, Kass PH: Effect of spironolactone on dialystolic function and left ventricular mass in Maine coon cats with familial hypertrophic cardiomyopathy, *J Vet Intern Med* 22:335-341, 2008.

Refsal KR, Mazaki-Tovi M: Baseline concentrations of progesterone, cortisol, and corticosterone in a laboratory survey of feline sera submitted for assay of aldosterone, Proceedings of the 19th ECVIM Companion Animals Congress, 2009, p 290 (abst).

Renschler JS, Dean GA: What is your diagnosis? Abdominal mass aspirate in a cat with an increased Na:K ratio, *Vet Clin Path* 38:69-72, 2009.

Rijnberk A et al: Hyperaldosteronism in a cat with metastasized adrenocortical tumor, *Vet Q* 23:38-43, 2001.

Rose SA et al. Adrenalectomy and caval thrombectomy in a cat with primary hyperaldosteronism, *J Am Anim Hosp Assoc* 43:209-214, 2007.

CHAPTER 55

Feline Idiopathic Hypercalcemia

JOAO FELIPE DE BRITO GALVAO, *Downers Grove, Illinois*
DENNIS J. CHEW, *Columbus, Ohio*
PATRICIA A. SCHENCK, *Lansing, Michigan*

Since the early 1990s unexplained hypercalcemia has been recognized increasingly in cats. The most common cause of hypercalcemia is thought to be *idiopathic hypercalcemia* (IHC), defined as abnormally elevated serum ionized calcium (iCa) concentration in which the cause remains unknown after extensive evaluation to rule out the known causes of hypercalcemia. This condition is widespread across the United States, and reports are also emerging from other parts of the world as well. The frequency of diagnosis for IHC is higher when screening for this disorder using iCa rather than with serum total calcium (tCa).

Differential Diagnosis

Hypercalcemia is typically noted on an initial analysis of tCa and is often a seemingly fortuitous discovery when a blood sample is taken for other reasons (e.g., wellness examinations, preanesthesia screening, evaluation of urolithiasis, evaluation of gastrointestinal signs). When an increase in serum tCa is noted, an iCa measurement should be obtained to determine if the increase in tCa is accompanied by an increase in the ionized component, which is biologically active. Serum iCa concentration needs to be measured because the prediction of iCa status from tCa measurement is not accurate, especially in cats with concomitant chronic kidney disease (CKD). Hypercalcemia is detected more commonly when iCa is used as the screening analyte compared with measurement of serum tCa.

Hypercalcemia may be parathyroid-independent or parathyroid-dependent (primary hyperparathyroidism). In parathyroid-independent hypercalcemia, the elevation of iCa results in *suppression* of parathyroid hormone (PTH)

BOX 55-1

Differential Diagnosis of Hypercalcemia: HARDIONS-G Acronym

H: Hyperparathyroidism (1°, 3°, hyperplasia), houseplants (e.g., *Cestrum diurnum* [the day-blooming jessamine], *Solanum malacoxylon, Trisetum flavescens*), hyperthyroidism

A: Addison's disease, aluminum toxicity, vitamin A toxicity, milk-alkali syndrome

R: Renal disease

D: Vitamin D toxicosis, drugs (calcitriol, calcitriol analogs, psoriasis cream, vitamin D–based creams, rodenticide [cholecalciferol], calcipotriene [Dovonex]), dehydration, DMSO (if used to treat calcinosis cutis), diet

I: Idiopathic (cats), infectious, inflammatory, immobilization

O: Osteolytic (osteomyelitis, immobilization, LOH, bone infarct)

N: Neoplasia (LOH and HHM), nutritional

S: Spurious, schistosomiasis, salts of calcium, supplements (vitamin D–based)

G: Granulomatous diseases (fungal)

DMSO, Dimethyl sulfoxide; *HHM*, humoral hypercalcemia of malignancy; *LOH*, local osteolytic hypercalcemia.

production. In cats with IHC, PTH values are usually undetectable to within the lower half of the normal reference range (see later).

There are many potential causes of hypercalcemia in the cat (Box 55-1). A list of differential diagnoses ensures that all possibilities for the development of hypercalcemia have been considered. However, such a list does not indicate the frequency of the diagnoses. The most common diagnoses in cats with persistent elevations in iCa are IHC and malignancy. CKD is estimated to be accompanied by elevations in serum tCa in about 10% to 15% of cases. iCa was increased in about 30% of cats with CKD in one series compared with about 10% of dogs with CKD. In some cases the cause of hypercalcemia is obvious on analysis of history and physical examination. In others the cause may not be evident, and further workup, including hematology, serum biochemistry, body cavity imaging, cytology, and histopathology, is necessary. In some cases, measurement of the calciotropic hormones 25(OH) vitamin D_3 and 1,25(OH)2 vitamin D_3 (i.e., calcitriol) may be needed to secure the diagnosis. A diagnosis of IHC is made when all other causes of hypercalcemia are excluded. Although IHC is the most frequent diagnosis in cats with hypercalcemia, it is an exceedingly uncommon finding in dogs following adequate diagnostic workup (see Web Chapter 11).

The magnitude of elevation of serum tCa cannot be used to make a diagnosis of the underlying cause since there is considerable overlap in the degree of hypercalcemia in cats with IHC or other conditions. Most cats with IHC present with mild increases in tCa and iCa concentrations (11 to 12 mg/dl [2.75 to 3.00 mmol/L] and 6 to 6.5 mg/dl [1.5 to 1.6 mmol/L], respectively), whereas some cats may have tCa and iCa concentrations greater than 15 to 20 mg/dl (3.75 to 5 mmol/L) and 8 to 11 mg/dl (2 to 2.7 mmol/L), respectively.

The possibility of malignancy as the cause of hypercalcemia in both dogs and cats is always a concern, but malignancy-associated hypercalcemia (MAH), which includes both humoral hypercalcemia of malignancy and local osteolytic hypercalcemia, is much less common in cats than in dogs (it is the number one cause of pathological hypercalcemia in dogs). Based on serum tCa, MAH ranks behind IHC and CKD in frequency in cats. Patients with MAH are usually "sick," as it takes a reasonably large tumor burden to synthesize the compounds (especially parathyroid-related peptide [PTHrP]) that result in hypercalcemia. Thus it is unlikely for a cat that feels well to have MAH, especially if the hypercalcemia persists for a long period without the cat showing more clinical signs. The less sick the cat is in the face of persistent hypercalcemia, the more likely the diagnosis will be IHC or primary hyperparathyroidism.

Cats have a higher frequency of PTH-independent hypercalcemia than do dogs. In cats with parathyroid-independent hypercalcemia, the next step in the diagnostic evaluation is to rule out MAH, which requires imaging of the thorax and abdomen. Full imaging with thoracic and abdominal radiographs along with abdominal ultrasound is the gold standard in the diagnosis of IHC. Chest radiographs are useful, especially to rule out mediastinal lymphoma that may be associated with hypercalcemia. However, unlike in dogs, hypercalcemia from mediastinal lymphoma rarely occurs in cats. Abdominal radiographs are most useful to rule out nephroliths and ureteroliths that may be associated with hypercalcemia, which may lead to postrenal azotemia. Cats should have an empty colon to enable interpretation of radiographs over the areas of interest. Ultrasound may also be used if available. Treatment recommendations and prognosis may change with the presence of stones. Furthermore, it is strongly recommended to treat hypercalcemia in cats considered to be stone formers, thus decreasing the likelihood of future stone formation.

Many clients are unable to afford the gold standard diagnostic evaluation. Lack of clinical signs in conjunction with low PTH and ionized hypercalcemia significantly increases suspicion of IHC. In these cases, it may be appropriate to presumptively diagnose IHC.

Clinical Presentation

Cats with IHC may have persistent elevations in iCa for months without apparent clinical signs, and no relationship has been noted between the magnitude of elevation and occurrence of clinical signs. In a review of 427 cats with IHC diagnosed at an endocrinology referral laboratory, the mean age at presentation was 9.8 years old (range 0.5 to 20 years old), and long-haired cats were overrepresented (27% of cases). Both genders were equally represented. Almost half of the cats had no clinical signs (46%), 18% had mild weight loss, 6% had inflammatory bowel disease, 5% had chronic constipation, 4% presented with vomiting, and 1% were anorectic. Uroliths were reported in 15% of cats with IHC, and calcium oxalate stones were specifically present in 10% of cases (Schenk, 2004).

Serum iCa is increased in cats with IHC, and the PTH concentration is typically in the lower half of the reference range; many affected cats have PTH concentration in the lower quartile of the reference range. Concentrations of both ionized magnesium and 25-hydroxyvitamin D are within the reference range in most cats. Calcitriol concentration is normal to low in most cats, although this has not been measured in a large number of cats. Some cats with IHC develop CKD secondary to persistent hypercalcemia, and cats with CKD may develop IHC over time. Measuring a PTH level is key to determining if the hypercalcemia is from CKD or idiopathic. If PTH is low and azotemia is present, the cat either has IHC and CKD or hypercalcemia from IHC that has led to CKD. If PTH is elevated and hypercalcemia is present, but azotemia is not severe, tertiary renal hyperparathyroidism is considered unlikely. Therefore such a cat likely has IHC and CKD. However, if azotemia is severe (i.e., creatinine >5 mg/dl), PTH is elevated, and hypercalcemia is present, IHC cannot be definitively diagnosed. A few cats may have both CKD and IHC on initial presentation. Serum phosphorus is usually in the normal range in cats with IHC unless it is increased as a result of concurrent CKD. Urine specific gravity is typically greater than 1.030, and it appears that many cats with hypercalcemia can still maximally concentrate their urine if they do not have concurrent CKD.

Treatment

The treatment of hypercalcemia usually targets the dysregulated mechanisms that are responsible; however, in IHC these mechanisms remain unknown. Thus treatments at this time are empiric. When monitoring therapy, it is important to measure iCa and not tCa.

Should All Cats with IHC Receive Treatment?

Minor elevations in serum iCa concentrations are often ignored because many of these cats have mild or no apparent clinical signs. The calcium may increase gradually or remain at the initial increased level for long periods. Excess calcium is toxic to cells, particularly in the central nervous system, gastrointestinal tract, heart, and kidneys. Mineralization of soft tissues is an important complication, and the serum phosphorus concentration when hypercalcemia develops is important in determining the extent of mineralization. When the calcium concentration (mg/dl) multiplied by the phosphorus concentration (mg/dl) is greater than 60, soft tissue mineralization is likely to be most severe, but the validity of this concept has been challenged (O'Neill, 2007).

The need for therapy in IHC increases when iCa continues to elevate or clinical signs become obvious (weight loss, depression, vomiting, constipation, urinary stones, emergence of CKD, development of less concentrated urine). The consequences of long-standing hypercalcemia can be devastating in those that develop CKD or urolithiasis, and aggressive treatment for hypercalcemia is warranted in these cases. Continued elevation of iCa leads to further development of renal lesions and development of new stones. An algorithm for decision to treat

BOX 55-2

Summary of Treatment Recommendations

1. Try dietary modification for 6 to 8 weeks if patient is clinically stable. May try different diets (e.g., high fiber, those designed for chronic kidney disease).
2. If diet is not successful, add alendronate and start with 10 mg by mouth once weekly.
   a. Fast for at least 12 hours.
   b. Butter cat's lips.
   c. Pill and follow with 6 ml of water.
   d. Fast for another 2 hours.
3. Recheck ionized calcium in 3-4 weeks.
   a. If normal, recheck in another 4-6 weeks.
   b. If low, decrease dose to 10 mg PO every other week.
   c. If high, increase dose to 20 mg per week. Alternatively, can increase to 10 mg and 20 mg on alternate weeks (consider this if iCa is only mildly elevated).
      i. Recheck iCa in 3-4 weeks. Consider recommendations above according to iCa concentration.
4. If ionized calcium remains elevated and if 30 mg of alendronate per week is not enough to control iCa, we recommend adding prednisolone. Before, we recommend rechecking diagnosis by repeating PTH, PTHrP, 25-hydroxyvitamin D level, abdominal ultrasound (with aspirates of liver and spleen for cytology to rule out mast cell disease and lymphoma), and chest radiographs.
   a. Prednisolone 5 to 10 mg PO q24h.
   b. Recheck iCa in 3-4 weeks.
   c. If still elevated, consider increasing prednisolone 10 to 20 mg PO q24h.

is presented in Figure 55-1. A treatment plan for hypercalcemia is presented in Figure 55-2 and Box 55-2.

Diet Therapy

Normocalcemia may be restored after a change to a different diet. One high-fiber veterinary diet was reported to restore normocalcemia in five cats with IHC and calcium oxalate urolithiasis. This high-fiber diet was similar to the original diet being fed to the cats in terms of urinary acidification and magnesium restriction (McClain et al, 1995). However, in another study there was no beneficial effect of high-fiber diets in cats with IHC (Midkiff et al, 2000). The effects of fiber on intestinal absorption are complex and depend on the type and amount of fiber in the diet and the interactions with other nutrients. High-fiber diets are considered acidifying in general, an effect that would lead to ionization of luminal calcium and subsequent increased intestinal absorption; normocalcemia can result despite this effect. High-fiber diets may decrease intestinal transit time, lessening the opportunity for intestinal absorption of calcium; however, most manufacturers increase the quantity of calcium in high-fiber diets to offset the potential for decreased absorption.

Feeding a veterinary renal diet may result in normocalcemia in some cats with IHC but how this benefit is achieved is not known. Veterinary diets designed for cats

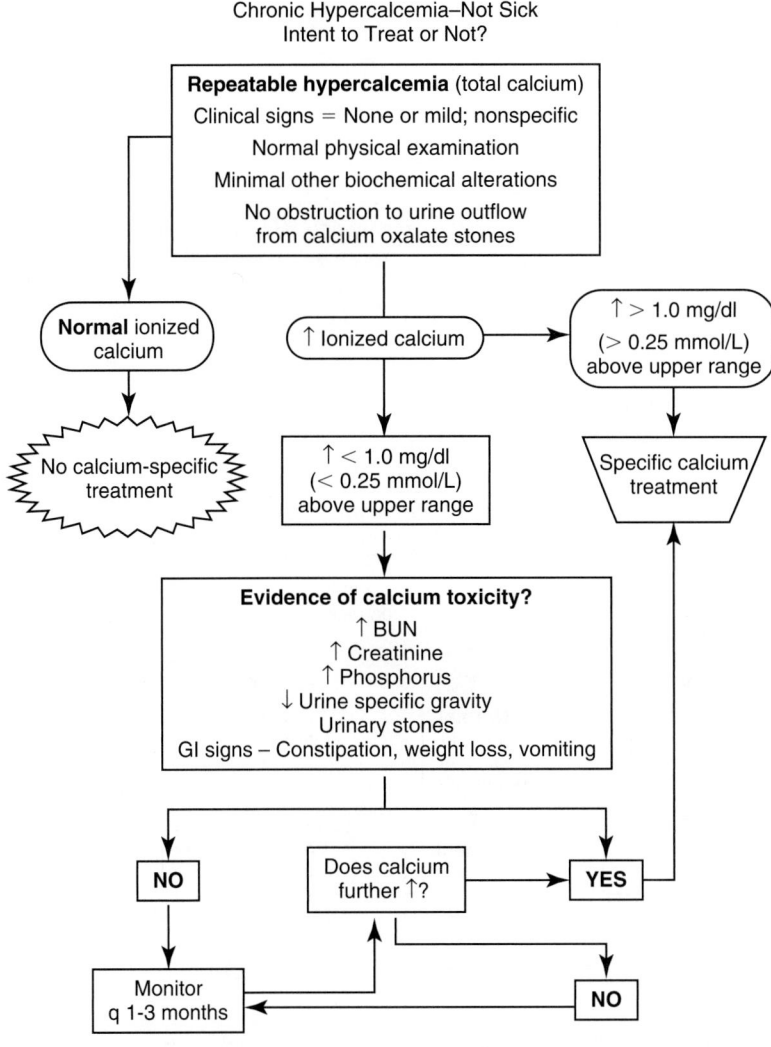

Chronic Hypercalcemia–Not Sick
Intent to Treat or Not?

Repeatable hypercalcemia (total calcium)
Clinical signs = None or mild; nonspecific
Normal physical examination
Minimal other biochemical alterations
No obstruction to urine outflow
from calcium oxalate stones

Normal ionized
calcium

↑ Ionized calcium

↑ > 1.0 mg/dl
(> 0.25 mmol/L)
above upper range

No calcium-specific
treatment

↑ < 1.0 mg/dl
(< 0.25 mmol/L)
above upper range

Specific calcium
treatment

Evidence of calcium toxicity?
↑ BUN
↑ Creatinine
↑ Phosphorus
↓ Urine specific gravity
Urinary stones
GI signs – Constipation, weight loss, vomiting

NO

Does calcium
further ↑?

YES

Monitor
q 1-3 months

NO

Figure 55-1 Diagnostic plan for initiation of treatment in hypercalcemic cats.

in renal failure are less acidifying than maintenance diets and are low in calcium and phosphorus. Canned diets are generally more restricted in calcium than dry diets. The decreased consumption of calcium could lead to a decrease in the amount of calcium undergoing intestinal absorption, and the effects of less acidification may decrease the release of calcium from bone. On the other hand, the feeding of veterinary renal diets could enhance renal calcitriol synthesis caused by the dietary restriction of phosphorus, an effect that could offset the advantage of the decreased calcium absorption in cats with IHC. In one study, 2 of 15 cats with CKD developed ionized hypercalcemia after being fed a diet low in phosphorus and protein. Ionized calcium normalized after discontinuing dietary phosphorus and protein restriction (Barber, 1998).

Veterinary diets developed to prevent calcium oxalate urolithiasis may be beneficial in the treatment of some cats with IHC. These diets are restricted in calcium and have less urinary acidification (production of urine with a neutral pH). Some are also restricted in oxalic acid and sodium and have increased moisture in the canned formulation. In two of three cats with IHC and calcium oxalate uroliths, hypercalcemia resolved after feeding a calcium oxalate–prevention diet. One cat did not become

normocalcemic but did have a reduction in the magnitude of hypercalcemia.

The addition of sodium chloride may be useful in cats with IHC as long as the added salt enhances calcium excretion without an increased risk of calcium oxalate urolith formation. Increased dietary sodium chloride increased urine volume but did not increase calcium oxalate relative supersaturation in a small number of young healthy cats. However, an increase in urinary calcium excretion does not always correlate to the development of calcium urolithiasis, since the concentration of calcium in the urine also depends on the degree of water excreted at the same time. The effects of additional dietary sodium chloride have yet to be reported in cats with IHC.

IHC is not the result of obvious excess dietary vitamin D intake since serum concentrations of 25-hydroxyvitamin D are within the reference range in most cats with IHC. However, the minimal dietary requirement for vitamin D in cats is debatable since reference ranges have been established in cats fed vitamin D–supplemented diets. Normal concentrations of 25-hydroxyvitamin D could still potentially be associated with IHC in cats if the cats have mutations in the vitamin D or calcitriol receptors.

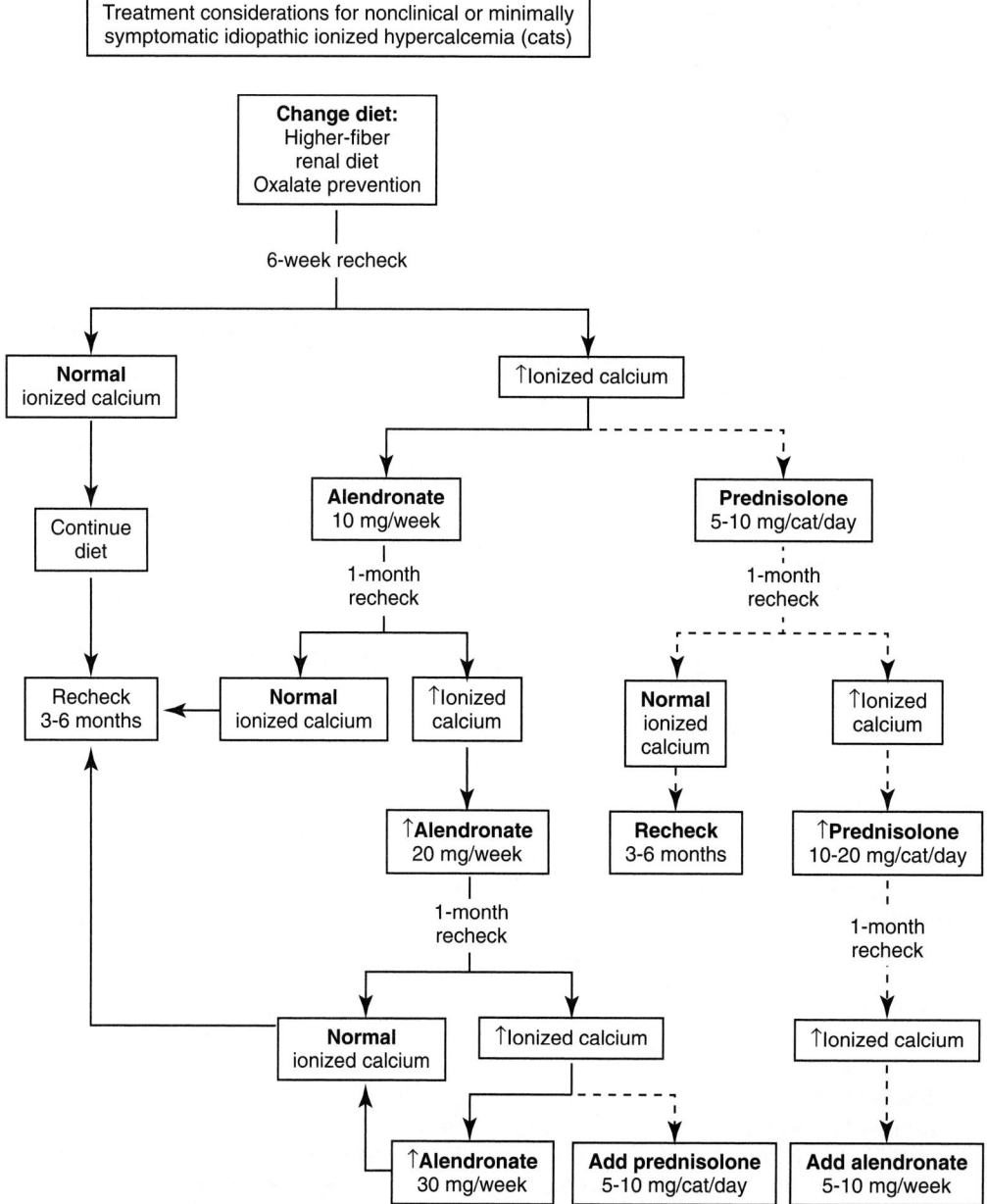

Figure 55-2 Treatment of minimally symptomatic ionized hypercalcemia in cats. Arrows represent alternate route.

These possibilities have not yet been investigated. Since the amount of vitamin D supplied in most diets is not listed on the diet label, it is difficult to choose a diet that is lower in vitamin D.

Hypercalcemia may return in some cats with IHC that previously have been successfully treated with a dietary change. In these cases changing to another diet or medical therapy should be considered.

Bisphosphonates

If normocalcemia has not been restored after a dietary feeding trial of 6 to 8 weeks, bisphosphonate treatment should be considered. Bisphosphonates reduce the activity and number of osteoclasts following binding to

hydroxyapatite. The bisphosphonates bind to hydroxyapatite and are engulfed by osteoclasts; in turn, they prevent osteoclasts from breaking down bone (decreasing bone turnover). Treatment with bisphosphonates may be useful for IHC. Even though not extensively reported, bisphosphonate therapy is now considered a safer alternative to glucocorticosteroid use in cats that failed dietary intervention.

The safety and efficacy of pamidronate at 1 to 1.5 mg/kg IV to two cats with hypercalcemia (one cat with IHC) have been reported. Adequate hydration is essential when treating with bisphosphonates because these drugs may cause nephrotoxicity, especially at higher doses given intravenously. We have successfully treated a small number of cats with IHC given 10 mg of alendronate orally once weekly for up to 1 year. Erosive esophagitis is noted as a possibility in women receiving oral bisphosphonates, an effect that has not been reported or observed by us. In one study in dogs, the presence of alendronate in the esophagus for 1 hour caused minor mucosal damage but esophagitis was exacerbated when gastric juice containing alendronate was refluxed into the esophagus (Mohn et al, 2009). It is thought that alendronate sodium is converted to free acid in the presence of gastric juice. No esophageal lesions and trivial gastric lesions (i.e., deemed not clinically significant by the pathologist) were reported from necropsy in cats undergoing treatment with relatively high doses (9 mg/kg twice a week in tuna juice) of oral alendronate for 49 weeks. Although the risk for development of esophagitis in cats is low, it is recommended to follow the weekly pill with 6 ml of water given with a dosing syringe and then to dab a small amount of butter on the cat's lips to increase licking and salivation, which further promotes decreased transit time of the pill to the stomach.

The oral bioavailability of alendronate administered in water to cats was recently reported to be about 3% and was reduced approximately tenfold when alendronate was formulated in tuna juice. To maximize intestinal absorption of alendronate, we recommend an overnight fast for 12 hours prior to the administration of medication, giving the pills in nothing else besides tap water, and then feeding the cat 2 hours later. Ideally, an 18-hour fast prior to administration of medication and 4-hour fast post-pill is recommended to achieve an oral bioavailability of 3%. It is not recommended administering alendronate that has been formulated by compounding pharmacies in flavored solution or suspension due to the severe decreases in intestinal absorption.

As seen with other therapies, hypercalcemia may return after a period of normocalcemia, requiring an increase in dose. Long-term bisphosphonate treatment in humans can lead to osteonecrosis of the jaw (ONJ) in a small number of patients. It is mostly reported in humans given high doses of intravenous bisphosphonates to treat cancer; it is far less frequently encountered following oral bisphosphonate treatment for postmenopausal osteoporosis. The alveolar bone region of the mandible has a high basal turnover rate for bone and so may be especially prone to necrosis of bone matrix following exposure to bisphosphonates. It is not clear if bisphosphonate exposure creates bone necrosis directly or if this is secondary to reduced bone turnover. Healthy male mongrel dogs treated with 5 mg oral alendronate daily for 23 weeks (35 mg weekly in an average weight dog of 35 kg) did not develop bone weakness or changes in structural and mechanical properties of bone (Allen and Burr, 2008). Daily oral alendronate at 0.2 mg/kg or 1 mg/kg given to skeletally mature female beagles for 3 years resulted in matrix necrosis of the mandible in 25% of the dogs treated with the lower dose and in 33% of the dogs treated with the higher dose. No dogs displayed gross, exposed bone lesions in this study. Intravenous zoledronate given to dogs at 0.06 mg/kg q24h for 6 months resulted in more osteonecrosis of the mandible than that encountered with oral alendronate. ONJ was not described in cats with dental lesions treated for 49 weeks with oral alendronate

(Mohn et al, 2009). We have not observed ONJ in cats treated with any form of bisphosphonate including some that have been on oral alendronate for several years.

Glucocorticosteroids

If normocalcemia has not been restored after a dietary feeding trial of 6 to 8 weeks and subsequent treatment with bisphosphonates (see Figure 55-2), glucocorticoid therapy should be considered. Administration of glucocorticoids is thought to decrease serum calcium concentration by decreasing intestinal absorption of calcium, renal tubular calcium resorption, and skeletal mobilization of calcium. Cats usually do not exhibit serious side effects from glucocorticoid treatment as do dogs. Prednisolone is given orally at 5 mg/cat/day for 1 month before reevaluation. If serum iCa concentration is normal, this dose is continued for several months. If serum iCa concentration is still increased, the dose is increased to 10 mg/cat q24h. Some cats may require as much as 15 to 20 mg of prednisolone per day to restore normocalcemia. Approximately 50% of cats with IHC become normocalcemic with 5 or 10 mg of prednisone per day, but some may require increasing doses to remain normocalcemic over time.

There is some concern that glucocorticoids may increase urinary excretion of calcium, contributing to calcium oxalate urolith formation. However, little is known regarding the effects of glucocorticoids on filtration and tubular resorption of calcium in the cat. In a few healthy cats that have been studied, oral prednisolone treatment did not result in diuresis or an increase in calcium oxalate excretion.

Miscellaneous Treatments

Fluid therapy is a possible treatment option in cats with IHC but has not been evaluated. The administration of subcutaneous fluids on a daily or every-other-day basis potentially could expand the extracellular fluid and promote calciuresis. Diuretics such as furosemide have been used effectively to decrease serum iCa during acute rescue protocols for hypercalcemia, usually in combination with intravenous fluids. Little is known about the effects of chronic furosemide administration regarding calcium status and the development of dehydration. It is a concern that cats receiving chronic diuretics will undergo diuresis but not increase their water intake, leading to dehydration.

Calcimimetics are a new class of drug that has emerged in human medicine. Calcimimetics interact with the calcium receptor directly and have been proven effective in lowering iCa, phosphorus, and PTH concentrations in human dialysis patients. The potential future use of calcimimetics in the treatment of IHC is an interesting treatment consideration for future study.

References and Suggested Reading

Allen MR, Burr DB: Mandible matrix necrosis in beagle dogs after 3 years of daily oral bisphosphonate treatment, *J Oral Maxillofac Surg* 66:987-994, 2008.

Barber PJ, Elliott J: Feline chronic renal failure: calcium homeostasis in 80 cases diagnosed between 1992 and 1995, *J Small Anim Pract* 39:108-116, 1998.

Burr DB, Allen MR: Mandibular necrosis in beagle dogs treated with bisphosphonates, *Orthod Craniofac Res* 12:221-228, 2009.

Geyer N et al: Influence of prednisolone on urinary calcium oxalate and struvite relative supersaturation in healthy young adult female domestic shorthaired cats, *Vet Ther* 8:239-246, 2007.

Graham-Mize CA, Rosser EG, Hauptman J: Absorption, bioavailability and activity of prednisone and prednisolone in cats, *Adv Vet Dermatol* 5:152-158, 2005.

Griffin B, Beard DM, Klopfenstein KA: Use of butter to facilitate the passage of tablets through the esophagus in cats, *J Vet Intern Med* 17:445, 2003.

Hostutler RA et al: Uses and effectiveness of pamidronate disodium for treatment of dogs and cats with hypercalcemia, *J Vet Intern Med* 19:29, 2005.

Lulich JP et al: Effects of diet on urine composition of cats with calcium oxalate urolithiasis, *J Am Anim Hosp Assoc* 40:185, 2004.

McClain HM, Barsanti JA, Bartges JW: Hypercalcemia and calcium oxalate urolithiasis in cats: a report of five cases, *J Am Anim Hosp Assoc* 35:297, 1995.

Midkiff AM et al: Idiopathic hypercalcemia in cats, *J Vet Intern Med* 14:619, 2000.

Mohn KL et al: Alendronate binds to tooth root surfaces and inhibits progression of feline tooth resorption: a pilot proof-of-concept study, *J Vet Dent* 26:74-81, 2009.

O'Neill WC: The fallacy of the calcium-phosphorus product, *Kidney Int* 72:792-796, 2007.

Schenck PA: Calcium metabolic hormones in feline idiopathic hypercalcemia, *J Vet Intern Med* 18:442, 2004.

Schenck PA: Chew DJ: Prediction of serum ionized calcium concentration by serum total calcium measurement in cats, *Can J Vet Res* 74:209-213, 2010.

Schenck PA et al: Disorders of calcium: hypercalcemia and hypocalcemia. In DiBartola SP, editor: *Fluid therapy in small animal practice*, St Louis, 2011, Elsevier, p 120-194.

Westfall DS et al: Evaluation of esophageal transit of tablets and capsules in 30 cats, *J Vet Intern Med* 15:467-470, 2001.

Whitney JL et al: Use of bisphosphonates to treat severe idiopathic hypercalcaemia in a young Ragdoll cat, *J Feline Med Surg* 13:129-134, 2011.

CHAPTER **56**

Approach to Hypomagnesemia and Hypokalemia

LEE E. PALMER, *Auburn, Alabama*
LINDA G. MARTIN, *Pullman, Washington*

Hypomagnesemia

Hypomagnesemia refers to low circulating concentrations of magnesium in the serum and occurs when total magnesium (Mg) concentrations are below 1.89 mg/dl in dogs and below 1.75 mg/dl in cats; ionized hypomagnesemia occurs when serum ionized Mg concentrations are below 0.43 mmol/L in both species. These values may vary slightly depending on the reference laboratory used. In veterinary medicine, hypomagnesemia is one of the most common electrolyte abnormalities detected in critically ill patients. In 48 dogs admitted to a veterinary teaching hospital intensive care unit, the incidence of hypomagnesemia at admission was 54%, and hypomagnesemic dogs had a higher incidence of concurrent hypokalemia and hyponatremia, as well as a longer length of hospitalization, compared with normomagnesemic counterparts (Martin et al, 1994). A prospective study of 57 cats admitted to an intensive care unit reported that hypomagnesemia developed in 28% during hospitalization (Toll et al, 2002); another study reported an incidence of hypomagnesemia of 62% and 57% in cats with diabetes mellitus and diabetic ketoacidosis, respectively (Norris, Nelson, and Christopher, 1999). Its high frequency of occurrence and impact on morbidity in veterinary patients have established hypomagnesemia as one of the most clinically significant electrolyte disorders in critically ill animals.

Physiologic Role and Function

Mg plays a pivotal role in many physiologic processes. One of its main contributions is serving as an essential cofactor and catalyst in over 300 intracellular enzymatic reactions, which makes it vital in regulating (1) synthesis and metabolism of carbohydrates, lipids, and proteins;

(2) synthesis, degradation, and stabilization of nucleic acids; (3) oxidative phosphorylation and anaerobic glycolysis; (4) neuromuscular activity, cardiac conduction, and excitability; (5) signal transduction; (6) intracellular potassium (K) and cytoplasmic calcium concentrations; and (7) immunologic function. Of greatest importance, Mg complexes with and stabilizes many polyphosphate compounds and therefore plays a vital role in facilitating most cellular phosphorylation reactions. For example, every molecule of adenosine triphosphate (ATP) must complex with Mg to be biologically active.

Distribution and Homeostasis

Mg is the second most abundant intracellular cation (second to K) and the most abundant free divalent cation in the body. Ninety-nine percent of total body Mg content is found intracellularly, with approximately 60% to 85% located in bone complexed with calcium and phosphorus. The remainder of intracellular Mg is located primarily within skeletal muscle and to a smaller degree within the liver, heart, and other soft tissues. Less than 1% of total body Mg content is located extracellularly in the serum. Approximately 60% to 70% of serum Mg is unbound or ionized and freely filterable across the glomerular filtration barrier, while the remainder is either bound to protein (primarily albumin) or complexed with anions such as phosphate, citrate, sulfate, lactate, or bicarbonate. The ionized portion is available for cellular use and physiologic processes and is therefore considered the biologically active portion.

The kidneys serve as the major regulatory organ for Mg homeostasis through glomerular filtration and tubular reabsorption. Secondary to the kidneys is the intestinal tract. The ileum followed by the jejunum and colon are responsible for most of the absorption. The amount of dietary Mg intake, along with the degree of complex formation or chelation of Mg within the intestinal lumen, influences absorption. During low dietary intake of Mg, intestinal absorption may be as high as 70%, compared with only 25% during periods of high dietary intake. Only ionized Mg is absorbed across the intestinal barriers; therefore any increase in complex formation or chelation of Mg reduces absorption.

Causes

The three causes of Mg deficiency are (1) decreased intake, (2) alterations in compartmental and cellular distribution, and (3) increased loss (Box 56-1). Realistically, hypomagnesemia results not from any one of these mechanisms but rather from a combination of all three. Poor dietary Mg intake does not usually cause clinically significant hypomagnesemia; however, chronic dietary Mg deficiency may lead to a significant depletion of body stores. Administration of Mg-deficient intravenous fluids or parenteral nutrition may also result in hypomagnesemia in hospitalized animals.

Cellular translocation, chelation, and sequestration account for redistribution of Mg between body compartments. Cellular translocation involves shifting from extracellular space to intracellular space, a result of

---

BOX 56-1

Etiologies of Hypomagnesemia

Decreased Intake
Chronic dietary magnesium (Mg) deficiency
Mg-deficient intravenous fluids, partial or total parenteral nutrition

Cellular Translocation
Transcellular shifts
    Insulin, glucose, or amino acid administration
Chelation
    Massive catecholamine release (e.g., sepsis, trauma, shock)
    Massive blood transfusion (e.g., citrate chelation)
Sequestration: Pancreatitis

Excessive Losses
Renal
Intrinsic renal tubular disorders
    Infectious
    Neoplastic
    Ischemic
    Drug-induced (e.g., NSAIDs, aminoglycosides, cyclosporine)
Extrinsic renal factors
    High tubular flow rate/diuresis
    Extracellular fluid volume expansion
    Diuretic therapy (e.g., mannitol, furosemide, thiazides)
    Hyperthyroidism (cats)
    Diabetic ketoacidosis
    Posturethral obstructive diuresis
    Hemodialysis (observed in humans)
Gastrointestinal
    Acute/chronic diarrhea
    Excessive vomiting
    Malabsorptive syndromes (e.g., protein-losing enteropathy, short-bowel syndrome)
    Inflammatory bowel disease
Lactation

---

catecholamine and insulin release as well as administration of amino acids. Disease states involving massive catecholamine release (e.g., sepsis, trauma, shock) can stimulate release of free fatty acids that chelate Mg. Massive transfusions can result in ionized hypomagnesemia due to chelation of Mg with citrate. Similar to calcium, Mg may undergo saponification and be sequestered in necrotic fat during acute pancreatitis. Lactation may influence Mg balance because the Mg content of both canine and feline milk tends to be higher in the first few days of lactation. In addition, lactation's influence on parathyroid hormone and circulating calcium concentrations most likely influences renal and intestinal handling of Mg.

Both increased renal excretion and gastrointestinal losses account for the major disturbances in circulating Mg concentrations. Various disorders such as acute or chronic diarrhea, malabsorptive syndromes (e.g., protein-losing enteropathy), short-bowel syndrome, or vomiting can lead to decreased intestinal absorption and excessive Mg loss from the body. Renal losses can occur with acquired intrinsic renal diseases (e.g., infections, nephrotoxins, ischemia) by causing renal Mg wasting through renal tubular dysfunction and decreased renal absorption. Renal Mg wasting may also result from a high tubular flow rate due to extracellular fluid volume expansion, diuretic therapy, or disease states such as feline hyperthyroidism. Diabetic ketoacidosis or posturethral obstructions result in profound diuresis and are commonly associated with hypomagnesemia.

Clinical Signs

The predominant clinical signs of hypomagnesemia result from abnormalities involving the cardiovascular, neuromuscular, and endocrine systems. Clinical signs depend on the degree and rate of decline, as well as on the temporal nature (acute versus chronic) of Mg deficiency.

The myocardial effects of Mg are linked to its role as a regulator of other ions, primarily calcium and K. For this reason, one of the most dramatic clinical signs associated with hypomagnesemia is cardiac arrhythmia such as atrial fibrillation, supraventricular tachycardia, and ventricular tachycardia or fibrillation. Prior to seeing overt arrhythmias, electrocardiographic (ECG) changes may occur, such as prolongation of the PR interval, widening of the QRS complex, depression of the ST segment, and peaking of the T wave.

Mg deficiency can result in various nonspecific neuromuscular signs caused by changes in the resting membrane potential, signal transduction, and smooth muscle tone. If present, concurrent hypocalcemia and hypokalemia may also contribute. Clinical manifestations of hypomagnesemia include skeletal muscle weakness or fasciculations, seizures, and ataxia. Esophageal or respiratory muscle weakness can manifest as dysphagia or dyspnea, respectively.

Metabolic complications of hypomagnesemia include concurrent hypokalemia, hyponatremia, hypocalcemia, and hypophosphatemia. Isolated Mg deficiency is uncommon. Mg's role as a cofactor for sodium-potassium (Na/K) and calcium adenosine triphosphatase (ATPase) pumps likely plays a role in the development of concurrent electrolyte disturbances. Reduced Na/K-ATPase function in states of Mg deficiency leads to extracellular K loss. In addition, hypomagnesemia impairs the function of the Na/K-chloride cotransport system, decreasing K reentry into the cell. Overall, K accumulates extracellularly and is subsequently lost from the body due to ineffective renal K reabsorption. Urinary sodium loss generally occurs concurrently with K. The most likely origin of concurrent hypocalcemia is renal loss via reduced calcium ATPase pump function with decreased bone mobilization from impaired parathyroid function. Hypophosphatemia is thought to occur from increased renal phosphate loss. Concurrent hypokalemia or hypocalcemia that is refractory to aggressive potassium or calcium supplementation may be due to hypomagnesemia.

Diagnostics

To date, no gold standard test exists for determining the extent of a total body Mg deficit. Total serum Mg concentrations do not accurately reflect total body stores; therefore low total Mg concentrations in serum only suggest that total body stores are depleted. Ionized Mg is the biologically active form and its measurement is the preferred method

for evaluating the presence of hypomagnesemia. However, serum ionized Mg only accounts for approximately 0.2% to 0.3% of total body stores; therefore, as with total Mg, it may not be reflective of the total body Mg deficit.

Both total and ionized Mg can be measured using serum or heparinized whole blood. Ionized Mg is measured via an ion-selective electrode, which can be accomplished on some models of the NOVA Critical Care Xpress analyzers. The authors are unaware of any commercial reference laboratories that currently measure ionized Mg. Mg may be measured in mEq/L or mmol/L; since it is a divalent cation the following conversions may be used:

$$2\,mEq/L = 1\,mmol/L = 2.43\,mg/dl.$$

Treatment

Treatment depends on the severity of hypomagnesemia, the rate of decline, and the patient's overall clinical condition and stability. Patients without clinical signs may have their Mg corrected by addressing the underlying disorder or via oral supplementation with chloride, gluconate, oxide, or hydroxide salts of Mg. The recommended daily oral dose of elemental Mg is 1 to 2 mEq/kg/day. Since each Mg salt formulation may contain differing amounts of elemental Mg, it is necessary to read the label and determine the amount of elemental Mg that is contained in each unit serving before prescribing or administering the medication to the patient. The main side effect of oral Mg supplementation is diarrhea.

Supplementation should be considered if serum Mg concentrations are below 1.5 mg/dl and at higher serum concentrations if clinical signs of hypomagnesemia (e.g., cardiac arrhythmias, muscle tremors, refractory hypokalemia) are present. Renal function and cardiac conduction should be assessed prior to Mg administration. Since Mg is primarily excreted by the kidneys, the Mg dose should be reduced by 50% in azotemic patients, and serum concentrations should be monitored to prevent the development of hypermagnesemia. Since Mg prolongs conduction through the atrioventricular (AV) node, patients with cardiac conduction disturbances (e.g., AV and bundle branch blocks) should have judicious Mg supplementation and continuous ECG monitoring.

The intravenous route is preferred for rapid repletion of serum Mg concentrations because the intramuscular route is generally painful. Both sulfate and chloride salts of Mg are available. Since parenteral administration of Mg sulfate may result in hypocalcemia due to chelation of calcium with sulfate, Mg chloride should be given if hypocalcemia is present.

For more rapid Mg repletion, a dose of 0.75 to 1 mEq/kg q24h can be administered for the first 24 to 48 hours by continuous rate infusion in normal saline or 5% dextrose in water. Once clinical signs abate and as ionized Mg concentrations improve, a lower dose of 0.3 to 0.5 mEq/kg q24h can be used for an additional 3 to 5 days. Mg supplementation can be discontinued once ionized Mg concentrations are within the reference range. Ionized Mg concentrations should be monitored at least daily until normal; however, rapid Mg repletion will require more frequent monitoring of ionized Mg concentrations (i.e., every 6 to 12 hours). For the treatment of life-threatening ventricular arrhythmias due to hypomagnesemia, a dose of 0.15 to 0.3 mEq/kg of Mg diluted in normal saline or 5% dextrose in water can be slowly administered IV over 5 to 60 minutes. Side effects of overzealous intravenous Mg therapy include hypocalcemia, respiratory muscle weakness, hypotension, and AV and bundle branch blocks; therefore evaluation of blood pressure, as well as continuous ECG monitoring, should be performed during intravenous supplementation. Adverse effects are usually associated with intravenous boluses rather than continuous rate infusions.

Hypokalemia

Hypokalemia is defined as low circulating serum concentrations of K (usually < 3.5 mEq/L) in dogs and cats, whereby moderate hypokalemia refers to serum concentrations between 2.5 and 3 mEq/L and severe hypokalemia lower than 2.5 mEq/L. Hypokalemia is also a common electrolyte disturbance encountered in critically ill veterinary patients. Hypokalemia also commonly occurs during postobstructive diuresis that follows relief of urethral obstruction in cats with idiopathic lower urinary tract disease. Although not always as life threatening as its counterpart hyperkalemia, hypokalemia has adverse effects that can be nearly as significant.

Physiologic Role and Function

Normal total body K concentrations are essential for many physiologic processes involved in cell growth, enzymatic functions, metabolic pathways, neuromuscular function, and cardiac conduction. As the major intracellular cation, K plays a large role in maintaining intracellular volume. The ratio of intracellular to extracellular K is the primary determinant of the cellular resting membrane potential and plays a pivotal role in cellular excitability.

Distribution and Homeostasis

Approximately 98% to 99% of total body K is located intracellularly. The skeletal muscle serves as the primary reservoir, with the liver and erythrocytes providing secondary contributions.

The kidneys play the pivotal role in maintaining K balance because over 90% of ingested K is excreted by the kidneys. The main driving mechanisms behind K excretion are (1) the amount of sodium delivered to and reabsorbed in the distal tubules and (2) the effects of aldosterone and antidiuretic hormone. The gastrointestinal tract plays a more minor role in regulation of K balance, with passive absorption of dietary K occurring within the stomach and small intestines. The small intestines absorb nearly all the dietary K ingested, with very little excreted in the feces. Normally, only about 5% to 10% of body K is excreted via the gastrointestinal tract. During some chronic disease states in which renal excretion of K is impaired, the colon's role may become more important at maintaining extrarenal K balance through increasing its active K secretion. Conversely, if K stores are depleted, the colon can decrease K excretion.

BOX 56-2

Etiologies of Hypokalemia

Decreased Intake
Chronic dietary potassium deficiency
Potassium deplete intravenous fluids (e.g., 0.9% saline)

Cellular Translocation
Metabolic alkalosis or administration of exogenous bicarbonate
Insulin administration
Dextrose administration
Catecholamines
Endogenous (e.g., trauma, rattlesnake envenomation, congestive heart failure, myocardial infarction, endotoxemia, stress, hypothermia, pheochromocytoma)
Exogenous (e.g., parenteral, oral, and inhalational formulations of β_2-adrenergic agonists such as albuterol, methylxanthines, terbutaline)

Renal Losses
Polyuric conditions
Diabetes mellitus
Loop and thiazide diuretics
Postobstructive diuresis
Sodium-losing nephropathies (e.g., pyelonephritis, tubular interstitial cystitis)
Ketonuria (i.e., acetoacetate and β-hydroxybutyrate)
Penicillin metabolites
Metabolic alkalosis
Renal tubular acidosis
Hyperaldosteronism
Amphotericin B
Chronic renal disease
Peritoneal dialysis with a potassium-free dialysate

Gastrointestinal losses
Excessive vomiting
Excessive diarrhea
Decreased intestinal absorption
Ingestion of potassium-binding clay (e.g., cat litter)

Causes

Similar to those of Mg deficiency, the causes of hypokalemia can be divided into decreased dietary intake, excessive renal and gastrointestinal losses, and compartmental translocation (extracellular to intracellular) (Box 56-2). Poor dietary intake is an unusual cause of clinically significant hypokalemia, except for cases involving chronic dietary deficiency with concurrent administration of K-deficient intravenous fluids or parenteral nutrition.

Increased renal and gastrointestinal K losses are most commonly responsible for inducing profound hypokalemia. Renal losses usually result from increased tubular flow rates associated with polyuric conditions such as diabetes mellitus, administration of loop and thiazide diuretics, postobstructive diuresis, or sodium-losing nephropathies (e.g., pyelonephritis, tubular interstitial cystitis). The ketone bodies acetoacetate and β-hydroxybutyrate may alter the electrochemical gradient to favor K excretion; penicillin metabolites have been reported to have this same effect. Marked loss of hydrochloric acid through vomiting of gastric contents alone (i.e., pyloric obstruction) results in metabolic alkalosis that subsequently increases renal K excretion through a mechanism similar to that of ketone bodies. Renal tubular acidosis, hyperaldosteronism, and administration of amphotericin B have also been associated with hypokalemia due to increased K secretion. Although the exact pathogenesis is not fully understood, cats suffering from chronic renal disease commonly develop hypokalemia.

Gastrointestinal losses may involve gastric loss of K-rich fluids from excessive vomiting or intestinal loss and decreased intestinal absorption of dietary K from diarrhea. Another less common cause of hypokalemia is ingestion of K-binding clay found in some cat litter. This may be of particular concern in anemic cats with pica or dogs that have ingested large quantities of cat litter.

Transcellular shifting of K from the extracellular to intracellular space may contribute significantly to the development of clinical hypokalemia. Metabolic alkalosis or administration of exogenous bicarbonate shifts K intracellularly in response to hydrogen ions shifting extracellularly. Additionally, insulin and catecholamines promote cellular K uptake through activation of the Na/K-ATPase pump. Thus administration of exogenous insulin as well as release of endogenous insulin may induce hypokalemia in an animal that initially presents with serum K concentrations within the reference interval. Hypokalemia due to endogenous catecholamine release has been reported in patients with trauma, rattlesnake envenomation, congestive heart failure, myocardial infarction, endotoxemia, illness-induced stress, hypothermia, and pheochromocytomas. Similarly, administration of β_2-adrenergic agonists (e.g., albuterol, methylxanthines, terbutaline) may cause hypokalemia.

Clinical Signs

Clinical signs depend on the degree, rate of decline, and cause of hypokalemia. The predominant physiologic features involve cardiovascular, neuromuscular, metabolic, and renal disturbances. Most hypokalemia-induced cardiovascular and neuromuscular disorders are related to K's pivotal role in maintaining the resting membrane potential. Hypokalemia causes cell membranes to become hyperpolarized (i.e., less excitable), therefore impairing electrical conduction at the cell membrane and neuromuscular junction. As a result, skeletal and smooth muscle weakness develops that may result in ventroflexion of the head and neck; plantigrade stance; stiff, stilted gaits; ataxia; respiratory muscle paralysis; gastric atony and intestinal ileus; and potentially death. Cervical ventroflexion and ataxia are the most commonly reported clinical signs of hypokalemia in cats (see Chapter 54). As a general rule, clinically significant neuromuscular disorders seldom become apparent until serum K concentrations fall below 2.5 mEq/L. Severe hypokalemia (< 2.0 mEq/L) has been associated with development of rhabdomyolysis and muscle cramps accompanied by marked increases in creatine kinase.

Marked hypokalemia (< 2.5 mEq/L) may impair cardiac conduction due to prolongation of the action potential, increased automaticity, and prolongation of ventricular repolarization, all factors that may predispose a patient to various atrial and ventricular dysrhythmias (e.g., sinus bradycardia, paroxysmal atrial tachycardia, atrioventricular dissociation, ventricular tachyarrhythmias, ventricular fibrillation). ECG findings may include increased P wave amplitude, prolongation of the PR interval, prolongation and widening of the QT interval, decreased T wave amplitude, and depression of the ST segment. Additionally, the presence of hypokalemia may predispose the myocardium to become refractory to class I antiarrhythmic drugs (e.g., lidocaine, quinidine, procainamide), as well as exacerbate digitalis-induced cardiotoxicity.

Hypokalemia-induced renal dysfunction may manifest as impaired urinary concentrating ability, increased ammonia production, increased bicarbonate reabsorption, altered sodium reabsorption, and hypokalemic nephropathy. Polyuria and polydipsia are commonly associated with hypokalemia and result from impairment of renal tubule responsiveness to antidiuretic hormone and medullary washout. All the aforementioned clinical manifestations, except hypokalemic nephropathy, are potentially reversible with correction of serum K. Conversely, hypokalemic nephropathy involves swelling and vacuolization of the proximal tubules and resultant tubulointerstitial nephritis. Persistence of interstitial nephritis can lead to fibrosis, tubular atrophy, and subsequent irreversible renal dysfunction. Hypokalemic nephropathy has primarily been reported in both dogs and cats exposed to chronic K-deficient diets.

Diagnostics

Serum K concentration tends to reflect total body K status when acid-base status is normal; thus as a general rule serum K concentration should be assessed in light of acid-base status. Serum K concentrations may shift proportionally in response to alterations in acid-base status. Metabolic alkalemia may be associated with a low normal to decreased serum K concentration, and a metabolic acidosis may be associated with normal to increased serum K concentration. In most instances, the changes in serum K that are associated with changes in serum pH are usually mild; therefore significant changes in serum K cannot be attributed to acid-base disturbances and require further investigation. Apparently paradoxical changes are important. For example, metabolic acidemia should be associated with hyperkalemia; thus the presence of hypokalemia in the face of acidosis (e.g., diabetic ketoacidosis) may suggest the presence of a total body K depletion requiring immediate therapeutic intervention. Hypokalemia associated with hypochloremia and metabolic alkalosis in a patient presenting for vomiting is generally suggestive of a pyloric outflow obstruction.

Treatment

For a K imbalance to be successfully resolved, the underlying cause must be identified and addressed. Even with the primary issue addressed, most cases of hypokalemia require K supplementation, particularly if it relates to an ongoing disorder such as chronic renal failure in cats. K

TABLE 56-1

Intravenous Potassium Supplementation

Patient's Serum Potassium (mEq/L)	Potassium Chloride Added to Fluids (mEq/L)
3.6-5	20
3.1-3.5	30
2.6-3	40
2.1-2.5	50
≤2	60

may be supplemented intravenously and orally, and the route of administration in part depends on the acuteness of onset, the extent and severity of imbalance, the presence of clinical signs of hypokalemia, and the underlying condition. Examples of patients requiring parenteral rather than oral supplementation are those with continued gastrointestinal and renal losses from vomiting or diarrhea, as well as anorexic patients that do not tolerate enteral nutrition.

As a general rule, oral K supplementation is considered the safest and preferred route of administration. It is used primarily for patients with mild hypokalemia (3 to 3.4 mEq/L) that are eating voluntarily. Potassium gluconate is the most commonly used oral salt and is available as a powder, elixir, and tablet. The recommended starting dose for daily K supplementation is 1 to 3 mEq/kg q24h but divided and given q12h. Based on the patient's response to therapy and ability to maintain normal serum K concentration, the dose can be adjusted to a maintenance level of 1 mEq/kg q24h divided q12h.

Parenteral K supplementation usually entails adding potassium chloride (KCl) to intravenous fluids. In cases involving concurrent hypophosphatemia, potassium phosphate may be used instead. A simple empiric approach is to use the patient's serum K concentration as the basis for how many milliequivalents (mEq) of K should be added per liter of intravenous fluids (Table 56-1). The concentration is then adjusted based on the patient's response. The addition of KCl to 0.9% saline solutions exposes the patient to a supraphysiologic dose of chloride that very likely can lead to a hyperchloremic acidosis. For conditions in which serum K concentration is in the reference range but K loss is expected or in cases in which hypokalemia has already been corrected into the reference range, supplementation of 10 to 20 mEq KCl per liter of intravenous fluid solution is typically sufficient for maintaining serum K concentrations; however, serum K concentration should be checked periodically.

Due to life-threatening adverse cardiac effects, the rate at which intravenous K is administered is more critical than the total amount. The intravenous rate should not typically exceed 0.5 mEq/kg/hr. The single exception involves cases of severe hypokalemia (< 2 mEq/L) with associated life-threatening clinical signs (e.g., respiratory muscle paralysis, cardiac arrhythmias), when the rate may be gradually increased to 1 to 1.5 mEq/kg/hr as long as continuous ECG monitoring is provided and urine output is adequate. Serum K concentrations should be checked every 1 to 4 hours, depending on aggressiveness of supplementation. KCl may be administered subcutaneously; however, it is recommended not to exceed concentrations higher than 35 mEq/L. The administration of K subcutaneously may be painful.

Cats in general appear to be more susceptible to the effects of hypokalemia; therefore K supplementation in cats may require special considerations. A typical feline diet should contain a minimum of 0.3% K on a dry weight basis. For cats on urinary acidifying diets, the risk of developing hypokalemia may be increased if the diet contains less than 0.4% K. Cats suffering from urinary tract obstructions or diabetic ketoacidosis most often present initially with hyperkalemia; however, K concentrations can drop precipitously following treatment, particularly if cats are treated with low K-containing fluid solutions. Therefore it is imperative to monitor serum K concentrations vigilantly in these patients. Finally, in cases of canine and feline refractory hypokalemia, consider hypomagnesemia as a potential underlying cause. If the patient is hypomagnesemic, supplement Mg as outlined earlier.

References and Suggested Reading

Bateman S: Disorders of magnesium: magnesium deficit and excess. In DiBartola SP, editor: *Fluid, electrolyte, and acid-base disorders in small animal practice*, ed 4, St Louis, 2012, Elsevier Saunders, pp 212-229.

Bateman SW: Magnesium: a quick reference, *Vet Clin Small Anim* 38:467-470, 2008.

DiBartola SP et al: Development of chronic renal disease in cats fed a commercial diet, *J Am Vet Med Assoc* 202:744-751, 1993.

DiBartola SP, de Morais HA: Disorders of potassium: hypokalemia and hyperkalemia. In DiBartola SP, editor: *Fluid, electrolyte, and acid-base disorders in small animal practice*, ed 4, St Louis, 2012, Elsevier Saunders, pp 92-119.

Kogika MM, de Morais HA: Hypokalemia: a quick reference, *Vet Clin Small Anim* 38:481-484, 2008.

Martin LG: Magnesium disorders. In Silverstein DC, Hopper K, editors: *Small animal critical care medicine*, St. Louis, 2009, Saunders Elsevier, pp 240-243.

Martin LG et al: Abnormalities of serum magnesium in critically ill dogs: incidence and implications, *J Vet Emerg Crit Care* 4:15-20, 1994.

Norris CR, Nelson RW, Christopher MM: Serum total and ionized magnesium concentrations and urinary fractional excretion of magnesium in cats with diabetes mellitus and diabetic ketoacidosis, *J Am Vet Med Assoc* 215:1455-1459, 1999.

Riordan LL, Schaer M: Potassium disorders. In Silverstein DC, Hopper K, editors: *Small animal critical care medicine*, St. Louis, 2009, Saunders Elsevier, pp 229-233.

Schaer M: Therapeutic approach to electrolyte emergencies, *Vet Clin Small Anim* 38:513-533, 2008.

Toll J et al: Prevalence and incidence of serum magnesium abnormalities in hospitalized cats, *J Vet Intern Med* 16:217-221, 2002.

Willard M: Therapeutic approach to chronic electrolyte disorders, *Vet Clin Small Anim* 38:535-541, 2008.

CHAPTER 57

Obesity

ANGELA LUSBY WITZEL, *Knoxville, Tennessee*
CLAUDIA A. KIRK, *Knoxville, Tennessee*

Prevalence and Risk Factors

The incidence of obesity is reaching epidemic proportions worldwide, and the impact of excessive body fat on overall health is a topic at the forefront of human medicine. Obesity in companion animals has similar health consequences and should receive the same attention from practitioners as other chronic diseases. In dogs and cats a general definition for obesity is exceeding ideal body weight by 15% to 20% because of excess adipose tissue. Based on recent studies, approximately 35% to 40% and 25% to 35% of adult dogs and cats, respectively, are either overweight or obese.

Several risk factors are linked to obesity in dogs and cats. In both species the peak incidence occurs at middle age and is often associated with gonadectomy. Several studies in cats suggest that weight gain after spaying or neutering is a combination of slower metabolic rate and increased food intake. The metabolic changes caused by gonadectomy in dogs are not clear, but increased food consumption and decreased activity levels are suggested mechanisms for weight gain. Gender can also influence weight gain, with spayed female dogs and neutered male cats having an increased risk for excess body fat. Breed also plays a significant role in the development of obesity in dogs. In particular, the golden retriever, dachshund, Shetland sheepdog, Labrador retriever, cocker spaniel, and dalmatian are more likely to become overweight. Finally, environmental factors such as sedentary lifestyles and ad libitum feeding regimens contribute to both canine and feline obesity.

Physiology

Weight gain occurs when energy intake exceeds energy output. Certain diseases such as hypothyroidism and Cushing's disease can contribute to weight gain by decreasing the metabolic rate and energy output. However, most overweight dogs and cats do not have underlying endocrine disease, and weight gain is caused by excessive caloric intake with inadequate physical activity.

Until recently, adipose tissue was thought to be involved only in energy storage and insulation. The role of adipose tissue as an endocrine organ is now established, and hormones and proteins secreted from adipose cells, termed *adipokines,* have roles in appetite, inflammation, insulin sensitivity, and metabolism. To date, over 100 adipokines have been identified; some of the most intensely studied ones are leptin, adiponectin, and tumor necrosis factor-α (TNF-α). Leptin was the first adipokine identified and its main function is to regulate body fat mass through appetite and energy metabolism. As adipose tissue increases, more leptin is secreted from adipocytes. Leptin inhibits neurotransmitters that increase appetite and slow metabolism and stimulates neurons that decrease appetite and increase energy expenditure. Therefore, as individuals gain body fat, leptin promotes weight loss. Adiponectin is the most abundantly secreted adipokine in circulation. Although adipocytes are responsible for secreting adiponectin, hormone levels become paradoxically lower with increased fat mass. Adiponectin is closely associated with insulin sensitivity, independent of body fat mass. Numerous clinical and epidemiologic studies in humans associate low levels of adiponectin with chronic inflammatory states such as obesity, insulin resistance, type 2 diabetes mellitus, and cardiovascular disease. Therefore, as individuals gain weight, they have lower concentrations of adiponectin and higher disease risk. While initial adiponectin studies in cats demonstrate characteristics similar to those for humans, canine studies are variable and further research is needed. TNF-α is an inflammatory cytokine expressed by many cell types including macrophages, adipocytes, mast cells, neuronal cells, and fibroblasts. Obesity increases macrophage migration into adipose tissue, causing increased TNF-α expression in overweight individuals. One theory behind recruitment of monocytes and macrophages to expanding adipose tissue is that increased levels of adipocyte apoptosis and necrosis produce chemoattractant agents. One of the primary actions of adipose TNF-α is induction of local insulin resistance. In addition to inhibiting glucose entry into cells, TNF-α decreases uptake of free fatty acids (FFA) into adipocytes and promotes lipolysis and release of FFA into circulation. As a result, FFA levels increase in circulation and negatively affect insulin sensitivity in peripheral tissues.

Obesity affects systemic health not only by releasing adipokines but also through mechanical compression of organs and excessive strain on joints. Obesity has also been implicated in the cause or progression of neoplasia, cardiorespiratory disease, urogenital disease, endocrinopathies, metabolic derangements, dermatologic disease, and orthopedic disorders (Box 57-1).

Diagnosis of Body Condition

Many methods are available to evaluate the body condition of dogs and cat, but not all are practical or cost effective. Body condition scoring (BCS) is a simple method for assessing a patient's body condition and correlates

BOX 57-1

Diseases Associated with Obesity in Dogs and Cats

Endocrinopathies
- Hypothyroidism
- Hyperadrenocorticism
- Diabetes mellitus

Orthopedic disorders
- Osteoarthritis
- Cranial cruciate ligament rupture
- Humeral condylar fractures
- Lameness

Metabolic alterations
- Insulin resistance
- Glucose intolerance
- Hepatic lipidosis (cats)
- Hyperlipidemia/dyslipidemia

Cardiorespiratory disease
- Tracheal collapse
- Laryngeal paralysis
- Brachycephalic airway obstruction syndrome
- Dyspnea
- Hypertension

Dermatologic abnormalities
- Dry, flaky skin
- Feline acne
- Alopecia
- Seborrhea

Neoplasia
- Mammary
- Transitional cell carcinoma

Urogenital system
- Urolithiasis (calcium oxalate)
- Urethral sphincter mechanism incompetence
- Dystocia
- Urinary tract infection

Functional alterations
- Decreased immune function
- Increased anesthetic risk
- Heat intolerance
- Decreased life span

strongly with other techniques used to estimate body fat. Using visual observation and palpation, a BCS is assigned using either a 5-point or a 9-point scale (Figure 57-1). The goals of assessing body condition are to estimate proportion of body fat, irrespective of weight; to help assess risk for obesity-related disease or physical dysfunction; and to monitor changes in body fat over time. BCS can also be used to estimate a patient's percent body fat, which is useful for determining weight-loss goals (see Figure 57-1). Unfortunately, the rising rate of obesity among dogs and cats has led to a higher proportion of morbidly obese pets. The 9-point and 5-point BCS systems were designed to assess animals below 45% and 40% body fat, respectively. It is not uncommon to see dogs and cats with body fat percentages up to 60%. This observation led to the development of a new method for assessing body fat percentage in veterinary patients. A body fat index system has

been designed that uses body descriptions and palpation methods similar to traditional BCS but extends to patients up to 70% body fat (Figures 57-2 and 57-3).

Treatment

The concept behind the treatment of obesity is simple: decrease caloric intake and increase physical activity. However, management of real-life cases is rarely so straightforward. Practical issues such as dietary restrictions, owner compliance, and multiple-animal households can make the process of weight loss more challenging. By taking a thorough history before prescribing a weight-loss strategy, the clinician addresses issues early and minimizes owner frustration. Also, having an accurate description of the current diet, including table scraps, helps in determining current caloric intake and understanding owners' perceptions and beliefs about food. Planning a weight-loss strategy has five main steps:

1. Estimate current body condition and body fat percentage (see Figures 57-1 to 57-3).
2. Estimate ideal body weight. This estimation is often based on clinical experience; a weight history can also be useful in determining ideal weight since most animals are close to ideal at the onset of maturity (approximately 1 year of age). The estimated body fat percentage from BCS can also be used to determine ideal body weight. For example, if a 100-pound dog is 45% body fat, then it is approximately 55% lean tissue. Take the current weight and multiply by the percent of lean tissue to estimate body weight at 0% body fat (100 pounds × 0.55 = 55 pounds). Ideally dogs and cats should be about 20% body fat (80% lean). The estimated body weight at 0% body fat is then divided by the percent lean mass you want to achieve. Using the example above, 55 pounds/0.80 = 68.75 pounds for ideal body weight for the dog in question.
3. Determine the current caloric intake through dietary history. This step is important because animals vary in their metabolic rate and those with a slow metabolism may already be eating less food than would be calculated. Calculate desired caloric intake (see later).
4. Implement an exercise plan.

Choosing an Appropriate Diet

Weight-loss diets for dogs and cats typically fall into two categories: over-the-counter light and lean products or prescription weight-loss diets. Although over-the-counter products may be sufficient in animals that are mildly overweight, prescription weight-loss diets are recommended for moderate to substantial weight loss. Owners often ask if they can simply reduce the amount fed of the animal's current diet. Switching to a diet designed for weight loss is more desirable. Maintenance diets are calorically denser, with higher levels of fat than calorie-restricted diets. In addition, the components of maintenance foods are balanced to provide adequate amounts of nutrients when standard feeding guidelines

5-pt scale	9-pt scale	% body fat	Body condition scoring	Dogs	Cats
1	1	≤5	**Emaciated**—ribs and bony prominences are visible from a distance. No palpable body fat. Obvious abdominal tuck and loss of muscle mass.	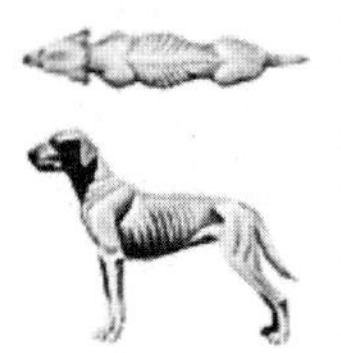	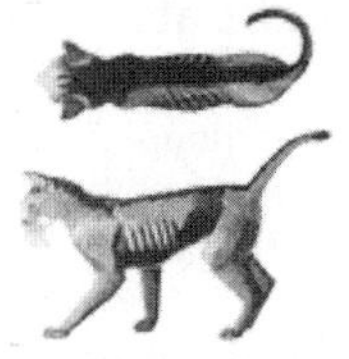
2	2	6-9	**Very thin**—ribs and bony prominences visible. Minimal loss of muscle mass, but no palpable fat.	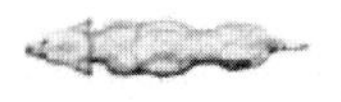	
	3	10-14	**Thin**—ribs easily palpable, tops of lumbar are visible. Obvious waist and abdominal tuck.	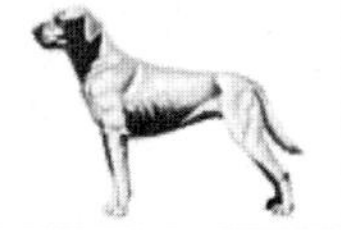	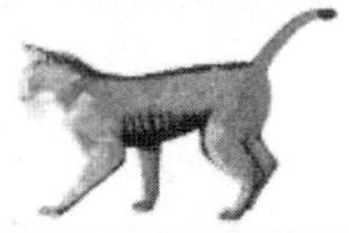
3	4	15-19	**Lean**—ribs easily palpable, waist visible from above. Abdominal tuck present. Abdominal fat pad is absent in cats.	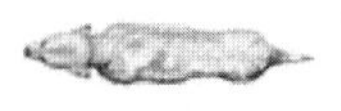	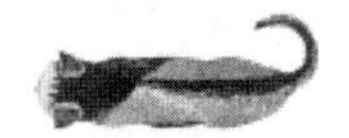
	5	20-24	**Ideal**—ribs palpable without excess fat covering. Waist and abdominal tuck present in dogs. Cats have a waist and a minimal abdominal fat pad.	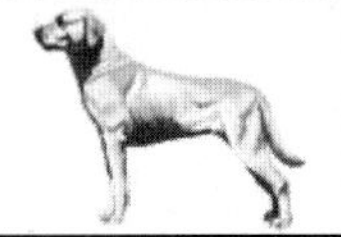	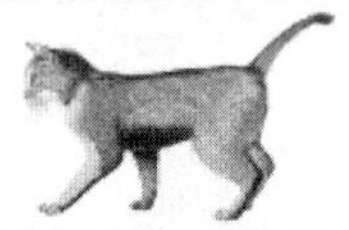
4	6	25-29	**Slightly overweight**—ribs have slight excess fat coverring. Waist is discernible from above, but not obvious. Abdominal tuck still present in dogs. Abdominal fat pad is apparent, but not obvious in cats.	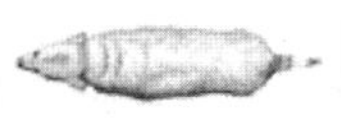	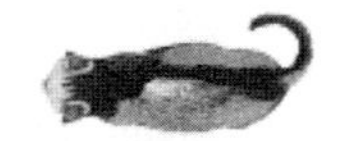
	7	30-34	**Overweight**—difficult to palpate ribs. **Dogs:** fat deposits over lumbar area and tail base. Abdominal tuck may be present, but waist is absent. **Cats:** moderate abdominal fat pad and rounding of the abdomen.	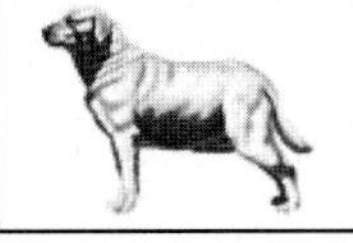	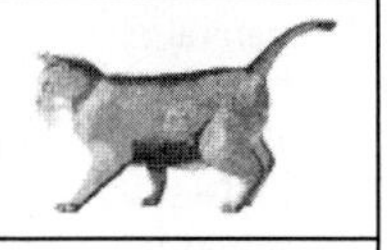
5	8	35-39	**Obese**—ribs not palpable and abdomen may be rounded. **Dogs:** heavy fat deposits over lumbar and base of tail. No abdominal tuck or waist. **Cats:** prominent abdominal fat pad and lumbar fat deposits.	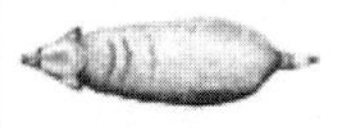	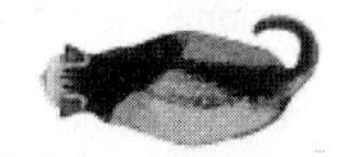
	9	40-45+	**Morbidly obese**—**Dogs:** large fat deposits over thorax, tail base, and spine with abdominal distension. **Cats:** heavy fat deposits over lumbar area, face, and limbs. Large abdominal fat pad and rounded abdomen.	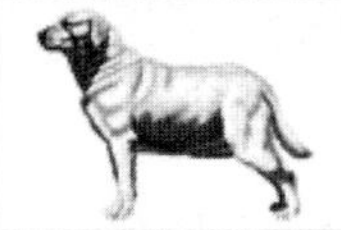	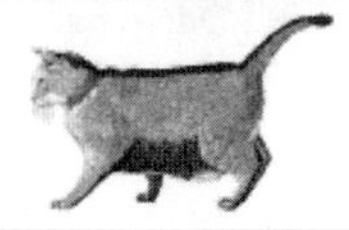

Figure 57-1 Description of body condition scoring systems and their relationship to body fat percentage. (Images in the table were reproduced and used by permission from Drs. Foster and Smith, Inc.)

are followed. When the amount of a maintenance diet is significantly reduced below feeding recommendations, deficiencies in protein and other nutrients can occur. Diets formulated for weight loss are balanced to provide both adequate nutrients and energy restriction. In cases in which the diet cannot be changed because of medical conditions, the quantity of the current diet can be reduced, but review of total intake should be done to ensure adequate nutrient intake.

Most canine weight-reduction diets rely on high levels of fiber, air, or moisture to reduce energy density. It has been proposed that high levels of fiber increase satiety by allowing the dog to ingest more food while receiving fewer calories. Although some evidence suggests that high levels of fiber do not affect satiety in dogs, other studies support the effect of diet bulk (i.e., fiber) in lowering total energy intake. Following the trend in human dieting, low-carbohydrate, high-protein diets have also been proposed for use in dogs. Current evidence suggests limited benefit to using these diets for weight loss in dogs. In general, it appears that weight loss occurs with caloric restriction, regardless of the protein or fiber content. However, the proportion of fat loss over lean tissue loss is greater in dogs when fed high-protein foods compared with maintenance protein levels.

In recent years there has been much debate about the most appropriate diets for feline weight control. Cats are strict carnivores and naturally consume very

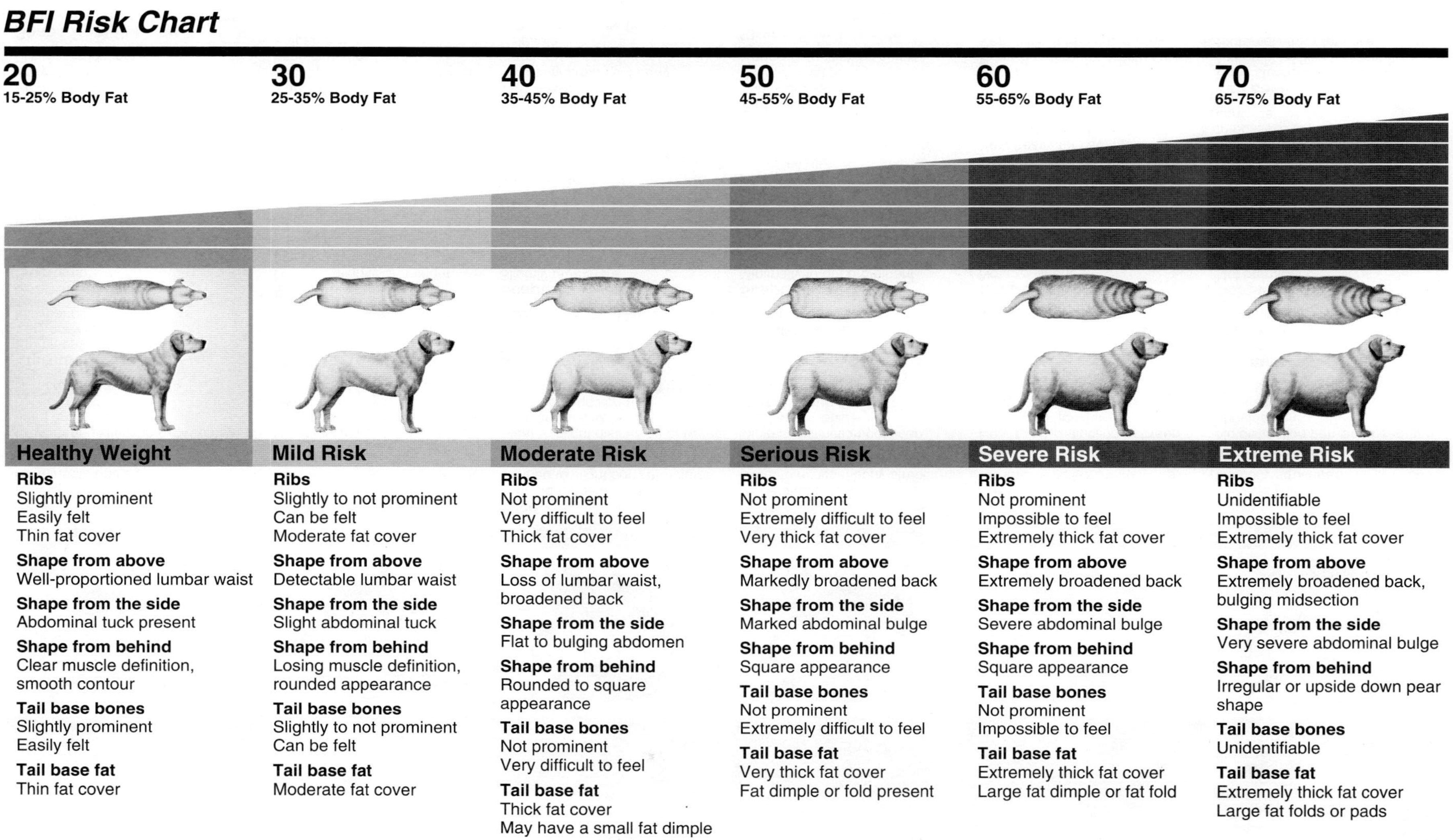

BFI Risk Chart

	20 15-25% Body Fat	**30** 25-35% Body Fat	**40** 35-45% Body Fat	**50** 45-55% Body Fat	**60** 55-65% Body Fat	**70** 65-75% Body Fat
	Healthy Weight	**Mild Risk**	**Moderate Risk**	**Serious Risk**	**Severe Risk**	**Extreme Risk**
Ribs	Slightly prominent Easily felt Thin fat cover	Slightly to not prominent Can be felt Moderate fat cover	Not prominent Very difficult to feel Thick fat cover	Not prominent Extremely difficult to feel Very thick fat cover	Not prominent Impossible to feel Extremely thick fat cover	Unidentifiable Impossible to feel Extremely thick fat cover
Shape from above	Well-proportioned lumbar waist	Detectable lumbar waist	Loss of lumbar waist, broadened back	Markedly broadened back	Extremely broadened back	Extremely broadened back, bulging midsection
Shape from the side	Abdominal tuck present	Slight abdominal tuck	Flat to bulging abdomen	Marked abdominal bulge	Severe abdominal bulge	Very severe abdominal bulge
Shape from behind	Clear muscle definition, smooth contour	Losing muscle definition, rounded appearance	Rounded to square appearance	Square appearance	Square appearance	Irregular or upside down pear shape
Tail base bones	Slightly prominent Easily felt	Slightly to not prominent Can be felt	Not prominent Very difficult to feel	Not prominent Extremely difficult to feel	Not prominent Impossible to feel	Unidentifiable
Tail base fat	Thin fat cover	Moderate fat cover	Thick fat cover May have a small fat dimple	Very thick fat cover Fat dimple or fold present	Extremely thick fat cover Large fat dimple or fat fold	Extremely thick fat cover Large fat folds or pads

Figure 57-2 Body fat index (BFI) system for estimating percentage of body fat in dogs. (Courtesy Hill's Pet Nutrition, Inc.)

BFI Risk Chart

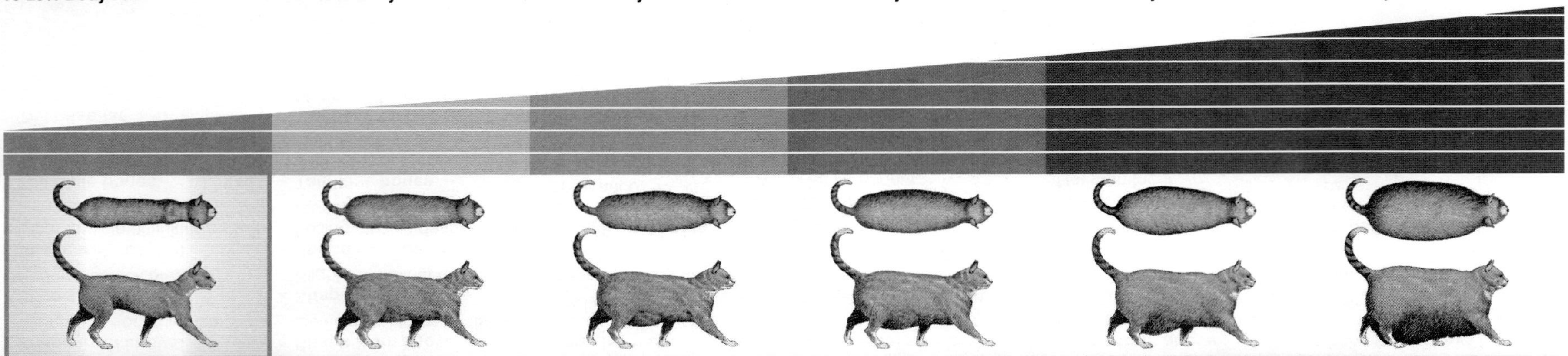

	Healthy Weight 20 (16-25% Body Fat)	Mild Risk 30 (26-35% Body Fat)	Moderate Risk 40 (36-45% Body Fat)	Serious Risk 50 (46-55% Body Fat)	Severe Risk 60 (56-65% Body Fat)	Extreme Risk 70 (65% Body Fat)
Face	Minimal fat cover; Prominent bony structures	Slight fat cover; Defined bony structures	Slight to moderate fat cover; Defined to slight bony structures	Moderate fat cover; Slight to minimal bony structures	Thick fat cover; Minimal to no bony structures	Very thick fat cover; No bony structures
Head and neck	Prominent distinction between head and shoulder; Loose scruff; No scruff fat	Clear distinction between head and shoulder; Loose scruff; Slight scruff fat	Clear to slight distinction between head and shoulder; Loose to snug scruff; Slight to moderate scruff fat	Minimal distinction between head and shoulder; Loose to snug scruff; Moderate scruff fat	Poor to no distinction between head and shoulder; Snug to tight scruff; Very thick scruff fat	No distinction between head and shoulder; Tight scruff; Very thick scruff fat
Sternum	Prominent; Very easy to palpate; Minimal pectoral fat	Defined, slightly prominent; Easy to palpate; Slight to moderate pectoral fat	Minimally prominent; Palpable; Moderate pectoral fat	Poorly defined; Difficult to palpate; Thick pectoral fat	Not prominent; Extremely difficult to palpate; Extremely thick pectoral fat	Not prominent; Impossible to palpate; Extreme pectoral fat
Scapula	Prominent; Very easy to palpate	Defined, slightly prominent; Easy / very easy to palpate	Slightly prominent; Easy to palpate	Minimally to not prominent; Palpable	Not prominent; Difficult to palpate	Not prominent; Impossible to palpate
Ribs	Prominent; Very easy to palpate	Not prominent; Easy to palpate	Not prominent; Palpable	Not prominent; Difficult to palpate	Not prominent; Extremely difficult to impossible to palpate	Not prominent; Impossible to palpate
Abdomen	Loose abdominal skin; Easy to palpate abdominal contents	Loose abdominal skin with minimal fat; Easy to palpate abdominal contents	Obvious skin fold with moderate fat; Easy to palpate abdominal contents	Heavy fat pad; Difficult to palpate abdominal contents	Very heavy fat pad; indistinct from abdominal fat; Impossible to palpate abdominal contents	Extremely heavy fat pad; indistinct from abdominal fat; Impossible to palpate abdominal contents
Tail base	Prominent bony structure; Easy to palpate; Minimal fat cover	Slightly to minimally prominent bony structure; Palpable; Slight fat cover	Minimally prominent bony structure; Palpable; Slight to moderate fat cover	Poorly defined bony structure; Difficult to palpate; Moderate to thick fat cover	Bony structure not prominent; Very difficult to palpate; Very thick fat cover	Bony structure not prominent; Extremely difficult to palpate; Extremely thick fat cover
Shape from the side	Moderate to slight abdominal tuck	No abdominal tuck	Slight abdominal bulge	Moderate abdominal bulge	Severe abdominal bulge	Very severe abdominal bulge
Shape from above	Marked hourglass	Slight hourglass / lumbar waist	Lumbar waist	Broadened back	Severely broadened back	Extremely broadened back

Figure 57-3 Body fat index (BFI) system for estimating percentage of body fat in cats. (Courtesy Hill's Pet Nutrition, Inc.)

high-protein diets with few carbohydrates. Therefore many are advocating low-carbohydrate weight-loss diets for cats instead of more traditional high-fiber diets. Dietary protein is a potent stimulator for the release of satiety hormones. Prescription diets currently marketed for feline weight loss all contain similar levels of protein but vary in their fat and carbohydrate content. Studies have shown that low-carbohydrate diets do have beneficial effects on insulin sensitivity and diabetic control (Bennett et al, 2006). However, a study evaluating only weight loss in cats did not detect any differences between low-carbohydrate and high-fiber diets (Michel et al, 2005). While canned diets appear to increase satiety in cats undergoing weight loss, a comparison of low-carbohydrate versus high-carbohydrate canned diets showed no difference in owner-perceived satiety (Cline et al, 2012). Therefore cats should ideally be fed a high-protein canned diet for weight loss. High-fiber diets for dogs also appear to increase satiety, although the benefits of canned versus dry diets are unclear.

Estimating Desired Caloric Intake

As stated previously, obesity is the consequence of energy intake exceeding energy output. Energy output can also be called the daily energy requirement (DER). It comprises several components, but the resting energy requirement (RER) and the exercise energy requirement (EER) are the two largest contributors. The RER is the energy needed to maintain normal metabolic functions (e.g., blood flow, cellular metabolism, respiration) and is closely correlated with lean body mass. The RER typically accounts for 60% to 80% of the total DER. The EER is the energy exerted through muscular activity and exercise and accounts for roughly 10% to 20% of DER in inactive humans. Compared with lean mass, fat mass is metabolically inactive and contributes little to the RER. Therefore estimations of RERs should be based on ideal rather than current weight using the following formula:

$$RER = 70 \, (BW_{kg}{}^{0.75})$$

If a scientific calculator is not available, the linear equation achieves similar results in animals over 2 kg and less than 30 kg:

$$RER = (30 \times BW_{kg}) + 70$$

The DERs needed to achieve weight loss are then estimated using the RER. The result is the total number of calories that should be fed in a 24-hour period. (Calculations are based on ideal weight.)

$$Canine \; DER \; for \; weight \; loss = 1 \; to \; 1.2 \times RER$$

$$Feline \; DER \; for \; weight \; loss = 0.8 \times RER$$

Careful monitoring of patients should occur during any weight loss program. The goal is to achieve 1% to 2% loss of body weight per week. Although the formulas above are useful for initial estimations, some animals, especially cats, may require further restriction to achieve

weight loss. Reducing energy by 10% of calories every 2 weeks until adequate weight loss is achieved may be required.

Case example: A 7-year-old, male, castrated beagle mix weighing 14 kg with a BCS of 8/9 and an ideal weight of approximately 11 kg arrives at your clinic for a weight loss program. First, his RER is calculated based on *ideal* weight (11 kg) = 70 $(11_{kg}{}^{0.75})$ = 422 kcal/day. You decide to feed at RER, so a lifestage factor of 1 is chosen. So then 422 kcal × 1 = 422 kcal/day = DER for weight loss. Two weeks later, the patient returns weighing 10.5 kg. To calculate the rate of weight loss, you take the amount lost (0.5 kg) and divide by the initial weight (0.5 kg/11kg = 0.04 × 100 = 4%). Next, divide by the number of weeks you are assessing (4%/2 weeks = 2% weight loss per week).

Role of Exercise

Increasing physical activity is an intuitive part of any weight loss program, yet exercise is often overlooked in companion animals. In dogs a 20- to 30-minute walk 3 to 4 days a week is a good method for burning calories. It may be necessary to address any medical issues that limit a pet's exercise, such as respiratory disease or osteoarthritis. Having owners play games such as fetch or hide-and-seek using toys or treats can also increase activity. Also, any limitations that owners may have that could affect exercising their pets should be discussed and creative, helpful suggestions offered. Creativity becomes even more valuable when trying to increase the physical activity levels of cats. Indoor cats lead more sedentary lives than outdoor cats, and special efforts must be made to increase their activity. Owners can begin by changing the cat's environment; window hammocks, platforms, and cat furniture provide more vertical space for cats to explore. Barriers such as baby gates force cats to exert more effort while moving around the house. Meals can be served on surfaces that require cats to climb. Toys that hide kibble that requires effort to extract can occupy some cats. In addition, owner interaction in the form of play can be very effective. Even increasing play or exercise for just 10 minutes a day can be highly effective in promoting weight loss.

Future Role of Pharmacotherapy in Veterinary Obesity Management

Pharmacologic therapies for the treatment of obesity can target several areas. They can decrease energy consumption through modulation of satiety signals or blocking of intestinal absorption, increase energy expenditure by increasing metabolic rates, or redistribute stored energy in adipose tissue to more metabolically active tissue such as muscle. Currently only a handful of drugs are approved for weight loss in humans. Sibutramine (Meridia) exerts anorectic effects by inhibiting serotonin/norepinephrine reuptake. Orlistat (Xenical) increases fecal fat excretion. Phentermine (Adipex-P) increases metabolism in a manner similar to amphetamines. In dogs and cats, drugs such as sibutramine that increase serotonin availability are associated with significant adverse side effects. Orlistat has not been studied in cats, but in dogs only modest weight loss was achieved and treatment complications included leakage of colonic contents with perianal soiling. Phentermine has not been evaluated in dogs or cats.

Pharmaceutical induction of canine weight loss is now possible following the 2007 introduction of dirlotapide (Slentrol) and mitratapide (Yarvitan). These drugs are classified as microsomal triglyceride transfer protein (MTP) inhibitors. MTPs are endoplasmic reticulum proteins expressed predominantly in intestinal and liver tissue where they play a pivotal role in the assembly of lipids to apoprotein B (apoB). Lipid assembly is required for export of lipoproteins across cell membranes and transport of lipids in the circulation. The MTP inhibitors for canine weight loss are selective for the intestine, thereby blocking intraluminal transport of fat across the enterocyte. Turnover of lipid-laden enterocytes results in loss of fat (and calories) into the feces. More importantly, intestinal lipid accumulation appears to increase release of potent satiety signals from the gut (e.g., pancreatic peptide YY [PYY]) and inhibition of voluntary food intake. Up to 90% of the canine weight loss has been attributed to appetite control. These drugs are an effective tool for canine weight loss. However, if feeding and exercise plans are not initiated, dogs will regain weight when treatment is stopped. Dirlotapide is most useful in cases in which owners cannot control their dog's food intake. It can also be an effective motivating tool for owners by demonstrating how much food their dog actually needs to eat and by allowing them to see their pet's improved quality of life following weight loss. The selectivity of MTP inhibitors varies by species. Dirlotapide and mitratapide are not to be used in humans or cats due to the possible risk of hepatic lipid accumulation.

References and Suggested Reading

Armstrong PJ, Lusby (Witzel) A: Clinical importance of canine and feline obesity. In Towell T, editor: *Practical weight management in dogs and cats*, Ames IA, 2011, Iowa State University Press.

Bennett N et al: Comparison of a low-carbohydrate–low-fiber diet and a moderate carbohydrate–high-fiber diet in the management of feline diabetes mellitus, *J Feline Med Surg* 8:73, 2006.

Butterwick RF, Markwell PJ: Effect of amount and type of dietary fiber on food intake in energy-restricted dogs, *Am J Vet Res* 58:272, 1997.

Cline M et al: Comparison of high fiber and low carbohydrate diets on owner-perceived satiety of cats during weight loss, *Am J Applied Vet Sci* 7:218, 2012.

Diez M et al: Weight loss in obese dogs: evaluation of a high protein, low-carbohydrate diet, *J Nutr* 132:1685S, 2002.

Fettman MJ: Effects of neutering on body weight, metabolic rate and glucose tolerance of domestic cats, *Res Vet Sci* 62:131, 1997.

Jeusette I et al: Effect of ovariectomy and ad libitum feeding on body composition, thyroid status, ghrelin, and leptin plasma concentrations in female dogs, *J Anim Physiol Anim Nutr* 90:12, 2006.

Kirk CA et al: Influence of dirlotapide, a microsomal triglyceride transfer protein inhibitor, on the digestibility of a dry expanded diet in adult dogs, *J Vet Pharmacol Ther* 30s1:66, 2007.

Koerner A, Kratzsch J, Kiess W: Adipocytokines: leptin—the classical, resistin—the controversial, adiponectin—the promising, and more to come, *Best Pract Res Clin Endocrinol Metab* 19:525, 2005.

Li J et al: Discovery of potent and orally active MTP inhibitors as potential anti-obesity agents, *Bioorg Med Chem Lett* 16:3039, 2006.

Lund EM et al: Prevalence and risk factors for obesity in adult cats from private US veterinary practices, *Intern J Appl Res Vet Med* 3:88, 2005.

Lund EM et al: Prevalence and risk factors for obesity in adult dogs from private US veterinary practices, *Intern J App Res Vet Med* 4:177, 2006.

Michel KE et al: Impact of time-limited feeding and dietary carbohydrate content on weight loss in group-housed cats, *J Feline Med Surg* 7:349, 2005.

Wei A et al: Influence of a high-protein diet on energy balance in obese cats allowed ad libitum access to food, *J Anim Physiol Anim Nutri* 95(3):359-367, 2011.

CHAPTER 58

Approach to Canine Hyperlipidemia

PANAGIOTIS G. XENOULIS, *College Station, Texas*

Hyperlipidemia refers to an increased concentration of lipids in the blood (serum or plasma). Specifically, an increased blood concentration of triglycerides is referred to as hypertriglyceridemia, while an increased blood concentration of cholesterol is referred to as hypercholesterolemia. In contrast to the condition in humans, hyperlipidemia in dogs has been traditionally considered relatively benign; therefore clinical experience with and research regarding canine hyperlipidemia are in their infancy. In the last decade, several studies in both humans and dogs have associated specific forms of hyperlipidemia with a much wider range of diseases than previously thought. Therefore canine hyperlipidemia has emerged as an important clinical condition that requires a detailed diagnostic approach and appropriate treatment.

Causes of Canine Hyperlipidemia

Table 58-1 presents a list of causes of canine hyperlipidemia (Xenoulis and Steiner, 2010). Postprandial hyperlipidemia is physiologic and typically resolves within 7 to 12 hours after a meal. Therefore determination of serum lipid concentrations should always follow a fast of at least 12 and ideally 15 hours.

Persistent fasting hyperlipidemia is abnormal and can be either primary or secondary to other conditions, diseases, or drug administration. Secondary hyperlipidemia is the most common pathologic form of hyperlipidemia in dogs. Most often, canine hyperlipidemia is the result of obesity or an endocrine disorder such as hypothyroidism, diabetes mellitus, or hyperadrenocorticism. Protein-losing nephropathy and cholestasis are relatively common causes of hypercholesterolemia. Hyperlipidemia has also been traditionally thought to be the result of naturally occurring pancreatitis in dogs, although this has not been convincingly shown.

Primary lipid abnormalities are usually, but not always, associated with certain breeds (see Table 58-1). Depending on the breed, the prevalence of a primary lipid abnormality can vary widely. Also, the geographic region of the canine population tested seems to play an important role due to genetic differences. Primary hyperlipidemia is very common in miniature schnauzers in the United States (with >30% of this breed being affected based on one study) and it was the first breed-related primary lipid disorder described in dogs. It is typically characterized by hypertriglyceridemia; hypercholesterolemia may also be

present, but it is not found in all affected miniature schnauzers and is always present in association with hypertriglyceridemia. Primary hyperlipidemia has also been reported to occur in other dog breeds (see Table 58-1).

Clinical Importance of Hyperlipidemia in Dogs

Although hyperlipidemia itself does not seem to lead directly to the development of any major clinical signs, it has been shown to be associated with the development of other diseases that are clinically important and potentially life threatening (Table 58-2).

Hyperlipidemia, and more specifically hypertriglyceridemia, has long been suspected as a causative factor of canine pancreatitis (see Chapter 137). Two recent clinical studies, each using a different methodologic approach, provided evidence that hypertriglyceridemia, especially if severe (>800 mg/dl in one study), is a risk factor for and may cause pancreatitis in miniature schnauzers (Xenoulis et al, 2010; Xenoulis et al, 2011b). Therefore, in dogs with severe hypertriglyceridemia and pancreatitis, the first disorder should be considered the cause of the latter rather than vice versa and treatment of pancreatitis in those cases should always include measures to control hypertriglyceridemia.

In a recent study, primary hypertriglyceridemia was found to be associated with increased serum hepatic enzyme activities in clinically healthy miniature schnauzers (Xenoulis et al, 2008). Although in that particular study the cause of the increased serum hepatic enzyme activities was not determined, clinical studies and anecdotal observations suggest that two hepatic disorders are associated with hypertriglyceridemia in dogs: diffuse hepatocellular steatosis and gallbladder mucocele. Hyperlipidemia-associated hepatocellular steatosis (or hepatic lipidosis) has been anecdotally reported and is characterized by hepatocellular accumulation of triglycerides. Gallbladder mucoceles (see Web Chapter 46) have been commonly reported in dog breeds that are predisposed to primary hyperlipidemia (e.g., miniature schnauzers and Shetland sheepdogs). Mature gallbladder mucoceles might lead to biliary obstruction, cholecystitis, or rupture of the gallbladder.

Another potential complication of hypertriglyceridemia in dogs is insulin resistance. Almost 30% of miniature schnauzers with primary hypertriglyceridemia had

261

TABLE 58-1

Causes of Hyperlipidemia in Dogs

	Type of Lipid Abnormality	Comments
Postprandial Hyperlipidemia*	HTG (rarely HCH)	Increases are typically mild and last < 15 hours Most common cause of hyperlipidemia
High-Fat Diets	HTG and/or HCH	Fat content must be very high (typically >50%) to cause fasting hyperlipidemia
Secondary Hyperlipidemia		
Endocrine disease		
Diabetes mellitus*	HTG (mainly) and/or HCH	HTG and HCH can range from mild to marked; present in >50% of cases
Hypothyroidism*	HTG and/or HCH	HTG and HCH can range from mild to marked; present in >75% of cases
Hyperadrenocorticism*	HTG and/or HCH	HTG and HCH can range from mild to marked
Pancreatitis*	HTG and/or HCH	Both HTG and HCH are typically mild if other causes of hyperlipidemia are not present; present in ~30% of cases
Obesity*	HTG and/or HCH	HTG and HCH can range from mild to marked; present in >25% of cases
Protein-losing nephropathy*	HCH	HCH is part of the nephrotic syndrome; HCH is usually mild
Cholestasis*	HTG and/or HCH	Increases are usually mild
Hepatic insufficiency*	HTG and/or HCH	Increases are usually mild
Lymphoma	HTG with or without HCH	Hyperlipidemia might persist despite treatment
Leishmania infantum infection	HTG and HCH	Increases are typically mild if present
Parvoviral enteritis	HTG	HTG is typically mild if present
Hypernatremia?	HTG and HCH	Based on a case report and evidence from human medicine
Drugs*		
Glucocorticoids	HTG and/or HCH	Increases can range from mild to marked
Phenobarbital	HTG	HTG can range from mild to marked; present in >30% of cases
Estrogen/progesterone?	HTG and/or HCH	Anecdotal
Primary Hyperlipidemia		
Miniature schnauzer*	HTG with or without HCH	HTG can range from mild to marked; HCH may be mild to moderate; present in >30% of all dogs in the United States; prevalence increases with age
Beagle*	HTG and/or HCH	Increases are usually mild to moderate
Shetland sheepdog*	HCH with or without HTG	HCH might be marked; HTG is typically mild; present in >40% of dogs in Japan
Doberman pinscher	HCH	HCH is usually mild
Rottweiler	HCH	HCH is usually mild
Briard	HCH	HCH in briards has only been reported in the United Kingdom
Rough-coated collie	HCH	Reported in a single family in the United Kingdom
Pyrenees mountain dog	HCH	HCH is usually mild

*Indicates common causes.
HTG, Hypertriglyceridemia; *HCH,* hypercholesterolemia; *?,* this cause is not well documented or is questionable.

evidence of insulin resistance in one study (Xenoulis et al, 2011a). This might have an implication on glycemic control in dogs with hypertriglyceridemia and concurrent diabetes mellitus or other diseases that cause insulin resistance.

Finally, several other conditions have been reported or suspected to be consequences of hyperlipidemia in dogs. These include atherosclerosis, ocular disease (e.g., lipemia retinalis, lipemic aqueous, lipid keratopathy,

solid intraocular xanthogranuloma), seizures, and cutaneous xanthomata or lipomas.

Diagnostic Approach to Canine Hyperlipidemia

Hyperlipidemia is typically diagnosed by measuring fasting serum triglyceride and cholesterol concentrations. Because hyperlipidemia is an important diagnostic clue

TABLE 58-2

Possible Consequences and Complications of Hyperlipidemia

Disorder	Type of Lipid Abnormality Responsible
Pancreatitis	HTG
Hepatobiliary disease	
Vacuolar hepatopathy	HTG
Lipidosis	HTG
Biliary mucocele	HTG/HCH
Insulin resistance	HTG
Ocular disease	
Lipemia retinalis	HTG
Lipemic aqueous	HTG
Lipid keratopathy	HTG
Intraocular xanthogranuloma	HTG
Arcus lipoides corneae	HTG/HCH
Seizures	HTG
Lipomas	HTG
Atherosclerosis	HCH

HTG, Hypertriglyceridemia; *HCH,* hypercholesterolemia.

for dogs with secondary hyperlipidemia and often the only abnormality in dogs with primary hyperlipidemia, measurement of serum triglyceride and cholesterol concentrations should be part of every routine chemistry panel. Moderate and severe hypertriglyceridemia (but not mild hypertriglyceridemia or hypercholesterolemia) can be diagnosed on the basis of inspection of serum or plasma that has turbid or lactescent appearance. However, even in those cases, measurement of serum triglyceride and cholesterol concentration is mandatory in order to get an accurate picture of the severity and spectrum of hyperlipidemia.

After hyperlipidemia has been diagnosed, it must be determined whether the patient has a primary or a secondary lipid disorder. If hyperlipidemia is secondary, the specific condition responsible for causing hyperlipidemia should be diagnosed and treated. Thus specific diagnostic investigations should be performed in order to diagnose or rule out specific diseases that can cause secondary hyperlipidemia. If secondary hyperlipidemia is excluded, a tentative diagnosis of a primary lipid disorder can be made.

In the diagnostic effort, a detailed history should be obtained and physical examination performed first. This is crucial because dogs with secondary hyperlipidemia typically show clinical signs of the primary disease (e.g., obesity, polyuria and polydipsia in dogs with diabetes mellitus or hyperadrenocorticism, hypoactivity and hair loss in dogs with hypothyroidism), which can prioritize the selection of diagnostic tests and lead the way toward an appropriate diagnostic plan. Dogs with primary

hyperlipidemia may or may not have clinical signs; as mentioned earlier, primary hyperlipidemia per se is unlikely to cause any clinical signs, and therefore many dogs with hyperlipidemia are asymptomatic. However, diseases that develop as a result of hyperlipidemia can lead to various clinical signs (see the section on Clinical Importance of Hyperlipidemia in Dogs). Dogs with hyperlipidemia should have at least a complete blood count (CBC), chemistry panel, and urinalysis performed. Additional tests that aid in the diagnostic investigation of dogs with hyperlipidemia include measurement of serum total and free thyroxine concentrations, serum thyroid-stimulating hormone (TSH) concentration, serum glucose concentration and urine glucose (if not previously performed), serum pancreatic-lipase immunoreactivity concentration, serum bile-acid concentrations, urine protein:creatinine ratio, and low-dose dexamethasone suppression test. The selection of tests to be performed is based on information from the history and clinical signs present and is tailored to each individual case. A more general and wide selection of tests might be necessary for patients that have vague or no clinical signs.

Ideally, an appropriate selection of the aforementioned tests should be used in every dog with hyperlipidemia as part of the diagnostic investigation of the condition. One possible exception is the miniature schnauzer, in which primary hyperlipidemia is well documented and more common than secondary hyperlipidemia. A detailed diagnostic investigation of hyperlipidemia might not be necessary in this breed in the absence of clinical signs, unless hypercholesterolemia seems to be the main abnormality (without or with only mild hypertriglyceridemia) because in this case it is more likely that the dog has some form of secondary hyperlipidemia. Also, all miniature schnauzers in the United States (and potentially other dog breeds that commonly develop primary hyperlipidemia) should be evaluated for hypertriglyceridemia on multiple occasions (to incorporate the possibility of age-related lipid metabolism disorders) while they are healthy because this information may help prevent misinterpretation of increased serum triglyceride concentrations when the dogs are presented for a clinical illness. In addition, by knowing the serum triglyceride status of the dog, the veterinarian might consider switching the affected dog to a low-fat diet to avoid possible complications of hypertriglyceridemia.

When an appropriate diagnostic investigation suggests a primary lipid disorder leading to hyperlipidemia is present, there is little more that can be done to diagnose the exact cause of hyperlipidemia. In the majority of cases the exact cause cannot be identified and such an investigation is usually only of academic and not therapeutic importance. Tests or methods that have been used to further characterize or investigate the cause of primary hyperlipidemia in dogs include the chylomicron test, lipoprotein electrophoresis, ultracentrifugation, and assessment of lipoprotein lipase activity. None of these tests or methods is used routinely in clinical cases and their availability is limited. Genetic testing for specific lipid disorders related to mutations of genes involved in lipid metabolism is currently not available.

Treatment of Canine Hyperlipidemia

Treatment of secondary hyperlipidemia relies on the successful treatment of the underlying disorder after which hyperlipidemia usually resolves. Resolution of secondary hyperlipidemia after treatment of the cause should always be confirmed by laboratory testing (typically 4 to 6 weeks after control of the primary disease). If hyperlipidemia has not resolved, an incorrect diagnosis, ineffective treatment, or concurrent primary or secondary hyperlipidemia due to other causes should be considered. In some dogs with secondary hyperlipidemia, especially those with hyperlipidemia due to diabetes mellitus, it might be difficult to optimally control their primary disease, and therefore hyperlipidemia might persist despite treatment. If persistent hyperlipidemia in such cases is severe, it may be necessary to take measures for its control. The management of persistent secondary hyperlipidemia relies on the same principles as for primary hyperlipidemia (see later).

It has been traditionally recommended that hypertriglyceridemia should be treated only when serum concentrations of triglycerides exceed 500 mg/dl or even 1000 mg/dl. However, recent studies have shown that insulin resistance, hepatobiliary disease, and possibly other complications of hypertriglyceridemia can exist even with serum triglyceride concentrations below 500 mg/dl. Therefore it is the author's opinion that even mild hypertriglyceridemia (i.e., serum triglyceride concentrations above 200 mg/dl) should be treated, at least with dietary management, to keep serum triglyceride concentrations as low as possible and reduce the risk for complications.

The initial treatment goal for severe hypertriglyceridemia should be to keep fasting serum triglyceride concentration below 500 mg/dl. Attempts to reach this goal should start with dietary management, while drug therapy can be initiated at a later point if deemed necessary. After this initial goal has been achieved, further reduction or even normalization of serum triglyceride concentration (typically with the addition of lipid-lowering drugs) should be considered on the basis of a risk-to-benefit ratio calculation for each individual case. Dogs with hyperlipidemia in which treatment does not seem necessary (e.g., when serum triglycerides or cholesterol are borderline above the reference range) or has been declined by the owner should be monitored periodically for potential worsening of hyperlipidemia.

Although the management of hypercholesterolemia seems to be of less clinical importance than that of hypertriglyceridemia in dogs, hypercholesterolemia should be treated appropriately at least with dietary management. Drug therapy should be considered in cases in which hypercholesterolemia is resistant to dietary therapy and exceeds 500 mg/dl. The following sections focus mainly on the treatment of hypertriglyceridemia unless otherwise indicated.

Dietary Management

The first step in the management of primary or persistent secondary hyperlipidemia is dietary modification. Dogs with primary hyperlipidemia should be offered a low-fat diet throughout their lives, while dogs with persistent secondary hyperlipidemia should be offered low-fat diets on the basis of repeated testing and the effectiveness of control of the primary disease. Diets that contain less than 25 g of total fat per 1000 kcal are generally recommended. Many commercially available diets are labeled "low-fat" but their fat content can vary widely. In addition, although many diets have low total fat content and in theory should be effective in the management of hyperlipidemia, several dietary aspects that might affect the response of dogs to specific diets are unknown. Published studies investigating the efficacy of low-fat diets in dogs with hyperlipidemia are lacking. Therefore the selection of the most effective low-fat diet for the treatment of hyperlipidemia is uncertain and quite challenging. In a recent unpublished study (Xenoulis et al, 2011c), miniature schnauzers with primary hyperlipidemia were put on the Royal Canin Gastrointestinal Low Fat diet for 8 weeks. By the end of the treatment period, there was a significant reduction in both serum triglyceride and cholesterol concentrations. Serum cholesterol concentrations returned to normal in all dogs, while serum triglyceride concentrations returned to normal in about 30% of dogs. However, all dogs that had serum triglyceride concentrations above 500 mg/dl at the beginning of the study had serum triglyceride concentrations below 500 mg/dl by the end of the trial.

Homemade low-fat diets are also suitable for the management of canine hyperlipidemia, but care should be taken to make sure that these diets are balanced, especially when used for long periods. Some of these diets (e.g., boiled lean turkey breast without the skin and rice) have even lower fat content than most commercially available low-fat diets and may be more effective in lowering serum lipid concentrations in dogs. Therefore, in dogs that do not sufficiently respond to commercially available low-fat diets, an ultra-low-fat home-prepared diet can be offered or medical treatment can be initiated. Treats and table scraps should be avoided unless they are low in fat. Fruits and vegetables typically constitute ideal treats for hyperlipidemic dogs.

Serum lipid concentrations should be reevaluated after feeding a low-fat diet for about 4 to 6 weeks. If the serum triglyceride concentration in hypertriglyceridemic dogs has decreased to below 500 mg/dl, dietary therapy should be continued and serum triglyceride concentrations should be reevaluated every 6 months. If serum triglyceride concentration remains above 500 mg/dl or if additional reduction of serum triglyceride concentration is desired, additional dietary modifications (if possible) or medical treatment should be considered.

Medical Management

Some dogs with primary hyperlipidemia do not respond sufficiently to being fed a low- or ultra-low-fat diet alone. In these cases, medical treatment is required in addition to the low-fat diet in an effort to effectively reduce serum lipid concentrations. Many lipid-lowering drugs are available and have been widely used in human medicine for decades. However, no studies have evaluated the efficacy and safety of lipid-lowering drugs in dogs, and therefore evidence-based recommendations cannot be made. Instead, recommendations in this chapter are based on clinical experience and extrapolation from human medicine. Also, lipid-lowering drugs are not approved for use in dogs and therefore owner consent is recommended when these drugs are used. The order of the discussion of the following drugs reflects the author's preferred order of medical treatment of hyperlipidemia in dogs.

Omega-3 Fatty Acids (Fish Oils)

Polyunsaturated fatty acids of the n-3 series (omega-3 fatty acids; eicosapentaenoic acid [EPA] and docosahexaenoic acid [DHA]) are abundant in marine fish. Omega-3 fatty acid supplementation has been shown to lower serum triglyceride concentrations in experimental animals, normal humans, and humans with primary hypertriglyceridemia. Specifically, omega-3 fatty acids have been shown to reduce serum triglyceride concentrations by up to 50% when used at high doses in humans with hypertriglyceridemia. The mechanisms of the lipid-lowering action of omega-3 fatty acids include reduced lipogenesis, increased β-oxidation, and activation of lipoprotein lipase. In a study of healthy dogs, fish oil supplementation led to a significant reduction of serum triglyceride concentrations, suggesting that this supplement may be helpful in the treatment of canine hypertriglyceridemia. No major side effects have been observed in humans or in dogs receiving omega-3 fatty acids, even when administered at high doses. However, studies evaluating the efficacy and safety of omega-3 fatty acid supplementation in dogs with hyperlipidemia are lacking and clinical experience is limited.

Because serious side effects are rarely reported and because omega-3 fatty acids are likely effective in lowering serum triglyceride concentrations, omega-3 fatty acid supplementation is recommended as a second-line therapy in dogs with primary hypertriglyceridemia that do not respond to a low-fat diet alone. The formulation of omega-3 fatty acids with the highest purity currently is Lovaza, which is FDA approved for use in humans as a lipid-lowering agent. Care should be taken to select products low in mercury because high concentrations of mercury and other environmental toxins may be present in fish oil products. Omega-3 fatty acids are used in dogs at doses ranging from 200 mg/kg to 300 mg/kg PO once a day, and their effect on serum triglyceride concentrations is dose-dependent. Their lipid-lowering effect typically requires doses at the high end of the recommended dose for dogs. An upper daily limit of 4 to 5 grams might be recommended. Periodic retesting of serum triglyceride concentrations is recommended during the treatment period.

Fibrates (Fibric Acid Derivatives)

Fibrates are weak agonists of peroxisome proliferator-activated receptor α (PPARα), a nuclear transcription factor that regulates lipid and lipoprotein synthesis and catabolism. Fibrates suppress fatty acid synthesis, stimulate fatty acid oxidation, activate lipoprotein lipase, and inhibit noncompetitively the enzyme diacylglycerol acyltransferase (the enzyme that catalyzes the conversion of diglycerides to triglycerides), therefore leading to an overall reduction in serum triglyceride concentration. In humans, fibrates typically reduce serum triglyceride concentrations by 25% to 50%. Fibrate use in humans is associated with a low incidence of myotoxicity and increases in serum liver enzyme activities.

Gemfibrozil is the most commonly used fibrate in humans and has also been used anecdotally in dogs with hypertriglyceridemia. It can be administered at 7.5 mg/kg q12h oral for dogs and cats. No side effects have been observed in dogs, although no studies have evaluated its safety in this species. Gemfibrozil may be recommended in dogs in which dietary modification and omega-3 fatty acids have failed to effectively reduce serum triglyceride concentrations. Periodic testing of serum triglyceride concentration and liver enzyme activities is recommended.

Niacin (Nicotinic Acid)

Niacin, a form of vitamin B_3, has been used successfully for the treatment of hyperlipidemia in humans for years. When used in pharmacologic doses, niacin is a broad-spectrum lipid-modifying drug and, in humans, it reduces both low-density lipoprotein (LDL)-cholesterol and serum triglyceride concentrations. The mechanism of action of niacin is complex and incompletely understood but includes inhibition of hormone-sensitive lipase and the enzyme diacylglycerol acyltransferase, both of which actions eventually lead to reduced triglyceride biosynthesis. In dogs, niacin treatment has been reported in very few patients with primary hypertriglyceridemia. In these patients, niacin reduced serum triglyceride concentrations for several months without causing any side effects. However, large clinical trials regarding the efficacy and safety of niacin in dogs with primary hypertriglyceridemia are lacking. As is often the case in humans, niacin administration in dogs is potentially associated with side effects such as erythema and pruritus, which usually require discontinuation of therapy. Long-term risk for myotoxicity and hepatotoxicity may also exist.

Niacin ER (extended release) has been recommended as the preferred choice of niacin in humans due to its purity, tolerability, and lower incidence of side effects. Niacin is usually administered to dogs at a dose of 50 to 200 mg/day. Both the therapeutic and side effects of niacin are dose dependent and it is therefore recommended that niacin is started at a low dose and slowly titrated upward (every 4 weeks) based on the results of follow-up lipid panels. It should be used with caution in diabetic patients because it can increase blood glucose concentration (especially when used at higher doses), and serum liver enzyme activities should be monitored with long-term use of niacin.

Other Drugs

A large number of other drug classes are available for use in humans with hyperlipidemia. However, the use of most of these drugs is currently not recommended in dogs. Statins (HMG-CoA reductase inhibitors) are among the most potent and commonly used lipid-lowering drugs in humans. They are reversible inhibitors of the enzyme HMG-CoA reductase, which is the rate-limiting step for cholesterol biosynthesis. Therefore statins are mainly cholesterol-lowering drugs with less potent effects on triglyceride metabolism. This makes them less than ideal drug choices when hypertriglyceridemia is the main lipid abnormality. Statin use has been associated with myopathy, rhabdomyolysis, and hepatotoxicity in humans, and there are anecdotal reports of hepatotoxicity in dogs. The potential for hepatotoxicity is probably higher when hepatic steatosis is present, a condition that likely occurs in at least a portion of dogs with severe hypertriglyceridemia (especially miniature schnauzers). When collectively considering the potential side effects of statins, the fact that hypercholesterolemia rarely needs to be treated medically in dogs, and the fact that statins are unlikely to be very effective in the treatment of canine hypertriglyceridemia, the routine use of statins is not recommended in hyperlipidemic dogs. If statins are to be used in dogs, it should be kept in mind that the pharmacokinetic profiles of the various statins are unknown in this species and therefore the dose and frequency of administration of these drugs can currently only be extrapolated from human medicine. Serum liver enzyme activities should be periodically monitored for potential hepatotoxicity. Concurrent administration of statins and fibrates (e.g., gemfibrozil) should be avoided because the latter has been shown to affect the pharmacokinetics of statins, leading to increased risk for toxicity.

Combination Drug Therapy

Some dogs, especially those with primary hypertriglyceridemia, can manifest serum triglyceride concentrations in the thousands. Serum triglyceride concentration in many of these dogs cannot be controlled with diet alone or monotherapy with lipid-lowering drugs, and a combination of more than one lipid-lowering medication and ultra-low-fat diet may be required. Experience with combination therapy is very limited in dogs. The author's preferred order of treatment trials in dogs with severe hypertriglyceridemia is the administration of a low- or ultra-low-fat diet, followed by the addition of omega-3 fatty acids, followed by gemfibrozil, and finally the addition of niacin if necessary. Statins may also be used when other medications have proven ineffective.

References and Suggested Reading

Toth PP: Drug treatment of hyperlipidemia: a guide to the rational use of lipid-lowering drugs, *Drugs* 70:1363-1379, 2010.

Xenoulis PG et al: Serum liver enzyme activities in healthy Miniature Schnauzers with and without hypertriglyceridemia, *J Am Vet Med Assoc* 232:63-67, 2008.

Xenoulis PG, Steiner JM: Lipid metabolism and hyperlipidemia in dogs, *Vet J* 183:12-21, 2010.

Xenoulis PG et al: Association between serum triglyceride and canine pancreatic lipase immunoreactivity concentrations in miniature schnauzers, *J Am Anim Hosp Assoc* 46:229-234, 2010.

Xenoulis PG et al: Association of hypertriglyceridemia with insulin resistance in healthy Miniature Schnauzers, *J Am Vet Med Assoc* 15:238:1011-1016, 2011a.

Xenoulis PG et al: Serum triglyceride concentrations in Miniature Schnauzers with and without a history of probable pancreatitis, *J Vet Intern Med* 25:20-25, 2011b.

Xenoulis PG et al: Effect of a low-fat diet on serum triglyceride, cholesterol, and pancreatic lipase immunoreactivity concentrations in Miniature Schnauzers with hypertriglyceridemia, *J Vet Intern Med* 25:687, 2011c.

SECTION IV

Oncology and Hematology

Chapter 59:   Immunosuppressive Agents   268
Chapter 60:   Management of Immune-Mediated Hemolytic
               Anemia in Dogs   275
Chapter 61:   Thrombocytopenia   280
Chapter 62:   von Willebrand Disease and Hereditary
               Coagulation Factor Deficiencies   286
Chapter 63:   Disseminated Intravascular Coagulation   292
Chapter 64:   Hypercoagulable States   297
Chapter 65:   Lymphocytosis in Dogs and Cats   301
Chapter 66:   Quality Control for the In-Clinic Laboratory   306
Chapter 67:   Transfusion Medicine: Best Practices   309
Chapter 68:   Bone Marrow Dyscrasias   314
Chapter 69:   Talking to Clients about Cancer   318
Chapter 70:   Tumor Biopsy and Specimen Submission   322
Chapter 71:   Chemotherapeutic Drug Handling and Safety   326
Chapter 72:   Treatment of Adverse Effects from Cancer Therapy   330
Chapter 73:   Cancer Immunotherapy   334
Chapter 74:   Advances in Radiation Therapy for Nasal Tumors   338
Chapter 75:   Malignant Effusions   341
Chapter 76:   Interventional Oncology   345
Chapter 77:   Nutritional Support of the Cancer Patient   349
Chapter 78:   Metronomic Chemotherapy   354
Chapter 79:   Drug Update: Toceranib   358
Chapter 80:   Drug Update: Masitinib   360
Chapter 81:   Oral Tumors   362
Chapter 82:   Perineal Tumors   366
Chapter 83:   Urinary Bladder Cancer   370
Chapter 84:   Mammary Cancer   375
Chapter 85:   Rescue Therapy for Canine Lymphoma   381
Chapter 86:   Plasma Cell Neoplasms   384
Chapter 87:   Osteosarcoma   388
Chapter 88:   Canine Hemangiosarcoma   392
Chapter 89:   Thyroid Tumors   397

**The following web chapters can be found on the companion website at
www.currentveterinarytherapy.com**

Web Chapter 25:   Anticancer Drugs: New Drugs
Web Chaptre 26:   Blood Typing and Crossmatching to Ensure Blood Compatibility
Web Chapter 27:   Soft Tissue Sarcomas
Web Chapter 28:   Collection of Specimens for Cytology
Web Chapter 29:   Nasal Tumors
Web Chapter 30:   Nonregenerative Anemias
Web Chapter 31:   Pulmonary Neoplasia
Web Chapter 32:   Surgical Oncology Principles

CHAPTER 59
Immunosuppressive Agents

CLARE R. GREGORY, *Santa Rosa, California*

Over the last half of the twentieth century immunosuppressive agents have evolved from nonspecific, myelotoxic drugs to agents that target specific enzymes catalyzing reactions required for normal immune function. Much of our current understanding of T-cell function has been provided by research performed to understand the mechanism of action of cyclosporine. As each element of antigen recognition, T-cell activation, cytokine synthesis, and T cell–dependent cytolysis is unraveled, investigators are devising specific, less toxic, and more efficacious agents for interrupting the immune response. This process, termed *rational drug development,* replaces the selection of potential immunosuppressive agents based on their ability to lyse or inhibit the activation of T and B cells *in vitro.* Although specific immunosuppression with the use of naturally induced and genetically engineered antibodies, soluble receptor fragments, and other biologic methods is available for the treatment of human diseases, most of these therapies are either inapplicable or unavailable for treatment of animal diseases. For the foreseeable future in veterinary medicine, immunosuppression will rely on chemotherapeutic agents. As new immunosuppressive agents become more available and clinicians become familiar with their indications, effects, and adverse effects, immunosuppressive therapy should become more specific, effective, and safe.

Myelotoxic Agents

Cyclophosphamide

The major effect of cyclophosphamide results from alkylation of DNA during the S phase of the cell cycle. The alterations in DNA structure can be lethal to the cell or can produce miscoding errors that inhibit cell replication or DNA transcription. Cyclophosphamide produces T- and B-cell lymphopenia and suppresses both T-cell activity and antibody production. Cyclophosphamide is administered to dogs for the treatment of corticosteroid-resistant immune-mediated hemolytic anemia (IMHA), corticosteroid-resistant immune-mediated thrombocytopenia (IMTP), rheumatoid arthritis (RA), and polymyositis (in conjunction with corticosteroids). Cyclophosphamide is administered to cats for the treatment of IMHA and RA. Myelosuppression, gastroenteritis, alopecia, and hemorrhagic cystitis are the major complications associated with cyclophosphamide therapy.

Azathioprine

Azathioprine is a purine analog that is metabolized to ribonucleotide monophosphates. Poor conversion to diphosphates and triphosphates leads to an intracellular accumulation of monophosphates that produces a feedback inhibition of the enzymes required for the biosynthesis of purine nucleotides. The triphosphate analogs that do form become incorporated into DNA and result in ribonucleic acid miscoding and faulty transcription. Azathioprine has a greater effect on humoral than on cell-mediated immunity. For the treatment of immune-mediated diseases in dogs, azathioprine generally is administered in conjunction with a corticosteroid or cyclophosphamide.

Azathioprine has been used for the treatment of IMTP, IMHA, autoimmune skin diseases, chronic hepatitis, myasthenia gravis, immune-mediated glomerulopathy, chronic atrophic gastritis, systemic lupus erythematosus, and inflammatory bowel disease. In recent studies azathioprine combined with prednisolone was no more effective than prednisolone administered alone in the treatment of IMHA, and azathioprine monotherapy was only moderately effective in the treatment of perianal fistulas. Azathioprine monotherapy was not effective enough to be recommended for general use in the treatment of atopic dermatitis in dogs. Although very myelotoxic in cats, azathioprine has been used for the treatment of feline autoimmune skin diseases. Azathioprine and prednisolone, when administered at maximally tolerated levels, do not effectively suppress the rejection response against canine renal allografts not matched for major histocompatibility complex (MHC) antigens. However, when administered on an every-other-day schedule (1 to 3 mg/kg PO) with cyclosporine, azathioprine has been used to maintain canine MHC-matched renal allografts successfully. In feline renal transplantation patients with suspected inflammatory bowel disease or following an allograft rejection episode, azathioprine is administered with cyclosporine at a dosage of 0.3 mg/kg every 3 days PO. The dose is decreased if the total white blood cell count falls below 3000 cells/µl or there is biochemical evidence of hepatotoxicity. The primary complication encountered with the administration of azathioprine is bone marrow suppression, which can result in leukopenia, anemia, and thrombocytopenia. Acute pancreatitis and hepatotoxicity may also occur.

Methotrexate

Methotrexate competitively inhibits folic acid reductase, which is necessary for the reduction of dihydrofolate to tetrahydrofolate and affects the production of both purines and pyrimidines. The effects of methotrexate manifest during the S phase of the cell cycle. Methotrexate is used occasionally as an antineoplastic agent in dogs and cats for the treatment of lymphomas, carcinomas, and sarcomas. In human medicine methotrexate is administered for the treatment of RA and psoriasis. Gastrointestinal toxicity is the most common complication encountered with the administration of methotrexate.

Glucocorticoids

Prednisolone

Glucocorticoids, and in particular prednisolone, have both direct and indirect effects on the immune response. Glucocorticoids stabilize the cell membrane of endothelial cells and inhibit the production of local chemotactic factors, thus decreasing infiltration of neutrophils, monocytes, and lymphocytes. In allogeneic tissues the secretion of destructive proteolytic enzymes such as collagenase, elastase, and plasminogen activator is inhibited. Glucocorticoids also inhibit the release of arachidonic acid from membrane phospholipids. This inhibition prevents the synthesis of prostaglandins, thromboxanes, and leukotrienes, which are major mediators of inflammation. Glucocorticoids redistribute monocytes and lymphocytes from the peripheral circulation to the lymphatics and bone marrow. This redistribution affects primarily T cells. T-cell activation and cytotoxicity also are reduced. Glucocorticoids suppress cytokine activity and alter macrophage function. Prednisolone and prednisone are considered to be the first-line immunosuppressive agents for the treatment of immune-mediated and chronic inflammatory diseases in dogs and cats because of their general efficacy and low cost. IMHA and IMTP, autoimmune and allergic skin diseases, myasthenia gravis, allergic pneumonitis and bronchitis, immune-mediated arthritis, and systemic lupus erythematosus are just some of the indications for corticosteroid therapy in animals. Prednisolone has been used in both dogs and cats to slow allograft rejection; however, when administered as a single agent, prednisolone is not capable of preventing allograft rejection. For the prevention of allograft rejection in cats, prednisolone is administered with cyclosporine at an initial dosage of 2.5 to 5 mg q12h PO. This dosage generally is reduced to 2.5 to 5 mg q24h PO 30 days following transplantation. Over the next several months, with monitoring serum creatinine and blood urea nitrogen concentrations, the prednisolone dosage is reduced to 2.5 mg q24h PO or discontinued.

Although corticosteroids are inexpensive and often effective, the long-term use of these drugs can result in severe complications, usually manifested as signs of iatrogenic hyperadrenocorticism. The potential for this complication, in addition to the fact that corticosteroids suppress multiple elements of the immune response, has led to the search for *steroid-sparing* immunosuppressive protocols.

Calcineurin Inhibitors

Cyclosporine

Cyclosporine is bound in the cytosol of lymphocytes by cyclophilins (cyclosporine-binding proteins). The cyclosporine-cyclophilin complexes associate with calcium-dependent calcineurin-calmodulin complexes to impede calcium-dependent signal transduction. Transcription factors that promote cytokine gene activation are either direct or indirect substrates of the serine-threonine phosphatase activity of calcineurin. This enzymatic activity is reduced by association of the cyclosporine-cyclophilin bimolecular complex with calcineurin. Via this mechanism of action, cyclosporine inhibits early T-cell activation (G_0 phase of the cell cycle) and prevents synthesis of several cytokines, in particular interleukin-2 (IL-2). Without stimulation by IL-2, further T-cell proliferation is inhibited, and T-cell cytotoxic activity is reduced. Cyclosporine also may exert an immunosuppressive effect because it stimulates mammalian cells to secrete transforming growth factor-β (TGF-β) protein. TGF-β is a potent inhibitor of IL-2–stimulated T-cell proliferation and generation of antigen-specific cytotoxic lymphocytes. Cyclosporine is not cytotoxic or myelotoxic and is specific for lymphocytes. This specificity spares other rapidly dividing cells and allows nonspecific host defense mechanisms to continue to function.

Cyclosporine has gained widespread use in veterinary medicine. Immunosuppression with a combination of cyclosporine and prednisolone has maintained normal function of non–MHC-matched feline renal allografts for longer than 12 years. Cyclosporine in combination with azathioprine, prednisolone, and antithymocyte serum has been used to maintain non–MHC-matched canine renal allografts. Bone marrow transplantation has been performed successfully in cats with the use of cyclosporine immunosuppression. Cyclosporine also has been used to control corticosteroid-resistant IMHA and IMTP in dogs. Cyclosporine is available in an ophthalmic preparation (Optimmune) for the control of keratoconjunctivitis sicca in dogs. An ophthalmic preparation of cyclosporine was shown to be an effective treatment for feline eosinophilic keratitis. Lifelong therapy is recommended. Cyclosporine (10 to 20 mg/kg q24h PO) was found to significantly reduce the size and depth of perianal fistulas in dogs (Mathews and Sukhiani, 1997). Most dogs did not require further therapy, either medical or surgical, after 6 to 8 weeks of treatment. In a more recent study (Hardie et al, 2005) cyclosporine resolved or reduced anal furuncular lesions in 25 of 26 dogs. However, residual or recurrent lesions were encountered that required long-term medical therapy or surgical resection. Cyclosporine (5 mg/kg q24h PO induction dose, reduced by 50% to 75% over weeks to months, depending on response) has been shown to be effective in the reduction of skin lesions and pruritus in dogs with atopic dermatitis (Steffan et al, 2006). Cyclosporine also has been shown to be effective in the treatment of atopic dermatitis in cats and is an alternative treatment to prednisolone (Wisselink and Willemse, 2009).

Cyclosporine has been used for the treatment of other dermatologic diseases such as pemphigus foliaceus (Guaguere et al, 2004). Cyclosporine also has been shown to be effective in the treatment of granulomatous meningoencephalitis (Adamo and O'Brien, 2004) and, combined with prednisolone, in the treatment of necrotizing meningoencephalitis. Cyclosporine has been used to treat steroid-refractory inflammatory bowel disease (5 to 10 mg/kg q24h PO for 10 weeks; Allenspach et al, 2006) and recently has been shown to control inflammatory colorectal polyps in miniature dachshunds when combined with prednisolone. Cyclosporine appears to be effective in the management of myasthenia gravis in dogs, especially when anticholinesterase medication fails and other immunosuppressive medications such as corticosteroids lead to deterioration in clinical signs. Very recently, feline idiopathic pure red cell aplasia was shown to be responsive to combination therapy with cyclosporine and glucocorticoids. Most cats required long-term low-dose therapy.

Cyclosporine is available in two oral formulations: Sandimmune and Neoral. Both contain cyclosporine at a concentration of 100 mg/ml, but the two solutions are not biologically equivalent. Sandimmune has an olive oil base, and adsorption of cyclosporine requires emulsification of the agent by bile salts and digestion by pancreatic enzymes. The absorption percentage can be as little as 4%, and there is a tremendous variation in dose-trough whole blood levels among individuals of the same species. Neoral (and now various generics) is a microemulsion preconcentrate of cyclosporine that becomes a microemulsion when in contact with gastrointestinal fluids. The microemulsion is absorbed directly through the gut epithelium, which results in more sustained and consistent blood levels of the drug. When Neoral replaces Sandimmune as treatment, most feline renal transplant recipients have had a reduction in the dosage level necessary to maintain the same trough whole blood levels. In addition, feline renal transplant patients have been administered Sandimmune at a dosage of 10 to 15 mg/kg q24h PO to initiate immunosuppression at the time of surgery. To achieve the same trough whole blood levels of cyclosporine (approximately 500 ng/ml), Neoral is administered at a dose of 1 to 4 mg/kg q24h PO. Neoral appears to be a more effective immunosuppressant than Sandimmune because of its more complete absorption, which results in a more sustained and predictable blood level. In addition, it is more economical to use. The various generic formulations of the microemulsion form of cyclosporine do not appear to be interchangeable; that is, the same dosage does not necessarily result in the same trough blood concentrations in patients. If one microemulsion form is exchanged for another, it is important to check whole blood trough concentrations to ensure both that adequate levels have been achieved and that the concentration of the drug in the blood has not become too high.

To achieve immunosuppression using cyclosporine in dogs, I recommend treating to attain a 12-hour whole blood trough level (measured just before the next oral dose) of at least 500 ng/ml. With Sandimmune, achieving this level requires an oral dosage of 10 to 25 mg/kg q24h divided into two doses. Neoral can be initiated at 5 to 10 mg/kg q24h divided into two doses. With either formulation the presence of gastrointestinal inflammation increases the dosage requirements, and blood levels of the agent must be measured starting 24 to 48 hours after initiation of therapy to ensure that adequate blood levels are achieved. Blood levels of cyclosporine should be measured at periodic intervals during the time of therapy. To reduce the cost of the cyclosporine necessary to treat medium-sized to large dogs, I administer ketoconazole at a dosage of 10 mg/kg q24h PO in addition to the cyclosporine. Ketoconazole interferes with the hepatic metabolism of cyclosporine, and it reduces the dosage requirement of cyclosporine by as much as 60%. I have not encountered toxic effects with the coadministration of these agents, but it has been reported that the long-term administration of ketoconazole to dogs may result in cataract formation.

To achieve immunosuppression with cyclosporine in cats, I recommend attaining a 12-hour whole blood trough level of 250 to 500 ng/ml. With Sandimmune, obtaining this level requires a dose of 4 to 15 mg/kg q24h PO divided into two doses. Neoral can be initiated at 1 to 5 mg/kg q24h PO divided into two doses. Again it is imperative to measure blood levels 24 to 48 hours after initiation of therapy to ensure that adequate blood levels have been achieved. Blood levels must also be measured periodically during the course of therapy. Based on pharmacokinetic studies in the cat, trough whole blood concentrations of cyclosporine may not correlate well with drug exposure (Mehl et al, 2003). The whole blood concentrations measured at 2 hours after administration of the drug may correlate better with drug exposure and give a better index for drug dosage and change in dose. The blood concentration of cyclosporine measured 2 hours after administration is recommended for therapeutic drug monitoring in human renal transplant patients.

Whole blood or plasma levels of cyclosporine can be determined by high-pressure liquid chromatography, fluorescence polarization immunoassay, and specific monoclonal antibody radioimmunoassay. Most medical centers that serve humans perform cyclosporine assays and will serve veterinary needs.

Unlike the situation in humans, cyclosporine does not appear to be hepatotoxic in dogs and cats unless extremely high blood levels are maintained (>3000 ng/ml). Although nephrotoxicity is not as frequently encountered in humans, cyclosporine can be nephrotoxic in the cat. Nephrotoxicity in the cat does not seem to be related to the level of the drug in whole blood and can occur at relatively low plasma concentrations. Cats with extremely high cyclosporine whole blood concentrations (>4000 ng/ml) often show no toxicity at all. In my years of practice I have seen cyclosporine nephrotoxicity develop in only one dog. This dog had a chylothorax that resulted in trough whole blood concentrations of cyclosporine of more than 3000 ng/ml. Levels higher than 1000 ng/ml can cause inappetence in cats. If levels of 1000 ng/ml are maintained for several weeks or months, opportunistic bacterial and fungal infections can occur. As in humans, cyclosporine can promote the development of neoplasia, particularly lymphomas, in cats and dogs. The administration of high levels of prednisolone (1 to 2 mg/kg q24h PO) with cyclosporine increases the likelihood of tumor formation. As in humans, cyclosporine has resulted in a marked increase in hair growth in several of my feline renal transplant recipients. When administered to dogs, cyclosporine can result in severe gingival hyperplasia, fibropapillomatosis, and severe or fatal pyodermas, especially when combined with azathioprine (Gregory et al, 2006).

Cyclosporine has a distinctly unpleasant taste to both humans and animals, which necessitates administration in gelatin capsules or mixed with other fluids. Novartis supplies capsules (Atopica) containing 10, 25, 50, or 100 mg of cyclosporine. Novartis now has an oral solution specifically marketed for cats that is deemed to be palatable. I still place the oral solution in No. 0 or No. 1 gelatin capsules. Some cats need only a very small dose of cyclosporine (1 to 3 mg per dose). Measuring and administering this small amount (0.01 to 0.03 ml) of a drug is very difficult and imprecise. Sandimmune can be diluted and stored in olive oil; I usually make a 1:10 dilution. Neoral can be diluted in any oral solution, but it must be administered immediately after it is diluted because it is a microemulsion concentrate. I dilute Neoral in tap water.

Cyclosporine also is available in an intravenous solution (Sandimmune IV) that must be diluted in 0.9% sodium chloride or 5% dextrose in water. For the treatment of acute renal allograft rejection, I administer a dose of 6 mg/kg over 4 hours in the calculated maintenance fluid requirement. Intravenous cyclosporine is administered to control organ rejection episodes, treat an acute hemolytic crisis, or provide therapy during periods when a patient cannot tolerate oral medications.

Tacrolimus

Although tacrolimus, or FK-506 (Prograf), is structurally different from cyclosporine, it shares a similar mechanism of action. Tacrolimus binds in the cytosol of lymphocytes with an immunophilin, FK-binding protein (FKBP). Like the cyclosporine-cyclophilin complex, the tacrolimus-FKBP complex binds to calcineurin and inhibits its phosphatase activity. This inhibition directly and indirectly inhibits de novo expression of nuclear regulatory proteins and T-cell activation genes. The transcription of cytokines responsible for lymphocyte activation (IL-2, IL-3, IL-4, IL-5, interferon-γ, tumor necrosis factor-α, and granulocyte-macrophage colony-stimulating factor) is suppressed, as is the expression of IL-2 and IL-7 receptors. Tacrolimus is 50 to 100 times more potent as an inhibitor of lymphocyte activation than cyclosporine *in vitro*. Tacrolimus also inhibits B-cell proliferation and production of antibody by unknown mechanisms. Tacrolimus decreases the hepatic damage associated with ischemia-reperfusion injury, perhaps by inhibiting production of tumor necrosis factor-α and IL-6 by hepatocytes, and stimulates hepatic regeneration following liver injury. Experimentally, allograft recipients of many species have been treated successfully with tacrolimus at dosages several times lower than those for cyclosporine. Tacrolimus has prolonged the survival of renal, liver, pancreas, heart, lung, and vascularized limb grafts in rodents, dogs, and nonhuman primates. In human organ recipients tacrolimus is superior to cyclosporine for the reversal of ongoing rejection. Also the steroid-sparing effect of tacrolimus seems to be greater than that of Sandimmune, but it may not be superior to that of Neoral. The toxicity of tacrolimus is similar to that of cyclosporine in humans.

Little if any systematic use of tacrolimus has occurred in veterinary patients, but based on its effectiveness in experimental animal trials, it could be very useful in controlling a wide range of immune-mediated conditions. Tacrolimus may be particularly effective in controlling IMHA, IMTP, and immune-mediated arthritis because of its inhibition of antibody synthesis and T-cell proliferation. Despite the potential benefits of tacrolimus for treating diseases in dogs, a major concern is the possible toxicity of the drug. A dosage of 0.16 mg/kg q24h IM or 1 mg/kg q24h PO has been reported to be effective in prolonging renal allograft survival in beagle dogs. The adverse effects included anorexia, vasculitis, and intestinal intussusception. In a study in mongrel dogs the same dosages were not effective in prolonging renal allograft survival, and most of the dogs developed severe vasculitis leading to fatal myocardial infarction, hepatic failure, and intussusception. Tacrolimus and cyclosporine administered as combination therapy appear to have an additive effect with less toxicity. Blood levels of tacrolimus are assayed at human medical centers with the use of monoclonal immunoassays. The effective serum trough level of tacrolimus in dogs is approximately 0.1 to 0.4 ng/ml, about 100 times lower than that of cyclosporine. Trough levels of 2 ng/ml or more can result in death. Used topically in a 0.1% solution, tacrolimus has safely controlled the lesions of discoid lupus erythematosus and pemphigus foliaceus in dogs (Rosenkrantz, 2004). The International Task Force on Canine Atopic Dermatitis included topical tacrolimus (Protopic) in the group of medications for which there is good evidence of high efficacy in the treatment of that disease. Tacrolimus in a topical 0.02% or 0.03% aqueous suspension is effective for the treatment of dogs with keratoconjunctivitis sicca and chronic superficial keratitis (Berdoulay et al, 2005). Tacrolimus has been shown to increase Schirmer's tear test values effectively in dogs unresponsive to cyclosporine therapy. Topical tacrolimus also is very effective in the control of perianal fistulas in dogs.

Inhibitors of Cytokine and Growth Factor Action

Sirolimus and Everolimus

Sirolimus, or rapamycin (Rapamune), and everolimus (Afinitor) are macrocyclic antibiotics with a structure similar to that of tacrolimus that also bind in the cell cytosol to FKBP. However, sirolimus and tacrolimus affect different and distinct sites in the signal transduction pathway. The immunosuppressive activity of sirolimus appears to be a consequence in part of the sirolimus-FKBP complex's blocking of the activation of the mammalian target of rapamycin (mTOR). A serine/threonine protein kinase, mTOR is involved in the regulation of cell proliferation through the initiation of gene translation in response to amino acids, growth factors, cytokines, and mitogens. The kinase activity of the additional cell cycle–regulatory proteins cyclin-dependent kinase 2 and cyclin-dependent kinase 4 also is inhibited by sirolimus. Sirolimus blocks IL-2 and other growth factor–mediated signal transduction (signal 3 of the allograft rejection response) and the calcium-independent CD28/B7 (CD80/CD86) costimulatory pathway. Cyclosporine and tacrolimus block T-cell cell cycle progression at the G_0 to G_1 stage; sirolimus prevents cells from progressing from G_1 to the S phase. Sirolimus blocks T-cell activation by IL-2, IL-4, and IL-6 and stimulation of B-cell proliferation by lipopolysaccharide. Sirolimus directly inhibits B-cell immunoglobulin synthesis caused by interleukins.

Sirolimus has been shown to prevent acute, accelerated, and chronic rejection of skin, heart, renal, islet, and small bowel allografts in rodent, rabbit, dog, pig, and nonhuman primate graft recipients. It also has been shown to be efficacious in models of autoimmunity, including insulin-dependent diabetes, and systemic lupus erythematosus. The antagonism of cytokine and growth factor action by sirolimus is not limited to cells of the immune system. It inhibits the proliferation of fibroblasts, endothelial cells, hepatocytes, and smooth muscle cells induced by growth factors such as platelet-derived growth factor and fibroblast growth factor. Sirolimus has been very effective in preventing intimal smooth muscle proliferation (arteriosclerosis) following mechanical or immune-mediated arterial injury. In human clinical trials supplementation of cyclosporine-based protocols with sirolimus is associated with a reduction in acute allograft rejection; however, the combination of the two drugs increases the risk of nephrotoxicity, hemolytic-uremic syndrome, and hypertension. Other reported adverse effects include hyperlipidemia, thrombocytopenia, delayed wound healing, delayed graft function, mouth ulcers, pneumonitis, and interstitial lung disease.

Signaling through the mTOR pathway has been shown to contribute to the growth, progression, and chemoresistance of several cancers. Accordingly, mTOR inhibitors are being studied as potentially valuable therapeutics. It has been demonstrated that rapamycin may be safely administered to dogs and can yield therapeutic exposures. *In vitro*, rapamycin has been effective in decreasing tumor cell survival in both canine osteosarcoma and melanoma cell lines. Investigations into the efficacy of mTOR inhibitors in treating naturally occurring osteosarcomas in dogs currently are under way.

Mycophenolate Mofetil

Mycophenolate mofetil (MMF), also known as *RS-61443* and *mycophenolic acid* (CellCept), is a prodrug hydrolyzed by liver esterases to mycophenolic acid. MMF is cytostatic for lymphocytes owing to its inhibition of inosine monophosphate dehydrogenase, an enzyme necessary for de novo purine biosynthesis. MMF is a relatively selective inhibitor of T- and B-cell proliferation during the S phase of the cell cycle via its ability to prevent guanosine and deoxyguanosine biosynthesis. MMF has been shown to reduce allograft rejection in multiple animal models, demonstrating the most effect when combined with cyclosporine, tacrolimus, or sirolimus. MMF was developed in part as a nonmyelotoxic replacement for azathioprine for treatment of human allograft patients. Early clinical trials in human renal allograft recipients showed a decrease in biopsy-proven acute rejection episodes in patients receiving MMF in place of azathioprine. At

therapeutic dosages MMF can be toxic to animals. The primary dose-limiting effects are anemia and weight loss in rats; leukopenia, diarrhea, and anorexia in monkeys; and gastrointestinal hemorrhage, anorexia, and diarrhea in dogs. To reduce the toxic effects, the dosage can be lowered, or mycophenolic acid can be given in combination with other immunosuppressive agents. MMF (10 mg/kg q12h PO) has been used in combination therapy in veterinary medicine to control renal allograft rejection in dogs (Broaddus et al, 2006).

There are anecdotal reports of the use of MMF for the treatment of RA and renal allograft rejection in the dog. In a study involving 27 dogs with myasthenia gravis, MMF was not found to be an effective treatment (Dewey et al, 2010). MMF (10 mg/kg q12h PO) was used to control primary IMHA in two cats that showed a lack of response to corticosteroid therapy (Bacek et al, 2011). MMF (20 mg/kg q12h PO, then reduced to 10 mg/kg q12h PO) with prednisolone was used to control subepidermal blistering autoimmune disease in a dog. In this dog, the dosage of 20 mg/kg q12h was well tolerated. In humans MMF has been used to treat scleroderma lung disease and Evans's syndrome. MMF also can inhibit growth factor–induced smooth muscle and fibroblast proliferation. Sirolimus and MMF in combination are extremely effective in preventing arterial intimal smooth muscle proliferation following mechanical injury. This may have implications for the control of chronic allograft rejection in humans.

Leflunomide and Leflunomide Analogs

Leflunomide is a synthetic organic isoxazole that the intestinal mucosa metabolizes to the active form, A77 1726. Leflunomide exerts at least part of its antiproliferative activity during the S phase of the cell cycle by inhibiting the pathway of de novo pyrimidine biosynthesis. The target of A77 1726 in this pathway is the enzyme dihydroorotate dehydrogenase. At higher concentrations leflunomide also is an inhibitor of tyrosine kinases associated with growth factor receptors. In addition to its effects on T and B lymphocytes, leflunomide also has an antiproliferative effect on smooth muscle cells and fibroblasts, which also results from inhibition of the pyrimidine biosynthetic pathway in these cells. Leflunomide currently is approved for the treatment of RA in humans. It has been shown to be an effective disease-modifying antirheumatic drug free from the side effects commonly associated with currently approved immunosuppressants.

In addition to showing efficacy in humans and animal models with autoimmune diseases, leflunomide has been found to control acute, ongoing, and chronic allograft rejection of the kidney, skin, heart, vessels, and lung in small and large animal models. I have used leflunomide successfully to treat steroid-resistant autoimmune hemolytic anemia, Evans's syndrome, IMTP, multifocal non-suppurative encephalitis-meningomyelitis, polyarthritis, pemphigus foliaceous, and systemic histiocytosis in dogs (Gregory et al, 1998). In combination with cyclosporine, leflunomide has completely prevented the rejection of canine non–MHC-matched renal allografts in both experimental and clinical studies. At dosages used in humans, leflunomide causes gastrointestinal toxicity in dogs as a result of the accumulation of a metabolite, trimethylfluoroanaline (TMFA). Fortunately, the canine lymphocyte is far more sensitive than the human lymphocyte to the effects of the active agent A77172, and much lower oral dosages are equally effective in achieving immunosuppression. I currently use a dosage of 4 mg/kg q24h PO and adjust the dose as needed to obtain a 24-hour serum trough level of 20 mg/ml. Early studies in the cat suggest that TMFA does not present the toxicity problem encountered in dogs. The recommended dosage for cats is 2 mg/kg q24h PO for two consecutive days and then a maintenance dosage of 2 mg/kg q48h PO. This dosage produces a mean blood concentration of 16 μg/ml and results in a 50% reduction in mitogen-stimulated lymphocyte proliferation (Mehl et al, 2012). Leflunomide serum concentrations can be measured by simple high-performance liquid chromatography assays.

Leflunomide (70 mg per cat once weekly PO) in combination with methotrexate (7.5 mg per cat once weekly PO) has been used to treat feline RA (Hanna, 2005). Leflunomide (3 to 4 g/kg q24h PO was effective in controlling immune-mediated polyarthritis in 14 dogs (Colopy et al, 2010).

Leflunomide is showing effectiveness in treating viral diseases and certain cancers. Leflunomide has been used successfully to treat primary cytomegalovirus infection and ganciclovir-resistant cytomegalovirus infection in human renal transplant patients. *In vitro,* leflunomide inhibits replication of herpesvirus type 1 in feline kidney cell cultures. Leflunomide may be useful in the treatment of reactivation of latent feline herpesvirus 1 infection that occurs secondary to the stress of illness, surgery, or pharmacologic immunosuppression. Leflunomide has cytostatic, antioxidant, and apoptotic effects in human transformed epithelial cells and may play a role in prostate cancer chemoprevention. In studies in mouse models investigating the treatment of melanoma, leflunomide significantly inhibited tumor growth. When leflunomide was combined with PLX4720, a new antimelanoma agent, in clinical trials, tumor growth was almost completely inhibited.

Both cats and dogs with diminished renal function may be subject to TFMA toxicity since TFMA is excreted by the kidneys. Leflunomide is marketed under the trade name Arava. The use of leflunomide in dogs has been very expensive; however, a generic form of the drug is now available, which has reduced the cost of therapy by approximately 80%.

Leflunomide analogs currently are under development for use in transplantation and other chemotherapeutic applications. A combination of cyclosporine and FK778, a leflunomide analog, has been found to prolong MHC-mismatched canine renal allograft survival significantly.

Investigational Compounds

FTY 720 is obtained from myriocin, a fungus-derived sphingosine analog. After phosphorylation, FTY 720 engages lymphocyte sphingosine-1-phosphate receptors and profoundly alters lymphocyte trafficking, acting as a functional sphingosine-1-phosphate antagonist. FTY 720 sequesters naïve and activated CD4+ and CD8+ T and B cells from the blood into lymph nodes and Peyer's patches without affecting their functional properties. It is important to note that FTY 720 does not impair cellular or humoral immunity to systemic viral infection nor does it affect T-cell activation, expansion-proliferation, or immunologic memory.

FTY 720 synergizes effectively with inhibitors of T-cell activation and proliferation to prevent allograft rejection in a wide range of animal models. In combination with subtherapeutic concentrations of cyclosporine, FTY 720 has been shown to delay or prevent the rejection of skin, heart, small bowel, liver, and kidney allografts in rats, dogs, and nonhuman primates. Similar results have been seen when FTY 720 is combined with sirolimus and tacrolimus. FTY 720 is metabolized extensively in the liver via cytochrome enzymes that are not involved in the metabolism of cyclosporine, sirolimus, or tacrolimus; therefore variations in drug concentrations are unlikely to occur when these agents are coadministered. The pharmacokinetic profile of FTY 720 is characterized by linear dose-proportional exposure over a wide range of doses, only moderate interpatient variability, and a prolonged elimination half-life (89 to 150 hours). These characteristics suggest that FTY 720 will be administered once daily without the need for monitoring blood concentrations or dose titration. Human renal transplant patients experienced a significant reduction in peripheral blood lymphocyte counts by up to 85%. In the initial clinical trials in human renal transplant patients, FTY 720 was well tolerated and did not cause any significant toxicity, allograft loss, increase in infection rates, or other complications such as diabetes. However, when administered in combination with cyclosporine or tacrolimus in later studies, it showed possible toxic side effects and was no more effective than MMF, which has slowed development for use in human transplantation. In cats a single dose of FTY 720 produced a marked (≥80%) and prolonged reduction in circulating lymphocytes within 12 hours of administration. A 30-day administration trial did not reveal any toxicity. In human medicine, FTY 720 is distributed as fingolimod and is used for the treatment of relapsing forms of multiple sclerosis.

Combination Therapy

Most of the currently used or soon to be available immunosuppressive agents have differing mechanisms of action and are effective at different stages of the cell cycle. Experimentally and clinically, combining agents often results in more effective immunosuppression with fewer drug-induced adverse effects. In human transplant patients cyclosporine and tacrolimus currently are considered to be the first line of immunosuppressive agents. To increase their effectiveness and decrease toxicity, azathioprine, sirolimus, prednisolone, MMF, or some combination of these is added to antirejection protocols. Few of the new nonmyelotoxic agents have been used in veterinary patients, but published results of many experimental animal trials investigating autoimmune disease and organ transplantation provide indications and insight into their use. Experimental and clinical experience in canine non–MHC-matched organ transplantation indicates that the combination of cyclosporine and leflunomide or cyclosporine and azathioprine is extremely effective in preventing renal allograft rejection. The major complication associated with immunosuppressive therapy in canine renal transplant patients remains the development of lethal infections.

References and Suggested Reading

Adamo FP, O'Brien RT: Use of cyclosporine to treat granulomatous meningoencephalitis in three dogs, *J Am Vet Med Assoc* 225:1211, 2004.

Allenspach K et al: Pharmacokinetics and clinical efficacy of cyclosporine treatment of dogs with steroid-refractory inflammatory bowel disease, *J Vet Intern Med* 20:239, 2006.

Bacek LM, Macintire DK: Treatment of primary immune-mediated haemolytic anemia with mycophenolate mofetil in two cats, *J Vet Emerg Crit Care* 21:45, 2011.

Berdoulay A, English RV, Nadelstein B: Effect of topical 0.02% tacrolimus aqueous suspension on tear production in dogs with keratoconjunctivitis sicca, *Vet Ophthalmol* 8:225, 2005.

Broaddus KD et al: Renal allograft histopathology in dog leukocyte antigen mismatched dogs after renal transplantation, *Vet Surg* 35:125, 2006.

Chiba K et al: Immunosuppressive activity of FTY720, sphingosine 1-phosphate receptor agonist. 1. Prevention of allograft rejection in rats and dogs by FTY720 and FTY720-phosphate, *Transplant Proc* 37:102, 2005.

Colopy SA, Baker TA, Muir P: Efficacy of leflunomide for treatment of immune-mediated polyarthritis in dogs: 14 cases (2006-2008), *J Am Vet Med Assoc* 236:312, 2010.

Dewey CW et al: Mycophenolate mofetil treatment in dogs with serologically diagnosed acquired myasthenia gravis: 27 cases (1999-2008), *J Am Vet Med Assoc* 15:236, 2010.

Gregory CR et al: Leflunomide effectively treats naturally occurring immune-mediated and inflammatory diseases of dogs that are unresponsive to conventional therapy, *Transplant Proc* 30:4143, 1998.

Gregory CR et al: Results of clinical renal transplantation in 15 dogs using triple drug immunosuppressive therapy, *Vet Surg* 35:105, 2006.

Guaguere E et al: Cyclosporin A: a new drug in the field of canine dermatology, *Vet Dermatol* 15:61, 2004.

Hanna FY: Disease modifying treatment for feline rheumatoid arthritis, *Vet Comp Orthop Traumatol* 18:94, 2005.

Hardie RJ et al: Cyclosporine treatment of anal furunculosis in 26 dogs, *J Small Anim Pract* 46:3, 2005.

Mathews KA, Sukhiani HR: Randomized controlled trial of cyclosporine for the treatment of perianal fistulas in dogs, *J Am Vet Med Assoc* 211:1249, 1997.

Mehl ML et al: Disposition of cyclosporine after intravenous and multi-dose oral administration in cats, *J Vet Pharmacol Ther* 26:349, 2003.

Mehl ML et al: Pharmacokinetics and pharmacodynamics of A77 1726 and leflunomide in domestic cats, *J Vet Pharmacol Ther* 35(2):139, 2012. Epub May 26, 2011.

Rosenkrantz WS: Pemphigus: current therapy, *Vet Dermatol* 15:90, 2004.

Steffan J et al: A systematic review and metaanalysis of the efficacy and safety of cyclosporin for the treatment of atopic dermatitis in dogs, *Vet Dermatol* 17:3, 2006.

Wisselink MA, Willemse T: The efficacy of cyclosporine A in cats with presumed atopic dermatitis: a double blind, randomised prednisolone-controlled study, *Vet J* 180:55, 2009.

CHAPTER 60

Management of Immune-Mediated Hemolytic Anemia in Dogs

VALERIE JOHNSON, *Fort Collins, Colorado*
STEVEN DOW, *Fort Collins, Colorado*

Immune-mediated hemolytic anemia (IMHA) is one of the most devastating and rapidly fatal diseases of domestic dogs worldwide. Interestingly, there are no reports of IMHA occurring in nondomestic dogs. Despite a large amount of research conducted over the past 20 years, the mortality rate for IMHA in dogs remains high, with mortality estimates ranging from 30% to 70% within 1 to 2 months of diagnosis (Scott-Moncrieff, 2001). Diagnosis of IMHA in dogs is relatively straightforward. The major diagnostic criterion for IMHA is the presence of strongly regenerative anemia with evidence of spherocytosis or autoagglutination. Other common abnormalities in dogs with IMHA include hyperbilirubinemia, leukocytosis, thrombocytopenia, and elevated liver enzymes. Mortality in dogs with IMHA is generally the result of euthanasia due to severe and persistent erythrocyte destruction or to rapid onset of widespread, severe thromboembolic disease (McManus and Craig, 2001).

Pathogenesis

The primary cause of erythrocyte destruction in dogs with IMHA is the presence of high concentrations of antierythrocyte autoantibodies. These autoantibodies bind to the surface of erythrocytes and target them for destruction by macrophages in the spleen (extravascular hemolysis) or by complement-mediated lysis in the bloodstream (intravascular hemolysis). Although autoantibodies produced by B cells are the immediate cause of erythrocyte destruction in IMHA, from the standpoint of therapy IMHA is primarily a CD4 T cell–driven disorder. Several erythrocyte antigens recognized by T cells from IMHA patients have been identified previously (Day, 1999).

Triggers for Development of IMHA

At present there is no convincing explanation as to what triggers the spontaneous production of high concentrations of antierythrocyte antibodies in dogs with IMHA. The disease has a genetic susceptibility component, as evidenced by the high prevalence of IMHA in certain breeds of dogs such as cocker spaniels. A number of potential initiating factors have been implicated, although not proven, including previous infection, tissue injury,

recent vaccination, and drug therapy (Duval and Giger, 1996). In many respects IMHA in dogs differs greatly from the disease in most other species. For one thing, IMHA in dogs appears to exhibit a slight predilection for certain seasons, with the highest number of cases reported in the spring and early summer. In addition, disease onset is also extremely rapid in dogs, with otherwise previously healthy-appearing animals succumbing within a few days of diagnosis. It is difficult to detect circulating antierythrocyte antibodies in the serum of affected dogs even though erythrocyte surface–bound immunoglobulin G (IgG) can be readily detected in the same animals using flow cytometry (Morley et al, 2008). The most puzzling aspect of all may be the strong association between IMHA and the extremely high risk of developing widespread and often fatal thromboembolic disease.

In the vast majority of cases, IMHA develops spontaneously, with no known inciting cause. The diagnosis of primary IMHA is based on exclusion of other obvious causes for development of antierythrocyte antibodies, such as infection with erythroparasites or hemoplasmas or certain species of rickettsia. Secondary IMHA is diagnosed in animals in which potential inciting causes for development of antierythrocyte antibodies can be identified, primarily neoplasia or infection with erythroparasites.

Immunologic Abnormalities

The presence of immunoglobulin molecules bound to the surface of erythrocytes is the primary immunologic abnormality in dogs with IMHA. When evaluated using flow cytometry, most animals were found to have either IgG only or IgG plus IgM antibodies bound to erythrocytes, whereas it was distinctly rare to find animals with only IgM antibodies bound to their erythrocytes (Morley et al, 2008). Surface-bound antibodies on erythrocytes target the cells for rapid destruction in the spleen via macrophage engulfment, whereas intravascular hemolysis may occur when IgM antibodies activate complement. However, dogs with IMHA also have a number of other immunologic abnormalities. For example, dogs with active IMHA have increased serum concentrations of proinflammatory cytokines, especially monocyte chemoattractant protein-1 (MCP-1) and granulocyte-macrophage colony-stimulating factor (GM-CSF) (Kjelgaard-Hansen et al,

2011). Platelet activation is also a common finding in dogs with IMHA, with up to 75% of these dogs having activated platelets in circulation (Weiss and Brazzell, 2006). The authors have also found that antierythrocyte antibodies are commonly detected in dogs with thrombocytopenia, suggesting that cross-reactive antigens may be present in dogs with immune-platelet destruction. T cells reactive to peptides derived from erythrocyte antigens such as glycophorin have also been detected in dogs with IMHA, suggesting that autoimmune recognition of self-antigens by T cells may be a key immunologic abnormality in IMHA.

Thromboembolism

One of the most perplexing aspects of IMHA in dogs is the high prevalence of thromboembolic disease. Although the prevalence of thromboembolism is estimated at 30% to 50% clinically, careful necropsy studies suggest that the prevalence of thromboembolism in IMHA may actually be much higher. In addition, while pulmonary symptoms are often the first sign of thromboembolism in IMHA, emboli are actually quite widespread throughout the body in nearly all dogs with IMHA-associated thromboembolic disease, including emboli in the brain, heart, liver, spleen, and kidneys.

Thromboembolism is generally thought to result from endothelial injury, low blood flow, and/or hypercoagulability. While the cause of thromboembolism in IMHA is not currently known, several hypotheses have been proposed and others recently discounted. For one, endothelial injury due to antiendothelial antibodies or complement deposition does not appear to be an important inciting factor for thromboembolism in dogs with IMHA (Wells et al, 2009). Moreover, since dogs with IMHA primarily develop emboli in the venous circulation, low blood flow in arteries also does not appear to be an important factor. However, coagulation abnormalities are quite common in dogs with IMHA and are thought to reflect a fundamental interruption in normal coagulation pathways. For example, a prospective study of 20 dogs with IMHA found disseminated intravascular coagulation was present at the time of diagnosis in more than half the animals (Scott-Moncrieff et al, 2001). What is not clear at present is whether coagulopathies represent the primary hemostatic abnormality in dogs with IMHA or are instead simply a manifestation of a more fundamental problem.

Studies to determine whether dogs with early-onset IMHA are hypercoagulable have not yet been reported. It is known that dogs with IMHA have increased numbers of activated platelets, as assessed by up-regulation of P-selectin expression. Activated platelets are much more likely to spontaneously form thrombi, and platelet activation may be driven by increased concentrations of proinflammatory cytokines in dogs with IMHA, as reported recently (Kjelgaard-Hansen et al, 2011).

The role of lupus anticoagulant activity or antiphospholipid antibodies in triggering spontaneous clot formation in dogs with IMHA has also recently been investigated because these syndromes in humans are associated with widespread spontaneous formation of venous thromboemboli. However, at present there is little evidence of increased lupus anticoagulant activity or antiphospholipid antibodies in dogs with IMHA. Thus it remains an open question as to the primary underlying abnormality that drives the high prevalence of thromboembolic disease in dogs with IMHA.

Prognostic Factors

Given the high morbidity and mortality associated with IMHA in dogs, it is not surprising that there have been multiple attempts to identify clinical factors that are associated with a poor prognosis. Interestingly, factors specifically associated with positive outcomes have not yet been identified. At present, the clinical parameters most consistently associated with poor prognosis in dogs with IMHA include hyperbilirubinemia, thrombocytopenia, and leukocytosis, especially with increased band neutrophils. Other factors that have been identified in at least one study each as negative prognostic factors include petechiation, azotemia, and hypoalbuminemia. Somewhat counterintuitively, the degree of anemia, the magnitude of the reticulocyte response, and the degree of spherocytosis were not associated with outcomes in dogs with IMHA.

There have also been attempts to identify biomarkers that accurately predict treatment outcomes in animals monitored in a critical care setting. The acute-phase proteins α-1-acid glycoprotein and C-reactive protein were both found to be significantly elevated early in dogs with IMHA, but neither was able to predict survival. It was also reported recently that higher serum lactate concentrations at diagnosis correlated with increased mortality in IMHA, although serial lactate measurements were not performed (Holahan et al, 2010). In general it is believed that the change in serum lactate concentration over time is more predictive of outcome than a single baseline value measurement. In a recent study in which serum cytokines were evaluated in dogs with IMHA, the cytokines interleukin-15 (IL-15), IL-18, GM-CSF, and MCP-1 were associated with poor outcomes (Kjelgaard-Hansen et al, 2011). We also found increased serum MCP-1 concentrations were associated with a higher risk of death in dogs with IMHA (Duffy et al, 2010).

Therapy

Anticoagulant Therapy

Development of massive thromboembolism in dogs with IMHA is often associated with either acute death or the need for prolonged intensive therapy. Thus the general consensus is that animals with newly diagnosed IMHA should be aggressively anticoagulated. However, there is certainly no consensus as to how to best accomplish this in the critically ill dog with IMHA (Table 60-1). At present, anticoagulation protocols can be classified as targeting either coagulation factors or platelet function. However, none of the anticoagulation protocols discussed in the next sections have been shown in properly designed clinical trials to significantly improve survival in dogs with IMHA.

TABLE **60-1**

Anticoagulant Therapy for Dogs with IMHA

Drug	Dose	Monitoring	Therapeutic Range
Heparin (SC)	300-500 IU/kg q6h SC (titrate to effect)	1. aPTT 2. Anti-factor Xa concentration	1. Increase aPTT to 1.5-2.5 X normal starting range 2. Maintain in range of 0.35-0.75 U/ml
Heparin (CRI)	Loading dose of 100 IU/kg then CRI 100-300 units/kg q6-8h	1. aPTT* 2. Anti-factor Xa concentration (*monitor closely and adjust dose as needed)	1. Increase aPTT to 1.5-2.5 times normal starting range 2. Maintain in range of 0.35-0.75 U/ml
Low-molecular-weight heparin (dalteparin, enoxaparin)	Enoxaparin: 0.8 mg/kg q6h* SC Dalteparin: 100 mg/kg q12h* SC (*dosage adjusted based on therapeutic response)	Anti-factor Xa concentrations	Maintain in range of 0.5-1.0 U/ml
Low-dose aspirin	5 mg/kg q24h PO	None	Not determined
Clopidogrel (Plavix, others)	10 mg/kg loading dose, then 2 mg/kg q24h PO maintenance	None	Not determined

Unfractionated Heparin

One protocol relies primarily on anticoagulation using heparin. For most dogs, unfractionated heparin is selected because of its relatively low cost and the ease of monitoring with common hematologic analyzers. Although unfractionated heparin is much cheaper than fractionated, low-molecular-weight heparin (LMWH), it is also associated with greater risk of iatrogenic coagulopathy. Heparin functions as an anticoagulant by binding to antithrombin (AT), which in turn greatly enhances the activity of AT and thereby leads to inhibition of factors II and Xa and overall inhibition of coagulation. The dosing recommendations for administration of unfractionated heparin vary widely, from 50 to 500 IU/kg q6-8h SC. However, more rapid and effective anticoagulation can be achieved by continuous IV infusion of heparin (loading dose of 100 IU/kg administered IV, followed by 300 to 900 IU/kg/hr as a continuous rate infusion [CRI]). One study evaluating heparin CRI dosing in critically ill dogs reported that CRI doses of 900 IU/kg/hr were needed to achieve therapeutic anti-Xa levels. In this study a small number of dogs experienced hemorrhage, but in all dogs the baseline anti-Xa level was obtained within 4 hours of discontinuing the infusion (Scott et al, 2009). The dose of heparin required to achieve adequate anticoagulation in dogs with IMHA therefore appears to vary widely, and thus it is prudent to closely monitor individual patients and adjust anticoagulant doses accordingly. The effectiveness of heparin therapy is typically monitored using activated partial thromboplastin time (aPTT), with the goal of increasing aPTT by 1.5 to 2.5 times the baseline value. In healthy dogs, doses of unfractionated heparin in the range of 200 to 250 IU/kg q6h SC were sufficient to increase aPTT values by at least 1.5 times. However, in animals with IMHA with preexisting coagulopathies, much higher SC heparin doses or CRI of heparin may be required.

Low-Molecular-Weight Heparin

LMWH is a more highly purified form of heparin that inhibits the function of factor Xa but does not block the activity of thrombin. As a consequence, the likelihood of inducing unintended hemorrhage with LMWH is much lower than with unfractionated heparin. LMWH exhibits much less protein binding and displays more stable pharmacokinetics than unfractionated heparin. The activity of LMWH is monitored by measuring anti-factor Xa activity. Studies in dogs suggest that higher doses and more frequent dosing may be necessary with LMWH to achieve similar reductions in factor Xa activity as observed following LMWH therapy in humans. Although use of LMWH for anticoagulation in IMHA is appealing, the drug is much more expensive than fractionated heparin and therefore cost prohibitive for many dogs, especially for prolonged therapy.

Platelet Inhibition

An alternative approach to prevention of thromboembolism in dogs with IMHA is to block platelet function, although as noted previously there is no evidence to suggest that this approach is any more effective than targeting coagulation factors with heparin. However, the fact that most dogs with active IMHA have high numbers of activated platelets does provide some rationale for considering this approach. At present, the two best options for inhibiting platelet function in dogs include use of aspirin or use of clopidogrel (Plavix). For aspirin therapy, ultralow doses have been recommended previously (0.5 mg/kg q24h PO) to avoid inducing gastrointestinal injury in animals concurrently receiving high doses of corticosteroids. However, recent studies have indicated that this ultralow dose of aspirin had no effect on platelet function in the majority of healthy dogs. It is thus unclear at present what dose of aspirin is safe and effective in dogs with IMHA that are concurrently receiving high-dose corticosteroid therapy. A single antiinflammatory dose of 10 mg/kg consistently inhibits platelet function in dogs (Dudley et al, 2013). Other unpublished studies have documented this effect at doses of 5 mg/kg. However, increasing the dose of aspirin also substantially increases the risk of gastrointestinal toxicity due to the potent interaction of nonsteroidal antiinflammatory drugs (NSAIDs) with corticosteroids and the gastrointestinal tract.

Clopidogrel (Plavix) is an antiplatelet drug that causes irreversible inactivation of a subtype of the adenosine diphosphate (ADP) receptor on the membrane of platelets and thereby blocks platelet aggregation. Studies in dogs indicate that a loading dose of 10 mg/kg PO followed by a maintenance dose of 2 mg/kg q24h PO is sufficient to significantly inhibit platelet function. In a recent small clinical trial, clopidogrel administered to dogs with IMHA was not found to be associated with increased survival compared with dogs treated with ultra-low-dose aspirin but was also not associated with adverse effects (Mellett, Nakamura, and Bianco, 2011). Thus at present there is no evidence to indicate that clopidogrel is more effective or safer than low-dose aspirin for prophylaxis of thromboembolism in dogs with IMHA. In summary, the relative efficacy of clopidogrel versus heparin versus aspirin for prevention of thromboembolism in dogs with IMHA remains to be determined.

Immunosuppressive Therapy

Glucocorticoid Therapy

High-dose corticosteroid therapy remains the primary treatment for correction of immune abnormalities in dogs with IMHA. The most important effects of glucocorticoids in IMHA include rapid suppression of cytokine production by neutrophils, macrophages, and T cells; suppression of macrophage function, especially phagocytosis; and induction of lymphocyte apoptosis. By suppressing macrophage function, corticosteroids reduce erythrocyte destruction in the spleen and liver. In addition, over longer periods, corticosteroids also suppress T cell function and ultimately suppress production of antierythrocyte antibodies by B cells. However, antibodies already present in animals with IMHA may be relatively unaffected by corticosteroid therapy due to their relatively long half-life (weeks to months).

There is currently little consensus on the optimal dose of prednisone or dexamethasone for inducing effective immunosuppression in dogs. Relatively little work has been done to establish effective steroid doses in dogs and a wide range of doses are reported in the literature. In species in which prednisone doses have been carefully evaluated for their ability to completely occupy the glucocorticoid receptor, doses in the range of 0.5 to 1 mg/kg q24h have been shown to induce 90% to 100% receptor occupancy, which is more than sufficient to induce functional immunosuppression. Therefore there is at present little scientific rationale for administration of doses of prednisone exceeding 1 to 2 mg/kg q24h to dogs for immunosuppression in IMHA. Current protocols suggest induction therapy with 1 to 2 mg/kg q24h of prednisone (or prednisolone) until disease remission is induced, as

assessed by inducing normal, stable packed cell volume (PCV) values for several weeks. At that point, tapering of prednisone begins over a period of several months, accompanied by careful monitoring of PCV values. For animals that cannot tolerate prednisone therapy, dexamethasone may be administered as an alternative at an initial dose of 0.125 to 0.25 mg/kg q24h.

Recently, an alternative approach to dosing corticosteroids (very-high-dose pulse steroid therapy) for rapid disease remission of IMHA has been under investigation. In this approach, very high doses (5 to 10 mg/kg q24h) of a water-soluble corticosteroid (e.g., prednisolone sodium succinate [Solu-Delta-Cortef]) are administered by rapid IV infusion once daily for 2 to 3 days. After the brief 2- to 3-day induction period, the corticosteroid dose is rapidly reduced to lower maintenance oral doses of prednisone (0.5 to 1 mg/kg q24h). The rationale for the very-high-dose approach is based on the fact that very high doses of corticosteroids induce "nongenomic" effects on immune cells, which are reflected by profound and rapid immunosuppression. Thus these very high doses of water-soluble corticosteroids block immune abnormalities in IMHA much more rapidly than conventional steroid therapy (Lowenberg et al, 2008; Whitley and Day, 2011). However, the effectiveness of the very-high-dose pulse steroid approach remains to be determined by carefully controlled clinical trials in dogs with IMHA.

Adjunctive Immunosuppressive Drugs

Although disease remission can be induced in some dogs with IMHA with corticosteroids alone, a number of dogs require the addition of adjunctive immunosuppressive drugs. These additional drugs are administered to achieve more complete immunosuppression and to allow more rapid tapering of corticosteroid therapy to ameliorate steroid adverse effects. At present, azathioprine and cyclosporine are the most widely administered adjunctive immunosuppressive drugs (Whitley and Day, 2011). Both azathioprine and cyclosporine have a relatively slow onset of action and generally require several days to a week for full activity. The advantages of azathioprine are its relatively low cost and low incidence of adverse effects. However, azathioprine is associated in some animals with acute hepatic toxicity, which can be life threatening if not recognized early (by serially monitoring liver enzymes) and rapidly discontinuing therapy. There have been no published clinical trials that have demonstrated the clinical effectiveness of azathioprine as an immunosuppressant in dogs, and a recent metaanalysis suggests that azathioprine does not provide any clinical benefit in dogs with IMHA (Piek et al, 2008).

The clinical benefits of adding cyclosporine to prednisone therapy for IMHA also have not been established by rigorous clinical trials. Side effects of cyclosporine therapy in dogs are primarily associated with gastrointestinal adverse effects, while nephrotoxicity is possible at higher doses. Dogs treated with cyclosporine may also develop reactivation of oral papillomatosis lesions. While monitoring of serum cyclosporine concentrations has been advocated, it should be noted that synergistic immunosuppression with prednisone may be achieved by serum concentrations below those typically required for suppression of transplant rejection. Once disease remission is achieved using combination therapy, it is generally recommended that prednisone therapy be tapered and discontinued first, followed by tapering of cyclosporine or azathioprine therapy.

Experimental Drugs for Immunosuppression

For particularly severe or refractory cases of IMHA, alternative immunosuppressive drugs may be considered. The two primary options at present are mycophenolate mofetil and leflunomide. In both cases, corticosteroid therapy is continued, while mycophenolate or leflunomide is substituted for azathioprine or cyclosporine.

Mycophenolate

Although mycophenolate has a similar mechanism of action as azathioprine, the drug is up to 10 times more potent and has a much more rapid onset of action. Recommended doses of mycophenolate are 5 to 12 mg/kg q12h PO. Intravenous administration of mycophenolate results in much more rapid onset of action than oral administration. Mycophenolate has been widely used previously as a potent immunosuppressive drug for dogs undergoing bone marrow transplantation. Side effects are related primarily to the gastrointestinal tract, including vomiting and diarrhea, which may be severe.

Leflunomide

Treatment with leflunomide has become more attractive recently now that generic versions of the drug are available. The currently recommended leflunomide dose is 2 to 6 mg/kg q24h PO. If serum concentrations are monitored, a recommended therapeutic serum trough concentration is 20 µg/ml. While leflunomide has been evaluated in small numbers of dogs with immune-mediated disorders, and in experimental animals undergoing renal transplantation, there have been no controlled clinical trials of leflunomide therapy for dogs with IMHA. It is therefore unclear whether leflunomide offers any particular advantage over azathioprine, cyclosporine, or mycophenolate for the management of IMHA in dogs.

Intravenous Immunoglobulin

Administration of intravenous immunoglobulin (IVIG) is a third option for the short-term management of IMHA, especially for dogs with life-threatening disease. High doses of pooled human immunoglobulins exert potent immunosuppressive effects, through still incompletely understood mechanisms that involve signaling through immunosuppressive receptors on macrophages. Thus intravenous administration of human immunoglobulins can induce rapid immunosuppression in dogs with immune-mediated diseases. A single dose of 0.5 to 1 gm/kg administered IV over 4 to 6 hours is recommended. Results from a randomized clinical trial suggest that administration of IVIG can be beneficial in dogs with refractory immune-mediated thrombocytopenia, although controlled studies of IVIG administration for dogs with IMHA have not been reported. Administration of IVIG is expensive, and presumed allergic reactions to the drug have been reported. To minimize administration reactions, animals may be premedicated with diphenhydramine.

References and Suggested Reading

Day MJ: Antigen specificity in canine autoimmune haemolytic anaemia, *Vet Immunol Immunopathol* 69:215-224, 1999.

Dudley A et al: Cyclooxygenase expression and platelet function in healthy dogs receiving low-dose aspirin, *J Vet Intern Med* 27:141, 2013.

Duffy AL et al: Serum concentrations of monocyte chemoattractant protein-1 in healthy and critically ill dogs, *Vet Clin Pathol* 39:302-305, 2010.

Duval D, Giger U: Vaccine-associated immune-mediated hemolytic anemia in the dog, *J Vet Intern Med* 10:290-295, 1996.

Holahan ML, Brown AJ, Drobatz KJ: The association of blood lactate concentration with outcome in dogs with idiopathic immune-mediated hemolytic anemia: 173 cases (2003-2006), *J Vet Emerg Crit Care* 20(4):413, 2010.

Kjelgaard-Hansen M et al: Use of serum concentrations of interleukin-18 and monocyte chemoattractant protein-1 as prognostic indicators in primary immune-mediated hemolytic anemia in dogs, *J Vet Intern Med J Vet Intern Med* 25:76-82, 2011.

Lowenberg MC et al: Novel insights into mechanisms of glucocorticoid action and the development of new glucocorticoid receptor ligands, *Steroids* 73:1025-1029, 2008.

McManus PM, Craig LE: Correlation between leukocytosis and necropsy findings in dogs with immune-mediated hemolytic anemia: 34 cases (1994-1999). *J Am Vet Med Assoc* 218:1308-1313, 2001.

Mellet AM, Nakamura RK, Bianco D: A prospective study of clopidogrel therapy in dogs with primary immune-mediated hemolytic anemia, *J Vet Intern Med* 25:71-75, 2011.

Morley P et al: Anti-erythrocyte antibodies and disease associations in anemic and nonanemic dogs, *J Vet Intern Med* 22:886-892, 2008.

Piek CJ et al: Idiopathic immune-mediated hemolytic anemia: treatment outcome and prognostic factors in 149 dogs, *J Vet Intern Med* 22:366-373, 2008.

Piek CJ et al: Lack of evidence of a beneficial effect of azathioprine in dogs treated with prednisolone for idiopathic immune-mediated hemolytic anemia: a retrospective cohort study, *BMC Vet Res* 7:15, 2011.

Scott KC, Hansen BD, DeFrancesco TC: Coagulation effects of low molecular weight heparin compared with heparin in dogs considered to be at risk for clinically significant venous thrombosis, *J Vet Emerg Crit Care* 19:74, 2009.

Scott-Moncrieff C: Immune-mediated hemolytic anemia: 70 cases (1988-1996), *J Am Anim Hosp Assoc* 37:11, 2001.

Scott-Moncrieff JC et al: Hemostatic abnormalities in dogs with primary immune-mediated hemolytic anemia, *J Am Anim Hosp Assoc* 37:220-227, 2001.

Stahn C, Buttgereit F: Genomic and nongenomic effects of glucocorticoids, *Nat Clin Pract Rheumatol* 4:525-533, 2008.

Weinkle TK et al: Evaluation of prognostic factors, survival rates, and treatment protocols for immune-mediated hemolytic anemia in dogs: 151 cases (1993-2002). *J Am Vet Med Assoc* 226:1869-1880, 2005.

Weiss DJ, Brazzell JL: Detection of activated platelets in dogs with primary immune-mediated hemolytic anemia, *J Vet Intern Med* 20:682-686, 2006.

Wells R et al: Anti-endothelial cell antibodies in dogs with immune-mediated hemolytic anemia and other diseases associated with high risk of thromboembolism, *J Vet Intern Med* 23:295-300, 2009.

Whitley NT, Day MJ: Immunomodulatory drugs and their application to the management of canine immune-mediated disease, *J Small Anim Pract* 52:70-85, 2011.

CHAPTER 61

Thrombocytopenia

JENNIFER A. NEEL, *Raleigh, North Carolina*
ADAM J. BIRKENHEUER, *Raleigh, North Carolina*
CAROL B. GRINDEM, *Raleigh, North Carolina*

Thrombocytopenia is the most common platelet disorder observed in dogs and cats. Of dogs and cats presenting to the authors' institution from 2006 to 2012, thrombocytopenia was found in 17.6% of dogs and 12% of cats, with 6.2% of dogs and 4.8% of cats having counts of less than 100,000 platelets/µl. Previous studies at this university have shown that in dogs the etiology of thrombocytopenia is 5% primary immune mediated, 13% neoplasia, 23% infectious or inflammatory disease, and 59% miscellaneous or multifactorial causes (Grindem et al, 1991). In cats causes of thrombocytopenia included 2% primary immune mediated, 20% neoplasia, 29% infectious diseases, 7% cardiac diseases, 22% multiple etiologies, and 20% unknown causes (Jordan, Grindem, and Breitschwerdt, 1993).

Pseudothrombocytopenia occurs when platelets present in a specimen are not counted. This must be eliminated as the cause of a low platelet count. Platelet aggregation that results from activation during blood sampling is a major cause of falsely decreased counts and occurs commonly in cats; one study found low automated platelet counts in 71% of feline samples (Norman et al, 2001). Large platelets are also a cause of low platelet counts on some automated impedance-based hematology analyzers when they overlap with the size of red blood cells (RBCs). Ethylenediaminetetraacetic acid (EDTA)–induced platelet clumping has rarely been reported. Some breeds such as cavalier King Charles spaniels and greyhounds normally have lower platelet counts than most dogs or established platelet reference intervals.

Mechanisms of Thrombocytopenia

Thrombocytopenia occurs by one of four general mechanisms: decreased production, increased consumption/destruction, sequestration, and excessive loss. Often more than one mechanism occurs in any single disease or disorder. Decreased production is seen with suppression or destruction of megakaryocytes caused by immune-mediated disease, drugs, infectious agents, whole body irradiation, and myelophthisic disorders. Increased consumption or destruction is a common cause of thrombocytopenia in dogs and cats; etiologies include primary or secondary immune-mediated disease, drugs, toxins, disseminated intravascular coagulation (DIC) (vascular damage, septicemia, endotoxemia, massive tissue necrosis/damage, or release of procoagulant substances), disseminated neoplasia, and infectious diseases. Thrombocytopenia resulting from sequestration or abnormal distribution of platelets can be caused by splenic congestion/splenomegaly, hepatomegaly, neoplasia, severe hypothermia in dogs, and experimentally induced endotoxemia. Marked thrombocytopenia is not typically noted, and the effect is often transient. Excessive loss can occur with massive blood loss and is observed in some cases of hemorrhage associated with rodenticide toxicity, but often platelet counts are normal to increased in these patients. This chapter focuses on causes and treatment of immune-mediated and infectious thrombocytopenia.

Immune-Mediated Thrombocytopenia

Immune-mediated thrombocytopenia (IMTP) can be primary, secondary, vaccine induced, or posttransfusion. *Primary,* or *idiopathic, IMTP* is reported most commonly in dogs but has also been reported in cats. This is a disease of exclusion; other potential causes of secondary IMTP must be eliminated before a diagnosis of primary IMTP can be made. Acquired amegakaryocytic thrombocytopenia is a rare form of either primary or secondary immune-mediated disease resulting from autoantibodies directed toward megakaryocytes and has been reported in both dogs and cats (Thomas, 2010).

Secondary IMTP occurs when antibody targets nonself antigens adsorbed onto the surface of platelets or when immune complexes become bound to platelet surfaces. Underlying mechanisms include systemic autoimmune diseases (systemic lupus erythematosus), neoplasia, infectious agents, and drugs; occasionally, however, additional causes are identified or suspected, such as pemphigus, juvenile-onset polyarthritis syndrome in Akitas, and possibly canine inflammatory bowel disease (Scott and Jutkowitz, 2010). Thrombocytopenia associated with neoplasia is often multifactorial, with secondary immune-mediated destruction representing one potential component. Lymphoma in dogs has been associated most commonly with secondary IMTP, but it can occur with any neoplasm. In one study 10% of dogs with neoplasia had concurrent thrombocytopenia, and of this group 61% did not have identifiable factors known to cause secondary IMTP (Grindem et al, 1994). As with neoplasia, thrombocytopenia in infectious diseases is often multifactorial and can include a secondary immune-mediated component. Antiplatelet antibodies have been detected in various infectious diseases, including *Ehrlichia canis* infections and Rocky Mountain spotted fever (RMSF). Drugs are rarely reported to cause a true primary IMTP; more typically it is secondary in nature. With this mechanism the drug acts as a hapten, allowing immune-mediated targeting of the platelets. A few drugs are capable of causing a secondary immune-mediated reaction without a history of prior exposure (e.g., heparin in horses), but most occur following extended use or prior exposure. Several documented cases involving trimethoprim sulfonamide/sulfamethoxazole have been reported in dogs, but it could potentially be caused by any number of drugs. Vaccine-induced thrombocytopenia has been reported in dogs following immunization with modified live vaccines (canine distemper). Typically thrombocytopenia is mild and develops within 3 to 10 days after vaccination, but marked thrombocytopenia can occur. Posttransfusional thrombocytopenia has been reported occasionally in dogs.

Infectious Etiologies Associated with Thrombocytopenia

Table 61-1 lists infectious agents associated with thrombocytopenia in dogs and cats (Greene, 2012). Thrombocytopenia associated with infectious causes is often multifactorial, involving increased consumption, destruction, vasculitis, or sequestration; in many cases the pathogenesis is incompletely understood. As mentioned previously, a number of agents are associated with secondary IMTP. Some are known to cause bone marrow suppression, including feline leukemia virus (FeLV) infection, feline immunodeficiency virus (FIV) infection, feline panleukopenia (parvovirus), canine parvovirus, and chronic monocytic ehrlichiosis (*E. canis*, *Ehrlichia*

TABLE **61-1**

Infectious Causes of Thrombocytopenia in Dogs and Cats

Disease	Species	Mechanism	Diagnostic Tests*	Therapy
Viral				
Canine distemper	C	U	Ag detection, PCR, serology	Supportive
Canine herpesvirus	C	V	Ag detection, serology, VI	Supportive
Canine parvovirus infection: canine parvovirus 2	C	P, U	Ag detection, EM feces, PCR, serology	Supportive
Infectious canine hepatitis: canine adenovirus 1	C	U, V	Serology, PCR, VI	Supportive
Feline immunodeficiency virus	F	P	Serology, PCR	Supportive
Feline infectious peritonitis: feline coronavirus	F	U, V	Ag detection, histopathology, PCR, serology	Supportive
Feline leukemia virus	F	P	Ag detection, PCR, serology	Supportive
Feline panleukopenia/feline parvovirus	F	P, U	Ag detection, EM, fecal VI, PCR, serology	Supportive
Rickettsial, Neorickettsial, Anaplasmal, Mycoplasmal				
Canine granulocytic anaplasmosis: *Anaplasma phagocytophilum*	C	D, U	Blood smear, PCR, serology	Doxycycline (10 mg/kg PO q24h for 28 days)
Canine granulocytic ehrlichiosis: *Ehrlichia ewingii*	C	D, U	Blood smear, PCR, serology	Doxycycline (10 mg/kg PO q24h for 28 days)
Canine monocytic ehrlichiosis: *Ehrlichia canis, Ehrlichia chaffeensis*	C	D, P, U	Blood smear, PCR, serology	Doxycycline (10 mg/kg PO q24h for 28 days)
Feline granulocytic anaplasmosis: *A. phagocytophilum*	F	D?	PCR, serology	Doxycycline (10 mg/kg PO q24h for 28 days)
Feline mononuclear ehrlichiosis *E. canis, Neorickettsia risticii* (?)	F	D?	PCR, serology	Doxycycline (10 mg/kg PO q24h for 28 days)
Hemotropic mycoplasmosis: *Mycoplasma haemofelis*	C, F	D, S	Ag detection, blood smear, PCR	Doxycycline (10 mg/kg PO q24h for 28 days), enrofloxacin (5 mg/kg PO q24h for 14 days)
Rocky mountain spotted fever: *Rickettsia rickettsii*	C	D, V	Ag detection (skin), PCR, serology	Doxycycline (10 mg/kg PO q24h for 28 days)
Salmon poisoning disease: *Neorickettsia helminthoeca*	C	D, U	Cytology, fecal examination	Doxycycline (10 mg/kg PO q24h for 28 days)
Thrombocytotropic ehrlichiosis: *Anaplasma platys*	C	D, U	Ag detection, blood smear, PCR, serology	Doxycycline (10 mg/kg PO q24h for 28 days)

Continued

TABLE 61-1

Infectious Causes of Thrombocytopenia in Dogs and Cats—cont'd

Disease	Species	Mechanism	Diagnostic Tests*	Therapy
Bacterial				
Bacteremia/septicemia	C, F	D, U, V	Blood, urine, body fluid culture	Ampicillin sulbactam (30 mg/kg IV q8h) and enrofloxacin (10 mg/kg IV q24h)
Bartonellosis: *Bartonella vinsonii, Bartonella henselae*	C	D, V	Culture, PCR, serology	Optimal treatment is unknown. Azithromycin (5 mg/kg PO q24h for 5 days, then EOD for 45 days) has been recommended
Endotoxemia: most often *Escherichia, Klebsiella, Enterobacter, Proteus, Pseudomonas*	C, F	S	Blood, urine, wound culture, often presumptive	Ampicillin sulbactam (30 mg/kg IV q8h) and enrofloxacin (10 mg/kg IV q24h)
Leptospirosis	C	D, U, V	Ag detection, histopathology, PCR, serology, urine dark-field microscopy, urine or blood culture	Ampicillin (22 mg/kg IV q8h for 2 weeks) followed by doxycycline (5 mg/kg PO q12h for 3 weeks). Some recommend doxycycline for initial therapy
Plague: *Yersinia pestis*	F	S, U	Ag detection, culture, PCR, serology	Doxycycline (10 mg/kg PO q24h for 21 days), enrofloxacin (5 mg/kg PO q24h for 14 days)
Salmonellosis	C, F	D, S, U, V	Culture, PCR	Enrofloxacin (5-10 mg/kg IV q24h) reserved for patients with septicemia
Tularemia: *Francisella tularensis*	C, F	D, U, V	Ag detection, culture, PCR, serology	Doxycycline (5 mg/kg PO q12h)
Protozoal				
Babesiosis: *Babesia canis, Babesia gibsoni, Babesia conradae, Babesia microti*-like sp. *Babesia* sp. (Coco)	C	U, S	Blood smear, PCR, serology	Imidocarb dipropionate (6.6 mg/kg IM twice, 2 weeks apart) for *B. canis*, atovaquone (13.5 mg/kg PO q8h for 10 days) and azithromycin (10 mg/kg PO q24h for 10 days) for *B. gibsoni*
Cytauxzoonosis: *Cytauxzoon felis*	F	U, S	Blood smear, cytology, PCR†	Imidocarb dipropionate (2-3 mg/kg IM twice 1 week apart) or atovaquone (15 mg/kg PO q8h for 10 days) and azithromycin (10 mg/kg PO q24h for 10 days)
Leishmaniasis	C	U	Ag detection, cytology, PCR, serology, Western blot analysis	Meglumine antimoniate (100 mg/kg SC q24h) and allopurinol (15 mg/kg PO q12h) for 3-4 months, allopurinol indefinitely
Toxoplasmosis: *Toxoplasma gondii*	C, F	U	Fecal (cats), serology, cytology	Clindamycin (12.5-25 mg/kg PO q12h)
Nemotodal				
Heartworm disease: *Dirofilaria immitis*	C	D, U, V	Ag detection, blood smear, Knott test, serology	Melarsomine (2.5 mg/kg IM)
Angiostrongylus vasorum	C	D, U, V	Fecal, direct, or Baermann	Fenbendazole (25-50 mg/kg PO q24h for 7-21 days)
Fungal				
Disseminated candidiasis	C, F	U	Culture, cytology	Itraconazole (5-10 mg/kg PO q12h)
Histoplasmosis: *Histoplasma capsulatum*	C, F	U	Ag detection, culture, cytology, serology	Itraconazole (5-10 mg/kg PO q12h)

Ag, Antigen; *C*, canine; *D*, destruction; *EM*, electron microscopy; *F*, feline; *PCR*, polymerase chain reaction; *S*, sequestration; *P*, immunosuppression; *U*, utilization; *V*, vasculitis; *VI*, virus isolation; *?*, uncertain.

*Refer to Greene CE: *Infectious diseases of the dog and cat*, ed 4, for more information on diagnostic tests, available test kits, specimens, and commercial diagnostic laboratories.

†Available at the North Carolina State University, Tick-Borne Disease Laboratory, Raleigh, NC.

chaffeensis). FeLV and FIV are of particular importance in feline thrombocytopenia. Viral diseases (FeLV, FIV, and feline infectious peritonitis [FIP]) are a major cause of or contributing factor to the development of thrombocytopenia in cats (Jordan, Grindem, and Breitschwerdt, 1993; Thomas, 2010).

DIC is commonly seen in gram-negative sepsis, infectious canine hepatitis (ICH), leptospirosis, salmonellosis, babesiosis (virulent strains), canine and feline parvovirus, cytauxzoonosis, and plague. Vascular damage occurs in endotoxemia, septicemia, heartworm disease, FIP, ICH, RMSF, and bartonellosis. Platelet sequestration within the spleen, liver, or lungs is noted in endotoxemia; plague; salmonellosis; babesiosis; cytauxzoonosis; and hemolytic crisis secondary to babesiosis, hemotropic mycoplasmosis (formerly hemobartonellosis), or cytauxzoonosis. Etiologic agents vary with geographic location and may be limited by the vector, intermediate host, or environmental requirements of the organism.

The degree of thrombocytopenia can vary. Although thrombocytopenia is most severe in IMTP and overwhelming sepsis (counts of less than 50,000/µl and often fewer than 10,000/µl), it can be moderate to severe in canine monocytic ehrlichiosis. In one report on prevalence of *E. canis* infection in thrombocytopenic dogs in an endemic region, infection was found in 63.1% of dogs with a platelet count of less than 100,000/µl but in only 21% of dogs with platelet counts between 100,000 and 200,000/µl; nonthrombocytopenic dogs had an infection rate of 1.4% (Bulla et al, 2004). Severe, cyclic thrombocytopenia is also seen with thrombocytotropic ehrlichiosis, but dogs are not systemically sick; clinically ill dogs with this disease should be evaluated for concurrent tick-borne diseases such as monocytic ehrlichiosis.

Tests used to diagnose infectious diseases include serology, polymerase chain reaction (PCR), antigen detection in fluids or tissues, cytology, blood smear evaluation, culture, virus isolation, electron microscopy, and histopathology (see Table 61-1; Greene, 2012).

Clinical Evaluation of Thrombocytopenia

Because thrombocytopenia typically is secondary to another disease or condition, signalment, history, and physical examination findings are extremely important. Primary IMTP is more commonly reported in middle-aged female dogs, especially cocker spaniels, German shepherds, poodles, and Old English sheepdogs, but can occur in any breed at any age. Most animals present for signs relating to the underlying disease, or the thrombocytopenia is found serendipitously on routine blood work. Risk of bleeding increases as platelet counts decrease below 20,000/µl, although spontaneous bleeding typically does not occur, even with marked thrombocytopenia. The authors have seen primary IMTP in dogs with platelet counts of fewer than 5000/µl that have no bleeding tendencies or clinical signs.

When present, signs directly related to thrombocytopenia can include petechiae; ecchymoses; prolonged bleeding after trauma, venipuncture, whelping, or surgical procedures; prolonged estrus; bruising; melena; hematemesis; intraocular hemorrhage or blindness;

hematuria; oral bleeding; neurologic signs associated with cerebral bleeding; and epistaxis. Petechiae and ecchymoses are easiest to identify on mucous membranes or thin-skinned regions such as the abdomen. Other signs related to the underlying cause of thrombocytopenia may include fever, weight loss, enlarged lymph nodes, splenomegaly, hepatomegaly, abdominal masses, stiffness, joint pain, neurologic signs, or edema.

A thorough history can provide valuable clues to the cause of thrombocytopenia. Vaccination history; FeLV and FIV status; exposure to drugs or toxins; travel history; exposure to infectious agents, ticks, or other animals; history of previous illnesses; tick/flea/heartworm preventive use; indoor/outdoor status; and clinical signs or changes noted by the owner should all be ascertained.

Diagnostic Approach to Infectious or Immune-Mediated Thrombocytopenia

The first step is to confirm the presence of thrombocytopenia by performing a complete blood count with an automated platelet count and examining a peripheral blood smear. Extremely high or low platelet counts may not be assessed accurately by automated instruments if they are outside instrument linearity, and platelet clumps or large platelets can result in spuriously low counts. For these reasons abnormal automated platelet counts must always be confirmed by examination of a blood smear. Platelet clumping is best appreciated along the feathered edge of the smear and, if present, indicates that a new sample must be collected. If repeated samples yield clumped platelets, blood can be collected into a syringe rinsed with EDTA. Alternatively, a needle can be inserted into a peripheral vein, and blood collected directly from the hub and immediately put into a 1% ammonium oxalate solution (1:100 dilution) for a manual platelet count. When clumps are found, platelets typically are present in sufficient numbers to prevent spontaneous hemorrhage. If clumps are not present, the platelet count can be estimated by multiplying the mean platelet count in ten 100× fields within the monolayer of the blood film by 15,000 to give the total platelet count per microliter. A patient with a normal or increased platelet count with signs of a primary hemostatic defect (petechia, ecchymosis) should be evaluated for platelet function defects or vascular disorders.

Platelet size and morphology should also be evaluated in the thrombocytopenic patient. Large platelets are an indication of increased platelet production and support a regenerative response by the bone marrow. Normal-size platelets may be seen in acute disorders in which the bone marrow has not had time to respond, or they can indicate a hyporesponsive or unresponsive marrow. Small platelets or platelet fragments can be associated with early or nonregenerative IMTP. *Anaplasma platys* may be identified as stippled blue morulae within platelets during clinical episodes.

Evaluation of the erythrogram, leukogram, and a peripheral blood smear can help distinguish decreased platelet production from increased use or destruction. Decreased production or suppression of only the megakaryocytic line is rare; most causes are associated with decreased production or suppression of the myeloid and erythroid series as well. Typically a peripheral neutropenia without a left shift is seen. A nonregenerative anemia may be present in long-standing conditions but is not expected in acute conditions or conditions of short duration because of the long life span of RBCs (110 days in dogs, 68 days in cats). Conditions or diseases causing increased platelet destruction or consumption are often associated with an inflammatory leukogram characterized by a neutrophilia or neutropenia with a left shift. Toxic change may also be seen in a variety of inflammatory conditions; when moderate to marked, it is most indicative of a bacterial infection. A mild, nonregenerative anemia (anemia of inflammatory disease) often accompanies inflammatory conditions. Although classically associated with chronic conditions, this anemia can develop within a week of the onset of significant inflammation. Evidence of hemolytic disease may be seen with some etiologic agents such as *Babesia, Cytauxzoon,* and *Mycoplasma*; these agents may also be identified in RBCs on a peripheral blood smear. Morulae may be found within neutrophils in acute canine granulocytic ehrlichiosis and anaplasmosis or in monocytes in monocytic ehrlichiosis. IMTP can also accompany primary or secondary immune-mediated hemolytic anemia, which is classically characterized by a regenerative anemia with spherocytosis and an inflammatory leukogram. Vasculitis and DIC often result in circulating schistocytes.

Examination of the bone marrow may be indicated if the cause of the thrombocytopenia is not apparent from the routine clinical evaluation. Other indications for bone marrow examination include suspicion of leukemia, multiple myeloma, or lymphoma or other myeloproliferative disorder, or the presence of multiple cytopenias of unknown origin. Collection of a bone marrow aspirate for cytology and a bone marrow core biopsy for histopathology is ideal; these provide the greatest amount of information when interpreted together. Even when thrombocytopenia is severe, it is not a contraindication for performing a bone marrow biopsy. Patients rarely have significant hemorrhage from the procedure; however, it is wise to choose a site without significant muscle mass such as the proximal humerus where hemorrhage can be more easily controlled. Transfusion (fresh whole blood, platelet concentrate, or lyophilized platelets) may be necessary before performing the biopsy if the patient is bleeding actively. Increased numbers and immaturity of megakaryocytes indicate a regenerative response; decreased numbers indicate an unresponsive or preregenerative marrow (a regenerative response should occur within 3 to 5 days of acute thrombocytopenia).

A coagulation profile consisting of prothrombin time (PT), activated partial thromboplastin time (aPTT), and fibrin degradation products (FDPs) should ideally be performed in all animals with thrombocytopenia. D-dimer levels may also be useful in dogs. Fulminant DIC is classically characterized by a prolonged PT and aPTT with significantly increased FDPs and D-dimer levels, but peracute or chronic DIC should not be ruled out if coagulation parameters are within reference intervals and clinical suspicion of DIC is high. DIC is a common secondary condition in a variety of infectious, inflammatory, and neoplastic diseases and is triggered by vascular damage, massive tissue damage, or release of activating substances (see Chapter 63). Hemorrhage caused by rodenticide toxicity is characterized by markedly prolonged PT and aPTT with normal FDPs or D-dimer levels. Selection of additional diagnostic tests is based on information provided by the patient's history, signalment, physical examination findings, and initial blood work. EDTA anticoagulated blood and a serum sample should be collected and saved for serology, PCR, and culture and antiplatelet antibody assays; these specimens must be collected before initiating therapy. Culture of blood or other fluids/tissues should be performed on any animal with suspected septicemia. Survey radiographs or ultrasonography may be indicated. Enlarged lymph nodes or organs, masses, and effusions should be examined via cytology or histopathology. Joint fluid should be collected and examined cytologically in animals with joint pain or swelling, and cerebrospinal fluid (CSF) collection and cytologic evaluation may be indicated in animals with neurologic disease. Titers for infectious diseases, PCR, and culture can also be performed on joint fluid or CSF. For animals with suspected systemic immune-mediated disease, antinuclear antibody testing, antierythrocytic antibody testing (Coombs' test), and potentially histopathologic and immunohistochemical examination of dermal lesions should be performed.

Tests to confirm IMTP are available, but it is important to remember that no test can distinguish primary from secondary disease; thus all causes of secondary immune-mediated disease must be ruled out before a diagnosis of primary IMTP can be made. Tests can detect platelet-bindable autoantibodies in patient serum or plasma (indirect assays) or antibody present on the surface of platelets or megakaryocytes (direct assays). Direct assays are preferred because they are more specific; indirect assays fail to differentiate autoimmune antibodies from alloantibodies, circulating immune complexes, or nonspecific immunoglobulin G aggregates formed in stored serum. Shipping and handling potentially can be problematic for direct antiplatelet antibody assays; thus it is advisable to contact the reference laboratory regarding sample handling before collection and shipping. The direct megakaryocytic immunofluorescence assay (D-MIFA) circumvents sample handling issues by using unstained, air-dried bone marrow smears. When this assay is used, it is important to remember that poorly cellular specimens or specimens with inadequate numbers of megakaryocytes preclude adequate evaluation. In addition, autoantibodies targeting platelets may not target megakaryocytes; thus a negative result cannot be used to rule out immune-mediated disease. Low sensitivity has been reported with this test.

Therapy

The goals of treatment are to stop hemorrhage, halt ongoing platelet destruction, and treat any underlying disorders. Treatment usually consists of a combination of both specific and supportive measures. Supportive measures include the use of blood products (whole blood or packed RBCs) or purified polymerized bovine hemoglobin solutions to maintain oxygen delivery to tissues and

TABLE 61-2

Adjunctive Immune Suppressive Therapies

Drug	Dose	Side Effects/Monitoring
Azathioprine	2 mg/kg PO q24h for 2 weeks, then 2 mg/kg PO every other day	Bone marrow suppression, hepatotoxicity, pancreatitis, complete blood counts, serum biochemical profiles
Cyclosporine	5-10 mg/kg PO q12h	Vomiting, diarrhea, therapeutic drug monitoring
Human γ-globulin	0.5-1 g/kg IV over 6-12 hours once	Anaphylaxis, thromboembolism
Mycophenolate mofetil	10-20 mg/kg PO q12h	Vomiting, diarrhea, pyoderma

IV, Intravenously; *PO,* orally.

crystalloid fluids to maintain hydration in patients that are anorexic and not drinking. Venous access may not be necessary in patients that are stable. When intravenous access is needed, catheterization of the jugular vein is contraindicated in patients with severe thrombocytopenia because of the difficulty in controlling hemorrhage at this site. The use of fresh frozen plasma is limited to patients with concurrent coagulopathies associated with decreased clotting factors such as rodenticide intoxication or DIC. Platelet transfusions have limited use because of difficulty in transfusing a large enough number of platelets to exert a clinical benefit combined with the short circulating half-life of transfused platelets in patients with destructive platelet disorders. Platelet transfusions may provide transient improvement in hemostasis but typically do not increase detectable platelet counts. They can be performed using platelet concentrates, platelet-rich plasma, or whole blood and should be reserved for patients with life-threatening hemorrhage. Since the gastrointestinal tract is the most common site of significant bleeding secondary to thrombocytopenia, gastroprotectants (sucralfate, H₂ blockers, proton pump inhibitors) are frequently used. However, since true ulceration is rarely present in dogs with IMTP, the use of these drugs for gastrointestinal bleeding secondary to thrombocytopenia is questionable.

If an underlying infectious cause of thrombocytopenia is identified or highly suspected, specific therapy should be instituted. Treatments for selected infectious causes of thrombocytopenia are listed in Table 61-1. In patients that are stable and not experiencing life-threatening hemorrhage, antimicrobial therapy alone may be sufficient to resolve the thrombocytopenia. However, specific therapy against infectious agents may not be sufficient to halt the immune-mediated destructive process, and concurrent immunosuppressive therapy may be indicated. When immunosuppressive therapy and antimicrobial therapy are started concurrently, worsening of infection from the immunosuppressive therapy is rare, except with systemic fungal infections or in cases in which immunosuppression has been ongoing for weeks to months before antimicrobial therapy. When instituted simultaneously in cases with IMTP secondary to infectious diseases, immunosuppressive therapy frequently can be weaned more quickly (i.e., 25% dose reductions every 2 weeks) than in dogs with primary IMTP.

When no underlying cause of IMTP can be identified, immunosuppressive therapy is the treatment of choice. Corticosteroids remain the backbone of therapy for the treatment of primary IMTP. Prednisone is usually administered at a dose of 1 to 2 mg/kg q12h PO for a minimum of 3 to 4 weeks or at least until the platelet count is greater than 200,000/µl. Vincristine (0.02 mg/kg IV once) or a single intravenous infusion of human immunoglobulin (0.5 gm/kg) has been used in patients with IMTP and has been associated with faster rises in platelet counts and shorter hospitalization times (Whitley and Day, 2011). If treatment with corticosteroids and vincristine or human immunoglobulin does not result in increased platelet counts within 5 to 7 days, one or more adjunctive immunosuppressive drugs should be used (Table 61-2; see Chapter 59).

Long-term immunosuppressive therapy (≥6 months) is necessary for most cases of primary IMTP, and client expectations should be set accordingly. Some patients may require lifelong therapy to maintain normal platelet counts. The main cause for the relapse of thrombocytopenia in the authors' experience is rapid corticosteroid taper (i.e., dose reductions at intervals equal to or less than 2 weeks) or failure to document the platelet count before each dose reduction. Tapering of the corticosteroid dose by approximately 25% of the current dosage every 3 to 4 weeks should only be attempted *after* the platelet count has returned to, and remained within, the reference interval. Steroids can usually be discontinued completely when the dose administered is similar to the physiologic amount of cortisol produced in a normal patient (0.2 mg/kg q24h of prednisone). If thrombocytopenia recurs during the tapering of the corticosteroids, the dose should be increased to the *original* dose, and adjunctive immunosuppressive drugs should be added if not already in use (see Table 61-2). Corticosteroids should then be tapered as before, down to the last dose at which a normal platelet count was detected. This dose is often maintained indefinitely or for a minimum of several months before tapering of corticosteroids is attempted again.

Splenectomy has been recommended as an adjunctive treatment for thrombocytopenia. This should typically be considered as a last resort, and thorough screening for infectious diseases, particularly babesiosis, should be performed before the procedure. Splenectomy can exacerbate hemoparasite infections and is associated with resistance to antiprotozoal treatments.

The prognosis for IMTP is guarded to good. In some university studies mortality rates have been 25% to 30%, but these often represent the most severe cases. Reported recurrence rates have varied from 9% to 58% (O'Marra, Delaforcade, and Shaw, 2011). Although formal studies of prognostic indicators for survival are minimal, most clinicians agree that clinically significant bleeding with anemia and intracranial hemorrhage are the worst prognostic indicators. In one dog study an elevated blood urea nitrogen (BUN) or the presence of melena at admission was associated with a poor prognosis (O'Marra, Delaforcade, and Shaw, 2011). The severity of the thrombocytopenia does not appear to be a significant prognostic indicator.

References and Suggested Reading

Bulla C et al: The relationship between the degree of thrombocytopenia and infection with *Ehrlichia canis* in an endemic region, *Vet Res* 35:141-146, 2004.

Callan MB, Appleman EH, Sachais BS: Canine platelet transfusions, *J Vet Emerg Crit Care* 19:401-415, 2009.

Greene CE: *Infectious diseases of the dog and cat*, ed 4, St Louis, 2012, Elsevier.

Grindem CB et al: Epidemiologic survey of thrombocytopenia in dogs: a report on 987 cases, *Vet Clin Pathol* 20:38-43, 1991.

Grindem CB et al: Thrombocytopenia associated with neoplasia in dogs, *J Vet Intern Med* 8:400-405, 1994.

Jordan HL, Grindem CB, Breitschwerdt EB: Thrombocytopenia in cats: a retrospective study of 41 cases, *J Vet Intern Med* 7:261-265, 1993.

Norman EJ et al: Prevalence of low automated platelet counts in cats: comparison with prevalence of thrombocytopenia based on blood smear estimation, *Vet Clin Pathol* 30:137-140, 2001.

O'Marra SK, Delaforcade AM, Shaw SP: Treatment and predictors of outcome in dogs with immune-mediated thrombocytopenia, *J Am Vet Med Assoc* 238:346-352, 2011.

Scott MA, Jutkowitz LA: Immune-mediated thrombocytopenia. In Weiss DJ, Wardrop KJ, editors: *Schalm's veterinary hematology*, ed 6, Ames, IA, 2010, Wiley-Blackwell, pp 586-595.

Thomas JS: Non-immune-mediated thrombocytopenia. In Weiss DJ, Wardrop KJ, editors: *Schalm's veterinary hematology*, ed 6, Ames, IA, 2010, Wiley-Blackwell, pp 596-604.

Whitley NT, Day MJ: Immunomodulatory drugs and their application to the management of canine immune-mediated disease, *J Sm Anim Pract* 52:70-85, 2011.

Wondratschek C, Weingart C, Kohn B: Primary immune-mediated thrombocytopenia in cats, *J Am Anim Hosp Assoc* 46:12-19, 2010.

CHAPTER 62

von Willebrand Disease and Hereditary Coagulation Factor Deficiencies

MARJORIE B. BROOKS, *Ithaca, New York*

Thrombocytopenia and acquired coagulation factor deficiencies are the most common hemostatic defects encountered in clinical practice. Nevertheless, numerous hereditary factor deficiencies have been identified in dogs and cats. von Willebrand disease (VWD) is the most common hereditary bleeding disorder in purebred dogs, whereas new cases of hemophilia continually arise in mixed breed and many different breeds of dogs and cats. The clinical signs and severity of hereditary factor deficiencies vary based on the physiologic role of the hemostatic protein involved. With the advent of veterinary blood banks and the availability of blood component products, many affected patients can be maintained with good quality of life.

Clinical Signs

Clinical signs overlap among the various factor deficiencies, with abnormal gingival hemorrhage at teething, prolonged hemorrhage after surgery or trauma, and recurrent episodes of hemorrhage being common to all (Brooks, 1999). The anatomic site and type of spontaneous hemorrhage may provide some diagnostic clues. Mucosal hemorrhage (e.g., epistaxis, hematuria, melena) is suggestive of VWD, whereas hemarthrosis, intramuscular and subcutaneous hematoma formation, and hemorrhage into body cavities are more typical of coagulation factor deficiencies. Severe forms of VWD and factor deficiencies usually manifest within the first few months of age and

PLATELET COUNT AND COAGULATION PANEL (APTT, PT, FIBRINOGEN, OR TCT)

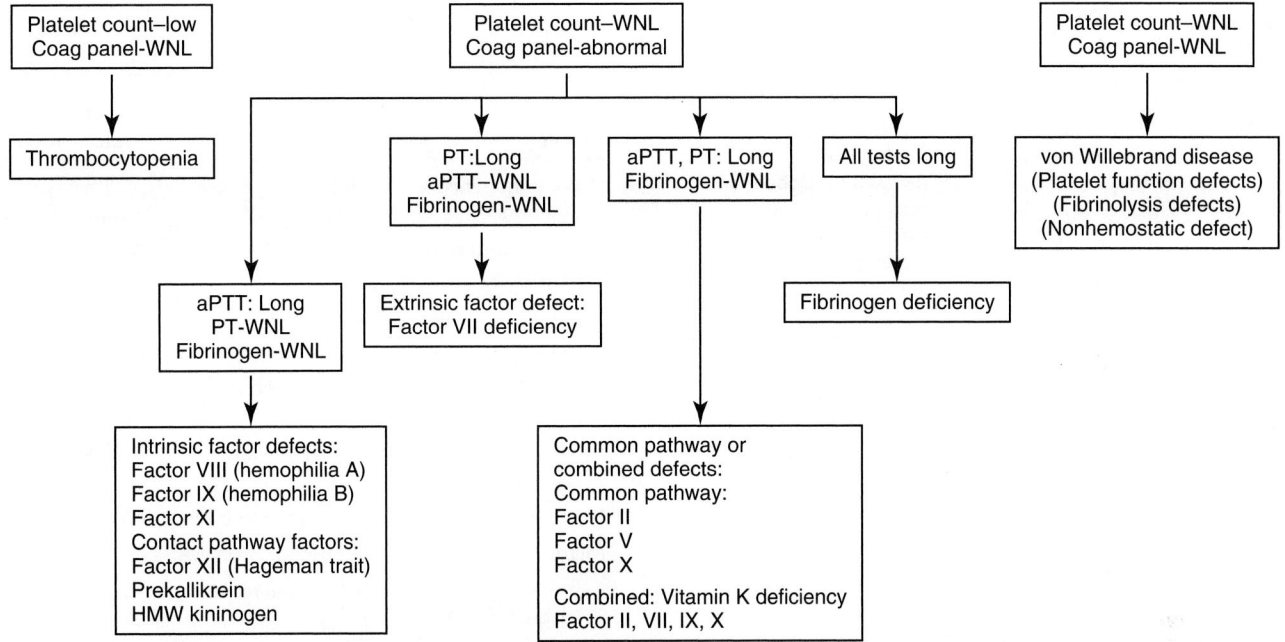

Figure 62-1 Preliminary screening for hereditary factor deficiencies.

BOX 62-1

Screening Questionnaire for Diagnosis of Bleeding Disorders

1. Has this patient had any previous evidence of spontaneous bleeding from the nose, mouth, or urinary or digestive tract? Any noticeable hemorrhage when teething?
2. Has this patient ever had surgery, dentistry, or trauma that required veterinary care? Was there any abnormal hemorrhage?
3. Has this patient ever had a transfusion?
4. Is this patient receiving any medication or dietary supplements?
5. Are you aware of any bleeding disorder in this breed or relatives of this patient?

patients are transfusion-dependent for survival. Fatalities result from hemorrhage into the central nervous system and respiratory tract or from acute blood loss anemia and hemorrhagic, hypovolemic shock. Milder forms may be unapparent until a patient undergoes surgery or major trauma.

Diagnostic Strategy

The initial workup of any patient suspected of having a bleeding diathesis should include platelet count and coagulation screening tests (Figure 62-1). Consistent use of a standard history questionnaire (Box 62-1) and collection of pretreatment citrate plasma samples facilitate early recognition of a hereditary hemostatic defect and provide the appropriate sample type for definitive testing. For patients with a normal platelet count, abnormal clotting times in one or more coagulation screening tests are compatible with a coagulation factor deficiency. In contrast, dogs and cats with VWD typically have normal coagulation panel results (Johnson, Turrentine, and Kraus, 1988). Buccal mucosal bleeding time is a point-of-care technique to assess von Willebrand factor (VWF) and platelet function. Prolonged bleeding time (> 6 minutes) is a typical feature of VWD. However, the bleeding time end point is also influenced by platelet count, hematocrit, and blood viscosity, and is subject to interoperator variability. The Platelet Function Analyzer (PFA100), a tabletop instrument, has replaced bleeding time determinations as a screening tool to assess primary hemostasis in medical settings. The PFA100 Collagen/ADP closure time is sensitive to VWF deficiency, and prolonged closure times (> 120 seconds) have been described in canine VWD (Mischke and Keidel, 2003). Many of the nonspecific factors that influence bleeding time also affect the closure time end point. Bleeding time and closure times are normal in patients with hereditary coagulation factor deficiencies.

Definitive diagnosis of VWD and hereditary coagulation factor deficiencies is based on specific quantitative and/or functional assays of the individual factors. Differences among species in the antigenic and procoagulant properties of hemostatic proteins require species-specific assays or specific validation of human assays for animals. Plasma VWF is primarily measured in immunologic assays that detect protein concentration, referred to as VWF antigen (VWF:Ag). Functional assays have also been developed to measure VWF protein's ability to bind collagen (VWF collagen-binding activity [VWF:CBA])

TABLE 62-1

von Willebrand Disease Subtype Classification

Type	VWF Defect	Affected Breeds
1	Partial quantitative deficiency; residual VWF has normal structure & function	Airedale, Akita, Bernese mountain dog, dachshund, Doberman pinscher, German shepherd, golden retriever, greyhound, Kerry blue terrier, Manchester terrier, miniature pinscher, papillon, Pembroke Welsh corgi, poodle, and others
2A	Selective loss of large VWF multimers, decreased platelet-VWF & collagen interactions	German shorthaired and wirehaired pointers
2B	Increased VWF-platelet binding	Not identified
2M	Decreased VWF-platelet binding with normal VWF multimers	Not identified
2N	Decreased VWF-factor VIII binding	Not identified
3	Complete VWF deficiency	Kooiker, Scottish terrier, Shetland sheepdog Sporadic cases: Border collie, Chesapeake Bay retriever, cocker spaniel, Labrador retriever, Maltese, Pomeranian

TABLE 62-2

Inheritance Pattern and Coagulation Screening Test Abnormalities for Hereditary Factor Deficiencies

Defect	Inheritance Pattern	Screening Test Prolongation
Hypofibrinogenemia, dysfibrinogenemia	Autosomal	ACT, aPTT, PT, TCT
Factor II (prothrombin deficiency)	Autosomal	ACT, aPTT, PT
*Factor V deficiency	Autosomal	ACT, aPTT, PT
Factor VII deficiency	Autosomal recessive	PT
Factor VIII deficiency (hemophilia A)	X-linked recessive	ACT, aPTT
Factor IX deficiency (hemophilia B)	X-linked recessive	ACT, aPTT
Factor X deficiency	Autosomal recessive	ACT, aPTT, PT
Factor XI deficiency	Autosomal recessive	ACT, aPTT
Factor XII deficiency (Hageman trait)	Autosomal recessive	ACT, aPTT

*Not yet identified in dogs or cats.
ACT, Activated clotting time; aPTT, activated partial thromboplastin time; PT, prothrombin time; TCT, thrombin clotting time.

(Callan, Giger, and Catalfamo, 2005). Coagulation factors are typically measured in functional clotting time tests that determine individual procoagulant activities (Brooks, 1999). By convention, results of VWF and coagulation factor assays are reported as a percentage of "normal." Results of each test sample are compared with a plasma standard that has an assigned value of 100%. Values below 50% of the standard indicate a factor deficiency. Canine and feline factor assays are routinely performed in the author's laboratory for clinical diagnosis of VWD and coagulation factor deficiencies (Comparative Coagulation Section, Cornell University). Information on the biologic basis and inheritance of these disorders is presented in the following sections and in Tables 62-1 and 62-2.

Specific Disorders

von Willebrand Disease

The bleeding tendency of VWD is caused by quantitative and functional deficiencies of VWF, a large, multimeric plasma glycoprotein that supports platelet adhesion and aggregation at sites of vascular injury under conditions of high shear (Johnson, Turrentine, and Kraus, 1988). Endothelial cells are the primary source of plasma VWF. In some species, platelets contain a secondary pool of circulating VWF. This pool is lacking in dogs. The highest-molecular-weight forms of VWF, consisting of more than 100 VWF subunits, are the most hemostatically active. Plasma VWF is also a carrier protein for coagulation factor VIII (FVIII), and the association between these two proteins may help localize coagulation to sites of platelet aggregate formation. In another species difference, canine FVIII appears more stable in the absence of VWF than does human FVIII.

A subtype classification scheme for VWD in people is applicable for characterizing VWD in animals (see Table 62-1). The classification criteria include VWF concentration, multimeric structure, and interactions with platelets, collagen, and FVIII. Although VWD is the most common hereditary bleeding disorder in dogs, only a few cases have been identified in cats. Type 1 VWD is a quantitative protein deficiency found in many individual canine breeds across many breed groups (see Table 62-1). The clinical expression of type 1 VWD varies and is generally related to the severity of protein deficiency. Dogs with low residual protein concentration (e.g., VWF:Ag < 25%) have the most risk of abnormal bleeding. Additional undefined factors influence clinical expression of this subtype, even among dogs with VWF:Ag below 10%. Types 2 and 3 VWD are more severe forms. Affected dogs often experience spontaneous hemorrhage and are at risk for severe, fatal hemorrhage if they undergo surgery without transfusion. To date, type 2 VWD has been identified only in German shorthaired and wirehaired pointers. Affected dogs have low VWF concentration and the residual protein lacks high-molecular-weight multimers. Dogs with type 3 VWD have essentially no detectable plasma VWF (VWF:Ag < 0.1%).

VWD is an autosomal trait. In this form of inheritance, males and females express and transmit the defect with equal frequency. Types 2 and 3 VWD demonstrate recessive expression patterns; homozygous dogs have a bleeding tendency, whereas heterozygous carriers are clinically normal. Type 1 VWD in people is usually a dominant, incompletely penetrant trait. Patients are typically heterozygous or compound heterozygous for VWF mutations. The variable expression of type 1 VWD in dogs is suggestive of this form of inheritance. Regardless of VWD subtype, dogs with VWF deficiency (i.e., VWF: Ag < 50%) can be considered carriers of the VWD trait; to reduce prevalence of VWD within a breed or line, these dogs can be used selectively or removed from breeding programs. However, the VWF:Ag values of carriers may overlap with clear dogs at the low end of normal range. Distinct VWF mutations have been described in Scottish terriers (Venta, Li, and Yuzbasiyan-Gurkan, 2000) and Kooiker dogs (van Oost, Versteeg, and Slappendel, 2004) with type 3 VWD. Direct DNA tests are commercially available for these mutations and for unreported mutations in other breed-variants of VWD (VetGen, http://www.vetgen.com/). Using these tests, dogs with a single copy of a VWF mutation are considered carriers, and dogs with two copies are considered affected with VWD.

Hereditary Coagulation Factor Deficiencies

The clinical severity of the various hereditary deficiencies depends on the presence of any residual factor activity and the factor's enzymatic or cofactor action in promoting fibrin formation. Prolongation of clotting time in point-of-care or laboratory coagulation screening tests is an indicator of factor deficiencies that can be differentiated based on specific factor assays (see Table 62-2).

X-Linked Factor Deficiencies: Hemophilia A and B

FVIII and factor IX (FIX) act as an essential cofactor and serine protease factor, respectively, to rapidly activate factor X in the amplification and propagation phase of coagulation. Hemophilia A (FVIII deficiency) and hemophilia B (FIX deficiency) are both X-linked, recessive traits. Consequently, the bleeding tendency of these disorders is primarily manifest by males, whereas carrier females are clinically normal. Unlike many hereditary defects, hemophilia is not found primarily in inbred lines. Hemophilia has been identified in mixed breed and more than 50 individual breeds of dog and in domestic and purebred cats. Hemophilia A is by far the more common form, presumably due to frequent de novo mutations in the FVIII gene. Severe hemophilia is characterized by factor activities below 2% of normal, and affected patients experience recurrent episodes of spontaneous hemarthrosis, hematoma formation, and severe, fatal hemorrhage if they undergo surgery or trauma. Residual FVIII or FIX activities of 2% to 20% are associated with mild to moderate forms of hemophilia. These patients have relatively few spontaneous bleeds and are often diagnosed because of prolonged hemorrhage after surgery.

Genetic analyses have revealed unique FIX mutations in different breeds of dog (Brooks, 1999). Carrier detection based on linkage analyses of FVIII markers has been successful in identifying carriers in different breed-variants of hemophilia A (Brooks, Barnas, and Fremont, 2005). Pedigree review and selective breeding also help prevent propagation of hemophilia. Males can be definitively classified as affected or clear based on factor assay results. Obligate carrier females are defined as the dams and daughters of affected males. The daughters of carrier dams have a 50% chance of being a carrier. These suspect carriers and obligate carriers can be safely spayed without risk of hemorrhage.

Autosomal Factor Deficiencies

The remaining factor deficiencies identified in animals are relatively uncommon compared with hemophilia. All are autosomal traits with apparent recessive expression patterns. Of these factors, deficiencies of fibrinogen and factors VII (FVII), XI (FXI), and XII (FXII) are best characterized in companion animals.

Fibrinogen deficiency includes quantitative defects (hypofibrinogenemia) and qualitative defects (dysfibrinogenemia). Although acquired fibrinogen defects are among the most common coagulopathies, hereditary hypofibrinogenemia and dysfibrinogenemia have been reported in only a few breeds of dog (borzoi, collie, bichon frise) and in domestic cats. The bleeding tendency in these and human cases is variable, including some with severe spontaneous or postsurgical hemorrhage.

FVII interacts with tissue factor to initiate coagulation; however, only trace amounts of its active form (FVIIa) are required for this reaction. Canine FVII deficiency was first characterized in beagles as a mild or subclinical bleeding tendency associated with residual FVII activities of approximately 2% to 10%. A missense FVII mutation was identified in affected beagles (Callan et al, 2006), and subsequently the same mutation was found in FVII-deficient Alaskan Klee Kai and deerhounds. More severe forms of FVII deficiency have also been identified in malamutes and domestic cats.

FXI participates in the early activation of FIX and deficiency of this factor is generally considered to cause a mild or variable bleeding disorder. The trait has been best characterized in Kerry blue terriers but has also been reported in springer spaniels and domestic cats. Spontaneous hemorrhage is rare and affected patients are typically diagnosed after surgery or trauma.

FXII deficiency (Hageman trait) is the most common factor deficiency in cats (Brooks and DeWilde, 2006). Factor XII is a contact pathway factor that activates the intrinsic pathway in vitro; however, FXII is not required for physiologic in vivo fibrin formation. Although FXII deficiency causes marked prolongation of the activated clotting time (ACT) and activated partial thromboplastin time (aPTT) (see Table 62-2), FXII-deficient cats have no clinical signs of a bleeding disorder. These patients can safely undergo major surgical procedures and do not require any special management or transfusion therapy.

TABLE 62-3

Blood Products for VWD and Factor Deficiencies

Products	Dosage Guidelines	Indications
Fresh frozen plasma	10 to 12 ml/kg	All coagulation factor deficiencies and VWD
Cryoprecipitate	1 unit*/10 kg	VWD, fibrinogen, and factor VIII deficiency
Cryosupernatant	10 to 12 ml/kg	Factor II, VII, IX, X, and XI deficiencies
Fresh whole blood	12 to 20 ml/kg	Anemia and VWD, factor deficiencies

*1 unit cryoprecipitate prepared from 200 ml fresh frozen plasma.

Treatment of VWD and Factor Deficiencies

Management of VWD and other hereditary factor deficiencies includes controlling hemorrhage and hypovolemia in patients with active bleeds and preventing abnormal bleeding in patients that require surgery or invasive procedures.

Transfusion Therapy

Blood component transfusion is the best means to provide hemostatic levels of VWF and coagulation factors (Table 62-3). The use of plasma components, rather than whole blood, replaces the deficient factor but minimizes the risk of volume overload or red cell sensitization (Abrams-Ogg and Schneider, 2010). Fresh whole blood or packed cells may be transfused to patients with acute anemia or hemorrhagic shock, but subsequent transfusion with plasma components may be needed to sustain hemostasis. Patients with severe forms of VWD, hemophilia, and other factor deficiencies invariably require transfusion to undergo surgery or control more than minor bleeds. The most successful strategy is early, high-dose transfusion to rapidly increase VWF or factors to levels capable of supporting platelet adhesion or effective thrombin generation. The most severely affected patients may require repeated transfusions, with lower dosages at longer intervals, to sustain hemostasis for 1 to 2 days after an initial hemostatic stress. Measurement of *in vitro* clotting time (for coagulation factor deficiencies) and the use of viscoelastic monitoring (such as thromboelastography) can aid in patient assessment; however, clinical status is the most important parameter for determining response to therapy (Koreth et al, 2004). Stabilization and increase in hematocrit and plasma protein levels, cessation of active hemorrhage, and resolution of swelling and bruising are signs of adequate transfusion support.

Fresh frozen plasma (FFP) refers to plasma stored frozen within 8 hours of collection and separation from whole blood. It retains essentially all the coagulation factors and VWF from the starting plasma. This product is appropriate for transfusing patients suspected of having VWD or factor deficiency pending a definitive diagnosis, or if other plasma components are unavailable.

Cryoprecipitate is prepared by slowly thawing FFP at 1° to 6° C (33.8° to 42.8° F) and then centrifuging the thawed plasma to sediment the large, cold, insoluble proteins. The resultant cryoprecipitate fraction is then refrozen for storage. The cryoprecipitate fraction contains VWF, FVIII, and fibrinogen (and fibronectin and factor XIII) in approximately one-tenth volume of the starting plasma (Stokol and Parry, 1998). The unit definition of cryoprecipitate is not standardized and may refer to the starting volume of FFP, fibrinogen, or factor content. Small volume is the major advantage of cryoprecipitate for treatment of VWD, hemophilia A, and fibrinogen defects. Hemostatic levels of these proteins can be attained within minutes of slow bolus cryoprecipitate infusion, and repeated doses can be given with little risk of volume overload.

Cryosupernatant refers to the plasma component remaining after centrifugation to remove cryoprecipitate. This plasma product does not contain VWF, FVIII, or fibrinogen but does retain activity of all other coagulation factors and contains albumin, globulins, and other plasma proteins. Cryosupernatants are administered at the same dosage as FFP (see Table 62-3) and are suitable for patients with hemophilia B or deficiencies of FII, FV, FVII, FX, and FXI.

Nontransfusion Therapy

Drug therapy and management practices may help reduce or replace transfusion requirements for patients with VWD and coagulation factor deficiencies. Due to the life-long bleeding tendencies of these patients, it is best to avoid antiplatelet agents (e.g., nonsteroidal antiinflammatory drugs, clopidogrel), anticoagulants, and plasma expanders (e.g., hetastarch), as well as invasive diagnostic procedures. Intravenous catheters should be placed in peripheral veins, and topical wound care (e.g., bandage, tissue glue, multilayer closure) may help limit cutaneous hemorrhage or hematoma formation.

Desmopressin (DDAVP) is a synthetic analog of arginine vasopressin that promotes hemostasis by inducing endothelial release of VWF stores (Callan, Giger, and Catalfamo, 2005). The drug is also believed to enhance platelet function by mechanisms independent of VWF. Desmopressin has been reported to improve surgical hemostasis in dogs with type 1 VWD. The empiric dosage for this use is 1 µg/kg given subcutaneously one half hour before surgery. The maximal increment in VWF occurs approximately 1 hour after administration, with no additional benefit of repeated doses. Blood products (e.g., FFP, cryoprecipitate) should be available to control hemorrhage in case of inadequate response.

The antifibrinolytic drugs aminocaproic acid (EACA) and tranexamic acid are used in human medicine to reduce postoperative transfusion requirements in patients with acquired or hereditary coagulopathies (Levy, 2008). These drugs are lysine analogs that delay fibrinolysis by inhibiting activation of plasmin and its subsequent interaction with fibrin. The drugs are given intravenously and orally. An initial loading dosage for EACA is 100 mg/kg IV, followed by IV infusion at 30 mg/kg/hr. Tranexamic acid is given at 10 mg/kg IV or 25 mg/kg PO q8h for up to 7 days postoperatively. The lysine analogs have few adverse side effects in human medicine but have not yet been investigated for safety or efficacy in veterinary patients.

Topical agents, classified as sealants, adhesives, and hemostats, have been developed for direct application to support local wound hemostasis at sites of surgical information or tissue trauma (Spotnitz and Burks, 2008). Some products (hemostats) contain gelatin, collagen, or polysaccharide spheres designed to act as mechanical barriers and enhance platelet activation and fibrin generation. Other products contain natural or recombinant thrombin, used alone or in combination with mechanical barriers and fibrinogen sealants, to further enhance local hemostasis. Although these agents may aid in cutaneous wound management, there is some risk of allergic reaction or sensitization to foreign proteins and potential for wound infection or delayed healing.

References and Suggested Reading

Abrams-Ogg AC, Schneider A: Principles of canine and feline blood collection, processing, and storage. In Weiss DJ, Wardrop KA, editors: *Schalm's veterinary hematology*, Ames, IA, 2010, Wiley Blackwell, p 731.

Brooks M: A review of canine inherited bleeding disorders: biochemical and molecular strategies for disease characterization and carrier detection, *J Hered* 90:112, 1999.

Brooks M, Barnas J, Fremont J: Cosegregation of factor VIII microsatellite marker with mild hemophilia A in golden retriever dogs, *J Vet Intern Med* 19:205, 2005.

Brooks MB, DeWilde LA: Feline factor XII deficiency, *Compendium* 28:148, 2006.

Callan M, Giger U, Catalfamo J: Effect of desmopressin on von Willebrand factor multimers in Doberman pinschers with type I von Willebrand disease, *Am J Vet Res* 66:861, 2005.

Callan MB et al: A novel missense mutation responsible for factor VII deficiency in research Beagle colonies, *J Thromb Haemost* 4:2616, 2006.

Johnson GS, Turrentine MA, Kraus KH: Canine von Willebrand's disease: a heterogeneous group of bleeding disorders, *Vet Clin North Am Small Anim Pract* 18:195, 1988.

Koreth R et al: Measurement of bleeding severity: a critical review, *Transfusion* 44:605, 2004.

Levy JH: Pharmacologic methods to reduce peri-operative bleeding, *Transfusion* 48:31S, 2008.

Mischke R, Keidel A: Influence of platelet count, acetylsalicylic acid, von Willebrand's disease, coagulopathies, and haematocrit on results obtained using a platelet function analyser in dogs, *Vet J* 165:43, 2003.

Spotnitz WD, Burks S: Hemostats, sealants, and adhesives: components of the surgical toolbox, *Transfusion* 48:1502, 2008.

Stokol T, Parry BW: Efficacy of fresh-frozen plasma and cryoprecipitate in dogs with von Willebrand's disease and hemophilia A, *J Vet Intern Med* 12:84, 1998.

van Oost B, Versteeg S, Slappendel R: DNA testing for type III von Willebrand disease in Dutch kooiker dogs, *J Vet Intern Med* 18:282, 2004.

Venta P, Li J, Yuzbasiyan-Gurkan V: Mutation causing von Willebrand's disease in Scottish terriers, *J Vet Intern Med* 14:10, 2000.

Websites

National Institutes of Health: OMIM, OMIA (On line Mendelian Inheritance in Man and Animals) database of hereditary defects in man and animals http://www.ncbi.nlm.nih.gov/omim; http://www.ncbi.nlm.nih.gov/omia

Comparative Coagulation Laboratory: Animal factor assays and mutation detection tests http://ahdc.vet.cornell.edu/sects/Coag/

PennGenn Laboratories: Mutation detection tests for factor deficiencies http://research.vet.upenn.edu/Default.aspx?alias=research.vet.upenn.edu/penngen

VetGen: Mutation detection tests http://www.vetgen.com/

CHAPTER 63

Disseminated Intravascular Coagulation

ELKE RUDLOFF, *Glendale, Wisconsin*
REBECCA KIRBY, *Gainesville, Florida*

Disseminated intravascular coagulation (DIC) is a syndrome characterized by systemic microthrombosis, which can progress to life-threatening hemorrhage. DIC is reported in dogs but is less commonly recognized in cats. The DIC syndrome occurs secondary to an underlying acute or chronic condition associated with one or more of the following: systemic inflammation, tissue necrosis, capillary stasis, loss of vascular integrity, red cell hemolysis, and the presence of particulate matter in the blood.

Pathogenesis

The pathogenesis of DIC is characterized by (1) increased thrombin production, (2) suppression of physiologic anticoagulant pathways, (3) impaired fibrinolysis, and (4) activation of inflammatory pathways (Figure 63-1). Tissue factor (TF) is expressed on monocytes and endothelial cells within the circulation during inflammation and on malignant cells in cancer patients. The TF:factor VIIa complex (extrinsic pathway), the main stimulus for thrombin formation in DIC, activates factor IX (intrinsic pathway) and factor X (common pathway) (Figure 63-2). In human cancer patients DIC also can involve the expression of a specific cancer procoagulant, a cysteine protease that has factor X–activating properties.

Impaired function of the normal physiologic anticoagulant pathways (see Figures 63-2 and 63-3) during DIC allows thrombin generation and the resultant fibrin formation to become exaggerated. Antithrombin (AT), a natural anticoagulant, binds to thrombin and inactivates thrombin and factors IXa, Xa, XIa, and TF:factor VIIa. During DIC, AT levels are reduced as a result of increased AT consumption by AT-thrombin complex formation, AT degradation by neutrophil elastase, impaired hepatic synthesis of AT, and loss of AT because of increased capillary permeability. Depression of endogenous anticoagulant protein C:protein S activity results from enhanced consumption, impaired hepatic synthesis, and capillary leakage. In addition, proinflammatory cytokines (tumor necrosis factor-α [TNF-α] and interleukin-1β [IL-1β]) can cause down-regulation of protein C–thrombomodulin expression on endothelial cell surfaces.

During DIC fibrin deposition typically surpasses fibrinolysis. The release of plasminogen activators from endothelial cells causes an initial rapid increase in fibrinolytic activity during sepsis. However, this usually is followed by a prompt suppression of fibrinolytic activity caused by endothelial release of plasminogen activators and increased plasma levels of plasminogen activator inhibitor type 1. In contrast, people with acute promyelocytic leukemia may exhibit a severe hyperfibrinolytic state associated with systemic coagulation activation.

The "cross talk" between the coagulation system and the inflammatory reaction is an important factor contributing to DIC pathogenesis (see Figure 63-1). Activated coagulation proteins stimulate the endothelial cells to release inflammatory cytokines. Recruited white blood cells release TNF-α (activating factor VII), IL-1, and IL-6 (activating factors VII and XII). Platelet-activating factor, a strong promoter of platelet aggregation, also is released from inflammatory cells. Additional activation of the inflammatory cascade is promoted by thrombin and other serine proteases interacting with protease-activated receptors on cell surfaces. The typical antiinflammatory effect of activated protein C is lost with depression of the protein C system during DIC, which enhances the proinflammatory state of DIC.

It is important to recognize that the hypercoagulable condition occurs early in the course of DIC and bleeding associated with prolongation of coagulation times occurs later in the course of DIC. As a consequence of coagulation activation, platelets, coagulation factors, and anticoagulants are consumed, degraded, or inhibited. A transition from accelerated coagulation to consumption of coagulants and anticoagulants corresponds with the clinical consequences of microthrombosis and vascular occlusion followed by uncontrolled hemorrhage. Therefore variations and combinations of the coagulation-anticoagulation-fibrinolytic-inflammatory derangements exist, depending on the underlying cause and coexisting disease processes. Diagnosis of an active DIC process is made through clinical findings and laboratory testing.

Clinical Findings

DIC should be an anticipated complication in any animal experiencing one or more of the following: hypotensive crisis, impaired blood flow to a major organ, systemic inflammatory response syndrome, or release of vasoactive agents into the vasculature (Box 63-1). The severity of clinical signs associated with DIC can range from no signs to life-threatening complications of vascular

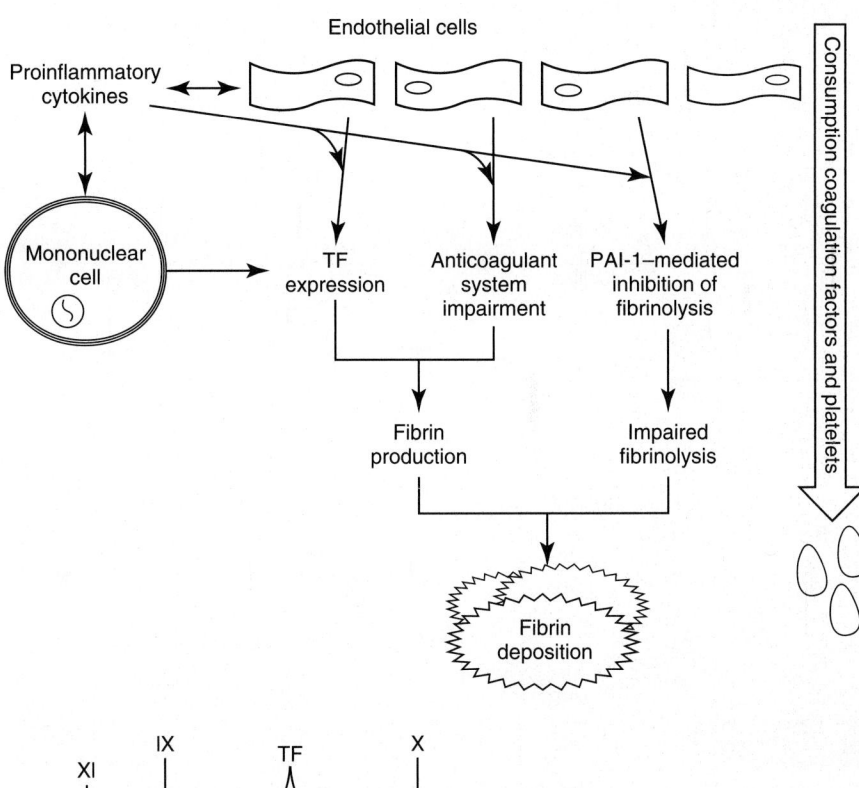

Figure 63-1 Alterations in coagulation and anticoagulation during systemic inflammation and disseminated intravascular coagulation. Fibrin deposition exceeds fibrinolysis when tissue factor (TF) expression is enhanced, the anticoagulation system is impaired, and levels of plasminogen activator inhibitor type 1 (PAI-1) are increased.

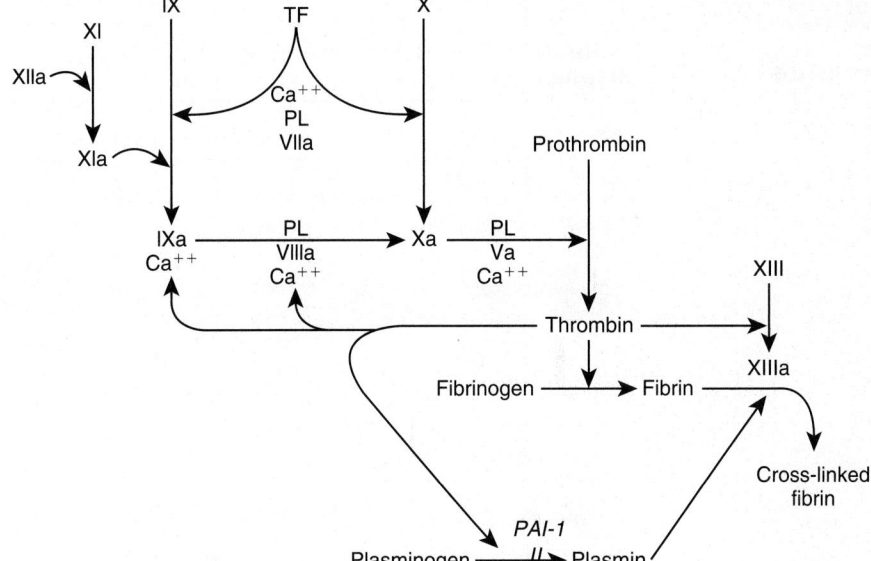

Figure 63-2 Coagulation during inflammation promoting thrombin and fibrin production. Tissue factor (TF) is the prime initiator of coagulation. Amplification of the coagulation scheme during disseminated intravascular coagulation occurs by activation of factor IX (cross talk) and continued activation of factors VIII and IX and platelet surfaces by thrombin (feedback). Plasminogen activator inhibitor type 1 (PAI-1) prevents plasmin activation and fibrinolysis. During inflammation there is inhibition of fibrinolysis when PAI-1 is up-regulated and promotion of fibrin deposition. Ca^{++}, Calcium; *PL*, phospholipase.

microthrombosis reflected by organ dysfunction or evidence of systemic bleeding. Clinical signs can vary as DIC progresses.

The earliest (peracute) phase of DIC typically is characterized by subtle abnormal laboratory findings (Table 63-1) without obvious clinical signs. Clinical signs more compatible with the acute phase of DIC (days to weeks) include evidence of organ dysfunction from microthrombosis or hemorrhage and laboratory findings suggestive of alterations in hemostasis. Animals experiencing consumption of endogenous coagulation proteins during this phase can demonstrate bleeding from venipuncture sites, bleeding along the gum line, petechiae, ecchymosis, purpura, hematomas, or hemarthrosis.

The chronic phase of DIC (weeks to months) can develop from low-grade or intermittent procoagulant release (see Box 63-1). In the compensated state of chronic DIC, time exists for replenishment of coagulation factors, anticoagulation proteins, and platelets. There may be abnormal laboratory findings without obvious clinical signs (see Table 63-1). Stress, concurrent disease, and disease progression can cause decompensation, abnormal laboratory findings, and clinical signs associated with microthrombosis or hemorrhage.

Laboratory Findings

No single laboratory test is sufficiently sensitive or specific to confirm a diagnosis of DIC. A diagnosis of DIC can be made when a clinical condition known to be associated with DIC and a combination of the following laboratory findings is present (also see Table 63-1):

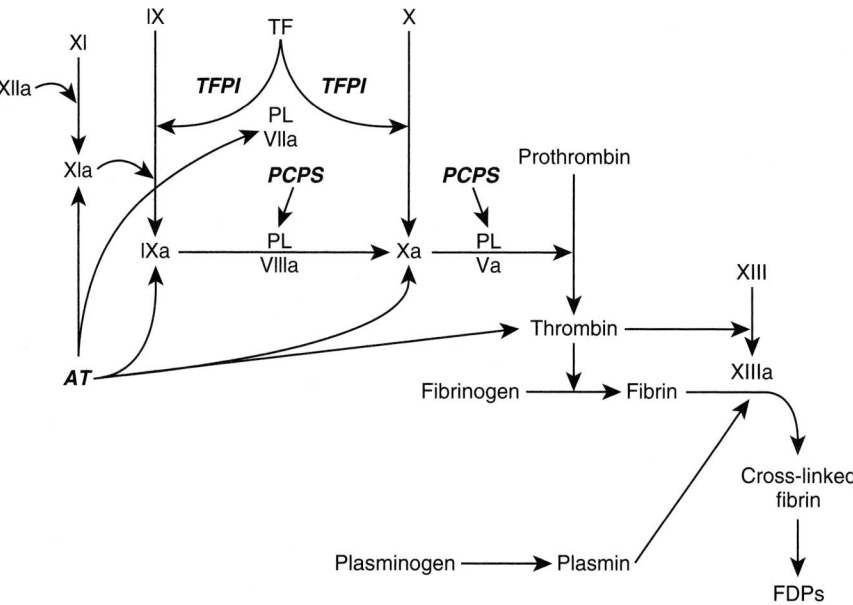

Figure 63-3 Anticoagulation process, which normally should balance coagulation. Tissue factor pathway inhibitor (TFPI) is a protease inhibitor of tissue factor (TF) complex. Bound to thrombin, antithrombin (AT) inactivates thrombin and factors IXa, Xa, XIa, and TF:factor VIIa. The protein C:protein S (PCPS) system irreversibly inactivates factors Va and VIIIa. Activation of plasminogen produces plasmin, which lyses fibrin and fibrinogen into fibrin degradation products (FDPs) and fibrin monomers. During inflammation there is consumption and inhibition of the anticoagulants and promotion of fibrin deposition. *PL,* Phospholipase.

BOX 63-1

Disease States Associated with Disseminated Intravascular Coagulation

Peracute
- Sepsis (bacterial, viral, fungal, protozoal)
- Severe gastroenteritis
- Vascular disorders
- Immune-mediated disorders
- Severe toxic or immunologic reactions (e.g., viper envenomation)
- Transfusion reaction
- Severe hepatic failure

Acute
- Sepsis (bacterial, viral, fungal, protozoal)
- Trauma or crush injuries
- Pancreatitis
- Burns or heatstroke
- Severe gastroenteritis
- Vascular disorders
- Immune-mediated disorders
- Severe toxic or immunologic reactions (e.g., viper envenomation)
- Transfusion reaction
- Severe hepatic failure
- Neoplasia

Chronic
- Neoplasia
- Protein-losing nephropathy
- Protein-losing enteropathy
- Heartworm disease
- Chronic hepatic disease
- Vascular disorders
- Hyperadrenocorticism

TABLE 63-1

Laboratory Values Supporting a Diagnosis of Disseminated Intravascular Coagulation

Test	Peracute	Acute	Chronic
Prothrombin time	N or ↓	N or ↑	N
Partial thromboplastin time	N or ↓	N or ↑	N
Activated clotting time	N or ↓	N or ↑	N
Platelet count	N or ↓	↓	N or ↓
Fibrinogen level	N or ↓	N or ↓ or ↑	N or ↓ or ↑
Level of fibrin degradation products	N or ↑	↑	N or ↑
D-dimer level	N or ↑	↑	↑
Antithrombin level	N or ↓	↓	N or ↓

N, Normal; ↑, above normal reference range; ↓ below normal reference range.

1. Prolongation of coagulation times
2. Reduction in platelet numbers
3. Elevated levels of D-dimer or fibrin degradation products
4. Decrease in AT activity
5. Clinical or postmortem evidence of thrombosis

Stokol and colleagues (2000) report that a negative D-dimer test result in dogs excludes DIC as a diagnosis with a confidence level of 95%.

A scoring algorithm is used in humans with an underlying condition known to be associated with DIC. The scoring system rates a decreased platelet count, prolongation of prothrombin time, decreased fibrinogen levels, and increasing plasma levels of a fibrin-related marker (D-dimer, soluble fibrin, or fibrin degradation products) as predictive of DIC. The use of fibrinogen level to predict DIC can be questioned because fibrinogen levels are influenced by many factors other than DIC. An alternate scoring system in humans evaluates a dynamic coagulopathy score in which changes in AT activity, prothrombin time, and D-dimer levels are used. A similar scoring system is under investigation in veterinary medicine to assist in the diagnosis of DIC and the categorization of DIC to predict mortality.

Treatment

Once a disease process associated with DIC has been identified, early recognition and aggressive therapy can improve outcome. Therapy is focused on promoting capillary blood flow, eliminating the underlying cause, supporting target organs, providing replacement therapy, and administering anticoagulants.

Promoting Capillary Blood Flow

Restoring capillary blood flow and tissue oxygenation requires rapid intravascular volume resuscitation to correct perfusion deficits. Administering a combination of crystalloids and synthetic colloids increases capillary fluid volume and improves microvascular flow. Dextran 70 and hetastarch may improve flow dynamics and reduce platelet aggregation during hypercoagulable states. Red blood cell transfusions are given when hemoglobin levels have dropped precipitously (<8 to 10 g/dl). Oxyglobin, a hemoglobin-based oxygen carrier approved for use in dogs, provides colloid osmotic pressure and oxygen-carrying molecules for the transport of oxygen to tissue beds experiencing maldistribution of blood flow. The vasoconstricting property of Oxyglobin can aid in reversing hypotension that is refractory to standard crystalloid and synthetic colloid infusion. Maintaining capillary flow depends on meeting ongoing fluid needs through continuous crystalloid and colloid infusions.

Eliminating the Underlying Cause

Identification and treatment of the underlying disease process is crucial to the elimination of DIC. When a septic process is suspected, tissue and fluid samples are collected for histopathologic evaluation, cytologic examination, culture and sensitivity testing, and serologic testing. Antimicrobial therapy for bacterial, protozoal, or fungal infections is initiated as early in the disease course as deemed appropriate. Removal or drainage of infected, torsed, ischemic, or necrotic tissue may be necessary. Antivenom and specific antidotes are used when indicated. Immune-mediated diseases require immunosuppressive medications. Neoplastic conditions may require surgical or medical treatment. Animals with medical conditions such as pancreatitis, severe gastroenteritis, or liver failure require aggressive cardiovascular support throughout hospitalization to minimize the effects of DIC during medical management.

Supporting Target Organs

Organs with high blood flow or high oxygen requirements are more susceptible to microthrombosis, hemorrhage, or tissue hypoxia secondary to DIC. Oxygen therapy, either with or without ventilatory support, may be necessary when hypoxemia or hypoventilation results from pulmonary disease. Early enteral nutrition supports gastrointestinal mucosal integrity.

Providing Replacement Therapy

Blood Products
Correction of coagulation times (prothrombin and partial thromboplastin time) to normal usually is not possible when DIC is ongoing. The volume of blood products required varies among patients. Factors used to determine the type and dose of transfusion include the degree of factor deficiency, the degree of anemia, and the patient's volume status.

Plasma transfusion can be administered to rebalance coagulant and anticoagulant proteins. Fresh whole blood and fresh frozen plasma contain all coagulation factors and AT. Stored whole blood and frozen plasma lack factors V and VIII. Fresh whole blood, platelet-rich plasma, or platelet concentrate is needed to provide platelets if bleeding attributed to thrombocytopenia is causing organ malfunction (e.g., ocular hemorrhage, myocardial arrhythmias, increased intracranial pressure). When significant anemia is present, fresh or stored whole blood, packed red blood cells, or Oxyglobin is given to improve oxygen-carrying capacity.

Antithrombin
AT activity accelerated by heparin inactivates thrombin and factors IXa, Xa, XIa, and TF:factor VIIa. In addition, AT binds to heparan sulfate proteoglycans on the endothelial surface, stimulating the production of antiinflammatory and antiplatelet prostacyclin. AT binds directly to cellular receptors on neutrophils and monocytes, which limits proinflammatory signaling. In phase III clinical trials high-dose recombinant AT has not been associated with a significant improvement in mortality in humans unless it is used without heparin (Warren et al, 2001). The use of recombinant human AT concentrate has not been investigated clinically in animal patients with DIC. Allogeneic AT can be infused in the form of plasma products when AT replacement is desired. The use of heparin in conjunction with AT supplementation is controversial (see the section on heparin later in the chapter).

Activated Protein C
Recent large-scale phase III clinical trials in humans with severe sepsis have shown a reduction in organ damage and mortality when recombinant human activated protein C is administered early in the course of disease. Additional benefits included a decrease in inflammatory cytokines and improved clotting times. The use of recombinant human activated protein C or allogenic plasma transfusion for activated protein C replacement has not yet been investigated clinically in veterinary patients.

Administering Anticoagulant Therapy

Aspirin

Aspirin is a nonreversible thromboxane A2 inhibitor that reduces platelet aggregation and adhesion. Aspirin is used to reduce thrombotic events in people with coronary artery disease. Administration of low-dose aspirin (0.5 mg/kg q24h PO) has been associated with reduced mortality in dogs with immune-mediated hemolytic anemia (a disease associated with DIC) that are receiving azathioprine and prednisone (see Chapter 60). Further studies still need to be performed to determine its use in other forms of DIC.

Heparin

Heparin is a glycosaminoglycan that exerts an antithrombotic effect by binding to and potentiating the inhibitory actions of AT on thrombin and factors IXa, Xa, XIa, and TF:factor VIIa. Heparin administration has been established as beneficial for the prevention of venous thrombosis in people. Heparin therapy has long been a mainstay of treatment for DIC, but its use has become controversial. A beneficial effect of heparin on DIC has not been demonstrated in controlled clinical trials in humans, and it can be detrimental when overt bleeding is occurring. Heparin is ineffective in patients with reduced plasma levels of AT. In critically ill dogs heparin administration has been shown to further decrease AT levels (Rozanski et al, 2001). Binding of heparin to AT can reduce the antiinflammatory effects of AT (see the section on Antithrombin earlier in the chapter).

Heparin cannot eliminate existing thrombi but can help prevent the formation of new thrombi or expansion of established thrombi. At this time there is insufficient information to advocate the use of heparin in the treatment of any phase of DIC. Heparin therapy may be most useful for patients with chronic DIC conditions in which there is predominantly a prothrombotic stage of DIC and no significant inflammatory stimulus.

Tissue Factor Pathway Inhibitors

A number of agents targeting the TF pathway currently are under study, including TF pathway inhibitor, recombinant nematode anticoagulant protein c2, recombinant hirudin, and inactivated factor VIIa. Phase III clinical trials in humans are lacking, and the use of these agents in veterinary medicine has not been investigated at this time.

References and Suggested Reading

Bateman S: Disseminated intravascular coagulation in dogs: review of the literature, *J Vet Emerg Crit Care* 8:29, 1998.

Bateman S et al: Diagnosis of disseminated intravascular coagulation in dogs admitted to an intensive care unit, *J Am Vet Med Assoc* 215:798, 1999.

Feldman B, Madewell B, O'Neill M: Disseminated intravascular coagulation: antithrombin, plasminogen, and coagulation abnormalities in 41 dogs, *J Vet Med Assoc* 179:151, 1981.

Maruyama H et al: The incidence of disseminated intravascular coagulation in dogs with malignant tumor, *J Vet Med Sci* 66:573, 2004.

Rozanski EA et al: The effect of heparin and fresh frozen plasma on plasma antithrombin III activity, prothrombin time and activated partial thromboplastin time in critically ill dogs, *J Vet Emerg Crit Care* 11:15, 2001.

Stokol T et al: D-dimer concentrations in healthy dogs and dogs with disseminated intravascular coagulation, *Am J Vet Res* 61:393, 2000.

Vincent J et al: Drotrecogin alfa (activated) treatment in severe sepsis from global open-label trial ENHANCE: further evidence for survival and safety and implications for early treatment, *Crit Care Med* 33:2266, 2005.

Warren BL et al: High-dose antithrombin III in severe sepsis: a randomized controlled trial, *J Am Med Assoc* 286:1869, 2001.

CHAPTER 64

Hypercoagulable States

BO WIINBERG, *Copenhagen, Denmark*
ANNEMARIE T. KRISTENSEN, *Copenhagen, Denmark*

A hypercoagulable state is an enhanced tendency to form venous or arterial thrombi. In 1845 a young German pathologist named Rudolf Virchow presented a novel and relatively simple concept of the pathogenesis of thromboembolic disease, which remains valid to this day. Virchow described three factors (Figure 64-1) that are the core reasons for the development of venous thrombosis: alterations of the blood (hypercoagulability), impairment of blood flow (stasis), and changes in the vessel wall (vascular injury). Research into the molecular basis of thrombosis has since enhanced our understanding of the pathophysiology of each of these concepts and thereby also our ability to diagnose and treat patients with thromboembolic disease. This chapter focuses primarily on the first of the three legs of Virchow's triad—hypercoagulable states—but briefly describes the effects of stasis and disruption of the intact endothelium.

Pathophysiology

Impairment of normal blood flow (stasis) leads to accumulation of procoagulant factors and facilitates increased interaction between the platelets and their receptors on the vessel and increased exposure to procoagulant factors released by the endothelium, which promotes thrombus formation. If prolonged or severe, stasis may cause acidosis and tissue hypoxia, which lead to vascular injury. Stasis, along with hypercoagulability, plays an important role in the development of venous thrombosis. The venous system is a low-pressure, low-flow, high-capacity system that is more susceptible to stasis. In contrast, the arterial system is less affected by vascular injury and hypercoagulable changes in the blood.

The endothelium protects against the development of thrombosis in several ways. The endothelial surface expresses thrombomodulin, which binds thrombin produced during activation of coagulation, and changes its conformation to allow it to activate protein C (APC). The activated protein C then associates with its cofactor protein S, and this complex exerts its anticoagulant effect via inactivation of coagulation factors Va and VIIIa. Importantly, thrombin bound to thrombomodulin is no longer available to activate fibrinogen or promote platelet aggregation. Thrombin activates endothelial production of prostacyclin, which in turn inhibits platelet aggregation. Heparin-like proteoglycans on the endothelial surface promote inactivation of thrombin via enhanced antithrombin (AT) activity. Activation of fibrinolysis via tissue-type plasminogen activator produced and released by the endothelium subsequently activates plasminogen to plasmin, which results in clot lysis. Vascular injury destroys these protective mechanisms of the endothelium and also exposes procoagulant subendothelial components such as collagen and tissue factor (TF) to the blood, which leads to fibrin formation and platelet aggregation. Inflammatory mediators such as interleukins and endotoxins also are released secondary to vascular injury, and these mediators in turn promote clot formation and, importantly, down-regulate normal protective mechanism such as the thrombomodulin receptor.

Causes

As diagnostic capabilities have evolved it has become clear that thrombosis is more prevalent in small animals than previously thought, and although its importance in relation to morbidity and mortality presently is unknown, it almost is certainly not insignificant.

Primary (hereditary) deficiencies, such as factor V Leiden, prothrombin G20210A mutation, deficiencies of natural anticoagulants (antithrombin, protein C, and protein S), and hyperhomocysteinemia, have not been described in animals, but there are a number of acquired underlying conditions or disease states that are associated with increased risk of thrombosis in dogs and cats. The causes of secondary hypercoagulable states often are unclear and may be multifactorial but can be divided into the following categories (Figure 64-2): (1) decreased levels of endogenous anticoagulants, (2) increased enzymatic activity, (3) increased fibrinogen levels, and (4) increased platelet activity.

Decreased Levels of Endogenous Anticoagulants

The most important endogenous anticoagulants are AT, protein C, and its cofactor protein S. Low levels of endogenous anticoagulants can be caused by (1) decreased production, which can be seen in hepatic disease or secondary to administration of certain drugs (e.g., L-asparaginase); (2) increased consumption, which can be seen secondary to major surgery, disseminated intravascular coagulation, sepsis, trauma, or cancer; or (3) enhanced clearance secondary to renal or intestinal disease. Endogenous anticoagulants limit activation of coagulation to the site of injury and thus inhibit the development of a clot into a thrombus. Most anticoagulant factors are released from, or are present on, the surface of endothelial cells, and normal endothelial cell function is of vital importance to these anticoagulation mechanisms.

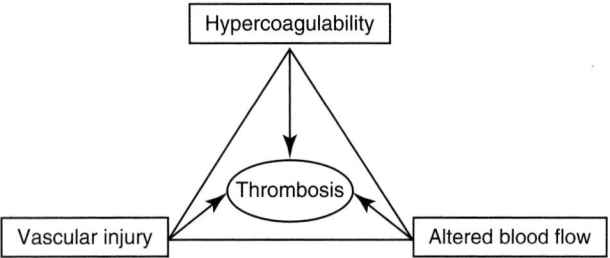

Figure 64-1 Virchow's triad, which describes the three factors contributing to the development of venous thrombosis.

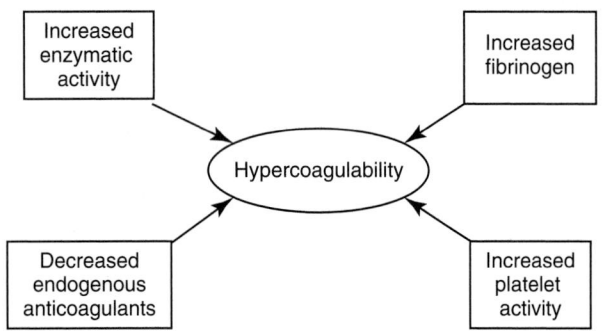

Figure 64-2 Common causes of secondary hypercoagulable states.

Increased Enzymatic Activity

Elevated levels of factor VIII and other coagulation factors, including XI and IX, have been implicated as independent risk factors for development of thrombosis in humans. Apart from increased factor VIII levels in Cushing's disease, elevated levels of coagulation factors have not been described in dogs or cats. Increased thrombin generation is more common, however, and is seen in several systemic disease states such as cancer, trauma, immune-mediated diseases, and sepsis. Normal *in vivo* activation of coagulation is triggered by binding of factor VIIa to exposed TF, which is constitutively expressed on the adventitial cells and pericytes surrounding the blood vessels; consequently, tissue injury that disrupts the endothelial lining of the vessels normally is needed to activate coagulation. However, in inflammatory or pathologic states such as the ones mentioned earlier, monocytes, endothelium, and perhaps even platelets can be stimulated to express TF. TF binding of factor VIIa and factor Xa in turn initiates intracellular signal transduction pathways, which induce production of transcription factors necessary for the synthesis of adhesion proteins, proinflammatory cytokines, and growth factors; this collectively leads to increased thrombin generation and fibrin formation.

Increased Fibrinogen Level

Fibrinogen is an acute phase reactant, and thus the most common cause of increased fibrinogen is an inflammatory response secondary to injury or infection. In the last decade it has become increasingly clear that inflammation and hemostasis are intricately linked and

that both play roles in host defense. Thus cells and inflammatory mediators of the immune system are capable of triggering coagulation pathways, and coagulation proteases, on the other hand, have significant immunomodulatory effects. Although it is beyond the scope of this chapter to discuss this complex subject in detail, the cross talk between inflammation and hemostasis is essential in the development of hypercoagulability. Because fibrinogen influences blood viscosity and red blood cell aggregation, elevated fibrinogen levels may lead to reduced blood flow in vessels, which in itself is a major risk factor for thrombosis. High fibrinogen levels also create a hypercoagulable state by increasing the velocity of platelet aggregation as well as platelet reactivity. In addition, the structure of the fibrin clot itself is affected by fibrinogen levels. Fibrin clots formed *in vitro* at high fibrinogen concentrations are denser than those formed at lower concentrations, have more dense fibers, and are more resistant to fibrinolysis.

Increased Platelet Activity

Thromboembolic complications have been described in relation to numerous diseases in which hyperactive platelets potentially play a significant causative role. In dogs the relevant diseases are neoplasia, hyperadrenocorticism, immune-mediated hemolytic anemia (IMHA), pancreatitis, disseminated intravascular coagulation, sepsis, cardiac disease, diabetes mellitus, and hypothyroidism. In cats the current relevant diseases are cardiac disease, IMHA, neoplasia, pancreatitis, and feline infectious peritonitis.

Laboratory Testing

Laboratory testing plays an important role in identifying a growing number of hypercoagulable states. The presence of multiple risk factors appears synergistically to increase the risk of thrombosis. Advances in our understanding of the molecular underpinnings of these hypercoagulable conditions have important implications not just for improving the performance of existing assays but also for identifying relevant new diagnostic targets. At present, the most relevant tests are plasma-based tests such as standard clotting assays (prothrombin time [PT], activated partial thromboplastin time [aPTT], fibrinogen level, and AT activity), viscoelastic tests such as thromboelastography (TEG or ROTEM device), and platelet function tests such as those provided by the Multiplate platelet function analyzer and flow cytometry. Although these tests can help determine whether a patient has a hypercoagulable condition and pinpoint the contributing components, the results cannot be used to guide treatment.

Management of Hypercoagulable States

It is evident that the causes of hypercoagulability are multifactorial and complex. The direct link to thrombosis has not been clarified, and difficulties in selecting appropriate therapy often arise due to the diverse causes and clinical manifestations. This means that a certain therapeutic approach may be suitable for one cause but not for another. Often treatment is based on expert opinion, and the use of heparin is an excellent example of this. Some clinicians give heparin in every case even though there is no objective scientific evidence to support its beneficial effect, whereas other clinicians strongly discourage the use of heparin although there also is no documentation of adverse effects. A logical approach to the treatment of hypercoagulable states involves the following three components: (1) individualization of the therapy, (2) treatment or removal of the underlying cause, and (3) prevention of the intravascular clotting process.

Individualized Therapy

It is clear from our understanding of the complex causes, pathophysiology, and diverse clinical picture of hypercoagulability that the therapy must be individualized for each patient. Only then can one develop both a logical and aggressive approach in case management.

Treatment of the Underlying Cause

Early intervention is needed for effective treatment of patients with hypercoagulability, and it is essential that the underlying cause be treated aggressively since hypercoagulability likely will persist until the initiating cause is eliminated. Specific treatments are beyond the scope of this chapter but may involve, for example, treatment of shock, fluid resuscitation, maintenance of blood pressure, surgery, antibiotics, or chemotherapy.

Prevention of Coagulation

Anticoagulation therapy includes administration of unfractionated heparin (UFH), low-molecular-weight heparin (LMWH), warfarin, and antiplatelet drugs such as aspirin or clopidogrel.

Heparin

Heparin is the drug most commonly used for the prevention and treatment of acute thromboembolic diseases. Heparin can prevent venous thromboembolism in human patients with trauma, and consequently it has been hypothesized that it also would be suitable as a prophylactic agent in other hypercoagulable conditions. Heparin should be avoided during AT replacement to permit AT to modulate sepsis-induced inflammatory responses. Treatment is not evidence based, and both the dosage ranges and methods vary widely depending on the clinician. The suggested dosage of UFH is 100 U/kg q6-8h SC. Dosing should be started low and increased until the aPTT measured 3 hours after injection is prolonged to 1.5 to 2 times the normal range. Treatment with UFH must be tapered over 48 hours to avoid a rebound hypercoagulability. Suggested dosage of the LMWH dalteparin (Fragmin) is 150 U/kg q8h SC. LMWH treatment cannot be monitored using aPTT, but the risk of adverse bleeding is lower than with UFH and the treatment does not need to be tapered.

Warfarin

Warfarin is an oral vitamin K antagonist that inhibits the formation of the vitamin K–dependent coagulation factors II, VII, IX, and X and the important anticoagulants protein C and S. Because of the effect on protein C and S, heparin usually is coadministered for the first few days to prevent hypercoagulability. Warfarin often is used in humans to treat patients at risk of developing arterial thromboembolism and cardiac patients. The effect of warfarin is irreversible, and there is large intraindividual and interindividual variation in the effect; the drug therefore should be dosed conservatively and the effect monitored closely by measurement of the international normalized ratio (INR), which is the ratio of the patient's PT to the PT of a normal control sample. Objective clinical trials in animals do not exist, but an INR of 1.5 to 2.5 is considered adequate by most clinicians. A common starting dosage is 0.2 mg/kg q12h PO in dogs and 0.1 to 0.2 mg/kg q24h PO in cats. Close monitoring is essential, and INR should be measured daily for the first week, then twice weekly for 1 month, then once weekly for 2 months, and then once monthly. Dose adjustment should be based on the total weekly dose because the effect is delayed 4 to 5 days. Even with close monitoring, there still is about a 20% risk of bleeding episodes.

Aspirin

Aspirin (acetylsalicylic acid, ASA) is the most widely used antiplatelet drug in both veterinary and human medicine. It is a nonselective cyclooxygenase inhibitor that exerts an antiplatelet effect through irreversible inhibition of thromboxane A_2 formation by inhibiting cyclooxygenase-1 for the lifetime of the platelet. Thromboxane mediates platelet activation through the G-protein signaling pathway. Studies have demonstrated that up to 70% of normal dogs have a defect in G-protein signaling, which calls into question the usefulness of aspirin as a general antiplatelet drug in dogs when empiric dosing is used. Prostaglandin depletion seems to be the main mechanism involved in the development of gastrointestinal adverse effects of aspirin, but the direct contact of aspirin with the gastroduodenal mucosa also can induce damage by disrupting the gastric epithelial cell barrier. Prostaglandin level recovers much more rapidly at low doses since deacetylation of aspirin takes place at first passage through the liver and therefore the systemic circulation is no longer exposed to the aspirin, whereas the platelets passing through the portal system continue to be exposed.

Aspirin is the most common antiplatelet drug used in cats for the prevention of acute thromboembolism (ATE). Although aspirin has been used in cats for 30 years, prospective, blinded, placebo-controlled clinical studies of the use of aspirin in cats with ATE are lacking. Multiple retrospective studies have evaluated the effect of aspirin therapy and report recurrence rates from 17% to 70%. A relatively high aspirin dose of 75 to 81 mg per animal q72h PO has been used routinely in cats. However, in 2003 a retrospective study of 127 cats with ATE that compared safety and recurrence rates for a high dose and a low dose (5 mg per cat q72h PO) of aspirin reported no difference in recurrence between groups and many fewer gastrointestinal adverse effects when the low dose was used (Smith et al, 2003). A recently published study compared the inhibitory effect of aspirin and meloxicam on whole blood aggregation (WBA) in healthy cats (Cathcart et al, 2012). The cats given aspirin received 5 mg/kg q48h PO and the effect was evaluated by measuring WBA, oral mucosal bleeding time, postaggregation serotonin plasma concentration, and thromboxane B_2 concentration in serum. Meloxicam did not have any measurable effect on any of the analyzed parameters, and although thromboxane B_2 concentrations were significantly lower in the cats treated with aspirin at all time points, there was no statistical difference in either WBA or oral mucosal bleeding time between the aspirin-treated and meloxicam-treated groups.

In dogs aspirin often is used empirically as thromboprophylaxis in diseases such as IMHA, glomerulopathies, pulmonary thromboembolism, and other conditions in which thromboembolism may be anticipated. The antithrombotic dosage in dogs recommended by most textbooks is 0.5 mg/kg q12-24h PO; however, the optimum antithrombotic dosage is unknown. The antithrombotic benefit of aspirin alone in dogs has not been evaluated in prospective clinical studies. In one retrospective study of dogs with IMHA, improved outcome was observed in the group of dogs receiving ultra-low-dose aspirin (ULDA; 0.5 mg/kg q24h PO) as adjunctive therapy to immunosuppression with prednisolone and/or azathioprine with or without concomitant heparin treatment (Weinkle et al, 2005). The inhibitory effect of aspirin on platelet function in dogs has been evaluated *ex vivo* in multiple studies with variable results, probably due to differences in methodology, natural breed variability, and resistance. Significantly reduced plasma thromboxane concentration in response to 5-mg/kg aspirin treatment in dogs was documented in one study, whereas the reduction in thromboxane concentration did not reach statistical significance in another study that administered 10 mg/kg aspirin (Brainard et al, 2007; Blois et al, 2010). The majority of the more recent studies have documented decreased whole blood and platelet-rich plasma aggregation in response to treatment with aspirin at dosages ranging from 0.5 mg/kg (ULDA) to 10 mg/kg; however, the study examining ULDA therapy could not detect any reduction in P-selectin platelet expression, a measure of activation (Weinkle et al, 2005). Prolongation of platelet function analyzer closure time in response to aspirin has been documented in some but not all studies, and the results of recent studies suggest that platelet closure time in dogs may be agonist dependent, as is the case in people. The development of gastric mucosal lesions secondary to aspirin treatment in dogs has been documented in several studies at aspirin dosages ranging from 10 mg/kg q12h to 25 mg/kg q8h. However, in a recent study evaluating gastric adverse effects of ULDA therapy in combination with prednisolone treatment, no significant increase in gastroduodenal lesions was documented compared with prednisolone treatment alone or placebo, although a mild self-limiting diarrhea was noted in the group receiving combination therapy (Graham and Leib, 2009).

Clopidogrel

Clopidogrel is a second-generation thienopyridine, and its pharmacokinetics and antiplatelet effect have been studied in both healthy cats and healthy dogs. In people clopidogrel is the most used $P2Y_{12}$ receptor antagonist and is recommended for prevention of further thrombotic events following acute coronary syndrome and ischemic stroke. Large studies have shown that clopidogrel provides significant protection against thrombotic episodes when administered to patients at risk of thrombosis, especially in combination with aspirin.

In cats dosages from 18.75 to 75 mg per cat q24h PO resulted in significantly reduced platelet aggregation and serotonin release and a significant prolongation of oral mucosal bleeding time. No significant difference between doses was identified, which indicates that a dose of 18.75 mg per cat q24h or lower should be adequate in cats (Hogan et al, 2004). The benefit of clopidogrel as an antiplatelet agent in cats has yet to be documented for any clinical indication. However, a prospective, double-blind, multicenter study on the efficacy of clopidogrel compared with aspirin in preventing arterial thromboembolism in cats that recently experienced a cardiogenic embolic event is ongoing.

In dogs thromboelastographic platelet mapping and whole blood aggregation measurements both have shown that clopidogrel produces a rapid inhibitory effect beginning 60 minutes after treatment, with a sustained significant reduction in optical platelet aggregation at 24 hours after a dose of 1.13 ± 0.17 mg/kg. Platelet function has been reported to return to normal values in most dogs within 7 to 8 days, although there is individual variation in duration of effect.

A small-scale prospective study in 24 dogs with IMHA compared the effect and safety of three drug regimens: clopidogrel alone at a 10-mg/kg PO loading dose followed by 2 to 3 mg/kg q24h PO for 89 days, clopidogrel in combination with ULDA at 0.5 mg/kg q24h PO, and ULDA alone for 90 days (Mellett et al, 2011). No hemorrhagic events were noted in any of the groups and the transfusion requirements were similar in all groups, as were the survival rates at discharge and at 90 days. Although this study showed no significant differences between groups, the groups were very small and there was no placebo group. Therefore larger randomized clinical studies must be performed before any conclusions can be drawn regarding the beneficial effects of clopidogrel or aspirin in dogs with IMHA.

References and Suggested Reading

Alwood AJ et al: Anticoagulant effects of low-molecular-weight heparins in healthy cats, *J Vet Intern Med* 21(3):378, 2007.

Blois SL et al: Effects of aspirin, carprofen, deracoxib, and meloxicam on platelet function and systemic prostaglandin concentrations in healthy dogs, *Am J Vet Res* 71(3):349, 2010.

Brainard BM et al: Changes in platelet function, hemostasis, and prostaglandin expression after treatment with nonsteroidal anti-inflammatory drugs with various cyclooxygenase selectivities in dogs, *Am J Vet Res* 68(3):251, 2007.

Cathcart CJ et al: Lack of inhibitory effect of acetylsalicylic acid and meloxicam on whole blood platelet aggregation in cats, *J Vet Emerg Crit Care* 22(1):99, 2012.

Goggs R et al: Pulmonary thromboembolism, *J Vet Emerg Crit Care* 19(1):30, 2009.

Graham HA, Leib MS: Effects of prednisone alone or prednisone with ultralow-dose aspirin on the gastroduodenal mucosa of healthy dogs. *J Vet Intern Med* 23(3):482, 2009.

Hogan DF et al: Antiplatelet effects and pharmacodynamics of clopidogrel in cats, *J Am Vet Med Assoc* 225(9):1406, 2004.

Lunsford KV, Mackin AJ: Thromboembolic therapies in dogs and cats: an evidence-based approach, *Vet Clin Small Anim* 37(3):579, 2007.

Mellett AM, Nakamura RK, Bianco D: A prospective study of clopidogrel therapy in dogs with primary immune-mediated hemolytic anemia, *J Vet Intern Med* 25(1):71, 2011.

Mischke R et al: Amidolytic heparin activity and values for several hemostatic variables after repeated subcutaneous administration of high doses of a low molecular weight heparin in healthy dogs, *Am J Vet Res* 62(4):595, 2001.

Smith SA et al: Arterial thromboembolism in cats: acute crisis in 127 cases (1992-2001) and long-term management with low-dose aspirin in 24 cases, *J Vet Intern Med* 17(1):73, 2003.

Weinkle TK et al: Evaluation of prognostic factors, survival rates, and treatment protocols for immune-mediated hemolytic anemia in dogs: 151 cases (1993-2002), *J Am Vet Med Assoc* 226(11):1869, 2005.

Wiinberg B et al: Diagnosis and treatment of platelet hyperactivity in relation to thrombosis in dogs and cats, *J Vet Emerg Crit Care* 22(1):42, 2012.

Wiinberg B, Kristensen AT: Thromboelastography in veterinary medicine, *Semin Thromb Hemost* 36(7):747, 2010.

CHAPTER 65

Lymphocytosis in Dogs and Cats

SUSAN E. LANA, *Fort Collins, Colorado*
CHRISTINE S. OLVER, *Fort Collins, Colorado*
ANNE AVERY, *Fort Collins, Colorado*

The term *lymphocytosis* refers to an absolute lymphocyte count above the reference range for the laboratory performing the count. For the majority of diagnostic laboratories, a lymphocyte count of more than 5000 cells/µl is considered above the reference range for dogs. It is clinically useful to distinguish isolated lymphocytosis, with minimal changes to other lineages, from mild and possibly artifactual lymphocytosis. The latter can be seen when there is marked leukocytosis secondary to severe inflammation or a significant response to other immunologic diseases such as hemolytic anemia. For example, practitioners should be cautious in overinterpreting a mild lymphocytosis in the context of a severe leukocytosis consisting primarily of neutrophils.

It also is important that clinicians not draw any conclusions from the presence of relative lymphocytosis when the total lymphocyte count is normal. When laboratories report differential counts, the results usually are accompanied by a normal range, and if the percentage of white cells that are lymphocytes is high, the result may be flagged as abnormal. However, there is no clinical significance to an increase in the percentage of lymphocytes in the blood when the total lymphocyte count is normal. Usually such an increase is the result of neutropenia, in which case the cause of the neutropenia should be addressed.

Although there are no published data systematically examining the incidence of lymphocytosis in a large population of dogs, analysis of 27,000 unique complete blood counts (CBCs) performed over a 4-year-period at the Veterinary Teaching Hospital at Colorado State University and over 100,000 CBCs performed through IDEXX Laboratories (Copland, n.d.) indicates that mild lymphocytosis occurs primarily in dogs that are 3 years old or younger. In the Colorado State University cases, only 0.6% of all CBCs performed showed lymphocytosis, and 45% of these cases were in dogs younger than 3 years. Although follow-up is not available presently for either of these two cohorts of patients, the data suggest that mild lymphocytosis in dogs is rare and is seen most commonly in younger patients.

Diagnosis

Differential Diagnoses

For mature dogs that have lymphocytosis but no evidence that other marrow elements are mobilized (i.e., no evidence of a strong erythroid regenerative response or marked neutrophilia) the list of differential diagnoses is short and can be investigated with readily available diagnostic tests. By far the most common reason for an adult dog to have isolated lymphocytosis is a lymphoproliferative disorder (lymphoma or leukemia). Additional but much less common differential diagnoses are thymoma, Addison's disease, and chronic infection with *Ehrlichia canis*. There is little evidence in the literature that, in an adult dog, other infectious or inflammatory diseases cause lymphocytosis in the absence of significant anemia (e.g., lymphocytosis has been reported in cases of babesiosis, but these dogs also are anemic, and lymphocytes may be mobilized as a part of the bone marrow response to anemia).

Diagnostic Testing

Because a lymphoproliferative disorder is the most common reason for a mature adult dog to develop lymphocytosis, in the absence of clear signs pointing to a different cause (e.g., electrolyte abnormalities signaling Addison's disease, or clinical signs suggesting a mediastinal mass), the most efficient diagnostic path begins with determining if the patient has lymphoma or leukemia. In canine patients a lymphocyte count higher than 20,000 cells/μl can be considered diagnostic for lymphoma or leukemia, and a presumptive diagnosis of neoplasia may be made on this observation alone. Further evaluation is warranted, however, because of the diverse outcomes and treatment differences associated with different categories of lymphoproliferative disorders.

The first step in evaluating a case of lymphocytosis, regardless of lymphocyte count, is cytologic review of the peripheral blood by a clinical pathologist. Such review is essential to verify lymphocytosis, especially if a differential count was obtained using automated equipment. Furthermore, the appearance of the cells provides essential information about the nature of the disease. Useful cytologic evaluations are descriptions of the size, uniformity, and nuclear and cytoplasmic characteristics, including cytoplasmic basophilia, granulation, chromatin texture, and the presence or absence of nucleoli. The presence of a predominant population of small mature lymphocytes is required for the diagnosis of chronic lymphocytic leukemia, whereas the presence of blasts and immature lymphocytes is more compatible with an acute leukemia.

Flow Cytometry

The second step in the evaluation of lymphocytosis is flow cytometry. Flow cytometry is performed on anticoagulated blood and provides information about the immunophenotype of the cells. The goal of a flow cytometry study is twofold: First, in cases in which the lymphocyte count is less than 20,000 cells/μl, flow cytometry can help determine if the lymphocyte population is homogeneous (i.e., consisting primarily of cells of a single phenotype), a finding that is most consistent with neoplasia. If the population is heterogeneous, other differential diagnoses listed earlier can be considered (the exception is *E. canis* infection, discussed later). Second, flow cytometry can determine the phenotype of the cells, which can help further classify the disease process and in some cases provide prognostic information.

A flow cytometry study involves staining peripheral blood leukocytes with antibodies against a variety of cell surface proteins (Wilkerson, 2012). At a minimum, most laboratories determine whether the lymphocytes express T-cell antigens (CD3, CD4, CD5, and CD8), B-cell antigens (CD21 and CD22), and CD34, an antigen expressed on immature lymphoid and myeloid precursors. The flow cytometry results indicate the concentration of each lymphocyte subset in the peripheral blood and should be accompanied by an interpretation from the laboratory carrying out the assay. Many different laboratories now provide flow cytometry services, and most use a similar panel of antibodies. Flow cytometry is not a standardized assay in veterinary medicine, however, and there are no universally accepted protocols, normal ranges, or standard reporting format. For a clinician to get the most out of flow cytometry as a diagnostic tool, it is suggested that the clinician consistently use the same laboratory so that he or she can become familiar with that laboratory's practices and reporting format.

Clonality Testing

A third step in evaluating an expanded lymphocyte population may be determination of clonality using the PARR (polymerase chain reaction for antigen receptor rearrangements) assay. This assay is used when the flow cytometry study and cytologic analysis do not give definitive results. For example, flow cytometry might reveal an expansion of more than one lymphocyte subset, but a lymphoproliferative disorder still is strongly suspected based on clinical signs. Detection of clonality relies on the fact that lymphocytes contain DNA regions that are unique in length and sequence. This is a result of the recombination of the V, D, and J gene segments (B cell) or the V and J segments (T cell) to produce the region that encodes the antigen-binding portion of the immunoglobulin heavy chain or T-cell receptor-γ. Current methodology uses polymerase chain reaction to detect antigen receptor rearrangements, with primers for conserved regions of the V and J genes used to amplify the intervening region (Avery, 2012). Detection of clonal lymphocyte populations by this method is well established in human medicine and is routinely used in several veterinary laboratories. It is important to note that the conditions under which the assay is performed can have a profound effect on the sensitivity and specificity of the results; therefore each laboratory conducting the assay should report these numbers when they report results to allow proper interpretation of the findings.

Lymphoproliferative Disease in Dogs

Lymphocytosis can occur in any type of lymphoproliferative disease, and traditionally there has been a distinction between leukemia (generally considered a disease of bone marrow origin that results in circulating lymphocytosis) and lymphoma (originating as a solid tumor). Recent developments in human medicine make this distinction less important. Rather, the contemporary human classification scheme describes more than 50 subtypes of leukemia and lymphoma, grouped instead by phenotype (B cell versus T cell) and by characteristic histologic, immunophenotypic, genetic, and epidemiologic features. Some of these diseases are classified as lymphoma, even though they commonly present with peripheral blood involvement, and others are classified as leukemia but may present primarily with nodal involvement. The clinically important diagnostic issue is determination of the subtype of neoplasia. For example, consider several B-cell lymphoproliferative disorders in people (Swerdlow, 2008). Mantle cell lymphoma is a B-cell tumor that presents with hepatic and splenic involvement, lymphadenopathy, and in most cases also lymphocytosis involving the neoplastic B cells. It is not thought to be curable. Diffuse large B-cell lymphoma also is a B-cell lymphoma that presents as a nodal or extranodal mass, but it only rarely includes lymphocytosis. The prognosis of this disease is different; it is associated with a longer median survival time and in some cases can be cured. These two diseases are distinguished by their characteristic histologic appearances, chromosomal abnormalities, and the constellation of cell surface antigens they express. They are both called *lymphoma* despite the fact that one of these diseases usually features blood involvement and the other one does not. As another example, chronic lymphocytic leukemia (CLL) and small lymphocytic lymphoma used to be considered two separate entities, one of which presents primarily as circulating lymphocytosis and one of which is primarily nodal. They are now considered a single disease that usually, but not always, features lymphocytosis and is characterized by mature B cells. The clinical course is indolent and can progress over many years, regardless of whether the patient has primarily nodal disease or blood disease at presentation.

As suggested by these examples, a canine patient with lymphocytosis may have any number of lymphoproliferative disorders, most of which are not yet well described in the veterinary literature. The majority of these cannot be distinguished by examination of the peripheral blood alone, but cytologic examination and immunophenotyping of peripheral blood can give important prognostic and diagnostic information.

Lymphocytosis Involving CD34+ Cells

The only lymphoproliferative disorder than can be diagnosed definitively by immunophenotype is acute leukemia expressing CD34. CD34+ cells are precursor cells whose normal counterpart is found in the bone marrow. CD34 is expressed on both myeloid and lymphoid precursors. In most cases of CD34+ acute leukemia no antigens are expressed on the cell surface that would further allow for the definitive distinction between B, T, and myeloid lineages. If such a distinction is considered clinically relevant, the cells can be permeabilized and stained for intracellular expression of CD3 (for T-cell leukemia), Pax5 (for B-cell leukemia), or myeloperoxidase protein (for myeloid origin). The cells in these cases generally will be described by the cytopathologist as immature cells or blasts but occasionally can have a more mature appearance. Almost all cases of CD34+ leukemia show evidence of bone marrow involvement (anemia, thrombocytopenia, neutropenia) and can also show involvement of lymph nodes and spleen as well as a mediastinal mass at presentation. Regardless of the presentation and lineage designation, this form of acute leukemia has been shown to have a poor prognosis (Villiers et al, 2006; Williams et al, 2008).

Lymphocytosis Involving Granular Lymphocytes

Some cases of lymphocytosis involve granular lymphocytes (sometimes called *large granular lymphocytes* or *LGLs*, but the cells are not necessarily large). These cells will be described by the cytopathologist as having azurophilic cytoplasmic granules, but it is important to note that the granules are not be visible with Diff-Quik or other water-based stains. The phenotype of these cells is almost always CD8+, and they are thought to originate in the spleen, with a slight majority of cases presenting with splenomegaly (McDonough and Moore, 2000). It is useful to specifically identify granular lymphocytes for two reasons: first, the prognosis for patients with LGL leukemia/lymphoma was reported as generally good, with 14 of 23 cases reported to live longer than a year when treated with prednisone alone or prednisone plus chlorambucil (McDonough and Moore, 2000). Second, the presence of granular lymphocytes suggests another differential diagnosis. Chronic *E. canis* infection also can involve an LGL lymphocytosis and a homogeneous expansion of CD8 T cells (Heeb et al, 2003). Thus *E. canis* infection should be considered if warranted by geographic factors.

B-Cell Leukemia/Lymphoma

Antibody to the surface antigen CD21 is used to identify canine B cells by flow cytometry and is expressed on all B cells except the earliest precursors (which are CD34+) and plasma cells. Thus immunophenotyping can establish whether lymphocytosis is due to a B-cell disorder but does not help in determining whether the disorder is an acute CD34− leukemia, blood involvement of a more mature B-cell lymphoma such as diffuse large B-cell lymphoma, or CLL. Furthermore, with the exception of CLL, the clinical utility of distinguishing these various entities has not been established in veterinary medicine as it has in human medicine.

Patients with CLL often are not treated until clinical signs develop. When they are treated, therapy typically consists of prednisone and chlorambucil. Therefore it is clinically useful to establish a diagnosis of CLL in a patient with expansion of B cells. Although there are no universally accepted criteria for making this diagnosis, CLL is the primary differential diagnosis for a patient with lymphocytosis involving small to intermediate-sized lymphocytes with mature chromatin and mild or no clinical signs. CLL can include lymphadenopathy (Comazzi et al, 2011). A bone marrow sample is not necessary to make the diagnosis of CLL in canine or human patients. In human patients, determination of bone marrow involvement is used for prognostic purposes, but there are no data addressing the usefulness of bone marrow evaluation in canine patients. Patients with B-cell CLL have a median survival of 480 days (Comazzi et al, 2011) compared with 930 days for those with CD8 T-cell CLL (discussed later).

If the cytologic appearance of the lymphocytes does not support a diagnosis of CLL, or if the patient has significant clinical signs (cytopenias, significant lymphadenopathy or visceral organ involvement, systemic illness), flow cytometry nonetheless can provide prognostic information. B-cell disorders involving the peripheral blood are associated with a median survival of 150 days if they involve large cells as determined by flow cytometry and more than 1000 days if the disease involves small cells; the latter category may include B-cell CLL (Williams et al, 2008). The B-cell disorder may be classified further as to the type of lymphoma by biopsying nodes, spleen, or another involved organ. Such classification would be useful only if it provides additional prognostic or treatment guidance for the practitioner. Currently there are two studies in the literature that correlate survival with the contemporary histologic classification of lymphoproliferative disorders: Ponce and colleagues (2004) demonstrated that B-cell lymphomas are associated with radical differences in survival depending on the histologic subtype, with Burkitt's lymphoma being unresponsive to chemotherapy (median survival, 15 days) and diffuse large B-cell lymphoma associated with a median survival of 17 months when treated. Flood-Knapik and colleagues (2012) found that marginal zone lymphoma, an indolent form of B-cell lymphoma, was associated with an overall survival time of 21 months.

Taken together, these findings indicate that if there is lymphadenopathy in a patient with peripheral B-cell lymphocytosis and a diagnosis of CLL is not obvious, biopsy of a node may be useful in determining prognosis. It is important to understand, however, that there is no universal agreement among pathologists about grading schemes. Thus a conversation with the pathology service that is going to examine the biopsy specimen is warranted before that step is taken.

T-Cell Leukemia/Lymphoma

Antibodies recognizing CD3 and CD5 identify all T cells. Antibodies recognizing CD4 and CD8 recognize helper T and cytotoxic T cell subsets, respectively, and their expression is mutually exclusive (with rare exceptions). Most laboratories that perform flow cytometry use a combination of these antibodies to investigate lymphocytosis in dogs.

Most T-cell lymphoproliferative disorders involving peripheral blood present with an expansion of CD8 T cells. These may be LGL disorders (discussed previously), CLL, or other forms of T-cell lymphoma/leukemia. The criteria for a diagnosis of CLL are the same for B cells and T cells (see earlier) and as stated previously, there is no evidence that bone marrow examination changes the diagnosis or prognosis. CD8 T-cell CLL is associated with a median survival of 930 days (Comazzi et al, 2011). As with B-cell disease, if a diagnosis of CLL cannot clearly be made, other features of the disease can provide prognostic information. In the case of CD8 T-cell lymphocytosis, the lymphocyte count at presentation, not the cell size, is prognostic. Patients with more than 30,000 lymphocytes/μl have poorer overall survival than those with fewer than 30,000 lymphocytes/μl (150 days versus >1000 days, respectively) (Williams et al, 2008).

As with B-cell disorders, biopsy of a lymph node may be warranted depending on the practitioner's clinical goals. One type of T-cell lymphoma, called *T-zone lymphoma,* presents with lymphocytosis in one half of cases (Flood-Knapik et al, 2012). The specific phenotype of these T cells has not yet been described. T-zone lymphoma is an indolent disease that responds as well to prednisone and chlorambucil as it does to more aggressive chemotherapy protocols. Currently the only way to make a definitive diagnosis of T-zone lymphoma is by histopathologic analysis, but given the prognostic and treatment implications of making this diagnosis, taking this additional step may be very useful clinically. This disease also provides an excellent illustration of the fact that the distinction between lymphoma and leukemia can be arbitrary and not clinically meaningful—in the absence of biopsy findings, many of these T-zone lymphomas may have been classified as cases of leukemia. Dogs with T-zone lymphoma that have lymphocytosis, however, have the same clinical characteristics and overall survival as those without lymphocytosis.

A smaller number of patients with T-cell lymphocytosis have a different phenotype: CD4 T cells or, more commonly, T cells that do not express CD4 or CD8. Few outcome data are available for either of these subtypes, but again, biopsy of lymph nodes, if they are enlarged, may be useful if the findings are classified appropriately by the pathologist.

Lymphocytosis Associated with Thymoma

Thymomas can cause lymphocytosis characterized by expanded populations of T cells. This is because the neoplastic thymic epithelium supports the differentiation of an increased number of CD4 and CD8 T cells, which exit to the peripheral circulation. The T cells are not neoplastic, but the prevalence of autoimmune diseases that are known to coexist with thymoma suggests that these cells do not necessarily differentiate normally.

Thymomas are discussed in the context of lymphocytosis because occasionally thymomas are clinically silent and are identified because of an incidental finding of lymphocytosis in the peripheral blood. In these cases, the lymphocytes will consist of increased numbers of CD4 and CD8 T cells (but usually not B cells). This result is not considered diagnostic for thymoma, simply suggestive. In addition, the cells will be described as small and mature on cytologic examination. In these cases, a diagnosis of thymoma then is made tentatively based on the presence of a mediastinal mass on thoracic radiographs.

The main differential diagnoses for a mediastinal mass accompanied by lymphocytosis are thymoma and T-cell lymphoma. In this situation, the most efficient diagnostic step for arriving at a definitive diagnosis is aspiration of the mass for cytologic analysis. Flow cytometry testing of the mass aspirate is an excellent means to distinguish thymoma from lymphoma if results of the cytologic evaluation are ambiguous (Lana et al, 2006). Thymomas consist of small T cells with an immunophenotype that reflect the normal stages of T-cell development. Thus the T cells from thymomas express only CD4, only CD8, or both CD4 and CD8 simultaneously. Since flow cytometry requires freshly aspirated material in cell suspension, it is useful to acquire samples for both cytologic analysis and flow cytometry at the same time to avoid the need for reaspiration if the cytologic results are not diagnostic.

Lymphocytosis Associated with Addison's Disease

Most patients with Addison's disease are identified readily by characteristic electrolyte abnormalities and are diagnosed using an adrenocorticotropic hormone stimulation test. The diagnosis can be more elusive when patients lack obvious electrolyte alterations and have vague clinical signs. Since lymphocytosis often is seen in Addison's disease, lymphoma or leukemia is sometimes considered in the list of differential diagnoses in cases without characteristic electrolyte abnormalities, and blood is submitted for immunophenotyping. In these cases, lymphocytes of all three major subsets (CD4 T cells, CD8 T cells, and B cells) will be expanded in number. The finding of heterogeneous expansion of lymphocytes is not diagnostic for Addison's disease, nor does it rule out lymphoproliferative disease, but it may suggest Addison's disease if this condition had not been considered previously.

Lymphoproliferative Disease in Cats

As in dogs, lymphocytosis in cats is not common, but cats appear to develop reactive lymphocytosis more frequently than dogs. Nonetheless, since neoplastic causes (lymphoma and leukemia) are more common, as with dogs, an efficient diagnostic approach is first to address the possibility of lymphoproliferative disease. This involves three steps (see earlier): (1) cytologic examination of the cells, (2) flow cytometry, and (3) clonality assays in some cases.

Lymphoproliferative Disease

The most common neoplastic cause of lymphocytosis in the cat is CLL. The majority of cases of feline CLL involve expansion of CD4 T cells. Information in the literature concerning clinical signs or prognosis for feline CLL is limited, although one study recently reported favorable outcomes in 18 cats (Campbell et al, 2012). These patients all had lymphocyte counts of more than 9000/µl, the median age was 12.5 years, and weight loss was the most common clinical sign. A combination of prednisone and chlorambucil was the most common treatment regimen, and 88% of the cats showed a response. The median remission time was 15.7 months. In contrast, LGL leukemia typically is CD8+, is seen accompanying cases of intestinal lymphoma, and is associated with very poor survival (median, 10 days after identification) (Roccabianca et al, 2006). These studies together demonstrate the importance of cytologic evaluation of lymphocytes coupled with immunophenotyping. There is no evidence that bone marrow evaluation is useful or necessary in most cases of feline leukemia/lymphoma.

Nonneoplastic Lymphocytosis

In the authors' anecdotal experience, approximately 20% of cases of feline lymphocytosis are the result of nonneoplastic lymphocyte expansion, as judged by immunophenotyping, clonality assessment, and clinical follow-up. Often, nonneoplastic B cells dominate reactive lymphocytosis, and the finding of homogeneous lymphocytosis may be interpreted inaccurately as B-cell neoplasia. Thus the finding of a homogeneous B-cell expansion in cats should be followed by ancillary testing such as clonality assays. On the other hand, homogeneous CD4 T-cell expansion, as noted earlier, is most likely due to T-cell leukemia/lymphoma.

Published studies indicate that nonneoplastic causes of feline lymphocytosis include hyperthyroidism treated with methimazole, hyperadrenocorticism and immune-mediated hemolytic anemia, and a number of infectious diseases. *Toxoplasma gondii* infection that is experimentally induced has been reported to cause lymphocytosis, but naturally occurring infection has not. Approximately 20% of cats infected with feline leukemia virus and feline immunodeficiency virus had lymphocytosis in one study, compared with 10% of all other cats (Gleich and Hartmann, 2009). In many and perhaps most cases, however, the underlying reason for lymphocytosis is not established. Further study of these cases would be very useful to determine whether the patients share an underlying disease process.

References and Suggested Reading

Avery AC: Molecular diagnostics of hematologic malignancies in small animals, *Vet Clin North Am Small Anim Pract* 42:97, 2012.

Campbell MW, Hess PR, Williams LE: Chronic lymphocytic leukaemia in the cat: 18 cases (2000-2010), *Vet Comp Oncol*, February 28, 2012 (epub ahead of print).

Comazzi S et al: Immunophenotype predicts survival time in dogs with chronic lymphocytic leukemia, *J Vet Intern Med* 25:100, 2011.

Copland M: Personal communication.

Flood-Knapik KE et al: Clinical, histopathological and immunohistochemical characterization of canine indolent lymphoma, *Vet Comp Oncol*, February 2, 2012 (epub ahead of print).

Gleich S, Hartmann K: Hematology and serum biochemistry of feline immunodeficiency virus-infected and feline leukemia virus-infected cats, *J Vet Intern Med* 23:552, 2009.

Heeb HL et al: Large granular lymphocytosis, lymphocyte subset inversion, thrombocytopenia, dysproteinemia, and positive *Ehrlichia* serology in a dog, *J Am Anim Hosp Assoc* 39:379, 2003.

Lana S et al: Diagnosis of mediastinal masses in dogs by flow cytometry, *J Vet Intern Med* 20:1161, 2006.

McDonough SP, Moore PF: Clinical, hematologic, and immunophenotypic characterization of canine large granular lymphocytosis, *Vet Pathol* 37:637, 2000.

Ponce F et al: Prognostic significance of morphological subtypes in canine malignant lymphomas during chemotherapy, *Vet J* 167:158, 2004.

Roccabianca P et al: Feline large granular lymphocyte (LGL) lymphoma with secondary leukemia: primary intestinal origin with predominance of a CD3/CD8αα phenotype, *Vet Pathol* 43:15, 2006.

Swerdlow DL, editor: *WHO classification of tumours of haematopoietic and lymphoid tissues*, ed 4, Lyon, France, 2008, International Agency for Research on Cancer.

Villiers E et al: Identification of acute myeloid leukemia in dogs using flow cytometry with myeloperoxidase, MAC387, and a canine neutrophil-specific antibody, *Vet Clin Pathol* 35:55, 2006.

Wilkerson MJ: Principles and applications of flow cytometry and cell sorting in companion animal medicine, *Vet Clin North Am Small Anim Pract* 42:53, 2012.

Williams MJ et al: Canine lymphoproliferative disease characterized by lymphocytosis: immunophenotypic markers of prognosis, *J Vet Intern Med* 22:596, 2008.

CHAPTER 66

Quality Control for the In-Clinic Laboratory

GLADE WEISER, *Fort Collins, Colorado*
LINDA M. VAP, *Fort Collins, Colorado*

Background

Why Quality Control: Rationale for Implementation

The concept of the in-clinic laboratory that consists of reagent kits and instrumentation originated in the mid-1970s. Today the concept has evolved to the use of complex instrumentation with capabilities in hematology and chemistry matching those of the central laboratory. More than 80% of veterinary facilities now have such in-clinic laboratory instrumentation. This trend has occurred with no regulatory oversight of either laboratory quality assurance or instrumentation performance claims. Any leadership in quality control recommendations or procedures has been left to the discretion of instrument suppliers.

Complex instruments perform a complicated series of functions to produce laboratory data. Mechanical components include pipetting mechanisms, addition of diluents and reagents, reaction-sample mixing, reagent stability, and sample movement to or through a measuring mechanism. Measuring components may include various transducer mechanisms or light sources that interact with the reacted sample. The physical elements may include tubing, valves, printed circuit boards, stepper motors, syringes, light-emitting sources, photodetectors, and data-reduction software. Most of these elements are variably subject to wear and eventual failure. Superimposed on this is user interaction with the sample and the system. In the in-clinic environment there is variable laboratory supervision and variable training in laboratory science among users.

The result is a complex operation that requires regular monitoring of performance accuracy. Because the in-clinic veterinary laboratory provides actionable patient data, it is regarded as equivalent to a professional diagnostic laboratory, perhaps with a limited list of services. Professional laboratories implement a standardized plan to monitor each instrument system with quality-control material at least once each shift. In high-volume settings, even more frequent monitoring may be interspersed with processing of patient samples. The authors believe this monitoring can be somewhat simplified for the veterinary practice facility. An analysis of a quality-control material once per day of use is the recommended minimum. The accumulation of daily data allows identification of a developing trend or pinpoints when system failure occurs. Analysis of quality-control material once per month or only when a problem is suspected does not allow identification of a trend or pinpointing of the time of failure.

Rather than trying to sell the merits of a quality-control program, it may be more convincing to present an example. A hematology quality-control material has a total white blood cell (WBC) target range of 12 to 14 × $10^3/\mu l$. On a given morning, someone is suspicious about the fact that WBC count has been low in an unusual fraction of tested patients and decides to analyze the control material. The system produces a value of $6.4 \times 10^3/\mu l$. The question then is, How do you feel about interpreting WBC values for your patients for the rest of the day? Further, do you have a concern about your interpretations over some number of preceding days? Implementation of a standardized program that analyzes quality-control material on a regular basis *before* patient testing minimizes such uncertainty. This provides confidence in the results obtained up to that point. It does not, however, guarantee results produced in the future.

Role of Animal Health Diagnostics Companies

Unfortunately, the companies marketing instruments have been variably informative about quality control. At one extreme is the lack of availability of quality-control sample material for some instrument systems. At the opposite extreme is a recommended program of daily control sample analysis with supporting data management software that is patterned after minimal standards for a professional laboratory, but with which compliance is optional and is not monitored. In the middle are numerous recommendations, an example being to analyze a quality-control sample once per month. Some systems claim to have various mechanisms of internal quality control. Although there are procedures for monitoring electronics, these are not a substitute for analysis of a quality-control material that consists of blood or serum, which also allows monitoring of operator technique and the reagent system. The absence of quality control in the diagnostic product offering plays to concerns about cost and the expertise required to implement a quality-control program. Ironically, some people believe that a system with a quality-control program is inferior to one without. Statements like "If it requires daily quality control, it must be unreliable or malfunction frequently" actually are heard. Companies with the product offerings may unknowingly reinforce the perception that quality control is not important. This creates the impression that sales are more important than the reliability of data for medical case management.

The veterinary community, acting as individuals and through organized veterinary medicine, should encourage diagnostics companies to provide and integrate quality-assurance programs. The opportunity now exists for companies to become responsible for monitoring, analysis, and preemptive technical support in the following way. Modern instrument systems have computing power and connectivity to enable bidirectional communication via a network and the Internet. With that capability, it is possible to automate analysis and monitoring of quality control by the supplier. The supplier's technical support personnel could then proactively intervene when quality-control analysis suggests a potential problem. With the supplier assuming much of the responsibility for the inherent complexity, this approach could standardize quality assurance across veterinary facilities. This approach has the potential to assert expertise that often is lacking or not consistent in veterinary facilities.

Implementations for Chemistry and Hematology Analyzers

The authors believe the quality-control program can be somewhat simplified for the veterinary practice facility. The most practical way to integrate quality control is to include it as part of daily start-up procedures, typically in the morning when the workday is begun. Most systems are in a stand-by mode when personnel arrive in the morning. Most benchtop units have a wake-up or start-up procedure. Analysis of a quality-control material at the conclusion of the start-up procedure verifies that the system is working properly and is ready to analyze patient samples. The procedure involves handling the quality-control material according to manufacturer directions. The material is accompanied by target values determined by repetitive reference procedures. These are expressed as a range for each measurement. Results from the analyzer are expected to fall within this range on a daily basis when all elements are functioning properly. The software of most benchtop instrument systems can store control range values and present control analysis results for inspection. The system also should be able to store control data in a way that can be retrieved for trend analysis. Additional background on quality-control procedures is available (Weiser and Thrall, 2007). More advanced treatment of quality-control data is discussed later in the chapter.

Adjunct Procedures That Supplement Routine Use of Quality-Control Material

Laboratory professionals use a variety of procedures to corroborate anomalies in laboratory data. These also may be used to evaluate data that do not fit a preconceived clinical impression when consulting with the clinician.

Some of these techniques may be used in the practice setting. These include the following:

- *Sample evaluation.* Occasionally, results may be obtained that do not fit the clinical picture or preconceived expectations. When this happens, the sample and sample handling should be evaluated. In blood chemistry analyzers, the presence of interfering substances such as those associated with lipemia or hemolysis, the presence of fibrin clots interfering with sample loading, and improper anticoagulant use are considerations for evaluation. In hematologic testing, the adequacy of sample mixing and the presence of microclots in the sample are considerations, as are hemolysis or lipemia. Instrumentation suppliers should provide guidelines for this evaluation, and their technical support personnel may provide additional help in the evaluation when needed. One should keep in mind that it may be appropriate to repeat the analysis when an unexplained aberrant value occurs.

- *Use of quality-control material outside the routine cycle.* In addition to performing regular analysis of quality-control material at the beginning of each day, occasionally it is appropriate to check system function with quality-control material whenever it is suspected that analytical failure may be occurring.

- *Blood film examination.* It is important to note that the capability of hematology analyzers to produce a differential distribution is not intended to replace blood film review of leukocytes. At best, it is intended to detect a reasonably normal hemogram. Furthermore, there is no good quality-control material for the differential analysis. Hematology analyzers cannot detect abnormalities such as left-shifted cells, leukemic cells, nucleated erythrocytes, and other abnormal cell types. When there is leukopenia, leukocytosis, an abnormality in the differential distribution, or any abnormality in the instrument's histogram or cytogram display, a blood film scan should be performed to corroborate the generated differential data as well as to evaluate erythrocyte morphology and screen for hemoparasites. A differential count should be performed by microscopy whenever a discrepancy or abnormal cells are detected by the scan.

- *Evaluation of mean corpuscular hemoglobin concentration (MCHC).* The relationship between hemoglobin concentration (Hb) and hematocrit (Hct) is a physiologic constant. These two values are used to calculate the MCHC: MCHC = (Hb × 100)/Hct. The MCHC is typically 32 to 36 g/dl, with minor variation among instrument systems. Because the two primary measurements are performed independently by taking separate measurements on two separate dilutions, they can be used to corroborate each other. Certain pathologic conditions, including iron deficiency and marked regeneration, may cause a minimal decrease in MCHC (e.g., to 30 g/dl). Certain sample abnormalities may variably increase MCHC by artifact, including marked lipemia, sample hemolysis, pathologic red blood cell (RBC) agglutination, and marked numbers of Heinz bodies. Occasionally an Hct value does not meet clinical expectations. There are two readily available means to evaluate this. One is to corroborate the Hct value with the Hb concentration. This is most easily done by examination of the MCHC value; if it is in the physiologic reference interval, the Hct and Hb are confirming each other. A nonsensically low MCHC value indicates an analytical malfunction. A very high MCHC value may indicate the same after sample abnormalities such as marked lipemia, marked sample hemolysis, prominent RBC agglutination, and marked numbers of Heinz bodes are ruled out. The second method is to compare the instrument-derived Hct with a manually obtained packed cell volume. Results for the two methods should match within a reasonable limit, provided the collection tube is filled properly. This limit may vary slightly with the instrument and the patient's disorder. Failure of the results to match can localize the source of the nonsense MCHC values to the RBC counting and sizing. In addition, the centrifuged microhematocrit tube provides a simple means of examining the supernatant for hemolysis and lipemia. If nonsense values are obtained repeatedly, analyzing the quality-control material or contacting technical support is warranted.

More Advanced Quality-Control Procedures

There are more advanced procedures for monitoring instrument performance with quality-control material. These are gaining visibility in central laboratories, and recommendations for the control of general analytical factors in veterinary diagnostic and research laboratories were published recently (Flatland et al, 2010). However, because of their complexity and the required expertise these procedures would need to be automated and managed over a network link by the diagnostics supplier in the clinic setting. Detailed recommendations intended for the point-of-care type of hematology analyzers typically used in veterinary clinics are available (Flatland and Vap, 2012). Familiarity with the guidelines is encouraged, particularly for the primary instrument operators. Over time, it is expected (hoped) that educational programs for veterinary allied health personnel will include comprehensive training in this area. Main concepts are discussed briefly here.

Running quality-control material on a regular basis is a crucial first step, but there is little value in doing so unless the acceptability of the results is evaluated and appropriate action is taken when results are deemed unacceptable. This can be accomplished by a primary operator with sufficient education and experience or deferred to the technical support personnel.

The definition of "unacceptable" is arguable; however, a practical recommendation applicable under certain circumstances was published recently in the veterinary literature (Rishiniw et al, 2012). This recommendation uses one of several possible Westgard decision criteria known as the 1_{3s} *rule* (Westgard, 2012). Understanding this rule requires familiarity with quality-control charts. The analyte concentration or enzyme activity value obtained by running the quality-control material is plotted over time. The data may be plotted automatically by the testing system. The resulting graph is known as a *Levey-Jennings control chart* and typically includes visual indicators of the expected mean (obtained from the package insert of the quality-control material) and 1, 2, and 3 standard deviation units (SDs) above and below the mean for each analyte evaluated. Examples are readily available (Flatland and Vap, 2012; Stockham and Scott, 2008; Westgard, 2012). These values may change slightly with each new lot number of quality-control material. Daily quality-control runs provide sufficient data points to assess the instrument visually for accuracy and reproducibility as well as for the presence of trends or shifts. Accurate results are indicated by closeness of obtained values to the expected mean, with results usually distributed evenly above and below the stated mean. Good reproducibility is indicated by minimal scatter around the average value, ideally within 2 SDs of the mean. A single value outside this range may occur spuriously for various reasons. The repeated occurrence of widely scattered data may indicate a major malfunction or, if the data are traceable to a single individual, operator error regarding sample handling. Trends are indicated by gradually increasing or decreasing values over time and suggest wear or decline of tubing, light sources, or reagents, or perhaps a slowly developing leak or plug. Shifts are indicated by a sudden significant change in results either upward or downward and suggest a change in the reagent or quality-control material lot number, a recent calibration adjustment, or perhaps sudden development of a leak or plug.

Instruments vary in their ability to be precise and accurate. To be able to use quality-control material to monitor analyzer function, one must determine if the analyzer in question meets necessary quality requirements for each analyte tested. Information to assist with this type of evaluation of several biochemistry analyzers has been published recently (Farr and Freeman, 2008; Rishiniw et al, 2012). If the instrument qualifies, performance can be monitored by using a single quality-control material with a reasonably high probability of detecting error (≥85%) and a low probability of falsely rejecting data (0%) when using the 1_{3s} rule. According to this rule, if the measurement for the quality-control material exceeds the ±3 SD limit on one occasion, investigation into the source of the problem is warranted. Similar information for hematology instruments is not yet available. Testing of patient samples should cease and the source of the problem should be investigated if the measurement value for the quality-control material falls outside ±3 SDs of the mean.

If a given analyzer cannot meet such requirements, there is no value in running quality-control material. In this case, the manufacturer may provide recommendations to improve analyzer performance. If it does not, participation in an external quality-assurance program (e.g., the VLA Quality Assurance System, http://vla.timelessveterinarysystems.com/) may be helpful. These programs provide a commercially prepared product several times a year. This material is tested by the participants as if it were a patient sample. Data are returned to the company and compiled in such a way as to allow comparison of the results provided with the results from all those in the same peer group based on instrumentation and methodology. One must ensure that there are sufficient participants within the peer group for the comparison to be meaningful. Unexplained values falling outside the peer group range indicates error involving sample handling, instrument operation, or instrument malfunction for which technical support may be required. Because of the low frequency of testing, participants receive only information related to the long-term performance of their system. Therefore this does not provide or replace the daily assessment of analyzer performance described earlier. How quality-control principles will be implemented for in-clinic diagnostics is yet to be determined.

Discussions are ongoing and recommendations are evolving. Ideally, instrument manufacturers, veterinary practitioners, allied health professionals, and their educators will work toward a consensus to ensure that laboratory diagnostics quality-assurance methods are expanded, adopted, and implemented.

References and Suggested Reading

Farr AJ, Freeman KP: Quality control validation, application of sigma metrics, and performance comparison between two biochemistry analyzers in a commercial veterinary laboratory, *J Vet Diagn Invest* 20:536, 2008.

Flatland B et al: ASVCP quality assurance guidelines: control of general analytical factors in veterinary laboratories, *Vet Clin Pathol* 39:264, 2010.

Flatland B, Vap LM: Quality management recommendations for automated and manual in-house hematology of domestic animals, *Vet Clin North Am Small Animal Pract* 32:11, 2012.

Rishiniw M, Pion PD, Maher T: The quality of veterinary in-clinic and reference laboratory biochemical testing, *Vet Clin Pathol* 41:92, 2012.

Stockham SL, Scott MA: Introductory concepts. In Stockham SL, Scott MA, editors: *Fundamentals of veterinary clinical pathology*, ed 2, Ames, IA, 2008, Blackwell Publishing, p 28.

Weiser MG, Thrall MA: Quality control recommendations and procedures for in-clinic laboratories, *Vet Clin North Am Small Animal Pract* 37:237, 2007.

Westgard J: "Westgard rules and multirules," updated November 20, 2012. Available at: www.westgard.com/westgard-rules-and-multirules.htm. Accessed January 6, 2012.

CHAPTER 67

Transfusion Medicine: Best Practices*

LAUREN SULLIVAN, *Fort Collins, Colorado*
TIMOTHY B. HACKETT, *Fort Collins, Colorado*

The positive and negative aspects of blood product administration, as further understood through recent developments in transfusion medicine, have significantly changed how and why veterinarians use these products. Practitioners have better access to a wider variety of blood products, which allows for more selective component therapy. This improved product availability has enhanced the level of care provided in the fields of surgery, medicine, and critical care. The ability to ensure donor-recipient compatibility, and thus patient safety, because of increased understanding of canine and feline erythrocyte antigens has made transfusion medicine

practical. However, the negative effects of blood products on the inflammatory, immune, and coagulation systems also have been further documented. Although blood products are a great resource when required, they also are often a finite resource and require a risk:benefit analysis before use. An understanding of current practices in transfusion medicine can help guide the practitioner to smart, safe, and successful use of blood products in the small animal patient.

Indications for Blood Products

Deciding on a "transfusion trigger" is patient dependent and requires careful review of historical, physical examination, and hematologic parameters. Factors to consider include the cause and chronicity of anemia, quantity and rapidity of blood loss, possibility of additional blood loss,

*Acknowledgment is extended to Maura Green, LHAT, Blood Donor Director, Colorado State University, for her critical review of this chapter.

and existing comorbidities. Although critically ill animals tend to tolerate anemia well, those with pulmonary or cardiac disease already may be at risk of hypoxemia. This may change the animal's ability to tolerate anemia and thus alter the transfusion trigger for that animal. Key points to assess on physical examination include markers of intravascular volume status and peripheral tissue perfusion (e.g., mucous membrane color, capillary refill time, heart rate, pulse quality, arterial blood pressure, respiratory rate, and the presence of weakness or lethargy). Additional markers of impaired oxygen delivery, such as blood lactate concentration or central venous oxygen saturation, also may be helpful in determining a transfusion trigger.

Which blood product to administer depends largely on the aforementioned parameters along with the patient's packed cell volume (PCV), hemoglobin concentration, total solids concentration, platelet count, and clotting profile. Blood products containing red cells should be considered if the hemoglobin concentration is 7 g/dl or less or the PCV is 20% or less. If surgery with significant blood loss is anticipated, the PCV transfusion trigger may be slightly higher. Products containing clotting factors should be considered if the prothrombin time or partial thromboplastin time is increased by 30% or more. Products containing platelets generally are indicated in animals with life-threatening hemorrhage due to severe thrombocytopenia or thrombocytopathia, in animals requiring massive transfusion, and in those with significantly decreased thrombopoiesis. When these general guidelines are used, it is important to remember that the entire clinical picture must be taken into account and that the decision to transfuse is highly patient dependent.

Types of Blood Products

Numerous blood products are available, and choice is based on the needs of the patient. Making an educated decision regarding which blood components are required helps conserve resources, limit transfusion reactions, and prevent other transfusion-related adverse effects. Categories of products to consider are discussed in the following sections.

Whole Blood

Fresh whole blood (FWB) and whole blood (WB) contain red blood cells (RBCs), white blood cells (WBCs), stable clotting factors, and plasma proteins. FWB also provides labile clotting factors (factor V and factor VIII) and some platelets if administered within a short time of collection. If FWB is not administered within the initial 24-hour time frame, it is termed whole blood. Both products are stored at 1° to 6°C (33.8° to 42.8°F). WB may be stored for up to 35 days but undergoes significant changes during this time. These changes include decreased concentrations of 2,3-diphosphoglycerate, which increases hemoglobin's affinity for oxygen and thereby decreases offloading of that oxygen to the tissue. Older RBCs also develop other "storage lesions" that alter their biochemical structure and the efficacy of oxygen delivery. With time, storage products (e.g., ammonia, hydrogen ions, proinflammatory cytokines, potassium) also accumulate within the blood unit. Another option for administration of WB is autotransfusion, defined as the collection and subsequent reinfusion of the patient's own shed blood. This can be a practical, cost-effective way to provide blood without placing a large demand on hospital resources. Autotransfusion should not be considered if the shed blood contains bacteria, urine, bile, or neoplastic cells. The recommended starting dose for WB is 10 to 20 ml/kg, or dose may be determined by using the formula that 2 ml/kg of WB will raise the PCV approximately 1%.

When clotting factors are not required and the total solids concentration is normal, packed red blood cells (pRBCs) may be considered in place of WB. Anemia is common in the critically ill due to decreased erythropoietin synthesis, resistance to erythropoietin, reduced RBC life span, blood loss, frequent blood sampling, and oxidative damage. Use of pRBCs should be considered in animals with normal total solids and clotting times (e.g., the critically ill, those with chronic anemia, those with hyperglobulinemia). Advantages of pRBCs include administration of less volume (6 to 10 ml/kg) without the unnecessary WBC and plasma proteins. pRBCs also tend to have a higher PCV than WB. Administration of lactated Ringer's solution through the same line as the blood product should be avoided because calcium within the fluid precipitates with anticoagulants present in WB and pRBCs (acid citrate dextrose or citrate phosphate dextrose adenine).

Plasma

Fresh frozen plasma (FFP) is frozen at −18°C (−0.4°F) or colder within 6 hours of collection and contains all clotting factors, albumin, antiproteases, and immunoglobulins. If it is frozen for a year or longer, the labile clotting factors are no longer present and the product is termed frozen plasma (FP). Either FFP or FP can be used in cases of rodenticide intoxication, other vitamin K deficiencies, and hemophilia B (factor IX deficiency). FFP is preferred for liver disease–associated coagulopathy, hemophilia A (factor VIII deficiency), von Willebrand's disease, and active hemorrhage associated with disseminated intravascular coagulation. To raise albumin levels significantly, plasma must be administered in large quantities (approximately 40 ml/kg to raise serum albumin 1 g/dl). The starting dose for plasma is 6 to 10 ml/kg; the product must be rewarmed slowly but temperature should not exceed 37°C (98.6°F).

FFP may be processed further to create cryoprecipitate, then stored at −18°C (−0.4°F) for up to 1 year. Cryoprecipitate contains von Willebrand's factor, factor VIII, factor XIII, fibrinogen, and fibronectin. Indications for cryoprecipitate include von Willebrand's disease, hemophilia A, and hypofibrinogenemia or dysfibrinogenemia. The dose is 1 unit per 10 kg. The portion of slowly thawed FFP that is not cryoprecipitate is termed cryo-poor plasma and contains factors II, VII, IX, and X. Cryo-poor plasma may be used for rodenticide intoxication, and the dose is 1 unit/10 kg.

Platelets

Although newer and rarely used in clinical practice, platelet-rich products are gaining attention and becoming available commercially. Clinical studies showing efficacy are in their infancy (Davidow et al, 2012), and therefore platelet component therapy should be considered clinically unproven in veterinary patients. As discussed previously, FWB contains a small number of platelets if administered shortly after collection. Platelet-rich plasma (PRP) is prepared from one unit of FWB and may be administered as PRP or further processed to obtain platelet concentrate (PC). PRP and fresh PC must be stored at room temperature with continuous gentle agitation and remain viable for up to 5 days, which makes their use cumbersome in clinical practice. Refrigeration quickly decreases platelet viability and results in rapid clearance from the circulation, and thus is not recommended.

A more practical alternative is cryopreserved platelets, which commonly are preserved in DMSO (dimethyl sulfoxide) at $-80°$ C $(-112°$ F) and have a shelf life of 6 months. Cryopreserved platelets are available commercially but demonstrate decreased viability and function compared with fresh PC. The dose is 1 to 2.5 units/10 kg, which may raise the platelet count as much as 20,000 to 40,000/μl. Due to the short platelet life span (5 to 7 days), repeat transfusions may be required and platelet alloantibodies may develop. Lyophilized platelets are freeze-dried in paraformaldehyde and can be stored at $-80°$ C $(-112°$ F) for several years. Unfortunately, they must be resuspended before use and have an extremely short half-life, so that their use is limited strictly to control of active hemorrhage.

Compatibility

Minimizing the possibility of a transfusion reaction is paramount to patient safety and is considered standard of care in veterinary practice. Important historical points to review before transfusion include the animal's blood group, any history of transfusion, and concurrent drug and fluid therapy.

Canine Blood Groups

Blood groups are based on the presence of particular antigens (glycoproteins or glycolipids) on the surfaces of red cell membranes. At least a dozen blood group systems have been recognized in dogs, with some involving naturally occurring but clinically insignificant alloantibodies. The most important red cell antigens that induce alloantibody formation on exposure to blood products are dog erythrocyte antigens (DEAs) 1.1, 1.2, and 7. The results of commercial blood-typing systems correlate well with standard laboratory test results, and such systems typically test for DEA 1.1, the most antigenic of canine erythrocyte antigens (see Web Chapter 26). Dogs can be DEA 1.1 positive or negative, and DEA 1.1–negative dogs can be either positive or negative for DEA 1.2. A new canine red cell antigen missing in some dalmatians (*Dal*) also has been described recently in the literature. *Dal*-negative dogs that are exposed to *Dal*-positive blood are at risk of formation of alloantibodies, which increases the risk of acute and delayed reactions after a subsequent transfusion. Therefore, due to the presence of antigens other than DEA 1.1, dogs for which appropriate blood typing has been done still can develop clinically significant alloantibodies after a blood transfusion because these other antigens are not identified in the commercial typing system. These formed alloantibodies can last for many years, which necessitates crossmatching for future red cell transfusions.

Feline Blood Groups

Feline blood groups include A, B, and AB. Unlike dogs, cats have clinically significant, naturally occurring alloantibodies. The recommendation therefore is to blood-type every cat before any transfusion (see Web Chapter 26). Cats with type B blood produce strong anti-A antibodies, predominantly of the immunoglobulin M (IgM) class, which fix complement and cause a severe acute intravascular hemolytic reaction. Approximately 20% of cats with type A blood produce weaker anti-B antibodies of the IgG and IgM classes, which commonly results in extravascular hemolysis. Cats with type AB blood do not produce alloantibodies but should be administered AB or A blood. As in dogs, blood typing does not identify all possible red cell antigens and therefore does not ensure serologic compatibility. A new feline red cell antigen (*Mik*) has been documented recently in the veterinary literature, and naturally occurring *Mik* antibodies in *Mik*-negative cats can result in an acute hemolytic transfusion reaction.

Crossmatching

Crossmatching identifies the presence of natural or induced alloantibodies (hemolysins or hemagglutins) in plasma. Crossmatching is not a substitute for blood typing but rather a way to help ensure serologic compatibility, avoid immediate transfusion reactions, and provide longer life span to the transfused RBCs (see Web Chapter 26). Commercial crossmatching systems are available for dogs and cats, and their use is recommended in any dog or cat that has received a blood transfusion 4 or more days after the initial transfusion. Given the presence of naturally occurring alloantibodies and the potential consequences of administering incompatible red cells, there is debate as to whether or not typed cats should undergo crossmatching before their first transfusion. A major crossmatch determines compatibility of the donor's red cells with the recipient's serum. A minor crossmatch determines compatibility of the donor's serum with the recipient's red cells. The major crossmatch is considered more important because it determines whether or not the transfused red cells will be tolerated in the recipient. Crossmatching does not guarantee the compatibility of donor leukocytes, platelets, or proteins in the recipient. Crossmatching also does not guarantee an absence of delayed transfusion reactions or normal RBC survival.

Allogeneic Blood Administration

Given the possible consequences of transfusion reactions in both dogs and cats, an alternative to allogeneic blood administration is autologous transfusion. For animals facing an anticipated surgical procedure that may require blood administration, predonation is performed up to 4 weeks beforehand. The animal's stored blood then is administered when needed during the perioperative period. Autotransfusion, as described previously, is another alternative to providing allogeneic blood products and also may be considered in select situations.

Optimization of Patient Safety

Safety when administering blood products can be enhanced in many ways. Ensuring a donor has undergone appropriate infectious disease testing, properly collecting and storing blood products, performing blood typing and crossmatching when indicated, administering only the blood components needed by the recipient, and using a detailed protocol for blood product administration and patient monitoring are all critical to transfusion success.

An increase in morbidity and mortality in transfusion recipients has received widespread attention in human medicine. Blood product administration in people has been associated with transfusion-related immunomodulation (e.g., decreased immune response and increased postoperative infections), acute lung injury, recurrence of cancer, and transfusion-related circulatory overload. This has led to a more conservative trend in blood product administration. In dogs administration of autologous stored pRBCs results in a profound inflammatory response, with increased levels of fibrinogen and C-reactive protein (McMichael et al, 2010). The inflammatory nature of stored blood products is one major factor in the development of transfusion-related adverse effects. Many of the inflammatory effects are caused by the transfusion of the donor's WBCs, which makes leukoreduction (removal of WBCs from the blood product before administration) an appealing method by which the practitioner can attenuate the inflammatory response, reduce the risk of immunosuppression, improve RBC survival, decrease transmission of infectious agents, and decrease the incidence of transfusion reactions. Acute life-threatening transfusion reactions also have been reported recently in dogs due to the inappropriate storage of RBC products (Patterson et al, 2011). As with most therapies, the risks of transfusion must be weighed against the benefits before administration of blood products.

Transfusion Reactions

One of the most serious risks of blood product administration is the development of transfusion reactions. These reactions are classified as either acute or delayed, and immunologic or nonimmunologic. This chapter focuses on acute reactions that are commonly seen during the transfusion period. Acute transfusion reactions are best detected by close patient monitoring throughout the transfusion. Most transfusions are initiated at a very slow rate (0.25 ml/kg/hr) and slowly increased to accomplish administration of the desired volume within a 4- to 6-hour period. Rectal temperature, pulse rate and quality, respiratory rate and effort, mucous membrane color, capillary refill time, mental status, and rate of the transfusion (milliliters per hour) should be recorded regularly. These parameters should be recorded every 15 minutes for the first hour, then every hour for the remainder of the transfusion. The clinician should be alerted if the patient develops an increased heart rate or respiratory rate, increased respiratory effort, a temperature change of 2°C (3.6°F) or more, shaking, restlessness, itching, urticaria, change in mentation, or change in urine color.

Immunologic Transfusion Reactions

The most common acute immunologic transfusion reactions are febrile nonhemolytic transfusion reaction (FNHTR) and acute hemolytic transfusion reaction (AHTR). FNHTR is defined as a temperature increase of more than 1°C (1.8°F) without any other recognized cause of the fever and occurs when recipient antibodies bind to donor platelets, WBCs, or plasma proteins. This antigen-antibody complex causes the release of endogenous inflammatory mediators. The reaction usually is self-limiting and is of little clinical significance. It is important to rule out bacterial contamination of the blood product and AHTR before continuing with the transfusion. Bacterial contamination can be ruled out by examining the blood product for discoloration and performing Gram staining on a blood sample from the bag. Blood culture can be performed, if needed, to confirm the presence of bacteria in the blood product. AHTR can be ruled out by centrifuging the patient's blood and looking for evidence of hemolysis. AHTR is the most life-threatening type of transfusion reaction. In AHTR transfused RBCs interact with preformed antibodies in the recipient's blood (typically IgG or IgM), which results in a type II hypersensitivity reaction. Intravascular hemolysis leads to hemoglobinemia, hemoglobinuria, and a systemic inflammatory response. Severe AHTRs can progress to organ dysfunction, disseminated intravascular coagulation, and death. Clinical signs of AHTR include fever, vomiting, tachycardia, hypotension, hemoglobinemia, and hemoglobinuria.

When identifying and treating an acute immunologic reaction, the clinician should take several steps to optimize patient safety. First, the transfusion should be discontinued and the patient's temperature, pulse, respiration, and blood pressure assessed. If fever or hypotension is present, a small crystalloid bolus (20 ml/kg) may be administered. The patient's and donor's blood type and crossmatch information should be reviewed. The blood product should be examined for any discoloration, and Gram staining and culture should be performed if there is suspicion of contamination. The date of expiration on the blood product and the temperature at which the product was being stored should be verified. Finally, the recipient's blood should be spun down in a hematocrit tube and evaluated for evidence of hemolysis. Although their efficacy is debatable, antihistamines (diphenhydramine 2 mg/kg IM) and glucocorticoids (dexamethasone sodium phosphate 0.2 mg/kg IV) can be administered. If FNHTR is suspected, the transfusion may be reinitiated at a much slower rate once clinical signs have resolved. If AHTR is suspected, then the transfusion should be discontinued and additional supportive care instituted as needed.

Nonimmunologic Transfusion Reactions

Acute nonimmunologic reactions include electrolyte disturbances, embolism, endotoxic shock, circulatory overload, and hypothermia. Hypocalcemia and hypomagnesemia occur most commonly due to complexing with citrate anticoagulant. Animals that have severe liver disease or undergo multiple transfusions may be at greater risk of these disturbances because of an inability to process large amounts of citrate. Signs of hypocalcemia include hypotension, facial pruritus, muscle fasciculations, and tremors; hypocalcemia can be treated by administration of calcium gluconate (50 to 100 mg/kg by slow IV infusion), which should be accompanied by electrocardiographic monitoring. Embolism most commonly occurs because of collections of WBCs, platelets, and fibrin in the blood product, and this risk is reduced if a filter (170 μm) is used during blood administration. Endotoxic shock may occur secondary to blood contamination. Circulatory overload is possible if colloids or crystalloids are administered concurrently with the transfusion, and the risk is highest in patients with underlying cardiac disease. These acute nonimmunologic reactions should be treated appropriately, and the possibility of their occurrence as a consequence of transfusion should not be ignored.

Expectations for Results

Transfused RBCs may live for up to 100 days in the dog and 70 days in the cat. After RBCs are administered, the PCV should be reassessed at 1, 12, and 24 hours after transfusion, unless a continued drop in PCV is expected. A recent publication (McDevitt, Ruaux, and Baltzer, 2011) found that the use of mechanical delivery systems (e.g., volumetric or syringe pumps) is associated with a high risk of early loss of transfused cells in dogs. In the future, additional recommendations regarding the method of

blood administration may be developed as part of the standard of transfusion practice.

After plasma administration, clotting times should be rechecked in keeping with the underlying reason for the coagulopathy or if ongoing hemorrhage is suspected. After platelet administration, the platelet count should be rechecked at 1 and 24 hours after transfusion. Transfused platelets may live for up to 5 days in the dog, and therefore multiple transfusions may be required because of the short platelet life span.

Use of blood products is a necessary, lifesaving part of veterinary practice and has allowed immeasurable enhancement of patient care. But because of the many possible reactions and mounting evidence that blood transfusions contribute to hospital morbidity, the clinician should carefully weigh the decision to use blood products before administration. A thoughtful, well-executed plan will optimize patient outcome and help achieve the desired goals of the transfusion, with minimal patient risk and appropriate allocation of blood resources.

References and Suggested Reading

Barfield D, Adamantos S: Feline blood transfusions: a pinker shade of pale, *J Feline Med Surg* 13(1):11, 2011.

Bracker K, Drellich S: Transfusion reactions, *Compend Contin Educ Vet* 7:500, 2005.

Callan MB, Appleman EH, Sachais BS: Canine platelet transfusions, *J Vet Emerg Crit Care* 19(5):401, 2009.

Davidow EB et al: Use of fresh platelet concentrate or lyophilized platelets in thrombocytopenic dogs with clinical signs of hemorrhage: a preliminary trial in 37 dogs, *J Vet Emerg Crit Care* 22(1):116, 2012.

Giger U, Bucheler J: Transfusion of type-A and type-B blood to cats, *J Am Vet Med Assoc* 198(3):411, 1991.

Lanevschi A, Wardrop KJ: Principles of transfusion medicine in small animals, *Can Vet J* 42:447, 2001.

McDevitt RI, Ruaux CG, Baltzer WI: Influence of transfusion technique on survival of autologous red blood cells in the dog, *J Vet Emerg Crit Care* 21(3):209, 2011.

McMichael MA et al: Effect of leukoreduction on transfusion-induced inflammation in dogs, *J Vet Intern Med* 24(5):1131, 2010.

Patterson J et al: In vitro lysis and acute transfusion reactions with hemolysis caused by inappropriate storage of canine red blood cell products, *J Vet Intern Med* 25(4):927, 2011.

Prittie JE: Controversies related to red blood cell transfusion in critically ill patients, *J Vet Emerg Crit Care* 20(2):167, 2010.

Tocci LJ: Transfusion medicine in small animal practice, *Vet Clin North Am Small Anim Pract* 40(3):485, 2010.

Tocci LJ, Ewing PJ: Increasing patient safety in veterinary transfusion medicine: an overview of pretransfusion testing, *J Vet Emerg Crit Care* 19(1):66, 2009.

CHAPTER 68

Bone Marrow Dyscrasias

CHRISTINE S. OLVER, *Fort Collins, Colorado*

The term *bone marrow dyscrasia* technically means any disease originating in the bone marrow. *Dysmyelopoiesis* is another term used to describe disorders stemming from bone marrow problems. This chapter describes bone marrow diseases that result in peripheral cytopenias and that require a bone marrow evaluation to determine the cause or classify the disorder. These diseases may be nonneoplastic (secondary dysmyelopoiesis) or neoplastic or "preneoplastic" (primary dysmyelopoiesis). Secondary dysmyelopoiesis includes immune-mediated or drug-induced phenomena, and preneoplastic or neoplastic diseases include myelodysplastic syndromes, acute and chronic myeloid leukemias, and acute and chronic lymphocytic leukemias. Determining the cause of the dyscrasia, whether it is primary or secondary, and its classification if it is myelodysplastic or leukemic influences treatment and prognosis. Clinical signs of bone marrow dyscrasias are related directly to the effects of the cytopenias or to the effects of proliferating hematopoietic cells (e.g., leukemia). For example, clinical signs in a dog with pure red cell aplasia may include nonspecific malaise progressing to exercise intolerance and severe lethargy related to the lack of oxygen-carrying capacity caused by anemia. Clinical signs of an acute leukemia that is infiltrating abdominal organs may be acute-onset lethargy, fever, anorexia, vomiting, cranial organomegaly, and biochemical abnormalities related to the organ that is infiltrated with neoplastic cells. An animal with drug-related neutropenia may have fever secondary to an opportunistic infection. Diagnosis of a bone marrow dyscrasia is based on a finding of one or more unexplained cytopenias or severe leukocytosis in a complete blood count, accompanied by characteristic features on cytologic evaluation of bone marrow. A flow chart for the diagnostic workup of unexplained cytopenias is presented in Figure 68-1.

Definitions

Myeloid: Adjective referring to commitment of a progenitor to erythroid, granulocytic, monocytic, or megakaryocytic lineage. These progenitors may differentiate into any blood cell other than a lymphoid cell. It also refers to the granulocytic component of the precursor cell population in the myeloid:erythroid ratio determined during bone marrow cytologic evaluation.

Lymphoid: Adjective referring to lineage commitment to any lymphoid cell line, including all B and T cells.

Dysplasia: Abnormalities in the cytologic appearance of any maturational stage of bone marrow cells.

Dyserythropoiesis: Dysplastic features of erythroid precursors. Includes binucleation, megaloblastosis (excess cytoplasm relative to nucleus), nuclear fragmentation, and asynchronous maturation (e.g., hemoglobinized cytoplasm with an immature nucleus).

Dysgranulopoiesis: Dysplastic features of myeloid precursors. Includes small myeloblasts and promyelocytes, giant metamyelocytes and band cells, asynchronous maturation, and hypersegmentation of mature neutrophils.

Primary myelodysplastic syndrome: One or more cytopenias, cell dysplasia, and maturation abnormalities in the marrow, not associated with infection, drug administration, a toxin, or other neoplasia. These are hematopoietic cell clonal disorders in human beings and are assumed to be clonal in dogs and cats.

Leukemia: Clonal proliferation of hematopoietic cells of any lineage in the blood or bone marrow.

Acute myeloid leukemia: Clonal proliferation of immature cells of erythroid, granulocytic, monocytic, or megakaryocytic lineage in the bone marrow.

Acute lymphoblastic leukemia: Clonal proliferation of immature cells of lymphoid lineage in the bone marrow.

Chronic myeloid leukemia: Clonal proliferation of hematopoietic cells that differentiate enough to appear mature in the peripheral blood. These cause extreme leukocytosis and are usually of a granulocytic, monocytic, or eosinophilic lineage.

Chronic lymphocytic leukemia (chronic lymphoid leukemia): Clonal proliferation of mature-appearing lymphoid cells arising from spleen or bone marrow.

Blast cell: Earliest recognizable precursor of a certain cell lineage. A rubriblast is the earliest erythroid precursor and a myeloblast is the earliest granulocytic precursor.

Bone Marrow Aspirate Cytologic Evaluation

The reader is encouraged to consult a recent excellent review on the evaluation of bone marrow, including collection techniques (Moritz et al, 2010). A brief description of bone marrow collection for smears is given here. Bone marrow evaluation is indicated any time there is a cytopenia that cannot be explained by other clinical or laboratory findings. Some examples are persistent neutropenia without evidence of sepsis and nonregenerative anemia

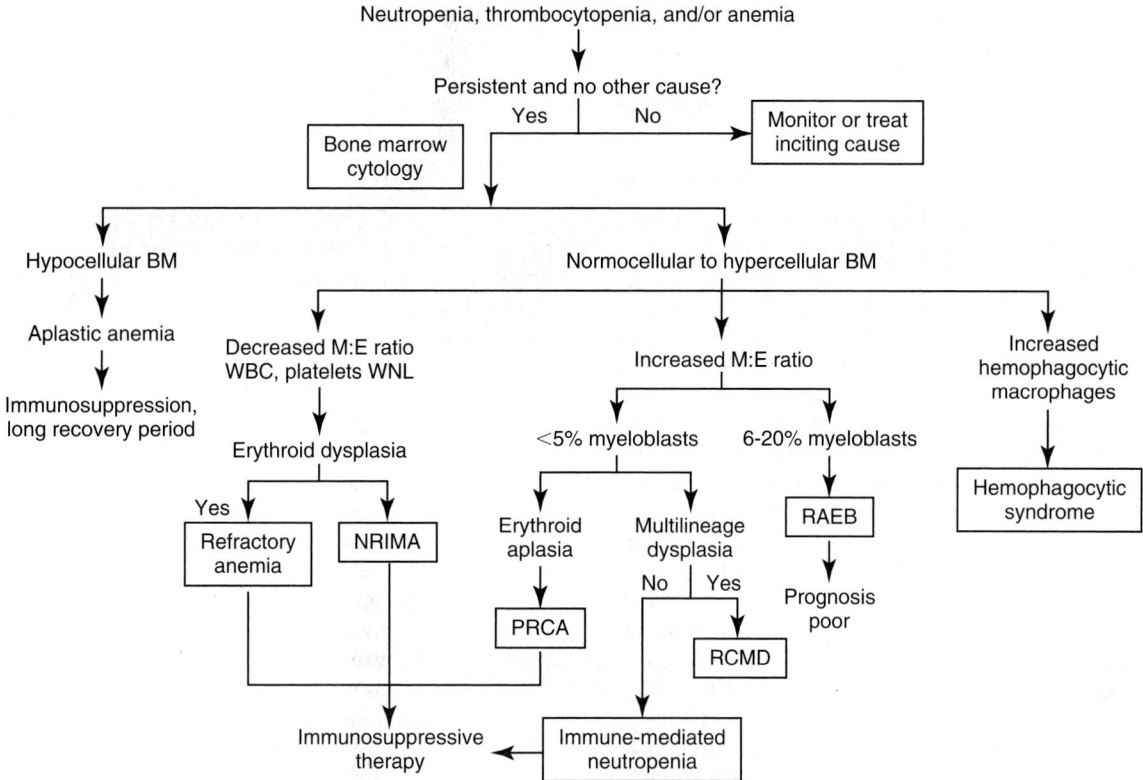

Figure 68-1 Diagnostic workup for unexplained cytopenias in peripheral blood. *BM,* Bone marrow; *M:E ratio,* myeloid to erythroid ratio; *NRIMA,* nonregenerative immune-mediated anemia; *PRCA,* pure red cell aplasia; *RAEB,* refractory anemia with excess blasts; *RCMD,* refractory cytopenia with multilineage dysplasia; *WBC,* white blood cell count; *WNL,* within normal limits.

without evidence of renal failure, neoplasia, infection, or inflammatory disease. Bone marrow may be collected from dogs at the iliac crest, the proximal femur, or the ribs, and from cats at the iliac crest, proximal humerus, or trochanteric fossa. The skin at the site is shaved and aseptically prepared. Two percent lidocaine solution is used to provide local anesthesia in all tissue layers, including deep infusion to the periosteum. A sterile 16- to 18-gauge bone marrow needle with an interlocking stylet is used, and in general the animal is at least heavily sedated. The needle, with the stylet in place, is inserted into the skin at the site of aspiration and is seated on the bone. Slow twisting is used to insert the needle through the cortex into the marrow cavity. The stylet is removed, and a 10- to 12-ml syringe is placed in the needle hub. Strong aspiration is used to remove marrow. Only a small amount of marrow should be collected; otherwise hemodilution will occur and a poor-quality sample will result. No more than about 250 μl of marrow should be aspirated. For best staining quality, no anticoagulant should be used, but the marrow should be smeared on glass slides immediately. The smears should be stained within 24 hours of collection and evaluated by a veterinary clinical pathologist. The evaluation will include assessment of overall cellularity, presence or absence of iron stores, quantification of megakaryocytes, differential count of myeloid (granulocytic) and erythroid precursors (producing the myeloid:erythroid ratio), evaluation of

the orderliness of precursor maturation, morphologic abnormalities, and the presence of abnormal (e.g., neoplastic) cells. A complete blood count must be performed within 24 hours of bone marrow collection.

Nonneoplastic Dyscrasias

Nonregenerative Immune-Mediated Anemia

Nonregenerative immune-mediated anemia (NRIMA), primarily described in dogs, is secondary to an immune response against erythroid precursors in the bone marrow. Affected dogs may have a short to several-month history of lethargy, anorexia, weight loss, and exercise intolerance, and show pallor, systolic heart murmurs, and tachycardia on physical examination; these signs all are referable to severe anemia. Laboratory abnormalities include a severe, nonregenerative anemia and reticulocytopenia. Leukocyte counts typically are normal, although platelet counts may be decreased in a minority of dogs. Spherocytes are present in many dogs, and Coombs' test yields positive results in over half of cases. The majority of bone marrow samples show erythroid hyperplasia, and there may be an expansion of immature erythroid precursors. Other cell lines are normal. Although over half of cases respond to immunosuppressive therapy, the mortality rate for this disease in one report was 28% (Stokol et al, 2000).

Hemophagocytic Syndrome

Hemophagocytic syndrome is associated with various primary causes, such as immune-mediated, infectious, and neoplastic disease. It is characterized by a bicytopenia or pancytopenia and more than 2% hemophagocytic macrophages on cytologic examination of a bone marrow aspirate. Clinical signs include lethargy, fever, icterus, splenomegaly, hepatomegaly, and diarrhea. The hallmark finding in these dogs is a hypercellular marrow accompanied by 3% to 14% hemophagocytic macrophages. A hemophagocytic macrophage in one that clearly is activated (has vacuoles) and contains cytoplasmic debris interpreted to be phagocytosed normal bone marrow elements. The prognosis for this condition is poor, with 75% of affected patients dead at 1 month from the time of diagnosis, although dogs with infectious primary causes have a better prognosis.

Pure Red Cell Aplasia

Dogs and cats with pure red cell aplasia have a severe nonregenerative (normocytic normochromic) anemia, reticulocytopenia, and a myeloid:erythroid ratio of more than 75:1 (selective erythroid aplasia). Other laboratory values are typically within normal limits, and infectious disease titers show negative results. Clinical signs include weakness, lethargy, pallor, tachycardia, tachypnea, and systolic murmur. Most of these dogs and cats respond completely to immunosuppressive therapy (prednisolone with or without other immunosuppressive agents). Notably, dogs may not show PCV increases until approximately 1 month after initiation of therapy and may not recover completely until up to 6 months after initiation of therapy. Animals should be monitored for relapse during their life span.

Aplastic Anemia

Aplastic anemia is a lack of production of all cell lines in the marrow (erythroid, granulocytic, megakaryocytic) resulting in a hypocellular marrow with cells replaced by fat and pancytopenia in the peripheral blood. Aplastic anemia in cats has been associated with chronic renal failure, feline leukemia virus infection, and griseofulvin or methimazole therapy, and in some the cause is undetermined. The response to therapy is poor, and prognosis is variable; however, some cats may live for years with pancytopenia, even without showing a response to therapy. Aplastic anemia is extremely rare in dogs. It has been associated with trimethoprim/sulfa or fenbendazole therapy and estrogen administration, or it can be idiopathic.

Secondary Bone Marrow Dyscrasia

Bone marrow abnormalities in response to phenobarbital administration and immune-mediated neutropenia are examples of secondary bone marrow dyscrasias. Neutropenia, thrombocytopenia, anemia, or some combination of the three can be seen idiosyncratically in dogs treated for at least 2 months with the anticonvulsant phenobarbital. Dogs may be asymptomatic or may have signs referable to the cytopenia present. These include fever (neutropenia), petechiae (thrombocytopenia), lethargy, and inappetence (anemia). The cytopenias invariably include neutropenia but may also include thrombocytopenia and anemia. The bone marrow is hypercellular, usually with hyperplasia of the granulocytic series, and there may be an expansion of immature myeloid cells (dysmaturation). These bone marrow findings suggest an immunologic attack against more mature cells of the granulocytic line. The presentation of a neutropenia along with a hypercellular marrow and dysmaturation must be distinguished from the preneoplastic condition of myelodysplastic syndrome (as discussed later), and the drug history is important in making this differentiation. Removal of the drug results in recovery within 2 weeks to 2 months. Additionally, rare cases of immune-mediated neutropenia have been reported that present with persistent neutropenia and a hypercellular marrow with dysmaturation. This condition can be difficult to differentiate from myelodysplastic syndrome, and response to immunosuppressive therapy may be the best way to confirm the diagnosis.

Clonal Bone Marrow Dyscrasias

Clonal disorders are those that result from a genetic abnormality of one cell and its progeny that manifests as either dysmaturation or cytopenias (myelodysplastic syndrome) or uncontrolled proliferation of one cell line (acute leukemia). All circulating blood cells are derived from hematopoietic stem cells in the bone marrow. These cells are multipotent and can divide into copies of themselves or into cells committed to specific blood cell lineages. The hematopoietic stem cell first divides into the common myeloid progenitor and common lymphoid progenitor. The common myeloid progenitor also is multipotent, although it can no longer differentiate into any lymphoid cells. The myeloid progenitor has the capability to differentiate into cells of the erythroid, granulocytic, monocytic, or megakaryocytic cell lines. These differentiation steps are sequentially limiting so that progenitors are formed that are restricted to one lineage. Any of these precursors can become deranged and clonally proliferate.

Classification of Clonal Bone Marrow Dyscrasias

Clonal bone marrow dyscrasias are classified by the character of the blood and bone marrow findings to aid the clinician in treating the disorder properly and understanding the prognosis. Specifically, clonal disorders are classified as either one of several types of myelodysplastic syndromes (preleukemias) or as one of several types of acute leukemias. Although a few cases of veterinary myelodysplastic syndromes have been assessed as definitively clonal, clonality usually is inferred based on the characteristics of similar entities described in the human literature. Thus some of the cases reported in the literature may not, in fact, be clonal diseases. Several systems have been used to classify clonal bone marrow dyscrasias.

History of the Classification System

The Animal Leukemia Study Group established a classification scheme for dog and cat leukemias in 1991 (Jain et al, 1991). This group modeled the French-American-British (FAB) cooperative group classification system to develop a scheme, with some modification, for cats and dogs (Bennett et al, 1976). Additionally, the World Health Organization modified the original FAB categories based on new information (Vardiman et al, 2002). Although there has not been a consensus revision of the dog-cat classification scheme, several individuals have proposed systems in the veterinary literature. The bulk of the implementation of the newer classification system for veterinary patients has been performed at one institution in retrospective studies sourcing medical records of hundreds of patients with bone marrow samples.

Myelodysplastic Syndromes

Myelodysplastic syndromes are characterized by one or more cytopenias, accompanied by a normocellular to hypercellular bone marrow, with dysplastic changes in one or more cell lines. The cytopenias should be persistent, and no other secondary condition, such as neoplasia, endocrine disease, renal failure, immune-mediated disease, drug administration, or toxin exposure, should be present. Myelodysplastic syndromes actually are heterogeneous in their blood, bone marrow, and clinical findings; two of the more common and recently described syndromes are discussed here. The number of myeloid blast cells present distinguishes one from the other and also dramatically affects prognosis. It is important to recognize that this terminology is not standardized; thus the nomenclature used in this chapter may not reflect the usage in what has been published previously or what may be published in the future. When one reads studies and case reports describing bone marrow dyscrasias, it is therefore important to review the hematologic abnormalities thoroughly because the names of the entities are somewhat fluid.

Refractory Anemia

Refractory anemia also is known as *myelodysplastic syndrome with erythroid predominance.* Dogs with refractory anemia have clinical signs associated with a moderate to severe nonregenerative anemia, including gradual onset of lethargy and exercise intolerance. Laboratory findings include a moderate to severe nonregenerative anemia with normal leukocyte and platelet counts. The bone marrow usually is normocellular to hypercellular with an increase in rubriblasts (5% to 30% of all nucleated cells, whereas typically they comprise fewer than <2% of all nucleated cells) and the dysplastic changes are restricted to the erythroid cell line. Myeloblasts, however, represent fewer than 5% of all nucleated cells. A few dogs with this syndrome have been described in the literature. Reported treatment regimens include aclarubicin, erythropoietin, prednisolone, and cyclophosphamide. Although myelodysplastic syndromes usually carry a grave prognosis, this type purports to have a good prognosis, with a possibility of survival for years after therapy.

Refractory Anemia with Excess Blasts

Normally the proportion of myeloblasts (blasts of the granulocytic series) in the bone marrow is less than 1% of all nucleated cells. Refractory anemia with an excess of blasts is diagnosed when the proportion of myeloblasts is 6% to 20% of all nucleated cells. This is the most frequent type of myelodysplastic syndrome in dogs and cats, and typically presents with more serious clinical signs than those in dogs with refractory anemia without excess blasts. Symptoms of lethargy, anorexia, fever, and diarrhea may appear acutely or progress over weeks. The hematologic findings include moderate to severe normocytic, normochromic anemia; neutropenia; and thrombocytopenia. The bone marrow is hypercellular with an increased myeloid:erythroid ratio and an increased myeloblast count. Dysplastic changes are seen in all three cell lineages (myeloid, erythroid, and megakaryocytic). Treatment typically is supportive, and expected survival ranges from days to months. A common sequel to myelodysplastic syndrome is development of acute leukemia. In cats this condition often is associated with feline leukemia virus positivity.

Refractory Cytopenias with Multilineage Dysplasia

Refractory cytopenias with multilineage dysplasia presents with one or more cytopenias and dysplastic changes in two or more lineages in the bone marrow. The number of reported cases is very low, and the prognosis is variable. Two of the reported cases progressed to acute leukemia, and two of the patients had prolonged survival (years). One long-lived patient was treated with aclarubicin, a cytotoxic anthracycline, and one was treated with cytarabine ocfosfate, a prodrug of cytosine arabinoside.

Leukemias

Leukemias may be of either myeloid (granulocytic, erythroid, megakaryocytic, or monocytic) lineage or lymphoid lineage, and may be acute or chronic. Lymphocytic leukemias are covered in Chapter 65, and thus only myeloid leukemias are discussed here.

Chronic Myeloid Leukemias

Chronic myeloid leukemias (CMLs) arise from a proliferation of myeloid cells that are maturing almost normally, so that there is a mature leukocytosis and normal maturation of this cell lineage in the bone marrow. The leukemias are named for the type of cell that is proliferating. For example, *chronic granulocytic leukemia* is the name given to a proliferation of neutrophils, with a mature neutrophilia in the peripheral blood. *Chronic eosinophilic leukemia* is the name for a clonal proliferation of eosinophils and a mature eosinophilia in the peripheral blood. With any CML, there can be a small number of circulating blast cells and other immature cells. The bone marrow usually shows an increased myeloid:erythroid ratio that reflects the clonal proliferation of myeloid cells. CML typically is treated with hydroxyurea. The reported average survival time for animals diagnosed with CML is approximately 1 year, although some patients live longer. Diagnosis of CML is accomplished by detecting marked and persistent leukocytosis (50,000 to 100,000 white blood cells/μl) in the absence of infection, inflammation, or other neoplasia. The animal may be asymptomatic or may show nonspecific signs such as lethargy, inappetence, and exercise intolerance. Organomegaly may or may not be present. Cats with CML are variably positive for feline leukemia virus. Other laboratory abnormalities usually are referable to organ involvement and therefore may include elevations in hepatocellular leakage or cholestatic enzymes.

Acute Myeloid Leukemias

Acute myeloid leukemias (AMLs) are leukemias with more than 20% blast cells (of whatever lineage is proliferating) in the blood and bone marrow. These leukemias are characterized by a leukocytosis with extreme dysmaturation in the blood and bone marrow. The Animal Leukemia Study Group has classified AMLs and named them after the cell that is proliferating. The details of this classification scheme are beyond the scope of this chapter. In general, however, the prognosis for these diseases is grave, and survival is usually measured in weeks.

References and Suggested Reading

Bennet JM et al: Proposals for the classification of the acute leukaemias. French-American-British (FAB) co-operative group, *Br J Haematol* 33:452, 1976.

Blue JT: Myelodysplasia: differentiating neoplastic from nonneoplastic syndromes of ineffective hematopoiesis in dogs, *Toxicol Pathol* 31(Suppl):44, 2003.

Jain NC et al: Proposed criteria for classification of acute myeloid leukemia in dogs and cats, *Vet Clin Pathol* 20:63, 1991.

McManus PM: Classification of myeloid neoplasms: a comparative review, *Vet Clin Pathol* 34:189, 2005.

Moritz A et al: Evaluation of bone marrow. In Weiss DJ, Wardrop JK, editors: *Schalm's veterinary hematology*, ed 6, Ames, IA, 2010, Blackwell Publishing, p 1039.

Raskin RE: Myelopoiesis and myeloproliferative disorders, *Vet Clin North Am Small Anim Pract* 26:1023, 1996.

Snyder LA: Acute myeloid leukemia. In Weiss DJ, Wardrop JK, editors: *Schalm's veterinary hematology*, ed 6, Ames, IA, 2010, Blackwell Publishing, p 475.

Stokol T, Blue JT, French TW: Idiopathic pure red cell aplasia and nonregenerative immune-mediated anemia in dogs: 43 cases (1988-1999), *J Am Vet Med Assoc* 216:1429, 2000.

Vardiman JW et al: The World Health Organization (WHO) classification of the myeloid neoplasms, *Blood* 122:2292, 2002.

Weiss DJ: Myelodysplastic syndromes. In Weiss DJ, Wardrop JK, editors: *Schalm's veterinary hematology*, ed 6, Ames, IA, 2010, Blackwell Publishing, p 467.

CHAPTER 69

Talking to Clients about Cancer

DOUGLAS H. THAMM, *Fort Collins, Colorado*

Cancer is being treated more and more frequently in the primary care setting. Furthermore, the primary care veterinarian often makes a diagnosis of cancer and performs initial client education. Critically important life-or-death decisions regarding euthanasia, treatment, pursuit of referral, and so on may be made based on information from the primary veterinarian. There is a stigma attached to a cancer diagnosis, and owners of pets with cancer may anthropomorphize and equate cancer treatment in animals with experiences they may have had. Being able to address these concerns succinctly and dispel some of the myths that owners may have is a critical component of cancer management in the primary care setting, whether the pet is to be treated in the primary care clinic or referred elsewhere. The following questions and answers between a pet owner and a veterinary caregiver illustrate some ways to discuss these issues with clients.

Is Cancer Really a Problem in Pets?

Unfortunately, cancer occurs in many pets. It is the leading natural cause of death in adult dogs, and the second or third most common cause of death in cats. Approximately 50% of dogs and 30% to 35% of cats will be affected by some type of tumor in their lifetime.

Why Does It Seem That There Is So Much More Cancer in Pets These Days?

Better health care for our pets has resulted in longer life, and cancer is primarily a disease of age. Management of other husbandry-related conditions in dogs and cats (better nutrition, control of infectious and parasitic disease, leash laws) has improved to the point that many more animals are now living long enough to develop geriatric conditions such as heart disease, kidney disease, endocrine disease, and cancer. Additionally, there is greater recognition and reporting of cancer by small animal veterinarians.

Did Something in the Environment Play a Role in My Pet's Cancer? Was I Feeding the Wrong Food?

Some weak associations have been proposed between certain types of cancer and environmental influences. These include an association between herbicide or insecticide exposure and transitional cell carcinoma risk in Scottish terriers, exposure to environmental tobacco smoke and gastrointestinal lymphoma risk in cats, and exposure to the herbicide 2,4-dichlorophenoxyacetic acid (2,4-D) and lymphoma risk in dogs. In the vast majority of cases, no such association can be made, and most of the studies reporting environmental associations with cancer have been small and their results have not been verified independently. Thus for the most part there are no confirmed strong associations between environmental or dietary factors and cancer risk in animals.

Why Should I Treat My Pet with Cancer?

The simple answer is because we can. We treat many animals with chronic disease that are never cured (diabetes, hyperadrenocorticism, chronic kidney disease, congestive heart failure), and cancer may be thought of as another chronic disease. Furthermore, cancer is a disease for which cure is sometimes possible. Even when cure is unlikely, there are many cancers in which we may be able to extend an excellent quality of life with treatment.

Do We Have to Do That for This Lump Now? Can't We Just Wait and See What Happens?

Owners may use such a phrase regarding initial diagnostic testing ("Let's wait and see if it grows"), additional surgery or other treatments to prevent local recurrence after incomplete excision ("Let's wait and see if it grows back"), or therapy to delay or prevent metastasis ("Let's wait and see if it spreads"). All of these statements may require discussion with owners to promote early and appropriate diagnostic testing and therapy.

Let's wait and see if it grows: In general, delay in reaching a diagnosis serves only to increase the difficulty of surgery and, potentially, the likelihood of metastasis. The lump that has been found may very well be nothing, but if it is a malignancy, the time to find that out is sooner rather than later.

Let's wait and see if it grows back: Locally recurrent tumors are associated statistically with a worse prognosis in certain diseases and suspected of carrying a worse prognosis in others. For this reason, the time to pursue aggressive local therapy is the very first time the tumor occurs.

Let's wait and see if it spreads: In general, treatment of gross metastatic disease is palliative at best. Asking drugs to treat bulky metastatic disease is asking a lot, but asking those same drugs to have an effect against microscopic tumor cells in the lung or lymph node may be much more reasonable.

Doesn't Performing Fine-Needle Aspiration or Biopsy Irritate the Tumor and Increase the Risk of Spread?

Fine-needle aspiration or biopsy does not make the tumor more likely to spread. Getting from the primary tumor into the bloodstream is only one of many steps in the "metastatic decathlon." Exceptions to this rule are the following: (1) Some mast cell tumors may become inflamed following fine-needle aspiration because of degranulation and histamine release, although this in no way hastens metastasis. This is rarely serious and can be treated or prevented by administering a histamine H1 blocker. (2) Transabdominal needle aspiration or needle-core biopsy of splenic and bladder masses is contraindicated because of the risk of local dissemination in the abdomen or seeding of the biopsy tract.

Why Don't We Just Remove the Tumor? Why Do We Need to Do a Fine-Needle Aspirate or Biopsy First?

Obtaining a diagnosis before surgery helps in planning the surgical approach and lets us know whether additional tests are indicated before surgery. This helps avoid situations like "Why didn't you take X-rays before surgery?" and "Why should I have to pay for a second surgery if you didn't get it all the first time?" If excisional biopsy is the first diagnostic test performed, it is wise to forewarn the owner that this procedure is being used only to obtain a diagnosis and that additional diagnostic testing and staging or treatment might be necessary based on the results.

Why Should I Pay for Histopathologic Evaluation? Why Don't You Just Remove the Tumor and Throw It Away?

If the tumor is worth removing, it is worth submitting for analysis. Many practices are incorporating the fee for histopathologic evaluation into the surgery package, so that it is not optional. See "Just wait and see" earlier for problems with the "We'll submit it for histopathologic analysis if it recurs" approach. Similarly, it is important to avoid submission of parts of excised tissue or a "representative section" of an excised mass. This cuts the information gleaned from the pathology report in half because surgical margins cannot be interpreted.

My Great Aunt Had Chemotherapy and Felt Miserable All the Time—I'd Never Do That to My Pet!

The drugs we use to treat cancer in animals generally are the same drugs used in humans, but considerably lower dosages are used and fewer drugs are given concurrently. These changes are made to minimize the risk of adverse effects. With most veterinary chemotherapy protocols in common use, fewer than one third of patients experience unpleasant adverse effects, and 5% or fewer experience a severe adverse effect. The rare adverse effect necessitating hospitalization usually can be treated in 24 to 72 hours. Should unpleasant adverse effects occur, dosages can be reduced, other drugs can be substituted, or prophylactic medications (e.g., antiemetics, antidiarrheals) can be dispensed to minimize the likelihood of subsequent adverse effects. These changes are effective 90% of the time.

I Don't Want My Pet to Go Bald!

It is true that certain dog breeds (the so-called nonshedding breeds) can experience substantial hair loss from chemotherapy. It is rarely complete. Most other breeds experience little or no hair loss, although the owners probably will find more hair around the house, and long-haired breeds have the potential for excessive matting. Hair loss from chemotherapy is nonpruritic and nonpainful—it is purely cosmetic. Cats may lose whiskers and the long, stiff guard hairs of their coats.

I Don't Want My Pet's Last Weeks/Months/ Years to Be Spent in and out of the Hospital, Like They Were for My Uncle When He Had Cancer

Almost all veterinary chemotherapy treatments are done in an outpatient setting, and the majority involve relatively rapid injections rather than prolonged infusions (although there are exceptions). Many protocols involve a series of treatments followed by a period of careful observation. Continuous, indefinite chemotherapy is not the norm.

I Don't Want My Family/Guests/House/ Other Pets to Be Contaminated

This is a legitimate concern, especially for women who may be pregnant or breastfeeding. However, urine and feces generally pose a minimal risk to owners—few drugs are excreted for longer than 48 to 72 hours. Using common sense (i.e., wearing gloves when handling urine or feces) usually is sufficient to minimize risk. Accidents in the house during this period should be cleaned using a detergent solution and the excreta flushed down the toilet. Normal daily interactions (grooming, playing, petting, handling food and water bowls) pose no real risk. It is important that owners be instructed to wear gloves when handling oral medications and that pills not be crushed or split nor capsules opened. Furthermore, chemotherapy drugs never should be formulated into oral solutions or suspensions.

But What about My Pet's Age? Isn't She Too Old for Treatment?

Age is not a disease! Most of the patients we treat with cancer are older pets. Statistics regarding efficacy, tolerability, and outcome of cancer therapy usually are generated in a population of older patients. Far more important than chronologic age are general health (e.g., cardiovascular and renal function) and performance status (e.g., how the pet is feeling).

So What Are Our Choices? We Either Do Chemotherapy or Put Him to Sleep?

Chemotherapy (and cancer therapy in general) usually is not an all-or-nothing proposition. For most tumor types, a spectrum of treatment options may be available depending on factors such as the owner's availability to bring the pet for treatment, owner finances, and owner willingness to tolerate adverse effects. These therapy options have different costs, carry different risks of adverse effects, require different numbers of trips for treatment, and have varying degrees of efficacy.

What about Radiation Therapy for My Pet's Tumor?

Radiation therapy (RT) can be very useful for certain tumor types. Since it is a local treatment, RT is most often used to treat local disease, such as tumors with a high likelihood of aggressive local infiltration but a relatively low risk of metastasis. Common examples are postoperative treatment of incompletely excised intermediate-grade mast cell tumors, soft tissue sarcomas, and oral tumors. It can be used before surgery in certain cases to render an inoperable tumor more amenable to surgery. It also can be used as the primary therapy for certain diseases such as nasal tumors, central nervous system tumors, and acanthomatous epulides. Finally, RT can be used to provide palliation in patients with some highly metastatic tumors such as osteosarcoma and malignant melanoma. The majority of definitive or full-course RT protocols in common use involve a series of 10 to 25 treatments delivered either Monday through Friday or 3 days per week. Most palliative or coarsely fractionated RT protocols involve 1 to 6 weekly treatments on an outpatient basis.

But Won't My Pet Be Horribly Sick from Radiation?

RT is a local form of therapy—the radiation is delivered only to the site of the disease. Thus systemic side effects (nausea, fatigue, bone marrow suppression) generally do not occur. However, each treatment does require very brief anesthesia or heavy sedation to ensure that the radiation is delivered accurately.

What about Radiation Burns?

It is true that animals receiving RT can develop varying degrees of a "sunburn-like" reaction at the site where the radiation is delivered. These can range from mild erythema and pruritus to moist, oozing or ulcerated, and painful skin. These effects typically do not start until the second or third week of treatment and generally resolve within 2 to 4 weeks after the completion of RT. The animal can be left with an area of irradiated skin that is permanently hairless, the hair may grow back only partially, and the hair may turn white within the radiation field. Long-term adverse effects are rare except for those involving the eyes of animals receiving RT for nasal, oral, or brain tumors.

Will My Pet Be Radioactive When He Comes Home?

The standard form of RT in animals is external beam irradiation; that is, radiation is shone down from an external source, and in practical terms the procedure is not that different from taking a diagnostic radiograph except that higher-energy particles are used. Animals undergoing RT pose no health risk to their owners.

What Can We Give My Pet Just to Make Him Feel Better for Whatever Time He Has Left?

Often we are called upon to provide palliative care for our cancer patients. Perhaps the most common clinical signs we are asked to address are pain and poor appetite.

Frequently a reflexive action is to reach for corticosteroids to address these signs. Corticosteroids can be very useful for certain tumor types in which they can have direct antitumor effects (e.g., lymphomas and leukemias, mast cell tumors, myeloma) or address specific clinical signs (e.g., hypoglycemia, hypercalcemia, neurologic signs). However, for other diseases, corticosteroids can be potentially harmful as a result of their adverse effects and theoretical negative impact on tumor progression (immunosuppression). For these conditions, alternative analgesics (nonsteroidal antiinflammatory agents, opiates) and alternative appetite stimulants (megestrol acetate, cyproheptadine, antiemetics) can be considered first, with corticosteroids used only as a last resort.

References and Suggested Reading

Chun R, Garrett LD, Vail DM: Cancer chemotherapy. In Withrow SJ, Vail DM, editors: *Withrow and MacEwen's small animal clinical oncology*, ed 4, St Louis, 2007, Saunders, p 163.

Green EM: Radiotherapy: basic principles and indications. In Bonagura JD, Twedt DC, editors: *Kirk's current veterinary therapy XIV*, St Louis, 2009, Saunders, p 315.

Harvey A et al: A bond-centered practice approach to diagnosis, treatment and euthanasia. In Withrow SJ, MacEwen EG, editors: *Small animal clinical oncology*, ed 3, Philadelphia, 2001, Saunders, p 672.

Lester P, Gaynor JS: Management of cancer pain, *Vet Clin North Am Small Anim Pract* 4:951, 2000.

Moore AS: Radiation therapy for the treatment of tumours in small companion animals, *Vet J* 164:176, 2002.

Thamm DH, Vail DM: Aftershocks of cancer chemotherapy: managing adverse effects, *J Am Anim Hosp Assoc* 43:1, 2007.

Withrow SJ: Why worry about cancer in pets? In Withrow SJ, Vail DM, editors: *Withrow and MacEwen's small animal clinical oncology*, ed 4, St Louis, 2007, Saunders, p xv.

CHAPTER 70

Tumor Biopsy and Specimen Submission

DEBRA A. KAMSTOCK, *Fort Collins, Colorado*
NICHOLAS J. BACON, *Gainesville, Florida*

Tumor biopsy specimens typically are submitted to obtain a diagnosis. This diagnosis, in conjunction with additional information in the pathology report, becomes the cornerstone on which therapeutic decisions and management of the patient are based. The information provided in the pathology report should be accurate, thorough, and reliable. Generation of such a report, in turn, relies upon the submission of quality specimens and necessary clinical information by the clinician requesting specimen analysis.

Tumor Biopsy and Tissue Procurement

Several biopsy techniques are available and the decision to use one over the others depends on specific details of the individual tumor and patient. These techniques, including incisional (needle-core, punch, wedge) and excisional biopsy, are addressed in Web Chapter 32. Specimens obtained endoscopically and via flushes or washes (e.g., nasal flush, traumatic catheterization) are also included.

Regardless of the technique employed, universal principles apply regarding tissue acquisition and handling. The fundamental purpose of a biopsy is to obtain a reliable diagnosis. This depends, at least in part, upon submission of quality diagnostic specimens. Acquiring viable tissue from representative regions and minimizing tissue artifact from time of acquisition to delivery at the laboratory help to ensure submission of a diagnostic sample.

Obtaining a Diagnostic Sample

Principles to follow to increase the potential for obtaining a viable and representative sample by incisional biopsy include the following (Box 70-1):

- Biopsy both mass and surrounding normal tissue— the *tumor-nontumor junction*. This region provides the highest diagnostic yield and in addition may provide information on invasion.
- Avoid obtaining tissue solely from the center of the mass. The center typically is the most necrotic, which often results in a nondiagnostic sample.
- Obtain ample tissue or, if possible, multiple samples from different areas. This increases the chance of obtaining a representative section.

- Biopsy an alternative area of the mass if the first specimen has the following characteristics:
  - It is poorly structured and appears mucinous, gelatinous, semisolid, or liquefied. This may reflect poor cellularity, inflammation or abscessation, or necrosis, and may be nondiagnostic.
  - It is red to dark red or black and the mass is not suspected to be a melanoma. Such coloration may indicate areas of tumor-associated hemorrhage, and the specimen may be nondiagnostic.

Minimizing Tissue Artifact: Handling and Fixation

Regardless of biopsy technique, minimizing tissue artifact during and after the procedure is critical. Principles to follow include the following (Box 70-2):

- Avoid excessive tissue trauma. For example, be aware of the negative effect of suction on biopsy quality, avoid crush artifact by gentle handling with forceps, and minimize the degree of palpation before biopsy or physical handling of the specimen afterward.
- Electrocautery or lasers should be not be used to cut the tissue because these compromise tissue architecture, which hinders evaluation of margins and excisional completeness. After excision with a scalpel blade, electrocautery can be used for hemostasis as long as no tissue from the tumor bed will be collected.
- Ensure proper fixation to preserve tissue architecture.
  - Specimens should be placed in 10% neutral buffered formalin, or other appropriate fixative, at a *1:10 tissue:formalin volumetric ratio.* This should be done immediately following excision unless the specimen requires tissue marking (inking or suture placement to denote surgical margins, orientation, areas of concern, or other features).
  - To aid fixation of larger specimens and prevent *ex vivo* autolysis, make parallel incisions approximately 1.0 cm apart ("bread loafing") if required. Incisions should not entirely transect the specimen nor should they compromise a surgical margin. Additional options for handling larger specimens are addressed later.

Principles for Obtaining a Diagnostic Sample

- Biopsy the *tumor-nontumor junction.*
- Avoid the center of the mass.
- Collect ample tissue or multiple samples from various regions if possible.
- Rebiopsy if specimen lacks conformation or is red to dark red or black and is not a suspected melanoma.

Principles for Minimizing Tissue Artifact

- Avoid excessive handling and instrument-induced crush artifact.
- Excise tissue with a sharp blade, reserving electrocautery and lasers for postexcisional hemostasis.
- Ensure proper, timely fixation of the specimen, which is critical to tissue preservation.
- Avoid freeze artifact.

- Avoid tissue freezing. Freezing causes *ex vivo* ice crystal formation, cell shrinkage, and lysis leading to extensive tissue artifact, which markedly compromises microscopic evaluation.
  - *Never* place specimens in a freezer. Refrigeration is acceptable.
  - Never ship specimens on dry ice. Ice packs and other cooling inserts are acceptable if needed.
  - To avoid freezing during shipment in cold environments, pack the specimen in an insulated container or add isopropyl alcohol to the formalin fixative (1 part alcohol to 10 parts formalin).

Sample Submission

Tissue specimens range from endoscopic biopsy samples to entire spleens and amputated limbs. There is no one way to handle all specimens, although the principles listed earlier universally apply. This section addresses methods of handling some unconventional biopsy specimens. Methods and principles of tissue marking (e.g., identifying surgical margins) as well as the benefits of providing thorough information on the submission form also are addressed. Further information on these topics is available in a recent consensus document (Kamstock et al, 2011), which readers are encouraged to review.

Fixation and Packaging

The most widely used fixative is 10% neutral buffered formalin. Others, such as Davidson's and Bouin's solutions, also are available and may be preferable for certain tissues (e.g., eyes, testes, brain). More recently, a number of low-hazard, formalin-free fixatives (e.g., ExCell Plus, FineFIX, RCL2), which also better preserve the tissue for molecular testing, are gaining interest. Many laboratories provide prefilled containers. The following principles apply to containers:

- The container should be a wide-mouthed plastic jar with a lid that seals securely.
- If the jar has a narrow neck, the neck must be wider than the specimen being submitted. Fresh tissue is malleable and can be squeezed through the neck easily; however, fixed tissue becomes rigid and will be impossible to retrieve without damage.
- The container (not lid) should be labeled with the patient's name, case number, and anatomic site from which the specimen was obtained (e.g., dermal mass, thorax). If multiple specimens are submitted in one jar, a numbered list of the specimens and respective anatomic sites should be provided and the specimens themselves should be identified so that they correlate with the list.
- The container should be placed in one, if not two, secured and sealed plastic bags to contain any leakage during shipping and should be surrounded by absorbent packing material.
- Glass should be avoided because it carries a greater risk of breaking in transit.

Oversized Specimens

For oversized specimens (e.g., limbs and spleens), options include the following:

- *Ship the fresh tissue.* Prerefrigerated fresh tissue specimens can be shipped overnight as long as refrigerated temperatures are maintained throughout. This can be achieved by placing the bagged specimen in an insulated container with cold packs or other cooling materials. Do not freeze and do not ship on dry ice.
- *Prefix the specimen.* Facilities permitting, specimens can be fixed in formalin for 48 to 72 hours (ensuring a 1:10 tissue:formalin volumetric ratio) then removed from the fixative, gently wrapped in formalin-soaked paper towels, double-bagged, and shipped chilled.
- *Section before shipping.* If the whole specimen is unable to be fixed on site, it can be carefully sectioned into portions and submitted in appropriately labeled formalin jars or prefixed as described earlier. An annotated digital image or sketch of the original specimen showing the sections made and their orientation should accompany the submission. Sections should be numbered 1, 2, 3, and so on, and the numbers on the jars should correspond with numbered sections on the sketch or image.
- *Submit a portion of the mass.* A diagnosis may be obtained from a portion of the specimen, but this method precludes assessment of excisional completeness. The remaining tissue should be held at the clinic until the pathology report is received.

Extremely Small Specimens

Minimal volumes of tissue may be obtained from endoscopic biopsy, pinch biopsy, needle-core biopsy, and flushing. The following practices are recommended:

- Tiny samples should be placed into screened cassettes and the cassette placed into the formalin container. Samples should not be free floating in formalin.
- To indicate the biopsy site (e.g., stomach, duodenum, colon) cassettes can be written on with a No. 2 pencil. Tissue from different sites should be placed in separate appropriately labeled cassettes.
- Gauze and surgical sponges should be avoided because specimens become entrapped in the fibers.
- Cardboard should be avoided because tissue may adhere and become damaged upon retrieval at the laboratory. Adherence also reduces the size of an already small sample.
- Surgical paper is acceptable; however, screened cassettes are preferred.
- Small tissue biopsy specimens often contain sampling artifacts, which may require that the lesion be biopsied again. Obtaining multiple samples per site at the outset therefore is strongly recommended.

Demarcation of Surgical Margins

If excisional biopsy is performed, the goal most likely is complete excision. Assessment of excisional completeness depends on microscopic evaluation for neoplastic cells at the surgical edge. This assessment is key because it may impact prognosis and additional therapeutic decisions. Although the surgical margins may be obvious to the clinician performing the surgery, this may not be true for personnel receiving the sample at the laboratory; hence the need for tissue marking. Of note, although a positive margin indicates incomplete excision, a negative (clean) margin does not guarantee a disease-free state but is the best determinant of the success of surgical treatment.

Before the specimen is placed in fixative, the surgical margins should be denoted either by surgical ink or placement of sutures. Surgical ink is superior to sutures because it can be seen at both the gross and microscopic level. Surgical ink viewed microscopically by the pathologist identifies the true surgical edges as distinguished from the artifactual edges created during tissue trimming. Additionally, it allows the pathologist to provide information relative to tissue orientation (e.g., the lateral margins are marked with yellow ink and the deep margins with black ink). Principles to follow when inking specimens include the following (Box 70-3):

- Use official surgical ink or waterproof drawing ink to ensure retention of the ink throughout tissue processing.
- Place the specimen on absorptive material and blot dry before inking.
- Use a cotton swab or wooden applicator stick and apply the ink only to areas of interest or true surgical margins. Do not submerge the specimen in the ink.

BOX 70-3

Principles for Inking Tissue Specimens

- Use official surgical ink or waterproof drawing ink.
- Ink specimens within 30 minutes of excision.
- Gently blot specimen dry before inking.
- Apply ink only to specific areas of interest.
- Allow ink to dry completely (5 to 10 minutes) before placement in fixative.
- Use yellow, black, or green ink if possible.

- Allow the ink to dry completely (approximately 5 to 10 minutes) before placing the specimen in fixative to prevent the ink from washing off or coating insignificant areas.
- Ink the specimen as soon as possible after removal, ideally within 30 minutes of excision.
- If the specimen cannot be inked within 30 minutes, place it in fixative and later remove it, blot it dry, and ink it. This is not ideal because postfixation tissue shrinkage and conformational changes may alter true margins.
- For larger specimens, first ink the specimen, allow the ink to dry, and *then* bread-loaf the specimen to prevent the ink from permeating inappropriate areas.
- Use yellow, black, or green surgical inks when possible because blue and red inks are more difficult to discern with routine hematoxylin and eosin staining.

Placement of sutures, identified either by number or color, can be used to denote surgical margins, relay tissue orientation (e.g., one suture dorsal, two sutures caudal), or identify individual masses when multiple specimens are placed in a single jar (e.g., blue suture indicates dermal mass from muzzle, purple suture indicates dermal mass from carpus). Information should not be relayed based on suture type (e.g., Prolene, Vicryl, braided) because laboratory personnel may not be familiar with these terms.

Regardless of whether inking, sutures, or both are used, it is imperative that a corresponding written explanation of these tissue demarcations be provided on the submission form (Box 70-4).

Submission Form

Unless a complete and thorough submission form is included, the effort to provide a quality diagnostic specimen will be undermined. This is the only written piece of communication from the clinician to the laboratory team, and if the clinician desires an accurate and relevant pathology report, it is paramount that sufficient detail be provided in the submission process. Submission forms typically are provided by the diagnostic laboratory and often are available online. The following are guidelines for filling out an ideal tumor biopsy submission form, including a listing of the basic (but not necessarily all) information that should be included (see Box 70-4):

BOX 70-4

The Submission Form: Help the Pathologist Help You!

- Type, or write legibly.
- Provide signalment (age, sex, reproductive status, breed).
- Provide all necessary patient and lesion information (see text).
- Indicate biopsy type (incisional, excisional, recut, other).
- Provide a working clinical diagnosis or list of differential diagnoses.
- Provide written explanation of any tissue markings (ink, suture, other demarcation).
- Relay any specific questions or concerns.
- Provide appropriate clinic information.
- Submit paperwork together with the samples but in a separate plastic bag or compartment.

- Ensure readability. The form ideally should be typed but must at least be handwritten legibly. An illegible form is equivalent to an incomplete form.
- Thoroughly fill in *all* requested areas.
- Include the following information regarding the patient and lesion:
  - Patient name or case identification number
  - Signalment (age, sex, reproductive status, breed)
  - Lesion-specific information (anatomic site, size, color, consistency, duration, rate of growth, other features; specify for each lesion if more than one is submitted)
  - Type of lesion (new, recurrent, possible metastasis subsequent to known primary)
  - Type of biopsy (incisional, excisional, recut following incomplete excision, other)
  - Results of prior diagnostic tests (e.g., cytologic analysis, prior biopsy if performed or if a recurrent lesion, imaging results—especially for bone and gingival tumors)
  - Potentially relevant or related clinical signs (e.g., vomiting, lameness)
  - Complete blood count (CBC) results, biochemical or hormonal abnormalities (e.g., hypercalcemia, hyperinsulinemia)
  - Patient's prior cancers (plus cancers in siblings and parental lines if a hereditary condition is suspected)
  - Treatment history, if any (e.g., corticosteroids, chemotherapy, radiation)
  - Previous unrelated treatments or potential carcinogenic events (e.g., prior radiation or surgery at the site; vaccination; implants, including microchips)
  - Any additional relevant patient information (strongly encouraged)
- Provide a working clinical diagnosis or list of differential diagnoses; it is often just as important for the pathologist to rule out certain diseases.
- Provide a complete and comprehensive *written explanation of any tissue demarcations.*
- Relay any additional questions or concerns you would like the laboratory or pathologist to address.
- Provide general clinic information including clinic name, address, telephone and fax numbers, and submitting clinician's name and possibly e-mail address.
- Send the submission form and additional paperwork if desired (e.g., other reports or diagnostic test results such as CBC or biochemistry results, cytology report, and imaging reports) together with the sample, but place them in a separate plastic bag (or compartment) to protect from potential formalin leakage in transit.

Postreport Options

If the final pathology report conflicts with clinical impression, the clinician should not hesitate to contact the laboratory or reporting pathologist directly. This communication may result in any number of outcomes, including clarification of information, correction of a clerical error or slide or case number error, or initiation of additional steps. There are a number of requests that can be made by the submitting clinician. Some may incur an additional charge but hopefully will add clarity in a complex or frustrating case.

- *Reevaluation of the original slide.* If the clinician is skeptical of the diagnosis or wants additional information not originally reported (e.g., vascular invasion, objective measurement of surgical margin) he or she may request that the original slide(s) be revaluated by the reporting pathologist. If there is concern about an alternative diagnosis, the clinical reasons should be explained to the pathologist so the specimen can be reevaluated with those factors in mind. Additional stains (see later) ultimately may be required. Reevaluation of the slide(s) may result in an amended report or an addendum if the case has already been closed.
- *Evaluation of additional wet tissue.* If the pathology report indicates "no evidence of neoplasia" or "nondiagnostic" (which suggests that the neoplastic process or viable tissue, respectively, may not have been captured during trimming), additional sections can be trimmed from different areas of the wet specimen, which may provide a new perspective.
- *Evaluation of deeper levels of the original block.* If there is no wet tissue, which suggests that all tissue submitted was processed (such as with needle-core biopsy), yet further evaluation is desired, examination of deeper levels or step sections, partially or through the block in its entirety can be requested.
- *Application of special stains.* If a tumor is poorly differentiated so that its origin cannot be determined on routine microscopy alone, histochemical or immunohistochemical stains may be available to assist in further classifying (e.g., round cell versus epithelial cell) or specifically identifying (e.g., lymphoma versus histiocytic sarcoma) the cell of

origin, which may have a significant impact on therapeutic decisions and prognosis.

- *Second opinion.* If the aforementioned options are exhausted and clinical concerns persist, the clinician can request a second opinion from an additional pathologist. Most commonly, second opinions are obtained internally; however, at the clinician's request, slides can be sent to a pathologist at a different laboratory or institution. More extensive information regarding second opinions is provided in a 2011 consensus paper (Kamstock et al, 2011).
- *Rebiopsy.* At times, repeated biopsy ultimately is the best option.

When working with the reporting pathologist or laboratory to address postreport options, it is useful to remember that pathology is not a perfect science and tumors are not black and white. Patience and professional respect should be shown by both parties and will help to ensure optimal patient care and service to the client.

References and Suggested Reading

Becker G: The many faces of surgical margins, *Am J Clin Oncol* 30:556, 2007.

Ehrhart NP, Withrow SJ: Biopsy principles. In Withrow SJ, Vail DM, editors: *Withrow and MacEwen's small animal clinical oncology*, ed 4, St Louis, 2007, Saunders, p 147.

Kamstock DA et al: Recommended guidelines for submission, trimming, margin evaluation, and reporting of tumor biopsy specimens in veterinary surgical pathology, *Vet Pathol* 48(1):19, 2011.

Kronz JD, Westra WH, Epstein JI: Mandatory second opinion surgical pathology at a large referral hospital, *Cancer* 86(11):2426, 1999.

Raab SS, Grzybicki DM: Quality in cancer diagnosis, *CA Cancer J Clin* 60(3):139, 2010.

Rassnick KM: Ten things you can do with tumor biopsies. In *Proceedings of the 24th Annual ACVIM Forum*, 2006, p 61.

Regan RC et al: Comparison of first-opinion and second-opinion histopathology from dogs and cats with cancer: 430 cases (2001-2008), *Vet Comp Oncol* 8(1):1, 2010.

CHAPTER 71

Chemotherapeutic Drug Handling and Safety

ANDREA FLORY, *San Marcos, California*
BRENDA PHILLIPS, *San Diego, California*
MARGO KARRIKER, *San Diego, California*

Chemotherapeutic drugs are considered *hazardous drugs*. Hazardous drugs (HDs) are defined as drugs that can have adverse health effects and significant toxicity at low doses. Drugs are classified as hazardous if studies in animals or humans indicate that exposures to them have a potential to cause cancer, developmental or reproductive toxicity, or harm to organs (National Institute for Occupational Safety and Health [NIOSH], 2004).

In the United States, an estimated 500,000 veterinary health care workers potentially are exposed to HDs or drug waste at their workplaces (NIOSH, 2010). Routes of exposure include skin absorption, inhalation, and ingestion. Most HDs used in veterinary species are antineoplastic (chemotherapeutic) agents.

Because knowledge about the effects of HD exposure is evolving continually and the degree of HD absorption is difficult to assess, a general procedure for creating and enforcing protocols to minimize exposure to HDs and drug waste should be a priority at veterinary hospitals. These protocols should protect all staff working in a veterinary hospital, not only those who administer chemotherapeutic drugs. Specialized equipment and work practices are required to protect veterinary health care workers from the dangers of HD exposure.

Equipment

Drug Preparation Equipment

Biological safety cabinets (BSCs) are the hallmark equipment for the safe preparation of hazardous and cytotoxic drugs. A BSC is a ventilated cabinet that provides personnel, product, and environmental protection via inward airflow, downward high-efficiency particulate air (HEPA) airflow, and HEPA-filtered exhausted air, respectively. BSCs must be vented to the outside environment with no recirculation (U.S. Pharmacopeial Convention, 2011).

The effectiveness of BSCs in containing drug contamination depends on user technique.

BSCs require initial certifications to assure proper airflow and function, as well as recertifications every 6 to 12 months, depending on manufacturer recommendations. HEPA filters may need to be replaced every 2 to 5 years depending on the level of contamination within the surrounding workspace.

Several styles of safety cabinets are available; however, the recommended cabinet type is class II, type B2. A class II, type B2 BSC can cost $8000 to $15,000 depending on size and installation charges. This type of cabinet offers the recommended level of protection for the preparation of all products used in veterinary practice when employed under the proper conditions; it is vital that the airflow and negative-pressure environment be maintained within the BSC at all times. The use of *closed-system drug-transfer devices* (CSTDs) to provide staff with two tiers of containment for HDs is recommended if BSCs are not located within a negative-pressure clean-room environment.

CSTDs are designed to mechanically prevent the transfer of environmental contaminants into the system and the escape of drug or vapor out of the system. Each multicomponent system has specific components for the preparation and administration of HDs, including components for drug vials, locking syringes, and administration sets. The choice of CSTD should be based on proven, independent, effectiveness data. There are several CSTD systems on the market; the authors currently use the PhaSeal system. Chemotherapy adjuncts and chemotherapy vial venting pins are not closed-system devices and should not be used in place of a closed system and proper environmental controls. CSTDs and chemotherapy adjuncts alone never should be used in place of proper two-tiered protection, such as a BSC in a clean room or a CSTD within a BSC (American Society of Health-System Pharmacists [ASHP], 2006).

When proper equipment is not available to prepare HDs, they may be sourced from pharmacies that are properly equipped in ready-to-use, unit-dose packaging. Other alternatives are sending patients to a facility where HDs can be prepared in a BSC and sharing a BSC among several private practices.

Drug Transport Equipment

When HDs are transported within the hospital, gloves always should be worn and care taken to prevent workspace exposure to drug residues. Stock bottles, commercial vials, dispensing containers, prepared doses, syringes, and administration devices containing HDs should be transported by hand in a secondary container, such as a rigid plastic closed-top bin (for stock bottles) or a clear zip-lock bag (for prepared doses), to reduce potential for spills. Transport containers never should be placed into a potentially contaminated area (such as the workspace in the BSC).

Drug Storage

Hospital areas that contain storage for HDs should be identified with distinct placards and signs that are easily recognizable, even to non-English speakers, to distinguish them from general product storage areas. Efforts should be made to store HDs in an area in close proximity to the area in which they will be used, and all HDs should be segregated from other drug inventory by physical means such as closed storage bins and boxes.

Personal Protective Equipment

In addition to physical barriers discussed earlier such as BSCs and CTSDs, all components of HD handling require some level of *personal protective equipment.*

Gloves

Gloves should be worn at all times during the receipt, transport, preparation, and administration of HDs, and in handling excreta from patients that have recently received HDs. Latex, nitrile, rubber, and polyurethane gloves all can provide protection against exposure to HDs. Glove packaging should note that the product meets the ASTM International standards for resistance to permeation of chemotherapeutic drugs. Generally, powder-free latex or nitrile gloves that are less than 8 mil (1 mil = 0.001 inch) in thickness should be used in a double-glove protocol, with one glove worn under the cuff of the gown and one glove over the cuff. Frequent exposure of gloves to isopropyl alcohol should be avoided. Gloves never should be worn for longer than 30 minutes and should be changed immediately if torn, punctured, or contaminated. Care always should be taken to avoid touching the contaminated outer surfaces when removing gloves. Hands always should be washed thoroughly with soap and water before gloves are donned and after removal.

Gowns

Gowns are required for preparation, administration, spill control, and waste management of HDs. Generally, gowns should be of a disposable, lint-free, closed-front style with long sleeves and tight-fitting elastic or knit cuffs. Washable cloth or reusable gowns or smocks never should be used when handling HDs. Polyethylene, polypropylene, or vinyl-coated gowns offer the best level of protection. Gowns never should be worn outside of the immediate drug preparation and administration area because they can be a source of contamination for other hospital areas and other staff members. Gowns should be disposed of immediately after use (ASHP, 2006).

Additional Personal Protective Equipment

Eye and face protection should be used whenever there is a risk of splashes or aerosols. The protective equipment of choice for eye and face protection are face shields, rather than safety glasses or goggles (ASHP, 2006). Surgical masks, even those with plastic face shields, do not offer adequate protection. Respiratory protection using a fit-tested respirator with an N95 rating (i.e., one that filters 95% of airborne particles) is required when engineering mechanisms cannot control exposure to an aerosolized drug (e.g., in a drug spill) (NIOSH, 2004). Use of shoe coverings should be considered during the preparation and administration of HDs to prevent cross contamination of other work areas.

Work Practices

Preparation of Hazardous Drugs

HDs should be prepared in a restricted, preferably centralized area that is posted with signs warning of possible contamination with cytotoxic drugs and to which the access of unauthorized personnel is limited. Eating, drinking, chewing gum, applying cosmetics, and storing personal items such as food, drinks, cosmetics, gum, and cigarettes within the HD preparation area should be strictly forbidden.

Only supplies and drugs essential to drug preparation should be placed in the BSC (ASHP, 2006). A plastic-backed absorbent pad should be placed under the preparation site to catch any spills; this pad should be replaced at least once daily. Syringes should be filled no more than three fourths full to minimize the risk of plunger separation from the syringe barrel. Locking fitted syringes and intravenous administration sets should be used for HD preparation. All syringes and intravenous fluids bags containing HDs should be appropriately labeled so that they are handled and disposed of properly.

Studies have shown that the workspace in and around the BSC often is contaminated with drug residues (Sessink et al, 2011). Final preparations of drugs should undergo surface decontamination after drug preparation is complete and before their removal from the BSC (ASHP, 2006). Tablets and capsules containing cytotoxic drugs should be counted in the BSC to avoid dispersal of hazardous dust (Lucroy, 2001). Tablets never should be split, broken, or crushed (Frimberger, 2011). If splitting of HD tablets is unavoidable, the splitting should be done only inside a BSC (European College of Veterinary Internal Medicine of Companion Animals [ECVIM-CA], 2007). Oral chemotherapeutic drugs ideally should be reformulated by a compounding pharmacy when necessary.

Decontamination, Deactivation, and Cleaning

Decontamination (or cleaning) is the process of transferring HDs from the surface of a nondisposable item to a disposable one such as gauze, wipes, or towels. Deactivating a hazardous substance is preferred; however, no single process has been found to deactivate all HDs (ASHP, 2006). BSCs should be cleaned before the day's operations begin and again when the day's work is completed. Additionally, trays under the work surface should be cleaned monthly, or any time there is a spill in the BSC.

Strong oxidizing agents such as sodium hypochlorite (a component of commercial bleach) are effective deactivators of many HDs (ASHP, 2006). A commercial product containing sodium hypochlorite, detergent, and thiosulfate neutralizer (Surface Safe) provides a system for decontamination and deactivation. Bleach solution, followed by a strong detergent and water rinse, may also remove most drug residues (NIOSH, 2010). Alcohol may be used for disinfection; however, it does not deactivate any HDs and may cause spread of contamination, and it should not be used to clean the BSC (ASHP, 2006).

Handling of Chemotherapy Waste

Regulations issued by the U.S. Environmental Protection Agency (EPA) as implementation of the Resource Conservation and Recovery Act (RCRA) require that hazardous waste be managed by following a strict set of regulatory requirements (EPA, n.d.). All HD waste should be stored in designated, clearly labeled, covered, leak-proof containers until disposal and should be disposed of separately from regular waste according to federal, state, and local regulations (NIOSH, 2010). Empty vials or those containing trace amounts of drug (less than 3% by weight of the original quantity of drug) can be discarded into containers clearly marked "cytotoxic waste" (not red sharps containers). Partially filled vials or undispensed products should be double-bagged for disposal. Licensed commercial waste disposal companies should be retained to dispose of drugs via incineration or internment into a licensed toxic waste landfill (Lucroy, 2001).

Spill Management

Veterinary hospitals that prepare and administer HDs must have emergency policies for handling spills readily available, including written procedures that specify who is responsible for spill management (ASHP, 2006). Spill kits should be placed in all areas where HDs are stored, handled, and administered. Spill kits should contain the following items: protective eyewear, disposable low-permeability gown, overshoes, latex gloves, utility gloves, NIOSH-approved respirator, multiple sheets of disposable absorbent material, cleaner such as strong alkaline detergent, approved container for cytotoxic waste and sharps, small scoop for picking up glass fragments, and large HD disposal bags (Frimberger, 2011; Lucroy, 2001).

All contaminated surfaces should be cleaned thoroughly three times with detergent and water. Spray bottles should not be used because of the potential for aerosolization. All contaminated absorbent sheets and other materials should be placed in an HD disposal bag. Spill cleanup materials should be disposed of according to local waste requirements but often must be separated from chemotherapy trace waste.

Handling of Excreta

Chemotherapeutic drugs may be excreted as metabolites or whole drug in the urine, feces, vomitus, and saliva of treated patients (Occupational Safety and Health Administration [OSHA], 2000). Specific recommendations based on peer-reviewed studies of the handling of urine, feces, vomitus, and saliva after chemotherapy have been scarce, but recent publications have begun to provide more concrete information about excretion of antineoplastic agents from veterinary species. Urine residues of some drugs (e.g., cyclophosphamide) are below detectable levels by 2 days after administration, whereas low levels of other drugs (e.g., doxorubicin) can be detected up to 21 days after dosing (Knobloch et al, 2010). Excreta from patients that have received chemotherapeutic drugs should be handled using the same personal protective equipment as that used in cleaning up spills. Sprayers or pressure washers should not be used to clean cages, kennels, or stalls of animals treated with HDs to avoid aerosolization. Bedding soiled with excreta from patients that recently have received HDs should be handled as contaminated.

Safety Program: Recommended Policies and Procedures

Written policies and procedures for the safe handling of HDs must be in place in any facility in which HDs are handled (ASHP, 2006). A key element of the safety program is the availability of Safety Data Sheets. These should be reviewed and updated regularly. Employees must be trained to understand the risks of working with HDs and the physical and health hazards of HDs in the work area, including the carcinogenic potential and reproductive hazards of these drugs (NIOSH, 2010; OSHA, 2000). Employees who are pregnant, breastfeeding, or of reproductive age must be warned of the potential health effects of handling HDs, especially during the first trimester, when a woman may not know she is pregnant (NIOSH, 2010).

A written Hazardous Drug Safety and Health Plan will help outline policies and diminish employee fear about working with these drugs (Lucroy, 2001; OSHA, 2000). Most importantly, this plan will assist in protecting employees and keeping exposures as low as is reasonably achievable. Components of the plan include procedures to be followed when personnel are exposed to HDs, provision for training and access to information, medical surveillance plan, establishment of a designated HD handling area, use of BSCs, procedures for safe removal of contaminated waste, procedures relating to cleaning of spilled HDs, decontamination procedures, requirement that ventilation devices and personal protective equipment function properly, and designation of personnel responsible for implementing the Hazardous Drug Safety and Health Plan (Frimberger, 2011; Lucroy, 2001; OSHA, 2000). Employees must be trained to recognize HDs by their required labeling with OSHA-standardized pictograms, a signal word, hazard and precautionary statements, the product identifier, and supplier information (OSHA, 2012).

Client Safety

Clients should be informed about the potential hazards of cytotoxic drugs and should be advised of necessary precautions for oral administration of chemotherapeutic drugs and for handling of bodily wastes (ECVIM-CA, 2007; Frimberger, 2011). Although there appear to be no legal guidelines mandating creation of client safety information, the authors recommend that written handouts detailing drug administration protocols and potential hazards to humans be provided to clients and that documentation of the provision of such handouts be included in the patient record.

Gloves should be provided to clients, and they should be instructed to use them when cleaning up excreta and when administering oral chemotherapeutic agents, and to wash the hands afterward. Accidents in the house should be cleaned up with detergent and bleach or other cleaner.

HDs dispensed for at-home administration should be marked with "cytotoxic" or an equivalent label and should be packaged in medication bottles, not in paper envelopes or plastic bags (Frimberger, 2011). At home, oral chemotherapeutic drugs should be kept away from children and should be kept separate from food items and other medications. Clients should be advised never to split or crush tablets or to open chemotherapy capsules (Frimberger, 2011). Women who are pregnant or breast-feeding should never handle chemotherapeutic medications (Frimberger, 2011). Empty bottles and used gloves should be returned to the hospital for appropriate disposal.

References and Suggested Reading

American Society of Health-System Pharmacists: ASHP guidelines on handling hazardous drugs, *Am J Health Syst Pharm* 63:1172, 2006.

European College of Veterinary Internal Medicine of Companion Animals (ECVIM-CA): *Preventing occupational and environmental exposure to cytotoxic drugs in veterinary medicine, 2nd version*, Munich, 2007, ECVIM-CA.

Frimberger A: Chemotherapy preparation and administration safety issues. In *Proceedings of the 29th Annual ACVIM Forum*, 2011.

Knobloch A et al: Cytotoxic drug residues in urine of dogs receiving anticancer chemotherapy, *J Vet Intern Med* 24;384, 2010.

Lucroy MD: Chemotherapy safety in veterinary practice: hazardous drug preparation, *Comp Cont Educ Pract Vet* 24:140, 2001.

National Institute for Occupational Safety and Health (NIOSH): NIOSH alert: preventing occupational exposure to antineoplastic and other hazardous drugs in health care settings, DHHS (NIOSH) Pub. No. 2004-165, September 2004. Available at www.cdc.gov/niosh/docs/2004-165/. Accessed October 27, 2011.

National Institute for Occupational Safety and Health: Safe handling of hazardous drugs for veterinary healthcare workers, DHHS (NIOSH) Pub. No. 2010-150, June 2010. Available at www.cdc.gov/niosh/topics/hazdrug/. Accessed October 27, 2011.

Occupational Safety and Health Administration: Communication standard, 2012. Available at www.osha.gov/dsg/hazcom/index2.html.

Occupational Safety and Health Administration: Controlling occupational exposure to hazardous drugs. In *OSHA technical manual*, Washington, DC, 2000, US Department of Labor, sect VI, chap 2. Available at www.osha.gov/dts/osta/otm/otm_vi/otm_vi_2.html. Accessed October 27, 2011.

Sessink PJ et al: Reduction in surface contamination with antineoplastic drugs in 22 hospital pharmacies in the US following implementation of a closed-system drug transfer device, *J Oncol Pharm Pract* 17:39, 2011.

US Environmental Protection Agency: RCRA online. Available at www.epa.gov/epawaste/inforesources/online/index.htm. Accessed October 27, 2011.

US Pharmacopeial Convention: General chapter 797: Pharmaceutical compounding—sterile preparations. In *United States Pharmacopeia and the National Formulary*, Rockville, Maryland, 2011, US Pharmacopeial Convention, p 336.

CHAPTER 72

Treatment of Adverse Effects from Cancer Therapy

DENNIS B. BAILEY, *Paramus, New Jersey*

One of the primary goals of cancer treatment in veterinary patients is to preserve quality of life. Every effort is made to minimize adverse effects of chemotherapy, but it is not possible to eliminate them completely. Chemotherapy is unique in that dosages are based on toxicity rather than efficacy. Dose-response curves tend to be very steep for most cancers, and to minimize treatment failures drugs are administered at the highest possible dosages that are tolerated by most patients. Some risk of toxicity has to be accepted; anticipation, early recognition, and prompt intervention can help minimize adverse effects and maintain patient quality of life.

Chemotherapy Dosages

Most chemotherapy dosages are based on body surface area (BSA) because it is thought that this parameter predicts biologic functions more closely than body weight; however, there is no direct evidence that BSA predicts drug absorption, distribution, metabolism, or excretion. Additionally, when chemotherapy drugs are dosed based on BSA, smaller patients receive a larger dose on a milligrams-per-kilogram basis. Doxorubicin (DOX), cisplatin, carboplatin, and melphalan all are associated with an increased prevalence of adverse effects in small dogs when dosed based on BSA. Consequently, melphalan often is dosed on a milligrams-per-kilogram basis for dogs of all sizes. For the other drugs listed, lower BSA-based dosages or milligrams-per-kilogram dosing schemes often are used in smaller dogs (usually <10 to 15 kg). In cats a carboplatin dosing equation has been derived based on patient glomerular filtration rate that predicts toxicity more accurately than dosing based on BSA.

A polymorphism in the gene that encodes the membrane-associated pump ABCB1 (adenosine triphosphate–binding cassette, subfamily B, member 1; also called *MDR-1* [multidrug resistance protein 1] and P-glycoprotein) increases the risk of adverse effects with drugs that are substrates of the pump (Mealey et al, 2008). The collie, Australian shepherd, long-haired whippet, McNab, and silken windhound are among the most commonly affected breeds. Dogs homozygous for the ABCB1-1Δ polymorphism experience a higher incidence of vincristine-associated neutropenia and thrombocytopenia, and computer-based pharmacokinetic modeling predicts that they cannot receive therapeutic dosages of DOX without unacceptable gastrointestinal (GI) toxicity. Other chemotherapy drugs that are substrates of ABCB1 are vinblastine, vinorelbine, mitoxantrone, dactinomycin, docetaxel, paclitaxel, and etoposide. Alkylating agents, antimetabolites, and platinum chemotherapy drugs are not impacted by ABCB1. Genetic testing for the ABCB1-1Δ polymorphism is available through Washington State University (www.vetmed.wsu.edu/depts-VCPL/index.aspx).

Management of Adverse Events

Hematologic Toxicity

One of the most common adverse effects associated with chemotherapy is *myelosuppression,* a decrease in blood cell counts. This should be distinguished from immunosuppression, inhibition of immune system function. *Neutropenia* is the most common manifestation of myelosuppression, followed by thrombocytopenia. Severe anemia is uncommon because of the prolonged life span of red blood cells, although a slow decline in hematocrit can be observed over the course of a protocol.

Bone marrow aspiration with cytologic evaluation should be considered before starting chemotherapy in patients with cancers that can infiltrate the marrow, such as lymphoma and leukemias, especially if the baseline complete blood count (CBC) shows abnormal cells in circulation or normal cell line cytopenias. Patients with substantial marrow involvement (>50% effacement) are at higher risk of chemotherapy-associated cytopenias, and occasionally it is necessary to administer chemotherapy when they are cytopenic. Using less myelosuppressive drugs (such as L-asparaginase) at the start of treatment in these patients is preferable whenever possible, and prophylactic antibiotic therapy should be considered.

A CBC should be performed on the day of each chemotherapy treatment. In a patient with a relatively healthy bone marrow, the neutrophil count should be at least 1500 to 2500/μl and platelet counts should be 50,000 to 100,000/μl or more on the day of treatment. If a patient is too cytopenic, chemotherapy treatment should be delayed by 3 to 7 days. A CBC should be repeated to ensure that the cytopenias have improved before treatment is resumed.

CBCs should be performed to assess blood cell counts at their nadirs (low points). With most drugs, nadirs typically occur around 5 to 10 days after treatment, and a CBC should be performed 1 week after the first treatment. Notable exceptions include carboplatin, which can cause neutropenia or thrombocytopenia anywhere from 7 to 14 days after treatment in dogs and neutropenia anywhere from 7 to 21 days after treatment in cats, and lomustine (CCNU), which can cause neutropenia anywhere from 7 to 28 days after treatment in cats. For these drugs, CBCs should be performed weekly to ensure that the nadir is identified accurately. Measurement of nadir CBCs is essential after the first dose of any myelosuppressive chemotherapy drug. Measurement of subsequent nadir CBCs is indicated only if severe cytopenias are identified that result in a dosage reduction.

Nadir neutrophil counts of 1000/µl or higher typically do not require any intervention. Patients with fewer than 1000 neutrophils/µl are at increased risk of systemic infections. Prophylactic treatment with antibiotics is recommended. Common choices include amoxicillin/clavulanic acid (13.75 mg/kg q12h PO), enrofloxacin (dogs: 10 mg/kg q24h PO; cats: 2.5 to 5.0 mg/kg q24h PO; high-dose treatment not recommended), or trimethoprim/sulfamethoxazole (15 mg/kg q12h PO). The dosage of the causative drug should be decreased by 10% to 25% in subsequent treatments, regardless of whether or not the patient develops an infection. The most common causative agents for systemic infections in neutropenic patients are normal gut and skin flora; however, neutropenic dogs and cats also should avoid groomers, pet stores, kennels, and public parks while their counts remain low. In most dogs and cats, the neutrophil count recovers within 3 to 5 days, although in the author's experience severe neutropenias can be slower to recover in cats.

Signs of systemic infection most commonly are acute-onset lethargy and anorexia. Vomiting and diarrhea occasionally are seen as well. Most patients are febrile, although this is not always the case since white blood cells are one of the primary sources of the inflammatory cytokines that cause fever (interleukin-1, tumor necrosis factor). *A patient with a neutrophil count of less than 1000/µl that is systemically ill should be considered to have a systemic infection until proven otherwise.* Systemic infections require prompt treatment with intravenous fluids and intravenous antibiotics. Common choices are ampicillin/sulbactam (30 mg/kg q8h IV) or a combination of ampicillin (22 mg/kg q8h IV) or cefazolin (22 mg/kg q8h IV) with enrofloxacin (dogs: 10 mg/kg q24h IV; cats: 2.5 to 5.0 mg/kg q24h IV). If needed, additional treatment for signs of septic shock (hypotension, hypoglycemia) should be implemented. In patients with uncomplicated systemic infections the fever should break within 24 hours, and temperature usually returns to the normal range within 24 to 48 hours of initiation of therapy. After temperature has been within normal limits for 24 hours, patients can be switched to the oral equivalents of their intravenous antibiotics and discharged from the hospital. If clinical signs do not improve, imaging of the thorax or abdomen should be considered to search for a nidus of infection. Blood cultures are not routinely performed; in most patients the infection is under control before results are available.

Thrombocytopenia is seen most commonly with carboplatin, lomustine, dacarbazine, melphalan, and occasionally DOX. It usually is not clinically significant, but patients with fewer than 25,000 to 50,000 platelets/µl should avoid trauma and be monitored for petechiae, ecchymoses, epistaxis, or GI bleeding. Also, lomustine and melphalan can be associated with cumulative and often irreversible thrombocytopenia. These drugs should be discontinued in patients with persistent platelet counts below 75,000 to 100,000/µl.

Gastrointestinal Toxicity

GI toxicity most commonly results from damage to the rapidly dividing cells in the crypts of the intestine but also can result from direct stimulation of the chemoreceptor trigger zone within the brain. Anorexia, vomiting, and diarrhea caused by the first mechanism typically occurs anywhere from 2 to 5 days after treatment. Acute vomiting caused by the second mechanism typically occurs during or within 24 hours of treatment. Almost all chemotherapy drugs have the potential to cause delayed GI toxicity. Drugs that can cause acute vomiting include cisplatin, dacarbazine, streptozocin, and occasionally mustargen and DOX.

Anorexia is managed most commonly by offering palatable foods. Appetite stimulants can be used on an as-needed basis. Choices include prednisone (dogs: 0.5 mg/kg q24h PO; cats: usually not effective), cyproheptadine (dogs: 0.3 mg/kg q12h PO; cats: 2 to 4 mg q12-24h PO), and mirtazapine (dogs: 0.6 mg/kg q24h PO; cats: 3.75 mg q3d PO). Nausea is difficult to assess in veterinary patients, but it can contribute to anorexia. Centrally acting antiemetics such as maropitant (Cerenia; dogs: 1 mg/kg q24h SC or 2 mg/kg q24h PO for up to 5 days; cats: 1 mg/kg q24h SC or PO) are indicated in patients thought to be nauseated, even if there is no concurrent vomiting. Similarly, vincristine can cause an ileus that manifests with anorexia or vomiting. Metoclopramide (0.4 mg/kg q8-12h SC or PO) often is beneficial because of its GI prokinetic effects.

Mild vomiting is controlled by restricting the patient to nothing by mouth for 12 to 24 hours, followed by introduction of small amounts of water and then small meals with a bland diet. Moderate to severe vomiting usually requires intervention with antiemetics with or without parenteral fluid support. Maropitant has been shown to reduce the frequency and severity of vomiting associated with cisplatin and DOX in dogs (Rau et al, 2010; Vail et al, 2007). Other antiemetic choices include metoclopramide, dolasetron (Anzemet; 0.6 mg/kg q12-24h SC or IV), and ondansetron (Zofran; 0.5 to 1.0 mg/kg q12-24h IV or PO). Severe vomiting can require subcutaneous or intravenous fluids. For drugs that routinely stimulate the chemoreceptor trigger zone, pretreatment with maropitant or another centrally acting antiemetic is recommended before chemotherapy administration.

Mild diarrhea usually is easily managed by feeding a bland, high-fiber diet. More severe or persistent diarrhea can be treated with loperamide (Imodium A-D; 0.08 mg/kg q8-12h PO), metronidazole (Flagyl; 15 mg/kg q12h PO), or tylosin (7 to 15 mg/kg q12h PO). Probiotics such as FortiFlora also can be considered as part of chronic therapy. Also, prevention of vomiting can have a positive impact on diarrhea. In dogs receiving DOX, treatment with maropitant also reduces the incidence and severity of diarrhea.

Mild adverse GI effects do not require dosage modification. Prophylactic GI support with bland diet, antiemetics, or subcutaneous fluids usually is adequate. A dosage reduction of 10% to 25% should be implemented if adverse GI effects are moderate to severe, especially if they necessitate hospitalization or do not resolve quickly with supportive care.

Cardiac Toxicity

In veterinary oncology, the cardiotoxic effects of DOX in dogs have been well established. The other anthracyclines and analogs used in small animals—epirubicin mitoxantrone, and liposomal DOX (Doxil)—are substantially less cardiotoxic.

Acute DOX cardiotoxicity manifests as transient arrhythmias resulting from transient increases in circulating histamines and catecholamines and usually is of little clinical significance. Cumulative cardiotoxicity manifests as a decrease in myocardial contractility with or without secondary arrhythmias, which often leads to congestive heart failure. The damage is irreversible and carries a grave prognosis. Cumulative cardiotoxicity is caused primarily by oxidative injury to the sarcoplasmic reticulum. The heart is particularly susceptible to oxidative injury because cardiac myocytes are rich in iron-containing proteins (such as myoglobin) that can donate their metal to catalyze strong oxidant formation. Additionally, cardiac tissue has limited ability to scavenge these free radicals: it has very low levels of catalase, and DOX causes a transient drop in the level of glutathione peroxidase.

In dogs with normal baseline myocardial function, the risk of cardiotoxicity increases with cumulative DOX doses above 180 to 240 mg/m^2. Clinical cardiotoxicity can occur at lower cumulative doses in dogs with underlying myocardial disease. A careful consideration of risk and benefit is warranted before administering DOX at high cumulative doses or to dogs with underlying myocardial disease. Dexrazoxane (Zinecard; 10 mg/1 mg of DOX IV) can be administered immediately before DOX to reduce its cardiotoxic effects substantially. In people, there is debate as to whether dexrazoxane can reduce the antitumor efficacy of DOX; results have been inconsistent.

Urinary Tract Toxicity

Cisplatin, ifosfamide, and streptozocin all are nephrotoxic and require intensive saline diuresis during administration. These drugs should not be administered to patients with renal insufficiency or failure. Serum creatinine concentration should be measured before each treatment, and these drugs should be discontinued if creatinine concentration becomes elevated. In cats specifically, DOX treatment is associated with cumulative nephrotoxicity.

However, the renal toxicity is neither as consistent nor as rapidly progressive as with the other nephrotoxic drugs mentioned. It can be used cautiously in cats with underlying renal disease as long as renal parameters are monitored closely. Carboplatin, although closely related to cisplatin, is not nephrotoxic. However, it is eliminated almost exclusively via passive glomerular filtration. Dosage modifications should be considered in patients with concurrent renal disease. Alternatively, in cats a dosing equation has been derived based on patient glomerular filtration rate.

Sterile hemorrhagic cystitis can occur secondary to treatment with cyclophosphamide or ifosfamide. Acrolein, an inactive metabolite, can cause direct contact irritation of the bladder mucosa. For dogs receiving standard doses of cyclophosphamide, concurrent administration of furosemide (2 mg/kg IV or SC) is recommended to dilute the acrolein and encourage frequent urination. For dogs receiving oral cyclophosphamide at home, owners should give the medication when they are able to take the dog outside regularly. Mesna (sodium 2-mercaptoethane sulfonate) binds to acrolein within the urinary bladder to help prevent irritation. It typically is not needed with standard cyclophosphamide dosages, but it is recommended with high-dose treatments (such as those used before whole body irradiation for canine lymphoma). Ifosfamide generates more acrolein than cyclophosphamide; administration of mesna is routinely recommended. Additionally, saline diuresis is required with ifosfamide to prevent nephrotoxicity. The risk of sterile hemorrhagic cystitis appears lower in cats than in dogs, likely due to differences in their urination behavior.

Treatment for sterile hemorrhagic cystitis is largely symptomatic. Clinical signs typically resolve over weeks to months, although they can be severe. Nonsteroidal antiinflammatory drugs are recommended to reduce inflammation and pain. Phenoxybenzamine (dogs: 0.25 mg/kg q8-12h PO) or oxybutynin (dogs: 0.2 to 0.3 mg/kg q8-12h PO) also can help alleviate muscle spasms. Additional pain medication should be used as needed. Cyclophosphamide and ifosfamide should be discontinued indefinitely in affected patients.

Hepatotoxicity

Lomustine is associated with hepatotoxicity. It usually is a cumulative toxicity, although acute hepatic failure can occur after a single treatment. In dogs with clinical hepatic failure, the most consistent and dramatic blood test abnormality is a marked elevation in the level of alanine aminotransferase (ALT). Therefore ALT should be measured before each lomustine treatment. Not every dog with an elevated ALT concentration develops clinical hepatic failure. However, if ALT level is four or more times the upper limit of the normal reference range, further treatment with lomustine should be discontinued unless there is a clear risk:benefit justification. Concurrent administration of Denamarin, a nutraceutical containing S-adenosylmethionine and silybin, decreases the risk that ALT will become elevated and reduces the magnitude of any elevations in ALT, aspartate aminotransferase, alkaline phosphatase, and bilirubin levels (Skorupski et al, 2011).

Hypersensitivity Reactions

Anaphylaxis can occur after administration of L-asparaginase, and the risk increases with sequential doses. Patients that have received L-asparaginase previously should be pretreated with diphenhydramine (2 mg/kg IM or SC) before each subsequent treatment, and they should be observed for at least 15 to 30 minutes after drug administration before being discharged from the hospital. DOX also can cause an anaphylactoid reaction. Rapid administration can cause non–immunoglobulin E–mediated mast cell degranulation. Pretreatment with diphenhydramine typically is not needed as long as the drug is administered over at least 20 to 30 minutes, although patients with a history of hypersensitivity should be premedicated.

Docetaxel, paclitaxel, and etoposide all can cause cutaneous hypersensitivities manifested by head shaking, flushing, pruritus, or urticaria. These reactions are mediated by the inert carriers polysorbate 80 (docetaxel and etoposide) and Cremophor EL (paclitaxel) needed to improve drug solubility. Cutaneous hypersensitivities can be reduced by pretreating with histamine-1 (H_1) and H_2 antagonists as well as glucocorticoids, and then administering the drugs as slow intravenous infusions over several hours. Docetaxel also can be administered orally (along with cyclosporine to improve oral bioavailability) to avoid cutaneous reactions, although the incidence of adverse GI effects increases.

Chemotherapeutic Drug Extravasation and Tissue Sloughing

Vincristine, vinblastine, vinorelbine, DOX, epirubicin, dactinomycin, and mustargen are vesicants. Mitoxantrone, cisplatin, dacarbazine, docetaxel, paclitaxel, and streptozocin are considered irritants. To minimize the risk of extravasation injuries, catheters must be placed cleanly on the first stick, using a vein that has not been punctured within the previous 24 hours. The patency of a catheter should be assessed by drawing back with a syringe, never by flushing since this can worsen an extravasation by depositing additional chemotherapy from the line into surrounding tissues. If an extravasation is suspected or confirmed, the chemotherapeutic drug should be aspirated as much as possible from the tissue, catheter, and line. Aspiration should continue while the catheter is removed. If a subcutaneous blister persists, additional aspirations can be performed using a new needle and syringe each time. Moist compresses and occlusive bandages should not be used because they can further spread the extravasated drug and worsen tissue damage. Drug-specific antidotes are listed in the following paragraphs.

It can take up to 1 to 2 weeks for the full extent of the tissue injury from an extravasation to become evident. A tissue slough should be treated like any other open wound with débriding as needed, pain medications, and antibiotic therapy. In severe cases, amputation might be required.

Vincristine, Vinblastine, Vinorelbine

Immediately after extravasation of vincristine, vinblastine, or vinorelbine, 6 ml of saline can be infused around the affected area, divided into four to six small injections and using a new needle for each one. The addition of sodium hyaluronidase (150 U/1 ml of extravasated drug) to the saline has been reported, but it is not widely available. Warm compresses should be applied to the affected site four times a day, 1 hour initially and then 20 minutes all subsequent times, for 3 to 5 days. A solution of dimethyl sulfoxide (DMSO) and fluocinolone acetonide (Synotic) mixed with 10 mg flunixin meglumine (Banamine) should be applied topically after each heat application.

Doxorubicin, Epirubicin, Dactinomycin

When the extravasated drug is doxorubicin, epirubicin, or dactinomycin, cold compresses should be applied to the affected site four times a day, 1 hour initially and then 20 minutes all subsequent times, for 3 to 5 days. Topical application of DMSO is of questionable benefit. Specifically for DOX, dexrazoxane (10 mg/1 mg DOX) substantially reduces the extent of tissue damage. It is administered intravenously immediately after the extravasation occurs and then ideally again 24 and 48 hours later.

Mustargen

For mustargen extravasation, sodium thiosulfate (0.17 mol/l, or 2.5%) should be administered through the catheter before it is removed, or it can be injected directly into the affected site after the catheter is removed. The volume injected should be equal to the volume of the intended mustargen dose.

Cat-Specific Toxicities

Cisplatin should not be given intravenously to cats because of the potential for fatal pulmonary edema. Intralesional administration is tolerated, but carboplatin is a more rational choice. The use of 5-fluorouracil is contraindicated because of the high incidence of fatal neurotoxicity with systemic or topical use.

References and Suggested Reading

Chun R, Garrett LD, Vail DM: Cancer chemotherapy. In Withrow SJ, Vail DM, editors: *Withrow and MacEwen's small animal clinical oncology*, ed 4, St Louis, 2001, Saunders, p 163.

Mealey KL et al: ABCB1-1Delta polymorphism can predict hematologic toxicity in dogs treated with vincristine, *J Vet Intern Med* 22:996, 2008.

Rau SE, Barber LG, Burgess KE: Efficacy of maropitant in the prevention of delayed vomiting associated with administration of doxorubicin to dogs, *J Vet Intern Med* 24:1452, 2010.

Skorupski KA et al: Prospective randomized clinical trial assessing efficacy of Denamarin for prevention of CCNU-induced hepatopathy in tumor-bearing dogs, *J Vet Intern Med* 25:838, 2011.

Vail DM et al: Efficacy of injectable maropitant (Cerenia) in a randomized clinical trial for prevention and treatment of cisplatin-induced emesis in dogs presented as veterinary patients, *Vet Comp Oncol* 5:38, 2007.

Veterinary Cooperative Oncology Group—common terminology criteria for adverse events (VCOG-CTCAE) following chemotherapy or biological antineoplastic therapy in dogs and cats v1.1, *Vet Comp Oncol*. Epub July 2011.

CHAPTER 73

Cancer Immunotherapy

LEAH ANN MITCHELL, *Fort Collins, Colorado*
AMANDA GUTH, *Fort Collins, Colorado*
STEVEN DOW, *Fort Collins, Colorado*

The field of cancer immunotherapy continues to evolve, and the past decade has witnessed several important breakthroughs in both the human and veterinary oncology fields. Monoclonal antibodies designed to block specific signaling pathways in tumor cells (e.g., trastuzumab [Herceptin]), to deplete malignant lymphoma cells (e.g., rituximab [Rituxan]), and to alter T-cell signaling (e.g., ipilimumab [Yervoy]) represent major advances in cancer immunotherapy. Although monoclonal antibodies are not yet available for targeted immunotherapy in veterinary medicine, a canine lymphoma–targeting antibody is expected soon. One notable recent advance in veterinary cancer immunotherapy is the development and approval of the first canine cancer vaccine (Oncept), which targets a melanoma antigen (tyrosinase) for immune recognition by T cells.

As the field of cancer immunotherapy advances, progress can be expected on several fronts. First, there is likely to be a continued focus on the development of new monoclonal antibodies targeting either tumor cells directly or key immune-regulatory molecules. Second, a number of new cancer vaccines currently are under development, most targeting tumor antigens that are shared by tumors of a certain histotype or in some cases by different tumor types. Third, there is also increasing emphasis on immune interventions designed to modify the immunosuppressive tumor microenvironment, including and especially tumor-associated macrophages.

Nonspecific Tumor Immunotherapy

Most cancer immunotherapeutics currently available in veterinary medicine are designed to activate multiple components of the innate immune system nonspecifically to generate antitumor immunity. Natural killer cells, macrophages, and dendritic cells are the primary effector cells responsible for generating antitumor activity following administration of nonspecific immune activators. Release of innate immune cytokines, especially interferon-α (IFN-α) and IFN-γ, also contributes significantly to antitumor activity by suppressing tumor cell growth and by inhibiting tumor angiogenesis. There is generally only a minor T-cell contribution to antitumor immunity following administration of nonspecific tumor immunotherapeutics.

Systemic Tumor Immunotherapy Using Toll-like Receptor and Nod-like Receptor Agonists

Most nonspecific cancer immunotherapeutics stimulate the innate immune system by activating Toll-like receptors (TLRs) or Nod (nucleotide-binding oligomerization domain)–like receptors (NLRs). The TLRs and their activating ligands with greatest relevance to cancer immunotherapy are TLR3 (activated by double-stranded RNA from viruses), TLR4 (activated by lipopolysaccharide), TLR7 and TLR8 (activated by viral nucleic acids and synthetic molecules such as imiquimod), and TLR9 (activated by bacterial DNA). NLRs are expressed primarily in the cytoplasm of immune and nonimmune cells and recognize bacterial cell wall peptides (Nod1 and Nod2) as well as viral nucleic acids (retinoic acid–inducible gene [Rig-I] and nucleotide-binding oligomerization domain, leucine-rich repeat, and pyrin domain containing [NLRP]), and in some cases eukaryotic DNA and uric acid and NACHT-, LRR-, and PYD-containing proteins (NALPs).

Liposome-encapsulated muramyl tripeptide phosphatidylethanolamine (L-MTP-PE) is a Nod2 agonist. L-MTP-PE has been evaluated previously as an immunotherapeutic for prevention of metastases from osteosarcoma and hemangiosarcoma (MacEwen et al, 1999). L-MTP-PE triggers activation of macrophages in the lungs and other tissues and generates production of tumor necrosis factor-α and other innate immune cytokines. Repeated intravenous administration of L-MTP-PE has been shown to prolong survival times significantly in dogs with osteosarcoma and hemangiosarcoma and is roughly equivalent to chemotherapy in overall effectiveness.

Systemic administration of cationic liposomes complexed to bacterial plasmid DNA (CLDC) triggers potent activation of innate immunity in dogs with cancer, presumably primarily by stimulating activation of TLR9. CLDC immunotherapy was shown to activate innate immunity in dogs with metastatic osteosarcoma and significantly improved overall survival times in treated dogs compared with untreated control animals (Dow et al, 2005). In addition, CLDC administration was associated with significant inhibition of tumor angiogenesis. Currently CLDC immunotherapy is being developed in Europe for the veterinary market.

Systemic administration of live attenuated bacteria (primarily engineered *Salmonella*) also has been evaluated as a novel cancer immunotherapy. The engineered *Salmonella* localizes to the hypoxic tumor environment following intravenous administration (Thamm et al, 2005). This approach, in some cases, generated local control of tumor growth or tumor regression, presumably mediated by local activation of innate immunity.

Recombinant Cytokine Therapy

Natural killer cells and T cells can be activated by systemic administration of high doses of immune-stimulatory cytokines, primarily interleukin-2 (IL-2) and IFN-α. Immunotherapy with recombinant IL-2 is approved for treatment of melanoma and renal cell carcinoma in humans. Infusions of human IL-2 have been assessed in clinical trials in dogs with advanced cancer and have been reported to produce systemic immune activation (fever) and some antitumor activity. Although human recombinant IFN-α (Roferon, others) is administered systemically at high doses for treatment of melanoma and renal cell carcinoma in humans, the drug rarely is administered at high doses in companion animals for treatment of cancer. However, recombinant IFN-α has been used for treatment of certain oral malignancies in cats, including squamous cell carcinoma.

Local Immunotherapy with Toll-like Receptor Agonists

Imiquimod (Aldara) is a recent example of a locally administered TLR agonist. For cancer immunotherapy, imiquimod is administered as a topical cream, which triggers activation of TLR7 and TLR8 receptors in the skin and thereby leads to stimulation of cutaneous innate immune responses. Imiquimod has demonstrated modest efficacy when applied topically in cats with cutaneous squamous cell carcinoma *in situ*. Acemannan, an immunotherapeutic agent prepared from the aloe plant, likely activates several TLRs, including TLR2 and possibly TLR4. The drug has been reported to induce partial tumor regression following injection into fibrosarcoma tumors in dogs. A live attenuated strain of *Mycobacterium bovis* (bacille Calmette-Guérin [BCG]) has been used extensively in humans as an intravesicular agent for the treatment of early bladder cancer. There are reports of the use of BCG in dogs with bladder cancer, mast cell tumors, and osteosarcoma. A heat-killed preparation of *Propionibacterium acnes* (ImmunoVet) induces nonspecific activation of innate immunity when injected locally and has been evaluated for the treatment of several different tumor types in dogs.

Tumor Vaccines

Unlike nonspecific immunotherapy, tumor vaccines are designed to activate populations of tumor-specific T cells, including both CD4 and CD8 T cells. The advantage of generating a strong T-cell response is the ability to control growth of both the local tumor and tumor metastases. However, there are a number of hurdles to overcome in developing successful tumor vaccines, including identification of immunogenic and widely expressed tumor antigens, development of effective vaccine adjuvant and delivery systems, and design of effective immunization protocols.

A canine DNA-based vaccine encoding the human tyrosinase 2 gene (Oncept) is the first approved veterinary vaccine for cancer. The Oncept vaccine is delivered by a series of four repeated intradermal injections of plasmid DNA encoding the human tyrosinase gene. Adverse effects related to vaccination have been reported to be mild, consisting primarily of bruising and pain at the vaccination site. Several studies have demonstrated the safety of the Oncept vaccine and have provided evidence of induction of humoral immunity in tumor-bearing dogs and cellular immunity in normal dogs. The vaccine was approved by the U.S. Department of Agriculture (USDA) based on safety studies and anecdotal reports of tumor regression in vaccinated dogs. A recent follow-up study compared survival times in dogs with melanoma receiving the Oncept vaccine with survival times in historical control populations. In this study, survival times were significantly improved in dogs that received the vaccine compared with historical controls (Grosenbaugh et al, 2011). The efficacy of the Oncept vaccine has yet to be demonstrated in a randomized clinical trial.

Lymphoma Vaccines and Immunotherapies in Development

In 1992 the USDA approved CL/mAb 231, a murine monoclonal antibody shown to bind to the surface of over 75% of canine lymphomas, for use in dogs with lymphoma as adjuvant therapy following chemotherapy-induced remission. However, subsequent studies found that administration of CL/mAb 231 did not increase survival times of dogs with lymphoma and production of the drug was discontinued. Nonetheless, production of the antibody recently has resumed, and CL/mAb 231 may reemerge as a new chemoimmunotherapy product in veterinary medicine. ImmuneFx was introduced in 2008 as an autologous lymphoma vaccine that uses lymphoma cells transfected with a bacterial antigen. Although ImmuneFx was found to be safe and to induce measurable antitumor humoral and cellular immune responses, studies have not demonstrated improvement in overall survival times. A second autologous lymphoma vaccine using lymphoma cells transfected with human granulocyte-macrophage colony-stimulating factor DNA also was evaluated in dogs and showed enhancement of antitumor immunity without improving survival times (Turek et al, 2007).

Macrophage Depletion Therapy

Recent studies suggest that tumor growth also can be controlled by selective removal of certain immune cell

TABLE 73-1

Immunotherapeutic Options for Veterinary Cancer Patients

Drug	Mechanism of Action	Indications	Manufacturer	Dosing	Adverse Effects
Biological Response Modifiers					
Bacille Calmette-Guérin (BCG)	Live attenuated *M. bovis* promotes inflammatory response	Mast cell tumor, osteosarcoma, bladder tumors	Tice	BCG 50-250 × 10⁶ CFU IV or intralesional, 0.2 ml q24h SC	Lethargy and fever, lymph node enlargement
Corynebacterium parvum (ImmunoRegulin)	Heat killed *Propionibacterium acnes*; nonspecific immunostimulant	Mammary carcinoma, melanoma, squamous cell carcinoma	Immunovet	0.03-0.06 ml/kg IV weekly or as needed	Fever
Salmonella typhimurium VNP20009 (Tapet)	Activation of innate immunity	Melanoma	Vion Pharmaceuticals	3 × 10⁷ CFU/kg IV weekly or as needed	Liver enzyme elevation, splenic enlargement
L-MTP-PE	Activation of innate immunity	Osteosarcoma, hemangiosarcoma, mammary carcinoma	Takeda	1-2 mg/m² IV twice weekly	Fever
Imiquimod (Aldara, others)	Activation of innate immunity	Squamous cell carcinoma	Meda, Graceway, iNova	5% Topical daily as needed	Skin irritation
Acemannan	Activation of innate immunity	Fibrosarcoma	Carrington Labs	IP (1 mg/kg) or intralesional (2 mg) weekly	Tissue necrosis
Cationic liposomes with TLR ligands	Activation of innate immunity	Soft tissue sarcoma, osteosarcoma lung metastases	In development	20 µg DNA/kg IV weekly to every other week	Lethargy and fever
Liposomal clodronate	Depletion of immunosuppressive macrophages; direct killing of MH cells	Soft tissue sarcoma, malignant histiocytosis	FormuMax	0.5 ml/kg IV weekly or every other week	Fever
Piroxicam (Feldene, others)	Immunomodulatory properties; direct antitumor effects	Transitional cell carcinoma, squamous cell carcinoma, hemangiosarcoma, prostatic carcinoma, rectal neoplasms	Pfizer	0.1-0.3 mg/kg q24h PO (dog)	GI ulceration, nephrotoxicity
Recombinant Cytokines/Growth Factors					
Hu rIFN α (Roferon-a, others)	Enhancement of cell-mediated immunity, NK and T cell activity	Mast cell tumor, preputial epitheliotropic lymphoma	Roche/Virbac	2.5 million units/kg SC weekly	Anemia, hepatotoxicity
Feline IFN-omega (Virbagen)	Activation of antiviral activity		Virbac	Cats: 1 million units/kg once IV daily for 5 consecutive days. Usually, 3 separate 5 day treatments are performed on day 0, 14, and 60 Dogs: 2.5 million units/kg, IV once daily for 3 consecutive days	Anemia
Hu rIL-2 (Proleukin, others)	T cell proliferation and survival	Soft tissue sarcoma, melanoma	Chiron/ Hoffman-La Roche, others	1-3 MU/m² IV weekly	Capillary leak, anemia, fever, hypotension
Cancer Vaccines					
Oncept	Induction of immunity to melanoma antigen	Melanoma	Merial	1 Vial IM once every 2 weeks	Bruising, pain at injection site

populations, especially immune-suppressive myeloid cells (Gabrilovich and Nagaraj, 2009). For example, tumor-associated macrophages and certain circulating myeloid cell populations are, in fact, potent inhibitors of tumor immunity. These myeloid cell populations are greatly expanded in patients with cancer and can suppress tumor immunity via a variety of different mechanisms, most of which affect T-cell responses. In addition, expanded populations of tumor-associated macrophages can stimulate tumor angiogenesis, trigger tumor genomic instability, and enhance tumor metastasis.

Our laboratory has shown recently that the myeloid cell–depleting agent, liposomal clodronate, can be used to deplete tumor-associated macrophages in dogs with soft tissue sarcoma (Guth et al, n.d.). We have also shown that liposomal clodronate kills malignant macrophages and can induce tumor regression in dogs with malignant histiocytosis (Hafeman et al, 2010). Thus depletion of phagocytic myeloid cells, or blocking of their entry into tumor tissues, represents a new approach to tumor immunotherapy.

Depletion of Regulatory T Cells

Regulatory T (Treg) cells normally function to suppress spontaneous autoimmunity, but in animals with cancer Treg populations are greatly expanded, which leads to marked suppression of tumor immunity. Dogs with cancer have significantly increased numbers of Treg cells in circulation and in tumor-draining lymph nodes (Biller et al, 2010). In addition, dogs with osteosarcoma with higher Treg numbers have reduced survival times compared with disease-matched dogs with lower Treg numbers.

Certain chemotherapy drugs can deplete Treg cells in addition to having direct antitumor effects. For example, metronomic dosing of cyclophosphamide can reduce circulating Treg populations in dogs with soft tissue sarcoma (Burton et al, 2011). In addition, the oral kinase inhibitor toceranib (Palladia) was reported recently to reduce circulating Treg cells in dogs with a variety of cancers (Mitchell et al, 2012). The reduction in Treg numbers in dogs treated with toceranib also correlated with increased concentrations of IFN-γ, which suggests that immune function was enhanced by depletion of Treg cells. Finally, dogs with lymphoma also had marked reductions in the number of circulating Treg cells after treatment with doxorubicin. The reduction of Treg numbers in doxorubicin-treated dogs with lymphoma was accompanied by evidence of improved cytotoxic T-cell activity.

Summary

These are exciting times for the field of veterinary cancer immunotherapy because advances in our understanding of tumor immunity have generated a variety of new potential approaches to cancer treatment. (Those discussed here are outlined in Table 73-1). Moreover, these new advances often are translated to clinical trials in veterinary patients sooner than in the past. The major advances in the field over the next decade are likely to come in several areas, including the implementation of canine monoclonal antibody therapy, the development of new cancer vaccines, and the use of drugs to selectively block or deplete immunosuppressive cell populations.

References and Suggested Reading

Biller BJ et al: Decreased ratio of CD8[+] T cells to regulatory T cells associated with decreased survival in dogs with osteosarcoma, *J Vet Intern Med* 24:1118, 2010.

Burton JH et al: Low-dose cyclophosphamide selectively decreases regulatory T cells and inhibits angiogenesis in dogs with soft tissue sarcoma, *J Vet Intern Med* 25:920, 2011.

Dow S et al: Phase I study of liposome-DNA complexes encoding the interleukin-2 gene in dogs with osteosarcoma lung metastases, *Hum Gene Ther* 16:937, 2005.

Gabrilovich DI, Nagaraj S: Myeloid-derived suppressor cells as regulators of the immune system, *Nat Rev Immunol* 9:162, 2009.

Grosenbaugh DA et al: Safety and efficacy of a xenogeneic DNA vaccine encoding for human tyrosinase as adjunctive treatment for oral malignant melanoma in dogs following surgical excision of the primary tumor, *Am J Vet Res* 72:1631, 2011.

Guth AM et al: Liposomal clodronate treatment for tumour macrophage depletion in dogs with soft-tissue sarcoma, *Vet Comp Oncol* 2012 epub.

Hafeman S et al: Evaluation of liposomal clodronate for treatment of malignant histiocytosis in dogs, *Cancer Immunol Immunother* 59:441, 2010.

MacEwen EG et al: Adjuvant therapy for melanoma in dogs: results of randomized clinical trials using surgery, liposome-encapsulated muramyl tripeptide, and granulocyte macrophage colony-stimulating factor, *Clin Cancer Res* 5:4249, 1999.

Mitchell L, Thamm DH, Biller BJ: Clinical and immunomodulatory effects of toceranib combined with low-dose cyclophosphamide in dogs with cancer, *J Vet Intern Med* 26:355, 2012.

Thamm DH et al: Systemic administration of an attenuated, tumor-targeting *Salmonella typhimurium* to dogs with spontaneous neoplasia: phase I evaluation, *Clin Cancer Res* 11:4827, 2005.

Turek MM et al: Human granulocyte-macrophage colony-stimulating factor DNA cationic-lipid complexed autologous tumour cell vaccination in the treatment of canine B-cell multicentric lymphoma, *Vet Comp Oncol* 5:219, 2007.

CHAPTER 74

Advances in Radiation Therapy for Nasal Tumors

JAMES T. CUSTIS III, *Fort Collins, Colorado*
SUSAN M. LARUE, *Fort Collins, Colorado*

Nasosinal tumors always have presented a therapeutic challenge. Surgery alone rarely is an option due to local macroscopic and microscopic extension to critical normal tissue structures, and combining surgery with radiation therapy has not uniformly improved treatment outcome. Chemotherapy, including the use of nonsteroidal antiinflammatory drugs, has been reported as a palliative option. Radiation therapy long has been considered the standard of care despite the significant acute effects associated with treatment. Disappointingly, the collective median survival times for patients treated with radiation therapy have not improved since early data were reported in the 1980s.

The introduction of two new radiation-associated technologies now available in veterinary medicine already has decreased acute radiation effects in these patients, and ongoing work is evaluating the impact on long-term tumor control. These technologies are (1) intensity-modulated radiation therapy (IMRT), which, by using inverse treatment-planning algorithms, allows for more precise application of radiation dose to the tumor and preferentially spares adjacent normal tissue structures in the region; and (2) stereotactic radiation therapy (SRT), which delivers curative-intent radiation therapy according to protocols that require only one to five fractions. This chapter focuses on treatment advances associated with these technologies.

Pathologic Features and Clinical Presentation

Nasosinal tumors represent 1% of all canine neoplasia. Carcinomas, including adenocarcinomas, solid tumors, and squamous cell carcinomas, represent 60% of these tumors; sarcomas, including fibrosarcomas, chondrosarcomas, and osteosarcomas, make up approximately 30% of all nasal tumors. Lymphoma, mast cell tumors, transmissible venereal tumors, hemangiosarcomas, neuroendocrine tumors, and histocytic sarcomas are seen less frequently. Most nasal tumors are locally invasive and generally have not metastasized at the time of diagnosis. These tumors occur most commonly in middle-aged to older dogs, and dolichocephalic breeds may be overrepresented. Clinical signs include intermittent and progressive history of unilateral or bilateral mucopurulent discharge or epistaxis. Stertorous breathing, sneezing, reverse sneezing, and dyspnea can be observed. Facial deformity caused by bone erosion and tumor extension outside of the bone as well as exophthalmos also can be seen. Neurologic signs may occur in cases with lysis of the cribriform plate and tumor extension into the cranial vault. Initial signs may respond to antibiotics or steroids, which can prolong the time until an accurate diagnosis is established.

Diagnostic Approach

Differential diagnoses include fungal or bacterial infection, lymphocytic-plasmacytic rhinitis, bleeding disorders, and foreign bodies. Nasal radiographs may define changes in the nasal cavities and sinuses, but cross-sectional imaging (computed tomography [CT] or magnetic resonance imaging [MRI]) is preferred. Histologic confirmation is required for definitive diagnosis, although classic changes observed on CT or MRI scans combined with history and clinical signs are highly suggestive. The patient should be evaluated for potential coagulopathies before biopsy because postprocedure bleeding can be significant. The CT or MRI should be performed before biopsy to identify the optimal site from which to procure a specimen and to prevent postbiopsy bleeding from complicating the interpretation of the imaging study. A number of biopsy techniques have been described in the literature. Transnostril techniques are advantageous because they do not create a biopsy track that will have to be addressed if the patient is to be treated with surgery or radiation therapy. When this technique is used, one should make sure that the biopsy instrument is marked so that it penetrates no further than the medial canthus, which minimizes the risk to the cribriform plate and brain. Rhinoscopic techniques are minimally traumatic; however, even experienced operators can be frustrated by the inability to obtain a sample of sufficient quality and quantity for diagnosis. Nasal hydropulsion was reported recently as a minimally invasive technique that yielded samples from which a definitive diagnosis could be made in 90.2% of attempts (Ashbaugh et al, 2011). Although these tumors are unlikely to have metastatic spread, thoracic radiographs should be included in staging if radiation therapy is being considered as a treatment option.

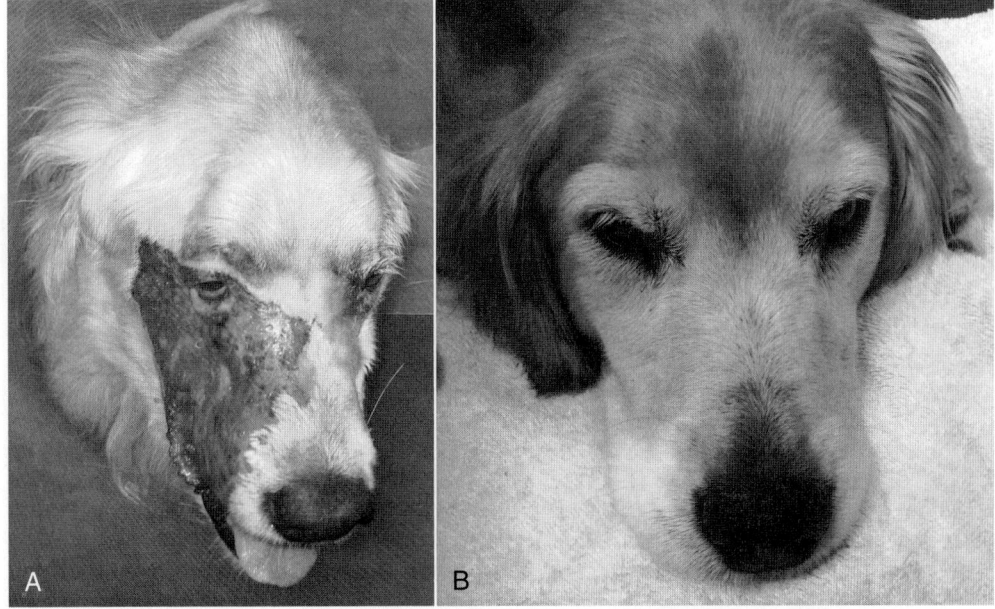

Figure 74-1 Two patients with similar-sized right-sided nasal tumors, each having completed a course of radiation therapy. The typical distribution of moist desquamation resulting from 3DCRT **(A)**, and the absence of observable clinical signs following IMRT **(B)**.

Treatment and Prognosis

Survival following treatment with traditional fractionated radiation therapy, including three-dimensional conformal radiation therapy (3DCRT), administered with curative intent ranges from 6 to 20 months. Given that the number of dogs evaluated in each study is small and the techniques vary dramatically (in type of radiation, fractionation schedule, immobilization device), it is hard to discern prognostic indicators. However, squamous cell carcinomas, undifferentiated carcinomas, and anaplastic carcinomas have been reported to be associated with survival times of 6 to 7 months. Any type of tumor that has eroded the cribriform plate and has extended into the brain likely is associated with poor long-term outcome. Although generally effective, conventionally fractionated 3DCRT is associated with severe acute radiation effects that require aggressive pain management and supportive care (Figure 74-1).

Two recent publications reported that dogs treated with IMRT experienced median survival times of over 420 days (Hunley et al, 2010; Lawrence et al, 2010). More significantly, the acute radiation toxicity was minimal. IMRT and related modalities such as tomotherapy allow sculpting of radiation dose by the use of inverse treatment-planning technology. Patient positioning and immobilization strategies are important to minimize interfractionation treatment error. IMRT controls the intensity of each beam through motorized collimator leaves that move during treatment, which allows the dose to be sculpted around important normal structures (Figure 74-2). Inverse planning requires that the tumor as well as critical normal tissue structures be identified. This is achieved by outlining (contouring) each structure of interest on each slice of the CT scan. Dose objectives for each structure are entered, and a sophisticated algorithm attempts to meet all objectives. With IMRT, the dose to adjacent normal tissue structures can be minimized, which dramatically reduces acute effects, while at the same time the radiation dose to the tumor can be increased, which improves the probability of tumor control.

SRT involves the use of high dose per fraction radiation but overcomes the radiobiologic limitations with stereotactically verified positioning and treatment delivery techniques that leave a minimal volume of normal tissue in the high-dose area. SRT, by definition, requires (1) a tumor for targeting (it is not acceptable for treatment of microscopic disease); (2) treatment planning and administration that will achieve a steep dose gradient between the tumor and the surrounding normal tissue structures; and (3) a method of stereotactically verifying patient positioning. The result is that normal late-responding tissue structures are spared through dose avoidance rather than by administration of small doses per fraction. However, the normal tissue structures still receive dose, and the dose per fraction is higher than with traditional radiation therapy. This technique is appealing because only one to five fractions of radiation are required, and treatments are generally well tolerated by the patient. A number of different systems have been developed for SRT including the Gamma Knife, the CyberKnife, and linear accelerator–based systems such as the Varian Trilogy. As with IMRT, acute radiation effects are minimized with this technique. For 29 dogs treated with three fractions of SRT, median survival exceeded 400 days (Custis, 2012). Long-term studies to evaluate tumor control and late effects are ongoing.

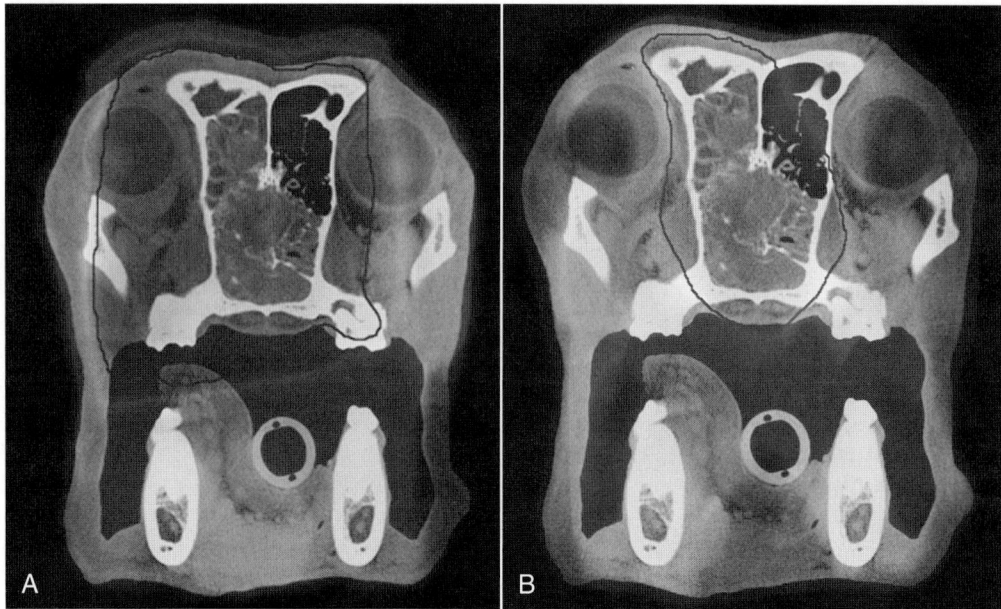

Figure 74-2 3DCRT **(A)** and IMRT **(B)** treatment plans of the same nasal tumor. The black line reflects the 100% isodose line. Note the preferential sparing of the·eyes achieved with IMRT.

Feline Tumors

Nasal lymphoma is the most commonly observed nasosinal tumor in the cat, followed by carcinoma and sarcoma. Clinical signs are similar to those seen in dogs and mimic signs associated with rhinitis. Small surgical curettes used intranasally or endoscopic techniques often are used to obtain biopsy specimens. These tumors are locally invasive but generally have not metastasized at the time of diagnosis; however, any enlarged regional lymph node should be aspirated, and thoracic radiography also should be part of staging. Radiation therapy is considered the standard of care; response rate is high and treatment is well tolerated (Theon et al, 1994). Systemic failure at nonnodal sites has been reported, but the role of systemic chemotherapy has not been determined.

Future Directions

The future for the treatment of nasal tumors in dogs and cats has arrived. Integration of positron emission tomography (PET) and CT into radiation therapy planning may improve tumor delineation and aid in monitoring response to therapy. Studies evaluating the usefulness and efficacy of PET and CT are under way. Currently IMRT and SRT offer the hope of better tumor control with fewer acute side effects.

References and Suggested Reading

Ashbaugh EA et al: Nasal hydropulsion: a novel tumor biopsy technique, *J Am Anim Hosp Assoc* 47:312, 2011.

Custis J: Unpublished data, 2012.

Hunley DW et al: Clinical outcome in dogs with nasal tumors treated with intensity-modulated radiation therapy, *Can Vet J* 51:292, 2010.

LaRue SM, Gordon I: Radiation therapy. In Withrow SJ, Vail DM, Page R, editors: *Withrow and MacEwen's small animal clinical oncology*, ed 5, St Louis, 2012, Saunders.

Lawrence JA et al: Proof of principle of ocular sparing in dogs with sinonasal tumors treated with intensity-modulated radiation therapy, *J Vet Radiol Ultrasound* 51:561, 2010.

Theon AP et al: Irradiation of nonlymphoproliferative neoplasms of the nasal cavity and paranasal sinuses in 16 cats, *J Am Vet Med Assoc* 204:78, 1994.

Turek MM, Lana SE: Nasosinal tumors. In Withrow SJ, Vail DM, Page R, editors: *Withrow and MacEwen's small animal clinical oncology*, ed 5, St Louis, 2012, Saunders.

CHAPTER 75

Malignant Effusions

ANTONY S. MOORE, *Wauchope, Australia*

Effusions that affect the pleural, abdominal, or pericardial spaces in cancer patients may be caused directly by the effects of the malignancy itself or indirectly by the exacerbation of cardiac disease or the occurrence of infection, bleeding, or rupture of an organ precipitated by the cancer. Malignant effusions are protein-rich exudates that occur in a variety of cancers; when malignant effusion is present it is a major cause of morbidity and mortality. Reported clinical signs include abdominal pain, inappetence and nausea, cachexia, fatigue, and dyspnea leading to decreased activity and reduced exercise intolerance. The types of cancer associated with malignant effusion are similar in dogs and cats. Effusions caused by lymphoma are common in both species; carcinoma-associated effusions (carcinomatosis) resulting from metastasis of mammary, ovarian, pulmonary, urothelial, hepatic, or gastrointestinal carcinomas are the next most common. Malignant effusions caused by sarcomas are rare but may be seen with metastatic lesions in the lungs or abdominal organs. Mesothelioma is another cause of malignant effusion in dogs and cats and may affect pleural, peritoneal, or pericardial spaces. In some veterinary patients, malignant effusions may be identified as the principal problem and a primary cancer may not be identified immediately (unknown primary). In a study of human patients with malignant ascites from an unknown primary tumor, laparoscopy with biopsy was able to disclose a primary site in 86% (Chu et al, 1994), so further investigation certainly is warranted in such patients because a definitive tissue diagnosis often allows more precise or targeted therapies.

Most malignant effusions are not the reason for initial presentation to a veterinarian but develop in the later stages of advanced malignancy and often signal metastatic disease that is advanced and incurable. In humans the average survival time for patients with malignant effusions is 5 months; patients with unknown primary tumors have the worst prognosis, and better survivals are reported for those who have chemotherapy-responsive neoplasia such as lymphoma and ovarian carcinoma. Similarly, in dogs and cats the most responsive malignant effusions are those associated with lymphoma, for which multiagent chemotherapy produces a response in the majority of patients, although true cures are rare. Responses to treatment leading to resolution or marked reduction in effusion, sometimes long term, also have been seen in patients with carcinomatosis and mesothelioma.

Pathophysiology

The traditional view of the physiology of malignant effusions is that invasion of lymphatic vessels by tumor cells leads to lymphatic obstruction, which in turn is exacerbated by increases in vascular and lymphatic permeability. The end result is increased fluid production with decreased fluid removal leading to accumulation. This view is supported by lymphoscintigraphy that demonstrates decreased lymphatic flow in such patients. Additionally, metastases to lymph nodes (e.g., hilar lymph nodes) may obstruct lymphatic flow, and direct implantation of tumor cells on the mesothelial surfaces results in inflammation as well as obstruction of drainage.

In addition to decreased removal of fluid by lymphatics, there is an increase in fluid production that is mediated by angiogenesis. In the early 1980s it was demonstrated that cell-free malignant ascitic fluid led to increased capillary permeability and increases in omental edema. The factor responsible (originally called *vascular permeability factor,* now known as *vascular endothelial growth factor* [VEGF]) is produced by tumor cells, mesothelial cells, macrophages, monocytes, and tumor-infiltrating T lymphocytes. Not only does VEGF induce the proliferation of new vasculature, which is more permeable than normal vessels, it also increases the permeability of existing vasculature. Therefore VEGF is responsible for both initiating and maintaining production of ascitic or pleural fluid in a wide range of cancers. When this is coupled with decreases in lymphatic drainage, it is easy to see how malignant effusions are able to arise and re-form so rapidly. It has been shown that the total volume of ascitic fluid correlates directly with the concentration of VEGF in that fluid. In addition, the concentration of VEGF in the effusion also is correlated with both response to therapy and survival in human studies (Rudlowski et al, 2006). In dogs with pleural, pericardial, and abdominal effusions, VEGF concentrations have been shown to be elevated in the effusions. Concentrations are similar in both malignant and nonmalignant effusions, so VEGF concentration is not helpful in distinguishing the *cause* of an effusion; however, the elevation in VEGF concentration substantiates the potential role of inhibitors of VEGF signaling in the palliation of malignant effusions (Clifford et al, 2002).

Diagnosis

In many patients the malignant effusion arises after the primary tumor has been diagnosed and possibly after surgery, radiation therapy, or chemotherapy. In such patients in which a histologic diagnosis already is confirmed, palliative measures to relieve symptoms associated with the effusion should be implemented, and then further treatment options appropriate to the primary tumor should be evaluated and discussed with the owner.

In patients in which the presentation with effusion precedes a definitive diagnosis, the primary objective should be to stabilize the patient's condition because many dogs and cats with pleural effusion are in a delicate state and may not tolerate manipulations even for imaging studies. This is less true of pets with abdominal effusion than of those with pericardial or thoracic effusion, although complete assessment of the circulatory and respiratory systems is important. Fluid removal by needle centesis may be needed before more specific investigations are undertaken; however, samples collected at the time should be put aside for analysis. Investigations should focus on obtaining a cytologic or histologic diagnosis, which can help in selecting therapeutic options, as well as palliation of the effusion itself. If there is diffuse involvement with implanted cancer cells on the parietal and visceral surfaces, the resulting effusion is more likely to contain malignant cells. Therefore cancer cells are more likely to be found in ascitic or pleural fluid of patients with carcinomatosis (97%) than in the fluid of patients with lymphoma and those with deep visceral (e.g., pulmonary or liver) metastases.

Once the patient with suspected malignant effusion is in stable condition, fluid can be submitted for evaluation by a veterinary cytopathologist. Chylous effusions may be present in lymphoma. Routine cytologic examination may not provide a definitive diagnosis, but immunocytochemical testing using markers such as CD3 and CD79a (or other B-lymphocyte markers), as well as stains for intermediate filaments (e.g., cytokeratins, which are markers for epithelium-derived cells), may allow at least a narrowing of the diagnosis to lymphoma or carcinoma. Reactive mesothelial cells are found in most malignant effusions, regardless of cause, and may be difficult to distinguish from malignant mesothelial cells (mesothelioma). Additional investigations include polymerase chain reaction testing for antigen receptor rearrangements or flow cytometry in patients with suspected lymphoma.

When fluid is present, particularly when there is a large volume, radiography may not be helpful in identifying a primary site, but ultrasonography can assist in guiding fluid sample collection, safe removal of a volume of fluid for palliation, and potentially identification of an underlying neoplasm. In the latter case, ultrasonographically guided needle aspiration or biopsy may allow a histologic diagnosis.

Thoracoscopy and laparoscopy may be minimally invasive methods of obtaining a specimen for tissue diagnosis when there are no obvious masses on ultrasonography and a parietal or visceral surface tumor is suspected. The advantage is minimal morbidity, although invasion of mesothelioma cells along a thoracoscopy tract has been reported in people and in one dog (Brisson et al, 2006). To put this in context, surgical exploration to obtain a biopsy specimen also would carry a risk of tumor cell seeding, and even centesis poses some risk of seeding of mesothelioma. Minimally invasive techniques also may allow concurrent therapeutic and palliative procedures (e.g., pericardectomy) to be performed.

Treatment

Palliative Treatment

The use of diuretics has been reported anecdotally in the treatment of ascites in humans, but to date there is no evidence that such therapy actually is palliative in humans or in veterinary patients.

Needle centesis is a simple, low-cost procedure that can be repeated as needed; however, as the disease progresses the frequency of centesis must be increased, which has a much greater impact on the patient's quality of life and the costs of therapy. The risks of centesis include bleeding, perforation of organs (e.g., lungs, liver, spleen, or urinary bladder), and infection. Some of these risks can be reduced by using ultrasonography to guide needle placement and sterile preparation of the centesis site. Less common is hypotension due to excessive fluid drainage. The latter problem is of particular concern if the patient is small or has compromised circulation. It probably is not wise to drain abdominal fluid completely without careful attention to the hydration status of the patient during and after the procedure. In patients with poor appetite, repeated removal of a high-protein fluid may exacerbate cachexia and result in a greater need for dietary protein.

Pleurodesis

In the thoracic cavity, the introduction of sclerosing agents may create attachment of the visceral and parietal pleural surfaces, which prevents fluid accumulation. This technique is successful in people, and asbestos-free sterilized talc slurry causes obliteration of the pleural space in 80% to 100% of patients. Less effective agents include bleomycin (70%), and tetracyclines are the least effective, often requiring multiple treatments for complete obliteration. With all these techniques, the pleural space must be essentially free of fluid before introduction of the sclerosing agent or else pleurodesis will not occur. Additionally, any loculated areas of pleural fluid will not be drained and will not be accessible to pleurodesis, so any adhesions should be broken down either manually (e.g., with thoracoscopy) or using hyaluronidase. Talc pleurodesis is not felt to be as successful in dogs as it is in people (at least for control of chylothorax) (Hawkins and Fossum, 2009). Such techniques obviously do not have a place in the management of pericardial or peritoneal effusions.

Surgery

Peritoneovenous shunts have been used in human patients with malignant ascites, but this technique has fallen out of favor due to the need for surgery in a terminally ill patient and the risks inherent in placement of a central shunt. Major complications reported include disseminated intravascular coagulopathy, pulmonary emboli, and infection. In human medicine, most publications have shown that quality of life is no better after this procedure than when repeated paracentesis is used, and there is no reason to believe that the situation would be different in veterinary patients.

Pleuroperitoneal shunt placement has been used in canine patients with chylothorax. Severe short-term complications were seen in 23% and resulted in euthanasia of 1 dog (7.6%). Control of the chylothorax was achieved for a median of 20 months in the remaining dogs, but complications were seen in 73% of dogs (Smeak et al, 2001). Although this may be a viable treatment for dogs with chylothorax, for patients that have confirmed malignant effusions, and therefore a poor long-term prognosis, such high rates of complications make this a less attractive option.

Pleurectomy has been used to control mesothelioma in human patients, but since there is a 10% mortality rate and a high rate of morbidity, it is unlikely to be acceptable in veterinary patients.

Chemotherapy

When there are confirmed tumor cells in the malignant effusion, intraperitoneal or intrathoracic chemotherapy may be used. Drugs used in human patients include cisplatin, bleomycin, 5-fluorouracil, thiotepa, and doxorubicin. Note that cisplatin cannot be used in cats due to the risk of severe fatal pulmonary edema. Intracavitary doxorubicin is not recommended in either cats or dogs because of the (at least theoretical) risk of tissue necrosis. Other drugs that have been reported to be used intracavitarily in canine patients are mitoxantrone and carboplatin.

The theoretical advantages of intracavitary chemotherapy rely on drug distribution modeling, which predicts that clearance of anticancer drugs from body cavities is slower than clearance when the drugs are given systemically. This also means that serosal surfaces (and any free-floating cells) are exposed to much higher drug concentrations. In a study that compared the intraperitoneal pharmacokinetics of cisplatin, carboplatin, and iproplatin in human patients, there were no differences between the drugs (Lind et al, 1991); but in rats, penetration of cisplatin (1 to 3 mm) was shown to be greater than that of carboplatin. Clinical comparison trials have not yet been performed, but many veterinarians prefer carboplatin for its ease of use and toxicity profile.

There is considerable experience in veterinary oncology with intracavitary (intraperitoneal or intrathoracic) chemotherapy, and the technique is similar regardless of the chemotherapy agent used. As with other types of chemotherapy, both the administrator and the restrainer should wear full personal protective equipment (see Chapter 71 for more information). The calculated chemotherapy dose is suspended in 0.9% NaCl (warmed to body temperature) at a volume of 250 ml/m^2 for intrathoracic and 1000 ml/m^2 for intraabdominal treatment in an intravenous bag *after* the fluid line is primed with plain 0.9% NaCl. This latter step reduces the chances for exposure to the chemotherapeutic agent during placement of the line and testing of fluid flow; the chemotherapeutic drug will not reach the patient until the primer fluid in the line has been exhausted. If effusion is present, there is little risk of puncture of any organ, but care always should be taken during catheter placement.

For intraabdominal administration, the dog is restrained in dorsal recumbency and a cannula placed as for abdominocentesis after clipping, scrubbing, and locally anesthetizing the site with lidocaine. An 18-gauge rigid plastic intravenous cannula is inserted on the midline caudal to the umbilicus; care is taken to avoid the spleen and urinary bladder, and ideally ultrasonographic guidance is used.

For intrathoracic (pleural) administration, the dog is restrained in lateral recumbency and a cannula is placed as for thoracocentesis after clipping, scrubbing, and locally anesthetizing the site with lidocaine. An 18-gauge rigid plastic intravenous cannula is inserted, usually in the area of the cardiac notch, using ultrasonographic guidance. When the volume of effusion present is threatening to cause respiratory impairment, a volume that is equal to, or somewhat more than, the volume to be infused should be removed using the catheter before the chemotherapeutic agent is infused. Once placement is confirmed by flushing with 0.9% NaCl, the chemotherapeutic agent is infused and should flow freely. If there is resistance to flow or if the dog appears uncomfortable (or coughs in the case of pleural administration), the cannula should be removed and replaced. The area should be monitored continuously for subcutaneous leakage. When the infusion has been completed, the cannula is covered with alcohol-moistened gauze and withdrawn, and the restrainer holds pressure on the site with gauze for several minutes to stop bleeding and prevent leakage of the drug. The patient can be rolled to and fro on its back to help distribute the chemotherapeutic agent and then should be allowed to move around freely.

Based on a preclinical study in which intraperitoneal administration of cisplatin to dogs led to greater concentration in abdominal visceral tissue than intravenous administration, we performed a pilot study using intracavitary cisplatin at the comparatively low dose of 50 mg/m^2. Five of six dogs (three with pleural mesothelioma and two with malignant ascites caused by carcinomatosis) achieved complete resolution of their effusion (four dogs after one treatment and one dog after two treatments) that lasted a median of 9.5 months (range, 4.2 to >26.5 months) (Moore et al, 1991). Since that time we have administered cisplatin intrathoracically and intraperitoneally to multiple patients and have encountered similar success in more than 50% of patients.

This technique uses a large volume of fluid to ensure complete contact with all affected parietal and visceral surfaces in the treated body cavity, and clinically there have been minimal problems with dyspnea or discomfort associated with this approach. On the other hand, 40 ml of fluid is reported to provide adequate pleural contact during pleurodesis in human patients, and smaller volumes of fluid containing chemotherapeutic agents may be effective for veterinary patients as well. One small study investigating the intracavitary administration of mitoxantrone and cisplatin in four dogs seems to support that contention, at least when malignant effusion already is present (Charney et al, 2005).

Our preference is to administer cisplatin to patients except when such treatment is contraindicated (e.g., in dogs with renal failure or cats) and to administer a large volume after removal of a similar volume from the effusion. In patients in which cisplatin administration is not advisable, carboplatin is used. For both drugs, dose and frequency should not exceed that used for systemic administration. If there is no resolution of effusion after two treatments, other intracavitary drugs or alternate measures may be used.

Investigational Possibilities

The role of VEGF in causing efflux of malignant effusion has led to speculation and some preclinical and clinical reports of the use of anti-VEGF antibodies intraperitoneally. In studies in mice with ascites caused by sarcomas or carcinomas, intraperitoneal administration of anti-VEGF antibodies led to remissions of fluid accumulations. This appeared to be due primarily to decreased permeability of vessels, although there was some suppression of tumor growth that led the authors to suggest that increases in vascular permeability and development of ascites may also hasten tumor dissemination in the affected cavity (Luo, Toyoda, and Shibuya, 1998). If true this would be another reason to control ascites and pleural effusion in veterinary patients. There have been clinical reports that intravenous or intraperitoneal administration of the humanized monoclonal VEGF antibody bevacizumab (Avastin) has led to resolution of pleural effusion and ascites in human patients with carcinoma of colorectal, ovarian, breast, and uterine origins, and these reports were reviewed recently (Kobold et al, 2009). Effusions resolved after a single dose, with the duration of control ranging from 2 to 6 months. Although bevacizumab is unlikely to work in veterinary patients (because it is a humanized antibody), these results suggest that there may be a potential role for other drugs that interfere with VEGF signaling, such as toceranib (Palladia) in palliation of malignant effusions.

References and Suggested Reading

Brisson BA, Reggeti F, Bienzle D: Portal site metastasis of invasive mesothelioma after diagnostic thoracoscopy in a dog, *J Am Vet Med Assoc* 229:980, 2006.

Charney SC et al: Evaluation of intracavitary mitoxantrone and carboplatin for treatment of carcinomatosis, sarcomatosis and mesothelioma, with or without malignant effusions: a retrospective analysis of 12 cases (1997-2002), *Vet Comp Oncol* 3:171, 2005.

Chu CM et al: The role of laparoscopy in the evaluation of ascites of unknown origin, *Gastrointest Endosc* 40:285, 1994.

Clifford CA et al: Vascular endothelial growth factor concentrations in body cavity effusions in dogs, *J Vet Intern Med* 16:164, 2002.

Hawkins EC, Fossum TW: Pleural effusion. In Bonagura JD, Twedt DC, editors: *Kirk's current veterinary therapy XIV*, St Louis, 2009, Saunders, p 675.

Kobold S et al: Intraperitoneal VEGF inhibition using bevacizumab: a potential approach for the symptomatic treatment of malignant ascites? *Oncologist* 14:1242, 2009.

Lind MJ et al: Comparative intraperitoneal pharmacokinetics of three platinum analogues, *Cancer Chemother Pharmacol* 28:315, 1991.

Luo JC, Toyoda M, Shibuya M: Differential inhibition of fluid accumulation and tumor growth in two mouse ascites tumors by an antivascular endothelial growth factor/permeability factor neutralizing antibody, *Cancer Res* 58:2594, 1998.

Moore AS, Kirk C, Cardona A: Intracavitary cisplatin chemotherapy experience with six dogs, *J Vet Intern Med* 5:227, 1991.

Rudlowski C et al: Prognostic significance of vascular endothelial growth factor expression in ovarian cancer patients: a long-term follow-up, *Int J Gynecol Cancer* 16(Suppl 1):183, 2006.

Smeak DD et al: Treatment of chronic pleural effusion with pleuroperitoneal shunts in dogs: 14 cases (1985-1999), *J Am Vet Med Assoc* 219:1590, 2001.

Interventional Oncology

WILLIAM T.N. CULP, *Davis, California*
CHICK WEISSE, *New York, New York*

Although surgery, chemotherapy, and radiation therapy (RT) are being offered in many practices and are the foundations of oncologic treatment, other options are emerging and rapidly gaining acceptance. Interventional radiology (IR) is a specialty that involves the use of image guidance to perform minimally invasive diagnostic and therapeutic procedures. IR techniques are being used more commonly in veterinary medicine to treat neoplastic disease, and this subspecialty of IR, interventional oncology (IO), is expanding. IO provides advanced options to improve the overall standard of care that can be offered to our veterinary patients and is steadily becoming a fourth pillar of oncologic treatment.

Principles

The goal of IO is to perform diagnostic and therapeutic procedures in a minimally invasive fashion. To accomplish this, different imaging modalities are used to allow a clinician to visualize and successfully access a lesion without needing to perform a more invasive procedure. Fluoroscopy is the most readily used imaging modality, and a thorough understanding of the anatomy as revealed by fluoroscopy is crucial to successful performance of IO procedures. Other imaging modalities commonly employed include ultrasonography, computed tomography, and magnetic resonance imaging.

A clinician performing IO procedures needs to have a fully developed understanding of the vast array of available IO instrumentation. Instruments including guidewires, sheaths, diagnostic and guiding catheters, stents, embolic agents, balloons, and various types of contrast are available, and knowing the advantages and disadvantages of the use of each of these items is essential to optimizing the outcome in a particular case.

With the goal of minimizing patient discomfort through the use of minimally invasive techniques, access to organs or regions of the body generally is obtained either percutaneously, through a natural orifice (mouth, nares, anus, or vestibule or penis), or through a blood vessel using the Seldinger technique. In veterinary patients venous approaches do not require vascular repair after the procedure due to the low pressure in the venous system; however, arterial approaches generally do require vessel ligation or repair.

Veterinary Interventional Oncology Treatment Categories

Although IO techniques can be used as supplementary diagnostic tools, IO generally is focused on therapy. The current indications for IO in veterinary medicine fall into three major categories: palliation, primary treatment, and neoadjuvant or adjuvant therapy. Some treatments can overlap across categories, and several different therapies may be offered to an individual patient.

Palliation

Stenting of Malignant Obstructions

Currently IO is used most commonly in veterinary medicine for the palliation of clinical signs associated with neoplastic obstructions. Luminal obstructions secondary to neoplasia occur commonly in veterinary patients and can cause significant morbidity and even mortality. Stents are regularly employed in human medicine for the purpose of opening or "recanalizing" obstructed lumens. The use of stents in veterinary patients is growing rapidly, and several stenting options for the palliative care of animals have been explored.

Urethra. Urethral stenting has been described in several human studies. Reports of the treatment of malignant urethral obstructions in both dogs and cats have been published (Christensen et al, 2010; Newman et al, 2009; Weisse et al, 2006), and this treatment is now available in many clinics (Figure 76-1). In the first veterinary case series (Weisse et al, 2006), 12 dogs underwent placement of urethral stents to relieve malignant urethral obstructions secondary to prostatic or urethra-bladder neoplasia; in all cases, the dogs were experiencing severe or complete obstruction. All dogs regained the ability to urinate after stent placement. Although urinary incontinence occurred in 25% of cases after stenting, the outcome was considered fair to excellent in 10 of 12 dogs (Weisse et al, 2006). Urethral stenting has been reported in two separate feline case reports of malignant obstruction as well (Christensen et al, 2010; Newman et al, 2009). Both cats were diagnosed with urothelial carcinoma and were noted to have successful urination after stent placement.

Urethral stents are placed through a natural orifice in both dogs and cats. In male dogs, access to the urethra and bladder is straightforward because a guidewire can be

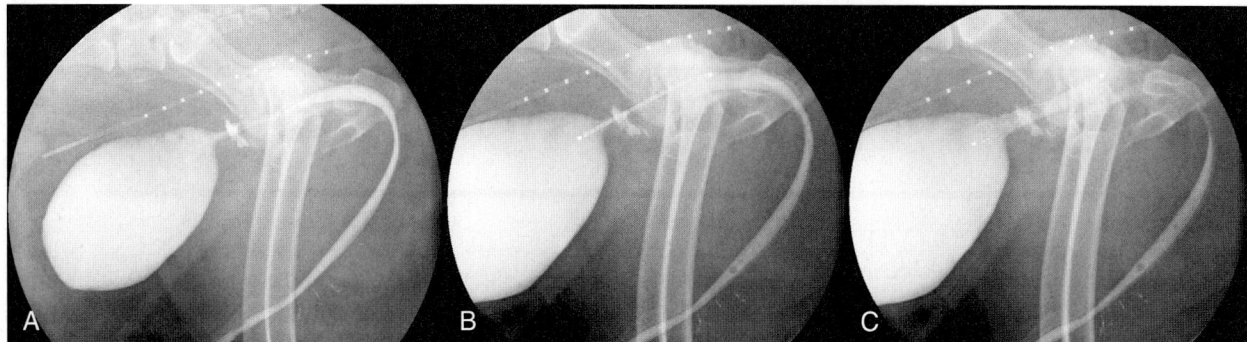

Figure 76-1 Urethral stenting: prostatic carcinoma. **A,** A positive-contrast cystourethrogram has been obtained, and a urethral obstruction in the region of the prostate is noted. **B,** A urethral stent has been placed over a guidewire and is positioned over the obstructed region of the urethra. **C,** The stent has been deployed, and the obstruction has been relieved.

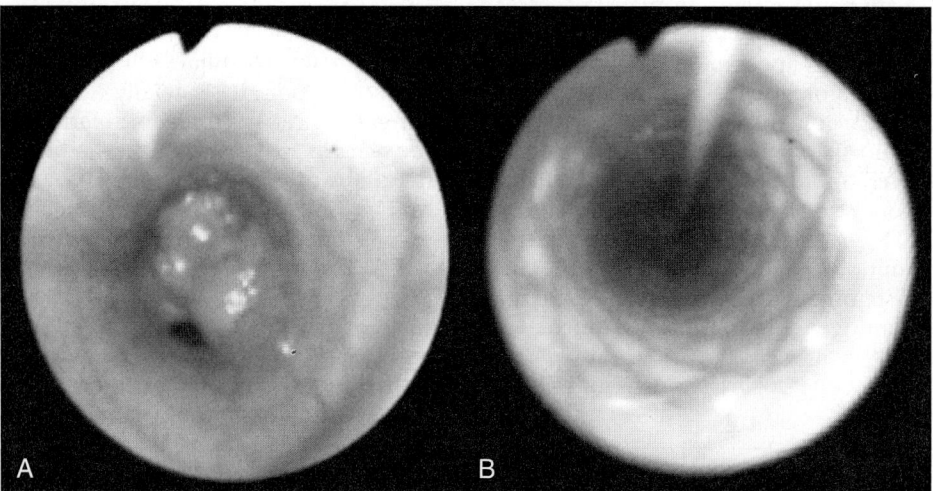

Figure 76-2 Tracheal stenting: tracheal carcinoma. **A,** Tracheoscopic image of an intraluminal tracheal carcinoma in a cat. **B,** A self-expanding stent has been placed, and the tracheal lumen is now open.

introduced easily into the penile urethra. In female dogs and cats, endoscopic or fluoroscopic guidance often is necessary to pass a guidewire into the urethra and bladder. In the authors' practices, access to the male cat urethra generally requires a surgical approach with a small incision in the bladder and antegrade placement of a stent.

Ureter. Ureteral obstruction secondary to neoplasia is rare. Primary ureteral tumors that occur cranial to the ureterovesicular junction generally are treated with surgical removal; however, ureteral obstruction secondary to a tumor originating in the bladder or urethra and encompassing the ureterovesicular junction often is not as amendable to resection. Non–urinary tract tumors also can cause extraluminal compression of the ureter. The use of ureteral stents to relieve ureteral obstruction is an important treatment option in humans, and both retrograde and antegrade techniques (using nephrostomy) have been described.

A technique for percutaneous placement of ureteral stents in dogs with malignant ureteral obstruction was reported recently (Berent et al, 2011). In this series of 12 dogs, the obstructed ureters were accessed in antegrade fashion through the placement of a needle within the renal pelvis (successful in 11 of 12 dogs); ultrasonographic guidance was used to position the needle appropriately. In all cases, a double-pigtail stent was placed with the goal of leaving the cranial pigtail in the renal pelvis and the caudal pigtail in the urinary bladder beyond the obstruction. All patients with azotemia demonstrated improvement in blood urea nitrogen and creatinine concentrations after stent placement. Of the 10 patients that underwent abdominal ultrasonography after stent placement, all were demonstrated to have decreased severity of hydronephrosis and hydroureter. Overall, ureteral stent placement was determined to be safe and well tolerated in that cohort of dogs.

Trachea. In dogs, tracheal stenting has been used most commonly to treat tracheal collapse. Although treatment of malignant tracheal obstruction has not been reported in dogs, stenting has been performed in several such cases in the authors' practices. In general, these patients experience immediate relief of clinical signs. Simultaneous tracheoscopy and fluoroscopy is helpful in performing these procedures to be certain that the stent is placed appropriately across the entire length of the tumor (Figure 76-2).

Stenting of a feline tracheal carcinoma has been reported (Culp et al, 2007). In this case, a self-expanding stainless steel stent was used and was placed with fluoroscopic guidance. The cat developed radiographically evident pulmonary metastasis 6 weeks after stent placement, and euthanasia was elected at that time (Culp et al, 2007).

Gastrointestinal System. Stenting of gastrointestinal lesions is pursued to provide an increased quality of life and relief or improvement of clinical signs, and in certain cases is done as a preparatory step before surgery. Many human patients with esophageal and colonic neoplastic disease initially are evaluated for complete obstruction, and unfortunately, surgical options may be limited at the time of initial presentation.

Surgery, when feasible, is the treatment of choice for esophageal neoplasia in companion animals. Esophageal stenting for the relief of malignant obstructions has not been reported in dogs and cats; however, the experience of the authors is that the procedure can be performed successfully and safely. Because clinical signs often do not resolve completely and the chance of adverse effects (e.g., stent migration, ptyalism, esophagitis) is high, proper case selection is critical.

Colonic stenting has been reported in two cats and one dog (Culp et al, 2011; Hume et al, 2006). In one cat, clinical signs were limited to mechanical obstruction of the colon, despite the presence of suspected pulmonary metastatic disease at the initial evaluation. The clinical signs improved after stent placement in this cat, and tenesmus was observed rarely; fecal incontinence was not reported. Despite the presence of multiorgan metastasis at the time of euthanasia (the colonic tumor was noted to be an adenocarcinoma), the cat survived for 274 days after stent placement (Hume et al, 2006). The second cat underwent successful colonic stent placement to relieve an obstruction secondary to a colonic adenocarcinoma and maintained fecal continence as well. However, the cat was euthanized due to progression of peritoneal effusion secondary to carcinomatosis 19 days after stent placement. In a single canine case report, stent placement was successful and clinical signs improved for just over 200 days. The tumor in that particular case underwent malignant transformation from adenoma (at the time of first biopsy) to carcinoma *in situ* (at the time of necropsy) (Culp et al, 2011).

Vascular System. Syndromes of vascular obstruction have been described in human medicine. Obstruction of the flow of venous blood from the upper body into the right atrium is known as *superior vena cava syndrome* and obstruction of hepatic venous flow is known as *Budd-Chiari syndrome*. A recent report described the endovascular placement of stents to relieve Budd-Chiari syndrome in three dogs. In all cases, obstruction was thought to be secondary to neoplasia. Procedural success and relief of clinical signs was achieved in all three dogs, and survival times varied from 7 to 20 months (Schlicksup et al, 2009).

Cavity Drainage
Percutaneous catheterization of body cavities often is successful in allowing minimally invasive drainage of malignant effusions. Placement of a drainage catheter into the thorax or chest has the benefit of allowing both drainage of the effusion and the administration of intracavitary treatments such as chemotherapy. Newer methods are focused on the placement of drainage catheters using a modified Seldinger technique to gain access into a body cavity; this prevents the need for a thoracotomy. Additionally, catheters can be attached to subcutaneous ports that permit easier drainage, minimize patient morbidity, and decrease the complications that may be noted with serial thoracocentesis or abdominocentesis.

Primary Tumor Treatment

The mainstay of treatment for bulky tumors is surgery. Whenever possible and practical, surgery is pursued because it provides the greatest opportunity for tumor control and, for certain tumor types, may result in a cure. Before the introduction of IO techniques into veterinary medicine, tumors that were nonresectable and resistant to RT or chemotherapy presented a therapeutic challenge. IO techniques such as intraarterial chemotherapy, embolization and chemoembolization, and tumor ablation are emerging as possible primary treatment options in veterinary patients and mirror procedures that are performed actively and regularly in human medicine. Although evidence supporting the use of these treatments is scant in the veterinary literature, much has been accomplished in humans to suggest that these options have efficacy. Additionally, for many nonresectable tumors in humans, these techniques are the first-line therapy that is pursued.

Intraarterial Chemotherapy
Chemotherapy often is used in veterinary oncology cases as a neoadjuvant or adjuvant treatment, and survival times for several tumor types have been shown to be prolonged when chemotherapy is given. Historically, in veterinary patients chemotherapeutic agents have been administered through a peripheral vein. The delivery of chemotherapeutic drugs directly into the arterial supply of a tumor has the potential benefit of increasing the concentration of drug that reaches the tumor. Additionally, adverse effects associated with the administration of chemotherapy may be decreased because less drug is delivered systemically. The technique of intraarterial chemotherapy is used regularly in human medicine, particularly to treat tumors of the head and neck.

To perform the procedure, a sheath is placed within the artery that has been chosen. Using various sizes and types of guidewires and catheters, the vascular supply of the affected organ is accessed via superselective catheterization. Once the desired vessel is selected, chemotherapy can be administered, which increases the locally delivered dose.

Urothelial carcinoma has been shown to be chemosensitive; however, tumor responses are variable and often not prolonged. For this reason, alternative therapies need to be pursued to determine if efficacy can be improved. In the authors' practices, intraarterial delivery of chemotherapeutic drugs is used most commonly to treat bladder and urethral transitional cell carcinoma and prostatic

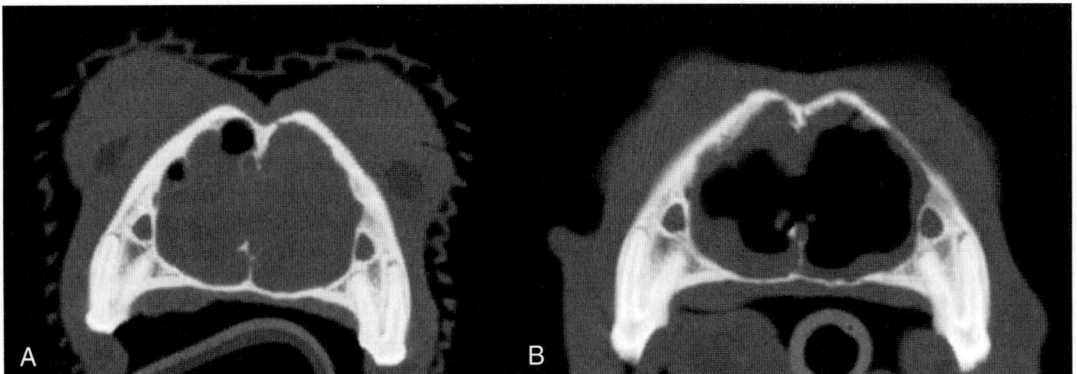

Figure 76-3 Chemoembolization: nasal carcinoma **A,** Pretreatment transverse computed tomographic (CT) image of a dog with a nasal carcinoma. **B,** Transverse CT image obtained at the same level 3 weeks after nasal chemoembolization.

carcinoma. These procedures can be performed via either the femoral or carotid artery, and treatment of both the right and left side of the affected organ is possible.

Embolization and Chemoembolization

Embolization is the local delivery of an embolic agent (particles, liquids, coils, or balloons) to the vascular supply of an organ or tumor. The goal of embolization is to cause vascular stasis in the tumor blood supply resulting in tumor cell ischemia and subsequent death. *Chemoembolization* refers to embolization that is performed with a mixture of an embolic agent and a chemotherapeutic drug. The proposed advantages of chemoembolization are related to the combination of altered blood flow to a tumor and direct intraarterial delivery of chemotherapy to the tumor blood supply. In addition, if blood flow to the tumor is interrupted, the chemotherapeutic drug theoretically will dwell within tumor cells for a longer period.

The effects of embolization and chemoembolization have been investigated most frequently in liver tumors. The blood supply of the liver is unique in that the venous system provides the vast majority of blood (from the portal vein) to the liver; studies have shown that 75% to 85% of the liver's blood supply comes from the portal vein. On the other hand, the blood supply to hepatic tumors is mostly from the hepatic artery (85% to 100%). The result of this unique situation is that the blood supply to a hepatic tumor can be interrupted and the normal liver can remain virtually unaffected.

There are a few reports of embolization or chemoembolization in dogs, and in the authors' practices, chemoembolization of liver and nasal tumors is being performed regularly. After surgical and RT options are reviewed and pursued, chemoembolization can be considered in certain cases. Initial results are promising, and computed tomographic scans performed after the procedure demonstrate a decrease in tumor size compared with preprocedure scans (Figure 76-3).

Tumor Ablation

Tumor ablation involves direct application of either a chemical agent or thermal energy to a tumor to produce tumor destruction. The most common form of chemical ablation is percutaneous ethanol injection. Several types of thermal ablation techniques are available including radiofrequency ablation, microwave ablation, laser ablation, and cryoablation. Use of these techniques for the treatment of many tumor types has been described, but the form of ablation chosen depends on the clinician and his or her experience. These different ablative techniques incorporate the principles of other types of IO procedures in that they are minimally invasive and are performed with image guidance.

Neoadjuvant and Adjuvant Therapy

The potential uses of IO techniques in the neoadjuvant and adjuvant setting are few, but new indications and techniques are evolving. Intraarterial chemotherapy can be used as a primary treatment, in combination with an embolic agent to perform chemoembolization, in the neoadjuvant setting to decrease tumor burden before surgical resection, or in the adjuvant setting to decrease tumor recurrence. Use of the latter two options has not been described in veterinary patients, but for certain malignancies, these treatments have been advocated in humans.

Intraarterial delivery of a radiosensitizing chemotherapeutic agent such as cisplatin directly to a tumor that is being irradiated may improve the efficacy of RT. A combination of intraarterial chemotherapy and RT has been described in several clinical reports (Heidner et al, 1991; McCaw et al, 1988; Withrow et al, 1993). In one study (McCaw et al, 1988), a chemotherapeutic agent was administered intraarterially at the level of the aortic bifurcation in two dogs with bladder carcinoma, and RT was performed the same day. Both dogs were evaluated for response by double-contrast cystourethrography, and the tumors were determined to be reduced in size. Both dogs improved clinically and adverse effects were minimal.

Intraarterial chemotherapy has been combined with RT to treat canine osteosarcoma as well (Heidner et al, 1991; Withrow et al, 1993). Results of these studies were promising; adverse effects were uncommon, and greater tumor necrosis was observed when combination therapy was used. The median survival times for the dogs in these studies ranged from 6.7 to 9.3 months.

Chemoembolization also has been advocated as both a neoadjuvant and adjuvant therapy in humans. Embolization of the portal vein blood supply of the liver segment containing a tumor has been performed in humans. The goal of this procedure is to atrophy the segment of liver affected by tumor and cause the remaining liver to hypertrophy. Although use of this treatment in clinical veterinary cases has not been reported, it may offer a potential option in the future in cases of large liver masses.

References and Suggested Reading

Berent AC et al: Use of indwelling, double-pigtail stents for treatment of malignant ureteral obstruction in dogs: 12 cases (2006-2009), *J Am Vet Med Assoc* 238:1017, 2011.

Christensen NI, Culvenor J, Langova V: Fluoroscopic stent placement for the relief of malignant urethral obstruction in a cat, *Aust Vet J* 88:478, 2010.

Culp WTN et al: Intraluminal tracheal stenting for treatment of tracheal narrowing in three cats, *Vet Surg* 36:107, 2007.

Culp WTN et al: Use of a nitinol stent to palliate a colorectal neoplastic obstruction in a dog, *J Am Vet Med Assoc* 239:222, 2011.

Heidner GL et al: Treatment of canine appendicular osteosarcoma using cobalt 60 radiation and intraarterial cisplatin, *J Vet Intern Med* 5:313, 1991.

Hume DZ, Solomon JA, Weisse CW: Palliative use of a stent for colonic obstruction caused by adenocarcinoma in two cats, *J Am Vet Med Assoc* 228:392, 2006.

McCaw DL et al: Radiation and cisplatin for treatment of canine urinary bladder carcinoma, *Vet Radiol* 29:264, 1988.

Newman RG et al: Use of a balloon-expandable metallic stent to relieve malignant urethral obstruction in a cat, *J Am Vet Med Assoc* 234:236, 2009.

Schlicksup MD et al: Use of endovascular stents in three dogs with Budd-Chiari syndrome, *J Am Vet Med Assoc* 235:544, 2009.

Weisse C et al: Evaluation of palliative stenting for management of malignant urethral obstructions in dogs, *J Am Vet Med Assoc* 229:226, 2006.

Withrow SJ et al: Intra-arterial cisplatin with or without radiation in limb-sparing for canine osteosarcoma, *Cancer* 71:2484, 1993.

CHAPTER 77

Nutritional Support of the Cancer Patient

GLENNA E. MAULDIN, *Calgary, Alberta, Canada*

Cancer cachexia is the unique form of protein-calorie malnutrition that may occur in both people and animals with neoplastic disease. Evidence of cancer cachexia is present in as many as 80% of people with cancer, although the reported incidence varies with the type of malignancy and the sensitivity of the means of nutritional assessment. The syndrome typically is characterized by one or more of three clinical findings: diminished host nutrient intake, progressive host weight loss, and the presence of distinctive clinicopathologic abnormalities.

The detrimental effects of protein-calorie malnutrition overall are well documented and include anemia, hypoproteinemia, delayed wound healing, decreased immunocompetence, and compromise of gastrointestinal, pulmonary, and cardiovascular function. Severe debilitation and death are possible in affected individuals. In addition, along with unfavorable tumor type, advanced stage of disease, and low performance score, weight loss has been shown repeatedly to have an independent and negative impact on prognosis in people with cancer. Thus the importance of accurate nutritional assessment and early nutritional intervention in malnourished patients with neoplastic disease cannot be overemphasized. This chapter briefly reviews the current understanding of the pathophysiology of cancer cachexia, discusses some practical methods of nutritional assessment for veterinary patients, and makes specific recommendations for the nutritional support of cats and dogs with cancer.

Theoretical Considerations

Cancer cachexia can be divided by underlying cause into two basic categories: primary and secondary. Secondary cancer cachexia is caused by reduced nutrient intake resulting from the physical effects of the tumor itself or the therapies used to treat it. It is intuitively obvious that many tumors have a negative impact on host nutritional status simply because of their location or size: for instance, large intraoral masses may prevent normal food intake, and diffuse neoplastic infiltration of the small bowel may significantly disrupt normal digestion or absorption of nutrients. It also is well established that decreased food intake may occur secondary to various anticancer therapies. Cancer treatment may be associated with important abnormalities in nutrient intake, digestion, and absorption because of the nausea, vomiting, mucositis, and diarrhea caused by radiation therapy or chemotherapy.

In contrast, primary cancer cachexia is not understood nearly as easily. It probably is best defined as a paraneoplastic syndrome in which various metabolic abnormalities lead to inefficient energy utilization by the host, which results in accelerated loss of both lean body mass and adipose stores. The presence of these underlying metabolic abnormalities means that, unlike secondary cancer cachexia, primary cancer cachexia cannot be reversed simply by increasing nutrient intake. Published work suggests that primary cancer cachexia is a complex systemic inflammatory syndrome caused by alterations in proinflammatory mediators that have wide-ranging effects on intermediary metabolism. Interleukin-1α (IL-1α), IL-1β, IL-6, tumor necrosis factor-α (TNF-α), and interferon-γ all have been implicated in the pathogenesis of this disorder, as have a number of eicosanoids. Changes in the production of these substances also may lead to neuroendocrine abnormalities, including variations in catecholamine and cortisol secretion and changes in the relative and absolute concentrations of plasma insulin and glucagon. The specific changes that occur vary from affected individual to individual but ultimately cause characteristic perturbations in the metabolism of all three energy substrates—carbohydrate, protein, and lipid. Classically, abnormalities in carbohydrate metabolism have been described most often and have included hyperlactatemia, increased rates of whole body glucose turnover and disposal, increased rates of gluconeogenesis from lactate and amino acids, abnormal glucose tolerance curves, hyperinsulinism, and insulin resistance. Documented changes in protein metabolism consist of altered serum amino acid profiles, increased rates of whole body protein turnover, decreased protein fractional synthetic rates in skeletal muscle, and increased protein fractional synthetic rates in liver. Finally, abnormalities in lipid metabolism include accelerated fat oxidation, increased lipolysis, hypertriglyceridemia, decreased lipoprotein lipase activity, increased synthesis of triacylglycerols and very low-density lipoproteins, and increased plasma concentrations of nonesterified or free fatty acids and ketone bodies (acetoacetate and β-hydroxybutyrate).

Theoretically, host energy expenditure should be increased as a consequence of futile cycling and the changes in flux through these varied metabolic pathways, with host weight loss being the ultimate result. Many investigators have attempted to prove this hypothesis by using indirect calorimetry to measure energy expenditure in tumor-bearing subjects. Unfortunately, the results of these studies are variable and difficult to interpret. Energy expenditure seems to vary with tumor type and stage of disease. It appears to be increased in some studies, to be apparently unchanged in others, and actually to be decreased in still others. One valid conclusion must be that significant variation exists in energy expenditure and the manifestations of cancer cachexia, not only among tumor types but also among individuals with the same tumor, depending on the stage of the disease. However, one must also consider several additional explanations for these findings. First, the methodology involved in indirect calorimetry is complex, and results may be difficult to reproduce consistently. Second, selection of the best controls for such studies is problematic: some authors compare their cachectic cancer patients with young, healthy, weight-stable control subjects, whereas others insist that the only appropriate comparison is between weight-losing cancer patients and weight-losing patients with nonmalignant disease. Finally, the analysis of results is complicated further in animals because the true energy requirements of even healthy cats and dogs are controversial and incompletely defined. Much more work is needed to define thoroughly the changes in energy expenditure that occur in people and animals with cancer.

Although cancer-associated weight loss has been studied most extensively in people and rodent models, work by veterinary investigators suggests that many of the metabolic changes typical of primary cancer cachexia also are present in dogs with naturally occurring neoplastic disease. Dogs with lymphoma have been studied in greatest detail, and this tumor has been proposed as a model of primary cancer cachexia. However, a convincing clinical association between documented metabolic abnormalities, actual weight loss, and poor prognosis has yet to be demonstrated in dogs with any type of cancer. Recent work shows that clinically relevant hyperlactatemia is uncommon in dogs with all types of neoplastic disease, including lymphoma. When hyperlactatemia is present, it almost always is related to decreased tissue perfusion and not to increased production by tumor cells (Touret et al, 2010). Furthermore, weight loss appears to be less common in dogs with cancer than in people with neoplastic disease. One study found that only 4% of dogs evaluated or treated for neoplastic disease by a large referral oncology practice were cachectic as defined by body condition scoring, whereas 29% were obese (Michel et al, 2004). Similarly, another group of investigators found that even though dogs with malignant tumors were somewhat less likely to be overweight than dogs without neoplastic disease, there was no difference in the proportion of underweight or very thin dogs in the two groups (Weeth et al, 2007). There are several possible explanations for the apparent discrepancy between the prevalence of weight loss in dogs and in people with cancer. The most common types of cancer diagnosed and treated in dogs and in people are not the same, and those treated most often in dogs (e.g., lymphoma) are relatively less likely to result in weight loss in people. In addition, it seems probable that people receive aggressive anticancer therapy despite facing a poor prognosis more often than do dogs, and this type of patient would be expected to be at increased risk of weight loss. Finally, dogs with cancer routinely are euthanized when their quality of life declines, and this is likely to decrease further the prevalence of cancer-associated weight loss in dogs compared with people. Regardless, the potential differences between dogs and people with respect to the prevalence of cancer-associated weight loss are intriguing and merit further confirmation and study.

It is interesting to note that published work suggests that the relationship between weight loss and the tumor-bearing state may be different in cats than in dogs. In one study, the effect of body condition score on prognosis was examined in cats with neoplastic disease (Baez et al, 2007). Almost half of the cats evaluated were underweight or very thin, and over 90% of them had evidence of muscle wasting. Body condition score was strongly correlated with survival time and prognosis: cats with decreased body condition scores had markedly shorter survival times. Other investigators also have shown that weight loss is a negative prognostic indicator for some cats with lymphoma (Krick et al, 2011). Further work is needed to determine if the relatively lower body condition that apparently exists in many cats with cancer is related specifically to the presence of underlying neoplastic disease or whether it represents a more generic feline response to illness. It seems possible that sick cats are simply more likely to experience weight loss than sick dogs, regardless of whether they have neoplastic disease or not.

Nutritional Assessment

Understanding the pathophysiology of cancer cachexia serves no practical purpose for the veterinary clinician unless affected animals can be recognized and treated. A systematic method to determine the cause and severity of malnutrition, identify individuals needing nutritional intervention, and predict animals at greatest risk of developing malnutrition and its related complications would permit the most appropriate and presumably successful nutritional therapy possible. In people, this process is called *nutritional assessment.* It incorporates a detailed dietary history, a complete physical examination, and morphometric, hematologic, and biochemical evaluations. Less is known about the application of some of these techniques in cats and dogs with cancer, but enough work has been done that some general recommendations can be made.

A detailed diet history and physical examination are the initial components of a complete nutritional assessment. The diet history must include specific information about the quantity and content of the animal's present diet as well as the diet before illness, with the recognition that these may differ significantly. Any medications or nutritional supplements currently being administered by the owner also are identified. A thorough physical examination is the next step, and the veterinarian must take care to look for evidence of malnutrition caused by both nutrient excess (i.e., obesity) and nutrient deficiency (i.e., cancer cachexia or protein-calorie malnutrition). The diagnosis of obesity obviously is straightforward, but the clinical signs associated with cancer cachexia and protein-calorie malnutrition often are subtle and nonspecific. One or more abnormalities including muscle wasting, pallor, poor hair coat, hepatomegaly or splenomegaly,

evidence of chronic infections, lymphadenopathy, or even peripheral edema may be present.

In people, lean body mass and body fat stores often are evaluated through morphometric measurements such as triceps skinfold thickness and midarm circumference. Adapting these specific techniques for use in cats and dogs is difficult because of the large variation in body size and conformation among different breeds. However, careful monitoring of body weight as well as consistent use of a standardized body condition scoring system provides the veterinarian with much of the same information. Body condition scoring systems generally use a five- or nine-point system in which each point corresponds to a particular body condition with defined criteria; for example, "cachectic" (no obvious body fat) through "optimal" (ribs easily palpable) to "obese" (large deposits of subcutaneous and abdominal fat). These classifications provide at least an initial assessment of a small animal's lean body mass and adipose stores.

Finally, although relatively insensitive as nutritional markers, several hematologic and biochemical parameters easily available to the veterinarian can provide additional information. Cancer-associated weight loss and the effects of protein-calorie malnutrition may result in anemia and decreased total lymphocyte counts. Animals with significant protein deficiency also may have decreased serum albumin concentrations. Hypoalbuminemia is a reliable indicator of protein deficiency and has been associated repeatedly with poor clinical outcome in people. However, the serum half-life of this protein is relatively long (approximately 8 days in the dog); thus an extended period of protein deprivation is required before concentrations fall below the normal range. A more sensitive means of nutritional assessment, at least in the cat, may be determination of serum creatine kinase concentrations. Serum creatine kinase concentrations increase rapidly in the cat during anorexia and decrease dramatically after initiation of assisted feeding. Further study is required to determine whether serum creatine kinase concentration is a useful marker of nutritional status in the dog.

Dietary Recommendations

Specifically targeted nutritional therapy is indicated for malnourished cats and dogs with cancer. Although treatment of presumed cancer cachexia has been the traditional focus in this area, it is important to remember that a substantial number of animals with neoplastic disease and concurrent malnutrition actually are overweight. A judicious reduction in caloric intake may be appropriate in such cases to gradually achieve an ideal body condition score and optimal nutritional status. However, aggressive weight reduction should not be attempted during critical illness, even in extremely obese animals. Severe caloric restriction could contribute to the rapid development of clinically significant protein-calorie malnutrition and its associated complications; initiation of a conservative weight-loss program once the animal's condition has stabilized is a better approach. Algorithms for successful weight loss in obese cats and dogs using a variety of prescription reducing diets have been described previously (Toll et al, 2010).

On the other hand, a palatable, highly digestible, or energy-dense diet may be advantageous in cats and dogs with either primary or secondary cancer cachexia. Potential benefits include improved ability to tolerate aggressive antineoplastic therapy, enhanced quality of life, and longer survival times. Rations also can be designed to take advantage of the metabolic differences between tumor cells and normal host tissues. Tumor cells have an obligate requirement for glucose and are incapable of significant fat oxidation: they derive virtually all of their energy from glycolysis. Diets with a relatively high fat content thus are preferred, in the hope that they will preferentially provide energy to the host. Diets high in carbohydrate are generally avoided since they may supply additional energy to the tumor; furthermore, utilization of carbohydrate calories may be inefficient in a tumor-bearing animal because of insulin resistance. Beneficial effects have been documented in people with cancer fed such diets, including improved weight gain, improved energy and nitrogen balance, improved preservation of body adipose stores, and decreased glucose intolerance.

The optimal dietary protein intake in cats and dogs with neoplastic disease is unknown. Obviously each animal must be evaluated carefully on an individual basis, but the protein content of any ration fed to a cat or dog with cancer needs to be adequate to meet the potentially increased requirements that may be encountered when neoplastic disease is complicated by systemic conditions such as sepsis. Investigators studying hospitalized dogs with a variety of critical illnesses have documented high rates of urinary nitrogen loss, a reflection of accelerated protein catabolism (Michel et al, 1997). Loss of lean tissue among many of the dogs in this study that had no food intake was over 200 g per dog per day. It seems probable that critically ill cats and dogs with cancer have equally high protein requirements, and thus they may require as many as 30% to 50% of their total daily calories as protein. This should be especially true in critically ill cats, which rapidly develop life-threatening protein-calorie malnutrition. Cats are less efficient at conserving lean body mass than dogs; the increased protein requirements of illness are superimposed on an unusually high basal protein requirement in this species. This requirement is the result, in part, of obligatory gluconeogenesis from amino acids and continuous cycling of hepatic transaminases and urea cycle enzymes. Based on these theoretical and practical considerations, a high-fat (i.e., >40% to 50% of calories from fat), restricted-carbohydrate, highly palatable and digestible ration that contains ample protein usually is recommended for weight-losing cats and dogs with cancer. Exceptions to this rule of thumb include animals with a history of fat intolerance or concurrent diseases such as renal or hepatic insufficiency that are managed with dietary protein restriction. Either canned or dry foods may be appropriate, although it is useful to remember that dry foods often are more energy dense than canned products. Rations should be complete and balanced. Use of a commercial pet food produced by a reputable manufacturer is the safest and most convenient way of avoiding micronutrient deficiencies or excesses. In general, the types of rations most likely to fit the outlined profile are canned or dry products designed for use during performance or critical illness, and dry or canned kitten or puppy foods.

For the most part, definitive recommendations regarding specific dietary intake of nutrients such as glutamine, arginine, and various antioxidants must await the publication of data from controlled studies. However, there are now an increasing number of studies that support the potential benefit of a diet enriched with n-3 (omega-3) fatty acids, at least in dogs with neoplastic disease. Since n-3 fatty acids alter eicosanoid production and can affect the inflammatory response by modifying the synthesis of cytokines such as IL-1, TNF-α, and IL-6, it is reasonable to hypothesize that supplementation could have a positive impact on an inflammatory condition such as primary cancer cachexia. Likewise, some abnormalities in carbohydrate metabolism resolved in dogs with lymphoma that were fed a test diet enriched with both n-3 fatty acids and arginine, and prolonged survival times were observed in a subset of animals in one study (Ogilvie et al, 2000); however, more work is needed to prove definitively that these findings were the result of n-3 fatty acid supplementation. In addition, the optimal dose and method of administration for n-3 fatty acids in tumor-bearing dogs remains unknown.

Assisted Feeding

It is vital to recognize that many of the cats and dogs that would benefit most from the types of dietary therapy outlined previously are unwilling or unable to eat for themselves and have inadequate voluntary food intake. Every effort should be made to encourage animals to eat on their own, including hand feeding of highly palatable foods. Provision of small, frequent meals also may improve food intake in animals with inconsistent appetites. However, despite these measures, caloric intake still will be marginal in many cases. Feeding tubes or catheters should be placed without hesitation in animals with persistent anorexia to ensure maintenance of optimal nutrient intake.

The use of pharmacologic appetite stimulants for anorectic cats and dogs with cancer is advised by some authors. Various benzodiazepine derivatives, most commonly diazepam (Valium), as well as the drug cyproheptadine (Periactin) have been reported to increase food intake in cats and dogs; however, objective evidence supporting the clinical efficacy of these compounds generally is lacking. Careful monitoring of actual food intake frequently reveals that although consumption may be transiently increased immediately after drug administration, the overall food intake over longer periods is unchanged. Furthermore, appropriate and necessary placement of feeding tubes frequently is delayed while a response to medication is awaited. For these reasons, these drugs should be used with care in anorectic cats and dogs with cancer, and then only when the clinician is committed to measuring food intake to confirm occurrence of the desired effect.

Assisted Enteral Feeding

Reviews have been published describing assisted enteral feeding in cats and dogs (Saker and Remillard, 2010). With few exceptions, enteral feeding is superior to parenteral or intravenous feeding. Enteral nutrition helps prevent intestinal mucosal atrophy and bacterial translocation from the gut, is cheaper and technically less complex than parenteral feeding, and has fewer potential complications. The potential disadvantages of enteral nutrition include the extended periods of transition and contraindication in situations in which the gastrointestinal tract is nonfunctional.

Several different types of feeding tubes are available for delivery of enteral nutrition in cats and dogs with cancer. Nasoesophageal tubes are indicated for relatively short-term support in animals that are anorectic but have normal gastrointestinal function, in animals that have oropharyngeal disease that prevents normal food intake, and in animals that are too critically ill to tolerate the general anesthesia required for placement of most other types of feeding tubes. Esophagostomy or gastrostomy tubes are a better choice when long-term nutritional support is needed because they often can be left in place indefinitely. They also are useful in animals that are anorectic but have normal gastrointestinal tract function and in animals with oropharyngeal disease. Jejunostomy tubes allow bypass of the entire upper gastrointestinal tract, including the stomach and pancreas, so they can be used to support animals with persistent vomiting, gastric outflow obstructions, and pancreatitis.

The ideal tube-feeding formula for cats and dogs with cancer has the same characteristics as the ideal commercial ration: it is high in fat, provides ample protein calories, is relatively restricted in simple carbohydrates, and is complete and balanced with regard to micronutrients. A very calorie-dense formula (i.e., high fat) also minimizes the volume that must be fed through the tube. Liquid commercial veterinary products specifically designed for tube feeding (e.g., CliniCare) generally are the best choices for use with nasoesophageal and jejunostomy tubes, whereas paste-type formulations (Iams Veterinary Formula Maximum-Calorie Plus, Hill's Prescription Diet a/d Canine/Feline Critical Care) or canned cat or dog food that has been put through a blender may be fed through esophagostomy and gastrostomy tubes. It is important to remember that human enteral feeding products are not complete and balanced for use in cats and dogs. Initial bolus feedings should be administered every 2 hours and should consist of a small volume of dilute formula. If this ration is well tolerated, the concentration and volume can be increased gradually until the animal finally is receiving the full target volume in four to six daily feedings. This process usually takes at least 3 to 4 days, and in some cases even longer. Constant-rate infusion, rather than bolus feeding, is preferred with jejunostomy tubes.

Assisted Parenteral Feeding

Parenteral nutrition is the only option for nutritional support in animals with cancer that cannot tolerate enteral feeding. The primary indication for parenteral nutrition is a nonfunctional intestinal tract, such as may occur with intractable vomiting, gastrointestinal obstruction, or severe ileus. Parenteral nutrition also is considered primary therapy for certain types of inflammatory gastrointestinal lesions, such as pancreatitis or severe inflammatory colitis. The major advantage of parenteral nutrition in these situations is that it permits complete bowel rest. Parenteral nutrition also can be used in animals that are too critically ill to tolerate the general anesthesia that may be required for the placement of some enteral feeding tubes. Finally, coma is another potential indication; the risk of aspiration is significantly decreased when intravenous feeding is used in such cases. The major disadvantages of parenteral nutrition are the development of significant intestinal mucosal atrophy after long-term use; an increased incidence of bacterial translocation from the gut; the need for specialized equipment, products, and care; and increased expense. In addition, there is a greater potential for complications with parenteral nutrition than with enteral feeding. The possible complications include an increased risk of sepsis, thrombophlebitis, mechanical complications such as catheter disconnection and twisted intravenous lines, and biochemical complications such as hyperglycemia and hyperlipidemia. A combination of parenteral nutrition and enteral support always should be considered for animals that will tolerate it, since even very small amounts of food within the gut help to prevent deterioration in gastrointestinal function.

The parenteral nutrition prescription for a cat or dog with cancer should be designed to follow the same principles as the enteral diets described previously. The dextrose content should be restricted as much as is reasonable, with fat providing at least 60% to 70% of nonprotein calories unless contraindicated. Sufficient protein must be supplied to meet requirements, and this level is currently estimated to be 2 to 3 g/100 kcal of energy per day in parenterally fed dogs with normal hepatic and renal function, and 3 to 4 g/100 kcal of energy per day in parenterally fed cats with normal hepatic and renal function. If parenteral nutrition is continued for longer than 5 to 7 days, appropriate vitamin and mineral supplements must be administered to ensure an adequate nutrient intake.

References and Suggested Reading

Baez JL et al: A prospective investigation of the prevalence and prognostic significance of weight loss and changes in body condition in feline cancer patients, *J Feline Med Surg* 9:411, 2007.

DeWys WD et al: Prognostic effect of weight loss prior to chemotherapy in cancer patients, *Am J Med* 69:491, 1980.

Fearon KCH, Barber MD, Moses AG: The cancer cachexia syndrome, *Surg Oncol Clin North Am* 10:109, 2001.

Krick EL et al: Prognostic significance of weight changes during treatment of feline lymphoma, *J Feline Med Surg* 13:976, 2011.

Michel KE, King LG, Ostro E: Measurement of urinary urea nitrogen content as an estimate of the amount of total urinary nitrogen loss in dogs in intensive care units, *J Am Vet Med Assoc* 210:356, 1997.

Michel KE, Sorenmo K, Shofer FS: Evaluation of body condition and weight loss in dogs presented to a veterinary oncology service, *J Vet Intern Med* 18:692, 2004.

Ogilvie GK et al: Effect of fish oil, arginine and doxorubicin chemotherapy on remission and survival time for dogs with lymphoma: a double-blind, randomized placebo-controlled study, *Cancer* 88:1916, 2000.

Saker KE, Remillard RL: Critical care nutrition and enteral-assisted feeding. In Hand MS et al, editors: *Small animal clinical nutrition*, ed 5, Topeka, KS, 2010, Mark Morris Institute, p 439.

Toll PW, Yamka RM, Schoenherr WD: Obesity. In Hand MS et al, editors: *Small animal clinical nutrition*, ed 5, Topeka, KS, 2010, Mark Morris Institute, p 501.

Touret M, Boysen SR, Nadeau ME: Prospective evaluation of clinically relevant type B hyperlactatemia in dogs with cancer, *J Vet Intern Med* 24:1458, 2010.

Weeth LP, Fascetti AJ, Kass PH: Prevalence of obese dogs in a population of dogs with cancer, *Am J Vet Res* 68:389, 2007.

CHAPTER 78

Metronomic Chemotherapy

ANTHONY J. MUTSAERS, *Guelph, Ontario, Canada*

Conventional cytotoxic chemotherapy agents have been the cornerstone of the medical oncologist's treatment arsenal for many decades. However, in the emerging era of newer targeted drugs such as receptor tyrosine kinase inhibitors, traditional chemotherapy agents are being reexamined to determine whether particular efficacy and resistance patterns may be explained, at least in part, through a different mechanism than solely the killing of highly proliferative cancer cell populations.

The design of conventional chemotherapy treatment protocols is based largely on the principle of administration of the maximum tolerated dose (MTD), which requires an obligatory "break" period to allow for the recovery of normal cell populations. Despite the use of these chemotherapy protocols for the treatment and outright cure of certain cancers, some oncologists believe that we may be nearing the limit of what cytotoxic chemotherapy regimens can accomplish. A different approach based on more continuous exposure time, with reduction or elimination of the break period between each dose, has come to be known as *metronomic* chemotherapy delivery. Not surprisingly, to provide a more continuous treatment schedule, a reduction in drug dose is required. The reduced toxicity profile, ease of administration when oral drugs are used, and relatively low cost make metronomic chemotherapy protocols appealing in veterinary oncology; however, an understanding of the mechanisms of action and rigorous clinical evaluation in veterinary patients are still at an early stage.

Antitumor Mechanisms

Antiangiogenesis

Cytotoxic chemotherapeutics achieve at least a portion of their therapeutic efficacy by inhibition of tumor angiogenesis, which is the process of new blood vessel growth in tumors. The basis for this notion likely originated with the observation that tumor endothelial cell populations are much more proliferative than the quiescent endothelial cells elsewhere in the body. These rapidly dividing endothelial cells are targets of chemotherapy, and for this reason other proliferative cells, such as intestinal epithelia and bone marrow precursors, are also damaged. When the antiangiogenic effects of MTD chemotherapy were evaluated in preclinical models, it was revealed that repair and repopulation of endothelial cells occurs during the break period, just as it does for other cell populations. Therefore the key to maximizing the antiangiogenic potential of chemotherapeutic drugs was considered to be the reduction or elimination of the break period between doses.

Like many aspects of physiology, angiogenesis is regulated through the relative balance of endogenous promoters and inhibitors of this process. Experimental evidence has suggested that up-regulation of the endogenous angiogenesis inhibitor thrombospondin-1 in the tumor microenvironment occurs during metronomic treatment with cyclophosphamide (CYC), and possibly other agents, leading to an antiangiogenic effect. This indirect antiangiogenic mechanism may complement the direct cytotoxicity to endothelial cells provided by chemotherapy.

The process of tumor angiogenesis also may involve recruitment of circulating cells from the bone marrow that travel to the tumor site and incorporate into endothelial walls or support vessel growth indirectly through cytokine production. Circulating endothelial progenitor cells (CEPs) from the bone marrow are an example. These cells, if they play a significant role in the growth of tumor blood vessels, may be most influential after the acute damage that occurs in the early break period of MTD chemotherapy schedules. Preclinical models have demonstrated that CEPs immediately decrease with MTD treatment (similar to other bone marrow progenitor populations), only to rapidly rebound during the break period, and potentially contribute to endothelial cell repopulation. In contrast, metronomic chemotherapy does not appear to be associated with a CEP rebound, leading instead to a sustained antiangiogenic effect.

Immunomodulation

In addition to tumor blood vessels, other components of the tumor microenvironment may be the target of metronomic chemotherapy drugs. Immune effector cells such as lymphocytes and macrophages influence tumor biology and may be affected by chemotherapy treatment. For this reason, the potential immunomodulatory mechanisms of metronomic chemotherapy, particularly that associated with using the alkylating agent CYC, are receiving significant research interest. Low doses of CYC alter the T-lymphocyte subset population by decreasing levels of $CD4^+CD25^+$ regulatory T (Treg) cells. Treg cells inhibit the immune response and thereby suppress tumor immune surveillance. In dogs with various malignancies, circulating Treg cells in the blood have been quantified by flow cytometry and have been found to decrease in dogs with soft tissue sarcoma during treatment with metronomic CYC (Burton et al, 2011). Further effects of metronomic CYC on tumor immunology are under investigation, and possible immunomodulatory mechanisms for other antineoplastic agents delivered metronomically may be revealed in future studies.

Direct Cancer Cell Targeting

Metronomic chemotherapy treatment likely retains a certain degree of direct cytotoxicity to cancer cells. Susceptible cancer cells still may sustain toxic damage at drug doses considerably lower than the MTD. Because of this, prolonged drug exposure protocols have merit for some agents, particularly those that display cell cycle phase–specific toxicity, and this type of schedule could be considered metronomic. Direct killing of cancer cells also has an indirect antiangiogenic effect, given that many potent proangiogenic growth factors, such as vascular endothelial growth factor (VEGF), are produced by tumor cells. Decreased VEGF levels in the tumor microenvironment may be accomplished through a reduction in tumor cell mass as a result of direct cancer cell killing

by chemotherapy. This explains why the antiangiogenic actions of metronomic chemotherapy may be enhanced when there is concomitant direct tumor cell kill; however, in theory, blood vessel targeting by chemotherapeutic drugs does not require drug sensitivity of the tumor cell population.

Clinical Application

Small retrospective and phase II metronomic chemotherapy trials involving a variety of drugs and drug combinations have been reported recently in the veterinary oncology literature. Most clinical trial evaluations to date have paired conventional chemotherapy drugs with noncytotoxic drugs that are meant to target angiogenesis directly or indirectly. This approach was based on preclinical experiments demonstrating that such combinations resulted in superior outcomes, likely because of more complete neutralization of induced prosurvival factors such as VEGF in the tumor endothelium. As a result of this approach, most clinical trials have evaluated combination protocols without necessarily having any clear prior documentation of single-agent clinical activity for each drug. Bevacizumab, the antibody targeting human VEGF, has been a popular choice to pair with human metronomic chemotherapy schedules and has been approved by the U.S. Food and Drug Administration for the treatment of multiple cancers; however, other, more readily available "targeted" drugs shown to have at least indirect antiangiogenic effects also are commonly used. Examples are cyclooxygenase (COX) inhibitors, tetracyclines, thalidomide, and glitazones.

Veterinary Trials of Alkylating Agents

Cyclophosphamide

CYC has been the drug most commonly studied in low-dose metronomic treatment protocols in both human and veterinary oncology. A protocol of low-dose CYC 15 mg per sq meter q24h (dogs), alternating after 21 days with etoposide and paired with continuous piroxicam (0.3 mg/kg q24h PO) was evaluated for adjuvant treatment of splenic hemangiosarcoma in dogs (Lana et al, 2007). The survival time of 9 dogs treated with this regimen was no different from that of a historical control group of 24 dogs treated with doxorubicin alone. The metronomic protocol was well tolerated over a 6-month period. Pharmacokinetic analysis of etoposide in three dogs revealed detectable drug levels, although this drug may have low and variable oral bioavailability in the dog.

A low-dose continuous CYC and piroxicam protocol also was evaluated for adjuvant treatment of incompletely resected soft tissue sarcoma in dogs (Elmslie et al, 2008). Unlike in the hemangiosarcoma study, in this trial the dosage of CYC was 10 mg/m^2 q24h or q48h PO. The disease-free interval was significantly longer in the treated group of 30 dogs than in an age-, site-, and grade-matched contemporary control group of 55 dogs treated with surgery alone. Again the protocol was well tolerated, although 40% of dogs experienced mild toxicity at some point in the treatment and one dog experienced grade 4 sterile hemorrhagic cystitis. The every-other-day dosing regimen was better tolerated than daily CYC dosing.

The use of metronomic CYC treatment also has been reported recently by Marchetti and colleagues (2012) for first-line therapy of metastatic canine tumors of varying histologic types. Fifteen dogs were treated with CYC at 25 mg/m² q24h PO combined with the COX-2 inhibitor celecoxib at 2 mg/kg q24h PO. One dog showed a complete response and five dogs had stable disease with a treatment protocol that was devoid of toxicity. All dogs were reported to have improved quality-of-life scores. Most of the tumors treated were carcinomas, and as in many other trials, what the relative contribution of each drug may have been to the overall response rate was not apparent because single-agent responses to COX inhibitors have been documented in cancer-bearing dogs.

CYC has become a popular drug choice for metronomic scheduling, but it is associated with the potential for sterile hemorrhagic cystitis. Currently it is not known whether cystitis occurs more frequently in metronomic administration protocols, but close urinary monitoring is recommended strongly for these patients.

Chlorambucil

Chlorambucil has been used in many veterinary treatment protocols, such as in first-line treatment of canine chronic lymphocytic leukemia, low-grade lymphoma, and mast cell tumors, and as a replacement for CYC in patients that develop sterile hemorrhagic cystitis. The protocols used in many of these applications involve frequent drug administration on a continuous schedule that could be considered metronomic. In a recent prospective clinical trial (Leach et al, 2012), single-agent metronomic chlorambucil therapy administered at a dosage of 4 mg/m² q24h PO to 36 dogs with tumors of varying histologic types and prior treatments resulted in a complete response of over 35 weeks' duration in 3 dogs, a partial response in 1 dog, and stable disease in 17 dogs. The median progression-free interval was 61 days, and there were no grade 3 or 4 toxicities noted.

Lomustine

Lomustine (CCNU) also has been evaluated in a metronomic protocol at a dosage of 2.84 mg/m² q24h PO, which corresponds to the conversion of a 60 mg/m² q3wk dosage into a daily schedule (Tripp et al, 2011). A total of 81 dogs with various primary and metastatic tumors were treated using this single-agent regimen for a median of 98 days. Lomustine has been associated with hepatotoxicosis and thrombocytopenia, and in this study azotemia also developed to some degree in eight cases. Treatment was discontinued in 22 dogs due to toxicosis of gastrointestinal, bone marrow, hepatic, or renal origin, although the treatment protocol generally was well tolerated.

Veterinary Trials of Platinum Compounds

Although not designed for metronomic administration per se, the various slow-release and oral formulations of platinum compounds that have been evaluated in veterinary oncology may represent metronomic application of these drugs. Administration of slow-release cisplatin using delivery systems such as an open-cell polylactic acid polymer impregnated with drug has been studied in a variety of settings, including treatment of canine osteosarcoma, soft tissue sarcoma, and nasal tumors, and has shown desirable efficacy and manageable toxicity. Carboplatin also has been evaluated recently using both a slow-release drug formulation and prolonged administration by a subcutaneously placed pump providing continuous drug release over 3 to 7 days. This latter protocol was effective in the treatment of canine osteosarcoma following amputation or limb-sparing surgery (Simcock et al, 2012). A dose-escalation and pharmacokinetic study of satraplatin, the first orally bioavailable platinum agent, has been reported recently (Selting et al, 2011). The aim of this study was to determine the MTD; however, the fact that this drug is administered orally makes possible the future investigation of the use of satraplatin in a metronomic dosing schedule. These studies with platinum compounds raise the general question of whether forms of slow-release delivery of chemotherapeutics, such as liposome encapsulation, may represent a form of metronomic drug delivery.

Patient Selection and Monitoring

The identification and application of biomarkers is becoming increasingly important as oncology moves further into clinical application of targeted therapeutics. The goals in the development of validated biomarkers are to (1) predict patient populations that will or will not respond to treatment, (2) monitor response to therapy on a cellular or molecular level, and (3) determine the proper therapeutic dosage for targeted agents, which often possess optimal biologic activity at dosages well below the traditionally defined MTD. The use of biomarkers in metronomic chemotherapy protocols can serve all three goals.

Measurements of tumor tissue expression and blood-based circulating growth factor levels have been the most popular approaches for predicting response to metronomic chemotherapy, and VEGF is the most studied molecule. For example, in an investigation of metronomic treatment with CYC and celecoxib (Marchetti et al, 2012), low baseline plasma VEGF level was predictive of response, as has been observed in human clinical trials of metronomic CYC. In many cases a comparison of pretreatment and posttreatment levels may provide the insight to be gained from such a surrogate marker, as has been demonstrated with urinary basic fibroblast growth factor and VEGF in piroxicam treatment of canine transitional cell carcinoma. The most important biomarker for metronomic chemotherapy protocols may be one that defines tumor response because inhibition of angiogenesis or modulation of immune surveillance may not necessarily correspond to a large reduction in tumor volume. Tumor stasis stands in sharp contrast to the measurable tumor shrinkage that results from MTD chemotherapy approaches. Systems for clinical evaluation of tumor response to therapy often are formally based on World Health Organization criteria or the Response Evaluation Criteria in Solid Tumors (RECIST), which equate tumor shrinkage with positive outcome. Therefore there may be a need both for recognition of sustained stable disease as a desirable clinical trial end point and for biomarkers to evaluate angiogenic or other functional changes during treatment. Imaging modalities such as dynamic contrast-enhanced magnetic resonance imaging and positron emission tomography that provide information about vascular function or tumor metabolism are potentially valuable tools for monitoring the effects of targeted therapy.

Dose optimization also represents an area of unmet need for biomarkers in the field of metronomic chemotherapy. This area of research addresses the obvious question of how great a reduction of dose from the MTD is optimal. Treg cells are providing insight in this regard. Recent results demonstrated a dose-dependent reduction in Treg cells with metronomic CYC treatment (Burton et al, 2011). This effect, as well as changes in microvessel density, were observed at a CYC dosage of 15 mg/m^2 q24h but not at a dosage of 12.5 mg/m^2 q24h, which led the investigators to conclude that 15 mg/m^2 may be a more appropriate dose for future clinical trials. In addition to Treg changes, temporal changes in other markers may be evaluated in future studies.

Combination of Metronomic Chemotherapy with Targeted Drugs

Generally speaking, in contrast to the drugs used in MTD chemotherapy protocols, targeted drugs such as receptor tyrosine kinase inhibitors often are given for longer periods of time at their optimal biologic dose. As a result, combining targeted drugs with metronomic chemotherapy may be an effective treatment strategy because the drugs follow a similar dosing and scheduling principle. For example, clinical evaluation of combination therapy using the receptor tyrosine kinase inhibitor toceranib and metronomic CYC was reported recently (Mitchell et al, 2012). In addition, it is possible that there may be a role for targeted antiangiogenic treatment or metronomic chemotherapy in combination with MTD chemotherapy protocols to neutralize rebound angiogenic responses that occur during the break period. This approach has been demonstrated successfully in preclinical studies; however, rigorous clinical trials are necessary to identify and optimize effective drug combination protocols.

References and Suggested Reading

Burton JH et al: Low-dose cyclophosphamide selectively decreases regulatory T cells and inhibits angiogenesis in dogs with soft tissue sarcoma, *J Vet Intern Med* 25:920, 2011.

Elmslie RE, Glawe P, Dow SW: Metronomic therapy with cyclophosphamide and piroxicam effectively delays tumor recurrence in dogs with incompletely resected soft tissue sarcomas, *J Vet Intern Med* 22:1373, 2008.

Kerbel RS, Kamen BA: The anti-angiogenic basis of metronomic chemotherapy, *Nat Rev Cancer* 4:423, 2004.

Lana S et al: Continuous low-dose oral chemotherapy for adjuvant therapy of splenic hemangiosarcoma in dogs, *J Vet Intern Med* 21:764, 2007.

Leach TN et al: Prospective trial of metronomic chlorambucil chemotherapy in dogs with naturally occurring cancer, *Vet Comp Oncol* 10:102, 2012.

Marchetti V et al: First-line metronomic chemotherapy in a metastatic model of spontaneous canine tumours: a pilot study, *Invest New Drugs* 30(4):1725, 2012.

Mitchell L, Thamm DH, Biller BS: Clinical and immunomodulatory effects of toceranib combined with low-dose cyclophosphamide in dogs with cancer, *J Vet Intern Med* 26:355, 2012.

Mutsaers AJ: Antiangiogenic and metronomic therapy. In Withrow SJ, Vail DM, Page RL, editors: *Withrow and MacEwen's small animal clinical oncology*, ed 5, St Louis, 2012, Saunders.

Pasquier E, Kavallaris M, Andre N: Metronomic chemotherapy: new rationale for new directions, *Nat Rev Clin Oncol* 7:455, 2010.

Selting KA et al: Evaluation of satraplatin in dogs with spontaneously occurring malignant tumors, *J Vet Intern Med* 25:909, 2011.

Simcock JO et al: Evaluation of a single subcutaneous infusion of carboplatin as adjuvant chemotherapy for dogs with osteosarcoma: 17 cases (2006-2010), *J Am Vet Med Assoc* 241:608, 2012.

Tripp CD et al: Tolerability of metronomic administration of lomustine in dogs with cancer, *J Vet Intern Med* 25:278, 2011.

CHAPTER 79

Drug Update: Toceranib

CHERYL A. LONDON, *Columbus, Ohio*

Toceranib phosphate (Palladia) is an orally bioavailable small-molecule inhibitor that blocks a variety of receptor tyrosine kinases (RTKs) expressed on the cell surface by acting as a reversible competitive inhibitor of adenosine triphosphate binding; it thereby prevents receptor phosphorylation and subsequent downstream signaling. The published inhibitory profile of toceranib includes the RTKs, vascular endothelial growth factor receptor 2 (VEGFR2), platelet-derived growth factor receptor β (PDGFRβ), and stem cell factor receptor (KIT) (London et al, 2003); however, it is very closely related to another TKI called *sunitinib* (Sutent) that blocks the activity of several members of the split RTK family, including VEGFR2, VEGFR3, PDGFRα/β, KIT, colony-stimulating factor receptor (CSF1R), FMS-like tyrosine kinase-3 (FLT3), and "rearranged during transfection" RTK (RET) (Papaetis and Syrigos, 2009). A recent kinome analysis (London et al, n.d.) supports the broad activity of toceranib against the split kinase RTKs, RET, and possibly Janus kinase (JAK) family members. Toceranib initially was developed as an antiangiogenic agent because inhibition of VEGFR and PDGFR family members blocks angiogenesis in several mouse tumor models; however, its broad target profile including KIT, FLT3, and RET results in direct antitumor activity in some cancer types as well. The combination of antiangiogenic and antitumor activity likely provides more extensive clinical activity than that observed with narrowly targeted TKIs.

Work with Toceranib before Food and Drug Administration Approval

The first evaluation of toceranib in dogs was a phase I clinical trial in 57 dogs with a variety of cancers (London et al, 2003). In this study, objective responses were observed in 16 dogs (objective response rate [ORR], 28%) consisting of 6 complete responses (CRs) and 10 partial responses (PRs), with stable disease (SD) achieved in an additional 15 dogs for an overall clinical benefit rate of 54%. Responding tumors included sarcomas, carcinomas, melanomas, myeloma, and mast cell tumors (MCTs). The highest ORR was in dogs with MCT, with 10 of 11 dogs with activating mutations in the c-*kit* gene exhibiting responses (n = 9) or SD (n = 1). This study also established the maximum tolerated dose (MTD) of toceranib as 3.25 mg/kg q48h PO. Adverse events were primarily gastrointestinal (GI), including loss of appetite, diarrhea, and less commonly vomiting, although these toxicities were

relatively well controlled with the addition of appropriate concomitant medications.

Based on the phase I trial results, a placebo-controlled randomized registration study of toceranib was performed subsequently in dogs with nonresectable grade II and III MCTs (London et al, 2009). During the blinded phase, the ORR in toceranib-treated dogs (n = 86) was 37.2% (7 CRs, 25 PRs) compared with 7.9% (5 PRs) in placebo-treated dogs (n = 63). Of 58 dogs that received toceranib following placebo failure, 41.4% (8 CRs, 16 PRs) experienced an objective response. The ORR for all 145 dogs was 42.8% (21 CRs, 41 PRs) with an additional 16 dogs experiencing SD for an overall clinical benefit rate of 60%. Dogs with MCTs harboring activating mutations in c-*kit* were roughly twice as likely to respond to toceranib than those with wild-type c-*kit* (69% versus 37%), and dogs without lymph node metastasis had a higher ORR than those with lymph node involvement (67% versus 46%). As expected, GI toxicity was the most common adverse effect and was generally manageable with symptomatic therapy, drug holidays, and dosage reductions.

Work with Toceranib after Food and Drug Administration Approval

Following its approval in 2009, toceranib was used off label to treat a variety of canine cancers, typically in the setting of failed primary or standard-of-care treatments. A retrospective analysis of the use of toceranib in this setting was reported recently, and biologic activity was observed in several solid tumors, including anal gland anal sac adenocarcinoma (AGASACA), metastatic osteosarcoma, thyroid carcinoma, head and neck carcinoma, and nasal carcinoma (London et al, 2012). Clinical benefit (CR, PR, plus SD of clinically relevant duration) was observed in 63 of 85 dogs (74%), including 28 of 32 dogs with AGASACA (8 PRs, 20 SD), 11 of 23 dogs with osteosarcoma (1 PRs, 10 SD), 12 of 15 dogs with thyroid carcinoma (4 PRs, 8 SD), 7 of 8 dogs with head and neck carcinomas (1 CR, 5 PRs, 1 SD), and 5 of 7 dogs with nasal carcinomas (1 CR, 4 SD). In dogs experiencing clinical benefit, the median dose of toceranib was 2.8 mg/kg; 36 of 63 (58.7%) dogs were dosed on Monday, Wednesday, and Friday, and 47 of 63 (74.6%) were treated for 4 months or longer. These data provide preliminary evidence that toceranib exhibits clinical benefit in dogs with certain solid tumors, although future prospective studies are necessary to define its true activity.

There is significant interest in the use of nonsteroidal antiinflammatory medications (NSAIDs) for the treatment of cancer in dogs and cats, not only for the management of cancer-related pain, but as part of multiagent protocols. Piroxicam, a mixed cyclooxygenase-1/cyclooxygenase-2 inhibitor, has demonstrated single-agent activity in some canine cancers, particularly carcinomas. Given that both toceranib and piroxicam exhibit dose-limiting GI toxicity, it was predicted that combining these drugs would result in a more unfavorable adverse effect profile that would preclude their concurrent use. Therefore a phase I trial was performed in dogs with tumors (non-MCT) to establish the safety of toceranib/piroxicam coadministration (Chon et al, 2012). Five escalating dosages, up to and including the approved label dosage for toceranib and the standard dosage for piroxicam, were tested and no increase was noted in the frequency of dose-limiting adverse effects necessitating drug discontinuation. Additionally, several antitumor responses were observed. Although the combination of standard dosages of both drugs (toceranib 3.25 mg/kg q48h PO and piroxicam 0.3 mg/kg q24h PO) was found to be generally safe, the dogs were not monitored long term to assess whether GI adverse effects occurred after long-term drug administration. Therefore it is generally recommended that the piroxicam be given q48h alternating with the toceranib to avoid potential GI issues.

Because the ability to combine toceranib with chemotherapy agents would be desirable, particularly in the setting of MCT, a phase I clinical trial was performed to identify an appropriate dosing regimen combining toceranib with vinblastine in canine MCT (Robat et al, 2012). These two drugs were chosen because both exhibit single-agent activity in MCT, and they have nonoverlapping primary toxicities. The dose-limiting toxicity for the toceranib/vinblastine combination was found to be neutropenia, and the MTD was vinblastine at 1.6 mg/m^2 every other week with toceranib 3.25 mg/kg q48h. The 50% reduction in dose intensity for vinblastine was required because of the enhanced myelosuppression when it was combined with toceranib. Despite the reduction in vinblastine dose intensity, the ORR was 71% for the drug combination. The enhanced myelosuppression and significant biologic activity suggests the possibility of additive or synergistic activity, although a prospective randomized evaluation of this drug combination will be necessary to confirm this.

In addition to combining toceranib with chemotherapeutic drugs, there is interest in combining it with radiation therapy (RT) for the treatment of MCT and other canine cancers (Carlsten et al, 2012). Dogs with nonresectable MCTs received prednisone, omeprazole, diphenhydramine, and toceranib at 2.75 mg/kg on a Monday-Wednesday-Friday schedule for 1 week before starting coarsely fractionated RT (24 Gy delivered in three or four treatments over 21 days). The ORR was 76.4%, with 58.8% of dogs achieving CR and 17.6% experiencing PR. The overall median survival time was not reached with a median follow-up of 374 days. Importantly, there was no evidence of enhanced radiation-induced toxicities in this clinical trial. Future clinical trials are necessary to determine the long-term activity of combined RT and toceranib treatment in dogs with cancer.

Toceranib Dosing and Clinical Management

The toceranib label indicates that dosing should be initiated at 3.25 mg/kg q48h and the dose reduced based on clinical adverse effects; the lowest recommended dose is 2.2 mg/kg; however, evidence exists that good biologic activity occurs when doses are initiated below the 3.25 mg/kg level, and flexible dosing schedules also may be effective. For example, in the phase I study, of 16 dogs treated with toceranib at 2.5 mg/kg q48h, 6 (37.5%) exhibited a response to therapy (4 CRs, 2 PRs). This compares favorably with the results in 20 dogs treated with 3.25 mg/kg q48h, of which 8 (40%) had objective responses (2 CRs and 6 PRs). Based on these data, it is possible that for many dogs lower doses of toceranib result in significant clinical activity. This is important because clinical experience with toceranib suggests that dosing at 2.5 to 2.75 mg/kg q48h is better tolerated than dosing at the MTD, which results in less toxicity, better owner compliance, and fewer drug holidays. This was recently confirmed in a prospective study in which dogs with solid tumors received lower doses of toceranib (London et al, unpublished data). Pharmacokinetic analysis of toceranib blood levels in these dogs showed good drug exposure across 2.4 to 2.8 mg/kg q48 hours, with all in what would be considered therapeutic range by day 21 of dosing. In this study, the adverse event profile was reduced with the lower dose of toceranib, and nearly all reported toxicities were either grade 1 or 2 in nature. With respect to the dosing regimen, the label indicates that the drug should be administered q48h. Data generated from the retrospective analysis of toceranib use in solid tumors found that the Monday-Wednesday-Friday schedule may be better tolerated by some dogs and may be particularly useful when toceranib is combined with other therapeutic drugs, such as NSAIDs.

Dogs with cancer may have underlying conditions that predispose them to some of the toxicities induced by toceranib. Because the use of toceranib may enhance the magnitude of clinical illness in patients that are already sick, it is highly recommended that every effort be made to improve the health status of dogs before initiation of treatment. This is particularly true for MCT patients, who may have subclinical (or clinical) GI ulceration making them more susceptible to vomiting, diarrhea, and GI bleeding. It is important to note that toceranib drug holidays, dose reductions, and schedule modifications are extremely useful tools in managing clinical toxicities and should be instituted as needed in conjunction with the concomitant use of appropriate medications. Anecdotal data suggest that dogs receiving toceranib may benefit from the use of famotidine or omeprazole to help prevent GI ulceration. Diarrhea remains the most common adverse effect and occurs in most dogs that receive toceranib. Intermittent use of metronidazole or loperamide can be effective in treating minor episodes, although some dogs require continual administration of one or both agents to manage this toxicity. Inappetence may occur in dogs receiving toceranib and often responds to standard antinausea therapies (metoclopramide, ondansetron, maropitant) or the addition of low-dose prednisone to the treatment regimen. Other toxicities that have been observed since toceranib's approval are hepatotoxicity, protein-losing nephropathy, and pancreatitis. In the author's experience, hepatotoxicity responds to the addition of Denamarin (a nutraceutical containing S-adenosylmethionine and silybin), which permits reinstitution of toceranib, often at a lower dose. The author has effectively managed protein-losing nephropathy in dogs receiving toceranib with both a dose reduction and the addition of enalapril/benazepril to the treatment regimen. Although toceranib-induced pancreatitis is an uncommon event in dogs, caution should be used in deciding whether toceranib therapy should be continued once the condition has resolved.

Summary

Toceranib has become an important asset in the management of several canine cancers. Clinical work is ongoing to help define the most appropriate use of toceranib as both a single agent and in combination therapies. Vigilant patient monitoring and rapid intervention at the first sign of clinical toxicities is critical for the successful use of toceranib in dogs.

References and Suggested Reading

Carlsten KS et al: Multicenter prospective trial of hypofractionated radiation treatment, toceranib, and prednisone for measurable canine mast cell tumors, *J Vet Intern Med* 26:135, 2012.
Chon E et al: Safety evaluation of combination toceranib phosphate (Palladia®) and piroxicam in tumor-bearing dogs (excluding mast cell tumors): a phase I dose-finding study, *Vet Comp Oncol* 10:184, 2012. Epub March 21, 2011.
London CA et al: Unpublished data.
London CA et al: Phase I dose-escalating study of SU11654, a small molecule receptor tyrosine kinase inhibitor, in dogs with spontaneous malignancies, *Clin Cancer Res* 9:2755, 2003.
London CA et al: Multi-center, placebo-controlled, double-blind, randomized study of oral toceranib phosphate (SU11654), a receptor tyrosine kinase inhibitor, for the treatment of dogs with recurrent (either local or distant) mast cell tumor following surgical excision, *Clin Cancer Res* 15:3856, 2009.
London C et al: Preliminary evidence for biologic activity of toceranib phosphate (Palladia®) in solid tumours, *Vet Comp Oncol* 10:194, 2012. Epub June 1, 2011.
Papaetis GS, Syrigos KN: Sunitinib: a multitargeted receptor tyrosine kinase inhibitor in the era of molecular cancer therapies, *Biodrugs* 23:377, 2009.
Robat C et al: Safety evaluation of combination vinblastine and toceranib phosphate (Palladia®) in dogs: a phase I dose-finding study, *Vet Comp Oncol* 10:174, 2012. Epub January 31, 2011.

CHAPTER 80

Drug Update: Masitinib

KEVIN A. HAHN, *Topeka, Kansas*

Masitinib is a tyrosine kinase inhibitor (TKI), an innovative class of drug that recently become has available to veterinary medicine. Masitinib was the first approved anticancer drug in veterinary medicine, receiving approval from the European Medicines Agency in 2008 under the name Masivet. Masitinib now also is registered for use in the United States under the name Kinavet-CA1 after receiving conditional approval from the U.S. Food and Drug Administration. Masitinib is indicated for the treatment of recurrent (postsurgery) or nonresectable grade II or III cutaneous mast cell tumors (MCTs) in dogs that have not previously received radiation therapy or chemotherapy except corticosteroids.

Targeted Therapies

TKI targeted therapies selectively inhibit protein tyrosine kinases, enzymes involved in cellular signaling pathways that regulate key cell functions and survival. Activation of these enzymes through mechanisms such as point mutations or overexpression can lead to various forms of cancer and nononcologic disorders. Masitinib has been designed specifically to optimize its selectivity against key tyrosine kinases that are implicated in various cancers (primarily KIT [stem cell factor receptor], platelet-derived growth factor receptor, and Lyn [an intracellular kinase of the Src family]) while not inhibiting, at therapeutic

TABLE **80-1**

Therapeutic Potential of Masitinib in Veterinary Medicine

Targets	Action	Therapeutic Potential
KIT PDGFR FAK pathway	Inhibition of proto-oncogenic targets	Mast cell tumor T-cell lymphoma Melanoma Hemangiosarcoma
PDGFR Lyn/FAK	Potentiation of chemotherapeutic agents	Tumors treated with chemotherapy
Mast cells via KIT/Lyn	Inhibition of mast cell activation	Atopic dermatitis Arthritis Asthma Atopy

NOTE: Masitinib has regulatory approval only for the treatment of canine mast cell tumors.
FAK, Focal adhesion kinase; *KIT,* stem cell factor receptor; *Lyn,* intracellular kinase of the Src family; *PDGFR,* platelet-derived growth factor receptor.

doses, those tyrosine kinases or tyrosine kinase receptors associated with possible toxicity (Dubreuil et al, 2009). This degree of specificity contrasts with the TKIs imatinib and toceranib, which inhibit a broader range of kinases as part of a more multitargeted strategy; for example, toceranib inhibits in excess of 50 kinases.

Indications in Veterinary Medicine

To date, masitinib has been evaluated in two pivotal phase III randomized controlled veterinary trials: the first in dogs with MCT (Hahn et al, 2008, 2010) and the second in dogs with atopic dermatitis (Cadot et al, 2011). Observations from these two studies showed that masitinib was effective in managing the disease condition and was generally well tolerated with medically manageable adverse effects. The most common adverse effects that may occur with masitinib are diarrhea and vomiting. To minimize the risk of adverse drug effects, and in particular protein-loss syndrome, regular evaluations that include a complete blood count, serum biochemical evaluation, and urine protein assessment are required.

Additional case studies of on- and off-label use in Europe, along with ongoing *in vitro* preclinical research, are driving development of further clinical application of masitinib in the treatment of other cancers and as a chemosensitizer for standard chemotherapies (Ogilvie et al, 2011; Thamm et al, 2012). Table 80-1 lists the various oncologic and immune-mediated diseases for which masitinib treatment is being evaluated, along with the associated kinase or cellular target and mechanism of action. Additionally, masitinib is being developed for the treatment of feline disorders, including asthma, injection site sarcoma, and melanoma (Ogilvie et al, 2011). It is interesting to note from a comparative standpoint that masitinib is being investigated for various indications simultaneously in veterinary and human medicine.

TABLE **80-2**

Response and Survival Rates with Masitinib Treatment of Canine Mast Cell Tumors

	Masitinib	Placebo	*P* value
Best response rate (first 6 mo)	50%	29%	0.020
12-mo survival rate (nonresectable tumors)	62%	36%	0.024
24-mo survival rate (nonresectable tumors)	40%	15%	0.040
Median overall survival (first-line use, nonresectable tumors)	803 days	322 days	0.045

Masitinib for Treatment of Mast Cell Tumors

Registration of masitinib was based on the successful outcome of a phase III randomized clinical trial that included 202 dogs with grade II or III cutaneous MCT recruited from 25 veterinary centers in the United States and France (Hahn et al, 2008). This trial, and its long-term follow-up study, reported that treatment with masitinib significantly increased survival rates at 6, 12, and 24 months compared with placebo (Hahn et al, 2008, 2010). Responses varied from complete disappearance of the tumor to no impact at all, with 62% of dogs treated with masitinib still alive after 12 months of therapy. Table 80-2 shows long-term survival data from the phase III study. The therapeutic benefits of masitinib were more pronounced when it was used as first-line therapy and occurred regardless of whether the tumors expressed mutant or wild-type KIT. This suggests that masitinib should be used before any other treatments, including conventional chemotherapies, when the tumor is nonresectable. Finally, analyses revealed that control of disease at 6 months of treatment correlated highly with long-term survival, which indicates that tumor stabilization also provides important clinical benefits (Hahn et al, 2008, 2010).

Masitinib for Treatment of Canine Atopic Dermatitis

The main cellular targets of masitinib are mast cells, which are capable of releasing large amounts of proinflammatory mediators that result in the triggering and sustaining of an inflammatory response. Masitinib therefore can provide therapeutic benefit in inflammatory or autoimmune diseases with mast cell involvement, such as atopic dermatitis, asthma, inflammatory bowel disease, and arthritis. The most advanced of these applications is the treatment of canine atopic dermatitis, for which a phase III study enrolling one of the largest cohorts tested to date showed a significant reduction of clinical signs following masitinib treatment (Cadot et al, 2011). In general, a positive response was evident for treatment-naïve dogs, dogs resistant to cyclosporin or corticosteroids, and dogs with severe pruritus; the latter two groups represent populations with high unmet medical need. More specifically, a reduction of 50% or more in the score on the Canine Atopic Dermatitis Extent and Severity Index (CADESI-02) at week 12 was observed in 61% of masitinib-treated dogs but in only 35% of control dogs. For dogs resistant to cyclosporin or corticosteroids, the response rate was 60% versus 31% in control dogs. Overall, 63% of investigators assessed masitinib efficacy as good to excellent versus 35% in control dogs.

Future Directions for Masitinib

Owing to its novel mechanism of action, masitinib holds therapeutic potential in veterinary medicine for both oncologic and immune-mediated conditions. There is grade 1 evidence of effectiveness in managing canine mast cell tumors and atopic dermatitis. Emerging clinical evidence also indicates that masitinib may be of benefit in the treatment of canine T-cell lymphoma, neurofibrosarcoma, and melanoma; in the treatment of feline asthma and injection site sarcoma; and as a chemosensitizer for standard chemotherapies (Ogilvie et al, 2011).

TKIs are now making inroads into veterinary medicine, with treatment of MCT being their first major success story. The evidence reviewed previously indicates that this remarkably versatile class of targeted therapeutic drugs will become an increasingly important tool in veterinary medicine.

References and Suggested Reading

Cadot P et al: Masitinib decreases signs of canine atopic dermatitis: a multicentre, randomized, double-blind, placebo-controlled phase 3 trial, *Vet Dermatol* 22(6):554, 2011.

Dubreuil P et al: Masitinib (AB1010), a potent and selective tyrosine kinase inhibitor targeting KIT, *PLoS One* 4:e7258, 2009.

Hahn KA et al: Masitinib is safe and effective for the treatment of canine mast cell tumors, *J Vet Intern Med* 22:1301, 2008.

Hahn KA et al: Evaluation of 12- and 24-month survival rates after treatment with masitinib in dogs with nonresectable mast cell tumors, *Am J Vet Res* 71:1354, 2010.

Ogilvie GK et al: Masitinib—a targeted therapy with applications in veterinary oncology and inflammatory diseases, *CAB Rev* 6(021):1, 2011.

Thamm DH et al: Masitinib as a chemosensitizer of canine tumor cell lines: proof of concept study, *Vet J* 191(1):131, 2012. Epub February 17, 2011.

CHAPTER 81

Oral Tumors

MICHAEL S. KENT, *Davis, California*
BERNARD SÉGUIN, *Corvallis, Oregon*

Tumors of the oral cavity are relatively common in both dogs and cats, representing approximately 6% of tumors in dogs and 3% of tumors in cats. They can be benign or malignant, and multiple histologic types have been described. The most commonly reported oral tumor in dogs is malignant melanoma, followed by squamous cell carcinoma (SCC), fibrosarcoma, and peripheral odontogenic fibroma. Many other tumor types have been reported and include chondrosarcoma, osteosarcoma, lymphoma, mast cell tumor, and plasmacytoma. In cats the most commonly reported tumors are SCC, fibrosarcoma, and osteosarcoma. Other types include odontogenic tumor, lymphoma, chondrosarcoma, salivary gland tumor, and melanoma.

Presenting Signs

Although oral masses may be found by owners or discovered incidentally on an oral examination by a

veterinarian as part of a routine physical examination or during a dental procedure, animals often are clinically affected. The most common clinical signs in dogs and cats with oral neoplasia are halitosis, dysphagia, ptyalism, facial deformity, pain on opening of the mouth, weight loss, and epistaxis. In cats, owners also may notice decreased grooming or unkempt hair coat.

Diagnosis

Biopsy is an essential part of the evaluation of a dog or cat with an oral mass. It is not possible to distinguish tumor type or degree of malignancy based on visual inspection. Aspiration cannot often be performed without anesthesia or heavy sedation and is less likely to give a definitive diagnosis, which limits the usefulness of this test. Incisional biopsy and histopathologic evaluation provides important information regarding additional staging needed, treatment approach, and prognosis. The biopsy procedure should be planned properly so that the biopsy tract can be included easily as part of the excision of the tumor at the time of curative-intent surgery or included in the field of radiation if radiation therapy (RT) is performed. For tumors that appear locally invasive on physical examination, ideally the biopsy should be performed following imaging (see section on staging). If a definitive surgical excision is attempted, margin assessment is important to check for completeness of excision and the need for adjuvant therapy (see later).

Staging

Staging of oral tumors in both dogs and cats evaluates for the extent and invasion of the local tumor as well as the presence of regional or distant metastasis. A clinical staging system has been described by the World Health Organization for use with oral tumors (Table 81-1). This staging system can be used to guide pretreatment assessment and also is important for treatment planning. Documenting the exact location and size of an oral mass helps assess the local extent of a tumor, although radiographs and computed tomography (CT) can provide more complete information as to extent and bony involvement. To assess local lymph node involvement, palpation and cytologic evaluation of mandibular lymph node aspirates is an essential first step. Because lymph node drainage is variable in the head, contrast CT studies and ultrasonography can be performed to further assess local and regional lymph nodes, which include the mandibular, parotid, retropharyngeal, and cervical lymph nodes. Ultrasonographic guidance may be necessary for sampling of all but the mandibular lymph nodes. For malignant tumors, either three-view thoracic radiography or CT of the thorax should be performed to assess for pulmonary metastasis.

Treatment—General Principles

Surgery

Surgery is the most commonly used treatment for oral tumors in dogs and cats. The aggressiveness of the surgery depends mostly on tumor type and the goal of the owner. Tumors that invade the mandible or maxilla require mandibulectomy or maxillectomy, respectively, for a chance at cure. The size of the margins required to obtain a complete excision has not been evaluated thoroughly, and cited margins therefore remain a recommendation. In dogs margins of at least 2 cm, and preferably 3 cm, are recommended for malignant tumors such as SCC, malignant melanoma, and fibrosarcoma. In cats surgical margins of more than 2 cm for SCC are recommended because of high local recurrence rates; however, this is seldom possible because these tumors usually are advanced. Benign tumors can be removed by marginal excision, for which a margin of 0.5 cm around the tumor is recommended. Acanthomatous ameloblastomas, although considered benign tumors, are locally invasive and require wide margins like a malignant tumor.

Peripheral odontogenic fibromas (previously known as *fibromatous epulides*) can be excised by cutting them at

TABLE 81-1

World Health Organization Staging System for Oral Tumors in Dogs and Cats

Primary Tumor (T)

Tis	Preinvasive carcinoma (carcinoma *in situ*)
T0	No evidence of tumor
T1	Tumor <2 cm maximum diameter
T2	Tumor 2-4 cm maximum diameter
T3	Tumor >4 cm maximum diameter
Subclassification a: Without bone invasion	
Subclassification b: With bone invasion	

Regional Lymph Nodes (N)

N0	No evidence of regional lymph node involvement
N1	Movable ipsilateral nodes
N2	Movable contralateral or bilateral nodes
N3	Fixed nodes
For N1 and N2 subclassification a: No histologic evidence of metastasis	
For N1 and N2 subclassification b: Histologic evidence of metastasis	

Distant Metastasis (M)

M0	No evidence of distant metastasis
M1	Distant metastasis (including distant lymph nodes) detected

Stage Grouping

	T	N	M
I	T1	N0, N1a, N2a	M0
II	T2	N0, N1a, N2a	M0
III	T3	N0, N1a, N2a	M0
	Any T	N1b	M0
IV	Any T	Any N2b or N3	M0
	Any T	Any N	M1

their base along the gingiva. Cautery or cryotherapy can be used at the base to help prevent local recurrence.

Benign tumors and small malignant tumors involving the mandible can be resected by mandibular rim excision. With this technique, the ventral cortex of the mandible is preserved and left intact. This avoids some of the adverse effects of a complete segmental mandibulectomy such as mandibular drift and malocclusion. Case selection for this technique is imperative. This procedure cannot be performed in a small-breed dog, and the tumor must be 10 mm dorsal to the mandibular canal. Dental radiography and CT with and without tumor contrast are necessary to ensure that a rim excision is appropriate (Arzi and Verstraete, 2010; Murray et al, 2010). If there are any doubts, it is best to perform a segmental mandibulectomy to ensure complete excision of the tumor, particularly with malignant tumors and acanthomatous ameloblastomas.

Tumors of the tongue can be excised by partial or complete glossectomy in dogs. Dogs can adapt to a complete glossectomy, but a feeding tube should be placed in animals in which more than 50% of the tongue is removed because it can take several weeks for the animal to adapt (Dvorak et al, 2004). Anecdotally, cats do not do well with significant (>50%) glossectomies.

Chemotherapy

The use of adjuvant chemotherapy in the treatment of oral tumors depends largely on tumor type, grade, local control, and goals of therapy. The use of systemic chemotherapy to treat gross disease and distant metastasis is of limited value in most cases and is considered palliative. In one study of dogs treated with carboplatin for oral melanoma, an objective response rate of 28% was reported. The responses were short-lived in most cases, with a median response duration of 165 days (Rassnick et al, 2001).

Radiation Therapy

The role of RT in the treatment of oral tumors depends on the species and histologic features of the tumor. It also depends on the goal of therapy. RT can be used alone as a primary therapy, the goal of which is either cure or palliation of clinical signs, or it can be used as an adjunctive therapy to surgery when a tumor is resected incompletely. The goals and course of therapy depend on the histologic characteristics of the tumor, the extent of local disease, the stage of disease, and the wishes of the owner. Dogs and cats not expected to live longer than 6 months, even with treatment, often are treated using palliative protocols, whereas those with a better prognosis are treated with curative-intent protocols to avoid unacceptable and life-threatening adverse effects.

The most significant acute effect associated with RT is mucositis, or inflammation of the mucous membranes. Although this tends to be worse with definitive protocols, it generally is well tolerated and resolves within a week or two of finishing a course of RT. Late effects, which can occur months to years after completion of a course of RT, occur more commonly with palliative protocols and can be life threatening. Because of the risk of late effects, particularly the increased risk of radiation-induced bone necrosis and fracture, any tooth extractions done in a previously irradiated area should be performed as atraumatically as possible with the alveolar bone smoothed. Other late effects of concern in dogs or cats that have undergone RT include necrosis of mucosal tissues and secondary tumor formation in the radiation field. It generally is recommended that a complete oral examination be performed and that any required dental work be done before RT is begun.

Targeted Therapy

The use of targeted therapies is growing in veterinary oncology. Probably the most studied and oldest drug in this category is the nonsteroidal antiinflammatory drug (NSAID) piroxicam. Expression of cyclooxygenase-2 has been identified in SCC in both dogs and cats. As a single agent, piroxicam (0.3 mg/kg q24h or q48h PO) has had limited efficacy in the treatment of SCC in dogs and cats (Schmidt et al, 2001). Caution is necessary in the use of NSAIDs in animals with renal insufficiency or renal failure. Increased toxicity has been seen when piroxicam is used in combination with chemotherapy agents such as cisplatin.

Toceranib phosphate, a multitargeted tyrosine kinase inhibitor, has been approved by the Food and Drug Administration for use in the treatment of canine mast cell tumors. The phase I trial of this drug included several dogs with oral melanoma (n = 3) and SCC (n = 2). Although no objective tumor responses were seen, stable disease was achieved for a period of time in two of the three dogs with oral melanoma and one of the two dogs with SCC, which indicates a possible role for this drug in the treatment of oral tumors (London et al, 2003). The use of toceranib in cats, alone or in combination with RT, currently is being investigated.

Immunotherapy

The use of immunotherapy for oral tumors is evolving rapidly. To date, immunotherapy has been limited largely to the treatment of malignant melanoma, although it is being investigated for treatment of other tumor types. In melanoma, multiple therapeutic vaccine strategies have been pursued and both preclinical and clinical trials have been reported (Grosenbaugh et al, 2011). Recently the U.S. Department of Agriculture has approved a xenogeneic plasmid DNA vaccine encoding the human tyrosinase gene for use in dogs with locally controlled stage I or II oral melanoma. Currently it is available only for use by board-certified oncologists, and full efficacy data for this vaccine in canine oral melanoma treatment still are pending; however, this vaccine may prove useful in at least a subset of dogs diagnosed with malignant melanoma. There have been anecdotal reports of the use of this vaccine in cats, but no efficacy data are available.

Specific Tumor Types

Oral Melanoma

Oral melanomas in dogs are highly aggressive. They can be pigmented, variably pigmented, or amelanotic in appearance. They are locally aggressive, invade underlying bone, and have a high metastatic rate, with local lymph nodes and the lungs being the most common sites of metastasis. Treatment for local control can include surgery and RT. The size of the tumor is important for prognosis, and tumors of less than 2 cm in diameter have a better prognosis. The reported median survival time for dogs with oral melanoma treated with surgery alone is 17 months for T1 tumors and approximately 5 months for T2 and T3 tumors. Most RT protocols are hypofractionated (palliative) protocols and are good at achieving local control, with 80% to 100% response rates for gross disease and reported median survival times of 5 to 12 months; most dogs die of metastatic disease (Proulx et al, 2003). The most commonly implemented chemotherapy protocols use carboplatin, although its efficacy in the adjuvant setting has not been well evaluated. Immunotherapy (see earlier) also has shown some promise as an adjuvant therapy to treat presumptive microscopic metastatic disease.

In the cat, oral melanoma also appears to be highly aggressive, although less has been published on this subject. There is a single published case series of five cats treated with RT for gross disease. Three of the five cats experienced at least a partial response to treatment, and median survival time was 146 days.

Squamous Cell Carcinoma

Nontonsillar oral SCC in dogs is a locally aggressive neoplasm that often invades bone. These lesions can appear as masses or areas of ulceration, most commonly over the gingiva. Although regional metastasis to local lymph nodes is relatively uncommon (roughly 10%), the reported pulmonary metastatic rates range from less than 5% to 36%. Surgery alone, RT alone, and surgery combined with RT all have been described in the treatment of this disease. With surgery alone, the reported local recurrence rates range from 8% to 29%. RT often is used as a single modality when surgery is not possible or when owners are resistant to having the pet undergo a mandibulectomy or maxillectomy. Median progression-free intervals of approximately 1 year have been reported, with dogs with smaller tumors doing better than those with larger tumors. In cases in which excision is incomplete, RT can be used as a successful adjuvant therapy, with reported median local control times of 36 months. The role of chemotherapy in this disease remains undefined.

Tonsillar SCC is a more aggressive and metastatic variant of this disease, with a higher rate of metastasis to local lymph nodes (>40%). Bilateral disease is relatively common, and treatment, such as tonsillectomy, can be performed bilaterally. Animals that receive combinations of surgery and RT seem to have superior outcomes, although there are limited numbers of reported cases in the literature. Median survival times with aggressive therapy range from 7 to 9 months. As with nontonsillar SCC, the role of chemotherapy in this disease remains undefined. The use of NSAIDs may have some benefit.

In cats SCC presents most commonly along the base of the tongue and next most commonly over the mandibular or maxillary mucosa. When SCC is present over bone, it is common to find bone invasion. Usually these tumors are diagnosed when they are already invasive and the cats are clinically affected. This tumor type is very locally invasive but is slow to metastasize, with regional lymph node metastasis reported in fewer than 10% of cases and pulmonary metastasis uncommon at presentation. One study reported a median survival time of about 1.5 months with supportive care alone. There are few reported effective treatments. Surgery and palliative RT may have roles in select cases. If the tumor is small and localized to the rostral mandible, partial mandibulectomy may be an effective treatment. Although these tumors often initially respond to RT, recurrence usually is rapid; median survival times in most reports range from 3 to 5 months, with very few cats living beyond 1 year. To date, chemotherapy has limited utility. NSAIDs may have a role in the treatment of feline oral SCC for control of pain, but they also may have some antitumor effect (see earlier).

Fibrosarcoma

Fibrosarcomas in dogs are locally invasive tumors that often affect underlying bone. The reported metastatic rate has been variable, ranging from 24% to 57%, with regional lymph nodes and lungs being the most commonly reported sites. There appear to be several histologic variants of this disease, with a histologically low-grade but biologically high-grade variant reported. Surgery alone has resulted in reported median survival times of 7 to 34 months depending on the study. The role of RT in the treatment of this tumor type has not been completely investigated. In the setting of gross disease, reported survival times of 7 to more than 26 months have been reported with RT. RT also may be used as an adjuvant therapy to surgery; one study reported a median survival of 18 months and another study 19 months after a definitive course of RT (Forrest et al, 2000; Frazier et al, 2011).

Although oral fibrosarcoma is the second most commonly reported oral cavity tumor in the cat, little clinical information is available. This tumor type is thought to have a low metastatic rate, although this may be because adequate treatment is lacking and local disease may cause patient death before the tumor has a chance to metastasize. In one study of cats that underwent mandibulectomy for mandibular fibrosarcoma, the 1- and 2-year survival rates were reported as 83%, although four of these six cats did have local recurrence.

Acanthomatous Ameloblastoma

Although acanthomatous ameloblastoma (previously known as *acanthomatous epulis*) can be a locally aggressive tumor with a component of bone invasion, metastasis has not been reported. Both wide surgical excision (requiring bone removal) and RT have been reported to be effective and curative treatments for this disease.

References and Suggested Reading

Arzi B, Verstraete FJ: Mandibular rim excision in seven dogs, *Vet Surg* 39:226, 2010.

Dvorak LD et al: Major glossectomy in dogs: a case series and proposed classification system, *J Am Anim Hosp Assoc* 40:331, 2004.

Forrest LJ et al: Postoperative radiotherapy for canine soft tissue sarcomas, *J Vet Intern Med* 14:578, 2000.

Fazier SA et al: Outcome of dogs with surgically resected oral fibrosarcoma (1997-2008), *Vet Comp Oncol* 10:33, 2012. Epub May 2, 2011.

Grosenbaugh DA et al: Safety and efficacy of a xenogeneic DNA vaccine encoding for human tyrosinase as adjunctive treatment for oral malignant melanoma in dogs following surgical excision of the primary tumor, *Am J Vet Res* 72:1631, 2011.

Liptak JM, Withrow SJ: Cancers of the gastrointestinal tract: oral tumors. In Withrow SJ, Vail DM, editors: *Withrow and MacEwen's small animal clinical oncology*, ed 4, St Louis, 2007, Saunders, p 455.

London CA et al: Phase I dose-escalating study of SU11654, a small molecule receptor tyrosine kinase inhibitor, in dogs with spontaneous malignancies, *Clin Cancer Res* 9:2755, 2003.

Murray RL, Aitken ML, Gottfried SD: The use of rim excision as a treatment for canine acanthomatous ameloblastoma, *J Am Anim Hosp Assoc* 46:91, 2010.

Proulx DR et al: A retrospective analysis of 140 dogs with oral melanoma treated with external beam radiation, *Vet Radiol Ultrasound* 44:352, 2003.

Rassnick KM et al: Use of carboplatin for treatment of dogs with malignant melanoma: 27 cases (1989-2000), *J Am Vet Med Assoc* 218:1444, 2001.

Schmidt BR et al: Evaluation of piroxicam for the treatment of oral squamous cell carcinoma in dogs, *J Am Vet Med Assoc* 218:1783, 2001.

CHAPTER 82

Perineal Tumors

MICHELLE M. TUREK, *Athens, Georgia*

Many types of neoplasia can affect the perineum of dogs and cats. These include tumors whose development is not specific to this area, including mast cell tumors, soft tissue sarcomas, lymphoma, and benign masses such as lipomas and sebaceous gland adenomas. Although these must be considered as differential diagnoses when a dog or cat has a perineal mass, this chapter focuses on the three tumor types that arise from specialized glandular tissue in the perineum.

The *perianal glands* are modified sebaceous glands that are abundant in the skin around the anus. They often are referred to as *circumanal glands* owing to the ring pattern that they form around the anus. They also can be found scattered on the prepuce, tail, and hind legs. Perianal glands are unique to the dog (absent in the cat), and their development is androgen dependent. Tumors that arise from these structures can be benign or malignant and are referred to as *perianal gland adenomas* and *adenocarcinomas,* respectively.

The *apocrine glands of the anal sac* are embedded within the stroma that lies between the internal and external anal sphincters. The anal sacs represent cutaneous diverticula at the 4- and 8-o'clock positions around the anus that are lined by squamous epithelium originating at the anocutaneous junction. The anal sacs serve as reservoirs for the secretions produced by their associated apocrine glands. Tumors affecting the apocrine glands of the anal sac are almost always malignant. Unlike perianal tumors, which occur only in dogs, anal sac apocrine gland carcinomas can affect both dogs and cats.

Of the three perineal neoplasms described here, the perianal adenoma is the most common in the dog. Of the two malignant tumors, anal sac apocrine gland carcinoma occurs more frequently than perianal adenocarcinoma.

Perianal Gland Tumors

Clinical Signs and Diagnosis

Perianal adenoma, the benign form of perianal gland neoplasia, is common in older intact male dogs because of its sex hormone dependence. Dogs usually have a slow-growing mass on the hairless skin around the anus. The tumor can also arise at the tail base, on the prepuce, or on the hind limbs. Perianal adenoma usually occurs as a single and well-circumscribed mass but can be multiple or appear as generalized hypertrophy of the perianal region. The tumors generally are nonpainful and asymptomatic. Rarely, large adenomas can become ulcerated and infected. Although it is unusual, perianal adenomas can affect females or castrated males. Androgen secretion from the adrenal glands in dogs with hyperadrenocorticism and lack of estrogen in ovariohysterectomized females are possible causes of perianal adenoma development in these dogs.

Perianal adenocarcinoma should be considered as a differential diagnosis in these cases. Contrary to its benign counterpart, perianal adenocarcinoma is less common and is not androgen dependent. It can develop in any sex and is characterized by faster tumor growth and clinical signs. Perianal adenocarcinoma is more invasive and adherent to underlying tissues. It may occur as one or multiple masses. Dogs typically are brought to the veterinarian because of the presence of a mass, which may be ulcerated, or discomfort in the perianal region. Dyschezia and tenesmus can occur with large tumors.

Cytologic analysis of a fine-needle aspirate of a perianal mass should be performed before a treatment plan is formulated. Differentiation between perianal adenoma and adenocarcinoma can be difficult by cytologic examination, but other conditions can be ruled out. A tissue biopsy is often needed to confirm malignancy, which greatly impacts the treatment approach. Because of their morphologic resemblance to hepatocytes, perianal adenomas are sometimes referred to as *hepatoid* tumors.

Cats do not have perianal glands and therefore are not affected by these tumors.

Biologic Behavior and Staging

Perianal adenoma has a benign clinical course. Metastasis does not occur. Removal of hormonal stimulation, combined with local therapy if needed to hasten relief of clinical signs, almost always is curative. Thoracic radiography and abdominal imaging for tumor staging are not cost effective unless needed to assess non–tumor-related problems before treatment. For cases in which perianal adenocarcinoma is high on the differential diagnosis list, such as in neutered males and females, tumor staging should be considered before a treatment plan is formulated.

Perianal adenocarcinoma is a more locally invasive tumor, and it grows at a faster rate. The risk of metastasis is low early in the course of disease (15%). When metastasis does occur, it progresses via the lymphatic system to regional lymph nodes (sacral, hypogastric, and iliac) and then to lungs, liver, spleen, bone, and other organs. Tumor staging should begin with a thorough rectal examination. It is important to identify the gross tumor margins accurately for surgical planning. Palpation of the ventral aspect of the lumbar vertebral bodies during a rectal examination may reveal enlargement of sacral lymph nodes. Distant metastasis should be ruled out by thoracic radiography and abdominal imaging. Abdominal ultrasonography is more sensitive than radiography for less advanced lymph node metastasis and allows for a thorough evaluation of other organs. Lymph nodes within the pelvic canal are not well visualized with ultrasonography, so rectal palpation remains important, and radiography may be helpful to show pelvic lymphadenopathy in large dogs. Although the likelihood of metastasis at diagnosis is low for this tumor type, complete staging is recommended so that an accurate prognosis and effective treatment plan can be formulated for each patient. Clinicians should keep in mind that the presence of lymph node enlargement or splenic or hepatic nodules is not specific for metastasis. Tissue sampling with cytologic analysis is necessary to rule out a reactive or hyperplastic process.

Treatment and Prognosis

Castration is the treatment of choice for *perianal adenoma* in intact male dogs. Most tumors regress, and recurrence is rare in the absence of androgenic stimulus. For ulcerated tumors, surgical excision can be considered to hasten relief. If surgical resection would be associated with a high risk of fecal incontinence, castration is recommended first, followed by surgery when the adenoma regresses to a more manageable size. When females or neutered males are affected, surgery is the treatment of choice. The surgical approach need not provide wide margins of normal tissue because these benign tumors are not highly invasive.

Perianal adenocarcinoma requires a more aggressive therapeutic approach. Tumor growth is more invasive and independent of hormonal influences, so castration is not effective. Surgical excision should include a margin of normal tissue to remove microscopic cancer cells that extend beyond the gross tumor margin. Completeness of excision should be reported in the histopathology report. In the author's practice, adjuvant radiotherapy (RT) is recommended when the microscopic margin of normal tissue is less than 5 to 10 mm and additional surgery is not possible. Incomplete or marginal tumor resections are common given the difficulty of surgery in this location. Local RT, targeting only the primary tumor bed, is justified for this tumor, which is associated with a low incidence of metastasis. The adjuvant radiation prescription used by the author is 2.7 Gy delivered daily (Monday through Friday) for 18 treatments. Information is lacking about the efficacy of RT, and variations on this prescription are common. Acute adverse effects related to RT with curative intent are self-limiting and include moist desquamation of the perianal region within the RT field. The benefit of chemotherapy is not known; often it is not recommended if RT is available since the risk of metastasis is low. For rare cases in which metastasis has occurred, chemotherapy is a logical treatment recommendation. Although efficacy information is lacking, doxorubicin and platinum-based protocols are reasonable to consider (see later for dosing information). Tumor recurrence often can be managed with multiple palliative surgeries; however, each recurrence generally is more difficult to resect. Early diagnosis followed by an aggressive first surgery is the best therapeutic approach. The reported median disease-free interval is approximately 2 years for dogs with tumors smaller than 5 cm treated with surgical resection. Prognosis worsens with more advanced disease, including larger tumors or metastasis.

For dogs with nonresectable tumors associated with dyschezia, discomfort, or tumor ulceration, palliative RT using a coarse-fraction radiation prescription is reasonable to consider. Common protocols include 6 to 8 Gy delivered once weekly for four treatments, or 4 Gy delivered daily for five treatments. Although the efficacy of RT in this setting has not been documented, responses have been observed anecdotally by the author, and acute adverse effects are minimal.

Tumors of the Apocrine Gland of the Anal Sac

Clinical Signs and Diagnosis

Anal sac apocrine gland adenocarcinoma (ASAC) occurs most commonly in older dogs (9 to 11 years), although dogs as young as 5 years can be affected. There appears to be no sex predilection. Cocker spaniels may be at increased risk. Dogs may be brought to the veterinarian because of perianal discomfort or because the owner detected a mass. In many animals, the primary tumor is small, does not protrude through the perineum, and is detectable only by rectal examination. In these cases, the presenting clinical signs are related to indirect effects of the primary tumor, such as the presence of regional lymph node metastasis that causes obstipation (dyschezia, tenesmus) or paraneoplastic hypercalcemia (associated with polyuria, polydipsia, or lethargy). Tumors also are found incidentally in asymptomatic dogs. This speaks to the importance of including a rectal examination as part of the routine physical examination. The presence of a firm subcutaneous mass palpable through the rectum at the 4- or 8-o'clock position around the anus is typical for ASAC. Usually only one anal sac is affected, although bilateral tumors can occur. Tumors range in size from a few millimeters to several centimeters. Differential diagnoses for small to moderate-sized masses include anal sacculitis, abscesses, and inspissated anal sac contents. ASAC often can be diagnosed by cytologic analysis of a fine-needle aspirate. Cytologically, tumor cells are uniform in appearance and organized in clusters. Notably, they lack many of the features usually associated with malignancy. Cytology reports specifying benign anal sac tumors should be interpreted with caution because truly benign tumors are exceedingly rare. A serum biochemistry panel and urinalysis should be performed to screen for hypercalcemia (approximately 30% of dogs are affected) and to evaluate renal function in hypercalcemic dogs.

ASAC is rare in the cat. Affected animals usually are older. Clinical signs and diagnostic procedures are similar to those described for the dog. Paraneoplastic hypercalcemia is not associated with this cancer in cats.

Biologic Behavior and Staging

ASAC is associated with a high risk of metastasis early in the course of disease. Fifty percent or more of dogs have metastasis along the regional lymph node chain (sacral, hypogastric, and/or iliac lymph node) at the time of diagnosis. A small primary ASAC may be associated with a greatly enlarged metastatic lymph node. Distant metastasis to lungs, liver, spleen, bone, or other sites develops later. Most dogs that succumb to this cancer are euthanized because of progressive disease at the primary tumor site (causing discomfort, tumor ulceration, and dyschezia), regional lymph node enlargement that results in obstipation, or uncontrollable hypercalcemia.

Tumor staging and treatment planning begin with a thorough rectal examination to assess the size and degree of fixation of the anal sac mass. Evaluation of the sacral lymph nodes located along the ventral aspect of the lumbar vertebrae should be performed. Affected lymph nodes can be millimeters in size or markedly enlarged. Asymmetry or narrowing of the pelvic canal usually represents severe lymph node involvement. Sublumbar lymph nodes, including the hypogastric and iliac nodes, may not be detected by digital palpation depending on the size of the dog. Abdominal imaging is used to assess lymph node size objectively. Ultrasonography is more sensitive than radiography for less advanced disease and also provides the opportunity to evaluate other organs. Mild to moderate lymph node enlargement and hepatic or splenic nodules should be evaluated by cytologic examination of a fine-needle aspirate to distinguish a reactive process from metastasis. Thoracic radiographs are recommended to evaluate for gross pulmonary metastasis, although distant metastasis is rare at the time of diagnosis.

The biologic behavior of this rare tumor type in cats has not been clearly defined. As in dogs, ASAC is locally invasive, and metastatic sites include regional lymph nodes and distant sites. The rate of metastasis reported is variable, from low to high. The approach to tumor staging is similar to that used in dogs: rectal palpation, thoracic radiography, and abdominal imaging (preferably ultrasonography).

Treatment and Prognosis

A treatment plan for ASAC should take into consideration (1) the invasive nature of the primary tumor, (2) the high risk of metastasis to regional lymph nodes that extend into the sublumbar region of the abdomen, and (3) the risk of distant metastasis later in the course of disease.

The surgical approach for ASAC is similar to that for an anal sacculectomy and involves sharp dissection of the anal sac and the associated mass. Because en bloc resection is not performed, histopathology reports suggesting complete excision of an ASAC should be interpreted with caution. Most tumor excisions are marginal or incomplete. Although bilateral tumors can occur, they are rare. The author generally does not advocate prophylactic removal of an unaffected anal sac. Metastatic regional lymph nodes accessible via laparotomy should be excised if an aggressive treatment plan is elected. Removal of nodes can be difficult owing to their sometimes friable texture and the proximity to large vessels. Changing instruments before closure of the abdomen is good surgical practice that prevents seeding of cancer cells in unaffected areas. To facilitate adjuvant RT planning, hemoclips should be placed at the borders of the sublumbar surgical field to delineate the extent of disease and tissue handling. Surgical resection of gross disease achieves palliation for dogs with clinical signs related to the primary tumor, metastatic lymph nodes, or hypercalcemia.

The risk of recurrence after surgery is high, so adjuvant therapy, including curative-intent RT and chemotherapy, is recommended. It must be acknowledged that the relative importance of chemotherapy versus RT in tumor control has not been defined. In the author's practice, both modalities are offered—RT to target the primary tumor and lymph node beds, and chemotherapy to address the risk of distant metastasis. Chemotherapy also may potentiate the effect of RT. Adjuvant RT can begin once surgical wounds are healed, usually 2 weeks after surgery. Curative-intent RT protocols involve total radiation doses of 48 to 54 Gy delivered daily (Monday to Friday) over approximately 4 weeks. The RT field should target both the primary site and the lymph node bed extending from the perineum to the sublumbar region in the abdomen. Since the rectum and colon commonly are included in the field, acute effects include loose stool and tenesmus as well as perianal moist desquamation. The dose per radiation treatment has an important impact on the risk of late effects, in particular rectal stricture. Daily RT doses should not exceed 3 Gy to minimize this risk. Optimal RT treatment planning for ASAC is performed using a computerized treatment planning system. This allows optimization of dose heterogeneity across the radiation field, ensuring adequate dosing to tumor targets and allowing for control of dose to normal tissues. A computed tomographic scan of the area undergoing treatment is required. Curative-intent RT may be considered if metastatic lymph nodes have not been excised. Although good tumor responses can occur, RT is most effective in treating microscopic disease. Until studies indicate that prior surgical excision is not beneficial, the most aggressive approach is to resect all gross disease including metastatic lymph nodes and follow with RT.

Commonly used single-agent chemotherapy protocols include carboplatin (300 mg/m² q21d IV), mitoxantrone (5 to 6 mg/m² q21d IV), or, less commonly, melphalan (7 mg/m² daily for 5 days repeated q21d PO). The relative biologic activity of these drugs is not known; however, carboplatin is favored anecdotally. In the author's experience, concurrent administration of RT and chemotherapy using mitoxantrone or carboplatin is well tolerated. Some clinicians prefer to treat sequentially, using chemotherapy after RT. Recurrent or progressive disease can be managed with repeated surgeries (when possible), or alternate chemotherapy. Toceranib phosphate (Palladia), a novel tyrosine kinase inhibitor (see Chapter 79), also is used currently as a second-line therapy for progressive disease or when traditional therapies are declined by the owner. As safety and efficacy information becomes available, its use as a first-line treatment in combination with standard therapies may become more frequent.

For dogs with nonresectable ASAC that have dyschezia or tumor ulceration, palliative RT is reasonable to consider. Common protocols include 6 to 8 Gy delivered once weekly for four treatments or 4 Gy delivered daily for five treatments. Although efficacy has not been documented, responses have been observed anecdotally by the author, and acute adverse effects are limited. Medical therapy, including toceranib, also may be useful in this setting. When surgical options, including partial debulking of gross disease, are not available to control paraneoplastic hypercalcemia, bisphosphonates such as pamidronate (1 to 2 mg/kg delivered in 250 ml 0.9% NaCl over 2 hours IV q21-28d) can be useful to manage chronic hypercalcemia.

An accurate estimate of prognosis is difficult to establish in dogs with ASAC. Reported survival times range from 6 to 31 months with varying treatments. The longest survival time is reported with RT and chemotherapy (mitoxantrone). Based on favorable results with platinum drugs, the author's approach to adjuvant therapy when aggressive treatment is elected is combination curative-intent RT and carboplatin as described earlier. Prognostic factors are not clearly defined. It appears that dogs with advanced-stage disease (large primary tumor and distant metastasis) and those that receive no treatment may have shorter survival times. Lymph node metastasis is controversial as a predictor of outcome and may not influence survival negatively. Clinical experience has led to the following two important observations. First, a subset of dogs will enjoy a long survival time without progressive disease following surgery alone. These dogs may not benefit from adjuvant therapies. Currently we do not have a way to identify these dogs at presentation, so adjuvant therapy is recommended for all patients. Second, distant metastasis often progresses slowly, so many dogs can live a long time with advanced disease. These two factors may contribute to the disparate outcome results in the literature. The author's approach to this uncertainty is to educate pet owners about the limitations of the information available and to inform them that the best survival time is reported with surgery followed by combination RT and chemotherapy. The owner is told that additional therapies may be needed to manage tumor recurrence (surgery, chemotherapy, or toceranib) and that disease progression can be slow, which may contribute to a prolonged survival. For cases in which combination therapy is not feasible following surgery, RT alone (preferred by the author), chemotherapy alone, and toceranib alone also are options that may be considered if adjuvant therapy is desirable. In general, early diagnosis and treatment may favor the best possible outcome.

Little information is available about treatment efficacy and prognosis of ASAC in cats. Estimates of prognosis range from poor to good. Because of the lack of information suggesting otherwise, the author's clinical approach to ASAC in cats is similar to that in dogs.

References and Suggested Reading

Arthur JJ et al: Characterization of normal tissue complications in 51 dogs undergoing definitive pelvic region irradiation, *Vet Radiol Ultrasound* 49:85, 2008.

Bennett PF et al: Canine anal sac adenocarcinomas: clinical presentation and response to therapy, *J Vet Intern Med* 16:100, 2002.

Elliott JW, Blackwood L: Treatment and outcome of four cats with apocrine gland carcinoma of the anal sac and review of the literature, *J Feline Med Surg* 13:712, 2011.

Emms SG: Anal sac tumours of the dog and their response to cytoreductive surgery and chemotherapy, *Aus Vet J* 83:340, 2005.

London C et al: Preliminary evidence for biologic activity of toceranib phosphate (Palladia®) in solid tumours, *Vet Comp Oncol* 10(3):194, 2012. Epub June 1, 2011.

Polton GA, Brearley MJ: Clinical stage, therapy, and prognosis in canine anal sac gland carcinoma, *J Vet Intern Med* 21:274, 2007.

Shoieb AM, Hanshaw DM: Anal sac gland carcinoma in 64 cats in the United Kingdom (1995-2007), *Vet Pathol* 46:677, 2009.

Turek MM et al: Postoperative radiotherapy and mitoxantrone for anal sac adenocarcinoma in the dog: 15 cases (1991-2001), *Vet Comp Oncol* 1:94, 2003.

Vail DM et al: Perianal adenocarcinoma in the canine male: a retrospective study of 41 cases, *J Am Anim Hosp Assoc* 26:329, 1990.

Williams LE et al: Carcinoma of the apocrine glands of the anal sac in dogs: 113 cases (1985-1995), *J Am Vet Med Assoc* 223:825, 2003.

CHAPTER 83

Urinary Bladder Cancer

DEBORAH W. KNAPP, *West Lafayette, Indiana*

Canine Urinary Bladder Tumors

Urinary bladder cancer comprises approximately 2% of all reported malignancies in the dog. With the pet dog population in the United States exceeding 70 million, this translates into several thousand cases of urinary bladder cancer annually.

Transitional cell carcinoma (TCC) is the most common form of canine urinary bladder cancer (Knapp, 2006, 2007). The vast majority of dogs with TCC have papillary infiltrative cancer of intermediate to high grade. TCC most often is located in the trigone region of the bladder. Papillary lesions and bladder wall thickening can lead to partial or complete urinary tract obstruction. In a series of 102 dogs with TCC, the tumor involved the urethra (as well as the bladder) in 56% of dogs and the prostate in 29% of male dogs (Knapp, 2007). TCC metastasizes to distant sites in approximately 50% of cases. Sites of metastasis include regional lymph nodes, lung, liver, spleen, and, less commonly, kidney, bone, and other organs.

The clinician should not assume that all bladder masses are TCC. Mass effects in the bladder can occur with polyps, other inflammatory lesions, and other tumor types. The latter can include squamous cell carcinoma, adenocarcinoma, undifferentiated carcinoma, lymphoma, rhabdomyosarcoma, hemangiosarcoma, fibroma, and other tumors.

Cause and Possible Prevention Strategies

The cause of canine bladder cancer is multifactorial. Risk factors include exposure to older-generation flea-control products (dips, powders, sprays), herbicides, insecticides, and possibly cyclophosphamide; obesity; female gender (female:male ratio, 1.7:1 to 1.95:1); and breed (Knapp, 2006, 2007). Breeds with increased risk of TCC are listed in Table 83-1.

Knowledge of the risk factors for TCC can be used to take steps that can reduce TCC risk or allow earlier detection if TCC develops. The owners of dogs in high-risk breeds should be informed of the risk and the clinical signs of TCC (hematuria, stranguria, inappropriate urination) and encouraged to seek timely veterinary care should these signs occur. Although it would appear appropriate to perform some form of TCC screening in older at-risk dogs (e.g., periodic urinalysis with sediment examination, abdominal ultrasonography), the benefit of this has not yet been determined. There is evidence that limiting exposure to lawn chemicals and older types of flea products can be important in reducing TCC risk,

especially in dogs in high-risk breeds. A significant association between herbicide exposure and TCC was identified in a case-control study in 166 Scottish terriers (Knapp, 2007). TCC risk was sevenfold higher (odds ratio, 7.19; 95% confidence interval, 2.15 to 24.07; $P < .001$) in dogs exposed to lawns or gardens treated with herbicides and insecticides than in dogs not exposed to these chemicals. An earlier case-control study of dogs of several breeds demonstrated the risk of older types of flea-control products (e.g., flea and tick dips). In the highest-risk group (overweight female dogs), the risk of TCC was 28 times that in normal-weight male dogs not exposed to the insecticides. It is important to note that the newer spot-on types of flea-control products appear safer. In a case-control study in Scottish terriers, spot-on products containing fipronil were not associated with increased risk of TCC (Knapp, 2007). In addition to avoiding certain exposures, adding vegetables to the diet can reduce TCC risk. In a study in Scottish terriers, dogs that ate vegetables at least three times a week, along with their normal diet, had a 70% reduction in TCC risk (odds ratio, 0.30; 95% confidence interval, 0.01 to 0.97; $P < .001$) (Knapp, 2007). The specific types of vegetable with the most benefit could not be determined, but carrots, given as treats, were the most frequently fed vegetable in the study.

Presentation, Diagnosis, and Clinical Staging

Typically, TCC is a disease of older dogs (median age at diagnosis, 11 years), with females affected more often than males. Common clinical signs include hematuria, dysuria, pollakiuria, and, less commonly, lameness caused by bone metastasis or hypertrophic osteopathy. It is important to note that the lower urinary tract signs observed with TCC are similar to those that occur with urinary tract infection or calculi. Factors that raise suspicion of TCC include persistent or recurrent lower urinary tract signs or infection, older age, and high-risk breed.

The physical examination of a dog with possible TCC should include a thorough rectal examination. Findings depend on the dog's size but could include a thickened urethra, an enlarged or irregular prostate, a trigonal mass, or enlarged lymph nodes. Bladder masses often are not detected on abdominal palpation. Normal physical examination findings do not rule out TCC.

When TCC is suspected, the clinician should pursue testing to (1) make a definitive diagnosis, (2) determine the cancer stage, and (3) assess the overall health of the patient. These tests include complete blood count, serum biochemistry panel, urinalysis, urine culture, thoracic radiography, abdominal ultrasonography, and bladder

TABLE 83-1

Breed and Risk of Urinary Bladder Cancer in Pet Dogs (Summary Data From Veterinary Medical Database)*

Breed	Odds Ratio	95% Confidence Interval
Mixed breed	1.0†	
All pure breeds	0.74	0.62-0.88
Scottish terrier	19.89	7.74-55.72
West Highland white terrier	5.31	2.51-11.63
Shetland sheepdog	4.46	2.48-8.03
Beagle	4.15	2.14-8.05
Wirehaired terrier	3.20	1.19-8.63
Miniature poodle	0.86	0.55-1.35
Miniature schnauzer	0.92	0.54-1.57
Doberman pinscher	0.51	0.30-0.87
Labrador retriever	0.46	0.30-0.69
Golden retriever	0.46	0.30-0.69
German shepherd	0.40	0.26-0.63

*Updated from results published previously (Knapp, 2007).
†Reference category.

BOX 83-1

World Health Organization Clinical Staging System (TNM) for Canine Urinary Bladder Cancer

T: Primary tumor
Tis: Carcinoma *in situ*
- T0 No evidence of primary tumor
- T1 Superficial papillary tumor
- T2 Tumor invading the bladder wall, with induration
- T3 Tumor invading neighboring organs (prostate, uterus, vagina, and pelvic canal)

N: Regional lymph node (internal and external iliac lymph node)
- N0 No regional lymph node involved
- N1 Regional lymph node involved
- N2 Regional lymph node and juxtaregional lymph node involved

M: Distant metastases
- M0 No evidence of metastasis
- M1 Distant metastasis present

imaging. Urine should be obtained by free catch or catheter sample and not by cystocentesis, which has been associated with TCC seeding of the needle tract.

A diagnosis of TCC requires histopathologic confirmation. Although neoplastic cells have been reported to be present in the urine of 30% of dogs with TCC, cancer cells often are indistinguishable from reactive epithelial cells associated with inflammation. Urine antigen tests have been found to be sensitive for TCC, but high numbers of false-positive results limit the value of these tests. It is essential to perform histopathologic examination of the abnormal tissues to determine if TCC is present. Methods of obtaining tissue for diagnosis include cystotomy, cystoscopy, and traumatic catheterization. If surgery is performed, great care must be taken to avoid TCC seeding. Similarly, percutaneous biopsy methods (e.g., transabdominal core biopsy or fine-needle aspiration) should be avoided because these can lead to tumor seeding.

Cystoscopy, using either a rigid or a flexible cystoscope, provides a means to visualize the mucosal surface of the urinary bladder and urethra, to determine tumor location and involvement of the ureteral orifices and urethra, and to collect tissues for diagnosis. Placing tissue samples in a histology cassette before processing helps prevent loss of small samples. In a recent study involving 92 dogs, diagnostic samples reportedly were obtained by cystoscopy in 96% of female dogs and 65% of male dogs that ultimately had histopathologically diagnosed TCC (Childress et al, 2011). The recent introduction of a wire basket designed to capture stones during cystoscopy allows collection of larger tissue samples and is expected to increase the yield of diagnostic biopsy samples.

Traumatic catheterization to collect tissues for diagnosis also has been performed, but samples usually are small and of limited diagnostic value. Percutaneous biopsy methods can lead to tumor seeding and are best avoided.

Thoracic radiography and abdominal ultrasonography are recommended to look for evidence of metastases. Lymph node and distant metastases were present in 16% and 14% of 102 dogs, respectively, at the time of diagnosis of TCC (Knapp, 2007). Distant metastases were detected in 50% of dogs at the time of death. Tumor stage can be assigned following the World Health Organization clinical staging system for canine bladder tumors (Box 83-1). Abdominal ultrasonography also is useful for detecting ureteral obstruction and hydronephrosis. Such findings could be an indication for the placement of one or more ureteral stents, especially if other therapies do not relieve the urinary obstruction (see Chapter 76).

Bladder imaging is used to determine the location of the tumor within the urinary tract and to obtain baseline measurements of the TCC to monitor response to subsequent therapy. Ultrasonography is the method most commonly used to image the bladder. Cystography is used less frequently because of the need for anesthesia, catheterization, and enemas to remove colonic contents that could obscure images of the bladder; risk of urinary perforation with catheterization; and production of inconsistent images when the bladder shifts in position or is imaged at different levels of distention. Computed tomography (CT) with intravesical and intravenous contrast provides the best images of bladder masses, but CT is pursued less commonly because of expense and the need for anesthesia and urinary catheterization.

Ultrasonography is an important imaging modality for the bladder. The degree of distention is important when imaging the bladder. When the bladder is minimally distended, it can be difficult to visualize some lesions accurately, and it is not possible to determine whether evident lesions are remote to the trigone (where surgical resection could be possible). When ultrasonography is used to measure bladder masses over the course of therapy, it is crucial to follow a consistent protocol from visit to visit with regard to bladder distention, patient positioning, and method of measuring masses and to have the same operator perform the examinations over the multiple visits.

Treatment

Surgery

Surgical excision of TCC should be considered for lesions in the bladder apex for which 3-cm margins of grossly normal bladder can be removed around the tumor mass. Unfortunately, most TCCs are trigonal and many involve the urethra, which precludes surgical excision. In addition, many dogs appear to develop multifocal TCC in the bladder. This is consistent with the proposed "field effect," in which the entire bladder lining is thought to undergo malignant change in response to exposure to carcinogens in urine. In the limited number of cases in which TCC has been removed "completely," local recurrence still is common.

If TCC is removed surgically from the bladder, there is some evidence that cyclooxygenase (COX) inhibitor treatment can reduce risk of recurrence. In a pilot study conducted at Purdue University, adjuvant deracoxib (Deramaxx) was given to nine dogs following surgical removal of TCC (McMillan et al, 2011). Three dogs had tumor-free margins, and six dogs had microscopic TCC present in surgical margins. Deracoxib (3 mg/kg q24h PO) was instituted postoperatively. In four of the dogs with microscopic residual TCC after surgery, there was no evidence of relapse at 345, 749, 963, and 2057 days, respectively. The other two dogs with residual microscopic TCC had recurrence at 140 and 231 days, respectively. Of the three dogs with tumor-free margins, one dog was disease free at death at 1437 days, and the other two dogs had recurrence at 210 and 332 days, respectively. The median survival time of the nine dogs was 749 days (range, 231 to 2581 days). Without a randomized trial comparing deracoxib with placebo, the true benefit of deracoxib in this setting is not known, but results to date have been encouraging.

Even if surgical removal of the TCC is not possible, surgery has a role as an emergency palliative procedure to bypass urinary obstruction through the placement of ureteral and urethral stents (see Chapter 76) and prepubic cystostomy tubes (Berent, 2011). Urethral stents, which can be placed nonsurgically with fluoroscopic guidance, are attractive because no external tubing or hardware is necessary (as is the case with cystostomy tubes). The use of ureteral and urethral stents has been very important in prolonging the life of some dogs with TCC.

Transurethral resection of bladder and urethral TCC has been attempted in a small number of dogs but has been limited by complications of the procedure and local disease recurrence. Laser ablation of TCC combined with medical therapy also has been reported, but it is not yet known if this offers an advantage over traditional surgery and medical therapy.

Radiation Therapy

Studies of the effects of radiation therapy (RT) on TCC are very limited. RT appears to kill TCC cells effectively, but complications (urinary incontinence, cystitis with accompanying pollakiuria and stranguria) have limited the use of traditional RT. In a report of RT in 10 dogs (Poirier et al, 2004), weekly coarse-fraction external beam RT plus mitoxantrone and piroxicam was tolerated, but results were no better than those with medical therapy alone. Recently, the use of intensity-modulated and image-guided radiation therapy for treatment of genitourinary carcinomas in dogs has been described with encouraging results (Nolan et al, 2012).

Medical Treatment of Transitional Cell Carcinoma

Medical management of TCC is indicated in dogs with nonresectable or metastatic tumors. Medical therapy for TCC consists of chemotherapy, COX inhibitors, and combinations of the two (Henry et al, 2003; Knapp, 2006, 2007, 2013).

Regardless of the treatment pursued, basic concepts apply in tailoring the therapy to the individual dog with TCC. Complete staging of the TCC to define the extent of the disease and size of lesions should be performed before and after approximately 6 weeks of treatment. After 6 weeks of treatment, if the tumor is smaller or stable in size, and if the treatment is acceptable with regard to any adverse effects, the same treatment should be continued. Restaging should be performed at 6- to 8-week intervals, and therapy adjusted as appropriate. If cancer progression or unacceptable toxicity occurs, different therapy could be considered.

COX Inhibitor Treatment. COX inhibitors offer a simple oral treatment for TCC that is associated with relatively few side effects and lower costs than chemotherapy. Although COX inhibitors induce remission less often than standard chemotherapy for TCC, some pet owners elect to use COX inhibitor therapy for their pets. The nonselective COX inhibitor piroxicam (0.3 mg/kg q24h PO) has been used to treat dogs with TCC since the 1980s. The quality of life in most dogs receiving piroxicam has been excellent. In 62 dogs treated with piroxicam (Knapp, 2007), tumor responses included complete remission (complete resolution of all evidence of cancer) in 3%, partial remission (≥50% reduction in tumor volume) in 14%, stable disease (<50% change in tumor volume) in 56%, and progressive disease (≥50% increase in tumor volume or the development of new TCC lesions) in 26% of dogs. The median survival time was 195 days. A compounding pharmacy must prepare piroxicam for use in small to medium-sized dogs because the commercially available 10-mg capsules are too large for dogs of this size. Although the majority of dogs tolerate piroxicam well, care must be taken to detect any gastrointestinal toxicity that could occur. If vomiting, melena, or anorexia occurs, it is important to withdraw piroxicam and give supportive care as needed until the toxicity resolves. If toxicity develops with piroxicam, a selective COX-2 inhibitor can be given instead.

There is evidence that selective COX-2 inhibitors have antitumor activity against TCC, and these drugs are associated with less risk of toxicity than piroxicam. In preliminary study results, firocoxib (Previcox) showed antitumor activity as a single agent and enhanced the activity of cisplatin (Knapp et al, 2013). The COX-2 inhibitor deracoxib also has been evaluated as a single agent at a dosage of 3 mg/kg q24h PO in 26 dogs with TCC (McMillan et al, 2011). Tumor responses included 17% partial remissions, 71% stable disease, and 12% progressive disease. The median time to disease progression was 133 days. The median survival following deracoxib treatment and subsequent therapies was 323 days. Mild gastrointestinal toxicity occurred in 20% of dogs, and 4% of dogs had renal or hepatic side effects. When deracoxib is prescribed for other conditions, dosages of 1 to 2 mg/kg q24h PO typically are used. Although it has not been studied to date, it is possible that deracoxib given at dosages lower than 3 mg/kg has antitumor activity against TCC. The 17% remission rate with deracoxib appears comparable to the remission rate with piroxicam; however, occasional complete remissions occur in dogs receiving piroxicam, whereas complete remissions were not noted in dogs treated with deracoxib.

Chemotherapy. The most commonly used chemotherapy protocol in dogs with TCC has been mitoxantrone (5 to 6 mg/m^2 q21d IV) combined with piroxicam. In a study of 55 dogs with TCC receiving this treatment, 35% of dogs experienced objective responses with minimal toxicity (Henry et al, 2003). The median progression-free interval was 194 days, and the median survival time was 291 days.

Three other chemotherapy protocols also have been shown to have antitumor activity against TCC with acceptable toxicity in dogs. The first, carboplatin combined with piroxicam, induced remission in 38% of dogs in one study (Knapp, 2007). Carboplatin has been a second choice behind mitoxantrone because carboplatin has been associated with more toxicity and relatively short progression-free interval and survival time in dogs with TCC. Although a higher remission rate (50% to 70%) has been noted with cisplatin combined with piroxicam, the use of this protocol has been limited by the frequency of renal damage (Knapp, 2007). Results of a recent trial of vinblastine in 28 dogs with TCC performed at Purdue University included partial remission in 35% of dogs and stable disease in 50% of dogs (Arnold et al, 2011). The starting vinblastine dosage in the trial (3 mg/m^2 q14d IV) was associated with neutropenia requiring dose reduction in the majority of dogs. Because of myelosuppression, it would be safer to start with a lower dose of vinblastine if using this drug in dogs with TCC. A third chemotherapeutic agent with a potential role in the treatment of TCC in dogs is gemcitabine. In a recent study, gemcitabine (800 mg/m^2 q7d IV) and piroxicam were given to 38 dogs with cytologic evidence of TCC or biopsy-confirmed TCC (Marconato et al, 2011). Reported responses included 5% complete remissions, 21% partial remissions, and 50% stable disease. The median survival time was 230 days.

Intravesical Therapy. Intravesical therapy commonly is used in humans with superficial TCC, and there has been interest in the potential of this approach to treat the higher-grade invasive TCC that occurs in dogs. A phase I clinical trial and pharmacokinetic study of intravesical mitomycin C (1-hour dwell time per day, 2 consecutive days per month, escalating concentrations) was conducted in dogs with TCC (Abbo et al, 2010). Tumor response was assessed in 12 dogs and included five partial remissions and seven cases of stable disease. The treatment was well tolerated by most dogs. The maximum tolerated dose based on local toxicity (bladder irritation of 1 to 2 days' duration) was 700 µg/ml. It was noted that care should be taken to prevent the drug from pooling in the prepuce because this could cause more severe irritation. Unfortunately, a much more serious toxicosis emerged. Marked myelosuppression and severe gastrointestinal upset were noted in two dogs, which suggested systemic drug absorption. This occurred after the first treatment cycle in one dog and the fourth cycle in another dog. Serum mitomycin C concentrations were minimal in dogs that provided samples for pharmacokinetic analyses, but neither of the two dogs with severe toxicity provided samples. Although both dogs recovered with supportive care, such toxicity raises great concern because, if a substantial amount of the intravesical dose is absorbed systemically, it could be lethal. Therefore intravesical therapy is not recommended for front-line use in dogs with TCC.

Other Therapies for TCC. Although substantial progress has been made in the treatment of canine TCC, there is much room for improvement. Clinical trials are important to define better treatment approaches for this deadly disease. By participating in a clinical trial, the pet dog with TCC could gain access to a new beneficial treatment, and information gained from that dog could be useful in developing better therapeutic approaches for other dogs and potentially for humans (Knapp, 2006). Websites posted by veterinary schools, the Veterinary Cancer Society, and veterinary oncologists can provide information to help veterinarians and pet owners learn about current TCC trials.

Supportive Care. Dogs with TCC are at high risk of secondary bacterial infections. Urinalysis and urine culture should be performed regularly, and antibiotics prescribed as needed. Antibiotic therapy should be based on results of urine culture and sensitivity testing, and the appropriate antibiotic should be given for 3 weeks or longer. Urination should be monitored closely. If urinary tract obstruction occurs, catheterization, definitive anticancer therapy, antibiotics to reduce inflammation associated with secondary bacterial infection, or placement of a stent or cystostomy tube to relieve obstruction could be considered.

Prognosis

The progress being made to help dogs with TCC is very encouraging. Multiple different treatments have been identified that result in remission or stable disease for several months, and the quality of life can be excellent. If TCC becomes resistant to one drug, it still is possible that the cancer will respond to other drugs. By taking advantage of multiple treatment protocols over time, veterinarians can enable many dogs with TCC to live well beyond a year. Unfortunately, most dogs with TCC still ultimately die of the disease. Survival has been correlated strongly with the TNM stage at the time of diagnosis.

Factors associated with a more advanced TNM stage at diagnosis include younger age (increased risk of nodal metastasis), prostate involvement (increased risk of distant metastasis), and higher tumor category (increased risk of nodal and distant metastasis).

Feline Urinary Bladder Tumors

Information concerning urinary bladder cancer in cats is very limited. Bladder tumors reported in 27 cats included 15 carcinomas, 5 benign mesenchymal tumors, 5 malignant mesenchymal tumors, and 2 lymphomas (Schwarz et al, 1985). There were 20 male and 7 female cats, and most were elderly. Partial cystectomy was performed in nine cats, and four cats (two with leiomyoma, one with hemangiosarcoma, and one with leiomyosarcoma) survived longer than 6 months.

A series of 20 cats with TCC included 13 neutered male and 7 spayed female cats (median age, 15.2 years) (Wilson et al, 2007). Clinical signs included hematuria, stranguria, and pollakiuria. Concurrent urinary tract infection was common. Various treatments were given to 14 of the 20 cats. The median survival time was 261 days. Regional and distant metastases were noted in some cats in the study, but the metastatic rate of TCC in cats has not yet been defined.

References and Suggested Reading

Abbo AH et al: Phase 1 clinical trial and pharmacokinetics of intravesical Mitomycin C in dogs with localized transitional cell carcinoma of the urinary bladder, *J Vet Intern Med* 24:1124, 2010.

Arnold EA et al: Phase II clinical trial of vinblastine in dogs with transitional cell carcinoma of the urinary bladder, *J Vet Intern Med* 25:1385, 2011.

Berent AC: Ureteral obstruction in dogs and cats: a review of traditional and new interventional diagnostic and therapeutic options, *J Vet Emerg Crit Care* 21:86, 2011.

Childress MO et al: Comparison of cystoscopy vs surgery in obtaining diagnostic biopsy specimens from dogs with transitional cell carcinoma of the urinary bladder and urethra, *J Am Vet Med Assoc* 239:350, 2011.

Henry CJ et al: Clinical evaluation of mitoxantrone and piroxicam in a canine model of human invasive urinary bladder carcinoma, *Clin Cancer Res* 9:906, 2003.

Knapp DW: Animal models: naturally occurring canine urinary bladder cancer. In Lerner SP, Schoenberg MP, Sternberg CN, editors: *Textbook of bladder cancer,* Oxfordshire, UK, 2006, Taylor & Francis, p 171.

Knapp DW: Tumors of the urinary system. In Withrow SJ, Vail DM, editors: *Withrow and MacEwen's small animal clinical oncology,* ed 4, St Louis, 2007, Saunders, p 649.

Knapp DW et al: Randomized trial of cisplatin versus firocoxib versus cisplatin/firocoxib in dogs with transitional cell carcinoma of the urinary bladder, *J Vet Intern Med* 27:126, 2013.

Marconato L et al: Toxic effects and antitumor response of gemcitabine in combination with piroxicam treatment in dogs with transitional cell carcinoma of the urinary bladder, *J Am Vet Med Assoc* 238:1004, 2011.

McMillan SK et al: Antitumor effects of deracoxib treatment in 26 dogs with transitional cell carcinoma of the urinary bladder, *J Am Vet Med Assoc* 239(8):1084, 2011.

Nolan MW et al: Intensity-modulated and image-guided radiation therapy for treatment of genitourinary carcinomas in dogs, *J Vet Intern Med* 26:987, 2012.

Poirier VJ et al: Piroxicam, mitoxantrone, and coarse fraction radiotherapy for the treatment of transitional cell carcinoma of the bladder in 10 dogs: a pilot study, *J Am Anim Hosp Assoc* 40:131-136, 2004.

Schwarz PD et al: Urinary bladder tumors in the cat: a review of 27 cases, *J Am Anim Hosp Assoc* 21:237, 1985.

Wilson HM et al: Clinical signs, treatments, and outcome in cats with transitional cell carcinoma of the urinary bladder: 20 cases (1990-2004), *J Am Vet Med Assoc* 231:101, 2007.

CHAPTER 84

Mammary Cancer

CAROLYN J. HENRY, *Columbia, Missouri*

Mammary tumors are among the most commonly encountered neoplasms in female dogs and cats, consistently reported as one of the top three tumors in both species. Despite steady improvement in the survival rates for women with breast cancer over the past several decades, there have been relatively few advances in the treatment of canine and feline mammary tumors. Perhaps the greatest progress has been in the area of public education regarding measures to prevent tumor development. It has long been established that spaying dogs before the age of 2½ years is protective against the development of mammary cancer, and work published to date suggests that ovariectomy at a young age (<1 year) has a similar protective effect in cats. Beyond educating clients regarding the potential benefits of ovariectomy, practitioners should alert clients to the relative frequency of mammary cancer development and the need for early detection and appropriate case management. This chapter summarizes what is known regarding the natural behavior and prognosis associated with canine and feline mammary tumors and provides guidelines for case management in both species.

Canine Mammary Tumors

Incidence, Causes, and Pathogenesis

The true incidence of mammary tumor development in dogs is difficult to determine since many small or benign-appearing tumors may go untreated and thus unreported. However, an insurance population study of female dogs in Sweden reported 111 mammary tumor claims per 10,000 dog-years at risk. Prior reports indicated that the annual incidence of canine mammary tumors (CMTs) in the United States approximates 200 per 100,000 dogs at risk. Breeds reported to be at increased risk include English springer spaniels, Brittany spaniels, cocker spaniels, toy and miniature poodles, English setters, pointers, German shepherds, Maltese, Yorkshire terriers, and dachshunds. Mammary tumors most commonly affect middle-aged (9 to 11 years) female dogs, with an increased incidence beginning at approximately 6 years of age. The influence of hormones on CMT development is supported by the early work showing that the risk of developing mammary tumors rises to 26% for dogs spayed after their second estrus, compared with 0.5% and 8% for dogs spayed before their first or second estrus, respectively. It is thought that sex steroid hormones have their primary effect on target cells during the early stages of mammary carcinogenesis, which accounts for the lack of protective effect with spaying beyond two estrous cycles. The use of products containing medroxyprogesterone acetate (progestin and estrogen combination) for the prevention of estrus or to treat pseudopregnancy has also been linked to an increased incidence of CMTs. Although CMTs are primarily a disease of female dogs, approximately 1% of CMTs are in males and can be associated with hormonal abnormalities such as estrogen secretion by a Sertoli cell tumor. Other factors reportedly associated with an increased risk of CMT development include obesity at a young age and feeding of homemade diets as opposed to commercial foods.

Clinical Presentation

Mammary tumors often are detected during routine wellness examinations in older female dogs or are discovered by conscientious owners. The median age of onset for benign tumors is reported to be lower than that for malignant tumors (8.5 years versus 9.5 years, respectively). In over half of all cases, dogs have more than one mammary mass at presentation; these may be simultaneous primary masses or may represent one primary lesion with regional extension or metastasis. Although some studies have suggested that the caudal mammary glands are the most commonly affected in the dog, other reports have not confirmed this. Either the axillary or inguinal lymph nodes may be palpably enlarged in dogs with nodal metastases, given the complex pattern of lymphatic drainage for canine mammary tissue. There are five pairs of mammary glands in the dog (two cranial-thoracic, two abdominal, and one caudal-inguinal). The thoracic glands generally drain to the axillary or sternal nodes, the inguinal glands drain to the inguinal nodes, and the two abdominal glands may drain to either site. The presence of lymph node enlargement, lymphedema, skin ulceration, and fixation to underlying tissue are characteristics that suggest malignancy.

Inflammatory mammary carcinoma (IMC) is a unique clinical entity that warrants an altered approach to diagnosis and case management. This tumor type may be mistaken for mastitis since affected dogs classically have warm, erythematous mammary tissue and associated lymphedema; ulceration and vesicles; and significant pain on any manipulation of the tissue. Alternatively, the diagnosis of IMC may become apparent when wound dehiscence occurs secondary to what was anticipated to be a routine mammary mass excision (referred to as *secondary IMC*).

Diagnosis and Staging

The diagnosis of CMTs relies on histologic examination of incisional or excisional biopsy samples. Fine-needle aspiration and cytologic examination of mammary nodules is recommended by some because it may help differentiate preoperatively between benign and malignant masses and between CMT and other tumors (such as mast cell tumor) or nonneoplastic lesions. However, a 2007 study showed that one in four cytologic specimens from CMT contain inadequate cellularity to be of diagnostic value; thus histopathologic analysis still is considered to be imperative for diagnosing CMT (Cassali et al, 2007). It is vital to bear in mind that benign and malignant nodules may coexist in canine mammary tissue. Therefore it is necessary to confirm the histologic diagnosis independently for each nodule rather than assume that one nodule is representative of all tumors present. Estimates vary in the literature, but a simple rule of thumb for CMTs is that approximately 50% are malignant and approximately 50% of the malignant tumors metastasize. Of these, sarcomas and IMCs are associated with the worst prognosis. Mixed malignant tumors and squamous cell carcinomas also are associated with poor survival times. Of the carcinomas, solid carcinomas are reported to have worse survival times than either tubular or papillary carcinomas. Carcinomas that have a better prognosis include carcinoma *in situ* and adenocarcinomas.

The original clinical staging for CMTs was based on a four-stage system developed by the World Health Organization (WHO) and reported in 1980. Since that time, a modified staging system has been reported and is described in Table 84-1. The primary differences are the addition of a stage V for dogs with distant metastatic disease and the designation of a stage IV (rather than stage II or III) for those with nodal metastasis. Either staging system necessitates evaluation of regional lymph nodes and assessment of potential distant sites of metastasis, especially distant lymph nodes and lungs. Preoperative cytologic examination of any palpable lymph nodes may aid in determining disease extent before surgery. Regardless of preoperative assessment, lymph node tissue removed at the time of surgery should be submitted for histologic examination. Although standard hematoxylin and eosin (H&E) staining of slides from nodal tissue permits accurate identification of micrometastasis in most cases, cytokeratin immunostaining using an antipancytokeratin antibody AE1/AE3 was reported to detect occult micrometastasis in 12 of 131 lymph nodes (9.2%) from dogs judged to have node-negative disease based on H&E results (Matos et al, 2006). The impact of the presence of micrometastatic disease on the prognosis for CMT is unknown at this time. Obtaining three-view thoracic radiographs before surgery is essential because pulmonary metastases are associated with a poor prognosis and may alter therapy decisions.

In addition to clinical staging, there is a histologic staging system outlined in Table 84-2. In this system stages 0, I, and II are based on histologic assessment, whereas stage III is based on clinical assessment of distant metastasis. This system is not to be confused with the clinical staging systems proposed in Table 84-1. Although the histologic staging system is not universally applied in veterinary medicine, it is highlighted in this chapter because of its correlation with clinical outcome in a report of 232 dogs undergoing mastectomy for CMTs.

TABLE 84-1

Comparison of the Original and Modified TNM Staging Systems for the Classification of Canine Mammary Tumors

Stage	Original WHO Staging	Modified WHO Staging
I	T1 (<3 cm), N0, M0	T1 (<3 cm), N0, M0
II	≤T2 (<5 cm), N1, M0 (histologically positive node, but not fixed to underlying tissues)	T2 (3-5 cm), N0, M0
III	Any T3 or any with fixed nodal involvement	T3 (>5 cm), N0, M0
IV	Distant metastasis (any T, any N, M1)	Regional node metastasis (any T, N1, M0)
V	No stage V	Distant metastasis (any T, any N, M1)

TNM, Tumor-node-metastasis system, where T is the size of the primary tumor, N is regional lymph node involvement, and M is distant metastasis (e.g., N0 indicates no lymph node involvement, and N1 indicates confirmed lymph node involvement); *WHO,* World Health Organization.

TABLE 84-2

Histologic Staging System for Canine Mammary Tumors (CMTs)

Stage	Features	Frequency of New or Recurrent CMT 2 Years after Surgery
0	Tumor cells are limited to ductal tissue	25%
I	Tumor cells invade stromal tissue	72%
II	Vascular/lymphatic invasion and/or regional lymph node metastasis	95%
III	Systemic metastasis	Not reported; dogs with stage III disease by definition have no disease-free interval

From Gilbertson SR et al: Canine mammary epithelial neoplasms: biologic implications of morphologic characteristics assessed in 232 dogs, *Vet Pathol* 20:127, 1983.

Treatment

Surgery

Surgery is the mainstay of therapy for most CMTs, with the exception of IMC (see following paragraphs). In their pivotal study published in 1985, MacEwen and colleagues demonstrated that type of surgery is not a major prognostic factor for CMTs provided resection is histologically complete (MacEwen et al, 1985). Thus they established that the surgical standard of care for CMTs includes minimal but adequate tumor excision, usually via lumpectomy or partial mastectomy. A more recent prospective study reported a 58% rate of new tumor development in the ipsilateral mammary tissue after local excision of CMT (Stratmann et al, 2008). This has prompted some to recommend a more radical surgery than previously thought necessary. However, given that roughly half of all CMTs are benign, this more aggressive approach may not be warranted in many cases.

The issue of whether or not to perform ovariohysterectomy (OHE) at the time of mammary tumor excision has long been debated. Given the high rate of estrogen receptor–positive tumors in dogs, it is reasonable to consider hormone ablation via OHE as an adjunctive therapy for treatment of CMT. However, early reports suggested that no benefit was derived from OHE at the time of tumor excision in dogs. Data from two more recent studies indicate that there is a survival advantage for dogs that undergo OHE (Chang et al, 2005; Sorenmo et al, 2000). Although one may not know the underlying diagnosis (malignant versus benign) at the time of surgery, these two latter studies certainly support a recommendation for OHE as an adjunct to complete tumor excision when feasible. If OHE is performed at the same time as tumor removal, one should excise the tumor *after* the OHE is completed to avoid seeding the abdomen with tumor cells.

Hormonal Therapy

Because of the relative difficulty of performing routine estrogen and progesterone receptor assays on CMTs, the use of hormonal therapy in dogs with mammary tumors has lagged behind that in human oncology. In addition to hormone ablation via OHE described previously, tamoxifen has been evaluated as hormonal therapy for CMTs. Tamoxifen has both estrogenic and antiestrogenic effects, and its use has been advocated for many years for the treatment of human patients with estrogen receptor–positive breast cancer. A pilot study evaluated outcome for 16 dogs with mammary carcinoma treated with 2.5 to 10 mg of tamoxifen (mean dose, 0.42 mg/kg q12h PO). Five of seven dogs with either metastatic or nonresectable mammary carcinoma experienced a decrease in tumor burden. In another report of 10 dogs with advanced mammary cancer treated with 0.7 mg/kg of tamoxifen q24h, no measurable responses were noted. Adverse effects, including vaginal discharge, vulvar swelling, urinary incontinence, urinary tract infection, mental dullness, signs of estrus, and partial alopecia, have been seen in dogs undergoing tamoxifen therapy. One quarter of the treated dogs in the aforementioned pilot study developed pyometra (one case of closed-cervix pyometra and three cases of stump pyometra). An identical rate of pyometra induction (20%) was noted in a 1988 report of 20 bitches treated with 1 mg/kg of tamoxifen q12h PO for 10 days for prevention or termination of pregnancy. Thus clients must be counseled regarding this potential adverse effect if tamoxifen therapy is to be considered.

Chemotherapy

Chemotherapy has not been clearly documented to provide a survival advantage for dogs with CMT. However, based on responses in women with breast cancer, various chemotherapy agents, including vincristine, paclitaxel, fluorouracil, cyclophosphamide, doxorubicin (DOX), docetaxel, mitoxantrone, gemcitabine, and carboplatin, have been used for treatment of high-grade or metastatic mammary carcinoma in dogs. In one prospective study comparing outcomes for eight dogs with CMT treated with fluorouracil (150 mg/m^2 IV) and cyclophosphamide (100 mg/m^2 IV) once weekly for 4 weeks with those for eight dogs treated with surgery alone, a significant improvement in survival was demonstrated for the dogs receiving chemotherapy (Karayannopoulou et al, 2001). Dogs in the chemotherapy group had a median survival time of 24 months compared with 6 months for dogs in the surgery-only group. A prospective study examining postoperative treatment with DOX or docetaxel (n = 12) versus surgery alone (n = 19) in dogs with invasive mammary cancer failed to demonstrate a significant impact of chemotherapy on recurrence-free interval, time to metastasis, or overall survival (Simon et al, 2006). Additional randomized prospective studies are necessary to determine the role of chemotherapy in the clinical management of dogs with mammary cancer.

Other Medical Therapy

The use of desmopressin (DDAVP) has been advocated by some for its ability to inhibit tumor metastasis in dogs with CMT. Although the exact mechanism of action is unknown, desmopressin is thought to inhibit tumor cell dissemination at the time of surgical excision via effects on cellular adherence to the microvasculature, perhaps by inducing release of multimeric forms of von Willebrand factor. In two studies, administration of desmopressin at 1 µg/kg IV 30 minutes before surgery and again 24 hours after was associated with significant increases in disease-free interval and overall survival time of dogs with CMT (Hermo et al, 2008; Hermo et al, 2011).

Although monoclonal antibody therapy is well established as a treatment modality for human breast cancer, commercial drug costs for such therapy and the paucity of information regarding antigen expression and homology have hindered the application of antibody-based immunotherapy for CMT to date. However, scientific interest in the comparative oncology of breast cancer has recently resulted in elucidation of some breed differences in hormone receptor and tumor antigen expression. For example, a study examining breed differences among Maltese, Yorkshire terrier, Shih Tzu, poodle, and mixed breeds of 139 dogs in Korea found that the Shih Tzu breed had a higher percentage of BRCA1 overexpression, which related to triple-negative phenotype, similar to BRCA1-related human breast cancer (Im et al, 2013). In addition to identifying potentially relevant animal models of human disease, these findings may lead to more individualized options for treatment of dogs with mammary cancer in the future.

Radiation Therapy

Although radiation therapy (RT) is an important component of breast cancer treatment in women, it remains largely unexplored for the treatment of CMTs. Anecdotal reports of palliation for nonresectable lesions or for IMC serve as the only current evidence to support the use of RT for CMTs. Given the efficacy of RT in women with breast cancer, further evaluation of this treatment modality for CMTs is warranted.

Therapy for Inflammatory Mammary Carcinoma

No therapy has been shown to be of significant long-term benefit for dogs with IMC, but there is general agreement among veterinary oncologists that surgery is contraindicated. Wound dehiscence, ventral and limb edema, and disseminated intravascular coagulation all are potential complications of IMC, which is unlikely to be amenable to complete surgical excision. There are anecdotal reports of disease palliation with various medical therapies or RT, but the prognosis remains poor despite all treatment attempts reported to date. One small retrospective study showed clinical improvement in seven of seven dogs with IMC treated with 0.3 mg/kg piroxicam daily PO (de M Souza et al, 2009). Median survival time was 185 days, which was significantly longer than that of three dogs treated with DOX.

Prognosis

Prognostic factors for CMTs have been examined in multiple prospective and retrospective studies. Factors correlating with prognosis in multivariate analysis are the most compelling since the interdependent effects of multiple factors are considered in such analyses. Reports give conflicting results regarding the impact of many factors on prognosis; those generally accepted to have a negative impact on prognosis are listed in Table 84-3.

Feline Mammary Cancer

Incidence, Causes, and Pathogenesis

Mammary cancer is the third most common feline tumor after skin tumors and lymphoma. As in dogs, mammary tumors may affect both male and female cats. Both estrogen and progesterone are thought to play important roles in the development of feline mammary cancer (FMC), although the underlying mechanisms are less clear than for CMTs. Intact females and cats exposed regularly to progestins have been shown to be at an increased risk of mammary cancer development. The literature also suggests that, as in dogs, early OHE may lower the risk of FMC. One published report demonstrated that cats ovariectomized at 6 months of age had an approximately sevenfold reduction in risk of FMC compared with intact cats (Dorn et al, 1968). A more recent study reported a 91% reduction in risk in those spayed before 6 months of age

and an 86% reduction in those spayed before 1 year of age (Overley et al, 2005). Parity was not significantly related to the risk of developing FMC. Thus there is justification for recommending OHE before 1 year of age in cats.

Clinical Presentation

As with mammary tumors in dogs, FMC generally presents as a palpable nodule detected by the owner or veterinarian. However, in contrast with CMTs, the majority (80% to 96%) of FMCs are malignant. Ulceration is not uncommon and is suggestive of malignancy. As in dogs, multiple lesions often are present at the time of diagnosis, although cats are less likely to have a combination of benign and malignant lesions.

Diagnosis and Staging

Complete evaluation of a cat with suspected mammary carcinoma should include an assessment of general health with urinalysis, complete blood count, and serum biochemical evaluation in anticipation of anesthesia and surgery. Thoracic radiography (right lateral, left lateral, and ventrodorsal views) and regional lymph node palpation and aspiration are critical, given that the reported metastatic rate for FMC ranges from 25% to as high as 100%, with the most common sites being the lymph nodes and lungs. Interestingly, cats have a very low rate of skeletal metastasis from mammary carcinoma compared with people and dogs.

Histopathologic examination is necessary to confirm a diagnosis of FMC. Often biopsy specimens are obtained at the time of definitive surgery rather than as a presurgical evaluation. The majority of mammary tumors in cats are diagnosed as adenocarcinomas, specifically of tubular, papillary, solid, or cribriform type. Less common malignant lesions are squamous cell carcinomas, sarcomas, and mucinous carcinomas. IMC was first described in cats in 2004, with three cats having lesions comparable in gross appearance to those of human and canine IMC and with a similarly poor prognosis (Pérez-Alenza et al, 2004).

As in dogs, fine-needle aspiration and cytologic examination of mammary lesions seldom is of clinical use but may be considered if cutaneous or subcutaneous lesions of nonmammary tissue origin such as mast cell tumors are suspected. Cytologic evaluation of pleural effusion fluid or of aspirates from enlarged lymph nodes is warranted when these conditions are present. As with dogs, the staging system for FMC has been modified from the original system proposed by Owen in 1980. The modified system classifies all nodal metastasis as stage III or IV, whereas the original system placed histologically confirmed nodal metastasis but without fixation of nodes to surrounding tissue into stage II. A comparison of the staging systems is outlined in Table 84-4.

Treatment

Surgery

Surgery, often with adjuvant chemotherapy, is the primary treatment for FMC. In contrast to the recommendations

TABLE **84-3**

Comparative Aspects of Canine and Feline Mammary Tumors

	Dog	Cat
Estimated annual incidence in the United States	199 per 100,000	25 per 100,000
Percent of tumors that are benign	50%-70%	10%-20%
Most common malignancy	Complex carcinoma	Tubulopapillary carcinoma
Hormone receptor expression in invasive carcinomas	Majority have been reported to be ER-α^+ and PR$^-$; in one report of high-risk breeds, 57% and 58% were ER-α and PR positive, respectively	Majority (57%) are ER-α^- and PR$^+$, although recent report had 41% ER-α^+ and 18% PR$^+$
HER2/neu expression	Up to 40% of samples have overexpression equivalent to "+++" grading on human HercepTest classification	Protein overexpressed in ~33%-55%
p53 overexpression	15%-75%	35%-45%
Metastatic behavior	32%-77% metastatic, depending on histologic type	>50% metastatic
Poor prognostic factors	Ductal carcinoma, IMC, or sarcoma Ulceration of skin Invasive/fixed tumor Older age at diagnosis ER negativity p53 mutations and protein overexpression Loss of PTEN expression German shepherd breed Heat shock protein expression Advanced stage Large tumor size (>3 cm) High histologic grade Increased MMP-9 expression in stromal cells High Ki-67 index (increased MIB-1 labeling index) Intact ovaries Male gender	High AgNOR count Tumor size >3 cm High Ki-67 index Lymphatic invasion Increased WHO stage HER2 overexpression p-AKT expression High histologic grade (Elston and Ellis method)
Overall prognosis	Reported MST is 439 days MST is 70 wk after surgery for malignant tumors vs. 114 wk for benign tumors	1-yr survival noted for ≈ ⅓ to ½ of cats treated with surgery alone; up to 59% with adjuvant chemotherapy 2-yr survival is ≈15%-20% with surgery alone; improves to ≈37% with addition of chemotherapy Complex carcinomas are associated with a more favorable prognosis (MST of 32.6 mo vs. 15.5 mo for other carcinomas)

AgNOR, Argyrophilic nucleolar organizer region; *ER,* estrogen receptor; *IMC,* inflammatory mammary carcinoma; *MST,* mean survival time; *PR,* progesterone receptor; *WHO,* World Health Organization.

for CMT, unilateral or bilateral chain mastectomy is considered the preferred surgical method for FMC. There are conflicting reports regarding whether chain mastectomy provides a survival advantage, although the procedure has been shown to decrease the recurrence rate of FMC significantly. When bilateral chain mastectomy is performed, it may be done as one surgical procedure or as a staged procedure, with the second unilateral mastectomy 2 to 6 weeks after the first. The inguinal lymph node is removed with the caudal mammary glands; however, axillary node excision is not a routine part of the radical mastectomy. Removal of the axillary node is recommended only if it is known to have metastatic disease since prophylactic axillary node excision is unlikely to benefit the patient.

Chemotherapy

Few studies have assessed the role of chemotherapy for the primary or adjuvant treatment of FMC. DOX-based protocols have been evaluated most frequently, and

TABLE 84-4

Comparison of the Original and Modified TNM Staging Systems for the Classification of Feline Mammary Carcinoma

Stage	Original WHO Staging	Modified WHO Staging
I	T1 (<1 cm), N0, M0	T1 (<2 cm), N0, M0
II	≤T2 (<3 cm), N1(+), M0 (histologically positive node, but not fixed to underlying tissues)	T2 (2 to 3 cm), N0, M0
III	Any T3 or any with fixed nodal involvement	Regional node metastasis or T3 (>3 cm) lesion or both, but no distant metastasis
IV	Distant metastasis (any T, any N, M1)	Distant metastasis (any T, any N, M1)

TNM, Tumor-node-metastasis system, where T is the size of the primary tumor, N is regional lymph node involvement, and M is distant metastasis (e.g., N0 indicates no lymph node involvement, and N1 indicates confirmed lymph node involvement); *WHO*, World Health Organization.

approximately one third to one half of cats with stage III or IV disease (see Table 84-4 for staging criteria) have a measurable response to the combination of DOX and cyclophosphamide. In a retrospective study of 67 cats with mammary adenocarcinoma that received adjuvant DOX chemotherapy (1 mg/kg q21d IV for an intended five treatments) beginning at the time of suture removal, the median survival time was 448 days, and the 1- and 2-year survival rates were 58.9% and 37.2%, respectively (Novosad et al, 2006). The author and others conducted a randomized, prospective clinical trial comparing mitoxantrone (5 mg/m^2 q21d IV for four total doses) to DOX treatment (four doses at 20 mg/m^2 q21d IV) for adjuvant treatment of FMC after chain mastectomy. Data analysis indicated no significant difference in survival times between the two treatment groups, with a median survival of 747 days for the group given mitoxantrone and 484 days for the group receiving DOX. The literature supports the use of adjuvant chemotherapy for advanced-stage FMC, although its role in the treatment of stage I tumors is less clear.

Prognosis

Tumor size and therefore T category according to the WHO staging system is the single most reliable prognostic indicator in cats. In one report, the median survival time for cats with tumors larger than 3 cm was 12 months compared with 21 months for cats with lesions smaller than 3 cm (Viste et al, 2002). Other prognostic factors and a summary of the literature reporting survival times are given in Table 84-3.

References and Suggested Reading

Cassali GD et al: Evaluation of accuracy of fine needle aspiration cytology for diagnosis of canine mammary tumours: comparative features with human tumours, *Cytopathology* 18:191, 2007.

Chang SC et al: Prognostic factors associated with survival two years after surgery in dogs with malignant mammary tumors: 79 cases (1998-2002), *J Am Vet Med Assoc* 227:1625, 2005.

de M Souza CH et al: Inflammatory mammary carcinoma in 12 dogs: clinical features, cyclooxygenase-2 expression, and response to piroxicam treatment, *Can Vet J* 50:506, 2009.

Dorn ER et al: Survey of animal neoplasms in Alameda and Contra Costa County, California. II: Cancer morbidity in dogs and cats from Alameda County, *J Natl Cancer Inst* 40:317, 1968.

Elston CW, Ellis IO: Pathological prognostic factors in breast cancer. I. The value of histological grade in breast cancer: experience from a large study with long-term follow-up, *Histopathology* 19:403, 1991.

Hermo GA et al: Perioperative desmopressin prolongs survival in surgically treated bitches with mammary gland tumours: a pilot study, *Vet J* 178:103, 2008.

Hermo GA et al: Effect of adjuvant perioperative desmopressin in locally advanced canine mammary carcinoma and its relation to histologic grade, *J Am Anim Hosp Assoc* 47:21, 2011.

Im K-S et al: Breed-related differences in altered BRCA1 expression, phenotype and subtype in malignant canine mammary tumors, *Vet J* 195:366, 2013.

Karayannopoulou M et al: Adjuvant post-operative chemotherapy in bitches with mammary cancer, *J Vet Med A Physiol Pathol Clin Med* 48:85, 2001.

Klopfleisch R et al: Molecular carcinogenesis of canine mammary tumors: news from an old disease, *Vet Pathol* 48:98, 2011.

MacEwen EG et al: Evaluation of effects of levamisole and surgery on canine mammary cancer, *J Biol Response Mod* 4:418, 1985.

Matos AJ et al: Detection of lymph node micrometastases in malignant mammary tumours in dogs by cytokeratin immunostaining, *Vet Rec* 158:626, 2006.

Millanta F et al: A case of feline primary inflammatory mammary carcinoma: clinicopathological and immunohistochemical findings, *J Feline Med Surg* 14(6):420, 2012. Epub March 9, 2012.

Novosad CA et al: Retrospective evaluation of adjunctive doxorubicin for the treatment of feline mammary gland adenocarcinoma: 67 cases, *J Am Anim Hosp Assoc* 42:110, 2006.

Overley B et al: Association between ovariohysterectomy and feline mammary carcinoma, *J Vet Intern Med* 19:560, 2005.

Pérez-Alenza MD et al: First description of feline inflammatory mammary carcinoma: clinicopathological and immunohistochemical characteristics of three cases, *Breast Cancer Res* 6: R300, 2004.

Simon D et al: Postoperative adjuvant treatment of invasive malignant mammary gland tumors in dogs with doxorubicin and docetaxel, *J Vet Intern Med* 20:1184, 2006.

Sleeckx N et al: Canine mammary tumours, an overview, *Reprod Domest Anim* 46:1112, 2011.

Sorenmo KU, Shofer FS, Goldschmidt MH: Effect of spaying and timing of spaying on survival of dogs with mammary carcinoma, *J Vet Intern Med* 14:266, 2000.

Stratmann N et al: Mammary tumor recurrence in bitches after regional mastectomy, *Vet Surg* 37:82, 2008.

Viste JR et al: Feline mammary adenocarcinoma: tumor size as a prognostic indicator, *Can Vet J* 43:33, 2002.

CHAPTER 85

Rescue Therapy for Canine Lymphoma

DAVID M. VAIL, *Madison, Wisconsin*

When lymphoma is being treated, the fundamental goals of chemotherapy are to induce a complete and durable (>6 months) first remission (termed *induction*), to reinduce a remission when the disease recurs (or the patient experiences relapse) following remission (termed *reinduction*), and, finally, to induce remission when the cancer fails to respond to induction or reinduction therapy using drugs not included in the initial protocols (termed *rescue*). Despite the plethora of induction chemotherapeutic protocols for dogs with lymphoma developed over the past 15 to 20 years, most are modifications of the regimen known as *CHOP*, initially designed for human oncologic use. CHOP consists of combinations of cyclophosphamide (C), doxorubicin (H, for hydroxydaunorubicin), vincristine (O, for Oncovin), and prednisone (P). Conventional CHOP-based chemotherapy induces remission in approximately 80% to 95% of dogs, with overall median survival times of 10 to 12 months. Eventually, the majority of dogs with lymphoma that achieve remission following induction with a CHOP-based protocol experience a relapse. This usually represents the emergence of tumor clones or tumor stem cells that are inherently more resistant to chemotherapy than the original tumor, so-called MDR clones that either were initially drug resistant or became so following exposure to selected chemotherapy agents. Reinduction or rescue therapy then becomes necessary and is the subject of this discussion.

Reinduction Chemotherapy

At the first recurrence of lymphoma, it is recommended that reinduction be attempted, first by re-treating with the induction protocol that was initially successful, provided the recurrence occurred far enough temporally from the conclusion of the initial protocol (e.g., ≥2 months) to make reinduction successful. Attention must be given to the cumulative dose of doxorubicin that will result from reinduction, and baseline cardiac assessment, the use of cardioprotectants, alternative drug choices, and client education all should be considered. In general, the length of the reinduction is half that experienced following the initial therapy; however, a subset of animals enjoy long-term responses following reinduction, especially dogs that completed the initial induction protocol and had not been receiving chemotherapy for several months when relapse occurred. Nearly 80% to 90% rates of

successful reinduction can be expected in dogs that have completed CHOP-based protocols and experience relapse while not currently receiving therapy (Flory et al, 2011; Garrett et al, 2002).

The duration of the remission with a reinduction CHOP-based protocol is predicted by the duration of the interval between protocols and the duration of the first remission (Flory et al, 2011). In their study, Flory and colleagues found that 78% of dogs achieved a complete response (CR) with the reinduction CHOP protocol, and the median second remission duration was 159 days. Furthermore, dogs that had at least a 4-month remission following their induction CHOP treatment experienced reinduction remissions that were approximately twice as long as those of dogs with induction remissions of less than 4 months (214 days versus 98 days, respectively), which suggests that time off chemotherapy is an important predictor of reinduction success. This implies that dogs that experience relapse quickly after completion of their initial CHOP protocol may be better served by initiating rescue therapy immediately and bypassing reinduction altogether; however, the absolute temporal cutoff for what constitutes a "quick" relapse currently is unknown.

Rescue Chemotherapy

If reinduction fails or the dog does not respond to the initial induction, the use of so-called rescue agents or protocols may be attempted. These are single drugs or drug combinations that typically are not found in standard CHOP protocols and are reserved for use in the setting of drug resistance. The most common rescue protocols used in dogs include single-agent or combination treatment with actinomycin D, mitoxantrone, doxorubicin (if doxorubicin was not part of the original induction protocol), dacarbazine, temozolomide, lomustine (CCNU), L-asparaginase, mechlorethamine, vinblastine, vinorelbine, procarbazine, prednisone, or etoposide. Some rescue protocols are relatively easy and convenient single-agent treatments, whereas others are more complicated (and expensive) multiagent protocols, such as MOPP (mechlorethamine, vincristine [Oncovin], procarbazine, prednisone). Overall rescue response rates of 40% to 90% are reported; however, responses usually are not durable, with median response durations of 1.5 to 2.5 months being typical, regardless of the complexity of the

TABLE 85-1

Summary of Response Data for Rescue Protocols in Dogs (Tested in a Minimum of 25 Animals)*

Protocol	Number of Animals	Overall Response	Complete Response	Median Response Duration†	Median Duration of Complete Response	Study
Actinomycin D	25	0%	0%	0 days	0 days	Moore et al, 1994
Actinomycin D	49‡	41%	41%	129 days	129 days	Bannink et al, 2008
Dacarbazine	40	35%	3%	43 days	144 days	Griessmayr et al, 2009
Dacarbazine or temozolomide with anthracycline	63	71%	55%	45 days	Not reported	Dervisis et al, 2007
DMAC (dexamethasone, melphalan, actinomycin D, cytosine arabinoside)	54	72%	44%	61 days	112 days	Alvarez et al, 2006
Lomustine (CCNU)	43	27%	7%	86 days	110 days	Moore et al, 1999
Lomustine, L-asparaginase, prednisone	48	77%	65%	70 days	90 days	Saba et al, 2009
Lomustine, L-asparaginase, prednisone	31	87%	52%	63 days	111 days	Saba et al, 2007
Lomustine, dacarbazine (DTIC)	57	35%	23%	62 days	83 days	Flory et al, 2008
Mitoxantrone	44	41%	30%	Not reported	127 days	Moore et al, 1994
MOPP (mechlorethamine, vincristine, procarbazine, prednisone)	117	65%	31%	61 days	63 days	Rassnick et al, 2002
MPP (mechlorethamine, procarbazine, prednisone)	41	34%	17%	56 days	238 days	Northrup et al, 2009

*Few of these studies tested protocols in sufficient numbers of subjects for adequate statistical power, and even fewer compared treatment protocols in a randomized prospective fashion. In addition, staging, inclusion, and response criteria varied considerably among studies listed. Therefore evaluations of efficacy between the various protocols are subject to bias, which makes direct comparisons difficult.
†Various temporal response end points were used, including disease-free interval, time to progression, and progression-free survival.
‡Prednisone often was used concurrently.

TABLE 85-2

First-Line Rescue Protocol Used by the Author

Cycle 1

Week 1	**Baseline ALT Measurement** L-Asparaginase 400 U/kg SC CCNU 70 mg/m² PO Prednisone 2 mg/kg once daily PO
Week 2	Prednisone 1.5 mg/kg once daily PO
Week 3	Prednisone 1.0 mg/kg once daily PO

Cycle 2

Week 1	**Optional ALT Measurement** L-Asparaginase 400 U/kg SC CCNU 70 mg/m² PO Prednisone 1.0 mg/kg every other day PO
Week 2	Prednisone 1.0 mg/kg every other day PO
Week 3	Prednisone 1.0 mg/kg every other day PO

Cycles 3-5

Week 1	**Mandatory ALT Measurement** CCNU 70 mg/m² PO Prednisone 1.0 mg/kg every other day PO
Week 2	Prednisone 1.0 mg/kg every other day PO
Week 3	Prednisone 1.0 mg/kg every other day PO

Treatment discontinuation criteria:
1. Completion of protocol, or completion of two treatments beyond complete remission, whichever is longer.
2. Progressive disease.
3. Increase in ALT activity to more than twice the upper limit of normal (or twice the baseline level if higher than baseline at initiation); discontinue drug and reinstitute/reduce dose depending on normalization of ALT activity.

ALT, Alanine aminotransferase; *CCNU*, lomustine; *PO*, orally; *SC*, subcutaneously.

protocol. A small subset of animals (<20%) experience longer rescue response durations. Table 85-1 provides a summary of canine rescue protocols for which results have been published. It is critical to note that current published studies of rescue protocols do not include sufficient numbers of subjects for adequate statistical power, nor do they compare protocols in a randomized prospective fashion. Therefore evaluations of efficacy for various protocols are subject to substantial bias, which makes direct comparisons difficult and indeed precarious. Therefore, at present, choice of a particular rescue protocol should depend on several factors, including cost, time commitment required, efficacy, adverse event profile (i.e., toxicity), and experience of the clinician with the protocols in question. Because the complexity of rescue protocols does not yet appear to be associated with significant gains in rescue durability, the author tends to choose simpler and less costly protocols (e.g., lomustine/L-asparaginase/prednisone) (Saba et al, 2007) (Table 85-2). That being said, the use of multiple varied rescue protocols, altering as needed based on response and continuing as long as clients are comfortable with the quality of life of their dog, is commonplace. This sequential application of several different rescue protocols can result in several months of extended survival with acceptable quality of life.

Strategies to Enhance the Effectiveness of Chemotherapy

Further advances in remission and survival durations await the development of new methods of delivering or targeting traditional chemotherapeutic drugs, new generations of chemotherapeutic agents, or novel nonchemotherapeutic treatment modalities. Mechanisms for avoidance or abrogation of multidrug resistance, enhancement of tumor apoptosis (programmed cell death), tumor ablation (e.g., bone marrow ablation and reconstitution), and immune-system reconstitution, as well as novel immunomodulatory therapies (e.g., monoclonal antibodies), all are active areas of investigation in veterinary oncology.

References and Suggested Reading

Alvarez FJ et al: Dexamethasone, melphalan, actinomycin D, cytosine arabinoside (DMAC) protocol for dogs with relapsed lymphoma, *J Vet Intern Med* 20:1178, 2006.

Bannink EO et al: Actinomycin D as rescue therapy in dogs with relapsed or resistant lymphoma: 49 cases (1999-2006), *J Am Vet Med Assoc* 233:446, 2008.

Dervisis NG et al: Efficacy of temozolomide or dacarbazine in combination with an anthracycline for rescue chemotherapy in dogs with lymphoma, *J Am Vet Med Assoc* 231:563, 2007.

Flory AB et al: Combination of CCNU and DTIC chemotherapy for treatment of resistant lymphoma in dogs, *J Vet Intern Med* 22:164, 2008.

Flory AB et al: Evaluation of factors associated with second remission in dogs with lymphoma undergoing retreatment with a cyclophosphamide, doxorubicin, vincristine and prednisone chemotherapy protocol: 95 cases (2000-2007), *J Am Vet Med Assoc* 238:501, 2011.

Garrett LD et al: Evaluation of a 6-month chemotherapy protocol with no maintenance therapy for dogs with lymphoma, *J Vet Intern Med* 16:704, 2002.

Griessmayr PB et al: Dacarbazine as single-agent therapy for relapsed lymphoma in dogs, *J Vet Intern Med* 23:1227, 2009.

Moore AS et al: Evaluation of mitoxantrone for the treatment of lymphoma in dogs, *J Am Vet Med Assoc* 204:1903, 1994.

Moore AS et al: Lomustine (CCNU) for the treatment of resistant lymphoma in dogs, *J Vet Intern Med* 13:395, 1999.

Moore AS, Ogilvie GK, Vail DM: Actinomycin D for reinduction of remission in dogs with resistant lymphoma, *J Vet Intern Med* 8:343, 1994.

Northrup NC et al: Mechlorethamine, procarbazine and prednisone for the treatment of resistant lymphoma in dogs, *Vet Comp Oncol* 7:38, 2009.

Rassnick KM et al: MOPP chemotherapy for treatment of resistant lymphoma in dogs: a retrospective study of 117 cases (1989-2000), *J Vet Intern Med* 16:576, 2002.

Saba CF et al: Combination chemotherapy with continuous L-asparaginase, lomustine and prednisone for relapsed canine lymphoma, *J Vet Intern Med* 23:1058, 2009.

Saba CF, Thamm DH, Vail DM: Combination chemotherapy with L-asparaginase, lomustine, and prednisone for relapsed or refractory canine lymphoma, *J Vet Intern Med* 21:127, 2007.

CHAPTER 86

Plasma Cell Neoplasms

RACHEL STERNBERG, *Urbana-Champaign, Illinois*
DAVIS M. SEELIG, *Madison, Wisconsin*
LAURA D. GARRETT, *Urbana-Champaign, Illinois*

Plasma cell neoplasms originate from terminally differentiated B lymphocytes that have undergone malignant transformation. These neoplasms are associated with a wide range of clinical syndromes including multiple myeloma, macroglobulinemia, solitary osseous plasmacytoma, and extramedullary plasmacytoma.

Multiple Myeloma

Pathology and Natural Behavior

Multiple myeloma (MM) is a B-cell malignancy characterized by the infiltration and proliferation of a clonal population of plasma cells in the bone marrow. MM is uncommon in animals, accounting for fewer than 8% of all canine hematopoietic tumors. No breed or sex predilections are seen, and older dogs are affected most commonly, with a mean age at onset of 8 to 9 years. MM is less common in cats than in dogs; the median age at presentation in cats is 12 to 14 years and there is a possible male predisposition. The cause of MM is largely unknown. Unlike in other hematopoietic diseases, there is no evidence that infection with feline immunodeficiency virus or feline leukemia virus is related to MM development in cats.

Myeloma cells produce large quantities of an identical immunoglobulin protein, called the *paraprotein* or *monoclonal (M) protein,* which often can be identified as a monoclonal spike on a serum or urine protein electrophoretogram. The paraprotein may represent a complete immunoglobulin or a portion of the immunoglobulin (light or heavy chain). Immunoglobulin G (IgG) and IgA gammopathies are the most common, whereas IgM gammopathy (macroglobulinemia) is rare. Although IgG and IgA gammopathies are equally common in dogs, in cats the proportions are reported to be 80% IgG gammopathies and 20% IgA gammopathies. Biclonal gammopathies occasionally are reported in veterinary patients. Production of pure light chains (κ or λ type), referred to as *light-chain myeloma* or *Bence Jones myeloma,* has been reported rarely in cats and dogs.

The pathologic conditions associated with MM are related to the effects of the circulating paraprotein as well as organ or bone marrow dysfunction caused by neoplastic infiltration. High serum paraprotein concentrations may result in hyperviscosity syndrome (HVS), manifesting in neurologic signs, retinopathy, and cardiomyopathy. Other pathologic conditions include osteolysis, hemorrhagic diathesis, cytopenias, hypercalcemia, renal disease, and increased susceptibility to bacterial infection.

Clinical Signs

Clinical signs associated with MM often are nonspecific and insidious in onset and include lethargy, weakness, and anorexia. Polyuria and polydipsia can occur secondary to hypercalcemia or MM-related renal disease. Lameness, paresis or paralysis, and pain occur secondary to osteolysis or spinal cord compression. Bleeding diatheses, including epistaxis, gingival bleeding, intraocular hemorrhage, and, less frequently, melena or hematuria, are common. Retinal abnormalities occur frequently secondary to HVS and include hemorrhage or tortuous, dilated vessels. Central nervous system deficits, including dementia and seizures, also may be present secondary to HVS, bleeding diathesis, or severe hypercalcemia. In dogs the median duration of clinical signs before presentation is 30 days.

Diagnosis

Diagnostic criteria for MM are adapted from those in human medicine. Establishing a diagnosis requires confirming the presence of at least two of the disease manifestations listed in Box 86-1. Recent studies suggest that these criteria should be reevaluated in cats because visceral organ infiltration (primarily of the liver or spleen) is common in cats at initial presentation (Mellor et al, 2006; Patel et al, 2005).

Initial diagnostic tests should include a complete blood count (CBC), serum chemistry panel, and urinalysis. Nonregenerative anemia is the most common CBC finding, reported in 55% to 68% of cases. Serum chemistry testing commonly reveals azotemia and hypercalcemia as well as hyperglobulinemia with secondary hypoalbuminemia and hypocholesterolemia. Urine culture is recommended since patients often have dilute urine and are immunologically compromised, and thus are prone to infection.

Serum and urine samples can be submitted for parallel protein electrophoresis. Serum protein electrophoresis generally reveals a monoclonal gammopathy with a peak in the β- or γ-globulin region or, less commonly, a biclonal gammopathy. Immunofixation electrophoresis or capillary zone electrophoresis may be used to detect M proteins in patients with normal protein and globulin concentrations and equivocal serum protein

Diagnostic Criteria for Multiple Myeloma

Diagnosis requires the presence of at least two of the following:
- Monoclonal gammopathy or paraproteinemia
- Radiographic evidence of osteolytic bone lesions
- >5% Neoplastic cells or >10% to 20% plasma cells in the bone marrow
- Immunoglobulin light-chain (Bence Jones) proteinuria
- Proposed for cats: Plasma cell infiltration of visceral organs

electrophoresis findings (Seelig et al, 2010). Urine electrophoresis can detect light-chain proteinuria that will not be detected with a urine dipstick. Bence Jones protein in the urine without a corresponding monoclonal gammopathy on serum electrophoresis is diagnostic for pure light-chain disease.

Abdominal imaging is useful to evaluate commonly affected organs such as the liver and spleen. In cats with MM, 85% of abdominal organs showing an abnormality on imaging had cytologically confirmed plasma cell infiltration (Mellor et al, 2006). Limb and spinal radiographs can help detect bone lesions. Importantly, bone lysis is rare in patients with macroglobulinemia, whereas hepatosplenomegaly and lymphadenopathy are common.

MM usually is diagnosed definitively by cytologic examination of a bone marrow aspirate; plasma cells are distributed unevenly among normal marrow elements. Optimal samples may be obtained by performing bone aspiration at the site of lytic lesions; however, multiple bone marrow aspirates or a core biopsy may be necessary for definitive diagnosis, especially when no lytic lesions are seen.

Treatment

When patients with MM are treated, not only the underlying cancer but also the secondary conditions associated with the disease must be treated.

Fluid Therapy
Intravenous fluid therapy often is needed initially to correct dehydration, improve cardiovascular status, and manage hypercalcemia and azotemia. Isotonic saline solution is preferred over other fluids in the initial management of hypercalcemic patients.

Antibiotics
Antibiotic therapy may be needed to treat concurrent infections, such as urinary tract infection or bacterial pyoderma because these can progress to life-threatening infections if left untreated.

Palliative Radiation Therapy
Neoplastic plasma cells are sensitive to radiation, and radiation therapy (RT) is a highly effective palliative treatment for MM since it can relieve discomfort and quickly decrease tumor burden. Indications for RT include painful bone lesions, spinal cord compression, pathologic fracture (after fracture stabilization), or a large soft-tissue mass.

Bisphosphonates
Bisphosphonates such as pamidronate may be useful in managing hypercalcemia as well as decreasing osteoclastic bone resorption and bone pain. The recommended dosage of pamidronate is 1 to 2 mg/kg IV in dogs and, anecdotally, 1 mg/kg IV in cats q21-28d. Pamidronate is diluted in saline solution (with the amount based on the size of the patient) and administered as a 2-hour infusion to minimize renal toxicosis.

Analgesics
Dogs and cats with MM may experience moderate to severe pain; treating this pain is a priority. Pain may be relieved by treating the underlying cancer and providing various analgesic therapies and supportive care.

Plasmapheresis
Plasmapheresis, an extracorporeal blood purification technique, is the best immediate treatment for HVS. This procedure, which is performed rarely in veterinary medicine, involves withdrawing anticoagulated blood, separating blood components, removing the plasma, and reinfusing the remaining components with crystalloid fluids.

Chemotherapy
Although a cure is unlikely, MM can be a rewarding disease to treat since chemotherapy can greatly increase the quality and duration of life. The chemotherapy drugs most often used are alkylating agents, usually melphalan, combined with corticosteroids. However, eventual relapse during therapy is anticipated.

Melphalan. In dogs the recommended treatment protocol is melphalan administered at a dosage of 0.1 mg/kg q24h PO for 10 days and then 0.05 mg/kg q24h until the disease relapses or myelosuppression occurs. Prednisone is given concurrently at a dosage of 0.5 mg/kg q24h PO for 10 days and then 0.5 mg/kg every other day for 30 to 60 days, at which time prednisone is discontinued (Matus et al, 1986). Pulse-dose therapy with melphalan also has been described in which melphalan, at a dose of 7 mg/m², is given q24h PO for five consecutive days every 21 days. The most common adverse effects associated with melphalan therapy are myelosuppression and *delayed thrombocytopenia*. A CBC should be performed every 2 weeks for the first 2 months of treatment and then monthly thereafter.

Combined melphalan and prednisolone therapy also can be used in cats; however, cats appear to be more susceptible to melphalan-induced myelosuppression. The recommended treatment protocol is melphalan 0.1 mg/kg (or 0.5 mg total dose) q24h PO for 10 to 14 days and then every other day until clinical improvement occurs or leukopenia develops. A maintenance dosage of 0.5 mg q7d then is recommended (Hanna, 2005). Prednisolone is given concurrently at a dosage of 0.5 mg/kg q24h PO. If leukopenia develops, melphalan therapy should be discontinued until white blood cell counts return to normal; then maintenance therapy may be attempted at the same or a lower dose.

Other Antineoplastic Drugs. Other alkylating agents used to treat MM include chlorambucil, cyclophosphamide, and lomustine. In sick MM patients, in which a faster response to treatment is needed, cyclophosphamide may be administered intravenously at a dosage of 200 mg/m² once (with furosemide or saline diuresis) at the time that oral melphalan treatment is initiated. The authors also have successfully used single-agent cyclophosphamide, administered weekly or biweekly, in the treatment of cats with MM.

In dogs with relapsing MM or resistance to alkylating agents, single-agent doxorubicin or the VAD protocol (vincristine 0.7 mg/m² IV on days 8 and 15, doxorubicin [Adriamycin] 30 mg/m² IV every 21 days, and dexamethasone 1 mg/kg IV on days 1, 8, and 15) can be considered. Although dexamethasone is not routinely used as a first-line treatment for MM in veterinary medicine, it should be noted that dexamethasone is the corticosteroid of choice for the treatment of MM in humans.

Outcome and Prognostic Factors

The overall response rate for dogs treated with melphalan and prednisone chemotherapy is 92%, with 43% of dogs achieving a complete response. The median survival time of dogs treated with this drug combination is 540 days. Negative prognostic factors in dogs include hypercalcemia, light-chain proteinuria, and extensive lytic bone lesions (Matus et al, 1986).

Response to therapy and duration of response appear to be more variable in cats. Negative prognostic factors include bone lesions with pathologic fracture, hypercalcemia, anemia, light-chain proteinuria, azotemia, and poor response to treatment (Hanna, 2005). When treated with melphalan and prednisolone chemotherapy, four cats classified as having aggressive disease had a median survival time of 5 days, whereas the median survival time of five cats with less aggressive disease was 387 days (Hanna, 2005). Other studies have shown less promising results overall, with a shorter duration of response to treatment and a survival time of 6 months or less in treated cats (Patel et al, 2005). In cats with MM and other related disorders, the degree of plasma cell differentiation is correlated significantly with survival. Cats with well-differentiated tumors (<15% plasmablasts) have a median survival of 254 days, whereas cats with poorly differentiated tumors (≥50% plasmablasts) have a median survival of 14 days (Mellor et al, 2008).

Monitoring of Response to Treatment

Clinical response to treatment is indicated by improvement or resolution of clinical signs and laboratory and imaging abnormalities. In patients that respond to treatment, improvement in clinical signs and findings on laboratory tests (CBC, serum chemistry panel, and protein electrophoresis) are expected within the first 4 to 8 weeks. When serum Ig is assessed, complete remission is defined as normal globulin concentrations or undetectable monoclonal immunoglobulin. Partial remission is defined as a 50% decrease in globulin concentrations. Repeated CBCs to evaluate for resolution of cytopenias as well as serum biochemistry panels to check for resolution of azotemia and hypercalcemia are important. Repeated assessments of bone marrow aspirates, serum viscosity, and light-chain proteinuria are less useful in gauging response to treatment. Bone marrow aspiration is indicated in patients with persistent or relapsing cytopenias to differentiate neoplastic bone marrow involvement from myelosuppression secondary to chemotherapy. Ultrasonography with or without fine-needle aspiration may be used to evaluate resolution of visceral organ infiltration. Although serial radiographs can be used to assess for improvement of bony changes, radiographic changes may not reflect current disease progression or remission adequately.

Plasmacytomas

Extramedullary Plasmacytoma

Extramedullary plasmacytomas (EMPs) comprise about 2.5% of all neoplasms in dogs and occur most commonly in middle-aged to older dogs (mean, 8 to 10 years). Overrepresented breeds include cocker spaniels, certain terrier breeds (West Highland white, Yorkshire, and Airedale terriers), boxers, and golden retrievers. The incidence of EMP in cats is low, and few cases have been reported. Affected cats usually are older, with a mean age of 8.5 years.

In a study evaluating 751 cases of canine EMP, the most frequent sites of origin were the skin (86%), mucous membranes of the oral cavity and lips (9%), and rectum and colon (4%) (Kupanoff et al, 2006). Other reports suggest that oral plasmacytomas are more common and comprise up to one fourth of EMPs. Frequently reported locations for cutaneous tumors include the trunk, limbs, and head, with the ear being the most common head location. Cutaneous EMPs can be seen with MM. The incidence of EMPs may be underestimated because of previous classification as reticulum cell sarcoma, neuroendocrine tumor, anaplastic round cell tumor, or lymphoma.

Clinical signs associated with EMP vary with tumor location. Tenesmus, rectal prolapse, hematochezia, and rectal bleeding are the most frequent clinical signs in dogs with colorectal EMPs. Clinical signs other than the visible mass (most often smooth, raised, red, and measuring 10 to 20 mm) or oral bleeding are uncommon in most dogs with localized mucocutaneous EMP. Globulin-secreting EMPs have been reported rarely, and in these few cases, clinical signs consistent with HVS may be present.

EMP most often is diagnosed by cytologic evaluation or immunohistochemical testing. Morphologically, the neoplastic cells usually resemble mature, well-differentiated plasma cells. The cells are round to oval with distinct cell borders and contain a moderate amount of deep blue to gray cytoplasm and a prominent perinuclear clear zone (the Golgi zone). Cellular and nuclear pleomorphism may be noted, and binucleate forms are common. Rarely, aggregates of amorphous, extracellular pink material representative of amyloid (immunoglobulin light chain) can be seen. There is no evidence correlating cytologic appearance with biologic behavior. Histologic findings for EMP reveal that these tumors are nonencapsulated. Neoplastic plasma cells have been described as positive for vimentin, CD45, CD45a, CD79a, CD18, and IgG, IgA, or IgM. Testing for the immunohistochemical marker multiple myeloma 1/interferon regulatory factor 4 (MUM1/IRF-4) also may assist in diagnosis (Ramos-Vara et al, 2007).

Imaging studies of oral EMPs, such as high-detail dental radiography or computed tomography, may improve assessment of tumor infiltration and optimize surgical planning. Staging is especially important for EMPs that tend to be associated with more aggressive disease, such as noncutaneous, nonoral EMPs and solitary osseous plasmacytoma (see later).

Unlike MM, EMP generally carries a favorable prognosis. These tumors tend to be locally invasive but have a low metastatic rate, and complete surgical removal often is curative. In compilations of reports of canine cutaneous and mucocutaneous EMPs, surgical excision was noted to be curative in about 90% to 95% of cases. Local recurrence rates of 5% to 8% were reported, most often after microscopically incomplete resection, and distant metastasis was present in fewer than 4% of cases. In cases of incomplete excision, additional surgery, adjunctive RT, or systemic chemotherapy may extend the disease-free interval. A syndrome of multiple cutaneous EMPs that are aggressive in behavior has been reported in dogs. Additionally, progression of EMP to MM in cats and dogs has been reported.

Noncutaneous, nonoral EMPs are reported to have a more aggressive behavior in dogs, with metastasis to local lymph nodes commonly seen. However, dogs treated with surgery alone or a combination of surgery and adjuvant therapy can have extended survival times. In a report of nine dogs treated surgically for colorectal plasmacytomas, the median survival time was 15 months (Kupanoff et al, 2006). Adjuvant chemotherapy (generally melphalan or chlorambucil) is recommended if metastatic disease is detected or if incomplete surgical margins are obtained.

Solitary Osseous Plasmacytoma

Solitary osseous plasmacytoma (SOP) is reported rarely in dogs and cats, and cases may progress to systemic plasma cell disease months to years after local tumor development. Reported sites include the vertebrae, zygomatic arch, and rib. The authors also have seen cases of SOP in which long bones are affected. Complete staging is indicated before definitive treatment is pursued. The optimal treatment for most patients with SOP is RT in a total dose of 40 to 50 Gy administered in daily fractions for 3 to 4 weeks. Depending on the location of the tumor, surgical excision also may be an option. Systemic chemotherapy can be considered at the time of local treatment of SOP, but its use is controversial in the absence of systemic involvement.

References and Suggested Reading

Hanna F: Multiple myelomas in cats, *J Feline Med Surg* 7(5):275, 2005.

Kupanoff PA, Popovitch CA, Goldschmidt MH: Colorectal plasmacytomas: a retrospective study of nine dogs, *J Am Anim Hosp Assoc* 42(1):37, 2006.

Matus RE et al: Prognostic factors for multiple myeloma in the dog, *J Am Vet Med Assoc* 188(11):1288, 1986.

Mellor PJ et al: Myeloma-related disorders in cats commonly present as extramedullary neoplasms in contrast to myeloma in human patients: 24 cases with clinical follow-up, *J Vet Intern Med* 20(6):1376, 2006.

Mellor PJ et al: Histopathologic, immunohistochemical, and cytologic analysis of feline myeloma-related disorders: further evidence for primary extramedullary development in the cat, *Vet Pathol* 45(2):159, 2008.

Patel RT et al: Multiple myeloma in 16 cats: a retrospective study, *Vet Clin Pathol* 34(4):341, 2005.

Ramos-Vara JA, Miller MA, Valli VE: Immunohistochemical detection of multiple myeloma 1/interferon regulatory factor 4 (MUM1/IRF-4) in canine plasmacytoma: comparison with CD79a and CD20, *Vet Pathol* 44(6):875, 2007.

Seelig DM et al: Monoclonal gammopathy without hyperglobulinemia in 2 dogs with IgA secretory neoplasms, *Vet Clin Pathol* 39(4):447, 2010.

Wright ZM, Rogers KS, Mansell J: Survival data for canine oral extramedullary plasmacytomas: a retrospective analysis (1996-2006), *J Am Anim Hosp Assoc* 44(2):75, 2008.

CHAPTER 87

Osteosarcoma

NICOLE P. EHRHART, *Fort Collins, Colorado*
TIMOTHY M. FAN, *Urbana-Champaign, Illinois*

Appendicular osteosarcoma (OSA) is the most common primary bone tumor in dogs, accounting for approximately 75% to 80% of focal malignant bone lesions. Arising from transformed osteoblasts, OSA frequently develops within the metaphyseal regions of long bones. OSA tends to affect middle-aged to older dogs (7 to 10 years); however, some reports describe an additional incidence peak at 2 years of age. Unlike some tumors, OSA shows an incidence that only subtly favors males, with a reported male:female ratio of 1.5:1. Specific breeds with large skeletal mass, including Saint Bernards, rottweilers, Great Danes, greyhounds, and Labrador retrievers, appear to be at increased risk of OSA development.

Diagnosis

History and Physical Examination

The most common sites of OSA development are the distal radius, proximal humerus, and proximal tibia. Given these anatomic sites, dogs with appendicular OSA commonly are brought to the veterinarian because of acute or chronic lameness and limb swelling. Clinical signs of lameness often are associated temporally with perceived traumatic events such as running, jumping, or rough play with other dogs. In addition to showing varying degrees of lameness, dogs also may have significant peritumoral soft tissue swelling. Following the onset of lameness, some dogs partially improve with symptomatic therapy, including rest, nonsteroidal antiinflammatory drugs, or other analgesics; however, recurrent and progressive bone pain refractory to conservative therapy is common. Dogs with OSA that have had long-standing chronic pain may demonstrate significant discomfort of the affected limb even after minimal or light manipulation.

Imaging Modalities

Despite the increasing availability of advanced imaging modalities such as computed tomography (CT), magnetic resonance imaging (MRI), and positron emission tomography, radiography remains the most commonly employed radiologic method for assessing the extent of disease in dogs with OSA. Given that appendicular OSA has the capacity not only for local bone destruction but also for distant metastasis, it is recommended that every dog suspected of having OSA undergo radiography of both the primary tumor site and the thorax. At presentation, the majority of affected dogs have radiographically evident disease at the primary tumor site, typically characterized by a mixed osteolytic-osteoproductive focal lesion arising from the metaphyseal region of long bones. Only a small percentage of dogs (~10%) have radiographic evidence of macroscopic pulmonary metastases at initial presentation; however, the vast majority (>90%) eventually develop radiographically evident pulmonary metastatic disease.

In addition to radiography, various advanced imaging modalities can be used for evaluating the size of the primary tumor or the extent of pulmonary metastasis. For more accurate characterization of primary tumor size and degree of intramedullary involvement, imaging modalities such as CT, MRI, nuclear scintigraphy, and single-photon emission CT can provide supplemental information to ensure that adequate surgical margins are achieved as required for successful limb-sparing surgery. Nuclear scintigraphy is useful not only for assessing the primary tumor but also for identifying additional skeletal lesions distant from the primary tumor. CT is more sensitive than conventional radiography in assessing for pulmonary metastasis and has the ability to identify small metastatic lesions (2 to 3 mm), which are undetectable by conventional radiography. The greater sensitivity of CT for detection of metastasis might allow for improved disease stratification and determination of prognosis in patients diagnosed with OSA (Eberle et al, 2011).

Differential Diagnoses

Differential diagnoses for OSA include other primary bone tumors, bacterial or fungal osteomyelitis, bone metastasis from other primary sites, and systemic diseases that affect bone such as multiple myeloma or lymphoma. Benign processes such as bone cysts and degenerative or active remodeling also can be considered. It is important that a complete history be obtained (including any history of travel to areas of endemic fungal infection) so that the clinician can take into account all factors when making a diagnosis. Radiographic appearance is helpful, especially when there is a classic appearance in a classic location. However, the classic radiographic features of OSA are not present in every case. In addition, other primary bone tumors may have a similar radiographic appearance. Involvement of multiple bones is uncommon in OSA; however, synchronous primary OSAs occasionally can occur. Metastatic disease affecting bone is usually in a diaphyseal location rather than in the metaphysis but can be either lytic or proliferative. The presence of multiple punched-out lesions in several bones suggests multiple myeloma.

The most accurate means to differentiate OSA from other bone diseases is through a bone biopsy. However, because bone biopsy is an invasive procedure and the results are not always available immediately, fine-needle aspiration and cytologic evaluation can be helpful initially to help rule out other differential diagnoses. Most bone tumors have a soft tissue component that yields cells on needle aspiration. A cytologic specimen devoid of inflammation and yielding a population of malignant mesenchymal cells supports the diagnosis of a primary bone malignancy. Osteosarcoma generally cannot be differentiated cytologically from other sarcomas using standard staining methods. Staining of bone tumor aspirates for alkaline phosphatase (AP) activity can be helpful in further characterizing malignant mesenchymal cells as OSA. In one study, AP staining of 61 bone lesion aspirates provided an accurate diagnosis of OSA with 100% sensitivity and 89% specificity (Barger et al, 2005).

The gold standard for diagnosis remains biopsy. There are several methods for obtaining bone tissue for analysis. The two most common techniques are closed biopsy using a Jamshidi bone marrow biopsy needle and open biopsy using a trephine or curette. Both methods require general anesthesia, and regional radiographs or fluoroscopy should be available to aid the clinician in selecting an appropriate area within the tumor from which to collect the specimen. Attempts should be made to obtain a sample from the center of the radiographic lesion. The advantages of needle biopsy are that the procedure can be done through a single tiny stab incision without a surgical approach. The resulting bone defect is small, typically involving a single cortex, and therefore is unlikely to initiate a pathologic fracture. The disadvantage of the closed technique is the relatively small sample obtained. An open biopsy using a trephine requires a surgical approach and creates a bigger defect through both cortices; however, the sample obtained is larger. The downside of this technique is that there is a higher potential risk of pathologic fracture. Regardless of the method used to obtain the specimen, it is important to send the tissue to an experienced pathologist with expertise in bone pathology.

It must be emphasized to clients that no diagnostic test is 100% accurate. A diagnosis of reactive bone is not uncommon on preoperative biopsy of an OSA, regardless of whether the specimen is obtained by needle or trephine. In cases in which the histopathologic interpretation does not match the clinical picture, OSA should not be ruled out. In some cases second, larger biopsy specimens still yield reactive bone; yet when the entire lesion is submitted following definitive surgery, the pathologist can readily make a diagnosis of OSA. Similarly, one should be cautious when interpreting bone biopsy results indicating the presence of a primary bone fibrosarcoma, chondrosarcoma, or hemangiosarcoma. Although these other primary tumors do occur on occasion, OSA is far more common.

Biologic Behavior

Appendicular OSA is associated with two distinct life-limiting pathologic processes: local invasion and distant metastases. Although OSA arises from the medullary cavity, it rapidly grows eccentrically, which results in the invasion and destruction of surrounding trabecular and cortical bone with eventual soft tissue involvement.

Although local tissue destruction is a hallmark of OSA, several effective management strategies can limit the morbidity associated with the localized invasive properties of OSA. For this reason, the major life-limiting barrier for dogs diagnosed with OSA is the development of distant metastases. The pulmonary parenchyma is the most common metastatic site, whereas involvement of regional lymph nodes appears relatively uncommon (Hillers et al, 2005). Pulmonary metastatic lesions usually appear as discrete soft tissue nodules, and multiple lesions are common. Additional sites of metastases include bone, skin, and other extraskeletal sites.

Client Education and Treatment Options

Many treatment options are available for OSA. Treatment choices fall into two major categories based on the pet owner's goals: palliative-intent treatments and curative-intent treatments. Palliative-intent treatments have as their main goal the relief of symptoms associated with OSA. With palliative treatment it is accepted that the disease will continue to progress during treatment. Curative-intent treatments have as their main goal prolonged symptom-free survival or cure. Although a true cure occurs in fewer than 10% of canine patients with OSA, survival can be greatly increased with the use of curative-intent therapy. Owners need to have an accurate understanding of a given treatment goal, possible adverse effects, benefits, costs, and lifestyle changes expected with each category of treatment (palliative or curative) and each specific treatment within that category.

Because OSA is an aggressive disease and can be considered to be systemic at the time of diagnosis, curative-intent therapy must be multimodal (including both local and systemic treatments) to improve survival. At a minimum, curative-intent therapy involves surgical removal of the tumor by amputation or limb salvage surgery and adjuvant chemotherapy. If no treatment is given, most owners seek euthanasia within 2 months after diagnosis.

Surgical Options

Amputation
Amputation remains the gold standard of surgical therapy for OSA. Amputation is by far the simplest, least expensive surgical solution with the fewest complications. In addition, for most common OSA locations, amputation affords generous bone and soft tissue margins, which makes the risk of local recurrence very low, and requires

no special surgical training to perform. Forequarter amputation (removal of the scapula en bloc with the limb) for forelimb tumors and disarticulation at the level of the coxofemoral joint for hind limb tumors is recommended. For OSA located in the proximal femur, partial hemipelvectomy (acetabulectomy) is required to prevent local recurrence.

Function, cosmesis, and patient acceptance following amputation have been excellent, even in very-large- and giant-breed dogs. Although deciding to move forward with an amputation in a large- or giant-breed dog with OSA often is difficult for owners, most are satisfied with the functional outcome. Keeping amputation patients comfortable during the period immediately after surgery is very important to ensure a rapid recovery. To this end, preemptive analgesia is recommended before surgery, and amputation patients should remain hospitalized and receive injectable pain medications for at least 15 to 24 hours following surgery to ensure comfort. If effective analgesia is administered, most dogs are ready for discharge the day after surgery. Oral analgesics can be administered by the owner at home for the first 5 to 7 days following discharge. Owners should be instructed to keep amputees away from slippery surfaces during the early postoperative period unless they can provide support using a sling. Most dogs are able to go upstairs immediately following discharge but have some apprehension about and difficulty going downstairs. Temporary use of a harness to help the animal navigate stairs and slippery floors often is very helpful. Commercial harnesses with handles for lifting and support are available (e.g., www.helpemup.com). Weight control, rehabilitation, and controlled physical activity are important for long-term mobility. Many large-breed OSA patients have concurrent preexisting degenerative joint disease in other limbs that requires lifelong management for the best functional outcome.

Limb Salvage Surgery
Several alternatives to amputation are available to salvage the OSA-affected limb. Limb salvage is a more costly and complicated option than amputation, and there is no survival advantage associated with limb salvage per se. The only advantage of limb salvage is that the patient retains the affected limb. Some dogs with severe concurrent arthritis or neurologic conditions are not able to ambulate on three limbs and therefore require limb salvage if curative-intent treatment is pursued. More commonly, owners choose limb salvage because an amputation seems like a less desirable option. Disadvantages of limb salvage are that it is a more complex surgery, requires specialized training and equipment to perform, involves dissection very near the tumor (and therefore is associated with a higher risk of local recurrence), and is associated with a high complication rate. Limb salvage surgery involves removal of the portion of bone affected by the tumor along with a margin of normal bone. Candidates for limb salvage surgery should have no known metastatic disease, no serious concurrent health issues other than the OSA, no pathologic fractures, and a tumor involving less than 50% of the length of the affected bone with a small soft tissue component. The most suitable

cases for limb salvage are those with tumors in the distal radius.

Methods of limb salvage include allograft reconstruction, metal endoprosthesis reconstruction, ulna rollover, vascularized ulna graft, and bone transport osteogenesis, a method of creating new bone in a defect by distraction using an external fixator. Choice of procedure depends on surgeon experience, case selection, and owner preference. All limb salvage procedures require an experienced surgical team and intensive aftercare. The most common complications associated with allograft and metal endoprosthesis reconstruction are bacterial infection and hardware failure (screw failure or backout). Interestingly, there seems to be a survival advantage for canine OSA patients that develop infection: limb salvage patients with OSA that develop infection survive 1.5 to 2 times longer than limb salvage patients without infection. Most infections in limb salvage patients can be managed with lifelong antibiotic therapy; however, periodic flare-ups occur, and occasionally amputation becomes necessary. Overall limb use is fair to good in 80% of limb salvage patients. Local recurrence rates are 10% to 20% and do not differ among techniques. Local recurrence does not automatically require amputation because revision surgery can be performed. Local recurrence does not negatively impact overall survival or rates of metastasis. Therefore, although more complicated, limb salvage is a viable surgical alternative to amputation for curative-intent treatment of canine OSA.

Other Ablative Surgery
OSA located in the pelvis, maxilla, mandible, or scapula often is amenable to ablative surgery. Scapulectomy, hemipelvectomy, maxillectomy, or mandibulectomy can be used to treat OSA successfully and obtain clear margins in many cases. Advanced imaging such as MRI and CT often is necessary to identify appropriate candidates for these types of procedures. Owners should seek the services of a surgical oncologist or board-certified surgeon who has specific experience with advanced oncologic surgeries such as these. Function and cosmesis can be excellent following scapulectomy, hemipelvectomy, maxillectomy, or mandibulectomy.

Systemic Chemotherapy

Given the high metastatic rate of OSA, the adjuvant use of systemic chemotherapy is necessary to extend the survival time of dogs following surgery. Chemotherapy is most effective in the microscopic disease setting because once metastatic foci have reached macroscopic volumes, the benefit derived from systemic chemotherapy appears minimal (Ogilvie et al, 1993). Although there is a definite consensus as to the added survival benefit that chemotherapy provides in the microscopic disease setting, it is not possible to state which anticancer agents, used alone or in combination, are most effective. Until large prospective studies are conducted, information regarding effective adjuvant treatment options will have to come from more limited sample populations. Current conventional adjuvant chemotherapy protocols are based on doxorubicin, platinum-based chemotherapy drugs, or

TABLE **87-1**

Adjuvant Chemotherapy Regimens for Canine Appendicular Osteosarcoma

Chemotherapy Protocols after Surgery	Study	Median Survival Time
Single-Agent Protocols		
cDDP 70 mg/m² q21d × 2 doses (n = 36)	Straw et al, 1991	262-282 days
DOX 30 mg/m² q2wk × 5 doses (n = 35)	Berg et al, 1995	366 days
DOX 30 mg/m² q2wk × 5 doses (n = 303)	Moore et al, 2007	240 days
Carbo 300 mg/m² q21d × up to 4 doses (n = 48)	Bergman et al, 1996	321 days
Carbo variable dose and schedule (n = 155)	Phillips et al, 2011	307 days
Carbo 300 mg/m² q21d × 4-6 doses (n = 65)	Saam et al, 2011	277 days
Concurrent Combination-Agent Protocols		
cDDP (50 mg/m² day 1) + DOX (15 mg/m² day 2) × 4 doses (n = 35)	Chun et al, 2005	300 days
Carbo (175 mg/m² day 1) + DOX (15 mg/m² day 2) × 4 doses (n = 24)	Bailey et al, 2003	235 days
Carbo (300 mg/m²) + GEM 2 mg/kg × 4 doses (n = 50)	McMahon et al, 2011	279 days
Alternating Combination-Agent Protocols		
DOX (30 mg/m² day 1) + cDDP (60 mg/m² day 21) × 2 doses (n = 35)	Mauldin et al, 1988	300 days
Carbo (300 mg/m²) + DOX (30 mg/m²) q21d × 3 doses (n = 32)	Kent et al, 2004	320 days
Carbo (300 mg/m²) + DOX (30 mg/m²) q21d × 3 doses (n = 50)	Bacon et al, 2008	258 days

Carbo, Carboplatin; *cDDP,* cisplatin; *DOX,* doxorubicin; *GEM,* gemcitabine.

combinations of the two. Results from select studies are summarized in Table 87-1.

Prognostic Factors

Although a large number of prognostic factors have been identified in individual studies, the two factors found to be associated most consistently with prognosis are an increase in serum total or bone-specific AP level and tumor volume. Dogs with serum AP concentrations outside of the normal range have outcomes two to three times worse than dogs with normal AP. Tumor volume, measured either directly or using surrogates such as tumor length or percentage of bone affected, has been correlated with outcome in multiple studies. Several studies have identified proximal humeral location as an independent prognostic factor, and this may be a surrogate for comparatively large tumor volume. A recent metaanalysis of 55 articles reporting canine OSA prognostic factors confirmed the prognostic value of serum AP level and humeral location (Boerman et al, 2012).

Palliative Therapies

In dogs with OSA, bone cancer pain is attributed to two specific host responses. First, the invasive growth of malignant osteoblasts in the bone microenvironment results in the release of chemical mediators by nonneoplastic stromal cells, which in turn stimulate nociceptors and lead to the generation of painful sensations. Second, the genesis, maintenance, and exacerbation of bone cancer pain are attributed directly to dysregulated and pathologic osteoclastic bone resorption. Because of this, the most effective management of malignant osteolytic pain requires a combination of eradication of malignant osteoblasts in bone matrix and inhibition of tumor-induced osteoclastic bone resorption.

Radiation Therapy

In terms of mechanism, the analgesic effects of ionizing radiation can be attributed to the induction of apoptosis in both malignant osteoblasts and resorbing osteoclasts, and in dogs this has been documented by assessment of percent tumor necrosis. Thus radiation therapy (RT) reduces overall tumor burden and attenuates the degree of osteoclastic resorption within the focal OSA microenvironment. Multiple palliative RT protocols been evaluated and reported in the veterinary literature, and the majority of dosing schemes use two to four individual treatments of 6- to 10-Gy fractions. Although variable and subjectively reported in these studies, improvement in the level of pain has been achieved in the majority of dogs treated (74% to 93%) and persists for a median of 2 to 4 months.

Aminobisphosphonates

The effective treatment of bone disorders by aminobisphosphonates (NBPs) is attributed to their differential effect on bone resorption and bone mineralization. The mechanism for the bone-protective effects exerted by NBPs is the induction of osteoclast apoptosis, which results in the net attenuation of pathologic bone resorption.

In general, NBPs such as pamidronate or zoledronate are tolerated extremely well by dogs with OSA and produce subjective improvements in bone pain control in approximately 25% to 50% of dogs treated for 4 to 8 months. Additionally, definitive beneficial bone biologic effects are observed in dogs receiving pamidronate or zoledronate as indicated by reductions in urine N-telopeptide levels and augmentation of relative bone mineral density in the primary tumor as assessed by dual-energy x-ray absorptiometry. Although NBPs exert activity as single agents, improved pain control is achieved when NBPs are combined with RT and oral analgesics.

Stereotactic Radiosurgery

Stereotactic radiosurgery (SRS) involves the precise delivery of a large dose of RT administered over one to three treatments to a designated tumor target. The use of SRS in dogs with OSA can provide impressive pain alleviation, long-term local tumor control, and improvement in limb function (Farese et al, 2004). The potent anticancer effects of SRS have been substantiated with percent necrosis assessment, with the majority of treated patients achieving more than 90% necrosis of the primary tumor following therapy. Combining systemic chemotherapy and NBPs with SRS appears to enhance response rates and durations.

Treatment of Metastatic Disease

Like the treatment of microscopic disease, the effective treatment of macroscopic distant metastases also remains a clinical dilemma; however, several preliminary studies have shown promise for improving disease control and prolonging overall survival time. Surgical resection of pulmonary metastatic disease can be considered in carefully selected cases (O'Brien et al, 1993). The receptor tyrosine kinase inhibitor toceranib phosphate (Palladia) has demonstrated preliminary activity in a number of tumor histologic types (see Chapter 79). In dogs with macroscopic pulmonary OSA metastases, toceranib appears to exert marginal therapeutic effects with a biologic response rate approaching 50% (partial response rate of 4.3% and stable disease rate of 43.5%) (London et al, 2012).

References and Suggested Reading

Barger A et al: Use of alkaline phosphatase staining to differentiate canine osteosarcoma from other vimentin-positive tumors, *Vet Pathol* 42:161, 2005.

Boerman I et al: Prognostic factors in canine appendicular osteosarcoma—a meta-analysis, *BMC Vet Res* 5:56, 2012.

Eberle N et al: Comparison of examination of thoracic radiographs and thoracic computed tomography in dogs with appendicular osteosarcoma, *Vet Comp Oncol* 9:131, 2011.

Farese JP et al: Stereotactic radiosurgery for treatment of osteosarcomas involving the distal portions of the limbs in dogs, *J Am Vet Med Assoc* 225:1567, 2004.

Hillers KR et al: Incidence and prognostic importance of lymph node metastases in dogs with appendicular osteosarcoma: 228 cases (1986-2003), *J Am Vet Med Assoc* 226:1364, 2005.

London C et al: Preliminary evidence for biologic activity of toceranib phosphate (Palladia®) in solid tumours, *Vet Comp Oncol* 10:194, 2012. Epub June 1, 2011.

O'Brien MG et al: Resection of pulmonary metastases in canine osteosarcoma: 36 cases (1983-1992), *Vet Surg* 22:105, 1993.

Ogilvie GK et al: Evaluation of single-agent chemotherapy for treatment of clinically evident osteosarcoma metastases in dogs: 45 cases (1987-1991), *J Am Vet Med Assoc* 202:304, 1993.

CHAPTER 88

Canine Hemangiosarcoma

CRAIG A. CLIFFORD, *Malvern, Pennsylvania*
LOUIS-PHILIPPE DE LORIMIER, *Brossard, Québec, Canada*

A highly malignant tumor of endothelial cells, hemangiosarcoma (HSA) is diagnosed more frequently in dogs than in any other domestic species and is associated with a high fatality rate. Accounting for approximately 2% of all canine tumors, HSA tends to affect older dogs of either gender, with a median age of 10 years at diagnosis. Although dogs of any breed can develop HSA, German shepherds, golden retrievers, and other large or giant breeds appear predisposed.

Causes

The definitive etiology of canine HSA remains uncertain, although the strong breed association suggests that heritable factors are present to explain this genetic predisposition, and in fact gene expression phenotypes were shown to vary in HSA cells from different breeds in a recent study (Tamburini et al, 2009). Long-term ultraviolet light exposure is a known risk factor for superficial (dermal) HSA in lightly pigmented short-haired breeds of dogs and appears also to be a risk factor for HSA in the conjunctival location.

Research has shown overexpression of the oncoprotein STAT3 (signal transducer and activator of transcription 3) to be common in canine HSA. Inactivating mutations in the tumor-suppressing genes *p53* and *PTEN* were demonstrated in canine HSA and also may contribute to the malignant transformation of vascular endothelial cells.

Angiogenesis, the formation of new blood vessels, is a tightly regulated and balanced process in homeostasis, involving both proangiogenic and antiangiogenic factors. Levels of vascular endothelial growth factor (VEGF), one of the most potent angiogenic factors, were higher in the plasma and effusions of dogs with HSA than in healthy dogs. Furthermore, increased expression of the VEGF receptor 1 (VEGFR1) gene recently was demonstrated in HSA cells obtained specifically from golden retrievers. Evidence derived from *in vitro* research suggests that HSA cells are capable of producing a plethora of angiogenic factors, including VEGF and basic fibroblastic growth factor (bFGF). Matrix metalloproteinases, which play a role in the breakdown of the extracellular matrix, have been shown to be active in canine HSA.

With the advent of platforms enabling evaluation of global gene expression, it soon may be possible to identify which genes and pathways are dysregulated in HSA. One recent study noted differences between HSA cells and nonmalignant endothelial cells in regard to increased expression of genes involved in inflammation, angiogenesis, adhesion, invasion, metabolism, cell cycle, signaling, and patterning. Importantly, this "signature" not only reflected a cancer-associated angiogenic phenotype but could distinguish HSA from other nonendothelial, angiogenic bone marrow–derived tumors such as lymphoma, leukemia, and osteosarcoma (Tamburini et al, 2009, 2010).

Biologic Behavior and Prognosis

Canine HSA can develop anywhere in the body. The four most common primary sites are the spleen, heart (right atrium or auricle), skin or subcutaneous tissues, and liver. Other reported primary sites include kidney, muscle, bone, oral cavity, bladder, and lung. Metastatic dissemination and local infiltration occur early in disease, either hematogenously or via local seeding following tumor rupture. The lungs, liver, and omentum are the most frequent sites of dissemination, but HSA also is recognized as the most common sarcoma to metastasize to the central nervous system (CNS). Certain primary tumor locations may predict a better prognosis, and dermal, conjunctival, and possibly subcutaneous HSA tend to have a lower metastatic rate than visceral locations. Studies have demonstrated that higher clinical stage (Box 88-1) results in earlier metastasis and shorter survival time for splenic and cutaneous HSA. When advanced metastatic disease is present, it is sometimes impossible to identify the primary site, and the prognosis is unsurprisingly poor to grave, even though occasional responses to therapy have been observed.

Diagnosis and Staging

Since clinical stage affects prognosis and HSA is a highly metastatic cancer, complete clinical staging is highly recommended at diagnosis when the patient is in sufficiently stable condition. In cases in which emergency surgical intervention is mandatory to save the patient's life, certain diagnostic tests may need to be postponed temporarily. As previously mentioned, metastatic disease

---

BOX 88-1

Clinical Staging System for Hemangiosarcoma (HSA)

Primary Tumor (T)
T0: No measurable tumor
T1: Tumor <5 cm in diameter, confined to primary site; does not invade beyond dermis (cutaneous HSA)
T2: Tumor ≥5 cm in diameter, or ruptured; invades subcutaneous tissues (cutaneous HSA)
T3: Tumor invades adjacent structures; invades into the underlying muscle (cutaneous HSA)

Regional Lymph Nodes (N)
N0: No regional lymph node involvement
N1: Regional lymph node involvement
N2: Distant lymph node involvement

Distant Metastasis (M)
M0: No measurable distant metastasis
M1: Detectable distant metastasis

Stage Grouping
Stage I: T0 or T1, N0, M0
Stage II: T1 N1 or T2 N0, M0
Stage III: T2 N1 or T3 N0, or N2, M1

---

frequently affects the lungs, liver, and omental surfaces and occasionally affects the soft tissues, adrenal glands, and CNS. Although it is not considered to be true metastatic dissemination, it is known that dogs occasionally may have HSA affecting multiple primary sites (e.g., spleen plus right atrium) at presentation, a condition known as *synchronous disease*.

As a result, complete clinical staging ideally should include three-view high-detail thoracic radiography, abdominal ultrasonography, and echocardiography, in addition to standard blood studies. Although the typical appearance of measurable pulmonary metastatic disease is that of a coalescing miliary pattern, nodular or generalized miliary interstitial patterns also can be observed on occasion (Figure 88-1). Abdominal ultrasonography is a fairly sensitive routine imaging technique permitting the detection of splenic or hepatic lesions (Figure 88-2) and occasionally of omental nodules as well, and in most cases will identify free abdominal fluid when present. Early experience of the use of contrast-enhanced ultrasonography suggest that this technique may become more common in the veterinary setting; when the echogenicity of hepatic nodules is evaluated during arterial and parenchymal phases of contrast enhancement, malignant tumors can be differentiated from benign nodules with high rate of accuracy. Echocardiography remains the method of choice to identify right atrial masses, and these are better observed when at least some amount of pericardial effusion is present. Although urinalysis and serum biochemical studies rarely help in the diagnosis of HSA, the complete blood cell count typically shows changes that may suggest a microangiopathic process, including regenerative anemia, thrombocytopenia, and fragmented

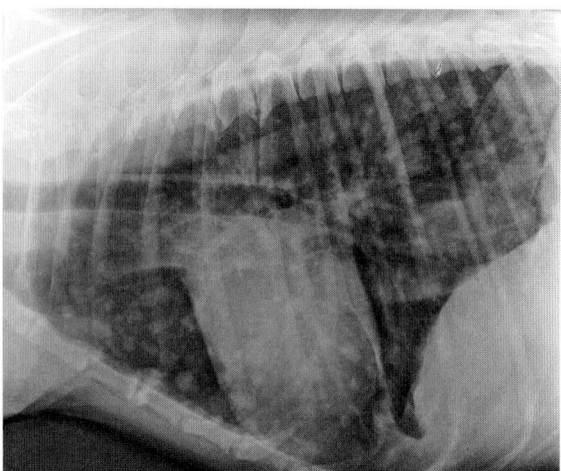

Figure 88-1 Left lateral thoracic digital radiograph of a 6-year-old Irish wolfhound, demonstrating a nodular pattern of pulmonary metastasis from intramuscular hemangiosarcoma.

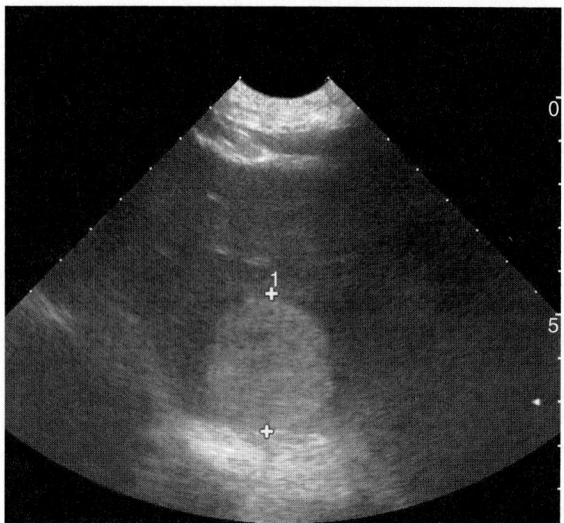

Figure 88-2 Abdominal ultrasonographic image of a 9-year-old Labrador retriever demonstrating a heterogeneous liver nodule, later confirmed histopathologically to be a primary liver hemangiosarcoma.

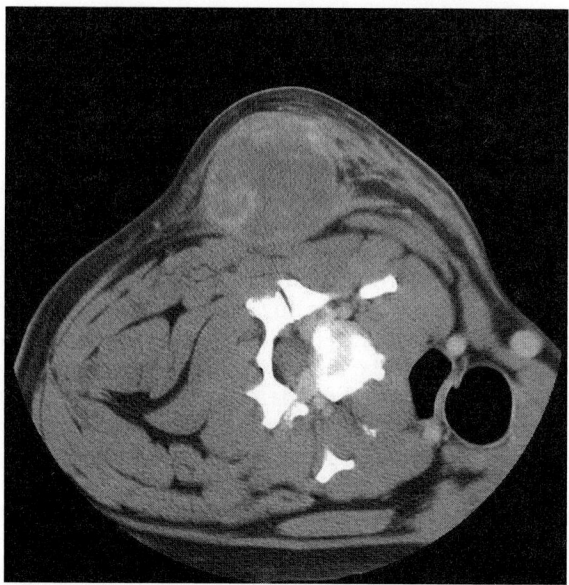

Figure 88-3 Computed tomographic image of a subcutaneous intramuscular hemangiosarcoma in the lateral cervical area in a 6-year-old Irish wolfhound (same dog as in Figure 88-1).

red blood cells (schistocytes). In addition, when the spleen is affected severely, a deficient reticuloendothelial system allows higher numbers of metarubricytes (nucleated red blood cells) to be observed in the circulation and on manual blood smears.

In selected cases, additional imaging techniques may be required for identification of suspect metastasis based on physical examination findings (e.g., suspected bone or CNS metastasis). Advanced sectional imaging, in the form of computed tomography (CT) (Figure 88-3) or magnetic resonance imaging (MRI), is recommended for invasive subcutaneous or intramuscular HSA to assess invasiveness and plan surgical resection and radiation therapy (RT), if indicated. In addition, studies of splenic and hepatic lesions have shown that MRI and CT have a high sensitivity and specificity in differentiating benign from malignant processes. Furthermore, the increased

sensitivity of thoracic CT for detection of early pulmonary metastasis has been reported. With the increasing use of such diagnostic modalities in veterinary medicine, they are being incorporated gradually into the thorough staging of HSA in dogs.

A definitive diagnosis of HSA is obtained through histopathologic evaluation. It is crucial to remember that no imaging technique can confirm with certainty that the observed lesion is in fact HSA. Therefore no patient with hemoabdomen should be euthanized based on the presence of a splenic mass that is "consistent with HSA," especially since nonmalignant splenic lesions, including hematomas and hemangiomas, appear identical in many cases, bear an excellent prognosis with splenectomy alone, and often are diagnosed in the same breeds as HSA. Several retrospective studies have shown that for splenic nodules, roughly a third of the patients are cured with splenectomy alone. Although cytologic evaluation is a noninvasive and clinically valuable technique for the diagnosis of cancer in general, the diagnostic yield for HSA is reported to be low. A few studies evaluating dogs with nontraumatic hemoabdomen noted that 65% to 70% were diagnosed with HSA. Interestingly, a recent study evaluating 65 dogs that underwent splenectomy, including 30 dogs (46%) with HSA, showed that larger splenic masses, or a higher ratio of mass to splenic volume, and heavier spleens (as a percentage of body weight) were more likely to be benign and less likely to be diagnosed as HSA (Mallinckrodt and Gottfried, 2011).

One possible way to improve the prognosis of canine HSA is earlier detection. Although the current standard for diagnosing HSA remains histopathologic analysis of measurable lesions, usually after metastatic dissemination already has occurred, new detection methods eventually may help in obtaining an early diagnosis in dogs at high risk. One such method is flow cytometry to identify cells of specific lineage that coexpress certain cell surface markers that are detected in higher numbers in the peripheral blood of dogs harboring HSA than in healthy control dogs or dogs that are free of measurable HSA following surgical excision.

The development of biomarkers with HSA specificity that can be obtained noninvasively would be clinically useful not only to enable early detection and treatment but also to monitor for progression of disease. Several recent studies have evaluated such markers in both the blood and effusion of dogs with HSA. Cardiac troponin I (cTnI) has proven to be a highly specific and sensitive marker for myocardial cellular damage in many mammalian species, and a recent study evaluated its ability to identify cardiac involvement in dogs with HSA, detect cardiac HSA in dogs with pericardial effusion, and exclude cardiac HSA in dogs with noncardiac HAS (Chun et al, 2010). The median plasma cTnI concentration in dogs with cardiac HSA was significantly higher than the concentration in each of the other groups. In addition, a specific plasma cTnI concentration (>0.25 ng/ml) could identify cardiac involvement in dogs with HSA at any site (sensitivity, 78%; specificity, 71%) and could identify cardiac HSA in dogs with pericardial effusion (sensitivity, 81%; specificity, 100%) (Chun et al, 2010).

A fragment of collagen XXVII was noted to be high in serum concentrations of dogs diagnosed with advanced-stage HSA. Furthermore, the finding of reductions after surgical resection of HSA and subsequent increases with tumor recurrence lends credence to the view that this peptide can act as a HSA biomarker. Its biologic significance still is unclear, although it has been proposed that elevations may be related to protein cleavage or degradation in surrounding tissue or may be associated with invasive or angiogenic processes.

Thymidine kinase (TK) is a cytosolic enzyme whose activity is closely correlated with DNA synthesis, and its expression is restricted to proliferating cells. Serum TK1 activity has been found to be significantly higher in dogs with HSA than in healthy dogs. In a prospective evaluation of TK1 activity in 62 dogs with hemoabdomen caused by either a benign splenic mass or HSA, the two conditions could not be distinguished based on mean TK1 activity level; however, differentiation of the two groups became possible when a specific two-tiered cutoff system was implemented (Thamm et al, 2011); this makes TK1 an attractive biomarker.

Traditional Therapy

Traditional therapy for HSA, as for other cancers, involves surgery, RT, and systemic cytotoxic chemotherapy, alone or in combination.

Surgery

Splenectomy, liver lobectomy, excision of a dermal or resectable subcutaneous nodule, and right auriculectomy all have been reported. Such surgeries are performed to remove all macroscopic tumor tissue and to prevent further risk of acute hemorrhage, disseminated intravascular coagulation, and death. Surgery alone for splenic, cardiac, subcutaneous or intramuscular, or hepatic HSA

has yielded unsatisfactory results and generally is considered purely palliative, with median survival times typically averaging 1 to 3 months with splenectomy alone. A study of 23 dogs with cardiac HSA reported a median survival time of 56 days in all dogs, but survival was significantly prolonged in 8 dogs receiving chemotherapy (175 days) compared with 15 dogs treated with surgery alone (42 days) (Weisse et al, 2005).

Pericardiectomy via thoracotomy or thoracoscopy can alleviate life-threatening cardiac tamponade but alone is unlikely to prolong survival significantly. Surgical resection of superficial dermal or conjunctival HSA often results in prolonged survival times because of the lower rates of metastasis observed with these primary locations. The median survival time of 94 dogs treated surgically for dermal HSA was reported to be 987 days. Dogs with subcutaneous or intramuscular HSA have survival times of less than 4 to 5 months with surgery alone in most studies, and thus adjuvant chemotherapy is warranted.

Conventional Chemotherapy

Doxorubicin (DOX)–based adjuvant chemotherapy, with or without the addition of cyclophosphamide or vincristine, has resulted in the best survival times to date. Common protocols include single-agent DOX, DOX and cyclophosphamide (AC protocol), and vincristine, DOX, and cyclophosphamide (VAC protocol). Survival times ranging from 140 to 202 days have been reported for the various DOX-based protocols; however, no protocol is regarded as clearly superior. In an attempt to extend survival time, a dose-intensive protocol with administration of DOX every other week has been evaluated, but no improvement was noted. A study evaluating adjuvant DOX therapy following surgery in 21 dogs with subcutaneous or intramuscular HSA recorded median survival times of 1189 and 273 days, respectively, for the two HSA types (Bulakowski et al, 2008; Shiu et al, 2011). The use of Doxil, a liposome-encapsulated form of DOX administered by the intravenous or intraperitoneal route, does not appear to improve outcome compared with conventional DOX (Teske et al, 2011). Ifosfamide, an alkylating agent with therapeutic activity in human sarcomas, was administered after splenectomy to six dogs with HSA, resulting in a median survival time of 147 days. When a combination of ifosfamide and DOX was evaluated in the adjuvant setting in 27 dogs with HSA, a disappointing median survival time of 149 days was obtained. Although the beneficial effects of adjuvant chemotherapy on survival times are well recognized, additional or alternative therapeutic modalities clearly are needed.

Conventional chemotherapy also has been evaluated for the treatment of macroscopic HSA. In 18 dogs with inoperable subcutaneous HSA treated with DOX monotherapy, the overall response rate was 38.8% to 44% depending on the criteria used for assessment, with an overall median response duration of 53 days (range, 13 to 190 days) (Wiley et al, 2010). An aggressive protocol combining dacarbazine, DOX, and vincristine (DAV protocol) was evaluated in 24 dogs with advanced-stage inoperable HSA and yielded a response rate approaching 50%, including five complete and four partial responses;

a median time to tumor progression of 101 days; and a reported median survival time of 125 days. Toxicities were encountered frequently with this protocol, however (Dervisis et al, 2011).

Radiation Therapy

There is a paucity of published information regarding the use of RT for treatment of canine HSA; however, clinical responses and quality-of-life improvements have been observed when large fractions of megavoltage RT are delivered (once or twice weekly) to invasive and nonresectable subcutaneous or intramuscular HSA lesions. A study of 20 dogs with measurable, histologically confirmed nonsplenic HSA treated with palliative RT showed subjective reduction in tumor size in 14 dogs (70%), with four complete responses and a median survival time of 95 days. In such cases, palliation is obtained through a decrease in pain and bruising, in addition to tumor shrinkage, and the RT generally is combined with systemic DOX-based chemotherapy.

Novel Therapy

Since results with a combination of traditional therapeutic modalities has reached a plateau unlikely to be surpassed, with median survival times averaging 6 to 7 months, new therapies are awaited impatiently. It is hoped that the growing body of knowledge regarding the molecular alterations observed in canine HSA cells will unveil numerous novel targets.

Immunotherapy has long been a field of active research, and an aggressive and rapidly progressing cancer such as HSA provides a great opportunity for even small improvements in treatment to be detected. Although initial studies evaluating nonspecific immunotherapy failed to provide positive outcomes in canine HSA patients, the combined AC protocol with liposome-encapsulated muramyl tripeptide phosphatidylethanolamine (L-MTP-PE), a synthetic macrophage activator derived from mycobacterial cell walls, resulted in the only published data showing a median survival time significantly superior to that with traditional chemotherapy alone (273 days). Although this study firmly established a role for immunotherapy in treating canine HSA, the clinical use of L-MTP-PE to benefit canine cancer patients has been slowed since the drug currently remains unavailable commercially (Teske et al, 2011). Recently, a study evaluated an intraperitoneally administered allogeneic HSA vaccine in 22 dogs, most of which also received conventional chemotherapy. Vaccinated dogs were found to mount antibody responses against canine HSA cells, and the median survival time of 13 dogs with stage II splenic HSA that received the tumor vaccine plus DOX chemotherapy was 182 days (U'Ren et al, 2007). Further studies are ongoing.

Antiangiogenic therapy is an important field of investigational cancer treatment in humans and is the subject of numerous ongoing clinical studies in canine HSA. Such studies, which are evaluating interleukin-12, interferon alfa-2a, thrombospondin-1, protease inhibitors, and thalidomide, eventually may demonstrate benefits in terms of improved survival time, and the results are highly anticipated. Although the novel humanized monoclonal antibodies directed against certain angiogenic proteins (e.g., bevacizumab, which targets VEGF-A) may not be practical for use in dogs, the ongoing basic and clinical research on small-molecule inhibitors targeting the same proteins (VEGF, bFGF, integrins) and their receptors raises cautious optimism regarding application in the veterinary field.

Unlike most canine carcinomas surveyed so far, canine HSA typically does not overexpress cyclooxygenase-2 (COX-2). However, because nonsteroidal antiinflammatory drugs have demonstrated clinical efficacy against certain tumors that do not overexpress COX-2, it could be conceivable to combine them with conventional therapy in an attempt to prolong the survival time of dogs with HSA. A recently published study of dogs with splenic HSA found no overall improvement in survival when a COX-2–selective inhibitor was coadministered with adjuvant DOX therapy.

The use of traditional chemotherapy agents is being revisited through the use of novel methods or schedules of administration. A pilot study evaluating inhalational therapy with DOX and paclitaxel demonstrated encouraging results in canine patients with pulmonary metastasis from HSA. The daily administration of low doses (metronomic dosing) of traditional cytotoxic chemotherapy agents is another new approach. The therapeutic target shifts from the cancer cells to the normal host endothelial cells when frequent low doses of chemotherapeutic drugs are administered. In this way, the common problems of toxicities and drug resistance largely can be avoided. A small pilot study evaluated a continuous low-dose protocol of cyclophosphamide, piroxicam, and etoposide in nine dogs with stage II splenic HSA in the adjuvant setting. When the median survival time of the dogs treated using this protocol was compared with that of historical controls treated with DOX, no statistical difference was observed. Two recent studies have documented responses of macroscopic HSA to continuous low-dose administration of lomustine (CCNU) and chlorambucil.

Finally, alternative therapies using natural products have become a novel source of study. Polysaccharopeptide (PSP) is the bioactive agent from the mushroom *Coriolus versicolor* with documented *in vitro* and *in vivo* antitumor effects. In a recent double-blind randomized multidose pilot study, high-dose PSP significantly delayed the progression of metastases, and improved survival times were reported when compared with historical data. Further studies with PSP as a single agent or in combination with standard therapy are warranted.

References and Suggested Reading

Bulakowski EJ et al: Evaluation of outcome associated with subcutaneous and intramuscular hemangiosarcoma treated with adjuvant doxorubicin in dogs: 21 cases (2001-2006), *J Am Vet Med Assoc* 233:122, 2008.

Chun R et al: Comparison of plasma cardiac troponin I concentrations among dogs with cardiac hemangiosarcoma, noncardiac hemangiosarcoma, other neoplasms, and pericardial effusion of nonhemangiosarcoma origin, *J Am Vet Med Assoc* 237:806, 2010.

Dervisis NG et al: Treatment with DAV for advanced-stage hemangiosarcoma in dogs, *J Am Anim Hosp Assoc* 46:170, 2011.

Kahn SA et al: Doxorubicin and deracoxib adjuvant therapy for canine splenic hemangiosarcoma: a pilot study, *Canadian Vet J* 54:237, 2013.

Mallinckrodt MJ, Gottfried SD: Mass-to-splenic volume ratio and splenic weight as a percentage of body weight in dogs with malignant and benign splenic masses: 65 cases (2007-2008), *J Am Vet Med Assoc* 239:1325, 2011.

Shiu KB et al: Predictors of outcome in dogs with subcutaneous or intramuscular hemangiosarcoma, *J Am Vet Med Assoc* 238:472, 2011.

Tamburini BA et al: Gene expression profiles of sporadic canine hemangiosarcoma are uniquely associated with breed, *PLoS One* 4:e5549, 2009.

Tamburini BA et al: Gene expression profiling identifies inflammation and angiogenesis as distinguishing features of canine hemangiosarcoma, *BMC Cancer* 10:619, 2010.

Teske E et al: A randomized controlled study into the efficacy and toxicity of pegylated liposome encapsulated doxorubicin as an adjuvant therapy in dogs with splenic haemangiosarcoma, *Vet Comp Oncol* 9:283, 2011.

Thamm DH, Kamstock DA, Sharp CR: Elevated serum thymidine kinase activity in canine splenic hemangiosarcoma, *Vet Comp Oncol* 10:292, 2012. Epub October 20, 2011.

U'Ren LW et al: Evaluation of a novel tumor vaccine in dogs with hemangiosarcoma, *J Vet Intern Med* 21:113, 2007.

Weisse C et al: Survival times in dogs with right atrial hemangiosarcoma treated by means of surgical resection with or without adjuvant chemotherapy: 23 cases (1986-2000), *J Am Vet Med Assoc* 226:575, 2005.

Wiley JL et al: Efficacy of doxorubicin-based chemotherapy for non-resectable canine subcutaneous hemangiosarcoma, *Vet Comp Oncol* 8:221, 2010.

CHAPTER **89**

Thyroid Tumors

SUZANNE MURPHY, *Kentford, Suffolk, Great Britain*

The thyroid gland is a bilobed structure in cats and dogs, sometimes with an isthmus connecting the two lobes; it spans a region from the fifth to the eighth tracheal ring, and the right lobe usually is more cranial than the left. In normal animals, the lobes are lateral to and closely associated with the trachea. The gland is extremely well vascularized in both cats and dogs, especially when neoplastic.

Ectopic thyroid tissue is common and can be found from the base of the tongue to the heart base, anywhere vestigial tissue may be present from embryologic development. Neoplasia can arise in this ectopic tissue.

The thyroid gland is composed mostly of two cell types, both of which can become neoplastic. Thyroid epithelial cells—the cells responsible for synthesis of the thyroid hormones—are arranged in thyroid follicles around a central space filled with colloid. In spaces between thyroid follicles are found the *parafollicular* or *C cells*, which secrete the hormone calcitonin.

Palpable masses can be caused by hyperplasia, adenoma, or adenocarcinoma of the thyroid gland. In cats, benign adenomatous hyperplasia is a common presentation in older animals, with the functional tissue giving rise to the signs associated with hyperthyroidism. In contrast, the vast majority of thyroid tumors in dogs are nonfunctional and malignant, with benign lesions usually being an incidental finding at postmortem.

In humans, thyroid tumors can be seen as part of two multiple endocrine syndromes referred to as *multiple endocrine neoplasia type 1 and type 2* (MEN1, MEN2). It is not clear that cats or dogs have shown evidence of a truly analogous syndrome; however, it is important to note that thyroid tumors have been seen in dogs that had developed tumors of other histologic types, and so it is especially important to examine the animal thoroughly at presentation for other masses. The additional distinct tumors were not in other endocrine organs.

Canine Thyroid Carcinoma

Thyroid cancer represents between 1% and 4% of all canine tumors. Tumors arising from the cells lining the follicles are known as *follicular carcinomas,* which are further subclassified as papillary, compact (solid), or anaplastic, whereas those arising from the parafollicular cells are called *medullary thyroid carcinomas* or *C-cell carcinomas* and are less common.

Affected dogs usually are 9 to 10 years or older. Boxers, beagles, golden retrievers, and Siberian huskies have been found to be more commonly affected in some studies. A mixed-breed family of dogs (three out of four littermates) with a significant pedigreed Alaskan malamute component in their breeding developed medullary

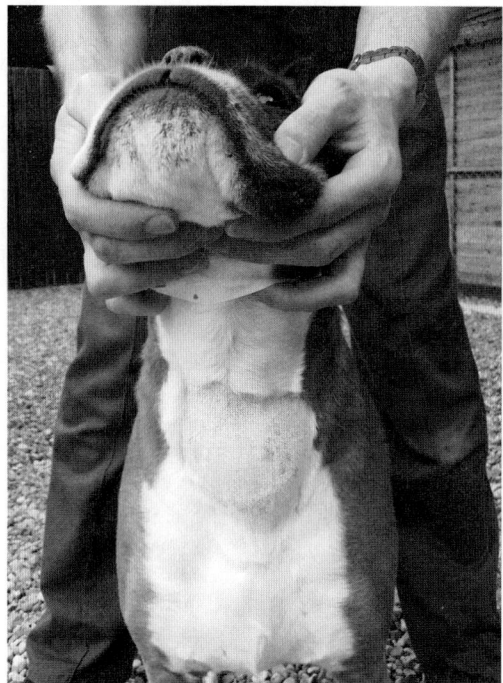

Figure 89-1 Ten-year-old boxer with an obvious mass in the thyroid area.

thyroid carcinomas (Lee et al, 2006). There is no reported sex predisposition.

Presentation

Clinical signs depend on where the tumor is located and whether the mass is functional. The vast majority of the lesions are nonfunctional and are situated in the area of the thyroid gland; therefore a noticeable mass is by far the most common presenting sign (Figure 89-1). The average time to diagnosis is 1 to 2 months from owner appreciation of the mass. It is important to assess mobility of the mass. Roughly one third to one half of thyroid carcinomas are freely moveable at presentation, and freely mobile thyroid carcinomas have different treatment options and different prognoses from fixed carcinomas.

Other clinical signs frequently reported are associated with the primary mass and include dysphonia, dysphagia, and cough. Dyspnea can be associated with either the primary mass, which may press on the trachea, or with lung metastases. Sometimes signs can be present that are consistent with laryngeal paralysis because the mass can damage the recurrent laryngeal nerves. Rarely, facial edema can be seen in association with impaired venous return.

Most dogs with thyroid carcinomas are euthyroid; however, thyroid function is affected in a small percentage of cases. Therefore a dog with clinical signs consistent with hyperthyroidism (polyuria, polydipsia, weight loss, increased appetite, muscle atrophy, hypertension, nervousness) should undergo routine thyroid function testing. Additionally, hypothyroidism may be diagnosed in some, which may precede the tumor's development or be caused by destruction of normal thyroid tissue.

Unfortunately, there are few studies that report thyroid hormone assay results in dogs with thyroid carcinoma so it is difficult to say with any accuracy what percentage of dogs are hypothyroid, euthyroid, or hyperthyroid at presentation.

Medullary carcinomas usually are nonfunctional, but calcitonin-producing tumors causing hypocalcemia have been reported.

Diagnosis

It has been suggested that a palpable mass in the thyroid of a dog has a 85% to 90% probability of being malignant. Differential diagnoses include abscess, granuloma, foreign body, lymphadenitis, lymph node metastases, lymphoma, and subcutaneous tumors such as soft-tissue sarcoma and mast cell tumor.

Thyroid tumors are extremely vascular, and thus the first approach to diagnosing such a mass may be fine-needle aspiration, without suction, followed by digital pressure after the needle is withdrawn. Because these lesions are well vascularized it is not surprising that blood contamination is a problem. Ultrasonographic guidance may be used to minimize the risk of sampling the most well-vascularized areas.

Surgical biopsy can be challenging due to the high risk of hemorrhage, and so a more pragmatic approach is to assess the mass for surgical resectability and obtain a diagnosis at the time of surgery. This assessment may involve palpation, ultrasonography, or computed tomography or magnetic resonance imaging to be sure that the mass is not attached to other structures.

Once histopathologic evaluation can be undertaken, any diagnostic dilemma as to tumor type can be resolved by immunohistochemical analysis. This may be especially useful if ectopic tissue is involved. Thyroid follicular tumors stain positive for thyroglobulin. Medullary tumors can be confused with compact follicular tumors, and an immunostain for calcitonin can be used to differentiate the two, with medullary tumors staining positive for calcitonin.

Tumor Behavior and Staging

For thyroid carcinomas the overall risk of metastatic disease at the time of diagnosis is 16% to 38%. Metastasis usually is to the lungs, with the retropharyngeal and submandibular lymph nodes the next most commonly affected. Because of the lymphatic drainage pattern of the thyroid gland, both ipsilateral and contralateral regional lymph nodes cranial and caudal to the gland can be affected. The larger the primary mass at presentation, the higher the likelihood of metastatic disease. If the tumor volume is 100 cm^3 or greater, the chance of metastasis is almost 100%. If the disease is in both lobes there is a considerably higher (sixteenfold) risk of metastatic disease. One study (Carver et al, 1995) suggested that medullary thyroid carcinomas are less likely to metastasize and less likely to be invasive. It also has been reported that freely mobile masses are less likely to have metastasized. It should be remembered that metastasis from thyroid carcinoma can be slow, with some dogs showing clinical signs associated with lung metastases up to 3 years after control of the primary tumor.

Staging therefore should include an evaluation of the primary mass to check for tumor volume and to assess whether the tumor is unilateral or bilateral and whether the mass is fixed or moveable. If the tumor is situated in ectopic tissue, then advanced imaging techniques may be necessary to delineate the lesion and could include the use of scintigraphy. Advanced imaging is necessary if the dog is a candidate for external beam radiotherapy to allow radiation planning. In all cases, thoracic radiography is necessary, as is fine-needle aspiration of any abnormal lymph nodes. The World Health Organization staging system for thyroid tumors is shown in Table 89-1.

Treatment

If no definitive therapy is undertaken, then reported survival times vary from 1 week to 38 weeks, with one study (Worth et al, 2005) reporting a median survival time of 3 months after diagnosis.

TABLE **89-1**

World Health Organization Staging System for Canine Thyroid Carcinoma

Primary Tumor (T)

T0	No evidence of tumor
T1	Tumor <2 cm maximum diameter T1a not fixed, T1b fixed
T2	Tumor 2-5 cm maximum diameter T2a not fixed, T2b fixed
T3	Tumor >5 cm maximum diameter T3a not fixed, T3b fixed

Regional Lymph Nodes (N)

N0	No evidence of lymph node involvement
N1	Ipsilateral regional lymph node involvement N1a not fixed, N1b fixed
N2	Contralateral regional lymph node involvement N2a not fixed, N2b fixed

Distant Metastasis (M)

M0	No evidence of distant metastasis
M1	Distant metastasis detected

Stage Grouping

	T	N	M
I	T1a, b	N0	M0
II	T0 T1a, b T2a, b	N1 N1 N0, N1	M0
III	T3	Any N	M0
IV	Any T	Any N	M1

Surgery

If the mass is freely moveable, then a surgical procedure to dissect out the tumor without wide margins but also without breaching the capsule will give local control, with a median survival time of between 2 and 3 years. Figure 89-2 shows the appearance at surgery of a unilateral thyroid carcinoma in which the capsule has not been breached. In the odd case in which both lobes of the thyroid are affected and surgery is feasible, bilateral thyroidectomy should be undertaken with care. A decision actively needs to be made as to whether the external parathyroid glands need to be sacrificed or can be saved because the loss of internal and external parathyroid glands may result in hypocalcemia.

If the tumor is fixed to adjacent tissue then it is inadvisable to attempt a surgical procedure for several reasons. First, because these masses are very vascular, there is a significant risk of severe hemorrhage during surgery. Second, often the recurrent laryngeal nerves are involved, and thus there is a risk that the dog will experience postoperative laryngeal paralysis. Finally, because the mass in such presentations usually adheres to important structures, the chance of complete excision is extremely low and thus the rate of recurrence is high.

Radiotherapy

External beam radiotherapy (EBRT) is successful in controlling local disease and is used either when there is residual tumor following an attempted thyroidectomy or, more commonly, when there is a fixed and therefore unresectable mass. EBRT is the modality of choice for dogs with fixed thyroid masses.

Several EBRT protocols have been described. Using 12 fractions of 4 Gy over 4 weeks gave progression-free survival rates of 80% at 1 year and 72% at 3 years. Time to maximum tumor volume reduction was long, from 8 to 22 months (Théon et al, 2000). At the other extreme, treating dogs with stage T3a or T3b tumors once weekly with 9-Gy fractions for four weeks resulted in a median survival time of 22 months from the first dose to death from either primary or metastatic disease (Brearley et al, 1999). In all studies, dogs went on to develop metastatic

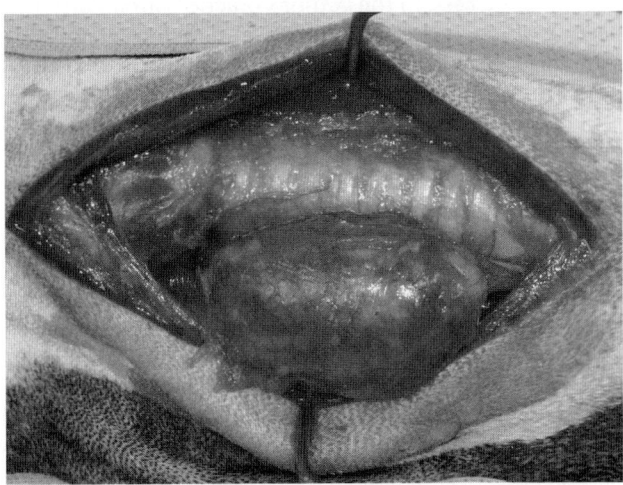

Figure 89-2 Resectable thyroid carcinoma at surgery. (Courtesy Daniela Murgia, Animal Health Trust, Kentford, Suffolk.)

disease in about 30% of cases. Adverse effects included suspected hypothyroidism in two dogs over a year after EBRT was administered.

Radioiodine Therapy

Iodine 131 (^{131}I) has been used to treat canine thyroid carcinoma. The advantages of using ^{131}I treatment rather than EBRT in cases that are unsuitable for surgery include the ability to target tumor tissue regardless of location and the potential to repeat treatment in dogs that develop tumor recurrence. There are limitations, however, including health and safety regulations regarding the handling of radioisotopes in veterinary patients, which vary from country to country. This affects the length of time that dogs need to be hospitalized after treatment and limits the number of facilities that can provide such therapy because they need to be capable of handling ^{131}I-contaminated waste from treated dogs and isolating dogs to minimize exposure of the public and veterinary personnel to radiation.

The other consideration is that of delivery of ^{131}I to the tumor. Most dogs with thyroid carcinomas are euthyroid, and therefore the gland may not take up an adequate dose of ^{131}I. Initially, therefore, this treatment was reserved for the minority of dogs with hyperthyroidism associated with a functional unresectable mass. One group has reported a technique for treating euthyroid dogs with thyroid cancer, feeding a low-iodine diet for several weeks before ^{131}I administration to increase uptake, and prolonged survival times have been associated with this modified technique (Turrel et al, 2006). Pretreatment nuclear scintigraphy with ^{125}I or technetium (^{99m}Tc), an iodine mimetic, can help to determine whether adequate ^{131}I uptake is likely to be obtained.

Systemic Therapy

The use of chemotherapy can be considered in cases where surgery, EBRT, and ^{131}I are not feasible because of either the location or extent of the mass or the client's circumstances. It is a poor third choice as a definitive treatment option.

Cisplatin, carboplatin, mitoxantrone, doxorubicin, and actinomycin D all have been used with varying degrees of success. In the author's practice carboplatin has been used as a first choice because it is well tolerated and frequently gives some reduction in tumor volume, palliating clinical signs. Clients should be counselled to expect a partial remission at best for a few months, although occasionally the author has seen a dog survive for over a year.

In a recent case series, toceranib phosphate, a receptor tyrosine kinase inhibitor, was used to treat 15 dogs with advanced thyroid tumors. In this study, dogs were administered a median dose of 2.75 mg/kg PO on Mondays, Wednesdays, and Fridays. This dosing regimen differs from the on-label dosing regimen of 3.25 mg/kg q48h PO for canine mast cell tumors. Of the 15 dogs in the study, four (26.7%) experienced partial remission and eight (53.3%) had stable disease. The median duration of therapy for these 12 dogs was 24.5 weeks (London et al, 2012).

Feline Thyroid Carcinoma

Feline thyroid carcinoma is a rare presentation. The presenting signs usually are identical to those in a cat with functional adenomatous hyperplasia, and the diagnosis often is a histopathologic one following surgical resection. Features causing concern at presentation include masses that are growing rapidly or are fixed, or are identified as multiple by palpation or scintigraphy. Attempts to differentiate carcinoma definitively from adenoma or hyperplasia using scintigraphy are not always rewarding, but an irregular margin of the gland or lack of uniform uptake of the radioisotope with "hot" and "cold" areas would be suggestive of carcinoma, as would the presence of overt metastatic disease. Cats that respond poorly to medical therapy or conventional ^{131}I therapy for presumed functional adenomatous hyperplasia also may have a thyroid carcinoma.

Treatment

Definitive surgery may not be feasible because of the invasive nature of the tumor. A debulking surgery may provide a transitory improvement in thyroxine levels and thus an amelioration of signs but is by no means a straightforward option. Even if surgery is feasible, thyroid carcinoma in this species carries a high risk of metastasis to the regional lymph nodes and lungs. ^{131}I therapy can be very successful in treating carcinoma, but much higher doses of ^{131}I need to be used than for adenoma or hyperplasia.

Chemotherapy has not been used in any studies, nor by the author, and medical management aimed at trying to control the hyperthyroidism usually is unsuccessful.

References and Suggested Reading

Brearley MJ, Hayes AM, Murphy S: Hypofractionated radiation therapy for invasive thyroid carcinoma in dogs: a retrospective analysis of survival, *J Small Anim Pract* 40:206, 1999.

Carver JR, Kapatkin A, Patnaik AK: A comparison of medullary thyroid carcinoma and thyroid adenocarcinoma in dogs: a retrospective study of 38 cases, *Vet Surg* 24:315, 1995.

Fineman LS et al: Cisplatin chemotherapy for treatment of thyroid carcinoma in dogs: 13 cases, *J Am Anim Hosp Assoc* 34:109, 1998.

Lee JJ et al: A dog pedigree with familial medullary thyroid cancer, *Int J Oncol* 29:1173, 2006.

London C et al: Preliminary evidence for biologic activity of toceranib phosphate (Palladia®) in solid tumours, *Vet Comp Oncol* 10:194, 2012. Epub June 1, 2011.

Pack L et al: Definitive radiation therapy for infiltrative thyroid carcinoma in dogs, *Vet Radiol Ultrasound* 42:471, 2001.

Théon AP et al: Prognostic factors and patterns of treatment failure in dogs with unresectable differentiated thyroid carcinomas treated with megavoltage irradiation, *J Am Vet Med Assoc* 216:1775, 2000.

Turrel JM et al: Sodium iodide I 131 treatment of dogs with nonresectable thyroid tumors: 39 cases (1990-2003), *J Am Vet Med Assoc* 229:542, 2006.

Worth AJ, Zuber RM, Hocking M: Radioiodide (131I) therapy for the treatment of canine thyroid carcinoma, *Aust Vet J* 83:208, 2005.

SECTION V

Dermatologic and Otic Diseases

Chapter 90:	Diagnostic Criteria for Canine Atopic Dermatitis	403
Chapter 91:	Treatment Guidelines for Canine Atopic Dermatitis	405
Chapter 92:	Cyclosporine Use in Dermatology	407
Chapter 93:	Allergen-Specific Immunotherapy	411
Chapter 94:	Systemic Glucocorticoids in Dermatology	414
Chapter 95:	Topical Therapy for Pruritus	419
Chapter 96:	Elimination Diets for Cutaneous Adverse Food Reactions: Principles in Therapy	422
Chapter 97:	Flea Control in Flea Allergy Dermatitis	424
Chapter 98:	Treatment of Ectoparasitoses	428
Chapter 99:	Canine Demodicosis	432
Chapter 100:	Staphylococci Causing Pyoderma	435
Chapter 101:	Treatment of Superficial Bacterial Folliculitis	437
Chapter 102:	Topical Therapy for Infectious Diseases	439
Chapter 103:	Methicillin-Resistant Staphylococcal Infections	443
Chapter 104:	Nontuberculous Cutaneous Granulomas in Dogs and Cats (Canine Leproid Granuloma and Feline Leprosy Syndrome)	445
Chapter 105:	Treatment of Dermatophytosis	449
Chapter 106:	Dermatophytosis: Investigating an Outbreak in a Multicat Environment	452
Chapter 107:	Disinfection of Environments Contaminated by Staphylococcal Pathogens	455
Chapter 108:	Principles of Therapy for Otitis	458
Chapter 109:	Topical and Systemic Glucocorticoids for Otitis	459
Chapter 110:	Topical Antimicrobials for Otitis	462
Chapter 111:	Systemic Antimicrobials for Otitis	466
Chapter 112:	Ototoxicity	468
Chapter 113:	Ear-Flushing Techniques	471
Chapter 114:	Primary Cornification Disorders In Dogs	475
Chapter 115:	Alopecia X	477
Chapter 116:	Actinic Dermatoses and Sun Protection	480
Chapter 117:	Drugs for Behavior-Related Dermatoses	482
Chapter 118:	Superficial Necrolytic Dermatitis	485
Chapter 119:	Cutaneous Adverse Drug Reactions	487

The following web chapters can be found on the companion website at www.currentveterinarytherapy.com

Web Chapter 33:	Acral Lick Dermatitis	
Web Chapter 34:	Avermectins in Dermatology	

Web Chapter 35:   Canine Papillomaviruses
Web Chapter 36:   Diseases of the Anal Sac
Web Chapter 37:   Feline Demodicosis
Web Chapter 38:   Feline Viral Skin Disease
Web Chapter 39:   House Dust Mites and Their Control
Web Chapter 40:   Interferons
Web Chapter 41:   Pentoxifylline
Web Chapter 42:   Pyotraumatic Dermatitis ("Hot Spots")
Web Chapter 43:   Therapy for Sebaceous Adenitis
Web Chapter 44:   *Malassezia* Infections
Web Chapter 45:   Topical Immunomodulators

CHAPTER 90

Diagnostic Criteria for Canine Atopic Dermatitis

CLAUDE FAVROT, *Zurich, Switzerland*

Canine atopic dermatitis (AD) is an inflammatory and pruritic disease driven most commonly by immunoglobulin E (IgE) antibody reactions to environmental, food, and microbial allergens. Numerous flare factors, such as microbial infections, psychologic factors, and climate, may contribute to the clinical signs. Furthermore, breed-associated phenotypes of canine AD have been described. Thus it is not surprising that the disease may present with highly variable clinical signs, none of which is pathognomonic.

The diagnosis of AD requires a meticulous workup and evaluation of historical and clinical information, and includes two different and complementary steps: the exclusion of similar diseases and confirmation of the suspected AD.

Differential Diagnosis: Exclusion of Similar Diseases

Exclusion of similar diseases is a mandatory first step, because many are readily manageable and straightforward to rule out. Practitioners should first exclude ectoparasitic infections, especially sarcoptic mange, flea infestation, and possibly cheyletiellosis and chigger bites.

Because the regional localization (face, ears, elbows, hocks) of pruritus and lesions in sarcoptic mange resembles those in canine AD, this disease is an important rule out. Numerous superficial skin scrapings should be examined. However, the sensitivity of skin scraping analysis is low, and "diagnostic treatment" (see Chapter 98) or IgG serologic testing (where available) should be performed if the clinical presentation is compatible with scabies and the superficial skin scrapings are negative for the mites.

Fleabite hypersensitivity usually affects the caudal dorsum and tail base initially; these are atypical sites for AD. However, many dogs also have lesions and pruritus of the abdomen, groin, medial thigh, and perineum, which can mimic AD. Thus fleabite hypersensitivity also should be ruled out in all dogs during the AD workup using trials of parasiticidal agents (see Chapter 97).

Bacterial and *Malassezia* (yeast) infections often develop secondary to canine AD, and it is critical that these disorders be identified and treated (see Chapters 100 to 102 and Web Chapter 44). Additionally, microbial hypersensitivity may play a role in some dogs with AD, in which significant clinical improvement may be anticipated with treatment of the infection.

Currently food allergy is considered a triggering factor for canine AD. Thus, in dogs with the typical clinical presentation of AD triggered by food allergens, the food allergy is regarded as a causal agent of AD, not as a separate entity. The role of diet should always be assessed in dogs with suspected AD that have a nonseasonal history of clinical signs (see Chapter 96). However, cutaneous adverse food reactions can be immune mediated or non–immune mediated and associated with a wide range of clinical signs (e.g., vomiting, diarrhea, urticaria)—signs that are dissimilar from those of typical AD.

In rare cases diseases such as epitheliotropic lymphoma or sebaceous adenitis demonstrate clinical signs with pruritus mimicking that of AD. If these diseases are suspected, skin biopsy for histopathologic analysis (a procedure rarely helpful in the diagnosis of AD) is indicated.

Clinical Signs of Canine Atopic Dermatitis

In a recent study of over 800 dogs, the frequency of each clinical sign of AD was studied. Data were collected from dogs with chronic or recurrent pruritus examined by veterinary dermatologists on four continents. Typical characteristics of AD in these dogs were identified as follows:

- Most dogs (68%) show the first clinical signs before 3 years of age.
- Fifty percent of dogs had chronic otitis; otitis was the first sign of disease in 43% of this group.
- Owners observed pruritus before lesions in 61% of cases.
- Pruritus was responsive to glucocorticoids in 78% of cases.
- Breed predispositions were identified but varied by geographical area.
- AD was seasonal in 24% of dogs, causing recurrent disease.
- The distributional pattern of lesions can be strongly suggestive of AD, with the following areas most frequently affected: front feet (79%), hind feet (75%), abdomen (66%), axillae (62%), ear pinnae (58%), genitalia (43%), lips (42%), eyelids (32%), and chest (32%).
- Secondary bacterial infection (66%) or yeast infection often develops, with some breed predispositions (German shepherd and West Highland white terrier) observed for yeast infections.

BOX 90-1

Sets of Criteria for the Diagnosis of Canine Atopic Dermatitis

Set 1
1. Age at onset <3 years
2. Mostly indoor living
3. Corticosteroid-responsive pruritus
4. Chronic or recurrent yeast infections
5. Affected front feet
6. Affected ear pinnae
7. Nonaffected ear margins
8. Nonaffected dorsolumbar area

Set 2
1. Age at onset <3 years
2. Mostly indoor living
3. Pruritus sine materia at onset
4. Affected front feet
5. Affected ear pinnae
6. Nonaffected ear margins
7. Nonaffected dorsolumbar area

Recognition of these clinical features of canine AD often is sufficient to confirm the diagnosis, especially when typical body regions are affected. In some patients, however, the diagnosis may still be troublesome.

Criteria for the Diagnosis of Canine Atopic Dermatitis

To facilitate the diagnosis of diseases with variable clinical features, sets of typical, although not pathognomonic, signs are often developed. This approach has been used for human atopic dermatitis and previously also in canine AD (Willemse's and Prélaud's criteria) for many years.

Recently we have used simulated annealing to determine the optimal sensitivity and specificity of sets of selected associated criteria. Two sets of criteria with both high sensitivity and high specificity were generated (Box 90-1). Although the primary use of these criteria is to establish inclusion criteria for clinical studies, these features are also useful for clinicians uncertain about a diagnosis of AD.

The first set of criteria is more useful for dogs with *chronic* disease, whereas the second set is better adapted for dogs with more *recent development* of clinical signs. When five criteria are met, the sensitivity and specificity of both sets of criteria for AD is about 80%. It is vital to remember that these sets of criteria should always be considered in conjunction with exclusion of similar diseases (see the earlier section on differential diagnosis). Additionally, as sets of criteria with an estimated sensitivity and specificity of 80%, these diagnostic sets (if used alone) lead to an incorrect diagnosis in every fifth patient.

Allergy Testing

Because canine AD is often associated with IgE-antibody reactions to allergens, it is tempting to use so-called allergy tests (which demonstrate the presence of allergen-specific IgE antibodies) for the diagnosis of AD. Unfortunately, numerous studies have demonstrated that this approach is invalid because dogs without AD may have high levels of allergen-specific IgE (subclinical hypersensitivity) whereas dogs with AD may not have demonstrable allergen-specific IgE (false-negative results). This latter group of dogs with AD but negative allergy test results have a condition called *atopic-like dermatitis*. Additionally, nonenvironmental allergens such as food or microbes (for which no validated tests or allergens are currently available) may also trigger AD; these patients also show nonreactivity on allergy tests (false-negative results).

In conclusion, atopic dermatitis in dogs is a very common disease, but the diagnosis is sometimes challenging. The first step in suspected cases of canine AD is completion of a thorough workup aimed at ruling out diseases with similar clinical signs. Diagnostic sets of criteria (see Box 90-1) can then be used to evaluate the probability of AD, but these criteria should not be used in isolation.

References and Suggested Reading

DeBoer DJ, Hillier A: The ACVD task force on canine atopic dermatitis (XV): fundamental concepts in clinical diagnosis, *Vet Immunol Immunopathol* 81:271, 2001.

Favrot C et al: A prospective study on the clinical features of chronic canine atopic dermatitis and its diagnosis, *Vet Dermatol* 21:23, 2010.

Griffin CE, Deboer DJ: The ACVD task force on canine atopic dermatitis (XIV): clinical manifestations of canine atopic dermatitis, *Vet Immunol Immunopathol* 81:255, 2001.

Halliwell R: Revised nomenclature for veterinary allergy, *Vet Immunol Immunopathol* 114:207, 2006.

Wilhem S, Kovalik M, Favrot C: Breed-associated phenotypes in canine atopic dermatitis, *Vet Dermatol* 22:143, 2011.

CHAPTER 91

Treatment Guidelines for Canine Atopic Dermatitis

THIERRY OLIVRY, *Raleigh, North Carolina*
PASCAL PRÉLAUD, *Paris, France*

Atopic dermatitis (AD) is a common chronic relapsing pruritic skin disease of dogs. In 2010 the International Task Force on Canine Atopic Dermatitis published guidelines recommending a multifaceted approach to the treatment of dogs with AD (Olivry et al, 2010). Treatment recommendations considered two main factors: whether the patient has an acute flare of disease or the AD is chronic, and whether skin lesions are localized or extensive. Not every intervention is suitable for every patient; neither are drugs equally effective for every dog. Pet owner preferences (based on cost and ease of compliance) and quality of life of each patient must always be considered.

Treatment of Acute Flares of Atopic Dermatitis

Identification and Avoidance of Flare Factors

Allergenic Flares
The clinician must consider whether any known cause of flares is present. Such causes can include flea exposure, ingestion of food allergens, and exposure to environmental allergens such as house dust mites, seasonal pollens, and mold spores. These causes should be eliminated or controlled if identified.

Evaluation of Use of Antimicrobial Therapy
Reemergence of bacterial or yeast infections frequently causes flares of disease and is identified based on clinical signs and cytologic examination. Infections are treated with topical or systemic antimicrobial therapy, or both (see Chapters 100 to 103 and 121 and Web Chapter 44).

Improvement of Skin and Coat Hygiene and Care

Bathing with a Nonirritating Shampoo
A complex-sugar, antiseptic, and lipid-containing shampoo (Allermyl, Virbac) helped reduce pruritus in 25% of dogs treated in one study. Currently there is a lack of evidence for a clinical benefit from other shampoos or conditioners that contain ingredients such as oatmeal, pramoxine, antihistamine, lipids, or glucocorticoids (see Chapter 95).

Reduction of Pruritus and Skin Lesions with Pharmacologic Agents

Pruritus in AD may be improved by short-term use of topical or systemic glucocorticoids.

Short-term Treatment with a Topical Glucocorticoid Formulation
There is evidence for high effectiveness of two medium-potency glucocorticoid sprays for treating acute flares of AD: triamcinolone (Genesis, Virbac) and hydrocortisone aceponate (Cortavance, Virbac). Caution is advised with long-term use because adverse effects, such as skin thinning, are likely to occur (see Chapter 95).

Short Course of Oral Glucocorticoids
Oral glucocorticoids are recommended if severe or extensive clinical signs are present or if there is concurrent stenotic otitis externa. Prednisone, prednisolone, or methylprednisolone can be given at antiinflammatory dosages (see Chapter 94) until clinical remission occurs.

Interventions Likely to Be of Little or No Benefit for Treatment of Acute Atopic Dermatitis

There is no conclusive evidence for the effectiveness of oral type 1 antihistamines for the treatment of active AD in dogs. Essential fatty acids, oral cyclosporine, and topical tacrolimus are also unlikely to be of any benefit for acute flares because their mode of action necessitates several weeks of treatment.

Treatment Options for Chronic Canine Atopic Dermatitis

Identification and Avoidance of Flare Factors

Food allergens may be triggers for AD in dogs; thus restriction-provocation dietary trials (i.e., "elimination diets") must be performed in all dogs with nonseasonal AD (see Chapter 96). Additionally, because dogs with AD are predisposed to developing fleabite hypersensitivity, all dogs with AD must be treated year-round with flea adulticides (see Chapter 97).

Allergen-Specific Intradermal and/or Immunoglobulin E Serologic Tests

Environmental allergens, such as house dust mites, have been shown to cause flares of AD in dogs hypersensitive to these allergens. Performing intradermal testing or immunoglobulin E serologic testing can help to identify hypersensitivity to environmental allergens. These tests are used for immunotherapy formulation (see Chapter 93) and may be of potential benefit in indicating the need for house dust mite allergen reduction or avoidance, although this is largely unproven.

Evaluation of Use of Antimicrobial Therapy

The skin and ears of dogs with AD are commonly infected or colonized with staphylococci and *Malassezia* species. Their contribution to the severity of clinical signs of AD often is determined only by an assessment of the response to antimicrobial therapy alone. The systematic prescription of antimicrobials to every dog with AD is not recommended, however, because the long-term use of these drugs is likely associated with the emergence of drug-resistant microbes (see Chapter 103 and Web Chapter 44).

Improvement of Skin and Coat Hygiene and Care

Weekly bathing with a mild nonirritating shampoo and lukewarm water is likely to be beneficial by providing a direct soothing effect, removing surface allergens and microbes, and increasing skin hydration. There is no evidence of superiority of any particular shampoo or protocol. Antiseborrheic shampoos are indicated for greasy/scaly skin, antiseptic shampoos should be used when infections are present, and moisturizers may alleviate the skin dryness that may occur after the baths.

In normal dogs, supplementation with *essential fatty acids* (EFA) or feeding of EFA-rich diets usually improves coat quality and gloss. At this time, there is no evidence of superiority of any particular EFA combination, dosage, ratio, or formulation (including enriched diets) for improving skin and coat quality in dogs with AD. In general, EFA-enriched diets provide higher amounts of EFA than oral supplements. The benefit of EFA supplementation might not be seen before 2 months of treatment.

There is insufficient evidence at this time to support the use of topical formulations containing EFA, essential oils, or complex lipid mixtures. These have not been documented as beneficial for dogs with AD.

Reduction of Pruritus and Skin Lesions with Pharmacologic Agents

Treatment of pruritus and skin lesions topically or systemically is an important component of AD therapy.

Treatment with Topical Glucocorticoids or Tacrolimus

There is good evidence supporting the efficacy of topical glucocorticoids for treatment of AD in dogs. Such formulations are best suited for focal (e.g., foot) or multifocal lesions and for relatively short treatment durations (e.g., less than 2 months). Alternatively, 0.1% tacrolimus ointment (Protopic, Astellas) has been shown to be effective in localized AD when used twice daily for 1 week, followed by less frequent application as needed. Mild irritation might follow its application (see Web Chapter 45).

Treatment with Oral Glucocorticoids or Cyclosporine

There is strong evidence for the efficacy of oral glucocorticoids and cyclosporine in the treatment of AD in dogs. Such oral medications are especially well suited for dogs with generalized AD. The onset of clinical benefit occurs earlier with glucocorticoids than with cyclosporine. Oral glucocorticoids (e.g., prednisone, prednisolone, methylprednisolone) should be started at a dosage of approximately 0.5 to 1.0 mg/kg per day and then reduced as signs decrease to the lowest dose and frequency (e.g., every other day) that maintains a good quality of life and controls signs while producing minimal side effects (see Chapter 94).

Modified cyclosporine (Atopica, Novartis) should be started at 5 mg/kg once daily and continued at this dosage until a satisfactory decrease in signs is achieved. Thereafter, the dose should be reduced either by increasing dosing intervals (e.g., from every day to every other day) or by decreasing the daily dose by half. If signs are reduced by 75% or more, dosing frequency may be reduced to twice weekly or the dose reduced to 25% of the original daily dose. Initially, satisfactory clinical benefit normally cannot be expected before 4 to 8 weeks. To increase the speed of clinical improvement, the administration of a short course of oral glucocorticoids during the first 1 to 3 weeks of cyclosporine treatment may be beneficial. Minor adverse effects (e.g., vomiting, diarrhea) are common after initiation of cyclosporine therapy; most improve spontaneously upon further administration of the drug (see Chapter 92).

Interventions Likely to Be of Little or No Benefit for Treatment of Chronic Atopic Dermatitis

Results from clinical trials suggest that, as a group, oral type 1 antihistamines are unlikely to be beneficial in dogs with chronic AD. Veterinarians wishing to use type 1 antihistamines should limit their prescriptions to those drugs that have been shown to have a real histamine-inhibiting effect in dogs (e.g., hydroxyzine at 2 mg/kg twice daily or cetirizine 0.5 to 1.0 mg/kg once daily). Finally, antihistamines may be more effective as a preventative—that is, to block histamine receptors before histamine is released—than as a treatment after the fact.

A systematic review of clinical trials provided evidence that EFA supplements, EFA-enriched diets, and nutritional or herbal supplements are unlikely to provide meaningful benefit if given alone for relief of inflammation and/or pruritus. EFAs might be useful to improve coat quality and ameliorate dry skin (see earlier).

Because of their low efficacy, high cost, or potential for adverse effects, oral pentoxifylline, misoprostol, and tepoxalin probably should not be used as first-line medications to treat dogs with AD.

Implementation of Strategies to Prevent the Recurrence of Signs

Avoidance of Flare Factors

Avoidance of known flare factors is the best strategy to prevent the recurrence of signs and may include maintenance of the dog on an elimination diet, maintenance of effective flea control, and reduction of contact with provocative environmental or microbial allergens whenever possible.

Implementation of Proactive (Preventive) Pharmacotherapy

The strategy of proactively applying topical glucocorticoids and tacrolimus to areas repeatedly affected during flares of AD has not been evaluated in dogs at this time. Because of the possible benefit, low risk, and low cost, regular but *intermittent* topical glucocorticoid application (i.e., twice weekly or "weekend" therapy) might be worth considering in dogs with moderate or severe AD.

Implementation of Allergen-Specific Immunotherapy

Subcutaneous allergen-specific immunotherapy (ASIT) appears effective and safe (see Chapter 93). It is expected that between 50% and 80% of dogs with AD treated with ASIT for 6 to 12 months will exhibit an improvement in signs or a decrease in the use of antiinflammatory medication. At this time, there appears to be no advantage to any particular ASIT protocol (traditional, rush, or low dose). Antiinflammatory drugs may be given temporarily as needed to maintain good quality of life until ASIT becomes effective. ASIT must be continued for at least 1 year before it is dismissed as ineffective.

References and Suggested Reading

Olivry T et al: Treatment of canine atopic dermatitis: 2010 clinical practice guidelines from the International Task Force on Canine Atopic Dermatitis, *Vet Dermatol* 21:233, 2010. *Note:* the English version of this article can be downloaded at http://www3.interscience.wiley.com/cgi-bin/fulltext/123371643/PDFSTART. Translations in multiple foreign languages can be found at http://onlinelibrary.wiley.com/doi/10.1111/j.1365-3164.2010.00889.x/suppinfo.

CHAPTER **92**

Cyclosporine Use in Dermatology

ANDREW HILLIER, *Columbus, Ohio*

Cyclosporine has been approved in the United States for use in the control of atopic dermatitis in dogs as Atopica since 2003 and for the control of allergic dermatitis in cats as Atopica for Cats since 2011.

Cyclosporine is a potent immunomodulatory agent whose primary mechanism of action is inhibition of T-cell activation. Additional affects on the function of dendritic cells, Langerhans cells, B cells, mast cells, eosinophils, and keratinocytes contribute to the immunomodulatory and antiinflammatory actions of cyclosporine.

Because cyclosporine use in dogs was discussed extensively in Chapter 84 of the previous edition of *Current Veterinary Therapy*, this chapter focuses on new information relevant to the treatment of canine atopic dermatitis, the use of cyclosporine in cats, and additional extralabel uses for cyclosporine in small animals.

Updates on Cyclosporine for Canine Atopic Dermatitis

Dose Adjustments by Body Weight

A recent unpublished study evaluated whether body weight was related to the final effective dose of cyclosporine. It was reported that a mean dose of 4.4 mg/kg of cyclosporine was necessary to control clinical signs of atopic dermatitis in dogs weighing more than 15 kg, which was 0.53 mg/kg less than the mean dose for dogs weighing less than 15 kg. Overall, a mean decrease of 0.04 mg/kg/day for each kilogram of body weight was reported. This author does not alter the initial target dose based on body weight; all dogs are treated with at least 5 mg/kg q24h for at least 30 days.

Dose Adjustments for Concurrent Administration with Ketoconazole

The effects of ketoconazole administered simultaneously with cyclosporine on skin and whole blood cyclosporine concentrations have been reported. In a study using normal adult laboratory dogs, it was determined that when dogs were administered 2.5 mg/kg q24h of keto-conazole and 2.5 mg/kg q24h of cyclosporine for 7 days, the adjusted mean whole blood and skin concentrations of cyclosporine were no different from the adjusted mean whole blood and skin concentrations achieved when cyclosporine was administered alone at the target dosage of 5 mg/kg q24h for 7 days (Gray et al, 2013). This suggests that administration of cyclosporine and ketoconazole concurrently at 2.5 mg/kg q24h each may be as effective as administration of cyclosporine alone at 5.0 mg/kg for treatment of canine atopic dermatitis. In practice the author usually administers cyclosporine at 5 mg/kg q24h without ketoconazole during the initial 30-day trial. If at any time the ongoing expense of cyclo-sporine becomes an issue for continued therapy, the cyclosporine dose is halved (to 2.5 mg/kg q24h) and ketoconazole is added at 2.5 mg/kg q24h. Typically, dogs that have responded favorably to the cyclosporine alone will continue to do well on the combination therapy, although some patients do experience some loss of effi-cacy, which usually is noticeable within a few days to a week.

Dose Adjustments for Concurrent Administration with Fluconazole

The effect of fluconazole on the cyclosporine dosage also has been investigated in dogs with renal transplants and normal dogs receiving cyclosporine-based immunosup-pressive therapy. Concurrent administration of flucon-azole (5 mg/kg q24h PO) significantly decreased the required cyclosporine dosage in both normal dogs and dogs with renal transplants, but a higher dosage of cyclosporine was needed in the transplanted dogs. In normal dogs, the cyclosporine requirements significantly decreased by 29% to 51% compared with initial cyclospo-rine dosages (Katayama et al, 2010). The effect of flucon-azole on skin levels of cyclosporine was not reported, and thus the effects of fluconazole on cyclosporine's effi-cacy in the treatment of canine atopic dermatitis are not known.

Urinary Tract Infections with Long-Term Cyclosporine Therapy

Another study assessed the frequency of urinary tract infections in dogs receiving cyclosporine with or without glucocorticoids (Peterson et al, 2012). The results suggest that routine urine culture and assessment of bacteriuria by cystocentesis should be part of the monitoring regimen for dogs receiving long-term cyclosporine therapy (>5 months) because 26 of 81 dogs (30%) had at least one positive urine culture result. However, 16 of the dogs also were being treated with glucocorticoids, and when the number of positive urine culture results in dogs receiving

cyclosporine alone was compared with the number of positive urine culture results in a control group (dogs with inflammatory skin disease), no significant difference was seen. Further prospective studies are needed before one can make a firm recommendations regarding routine urine culture in dogs receiving long-term cyclosporine treatment. The author does not perform routine urine culture in dogs receiving long-term cyclosporine therapy unless they also are receiving long-term corticosteroid therapy or show clinical signs of cystitis.

Management of Gastrointestinal Adverse Effects

A variety of management strategies are available for dogs that develop gastrointestinal symptoms with cyclospo-rine administration, as occurs in approximately 30% of patients. In dogs with a history of gastrointestinal disease or upset, the author starts cyclosporine therapy at a lower dose (e.g., 2 to 3 mg/kg) and increases to the target dose over 7 to 10 days. Some dogs do better when administered frozen capsules or when given the cyclosporine with a small amount of food, which does not seem to diminish the clinical effect despite the slightly decreased gastroin-testinal absorption. Metoclopramide (0.2 to 0.4 mg/kg q12h) or maropitant citrate (Cerenia; 2 mg/kg q24h PO for 5 days) also can be administered to help control vom-iting. For soft stools, use of a high-fiber supplement (e.g., canned pumpkin) or high-fiber diets or probiotics may be helpful in dogs.

Management of Gingival Hyperplasia and Papillomatosis

Gingival hyperplasia is a recognized but uncommon adverse effect of cyclosporine therapy that can be treated either by the use of azithromycin toothpaste or by dental prophylactic treatment and surgical debulking of the hyperplasia. Azithromycin may be administered systemi-cally (10 mg/kg q24h PO) to treat papillomatosis, which is another uncommon adverse effect of cyclosporine treatment.

Cyclosporine for Feline Allergic Dermatitis

Atopica for Cats is indicated for the control of feline allergic dermatitis as manifested by excoriations (includ-ing facial and neck), miliary dermatitis, eosinophilic plaques, and self-induced alopecia. The initial dosage of Atopica for Cats is 7 mg/kg q24h as a single daily dose for a minimum of 4 to 6 weeks or until resolution of clinical signs.

Atopica for Cats may be tapered by decreasing the frequency of dosing to every other day or twice weekly to maintain the desired therapeutic effect. Before the availability of Atopica for Cats, the author used modified cyclosporine in cats at an initial dosage of 5 mg/kg q24h with excellent results. However, the author now uses the dosage of 7 mg/kg q24h because the brand-name drug is supplied with a dispensing system that includes an oral dosing syringe graduated in 1-lb increments, which creates confusion for some owners if they are instructed to dose differently than indicated by the label and syringe. It is important always to provide the owner with the manufacturer's "Instructions for Assembling the Dispensing System and Preparing a Dose of Atopica for Cats," which contains information on assembling the system, fitting the adaptor into the bottle, and preparing a dose, as well as answers to questions asked frequently by owners.

Anticipated Efficacy of Cyclosporine for Feline Allergic Dermatitis

There is good evidence for the efficacy of cyclosporine in the control of allergic dermatitis lesions in cats; the practitioner can anticipate that the majority of patients will experience at least a 50% decrease in pruritus and lesions after 6 weeks of therapy. If there is a satisfactory response at this time, dosing is reduced to q48h for 4 weeks, and if control of disease is maintained, dosing is further reduced to twice weekly. The majority of cats treated continue to have good control of their allergic dermatitis with q48h dosing, and many do well with twice weekly dosing. The author has treated several cats in which maintenance dosing has been reduced to once weekly, and the overall impression of Atopica for Cats is that it is a highly effective drug and appears to be more effective in cats than in dogs in general.

Contraindications for Cyclosporine Use in Cats

Cyclosporine is contraindicated for use in cats with known or suspected malignant neoplasia and in cats that test positive for feline leukemia virus or feline immunodeficiency virus (cats should be tested before treatment). Cats that are seronegative for *Toxoplasma gondii* may be at risk of developing potentially fatal clinical toxoplasmosis if they become infected while receiving cyclosporine. This is more likely to be a problem in cats that develop very high serum levels of cyclosporine, so that monitoring of serum cyclosporine levels may be of value in seronegative cats. In a controlled laboratory study (Novartis FOI, 2001), cats seronegative for *T. gondii* were administered cyclosporine and subsequently infected with *T. gondii*. Cyclosporine administration resulted in increased susceptibility to infection and subsequent expression of toxoplasmosis. Cyclosporine did not increase *T. gondii* oocyst shedding. Potential exposure of seronegative cats to *T. gondii* should be avoided by keeping treated cats indoors, not feeding raw meat, and not allowing scavenging or hunting.

Adverse Effects of Cyclosporine Use in Cats

Adverse effects of cyclosporine in cats are similar to those in dogs. Progressive weight loss associated with hepatic lipidosis has been reported in 1% to 2% of cyclosporine-treated cats; thus close monitoring of body weight and appetite are necessary. Clinical signs associated with herpesvirus and calicivirus infections may occur in some cats that had inactive viral infections before cyclosporine therapy. These signs typically are mild but may become more severe and debilitating in some patients.

Other Uses for Cyclosporine

Cyclosporine for Perianal Fistulas

Numerous treatment and dosing protocols for the use of cyclosporine in the treatment of perianal fistulas have been evaluated and published. When used alone, cyclosporine dosed at 5 to 7.5 mg/kg q24h provides the best responses. Alternatively, the combination of cyclosporine (1 to 2.5 mg/kg q24h) plus ketoconazole (5 to 10 mg/kg q24h) seems to be effective. Note that the dose of each drug is different from the doses given when this combination is used to treat atopic dermatitis. Most studies of the use of cyclosporine to treat perianal fistulas indicate that relapse occurs in the majority of dogs if therapy is discontinued. Thus, once remission of clinical signs is achieved, the frequency of administration of the combination of cyclosporine and ketoconazole should be reduced by 1 day per week every 2 weeks until clinical signs start to recur, which indicates the likely maintenance dose for the patient.

Cyclosporine for Sebaceous Adenitis

A recent placebo-controlled study (Lortz et al, 2010) involving 34 dogs with sebaceous adenitis treated for 4 to 6 months compared the use of oral cyclosporine alone (5 mg/kg q24h), cyclosporine (at the same dosage) combined with topical therapy, and placebo capsules combined with topical therapy. Both topical therapy and cyclosporine were effective in reducing alopecia and inflammation, but topical therapy was more effective in reducing scaling and cyclosporine was more likely to be associated with regeneration of sebaceous glands on histopathologic examination. Improvement generally is seen within 4 months, at which time reduction of bathing or cyclosporine administration can commence.

Cyclosporine for Pemphigus Foliaceus

Earlier reports of the use of cyclosporine for the treatment of pemphigus foliaceus in dogs were not promising, and indications are that dosages of 5 to 10 mg/kg q24h of cyclosporine alone are ineffective. However, combination of cyclosporine (5 to 18 mg/kg q24h) with prednisone (1 to 2.6 mg/kg q24h) induced remission of pemphigus foliaceus in 5 dogs in a recent unpublished study (Maeda et al, 2008). Thereafter, first the prednisone was tapered to 0.5 mg/kg q48h and then the cyclosporine was tapered to 3 to 4 mg/kg q48h.

Cyclosporine is likely more effective in treating pemphigus foliaceus in cats than in dogs. A recent report (Irwin et al, 2012) compared outcomes in cats with pemphigus foliaceus treated with cyclosporine (4.4 to 5.6 mg/kg q24h) or chlorambucil (0.17 to 0.38 mg/kg q48h) (six cats in each group). Most cats in both groups received corticosteroids as well (dexamethasone, triamcinolone, or prednisolone). There was no difference in time to remission or disease response between the two

BOX 92-1

Conditions for Which Cyclosporine Has Potential Use as Adjunctive Therapy in Dogs and Cats

Dogs
- Sterile nodular panniculitis
- Alopecia areata
- Exfoliative cutaneous lupus erythematosus
- Pedal furunculosis
- German shepherd dog pyoderma
- Metatarsal sinus tracts
- Sterile granuloma syndrome
- Erythema multiforme
- Primary seborrhea
- Cutaneous and systemic reactive histiocytosis
- Nasal arteritis
- Discoid lupus erythematosus
- Juvenile cellulitis

Cats
- Plasmacytic stomatitis
- Sebaceous adenitis
- Facial dermatitis of Persian cats
- Pseudopelade
- Urticaria pigmentosa
- Plasma cell pododermatitis

groups. However, six of six cats in the cyclosporine-treated group were weaned off corticosteroids totally, whereas this was achievable in only one of six cats treated with chlorambucil; this indicates a significant corticosteroid-sparing effect of cyclosporine.

Cyclosporine as Secondary or Tertiary Therapy in Other Conditions

Evidence for the efficacy of cyclosporine in the treatment of a variety of other dermatologic diseases is anecdotal and typically weak. Box 92-1 lists diseases for which cyclosporine treatment has been used. Note that for many of the diseases listed, several other therapeutic options are available for which there is better evidence of efficacy and which may have advantages over cyclosporine (e.g., a better safety profile, lower cost, fewer adverse effects).

References and Suggested Reading

Gray LL et al: The effect of ketoconazole on whole blood and skin ciclosporin concentrations in dogs, *Vet Dermatol* 24(1):118-e28, 2013.

Heinrich NA, McKeever PJ, Eisenschenk MC: Adverse events in 50 cats with allergic dermatitis receiving ciclosporin, *Vet Dermatol* 6:511, 2011.

Irwin KE, Beale KM, Fadok VA: Use of modified ciclosporin in the management of feline pemphigus foliaceus: a retrospective analysis, *Vet Dermatol* 23:403-e76, 2012.

Katayama M et al: Fluconazole decreases cyclosporine dosage in renal transplanted dogs, *Res Vet Sci* 89(1):124, 2010.

King S et al: A randomized double-blinded placebo-controlled study to evaluate an effective ciclosporin dose for the treatment of feline hypersensitivity dermatitis, *Vet Dermatol* 23(5):440-e84, 2012.

Lortz J et al: A multicentre placebo-controlled clinical trial on the efficacy of oral ciclosporin A in the treatment of canine idiopathic sebaceous adenitis in comparison with conventional topical treatment, *Vet Dermatol* 21(6):593, 2010.

Maeda H et al: Treatment of five dogs with pemphigus foliaceus with cyclosporine and prednisone, *Vet Dermatol* 19(S1):51, 2008.

Novartis FOI: Freedom of information summary, Novartis Animal Health; Atopica for Cats, *NADA* 141; 19, 2001.

Peterson AL et al: Frequency of urinary tract infection in dogs with inflammatory skin disorders treated with ciclosporin alone or in combination with glucocorticoid therapy: a retrospective study, *Vet Dermatol* 23:240, 2012.

CHAPTER 93

Allergen-Specific Immunotherapy

DOUGLAS J. DEBOER, *Madison, Wisconsin*

Allergen-specific immunotherapy (ASIT) is a treatment for atopic dermatitis (AD) in dogs and cats in which allergenic substances to which the patient is sensitive are administered in gradually increasing amounts to lessen the hypersensitivity state. It is the only proven treatment for allergies that reverses the underlying immunopathogenesis of the disease instead of covering up clinical signs, as with antiinflammatory therapies. ASIT is nearly free of serious adverse effects in the great majority of dogs and cats, and can produce substantial, long-lasting relief in many patients. In human beings, ASIT is recommended as early as possible in the course of the disease because it may prevent development of additional sensitivities as well as progression of disease severity. These factors have not been studied in animals, but nevertheless, the potential lifelong benefits of ASIT make it a preferred treatment for AD that should be discussed with owners earlier rather than later in the management process.

The mechanisms of action of ASIT still are not completely understood but likely include downregulation of effector cells (mast cells, basophils, eosinophils), immune deviation of lymphocytes away from a proallergic response, production of immunoglobulin G (IgG) blocking antibodies, and induction of immunologic tolerance or nonreactivity.

Allergen Selection and Formulation

Most effects of ASIT are known to be allergen specific, and thus accurate testing to identify the offending allergens is of paramount importance. In general practice, serologic tests are often used as a basis for ASIT. The results of such tests should be interpreted in light of the individual patient's clinical history; if the results do not fit the clinical picture (e.g., positive results are obtained for only a few seasonal allergens in a dog with year-round disease), then referral for an intradermal test should be considered.

Choosing which allergens to include in a treatment mixture is part art and part science. Effective ASIT is dose dependent; thus it is generally recommended that no more than 10 to 12 allergens be included in a single treatment set. This recommendation is controversial, and some clinicians routinely include more than this number in their formulations. When a large number of test reactions are positive in a given animal, selection of allergens

for inclusion in the treatment set is based on known allergen cross-reactivities, botanical relationships of allergenic plants, exposure history, and strength of the test reaction. In practical terms, these decisions are facilitated by the company performing the serologic testing.

Conventional ASIT for animals in the United States has typically involved administration of aqueous extracts via subcutaneous injection. Extracts contain a phenol preservative and require refrigeration to maintain potency. Proteases in a treatment solution may degrade the allergens; it is well established that mold extracts contain proteases and, if mixed with pollen extracts in the same vial, accelerate degradation of the pollen allergens. Thus, if there is notable mold allergy, mold extracts should be formulated in a separate vial and administered by separate injection.

Treatment solutions for injection are provided as a series of two or three vials of gradually increasing concentration. The concentration of the vial is expressed in units that are somewhat archaic and unique to allergen extracts. The most common is *protein nitrogen units per milliliter* (PNU/ml; 100,000 PNU = 1 mg protein and therefore a solution of 20,000 PNU/ml contains 0.2 mg/ml of allergen protein). Alternatively, the strength may be expressed as *weight/volume* (w/v; a solution of 1/10 w/v simply means that 1 g of starting material was extracted with 10 ml of buffer to produce the solution).

Protocols and Injection Schedules

The treatment set manufacturer will provide an injection schedule, and no particular schedule has been shown to be superior to another. An initial buildup or *escalation phase* (in which injections are given every 2 to 7 days, gradually increasing in volume and concentration over a period of several weeks) is followed by a prolonged *maintenance phase* (in which a uniform dose is given less frequently, e.g., every 7 to 30 days, with gradual tapering of frequency as response occurs). (Examples of typical schedules can be found in Chapter 92 of the previous edition of *Current Veterinary Therapy*.) Protocols are similar for dogs and cats.

Injections are administered using 1-ml syringes and fine-gauge (e.g., 27-gauge) needles, which cause negligible injection pain to the pet. After proper instruction, most owners are able to give the injections at home with relative ease. An office visit should be scheduled at which the

Important Elements of Client Education Regarding Allergen-Specific Immunotherapy (ASIT)

Discuss each of the following points with the client, and ideally provide a printed explanatory handout for the client's later reference:
- **Explain that ASIT is only part of an overall management plan.**
Emphasize the lifelong nature of atopic dermatitis and the necessity of developing a long-term management plan that will be based on ASIT but also may include periodic use of concurrent medications, avoidance strategies, topical therapies, infection prevention strategies, and other measures as appropriate to the patient.
- **Explain the administration schedule.**
Outline the specific injection or oral administration schedule and progression through escalating vial series. Emphasize the importance of consistent administration. Stress that, even if benefits occur quite rapidly, for lasting benefit a full therapy course of several years will be necessary and that some patients require lifetime maintenance treatment.
- **Provide proper instruction on administration technique.**
For injections, describe the need for refrigerated storage and the way to fill and measure with syringes, and make the client practice injection in the office. For sublingual ASIT, demonstrate the use of the dispenser and administration; remind the client that the solution cannot be mixed with food.
- **Explain the necessity and schedule for follow-up examinations.**
Plan routine follow-up examinations for 3 months, 6 months, and 12 months after starting therapy. Emphasize the importance of

rechecks to adjust the injection schedule, adjust concurrent medication use, and identify flare factors such as infections before they become severe.
- **Explain possible adverse effects of ASIT and how to recognize them.**
Advise the client to watch for mild localized or transient reactions and report them if concerned. Describe signs associated with systemic anaphylaxis and note that these typically occur within an hour or so after administration.
- **Explain the response that is expected to occur.**
Clarify that the expected response is a gradual diminution of itch, episodes of infections, and other clinical signs. Instruct the client to be patient—response occurs gradually over a period of months, and it may take 6 to 12 months or more for the treatment to reach maximum benefit.
- **Explain when to call for advice.**
Advise an initial call after 4 weeks of treatment to report grade of itching, any problems with administration, and any possible mild reactions. Instruct the client always to call immediately in the case of suspected anaphylactic reaction. Communicate that the overall management plan should result in a comfortable, minimally symptomatic pet.

injection schedule and technique are explained to the owner (Box 93-1).

Injection Schedule Adjustments

Most patients progress satisfactorily through the injection series without modification. However, the standard protocol should be viewed as a reference point; in some situations, it will be necessary to modify the frequency or volume of injection (Box 93-2). It is best to consult with medical-technical advisers at the supplier for their recommendation as to the best method for schedule adjustment.

Alternatives to Conventional Injection Protocols

Some European manufacturers provide extracts that are adsorbed to an aluminum hydroxide adjuvant (*alum-precipitated extract*) that provides a constant slow release of allergen from the injection site, and therefore injections can be given less frequently (every 2 to 4 weeks).

Rush immunotherapy is a less common protocol occasionally used by specialists. Using standard extracts delivered by subcutaneous injection, the escalation phase is performed very rapidly in a hospitalized patient, with the allergen dose increased every 30 minutes so that the entire escalation phase lasts a matter of hours rather

than weeks. Thereafter, the maintenance phase is carried out as for the conventional protocol. Generally, response rates are comparable to those with conventional protocols, although response may occur more rapidly. Rush ASIT avoids the necessity for the owner to give frequent injections at home during escalation; thus it may be appropriate for animals to which administering injections is difficult. Theoretically there may be an increased risk of anaphylactic reactions with rush protocols, although this has not proven to be a major concern. However, the author recommends use of the more standard protocols in general-practice situations.

Some authors administer a uniform, noncustomized mixture of allergens to every patient, regardless of their sensitivities (i.e., without performing any allergy tests). Every allergic patient thus gets the same mixture *(blind immunotherapy)* or else a standard mixture that includes common allergens present in a specific geographic region *(regionally specific immunotherapy)*. Since it is known that the effects of ASIT are in large part allergen specific, this approach is less desirable, although it eliminates the expense of allergy testing. The presence of allergens in the mixture to which the patient is *not* sensitive probably is not harmful, although their inclusion may dilute the mixture and result in a lower dose of the relevant allergens. This approach may result in failure to include one or more allergens to which the patient is sensitive, which may lessen efficacy. Current (albeit limited) studies

BOX 93-2

Typical Situations Requiring Adjustment of Treatment Schedule for Allergen-Specific Immunotherapy (Injection or Sublingual Formulations)

Worsening of clinical signs after administration. Particularly when the animal is small or when the allergen mixture has larger amounts of only a few allergens, the animal may not be able to tolerate the maximum specified "standard" dosage, in which case the dosage should be reduced.

Rubbing at the face or mouth, or vomiting, after SLIT administration. These effects are uncommon, typically occur only with the first few doses and usually will disappear with continued administration. Dosage adjustment is not necessary unless the effects worsen or persist.

Benefit of an injection seems to wear off before the next scheduled dose is due. In this case, the injections can be given more frequently.

Anaphylactic reaction. Although anaphylaxis to injections is rare (<1% of cases), if systemic anaphylaxis is suspected, treatment should be stopped immediately. Options include continuing injections at a lower dose; switching to SLIT, which is not likely to induce such reactions; or referring the patient to a specialist. In all cases, contact the treatment supplier for advice.

Modification when pet is doing very well on maintenance treatment. The frequency of injections can be gradually reduced. With most SLIT protocols, frequency is *not* tapered during maintenance.

SLIT, Sublingual immunotherapy.

BOX 93-3

Shots or Drops? Considerations in the Selection of Injection versus Sublingual Formulations of Allergen-Specific Immunotherapy (ASIT)

Client schedule and convenience factors. Some clients find it easier to give an injection every 14 days or so than to administer SLIT one or two times daily; others prefer regular daily administration. Some SLIT formulations do not require refrigeration (injection formulations do).

Client aversion to needles. Some clients find injections very easy to give to their pets; others are fearful of needles and are delighted to have the option of oral SLIT administration.

Patient cooperation factors. Most pets tolerate injections at home quite well, although some may be extremely resistant. Most pets find SLIT formulations palatable and view administration as a "treat," although some head-shy animals may be difficult to medicate.

Importance of mold/fungal allergens. If molds are an important allergen, fungal extracts for injection should not be mixed with other allergens but rather given by separate injection. In contrast, fungal extracts can be included within the same vial for some suppliers' SLIT formulations.

Anaphylactic reactions to injections. In humans, anaphylactic reactions to SLIT formulations are much less common than reactions to injections. In animals, SLIT formulations can be safely used even in pets that have had reactions to injection ASIT; the supplier should be advised of this history, because a modified administration schedule may be recommended for such patients.

History of failure of injection ASIT. For pets that have experienced no clinical benefit from injection immunotherapy, SLIT still can be considered. A substantial number of "injection failure" dogs improve with SLIT.

SLIT, Sublingual immunotherapy.

suggest that individualized ASIT based on specific allergy testing is associated with a higher success rate than other approaches.

Sublingual Immunotherapy

Sublingual immunotherapy (SLIT) involves administration of allergen extract into the oral cavity, under the tongue, instead of by injection. It is commonly used in Europe for treatment of human allergy, atopic rhinitis, and asthma, and response rates are similar to those with subcutaneous ASIT. Conflicting reports of efficacy may be explained in part by the extreme variation in protocols used for dose, dosing interval, administration method, and vehicle in the different studies reported. Its use in animals is very new, and only recently has it become widely available for veterinary use.

SLIT protocols often use glycerin-preserved extracts (not phenol-saline extracts) or special vehicles that protect and preserve allergen molecules from degradation at room temperature and from degradation by proteases. The extract is dispensed into the mouth or under the tongue to provide contact with oral mucosa. Typical protocols involve very frequent administration, even several times daily.

The mechanism of SLIT differs from that of injection immunotherapy because of the unique characteristics of oromucosal dendritic cells and induction of immunologic tolerance. SLIT has the additional benefit of nearly complete freedom from the dangers of anaphylactic reactions.

Recent trials of SLIT in dogs have demonstrated that this treatment holds great promise; its use has not yet been studied in cats, although it is likely to be beneficial in this species. An initial pilot study by the author in mite-sensitive dogs found that clinical improvement occurred in the majority of dogs and was accompanied by reductions in mite allergen–specific IgE and increases in allergen-specific IgG. Further experience in several hundred atopic dogs has led the author to conclude that SLIT is effective in approximately 60% of patients, comparable to expectations for injection ASIT. SLIT is effective in a substantial percentage of patients who have experienced no improvement from traditional allergy shots and can be used safely in patients that have had anaphylactic reactions to subcutaneous ASIT. SLIT is well accepted by dogs and owners, and ease of administration will make SLIT an attractive treatment option (Box 93-3).

Success, Monitoring, and Follow-up Examinations

Regardless of the protocol chosen, it is critical to perform regular recheck examinations during the first year of ASIT. During these examinations, flare factors (infections, parasites, potential for exposure to food allergens, and seasonal increases in exposure) should be identified and addressed. Additionally, potential adverse reactions should be evaluated and the injection schedule and any concurrent medications adjusted as necessary. Successful ASIT is a long-term project, and it is important to set the client's expectations appropriately. ASIT takes time to work and typically is only part of an overall management plan.

Because response to ASIT occurs gradually over months, it is often necessary to provide temporary concurrent medication to provide immediate relief. Treatment with topical or oral corticosteroids or cyclosporine can be instituted along with ASIT without fear of interference with efficacy. At each recheck examination, as response to ASIT occurs, concurrent medication should be tapered and eventually discontinued.

The total length of ASIT treatment varies; many patients show improvement within 3 to 6 months, although 12 months is recommended to assess efficacy completely. If after 12 months of treatment there has been no improvement, therapy can be stopped. If treatment is effective, treatment is continued for 2 to 3 years before stopping is considered. In some cases, treatment can be stopped with prolonged benefit; other patients may require lifelong maintenance dosing.

References and Suggested Reading

Akdis CA, Akdis M: Mechanisms of allergen-specific immunotherapy, *J Allergy Clin Immunol* 127(1):18, 2011.

Loewenstein C, Mueller RS: A review of allergen-specific immunotherapy in human and veterinary medicine, *Vet Dermatol* 20(2):84, 2009.

Olivry T et al: Treatment of canine atopic dermatitis: 2010 clinical practice guidelines from the International Task Force on Canine Atopic Dermatitis, *Vet Dermatol* 21(3):233, 2010.

CHAPTER 94

Systemic Glucocorticoids in Dermatology

LAUREN RIESTER PINCHBECK, *Wilton, Connecticut*

Glucocorticoids (GCs) have a pivotal role in the effective treatment of many dermatologic diseases, but indiscriminate use and misuse of these drugs is common. Every effort should be made to use GCs judiciously and strategically to minimize the risk of adverse effects. Clinical benefits should be considered in light of the potential risks.

Effects of Glucocorticoids on the Immune System

Antiinflammatory actions are the most important therapeutic benefit of GCs; they decrease tissue *responses* to inflammation without affecting the *cause* of inflammation. GCs affect humoral and cell-mediated immune systems, but immunosuppressive actions are more pronounced on cell-mediated immunity. GCs inhibit phospholipase A_2 and the conversion of arachidonic acid to prostaglandin and leukotriene metabolites, suppress bacteriocidal and fungicidal actions of macrophages, decrease production of intracellular signaling cytokines, decrease expression of inflammatory cytokines, and increase expression of antiinflammatory cytokines.

Structure of Glucocorticoids

Orally administered GCs are formulated as a free base or an ester that is converted to a free base. The free base is absorbed, and its structure determines duration of action. Biologic half-life and duration of action are longer for high-potency GCs and for higher doses of administered GCs. These factors increase the risk of adverse effects. Injectable GCs are esters of acetate, diacetate, sodium phosphate, or sodium succinate. Parenteral sodium phosphate and sodium succinate esters are very soluble, attain serum levels quickly, and are metabolized rapidly. Acetate or diacetate esters are poorly water soluble and are absorbed and metabolized slowly; such repositol formulations provide prolonged therapeutic benefits but increase the risk of adverse effects.

Cortisone is converted in the liver to its active form, cortisol. Hydrocortisone is identical to cortisol and has a short duration of action (<12 hours) and low potency. The relative potency of synthetic GCs traditionally is compared with that of hydrocortisone. Prednisone, which is four times as potent as cortisol, is inactive and requires hydroxylation in the liver to the active form, prednisolone, which has an intermediate duration of action (12 to 36 hours). Methylprednisolone is formed by the addition of a methyl group to prednisolone at the C-6 position, which decreases salt-retaining effects and increases GC effects. Methylprednisolone is five times as potent as hydrocortisone and has an intermediate duration of action (12 to 36 hours). When given as the injectable acetate salt, the duration of effect is 3 to 6 weeks. Triamcinolone acetonide is a fluorinated synthetic GC with four to five times the potency of hydrocortisone but has no appreciable mineralocorticoid activity because of methylation at position C-16. Its duration of action is longer than 48 hours. Dexamethasone (30 times as potent as hydrocortisone) and betamethasone (25 to 30 times as potent as hydrocortisone) are other fluorinated synthetic GCs with potent GC effects and prolonged duration of action (48 hours). They demonstrate low mineralocorticoid activity.

Use of Glucocorticoids

Table 94-1 is a guideline to dosages of synthetic GCs commonly used in veterinary dermatology. Although sources often suggest twice-daily administration, the author prescribes oral GCs once daily in dogs and cats. It may be common to use injectable GCs in primary care practice, but the author rarely recommends this route because it does not allow for dosage adjustments or withdrawal in the event of severe adverse effects. Injectable GCs should be used only after careful consideration and when a patient shows no response to oral GCs.

Cats seem to tolerate GCs better than dogs. Dosages for cats also generally are higher because cats have fewer GC receptors and weaker receptor-binding affinity. In addition, cats may differ from dogs in the rate of GC metabolism or extent of oral absorption. A recent study demonstrated that cats do not absorb prednisone or do not convert prednisone to prednisolone effectively. Thus *prednisolone,* not prednisone, should be used in cats. In cats, the author finds dexamethasone to be effective for pruritic and inflammatory skin diseases.

In dogs, oral methylprednisolone often is substituted for prednisone if polyuria and polydipsia become problematic. These adverse effects seemingly are less dramatic with oral methylprednisolone. If a cat does not tolerate oral administration of prednisolone or dexamethasone, methylprednisolone acetate may be considered for pruritic or inflammatory skin diseases. It is recommended that this GC be administered no more often than every 2 months, with a maximum of three or four injections per year.

Common Indications for Glucocorticoid Use in Dermatology

Pruritus is a very common presenting problem, and there are numerous diseases for which it is the primary symptom. To manage pruritus in the dog or cat, one must identify, treat, and manage the primary disease(s). However, systemic GCs may be necessary to provide the patient relief from pruritus while one works toward a definitive diagnosis.

Acute-Onset Severe Pruritus

Examples of acute-onset severe pruritus are pyotraumatic dermatitis and by fleabite hypersensitivity. An initial reduction of inflammation may be achieved with an antiinflammatory dose of prednisone every 24 hours for 3 to 7 days with tapering over 2 weeks.

Canine Atopic Dermatitis

Treatment of Exacerbations
Patients with canine atopic dermatitis (CAD) may experience acute or seasonal flares in pruritus. For flares that are not attributable to other causes (such as secondary bacterial or yeast infections), a short antiinflammatory "crisis buster" course of prednisone every 24 hours for 3 days typically results in 7 to 14 days of relief from pruritus. Some dogs require 1 to 4 weeks of alternate-day antipruritic doses of prednisone following the initial 3 days of treatment to get through a seasonal exacerbation. The author also uses the combination of trimeprazine and prednisolone (Temaril-P) for similar purposes; the dosage is based on the prednisolone component (2 mg/tablet).

Long-Term Management
Numerous studies have demonstrated the effectiveness of low-dose oral GCs for control of pruritus and lesions in CAD. The effectiveness of long-acting injectable GC formulations for treatment of CAD has not been established in controlled trials, and such formulations should not be used for long-term management. For dogs with moderate to severe CAD, a comprehensive management plan should be devised, but systemic GCs may be one component. Antipruritic dosages of prednisone should be given orally every 24 hours and should be tapered to the lowest effective alternate-day dose. Oral methylprednisolone is another option but typically is more costly. Temaril-P also may be used for this purpose.

Pruritus Associated with Cutaneous Infection

If bacterial folliculitis or yeast dermatitis is a concurrent problem, the aim should be to treat the secondary infection without the use of GCs. This will establish whether treating the infection alone reduces pruritus. If GCs are administered concurrently with antimicrobials and pruritus is reduced, one does not know if the improvement is due to the GC or to satisfactory treatment of infection. If the situation warrants, a short 3-day course of prednisone (prednisolone in cats) at an antiinflammatory dosage may be prescribed to alleviate pruritus while topical and

TABLE 94-1
Canine and Feline Dosages of Glucocorticoids Commonly Used in Veterinary Dermatology

Glucocorticoid (Species)	Antipruritic	Taper	Antiinflammatory	Taper	Immunosuppressive	Taper
Prednisone/prednisolone (dog)	0.5-1 mg/kg q24h PO for 3-10 days	Over days to weeks to 0.25-0.5 mg/kg or lowest effective q48h PO	1-1.5 mg/kg q24h PO for 7-14 days	Over days to weeks to lowest effective q48h	2.2-6.6 mg/kg q24h PO to remission (2-3 wk)	Over weeks to months to 0.5-1 mg/kg q48h PO
Prednisolone (cat)	1-2 mg/kg q24h PO for 3-10 days	Over days to weeks to lowest effective q48-72h	2-3 mg/kg q24h PO for 7-14 days	Over days to weeks to lowest effective q48-72h	2-4 mg/kg q24h PO to remission (2-3 wk)	Over weeks to months to lowest effective q48-96h
Methylprednisolone (dog)	0.4-0.8 mg/kg q24h PO for 3-10 days	Over days to weeks to lowest effective q48h	1-2 mg/kg q24h PO	Over days to weeks to lowest effective q48h	0.8-2.4 mg/kg q24h PO to remission (2-3 wk)	Over weeks to months 0.4-0.8 mg/kg q48h PO
Methylprednisolone (cat)	2-4 mg per cat (or 0.8-2.0 mg/kg) q24h PO for 3-10 days	Over days to weeks to lowest effective q48-72h	2-4 mg per cat (or 0.8-2.0 mg/kg) q24h PO	Over days to weeks to lowest effective q48-72 h	Not recommended	
Methylprednisolone acetate (cat)	5 mg/kg SC (20 mg per cat)	Not applicable	5 mg/kg SC (20 mg per cat)	Not applicable	Not recommended	Not applicable
Dexamethasone (dog)	0.25-0.5 mg IV or IM or 0.25-0.5 mg PO q24h	Not applicable	0.5-1 mg IV/IM or 0.25-1 mg PO q24h	Not applicable	0.1-0.2 mg/kg q24h PO to remission (2-3 wk)	Over weeks to months to 0.05-0.1 mg/kg q2-7d
Dexamethasone (cat)	0.125-0.5 mg per cat q24h PO	Over days to weeks to q72h	0.1-0.2 mg/kg q24h PO (up to 1 mg per cat q24h PO)	Over days to weeks to q48-72h	0.1-0.2 mg/kg q12-24h PO to remission (2-3 wk)	Over weeks to 0.05-1 mg/kg q2-7d PO
Triamcinolone (dog)	Not recommended	Not applicable	0.05-0.1 mg/kg q24h PO	To 0.028 mg/kg q24-72h	0.1-0.3 mg/kg q24h PO to remission (2-3 wk)	Over weeks to 0.1-0.2 mg/kg q48-72h PO
Triamcinolone injectable (dog)	0.11-0.22 mg/kg SC/IM	Not applicable	0.11-0.22 mg/kg SC/IM	Not applicable	Not recommended	Not applicable
Triamcinolone (cat)	0.25-0.4 mg/kg PO for 3-10 days	Over days to weeks to q72h or less	0.25-0.75 mg/kg PO for 3-10 days	Over weeks to q72h or less	0.3-1 mg/kg q24h PO to remission (2-3 wk)	Over weeks to 0.6-1 mg/kg q2-7d PO
Triamcinolone injectable (cat)	0.11-0.22 mg/kg SC/IM	Not applicable	0.11-0.22 mg/kg SC/IM	Not applicable	Not recommended	Not applicable

PO, Orally; IM, intramuscularly; IV, intravenously; SC, subcutaneously.

systemic antimicrobials are instituted and then continued beyond the completion of GC treatment.

Nonpruritic Inflammatory Skin Disease

Nonpruritic inflammatory skin conditions include sterile nodular panniculitis, idiopathic sterile granulomapyogranuloma syndrome, cutaneous cellulitis or vasculitis, eosinophilic folliculitis and furunculosis, and juvenile cellulitis. Systemic GC administration typically is required to achieve remission of disease. Treatment should start with antiinflammatory dosages of prednisone every 24 hours for 2 to 3 weeks and then the patient should be reevaluated. If remission is achieved in that time, the GC should be tapered until signs resolve or until the patient is on the lowest alternate-day dosage that can be sustained. If remission is not achieved in that time, one should ensure that the diagnosis is correct and consider increasing the dose of GC or adding a second antiinflammatory medication.

Autoimmune Skin Diseases

Systemic GCs almost always are required for the treatment of autoimmune diseases such as pemphigus foliaceus. The goal is to induce remission with orally administered GCs and taper to the lowest alternate-day dosage that maintains lesion control and is tolerated by the patient. Treatment should be initiated with immunosuppressive dosages of prednisone (prednisolone in cats) every 24 hours for 2 to 3 weeks and then the patient should be reevaluated. If remission is achieved within that time, the dosage should be decreased by 25% to 50% on alternate days every 7 to 14 days until the immunosuppressive dosage is being administered every 48 hours. Then this dosage should be tapered further until the lowest effective alternate-day dose that controls lesions or a target dose of 0.5 mg/kg of prednisone every 48 hours is reached. If remission is not achieved with prednisone monotherapy within this period, the diagnosis should be confirmed and the addition of a second immunosuppressive agent (see Chapter 59) should be considered. Rarely, a different GC may be selected; oral dexamethasone would be the author's second choice in these circumstances.

Otitis

In dogs, systemic GCs have a role in the initial management of severe acute inflammatory or infectious otitis externa, and antiinflammatory dosages of prednisone to reverse inflammation over 3 to 7 days may be prescribed. At the recheck, the ear canal should be examined by otoscope for masses, foreign bodies, and so on. Reduction of inflammation increases the likelihood that pet owners will be able to instill topical otic therapies successfully. The author also routinely prescribes a systemic GC for its value as a prognostic indicator in dogs that have chronic otitis externa with severe canal stenosis to help assess the reversibility of pathologic changes in the ear. Antiinflammatory dosages of prednisone should be prescribed for 2 to 3 weeks followed by reevaluation. If this dosage does

not reduce the severity of stenosis and otoscopic examination is still impossible, medical therapy will be unlikely to reverse the pathologic changes sufficiently to allow for effective medical management. Total ear canal ablation with bulla osteotomy is the preferred treatment option in this case. Systemic GCs also may be prescribed in patients with chronic otitis that are going to be evaluated for otitis media; if the canal epithelium is severely inflamed, passage of a handheld or video otoscopy unit for an extended time to clean, flush, and evaluate the ear may result in epithelial swelling that limits visualization of the tympanic membrane.

Adverse Effects

Systemic adverse effects attributable to GC administration (e.g., Cushing's syndrome) are described at length elsewhere. In the skin, GCs cause dermal, epidermal, and follicular atrophy; predisposition to bruising; and poor wound healing. Effects on adnexal structures may result in a dull and coarse hair coat, alopecia, comedones, milia, and calcinosis cutis. Localized dermal and adnexal atrophy following subcutaneous and intramuscular administration of repositol GCs also have been reported, especially when the drugs are administered subcutaneously. GCs may facilitate the establishment and spread of opportunistic infections (e.g., dermatophytosis and deep fungal infections) or increase susceptibility to bacterial infections. If symptoms or lesions change during GC use, the pet should be evaluated for new infections or the development of iatrogenic demodicosis.

Although, as noted earlier, cats are perceived to tolerate GCs better than dogs, they may experience transient or severe life-threatening adverse effects. Feline skin fragility syndrome is a characteristic cutaneous sign of hyperadrenocorticism. The skin becomes paper thin, translucent, and friable and is easily damaged or bruised. Exogenous GC administration has been associated with induction of diabetes mellitus because as GCs are hyperglycemic agents and cause insulin resistance in cats. In cats with subclinical or undiagnosed cardiomyopathy administration of GCs, especially repositol GC preparations, may cause an increase in plasma volume resulting in heart failure.

Contraindications

GC administration should be avoided when ulcerogenic nonsteroidal antiinflammatory drugs (NSAIDs) are being used (e.g., to treat arthritis). The use of GCs in patients with the following conditions is either contraindicated or relatively contraindicated (i.e., reference sources should be consulted and GCs used with caution): diabetes mellitus, pancreatitis, certain cardiovascular diseases (e.g., feline cardiomyopathies), certain infections (e.g., dermatophytosis or deep fungal diseases), some parasitic diseases (e.g., demodicosis), some ocular diseases (e.g., corneal ulceration, glaucoma, cataracts), renal insufficiency, systemic hypertension, pulmonary hypertension, and hyperadrenocorticism. Caution should be taken in patients with seizure disorders because GCs may lower the seizure threshold. GCs should be used sparingly in puppies and kittens and should be avoided in pregnant females.

Monitoring

For most patients that are otherwise healthy, physical examination and review of concurrent medications are sufficient before short-term administration of oral GCs at antipruritic or antiinflammatory dosages. If the primary disease necessitates long-term administration of antipruritic or antiinflammatory dosages of an oral GC, at least quarterly examination of the patient and evaluation by performing a complete blood count (CBC) and serum biochemistry studies is indicated. For patients that require immunosuppressive dosages of oral GCs, physical examination, CBC, and serum biochemistry panel are indicated before GC therapy is initiated and every 2 to 3 weeks during induction. Once the GC dosage is reduced (maintenance), the monitoring interval can be lengthened to every 3 months.

For all patients receiving long-term GC therapy, urine culture is indicated every 6 months to ensure that a subclinical urinary tract infection (UTI) has not developed. The author generally does not perform urinalysis unless indicated by the results of the serum biochemistry testing (e.g., hyperglycemia or azotemia). The antiinflammatory properties of GCs make identification of UTI by urinalysis alone difficult. In one study, 39% of dogs receiving long-term GC therapy developed UTIs. Dogs with infection had minimal to no clinical signs, and urinalyses did not necessarily reveal pyuria or bacteriuria. In another study evaluating pruritic dogs that received GCs for longer than 6 months, 18.1% were identified as having a UTI at least once based on culture results. None exhibited clinical signs. Overall, 12.1% of urine cultures demonstrated bacterial growth. The authors concluded that UTIs would be missed in 5% to 10% of dogs receiving

long-term GC treatment if urinalysis alone were used for detection.

Monitoring protocols are similar for cats. However, before medium- to long-term GC therapy is instituted, the cat should be evaluated to make sure it does not have preexisting cardiovascular disease and is not at risk of diabetes mellitus, pancreatitis, or hepatic lipidosis. If signs develop that suggest the emergence of a previously latent infectious disease (e.g., toxoplasmosis, herpesvirus infection), the cat should be evaluated fully. CBC and serum biochemistry studies should be performed quarterly if GCs are used for extended periods.

References and Suggested Reading

Boothe DW: *Small animal clinical pharmacology and therapeutics,* ed 2, Philadelphia, 2011, Saunders.
Freedman ND, Yamamoto KR: Importin 7 and importin α/importin β are nuclear import receptors for the glucocorticoid receptor, *Mol Biol Cell* 15:2276, 2004.
Graham-Mize CA, Rosser EJ, Hauptman J: Absorption, bioavailability and activity of prednisone and prednisolone in cats. In Hillier A, Foster AP, Kwochka KW, editors: *Advances in veterinary dermatology,* vol 5, Oxford, UK, 2005, Blackwell, p 152.
Ihrke PJ et al: Urinary tract infection associated with long-term corticosteroid administration in dogs with chronic skin disease, *J Am Vet Med Assoc* 186:43, 1985.
Lowe AD et al: A pilot study comparing diabetogenic effects of dexamethasone and prednisolone in cats, *J Am Anim Hosp Assoc* 45:215, 2009.
Lowe AD, Campbell KL, Graves TK: Glucocorticoids in the cat, *Vet Dermatol* 19:340, 2008.
Ployngam T et al: Hemodynamic effects of methylprednisolone acetate administration in cats, *Am J Vet Res* 67(4):583, 2006.
Torres SMF et al: Frequency of urinary tract infection among dogs with pruritic disorders receiving long-term glucocorticoid treatment, *J Am Vet Med Assoc* 227:239, 2005.
Van den Broek AH, Stafford WL: Epidermal and hepatic glucocorticoid receptors in cats and dogs, *Res Vet Sci* 52(3):312, 1992.

CHAPTER 95

Topical Therapy for Pruritus

WAYNE S. ROSENKRANTZ, *Tustin, California*

The use of topical therapeutics for pruritus in the form of shampoos, lotions, rinses, soaks, and spot-on products has gained increasing popularity. Topical treatment for pruritus can be used as sole therapy or as an adjunctive therapy, reducing the need for systemic treatment. Owner compliance can be a problem, although many owners want to participate actively in the management of their pet's skin condition.

Familiarity with available products is important, and personal use of products on one's own pets provides experience and insight, and constitutes a powerful recommendation to your clients. The frequency of application is patient and disease dependent; typically, applications as often as once daily are required. Contact time may be important for the best efficacy, and it is critical to know which products can be left on and which require complete rinsing to avoid irritation.

Specific Antipruritic Agents

Water

Water has therapeutic antipruritic properties, it moisturizes the skin, and when combined with emollients and moisturizing agents it can help maintain skin hydration and prevent transepidermal water loss. However, if used repeatedly without proper emollients and moisturizing agents, water also can dry out the skin by stripping its natural barriers. Decreased barrier function can lead to increased penetration of allergens, irritants, and infectious agents resulting in increased pruritus. In general, cool water is recommended for shampoo therapy, especially in cases of pruritic allergic skin disease.

Protectants and Moisturizing Agents

Protectants and moisturizing agents include oils and hygroscopic agents (vegetable oils, lanolin, phytosphingosine, propylene glycol, glycerin, colloidal oatmeal, urea, and lactic acid). Moisturizers increase the water content of the stratum corneum, are useful in hydrating and softening the skin, and work best if applied immediately after saturation of the stratum corneum with water. Formulations such as sprays and rinses that are left on are generally more effective than shampoos that are washed off (Table 95-1).

Substitution of Sensation and Topical Anesthetic Agents

Substituting another sensation such as heat or cold for pruritus is sometimes effective. Heat initially lowers the pruritic threshold, but if the heat is high enough and of sufficient duration, itching abates and a short-term antipruritic effect is induced. Examples of agents than can temporarily increase local heat are menthol 0.12% to 1% (Dermacool), camphor 0.12% to 5% (Caladryl), thymol 0.5% to 1%, and warm soaks. Cooling (cool or cold water baths, ice packs, cool dressings) also tends to decrease pruritus.

The peripheral nerves can be anesthetized by using local anesthetics such as pramoxine, benzocaine, tetracaine, lidocaine, benzoyl peroxide, and tars (see Table 95-1). These products generally have a short duration of action and rarely are effective in chronic pruritus.

Topical Antihistamines

Topical antihistamines have low efficacy for reduction of pruritus. A report of topical diphenhydramine treatment in dogs with atopic dermatitis showed reductions of 20.7% for pruritus, 27.6% for excoriation, 24.1% for erythema, and 24.1% for alopecia (Iwasaki and Hasegawa, 2006). Often topical antihistamines are combined with a colloidal oatmeal shampoo vehicle (Histacalm) or lotion (ResiHIST Leave-On Lotion; Caladryl [1% diphenhydramine with calamine and camphor]).

Topical Glucocorticoids

Topical glucocorticoids are valuable for treating localized pruritus. The potency of topical glucocorticoids depends on the class of glucocorticoid and the vehicle; the most potent are ointments, followed by creams, lotions, and gels. Glucocorticoids are typically rated on their antiinflammatory activity (Table 95-2).

In general, treatment should begin with a mid- to high-potency product applied twice daily until the pruritus is controlled, and then a less potent product should be used once daily. The author has used 1% hydrocortisone sprays (CortiSpray, CortiCalm, CLEAN 'N COOL) and leave-on conditioners, (ResiCORT) effectively. A low-dose 0.015% triamcinolone spray (Genesis) has been

TABLE 95-1

Selected Topical Nonsteroidal Antipruritic Agents

Active Ingredient	Formulation	Brand Name
Diphenhydramine 1%, calamine 8%, camphor	Lotion	Caladryl
Hamamelis extract, menthol	Spray	Dermacool
Aluminum sulfate, calcium acetate	Soak	Domeboro
Diphenhydramine 2%	Spray	Histacalm
Pramoxine 1%	Spray, lotion, shampoo, rinse	Relief Dermal-Soothe ResiPROX
Fatty acids (hemp seed and neem seed oils), emollients	Spot-on	Dermoscent Essential 6
Ceramides and fatty acids	Spot-on	Allerderm Spot-on
Phytosphingosine	Spot-on	Douxo Seborrhea Spot-on
Pimecrolimus	Cream	Elidel
Tacrolimus 0.1%	Cream	Protopic
Moisturizers, ceramides, and rhamnose	Shampoo	Allergroom Allermyl
Moisturizers and fatty acids	Shampoo, rinse	HyLyt efa
Encapsulated moisturizers	Shampoo, rinse	Hydra-Pearls
Moisturizers, coconut oil, and safflower oil	Shampoo, rinse	DermaHypoCS
Colloidal oatmeal	Shampoo, rinse, soak	Epi-Soothe Allay Oatmeal ResiSOOTHE Aveeno
Phytosphingosine, hinokitiol	Shampoo, spray	Douxo Calm
Diphenhydramine	Shampoo, spray	Histacalm

TABLE 95-2

Selected Topical Glucocorticoids

Active Ingredient and Formulation	Formulation	Brand Name
Group I: Ultrapotent		
Augmented betamethasone dipropionate 0.05%	Gel, ointment	Diprolene
Clobetasol propionate 0.05%	Gel, cream, ointment	Temovate
Group II: Potent		
Betamethasone dipropionate 0.05%	Ointment	Diprosone
Amcinonide 0.1%	Ointment	Cyclocort
Group III: Upper-Medium Strength		
Triamcinolone acetonide 0.5%	Cream	Kenalog
Amcinonide 0.1%	Lotion, cream	Cyclocort
Mometasone furoate 0.1%	Ointment	Mometamax* Posatex*
Group IV/V: Medium to Low Strength		
Fluocinolone acetonide 0.025%	Cream, ointment	Synalar*
Fluocinolone acetonide 0.01%	Solution	Synotic*
Triamcinolone acetonide 0.1%	Lotion, cream Ointment	Vetalog* Kenalog Animax* Derma-Vet* Forte Topical* Panolog*
Hydrocortisone aceponate 0.0584%	Solution	Cortavance*
Group VI: Low Strength		
Fluocinolone acetonide, 0.01%	Shampoo	FS Shampoo
Triamcinolone acetonide 0.015%	Spray	Genesis*
Dexamethasone 0.1%	Lotion	Tresaderm*
Group VII: Least Potent		
Hydrocortisone 1%	Spray Gel Shampoo Lotion Cream	CortiSpray* CLEAN 'N COOL* Dermacool HC* Hydro-Plus* Hydro-10 Mist* CortiCalm* Cortisoothe* SOOTHE 'N MOIST* ResiCORT* HEAL 'N SEAL*

*Veterinary formulation.

reported as more effective than the hydrocortisone-based products (DeBoer et al, 2002). However, when it is applied to the flanks and medial thighs, localized cutaneous atrophy reactions have been seen. Recently a hydrocortisone aceponate (HCA) product (Cortavance) has been released for use in dogs. HCA is a lipophilic diester with enhanced skin penetration but low plasma availability, which results in high local activity with reduced systemic secondary effects. However, visible skin atrophy in the axillary and inguinal regions with a significantly reduced dermal thickness has been reported (Bizikova et al, 2010). Initial studies show little impact of HCA on adrenocortical suppression.

Application of a more potent topical glucocorticoid (e.g., triamcinolone acetonide, dexamethasone) may cause iatrogenic Cushing's disease, adrenal suppression, and elevated liver enzyme levels. Thus client education and regulation of refills is important. Localized adverse reactions include cutaneous atrophy, comedone formation, folliculitis, poor healing, pigment changes, and suppression of local immune responses. Owners should wear gloves or use an applicator when treating their pets and immediately wash exposed skin after applying the medication. It is especially important to avoid contact with human facial skin because it is particularly sensitive to the effects of more potent topical glucocorticoids.

Topical Fatty Acids

Fatty acids are important in hydration and control of transepidermal water loss. The Dermoscent Essential 6 spot-on skin care product contains fatty acids, essential oils, and emollients that restore the epidermal barrier and thus maintain hydration and control transepidermal water loss. Preliminary evaluations indicate that this product may be useful for canine atopic dermatitis (Tretter and Mueller, 2010), and a recent double-blind placebo-controlled trial examining its use in the treatment of canine atopic dermatitis showed a significant difference in pretreatment and posttreatment Canine Atopic Dermatitis Extent and Severity Index (CADESI) and Pruritus Visual Analogue Scale (PVAS) scores (Blaskovic et al, 2012).

Allerderm Spot-On contains a skin lipid complex consisting of a blend of ceramides and fatty acids. Reports on this product suggest benefits in the treatment of allergic skin conditions due to its effects in improving epidermal barrier function by stimulating the production and secretion of endogenous stratum corneum lipids (Piekutowska et al, 2008).

Phytosphingosine is a component of ceramides (key lipids in the skin), which maintain stratum corneum cohesion, control local flora, and maintain the correct moisture balance. Ceramide-based products are used effectively to treat human atopic dermatitis (Na et al, 2010). A product with phytosphingosine (Douxo Seborrhea Spot-on) is available for animals, but blinded controlled studies of its efficacy have yet to be reported.

Topical Immunomodulating Agents

Tacrolimus (Protopic) is a calcineurin inhibitor similar in action to cyclosporine (see Chapter 92) and is approved for treatment of atopic dermatitis in humans. In canine atopic dermatitis, one study reported a decrease in severity of symptoms, and dogs with localized disease responded better than dogs with generalized disease (Marsella et al, 2004). In another study in atopic dogs, tacrolimus ointment decreased the severity of localized lesions of canine atopic dermatitis by 50% or more in 15 of 20 dogs (Bensignor and Olivry, 2005). A black box warning from the U.S. Food and Drug Administration regarding the potential risk of neoplasia has made patients and physicians uncertain about its safety, although current data do not support increased concern regarding risk of malignancy (Thaci and Salgo, 2007). Because of this concern, it is recommended that veterinary clients apply the product with gloves.

Pimecrolimus (Elidel) is an ascomycin macrolactam derivative that acts similarly to tacrolimus (see Chapter 59). In human patients, pimecrolimus is less skin permeable than tacrolimus and much less so than corticosteroids, which results in a lower risk of systemic effects. Anecdotal reports have suggested efficacy similar to or lower than that of tacrolimus. As with tacrolimus, there is some controversy about whether pimecrolimus promotes malignancies in humans, and it is recommended that owners wear gloves when applying it.

References and Suggested Reading

Bensignor E, Olivry T: Treatment of localized lesions of canine atopic dermatitis with tacrolimus ointment: a blinded randomized controlled trial, *Vet Dermatol* 16(1):52, 2005.

Blaskovic M et al: The effect of a spot on formulation containing fatty acids and essential oils (Essential 6, Dermoscent, LDCA, France) on dogs with canine atopic dermatitis, *Vet Dermatol* 23(Suppl 1):4, 2012.

Bizikova P et al: Effect of a novel topical diester glucocorticoid spray on immediate- and late-phase cutaneous allergic reactions in Maltese-beagle atopic dogs: a placebo-controlled study, *Vet Dermatol* 21(1):70, 2010.

DeBoer DJ et al: Multiple-center study of reduced-concentration triamcinolone topical solution for the treatment of dogs with known or suspected allergic pruritus, *Am J Vet Res* 63(3):408, 2002.

Iwasaki T, Hasegawa A: A randomized comparative clinical trial of recombinant canine interferon-gamma (KT-100) in atopic dogs using antihistamine as control, *Vet Dermatol* 17(3):195, 2006.

Marsella R: Calcineurin inhibitors: a novel approach to canine atopic dermatitis, *J Am Anim Hosp Assoc* 41(2):92, 2005.

Marsella R et al: Investigation on the clinical efficacy and safety of 0.1% tacrolimus ointment (Protopic) in canine atopic dermatitis: a randomized, double-blinded, placebo-controlled, cross-over study, *Vet Dermatol* 15(5):294, 2004.

Na JI et al: A new moisturizer containing physiologic lipid granules alleviates atopic dermatitis, *J Dermatolog Treat* 21(1):23, 2010.

Piekutowska A et al: Effects of a topically applied preparation of epidermal lipids on the stratum corneum barrier of atopic dogs, *J Comp Pathol* 138(4):197, 2008.

Reme C: Introduction to Cortavance: a topical diester glucocorticoid developed for veterinary dermatology. Paper presented at the Virbac International Derm Symposium: Advances in Topical Glucocorticoid Therapy, Nice, France, 2007.

Shimada K et al: Transepidermal water loss (TEWL) reflects skin barrier function of dog, *J Vet Med Sci* 70(8):841, 2008.

Thaci D, Salgo R: The topical calcineurin inhibitor pimecrolimus in atopic dermatitis: a safety update, *Acta Dermatovenerol Alp Panonica Adriat* 16(2):58, 2007.

Tretter S, Mueller R: The influence of topical unsaturated fatty acids and essential oils on normal and atopic dogs—a pilot study. Paper presented at the North American Veterinary Dermatology Forum, Portland, Oregon, 2010.

CHAPTER 96

Elimination Diets for Cutaneous Adverse Food Reactions: Principles in Therapy

HILARY A. JACKSON, *Glasgow, Scotland*

Indications for and Use of Elimination Diets

Elimination diets are designed primarily for the diagnosis and management of adverse reactions to food ingredients in dogs and cats. The following definitions are used in this discussion:

- *Adverse food reaction:* any clinically abnormal response attributable to the ingestion of food or food additive
- *Food intolerance:* an abnormal physiologic response to food with no immunologic basis
- *Food allergy:* an immunologically mediated adverse food reaction

The ideal elimination diet used in the diagnosis and management of adverse food reactions should contain an ingredient that is either novel to the animal or in a form that does not incite an adverse response. Commercially available diets generally are designed for the management of true food allergy and thus often are referred to as *hypoallergenic diets,* although the incidence of immunologically mediated disease in the dog and cat currently is unknown. In humans most food allergies are mediated by immunoglobulin E (IgE) antibodies (Sampson, 2004), and many food allergens have been characterized at the molecular level; however, those inciting specific reactions in dogs and cats are largely unknown. Food allergens in humans generally are glycoproteins with a molecular weight of more than 10,000 D because smaller molecules are less likely to bridge IgE molecules on the mast cell surface and incite a hypersensitivity reaction. The currently available commercial elimination diets contain either novel or hydrolyzed proteins with added carbohydrate and nutrients to balance the diet for long-term feeding. It is assumed that the dietary protein is the allergenic substance, although there is a report of dogs with spontaneous food allergy reacting to cornstarch (Jackson et al, 2003). This chapter considers a number of key issues related to elimination diets.

Novel Protein Diets

Most novel protein diets have one carbohydrate and one protein source. After a detailed history of the patient's diet is reviewed, a trial diet with a novel protein is selected on the assumption that the protein has not been fed before. This approach does assume complete recall by the owner of all diets, foods, and treats to which the patient has been exposed. It also assumes that commercial diets are not contaminated with foreign proteins, which may not necessarily be the case (Raditic et al, 2011). A recent study found that three out of three over-the-counter limited-antigen diets tested positive for soy protein and one quarter tested positive for beef protein; neither soy nor beef was on any of the diet ingredient lists (Raditic et al, 2011). The presence of cross-reacting protein epitopes in different foods may also be a factor. For example, if the author is treating a patient with chicken intolerance, then intolerance to other poultry meats is considered possible, and turkey- or duck-based diets also are avoided.

Hydrolyzed Protein Diets

Hydrolyzed protein diets are available for humans, specifically for the management of infants with milk allergy. Hydrolyzed protein is available as either a partial or a complete hydrolysate. Before a claim of hypoallergenicity can be made, the complete hydrolysate formula should be demonstrated to be tolerated by 90% or more of infants with milk allergy in double-blind, placebo-controlled conditions (Baker et al, 2000). Complete milk protein hydrolysates have free amino acids and peptides of less than 1500 D, whereas partially hydrolyzed formulations are not hydrolyzed as extensively. The hydrolyzed veterinary diets available at the time of this writing would be classified as partial hydrolysates. Typically these include common sources of protein such as chicken or soy. A newer product on the market based on feather protein represents both a novel and a highly hydrolyzed protein source.

Only a small number of studies have been performed to address the issue of whether these diets are clinically effective and have reduced immunogenicity in the food-allergic animal. These studies have been reviewed by Olivry and Bizikova (2009), who concluded that there was limited evidence of reduced immunologic and clinical allergenicity in dogs with suspected adverse food reactions; furthermore, between 20% and 50% of dogs actually experienced a worsening of clinical signs when fed these diets.

Additionally, these diets are recommended for the treatment of canine and feline adverse food reactions based on the assumption that most adverse food reactions in these species are mediated by IgE, as they are in humans. Since this is not necessarily the case, the size of the protein hydrolysate may not be critical or, paradoxically, hydrolysis could enhance uptake and presentation to the immune system.

Home-Cooked Diets

Home-cooked diets often are advocated to avoid pet food additives that may cause adverse reactions, although there are no well-documented reports to support this idea. Home-cooked diets usually include a single novel protein and a single carbohydrate source, which have been selected on the basis of a dietary history. Home-cooked diets often are nutritionally inadequate for maintenance or growth, and clinicians must use recipes available in textbooks (Remillard and Crane, 2010) or the services of a diplomate in veterinary nutrition (see www.acvn.org) to create balanced diets. In one study, 36% of clients preparing home-cooked food for their dogs discontinued the diet trial prematurely (Tapp et al, 2002). Another study documented a failure rate of 52% of clients, although the failure rate dropped to 27% after better client education was instituted (Chesney, 2002), which emphasizes the importance of client communication if home-cooked diets are used.

A small number of animals may tolerate a home-cooked diet but not a commercial equivalent (White, 1986; White and Sequoia, 1989). The reasons for this are unknown but may relate to processing, which may render proteins more or less allergenic. Food additives or the presence of vasoactive amines in commercial diets also might be causative. There has been recent interest on the part of the pet-owning public in the feeding of raw-meat diets to their pets. There is no justification for the use of these diets from the standpoint of diagnosis or management of the pet with food allergies. Furthermore, the use of these diets raises significant public health concerns related to the high bacterial burden often present in raw meat.

Diet Selection

Selection of the diet for the trial is based on a thorough dietary history, including the main diet and any treats, table scraps, and flavored toothpaste or toys to which the animal is exposed. The selected protein should be one to which the animal has had little or no previous exposure. Clients often must be informed that they cannot hide pills in food unless the food is part of the selected dietary trial.

For giant-breed dogs younger than 12 months of age, the advice of a nutritionist should be sought to ensure that calcium:phosphorus ratios adequately support rapid skeletal growth. Elimination diets specially formulated for the growing dog are available, and these should be fed preferentially. In the feline patient, home-cooked diets usually are inadequate in taurine and rarely are balanced for minerals and vitamins; thus advice should be sought if long-term feeding is required.

Duration of the Trial Diet

An elimination diet trial of 6 weeks is appropriate in many cases, but a longer trial may be required. In a study performed by Rosser (1993) 13 of 51 dogs required longer than 6 weeks on an elimination diet to achieve maximal improvement. The majority of published studies have included dogs with additional hypersensitivities such as atopic dermatitis or flea allergies in which pruritus and clinical signs might be expected to fluctuate daily or seasonally, and resolution of pruritus is unlikely to occur in these cases. These factors confound evaluation of a diet trial in a clinical setting, and in practice the length of the diet trial will vary in individual cases. Thus, in patients with additional hypersensitivities, only a partial response to an elimination diet may occur. Notwithstanding, a diagnosis of an adverse food reaction can be made only if the animal shows relapse in response to challenge with previously fed foods.

Additional Benefits of Elimination Diets

Since most of the commercially available hypoallergenic diets have an enhanced omega-3 and omega-6 essential fatty acid content, they can be useful in the management of dogs with impaired epidermal barrier structure or function such as has been found in some dogs with atopic dermatitis. Thus supplementation with omega-6 fatty acid has the potential to enhance skin health in dogs with atopic dermatitis. Omega-3 essential fatty acids have anti-inflammatory potential, although a definitive reduction in pruritus associated with their supplementation has not been demonstrated.

References and Suggested Reading

Baker SS et al: Elimination infant formulas, *Pediatrics* 106:346, 2000.

Chesney CJ: Food sensitivity in the dog, a quantitative study, *J Small Anim Pract* 43:203, 2002.

Jackson HA et al: Evaluation of the clinical and allergen specific serum IgE responses to oral challenge with cornstarch, corn, soy and a soy hydrolysate in dogs with spontaneous food allergy, *Vet Dermatol* 14:181, 2003.

Olivry T, Bizikova P: A systematic review of the evidence of reduced allergenicity and clinical benefit of food hydrolysates in dogs with cutaneous adverse food reactions, *Vet Dermatol* 21:32, 2009.

Raditic DM, Remillard RL, Tater KC: ELISA testing for common food antigens in four dry dog foods used in dietary elimination trials, *J Anim Physiol Anim Nutr (Berl)* 95(1):90, 2011.

Remillard RL, Crane S: Making pet foods at home. In Hand MS et al, editors: *Small animal clinical nutrition*, Topeka, KS, 2010, Mark Morris Institute, p 207.

Rosser EJ: Diagnosis of food allergy in dogs, *J Am Vet Med Assoc* 203:259, 1993.

Sampson HA: Update on food allergy, *J Allergy Clin Immunol* 113:805, 2004.

Tapp TC et al: Comparison of a commercial limited-antigen diet versus home-prepared diets in the diagnosis of canine adverse food reaction, *Vet Ther* 3:244, 2002.

White SD: Food hypersensitivity in 30 dogs, *J Am Vet Med Assoc* 188:695, 1986.

White SD, Sequoia D: Food hypersensitivity in cats: 14 cases (1982-1987), *J Am Vet Med Assoc* 194:692, 1989.

CHAPTER 97

Flea Control in Flea Allergy Dermatitis

ROBERT ALLEN KENNIS, *Auburn, Alabama*
ANDREW HILLIER, *Columbus, Ohio*

Flea infestations within a home or outdoor environment can be a constant or recurring problem for humans and their pets. Although many pets experience flea bite dermatitis, some also may develop flea allergy dermatitis. The most common flea found in North America is the cat flea, *Ctenocephalides felis felis,* which affects dogs and cats as well as nondomestic wildlife such as opossums, raccoons, skunks, foxes, and coyotes. Wildlife can be a problematic continual reservoir of fleas for domestic pets that may be challenging to eliminate or control. The purpose of this chapter is to provide guidance for the practitioner regarding the important factors to consider when designing a flea-control strategy for a patient.

Flea Biology

The adult flea spends its entire life on the dog or cat host, with the female laying up to 50 eggs per day and potentially several thousand eggs over a lifetime. Eggs are shed into the environment when laid on the host and hatch in 1 to 10 days into larvae, which move deep into carpet fibers or soil. Larvae are susceptible to desiccation at low humidity and extreme temperatures and survive outdoors only in shady moist areas protected from sunlight or heavy rain. Carpeted areas within the home can provide optimum conditions for larval survival. Larvae molt twice before spinning a cocoon that is impervious to chemicals or environmental hazards. Within the cocoon, the larva

pupates and becomes a preemergent adult until a suitable host is present. Pupae can remain dormant for several months; however, in ideal conditions, the flea life cycle can be completed in about 2 to 3 weeks. Adult fleas feed within minutes of finding a host, may mate within 8 hours, and can begin egg production within 24 hours of acquiring a host.

Flea Allergy Dermatitis

A variety of flea salivary proteins have been identified that elicit positive intradermal skin test results and elevated immunoglobulin E antibody responses detectable on enzyme-linked immunosorbent assay. In dogs, the disease is characterized by pruritus and a papular dermatitis affecting the caudodorsal trunk, tail base, perineum, caudomedial thighs, flanks, or ventral abdomen. Pyotraumatic dermatitis ("hot spots") on the rump is a feature in some affected dogs, as is a secondary staphylococcal pyoderma or yeast *(Malassezia)* dermatitis. In cats, a similar regional localization of pruritus and lesions may occur. However, cats additionally may have lesions and pruritus in other body locations including the head, neck, and trunk, and this may manifest as miliary dermatitis. Further, some flea-allergic cats have eosinophilic granuloma complex lesions such as indolent ulcers of the upper lip, eosinophilic plaques of the ventral abdomen, and eosinophilic granulomas. Thus the clinical signs are significantly more varied and less distinctive in the cat than in the dog. For both dogs and cats, a diagnosis of flea allergy dermatitis (FAD) is confirmed upon resolution of clinical signs following institution of an aggressive flea-control therapeutic trial.

Flea-Control Strategies

General Points

The term *flea control* may be interpreted in several ways by pet owners. Clients may be content with seeing just a few fleas on their pet, which may be adequate for pets without FAD. However, for pets with FAD, reduction of flea exposure to zero is the goal whenever possible, and this must be communicated clearly to the client. Achieving this goal may require frequent application of possibly more than one product to the affected pet, at least initially. Routine flea control for all pets should be implemented continuously throughout the year in households with a flea-allergic pet.

Clients often buy over-the-counter (OTC) products that may look similar to prescription products and have names that sound familiar. Unfortunately, many OTC products have active ingredients whose properties are not as favorable, nor are they are as effective as the prescription products. Furthermore, even when products are purchased OTC that previously were prescription products, owners are unlikely to obtain professional advice and expertise regarding proper dosing, dosing intervals, treatment of other pets, and management of the environment, which puts them at risk of failed flea control and apparent flea resistance.

Factors That Influence the Strategy

Flea eradication is essential for those pets exhibiting FAD; the goal must be zero flea exposure, at least for the initial 4 to 8 weeks of the flea-control therapeutic trial. This can be challenging considering the variety of environments in which pets reside, which necessitates customized flea-eradication plans for each household; that is, strategy will vary significantly depending on the specific circumstances. The following factors should be considered:

- *Speed of flea kill:* The more rapidly fleas are killed, the less they feed and the less salivary allergens are injected to continue the allergic reaction. Although most products kill fleas fairly rapidly when first applied, this effect may be diminished significantly 3 or 4 weeks later, so residual speed of kill also is important. This is why many dermatologists will apply spot-on formulations every 2 weeks during the flea-control therapeutic trial to ensure maximal residual speed of kill.
- *Compliance:* There may be large differences in owner compliance with regimens requiring a daily tablet, a monthly spot-on formulation, and a 6- to 8-month collar.
- *Spectrum of activity:* Treatment may be directed solely at flea control or there may be a need for tick control, heartworm prevention, or activity against other parasites (such as mites, lice, or mosquitoes).

- *Route of administration:* Some owners prefer oral medications over topicals, whereas some dogs or cats tolerate topicals better than oral medication.
- *Product characteristics:* Consideration of whether frequent bathing or wetting is likely to occur may favor oral or systemic agents. If the patient is undergoing a food trial for a possible adverse food reaction at the same time, the use of many oral medications (including some flea-control products and heartworm preventives) is precluded because of the presence of flavorings in the medications that may negate the food trial. Some owners find the odor of topical spot-on formulations unacceptable and thus prefer oral medication.
- *Pet's environment and all possible sources of flea exposure:* Wildlife, neighboring animals, and feral cats are major sources of exposure to fleas.
  - Does the pet visit other animals or homes (e.g., boarding facilities, grooming parlors)?
  - Do other animals visit this pet's household (pets of family, friends, neighbors)?
  - Does the pet go outdoors, and if so is there access to areas that wildlife or other animals may frequent (a space under porches, a crawl space, a shed, a shady mulched area under bushes)?
  - Are there bird feeders in the yard? These attract opossums and raccoons.

  Eliminating access to locations harboring fleas is important. In cases in which this may be difficult to achieve, confining all pets in the household indoors may be necessary, at least during the initial flea-control therapeutic trial to confirm the diagnosis of FAD.
- *Communication:* Failure of flea control most frequently is a result of failure to communicate the details and importance of prescribed flea-control measures or failure to understand all the factors within the pet's environment that may contribute to the flea burden and flea exposure. Resistance of fleas to parasiticidal agents is known to occur but is not commonly the problem when flea infestations persist.
- *Expense:* Especially in households with multiple pets, implementation of flea control for all pets may be costly, particularly during the initial aggressive flea-control therapeutic trial.

Sometimes it is recommended that more than one product with more than one mechanism of action be used. This is commonly referred to as *integrated pest management* and is recommended by some parasitologists. Thereafter, the pet with FAD will need a more aggressive ongoing protocol for flea prevention than will other pets in the household. Too often, achievement of flea eradication is neither cheap nor easy. It is imperative that the owner understand the goals and time frames to achieve success. Depending on the severity of the flea infestation, it might take several months to achieve eradication.

Products and Protocols for Dogs

Table 97-1 provides a list of active ingredients and products that may be considered for flea control in dogs, with

426 SECTION V Dermatologic and Otic Diseases

TABLE 97-1

Flea-Control Products for Dogs with Specific Indications*

FLEA CONTROL ONLY		FLEA + TICK CONTROL	
Topical	**Oral**	**Topical**	**Collar**
Dinotefuran (Vectra)	Nitenpyram (Capstar)	Dinotefuran/permethrin/pyriproxyfen (Vectra 3D)	Deltamethrin (Scalibor)
Fipronil (Frontline and many generics)	Spinosad (Comfortis)	Fipronil (Frontline and many generics)	Imidacloprid/flumethrin (Seresto)
Imidacloprid/pyriproxyfen (Advantage II)		Fipronil/methoprene/amitraz (Certifect)	
Indoxacarb (Activyl)		Imidacloprid/permethrin/pyriproxyfen (K9 Advantix II)	
		Indoxacarb/permethrin (Activyl Tick Plus)	
		Selamectin (Revolution)	

FLEA CONTROL + HEARTWORM PREVENTION		FLEA CONTROL + SCABIES TREATMENT
Topical	**Oral**	Fipronil (Frontline and many generics)
Imidacloprid/moxidectin (Advantage Multi)	Spinosad/milbemycin (Trifexis)	Selamectin (Revolution)
Selamectin (Revolution)		

FLEA CONTROL + ELIMINATION FOOD TRIAL + HEARTWORM PREVENTION	FLEA CONTROL + INTENSIVE BATHING
Imidacloprid/moxidectin (Advantage Multi)	Nitenpyram (Capstar)
Selamectin (Revolution)	Selamectin (Revolution)
	Spinosad (Comfortis)
	Spinosad/milbemycin (Trifexis)

NOTE: Several products have additional label claims (control of intestinal parasites, fly and mosquito repellency, lice treatment) that have not been discussed here because they are not usually significant factors to consider when designing flea-control strategies for patients with flea allergy dermatitis.
*Listed in alphabetical order by active ingredient.

TABLE 97-2

Flea-Control Products for Cats with Specific Indications*

FLEA CONTROL ONLY		FLEA + TICK CONTROL	
Topical	**Oral**	**Topical**	**Collar**
Dinotefuran (Vectra)	Nitenpyram (Capstar)	Dinotefuran/permethrin/pyriproxyfen (Vectra 3D)	Imidacloprid/flumethrin (Seresto)
Fipronil (Frontline and many generics)	Spinosad (Comfortis)	Fipronil (Frontline and many generics)	
Imidacloprid/pyriproxyfen (Advantage II)		Selamectin (Revolution)	
Indoxacarb (Activyl)			

FLEA CONTROL + HEARTWORM PREVENTION	
Topical	**Oral**
Imidacloprid/moxidectin (Advantage Multi)	
Selamectin (Revolution)	

NOTE: Several products have additional label claims (control of intestinal parasites, fly and mosquito repellency, lice treatment) that have not been discussed here because they are not usually significant factors to consider when designing flea-control strategies for patients with flea allergy dermatitis.
*Listed in alphabetical order by active ingredient.

specific indications that influence the authors' selection of products for individual patients. Multiple products can be used simultaneously (see sample protocols later).

Because most ectoparasiticides are regulated by the Environmental Protection Agency these agents must be prescribed according to label instructions. It is a violation of federal law to recommend extralabel protocols. If veterinarians wish to prescribe parasiticides off label, they should use Food and Drug Administration (FDA)–regulated products for which the Animal Medicinal Drug Use Clarification Act of 1994 allows extralabel prescription. Parasiticides for flea control that are FDA approved include (in alphabetical order): imidacloprid/moxidectin (Advantage Multi), nitenpyram (Capstar), selamectin (Revolution), spinetoram (Assurity), spinosad (Comfortis), and spinosad/milbemycin (Trifexis).

One further concern is exposure of other pets—especially cats, because they are more susceptible to the possible toxic adverse effects associated with amitraz and permethrin. In multiple-pet households where cats and dogs are well socialized, the relationship among the pets should be considered. If the cat grooms the dog or has friendly contact, it would be best to avoid products with permethrin or amitraz.

Sample Protocols for Dogs
1. Heavy flea burden
   - Nitenpyram every 48 hours for 2 weeks then twice weekly or after known flea exposure.
   - One of the topical preventatives (fipronil, imidacloprid, selamectin, dinotefuran, indoxacarb) applied monthly. Formulations that include an insect growth regulator, such as those with pyriproxyfen or methoprene, should be selected.
2. Mild to moderate flea burden
   - Spinosad monthly.
   - One of the topicals (fipronil, imidacloprid, selamectin, dinotefuran, indoxacarb) used monthly (applied between spinosad treatments). Selection of a specific product is based on additional requirements such as the need for tick control or heartworm prevention.
   - Nitenpyram as necessary if flea exposure is known or anticipated.
3. Possible FAD and scabies
   - Nitenpyram twice weekly.
   - Selamectin or imidacloprid/moxidectin every 2 weeks.

Products for Cats

A most important step in attaining flea control in cats with FAD is to keep the cat indoors. Other factors that influence selection of flea-control products in cats include the following: ticks are less of a problem, oral medications are more challenging to administer in some cats, and the need for heartworm prevention in cats is more geographically limited. Table 97-2 provides a listing of active ingredients and products that may be considered, with specific indications that influence the authors' selections of products for individual patients.

Treatment of the Indoor and Outdoor Environment

In households with a pet with FAD, it is the authors' recommendation to seek out a licensed pest management expert for assistance. Reputable companies will provide a guarantee and assume responsibility for any liability involving people, pets, and other animals that may be exposed to these chemicals. Frequent vacuuming helps to remove flea eggs, larvae, pupae, and flea feces from the indoor environment; the vacuum bags should be thrown away frequently.

The elimination of fleas from the outside environment usually is best left to licensed exterminators. The pet owner should exclude nondomestic animals, feral cats, and pets not receiving flea-control products from the yard.

References and Suggested Reading

Blagburn BL et al: Effects of orally administered spinosad (Comfortis) in dogs on adult and immature stages of the cat flea (*Ctenocephalides felis*), *Vet Parasitol* 168(3-4):312, 2010.

Blagburn BL, Dryden MW: Biology, treatment, and control of flea and tick infestations, *Vet Clin North Am Small Anim Pract* 39:1173, 2009.

Dryden MW: Flea and tick control in the 21st century: challenges and opportunities, *Vet Dermatol* 20(5-6):435, 2009.

Dryden MW et al: Efficacy of dintoefuran-pyriproxyfen, dinotefuran-pyriproxyfen-permethrin, and fipronil-(S)-methoprene topical spot-on formulations to control flea populations in naturally infested pets and private residencies in Tampa FL, *Vet Parasitol* 182(2-4):281, 2011.

CHAPTER 98

Treatment of Ectoparasitoses

RANDALL C. THOMAS, *Mount Pleasant, South Carolina*

Diagnosis and management of ectoparasitoses is a common part of small animal practice. This chapter discusses the clinical aspects and treatment of several less common ectoparasites. Chapter 97 considers flea control.

Lice Infestation (Pediculosis)

Lice species are divided into two orders, the Mallophaga or biting lice, and the Anoplura or sucking lice (Table 98-1). Lice are obligate parasites, completing the entire life cycle on one host in 3 to 5 weeks. Lice are transmitted from host to host primarily by direct contact. However, infestation by contact with infested bedding or grooming tools also can occur.

Clinical Signs and Diagnosis

Most of the symptoms of lice infestation are secondary to skin irritation, including nonspecific pruritus, excoriations, an unkempt hair coat, seborrhea, and self-induced alopecia. In severe cases, anemia and weakness may occur, especially in young animals. In cats, a crusted papular dermatitis (miliary dermatitis) may develop. Pediculosis in both dogs and cats can be asymptomatic. The diagnosis is made by careful observation and visualization of adult lice on the skin or eggs (nits) attached to hair shafts. In some instances, taking an acetate tape impression of hair and debris may be necessary.

Treatment

Table 98-2 lists the various treatment options for pediculosis in dogs and cats. Pruritus may persist for 2 to 4 weeks after treatment. Environmental treatment usually is not required because lice do not survive off the host; however, thorough cleansing of bedding and grooming tools is recommended. Treatment of contact animals is recommended since some may be asymptomatic carriers. Lice are species specific and do not present a significant zoonotic risk to owners.

Canine Scabies

Canine scabies, or sarcoptic mange, results from infestation by the mite *Sarcoptes scabiei* var. *canis*. The life cycle occurs entirely on the host and is completed in approximately 10 to 14 days. Although *S. scabiei* var. *canis* has a preference for dogs, it also has been reported to cause dermatitis in cats, foxes, and humans. In aberrant hosts, infestation usually is transient, with lesions lasting approximately 2 weeks. Most cases of sarcoptic mange are caused by direct contact with an infested host, but transmission may occur from infested environments.

Clinical Signs and Diagnosis

Canine scabies is characterized by intense pruritus. It classically affects the pinnae, elbows, and hocks but also can affect sparsely haired areas of the body such as the ventral abdomen and limbs. Early erythematous papules progress rapidly to yellowish crusts, alopecia, excoriations, lichenification, hyperpigmentation, and seborrhea. Secondary bacterial pyoderma is common.

In some instances, dogs may have intense nonseasonal pruritus but minimal lesions (scabies incognito) at presentation. Minimally pruritic, crusted scabies (Norwegian scabies) caused by *S. scabiei* var. *canis* also has been reported in rare cases in immunosuppressed patients.

Demonstration of scabies mites on superficial skin scrapings is diagnostic of canine scabies. However, finding mites on scrapings often is difficult. Taking multiple wide, superficial scrapings from areas with crusting provides the best chance of observing adult mites, eggs, or feces. However, because adults may be present in very low numbers, negative findings on scrapings do not rule out this disease. The pinnal-pedal reflex (rubbing the convex portion of the pinna or ear margin against itself causes scratching with the back leg) may be present in more than 75% of dogs with scabies. An enzyme-linked immunosorbent assay for canine scabies antibodies has been evaluated and shown to have high sensitivity and specificity. Dogs with persistent intense pruritus should be considered for empirical treatment. In some studies, 30% of dogs with scabies have shown some response to corticosteroid treatment, so steroid responsiveness should not be considered to rule out scabies.

Treatment

In the author's experience, systemic treatments are generally safe, highly effective, and easier for owners to administer than topical treatments. Only selamectin has a label claim for the treatment of sarcoptic mange in the dog. See Table 98-3 for treatment options for canine scabies.

In cases of confirmed or suspected sarcoptic mange, all contact dogs also should be treated to avoid reinfestation. Treatment of secondary bacterial and yeast infections often is necessary to completely resolve clinical signs. Sarcoptic mange is highly contagious to humans, and approximately 33% to 50% of humans in contact

TABLE 98-1

Lice Species Affecting Dogs and Cats

Species	Classification	Hosts
Linognathus setosus	Anoplura (sucking)	Dogs
Trichodectes canis	Mallophaga (biting)	Dogs, wolves, foxes, other canids
Heterodoxus spiniger	Mallophaga (biting)	Dogs
Felicola subrostratus	Mallophaga (biting)	Cats

with affected dogs develop a self-limiting erythematous, papular eruption, often on the trunk and hands. This dermatitis may persist for 10 to 14 days. Skin scrapings in humans typically are negative for the mite. In rare cases, infestation may be established and scabicidal treatment becomes necessary.

Feline Scabies

Feline scabies is caused by *Notoedres cati*, which also has been reported in foxes, civets, raccoons, coatis, and humans. The life cycle of *N. cati* is very similar to that of *S. scabiei* var. *canis* (see earlier).

TABLE 98-2

Treatment Options for Pediculosis in Dogs and Cats

Treatment	Dose	Frequency	Comments
Lime sulfur dip	4-6 oz/gal water	q14d for 2-3 treatments	Safe for puppies and kittens; use Elizabethan collar on cats and kittens until dry
Pyrethrins (various shampoos, dips)	Per label instructions	q7-14d for 2-3 treatments	Safe for puppies and kittens
Ivermectin 1%	0.2 mg/kg PO or SC	q14d for 2-3 treatments	Extralabel use; caution owners of potential adverse effects
Imidacloprid 10% (Advantage II for dogs or K9 Advantix)	Per label instructions	Single application	Label approved for treatment of pediculosis in dogs
Fipronil (Frontline Spray, Frontline Top Spot)	Per label instructions	Single application	Labeled for treatment of chewing lice in dogs and cats
Selamectin (Revolution)	Per label instructions	Single application	Extralabel use both dogs and cats
Dinotefuran/pyriproxyfen/permethrin (Vectra 3D for Dogs)	Per label instructions	Single application	Labeled for treatment of lice in dogs and puppies

PO, Orally; *SC*, subcutaneously.

TABLE 98-3

Treatment Options for Sarcoptic and Notoedric Mange in Dogs and Cats

Treatment	Dose	Frequency	Dog or Cat	Comments
Selamectin (Revolution)	Per label instructions	Two applications at 30-day interval (dermatologists recommend q14d for 3 applications	Dog and cat	Label claim for canine scabies
Moxidectin 1%/imidacloprid 10% (Advantage Multi)	Per label instructions	Two applications at 30-day interval; many recommend treating q14d for 3 applications	Dog	Should be effective in both dogs and cats
Ivermectin 1%	0.2-0.3 mg/kg PO or SC	q2wk for 3 treatments	Dog	Extralabel use, possible adverse effects
Ivermectin 1%	0.3 mg/kg SC	q2wk for 3 treatments	Cat	Extralabel use
Milbemycin oxime	2 mg/kg PO	q7d for 4 treatments	Dog	Extralabel use; well tolerated by ivermectin-sensitive breeds
Fipronil 0.25% spray (Frontline Spray)	12-39 mg/kg per application	q7d for 4 treatments	Dog	This dose is higher than label dose of Frontline Spray
Fipronil 10% spot-on (Frontline Plus)	Per label instructions	Twice at 28-day interval	Dog	Label claim for "control of sarcoptic mange infestations"
Lime sulfur dip	4-6 oz/gal water	q7d for 4-6 dips	Dog and cat	Use Elizabethan collar on cats and kittens until dry

PO, Orally; *SC*, subcutaneously.

TABLE 98-4

Treatment Options for Cheyletiellosis in Dogs and Cats

Treatment	Dose	Frequency	Dog or Cat	Comments
Lime sulfur dip	4-6 oz/gal water	q7d for 6 dips	Dog and cat	Use Elizabethan collar on cats and kittens until dry
Ivermectin 1%	0.2-0.3 mg/kg PO or SC	q14d for 4 treatments	Dog and cat	Extralabel
Fipronil (Frontline Top Spot)	Per label instructions	Two applications at 30-day interval	Dog and cat	No label claim
Selamectin (Revolution)	Per label dose	q2-4wk for 3-4 treatments	Dog and cat	No label claim
Moxidectin 1%/imidacloprid 10% (Advantage Multi)	Per label instructions	q30d for 2 applications	Dog (cat not evaluated)	No label claim; should be effective in cat as well

PO, Orally; *SC,* subcutaneously.

Clinical Signs and Diagnosis

Intense pruritus, erythema, and a progressive crusting dermatitis start on the head and ears and progress to the periocular regions, face, and neck. Alopecia, lichenification, and tightly adherent crusts occur as the symptoms progress. This mite is highly contagious, so involvement of multiple contact cats or kittens is common. Unlike canine mites, *Notoedres* mites usually are numerous on superficial skin scrapings. Although the absence of mites on skin scrapings is rare, it does not rule out *Notoedres* infestation entirely.

Treatment

Table 98-3 shows various treatment options for notoedric mange in cats and kittens. Symptomatic treatment such as clipping of matted hair, physical removal of severe crusts, and corticosteroid therapy may be necessary. All contact cats and kittens should be treated concurrently to avoid reinfestation. *Notoedres* is highly contagious to humans, so transient zoonotic spread is possible, although clinical signs usually are self-limiting once the affected pets have been treated.

Cheyletiellosis

Cheyletiella spp. are highly contagious mites affecting dogs (*Cheyletiella yasguri*), cats (*Cheyletiella blakei*), and rabbits (*Cheyletiella parasitovorax*). The mites have host preferences but can cause infestation across species. Transmission is either by direct contact or contact with fomites. *Cheyletiella* mites are obligate parasites, completing their entire life cycle on the host in 21 to 35 days.

Clinical Signs and Diagnosis

Younger dogs and cats are more likely to be affected. Clinical signs in dogs and cats can be highly variable (some adults may be asymptomatic carriers) but typically include dorsal truncal scaling. Pruritus often is minimal but can be severe in some instances. Miliary dermatitis with substantial pruritus also has been reported in cats.

The diagnosis of cheyletiellosis is confirmed by the observation of adult mites on the skin or eggs (nits) attached to hair shafts. Microscopic examination of plucked hairs (trichogram) should allow visualization of nits attached to hair shafts. Mites or nits also may be found by examining debris collected by flea combing or acetate tape preparations. Cats are notoriously efficient groomers and may make it difficult to find this superficial mite. Eggs and adult mites may be observed in fecal flotations in affected pets.

Treatment

Cheyletiella mites are susceptible to many of the commonly used parasiticides, Table 98-4 shows treatment options for dogs and cats. All contact animals should be treated to prevent reinfestation since the mites are highly contagious and carriers can be asymptomatic. Total body clipping to remove nits that might be shed can help prevent reinfestation. Secondary infections should be identified and treated with an appropriate antibiotic or topical therapy. If pruritus is significant, symptomatic treatment with corticosteroids may be indicated. Environmental treatment should be instituted to speed resolution and prevent reinfestation. Bedding should be thoroughly washed. Carpeting, rugs, and furniture should be vacuumed and a flea adulticide product applied, preferably by a licensed pest exterminator.

Cheyletiella is considered highly contagious to humans, causing erythematous macules and vesicles on the arms, abdomen, or other areas of contact that may persist for up to 3 weeks.

Otodectes cynotis Infestation

Otodectes cynotis, the ear mite, is an obligate parasite of the host but is not host specific. The life cycle is typically completed in about 3 weeks.

Clinical Signs and Diagnosis

Ear mites primarily infest the external ear canal of dogs and cats causing accumulation of a dark, granular

TABLE **98-5**

Treatment Options for *Otodectes* Infestation in Dogs and Cats

Treatment	Dose	Frequency	Dog or Cat	Comments
Thiabendazole/neomycin/ dexamethasone (Tresaderm)	Sufficient drops to treat each affected ear	Twice daily for at least 10 days	Dog and cat	Treatment must extend at least 10 days to ensure adequate treatment.
Pyrethrin (Otomite)	Sufficient drops to treat each affected ear	Twice daily for at least 10 days	Dog and cat	Treatment must extend at least 10 days to ensure adequate treatment.
Milbemycin 0.1% (MilbeMite)	Single dose per ear	Single treatment recommended	Labeled for cat and kitten	99%-100% effective with single dose; redosing may be indicated rarely.
Ivermectin 1%	1:9 dilution in propylene glycol	Once daily for 21 days	Dog and cat	Extralabel use in both dog and cat.
Fipronil 10% (Frontline Top Spot)	2 drops	Single application	Dog and cat	No label claim made by manufacturer.
Selamectin (Revolution)	Per label instructions	Single application	Dog and cat	Labeled for treatment of *Otodectes* infestation.
Moxidectin 1%/imidacloprid 10% (Advantage Multi)	Per label instructions	Single application	Cat and kitten	Label claim for cats and kittens older than 7 wk; should work for dogs.
Ivermectin 1%	0.2-0.3 mg/kg PO or SC	Two treatments at 14-day intervals	Dog and cat	Extralabel use.

PO, Orally; *SC,* subcutaneously.

otic discharge ("coffee ground" appearance), most commonly in kittens and cats. Pruritus and self-trauma are common but may be minimal. Mites uncommonly may leave the external ear canal and cause pruritus of the head, neck, tail head, and trunk or produce no symptoms. Miliary dermatitis has been reported in feline patients.

Direct examination of otic discharge results in visualization of mites at all stages of the life cycle. "Occult" infestations, in which low numbers of mites cause clinical signs, have been reported, so empirical treatment may provide a diagnosis in some instances.

Treatment

Table 98-5 shows the treatment options for *Otodectes* infestation in dogs and cats. Physical removal of as much otic debris as possible is recommended to increase direct drug contact with mites. All contact animals should be treated concurrently to avoid reinfestation. *Otodectes* mites are not host specific, and they can cause a transient papular dermatitis, and rarely otitis, in humans.

Cat Fur Mite Infestation

Lynxacarus radovskyi is a small mite reported to infest in cats in Australia, Brazil, Hawaii, Florida, and Texas. These mites are not particularly contagious, so infestation throughout a household may not always be seen.

Clinical Signs and Diagnosis

Clinical signs are variable, the most common being a dull, dry hair coat, self-induced alopecia on the dorsal and lateral aspects of the hind limbs, and variable pruritus. Diagnosis is made by direct visualization of mites on scrapings or hair plucks.

Treatment

Cat fur mites are susceptible to most of the topical and systemic insecticides used in cats, with reports of efficacy of a single application of fipronil (Frontline Top Spot), weekly lime sulfur dips, and ivermectin (0.2 to 0.3 mg/kg PO or SC).

Trombiculiasis

Several species of chigger mites (harvest mites) can cause skin disease, but only four species have been reported in detail: *Eutrombicula alfreddugesi*, *Neotrombicula autumnalis*, *Walchia americana*, and *Straelensia cynotis*. The clinical features of infestation by these mites have similarities.

Cutaneous manifestations related to infestation with chigger mites (harvest mites) are rare. Adult mites live off the host, feeding on decaying vegetation. Eggs are laid in moist soil and hatch into bright orange-red larvae, which are the cause of skin lesions. Symptoms tend to occur in late summer and fall when the larval form is prevalent. Infestation has been reported in dogs, cats, and humans, as well as in other hosts.

Clinical Signs and Diagnosis

The larval stage of the chigger mite feeds on the host, creating intense pruritus and inflammation of the ventrum, feet, legs, and head after direct contact with the larvae-infested soil. Secondary bacterial infections are common. Diagnosis typically is made by direct visualization of bright orange-red, six-legged larvae on the skin surface or on skin scrapings.

Treatment

These mites are susceptible to a variety of topical and systemic parasiticides, including lime sulfur dips, thiabendazole, and permethrin/pyrethrin products. Topical application of fipronil (Frontline Spray Treatment) may be an effective treatment but has variable success in the prevention of reinfestation. Prevention of future outbreaks can be accomplished reliably only by avoiding exposure to infested areas outdoors. Zoonotic spread from affected dogs or cats has not been reported.

References and Suggested Reading

Curtis CF: Current trends in the treatment of *Sarcoptes, Cheyletiella* and *Otodectes* mite infestations in dogs and cats, *Vet Dermatol* 15:108, 2004.
Durden L: Biting and sucking lice. In Meyer RP, Madon MB, editors: *Arthropods of public health significances in California,* Sacramento, CA, 2002, Mosquito and Vector Control Association of California, p 37.
Scott DW, Miller WH Jr, Griffin CE: Parasitic skin diseases. In *Muller and Kirk's small animal dermatology,* ed 6, Philadelphia, 2001, Saunders, p 423.
Sosna CB, Medleau L: External parasites: life cycles, transmission, and the pathogenesis of disease, *Vet Med* 87:538, 1992a.
Sosna CB, Medleau L: The clinical signs and diagnosis of external parasite infestation, *Vet Med* 87:548, 1992b.
Sosna CB, Medleau L: Treating parasitic skin conditions, *Vet Med* 87:573, 1992c.

CHAPTER 99
Canine Demodicosis

RALF S. MUELLER, *Munich, Germany*

Canine demodicosis is a disease encountered commonly in small animal practice. Although in the past severe generalized demodicosis may have prompted euthanasia, current miticidal therapy allows the disease to be cured, or at least managed, in almost every patient.

Demodex mites are part of the normal cutaneous fauna in dogs. They live in the hair follicles and cause a problem only when they proliferate abnormally. The predisposition to develop canine demodicosis is an inherited trait (presumably a defect in cell-mediated immunity); thus dogs with generalized demodicosis must not be bred, and the author strongly advocates neutering of all affected dogs. Other predisposing factors in young dogs include nutritional deficiencies, endoparasites, and stress. Adult-onset demodicosis is associated with neoplastic disease, chemotherapy, hyperadrenocorticism, and hypothyroidism. Diagnosis and treatment of these predisposing factors results in improved treatment outcome for demodicosis.

Demodicosis may occur as localized or generalized disease. Up to four small lesions in any body location are considered to be localized disease by the author. Involvement of a large area on the trunk or any affected paw always constitutes generalized disease. Spontaneous remission is seen in the vast majority of dogs that develop localized demodicosis; thus specific miticidal therapy is not indicated. Use of antiseptic shampoos or gels minimizes the chance of a secondary bacterial infection. Dogs with localized demodicosis that do not achieve spontaneous remission without miticidal therapy also should not be bred.

Clinical Signs and Diagnosis

Initially, the only clinical signs may be any combination of multifocal alopecia, comedones, mild erythema, and scaling. These are followed later by follicular papules and pustules. Furuncles, crusts, and draining tracts may develop if furunculosis results from the folliculitis. Lesions typically start on the face and feet and gradually generalize. Otitis externa can be caused by *Demodex* mites and infrequently is the only clinical sign in dogs. Secondary bacterial pyoderma is common; typically it is caused by *Staphylococcus pseudintermedius,* but *Pseudomonas aeruginosa* or other gram-negative rods also may be involved, particularly with deep furunculosis. Lymphadenopathy and fever may develop.

Demodicosis is diagnosed easily by deep skin scrapings. If three scrapings are negative for the mites, demodicosis typically is ruled out. False-negative results on scrapings have been reported in dogs with pododemodicosis and in shar-pei dogs. Because *Demodex* mites are part of the normal fauna, a single mite on a deep skin scraping may be an incidental finding. However, two or more mites on three scrapings usually are diagnostic of the disease. Trichography (in which hairs are plucked with a hemostat, placed in a drop of mineral or paraffin oil on a slide, and inspected under a coverslip) is an alternative diagnostic technique that is useful for lesions around the eyes or on the paws. In rare cases demodicosis may be diagnosed only on histopathologic examination of affected skin.

Secondary Infections in Dogs with Demodicosis

Cytologic evaluation to identify secondary bacterial infection usually is necessary. Systemic antibiotics are recommended for dogs with demodicosis and severe secondary bacterial pyoderma. Bacterial culture and susceptibility testing is recommended when rods are found on cytologic examination or in dogs with staphylococcal infections that have failed to respond to prior antibiotic treatment (see Chapters 101 through 103). However, recent evidence indicates that in many dogs with demodicosis and pyoderma antimicrobial shampoos are sufficient to treat the bacterial infection. Antimicrobial therapy should be continued until clinical and microscopic resolution of the pyoderma is achieved.

Miticidal Therapies

A number of successful miticidal therapies for canine demodicosis have been reported (Table 99-1). Amitraz and the macrocyclic lactones are the most commonly used, and their efficacy has been evaluated in numerous open-label studies.

Amitraz initially was introduced as a rinse. It is an acaricidal and insecticidal formamidine and is licensed for the treatment of canine demodicosis in the United States. The recommended concentration is 0.025% applied as a rinse to the whole body every other week. Medium- and long-haired dogs should be clipped before rinsing. Rinsing should take place in a well-ventilated area. The rinse should be worked into the dog's coat and skin with a sponge. Standing the dog in a small plastic

TABLE 99-1

Recommended Treatment Options for Canine Demodicosis

Drug	Trade Name	Dosage
Amitraz	Mitaban	0.025% rinse q14d
Ivermectin*	Ivomec	0.3 (up to 0.6) mg/kg q24h PO
Milbemycin oxime*	Interceptor	1-2 mg/kg q24h PO
Moxidectin*	Cydectin	0.2-0.4 mg/kg q24h PO

*Treatment of demodicosis is an extralabel use of these drugs; appropriate education should be provided and consent should be obtained. Extralabel use of drugs should take into account local and regional restrictions on their use.
PO, Orally.

bathtub facilitates the rinsing. Dogs should be air-dried or blow-dried after the rinse. Dogs must not be bathed or allowed to swim between rinses to avoid washing off the miticidal agent. This may be particularly difficult for paws and distal legs, which may have to be treated more frequently. Adverse effects seen with amitraz include lethargy, depression, sleepiness, ataxia, bradycardia, vomiting, diarrhea, and polyphagia-polydipsia. The success rate of amitraz treatment is higher in juvenile dogs than in dogs with adult-onset demodicosis. Higher concentrations and more frequent applications have been reported to be more effective but also carry higher risk of adverse effects. Rinsing half the body on alternate days has cured some dogs previously unresponsive to conventional treatment. Similarly, a high concentration of amitraz (1.25%) has been used in conjunction with intramuscular atipamezole (0.1 mg/kg once) and oral yohimbine (0.1 mg/kg q24h for 3 days) administered after the rinse to counteract the α_2-adrenergic effects and associated bradycardia and hyperglycemia. These protocols should be reserved for dogs resistant to conventional therapy.

A spot-on product containing amitraz in combination with metaflumizone applied every other week was effective in pilot studies in dogs with generalized demodicosis. However, due to pemphigus foliaceus–like drug eruptions following application, the product has been withdrawn from the market in the United States, although currently it is still available in some other countries.

Macrocyclic lactones as a group have strong acaricidal activity. Avermectins such as ivermectin and doramectin and milbemycins such as milbemycin oxime and moxidectin have been evaluated for the treatment of demodicosis. These drugs cause paralysis and death of the *Demodex* mites by binding to chloride channels and increasing cell permeability as well as interacting with γ-aminobutyric acid (GABA). In mammals GABA is a neurotransmitter in the central nervous system, and there are no glutamate-gated chloride channels in the peripheral nervous system; thus these agents normally are safe to use in mammals. However, the macrocyclic lactones may cause neurologic adverse effects such as ataxia, tremors, mydriasis, blindness, and even coma and death in some dogs, particularly collies and Old English sheepdogs, although other breeds may be affected occasionally. An ABCB1 (MDR1) gene mutation is responsible for the acute and peracute neurologic adverse effects, although other mechanisms of neurotoxicity appear to be present because neurologic adverse effects have been reported in dogs with normal ABCB1 genes.

Studies of ivermectin at dosages of 0.3 to 0.6 mg/kg (300 to 600 µg/kg) q24h PO have demonstrated that the efficacy of ivermectin is comparable to that of amitraz rinses. The author always increases the dose gradually from 0.05 mg/kg (50 µg/kg) on day 1 to 0.1 mg/kg on day 2, 0.15 mg/kg on day 3, 0.2 mg/kg on day 4, and finally 0.3 mg/kg on day 5; the latter dose then is continued q24h thereafter. Ivermectin can lead to rapid killing of heartworm microfilaria, which causes a shocklike reaction in 8% to 10% of microfilaria-positive dogs; therefore heartworm status should be known in endemic areas. Owner education and awareness of early adverse clinical signs (lethargy, mydriasis, ataxia, and tremors) is important; immediate discontinuation of therapy is essential to avoid potentially lethal complications. If adverse effects occur later in the treatment period, halving the dose may be sufficient in some dogs to resolve those effects and still achieve remission of the demodicosis. Early adverse effects are reversible and typically resolve within 1 or 2 days. Ivermectin has an unpleasant taste and may be diluted in cordial or ice cream to facilitate oral administration. The average time to negative results on skin scrapings is approximately 2 to 3 months, although individual dogs may need treatment for much longer. Subcutaneous weekly ivermectin injections are not effective in most cases of canine generalized demodicosis.

Milbemycin oxime is administered at a dosage of 0.5 to 2 mg/kg q24h PO. The higher dose is more effective. Adult dogs respond to treatment less favorably than young dogs. Milbemycin oxime has a wider safety margin than other macrocyclic lactones and neurologic adverse effects are less common than with ivermectin. Nevertheless, adverse effects may occur, and a gradual dose increase over 2 to 3 days is recommended, particularly in herding breeds. Additionally, at the dosage used, milbemycin oxime can cause a similar rapid microfilaria kill in dogs with heartworm, and heartworm status therefore should be known.

Moxidectin is administered at a dosage of 0.2 to 0.4 mg/kg q24h PO. The adverse effects are similar to those seen with ivermectin but may occur more frequently. A gradual dose increase similar to the increase described for ivermectin is recommended for moxidectin.

Doramectin has been used with success at higher dosages of 0.6 mg/kg weekly PO or SC in a few studies. The author has not had extensive experience with this particular drug. Adverse effects are similar to those of other macrocyclic lactones, and a gradual dose increase to identify a dog that is not tolerating the drug is recommended for doramectin as well. Severe adverse effects may be life threatening. Recent reports of treatment with intravenous lipid emulsions and supportive care provide hope for management of these effects.

A number of other drugs have been evaluated for treatment of demodicosis. Based on current knowledge, topical or oral selamectin, pour-on ivermectin, lufenuron, ronnel, amitraz spot on, and levamisole cannot be recommended for treatment of canine demodicosis.

Treatment Duration and Monitoring

Regardless of the specific treatment, reevaluations should occur monthly and should include physical examination, evaluation for secondary pyoderma, and examination of skin scrapings taken from the same locations sampled previously to identify changes in the number and life stage of mites present. Deterioration in clinical signs between visits or failure to improve over three visits should prompt consideration of a change of miticidal therapy. If steady improvement occurs, acaricidal therapy should be continued for 8 weeks past the first set of negative skin scraping results (all locations negative for mites) and 4 weeks past the second set of negative results to minimize recurrences. In dogs with a history of demodicosis, glucocorticoid and immunosuppressive therapy should be avoided if at all possible. If the disease recurs, treatment should be repeated and again extended at least 8 weeks past the first negative scraping result. In some rare cases of canine demodicosis, clinical remission is possible, but skin scrapings always show a few mites. In other dogs the disease recurs every time the treatment is discontinued. In those patients, long-term therapy with oral ivermectin or moxidectin or topical amitraz or moxidectin at extended intervals may be necessary.

References and Suggested Reading

Bissonnette S et al: The ABCB1-1Delta mutation is not responsible for subchronic neurotoxicity seen in dogs of non-collie breeds following macrocyclic lactone treatment for generalized demodicosis, *Vet Dermatol* 20:60, 2009.

Duclos DD, Jeffers JG, Shanley KJ: Prognosis for treatment of adult-onset demodicosis in dogs: 34 cases (1979-1990), *J Am Vet Med Assoc* 204:616, 1994.

Fernandez AL et al: The use of intravenous lipid emulsion as an antidote in veterinary toxicology, *J Vet Emerg Crit Care* 21(4): 309, 2011.

Kusnetsova E et al: Influence of systemic antibiotics on the treatment of dogs with generalized demodicosis, *Vet Parasitol* 188:148, 2012.

Mueller RS: Treatment protocols for demodicosis: an evidence-based review, *Vet Dermatol* 15:75, 2004.

Mueller RS et al: Treatment of demodicosis in dogs: 2011 clinical practice guidelines, *Vet Dermatol* 23(2):86, 2012. Epub February 13, 2011.

Mueller RS, Bettenay SV: A proposed new therapeutic protocol for the treatment of canine mange with ivermectin, *J Am Anim Hosp Assoc* 35:77, 1999.

Paterson TE et al: Treatment of canine-generalized demodicosis: a blind, randomized clinical trial comparing the efficacy of Advocate (Bayer Animal Health) with ivermectin, *Vet Dermatol* 20:447, 2009.

Plant JD, Lund EM, Yang M: A case-control study of the risk factors for canine juvenile-onset generalized demodicosis in the USA, *Vet Dermatol* 22:95, 2011.

CHAPTER 100

Staphylococci Causing Pyoderma

LINDA A. FRANK, *Knoxville, Tennessee*

Staphylococcus species are both normal resident cutaneous microflora and opportunistic pathogens frequently associated with pyoderma in dogs and cats. *Staphylococcus* species usually are divided into coagulase-positive and coagulase-negative species, with the former most often associated with skin infections. Recently, *Staphylococcus intermedius* has been reclassified, with *Staphylococcus pseudintermedius* being recognized as the common coagulase-positive canine staphylococcus (Sasaki et al, 2007). *Staphylococcus aureus, Staphylococcus schleiferi,* and coagulase-negative staphylococci occasionally are isolated from skin infections of animals. Often these isolates are methicillin- and multidrug resistant, which most likely is attributable to empiric treatment with multiple classes of antibiotics before culture (see Chapter 103). Methicillin resistance implies resistance to all β-lactam antibiotics including cephalosporins and amoxicillin/clavulanic acid. *S. aureus, S. schleiferi,* and coagulase-negative staphylococci, unlike *S. pseudintermedius,* also are human pathogens or opportunistic invaders. Identification of the causative organism is important to determine the likelihood of resistance as well as the source and possible human risk.

Staphylococcus pseudintermedius

Formerly known as *S. intermedius, S. pseudintermedius* is now accepted as the organism that colonizes canine and feline skin and is the organism within the *S. intermedius* group that is associated mainly with canine and feline skin and ear infections; *S. intermedius,* in the strict sense, is associated primarily with pigeons. The *S. intermedius* group consists of *S. intermedius, S. pseudintermedius,* and *S. delphini.* In recent years there has been an increase in methicillin and multidrug resistance in *S. pseudintermedius,* which makes treating skin infections associated with this organism a therapeutic challenge (see Chapter 103). *S. pseudintermedius* is an infrequent pathogen in people and most often is associated with dog bite wounds.

Staphylococcus aureus

S. aureus is a resident organism and the predominant pathogenic staphylococcus of humans. *S. aureus* also colonizes healthy cats and has been associated uncommonly with skin infections in dogs and cats. In addition, wound infections, surgical site infections, otitis, and urinary tract infections caused by *S. aureus* all have been reported. Animals are thought to acquire the infection from people and then may serve as a source for human infections. When methicillin-resistant *S. aureus* (MRSA) is isolated from dog or cat skin infections, it usually is genetically related to the human hospital-acquired MRSA isolates for that region based on genetic typing. Although deep concern often follows a diagnosis of MRSA in a pet, the organism was likely acquired from the owner or another resident of the household. Because the numbers of dogs or cats infected with *S. aureus* have remained low, it is unlikely that permanent colonization occurs, which makes pets unlikely true reservoirs for the bacteria. MRSA carriage in a dog is not maintained for long periods when the dog is moved to a clean environment, which suggests that attempts at decolonization are not necessary. *S. aureus* has been shown to preferentially colonize human keratinocytes, whereas *S. (pseud)intermedius* preferentially colonizes canine keratinocytes (Simou et al, 2005).

Staphylococcus schleiferi

S. schleiferi now is recognized as a cause of pyoderma and otitis in dogs. *S. schleiferi* has only rarely been isolated from cats. Two subspecies have been identified: *S. schleiferi* subsp. *schleiferi,* a coagulase-negative staphylococcus, and *S. schleiferi* subsp. *coagulans,* a coagulase-positive staphylococcus. A recent publication shows that the coagulase-positive and coagulase-negative isolates are genotypically similar and may represent a single species with variable coagulase production rather than two distinct subspecies (Cain et al, 2011). It is important that microbiology laboratories identify *S. schleiferi* regardless of its coagulase status because both are recognized human and animal pathogens.

The number of canine and feline infections caused by *S. schleiferi* apparently is low; however, this could be due to underreporting of the organism because of its similarity to *S. aureus* and *S. pseudintermedius.* Presumptive identification of bacterial colonies as *S. pseudintermedius* is based on classic colony characteristics (double zone of hemolysis, large diameter, and opaque off-white color) and biochemical reactions (positive catalase and coagulase test findings and no or delayed fermentation of maltose and mannitol). However, *S. schleiferi* subsp. *coagulans* would be indistinguishable from *S. pseudintermedius* on the basis of these characteristics, and *S. schleiferi* subsp.

schleiferi can give false-positive coagulase test results because of production of pseudocoagulases. Simple biochemical tests to distinguish *S. pseudintermedius* from *S. schleiferi,* such as additional carbohydrate fermentation tests, therefore are needed but often are not done. *S. pseudintermedius* ferments trehalose and lactose, whereas most *S. schleiferi* strains do not. In addition, *S. schleiferi* produces acetoin from glucose or pyruvate (positive Voges-Proskauer test result) but *S. pseudintermedius* does not. In some larger or reference laboratories molecular methods are being used to distinguish these *Staphylococcus* species.

Both *S. schleiferi* subsp. *schleiferi* and *S. schleiferi* subsp. *coagulans* have been isolated from the ear canals of healthy dogs, dogs with otitis, and dogs with recurrent pyoderma. Many of the isolates from dogs with otitis and recurrent pyoderma are methicillin resistant and contain the *mecA* gene, similar to most methicillin-resistant staphylococci. The fact that the organism is seen more frequently in dogs with recurrent infections suggests that it is an opportunistic pathogen. Recurrent skin infections usually are associated with an underlying cause such as allergies or endocrinopathies. *S. schleiferi* frequently develops resistance to fluoroquinolones but remains susceptible to many other classes of antibiotics.

Coagulase-Negative Staphylococci

Coagulase-negative *Staphylococcus* (CNS) species frequently are isolated in the veterinary clinical microbiology laboratory. Many times further speciation is not performed. The clinical significance of these organisms frequently is questioned, with some laboratories disregarding any CNS isolate. Because *S. schleiferi* is a known pathogen and has variable coagulase production, it should be identified fully and not grouped with other CNS organisms.

In people CNS organisms are known to be opportunistic pathogens, with infections most often associated with hospitalization, indwelling catheters, prosthetics, and immunocompromise. CNS species often are methicillin and multidrug resistant. There are very few reports in the veterinary literature regarding CNS infections in animals. *Staphylococcus epidermidis, Staphylococcus hominis, Staphylococcus hemolyticus,* and *Staphylococcus xylosus* have been isolated from various dog specimens either alone or in combination with coagulase-positive staphylococci; however, their role as a primary pathogen is unknown. Methicillin-resistant *S. epidermidis* and other CNS organisms have been isolated from skin infections of dogs

with hypercortisolemia, and treatment has required choosing antibiotics directed at these organisms. Therefore, although their pathogenicity remains uncertain, in cases in which CNS organisms are cultured in large numbers and show resistance to the current antibiotic, choosing an antibiotic based on the susceptibility pattern identified would be warranted.

In summary, *S. pseudintermedius* is an opportunistic staphylococcus commonly associated with skin infections in dogs and cats, whereas *S. aureus, S. schleiferi,* and CNS species are uncommon causes of infections in animals. The challenge with these infections lies with the emerging methicillin and multidrug resistance of the causative organisms and the potential risk these bacteria may have to the people who are in contact with affected pets. Administration of antimicrobials appears to be a major risk factor for the selection of methicillin- and multidrug-resistant staphylococci in dogs and cats. Therefore identification of these organisms from culture can aid the veterinarian in choosing the appropriate antibiotic based on susceptibility results so as to prevent selection of resistant bacteria from inappropriate antibiotic use.

References and Suggested Reading

Bemis DA et al: Evaluation of susceptibility test breakpoints used to predict *mecA*-mediated resistance in *Staphylococcus pseudintermedius* isolated from dogs, *J Vet Diagn Invest* 21:53, 2009.

Cain CL et al: Genotypic relatedness and phenotypic characterization of *Staphylococcus schleiferi* subspecies in clinical samples from dogs, *Am J Vet Res* 72:96, 2011.

Faires MC et al: Methicillin-resistant and -susceptible *Staphylococcus aureus* infections in dogs, *Emerg Infect Dis* 16:69, 2010.

Jones RD et al: Prevalence of oxacillin- and multidrug-resistant staphylococci in clinical samples from dogs: 1,772 samples (2001-2005), *J Am Vet Med Assoc* 230:221, 2007.

Loeffler A, Lloyd DH: Companion animals: a reservoir for methicillin-resistant *Staphylococcus aureus* in the community? *Epidemiol Infect* 138:595, 2010.

Morris DO et al: Screening of *Staphylococcus aureus, Staphylococcus intermedius,* and *Staphylococcus schleiferi* isolates obtained from small companion animals for antimicrobial resistance: a retrospective review of 749 isolates (2003-04), *Vet Dermatol* 7:332, 2006.

Sasaki T et al: Reclassification of phenotypically identified *Staphylococcus intermedius* strains, *J Clin Microbiol* 45:2770, 2007.

Simou C et al: Species specificity in the adherence of staphylococci to canine and human corneocytes: a preliminary study, *Vet Dermatol* 16:156, 2005.

Weese JS, van Duijkeren E: Methicillin-resistant *Staphylococcus aureus* and *Staphylococcus pseudintermedius* in veterinary medicine, *Vet Microbiol* 140:418, 2010.

CHAPTER 101

Treatment of Superficial Bacterial Folliculitis

ANDREW HILLIER, *Columbus, Ohio*

Superficial bacterial folliculitis (SBF) is diagnosed frequently in dogs and can develop secondary to almost any primary skin disease. SBF is most commonly encountered as a complication of primary allergic, parasitic, or metabolic disease. Staphylococci, and in particular *Staphylococcus pseudintermedius,* are the most important pathogens causing SBF (see Chapter 100).

Diagnosis

Clinical Lesions

Common lesions of SBF are papules and pustules, typically arising from a hair follicle. Pustules, which may be transient, are usually small but may on occasion be large, expansile, or flaccid. Crusts and variable alopecia, hypopigmentation and hyperpigmentation, and erythema may be present. Epidermal collarettes and target lesions can be prominent lesions in some patients.

Cytologic Analysis

Cytologic demonstration of cocci is helpful if there is any doubt that lesions represent SBF. However, if classic lesions of SBF are present and if similar lesions have responded to antimicrobial drug (AMD) therapy in the past, then cytologic examination is unnecessary. Cytologic analysis for cocci is never a poor diagnostic test and is mandatory in the following circumstances:

- When typical lesions are not present.
- When typical lesions are present but there has been a poor response to AMDs.
- When bacterial culture is performed (in the case of a negative culture result, a positive cytologic finding would prompt repeated culture, whereas a negative culture and negative cytologic finding would suggest a sterile pustular disease for which biopsy may be indicated).

The absence of bacteria on cytologic analysis does not rule out SBF, and the absence of inflammatory cells does not rule out infection (these cells may be absent in the presence of immunosuppressive diseases or in patients treated with immunosuppressive drugs).

Bacterial Culture and Susceptibility Testing

When to Culture

Bacterial culture is never contraindicated. Culture of SBF lesions is mandatory in the following circumstances:

- When there is less than 50% improvement in lesions after 2 weeks of systemic antibiotic therapy.
- When new lesions emerge 2 weeks or more after the initiation of systemic AMD therapy.
- When residual lesions remain after 6 weeks of AMD treatment.
- If there is a prior history of multidrug-resistant infection in the patient or in a pet from the same household.

What to Culture

Pustules are the preferred lesion because they have the highest reported rate for positive growth. Performing a diligent search, clipping hair with scissors to obtain "windows of the skin," and using a magnifying lens are encouraged. Do NOT disinfect the pustule surface. Lance the lesion with a sterile needle and apply a culturette to the purulent exudate.

Crusts, especially if fresh with pus on the underneath surface, are also suitable lesions to culture. Do NOT disinfect the surface; lift the edge of the crust with a sterile needle or forceps and touch a culturette to the exposed skin surface.

Epidermal collarettes may be cultured, but this is not as sensitive a technique as pustule culture. Do NOT disinfect; rub a culturette across the center of the lesion and under the leading edge of the collarettes.

Finally, papules also may be cultured; however, the technique is more invasive, time consuming, and expensive. After subcutaneous injection of local anesthesia, wipe the lesion once with 70% alcohol, then collect a tissue sample with a 3-mm sterile punch and submit the sample in a sterile container. Suture the biopsy site.

Antimicrobial Susceptibility Testing

The following AMDs should be tested with all staphylococcal isolates: erythromycin, clindamycin, tetracycline (doxycycline), trimethoprim/sulfamethoxazole, gentamicin, cephalothin (cefazolin), cefpodoxime, cefovecin, cefoxitin, amoxicillin/clavulanic acid, oxacillin (methicillin), enrofloxacin, and marbofloxacin. With the emergence of multidrug-resistant staphylococcal infections as a significant problem in recent years, it is mandatory that all clinical microbiology laboratories test for methicillin resistance using the correct guidelines for assessment of *S. pseudintermedius* as mandated by the Clinical and Laboratory Standards Institute.

Treatment

Before deciding on specific therapy, the clinician should consider the following factors: severity of lesions, extent of lesions, concurrent disease, local (regional) prevalence of methicillin-resistant staphylococci, and ability to perform topical therapy (and other drug therapy). Owner compliance with instructions and completion of treatments is critical to the resolution of infection and prevention of recurrence. Careful explanation of the rate of lesion resolution, expected duration of treatment, and necessity for treatment beyond lesion resolution are all very important in combating recurrence and the emergence of resistant infections. When recurrence of infection occurs, a diagnostic plan for evaluation of underlying primary disease is the best means to control recurrence and reduce AMD use.

Systemic Antimicrobial Therapy

Selection of systemic AMDs is based on availability, safety, cost, local prevalence of resistant staphylococci, and any patient-specific factors (e.g., concurrent disease or drug administration, previous drug reactions) (Table 101-1).

TABLE 101-1

Recommended Antimicrobial Drug Dosages for Use in Canine Superficial Bacterial Folliculitis

Amikacin	15 mg/kg q24h SC
Amoxicillin/clavulanic acid	12.5-20 mg/kg q12h PO
Cephalexin	22-30 mg/kg q12h PO
Cefadroxil	22-30 mg/kg q12h PO
Cefpodoxime	5-10 mg/kg q24h PO
Cefovecin	8 mg/kg q14d SC
Chloramphenicol	30-50 mg/kg q8h PO
Clindamycin	10 mg/kg q12h PO
Doxycycline	10 mg/kg q12h PO
Enrofloxacin	5-20 mg/kg q24h PO
Erythromycin	10-20 mg/kg q8h PO
Lincomycin	15-25 mg/kg q12h PO
Marbofloxacin	2.75-5.5 mg/kg q24h PO
Orbifloxacin	7.5 mg/kg q24h PO
Ormetoprim/sulfadimethoxine	27.5 mg/kg PO q24h
Rifampin	5-10 mg/kg q12h PO
Trimethoprim/sulfonamide	15-30 mg/kg PO q12h

PO, Orally; *SC,* subcutaneously.

Suggested (first-tier) antimicrobials for empiric therapy (in no particular order) include the following: clindamycin, cephalosporins (cephalexin, cefadroxil, cefpodoxime, cefovecin), and amoxicillin/clavulanic acid. Despite reports of the clinical efficacy of once-daily administration of some time-dependent antimicrobials (e.g., cephalexin, clindamycin, amoxicillin/clavulanic acid) it is recommended that these drugs be administered every 12 hours.

Additional first-tier AMDs may be appropriate for empiric therapy if local susceptibility is known (and disadvantages of the drugs are appreciated). These include trimethoprim- and ormetoprim-potentiated sulfonamides (frequent and varied adverse effects—consult a formulary); erythromycin (a rarely used drug due to the frequent vomiting and the need for administration every 8 hours); lincomycin (use is limited by significant expense); and doxycycline (use is limited by regionally variable susceptibility of microorganisms).

Second-tier AMDs may be necessary in situations in which first-tier AMDs are unable to be administered based on susceptibility or patient factors. These second-tier AMDs should always be prescribed based on culture and susceptibility testing and include doxycycline, chloramphenicol, rifampin (when used in combination with another drug to which the organism is susceptible, such as with a second-tier drug), fluoroquinolones (e.g., enrofloxacin, marbofloxacin), and amikacin. In addition, any non–β-lactam first-tier AMD (clindamycin, potentiated sulphas, doxycycline, minocycline) may also be considered when they have not previously been administered to the patient and culture and sensitivity results indicate susceptibility.

Second-tier AMDs typically are necessary only in multidrug-resistant infections (see Chapter 103).

Duration of Systemic Therapy

Although rapid improvement in lesions is seen in most cases, few patients have resolution of lesions within 2 weeks, and numerous studies indicate that most dogs need at least 3 weeks of systemic AMDs before the lesions are resolved. Continuation of treatment for at least 7 days beyond clinical resolution of lesions is recommended. A small number of dogs may require up to 6 weeks of treatment for resolution of SBF.

Topical Antimicrobial Therapy

Advantages of topical AMD therapy (see Chapter 102) include the following:

- High concentrations of antimicrobial agents are delivered directly to the site of infection on the skin surface.
- There is the potential to decrease the duration of systemic AMD therapy or even to eliminate it.
- Resistance to topical antimicrobials and antiseptics is rare.
- Methicillin-resistant staphylococci are killed.
- Adverse effects are minimal.
- Organisms are removed from the skin surface.

- There is minimal exposure of nonskin microbiota to AMDs (which reduces the risk of inadvertent emergence of resistant strains).

For *generalized disease,* topical formulations such as shampoos, conditioners, sprays, and rinses may incorporate chlorhexidine, benzoyl peroxide, ethyl lactate, povidone-iodine, and triclosan.

For more *focal and localized infections,* in addition to the aforementioned agents, the following have excellent efficacy against staphylococci: aminoglycosides, bacitracin, fusidic acid, a variety of hydroxyl acids (e.g., acetic acid, lactic acid, malic acid), novobiocin, silver sulfadiazine, pristinamycin, tea tree oil, and others. Mupirocin is another topical AMD with excellent activity against staphylococci.

Prevention of Superficial Bacterial Folliculitis

The most effective measure to prevent recurrence is to identify and control the underlying primary disease. Numerous protocols for the use of systemic AMDs to aid in the prevention of SBF, or to delay recurrence, have been published and advocated in public. Such protocols include pulse therapy (intermittent administration of therapeutic doses of AMD) and subminimal/subtherapeutic dosing (continuous use of AMDs at subtherapeutic dosages). There is significant concern about the selection of resistance with these protocols; accordingly, these approaches are discouraged. The use of autogenous bacterins or commercial bacterial antigens (e.g., Staphage Lysate in the United States) is encouraged. However, very few studies of the efficacy and usefulness of these measures have been reported, and further research is needed. If pulse or subminimal AMD therapy is considered, the patient should first be referred to a specialist for further evaluation and treatment.

References and Suggested Reading

Fitzgerald JR: The *Staphylococcus intermedius* group of bacterial pathogens: species re-classification, pathogenesis and the emergence of methicillin resistance, *Vet Dermatol* 20:490, 2009.

Jones RD et al: Prevalence of oxacillin- and multidrug-resistant staphylococci in clinical samples from dogs: 1,772 samples (2001-2005), *J Am Vet Med Assoc* 230(2):221, 2007.

Loeffler A et al: In vitro activity of fusidic acid and mupirocin against coagulase-positive staphylococci from pets, *J Antimicrob Chemother* 62:1301, 2008.

Monnet DL, Frimodt-Moller N: Antimicrobial drug use and methicillin-resistant *Staphylococcus aureus, Emerg Infect Dis* 7:1, 2001.

White SD et al: Evaluation of aerobic bacteriologic culture of epidermal collarette specimens in dogs with superficial pyoderma, *J Am Vet Med Assoc* 226(6):904, 2005.

CHAPTER **102**

Topical Therapy for Infectious Diseases

KENNETH W. KWOCHKA, *St. Joseph, Missouri*

In recent years, there has been a disturbing trend toward less use of topical therapy in patients with infectious skin diseases in favor of sole use of veterinary and human systemic antibiotics. Combined use of systemic antibiotics *and* topical antimicrobial therapy is preferred because it produces more rapid resolution of infection, causes less microbial resistance from overuse of systemic antibiotics, and yields possible cost savings. Because staphylococcal resistance has emerged as a significant problem, treatment programs to slow this process (such as judicious use of systemic and topical antibiotics, and more frequent use of antiseptics in shampoo, spray, rinse, and wipe formulations) are critical parts of the treatment plan.

Currently a very large number of topical antimicrobial ingredients in many formulations are available for veterinary use. Most are not licensed by the Food and Drug Administration and have not undergone the same rigorous approval process as drugs. Therefore, there is a great deal of product variability, and more companies are encouraged to provide adequate efficacy, safety, and manufacturing quality data for claims associated with their products.

This chapter reviews current recommendations for the topical management of bacterial and yeast skin infections.

Basic Guidelines for Topical Antimicrobials

- Demonstration and written instructions should be provided to clients on the proper use of prescribed topical products: the reason to use them, the way to use them, the desired response, the duration of treatment, and the need for a recheck to follow progress.
- A gentle, general cleansing shampoo should be used before an antimicrobial shampoo to clean the skin and hair coat and minimize the amount of the more expensive medicated product.
- The hair coat should be kept short for easier and more successful management of recurrent infections.
- The client should be instructed to ensure *at least 10 minutes of contact time* with gentle lathering for antimicrobial shampoos.
- Tepid or cool water should be used and the animal should be rinsed very well, especially when skin is inflamed and pruritic.
- The animal should be bathed *at least twice weekly* to treat a cutaneous infection and then as needed for maintenance.
- Antimicrobial sprays, rinses, or wipes should be used between shampoos for continual and residual activity.
- *Cytologic examination is extremely important* before, during, and after treatment to gauge response.

Bacterial Pyoderma

Bacterial pyoderma caused by staphylococcal infections is the most common and important indication for combined therapy with systemic antibiotics and topical therapy. Vigilant use of topical antimicrobial formulations can successfully treat and control recurrent infections, while minimizing use of the systemic drugs. Bacterial skin infections are secondary to primary dermatoses such as those caused by allergies, parasites, endocrinopathies, autoimmune skin diseases, and immunosuppressive therapy; control of these diseases lessens the likelihood of recurrent infections.

The most common organism isolated from pyoderma lesions in dogs is *Staphylococcus pseudintermedius* (see Chapter 100). Several topical antiseptics and antibiotics are used to treat staphylococcal infections, including benzoyl peroxide, chlorhexidine, miconazole, ethyl lactate, and mupirocin, either alone or in combination. New products and technologies are needed to address emerging bacterial resistance in a safe and effective manner.

Benzoyl Peroxide

Benzoyl peroxide is metabolized in the skin to benzoic acid, which alters pH and acts as an oxidizing agent to damage bacterial cell membranes. It is clinically effective in staphylococcal pyoderma, has demonstrated superior prophylactic activity compared with complexed iodine and triclosan, and is used in shampoos and a gel (Table 102-1). Benzoyl peroxide has been formulated with sulfur and salicylic acid for enhanced keratolytic, degreasing, and antibacterial activity.

Because of its follicular flushing, comedolytic, keratolytic, and degreasing activity, benzoyl peroxide has most commonly been used in greasy dogs with pyoderma, with deep pyoderma, and with pyoderma associated with demodicosis. Repeated use of benzoyl peroxide shampoos on dogs with atopic skin disease may cause further disruption of epidermal barrier function and increased percutaneous penetration of potential allergens. Moisturizing agents and fatty acids have been added to some benzoyl peroxide shampoos to offset the epidermal lipid loss and excessive drying that might occur with frequent use. However, if repeated use is necessary, chlorhexidine, chlorhexidine and miconazole, chlorhexidine and phytosphingosine, or ethyl lactate–containing shampoos are preferred.

Chlorhexidine

Chlorhexidine is a cationic biguanide antiseptic with activity against most of the common bacteria causing cutaneous infections. It is bactericidal by disrupting and increasing permeability of cell membranes of susceptible organisms. Chlorhexidine may have up to 48 hours of residual activity by adherence to the skin surface and hair coat because of its positive charge. It is generally nonirritating and rarely sensitizing, but may cause problems at high concentrations on mucous membranes and if ingested by puppies, kittens, and cats. Stability, bioavailability, and adherence characteristics of chlorhexidine can be significantly affected by the formulation into which it is incorporated. Chemical formulation of chlorhexidine is a challenge, and some marketed products may not meet label claims for potency and clinical efficacy. Unfortunately, comparative clinical efficacy studies and residual activity studies are lacking for most of the current veterinary formulations.

Dermatologists typically use 3% or 4% chlorhexidine shampoos (see Table 102-1). A recent clinical study documented better efficacy of a 3% chlorhexidine gluconate shampoo than of a 2.5% benzoyl peroxide shampoo used as sole therapy for canine *superficial* pyoderma (Loeffler et al, 2011). A Japanese study (Murayama et al, 2010) revealed comparable clinical activity for a 2% chlorhexidine acetate surgical scrub and a 4% chlorhexidine gluconate shampoo in 10 dogs with superficial pyoderma when treated twice per week. Additionally, in a population of seven dogs with methicillin-resistant staphylococcal (MRS) pyoderma treated with the 2% scrub every 2 days for 2 weeks, five dogs responded completely and one partially. Clinical efficacy may be more contingent on frequency of treatment than concentration of the active ingredient. For more residual activity, a chlorhexidine leave-on conditioner/rinse, spray, or wipe should be used between shampoos (see Table 102-1).

Miconazole

Miconazole is a topical imidazole antifungal agent that works by inhibiting the synthesis of ergosterol,

TABLE **102-1**

Topical Antimicrobial Formulations

Active Ingredient(s)	Product	Formulation(s)	Primary Indication(s)
Acetic acid 2%, boric acid 2%	MalAcetic	Shampoo, spray, wipes	*Malassezia* dermatitis
Benzoyl peroxide 3%/5%	Pyoben	Shampoo, gel	Bacterial pyoderma
Benzoyl peroxide 2.5%	Benzoyl-Plus	Shampoo	Bacterial pyoderma
Benzoyl peroxide 3%, sulfur 2%, salicylic acid 2%, phytosphingosine 0.05%	Oxiderm Shampoo +PS	Shampoo	Bacterial pyoderma, greasy scale
Benzoyl peroxide 2.5%, sulfur 1%, salicylic acid 1%	DermaBenSs	Shampoo	Bacterial pyoderma, greasy scale
Chlorhexidine gluconate 4%	ChlorhexiDerm 4%	Shampoo, spray	Bacterial pyoderma
Chlorhexidine gluconate 4%	TrizCHLOR 4	Shampoo, spray, wipes	Bacterial pyoderma
Chlorhexidine gluconate 3%	Hexadine	Shampoo	Bacterial pyoderma
Chlorhexidine gluconate 3%, phytosphingosine 0.05%	Douxo Chlorhexidine PS	Shampoo, spray, pads	Bacterial pyoderma
Chlorhexidine gluconate 2.3%, ketoconazole 1%	KetoChlor	Shampoo	Bacterial pyoderma, *Malassezia* dermatitis
Chlorhexidine gluconate 2.3%, ketoconazole 1%	Resi KetoChlor	Leave-on lotion	Bacterial pyoderma, *Malassezia* dermatitis
Chlorhexidine gluconate 2%, miconazole nitrate 2%	Malaseb	Shampoo, spray, flush	Bacterial pyoderma, *Malassezia* dermatitis
Chlorhexidine gluconate 2%, ketoconazole 1%, acetic acid 2%	Mal-A-Ket	Shampoo, wipes	Bacterial pyoderma, *Malassezia* dermatitis
Ethyl lactate 10%	Etiderm	Shampoo	Bacterial pyoderma
Hypochlorous acid, sodium hypochlorite	Vetericyn VF	Spray, spray gel	Bacterial pyoderma
Lactoferrin, lysozyme, lactoperoxidase	Zymox	Shampoo, rinse	Bacterial pyoderma
Miconazole nitrate 2%, chloroxylenol 1%	Sebozole	Shampoo	Bacterial pyoderma, *Malassezia* dermatitis
Miconazole nitrate 1%-2%	Generics	Spray, cream	Bacterial pyoderma, *Malassezia* dermatitis
Mupirocin 2%	Muricin	Ointment	Reserve for methicillin-resistant staphylococcal pyoderma
Nisin 25 µg/ml	Preva	Wipes	Bacterial pyoderma

a critical component of fungal cell membranes. It also has activity against some gram-positive bacteria, including methicillin-sensitive and methicillin-resistant staphylococci. Minimal inhibitory concentrations (MICs) in the range of 1 to 2 µg/ml have been reported for methicillin-resistant *Staphylococcus aureus* (MRSA) isolates from humans. Results of a study of 112 methicillin-resistant *Staphylococcus pseudintermedius* isolates from dogs showed a range of 1 to 4 µg/ml with the majority at 2 µg/ml (Weese et al, 2012). These MICs are well below concentrations achievable with topical therapy at 2% miconazole nitrate (20,000 µg/ml). Additionally, miconazole is narrow spectrum, safe, readily available, and of low priority for use in human patients with MRS infections.

The antibacterial activity of miconazole appears to be related to induction of intracellular reactive oxygen species and direct cell membrane damage by mechanisms other than inhibition of ergosterol. These actions also appear to be miconazole specific, since ketoconazole has

MICs that are tenfold higher than those demonstrated for miconazole (Sud and Feingold, 1982).

Miconazole is available alone in shampoo, spray, and cream formulations (see Table 102-1), but most commonly is used at 2% in combination with 2% chlorhexidine (Malaseb). Synergistic antifungal activity (Perrins and Bond, 2003) and antibacterial activity (Kwochka, 2005) have been demonstrated with chlorhexidine and miconazole at equal concentrations.

Ethyl Lactate

Ethyl lactate (Etiderm) is hydrolyzed in the skin to ethanol and lactic acid, thus lowering the skin pH and acting similarly to benzoyl peroxide. One study demonstrated comparable clinical efficacy to benzoyl peroxide in dogs with *superficial* pyoderma (Ascher et al, 1990), but repeated use is less drying and irritating. For severe infections, ethyl lactate usually is not as clinically effective and is reserved for those patients with sensitive, inflamed, and pruritic skin that cannot tolerate more potent formulations.

Mupirocin

Mupirocin (Muricin) is an antibiotic isolated from *Pseudomonas fluorescens* with more than 90% of the formulation comprised of pseudomonic acid A. It is an excellent ointment formulation for localized staphylococcal skin infections that is bactericidal, has enhanced activity at an acid pH, shows no cross-resistance with other classes of antibiotics, and has virtually no systemic penetration but excellent local penetration. Mupirocin is used twice daily for focal skin infections such as impetigo, focal superficial or deep pyoderma, callus/pressure point pyoderma, infected chin acne, fold pyoderma, mucocutaneous pyoderma, and interdigital abscesses.

A recent study (Fulham et al, 2011) demonstrated that 86.6% of MRS field isolates from dogs with pyoderma were susceptible to mupirocin. Mupirocin is the most commonly used topical antibiotic for treatment of humans with MRS infections and for decolonization of human MRS carriers who are at risk of recurrent severe infections and potential transmission to susceptible individuals with whom they are in contact. However, resistance is increasing with widespread continual use in human hospitals and other health care facilities, with the result that over 60% of MRS isolates also are resistant to mupirocin.

For these reasons, it is medically and ethically prudent to reserve use of mupirocin in veterinary patients to those with MRS skin or ear infections that are documented by culture and susceptibility testing and are not responsive to conventional topical antiseptics and antibiotics. The use of mupirocin to treat interdigital abscesses is also justified given the usually slow and incomplete response of these infections to systemic antibiotics and other forms of topical therapy.

Methicillin-Resistant Staphylococcal Pyoderma

MRS skin infections are dramatically increasing in general and specialty practice. Two websites provide excellent clinical information on this complex subject (British Small Animal Veterinary Association, 2011; Weese and Anderson, n.d.).

Many MRS isolates are now multidrug resistant, and systemic antibiotics are no longer a viable option for some patients. Aggressive topical therapy is required. Clinical efficacy studies are needed to substantiate these recommendations. However, diligent owners and their veterinarians are successfully treating these resistant infections by managing the underlying primary dermatosis, following hygienic practices reviewed in the websites referenced earlier and doing the following:

- Keeping the patient's hair coat short
- Using antimicrobial shampoos with *at least a 10-minute contact time every 2 or 3 days initially*
- Applying antimicrobial rinses, sprays, lotions, wipes, or ointments on focally affected areas *two or three times a day on the nonshampoo days*

The most commonly used products available at this time are the following:

- 3% or 4% chlorhexidine shampoo or 2% chlorhexidine/2% miconazole combination shampoo
- 4% chlorhexidine sprays and wipes
- 2% mupirocin ointment
- 25 µg/ml nisin wipes (Preva)

Other topical options include the following:

- Hypochlorous acid and sodium hypochlorite spray and hydrogel (Vetericyn VF)
- Soakings with diluted sodium hypochlorite (bleach)
- Lactoferrin, lysozyme, and lactoperoxidase shampoo and rinse (Zymox)
- 1% amikacin sprays (compounded), reserved for patients with unresponsive infections
- Fusidic acid cream used as indicated for mupirocin (not available in the United States)

Treatment is continued until full clinical resolution is achieved and cytologic results are negative. For patients with recurrent infections, long-term maintenance may be indicated with topicals applied as frequently as needed to prevent flare-ups.

Malassezia Dermatitis

Malassezia dermatitis is similar to bacterial pyoderma in that it tends to be recurrent and caused by the same underlying primary dermatoses. Generalized infection warrants both systemic and topical treatment, whereas the latter alone may be effective for yeast otitis and pododermatitis, and for prevention of recurrent infections (see Web Chapter 44).

Chlorhexidine, Miconazole, Ketoconazole

Chlorhexidine used alone at 3% or 4% and miconazole used alone at 1% or 2% may be effective in many cases of yeast dermatitis. However, when chlorhexidine is combined with a topical azole antifungal agent, efficacy is more consistent. Examples of such combinations include 2% chlorhexidine and 2% miconazole (Malaseb), 2.3% chlorhexidine and 1% ketoconazole (KetoChlor), and 2% chlorhexidine, 1% ketoconazole, and 2% acetic acid (Mal-A-Ket). In a published evidence-based review of treatments for *Malassezia* dermatitis in dogs, only a 2% chlorhexidine and 2% miconazole shampoo could be recommended with good evidence for efficacy (Negre et al, 2009). Twice-weekly shampoos are recommended with rinses, lotions, sprays, or wipes applied to focally severe lesions between shampoos (see Table 102-1).

Acetic Acid, Boric Acid

The combination of 2% acetic acid and 2% boric acid is effective in the treatment and control of *Malassezia* dermatitis. These active ingredients are incorporated into shampoo, spray, and wipe formulations (MalAcetic). Because of their acidity, more irritation may be seen with these ingredients, especially when used on inflamed irritated skin. Acetic acid also has excellent antibacterial activity against *Pseudomonas aeruginosa* and is commonly used to treat resistant ear infections as a vehicle with other antibiotics. Results of a recent *in vitro* study demonstrated inactivation of two *S. pseudintermedius* isolates from the uterus of a dog with pyometra after 30 minutes of exposure to a 2% acetic acid and 2% boric acid aqueous solution (Haesebrouck et al, 2009). More work is needed to determine how this finding may relate to clinical efficacy of bacterial infections of the skin.

References and Suggested Reading

Ascher F et al: Controlled trial of ethyl lactate and benzoyl peroxide shampoos in the management of canine surface pyoderma and superficial pyoderma. In Von Tscharner C, Halliwell REW, editors: *Advances in veterinary dermatology,* vol 1, London, 1990, Baillière Tindall, p 375.

British Small Animal Veterinary Association: BSAVA practice guidelines—reducing the risk from MRSA and MRSP, updated August 23, 2011. www.bsava.com/Advice/MRSA/tabid/171/Default.aspx. Accessed December 2, 2012.

Fulham KS et al: *In vitro* susceptibility testing of methicillin-resistant and methicillin-susceptible staphylococci to mupirocin and novobiocin, *Vet Dermatol* 22:88, 2011.

Haesebrouck F et al: Antimicrobial activity of an acetic and boric acid solution against *Staphylococcus pseudintermedius, Vlaams Diergen Tijdschr* 78:89, 2009.

Kwochka KW: *In vitro* placebo-controlled time-kill comparison of an aqueous rinse formulation containing miconazole nitrate and chlorhexidine gluconate against bacterial and fungal cutaneous pathogens, *Vet Dermatol* 16:200, 2005.

Loeffler A, Cobb MA, Bond R: Comparison of a chlorhexidine and a benzoyl peroxide shampoo as sole treatment in canine superficial pyoderma, *Vet Rec* 169:249, 2011.

Murayama N et al: Efficacy of a surgical scrub including 2% chlorhexidine acetate for canine superficial pyoderma, *Vet Dermatol* 21:586, 2010.

Negre A, Bensignor E, Guillot J: Evidence-based veterinary dermatology: a systematic review of interventions for *Malassezia* dermatitis in dogs, *Vet Dermatol* 20:1, 2009.

Perrins N, Bond R: Synergistic inhibition of the growth *in vitro* of *Microsporum canis* by miconazole and chlorhexidine, *Vet Dermatol* 14:99, 2003.

Sud IJ, Feingold DS: Action of antifungal imidazoles on *Staphylococcus aureus, Antimicrob Agents Chemother* 22:470, 1982.

Weese S, Anderson M: Worms & germs blog, www.wormsandgermsblog.com. Accessed December 2, 2012.

Weese JS, Walker M, Lowe T: *In vitro* miconazole susceptibility of methicillin-resistant *Staphylococcus pseudintermedius* and *Staphylococcus aureus, Vet Dermatol* 23:400, 2012.

CHAPTER 103

Methicillin-Resistant Staphylococcal Infections

CARLO VITALE, *San Francisco, California*

The rapid and widespread emergence of methicillin-resistant *Staphylococcus* spp. has led to infections that are among the more difficult diseases to treat in veterinary dermatology. *Staphylococcus pseudintermedius* is by far the most common species encountered in veterinary medicine. In dogs, the most common presentation of *S. pseudintermedius* infection is superficial pyoderma (and, less frequently, otitis, deep pyoderma, and surface pyoderma). These infections have been linked to poorly controlled allergic dermatitis, predominantly canine atopic dermatitis and other primary diseases that compromise the skin integrity and defense mechanisms.

Methicillin is a penicillin-type antibiotic that no longer is used in the treatment of patients. It also has been replaced in the laboratory by oxacillin for culture and susceptibility testing because it is unstable; thus oxacillin resistance is used as a marker for methicillin resistance of staphylococci. By convention, *in vitro* resistance to oxacillin implies resistance to all penicillins and cephalosporins (β-lactams), with the exception of some new-generation cephalosporins such as ceftobiprole and ceftaroline. Production of penicillin-binding protein 2a (PBP2a) by staphylococci confers methicillin resistance. These staphylococci carry the gene *mecA* that encodes the protein PBP2a.

Incidence

Historically, *Staphylococcus intermedius* was the most common bacteria isolated from cases of pyoderma. It has been shown, however, that most strains previously identified as *S. intermedius* actually are *S. pseudintermedius,* as shown through multilocus sequence typing (Bannoehr et al, 2007) (see Chapter 100).

The clinical presentation of superficial pyoderma caused by methicillin-resistant organisms generally does not differ from that of routine cases. However, it is the author's experience that pyoderma caused by methicillin-resistant *Staphylococcus aureus* (MRSA) in dogs and cats differs markedly and characteristically is severe and deep. Articles have been published documenting methicillin resistance in cases of *S. pseudintermedius* infection (Cole et al, 2004; Gortel et al, 1999; Morris et al, 2006; Ruscher et al, 2010; Bryan et al, 2012). Interestingly, in another study only 2 of 57 *S. intermedius* isolates were resistant to methicillin; however, about half of the total expressed PBP2a, which indicates that the genetic capability was present to be resistant under more optimal conditions (Kania et al, 2004).

Since most of the public's attention has been given to MRSA in animals, it is clear that there has been a definite increase in the number of reports of MRSA infections in pets (Baptiste et al, 2005; Gortel et al, 1999; Kania et al, 2004; Loeffler et al, 2005; Morris et al, 2006; Weese et al, 2010; Vitale et al, 2005). In addition to MRSA, *Staphylococcus schleiferi* recently has been associated with cases of canine pyoderma and has demonstrated methicillin resistance (May et al, 2005; Morris et al, 2006). MRSA and methicillin-resistant *S. schleiferi* infections appear to be uncommon in dogs. Many strains of methicillin-resistant *Staphylococcus* are not multidrug resistant.

Zoonosis

MRSA is considered to be a reverse zoonosis (human to animal transmission). There have been several documented cases of likely transmission of MRSA from humans to animals (Manian, 2003; O'Mahony et al, 2005; Tomlin et al, 1999; van Duijkeren et al, 2004; Weese et al, 2006). Transmission of MRSA to pets via contact with infected humans likely results in colonization (primarily nasal and rectal), infection, or both in dogs and cats. In addition, some of these reports have shown that pets can serve as a colonized or infected reservoir, which allows transmission back to the humans. The author has seen several cases of nasal colonization with MRSA in dogs that acted as a source of reinfection of humans who had intimate contact with the affected pet.

Management and Therapy

The following recommendations may be useful to achieve treatment success and possibly reduce the risk of further antibiotic resistance. Less commonly prescribed antibiotics have been recently reviewed with updated treatment recommendations (Papich, 2012).

The most common first-line antibiotic prescribed empirically for proven or suspected non–methicillin-resistant *S. pseudintermedius* (non-MRSP) canine pyoderma is cephalexin (22 mg/kg q12h) or another similar antibiotic. The American College of Veterinary Internal Medicine and several university teaching hospitals have developed guidelines for the general use of antibiotics (Weese, 2006). In all cases of poorly responsive pyoderma, bacterial culture and susceptibility testing is recommended, and treatment is based on results. Culture is also recommended in patients with deep pyoderma because these cases may have additional gram-negative bacteria

or may have dermal fibrosis and thus can be a pharmacologic challenge. Interpretation of susceptibility results generally is not difficult. Not all MRSP organisms are also multidrug resistant. In cases of MRSP pyoderma, clindamycin (11 mg/kg once daily or divided q12h) is recommended (as long as the isolate shows susceptibility to erythromycin as well). Doxycycline (5 mg/kg q12h) is a good alternative, but the author has found that in some cases resistance develops while the patient is receiving treatment. Additionally, for the two aforementioned antibiotics resistance can develop after a second or third period of treatment. Potentiated sulfonamides also are a good choice, but they have lost favor because of historical resistance and concerns about more serious adverse effects. Use of chloramphenicol (50 mg/kg q8h) has gained popularity, and in most cases this drug is superior to other antibiotics because of its reliability in treating dogs with MRSP pyoderma. Certain undesirable adverse effects have limited its use. These include vomiting, anorexia, diarrhea, mild anemia (particularly after several weeks of treatment), and rarely limb weakness or myositis. Owners are usually advised to wear gloves because published data describe aplastic anemia as an adverse event when administered to human patients.

Recommended duration of treatment generally is 2 to 3 weeks for superficial pyoderma and 4 to 6 weeks for deep pyoderma. In cases of recurrent pyoderma, and particularly in infections caused by multidrug-resistant MRSP, topical therapy is recommended. This can include shampoo therapy (2% to 4% chlorhexidine or benzoyl peroxide based) several times weekly or daily application of leave-on rinses or sprays such as chlorhexidine with or without tromethamine and edetate disodium dihydrate or dilute bleach. Consultation with a microbiologist or dermatologist may be useful to confirm proper interpretation of susceptibility test results and ensure treatment success. Less commonly prescribed antibiotics for MRSP pyoderma include rifampicin (10 mg/kg usually divided q12h) and injectable amikacin (15 mg/kg once daily). Careful monitoring of all hepatic enzymes every 3 to 4 days is recommended for patients treated with rifampicin, and performing urinalyses (monitoring casts) and monitoring renal values every 3 to 4 days are advised with amikacin.

As in all cases of infectious disease, it is extraordinarily important to wash hands thoroughly and frequently after touching each patient or contaminated objects. Proper hand hygiene (frequent washing with warm water and soap or use of waterless alcohol-based rubs) is the single most important factor in reducing cross contamination as well as infections. The use of clean latex gloves can be helpful. All patients suspected or proven to be infected with MRSA should be managed in a proper isolation ward.

References and Suggested Reading

Bannoehr J et al: Population genetic structure of the *Staphylococcus intermedius* group: insights into *agr* diversification and the emergence of methicillin-resistant strains, *J Bacteriol* 189:8685, 2007.

Baptiste KE et al: Methicillin-resistant staphylococci in companion animals, *Emerg Infect Dis* 11:1942, 2005.

Bryan J et al: Treatment outcome of dogs with methicillin-resistant and methicillin-susceptible *Staphylococcus pseudintermedius* pyoderma, *Vet Dermatol* 23:361, 2012.

Cole LK et al: Methicillin-resistant *Staphylococcus intermedius* organisms from the vertical ear canal of dogs with end stage otitis externa, *Vet Dermatol* 15:35, 2004.

Gortel K et al: Methicillin resistance among staphylococci isolated from dogs, *Am J Vet Res* 60:1526, 1999.

Kania SA et al: Methicillin resistance of staphylococci isolated from the skin of dogs with pyoderma, *Am J Vet Res* 65:1265, 2004.

Loeffler A et al: Prevalence of methicillin-resistant *Staphylococcus aureus* among staff and pets in a small animal referral hospital in the UK, *J Antimicrob Chemother* 56:692, 2005.

Manian FA: Asymptomatic nasal carriage of mupirocin-resistant, methicillin-resistant *Staphylococcus aureus* (MRSA) in a pet dog associated with MRSA infection in household contacts, *Clin Infect Dis* 36:e26, 2003.

May ER et al: Isolation of *Staphylococcus schleiferi* from healthy dogs and dogs with otitis, pyoderma, or both, *J Am Vet Med Assoc* 227:928, 2005.

Morris DO et al: Screening of *Staphylococcus aureus, Staphylococcus intermedius,* and *Staphylococcus schleiferi* isolates obtained from small companion animals for antimicrobial resistance: a retrospective review of 749 isolates (2003-04), *Vet Dermatol* 17: 332, 2006.

O'Mahony R et al: Methicillin-resistant *Staphylococcus aureus* (MRSA) isolated from animals and veterinary personnel in Ireland, *Vet Microbiol* 109:285, 2005.

Papich M: Selection of antibiotics for methicillin-resistant *Staphylococcus pseudintermedius*: time to revisit some old drugs? *Vet Dermatol* 23:352, 2012.

Ruscher C et al: Widespread rapid emergence of a distinct methicillin- and multidrug-resistant *Staphylococcus pseudintermedius* (MRSP) genetic lineage in Europe, *Vet Microbiol* 144:340, 2010.

Tomlin J et al: Methicillin-resistant *Staphylococcus aureus* infections in 11 dogs, *Vet Rec* 144:60, 1999.

van Duijkeren E et al: Human-to-dog transmission of methicillin-resistant *Staphylococcus aureus, Emerg Infect Dis* 10:2235, 2004.

Vitale C et al: Methicillin-resistant *Staphylococcus aureus* in cat and owner, *Emerg Infect Dis* 12:1998, 1995.

Weese JS: Investigation of antimicrobial use and the impact of antimicrobial use guidelines in a small animal veterinary teaching hospital: 1995-2004, *J Am Vet Med Assoc* 228:553, 2006.

Weese JS et al: Suspected transmission of methicillin-resistant *Staphylococcus aureus* between domestic pets and humans in veterinary clinics and in the household, *Vet Microbiol* 115:148, 2006.

Weese JS et al: Methicillin-resistant *Staphylococcus aureus* and *Staphylococcus pseudintermedius* in veterinary medicine, *Vet Microbiol* 140:418, 2010.

CHAPTER 104

Nontuberculous Cutaneous Granulomas in Dogs and Cats (Canine Leproid Granuloma and Feline Leprosy Syndrome)

ANNE FAWCETT, *Sydney, New South Wales, Australia*
JANET A.M. FYFE, *Melbourne, Victoria, Australia*
RICHARD MALIK, *Sydney, New South Wales, Australia*

Canine leproid granuloma and feline leprosy syndrome are relatively uncommon nodular dermatoses caused by saprophytic mycobacterial species that are extremely fastidious and difficult to culture. Infection may be self-limiting, particularly in dogs with CLG, but that is rarely the case in cats. Because differential diagnoses for cutaneous nodules include potentially life-threatening conditions (e.g., neoplasia and tuberculosis), it is critical to make a definitive diagnosis.

Canine Leproid Granuloma

Canine leproid granuloma (CLG) is a cutaneous or subcutaneous, typically self-limiting nodular mycobacteriosis caused by a novel mycobacterium yet to be fully characterized. The causal organism is distributed worldwide and is common in Australia and Brazil, as well as parts of Europe and the United States (Foley et al, 2002).

Causes

The route of inoculation is unknown, but biting flies, midges, mosquitoes, or other arthropods may introduce mycobacteria into the host based on the following evidence: the presence of potential vectors around affected dogs, lesions occurring at sites favored by such vectors (e.g., the dorsal fold of the ears), and the prevalence of

CLG in short-coated breeds and dogs housed outdoors (Malik et al, 1998).

Signalment and Clinical Findings

CLG occurs almost exclusively in short-coated breeds, with boxers and boxer crosses remarkably overrepresented. Staffordshire bull terriers and Doberman pinschers also are commonly affected (Malik et al, 2001). The finding of multiple characteristic lesions in typical locations in a short-coated breed suggests the diagnosis of CLG.

CLG usually is manifest as single or multiple firm, granulomatous to pyogranulomatous, well-circumscribed nodules in the skin or subcutis (Figure 104-1). Nodules typically are located on the head, particularly the dorsal fold of the ears. Some nodules ulcerate and are usually painless, but may be pruritic when secondary infection with *Staphylococcus pseudintermedius* occurs. Affected dogs are otherwise healthy.

Diagnosis

The differential diagnoses include infectious, inflammatory, and neoplastic diseases of the subcutis and skin. When samples are collected, the skin surface should be disinfected first because environmental mycobacteria may be present on the epidermis and can cause erroneous results in both culture and polymerase chain reaction (PCR) studies.

On cytologic examination, mycobacteria appear as bacilli that do not stain with Romanowsky-type stains (e.g., Diff-Quik) but do stain with a modified acid-fast procedure such as the Ziehl-Neelsen method, and thus are so-called acid-fast bacilli (AFB). Organisms appear in variable numbers either within the macrophages or giant cells, or extracellularly. Absence of visible AFB organisms on cytologic examination does not rule out CLG.

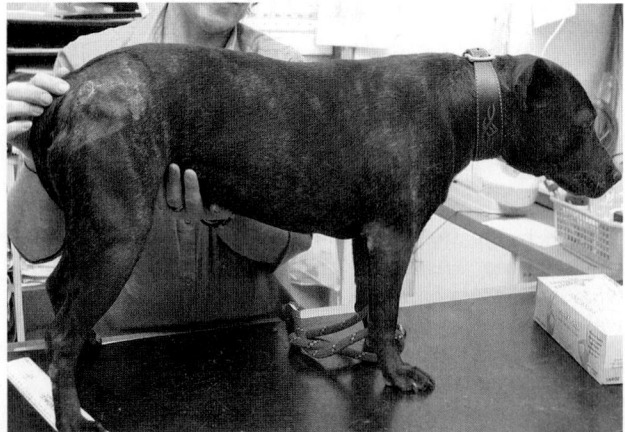

Figure 104-1 A single cutaneous nodule in a Staffordshire terrier with canine leproid granuloma (CLG) and secondary *Staphylococcus pseudintermedius* infection. The dog made a complete recovery following surgical excision with wide margins. Note the majority of CLG locations are found around the head and ears, but they can occur elsewhere on the body as in this case. (Photo courtesy Anne Fawcett.)

Histopathologic analysis reveals pyogranulomatous dermatitis with AFB. The bacteria are highly variable in appearance, ranging from long, slender filaments to short, variably beaded bacilli to coccoid forms. Sections may require a lengthy search, even by experienced pathologists, to locate foci in which AFB organisms are evident. A histologic diagnosis of "sterile" pyogranuloma syndrome should prompt a search for an infectious agent.

The CLG organism is not possible to culture because its growth requirements have not been determined. Other organisms that can be cultured, particularly *S. pseudintermedius,* can secondarily infect leproid granulomas.

PCR testing provides a definitive diagnosis by amplifying regions of the bacterial 16S ribosomal RNA gene using mycobacterium-specific primers. The test is more sensitive when performed on DNA extracted from fresh tissue; however, published PCR protocols generally are successful even when used on paraffin-embedded, formalin-fixed tissue, although false-negative results may occur when contact time with formalin is over 48 hours. Retrospective studies using PCR have demonstrated the presence of microbial DNA (e.g., from mycobacteria and *Leishmania* spp.) in specimens previously diagnosed as sterile. Recently, one of the authors (JF) has developed a real-time PCR test for the CLG organism that is sensitive and specific and improves the availability and accuracy of molecular diagnostics (Smits et al, 2012).

Feline Leprosy Syndromes

The term *feline leprosy syndromes* (FLS) refers to a group of cutaneous or subcutaneous granulomas caused by mycobacteria that usually do not grow on routinely used laboratory media and that cannot be distinguished clinically or microscopically from lesions caused by tuberculosis bacteria (*Mycobacterium bovis, Mycobacterium microti*) and members of the *Mycobacterium avium-intracellulare* complex (MAC) group. FLS should not be confused with infection caused by rapidly growing mycobacteria (*Mycobacterium fortuitum* group, *Mycobacterium phlei, Mycobacterium smegmatis* group, and *Mycobacterium chelonae/abscessus* group) characterized by chronic fistulous tracts, ulcerative nodules, and fasciitis or panniculitis in the fatty subcutaneous tissues of the ventral abdomen.

Causes

The location of lesions on cats suggests inoculation of organisms through insect bites, rodent bites, or fight wounds and hematogenous spread. Mycobacterial species associated with FLS include *Mycobacterium lepraemurium, Mycobacterium visibilis* (Appleyard and Clark, 2002), *Mycobacterium* sp. strain Tarwin (Fyfe et al, 2008), and a novel species common on the east coast of Australia related to *Mycobacterium leprae* and *Mycobacterium haemophilum* (Hughes et al, 2004).

Signalment and Clinical Findings

FLS is seen in cats with outdoor access; young males are overrepresented. Single or multiple cutaneous nodules of the head, limbs, or trunk typically are accompanied by

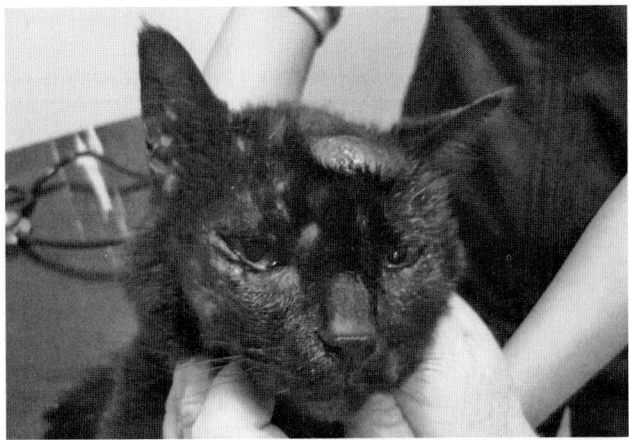

Figure 104-2 A domestic shorthair cat with lesions typical of feline leprosy syndrome (FLS). Clinical improvement was seen following treatment with clarithromycin and rifampicin. (Photo courtesy Sue Cook.)

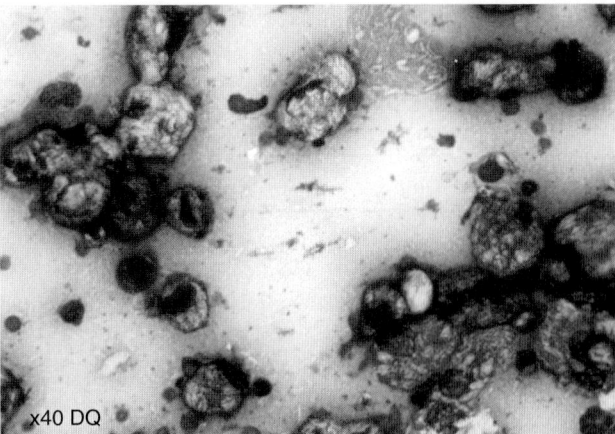

Figure 104-3 Negative staining bacilli on a Diff-Quik–stained fine-needle aspirate of feline leprosy lesions in a 14-year-old domestic shorthair cat. (Photo courtesy George Reppas.)

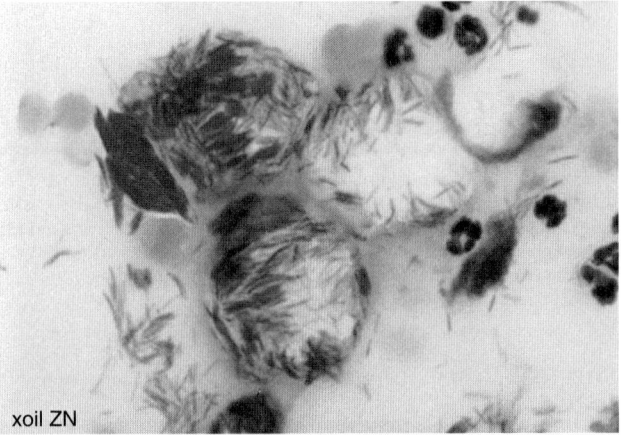

Figure 104-4 Acid-fast bacilli on a Ziehl-Neelsen–stained fine-needle aspirate of feline leprosy lesions in a 14-year-old domestic shorthair cat. (Photo courtesy George Reppas.)

peripheral lymphadenomegaly (Figure 104-2). FLS typically is divided into two syndromes: the first occurs in young cats and is characterized by localized, ulcerated, nodular lesions on the limbs with tuberculoid pathologic features and is associated with *M. lepraemurium;* the second is seen in older cats and is characterized by generalized, nonulcerated, and less rapidly progressive lesions with lepromatous pathologic features and is caused by either the novel species on the east coast of Australia or *M. visibilis.* Such division recently has been questioned by Davies and colleagues (2006), who noted both tuberculoid and lepromatous histologic features in cats of all ages. A better way to think about the pathologic process is that lepromatous features (linked to *M. visibilis* and the novel east coast species) are associated with immune deficiency. Unlike CLG, FLS almost invariably has a progressive clinical course.

Diagnosis

Hematologic and biochemical testing demonstrate nonspecific changes but are worth pursuing because some older cats have comorbidities such as liver or kidney disease that affect drug choices and prognosis. Testing for feline immunodeficiency virus and feline leukemia virus should be considered, although feline immunodeficiency virus positivity does not preclude effective treatment. Major differential diagnoses are similar to those described for CLG. Techniques and precautions for specimen collection are as described earlier for CLG, except that organisms are seen easily and are numerous on cytologic examination (Figure 104-3).

Histopathologic Analysis

Lesions are characterized by pyogranulomatous inflammation (either lepromatous or tuberculoid form) with macrophages containing many AFB organisms in sections stained using the Ziehl-Neelsen or Fite method (Figure 104-4). Histologically, FLS is not distinguishable from potentially zoonotic tuberculous infections; hence the importance of PCR and sequence analysis performed at a mycobacterial reference laboratory (see CLG earlier). Culture results typically are negative.

Treatment of Canine Leproid Granuloma and Feline Leprosy Syndromes

Most CLG infections are self-limiting, with spontaneous lesion regression occurring within 1 to 3 months regardless of treatment, likely due to the mounting of an effective adaptive cell-mediated immune response by the host. This complicates assessment of the efficacy of empiric antimicrobial regimens. For example, in one study a favorable response was seen in 57% of cases treated with doxycycline and 63% treated with amoxicillin/clavulanic acid, whereas spontaneous regression occurred in 86% of untreated dogs (Malik et al, 1998). Persistence of lesions for longer than 3 to 6 months warrants further treatment because cell-mediated immunity may be compromised.

In contrast, FLS syndromes generally have a progressive clinical course and can recur following surgical excision, especially when inadequate margins are obtained and appropriate antimycobacterial agents are not given postoperatively. Thus medical treatment should be instituted immediately after diagnosis.

TABLE **104-1**

Antimicrobial Agents Used in the Treatment of Canine Leproid Granuloma and Feline Leprosy Syndromes

Drug	DOSE (mg/kg) Dog	Cat	Route of Administration	Dosing Interval (hours)	Comments
Pradofloxacin*	3-5 (tablets) once daily	5-7.5 (suspension) once daily	Oral	24	Most effective veterinary fluoroquinolone; devoid of retinotoxicity
Rifampicin	10-15 (maximum 600 mg q24h)	10-15	Oral	24	May cause hepatotoxicity, generalized erythema and pruritus, dyspnea, central nervous system signs; teratogenic
Clarithromycin	15-25		Oral	12	May cause pinnal erythema, generalized erythema, hepatotoxicity
		10-15 mg/kg	Oral	12	
		62.5-125 mg per cat	Oral	12	
Azithromycin	5-10	5-10	Oral	24	May cause GI signs
Clofazimine	NA	4-10	Oral	24	May cause hepatotoxicity, GI signs, photosensitization, pitting corneal lesions
		25-50 mg per cat	Oral	24-48	
Doxycycline	5-7.5	5-10	Oral	12	May cause GI signs, esophagitis
Amikacin	10-15	10-15	Intravenous, intramuscular, subcutaneous	24	May cause nephrotoxicity, ototoxicity

A combination of rifampicin (10-15 mg/kg q24h PO) and clarithromycin (7.5-12.5 mg/kg q8-12h PO) is recommended for treating severe or refractory canine leproid granuloma (Malik et al, 2001), in concert with topical silver sulfasalazine. Feline leprosy syndromes can be treated with combinations of two or three drugs from this table, typically (1) clarithromycin, (2) pradofloxacin, and (3) rifampicin or clofazimine.
*Where pradofloxacin is unavailable the human drug moxifloxacin may be substituted at a dosage of 10 mg/kg once daily PO; because of the large tablet size, this drug needs to be compounded for use in cats and small dogs.
GI, Gastrointestinal; *NA,* not applicable.

Surgical Resection of Nodules

In dogs with CLG, marginal surgical resection of nodules typically is curative. Although lesions can recur after surgery in cats with early FLS lesions, if antimicrobials are administered before, during, and after resection, recurrence is rare. In animals with large or multifocal lesions, medical treatment alone may be a better first-line option.

Medical Therapy

Because of the intracellular infection, the wide range of tissues affected, a sometimes inadequate host immune response, and potentially rapid development of antimicrobial resistance, combination antimicrobial therapy generally is indicated with agents such as rifampicin (also known as rifampin), clarithromycin, and pradofloxacin (Table 104-1).

Treatment should be continued until lesions have resolved completely and then for an additional 2 to 3 months to reduce the risk of recurrence. Some cats with FLS may require lifelong treatment with clarithromycin to prevent recurrence of lesions.

Some medications, for example rifampicin, may have serious adverse effects, specifically hepatotoxicity. Animals should be monitored closely for signs of liver dysfunction, including inappetence, vomiting, and jaundice. Rifampicin hepatopathy can be fatal. Because clofazimine can cause photosensitization, cats should be housed indoors for the duration of therapy.

References and Suggested Reading

Appleyard GD, Clark EG: Histologic and genotypic characterisation of a novel *Mycobacterium* species found in three cats, *J Clin Microbiol* 40:2425, 2002.
Charles J et al: Cytology and histopathology of canine leproid granuloma syndrome, *Aust Vet J* 77:799, 1999.
Davies JL et al: Histological and genotypical characterisation of feline cutaneous mycobacteriosis: a retrospective study of formalin-fixed paraffin-embedded tissues, *Vet Dermatol* 17:155, 2006.
Foley JE et al: Clinical, microscopic, and molecular aspects of canine leproid granuloma in the United States, *Vet Pathol* 39:234, 2002.
Fyfe JA et al: Molecular characterization of a novel fastidious mycobacterium causing lepromatous lesions of the skin, subcutis, cornea, and conjunctiva of cats living in Victoria, Australia, *J Clin Microbiol* 46:618, 2008.
Gunn-Moore D, Dean R, Shaw S: Mycobacterial infections in cats and dogs, *In Practice* 32:444, 2010.
Hughes MS et al: Identification by 16S rRNA gene analyses of a potential novel mycobacterial species as an etiological agent of canine leproid granuloma syndrome, *J Clin Microbiol* 38(3):953, 2000.
Hughes MS et al: PCR studies of feline leprosy cases, *J Feline Med Surg* 6:235, 2004.
Malik R et al: Mycobacterial nodular granulomas affecting the subcutis and skin of dogs (canine leproid granuloma syndrome), *Aust Vet J* 76:403, 1998.
Malik R et al: Treatment of canine leproid granuloma syndrome: preliminary findings in seven dogs, *Aust Vet J* 79:30, 2001.
Smits B et al: Case clusters of leproid granulomas in foxhounds in New Zealand and Australia, *Vet Dermatol* 23(6):465-e88, 2012.

CHAPTER 105

Treatment of Dermatophytosis

KAREN A. MORIELLO, *Madison, Wisconsin*
DOUGLAS J. DEBOER, *Madison, Wisconsin*

Dermatophytosis is caused by a superficial fungal disease that infects keratinized tissues (hairs, claws, or stratum corneum). It is a skin disease of zoonotic importance. The most common cause of dermatophytosis in cats is *Microsporum canis;* dogs may be infected with *M. canis, Microsporum gypseum,* or *Trichophyton mentagrophytes.* Recently, infections in cats with *Microsporum persicolor* or *Trichophyton* spp. have been reported.

Dermatophytosis is more common in cats than in dogs. Hair loss, scaling, and crusting are frequent clinical findings. In cats the disease can mimic many skin diseases; therefore fungal cultures are a reasonable core diagnostic test. In dogs the typical circular alopecic lesions of bacterial pyoderma often are mistaken for dermatophytosis. Dermatophytic *kerion reactions* appear as nodular or draining lesions that may mimic deep bacterial pyoderma. Infections may be subtle, especially in long-haired cats and small dogs such as Jack Russell terriers and Yorkshire terriers.

Important Points to Remember about Diagnostic Tests

Wood's lamp examination is most useful to identify potentially infected hairs (which show bright apple-green fluorescence) for culture or for direct examination. *Direct microscopic examination* of hairs for ectothrix spores is recommended only for hairs that show fluorescence under Wood's lamp. *Skin biopsy* is necessary only for confirmation of fungal kerion reactions or pseudomycetoma. *Fungal culture* must still be performed to confirm the presence of dermatophytes. The most widely used fungal culture medium is dermatophyte test medium (DTM), which contains inhibitors of bacterial and saprophyte growth and a color indicator. A toothbrush is most commonly used for obtaining diagnostic specimens. The toothbrush is combed over the hair coat until the bristles are full of hair; comb lesional areas last. Cultures should be incubated between 24° and 30°C (75° and 86°F). Daily visual examination of inoculated plates allows rapid identification of highly suspicious colonies. On DTM, suspect pathogenic colonies are pale or white with a red ring of color developing around them as they grow. Microscopic confirmation is required (using either lactophenol cotton blue or new methylene blue stain) because some nonpathogenic fungi can turn DTM red. The reader can find help with microscopic identification in mycology textbooks or on websites such as www.doctorfungus.com. Most *Microsporum* pathogens grow within 7 to 14 days; however, cultures from animals undergoing treatment should be held for 21 days because treatment slows the growth of the organisms.

Treatment Principles and Options

In most healthy animals dermatophytosis is a self-curing disease. However, dermatophytosis is a public health concern and treatment is recommended to shorten the course of infection and minimize the chances of transmission. Treatment includes three key aspects:

- Antifungal treatment for the pet (systemic therapy and adjuvant topical therapy)
- Reasonable confinement to limit contagion
- Cleaning of the environment to remove infective spores

Limiting and Controlling Contamination of the Environment

The authors recommend *starting* treatment discussion with instructions on how to limit the spread of spores because then it is easier for clients to understand and comply with treatment recommendations. It is critical to explain to clients that these spores do not multiply in the environment unlike mildew or other mold overgrowth and repeat cleaning minimizes the amount of infective material in the environment. Homes are readily decontaminated once the animal is cured or removed. The use of reasonable cleaning practices minimizes spore contamination (Box 105-1). The *most important cleaning steps* are gross removal of debris and aggressive detergent cleaning followed by rinsing with water (i.e., hard cleaning); disinfectants do not work in the presence of organic debris and can be inactivated in detergent residue.

Older studies investigating disinfection against *M. canis* tested products in heavily contaminated environments (i.e., gross debris was present) and only undiluted bleach and enilconazole were reported as effective. However, now that the importance of hard cleaning is known, studies have shown that disinfectants labeled as effective against *Trichophyton* spp. are effective against *M. canis* spores when surfaces have been properly prepared by hard cleaning. Clients need to be cautioned against relying on "one-step" cleaners as short cuts because invariably labels recommend hard cleaning before use. Ready-to-use products include many household bathroom disinfectants that contain, for example, quaternary ammonia 0.3%, sodium hypochlorite 1.84% (Clorox Clean-Up), lactic acid 2%, ethoxylated alcohol mixture

BOX 105-1

Recommended Environmental Control Measures in the Treatment of Dermatophytosis

For Households with One or a Few Animals

Confine pets to easily cleaned rooms. Close closets and drawers, and remove knick-knacks.

Thoroughly dust surfaces with Swiffer-type dusters and vacuum or use Swiffer-type sweepers on floors as often as possible but at least twice a week.

Wash hard surfaces with detergent and water as often as possible but at least twice a week.

Launder (hot water/hot dryer) rugs, animal bedding, and other pet contact bed linens.

Launder, disinfect, or discard pet toys and grooming aids.

If possible, disinfect hard floor surfaces with a product labeled as effective against *Trichophyton* spp.; allow 10 minutes of wetting time.

Vacuum (and disinfect if possible) any vehicles and transport cages used for animals.

After cure or removal of the animal, obtain culture specimens to check for contamination by wiping small squares of Swiffer cloths over exposed areas and using the surfaces of the cloths to inoculate fungal culture plates.

TABLE 105-1

Recommended Adjunct Topical Products for Treatment of Dermatophytosis in Dogs and Cats

Treatment	Use and Comments
Lime sulfur rinse (sulfurated lime solution) NOTE: Agricultural formulations that list "calcium polysulfide 29%" as the active ingredient are equivalent to veterinary products listing "90% sulfurated lime solution" on the label, and the dilutions are exactly the same, i.e., 4-8 oz of either solution per gallon of water.	Mix 8 oz in 1 gal warm water. Saturate hair by sponging or drenching with a watering can or garden sprayer. Do not rinse off, towel dry. Discard excess solution. Treat twice weekly. Will stain jewelry or porous surfaces. Temporarily discolors light hair coats.
Enilconazole topical rinse (Imaverol)	Per label, dilute in water to a 0.2% solution. Apply as for lime sulfur, twice weekly. If used on cats, place Elizabethan collar until hair coat is dry. Not available in United States.
Antifungal shampoos: miconazole/chlorhexidine (Malaseb), ketoconazole/chlorhexidine (KetoChlor)	Optional treatment; does not replace use of whole body rinses above. Use twice weekly, towel dry before applying antifungal rinse.

3% (Simple Green), and potassium peroxymonosulfate (Trifectant). One of the most recent products available for use is accelerated hydrogen peroxide (Accel TB). Of course, household bleach diluted 1:100 is effective, but it is important to prepare it fresh prior to use and store it in a dark bottle. The key to disinfection is frequent, aggressive hard cleaning with once- or twice-weekly application of a disinfectant safe for use on the intended surface.

Clipping the Hair Coat

Removing infected hairs by clipping reduces environmental contamination and spread of the infection but is not always necessary. For early-stage disease, clipping or plucking of the hair from around the lesions with scissors can be done. Alternately, a flea comb can be used to remove shed and broken hairs. Whole body clipping requires sedation, can lead to thermal injuries that are not visible until several weeks later, and is advised when there is evidence of prolonged treatment. However, if the hair coat is matted it may be advisable to clip the coat at the start of treatment. Clipping may worsen the infection temporarily by mechanical spread of the spores and microtrauma to the skin.

Adjunct Topical Treatments

Topical therapy is required to kill spores that are present on the hair shafts. Systemic antifungal therapy will not kill these spores. Topical therapy helps shorten the course of infection and limits the spread of infective material. Localized spot treatment is not recommended: it is messy, the medication is removed easily by grooming, its use encourages owners to perform only spot treatment, and treatment efficacy is unproven. Whole body treatment is recommended: lime sulfur, enilconazole, and miconazole

are effective (Sparkes et al, 2000). Miconazole or ketoconazole plus chlorhexidine act synergistically, and combination shampoos or rinses (Malaseb, KetoChlor) are more effective than the single ingredients. Currently favored topical whole body rinses for treatment of dermatophytosis are listed in Table 105-1. The authors believe that lime sulfur or enilconazole rinses are the most effective adjunct topical treatments..

Systemic Treatment Options

Recommended systemic treatment options are listed in Table 105-2.

Griseofulvin

Griseofulvin was the most common systemic antifungal drug for many years, although it is used less frequently today. It needs to be given with a fatty meal, it is teratogenic, and common, potentially lethal adverse effects include vomiting, diarrhea, and bone marrow suppression (in cats).

Ketoconazole

The true clinical efficacy of ketoconazole in dermatophytosis is unknown. The drug is not recommended in cats because of frequent hepatotoxicity and the authors do not recommend its use in dogs due to better alternatives. The dosage in dogs is 10 mg/kg q24h PO; however, the documented efficacy of itraconazole and terbinafine make them superior therapeutic options.

TABLE **105-2**

Recommended Systemic Products for Treatment of Dermatophytosis in Dogs and Cats

Treatment	Use and Comments
Itraconazole (Sporanox [100-mg capsule], Itrafungol [10-mg/ml oral solution]) (always use with concurrent topical therapy)	*First-time infection:* 5 to 10 mg/kg once daily PO on a 7 days on/ 7 days off treatment cycle until cured. *Multiple affected pet cats or dogs:* 5 to 10 mg/kg PO for 21 to 28 days with twice-weekly lime sulfur rinse. Thereafter, continue twice-weekly lime sulfur rinse until cured. *Chronic, recurrent, or severe generalized infection:* 5 to 10 mg/kg daily PO until cured.
Terbinafine 250-mg/ tablet	*Dogs:* 30-35 mg/kg once daily PO *Cats:* <2.7 kg (6 lb), ¼ tablet once daily 2.7 to 5.45 kg (6-12 lb), ½ tablet once daily >5.45 kg (>12 lb), 1 tablet once daily Use daily or as for multiple affected cats or dogs in home (see above)

Itraconazole

Itraconazole (10-mg/ml oral solution [Itrafungol] or 100-mg capsules [Sporanox]) currently is the most commonly used drug. Because of persistence in hair and epidermis it is suitable for pulse therapy or limited-therapy protocols, in addition to daily treatment regimens. Pulse therapy reduces the total number of doses and treatment costs. Adjunct topical therapy (lime sulfur or enilconazole) always is indicated. Outside of the United States, the veterinary formulation is licensed for use at a dosage of 5 mg/kg q24h PO for 1 week followed by 1 week without treatment; the 2-week cycle is repeated until mycological cure. Currently, the authors do not routinely monitor serum chemistry values in cats.

For cats the 100-mg capsules can be divided into smaller doses and repackaged in empty gelatin capsules or mixed with a small amount of food; alternatively, the 10-mg/ml oral solution can be used. The authors are aware that some owners have obtained bulk itraconazole powder inexpensively in foreign countries; anecdotally this treatment often fails. Itraconazole requires careful formulation in appropriate vehicles to ensure its absorption, and use of any material other than registered products is not recommended.

Fluconazole

The authors have used fluconazole (dosed at 10 mg/kg once daily PO) with success as the sole therapy in a group of kittens; disease resolution occurred within 56 to 70 days. Fluconazole is not well studied for animal use, and recent studies indicate that it is probably less active against animal dermatophytes than itraconazole. Current evidence and clinical anecdotes suggest that there is no advantage of this drug over the more proven itraconazole or terbinafine.

Terbinafine

Terbinafine is an allylamine that is fungicidal (see Table 105-2 for dosing). In countries where it is available as a generic it is an alternative to itraconazole. One author (KM) found it ineffective when used as a 14-day pulse with twice weekly lime sulfur rinses even though one study found it had fungicidal MIC for 5.3 weeks after discontinuance of therapy (Foust et al, 2007). It was effective when used for 21 days with twice-weekly lime sulfur rinses. The most common adverse effect with terbinafine is vomiting. Serum alanine transaminase levels may increase, although clinical toxicity is not reported.

Lufenuron

Controlled studies have shown that lufenuron is ineffective as a treatment and preventive drug (DeBoer et al, 2006), despite early reports of efficacy. The authors do not recommend use of lufenuron.

End Point of Therapy

All infected animals should be treated until negative results are obtained on at least two fungal cultures performed 1 week apart. Culturing should be started as soon as therapy is initiated. This will identify the first and second negative fungal culture sooner than any other schedule. In addition, it will minimize unnecessarily long confinement of a pet and unnecessary treatment of animals with topical and systemic therapy. It is important to remember that treatment must continue pending culture result. If culture results shift from negative to positive, this indicates environmental contamination or development of new lesions.

References and Suggested Reading

DeBoer DJ et al: Lufenuron does not augment effectiveness of terbinafine for treatment of *Microsporum canis* infections in a feline model. In Hillier A, Foster AP, Kwochka KW, editors: *Advances in veterinary dermatology,* vol 5, Oxford, UK, 2006, Blackwell, p 123.

Foust AL et al: Evaluation of persistence of terbinafine in the hair of normal cats after 14 days of daily therapy, *Vet Dermatol* 18:246, 2007.

Kunder K, Moriello KA: Efficacy of eight commercial disinfectants against *Microsporum canis* spores on textile swatches, *Vet Dermatol* 23(S1):85 (Abstract), 2012.

Moriello KA: Treatment of dermatophytosis in dogs and cats: review of published studies, *Vet Dermatol* 15:99, 2004.

Moriello KA, DeBoer DJ: Dermatophytosis. In Greene CG, editor: *Infectious diseases of the dog and cat,* ed 4, St Louis, 2011, Elsevier Saunders, p 588.

Newbury S et al: Use of itraconazole and either lime sulphur or Malaseb Concentrate Rinse® to treat shelter cats naturally infected with *Microsporum canis:* an open field trial, *Vet Dermatol* 22:75, 2011.

Sparkes AH et al: A study of the efficacy of topical and systemic therapy for the treatment of feline *Microsporum canis* infection, *J Feline Med Surg* 2:135, 2000.

CHAPTER 106

Dermatophytosis: Investigating an Outbreak in a Multicat Environment

SANDRA NEWBURY, *Madison, Wisconsin*
KAREN A. MORIELLO, *Madison, Wisconsin*

This chapter focuses on the response to a suspected or confirmed outbreak of *Microsporum canis* dermatophytosis in a multicat environment. Such environments include multicat homes, catteries, pet stores, research facilities, feline rescue operations, and cat shelters. The recommendations given here are the result of collaborative work of the authors and include shelter-specific information published as a web seminar by one of the authors (Newbury, n.d.). The suggested response is organized in terms of steps. "Days" have been associated with the steps to offer the clinician and shelter staff a possible timetable for the investigation and response. Timelines may vary for each organization or for each case depending on the time and resources available. In some cases several steps may be accomplished in one day or in just a few days. Details regarding clinical signs, diagnostic testing, treatment, and monitoring of dermatophytosis can be found in Chapter 105 of this book and in the reference sources given at the end of that chapter.

Step 1: Initial Assessment (Day 1)

When the veterinarian initially is contacted by someone with multiple cats about a possible dermatophytosis problem the *first goal is to confirm suspicions that dermatophytosis is contributing to the problem*. This initial evaluation collects the history of the current concerns and reviews any prior diagnostic testing. During the initial history taking, as much information as possible should be collected to assess the level of suspicion for dermatophytosis. The clinician can begin with the following 11 questions:

1. What clinical signs are present?
2. How many cats are affected?
3. What are their ages?
4. Did a veterinarian examine these animals?
5. Have any animals been treated?
6. What diagnostic tests were performed previously (when, where, and by whom)?
7. Was a Wood's lamp used?
8. Was hair trichography performed?
9. If the diagnosis was based on results of a fungal culture, what medium was used and how and where was it incubated?
10. Were culture results reported as "positive" or "negative"?
11. Were color changes in the dermatophyte medium confirmed by microscopic examination?

It also is useful to have the facility operator make a list of the animals with suspected skin lesions, map the facility, and gather as much history as possible about these animals and any treatments they may have received. The clinician should remember that he or she may not be the first veterinarian involved in the evaluation.

Step 2: Provide an Appropriate Temporary Action Plan (Day 1 or 2)

A high level of suspicion for dermatophytosis may emerge based on the clinical history, or more information may be needed. A site visit (e.g., to an animal shelter or cattery) and/or further diagnostics may be necessary. If any concerns about infectious disease exist, the owner or operator of the facility should be instructed to take steps to minimize spread.

To prevent the spread of disease until more information is available and a comprehensive plan can be implemented, the owner or operator should be instructed to stop further movement of cats from section to section or cage to cage within the shelter as much as possible.

Mechanical removal of hair and debris and a detergent cleaning afterward are the most important steps in minimizing environmental contamination. Disinfectant is applied only to kill remaining spores not removed by mechanical cleaning.

In most cases the environment is sampled for contamination after enhanced cleaning has been initiated as part of an assessment of cleaning (with evaluation of the sample cultures in Step 9). If information is needed to evaluate the initial level of environmental contamination, then samples should be taken prior to cleaning.

Step 3: Assessing Affected Animals and the Environment: Collection of Diagnostic Specimens (Day 2)

For the site visit, the veterinarian should bring a microscope, Wood's lamp, and extension cords or ensure that these are available. Unless the investigation is occurring in a research facility, it should be assumed to be necessary to bring gloves/gowns, new toothbrushes for obtaining culture specimens, forceps for plucking hairs, a skin spatula to lift crusts, sterile containers for material, mineral oil, new methylene blue or lactophenol cotton blue stain, plastic sandwich bags, and pens and paper. Any recent fungal cultures declared to be positive should be examined under a microscope to confirm that the interpretation was correct.

Ideally, affected cats are examined where they are housed; however, the assessment area should be located in a site where Wood's lamp examination is possible. Appropriate care must be taken to minimize cross contamination of specimens and cats. Cats should be examined in white light and in a darkened room with a Wood's lamp; examination with a Wood's lamp often reveals lesions not visible under white light. *The authors stress the value of Wood's lamp examinations in these investigations.* Crusts should be lifted to look for glowing hairs, if necessary. Fluorescing hairs should be mounted in mineral oil (clearing agents such as KOH are not needed for this) and examined for the presence of ectothrix spores. The toothbrush technique should be used to obtain samples of inflammatory lesions for fungal culture. It may be possible to examine and take samples from all affected cats at this visit or, if large numbers of cats are involved, examination and sampling may take several days.

If an adequate isolation area is already established for affected animals, those animals with highly suspicious clinical signs may be moved there as they are identified. If not, cats should remain in their current location until the first shuffle (see Step 8 below).

The clinician must also make an assessment of any management or structural environmental risks, such as crowding, random comingling, lack of separation/ segregation of affected or ill animals, or potential difficulties with decontamination or transmission reduction. Also at this visit, environmental samples should be collected using Swiffer-type cloths to determine if environmental contamination is present after cleaning.

Step 4: Planning (Day 2 or 3)

If an outbreak is present, a situation-specific plan should be formulated. No matter how many cats are involved two key issues must be discussed. The first consideration is the capacity of the owner or organization to respond to the disease. The second is the potential impact on the animals, operations, and public image of the facility. Because dermatophytosis is a treatable curable disease, treatment, for at least some set of cats, is often an important part of this plan. A long-term plan to prevent recurring outbreaks of dermatophytosis should be included in the planning process.

Step 5: Establishment of a "Clean Break" Area (Day 3 or 4)

Defining a clear separation between "clean" and "exposed" areas stops the cycle of transmission and allows for safe continuation of animal intake. A "clean break" area should be established that will *not* house any animals that may have been exposed. If the site selected previously contained exposed or infected cats, the room must be cleaned and disinfected thoroughly.

If new, unexposed animals will be entering the facility, initially, the clean break area should be reserved only for new, incoming animals. New cats brought to this "clean" area should be examined for lesions in white light and under a Wood's lamp; direct examinations of glowing hairs should be carried out, and fungal cultures should be performed. In some cases, where risk is low, the clean break area may have some animals that have been in the facility but are considered to be unexposed.

Step 6: Screening of the Full or Exposed Population for Dermatophytosis (Day 3 or 4)

All potentially exposed cats should be kept in their current locations pending screening. As described above, screening consists of physical examination in white light, Wood's lamp examination, direct examination of fluorescing hairs, and fungal culture. As noted earlier, and contrary to previous suggestions by others, Wood's lamp examination is invaluable in detecting lesions that would be missed on clinical examination in room lighting alone. A positive Wood's lamp examination and a direct examination that reveals ectothrix spores should be seen as a temporary confirmation of infection pending culture results.

Step 7: Use of Clinical Data to Group Cats Based on Risk (Day 4 or 5)

Considerable clinical information has been collected to help define risk groups and make treatment decisions. This allows cats to be placed into one of three groups:

- Truly infected/high risk: Lesions present, positive findings on Wood's lamp examination, positive findings on direct examination of hairs
- Infection suspected/moderate risk: Lesions present, negative findings on Wood's lamp examination, fungal culture results pending
- Nonlesional/low risk: No apparent lesions present, negative findings on Wood's lamp examination

Although confirmed culture results may not be available for 7 to 14 days, if fungal cultures are examined daily, suspicious growth may be noted as early as 3 to 4 days. Animals may be identified as "suspect" pending microscopic confirmation, which may be possible as early as day 4 or 5.

Step 8: First Cat Shuffle (Day 4 or 5)

In this step, high-risk cats (or those known to be infected) are separated from the general population to stop further transmission of the disease pending fungal culture results. The ideal situation is to isolate these cats from other cats by placing them in a separate area or room.

Step 9: Assessment of the Efficacy of Environmental Cleaning (Day 8)

Cultures of environmental samples from areas that are contaminated may show evidence of pathogen growth within the first week of incubation; if not, the plates should be watched carefully during week 2 because environmental cultures may also contain contaminants that can swarm the plate. In general, when finances are limited it is more important to know the current level of cleanliness than to have documentation of the initial contamination. Positive results on environmental fungal cultures suggest some combination of poor cleaning or active infection with cats shedding spores into the environment. Risk is increased for lesion-free cats being culture-positive because of fomite contamination. Contaminated environments can lead to false-positive culture results, which may confound the diagnosis of true infection.

Step 10: Evaluation of Culture Results (Days 5 to 14)

An important reason to perform fungal cultures in-house is that it provides the ability to observe the cultures daily, count colony-forming units (CFUs), and have results available on a daily or weekly basis. The number of CFUs per plate is assessed for cultures from samples of individual cats. The number of CFUs, along with the presence or absence of lesions, is used to determine the final risk assessments and to make treatment decisions. (Colony-forming unit counts can only be done on toothbrush fungal cultures.)

Step 11: Second Cat Shuffle (Days 7 to 14)

In Step 7, cats were divided into three groups based on the initial screening. In this step, culture results are used to confirm the presence or absence of disease. A thorough examination should be made for lesions in any cat with a positive fungal culture even if none were originally identified at the time samples were collected. Any cat for which culture results are positive is examined again in white light and under a Wood's lamp. Cats that currently have no lesions, show no evidence of infection on Wood's lamp examination, and have fewer than 10 CFUs per culture plate are treated as fomite carriers. A prophylactic topical treatment with lime sulfur or enilconazole is advisable. Culture-positive cats with lesions and cats without lesions but with more than 10 CFUs per plate are considered to have true infections and are treated (see Chapter 105 for details).

Step 12: Implementation of a Long-Term Response Plan

Unless a long-term response plan is implemented, a future outbreak is almost inevitable. New cats brought into homes, catteries, pet shops, and research facilities should be examined for lesions in white light and under a Wood's lamp; direct examinations should be carried out; and fungal cultures should be performed. Depending on the situation, isolation of these cats from others in the facility is recommended until fungal culture results are known. For shelters, ideally both a treatment and a screening program should be implemented; however, this may not be within the organization's capabilities. Screening is cost effective, and staff can be trained to perform thorough examination of the skin in the intake room. The examinations described earlier should be performed before cats are moved to community housing or foster care or anytime suspicious lesions are noted on a cat. Funds should be allocated to permit fungal cultures to be performed on specimens from all cats with inflammatory skin lesions.

References and Suggested Reading

Newbury S: Webinar: ringworm outbreak management. Available at www.aspcapro.org/webinar-ringworm-outbreak-management.php.

CHAPTER 107

Disinfection of Environments Contaminated by Staphylococcal Pathogens

ARMANDO E. HOET, *Columbus, Ohio*

Environmental contamination with pathogens commonly occurs in veterinary hospitals. Rooms in which dermatologic patients are examined are considered high-risk areas because patients frequently have infected lesions or open wounds, are immunocompromised, or are receiving antimicrobial treatment. Of particular concern are methicillin-resistant *Staphylococcus pseudintermedius* (MRSP) and methicillin-resistant *Staphylococcus aureus* (MRSA) because they cause health care–associated and nosocomial infections in dogs and cats, and MRSA is an important occupational health risk for veterinary personnel. Studies have documented transmission of such pathogenic organisms through contact with contaminated surfaces. Therefore, in locations frequented by patients with dermatologic disease, intensive and detailed cleaning and disinfection protocols are critical to prevent potential transmission to humans and other patients. The purpose of this chapter is to summarize the human and animal contact surfaces most commonly contaminated with *S. pseudintermedius* and *S. aureus* in dermatologic areas and provide recommendations on how to clean and disinfect them to decrease the risk of transmission.

MRSP and MRSA

S. pseudintermedius is an opportunistic pathogen that is part of the normal flora of dogs and cats whereas *S. aureus* is not, although dogs and cats can acquire this pathogen from humans (see Chapter 100). Both *S. pseudintermedius* and *S. aureus* frequently are methicillin resistant; however, MRSP and MRSA strains are not more resistant to detergents or disinfectants, nor do they survive longer on contaminated surfaces than methicillin-susceptible strains.

Surfaces Commonly Contaminated by Staphylococci

Contaminated surfaces are important sources of hand exposure to pathogens for veterinary personnel, increasing the chances that they may become infected themselves or transfer the infection to other patients. During 5 years of active monthly surveillance at the Ohio State University Veterinary Medical Center (Hoet et al, 2011), over 90% of all MRSP and MRSA strains in the dermatology service areas came from 10 major surfaces (Table 107-1). Similar surfaces have been reported in other studies to be "hot spots" of environmental contamination in veterinary hospitals (Heller et al, 2009; Weese et al, 2004). In addition to focusing on surfaces listed in the table, it is recommended that a staff member observe animal and human flow through the veterinary clinic to identify additional hot spots in the facility.

Selection and Proper Use of Disinfectants for Specific Surfaces

Antimicrobial-resistant pathogens can persist on environmental surfaces for weeks or months if regular cleaning and disinfection are not performed. In our active surveillance, we have detected the same clone of staphylococcus at the same location for as long as 5 months when cleaning and disinfection protocols were not properly followed. Surfaces such as computer keyboards, drawer handles, and paper towel and alcohol gel dispensers frequently are touched by veterinary personnel and often are cleaned and disinfected inadequately. Some surfaces are very difficult to disinfect, such as leather or nylon muzzles, which may be persistently contaminated.

To avoid long-term contamination and decrease potential sources of exposure, our recommendations are the following.

Gurneys, Examination Tables, and General Surfaces

Use of quaternary ammonium–based disinfectants (quats), which have detergent (cationic) properties and are active against most bacteria, is efficacious and cost effective. Chlorhexidine is a good alternative, but it does not confer any advantages over quats for the destruction of staphylococci, and some formulations are not labeled as active against other gram-positive cocci or *Pseudomonas*, also important dermatologic pathogens. Both disinfectants may be inactivated by the minerals found in hard water. Whether quats or chlorhexidine solutions are used, we recommend the following procedures:

- Remove all organic material (such as hair and dander) using paper towels.
- Wash surfaces that are soiled (e.g., with blood, pus, sebum) using water and soap or detergent, rinse per product label, and dry before applying the

455

TABLE 107-1

Contact Surfaces in Dermatology Service Areas That Frequently Are Contaminated with MRSP and MRSA

Human Contact Surfaces	Animal Contact Surfaces
Doors*	Gurneys or carts
Computers, keyboards, and mice	Examination tables
Drawer handles on storage cabinets	Areas of the floor where animals are examined†
Paper towel and alcohol gel dispensers‡	Water bowls and muzzles
Microscope knobs, fax and telephone keypads, otoscope handles, examination light handles	Cages

*The screening included the doorknobs and an area up to 1 ft in radius from the door knobs, which are frequent areas of hand contact.
†These are areas of the floor on which regular examination and interventions are performed on large dogs and nervous animals, instead of using the examination tables.
‡The screening only included the handles, levers, or wheels of the dispensers.
MRSA, Methicillin-resistant *Staphylococcus aureus; MRSP,* methicillin-resistant *Staphylococcus pseudintermedius.*

disinfectant. Organic material must be removed; otherwise, the effectiveness of disinfectants may be compromised.

- Anionic detergents (e.g., most laundry detergents) or soaps must be properly rinsed because they can inactivate these disinfectants, reducing their biocidal activity.
- Generously apply disinfectant, saturating the entire surface and allowing 10 minutes wet contact time for maximum effect (unless otherwise specified on the product label). Because this practice may be difficult to achieve during regular clinic activities, the solution should be left to dry before the next use. If there is suspected contamination with MRSP or MRSA, a full 10 minutes of wet contact time is essential. Note that rewetting with disinfectant may be necessary to achieve 10 minutes of wet contact time. Contact surfaces should be cleaned once daily at least.

We recommend that each room and gurney have its own dedicated bottles of disinfectant, with the solution refreshed as frequently as indicated in the label. The bottle never should be replenished with new solution without discarding the residual solution.

Doors

Multiple reports and our surveillance data show that doors frequently are contaminated (Heller et al, 2009; Hoet et al, 2011; Loeffler et al, 2005; Weese et al, 2004) and often are not cleaned and disinfected as frequently as other surfaces. Quats and chlorhexidine solutions are effective in minimizing contamination on doors when used at least once weekly. Immediate cleaning or

disinfection is necessary when known or suspected MRSP or MRSA patients have been handled in a nearby area. The doorknob and its surrounding surfaces up to a 1-foot radius, as well as any other known human or animal contact areas on the door, must be disinfected. Sticky residue or grease should be removed regularly with a commercial water-soluble degreasing agent; the surface should be allowed to dry before disinfectant is applied because degreasers may interfere with the activity of disinfectants. Many degreasers have an alkaline pH and thus may discolor or stain doors with repeated use. The product label always should be read to ensure safe use on various materials.

Examination Floors

Dogs lie down and may be examined on the floor, which results in contamination of that surface. Personnel therefore are likely to spread pathogens around the hospital (and even to their homes) on their shoes. We have observed that floor areas used for examination purposes frequently are contaminated by MRSP, MRSA, or both, becoming a source of exposure for other patients. As a result, we strongly recommend that all patients be examined on stainless steel examination tables, which are more easily cleaned and disinfected (hydraulic lift tables should be used for larger dogs). Further, it is very difficult to clean or disinfect floors during work hours because the floor becomes wet, which creates a hazard for personnel and patients. If patients must be examined on the floor, provide a designated area that may be more easily cleaned and disinfected after a floor examination. The floors must be cleaned of debris and organic material first, and then mop disinfected with sodium hypochlorite (household bleach) diluted 1:10 (to 5000 ppm) in clean high-quality water, with the solution prepared fresh for each use. Solutions remain effective for up to 24 hours when stored in a sealed container; however, the chlorine will dissipate as a gas within just a few hours of preparation when exposed to the air in open containers. Typically, dilutions of bleach do not leave residues or contaminate the environment; however, when they are mixed with urine or detergents containing ammonia, a significant release of free chlorine gas and other irritants may occur. At higher concentrations, bleach can cause deterioration of rubber instruments, discolor garments and clothing, and corrode surfaces that contain copper, aluminum, and iron.

Computer Keyboards and Other Small Contact Surfaces

Computer keyboards and mice, as well as the dialing pads of telephones and fax machines, faucets, lamp handles, microscope knobs, otoscopes, stethoscopes, and other handheld devices frequently are contaminated and touched by multiple people, which permits rapid spread of organisms. The levers of paper towel dispensers and alcohol gel dispensers, as well as the handles of drawers and cabinets, are especially important because they frequently test positive for MRSP and MRSA and they rarely are cleaned or disinfected. Alcohol can be used to disinfect surfaces because it is active against *Staphylococcus* spp. and other bacteria, as well as some enveloped viruses. However, because of the potential fire hazards when it used in large volumes, it is recommended that application of alcohol be limited to small surfaces such as the ones described here. Alcohol can be applied carefully to the surfaces of electronic equipment (e.g., keyboards, keypads, and computer mice) by wiping them with alcohol wipes for at least 30 seconds as well as by spraying less sensitive areas. The alcohol should be allowed to air-dry, ideally with 1 to 2 minutes of contact time. Use of quats or chlorhexidine may result in residue buildup affecting the aesthetics of the equipment or surfaces. Specific manufacturer's instructions should be consulted for alternative methods of disinfection.

Otoscope Tips

Pathogens have been detected on otoscopic cones, and the cones should be prewashed with detergent (after ensuring that all organic matter has been eliminated) and generously rinsed before being submerged in 2.4% alkaline glutaraldehyde solution (cold sterilization). At least 20 minutes' contact at room temperature is required to kill *S. aureus*. Some commercial alkaline glutaraldehyde solutions last up to 30 days; strips that check effectiveness should be used on a regularly basis.

Hand Hygiene

Good hand hygiene is essential to prevent the transmission of pathogens to and from environmental surfaces. Regular hand washing and the use of alcohol-based hand rubs are the most important means of preventing the spread of MSRP and MRSA.

Safety, Protocols, and Conclusion

Some disinfectants, such as glutaraldehydes, are potentially toxic or can produce sensitization and later allergic reactions. Similarly, chlorhexidine and chloride solutions can produce severe eye irritation. Therefore it is strongly recommended that appropriate precautions be used, such as wearing gloves when these disinfectants are prepared or when extended skin contact is expected. Personnel using these products should be aware of the associated risks and should be familiar with the contents and location of the Material Safety Data Sheet for each product. Practice protocols should be in writing, updated regularly, and readily available to all staff. Staff must receive hands-on training and regular supervision. Regular quality-control assessments that sample the same environmental surfaces are critical. Based on our experience, sampling selected hot spot areas every 3 months is feasible and cost effective. The results of these quarterly screenings can be compared with a standard baseline for the hospital. This allows clinics to assess the effectiveness of their current cleaning and disinfection protocols and to evaluate any changes made. Although it is impossible to sterilize all surfaces, adequate cleaning and disinfection practices can significantly decrease the risk of infection of other patients as well as occupational infections.

References and Suggested Reading

Canadian Committee on Antibiotic Resistance: Infection prevention and control best practices for small animal veterinary clinics, Ontario, Canada, 2008, Canadian Committee on Antibiotic Resistance, p 1.

Heller J et al: Prevalence and distribution of methicillin-resistant *Staphylococcus aureus* within the environment and staff of a university veterinary clinic, *J Small Anim Pract* 50:168, 2009.

Hoet AE et al: Environmental methicillin-resistant *Staphylococcus aureus* in a veterinary teaching hospital during a nonoutbreak period, *Vector Borne Zoonotic Dis* 11:609, 2011.

Loeffler A et al: Prevalence of methicillin-resistant *Staphylococcus aureus* among staff and pets in a small animal referral hospital in the UK, *J Antimicrob Chemother* 56:692, 2005.

Scheftel JM et al: Compendium of veterinary standard precautions for zoonotic disease prevention in veterinary personnel: National Association of State Public Health Veterinarians Veterinary Infection Control Committee 2010, *J Am Vet Med Assoc* 237:1403, 2010.

Weese J et al: Isolation of methicillin-resistant *Staphylococcus aureus* from the environment in a veterinary teaching hospital, *J Vet Intern Med* 18:468, 2004.

Website

British Small Animal Veterinary Association: www.bsava.com.

CHAPTER 108

Principles of Therapy for Otitis

LYNETTE K. COLE, *Columbus, Ohio*

This chapter emphasizes the general principles essential to the successful diagnosis, treatment, and management of otitis. Additional information regarding specific therapeutic methods for otitis is found in other chapters within this section.

Primary Causes and Predisposing and Perpetuating Factors of Otitis

The initial goal in the management of otitis is determining the primary cause of the otic disease and controlling any predisposing and perpetuating factors. The primary cause of otitis externa must be diagnosed, treated, and controlled or the condition is likely to become chronic or recurrent, which makes the ear disease much more difficult to manage. In a retrospective study of 100 dogs with acute (37%) or chronic (63%) otitis externa, the most common primary cause of the otitis was underlying allergic disease. This may include cutaneous adverse food reaction (CAFR), atopic dermatitis, or both. This point was emphasized in another retrospective study of 130 dogs in which 10 of 16 dogs (62.5%) diagnosed with CAFR had bilateral otitis externa, a prevalence that was significantly higher than in study dogs without CAFR. In addition to allergic diseases, other primary causes of otitis externa include parasitic diseases (e.g., *Otodectes cynotis* infestation), keratinization disorders, juvenile cellulitis, foreign bodies, autoimmune disease, endocrine disease, otic neoplasms, and nasopharyngeal polyps.

Predisposing factors facilitate inflammation of the ear by altering the microenvironment of the ear canal, allowing for establishment of secondary infections. Once these factors are identified, as many as possible should be eliminated. Predisposing factors include otic conformation (e.g., stenotic ear canals, pendulous pinna), excessive moisture (e.g., swimming), and injury due to treatment effects. The latter can include hair plucking, trauma from the use of cotton-tipped applicators, improper antibiotic use, and application of irritant solutions.

Perpetuating factors sustain and aggravate the inflammatory process, preventing resolution of or even worsening the otitis. Bacterial and yeast infections are the most common perpetuating factors. But undoubtedly in chronic recurrent otitis externa, there also will be progressive pathologic changes such as hyperplasia or stenosis in the ear canal as well as a high probability of a concurrent otitis media. The otic examination allows assessment of the degree of hyperplasia, erythema, ulceration, and stenosis present in the ears. It is also important to palpate the ear canals to identify thickening or even calcification of the canals.

Identification of Active Otic Infection

After the otic examination is performed, a sample of the otic exudate is obtained for cytologic analysis to determine if there is active infection in the ear. Cytologic specimens revealing numerous rod bacteria should raise suspicion of an infection due to *Pseudomonas aeruginosa*, and bacterial culture and susceptibility testing would be indicated for positive identification of the organism as well for guidance of antimicrobial choices for systemic treatment.

Treatment of Otitis

The principles of treatment of otitis can be summarized as follows: (1) cleaning the ear, (2) decreasing inflammation, (3) treating otic infections, (4) treating any concurrent skin disease, and (5) prescribing a maintenance otic therapy plan to prevent recurrence.

Cleaning the Ear and Decreasing Inflammation

In cases of acute otitis or in animals with occasional otitis, at-home cleansing with a cleaning and drying agent should be sufficient to remove exudate from the ears. However, in animals with chronic recurrent otitis and possible otitis media, an in-hospital deep ear flush is usually necessary to completely clean the ear, visualize the entire ear canal, and evaluate the tympanic membrane (see Chapter 113). Glucocorticoids are indicated in most cases of otitis, especially in animals with chronic recurrent otitis or before a deep ear flush (see Chapter 109).

Radiographic Imaging of the Ear

In dogs with chronic recurrent otitis externa, radiographic imaging of the ears is useful for identification of changes consistent with otitis media. Radiographs also aid in determining the prognosis associated with medical management of the ear disease. Examples of imaging abnormalities are soft tissue opacity in the lumen of the bulla, sclerosis and thickening of the bulla wall, sclerosis and bony proliferation of the petrous temporal bone, bone lysis of the bulla and petrous temporal bone, irregular bulla wall, and mineralization of the external auditory canal. It is emphasized that normal findings on images, whether obtained by conventional radiography, computed tomography, or magnetic resonance imaging, do not rule out otitis media.

Treatment of Infectious Otitis

All cases of infectious otitis, both otitis externa and otitis media, should be treated with topical antimicrobial agents. Therapy should be based on the results of otic cytologic analysis (see Chapter 110). When animals have otitis media and a ruptured tympanic membrane, or have undergone myringotomy, owners should be informed of the possibility of ototoxicity related to the use of topical antimicrobial agents. Unfortunately, data are sparse regarding topical drug ototoxicity in animals, so it is difficult to derive a precise risk from the veterinary literature (see Chapter 112). In cases of otitis media or severe otitis externa, systemic antimicrobial agents should be dispensed based on the results of a bacterial culture and susceptibility tests (see Chapter 111).

Maintenance Otic Therapy

Maintenance otic therapy is indicated in cases of otitis for which the primary cause has not been identified or controlled, in patients previously diagnosed with *Pseudomonas* otic infections, and in those cases with chronic or recurrent otitis. For maintenance otic therapy, a product is dispensed for the client to use at home (see Chapter 113). These products will accomplish the following, with the overall goal of preventing recurrent infections:

1. Keep the ear clean and free of excess wax and ceruminous exudate (e.g., squalene, propylene glycol)
2. Dry the ear (e.g., propylene glycol, glycerin)
3. Decrease the canal pH (e.g., acetic acid)
4. Exert antimicrobial effects (e.g., tromethamine/ethylenediaminetetraacetic acid [Tris-EDTA], parachlorometaxylenol [PCMX])
5. Promote normalization of the epithelium (e.g., ceramides, phytosphingosine, α-hydroxy acids)

Since most otic flushing products contain multiple ingredients, one product, or two at most, should suffice. The frequency of use of these products depends on the severity of the otitis and may range from daily to bimonthly.

References and Suggested Reading

Garosi LS, Dennis R, Schwarz T: Review of diagnostic imaging of ear diseases in the dog and cat, *Vet Radiol Ultrasound* 44:137, 2003.

Proverbio D et al: Prevalence of adverse food reactions in 130 dogs in Italy with dermatological signs: a retrospective study, *J Small Anim Pract* 51:370, 2010.

Rosser EJ: Causes of otitis externa, *Vet Clin Small Anim* 34:459, 2004.

Saridomichelakis MN et al: Aetiology of canine otitis externa: a retrospective study of 100 cases, *Vet Dermatol* 18:341, 2007.

CHAPTER **109**

Topical and Systemic Glucocorticoids for Otitis

TIM NUTTALL, *Roslin, Scotland, United Kingdom*

Glucocorticoids are helpful in almost any animal with otitis, regardless of the underlying cause. This chapter considers the why and how of glucocorticoid use for management of otitis in canine and feline patients.

Why Use Glucocorticoids for Otitis?

Drugs of the glucocorticoid class work by reducing pruritus, pain, swelling, exudation, tissue proliferation, and stenosis. In addition, glucocorticoids (particularly dexamethasone) appear to reverse the ototoxicity associated with *Pseudomonas* infections (Takeuchi and Anniko, 2000). The clinical decision is not whether to use glucocorticoids, but how their use should be combined with ear cleaning and antimicrobial therapy to ensure a successful outcome (see Chapters 110, 111, and 113). Long-term maintenance therapy with glucocorticoids is often required to prevent recurrence in animals with underlying conditions such as atopic dermatitis.

Should Topical or Systemic Glucocorticoids Be Used?

The choice between topical and systemic glucocorticoids depends largely on the severity of the otitis. It is important carefully to assess the degree of pain, firmness, mobility, erythema, swelling, fibrosis, hyperplasia, and stenosis of the ear canals by palpation and otoscopy (see Chapter 108). Topical therapy is preferred because it delivers the drug to the affected site, avoiding systemic exposure. The ear canal is a self-contained unit ideally suited to topical treatment, and most polyvalent ear products contain a glucocorticoid. Systemic treatment is necessary if the ear canals are stenosed, if there is severe fibrosis or hyperplasia, if topical therapy cannot be administered safely, and/ or with some cases of otitis media. Once the ear canals have opened it is usually possible to switch to topical therapy. Animals may also tolerate topical therapy better once the pain and inflammation have decreased.

Which Topical Glucocorticoids Should Be Used?

The antiinflammatory potency of topical glucocorticoids varies widely (Table 109-1 and Figure 109-1). Lotions and gels are easier and less messy to apply and dry quickly, leaving fewer residues. Oils, creams, and ointments may moisten and soothe dry and inflamed skin but can be occlusive and are contraindicated for use in exudative or seborrheic ears.

The topical glucocorticoids incorporated in most polyvalent ear medications are appropriate for managing the

TABLE 109-1

Relative Potency of Topical Glucocorticoids Commonly Used in Veterinary Medicine

Potency	Glucocorticoid
Very potent glucocorticoids (up to 100× hydrocortisone)	Fluocinolone
Potent glucocorticoids (25×-100× hydrocortisone)	Betamethasone Dexamethasone Hydrocortisone aceponate Mometasone furoate
Moderate glucocorticoids (2×-25× hydrocortisone)	Prednisolone Triamcinolone
Mild glucocorticoids	Hydrocortisone

This table should be used for guidance only, because the relative potency of topical glucocorticoids also can vary with the concentration, formulation, and preparation (see Figure 109-1). For example, in human dermatology, for the same steroid, occlusive preparations (e.g., ointments, creams) and certain esters (e.g., propionates and valerates) are more potent.

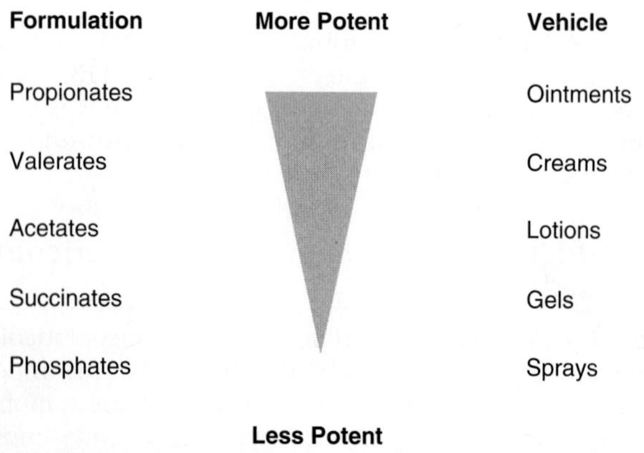

Formulation	More Potent	Vehicle
Propionates		Ointments
Valerates		Creams
Acetates		Lotions
Succinates		Gels
Phosphates		Sprays

Less Potent

Figure 109-1 Effect of vehicle and formulation on the potency of topical steroid preparations.

mild to moderate inflammation in acute otitis externa. Use of antimicrobial-containing products, however, is not indicated in the absence of infection.

A variety of glucocorticoid-containing eyedrops, eardrops, and ear cleaners are available, although some of these are human products not licensed for use in animals. Soluble glucocorticoid preparations also can be added to tromethamine/ethylenediaminetetraacetic acid (Tris-EDTA) solutions or compounded with sterile saline to create solutions with an appropriate glucocorticoid concentration (e.g., 0.02% to 0.1% dexamethasone).

Mild inflammation responds rapidly to low-potency topical glucocorticoids, but progressively more severe inflammation requires longer courses of more potent products. Fluocinolone acetonide in 60% dimethylsulfoxide (DMSO) is particularly effective at reducing tissue hyperplasia.

Products should be applied once or twice daily until remission occurs; efficacy may be greater with more frequent administration, but compliance with treatment may be lower. Once the otitis has resolved, topical glucocorticoids should be used at the lowest frequency that controls the inflammation or discontinued if possible. When continued use is required, data on owner compliance from studies of atopic dermatitis and recurrent pyoderma suggest that a regimen of treatment on 2 or 3 consecutive days each week (i.e., "weekend therapy") is better adhered to than therapy every other day or twice weekly (Carlotti et al, 2004; Martins et al, 2012).

Which Systemic Glucocorticoids Should Be Used?

Table 109-2 summarizes the typical dosages, glucocorticoid potency, and potential for mineralocorticoid activity–associated adverse effects of commonly used systemic glucocorticoids. Prednisolone (or, in dogs only, prednisone) or methylprednisolone for 1 to 3 weeks is sufficient to control inflammation and stenosis in most cases. Patients with severe fibrosis and stenosis may respond better to triamcinolone, betamethasone, or dexamethasone, although these are much more potent glucocorticoids. Once the swelling and inflammation have subsided and the lumen has returned to a normal diameter, therapy should be tailed off gradually to avoid a hypoadrenocortical crisis. Animals with long-term underlying conditions may need ongoing treatment to maintain remission. The drugs most suited for long-term administration are prednisolone, prednisone, and methylprednisolone. Treatment should be tapered to the lowest dose that prevents recurrence of the otitis, preferably given at least every other day.

Parenteral glucocorticoids should be used only when oral medication cannot be safely administered. Parenteral treatment is as effective as oral medication, but the dose or frequency cannot be as easily altered and there is more potential for adverse effects with long-term therapy. Severe fibrosis and stenosis can be treated by injecting 0.05 ml triamcinolone acetonide (using a suspension of 10 mg/ml) into the dermis in a spiral pattern around the vertical canal in an anesthetized dog at three or four sites to a maximum total dose of 0.1 mg/kg. Triamcinolone

TABLE **109-2**

Systemic Glucocorticoids Commonly Used in Veterinary Medicine

Glucocorticoid	Initial Dosage in Otitis	Antiinflammatory Potency	Mineralocorticoid Activity	Duration of Activity	Species
Prednisone	0.5 mg/kg q12-24h	Moderate	High	12-24 hr	Dog
Prednisolone	0.5 mg/kg q12-24h	Moderate	High	12-24 hr	Dog and cat (may need to double dose in cat)
Methylprednisolone	0.8 mg/kg q12-24h	Moderate	Low to moderate	12-24 hr	Dog and cat
Triamcinolone	0.11 mg/kg q24h	Moderate to high	Negligible	18-36 hr	Dog and cat
Betamethasone	0.15 mg/kg q24h	High	Negligible	36-54 hr	Dog and cat
Dexamethasone	0.15 mg/kg q24h	High	Negligible	36-54 hr	Dog and cat

The duration of activity is indicative only—there can be considerable individual variation, and the dose and frequency should be tailored to the clinical response in the individual animal. For instance, in dogs with severe otic stenosis and hyperplasia, the initial starting dosage of an oral glucocorticoid, such as prednisolone, may need to be doubled for a few days (e.g., to 1 mg/kg q12h), then reduced to 0.5 to 1 mg/kg q24h. In addition, the table refers to oral medication; parenteral depot preparations may have a considerably longer duration of activity.

inhibits fibroblast activity and collagen synthesis, which may help to open up the vertical canal, but this technique causes hemorrhage and is not appropriate if severe changes also affect the horizontal canal.

Adverse Effects of Systemic Glucocorticoids
Systemic glucocorticoids cause a variety of acute adverse effects such as polyuria/polydipsia, polyphagia, weight gain, behavioral changes, muscle weakness, and panting. Glucocorticoids may also suppress total thyroxine levels, which potentially can lead to a misdiagnosis of hypothyroidism. These effects can be managed by reducing the dose or frequency of treatment. Some polyphagic animals may need a calorie-controlled diet. Switching to methylprednisolone, triamcinolone, dexamethasone, or betamethasone may be necessary in animals with severe polyuria/polydipsia. The onset of long-term adverse effects such as iatrogenic hyperadrenocorticism, steroid hepatopathy, hypertension, and demodicosis is dose and duration dependent, but there is individual variation and animals receiving long-term systemic treatment should be monitored carefully. Urinary tract infections are a particular concern, and urine samples should be obtained by cystocentesis for culture at 3- to 12-month intervals.

Adverse Effects of Topical Glucocorticoids
Topical glucocorticoid treatment is generally safer than systemic therapy, but hypothalamus-pituitary-adrenal axis function can be affected for up to 2 to 4 weeks after otic administration (Ghubash et al, 2004; Moriello et al, 1988; Zenoble and Kemppainen, 1987). One study reported that dexamethasone suppressed adrenocorticotropic hormone responses more than betamethasone, triamcinolone, or mometasone, but the differences were not significant (Reeder et al, 2008). Two weeks of otic application of 0.1% dexamethasone resulted in elevated liver enzyme levels and adrenal suppression in healthy dogs (Aniya and Griffin, 2008), although no effects were seen with 0.01% dexamethasone. The diester topical glucocorticoid hydrocortisone aceponate has a better safety profile than traditional glucocorticoids by virtue of its metabolism into cortisol in the skin, which reduces the likelihood of cutaneous atrophy and iatrogenic hyperadrenocorticism. Safety studies and clinical trials did not report any local or systemic adverse effects (Nuttall et al, 2009; Reme and Dufour, 2010; Rigaut et al, 2011), although one study did demonstrate some effect on intradermal allergy testing at untreated sites and atrophy of the ventral abdominal skin following topical application of a 0.0584% spray to the flanks and ventral body (Bizikova et al, 2010). Mometasone is another topical glucocorticoid with minimal systemic effects in healthy animals.

Absorption of topical glucocorticoids is related to the thickness of the epidermis and stratum corneum, and may be higher across the thin lining of the ear canals. In addition, absorption of topical glucocorticoids is increased in inflamed skin (Ahlstrom et al, 2011). Treatment with topical glucocorticoids, particularly potent products, could therefore cause adverse effects similar to those seen with systemic treatment. Atrophic effects early in treatment can be useful in reversing fibrosis and stenosis, which helps restore normal ear canal anatomy and function, including epithelial cell migration and clearance. In theory, however, pronounced epidermal and dermal atrophy could interfere with epidermal migration, allowing debris and desquamated cells to accumulate in the ear canals. It is possible that local immunosuppression could facilitate microbial colonization, but in the author's experience long-term control of inflammation is important in reducing microbial colonization and infection. Contact reactions to topical glucocorticoids are well recognized in humans, but reactions in animals have not been reported. In the author's experience, contact reactions are more commonly due to other ingredients in topical ear preparations. Finally, there are anecdotal reports of loss of efficacy (steroid tachyphylaxis) following long-term regular use of topical glucocorticoids. In humans this can be minimized by using intermittent treatment with less potent preparations for long-term maintenance.

Long-term topical glucocorticoid therapy therefore should be monitored carefully. Potent glucocorticoids can be used initially, but less potent products are preferred for maintenance treatment. Alternatively, effective topical glucocorticoids with less potential for adverse effects such as hydrocortisone aceponate can be considered if available.

References and Suggested Reading

Ahlstrom LA, Cross SE, Mills PC: The effects of skin disease on the penetration kinetics of hydrocortisone through canine skin *in vitro*, *Vet Dermatol* 22:482, 2011.

Aniya JS, Griffin CE: The effect of otic vehicle and concentration of dexamethasone on liver enzyme activities and adrenal function in small breed healthy dogs, *Vet Dermatol* 19:226, 2008.

Bizikova P et al: Effect of a novel topical diester glucocorticoid spray on immediate- and late-phase cutaneous allergic reactions in Maltese-beagle atopic dogs: a placebo-controlled study, *Vet Dermatol* 21:70, 2010.

Carlotti DN et al: Evaluation of cephalexin intermittent therapy (weekend therapy) in the control of recurrent idiopathic pyoderma in dogs: a randomized, double-blinded, placebo-controlled study, *Vet Dermatol* 15:8, 2004.

Ghubash R, Marsella R, Kunkle G: Evaluation of adrenal function in small-breed dogs receiving otic glucocorticoids, *Vet Dermatol* 15:363, 2004.

Laurenço-Martins AM et al: Long-term maintenance therapy of canine atopic dermatitis with a 0.0584% hydrocortisone aceponate spray (Cortavance®) used on two consecutive days each week, *Vet Dermatol* 23(suppl 1):39, 2012.

Moriello KA et al: Adrenocortical suppression associated with topical otic administration of glucocorticoids in dogs, *J Am Vet Med Assoc* 193:329, 1988.

Nuttall TJ et al: Efficacy of a 0.0584% hydrocortisone aceponate spray in the management of canine atopic dermatitis: a randomised, double blind, placebo controlled trial, *Vet Dermatol* 20:191, 2009.

Reeder CJ et al: Comparative adrenocortical suppression in dogs with otitis externa following topical otic administration of four different glucocorticoid-containing medications, *Vet Ther* 9:111, 2008.

Reme C-A, Dufour P: Effects of repeated topical application of a 0.0584% hydrocortisone aceponate spray on skin thickness in beagle dogs, *Int J Appl Res Vet Med* 8:1, 2010.

Rigaut D et al: Efficacy of a topical ear formulation with a pump delivery system for the treatment of infectious otitis externa in dogs: a randomized controlled trial, *Int J Appl Res Vet Med* 9:15, 2011.

Takeuchi N, Anniko M: Dexamethasone modifies the effect of *Pseudomonas aeruginosa* exotoxin A on hearing, *Acta Otolaryngol* 120:363, 2000.

Zenoble RD, Kemppainen RJ: Adrenocortical suppression by topically applied corticosteroid in healthy dogs, *J Am Vet Med Assoc* 191:685, 1987.

CHAPTER 110

Topical Antimicrobials for Otitis

COLLEEN L. MENDELSOHN, *Tustin, California*

Canine ear disease is a prevalent and persistent problem and accounts for up to 15% of all canine veterinary case presentations. The large variety and quantity of veterinary topical otic preparations available demonstrate the demand for a wide range of therapeutics for this condition. Otic preparations that address bacterial, yeast, or mixed infections are usually combinations of corticosteroids and antimicrobials. Preparations designed for long-term control are mixtures of mild cleansers, drying agents, or disinfectants, and may contain antimicrobial agents.

Each case represents a different level of proliferation and exudate with a different degree of infection versus inflammation. Therapy needs to be targeted at each aspect of the condition. Becoming familiar with the products available and their effects is essential to formulating the best therapeutic plan for each patient. Since new products are continually introduced, some with familiar ingredients and some with newer antimicrobial agents, it is important to be aware of new products and new active ingredients that already may have been used by the client or by other veterinarians to treat the patient. Clients also may inquire about newer products that might be used to treat their pets.

General Properties of Topical Antimicrobial Formulations

The Vehicle

As with all forms of topical therapy, both multiple formulations and multiple vehicles are used in otic products.

Each demonstrates specific properties that must be considered when selecting an appropriate product. The various vehicles use different mechanisms for delivery of active ingredients and also have different therapeutic, irritant, or cosmetic properties that determine their efficacy in practice. Formulations used for veterinary topical otic therapy include both solutions and suspensions. Different types of suspensions are lotions, creams, emulsions, and ointments. Solutions are homogenous mixtures in which the active ingredient is dissolved. In contrast, suspensions disperse fine particles within a less dense liquid.

Lotions tend to be liquids that evaporate leaving a thin layer of active ingredient (such as miconazole or another antimicrobial) in the ear. Lotions are likely to be drying because of their alcohol or propylene glycol content. Generally a "cooling" lotion or solution tends to contain alcohol, whereas a "soothing" one does not.

Creams, emulsions, and ointments are occlusive and prevent contact with the environment. These agents do not "dry" like lotions, but rather leave a moist layer with the active ingredient contained within. Creams create the least occlusive barrier and ointments are the most occlusive; emulsions share characteristics of each delivery system. In cases of exudative otitis, the use of an ointment may be contraindicated because increased water loss and drying are desired therapeutic outcomes.

Active Ingredients

Antibiotics, antifungals, and antiparasitics can be delivered using topical otic preparations. Additionally, various combinations of soothing agents, acidifiers, alkalinizing agents, keratolytic agents, keratoplastic agents, and astringents can be found in the range of available preparations. When a topical otic product is being selected, the patient's specific infection, as well as the practitioner's familiarity with the product, must be considered. Some practitioners and dermatologists prepare in-house otic remedies from injectable antibiotics or antifungal agents, or combine a variety of available otic products to create a single mixture to target a patient's specific needs. This practice is a controversial and extralabel use of these drugs and is a topic beyond the scope of this chapter. However, if this approach is taken, it is important to remember that the stability and efficacy of the active ingredients may be affected. Additionally, the client must be clearly informed of the off-label formulation.

Treatment of Infections

Initial Approach

Cytologic Analysis
Cytologic analysis is an inexpensive procedure that can be performed easily in-house and allows the practitioner to make immediate decisions regarding treatments or further diagnostics. This procedure should be performed with every reevaluation of the ear. Often, the character of the infection or the degree of inflammation changes over time. Serial cytologic examinations may reveal a change in the infectious organisms and indicate that an antimicrobial treatment change is in order. In addition, the presence of various inflammatory cells could be a sign that an irritant, allergic, or immune-mediated reaction might be present.

Culture and Sensitivity Testing
Obtaining samples for culture is often necessary when there is concern for antimicrobial resistance; for example, when gram-negative organisms are suspected based on cytologic findings, or when bacteria are identified from an ear currently under treatment. However, the interpretation of these tests can be challenging. Studies have demonstrated that the isolates can differ depending on the area of the ear sampled. Furthermore, the concentration of antibiotic applied to the ear is much higher than the plasma levels on which the sensitivity results are based. Thus in some instances a topical antimicrobial may effectively treat an ear infection, even when the susceptibility test indicated bacterial resistance to that agent.

Antibacterial Therapy

Topical treatment of active infections is imperative to success. Systemic (oral or injectable) therapy is sometimes indicated but is unlikely to achieve therapeutic concentrations within the ear when used as a sole treatment modality (see Chapter 111). The topical antimicrobial agent is often chosen empirically based on cytologic examination of ear canal exudate and otoscopic evaluation of the ear canal.

Several veterinary topical otic formulations contain antibacterial agents (Table 110-1). In selecting these drugs the clinician should consider previous therapies, the type of bacteria encountered, the degree of inflammation, and the amount of exudate evident in the ear canal. For more resistant bacterial infections, especially infection with gram-negative bacteria such as *Pseudomonas aeruginosa*, pretreatment of the canal with a product containing tromethamine/ethylenediaminetetraacetic (Tris-EDTA) before application of a topical antibiotic is recommended.

Antiyeast Therapy

Numerous products are available to address yeast otitis (Table 110-2). Many of these contain potent broad-spectrum antibiotics; however, the included antifungal agent is sometimes less potent against the commonly encountered yeast *Malassezia pachydermatis*. Generally miconazole solutions are beneficial against *M. pachydermatis* and in some cases have activity against *Staphylococcus pseudintermedius*. Additionally, in resistant cases, posaconazole has been demonstrated to be effective, but it is currently available only in the proprietary product Posatex. The disadvantage of this product is

TABLE **110-1**

Selected Veterinary Topical Otic Products with Antibacterial Agents

Antibacterial Agent	Uses/Comments	Product/Formulation
Enrofloxacin, marbofloxacin, and orbifloxacin	Fluoroquinolone: bactericidal Gram-negative or gram-positive bacteria Disrupt DNA synthesis by interfering with DNA gyrase or topoisomerase II	1. Baytril Otic Emulsion: enrofloxacin and silver sulfadiazine 2. Aurizon Suspension: marbofloxacin, clotrimazole, and dexamethasone 3. Posatex Suspension: orbifloxacin, posaconazole, and mometasone furoate monohydrate
Gentamicin	Aminoglycoside: bactericidal Gram-negative or gram-positive bacteria Attaches to the 30S ribosomal subunit and disrupts protein synthesis	1. Otomax Ointment: gentamicin sulfate, betamethasone valerate, and clotrimazole 2. Mometamax Ointment: gentamicin sulfate, mometasone furoate monohydrate, and clotrimazole 3. easOtic Suspension: gentamicin sulfate, hydrocortisone aceponate, and miconazole nitrate
Neomycin	Aminoglycoside: bactericidal Similar to gentamicin, but less potent; often chosen for gram-positive bacteria Contact/irritant reactions reported	1. Panolog Ointment: neomycin sulfate, nystatin, thiostrepton, and triamcinolone acetonide 2. Tresaderm Solution: neomycin sulfate, thiabendazole, and dexamethasone
Polymyxin	Broad-spectrum polypeptide antibiotic with activity against all gram-negative bacteria (except *Proteus*) Synergistic with miconazole against gram-negative bacteria (*Pseudomonas aeruginosa*, *Escherichia coli*) and *Malassezia pachydermatis* Binds to lipopolysaccharide in the outer membrane of bacteria; disrupts both the outer and inner membranes	Surolan Suspension: polymyxin B, miconazole nitrate, and prednisolone acetate
Silver sulfadiazine	Structural and metabolic cell disruptor Mechanisms not completely understood Broad-spectrum antibacterial and some antiyeast activity	Baytril Otic Emulsion: silver sulfadiazine and enrofloxacin
Tromethamine/ ethylenediaminetetraacetic acid (Tris-EDTA)	Alkalinizing chelating agent Gram-negative infections Usually used as a pretreatment flush followed by a topical antibiotic	1. TrizEDTA Aqueous Flush Solution: Tris-EDTA 2. TrizChlor Flush Solution: Tris-EDTA and chlorhexidine gluconate 3. TRIS Flush Solution: Tris-EDTA

that it combines the antifungal with a potent fluoroquinolone antibiotic that may not be needed and could potentially induce resistant bacterial organisms if used inappropriately.

It should be noted that in cases of mild allergic yeast otitis, simply decreasing the otic inflammation with a topical glucocorticoid can aid in the elimination of a yeast infection or overgrowth by controlling many of the inflammatory by-products on which yeast survive. In chronic recurrent yeast otitis the use of boric acid– or acetic acid–containing products is often effective in preventing recurrence of infection.

Topical Ototoxicity

Ototoxicity is defined as the tendency of certain therapeutic agents to cause functional impairment and cellular degeneration of the inner ear and the eighth cranial nerve. It may be reversible or irreversible. Patients with otitis commonly present with ruptured tympanic membranes, and some otic products contain ingredients that may be ototoxic and are contraindicated when a ruptured tympanum is present (see Chapter 112). Dermatologists may recommend these products in resistant cases; however, the client must be informed of the risks and benefits of pursuing this therapy.

TABLE **110-2**

Selected Veterinary Topical Otic Products with Antifungal Agents

Antifungal Agent	Uses/Comments	Product/Formulation
Boric acid	Detergent with activity against yeast otic organisms	Maxi/Guard Zn 4.5 Otic Solution: boric acid and zinc complexed with two amino acids, taurine and l-lysine
Clotrimazole	Imidazole antifungal: disrupts ergosterol synthesis Mild to moderate potency against *Malassezia pachydermatis*	1. Otomax Ointment: clotrimazole, gentamicin sulfate, and betamethasone valerate 2. Mometamax Ointment: clotrimazole, gentamicin sulfate, and mometasone furoate monohydrate 3. Aurizon Suspension: clotrimazole, marbofloxacin, and dexamethasone
Ketoconazole	Imidazole antifungal: disrupts ergosterol synthesis	1. Keto-TRIS Flush Solution: ketoconazole and Tris-EDTA 2. Keto-TRIS Flush + PS Solution: ketoconazole and Tris-EDTA 3. TrizULTRA + KETO Otic Flush Solution: ketoconazole and Tris-EDTA 4. Mal-A-Ket Plus TrizEDTA Flush Solution: ketoconazole, chlorhexidine gluconate, and Tris-EDTA
Miconazole	Imidazole antifungal: disrupts ergosterol synthesis	1. Surolan Suspension: miconazole nitrate, polymyxin B, and prednisolone acetate 2. Generics Lotion: miconazole nitrate, polyethylene glycol 400, and ethyl alcohol 55%
Nystatin	Polyene antifungal: binds sterols in the fungal cell membrane Relatively weak activity against *M. pachydermatis*	Panolog Ointment: nystatin, thiostrepton, neomycin sulfate, and triamcinolone acetonide
Thiabendazole	Benzimidazole antifungal: disrupts ergosterol synthesis	Tresaderm Solution: thiabendazole, neomycin sulfate, and dexamethasone

Tris-EDTA, Tromethamine/ethylenediaminetetraacetic acid.

References and Suggested Reading

Cole LK et al: In vitro activity of an ear rinse containing tromethamine, EDTA, benzyl alcohol and 0.1% ketoconazole on *Malassezia* organisms from dogs with otitis externa, *Vet Dermatol* 18(2):115, 2007.

Mendelsohn CL et al: Efficacy of boric-complexed zinc and acetic-complexed zinc otic preparations for canine yeast otitis externa, *J Am Anim Hosp Assoc* 41(1):12, 2005.

Mendelsohn CL, Rosenkrantz WS, Griffin C: Practical cytology for inflammatory skin diseases, *Clin Tech Small Anim Pract* 3:17, 2006.

Morris DO: Medical therapy of otitis externa and otitis media, *Vet Clin North Am* 34(2):591, 2004.

CHAPTER 111

Systemic Antimicrobials for Otitis

LYNETTE K. COLE, *Columbus, Ohio*

Topical antimicrobial therapy is the most common and important treatment for infectious otitis. The use of systemic antimicrobial therapy for infectious otitis externa and otitis media is controversial. However, there are indications for the use of systemic antimicrobial agents for the treatment of otitis.

One indication in dogs is chronic, recurrent, or end-stage otitis externa complicated by otitis media. In these cases, not only is infection present within the lumen of the canal but the epithelium of the ear canal and middle ear can be infected as well. Additionally, the ear canal epithelium can be involved with infections and ulcerations caused by gram-negative organisms such as *Pseudomonas aeruginosa*. Epithelial involvement also is likely when inflammatory cells are identified cytologically, because this finding indicates deeper skin involvement. Another situation where systemic antimicrobial agents may be needed is one in which the owner is incapable of treating the otitis topically in the home setting.

The selection of a systemic antimicrobial agent must be based on the results of culture and susceptibility (C/S) testing of specimens from the external ear (for otitis externa) or middle ear (for otitis media). However, therapy may be initiated based on cytologic findings while the C/S results are awaited.

Indications for systemic antifungal agents are similar to those mentioned previously for antibacterial medications. These include yeast otitis media, severe yeast otitis externa, and inability of the owner to administer topical therapy.

Systemic Treatment of Staphylococcal Otitis

The most common coccoid bacterium isolated from dogs with otitis externa or otitis media is *Staphylococcus pseudintermedius*. Good empiric choices while C/S results are awaited include cephalexin (22 mg/kg q12h PO) or amoxicillin trihydrate/clavulanate potassium (Clavamox; 13.75 to 22 mg/kg q12h PO).

Systemic Treatment of *Pseudomonas* Otitis

Probably the most challenging bacterial otic infections are those associated with *P. aeruginosa* (Table 111-1). Although there is insufficient evidence for the use of systemic antimicrobial agents for the treatment of *Pseudomonas* otitis, the cause is mainly the lack of published reports of randomized controlled studies in the veterinary

TABLE 111-1

Systemic Drugs and Suggested Dosages for the Treatment of *Pseudomonas aeruginosa* Otitis Externa and Otitis Media

Drug Name (Trade Name)	Dosage
Fluoroquinolone Antibiotics	
Ciprofloxacin	Dog: 25 mg/kg q24h PO
Enrofloxacin (Baytril)	Dog: 20 mg/kg q24h PO Cat: 5 mg/kg q24h PO
Marbofloxacin (Zeniquin)	Dog: 5.5 mg/kg q24h PO Cat: 2.75 mg/kg q24h PO
β-Lactam Antibiotics	
Ticarcillin disodium/ clavulanate potassium (Timentin)	Dog: 15 to 25 mg/kg q8h IV
Imipenem (Primaxin)	Dog and cat: 10 mg/kg q8h, diluted in 100 ml suitable IV solution, administered IV over 30 to 60 min
Meropenem (Merrem)	Dog: 12 mg/kg q8h SC or 24 mg/kg q8h IV
Ceftazidime sodium (Fortaz)	Dog and cat: 30 mg/kg q6h IV, IM Dogs only: 30 mg/kg q4h SC Dogs only: constant IV infusion: loading dose of 4.4 mg/kg, followed by 4.1 mg/kg/hr, delivered in IV fluids
Aminoglycoside Antibiotics	
Amikacin	Dog: 15 to 30 mg/kg q24h IM, SC, IV Cat: 10 to 15 mg/kg q24h IM, SC, IV
Gentamicin	Dog: 10 to 14 mg/kg q24h IM, SC, IV Cat: 5 to 8 mg/kg q24h IM, SC, IV

IM, Intramuscularly; *IV,* intravenously; *PO,* orally; *SC,* subcutaneously.

literature evaluating systemic treatments in this setting. At the present time the fluoroquinolones are the only oral systemic antibiotic available for the treatment of *P. aeruginosa* infection. Most veterinary dermatologists recommend starting treatment with an oral fluoroquinolone while the C/S results are awaited. When the fluoroquinolones are used in dogs, a dosage at the upper end of the dosage range should be administered. Blindness caused by retinal degeneration has been reported in rare cases in cats given enrofloxacin; therefore a dosage at the low end of the range for an oral fluoroquinolone should be administered in cats. In one multicenter trial, 54 dogs with *Pseudomonas* otitis externa were administered marbofloxacin at a dose of 5 mg/kg PO once daily for 21 or 42 days, with an overall improvement in 38 of 54 dogs: 15 were cured and 23 partially improved, whereas 16 did not improve (Carlotti et al, 1998).

In multidrug-resistant *P. aeruginosa* infections, aggressive antibiotic therapy with systemic β-lactam antibiotics can be considered. However, these agents should be used only after deep cleaning of the external ear canal and middle ear (if indicated) under anesthesia, the use of topical cleaning and drying agents at home, and the application of tromethamine/ethylenediaminetetraacetic acid (Tris-EDTA)–containing topicals and topical antimicrobial agents have been ineffective. Systemic β-lactam antibiotics include ticarcillin disodium/clavulanate potassium (Timentin), imipenem (Primaxin), meropenem (Merrem), and ceftazidime sodium (Fortaz). These agents are very expensive, must be administered parenterally, and should be considered *only* as a last resort. A potential adverse effect of imipenem and meropenem is seizures, and these drugs should be used cautiously if at all in patients prone to seizure disorders.

Aminoglycoside antibiotics such as gentamicin and amikacin are less commonly prescribed but remain potentially effective drugs for the treatment of *P. aeruginosa* otic infections. These drugs also are administered parenterally and have a limited potential for nephrotoxicity. A recent letter to the editor in *Veterinary Dermatology* (Noli and Morris, 2011) describes the International Renal Interest Society guidelines for the prevention of aminoglycoside-induced acute kidney injury.

Systemic Treatment of Yeast Otitis

In one study neither pulse-dose nor daily-dose itraconazole alone significantly decreased the number of yeast organisms identified cytologically from otic exudate in dogs with yeast otitis externa, which suggests that otic yeast infections may require topical therapy in addition to systemic therapy for resolution (Pinchbeck et al, 2002). Both ketoconazole (5 mg/kg q24h) and itraconazole (Sporanox; 5 mg/kg q24h PO or pulse-dosed 2 days on and 5 days off) have been used in dogs, whereas itraconazole (5 mg/kg q24h PO) is recommended for use in cats.

References and Suggested Reading

Carlotti DN et al: Marbofloxacin for the systemic treatment of *Pseudomonas* spp. suppurative otitis externa in the dog. In von Tscharner C, Kwochka KW, Willemse T, editors: *Advances in veterinary dermatology,* vol 3, Oxford, 1998, Butterworth-Heinemann, p 463.

Cole LK et al: Comparison of bacterial organisms and their susceptibility patterns from otic exudate and ear tissue from the vertical ear canal of dogs undergoing a total ear canal ablation, *Vet Ther* 6:252, 2005a.

Cole LK et al: Comparison of bacterial organisms from otic exudates and ear tissue from the middle ear of untreated and enrofloxacin-treated dogs with end-stage otitis. In Hillier A, Foster AP, Kwochka KW, editors: *Advances in veterinary dermatology,* vol 5, Oxford, 2005b, Blackwell, p 147.

Moore KW, Trepanier LA, Lautzenhiser SJ: Pharmacokinetics of ceftazidime in dogs following subcutaneous administration and continuous infusion and the association with in vitro susceptibility of *Pseudomonas aeruginosa,* Am J Vet Res 61:1204, 2000.

Noli C, Morris D: Guidelines on the use of systemic aminoglycosides in veterinary dermatology, *Vet Dermatol* 22:379, 2011.

Nuttal TJ: Use of ticarcillin in the management of canine otitis externa complicated by *Pseudomonas aeruginosa, J Small Anim Pract* 39:165, 1998.

Nuttal T, Cole LK: Evidence-based veterinary dermatology: a systematic review of interventions for treatment of *Pseudomonas* otitis in dogs, *Vet Dermatol* 18:69, 2007.

Papich MG: Solving problems in therapy: new drugs, new approaches. In *Just the FAQs: managing microbes/pain management,* proceedings of the North American Veterinary Conference, Orlando, FL, 2005, and Western Veterinary Conference, New York, 2005, Pfizer Animal Health, p 15.

Papich MG: *Saunders handbook of veterinary drugs,* Philadelphia, 2002, Saunders.

Pinchbeck LR et al: Comparison of pulse administration versus once-daily administration of itraconazole for the treatment of *Malassezia pachydermatis* dermatitis and otitis in dogs, *J Am Vet Med Assoc* 220:1807, 2002.

CHAPTER 112

Ototoxicity

MICHAEL PODELL, *Chicago, Illinois*
CECILIA FRIBERG, *Chicago, Illinois*

The impact of ototoxicity on veterinary patients' quality of life is significant. Dogs and cats have an almost threefold greater frequency hearing range than people. Auditory cues are essential both from the evolutionary perspective of predator survival and as a daily method of interaction with their domestic owners. Hearing is often taken for granted, and the effect of hearing loss is typically not apparent until almost complete deafness is present, when pets no longer respond to an owner's voice or surrounding environmental noise. Because of this, early detection of ototoxicity-induced deafness (OID) through subjective evaluation is difficult for veterinarians, a problem that can translate into irreversible deafness by the time the condition is noted. Moreover, the majority of OID cases are iatrogenic and thus potentially preventable. The purpose of this chapter is to enhance awareness of the potential causes of ototoxicity, to develop a strategy for its early evaluation and detection, and ultimately, to prevent the progression to irreversible hearing loss.

Causes

Deafness can result from either failure of conduction of sound waves through the outer and middle ear structures (conduction deafness) or failure of transformation of mechanical to electrical energy for signal generation through the auditory nerve to the brain (sensorineural deafness). The true prevalence or incidence of either cause of deafness in veterinary medicine is poorly documented. A summary of potential causes of deafness is listed in Box 112-1; some of these causes have been reported in the dog and cat.

The most common cause of *conductive hearing loss* in the dog is chronic otitis externa and otitis media, with associated ceruminous or purulent exudates; mucoid effusions; canal stenosis and hyperplasia; and changes to the bony and epithelial structures of the middle ear. Mild conductive hearing loss of up to 20 dB may occur with tympanic membrane rupture from acute effusions or trauma, or after myringotomy, but hearing should return as the membrane heals (Steiss et al, 1990).

Sensorineural hearing loss occurs most commonly as a congenital, and suspected inherited, disease (Strain, 2011). Congenital deafness is apparent early in a dog's life, usually within the first months of life. The most common condition is a complete unilateral hearing loss, but may affect both ears. The cause of this hearing loss is a lack of formation or degeneration of small receptors in the inner part of the ear. Certain breeds are predisposed to congenital deafness, including, but not

BOX 112-1   Causes of Deafness

Conduction Deafness
1. Otitis externa (excessive cerumen, purulent exudate)
2. Otitis media (infectious or primary [i.e., primary secretory otitis media in the cavalier King Charles spaniel])
3. External ear canal stenosis (congenital or acquired)
4. Occlusive otic pastes, ointments, or powders
5. Presbycusis (mechanical form)

Sensorineural Deafness
1. Congenital or hereditary disorders
2. Acquired disorders
   a. Autoimmune disorders (e.g., immune-mediated neuropathy)
   b. Metabolic disorders (e.g., metabolically induced neuropathy)
   c. Neoplasia
      i. Benign (polyps)
      ii. Malignant (e.g., squamous cell carcinoma)
3. Ototoxicity
   a. Systemic
      i. Antibiotics
         (1) Aminoglycoside (gentamicin: B)
         (2) Macrolide (erythromycin, minocycline)
         (3) Chloramphenicol
      ii. Chemotherapy
         (1) Platinum compounds (carboplatin cisplatinum)
         (2) Nitrogen mustard compounds
      iii. Salicylates (aspirin products)
      iv. Loop diuretics (furosemide: A, B)
   b. Topical
      i. Antibiotics
         (1) Aminoglycoside (neomycin: B)
         (2) Chloramphenicol
         (3) Polymyxin
      ii. Antiseptics
         (1) Quaternary ammonium compounds: benzalkonium/benzethonium chloride
         (2) Ethanol
         (3) Chlorhexidine: B
         (4) Iodine compounds
         (5) Acetic acid
         (6) Propylene glycol
   c. Environmental
      i. Heavy metals (lead, mercury, arsenic)
      ii. High-decibel sounds
4. Presbycusis

The letters indicate the animal species (dog = A, cat = B) in which ototoxicity has been documented or research studies have been done.

limited to, dalmatians, English setters, bull terriers, and Jack Russell terriers.

Ototoxicity is the result of chemical- or noise-induced toxic changes to inner and/or outer hair cells. Close to 200 ototoxic drugs and chemicals have been identified in a variety of mammalian species. In most cases, the hearing loss is irreversible and often progressive even after cessation of exposure to the toxic agent. The more common ototoxic agents include aminoglycoside antibiotics, loop diuretics, anticancer drugs, topical cerumenolytics (Mansfield et al, 1997), antiseptic preparations (Mills et al, 2005), and heavy metals (Merchant, 1994). Further insight into the molecular pathogenesis of ototoxicity may help lead to clinical management (Yorgason et al, 2006). Reversible noise-induced hearing loss also occurs after brief exposure to extremely loud sounds (over 100 dB), but hearing loss can become permanent with repeated and long-lasting exposure. Typically, the hearing loss is in the range of normal speech.

Presbycusis is an age-related hearing loss that is not associated with a specific pathologic process. Six categories of presbycusis have been described in people depending on the site of degeneration: sensory (predominant loss of outer hair cells), neural (loss of afferent neurons), metabolic (atrophy of the stria vascularis), mechanical (i.e., cochlear conductive), mixed (sensory, neural, and metabolic), and indeterminate. Sensorineural presbycusis is thought to be the most common form to occur in small animals, although in one study of 10 aged dogs age-related hearing loss was identified as a mixed type of presbycusis (ter Harr et al, 2009). Documentation on a larger-scale population is lacking.

In a longitudinal study of age-related hearing loss in dogs, frequency-specific brainstem auditory evoked response thresholds were determined once yearly or every other year for 7 years starting at around age 6. Age-related hearing loss was found to begin at around 8 to 10 years of age and was most pronounced in the middle to high frequency (8- to 32-kHz) range (ter Harr et al, 2008). Many owners of older dogs with suspected presbycusis-related hearing loss describe acute-onset deafness. A recent study of postanesthetic deafness reported a low prevalence based on data gathered from owners' telephone communications, cases discussed on a veterinary information website, and a survey of general practice and dental specialists. Although prevalence was low, deafness was permanent in dogs and cats following anesthesia and occurred mainly in older dogs and cats undergoing dental and ear-cleaning procedures (Stevens-Sparks and Strain, 2010). This has been the author's experience as well. Prospective studies should be conducted using brainstem auditory evoked response testing before and after ear cleanings and dental work performed under anesthesia to validate the prevalence of this hearing loss and identify the cause.

Clinical Evaluation

History

Evaluation of hearing loss begins by taking a history of owner awareness of a problem. Owners need to be questioned regarding their pets' hearing response to voice and routine sounds, as well as any prior ear disease. Early recognition often occurs when a pet no longer greets the owner or has to be physically awakened. A complete list should be made of all topical ear products used, because owners now have more access to medications and may have administered home remedies of which the attending veterinarian is unaware.

Otoscopic Evaluation

An otoscopic examination is the first step in evaluation of patients who are suspected to have a hearing loss. Animals that are uncomfortable may need chemical restraint to allow evaluation of the status of the canal. If the ear canal is not patent and swollen tissues obstruct the view, then this inflammation must be controlled with glucocorticoids (see Chapter 109). Cytologic analysis and, in some cases, bacterial culture are essential to guide appropriate antimicrobial therapy (see Chapters 110 and 111).

Audiometry

Evoked potential audiometry is based on evaluation of an evoked potential as an electrical manifestation of the brain's reception of and response to an external stimulus. Auditory evoked responses are signal-averaged recordings of brain activity in response to acoustic stimuli. Auditory evoked responses have the advantage of providing objective, quantifiable data that does not require patient cooperation and is highly resistant to the effects of sedatives and anesthetic agents.

Evoked potential audiometry measures very specific components of the auditory pathway. Early-latency (0- to 10-ms) components are the result of activation of the peripheral receptor, nerve, and brainstem structures, and thus are often referred to as *brainstem auditory evoked responses* (BAERs). The BAER test can be used to characterize both conductive and sensorineural deafness. Changes in latency of onset, amplitude, and interval between waveforms can be analyzed to evaluate for site-specific abnormalities of the auditory pathway. Either clicks (2 to 4 kHz) or frequency-specific tones can be introduced as acoustic stimuli. Broadband clicks generate a robust, highly repeatable pattern of six identifiable waves, each correlating with a specific anatomic, or neural, generator from the cochlear receptors to the thalamus.

Hearing threshold can be assessed by evaluating the presence of wave V at progressively lower decibel levels. The presentation of frequency-specific tones at varying intensities (tone-burst BAER) provides the ability to distinguish hearing loss at specific frequencies. This test is useful as a screening method for early hearing loss caused by ototoxic agents and for correlating hearing loss with behavioral response patterns such as speech recognition (Mills et al, 2005).

Otoacoustic Emissions

Otoacoustic emissions (OAEs) are spontaneous or acoustic stimulated sounds generated within the normal cochlea. These sounds can be measured when the middle ear and cochlea are functioning normally. The reemitted sounds of OAEs are thought to originate from active feedback of sound energy into the cochlea, a function attributed to outer hair cells. Decrease in the amplitude of OAEs is found in pathologic conditions that result in the loss of outer hair cells, such as noise exposure, anoxia, and aminoglycoside intoxication. Two types of OAEs are commonly evaluated: transient evoked otoacoustic emissions (TEOAEs) and distortion product otoacoustic emissions (DPOAEs). TEOAEs are assessed by presenting a broadband click to the ear and measuring the magnitude of the emissions. This test is a highly sensitive, rapid screen for congenital sensorineural deafness in puppies (McBrearty and Penderis, 2011). Two tones of overlapping frequencies are used to stimulate the basilar membrane to evoke DPOAEs. Distortion is generated where the two frequencies interact on the basilar membrane. The distortion product signals are propagated along the basilar membrane to appropriate and predictable frequency locations for the separate distortion components. Responses to these signals can be recorded as if they had been presented as pure tones to the ear. DPOAEs are highly sensitive in detecting early altered hearing threshold within 4 days of cisplatin administration (Sockalingam et al, 2002).

Treatment and Prevention

Conduction Deafness: Otitis Externa and Otitis Media

A number of steps can be taken to treat and prevent conduction deafness related to otitis externa and otitis media. These can be summarized as follows.

Step 1: Obtain an Accurate Diagnosis and Treat

Otitis externa/otitis media infections must be treated aggressively. Cytologic analysis of otic discharge must be performed to identify bacterial and yeast infections. Bacterial and yeast infections must be treated with appropriate long-term antimicrobial therapy until resolved. Antiinflammatory therapy, in the form of a systemic agent given alone or in combination with topical corticosteroids, can be an essential component in managing the episode. Caution should be used when vestibular signs are present, however, because progression to extensional otogenic brain abscess has been associated with steroid use.

Step 2: Treat until Resolution Occurs

It is imperative that therapy be maintained for at least 1 week beyond the point at which all signs of infection have resolved. This treatment period is often a minimum of 2 weeks, but prolonged therapy for up to 4 to 6 weeks or longer is common. Resolution must be confirmed with normal findings on otoscopic examination and otic cytologic analysis. Early cessation of treatment can result in drug-resistant bacterial infections, recurrent yeast infections, progressive accumulation of middle ear fluid or exudate, and advancement to otitis interna.

Step 3: Avoid Topical Compounds with Potential for Ototoxic Reactions

It is important when scrutinizing the list of potentially ototoxic drugs in the dog and the cat to note that many

of the reports on which this list is based are of studies in species other than the dog or cat. Additionally, some reports describe infusion into a closed middle ear, are anecdotal, or involve concentrations of a drug that far exceed those found in commonly used topical medications. Solutions introduced into an inflamed or infected ear are less likely to diffuse into the inner ear because of decreased penetration through the swollen inflamed tissue. Use of topical otic preparations is highly unlikely to be responsible for toxicity in most practical clinical situations; however, subclinical or latent toxicity may not be appreciated, and this is not a justification for frivolous use of these agents. Furthermore, even though it is rare for a commercially available topical otic product to cause hearing loss, transient hearing loss is a label-listed possible adverse reaction; accordingly, owners should be made aware of this risk before using these products. Application of high concentrations of nonototoxic agents (i.e., ear packing medications) can cause physical damage to ear structures if ear canal impaction occurs.

Step 4: Work toward Prevention of Recurrence

The allergic component contributing to the inflammation should also be addressed. This involves educating dog owners about both proper maintenance and identification of a progressing problem (e.g., atopic dermatitis, cutaneous adverse food reaction) for which they must seek veterinary counsel. Dogs with a history of otitis should have the ears cleaned at regular intervals, based on the individual dog's needs. Dog owners who clean their pets' ears must be carefully instructed and reminded about the appropriate procedures, since inappropriate cleaning can exacerbate the situation or even create further problems (see Chapter 113).

Sensorineural Deafness: Iatrogenic Ototoxicity

Once sensorineural deafness occurs, the prognosis is often guarded, even with treatment. Therefore the goal is to avoid clinical situations that place the patient at risk of OID.

Step 1: Assess Patient Risk

Patients at higher risk of OID include those that are older, have reduced renal function, or are receiving multiple drugs that may interfere with drug metabolism. Additional risk factors include a history of chronic ear disease, chemotherapy, and any history of abnormal hearing function. BAER threshold testing is the most accurate method of hearing threshold assessment and can be done in serial fashion to evaluate for progressive hearing loss.

Step 2: Determine If a Treatment Has Potential Ototoxicity

Clinicians should be aware of the potential adverse effects of a given treatment and warn owners accordingly. Avoidance of known ototoxic drugs is recommended whenever possible (see Box 112-1).

Step 3: Avoid Concomitant Use of Drugs with Synergistic Ototoxicity

Coadministration of loop diuretics and aminoglycosides or platinum-based chemotherapy agents should be avoided at all costs due to the high risk of rapid OID (Li et al, 2011). Caution should be exercised in the prolonged use of macrolide antibiotics and aspirin, especially in older patients with decreased renal function.

Step 4: Avoid Confounding Variables

Synergistic exposure to high-intensity or prolonged noise in conjunction with aminoglycoside therapy should be avoided to prevent irreversible cochlear damage (Li and Steyger, 2009). These patients should not be placed in closed rooms with other loud, barking dogs. When possible, avoid anesthesia in patients receiving potentially ototoxic drugs and, in particular, avoid aggressive ear cleaning that could introduce excessive fluid under pressure into the middle ear.

References and Suggested Reading

Li H, Steyger PS: Synergistic ototoxicity due to noise exposure and aminoglycoside antibiotics, *Noise Health* 11:26, 2009.

Li Y et al: Co-administration of cisplatin and furosemide causes rapid and massive loss of cochlear hair cells in mice, *Neurotox Res* 20:307, 2011.

Mansfield PD et al: The effects of four, commercial ceruminolytic agents on the middle ear, *J Am Anim Hosp Assoc* 33:479, 1997.

McBrearty A, Penderis J: Transient evoked otoacoustic emissions testing for screening of sensorineural deafness in puppies, *J Vet Intern Med* 25:1366, 2011.

Merchant S: Ototoxicity, *Vet Clin North Am Small Anim Pract* 24:971, 1994.

Mills PC et al: Ototoxicity and tolerance assessment of TrisEDTA and polyhexamethylene biguanide ear flush formulation in dogs, *J Vet Pharmacol Ther* 28:391, 2005.

Sockalingam R et al: Cisplatin-induced ototoxicity and pharmacokinetics: preliminary findings in a dog model, *Ann Otol Rhinol Laryngol* 111:745, 2002.

Steiss JE et al: Alterations in the BAER threshold and latency-intensity curve associated with conductive hearing loss in dogs, *Prog Vet Neurol* 1:205, 1990.

Stevens-Sparks CK, Strain GM: Post-anesthesia deafness in dogs and cats following dental and ear cleaning procedures, *Vet Anaesth Analg* 37:347, 2010.

Strain GM: *Deafness in dogs and cats*, Wallingford, UK, 2011, CAB International.

ter Harr G et al: Effects of aging on brainstem responses to tone-burst auditory stimuli: a cross-sectional and longitudinal study in dogs, *J Vet Intern Med* 22:937, 2008.

ter Harr G et al: Effects of aging on inner ear morphology in dogs in relation to brainstem responses to toneburst auditory stimuli, *J Vet Intern Med* 23:536, 2009.

Yorgason JG et al: Understanding drug ototoxicity: molecular insights for prevention and clinical management, *Expert Opin Drug Saf* 5:383, 2006.

CHAPTER **113**

Ear-Flushing Techniques

DAWN LOGAS, *Maitland, Florida*

One of the most important components in the management of acute and chronic otitis externa is proper ear flushing, both in the office and at home. In a discussion of ear flushing it is essential to incorporate information on both the physical flushing techniques and the various types of cleansing solutions available.

In-Office Ear Flushing (Under General Anesthesia)

A bulb syringe or a No. 3 to No. 12 Fr red rubber feeding tube attached to a 6- to 12-ml syringe is an excellent and relatively safe flushing apparatus for in-office use. The wide end of the tube must be trimmed to accommodate the syringe hub. The tip is then cut off the other end so the final length of the tube is 4 to 6 inches or one to two times the length of the ear canal. Both straight and curved dull Buck ear curettes can be used to remove large pieces of wax and debris. Once the horizontal canal has been cleared, it is usually easier to assess the status of the tympanic membrane. In many cases of chronic otitis, the tympanum is still difficult to visualize because the canal is stenotic secondary to hyperplasia and fibrosis. If the tympanum cannot be visualized, its status can be assessed indirectly by noting the disappearance of the feeding tube tip from view, the need for an excessive length of tubing, and the exiting of fluid from the nares. Any of these observations indicates a false middle ear or imperforate tympanum. If the tympanum is visually intact but this is a case of chronic otitis (>3 months' duration), performing a myringotomy using a dull Buck curette, tomcat catheter, or 5 Fr polypropylene urinary catheter may be necessary. A specimen for culture should always be taken from the middle ear if there is any evidence of fluid behind the membrane or if there is membrane opacity and fibrosis.

The hazards of deep ear cleaning include inadvertent rupture of the tympanum, vestibular dysfunction, auditory dysfunction, contact irritation and allergy, and introduction of other pathogens.

At-Home Ear Flushing

In many cases a commercial solution in a squeeze bottle is all that is necessary for at-home ear flushing. If there is a great deal of purulent material, a bulb syringe should be used, and the owners instructed in its appropriate use.

The frequency of flushing prescribed for home care depends on the severity of infection, consistency of the discharge, chronicity of the otitis, presence of yeast or bacteria, and presence or absence of a tympanum. Initially the frequency of flushing in severe cases, especially resistant *Pseudomonas* infections, can be three to four times daily. In most cases of less severe otitis, twice daily suffices. As therapy continues, the frequency should decrease to several times per week and then once weekly to every other week prophylactically.

It is particularly important that dogs with chronic ear canal changes such as fibrosis, stenosis, and lichenification be placed on a maintenance at-home flushing program to help to remove the debris and acidify the canal, which helps prevent recurrence of active infections. The frequency of flushing ranges from two to three times weekly to once every other week.

Although flushing is extremely important in the management of both chronic and acute otitis, it is imperative that the clinician remember that flushing too vigorously and too frequently can also be detrimental to the otic epidermis. If excessive white ceruminous exudate is noted on otic examination, and otic cytologic analysis reveals only keratinocytes, the flushing frequency should be decreased.

Cleansing Solutions

Currently there are a multitude of veterinary ear-cleansing solutions, which contain many similar ingredients. Most of these ingredients are purported to fulfill one or more of the following functions: dissolve discharge, lubricate the canal, remove excess water from the canal, kill infectious organisms, and decrease inflammation (Table 113-1). The type of discharge, the degree of inflammation, the chronicity of the disease, and the status of the tympanic membrane all should be taken into consideration when selecting which solution to use in a particular case. Different solutions may also be recommended for at-home versus in-office use. In general, milder solutions are recommended for use at home to minimize the chances of contact irritation. Antiinflammatory agents

TABLE 113-1

Common Veterinary Ear Cleanser Ingredients and Their Functions*

Ingredient	Function
Sodium lauryl sulfate	Break up debris
Carbamate peroxide	Break up debris
Cocamidopropyl betaine	Break up debris
Sodium tetraborate pentahydrate (borax)	Break up debris, antimicrobial
Docusate sodium (dioctyl sodium sulfosuccinate, DSS)	Ceruminolytic
Triethanolamine polypeptide oleate	Ceruminolytic
Squalene	Lubricant
Propylene glycol	Lubricant, drying agent, antimicrobial
Glycerin	Lubricant, drying agent
Salicylic acid	Ceruminolytic
Natural and synthetic oils	Lubricant, drying agent
α-Hydroxy acids such as lactic, malic, and citric acids	Normalize skin
Organic and inorganic alcohols	Drying agent, antimicrobial
Menthol (alcohol)	Counterirritant, antipruritic, antimicrobial, drying agent
Chlorothymol (phenol derivative)	Antimicrobial
Organic and inorganic acids such as boric and acetic acids	Antimicrobial
Parachlorometaxylenol (PCMX)	Antimicrobial
Tromethamine/ ethylenediaminetetraacetic acid (Tris-EDTA)	Antimicrobial

*Many of the functions have not been verified by *in vitro* and *in vivo* veterinary studies.

are described elsewhere in this section (see Chapters 94 and 109). Some specific recommendations follow.

Debris Removal Agents

The physical removal of debris and microorganisms from the ear canal is one of the primary functions of most ear cleansers. Many antibiotics are inactivated by contact with debris and purulent exudate; therefore cleaning the ear canal before application of medication is important. Surfactants in the form of emulsifiers, detergents, or foaming agents usually are incorporated for this purpose. These agents decrease the surface tensions between water and lipids or organic solids to break up and help remove purulent debris when mixed with water. Sodium lauryl sulfate, carbamate peroxide, and cocamidopropyl betaine are examples of these agents.

Cerumenolytics and lubricants are added to ear cleansers to remove excess cerumen. Ceruminolytic agents, with the exception of squalene, should be considered ototoxic (Mansfield et al, 1997). Cerumenolytics, many of which are also considered surfactants, accomplish cerumen removal by hydrating the desquamated sheets of corneocytes and inducing keratolysis, whereas lubricants soften wax by hydration. Docusate sodium (dioctyl sodium sulfosuccinate, DSS) and triethanolamine polypeptide oleate are commonly used cerumenolytics. Squalene, mineral oil, propylene glycol, and glycerin all act primarily as lubricants. Each of these ingredients is fairly gentle to the aural epidermis and can be used in most cases of otitis externa. Salicylic acid is added to many preparations because of its potent keratolytic and ceruminolytic activity. In one *in vitro* study that examined 13 veterinary cleansers, only the product with the highest concentration of salicylic acid (0.23%) demonstrated an ability to remove over 80% of the cerumen compared with water (Sanchez-Leal et al, 2006). At these higher concentrations, salicylic acid can be irritating, particularly to already inflamed aural skin. Products containing high concentrations of salicylic acid should be used for in-office flushing and in cases of chronic ceruminous otitis without inflammation.

Normalizing Agents

Another purpose of an ear cleanser is to protect and maintain the normal function of the epidermis of the ear canal. Drying agents are added to ear preparations to prevent maceration of the aural epidermis. Alcohols are one of the most commonly used and most potent drying agents. They are particularly useful in noninflamed canals that are moist and waxy. Propylene glycol, glycerin, and natural or synthetic oils act as milder drying agents whose major advantage over alcohols is their less irritating nature. However, propylene glycol, which is extremely common in canine ear cleansers, has been implicated in causing contact reactions in some dogs with otitis externa. These milder drying agents also lubricate and protect the aural epidermis. This helps minimize excessive epidermal water loss and epidermal irritation caused by topical medications and purulent debris.

α-Hydroxy acids such as lactic, malic, and citric acids are added for their beneficial effects on the epidermis and dermis. Although the exact mechanisms of action remain unclear, α-hydroxy acids appear to normalize the skin, which leads to a smoother, fuller epidermis and dermis with fewer crevices and a more normal barrier that decreases adherence of microbes to the aural epidermis. α-Hydroxy acids are generally not irritating at the concentrations used except in severely inflamed ears.

Antiseptics

The control of bacteria and yeast is another important function of many ear cleansers. Antiseptics commonly found in veterinary preparations include alcohols, organic and inorganic acids, parachlorometaxylenol (PCMX), and tromethamine/ethylenediaminetetraacetic acid (Tris-EDTA). In addition to being potent drying agents, alcohols are also potent antiseptics. The alcohols most commonly found in veterinary preparations are benzyl and isopropyl alcohols; ethyl alcohol is found in a few. *In vitro* studies have shown that veterinary otic preparations containing benzyl or isopropyl alcohol have better antimicrobial activity against *Staphylococcus pseudintermedius*, *Pseudomonas aeruginosa*, *Streptococcus*, *Proteus*, and *Malassezia pachydermatis* than preparations that do not (Cole et al, 2006; Swinney et al, 2008).

Organic and inorganic acids are commonly found in veterinary ear cleansers. Some examples are acetic, lactic, salicylic, and citric acids, which are organic acids, and boric acid, which is an inorganic acid. *In vitro*, both 2% to 3% acetic acid and 2% boric acid alone or in specific veterinary otic preparations are effective against various bacteria, including *S. pseudintermedius*, *Staphylococcus aureus*, *Proteus mirabilis*, and *P. aeruginosa* as well as *M. pachydermatis* (Swinney et al, 2008). In an *in vivo* study, boric acid significantly reduced the number of *M. pachydermatis* organisms compared with acetic acid and placebo (Mendelsohn et al, 2005). Some of these acids, in particular acetic acid, can be irritating in inflamed ears, especially at higher concentrations and if the product has an acidic pH. At higher concentrations (usually those >2%) these acids are more useful in cases of less inflamed acute and chronic otitis.

PCMX is a phenolic antiseptic found in several veterinary ear cleansers. *In vitro*, PCMX-containing ear preparations are effective against *Escherichia coli*, *Staphylococcus* species, and *P. aeruginosa* (Swinney et al, 2008). In one *in vivo* study, approximately 70% of infected ears were cleared of their infection within 2 weeks when an ear preparation containing PCMX, lactic acid, and salicylic acid was used (Cole et al, 2003). Both *S. pseudintermedius* and *P. aeruginosa* infections were cleared along with *M. pachydermatis* infections, although the antiyeast activity may be due more to the lactic and salicylic acids than the PCMX. PCMX does not appear to be irritating, so it may be useful in inflamed ears.

Another antiseptic commonly added to veterinary ear cleansers is Tris-EDTA. Tris-EDTA is best known for its ability to increase the permeability of the outer membranes of gram-negative bacteria such as *Pseudomonas*, which allows increased penetration by antibiotics. Studies report varying degrees of antimicrobial activity of Tris-EDTA by itself. One *in vitro* study showed no effect of one Tris-EDTA preparation against *S. pseudintermedius*, *P. aeruginosa*, or *M. pachydermatis*, whereas another study showed that a different Tris-EDTA preparation alone significantly decreased the number of *Pseudomonas* organisms but not *Streptococcus*, *Staphylococcus*, or *Proteus* (Cole et al, 2006; Swinney et al, 2008). In another *in vitro* study, a different ear preparation containing Tris-EDTA and 0.15% chlorhexidine was tested. The combination was very effective against both methicillin-resistant and methicillin-sensitive *S. aureus* and *S. pseudintermedius*, *E. coli*, *P. aeruginosa*, and *M. pachydermatis*. *P. mirabilis* was the organism most resistant to the combination (Guardabassi et al, 2010; Swinney et al, 2008). Chlorhexidine is no longer commonly incorporated into cleansers specifically labeled for use in the ear because of the potential for ototoxicity, although at the low concentrations used (0.15%) biguanide compounds like chlorhexidine have not demonstrated ototoxic effects in dogs (Mills et al, 2005). Tris-EDTA is usually nonirritating, so it can be used in very inflamed ears with little problem; however, the author has seen a small number of dogs develop a significant contact reaction characterized by a very watery brown discharge and moderate erythema. Tris-EDTA is not good at removing debris, so it should be used in combination with another agent if the ears are very waxy or contain thick, purulent debris.

Unique Ingredients

Several veterinary ear cleansers are available that contain ingredients with unique properties, but unfortunately there are few *in vivo* studies confirming their efficacy. The first of these ingredients is phytosphingosine. Phytosphingosine is one of the most widely distributed natural sphingoid bases found in plants, fungi, and animals. *In vitro* it has good antiinflammatory and antimicrobial activity against *Staphylococcus* and *Pseudomonas* as well as mild activity against *M. pachydermatis*. No *in vivo* otic studies have been done with phytosphingosine-containing products. Phytosphingosines are also the base for ceramides, one of the components of the stratum corneum lipid barrier. Besides helping to maintain normal barrier function, ceramides are important in normal cell turnover since they can arrest epidermal proliferation.

Stabilized hypochlorous acid is another ingredient that has been introduced into a veterinary otic cleanser for its antimicrobial activity. Hypochlorous acid is a weak acid formed by acidification of hypochlorite or by electrolysis of a salt solution. *In vitro* studies have shown excellent antibacterial, antiviral, and antifungal activity, but these types of studies have not been published for veterinary pathogens. The only *in vivo* studies published are human case reports. No reports of randomized placebo-controlled human or veterinary studies have been published at this time using stabilized hypochlorous acid.

Bioactive enzymes (lactoperoxidase, lactoferrin, and lysozyme) have been added to a veterinary ear cleanser for their antimicrobial activity. In a single *in vitro* study the product containing all three of these enzymes demonstrated antimicrobial activity against several laboratory strains of bacteria and yeast (Atwal, 2003). At this time no *in vivo* veterinary studies have been performed using these enzymes topically in the ear.

Monosaccharide and polysaccharide sugars have been added to a veterinary otic cleanser to decrease microbial adherence to the epidermis and reduce the release of proinflammatory cytokines. *In vitro* studies have demonstrated a decrease in the adherence of both *P. aeruginosa* and *S. pseudintermedius* to cultured canine corneocytes (McEwan et al, 2006, 2008). An *in vivo* study found that the sugar-containing ear cleanser was effective in controlling the clinical signs of otitis externa and dramatically reducing the number of bacteria and yeast in dogs with otitis externa (Reme et al, 2006).

Ototoxicity

Many ingredients found in veterinary ear cleaners are considered ototoxic to the middle and inner ear (see Chapter 112), although most of these ingredients have not been examined in clinical settings and there are very few studies reported in the veterinary literature evaluating the ototoxicity of topical otic products. However, products containing squalene (Mansfield et al, 1997) or Tris-EDTA and polyhexamethylene biguanide (Mills et al, 2005) were found to be nonototoxic in the dog.

The integrity of the tympanic membrane should be ascertained if possible before any ear cleanser is used. If the status of the tympanic membrane cannot be determined or if the tympanic membrane is found to be ruptured after cleaning, the canal should be flushed with saline to remove any residue of the cleanser. If it is necessary to use a cleanser in an ear with a known ruptured tympanic membrane, a product without known ototoxic ingredients should be used if possible and the owners should be warned of the chance of ototoxicity.

References and Suggested Reading

Atwal R: *In vitro* antimicrobial activity assessment of Zymox otic solution against a broad range of microbial organisms, *Int J Appl Res Vet Med* 1:240, 2003.
Cole LK et al: Evaluation of an ear cleanser for the treatment of infectious otitis externa in dogs, *Vet Ther* 4:12, 2003.
Cole LK et al: *In vitro* activity of an ear rinse containing tromethamine, EDTA and benzyl alcohol on bacterial pathogens for dogs with otitis, *Am J Vet Res* 67:1040, 2006.
Guardabassi L, Ghibaudo G, Damborg P: *In vitro* antimicrobial activity of a commercial ear antiseptic containing chlorhexidine and Tris-EDTA, *Vet Dermatol* 21:282, 2010.
Mansfield PD et al: The effects of four, commercial ceruminolytic agents on the middle ear, *J Am Anim Hosp Assoc* 33:479, 1997.
McEwan NA et al: Monosaccharide inhibition of adherence by *Pseudomonas aeruginosa* to canine corneocytes, *Vet Dermatol* 19:221, 2008.
McEwan NA, Mellor D, Kalna G: Sugar inhibition of adherence by *Staphylococcus intermedius* to canine corneocytes, *Vet Dermatol* 17:151, 2006.
Mendelsohn CL et al: Efficacy of boric-complexed zinc and acetic-complexed zinc otic preparations for canine yeast otitis externa, *J Am Anim Hosp Assoc* 41:12, 2005.
Mills PC, Ahlstrom L, Wilson WJ: Ototoxicity and tolerance assessment of a TrisEDTA and polyhexamethylene biguanide ear flush formulation in dogs, *J Vet Pharmacol Ther* 28:391, 2005.
Reme CA et al: The efficacy of an antiseptic and microbial anti-adhesive ear cleanser in dogs with otitis externa, *Vet Ther* 7:15, 2006.
Sanchez-Leal J et al: *In vitro* investigation of cerumenolytics activity of various otic cleansers for veterinary use, *Vet Dermatol* 17:121, 2006.
Swinney A et al: Comparative in vitro antimicrobial efficacy of commercial ear cleaners, *Vet Dermatol* 19:373, 2008.

CHAPTER 114

Primary Cornification Disorders in Dogs

ELIZABETH A. MAULDIN, *Philadelphia, Pennsylvania*

The term *cornification* (keratinization) refers to the process by which epidermal cells undergo terminal differentiation from basal keratinocytes to the highly specialized corneocytes. Traditionally, disorders of cornification have been divided into those with primary and those with secondary causes. In primary cornification disorders, the excessive scale is due to a direct defect in one or more steps involved in the formation of the stratum corneum. Some authors include abnormalities of sebaceous gland function (e.g., sebaceous adenitis, sebaceous gland dysplasia) as primary cornification disorders as well. Secondary disorders are those in which excessive scaling develops as a result of another condition such as fleabite hypersensitivity, sarcoptic mange, hypothyroidism, or epitheliotropic lymphoma. More than 80% of scaling disorders arise from *secondary* causes.

Primary disorders of cornification are generally diagnosed by ruling out secondary causes. The signalment, age of onset, and presence or absence of pruritus aid in the formation of differential diagnoses and determination of the diagnostic approach. In a standard veterinary practice, a minimal dermatologic data set (e.g., skin scrapings, acetate tape preparations, impression smears, trichograms, dermatophyte culture) along with routine blood work can effectively rule out secondary disorders. Skin biopsies are often needed to establish a definitive diagnosis. Primary cornification disorders are generally nonpruritic and arise in young animals. These disorders have strong breed predilections; however, it should be kept in mind that spontaneous mutations can arise in any breed or mixed-breed animal.

Ichthyosis

In veterinary medicine, the term *ichthyosis* has been limited to rare congenital or hereditary disorders believed to be due to primary defects in the formation of the stratum corneum. A skin biopsy is invaluable in establishing a definitive diagnosis. For breeding dogs, molecular testing may be needed to further characterize the defect and identify carrier dogs.

Epidermolytic Ichthyosis

Epidermolytic ichthyosis (epidermolytic hyperkeratosis) can be diagnosed on light microscopic examination by an experienced dermatopathologist. The main histopathologic features (suprabasal keratinocyte vacuolation and lysis, hypergranulosis, and hyperkeratosis) are uniquely correlated with mutations in epidermal keratins. This disorder has been identified in a few dog breeds (Rhodesian ridgeback, Labrador cross), but has been well characterized only in Norfolk terriers. The affected dogs have regions of mild pigmented scale with alopecia and roughening of the skin.

Nonepidermolytic Ichthyosis

Nonepidermolytic ichthyosis in golden retrievers appears to be common, relatively mild, and unique in its variable presentation and onset. An autosomal-recessive mode of inheritance has been shown. Affected dogs develop large, soft, white to gray adherent scale that is prominent on the trunk and may be associated with ventral hyperpigmentation. A definitive diagnosis can be achieved by skin biopsy. Histologically, affected dogs have diffuse lamellar orthokeratotic hyperkeratosis in the absence of epidermal hyperplasia and dermal inflammation. Dogs are typically diagnosed at younger than 1 year of age; however, adult-onset cases are not uncommon. Some dogs develop secondary bacterial folliculitis, which may lead to pruritus. The disease may wax and wane with periodic bouts of exacerbation and remission.

Nonepidermolytic ichthyosis has been characterized in American bulldogs at the author's institution. Unlike golden retrievers, bulldogs consistently develop clinical signs before weaning. Extensive pedigree analysis suggests an autosomal mode of inheritance. Young puppies have a disheveled hair coat compared with normal littermates. In puppies as young as 1 to 2 weeks of age, the glabrous skin becomes erythematous with tightly adherent brown scale, which gives the abdominal skin a "wrinkled" appearance. The remainder of the pelage has widely distributed large white scale. *Malassezia* overgrowth may be severe. In the absence of yeast infection, the histologic features are similar to those seen in the golden retriever. The development of otitis externa, intertrigo, and pododermatitis corresponds with the yeast proliferation and the onset of pruritus. In adult dogs, this clinical presentation can be easily confused with atopic skin disease. Occasionally adult dogs may have footpad hyperkeratosis. Unlike in golden retrievers, the skin lesions in bulldogs do not wax or wane and are generally more severe.

Nonepidermolytic ichthyosis in Jack Russell terriers appears to be less common and has a more severe phenotype than that in golden retrievers and American bulldogs. Affected dogs have large, thick, adherent parchment paper–like scales that have the histologic appearance of marked, tightly laminated, orthokeratotic hyperkeratosis. The dogs develop severe *Malassezia* infections.

A congenital and autosomal-recessive form of keratoconjunctivitis sicca with scaling has been documented in cavalier King Charles spaniel dogs. The dogs have a syndrome that includes the following features: keratoconjunctivitis from the time the eyelids open, roughened curly pelage, scaling with abdominal hyperpigmentation, footpad hyperkeratosis, nail dystrophy, and periodic nail sloughing.

Treatment

In both human and veterinary medicine, the therapy for ichthyosiform disorders has not kept pace with the research into the pathogenesis and molecular characterization. Topical therapy remains the treatment of choice for all forms of ichthyosis. The importance of ruling out secondary forms of scaling cannot be overemphasized. One should keep in mind that the skin barrier is abnormal. Dogs with primary cornification defects have excessive water loss through the skin and are susceptive to skin infections (bacterial and yeast), and are theoretically prone to allergen penetration and sensitization (i.e., atopic dermatitis and cutaneous adverse food reaction). The goal of therapy should be to restore the skin barrier, remove excessive scale, and keep the skin subtle and pliable.

Initially, baths may be required every other day to twice weekly. Shampoos containing 2% sulfur and salicylic acid help soften the scale and break apart the keratin squames. The shampooing should always be followed by application of a good moisturizer. Products containing humectants such as propylene glycol (e.g., Humilac) may be helpful between baths. One should avoid the use of harsh topical products that may further harm the skin barrier (e.g., tar-based shampoos) and ensure that the product does not cause erythema or pruritus. Topical lipid-based spot-ons such as Duoxo Seborrhea Spot-on or micro-emulsion spray, which contains 1% phytosphingosine (a major component of ceramides), and Allerderm spot-on, which contains a combination of ceramides and fatty acids, are helpful products that can be administered between baths and may prolong the required bathing intervals. Severe cases may require a treatment regimen similar to that for sebaceous adenitis: pretreatment with bath oil soaks to remove excessive thick scale, followed by a keratolytic shampoo and generous application of a moisturizer. Oral omega-3 and omega-6 fatty acids may also be beneficial, but the true efficacy is difficult to quantify.

The topical regimen is tailored to the degree of scale and then tapered based on the clinical response. Periodic rechecks (e.g., impression smears, acetate tape preparations) are warranted to assess scale production and secondary infection. American bulldogs and Jack Russell terriers are more likely to need oral antifungal therapy (e.g., ketoconazole 5 to 8 mg/kg/day for 21 days) for secondary yeast infections. In refractory cases, retinoids can be considered; however, the use of retinoids by veterinarians has become problematic, because some pharmacies will dispense only with permission from an authorized physician and a patient consent form. The retinoid currently on the market is acitretin (dosed at 0.5 to 1 mg/kg q24h); however, it may not be as effective as etretinate, which is currently off the market. If retinoids are used, the dog should be monitored for keratoconjunctivitis sicca and liver toxicity, and the drugs should not be used in intact females due to the threat of teratogenicity. Oral vitamin A is unlikely to be beneficial.

Immunomodulatory-lacrimostimulant therapy may decrease progression of keratitis in cavalier King Charles spaniels; however, the therapy does not result in a clinical cure.

Vitamin A–Responsive Dermatosis

Vitamin A–responsive dermatosis is most commonly seen in adult cocker spaniels although it reportedly occurs in Labrador retrievers, miniature schnauzers, and Gordon setters as well. Clinical lesions consist of hyperkeratotic plaques with follicular plugging and follicular casts on the ventral and lateral chest and abdomen. The dogs may have greasy hair coat with ceruminous otitis. The diagnosis is achieved by skin biopsy findings and observation of a response to vitamin A supplementation. The major histologic feature is marked follicular orthokeratotic hyperkeratosis, which is more severe than the epidermal surface hyperkeratosis. The standard vitamin A dosage for a cocker spaniel is 10,000 IU/day or 500 to 800 IU/kg/day. A clinical response is typically seen in 3 to 8 weeks, and dogs may require lifelong therapy.

Labrador Retriever Nasal Parakeratosis

Nasal parakeratosis arises in Labrador retrievers at less than 1 year of age and is thought to have an autosomal-recessive pattern of inheritance. The dogs develop thick, slightly verrucous, brown scale on the nasal planum with variable depigmentation. The disorder has characteristic histologic features: marked parakeratotic hyperkeratosis with serum lake formation and a variable band of lymphocytes and plasma cells in the superficial dermis. Topical emollients are generally all that is needed for treatment. Daily applications of white petrolatum (petroleum jelly) or propylene glycol in water are effective; however, the hyperkeratosis will recur if the therapy is stopped.

Generalized Sebaceous Gland Hyperplasia of Terriers

Idiopathic generalized sebaceous gland hyperplasia has been reported in both Border terriers and wirehaired terriers. This disorder is different from the nodules of sebaceous gland hyperplasia seen in aging dogs. The terriers have a greasy hair coat that is most severe on the dorsum. Some dogs, particularly wirehaired terriers, have been documented with *Demodex injai* infestation. These long-bodied *Demodex* mites are often found in sebaceous gland ducts in addition to hair follicles. Skin biopsy specimens reveal diffuse sebaceous gland hyperplasia independent of the mite infestation. The true relationship of the sebaceous gland hyperplasia to the *Demodex* mites is unknown. Treatment of mite infestation improves the skin but does not reverse the sebaceous gland hyperplasia. It is plausible that the sebaceous gland hyperplasia is the primary lesion and predisposes the dogs to *Demodex* infestation.

References and Suggested Reading

Credille KM: Primary cornification defects. In Guaguère E, Prélaud P, editors: *A practical guide to canine dermatology*, Paris, 2008, Kalianxis, pp 425-438.

Credille KM et al: Mild recessive epidermolytic hyperkeratosis with a novel keratin 10 donor splice-site mutation in a family of Norfolk terrier dogs, *Br J Dermatol* 153(1):51, 2005.

Credille KM et al: Transglutaminase 1-deficient recessive lamellar ichthyosis associated with a LINE-1 insertion in Jack Russell terrier dogs, *Br J Dermatol* 161:265, 2009.

Dedola C et al: Idiopathic generalized sebaceous gland hyperplasia of the Border terrier: a morphometric study, *Vet Dermatol* 21:494, 2010.

Hartley C et al: Congenital keratoconjunctivitis sicca and ichthyosiform dermatosis in 25 Cavalier King Charles spaniel dogs. Part I: clinical signs, histopathology, and inheritance, *Vet Ophthalmol* 15:315, 2012. Epub December 29, 2011.

Marsella R, Olivry T, Carlotti DN; for the International Task Force on Canine Atopic Dermatitis: Current evidence of skin barrier dysfunction in human and canine atopic dermatitis, *Vet Dermatol* 22:239, 2011.

Mauldin EA et al: The clinical and morphologic features of non-epidermolytic ichthyosis in the golden retriever, *Vet Pathol* 45:174, 2008.

Ordeix L et al: *Demodex injai* infestation and dorsal greasy skin and hair in eight wirehaired fox terrier dogs, *Vet Dermatol* 20:267, 2009.

Pagé N et al: Hereditary nasal parakeratosis in Labrador retrievers, *Vet Dermatol* 14:103, 2003.

CHAPTER 115
Alopecia X

ROSARIO CERUNDOLO, *Six Mile Bottom, Suffolk, United Kingdom*

Alopecia X is a form of canine adult-onset alopecia that was formerly known by various names (Box 115-1). However, this diversity in names is merely descriptive and is based on the differences in endocrine findings or clinical responses to various therapeutic modalities. Alopecia X mainly affects Nordic breeds (Samoyed, Siberian husky, spitz, and Alaskan malamute) but may also affect the chow-chow, Pomeranian, and miniature poodle. Alopecia X is probably a clinical spectrum of different conditions. It is not yet proven that Alopecia X in the aforementioned breeds actually is a single disease entity with similar causes and pathogenesis.

Alopecia X usually starts in dogs between 1 and 3 years of age, although cases have been reported in 9-month-old puppies and 11-year-old dogs. Intact males seem to be predisposed.

Pathogenesis

The pathogenesis of alopecia X remains poorly understood. A genetic predisposition to a hormone production defect or abnormal hormone action on the hair follicle is suspected. Arguments in favor of a defect in sex hormone production include hair regrowth in affected dogs following neutering or treatment with products that affect sex hormone production and elevated levels of certain sex hormones, especially 17-hydroxyprogesterone (17-OHP), following adrenocorticotropic hormone (ACTH) stimulation in some affected dogs. It has been proposed that alopecia X in miniature poodles and Pomeranians may be a variant of pituitary-dependent hyperadrenocorticism (Cerundolo et al, 2007).

Clinical Signs

Alopecia X is a disease that exclusively affects the hair coat and skin of dogs. Dogs are normally healthy. If there are signs of systemic disease, other endocrine diseases should be suspected.

Initially there is sparse loss of guard hairs resulting in a dull, dry coat. Sometimes a more generalized loss of guard hairs gives the coat a "puppy" appearance. The hair coat may also appear lighter or a different color with the loss of guard hairs. Hair loss may be noted first in frictional areas such as around the neck, tail head region, and caudal thighs, and these areas become more severely involved with time. The progression from early changes in hair coat to complete hair loss may take several years in some dogs. The retained secondary hairs are also lost with time, which results in complete alopecia of the affected areas. The exposed skin may become hyperpigmented. It is likely that the increased pigmentation is the

BOX 115-1   Synonyms of Alopecia X

1. Pseudo–Cushing's syndrome
2. Growth hormone deficiency of the adult dog
3. Hyposomatotropism of the adult dog
4. Growth hormone–responsive dermatosis
5. Castration-responsive dermatosis
6. Sex hormone dermatosis
7. Estrogen-responsive dermatosis
8. Testosterone-responsive dermatosis
9. Biopsy-responsive alopecia
10. Adrenal sex hormone disorder
11. Congenital adrenal hyperplasia
12. o,p'DDD-responsive dermatosis
13. Nordic breed follicular dysplasia
14. Follicular dysplasia of the Siberian husky and malamute
15. Malamute coat funk
16. Woolly syndrome
17. Black skin disease
18. Hair cycle arrest

o,p'DDD, Mitotane.

BOX 115-2   Criteria Commonly Used by the Author to Confirm a Diagnosis of Alopecia X

1. Predisposed breed
2. Age of onset between 1 and 6 years
3. Clinical pattern of alopecia: truncal progressive hair loss and/or woolly coat quality, with or without cutaneous hyperpigmentation
4. Absence of systemic clinical signs
5. Normal hematologic and biochemical findings
6. Normal thyroid function
7. Increase in concentration of 17-hydroxyprogesterone before and/or after stimulation with adrenocorticotrophic hormone (often present)
8. Increase in cortisol:creatinine ratio in morning urine samples (often present)
9. Mild or moderate suppression of cortisol:creatinine ratio by intravenous or oral low-dose dexamethasone suppression test
10. Histologic findings of hair follicle cycle arrest

and anagen effluvium, should be ruled out. Sometimes affected dogs have thyroid test results suggestive of hypothyroidism (low total thyroxine level), but other thyroid test results are normal. In those cases thyroid supplementation fails to cause hair regrowth.

Skin biopsies are helpful to support the diagnosis of alopecia X and are useful to rule out inflammatory causes of the alopecia. Histologically, there is orthokeratotic hyperkeratosis, epidermal melanosis, follicular keratosis, and follicular dilatation. Hairs have excessive trichilemmal keratinization (flame follicles), a sign of late catagen suggesting catagen arrest. Hair regrowth may occur at the site of the biopsy.

Evaluation of the steroids produced by the adrenal gland may be supportive in the diagnosis of alopecia X and can be assessed by performing an ACTH stimulation test, but the test results can be inconclusive. The classic ACTH stimulation test is performed; however, the prestimulation and poststimulation test samples must be sent to a laboratory that is capable of measuring concentrations of adrenal and sex hormones, including cortisol, 17-OHP, estrogen, progesterone, and testosterone. Results may demonstrate increased levels of progesterone or 17-OHP in both males and females, intact or neutered, which suggests abnormal steroid production or conversion, although this should not be considered pathognomonic of alopecia X.

Additional diagnostic testing that may be useful in the workup of alopecia X includes the oral or intravenous low-dose dexamethasone suppression test (LDDST) and the urinary cortisol:creatinine ratio (UCCR). A normal oral or intravenous LDDST result can help rule out alopecia X because most dogs with alopecia X show abnormal suppression. This was demonstrated in Pomeranians with alopecia X, which showed lack of complete suppression when compared with healthy dogs of other breeds and with healthy Pomeranians (Cerundolo et al, 2007).

The UCCR can be determined for urine samples collected on several days, and subsequently the average of the ratios can be calculated (Cerundolo et al, 2007). Dogs with alopecia X should have ratios higher than those commonly found in normal dogs, whose UCCRs range from 0.3 to 8.3×10^{-6} with a mean ± 1 standard deviation of $2.9 \pm 1.4 \times 10^{-6}$ (Van Vonderen et al, 1997). However, overlap of UCCRs may occur between dogs affected with alopecia X and normal dogs (Cerundolo et al, 2007), and dogs with other illnesses can have elevated UCCRs.

It is reemphasized that this disease is one in which diagnosis can be difficult because none of the tests described earlier is pathognomonic for alopecia X. However, the aforementioned battery of tests should be useful in the workup and help to rule out other causes of the alopecia.

result of sun exposure and can be minimized with sun restriction or use of clothing. Owners may first become aware of the problem when the dog's hair coat fails to regrow after clipping. This can also be seen in endocrine diseases or in Nordic or plush-coated breeds that were shaved during the normal telogen phase of the hair cycle. Hair regrowth is often seen in areas of trauma (e.g., skin scraping or biopsy sites). Secondary skin infections are rare in this condition.

Diagnosis

There is no test that can definitively diagnose alopecia X in a dog. The diagnosis is often made by exclusion (Box 115-2). Other endocrine diseases such as hyperadrenocorticism, hypothyroidism, and hyperestrogenism, as well as breed-specific hair cycle abnormalities, color dilution alopecia, black hair follicular dysplasia, telogen effluvium,

Treatment

The pros and cons of each therapeutic option listed in the following sections must be explained to the owner because alopecia X is a cosmetic disorder. "Benign neglect" could be an option and may be the best treatment. The various medical and surgical treatments, sometimes contradictory, reflect the difficulty in treating this type of hair loss. The following therapeutic options are currently recommended to the owners of affected dogs.

Neutering

Castration may lead to hair regrowth in a few weeks (Rosser, 1990). Although response may be complete, the owner should be warned that some animals relapse and lose their hair again after a few years. Although less well documented, hair may also regrow in females following ovariohysterectomy.

Melatonin

Melatonin treatment results in partial to complete hair regrowth in approximately 40% of cases. It is very safe, although it is contraindicated in dogs with diabetes mellitus because melatonin can cause insulin resistance at high doses. The mode of action is unknown, but melatonin may affect the metabolism of sex hormones (Ashley et al, 1999). The recommended dosage of melatonin is 3 mg q12h PO for small breeds and 6 to 12 mg q12h PO for large breeds. Many dogs subsequently lose hair even if current treatment is maintained; therefore it is recommended to stop treatment once hair regrowth is established and to restart treatment only if the hair loss recurs. There appear to be no adverse effects apart from mild sedation.

Mitotane and Trilostane

Two drugs used to treat hyperadrenocorticism, mitotane and trilostane, have been used to manage dogs with alopecia X. The exact mechanisms by which mitotane or trilostane causes hair regrowth in dogs with alopecia X are unknown. These drugs may work through manipulation of the adrenal-gonadal steroids, since these hormones are known to have both stimulatory and inhibitory effects on the hair follicle cycle.

Mitotane
Mitotane (Lysodren) causes selective necrosis and atrophy of the zona fasciculata and zona reticularis of the adrenal cortex. It has been used to treat dogs with alopecia X at induction dosages of 15 to 25 mg/kg q24h PO followed by twice weekly dosing (Frank et al, 2004; Rosenkrantz and Griffin, 1992). Routine ACTH stimulation tests should be performed to monitor cortisol concentrations and prevent hypocortisolemia or iatrogenic Addison's disease. Unfortunately, some dogs may subsequently lose hair again despite achievement of good hormonal control and continued therapy. Therefore it is best not to continue therapy once hair regrowth is achieved and to restart only if hair loss recurs. Mitotane should be used only after other treatments have failed and, in view of the potential adverse effects (e.g., vomiting and weakness due to hypoadrenocorticism), with consent of a fully informed owner.

Trilostane
Trilostane (Vetoryl), an inhibitor of 3β-hydroxysteroid dehydrogenase, has been used with success to treat Pomeranians, miniature poodles, and Alaskan malamutes with alopecia X (Cerundolo et al, 2004; Leone et al, 2005). The dosages used by the authors include 3.0 to 3.6 mg/kg q12h PO in Alaskan malamutes and 2.5 to 5.0 mg/kg q24h PO in Pomeranians and miniature poodles. Complete hair regrowth within 4 months has been reported in Alaskan malamutes, miniature poodles, and Pomeranians. Once full hair regrowth has been achieved the trilostane can be given two or three times a week to maintain a good coat because withdrawing it completely results in hair loss after a few months. Adverse effects (e.g., vomiting, diarrhea) are rare, and dogs should be reexamined routinely and monitored for signs of hypoadrenocorticism. An ACTH stimulation test is normally performed 10 days after beginning the treatment, then after 4 weeks, 12 weeks, and 6 months, and finally twice yearly. Large-scale trials are still needed to further evaluate the exact dosage needed to treat affected dogs of various breeds.

Antiandrogens

Recently antiandrogens have been used in an attempt to stimulate hair regrowth in dogs with alopecia X. These include the oral antiandrogen finasteride (Propecia), which has been anecdotally reported to result in partial to complete hair regrowth in alopecic Pomeranian dogs, and a deslorelin-based implant (Suprelorin) used to reversibly induce infertility in male dogs. To the author's knowledge no studies have been conducted evaluating the efficacy or side effects of these treatments for alopecia X.

References and Suggested Reading

Ashley PF et al: Effect of oral melatonin administration on sex hormone, prolactin, and thyroid hormone concentrations in adult dogs, *J Am Vet Med Assoc* 215:1111, 1999.

Cerundolo R et al: Treatment of canine Alopecia X with trilostane, *Vet Dermatol* 15:285, 2004.

Cerundolo R et al: Alopecia in Pomeranians and miniature poodles in association with high urinary corticoid:creatinine ratios and resistance to glucocorticoid feedback, *Vet Rec* 160:393, 2007. Erratum in *Vet Rec* 160:547, 2007.

Frank LA: Oestrogen receptor antagonist and hair regrowth in dogs with hair cycle arrest (Alopecia X), *Vet Dermatol* 18:63, 2007.

Frank LA, Hnilica KA, Oliver JW: Adrenal steroid hormone concentrations in dogs with hair cycle arrest (Alopecia X) before and during treatment with melatonin and mitotane, *Vet Dermatol* 15:278, 2004.

Leone F et al: The use of trilostane for the treatment of alopecia X in Alaskan malamutes, *J Am Anim Hosp Assoc* 41:336, 2005.

Rosenkrantz WS, Griffin C: Lysodren therapy in suspect adrenal sex hormone dermatosis. In *Proceedings of the 2nd World Congress of Veterinary Dermatology*, 1992, p 121.

Rosser EJ: Castration responsive dermatosis in the dog. In von Tscharner C, Halliwell REW, editors: *Advances in veterinary dermatology*, vol 1, Philadelphia, 1990, Baillière Tindall, p 34.

Shibata K, Koie H, Nagata M: Clinicopathologic and morphologic analysis of the adrenal gland in Pomeranians with nonillness alopecia, *Jpn J Vet Dermatol* 11:115, 2005.

Van Vonderen IK, Kooistra HS, Rijnberk A: Intra- and interindividual variation in urine osmolality and urine specific gravity in healthy pet dogs of various ages, *J Vet Intern Med* 11:30, 2007.

CHAPTER 116

Actinic Dermatoses and Sun Protection

AMANDA K. BURROWS, *Perth, Australia*

Solar-induced lesions in dogs and cats occur on skin with no or light pigmentation and sparsely haired regions that are exposed frequently to sun. Lesions are more common in dogs and cats that spend substantial time outdoors or sunbathe (lying in dorsal or lateral recumbency for extended periods), or are housed where there is reflective ground cover (including snow) and little sun protection. The most commonly affected dog breeds are white English bull terriers, dalmatians, beagles, fox terriers, whippets, white boxers, American Staffordshire bull terriers, basset hounds, and American bulldogs. White-haired areas of short-haired cats are most at risk. Blue-eyed white cats are most susceptible.

Clinical Features of Actinic Dermatoses in Dogs and Cats

Canine Disease

In dogs lesions range from patchy or confluent erythema and scaling affecting nonpigmented thickened skin to scaly erythematous papules or crusted indurated linear plaques and nodules with erosions and ulcers and hemorrhagic crusts. Actinic comedones may be present, filled with darkly colored keratinous or caseous debris in non-pigmented lightly haired skin and may be irregularly thickened and firm on palpation. Lesions may be discrete pigmented subepidermal foci or small nodules. Comedones may rupture, eliciting a foreign body response and furunculosis. Intact hemorrhagic bullae are a distinctive feature secondary to actinic comedone rupture with crusted erythematous nodules that may be intact or fistulated. A coexistent bacterial pyoderma may make the clinical diagnosis more difficult.

Actinic keratoses are premalignant epithelial lesions that can transform into invasive squamous cell carcinoma. These lesions are either single or multiple and are erythematous, scaly red to reddish-brown, ill-defined macules that progress to indurated, crusted plaques and are rough on palpation. Induration, erosion, ulceration, or increasing diameter should raise the suspicion of evolution into squamous cell carcinoma. Lesions often are found abruptly adjacent to normal pigmented skin. In dogs that sunbathe lesions commonly are observed on the glabrous skin of the ventral and lateral abdomen, flank folds, inner thighs, scrotum, and perineum. The hock and distal hind limb, bridge of the nose, pinnae, dorsal muzzle, periorbital regions, and tail tip also may be affected.

Feline Disease

In cats early lesions appear on the margins of the sparsely haired pinnae and are characterized by mild erythema and fine scaling. These progress to erythematous plaques, crusting, erosions and superficial ulceration with pain, scratching, and twitching of the pinnae. The margins of the lower eyelids, lips, nasal planum, preauricular region of the face, and dorsal muzzle may be affected similarly.

Diagnosis of Actinic Dermatosis

The diagnosis of actinic dermatitis is based on the correlation of breed, coat color, coat length, ultraviolet (UV) light exposure, and lesion localization to body sites commonly affected by solar damage. Comedones in sun-exposed skin, with or without evidence of other solar-induced lesions, should increase suspicion of actinic dermatosis. The lesions of actinic furunculosis need to be differentiated from deep bacterial folliculitis and furunculosis, demodicosis with deep pyoderma, systemic or opportunistic fungal infections, and neoplasia.

Actinic dermatitis is diagnosed by histopathologic analysis. It is important to resolve any secondary infections before collection of biopsy samples. Biopsy specimens should be obtained from different types of lesions and different stages of the disease. A complete history should be provided with the biopsy submission, including signalment, degree of solar exposure, and distribution and clinical description of lesions, and the specimens should be examined by a veterinary dermatohistopathologist if possible. Characteristic microscopic lesions include vacuolated keratinocytes with pyknotic nuclei and eosinophilic cytoplasm ("sunburn cells"), epidermal hyperplasia, follicular keratosis, laminar alteration of collagen in the superficial dermis (dogs) with superficial laminar fibrosis, perivascular to lichenoid inflammation, solar elastosis, and actinic comedones with pyogranulomatous folliculitis and furunculosis as common sequelae to comedonal rupture.

Sun Protection

The best treatment for solar dermatitis is prevention, and owners should be educated to practice sun avoidance and protection for their pets at an early age. Once chronic actinic dermatitis is present, the disease is incurable.

Sun Avoidance

Dogs and cats should be kept inside from 9 AM to 3 PM and should not be permitted to sunbathe near open doors and windows (normal window glass does not block UV radiation). For animals that cannot be kept inside, providing generous shade is highly recommended. White concrete floors should be avoided because they reflect sunlight.

Sun-Protective Clothing

Cotton T-shirts may assist in decreasing sun exposure; however, they rarely cover all at-risk areas of the skin. Body suits made from synthetic fabrics (Lycra, Dacron) with a high sun protection factor (SPF) (www. designerdogwear.com) are recommended, or owners may be able to make sunsuits for their pets using sun-protective fabric. In the author's experience, most dogs tolerate the flexible and comfortable protection suits.

Sunscreens

Sunscreen should be applied 10 to 15 minutes before sun exposure and, if solar exposure is unpredictable, should be applied twice daily. Titanium or zinc oxide products should not be rubbed in because they work best when applied as a thin smear. A waterproof SPF 30 (or higher) sunscreen containing a broad-spectrum UV-absorbing chemical in combination with titanium or zinc oxide should be used for maximal efficacy. Ingestion of some ingredients may cause adverse gastrointestinal effects, and zinc toxicity may result from ingestion of zinc-based products; excessive ingestion should be prevented. Colorants absorb or reflect visible light *but offer no protection against UV rays.* Thus recommendations to apply black ink and tattoo skin surfaces should be disregarded.

Treatment of Actinic Dermatoses

Topical Treatments

Topical therapy for actinic dermatoses can include glucocorticoids, diclofenac, imiquimod, and retinoids.

Glucocorticoids

For acute solar dermatitis 1% to 5% hydrocortisone ointment or cream is applied q12-24h for 7 to 10 days. If systemic therapy is required to reduce erythema, oral prednisolone (1 mg/kg q24h for 7 to 10 days) is used.

Diclofenac

Topical 3% diclofenac in 2.5% hyaluronan gel (Solaraze Gel), developed for humans with actinic keratoses, has been used in dogs and cats with actinic dermatitis and is effective and well tolerated. The adverse effects are limited to mild pruritus and irritation at the site of application.

Imiquimod

Five percent imiquimod (Aldara cream) has good efficacy with moderate morbidity in the treatment of human actinic keratosis. Recently pinnal lesions in a cat were treated with topical 5% imiquimod three times weekly for 12 weeks, which resulted in resolution of the lesions. Adverse effects were limited to erythema, crusting, alopecia, and mild discomfort at the sites of application during the first 3 weeks. These results suggest that topical imiquimod might be a therapeutic option for cats for which surgery and radiation therapy are not feasible.

Retinoids

Tretinoin is a topical retinoid considered to be of low efficacy for the treatment of actinic keratoses in humans, but there are anecdotal reports of its use to treat actinic dermatitis in dogs and cats.

Oral Treatments

Synthetic Retinoids

Partial to complete resolution of actinic keratoses in dogs was achieved with the administration of etretinate 1 mg/kg q12h PO for 3 months. Etretinate is no longer available, but acitretin administered at 0.5 to 1 mg/kg q24h PO for 4 to 6 weeks, with the frequency then reduced to q48h for 4 to 6 weeks and finally to twice a week, is effective in dogs with actinic dermatitis in the author's experience. Potential adverse effects include keratoconjunctivitis sicca, vomiting, diarrhea, elevation in triglyceride levels, and hepatotoxicity; regular monitoring for these adverse effects is critical. Retinoids are teratogenic and very expensive, which limits their use, particularly in larger-breed dogs.

Vitamin A

Oral vitamin A has been recommended for canine and feline actinic dermatitis, but controlled clinical trials are lacking. The recommended dosage is 800 to 1000 IU/kg q24h for 3 months, with frequency then tapered to three times a week.

Other Treatment Options

The principal surgical therapeutic options for actinic keratosis in dogs and cats are excisional surgery, cryosurgery, and carbon dioxide laser ablation of the affected epidermis. For optimal success with cryosurgery, temperature probes should be used to ensure adequate freezing time. Laser ablation with a carbon dioxide laser is an effective treatment modality in human actinic keratosis and is used by some veterinary dermatologists. Cutaneous dermabrasion and chemical peeling with 35% trichloroacetic acid, α-hydroxy acid, and liquid nitrogen spray also are treatment options for diffuse actinic keratoses in humans and their use has been advocated in dogs.

References and Suggested Reading

Frank LA, Calderwood Mays MB: Solar dermatitis in dogs, *Compend Contin Educ Pract Vet* 16:465, 1994.

Gross TL, Ihrke PJ, Walder EJ: *Veterinary dermatopathology: a macroscopic and microscopic evaluation of canine and feline skin disease*, St Louis, 2005, Mosby Year Book.

Peters-Kennedy J, Scott DW, Miller WH Jr: Apparent clinical resolution of pinnal actinic keratoses and squamous cell carcinoma in a cat using topical imiquimod 5% cream, *J Feline Med Surg* 10(6):593, 2008.

Power HT, Ihrke PI: The use of synthetic retinoids in veterinary medicine. In Bonagura JD, editor: *Kirk's current veterinary therapy XII: small animal practice*, Philadelphia, 1995, Saunders, p 585.

Rosenkrantz WS: Solar dermatitis. In Griffin CE, Kwochka KW, Macdonald JM, editors: *Current veterinary dermatology: the science and art of therapy*, St Louis, 1993, Mosby Year Book, p 309.

CHAPTER 117

Drugs for Behavior-Related Dermatoses

MEGHAN E. HERRON, *Columbus, Ohio*

Common behavior problems that manifest with dermatologic disease include overgrooming (i.e., feline psychogenic alopecia), repetitive licking (i.e., lick granulomas), and self-mutilating behaviors. Differentiation between dermatologic and psychologic disease is a complex process. These behaviors can be a response to underlying pain or pruritus, or the symptoms of anxiety and compulsive disorders. Recent studies suggest that a behavioral cause for self-inflicted dermatologic disease may be overdiagnosed. Despite the repetitive and seemingly compulsive nature of self-injurious behavior disorders, often the initial trigger is pruritic disease, such as atopic dermatitis, cutaneous adverse food reactions, or flea allergy dermatitis.

Many patients have comorbidities, and special care should be taken to address the underlying medical conditions before or simultaneously with the treatment of behavior disorders. A thorough medical and behavioral history should be obtained and a full dermatologic workup performed before diagnosing and treating a patient for a behavior disorder. Psychotropic medications often are indicated for patients with primary behavior disorders or for those with behavior that may be complicating or caused by an underlying dermatologic disease. These medications can mitigate the behavioral aspects of primary dermatologic disease as well as allow medical treatment to be more effective when both dermatologic and behavioral conditions are suspected. This chapter offers an overview and clinical insight into the use of psychotropic medications to treat behavior-related dermatoses.

Psychotropic medications are used for their ability to mitigate anxiety and the animal's response to external stressors. Several classes of drugs offer these benefits, some of which also have antipruritic properties, which makes them especially helpful when both dermatologic and behavioral problems are present. Before the patient begins treatment, baseline laboratory testing should be performed to ensure that it is safe to administer hepatically metabolized and renally excreted medications long term. Typically this includes a complete blood count, chemistry profile, total thyroxine level, and urinalysis. These tests should be performed every 6 to 12 months during treatment, depending on the age and health status of the pet. The initial goal should be to achieve therapeutic effects and to minimize adverse effects. This is best accomplished by starting the patient at the low end of the dosage range for the first 2 weeks of treatment, then titrating up to effect, while keeping in mind that therapeutic effects of some medications may take 4 to 6 weeks to appear. In mild to moderate cases, particularly those in which an instigating medical disease can be identified and treated, the patient can be weaned from medications by decreasing the dose by 25% every 2 weeks beginning 3 to 6 months after the cessation of clinical signs. In patients with severe compulsive disorders, however, treatment with psychotropic medications may be lifelong.

Classes of Psychotropic Medications

Tricyclic Antidepressants

The tricyclic antidepressants (TCAs) are named for their three-ringed molecular structure. Commonly used TCAs in veterinary medication include clomipramine (Clomicalm), doxepin, and amitriptyline (Elavil). Clomipramine, under the brand name Clomicalm, is approved by the U.S. Food and Drug Administration for use in dogs with separation anxiety and carries a veterinary label. The author recommends the use of the brand name drug Clomicalm, rather than the generic drug clomipramine, unless an allergy to the meat flavoring is suspected, because anecdotally many patients seem not to respond as well to the generic product. Each TCA has properties that block the reuptake pumps for the neurotransmitters serotonin, norepinephrine, and, to a lesser extent, dopamine. The blockade of neurotransmitter reuptake pumps results in greater neurotransmitter availability, which leads to receptor changes that allow for therapeutic anxiety relief within approximately 4 to 6 weeks. Specifically, activation of the serotonin 1A (5-HT$_{1A}$) receptor because of the persisting increase in serotonin levels is responsible for the anxiety-relieving effects. Clomipramine has the greatest specificity for serotonin, which makes it more effective for anxiety relief. Amitriptyline tends to be heavily sedating and to have poorer anxiety-relieving effects and is therefore rarely used by the author. Furthermore, this class of drugs also exerts anticholinergic (muscarinic), antiadrenergic (α_1), and antihistaminic (H$_1$) properties and can block sodium channels in the brain and heart. These additional properties are responsible for adverse effects, such as sedation, dry mouth, constipation, urine retention, increased seizure potential, and arrhythmias. In cats the sedative effect can be profound and often leads to owner dissatisfaction and noncompliance. Preparing owners about the potential for these adverse effects may increase compliance and encourage communication about the pet's response. In animals with a history of obstipation, seizures, or cardiovascular disease, this class of drugs should be avoided.

When a concurrent pruritic disease is being treated, the antihistamine properties of TCAs offer an additional benefit. Doxepin has the most potent antihistamine properties of any of the TCAs and, in fact, has 600 to 800 times the antihistamine effects of diphenhydramine. Unfortunately, the serotonin-enhancing effects of doxepin are the lowest in its class, which makes it a poor choice when anxiety or compulsion is the primary cause for the dermatosis. Each clinician should weigh the effects of both anxiety/compulsion and pruritus when choosing a TCA that will affect skin and behavior. See Table 117-1 for dosing recommendations.

Selective Serotonin Reuptake Inhibitors

The selective serotonin reuptake inhibitors (SSRIs) are a class of drugs that produce potent and selective blockade of the serotonin reuptake pump. This is a property shared with the TCAs, but this class is much more specific for serotonin and has little to no effect on reuptake of other neurotransmitters. The specificity of this class of drugs for the treatment of anxiety often makes them a better choice when treating a primary anxiety or compulsive disorder when little to no pruritus is present. As with the TCAs, therapeutic effects of SSRIs take 4 to 6 weeks to manifest and occur primarily through activation of the 5-HT$_{1A}$ receptors. Commonly used SSRIs in the treatment of compulsive, self-directed behaviors are fluoxetine (Reconcile,

TABLE **117-1**

Systemic Drugs and Suggested Dosages for the Treatment of Behavioral Dermatoses

Drug Name (Trade Name)	Dog	Cat
Tricyclic Antidepressants (TCAs)		
Allow 4-6 wk for therapeutic effects to manifest.		
This class of drugs has antihistamine properties and may be useful if allergic disease is also suspected.		
Clomipramine (Clomicalm)	1.0-3.0 mg/kg q12h PO	0.25-1.0 mg/kg q24h PO
Doxepin	3.0-5.0 mg/kg q12h PO	0.5-1.0 mg/kg q12-24h PO
Selective Serotonin Reuptake Inhibitors (SSRIs)		
Allow 4-6 wk for therapeutic effects to manifest.		
Fluoxetine (Reconcile)	0.5-2.0 mg/kg q24h PO	0.25-1.5 mg/kg q24h PO
Paroxetine	0.5-1.5 mg/kg q24h PO	0.25-1.0 mg/kg q24h PO
Sertraline	1.0-4.0 mg/kg q24h PO	0.25-0.5 mg/kg q24h PO
Serotonin Antagonist Reuptake Inhibitors (SARIs)		
May see some immediate effect with greater effect over 4-6 weeks. This class of drugs has antihistamine properties and may be useful if allergic disease is also suspected and can be used to augment the effects of TCAs or SSRIs.		
Trazodone	1.0-10.0 mg/kg q12h, not to exceed 600 mg per 24h	No published dose
Benzodiazepines		
Allow 30-60 min for onset of therapeutic effects.		
Alprazolam	0.05-0.25 mg/kg q4h PO	0.025-0.2 mg/kg q8h PO
Diazepam	0.5-2.2 mg/kg q4-6h PO	Avoid
Clorazepate	0.5-2.2 mg/kg q8-12h PO	Avoid
Clonazepam	0.1-0.5 mg/kg q12h PO	0.025-0.2 mg/kg q12h PO
Lorazepam*	0.1-0.5 mg/kg q12h PO	0.025-0.25 mg/kg q12h PO
Oxazepam*	0.2-1.0 mg/kg q121h PO	0.2-1.0 mg/kg q12h PO

*No active hepatic metabolites—may be safer in geriatric and feline patients.
PO, Orally.

Prozac), paroxetine (Paxil), and sertraline (Zoloft). Unlike the TCAs, SSRIs have minimal anticholinergic, antiadrenergic, and antihistaminic effects, which gives them a lower side effect profile. This also means that there are little to no antipruritic benefits to this class of drugs. Fluoxetine is the most frequently used SSRI in behavioral medicine, has been the subject of the most published reports of SSRI use in companion animals, and carries a veterinary label for treatment of separation anxiety (Reconcile). The most common adverse effects of fluoxetine are decreased appetite and mild lethargy, both of which resolve over the course of a few weeks. For animals with finicky appetites, especially cats, this medication may be problematic. Owners seem to have little tolerance for inappetence in their pets, and an SSRI such as paroxetine or sertraline may be a better option, despite the lower availability of published information on their use in animals. Of the SSRIs, paroxetine has the highest potential for anticholinergic effects, although still lower than that of the TCAs. Although typically the use of paroxetine allows the avoidance of anorexigenic effects, the potential for constipation, urine retention, and dry mouth persists. Sertraline is the newest of the SSRIs to come off patent and tends to have the fewest adverse effects. Another potential benefit of sertraline is that its excretion is primarily fecal, and therefore it may be safer in patients with renal compromise. See Table 117-1 for dosing recommendations.

Serotonin Antagonist Reuptake Inhibitors

Serotonin antagonist reuptake inhibitors (SARIs) are relatively new to veterinary medicine. Their primary mode of action is potent blocking of the 2A serotonin receptor (5-HT$_{2A}$). Active 5-HT$_{2A}$ receptors have inhibitory effects on 5-HT$_{1A}$ receptors. Since 5-HT$_{1A}$ receptor activation caused by increased serotonin is what is responsible for the anxiety-relieving effects of SSRIs and TCAs, active 5-HT$_{2A}$ receptors can prevent other serotonin-enhancing drugs from working to their full capacity. Therefore the use of a SARI to block 5-HT$_{2A}$ receptors in combination with an SSRI or TCA should lead to synergistic effects. Trazodone (Desyrel) is the only SARI with reported use in dogs, and there are no published reports of its use in cats. This drug can be added to the treatment plan of canine patients whose compulsive or anxious behaviors have been minimally responsive to SSRI or TCA monotherapy. Some immediate improvement may occur, and more can be expected over 4 to 6 weeks of therapy. Trazodone and other SARIs also have mild serotonin reuptake inhibition properties, which makes them a reasonable choice for monotherapy if needed. Unique to trazodone within this class are its antihistamine properties. The use of this medication alone or in combination with other medications may therefore provide additional relief of pruritus when underlying dermatologic disease is also suspected. For dogs with marked anxiety-related and pruritic disease, perhaps the combination of an SSRI and trazodone may provide the greatest relief. Adverse effects are uncommon but may include sedation, gastrointestinal upset, and agitation. See Table 117-1 for dosing recommendations.

Benzodiazepines

Benzodiazepines are part of a group of drugs known as *anxiolytic sedatives-hypnotics*. Their primary effects on behavior include an almost immediate relief of anxiety, but they also produce appetite stimulation, sedation, and muscle relaxation. The effects are a result of the drug's binding to a site on the γ-aminobutyric acid A (GABA-A) receptor complex. This then potentiates the effects of GABA when binding to this complex, causing an immediate and potent reduction in firing of the corresponding neuron. This is the only class of drugs discussed in this chapter with the ability to quickly halt the cascade of anxiety and panic in animals. These drugs have no effect on the reuptake of serotonin or other neurotransmitters and have no antihistaminic properties; therefore they are best used in patients with primary anxiety or compulsive behaviors as opposed to those resulting from underlying dermatologic disease. This class of drugs is most often reserved for patients whose self-directed behaviors occur at predictable times or in predictable contexts. For example, this medication can be administered as needed when the behavior is predicted to occur in response to experiencing a thunderstorm or loud noise, being home alone, traveling by car, or boarding. The onset of action is approximately 30 to 60 minutes and effects persist as long as the active drug remains in the system. In some cases in which marked generalized anxiety or compulsive behaviors are constant, daily use in combination with serotonin-enhancing drugs (SSRIs, TCAs) may be helpful. Behavioral clinicians frequently augment treatment of anxiety-based overgrooming or self-directed behaviors with 24-hour dosing of a benzodiazepine when SSRIs or TCAs alone have provided only marginal relief. Although around-the-clock use of a benzodiazepine provides substantial relief in many cases, as-needed dosing is often preferred because both drug dependence and tolerance develop with prolonged daily use. There is also a significant potential for drug diversion and human drug abuse. Accordingly, caution must be exercised when prescribing benzodiazepines to animal patients.

Commonly used benzodiazepines are alprazolam (Xanax), diazepam (Valium), clorazepate (Tranxene), clonazepam (Klonopin), lorazepam (Ativan), and oxazepam (Serax). The choice among various benzodiazepines is based on the required duration of action and the health status of the patient. For patients taking constant daily doses of benzodiazepines, drugs such as lorazepam, clonazepam, and oxazepam may be better options because they provide 12 hours of relief. In contrast, alprazolam would need to be dosed six times daily to provide 24-hour relief. Caution should be used when administering benzodiazepines to feline patients because acute hepatic necrosis has been reported after oral administration of diazepam. The author has observed this toxicosis with the use of clorazepate in cats as well. If benzodiazepine use is indicated in a cat, lorazepam and oxazepam may be safer options because they lack active hepatic metabolites. These two drugs also may be more appropriate for geriatric dogs or those with known hepatic disease. Table 117-1 summarizes dosing recommendations.

Other Considerations

When treating behavioral dermatoses, the clinician should keep in mind that many of these compulsive or anxiety-driven behaviors are a result of underlying stressors in the animal's environment. The clinician should talk to owners about identifying triggers for the behavior.

Owners should be assisted in finding ways to remove the pet from such situations or to provide the pet with other coping mechanisms. Emphasis should be placed on managing the home environment and training new behaviors that are incompatible with self-injury. For example, dogs can be taught to engage with food enrichment toys to redirect their behavior and to prevent them from licking and traumatizing their skin. Food enrichment, in the form of puzzle toys that have been stuffed with canned food and frozen or rolling toys that dispense dry kibble or treats, can be especially helpful in directing pets to other oral behaviors. Time spent interacting with puzzle toys means less time spent on self-directed behaviors that can perpetuate dermatologic disease. However, if the underlying dermatologic disease is due to cutaneous adverse food reactions, care must be taken to select a food that is compatible with the restricted diet.

Pheromone enrichment in the form of feline facial pheromones (Feliway) and canine appeasing pheromones (DAP, Adaptil, Comfort Zone) can also help to create a sense of safety and comfort in the pet's home environment. Close follow-up with owners and frequent monitoring of both medical and behavioral progress is essential in any successful treatment plan.

References and Suggested Reading

Crowell-Davis SL, Murray T: *Veterinary psychopharmacology*, ed 1, Ames, IA, 2006, Blackwell.

Landsberg G, Hunthausen W, Ackerman A: *Handbook of behavior problems of the dog and cat*, ed 2, New York, 2003, Saunders.

Stahl SM: *Essential psychopharmacology: neuroscientific basis and practical applications*, ed 2, Cambridge, UK, 2000, Cambridge University Press.

Virga V: Behavioral dermatology, *Vet Clin North Am Small Anim Pract* 33:231, 2003.

Waisglass SE et al: Underlying medical conditions in cats with presumptive psychogenic alopecia, *J Am Vet Med Assoc* 228:1705, 2006.

CHAPTER 118

Superficial Necrolytic Dermatitis

KEVIN BYRNE, *Bensalem, Pennsylvania*

Superficial necrolytic dermatitis (SND) was initially reported in dogs as "diabetic dermatopathy" because of the association of the disorder with diabetes mellitus (Walton et al, 1986). There is a similar skin disorder in humans: necrolytic migratory erythema. Necrolytic migratory erythema is usually associated with a malignant neuroendocrine tumor called a *glucagonoma*. Most cases of SND in dogs are associated with liver disease, are termed the *hepatocutaneous syndrome* (HS) form of SND, and are not associated with a glucagonoma. However, there have been a few reported cases of the glucagonoma syndrome (GS) form of SND in dogs. A small number of cases of SND have been associated with medications (phenobarbital, primidone) and mycotoxin ingestion. The number of reported cases of SND in cats is relatively low.

Clinical Findings in Dogs

The disease is more common in middle-aged or older dogs. Primary complaints of SND in dogs include soreness of the dog's paws and lethargy or anorexia. The most useful clinical findings in dogs are abnormalities of the paws, including crusts, erythema, and oozing. Usually all paw pads exhibit varying degrees of hyperkeratosis with subsequent crusting and fissuring of the pads. Lesions including erythema, erosions or ulcerations, serous to purulent discharge, crusts, and hyperkeratotic plaques may occur in other sites such as perioral, perianal, perivulvar, preputial, and scrotal skin. Differential diagnoses of the lesions of SND include zinc-responsive dermatosis, pemphigus foliaceus, erythema multiforme, epidermolysis bullosa acquisita, and bullous pemphigoid. Impression cytologic analysis of SND lesions is usually helpful in revealing the presence of secondary infections, which are commonly associated with this disease. Complete blood count (CBC) may reveal mild nonregenerative anemia and leukocytosis.

Dogs with SND (HS) have elevated levels of liver enzymes (serum alkaline phosphatase, alanine transaminase) and increased bile acids; some have hyperglycemia with or without other features of diabetes mellitus. Abdominal ultrasonography is useful to check for the presence of the hyperechoic and hypoechoic pattern within the liver often seen in dogs with SND (HS). This pattern is sometimes described as having a "Swiss cheese" or "honeycomb" appearance.

The absence of abnormal results on the serum chemistry panel makes it more likely that the dog may have the GS form of SND. Thus, in cases of SND without evidence of liver disease, thought needs to be given to the possibility of SND (GS). Abdominal ultrasonography may not be able to detect small pancreatic tumors. Magnetic resonance imaging might be able to distinguish small tumors, although contrast enhancement may be necessary. It is recommended that the owners of dogs suspected of having SND (GS) submit a sample of the dog's plasma for glucagon measurement and that the results be compared with published information on canine plasma glucagon. High levels of plasma glucagon support the possibility that a glucagon-secreting tumor is present. Unfortunately, assays for canine plasma glucagon usually are not available, and the sample must be submitted to a human endocrinology laboratory that measures human plasma glucagon level. It may be beneficial to consult a specialist in internal medicine or endocrinology.

Clinical Findings in Cats

Cats are likely to manifest lethargy, anorexia, or weight loss. Clinical findings of SND (HS) in cats include ulceration and crusting of oral mucocutaneous junctions, and ulceration of the pinnae, periocular areas, interdigital areas, ventral abdomen, and inguinal areas with or without crust formation. Lesions may not appear on the footpads, unlike in SND in dogs. Secondary bacterial infection may be present. The CBC may reveal neutropenia, and results of a serum biochemistry profile may show elevations in alanine transaminase, aspartate transaminase, or bilirubin. Abdominal ultrasonography may reveal a diffusely coarse echotexture with reticular pattern of the liver and may or may not reveal discrete nodules.

Dermatohistopathologic Analysis

Once any secondary pyoderma has been treated, skin punch biopsy with dermatohistopathologic analysis is usually adequate to diagnose the condition. Collection of three or four biopsy specimens is more likely to produce at least one specimen with the findings required for diagnosis. Specimens must contain epidermis and so should be from areas where there is no ulceration. A good practice is to collect at least one specimen from a paw pad in each patient suspected of having SND. Biopsy specimens from perioral or perianal areas seem to carry a higher risk of secondary bacterial pyoderma even with appropriate antibiotic therapy, so these sites are used only if there are no better choices. In dogs, classic lesions of SND reveal epidermal hyperplasia, parakeratosis, and variable pallor of the upper epidermal keratinocytes. Pallor may not be present at all sites biopsied, which may lead to difficulty in distinguishing the condition from zinc-responsive dermatosis. In cats, lesions of SND show epidermal hyperplasia with focal compact hyperkeratosis or parakeratosis, acanthosis, and spongiosis, and may also reveal basal cell hyperplasia. Once dermatohistopathologic diagnosis of SND is made, diagnostic tests can be ordered to differentiate the HS form from the GS form in individual patients.

Treatment

The prognosis for SND is poor, and therapy is palliative. Debilitation caused by painful crusting lesions, especially lesions of the paws, must be addressed. Bacterial pyoderma should be treated with antibiotics that are expected to be effective against *Staphylococcus* and are not contraindicated in dogs with compromised liver function. Topical therapy with shampoos that contain chlorhexidine may help reduce the numbers of bacterial and yeast organisms.

Since patients with SND usually have low levels of plasma amino acids, nutritional therapy centers on giving foods that provide high-quality protein. However, partial to complete anorexia is common in pets with SND, and coaxing the pet to eat may be difficult. Any prescription food designed for critical-care patients can be used as a base diet. To this are added hard-boiled egg yolks, three to six per day, and a protein powder supplement. There are many over-the-counter protein powder supplements, but all are flavored for people. The use of chocolate flavors should be avoided. Optimum Nutrition 100% casein protein powder provides 24 g of protein per scoop. The recommended dosage is $\frac{1}{4}$ scoop per 10 lb body weight per day, mixed with food. Palatability is a problem with protein powders, and some dogs eventually lose interest in eggs. If the pet refuses prescription critical-care diets, feeding any food that is high in protein, especially meat proteins, may be an option. The prognosis worsens when it becomes difficult to coax the pet to eat. It is also recommended that pets with SND be given an essential fatty acid supplement such as Allerderm Efa-Caps and a zinc supplement such as NutriVed Zinpro chewable tablets.

Although intravenous amino acid therapy using a product such as Aminosyn has been reported to be helpful in some cases of canine SND, the author has treated numerous animals that did not respond to this therapy. Administration via a catheter inserted into a larger vein, such as the jugular vein, reduces the likelihood of phlebitis. For Aminosyn 10% solution a suggested dosage is 25 ml/kg of body weight administered over 6 to 8 hours. For Aminosyn 8.5% solution the dosage is 30 ml/kg of body weight administered over 6 to 8 hours. Two to three administrations should be given at weekly intervals before a decision is made as to whether continuation of the treatment is worthwhile. For many dogs with SND (HS), the condition progresses and the pet's condition deteriorates. At this point many pet owners understandably elect euthanasia for their pets.

Treatment of Superficial Necrolytic Dermatitis with Glucagonoma

Ideally, excision of a glucagon-secreting pancreatic tumor should result in resolution of lesions of SND as is the case in many humans with necrolytic migratory erythema. Unfortunately, the mortality rate for pancreatic tumor excision in dogs is high. Also, glucagonomas are quick to metastasize, and smaller tumors may be difficult to find.

For patients with GS in which excision of the glucagonoma is not feasible, temporary improvement of clinical signs may be possible with the use of octreotide.

Use of Octreotide

Octreotide is a somatostatin-like drug that inhibits multiple hormones, including glucagon. It has been reported to result in improvement of skin lesions in a dog with SND (GS) (Oberkirchner et al, 2010). The author treated a 10-year-old male beagle dog with SND (GS) using generic octreotide at a dosage of 2 to 3 µg/kg q12h by SC injection. Two weeks after octreotide treatment began, significant improvement was observed in the skin and paw pads and the dog was feeling much better. Six weeks after the initiation of octreotide therapy there were no ulcerated areas of the skin and paw pads and only a small number of crusts.

There might be some benefit to using octreotide in patients with SND (HS). However, adverse effects of octreotide in humans include hepatic/biliary problems. Adverse effects of octreotide injection therapy in dogs include decreased appetite. Given the debilitation that SND causes in the patient and the lack of consistently beneficial therapies, octreotide might be considered in

SND (HS) patients whose owners are willing to try this therapy with the understanding that it is not an approved treatment in dogs and also that there is the potential for adverse effects, including the theoretical possibility that it could make liver disease worse.

References and Suggested Reading

Byrne KP: Metabolic epidermal necrosis—hepatocutaneous syndrome, *Vet Clin North Am Small Anim Pract* 29:1337, 1999.

Kimmel SE, Christiansen W, Byrne KP: Clinicopathologic, ultrasonographic, and histopathological findings of superficial necrolytic dermatitis with hepatopathy in a cat, *J Am Anim Hosp Assoc* 39:23, 2003.

Oberkirchner U et al: Successful treatment of canine necrolytic migratory erythema (superficial necrolytic dermatitis) due to metastatic glucagonoma with octreotide, *Vet Dermatol* 21:510, 2010.

Outerbridge CA, Marks SL, Rogers QR: Plasma amino acid concentrations in 36 dogs with histologically confirmed superficial necrolytic dermatitis, *Vet Dermatol* 13:177, 2002.

Torres S et al: Superficial necrolytic dermatitis and a pancreatic endocrine tumour in a dog, *J Small Anim Pract* 38:246, 1997.

Walton DK et al: Ulcerative dermatosis associated with diabetes mellitus in the dog: a report of four cases, *J Am Anim Hosp Assoc* 22:79, 1986.

CHAPTER 119

Cutaneous Adverse Drug Reactions

IAN BRETT SPIEGEL, *Levittown, Pennsylvania*

Adverse drug reactions are due to interactions between a pharmacologic agent, such as an antimicrobial, and the immune system. Common cutaneous clinical signs associated with cutaneous adverse drug reactions (CADRs) are listed in Table 119-1 along with the associated pharmacologic agents. These cutaneous signs may develop coincident with other clinical signs involving the gastrointestinal, respiratory, or cardiovascular systems. Signs can vary from lethargy and depression to fever, anemia, systemic hypotension, and shock.

Reactions can develop within hours to months of exposure, but CADRs usually occur within 1 to 3 weeks. Many of the cutaneous clinical signs can persist for up to a month, even with medical intervention, and as well as

removal and avoidance of a known or suspected offending agent. Diagnosis of CADR is often supported by the results from a skin biopsy.

Principles of management include (1) avoidance or discontinuation of the suspected causative agent(s), (2) supportive symptomatic care as necessary, and (3) client education regarding prevention of future similar reactions.

There are several specific drug eruption syndromes that warrant a more detailed discussion. These were selected for discussion in this chapter. These are erythema multiforme, Stevens-Johnson syndrome, toxic epidermal necrolysis, itraconazole-associated reactions, methimazole reactions, injection site reactions (vasculitis/

TABLE 119-1

Clinical Presentations of Cutaneous Adverse Drug Eruptions and Associated Pharmacologic Agents

Clinical Presentation	Selected Pharmacologic Agents
Erythema/erythroderma/ violaceous lesions	Sulfonamides, cephalosporins, penicillins, macrolides, fluoroquinolones, tetracyclines, levothyroxine, acepromazine, levamisole, ivermectin, hydroxyzine, chlorpheniramine, shampoo (e.g., D-limonene), itraconazole, neomycin, propylene glycol
Wheals/hives (urticaria) and angioedema	Sulfonamides, cephalosporins, penicillins, tetracycline, allergen-specific immunotherapy, barbiturates, insecticides (e.g., avermectins and amitraz), transfusions
Scaling/exfoliative dermatitis	Sulfonamides, cephalosporins, penicillins, macrolides, acepromazine, levamisole, hydroxyzine, chlorpheniramine, shampoo (e.g., tar)
Erosion/ulceration	Sulfonamides, cephalosporins, penicillins, retinoids, moxidectin, spironolactone (cats)
Pruritus	Sulfonamides, cephalosporins, penicillins, methimazole, propylthiouracil, gentamicin, chloramphenicol, acepromazine, griseofulvin, niacinamide, tetracyclines, doxorubicin, clopidogrel, propranolol, cyclosporine
Vesicles and bullae (blisters), pemphigus-like lesions	Sulfonamides, cephalosporins, penicillins, amitraz, diethylcarbamazine, thiabendazole, phenytoin, triamcinolone, neomycin
Papules and macules (maculopapular lesions)	Sulfonamides, cephalosporins, penicillins, 5-fluorocytosine, diethylcarbamazine, shampoo, cimetidine, hydroxyzine, procainamide
Petechiae/ecchymosis (purpura)	Sulfonamides, cephalosporins, penicillins
Alopecia	Sulfonamides (follicular necrosis/atrophy), cephalosporins, penicillins, chemotherapy, corticosteroids, levamisole (follicular necrosis/atrophy)
Otitis (contact dermatitis)	Sulfonamides, cephalosporins, penicillins, neomycin, propylene glycol, thiabendazole

ischemic dermatopathy caused by rabies vaccine), reactions associated with flea and tick products, nonsteroidal antiinflammatory subcorneal to follicular neutrophilic dermatitis, cyclosporine-induced psoriasiform-lichenoid dermatosis, and corticosteroid-induced calcinosis cutis.

Erythema Multiforme and Stevens-Johnson Syndrome

Erythema Multiforme

Erythema multiforme (EM) is an uncommon skin disease that is often sudden in onset and can affect skin, mucous membranes, and the mucocutaneous junctions. The condition can wax and wane, and can be self-limiting or require diagnostic workup and therapeutic intervention. It is currently believed that with EM a cell-mediated hypersensitivity reaction is directed against infectious organisms (viral and bacterial), medications (griseofulvin, aurothioglucose, cephalosporins, penicillins, macrolides, gentamicin, tetracyclines, sulfonamides, polythiouracil), foods, antiparasitic agents (ivermectin, levamisole), levothyroxine, or various nutraceutical products (e.g., Glyco-Flex). This disorder also may be associated with neoplasia (paraneoplastic syndrome) or connective tissue disorders. Usually the underlying cause is unknown and the disorder is categorized as idiopathic.

The classic finding is a target lesion that is raised on the borders with erythema centrally. Other lesions include hyperpigmented macules, raised erythematous papules, plaques, scaling, crusting, and oozing. Areas of the skin most affected include the ventral abdomen,

inguinal, and axillary regions; oral cavity; pinnae; and footpads. Almost 50% of cases have a mucocutaneous involvement.

Management includes stopping current medications (oral, injectable, and topical) and supplements. The diet may need to be changed as well. More severe cases require corticosteroids and other medications. Treatments have included cyclosporine (5 to 10 mg/kg daily PO), tacrolimus (topical), leflunomide (3 to 4 mg/kg daily PO), pentoxifylline (25 mg/kg twice daily PO), retinoids (e.g., isotretinoin 2 to 3 mg/kg daily PO), chemotherapy medications (azathioprine 2 mg/kg daily PO initially, chlorambucil 0.2 mg/kg daily PO initially), vitamin E (400 to 800 IU daily PO), and the combination of vitamin B (niacinamide 500 mg two or three times daily for ≥15 kg body weight and 250 mg two or three times daily for <15 kg body weight) and doxycycline (5 mg/kg twice daily PO initially). Practicing veterinarians are advised to consult with a dermatologist regarding the best treatment options.

Stevens-Johnson Syndrome

The pathogenesis of Stevens-Johnson syndrome (SJS) is similar to that described earlier for EM, and both disorders may be a variant of the same disease complex. SJS may even be a less aggressive version of toxic epidermal necrosis (next section) or a more aggressive form of EM. There is erythroderma without the target-shaped lesions seen in EM. Mucosal involvement is generally more severe than in EM. Management is similar to that for EM or TEN depending on the severity.

Toxic Epidermal Necrolysis (Lyell's Syndrome)

Toxic epidermal necrolysis (TEN) is a very rare and usually lethal disease that is more often than not associated with adverse drug reactions. More than 50% of the body surface area is involved. As in EM and SJS there is erythroderma and mucosal involvement, but more severe ulceration of the epidermis with detachment is seen. Vesicles and bullae are also present. TEN is usually considered the most severe form of EM. Systemic signs are also quite severe.

The management of TEN usually includes aggressive fluid therapy and supportive care. Immunomodulators also are incorporated, including corticosteroids (controversial) for no more than 5 days because this can delay wound healing. Other options include cyclosporine, cyclophosphamide, and human intravenous immunoglobulin. Secondary bacterial infections (of the skin and potentially systemic infection or sepsis) also need to be addressed.

Injection Site Reactions: Vasculitis/ Ischemic Dermatopathy in Response to Rabies Vaccine

The clinical signs observed in rabies vaccine injection site reactions usually start 3 to 6 months after vaccination and can include crusting, dry silvery scaling, and erosion, with or without ulceration. There is also hyperpigmentation of the pinnae (apices), tail tip, scrotum, and footpads (central punctate lesions). In some cases, the injection site may develop dark nodular lesions (panniculitis) with or without alopecia, erythema, and hyperpigmentation.

For future vaccinations the rabies vaccine should come from a different manufacturer because the adjuvant may be the actual cause of the ischemic dermatopathy. Alternatively, the clinician may wish to measure the rabies titers instead of revaccinating if this is permitted by local laws. Treatment options for the skin disease include pentoxifylline (25 mg/kg twice daily PO), topical tacrolimus, and oral cyclosporine (5 to 10 mg/kg daily PO). Even with treatment, in some cases alopecia may be permanent.

Reactions Associated with Specific Drugs

In addition to the syndromes described earlier, a number of CADRs have been reported in response to specific drugs, including antifungal agents, methimazole, flea and tick products, carprofen, cyclosporine, and corticosteroids.

Antifungal (Itraconazole)–Associated Reactions

Itraconazole has been associated with a dose-related (10 mg/kg/day) necroulcerative dermatitis secondary to a cutaneous vasculitis. This is reported in about 5% to 10% of the dogs administered this dosage. Decreasing the dosage or stopping the medication leads to resolution.

Methimazole-Associated Reactions

The antithyroid medication methimazole has been associated with severe facial pruritus in the cat that leads to excoriations, especially in the preauricular area. The neck is sometimes involved as well. The best option for these cats is stopping the medication and considering iodine 131 treatment for the hyperthyroidism.

Flea and Tick Product–Associated Reactions

Use of metaflumizone/amitraz (ProMeris) has been associated with spontaneously occurring pemphigus foliaceus. It is unknown whether the causative agent for the pemphigus foliaceus is the carrier vehicle, amitraz, or metaflumizone. This product is currently unavailable.

Other topical flea and tick preventives (e.g., fipronil, imidacloprid, dinotefuran, permethrins) have been associated with focal adverse reactions, including irritation, erythema, crusting, erosion, and ulceration. Focal mild alopecia is the most commonly reported adverse effect.

Nonsteroidal Antiinflammatory-Induced Subcorneal to Follicular Neutrophilic Dermatitis

Carprofen therapy has been associated in dogs with a Sweet's-like syndrome, a relatively rare disease also referred to as *sterile neutrophilic dermatosis*. Skin lesions include pustules, erythema, crusts, and erosions. Histopathologically, there is a neutrophilic dermatitis. The drug should be discontinued.

Cyclosporine-Induced Psoriasiform-Lichenoid Dermatosis

Cyclosporine has been used to treat many disorders in dogs and cats (see Chapter 92). Adverse reactions are usually limited to gastrointestinal tract disturbances, gingival hyperplasia, hirsutism, and papillomas. However, there is also an antimicrobial-responsive cutaneous reaction that occurs in dogs. Clinically, the lesions are usually erythematous with honey-colored, adherent, keratinaceous material and serous hyperkeratotic crusted papules that coalesce to form multiple well-demarcated lichenoid plaques. The extremities, ventral abdomen, and inguinal and axillary areas are predisposed, but the lesions also have been noticed on the pinnae and feet. This is an atypical staphylococcal infection because these patients respond to antimicrobial treatment and reduction or stopping of the cyclosporine. This is more likely to occur when ketoconazole is used concurrently.

Corticosteroid-Induced Calcinosis Cutis

Calcinosis cutis is an uncommon syndrome of mineralization characterized by deposition of calcium salts in soft tissues. The mineralization can be considered ectopic, idiopathic, dystrophic, metastatic, or iatrogenic. Clinically, these patients often have dome-shaped salmon-colored to erythematous papules that are firm and gritty when palpated. These lesions appear chalky and are surrounded by white to pink material with uneven margins. The lesions are often crusted and can be eroded or ulcerated. The most common anatomic areas affected are the back of the neck, axillary region, groin, perivulvar region, dorsum, elbows, footpads, skin around the tail base, and preauricular area.

In veterinary medicine, the most common cause of calcinosis cutis is exogenous corticosteroid administration (injected, oral, or topical). Discontinuation of the corticosteroid or lowering of the dose, management of secondary infections, and, if necessary, switching the type of corticosteroid used generally lead to resolution. Medical-grade (60% to 90%) DMSO (dimethyl sulfoxide) gel can be applied topically to the lesions one to two times daily to hasten resolution. Serum calcium levels should be monitored monthly because hypercalcemia has been reported when this product is used in calcinosis cutis. Also, owners should be warned of the risks of DMSO exposure (it is classified as a carcinogen at high dosages).

References and Suggested Reading

Hinn AC et al: Erythema multiforme, Stevens-Johnson syndrome, and toxic epidermal necrolysis in the dog: clinical classification, drug exposure, and histopathological correlations, *Vet Allergy Clin Immunol* 6:13, 1998.

Mellor PJ et al: Neutrophilic dermatitis and immune-mediated haematological disorders in a dog: suspected adverse reaction to carprofen, *J Small Anim Pract* 46:237, 2005.

Oberkirchner U et al: Metaflumizone-amitraz (Promeris)–associated pustular acantholytic dermatitis in 22 dogs: evidence suggests contact drug-triggered pemphigus foliaceus, *Vet Dermatol* 22(5):436, 2011.

Riedl MC, Casillas AM: Adverse drug reactions: types and treatment options, *Am Fam Physician* 68(9):1781, 2003.

Robson DC, Burton GG: Cyclosporin: applications in small animal dermatology, *Vet Dermatol* 14(1):1, 2003.

Scott DW: Erythema multiforme in a dog caused by a commercial nutraceutical product, *J Vet Clin Sci* 1(3):16, 2008.

Scott DW, Miller WH Jr: Erythema multiforme in dogs and cats: literature review and case material from the Cornell University College of Veterinary Medicine (1988-1996), *Vet Dermatol* 10:297, 1999.

Scott DW, Miller WH Jr, Griffin CD: *Muller and Kirk's small animal dermatology*, ed 6, Philadelphia, 2001, Saunders, p 729.

Trotman TK et al: Treatment of severe adverse cutaneous drug reactions with human intravenous immunoglobulin in two dogs, *J Am Anim Hosp Assoc* 42(4):312, 2006.

Werner AH: Psoriasiform-lichenoid–like dermatosis in three dogs treated with microemulsified cyclosporine A, *J Am Vet Med Assoc* 223:1013, 2003.

SECTION VI

Gastrointestinal Diseases

Chapter 120:	Feline Caudal Stomatitis	492
Chapter 121:	Oropharyngeal Dysphagia	495
Chapter 122:	Gastroesophageal Reflux	501
Chapter 123:	Antacid Therapy	505
Chapter 124:	Gastric *Helicobacter* spp. and Chronic Vomiting in Dogs	508
Chapter 125:	Gastric and Intestinal Motility Disorders	513
Chapter 126:	Current Veterinary Therapy: Antibiotic Responsive Enteropathy	518
Chapter 127:	Cobalamin Deficiency in Cats	522
Chapter 128:	Probiotic Therapy	525
Chapter 129:	Protozoal Gastrointestinal Disease	528
Chapter 130:	Canine Parvoviral Enteritis	533
Chapter 131:	Inflammatory Bowel Disease	536
Chapter 132:	Protein-Losing Enteropathies	540
Chapter 133:	Feline Gastrointestinal Lymphoma	545
Chapter 134:	Canine Colitis	550
Chapter 135:	Laboratory Testing for the Exocrine Pancreas	554
Chapter 136:	Exocrine Pancreatic Insufficiency in Dogs	558
Chapter 137:	Treatment of Canine Pancreatitis	561
Chapter 138:	Feline Exocrine Pancreatic Disorders	565
Chapter 139:	Diagnostic Approach to Hepatobiliary Disease	569
Chapter 140:	Drug-Associated Liver Disease	575
Chapter 141:	Acute Liver Failure	580
Chapter 142:	Chronic Hepatitis Therapy	583
Chapter 143:	Copper Chelator Therapy	588
Chapter 144:	Ascites and Hepatic Encephalopathy Therapy for Liver Disease	591
Chapter 145:	Portosystemic Shunts	594
Chapter 146:	Portal Vein Hypoplasia (Microvascular Dysplasia)	599
Chapter 147:	Extrahepatic Biliary Tract Disease	602
Chapter 148:	Idiopathic Vacuolar Hepatopathy	606
Chapter 149:	Feline Hepatic Lipidosis	608
Chapter 150:	Feline Cholangitis	614

The following web chapters can be found on the companion website at www.currentveterinarytherapy.com

Web Chapter 46:	Canine Biliary Mucocele
Web Chapter 47:	Canine Megaesophagus
Web Chapter 48:	Copper-Associated Hepatitis
Web Chapter 49:	Esophagitis
Web Chapter 50:	Evaluation of Elevated Serum Alkaline Phosphatase in Dogs
Web Chapter 51:	Flatulence
Web Chapter 52:	Gastric Ulceration
Web Chapter 53:	Hepatic Support Therapy
Web Chapter 54:	Oropharyngeal Dysphagia
Web Chapter 55:	Tylosin-Responsive Diarrhea

CHAPTER 120

Feline Caudal Stomatitis

LINDA J. DEBOWES, *Seattle, Washington*

The most common cause of oral inflammation in cats is periodontal disease (gingivitis, periodontitis). Inflammation of the buccal mucosa (stomatitis) also may be associated with severe periodontal disease. Eosinophilic complex–related disorders, neoplasia, trauma, irritation caused by ingestion of noxious materials, immune-mediated diseases, and metabolic abnormalities also are potential causes of oral inflammation. Caudal stomatitis is a problem seen in cats and should not be confused with inflammation in other areas of the mouth.

Infectious diseases have been associated with oral inflammation. Cats with altered immune function from infection with feline leukemia virus or feline immunodeficiency virus may have more severe periodontal disease or oral inflammation. Chronic calicivirus infection has been implicated as a factor in severe oral inflammation, especially in cats with inflammation in the area of the palatoglossal fold (caudal stomatitis). In one study, 81% of 25 cats with caudal stomatitis were shedding both feline calicivirus and feline herpesvirus 1 compared with 21% of a similar number of cats with periodontal disease (Lommer and Verstraete, 2003). The role of bacteria in caudal stomatitis is unknown. *Pasteurella multocida* subsp. *multocida* was identified more frequently in cats with caudal stomatitis than in normal cats in one study, which suggests that it may play a role in the disease (Dolieslager et al, 2011). *Bartonella henselae* infection has been suggested as a possible factor in the development of feline caudal stomatitis (Hardy et al, 2002). However, there is a high prevalence of *B. henselae* antibody positivity in healthy cats, which makes it difficult to determine the significance of an antibody-positive test result in a cat with caudal stomatitis. A recent study of 34 cats with chronic stomatitis and 34 age-matched healthy control cats reported no significant differences between the two groups in the prevalence of positivity for *Bartonella* spp. by polymerase chain reaction testing and antibody positivity for *B. henselae*. More recent studies evaluating potential causative agents have found that calicivirus and not *Bartonella* is associated with caudal stomatitis in cats (Belgard et al, 2010; Dowers et al, 2010).

Cats with chronic caudal stomatitis have decreased salivary immunoglobulin A (IgA) levels compared with healthy cats; however, the significance of this in the development of disease is unknown (Harley et al, 2003). Cats with chronic caudal stomatitis also have higher serum IgG, IgM, and IgA concentrations than healthy cats.

Oral inflammatory disease of unknown cause is a common problem in cats. The degree of inflammation is variable and may be severe. These cats present a diagnostic and therapeutic challenge, and management frequently is frustrating for both the veterinarian and owner. Inflammation may involve the gingiva (gingivitis), buccal mucosa (stomatitis), or tissues of and adjacent to the palatoglossal fold (caudal stomatitis) or pharyngeal area (pharyngitis). Current knowledge about the cause of caudal stomatitis unrelated to periodontal disease in cats is limited. The condition has been referred to as *lymphocytic-plasmacytic stomatitis* based on the major cellular infiltrate present on histologic examination. The histologic features are compatible with a chronic inflammatory or immunologic response but do not provide a definitive diagnosis as to the primary cause. Immunohistochemical studies have demonstrated a predominance of CD8+ cells over CD4+ cells, which could be consistent with a viral cause (Harley et al, 2011). Cats with severe caudal stomatitis often are grouped together as all having the same unknown problem; yet based on clinical presentation and variable response to treatment, it is more likely that multiple factors are involved.

Historical and Clinical Signs

Cats with caudal stomatitis frequently have a history of dysphagia, inappetence, or anorexia and of pain when eating is attempted. The cat may appear interested in food but is unwilling to eat or may attempt to eat but drops the food from its mouth or paws at its muzzle. The affected cat usually is reluctant to eat hard food but may eat soft food. As the severity of the inflammation increases, the cat becomes pickier about what it will eat, or blood-tinged saliva may be noted after eating. In severe cases the cat may be in a great deal of pain, which causes a reluctance to swallow and drooling (pseudoptyalism). Weight loss may be a significant problem, depending on the severity and duration of inflammation. Affected cats may exhibit altered behavior such as reduced activity, demonstrate aggressive behavior toward other pets or persons, or show an aversion to having the face or head touched. These cats may have an unkempt appearance resulting from a reluctance to groom because of oral pain. Owners may notice that the cat no longer yawns.

Oral Examination

Before the oral cavity is examined, the regional lymph nodes should be palpated and the mandible and maxilla examined for swelling or pain. It may not be possible to complete the initial oral examination if the cat has severe oral pain. In severe cases the inflamed tissues may be ulcerated and bleed readily. Proliferation of oral tissues may make it difficult to visualize the teeth. Cats with severe caudal stomatitis may have extreme pain on opening the mouth; thus the initial examination should be performed with the mouth closed while the lips are gently retracted. This examination is performed slowly to minimize pain. The mouth then is opened gently if possible. Lesions of the oral cavity may include inflammation of the gingiva (gingivitis), oral buccal mucosa (stomatitis), and tissues lateral to the palatoglossal fold (caudal stomatitis). Often a complete oral examination is not possible without benefit of sedation or general anesthesia.

Diagnostic Evaluation

A complete blood count, biochemical panel, and urinalysis are performed to identify concurrent or contributory diseases. The complete blood count usually is unremarkable. Hyperglobulinemia has been identified in some cats with chronic caudal stomatitis. Serologic evaluation for feline leukemia virus antigen and feline immunodeficiency virus antibody should be performed. It is ideal to include virus isolation studies on specimens obtained from oral swabs of inflamed tissues in cats with caudal stomatitis. Although bacterial cultures are not part of a basic evaluation in most cases, bacterial culture and sensitivity testing may be helpful in chronic cases that do not respond to the antibiotics commonly used for oral infections. A biopsy specimen should be obtained from any lesion that appears neoplastic or is of unknown cause and should be submitted for histopathologic examination.

A complete oral and dental examination is performed with the cat under general anesthesia. The animal is evaluated for periodontal disease, tooth resorption, and other problems that may cause oral inflammation. Dental radiographs are obtained to evaluate for alveolar bone loss (indicating periodontitis), tooth resorption, and retained roots.

Management

The goals of management are to control plaque bacteria and decrease the inflammatory and immunologic response. Control of plaque bacteria can be attempted by several methods, including scaling, topical antimicrobial application, systemic antimicrobial therapy, and tooth removal.

Cats with caudal stomatitis are best treated with extraction of all premolars and molars. This includes the extraction of any retained roots. Extraction of the teeth removes the surfaces that are available for plaque retention and consequently decreases plaque and the associated inflammation. Extractions are successful in decreasing inflammation when the plaque is initiating the excessive inflammatory response. Retained roots may be a source of residual bacteria and, if found in association with oral inflammation, should be extracted as well.

When an owner is not willing or able to proceed with extractions of premolars and molars, the cat should be managed with plaque removal, plaque control, and medications to suppress the inflammatory response. The first step is a complete scaling and polishing along with extraction of teeth that show evidence of periodontitis or tooth resorption. Oral antibiotic administration for 4 to 6 weeks following the dental surgery is recommended. In severe cases, when the patient is not eating, it is necessary to decrease the inflammation quickly so the patient will resume eating. To manage the inflammation and maintain appetite initially, most cats require methylprednisolone administration every 4 to 6 weeks and over time possibly as frequently as every 3 weeks. Potential complications including diabetes mellitus are a concern with long-term glucocorticoid administration; therefore oral triamcinolone 1.5 mg administered every day for 3 to 5 days during acute flare-ups then decreased to every second or third day is recommended rather than injections of methylprednisolone. Alternatively, other antiinflammatory or immunosuppressive drugs can be considered. Once the inflammation has decreased and the cat is eating, toothbrushing or wiping the teeth with a gauze pad is instituted if the owners are able to adequately perform this and the cat is cooperative. Many owners are not able to brush the cat's teeth sufficiently to decrease plaque accumulation and prevent inflammation. A topical rinse using a 0.12% chlorhexidine product is an adjunctive treatment in management of plaque accumulation. The author informs the owners on the initial visit that extractions of all premolars and molars provides the best long-term results. Medical management with antibiotics and glucocorticoids generally loses effectiveness over time, and severe clinical signs return, requiring more aggressive medical management or extractions. For these reasons, the author believes that extraction of all premolars and molars provides the best long-term management for the majority of affected cats.

Extractions

Extractions are indicated when there is severe periodontitis or when teeth have type 1 tooth resorption. In addition to extractions for treatment of related periodontal disease and tooth resorption, removal of healthy teeth is an option for cats with caudal stomatitis. Plaque bacteria attach to the tooth surfaces (crowns and roots), eliciting an inflammatory response. Oral hygiene directed at plaque control is difficult in cats with severe inflammation and oral pain. Extraction of the premolars and molars removes the surfaces to which plaque attaches and therefore decreases the plaque in the cat's mouth. Dental radiographs are needed to confirm removal of all premolar and molar roots in these cats.

When inflammation is present adjacent to the incisors, they also should be extracted. It is rarely necessary to extract the canine teeth unless they have severe periodontitis or resorptive lesions. The response to extractions is variable, ranging from complete resolution of the inflammation to no improvement, and clients should be so advised. Cats tolerate extractions, even full-mouth extractions, very well and can eat dry and moist cat food without teeth. After extractions some cats may show significant improvement, and medical management may not be required to keep the cat free of clinical signs. Other cats may exhibit a partial response, requiring less aggressive medical management than that required before extractions. Another group of cats appears to have minimal response to extractions, and medical management is continued as before the extractions. In the author's practice cats that responded poorly to full-mouth extractions often were those in which calicivirus was isolated from the oral cavity or cats that had received long-term (months to years) medical management. In a report of 30 cats with gingivitis, stomatitis, and caudal stomatitis, the response to periodontal treatment and extraction of selected teeth, including retained root tips, generally was favorable (Hennet, 1994). Oral inflammation resolved completely in 60% (18 of 30 cats), with an additional 20% (6 of 30 cats) responding with minimal residual inflammation and no oral pain. None of these 24 cats required medical therapy to manage oral inflammation after the treatment. Initial improvement requiring continued medical therapy to control clinical signs was seen in 13% (4 of 30 cats), and no improvement occurred in 7% (2 of 30 cats).

When long-term medical management becomes ineffective, or when the adverse effects of drug therapy are unacceptable, extractions of the premolars and molars offer the next option. The maximal clinical improvement may not be reached for several weeks in cats with severe and chronic inflammation. Some of these cats may benefit from enteral feeding to maintain an adequate caloric intake and balanced nutrition.

Appropriate pain management also should be provided. Buprenorphine HCL at 0.01 to 0.03 mg/kg administered in the cheek (buccal mucosal absorption) q6-12h for 3 days usually is adequate for postoperative pain control. Buprenorphine also may be beneficial for pain control in cats with owners who have chosen medical management.

Scaling and Polishing

The teeth should be scaled to remove plaque bacteria and calculus. Plaque bacteria may be a factor in the excessive inflammatory response present in these cats. The teeth should be polished after any scaling to smooth the tooth surface. Plaque attaches and becomes established on the tooth surfaces within several hours after the scaling and polishing procedures; therefore continued control measures should be undertaken. Cats with severe oral inflammation are usually in too much pain for toothbrushing to be practical; thus plaque control must be maintained initially with topical or systemic antimicrobial therapy. Once the oral inflammation is well controlled, the owner may attempt plaque control with toothbrushing. A finger toothbrush or small toothbrush designed for cats is used with an acceptably flavored veterinary dentifrice.

Antimicrobial Therapy

Antimicrobial therapy is best accomplished with systemic antibiotic administration. A variable response is observed with antibiotic therapy, although treatment for 4 to 6 weeks may result in improvement of clinical signs in some cats. Antibiotics as a single treatment rarely are effective in the initial management of inflammation, and combined treatment with both antibiotics and glucocorticoids usually is required. Amoxicillin/clavulanic acid (Clavamox), clindamycin (Antirobe), and metronidazole are useful antibiotics in managing inflammation in these cats. Repeated treatment with antibiotics may be necessary. Complete resolution of clinical signs is unlikely, and relapses are common. Topical chlorhexidine may be used for adjunctive antimicrobial therapy.

Antiinflammatory and Immunosuppressive Therapy

Immunosuppressive doses of glucocorticoids are required in most cats to decrease the inflammation and reduce pain sufficiently so that the cat will eat. Methylprednisolone acetate (Depo-Medrol) at 15 to 20 mg total dosage intramuscularly or subcutaneously, or triamcinolone 1.5 mg once daily for 3 to 5 days generally is adequate, and cats usually demonstrate a decrease in oral inflammation and a willingness to eat within 1 to 2 days. Triamcinolone 1.5 mg every second or third day generally is adequate following the initial daily dose. Satisfactory results are less common with oral prednisone administration in cats with severe inflammation. For cats demonstrating moderate improvement after extractions and requiring further control of residual inflammation, triamcinolone 1.5 mg every third day may be sufficient; however, higher dosages may be required, and the ultimate dosage is determined by the response. Clients should be cautioned about potential adverse effects of corticosteroid use in cats, including diabetes mellitus and precipitation of congestive heart failure in cats with cardiomyopathy. Recombinant feline interferon-ω administered orally for 90 days has been shown to improve clinical lesions and decrease pain in cats that have undergone extractions and have refractory chronic caudal stomatitis (Hennet et al, 2011). Oral administration of cyclosporine to cats with a poor response to extractions also has been show to improve oral inflammation significantly when trough whole blood levels are greater than 300 ng/dl (Lommer, 2013). The initial recommended dose of cyclosporine is 2.5 mg/kg twice daily PO; however, there is significant variability in absorption so the trough whole blood levels must be measured so the dose can be adjusted to maintain the level above 300 ng/dl.

Miscellaneous Treatments

A trial treatment of coenzyme Q_{10} (CoQ_{10}) supplementation at 30 to 100 mg daily for 4 months is recommended in cats with residual inflammation following extractions or as a supplement to medical management. There is anecdotal evidence of improvement in cats with caudal stomatitis and humans with chronic periodontitis after 3 to 4 months of supplementation with CoQ_{10}. Prospective studies are needed to prove efficacy.

References and Suggested Reading
Belgard S, Truyen U, Thibault JC: Relevance of feline calicivirus, feline immunodeficiency virus, feline leukemia virus, feline

herpesvirus and *Bartonella henselae* in cats with chronic gingivostomatitis, *Berl Munch Tierarztl Wochenschr* 123:369, 2010.

Dolieslager SM et al: Identification of bacteria associated with feline chronic gingivostomatitis using culture-dependent and culture-independent methods, *Vet Microbiol* 148(1):93, 2011.

Dowers KL et al: Association of *Bartonella* species, feline calicivirus, and feline herpesvirus 1 infection with gingivostomatitis in cats, *J Feline Med Surg* 12:314, 2010.

Hardy WD, Zuckerman E, Corbishley J: Serological evidence that *Bartonella* causes gingivitis and stomatitis in cats. In *Proceedings of the 16th Annual Veterinary Dental Forum*, Savannah, Ga, October 3-6, 2002, p 79.

Harley R, Gruffydd-Jones TJ, Day MJ: Salivary and serum immunoglobulin levels in cats with chronic gingivostomatitis, *Vet Rec* 152:125, 2003.

Harley R, Gruffydd-Jones TJ, Day MJ: Immunohistochemical characterization of oral mucosal lesions in cats with chronic gingivostomatitis, *J Comp Pathol* 144(4):239, 2011.

Hennet P: Results of periodontal and extraction treatment in cats with gingivo-stomatitis. In *Proceedings of the World Veterinary Dental Congress*, Philadelphia, 1994, p 49.

Hennet PR et al: Comparative efficacy of a recombinant feline interferon omega in refractory cases of calicivirus-positive cats with caudal stomatitis: a randomised, multi-centre, controlled, double-blind study in 39 cats, *J Feline Med Surg* 13:577, 2011.

Lommer MJ: Efficacy of cyclosporine for chronic, refractory stomatitis in cats: a randomized, placebo-controlled, double-blinded clinical study, *J Vet Dent* 30:8, 2013.

Lommer MJ, Verstraete FJ: Concurrent oral shedding of feline calicivirus and feline herpesvirus 1 in cats with chronic gingivostomatitis, *Oral Microbiol Immunol* 18:131, 2003.

CHAPTER **121**

Oropharyngeal Dysphagia

STANLEY L. MARKS, *Davis, California*

Oropharyngeal dysphagia (OPD) occurs when the elaborate mechanism of bolus transit from the oral cavity into the esophagus becomes compromised. The swallowing mechanism is complex and involves the action of 31 paired striated muscles and five cranial nerves (sensory and motor fibers of the trigeminal, facial, glossopharyngeal, and vagus nerve, and motor fibers of the hypoglossal nerve), their nuclei in the brainstem, and the swallowing center in the reticular formation of the brainstem. The normal swallowing reflex is a four-stage process, characterized by the oral preparatory phase, oral phase, pharyngeal phase, and esophageal phase. Esophageal and gastroesophageal dysphagias are described elsewhere (see Web Chapter 54).

Dysphagia is relatively common in dogs, and the list of possible causes is extensive (Box 121-1). Dysphagia is far less common in cats, and most of the causes of OPD in this species are structural (oral tumors, ulcers, stomatitis).

Phases of Swallowing

The *oral preparatory phase* is voluntary and begins as food or liquid enters the mouth. Mastication and lubrication of food are the hallmarks of this phase, as the bolus is modified and prepared for swallowing. Abnormalities of the oral preparatory phase usually are associated with dental disease, xerostomia, weakness of the lips (cranial nerves V and VII), tongue (cranial nerve XII), and cheeks (cranial nerves V and VII). The *oral phase* of swallowing consists of the muscular events responsible for movement of the bolus from the tongue to the pharynx and is facilitated by the tongue, jaw, and hyoid muscle movements. The *pharyngeal phase* begins as the bolus reaches the tonsils and is characterized by elevation of the soft palate to prevent the bolus from entering the nasopharynx, elevation and forward movement of the larynx and hyoid, retroflexion of the epiglottis and closure of the vocal folds to close the entrance into the larynx, synchronized contraction of the middle and inferior constrictor muscles of the pharynx, and relaxation of the cricopharyngeus muscle that makes up much of the proximal esophageal sphincter (PES) to allow passage of the bolus into the esophagus (Figure 121-1). Respiration is briefly halted (apneic moment) during the pharyngeal phase. Abnormalities of the pharyngeal phase of swallowing are associated with pharyngeal weakness secondary to neuropathies or myopathies, pharyngeal tumors or foreign bodies, and obstruction of the PES secondary to hypertrophy of the cricopharyngeus muscle. Synchrony between constriction of the pharyngeal muscles and relaxation of the cricopharyngeus muscle is essential to allow passage of the bolus into the esophagus. The *esophageal phase* is involuntary and begins with the relaxation of the PES and movement of the bolus into the esophagus. Despite the myriad causes of OPD, the pathophysiologic end results

BOX 121-1

Causes of Oropharyngeal Dysphagia in Dogs

Central Nervous System
Cerebrovascular accident
Brainstem tumor

Iatrogenic
Antihistamines
Anticholinergics
Phenothiazines
Chemotherapy
Postsurgical muscular or neurogenic damage
Radiation exposure
Ingestion of a corrosive substance

Infectious
Botulism
Tetanus
Candidiasis
Rabies
Abscess
Calicivirus infection (cats)
Rhinotracheitis virus infection (cats)

Metabolic
Cushing's disease
Thyrotoxicosis-associated myopathy (humans)

Myopathic/Neuropathic
Peripheral neuropathies
Inflammatory myopathies
Polymyositis
Dermatomyositis
Muscular dystrophies
Myasthenia gravis

Structural
Oropharyngeal tumor
Cricopharyngeal bar
Proximal esophageal webs
Foreign body
Congenital anomaly (cleft palate, diverticula)
Fracture of the mandible
Tooth fracture
Glossal ulcer or inflammation
Glossal hypertrophy (muscular dystrophy)

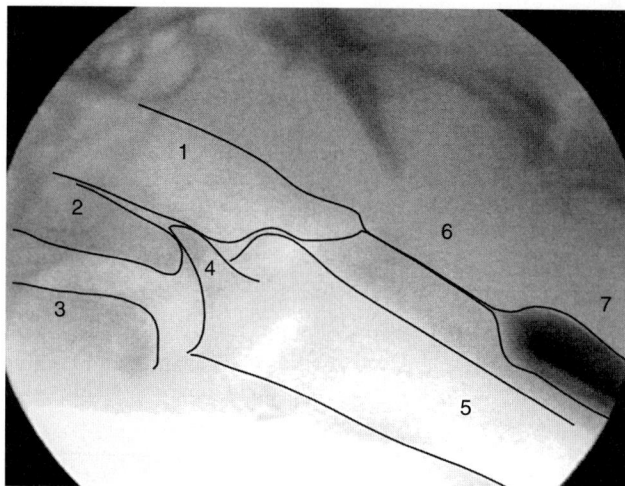

Figure 121-1 Normal lateral fluoroscopic view of the pharynx at rest. Note that the radiodensity is reversed on fluoroscopic images compared with conventional radiographic images (i.e., air is white, bone is black). *1,* Nasopharynx. *2,* Soft palate. *3,* Base of tongue. *4,* Epiglottis. *5,* Trachea. *6,* Proximal esophageal sphincter. *7,* Proximal esophagus with barium in the lumen. (From Pollard RE et al: Quantitative videofluoroscopic evaluation of pharyngeal function in the dog, *Vet Radiol Ultrasound* 41[5]:409, 2000.)

BOX 121-2

Clinical Signs of Oropharyngeal Dysphagia

Difficulty swallowing water or solids
Nasal regurgitation
Frequent repetitive swallowing
Falling of food from the mouth
Dysphonia
Coughing
Gagging
Retching
Syncope

fall into one of two interrelated categories: (1) abnormalities of bolus transfer and (2) abnormalities of airway protection. Abnormalities of bolus transfer can be further grouped into those caused by (a) oropharyngeal pump failure (pharyngeal weakness), (b) oropharyngeal and pharyngo-PES discoordination (neuropathies), and (c) pharyngeal outflow obstruction (cricopharyngeal achalasia, tumors of the pharynx, foreign bodies).

Diagnostic Approach

The diagnosis of disorders affecting the oropharyngeal phase of swallowing can be extremely challenging in dogs; however, a history of repetitive swallowing, gagging,

and retching associated with meals, nasal regurgitation with meals, swallow-related coughing, falling of food from the mouth during swallowing, and recurrent pneumonia should cause the clinician to suspect OPD (Box 121-2). Dysphagia may be the sole presenting sign in an animal or may be associated with myriad clinical abnormalities. It should be emphasized that OPD may be part of a systemic disease in dogs manifesting signs of dysphagia only, which underscores the importance of a comprehensive systemic evaluation in affected animals. The assessment of dogs with signs of OPD encompasses multiple dimensions that include (1) review of the signalment, (2) review of medication history and inquiry regarding recent anesthesia (Box 121-3), (3) physical examination (prefeeding assessment), (4) neurologic examination, (5) clinical feeding and swallowing evaluation, and (6) laboratory and other testing to provide a basic data set for neurologic evaluation, including imaging studies and endoscopic evaluation of swallowing.

History-Based Evaluation of the Dysphagic Animal

Age of onset?
Sudden onset or gradual onset?
Dysphagia while eating or between meals?
Difficulty with solids or liquids or both?
Intermittent or progressive dysphagia?
Temporal pattern of dysphagia (OPD occurs within seconds following swallowing)?
History of coughing?
History of medication administration?
Dysphonia?
Recent general anesthesia?
Odynophagia?

Signalment

Age and breed associations with OPD have been well documented in dogs. Causes of OPD in puppies include cleft palate, cricopharyngeal achalasia, glossal hypertrophy secondary to muscular dystrophy, and pharyngeal weakness. Breeds that have a hereditary predisposition or a high incidence of OPD include the golden retriever (pharyngeal weakness), cocker and springer spaniels (cricopharyngeal dysphagia), Bouvier des Flandres and cavalier King Charles spaniel (muscular dystrophy), and boxer (inflammatory myopathy). In addition, large-breed dogs are predisposed to masticatory muscle disorders.

Physical and Neurologic Examination

Physical examination of the animal must include careful examination of the oropharynx using sedation or anesthesia if necessary to help rule out morphologic abnormalities such as dental disease, foreign bodies, cleft palate, glossal abnormalities, and oropharyngeal tumors. The pharynx and neck should be palpated carefully for masses, asymmetry, or pain. The chest should be auscultated carefully for evidence of aspiration pneumonia. Evaluation of cranial nerves should be performed, including assessment of tongue and jaw tone, and abduction of the arytenoid cartilages with inspiration. A complete physical and neurologic examination may identify clinical signs supporting a generalized neuromuscular disorder, including muscle atrophy, stiffness, or decreased or absent spinal reflexes. The gag reflex should be evaluated by placing a finger in the pharynx; however, the presence or absence of a gag reflex does not correlate with the efficacy of the pharyngeal swallow nor the adequacy of deglutitive airway protection.

Observation of Eating and Drinking

The importance of the clinician's carefully observing the dysphagic animal while it is eating (kibble and canned food) and drinking in the hospital cannot be overemphasized, and such observation helps to localize the problem to the oral cavity, pharynx, or esophagus. Dogs with an abnormal oral phase of swallowing typically have difficulty with prehension or aboral transport of a bolus to the tongue base, and these disorders often can be diagnosed by watching the animal eat. OPDs affecting the pharyngeal phase of swallowing can be more challenging to diagnose and often present with nonspecific signs such as gagging, retching, and the necessity for multiple swallowing attempts before a bolus is moved successfully into the proximal esophagus. These patients have abnormal transport of bolus from the oropharynx to the hypopharynx or from the hypopharynx to the proximal esophagus. Cricopharyngeal dysphagia is associated with the abnormal transport of a bolus through the PES, and signs are similar to those seen with pharyngeal disorders.

Laboratory Testing to Provide a Minimum Neuromuscular Data Set

Comprehensive laboratory testing is warranted in animals with OPD to provide a minimum neuromuscular data set and should consist of a complete blood count, serum chemistry panel including creatine kinase (CK) and electrolyte concentrations, urinalysis, evaluation of thyroid function, and acetylcholine receptor (AChR) antibody titer for acquired myasthenia gravis. A persistently elevated CK level could be an indication of an inflammatory myopathy, whereas markedly elevated CK concentrations may suggest a necrotizing or dystrophic myopathy. A normal CK level does not rule out a myopathy, particularly when the myopathy is focal (masticatory muscle myositis) or in the chronic stage of disease. Acquired myasthenia gravis is an important neuromuscular cause of OPD and can be associated with focal signs including pharyngeal, esophageal, and laryngeal weakness without clinically detectable limb muscle weakness. Pharyngeal weakness as the only clinical sign of myasthenia gravis has been described in 1% of myasthenic dogs.

Cervical and Thoracic Radiography

The pharynx of healthy animals is evident on radiographs because it is air filled. The size of the air-filled space can be decreased by local inflammation or neoplasia, laryngeal edema, or elongation of the soft palate. Pharyngeal size also can appear increased with dysfunction of the pharynx or upper esophageal sphincter, chronic respiratory (inspiratory) disease, and chronic severe megaesophagus. The normal esophagus is not visible on survey radiographs. An exception occurs following aerophagia due to excitement, nausea, dyspnea, or anesthesia.

Videofluoroscopic Swallow Study

Contrast videofluoroscopy involves real-time capture of images of the animal as it is swallowing liquid barium or barium-soaked kibble and is one of the most important procedures for assessing the functional integrity of the swallow reflex (Figure 121-2). Videofluoroscopy is used to determine the normal sequence of events that make up a swallow and to measure the timing of these events in relation to one another. Additionally, the movement of certain anatomic structures is measured in relation to a

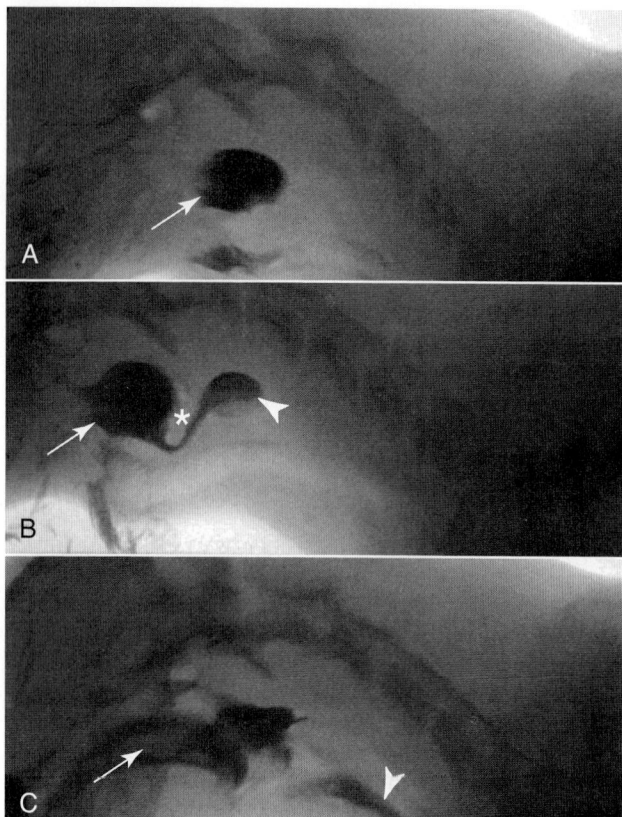

Figure 121-2 Fluoroscopic swallow study in a 7-month-old spayed female miniature dachshund with severe dysphagia secondary to cricopharyngeal achalasia. **A,** Pharynx *(arrow)* filled with liquid barium. **B,** Hypertrophied cricopharyngeus muscle (cricopharyngeal bar) *(asterisk)* obstructing the movement of the bolus from the pharynx *(arrow)* into the proximal esophagus *(arrowhead)*. Notice the attenuated column of barium being squeezed through the narrow opening of the proximal esophageal sphincter (PES). **C,** Retrograde movement of liquid barium into the oropharynx *(arrow)* caused by obstruction of the PES, and subsequent aspiration of barium into the trachea *(arrowhead)*.

fixed point to assess function further. Swallowing events that occur out of sequence, at inappropriate times, or with reduced vigor can cause significant morbidity. One problem with videofluoroscopy is that animal positioning is not standardized in veterinary medicine. Alterations in body position (sternal versus lateral recumbency) do not appear to affect measurements of pharyngeal constriction ratio or the timing of swallowing in healthy dogs; however, cervical esophageal transit is significantly delayed when dogs are imaged in lateral recumbency. Swallow studies performed with the dog in sternal recumbency are significantly more likely to result in generation of a primary peristaltic wave for both liquid and kibble boluses. Thus it is important to recognize that the retention of liquid or kibble boluses in the cervical esophagus may not be considered abnormal when clinically ill dogs are imaged in lateral recumbency because this may be related to body position. The fluoroscopic swallow study typically involves assessment of five swallows each of 5 to 10 ml of liquid barium (60% weight per volume) followed by five swallows of kibble soaked in barium.

The timing of the swallow can be determined easily when the swallow video is viewed frame by frame, with each frame representing $\frac{1}{30}$th of a second in the National Television System Committee (NTSC) system, the analog television system used in the United States. The frame in which the epiglottis is observed to close over the larynx is considered as the starting point for all time measurements, and frames are counted until the observation of maximal contraction of the pharynx, opening of the PES, and closing of the PES. The swallow is considered completed when the epiglottis is observed to reopen, which usually takes five or six frames in healthy dogs.

More recently, a contrast videofluoroscopy method for quantifying pharyngeal contractility in the dog has been described (Pollard et al, 2007). The pharyngeal constriction ratio is calculated by dividing the pharyngeal area at maximum contraction by the pharyngeal area at rest. As pharyngeal contractility diminishes, the ratio approaches 1.0. This simple procedure provides important information regarding the strength of pharyngeal contraction in dysphagic dogs and facilitates the improved selection of dogs diagnosed with cricopharyngeal dysphagia for surgical intervention.

Laryngoscopy and Pharyngoscopy

Thorough laryngeal examination is important in all animals with OPD to rule out laryngeal paralysis associated with a polyneuropathy. Geriatric large-breed dogs can experience a progressive generalized neuropathy with associated pharyngeal weakness, OPD, and esophageal dysmotility. Pharyngoscopy and esophagoscopy provide anatomic information about the structures involved in the oropharynx and esophagus, but both procedures are of limited diagnostic utility for evaluating functional disorders in anesthetized animals. Unsedated transnasal videoendoscopy is an easily accomplished and useful procedure in people that often is performed as an outpatient procedure. The author has assessed the feasibility of fiberoptic endoscopic evaluation of swallowing via transnasal intubation in fully awake dogs; however, the procedure is limited to larger dogs that can be restrained readily for the procedure.

Electrodiagnostic Testing

Electrodiagnostic evaluation, including electromyography and measurement of motor and sensory nerve conduction velocities, does not provide a specific diagnosis in most cases but can supply important information as to the severity, distribution, and character of a myopathic or neuropathic disease process and assist in selecting the optimal anatomic site for biopsy. Electrodiagnostic testing also should include evaluation of the pharyngeal muscles and tongue. The health status of the animal must be taken into consideration because the procedure is performed under general anesthesia.

Muscle and Nerve Biopsies

Muscle and nerve biopsies usually are integral to reaching a specific diagnosis. The biopsy procedure should be performed after the serum AChR antibody titer has been determined to be negative. If the onset of clinical signs is recent and the antibody test is negative, retesting in 4 to 6 weeks is suggested because a significant number of dogs with early clinical signs have antibody titers below the detection limits of the assay at initial testing but test positive 4 to 6 weeks later. Muscle biopsy specimens usually are obtained from a large proximal pelvic limb such as the vastus lateralis or a thoracic limb such as the triceps muscle; however, biopsy specimens from the pharynx and cricopharyngeus muscle also should be obtained in dogs with OPD. Muscle biopsy, when warranted, ideally should be performed relatively early in the disease process before irreversible muscle fibrosis and myofiber loss is extensive.

Magnetic Resonance and Computed Tomographic Imaging

Magnetic resonance and computed tomographic imaging of the head and neck have been used to diagnose inflammatory myopathies, particularly masticatory muscle myositis in dogs, and the imaging can be used to help select sites for diagnostic muscle biopsy. Common findings include changes in size (atrophy or swelling) of all masticatory muscles except the digastricus muscles and contrast enhancement with a predominantly inhomogeneous distribution pattern in the temporalis, masseter, and pterygoid muscles. Magnetic resonance imaging also can be used to detect neoplasia involving the cranial nerves.

Treatment

The treatment of OPD depends on what the underlying cause is and whether the condition is structural or functional.

Functional Disorders Associated with Oropharyngeal Dysphagia

Cricopharyngeal dysphagia is a swallowing disorder of the PES characterized by either cricopharyngeal dyssynchrony (functional) or cricopharyngeal achalasia (structural). *Cricopharyngeal dyssynchrony* is essentially a pump problem in which the weak pharyngeal muscles are unable to propel the bolus through the PES (see Figure 121-2). Early evidence in the author's laboratory points toward a neuropathy in these dogs. On videofluoroscopy, there is evidence of incoordination between the contraction of the dorsal cranial and middle pharyngeal contractor muscles (hyopharyngeus, pterygopharyngeus, and palatopharyngeus muscles) and opening of the PES (cricopharyngeus and thyropharyngeus muscles). A comprehensive workup should be completed in an effort to find a treatable cause of the suspected neuropathy (complete blood count and serum chemistry panel, AChR antibody titer, CK measurement, muscle and nerve biopsy). The prognosis for these dogs generally is extremely poor, and surgical intervention (cricopharyngeus myotomy or myectomy) is contraindicated because the procedure can exacerbate the dysphagia. An effort should be made to identify the optimal consistency of food and water that these dogs will tolerate (by adding commercial food thickeners such as Thick-It), although these animals will ultimately succumb to repeated bouts of aspiration pneumonia and malnutrition. Enteral feeding via a percutaneous endoscopic gastrostomy tube is a viable alternative in these animals; however, silent aspiration and pneumonia can occur despite the use of enteral feeding devices.

Pharyngeal weakness can be a primary disorder secondary to an underlying neuropathy (see earlier) or myopathy, or it can be seen in association with an obstructing cricopharyngeal bar that prevents the pharynx from contracting properly. Pharyngeal function usually can be restored following surgical correction of the obstructing bar (see later).

Structural Disorders Associated with Oropharyngeal Dysphagia

Structural causes of OPD in dogs include penetrating foreign bodies, cleft palate, cricopharyngeal achalasia, and iatrogenically shortened soft palate. *Cricopharyngeal achalasia* is the inability of the cricopharyngeus muscle to open during the cricopharyngeal phase of swallowing. The exact underlying causes have not been determined, although the disorder can be reproduced by transection of the pharyngeal branch of cranial nerve X. Cricopharyngeal dysphagia and achalasia are diagnosed via contrast videofluoroscopy. Cricopharyngeal achalasia has been well documented in miniature dachshunds and a variety of other small breeds in the author's laboratory, and all dogs had marked hypertrophy of the cricopharyngeus muscle (cricopharyngeal bar) causing severe obstruction to propulsion of the bolus through the PES.

In dogs with cricopharyngeal dysphagia a comprehensive workup must be undertaken before surgical intervention to ensure that systemic disorders (myopathies, polyneuropathies) are ruled out and aspiration pneumonia is managed properly. A fluoroscopic swallow study must be performed in dogs suspected of having cricopharyngeal dysphagia to assess pharyngeal function before surgical intervention. Dogs that are diagnosed with underlying neuropathies or myopathies are managed conservatively with alterations of feeding practice or the use of low-profile gastrostomy devices if specific management of the underlying neuropathy or myopathy is not possible.

Definitive treatment of cricopharyngeal achalasia involves surgical myotomy or myectomy of the cricopharyngeal muscle. In veterinary medicine, the standard surgical approach for myotomy or myectomy has remained constant over the years, and the cricopharyngeal and thyropharyngeal muscles are approached either by a standard ventral midline approach with 180-degree rotation of the larynx on its longitudinal axis or by a lateral approach with 90-degree rotation of the larynx. Cricopharyngeal myotomy involves transection of the cricopharyngeal muscle to the level of the pharyngeal mucosa. A closed endoscopic procedure employing a carbon dioxide laser increasingly is being used for cricopharyngeal myotomy in people and dogs and is associated with shorter anesthesia time and reduced morbidity compared with the more traditional transcervical cricopharyngeal myotomy.

An alternative and less invasive procedure involves the injection of botulinum toxin into the cricopharyngeus muscle. Botulinum toxin A is a neurotoxin synthesized from the bacillus *Clostridium botulinum*. It acts at the presynaptic cholinergic nerve terminals to block the release of acetylcholine at the myoneuronal junction. In a dose-related manner, it weakens contraction when injected into the target muscle. The toxin has been used successfully in people for the treatment of esophageal achalasia, a condition characterized by hypertonicity of the lower esophageal sphincter, and has been used successfully in people and dogs for the management of cricopharyngeal achalasia. Because of its short half-life (4 hours), the toxin is reconstituted shortly before injection with 0.9% sterile saline to a concentration of 25 U/ml. The author uses a transbronchial needle to inject the cricopharyngeus muscle in three sites, administering a dose of 10 U per site. The limited duration of effect of botulinum toxin (approximately 3 to 4 months) is a benefit because animals that respond favorably to the toxin should do well following surgical myotomy or myectomy. In contrast, animals that do poorly following botulinum injection can be supported with an enteral feeding device until the effects of the toxin have worn off. These animals should not undergo surgical correction of their cricopharyngeal disease because the disorder will be exacerbated.

The veterinary profession has made tremendous strides in our ability to evaluate and diagnose disorders causing OPD in dogs and has refined the surgical procedures for managing some of the structural disorders such as cricopharyngeal achalasia in dogs. The diagnostic utility of observing the dysphagic animal eating and drinking cannot be overemphasized because this approach will help localize the phase of swallowing affected. Future efforts should be concentrated on better understanding the functional disorders causing dysphagia because the prognosis for these animals unfortunately is poor. The observed association between certain dog breeds and a variety of causes of dysphagia warrant a comprehensive effort to perform genetic screening and modify breeding practices to help eradicate these disorders.

References and Suggested Reading

Cook IJ: Investigative techniques in the assessment of oral-pharyngeal dysphagia, *Dig Dis* 16:125, 1998.

Dauer E et al: Endoscopic laser vs. open approach for cricopharyngeal myotomy, *Otolaryngol Head Neck Surg* 134:830, 2006.

Davidson AP et al: Inheritance of cricopharyngeal dysfunction in Golden Retrievers, *Am J Vet Res* 65:344, 2004.

Dodds WJ, Stewart ET, Logemann JA: Physiology and radiology of the normal oral and pharyngeal phases of swallowing, *Am J Roentgenol* 154:953, 1990.

Dua KS et al: Coordination of deglutitive glottal function and pharyngeal bolus transit during normal eating, *Gastroenterology* 112:73, 1997.

Moerman MBJ: Cricopharyngeal Botox injection: indications and technique, *Curr Opin Otolaryngol Head Neck Surg* 14:431, 2006.

Pollard RE et al: Quantitative videofluoroscopic evaluation of pharyngeal function in the dog, *Vet Radiol Ultrasound* 41:409, 2000.

Pollard RE et al: Preliminary evaluation of the pharyngeal constriction ratio (PCR) for fluoroscopic determination of pharyngeal constriction in dysphagic dogs, *Vet Radiol Ultrasound* 48:221, 2007.

Shelton GD, Schule A, Kass PH: Risk factors for acquired myasthenia gravis in dogs: 1,154 cases (1991-1995), *J Am Med Vet Assoc* 211:1428, 1997.

Stanley B et al: Esophageal dysfunction in dogs with idiopathic laryngeal paralysis: a controlled cohort study, *Vet Surg* 39:139, 2010.

Walmsley G et al: A Duchenne muscular dystrophy gene hot spot mutation in dystrophin-deficient cavalier King Charles spaniels is amenable to exon 51 skipping, *PLoS One* 5(1):e8647, 2010.

Warnock JJ et al: Surgical management of cricopharyngeal dysphagia in dogs: 14 cases (1989-2001), *J Am Vet Med Assoc* 223 (10):1462, 2003.

CHAPTER 122

Gastroesophageal Reflux

PETER HENDRIK KOOK, *Zurich, Switzerland*

Esophagitis denotes a localized or diffuse inflammation of the esophageal mucosa. It generally is thought to result from a caustic (e.g., acid, alkali, bile salts) or chemical (e.g., drug-induced) injury that starts at the luminal surface and progresses to the deeper layers of the tissue. In people, gastroesophageal reflux disease (GERD) results from a failure of the normal antireflux barrier to protect against frequent and abnormal amounts of gastroesophageal reflux (GER). Although GER is not a disease, but a normal physiologic process occurring multiple times a day, GERD is regarded as a multifactorial process usually producing symptoms of heartburn and acid regurgitation. The most frequent mechanism for reflux is thought to result from lower esophageal sphincter (LES) incompetence. However, esophageal inflammation also may cause esophageal hypomotility and LES weakness by impairing the excitatory cholinergic pathways to the LES. In cats, these changes have been shown to be reversible with healing of the esophagus (Zhang et al, 2005).

GER occurs spontaneously in healthy dogs and is not associated with exercise, positioning of the animal, or sleeping. GER also has been evaluated in anesthetized patients and is affected by positioning of the animal during anesthesia and the type of surgical procedure. It has been reported that intraabdominal procedures have a higher risk for GER, and the duration of preoperative fasting and choice of preanesthetic drugs influence the incidence of GER during anesthesia (Galatos and Raptopoulos, 1995). No information exists on quantification of intraoperative GER and the risk for subsequent esophageal inflammation.

Hiatal hernias may predispose to GER in dogs and cats because of the altered functional anatomy of the gastroesophageal pressure barrier (losing the intrinsic support of the crural diaphragm) and impaired esophageal acid clearance. Reflux esophagitis resulting from upper airway obstruction can become a problem in brachycephalic dogs (Lecoindre and Richard, 2004; Poncet et al, 2005), but non–breed-specific upper airway obstruction may cause GER. The supposed pathomechanism is the negative intrathoracic pressure generated by increased inspiratory effort.

In veterinary medicine GERD secondary to a primary LES abnormality is poorly understood. Diagnosing GERD based on history and observed symptoms, as it often is done in human medicine, is not applicable. Esophagitis secondary to presumed GER has been reported in cats (Gualtieri and Olivero, 2006; Han et al, 2003); however, the diagnosis was based on a combination of presumably typical historical and clinical signs, as well as radiographic, endoscopic, or histopathologic findings without actual demonstration of acidic esophageal pH. At present it is not clear if GERD also represents a relevant problem in small animals. More common scenarios for increased esophageal acid exposure in dogs and cats are lodged foreign bodies, frequent vomiting, malpositioned esophageal feeding tubes, potentially aggressive gastric factors such as gastric volume, and duodenal contents associated with delayed gastric emptying. In chronic esophagitis cases, histologic changes comparable with Barrett's esophagus (replacement of the normal squamous epithelium of the distal esophagus with metaplastic columnar epithelium) rarely can be found.

Historical and Clinical Signs

Animals with mild esophagitis may show no clinical signs, whereas animals with severe esophagitis can show reduced appetite, anorexia, odynophagia or dysphagia, ptyalism, coughing, and regurgitation. Clinical signs noted by the author include retching, gagging, repeated swallowing motions, smacking, discomfort at night (or bedtime), and refusal to eat despite apparent interest in food. Although it would appear plausible that severity of clinical signs depends on the extent and depth of esophageal lesions, they do not always correlate and may vary greatly. Hoarseness, stridor or change of phonation, and dyspnea suggest injury to the epiglottis, larynx, and upper airway (Lux et al, 2012). Onset of anesthesia-associated reflux esophagitis varies from days to weeks after a causative anesthetic event. On physical examination, patients may have evidence of halitosis and laryngeal signs with redness, hyperemia, and edema of the vocal folds and arytenoids. However, the majority of patients have normal physical examinations.

Care should be taken to evaluate the respiratory system, because pulmonary manifestations of GERD potentially may include aspiration pneumonia, chronic bronchitis, and interstitial pulmonary fibrosis. Concerning this aspect, idiopathic pulmonary fibrosis is seen nearly exclusively in older West Highland white terriers, a breed that is also notoriously famous for lodged esophageal foreign bodies. Chronic intermittent microaspiration of gastric acid secondary to primary esophageal motility problem could be the causative event in this breed.

Diagnosis

Although historical and clinical findings may be suggestive of esophagitis, results of routine laboratory testing are usually normal. Survey thoracic radiographs are seldom diagnostic for esophagitis, but compatible findings may be mild esophageal dilations or fluid accumulation in the distal esophagus. However, foreign bodies, hiatal hernias, esophageal dilation, ring anomalies, or masses could be detected, and a pathologic lung pattern may reflect aspiration injury to the lungs. Mediastinal or pleural air or liquid accumulation may indicate esophageal perforation. If a perforation is considered likely, an iodinated contrast medium should be used instead of barium. A contrast esophagram is an inexpensive, readily available, and noninvasive test that is most useful in demonstrating stenotic narrowing of the esophagus. No veterinary study has evaluated the ability of barium esophagram to detect esophagitis. However, mucosal irregularities and a prolonged retention of the contrast medium can be seen with moderate to severe inflammation, whereas mild esophagitis most likely will be missed. The benefit of fluoroscopic swallow studies is assessing the esophageal motility during the whole swallow with less chance to miss the moment when the contrast medium passes a narrow point, as could be the case with static images. It is important to perform wet swallows with liquid contrast medium and dry swallows with a barium-food mixed bolus, because liquids sometimes can pass a partial stricture, whereas a food bolus may be retained.

With the exception of detecting strictures, these procedures cannot diagnose GER. Hiatal hernias may be seen during fluoroscopic contrast studies of the LES area by applying pressure on the cranial abdomen. In health the gastroesophageal junction should lie caudal to the hiatus, and no stomach or other viscera should lie cranial to the gastroesophageal junction. However, it can still be difficult to assess the clinical significance of small sliding hiatal hernias.

Endoscopic examination is the most sensitive method to diagnose esophagitis, although reliable diagnostic endoscopic criteria and grading schemes for severity of esophagitis have not been established in small animals. No descriptive endoscopic work larger than case reports has been published on canine or feline esophagitis. Early signs of esophagitis are erythema and edema, but these findings are nonspecific and depend on the quality of endoscopic equipment. More reliable signs include increased vascularity because enlarged capillaries develop in response to acid near the mucosal surface. Mucosal striations with visible submucosal vascularity may be seen in the distal third of the esophagus. Another common sign is increased granularity; the mucosal surface appears rough and puckered. Findings compatible with severe esophagitis are areas of exudative pseudomembranes and ulcerative mucosa. In contrast to people, linear mucosal breaks (erosions) with a sharp demarcation line from adjacent normal mucosa uncommonly are seen. Although typical for reflux esophagitis, circular inflammation just above the LES should not be confused with the squamocolumnar junction (demarcation line between the squamous esophageal lining and the columnar gastric lining), which can appear sharply delineated in cats and dogs with reddened gastric mucosa. This is especially the case with esophageal overinsufflation.

It could be argued that esophagoscopy without biopsy is insufficient to rule out esophagitis, as are cases with grossly normal appearing mucosa on endoscopy and necropsy, but histopathologic evidence of esophagitis has been reported (Dodds et al, 1970; Han et al, 2003). This is in accordance with findings in humans, in which endoscopic results in patients with GERD vary from no visible mucosal damage to esophagitis, peptic strictures, or Barrett's esophagus (a metaplastic change of normal squamous epithelium to columnar epithelium associated with chronic acid exposure). Because of the composition of the esophageal mucosa with its tough stratified squamous epithelium, it is difficult to obtain adequate esophageal biopsies; however, adequate endoscopic biopsy specimens from the lower canine esophagus showing the stratified squamous epithelium with basal cell layer, as well as the lamina propria with papillae, can be obtained by experienced endoscopists (Münster et al, 2012). The endoscopic examination always should include a full gastric inspection with special attention to the cardia and pylorus; this excludes underlying abnormality, such as obstructive lesions or radiolucent foreign bodies, and confirms that the esophagitis is a primary problem.

All aforementioned diagnostics may aid in the diagnosis of esophagitis but still fail to detect GER. Approaches other than endoscopy are needed. In humans, catheter-free esophageal pH monitoring has become the gold standard for diagnosing GERD. This technique provides information on distal esophageal acid exposure and also is able to assess symptoms associated with acid reflux episodes. A widely used system in humans is the Bravo system. It includes a small capsule (26 mm × 5.5 mm × 6.5 mm) containing an antimony pH electrode with internal reference, miniaturized electronics with radiofrequency transmitter and battery, a capsule delivery system, as well as an external receiver to monitor intraesophageal pH. The capsule is positioned approximately 3 cm above the LES and attached (i.e., pierced) to the mucosa. Once released from the delivery system, pH data are recorded by a receiver attached to the dog's harness. Owners are instructed to maintain a logbook to record all events presumed to be related to GER. Our experience with the Bravo Capsule pH test indicates that this technique can be used safely in patients from 5 kg to 50 kg bodyweight, and all dogs tolerate the measurements well. Our preliminary results contradict the previous hypothesis that minute amounts of acid could damage severely the canine esophagus. In healthy dogs with normal upper gastrointestinal endoscopy, the number of refluxes (defined as esophageal pH <4) and the duration of long refluxes (>5 min) vary considerably over the course of 96 hours. Although single reflux episodes lasting as long as 20 minutes rarely can be recorded, the overall fraction time pH less than 4 remains low and usually ranges between 0 and 3.2% (median 0.3%). These numbers actually are lower than the established norm in humans. First results in dogs with clinical signs commonly attributed to reflux esophagitis are surprising, because clinically relevant reflux episodes could not be demonstrated in the majority of suspected dogs and a temporal relationship between presenting signs observed by owners and reflux episodes lacked overall agreement. Because this is an ongoing study, more dogs must be evaluated before definitive conclusions can be made. Current disadvantages of the system are the high cost and need of upper endoscopy for accurate placement.

Therapy

Treatment ideally should be directed at the underlying causes of the gastroesophageal reflux; it is important to eliminate predisposing factors (e.g., hiatal hernia). Because anesthesia is the most common cause for reflux esophagitis in dogs and cats, it would appear desirable to prevent GER in patients undergoing anesthesia. Pretreatment with high doses of metoclopramide yielded conflicting results, and the administration of ranitidine prior to surgery also did not reduce the incidence of GER (Favarato et al, 2011; Wilson et al, 2006). Similarly, another study failed to demonstrate consistent intraoperative GER prevention with omeprazole given orally 4 hours prior to surgery (Panti et al, 2009).

As pointed out above, the primary underlying mechanism for GER in people is believed to be impaired LES function resulting in prolonged esophageal exposure to acid. Therefore treatments for GER have focused on increasing LES pressure or decreasing acid production. Prokinetic drugs increase the pressure of the LES and enhance gastric motility; they therefore influence a possible underlying motility disturbance of the disease (also see Chapter 125). Metoclopramide, a dopamine antagonist, and cisapride, a serotonin receptor agonist that increases acetylcholine release in the myenteric plexus, are available prokinetic drugs for treating presumed GER. Although experimental pharmacodynamic studies showed a positive strengthening effect of metoclopramide on the canine LES, these effects were of short duration; high doses potentially leading to extrapyramidal signs and sedation are needed (Wilson et al, 2006). Our own studies have failed to document a positive strengthening effect on the LES in healthy dogs. In people, cisapride was the best prokinetic drug before its withdrawal from the market. It is still available in many countries for use in small animals through compounding veterinary pharmacies. Even if the significance of a primary LES incompetence is still uncertain in animals with esophagitis, the use of cisapride seems warranted because esophagitis may lead to a reflex decrease in LES tone. The author uses 0.5 to 0.75 mg/kg q8h PO.

Sucralfate, an aluminum salt of a sulfated disaccharide, is considered a mucosal protectant that binds to inflamed tissue to create a protective barrier. It is supposed to block diffusion of gastric acid and pepsin across the esophageal mucosa and inhibit the erosive action of pepsin and possibly bile. Sucralfate stimulates secretion of growth factors implicated in ulcer healing and of mucus and bicarbonate. The efficacy of administrating sucralfate for the treatment of esophagitis has been questioned, because the rationale for its effectiveness is based on its protective adherence to denuded mucosal surface in an acidic environment. Our ambulatory wireless esophageal pH measurements indicate a weakly alkaline canine esophageal milieu in more than 90% of the time recorded. In humans with advanced-grade corrosive esophagitis caused by ingestion of chemical agents, intensive high-dose sucralfate therapy has been shown to be beneficial in enhancing mucosal healing and preventing stricture formation.

The most clinically effective drugs for treatment of reflux esophagitis in humans are acid suppressive drugs (also see Chapter 123). Proton pump inhibitors (PPI) are the most potent gastric acid suppressants because of their ability to inhibit the proton pump H+, K+-ATPase, which is the final common pathway of gastric acid secretion. In dogs, PPIs (e.g., omeprazole) provide superior gastric acid suppression compared with H_2 receptor antagonists (ranitidine or famotidine) and therefore should be considered more effective for the treatment of acid-related disorders (Bersenas et al, 2005; Tolbert et al, 2011). The same is probably true in cats, but objective data are lacking. PPIs ideally are given before feeding the first meal of the day, when most proton pumps become active. Because not all pumps are active at any given time, a single PPI dose does not inhibit all pumps. For this reason a second dose may be necessary before feeding 12 hours later; the author prefers administration of 1 mg/kg q12h PO. Because the enteric-coated tablets and microspheres should not be broken or crushed for dosing purposes, the use of reformulated omeprazole paste for horses diluted to 40 mg/ml in sesame oil has been evaluated recently and can be considered as an efficacious alternative (Tolbert et al, 2011). However, twice-daily dosing was advised in that study for the reformulated paste because of a reduced duration of effect. Important shortcomings of PPIs include the dependence on food consumption for maximal efficacy, a delayed onset of action compared with H_2 receptor antagonists, and soft to liquid feces.

Lifestyle changes are part of the initial management of reflux esophagitis in people and include losing weight if overweight, avoiding bedtime snacks, and elevating the head at night. Although this therapy intuitively makes sense, no data are available in small animals.

In cases in which a primary LES abnormality clearly has been identified manometrically, surgical fundoplication can correct the physiologic factors contributing to GER. Nissen fundoplication has been shown to be highly effective in reducing reflux by achieving a constant external pressure on the gastroesophageal junction in canine models. Similarly, in case of a chronic obstructive upper respiratory problem, corrective surgery minimizing or eliminating the obstruction also may resolve inflammatory esophageal lesions. The same applies to hernias.

Benign esophageal strictures must be addressed if they are causing clinical problems. The two nonsurgical techniques used to widen the narrowed lumen are ballooning and bougienage. Esophageal balloon dilation is performed with a catheter involving an inflatable balloon. The balloon has to be positioned in the stricture and then expanded either with insufflated fluid or air. Bougienage involves the use of rigid instruments in different diameters (depending on the stricture) pushed longitudinally through the narrow point. Bougienage allows more force to be applied to the stricture than is possible with a balloon, which may be important for patients with tough, fibrous strictures or strictures so small that balloons cannot be inserted through them. Outcomes of esophageal bougienage for the treatment of benign esophageal strictures are similar to those reported for balloon dilation (Bissett et al, 2009). Corticosteroids sometimes are administered to inhibit healing-associated fibroblastic proliferation and contraction and therefore to avoid esophageal stricture formation. Although oral corticosteroids are not considered effective in humans, endoscopically guided submucosal triamcinolone injections at the stricture site prior to ballooning are likely effective for preventing reformation of strictures; however, controlled studies are lacking. The author uses a 23-gauge through-the-channel flexible injection needle and injects approximately 0.5-cc (10 mg triamcinolone) into each site in a four-quadrant pattern before widening the narrowed lumen. The chest should be radiographed after difficult procedures or if there is evidence of respiratory compromise to check for pneumomediastinum secondary to esophageal tearing. Following a dilation procedure the author allows oral feeding with a watery food consistency after 24 hours.

References and Suggested Reading

Bersenas AM et al: Effects of ranitidine, famotidine, pantoprazole, and omeprazole on intragastric pH in dogs, *Am J Vet Res* 66:425, 2005.

Bissett SA et al: Risk factors and outcome of bougienage for treatment of benign esophageal strictures in dogs and cats: 28 cases (1995-2004), *J Am Vet Med Assoc* 235(7):844, 2009.

Dodds WJ et al: Sequential gross, microscopic, and roentgenographic features of acute feline esophagitis, *Invest Radiol* 5:209, 1970.

Favarato ES et al: Evaluation of metoclopramide and ranitidine on the prevention of gastroesophageal reflux episodes in anesthetized dogs, *Res Vet Sci* 2011, doi:10.1016/j.rvsc.2011.07.027.

Galatos AD, Raptopoulos D: Gastro-oesophageal reflux during anaesthesia in the dog: the effect of age, positioning and type of surgical procedure, *Vet Rec* 137:513, 1995.

Gualtieri M, Olivero D: Reflux esophagitis in three cats associated with metaplastic columnar esophageal epithelium, *J Am Anim Hosp Assoc* 42:65, 2006.

Han E, Broussard J, Baer KE: Feline esophagitis secondary to gastroesophageal reflux disease: clinical signs and radiographic, endoscopic, and histopathological findings, *J Am Anim Hosp Assoc* 39:161, 2003.

Lecoindre P, Richard S: Digestive disorders associated with the chronic obstructive respiratory syndrome of brachycephalic dogs: 30 cases (1999-2001), *Revue Méd Vét* 155(3):141, 2004.

Lux CN et al: Gastroesophageal reflux and laryngeal dysfunction in a dog, *J Am Vet Med Assoc* 240(9):1100, 2012.

Münster M et al: Assessment of the histological quality of endoscopic biopsies obtained from the canine gastro-esophageal junction, *Tierarztl Prax Ausg K Kleintiere Heimtiere* 40(5):318, 2012.

Panti A et al: The effect of omeprazole on oesophageal pH in dogs during anaesthesia, *J Small Anim Pract* 50:540, 2009.

Poncet CM et al: Prevalence of gastrointestinal tract lesions in 73 brachycephalic dogs with upper respiratory syndrome, *J Small Anim Pract* 46:273, 2005.

Tolbert K et al: Efficacy of oral famotidine and 2 omeprazole formulations for the control of intragastric pH in dogs, *J Vet Intern Med* 25:47, 2011.

Wilson DV, Evans AT, Mauer WA: Influence of metoclopramide on gastroesophageal reflux in anesthetized dogs, *Am J Vet Res* 67(1):26, 2006.

Zhang X et al: Effect of repeated cycles of acute esophagitis and healing on esophageal peristalsis, tone, and length, *Am J Physiol Gastrointest Liver Physiol* 288(6):G1339, 2005.

CHAPTER 123

Antacid Therapy

ALEXA M.E. BERSENAS, *Guelph, Ontario, Canada*

Pathogenesis of Ulcer Disease

Ulcer disease results from an imbalance between gastric acid secretion and the gastric mucosal defense mechanisms. The pathogenesis is multifactorial. The amount of acid in gastric contents is determined by the rate of gastric acid secretion, the neutralization of acid by bicarbonate, the dilution by food and other digestive enzymes, and back diffusion of acid through the gastric mucosa. Gastric acidity plays a role in ulcerogenesis; human studies have established that the healing of acid-related disorders (gastric and duodenal ulcers and erosive esophagitis) is correlated highly with the degree of gastric acid suppression. These studies also have identified that the optimal degree of acid suppression varies with the underlying disease process. However, the degree of gastric acidity is not the only cause of mucosal injury: erosions and ulcers can occur in areas of anacidity. Other factors include increased bile reflux, decreased mucosal perfusion, and decreased delivery of bicarbonate to the protective mucous layer.

The key cell in gastric acid secretion is the parietal cell. The parietal cell secretes hydrogen ion via a H^+/K^+-ATPase pump. Based on gastric stimulation, the proton pump proceeds from an inactive to an active state such that over a period of hours, essentially all the ATPase molecules cycle through an acid-producing state. Secretion of hydrochloric acid is initiated via three systems: endocrine, neurocrine, and paracrine. These systems are mediated by three separate chemical messengers; gastrin, acetylcholine, and histamine, respectively.

The goals of antisecretory therapy are to reduce gastric acid secretion, prevent damage to the gastric mucosa, and allow regenerative mucosal mechanisms to prevail (Box 123-1).

Gastric Acid Suppressants

H₂ Receptor Antagonists

Cimetidine, ranitidine, famotidine, and nizatidine are reversible H_2-specific receptor antagonists that competitively inhibit binding of histamine, thereby reducing gastric acid secretion. Formulations are available for oral and parenteral administration (IV, IM, and SC). Intravenous continuous rate infusions have been used in human medicine but have not been investigated in veterinary medicine.

H_2 receptor antagonists (H₂RAs) differ in their potency (famotidine > ranitidine = nizatidine > cimetidine); however, clinically increased potency does not necessarily correlate to increased efficacy. In developmental studies using the dog model, H₂RAs have been shown to have an effect on canine gastric pH, where they produce an effect on gastric acidity for 6 to 7 hours. Cimetidine, the first H₂RA, because of its increased frequency of administration and its interaction with the cytochrome P450 system, has been replaced by later-generation H₂RAs. Unfortunately, in the last decade, several veterinary studies have demonstrated underwhelming acid suppression with later-generation H₂RAs in dogs. In one veterinary study investigating the effects of different H₂RAs on gastric pH in healthy dogs, ranitidine at a clinically recommended dose (2 mg/kg IV q12h) offered no change in gastric pH compared with saline (Bersenas et al, 2005). Results using famotidine at 0.5 mg/kg IV (q12h) were also underwhelming. Famotidine's ability to raise substantially intragastric pH in dogs is limited (Tolbert et al, 2011). Clinically, oral famotidine has been shown to be efficacious for reducing the severity but not the prevalence of gastric lesions in racing sled dogs when used as a preventive (Williamson et al, 2007). Attempts at increasing the dose or dosing frequency of famotidine also have failed to show an improved outcome. It is unlikely that famotidine at the commonly used dose of 0.5 mg/kg q12h is very effective, and the once-daily dosing that has been recommended previously may not be as effective as suggested.

Overall, the acid suppression provided by H₂RAs at current veterinary doses is low. Some evidence suggests that famotidine should be selected over ranitidine for improved effect (Bersenas et al, 2005). Famotidine appears to help primarily animals that are at lesser risk for gastric lesions or are at risk for less severe gastric lesions. Famotidine remains an excellent drug for routine prophylaxis when cost is a concern or when an injectable drug is preferred.

In addition to the H₂RAs antisecretory effects, some of these drugs have a prokinetic effect on gastrointestinal motility. Ranitidine and nizatidine have prokinetic properties mediated by inhibition of acetylcholinesterase activity.

The H₂RAs are metabolized in the liver and excreted unchanged in urine. In renal failure the half-life is increased; therefore a decreased dose or decreased dosing frequency (q24h) is recommended. Otherwise H₂RAs have minimal adverse reactions and are considered very safe in humans and small animals.

Proton Pump Inhibitors

Omeprazole, pantoprazole, lansoprazole, rabeprazole, esomeprazole, and dexlansoprazole are proton pump inhibitors (PPIs) that block the H^+/K^+-ATPase enzyme

Dosages for Acid Control in Dogs and Cats

H₂ Receptor Antagonists
Cimetidine: 5-10 mg/kg q6-8h, PO, SC, IM, IV
Ranitidine: 1-2 mg/kg q8-12h, PO, SC, IM, IV
Famotidine: 0.5-1 mg/kg q12-24h, PO, SC, IM, IV
Nizatidine: 2.5-5 mg/kg q24h PO (dog) (dose not well established)

Proton Pump Inhibitors
Omeprazole: 0.7-1 mg/kg q24h PO; 1 mg/kg q12h for 3-5 days for quicker onset and greater efficacy
Pantoprazole: 0.5-1 mg/kg q24h PO, IV (dog and cat); 1 mg/kg bolus IV followed by 0.1 mg/kg/hr for 72 hours CRI (used only in dogs)

Cytoprotective Agents
Misoprostol: 2-5 μg/kg q8-12h PO (dog); (cat: no dose established)
Sucralfate: 0.5-1 g q8-12h PO (dog); 0.25 g q8-12h PO (cat)

Antacids
Aluminum hydroxide tablets: 10-30 mg/kg q8h PO, alternatively, ½-1 tablet q6h PO (dog), ¼ tablet q6h PO (cat)
Aluminum hydroxide or aluminum hydroxide/magnesium hydroxide suspensions: 2-10 ml q2-4h PO (dog)
Magnesium hydroxide: 5-10 ml q4-6h PO (dog and cat)

pump on the apical surface of the parietal cell. In contrast to receptor antagonists, PPIs block histamine-2, gastrin- and cholinergic-mediated sources of acid production and inhibit gastric acid secretion at the final common pathway of the H^+/K^+-ATPase proton pump. PPIs provide the most profound acid inhibition of the antisecretory drugs and are indicated for gastric and duodenal ulcers and erosive esophagitis and for the long-term treatment of pathologic hypersecretory conditions.

PPIs are substituted benzimidazoles, acid-activated sulfhydryl (SH) agents. All PPIs are available in oral formulation. These are unstable in the acidic environment of the stomach. Enterically administered PPIs are compounded as enteric-coated capsules or tablets and should not be crushed or split. Adjusted doses for smaller patients should be repackaged into new capsules; alternatively, a 2 mg/ml omeprazole suspension using 8.4% sodium bicarbonate as a base (one 20-mg tablet with 10 ml 8.4% NaHCO₃) is recommended (Phillips et al, 1996). More recently, a 40 mg/ml omeprazole suspension using an approved equine oral paste formulation (Gastrogard, AstraZeneca) in sesame oil at a ratio of 1:9 has been used (the formulation should be made up daily until further testing is performed) (Tolbert et al, 2011).

PPIs are irreversible inhibitors of the ATPase pump that lead to long-term acid suppression (up to 36 hours) despite very short plasma half-lives (0.5 to 2 hours). PPIs routinely are administered once daily and should be administered 1 hour before a meal to coincide with maximal proton pump activity. PPIs take several days to reach steady state because they bind only to the proton pumps that are actively secreting acid, sparing inactive pumps that are resting in the cytosol. Higher doses of omeprazole provide a more predictable inhibition of gastric acid, and short-term, twice daily dosing is recommended for more efficient acid suppression.

Intravenous formulations of PPIs, in North America, are limited to pantoprazole and lansoprazole. Pantoprazole administered once a day has been shown to have similar antisecretory efficacy to injectable famotidine in healthy dogs (Bersenas et al, 2005). Intravenous PPI use should be reserved for patients unable to take oral medications and have active bleeding ulcers requiring hemostasis (Pang and Graham, 2010) or are at very high risk of developing stress related ulcers (e.g., coagulopathic, mechanically ventilated more than 48 hours) (Cook et al, 1994). Acute gastrointestinal bleeding requires a pH greater than 6 to achieve hemostasis. The most potent acid suppression is achieved by using a constant rate infusion of a PPI after a high–dose bolus (infusions provide a steady state of the drug to inactivate any newly recruited or synthesized proton pumps). Infusional PPIs are endorsed in human medicine at a conventional rate of 80 mg bolus followed by 8 mg/hr for 72 hr (Pang and Graham, 2010). Pantoprazole infusion has been used in dogs when aggressive acid inhibition is required, and the dose extrapolated from the human dose with no negative effects noted; no veterinary studies have evaluated its efficacy.

Long-term use of PPIs has demonstrated an excellent safety profile and commercially available PPIs are equally effective with minimal side effects. Earlier concerns of hypergastrinemia and the development of gastric carcinoids with the long-term use of these drugs have not been substantiated clinically in people or animals. PPIs are metabolized by varying degrees by the cytochrome P450 enzyme system, with omeprazole and esomeprazole more actively reliant on this system. Current recommendations indicate that the use of omeprazole or esomeprazole with clopidogrel should be avoided because of competitive inhibition of clopidogrel metabolism (reducing clopidogrel's efficacy). Other drug interactions include decreased absorption of coadministered medications dependent on gastric acidity (e.g., ketoconazole, ampicillin esters, iron salts, and digoxin).

Cytoprotective Agents

Misoprostol

Misoprostol (Cytotec) is a synthetic prostaglandin (PGE₁) analog that has cytoprotective effects by enhancing gastric mucosal defense mechanisms (increasing bicarbonate and mucus production and increasing turnover and blood supply of gastric mucosal cells). Misoprostol also has acid inhibitory properties with direct action on the parietal cell causing decreased activity of the proton pump; this effect results in only modest decreases in gastric acid secretion.

The main indication for misoprostol use is the prevention of NSAID-induced gastric damage. Misoprostol is not recommended routinely for patients receiving NSAIDs but should be considered for select patients with high risk of GI ulceration. It is uncertain whether misoprostol improves healing of established ulcers, and it does not have any benefit in treating ulcers not associated with NSAIDs (e.g., corticosteroid administration in dogs with intervertebral disk disease) (Hanson et al, 1997; Neiger et al, 2000).

Unfortunately, misoprostol has a very short half-life (30 minutes), which requires frequent dosing (q6-8h); unexpectedly, one canine study found twice-daily dosing to be as effective as q8h administration (Ward et al, 2003). The drug also is associated with gastrointestinal distress, manifested as nausea, vomiting, diarrhea, and abdominal pain that frequently prevents the routine use of this drug. Misoprostol should be avoided in pregnant animals because of stimulation of uterine contractions and risk of abortion.

Sucralfate

Sucralfate is an oral antiulcer agent, an anionic sulfated disaccharide that, in the stomach, is broken down into sucrose sulfate and aluminum salt. The negatively charged sulfate binds electrostatically to positively charged protein molecules exposed in damaged mucosa of the GI tract to form an adhesive paste-like substance that physically protects the ulcer site from pepsin, acid, and bile, and prevents back diffusion of hydrogen ions. In addition, sucralfate stimulates mucus and bicarbonate secretion and stimulates the increase of prostaglandin E$_2$ and epidermal growth factor. Sucralfate is indicated for the treatment of erosions and ulcers in the stomach and upper duodenum and can treat esophageal lesions if gastroesophageal reflux is suspected. Its efficacy as a prophylactic for GI ulceration is not as well known, but no benefit has been attributed to its use with GI hemorrhage in dogs with IVDD administered corticosteroids (Hanson et al, 1997). In stress-related mucosal injury in humans, some studies have found that sucralfate administered prophylactically may be at least as effective as antacids and H$_2$RAs; however, conflicting studies report decreased GI bleeding with the use of acid-lowering therapies (H$_2$RAs).

Sucralfate is not absorbed systemically. Within the stomach it may bind to and decrease the absorption of concomitantly administered medications, such as fluoroquinolones, H$_2$RAs, levothyroxine, theophylline, tetracyclines, digoxin, phenytoin, and ketoconazole. Oral drugs should be administered 2 hours prior to sucralfate administration. Sucralfate should not be administered through duodenal or jejunal feeding tubes because its site of action is bypassed. Sucralfate is very safe with very few adverse effects. Patients with advanced renal failure and impaired aluminum excretion who take sucralfate have the potential for aluminum toxicity.

Antacids

Antacids work by directly buffering or neutralizing the acidic contents of the stomach. Many over-the-counter antacids are available; these are bases of aluminum, magnesium, calcium, or combinations of these. Some mixtures contain sodium and should be used with caution in patients in whom fluid retention is contraindicated.

Familiar antacid product names include Tums (calcium carbonate), Amphojel (aluminum hydroxide), Gaviscon (alginic acid/aluminum/magnesium/sodium bicarbonate), to name only a few. Antacids containing aluminum or magnesium neutralize stomach acid to form water and a neutral salt. In addition to neutralizing stomach acid, aluminum-containing antacids have additional beneficial effects, including decreasing pepsin activity, binding to bile acids in the stomach, and stimulating local prostaglandin (PGE$_1$). Products combining magnesium and aluminum salts take advantage of different buffering capacities of the individual cations and reduce side effects of any cation alone.

Antacids are the least therapeutic option for ulcer treatment. Dosages in veterinary medicine are empiric. Antacids are not considered sufficiently effective and, because of a very short duration of action, have labor-intensive dosing frequency (q4h) of rather large volumes. Moreover, administration of high doses of antacids may increase the risks of aspiration pneumonia and toxicity related to cation accumulation (particularly in patients with renal dysfunction).

Summary

Gastric acid suppression must be evaluated in light of its necessity for prophylaxis versus ulcer healing. Antacid therapy is extensive and has been recommended in all conditions in which gastrointestinal ulceration previously has been documented in human and veterinary patients. Potent antisecretory drugs are indicated for patients with overt ulceration. However, as in people, animals with low risk of bleeding may not derive benefit from prophylactic measures to protect the gastric mucosa from acid, and the costs associated with widespread use of antisecretory drugs may be unnecessary. Further studies in veterinary medicine investigating the benefits of acid-lowering therapies are necessary to evaluate whether their widespread use is warranted or beneficial.

References and Suggested Reading

Bell NJV et al: Appropriate acid suppression for the management of gastroesophageal reflux disease, *Digestion* 51(suppl):59, 1992.

Bersenas AME et al: Effects of ranitidine, famotidine, pantoprazole, and omeprazole on intragastric pH in dogs, *Am J Vet Res* 66:425, 2005.

Cook DJ et al: Risk factors for gastrointestinal bleeding in critically ill patients. Canadian Critical Care Trials Group, *N Engl J Med* 330:377, 1994.

Hanson SM et al: Clinical evaluation of cimetidine, sucralfate, and misoprostol for prevention of gastrointestinal tract bleeding in dogs undergoing spinal surgery, *Am J Vet Res* 58:1320, 1997.

Henderson AK, Webster CRL: The use of gastroprotectants in treating gastric ulceration in dogs, *Compendium* 28:358, 2006.

Madanick RD: Proton pump inhibitor side effects and drug interactions: much ado about nothing? *Cleve Clin J Med* 78:39, 2011.

Neiger R et al: Gastric mucosal lesions in dogs with acute intervertebral disc disease: characterization and effects of omeprazole or misoprostol, *J Vet Intern Med* 14:33, 2000.

Pang S, Graham D: Review: a clinical guide to using intravenous proton-pump inhibitors in reflux and peptic ulcers, *Therap Adv Gastroenterol* 3:11, 2010.

Phillips JO et al: A prospective study of simplified omeprazole suspension for the prophylaxis of stress-related mucosal damage, *Crit Care Med* 24:1793, 1996.

Tolbert K et al: Efficacy of oral famotidine and 2 omeprazole formulations for the control of intragastric pH in dogs, *J Vet Intern Med* 25:47, 2011.

Ward DM et al: The effect of dosing interval on the efficacy of misoprostol in the prevention of aspirin-induced gastric injury, *J Vet Intern Med* 17:282, 2003.

Williamson KK et al: Efficacy of famotidine for the prevention of exercise-induced gastritis in racing Alaskan sled dogs, *J Vet Intern Med* 21:924, 2007.

CHAPTER **124**

Gastric *Helicobacter* spp. and Chronic Vomiting in Dogs

MICHAEL S. LEIB, *Blacksburg, Virginia*

Spiral bacteria were identified in the stomachs of humans and animals in the late 1800s. However, it was not until the early 1980s that Warren and Marshall proposed a relationship between *Helicobacter pylori* and gastric disease in humans. Soon after, studies demonstrated that spiral bacteria were common in the stomachs of clinically normal dogs and cats, as well as those with signs of gastrointestinal (GI) disease. Experimental infection in dogs and cats resulted in lymphoid follicular gastritis; however, clinical signs were absent or very mild.

Currently a direct causal relationship between spiral bacteria and chronic gastritis and vomiting or with gastric neoplasia has not been established firmly in dogs or cats. However, based on clinical experience and several clinical studies evaluating dogs and cats treated for *Helicobacter* spp. and identifying improvement or resolution of clinical signs, the author believes that gastric *Helicobacter* spp. can cause or contribute to the clinical signs in some dogs and cats with chronic gastritis and vomiting (Happonen et al, 2000; Jergens et al, 2009; Leib et al, 2007). In addition, a potential relationship between gastric lymphoblastic lymphoma and *Helicobacter heilmannii* in cats has been proposed (Bridgeford et al, 2008).

The author routinely determines whether gastric *Helicobacter* spp. are present in all dogs and cats with chronic vomiting that undergo upper GI endoscopy in his clinic. In most instances, dogs and cats with gastric *Helicobacter* spp. and gastritis, with and without inflammatory bowel disease (IBD), are treated initially for *Helicobacter* spp. If clinical signs continue, dietary or antiinflammatory therapies for gastritis and IBD are instituted. Although the potential pathogenic role of gastric *Helicobacter* spp. in dogs and cats is being investigated, a thorough diagnostic evaluation to search for other potential causes of chronic vomiting always should be performed before considering *Helicobacter* spp. to be the primary etiologic agent. The purpose of this chapter is to describe the commonly used methods of identifying gastric spiral bacteria in dogs and cats and to review the evidence behind current treatment recommendations. Recommendations for humans with *H. pylori* have been modified by the results of hundreds of clinical studies. Treatment recommendations in dogs and cats no doubt also will change as further studies are performed.

Pathogenesis

Helicobacter spp. are gram-negative, microaerophilic, motile, curved-to-spiral bacteria with multiple terminal flagella. They contain large quantities of the enzyme urease, which results in the production of ammonia and bicarbonate when in contact with urea that is present in gastric juice. This reaction alters the pH immediately surrounding the bacteria and helps them colonize the acidic environment of the stomach.

More than 35 *Helicobacter* spp. have been identified in humans and animals. At least seven species have been identified in the stomachs of dogs and cats. In addition to the gastric species, others also have been identified in the intestine and liver. *H. pylori* is the most common gastric species in humans. *H. pylori* has been shown to be a major cause of gastritis and peptic ulcers and to increase the risk of gastric cancer. Infection rates can approach 100% in developing countries and 25% to 60% in developed countries. Infection usually is acquired in childhood and most often persists for life; natural immunity does not clear the infection. Most infected humans remain asymptomatic, but peptic ulcers may occur in approximately 16% of those infected, whereas gastric cancer may develop in 1% to 2% of infected humans. Symptomatic disease usually takes decades to develop in humans. Development of clinical signs is related to bacterial virulence, environmental factors, and host genetics, especially relating to the cytokine response to infection. Eradication of *H. pylori* usually results in healing of gastric and duodenal ulcers and remission of low-grade gastric mucosa–associated lymphoid tissue (MALT) lymphoma.

Although *H. pylori* has been identified in a research colony of cats, infections in pet dogs and cats with other species of *Helicobacter* is more common. Gastric *Helicobacter* spp. usually found in dogs and cats are larger than *H. pylori* (1.5 to 3 μm). Initially these large spiral bacteria (4 to 10 μm) were called *Gastrospirillum hominis* but were later reclassified as *Helicobacter heilmannii*. Other large gastric spiral bacteria such as *Helicobacter felis, Helicobacter bizzozeronii,* and *Helicobacter salomonis* are found and are indistinguishable from *H. heilmannii* using routine light microscopy. Multiple species also can be present within an individual animal. Gastric or duodenal ulceration associated with *Helicobacter* spp. is rare in dogs and cats, demonstrating a major pathophysiologic difference between *H. pylori* and the gastric spiral bacteria commonly found in dogs and cats. In addition to the role of *Helicobacter* spp. in the pathogenesis of gastritis and chronic vomiting in dogs and cats is the potential for zoonotic transmission. Most evidence indicates zoonotic transmission to be very low, but the potential is real. *H. heilmannii* is a rare cause of gastritis in humans, accounting for approximately 0.1% of cases. An epidemiologic survey of humans with *H. heilmannii* gastritis showed that contact with dogs and cats was a significant risk factor (Meining et al, 1998). In addition, there was an association between *H. heilmannii* gastritis and gastric lymphoma, although this relationship could be coincidental (Stolte et al, 1997). Some studies have identified cat ownership as a risk factor for *H. pylori* infection in humans, whereas others have found contact with dogs or cats not to be a risk factor for *H. pylori* infection. Although the potential for zoonotic transmission appears slight, until this issue is resolved conclusively, it seems prudent to identify the presence of gastric *Helicobacter* spp. in dogs

and cats during the diagnostic evaluation of chronic vomiting.

Diagnostic Tests

Invasive methods of diagnosis of gastric *Helicobacter* infection in humans include bacterial culture, routine microscopic or ultrastructural examination, polymerase chain reaction, or rapid urease testing of gastric mucosal biopsy specimens, usually obtained via endoscopy. Noninvasive methods of diagnosis include urea breath testing, fecal antigen determination, and serology. Although many of these noninvasive tests have been investigated in dogs and cats, they are not routinely available. Presently the clinical diagnosis of gastric *Helicobacter* spp. in dogs and cats requires endoscopic examination or exploratory celiotomy for retrieval of gastric biopsy samples. Recently, gastric washing with saline has identified spiral bacteria in a small group of cats. In the author's clinic, spiral bacteria are identified on gastric biopsy, from gastric brush cytology specimens, or indirectly by a positive rapid urease test using a gastric mucosal sample. Results from a rapid urease test and gastric brush cytology are available much sooner than results from histopathology. For reasons discussed in the following paragraphs, gastric brush cytology and histologic evaluation of biopsy samples are considered to be the most practical diagnostic tests available to the practicing veterinarian.

Brush Cytology

Gastric brush cytology is the least expensive and most practical diagnostic method with the quickest turnaround time. After completion of an endoscopic examination and collection of biopsy samples from the duodenum and stomach, a brush cytology specimen is collected. A guarded cytology brush is passed through the biopsy channel of the endoscope into the gastric body along the greater curvature. The cytology brush is extended from the sheath and gently rubbed along the mucosa from the antrum toward the fundus, along the greater curvature. Hemorrhagic areas associated with previous biopsy sites should be avoided. The brush is retracted into the protective sheath and withdrawn from the endoscope. The brush is extended from the sheath, gently rubbed across several glass microscope slides, which are air dried, and stained with a rapid Wright stain (Dip Quick stain). The slide is examined under 100× oil immersion. Areas with numerous epithelial cells and large amounts of mucus are examined initially for *Helicobacter* spp. If present, the spiral bacteria are seen easily. They are usually at least as long as the diameter of a red blood cell, and their classic spiral shape is obvious (Figure 124-1). The number of spiral bacteria can be highly variable, from one every several fields to massive numbers in most fields. At least 10 oil immersion fields are examined on two slides before the specimen is considered negative. Unlike diagnostic tests that involve using a single or several small biopsy samples, brush cytology gathers surface mucus and epithelial cells from a much larger area, increasing the chances for identification of bacteria. Brush cytology was found to be more sensitive than urease testing or histopathologic examination of gastric tissues in identifying *Helicobacter* spp. organisms in dogs and cats (Happonen et al, 1996).

Rapid Urease Test

The rapid urease test detects the presence of bacterial urease, produced by the *Helicobacter* spp., in a gastric biopsy sample. A commercially available test, the CLOtest, is used in the author's clinic (Figure 124-2). Individual tests cost less than $10. The test consists of an agar gel with urea and a pH indicator, phenol red, within a small plastic well. The tests should be kept refrigerated before

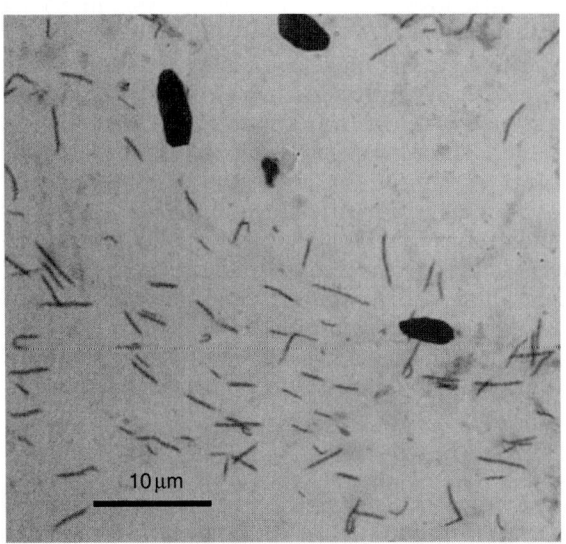

Figure 124-1 Gastric brush cytology specimens stained with Dip Quick stain. Large numbers of spiral bacteria are visible. Cellular debris is scattered throughout the photograph. (With permission from Leib MS, Duncan RB: *Compend Contin Educ Pract Vet* 27:221, 2005.)

use. A routine microbiologic urea slant tube also can be used for this same purpose. An endoscopic biopsy sample obtained from the angularis incisura of the stomach is pushed into the gel. The test is maintained at room temperature and examined frequently for a 24-hour period. If bacterial urease is present, urea is hydrolyzed to ammonia, which changes the pH of the gel. The color of the gel turns from yellow to magenta. The rate at which the gel changes color is proportional to the number of *Helicobacter* spp. present in the sample. When large numbers of bacteria are present in the biopsy sample, the rapid urease test quickly changes color, often within 15 to 30 minutes. If the color of the gel has not changed within 24 hours, the test is interpreted as negative.

Occasionally, false-positive tests occur, perhaps because of contamination of other urease-producing pharyngeal or intestinal bacteria. False-negative tests may occur because of the patchy distribution of bacteria within the stomach or the use of drugs that decrease acid secretion (increase in pH alters the activity of urease). Because of false positives and negatives, the cost of the tests, the turnaround time for results (especially if negative), and the ease and reliability of brush cytology, the author finds the rapid urease test to be a less valuable diagnostic method.

Histopathologic Identification

Histopathologic identification of *Helicobacter* spp. within gastric biopsy samples, using hematoxylin and eosin (H&E) or special stains, has a specificity of 100% and a sensitivity of greater than 90% in studies in humans. Because of the patchy distribution of organisms within the stomach, examination of samples from multiple gastric locations increases sensitivity. In the author's clinic, samples from the pylorus, angularis incisura, gastric body along the greater curvature, and cardia are examined routinely. Spiral bacteria can be seen within the mucus covering the surface epithelium, the gastric pits, glandular lumen, and the parietal cells (Figure 124-3). In

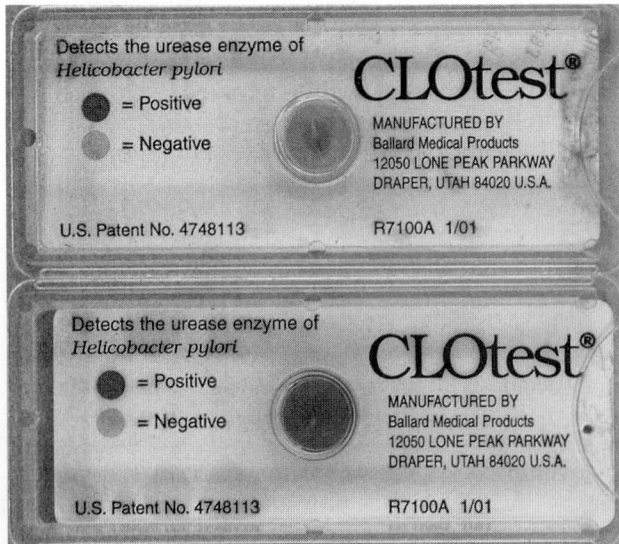

Figure 124-2 CLOtest. The top well is negative. The bottom well has changed color and is positive. (With permission from Leib MS, Duncan RB: *Compend Contin Educ Pract Vet* 27:221, 2005.)

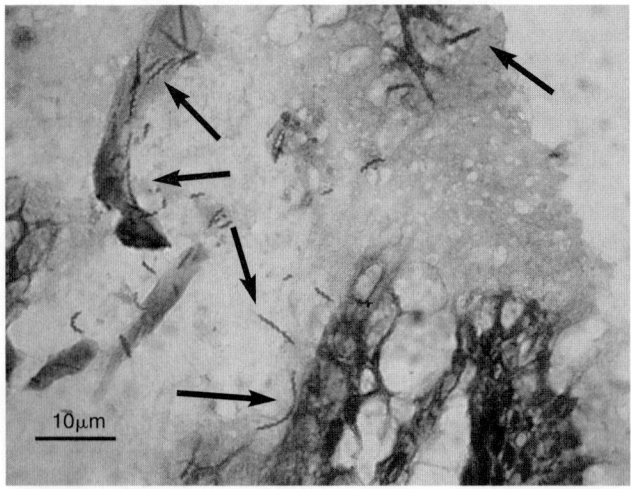

Figure 124-3 Photomicrograph of gastric mucosal samples stained with H&E showing spiral bacteria along the mucosal surface *(arrows)*. (With permission from Leib MS, Duncan RB: *Compend Contin Educ Pract Vet* 27:221, 2005.)

TABLE **124-1**

Treatment Protocols for Gastric *Helicobacter* Species in Dogs

Protocol	Drugs	Dosage mg/kg	Frequency/day	Duration (days)
Happonen, 2000	Amoxicillin	20	q12h	10-14
	Metronidazole	10	q12h	10-14
	Bismuth subcitrate	6	q12h	14-28
Leib, 2007	Amoxicillin	15	q12h	14
	Metronidazole	10	q12h	14
	Bismuth subsalicylate	<5 kg-65.5 mg	q12h	14
		5-9.9 kg-131 mg		
		10-24.9 kg-262 mg		
		>25 kg-524 mg		
	Famotidine	0.5	q12h	14
Jergens, 2009	Amoxicillin	22	q12h	21
	Metronidazole	11-15	q12h	21
	Bismuth subsalicylate suspension	0.22 ml/kg	q6-8h	21
	Clarithromycin	7.5	q12h	14
Cornetta, 1998; Simpson, 1999	Amoxicillin	20	q12h	14
	Metronidazole	20	q12h	14
	Famotidine	0.5	q12h	14
Anacleto, 2011	Amoxicillin	50	q12h	7
	Clarithromycin	25	q12h	7
	Lansoprazole	1	q12h	7

cats, bacteria have been identified submucosally within gastric lymphoid follicles. Spiral bacteria associated with the mucosal surface or within gastric pits are relatively easy to detect with routine H&E staining of tissues. However, if the distribution of bacteria favors gastric glands and glandular epithelial cells, bacteria are detected much more readily with a modified Steiner's silver stain. Because of similarities in morphologic characteristics it is not possible to identify specific species using routine histologic staining techniques. Histopathologic evaluation of biopsy samples also allows assessment of inflammation in the stomach and duodenum or identification of neoplasia that may be the cause of the animal's clinical signs.

Treatment

Many studies evaluating therapy have been performed in humans with *H. pylori*. The most effective treatment regimens contain two or three antimicrobials combined with a proton pump antagonist, given for 1 to 2 weeks. Multiple antibiotics are used because treatment with a single antibiotic has resulted in eradication rates less than 20%. Studies in humans not only have demonstrated effective regimens but also have evaluated protocols associated with the highest treatment compliance: those with the fewest side effects, the least number of tablets/day, and the shortest duration of therapy. Treatment protocols with eradication rates determined 4 weeks after completion of therapy that are higher than 80% to 90% are considered clinically effective. Reappearance rates after eradication of approximately 1% have been

demonstrated, thought mostly to be the result of recrudescence. Successful treatment of bacteria within the gastric lumen is difficult. Antibiotics must penetrate the thick mucus layer within the gastric lumen and be active at an acid pH. The volume of gastric contents is changing constantly as a meal is ingested and because of acid secretion and gastric emptying. In addition, metronidazole and clarithromycin, and rarely amoxicillin, resistance has been detected in strains of *H. pylori*.

Table 124-1 lists treatment protocols described in the veterinary literature and used in the author's hospital. In one study the author (Leib et al, 2007) treated 24 pet dogs with gastric *Helicobacter* spp. and chronic vomiting with either amoxicillin, metronidazole, and bismuth subsalicylate (triple therapy) or triple therapy and famotidine (quadruple therapy). The median duration of vomiting before therapy was 19 weeks, and the median frequency of vomiting was 3.5 episodes per week. The presence of gastric *Helicobacter* spp. was determined by histologic assessment of gastric biopsy specimens obtained before therapy, 4 weeks, and 6 months after completion of therapy. Eradication rates were 70% and 78.5% 4 weeks after therapy for the triple and quadruple therapy, respectively. Eradication rates decreased to 44.4% and 41.7% 6 months after therapy for the triple and quadruple therapy groups, respectively. Eight dogs that were negative at 4 weeks were positive at 6 months because of either reinfection or recrudescence of infection.

Both treatments reduced the vomiting frequency compared with the historical vomiting frequency. The median reduction in the frequency of vomiting episodes during the first 4-week period after therapy was 91.8% for triple-therapy dogs and 72% for quadruple-therapy dogs. After completion of therapy, the median reduction in the frequency of vomiting episodes for the entire 6-month period was approximately 86% for both groups. Almost 78% of dogs that were *Helicobacter* spp. negative at 6 months had at least a 90% reduction in vomiting frequency. In addition, dogs negative at 6 months had a significant improvement in the severity of their histologic gastritis scores. These data suggest that gastric *Helicobacter* spp. caused or contributed to clinical signs in some of the dogs in this study, and successful treatment dramatically decreased the incidence and severity of clinical signs. Because it often is presumed that treatment compliance may decrease as the number of drugs administered increases, omitting acid suppressors in treatment protocols might improve client compliance and treatment success in some cases. Acid suppression may not be necessary in dogs and cats with gastric *Helicobacter* spp. because peptic ulceration is very uncommon when compared with its incidence in humans. However, proton pump antagonists such as omeprazole have proven to have other potential benefits in humans with *H. pylori*, including bacteriostatic effects *in vitro,* facilitation of bacterial clearance from the stomach when combined with antibiotics, and inhibition of bacterial urease. Further study of the potential role of acid suppression in dogs and cats with gastric *Helicobacter* spp. is warranted.

The high infection rates 6 months after therapy in the Leib study (2007) were thought to be caused by initial treatment failure (25%), reinfection from the environment, or recrudescence of infection. High rates of treatment failure and potential recrudescence indicate that more effective treatment regimens should be developed to reach higher than 80% to 90% eradication rates. In the author's study it was not possible to differentiate between reinfection and recrudescence. It is possible that both treatments were effective initially, and reinfection from the environment occurred. Because of canine social habits and the relatively unsanitary nature of the environment in which they live, reinfection after successful eradication therapy seems more likely to occur in dogs than in humans. If further research confirms that reinfection commonly occurs, treatment strategies should include minimizing environmental contamination and exposure (Anacleto et al, 2011), treatment of asymptomatic animals within the household, and possibly periodic retreatment if clinical signs recur.

Only two other published studies are known to evaluate the effects of triple antimicrobial therapy on gastric *Helicobacter* spp. in pet dogs with upper GI signs (Happonen et al, 2000; Jergens et al, 2009). In the first study, seven of nine dogs that received amoxicillin, metronidazole, and bismuth subcitrate (see Table 124-1) became negative for *Helicobacter* spp. Clinical signs improved in all treated dogs, including two that remained positive. However, complete resolution of clinical signs required additional therapies. Four of these dogs were reevaluated a mean of 2.5 years after therapy, and all were found to be positive for gastric *Helicobacter* spp. However, these four dogs remained normal or only occasionally had mild clinical signs. In the second study (Jergens et al, 2009),

three dogs and two cats with chronic vomiting were treated with amoxicillin, metronidazole, and bismuth subsalicylate for 3 weeks (see Table 124-1) and fed an elimination diet. All five became *Helicobacter* spp. negative and vomiting also resolved after treatment. The results of these studies also provide evidence that gastric *Helicobacter* spp. contributed to the clinical signs in these dogs.

Because of the need to identify more effective treatment protocols, the author recently investigated the effectiveness of a dual antibiotic protocol using clarithromycin and amoxicillin for 2 weeks. The combination of clarithromycin and amoxicillin with a proton pump antagonist has been very effective in eradicating *H. pylori* in humans with peptic ulceration. Because famotidine did not improve results in previous study and because of the additional cost of such therapy and the potential for decreased client compliance, a proton pump antagonist was not used. Only preliminary results are available for the 14 dogs treated. The median duration of vomiting was 47 weeks, and the median frequency of vomiting was 2.5 episodes per week. Approximately 71% (10 of 14) of dogs were *Helicobacter* spp. negative 4 weeks after therapy and only 50% (5 of 10) after 6 months. The median reduction in the vomiting frequency was 79.4%, although there was considerable variation. However, only 40% of dogs negative 6 months after treatment had at least a 90% reduction in vomiting frequency.

Experimental studies in dogs cannot be compared directly to studies in pets with clinical signs but can provide assessment of bacterial eradication rates. Two studies evaluated the 2-week treatment of asymptomatic beagles naturally infected with gastric *Helicobacter* spp. with famotidine, amoxicillin, and metronidazole (see Table 124-1) (Cornetta et al, 1998; Simpson et al, 1999). In both reports all dogs were positive for gastric *Helicobacter* spp. 29 days after completion of therapy. These studies included bismuth as a third antimicrobial agent. Besides its beneficial effects in healing peptic ulcers in humans, bismuth compounds have antimicrobial effects and can suppress but not eliminate *H. pylori* from humans. Bismuth compounds have been shown to decrease the adherence of *H. pylori* from the gastric epithelium, distort bacterial structure by causing vacuolization, and be present within the cell wall and on the external surface of the bacteria. A recent study (Anacleto et al, 2011) treated 10 naturally infected dogs with amoxicillin, clarithromycin, and lansoprazole BID for 7 days. Dogs housed individually remained *Helicobacter* spp. negative after 60 days, but 80% of those housed with infected dogs became reinfected. However, only five dogs in this study were housed individually. Crowded housing conditions were associated commonly with reinfection, which may have contributed to disappointing eradication rates 6 months after treatment in these experimental studies.

In summary, although the role of gastric *Helicobacter* spp. as a cause of chronic vomiting in dogs and cats remains speculative, enough clinical and experimental evidence suggests that gastric spiral bacteria cause or contribute to chronic vomiting and gastritis in many dogs and cats. In the author's studies between 40% and 78%

of dogs with chronic vomiting, chronic gastritis, and *Helicobacter* spp. dramatically improve after successful treatment. It seems prudent to determine if gastric spiral bacteria are present in dogs and cats with chronic vomiting. This can be accomplished easily with brush gastric cytology specimens or routine histologic assessment of gastric biopsy samples. If other etiologies of chronic vomiting are not identified, a treatment protocol for gastric *Helicobacter* spp. is indicated. If clinical signs do not improve after treatment, dietary trials or antiinflammatory drugs should be considered. Based on all the studies performed and the author's clinical experience, the author's current treatment recommendation is amoxicillin and clarithromycin given q12h PO and omeprazole given q24h PO for 3 weeks. However, this combination has not been tested in a large number of dogs or cats with chronic vomiting.

Additional studies will further define the potential pathogenic role of gastric *Helicobacter* spp. in dogs, and more effective treatment recommendations no doubt will emerge.

References and Suggested Reading

Anacleto TP et al: Studies of distribution and recurrence of *Helicobacter* spp gastric mucosa of dogs after triple therapy, *Acta Cirugica Brasileira* 26:82, 2011.
Bridgeford EC et al: Gastric *Helicobacter* species as a cause of feline gastric lymphoma: a viable hypothesis, *Vet Immunol Immunopathol* 123:106, 2008.
Cornetta AM et al: Use of [13 C] urea breath test for detection of gastric infection with *Helicobacter* spp in dogs, *Am J Vet Res* 59:1364, 1998.
Flatland B: *Helicobacter* infection in humans and animals, *Compend Contin Educ Pract Vet* 24:688, 2002.
Geyer C et al: Occurrence of spiral-shaped bacteria in gastric biopsies of dogs and cats, *Vet Rec* 133:18, 1993.
Happonen I et al: Comparison of diagnostic methods for detecting gastric *Helicobacter*-like organisms in dogs and cats, *J Comp Pathol* 115:117, 1996.
Happonen I, Linden J, Westermarck E: Effect of triple therapy on eradication of canine gastric *Helicobacters* and gastric disease, *J Small Anim Pract* 41:1, 2000.
Jergens AE et al: Fluorescence in situ hybridization confirms clearance of visible *Helicobacter* spp. associated with gastritis in dogs and cats, *J Vet Intern Med* 23:16, 2009.
Leib MS, Duncan RB: Diagnosing gastric *Helicobacter* infections in dogs and cat, *Compend Contin Educ Pract Vet* 27:221, 2005.
Leib MS, Duncan RB, Ward DL: Triple antimicrobial therapy and acid suppression in dogs with chronic vomiting and gastric *Helicobacter* spp, *J Vet Intern Med* 21:1185, 2007.
Meining A, Kroher G, Stolte M: Animal reservoirs in the transmission of *Helicobacter heilmannii*, *Scand J Gastroenterol* 33:795, 1998.
Neiger R, Simpson K: *Helicobacter* infection in dogs and cats: facts and fiction, *J Vet Intern Med* 14:125, 2000.
Simpson K et al: Gastric function in dogs with naturally acquired gastric *Helicobacter* spp. infection, *J Vet Intern Med* 13:507, 1999.
Stolte M et al: A comparison of *Helicobacter pylori* and *H. heilmannii* gastritis: a matched control study involving 404 patients, *Scand J Gastroenterol* 32:28, 1997.

CHAPTER 125

Gastric and Intestinal Motility Disorders

FRÉDÉRIC P. GASCHEN, *Baton Rouge, Louisiana*

The prevalence of canine and feline nonobstructive gastrointestinal (GI) motility disorders cannot be documented precisely. They may go unnoticed by the animal's owner because of subtle clinical signs that are difficult to recognize until the problem is severe. However, these disorders likely are of significant clinical importance. They may result from primary segmental or diffuse inflammatory or neoplastic infiltration of the GI wall. GI motility also may be influenced by a variety of diseases affecting other organs, such as abdominal inflammation (e.g., pancreatitis, postoperative ileus) or diseases such as endocrinopathies, electrolyte abnormalities (e.g.,

hypokalemia, hypocalcemia), and uremic syndrome. Moreover, diseases affecting the autonomous nervous system (e.g., dysautonomia) often significantly affect GI motility.

Most available information on canine and feline GI motility has been obtained from studies using dogs and cats as animal models; only a few studies focus on spontaneous canine and feline GI motility disorders.

In dogs and cats, motility disorders resulting from obstruction of gastric outflow, of the small intestine or colon by foreign bodies, or by space-occupying lesions are a common occurrence. Their diagnosis generally is straightforward, and their treatment is surgical. Therefore they will not be further discussed in this chapter.

Disorders of Gastric Emptying

Physiology

After ingestion of solid food, the gastric antrum acts as a pump from which peristaltic waves originate, while the gastric body acts as a high compliance reservoir. The mechanical action of the antral pump is divided into three phases: (1) propulsion, (2) emptying of fine particles and mixing, and (3) retropulsion of particles larger than 1 mm for continued grinding. In healthy animals, the rate of gastric emptying is modulated by the composition of the diet (e.g., moisture and fat, protein and carbohydrate content) and is under the influence of neural and endocrine factors. Complete emptying of the stomach is followed by synchronized housekeeping contractions (migratory motor complexes [MMC] phase III).

Clinical Signs

Signs associated with disorders of gastric motility in dogs and cats are listed in Box 125-1. However, the signs may be difficult to recognize before the problem becomes severe.

Etiology

Primary Disorders of Gastric Motility

Primary functional disorders appear to be rare in small animals. Slower gastric emptying occurs in dogs following circumcostal gastropexy performed after gastric dilation-volvulus (GDV). Gastric motility is impaired in the fasting and postprandial phases in these dogs (Hall et al, 1992). However, it has not been established whether this abnormal motility is involved in the etiology of GDV or simply a consequence of surgical treatment. The exact role of gastric dysmotility in canine GDV has not been elucidated to date.

Dysautonomia is discussed in further detail later; it also may influence gastric emptying. The diagnosis of duodenogastric reflux (DGR) in dogs has been the subject

of controversy because this reflux may occur as a physiologic event. Moreover, most instances of vomiting are accompanied by some degree of DGR. However, a syndrome characterized by bilious vomiting, often before the morning meal, has been observed in apparently healthy dogs and attributed to DGR. Initial treatment consists of a late evening meal and may require addition of drugs lowering gastric acidity (H_2-receptor antagonist, proton-pump inhibitor) and/or prokinetics.

Secondary Disorders of Gastric Motility

Inflammation of the GI tract or other abdominal organs, abdominal surgery, or metabolic disorders may cause secondary gastric motility abnormalities.

Gastric or Intestinal Inflammation. GI inflammation is a common cause of gastric motility changes. Therefore it is hardly surprising that GI parasites, gastric ulcers, parvovirosis, adverse food reactions, dysbiosis, and inflammatory bowel disease (IBD) often are accompanied by abnormal gastrointestinal motility.

Acute canine pancreatitis also is associated commonly with decreased gastric and intestinal motility. This can complicate treatment significantly and probably is caused by extension of the inflammatory process to stomach and duodenum, which are in close proximity of the pancreas. In a similar manner peritonitis also affects gastric motility, and postoperative ileus is a frequent occurrence (see later).

Diseases Affecting Multiple Organ Systems. Systemic disorders also may affect GI motility. Hypoadrenocorticism often is accompanied by decreased gastric motility. Furthermore, abnormal small intestinal and colonic motility have been shown in dogs with ablation of 66% of renal mass and chronic renal disease, whereas gastric emptying seemed normal. However, it is not known if a larger reduction of functional renal mass, as is observed in clinical cases (>75%), may have negative effects on gastric motility. Finally, delayed gastric emptying may be induced by various medications; opioid analgesics and anticholinergics may interfere with GI neurotransmitters and cause impaired smooth muscle function. Vincristine, a frequently used chemotherapy agent, recently has been shown to decrease gastric antral motility transiently (Tsukamoto et al, 2011).

Diagnostic Approach

A detailed history and physical exam may help identify subtle changes suggestive of GI dysmotility. However, the initial approach of the dog or cat with suspected GI motility disorder consists of first ruling out obstructive GI disease with abdominal radiographs. Presence of food in the stomach after prolonged fasting (i.e., more than 10 to 12 hours) suggests delayed gastric emptying. In addition, an abdominal ultrasound exam may reveal severely decreased gastric and duodenal motility. Once GI obstruction has been ruled out, CBC, chemistry panel, and urinalysis are necessary to look for underlying disorders that may secondarily influence motility.

Evaluation of Gastrointestinal Motility

The various methods available to investigate gastric emptying have been reviewed in detail (Wyse et al, 2003).

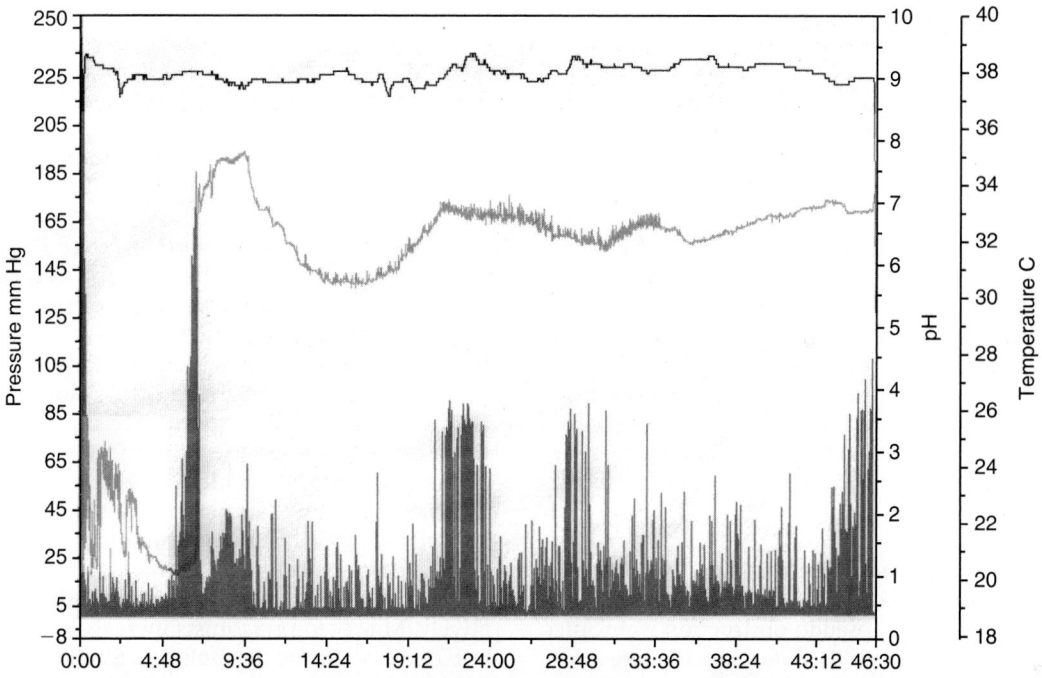

Figure 125-1 Wireless motility capsule recording in a young healthy male mixbreed dog. The top line reflects the temperature (in degrees Celsius), the line below represents the pH, while the bottom line shows the pressure profile (in mm Hg). Time is shown on the X axis (in hours [h] and minutes [min]). The massive rise in pH at 6 h 42 min indicates exit of the capsule from the stomach. The slight decline in pH at 9 h 20 min indicates entry into the large bowel. Gastric emptying time was 6 h 38 min, small bowel transit time was 2 h 38 min, and large bowel transit time was 36 h 57 min.

They aim at evaluating the gastric emptying or intestinal transit time of solid food and include radionuclide scintigraphy, radiographic contrast studies (barium meals and barium impregnated polyethylene spheres, or BIPS), and abdominal ultrasound. Gastric emptying also can be measured using indirect techniques relying on duodenal absorption of compounds that subsequently can be detected in the breath (e.g., ^{13}C-octanoid acid) or in the blood (e.g., acetaminophen). Recently, a wireless motility capsule (SmartPill) has been validated for use in dogs (Boillat et al, 2010) (Figure 125-1).

These noninvasive methods may be very useful, but all have potential pitfalls. Some require special equipment that can be found only at referral centers. Potential exposure of the veterinary staff to radiation may represent a problem. Some techniques can be performed only after the animals have been manually or chemically restrained, a potential source of interference with gastric motility. Radionuclide scintigraphy is recognized as the current gold standard in dogs and cats.

Radiographic studies are accessible in clinical veterinary practice. Liquid barium has been used widely to assess GI transit times. The dose of barium suspension is 6 to 12 ml/kg in dogs and 12 to 16 ml/kg in cats and should be administered when the stomach is empty. Barium sulfate should be present in the duodenum by 15 minutes in the dog and by 5 minutes in the cat. The stomach should be free of barium after 1 to 4 hours in the dog and after 20 minutes in the cat. However, assessment of gastric emptying of liquids is an insensitive technique, with the exception of mechanical obstructions resulting from foreign bodies or other space-occupying lesions obstructing the gastric or intestinal lumen. Mixing barium with food may allow better evaluation of the solid phase of gastric emptying. Unfortunately, barium can dissociate easily from the test meal and cause the study to be unreliable. Barium-impregnated polyethylene spheres (BIPS) have been used for evaluation of GI transit times in dogs and cats. They come in two sizes (1.5- and 5-mm diameter) and can be used easily in practice. However, correlation between gastric emptying of BIPS and the gold standard has been disappointing in dogs and in cats, and the use of these spheres has been limited.

Treatment

Therapy of functional, nonobstructive disorders of gastric motility is based on two main axes: dietary modification and judicious use of prokinetic drugs. Proper diagnosis and treatment of any underlying disease that might affect gastric motility is an essential premise.

Dietary modifications designed to facilitate gastric emptying are based on important facts from digestive physiology. For example, gastric emptying of liquid food is faster than that of solid foods. Diets with high caloric density tend to remain longer in the stomach. Gastric emptying of fat is slower than that of proteins, which is slower than that of carbohydrates. Consequently, feeding liquid or semi-liquid diet of low caloric density, low in fat and protein, should maximize gastric emptying. Increased feeding frequency and small meal size also are useful. In addition, prokinetic drugs may be beneficial in nonobstructive disorders of gastric emptying. Their properties are discussed at the end of this chapter.

Small and Large Intestinal Motility

Physiology

Three physiologic motility patterns are described in the small intestine: peristaltic waves (aboral movement of chyme over long intestinal segments), stationary contractions (leading to intestinal segmentation), and clusters of contraction (mixing and aboral movement of chyme over short segments). Diarrhea usually is associated with the occurrence of pathologic giant aboral contractions. The colon also exhibits several contraction types. The individual phasic contractions and the migrating and nonmigrating motor complexes produce extensive mixing and kneading of fecal material and slow net aboral propulsion. The giant motor complexes (GMC) occur at 10-hour intervals and produce mass movements of feces, ending in defecation.

Primary Disorders of Small or Large Bowel Motility

Primary disorders of small or large bowel motility include dysautonomia, intestinal pseudo-obstruction, chronic constipation, and megacolon. *Dysautonomia* is a rare idiopathic disease affecting the autonomic nervous system that occurs in specific regions such as the midwestern United States, Great Britain, and parts of continental Europe. Feline dysautonomia has been reported from many countries without breed, gender, or age predisposition, and its prevalence has decreased over the last 20 years. Canine dysautonomia affects most frequently young, midsize to large dogs that roam freely in rural areas in the midwestern United States. Toxic, infectious, or immune-mediated causes have been suspected, but the etiology remains unknown. Histopathology reveals widespread degeneration of autonomic neurons and ganglions. Dysautonomia is a systemic disease with dire consequences. GI signs represent only a part of the clinical picture. In dogs, they include vomiting, diarrhea, constipation, tenesmus, and regurgitation (Harkin et al, 2002). In cats, regurgitation and constipation are described as the most frequent GI signs (Sharp et al, 1984). Mortality is 70% in cats and 90% in dogs.

Several reports of *chronic intestinal pseudo-obstruction* have been published. The disorder is defined by the presence of segmental or diffuse chronic intestinal dilatation and dysmotility in the absence of mechanical obstruction. Most animals were diagnosed initially with GI obstruction based on abdominal imaging findings; however, surgery revealed dilated intestinal loops with no obstruction. All dogs were euthanized, but one cat was treated with cisapride and prednisolone and survived. Histopathology revealed fibrosing leiomyositis affecting the small intestinal *tunica muscularis*. No breed or age predilections were reported.

Nonobstructive chronic constipation may occur in older dogs and cats; however, it appears to be most prevalent in the feline species. *Feline idiopathic megacolon* is associated with colonic smooth muscle dysfunction that may be primary or secondary. A detailed discussion of the disease can be found elsewhere (Washabau and Holt, 1999). Prokinetics are an important part of treatment. The existence of a syndrome comparable to IBS in dogs has been a subject of controversy. The term *chronic idiopathic large bowel diarrhea* has been suggested for dogs without histologic evidence of mucosal inflammation. Some of these dogs appear to respond to dietary fiber supplementation, whereas others do not and require behavior-modifying drugs (Lecoindre and Gaschen, 2011).

Secondary Disorders of Small or Large Bowel Motility

Intestinal motility can be affected secondarily by a wide variety of disease processes. *Intestinal inflammation* (enteritis, colitis) may result in shortened transit times. In an experimental model, dogs with acute colitis had a decrease in nonpropulsive motility and an increase in GMCs, resulting in frequent defecation and tenesmus. Decreased nonpropulsive motility may be explained by disturbances of the circular colonic smooth muscle cells associated with inflammation. *Abdominal inflammation* also may delay intestinal motility (e.g., pancreatitis, peritonitis, postsurgical ileus).

Medications also may influence intestinal motility negatively. Mu-receptor agonists increase antral contractions but decrease antral propulsion. Similarly they increase intestinal tone and segmentation but decrease intestinal propulsion. Furthermore, they strengthen the activity of the ileocolic and anal sphincters. The mu-receptor agonist loperamide or diphenoxylate combined with the anticholinergic atropine is used in the treatment of acute episodes of diarrhea. They may lead to dysmotility if administered for more than a few days.

Postoperative ileus (POI) has been documented to occur in humans, dogs, and cats. Four major pathways have been identified:

1. *Neurogenic:* stimulation of inhibitory neural pathways associated with surgical stress
2. *Inflammatory:* stimulation of macrophages and neutrophils upon bowel manipulation, and release of proinflammatory mediators that reduce GI motility
3. *Hormonal:* release of corticotrophin-releasing factor and stimulation of proinflammatory cytokines in the bowel
4. *Pharmacologic:* in particular by the use of exogenous opioids as analgesics and their general inhibitory effect of GI motility

In dogs, POI caused reduced duration of MMC phase III activity and motility index. These changes were reversed after administration of metoclopramide at 0.4 mg/kg IV q6h (Graves et al, 1989). Constant-rate infusion (CRI) of lidocaine (0.025 to 0.05 mg/kg/min IV after loading bolus of 0.5 to 1 mg/kg IV, use low end of doses for cats) during the surgical intervention is thought to decrease the severity of POI because of the drug's antinociceptive, antihyperalgesic, and antiinflammatory properties. However, the current consensus is that lidocaine CRI does not have any direct effect on GI motility.

Prokinetic Drugs

Prokinetic drugs and their mode of action have been reviewed in detail elsewhere (Washabau, 2003) and are summarized in this paragraph and in Table 125-1.

TABLE **125-1**

Mode of Action and Posology of Commonly Used Prokinetics in Small Animals

Name	Mode of Action	Site of Action	Other Effects	Dose*
Metoclopramide	Serotoninergic ($5-HT_4$ receptors)	Pyloric antrum Duodenum (?)	Antiemetic (D_2 receptor antagonist)	0.2-0.5 mg/kg q8h PO, SC CRI: 1-2 mg/kg/24 hr
Cisapride	Serotoninergic (principally $5-HT_4$ receptors)	Lower esophagus (C) LES Pyloric antrum Small intestine Colon		0.1-0.5 mg/kg PO q8-12h
Mosapride (Pronamid, DS Pharma)	Serotoninergic ($5-HT_4$ receptor-specific)	Pyloric antrum		0.5-2 mg/kg PO q12-24h (D) Available only in Japan
Prucalopride (Resolor, Movetis)	Serotoninergic ($5-HT_4$-receptor-specific)	Pyloric antrum Small intestine (?) Colon		0.02-0.6 mg/kg PO q12-24h Available only in Europe
Erythromycin	Motilin analog	Pyloric antrum Small intestine Colon	Antibiotic (at 10-20× higher dose)	0.5-1.0 mg/kg PO q8h
Ranitidine	Acetyl-cholinesterase inhibitor (stimulation of M3 receptors)	Pyloric antrum (small intestine, colon)	H_2-antagonist (decreases gastric acid production)	1-2 mg/kg q12h PO or slowly IV (after dilution)
Nizatidine	Same as ranitidine	Same as raniditine	Same as ranitidine	2.5-5 mg/kg q24h PO

*For dogs and cats, unless otherwise specified.
D, Dog; *GMC,* giant migrating contraction (colon); *LES,* lower esophageal sphincter.

Serotonergic drugs (cisapride, metoclopramide, mosapride, and prucalopride) act on 5-hydroxytryptamine (5-HT) receptors of different types. Metoclopramide (MCP) often is used as an antiemetic for its inhibitory effects on dopamine receptors in the chemoreceptor trigger zone (CRTZ) of the medulla oblongata. MCP acts on $5-HT_3$ receptors (antagonist) and $5-HT_4$ (agonist). These effects stimulate contraction of smooth muscle cells of the stomach and intestine. Cisapride (CSP), another serotonergic drug, binds to $5-HT_4$ receptors and stimulates smooth muscle contractions. CSP was withdrawn from the pharmaceutic market because of its cross-reactivity with serotoninergic receptors in the myocardium and the risk of lethal cardiac arrhythmias in people. It currently is available as a generic substance from compounding pharmacies; however, generic cisapride may not be consistently available in all countries. Mosapride (Pronamid) is a highly selective $5-HT_4$ agonist that has been approved recently for use in dogs in Japan. Its activity has been documented in several studies and appears limited to the pyloric antrum in dogs. However, it may be of benefit in constipated cats. Prucalopride (Resolor) is another highly selective $5-HT_4$ agonist recently approved for use in people in Europe. It has been shown to stimulate gastric contractions in dogs and colonic motility in cats and dogs. *Motilin agonists* include erythromycin (EMC), a macrolide antibiotic with gastrokinetic properties at low doses. EMC triggers MMC phase III, a motility pattern responsible for cleaning the stomach during the interdigestive phase. The administration of EMC stimulates gastric emptying without any attention to particle size. This early release of gastric contents can lead to "dumping" of insufficiently processed food in the small intestine. Furthermore, in cats EMC increases the lower esophageal sphincter pressure. Beside their role in decreasing gastric acid production, ranitidine and nizatidine are *acetylcholinesterase inhibitors* that increase the concentration of acetylcholine in the synaptic cleft between postganglionic myenteric neurons and smooth muscle cells of the stomach and intestine. They stimulate the activity of GI smooth muscle. All other H_2 receptor antagonists lack this prokinetic effect. Domperidone (Motilium) is available in several countries outside the United States. It is a potent antiemetic (D_2 receptor inhibitor). Its prokinetic effects are mediated by antagonism of α_2- and β-adrenoreceptors, but their potency is questioned in dogs and cats.

Other compounds recently have been shown to have prokinetic effects in dogs, but their clinical use has not been established yet. Yohimbine (Yobine) is an α_2-adrenergic receptor antagonist used in reversal of xylazine sedation in dogs. Intravenous doses of 0.5 to 3 mg/kg IV have been shown to induce GMC in dogs (Nagao et al, 2007). This property may be interesting in the treatment of postoperative ileus (see earlier). However, the package insert mentions that doses of 0.55 mg/kg may occasionally induce "brief seizures" and muscle tremors; therefore caution is recommended. It is not known if other α_2-adrenergic receptor antagonists such as atipamezole exert similar direct prokinetic activities. Acotiamide, a novel specific acetylcholinesterase inhibitor, recently has been shown to increase gastric, small intestinal, and colonic motility in dogs after oral administration. Capsaicin is the major pungent ingredient of hot peppers. It has been shown to stimulate the release of peptides, including the prokinetic molecule calcitonin gene-related peptide (CGRP). In dogs, intragastric capsaicin induced contractions in the antrum, small intestine, and colon within 15 minutes. Once in the small bowel, the compound had inhibitory effects on GI motility. Finally, intracolonic application of 5 to 10 mg capsaicin stimulated colonic motility and defecation. Research in new prokinetic agents is ongoing. Dogs likely will be used as an animal model for new substances to be developed in the future.

References and Suggested Reading

Boillat CS et al: Variability associated with repeated measurements of gastrointestinal tract motility in dogs obtained by use of a wireless motility capsule system and scintigraphy, *Am J Vet Res* 71:903, 2010.

Graves GM, Becht JL, Rawlings CA: Metoclopramide reversal of decreased gastrointestinal myoelectric and contractile activity in a model of canine postoperative ileus, *Vet Surg* 18:27, 1989.

Hall JA et al: Gastric emptying of nondigestible radiopaque markers after circumcostal gastropexy in clinically normal dogs and dogs with gastric dilatation-volvulus, *Am J Vet Res* 53:1961, 1992.

Harkin KR, Andrews GA, Nietfeld JC: Dysautonomia in dogs: 65 cases (1993-2000), *J Am Vet Med Assoc* 220:633, 2002.

Lecoindre P, Gaschen FP: Chronic idiopathic large bowel diarrhea in the dog, *Vet Clin North Am Small Anim Pract* 41:447, 2011.

Nagao M et al: Role of alpha-2 adrenoceptors in regulation of giant migrating contractions and defecation in conscious dogs, *Dig Dis Sci* 52:2204, 2007.

Sharp NJH, Nash AS, Griffiths IR: Feline dysautonomia (the Key-Gaskell syndrome): a clinical and pathological study of forty cases, *J Small Anim Pract* 25:599, 1984.

Tsukamoto A et al: Ultrasonographic evaluation of vincristine-induced gastric hypomotility and the prokinetic effect of mosapride in dogs, *J Vet Intern Med* 25:1461, 2011.

Washabau RJ: Gastrointestinal motility disorders and gastrointestinal prokinetic therapy, *Vet Clin North Am Small Anim Pract* 33:1007, 2003.

Washabau RJ, Holt D: Pathogenesis, diagnosis, and therapy of feline idiopathic megacolon, *Vet Clin North Am Small Anim Pract* 29:589, 1999.

Wyse CA et al: A review of methods for assessment of the rate of gastric emptying in the dog and cat: 1898-2002, *J Vet Intern Med* 17:609, 2003.

CHAPTER 126

Current Veterinary Therapy: Antibiotic Responsive Enteropathy

ALBERT E. JERGENS, *Ames, Iowa*

*A*ntibiotic-responsive enteropathy (ARE) denotes a clinical syndrome characterized by acute or chronic diarrhea in animals that responds to antibiotic treatment (Hall, 2011). Well-recognized gastrointestinal (GI) disorders broadly responsive to antibiotics may be found in Box 126-1. Previously, this clinical disorder was termed *idiopathic small intestinal bacterial overgrowth* (SIBO), which implied that an absolute increase in bacterial numbers of the small intestine was responsible for disease pathogenesis. The term ARE is more appropriate than SIBO, given the unreliable nature of culture-dependent assays in quantifying intestinal bacterial numbers and the misunderstanding of what constitutes normal versus abnormal microbial densities and composition mediating GI disease.

Host-Microbiota Interactions in Healthy Animals

The GI tract in dogs and cats is colonized with a vast microbiota that is estimated to range between 10^{12} to 10^{14} organisms from 10 to 12 different bacterial phyla (Suchodolski, 2011). These bacteria play a crucial role in immune system development and help to maintain gut health through regulatory signals delivered to the epithelium that mediate mucosal homeostasis. Major functions of the intestinal microbiota affecting GI health include metabolic activities that cultivate energy and nutrients (e.g., short-chain fatty acids [SCFA], folate, and vitamin K), the trophic effects on intestinal epithelia and immune structure/function (i.e., bacterial-induced

Gastrointestinal Disorders Responsive to Antibiotics

- Infection with enteropathogenic bacteria
- Small intestinal bacterial growth (SIBO)
  - Idiopathic SIBO?
  - Secondary causes of SIBO
- Inflammatory bowel disease (IBD) associated with dysbiosis
  - IBD responsive to metronidazole
- Tylosin-responsive diarrhea
- Granulomatous colitis in boxer dogs

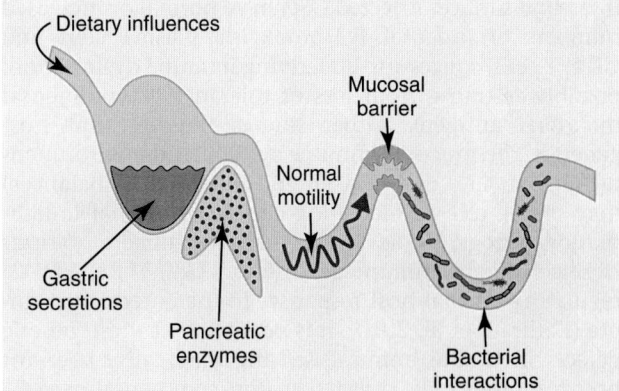

Figure 126-1 Host mechanisms contributing to microbial homeostasis. A variety of factors may affect the numbers and diversity of the gastrointestinal microbiota, including *environmental factors* (diet), *host factors* (gastric acid secretion, pancreatic digestive proteases, normal intestinal peristalsis, functional innate immunity, secretory immunoglobulins), and *bacterial factors* (immune modulation, competition for substrate and binding sites, interaction ["crosstalk"] with enterocytes, production of antibacterial substances).

host gene expression and regulation of T-cell repertoires), and protection against invasion by pathogenic microbes via the production of antimicrobial substances, such as bacteriocins.

Fecal bacterial culture useful for identifying a specific enteric pathogen (e.g., *Campylobacter jejuni*) has given way to culture-independent molecular techniques for in-depth analysis of complex bacterial communities. Contemporary studies using molecular microbiology have determined that the majority (>70%) of the GI microbiota is uncultivable, and composition and total bacterial numbers in different GI segments and luminal contents differ considerably as compared with the mucosa. It now is realized that the composition of gut flora in healthy dogs and cats is distinctly different. Healthy cats were shown to have a large number of total and anaerobic bacteria in the small intestines, which appear to be stable before and after antibiotic (metronidazole) administration (Johnston et al, 2000). A separate investigation similarly found high (10^4 to 10^8 CFU/ml) numbers of obligate anaerobes in the duodenum of cats but showed no differences in bacterial composition between healthy cats and cats with signs of GI disease (Johnston et al, 2001).

Traditional bacterial culture techniques have shown that the canine duodenal microflora typically harbors a bacterial count of greater than 10^5 CFU/ml of duodenal juice; however, significantly higher counts have been observed in some breeds and in dogs with no signs of intestinal disease. Moreover, marked variation in the enteric microbiota may occur among individual healthy dogs and among the intestinal compartments within individual dogs.

Pathogenic Mechanisms

Several different pathogenic mechanisms may contribute to the development of ARE. Aberrant host-microbial interactions have been associated with enteropathogenic bacterial infection, quantitative increases in total microbial numbers (SIBO), imbalances in enteric microbial composition (i.e., dysbiosis), and/or secondary to defects in mucosal barrier integrity (Hall, 2011). Colonization of the GI tract by pathogenic bacteria (i.e., *infectious diarrhea*) may induce gastroenteritis by direct mucosal invasion (e.g., invasive *Salmonella* spp.) or the secretion

of enterotoxins, which are directly injurious to intestinal epithelia (e.g., *Clostridium difficile*) or which stimulate the secretion of fluid and electrolytes (*Clostridium perfringens*), causing secretory diarrhea. Still other bacteria may produce diarrhea in dogs and cats through bacterial attachment to the intestinal epithelial surfaces (i.e., enteroadherent streptococci). Adherent and invasive *Escherichia coli* (AIEC) now are associated with the development of granulomatous colitis in susceptible boxer dogs (Simpson et al, 2006).

Canine SIBO traditionally is defined on the basis of increased numbers of total bacteria in duodenal juice, but controversy exists as to what bacterial quantity constitutes normal. Under physiologic conditions, the bacterial population of the small intestine is controlled by several host mechanisms (Figure 126-1). Although the numeric limits of bacteria found within asymptomatic dogs may vary by breed and within individuals of the same breed, there is general consensus that SIBO may occur secondary to exocrine pancreatic insufficiency, impaired clearance of bacteria (e.g., intestinal obstruction, motility disorder), and morphologic injury to the mucosa (e.g., infiltrative mucosal disease). Increased numbers of intestinal bacteria (i.e., SIBO) may cause malabsorption and diarrhea through (1) competition for nutrients (the bacterial binding of cobalamin, which impairs its intestinal absorption); (2) bacterial metabolism of nutrients into secretory products (e.g., hydroxylated fatty acids, deconjugated bile salts) that promote colonic secretions; and (3) biochemical injury to the intestinal brush border, which decreases enzyme activity causing maldigestion (Hall, 2011).

Antibiotic-responsive diarrhea also may develop secondary to *disrupted barrier function*, *aberrant mucosal immunity*, or *qualitative changes in the intestinal microbiota* (i.e., dysbiosis). Studies show that some dogs (i.e., German shepherd dogs [GSD]) with ARE have selective IgA deficiency caused by a defect in IgA secretion at the small intestinal surface. Affected GSD have normal or increased numbers of mucosal IgA-producing plasma cells and CD4+ T cells, suggesting underlying immune dysfunction, possibly resulting from loss of tolerance to commensal microbial antigens. Other studies indicate that host genetics, the mucosal immune system, and environmental factors (i.e., diet and enteric microbial imbalances) may play a role in mediating chronic intestinal inflammation in dogs. Studies in GSD have identified mutations in select innate immune genes (i.e., TLR2, TLR5, NOD2) regulating normal host responses to the enteric microbiota (Kathrani et al, 2010). It is possible that these genetic defects in innate immune sensing may cause aberrant host responses to be directed against commensal bacteria as if they were pathogens. Molecular studies have shown imbalances in microbial abundance and composition (i.e., enriched mucosal association with members of *Enterobacteriaceae* and *Clostridiaceae*) in diseased intestines of dogs with chronic enteropathy, including inflammatory bowel disease (IBD) (Suchodolski et al, 2010). Increased numbers of mucosal-associated Enterobacteriaceae also have been associated with clinical signs, up-regulated cytokine expression, and histopathologic lesions in cats with IBD (Janeczko et al, 2008).

Specific Gastrointestinal Disorders Responsive to Antibiotics

Enteropathogenic Bacterial Infection

A variety of bacterial enteropathogens (e.g., *Clostridium difficile*, *Clostridium perfringens*, *Salmonella* spp., *Campylobacter jejuni*, and *Escherichia coli* causing granulomatous colitis in boxers) may cause enteritis or enterocolitis in dogs and cats. Diagnosis of bacterial enteritis is particularly troublesome for clinicians because of the high prevalence of most of these bacteria in healthy animals and the technical difficulties related to successful isolation and identification of pathogenic species. Several of these bacteria (e.g., *C. jejuni*, *Salmonella* spp.) have important zoonotic implications.

Clinical Findings
Animals with bacterial-associated diarrhea may present with clinical signs of small or large intestinal disease or both. Clinical signs are not pathognomonic for a specific bacterial species and they may vary considerably (i.e., from mild, self-limiting diarrhea to fatal hemorrhagic diarrhea) with the same infection in different animals. Large-bowel diarrhea is observed most frequently with active infection. Physical findings often are normal with the exception of rectal examination, which confirms diarrhea, mucoid feces, and fresh blood.

Diagnosis
Diagnostic strategies for bacterial enterocolitis vary but may include fecal culture, fecal cytology, detection of fecal toxins, ELISA for detection of bacterial antigens, and/or molecular testing (i.e., fecal RT-PCR). Cytologic examination of fecal smears is easy and may be useful to detect bacteria with specific morphology (i.e., curved rod appearance of *Campylobacter* spp.), *C. perfringens*

TABLE 126-1

Treatment Options for Antibiotic-Responsive Enteropathy

GI Disorder	Antibiotic	Dosage
Campylobacteriosis	Erythromycin	(D) 10-15 mg/kg PO q8h
		(C) 10 mg/kg PO q8h
	Tylosin	10 mg/kg PO q8h
C. perfringens infection	Metronidazole	(D) 10 mg/kg PO q12h
		(C) 62.5 mg PO q12h
	Amoxicillin-clavulanic acid	12.5-22 mg/kg PO q12h
SIBO/idiopathic ARE	Oxytetracycline	10-20 mg/kg PO q8h
	Metronidazole	10 mg/kg PO q12h
	Tylosin	10 mg/kg PO q8h
Idiopathic IBD	Metronidazole	10 mg/kg PO q8h
	Tylosin	10 mg/kg PO q8h
Tylosin-responsive diarrhea in dogs	Tylosin	25 mg/kg PO q24h
Granulomatous colitis in boxer dogs	Enrofloxacin	5-10 mg/kg PO q24h for 6 weeks

ARE, Antibiotic-responsive enteropathy; *D,* dogs; *C,* cats; *GI,* gastrointestinal; *IBD,* inflammatory bowel disease; *PO,* by mouth; *SIBO,* small intestinal bacterial overgrowth.

endospores, or increased fecal leukocytes suggestive of active infection. A summary of the most useful diagnostic tests for enteropathogenic bacteria include the following:

- *C. jejuni:* fecal culture
- *C. difficile:* toxin testing by ELISA and organism detection (i.e., culture, antigen ELISA, or RT-PCR)
- *C. perfringens:* enterotoxin ELISA
- *Salmonella:* fecal culture

Diagnostic panels in which feces are screened for multiple organisms may be most cost effective and detect coinfections (Weese, 2011).

Treatment
Treatment recommendations for enteropathogens are largely empiric. For clostridial infections, metronidazole is a convenient and useful antibiotic choice (Table 126-1). Campylobacteriosis in animals with clinical signs may be treated with erythromycin or fluoroquinolone antibiotics. Antibiotic use in salmonellosis is controversial and is indicated only in animals with severe GI disease. The efficacy of probiotics or prebiotics as adjunctive treatments for infectious diarrhea remains unclear.

Small Intestinal Bacterial Overgrowth

The original culture-dependent techniques for determination of small intestinal bacterial overgrowth (SIBO) (i.e., $\geq 10^5$ total CFU/ml or $\geq 10^4$ anaerobic CFU/ml) revealed results of questionable validity. Now it is realized that much higher numbers of enteric bacteria are present in clinically healthy dogs and cats. It is reasonable to assume that GI disorders that diminish host defenses via decreased intestinal motility, decreased gastric acid secretion, or exocrine pancreatic function (e.g., exocrine pancreatic insufficiency [EPI]) may favor bacterial proliferation and the development of secondary SIBO. SIBO is a well-recognized complication of EPI in dogs unresponsive to enzyme supplementation alone.

Clinical Findings
Clinical signs in dogs with SIBO include small intestinal diarrhea characterized as watery, fetid, and of large volume, which may be accompanied by alterations in appetite and weight loss. Clinical signs involving extra-pancreatic disorders besides EPI reflect the primary organ of involvement.

Diagnosis
A definitive diagnosis of SIBO is difficult because quantification of bacterial numbers is flawed and indirect tests for microbial growth/metabolism are unreliable (German et al, 2003). Serum cobalamin is the most useful assay because it may detect distal small intestinal (i.e., ileum) disease and the need to treat for this vitamin deficiency. A presumptive diagnosis of SIBO may be made by ruling out other causes for chronic small bowel diarrhea and by showing resolution of clinical signs following antibiotic administration.

Treatment
The primary treatment for secondary SIBO is correction of the underlying disorder causing enteric microbial imbalances. Bacterial alterations should be assumed polymicrobial and treated with a broad-spectrum antibiotic such as oxytetracycline, metronidazole, or tylosin, which have good efficacy against anaerobic bacteria. The optimal duration of therapy is unknown, but 4 to 6 weeks of antibiotic treatment generally is recommended.

Inflammatory Bowel Disease Associated with Dysbiosis

Idiopathic IBD likely results from complex interplay between the mucosal immune system and environmental factors (including the enteric microbiota) in a genetically susceptible host. Direct interaction of the intestinal microbiota with components of the innate immune system is believed to evoke pathologic host responses and intestinal inflammation in humans and animals.

Alterations in microbial abundance and composition characterized by reductions in microbial diversity and increased mucosa-associated Enterobacteriaceae have been associated with IBD in dogs and cats (Suchodolski et al, 2010; Janeczko et al, 2008). It is unknown whether these noninvasive microbial perturbations are a cause or consequence of chronic immune-mediated intestinal inflammation.

Clinical Findings
Clinical signs in affected animals include chronic vomiting, diarrhea, inappetence, or weight loss, and the clinical course may be progressive or intermittent with periodic flares.

Diagnosis
A diagnosis of IBD is one of exclusion and includes careful integration of patient history, physical examination findings, diagnostic testing to detect GI versus non-GI diseases, and intestinal biopsy for histopathology. Molecular studies for microbial abundance (i.e., 454 pyrosequencing of the 16S rRNA bacterial gene) and mucosal association (i.e., fluorescence *in situ* hybridization [FISH] performed on endoscopic biopsy specimens) have demonstrated microbial imbalances in association with histopathologic inflammation in the intestines of dogs and cats with IBD.

Treatment
Treatment for IBD is aimed at reducing mucosal inflammation and correcting microbial imbalances contributing to disease pathogenesis. In general, an approach using sequential treatment with diet, select antibiotics, and/or glucocorticoids has proven successful in most case studies. Metronidazole (MTZ) may be used along with steroids or immunosuppressive drugs in animals having moderate-to-severe clinical disease.

Tylosin-Responsive Diarrhea in Dogs

The term tylosin-responsive diarrhea (TRD) refers to a specific diarrheal syndrome in dogs that responds to tylosin therapy within a few days (Westermarck et al, 2005). In TRD, the stool remains normal as long as treatment continues, but diarrhea may reappear several weeks after discontinuing the antibiotic. Most affected dogs are young to middle-aged and are medium-sized to giant breeds. The etiology of the diarrhea remains unknown.

Clinical Findings
Dogs with TRD usually have large bowel diarrhea characterized by increased frequency of defecation, mucus, and fresh blood in the feces. Physical findings are unremarkable.

Diagnosis
A diagnosis of TRD is made on rapid resolution of GI signs following the administration of tylosin.

Treatment
Tylosin administered at 25 mg/kg once daily for 7 days has proven effective in one study (Kilpinen et al, 2011). Intermittent drug therapy may be required in some dogs having recurring GI signs. Long-term diarrhea may be controlled using daily doses of 25 mg/kg.

Granulomatous Colitis

AIEC is involved in the pathogenesis of granulomatous colitis in susceptible boxer dogs as well as some other breeds. Identification and appropriate antibiotic therapy are effective in resolution of the disease in most cases (see Chapter 134).

References and Suggested Reading

German AJ et al: Comparison of direct and indirect tests for small intestinal bacterial overgrowth and antibiotic-responsive diarrhea in dogs, *J Vet Intern Med* 17:33, 2003.

Hall E: Antibiotic-responsive diarrhea in small animals, *Vet Clin North Am Small Anim Pract* 41:273, 2011.

Janeczko S et al: The relationship of mucosal bacteria to duodenal histopathology, cytokine mRNA, and clinical disease activity in cats with inflammatory bowel disease, *Vet Microbiol* 128:178, 2008.

Johnston KL et al: Effects of oral administration of metronidazole on small intestinal bacteria and nutrients of cats, *Am J Vet Res* 61:1106, 2000.

Johnston KL et al: Comparison of the bacterial flora of the duodenum in healthy cats and cats with signs of gastrointestinal tract disease, *J Am Vet Med Assoc* 218:48, 2001.

Kathrani A et al: Polymorphisms in the TLR4 and TLR5 gene are significantly associated with inflammatory bowel disease in German shepherd dogs, *PLoS ONE* 5:e15740, 2010.

Kilpinen S et al: Effect of tylosin on dogs with suspected tylosin-responsive diarrhea: a placebo-controlled, randomized, double-blinded, prospective clinical trial, *Acta Vet Scand* 53:26, 2011.

Simpson K et al: Adherent and invasive *Escherichia coli* is associated with granulomatous colitis in boxer dogs, *Infect Immun* 74:4778, 2006.

Suchodolski JS et al: Molecular analysis of the bacterial microbiota in duodenal biopsies from dogs with idiopathic inflammatory bowel disease, *Vet Microbiol* 142:394, 2010.

Suchodolski JS: Companion animals symposium: microbes and gastrointestinal health of dogs and cats, *J Anim Sci* 89:1520, 2011.

Weese JS: Bacterial enteritis in dogs and cats: diagnosis, therapy, and zoonotic potential, *Vet Clin North Am Small Anim Pract* 41:287, 2011.

Westermarck E et al: Tylosin-responsive chronic diarrhea in dogs, *J Vet Intern Med* 19:177, 2005.

CHAPTER **127**

Cobalamin Deficiency in Cats

KENNETH W. SIMPSON, *Ithaca, New York*
PAUL A. WORHUNSKY, *Ithaca, New York*

Gastrointestinal disease may decrease the availability of a number of micronutrients, such as vitamins and minerals, with important consequences for the pathogenesis, diagnosis, and treatment of gastrointestinal disease. Measuring the serum concentration of cobalamin (CBL) aids in the detection of gastrointestinal disease, guides therapeutic intervention, and informs prognosis in cats.

Cobalamin Absorption

Metabolism of CBL in cats is very different from that in people. CBL homeostasis is a complex, multistep process that involves participation of the stomach, pancreas, intestines, and liver (Figure 127-1).

After ingestion, CBL is released from food in the stomach. It then is bound to a nonspecific CBL-binding protein of salivary and gastric origin called haptocorrin. Intrinsic factor (IF), a CBL-binding protein that promotes CBL absorption in the ileum, is produced by the pancreas, not the stomach, in cats. In contrast, humans produce only gastric IF, and deficiency usually is associated with atrophic gastritis and the resultant lack of gastric IF production. The affinity of CBL for haptocorrin is high at acid pH, so most CBL is bound to haptocorrin in the stomach. Upon entering the duodenum, haptocorrin is degraded by pancreatic proteases, and CBL is transferred from haptocorrin to IF, a process facilitated by the high affinity of IF for CBL at neutral pH. Cobalamin-IF complexes traverse the intestine until they bind to specific receptors (previously called intrinsic factor cobalamin receptor [IFCR] but recently dubbed cubilin) located in the microvillus pits of the apical brush-border membrane of ileal enterocytes. CBL then is transcytosed to the portal bloodstream bound to a protein called transcobalamin 2 (TC II), which mediates CBL absorption by target cells. A portion of CBL taken up by hepatocytes is thought to be reexcreted rapidly in bile bound to haptocorrin. CBL of hepatobiliary origin, in common with dietary-derived CBL, is thought to undergo transfer to IF and receptor-mediated absorption, thus establishing enterohepatic recirculation of the vitamin. This situation of rapid turnover means that cats with CBL malabsorption can deplete totally their body CBL stores within 1 to 2 months. The half-life of exogenous parenteral CBL was 13 days in healthy cats as compared with 5 days in cats with GI disease. This is completely different from people, in whom CBL depletion may take several years, possibly because of the presence of long-term storage enabled by the CBL-binding protein TCI, which is absent in cats.

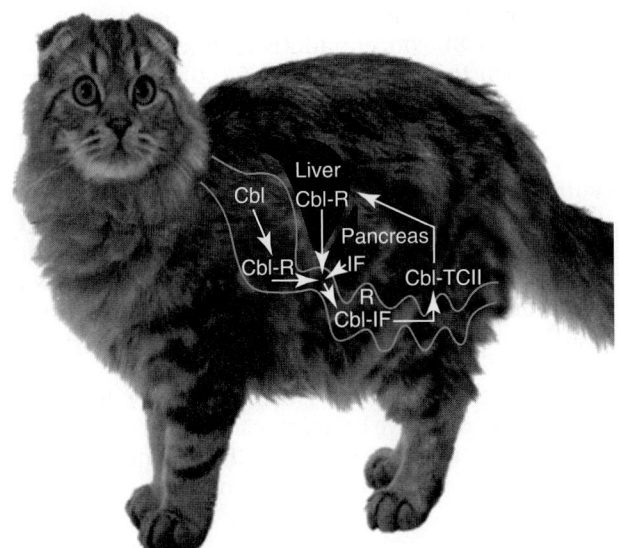

Figure 127-1 The pathway of cobalamin absorption involving the gastrointestinal tract, pancreas, and liver. *Cbl,* Cobalamin; *Cbl-R,* cobalamin bound to haptocorrin; *Cbl-IF,* cobalamin bound to intrinsic factor; *Cbl-TCII,* cobalamin bound to transcobalamin 2; *IF,* intrinsic factor.

TABLE **127-1**

Factors Influencing Serum Concentrations of Cobalamin in Cats

Increase	Decrease
High dietary content	Dietary deficiency
Parenteral supplementation	Inflammatory bowel disease
*Cholestatic liver disease	Alimentary lymphoma (multicentric lymphoma†)
	Exocrine pancreatic insufficiency
	Pancreatitis*
	Cholangitis*
	Hyperthyroidism*
	Intestinal bacterial utilization†
	Receptor abnormality†

*Recognized disease association, pathomechanism unclear.
†Theoretic cause not adequately documented in cats.

Serum concentrations of CBL are labile and reflect the balance between dietary intake, bacterial use and production, intestinal absorption, and body losses. Factors influencing serum CBL in cats are summarized in Table 127-1.

Measurement of Serum Cobalamin

CBL can be measured using a bioassay, radioimmunoassay (RIA), or an Immulite assay. The bioassay was the original method used and has been shown to correlate with RIA. In the RIA method an assay must be used that denatures endogenous CBL-binding proteins, usually by boiling the sample. The Immulite assay also has been shown to correlate with the RIA. Hemolyzed blood samples also affect test performance.

Interpretation of Serum Cobalamin Concentrations

Normal reference ranges for CBL in cats may differ greatly between laboratories. This can have a substantial impact on diagnosing the presence of subnormal CBL and determining the prevalence of subnormal CBL in cats (see below).

The interpretation of circulating CBL concentrations with regard to small intestinal disease is valid only if exocrine pancreatic insufficiency, dietary CBL supplementation, or parenteral administration has been excluded. Furthermore, dietary vitamin content of the diet warrants attention. Finding a low CBL concentration is useful in supporting the presence of an intestinal disorder. When low CBL is detected and exocrine pancreatic insufficiency (EPI), intestinal obstruction, or a stagnant loop has been excluded, localization of the problem to the ileum can be inferred. Simultaneous evaluation of CBL and folate do not distinguish reliably the type of intestinal disease in cats. Concomitant increases in folate and CBL are most consistent with high dietary intake, supplementation, and hemolysis. The authors have observed high CBL concentrations in some cats with cholestatic liver disease in the absence of parenteral supplementation. Finally, normal serum concentrations of CBL neither exclude nor support a diagnosis of intestinal disease.

Diseases Associated with Subnormal Serum Cobalamin

Gastrointestinal Disease

Subnormal serum CBL concentrations have been reported most frequently in middle-aged cats presented for investigation of suspected gastrointestinal disease. Predominant clinical findings associated with low serum CBL concentration are weight loss, diarrhea, vomiting, anorexia, lethargy, and thickened intestines. Low serum CBL was linked to body condition score and abnormalities in hematologic and serum biochemical variables such as increased mean corpuscular volume (MCV) and reduced serum phosphorous in some studies (Reed, Gunn-Moore, and Simpson, 2007; Simpson et al, 2001). The types of gastrointestinal disease associated with subnormal serum CBL concentrations include inflammatory bowel disease (IBD), intestinal lymphoma, cholangiohepatitis or cholangitis, pancreatitis, and exocrine pancreatic insufficiency. This diverse spectrum of diseases is thought to reflect the involvement of pancreas, intestine, and liver in feline CBL homeostasis as depicted in Figure 127-1.

The prevalence of low serum CBL reported in cats with signs of gastrointestinal disease ranges from 0.1% to 78%. This large variation is potentially a consequence of the assay used, the reference intervals for normal values, the patient population, and the geographic location. In single-disease studies, prevalence of low CBL concentration is particularly high in cats with EPI (10/10 evaluated) and 78% of 32 cats with GI lymphoma. In the first study to examine CBL deficiency in cats, 49 out of 80 cats (61%) had a serum CBL concentration below the reference range (900 to 2800 pg/ml; mean ± SD = 1775 ± 535 pg/ml SD; n = 33) using a RIA that correlated with the bioassay (Simpson et al, 2001). Conversely, in a recent British study only 11 out of 39 cats (28.2%) had a CBL concentration below the reference range (290 pg/ml) using an Immulite assay (Maunder et al, 2012). To examine the source of this variability, the authors reanalyzed the original data set from U.S. cats using the 290 pg/ml cutoff. This yielded a prevalence of 27%. Given the correlation between the RIA and Immulite assays, this suggests that differences in reference ranges between different studies using validated CBL assays have a major impact on the identification of cats with subnormal CBL concentrations. The cause of this variation in reference intervals (e.g., age of cats, presence or absence of occult GI disease, and geographic location [northern vs. southern United States, or Australia vs. United Kingdom]) remains to be determined.

Nongastrointestinal Disease

Low serum CBL recently has been described in cats with hyperthyroidism. Whether hyperthyroidism alone or with concurrent GI disease is responsible for low levels remains to be determined. In people and dogs multicentric lymphoma has been associated with low CBL. This may reflect use of CBL by rapidly dividing cells. Whether this occurs in cats has not been determined.

Relationship Between Low Serum Cobalamin and Cobalamin Deficiency

CBL is an essential cofactor for the activity of methylmalonyl-CoA mutase and methionine synthase. In people, reduced activity of these two enzymes causes the biochemical signatures of CBL deficiency, methylmalonicacidemia/methylmalonicaciduria (MMA) and homocysteinemia/homocysteinuria. Cats with undetectable or subnormal serum CBL concentrations have increased serum concentrations of MMA but not homocysteine. In one study, 68% of cats with a CBL less than 290 pg/ml had elevated MMA concentrations but normal homocysteine. Cats with elevated MMA also had substantial disturbances in amino acid metabolism, compared with healthy cats, with significantly increased serum concentrations of methionine (133.8 versus 101.1 μmol/L) and significantly decreased serum concentrations of cystathionine (449.6 versus 573.2 nmol/L) and cysteine (142.3 versus 163.9 μmol/L). Furthermore, treatment of CBL-deficient cats having high MMA concentrations with parenteral CBL resulted in a reduction in MMA concentrations and weight gain. Cats with the largest decrease in MMA concentration gained the most weight.

These studies illustrate that measurement of serum CBL is a useful marker of GI disease and that treatment of cats with CBL deficiency diagnosed on the basis of elevated MMA is of therapeutic benefit. Because MMA is not measured routinely in most clinical laboratories, it would be of practical value to know the serum CBL concentration at which CBL deficiency develops (i.e., the

point at which cats would benefit from treatment with parenteral CBL). Initial studies conducted in cats with subnormal CBL concentrations (defined as <290 pg/ml) have shown that a serum CBL of 160 ng/L or less has a 74% sensitivity and 80% specificity for detecting MMA greater than 867 nmol/L (Ruaux, Steiner, Williams, 2009). However, MMA has not been correlated with CBL concentrations outside of this range; this is important, given that the normal lower reference range limit of 290 is significantly lower than 900 pg/ml reported by others. From a clinical perspective it would be useful to know the spectrum of GI disease associated with CBL deficiency and the impact of CBL deficiency on clinicopathologic variables, but this has not been determined. In people, diseases such as renal failure, cholestatic liver disease, and diabetes mellitus have been associated with high MMA in the face of normal or elevated CBL concentrations. This possibility has not been explored in cats.

Treatment

In the absence of clear guidelines on the serum concentration of CBL that predicts CBL deficiency and the lack of adverse affects associated with CBL supplementation, most clinicians choose to treat all cats with subnormal CBL concentrations. Treatment recommendations are based largely on knowledge of the half-life of parenteral CBL in cats with GI disease (approximately 5 days) and measurement of serum CBL after supplementation. Current recommendations are to administer cyanocobalamin 0.25 to 0.5 mg q14d SC or IM. The interval between doses can be extended by a week if serum CBL concentration is within the reference range 14 days after administration. Further interval extension would be determined by measurement of serum CBL before the next dose. In the authors' experience most cats with low CBL require long-term CBL therapy despite treatment of their underlying disease.

References and Suggested Reading

Barron PM et al: Serum cobalamin concentrations in healthy cats and cats with non-alimentary tract illness in Australia, *Aust Vet J* 87(7):280, 2009.

Carmel R: Biomarkers of cobalamin (vitamin B-12) status in the epidemiologic setting: a critical overview of context, applications, and performance characteristics of cobalamin, methylmalonic acid, and holotranscobalamin II, *Am J Clin Nutr* 94(1):348S, 2011.

Cook AK et al: The prevalence of hypocobalaminaemia in cats with spontaneous hyperthyroidism, *J Small Anim Pract* 52(2):101, 2011.

Ibarrola P et al: Hypocobalaminaemia is uncommon in cats in the United Kingdom, *J Feline Med Surg* 7(6):341, 2005.

Kiselow MA et al: Outcome of cats with low-grade lymphocytic lymphoma: 41 cases (1995-2005), *J Am Vet Med Assoc* 232(3):405, 2008.

Maunder CL et al: Serum cobalamin concentrations in cats with gastrointestinal signs: correlation with histopathological findings and duration of clinical signs, *J Feline Med Surg* 14(10):686, 2012.

Reed N, Gunn-Moore D, Simpson K: Cobalamin, folate and inorganic phosphate abnormalities in ill cats, *J Feline Med Surg* 9(4):278, 2007.

Ruaux CG, Steiner JM, Williams DA: Early biochemical and clinical responses to cobalamin supplementation in cats with signs of gastrointestinal disease and severe hypocobalaminemia, *J Vet Intern Med* 19(2):155, 2005.

Ruaux CG, Steiner JM, Williams D: Metabolism of amino acids in cats with severe cobalamin deficiency, *Am J Vet Res* 62(12): 1852, 2001.

Ruaux CG, Steiner JM, Williams DA: Relationships between low serum cobalamin concentrations and methylmalonic acidemia in cats, *J Vet Intern Med* 23(3):472, 2009.

Simpson KW et al: Subnormal concentrations of serum cobalamin (vitamin B12) in cats with gastrointestinal disease, *J Vet Intern Med* 15(1):26, 2001.

Thompson KA et al: Feline exocrine pancreatic insufficiency: 16 cases (1992-2007), *J Feline Med Surg* 11(12):935, 2009.

CHAPTER 128

Probiotic Therapy

CRAIG B. WEBB, *Fort Collins, Colorado*
JAN S. SUCHODOLSKI, *College Station, Texas*

The popularity of probiotics as an adjunct therapy in the treatment of diarrhea in humans also has raised the interest in their use in small animal gastroenterology. A critical appraisal of the human literature tempers the expectations, if not the enthusiasm, for the applicability of probiotics to patients with a number of conditions. However, solid clinical evidence supports the use of probiotics in some specific human diseases, and strong theoretic arguments advocate this burgeoning area of research in veterinary medicine. Regardless of the research, a recent study showed that up to 26% of dogs presented to veterinarians for diarrhea end up on alternative therapies such as probiotics (German, Halladay, and Noble, 2010). Of importance to the selection of probiotics is the fact that the majority of available products do not meet minimum quality standards (Weese and Martin, 2011). Furthermore, the health effects of probiotics are strain specific (i.e., not all strains of bacterial species have the same functional characteristics). Therefore knowing the probiotic strain designation and dosage is critical to compare products and to be able to link the strains to clinical studies published in the literature.

Definition

As defined by the World Health Organization, probiotics are "live microorganisms which when administered in adequate amounts confer a health benefit on the host" (FAO/WHO, 2001). Key components to this current definition are that the microorganisms are alive and that they are administered in sufficiently high amounts. Theoretically any bacterial strain that fulfills this definition can be classified as a probiotic. The microorganisms found most frequently in various products are lactic acid bacteria (i.e., *Lactobacillus* spp., *Enterococcus* spp., *Streptococcus* spp., and *Bifidobacterium* spp.). These traditionally have been associated with health benefits, although probiotic products feature a range of bacteria and yeasts (e.g., *Escherichia coli* strain Nissle 1917, *Bacillus coagulans, Saccharomyces boulardii*).

Many products on the market now are offered as a combination of probiotics and prebiotics (undigestible food ingredients added to diets to stimulate the growth of native probiotic bacteria). In such a case the product is named a symbiotic. The U.S. Food and Drug Administration does not regulate probiotics, and currently no governing agency oversees quality control, product content, or label claims.

Intestinal Microbiota

The intestinal microbiota constitutes a highly complex ecosystem composed of several hundreds to thousands of phylotypes. The total microbial load in the intestine is estimated to contain 10^{12} to 10^{14} microbial cells. This bacterial population represents a huge degree of antigenic diversity containing approximately 100 times as many genes as the host genome. The microbiota is absolutely essential to the physiologic development and function of the GI tract. Studies of the GI tract in germ-free rodents show a decrease in vascularity, digestive enzyme concentration, and muscle wall thickness, decreased cytokine and immunoglobulin production, reduced lymphocyte numbers, and abnormal development of Peyer patches when compared with conventionally raised animals. In addition to normal development, the microbiota plays a key role in maintaining immunologic homeostasis within the GI tract, protecting the mucosa from pathogenic bacteria, and when necessary, coordinating the immunologic and inflammatory response to commensal and pathogenic organisms. It is this range of properties, central to maintaining GI health and function, that make the microbiota such a potent target for therapeutic intervention in cases of GI disease.

Mechanism of Action

Proper selection of probiotics requires an understanding that every bacterial strain, even if it is derived from the same bacterial species, can be different in its phenotypic, functional, and immunologic properties. This is one reason for the disparity in clinical reports: one study may report that a specific bacterial species caused clinical disease, whereas another study suggests that this same bacterial species may have beneficial properties. For example, *Bifidobacterium animalis* AHC7 significantly reduced duration of diarrhea in dogs (Kelley et al, 2009), whereas *B. animalis* ATCC 25527(T) caused duodenitis in interleukin-10–deficient mice (Moran et al, 2009). How probiotic strains impart beneficial effects remains poorly understood. Some probiotic strains have been shown to modulate the immune system and, in doing so, enhance IgA production and pathogen phagocytosis as well as stimulate the release of a variety of antiinflammatory cytokines. Other probiotic strains help restore or normalize the function of a leaky mucosal barrier and reduce abnormal intestinal permeability. Probiotics help protect the normal microbiota from pathogenic bacteria through the production of antimicrobial substances called bacteriocins and through competitive exclusion of pathogens by preventing adhesion, occupying binding sites, or consuming vital nutrients. Recent studies suggest that probiotics have no appreciable effect on the overall composition of the intestinal microbiota but are able to alter its metabolic function (Garcia-Mazcorro et al, 2011; McNulty et al, 2011).

To impart a health benefit to the host, a probiotic must be able to survive passage into the gut, be able to adhere to epithelial cells, and be able to proliferate within the GI tract. Even those probiotic strains that fulfill these criteria appear to colonize the GI tract for only relatively brief periods of time and usually are eliminated within a few days after the end of administration. Therefore, if the goal of therapy is to have a long-term impact on the patient, long-term daily administration of probiotics in high doses is required. Interestingly, colonization with probiotic strains does not occur in a subset of animals, most likely because of interindividual differences in microbiota composition at baseline that lead to competitive exclusion of probiotic strains and therefore potentially therapeutic failure.

Current Knowledge

Current Human Literature

A survey of the human literature regarding the use of probiotics in patients with gastrointestinal disease appears to support the principle that certain probiotic strains have the ability to affect positively the clinical outcome of patients. These outcomes are defined as the prevention, the treatment, or the maintenance of remission of certain specific diseases. Again, these results appear to depend on the specific disease, the probiotic strain employed, and the number of organisms administered. For example, the probiotic strains *Lactobacillus rhamnosus* GG and *Bifidobacterium lactis* BB-12 have been used successfully to prevent and treat acute rotavirus diarrhea in children. Specific probiotic strains appear useful as a prophylactic treatment to avoid antibiotic-associated diarrhea and to decrease the signs of *C. difficile* infection, whereas other strains frequently are used to prevent or treat "travelers' diarrhea." *L. rhamnosus* GG delayed the onset of pouchitis in postoperative ulcerative colitis patients, and *E. coli* Nissle 1917 helped maintain remission for patients with the same condition. Further studies in human patients are addressing the question of whether single-strain or multispecies probiotics are more likely to be beneficial. The potential advantages of multispecies probiotics (containing strains that belong to one or more bacterial genera; for example, different *Lactobacillus* and *Bifidobacterium* spp.) include the greater possibility that at least one species will colonize the gut and that each strain may have different probiotic properties, leading to synergistic effects. A well-described probiotic for human use is VSL#3, which contains a mixture of eight probiotic strains (a total of 450 billion live bacteria, including *Lactobacillus* spp., *Bifidobacterium* spp., and *Streptococcus thermophilus*). In cases of ulcerative colitis, VSL#3 treatment resulted in a significantly greater number of patients achieving remission and a decrease in the Ulcerative Colitis Disease Activity Index compared with a placebo group (Turcotte and Huynh, 2011).

Current Veterinary Literature

Because of the current paucity of studies specifically directed at the use of probiotics in companion animals, the veterinary profession must draw much of what is known from the human literature. Other sources of potentially relevant information include *in vitro* studies. For example, some studies demonstrate that specific probiotic strains inhibit the growth of pathogens or studies in animal models, which shows a beneficial effect against *Salmonella* spp., an organism of obvious interest for veterinary patients.

A number of studies also have been performed in healthy dogs to confirm the passage and survival of several potential probiotic bacteria as well as document some of the potential benefits of probiotic administration already discussed. However, the most relevant studies, those that examine probiotic supplementation in patients with signs of gastrointestinal disease, are few.

In a large, double-blind, placebo-controlled study of shelter animals, significantly fewer cats (7.4% vs. 20.7% in the placebo group) that received *Enterococcus faecium* SF68 (2.1×10^9 CFU/day) developed diarrhea for greater than a 2-day duration (Bybee, Scorza, and Lappin, 2011). A randomized, double-blind, placebo-controlled trial demonstrated that administration of a multispecies probiotic containing *Lactobacillus acidophilus* MA 64/4E, *Lactobacillus farciminis*, *Bacillus subtilis*, *Bacillus licheniformis*, and *Pediococcus acidilactici* significantly shortened the duration of acute diarrhea in dogs from 48 to 24 hours when given approximately 4.2×10^9 cfu/10 kg three times daily (Herstad et al, 2010). Similarly, administration of *Bifidobacterium animalis* strain AHC7 (at 2×10^{10} per day) to dogs with acute idiopathic diarrhea significantly reduced the time to resolution by $2\frac{1}{2}$ days and decreased the percentage of dogs that required adjunctive use of metronidazole (38.5% vs. 50.0% in the placebo group) (Kelley et al, 2011).

Less data are available about the clinical use of probiotics in animals with infectious organisms or chronic enteropathies. *Enterococcus faecium* SF68 (5×10^8 CFU twice daily) given to dogs with naturally acquired giardiasis failed to reduce fecal shedding or antigen content and did not increase fecal IgA concentration or leukocyte phagocytic activity compared with treatment with a placebo (Simpson et al, 2009). In a prospective double-blind, randomized placebo-controlled study, dogs with food-responsive diarrhea were treated with an elimination diet and either a probiotic cocktail containing three *Lactobacillus* spp. strains or placebo (Sauter et al, 2006). Probiotic administration failed to show a clinical benefit beyond the substantial improvement seen in both groups presumed to be due to the use of an elimination diet.

Recommendations for Probiotic Selection

Probiotics quickly are becoming an integral part of the therapeutic plan for many cats and dogs presenting to veterinarians for diarrhea. Owners often are aware of this nutraceutical approach. In a recent open-label study of a multistrain product, 70% of cat owners reported improvement in their pets' clinical condition with supplementation of multispecies probiotic (Proviable-DC, 5×10^9 CFU/day for 21 days; Hart et al, 2012). Currently, specific recommendations for the use of particular probiotic products are beyond our level of understanding in veterinary medicine. Several general principles, however, can be used to guide probiotic therapy in cats and dogs with gastrointestinal disease. When choosing a particular probiotic product, clinicians must consider that the organisms are alive and that they are administered at sufficiently high doses to compensate for losses during passage through the GI tract and competitive exclusion by the resident microbiota. The product should contain a probiotic strain that has shown beneficial effects in clinical studies, and the product should be administered at the dose as reported. It is crucial to select a product with a known strain designation to be able to link it to published studies. Providing a proper dosage for probiotics is difficult, because no dose-response studies have been performed in clinical patients. Based on the review of veterinary literature, doses between 5×10^8 and 2×10^{10} have been used and shown to have clinical benefits. By comparison, in a recent trial of the multispecies probiotic VSL#3 in adults with ulcerative colitis, the prescribed dosage was 3.6×10^{12} bacteria per day (Sood et al, 2009).

Significant discrepancies have been found between the claims made on the label of commercially available probiotic products and actual ingredients in the product; only a few selected probiotics from reputable manufacturers met the standard quality criteria (Weese and Martin, 2011).

Different probiotics likely have differing levels of efficacy in different diseases and with individual patients; therefore the success or failure of one probiotic strain in a particular patient does not predict its efficacy in other patients. Perhaps probiotics should be species specific (i.e., the probiotic strain has been isolated from the same animal species that it will be used in); however, no clear data support this assumption. Studies have shown that probiotic strains of human origin can adhere to intestinal mucosa of dogs and other species. Furthermore, probiotic strains derived from humans or dogs have shown beneficial effects in other animal species.

Probiotics probably are best suited for cases of acute diarrhea and stress-related diarrhea and may work particularly well as a prophylactic for cases at risk of developing antibiotic-associated diarrhea. Probiotics also may be useful in younger patients suspected of having viral diarrhea or that undergo stressful periods because of weaning or home transitions. For such cases it seems prudent to use probiotics in a prophylactic fashion and start administration a few weeks ahead of the event. Although not many studies have been performed in animals with chronic enteropathies, based on human studies probiotics likely may be useful as an adjunct to standard therapy until disease remission occurs. Furthermore, in such chronic diseases, long-term administration may beneficially influence the immune system.

Fortunately, as with many nutraceuticals, probiotic administration seems to have minimal adverse side effects, but it is best to avoid probiotic use in significantly immunocompromised patients. Probiotics, like any other bacteria, can be either susceptible or resistant to concurrently administered antibiotics. For the prevention of antibiotic-associated diarrhea, antibiotics and probiotics are prescribed concurrently. Generally, many probiotic strains are resistant to commonly used antibiotics, but clinicians should contact the manufacturers to obtain information about the susceptibility patterns of their products.

References and Suggested Reading

Bybee SN, Scorza AV, Lappin MR: Effect of the probiotic *Enterococcus faecium* SF68 on presence of diarrhea in cats and dogs housed in an animal shelter, *J Vet Intern Med* 25:856, 2011.

FAO/WHO Expert Consultation: *Health and nutritional properties of probiotics in food including powder milk with live lactic acid bacteria*. Report of a Joint FAO/WHO Expert Consultation, American Córdoba Park Hotel, Córdoba, Argentina, October 2001.

Garcia-Mazcorro JF et al: Effect of a multi-species synbiotic formulation on fecal bacterial microbiota of healthy cats and dogs as evaluated by pyrosequencing, *FEMS Microbiol Ecol* 78:542, 2011.

German AJ, Halladay LJ, Noble PJ: First-choice therapy for dogs presenting with diarrhea in clinical practice, *Vet Rec* 21:810, 2010.

Hart ML et al: Open-label trial of a multi-strain synbiotic in cats with chronic diarrhea, *J Fel Med Surg*, 14(4):240, 2012.

Herstad HK et al: Effects of a probiotic intervention in acute canine gastroenteritis—a controlled clinical trial, *J Small Anim Pract* 51:34, 2010.

Kelley RL et al: Clinical benefits of probiotic canine-derived *bifidobacterium animalis* strain AHC7 in dogs with acute idiopathic diarrhea, *Vet Ther* 10:121, 2009.

McNulty NP et al: The impact of a consortium of fermented milk strains on the gut microbiome of gnotobiotic mice and monozygotic twins, *Sci Transl Med* 3:106, 2011.

Moran JP et al: *Bifidobacterium animalis* causes extensive duodenitis and mild colonic inflammation in monoassociated interleukin-10-deficient mice, *Inflamm Bowel Dis* 15:1022, 2009.

Sauter SN et al: Effects of probiotic bacteria in dogs with food responsive diarrhoea treated with an elimination diet, *J Anim Physiol Anim Nutr* 90:269, 2006.

Simpson KW et al: Influence of *Enterococcus faecium* SF68 Probiotic on giardiasis in dogs, *J Vet Intern Med* 23(3):476, 2009.

Sood A et al: The probiotic preparation, VSL#3 induces remission in patients with mild-to-moderately active ulcerative colitis, *Clin Gastroenterol Hepatol* 7:1202, 2009.

Turcotte JF, Huynh HQ: Treatment with the probiotic VSL#3 as an adjunctive therapy in relapsing mild-to-moderate ulcerative colitis significantly reduces ulcerative colitis disease activity, *Evid Based Med* 16:108, 2011.

Weese JS, Martin H: Assessment of commercial probiotic bacterial contents and label accuracy, *Can Vet J* 52:43, 2011.

CHAPTER 129

Protozoal Gastrointestinal Disease

JODY L. GOOKIN, *Raleigh, North Carolina*
MICHAEL R. LAPPIN, *Fort Collins, Colorado*

Tritrichomonas foetus

Dietary trials, homeopathic remedies, corticosteroids, and most classes of antimicrobial drugs have been ineffective in ameliorating signs of diarrhea or eliminating *T. foetus* from infected cats (Foster et al, 2004; Gookin et al, 2010). Trichomonads generally are susceptible to the effects of 5-nitroimidazoles, because the organisms use anaerobic metabolic pathways that reduce these drugs to cytotoxic nitro anions capable of disrupting protozoal DNA. Prevalent resistance of feline *T. foetus* to metronidazole is presumed on the basis of common treatment failures with this drug, which has prompted investigation of related 5-nitroimidazoles such as tinidazole and ronidazole for treatment of the infection (Gookin et al, 1999, 2006; Kather et al, 2007). Tinidazole at high doses fails to consistently eradicate the infection from experimentally infected cats (Gookin et al, 2007) and has not been rewarding for treatment of naturally infected cats.

Ronidazole

Ronidazole (RDZ) is the only antimicrobial for which convincing efficacy for treatment of *T. foetus* infection has been demonstrated both *in vitro* and *in vivo* (Gookin et al, 2006). Pharmacokinetic studies of RDZ after oral administration to healthy cats demonstrate rapid drug absorption, high bioavailability, and a slow elimination half-life

consistent with once-a-day dosing recommendations (LeVine et al, 2011). Experientially, RDZ has a narrow margin of safety between the minimum therapeutic dose and minimum toxic dose, leading to strict recommendations that cats be treated with 30 mg/kg administered orally once a day. It is recommended that cats be treated for a maximum of 14 days; however, the possibility that shorter durations of treatment may be equally effective has not been examined. The most common adverse effect of RDZ is dose-dependent neurotoxicity that ranges in severity from lethargy and inappetence to ataxia and seizures (Rosado et al, 2007). The most common preventable causes of toxicity are the administration of higher-than-recommended doses of RDZ and continued administration of RDZ despite subtler signs of toxicity. RDZ should be avoided in cats with systemic illness that could confound recognition of adverse drug effects and should not be given to pregnant or nursing queens or their unweaned kittens. RDZ is not registered for human or veterinary use in the United States. Therefore treatment with RDZ should be considered only in cases of confirmed *T. foetus* infection, in which informed consent has been obtained. Several pharmacies compound chemical grade RDZ for veterinary use. Because of its foul taste and undetermined stability, compounding into gelatin capsules rather than flavored liquids is recommended. Several drug formulations for treatment of birds can be obtained online without prescription from pigeon supply

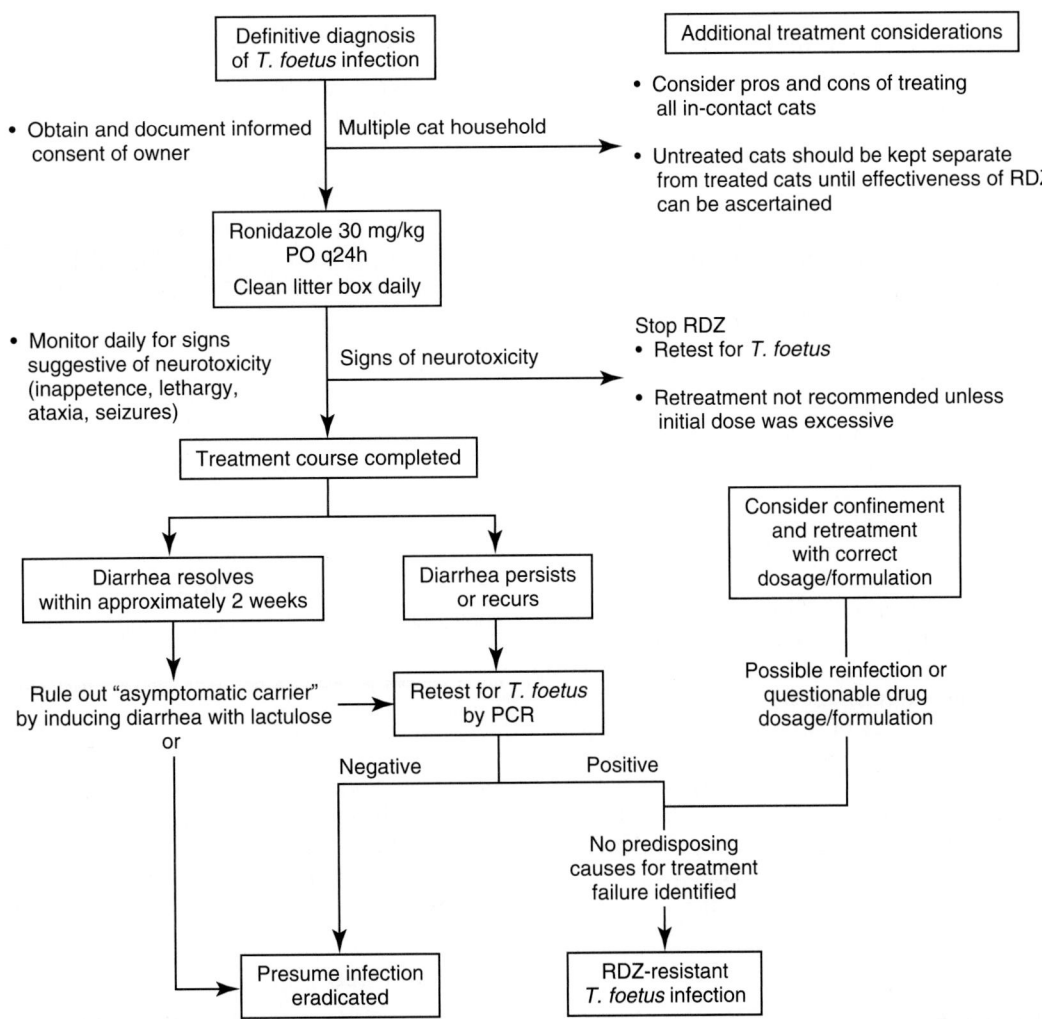

Figure 129-1 Approach to therapy and outcome assessment in cats receiving ronidazole (RDZ) for treatment of *T. foetus* infection.

warehouses. Because of their undetermined quality, composition, and low active-drug concentration, these products are not recommended.

Establishing Treatment Efficacy

Determining whether RDZ has eradicated or merely concealed *T. foetus* infection in any given cat remains an area of frustration (Figure 129-1). If diarrhea persists or recurs at 2 weeks or more after completion of RDZ, the author recommends that cats be retested for *T. foetus* by means of PCR performed on a fecal sample collected by the colon saline flush technique (www.JodyGookin.com). If this test result is negative in a cat with diarrhea, then persistent infection is considered unlikely. Repeat testing with confirmatory negative results would further support this conclusion. The greatest difficulty arises in confidently ruling out persistent infection in a cat that no longer has diarrhea after treatment with RDZ. In the author's experience, periods of asymptomatic infection are not uncommon in *T. foetus*–infected cats and can be difficult to diagnose. In cases in which confirmation of *T. foetus* eradication is particularly relevant (e.g., reintroduction of a treated cat into a cattery), the author treats the cat with lactulose "to

effect" to induce a soft diarrhea and then tests a colon saline flush sample for *T. foetus* by means of PCR. Negative test results in this instance would come as close as possible to confirming the absence of infection.

Causes and Prevention of Treatment Failure

Treatment failure with RDZ should be established by reconfirmation of *T. foetus* infection and not presumed on the basis of failure to resolve diarrhea. Many cats with persistent or recurrent diarrhea after treatment no longer have *T. foetus* infection. The cause of diarrhea and its clinical course in these cats remains undocumented. In such cases a search for other infectious and noninfectious causes of diarrhea may be warranted, as well as empiric treatment with fenbendazole for occult parasitism. If *T. foetus* infection is confirmed, three possibilities must be considered:

1. The cat was not effectively administered the recommended dose, duration, or formulation of RDZ. Treatment of cats with gel capsule–compounded pure RDZ at the recommended dosage typically prevents any second-guessing about drug quality and delivery.

2. Treatment failure could be attributed to reinfection during or after treatment with RDZ. A common misconception is that asymptomatic cats are not infected with *T. foetus*. When presumably uninfected cats are allowed contact with cats that later fail treatment with RDZ, reinfection (whether likely or unlikely) can never be ruled out. This possibility can be prevented by confining *T. foetus*–infected cats during treatment and until their treatment outcome can be assessed.

3. Treatment failure can be attributed to infection with a strain of *T. foetus* that is resistant to RDZ (Gookin et al, 2010). The prevalence of RDZ-resistant *T. foetus* infection in cats is unknown but is suspected to be significant. Although resistance can be documented in the laboratory, it can be assumed if treatment failure is observed in a cat that receives the appropriate dosage of RDZ and has not been exposed to other cats during or after treatment. In the author's experience, higher doses, more frequent administration, or longer durations of treatment with RDZ have been ineffective in eradicating *T. foetus* from such cats and directly increase the risk of neurotoxicity. The high level of existing clinical resistance of feline *T. foetus* to metronidazole, low efficacy of tinidazole, and documentation of resistance to ronidazole in some cats are consistent with a high level of cross-resistance to 5-nitroimidazole drugs among feline *T. foetus*. The current lack of alternative drugs with clinical efficacy against feline *T. foetus* infection suggests that active investigation of other treatment approaches is warranted.

Ramifications of Not Treating

When left untreated, 23 out of 26 (88%) cats with *T. foetus* infection were reported to undergo spontaneous resolution of diarrhea within 2 years (median 9 months; range 5 months to 2 years) (Foster et al, 2004); however, most remained infected based on PCR results when retested as long as 2 to 5 years after initial diagnosis. The role of these "asymptomatic carriers" in disease transmission is unclear; however, such cats can undergo a full relapse of clinical trichomonosis as long as 6 or more years after onset of clinical remission. Accordingly, any cat harboring *T. foetus* should be considered a liability for transmission of infection, and detection of such cats for the sake of preventing disease transmission appears warranted. At present no evidence or studies have been conducted to examine for any long-term adverse health effects of asymptomatic *T. foetus* infection in the cat.

Giardia Species

Although there are many *Giardia* spp., *Giardia duodenalis* (syn. *Giardia intestinalis* or *Giardia lamblia*) is the species that infects people, dogs, and cats. Based on genetic analyses, there are at least seven distinct assemblages (A through G) within *G. duodenalis*. Assemblage A has been amplified from feces of infected humans, dogs, and cats as well as many other mammals. Assemblage B most commonly is amplified from feces of humans but also is amplified occasionally from dog feces. Overall, most dogs

TABLE 129-1

Drugs Used for the Treatment of *Giardia* Species Infections

Drug	Species	Dosage
Albendazole	B	15 mg/kg q12h PO for 2 days (less commonly used because of bone marrow toxicity)
Febantel, pyrantel, praziquantel	C	Label dose for 3 days
	F	Feline dose: 56 mg/kg (based on the febantel) q24h PO for 5 days
Fenbendazole	B	50 mg/kg q24h PO for 3-5 days
Ipronidazole	C	126 mg/L of water ad libitum PO for 7 days
Metronidazole	B	15-25 mg/kg q12-24h PO for 5-7 days
Tinidazole	C	44 mg/kg q24h PO for 3 days
	F	30 mg/kg q24h PO for 3 days

B, Canine and feline; *C,* canine; *F,* feline.

are infected with the species-specific assemblages C and D, and cats are infected with assemblage F (Scorza et al, 2012). Although assemblages A and B occasionally infect dogs and cats, whether these *Giardia* spp. commonly are transmitted to people from dogs or cats is unknown.

Giardia Therapy

Giardia spp. have specific antimicrobial sensitivity patterns like bacteria; therefore predicting which anti-*Giardia* drug will be effective in individual dogs or cats is impossible. Because *Giardia* spp. of dogs and cats can be difficult to cultivate, little *in vitro* susceptibility test result information is available. Although multiple drugs have been used for the treatment of giardiasis in dogs and cats, few studies used dose titrations and evaluation of drugs in experimentally infected animals. In most studies, fecal samples were assessed only for short periods of time after treatment, and immune suppression was not induced to evaluate whether infection was eliminated or merely suppressed. Infection with *Giardia* spp. does not appear to cause permanent immunity and so reinfection can occur, a finding that also hampers assessment of treatment studies.

Treatment options currently available or used historically for dogs or cats with diarrhea suspected to be from *Giardia* spp. infection include albendazole, febantel/pyrantel/praziquantel, fenbendazole, furazolidone, ipronidazole, metronidazole, quinacrine, ronidazole, and tinidazole (Table 129-1). Newer drugs being studied or those with minimal information available for dogs and cats include azithromycin, nitazoxanide, paromomycin, and secnidazole.

If spore-forming rods morphologically consistent with *Clostridium perfringens* are detected concurrently with *Giardia* spp. on assessment of fecal cytology in dogs or cats with diarrhea, administration of metronidazole is indicated because this drug is an antibiotic with activity against *C. perfringens*. In cats, metronidazole benzoate is preferred to metronidazole USP because it is better tolerated by most cats. Ipronidazole, ronidazole, secnidazole, and tinidazole are other drugs within this class that have been used for the treatment of giardiasis in dogs or cats. Ipronidazole added to the drinking water could be considered if a large number of dogs were affected clinically. Ronidazole was used recently with hygiene management to control giardiasis in a dog kennel (Fiechter, Deplazes, and Schnyder, 2012). However, ronidazole is one of the only effective treatments for *T. foetus* infections in cats, and resistance already is recognized. Thus reserving ronidazole for treatment of confirmed *T. foetus* cases may be prudent. Tinidazole should be considered as a secondary *Giardia* spp. treatment for dogs and cats if metronidazole is not tolerated, but optimal protocols are not known. Secnidazole was evaluated in one small study of cats with minimal recognized toxicity (elevated liver enzyme activity in one cat) and apparent efficacy after one dose. However, further data should be collected before routinely using this drug.

If clinical evidence such as eosinophilia suggests concurrent nematode infestation, albendazole, febantel/pyrantel/praziquantel, and fenbendazole may be the most effective anti-*Giardia* drugs. Albendazole has been associated with bone marrow suppression in some dogs and cats, so some clinicians avoid use of this drug. Febantel/pyrantel/praziquantel is licensed for treatment of *Giardia* spp. infection in dogs of some countries and can be effective when administered daily for 3 days (Montoya et al, 2008). This combination also has been studied in small numbers of experimentally infected cats (Scorza, Radecki, and Lappin, 2006). Data from an experimental model suggested that the combination of febantel with pyrantel is synergistic (Olson and Heine, 2009). Many clinicians currently prescribe fenbendazole once daily for 5 days as initial therapy for dogs or cats with diarrhea and *Giardia* spp. because of minimal expense and wide safety margin.

Giardia spp. can have resistant patterns; therefore, if the first drug fails to clear the infection (cysts) or resolve the diarrhea, a second drug from an alternate class is indicated. Some clinicians currently recommend the concurrent administration of metronidazole and fenbendazole (www.capcvet.org). Others resort to combination therapy only in cases of evidence of a persistent infection not cleared by monotherapy.

Azithromycin was used successfully in the management of giardiasis in one dog (Zygner et al, 2008). Paromomycin has anti-*Giardia* properties but has been absorbed across the gastrointestinal (GI) epithelium and has been associated with reversible acute renal failure in cats. Nitazoxanide is labeled for the treatment of giardiasis and cryptosporidiosis in humans in some countries and has been studied in some dogs and cats, but optimal protocols for the treatment of giardiasis are unknown. In addition, nitazoxanide commonly is associated with vomiting in dogs and cats. The author (MRL) administers nitazoxanide at 10 mg/kg q12h PO with food for 7 days for the treatment of dogs or cats with small bowel diarrhea and coinfections with *Giardia* spp. and *Cryptosporidium* spp. Longer duration of therapy is required for some dogs and cats.

Supplemental Management Strategies

The addition of fiber to the diet may help control clinical signs of giardiasis in some animals by helping with bacterial overgrowth or by inhibiting organism attachment to microvilli. Feeding a restricted fat diet also may be effective. In one study, administration of the probiotic *Enterococcus faecium* SF68 (FortiFlora) lessened *Giardia* spp. shedding in mice when fed before infection and enhanced *Giardia* spp. immune responses. In contrast, administration of this probiotic to dogs with chronic subclinical giardiasis had no measureable effect on cyst shedding (Simpson et al, 2009). In a current study by the author (MRL), dogs with acute diarrhea housed in shelters had faster speed to response if this probiotic was administered with metronidazole than if metronidazole was administered alone; many of these dogs were infected with *Giardia* spp.

In one study, bathing the dog on the last day of treatment was a beneficial adjunct therapy. In dogs and cats with persistent diarrhea and *Giardia* spp. infection, a more extensive workup to attempt to diagnose other underlying diseases is indicated if several therapeutic trials fail to control the diarrhea. Common underlying disorders include cryptosporidiosis, *T. foetus* in cats, inflammatory bowel disease, bacterial dysbiosis, exocrine pancreatic insufficiency, and immunodeficiencies.

Treatment Outcomes

The primary goal of *Giardia* spp. treatment is to stop diarrhea. It is controversial whether to treat healthy dogs and cats with *Giardia* spp. cysts in feces. Healthy pets generally are not considered significant human health risks by the Centers for Disease Control (www.cdc.gov/hiv/pubs/brochure/oi_pets.htm), because infection can recur rapidly or not be cleared, and because all drugs have side effects. For example, in Lappin's recent study of naturally infected dogs, approximately 50% of dogs had adverse events associated with treatment, and more than 60% of treated dogs were still infected with *Giardia* spp. when rechecked 34 days after treatment. However, because clinical signs induced by *Giardia* spp. can be intermittent and some *Giardia* spp. may be zoonotic, treatment of healthy infected animals should be considered with each owner. If treatment is deemed indicated by the clinician and owner, many clinicians currently recommend that a 5-day course of fenbendazole be administered for apparently healthy dogs and cats that test positive for *Giardia* spp. cysts in feces. After treatment, if the animal is healthy and negative for cysts, retesting is not indicated again until the next scheduled fecal flotation. *Giardia* spp.–infected dogs or cats should not be tested for *Giardia* spp. antigen in feces because it is unknown how long positive assay results persist.

A common question is how to manage dogs or cats that have normal stool and are *Giardia* spp. antigen positive, *Giardia* spp. cyst negative. These animals have a low-grade infection, or a low percentage of animals (approximately 2% to 5%) have false-positive antigen test results. To further evaluate for cyst shedding, the veterinarian can perform an IFA test or two additional fecal flotations (three negative centrifugal flotation assays run within 5 days is considered adequate to rule out a *Giardia* spp. infection in animals and humans); if these other test results are negative, the antigen test was likely falsely positive. If cysts still are identified after fecal centrifugal flotation performed 2 to 4 weeks after appropriate administration of a drug with anti-*Giardia* activity, then a second course of therapy may be indicated using a drug from an alternate class. It is not recommended that apparently well animals be treated beyond two courses of therapy (www.capcvet.org). No further diagnostics are indicated until GI signs occur or the animal is again due for routine fecal screening (once to twice annually as a minimum for all dogs and cats).

Prevention of Giardiasis

Prevention of *Giardia* spp. infection involves boiling or filtering of water collected from the environment before drinking and disinfection of premises contaminated with infected feces with steam cleaning or quaternary ammonium compounds (1 minute contact time). Transport hosts should be controlled, and treatment and bathing of all animals in the environment could be considered. Feces from infected animals should be removed from the environment promptly. To date, no study has shown the *Giardia* spp. vaccines licensed for dogs and cats to have lessened *Giardia* spp. infections in the field, so both vaccines have been discontinued.

References and Suggested Reading

Fiechter R, Deplazes P, Schnyder M: Control of *Giardia* infections with ronidazole and intensive hygiene management in a dog kennel, *Vet Parasitol* 187:93, 2012.

Foster DM et al: Outcome of cats with diarrhea and *Tritrichomonas foetus* infection, *J Am Vet Med Assoc* 225:888, 2004.

Gookin JL et al: Diarrhea associated with trichomonosis in cats, *J Am Vet Med Assoc* 215:1450, 1999.

Gookin JL et al: Documentation of *in vivo* and *in vitro* aerobic resistance of feline *T. foetus* isolates to ronidazole, *J Vet Intern Med* 24:1003, 2010.

Gookin JL et al: Efficacy of ronidazole for treatment of feline *Tritrichomonas foetus* infection, *J Vet Intern Med* 20:536, 2006.

Gookin JL et al: Efficacy of tinidazole for treatment of cats experimentally infected with *Tritrichomonas foetus*, *Am J Vet Res* 68:1085, 2007.

Kather EJ, Marks SL, Kass PH: Determination of the in vitro susceptibility of feline *Tritrichomonas foetus* to 5 antimicrobial agents, *J Vet Intern Med* 21:966, 2007.

LeVine DN et al: Ronidazole pharmacokinetics after intravenous and oral immediate-release capsule administration in healthy cats, *J Fel Med Surg* 13:244, 2011.

Montoya A et al: Efficacy of Drontal Flavour Plus (50 mg praziquantel, 144 mg pyrantel embonate, 150 mg febantel per tablet) against *Giardia* sp in naturally infected dogs, *Parasitol Res* 103:1141, 2008.

Olson ME, Heine J: Synergistic effect of febantel and pyrantel embonate in elimination of *Giardia* in a gerbil model, *Parasitol Res* S135, 2009.

Rosado TW et al: Neurotoxicosis in 4 cats receiving ronidazole, *J Vet Intern Med* 21:328, 2007.

Scorza AV et al: Comparisons of mammalian *Giardia duodenalis* assemblages based on the β-giardin, glutamate dehydrogenase and triose phosphate isomerase genes, *Vet Parasitol* 189(2-4):182, 2012.

Scorza AV, Radecki SV, Lappin MR: Efficacy of a combination of febantel, pyrantel, and praziquantel for the treatment of kittens experimentally infected with *Giardia* species, *J Feline Med Surg* 8:7, 2006.

Simpson KW et al: Influence of *Enterococcus faecium* SF68 probiotic on giardiasis in dogs, *J Vet Intern Med* 23:476, 2009.

Zygner W et al: Azithromycin in the treatment of a dog infected with *Giardia intestinalis*, *Pol J Vet Sci* 11:231, 2008.

CHAPTER 130

Canine Parvoviral Enteritis

JULIA K. VEIR, *Fort Collins, Colorado*

Cause and Pathogenesis

Parvoviruses are single-strand, nonenveloped DNA viruses. Because of their lack of an envelope, they are extremely environmentally hardy and resistant to disinfection. Until the late 1970s, feline panleukopenia was the major disease associated with parvoviral infection in small animal medicine, and canine parvovirus-1 (CPV-1) was a relatively nonpathogenic virus most commonly associated with illness in neonatal dogs. However, after the emergence of canine parvovirus-2 (CPV-2) from a carnivore parvovirus (likely cats, mink, or other closely related hosts) the infectious enteritis associated with CPV-2 infection became a significant disease in dogs. Canine parvovirus-2 evolved in a relatively short time into two variants, CPV-2a and CPV-2b, both of which are geographically widespread and associated with similar clinical signs and significant pathogenicity. CPV-2b is capable of infecting and causing disease in the cat; therefore cross-species exposure of ill animals should be avoided. A new variant, CPV-2c, was reported first in Italy in 2000, with subsequent reports of detection in the United States starting in 2005. This newer variant is related closely to CPV-2a and CPV-2b and therefore should, in theory, be similar in pathogenicity and virulence. Some anecdotal reports indicate failure of current vaccines to protect adequately from disease associated with CPV-2c; however, most published reports suggest adequate protection.

Diagnosis

Diagnosis is based on presence of the appropriate clinical syndrome and, ideally, demonstration of recent parvoviral infection.

Clinical Syndrome

Inoculation most often occurs via the fecal-oral route; large numbers of viral particles are shed in the feces of infected animals. Because of the tremendous environmental hardiness of the virus, fomites and contaminated environmental surroundings are a major source of infection. After ingestion of viral particles by the host, the virus replicates in the lymphoid tissue of the tonsils, oropharynx, and intestinal tract and then progresses to viremia, occurring approximately 3 days after inoculation. During the viremic phase, signs of systemic illness such as fever, malaise, and lethargy may be present, along with fecal shedding. Progression of infection to rapidly dividing cells, such as those found in the intestinal crypts

and bone marrow, occurs 5 to 7 days after inoculation. As a result, damage to the intestinal tract becomes severe enough to cause the hemorrhagic diarrhea and vomiting characteristic of CPV enteritis in the dog. Intestinal hypermotility is common, and animals should be monitored closely for development of intussusceptions, a potentially fatal complication.

Leukopenia is a consistent clinical finding in infected animals. Neutropenia and lymphopenia are a result of direct infection and destruction of white cell lines in the bone marrow; however, lymphocyte counts frequently rebound in the face of persistent neutropenia. This is explained in part by the continued demand for neutrophils in the gastrointestinal tract as well as direct viral effect on the bone marrow.

Less consistent secondary findings in the hematologic and biochemical picture are anemia and thrombocytopenia, often associated with loss and consumption in the gastrointestinal tract. In theory, direct infection of the bone marrow can contribute as well, but the impact is less severe than on the white blood cell line. Biochemical findings are also more commonly a consequence of the body's reaction to infection rather than direct viral effect. Hypoglycemia can occur secondary to poor glycogen reserves of young animals with concurrent decreased oral intake of nutrients as well as sepsis secondary to bacterial translocation across the severely compromised gastrointestinal mucosa. Electrolyte abnormalities (i.e., hyponatremia, hypokalemia, and hypochloremia) are a result of the protracted vomiting and diarrhea and concurrent dehydration and metabolic acidosis.

Demonstration of Recent Parvoviral Infection

The most clinically useful method of detection of virus in the ill animal is via point-of-care enzyme-linked immunosorbent assays (ELISAs). These assays detect viral antigen in feces or rectal swabs and results are relatively sensitive and specific; however, false negatives and false positives can occur. False negatives can occur with infection of any CPV-2 variant secondary to relatively low concentrations of viral particles because of either decreased shedding in the later stages of the disease or dilutional effects from voluminous diarrhea. The impact of infection with CPV-2c on point-of-care ELISA results is controversial at this time. There are reports of CPV-2c causing clinical disease but negative point-of-care ELISA results. However, other studies have demonstrated similar results using such assays for CPV-2c as for CPV-2a and -2b (Decaro et al, 2010). Preliminary work in the author's laboratory has identified three animals in a series of 49

533

dogs with a clinical diagnosis in which CPV was not detected in feces using point-of-care ELISAs, but CPV was detected using quantitative polymerase chain reaction (PCR). All three of these isolates were later determined to be the CPV-2c variant (Veir, unpublished data). However, because a complete history and clinical illness were not available for all of these animals, the same reasons for any false negative may be the cause. In another study, there was no statistical difference in the sensitivity of a point-of-care ELISA for detection of CPV-2b and CPV-2c (Markovich et al, 2012). False positives have been reported in association with recent vaccination with modified live parvoviral diseases. One manufacturer of point-of-care assays has an unpublished study demonstrating lack of reaction after vaccination in a group of 60 beagles vaccinated with modified live parvoviral vaccines (MLV). In a study performed in the author's laboratory of 12 puppies vaccinated with a MLV parvoviral vaccine, feces from one puppy produced a positive result on a point-of-care ELISA 5 days after vaccination (Burton et al, 2008).

With the advent of PCR "panels" available from major diagnostic laboratories, PCR may be used more commonly in the diagnosis of CPV enteritis. Unfortunately, qualitative PCR using whole blood was frequently positive in the above study of 12 puppies as soon as 2 days after vaccination and continued until the study end point at 14 days after vaccination. The author's laboratory has attempted to decrease the frequency of false positives caused by recent vaccination via PCR using quantitative, instead of qualitative, PCR assays. Using samples from the same 12 puppies and an additional 8 naturally infected puppies positive for CPV using a point-of-care ELISA, a significantly higher viral load was detected via quantitative PCR in the naturally infected group (Veir et al, 2009). Although not yet commercially available, qPCR may prove useful in differentiating naturally infected and recently vaccinated animals. Virus isolation, hemagglutination inhibition, and electron microscopy can be used to demonstrate recent infection; however, because of the turnaround time, these often are reserved for confirmation of disease or in group health situations.

Treatment

Supportive and Symptomatic Care

Maintenance of hydration is at the core of supportive care because severe ongoing fluid losses resulting from vomiting and diarrhea are common in CPV enteritis. Intravenous crystalloids (e.g., lactated Ringer's solution [LRS], Normosol-R, Plasmalyte) are the preferred replacement fluids for the overwhelming majority of cases. At presentation, many animals are severely dehydrated; therefore absorption of fluids from the subcutaneous space is impaired. Intravenous access improves care tremendously, but if peripheral vasoconstriction prevents placement of an intravenous catheter, an intraosseous catheter allows for fluid replacement until peripheral vasoconstriction is corrected and intravenous access is restored. Once dehydration is corrected, attention must be paid to electrolyte balance and glucose levels. Hypokalemia is common and at minimum, maintenance fluids should be supplemented to a level of 20 mEq/L. If hypokalemia is present or develops in the face of fluid therapy, additional supplementation based on tables available in veterinary texts is recommended. Some authors suggest supplementing all maintenance fluids with 2.5% to 5% dextrose regardless of levels; however, in the author's hospital, dextrose is not added commonly to maintenance fluids unless glucose levels start to trend toward the lower end of the reference intervals. For ease of fluid rate adjustment, a maintenance bag of fluids with electrolyte supplementation and, if used, dextrose supplementation is run at a calculated maintenance rate to account for baseline needs and insensible losses. A second bag of a plain, nonsupplemented crystalloid fluid then is used to replace sensible losses (most commonly gastrointestinal losses, estimated by nursing staff on an hourly basis; more frequently if animal is critically ill) over the following hour.

Oncotic Support

The fluids lost in CPV enteritis can be high in protein; therefore hypoproteinemia can develop in affected animals. The author administers colloidal support if the dog develops peripheral edema or evidence of third spacing, total solids decrease below 3.5 mg/dl, or albumin approaches 1.5 mg/dl. Two types of colloids are available for administration. Naturally occurring colloids include fresh frozen plasma, whole blood, human albumin, and canine albumin. Traditionally, fresh frozen plasma has been espoused as the preferred treatment because of the possibility of additional benefits such as coagulation factors and CPV specific antibodies. However, in the absence of a coagulopathy, fresh frozen plasma may not be the best choice for colloidal support. Plasma has a relatively low oncotic pressure and actually may be associated with an increase in proinflammatory cytokines. Even in plasma taken from a recently recovered animal, anti-CPV antibody concentrations are minimal, and large volumes are required to bring albumin into a more acceptable range. Concentrated sources of albumin, either human or canine, now are commercially available. In theory, 25% human albumin or canine albumin provides natural colloidal support without the volume required for fresh frozen plasma. Expense can be a significant issue and no studies have been published evaluating efficacy of albumin in CPV enteritis as compared with the more affordable alternative, synthetic colloids. If significant anemia develops, whole blood transfusions or packed red blood cell transfusions can be used but provide little oncotic support.

The most commonly used synthetic colloids in veterinary medicine are hetastarch and dextran 70. Both provide a much greater oncotic pull per unit volume than the naturally occurring colloids yet remain relatively affordable and with a long shelf life. For these reasons, the author prefers synthetic colloids if colloidal support alone is needed. Because of dilution of coagulation factors, excessive administration of any synthetic colloids can be associated with coagulopathies. Judicious use (maintenance rate of 20 ml/kg q24h) avoids this hypocoagulable state, but periodic monitoring of coagulation parameters is recommended if prolonged use is needed.

Nutrition

Enteral nutrition is associated with improved mucosal integrity and repair, and starvation is associated with small intestinal mucosal atrophy. Early enteral nutrition starting 12 hours after admission, regardless of status, was associated with improved weight gain and clinical signs when compared with the more traditional approach of withholding food until 12 hours after cessation of vomiting (Mohr et al, 2003). In the study referenced, the authors used nasoesophageal feeding of a balanced liquid canine diet, although syringe feedings of a low-residue, easily digestible diet also can be attempted.

Antiemetics

As noted, many of the complications of CPV enteritis are at least in part associated with vomiting and anorexia. Maropitant (Cerenia) is a recently released, centrally acting antiemetic that acts via neurokin-1 (NK-1) receptor antagonism. In a placebo-controlled clinical trial in dogs with CPV enteritis, administration of maropitant (1 mg/kg q24h, IV) as compared with ondansetron (0.5 mg/kg q8h IV) was associated with weight gain while in hospital compared with weight loss in the ondansetron group (Lenberg et al, 2012). The maropitant was administered daily in dogs as young as 9 weeks of age with no adverse effects. Metoclopramide, a centrally and peripherally acting antiemetic, also has been used (2 mg/kg q24h as a constant rate infusion). Metoclopramide can increase intestinal motility, which, in theory, could increase the risk of intussusception. For this reason, maropitant is the preferred antiemetic in the author's hospital.

Antibiotics

Gastrointestinal mucosal barrier disturbances leading to increased bacterial translocation as well as the leukopenia common in many cases lead to an increased risk of sepsis. Mildly affected animals without leukopenia may not need antibiotic therapy. The author uses cefoxitin (22 mg/kg q8h IV) for moderately affected animals, and a combination of penicillin (ampicillin 22 mg q8h IV) and fluoroquinolone (enrofloxacin 5 mg/kg q24h IV) is used for animals that are felt to need broader gram-negative coverage. Cartilage abnormalities have been associated with use of enrofloxacin in young large-breed dogs, and clients are warned of this possibility. An alternative to enrofloxacin is an aminoglycoside (gentamicin, 6 mg/kg q24h IV), but avoidance of nephrotoxicity requires animals to be volume replete, which is difficult to guarantee early in the disease.

Miscellaneous Treatments

The use of equine endotoxin antiserum in animals affected by CPV enteritis to reduce the effects of gram-negative bacterial toxins has been reported with mixed results. At this time, because of the lack of proven efficacy and the possibility of ill effects, the use of the endotoxin antiserum in CPV enteritis is not supported in the author's hospital. Recombinant human granulocyte colony-stimulating factor (rhG-CSF) was evaluated for use in puppies with CPV enteritis but has not been shown to improve outcome (Rewerts et al, 1998). Empiric administration of anthelmintics, proton pump inhibitors or

H_2 blockers, pain medications, and gastrointestinal protectants may be used in animals with CPV enteritis at the discretion of the practitioner. There are no case-controlled studies supporting or discrediting the use of these therapies.

Antiviral Treatments

Immunotherapy. Passive immunotherapy using convalescent plasma collected from recently recovered dogs has been reported anecdotally to improve clinical outcome. However, in a recent blind, placebo-controlled study of naturally infected dogs in the author's hospital, the administration of an average of 2.2 ml/kg IV once on admission did not improve significantly any measured parameters, including survival, cost or duration of hospitalization, severity of clinical signs, or viral load. The dose was chosen empirically but closely corresponds to that which is recommended for passive immunotherapy in the human population. Recombinant feline interferon-ω (Virbagen) showed promise in two small placebo-controlled trials. Mortality and clinical signs were decreased in the treatment group (deMari et al, 2003). The product is not commercially available in the United States and can be cost prohibitive when available. It therefore is not used commonly; however, if the agent becomes more widely available, it may warrant further investigation.

Antiviral Medications. Oseltamivir (Tamiflu) is a neuraminidase inhibitor commonly used for treatment of influenza infections because of the heavy reliance of influenza viruses on neuraminidases. It has been proposed as a treatment in animals infected with CPV but is not yet showing significant clinical signs. In a published placebo-controlled study, an improvement in weight gain and maintenance of white blood cell counts was noted in the treatment group as compared with the control group; however, no significant difference was noted in survival or clinical signs. Based on these data, it is unclear the role that oseltamivir may play in treatment of CPV enteritis; however, oseltamivir resistance is on the rise in humans with influenza infections. For this reason, use of the drug in veterinary patients without a clearly documented advantage must be considered carefully.

References and Suggested Reading

Burton JH et al: Detection of canine parvovirus DNA from blood and antigen in feces collected from healthy puppies after administration of modified live vaccine, *J Vet Intern Med* 22: 703, 2008.

Decaro N et al: Detection of canine parvovirus type 2c by a commercially available in-house rapid test, *Vet J* 184:373, 2010.

deMari K et al: Treatment of canine parvoviral enteritis with interferon omega in a placebo-controlled field trial, *Vet Record* 152:105, 2003.

Lenberg J et al: The effects of maropitant versus ondansetron on the clinical recovery of dogs with parvoviral gastroenteritis, *J Vet Intern Med* 26:795, 2012.

Markovich JE et al: Effects of canine parvovirus strain variations on diagnostic test results and clinical management of enteritis in dogs, *J Am Vet Med* 241:66, 2012.

Mohr AJ et al: Effect of early enteral nutrition on intestinal permeability, intestinal protein loss, and outcome in dogs with severe parvoviral enteritis, *J Vet Intern Med* 17:791, 2003.

Rewerts JM et al: Recombinant human granulocyte colony-stimulating factor for treatment of puppies with neutropenia secondary to canine parvovirus infection, *J Am Vet Med* 213: 991, 1998.

Savigny MR, Macintire DK: Use of oseltamivir in the treatment of canine parvoviral enteritis, *J Vet Emerg Crit Care* 20:132, 2010.

Veir JK et al: Comparison of quantitative PCR and conventional endpoint PCR for amplification of parvovirus DNA in blood from naturally infected and recently vaccinated dogs, *J Vet Intern Med* 23:769, 2009.

CHAPTER 131

Inflammatory Bowel Disease

KARIN ALLENSPACH, *Hatfield, Hertfordshire, Great Britain*
AARTI KATHRANI, *Hatfield, Hertfordshire, Great Britain*

Inflammatory bowel disease (IBD) describes a group of idiopathic disorders characterized by chronic persistent or recurrent gastrointestinal (GI) signs, with histologic evidence of inflammation in the lamina propria of the small intestine, large intestine, or both. The diagnosis of IBD is one of exclusion, and a full diagnostic workup is necessary to rule out all known causes of GI inflammation. Currently, endoscopic evaluation and histopathology of intestinal biopsies is the preferred way to diagnose IBD definitively. Although the exact etiology of IBD is unknown, it is widely accepted that the pathogenesis involves a complex interplay among host genetics, the intestinal mucosal immune system, the environment, and the intestinal microbiota. This chapter briefly examines the current understanding of the pathogenesis and diagnosis of IBD and then concentrates in more detail on the current therapeutic practice, drawing from the most recent work conducted in this field.

Classification

IBD is classified according to the inflammatory cell infiltrate present, the most common of which is lymphoplasmacytic enteritis in dogs and cats. Eosinophilic enteritis is thought to be the second most common, whereas granulomatous enteritis is rare and most commonly diagnosed in young boxers and French bulldogs. Neutrophilic infiltration also is rare in canine and feline IBD. Furthermore, IBD patients can be classified retrospectively depending on their response to treatment. Those responding to an elimination diet or hydrolyzed diet are diagnosed with food-responsive diarrhea (FRD), whereas those responding to antibiotic treatment are diagnosed with antibiotic-responsive diarrhea (ARD). IBD patients that do not fall into either of the two latter categories require immunosuppressive medication to treat their clinical

signs and are classified commonly as having steroid-responsive diarrhea. Finally, certain breeds are highly susceptible to developing specific unique forms of IBD; examples include the immunoproliferative enteropathy of basenjis, the protein-losing enteropathy (PLE) and protein-losing nephropathy (PLN) complex in soft-coated wheaten terriers, IBD in Norwegian lundehunds, and granulomatous colitis in boxer dogs.

Etiopathogenesis

In the last few decades the study of human IBD and animal models of this disease has led to many significant advances in understanding the pathogenesis of IBD. These studies have shown that the pathogenesis of IBD is complex, involving an overly aggressive cell-mediated response resulting from the loss of tolerance to antigens of the microbiome in genetically susceptible hosts.

Genetics

The genetic inheritance of human IBD is not understood fully. A classical Mendelian inheritance attributable to a single locus has not been demonstrated, but rather a more complex polygenic model of inheritance with evidence of epistasis between genetic loci. Mutations in pattern-recognition receptors of the innate immunity, such as Toll-like receptors and NOD-like receptors as well as in genes coding for autophagy proteins, have been associated with the development of IBD in people.

A number of breed predispositions have been described in canine IBD, thus strongly supporting a role for host genetics. Using candidate gene analysis, polymorphisms in Toll-like receptor (TLR) 4 and TLR5 were shown recently to be significantly associated with IBD in German shepherds. Furthermore, the same polymorphisms in

TLR5 were associated with IBD in a heterogeneous population of dogs consisting of 38 different breeds. These mutations could well play an important role in the pathogenesis of IBD in dogs: a mutated receptor leads to misrepresentation of commensal bacteria as pathogens, therefore signaling "danger" to the host and initiating the characteristic inflammatory response seen in this disease. Further studies must focus on genome-wide association studies in specific breeds of dogs and cats and take into account environmental factors likely to be instrumental in the development of disease in individual susceptible animals.

Intestinal Mucosal Immune System

The concept of impaired immunoregulation in IBD is supported by observations of increased numbers of CD4+ T cells in people and increased numbers of immunoglobulin-producing plasma cells and T cell subsets in canine and feline IBD. Inflammation seen in IBD is thought to result from the inappropriate cytokine production by these different T cell subsets. Specifically, Crohn's disease (CD) is associated with a Th1 and Th17 cytokine profile and ulcerative colitis (UC) with a Th2 profile. In cats, a similar cytokine profile skewed toward a Th1 profile has been found. However, in dogs, no specific pattern of cytokines has been detected using real-time PCR on intestinal biopsies. It therefore is plausible that other immunologic components may play a role in the inappropriate inflammation seen in a subset of dogs with IBD. Indeed one study demonstrated that CD11c-positive dendritic cells (DCs) were decreased significantly in the intestinal mucosa of dogs with IBD. DCs are important in regulating the immunologic balance and are responsible for eliciting either an inflammatory or a tolerant immune response to an antigen. Thus a decrease in the number of DCs in the inflamed mucosa of dogs with IBD may explain the exaggerated inflammation seen in this disease. Moreover, cytokines such as the Th17 cytokine family have not been evaluated in dogs and cats with IBD and could, similarly to IBD in people, play a significant role in the pathogenesis of the disease.

Alterations of expression of TLR3 and TLR4 by intestinal epithelial cells have been described in human IBD. Similarly, TLR 2, 4, and 9 have been shown to be upregulated in the duodenum and colonic mucosa in dogs with IBD at the mRNA level, and TLR2 expression specifically was shown to be correlated with the severity of disease. This dysregulation of TLRs in human and canine IBD patients may be a pathologic consequence or the underlying cause of inflammation. However, if the latter applies, this may explain the chronic inflammation seen in these diseases.

Intestinal Microbiota

The importance of the commensal bacteria in the pathogenesis of IBD has been well documented in animal models and in people with IBD. Chronic intestinal inflammation does not develop in mice reared in germ-free environments; however, reconstitution of germ-free mice with commensal bacteria can be enough to induce IBD in several gene-deficient as well as T cell transfer models of IBD. The role of luminal bacteria in the pathogenesis of human IBD is supported strongly by the fact that clinical symptoms of CD improve after intestinal washes and antibacterial treatment. Similarly, a subset of canine IBD patients (ARD patients) responds solely to antibiotics with subsequent relapse of clinical signs on withdrawal of treatment.

Investigating DNA libraries of mucosal-associated microbiota using molecular methods has revolutionized our understanding of the microbiome in animals and human beings. In patients with CD and UC, a decreased complexity of the microbiome has been found. Most notably, members of the phyla Bacteroidetes and Firmicutes are reduced significantly in CD and UC, whereas *E. coli* is abundant in CD. Similarly, the species richness within the microbiome in the duodenal lumen of dogs with IBD was reduced. Dogs with IBD also exhibit dysbiosis, with an abundance of members belonging to the Enterobacteriaceae family and a significantly lower number of *Clostridia* spp. Such dysbiosis may well be breed specific because German shepherds with IBD have been shown to harbor increased numbers of sequences belonging to Erysipelotrichaceae and Lactobacillales. In cats, the number of Enterobacteriaceae, *E. coli*, and *Clostridium* spp. correlates with abnormalities in mucosal architecture, up-regulation of Th1-cytokines, and the number of clinical signs exhibited by the affected cats. Such dysbiosis is thought to contribute to the inflammation seen in dogs and cats with IBD, in that inflammatory signals from the microbes (so-called pathogen-associated patterns) are recognized by the innate immune system of the host (such as Toll-like receptors) and could lead to an exaggerated adaptive immune response in the lamina propria of the mucosa, therefore leading to clinical signs.

Diagnosis

The diagnosis of IBD is one of exclusion, and a full diagnostic workup is necessary to rule out all known causes of GI inflammation. Commonly this involves complete blood cell count, serum biochemical analysis, urinalysis, fecal analysis, further blood tests (e.g., trypsin-like immunoreactivity, pancreatic lipase immunoreactivity, ACTH test or basal cortisol concentration and folate and cobalamin concentrations, total thyroxine [T_4], feline leukemia virus/feline immunodeficiency virus [FeLV/FIV], and abdominal ultrasound). If the results of these tests do not point to an obvious cause for the clinical signs and the patient is stable (i.e., has a normal appetite, good attitude, not lethargic, no to minimal weight loss, normal serum protein concentration), then a well-conducted therapeutic trial first with diet and then antimicrobials can be attempted. Intestinal biopsies for histopathology are collected from those patients that either fail to respond to empirical therapy or experience worsening of their clinical signs. In stable patients with subnormal serum cobalamin or serum albumin concentrations, it is recommended to pursue endoscopic evaluation and intestinal biopsy rather than empiric treatment trials. Decreased serum albumin concentrations in particular have been shown to be associated with a poor prognosis in dogs with IBD. In addition, cobalamin deficiency may have systemic metabolic consequences, and response to specific therapy may be suboptimal if supplementation is not started early on. This is true especially for feline GI disorders.

Recent Advances in Laboratory Testing

C-reactive protein (CRP) has been shown to be increased significantly in some dogs with moderate to severe IBD. Although CRP is not specific to the intestinal tract, one study demonstrated that serum concentrations may decrease significantly after treatment. Currently, an ELISA for CRP exists only for dogs, and this assay may be beneficial in evaluating the response to treatment in canine IBD using a serologic test.

Perinuclear antineutrophilic cytoplasmic antibodies (pANCAs) are serum autoantibodies that result in a characteristic perinuclear staining pattern in neutrophils. They can be visualized with immunofluorescence detection methods. In human IBD, pANCAs have been used as serologic markers of disease and can be found in 50% to 80% of UC patients, whereas 70% to 90% of CD patients are negative (van Schaik et al, 2012). Assays for the measurement of pANCAs in canine IBD have poor sensitivity and therefore are not recommended as a screening test for IBD. However, the assay has good specificity when used in dogs with acute or chronic diarrhea and may therefore help identify which animals need further investigation, including endoscopy.

Calprotectin is a calcium-binding protein that is highly abundant in neutrophils. Fecal calprotectin has been shown to be increased in human IBD patients compared with healthy controls. An immunoassay for the measurement of serum and fecal canine calprotectin recently has been developed and analytically validated. This assay currently is being evaluated in dogs with various GI diseases, and if the clinical relevance is confirmed, it may become a valuable diagnostic tool for clinicians.

Genetic tests evaluating mutations in Toll-like receptors may become a useful tool in certain breeds that are predisposed to IBD, such as German shepherds. Subtypes of disease with different response to treatment possibly could be identified with specific genetic tests; however, studies specifically correlating outcome with genotype in subtypes of the disease or specific breeds are necessary before general recommendations on the use of these tests can be made.

Histopathology

Intestinal biopsy is essential to prove the presence of intestinal inflammation and confirm a diagnosis of IBD. Several studies have failed to reveal any significant correlation between histopathology and severity of clinical signs in canine IBD. The WSAVA guidelines were introduced in an attempt to reduce interpathologist variation in the interpretation of endoscopic biopsy samples. These guidelines are taking architectural changes into account, which seem to be more important than solely interpreting the inflammatory infiltrate present; this is especially true in cats. However, variation between pathologists still

exists when using these new guidelines, and clinical severity does not correlate with the WSAVA histology score. Furthermore, recent studies indicate that tissue processing at the laboratory can affect significantly interpathologist variation in interpreting biopsies (Willard et al, 2010). The site of endoscopic biopsies can be important in reaching the correct diagnosis. One study compared the histology of canine duodenal and ileal biopsies and found that ileal biopsies often revealed lesions not apparent in the duodenum and that feline lymphoma was much more likely to be found in the ileum than the duodenum (Casamian-Sorrosal et al, 2010). Therefore, in the author's opinion, the WSAVA histopathology guidelines currently cannot be recommended to assess severity of disease or response to treatment.

Treatment

IBD patients that have mild to moderate clinical disease activity and normal serum albumin concentration first are treated sequentially with a dietary and antibiotic trial (see Chapter 126). If they fail to respond to either of these trials, immunosuppressive therapy is initiated.

Diet

A positive response to a dietary trial allows the patient's IBD to be classified as FRD, a term that includes dietary allergy and intolerance. The main options for a dietary trial include switching to a diet that optimizes assimilation (e.g., highly digestible diet, a fat-restricted diet, or a restricted fiber diet), a diet that leads to antigenic modification (e.g., novel protein source or protein hydrolysate) or a diet that is immunomodulatory (e.g., prebiotics, omega-3 or omega-6 fatty acids). In dogs with FRD, a clinical response usually is observed within 1 to 2 weeks of changing the diet. One study demonstrated that dogs that respond to diet tended to be younger and had higher serum albumin concentrations and predominantly signs of large bowel diarrhea than dogs that did not respond to diet. If a dog responds to a dietary trial, then continuing strictly with the diet for 10 to 12 weeks is recommended. Most dogs can be switched back to the diet they were previously fed without showing any relapse. Only a small percentage of dogs with GI signs (8%) relapse on challenge and are therefore truly food allergic. If a diet trial is unsuccessful (no improvement in clinical signs after 10 to 14 days), the next step is usually an antibiotic trial.

Antibiotics

An antibiotic trial typically involves oral administration of tylosin 10 to 15 mg/kg q8h PO, oxytetracycline 20 mg/kg q8h PO, or metronidazole 10 mg/kg q8h PO. A positive response suggests ARD. The dog typically is maintained on antibiotics for 28 days. If signs reoccur after stopping, then long-term antibiotic therapy with tylosin 5 mg/kg q24h PO is used, or low-dose metronidazole (1 to 2 mg/kg q12h PO). If the response to antibiotics is poor, then the patient may need steroids or other immunosuppressives to control the clinical signs. Treatment of granulomatous colitis in boxer dogs consists of enrofloxacin therapy at 5 mg/kg q12h PO for 6 to 8 weeks that eradicates the adherent-invasive *E. coli* strains that seem in part responsible for the development of the disease (see Chapter 134).

Antiinflammatory and Immunosuppressive Therapy

Patients that do not respond to a diet or antibiotic trial usually are administered oral prednisolone 2 mg/kg q24h PO for at least 10 days that is tapered over an 8-week period. However, side effects of glucocorticoids usually are marked, especially in large-breed dogs, and studies have shown that only about 30% of dogs that failed diet and antibiotic treatment respond to steroids. If response to immunosuppression with steroids is poor after the first 3 to 4 weeks of treatment, then oral cyclosporine at 5 to 10 mg/kg q24h PO for at least 8 to 10 weeks should be given. In cats, the use of chlorambucil 2 to 6 mg/m^2 q24h PO with prednisolone is preferable if there is inadequate response to glucocorticoid treatment alone. Hematologic parameters should be monitored regularly if chlorambucil is used. Cyclosporine blood concentrations do not have to be monitored regularly, unless side effects induced by the cyclosporine treatment are suspected or an inadequate response to treatment is seen. To measure cyclosporine serum concentrations, it is recommended to take blood samples 1 to 2 hours after giving the medication to ensure that peak concentrations are measured. If the cyclosporine serum concentration is above 700 ng/ml at peak level, then halving the dosage for the first 2 weeks of treatment can reduce the side effects. If the patient responds to cyclosporine, then the medication can be tapered slowly or stopped after 10 weeks. Budesonide is a glucocorticoid medication that preliminarily has shown to be successful in the treatment of canine IBD. However, further studies on the use of this drug are needed because hypothalamic-pituitary-adrenal suppression and development of a steroid hepatopathy have been demonstrated in dogs. An optimal dose has not yet been determined, although anecdotally a dose of 0.3 mg/m^2 q24h PO has been recommended. Sulfasalazine (20 to 50 mg/kg q8h PO for 3 to 6 weeks), and related drugs are used often in dogs when IBD is limited to the large intestine. However, side effects include keratoconjunctivitis sicca; therefore tear production should be monitored regularly when using these drugs.

Treatment for Severe Protein Losing Enteropathy

Canine patients with serum albumin concentrations below 1.5 g/dl are at risk of developing ascites, pleural effusion, subcutaneous edema, and thromboembolism (see Chapter 132). Hypercoagulability has been shown to occur in a high percentage of dogs with PLE, and prophylactic treatment with low-dose aspirin is recommended (0.5 mg/kg q24h PO), especially when treating the dogs with immunosuppressive doses of steroids. Cyclosporine may be a better treatment option for dogs with PLE because some dogs with steroid-resistant IBD were rescued by sole treatment with cyclosporine for 10 weeks. In addition, the use of enteral nutrition via feeding tubes

can help in anorexic animals, and elemental diets and partial parenteral nutrition may be indicated at the beginning of the treatment in some dogs with severe PLE. Finally, these patients also may be at risk of complications associated with intestinal biopsy by celiotomy; therefore plasma transfusion, human albumin infusion, or synthetic colloid may be indicated during the perioperative period, and endoscopic biopsies should be obtained instead of full-thickness biopsies whenever possible.

Adjunctive Therapy

Hypocobalaminemia should be corrected by parenteral supplementation. A dose of 20 μg/kg every 7 days SC for 6 weeks followed by the same dose every 28 days for a further 3 months can be used. It is recommended to assess the serum cobalamin concentration to verify the efficacy of treatment. Prophylactic administration of an anthelmintic such as oral fenbendazole 50 mg/kg q24h for 5 days is warranted in all patients diagnosed with IBD.

The use of probiotics in people with IBD has led to some promising results, although there is still a lack of clinical trials assessing the usefulness of probiotics in canine IBD, despite promising initial reports for acute diarrhea.

Prognosis

One retrospective study demonstrated that only 26% of canine IBD cases progress to complete remission, with intermittent clinical signs remaining in approximately half of cases; 4% were completely uncontrolled, with 13% euthanized because of poor response to treatment (Craven et al, 2004). This suggests that the prognosis of IBD patients can be poor. The main negative prognostic indicator for IBD was identified to be hypoalbuminemia. Other factors associated with poor outcome are severity of disease, severe lesions detectable on endoscopy in the duodenum, and hypocobalaminemia. Furthermore, increased pancreatic lipase immunoreactivity concentrations in dogs with IBD have been shown to be associated with a poor response to steroid treatment and a negative outcome.

References and Suggested Reading

Allenspach K et al: Chronic enteropathies in dogs: evaluation of risk factors for negative outcome, *J Vet Intern Med* 21(4):700, 2007.

Allenspach K et al: Pharmacokinetics and clinical efficacy of cyclosporine treatment of dogs with steroid-refractory inflammatory bowel disease, *J Vet Intern Med* 20(2):239, 2006.

Casamian-Sorrosal D et al: Comparison of histopathologic findings in biopsies from the duodenum and ileum of dogs with enteropathy, *J Vet Intern Med* 24:80, 2010.

Craven M et al: Canine inflammatory bowel disease: retrospective analysis of diagnosis and outcome in 80 cases (1995-2002), *J Small Anim Pract* 45:336, 2004.

Day MJ et al: Histopathological standards for the diagnosis of gastrointestinal inflammation in endoscopic biopsy samples from the dog and cat: a report from the World Small Animal Veterinary Association Gastrointestinal Standardization Group, *J Vet Intern Med* 24(1):10, 2010.

Goodwin LV et al: Hypercoagulability in dogs with protein-losing enteropathy, *J Vet Intern Med* 25(2):273, 2011.

Heilmann RM et al: Development and analytic validation of an immunoassay for the quantification of canine S100A12 in serum and fecal samples and its biological variability in serum from healthy dogs, *Vet Immunol Immunopathol* 144(3-4):200, 2011.

Janeczko S: The relationship of mucosal bacteria to duodenal histopathology, cytokine mRNA, and clinical disease activity in cats with inflammatory bowel disease, *Vet Microbiol* 128(1-2):178, 2008.

Jergens AE et al: A scoring index for disease activity in canine inflammatory bowel disease, *J Vet Intern Med* 17(3):291, 2003.

Jergens AE et al: Intestinal cytokine mRNA expression in canine inflammatory bowel disease: a meta-analysis with critical appraisal, *Comp Med* 59(2):153, 2009. Erratum in: *Comp Med* 59(3):220, 2009.

Kathrani A et al: Polymorphisms in the TLR4 and TLR5 gene are significantly associated with inflammatory bowel disease in German shepherd dogs, *PLoS One* 5(12):e15740, 2010.

Schreiner NM et al: Clinical signs, histology, and CD3-positive cells before and after treatment of dogs with chronic enteropathies, *J Vet Intern Med* 22(5):1079, 2008.

van Schaik FD et al: Serological markers predict inflammatory bowel disease years before the diagnosis, *Gut* 2012. [Epub ahead of print.]

Willard MD et al: Effect of tissue processing on assessment of endoscopic intestinal biopsies in dogs and cats, *J Vet Intern Med* 24:84, 2010.

Xenoulis PG et al: Molecular-phylogenetic characterization of microbial communities imbalances in the small intestine of dogs with inflammatory bowel disease, *FEMS Microbiol Ecol* 66(3):579, 2008.

CHAPTER **132**

Protein-Losing Enteropathies

DEBRA L. ZORAN, *College Station, Texas*

Protein-losing enteropathies (PLE) are a complex group of enteropathies associated with increased loss of albumin and other proteins across the gastrointestinal (GI) mucosa. Because hypoalbuminemia and/or hypoproteinemia also can be caused by renal loss (protein-losing nephropathy), third space loss (high protein ascites or pleural effusion), loss across skin (burns), or lack of production of proteins (liver failure), the diagnosis of PLE must be made after evaluation of the patient for these other conditions.

Cause of Protein-Losing Enteropathies

Classification of PLE in dogs is not based on the same system used in humans, in which the diseases are placed into one of three groups: (1) erosive GI diseases resulting in protein leakage across an abnormal barrier (e.g., Crohn's disease), (2) nonerosive GI diseases associated with protein leakage across tight junctions or changes in protein uptake (e.g., intestinal parasites, cobalamin deficiency), and (3) diseases associated with increased lymphatic pressure and leakage of high protein lymph (e.g., lymphangiectasia, neoplasia) (Dossin and Lavoue, 2011). However, classification can be useful in consideration of therapeutic options and prognosis, and as such canine PLE generally are grouped according to their primary causes: (1) lymphangiectasia or crypt disease (e.g., Yorkshire terriers, rottweilers), (2) IBD (e.g., lymphoplasmacytic, eosinophilic, or granulomatous forms in many breeds),

(3) breed-associated forms of PLE (e.g., enteropathies of basenjis, soft-coated wheaten terriers, and Norwegian lundehunds), and (4) miscellaneous diseases of the GI tract, many of which are associated with GI hemorrhage (e.g., infectious diseases such as histoplasmosis or parvovirus, severe parasitism with hookworms or giardiasis, and neoplastic diseases such as lymphoma). Lymphangiectasia is a relatively well described, if poorly understood, cause of PLE associated with dilation of lacteals, crypts, and lymphatic ducts that appears to be due to an inflammatory process but also may be idiopathic. A newly described but specific disease associated with PLE in dogs is crypt disease, a dilation of the intestinal crypts with mucus, sloughed epithelial cells, and sometimes inflammatory cells, which is not associated with histologic signs of IBD or lymphangiectasia. Further, the lesions may be isolated or patchy in distribution. They often are separated by large areas of normal mucosa and appear to be more common in Yorkshire terriers and rottweilers (Willard et al, 2000). PLE secondary to infiltration of the bowel wall or other diseases, such as IBD, lymphoma, or infectious agents, are the most common forms of the disease and can be variable in severity and presentation. However, German shepherd dogs appear predisposed to development of PLE secondary to these conditions. Primary (idiopathic or breed associated) PLE occurs in just a few canine breeds (i.e., Norwegian lundehunds, Maltese, and shar-peis) and causes the most severe changes in the lymphatic vessels, including development of lymphogranulomas around

lymphatic vessels (Berghoff et al, 2007). Breed-associated severe IBD with concurrent PLE occurs in soft-coated wheaten terriers, and a rare immunoproliferative enteropathy affects basenjis; however, both represent severe forms of disease that can present a significant therapeutic challenge. The key feature of PLE is its wide variety of causes; the resultant clinical variability leads to an unpredictable clinical course and outcome.

Clinical Presentation and Diagnosis

The most consistent clinical feature of dogs with PLE is weight loss, especially loss of muscle mass, and may or may not be associated with diarrhea at the time of diagnosis. Diarrhea, either persistent small bowel diarrhea or chronic, relapsing, and intermittent diarrhea, is the next most prevalent clinical sign. Vomiting and inappetence, the other signs indicative of GI disturbance, are much less common and are unreliable indicators of PLE. Other signs of PLE occur as a result of the severe hypoproteinemia and include edema of limbs or ventrum, ascites, chylothorax, or pleural effusion; each of which may be present to a variable degree. Gut wall edema likely occurs in most dogs with PLE. It contributes to additional GI protein loss and increases the difficulty of getting high-quality intestinal biopsies. Other complications of severe PLE or IBD in dogs is malabsorption of fat-soluble vitamins (e.g., A, D, E, K) and decreased absorption of both divalent cations, calcium and magnesium, which in severe cases can lead to clinical hypocalcemia and resultant hypocalcemic tetany or seizures. Severe bleeding resulting from lack of vitamin K clotting factors has not been reported but is reasonable to consider. In addition to loss of albumin, other proteins of similar size and significance are lost from the GI tract. One protein in particular known to become deficient in PLE is antithrombin. Low antithrombin concentrations in dogs with PLE increase the risk of thromboembolism, a clinical complication reported in several separate case reports and studies of clotting profiles in dogs with PLE (Goodwin et al, 2011). However, the loss of antithrombin appears to explain only part of the process. Even dogs with PLE that have improved clinical values after treatment continue to have abnormal thromboelastograms. Furthermore, in a group of Yorkshire terriers with crypt disease and PLE, several had pulmonary thromboembolic events (Goodwin et al, 2011).

The diagnosis of PLE is a multistep process that requires a careful review of the patient's history and signalment, including characterization of the diarrhea, review of any and all diet changes and therapy, and a thorough physical examination, followed by laboratory confirmation of panhypoproteinemia, hypocholesterolemia, hypocalcemia, and lymphopenia, the laboratory hallmarks of PLE. Once hypoproteinemia is confirmed, the first step is to rule out other causes of protein loss as previously noted. This evaluation should include a urinalysis and urine protein-to-creatinine ratio to rule out protein-losing nephropathy; assessment of liver function, either via bile acid assays, ammonia testing, or possibly liver biopsy; and imaging studies. Imaging may be used to assess cardiovascular function, if indicated, and to collect a sample of

fluid accumulated to determine the type of effusion (particularly pleural, but also abdominal) and to rule out a septic or inflammatory fluid. Abdominal ultrasound also is important to complete the diagnostic picture and to rule out other causes of protein loss (e.g., lymphoma or histoplasmosis can be found on FNA of liver or spleen in many cases). Furthermore, ultrasound can be the ideal means of determining whether endoscopy is indicated. For example, if the lesions appear to be focal or located in a region of the intestinal tract not reachable by the endoscope, planning for possible surgical biopsies can be initiated. Imaging also documents the degree of effusion and is useful in guiding the operator when performing pleurocentesis. In addition to the above, measurement of serum cobalamin and folate levels is indicated to assess the need for cobalamin replacement therapy, which is a common complicating factor. Finally, all dogs should have coagulation parameters measured (especially antithrombin, D-dimers and, if possible, a thromboelastogram) to assess clotting status and serum vitamin D status assessed, particularly if iCa^{2+} levels are low.

Ultimately, collection of biopsies from the GI tract, either via endoscopy or full-thickness biopsies obtained in surgery, is necessary to make a definitive diagnosis, determine the cause, evaluate the extent and severity of the disease, and provide prognostic information. There is an ongoing unresolved discussion about the best approach for obtaining biopsies. Although surgical biopsies are necessary in a small number of cases, the author prefers endoscopic examination and procurement of biopsies because they allow visualization of mucosa, are less invasive, and require shorter recovery time. In addition, in the author's practice, endoscopy of the upper and lower GI tract is the standard method to obtain biopsies from the stomach, upper small intestine, and ileum. As has been reported recently in cats with lymphoma, lymphangiectasia in dogs can be found more commonly in the ileum. Therefore, if biopsies are not taken from the duodenum and ileum, the diagnosis may be missed or in error (e.g., IBD found in the duodenum with lymphangiectasia only present in the ileum) (Casamian-Sorrosal et al, 2010). The key in using endoscopy is collection of appropriate samples for biopsy (e.g., samples that are of sufficient depth to include the submucosa) so that crypt lesions and other structural changes can be identified adequately. This, of course, requires a skill set that must be developed and also requires appropriate patient preparation. For example, before the endoscopic procedure, the degree of gut edema must be reduced by use of colloid therapy so that the operator can grasp mucosal and submucosal tissue with the biopsy forceps and not just edematous tips of villi. In addition, to maximize the lacteal dilation for diagnostic purposes, administration of 1 tsp (5 cc) corn oil (or another liquid fat source) per 10 kg body weight 3 to 4 hours before the procedure is recommended. In cases in which a surgical approach is deemed most appropriate or endoscopy has failed to make the definitive diagnosis, one or two biopsies should be taken from each of the same sites. Despite concerns for hypoalbuminemia being a risk factor for suture site dehiscence, two separate studies did not document this complication (Shales et al, 2005). Thus, in PLE cases in which an exploratory is indicated, the clinician should proceed using the same preanesthetic and procedure preparation and careful attention to surgical detail.

Therapy

The treatment of PLE is complicated by the variety of different diseases that can cause it and by the differing degrees dogs are affected by it. Thus the focus of treatment is to identify and correct or control (if possible) any underlying cause (e.g., lymphoma, IBD, histoplasmosis, giardiasis) and then to reduce the leakage of lymph and protein across the gut wall through nonspecific but appropriate diet or drug therapy. Treatment of specific diseases that may cause PLE, such as histoplasmosis or GI lymphoma, are beyond the scope of this chapter. The focus of this section on treatment of PLE is directed at nonspecific therapy of idiopathic cases. The nonspecific therapy of PLE is based on four basic areas of focus: (1) providing nutritional support and selecting the most appropriate diet, (2) reversing edema and ascites by increasing oncotic pressure, (3) reducing inflammation associated with leakage of lymph and crypt lesions, and (4) addressing or preventing any associated complications, especially thromboembolic events.

All dogs with PLE carry a guarded prognosis, because the response to treatment cannot be predicted accurately, and relapses in well-controlled dogs are common. Therefore owners must understand that treatment of PLE may be intermittent or continuous but often is required for the duration of the dog's life.

Nutritional Therapy

Two aspects of nutritional support must be addressed: (1) replenishment of the proteins lost to allow recovery of protein functions (e.g., albumin, clotting proteins) and of lost muscle mass (a key controller of metabolism, energy, and overall health) and (2) to provide energy in the diet while avoiding fats that the GI tract is unable to digest and absorb efficiently or effectively. In the most severely affected dogs and especially those unwilling or unable to eat, total parenteral nutrition (TPN) may be necessary in the initial phase of therapy to provide immediate nutritional and oncotic support and increase plasma protein levels to safer levels. In hospitals with no option for TPN, partial parenteral nutrition (IV administration of amino acid solutions with dextrose) or administration of canine albumin intravenously are also alternative approaches to increase plasma proteins in critically ill PLE dogs while other supportive care mechanisms are initiated. These therapeutic interventions are not curative nor do they stabilize the oncotic crisis alone. However, in dogs at risk of imminent death resulting from hypoalbuminemia, this can be used as life support until other therapy is initiated.

No available studies support the nutritional recommendations that are made most frequently, but anecdotally there is general agreement that diets fed to dogs with PLE should be highly digestible (highly digestible is generally understood to mean the following: 88% to 90% protein digestibility, >95% for carbohydrates and fat in the diet) and contain more than 20% to 25% protein (on a dry matter [DM] basis, not necessarily novel, but may be considered if IBD is a component), less than 10% to 15% fat (this number may have be to significantly lower in severely affected dogs), and less than 5% insoluble dietary fiber. Soluble fibers (e.g., fructooligosaccharides, inulin, guar gum) may be beneficial to the GI tract in typical amounts and should not be excluded, but insoluble fibers, such as cellulose or other poorly digestible fibers intended for weight loss or fecal bulking purposes, should not be a major component of the diet because they reduce nutrient digestibility. Commercially available veterinary prescription products vary widely in amount of protein and fat in the diet; this is especially true in novel or hydrolyzed diets that are not formulated specifically for severe intestinal disease. Currently, Royal Canin's Gastrointestinal Low Fat diet, which contains 7% fat DM and chicken as the protein source, is the diet lowest in fat and most highly digestible that is available commercially. See Table 132-1 for a comparison of the protein and fat levels of selected diets used in dogs with PLE.

In many dogs with PLE, a commercially available, highly digestible diet often works well for dietary control of the disease. However, in the most severely affected dogs, nontraditional therapy using homemade diets or adding nutritional modules (elemental diets developed for human enteral nutrition) may be needed. Human elemental diets are not complete and balanced for dogs, so they can be used only short term or in addition to other diets. However, these can be very effective during the initial stages of therapy, because they require minimal digestive function for the nutrients to be absorbed. Once the dog's albumin is stabilized (not necessarily normal), a gradual transition back to a commercial diet or a combination of commercial food and special diet can be made for long-term control.

Although many elemental diets are on the market, only a few are low in fat and moderate to high in protein. (Note: There are many high-protein modules, but most are also high-fat recovery diets and therefore are not acceptable for dogs with PLE.) The one most commonly used product in the author's practice is Vivonex TEN (15% protein, 3% fat) (www.Nestle-nutrition.com), but other products in that same line also may be considered: Vivonex Plus (18% protein, 6% fat), Vivonex RTF (20% protein, 10% fat), or Tolerex (8% protein, 2% fat). All of these elemental diets have 100% free amino acids as the protein source, all are lactose and gluten free, and all have added glutamine and arginine for gut health. However, they are not complete and balanced diets for dogs, so they must be used short term (a few weeks) if they are fed alone (uncommon in the author's practice), or they must be fed as a supplement with a balanced diet to prevent development of vitamin and mineral imbalances. None of these diets contain an adequate amount of protein, amino acids (e.g., taurine, arginine), and fatty acids (arachidonic acid) to meet the nutritional needs of cats and should *NOT* be used in cats.

An alternative approach is to feed a homemade diet containing highly digestible but very low-fat protein sources, such as low-fat turkey breast, cooked egg whites, and nonfat cottage cheese. There are many potential options for this approach. Seeking the advice and counsel of a nutrition specialist is important to help with recipe

TABLE 132-1

Comparisons of Selected Highly Digestible, Hypoallergenic, and Hydrolyzed Diets Used in the Management of Protein-Losing Enteropathies in Dogs

	% Protein Dry*	% Protein Can*	% Fat Dry*	% Fat Can*	Protein Source
Royal Canin Digestive Low Fat	20.5	16.7	5.0	3.4	Chicken, pork
Hill's Prescription Diets i/d	26.5	27.8	14.1	14.3	Chicken, egg
Hill's Prescription Diets i/d low fat	25.9	25.1	7.4	8.5	Chicken/turkey, pork
Purina Veterinary Diets EN	23	—	10.5	—	Chicken
P&G Iams Low Residue	24.6	33	10.7	18.9	Chicken
Royal Canin Hypoallergenic HP	19	—	17	—	Soy protein isolate
Hill's Prescription Diet z/d	19	19.5	13.9	13.9	Chicken
Purina Veterinary Diets HA	18	—	8.0	—	Soy protein isolate
Royal Canin Hypoallergenic PD	19	17.7	10.5	16.7	Duck
Royal Canin Hypoallergenic PV	19.5	16.7	10	11.7	Venison
Royal Canin Hypoallergenic PR	19.5	18.4	10.5	13.3	Rabbit
Hill's Prescription Diet d/d duck	18	17.4	16.7	16.6	Duck
Hill's Prescription Diet d/d salmon	18.4	18.9	15.5	14.8	Salmon
Purina Veterinary Diets DRM	24	—	12	—	Salmon/trout

*Dry matter basis.

planning and evaluation of any homemade diets, especially if the diet is needed long term or as a primary source of nutrition for the dog. Another approach is to use recipes published for these specific purposes that have been generally approved by nutrition specialists. One such book containing a number of user-friendly and easy-to-prepare recipes for dogs with GI disease is *Home-Prepared Dog and Cat Diets*, second edition, by P. Schenck (Wiley Blackwell, 2010).

Finally, in addition to the above considerations, many dogs are hypocobalaminemic and require cyanocobalamin injections to replenish and maintain their vitamin B_{12} levels using well-established doses for lifelong supplementation. Other vitamins, particularly the fat-soluble vitamins D, E, and K, may become deficient in dogs with severe PLE. Measuring serum retinol, ionized calcium, and calcitriol levels before starting vitamin A or calcitriol therapy is recommended, because oversupplementation can be very harmful. Supplementation of vitamin E is unlikely to be harmful; 300 IU vitamin E can be injected IM and is sufficient for 2 to 3 months. Vitamin K is required for proper functioning of clotting factors 2, 7, 9, and 10 of the clotting cascade and can be assessed by measurement of the prothrombin time (PT). If the PT is prolonged in dogs with severe PLE, injections of vitamin K_1 (Mephyton, 1 mg/kg/day SC once every 3 to 5 days) are sufficient to prevent bleeding until the GI disease is stabilized.

Oncotic Support

Improvement of the dog's nutritional status and use of high-protein, low-fat diets help tremendously to increase serum protein levels and provide oncotic support to reverse the leakage of fluid out of vessels. However, in many severely affected dogs, the hypoproteinemia has been so severe and chronic that stabilization of the dog is essential before diagnostic evaluation or further treatment. In those dogs, colloid therapy using hydroxyethyl starches (Hetastarch or the new veterinary product Vetstarch) at a dose of 5 to 20 ml/kg/day IV infusion can be effective in pulling edema fluid back into the vascular space and holding it there for short periods of time (Chan, 2008). This can be especially helpful before endoscopic procedures in reducing the gut mucosal edema that often can complicate the anesthetic and biopsy process and help improve the digestive process by reducing the barrier to uptake of nutrients from the GI lumen. Alternatives to synthetic colloids, such as administration of plasma as a source of albumin and a colloid to increase colloid oncotic pressure, have been advocated in the past. However, the volume of plasma required to have any impact on the serum albumin level at all is substantial. In an example, a dog weighing 20 kg and having a serum albumin of less than 1.0 g/dl received more than 10 units (100 ml/unit, 1000 ml plasma) of canine plasma over a 36-hour period, more than 2.5 times the recommended amount of plasma. The albumin reached only 1.0 g/dl and then dropped immediately after the plasma was discontinued. Further, recent studies have shown that plasma administration in dogs with severe panhypoproteinemia does not substantially improve oncotic pressure compared with synthetic colloids (Chan, 2008). However, although improving oncotic pressure is important in the short term, ultimately it requires stabilization of the GI tract to reduce ongoing losses and increase protein uptake to reverse the disease effects and stabilize the dog. This involves finding the appropriate diet and using antiinflammatory drug therapy.

Reducing Intestinal Inflammation

Whether or not PLE in a particular dog is associated with IBD (see Chapter 131), which it often is, the leakage of lymph and protein into villous spaces surrounding the lacteals causes inflammation and granuloma formation. Lipogranulomas may cause further lymphatic obstruction and thus increased lymph leakage through the gut wall. Aggressive antiinflammatory therapy is the only known treatment for the inflammation associated with lymphatic leakage and granuloma formation, and immunosuppressive doses of prednisone (2 to 4 mg/kg q48h PO) have been the standard approach. Unfortunately, high-dose steroid therapy has a number of potential adverse effects that are detrimental, and in the case of hypoproteinemic patients with poor oncotic support, addition of a drug that causes significant polydipsia and its resultant increases in free water can result in dramatic worsening (or lack of improvement) in edema or ascites. As a result, use of other immunosuppressive or antiinflammatory drug therapies has been considered more often. To date, no controlled studies in dogs with PLE compare the therapeutic effectiveness of azathioprine to cyclosporine or mycophenolate; however, each of these drugs has been used with varying degrees of success in dogs with PLE. The drug currently recommended most commonly as the next drug of choice, based on its effectiveness in a small number of dogs with PLE and IBD and its relative lack of severe side effects, is cyclosporine at a dose of 5 mg/kg q12h PO (Allenspach et al, 2006). Azathioprine also is used for its multimodal immunosuppressive effects but must be started together with prednisone, because a period of 2 to 3 weeks on the drug is needed to achieve steady state therapeutic levels. The most commonly recommended dose is 1 mg/kg q24h PO for 5 days then q48h PO thereafter. The most common side effects associated with the use of azathioprine are development of a hepatopathy, bone marrow suppression, or pancreatitis. The most common adverse effect of cyclosporine therapy is development of a secondary infection (often times fungal). Because many dogs require long-term therapy to control their disease, this can be a significant factor.

As in humans with PLE, dogs may develop dysbiosis (disruption of the enteric microbiota) as either a trigger for the disease or as a result of the disease. However, it is unusual for antibiotic therapy alone to be effective in the management of PLE without appropriate dietary and antiinflammatory therapies already in place. Further, dysbiosis frequently can be resolved with improvement in gut function, reduction of protein leakage, and feeding highly digestible diets that minimize maldigestion. The most commonly used antibiotics in dogs with chronic enteropathies are metronidazole (10 to 15 mg/kg q12h PO) or tylosin (10 to 20 mg/kg q12h PO), and these remain appropriate choices. Other antibiotics should be used judiciously and only when cultures, antigen, or PCR testing indicates pathogen overgrowth requiring intervention. Finally, to date, no studies have been published using probiotic therapy as an adjunct to the overall management of dogs with PLE, but the use of probiotics would seem reasonable and prudent (see Chapter 128).

Preventing Complications of Protein-Losing Enteropathies

The most important complication of dogs with PLE is their tendency to be hypercoagulable (because of antithrombin deficiency and other factors) and prone to development of thromboembolic disease. Because there is no effective clot removal therapy in dogs, the best approach is to use preventive therapy when indicated to lessen the risk of clot formation. In hospitalized dogs with severe antithrombin deficiency, administration of fresh frozen plasma and heparin may provide temporary replacement of the anticlotting proteins to prevent development of massive thrombosis. However, for long-term therapy, this is completely impractical. Thus, in all dogs with PLE and especially those with thrombocytosis (such as many Yorkshire terriers) and decreased levels of antithrombin, anticoagulant therapy with aspirin (10 mg/kg q24h PO) or clopidogrel (2 to 4 mg/kg q24h PO) is indicated. The dose for aspirin indicated above is higher than previously reported but results from new studies that reveal a higher dose is required to achieve consistent antiplatelet effects. Gastroprotection is indicated because this dose may cause GI ulceration (Goodwin et al, 2011).

Because dogs with PLE often have disease recurrence or fluctuations in their level of control, all dogs with PLE should have frequent reassessment (every 3 to 6 months) of their protein values, coagulation status, fat-soluble vitamin and cobalamin levels, and overall health because this is the best way to make appropriate adjustments in therapy.

References and Suggested Reading

Allenspach K et al: Pharmacokinetics and clinical efficacy of cyclosporine treatment of dogs with steroid-refractory inflammatory bowel disease, *J Vet Intern Med* 20:239, 2006.
Berghoff N et al: Gastroenteropathy in Norwegian Lundehunds, *Compend Contin Educ Vet* 29:456, 2007.
Casamian-Sorrosal D et al: Comparison of histopathologic findings in biopsies from the duodenum and ileum of dogs with enteropathy, *J Vet Intern Med* 24: 80, 2010.
Chan DL: Colloids: current recommendations, *Vet Clin North Am Small Anim Pract* 38:587, 2008.
Dossin O, Lavoue R: Protein losing enteropathies in dogs, *Vet Clin North Am Small Anim Pract* 41:399, 2011.
Gaschen L et al: Comparison of ultrasonographic findings with clinical activity index (CIBDAI) and diagnosis in dogs with chronic enteropathies, *Vet Radiol Ultrasound* 48:51, 2007.
Goodwin LV et al: Hypercoagulability in dogs with protein losing enteropathy, *J Vet Intern Med* 25:273, 2011.
Littman MP et al: Familial protein losing enteropathy and protein losing nephropathy in Soft Coated Wheaten Terriers: 222 cases, (1983-1997), *J Vet Intern Med* 14:68, 2000.
Shales CJ et al: Complications following full thickness small intestinal biopsy in 66 dogs: a retrospective study, *J Small Anim Pract* 46:317, 2005.
Willard MD et al: Intestinal crypt lesions associated with protein losing enteropathy in a dog, *J Vet Intern Med* 14:298, 2000.

CHAPTER 133

Feline Gastrointestinal Lymphoma

KEITH P. RICHTER, *San Diego, California*

Epidemiology

Lymphoma is the most frequently diagnosed feline cancer and the most common gastrointestinal (GI) neoplasm in cats (Rissetto et al, 2011). Lymphoma occurs in several anatomic locations; the GI tract is the most common site, accounting for 32% to 72% of total cases. Discrepancies in the reported incidence of the various forms of lymphoma may be the result of the differences in classification schemes used, a change in incidence over time, differences in feline leukemia virus (FeLV) subtypes in various geographic areas, and a decreased incidence of non-GI forms since the introduction of an FeLV vaccine. An increase in the proportion of lymphoma of the GI tract over time is apparent by comparing incidences in the same institutions over different time periods. For example, in the New England area the percentage of lymphomas in cats that occurred in the GI tract increased from 8% in 1979 to 18% in 1983 and to 32% in 1996 (Francis et al, 1979; Cotter, 1983; Moore et al, 1996). Likewise, in the New York City area the percentage increased from 27% in 1989 to 72% in 1995 (Mooney et al, 1989; Mauldin et al, 1995). This increased incidence in the GI form over time could be due to a decreased incidence of FeLV infection, and therefore fewer cats died at a young age secondary to FeLV-induced diseases. Thus more cats are living longer, and they may then develop the GI form. Another explanation is that cats may be undergoing more complete evaluations more recently than in the past.

The association between FeLV and lymphoma in cats is well established. The incidence of FeLV antigenemia in cats with GI lymphoma ranges from 0 to 38%. However, such estimation of FeLV infection rate is influenced significantly by the method of testing. Underestimation of FeLV incidence with immunohistochemistry (IHC) versus polymerase chain reaction (PCR) has been suggested. In one study PCR testing detected FeLV viral nucleic acid sequences in up to 63% of cats with GI lymphoma, whereas only 38% of cats were positive by IHC (Jackson et al, 1993). Generally cats with leukemia or mediastinal lymphoma tend to be young and FeLV positive, whereas those with GI lymphoma typically are older and FeLV antigen negative. An association between lymphoma and feline immunodeficiency virus (FIV) also has been proposed, especially when coinfected with FeLV, although most cats with GI lymphoma in the author's experience are negative for FIV exposure.

Gross Pathologic Findings

The gross appearance of feline GI lymphoma varies with the specific anatomic location. Many segments of the GI tract, including the liver, may be involved. There can be a focal mass or diffuse infiltration. In some cases, especially with low-grade lymphocytic lymphoma, the gross appearance may be normal. When a focal alimentary tract mass is present, there is usually transmural thickening with or without mucosal ulceration. Mural thickening is often eccentric, resulting in preservation of the lumen, although a functional obstruction may develop. This contrasts with intestinal carcinoma, which often results in a mechanical obstruction from decreased luminal diameter, often appearing as a "napkin ring." With diffuse infiltration the intestinal wall may be visibly and/or palpably thickened. Mesenteric lymphadenopathy is often obvious grossly or on ultrasonographic examination. Intussusception can develop secondary to intestinal lymphoma; the jejunum is the most common location. Hepatic involvement can have a variable appearance. In some cases the liver appears to be grossly normal, whereas in others there may be an enhanced lobular pattern, a mottled appearance, or a gross nodular appearance. In summary, the appearance of lymphoma is extremely variable in all regions of the GI tract. In light of how commonly this neoplasm develops in cats, lymphoma should be considered as a differential diagnosis for GI illness with normal or grossly abnormal organ appearance.

Histopathology and Immunohistochemistry

There are different grades of GI lymphoma, commonly referred to as low grade (lymphocytic or small cell), high grade (lymphoblastic, immunoblastic, or large cell), and intermediate grade. Less common descriptions such as large granular lymphocytic lymphoma also exist (which behave in a manner similar to high-grade lymphoma). Many published reports are either of undetermined grade or predominantly high-grade lymphomas, although low-grade lymphocytic lymphomas have been described more recently in large case series (Fondacaro et al, 1999; Kiselow et al, 2008; Moore et al, 2012; Stein et al, 2010). In the study by Fondacaro et al (1999) 50 of 67 cats (75%) diagnosed with GI lymphomas had low-grade lymphocytic lymphoma. Criteria used to classify lymphoma as lymphocytic have been described (Fondacaro et al, 1999; Moore et al, 2012). In marked contrast to palpable masses of lymphoblastic lymphoma, masses formed by lymphocytic lymphoma are not distinct microscopically, because the mucosa beyond the apparent mass also is involved. The use of a standard grading scheme for GI lymphoma may lead to a greater recognition of low-grade lymphocytic lymphoma. However, criteria have been difficult to establish because of the difficulty in interpreting small endoscopic biopsies, differences in pathologists' opinions, a lack of characterization using IHC, and only recent availability of polymerase chain reaction (PCR) clonality studies (see Chapter 65). Consequently further studies are needed to define specific criteria for differentiating lymphocytic lymphoma, lymphocytic inflammation, and T-cell infiltrative disease and to correlate such classifications with clinical outcome. In addition, the role of endoscopic biopsies versus full-thickness biopsies must be better defined. The results of one study suggested that surgical biopsies are superior to endoscopic biopsies for the detection of GI lymphoma (Evans et al, 2006). However, many cats in that study did not have their duodenum entered endoscopically (many were blind biopsies), few biopsies were obtained, the quality of the biopsies were not described, histologic grading was not reported, and clonality studies were not performed. Many pathologists are comfortable making the diagnosis on endoscopic biopsy analysis, whereas others believe that full-thickness biopsies are necessary. The author relies heavily on the analyses of endoscopic biopsies in his practice. Although it is customary to consider a continuum from inflammatory bowel disease to lymphoma, there are little supporting data.

Recently IHC has been used to better characterize feline lymphoma. In some studies GI lymphomas were more likely to be of B cell rather than T-cell phenotype, whereas other studies describe a predominantly T-cell phenotype. Notably, most cats with low-grade GI lymphoma have a T-cell phenotype. In a limited number of studies immunophenotype did not appear to correlate with response to chemotherapy treatment or survival, although more recently one study reported a better outcome in cats having the T-cell phenotype (Moore et al, 2012). Thus further study is necessary to determine the clinical value of immunophenotyping.

More recently, detection of lymphoid neoplasia has been accomplished by detecting antigen receptor gene rearrangements. This method is especially useful to determine if the lymphocyte population is monoclonal or oligoclonal (thus suggestive of lymphoma) versus polyclonal (which is more suggestive of inflammation). It is especially helpful to detect the presence of low-grade lymphoma when present concurrently with inflammatory disease. This technique employs PCR to amplify the hypervariable regions of immunoglobulin or T-cell receptor genes. In the absence of neoplasia, this region differs from cell to cell. Amplifying this region can help determine if the products are monoclonal (or oligoclonal) or polyclonal based on their appearance on polyacrylamide gel electrophoresis. This method has been named PARR (PCR for antigen receptor rearrangements) or TCRG (T-cell receptor gamma gene rearrangements). This appears to be a more sensitive and objective method for detection of lymphoma (especially the low-grade form or in less severe lesions) compared with conventional histopathology (Moore et al, 2005; Moore et al, 2012). In one study, detection of TCRG rearrangements had a 91% sensitivity in detecting mucosal T-cell lymphoma regardless of the severity of the lesion (Moore et al, 2012).

Clinical Findings

Signalment

In some studies, males appear to be predisposed to GI lymphoma. Although a breed predilection is not apparent, most cats are domestic shorthair. The median age ranges from 9 to 13 years in different studies, with an age range spanning from 1 to 18 years (although most cats are older than 6 years).

Clinical Signs and Physical Examination Findings

Regardless of the histologic grade, clinical signs include weight loss, anorexia, vomiting, diarrhea, lethargy, and polydipsia/polyuria. Importantly, many cats have minimal or no vomiting and/or diarrhea, with anorexia, weight loss, or both as the only historical findings. Therefore, when confronted with these signs in a geriatric cat with an otherwise unrewarding initial evaluation, clinicians should consider GI lymphoma as a differential diagnosis. Physical findings may include poor body condition, thickened intestinal loops, and/or a palpable abdominal mass. The presence of an abdominal mass is more suggestive of high-grade lymphoma. Notably many cats may have a normal abdominal palpation.

Ancillary Test Findings

Laboratory findings generally are noncontributory, with mild anemia and/or hypoalbuminemia most commonly seen. Up to 78% of cats with low-grade GI lymphoma have hypocobalaminemia, so measurement of serum cobalamin concentrations should be included in the database of cats with suspected lymphoma (Kiselow et al, 2008). Abnormalities on plain abdominal and thoracic radiographs are also uncommon and usually nonspecific. An abdominal ultrasound examination may be helpful in many cases and is considered more sensitive than radiography. Lesions can be nodular (focal or multifocal) or diffuse. Although the most common ultrasonographic abnormality observed is thickening of the gastric or intestinal wall, other important findings include loss of normal intestinal wall layering, localized mass effects associated with the intestine, decreased intestinal wall echogenicity, regional hypomotility, regional lymphadenopathy, and rarely ascites. The finding of a thickened and prominent muscularis layer of the intestine is also a feature suggestive of lymphoma and less commonly seen with inflammation. Because ultrasonography provides information about the specific site of involvement of the lesion as well as other abdominal organs, it assists in staging the regional extent of disease and in screening for concurrent disorders. It also allows for precise guidance of fine-needle aspiration or biopsy for cytologic or histopathologic sampling, and it can be used to assess response to therapy noninvasively and objectively. A limitation of ultrasonography is the difficulty in assessing the exact anatomic location and extent of certain lesions, possibly because of the inability of ultrasound waves to penetrate gas-filled structures, such as the bowel, and lack of distinct fixed anatomic landmarks. Furthermore, ultrasonography results depend on the operator, operator's level of experience, and ultrasound system. Findings also may be normal, especially in cases of low-grade lymphoma.

Endoscopy can be an effective tool for diagnosing GI mucosal lymphoma when involved areas are within reach of an endoscope. It is critical that the small intestine be examined with endoscopy because there is significant evidence for a predisposition for the small intestine for lymphoma compared with the stomach or large intestine (Fondacaro et al, 1999; Moore et al, 2012; Rissetto et al, 2011). The results of one retrospective study suggested that simultaneous sampling of the upper small intestine and the ileum (rather than just upper GI endoscopy alone) may increase the detection rate for low-grade lymphoma (Scott et al, 2011). Another study showed a higher incidence of mucosal T-cell lymphoma in the jejunum compared with the duodenum or ileum (Moore et al, 2012). Most gross endoscopic findings are nonspecific, with considerable overlap with inflammatory bowel disease and other GI diseases. In many cases the endoscopic appearance can be grossly normal.

Treatment

Reports of treatment strategies for feline GI lymphoma are fairly limited, and only a few of these reports give detailed results in cats specifically with GI lymphoma. In addition, the outcome for different forms of GI lymphoma remains ill-defined because many reports do not describe histologic grade or the results of complete anatomic staging; they report various anatomic locations collectively, and different combinations of chemotherapeutic agents were used.

A summary of reported treatments and outcomes in cats with GI lymphoma is provided in Table 133-1. Few studies have evaluated outcome by histologic grade; however, those evaluating high-grade lymphomas only generally report poor outcomes (Fondacaro et al, 1999; Mahony et al, 1995; Moore et al, 2012). In general, response rates for high-grade GI lymphoma are in the 25% to 50% range, with reported median survival times (MSTs) of 2 to 9 months. The poor outcomes reported in some older studies for which grades were not specified likely were for high-grade lymphomas. For cats with high-grade GI lymphoma, combining doxorubicin with other agents in a multiagent protocol such as cyclophosphamide/vincristine (Oncovin)/prednisolone (CHOP) and L-asparaginase is associated with longer remission and survival times when compared with single-agent doxorubicin or COP alone.

A few large case series describe outcomes in cats with just the low-grade form of the disease, demonstrating a much better outcome compared with the high-grade form (Fondacaro et al, 1999; Kiselow et al, 2008; Moore

et al, 2012; Stein et al, 2010). In these studies, cats were treated with a relatively low-grade chemotherapy protocol of prednisone and chlorambucil (Leukeran). Depending on the study, prednisone generally was given at doses ranging from 5 to 10 mg per day. Chlorambucil was administered at a high pulse dose of 15 mg/m^2 of body surface area PO q24h for 4 days, repeated every 3 weeks (Fondacaro et al, 1999), at a low every-other-day dose of 2 mg/cat (Kiselow et al, 2008), or at a lower pulse dose of 20 mg/m^2 of body surface area PO once every 2 weeks. For all these regimens, the results were similar. Remission rates for the low-grade form vary from 69% to 96%, with median remission duration varying from 23 to 30 months for those cats that achieve a complete remission. However, it is unknown whether these cats would do better with a more aggressive multiagent protocol. Adverse reactions to chlorambucil are uncommon but can include self-limiting vomiting, diarrhea, anorexia, lethargy, and neutropenia. It may be difficult to distinguish some of these chemotherapy-related side effects from active or progressive lymphoma. Cats rarely require hospitalization or discontinuation of therapy. Neurologic side effects (including myoclonus and seizures) also have been described in cats receiving chlorambucil, but these are rare.

The author currently recommends 10 mg prednisolone (because of more reliable pharmacokinetics in cats compared with prednisone) q24h PO and 2 mg chlorambucil q48h PO (which is much simpler for clients to understand than pulse dose therapy). For smaller cats or those that do not tolerate chlorambucil well, the author decreases the frequency of administration to every 3 days. For cats in which administration of oral medication is difficult, the high pulse dose regimen of chlorambucil (or even cyclophosphamide; see below) can be used to decrease the frequency of oral medications. In addition, the author has used injections of methylprednisolone acetate (Depo Medrol) at a dose of 10 to 20 mg IM every 10 to 11 days in place of oral prednisolone for those cats that do not accept oral medication readily. Parenteral cobalamin supplementation should be administered to cats with hypocobalaminemia.

Rescue therapy with cyclophosphamide also has been described for cats with low-grade GI lymphoma (Fondacaro et al, 1999; Stein et al, 2010). It can be given at a dose of 200 to 250 m^2 of body surface area PO once every 3 weeks or dividing this dose on days 1 and 3 every other week. Second remissions are common and can result in prolonged survival.

The role of surgery in the treatment of GI lymphoma has been evaluated. Studies have shown either no effect or a negative effect of surgical intervention on disease-free interval and survival. However, this effect is most likely not caused by the surgical intervention itself but is more likely because cats requiring surgery (i.e., those with GI obstruction) have shorter survival periods because of the severity of their disease. The main indications for surgery are partial or complete intestinal obstruction, intestinal perforation, or obtaining biopsy specimens for definitive diagnosis. Some patients with solitary masses that are surgically resected and subsequently receive chemotherapy can have long survival times.

TABLE **133-1**

Reported Outcomes Following Treatment for Cats with Gastrointestinal Lymphoma

Authors	Number of Cats (Number of GI Lymphoma Cases)	Protocol	Percent with Complete Response	Median Survival Time (or Disease-Free Interval)	Comments
Cotter, 1983	7 (7)	COP	86	26 weeks ST	Grade not reported
Jeglum, Whereat, and Young, 1987	14 (14)	COP + M	NR	12 weeks ST	Grade not reported
Mooney et al, 1989	103 (28)	COP + M + LA	62	30 weeks ST if CR	Outcome in GI LSA not reported separately; grade not reported
Mauldin et al, 1995	132 (95)	COP + M + DOX + LA	67	30 weeks ST	Outcome in GI LSA not reported separately but location did not affect outcome; grade not reported
Zwahlen et al, 1998	21 (21)	COP + M + DOX + LA	38	40 weeks ST (41.5 weeks if CR)	Grade not reported
Malik et al, 2001	60 (14)	COP + M + DOX + LA	80	17 weeks ST (27 weeks if CR)	Outcome in GI LSA not reported separately; grade not reported
Kristal et al, 2001	19 (7)	DOX	26	12 weeks ST (64 weeks if CR)	Outcome in GI LSA not reported separately; grade not reported
Mahony et al, 1995	28 (28)	COP	32	7 weeks ST (30 weeks DFI if CR)	25 high grade; 3 low grade
Fondacaro et al, 1999	11 (11)	COP or COP + DOX + LA	18	11 weeks ST	All high grade
Fondacaro et al, 1999	29 (29)	Chlorambucil, prednisone	69	74 weeks/17 months ST (99 weeks/23 months if CR)	All low grade
Kiselow et al, 2008	41	Chlorambucil, prednisone	56 (+ 39% PR)	101 weeks/23 months ST (DFI = 128 weeks/30 months if CR)	All low grade
Stein et al, 2010	28 (29)	Chlorambucil, prednisone/ prednisolone	96	112 weeks/26 months DFI	All low grade

COP, Cyclophosphamide/vincristine/prednisone; *CR,* complete response; *DFI,* disease-free interval; *DOX,* doxorubicin; *GI,* gastrointestinal; *LA,* L-asparaginase; *LSA,* lymphosarcoma; *M,* methotrexate; *NR,* not reported; *PR,* partial response; *ST,* survival time.

Some patients with transmural focal disease may be at risk for perforation when treated with cytotoxic chemotherapy that induces a rapid response, although this is rare in the author's experience. Surgery may result in dehiscence at intestinal anastomosis sites and may require a delay in initiation of chemotherapy to allow proper wound healing. After resection of a focal GI or mesenteric mass, chemotherapy is still warranted because most cases have diffuse or multifocal microscopic involvement, and lymphoma should be considered a systemic disease in most cases.

Prognostic Factors

Few prognostic factors have been defined for cats with GI lymphoma. Histologic grade is a strong indicator of outcome. Compared with cats with high-grade lymphoma treated with a multiagent chemotherapy regimen, cats with low-grade lymphoma treated with oral prednisolone and chlorambucil have a significantly better remission rate and survival time. Therefore low- and high-grade GI lymphomas in many ways represent different disease entities and must be considered separately.

In a majority of studies the most significant prognostic indicator for a positive outcome is initial response to chemotherapy. In general cats that survive the initial induction period and achieve remission also have a better long-term outcome. Although this may seem intuitively obvious, it may give clinicians and owners encouragement to continue chemotherapy treatment in cats that attain a CR. Otherwise there is no consistent association with any patient or tumor characteristic that is predictive of outcome (including sex, immunophenotype, clinical stage, age, and body weight). In most recent studies, FeLV virus antigenemia was not a negative prognostic factor. Some studies also showed little benefit of an exhaustive "staging evaluation" because very few factors have enough impact on prognosis to make their determination helpful. Investigators have looked at molecular markers as prognostic factors. However, argyrophilic nucleolar organizer region (AgNOR) frequency and proliferating cell nuclear antigen labeling index (PCNA-LI) showed no correlation with response to chemotherapy or survival (Rassnick et al, 1999; Vail et al, 1998). Similarly the immunophenotype of tumor cells also does not seem to correlate with outcome in cats, although more recently one study reported a better outcome in cats having the T-cell phenotype (Moore et al, 2012). This is in contrast to dogs, in which a T-cell phenotype has long been recognized as a negative prognostic factor for response to therapy and survival. Concentration of serum α1-acid glycoprotein, an acute-phase protein, has been evaluated in cats with lymphoma, and was not shown to be useful in predicting response to treatment or survival. Limitations of many studies published include incomplete staging, inconsistent grading, multiple unsampled GI locations, lack of prospective randomization to different chemotherapy protocols, lack of control (untreated) patients, and lack of confirmation of remission through follow-up biopsies. Prospective, controlled, and randomized cohort studies with large numbers of cats aimed at investigating the response of each grade of GI lymphoma to uniform chemotherapeutic regimens seem warranted. Furthermore, additional studies to correlate clinical outcome with immunophenotype and molecular markers are needed.

References and Suggested Reading

Cotter SM: Treatment of lymphoma and leukemia with cyclophosphamide, vincristine, and prednisone. II. Treatment of cats, *J Am Anim Hosp Assoc* 19:166, 1983.

Evans SE et al: Comparison of endoscopic and full-thickness biopsy specimens for diagnosis of inflammatory bowel disease and alimentary tract lymphoma in cats, *J Am Vet Med Assoc* 229:1447, 2006.

Fondacaro JV et al: Feline gastrointestinal lymphoma: 67 cases (1988-1996), *Eur J Comp Gastroenterol* 4:5, 1999.

Francis DP et al: Comparison of virus-positive and virus-negative cases of feline leukemia and lymphoma, *Cancer Res* 39:3866, 1979.

Jackson ML et al: Feline leukemia virus detection by immunohistochemistry and polymerase chain reaction in formalin-fixed, paraffin-embedded tumor tissue from cats with lymphosarcoma, *Can J Vet Res* 57:169, 1993.

Jeglum KA, Whereat A, Young K: Chemotherapy of lymphoma in 75 cats, *J Am Vet Med Assoc* 190:174, 1987.

Kiselow MA et al: Outcome of cats with low-grade lymphocytic lymphoma: 41 cases (1995-2005), *J Am Vet Med Assoc* 232:405, 2008.

Kristal O et al: Simple agent chemotherapy with doxorubicin for feline lymphoma: a retrospective study of 19 cases (1994-1997), *J Vet Intern Med* 15:125, 2001.

Mahony OM et al: Alimentary lymphoma in cats: 28 cases (1988-1993), *J Am Vet Med Assoc* 207:1593, 1995.

Malik R et al: Therapy for Australian cats with lymphosarcoma, *Aust Vet J* 79:808, 2001.

Mauldin GE et al: Chemotherapy in 132 cats with lymphoma: 1988-1994, Proceedings of the 15th Annual Conference of the Veterinary Cancer Society, Tucson, Ariz, 1995, p 35.

Mooney SC et al: Treatment and prognostic factors in lymphoma in cats: 103 cases (1977-1981), *J Am Vet Med Assoc* 194:696, 1989.

Moore AS et al: A comparison of doxorubicin and COP for maintenance of remission in cats with lymphoma, *J Vet Intern Med* 10(6):372, 1996.

Moore PF et al: Characterization of feline T cell receptor gamma (TCRG) variable region genes for the molecular detection of feline intestinal T cell lymphoma, *Vet Immunol Immunopathol* 106:167, 2005.

Moore PF et al: Feline gastrointestinal lymphoma: mucosal architecture, immunophenotype, and molecular clonality, *Vet Pathol* 49(4):658, 2012.

Rassnick KM et al: Prognostic value of argyrophilic nucleolar organizer region (AgNOR) staining in feline intestinal lymphoma, *J Vet Intern Med* 13:187, 1999.

Rissetto K et al: Recent trends in feline intestinal neoplasia: an epidemiologic study of 1,129 cases in the Veterinary Medical Database from 1964 to 2004, *J Am Anim Hosp Assoc* 47:28, 2011.

Scott KD et al: Utility of endoscopic biopsies of the duodenum and ileum for diagnosis of inflammatory bowel disease and small cell lymphoma in cats, *J Vet Intern Med* 25:1253, 2011.

Stein TJ et al: Treatment of feline gastrointestinal small-cell lymphoma with chlorambucil and glucocorticoids, *J Am Anim Hosp Assoc* 46:413, 2010.

Vail DM et al: Feline lymphoma (145 cases): proliferation indices, cluster of differentiation 3 immunoreactivity, and their association with prognosis in 90 cats, *J Vet Intern Med* 12:349, 1998.

Zwahlen CH et al: Results of chemotherapy for cats with alimentary malignant lymphoma: 21 cases (1993-1997), *J Am Vet Med Assoc* 213:1144, 1998.

CHAPTER 134
Canine Colitis

KENNETH W. SIMPSON, *Ithaca, New York*
ALISON C. MANCHESTER, *Ithaca, New York*

The term *colitis* frequently is used to describe the clinical syndrome characterized by bloody mucoid diarrhea and tenesmus, or dyschezia, presumed to be caused by inflammation of the colonic mucosa. The modifiers *acute* and *chronic* are used to describe the chronicity of clinical signs. However, a definitive diagnosis of colitis requires histopathologic examination of the colonic mucosa. Thus a clinical diagnosis of "acute colitis" rarely is confirmed by colonic biopsy because most patients do not require endoscopy and respond to conventional therapy. Conversely, a clinical diagnosis of "chronic colitis" always should be confirmed by histopathology, because the success of treatment is related closely to the histopathologic appearance. This chapter reviews the diagnosis and treatment of canine colitis with an emphasis on the management of lymphoplasmacytic and granulomatous colitis.

Diagnostic Approach

The diagnostic approach to dogs presenting with signs of colitis is directed at detecting or ruling out extracolonic causes of tenesmus, dyschezia, or fresh blood in the feces, such as prostatomegaly, perineal hernia, constipation, pelvic canal abnormalities, anal sac and perianal problems, and the various causes of large bowel diarrhea (Table 134-1).

In dogs with acute signs of large bowel diarrhea, the diagnostic plan typically consists of fecal examination for parasites (*Giardia* spp., whipworms), fecal culture (*Campylobacter* and *Salmonella* spp., with or without *Clostridium* spp.), and possibly fecal ELISA for *Clostridium* toxins. Acute colitis frequently responds to symptomatic therapy with anthelminthics (e.g., fenbendazole) or diet.

If the dog is systemically unwell, or large bowel diarrhea is severe or chronic, a biochemical profile, urinalysis, and complete blood count should be submitted to screen for systemic disease. Rectal cytology can be informative in detecting fungi (*Histoplasma* spp.) and ingested bacteria within neutrophils. Survey radiographs of the abdomen often yield little information about primary colonic disease but can be performed to screen for masses or foreign bodies and to evaluate the relationship of the colon to other viscera and the pelvic canal. Ultrasonography is useful for ruling out extracolonic causes of large bowel diarrhea, detecting ileocecocolic lesions, and assessing mural infiltration of masses and regional lymph nodes. In many animals with large bowel diarrhea the physical exam, fecal exam, laboratory testing, and imaging are normal, enabling the problem to be localized to the large bowel. The next step in the investigation of large bowel diarrhea is colonoscopic examination of the rectum, colon, and cecum and, if indicated, the terminal ileum (e.g., concurrent signs of small bowel diarrhea or low serum cobalamin). Principal differential diagnoses at this stage include inflammatory bowel disease, polyps, and neoplasia. At least 8 to 10 endoscopic biopsies of normal and abnormal mucosa should be acquired for histopathologic evaluation because lesions can be patchy. Where granulomatous colitis is suspected (see granulomatous colitis later), biopsies should be obtained for bacterial culture. Rigid proctoscopy is an alternative to flexible endoscopy for investigating and biopsying the distal colon and rectum.

Histopathologic Features of Colitis

A definitive diagnosis of colitis is based on histopathologic evaluation of colonic biopsies. Colitis falls under the umbrella term *inflammatory bowel disease* (IBD), which usually is defined by increased cellularity of the lamina propria. The extent of colonic inflammation varies from focal to diffuse involvement. The type and degree of cellular accumulation is also variable and is categorized subjectively as normal, mild, moderate, or severe.

Increased numbers of lymphocytes and plasma cells, so-called "lymphoplasmacytic enteritis," is the most frequently reported form of colitis.

Colonic infiltration with macrophages or neutrophils is less common and raises the possibility of an infectious process, and culture, special staining, and fluorescence *in situ* hybridization (FISH) are indicated. The presence of moderate-to-large numbers of eosinophils in intestinal biopsy samples, often accompanied by circulating eosinophilia, suggests possible parasitic infestation or dietary intolerance.

The emphasis on cellularity has meant that abnormalities in mucosal morphology have been somewhat overlooked. Crypt hyperplasia often is interpreted as a regenerative response to an inflammatory stimulus. Erosions, ulcers, and fibrosis are interpreted to infer colitis of increased severity. A major problem of histopathologic evaluation is the subjectivity and variability of reporting. The recent finding that the WSAVA standardization of pathology scheme, like previous standardized photographic schemes, has poor agreement among pathologists, questions further the ability of standardized grading in its current form to translate to improved diagnosis and

TABLE **134-1**

Causes of Large Bowel Diarrhea

Etiologic Category	Cause
Infectious/ parasitic	*Salmonella, Campylobacter, Clostridium* spp., invasive *E. coli, Trichuris vulpis, Giardia, Histoplasma, Prototheca* spp.
Dietary	Indiscretion, intolerance, allergy
Metabolic	Pancreatitis, uremia, hypoadrenocorticism, hypothyroidism
Inflammatory	Lymphoplasmacytic, granulomatous, neutrophilic, eosinophilic
Neoplasia	Adenocarcinoma, lymphosarcoma, polyps
Anatomic	Stricture, ileocolic or cecocolic intussusception, cecal eversion, foreign bodies
Functional	Motility disorders, idiopathic, "irritable bowel syndrome" Secondary to small intestinal disease

BOX **134-1**

Medical Management of Colitis

Dietary Options
Highly digestible
Restricted antigen/novel protein
Hydrolyzed protein

Fiber Supplementation
Psyllium: 1T small, 2T medium, 3T large breed with each meal

Anthelminthics
Fenbendazole: 50 mg/kg q24h PO for 3 days, repeat in 21 days

Antimicrobials
Metronidazole: 10-15 mg/kg q24h PO for 5 days
Tylosin: 10-15 mg/kg q8h PO for 14-28 days, maintenance 5 mg/kg q24h PO
Enrofloxacin: use in biopsy proven GC, 7.5 mg/kg q24h PO for at least 6 weeks

Antiinflammatory
Sulfasalazine: 20-30 mg/kg q8-12h PO
Mesalamine: 10-20 mg/kg q12h PO

Immunosuppressive
Prednisolone: 2 mg/kg q24h PO, maintain remission for 10-14 days then taper over 6-8 weeks
Azathioprine: 2 mg/kg q24h PO for 7 days, then 2 mg/kg q48h PO
Cyclosporine: 5 mg/kg q24h PO 10 wks

Motility Modifiers and Spasmolytics
Diphenoxylate or loperamide: 0.1-0.2 mg/kg q8h PO
Dicyclomine HCl (Bentyl): 0.2 mg/kg q6-8h PO if severe straining

management of patients with IBD. A further limitation of the WSAVA scheme in respect to colitis is that it does not consider goblet cells, which correlate with the presence of granulomatous colitis and severity of lymphoplasmacytic colitis and show dramatic increases after treatment. Clearly, the emphasis on histopathologic evaluation has to shift from the subjective reporting of cellularity toward identifying and reporting features that correlate with presence of disease and its outcome. Although histopathologic changes can be helpful, they frequently represent a common endpoint of many different diseases.

Management of Chronic Colitis

Lymphocytic Plasmacytic Colitis

The predominant form of chronic colitis in dogs is characterized by mucosal infiltration with lymphocytes and plasma cells and frequently is referred to as *lymphocytic plasmacytic colitis*. The cause of lymphocytic plasmacytic colitis has not been determined, but it is suspected that intestinal inflammation in dogs, like people, is a consequence of uncontrolled intestinal inflammation in response to a combination of elusive environmental, enteric microbial, and immunoregulatory factors in genetically susceptible individuals.

Analysis of mucosal immunopathology has shown canine lymphocytic plasmacytic colitis is associated with an increase in CD3+ T cells, IgA and IgG, plasma cells, and up-regulation of proinflammatory cytokines interleukin-2 (IL-2) and tumor necrosis factor-α (TNF-α). There is currently no information on genetic susceptibility of dogs to lymphocytic plasmacytic colitis. In a recent study the authors sought to examine the relationship of mucosal bacteria to lymphocytic plasmacytic colitis in 23 dogs (unpublished observations). The authors observed

numerous spiral bacteria inhabiting the mucus and glands of the healthy and inflamed colon that were consistent with enterohepatic *Helicobacter* spp. Findings included no evidence of *Brachyspira* spp., a decrease in the total number of mucosal bacteria, and a reduction in the proportion of *Clostridium* spp. relative to total bacteria and Enterobacteriaceae. These findings parallel the "dysbiosis" that is described in small intestinal IBD in dogs and establish that the density and composition of the colonic mucosal flora is related to the presence and severity of lymphocytic plasmacytic colitis in dogs (see Chapter 131). The authors observed a correlation between goblet cells, mucosal bacteria, and the histologic severity of colitis. The loss of mucus and goblet cells may be related to the dysbiosis associated with colitis. However, it is not clear if the microbial shifts are a cause or a consequence of inflammation, and their role in the etiopathogenesis of colitis has not been established.

Treatment

Studies in dogs with lymphocytic plasmacytic colitis provide reasonable evidence that various subsets of dogs respond to treatment with diet, antibiotics, or immunosuppressive therapy (Box 134-1). At present, because there is no reliable means for predicting which dogs will respond to which treatment, standard treatment consists of a series of therapeutic trials.

Most dogs with lymphocytic plasmacytic colitis usually have been trial treated with fenbendazole or metronidazole before the definitive diagnosis is obtained. Dogs that have not received these drugs typically are treated with them before embarking on sequential therapeutic trials with diet, antibiotics, and immunosuppressive agents.

Diet. Several clinical studies indicate that dogs with lymphocytic plasmacytic colitis and idiopathic colitis with minimal histologic change can respond to dietary modification. In a study of 13 dogs with lymphocytic plasmacytic colitis, clinical signs resolved in all 13 dogs (with a 2- to 28-month follow-up) after they were fed a cottage cheese and rice diet. In 11 dogs, two commercial diets (antigen restricted and low residue) not previously fed to these dogs were substituted successfully for the initial test diet, without causing recurrence of signs. Only 2 of these 11 dogs subsequently tolerated a switch to diets that had been fed at the time of onset of signs of colitis (Nelson, Stookey, and Kazacos, 1988).

In a subsequent study, 11 dogs with idiopathic chronic colitis were treated for 4 months with a commercial antigen–restricted diet. Within 1 month, four key signs associated with colitis (straining, fecal blood, fecal mucus, and fecal consistency) were improved significantly and remained so for the subsequent 3 months. Sulfasalazine also was used in the initial stages of management to control presenting signs. However, within 1 month 60% of the dogs required either no sulfasalazine (or less than when originally presented); within 2 months 90% were stabilized with no drug therapy (Simpson, Maskell, and Markwell, 1994).

In a third study, 27 dogs with idiopathic colitis had soluble fiber (psyllium) added to a highly digestible intestinal diet, with a good to excellent response observed in most dogs. In some dogs, the fiber dosage was reduced or eliminated, or a grocery store brand of dog food was substituted, without causing the diarrhea to return (Leib, 2000).

Taken as a whole, these studies indicate that a large proportion of dogs with lymphocytic plasmacytic colitis and idiopathic colitis with minimal histologic change respond to diets that are easily assimilable, antigen restricted, or hydrolyzed, with or without the addition of psyllium. Treatment responses typically occur within 2 weeks.

Additional Therapy. In patients that fail dietary modification and psyllium, the author adds an antibiotic, usually tylosin or metronidazole (if not previously treated) for 2 weeks. Dogs that respond to tylosin but relapse after cessation of treatment can be maintained on it chronically at a reduced dose (5 mg/kg q24h PO). In patients in which diet and antimicrobials fail, a treatment trial with sulfasalazine or aminosalicylic acid can be considered. However, these drugs are associated with keratoconjunctivitis sicca, and tear production should be measured before and during their use.

The next line of treatment is corticosteroid therapy, typically prednisolone 1 to 2 mg/kg q12h PO for 10 to 14 days and then tapered over 6 to 8 weeks. In dogs that exhibit severe side effects of steroids, require long-term steroid therapy, or are refractory to steroids, the author typically introduces azathioprine. If azathioprine is unsuccessful, cyclosporine (5 mg/kg q24h PO for 10 weeks) may be used.

The majority of dogs with lymphocytic plasmacytic colitis have favorable clinical responses to combinations of diet, antimicrobials, and prednisolone. When treatment failure occurs, it is important to reevaluate the patient carefully to determine if the diagnosis is accurate. Weight loss, frequent vomiting, hypoalbuminemia, hypocobalaminemia, and lymphadenopathy are inconsistent with lymphoplasmacytic colitis. Therefore another review of the histopathology is warranted to ensure the diagnosis is lymphocytic plasmacytic colitis and that infectious agents have been ruled out before escalating to more aggressive immunosuppressive therapy. This should include comprehensive fecal analysis, rectal cytology, and special stains of intestinal biopsies.

Granulomatous Colitis

Granulomatous colitis (also called histiocytic colitis) is much less common than lymphocytic plasmacytic colitis and is characterized by mucosal infiltration of macrophages with variable concurrent infiltrates of neutrophils, lymphocytes, and plasma cells. Granulomatous colitis raises the probability of an underlying infectious etiology, such as *E. coli* (e.g., boxer dogs and French bulldogs); *Streptococcus*, *Campylobacter*, *Yersinia*, and *Mycobacteria* spp.; or fungal (e.g., *Histoplasma* spp.) or algal (e.g., *Prototheca* spp.) infections. Culture of mucosal biopsies, intestinal lymph nodes, and other abdominal organs and imaging of chest and abdomen should be undertaken in cases of granulomatous or neutrophilic colitis to detect infectious organisms and systemic involvement. Special stains such as Gomori methenamine silver (GMS), periodic acid-Schiff (PAS), Gram, and modified Steiner are traditional cytochemical methods used to search for infectious agents in fixed tissues. Fluorescence *in situ* hybridization (FISH) with a probe directed against eubacterial 16S rRNA is a more contemporary and sensitive method of detecting bacteria within formalin fixed tissues (www.vet.cornell.edu/labs/simpson). It is imperative not to immunosuppress patients with granulomatous or neutrophilic infiltrates until infectious agents have been excluded. The prognosis for idiopathic granulomatous or neutrophilic enteropathies is guarded to poor if an underlying cause is not identified.

Granulomatous Colitis of Boxer Dogs

Granulomatous colitis of boxer dogs (GCB), also known as histiocytic ulcerative colitis (HUC), was described first by Van Kruiningen in a kennel of boxer dogs in 1965. The clinical hallmarks of the disease are severe large bowel diarrhea often accompanied by profound weight loss, anemia, and hypoalbuminemia. Granulomatous colitis of boxer dogs, although rare, occurs worldwide with reported cases originating from Australia, Japan, North America, and Europe. The pathognomonic lesion of GCB for the pathologist is mucosal infiltration with large numbers of macrophages staining positively with

PAS and usually is accompanied by mucosal ulceration and loss of goblet cells.

The poor response of GCB to empiric therapy and immunosuppression led to a reappraisal of antibiotic therapy. Multiple independent studies have documented dramatic clinical responses to enrofloxacin and an association between GCB and intramucosal *E. coli*. In the first study to link definitively invasive *E. coli* to GCB, colonic biopsies from affected boxer dogs (*n* = 13) and controls (*n* = 38) were examined by FISH with a eubacterial 16S rDNA probe (Simpson et al, 2006). Culture, 16S ribosomal DNA sequencing, and histochemistry were used to guide subsequent FISH. Intramucosal gram-negative coccobacilli were present in 100% of GCB but not in controls, and invasive bacteria hybridized with FISH probes to *E. coli*. Independent support for these findings was provided by the immunolocalization of *E. coli* to macrophages within the colons of 10 out of 10 GCB. *E. coli* strains isolated from affected boxer dogs are novel in phylogeny and have an adherent and invasive pathotype (AIEC) similar to strains isolated from people with Crohn's disease.

Subsequent studies have examined further the relationship of intramucosal *E. coli* to clinical and histologic outcome in boxer dogs with GC. In one study, clinical response to enrofloxacin was noted in seven out of seven dogs within 2 weeks (mean dose of 7 mg/kg/day for a mean duration of 9½ weeks) and was sustained in six dogs (mean disease-free interval = 45 months). Post-enrofloxacin FISH was negative for *E. coli* in four out of five dogs. *E. coli* resistant to enrofloxacin were present in the FISH-positive dog that relapsed clinically. Antibiotic resistance is an increasing problem, and enrofloxacin-resistant *E. coli* were isolated from 6 out of 14 GCB in a recent study. Of the enrofloxacin-resistant cases, four out of six also were resistant to macrophage-penetrating antimicrobials such as chloramphenicol, rifampicin, and trimethoprim sulfamethoxazole. Enrofloxacin treatment before definitive diagnosis was associated with antimicrobial resistance and poor clinical outcome (Craven et al, 2010).

Taken as a whole, these findings indicate that invasive *E. coli* play a critical role in the initiation and/or progression of GCB. Unfortunately, antimicrobial resistance is becoming common among GCB-associated *E. coli* and affects clinical response. To optimize outcome in GCB the authors recommend that antimicrobial therapy should be guided by mucosal culture and antimicrobial susceptibility testing rather than by empiric wisdom.

Granulomatous Colitis of Non-Boxer Dogs

Isolated cases of granulomatous colitis with clinical and histologic similarity to boxer dogs (i.e., PAS-positive macrophages) have been described in the mastiff, Alaskan malamute, Doberman pinscher, English bulldog, and French bulldog. A recent study of six French bulldogs (age 5 to 12 months; 5 male, 1 female) has demonstrated that GC in French bulldogs is phenotypically, histologically, and microbiologically analogous to GC in boxer dogs. FISH of colonic mucosa revealed multifocal accumulations of intramucosal *E. coli* in colonic biopsies of six out of six dogs. Treatment with enrofloxacin (5 out of 6 dogs) or marbofloxacin (1 out of 6 dogs) at 4.4 to 10 mg/kg

(median 10 mg/kg) q24h PO 6 to 10 weeks was associated with rapid clinical remission. All dogs remained free of clinical signs over a 3- to 30-month follow-up period (Manchester et al, 2012).

Boxers, bulldogs, and mastiffs cluster in the group of mastiff-type dogs, along with bull terriers, rottweilers, and bullmastiffs based on genetic similarity using microsatellite markers, suggesting a potential shared genetic predisposition to this form of colitis. However, at this time it is not clear if GC in breeds other than boxers and French bulldogs is associated with invasive bacteria in general or *E. coli*. In dogs with confirmed or suspected GC or neutrophilic colitis, the authors recommend FISH analysis and culture of colonic biopsies to help evaluate the presence and type of adherent or invasive bacteria and their susceptibility to antimicrobial agents. Absence of bacteria would prompt a search for other infectious agents. Because treatment successes are predicated on the judicious selection of appropriate antimicrobial drugs, the authors caution against empiric use of macrophage-penetrating antimicrobial drugs in dogs with suspected but not proven *E. coli*–associated granulomatous colitis.

References and Suggested Reading

Craven M et al: Antimicrobial resistance impacts clinical outcome of granulomatous colitis in boxer dogs, *Vet Intern Med* 24:819, 2010.

Davies DR et al: Successful management of histiocytic ulcerative colitis with enrofloxacin in two boxer dogs, *Aust Vet J* 82:58, 2004.

Day MJ et al: Histopathological standards for the diagnosis of gastrointestinal inflammation in endoscopic biopsy samples from the dog and cat: a report from the World Small Animal Veterinary Association Gastrointestinal Standardization Group, *J Comp Pathol* 138(suppl1):S1, 2008.

Hostutler RA et al: Antibiotic-responsive histiocytic ulcerative colitis in 9 dogs, *J Vet Intern Med* 18:499, 2004.

Jergens AE et al: Colonic lymphocyte and plasma cell populations in dogs with lymphocytic-plasmacytic colitis, *Am J Vet Res* 60:515, 1999.

Kleinschmidt S et al: Characterization of mast cell numbers and subtypes in biopsies from the gastrointestinal tract of dogs with lymphocytic-plasmacytic or eosinophilic gastroenterocolitis, *Vet Immunol Immunopathol* 120:80, 2007.

Leib MS: Treatment of chronic idiopathic large-bowel diarrhea in dogs with a highly digestible diet and soluble fiber: a retrospective review of 37 cases, *J Vet Intern Med* 14:27, 2000.

Manchester AC et al: Association between granulomatous colitis in French Bulldogs and invasive *Escherichia coli* and response to fluoroquinolone antimicrobials, *J Vet Intern Med* 27(1):56, 2012.

Mansfield CS et al: Remission of histiocytic ulcerative colitis in Boxer dogs correlates with eradication of invasive intramucosal *Escherichia coli*, *J Vet Intern Med* 23:964, 2009.

Nelson RW, Stookey LJ, Kazacos E: Nutritional management of idiopathic chronic colitis in the dog, *J Vet Intern Med* 2:133, 1988.

Ridyard AE et al: Apical junction complex protein expression in the canine colon: differential expression of claudin-2 in the colonic mucosa in dogs with idiopathic colitis, *J Histochem Cytochem* 55:1049, 2007.

Ridyard AE et al: Evaluation of Th1, Th2 and immunosuppressive cytokine mRNA expression within the colonic mucosa of dogs with idiopathic lymphocytic-plasmacytic colitis, *Vet Immunol Immunopathol* 86:205, 2002.

Roth L et al: A grading system for lymphocytic plasmacytic colitis in dogs, *J Vet Diagn Invest* 2:257, 1990.

Simpson JW, Maskell IE, Markwell PJ: Use of a restricted antigen diet in the management of idiopathic canine colitis, *J Small Anim Pract* 35:233, 1994.

Simpson KW et al: Adherent and invasive *Escherichia coli* is associated with granulomatous colitis in boxer dogs, *Infect Immun* 74:4778, 2006.

Simpson KW, Jergens AE: Pitfalls and progress in the diagnosis and management of canine inflammatory bowel disease, *Vet Clin North Am Small Anim Pract* 41:381, 2011.

Suchodolski JS et al: Molecular analysis of the bacterial microbiota in duodenal biopsies from dogs with idiopathic inflammatory bowel disease, *Vet Microbiol* 142:394, 2010.

van der Gaag I: The histological appearance of large intestinal biopsies in dogs with clinical signs of large bowel disease, *Can J Vet Res* 52:75, 1988.

Westermarck E et al: Tylosin-responsive chronic diarrhea in dogs, *J Vet Intern Med* 19:177, 2005.

Willard MD et al: Effect of tissue processing on assessment of endoscopic intestinal biopsies in dogs and cats, *J Vet Intern Med* 24(1):84, 2010.

Willard MD et al: Interobserver variation among histopathologic evaluations of intestinal tissues from dogs and cats, *J Am Vet Med Assoc* 220:1177, 2002.

CHAPTER 135

Laboratory Testing for the Exocrine Pancreas

ROMY M. HEILMANN, *College Station, Texas*
JÖRG M. STEINER, *College Station, Texas*

Diseases of the exocrine pancreas are important and occur frequently in dogs and cats. Recent studies that established a far higher prevalence of exocrine pancreatic disease in both species than was estimated about 30 years ago suggest that exocrine pancreatic disease in general, and more specifically pancreatitis, have long been underdiagnosed in both species. Because of the relative inaccessibility of the pancreas, the diagnosis of exocrine pancreatic disease can pose a challenge and requires a combination of patient history, thorough clinical examination, evaluation of biochemical markers that are highly sensitive and specific for exocrine pancreatic disease, and the use of diagnostic imaging techniques.

Laboratory Tests for Pancreatitis

Pancreatitis is a common and important disease in dogs and cats; antemortem diagnosis of pancreatitis can be challenging. Depending on the severity, patients may or may not exhibit classical clinical signs, nonspecific signs, or signs of severe systemic complications. Particularly cats often show only mild clinical signs that can be masked by other disease processes commonly associated with feline chronic pancreatitis (i.e., cholangitis and or inflammatory bowel disease). Thus the diagnosis of pancreatitis can be elusive, and probably a significant number of especially mild or subclinical cases remain undiagnosed.

Clinical pathology findings (e.g., leukocytosis or leukopenia, hyper- or hypoglycemia, hypocalcemia and hypophosphatemia, increased liver enzyme activities, hypercholesterolemia) are seen commonly but are nonspecific and do not help to arrive at a diagnosis of pancreatitis. However, routine blood work is essential to rule out major differential diagnoses and to assess the patient with pancreatitis for systemic complications. Abdominal radiography is not useful for diagnosing patients with pancreatitis but, like routine laboratory data, abdominal radiographs are important in ruling out other differential diagnoses. Abdominal ultrasonography can be useful for diagnosing pancreatitis, but stringent diagnostic criteria are crucial (see Chapter 137).

For many years, serum amylase activity alone or in combination with serum lipase activity was used as an indicator for acute pancreatic acinar cell damage and biomarker for pancreatitis. Today more sensitive and specific laboratory tests for diagnosing pancreatitis, most importantly pancreatic lipase immunoreactivity (Spec cPL, Spec fPL), are available.

Other tests that have been evaluated for the diagnosis of pancreatitis include systemic and urinary concentrations of trypsinogen-activation peptide (TAP), a by-product of the activation of trypsinogen that is undetectable in the circulation unless trypsinogen is activated prematurely within the pancreas because of pancreatitis. However, TAP is not clinically useful for the diagnosis of pancreatitis in dogs and cats. The concentration of serum trypsin-alpha$_1$-proteinase inhibitor (α_1PI) complex, derived from prematurely activated trypsin leaking from the inflamed pancreas and scavenged by α_1PI, and serum α_2-macroglobulin as a scavenger for prematurely activated trypsin are also not useful for the diagnosis of pancreatitis. Serum C-reactive protein (CRP), an acute-phase protein, has been measured in dogs with acute pancreatitis. Because CRP is not specific for the pancreas and may increase with any inflammatory disease, infection, or trauma, CRP is not useful to diagnose pancreatitis but may be useful as a marker of disease severity.

Serum Amylase and Lipase Activities

Amylase and lipase are digestive enzymes produced by pancreatic acinar cells. Damage to these cells as occurs with pancreatic necrosis and inflammation during pancreatitis leads to increased amounts of both enzymes in the systemic circulation. Because many different lipases and amylases originate from a wide range of tissues, their activities that are measured by catalytic assays are not pancreas specific. An increased serum amylase activity can be found in patients with conditions other than pancreatitis; conversely, a normal serum amylase activity does not rule out pancreatitis. Similarly, the sensitivity and specificity of serum lipase activity for canine pancreatitis are low. To be suggestive of pancreatitis in dogs, serum amylase or lipase activities must be increased at least threefold to fivefold above the upper limit of the reference range, but both are of low diagnostic value. In cats, serum amylase and lipase activities have a very low sensitivity for pancreatitis and thus are of no diagnostic value in this species.

Serum Trypsin-like Immunoreactivity

Assays for serum trypsin-like immunoreactivity (TLI) measure cationic trypsinogen, trypsin (if present), and some trypsin molecules complexed with proteinase inhibitors. Serum TLI reflects the amount of functional pancreatic tissue present and is highly sensitive and specific for the diagnosis of exocrine pancreatic insufficiency (see later) but lacks sensitivity in the diagnosis of pancreatitis in dogs and cats.

Increased serum TLI concentrations can be measured in dogs and cats with pancreatitis, presumably because of leakage of trypsinogen and prematurely activated trypsin from the inflamed pancreas. However, the half-life of TLI in serum is thought to be very short, and a significant degree of inflammation is required for serum TLI concentrations to be increased. In dogs, the sensitivity and specificity of serum cTLI concentration for pancreatitis have been reported as less than 40% and 65% to 100%, respectively. In cats, serum fTLI concentration appears to be more useful clinically, but the increase of serum fTLI above the diagnostic cutoff value used for pancreatitis was of much shorter duration than that of serum fPLI in

mild experimentally induced feline pancreatitis. The sensitivity and specificity of serum fTLI concentration for the diagnosis of pancreatitis in cats range between 33% and 86% and 56% and 90%, respectively. TLI also may be increased in patients with renal failure, and thus a serum chemistry profile and urinalysis should be performed to rule out renal disease if the serum TLI concentration is increased. With the availability of newer, more sensitive and specific diagnostic tests (Spec cPL and Spec fPL), serum TLI concentration should no longer be employed for the diagnosis of pancreatitis in either species.

Serum Pancreatic Lipase Immunoreactivity

In contrast to serum lipase activity, immunoassays for pancreatic lipase immunoreactivity (PLI) measure lipase that originates exclusively from the exocrine pancreas. Increased amounts of pancreatic lipase escape into the systemic circulation during pancreatic inflammation and necrosis and can be measured using species-specific immunoassays.

Sensitivities of 82% to 94% have been reported for the diagnosis of clinically significant pancreatitis by serum cPLI concentration. In a study that evaluated the sensitivity of various serum markers in dogs with less severe pancreatitis, measurement of serum cPLI concentration showed the highest sensitivity of any diagnostic test evaluated with 64% (Steiner et al, 2008). However, a single measurement of cPLI in serum cannot predict the histopathologic severity of pancreatitis. In cats, sensitivities of serum fPLI for diagnosing patients with pancreatitis range from 54 (subclinical or mild disease) to 100% (moderate to severe pancreatitis). Unlike serum fTLI, serum fPLI was increased persistently in cats with experimentally induced pancreatitis, presumably because of a delayed renal elimination of the larger negatively charged protein measured.

Measurement of serum PLI is a practical test that requires a serum sample after withholding food for 8 to 12 hours. Commercially available tests that measure PLI in dogs (Spec cPL) and cats (Spec fPL) are reported to perform similarly to the originally developed assays. Concentrations of at least 400 µg/L (Spec cPL) in dogs and at least 5.4 µg/L (Spec fPL) in cats are consistent with a diagnosis of pancreatitis. Equivocal test results (Spec cPL: 201 to 399 µg/L; Spec fPL: 3.6 to 5.3 µg/L) require further evaluation of the patient or repeated testing. Recently, patient side tests (SNAP cPL and SNAP fPL) for use in the clinic have been introduced. In these tests, a color intensity of the sample spot that is lighter than the reference spot indicates that pancreatitis is very unlikely and other differential diagnoses should be considered. In contrast, a sample spot that is equal to or darker than the reference spot indicates an abnormal cPL or fPL concentration, suggesting pancreatitis. As a positive SNAP cPL/SNAP fPL indicates a Spec cPL/Spec fPL in the equivocal or diagnostic range for pancreatitis, Spec cPL/Spec fPL should be measured to verify the diagnosis of pancreatitis and to obtain a baseline concentration that then can be used to monitor the progression of disease in the patient.

Studies in dogs and cats with induced chronic renal failure (CRF) suggest that serum cPLI and fPLI can be used as diagnostic tests in patients with CRF because serum PLI is either not affected or only minimally affected. Also serum cPLI was not affected by long-term administration of prednisone (Steiner et al, 2009). Serum PLI is specific for the exocrine pancreas and is the most sensitive serum test that currently is available for the diagnosis of pancreatitis in dogs and cats. However, as for other diseases, the integration of all clinically available data, especially abdominal ultrasonography and serum PLI, are expected to yield the best diagnostic accuracy.

Laboratory Tests for Exocrine Pancreatic Insufficiency

Exocrine pancreatic insufficiency (EPI) is a deficiency of enzyme and fluid secretion from the exocrine pancreas. As a result of deficiency of digestive enzymes in the small intestine (SI), the syndrome is characterized by clinical signs of maldigestion. Because of the large secretory reserve capacity of the exocrine pancreas and a high degree of metabolic pathway redundancy for the digestion of some nutrients, clinical signs of maldigestion may not occur until the vast majority of the functional pancreatic mass has been lost. Although EPI may be suspected based on clinical signs, medical history, and patient signalment, the clinical signs are usually nonspecific and EPI must be differentiated from other causes of maldigestion and malabsorption.

Routine blood work (i.e., complete blood count [CBC] and chemistry profile) is often within normal limits or shows nonspecific changes that may be due to concurrent disease. Serum cobalamin concentration is decreased severely in most dogs (Batchelor et al, 2007) and cats (Thompson et al, 2009) with EPI (in >80% of cases in both species). In fact, EPI is an important reason for cobalamin deficiency in both species, because the exocrine pancreas is an important source of intrinsic factor in dogs and cats. Decreased serum cobalamin and increased serum folate concentrations also may reflect secondary SI dysbiosis; a decrease in both may indicate concurrent chronic small intestinal disease (e.g., inflammatory bowel disease). Serum glucose concentration is usually normal but may be increased in patients with concurrent diabetes mellitus (most commonly seen in patients in which EPI is due to chronic pancreatitis destroying endocrine and exocrine portions of the pancreas). Diagnostic imaging studies (i.e., abdominal radiography and ultrasonography) are not sensitive or specific and thus not useful for diagnosing EPI. In clinical practice, exocrine pancreatic function testing is the method of choice to confirm or rule out EPI before proceeding with further evaluation of the patient.

Laboratory techniques used in the past to diagnose EPI include the microscopic examination of feces for the presence of undigested food, the assessment of oral fat absorption by measuring plasma turbidity, the starch tolerance test, and the *in vivo* assessment of pancreatic enzyme activity in the intestinal juice after oral administration of the synthetic chymotrypsin substrate bentiromide. These tests are of limited usefulness because of practical constraints and are affected by the gastrointestinal transit time and other causes of malassimilation. A test that is more applicable in the clinical setting and that measures primarily the activity of pancreatic trypsin and chymotrypsin in feces is the determination of fecal proteolytic activity (FPA) by either qualitative gelatin digestion methods or semiquantitative azocasein hydrolysis or radial enzyme diffusion into agar containing a casein substrate. However, false-negative and false-positive test results occur frequently, and more sensitive and specific tests for the diagnosis of EPI in dogs and cats are available. Thus FPA can no longer be recommended for the diagnosis of EPI in both species.

Fecal Pancreatic Elastase-1

Elastase-1 is a digestive protease exclusively synthesized and secreted by the pancreas in the form of an inactive zymogen, proelastase. After its release and transport into the duodenum via the pancreatic ductal system, pancreatic proelastase-1 is activated in the intestinal lumen, where it resists proteolytic degradation and withstands the intestinal passage virtually undegraded. Thus the concentration of pancreatic elastase-1 (pE1) in feces theoretically should reflect the functional capacity of the exocrine pancreas.

Fecal pE1 can be measured in dogs by a species-specific enzyme-linked immunosorbent assay (ELISA) and has been reported to be sensitive and specific (95% and 92%, respectively) for clinical EPI when associated with typical clinical signs and using a cutoff value for EPI of 10 μg/g or less in a single fecal sample (Spillmann et al, 2000). Despite its lack of cross-reactivity with pE1 from other species (that may be contained in pancreatic enzyme supplements) and its potential to distinguish exocrine pancreatic disease from primary intestinal disorders (with potentially high luminal amounts of neutrophil elastase), a remarkable day-to-day variation and significant overlap between healthy dogs and dogs with EPI exist. A high false-positive rate renders the test unreliable and poses a risk for unnecessary treatment costs. Although fecal pE1 may aid in ruling out EPI, a positive result always should be confirmed by a more sensitive test (i.e., measurement of serum TLI). A situation in which fecal pE1 measurement could be useful is EPI resulting from occlusion or obstruction of the pancreatic duct, in which serum cTLI will likely be normal (which has not been reported and is probably extremely rare).

Serum Trypsin-like Immunoreactivity

Assays for TLI concentration in serum measure cationic trypsin (if present) and its zymogen form (trypsinogen) in the circulation, presumably of leakage of trace amounts into the pancreatic venous or lymphatic vessels and to some degree also trypsin complexed by scavenging proteins. Because the analyte measured as serum TLI originates only from the pancreas and reflects the amount of functional pancreatic tissue present, serum TLI is highly sensitive and specific for the diagnosis of EPI in dogs and cats. Normal ranges used at the authors' laboratory are 5.7 to 45.2 μg/L, with a cutoff value for diagnosing EPI of at least 2.5 μg/L for dogs, and 12.0 to 82.0 μg/L, with a cutoff for EPI of at least 8.0 µg/L for cats. An abnormally low serum TLI (dogs: ≤2.5 µg/L; cats: ≤8.0 µg/L) associated with clinical signs is considered diagnostic for EPI.

An equivocal serum cTLI concentration (i.e., between 2.5 and 5.7 µg/L) can be seen in patients with chronic SI disease but also in dogs in the process of developing EPI. Equivocal cTLI results may be found in dogs with autoimmune atrophic pancreatitis (see Chapter 136) tested early in the disease course and may precede the onset of clinical EPI. Conversely, a normal serum cTLI, especially when low normal, does not preclude the evolution of mild to moderate pancreatic dysfunction. In patients with EPI secondary to chronic intermittent or recurrent acute pancreatitis a normal serum cTLI could be due to an acute exacerbation of inflammation in the residual glandular tissue of the pancreas. If serum cTLI measures between 2.5 and 5.7 µg/L, retesting the patient in approximately 4 weeks is recommended to rule out subclinical EPI. Also, although TLI reflects the functional pancreatic mass, repeated testing is not predictive for the disease, and the need for dietary enzyme replacement therapy cannot be inferred from the TLI concentration alone but has to be based on the clinical evaluation of the patient.

Concurrent renal disease or a decreased rate of glomerular filtration may result in a slightly higher serum TLI concentration than reflected by the amount of functional pancreatic acinar tissue and thus in a falsely normal serum TLI. A normal serum TLI also is assumed to occur in patients with a pancreatic duct obstruction, congenital deficiency of intestinal enteropeptidase, or a selective pancreatic enzyme deficiency not involving trypsin. Measurement of serum TLI requires a single serum sample after withholding food for 8 to 12 hours. Postprandially, serum TLI may increase slightly and transiently. Serum TLI is the most sensitive and specific pancreatic function test currently available and remains the gold standard for diagnosing EPI in dogs and cats. Determination of the underlying disease process may require morphologic evaluation of the pancreas by pancreatic biopsy, but histologic pancreatic atrophy does not reflect the remaining functional pancreatic reserve.

Serum Pancreatic Lipase Immunoreactivity

The analyte measured as pancreatic lipase immunoreactivity (PLI) in serum is of exclusively pancreatic origin. Low concentrations of serum cPLI can be detected in dogs with EPI, but the overlap between healthy dogs and dogs with EPI renders the TLI assay superior for the diagnosis of EPI. Also, the PLI assays commercially available today (Spec cPL, Spec fPL) have been optimized for diagnosing patients with pancreatitis and are not useful for the diagnosis of EPI.

Exocrine Pancreatic Neoplasia

Lymphoma and pancreatic adenocarcinoma (AC) are the most common neoplasias of the exocrine pancreas in dogs and cats but are rare in both species. Clinical signs usually are nonspecific but can be severe. A local inflammatory response to avascular tumor necrosis may cause clinical signs of pancreatitis. Clinical pathology findings are unremarkable or nonspecific. Serum lipase activity may be extremely high in dogs with pancreatic AC, but serum amylase and lipase activities are reported not commonly in patients with pancreatic adenocarcinoma. Serum TLI or PLI concentrations have not been reported in dogs or cats with primary pancreatic neoplasia. Thus currently there is no laboratory test for the diagnosis of pancreatic AC.

References and Suggested Reading

Batchelor DJ et al: Prognostic factors in canine exocrine pancreatic insufficiency: prolonged survival is likely if clinical remission is achieved, *J Vet Intern Med* 21:54, 2007.

Forman MA et al: Evaluation of serum feline pancreatic lipase immunoreactivity and helical computed tomography versus conventional testing for the diagnosis of feline pancreatitis, *J Vet Intern Med* 18:807, 2004.

Holm JL et al: C-reactive protein concentrations in canine acute pancreatitis, *J Vet Emerg Crit Care* 14:183, 2004.

McCord K et al: A multi-institutional study evaluating the diagnostic utility of the Spec cPL™ and SNAP® cPL™ in clinical acute pancreatitis in 84 dogs, *J Vet Intern Med* 26(4):888, 2012.

Spillmann T et al: Canine faecal pancreatic elastase (cE1) in dogs with clinical exocrine pancreatic insufficiency, normal dogs and dogs with chronic enteropathies, *Eur J Comp Gastroenterol* 5:1, 2000.

Steiner JM, Williams DA: Serum feline trypsin-like immunoreactivity in cats with exocrine pancreatic insufficiency, *J Vet Intern Med* 14:627, 2000.

Steiner JM et al: Sensitivity of serum markers for pancreatitis in dogs with macroscopic evidence of pancreatitis, *Vet Ther* 9:263, 2008.

Steiner JM et al: Stability of canine pancreatic lipase immunoreactivity concentration in serum samples and effects of long-term administration of prednisone to dogs on serum canine pancreatic lipase immunoreactivity concentrations, *Am J Vet Res* 70:1001, 2009.

Steiner JM, Rehfeld JF, Pantchev N: Evaluation of fecal elastase and serum cholecystokinin in dogs with a false positive fecal elastase test, *J Vet Intern Med* 24:643, 2010.

Thompson KA et al: Feline exocrine pancreatic insufficiency: 16 cases (1992-2007), *J Feline Med Surg* 11:935, 2009.

Wiberg ME, Nurmi AK, Westermarck E: Serum trypsin-like immunoreactivity measurement for the diagnosis of subclinical exocrine pancreatic insufficiency, *J Vet Intern Med* 13:426, 1999.

Williams DA, Batt RM: Sensitivity and specificity of radioimmunoassay of serum trypsin-like immunoreactivity for the diagnosis of canine exocrine pancreatic insufficiency, *J Am Vet Med Assoc* 192:195, 1988.

CHAPTER 136

Exocrine Pancreatic Insufficiency in Dogs

MARIA WIBERG, *Helsinki, Finland*

Chronic diseases of the exocrine pancreas may affect pancreatic function and lead to inadequate production of digestive enzymes with associated maldigestion signs of exocrine pancreatic insufficiency (EPI). The exocrine pancreas has a large reserve in terms of secretory capacity, and clinical signs do not occur until about 90% of secretory capacity is lost. EPI in dogs can be the result of pancreatic acinar atrophy, chronic pancreatitis, pancreatic hypoplasia, and pancreatic neoplasia. EPI has been found in many different breeds, and breed-specific pathogenetic differences have been reported.

Etiopathogenesis

Pancreatic acinar atrophy is by far the most common reason for the clinical signs of EPI. The breeds most commonly affected with the acinar atrophy are German shepherds, rough-coated collies, and Eurasians. In these breeds, an autosomal-recessive inheritance model has been suggested. Thus far genetic studies have not been able to identify the genes involved (Clark et al, 2005; Proschowsky and Fredholm, 2007). Females and males usually are affected equally.

Studies with German shepherds and collies suggest that pancreatic atrophy is a result of an *autoimmune-mediated atrophic lymphocytic pancreatitis*, which gradually may lead to almost total destruction of pancreatic acinar tissue (Wiberg, Saari, and Westermarck, 2000). Typically the endocrine part of the pancreas is unaffected. A long-term follow-up study of a German shepherd litter revealed that the disease was not congenital, and a polygenic inheritance pattern has been suggested (Westermarck, Saari, and Wiberg, 2010). Genetic predisposition to the disease and the typical histologic findings during the progression of acinar atrophy have been taken as primary evidence of the autoimmune nature of the disease.

Wiberg, Saari, and Westermarck (1999b) divided the progression of acinar atrophy into subclinical and clinical phases. The subclinical phase is characterized by marked lymphocytic inflammation into a partially atrophied acinar parenchyma. Cytotoxic T cells are predominant when the tissue destruction is in progress. When the disease progresses to end-stage atrophy, the clinical phase of EPI develops. An atrophied pancreas is thin and transparent with no increase of fibrotic tissue.

The natural progression of the atrophic pancreatitis can vary markedly. Clinical signs of EPI usually appear at 1 to 5 years of age but also can be seen in older dogs. Dogs may remain in the subclinical phase for years and sometimes for life (Wiberg and Westermarck, 2002). Markers that predict which dogs are likely to develop clinical disease or environmental factors that trigger disease have not been identified thus far.

Chronic pancreatitis is the most common cause of EPI in cats and humans. In dogs, chronic pancreatitis has been recognized increasingly as a cause of EPI. Chronic pancreatitis usually affects older dogs, and breed-specific clinical and histopathologic features have been reported (Batchelor et al, 2007b; Watson et al, 2011). Unlike the situation of atrophic pancreatitis, in chronic pancreatitis usually a progressive destruction of the exocrine and endocrine pancreas is accompanied by fibrosis. Clinical signs are nonspecific gastrointestinal signs and sometimes are related to the development of diabetes mellitus. The congenital form of exocrine or exocrine and endocrine pancreatic hypoplasia sometimes is found in young puppies. EPI is reported rarely in association with pancreatic neoplasia.

Clinical Signs

Typical clinical signs of EPI include increased fecal volume and defecation frequency, yellow or gray feces, weight loss, and flatulence. Other common signs are polyphagia; poorly digested, loose, and pulpy feces; or coprophagia. Signs of nervousness or aggressiveness may occur possibly because of abdominal discomfort caused by increased intestinal gas. Severe watery diarrhea is usually only temporary. Skin disorders also have been reported. Although the signs of EPI are considered typical, they are not pathognomonic for pancreatic dysfunction, because similar maldigestion signs may be observed in other small intestinal disorders.

Diagnosis

Diagnosis of exocrine pancreatic dysfunction is based on typical clinical findings and confirmed with abnormal pancreatic function testing. Routine serum biochemistry profile and complete blood count often show unremarkable changes. Serum amylase and lipase activities are not useful in the diagnosis of EPI. Various pancreatic function tests that measure pancreatic enzymes in the blood and feces have been used to diagnose canine EPI. The diagnostic value of the tests has relied mostly on their ability to distinguish whether the clinical maldigestion signs are caused by EPI or a disease of the small intestine.

Serum Trypsin-like Immunoreactivity

The measurement of serum canine trypsin-like immunoreactivity (TLI) has become one of the most commonly used pancreatic function tests to diagnose canine EPI (see Chapter 136). Serum TLI measurement is species and pancreas specific, with high sensitivity and specificity for diagnosing EPI. The reference range for canine TLI (cTLI) in healthy dogs is greater than 5.7 to 45.2 μg/L (RIA). In dogs showing clinical maldigestion signs of EPI, cTLI concentrations are usually very low (<2.5 μg/L), indicating severe loss of digestive enzyme–producing acinar tissue. However, the interpretation of cTLI values is not always straightforward. Pathologic processes affecting exocrine pancreatic function are gradually progressive, and cTLI levels can vary from normal to abnormal, depending of the degree of pancreatic tissue lost. Overlapping results between normal and affected dogs can be expected, and a normal cTLI greater than 5 μg/L does not necessarily exclude the possibility of mild-to-moderate pancreatic dysfunction. In general, the lower the cTLI value, the more valuable a single measurement is in assessing the pancreatic dysfunction. Dogs with serum cTLI concentrations in the range of 2.5 to 5 μg/L and gastrointestinal signs can be a diagnostic challenge. Whether the signs are caused by a decreased exocrine pancreatic function or disease of the small intestine may be difficult to assess, and further diagnostic procedures repeating the cTLI measurement or treatment trials are needed. In breeds predisposed to autoimmune atrophic pancreatitis, repeatedly subnormal cTLI values (2.5 to 5 μg/L) in dogs showing no typical signs of EPI indicate subclinical EPI and suggest partial atrophy (Wiberg, Nurmi, and Westermarck, 1999a).

Fecal Enzyme Measurements

Canine fecal elastase is a species- and pancreas-specific test with high sensitivity but relatively low specificity. It has been shown that a single fecal elastase concentration greater than 20 μg/g is valuable for excluding EPI in dogs with chronic diarrhea. Values less than 20 μg/g in association with typical clinical signs of EPI are suggestive of severe pancreatic dysfunction (Battersby et al, 2005; Spillmann et al, 2000).

Treatment

Enzyme Replacement Therapy

When clinical maldigestion signs of EPI appear, enzyme replacement therapy is indicated. Basic treatment involves supplementation of the dog's ordinary food with pancreatic enzyme extracts. Various pancreatic enzyme extracts are available. The highest enzyme activity in the duodenum has been achieved by using non–enteric-coated supplements such as powdered enzymes or raw chopped pancreas, and these supplements have proved equally effective in controlling clinical signs.(Wiberg, Lautala and

Westermarck, 1998). A recent study revealed that a positive treatment response can also be achieved with enteric-coated pancreatic enzyme preparations (Mas et al, 2012). The maintenance dosage for enzyme supplementation depends on the preparation used as well as the individual animal variation. The dosage for raw frozen pancreas is 50 to 100 g/meal (for dogs that weigh 20 to 35 kg). The use of raw pig's pancreas should be avoided in areas endemic with Aujeszky's disease because of the danger for dogs acquiring pseudorabies. The enzyme preparation has to be given with the meal, and two or more meals a day should be fed to meet the animal's caloric requirements. Once clinical improvement and weight gain is achieved, the dose of enzyme supplementation can be tapered slowly to effect. In a small percentage of dogs treated with the non–enteric-coated enzymes gingival bleeding can occur, which generally resolves by reducing the amount of enzymes supplemented and by moistening the food. Dogs with partial acinar atrophy but no clinical signs of EPI do not require treatment. In autoimmune atrophic pancreatitis the value of early immunosuppressive treatment in slowing the progression of the autoimmune-mediated tissue destruction was found to be questionable; thus it is not recommended (Wiberg and Westermarck, 2002).

Supportive Treatments

Supportive treatments should be considered when the treatment response to enzyme replacement therapy is not satisfactory. Orally administered enzymes may be destroyed largely by gastric acid, and despite accurate enzyme administration, the digestive capacity does not return to normal. In some dogs the increase of enzyme dosage or change to another supplement may be beneficial. EPI also may be associated with secondary problems that may worsen the clinical signs. These include small intestinal dysbiosis, malabsorption of cobalamin, and the coexistence of a small intestinal disease.

Antibiotics

Antibiotics are the most commonly used supportive treatment. An increased amount of substrates for bacteria in the small intestine, a lack of bacteriostatic factors of the pancreatic juice, and changes in intestinal motility and immune functions are possible reasons for accumulation of bacteria in the small intestine of dogs with EPI. Antibiotics have been used during the initial treatment when clinical signs such as diarrhea, increased intestinal gas, and flatulence have not resolved with enzyme therapy or when these signs have recurred during long-term treatment. Commonly used antibiotics are tylosin and metronidazole (Wiberg, Lautala, and Westermarck, 1998).

Dietary Modification

Clinical feeding studies during long-term treatment of EPI have shown that the need for special diets is minimal and the dogs may continue to be fed with their original diet (Wiberg et al, 1998; Westermarck and Wiberg, 2006). However, radical dietary changes should be avoided, and special attention should be paid to individual needs because responses to different diets varied among dogs. Furthermore, the severity of some clinical signs of EPI can be decreased with dietary modification (Westermarck, Wiberg, and Junttila, 1990; Westermarck and Wiberg, 2006). A highly digestible, low-fiber, and moderate-fat diet can alleviate clinical signs such as defecation frequency, increased fecal volume, and flatulence. Highly digestible diets may be of particular value in the initial treatment until the nutritional status has improved and possible mucosal damage has been repaired. A low-fat diet has been recommended because enzyme supplements alone are incapable of restoring normal fat absorption. Fat absorption also may be affected by bacterial deconjugation of bile salts in a small intestinal disease, producing metabolites that in turn may result in diarrhea. Dietary sensitivities may be a consequence of EPI; therefore hypoallergic diets may benefit some dogs, especially those with concurrent skin problems.

Cobalamin

Cobalamin deficiency in dogs with EPI is partly the result of increased uptake of cobalamin by intestinal bacteria and partly because of the lack of the pancreatic intrinsic factor, shown to have a major role in the absorption of cobalamin. Because cobalamin deficiency has been found with 82% of dogs with EPI (Batchelor et al, 2007a), serum cobalamin should be measured in dogs that are clinically suspicious for EPI or do not respond satisfactorily to the enzyme treatment. Cobalamin is given subcutaneously, and the dosage currently used is 250 to 1000 μg once a week, depending on the size of the dog. The treatment should be repeated based on the serum levels.

Other Supportive Treatments

Inhibition of gastric acid secretion by H_2-antagonist may be indicated, especially when clinical signs such as vomiting or inappetence appear. Malabsorption of fat-soluble vitamins may be expected with EPI; however, the clinical importance of vitamin A, D, E, or K deficiency has not been reported. When the treatment response to enzymes and supportive therapies is still unsatisfactory, concomitant disease of the small intestine should be suspected.

Prognosis

When the clinical signs of EPI appear, the loss of pancreatic tissue is already almost total. The changes are considered to be irreversible, and lifelong enzyme treatment usually is required. Response to enzyme treatment usually is seen during the first weeks of treatment, with weight gain, cessation of diarrhea, and decrease in fecal volume. The level of treatment response achieved during the initial treatment period seems to remain fairly stable, with favorable long-term prognosis (Wiberg, Lautala, and Westermarck, 1998; Batchelor et al, 2007). Although some dogs experience short relapses with associated clinical signs, the permanent deterioration of the clinical

condition during long-term treatment is uncommon. During long-term treatment with non–enteric-coated enzyme supplements, the gastrointestinal signs considered typical for dogs with EPI were controlled almost completely in half of the dogs (Wiberg, Lautala, and Westermarck, 1998). Although it was not always possible to eliminate all signs, acceptable resolution of signs was achieved, especially in more serious signs. Poor response to treatment was observed in 20% of the dogs despite similar treatment regimens. Furthermore, about 20% of dogs diagnosed with EPI were euthanized during the first year of diagnosis. The most common reason for euthanasia was poor treatment response. Another reason was owner reluctance for expensive and lifelong treatment.

References and Suggested Reading

Batchelor DJ et al: Breed associations for canine exocrine pancreatic insufficiency, *J Vet Intern Med* 21:207, 2007b.
Batchelor DJ et al: Prognostic factors in canine exocrine pancreatic insufficiency: prolonged survival is likely if clinical remission is achieved, *J Vet Intern Med* 21:54, 2007a.
Battersby IA et al: Effect of intestinal inflammation on fecal elastase concentration in dogs, *Vet Clin Pathol* 34:49, 2005.
Clark LA et al: Linkage analysis and gene expression profile of pancreatic acinar atrophy in the German shepherd dog, *Mamm Genome* 16:955, 2005.
Mas A et al: A blinded randomised controlled trial to determine the effect of enteric coating on enzyme treatment for canine exocrine pancreatic insufficiency, *BMC Vet Res* 8:127, 2012.
Proschowsky HF, Fredholm M: Exocrine pancreatic insufficiency in the Eurasian dog breed—inheritance and exclusion of two candidate genes, *Anim Genet* 38:171, 2007.
Spillmann T et al: Canine faecal pancreatic elastase (cE1) in dogs with clinical exocrine pancreatic insufficiency, normal dogs and dogs with chronic enteropathies, *Eur J Comp Gastroenterol* 2:5, 2000.
Watson PJ et al: Characterization of chronic pancreatitis in English Cocker Spaniels, *J Vet Intern Med* 25:797, 2011.
Westermarck E, Wiberg M, Junttila J: Role of feeding in the treatment of dogs' pancreatic degenerative atrophy, *Acta Vet Scand* 31:325-331, 1990.
Westermarck E, Wiberg ME: Effects of diet on clinical signs of exocrine pancreatic insufficiency in dogs, *J Am Vet Med Assoc* 228:225, 2006.
Westermarck E, Saari SAM, Wiberg ME: Heritability of exocrine pancreatic insufficiency in German shepherd dogs, *J Vet Intern Med* 24:450, 2010.
Wiberg ME, Westermarck E: Subclinical exocrine pancreatic insufficiency in dogs, *J Am Vet Med Assoc* 220:1183, 2002.
Wiberg ME, Lautala H-M, Westermarck E: Response to long-term enzyme replacement treatment in dogs with exocrine pancreatic insufficiency, *J Am Vet Med Assoc* 1:86, 1998.
Wiberg ME, Nurmi A-K, Westermarck E: Serum trypsin-like immunoreactivity measurement for the diagnosis of subclinical exocrine pancreatic insufficiency in dogs, *J Vet Intern Med* 13:426, 1999a.
Wiberg ME, Saari SAM, Westermarck E: Cellular and humoral immune responses in atrophic lymphocytic pancreatitis in German shepherd dogs and rough-coated collies, *Vet Immunol Immunopathol* 76:103, 2000.
Wiberg ME, Saari SAM, Westermarck E: Exocrine pancreatic atrophy in German shepherds and rough-coated collies: an end-result of lymphocytic pancreatitis, *Vet Pathol* 36:530, 1999b.

CHAPTER 137

Treatment of Canine Pancreatitis

CRAIG G. RUAUX, *Corvallis, Oregon*

Pancreatic inflammation is a common, potentially challenging, and frustrating problem in canine internal medicine. In recent years interest in diseases of the pancreas has intensified. New diagnostic tests and imaging modalities have allowed unprecedented ability to detect pancreatic disease in canine patients. However, with this comes increasing evidence that canine pancreatic disease is far more common, and far more heterogeneous, than originally thought. With recognition of pancreatic pathology in increasing numbers of patients, determination of the correct therapeutic approach has become even more challenging. This is particularly the case in dogs with chronic pancreatic inflammation that may be either a primary disease or secondary to other gastrointestinal inflammatory disease. In some cases of chronic gastrointestinal disease with comorbid pancreatitis, the therapeutic approach may seem to be in conflict with accepted dogma regarding the treatment of pancreatitis.

Recognition of Acute Pancreatitis in the Canine Patient

The conclusive diagnosis of acute pancreatitis can be difficult. The presence of compatible clinical signs, such as vomiting, abdominal pain, dehydration, and pyrexia, increases the index of suspicion for the disease; however, no clinical findings are specific for pancreatitis.

Plain Radiography

The effects of acute pancreatitis on closely related organs and the peritoneum establish a localized peritonitis. This localized peritonitis is then the cause of most of the plain radiographic signs associated with acute pancreatitis in dogs, such as loss of contrast in the cranial abdomen, that is, the "ground glass appearance." Plain radiographic findings are nonspecific and at best only supportive of a clinical diagnosis of acute pancreatitis. A retrospective survey of 70 fatal cases of acute pancreatitis in dogs reported radiographic findings consistent with acute pancreatitis in only 10 of 41 cases (24%) for which radiographs were available (Hess et al, 1998). Because these cases were all fatal they likely represent a biased selection toward high-severity disease (Ruaux and Atwell, 1998). The frequency of radiographic abnormalities in lower-severity cases of acute pancreatitis is likely to be low. This suggests that the negative predictive value, or the ability

of negative findings on plain radiography to rule out the presence of acute pancreatitis, is low.

Ultrasonography

Ultrasonographic examination of the abdomen often yields useful information in the assessment of dogs with vomiting and abdominal pain. As a diagnostic modality, ultrasonography depends heavily on operator skill and experience. Ultrasonographic findings consistent with acute pancreatitis were noted in 23 of 34 cases of fatal pancreatitis (68%) in which ultrasonography was available (Hess et al, 1998). Although this was a better performance than plain radiography for this group of dogs, the sensitivity of ultrasonography was still low even for objectively severe disease; therefore abdominal ultrasound cannot rule out reliably the presence of pancreatitis.

Measurement of Pancreatic Lipase

The broad availability of immunoassays for canine pancreas-specific lipase, in the form of the quantitative Spec cPL assay and bedside Snap cPL tests, has advanced dramatically the ability to diagnose pancreatic disease in dogs (see Chapter 135). Canine pancreas-specific lipase as a diagnostic marker for pancreatitis has received a remarkable degree of investigation in the peer-reviewed literature and has been shown to have high sensitivity and specificity by several different groups and in a variety of contexts (Neilson-Carley et al, 2011; Trivedi et al, 2011). In an animal with compatible clinical signs, the presence of an elevated pancreas-specific lipase concentration provides strong evidence to support the clinical diagnosis of pancreatitis, whereas a normal concentration in a dog with similar signs is a strong indication that pancreatic disease is not present and should prompt investigation for other differential diagnoses.

Pathophysiology of Acute Pancreatitis

The pathophysiology of acute pancreatitis at the level of the exocrine cell, including changes in digestive enzyme handling and secretion, has been reviewed earlier (see page 534 of the previous edition of *Current Veterinary Therapy*). Although changes in the exocrine cell are important and have been investigated extensively in a variety of canine and rodent models of the disease, the relationship between these changes and the clinical outcome of naturally occurring pancreatic disease is tenuous at best. A growing body of evidence suggests that the exocrine pancreas is a source of numerous inflammatory cytokines during a bout of acute pancreatitis, and the systemic effect of these cytokines is the major determinant of overall severity and likelihood of complications in these cases. Severe acute pancreatitis puts the patient at a high risk for systemic inflammatory response syndrome (SIRS), which can then lead to multiple organ dysfunction syndrome (MODS) and death. The processes of SIRS and MODS, once initiated, tend to continue independent of the triggering factor. A rational therapeutic approach to these cases, then, is aimed at preempting complications and managing complications that can arise as a result of systemic inflammation. Early, aggressive therapy is important to prevent complications from acute pancreatitis. It is important to articulate to dog owners the need for this early, aggressive therapy and the likelihood of severe and significant complications early in the course of treating the disease.

Therapy of Acute Pancreatitis

Fluid Therapy

Fluid therapy is absolutely central to the management of most cases of acute pancreatitis in dogs, particularly those judged to be sufficiently severe to warrant hospitalization. For most cases of uncomplicated pancreatitis (those without accompanying organ failures), therapy with a replacement-type crystalloid intravenous fluid (typically supplemented to contain 20 to 30 mEq/L potassium) is sufficient. The volume of fluid given should be based on careful estimation and calculation of fluid deficits and maintenance needs. A typical aim is to replace calculated deficits over 8 to 12 hours, following a 30-minute to 1-hour period of shock rate fluid delivery (70 to 90 ml/kg/hr). The patient then is maintained at up to twice the calculated maintenance rate with crystalloid fluids once the fluid deficit is replaced, while urine output is monitored. This rate of fluid administration is continued until the animal is drinking and decreased to the maintenance rate at this point. Dogs with acute pancreatitis commonly are potassium depleted because of losses from vomiting, effective loss of circulating volume in bowel loops because of ileus, and enhanced renal potassium losses. Close monitoring of electrolytes (typically every 12 hours) and judicious supplementation are indicated in the initial period of fluid resuscitation.

In dogs with more severe acute pancreatitis the impact of systemic circulation of pancreas-derived inflammatory mediators becomes important. Although severe cases still demonstrate the fluid losses and electrolyte disturbances common in the less severe examples of pancreatitis, additional complicating factors arise as a result of vascular endothelial dysfunction.

Systemic vascular endothelial dysfunction from inflammation is associated with an increased rate of fluid loss into the extracellular spaces of tissues. This deterioration in endothelial function means a tendency for losses of albumin and lower-molecular-weight plasma proteins from circulation and into the extracellular space. The net effect of this is a loss of the plasma's colloid oncotic pressure and thus a declining ability to maintain circulating fluid volume and cardiac output. Colloid replacement, as part of the initial fluid resuscitation and for ongoing maintenance, commonly is indicated in more severe cases of acute pancreatitis.

Fresh frozen plasma (aiming for 10 to 15 ml/kg in the initial transfusion) is the author's preferred colloid fluid in the management of severe acute pancreatitis, particularly in the initial stages of volume replacement and fluid resuscitation. Fresh frozen plasma provides colloid support via replacement of albumin and other high-molecular-weight proteins, as well as replacing clotting factors and anti-thrombin III. Dogs with severe acute pancreatitis are at risk for the development of disseminated intravascular coagulation, and preemptive replacement of clotting factors and clotting cascade moderators is indicated. Although the use of fresh frozen plasma is the author's first choice for colloid support in dogs with severe acute pancreatitis, there is a lack of well-controlled studies demonstrating efficacy in canine patients with pancreatitis, and some retrospective studies have called into question the usefulness of this therapy (Weatherton and Streeter, 2009).

For cases requiring longer-term colloid support, particularly in which owner finances are limiting, synthetic colloids such as hetastarch can be administered (a total of 10 to 20 ml/kg q24h IV, with an initial bolus of half this volume given over 30 minutes followed by the balance as a continuous rate infusion [CRI]).

Pain Control

Pancreatitis is a painful condition, and aggressive pain control is centrally important in these cases. Given the questionable hemodynamic state of many patients at initial presentation, nonsteroidal antiinflammatory drugs (NSAIDs) are best avoided. Narcotic pain control is indicated in any patient with sufficiently severe disease to warrant hospitalization. The choice of agent obviously depends on availability; the author's preference is to use either buprenorphine (0.01 to 0.02 mg/kg q6-8h IV or IM) as a single agent or multimodal approaches using CRIs of fentanyl and lidocaine, in the first 24 to 48 hours of hospitalization followed by a transition to buprenorphine.

Control of Emesis

Severe vomiting and ongoing nausea are common presenting problems and complicating factors in the management of many dogs with pancreatitis. Control of vomiting is an important aim because this reduces or eliminates fluid and electrolyte losses. Ongoing nausea negatively affects the willingness of patients to eat, and the presence of vomiting impedes the ability to provide routine enteral nutrition.

Several different families of antiemetic and antinausea medications now are available, acting through a variety of mechanisms. These include antagonism of neurokinin-1 receptors (maropitant, Cerenia), antagonism of serotonin 5-HT$_3$ receptors (ondansetron and dolasetron), and antagonism of dopamine receptors (metoclopramide, chlorpromazine). Because these compounds work through differing and potentially complementary mechanisms a multimodal approach can be used for the management of vomiting in canine patients. Typically the author begins with maropitant, 1 mg/kg q24h SC. In many patients, vomiting has stopped by the time they are presented for veterinary care, and in these patients maropitant is often sufficient for control of nausea and reducing the risk of ongoing vomiting. Patients that continue to vomit after admission are treated with maropitant initially, and if vomiting continues after 1 to 2 hours, the author adds an HT_3 receptor antagonist, usually dolasetron (0.5 to 0.6 mg/kg q24h IV). Patients with ileus or that have failed to respond to the combination of maropitant and dolasetron are treated with metoclopramide (CRI of 1 to 2 mg/kg/ q24h IV), in addition to maropitant and dolasetron at previously described doses. Theoretic concerns have been raised regarding the effect of dopamine antagonism on pancreatic blood flow in patients with pancreatitis; however, there are no reports in peer-reviewed literature linking metoclopramide to poorer outcomes in either human or canine patients with pancreatitis.

A recent publication using a rodent model of caerulein-induced pancreatitis has shown that the pancreas secretes both substance P, the ligand for neurokinin-1 receptors, and the neurokinin-1 receptor when the pancreas becomes inflamed (Koh et al, 2011). If this finding holds true in naturally occurring disease, it may explain the significant efficacy observed for maropitant in many cases of canine pancreatitis.

Antibiotic Therapy

Like most aspects of therapy for pancreatitis, the use and selection of antibiotics is controversial at best. There is little to no evidence of bacterial involvement in the initiation of pancreatitis. However, septic complications of pancreatitis, particularly infection of necrotic pancreatic tissue and the formation of pancreatic abscesses, can be devastating. During pancreatitis the integrity, barrier function, and permeability of the gastrointestinal mucosa can become compromised; however, molecular studies in human beings have failed to demonstrate bacterial translocation in patients with severe pancreatitis (Ammori et al, 2003). A Cochrane review of the human literature found no evidence of benefit from antibiotic therapy in humans with acute pancreatitis; however, they did provide the caveat that "none of the studies were adequately powered" (Villatoro, Mulla, and Larvin, 2010).

Glycemic Regulation

Many canine patients have significant hyperglycemia in the early stages of severe acute pancreatitis, and in some cases patients demonstrate convincing evidence of acute pancreatitis and diabetic ketoacidosis (DKA). Canine patients with DKA and pancreatitis are highly challenging, bringing with them the additional complications of significant and rapid intracellular shifts of potassium and phosphate ions with the use of insulin therapy. Here the

therapeutic goals for one condition (the resumption of voluntary food intake as soon as possible with DKA) are apparently at odds with goals for the other condition, in which traditionally the approach to severe acute pancreatitis has been to withhold feeding. Typically these cases are treated in exactly the same manner as DKA related to other complicating disease, including the early resumption of oral feeding once control of emesis has been obtained (see Nutritional Support).

Early use of insulin therapy often is counterproductive in DKA patients and in patients with transient hyperglycemia secondary to pancreatitis. Insulin therapy should be withheld until the patient has had at least 8 to 12 hours of crystalloid fluid therapy and effective pain control. Many patients become normoglycemic during this initial period of stabilization and are found not to require insulin therapy.

Nutritional Support

The veterinary profession's approach and attitudes toward the nutritional support of pancreatitis in the canine patient is undergoing a paradigm shift. Traditionally, recommendations suggest that canine patients with pancreatitis should be kept *nil per os* for a minimum of 24 hours after vomiting ceases. Some authors even have recommended that dogs with pancreatitis be hospitalized "away from the sight and smell of food," a difficult prescription to follow for patients that require critical care.

A growing body of evidence demonstrates that an early return to enteral nutrition is associated with improved outcomes in human patients with severe acute pancreatitis and that nasogastric (prepyloric) and nasojejunal feeding appear to be safe (Olah and Romics, 2010). With access to highly efficacious antiemetics and use of a multimodal antiemetic approach, early introduction of food to canine patients with acute pancreatitis is feasible and desirable. The author's approach now is to "feed through" most cases of acute pancreatitis, once control of vomiting has been obtained for at least 6 hours. Patients that vomit after food is offered have another antiemetic added to their therapy, followed by further offering of food 1 hour later. Food is offered free choice initially (usually a lower-fat, "intestinal" formula such as Purina EN Gastroenteric or Hills Prescription i/d). When patients are unwilling to eat after 48 hours of hospital care, particularly if they already are receiving more than one antiemetic medication, placement of some form of nutritional support device is recommended, typically a nasoesophageal or esophagostomy feeding tube. Cases that undergo surgery routinely receive jejunostomy tubes, and these patients are fed with liquidized, high-calorie "recovery" diets such as CliniCare or IAMS Recovery Formula to meet approximately half of their metabolic energy requirement, with the balance offered via free choice oral feeding. Minimally invasive methods for providing enteral nutritional support, including the fluoroscopic placement of nasojejunostomy tubes and endoscopic placement of percutaneous gastrostomy/jejunostomy tubes have been reported in dogs. As experience with these techniques increases, their level of efficacy in management of acute pancreatitis patients will become apparent. One recent publication investigated the use of early enteral nutrition specifically in dogs with pancreatitis and found that dogs receiving early enteral nutrition via esophagostomy tube experienced fewer vomiting and regurgitation events than those receiving total parenteral nutrition (Mansfield et al, 2011). The outcome between the enteral-fed versus total parenteral nutrition groups did not differ; however, the study was not powered sufficiently to detect a difference, and further, larger-scale studies definitely are warranted.

Postbout and Postdischarge Management

Desirable parameters before discharge include cessation of vomiting for a minimum of 24 hours (including time elapsing before admission if the dog does not vomit once hospitalized), resolution of fluid and electrolyte abnormalities, and return of voluntary appetite. Serial determination of enzyme activities or serum Spec cPL concentrations to determine readiness for discharge is not beneficial. Spec cPL can remain elevated for extended periods (10 to 12 days or more) after the onset of a bout, and many animals recover to the point of discharge in substantially less time than that. Traditional recommendations are that the dog be transitioned to a lower-fat maintenance diet and that the feeding of table scraps, human food, and high-fat treats be avoided. There is no need to discharge these patients with antibiotic therapy.

Chronic Pancreatitis in Dogs

In humans chronic pancreatitis is well recognized as a distinct condition from acute pancreatitis, with familial predispositions and a variety of underlying genetic disorders recognized. Within the veterinary literature is a relative paucity of publications addressing chronic pancreatitis, with the exception of the breed-specific disorder recognized in the miniature schnauzer. However, a growing body of evidence suggests that chronic pancreatitis is an important, underrecognized disorder in the domestic dog. One published report, defining chronic pancreatitis as the presence of predominantly monocellular infiltrates, fibrosis, and sporadic neutrophil infiltrates, detected chronic pancreatitis in 34% of nonautolyzed pancreata from first-opinion practice dogs at necropsy (Watson et al, 2007). The same group subsequently characterized the clinical findings and histories of a group of 14 dogs with histologically confirmed disease and reported that most dogs showed "low grade gastrointestinal signs and abdominal pain" (Watson et al, 2010). Many of these dogs present with primary complaints that are attributable to small intestinal or pancreatic disease, such as poor appetite, weight loss, abdominal pain, and vomiting. Often routine biochemistry is unremarkable, although elevations in liver enzyme activities and mild inflammatory leukograms are not uncommon. Serum concentrations of Spec cPL often are elevated above 400 µg/L (the current cutoff value recommended for the diagnosis of pancreatitis using this test). However, clinical signs and Spec cPL concentrations either do not resolve or wax and wane over relatively short times (clinical signs seen daily to two to three times per week in many cases).

Recognition of this condition is hampered by a lack of well-defined diagnostic criteria in the absence of pancreatic biopsies. The author's criteria for increased index of suspicion are recurrent signs of poor appetite and abdominal pain occurring at least twice weekly for a period of at least 4 weeks. Cases presented with compatible histories usually are examined for gastric and small intestinal disease as well as further investigations of the pancreas. Serum concentrations of cobalamin and folate are measured, as well as serum Spec cPL. Biopsy of stomach and small intestine are recommended and often reveal mononuclear infiltrates compatible with chronic enteropathy (see Chapter 131). The therapeutic approach used in these cases is as recommended for canine chronic enteropathies, with the exception of first recommending a dietary change to an ultra-low-fat diet (Royal Canin Gastrointestinal Low Fat LF) in dogs that do not have mononuclear infiltrates in the stomach or small intestine. Dogs that fail therapy with ultra-low-fat diets undergo an elimination diet trial, followed by immune-modulating therapy if the dog fails the second dietary trial. Prednisone is the author's first choice for immune modulation, given initially at immune suppressive doses (1.5 to 2 mg/kg q24h) for 14 days, followed by a gradual taper with a goal either to taper completely or to maintain the dog at the lowest tolerable dose that demonstrates efficacy.

Some dogs with chronic pancreatitis have overt diabetes mellitus or rapidly develop this condition on exposure to glucocorticoids. Dogs with chronic pancreatitis and diabetes mellitus are often difficult to regulate with insulin therapy because of poor or variable appetite and presumably varying degrees of insulin resistance and endogenous insulin production that varies with waxing and waning pancreatic inflammation. Dogs with presumptive diagnoses of chronic pancreatitis and concurrent diabetes mellitus first are transitioned to an ultra-low-fat diet while attempting initial glycemic regulation. Those that continue to be difficult to regulate, particularly in which clinical signs attributable to chronic pancreatitis continue and serum concentrations of Spec cPL remain greater than 400 µg/L for extended periods, are likely to benefit from further immune modulation. In a relatively small number of cases to date, the author has used cyclosporine (Atopica) at standard dosages (approximately 5 mg/kg SID) in dogs with convincing evidence of chronic pancreatitis and difficult glycemic regulation, with marked improvement in insulin sensitivity and gastrointestinal signs. This is an area of significant interest, particularly if chronic pancreatitis is as common as Watson's (2007) paper would suggest; well-documented and well-controlled studies of this emerging condition are necessary.

References and Suggested Reading

Ammori BJ et al: The early increase in intestinal permeability and systemic endotoxin exposure in patients with severe acute pancreatitis is not associated with systemic bacterial translocation: molecular investigation of microbial DNA in the blood, *Pancreas* 26(1):18, 2003.

Hess RS et al: Clinical, clinicopathologic, radiographic, and ultrasonographic abnormalities in dogs with fatal acute pancreatitis: 70 cases (1986-1995), *J Am Vet Med Assoc* 213(5):665, 1998.

Koh YH et al: Activation of neurokinin-1 receptors up-regulates substance P and neurokinin-1 receptor expression in murine pancreatic acinar cells, *J Cell Mol Med* 16(7):1582, 2011.

Mansfield CS et al: A pilot study to assess tolerability of early enteral nutrition via esophagostomy tube feeding in dogs with severe acute pancreatitis, *J Vet Intern Med* 25(3):419, 2011.

Neilson-Carley SC et al: Specificity of a canine pancreas-specific lipase assay for diagnosing pancreatitis in dogs without clinical or histologic evidence of the disease, *Am J Vet Res* 72(3):302, 2011.

Olah A, Romics L Jr: Evidence-based use of enteral nutrition in acute pancreatitis, *Langenbecks Arch Surg* 395(4):309, 2010.

Ruaux CG, Atwell RB: A severity score for spontaneous canine acute pancreatitis, *Aust Vet J* 76(12):804, 1998.

Trivedi S et al: Sensitivity and specificity of canine pancreas-specific lipase (cPL) and other markers for pancreatitis in 70 dogs with and without histopathologic evidence of pancreatitis, *J Vet Intern Med* 25(6):1241, 2011.

Villatoro E, Mulla M, Larvin M: Antibiotic therapy for prophylaxis against infection of pancreatic necrosis in acute pancreatitis, *Cochrane Database Syst Rev* 5:CD002941, 2010.

Watson PJ et al: Observational study of 14 cases of chronic pancreatitis in dogs, *Vet Rec* 167(25):968, 2010.

Watson PJ et al: Prevalence and breed distribution of chronic pancreatitis at post-mortem examination in first-opinion dogs, *J Small Anim Pract* 48(11):609, 2007.

Weatherton LK, Streeter EM: Evaluation of fresh frozen plasma administration in dogs with pancreatitis: 77 cases (1995-2005), *J Vet Emerg Crit* 19(6):617, 2009.

CHAPTER 138

Feline Exocrine Pancreatic Disorders

MARNIN A. FORMAN, *Stamford, Connecticut*

With advances in serology and diagnostic imaging, disorders of the exocrine pancreas in cats are detected more frequently. Pancreatitis has been recognized as a relatively common disorder causing significant morbidity and, infrequently, mortality. Less-common disorders of the exocrine pancreas include exocrine pancreatic insufficiency (EPI), pancreatic cancers (adenocarcinoma, lymphoma), pancreatic pseudocyst, abscess, parasites, and nodular hyperplasia. This chapter focuses on diagnostic confirmation and therapeutic management of mild to moderate and severe pancreatitis, complications of pancreatitis, and areas of uncertainty in the management of pancreatitis, including the use of antibiotics and corticosteroids.

Pancreatitis is characterized histologically as acute (primarily neutrophilic), chronic (primarily lymphocytic or lymphoplasmacytic with fibrosis), or acute component with chronic disease (both neutrophilic and lymphocytic). The prevalence of cats with clinical pancreatitis is unknown; pancreatic inflammation is a relatively common necropsy finding (very mild to severe lesions in 67% of cats evaluated). In contrast to dogs, the two most frequent clinical signs of pancreatitis in cats are lethargy (88% to 100%) and anorexia (95% to 97%).

Less commonly, cats display weight loss (47%), vomiting (35% to 52%), and infrequently diarrhea (11% to 38%), labored breathing (20%), or polyuria/polydipsia (20%). Common physical examination findings include dehydration (92%), hypothermia (68%), and less frequently icterus (37%), palpable abdominal mass (23%), apparent abdominal pain (15%), and rarely fever (7%). Unlike dogs, many cats with pancreatitis have a normal complete blood count (CBC) with abnormalities such as neutrophilia (46%), nonregenerative anemia (38%), hemoconcentration (17%), and leukopenia (15%). Hypercholesterolemia (72%) frequently is noted on a biochemical panel with less common findings of hyperbilirubinemia (58%), increased liver enzymes (alanine transaminase [ALT] 57%, alkaline phosphatase [ALP] 49%), hypokalemia (56%), hyperglycemia (45%), and hypoalbuminemia (36%). Hypoglycemia and ionized hypocalcemia (65%) are a frequent finding in cats with severe, necrotizing pancreatitis, and these patients require more aggressive supportive care with a guarded prognosis. Despite these nonlocalizing clinical signs, physical examination findings and laboratory abnormalities, the frequency of the antemortem diagnosis of pancreatitis in cats has increased with advances in pancreatic serology and imaging.

Diagnosis of Feline Pancreatitis

Accurate diagnosis of pancreatitis involves a combination of appropriate clinical signs and physical examination findings, laboratory abnormalities including elevated pancreatic-specific lipase, and ultrasonographic changes. Pancreatic cytology or histopathology infrequently is needed for confirmation but can be beneficial in the treatment of pancreatitis, in particular if severe or with complications. Multiple generations of pancreatic enzyme serology testing have resulted in improvements in the diagnostic accuracy for feline pancreatitis. Serum amylase, lipase, and trypsin-like immunoreactivity (TLI) concentrations are of limited diagnostic value for pancreatitis; however, TLI is the preferred diagnostic test for EPI. Although not evaluated by a research study, higher ascites lipase concentrations compared with serum lipase concentrations have been associated with pancreatitis, in the author's experience. The current assay (Spec fPL) measures pancreatic-specific lipase by a monoclonal antibody sandwich enzyme-linked immunosorbent assay (ELISA) with a moderate sensitivity and specificity, 79.4% and 79.7%, respectively. Transabdominal pancreatic ultrasound is a moderately sensitive test (73%) for pancreatitis in cats; however, it has a variable specificity (24% to 67%) and depends on available equipment and sonographer skill level. However, unlike serology, ultrasound imaging permits detection of nonpancreatic concurrent disorders, screening for causes of pancreatitis, and ultrasound-guided fine-needle aspiration cytology of the pancreas and peripancreatic fluid accumulations. Using pancreatic-specific lipase and ultrasound imaging in the diagnosis of pancreatitis provides the highest positive predicative value, 69% and 80%, respectively, and negative predictive value, 87% and 57%, respectively.

Ultrasonographic changes associated with pancreatitis include pancreatomegaly, hypoechoic pancreatic parenchyma, hyperechoic peripancreatic fat or mesentery, dilated pancreatic or bile duct(s), dilation of the gallbladder, thickened gastric wall, and corrugated, thickened duodenal wall and peripancreatic fluid accumulation (ascites). The minimum requirements for the ultrasonographic diagnosis of pancreatitis in cats have not been determined. Certain abnormalities, including increasing pancreatic duct size and, potentially, pancreatic parenchyma hyperechogenicity, may occur in older cats without pancreatitis. Pancreatic computed tomography (CT), the standard diagnostic test for certain types of pancreatitis in humans, has poor specificity and sensitivity in cats.

Treatment of Mild to Moderate Feline Pancreatitis

Clinical signs of pancreatitis range in severity from mild and self-limiting to severe, life-threatening disease with an acute or chronic presentation. In contrast to dogs, the cause of pancreatitis in cats is not associated with dietary fat intake, obesity, or drugs. Specific causes include cancer, infections (viral [feline infectious peritonitis (FIP), feline immunodeficiency virus (FIV), calicivirus], *Toxoplasma gondii, Amphimerus pseudofelineus*), and organophosphates. In addition, up to two thirds of cats with pancreatitis have concurrent disorders, including hepatic lipidosis, cholangitis, obstructive jaundice, inflammatory bowel disease, diabetes mellitus, interstitial nephritis, and pleural effusion. It is important to consider these concurrent disorders with persistent or progressive clinical signs despite therapy.

The core therapy for pancreatitis without complications is supportive and symptomatic. Intravenous fluid is used to restore circulating blood volume, antiemetic medications are used to control nausea and vomiting, and pain relief is provided as needed (Table 138-1). Although less frequently detected than in dogs, potentially because cats have less definitive indicators of pain, abdominal pain can contribute to persistent inappetence, and these cats improve with therapy. The author uses buprenorphine or butorphanol as first-line pain relief medication in cats with mild to moderate pancreatitis. Nutritional support is an important component of therapy. Restriction of oral food and water intake in a nonvomiting cat is not considered necessary; rather, oral intake of food is encouraged. Fasting cats with pancreatitis can lead to development of malnutrition, intestinal atrophy, bacterial translocation, and hepatic lipidosis. With mild to moderate pancreatitis, appetite stimulants are often effective to encourage voluntary intake of food. However, with persistent inappetence for more than 3 to 4 days, placement of an esophageal or gastric feeding tube (percutaneous endoscopic gastrostomy [PEG]) should be considered. The ideal dietary composition to feed cats with pancreatitis has not been determined; however, in contrast to dogs, marked fat restriction is likely not necessary. Easily digested, enteral diets currently are recommended. Furthermore, for cats with mild to moderate pancreatitis, the author does not treat with antibiotics or corticosteroids (see section on Areas of Uncertainty later in the chapter).

Treatment of Severe Feline Pancreatitis

In addition to the supportive and symptomatic care listed above, cats with severe and acute, necrotizing pancreatitis with complications or concurrent disorders require intensive and specific care. Indicators of severe pancreatitis include marked dehydration (8% to 10%), persistent clinical signs despite medical management (tachycardia or bradycardia, tachypnea, hypothermia or pyrexia) or labwork abnormalities (leukocytosis or leukopenia, hypotension, hypoglycemia, and ionized hypocalcemia). In addition to correction of dehydration and maintenance fluid support with crystalloids, colloid therapy is beneficial to maintain and support normal colloid osmotic pressure and prevent fluid imbalance and edema formation. Fresh frozen plasma (FFP) provides colloid support by supplementing albumin and is therapeutic for correction of coagulopathies secondary to disseminated intravascular coagulation or vitamin K deficiency, a potential complication of necrotizing pancreatitis and secondary cholestatic disease, respectively. However, FFP does not alter significantly serum albumin concentrations and is controversial in providing proteinase inhibitors to scavenge activated pancreatic enzymes. Alternatively, synthetic colloids (Hetastarch, Dextran 70) are a cost-effective alternative to FFP; however, they provide only colloid support. In patients receiving aggressive fluid support,

TABLE **138-1**

Medical Therapies for Feline Pancreatitis

Treatment	Dosage
Fluid Therapy	
Isotonic crystalloids: lactated Ringer's solution, 0.9% NaCl	Shock 45-55 ml/kg/hr IV; correct dehydration; maintenance 40-45 ml/kg/day IV
Synthetic colloids: hetastarch, dextran 70	5 ml/kg IV
Fresh frozen plasma transfusion	10-40 ml/kg IV over 24h
Nausea and Vomiting Therapy	
Ranitidine	0.5-2 mg/kg PO, IV q12h
Famotidine	0.5-1 mg/kg PO, IV, SC, IM q12-24h
Metoclopramide	0.2-0.4 mg/kg PO, SC, IM q8h* 1-2 mg/kg/day CRI
Chlorpromazine	0.5 mg/kg IV, IM, SC q6-8h
Dolasetron mesylate	0.6-1 mg/kg PO q12h
Ondansetron	0.1-0.15 mg/kg slow IV q6-12h
Maropitant citrate	1 mg/kg PO, IV, SC q24h, 2 mg/kg PO q24h
Pain Management	
Buprenorphine	0.005-0.01 mg/kg IV, IM q4-8h
Butorphanol	0.2-0.4 mg/kg IM q2-4h
Lidocaine	20 µg/kg/min IV CRI
Ketamine	2-20 µg/kg/min IV CRI
Assorted Medications	
Ampicillin–sulbactam	20-40 mg/kg IV q8-12h
Ticarcillin–clavulanate	40-60 mg/kg IV q6-8h
Amoxicillin–clavulanic acid	10-20 mg/kg PO q8h
Clindamycin	5-11 mg/kg PO, SC, IV q12h
Enrofloxacin	2.5-5 mg/kg PO, IV q12h
Dalteparin	100 U/kg SC q12-24h
Enoxaparin	0.8 mg/kg SC q6h
Dopamine HCl	5-15 µg/kg/min IV CRI
Dobutamine HCl	0.2-2 µg/kg/min IV CRI
Epinephrine	0.5-2 µg/kg/min IV CRI
Norepinephrine	0.5-2 µg/kg/min IV CRI
Vasopressin	0.5 mU/kg/min IV CRI
Pancrelipase	0.5-0.75 teaspoonsful mixed with each meal
Cobalamin (vitamin B_{12})	250 µg/cat SC weekly
Prednisone	0.5 mg/kg PO q12h

*Consider alternative therapy, less efficacious in cats.
CRI, Constant rate infusion; *IM*, intramuscular; *IV*, intravenous; *PO*, by mouth; *SC*, subcutaneous.

it is important to avoid volume overload by monitoring respiratory rate and effort, pulmonary auscultatory sounds, and central venous pressure.

Tachypnea and labored breathing are common complications of severe pancreatitis. Possible etiologies include pleural effusion or pulmonary edema (secondary to acute lung injury [ALI], acute respiratory distress syndrome [ARDS], volume overload, and congestive heart failure [CHF]), aspiration pneumonia, pulmonary thromboembolism (PTE), and pain. Thoracic radiographs and Doppler echocardiography often permit a rapid diagnosis to guide therapy. Thoracocentesis with pleural fluid analysis is indicated with effusions. Although the finding of simultaneous pleural and peritoneal effusions has been reported to indicate a poor to grave prognosis, this is not necessarily the author's experience. A differentiation of CHF from pleural effusions secondary to pancreatitis is critical for accurate modifications of fluid therapy and initiation of diuretic therapy. Antibiotics (see Table 138-1) and, if hypoxemia is present, oxygen therapy are indicated to treat aspiration pneumonia. The optimal therapy, including indications to initiate antithrombotic therapy in cats with pancreatitis, has not been determined; however, use of thromboelastography (TEG) is a potential tool in guiding this complicated decision. Prevention of thrombotic complications, rather than reduction of the progression of existing hyperthrombotic complications, is beneficial. Low-molecular-weight heparins (dalteparin, enoxaparin) are tolerated well by cats with infrequent bleeding complications and have been recommended for use in cats with systemic inflammatory response syndrome (SIRS). In cats with persistent pain, despite buprenorphine or butorphanol, addition of titratable constant-rate infusions of lidocaine and ketamine rapidly leads to pain relief; however, monitoring for any signs of toxicity is important. Because of a concern for spasm of the pancreatic duct morphine should be avoided. Although uncommon, if postprandial pain is detected, supplementing pancreatic enzymes (twice the dose used in treating EPI dose) mixed with food may provide pain relief secondary to a proposed reduction in pancreatic sections.

In cats with hypotension, despite crystalloid and colloid fluid therapy, vasopressors are indicated. Dopamine is a vasopressor that also may increase pancreatic blood flow and reduce microvascular permeability; however, the pancreatic benefit is transient and may induce vomiting. Alternative vasopressors include epinephrine, norepinephrine, and vasopressin. Although less frequently detected in cats than dogs, gastroduodenal ileus can result in persistent vomiting and inappetence. Gastric decompressive therapy with a nasogastric or gastric tube is beneficial. Ranitidine, metoclopramide, and/or cisapride provide prokinetic activity. Traditional enteral nutrition, even with use of an esophageal or gastric feeding tube, is not possible in cats with persistent gastroduodenal ileus or drug-resistant vomiting. In these cats, short-term benefit can be provided from partial or total parental nutrition (P/TPN). With advances in intravenous catheters and intensive care, mechanical and septic complications with parental nutrition are infrequent; however, hyperglycemia after P/TPN administration is a significant concern and a poor prognosis indicator in cats receiving TPN. Cats with severe pancreatitis, whether receiving P/TPN or not, must be monitored for persistent hyperglycemia and treated with regular insulin if noted. The lower osmolarity of PPN permits administration via a peripheral, dedicated catheter; however, it provides only 50% of the daily energy needs. Therefore it is indicated as a sole nutritional support for only a few days. In addition, animals that receive supplemental enteral nutrition survived more often than those receiving PPN exclusively.

Jejunostomy feeding tubes (J-tubes) provide enteral nutrition in cats with persistent gastroduodenal ileus and drug-resistant vomiting and avoid pancreatic stimulation associated with gastric feeding. These tubes can be placed endoscopically or surgically, and tubes are available to allow gastric drainage (and later feedings) as well as jejunal feedings. Complications associated with J-tubes include premature removal, local pain or inflammation, retrograde tube migration, tube occlusion, and diarrhea. Surgical management is indicated rarely (4.4% of cases) in cats with acute pancreatitis, and clear indications to perform surgical management have not been determined. The most common indicator is progressive hyperbilirubinemia secondary to an obstructive jaundice from pancreatitis-associated extrahepatic biliary tract obstruction (EHBO). Diversionary surgical options, including cholecystoduodenostomy and cholecystojejunostomy, resolve the biliary tract obstruction but have been associated with multiple complications including cholangiohepatitis, stricture of the stoma, recurrence of EHBO, EPI, and chronic vomiting. Choledochal stenting uses a section of red rubber catheter (3.5 to 5 French, approximately 4 to 8 cm in length) to resolve the EHBO without performing a diversionary surgery. Initial experience with stenting involved complications, including ascending cholangitis, recurrence of EHBO, and chronic vomiting. However, with endoscopic removal of stents after resolution of pancreatitis, these complications appear to be less frequent. Cats with recurrent episodes of pancreatitis, pancreatic necrosis, or pancreatic diversionary surgery may develop EPI. The most common clinical sign of feline EPI is weight loss followed by diarrhea, polyphagia, and vomiting; cobalamin deficiency frequently is present. Therapy involves pancreatic enzyme replacement and, if required, cobalamin supplementation (see Table 138-1).

Areas of Uncertainty

Based on the inability to detect microbial growth on routine bacteria growth media, bacteria have not been considered a primary cause of pancreatitis, and antibiotics for noncomplicated cases of pancreatitis have not been recommended. Bacterial infections are common with certain concurrent pancreatic disorders (e.g., cholangitis and cholangiohepatitis) and complications of pancreatitis (e.g., pancreatic abscesses, pseudocyst and necrosis, and aspiration pneumonia). In a feline research model, *Escherichia coli* was shown to hematogenously spread to the pancreas following colonic transmigration, and by reflux into the pancreatic duct. The organisms most likely to colonize the severely diseased pancreas were gram-negative and anaerobic bacteria from the gastrointestinal tract. With these infectious disorders, broad-spectrum antibiotics with good penetration into the pancreas (ampicillin and sulbactam, ticarcillin and clavulanate, amoxicillin and clavulanic acid, and clindamycin) are indicated, ideally guided by culture and sensitivity testing.

Ongoing research using a novel mechanism to detect bacterial infections, fluorescence *in situ* hybridization (FISH) with a 16S rDNA probe that recognizes bacteria, is challenging the belief that bacterial infections are not a primary cause of pancreatitis and may result in a change in recommendations of management of cats with pancreatitis.

Similar to antibiotics, corticosteroids are beneficial in certain concurrent pancreatic disorders, including inflammatory bowel disease and sterile cholangiohepatitis and should be considered if these disorders are present. However, corticosteroids are associated with significant adverse effects, for which cats with pancreatitis are already at risk, including insulin antagonism and unmasking or worsening diabetes mellitus, immunosuppression with worsening of preexisting infections, or the development of opportunistic infections, and thromboembolism. To add to this complexity, autoimmune pancreatitis is an established cause of pancreatitis in humans and also may occur in cats. In the author's practice, corticosteroids (prednisolone, prednisone) are used in cases of chronic pancreatitis, frequently guided by pancreatic (and if indicated hepatic or intestinal) cytology or biopsy to screen for infectious complications or neoplasia and to confirm the type of inflammation present.

References and Suggested Reading

De Cock HE et al: Prevalence and histopathologic characteristics of pancreatitis in cats, *Vet Pathol* 44:39, 2007.

Ferreri JA et al: Clinical differentiation of acute necrotizing from chronic nonsuppurative pancreatitis in cats: 63 cases (1996-2001), *J Am Vet Med Assoc* 223:469, 2003.

Forman MA et al: Evaluation of serum feline pancreatic lipase immunoreactivity and helical computed tomography versus conventional testing for the diagnosis of feline pancreatitis, *J Vet Intern Med* 18:807, 2004.

Forman MA et al: Evaluation of feline pancreas-specific lipase (Spec fPL™) for the diagnosis of feline pancreatitis, *unpublished manuscript* 2011.

Gerhardt A et al: Comparison of the sensitivity of different diagnostic tests for pancreatitis in cats, *J Vet Intern Med* 15:329, 2001.

Hill RC, Van Winkle TJ: Acute necrotizing pancreatitis and acute suppurative pancreatitis in the cat. A retrospective study of 40 cases (1976-1989), *J Vet Intern Med* 7:25, 1993.

Kimmel SE, Washabau RJ, Drobatz KJ: Incidence and prognostic value of low plasma ionized calcium concentration in cats with acute pancreatitis: 46 cases (1996-1998), *J Am Vet Med Assoc* 219:1105, 2001.

Saunders HM et al: Ultrasonographic findings in cats with clinical, gross pathologic, and histologic evidence of acute pancreatic necrosis: 20 cases (1994-2001), *J Am Vet Med Assoc* 221:1724, 2002.

Swift NC et al: Evaluation of serum feline trypsin-like immunoreactivity for the diagnosis of pancreatitis in cats, *J Am Vet Med Assoc* 217:37, 2000.

Zoran DL: Pancreatitis in cats: diagnosis and management of a challenging disease, *J Am Anim Hosp Assoc* 42:1, 2006.

CHAPTER 139

Diagnostic Approach to Hepatobiliary Disease

CYNTHIA R.L. WEBSTER, *Grafton, Massachusetts*
JOHANNA C. COOPER, *Walpole, Massachusetts*

This chapter provides a rational approach to the diagnosis of hepatobiliary disease in small animal patients. The diagnosis of a primary hepatobiliary disorder can be a challenge; therefore a logical approach is necessary, incorporating all aspects of the case from signalment to diagnostic imaging and histopathology. The clinical signs of hepatobiliary disease generally reflect deficiencies in the varied functions of the liver. These diverse metabolic and biochemical activities include carbohydrate, lipid, and protein metabolism; fat digestion; detoxification of endogenous and exogenous substances; and immune surveillance. However, the clinical signs that develop with liver disease are seldom specific for that organ. Furthermore, the high blood flow of the liver, its dual blood supply (systemic and portal), and its role in detoxification render the liver sensitive to injury from systemic disorders and diseases in organs drained by the portal circulation (Box 139-1). To complicate the situation, the tremendous hepatic reserve capacity makes the appearance of relatively specific signs of hepatobiliary dysfunction such as icterus, hypoglycemia, bleeding tendencies, hepatic encephalopathy (HE), and ascites occur only in late-stage disease.

The first step in the diagnosis of hepatobiliary disease is to obtain an accurate history. Pertinent information includes the use of potentially hepatotoxic drugs, supplements, or nutraceuticals; exposure to environmental toxins, infectious agents, or recent anesthetic events; and details on housing, supervision outdoors, and travel and vaccine status (leptospirosis, canine adenovirus). Recognition of an agent's hepatotoxic potential (Box 139-2) and prompt withdrawal can prevent further liver damage (see Chapters 140 and 141). Often a sequence of events may increase the suspicion for hepatobiliary disease. A history of inappetence and weight loss in a previously over-conditioned feline is suggestive of hepatic lipidosis. Anesthetic intolerance, failure to thrive, and postprandial behavioral abnormalities in a predisposed canine breed should increase suspicion of a portosystemic vascular anomaly (PSVA) (Berent and Tobias, 2009). Primary hepatobiliary disease always should be considered in breeds predisposed to inflammatory/fibrotic hepatopathies (Box 139-3).

Patients with hepatobiliary disease may exhibit nonspecific clinical signs referable to the gastrointestinal (intermittent anorexia, vomiting, diarrhea, and/or weight loss), urinary (polyuria, polydipsia, stranguria, and dysuria), or central nervous system (lethargy and depression). More specific signs of hepatobiliary disease include the diffuse cerebral signs that accompany HE (blindness, head pressing, stupor, coma, and ptyalism [cats]), jaundice, bleeding tendencies, or dermatologic abnormalities (superficial necrolytic dermatitis).

Physical examination in patients with primary hepatobiliary disease may reveal jaundice, hepatomegaly, a poor body condition score, abdominal pain, or a fluid wave. Additional findings may include abnormalities on fundic examination (iridocyclitis or chorioretinitis) from an infectious etiology or pyrexia from infectious or inflammatory disease.

Laboratory Evaluation of Hepatobiliary Disease

Clinicopathologic evaluation helps to verify the presence of liver disease and determine the degree to which other organ systems are affected. The initial database should include a complete blood count (CBC), biochemical profile, and urinalysis.

The most consistent CBC abnormalities include changes in erythrocyte size and morphology, including microcytosis, target cells, poikilocytes, and Heinz body formation (cats). Microcytosis without anemia, most likely associated with impaired iron transport, occurs in dogs and cats with congenital PSVA and in dogs with acquired shunting secondary to portal hypertension. Target cells and poikilocytes result from alteration in the erythrocyte plasma membrane lipoprotein content, causing altered cell deformability. Anemia may accompany hepatic disease from a bleeding gastric ulcer, a coagulopathy, or the anemia of chronic disease. Some dogs with hepatobiliary disease have a mild thrombocytopenia, reflecting a systemic infectious disorder, synthetic failure from decreased hepatic thrombopoietin production, or secondary to a thrombotic episode.

Alanine aminotransferase (ALT), aspartate aminotransferase (AST), alkaline phosphatase (ALP), and γ-glutamyl transferase (GGT) are serum enzymes used as screening tests for hepatobiliary disease (Center, 2007). Increases occur as a result of (1) leakage from damaged hepatobiliary cells (ALT, AST); (2) elution from damaged membranes (ALP, GGT); or (3) increased synthesis (ALP). Although

BOX 139-1

Extrahepatic Disease Associated with Elevation in Serum Hepatobiliary Enzymes

- Gastrointestinal
  - Inflammatory bowel disease
  - Pancreatitis
- Vascular
  - Severe anemia
  - Congestive heart failure
  - Postcaval syndrome
- Cholestasis of sepsis
- Systemic infections
- Muscle injury
- Endocrine
  - Hyperadrenocorticism
  - Adrenal hyperplasia syndromes
  - Diabetes mellitus
  - Hyperthyroidism
  - Hypothyroidism
- Paraneoplastic
  - Bone disorders

BOX 139-2

Agents Associated with Hepatotoxicity

Chemicals
- Arsenic
- Carbon tetrachloride
- Chlorinated hydrocarbon
- Dimethylnitrosamine
- Heavy metals
- Pine oil
- Selenium
- Tannic acid

Food Additives
- Xylitol

Drugs
- Acetaminophen
- Amiodarone
- Asparaginase
- Carprofen
- Diazepam
- Doxycycline
- Griseofulvin
- Halothane
- Ketoconazole
- Lomustine
- Mebendazole
- Methotrexate
- Oxibendazole-DEC
- Phenobarbital
- Stanozolol
- Tetracycline
- Thiacetarsemide
- Potentiated sulfonamides
- Zonisamide

Alternative Medicines
- Chaparral leaf
- Comfrey
- Germander
- Jin Bu Huan
- Kava
- Pennyroyal oil

Environmental Agents
- Aflatoxins
- *Amanita* mushroom
- Blue-green algae toxins
- Cycad seeds

elevations in these serum enzymes have a high sensitivity for the detection of hepatobiliary damage, increases also occur in the absence of clinically important primary hepatobiliary disease.

This discordance occurs for several reasons. First, increases in serum hepatobiliary enzymes can originate from nonhepatic tissues. Second, in the dog endogenous or exogenous corticosteroids and phenobarbital can induce the production of excess hepatobiliary enzymes in the absence of liver damage. Finally, the liver is uniquely susceptible to secondary injury from primary disease in other organs, particularly the pancreas and gastrointestinal tract (see Box 139-1).

Elevations in ALT and AST result secondary to leakage from damaged hepatocytes. ALT is a liver-specific cytosolic enzyme; however, increases also may occur with severe muscle necrosis in the dog. The half-life ($T\frac{1}{2}$) of ALT is $2\frac{1}{2}$ days in dogs. No published values are available for cats; however, the $T\frac{1}{2}$ is presumed to be much shorter (around 6 hours). The largest elevations in ALT occur with acute hepatocellular necrosis and inflammation. Mild-to-moderate elevations occur with primary hepatic neoplasia. AST, which is present in the cytosol and mitochondria, is more sensitive but somewhat less specific for liver disease than ALT. Increases in AST typically parallel those of ALT but are of a smaller magnitude. AST elevations in excess of ALT indicate either a muscle source or the release of mitochondrial AST caused by severe irreversible hepatocellular injury. The $T\frac{1}{2}$ of AST is 22 hours in the dog and 77 minutes in the cat.

ALP is a membrane-bound enzyme (see Web Chapter 50). In dogs ALP has a high sensitivity (80%) but low specificity (51%) for hepatobiliary disease. Its low specificity is caused by the presence of several isoenzymes and its sensitivity to drug induction. In the dog three isoenzymes make up the total serum ALP (T-ALP), including a bone (B-ALP), liver (L-ALP), and corticosteroid (C-ALP) isoenzyme. B-ALP makes up one third of the T-ALP in dogs and is elevated in conditions with increased osteoblastic activity such as bone growth, osteomyelitis, osteosarcoma, and secondary renal hyperparathyroidism. L-ALP is present on the luminal surface of biliary epithelial cells and the hepatocyte canalicular membrane. L-ALP $T\frac{1}{2}$ is 70 hours in dogs and 6 hours in cats. Because of the cats' short $T\frac{1}{2}$ and the fact that feline hepatocytes contain less ALP, increases typically do not approach those seen in canine patients. These characteristics and

BOX 139-3

Feline and Canine Breeds Predisposed to Hepatobiliary Disease

Congenital Portosystemic Vascular Anomalies
- Australian cattle dog
- Cairn terrier
- Dachshund
- Golden retriever
- Irish wolfhound
- Labrador retriever
- Maltese terrier
- Miniature schnauzer
- Shih tzu
- Yorkshire terrier
- Himalayan
- Persian

Hepatic Amyloidosis
- Chinese shar-pei
- Abyssinian
- Siamese

Copper-Associated Hepatopathy
- Bedlington terrier
- Dalmatian
- Skye terrier
- West Highland white terrier
- Siamese

Idiopathic Inflammatory
- American and English cocker spaniel
- English springer spaniel
- Doberman pinscher
- Labrador retriever
- Standard poodle

Vacuolar
- Scottish terrier

Gallbladder Disease
- Shetland sheepdog

the fact that cats lack C-ALP make T-ALP less sensitive (50%) but more specific (93%) for liver disease than in the dog. The largest increases in L-ALP are associated with focal or diffuse cholestatic disorders and primary hepatic neoplasms. Less dramatic increases are found in chronic hepatitis, hepatic necrosis, and canine nodular hyperplasia. C-ALP is located on the hepatocyte canalicular membrane. C-ALP increases in dogs exposed to exogenous corticosteroids or in cases of spontaneous hyperadrenocorticism; however, increases also are associated with chronic illness, possibly secondary to increases in endogenous glucocorticoid secretion.

Hepatic GGT is located on the hepatocyte canalicular membrane. In dogs GGT has a lower sensitivity (50%) but higher specificity (87%) for hepatobiliary disease than T-ALP. If an elevated ALP is noted with a concurrent increase in serum GGT, specificity for liver disease

increases to 94%. The most marked elevations in GGT result from diseases of the biliary epithelium such as bile duct obstruction, cholangiohepatitis, and cholecystitis. Moderate elevations accompany primary hepatic neoplasia, whereas mild elevations result from hepatic necrosis. In cats GGT has a higher sensitivity (86%) but lower specificity (67%) for hepatobiliary disease than T-ALP. Serum GGT may be considerably greater than ALP in some cats with cirrhosis, extrahepatic bile duct obstruction (EHBDO), or cholangitis. In feline idiopathic hepatic lipidosis GGT is typically only mildly elevated.

In dogs substantial increases in hepatobiliary enzymes can result secondary to corticosteroid and phenobarbital therapy. These increases may result from hepatobiliary enzyme induction and/or hepatocyte damage. Exogenous or endogenous excess of corticosteroids increases serum enzyme activity (L-ALP, C-ALP, ALT, and GGT) secondary to induction. In general, the most marked increases occur in ALP and GGT, with lesser elevations in ALT. Typically induction of AST is minimal. Cessation of corticosteroid therapy in the absence of liver damage results in a gradual normalization of enzyme values over a period of 2 to 3 months. Corticosteroids induce morphologic vacuolar change in hepatocytes and have resulted in focal areas of hepatic necrosis in experimental studies; therefore hepatocyte damage may be the cause of some of the increased enzyme activity.

Idiosyncratic hepatotoxic reactions to phenobarbital may occur in dogs, leading to chronic inflammatory disease or the hepatocutaneous syndrome. In both of these disorders moderate-to-marked increases in ALP, moderate increases in ALT, and mild increases in AST typically are seen. Phenobarbital therapy in the dog has been reported to induce the production of hepatobiliary enzymes (primarily ALP). Prospective studies to assess the relative role of induction versus damage in dogs on phenobarbital therapy have resulted in conflicting results. One study demonstrated no increase in ALT and ALP enzyme activity in whole-liver homogenates from phenobarbital-treated dogs, suggesting that induction was not occurring (Gaskill et al, 2005). However, another study found increased T-ALP activity in the liver of phenobarbital-treated dogs, supportive of induction (Unakami et al, 1987). Overall the available literature suggests that mild-to-moderate increases in ALP (up to five times the upper limit of normal) and ALT (usually less than two times the upper limit of normal) may reflect enzyme induction. However, increases in GGT and AST seldom are caused by induction and may be suggestive of primary liver disease.

The magnitude of serum hepatobiliary enzyme elevation is usually proportional to the severity of active hepatobiliary damage; however, the degree of elevation is not predictive of hepatobiliary functional capacity. Marked increases in these enzymes may indicate substantial hepatobiliary injury but are not necessarily indicative of a poor prognosis because of the tremendous regenerative capacity of the liver. Alternatively, normal or only mildly increased serum hepatobiliary enzymes may be seen in end-stage chronic liver disease because of replacement of hepatocytes by fibrosis and/or prolonged enzyme leakage, resulting in depletion of hepatic stores. Thus a single determination of serum hepatobiliary enzyme values has little prognostic significance. Prognostic value increases with sequential evaluation in conjunction with liver function testing and biopsy.

Assessment of liver function requires evaluation of parameters that reflect the synthetic and excretory capacity of the liver. Several hepatic function tests are included on routine biochemical testing, including bilirubin, glucose, cholesterol, blood urea nitrogen (BUN), and albumin. Although these tests are not particularly sensitive or specific, they are obtained easily and may help build a case for primary hepatobiliary disease. Hyperbilirubinemia, the most sensitive and specific of these parameters, in the face of a normal hematocrit is caused by hepatic disease resulting in inadequate uptake, conjugation and/or excretion of bilirubin, posthepatic disease interfering with biliary excretion of bilirubin, or the cholestasis of sepsis. In cholestasis of sepsis, cytokines released during sepsis inhibit the expression of hepatocyte transporters necessary for bilirubin transport. Cholestasis of sepsis may occur in the presence or absence of hepatobiliary damage and appears to be common in the septic cat.

Hypoglycemia occurs only when 75% of hepatic mass is nonfunctional as a result of decreased gluconeogenesis and clearance of insulin. Hypoglycemia also occurs periodically in dogs with congenital PSVA, possibly secondary to impaired glucose production, reduced glycogen stores, decreased responsiveness to glucagon, or a combination of these factors. Serum cholesterol levels in hepatobiliary disease are variable; cholestatic disease frequently is associated with hypercholesterolemia, whereas hypocholesterolemia is seen most often in end-stage liver disease. The BUN may be low in dogs with chronic liver disease or PSVA because the hepatic conversion of ammonia to urea decreases with decreasing hepatic mass or shunting of blood past the liver. The liver is responsible for the synthesis of albumin; therefore hypoalbuminemia may accompany chronic hepatic disease. Synthetic failure occurs only when 70% of hepatic functional mass has been lost. However, serum hypoalbuminemia also may occur with protein-losing nephropathies or enteropathies, vasculitis, blood loss, or from third spacing in ascitic patients.

Urinalysis in cases of hepatobiliary disease may reveal bilirubinuria or ammonium biurate crystals. The canine renal threshold for bilirubin is low and dogs are capable of tubular secretion of bilirubin; therefore bilirubinuria may be present in the absence of bilirubinemia. However, cats have a high threshold for bilirubin and are not bilirubinuric unless also bilirubinemic. Freshly collected urine samples may reveal ammonia biurate crystalluria in dogs and cats with PSVA.

Ancillary Diagnostic Tests

Hepatobiliary disease may result in ascites formation secondary to portal hypertension (Buob et al, 2011). Portal hypertension occurs as a result of obstruction at the level of the right atrium/cranial vena cava, hepatic parenchyma, or portal vein. Portal hypertension from the latter two causes typically results in a low-protein ascites, whereas posthepatic portal hypertension is associated with a high-protein ascites. Generally ascitic fluid caused by hepatic disease is a pure transudate but with chronicity may have characteristics of a modified transudate. An effusion bilirubin value in excess of serum bilirubin is consistent with bile duct/gallbladder rupture. Ascites is rare even in cats with end-stage liver disease.

Other ancillary clinicopathologic tests that may be indicated include serology for infectious disease (leptospirosis, ehrlichiosis, Rocky Mountain spotted fever, toxoplasmosis, neosporosis, dirofilariasis, systemic mycosis), autoantibody testing (Coombs' or antinuclear antibody), and a coagulation profile (prothrombin time [PT], partial thromboplastin time [PTT], fibrinogen levels, and fibrinogen degradation products). Coagulation test abnormalities are common in dogs and cats with hepatobiliary disease, although spontaneous bleeding is rare. These abnormalities may be caused by hepatic synthetic failure, vitamin K deficiency, or the presence of a consumptive coagulopathy.

In cases in which secondary hepatobiliary disease is suspected, assessment for pancreatitis (serum lipase levels/pancreatic lipase immunoreactivity) and evaluation for an underlying endocrinopathy (hypothyroidism, hyperthyroidism, hyperadrenocorticism, and adrenal hyperplasia syndromes) or gastrointestinal disease (inflammatory bowel disease) may be pursued (see Box 139-1).

Hepatobiliary Function Tests

When a minimum database suggests the presence of hepatobiliary disease, the next step generally includes specific liver function tests and abdominal imaging. In many cases a definitive diagnosis requires hepatic biopsy.

Total serum bile acids (TSBAs) are common hepatic function tests. Bile acids are synthesized from cholesterol exclusively in the liver. Once conjugated to either glycine or taurine, they are secreted into the bile and subsequently stored and concentrated within the gallbladder. After a meal cholecystokinin (CCK) release initiates gallbladder contraction; bile acids are transported to the intestine, where they aid in the emulsification and digestion of fats. At the terminal ileum bile acids are resorbed and returned to the liver via the blood (enterohepatic circulation), where they are reextracted by hepatocytes. Normally enterohepatic circulation of bile acids occurs with 95% to 98% efficiency. Disruption of this enterohepatic circulation results in increases in TSBAs and occurs in the presence of acquired or congenital PSVA or cholestatic hepatobiliary disease. An endogenous challenge to assess the enterohepatic circulation of bile acids is used clinically by determining TSBAs after a 12-hour fast (preprandial) and then 2 hours after a test meal (postprandial).

TSBAs have a high specificity for hepatobiliary disease. In dogs the specificity of fasting and postprandial TSBAs for hepatobiliary disease is 95% and 100% when cutoff values greater than 15 μmol/L and 25 μmol/L are used, respectively. In cats, using similar cutoff values, fasting and postprandial TSBAs have a specificity of 96% and 100%, respectively. The sensitivity of TSBAs for hepatobiliary disease (ranging from 54% to 74%) is not high enough to support the routine use of TSBAs as screening tests for hepatobiliary disease. The two exceptions are congenital PSVA in dogs and cats and cirrhosis in dogs, in which the sensitivity of postprandial TSBAs at the above cutoff value is 100%.

A number of factors can influence the interpretation of TSBA testing. Higher fasting than postprandial values may result secondary to interdigestive gallbladder contraction or as a result of variations in gastric emptying, intestinal transit, or response to CCK release. Inaccurate postprandial values may occur because of failure of CCK release or gallbladder contraction if the test meal is inadequate in fat or amino acid content or if an insufficient amount is consumed. In addition, 2 hours may not represent the optimal time for postprandial sample collection in some animals. Furthermore, severe ileal disease or resection can decrease the bile acid resorption, thereby decreasing postprandial TSBAs.

Interpretation of abnormal TSBAs must occur with an understanding of the test limitations. TSBAs cannot be used to discriminate one hepatobiliary disease from another or to predict the severity of the histologic lesion or degree of portosystemic shunting. When monitoring disease progression or response to therapy using sequential TSBAs, clinicians can use only a return to normal to indicate clinical remission.

Urinary bile acids have been evaluated as a diagnostic test for hepatobiliary disease. The urinary excretion of water-soluble bile acids reflects the TSBA concentration during the period of urine formation so that persistently elevated TSBAs result in elevated urine bile acid levels. The normalized urine nonsulfated bile acids (UNSBAs) to urine creatinine ratio and the ratio of combined normalized urine sulfated (USBAs) and UNSBAs to urine creatinine have a higher specificity (100% vs. 67%) but lower sensitivity (62% vs. 78%) than TSBAs for the diagnosis of hepatobiliary disease in dogs. In the cat these urinary values were equivalent to TSBAs with respect to sensitivity (87%) and specificity (88%) for hepatobiliary disease. However, in both species urine bile acids appear to have a lower sensitivity for the detection of PSVA than postprandial TSBAs.

The liver detoxifies ammonia, primarily from the gastrointestinal tract, to urea. Elevations in blood ammonia concentrations result secondary to (1) portosystemic shunting, (2) greater than 70% reduction in liver parenchyma, and (3) inborn errors of metabolism in the urea cycle. Transient hyperammonemia has been reported in young Irish wolfhounds and with deficiencies of cobalamin and arginine in the dog and cat, respectively. Elevated fasting blood ammonia levels (>46 μmol/L) have been shown to be a sensitive (98%) and specific (89%) test for the detection of congenital or acquired PSVA in dogs (Gerritzen-Bruning, van den Ingh, and Rothuizen, 2006). Currently ammonia is the only toxin that can be measured clinically for the diagnosis of HE. The diagnostic use of blood ammonia is limited by the need for meticulous sample handling, including avoidance of hemolysis, use of cold heparinized tubes, transfer on ice, and refrigerated centrifugation and assay, all ideally within an hour of collection (Ruland, Fischer, and Hartmann, 2010.).

Diagnostic Imaging in the Evaluation of Hepatobiliary Disease

The size, shape, position, opacity, and margins of the liver can be assessed on standard radiographs of the cranial abdomen. Hepatomegaly is associated with congestion (right-sided heart failure), vacuolar hepatopathy (glycogen, lipid, amyloid), infiltrative disease (neoplasia), extramedullary hematopoiesis, and inflammatory liver disease. Microhepatica may be seen with PSVA or chronic hepatitis/cirrhosis (dogs). Increased opacity may be noted secondary to mineralization within the biliary system (49% of choleliths) or hepatic parenchyma (granulomas, long-term hematomas, abscesses, neoplasia, chronic hepatopathies, or regenerative nodules). Gas may be within the biliary tree (emphysematous cholecystitis, cholangitis), portal vessels (severe necrotizing gastroenteritis), or hepatic parenchyma (hepatic abscesses).

Ultrasonography enables differentiation among focal, multifocal, and diffuse disease; evaluation of the biliary system and portal vasculature; and procurement of tissue for hepatic histopathology (Gashen, 2009). Focal hepatic diseases include cysts, hematomas, abscesses, granulomas, regenerative nodules, primary and metastatic neoplasms, infarcts, and biliary pseudocysts. A large liver with diffuse hyperechoic parenchyma may be noted with fatty change (hepatic lipidosis) and vacuolar hepatopathy, whereas a small, hyperechoic liver may be seen with cirrhosis. Diffuse hypoechoic parenchyma may be noted in cases of hepatic congestion and suppurative hepatitis. Evaluation of the biliary tree and gallbladder may reveal a gallbladder mucocele, choleliths, and intrahepatic or extrahepatic bile duct dilation. A diffusely thick gallbladder wall is consistent with cholecystitis. A normal ultrasound scan does not preclude a diagnosis of hepatobiliary disease.

In many cases of PSVA ultrasonography permits direct visualization of the shunting vessel. Ultrasonography is more sensitive for the detection of intrahepatic shunts (100%) than extrahepatic shunts (80% to 98%). The sensitivity of ultrasound for the diagnosis of PSVA is enhanced by duplex-Doppler or color-flow Doppler, although this requires a cooperative patient and operator patience for accurate interpretation. Reduced or reversed portal flow is seen with multiple acquired shunts secondary to portal hypertension. When combined, findings of a small liver, enlarged kidneys, and uroliths had a positive predictive value of a 100% for a congenital PSVA in dogs. Portal vein/aorta and portal vein/caudal vena cava values of greater or equal to 0.8 and 0.75, respectively, consistently ruled out an extrahepatic PSVA (d'Anjou et al, 2004). Ultrasound can be used to detect vascular complications of hepatic disease such as portal hypertension and portal venous thrombosis. Ultrasonographic signs of portal hypertension include the presence of ascites, multiple acquired shunts, and reduced or reversed portal blood flow (Buob et al, 2011). Ultrasonography is currently the best imaging modality to evaluate for EHBDO. Ultrasonographic signs of EHBDO include dilation of the cystic duct, common bile duct (>5 mm in cats), or intrahepatic bile ducts and identification of an intraluminal or extraluminal mass obstructing the biliary tract (Gaillot et al,

2007). The degree of gallbladder distention appears to be variable and thus should not be used as a sole criterion to diagnose EHBDO, particularly in cats.

Scintigraphy may be a useful adjunct in cases of suspected EHBDO or PSVA. In scintigraphic imaging of the biliary tract, an intravenous ^{99m}Tc-iminodiacetic acid (technetium 99m) derivative is taken up by hepatocytes and subsequently undergoes biliary excretion. Using a cutoff of 180 minutes for the dye to enter the small intestine, the sensitivity of scintigraphy to identify complete EHBDO is high (83% to 100%), but the specificity is lower because partial bile duct obstruction also may slow dye excretion. Sensitivity remains similar, whereas specificity is increased markedly when the cutoff time is increased to 24 hours after injection. High serum bilirubin concentration did not reduce the diagnostic usefulness of scintigraphy.

Transcolonic pertechnetate scintigraphy (TCPS) is used for the detection of PSVA. In TCPS ^{99m}Tc pertechnetate is administered rectally and is absorbed subsequently into the portal venous system. In normal animals radioisotope activity is detected in the liver before its detection in the heart. In animals with PSVA the radioisotope activity is detected in the heart before the liver. In dogs TCPS has a high positive predictive value for the diagnosis of PSVA and discriminates dogs with macroscopic PSVA from those with primary hypoplasia of the portal vein because TCPS is abnormal only in the former.

Transplenic portal scintigraphy (TSPS) also can be used to diagnose PSVA. Ultrasound-guided TSPS results in higher radioisotope count densities, more consistent splenic and portal venograms, and a significant decrease in radiation exposure when compared with TCPS. TSPS misses cases of PSVA when the shunt originates distal to the splenic vein.

The value of magnetic resonance imaging (MRI) and helical computed tomography in the diagnosis of hepatobiliary disease is currently under evaluation (Gashen, 2009). MRI has shown promise in the differentiation of benign from malignant focal hepatic lesions in canine patients. Magnetic resonance angiography and helical computed tomography angiography have been used in dogs for the diagnosis of PSVA and offer the added advantage of accurate anatomic characterization of the shunt. The diagnostic use of these modalities currently is limited by availability and cost.

Hepatic Biopsy Acquisition and Interpretation

Indications for hepatic biopsy include persistent serial increases in liver enzymes, abnormal hepatic function tests, hepatomegaly of undetermined cause, ultrasonographic abnormalities in hepatic parenchyma, and evaluation for the presence of a breed-specific hepatopathy. Hepatic biopsy can be obtained by ultrasound guidance (needle biopsy) or exploratory or laparoscopy (wedge biopsy). The advantages of the latter two methods are the ability to grossly evaluate the liver, acquire large tissue samples, and quickly identify and control postbiopsy hemorrhage. When wedge biopsy is used as the standard, discordance between wedge and Tru-Cut biopsies may be

as high as 48% (Cole et al, 2002). However, the standard for any study evaluating the accuracy of hepatic biopsies is histopathologic assessment of the whole liver at necropsy. Thus any hepatic biopsy, no matter how it is obtained, must be interpreted in light of sampling error.

Prebiopsy considerations should include the patient's overall clinical status and the risk of hemorrhage. Acquisition of hepatic tissue is contraindicated in the presence of a hemodynamically unstable patient, coagulopathy, and encephalopathy. A PT, PTT, and platelet count should be performed. Tru-Cut biopsy should be avoided with elevations in PT and PTT of greater than 1.5 times normal and a platelet count of less than 80,000. A buccal mucosal bleeding time may improve the sensitivity of detecting bleeding deficiencies in cases of mild thrombocytopenia. Vitamin K is administered routinely 24 hours before hepatic biopsy. Fresh frozen plasma may be considered before biopsy in cases in which mild elevations in PT and PTT are noted.

The method of biopsy acquisition is influenced by the size of the liver, the suspected diagnosis, and the clinical condition of the patient. Microhepatica and large-volume abdominal effusion are contraindications for percutaneous ultrasound-guided biopsy. In some conditions, such as primary hypoplasia of the portal vein and nodular hyperplasia, a wedge biopsy is often necessary to obtain a definitive diagnosis. In cases of diffuse vacuolar hepatopathy, inflammatory disease, or neoplasia, a diagnosis can be obtained with a percutaneous ultrasound-guided Tru-Cut biopsy (a 16-gauge needle in dogs and an 18-gauge needle in cats). Multiple biopsy samples (three to five) should be taken from different areas of the liver.

In general hepatic biopsy is preferred over fine-needle aspiration (FNA) to characterize liver disorders. When compared with hepatic biopsy, discordance rates with FNA may be as high as 70%. However, in animals with bleeding disorders or large cavitary lesions or abscesses, ultrasound-guided FNA can be performed safely. In focal or diffuse hepatic disease (vacuolar or neoplastic) FNA may yield diagnostic samples. Occasionally FNA may identify an infectious agent that can be missed easily on histopathology. However, FNA cannot diagnose reliably necroinflammatory or vascular disease. Percutaneous cholecystocentesis has been shown to be a safe technique by which to obtain bile for cytology and culture.

The clinician must understand the benefits and limitations of hepatic histopathology. The purposes of obtaining hepatic tissue are to (1) determine the category of disease (inflammatory, neoplastic, vascular, or vacuolar); (2) define the extent of the disease; (3) assess the duration of illness; and (4) provide tissue for special stains and culture to aid in the diagnosis of metabolic and infectious causes. Although histopathology may result in a definitive diagnosis in the case of metabolic disease (hepatic lipidosis) and neoplasia, more often certain reaction patterns are described, which then provide clues to the underlying etiology. Correct interpretation of the biopsy results requires dialogue with the pathologist and reevaluation of the patient's history and clinical picture. A liver biopsy specimen represents only a small portion of the entire liver, and frequently even diffuse disorders have an uneven distribution; therefore the clinician always should be critical of whether the histopathologic diagnosis fits with the clinical picture.

Several breeds of dogs have copper-associated hepatopathies (Hoffman, 2009). Evaluation of hepatic biopsy for diagnosis of copper-associated hepatic disease ideally requires semiquantitative staining of the biopsy material and quantitative analysis of hepatic copper content. Hepatic wedge biopsies are ideal, although adequate material can be obtained to carry out these measurements in needle biopsy samples. Normal hepatocytes do not take up much copper stain, and hepatic copper values are 200 to 400 PPM. Dogs with copper-associated hepatopathies have quantitative copper values in excess of 1500 PPM with copper deposits in many hepatocytes, particularly those away from areas of inflammation or in the centrolobular area.

References and Suggested Reading

Berent AC, Tobias KM: Portosystemic vascular anomalies, *Vet Clin North Am Small Anim Pract* 39:513, 2009.
Buob S et al: Portal hypertension: pathophysiology, diagnosis, and treatment, *J Vet Intern Med* 25:169, 2011.
Center SA: Interpretation of liver enzymes, *Vet Clin North Am Small Anim Pract* 37:297, 2007.
Cole TL et al: Diagnostic comparison of needle and wedge biopsy specimens of the liver in dogs and cats, *J Am Vet Med Assoc* 220:1483, 2002.
d'Anjou MA et al: Ultrasonographic diagnosis of portosystemic shunting in dogs and cats, *Vet Radiol Ultrasound* 45:424, 2004.
Gaillot HA et al: Ultrasonographic features of extrahepatic biliary obstruction in cats, *Vet Radiol Ultrasound* 48:439, 2007.
Gashen L: Update on hepatobiliary imaging, *Vet Clin North Am Small Anim Med* 39:439, 2009.
Gaskill CL et al: Liver histopathology and liver and serum alanine aminotransferase and alkaline phosphatase activities in epileptic dogs receiving phenobarbital, *Vet Pathol* 42:147-160, 2005.
Gerritzen-Bruning MJ, van den Ingh TSGAM, Rothuizen J: Diagnostic value of fasting plasma ammonia and bile acid concentrations in the identification of portosystemic shunting in dogs, *J Vet Intern Med* 20:13, 2006.
Hoffman G: Copper associated liver disease, *Vet Clin North Am Small Anim Pract* 39:489, 2009.
Ruland K, Fischer A, Hartmann K: Sensitivity and specificity of fasting ammonia and serum bile acids in the diagnosis of portosystemic shunts in dogs and cats, *Vet Clin Pathol* 39:57, 2010.
Unakami S et al: Molecular nature of three liver alkaline phosphatases detected by drug administration in vivo: differences between soluble and membranous enzymes, *Comp Biochem Physiol B* 88:111, 1987.

CHAPTER 140

Drug-Associated Liver Disease*

LAUREN A. TREPANIER, *Madison, Wisconsin*

The liver is a common target of drug toxicity. It receives 25% to 30% of cardiac output and is the site of first-pass clearance of many orally administered drugs. Hepatic cytochrome P450s and other biotransformation enzymes can generate reactive metabolites, which may lead to local cytotoxicity, or haptenize liver proteins and trigger an immune response. Drugs also can inhibit transporter pumps in the sinusoidal or canalicular membranes, thus interfering with hepatocyte function and bile salt efflux. Two major patterns of drug-induced hepatotoxicity are recognized: cytotoxic (associated with hepatocyte necrosis) and cholestatic (which can be attributed to inhibition of biliary transporters, or mitochondrial injury with resulting steatosis). In humans, an R value is calculated to characterize hepatotoxicity by biochemical pattern, where

$$R = \frac{(\text{ALT/Upper limit of normal})}{(\text{ALP/Upper limit of normal})}$$

An R value greater than 5 indicates hepatocellular injury, an R less than 2 indicates cholestatic injury, and an R of 2 to 5 represents a mixed pattern.

Dose-Dependent Hepatotoxic Drugs

For dose-dependent, or intrinsic, hepatotoxicity, toxicity increases with increasing dose in one or more species, and virtually all members of a population or species are affected at high enough doses. Dose-dependent hepatotoxicity may be caused by the parent drug or by a metabolite generated reliably in the treated species (Figure 140-1). These reactions are relatively predictable, and therapeutic drug monitoring may be helpful in prevention. They

---

*Data included in this chapter were supported in part by grants from Miravista Laboratories, the Waltham Foundation, and the Companion Animal Fund at the University of Wisconsin-Madison.

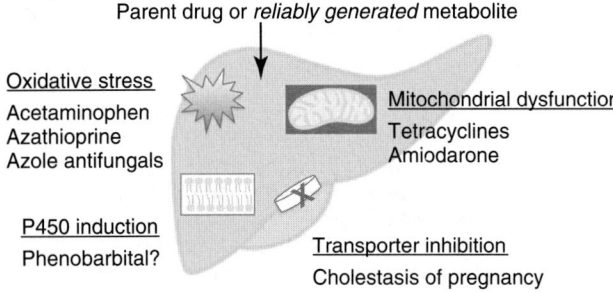

Parent drug or *reliably generated* metabolite

Oxidative stress
Acetaminophen
Azathioprine
Azole antifungals

Mitochondrial dysfunction
Tetracyclines
Amiodarone

P450 induction
Phenobarbital?

Transporter inhibition
Cholestasis of pregnancy

Figure 140-1 Dose-dependent, drug-associated hepatotoxicity typically is caused by either the parent drug or a consistently generated metabolite. Drugs can inhibit transporter pumps and lead to a functional cholestasis; this occurs with endogenous hormone metabolites during pregnancy. Many drugs yield reactive metabolites that cause oxidative stress; examples include acetaminophen, azathioprine, and azole antifungals. For these compounds, antioxidant supplementation may be effective. Drugs that interfere with mitochondrial function can lead to steatosis from inhibition of fatty acid β-oxidation or may lead to more severe hepatocellular damage because of impaired cellular respiration. Finally, drugs that act as P450 inducers, such as phenobarbital, may mediate hepatotoxicity by chronic bioactivation of environmental toxins.

require a dose reduction but usually not permanent drug discontinuation.

Phenobarbital

Hepatotoxicity from phenobarbital can range from subclinical increases in serum bile acids to clinical hepatopathy to fulminant liver failure (Dayrell-Hart et al, 1991). Signs typically develop after a year or more of phenobarbital treatment, and prolonged duration of administration is associated with degree of histologic injury in epileptic dogs. Typical histologic findings in dogs with clinical signs are bridging portal fibrosis, bile duct hyperplasia, and nodular regeneration. Dogs with phenobarbital hepatotoxicity improve clinically after phenobarbital dose reduction (Dayrell-Hart et al, 1991). However, liver enzyme abnormalities can develop in phenobarbital-treated dogs without histologic liver injury, and higher phenobarbital dosages and serum drug concentrations have not been correlated with the development of abnormal serum bile acids in epileptic dogs. These findings suggest that phenobarbital hepatotoxicity is dose dependent, with modifying factors that are not understood.

One hypothesized mechanism of phenobarbital hepatotoxicity is induction of cytochrome P450 enzymes, with secondary bioactivation and hepatotoxicity of other drugs, dietary components, or environmental toxins. For example, phenobarbital increases the hepatotoxicity of carbon tetrachloride in dogs, of chloroform in mice, and of acetaminophen in human hepatocytes. Phenobarbital hepatotoxicity therefore could be modulated by environmental exposures in individual dogs. Phenobarbital does not lead to either enzyme induction or hepatotoxicity in cats.

Azathioprine

Azathioprine can lead to increases in ALT and/or ALP activities in some dogs; these abnormalities commonly are subclinical but may be accompanied by jaundice and clinical signs. Azathioprine liver injury is associated with the generation of oxidative metabolites and depletion of hepatic antioxidants in rodent models and can be prevented by pretreatment with N-acetylcysteine.

Dogs treated with azathioprine should be monitored routinely for increases in liver enzyme activities. If glucocorticoids also are administered, liver enzyme interpretation can become clouded; discordant increases in ALT relative to SAP, or early increases in serum bilirubin, are cause for concern. Risk factors for azathioprine hepatotoxicity in dogs are not clear, but increases in ALT or ALP typically are reversible with simple dosage reduction. Based on what is known about azathioprine hepatotoxicity in other species, supplementation with glutathione precursors may be effective in preventing or reversing azathioprine hepatotoxicity in dogs, but this has yet to be evaluated.

Azole Antifungals

Ketoconazole, itraconazole, and fluconazole can lead to increases in serum ALT in dogs, although clinical signs such as jaundice are uncommon. Mild, clinically insignificant increases in ALT also have been reported in cats treated with itraconazole and fluconazole. In dogs with blastomycosis, higher dosages of itraconazole (10 mg/kg/day) were associated with a greater risk of ALT abnormalities than 5 mg/kg/day, with no difference in efficacy (Legendre et al, 1996). Further, increases in ALT and ALP were correlated with itraconazole plasma concentrations, which supports a dose-dependent mechanism.

In animal models, ketoconazole hepatotoxicity has been attributed to an oxidative metabolite, N-deacetyl ketoconazole, which leads to covalent binding to liver proteins and glutathione depletion. Fluconazole appears to be less hepatotoxic overall than either ketoconazole or itraconazole in humans and animal models. In dogs with blastomycosis, the author observed increases in serum ALT in 26% of dogs treated with itraconazole (median fold increase 2.7), and in 17% of dogs on fluconazole (median fold increase 1.5). The author has observed anecdotally increases in serum ALT during treatment with itraconazole, which have resolved after a switch to fluconazole during treatment for blastomycosis in dogs.

Acetaminophen

Acetaminophen is a classic dose-dependent hepatotoxin in humans and dogs; doses greater than 150 to 250 mg/kg lead to acute centrilobular hepatic necrosis. In cats, hematologic toxicity predominates over direct liver toxicity. Acetaminophen is bioactivated to the reactive oxidized metabolite, NAPQI (N-acetyl-p-benzoquinone imine), which is detoxified by glutathione conjugation. This provides the rationale for treatment of overdoses with the glutathione precursor N-acetylcysteine (140 mg/kg loading IV, then 70 mg/kg q6h for 7 treatments).

Although *N*-acetylcysteine is most effective in humans when given within 8 hours of acetaminophen ingestion, this antidote still has beneficial effects on survival when given much later in the course of intoxication.

S-adenosylmethionine (SAMe) also can be used for acetaminophen intoxication in dogs that can tolerate oral medications; the protocol that has been used successfully is a 40 mg/kg loading dose, followed by 20 mg/kg q24h for 7 days. Cimetidine has been recommended to inhibit oxidation of acetaminophen to NAPQI; however, this drug has no effect on NAPQI generation *in vitro* and is not effective in humans with acetaminophen overdose; cimetidine therefore is not recommended.

Amiodarone

Amiodarone leads to clinically significant hepatotoxicity in about 45% of dogs treated for refractory atrial fibrillation and ventricular arrhythmias, a median of 16 weeks after starting maintenance therapy (Jacobs et al, 2000; Kraus et al, 2009). Predominant increases in ALT typically are observed, with or without hyperbilirubinemia and neutropenia. These abnormalities slowly resolve over 1 to 3 months after drug discontinuation. Toxicity in animal models has been attributed to two oxidative metabolites, mono-*N*-desethylamiodarone (MDEA) and di-*N*-desethylamiodarone (DDEA), which generate reactive oxygen species that uncouple oxidative phosphorylation and lead to mitochondrial damage.

Because of the prevalence of hepatotoxicity and neutropenia, a baseline CBC and biochemical panel is recommended in all dogs before amiodarone initiation, with a recheck of liver enzymes after a loading period and monthly during treatment. The development of substantial increases in serum ALT is an indication for dose reduction or drug discontinuation.

Lomustine

The alkylating agent lomustine, or CCNU, is associated with substantial increases in serum ALT (> fivefold baseline) in about 29% of dogs (Hosoya et al, 2009; Rassnick et al, 2010). Enzyme elevations can occur suddenly and are most common after 1 to 3 monthly doses of CCNU. Dogs also may develop modest hyperbilirubinemia. The risk of ALT elevations is greatest in the boxer breed and in younger dogs (≤5 years old).

Clinical signs of hepatotoxicity occur in an estimated 6% of CCNU-treated dogs, are noted after a median of four doses, and are associated with a higher cumulative dosages (median 350 mg/m²) (Kristal et al, 2004). Liver histopathology shows portal aggregates of hemosiderin-laden Kupffer cells, enlargement of hepatocyte nuclei, and hepatocyte vacuolization. Dose reduction or drug discontinuation (for severe enzyme elevations) is associated with improvement in ALT activities in most dogs. However, some dogs that were not identified until clinical signs developed have been euthanized as a result of progressive liver disease.

The mechanism(s) for CCNU hepatotoxicity are not known. Because of the high incidence of biochemical hepatotoxicity associated with CCNU and the risk for

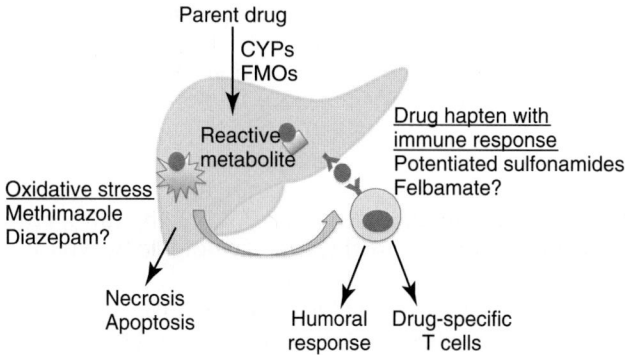

Figure 140-2 Although the pathogeneses of many idiosyncratic hepatotoxins are not understood, the most common demonstrated mechanism is the generation of reactive metabolites that lead to oxidative stress and/or hapten formation. Reactive metabolites typically are generated locally in the liver by cytochrome P450s (CYPs), flavin monooxygenases (FMOs), or other pathways. These metabolites may bind to critical proteins and impair hepatocyte function or generate reactive oxygen species than damage hepatocyte membranes. Drug-protein adducts also can be processed and presented to the immune system in association with MHC molecules. In the presence of a "danger" signal such as oxidative stress, this antigen presentation may lead to clonal expansion of drug-specific T cells, and/or the generation of drug-specific antibodies that target hepatocyte proteins.

progression to hepatic failure it is critical to monitor liver enzymes and bilirubin in all dogs treated with CCNU, at a minimum before each subsequent dosage. Concurrent SAMe and silybin (Denamarin) therapy given to dogs treated with CCNU led to lower liver enzyme elevations and less clinical toxicity (Skorupski et al, 2011).

Idiosyncratic Hepatotoxicity

Idiosyncratic hepatotoxicity reactions are more difficult to predict because they lead to toxicity in only a small proportion of patients at therapeutic dosages. Toxicity does not increase with dose in the general population (therefore they are not considered dose dependent), but toxicity probably does increase with dose in susceptible individuals. Idiosyncratic hepatotoxicity often is caused by reactive metabolites that are variably generated among individuals (Figure 140-2). These reactive metabolites may cause oxidative stress, mitochondrial damage, or form haptens that trigger a humoral or T cell–mediated immunologic response. Although idiosyncratic drug reactions sometimes are called drug hypersensitivity reactions, they may or may not involve an adaptive immune response. Idiosyncratic drug reactions usually require discontinuation of the suspect drug, and structurally related drugs may cause a similar reaction.

Potentiated Sulfonamides

Potentiated sulfonamides are the most common antimicrobials associated with idiosyncratic hepatotoxicity in the dog. All commercially available formulations have been implicated. Clinical signs usually are seen 5 to 30 days after starting sulfonamides, with a mean of 12 days. A hepatocellular pattern may progress over several days to cholestasis in some dogs; hepatic necrosis is the predominant histologic lesion initially. Signs also may include fever (55% of cases), transient neutropenia, thrombocytopenia, hemolytic anemia, polyathropathy, proteinuria, keratoconjunctivitis sicca, skin lesions, or uveitis. Dobermans are overrepresented among dogs with idiosyncratic sulfonamide toxicity, although arthropathy and glomerulonephropathy, not hepatotoxicity, typically are reported in this breed.

Sulfonamide antimicrobials are oxidized to form nitroso metabolites that covalently bind to proteins and act as haptens. Idiosyncratic sulfonamide toxicity is convincingly immune mediated in humans, with antidrug antibodies and drug- and metabolite-specific T cells documented. If potentiated sulfonamides must be prescribed, the client should be educated to look for any subtle signs of illness. Failure to discontinue sulfonamides at the time of initial development of adverse signs can lead to fatal outcomes. Although specific antidotes for sulfonamide hypersensitivity have not been evaluated, this author recommends supplementation with a glutathione precursor (SAMe or N-acetylcysteine, using the same protocols as for acetaminophen toxicity) and ascorbate (30 mg/kg q6-8h IV, empiric dosage), based on the finding that glutathione and ascorbate can reverse haptenization of the nitroso metabolite to canine liver microsomes *in vitro* (Lavergne and Trepanier, unpublished observations). Glucocorticoids may be considered in the subacute setting, particularly if a cholestatic pattern persists after drug discontinuation and support.

Carprofen

Potential hepatoxicity from carprofen is well recognized among veterinary clinicians, with an estimated incidence of 1.4 cases per 10,000 dogs treated (0.05%). Clinical signs of acute hepatic failure are noted 5 to 30 days after drug initiation, with a median of 19 days (MacPhail et al, 1998). A predominant hepatocellular or mixed pattern is found. No dogs with carprofen toxicity have been reported with increased ALP activities in the absence of clinically significant concurrent increases in ALT. Bridging hepatic necrosis is the predominant histopathologic finding. Although Labrador retrievers were overrepresented in the initial report, this may reflect the high ownership of this breed because the syndrome could not be reproduced in Labradors under controlled conditions (personal communication, Pfizer Animal Health).

Given the low incidence and abrupt onset of idiosyncratic hepatotoxicity from carprofen in dogs, routine monitoring of liver enzymes is not an efficient approach to preventing clinical toxicity. Owners should be advised to watch for subtle signs of illness during NSAID administration, to include inappetence, vomiting, diarrhea, lethargy, or dark urine. A normal ALT in the face of clinical illness essentially rules out carprofen hepatotoxicity.

Felbamate

The antiepileptic drug felbamate can lead to marked increases in serum ALT in dogs concurrently treated with phenobarbital (Dayrell-Hart et al, 1991). Four of 16 dogs developed clinical hepatopathies; in addition, serum phenobarbital concentrations increased in felbamate-treated dogs. This likely is due to an impairment of phenobarbital clearance by felbamate.

Felbamate generates an oxidative metabolite, 2-phenylpropenal (also called atropaldehyde), which is detoxified by glutathione. This metabolite is cytotoxic to hepatocytes *in vitro*, can bind tissues covalently, and leads to T cell stimulation in animal models. Based on the unfavorable safety profile, felbamate is not recommended, particularly in combination with phenobarbital, in dogs.

Zonisamide

Acute hepatotoxicity recently has been reported in two dogs treated with the anticonvulsant zonisamide (Miller et al, 2011; Schwartz et al, 2011). In one dog, clinical signs began 3 weeks after drug initiation, with a mixed biochemical pattern. Abnormalities resolved with drug discontinuation. In a second dog, marked increases in ALT with hyperbilirubinemia were noted 10 days after zonisamide was started. This dog was euthanized because of hepatic failure; histopathology showed massive panlobular hepatic necrosis with marked periportal microvesicular steatosis.

Further clinical experience is needed before the incidence of zonisamide hepatotoxicity is clear; however, dog owners and veterinary colleagues should be informed of this potential adverse drug reaction when zonisamide is prescribed. Clients should be alerted to watch for acute signs of illness; if noted, zonisamide should be discontinued and serum ALT should be evaluated.

Diazepam

Diazepam represents a classic idiosyncratic hepatotoxin in cats, first recognized and reported in the mid-1990s (Center et al, 1996). Cats develop clinical signs with sedation 5 or more days after drug initiation, with progression to jaundice and overt hepatic failure. Blood work shows dramatic increases in ALT activities in all cats. Marked centrilobular hepatic necrosis, with mild to marked biliary hyperplasia, is seen on liver biopsies. The syndrome of diazepam hepatotoxicity in cats has been reported with generic and brand name diazepam (Center et al, 1996) but has not been observed with parenteral diazepam administration as a premedicant. Unfortunately, the mechanism for this potentially fatal adverse drug reaction has not been explored.

Subsequent reports of diazepam hepatotoxicity have since appeared on veterinary message boards (Veterinary Information Network) in cats prescribed oral diazepam for seizures or urethral spasm. Although toxicity appears to be relatively rare, there are safer alternative drugs for behavioral problems, seizures, and urethral spasm in cats.

Methimazole

About 1% to 2% of hyperthyroid cats administered the antithyroid drug methimazole develop clinical evidence of hepatopathy with jaundice, typically in the first month of treatment (Peterson, Kintzer, and Hurvitz, 1988). These changes are distinct from "innocent" increases in ALT and ALP seen with untreated hyperthyroidism. Hepatopathies can demonstrate a predominantly hepatocellular or cholestatic pattern, with or without hyperbilirubinemia. These reactions usually are reversible with drug discontinuation but can be fatal if not detected promptly.

Methimazole hepatotoxicity in animal models presents as dose-dependent centrilobular hepatic necrosis, which is manifested in the presence of glutathione depletion. Hepatotoxicity has been attributed to an oxidative metabolite, *N*-methylthiourea, which is generated by flavin monooxygenases. This pathway has yet to be evaluated in cats.

Management of idiosyncratic methimazole toxicity in cats is focused ideally on prevention. Cats treated with methimazole should be screened for increases in ALT and ALP at a recheck visit during the first 4 weeks of treatment and at subsequent rechecks if clinical signs of lethargy or anorexia are noted. If cats develop adverse clinical signs, idiosyncratic toxicity (hepatopathy, blood dyscrasias, or facial excoriation) should be ruled out. The transdermal route does not seem beneficial in preventing idiosyncratic methimazole toxicity, including hepatotoxicity. Given the role of glutathione depletion in methimazole hepatoxicity in experimental models, the efficacy of glutathione precursors must be evaluated in the management of this adverse drug reaction.

Monitoring and Prevention

Client education and clinician index of suspicion are the mainstays of monitoring for, and recognizing, drug-induced hepatotoxicity. For dose-dependent reactions, periodic clinical monitoring such as serum drug concentrations, liver enzymes, serum bilirubin, and bile acids are useful in detecting hepatopathies before clinical signs develop. For idiosyncratic drug-induced hepatopathies, routine blood work is an inefficient monitoring tool. Hundreds of patients would have to be screened to detect a single rare adverse reaction, and more importantly, recent normal blood work may not predict an acute onset of hepatic necrosis a few days later. Clinicians always should consider the possibility of an adverse drug reaction in ill patients that have started a new drug, especially within the previous 4 weeks. Although any drug potentially could cause an adverse event in a given patient,

the clinician should focus on drugs with a high prior probability of toxicity (i.e., those drugs previously associated with idiosyncratic hepatotoxicity in dogs, cats, or humans). Most cases of drug-associated liver disease are reversible with drug discontinuation; for severe fulminant cases, rapid recognition of a possible drug-induced etiology, followed by aggressive support appropriate to the drug in question, is essential to a good outcome.

References and Suggested Reading

Center SA et al: Fulminant hepatic failure associated with oral administration of diazepam in 11 cats, *J Am Vet Med Assoc* 209:618, 1996.

Dayrell-Hart B et al: Hepatotoxicity of phenobarbital in dogs: 18 cases (1985-1989), *J Am Vet Med Assoc* 199:1060, 1991.

Hosoya K et al: Prevalence of elevated alanine transaminase activity in dogs treated with CCNU (Lomustine), *Vet Comp Oncol* 7:244, 2009.

Jacobs G, Calvert C, Kraus M: Hepatopathy in 4 dogs treated with amiodarone, *J Vet Intern Med* 14:96, 2000.

Kraus MS et al: Toxicity in Doberman Pinchers with ventricular arrhythmias treated with amiodarone (1996-2005), *J Vet Intern Med* 23:1, 2009.

Kristal O et al: Hepatotoxicity associated with CCNU (lomustine) chemotherapy in dogs, *J Vet Intern Med* 18:75, 2004.

Legendre AM et al: Treatment of blastomycosis with itraconazole in 112 dogs, *J Vet Intern Med* 10:365, 1996.

MacPhail CM et al: Hepatocellular toxicosis associated with administration of carprofen in 21 dogs, *J Am Vet Med Assoc* 212:1895, 1998.

Miller ML et al: Apparent acute idiosyncratic hepatic necrosis associated with zonisamide administration in a dog, *J Vet Intern Med* 25:1156, 2011.

Peterson ME, Kintzer PP, Hurvitz AI: Methimazole treatment of 262 cats with hyperthyroidism, *J Vet Intern Med* 2:150, 1988.

Rassnick K et al: A phase II study to evaluate the toxicity and efficacy of alternating CCNU and high-dose vinblastine and prednisone (CVP) for treatment of dogs with high-grade, metastatic or nonresectable mast cell tumours, *Vet Comp Oncol* 8:138, 2010.

Schulz BS et al: Suspected side effects of doxycycline use in dogs—a retrospective study of 386 cases, *Vet Rec* 169:229, 2011.

Schwartz M et al: Possible drug-induced hepatopathy in a dog receiving zonisamide monotherapy for treatment of cryptogenic epilepsy, *J Vet Med Sci* 73:1505, 2011.

Skorupski KA et al: Prospective randomized clinical trial assessing the efficacy of Denamarin for prevention of CCNU-induced hepatopathy in tumor-bearing dogs, *J Vet Intern Med* 25:838, 2011.

CHAPTER 141

Acute Liver Failure

SHARON A. CENTER, *Ithaca, New York*

Acute liver failure (ALF) is an uncommon, rapidly progressive, often lethal condition reflecting sudden, or perceptively sudden, severe hepatocellular necrosis or dysfunction associated with hyperbilirubinemia, coagulopathy, and evidence of hepatic encephalopathy (HE) (Nguyen and Vierling, 2011). As characterized in humans, HE manifests as a breadth of neurobehavioral or psychologic abnormalities ranging from overt to mild encephalopathy. No subjective or objective scoring system has been validated in companion animal patients, similar to criteria used in humans (Riordan and Williams, 1997). In humans with ALF, high-grade HE has a poor prognostic implication.

Causal Factors

Identifying the cause of ALF has prognostic and therapeutic implications but often remains enigmatic. However, a number of well-substantiated causes have been recognized (Boxes 141-1 and 141-2). Hepatotoxic and idiosyncratic drug reactions are most common, with environmental and plant toxins, infectious diseases, rare neoplastic disorders, and other conditions less common. The indiscriminant appetite of many dogs results in a greater risk of environmental toxin, hepatotoxic plant, or mycotoxin ingestion compared with cats.

Pathophysiology

The liver has a high susceptibility to toxicity because of its location and central role in metabolic and detoxification pathways. Susceptibility and severity of hepatobiliary injury is influenced by age, species, patient nutritional status, concurrent drug administration, antecedent disease, the presence of excessive hepatocellular transition metal storage, antioxidant status, hereditary factors, and current or prior exposure to the same or similar compounds. Hepatic toxicity is the most commonly reported organ system toxicity associated with true adverse drug reactions that may be intrinsic or idiosyncratic (see Chapter 140). Metabolically generated toxins often derive from reactions catalyzed by the cytochrome P-450 system. Such toxins may be potentiated by microsomal enzyme inducers (e.g., phenobarbital, omeprazole), whereas toxicity of some is impaired by microsomal enzyme blockers (e.g., cimetidine, chloramphenicol, ranitidine). Although pathophysiologic mechanisms leading to ALF vary depending upon the causal agent, oxidative injury often plays a critical role. Many toxins are metabolized to a secondary injurious product generating toxic electrophilic adducts that interact with structural proteins,

enzymes, or nucleoproteins (aflatoxin, cycad, sulfonamides) or that induce lymphocytotoxic responses or FAS-induced apoptosis (Box 141-3). The capacity of the hepatic microenvironment to terminate injury and regenerate perfused nonfibrosed hepatic parenchyma varies with the inciting cause, whether the toxin incapacitates protein transcription, the nutritional status of the patient (inappetence reduces glutathione [GSH] concentrations), presence of antecedent liver injury, and for dogs the status of transition metal accumulation (iron, copper). In humans, genetic polymorphisms in keratins 8 and 18 that confer antiapoptotic effects in liver injury increase susceptibility to ALF; these are known to segregate with ethnicity (Strnad et al, 2010). There is no information regarding this phenomenon in dogs or cats. Susceptibility to certain drugs and toxins having a narrow therapeutic or exposure window may reflect innate (individual or species related) or acquired low hepatic GSH. The increasing causal role of complementary alternative medications in ALF in humans is relatively uninvestigated in companion animals. All supplements or complementary alternative medications have risk for contamination with other undeclared botanicals or chemicals (Nguyen and Vierling, 2011).

Clinical and Clinicopathologic Features

Progressive clinical features of ALF include abrupt onset of lethargy, inappetence, vomiting, weakness, dehydration, hypothermia, jaundice, bleeding tendencies, and hypotension. Clinicopathologic tests reflect the type, rate, and zonal location of hepatocellular injury, development of acute splanchnic hypertension, and synthetic failure. Acute severe necrosis accompanied by zone 3 parenchymal collapse (perivenous, adjacent to hepatic venule) causes remarkable transaminase release (alanine aminotransferase [ALT] from hepatocellular cytosol, aspartate aminotransferase [AST] from mitochondria), whereas injury focused on zone 1 (periportal region) can lead to a combined early induction of alkaline phosphatase (ALP) and γ-glutamyl transferase (GGT) and transaminase activities. Cats with diazepam-induced ALF also demonstrate markedly increased CK activity attributable to skeletal and cardiac muscle necrosis (Center et al, 1996). Toxins binding with nucleoproteins can disrupt liver enzyme synthesis (block protein transcription), muting their diagnostic utility in detection of liver injury (e.g., aflatoxin, cyanobacteria [microcystin], cycad toxicity). Panlobular hepatic injury leads to rapid development of hypocholesterolemia, low protein C and antithrombin activities, low coagulation proteins, and prolonged

Drugs That May Cause Hepatic Injury in Dogs and Cats*

Acetaminophen[d,c]	Ketoconazole[d,c]
Acetylsalicylic acid[c]	Mebendazole[d]
Androgenic anabolic steroids[c]	Methimazole[c]
(methyltestosterone,	Methoxyflurane[d]
mibolerone)	Mitotane (*OP' DDD*)[d]
Antineoplastic drugs	Oxibendazole[d]
(methotrexate,	Phenols: in cats[c]
6-mercaptopurine	(aspirin, benzoic acid,
[azathioprine][d],	benzyl alcohol,
L-asparaginase,	hexachlorophene)
mithramycin,	Phenazopyridine
doxorubicin)	Phenobarbital[d]
Amiodarone[d]	Phenothiazines[d]
Chloroform[d]	Phenylbutazone[d]
Chlortetracycline[c]	Phenytoin[d]
CCNU (lomustine,	Primidone[d]
chemotherapy)[d]	Rimadyl (carprofen)[d]
Danazol (an impeded	Tetracycline[c]
androgen)[c]	Thiacetarsamide[d]
Diazepam[c]	Tolbutamide
Erythromycin	Trimethoprim/sulfa[d]
Glucocorticoids	Xylitol[d]
Griseofulvin[c]	Zonisamide[d]
Halothane[d]	

*Note that the superscript d in the table refers to dogs; the superscript c refers to cats.

clotting times. Acute onset of transudative abdominal effusion reflects intrahepatic and splanchnic hypertension that may worsen upon administration of polyionic fluids necessary to maintain hydration and perfusion pressure. Albumin lost with bleeding into the intestinal lumen and transudation into the abdominal cavity results in progressive hypoproteinemia and hypoalbuminemia. Administration of packed RBCs can rapidly escalate (by fivefold to tenfold) hyperbilirubinemia by delivery of pigment that must be conjugated and eliminated by the liver. Glucosuria discordant with hyperglycemia usually incriminates an acquired Fanconi's injury (e.g., severe copper hepatotoxicosis, NSAID injury [carprofen], leptospirosis) associated with proximal renal tubular necrosis; this usually is accompanied by the appearance of granular casts.

Prognosis

The ability to predict survival in ALF is limited with noninvasive assessments. The best noninvasive predictive measures include sequential assessment (every few days) of liver enzyme activity and concentrations of albumin, fibrinogen, cholesterol, blood urea nitrogen (BUN), total bilirubin, and monitoring for appearance and abatement of ammonium biurate crystalluria, specific drug- or toxin-related crystalluria, glucosuria, and granular casts. Provision of fresh frozen plasma to abate bleeding tendencies complicates interpretation of coagulant and anticoagulant proteins. During the regenerative phase of recovery, increased activity in ALP and GGT may reflect oval

Toxins and Conditions That May Cause Severe Acute Hepatic Injury to Dogs and Cats*

Environmental Toxins
Amanita mushrooms[d]
Aflatoxins[d]/mycotoxins[d]
Blue-green algae
(Cyanobacteria)[d]
Chlorinated compounds
Cycad (sago palm)[d]
Heavy metals (Pb, Zn, Mn, Ar, Fe, Cu)[d,c]
Phenolic chemicals (especially cats)[c]
Gossypol from cottonseed

Endotoxins/Infectious Agents
Enteric organisms
Clostridium perfringens
Clostridium difficile gram-negative enteric bacteria
Food poisoning bacteria
E. coli
Staphylococcus spp.
Salmonella spp.
Bacillus cereus (emetic toxin)
Leptospirosis
Toxoplasmosis
Disseminated fungal infections
Leishmaniasis

Nutritional/Herbal Products
Atractylis gummifera
Black cohosh
Callilepis laureola
Chaparral
Comfrey extracts
(pyrrolizidine alkaloids)[d]
Chinese herbal medicines
(difficult to characterize)
Germander
Greater celandine
Green tea extract
Herbalife (not all products)
Hydroxycut (not all products)
Lipoic acid[c,d]
Kava Kava[d]
Licorice
Mistletoe
Pennyroyal senna
Usnic acid
Valerian
Xylitol[d]

Neoplasia
Histocytocytic sarcoma[d]
Lymphosarcoma[d,c]
Massive hepatocellular carcinoma[d]
Leukemia[d,c]
Mast cell neoplasia[c]

*Note that the superscript d in the table refers to dogs; the superscript c refers to cats.

Mechanisms of Hepatotoxic Injury

1. Altered physicochemical properties of membranes: cell or organelles
2. Inhibition of membrane and cellular enzymes
3. Impaired hepatic uptake or export processes
4. Altered cytoskeletal function
5. Precipitation of insoluble complexes in bile
6. Altered cell calcium homeostasis
7. Metabolic conversion to reactive intermediates causing oxidative injury augmented by antecedent excessive hepatic copper or iron stores
8. Toxic adducts binding to nucleoproteins:
   Prohibits protein transcription
   Prohibits cell replication and tissue repair
9. Initiation of FAS-induced apoptosis
10. Molecular mimicry: leads to immunologic injury
11. Lymphocytotoxic responses

cell hyperplasia and development of so-called reactive cholangioles. With toxins causing zone 3 collapse (e.g., aflatoxicosis, cycad poisoning, acute severe copper hepatotoxicosis), acute onset intrahepatic portal hypertension can lead to splanchnic hypertension before formation of acquired portosystemic shunts. This may lead to critical and fatal diapedesis of blood into the alimentary canal in the absence of ulcerative lesions (Dereszynski et al, 2008). Persistent or recurrent severe hypoglycemia portends a grave prognosis; this indicates compromised gluconeogenesis and depletion of tissue glycogen stores. Abdominal ultrasound often demonstrates only abdominal effusion in animals with ALF but can disclose massive hepatocellular carcinoma, inducing the syndrome or parenchymal nodules or hypoechoic parenchyma associated with diffuse lymphosarcoma. A liver biopsy is more helpful in predicting chance for recovery than noninvasive assessments but is hazardous during the coagulopathic stage. Despite the diagnostic limits of small sample size, core needle biopsy samples are most appropriate owing to short anesthetic and collection time and limited tissue trauma. Needle aspirates of liver are used to rule out disseminated hepatic neoplasia. Needle aspirates or core biopsies require anticipatory treatment with vitamin K_1 (see below) and DDAVP (dose of 0.5 to 5.0 µg/kg SC or diluted in 10 to 20 ml of saline and given IV slowly over 10 minutes during the perioperative period [e.g., before liver biopsy or during a bleeding crisis]).

Supportive Care

Supportive care should include crystalloid fluid support with caution given to the patient's tolerance and proclivity for third space fluid transudation. Causal factors of ALF concurrently may impair endothelial integrity, promoting formation of edema and abdominal effusions. Propriety of hetastarch administration must be considered carefully in light of its antiaggregatory platelet effect that can heighten risk for critical hemorrhage. The recently introduced Vetastarch colloid seemingly does not impose similar marked coagulative influence. Rather, infusion of canine fresh frozen plasma is preferred, although cost can be prohibitive in large-breed dogs. Vitamin K_1 should be provided initially at three doses of 0.5 to 1.5 mg/kg q12h SC or IM. After that, it is administered as perceived necessary in one of two ways: (1) (optimal method) based on PIVKA testing (more sensitive than routine bench coagulation tests) or the dependent coagulation factors or (2) (more common method) assessed with routine prothrombin or partial thromboplastin coagulation bench tests. Judicious supplementation of B-soluble vitamins and KCl in fluids thwarts development of thiamine deficiency (can resemble neurologic signs confused with HE, and promotes lactic acidosis and hypoglycemia) and hypokalemia (that may promote hyperammonemia). Glucose supplementation should be provided as needed in fluids to abate hypoglycemia; a 2.5% or 5.0% dextrose supplement is usually sufficient. Because splanchnic hypertension increases risk for enteric bacterial translocation, which can contribute to HE, broad-spectrum antimicrobials are administered parenterally. A combination of ticarcillin, enrofloxacin, and metronidazole often is used initially, if septicemia, suppurative hepatitis, leptospirosis, or other infectious bacterial agents are considered possible causes of the ALF. Acute splanchnic hypertension is not associated with gastric ulceration in humans or companion animals. Although hypergastrinemia can accompany hepatic splanchnic hypertension, in humans this is not associated with increased gastric acid production but rather reflects gastric mucosal edema and reduced gastric acid production. Consequently, routine administration of H_2 or HCl pump blockers is not endorsed. Rather, this treatment should be defined by examining vomitus for pH and blood. Control of emesis with centrally acting antiemetics is recommended; metoclopramide using constant rate infusion (customary dosing) has been used successfully. There is less experience with maropitant in ALF; this drug is partially metabolized in the liver, so the conventional dose recommendations are reduced. Sucralfate (slurry preparation) should be prescribed for patients demonstrating hematemesis (1 to 2 g mixed with water q8-12h). Because ALF is associated with high risk for hepatic oxidant damage, N-acetylcysteine (NAC) should be administered IV over 20 minutes up to q6h (10% solution, nonpyrogenic filter, loading dose of 140 mg/kg, thereafter at a dose of 70 mg/kg). Chronic constant rate infusion of NAC should not be used to avoid interfering with urea cycle ammonia detoxification (protonation of carbomyl phosphate). Current studies of NAC utility in ALF because of a variety of toxins suggest antioxidant and antiinflammatory benefits. When oral medications are tolerated, administration of vitamin E (10 U/kg of α-tocopherol q24h PO), bioavailable S-adenosylmethionine (SAMe) (20 mg/kg q24h PO), and a silibinin/phosphatidylcholine (PPC) combination (2 to 5 mg/kg q24h PO) are recommended, primarily for their antioxidant properties. However, vitamin E, SAMe, and silibinin/PPC also may modulate beneficially NF-κB and cell apoptosis signaling, and reduce hepatofibrogenesis; SAMe and silibinin/PPC may stimulate cell repair and DNA replication and improve membrane fluidity (enhancing cell signaling), and SAMe may provide a choleretic response that may hasten biliary elimination of infectious organisms or toxins. Whether there is a role for ursodeoxycholate in ALF remains unclear. Treatment of HE by oral administration of nonabsorbable antimicrobials (e.g., neomycin, rifaximin) may modify beneficially the enteric biome reducing generation of HE toxins (Rivkin and Gim, 2011; Bajaj et al, 2012).

Cleansing water enemas followed by a lactulose retention enema may reduce production and uptake of enteric ammonia. Activated charcoal by oral dose or enema may be warranted if a specific toxin potentially persists in the alimentary lumen. Elimination of some toxins may be escalated by oral administration of cholestyramine, a binding resin. Nutritional support containing adequate protein levels for tissue repair should be provided. Parenteral alimentation may be needed in the recumbent, lethargic, and neuroencephalopathic animal unwilling or unable to eat. Use of an amino acid solution designed for support of humans with ALF (rich in branched-chain amino acids [BCAA]) can improve nitrogen balance and reduce the passage of aromatic amino acids (AAA) across the blood-brain barrier, where they function as false neurotransmitters (competition between BCAA and AAA at the blood-brain barrier). Special considerations are necessary when parenteral nutrition is designed for a feline ALF patient owing to the unique carnivore requirements of cats (Morris, 2002). Clinicians should keep animals with progressive neurologic signs leading to confusion, lethargy, recumbency, seizures, and coma in a head-up posture (45 degrees), give them mannitol, and induce mild hypothermia to reduce critical brain edema that may lead to herniation. Severe, acute HE in ALF reflects acute astrocyte swelling secondary to accumulation of metabolic milliosmoles (e.g., alanine, lactate, glucose, glutamine, glycine), impaired mitochondrial function (by ammonia), increased permeability of the blood-brain barrier, oxidative injury, and inflammatory cytokines. Although salvage interventions are described in experimental animal models of ALF, there is no information regarding their success in companion animals with ALF. Recent interest in development of extracorporeal hepatic-bridge modules offer potential therapeutic options in the future that may sustain life until hepatocellular regeneration initiates. For cats with ALF the following treatment is warranted: L-carnitine (250 mg q24h PO), taurine (250 to 500 mg q24h PO), vitamin B_1 (100 mg q12h PO initially × 3 days, then q24h), and vitamin B_{12} (cobalamin). (B_{12} is first tested in plasma, administered 500 µg once, SC or IM before test results are available and then judiciously repeated weekly based on test findings.) Vitamin K is given as previously recommended (see earlier). These supplements are recommended based on successful resuscitative experience in cats with severe hepatic lipidosis (Center, 2005).

References and Suggested Reading

Albretsen JC, Khan SA, Richardson: Cycad palm toxicosis in dogs: 60 cases (1987-1997), *J Am Vet Med Assoc* 213(1):99, 1998.

Bajaj JS et al: Linkage of gut microbiome with cognition in hepatic encephalopathy, *Am J Physiol Gastrointest Liver Physiol* 302(1):G168, 2012.

Bémeur C et al: N-acetylcysteine attenuates cerebral complications of non-acetaminophen-induced acute liver failure in mice: antioxidant and anti-inflammatory mechanisms, *Metab Brain Dis* 25(2):241, 2010.

Center SA: Feline hepatic lipidosis, *Vet Clin North Am Small Anim Pract* 35(1):225, 2005.

Center SA et al: Fulminant hepatic failure associated with oral administration of diazepam in 11 cats, *J Am Vet Med Assoc* 209 (3):618, 1996.

Dereszynski DM et al: Clinical and clinicopathologic features of dogs that consumed foodborne hepatotoxic aflatoxins: 72 cases (2005-2006), *J Am Vet Med Assoc* 232(9):1329, 2008.

Dunayer EK, Gwaltney-Brant SM: Acute hepatic failure and coagulopathy associated with xylitol ingestion in eight dogs, *J Am Vet Med Assoc* 229(7):1113, 2006.

Miller ML et al: Apparent acute idiosyncratic hepatic necrosis associated with zonisamide administration in a dog, *J Vet Intern Med* 25(5):1156, 2011.

Morris JG: Idiosyncratic nutrient requirements of cats appear to be diet induced evolutionary adaptations, *Nutr Res Rev* 15:153, 2002.

Nguyen NTT, Vierling JM: Acute liver failure, *Curr Opin Organ Transplant* 16:289, 2011.

Riordan SM, Williams R: Treatment of hepatic encephalopathy, *N Engl J Med* 337:473, 1997.

Rivkin A, Gim S: Rifaximin: new therapeutic indication and future directions, *Clin Ther* (7):812, 2011.

Strnad P et al: Keratin 8 and 18 variants are associated with ethnic background, *Gastroenterology* 139:828, 2010.

CHAPTER **142**

Chronic Hepatitis Therapy

PENNY J. WATSON, *Cambridge, Cambridgeshire, Great Britain*

Canine chronic hepatitis (CH) is defined by the World Small Animal Veterinary Association (WSAVA) Liver Standardization Group histologically as being characterized by hepatocellular apoptosis or necrosis, a variable mononuclear or mixed inflammatory cell infiltrate, and regeneration and fibrosis. This definition says nothing about temporal chronicity. Some authors suggest the same criteria for the term *chronic hepatitis* be used in animals as it is in humans: clinical or biochemical evidence of hepatocellular dysfunction in animals without improvement for at least 6 months. However, clinical and biochemical evidence of hepatic dysfunction alone in the absence of hepatic histopathology is never sufficient to diagnose CH. Unfortunately, none of the clinical and biochemical tests available in dogs differentiates primary from secondary liver disease, and in fact secondary and reactive hepatopathies are much more common than primary hepatitis in dogs. Serum liver enzymes and even ultrasound imaging and liver function tests can be altered secondary to a variety of other diseases, particularly those in the splanchnic bed drained by the portal vasculature. These diseases can produce similar clinical signs to CH, with vomiting, diarrhea, and even ascites and posthepatic jaundice in some cases. Some form of liver biopsy is therefore essential for definitive diagnosis and most appropriate treatment of CH in dogs.

Etiology

The most effective treatment for CH is to treat the primary etiology. However, although canine CH is common, it is a frustrating disease in dogs because the cause is often unknown. One recent pathology study suggested as many as 12% of dogs from first opinion veterinary practices had histologic lesions in the liver consistent with CH by the time of death from any disease (Watson et al, 2010). Any breeds and crossbreeds can suffer from CH, but studies of CH from various countries in various decades have noted increased breed prevalence, some of which are consistent between countries and decades and some of which have changed. Although not definitively proving an inherited basis for CH in certain dog breeds, these findings certainly are suggestive of a genetic basis to the disease.

Potential and proven causes of canine CH are detailed in Table 142-1 and include copper storage disease, chronic drug toxicities, and a number of proven or suggested infectious agents. However, many cases remain idiopathic, and a number of these may have autoimmune hepatitis. This has not been proven conclusively in canine CH; however, it is suspected from recent work in Doberman pinschers in Scandinavia and also may occur in other breeds. Some of the other idiopathic cases may have a currently unknown canine chronic hepatitis virus. This has been suspected for a number of years, since the first description of a transmissible "acidophil cell hepatitis virus" in Glasgow in the 1980s (Jarrett and O'Neil, 1985). Some canine CH cases look clinically and histologically similar to chronic viral hepatitis in humans, but the putative virus has yet to be identified. Therefore currently it is difficult if not impossible for a clinician or pathologist to determine whether a particular non-copper-associated canine CH case is potentially viral or autoimmune, which obviously has profound implications for treatment, particularly with immunosuppressive drugs.

Treatment Goals

The approach to treatment of canine CH is outlined in Figure 142-1. The aims of treatment of any dog with CH are the following:

- To treat the underlying cause, if this can be identified
- To try to slow progression of the disease even if the cause is not identified
- To support liver function as long as possible and support the dog in positive calorie and nitrogen balance
- To treat the complications of liver disease that affect quality and length of life

The underlying goal in all cases is to try to prevent the progression of disease to the end stage (i.e., cirrhosis). The WSAVA Liver Standardization Group defines cirrhosis as a diffuse process characterized by fibrosis of the liver

TABLE 142-1

Known and Potential Causes of Chronic Hepatitis in Dogs

Potential Cause	Evidence in Dogs
Copper storage disease	Proven and suspected in a number of breeds
Iron storage disease (hemochromatosis)	Recognized in humans. Anecdotally reported in dogs but no published evidence except in association with massive iron overload
Other storage disease	The liver is involved in a number of rare but recognized storage diseases, which have predominant metabolic and CNS signs α-1 antitrypsin deficiency is a locally common cause of chronic hepatitis in humans and has been suspected but not proven in Cocker spaniels
Autoimmune disease	Suspected but not clearly proven. Recent work in Doberman pinschers in Scandinavia supportive of a role in this breed
Chronic bacterial disease	*Bartonella* spp. have been identified in a small number of cases of chronic granulomatous hepatitis in dogs; other chronic bacterial infections could be possible, including chronic biliary tract infection with resistant organisms. There are two old reports of CH associated with hepatic infection with atypical leptospira and a single recent case report of CH associated with *Ehrlichia canis*
Chronic viral disease	Suspected but not proven. There may be variation in breed susceptibility to viral hepatitis, as in humans
Chronic toxic hepatopathy	Chronic alcoholism is a clear example in humans. Phenobarbital toxicity is a documented cause in dogs. Other chronic toxicities from environmental toxins or drugs should be considered, although most reported canine toxic hepatopathies are acute

and the conversion of normal liver architecture into structurally abnormal nodules. The liver has a high reserve capacity, but when loss of hepatocytes and fibrosis reduces liver function to less than 25% of normal, hepatic failure ensues, which is incompatible with life. Cirrhosis often is accompanied by the development of portal hypertension, where increased resistance to flow through the hepatic vasculature raises portal pressure, resulting in splanchnic congestion, development of ascites, and often acquired portosystemic shunts and hepatic encephalopathy (HE) (see Chapter 144). In humans, the development of portal hypertension in end-stage liver disease is a poor prognostic indicator. This has not been demonstrated specifically in dogs, although it is

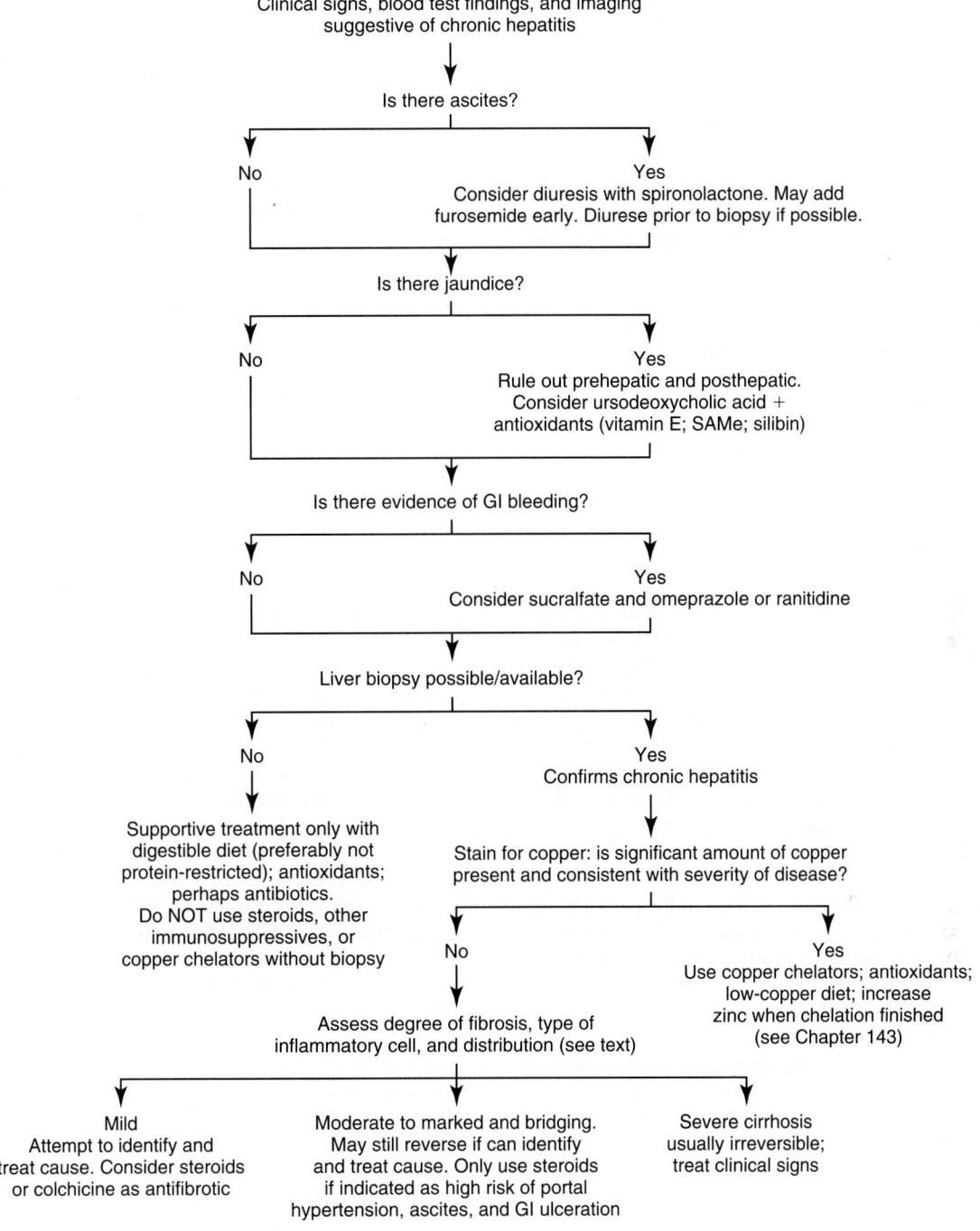

Clinical signs, blood test findings, and imaging
suggestive of chronic hepatitis

↓

Is there ascites?

No | Yes
Consider diuresis with spironolactone. May add
furosemide early. Diurese prior to biopsy if possible.

Is there jaundice?

No | Yes
Rule out prehepatic and posthepatic.
Consider ursodeoxycholic acid +
antioxidants (vitamin E; SAMe; silibin)

Is there evidence of GI bleeding?

No | Yes
Consider sucralfate and omeprazole or ranitidine

Liver biopsy possible/available?

No | Yes
Confirms chronic hepatitis

Supportive treatment only with
digestible diet (preferably not
protein-restricted); antioxidants;
perhaps antibiotics.
Do NOT use steroids, other
immunosuppressives, or
copper chelators without biopsy

Stain for copper: is significant amount of copper
present and consistent with severity of disease?

No | Yes
Use copper chelators; antioxidants;
low-copper diet; increase
zinc when chelation finished
(see Chapter 143)

Assess degree of fibrosis, type of
inflammatory cell, and distribution (see text)

Mild
Attempt to identify and
treat cause. Consider steroids
or colchicine as antifibrotic

Moderate to marked and bridging.
May still reverse if can identify
and treat cause. Only use steroids
if indicated as high risk of portal
hypertension, ascites, and GI ulceration

Severe cirrhosis
usually irreversible;
treat clinical signs

Figure 142-1 Logical approach to treatment of canine chronic hepatitis.

known that ascites is a negative prognostic indicator in
canine CH (Raffan et al, 2009).

The overarching aim in treating canine CH is therefore
to diagnose it early and prevent progression to end-stage
cirrhosis because liver transplantation is not as yet an
option. However, fibrosis of the liver is not inevitably
progressive in one direction, and even early cirrhosis
can be reversible if the underlying cause is removed, as
has been demonstrated clearly in humans with alcoholic
and viral hepatitis. The goal in treating canine CH therefore should be to identify and treat the cause wherever
possible.

Initial Treatment Considerations

Canine CH is not one single disease but a syndrome
caused by a number of known or potential etiologic
agents. Therefore no one treatment is effective for all
cases of canine CH. Optimal treatment of the individual
case of canine CH requires careful analysis of all the evidence available to the clinician: history, clinical findings,
diagnostic imaging, and blood test results, in addition to
biopsy results if available. It is impossible and potentially
dangerous to give specific treatments for CH (such as
copper chelators and steroid or other immunosuppressive

therapy) without biopsy confirmation of disease. If the owner does not permit a liver biopsy or the clinician believes it is too risky for that patient, therapy cannot be optimized for the disease and should be supportive only. In those cases, nonspecific supportive therapies and treatment of clinical signs as outlined at the end of this chapter are the goal.

The clinician should use all the information available to optimize treatment for an individual case. In the clinical examination, blood results, and imaging, the clinician must assess the degree of loss of liver function and identify signs of biliary stasis, portal hypertension, acquired portosystemic shunts, ascites, gastrointestinal edema or ulceration, or protein-calorie malnutrition. In the liver biopsy, if available, the clinician should assess the amount and distribution of inflammation and the types of inflammatory cells involved, the degree and distribution of fibrosis, and the presence of any obvious cause including buildup of copper. Combining all this information allows optimal treatment of the patient.

Specific Therapy

Every effort should be made to understand the cause of the disease because this allows optimal treatment. This is possible only if a liver biopsy is available. The history may suggest a cause: for example, elevated liver enzymes in a young Bedlington terrier would suggest copper storage disease, but other causes remain possible. Abnormal liver function tests in a dog on chronic phenobarbital therapy suggest phenobarbital hepatotoxicity, but other causes are possible or hepatotoxicity could be predisposed by an underlying copper storage disease or other hepatopathy. Therefore a liver biopsy always should be obtained if considered to be safe for the patient. The clinician should try to get the most representative biopsy possible in that patient. As discussed in Chapter 139, a wedge biopsy at laparotomy or laparoscopy is usually more representative than a needle biopsy, and a fine-needle aspirate is rarely helpful and should not be used to make a diagnosis of chronic hepatitis. The liver biopsy always should be stained for copper if CH is described on the hematoxylin-eosin stain. A section of liver also may be sent off for quantitation of hepatic copper concentration (see Chapter 143). The pathologist may elect to undertake a variety of other stains to try to elucidate the etiology of the disease. In some cases a discussion between the clinician and pathologist is ideal to come to a consensus for a logical course of action.

If a significant amount of copper is found in the biopsy, in proportion to the severity of the disease, copper storage disease should be suspected strongly and treated with chelation and dietary therapy as described in Chapter 143. If copper storage disease is ruled out, the type and distribution of inflammation present may suggest a cause for the disease. A strong neutrophilic component, particularly if it is periportal, may indicate a chronic hepatic or biliary tract infection, and consideration should be given to culturing bile or liver and ruling out chronic partial extrahepatic biliary obstruction or cholecystitis. A granulomatous inflammatory response may warrant

consideration of polymerase chain reaction (PCR) for *Bartonella* spp. or fluorescence *in situ h*ybridization (FISH) analysis for a bacterial etiology. A dense lymphoplasmacytic inflammatory component indicates consideration of an autoimmune cause. However, lymphoplasmacytic infiltration is nonspecific chronic inflammation occurring with a number of causes. Currently differentiating autoimmune hepatitis from other causes is impossible, so the most difficult decision to make may be over the use of steroids or immunosuppressive agents. In viral disease, steroid treatment may reduce temporarily the amount of inflammation but also increases the viral load. In humans with viral hepatitis, the amount of liver damage is proportional to viral load, so immunosuppressive therapy is avoided. In veterinary medicine, with the exception of adenovirus, viral hepatitis has not been documented; as yet it is impossible to rule out clinically viral disease as a cause.

Use of steroids requires a liver biopsy because there is no indication for use in noninflammatory fibrosis and cirrhosis. If steroids are used in these cases in the presence of portal hypertension, they increase the risk of serious consequences, including increased water retention and gastrointestinal ulceration. The evidence base for the efficacy of steroids in CH is small and relies almost entirely on one retrospective study, in which immunosuppressive doses of steroids improved survival time in 58 treated dogs compared with 37 untreated dogs (Strombeck, Miller, and Harrold, 1988). However, like all retrospective studies, this study had many sources of potential bias, including preexclusion of cases that survived less than a week, clinician selection of treatment option, and a high proportion of Doberman pinschers and cocker spaniels, which are breeds perhaps most likely to have autoimmune hepatitis. The question still remains as to whether corticosteroids are indicated in all dogs with CH and whether the ideal dose is immunosuppressive or antiinflammatory. Nonetheless, corticosteroid therapy should offer the best chance of survival in dogs with true autoimmune CH and so should not be withheld if the clinician and pathologist believe on the basis of liver biopsies that this is the most likely cause of disease in a particular dog. The author would start with 0.5 to 1 mg/kg per day in these cases and taper the dose over the following 2 to 4 weeks, while carefully monitoring clinical signs and hepatocellular enzymes. This author does not routinely use additional immunosuppressive drugs in CH because the evidence for immune-mediated disease remains weak, immunosuppressive agents may reduce hepatic regenerative ability, and there is potential increased risk of infectious complications. Furthermore, no evidence supports the use of antiviral drugs in dogs with CH as are used in humans with viral hepatitis. Nonspecific use of antivirals is very unlikely to be of benefit because specific antiviral therapy should be targeted at the virus involved.

Supportive Therapy

Slowing Progression of Disease

In most cases, the cause of canine CH is unknown. In these cases, the clinician still can attempt to slow progression of disease. The most important aim in slowing disease progression is to slow fibrosis. In addition, care should be taken to support liver function long term by feeding an appropriate diet and avoiding hepatotoxic drugs wherever possible in specific treatment of the liver disease and in the treatment of other, unrelated diseases. For example, all nonsteroidal antiinflammatory drugs should be avoided in dogs with CH. Therefore, if they have concurrent life-limiting chronic joint disease, alternatives will have to be found.

Slowing fibrosis remains a challenge. After many years of research in humans and rodents the development of a truly effective antifibrotic drug for humans is lacking. The source of hepatic fibrosis is the hepatic stellate cell or Ito cell that transforms when stimulated from a quiescent vitamin A–storing cell to a collagen-secreting myofibroblast with contractile properties. These cells may be stimulated directly or indirectly by cytokines from inflammatory cells. One of the arguments for the use of steroids in canine CH is that their antiinflammatory properties reduce cytokine release and stellate cell activation. Hepatic fibrosis also can be a protective strategy, attempting to wall off an insult (such as infectious agent or toxin), so reducing fibrosis without treating the cause may not always be ideal (e.g., it could allow more widespread dissemination of an infectious organism). Therefore treating the cause is the most effective way of treating fibrosis. Some limited anecdotal evidence suggests that colchicine used at a dose of 0.03 mg/kg q24h PO in early hepatic fibrosis in dogs may be beneficial, but many dogs develop anorexia and gastrointestinal signs on this drug, in which case it should be stopped because the efficacy remains uncertain. In many placebo-controlled studies treating fibrotic-associated liver disease in humans, colchicine has failed to show a benefit. Colchicine never should be used in cats. Angiotensin-receptor blockers are being tested in humans for treatment of hepatic fibrosis but with conflicting results in different studies. A recent study in rodents suggests spironolactone treatment reduces fibrosis and portal hypertension, so this drug may be having more than just a diuretic effect in dogs with chronic hepatitis (Luo et al, 2012). In addition, supportive therapy with antioxidants (S-adenosylmethionine, silybin, and vitamin E) and ursodeoxycholic acid may help reduce fibrosis (see later).

Treating Clinical Signs

Treating the clinical signs of disease nonspecifically is a worthwhile aim in CH because it improves the quality of life of the patient. Ultimately, most dogs with CH die because the owners request euthanasia because of poor quality of life, so improving the quality of life also should improve life expectancy in these patients. The factors to consider and treat are the following:

- Ascites: If present, this should be treated as detailed in Chapter 144 with spironolactone as the primary diuretic and addition of loop diuretics as necessary.
- Vomiting, diarrhea, and evidence of GI ulceration: These are common in animals with portal hypertension and should be treated predominantly by careful feeding of frequent, small amounts to provide nutrition for gut wall healing and avoidance of potentially ulcerogenic drugs such as steroids. H_2 antagonists such as ranitidine or proton pump inhibitors such as omeprazole could be used, together with sucralfate, although evidence for their efficacy in ulceration resulting from portal hypertension is lacking. If an antiemetic is required, metoclopramide would be preferred to maropitant because the latter is metabolized in the liver.
- Jaundice: When prehepatic causes and posthepatic obstruction have been ruled out, this should be treated with ursodeoxycholic acid and antioxidants. Ursodeoxycholic acid (4 to 15 mg/kg q24h PO total dose that can be divided q12h) has a large number of potential benefits in animals with CH including choleresis, displacement of toxic bile acids, and antioxidant properties. There are no contraindications to its use but, like all other therapies in canine CH, the evidence for its efficacy is sparse. However, it makes sense to use it. Use of antioxidants also is logical in this circumstance because refluxed bile damages mitochondrial membranes and is a strong oxidant toxin. A combination of S-adenosylmethionine, silybin, and vitamin E is advised. The clinician should try to choose nutraceuticals with proven bioavailability in dogs. A dosage of 20 mg/kg/day has been suggested for S-adenosylmethionine and 50 to 200 mg of silybin per dog per day, although the ideal dose for chronic liver disease is unknown. Vitamin E is usually dosed at 400 IU for a 30-kg dog, titrating accordingly to other sizes.
- Hepatic encephalopathy (HE): This is not as prominent or easily recognized in dogs with CH as it is in young dogs with congenital portosystemic shunt. Nonetheless, it can be an important cause of confusion and unusual behavior in these animals because of the development of acquired portosystemic shunts secondary to portal hypertension. It should be treated carefully: marked protein restriction is not indicated in these dogs because they are likely to be suffering from protein-calorie malnutrition already. HE can be addressed by treating any underlying inflammatory trigger and also any precipitating gastrointestinal bleeding and giving a highly digestible, high-quality diet in small, frequent amounts. Antibiotic and lactulose therapy also may be considered. Dietary protein restriction is rarely necessary in these cases. More details of treatment of HE are given in Chapter 144.
- Treatment of protein-calorie malnutrition: Many dogs with CH present in negative nitrogen balance. They are often thin with partial anorexia and vomiting and diarrhea, which contribute to nutrient malabsorption. It is therefore important to prioritize nutrition in the treatment of these patients. Ideally, they should be fed a highly digestible, high-quality diet in frequent, small amounts, and this diet should not be protein restricted. Prescription diets recommended for liver disease may be too low in protein in this context. Diets manufactured for intestinal disease are preferred because they are very

digestible. However, ultimately, it may be a matter of feeding whatever the dog will eat, which is preferable to no food at all.

References and Suggested Reading

Andersson M, Sevelius E: Breed, sex and age distribution in dogs with chronic liver disease: a demographic study, *J Small Anim Pract* 32:1, 1991.

Bexfield NH et al: Breed, age and gender distribution of dogs with chronic hepatitis in the United Kingdom, *Vet J* 193:124, 2012.

Friedman SL: Evolving challenges in hepatic fibrosis, *Nat Rev Gastroenterol Hepatol* 7:425, 2010.

Jarrett WF, O'Neil BW: A new transmissible agent causing acute hepatitis, chronic hepatitis and cirrhosis in dogs, *Vet Rec* 116: 629, 1985.

Luo W et al: Spironolactone lowers portal hypertension by inhibiting liver fibrosis, ROCK-2 activity and activating NO/ PKG pathway in the bile-duct-ligated rat, *PlosOne* 7:e34230, 2012.

Poldervaart JH et al: Primary hepatitis in dogs: a retrospective review (2002-2006), *J Vet Intern Med* 23:72, 2009.

Raffan E et al: Ascites is a negative prognostic indicator in chronic hepatitis in dogs, *J Vet Intern Med* 23:63, 2009.

Strombeck DR, Miller LM, Harrold D: Effects of corticosteroid treatment on survival time in dogs with chronic hepatitis: 151 cases (1977-1985), *J Am Vet Med Assoc* 9:1109, 1988.

Watson PJ: Canine chronic liver disease: a review of current understanding of the aetiology, progression and treatment of chronic liver disease in the dog, *Vet J* 167:228, 2004.

Watson PJ et al: Prevalence of hepatic lesions at post-mortem examination in dogs and association with pancreatitis, *J Small Anim Pract* 51:566, 2010.

WSAVA Liver Standardization Group: *WSAVA standards for clinical and histological diagnosis of canine and feline liver diseases*, ed 1, Philadelphia, 2006, Saunders-Elsevier.

CHAPTER 143

Copper Chelator Therapy

ALLISON BRADLEY, *Fort Collins, Colorado*
DAVID C. TWEDT, *Fort Collins, Colorado*

Pathophysiology of Copper-Associated Liver Disease

Copper is an essential component of metalloenzymes used in many metabolic functions, and the liver is central in regulating copper body stores. Copper enters the body through the diet, with approximately 30% to 60% absorbed in the small intestine, and the rest passing out through the feces. After hepatic uptake, it is complexed with the transport protein ceruloplasmin, incorporated into hepatic cellular pathways, or bound to hepatic metallothioneins. Metallothioneins are cytosolic proteins that store copper, thereby protecting the surrounding cell from its toxic effects. Biliary excretion is the major determinant of copper homeostasis, with about 80% of absorbed copper excreted in bile.

When copper concentrations exceed hepatic metallothionein–complexing capabilities, hepatic injury results from free radical–induced hepatocellular necrosis or apoptosis. Abnormal accumulation of hepatic copper can be caused by a metabolic defect of copper metabolism, secondarily from cholestatic or hepatocellular disease resulting in decreased biliary excretion of copper, or from increased dietary intake of copper.

Reduction of hepatic copper levels is fundamental to treatment of copper-associated hepatic disease. The mainstay of treatment for primary copper hepatopathy is typically a chelating agent, which is a ligand (or drug) that binds to a metal ion for the purpose of removing the metal from the body, generally by renal excretion. Adjunctive therapies include zinc, antioxidants, hepatoprotectants, and dietary restriction of copper intake.

Copper Chelating Agents

Indications for Chelating Agents

Therapy is indicated in cases with significant increases in hepatic copper concentrations. Ideally, quantification of hepatic copper should be performed; normal canine concentrations range from 200 to 400 µg/g of dry weight liver. A semiquantitative histochemical grading scheme estimating the amount of hepatic copper also has been described, with the amount of copper accumulation graded on a scale of 0 to 5+. The scoring system tends to approximate the magnitude of copper concentration in the liver.

Chelation therapy given to patients incorrectly diagnosed with copper-associated liver disease is detrimental. Therefore it is important to determine whether the hepatic copper accumulation is a primary condition leading to liver damage or secondary to cholestasis.

Secondary hepatic copper accumulation using histochemical staining is located predominantly in zone 1 (periportal), whereas in dogs with primary copper hepatotoxicity it is found in zone 3 (centrilobular). Generally, copper concentrations from cholestatic or hepatocellular disease are lower (e.g., <1000 µg/g or a grade of +2 or less) and located in zone 1 (Spee, Arends, and van den Ingh, 2006). The authors believe that most cases having secondary hepatic copper accumulation may not require chelator therapy, but rather treatment is directed at the primary liver disease and prevention of hepatic copper accumulation. However, the authors and others recommend chelation therapy if copper concentrations exceed 1500 µg/g regardless of the cause, believing concentrations at that level are hepatotoxic.

Dogs having primary copper-associated liver disease based on breed, hepatic copper concentrations (e.g., >750 to 1000 µg/g or >3+ grade), and location (zone 3) should have chelation therapy directed at lowering hepatic copper. If the suspected primary copper deposition is mild, other therapies, such as oral zinc supplementation and low-copper diets, may be sufficient.

Commonly Used Chelators

Penicillamine is the treatment of choice for humans with Wilson's disease, a primary metabolic disease associated with abnormal hepatic copper accumulation (Wiggelinkhuizen et al, 2009). Given the available veterinary data and experience, it should also be the first-line treatment for dogs with primary copper storage disease. Penicillamine is a thiol, a compound with a sulfhydryl (SH) group, making the molecule an active metal chelating agent with a high affinity for copper. It forms a stable water-soluble complex with copper that is then excreted through the kidneys. Additional mechanisms of action may include formation of a nontoxic hepatic chelate; induction of synthesis of metallothionein, which will bind to free copper; weak antifibrotic activity via interference with procollagen cross-linking; and immunomodulatory effects. The latter two mechanisms may be of additional benefit in chronic hepatitis.

The recommended initial dosage of penicillamine is 10 to 15 mg/kg q12h PO. It should be given on an empty stomach at least 1 hour before or 2 hours after meals to maximize absorption and reduce inactivation by chelating substances within the gastrointestinal tract. The most common side effect in dogs is nausea and vomiting, which is observed in about 30% of patients. The side effects often can be avoided by either reducing the dose or giving the medication with a small amount of food until the patient becomes accustomed to the medication. Dermatologic reactions have been observed occasionally in the dog. Penicillamine is reported to cause depletion of vitamin B_6 in people. Although not reported in dogs, B vitamin supplementation with long-term use may be advisable. Because penicillamine is related to penicillin, patients with a known penicillin allergy should not be treated with this chelator. Finally, because of potential teratogenic effects, penicillamine should not be given to pregnant animals, and pregnant women should avoid contact with the drug. Penicillamine is relatively

expensive, and using less-expensive compounding pharmacies is appealing; however, the purity and efficacy of the drug cannot be ensured.

Trientine is a triethylene tetramine or 2,2,2-tetramine used as an alternative copper chelator in humans that do not tolerate penicillamine. Similarly, it may be an alternative in dogs that do not tolerate penicillamine. The exact mechanism of trientine is poorly understood, but it appears to have a copper-lowering effect similar to that of penicillamine when given to affected Bedlington terriers and normal dogs. Because it may lower serum copper levels more rapidly it is the preferred treatment in cases of hemolysis resulting from copper toxicity.

The recommended dosage in dogs is 10 to 15 mg/kg q12h PO given on an empty stomach. Trientine appears to be well-tolerated by dogs, with rare cases of renal toxicity and vomiting being uncommon. Trientine also should be regarded as a potential teratogen.

Other Chelators

2,3,2-tetramine is similar in structure to trientine but is reported to be more four to nine times more potent than trientine in normal dogs without reported toxicity (Allen, Twedt, and Hunsaker, 1987). It has been used successfully in treating a number of affected Bedlington terriers, including two with copper-associated hemolysis (Twedt, Hunsaker, and Allen, 1988). It is not commercially available at this time. Tetrathiomolybdate has been used in the treatment of Wilson's disease and copper-associated neurologic signs. This chelator has four sulfur groups that bind copper, and its mechanism relies in part on biliary copper excretion, which could be defective in hepatic disease. It is unknown how effective this chelator would be in dogs with copper-associated hepatotoxicity. Other chelators used in veterinary medicine, such as disodium calcium ethylenediaminetetraacetic acid (EDTA), dimercaprol, and deferoxamine, are not beneficial in copper-associated hepatotoxicity.

Monitoring and Duration of Therapy

Only general guidelines can be made regarding chelation therapy, and each case should be monitored carefully, because hepatic copper deficiency is deleterious to the patient. Affected Bedlington terriers and some Dalmatians have high copper concentrations (>3000 to 10,000 µg/g) and often require prolonged (years) or lifetime therapy because hepatic copper concentrations rarely return to normal in these dogs. One study found that hepatic copper levels in Bedlington terriers decreased an average of 900 µg/g per year. The authors generally treat until liver enzymes approach normal and then decrease chelation to once a day or every 48 hours. Other breeds with elevated hepatic copper may require only a short course of chelation therapy before beginning zinc and or diet therapy. For example, Labrador retrievers and Doberman pinschers with copper concentrations ranging from 1000 to 2000 µg/g hepatic copper may require only 3 to a maximum of 6 months of therapy. Quantitation of hepatic copper during therapy can provide important objective information of when to transition from active chelation to preventive maintenance therapy. Normalization of alanine aminotransferase (ALT) concentrations during chelation therapy may indicate that hepatic copper concentrations are below the hepatotoxic threshold. Following clinical improvement and proof of sufficient copper removal, either intermittent chelation or oral zinc (see below) may be sufficient.

Dogs with chronic liver disease considered to have moderate secondary hepatic copper accumulation generally are not treated with chelation therapy but managed with specific therapy for the liver disease, low-copper diets, and possibly zinc therapy.

Adjunct Therapeutic Options

Diet

All dogs with moderate or greater copper accumulation should be placed on a low-copper diet. Most commercial diets contain too much copper for these affected dogs. Diets created specifically for liver disease typically contain appropriately restricted copper levels (approximately 4 mg/kg diet), but this should be verified for the exact formulation being prescribed. Most commercial dog foods contain ranges of 10 to 25 mg/kg diet. Copper-containing treats or vitamin-mineral supplements and high-copper foods, such as eggs, shellfish, liver and other organ meats, beans, mushrooms, nuts, and cereals, should be avoided.

Zinc

Zinc decreases intestinal absorption of dietary copper by competing directly for uptake and by inducing synthesis of enterocyte metallothionein. The zinc-induced metallothionein preferentially binds to copper, becomes sequestered within the enterocyte, and is lost into the feces when the enterocyte is sloughed into the lumen during normal cell turnover. Zinc also induces production of hepatic metallothionein, which sequesters the copper in an innocuous form. Zinc therapy has been shown to reduce hepatic copper concentrations in dogs with breed-associated copper hepatopathy; however, its effect is slower than that of chelation, with several months required to achieve any reduction and several years for maximal therapeutic response. Accordingly, zinc is likely better as a maintenance therapy.

Concurrent zinc and chelation therapy traditionally has been avoided because the chelators likely bind zinc in the intestinal tract, leading to decreased activity of both substances. More recently, patients with Wilson's disease reportedly have been treated successfully with trientine and zinc in combination. However, the authors' current recommendation is to initiate treatment of affected dogs with a faster-acting chelator and transition to prophylactic zinc once hepatic copper concentrations approach normal levels. If concurrent therapy is elected, the zinc and chelator should be staggered to allow for adequate chelator absorption. Zinc also may be considered in cases when cost or side effects preclude the use of chelator therapy. Reported induction dosages are 100 mg/dog or 5 to 10 mg/kg of elemental zinc q12h PO for approximately 1 month, and then the dose or frequency is halved. Because hemolysis can occur when serum zinc concentrations are greater than 750 µg/dl, serum zinc levels should be monitored several weeks into the induction phase. Dosing should be adjusted to target a therapeutic level of about 200 µg/dl. Gastrointestinal upset is common; the zinc salt may affect tolerability, with gluconate being the most favorable.

References and Suggested Reading

Allen KG, Twedt DC, Hunsaker HA: Tetramine cupruretic agents: a comparison in dogs, *Am J Vet Res* 48(1):28-30, 1987.

Center SA: Pathophysiology of liver disease: normal and abnormal function. In Guilford WG, Strombeck DR, editors: *Strombeck's small animal gastroenterology*, ed 3, Philadelphia, 1996, Saunders, p 597.

Hoffmann G: Copper associated liver diseases, *Vet Clin North Am Small Anim Pract* 39:489, 2009.

Rothuizen J: General principles in the treatment of liver disease. In Ettinger SJ, Feldman EC, editors: *Textbook of veterinary internal medicine*, ed 7, Philadelphia, 2010, Saunders, p 1629.

Scherk MA, Center SA: Toxic, metabolic, infectious, and neoplastic liver disease. In Ettinger SJ, Feldman EC, editors: *Textbook of veterinary internal medicine*, ed 7, Philadelphia, 2010, Saunders, p 1679.

Spee B, Arends B, van den Ingh T: Copper metabolism and oxidative stress in chronic inflammatory and cholestatic liver diseases in dogs, *J Vet Intern Med* 20:1085, 2006.

Twedt DC, Hunsaker MS, Allen KGD: Use of 2,3,2-tetramine as a hepatic copper chelating agent for treatment of copper hepatotoxicosis in Bedlington terriers, *J Am Vet Med Assoc* 192:52, 1988.

Wiggelinkhuizen M et al: Systematic review: clinical efficacy of chelator agents and zinc in the initial treatment of Wilson disease, *Aliment Pharmacol Ther* 29:947, 2009.

CHAPTER 144

Ascites and Hepatic Encephalopathy Therapy for Liver Disease

NICK BEXFIELD, *Cambridge, Great Britain*

Ascites

Pathophysiology

Ascites is the accumulation of fluid within the peritoneal cavity, and in liver disease this is usually a result of portal hypertension (PH). Hypoalbuminemia also can contribute to ascites formation in animals with reduced hepatic function, although it is unusual for hypoalbuminemia alone to cause ascites. PH, the sustained increase in blood pressure in the portal system, results from an increased intrahepatic resistance combined with increased portal blood flow. Increased intrahepatic resistance results from architectural distortion (fibrous tissue, regenerative nodules), sinusoidal endothelial dysfunction leading to impaired intrahepatic sinusoidal relaxation, and intra-hepatic vascular shunts. With the development of PH, fluid is driven into the interstitial space, and when the capacity of the regional lymphatics is overwhelmed, ascites develops. The development of ascites is worsened by the splanchnic vasodilation that accompanies PH. This vasodilation results in pooling of blood in the abdomen, leading to a decrease in circulating volume, and when ionotrophic and chronotropic compensation fails, systemic hypotension results. This cumulates in activation of the renin-angiotensin-aldosterone system (RAAS), and volume expansion, which further increases hydrostatic pressure in the portal vasculature. PH is seen most commonly in dogs with chronic liver disease, although it occasionally occurs with acute liver disease; therefore the most common cause in dogs is chronic hepatitis progressing to cirrhosis. The presence of ascites is a poor prognostic indicator in dogs with chronic hepatitis, with a survival from the time of diagnosis of 0.4 months, compared to 24.3 months for nonascitic dogs. Because cats rarely get advanced liver fibrosis or cirrhosis, the development of PH and therefore ascites is uncommon in this species.

Therapy for Ascites

Diuretics

Despite PH, ascitic animals actually have systemic hypotension and increased renal sodium retention because of reduced glomerular filtration rate and increased activation of the RAAS. Activation of the RAAS results in the release of aldosterone and increased sodium retention in the distal renal tubules. The aldosterone antagonist spironolactone is the diuretic of choice for the treatment of hepatogenic ascites. Spironolactone competes with aldosterone for its intracellular receptor sites, thus promoting sodium excretion and potassium retention in the renal tubules. Therapy with spironolactone at a dose of 2 mg/kg q24h PO is the initial therapy for animals with ascites resulting from PH (Figure 144-1). The dose of spironolactone can be increased gradually every few days to a maximum of 4 mg/kg q24h PO. Some animals may benefit from twice-daily therapy. Spironolactone can have a relatively slow onset of activity in humans, taking up to 14 days to cause diuresis; this also may occur in cats and dogs. In cases that are refractory to spironolactone, or when a more rapid resolution of ascites is required, furosemide (1 to 2 mg/kg q12h PO) also can be used. If there is no response to this dose of furosemide, it can be increased incrementally. Therapy with furosemide rather than spironolactone has been shown to precipitate more complications in humans with ascites, however. Importantly, serum electrolyte concentrations, especially sodium and potassium, should be monitored daily during the first few days of diuretic therapy, and every few weeks to months thereafter. Hypokalemia should be addressed as soon as possible as it can precipitate hepatic encephalopathy (HE) (see later). Body weight, abdominal girth (measure girth at level of the second lumbar vertebra with a tape measure), and hydration status as well as hematocrit and serum creatinine also should be monitored when on diuretic therapy. A safe loss of 0.5% to 1.0% body weight per day has been suggested for humans. Body weight reductions of 5% per day are dangerous and indicate the need for veterinary examination. When ascites has been mobilized adequately, intermittent use of diuretics is advised and guided by fluid reaccumulation. Administration of a diuretic two or three times per week is often sufficient to control fluid accumulation.

Abdominocentesis

Abdominocentesis should be avoided if possible because the removal of large volumes of relatively protein-rich fluid can cause significant hypoalbuminemia, potentially leading to worsened fluid re-formation. Hypoalbuminemia also may lead to protein catabolism and HE.

591

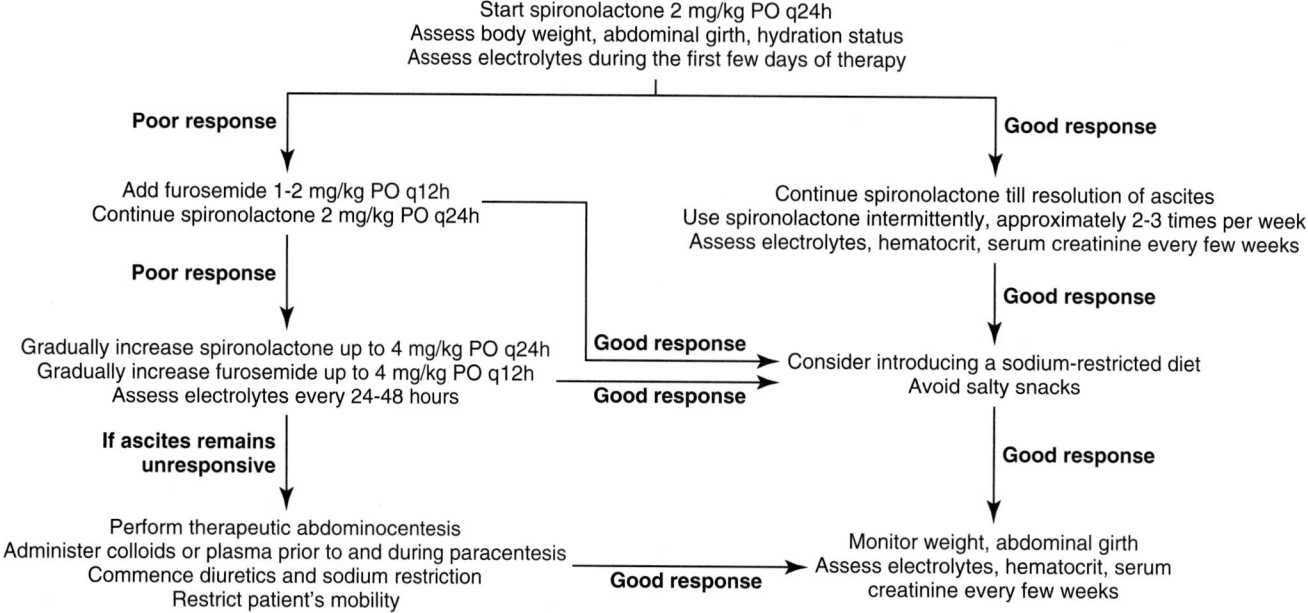

Figure 144-1 A flow diagram describing the management of ascites in patients with liver disease.

Therapeutic abdominocentesis is indicated if significant ascites is impairing mobility or causing respiratory compromise and is refractory to medical management. Fluid removal has the beneficial effects of improving cardiac function and stimulation diuresis. These effects are due to reductions of intraabdominal pressure, which compromises venous return. Administration of colloids or plasma before and during abdominocentesis is also advisable; this helps to prevent hypovolemia and worsening hypoalbuminemia as fluid shifts back into the abdomen. An infusion of 10 ml/kg of hetastarch over 3 hours is required, with abdominocentesis performed after the first 30 minutes of the infusion. Fluid removal is completed over 30 to 60 minutes.

Dietary Sodium Restriction

Dietary sodium restriction also is advocated in the management of ascites, although in humans this alone is inadequate. Recommendations for sodium restriction in the diet vary from 0.1% to 0.3%, or less than 0.05 g/100 kcal; this can be established by feeding a prescription or homemade diet. However, dietary sodium restriction can result in several complications, including hypovolemia, renal hypoperfusion, and compensatory polydipsia, which may worsen hyponatremia. Salt restriction, if performed, should be gradual, and patients should be monitored for complications of azotemia and hyponatremia.

Hepatic Encephalopathy

Pathophysiology

Hepatic encephalopathy (HE) is a neurophysiologic disorder of the central nervous system (CNS) that develops as a result of hepatic dysfunction. HE is usually a result of congenital and acquired portosystemic shunting of blood, and the reserve capacity of the liver in dogs is usually enough to prevent HE in liver disease without collateral circulation. Cats cannot make the essential amino acid arginine, an intermediate of the hepatic urea cycle, and deficiency causes inadequate detoxification of ammonia. HE therefore may occur in cats without shunting and as a result of fasting. Clinical signs are variable, from those of acute HE, which can lead to cerebral edema, increased intracranial pressure, and brain herniation, to those of chronic HE, which may include behavioral changes, or subtle signs such as depression, anorexia, and lethargy. Most signs are consistent with neuroinhibitory effects, although excitatory signs such as aggression and hyperexcitability also develop.

The pathogenesis of HE is multifactorial and still not understood completely. When portosystemic shunting exists, a number of toxic substances gain entry into the peripheral and cerebral circulation. In liver failure, the permeability of the blood-brain barrier also may be increased, allowing normally excluded substances to access the brain. The most commonly implicated and studied encephalopathic agent is ammonia. The effects of increased CNS ammonia are inhibitory and are due to glutamate depletion, altered glutamate receptors, blockade of GABA receptors, altered amino acid membrane transport, inhibition of Na/K-dependent ATPase, and impaired cerebral energy metabolism. A variety of other substances have been implicated in the pathogenesis of HE including short-chain fatty acids, aromatic and branched-chain amino acids, abnormal or false neurotransmitters, tryptophan, methionine, phenols, and bile acids.

Therapy

The main goals of therapy are to decrease the formation of gut-derived encephalotoxins, especially ammonia, with the hypothesis that the colon is the main source of this ammonia production. Therefore the mainstays of current therapy are a combination of protein-restricted diets, oral antibiotics to suppress bacterial populations that produce encephalopathic toxins, and local-acting agents to reduce gastrointestinal uptake of ammonia. However, emerging evidence from human medicine questions the efficacy of these commonly used treatment recommendations. For instance, studies suggest that the colon is not the main source of ammonia production, but in fact it originates from the obligate intestinal catabolism of glutamine by small intestinal enterocytes. Moreover, if dietary protein is highly digestible and not in excessive amounts, it should be digested in the small intestine and so not reach the colon. Controlled trials have not been performed in animals to determine the optimal treatment for HE and so current recommendations are based on anecdotal evidence. However, correction of acid-base abnormalities and the elimination of precipitating factors (Box 144-1) are a vital part of successful therapy. Emerging evidence also suggests that inflammatory cytokines are synergistic with ammonia in precipitating HE and that controlling inflammation in

other organs is an important part of managing the patient with HE.

Diet

Dietary manipulation is the key to the successful management of HE. Studies in humans and animals with acquired portosystemic shunts (PSSs) and dogs with experimental PSSs have shown a higher protein requirement than normal subjects. The current recommendation is therefore to feed patients with congenital or acquired PSSs with normal to slightly increased amounts of protein. Feeding a protein-restricted diet results in protein-calorie malnutrition, resulting in the breakdown of endogenous protein, which may worsen HE. The protein source should be high quality and highly digestible to minimize the amount of undigested protein reaching the colon to be converted into ammonia. High-quality proteins include dairy products, chicken, or soya. Diets manufactured for dogs with liver disease may be protein restricted and should be supplemented with high-quality protein. Alternatively, a veterinary diet designed for intestinal disease can be used because these contain high-quality and highly digestible protein. Animals also should be fed several times per day and with small amounts of food. Fat should be fed in normal amounts unless clinical steatorrhea develops, and the carbohydrate source should be highly digestible. Zinc supplementation also may be beneficial in the dietary management of HE because zinc is a vital component of many enzymes in the urea cycle and in muscle metabolism of ammonia.

Lactulose

Lactulose (β-galactosidofructose) is a semisynthetic disaccharide that passes into the colon, where it is degraded by bacteria into short-chain fatty acids (SCFAs). The SCFAs, primarily acetic and lactic acid, acidify the colon, trapping ammonia as ammonium ions (NH_4^+). Lactulose also promotes an osmotic diarrhea, so reducing the time colonic contents are acted on by intestinal bacteria. SCFAs also are used as an energy source by colonic bacteria, causing them to incorporate more ammonia into their own bacterial proteins. Lactulose (cats 2.5 to 5.0 ml q8-12h PO; dogs 2.5 to 15 ml q8-12h PO) is used with dose adjustment to produce two to three soft stools per day. Lactulose is sweet tasting and so not tolerated by some cats and dogs. An alternative is lactitol (β-galactosidosorbitol), available in some countries as a powder to add to food (500 mg/kg q6-8h PO, adjusted to produce two to three soft stools per day), although its efficacy in the management of HE has not been evaluated extensively.

Antibiotics

Antibiotics can be used if dietary therapy alone or in combination with lactulose does not control the signs of HE. Drugs effective against anaerobic organism such as metronidazole 7.5 mg/kg PO q12h, or amoxicillin 10 mg/kg PO q8-12h should be selected. The dose of metronidazole is lower than that normally suggested because excretion of this drug may be compromised in patients with liver disease. Antibiotics effective against gram-negative, urea-splitting bacteria, such as neomycin

---

BOX 144-1

Precipitating Factors for Hepatic Encephalopathy

Increased production of ammonia in the gastrointestinal tract
- A high-protein meal
- Undigested protein in the colon
- Constipation
- Gastrointestinal bleeding or ingestion of blood
- Azotemia

Increased systemic generation of ammonia
- Blood transfusions, especially of stored blood
- Protein-calorie malnutrition leading to breakdown of endogenous body protein
- Feeding a poor-quality protein

Factors affecting the uptake and metabolism of ammonia in the CNS
- Metabolic alkalosis (only the nonionized form of ammonia penetrates neuronal membranes. In alkalosis, the reaction equilibrium [$NH_3 + H^+ \leftrightarrow NH_4^+$] shifts to the left, making more nonionized ammonia available)
- Hypokalemia (potassium shifts from cells in exchange with H+. The resulting H+ shift causes alkalosis and the production of more nonionized ammonia)
- Hypoglycemia (potentiates the activity and production of other neurotoxins)
- Inflammation (inflammatory cytokines can be directly neurotoxic and synergistic with ammonia)
- Infections (fever and increased protein catabolism)
- Sedative and anesthetic drugs (interact with various neurotransmitters)

sulfate 20 mg/kg PO q8-12h also may be used. The latter drug is probably best reserved for acute, rather than long-term, management of HE as intestinal bacteria become resistant to neomycin. Moreover, neomycin's adverse effects include nephrotoxicity and ototoxicity. Metronidazole and amoxicillin have an added advantage over neomycin because they are absorbed systemically and therefore may protect against bacteremia. In human medicine, rifaximin, an oral rifamycin-based antibiotic, is the currently preferred antibiotic because of its superior safety profile, although it has not been studied in dogs or cats with HE.

References and Suggested Reading

Buob S, Johnston AN, Webster CRL: Portal hypertension: pathophysiology, diagnosis, and treatment, *J Vet Intern Med* 25:169, 2011.

Sanyal AJ et al: Portal hypertension and its complications, *Gastroenterology* 134:1715, 2008.

Shawcross DL et al: Ammonia and the neutrophil in the pathogenesis of hepatic encephalopathy in cirrhosis, *Hepatology* 51:1062, 2010.

Shawcross D, Jalan R: Dispelling myths in the treatment of hepatic encephalopathy, *Lancet* 365:431, 2005.

CHAPTER 145
Portosystemic Shunts

KAREN M. TOBIAS, *Knoxville, Tennessee*

Portosystemic shunts (PSS) are vascular anomalies that divert blood from the abdominal to the systemic venous circulation while bypassing the hepatic sinusoids. Products absorbed from the intestines are delivered to the heart without undergoing the extraction and detoxification processes normally performed by hepatocytes. This reduction in hepatic blood flow and function leads to decreases in protein production and glycogen storage, reticuloendothelial dysfunction, and altered metabolism of ammonia and other toxins. PSS can occur as congenital anomalies or may develop secondary to liver disease and portal hypertension. Although clinical signs from multiple acquired shunts must be managed medically, congenital PSS have been treated successfully with surgery in many dogs and cats.

Congenital portosystemic shunts (CPSS) usually occur as single large vessels, although some animals have two or more shunts. Common types of CPSS include intrahepatic portocaval shunts, such as a patent ductus venosus and extrahepatic portocaval or portal-azygos shunts. In a small percentage of dogs with CPSS, the prehepatic portal vein is absent. CPSS are considered heritable in many breeds. Multiple acquired shunts develop secondary to liver disease and/or causes of portal hypertension. They are small, tortuous vessels that frequently join the caudal vena cava around the base of the mesentery or the renal veins.

Signalment, History, and Clinical Signs

CPSS usually are diagnosed in immature animals, although a few animals are diagnosed at 10 years of age or older.

Breeds most commonly affected with extrahepatic CPSS are Yorkshire terriers, Havanese, Maltese, Dandie Dinmont terriers, pugs, and miniature schnauzers. Intrahepatic CPSS are found primarily in large-breed dogs such as Irish wolfhounds and in medium-sized breeds such as Australian shepherds and Australian cattle dogs.

General clinical signs of CPSS include small stature, weight loss or failure to gain weight, polydipsia, and anesthetic or tranquilizer intolerance. Neurologic dysfunction from hepatic encephalopathy (HE) is seen in most animals with CPSS and may include lethargy, restlessness or pacing, ataxia, head pressing, circling, seizures, behavioral changes, and amaurotic blindness. Precipitating factors of severe neurologic signs (HE) include protein overload, hypokalemia, alkalosis, hypovolemia, hypoxia, gastrointestinal hemorrhage, infection, azotemia, constipation, drugs, and transfusion of stored red cells. Gastrointestinal clinical abnormalities may include anorexia, vomiting, diarrhea, or pica and, in large-breed dogs, evidence of gastrointestinal bleeding such as melena or hematemesis. Some dogs have no apparent signs or signs of only lower urinary tract disease or urinary tract obstruction. Many cats have hypersalivation and seizures, and some have unusual copper-colored irises.

Diagnosis

Routine Laboratory Tests

In dogs, common blood work abnormalities include microcytosis and decreases in blood urea nitrogen, protein, albumin, glucose, and cholesterol. Serum alanine aminotransferase and alkaline phosphatase may be increased. Increase in alkaline phosphatase is most likely from bone growth because cholestasis is not usually a feature in animals with CPSS. Cats with CPSS may have normal albumin, glucose, total protein, and cholesterol concentrations but usually have increased liver enzymes. Up to half of dogs with CPSS have prolonged partial thromboplastin times; however, this usually does not result in a clinically significant problem.

Urine abnormalities include low urine specific gravity, ammonium biurate crystalluria, and occasionally abnormal urine sediment suggestive of cystitis secondary to crystalluria or (urate) urolithiasis. Some dogs may have silent urinary tract infections; therefore urine culture is performed routinely in many animals.

Common hepatic histologic changes in animals with CPSS include lobular atrophy, increased numbers of hepatic arterioles and bile ductules because of proliferation or tortuosity, decreased number or size of intrahepatic portal tributaries, and deposition of lipid and pigment within cytoplasmic vacuoles (lipogranulomas). These pathologic changes are variable and also can be seen in dogs with congenital portal vein hypoplasia with secondary microvascular dysplasia (PVH-MVD) that do not have CPSS and in dogs with other hepatic diseases such as noncirrhotic portal hypertension (see Chapter 146).

Liver Function Tests

Results of bile acids, ammonia, and protein C activity provide additional information about liver function. Serum bile acids are measured after a 12-hour fast and again 2 hours after a meal. Bile acid concentrations are usually greater than 75 μmol/L in dogs with CPSS but also can be increased with any significant liver disease. Occasionally postprandial bile acid concentrations are less than the prefasting sample (in approximately 20% of dogs) because of spontaneous interdigestive gallbladder contraction.

Most animals with CPSS also have increased ammonia concentrations, particularly if measured 6 hours after feeding or after oral or rectal administration of ammonia (ammonia tolerance test). Concentrations of blood ammonia are not well correlated with severity of hepatic encephalopathy, and ammonia concentrations may be normal with effective medical treatment. Ammonia can be increased falsely with improper sample handling.

Protein C is a component of the coagulation cascade that decreases clot formation. In normal dogs, protein C activity is at least 70%. Protein C activity is decreased in many dogs with severe liver disease and in most dogs with CPSS but is usually normal (>70%) in most dogs with PVH-MVD.

Diagnostic Imaging

Common findings on survey radiographs include a small liver and enlarged kidneys. Urate calculi are usually not visible unless combined with other compounds such as struvite or calcium.

Often CPSS can be identified on ultrasonography by experienced operators, particularly if color-flow Doppler is available. The combination of small liver, large kidneys, and uroliths is highly suggestive of shunting in dogs, and dogs and cats with extrahepatic shunts have reduced portal vein-to-aorta ratios. Extrahepatic CPSS can be more difficult to diagnose with ultrasonography because the patient is usually small and structures such as ribs and intestines can obscure the vessel.

Nuclear scintigraphy with technetium 99m provides a diagnosis of shunt or no shunt. If the radionuclide is injected directly into the spleen, the operator often can tell where the shunt terminates, how many shunts are present, and whether they are likely to be congenital or acquired. Normal shunt fraction is less than 5% for transsplenic scintigraphy and less than 15% for per rectal. Isolation for 12 to 24 hours usually is required in animals undergoing rectal scintigraphy.

Direct injection of contrast into the splenic or jejunal veins (portovenography) usually provides excellent information regarding the presence, number, and location of shunts; however, at most practices a celiotomy is required to obtain the images. In addition, some CPSS are not visible on portograms performed in dorsal or right lateral recumbency.

Computed tomographic (CT) angiography is considered the standard for definitive diagnosis of CPSS and is particularly useful for preoperative planning in animals with intrahepatic CPSS and hepatic arteriovenous malformations. Magnetic resonance angiography also can be used to detect shunts, but it is more expensive and image quality is not as good.

Differential Diagnoses

Single congenital portosystemic shunts must be differentiated from neurologic conditions such as hydrocephalus and epilepsy and from other primary hepatic diseases, including congenital PVH-MVD and multiple acquired shunts secondary to portal hypertension. Differentiation usually is based on results of advanced imaging; however, history, clinical signs, and results of blood work also may be helpful. Conditions other than CPSS should be suspected when neurologic or other clinical signs do not resolve with medical management of the HE.

Unlike animals with CPSS, ascites is a common finding on physical examination or ultrasonography in dogs with portal hypertension secondary to severe hepatocellular disease or hepatic arteriovenous malformations. With development of multiple acquired PSS, these animals have increased shunt fractions on scintigraphy.

Congenital portal vein hypoplasia is found in many small breeds predisposed to CPSS. Although results of liver biopsy are the same for both conditions, laboratory changes are usually less severe in dogs with PVH-MVD, unless noncirrhotic portal hypertension is present (see Chapter 146). Dogs with PVH-MVD are more likely to have normal red cell size (MCV); glucose, albumin, total protein, and cholesterol concentrations; and urine specific gravity and fewer if any at all clinical signs than dogs with CPSS. In addition, 90% to 95% of dogs with PVH-MVD have normal protein C activity and 81%

have postprandial bile acids less than 75 μmol/L at the author's institute. Results of scintigraphy, portography, and CT angiography are usually normal in dogs with PVH-MVD.

Medical Management of Portosystemic Shunts

All animals with CPSS should receive medical management to improve their physical condition and treat or prevent hepatic encephalopathy (see Chapter 144). Dietary protein is restricted moderately to reduce substrates for ammonia formation by colonic bacteria. Caloric requirements should be calculated based on ideal body weight because patients with shunts may be thin or have poor muscle development. At least 30% to 50% of dietary calories should be provided as easily digested, complex soluble carbohydrates; and diets for dogs and cats should contain 15% to 30% and 20% to 40% fat, respectively, on a dry matter (DM) basis. Crude protein requirements in dogs with liver disease are approximately 2.11 g per kilogram of body weight per day. On a dry matter basis, commercial liver diets range from 14% to 18% protein for dogs and 31% to 32% for cats, respectively. Soybean meal and dairy proteins often are recommended protein sources because of their high digestibility. If homemade diets are used, zinc, fat-soluble vitamins, and vitamins B and C should be supplemented and components that precipitate hepatic encephalopathy (e.g., manganese) should be limited.

Lactulose is given to animals showing signs referable to hepatic encephalopathy. Dosages should be regulated so that feces are soft but formed; in toy breed dogs a common dose is 1 to 2 ml q8-12h PO. Although usually administered orally, lactulose can be given by enema in obtunded or seizing animals. Yogurt with active cultures can be substituted in place of lactulose to alter colonic flora. Nutraceuticals used to treat animals with CPSS include S-adenosylmethionine (SAMe), vitamin E, and milk thistle (silymarin). Benefits of these compounds may include hepatoprotective, antioxidant, and antiinflammatory effects and improved hepatic function. Unfortunately, no controlled studies describe effectiveness of yogurt or nutraceuticals in the management of CPSS in dogs or cats.

Gastrointestinal hemorrhage (see Chapter 123), intestinal parasites, and cystitis should be treated appropriately. Gastrointestinal ulcers have been reported preoperatively, particularly in large-breed dogs with intrahepatic CPSS, and even after successful closure of a shunt and may require long-term management with proton pump inhibitors. Urate uroliths may respond to low-protein diets; renal calculi reportedly have dissolved after shunt ligation.

In severely encephalopathic animals, medical management includes correction of fluid, electrolyte, and glucose imbalances as needed. Enemas with water and lactulose may be used to reduce colonic bacteria and substrates. Fresh frozen plasma or hetastarch may be required in patients with coagulopathy or decreased oncotic pressure, respectively. Once animals can swallow, oral antibiotics effective against urease-producing bacteria (e.g., neomycin or metronidazole) can be administered to

decrease colonic bacterial populations; clinicians should be aware of the potential toxicity of these drugs. Seizures unrelated to hypoglycemia or hyperammonemia are treated initially with intravenous benzodiazepines. Some clinicians prefer low-dose midazolam over intravenous diazepam, which contains a propylene glycol–carrying agent that requires liver metabolism. However, at the author's institute, diazepam is used successfully to acutely halt seizures in dogs with CPSS. Once seizures are controlled, loading doses of, and continued treatment with, anticonvulsants such as phenobarbital, levetiracetam, zonisamide, or potassium or sodium bromide are recommended, particularly if continued seizure activity is anticipated. In a retrospective study by Fryer et al, postoperative seizures were reported in 4 of 84 dogs that did not receive preoperative levetiracetam before extrahepatic CPSS attenuation compared with 0 of 42 that received preoperative levetiracetam. Preoperative seizures are reported in 23% of cats; those with a history of frequent seizures are placed on levetiracetam, zonisamide, or phenobarbital for several weeks before surgery.

Prognosis with Medical Management

With proper medical management, weight and quality of life stabilizes or improves with treatment in most animals; however, long-term mortality rates of medically treated animals are higher than those of animals undergoing shunt attenuation. In a study by Watson and Herrtage (1998), 52% of dogs were euthanized with a median survival time of 10 months. At least one third of dogs did well with medical management as the sole method of treatment, however, with many living to 7 years of age or older. Shorter duration of survival was correlated with intrahepatic shunt location, younger age at onset initial signs, greater severity of clinical signs (e.g., hepatic encephalopathy), and lower blood urea nitrogen (BUN) concentration. Some dogs developed progressive hepatic fibrosis and subsequent portal hypertension.

In a more recent report by Greenhalgh et al (2010), 52% of dogs receiving medical treatment were still alive at the completion of the study, and 30% of medically treated dogs died of shunt-related causes. In comparison, 88% of surgically treated dogs were alive at the end of the study, and 10% of surgically treated dogs died of shunt-related causes. Median survival time for medically or surgically treated dogs that died was 164 days. Age at the time of diagnosis was not correlated with survival.

With medical management alone, survival time of cats with CPSS, particularly those that are neurologic, is usually less than 2 years. Dogs and cats with multiple acquired PSS are managed medically.

Surgery

Once patients have been managed medically for several weeks, attenuation of CPSS is recommended to improve long-term outcome. Options include acute ligation with suture; gradual occlusion with ameroid constrictors, cellophane banding, or hydraulic occluders; or embolization with coils (most commonly for intrahepatic CPSS). Because shunt closure with ameroid constrictors or cellophane bands relies on inflammatory reaction and subsequent scar tissue formation, use of antiinflammatory or immunosuppressive doses of glucocorticoids should be avoided after surgery.

Complication and mortality rates are highest in animals that undergo shunt ligation; therefore gradual occlusion or coil embolization is preferred. Excellent outcomes are seen in 80% to 85% of dogs undergoing gradual shunt occlusion, although bile acids remain mildly to moderately increased in many dogs because of concurrent PVH-MVD. Prognosis for successful surgical treatment is best for dogs with extrahepatic shunts, for animals that undergo complete shunt occlusion, and for those that present with urinary tract signs and no hepatic encephalopathy. Prognosis is not related to age but is poorer in animals with severe preoperative hypoalbuminemia, hypoproteinemia, anemia, or leukocytosis. Perioperative complications are reported in less than 15% of dogs undergoing coil embolization of intrahepatic CPSS, and long-term survival rate is more than 87%, as long as the dogs are maintained on lifelong antacid (e.g., omeprazole) therapy to prevent gastrointestinal ulceration.

Good or excellent long-term outcome is reported in about 75% of cats that survive surgery; however, many have postoperative complications. The most common is neurologic dysfunction, including generalized seizures and central blindness in up to 28% and 44% of cats, respectively. Blindness usually resolves in 2 months.

Postoperative Care

Portal hypertension is uncommon when gradual attenuation is performed. Most animals need analgesics, such as opioids, for the first 24 to 48 hours. Sedation with dexmedetomidine or a low dose (0.01 to 0.02 mg/kg IM) of acepromazine may be necessary if dogs are vocalizing or abdominal pressing because these activities increase portal pressure and hyperexcitability. Acepromazine does not appear to lower seizure threshold in PSS patients, but its effects may be prolonged, so careful dosing is critical. About 25% of toy breed dogs develop hypoglycemia despite concurrent intravenous treatment with dextrose-containing fluids. Patients with nonresponsive hypoglycemia, poor anesthetic recovery, or signs of circulatory disturbances (decreased systolic pressure, increased capillary refill time, poor peripheral pulses, pale mucous membranes) may require treatment with one or more doses of steroids (0.02 to 0.1 mg/kg dexamethasone sodium phosphate IV).

Seizures have been reported in 3% to 18% of dogs and 8% to 22% of cats after shunt attenuation. They usually are seen within 48 hours after surgery but may occur as late as 96 hours. Lethargy, restlessness, frantic or aggressive behavior, facial twitching, ataxia, muscle fasciculation, blindness, and abnormal vocalization are often apparent before generalized seizure activity. Etiology is unknown, and affected animals usually do not respond to fluids, dextrose, lactulose, or enemas. Single seizures are treated with a bolus of diazepam or midazolam to effect, correction of any hypoglycemia, and administration of lactulose retention enemas in case there is an underlying encephalopathy. If seizures recur, the animal

is given an additional bolus of benzodiazepine, anesthetized with propofol (5 to 8 mg/kg), and maintained on a propofol continuous rate infusion (0.1 to 1 mg/kg/min). Intubation may be required in some dogs. Phenobarbital can be started concurrently (3 to 8 mg/kg IV loading dose, then 2 to 2.5 mg/kg IV or IM q12h); patients are switched to oral phenobarbital (2 mg/kg q12h) once awake. Alternatively, levetiracetam can be administered intravenously (20 mg/kg) followed by oral administration (20 mg/kg q8h) once the patient is awake. Mannitol (1 g/kg IV) is administered every 6 hours to reduce intracranial swelling. Electrolyte and glucose abnormalities are corrected, and supportive care (e.g., maintenance fluids, body rotation, eye lubrication, oral cleansing) is provided. Partial or total parenteral nutrition should be considered in patients that have been fasted more than 48 hours. Lactulose can be administered as a retention enema if hepatic encephalopathy cannot be ruled out. Propofol infusion is discontinued after 12 to 24 hours; if the animal seizes during recovery, it is reanesthetized for another 12 to 24 hours and supportive care is continued. Differentiating anesthetic recovery from fulminant seizures can be difficult during the propofol weaning process, and sedation may be required to reduce anxiety. In a few cases, the author has used successfully an acepromazine or dexmedetomidine continuous-rate infusion during propofol recovery or in place of propofol to prevent seizure reoccurrence. Prognosis is poor for animals with persistent postoperative seizures. Those that survive usually improve neurologically over weeks to months, although incoordination and partial visual deficits may persist.

Portal hypertension occurs most frequently after acute ligation or overly aggressive coil embolization. Treatment includes intravenous fluids, hetastarch, broad-spectrum systemic antibiotics, and fresh frozen plasma and low-molecular-weight heparin if coagulation times are prolonged. For some dogs, clinical signs resolve with supportive therapy; others may require removal of the attenuating device.

Medical management is continued after surgery until liver function improves. Frequently animals can be gradually weaned off of lactulose 2 to 6 weeks after the surgery unless they are constipated or clinical signs recur. Bile acids, protein C activity, complete blood count, serum chemistry, and urinalysis are evaluated 3, 6, and 12 months after the surgery to assess liver function. Protein in the diet can be increased gradually once bile acids are near normal. In dogs with mildly increased bile acids and normal albumin, it may be necessary to monitor clinical response to diet change to determine whether protein content can be increased gradually. Animals with persistently increased bile acids or ammonia concentrations can be treated with a combination of silymarin and SAMe to improve hepatic function and regeneration. Animals with persistent clinicopathologic abnormalities may require further workup (e.g., scintigraphy or CT angiography and liver biopsy) to determine the underlying cause (Figure 145-1). For many dogs, bile acids never normalize after CPSS attenuation because of concurrent PVH-MVD. In those dogs, measurement of bile acids is discontinued and liver function instead is monitored by evaluation of albumin, total protein, BUN, liver

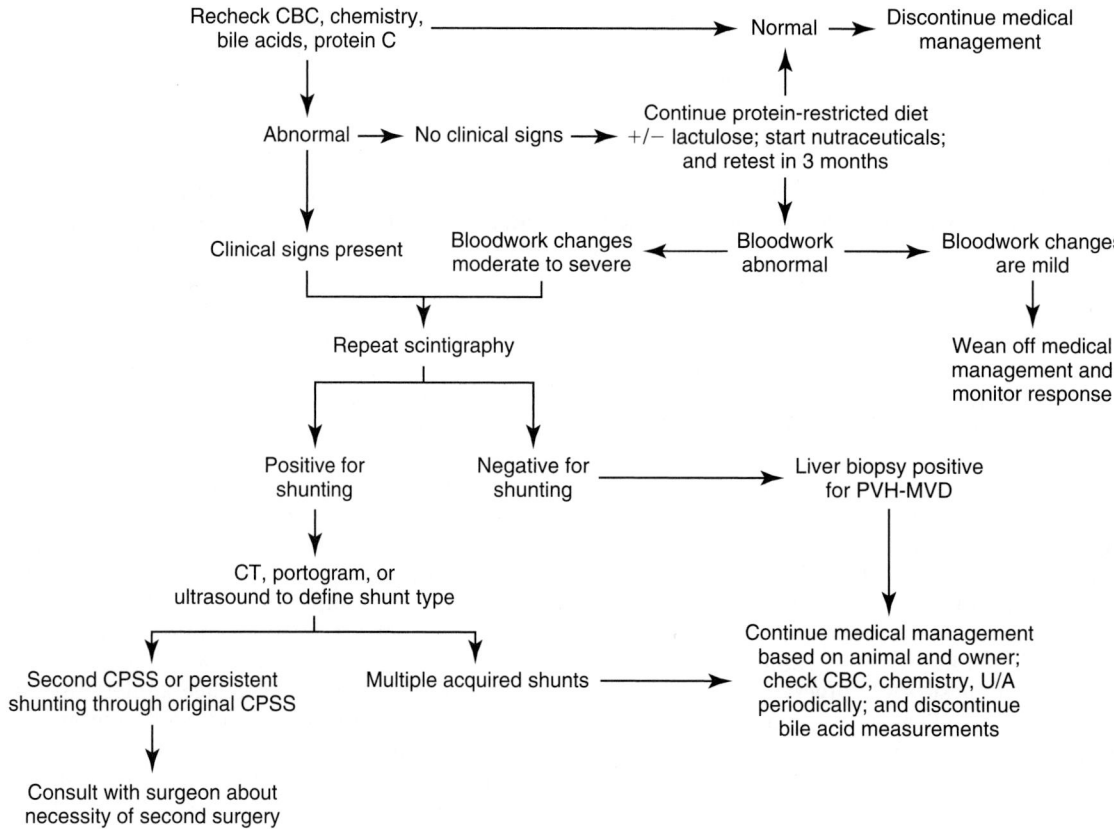

Figure 145-1 Algorithm for evaluation of animals with single congenital shunts 3 months after surgery.

enzyme, glucose, and cholesterol concentrations; MCV; urinalysis; and protein C activity. Controlled studies comparing effects of various medical treatments on long-term outcome of animals after CPSS attenuation are lacking; therefore management of asymptomatic animals with mild to moderate increases in bile acids is determined on a case-by-case basis and often is based on response to therapy and owner preference.

References and Suggested Reading

Bajaj JS et al: Probiotic yogurt for the treatment of minimal hepatic encephalopathy, *Am J Gastroenterol* 103:1707, 2008.

Berent A, Tobias K: Hepatic vascular anomalies. In Tobias KM, Johnston SA, editors: *Veterinary surgery: small animal*, St Louis, 2011, Elsevier, p 1624.

Berent A, Tobias K: Portosystemic vascular anomalies, *Vet Clin North Am Small Anim* 39:513-541, 2009.

Flatland B: Botanicals, vitamins, and minerals and the liver: therapeutic applications and potential toxicities, *Compend Contin Educ Pract Vet* 25:514, 2003.

Fryer KJ et al: Incidence of postoperative seizures with and without levetiracetam pretreatment in dogs undergoing portosystemic shunt attenuation, *J Vet Intern Med* 25:1379, 2011.

Greenhalgh SN et al: Comparison of survival after surgical or medical treatment in dogs with a congenital portosystemic shunt, *J Am Vet Med Assoc* 236:1215, 2010.

Proot S et al: Soy protein isolate versus meat-based low-protein diet for dogs with congenital portosystemic shunts, *J Vet Intern Med* 23:794, 2009.

Tobias KM, Rohrbach BW: Association of breed with the diagnosis of congenital portosystemic shunts in dogs: 2,400 cases (1980-2002), *J Am Vet Med Assoc* 223:1636-1639, 2003.

Toulza O et al: Evaluation of plasma protein C activity for detection of hepatobiliary disease and portosystemic shunting in dogs, *J Am Vet Med Assoc* 229:1761, 2006.

Watson PJ, Herrtage ME: Medical management of congenital portosystemic shunts in 27 dogs—a retrospective study, *J Small Anim Pract* 39:62, 1998.

CHAPTER 146

Portal Vein Hypoplasia (Microvascular Dysplasia)

ANDREA N. JOHNSTON, *Ithaca, New York*
CYNTHIA R.L. WEBSTER, *Grafton, Massachusetts*

In normal dogs approximately 70% of the blood flow to the liver is delivered by the portal circulation, with the remaining 30% derived from the hepatic artery. Hepatopetal blood flow from the portal system enters the portal triad, traverses the sinusoids, and returns to the systemic circulation via the hepatic veins. A spectrum of congenital hepatic vascular anomalies involving the hepatic portal vasculature exists in the dog. Macroscopic portosystemic vascular anomalies (PSVA) occur as single vessels within (intrahepatic) or outside (extrahepatic) the liver that shunt blood from the portal to the systemic circulation (see Chapter 145). Hypoplasia of the portal vein (also known as microvascular dysplasia, or MVD) is a microscopic intrahepatic vascular abnormality in which portal venous blood is diverted into the hepatic veins within the intrahepatic microcirculation (Allen et al, 1999; Center, 2008; Christiansen et al, 2000; Rothuzien et al, 2006; Schermerhorn et al, 1996). Originally called MVD, in 2004 the World Small Animal Veterinary Association (WSAVA) Liver Standardization Group renamed the syndrome primary hypoplasia of the portal vein (PHPV) (also referred to as portal vein hypoplasia [PVH]) because the association felt MVD was part of a group of congenital disorders (excluding PSVA) associated with the PVH resulting in hepatic parenchymal hypoperfusion. Although it is clear that some dogs with congenital portovascular disease have true hypoplasia (atresia) of the extrahepatic portal vein, it is not clear whether all dogs with the syndrome recognized as MVD have hypoplastic vessels.

PVH/MVD may occur independently or concurrently with PSVA. Multiple small-breed dogs are at increased risk for PVH/MVD, including many of the same breeds predisposed to PSVA. These breeds include Cairn terriers, Tibetan spaniels, Maltese, Havanese, Yorkshire terriers, Norfolk terriers, and miniature schnauzers. A small-breed genotyping initiative underway at Cornell University in these breeds has established that macroscopic or microscopic portovascular anomalies occur in 30% to 80% of those breeds (Center S, personal communication). They found the incidence of PVH/MVD exceeds PSVA 30:1 in all breeds that were studied. Genotyping data suggest that the PSVA/PVH/MVD trait is allelic and may represent an ancestral founder mutation. An autosomal incomplete penetrant or polygenic mode of inheritance is most consistent with trait transmission.

Clinical Features

Dogs with PVH/MVD are typically asymptomatic. They have none of the clinical features seen in dogs with PVSA, such as small body stature, neurobehavioral signs consistent with hepatic encephalopathy (amaurosis, head pressing, staring, vocalizing, seizures, lethargy, and coma), intermittent gastrointestinal signs (anorexia, vomiting, diarrhea), or urinary signs (polyuria/polydipsia, stranguria, hematuria, pollakiuria). Rarely dogs may exhibit drug intolerance to substances metabolized or extracted by the liver. These drug sensitivities often are noted initially at the time of neutering.

Reports of PVH/MVD dogs with neurobehavioral and gastrointestinal signs can be found in the veterinary literature (Allen et al, 1999; Christiansen et al, 2000). Although initial clinical impressions were that dogs with PVH/MVD could be subdivided into asymptomatic and symptomatic groups, some symptomatic PVH/MVD dogs actually may represent PSVA dogs in which the vascular anomaly escaped detection or dogs with other disorders such as noncirrhotic portal hypertension (NCPH) (see later) or ductal plate abnormalities, which share some clinical and histologic features with PSVA/PVH/MVD. The latter is differentiated from primary vascular disease by the presence of intense cytokeratin positive bile duct profiles on hepatic biopsy.

Clinical Pathology

The hallmark of PVH/MVD is the presence of increased total serum bile acids in a dog that is otherwise clinically normal. Diagnosis requires ruling out the presence of a PSVA. Although increases in total serum bile acids are relatively lower in dogs with PVH/MVD as compared with PSVA, the degree of elevation cannot be used to differentiate the two disorders because of the potential for overlap in bile acid values. Complete blood count, serum biochemistry, and urinalysis typically are normal in dogs with PVH/MVD, with occasional mild increases in serum aminotransferases. In contrast, dogs with PSVA may have an RBC microcytosis, hypocholesterolemia, low BUN and creatinine, hypoglycemia, and ammonium biurate crystalluria. If readily available, plasma protein C level may aid in the differentiation of PSVA and PVH/MVD because it typically is subnormal with PSVA (protein C < 70% in

88% of dogs) and normal with MVD (protein C ≥ 70% in 95% of dogs) (Toulza et al, 2006). The low protein C levels in PSVA likely reflect hepatic hypoperfusion and not synthetic failure; attenuation of the anomalous vessel results in normalization of these values.

Diagnostic Imaging

Abdominal ultrasound is an easily accessible imaging modality that can identify features consistent with PSVA. Dogs with PVH/MVD typically have normal abdominal ultrasound examinations. With an experienced operator, the use of color-flow Doppler, and adequate restraint of the patient (which often requires sedation), the sensitivity of ultrasound to identify a macroscopic extra- or intra-PSVA can be as high as 98% (d'Anjou et al, 2004). In addition to visualization of the anomalous vessel, other signs suggestive of a PSVA on ultrasound include the presence of a small hypovascular liver, turbulence in the portal vascular, renomegaly, urolithiasis, and a portal vein-to-aorta ratio less than 0.65 in a dog without portal hypertension. Unfortunately, a normal ultrasound examination does not definitively exclude PSVA, so additional imaging may be necessary to make a diagnosis of PVH/ MVD.

Transplenic portal or per rectal portal scintigraphy can be used to confirm the presence of portosystemic shunting (either congenital or acquired) with a sensitivity and specificity approaching 100% (Sura et al, 2007). In these procedures, small volumes of technetium 99m pertechnetate are administered to the sedated patient per rectum or transcutaneously into the spleen, and distribution of the radioactivity within the portal and systemic circulation is monitored with a computer-linked gamma camera. Dogs with PVH/MVD have a normal or mildly increased shunt fraction with these techniques, whereas dogs with PSVA usually have a shunt fraction greater than 60% (Center, 2008). Transplenic scintigraphy is a minimally invasive and relatively cost-effective secondary imaging modality often used by the authors as a second-line modality after ultrasound has failed to find a PSVA. In the authors' (CRLW) hospital a clinically normal dog with increased total serum bile acids but normal CBC, biochemical profile, urinalysis, abdominal ultrasound, and transplenic portal scintigraphy routinely is given a diagnosis of PVH/MVD without pursuing additional diagnostics (Box 146-1).

BOX 146-1

Typical Findings in Dogs with Microvascular Dysplasia

Absence of clinical signs
Increased total serum bile acids
Normal CBC, biochemistry panel, and urinalysis
Normal protein C activity
Normal abdominal ultrasound
Normal transplenic and per rectal scintigraphy

Additional imaging modalities to aid in the identification of a PSVA include contrast-enhanced multiphase magnetic resonance angiography and three-dimensional multidetector computed tomography angiography. Both techniques are noninvasive and accurate methods of visualizing PSVA; however, both require patient sedation or anesthesia, have limited availability in general practice, and are relatively expensive. It is presumed that the appearance of a liver with PVH/MVD would be normal; however, no large-scale studies have described the computed tomography (CT) or magnetic resonance imagery (MRI) appearance of PVH/MVD.

Normal radiographic mesenteric portography is the standard for excluding the presence of a PSVA. This requires abdominal exploratory and direct mesenteric injection of an iodinated contrast agent. Portography in dogs with MVD is essentially normal, although there may be failure of some regions of the liver to opacify with contrast or abnormally long retention of contrast in other areas.

Hepatic Biopsy

A diagnosis of MVD cannot be made by evaluation of hepatic histopathology (Rothuizen et al, 2006). The histopathologic changes associated with MVD are identical to those seen with PSVA and reflect chronic hypoperfusion of the liver (Figure 146-1). These features include juvenile or underdeveloped portal triads with hepatic arteriolar reduplication (increased number of profiles), small or absent portal veins, prominent central venous musculature, lobular atrophy, dilation of perivenular lymphatics, disorganized hepatic sinusoids, and multifocal lipogranulomas surrounding hepatic venules. Accurate histopathologic diagnosis of PSVA/PVH/MVD often requires surgical or laparoscopic wedge biopsy specimens collected from multiple liver lobes. Because the microscopic lesions can be inconsistent among liver lobes and subtle in dogs with PVH/MVD, lesions may be missed with single-lobe or small-needle biopsies. At least three liver biopsies should be taken from three different liver lobes to better identify this condition histologically. In general the workup to differentiate MVD from PSVA usually does not require hepatic biopsy.

Treatment and Prognosis

Because dogs with MVD typically are asymptomatic and nothing suggests that PVH/MVD is progressive, dogs with the disorder generally do not require any therapy. Caution should be exercised with use of drugs that require extensive hepatic metabolism. Occasionally, in the dog with increases in serum transaminases, treatment can be initiated with hepatic cytoprotective agents such as ursodeoxycholate or S-adenosylmethionine, and liver enzymes should be monitored periodically. Although studies with long-term follow-up in dogs with PVH/MVD are lacking, anecdotal experience suggests that the disease is not progressive. This is supported by the diagnosis of the condition in asymptomatic Cairn terriers at up to 8 years of age (Schermerhorn et al, 1996).

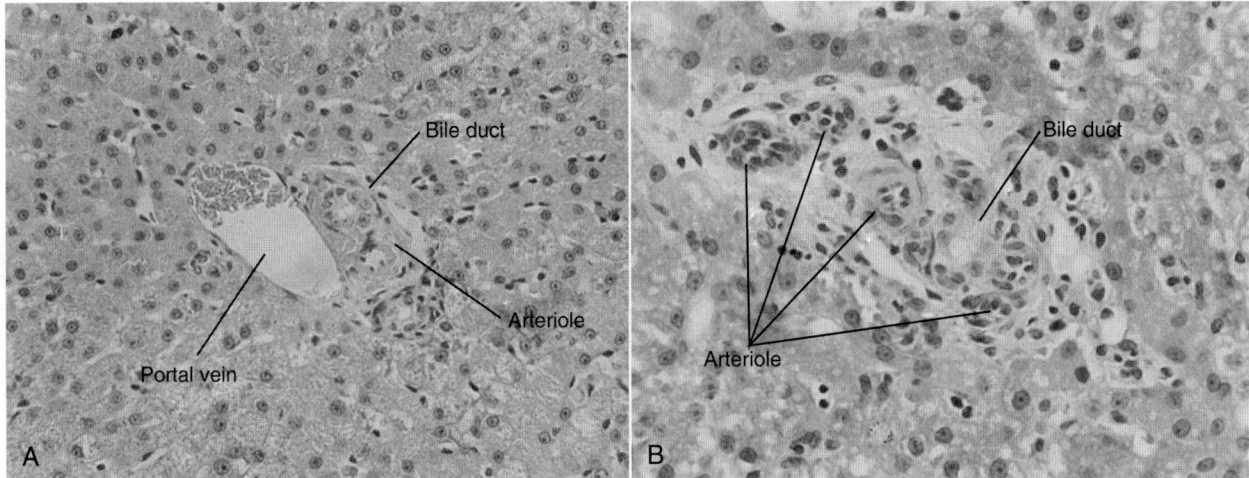

Figure 146-1 Hepatic histopathology in dogs with chronic hypoperfusion. **A,** A normal portal triad with one portal vein, hepatic artery, and bile duct. **B,** A typical portal triad from a dog with chronic hepatic hypoperfusion that shows portal vein attenuation and hepatic arteriolar reduplication.

Portal Vein Hypoplasia and Microvascular Dysplasia Versus Vascular Disease with Portal Hypertension

Within the WSAVA classification of PHPV, some symptomatic dogs show the stereotypical histologic picture of chronic hypoperfusion seen with PSVA/PVH/MVD but also have portal hypertension. Some of these dogs have true hypoplasia (atresia of the portal vein). Others have a clinical syndrome that has been referred to as noncirrhotic portal hypertension (NCPH), idiopathic hepatic fibrosis, hepatoportal fibrosis, and PHPV in the veterinary literature (Bunch, Johnson, and Cullen, 2011; Buob, Johnston, and Webster, 2011; Rothuizen et al, 2006; van dan Ingh, Rothuizen, and Meyer, 1995). In humans NCPH is an acquired vasculopathy of the small and medium branches of the portal vein associated with exposure to toxins absorbed from the gastrointestinal tract (e.g., lipopolysaccharide, some drugs), autoimmune disorders, and prothrombotic states. Veterinary cases of NCPH/PHPV may be due to primary hypoplasia of the intrahepatic portal vasculature or may be a consequence of a similar congenital or acquired disorder in hepatic perfusion.

The clinical features in dogs with NCPH/PHPV are different than those seen in PSVA/PVH/MVD. Typically dogs with this disorder are young (<2 years of age) large-breed dogs with polyuria/polydipsia, ascites, HE, and gastrointestinal signs. Rottweilers, cocker spaniels, and Doberman pinschers appear to be overrepresented. These dogs have moderate to severe increases in serum liver enzymes, mild to moderate hyperbilirubinemia, increased total serum bile acids and blood ammonia, hypoalbuminemia, and a low-protein ascitic fluid. Ultrasound shows microhepatica with evidence of portal hypertension including ascites, multiple acquired portosystemic shunts, and an enlarged portal vein with hepatofugal flow. Although this clinical presentation must be differentiated from acquired inflammatory or fibrotic disease, the presence of portal hypertension excludes a diagnosis of PSVA/MVD because these disorders are never associated with increased resistance to portal blood flow. In NCPH/PHPV hepatic histopathology has the classic lesions associated with chronic hypoperfusion (see earlier) with the additional findings of varying degrees of periportal and/or centrilobular fibrosis. Noteworthy is the absence of inflammation and regenerative nodules. Treatment of NCPH/PHPV is directed at the clinical signs, including management of hepatic encephalopathy and ascites, gastric protectants to prevent gastrointestinal ulceration, and the use of nonspecific hepatoprotective agents (see Chapter 144). Some dogs appear to stabilize after a period of time and can have extended survival times. Additional characterization of this disorder is necessary before its place in the spectrum of canine hepatic vascular disease can be defined.

Conclusion

PVH/MVD is an asymptomatic, inherited vasculopathy of the hepatic microcirculation, which occurs primarily in small-breed dogs. Accumulating evidence suggests that PSVA and PVH/MVD may represent the same genetic trait at opposite ends of the spectrum. Predisposed breeds must be screened for PVH/MVD so that the disorder can be identified early in life and confusion avoided in future diagnostic evaluations. If elevated total serum bile acids are identified in these dogs, additional testing (see Box 146-1) to rule out the presence of a PSVA is indicated. Performing invasive testing (portography, hepatic biopsy) seldom is necessary to make a diagnosis of MVD with a high level of confidence. Hepatic biopsy alone does not allow discrimination between PSVA and PVH/MVD.

In young symptomatic dogs with elevated total serum bile acids, congenital/acquired vascular (NCPH, portal vein atresia/obstruction, hepatoarteriovenous fistula, venoocclusive disease), biliary (ductal plate abnormalities), or inflammatory disorders must be considered. The presence of portal hypertension (most easily recognized by detection of abdominal effusion) differentiates these disorders clinically from simple PVH/MVD or PSVA. A review of how to approach the diagnostic workup of this complex series of hypertensive disorders may be helpful (Buob et al, 2011).

References and Suggested Reading

Allen L et al: Clinicopathologic features of dogs with hepatic microvascular dysplasia with and without portosystemic shunts: 42 cases (1991-1996), *J Am Vet Med Assoc* 214:218, 1999.
Bunch SE, Johnson SE, Cullen JM: Idiopathic noncirrhotic portal hypertension in dogs: 33 cases (1982-1998), *J Am Vet Med Assoc* 218:392, 2001.
Buob S, Johnston A, Webster CRL: Portal hypertension: pathophysiology, diagnosis and treatment, *J Vet Intern Med* 5:169, 2011.
Center SA: In Bonagura JD, Twedt DC, editors: *Kirk's current veterinary therapy XIV*, Philadelphia, 2008, Elsevier (Saunders).
Christiansen JS et al: Hepatic microvascular dysplasia in dogs: a retrospective study of 24 cases (1987-1995), *J Am Anim Hosp Assoc* 36:385, 2000.
d'Anjou MA et al: Ultrasonographic diagnosis of portosystemic shunting in dogs and cats, *Vet Radiol Ultrasound* 45:424, 2004.
Rothuizen J et al: *WSAVA standards for clinical and histological diagnosis of canine and feline liver disease*, New York, 2006, Saunders (Elsevier).
Schermerhorn T et al: Characterization of hepatoportal microvascular dysplasia in a kindred of cairn terriers, *J Vet Intern Med* 10:219, 1996.
Sura PA et al: Comparison of 99mTcO4(-) trans-splenic portal scintigraphy with per-rectal portal scintigraphy for diagnosis of portosystemic shunts in dogs, *Vet Surg* 36:654, 2007.
Toulza O et al: Evaluation of plasma protein C activity for detection of hepatobiliary disease and portosystemic shunting in dogs, *J Am Vet Med Assoc* 229:1761, 2006.
van den Ingh TSGAM, Rothuizen J, Meyer HP: Portal hypertension associated with primary hypoplasia of the portal vein in dogs, *Vet Rec* 137:424, 1995.

CHAPTER 147

Extrahepatic Biliary Tract Disease

KEITH P. RICHTER, *San Diego, California*
FRED S. PIKE, *San Diego, California*

The extrahepatic biliary tract (EHBT) consists of hepatic ducts, the common bile duct (CBD), the gallbladder (GB), cystic duct, and the duodenal papillae. In general the clinical presentations for diseases of the EHBT are the result of alteration in or obstruction of the normal passage of bile. Biliary diseases can be categorized as (1) biliary cystic disease, (2) cholestatic disease, (3) cholangitis, and (4) disorders of the GB. Clinical presentations of patients with extrahepatic biliary obstruction (EHBO) are varied, and the onset of clinical signs can be acute or chronic and insidious. Recent veterinary literature suggests that the prevalence of diseases of the EHBT is increasing.

Anatomy

In the liver, bile canaliculi unite to form plexiform interlobular ducts. Interlobular ducts congregate to form lobar ducts, which unite to form hepatic ducts. Three or four hepatic ducts terminate in the CBD. The order and location of termination of the hepatic ducts is varied and has been documented. The GB is a vesicle that stores bile.

Duplex GB and duplex cystic ducts have been reported in cats. The GB is lined by columnar epithelial cells that reabsorb water and electrolytes, resulting in concentrated bile with increased viscosity. Submucosal mucous glands secrete mucus that acts as a bile lubricant. The GB is nestled in a fossa between the right medial and quadrate liver lobes. The GB has a blind-end, rounded base termed the fundus, a large middle portion termed the body, and a slender tapered region termed the neck. The cystic duct extends from the neck of the GB to the junction with the first hepatic duct. The GB has an end-artery vascularity via the cystic artery. The lack of collateral arterial supply may contribute to vascular compromise during marked distention. The CBD begins at the junction of the last hepatic duct and ends on the major duodenal papilla; its length is approximately 5 cm in the medium-size dog. The normal CBD diameter is 2 to 2.5 mm in the cat and 3 mm in the dog. The canine CBD has a duodenal intramural length of 1.5 to 2 cm and terminates at the sphincter of the major duodenal papilla (commonly called the sphincter of Oddi or sphincter of ampulla). The orifice of the CBD shares the major duodenal papilla with the orifice of the accessory pancreatic duct in approximately 75% of dogs. In the cat the CBD unites with the major pancreatic duct before the duodenal papilla; manipulation and catheterization of the major duodenal papilla in cats may increase the risk of pancreatitis.

GB filling is passive; it is the result of retrograde flow into the GB caused by increased intraluminal CBD pressure that occurs when the sphincter of the major duodenal papilla is closed. GB contraction is induced by cholecystokinin synthesized by I cells in the mucosal epithelium of the duodenum. Cholecystokinin also causes increased production of bile and causes relaxation of the sphincter of the major duodenal papilla resulting in excretion of bile into the duodenum. Vagal parasympathetic innervation also contributes to GB contraction.

Diagnostic Imaging

Radiographic findings generally are insensitive for diseases of the EHBT with the exception of radiodense choleliths and emphysematous cholecystitis. Decreased serosal detail indicative of ascites may be identified radiographically in patients with bile peritonitis. Radiographic contrast studies (percutaneous transhepatic cholangiocystography) have been described for imaging the EHBT but largely have been replaced by ultrasonography. The ultrasonographic findings for EHBT diseases such as cholecystitis, cholelithiasis, and GB mucocele are well documented in the literature with abdominal ultrasound considered the standard imaging modality. A skilled ultrasonographer can evaluate the size and shape of the GB lumen, evaluate the integrity of the GB wall, measure the diameter of the CBD, evaluate the intrahepatic lobar ducts, and evaluate the region of the duodenal papillae. Evaluation for ascitic fluid during sonography is critical and fluid analysis can be a valuable diagnostic tool. (Cytologic evaluation includes evaluation for bile pigment, neutrophilic inflammation, and intracellular bacteria.) Dilation of the EHBT is time dependent after obstruction, and thus lack of dilation does not rule out biliary obstruction. In an experimental model in dogs, complete occlusion of the CBD resulted in GB distention within 24 hours, extrahepatic bile duct distention within 48 to 72 hours, and intrahepatic ductal dilation within 5 to 7 days. Chronic, partial CBD obstructions can provide a diagnostic dilemma because ultrasonographic findings can be subtle; the diagnosis is often presumptive.

Other diagnostic modalities infrequently used for the evaluation of the EHBT include cholecystography, hepatobiliary scintigraphy, endoscopic retrograde cholangiopancreatography, computed tomography, and magnetic resonance cholangiopancreatography. Cost, availability, patient size limitations, and the sensitivity of abdominal ultrasound generally preclude the use of these modalities.

Diseases

Cholecystitis

Cholecystitis can be categorized as necrotizing (type I), acute (type II), and chronic (type III) or emphysematous.

Ultrasound may identify a thickened GB wall, intraluminal echogenic debris, choleliths, EHBO, and emphysema of the GB wall. Ultrasound is highly sensitive for the identification of GB rupture (85% sensitivity). Loss of the GB wall continuity, hyperechoic fat in the cranial peritoneal cavity, and free abdominal fluid are supportive for GB rupture. Nonsurgical management of cholecystitis may be appropriate in select cases when the GB wall integrity is not compromised. Medical management includes antibiotic and analgesic therapy, choleretics (contraindicated preoperatively in patients with EHBO), and the treatment of any underlying comorbidities. Antibiotic therapy ideally should be guided by culture and sensitivity. In nonsurgical cases this would necessitate cholecystocentesis with the transhepatic method preferred to limit and contain leakage. Without samples for culture, empiric parenteral antibiotic therapy effective against gram-negative bacteria and anaerobic bacteria is advised. Cefoxitin, metronidazole, and/or enrofloxacin are appropriate antibiotic choices. *Escherichia coli*, *Enterococcus* spp., *Bacteroides* spp., and *Clostridium* spp. are among the most common isolates.

In patients with ultrasonographic evidence of severe GB wall compromise or GB rupture, cholecystectomy is advised. Histopathology and culture of the GB wall and luminal contents are imperative, and liver biopsies also are advised. Intraoperative evaluation of the patency of the CBD is mandatory and generally is performed via normograde catheterization of the CBD via the transected cystic duct. A red rubber (Brunswick) catheter generally is used. The surgeon must be certain to advance the catheter into the duodenum to confirm patency of the sphincter of the major duodenal papilla. Patients with cholecystitis can be compromised cardiovascularly with the need for aggressive perioperative crystalloid and colloid therapy. Pressor therapy also is needed frequently. Patients with chronic EHBO may be coagulopathic because of a relative deficiency in vitamin K from altered hepatobiliary excretion of bile acids required for vitamin K absorption. Coagulation profiles are advised perioperatively. Elevations in partial thromboplastin time (PTT) have been associated with a worse short-term outcome in dogs. Vitamin K_1 (0.5 mg/kg to 1.5 mg/kg IM or SC) can be administered with or without fresh frozen plasma. Chronic EHBO has been associated with septicemia, endotoxemia, and down-regulation of the reticuloendothelial system in humans and dogs.

A theoretic concern regarding perioperative analgesic therapy is the effect of pure mu-agonists, such as morphine, on smooth muscle tone. In humans, pure mu-agonists can increase the tone of the sphincter of the major duodenal papilla, resulting in a functional obstruction and increase in visceral pain. The effect in companion animals is documented poorly. Maropitant (Cerenia), a neurokinin-1 receptor antagonist, should be considered for managing visceral pain management and combating the nausea that can accompany distention of the EHBT.

Cholelithiasis

Cholelithiasis in companion animals is identified frequently as an incidental finding, and intervention in

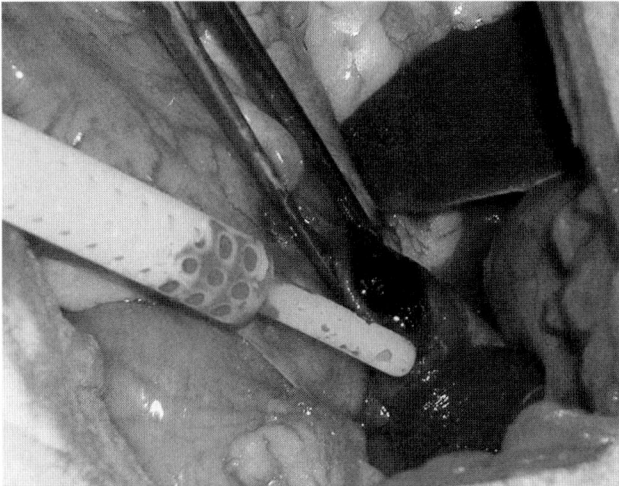

Figure 147-1 Intraoperative picture of a choledochotomy for cholelith removal. Note the cholelith (7 mm diameter) between the DeBakey forceps and the Poole suction tip. The choledochotomy site was created at the level of the cholelith slightly proximal to the duodenum.

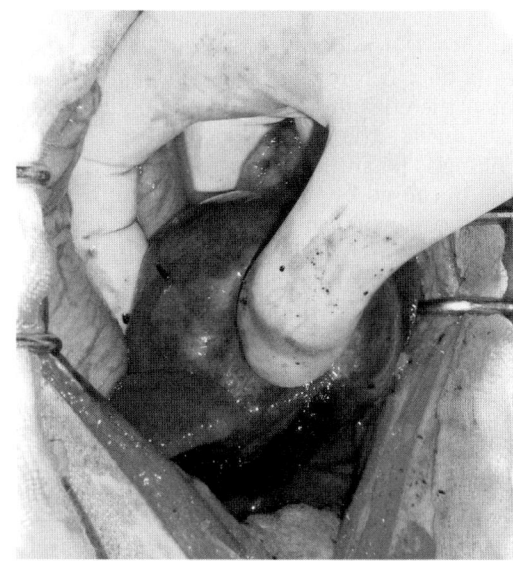

Figure 147-2 Intraoperative picture of a ruptured gallbladder (GB) mucocele before cholecystectomy. Note the extraluminal mucinous material (black) at the GB neck.

asymptomatic patients generally is not warranted. Most choleliths in companion animals contain calcium carbonate, bilirubin (pigment stones), and cholesterol. Although the exact mechanism is unknown, cholelith formation is a multifactorial process involving bile stasis, bile supersaturation, nidus formation, and alterations in crystallization inhibitors. Choleliths generally are formed in the GB; however, formation can occur within bile ducts or the CBD (choledocholithiasis) as a consequence of bile stasis, inflammation, or infection. Medical treatment of cholelithiasis includes broad-spectrum antibiotics (see antibiotic therapy for cholecystitis) and choleretic therapy to facilitate clearance of biliary aggregates (by promoting flow of lower viscosity bile). Treatment with ursodeoxycholic acid (UDCA, 10 to 20 mg/kg q24h PO) may have an advantage for choledocholiths lodged in small intrahepatic bile ducts that are not amenable to surgical intervention. Clinical signs associated with symptomatic cholelithiasis include progressive vomiting, dehydration, anorexia, icterus, and lethargy. The clinical signs may be indicative of obstructive disease or secondary cholecystitis and warrant surgical intervention. Cholecystectomy is reported to have a low morbidity with good clinical outcomes if choleliths are limited to the GB proper. Caution is warranted with patients with choledocholithiasis: cholecystectomy alone does not address the biliary obstruction. Such patients may require choledochostomy (Figure 147-1) or cholecystoenterostomy to reestablish bile flow. Cholecystotomy for cholelith removal rarely is indicated unless preservation of the GB is required for biliary diversion.

Gallbladder Mucoceles

It recently has been suggested that GB mucocele is the most common cause of EHBO in dogs (see Web Chapter 46). GB mucoceles are characterized histologically by hyperplasia of mucus-secreting glands within the GB mucosa, which results in an abnormal accumulation of mucus within the GB lumen. Extension of bile-laden mucus into the EHBT may result in various degrees of EHBO. Marked GB distention can result in GB rupture, which usually occurs at the fundus or junction of the cystic duct and hepatic ducts (Figure 147-2). Ultrasonographically, GB mucoceles are characterized by the presence of immobile, echogenic bile with a stellate pattern within the GB lumen. The pathogenesis remains unknown; however, a mutation in the canine gene *ABCB4* (which functions exclusively as a phospholipid translocator) has been identified recently in Shetland sheepdogs (and other breeds) with confirmed mucoceles. A weak association exists between mucocele formation and endocrine disease (hyperadrenocorticism and hypothyroidism) and exogenous steroid administration.

Dogs lacking clinical signs and with serum biochemical and ultrasonographic findings not supportive of EHBO or GB compromise may be candidates for medical management. Case reports in the literature have documented mucocele resolution with medical management. A combination of choleretic therapy (UDCA) and antibiotic therapy has been suggested. *S*-adenosylmethionine (SAMe; Denosyl) can provide hepatoprotective and antioxidant benefits. Sequential biochemical and ultrasound evaluations are necessary to monitor response to therapy. Prospective studies documenting medical therapy are warranted and currently ongoing.

Surgical intervention is necessary in patients exhibiting clinical signs attributed to mucocele formation or in patients with ultrasonographic or biochemical alterations consistent with EHBO or GB wall compromise. Cholecystoenterostomy and cholecystectomy have been reported in the surgical management of GB mucoceles. Cholecystectomy is preferred in the literature because of the excellent long-term results in patient's survival of the perioperative period (Figure 147-3). Concerns regarding the potential for mucocele recurrence and concerns

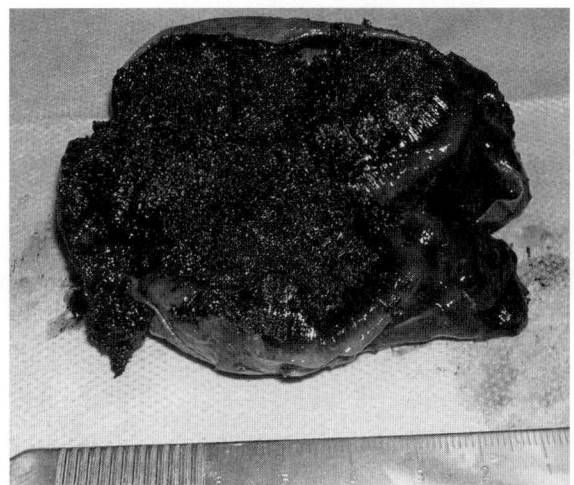

Figure 147-3 Cross-section of the gallbladder (GB) mucocele in Figure 147-2 after cholecystectomy. Striations in the organized luminal contents can be seen adjacent to the GB wall.

regarding the integrity of the GB wall also question the validity of cholecystoenterostomy in the management of GB mucoceles. At surgery, the CBD and visualized hepatic ducts must be cleared of obstructing mucinous debris. Patency of the sphincter of the major duodenal papilla also must be confirmed by catheterization. Normograde catheterization from the base of the cystic duct after cholecystectomy (but before cystic duct ligation) can accomplish confirmation of patency and avoid the need for a duodenotomy. The lack of a duodenotomy minimizes anesthetic time (which can be desirable in unstable anesthetic patients) and avoids the potential risk of enterotomy dehiscence. The potential value of a full-thickness small intestinal biopsy from the duodenotomy site should be considered in patients with a history suggestive of intestinal disease. Patients with ascites should have intraoperative samples collected for culture and warrant the consideration for peritoneal drainage (active suction Jackson-Pratt drains are the author's preference).

Long-term complications after cholecystectomy are uncommon. Clinicopathologic abnormalities are expected to normalize after GB excision; persistent clinicopathologic abnormalities are indicative of hepatopathy, cholangiohepatitis, or untreated endocrinopathies (emphasizing the value of a liver biopsy at the time of cholecystectomy). Persistent CBD dilation has been documented in approximately 25% of dogs after cholecystectomy, the cause of which is unknown. Recent studies of cholecystectomy in healthy dogs suggest that an increase in luminal pressure of the CBD after cholecystectomy and altered contraction of the sphincter of the major duodenal papilla are likely contributing factors to persistent CBD dilation.

Surgical Considerations

The veterinary literature over the past 15 years suggests survival in dogs and cats undergoing surgery of the EHBT is 64% and 41%, respectively (Mehler, 2011). The mortality rate for surgical intervention in cats with EHBO resulting from a neoplastic cause is nearly 100%. These extremely high mortality rates highlight the complex pathophysiology of hepatobiliary disease and highlight the systemic effects of EHBO.

With any biliary surgery, confirmation of patency of the CDB and duodenal papilla are of primary importance. Unfortunately, surgical determination of patency is subjective and visualization and palpation of the CBD alone is inadequate to determine patency. Evaluation of patency of the CBD via catheterization (normograde or retrograde) is critical for patients with biliary obstruction. Because of the anatomic considerations discussed retrograde catheterization (after duodenotomy) must be attempted with caution to avoid iatrogenic trauma to the duodenal papilla and pancreatic duct. Biliary stenting should be considered in patients at risk for recurrent obstruction (cholangitis or cholelithiasis) or patients with a persistent functional CBD obstruction (pancreatitis). With appropriate case selection, choledochal tube stenting can be an effective method to decompress the EHBT and is reported to have a lower morbidity than cholecystoenterostomy. Red rubber catheters (feeding or urethra) are the most commonly used luminal stents. Temporary stent position is maintained by suturing the stent to the duodenal mucosa with absorbable suture. After hydrolysis of the suture material, the stent is passed with intestinal luminal contents months later. The author has used human pediatric, self-expanding metallic stents in two clinical cases with excellent intermediate-term results. Such stents may have an advantage in that they expand the CBD rather than fill the lumen (as occurs with indwelling luminal catheters); further veterinary experience is needed. The reported morbidity of choledochal stenting is significantly greater in cats than in dogs. As veterinary experience with choledochal stenting evolves, endoscopic biliary stenting likely will become more common with limiting factors including patient size, biliary anatomy, and the need for specialized equipment.

The popularity of laparoscopic cholecystectomy (LC) has increased recently because of advances in surgical technique and improved availability. In the veterinary literature, LC has been described for the treatment of necrotizing cholecystitis, GB trauma, GB neoplasia, symptomatic cholelithiasis, and GB mucocele. The primary limitation of LC is the inability to evaluate completely patency of the CBD, restricting its use to diseases of the GB in patients that do not have ultrasonographic or biochemical evidence of CBD involvement.

References and Suggested Reading

Buote NJ et al: Cholecystoenterostomy for treatment of extrahepatic biliary tract obstruction in cats: 22 cases, *J Am Vet Med Assoc* 228:1376, 2006.

Center SA: Diseases of the gallbladder and biliary tree, *Vet Clin North Am Small Anim Pract* 39(3):543-598, 2009.

Mayhew PD et al: Choledochal tube stenting for decompression of the extrahepatic portion of the biliary tract in dogs: 13 cases, *J Am Vet Med Assoc* 228:1209, 2006.

Mehler SJ: Complications of the extrahepatic biliary surgery in companion animals, *Vet Clin North Am Small Anim Pract* 41(5):949-967, 2011.

Pike FS et al: Gallbladder mucocele in dogs: 30 cases, *J Am Vet Med Assoc* 224:1615, 2004.

CHAPTER 148

Idiopathic Vacuolar Hepatopathy

DAVID C. TWEDT, *Fort Collins, Colorado*

Hepatic vacuolar change is a common histologic diagnosis in dogs but not cats. In the author's review of 150 consecutive liver biopsies performed at Colorado State University approximately 12% of the cases had predominantly a vacuolar hepatopathy (VH) as the major histologic finding. By definition according to the World Small Animal Veterinary Association (WSAVA) Liver Standardization Group, VH refers to a reversible parenchymal change characterized by swollen hepatocytes with clear cytoplasm resulting from glycogen without displacement of the nucleus from the center (Cullen et al, 2006). The distribution and the extent of the lesion can be diffuse or zonal or involve individual cells. VH is a relatively easy histologic diagnosis to make; however, periodic acid-Schiff (PAS) staining with or without diastase can be used to demonstrate glycogen accumulation. Vacuolated hepatocytes also can result from fat accumulation secondary to abnormal fat metabolism and is referred to as hepatic steatosis or lipidosis. Hepatic steatosis is a distinct histologic vacuolar classification associated with abnormal fat metabolism and is not discussed in this chapter.

Cause

VH in dogs is associated most often with hyperadrenocorticism (HAC). The dog is particularly sensitive to the effects of glucocorticoids that induce serum alkaline phosphatase (ALP) steroid isoenzyme activity and cause hepatic glycogen accumulation (see Web Chapter 50). Congenital glycogen storage disorders, breed-specific disorders, hepatic nodular hyperplasia, and a variety of stress-associated secondary diseases are conditions that can cause this typical hepatic vacuolar change. A large study of 336 histologic liver specimens having VH (defined as making up greater than 25% of the hepatocytes) were reviewed retrospectively for an underlying etiology (Hill et al, 2006). The authors reported 55% of the cases were associated with either endogenous or exogenous glucocorticoids and 45% had no known glucocorticoid exposure. Most of the dogs with no glucocorticoid exposure had other identifiable concurrent illness. Conditions such as renal, immune-mediated, cardiac, hepatic, or gastrointestinal disease or neoplasia accounted for many cases. The author's hypothesis was that stress-induced hypercortisolemia associated with acute or chronic illness likely contributed to the

development of the VH. A second *in vivo* study showed that experimentally inducing chronic fourfold to fivefold elevations in plasma cortisol concentrations to simulate a stresslike state in normal dogs resulted in inhibited nonhepatic glucose use and increased hepatic gluconeogenesis and glycogen formation through enhanced substrate delivery to the liver (Goldstein et al, 1993).

A rare cause of VH is glycogen storage disease. These are groups of congenital disorders with deficient or defective activity of the enzymes responsible for metabolizing hepatic glycogen (Specht et al, 2011). Affected dogs are young, exhibit signs of hypoglycemia, and have large livers with marked glycogen accumulation. Hepatic nodular hyperplasia is a common, benign intrahepatic event; it causes an increase in liver enzymes and histologic changes, which include macroscopic or microscopic hepatic nodules that often contain a VH. VH also is observed in the regenerative nodules of dogs with the hepatocutaneous syndrome.

Idiopathic Vacuolar Hepatopathy

However, a subset of dogs have elevations in serum ALP and excessive hepatic glycogen accumulation that do not have evidence of a stress-induced illness or HAC based on cortisol testing, a history of recent glucocorticoid administration, or a specific hepatic disease. These dogs are referred to as having an idiopathic vacuolar hepatopathy (IVH). They generally have no clinical signs and usually are identified during investigation of unexplained elevations in serum ALP found on routine health screens. Several theories have been proposed regarding the cause of IVH. Some believe adrenal progestagens are the cause; most likely increases in 17-hydroxyprogesterone and progesterone are responsible as these abnormalities are frequently identified when using a commercial adrenal steroid panel. However, critical evaluation and validation of adrenal steroid panels (measuring 17-hydroxyprogesterone, progesterone, estradiol, testosterone, and androstenedione) are still lacking, and a direct association to IVH has not been made. To confuse matters further, the author and others have observed similar abnormalities in noncortisol adrenal steroids in dogs without IVH or having increases in serum ALP, which casts doubt on the relationship of these specific progestagens in this condition. Progestagens are reported to bind to glucocorticoid receptors, but whether they can induce a glucocorticoid response is unknown. One *in vitro* study found that sex hormones do not induce ALP production in isolated hepatocytes (see Chapter 50 for more detail). Some suggest that progestagens may act by increasing the bioavailability of cortisol by competing for the same binding receptors; this results in an increase in endogenous cortisol, which causes the VH. However, IVH dogs by definition have normal serum cortisol concentrations (see Chapter 50). Because the VH changes are typical of glucocorticoid excess, an adrenal steroid yet to be identified could be responsible for the VH. Obviously future research is necessary to delineate this syndrome and the relationship to adrenal steroids.

Scottish terriers also are reported to have a breed-specific syndrome associated with a VH and elevated serum ALP (Zimmerman et al, 2010). These affected dogs generally have no clinical signs. The authors of this study found that the elevated ALP was predominantly the corticosteroid isoform and following ACTH stimulation test in conjunction with an adrenal steroid panel found increases in one or more noncortisol steroid hormones. The authors concluded that affected Scottish terriers have a type of HAC on the basis of exaggerated adrenal hormone response. The author of this chapter also has observed similar noncortisol steroid hormone increases in Scottish terriers but also in Scottish terriers without VH or increases in ALP, adding more confusion to this syndrome. See Chapter 51 for further information on adrenal steroids.

Clinical Findings

Dogs with IVH generally have no clinical signs. They usually are identified serendipitously on a biochemical profile identifying elevations in serum ALP concentrations, which subsequently initiates a diagnostic workup. Most affected dogs are middle-aged or older at the time of diagnosis. No breed or sex predisposition is apparent other than the syndrome described above in the Scottish terrier. A small percentage of dog owners may have reported polyuria and polydipsia (PU/PD) in their dogs, but the other signs typical of HAC generally are absent.

Diagnosis

The workup of the asymptomatic dog with an IVH usually begins after the identification of an elevation in serum ALP. The ALP increases are often 5 to 10 times normal concentrations; the other liver enzymes are usually normal, or occasional mild elevations in alanine aminotransferase (ALT) and γ-glutamyltransferase (GGT) occur. Marked elevations in liver enzymes other than ALP are not typical of this syndrome, and if present other types of liver disease should be investigated. The workup first should rule out common causes for an elevated ALP such as drug administration (including topical or systemic steroids, phenobarbital, or herbal medications), cholestatic liver disease, or bone disorders. Next adrenal testing (ACTH stimulation or low-dose dexamethasone suppression) would be prudent to eliminate the possibility of HAC. Determining the percentage of ALP steroid isoenzyme is generally not helpful. Dogs with IVH have predominantly a steroid-induced ALP isoenzyme. However, this is specific for neither HAC nor IVH. Furthermore, other nonadrenal illness also may have similar increases in the steroid-induced ALP isoenzyme. Basic tests of liver function tend to be normal; however, the author has seen a few cases having mild elevations in serum bile acids. Abdominal ultrasound of the liver is helpful to rule out hepatic nodular hyperplasia, occult hepatic neoplasia, or cholestatic disorders, which all could be differentials for an elevated ALP. Affected IVH dogs generally have an enlarged, uniformly hyperechoic liver with rounded borders. Adrenal glands are generally normal. Fine-needle aspiration of the liver with cytology supports a diffuse vacuolar change. A PAS stain of the cytology sample can help confirm the presence of hepatic glycogen. A liver biopsy confirms diffuse vacuolar change but rarely is necessary. The author generally makes the diagnosis of IVH based on the above diagnostic findings and after exclusion of HAC, drugs, hepatic nodular hyperplasia, hepatic neoplasia, or cholestatic liver disease.

The author believes adrenal sex steroid panel testing for most cases is not necessary for two reasons: (1) the inability to interpret adequately the test results and (2) almost all IVH dogs generally are asymptomatic and information obtained from the testing offers little important diagnostic or therapeutic information. Several labs offer adrenal hormone analysis. Currently the most extensive adrenal steroid hormone profile is offered by the Clinical Endocrinology Laboratory at the University of Tennessee. The protocol for running the test is identical to that for a standard ACTH stimulation test.

Complicating Factors

Proteinuria and hypertension occasionally are identified in cases of IVH, and the affected dog should be monitored periodically for these complications and, if identified, managed appropriately. Dogs with IVH also are thought to have an increased risk for developing biliary mucoceles. Some anecdotal evidence suggests that some Scottish terriers with VH are at an increased risk of development of hepatic neoplasia (hepatocellular adenoma or carcinoma). Consequently, it would be prudent to monitor IVH dogs every 6 to 12 months with an ultrasound of the liver and biliary system.

Treatment

The management of IVH is controversial and no studies critically evaluate therapy for this syndrome. The author believes that specific therapy is unnecessary unless complicating factors such as hypertension, proteinuria, or significant PU/PD exist. Problems associated with therapy arise from the fact that the desired end point of therapy is unknown. Is the desired result normalization of adrenal hormones, return of ALP into the normal range, or histologic resolution of the VH? In anecdotal reports dogs with IVH were treated successfully using low doses of mitotane; monitoring clinical parameters; and measuring adrenal steroid concentrations, including cortisol, to ensure hypoadrenocorticism does not result. Trilostane often shows a similar clinical response; however, concentrations of 17-hydroxyprogesterone and progesterone are frequently higher after this therapy. Anecdotal reports of clinical improvement in dogs with IVH using either therapy suggest that abnormal adrenal steroid production may be involved in the pathogenesis of this syndrome. However, these treatments cast doubt on whether therapy is warranted because of (1) the expense of medication and monitoring and (2) the potential complications associated with the therapy. Until more is known about this syndrome this author cannot recommend specific adrenal therapy unless significant clinical findings warrant a trial therapy.

Alternative therapies suggested include melatonin and flaxseed products. Melatonin has been shown to decrease sex hormone concentrations in normal dogs. It is reportedly beneficial in some dogs with alopecia X syndrome and has been suggested for IVH. Dosages of 3 mg/15 kg q24h PO have been recommended; however, no published data demonstrate effectiveness for dogs with IVH. Flaxseed hull products with lignans also have been suggested because they compete with estradiol production; however, there is no reported evidence of benefit for IVH syndrome.

Liver support therapy using products such as S-adenosylmethionine (SAMe), the milk thistle products, or other antioxidants may have some beneficial effects. One study showed dogs given glucocorticoids and treated with SAMe failed to show a decrease in serum ALP or amount of VH but did have improvement in hepatocyte oxidative status through increased glutathione concentrations (Center et al, 2005). The above products are generally safe for liver support but are unlikely to have any effect in the resolution of IVH.

Prognosis

The prognosis for most dogs with IVH is generally good, and most remain asymptomatic for years without specific therapy. However, the author has observed a small number of dogs developing overt HAC requiring specific therapy.

References and Suggested Reading

Behrend EN et al: Serum 17-α-hydroxyprogesterone and corticosterone concentrations in dogs with nonadrenal neoplasia and dogs with suspected hyperadrenocorticism, *J Am Vet Med Assoc* 227:1762, 2005.

Benitah N et al: Evaluation of serum 17-hydroxyprogesterone concentrations after administration of ACTH in dogs with hyperadrenocorticism, *J Am Vet Med Assoc* 227:1095, 2005.

Center SA et al: Evaluation of the influence of S-adenosylmethionine on systemic and hepatic effects of prednisolone in dogs, *Am J Vet Res* 66:330, 2005.

Cullen JM et al: Normal histology, reversible hepatocytic injury and hepatic amyloidosis. In Rothuizen J et al, editors: *WSAVA standards for clinical and histological diagnosis of canine and feline liver diseases*, Edinburgh, 2006, Saunders/Elsevier, p 77.

Goldstein RE et al: Effects of chronic elevation in plasma cortisol on hepatic carbohydrate metabolism, *Am J Physiol* 264:E119, 1993.

Hill KE et al: Secretion of sex hormones in dogs with adrenal dysfunction, *J Am Vet Med Assoc* 226:556, 2005.

Hill KE et al: Vacuolar hepatopathy in dogs: 336 cases (1993-2005), *J Am Vet Med Assoc* 229:246, 2006.

Specht A et al: Glycogen storage disease type Ia in canines: a model for human metabolic and genetic liver disease, *J Biomed Biotechnol* ID 646257, 2011.

Zimmerman KL et al: Hyperphosphatasemia and concurrent adrenal gland dysfunction in apparently healthy Scottish Terriers, *J Am Vet Med Assoc* 237:178, 2010.

CHAPTER 149

Feline Hepatic Lipidosis

STEVE L. HILL, *San Diego, California*
P. JANE ARMSTRONG, *St. Paul, Minnesota*

Hepatic lipidosis (HL) is an intrahepatic cholestatic syndrome resulting from excessive accumulation of lipid within hepatocytes that can lead to severe hepatic dysfunction. Since the initial description in 1977 (Barsanti et al, 1977), HL has emerged as the most common liver disease diagnosed in cats in North America. It is seen in other parts of the world, although anecdotally not as commonly in some regions (Armstrong and Blanchard, 2009). HL may occur secondary to any disease process that results in protracted partial or complete anorexia. Decreased food intake may be for a period of time as short as 2 days (Center, 2005a). Common

concurrent diseases associated with the development of HL include pancreatitis, other hepatic disorders such as cholangitis (see Chapter 150), small intestinal disease, neoplasia, kidney disease, and diabetes mellitus. Concurrent diseases are reported to occur in more than 95% of HL cases (Center, 2005a). HL also occurs less commonly as an idiopathic (primary) condition in an otherwise healthy cat with inadequate food intake. Decreased food intake may occur with forced overly rapid weight loss, unintentional food deprivation, a change to a diet unacceptable to the cat, a sudden change in lifestyle, or stress (e.g., boarding). Early consideration of a diagnosis of HL, identification of any underlying disease process, and prompt initiation of medical and nutritional therapy are essential for the successful management of cats with HL.

Pathogenesis

Prolonged protein and/or calorie malnutrition in cats can result in derangement in all aspects of normal lipid metabolism including mobilization of fatty acids from adipocytes, fatty acid metabolism within hepatocytes, and removal of lipid from hepatocytes. Anorexia is the major clinical aspect of the disease; however, the cause for anorexia in the idiopathic form is undetermined. During a period of anorexia, peripheral lipolysis occurs through the stimulation of hormone-sensitive lipase, resulting in a dramatic increase in the concentration of free fatty acids in the blood. Circulating fatty acids taken up by the liver are either metabolized for energy or converted to triglycerides and stored or secreted back into the circulation as very-low-density lipoproteins (VLDL). If fatty acid delivery exceeds the capacity of the liver to oxidize or secrete them, excessive storage occurs and the clinical syndrome of lipidosis develops. The triglyceride content in the liver of cats with HL averages 43% compared with 1% in the liver of healthy cats (Hall et al, 1997). Although still incompletely understood, the pathogenesis of HL is probably multifactorial, involving factors that affect fatty-acid mobilization to liver, mitochondrial or peroxisomal oxidation of fatty acids in hepatocytes, and the synthesis and possibly secretion of VLDL. Several theories on the pathogenesis of HL have been proposed and have been the topic of some investigations. Hepatic accumulation of fatty acids has been proposed to be due to L-carnitine or apolipoprotein deficiency, but research has failed to substantiate these as primary mechanisms (Armstrong and Blanchard, 2009). Systemic oxidative injury, to which cats are particularly susceptible under normal conditions, also is augmented greatly in cats with HL (Center et al, 2005b) and is reflected by the characteristic presence of Heinz bodies on a complete blood count (CBC).

History and Clinical Signs

Most cats affected with HL are middle-aged, obese, or overweight adults. Although the condition has been reported in a wide age range of cats (Center, 2005a), the median age at presentation is 7 years, which tends to overlap the peak prevalence of obesity. Most reports have failed to show a gender or breed predilection. Most cats are obese or overweight at presentation or historically. Anorexia is the most common and sometimes is the only presenting complaint, with the period of anorexia ranging from 2 days to several weeks. Weight loss is common and can be profound, with concurrent sarcopenia (loss of muscle mass). Other common historical findings are lethargy, jaundice, vomiting, diarrhea or constipation, and an unkempt, poor-quality haircoat. Observant owners may report jaundice. In the absence of signs associated with an underlying disease or complicating factors such as severe hypokalemia or hepatic encephalopathy (HE), HL cats may be bright and alert despite profound anorexia and the presence of marked jaundice.

Physical examination commonly reveals lethargy, dehydration, and jaundice (about 70% of cases). Non-painful smooth hepatomegaly is common but not always present. Loss of muscle mass despite retention of fat stores can make assigning a BCS difficult. The falciform and inguinal fat pads characteristically are retained and can be seen radiographically and ultrasonographically. Severe electrolyte abnormalities, especially hypokalemia and/or hypophosphatemia, and potentially thiamine deficiency, can result in marked muscle weakness and ventroflexion of the neck. Although spontaneous bleeding is uncommon, bruising or hemorrhage from venipuncture or cystocentesis sites may reflect an underlying coagulopathy. Signs of HE, most notably ptyalism and mental dullness, occur in a minority (<5%) of cases (Center, 2005a). Ptyalism also may reflect nausea. Any concurrent disease resulting in anorexia, especially in an overweight cat, can trigger secondary HL. With this in mind any clinical findings related to a concurrent disease can be superimposed on the above clinical signs of HL (e.g., weakness, abdominal pain, or mass).

Diagnostic Evaluation

The diagnostic goal in cats with HL is twofold: establishing a diagnosis of lipidosis and a simultaneous workup for the presence of an underlying disease process. The diagnosis of HL is based on a compatible history, clinical signs, and biochemical and ultrasonographic abnormalities with cytologic or histopathologic confirmation. Additional tests to identify concurrent disease processes include feline pancreatic lipase immunoreactivity (Spec fPL, Snap fPL) and thoracic radiographs. A total T_4 and testing for feline leukemia virus antigen and feline immunodeficiency virus antibody also may be advisable.

Clinicopathologic Findings

The CBC is most commonly within normal limits with primary HL. There may be nonspecific abnormalities such as mild to moderate normocytic, normochromic nonregenerative anemia, poikilocytosis (erythrocytes with an abnormal shape), large numbers of Heinz bodies, lymphopenia, and a mild leukocytosis. The clinician should be aware that because of susceptibility to oxidative stress that occurs with HL poikilocytosis, Heinz bodies and anemia may develop during treatment. The presence of an inflammatory leukogram is uncommon in the idiopathic form of HL and when present should trigger a search for an underlying disorder.

Serum biochemical abnormalities in HL are typical of an intrahepatic cholestatic disorder. The most consistent abnormalities are an increase in serum bilirubin concentration and increased liver enzyme activities. Serum alkaline phosphatase (ALP) activity is increased more consistently than alanine aminotransferase (ALT) and aspartate aminotransferase (AST) activities. Increased γ-glutamyltransferase (GGT) activity is elevated inconsistently. Although the magnitude of increase in GGT tends to parallel the magnitude of increase in ALP in other forms of liver disease with HL, the GGT tends to be minimally increased or remains within the reference range (Center et al, 1993). Hypokalemia, hypophosphatemia, and/or hypomagnesemia are seen in some cases at presentation or may develop during treatment. Hypokalemia has been reported to be a negative prognostic indicator along with advanced age and lower PCV (Center et al, 1993). Hypertriglyceridemia, hypercholesterolemia, and transient hyperglycemia also may be observed. Hypoglycemia, hypoalbuminemia, and low blood urea nitrogen may occur and are indicators of significant altered hepatic dysfunction.

The urine of cats with HL commonly reveals bilirubinuria, and lipiduria may be noted on sediment examination or during sonographic evaluation (Armstrong and Blanchard, 2009).

Abnormalities in coagulation tests are reported to be common but resulted in clinically recognized bleeding in less than 4% of cats with severe HL. One or more coagulation abnormalities occurred in 45% of cats with severe HL, with the most common being a prolongation of the prothrombin time (PT) (Center et al, 1993). Response to vitamin K supplementation in cats with HL suggests that the coagulopathy is the result of vitamin K deficiency rather than decreased coagulation factor production because of hepatocellular failure. Intrahepatic cholestasis leading to reduced enterohepatic circulation of bile acids resulting in reduced absorption of fat-soluble vitamins is the suspected mechanism. Although the PIVKA test (proteins invoked by vitamin K antagonism or absence, Thrombotest) may be a more sensitive indicator of prolonged clotting times in cats with HL, this test is not always readily available. Specific liver function testing is not necessary in most cases of HL. Bile acid testing is not indicated if the cat is bilirubinuric or hyperbilirubinemic. Although HE is an uncommon metabolic consequence in HL, if HE is suspected, fasting ammonia measurement can help support the diagnosis of HE and guide therapeutic intervention.

Diagnostic Imaging

Ultrasonography is the most useful modality available for abdominal imaging. In addition to hepatobiliary evaluation, ultrasonography permits imaging of other abdominal organs to detect abnormalities associated with diseases that accompany HL. Evaluation of the gastrointestinal tract, pancreas, and lymph nodes is particularly important; ultrasonography readily allows detection of ascites, abdominal organ masses, and other abnormalities. Hepatomegaly is a frequent finding. Diffuse hyperechogenicity of the liver is a characteristic finding with HL; however, it is not pathognomonic and may be seen with other liver diseases and in obese cats or diabetic cats without the clinical syndrome of HL (Nicoll et al, 1998; Yeager and Mohammed, 1992). Although the overall accuracy of ultrasonographic evaluation as the sole criterion for discriminating among categories of diffuse liver disease in cats has been shown to be less than 60% regardless of biochemical or hematologic variables, the exception to this finding was HL. Greater than 70% of HL cases were classified correctly by radiologists in this study (Feeney et al, 2008).

Liver Cytology and Biopsy

Ultrasonographically guided fine-needle aspiration provides samples that in most cases are adequate for establishing a presumptive diagnosis of HL, especially when the index of suspicion is high based on the history, clinical, clinicopathologic, and diagnostic imaging findings. With HL, cytologic examination of the liver reveals cytosolic vacuolization of the majority (80% or more) of sampled hepatocytes. Vacuoles may be large, small, or a mixture of sizes. Aspiration cytology may confirm cytosolic vacuolar change in the liver but may fail to identify other important diagnoses, such as inflammatory or infiltrative disease. An advantage of liver aspiration is that it almost always can be performed without sedation or anesthesia during the initial diagnostic ultrasound and complications are uncommon.

A liver biopsy is not recommended or necessary for all cats with suspected HL. The potential risks must be considered carefully before deciding to biopsy the liver. At presentation, many HL cats are not candidates for general anesthesia, which is required for biopsies. Stabilization by correcting fluid, electrolyte, metabolic, and coagulation abnormalities is essential before pursuing general anesthesia. Biopsy confirmation is indicated if the number of inflammatory cells observed cytologically is judged to be excessive relative to the peripheral neutrophil count or if the cat fails to respond to appropriate nutritional support by showing an approximately 50% reduction in serum bilirubin concentration within about a week of initiation of therapy (Center, 2005a). Liver biopsies can be obtained percutaneously with ultrasonographic guidance, laparoscopically, or at laparotomy. Laparoscopic biopsies are preferred by many experienced operators. Laparoscopy is minimally invasive and allows for direct visualization of the liver, sampling of multiple liver lobes, and control of hemorrhage should it occur. Laparoscopic samples also minimize the risk of discordance between core needle and larger tissue samples (Cole et al, 2002). If indicated, ultrasonographically guided fine-needle aspirates of the pancreas or laparoscopic pancreatic biopsies also can be obtained.

Treatment

Treatment of HL initially requires correction of fluid and electrolyte abnormalities, but the cornerstone of therapy is enteral nutritional support with a focus on meeting protein and caloric needs via a feeding tube. Complications of HL such as vomiting, HE, or bleeding tendencies also must be managed. An important component of treatment is the diagnosis and concurrent management of any underlying disease process. Client education and encouragement is important; significant owner participation is necessary for a successful outcome of this reversible condition.

Fluid and Electrolyte Therapy

Most HL cats are dehydrated at the time of presentation primarily from vomiting and lack of intake. In most cases, intravenous therapy is the route of choice for fluid administration. Subcutaneous fluids may be adequate for mildly affected cats and also can be used when financial constraints are imposed. A balanced polyionic crystalloid fluid is recommended. Impaired lactate metabolism is suspected in cats with severe HL, leading some authors to advise against using lactated Ringer's solution (Center, 2005a). Although a theoretical concern, lactated Ringer's solution commonly is used with success by many clinicians. Unless hypoglycemia is present, dextrose-containing fluids are contraindicated in cats with HL because they are glucose intolerant, and glucose may potentiate hepatic triglyceride accumulation, inhibit fatty acid oxidation, and worsen electrolyte depletion.

Electrolyte abnormalities, especially hypokalemia and hypophosphatemia, are an important cause of morbidity and mortality in HL cats. These abnormalities may be present at admission or develop as a result of fluid therapy or secondary to a refeeding syndrome. Refeeding syndrome is a condition characterized by severe electrolyte and fluid shifts in malnourished patients undergoing initial feeding. With refeeding, insulin release stimulates cellular uptake of glucose, phosphate, potassium, magnesium, and water as well as enhanced protein synthesis. As noted above, enteral feeding is critical to the recovery of HL cats, but the clinician must monitor carefully for components of the refeeding syndrome and treat accordingly. Hypokalemia is the most common electrolyte disturbance. Lethargy, muscle weakness, ventroflexion of the neck, gastrointestinal stasis, cardiac arrhythmias, and inability to concentrate urine can develop when serum K+ is 2.5 mEq/L or less. Supplemental potassium chloride (KCl) is added to fluids using the conventional sliding scale at a rate of no more than 0.5 mEq/kg body weight per hour. Enteral supplementation with potassium gluconate syrup, gel, or granules (starting dose of 2 mEq per day) can be used if necessary when parenteral supplementation is discontinued. Hypokalemia may persist in the face of appropriate supplementation if there is concurrent hypomagnesemia (see Chapter 56). Enteral feeding usually is sufficient to resolve hypomagnesemia.

Hypophosphatemia is another potentially serious electrolyte abnormality that may be evident at presentation but more commonly develops secondary to refeeding syndrome. Phosphorus deficiency can result in hemolytic anemia, but other complications include muscle weakness and nonspecific gastrointestinal signs. When levels fall below 1.5 to 2 mg/dl, the clinician should add potassium phosphate or sodium phosphate (both contain 3 mmol phosphate/ml) to the intravenous fluids and administer at 0.03 to 0.12 mmol/kg/hr with careful monitoring. Phosphate should be administered in calcium- and magnesium-free solutions to prevent precipitation. If using potassium phosphate, clinicians must consider the potassium content to avoid potassium oversupplementation (one may need to reduce the amount of potassium chloride supplementation). After correction of hypophosphatemia with parenteral supplementation and provision of a balanced diet, continued phosphorus supplementation is rarely necessary.

Hypocalcemia is an uncommon finding in HL and should be confirmed with measurement of an ionized

calcium concentration. Low ionized calcium concentration should alert the clinician to the possibility of acute necrotizing pancreatitis. Calcium therapy would be indicated if clinical signs of hypocalcemia occur.

Enteral Feeding

Enteral feeding must be initiated as early as possible in HL cases and be sustained until adequate voluntary food intake resumes. Oral forced feeding may be tolerated by some cats but it generally is inadequate to provide enough calories to reverse HL. Force feeding also can be stressful and may exacerbate nausea and vomiting and could result in aversion to food, which may delay the return to self-alimentation. Appetite stimulants generally are not recommended in cats with HL. Although they may increase appetite transiently, they are unreliable for ensuring adequate caloric intake and may encourage a false sense of nutritional support success. In addition, drug metabolism may be impaired in cats with HL, making dosing and side effects unpredictable. The authors prefer to use mirtazapine (1.875 to 3.75 mg per cat q72h PO) for an appetite stimulant because it likely has appetite-stimulating and antiemetic effects (Quimby et al, 2010). A second choice of appetite stimulant is cyproheptadine (1 to 2 mg/cat q12-24h PO). Oral forced feeding and appetite stimulants usually are reserved for very early or mild cases or for cases with financial constraints and when tube feeding is declined.

Provision of adequate calories to reverse the progression of HL almost always requires placement of a feeding tube. Nasoesophageal (NE) and esophagostomy tubes are most commonly used; however, gastrostomy tubes are also an option (see Chapter 136 in the previous edition of *Current Veterinary Therapy*). One option is initially to place an NE tube and begin feeding until the cat is judged to be sufficiently metabolically stable for general anesthesia. An NE tube is inexpensive, is placed under local anesthesia, and is easy to use and remove. It requires close observation of the patient and usually an Elizabethan collar to prevent tube removal by the cat. A liquid diet (e.g., CliniCare) is required (see Dietary Considerations later in this chapter).

An esophagostomy tube (e.g., 19 French [Fr] Feline Esophagostomy Tube; 19 Fr Small Animal Esophagostomy Tube; 18 Fr red rubber tube) is a good choice for longer-term feeding. In some cats, placement of a primary esophagostomy feeding tube is possible within the first 24 hours of admission. Placement of either an esophagostomy or gastrostomy tube allows feeding of a blended solid (canned) food diet in the home environment until the HL is resolved and self-alimentation is resumed. Multiple anesthetic protocols suitable for patients with hepatic disease may be considered. Despite some controversy, propofol appears to be safe to induce anesthesia in cats with primary HL for placement of a feeding tube (Posner, Asakawa, and Erb, 2008) and commonly is used by both authors for that purpose. Use of the non–preservative-containing propofol (PropoFlo) is recommended. PropoFlo 28 is not recommended until further safety information is available because the product contains added benzyl alcohol as a preservative, which could have deleterious effects in cats with HL.

Dietary Considerations

Protein is the nutrient class most efficient at reducing hepatic lipid accumulation in cats with negative nitrogen balance, and when adequate energy must be provided to reverse HL, fat efficiently provides those calories. Consequently diets that derive the majority of their calories from protein and fat should be used. Carbohydrates are less well tolerated than lipids as a source of calories and diets too high in carbohydrates may cause diarrhea, abdominal cramping, borborygmus, and hyperglycemia (Armstrong and Blanchard, 2009). Many commercially available diets meet these requirements including CliniCare (good for NE tube feeding), Maximum Calorie, and Prescription Diets a/d, m/d, c/d, or p/d. The exception to feeding a high-protein diet is in the few HL cats (less than 5%) that develop HE. In these cases, feeding a diet moderate in protein such as Prescription diet l/d or k/d or CliniCare RF is indicated.

Feeding Protocol

Cats with HL are often volume intolerant when feeding is begun, necessitating slow implementation of the feeding plan. Cats recovering from HL generally are fed at calculated resting energy requirement (RER) (see Chapter 136 in the previous edition of *Current Veterinary Therapy*). Reaching RER may take 3 to 7 days. During the initial period of volume intolerance, a continuous rate infusion (CRI) of a liquid diet may be more practical than multiple small bolus feedings per day. Administration of a prokinetic agent and pharmacologic control of apparent nausea and vomiting are recommended. Persistence with feeding is necessary, even when some vomiting or other signs of volume intolerance occurs. For feeding via esophagostomy or gastrostomy tube, Maximum Calorie is preferred by the authors because of its high caloric density (2.1 kcal/ml) compared with most other commercial recovery-formula foods, which typically provide about 1 kcal/ml. Canned foods usually are diluted with water (30 to 90 ml for a 5.5 to 6 oz can) to achieve a consistency that flows easily through the tube and helps meet patient fluid requirements. A higher caloric density food allows energy requirements to be met with a lower total food volume. This helps improve patient tolerance and may increase client compliance as feeding frequency generally can be three to four times daily.

Other Therapeutic Considerations

Antiemetic and Prokinetic Therapy

Vomiting is a common clinical problem in cats with HL and often persists during the first week of refeeding despite gradual introduction of increasing meal volumes or use of a CRI. Control of emesis usually is achieved in cats with maropitant citrate (Cerenia) 1 mg/kg q24h SC or PO (Hickman et al, 2008). Because maropitant is metabolized by the liver a dosage of 0.5 mg/kg is sometimes used. Because SC administration is associated with irritation on injection, maropitant commonly is administered (off-label) intravenously at the same dose and interval. Increasing evidence suggests maropitant also provides visceral analgesia (Boscan et al, 2011). This would be useful in an HL cat with concurrent pancreatitis. Metoclopramide (CRI 1 to 2 mg/kg/day or 0.2 to 0.5 mg/kg q8h SC or PO 30 minutes before feeding) commonly is used for its prokinetic effects, even though it is a weak antiemetic in cats. Cisapride (obtained from a compounding pharmacy) at a dosage of 3 mg/kg/day divided based on the frequency of feeding (1.0 mg/kg if feeding q8h, 0.75 mg/kg if feeding q6h, 0.5 mg/kg if feeding q4h) administered 30 minutes before feeding PO is preferred as it may be a more effective prokinetic drug than metoclopramide (see Chapter 125). If emesis persists, ondansetron 0.1 to 1 mg/kg q12-24h IV or PO or dolasetron 0.5 to 1 mg/kg q12-24h IV also can be prescribed. If mirtazapine is used as an appetite stimulant, it also likely has an antiemetic effect. An H_2 receptor antagonist (famotidine 0.5 to 1.0 mg/kg q12-24h IV or PO) often is prescribed nonspecifically in vomiting animals to protect the lower esophagus from acid damage.

Cobalamin Therapy

Cobalamin (B_{12}) deficiency may occur in cats with HL, especially when there is underlying gastrointestinal disease (see Chapter 127). Hypocobalaminemia can impair nutrient absorption and is occasionally severe enough to produce neuromuscular signs. It is recommended that serum cobalamin be measured in cats with HL, especially if concurrent intestinal disease is suspected. The preferred route for cobalamin supplementation is parenteral at a dosage of 250 µg/injection every 7 days SC for 6 weeks, then one dose after 30 days, then reevaluate a serum cobalamin 30 days later. Cobalamin also may have a pharmacologic effect as an appetite stimulant.

Treatment of Coagulation Disorders

Apparent Vitamin K deficiency makes parenteral supplementation of vitamin K_1 necessary for cats with demonstrated coagulopathy and provides the rationale for empiric administration, especially if a liver biopsy is planned. Vitamin K_1 is administered at a dose of 0.5 to 1.5 mg/kg q12h SC for 2 to 3 doses. If necessary, coagulation disorders can be managed with fresh frozen plasma or fresh blood, as indicated.

Specific Micronutrient and Other Supplements

Supplementation with specific micronutrients has been suggested by some authors (Center, 2005a). Recommendations usually are based on the physiologic role of specific nutrients in lipid metabolism, in the urea cycle, or as antioxidants. To date, no prospective clinical trials have been conducted to evaluate specific nutrients or supplements in cats with spontaneously occurring HL. Based on uncontrolled retrospective case review, one author has reported improved survival rates in HL cats treated with multiple supplements (Center, 2005a). Until evidence becomes available, the use of supplements will continue to be based on clinician preference and experience. The most commonly prescribed supplements are

L-carnitine, taurine, *S*-adenosylmethionine (SAMe) and silybin (extract from milk thistle). The clinician must consider that prescribing multiple supplements and medications may risk decreasing client compliance with feeding instructions.

L-carnitine is necessary for the transport of long-chain fatty acids into the mitochondria for oxidation and energy production. L-carnitine has been studied in cats during experimental weight gain and loss (Blanchard et al, 2002; Center et al, 2000; Ibrahim et al, 2003). L-carnitine helps protect against loss of lean body tissue during weight loss. Supplementation with L-carnitine may improve fatty acid oxidation, decrease ketosis, and protect against hepatic lipid accumulation in overweight cats during rapid weight loss. However, one report failed to show carnitine deficiency in cats with spontaneous HL (Jacobs et al, 1990). Despite this, many clinicians provide L-carnitine to HL cats (250 mg added to the food q12-24h) with the goal of promoting fatty acid oxidation and retention of lean body mass but evidence is lacking that it provides any benefit for recovery from HL. To ensure bioavailability, medical grade L-carnitine should be used whenever possible (Quinicarn, Carnitor).

Taurine is used obligatorily by cats for bile acid conjugation. It increases water solubility, reduces cellular toxicity, and facilitates circulation and renal elimination. Taurine is an essential amino acid for cats, and a small study suggested that cats with HL have low plasma taurine concentrations (Trainor et al, 2003). Taurine can be added to the food at a dose of 250 mg q12-24h. Some recovery formula diets are high in taurine; for example, Hill's a/d provides 132 mg/100 kcal of taurine (caloric density 1.2 kcal/ml). Taurine analysis is not available for many other diets (including Iams Maximum Calorie), which suggests that supplementation may be prudent when this information is not available.

S-adenosylmethionine (SAMe) is an important hepatocellular metabolite and glutathione (GSH) donor with hepatic and systemic antioxidant effects. Low hepatic glutathione concentrations in the liver of cats with HL compared with healthy feline liver is consistent with a reduction in tissue antioxidant availability and provides the rationale to recommend SAMe for treating HL. In healthy cats, orally administered SAMe increases plasma SAMe and liver GSH (Center et al, 2005b). The benefit of SAMe or other antioxidants in cats with HL, however, is unproven. The commonly used dosages of SAMe are 90 mg/cat for cats weighing less than 5 kg and 225 mg/cat for cats larger than 5 kg PO q24h. Medical grade SAMe (Denosyl) is recommended. SAMe must be given as an intact tablet on an empty stomach (ideally 1 hour before feeding) for optimal absorption. Another antioxidant used with hepatic disease is milk thistle or its extract, silymarin. The active isomer silybin is available as silybin-phosphatidylcholine complex, which has increased oral bioavailability compared with silymarin. Silybin-phosphatidylcholine is available in combination with SAMe (Denamarin).

Treatment of Hepatic Encephalopathy

Although signs of HE (most notably ptyalism and depressed mentation) occur in a minority of cats with HL, HE can be a significant complication requiring therapeutic intervention. Cats with HE are treated by feeding a reduced-protein diet (see Dietary Considerations), and, if necessary, by administration of lactulose and or antibiotics by mouth or through a feeding tube. Lactulose is not absorbed in the small intestines and is degraded into volatile free fatty acids in the colon. The resulting acidification results in a shift to nonabsorbable ionized ammonia and less ammoniagenic flora and increased colonic transit. Lactulose is administered orally at a starting dose of 0.5 ml/kg q6-8h. If HE is severe, lactulose can be administered by retention enema at a total enema volume of 10 to 20 ml/kg q4-6h (3 parts lactulose and 7 parts water) aiming for 30-minute retention in the colon. Ampicillin 22 mg/kg q8h, amoxicillin 22 mg/kg q12h, metronidazole 7.5 mg/kg q12h, or neomycin 22 mg/kg q8-12h are administered orally to reduce colonic bacteria responsible for ammonia production. If blood transfusions are needed, fresh blood products are optimal because they have a lower ammonia concentration than do stored blood products.

Prognosis

Cats making a successful clinical recovery from HL demonstrate a gradual reduction in laboratory abnormalities over time. Total bilirubin concentration is expected to decrease by at least 50% within 7 to 10 days, although serum liver enzyme activities often require longer to decrease (Center, 2005a). Clinically, the two most important factors affecting the outcome in HL appear to be the presence of a serious and irreversible concurrent disease (more likely in an older cat) and how early enteral nutritional support is begun. In the absence of a fatal concurrent disease, recovery rates of 80% or higher can be expected if enteral feeding is initiated early in the course of disease and is sustained until voluntary food intake resumes. Lower serum and potassium concentration and lower hematocrit are negative prognostic indicators (Center et al, 1993). Tube feeding usually is required for several (3 to 6) weeks, which requires clients to be active participants in their cats' recovery. Once a cat recovers from HL, recurrence is unlikely.

References and Suggested Reading

Armstrong PJ, Blanchard G: Hepatic lipidosis in cats, *Vet Clin Small Anim* 39:599, 2009.

Barsanti JA et al: Prolonged anorexia associated with hepatic lipidosis in three cats, *Feline Pract* 7:52, 1977.

Blanchard G et al: Dietary L-carnitine supplementation in obese cats alters carnitine metabolism and decreases ketosis during fasting and induced hepatic lipidosis, *J Nutr* 132:201, 2002.

Boscan P et al: Effect of maropitant, a neurokinin 1 receptor antagonist, on anesthetic requirements during noxious visceral stimulation of the ovary in dogs, *Am J Vet Res* 72:1576, 2011.

Center SA: Feline hepatic lipidosis, *Vet Clin Small Anim* 35:225, 2005a.

Center SA et al: The clinical and metabolic effects of rapid weight loss in obese pet cats and the influence of supplemental L-carnitine, *J Vet Intern Med* 14:598, 2000.

Center SA et al: Liver glutathione concentrations in dogs and cats with naturally occurring liver disease, *Am J Vet Res* 63:1187, 2002.

Center SA et al: Retrospective study of 77 cats with severe hepatic lipidosis: 1975-1990, *J Vet Intern Med* 7:349, 1993.

Center SA, Randolph JF, Warner KL: The effects of S-adenosylmethionine on clinical pathology and redox potential in the red blood cell, liver and bile of clinically normal cats, *J Vet Intern Med* 19:303, 2005b.

Cole TL et al: Diagnostic comparison of needle and wedge biopsy specimens of the liver in dogs and cats, *J Am Vet Med Assoc* 220:1483, 2002.

Feeney DA et al: Statistical relevance of ultrasonographic criteria in the assessment of diffuse liver disease in dogs and cats, *Am J Vet Res* 69:212, 2008.

Hall JA, Barstad LA, Connor WE: Lipid composition of hepatic and adipose tissues from normal cats and cats with idiopathic hepatic lipidosis, *J Vet Intern Med* 11:238, 1997.

Hickman MA et al: Safety, pharmacokinetics and use of the novel NK-1 receptor antagonist maropitant (Cerenia™) for the prevention of emesis and motion sickness in cats, *J Vet Pharmacol Therap* 31:220, 2008.

Ibrahim WH et al: Effects of carnitine and taurine on fatty acid metabolism and lipid accumulation in the liver of cats during weight gain and weight loss, *Am J Vet Res* 64:1265, 2003.

Jacobs G et al: Comparison of plasma, liver, and skeletal muscle carnitine concentrations in cats with idiopathic hepatic lipidosis and in healthy cats, *Am J Vet Res* 51:1349, 1990.

Nicoll RG, O'Brien RT, Jackson MW: Qualitative ultrasonography of the liver in obese cats, *Vet Radiol Ultrasound* 39:47, 1998.

Posner LP, Asakawa M, Erb HN: Use of propofol for anesthesia in cats with primary hepatic lipidosis: 44 cases (1995-2004), *J Am Vet Med Assoc* 232:1841, 2008.

Quimby JM et al: Studies on the pharmacokinetics and pharmacodynamics of mirtazapine in healthy young cats, *J Vet Pharmacol Therap* 34:388, 2010.

Trainor D et al: Urine sulfated and nonsulfated bile acids as a diagnostic test or liver disease in cats, *J Vet Intern Med* 17:145, 2003.

Yeager AE, Mohammed H: Accuracy of ultrasonography in the detection of severe hepatic lipidosis in cats, *Am J Vet Res* 53:597, 1992.

CHAPTER 150

Feline Cholangitis

DAVID C. TWEDT, *Fort Collins, Colorado*
P. JANE ARMSTRONG, *St. Paul, Minnesota*
KENNETH W. SIMPSON, *Ithaca, New York*

Liver disease is a common clinical finding in the cat. The disorders that occur most frequently are hepatic lipidosis, chronic inflammatory disease (cholangitis), neoplasia, and hepatocellular necrosis (such as toxic or drug-related conditions). Based on a 10-year retrospective study of feline liver biopsy data from the University of Minnesota, inflammatory liver disease is the second most common category of liver disease in cats in the United States after hepatic lipidosis (Gagne et al, 1996). This chapter covers only liver disorders associated with cholangitis.

The Cholangitis Complex

In 2006 the World Small Animal Veterinary Association (WSAVA) Liver Standardization Group published a simplified classification scheme for inflammatory liver disease in cats (van den Ingh et al, 2006). Inflammatory liver disease was grouped into three different types of cholangitis based on histopathologic findings: neutrophilic cholangitis ([NC], subdivided into acute and chronic

forms), lymphocytic cholangitis (LC), and cholangitis associated with liver flukes (see Chapter 133 in the previous edition of *Current Veterinary Therapy*). The term *cholangitis* was adopted in preference to cholangiohepatitis because, unlike in dogs, the primary inflammatory changes in cats are centered on bile ducts and ductules. The categories are based on the type of cellular infiltrate, degree of periportal fibrosis, presence of destructive lesions in the bile ductules, and evidence of fluke infestation. In some cases of feline cholangitis, inflammatory changes may disrupt the limiting plate of the portal triad and extend into hepatic parenchyma. When this occurs, the term *cholangiohepatitis* is appropriate. Chronic inflammatory disease of the hepatic parenchyma, unrelated to specific infectious diseases such as feline infectious peritonitis or toxoplasmosis, is rare in cats and unlike that in dogs, in which chronic hepatitis represents the major class of inflammatory liver disease.

Although the histopathologic classification of cholangitis is now well described, good clinical characterization of the various forms of cholangitis has lagged necessarily behind the pathologic description. What has become clear is the clinical syndromes of NC and LC overlap considerably, and few clinical distinctions can be made between the acute and chronic forms of NC.

Pathologists also describe *lymphocytic portal hepatitis* in some feline hepatic biopsies. Lymphocytic portal hepatitis is no longer classified as a primary inflammatory hepatobiliary disease. This pathologic change seems to represent a nonspecific reaction to disease occurring in an extrahepatic location or as an aging change. As opposed to cholangitis (inflammation centered on bile ducts), lymphocytic portal hepatitis lacks bile duct involvement, infiltration of inflammatory cells into hepatic parenchyma, and periportal necrosis. Liver enzymes in cats with this histopathologic change are variable or normal, icterus is uncommon, and most cats with lymphocytic portal hepatitis have prolonged survival, bringing into question the rationale for corticosteroid or other therapy, which has been suggested in the past.

Neutrophilic Cholangitis

NC previously has been referred to as suppurative or exudative cholangitis or cholangiohepatitis. It is the most common type of biliary tract disease observed in cats in North America in one study (Callahan Clark et al, 2011) but was identified with approximately equal frequency to LC in another (Marolf et al, 2012). NC can be subdivided pathologically into an acute neutrophilic form (predominantly neutrophilic infiltration) and a chronic neutrophilic form (having a mixed cellular infiltrate of neutrophils, lymphocytes, and plasma cells). The classical histologic description of the acute form of NC is neutrophils within the walls and lumen of biliary ducts and surrounding the portal areas. Sometimes bacteria can be seen in the bile duct lumen or walls. Biliary hyperplasia, a sign of chronicity, is common in the chronic form, and occasionally periductal (sclerosing) fibrosis and bridging fibrosis may develop. The cause of the acute form is thought to be bacterial from gastrointestinal origin, whereas the chronic form may represent a later stage of the same disease process, possibly triggered by persistent infection or inflammation. Bacterial entry either by the biliary system or hematogenous uptake is possible. Protozoal infections have been identified rarely, including toxoplasmosis, coccidiosis, and hepatozoonosis. Despite being somewhat distinct histologically, almost complete overlap is seen in clinical findings between the two NC subtypes (Callahan Clark et al, 2011; Marolf et al, 2012). For this reason, they are discussed together in this chapter. NC has been described in a wide age range of cats, but the median age is about 9 years. Affected cats with either form of NC show anorexia, weight loss, lethargy, and vomiting. Cats with LC also have these same presenting signs. Physical examination findings are identical in cats with the acute and chronic forms of NC and may include fever, dehydration, icterus, abdominal pain, and hepatomegaly. A majority of cats (55%) demonstrate peripheral neutrophilia. One report indicated that cats with the acute form were more likely to exhibit neutrophilia (50%) than cats with the chronic

form (30%) (Callahan Clark et al, 2011). Band neutrophils, neutropenia, and anemia also may be present. Other laboratory findings include increases in serum activities of alanine aminotransferase (ALT), aspartate aminotransferase (AST), γ-glutamyltranspeptidase (GGT), alkaline phosphatase (ALP), and hyperbilirubinemia. Surprisingly, serum liver enzyme activities are within reference range in many cats. Signs of hepatic dysfunction, such as hepatic encephalopathy, abnormal coagulation parameters, hypoalbuminemia, low blood urea nitrogen (BUN), and hypocholesterolemia, are uncommon. With the exception of frequency of neutrophilia, these laboratory findings do not differ regardless if the histopathologic diagnosis is either the NC or LC form.

Routine abdominal radiographs rarely contribute to making a diagnosis of NC but may help exclude other diseases that can cause similar clinical signs. Somewhat surprisingly, it has been reported recently that most cats with cholangitis of any form have normal sonographic findings, including liver size, echogenicity, and biliary systems (Marolf et al, 2012). When abnormalities are present, they include hepatomegaly, hyperechoic hepatic parenchyma, dilated common bile duct (reference range <4 mm), and echogenic gallbladder contents. Identifying gallbladder debris in cats currently is somewhat confounding because it cannot be considered necessarily an incidental finding as it often is in dogs. Increased gallbladder wall thickness (reference range <1 mm) was not statistically significant in Marolf's study. However, bacterial cholecystitis can be associated with NC, and such cases may have a thickened gallbladder wall (Brain et al, 2006). Cystic and common bile ducts may be tortuous and dilated. Inspissated bile may cause partial or complete obstruction of the common bile duct. Biliary obstruction is suggested sonographically by a dilated gallbladder, tortuous bile ducts, and a dilated common bile duct.

Enteric bacteria, most often *Escherichia coli* alone or, less commonly, in combination with other organisms, may be cultured from the bile or liver of cats with cholangitis, especially acute NC. Other reported bacterial isolates include *Enterococcus* spp., *Bacteroides* spp., *Clostridia* spp., *Staphylococcus*, and α-hemolytic *Streptococcus* spp. One reported case with NC and cholecystitis had *Salmonella enterica* serovar Typhimurium isolated from bile and feces (Brain et al, 2006). Although most reported organisms are aerobes, anaerobic organisms also may be found, so aerobic and anaerobic cultures should be requested on biliary and hepatic cultures.

In the authors' experience, the rate of positive bile cultures is low in NC, even in untreated cats, but culture-independent studies on bile provide further support for the role of enteric bacteria in pathogenesis. Using a florescence *in situ* hybridization (FISH) assay, the authors (Twedt et al, 2013) have observed intrahepatic bacteria in 33% of cats with inflammatory liver disease they examined. The highest bacterial numbers in cats with *E. coli* were associated with NC, and intrahepatic bacteria were much more prevalent in cats with NC than the nonsuppurative LC.

Cats affected with cholangitis commonly have comorbidities, most often pancreatitis and inflammatory bowel disease (IBD). In addition, anorexia induced by cholangitis may precipitate a secondary hepatic lipidosis (see Chapter 149). Concurrent inflammation in the liver, pancreas, and small intestine of cats has been referred to as the *feline triaditis syndrome*. In the first report of feline triaditis, 83% of cats with cholangitis also had histologic evidence of IBD and 50% had concurrent chronic pancreatitis (Gagne et al, 1999). When pancreatitis was present, it was generally chronic and described predominantly as ductal inflammation and fibrosis. The authors (DT and KS) found that culture-independent *in situ* methods (FISH) in the evaluation of cats having pancreatitis indicated 35% (11 of 31) with moderate to severe forms had bacteria present (Twedt et al, 2013). The *common channel theory*, according to which the pancreatic ducts and bile ducts join as a common duct before entering the duodenum, may explain partially the relationship of cholangitis and chronic pancreatitis, in which bacterial infections in the biliary system are likely to involve the pancreatic ducts as well. This is supported by the fact that bile cultures are more frequently positive than liver cultures. However, the authors using FISH for bacterial localization found few bacteria were in the pancreatic or hepatic bile ducts but rather in the parenchyma, suggesting also possible portal translocation. With concurrent IBD and gastrointestinal dysbiosis along with the inflamed and leaky gut, enterohepatic translocation of bacteria such as *E. coli*, enterococcus, and *Clostridium* spp. could result. Anatomic abnormalities of the gallbladder or common bile duct or the presence of inspissated bile or choleliths also may predispose to, or accompany, cholangitis. Marolf found that cats with NC are more likely than cats with LC to have evidence of pancreatic disease detected on sonographic examination. These changes included diffuse pancreatic enlargement and hypoechoic pancreatic parenchyma. Callahan Clark (2011) also described sonographic changes in the pancreas in 81% of cats with cholangitis, with no difference in frequency between types of cholangitis. Feline pancreatic lipase (Spec fPL) concentration may be abnormal in cholangitis cats and may help support the diagnosis of concurrent pancreatitis.

Definitive diagnosis of NC requires a liver biopsy or biliary cytology and positive culture, but a tentative diagnosis often is made based on the clinical and laboratory findings coupled with a response to appropriate antibiotic therapy. Cytologic examination of fine-needle liver aspirates showing suppurative inflammation may help support the diagnosis, but liver aspiration cytology has a poor correlation with histopathology, especially in inflammatory liver disease. When peripheral neutrophilia is present, the inevitable blood contamination of the liver aspirate may be difficult to distinguish from neutrophilic inflammation in the liver. Whenever possible, a percutaneous ultrasound-guided gallbladder aspirate for bile cytology and culture should be performed, along with liver biopsies. Bile aspirates are relatively safe if a 20- or 22-gauge needle is directed through the right medial liver lobe and into the gallbladder lumen. With this approach, any bile leakage drains back into the liver and not into the peritoneal cavity. Suppurative inflammation and bacteria may be observed in the bile cytology and is

diagnostic for NC. Occasionally, cytologic examination reveals many bacteria but few inflammatory cells. Techniques for biopsy include ultrasound-guided needle biopsy, laparoscopy, or laparotomy. The latter two techniques also make it possible to examine the extrahepatic biliary system, pancreas, and other intraabdominal structures. Surgery allows culture of the liver and gallbladder contents, gallbladder wall, and material obstructing the bile duct (if found) as well as biopsy of the liver, gallbladder wall, and extrahepatic biliary system.

Treatment of Neutrophilic Cholangitis

Primary treatment of acute cholangitis centers around appropriate antibiotic therapy based ideally on culture and sensitivity. If cultures are negative or empiric antibiotic selection is necessary, the clinician should select an antibiotic based on the most common bacterial isolates from bile. A good choice is an antibiotic that is effective against most enteric gram-negative aerobes and that has good hepatic and biliary penetration, such as cephalosporins, amoxicillin, or amoxicillin-clavulanic acid (Box 150-1). Some cases require a fluoroquinolone. Metronidazole (7.5 mg/kg q12h PO) may be added to extend the spectrum to anaerobes and more coliforms. Based on reports of successful treatment with long-term follow-up (Brain et al, 2006), treatment should be continued for 4 to 6 weeks, even though most cats improve within a week with an appropriate antibiotic selection.

Corticosteroid therapy is considered in NC cases in which the biopsy sections contain relatively few neutrophils with a predominance of lymphocytic and plasmacytic inflammation and response to appropriate antimicrobial therapy is poor or incomplete. Some cases clinically improve but it is uncertain if clinical response is the result of resolution of liver disease or perhaps improvement in the frequently concurrent inflammatory bowel disease or pancreatitis.

Cats with NC frequently are acutely ill and require intensive supportive care. Successful recovery requires correction of fluid and electrolyte abnormalities (especially hypokalemia and hypophosphatemia) with frequent reassessment. Appropriate intravenous crystalloid fluid therapy correcting electrolyte deficits is recommended. If coagulation abnormalities are present, administer vitamin K_1 (0.5 to 1.5 mg q12h SC or IM using a 25-gauge needle) before performing a biopsy.

Nutritional support, concentrating on meeting protein and caloric needs, is important to aid in recovery, treat any concurrent hepatic lipidosis, and prevent fatty change from occurring.

Assisted oral feeding should be tried for no longer than 12 to 24 hours, after which a nasoesophageal tube should be placed if voluntary intake is inadequate. Ensuring that resting energy requirement (see Chapter 149) is met through intake of a high-energy, high-protein diet is a high priority throughout treatment. Protein is an important nutrient for liver repair and regeneration and should not be restricted unless hepatic encephalopathy occurs; however, it is unusual for biliary tract disease to result in sufficient parenchymal damage to cause encephalopathy. If present, hepatic encephalopathy is manifest

---

BOX 150-1

Therapy for Cats with Different Forms of Cholangitis*

Neutrophilic Cholangitis
- Antimicrobial therapy (ideally based on culture and sensitivity)
  - Cephalosporin (several options)
  - Amoxicillin
  - Amoxicillin-clavulanic acid
  - Enrofloxacin
  - Marbofloxacin

Lymphocytic Cholangitis
- Prednisolone

Supportive Therapy†
- Ursodeoxycholic acid (Ursodiol)
- Pain control:
  - Buprenorphine
  - Butorphanol
  - Hydromorphone
  - Meperidine
  - Fentanyl patch
- Antiemetics:
  - Maropitant
  - Ondansetron
  - Dolasetron
- Nutraceuticals:
  - Denamarin
  - Silymarin
  - SAMe
- Cobalamin (vitamin B$_{12}$)
- Dietary manipulation (for inflammatory bowel disease)
- Vitamin K$_1$
- Lactulose (for hepatic encephalopathy)
- Neomycin (for hepatic encephalopathy)

*Consult Appendix I and this chapter for recommended doses.
†Given as indicated regardless of form of cholangitis.

---

most frequently by excessive salivation and can be managed by administering lactulose (0.5 to 1.0 ml/kg q8h PO) with or without addition of enteric antibiotics (neomycin 20 mg/kg q8-12h PO), along with feeding a lower-protein diet.

Pain management is indicated in many cats with cholangitis, especially those with acute signs. Pain control usually can be accomplished through the parenteral administration of buprenorphine (this drug also can be administered sublingually and is well absorbed through the buccal mucous membranes), hydromorphone, meperidine, or butorphanol. For longer-duration pain control, a 25 µg/hr fentanyl patch reaches effective blood levels within 3 to 12 hours in cats, during which time one of the above opioids is administered concurrently.

The antiemetic maropitant (Cerenia) an NK-1 receptor antagonist, administered at 1 mg/kg q24 PO, SC, or IV (IV is off label but used by the authors) is useful in controlling emesis. Because maropitant undergoes hepatic metabolism, cases having advanced hepatic dysfunction

lower doses should be used (e.g., 0.5 mg/kg q24h PO, SC, IV). Alternatives are 5-HT$_3$ antagonists (ondansetron 0.1 to 1.0 mg/kg or dolasetron 0.5 to 1.0 mg/kg q12-24h PO, IV). The dopaminergic antagonist metoclopramide may be useful to enhance motility in the upper gastrointestinal tract, but its action as a centrally acting antiemetic is questionable; cats are reported to have few if any central nervous system (CNS) dopamine receptors in the chemoreceptor trigger zone.

Surgical therapy is uncommon but may be required for gallbladder rupture, cholelith removal, or bile duct decompression if biliary obstruction is present (see Chapter 147). Cholecystectomy is occasionally necessary in cases of acute cholecystitis, gallbladder rupture, or concern regarding gallbladder wall integrity. Occasionally the bile becomes the consistency of a thick sludge to the point of obstruction, and this requires vigorous flushing of the extrahepatic biliary system. This is best accomplished by opening the gallbladder and flushing antegrade down the common bile duct. Sometimes it also is necessary to open the duodenum and flush retrograde from the duodenal papilla. The authors advise preserving normal biliary anatomy and avoiding biliary bypass surgical techniques (cholecystoduodenostomy or cholecystojejunostomy) whenever possible because they often are associated with chronic postoperative problems.

Because cats with NC may concurrently have pancreatitis and IBD these other conditions may warrant additional therapy, such as cobalamin supplementation and limited antigen diet (see Chapters 127, 131, and 138).

Ursodeoxycholic acid (Ursodiol, Actigal, 10 to 15 mg/kg q24h PO) may be beneficial in cats with cholangitis. Among its effects include amelioration of damage to cell membranes caused by retained toxic bile acids. Ursodeoxycholic acid also improves biliary secretion of bile acids, improves bile flow (choleresis), helps prevent mitochondrial damage, and has antifibrotic and immunomodulatory properties. Clinical trials in human patients with primary sclerosing cholangitis and some other forms of hepatitis support improved quality of life. Adverse effects in cats are uncommon and usually limited to mild diarrhea. Some clinicians avoid using ursodeoxycholic acid when bile duct obstruction is a possibility, fearing that ursodeoxycholic acid could make the damage worse or even potentiate rupture of the ducts or gallbladder from the choleretic action of the drug. This theory is unfounded and not supported in experimental studies. For example, one study in rats with surgical obstruction of the common bile duct treated with either placebo or ursodeoxycholic acid found that the ursodeoxycholic acid–treated rats had less hepatocellular damage than the placebo group (Frezza et al, 2003). However, if an obstruction is identified in a cat with cholestatic liver disease, surgery is indicated.

Interest is increasing in the use of nutraceuticals in the treatment of feline liver disease, but controlled clinical trials are lacking. They generally are given for their antioxidant effects because oxidative damage from free radical formation is one potential mechanism of cellular damage. High concentrations of bile acids, accumulation of heavy metals, and inflammation cause free radical generation in the liver. Vitamin E and SAMe are used commonly; vitamin C and phosphatidylcholine also may be considered. The herb milk thistle, or its extract, silymarin, is used for its hepatoprotective effects. The active isomer, silybin, has increased oral bioavailability compared to silymarin. Silybin is available in combination with SAMe (90 mg SAMe and 9 mg silybin A+B [Denamarin]).

Lymphocytic Cholangitis

LC is a chronic disease that affects the biliary tree and is slowly progressive. Hepatic lesions include lymphocytic inflammation directed at bile ducts with some cases having ductopenia, peribiliary fibrosis, portal B-cell aggregates, or portal lipogranulomas. Preliminary immunologic studies suggest that LC could have an immune-mediated cause. In one study by Warren et al (2010) investigating 51 cats with LC, researchers found the majority of cases (68.6%) had a predominant dense T cell population, with fewer cases having B cells randomly distributed. These histologic findings tend to support an immunologic disorder. Studies also have focused on possible infectious causes using either FISH or through bacterial DNA analysis (Greiter-Wilke et al, 2006; Otte et al, 2012a; Warren et al, 2010), and all have failed to support a primary infectious cause. However, researchers have induced experimentally an LC with *Bartonella* spp. infection. In some cases it is difficult to differentiate LC from lymphoma, and additional diagnostics including polymerase chain reaction for T-cell receptor (TCR) gene rearrangement may be helpful (see Chapter 65). However, the relationship of LC with hepatic lymphoma has not been well elucidated.

Clinical Findings

Cats with LC tend to be older than those with NC at the time of the diagnosis (Weiss, Gagne, and Armstrong, 1996). A median age of 11.5 years, with a range of 4 to 11 years, has been reported (Marolf et al, 2012). No sex or breed predilection has been shown in North American cats. The clinical signs include vomiting, lethargy, anorexia, and weight loss; the same signs are seen in NC. Signs are often intermittent and tend to wax and wane over months. In one study 33% of the cats with LC had leukocytosis, a lower percentage than for cats with NC (Marolf et al, 2012). As in NC, most cases have increases in ALP, ALT, AST, and total bilirubin with variable increases in GGT. Sonographic changes in the liver and biliary system do not differ from those seen in NC cats, but LC cats were less likely to have concurrent pancreatic changes detected sonographically (Marolf et al, 2012).

Reports on cats diagnosed with LC in Europe and Japan describe a form of LC that is insidiously progressive over years (Lucke and Davies, 1984; Nakayama et al, 1992). In one report, young cats (<4 years), especially of the Persian breed, appeared overrepresented (Lucke and Davies, 1984). This has not been confirmed in subsequent reports. A median age at diagnosis of 12.3 years was reported, a male predisposition was found, and Norwegian Forest cats were overrepresented compared with the hospital population (Otte et al, 2012b). Clinical features included hyperglobulinemia and ascites, signs that differ from LC described in North American cats. This

difference remains unexplained. LC bears many similarities to primary sclerosing cholangitis in human patients, which also shows geographic differences.

Treatment

Cats diagnosed with LC are treated similarly to cats with NC (see treatment of NC and Box 152-1), except that corticosteroids usually are given to control the inflammatory component of the disease. In practice, antibiotic therapy usually is started while awaiting biopsy results, and corticosteroids added if cats fail to respond or if the biopsy shows LC. Prednisolone at a dosage of 1 to 2 mg/kg q24h PO is used initially. Prednisolone is well absorbed after oral administration in cats and hence is the corticosteroid of choice. If successful in improving clinical signs and biochemical changes, the dosage of prednisolone slowly is tapered after 4 to 6 weeks. A schedule commonly used for tapering is to reduce the dosage by 50% every 2 weeks, until 0.5 mg/kg q24h is reached; biochemical values and clinical response should be monitored before each reduction in dosage. A dosage of 0.5 mg/kg q48h may be administered for 4 weeks or long term, as needed, to control clinical signs. Ideally treatment decisions are based on repeat liver biopsies. One study retrospectively using prednisolone or ursodeoxycholic acid therapy showed an overall median survival time of 755 days in 26 LC cats; prednisolone therapy was associated with better survival (Otte et al, 2012b). Long-term corticosteroid treatment is well tolerated by most cats, although the cat should be observed carefully for signs consistent with diabetes mellitus or congestive heart failure. No reported studies use other types of immunosuppressive therapy. There are also anecdotal reports of using chlorambucil in conjunction with prednisolone in severe cases. Corticosteroid therapy may not be contraindicated in cats with concurrent chronic pancreatitis or IBD and actually may be beneficial.

References and Suggested Reading

Brain PH et al: Feline cholecystitis and acute neutrophilic cholangitis: clinical findings, bacterial isolates and response to treatment in six cases, *J Fel Med Surg* 8:91, 2006.
Callahan Clark JE et al: Feline cholangitis: a necropsy study of 44 cats (1986-2008), *J Fel Med Surg* 13:570, 2011.
Frezza EE et al: Effect of ursodeoxycholic acid administration on bile duct proliferation and cholestasis in bile duct ligated rat, *Dig Dis Sci* 38:1291, 1993.
Gagne JM et al: Clinical features of inflammatory liver disease in cats: 41 cases (1983-1993), *J Am Vet Med Assoc* 214:513, 1999.
Gagne JM et al: Histopathologic evaluation of feline inflammatory liver disease, *Vet Pathol* 33:521, 1996.
Greiter-Wilke A et al: Association of *Helicobacter* with cholangiohepatitis in cats, *J Vet Intern Med* 20:822, 2006.
Lucke VM, Davies JD: Progressive lymphocytic cholangitis in the cat, *J Small Anim Pract* 25:249, 1984.
Marolf AJ et al: Ultrasonographic findings of feline cholangitis, *J Am Anim Hosp Assoc* 48:36, 2012.
Nakayama H et al: Three cases of feline sclerosing lymphocytic cholangitis, *J Vet Med Sci* 54:769, 1992.
Otte CMA et al: Detection of bacterial DNA in bile of cats with lymphocytic cholangitis, *Vet Microbiol* 156:217, 2012a.

Otte CMA et al: Retrospective comparison of prednisolone and ursodeoxycholic acid for the treatment of feline lymphocytic cholangitis, *Vet J* 195(2):205, 2012b.

Twedt DC et al: Evaluation of fluorescence in situ hybridization for the detection of bacteria in feline inflammatory liver disease, *J Feline Med Surg*, 2013 [Epub ahead of print].

van den Ingh TSGAM et al: Morphological classification of biliary disorders of the canine and feline liver. In Rothuizen J et al, editors: *WSAVA standards for clinical and histological diagnosis of canine and feline liver diseases*, Edinburgh, 2006, Saunders/Elsevier, p 61.

Warren A et al: Histopathologic features, immunophenotyping, clonality, and eubacterial fluorescence in situ hybridization in cats with lymphocytic cholangitis/cholangiohepatitis, *Vet Path* 48:627, 2010.

Weiss DJ, Gagne JM, Armstrong PJ: Relationship between inflammatory hepatic disease and inflammatory bowel disease, pancreatitis, and nephritis in cats, *J Am Vet Med Assoc* 209:1114, 1996.

SECTION VII

Respiratory Diseases

Chapter 151: Respiratory Drug Therapy   622
Chapter 152: Feline Upper Respiratory Tract Infection   629
Chapter 153: Canine Infectious Respiratory Disease Complex   632
Chapter 154: Rhinitis in Dogs   635
Chapter 155: Rhinitis in Cats   644
Chapter 156: Brachycephalic Airway Obstruction Syndrome   649
Chapter 157: Nasopharyngeal Disorders   653
Chapter 158: Laryngeal Diseases   659
Chapter 159: Tracheal Collapse   663
Chapter 160: Chronic Bronchial Disorders in Dogs   669
Chapter 161: Chronic Bronchitis and Asthma in Cats   673
Chapter 162: Pneumonia   681
Chapter 163: Eosinophilic Pulmonary Diseases   688
Chapter 164: Pleural Effusion   691
Chapter 165: Pneumothorax   700
Chapter 166: Pulmonary Thromboembolism   705
Chapter 167: Pulmonary Hypertension   711

The following web chapters can be found on the companion website at www.currentveterinarytherapy.com

Web Chapter 56: Interstitial Lung Diseases
Web Chapter 57: Respiratory Parasites

CHAPTER 151
Respiratory Drug Therapy

ELEANOR C. HAWKINS, *Raleigh, North Carolina*
MARK G. PAPICH, *Raleigh, North Carolina*

Drugs are the "go to" therapy for respiratory diseases for most clinicians and are the focus of this chapter. However, other therapies can be equally or more important and should not be overlooked: for example, oxygen supplementation; physical therapy; maintenance of hydration, healthy body weight, and oral hygiene; improvement of environmental air quality (reduction of irritants); stenting procedures; and surgical intervention. Drugs used to treat respiratory conditions fall into several classes, including antitussives, bronchodilators, antiinflammatory drugs, expectorants and mucolytic drugs, decongestants, and antimicrobials. This chapter provides a brief overview of therapeutic agents in these classes. Dosage regimens not listed in this chapter are found in the Appendix of Commonly Used Drugs at the back of this book or in a separate formulary (Papich, 2011). The discussion of specific antimicrobial treatments is limited because the area is too large for exhaustive coverage in this brief chapter.

Antitussive Drugs

Cough suppression does not produce a cure and should not be used as primary treatment for undiagnosed respiratory disease because it may mask clinical signs and allow disease to progress unchecked. Cough suppression is rarely indicated for cats, in which the primary disease (often bronchitis) should be addressed directly. However, it may provide relief in dogs with acute airway diseases, may lessen tracheal irritation associated with repetitive and prolonged coughing episodes, and is a primary treatment for dogs with tracheobronchomalacia (tracheal and/or bronchial collapse) that do not have an active inflammatory or infectious component to their disease.

Unfortunately, except for early studies of butorphanol, there are no reliable clinical trials in small animals that have evaluated the effectiveness of antitussive agents, and the mechanism of action of antitussive drugs is not completely understood. There are both opiate and nonopiate antitussive drugs, although growing evidence suggests that the nonopiate drug dextromethorphan is less effective than once thought.

The most commonly used and seemingly most effective antitussives are opiate derivatives. These drugs directly depress the cough center in the medulla, possibly through either mu or kappa opiate receptors. There is evidence that either receptor may be responsible inasmuch as butorphanol (a kappa receptor agonist) and codeine or morphine (mu receptor agonists) can suppress cough (Gingerich et al, 1983; Takahama and Shirasaki,

2007), and naloxone is capable of antagonizing this effect. It has also been proposed that sedative effects produced from opiates may contribute to the reduced coughing.

The β_2-receptor agonists suppress cough in some animals. The effect of these drugs is mediated via bronchodilation, and discussion of these agents is presented later.

Codeine (Methylmorphine)

Morphine is not regularly used as an antitussive because of its side effects and potential for abuse, but its derivatives are commonly used. Codeine phosphate and codeine sulfate are found in many preparations, including tablets, liquids, and syrups. Codeine has analgesic effects that are approximately one tenth those of morphine but antitussive potency similar to that of morphine. Although codeine administered orally to dogs attains systemic levels of only 4% (KuKanich, 2010), other metabolites may be responsible for the antitussive effect. Despite its occasional use in dogs, its clinical efficacy for treating cough has not been studied. Important side effects include sedation and constipation. In people, the side effects of codeine at antitussive dosages are significantly less than those experienced with morphine. The potential for addiction and abuse is also considerably lower than for other opiates.

Hydrocodone

Hydrocodone is similar to codeine in mechanism of action, but it is more potent. Hydrocodone is combined with an anticholinergic drug (homatropine) in the preparation Hycodan, which has been prescribed for small animals. Pharmacokinetic studies have shown that it is absorbed following oral administration in dogs, and active metabolites may persist for several hours. Some veterinarians consider it their drug of first choice for symptomatic treatment of cough in dogs. The anticholinergic component (homatropine) is added to discourage abuse rather than for a respiratory indication. Oral dosages administered to dogs are approximately 0.22 to 0.25 mg/kg, q6-8h (~1 tablet per 20 kg). Higher dosages may be needed for patients with tracheobronchomalacia that have been treated with this drug for years. The side effect of sedation becomes the limiting factor, because it affects quality of life.

Formulation note: Hycodan is formulated as 5 mg of hydrocodone plus 1.5 mg homatropine. Only in Canada is hydrocodone (5 mg) available without an anticholinergic added. Hydrocodone (5 mg) and acetaminophen (500 mg) are combined in a tablet (Vicodin) and used for analgesia, which is safe for dogs but not for cats because of cats' sensitivity to acetaminophen toxicity.

Dextromethorphan

Routine use of dextromethorphan is not recommended in dogs, and its efficacy in people has been recently questioned. Further, pharmacokinetic studies in dogs indicate that dextromethorphan does not attain effective concentrations after oral administration (KuKanich and Papich, 2004). Dextromethorphan caused adverse central nervous system (CNS) effects after intravenous injection and vomiting after oral administration. Even after intravenous administration, concentrations of the parent drug and active metabolite persisted for only a short time after dosing. Therefore, routine use in dogs is not recommended until more data are available to establish safe and effective doses.

Butorphanol

Butorphanol (Torbutrol, Torbugesic) is an opioid agonist-antagonist that has been used as both an analgesic and a potent antitussive. High doses may induce sedation, the most significant side effect. Butorphanol is poorly bioavailable because of oral first-pass metabolism. Therefore, in dogs the oral dose is much higher (0.55 to 1.1 mg/kg) than the intravenous or subcutaneous dose (0.05 to 0.1 mg/kg). Butorphanol is administered as frequently as needed to control cough—usually every 6 to 12 hours. In clinical studies the peak effect was rapid after an injection. After oral administration in dogs, maximum effects were observed for 4 hours but effects persisted for up to 10 hours (Gingerich et al, 1983).

Bronchodilators

The primary indication for bronchodilators is treatment of cats with bronchial inflammation, regardless of cause (e.g., allergic, infectious, or idiopathic bronchitis), in which bronchoconstriction can be a major feature of disease. Dogs with bronchial disease rarely develop clinically apparent bronchoconstriction but may show clinical improvement when given these drugs because of effects beyond bronchodilation. Bronchodilators are sometimes used in cats or dogs in respiratory distress that have primarily parenchymal disease, such as aspiration pneumonia, because airways are often concurrently affected. A therapeutic trial is indicated to be sure that clinical status is not worsened in patients in distress. Bronchodilators have effects on vascular smooth muscle, as well as airway smooth muscle, and may interfere with the matching of perfusion to ventilation.

β-Adrenergic Receptor Agonists

Bronchial smooth muscle is innervated by β₂-adrenergic receptors. Stimulation of β₂-receptors leads to increased activity of the enzyme adenylate cyclase, increased intracellular cyclic adenosine monophosphate (cAMP), and relaxation of bronchial smooth muscle. In addition to bronchodilation, other effects may contribute to efficacy. Activation of the β-receptors on mast cells produces a stabilizing effect (inhibition of mediator release), even though there is little effect on other inflammatory cells. Also, there is some evidence that β-adrenergic receptor agonists increase mucociliary clearance in the respiratory tract.

Epinephrine is the prototype of adrenergic agonists and it has been used in emergency situations, but repeated and prolonged use for airway disease would be detrimental. Instead, β₂-receptor–specific agonists are preferred. Terbutaline is most often used and is similar to isoproterenol in its β₂ activity, but it is longer acting (6 to 8 hours). It may be injected subcutaneously or intravenously to relieve an acute episode of bronchoconstriction. It is also available in oral formulations. Dosages for this and other bronchodilators can be found in the appendix. Albuterol (called *salbutamol* in some countries) is similar to terbutaline. It can be given orally as a tablet or liquid up to four times daily.

Inhalant Administration: Nebulizers and Metered Dose Inhalers

Inhaled aerosols of β₂-agonists, particularly albuterol, are important drugs for treatment of acute bronchospasm (asthma attacks) in cats, usually seen in association with idiopathic, allergic, or infectious bronchitis but also occasionally with aspiration pneumonia and during performance of tracheal wash, bronchoscopy, or bronchoalveolar lavage. The β-agonists can be administered topically to the airways via inhalation using wet nebulization or metered dose inhalers (MDIs). Nebulization is the process by which small droplets are created from solutions of drug, resulting in a visible fog. To be effective, the particles must be within a size range that can reach the affected airways. Nebulization of a drug solution is carried out by jet or ultrasonic nebulizers. For best results, the drug is administered via a snug anesthetic face mask attached to connecting tubes. Delivery of drug by nebulizer is time consuming, usually requiring 10 to 15 minutes per treatment every 4 to 8 hours, not including time for setup. One method for nebulization in veterinary medicine is administration of drug directly into a small incubator or oxygen cage for treatment of fractious or easily stressed patients, although this does result in a damp patient. Bacterial colonization of the nebulization apparatus and solutions should be prevented, and instructions for care, cleaning, and disposal of parts should be followed carefully.

Administration of bronchodilators by MDI, delivered using a dedicated spacer, has largely replaced nebulization of albuterol in human medicine. Although scientific studies are limited, several reports in the literature and years of clinical experience have made the use of MDIs commonplace in veterinary medicine. It is critical that a spacer specifically designed for MDIs be used. Old practices such as using toilet paper rolls greatly diminish the already small percentage of drug that actually reaches the lower airways. In addition, the spacer must have a sensitive valve that will open during the relatively low pressures generated by tidal respirations of a cat or small dog. Spacers that have been used successfully in veterinary patients are the AeroKat and AeroDawg and OptiChamber devices. The AeroKat and AeroDawg spacers include a face mask, whereas an anesthetic face mask must be attached to the OptiChamber. The inconvenience of adapting a face mask may be worthwhile in some patients to achieve the best fit. Cleaning instructions provided by the manufacturer should always be followed. The primary bronchodilator used in the United States is albuterol (Ventolin). Administration of this drug by inhalation is indicated only for short-term use to treat acute exacerbations of bronchoconstriction.

Adverse Effects of and Tolerance to β-Agonists

The most common adverse effects of β-agonists occur at high doses and affect the cardiovascular system (tachycardia) and skeletal muscles (muscle tremors or twitching). The muscle activity, in turn, can produce hyperthermia. The β_2-receptor agonists also inhibit uterine motility and should not be used late in pregnancy. High doses of β_2-agonists also can produce hypokalemia.

Inhaled administration of albuterol by MDI can induce airway inflammation. Its use is best limited to treatment of acute bronchoconstriction, such as in exacerbations of feline bronchitis or respiratory distress accompanied by clinical signs supporting the presence of obstructive disease (marked expiratory effort, wheezing, and/or hyperinflation).

Regular administration of β-agonists can cause tolerance, which is a loss in the sensitivity of β-adrenergic receptors owing to down-regulation of receptors. This effect occurs when β-adrenergic drugs are administered regularly for several weeks. Therefore it is best to rely on these drugs intermittently (as rescue inhalation therapy) and allow drug-free breaks in treatment. Regular use of corticosteroids can mitigate the loss of β-receptor sensitivity caused by chronic use of β-agonists.

Methylxanthines (Xanthines)

The methylxanthines include theobromine, caffeine, and theophylline. Once a mainstay in the treatment of human asthma and chronic obstructive pulmonary disease, theophylline use in people has diminished because of a high incidence of adverse effects, primarily nausea, and the availability of better-tolerated and more effective drugs. However, its therapeutic effectiveness has led to ongoing development of more targeted phosphodiesterase 4 inhibitors, which are hoped to have fewer side effects.

In dogs and cats, theophylline is used for the treatment of bronchitis and may be of benefit to some dogs with tracheobronchomalacia. Unlike in people, the drug is well tolerated in these species, and oral dosing is convenient. As for most respiratory therapies for dogs and cats, well-controlled clinical studies of efficacy have not been performed. Anecdotally, marked clinical improvement is seen in some patients. In cats, the bronchodilatory effects may predominate. In dogs, it is quite possible that other effects contribute to improvement in clinical signs.

The methylxanthines relax bronchial smooth muscle and hence are known as bronchodilators. However, there is evidence that they have antiinflammatory effects, including possible enhancement of the activity of corticosteroids, which may occur at lower concentrations than those producing the bronchodilating effects. As described for terbutaline, there is evidence that methylxanthines improve mucociliary clearance in dogs. Nonrespiratory effects of methylxanthines include CNS stimulation, urinary diuresis (mild), and cardiac stimulation (mild).

The cellular basis of action of the methylxanthines is still not completely understood, although adenosine receptor antagonism is thought to play a role in humans because adenosine triggers bronchoconstriction in asthmatic individuals. Another probable action is inhibition of phosphodiesterase types 3 and 4. (Other drugs such as pimobendan and sildenafil target more specific inhibition of phosphodiesterase enzymes 3 and 5.) Phosphodiesterases are enzymes that catalyze the breakdown of cAMP and cyclic guanosine monophosphate to inactive products. Inhibition of the phosphodiesterase enzyme increases intracellular concentrations of the cyclic nucleotide cAMP. In turn, cAMP inhibits the release of inflammatory mediators from mast cells, has antiinflammatory effects, and produces bronchial smooth muscle relaxation.

Theophylline Formulations

Theophylline has been available in several formulations, including injectable aqueous solutions, elixirs, and immediate-release and extended-release tablets and capsules. All available formulations are designed for people; there are no veterinary preparations. Pharmacokinetic studies have been performed on both immediate-release and sustained-release formulations in dogs and cats that help to guide dosing; however, the sustained-release products that have been tested are not currently on the market. Because there are no approved animal formulations, the veterinarian is left to prescribe any formulation available. Our recommendation is to begin dosing using the guidelines listed in this chapter and to be prepared to increase or decrease the dose, or dosing interval, based on the patient's clinical response and tolerance. Dose adjustments are best made by measuring the patient's plasma/serum concentration and adjusting the dose to an appropriate plasma/serum concentration, as well as observing for adverse effects of this drug. Immediate-release theophylline and aminophylline are interchangeable. Aminophylline (theophylline ethylenediamine) is 80% theophylline.

Pharmacokinetics and Dosing

After oral administration, theophylline is rapidly and completely absorbed. Systemic availability is 91% in dogs and 96% to 100% in cats. Theophylline is metabolized primarily by the liver in all species; only 10% of the dose is eliminated unchanged in the urine. More complete dosing information is available in the appendix of this book as well as another formulary (Papich, 2011). A recommended initial dosage in dogs (which should be adjusted to individual patients) is 10 mg/kg q12h PO (Bach et al, 2004). In cats, the recommended dosage is

15 mg/kg (tablet) q24h PO in the evening, which is approximately equivalent to 50-100 mg per cat of the tablet form (Guenther-Yenke et al, 2007). These intervals can be extended to every 24 hours in dogs and every 48 hours in cats if there are documented benefits or sustained trough concentrations with reduced intervals.

Theophylline drug plasma assays are available in many laboratories. When theophylline is used for managing chronic disease, measurement is recommended to establish the optimum dose. This is particularly useful if a therapeutic effect was not appreciated by the client. The best time to sample when monitoring a patient is right before the next scheduled dose (trough). Maintaining the trough concentration above a minimum threshold level that is believed to be therapeutic will ensure that patients are receiving a correct dose. In dogs and cats, a cited therapeutic plasma concentration is 10 to 20 µg/ml, but these values were extrapolated from human studies. Antiinflammatory action may occur in patients at concentrations that are below the concentrations usually considered for bronchodilation. In the review by Barnes (2003) the antiinflammatory effects were reported to occur in people at concentrations of 5 to 10 µg/ml, which is approximately half of the concentration needed to produce bronchodilation. There is no need to exceed peak plasma concentrations of 20 µg/ml in small animals.

Side Effects and Adverse Effects

Despite the reported occurrence of adverse effects in people, such effects are observed infrequently in dogs and cats. The most common adverse effect is nausea, manifesting as anorexia. The nonspecific inhibition of phosphodiesterase also can produce vomiting. Anxiety and restlessness also have been observed in dogs. With good client communication when theophylline is prescribed to patients, adverse effects can generally be recognized early. Immediate discontinuation of the drug is generally sufficient for adverse effects to abate. If clinically indicated, the drug can be reinstituted after several days using a lower dosage.

Much less common, but more important, is the potential for adverse effects attributed to cardiac stimulation. In this regard, theophylline is more potent than caffeine or theobromine. The cardiac adverse effects include increased heart rate, increased myocardial contractility (mild), improved right and left systolic function, vasodilation (mild), and diuretic effect (weak). At high doses (>100 mg/kg), cardiac arrhythmias are possible. The adverse effects may be both dose and route dependent. If the drug is injected intravenously, CNS effects are more likely because of rapid and high blood concentrations.

The metabolism of theophylline may be inhibited by erythromycin, enrofloxacin, and cimetidine. Interactions with fluoroquinolones other than enrofloxacin have not been investigated. At our institution, the dosage interval is generally doubled for patients treated with enrofloxacin. The metabolism of theophylline may be increased by rifampin and phenobarbital, which may necessitate increasing the dose if these drugs are used together. As a phosphodiesterase inhibitor, theophylline shares a mechanism with the cardiac drugs pimobendan and sildenafil. Potentiation of effects is possible if these drugs are used together, but we are not aware of any clinical reports documenting that such interactions have occurred. Activated charcoal increases the clearance of theophylline and other methylxanthines and is useful for treatment of a toxic overdose.

Antiinflammatory Drugs

Glucocorticoids

Glucocorticoids are used most often to decrease inflammation associated with inflammatory airway diseases, particularly allergic or idiopathic feline or canine bronchitis. Their role in the treatment of asthma and chronic bronchitis in people continues to be studied extensively, and although few in number, reports in veterinary medicine support their use. For treatment of asthma in people, inhaled corticosteroids are recognized as the most effective maintenance therapy available. Glucocorticoids are also used in the treatment of other inflammatory respiratory diseases such as eosinophilic bronchopneumopathy, tracheobronchomalacia, and chronic (lymphoplasmacytic) rhinitis. Although they are not a direct treatment, they may also improve clinical signs related to inflammation associated with diseases such as dirofilariasis or neoplasia.

Mechanism of Action

In patients with inflammatory airway diseases, glucocorticoids have potent antiinflammatory effects on the bronchial mucosa. Glucocorticoids bind to receptors on cells and inhibit the transcription of genes for the production of mediators involved in airway inflammation (cytokines, chemokines, adhesion molecules). The result is a decrease in the synthesis of inflammatory mediators such as prostaglandins, leukotrienes, and platelet-activating factor. Although these inflammatory mediators are significantly suppressed, mast cells are not affected by glucocorticoids. Glucocorticoids also enhance the action of adrenergic agonists on β_2-receptors in the bronchial smooth muscle, either by modifying the receptor or augmenting muscle relaxation after a receptor has been bound. Corticosteroids prevent down-regulation of β_2-receptors and may be synergistic when used with β_2-agonists. Glucocorticoids and theophylline used together also appear to be synergistic.

Clinical Use

The clinical effectiveness of glucocorticoid therapy for chronic respiratory disease is enhanced by treating with a sufficient dose for a sufficient period of time before beginning to taper the dosage to low-dose, alternate-day therapy. Once inflamed, the respiratory mucosa is sensitized to react with a greater inflammatory response to subsequent insults, which may include simply irritants in the air. When the initial course of treatment is continued for 2 to 3 weeks before tapering is begun, the ultimate dose of glucocorticoids needed for good control of signs long term is often much less than that that required for moderate control of signs with a more rapid taper.

Dogs. Oral prednisolone or prednisone is usually the drug of choice for dogs. A typical antiinflammatory dosage is 0.5 to 1.0 mg/kg twice daily. Improvement in clinical signs is expected within a week. If improvement is seen, this dosage is continued for 2 to 3 weeks and then gradually tapered by 25% to 33% every 1 to 2 weeks, as long as signs remain controlled. The ultimate goal is an every-other-day schedule at the minimum effective dose.

Cats. Because cats are somewhat resistant to glucocorticoids, higher dosages have been used than in dogs. Oral prednisolone at initial dosages of 2 to 4 mg/kg/day has been used for inflammatory diseases, with expected response and tapering of dose as described earlier for dogs. For cats, prednisolone is often recommended instead of prednisone because of concern that either prednisone is not well absorbed or there is a deficiency in the conversion of prednisone to the active form prednisolone; however, supportive data have been reported only in preliminary form. Because of difficulty in giving oral medications to cats, many veterinarians have administered 20 mg per cat of a long-acting formulation, methylprednisolone acetate (Depo-Medrol) intramuscularly. The effects of one injection may persist for 3 weeks. The negative aspect of this approach is the inability to achieve stable remission and minimize long-term exposure to systemic glucocorticoids. Adverse effects are common with long-term treatment, and those of particular concern for patients with respiratory disorders include weight gain, muscle weakness, and potential predisposition to pulmonary thromboembolism or infection. In addition, glucocorticoids may exacerbate or increase the risk of congestive heart failure in cats, possibly through increased plasma glucose concentrations and an increase in plasma volume leading to cardiac overload (Ployngam et al, 2006), and the development of diabetes mellitus.

Topical Corticosteroids (Metered Dose Inhalers)

Glucocorticoids are among the most valuable drugs for managing asthma in people. For people, an MDI is used to deliver the drug topically to avoid systemic adverse effects. Examples of aerosolized corticosteroids are listed in Table 151-1. Fluticasone is the most potent (18 times the potency of dexamethasone) and is the one used most often in veterinary medicine. When glucocorticoids are delivered topically with these devices, systemic adverse effects are minimized but not eliminated.

Cats with bronchitis given inhaled corticosteroids twice a day and allowed 5 to 7 breaths from the spacing chamber (10 seconds) have reduced need for oral prednisolone. In one study, inhaled fluticasone reduced bronchial hyperresponsiveness and bronchoconstriction in cats with bronchitis (Kirschvink et al, 2006). Inflammatory cells and prostaglandins in bronchoalveolar lavage fluid were also reduced. Inhaled steroids also have been effective in the management of bronchitis in dogs.

Delivery options for MDI drugs in veterinary patients were described earlier in the discussion of inhalant therapy using the bronchodilator albuterol. Fluticasone is the agent most often administered because of its high potency and low systemic effects. MDIs can deliver fluticasone doses that range from 220 μg to 44 μg. For example, a 110-μg dose of fluticasone for a cat is delivered in one puff from a 110-μg MDI. In a study comparing dosages in cats, lower dosages of 44 μg twice daily were as effective as higher dosages (Cohn et al, 2010). However, this study used a mild, allergy-induced model of feline airway disease that may not reflect typical clinical cases. Our institution usually initiates therapy at a dosage of 110 to 220 μg of fluticasone twice daily in cats or dogs. Cats with marked signs are concurrently prescribed systemic prednisolone for 2 weeks. As with systemic glucocorticoids, the initial MDI dosage is continued for at least 2 to 3 weeks, and signs should be in remission before tapering (decreasing frequency or dose) is attempted.

In people, fluticasone has a systemic absorption of only 18% to 26%, and there are extensive first-pass effects and high protein binding that prevents significant systemic active blood concentrations if it is swallowed after delivery. Therefore, clinical effects are mostly confined to the airways, and the systemic action is minimized. In cats, flunisolide was studied for its systemic effects after administration by inhalation (Reinero et al, 2006). Although there was some suppression of the hypothalamic-pituitary-adrenal axis (indicating some systemic absorption), systemic effects on immune cells (lymphocytes and lymphocyte function) were not observed, which demonstrated that inhaled flunisolide is capable of producing a local effect in the airways with minimal effects on the systemic immune system. Another adverse effect is the development of localized dermatitis either from the mask or from the topical effects of the potent steroid. Demodectic mange mites and dermatophytes have been identified in some cases, but simply discontinuing the glucocorticoid by inhaler generally results in rapid resolution. In these patients, systemic glucocorticoids are instituted.

The canisters of MDI glucocorticoids are much more expensive than prednisone or prednisolone. There is also the investment in the spacer and mask. For patients without a contraindication for systemic steroids, it is reasonable to carry out a therapeutic trial with an oral glucocorticoid before transitioning to MDI administration.

Leukotriene Inhibitors

Leukotrienes, such as leukotriene D_4, contribute to airway inflammation, produce bronchoconstriction, and increase airway wall edema in people but have not been demonstrated to be important mediators in feline asthma.

TABLE 151-1

Examples of Corticosteroids Available in Metered Dose Inhalers

Drug	Brand Name	Dose Delivered
Beclomethasone dipropionate	Vanceril	40 or 80 μg per puff
Flunisolide	AeroBid	250 μg per puff
Fluticasone propionate (most potent)	Flovent	44, 110, or 220 μg per puff
Triamcinolone acetonide	Azmacort	75 μg per puff

Therefore, the leukotriene inhibitor class of drugs may not have a role in treatment of feline respiratory disease. Their use has not been explored in dogs.

Other Antiinflammatory Drugs

Nonsteroidal antiinflammatory drugs are not recommended for the treatment of inflammatory airway and parenchymal diseases in people, and there is no evidence to support their use for these diseases in dogs or cats. Traditionally *N*-acetylcysteine has been considered a mucolytic drug (discussed further later), but it has been investigated for the treatment of respiratory diseases such as idiopathic pulmonary fibrosis in people because of its effects as an antioxidant and its possible effects on remodeling. No clear indication for this drug exists to date. Azithromycin and other newer macrolide antibiotics are being studied in human medicine based on trials showing improvement in some chronic inflammatory airway diseases (bronchitis, asthma, bronchiectasis, cystic fibrosis) with long-term use. It is unclear whether antiinflammatory properties of these drugs or antimicrobial effects against poorly characterized organisms are playing a role. Omega-3 fatty acid supplementation may also be of nonspecific benefit through its role in dampening inflammation.

Expectorants and Mucolytic Drugs

The expectorants comprise a diverse group of compounds. Their proposed benefits include increased output of bronchial secretions, enhanced clearance of bronchial exudate, and promotion of a more productive cough. Unfortunately, few clinical studies have documented efficacy for any of these drugs in people. The mechanism of action for stimulation of mucous secretions is via a vagally mediated reflex action on the gastric mucosa. Examples of expectorants are various salts of iodide. Volatile oils such as eucalyptus oil and oil of lemon are believed to increase respiratory tract secretions directly. Their clinical efficacy in veterinary medicine is unknown.

Guaifenesin is typically classified as a muscle relaxant in anesthesia and as an anesthetic adjunct but at appropriate doses it also may have an expectorant effect. The mechanism of action is uncertain, but it is possible that guaifenesin stimulates bronchial secretions via vagal pathways or accelerates particle clearance from the airways. Although many over-the-counter cough remedies contain guaifenesin, efficacy has been questioned because most preparations do not contain a large enough dose. Formulations now used in people (but not evaluated in animals) employ higher doses than older over-the-counter drugs. Most older over-the-counter formulations contain doses of 100 mg; higher-dose formulations for people include Mucinex (600- and 1200-mg tablet), Mucinex D (with pseudoephedrine), and Mucinex DM (with dextromethorphan).

Mucolytic agents are desirable for patients with voluminous, tenacious mucous secretions that cannot be cleared with mucociliary transport and cough. Because there are no proven, safe, effective drugs to accomplish this goal, the primary means of treatment include maintenance of systemic hydration, nebulization with physiologic saline solution (which has mucolytic properties), and physical therapy.

Acetylcysteine is a mucolytic agent available as a 10% solution that can be nebulized for administration to patients. Its mucolytic effect is caused by an interaction of the exposed sulfhydryl groups on the compound with disulfide bonds on mucoprotein. However appealing its mucolytic potential may be, its use is greatly limited by its irritant effects on the respiratory mucosa. When administered in nebulized form to cats, it may induce bronchoconstriction.

Anecdotally reported uses of systemically administered acetylcysteine in veterinary medicine include intravenous administration to dogs with severe bronchopneumonia, particularly small puppies or bulldogs with a hypoplastic trachea, in which mucus appears to repeatedly obstruct the trachea. It has also been administered orally to dogs or cats with idiopathic pulmonary fibrosis based on some studies in people. Although there is no clear benefit to this treatment in people, and no studies in dogs or cats, there is little else to offer these patients. In people, a dose of 600 mg PO three times daily has been used, which is approximately 8 to 9 mg/kg. For both these indications, it is quite possible that antioxidant properties account for any benefit that may be seen. Oral acetylcysteine can be obtained from nutrition or health food stores.

Decongestants

Decongestants are used to "dry up" mucous membranes. They have few indications in veterinary medicine. Decongestants are sympathomimetic drugs that stimulate the α-adrenergic receptors, causing local vasoconstriction and a decongestant effect. Short-acting topical agents include phenylephrine and phenylpropanolamine, which are common ingredients in over-the-counter nasal sprays (e.g., Neo-Synephrine). In veterinary medicine, these products are applied topically to decrease bleeding associated with some surgical procedures (e.g., nasal turbinate surgery in dogs) and rhinoscopy, and for short-term management of severe congestion associated with feline upper respiratory tract infections. Some topical decongestants, such as oxymetazoline (Afrin) and xylometazoline (Dristan), are particularly long-acting. Caution should be exercised when using the topical products for long periods. Rebound inflammation and hyperemia may occur when the action of the drug diminishes, resulting in a worsening of the problem. The systemic use of adrenergic agonists as decongestants has been a common practice in human medicine for decades. The systemic decongestant phenylpropanolamine hydrochloride is used for treating urinary incontinence in dogs and approved formulations are available for dogs (Proin Chewable Tablets). However, a beneficial effect is rarely seen in dogs or cats with rhinitis, and their use is not recommended.

Antibacterial Drugs

Antimicrobial therapy for bacterial respiratory infections includes treatment for conditions such as pneumonia (airway origin or hematogenous), aspiration pneumonia, bacterial bronchitis or tracheobronchitis, pyothorax, and rhinitis/sinusitis. An accurate diagnosis is essential, because a common error is to administer antibiotics for conditions that do not require an antibiotic.

Diffusion of antibiotics to the airways has been the subject of considerable discussion and controversy. Antibiotic concentrations in interstitial (tissue) fluid predict the active concentration necessary for treating most infections. These concentrations are equivalent to the protein-unbound (free) drug concentrations in plasma. However, the respiratory tract presents another challenge—the diffusion of antibiotics across the blood-alveolar barrier (also referred to as the *blood-bronchus barrier* in some publications). The concentration of drug that penetrates the blood-alveolar barrier is represented by the concentrations in the epithelial lining fluid (ELF), which may be an important site of infection in pneumonia. Although drug concentration in the ELF may be better for predicting efficacy than lung or plasma concentrations, this assumption has some flaws. Healthy ELF assessed in experimental animals may not represent the actual environment during clinical infection. The importance of adequate antibiotic concentrations in ELF notwithstanding, lung infection can disrupt the alveolar wall and invade the interstitial space. Some lung infections are also borne hematogenously and invade the airway via the interstitium. After pneumonia is established, the drug concentration in the area of consolidation may be more equivalent to that in the interstitial (tissue) fluid than the ELF. In reality, both concentrations may be important to evaluate: interstitial fluid drug concentrations may be predictive of respiratory tissue concentrations during infection, but drug concentrations in ELF may be more predictive of drug concentrations in airway secretions and may be helpful in eradicating infecting agents that colonize the airways. Drug concentrations in ELF are probably more important for macrolide antibiotics (e.g., azithromycin) for which ELF concentrations far exceed concentrations in plasma. Properties that favor penetration to the ELF include high lipophilicity, high potency of the drug (low minimal inhibitory concentration), and the concentration of free (unbound) drug in the interstitial fluid.

Drugs such as macrolides (erythromycin, azithromycin), tetracyclines, and fluoroquinolones appear to achieve adequate concentrations in ELF. The β-lactam antibiotics, especially the highly protein-bound drugs, and aminoglycosides do not reach high concentrations in the ELF but may diffuse into the interstitial space to achieve effective concentrations in the presence of infection. Inflammation that occurs in pneumonia produces leakage of drugs into the ELF regardless of which drug is selected.

Another approach for enabling drugs to reach infections colonizing the airways is nebulization. There is no evidence supporting the benefit of this route of antibiotic treatment in veterinary medicine, and its use is based on anecdotal reports. Potential indications for this route are limited to bacterial tracheal or bronchial infection and adjunctive treatment for management of bacterial pneumonia. It is not sufficient treatment alone for pneumonia.

In veterinary medicine, nebulization of antibiotics is generally used for administration of aminoglycosides to the airways, which minimizes concerns of systemic toxicity. Treatment for *Bordetella bronchiseptica* has been suggested using gentamicin 50 mg in 3 ml of sterile water, nebulized for 10 minutes, and delivered by face mask twice daily for 3 days (Bemis and Appel, 1977). Although this treatment resulted in decreased numbers of *Bordetella* in the airways for up to 3 days, numbers returned to pretreatment levels by 7 days. It is not known if the formulation of the drug is important in veterinary patients. Typically in veterinary patients the injectable solutions are used. But in human medicine, antibiotics for nebulization are specifically formulated without preservatives or other excipients that might produce airway inflammation or bronchoconstriction and are matched to particular nebulizers. These human medications are more expensive than injectable solutions. Risks of antibiotic administration via nebulization include bronchospasm and environmental contamination, with potential exposure of the administrator. Bronchodilators should be on hand in case of acute distress. The nebulizer unit must be properly cleaned and the sterility of administered fluids maintained to avoid nebulizing additional pathogens into the airways.

Treatment of specific respiratory tract infections is reviewed in other chapters in this section.

References and Suggested Reading

Bach JE et al: Evaluation of the bioavailability and pharmacokinetics of two extended-release theophylline formulations in dogs, *J Am Vet Med Assoc* 224:1113, 2004.

Barnes PJ: Theophylline: new perspectives for an old drug, *Am J Respir Crit Care Med* 167:813, 2003.

Bemis DA, Appel MJG: Aerosol, parenteral, and oral antibiotic treatments of *Bordetella bronchiseptica* infections in dogs, *J Am Vet Med Assoc* 170:1082, 1977.

Cohn LA et al: Effects of fluticasone propionate dosage in an experimental model of feline asthma, *J Feline Med Surg* 12:91, 2010.

Gingerich DA, Rourke JE, Strom PW: Clinical efficacy of butorphanol injectable and tablets, *Vet Med Small Anim Clin* 78:179, 1983.

Guenther-Yenke CL et al: Pharmacokinetics of an extended release theophylline product in cats, *J Am Vet Med Assoc* 231:900, 2007.

Kirschvink N et al: Inhaled fluticasone reduces bronchial responsiveness and airway inflammation in cats with mild chronic bronchitis, *J Feline Med Surg* 8:45, 2006.

KuKanich B: Pharmacokinetics of acetaminophen, codeine, and the codeine metabolites morphine and codeine-6-glucuronide in healthy Greyhound dogs, *J Vet Pharmacol Ther* 33:15, 2010.

KuKanich B, Papich MG: Plasma profile and pharmacokinetics of dextromethorphan after intravenous and oral administration in healthy dogs, *J Vet Pharmacol Ther* 27:337, 2004.

Papich MG: *Handbook of antimicrobial therapy for small animals*, St Louis, 2011, Saunders.

Ployngam T et al: Hemodynamic effects of methylprednisolone acetate administration in cats, *Am J Vet Res* 67:583, 2006.

Reinero CR et al: Inhaled flunisolide suppresses the hypothalamic-pituitary-adrenal axis, but has minimal systemic immune effects in healthy cats, *J Vet Intern Med* 20:57, 2006.

Takahama K, Shirasaki T: Central and peripheral mechanisms of narcotic antitussives: codeine-sensitive and -resistant coughs, *Cough* 3:1, 2007.

CHAPTER 152

Feline Upper Respiratory Tract Infection

JYOTHI V. ROBERTSON, *Davis, California*
KATE HURLEY, *Davis, California*

Feline upper respiratory tract infection (URI) is frequently identified in high-density populations, including those in breeding catteries and animal shelters. This clinical syndrome is inextricably linked to stress, crowding, and poor husbandry. Consequently, adopting effective preventive strategies is essential to combatting this disease in both household pets and large feline populations.

Causes and Primary Agents

Feline URI is a multifactorial disease with a primarily viral origin and secondary bacterial components. *Feline herpesvirus type 1* (FHV-1) and *feline calicivirus* (FCV) cause approximately 80% of all URIs in cats, but the relative importance of each contributing pathogen varies with context. FHV-1 is an antigenically stable DNA virus, whereas FCV is an RNA virus with multiple strains of varying virulence. Both viruses maintain carrier states, both are readily spread by fomites, and droplets can be transmitted up to 5 ft by forceful sneezing.

FHV-1 shedding is closely associated with stress. In the United States, FHV-1 is the principal pathogen causing most shelter-acquired URIs, and once infected, most cats develop latent chronic infections. In one study, the percentage of cats shedding FHV-1 increased from 4% of cats on day 1 to more than 50% on day 7 of their shelter stay (Pedersen et al, 2004). Accordingly, cats are most commonly diagnosed with URI during their second week in a shelter. Intermittent shedding occurs after stress-induced reactivation of FHV-1. URI signs are manifest during recrudescence in 50% of cats.

In contrast, FCV shedding is not linked to stress and has greater prevalence in long-term sanctuaries and large, stable populations, including hoarding situations. One recent study documented the prevalence of FCV in long-term sanctuary cats with and without clinical signs to be more than double that in shelter cats with and without clinical signs (McManus et al, 2011). The relative importance of FCV in sanctuary settings is likely due in part to dissemination of multiple mutating strains in a constant population.

Less commonly, the bacterial agents *Chlamydophila felis*, *Bordetella bronchiseptica*, *Mycoplasma* spp., and *Streptococcus canis* have been implicated in primary disease. Respiratory pathogens have a synergistic effect, and there is increased likelihood that cats harbor multiple pathogens when clinically ill. However, all pathogens associated with URI have been isolated from both healthy and clinically affected cats, so identification of a microorganism does not necessarily implicate it as the primary cause of illness.

Risk Factors

Any factor that elicits stress has the potential cause clinical signs of URI by reactivating latent feline herpesvirus. For the household pet, the addition of a new animal, a recent move, or a trip to the veterinarian could be enough to cause recrudescence.

For cats entering animal shelters, the cumulative effect of many stressors compounded with a new environment, can lead to viral shedding. A cat's length of stay, or time spent in the shelter, is directly linked to development of URI, and, conversely, development of URI leads to increased lengths of stay. Crowded conditions, poor housing, loud noises, and new foods make cats more susceptible to illness. Notably, the single-compartment feline cages commonly used in shelters are directly linked to stress and, by extension, illness (Kessler and Turner, 1999). These housing units provide insufficient floor space, which limits a cat's ability to exhibit normal feline behaviors (e.g., stretching, hiding, grooming), and lack sufficient separation of bedding, food, and litter.

Cats in animal hoarding situations often manifest clinical signs of feline URI. When multiple cats from a single household are diagnosed with severe or chronic URI over an extended period, the clinician should obtain a thorough history and evaluate the housing environment.

Clinical Signs

The magnitude of evidenced clinical signs depends on the immune status of the cat, the specific pathogens or strains involved, infecting dose, presence of coinfections, and the environment. A list of clinical signs associated with the most common URI pathogens is provided in Table 152-1. The organisms listed in this table can cause overlapping clinical signs. Thus a particular clinical manifestation does not implicate a specific pathogen as the cause of disease. Synergism among pathogens may lead to more severe clinical signs in cats harboring multiple pathogens.

Clinical Signs Associated with Major Pathogens

Pathogen	Clinical Signs
Feline calicivirus	Rhinitis, stomatitis, oral ulceration, conjunctivitis, polyarthritis, lower airway disease, virulent systemic disease—systemic vasculitis
Feline herpesvirus type 1	Rhinitis, stomatitis, conjunctivitis, keratitis, facial dermatitis, corneal ulcerations, corneal sequestrum
Bordetella bronchiseptica	Conjunctivitis, tracheobronchitis, pneumonia
Chlamydophila felis	Conjunctivitis, mild upper airway signs; can cause severe disease in conjunction with other respiratory pathogens

Diagnosis

The diagnosis of acute feline URI is based on clinical signs often coupled to a triggering event. Diagnostic testing is warranted in individual cats, in cases of chronic disease, and in populations in which disease manifestations are unusually severe or frequent. It is important to consider noninfectious differential diagnoses for URI signs, including neoplasia, inflammatory polyp, foreign body, trauma, cleft palate, chronic rhinosinusitis, oronasal fistula, and fungal infection. Preexisting immunosuppression caused by feline leukemia virus or feline immunodeficiency virus infection should be considered in previously untested cats. It is also emphasized that although viral or bacterial culture or DNA detection can be used to confirm the presence of a potential pathogen, a positive test result does not confirm causality. Additionally, oculonasal or oropharyngeal swabs submitted for sampling are likely to contain some normal flora.

Real-time polymerase chain reaction (RT-PCR) is one test used to evaluate potential infectious primary causes of URI. However, RT-PCR results must be interpreted with caution, especially in individual cases. Currently, a positive PCR test result cannot distinguish between the inciting cause of disease, commensals, and vaccine strains. In the future, quantitative RT-PCR tests may be available to differentiate acute infection from carrier states. A negative test result helps rule out an acute infection with a particular infective agent but not a carrier state, because shedding can be sporadic.

In group settings, sampling a minimum of 5 to 10 affected cats or 10% of the population early in the course of disease should be considered. Positive test results should be interpreted in the context of the expected prevalence of the organism in that population. In severe outbreaks, in which cats are euthanized or are dying from disease, histopathologic analysis and necropsy should be performed to determine the underlying cause and guide risk assessment. Monitoring of disease prevalence, incidence, duration, and severity is critical for assessing the success of URI control measures. These data also provide a baseline for comparison. In this manner, URI incidence, prevalence, and rates serve as overall indicators of the welfare of a cat population (Hurley, 2004).

Treatment

Most cases of feline URI are self-resolving within 2 weeks. Because of the disease's viral origin, blanket application of antibiotics in group settings is not recommended. Rather, the instigating risk factors should be remedied to prevent cats from acquiring illness through exposure or reinfection. Supportive treatment that may be provided includes fluid rehydration therapy, humidification of the environment, and administration of appetite stimulants such as cyproheptadine HCl (1 to 2 mg per cat, q12-24h PO).

Antibiotics

Antibiotics are often administered to treat secondary bacterial infection or to target known or suspected primary or coinfecting bacteria. Doxycycline (5 mg/kg q12h PO or 10 mg/kg q24h PO) is commonly chosen to treat suspected infection with *Bordetella, Chlamydophila,* and *Mycoplasma* spp. Doxycycline (in particular doxycycline hyclate) should be compounded into a liquid form, since it has been linked to esophagitis and esophageal strictures in cats. Dry pills can be crushed and suspended in a variety of products, including milk or corn syrup or other sweet-tasting liquid. Formulations should be used within 7 days. Pills (and possibly even liquids) should be followed with a bolus of liquid (6 ml). Other commonly chosen antibiotics with dosages are listed in Table 152-2.

A broad-spectrum antibiotic that includes gram-negative coverage may be administered when there is no response to initial therapy or when secondary bacterial infection is the main target of treatment. If the patient does not improve after 5 to 7 days of treatment, treatment plans should be adjusted and a change in antibiotics considered. In general, antibiotics should be administered until resolution of clinical signs, rather than for a specified duration. An exception to this rule is chronic cases of URI or disease known to be caused by *Chlamydophila* infection, which will require a longer treatment course (2 to 3 months) beyond the resolution of clinical signs. If antibiotic therapy fails after two courses of antibiotic treatment, further diagnostic testing may be warranted to rule out other causes of illness or underlying immunosuppression.

Antivirals

Lysine is an essential amino acid that interferes with FHV replication in vitro. When used as adjunctive or palliative therapy in client-owned cats, it is administered as a bolus of 500 mg twice daily (Maggs, 2010). Lysine was found to be ineffective as a preventative in shelter populations when administered in food (Maggs et al, 2007; Rees and Lubinski, 2008). Treatments specifically targeting FHV-1 and FCV are currently under study but are beyond the scope of this chapter.

TABLE 152-2

Commonly Administered Antibiotics for Feline Upper Respiratory Tract Infection

Antibiotic	Dose	Comments
Amoxicillin/clavulanate	13.75 mg/kg q12h PO or 62.5 mg per cat q12h PO	Broad spectrum; disrupts cell wall; not effective against *Mycoplasma*
Azithromycin	15 mg/kg q24h PO	Relatively broad spectrum
Doxycycline	5 mg/kg q12h PO or 10 mg/kg q24h PO	Provides good coverage for primary bacterial respiratory pathogens including *Bordetella, Chlamydophila, Mycoplasma* spp. Administer as liquid suspension, or flush with water after administration
Cephalexin	22 mg/kg q8h PO	First-generation cephalosporin; active against gram-positive organisms; not effective against *Mycoplasma*
Clindamycin	10 mg/kg q24h PO	Lincosamide antibiotic; active against anaerobes; penetrates bone; effective against *Bordetella, Mycoplasma, Chlamydophila* Administer as liquid suspension, or flush with water after administration
Enrofloxacin	2.5-5.0 mg/kg q24h PO	Broad spectrum; effective against *Chlamydophila, Mycoplasma* Do not exceed 5 mg/kg/day
Minocycline	5 mg/kg q12h PO	Similar to doxycycline, less commonly used
Pradofloxacin	7.5 mg/kg (liquid suspension) q24h PO	Similar to enrofloxacin but better coverage of *Mycoplasma* spp. and anaerobes; less ophthalmic concerns

PO, Orally.

Prevention

Strategies to Combat Crowding

Since crowding is a primary cause of illness in animal shelters, adopting strategies that maintain the population at a number that is appropriate for the facility size and staffing capacity are critical to reducing the incidence of URI. Shelters must have sufficient staff, housing units, and time to care for all animals in their facility. Decreasing the length of stay for each individual cat by ensuring that it is moved through the facility quickly will decrease exposure to disease and increase the organization's ability to save more animals. Decreasing lengths of stay will notably also reduce the overall shelter population and further combat crowding.

Housing Solutions to Reduce Stress

Housing impacts many aspects of the health and well-being of those cats in confinement; therefore, simple improvements can greatly reduce disease in multicat facilities. Purchasing double-compartment housing units or installing portholes in existing cages allows separation of litter from food and bedding and increases the overall square footage of living space while minimizing animal handling (Figure 152-1). Hiding boxes or a simple towel draped over a cage can greatly reduce stress in cats and thereby decrease the incidence of disease (a towel or cage cover is preferred if floor space is limited). Cats should be housed away from dogs, and cats in different age groups should not be mixed in housing units.

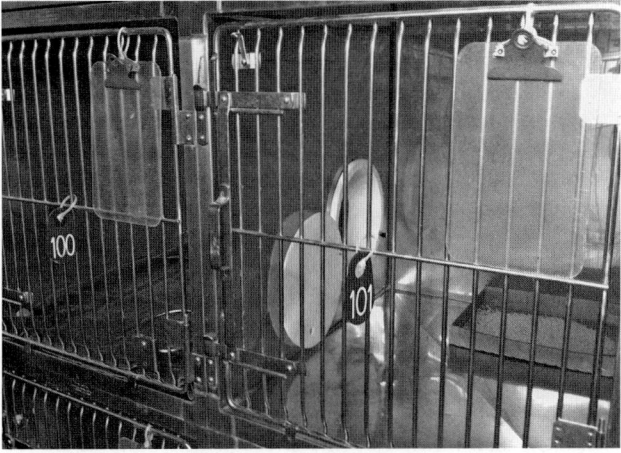

Figure 152-1 Example of a porthole between cages that allows separation of litter from food and bedding.

Vaccination

Natural infection does not create long-term immunity for any of the common URI pathogens. Therefore, while vaccination may diminish the severity of clinical signs and reduce pathogen shedding, it does not prevent infection or development of the carrier state. Both modified live virus (MLV) and inactivated virus subcutaneously administered vaccines are available for FHV-1 and FCV, formulated as combination vaccines with and without feline panleukopenia vaccine (feline viral rhinotracheitis and calicivirus [FVRC] and feline viral rhinotracheitis, calicivirus, and panleukopenia [FVRCP], respectively.

Intranasal MLV two-way (FVRC) or three-way (FVRCP) vaccines also are available.

A modified live intranasal vaccine is available for feline *Bordetella* and both modified live and inactivated vaccines are available for *Chlamydophila felis* in conjunction with the FVRCP vaccine. Use of these vaccinations is not recommended unless those pathogens have been diagnosed specifically in a feline population or a pet is at known risk of exposure. Cats living in high-density populations such as animal shelters should receive an MLV FVRCP vaccination (first vaccination at 4 to 6 weeks, then q2wk until 16 to 18 weeks). The intranasal MLV FVRC (two-way) vaccine may be administered to kittens as early as 2 weeks of age in animal shelters or other high-risk facilities where there is rampant URI.

References and Suggested Reading

Hurley KF: Implementing a population health plan in an animal shelter: goal setting, data collection and monitoring, and policy development. In Miller L, Zawistowski S, editors: *Shelter medicine for veterinarians and staff*, Ames, IA, 2004, Blackwell Publishing, p 211.

Kessler MR, Turner DC: Effects of density and cage size on stress in domestic cats (*Felis silvestris catus*) housed in animal shelters and boarding catteries, *Anim Welf* 8(3):259, 1999.

Maggs DJ: Antiviral therapy for feline herpesvirus infections, *Vet Clin North Am Small Anim Pract* 40(6):1055, 2010.

Maggs DJ et al: Effects of dietary lysine supplementation in cats with enzootic upper respiratory disease, *J Feline Med Surg* 9(2):97, 2007.

McManus CM et al: Prevalence of upper respiratory pathogens in four management models for unowned cats in the southeast United States, Research Abstract Program of the 2011 ACVIM Forum, Denver, CO, June 15-18, 2011 (abstr).

Pedersen NC et al: Common virus infections in cats, before and after being placed in shelters, with emphasis on feline enteric coronavirus, *J Feline Med Surg* 6(2):83, 2004.

Rees TM, Lubinski JL: Oral supplementation with l-lysine did not prevent upper respiratory infection in a shelter population of cats, *J Feline Med Surg* 10:510, 2008.

CHAPTER 153

Canine Infectious Respiratory Disease Complex

JANE E. SYKES, *Davis, California*

Canine infectious respiratory disease is a widespread problem where large numbers of dogs are collectively housed indoors, as in shelters, commercial dog colonies, and breeding facilities. In shelter environments, canine infectious respiratory disease complex (CIRDC), also known as *kennel cough* or *canine infectious tracheobronchitis,* delays rehoming and may result in unmanageable costs related to treatment, quarantine, and isolation. CIRDC can develop in pet dogs after contact with large numbers of other dogs at dog parks, at canine sporting events such as fly ball, or during dog behavior classes. It also can occur after dogs (or their owners) visit veterinary hospitals, boarding facilities, or pet daycare centers.

With the widespread clinical application of molecular diagnostic assays, it has become increasingly apparent that the number of infectious agents that can damage the canine respiratory tract is much larger than previously recognized. Most cases are viral in origin. Viruses believed to play a role in canine contagious respiratory disease include canine herpesvirus (CHV), canine adenovirus type 2 (CAV-2), canine distemper virus (CDV), canine parainfluenza virus (CPiV), canine respiratory coronavirus (CRCoV), and canine influenza virus (CIV). CIV appears to have originated from an equine H3N8 influenza virus that first emerged in racing greyhounds in Florida and has spread across the United States through dog-to-dog transmission. CRCoV was first identified in a rehoming kennel in the United Kingdom and also appears to be widespread in the United States. It is distinct from canine enteric coronavirus. Finally, a pneumovirus (canine pneumovirus) also may be involved in CIRDC, but more research is required to determine the significance of this agent.

Coinfections with multiple viruses and bacteria such as *Mycoplasma* spp., *Bordetella bronchiseptica,* and *Streptococcus equi* subspecies *zooepidemicus* are common and contribute to an increased severity of disease. Studies in England have suggested that *Mycoplasma cynos* may be a primary pathogen (Rycroft et al, 2007), but whether this is true in other countries is unclear. Other *Mycoplasma* spp. may be more likely to represent normal flora that invade opportunistically. Although the majority of the canine respiratory pathogens have a worldwide distribution, their relative prevalence varies from year to year and among geographic locations. Even within a state or city, predominant pathogens may differ from one shelter and boarding kennel to another.

Mycoplasma spp. and the enveloped viruses CDV, CHV, CPiV, CRCoV, and CIV survive poorly in the environment and are susceptible to a variety of disinfectants. Despite this relative fragility, direct contact with organisms that persist even for a short time in the environment may be important for transmission in densely housed canine populations. CAV-2 is a nonenveloped virus and has the potential to survive several weeks on fomites. Other microorganisms that may persist in the environment and may be transmitted on fomites include *B. bronchiseptica* and *S. equi* subspecies *zooepidemicus*.

There are a large number of strains of *B. bronchiseptica*, varying in virulence and in host specificity. Nevertheless, strains that infect dogs can be passed to cats and vice versa. Shedding of *B. bronchiseptica* by both dogs and cats may continue intermittently for at least a month and sometimes several months after infection. Survival inside of phagocytes may allow for evasion of the immune system and help to explain persistent infections. *S. equi* subspecies *zooepidemicus* has been isolated from shelter dogs in outbreaks of severe pneumonia and may contribute to an increased severity of disease when present in coinfections with respiratory viruses. Both *B. bronchiseptica* and *S. equi* subspecies *zooepidemicus* have been uncommonly reported to infect humans. *B. bronchiseptica* has caused primary respiratory illness in immunocompromised people.

Diagnosis

Generally it is not possible to identify the cause of transmissible respiratory disease in dogs based solely on clinical features. Each pathogen produces a similar spectrum of clinical signs. Occasionally, a specific causative diagnosis may be strongly suspected based on the presence of particular clinical signs, such as footpad hyperkeratosis or chorioretinitis in dogs with distemper, or dendritic corneal ulceration in dogs infected with CHV. However, the high prevalence of coinfections and increased severity of disease when multiple pathogens are present complicates diagnosis. In addition, other noncontagious causes of respiratory disease in dogs (such as inflammatory airway disease, respiratory tract neoplasia, or fungal pneumonia) can produce signs that resemble transmissible respiratory disease. A history of exposure to other dogs can increase suspicion for a diagnosis of CIRDC.

Most dogs experience self-limiting disease. Attempts to obtain a causative diagnosis should be made when disease persists for longer than 7 to 10 days or is complicated by secondary bacterial pneumonia. The latter may be accompanied by mucopurulent ocular or nasal discharge, fever, lethargy, and inappetence. When only one pet dog is affected, the diagnosis is further complicated by the fact that pathogens associated with CIRDC also can be isolated from healthy dogs. Thus the clinical significance of a positive test result for one of these pathogens may be unclear. When outbreaks occur in shelters or the pattern of endemic respiratory disease changes, attempts to make a causative diagnosis are indicated. Oropharyngeal, conjunctival, and nasal swabs or airway lavage specimens may be submitted for aerobic bacterial culture, for *Mycoplasma* culture, and for molecular diagnostic testing. In an outbreak situation, collection of multiple specimens from both affected and healthy dogs in the affected area facilitates diagnosis and interpretation of positive test results. Virus isolation also is available from some specialized veterinary diagnostic laboratories. Organism detection methods, such as polymerase chain reaction (PCR) assay or virus isolation, are best used early in the course of illness (e.g., the first 1 to 3 days) or in exposed dogs that have not yet developed clinical signs. Use of a combination of serologic and organism detection methods may also facilitate diagnosis when outbreaks occur. In shelter situations or in outbreaks in which severe disease occurs, necropsies can provide valuable information and should be performed by a veterinary pathologist as soon as possible after death or euthanasia. Tissues should be submitted for histopathologic analysis (in formalin), bacterial and viral cultures (fresh tissue), and PCR testing for respiratory viruses and bacteria (fresh or frozen tissue).

For dogs that develop chronic bronchitis or bronchopneumonia, a full physical examination, complete blood count, and thoracic radiographs are indicated, and if possible, specimens for aerobic bacterial culture and susceptibility testing, *Mycoplasma* culture, and molecular diagnostic testing should be collected using bronchoscopy and bronchoalveolar lavage. Tracheal lavage is acceptable if bronchoscopy is not possible or affordable; in some cases collection of an airway specimen may not be possible because of patient condition, and empiric antimicrobial drug therapy must be used.

Treatment and Prognosis

Uncomplicated CIRDC in dogs resolves without treatment in most cases, regardless of the underlying cause. Thus if a dog has signs of respiratory disease that have been present for fewer than 7 to 10 days and remains bright and has good appetite, no treatment may be necessary. In some patients (such as those with bordetellosis), cough may persist for as long as 10 to 30 days. Cough suppressants such as hydrocodone could be used in dogs with a nonproductive, honking cough that occurs throughout the day and night, but these drugs are not indicated for all dogs because they can suppress normal clearing mechanisms and contribute to pneumonia. Cough suppressants should not be used in dogs with a productive cough. Use of a harness or gentle leader rather than a neck collar for leash walking also may reduce cough. Removing affected animals to reduce stress and coinfections may be beneficial, especially in overcrowded environments with poor hygiene.

Antimicrobial treatment is indicated when there is evidence of bacterial infection, such as mucopurulent ocular and nasal discharge, lethargy, decreased appetite, and radiographic evidence of bacterial bronchopneumonia, such as pulmonary alveolar infiltrates and consolidation. Young puppies (<6 to 8 weeks of age) should also be considered candidates for early initiation of treatment, because disease may progress rapidly to pneumonia and death in neonates. For dogs with acute disease and clinical signs suggestive of primary or secondary bacterial infection, empiric treatment with amoxicillin/clavulanic acid or doxycycline could be considered. The optimal duration of treatment is unknown, but 7 to 10 days is a reasonable choice. When *B. bronchiseptica* or *Mycoplasma* infection is suspected, doxycycline is the best first choice. Isolates of *B. bronchiseptica* from dogs and cats have the propensity to exhibit multidrug resistance (i.e., resistance to three or more antimicrobial drug classes). Resistance to amoxicillin and trimethoprim/sulfamethoxazole appears to be common. Fluoroquinolones and azithromycin have activity against *Mycoplasma* spp. and many of the other bacteria associated with infectious bronchitis and pneumonia, and may be effective if doxycycline or amoxicillin/clavulanate fails. Treatment of dogs with CIRDC and evidence of bacterial infection is optimally based on the results of culture of an airway lavage specimen and antimicrobial susceptibility testing.

For dogs with severe bronchopneumonia, initial treatment should involve the use of broad-spectrum parenteral antimicrobial drugs that effectively penetrate the blood-bronchus barrier, such as a combination of a fluoroquinolone (such as enrofloxacin) and clindamycin. This treatment should be administered while the results of culture and susceptibility testing are awaited. Fluoroquinolones are generally active against *B. bronchiseptica* and *Mycoplasma* spp., and clindamycin is active against *Streptococcus* spp. as well as most anaerobes. Once culture and susceptibility results are available, treatment should be tailored to the *in vitro* susceptibility the organism(s) demonstrate (*de-escalation*); if there is resistance to one of the drugs, that drug could be discontinued. If there is resistance to both drugs, a different drug that has adequate penetration of the blood-bronchus barrier should be used, according to the results of culture and susceptibility testing.

Dogs with pneumonia also may require treatment with intravenous fluids, oxygen, nebulized agents, and coupage. A feeding tube may be required to provide nutritional support in dogs that are inappetent. Dogs with refractory *B. bronchiseptica* bronchopneumonia may respond to a short course of treatment with nebulized aminoglycoside solutions (5 days of 3 to 5 mg/kg/day), in addition to parenteral antimicrobial drugs. However, nebulized aminoglycosides also can irritate the airways, and so they should be used with caution and only if the presence of *Bordetella* has been confirmed and an adequate response does not occur to parenteral antimicrobial drugs. The optimum duration of oral antimicrobial drug treatment is unknown, but a minimum of 4 weeks of treatment is currently recommended. It is possible that shorter courses of treatment, as used to treat human patients, may be effective, but more research is required in this arena. Drugs that can be administered orally for outpatient treatment of bacterial pneumonia should be selected on the basis of culture and antimicrobial susceptibility results for organisms isolated from the lower airways. If culture and susceptibility testing was not performed, the antimicrobial drug class associated with clinical response is chosen for long-term oral therapy.

Given the large number of viruses involved in CIRDC, antiviral drugs also hold promise for treatment of severe or persistent CIRDC. For dogs with confirmed ocular CHV infections that are associated with corneal ulceration, topical antiviral ophthalmic preparations such as idoxuridine could be considered. The efficacy and optimal dosage of neuraminidase inhibitors used to treat influenza virus infections in humans, such as oseltamivir, is unknown. Because of this, and because oseltamivir is a first-line treatment for pandemic influenza in humans, it should not be used to treat dogs with respiratory disease, even when CIV infection is known to be present.

Prognosis depends on the virulence of the causative agent(s), the presence of coinfections, and other factors associated with host immunosuppression. Prognosis is generally excellent for dogs with uncomplicated infections caused by a single pathogen. For CIV infection, mortality rates have been less than 8% and could be lower with rapid diagnosis and appropriate treatment. In one study, bronchopneumonia associated with *B. bronchiseptica* infection was more severe than that associated with other bacterial agents, and affected dogs also had higher values of partial carbon dioxide pressure in mixed venous blood, were more likely to require supplemental oxygen, and had significantly longer hospitalization times (mean of 7.2 days compared with 4.9 days; Radhakrishnan et al, 2007).

Prevention

A variety of vaccines are available for CIRDC pathogens, including *B. bronchiseptica*, CDV, CPiV, CAV-2, and CIV. Except for the vaccine for CDV, none of the available vaccines completely prevents infection and shedding, but they can lessen the severity of disease, provided other factors such as overcrowding and appropriate disinfection and reduction of other stressors also are addressed. Vaccines for canine transmissible respiratory disease are considered to be noncore vaccines, so they should be administered to dogs at risk of exposure, such as those that enter shelters, boarding kennels, shows, sporting competitions, popular dog parks, or pet daycare facilities. Shedding of *B. bronchiseptica*, *Mycoplasma* spp., and CDV may continue despite resolution of clinical signs, so affected dogs and cats should remain in isolation from other animals whenever possible for at least 2 months after treatment. The remaining viruses are generally shed for short periods (<2 weeks).

Parenteral and intranasal attenuated live vaccines are available for CPiV and CAV-2. Inactivated, parenteral vaccines are available for reduction of disease caused by CIV and viral shedding. One CIV vaccine also reduced the severity of illness caused by co-challenge with CIV and *S. equi* subspecies *zooepidemicus*. Several avirulent live, intranasal *B. bronchiseptica* vaccines are available for dogs worldwide, some of which also contain CPiV with or without CAV-2. Intranasal vaccines stimulate mucosal immunity and provide protection as soon as 3 days after a single dose of vaccine. Protection with intranasal vaccines also occurs in the face of maternal antibody and has been shown to last at least 1 year. Inactivated parenteral *B. bronchiseptica* vaccines are also available for dogs, but two doses administered 3 to 4 weeks apart are required to stimulate maximal immunity, which occurs 1 week after the second dose. The rapid onset of protection that follows the use of intranasal vaccines makes them the vaccine type of choice for puppies and animals introduced into heavily contaminated environments, such as shelters, when immunization in advance of entry usually is not possible. Intranasal *B. bronchiseptica* vaccines should not be given to animals treated with antimicrobial drugs, and administration to aggressive animals without sedation may not be feasible. Transient signs of mild to moderate respiratory disease can occur in a small percentage of dogs (and cats) several days after vaccination with intranasal vaccines.

Inadvertent parenteral administration of intranasal vaccines can lead to severe injection site reactions, hepatic necrosis, and even death in some dogs. In this situation, subcutaneous fluids should be administered at the site of vaccination, and immediate treatment with antimicrobial drugs is indicated. A gentamicin sulfate solution should be instilled into the affected area (2 to 4 mg/kg gentamicin sulfate in 10 to 30 ml of saline), and dogs then should be treated with oral doxycycline for 5 to 7 days. Some dogs may need more aggressive supportive care. Special packaging has been developed by some vaccine manufacturers in an attempt to prevent inadvertent parenteral administration of the intranasal vaccine.

Concerns have also been raised that intranasal *B. bronchiseptica* vaccines may cause respiratory disease in immunosuppressed humans who inhale the vaccine directly during administration or who contact vaccine organisms shed by recently immunized dogs. However, there has been no molecular proof thus far that the *B. bronchiseptica* strains isolated from affected human patients match the vaccine strain. Fewer scientific data are available on the efficacy of parenteral vaccines in dogs compared with *B. bronchiseptica* intranasal vaccines, although parenteral vaccines are used in human medicine for prevention of pertussis. One study showed that an intranasal vaccine was more effective than a parenteral antigen extract vaccine (Davis et al, 2007). Additional challenge studies are required that directly compare the efficacy of intranasal and parenteral *B. bronchiseptica* vaccines for dogs.

References and Suggested Reading

Buonavoglia C, Martella V: Canine respiratory viruses, *Vet Res* 38:355, 2007.

Davis R et al: Comparison of the mucosal immune response in dogs vaccinated with either an intranasal avirulent live culture or a subcutaneous antigen extract vaccine of *Bordetella bronchiseptica*, *Vet Ther* 8:32, 2007.

Erles K et al: Longitudinal study of viruses associated with canine infectious respiratory disease, *J Clin Microbiol* 42:4524, 2004.

Radhakrishnan A et al: Community-acquired infectious pneumonia in puppies: 65 cases (1993-2002), *J Am Vet Med Assoc* 230:1493, 2007.

Renshaw RW et al: Pneumovirus in dogs with acute respiratory disease, *Emerg Infect Dis* 16:993, 2010.

Rycroft AN, Tsounakou E, Chalker V: Serological evidence of *Mycoplasma cynos* infection in canine infectious respiratory disease, *Vet Microbiol* 120:358, 2007.

Speakman AJ et al: Antibiotic susceptibility of canine *Bordetella bronchiseptica* isolates, *Vet Microbiol* 71:193, 2000.

CHAPTER **154**

Rhinitis in Dogs

NED F. KUEHN, *Southfield, Michigan*

Sneezing and nasal discharge usually are associated with diseases of the nose, paranasal sinuses, and nasopharynx. Sneezing frequently precedes the onset of notable nasal discharge. The severity and frequency of sneezing may diminish over time, whereas the nasal discharge frequently worsens in severity and changes in character. Therefore dogs with chronic rhinitis frequently have chronic nasal discharge rather than persistent sneezing. The nature of sneezing may aid in localizing the region of the problem. Expiratory sneezing typically is associated with sinus or intranasal disease. Reverse or inspiratory sneezing (aspiration reflex) is a normal response to mechanical irritation of the dorsal nasopharyngeal mucosa. The presence of reverse sneezing is usually correlated with caudal nasal, nasopharyngeal, or sinus disease. Some dogs may have posterior rather than anterior nasal discharge, and the only indication of primary nasal disease may be obstructive nasal breathing.

The causes of nasal discharge and obstructive nasal breathing in the dog are listed in Box 154-1. The principal diseases associated with chronic rhinitis are sinonasal neoplasia, idiopathic lymphoplasmacytic rhinitis, and fungal rhinitis (Lefebvre et al, 2005). Nasal discharge is not limited to primary nasal disease but also may occur with systemic and extranasal disorders. Extranasal disorders

BOX 154-1

Differential Diagnosis for Nasal Discharge or Obstructive Nasal Breathing

Nasal and Paranasal Sinus Disorders
- Allergic rhinitis
- Bacterial rhinitis (*Bordetella bronchiseptica*, *Pasteurella multocida*)
- Ciliary dyskinesia
- Dental disease
- Foreign body
- Fungal rhinitis (*Aspergillus fumigatus*, *Penicillium* spp., *Rhinosporidium seeberi*, *Cryptococcus neoformans*)
- Hyperplastic rhinitis (Irish wolfhounds)
- Idiopathic lymphoplasmacytic rhinitis
- Nasal polyps
- Nasopharyngeal stenosis
- Nasopharyngeal turbinates
- Neoplasia
- Nasal parasites (*Pneumonyssus caninum*, *Eucoleus [Capillaria] boehmi*, *Cuterebra* spp.)
- Oronasal fistula
- Palatine defects
- Trauma
- Viral rhinitis (canine distemper)

Viral Infection and Extranasal Disorders
- Coagulopathies
- Cricopharyngeal disease
- Environmental agents (dusts, smoke)
- Esophageal stricture
- Hypertension
- Hyperviscosity syndrome
- Immunoglobulin A immunodeficiency
- Megaesophagus
- Oropharyngeal diseases
- Pneumonia
- Polycythemia
- Thrombocytopenia
- Vasculitis
- Vomiting
- Xeromycteria

often have systemic signs (e.g., depression, pyrexia, hemorrhage) and a history of acute onset, whereas primary nasal disorders have a more chronic nature. Important extranasal disorders that may manifest with nasal discharge include coagulopathies, vasculitis, hypertension, hyperviscosity syndrome, and pneumonia.

The character and type of nasal discharge may be helpful in developing a list of potential causes, but these findings are not characteristic for specific diseases. Unilateral discharge is often associated with neoplasia, fungal and foreign body rhinitis, and dental disease. Bilateral discharge is typical of systemic disorders, advanced neoplasia or fungal rhinitis, idiopathic lymphoplasmacytic rhinitis, and allergic rhinitis. However, it also is possible for systemic disorders and idiopathic lymphoplasmacytic rhinitis to present with only unilateral nasal discharge. Serous nasal discharge may be seen initially in a variety of nasal diseases but often becomes mucopurulent as disease progresses and secondary bacterial invasion

occurs. Mucopurulent nasal discharge is most common and indicates bacterial infection *secondary* to an underlying disorder that has damaged the nasal mucosa with resultant bacterial invasion. Primary bacterial infection is an exceedingly rare cause of rhinitis in dogs. Mucopurulent and serous discharges may be blood tinged as a result of mucosal erosion. Epistaxis usually results from an underlying nasal disorder causing erosion of a major blood vessel but also may be seen with systemic disorders such as coagulopathies, hypertension, vasculitis, or hyperviscosity syndrome.

Diagnosis

Clinical history and physical examination findings generally offer an indication of primary nasal disease as opposed to systemic or extranasal disease. Routine laboratory tests (complete blood count, serum chemistry panels, urinalysis), coagulation profile, blood pressure, and thoracic radiographs are important to rule out most of the systemic or extranasal causes of nasal discharge. Cytologic evaluation of nasal discharge is rarely helpful except possibly for identification of *Eucoleus (Capillaria) boehmi* parasitic ova. Performing bacterial and fungal cultures of nasal discharge is not recommended because results are nonspecific and simply represent resident bacteria and fungi. Serologic testing for aspergillosis should be considered, because a positive result is highly suggestive of disease, although a negative result does not rule out nasal infection (Pomrantz et al, 2007). Empiric antimicrobial treatment is not advised and merely delays definitive diagnosis unless chronic *Bordetella bronchiseptica* or *Pasteurella multocida* rhinitis (both very rare) or pneumonia is present.

Diagnostic imaging studies are performed with the patient under anesthesia. Imaging studies often are essential in dogs with chronic rhinitis to help reach a diagnosis. It is critical that imaging studies be completed *before* rhinoscopy or collection of intranasal samples so that blood from secondary hemorrhage does not obscure subtle lesions or affect the quality of diagnostic images. If dental disease is suspected, dental radiographs are recommended to evaluate teeth and surrounding structures. Radiographic images of the nose and sinuses may provide some insight but often do not reveal a specific cause of the nasal disease. Radiographs often lack sufficient resolution to identify or localize early nasal disease. Computed tomography (CT) is vastly superior to plain radiography of the nasal cavity (Lefebvre et al, 2005). Nasal CT provides a thorough assessment of the nasal cavities and paranasal sinuses and provides superior insight into the nature and extent of disease. Contrast-enhanced CT images are useful to distinguish between vascularized soft tissue and mucus accumulation. Because nasal CT clearly demonstrates the location and extent of nasal disease, it is often used to help guide postimaging rhinoscopic and biopsy procedures and delineate nasal tumors for radiation therapy. If routine diagnostic steps do not provide a cause for rhinitis, referral to an institution providing CT imaging is advised. Although magnetic resonance imaging (MRI) is often considered superior to CT for delineation of tumor borders, a recent study failed to document an advantage of MRI over CT in detecting intracalvarial changes in dogs with nasal neoplasia (Dhaliwal et al, 2004).

Rhinoscopy should be performed only after all imaging studies are completed and with the patient still under anesthesia. The nasopharynx is examined before the nasal cavity, because if hemorrhage is induced by examination of the nasal cavities, blood frequently pools in the nasopharynx and obscures visualization of this area. Retroflex nasopharyngoscopy is performed by turning a small flexible scope 180 degrees around the caudal margin of the soft palate to evaluate the caudal nares, dorsal soft palate, and nasopharynx. Tumors or foreign bodies lodged within the caudal nares or within the nasopharynx occasionally cause rhinitis in dogs. Anterior rhinoscopy may be limited by the size of the nasal cavity compared with the size of the scope, lesion location, and difficulty in visualizing intranasal structures because of mucus or hemorrhage. The convoluted nature of the nasal passages does not allow for evaluation of the entire nasal cavity; thus foreign bodies and neoplastic masses may be overlooked. The mucosa should be evaluated for color, vascularity, friability, edema, and presence of parasites or fungal plaques. The nasal passages should be evaluated for obstruction by tissue masses, foreign bodies, and secretions. A loss of normal nasal turbinates indicates the presence of a destructive rhinitis secondary to fungal infection or severe idiopathic lymphoplasmacytic rhinitis. Rhinoscopy is especially helpful in the diagnosis of fungal rhinitis and rostrally positioned nasal foreign bodies. Fungal rhinitis often is associated with widespread turbinate destruction, and rhinoscopy may reveal a cavernous nasal cavity with off-white to gray fungal plaques scattered across the surface of the nasal mucosa.

Procurement of nasal specimens and biopsy of nasal tissue should be performed only after imaging and visual examinations are completed and while the patient is still under anesthesia. Tissue from lesions visualized during rhinoscopy may be obtained by direct biopsy with forceps passed either adjacent to or through the endoscope. Analysis of specimens obtained by rhinoscopically directed biopsy of masses identified within the nose can be limited by the size of the tissue samples recovered and inflammation surrounding the mass. Lymphoplasmacytic inflammation often is present with intranasal neoplasms, whereas idiopathic lymphoplasmacytic rhinitis is not associated with mass lesions in the nose. I prefer to use nasal CT images to guide instrumentation for procurement of biopsy samples. Depending on the size of the nose, either small (2- to 4-mm) clamshell or colonic biopsy forceps are advanced to the site of disease as identified from CT images, and multiple biopsy specimens are then obtained. During the biopsy procedure it is recommended that the dog be in sternal recumbency with the rostral end of the nose directed downward to facilitate drainage of escaping blood away from the nasopharynx and oropharynx. Following biopsy, the tip of the nose remains positioned downward, and the oropharynx and cranial esophagus are suctioned to remove blood clots. Nasal lavage may be required to dislodge foreign material identified or suspected to be present within the nose. The rostral aspect of the nose should be directed downward while copious amounts of saline are flushed vigorously through the nostrils. The endotracheal tube cuff should be inflated to prevent aspiration pneumonia. Some clinicians surround the glottis with surgical sponges or gauze.

Tissue samples are not submitted routinely for bacterial or fungal culture except when fungal plaques are detected (Pomrantz et al, 2007) or sometimes when a foreign body is identified. To confirm a diagnosis of aspergillosis, a positive result on fungal culture should be supported by diagnostic imaging, cytologic, rhinoscopic, or histologic evidence of infection. Primary bacterial rhinitis is exceedingly rare in the dog, and almost all bacterial infections develop secondary to underlying primary nasal disease. A heavy growth of even one or two bacterial isolates may merely be indicative of bacterial colonization; however, pure isolates of *B. bronchiseptica* and possibly of *P. multocida* may be significant if the clinical history is supportive. If tissue cultures are performed, the results must be interpreted carefully in light of histopathologic and other diagnostic information.

A thorough oral examination with inspection of the hard palate, oropharynx, and dental structures should be performed. A periodontal probe should be used to inspect the gingival sulci of maxillary teeth. Oronasal fistulae are often associated with the maxillary third incisors, first and second premolars, and mesial root of the third premolar.

Treatment of Common Causes of Rhinitis

Geographic locality plays a role but, excluding nasal foreign bodies (Aronson, 2004) and dental disease, the most common causes of chronic rhinitis in dogs are neoplasia, idiopathic chronic (lymphoplasmacytic) rhinitis, and fungal rhinitis. Parasitic rhinitis is uncommon. The treatment for nasal mites (*Pneumonyssus caninum*) is ivermectin 0.2 mg/kg PO, with the dose repeated in 2 to 3 weeks. Selamectin has been reported effective at 6 to 24 mg/kg for three doses at 2-week intervals, and milbemycin is recommended for use in dogs with possible MDR-1 (multidrug resistance protein 1) mutations using a dosage of 0.5 to 1.0 mg/kg body weight PO once a week for 3 weeks. The treatment for nasal nematodes (*E. [Capillaria] boehmi*) is not clearly defined, although ivermectin 0.2 mg/kg PO once or fenbendazole for 2 weeks reportedly have been effective. Allergic rhinitis often is mild, but if it is severe, antihistamines such as diphenhydramine, chlorpheniramine, or trimeprazine/prednisone (Temaril-P) may be prescribed to control clinical signs. In the rare situation of bacterial rhinitis caused by *B. bronchiseptica,* doxycycline 5 to 10 mg/kg every 12 hours PO for 2 weeks may be effective.

Fungal Rhinosinusitis

Fungal rhinitis is a relatively common cause of chronic rhinitis in the dog in various geographic regions throughout the world. *Aspergillus fumigatus* is the most common cause of fungal rhinitis in dogs, but occasionally *Penicillium* spp., *Rhinosporidium seeberi,* and very rarely *Cryptococcus neoformans* may cause disease in dogs. *R. seeberi* is associated with the growth of a granulomatous mass within the rostral nasal cavity. Cytologic examination of tissue from these granulomatous masses often is diagnostic. Treatment for rhinosporidiosis is best accomplished by aggressive surgical resection of the granulomatous mass.

Nasal aspergillosis is most commonly seen in young to middle-aged dolichocephalic dogs, although older-aged dogs should not be excluded. Sinonasal aspergillosis is a noninvasive disease in dogs with fungal hyphae confined to the surface of the mucosa and not within or below the surface mucosa. The bony destruction seen with this disease is not caused by the fungus itself but appears to result from the host inflammatory response due to an aberrant dysregulation of innate and adaptive immune responses. Systemic immunosuppression is not present in affected dogs. Local immune-dysfunction owing to imbalance between proinflammatory and antiinflammatory signals is likely involved in the pathogenesis of this disease. Dysregulation of genes encoding Toll- and Nod-like pattern recognition receptors involved in the innate immune response in the nasal mucosa of dogs with sinonasal fungal rhinitis has recently been described (Mercier et al, 2012).

Affected dogs often have copious unilateral or bilateral mucopurulent nasal discharge. The volume of nasal discharge is often less in dogs with primary fungal frontal sinusitis. Sneezing is common and may be accompanied by mild to severe epistaxis. Facial pain and depigmentation and ulceration of the nasal planum may be present. Unlike in nasal neoplasia, facial distortion is unusual in all but advanced cases of fungal rhinitis. Nasal CT images (Figure 154-1) along with rhinoscopy findings are noteworthy for the presence of dramatic turbinate loss within the nasal cavity (Saunders et al, 2004). Frontal sinus involvement may be present and is characterized on CT by an irregularly marginated soft tissue attenuating density within the affected sinus (see Figure 154-1). Mucosal thickening and bone remodeling of the affected sinus may also be seen. Invasion through the maxillary or palatine bones with extension into surrounding soft tissue structures is seen occasionally. Nasal CT is preferred over radiography so that the integrity of the cribriform plate can be evaluated before local antifungal therapy is initiated. Diagnosis of nasal aspergillosis is confirmed by visualization of fungal plaques on nasal or sinus mucosa and demonstration of branching septate hyphae on cytologic or histologic examination of samples from affected regions within the nose. Serologic tests positive for aspergillosis also support the diagnosis, although negative results may occur even with extensive disease. Occasionally special staining methods for fungi may be useful for identifying fungal elements in tissue biopsy samples. Repeated sampling or a trial of antifungal drugs may well be indicated in dogs for which the index of suspicion for nasal aspergillosis is high; however, extensive débridement of fungal plaques should be performed before treatment.

The prognosis after treatment of nasal aspergillosis is fair to good, but relapses are not uncommon, which necessitates retreatment. Treatment of nasal aspergillosis is best performed with topical infusion of either clotrimazole or enilconazole provided that the cribriform plate is intact. Topical therapy is more effective than orally administered antifungal agents, but multiple treatments are often required. When all topical treatments are considered together, approximately 46% of dogs have a successful first treatment and 69% respond successfully following multiple treatments (Sharman et al, 2010). Clotrimazole (Lotrimin solution) is available over the counter as a 1% solution, although the propylene glycol vehicle used in this preparation is more irritating to the nasal mucosa than prescription clotrimazole 1% solutions containing a polyethylene glycol vehicle. Enilconazole is provided as 13.8% emulsifiable concentrate (Clinafarm-EC) or 10% solution (Imaverol Concentrated Solution), which is diluted to a 1%, 2%, or 5% solution before instillation into the nasal cavity. Topical therapy with either drug alone is ineffective in dogs when the organism has invaded soft tissue structures adjacent to the nose. In these cases it is recommended that topical therapy be combined with administration of systemic antifungal agents. Rhinotomy and turbinectomy before topical treatment or oral antifungal therapy are often detrimental and are not recommended.

The topical application of antifungal agents is accomplished through catheters placed surgically or endoscopically into the nasal chambers and frontal sinuses. Trephination or exploration of the frontal sinuses may be required for débridement or for catheter placement. The antifungal solution is applied as a soak, with the solution maintained in the nasal cavities for 1 hour with the patient under anesthesia (Mathews et al, 1998; Zonderland et al, 2002). A nasopharyngeal Foley catheter and sponges placed in the caudal pharyngeal region are positioned before the procedure to minimize leakage of the infusate caudally, and the external nares are also obstructed with Foley catheters. A total volume of 60 ml is infused slowly through catheters placed into the right and left nares. The head is rotated every 15 minutes to ensure contact with all nasal surfaces. Adverse effects of local therapy include severe pharyngitis and pharyngeal edema.

Recently another approach with an excellent success rate, shorter treatment time, and low patient morbidity has been reported using a combination of clotrimazole irrigation and depot therapy (Sissener et al, 2006). Frontal sinus trephination is followed by a short, 5-minute flushing of 1% topical clotrimazole solution followed by instillation of a 1% clotrimazole cream as a depot agent into the frontal sinuses. The procedure includes a number of steps. The anesthetized dog is positioned in sternal recumbency with the pharynx packed with cotton gauze to prevent aspiration of fluid debris, and the head is tilted downward to allow fluid from the nasal sinuses to drain rostrally. The frontal bone is trephined to permit passage of a 10 Fr Jacques urethral catheter or a trimmed catheter-tipped red rubber catheter into each sinus. The sinuses are first irrigated with 500 to 1000 ml of warm saline over 5 minutes to establish appropriate catheter placement and patency of the nasofrontal ostium (which links the frontal sinus to the nasal cavity). The sinuses are then irrigated with 1% clotrimazole solution. For dogs weighing more than 10 kg, a total of 1 g (50 ml per side) is used, and for dogs weighing less than 10 kg a total of 500 mg (25 ml per side) is applied. Clotrimazole 1%

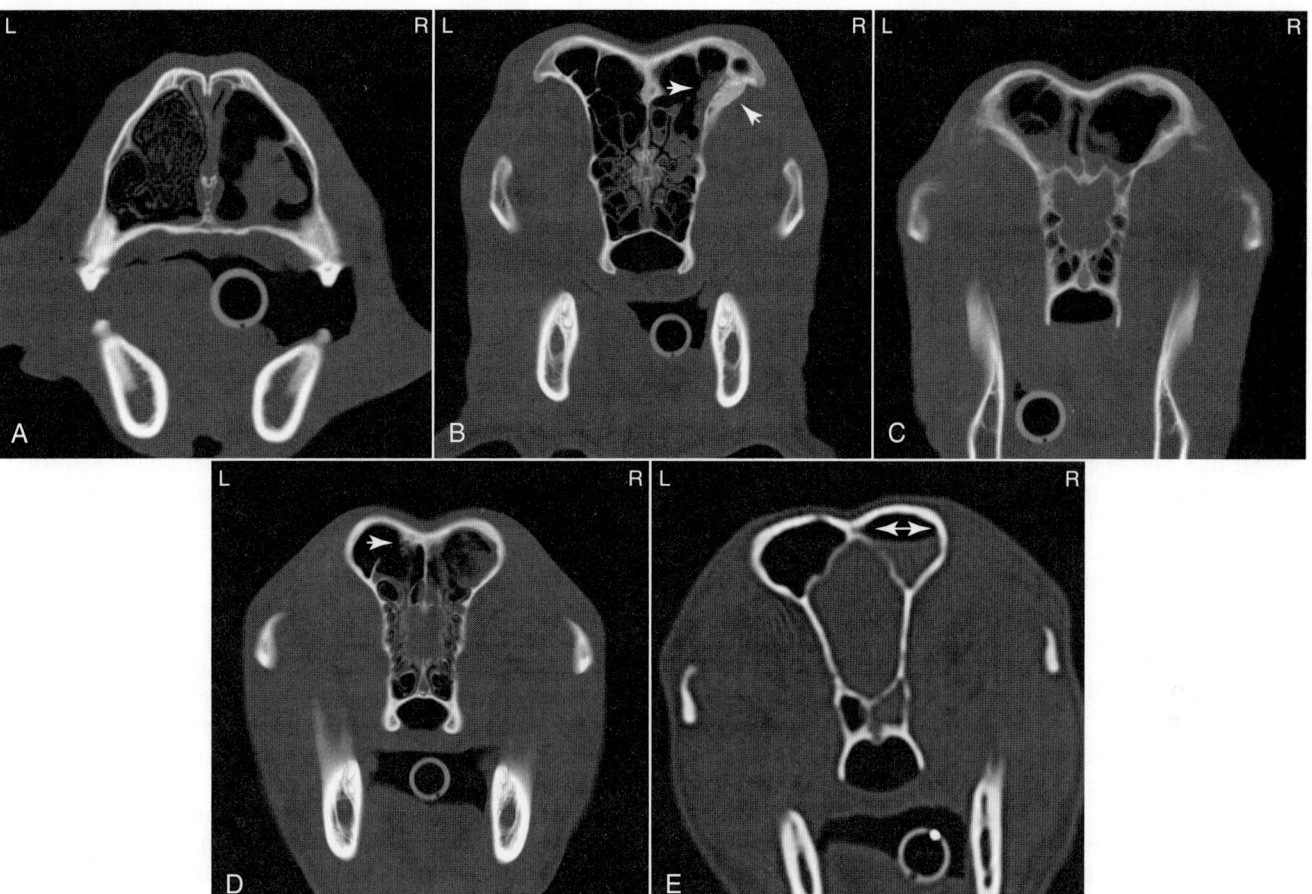

Figure 154-1 A, Computed tomographic (CT) scan of the middle region of the nasal cavity in a dog with nasal aspergillosis involving the right nasal cavity and right frontal sinus. The right nasal cavity is largely devoid of turbinate structures with scattered regions of soft tissue attenuating densities (mucopus) present. The left nasal cavity has normal turbinate structures present. **B,** CT scan for the same patient at the level of the rostral frontal sinuses. There is a fungal plaque in the right ventrolateral frontal sinus (*arrow* in sinus) characterized by an irregularly marginated amorphous soft tissue attenuating density along the frontal bone. Adjacent to the fungal plaque, periostitis of the ventrolateral aspect of the right frontal bone is present. **C,** CT scan in another patient at the level of the midregion of the frontal sinuses with bilateral fungal sinusitis. Within both sinuses the fungal plaques are seen irregularly marginated amorphous soft tissue attenuating material. Mucosal thickening of the frontal sinuses bilaterally is present. Mild periostitis of the ventrolateral aspect of the left frontal bone is present. **D,** CT scan in another patient with fungal sinusitis. A large irregularly shaped heterogenous representing a fungal plaque is present in the right frontal sinus. Mucosal thickening of the right frontal sinus is present. A small fungal plaque is present in the dorsal aspect of the left frontal sinus (*arrow*). The structure is irregularly marginated and associated with mild periostitis adjacent to the fungal plaque. **E,** CT scan showing a meniscus in the right frontal sinus, which is consistent with fluid caused by obstruction rather than the irregularly marginated amorphous soft tissue attenuating densities seen with fungal sinusitis.

cream is then introduced into the frontal sinuses. For dogs larger than 10 kg a total of 40 g (20 g per side) is used, and for dogs weighing less than 10 kg a total of 20 g (10 g per side) is applied. The catheters are then removed, the skin incisions are closed, and excess fluid is allowed to drain from the sinuses before the pharyngeal gauze is removed.

Oral antifungal agents have relatively poor efficacy against *Aspergillus* infection but are recommended if imaging demonstrates that the cribriform plate has been penetrated. Oral antifungal agents are used in combination with topical agents if invasion of local bone and soft tissue structures is present. The newer azole derivatives offer the best results. Adverse effects of the azole antifungal agents include anorexia, vomiting, lethargy, elevated blood urea nitrogen level, skin ulcerations, fever, and hepatotoxicity. Itraconazole (Sporanox) is recommended because of its low toxicity. Itraconazole 5 mg/kg every 12 hours PO given for 3 to 6 months may cure aspergillosis in up to 60% to 70% of dogs, although some studies have shown marginal effects of the drug on this disease. Terbinafine (Lamisil) is another option; it is well tolerated. Terbinafine 15 to 20 mg/kg every 12 hours PO appears to have similar efficacy to itraconazole when given for 3 to 6 months. The combination of terbinafine and triazoles has been shown to display a potent synergistic action and fungicidal activity against various *Aspergillus* spp. isolates *in vitro*. I routinely use oral terbinafine therapy for 3 to 6 months following topical clotrimazole irrigation and depot treatment, an approach that appears to minimize the necessity for repeated topical therapy. Voriconazole (Vfend) is a new-generation broad-spectrum antifungal agent that shows activity against a wide range of yeasts and filamentous fungi. Voriconazole demonstrates both fungicidal and fungistatic activities *in vitro* against *Aspergillus* spp. that is superior to that of fluconazole. Initial clinical experience in dogs suggests an oral dosage of 5 mg/kg every 12 hours for voriconazole. I have used voriconazole (5 mg/kg every 12 hours) in combination with terbinafine (15 to 20 mg/kg every 12 hours) for 1 month with success; however, liver enzyme activities must be closely monitored, because acute liver failure may occur.

Idiopathic Lymphoplasmacytic (Chronic) Rhinitis

Idiopathic lymphoplasmacytic rhinitis is a relatively common cause of chronic nasal disease in the dog. The definitive cause of lymphoplasmacytic rhinitis remains undetermined; however, it is likely an aberrant innate and adaptive immune response to multiple precipitating factors. Dysregulation of genes encoding Toll- and Nod-like pattern recognition receptors involved in the innate immune response in the nasal mucosa of dogs with lymphoplasmacytic rhinitis has recently been described (Mercier et al, 2012). Inhaled aeroallergens and irritants probably play a primary role in the development of this disease. Hypersensitivity to native commensal fungal

organisms within the nose also may play a role in some patients.

Young to middle-aged dolichocephalic and mesaticephalic large-breed dogs and dachshunds typically are affected. Chronic unilateral or bilateral mucoid to mucopurulent nasal discharge often is present, although some dogs may have mucohemorrhagic discharge or epistaxis. Obstruction to airflow through the nose may occasionally result from excessive mucus within nasal passages and turbinate mucosal edema. Since lymphoplasmacytic inflammation may be present with nasal neoplasia, fungal rhinitis, or foreign body rhinitis, it is imperative that these diseases be thoroughly excluded before a diagnosis of idiopathic lymphoplasmacytic (chronic) rhinitis is entertained.

Nasal radiography can reveal similar changes in dogs with chronic inflammatory rhinitis, neoplasia, and fungal rhinitis, including turbinate destruction and soft tissue opacification of the nasal passages and frontal sinus. Nasal CT is preferred because it greatly enhances the ability to define the extent and nature of disease. Nasal CT in idiopathic chronic rhinitis may show lesions that are completely unremarkable or disclose unilateral or bilateral mild to moderate turbinate destruction with mucus accumulation within air passages and sinuses (Figure 154-2). Occasionally the turbinate destruction may be severe, mimicking that seen with fungal rhinitis. Destruction of the nasal septum, frontal sinuses, or cribriform plate; mass lesions; and extension of soft tissue density into the nasopharynx or periorbital region are not expected with idiopathic chronic rhinitis. These findings should prompt investigation into the possibility of fungal rhinitis or neoplastic disease.

The most common rhinoscopic abnormalities seen are unilateral or bilateral erythema or hyperemia and edema of the nasal mucosa with the presence of mucus within air passages. Turbinate atrophy or loss is appreciated

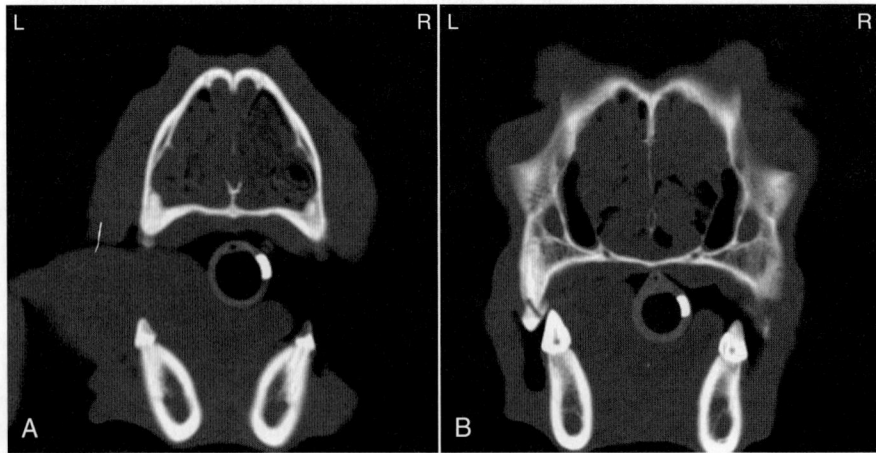

Figure 154-2 A, Computed tomographic scan of the midregion of the nose of a dog with lymphoplasmacytic rhinitis. Mucosal edema as seen with thickening of the turbinates and scattered soft tissue attenuating material (mucopus) is present within both sides of the nasal cavity (left side more severely affected than the right at the level of this image). **B,** Further caudal a large amount of soft tissue attenuating material (mucopus) admixed with air is present bilaterally. The soft tissue material was not contrast enhancing, confirming the presence of fluid rather than tissue density.

occasionally. Microbial culture of nasal samples is neither informative nor recommended. Histologic changes include mild to severe lymphoplasmacytic inflammation with occasional infiltration of neutrophils or eosinophils. Turbinate remodeling or destruction may be absent or vary from mild to severe. The severity of histologic changes may be discordant between the right and left sides of the nasal cavity.

Treatment of idiopathic lymphoplasmacytic rhinitis is extremely frustrating, with cure rarely achieved. Although this is not a life-threatening disease, owners of dogs so affected are often distraught at the pet's nasal obstruction or the need to clean up nasal discharge or nasal blood frequently in the house. Allergen avoidance is rarely helpful; however, avoidance of secondhand smoke can substantially reduce signs in some dogs. Despite earlier reports in the literature, systemic or topical corticosteroids are seldom effective in controlling clinical signs and actually may worsen them. Antihistamine medications rarely are effective, but they occasionally slightly reduce the severity of nasal discharge. Long-term administration of antibiotics with immunomodulatory effects combined with nonsteroidal antiinflammatory agents can be helpful in some dogs. Doxycycline 3 to 5 mg/kg every 12 hours PO or azithromycin 5 mg/kg every 24 hours PO in combination with piroxicam 0.3 mg/kg every 24 hours PO is recommended, if systemic health allows use of a nonsteroidal agent. If distinct clinical improvement is observed in 4 to 8 weeks, daily piroxicam therapy is continued, but the frequency of administration of the antibiotic is reduced to once daily for doxycycline and twice weekly for azithromycin. Therapy likely will be required for a minimum of 6 months if not indefinitely.

Oral itraconazole therapy in dogs whose disease is refractory to other therapeutic modalities may occasionally be effective. Nasal biopsy specimens from dogs with lymphoplasmacytic rhinitis have been reported to display higher transcription of fungal genes than those from dogs with nasal neoplasia when measured using polymerase chain reaction techniques (Windsor et al, 2006). Whether hypersensitivity to commensal nasal fungal organisms is involved or molecular techniques are detecting entrapment of fungal organisms is unclear. Preliminary experience with the administration of itraconazole 5 mg/kg every 12 hours PO for a minimum of 3 to 6 months occasionally has led to dramatic improvement and even resolution of signs in some dogs with this disease.

Nasal Neoplasia and Nasal Polyps

Nasal neoplasia is an important cause of chronic nasal disease in middle-aged to older dolichocephalic and mesaticephalic dogs. Nasal neoplasia accounts for approximately one third of all cases of chronic nasal disease in dogs, and tumors of epithelial origin cause about two thirds of these neoplasms. The majority of canine nasal tumors are malignant and primarily arise within the nasal cavity (Figure 154-3), although occasionally they originate in the paranasal sinuses (Figure 154-4). Nasal tumors tend to be invasive, with local to widespread destruction of nasal turbinates seen initially and invasion of septal, cribriform, or facial bones observed later in the course of

disease. Metastasis to regional lymph nodes or lung may occur, but this is rare and generally occurs in the late stages of disease. Clinical signs are related primarily to obstruction of airflow through the nasal cavities, mucopurulent nasal discharge, epistaxis, sneezing, and sometimes reverse sneezing. Facial deformity or swelling, exophthalmia, or neurologic signs may stem from tumor destruction of facial bones or the cribriform plate. Facial pain and head shyness are seen rarely (unlike in fungal rhinitis). In some patients initial clinical signs may be very subtle, with unexplained onset of snoring, obstructive nasal breathing, and occasional reverse sneezing reported.

For dogs that have primarily epistaxis at presentation, a coagulation profile, complete blood count with platelet count, blood pressure measurement, and serum protein levels should be obtained initially to rule out coagulopathy, hypertension, and hyperviscosity syndromes as causes of epistaxis. Nasal radiographs are insensitive for detection of subtle lesions, and radiographic changes seen with nasal tumors often overlap with those seen in lymphoplasmacytic and fungal rhinitis. Nasal CT images are far better for evaluating neoplastic disease and detecting bone destruction and neoplastic extension into surrounding structures (see Figure 154-3). Nasal CT also is needed for staging the tumor, delineating tumor boundaries, and planning radiation therapy. Retroflex nasopharyngoscopy is useful to evaluate the nasopharyngeal region and identify tumor extension through the caudal nares. Anterior rhinoscopy in dogs with nasal neoplasia may reveal a mass lesion protruding within and occluding nasal air passages. Multiple biopsies of masses should be performed to increase the likelihood of diagnosis, because severe inflammation often surrounds nasal tumors and can create a false-negative biopsy result. Frequently nasal tumors cannot be visualized during rhinoscopy because of hemorrhage or because the origin is inaccessible. In these situations nasal CT studies provide direction and help to determine the location for blind biopsy sampling of the affected region of the nose.

Radiation therapy is the treatment of choice for most nasal tumors, and a radiation oncologist or medical oncologist should be consulted. Fine-needle aspiration of regional lymph nodes with cytologic analysis and thoracic radiography are recommended to rule out metastatic disease before radiation therapy. Surgery alone is ineffective, with survival times similar to those observed in untreated dogs. Cytoreductive surgery is recommended before orthovoltage radiation therapy but not before cobalt or linear accelerator therapy. There is evidence suggesting that exenteration of the nasal cavity significantly prolongs the survival time in dogs with intranasal neoplasia that have previously undergone accelerated radiotherapy (Adams et al, 2005). However, exenteration after radiotherapy may increase the risk of chronic complications, including development of chronic or recurrent rhinitis and osteomyelitis. Cisplatin is used occasionally as a radiation sensitizer in radiotherapy protocols. Depending on the mode of radiation therapy available, approximate median survival times are between 16.5 and 23 months, and approximate 1-year survival rates are around 54% to 60%. Results with cryosurgery, either

Figure 154-3 A, Computed tomographic (CT) scan of the midregion of the nose of a dog with adenocarcinoma. A homogenous destructive soft tissue attenuating density is present within the right nasal cavity (note absence of turbinate structures). The nasal septum is deviated leftward and the midportion of the septal bone is lytic *(arrow)* with extension of disease into the adjacent right nasal cavity. **B,** CT scan at the same level but with contrast. There is contrast enhancement of the soft tissue attenuating density, indicating this is a tissue mass. **C,** CT scan for the same patient at the level of the eyes. There is lysis of the vomer bone *(angled arrow)* and ventrolateral aspect of the right maxillary bone *(horizontal arrow).* The mass extends into and completely obstructs the nasopharyngeal meatus. **D,** CT scan at the same level but with contrast. The mass is contrast enhancing and the borders of the mass can be clearly delineated.

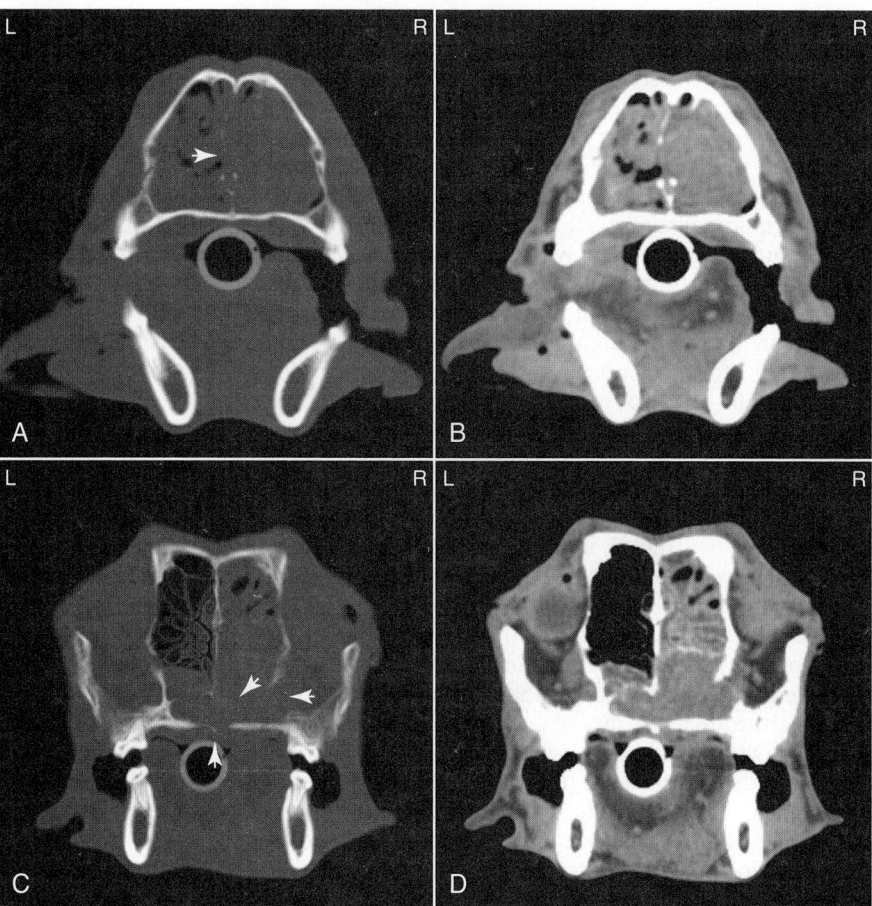

Figure 154-4 A, Computed tomographic scan of the midregion of the nose of a dog with right frontal sinus adenocarcinoma. The nasal cavity at this level is normal. **B,** CT scan of the same dog at the level of the frontal sinuses. A soft tissue attenuating structure is completely filling the right frontal sinus. **C,** CT scan at the same level but with contrast. The soft tissue structure in the right frontal sinus is contrast enhancing *(arrow* at ventral margin of the mass) with a small amount of noncontrasting fluid ventral to the mass. **D,** CT scan at the caudal aspect of the frontal bone showing lysis and cortical thinning *(arrow)* due to the mass.

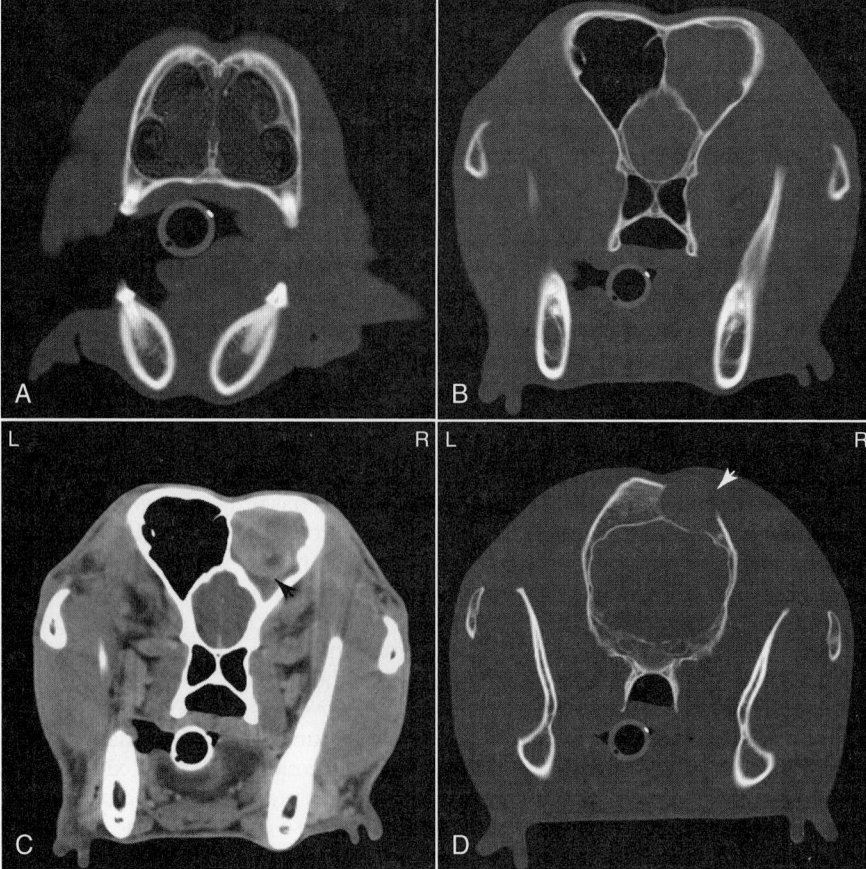

alone or in combination with radiation therapy, have been disappointing; therefore it is not recommended. There is limited information on the response of nasal tumors to chemotherapy alone. The median survival in a very small group of dogs with nasal adenocarcinoma given cisplatin alone was 20 weeks (Hahn et al, 1992), which is comparable to survival with no treatment. Some nonsteroidal antiinflammatory drugs can reduce nasal tumor volume or slow tumor growth. Meloxicam 0.1 mg/kg PO once daily or piroxicam 0.3 mg/kg PO once daily may induce clinical improvement in some patients having nasal carcinoma, with reduction in epistaxis and obstructive nasal breathing for periods of 6 to 12 months.

Polyps within the nasal cavity are very rare in dogs. These are usually unilateral, although extension through the nasal septum may occur. Histologically the polypoid lesions are covered with normal ciliated epithelium with edematous stroma with mucous accumulation, lymphangiectasia, and mixed inflammation. Nasal CT findings are similar to that seen with nasal neoplasia. Rhinotomy is required for removal of the polypoid tissue and surrounding conchae. Recurrence 1 to 2 years later is possible. To date in the vast majority of dogs I have seen with an initial diagnosis of a polyp, careful review of nasal CT images has demonstrated localized turbinate destruction, and the subsequent histologic diagnosis following surgical resection of the polypous tissue has been low-grade fibrosarcoma associated with moderate to severe chronic inflammation.

Xeromycteria

Xeromycteria (dry nose) can be unilateral or bilateral and is due to parasympathetic neurogenic loss of secretions from the lateral nasal gland. The lateral nasal gland provides moisture to the lining of the nose, and moisture translocates over the surface of the nasal planum. Otitis media can lead to transient or complete loss of parasympathetic innervation to the lateral nasal gland, because postganglionic parasympathetic innervation to the lateral nasal gland is via fibers coursing with the facial nerve through the petrous temporal bone. Clinically patients have unilateral or bilateral hyperkeratosis and dryness of the nasal planum and mild thick nasal secretions within the nostril(s). Tear production is often normal as long as there is no damage to the preganglionic parasympathetic nerve proximal to the pterygopalatine ganglion. Successful treatment of the otitis media may lead to restoration of normal secretions from the lateral nasal gland.

References and Suggested Reading

Adams WM et al: Outcome of accelerated radiotherapy alone or accelerated radiotherapy followed by exenteration of the nasal cavity in dogs with intranasal neoplasia: 53 cases (1990-2002), *J Am Vet Med Assoc* 227:936, 2005.

Aronson LR: Nasal foreign bodies. In King LG, editor: *Respiratory disease in dogs and cats*, Philadelphia, 2004, Saunders, p 302.

Dhaliwal RS et al: Subjective evaluation of computed tomography and magnetic resonance imaging for detecting intracalvarial changes in canine neoplasia, *Int J Appl Res Vet Med* 2:201, 2004.

Hahn KA et al: Clinical response of nasal adenocarcinoma to cisplatin chemotherapy in 11 dogs, *J Am Vet Med Assoc* 200:355, 1992.

Lefebvre J, Kuehn NF, Wortinger A: Computed tomography as an aid in the diagnosis of chronic nasal disease in dogs, *J Small Anim Pract* 46:280, 2005.

Mathews KG et al: Comparison of topical administration of clotrimazole through surgically placed versus nonsurgically placed catheters for treatment of nasal aspergillosis in dogs: 60 cases (1990-1996), *J Am Vet Med Assoc* 213:501, 1998.

Mercier E et al: Toll- and NOD-like receptor mRNA expression in canine sino-nasal aspergillosis and idiopathic lymphoplasmacytic rhinitis, *Vet Immunol Immunopathol* 145:618, 2012.

Pomrantz JS et al: Use of serologic evaluation via agar gel immunodiffusion and fungal culture of tissue for diagnosis of nasal aspergillosis in dogs, *J Am Vet Med Assoc* 230:1319, 2007.

Saunders JH et al: Radiographic, magnetic resonance imaging, computed tomographic, and rhinoscopic features of nasal aspergillosis in dogs, *J Am Vet Med Assoc* 225:1703, 2004.

Sharman M et al: Multi-centre assessment of mycotic rhinosinusitis in dogs: a retrospective study of initial treatment success (1998-2008), *J Small Anim Pract* 51:423, 2010.

Sissener TR et al: Combined clotrimazole irrigation and depot therapy for canine aspergillosis, *J Small Anim Pract* 47:312, 2006.

Windsor RC, Johnson LR, Sykes JE: Molecular detection of microbes in nasal biopsies of dogs with idiopathic lymphoplasmacytic rhinitis, *J Vet Intern Med* 20:250, 2006.

Zonderland JL et al: Intranasal infusion of enilconazole for treatment of sinonasal aspergillosis in dogs, *J Am Vet Med Assoc* 221:1421, 2002.

CHAPTER 155

Rhinitis in Cats

LYNELLE R. JOHNSON, *Davis, California*
VANESSA R. BARRS, *Sydney, Australia*

Sneezing and nasal discharge in the cat can result from infectious, inflammatory, or neoplastic disease. The most common syndrome is likely chronic rhinosinusitis (CRS), a disease with high morbidity in the feline population but uncertain etiopathogenesis. Multiple clinical reports have implicated a role for feline herpesvirus type 1 (FHV-1) in CRS; however, the high prevalence of infection with this virus and the ability of the virus to cause latent infection in the feline population have made it difficult to demonstrate a causal relationship between the presence of the virus and disease (Johnson et al, 2005). In addition, cats with CRS often demonstrate improvement in response to antibiotics, which suggests that bacterial infection plays a role in this disease. It is possible that severe early viral infection, viral persistence within nasal epithelium, or chronic reactivation of FHV-1 in nasal tissues damages the respiratory epithelium and results in mucus accumulation, sneezing, and ultimately turbinate destruction with subsequent bacterial invasion of nasal tissue.

Nasal tumors represent a small percentage of neoplasms in cats; however, the majority of cases exhibit malignant behavior through local invasion. Tumor types include lymphoma, adenocarcinoma, squamous cell carcinoma, undifferentiated carcinoma, and fibrosarcoma. These tumors cause clinical disease primarily through local extension, although systemic manifestations of lymphoma can accompany nasal lymphoma or can develop subsequent to local control of disease.

Fungal infection most commonly is caused by cryptococcal species (*Cryptococcus neoformans–Cryptococcus gattii* species complex), although more recently, *Aspergillus felis* in the *Aspergillus fumigatus* complex has been recognized as causing nasal and orbital infections in cats (Barrs et al, 2012). Secondary bacterial infection due to tooth root disease or an oronasal fistula can be a cause of nasal discharge, and foreign body impaction should be considered as a cause of unilateral nasal disease, although this is much less common in cats than in dogs. Finally, nasal discharge can result from systemic or pulmonary disease, particularly with nasal regurgitation of material associated with either chronic vomiting or pneumonia, or with epistaxis due to systemic hypertension, hyperviscosity, or a coagulopathy.

Diagnosis

CRS affects cats of all ages, whereas fungal infections tend to occur primarily in younger cats and neoplasia tends to be seen in older cats. Nasal discharge is often bilateral in cats with CRS, in contrast to cats with fungal infection, neoplasia, or dentally related disease; however, some cases are remarkably unilateral. Nasal airflow is generally preserved in cats with CRS and dentally related nasal disease; in contrast, it is often absent in cases of neoplasia or fungal infection because of a mass effect. Polypoid masses in the nares and ulcers or nodules on the nasal planum or nasal bridge are common in cryptococcal rhinitis. Exophthalmos is a presenting sign in cats with fungal or neoplastic lesions invading from the nasal cavity into the orbit and may be accompanied by prolapse of the nictitating membrane, exposure keratitis, a mass or ulcer in the pterygopalatine fossa, and stertor. Other examination findings suggestive of a space-occupying mass include loss of ocular retropulsion, facial asymmetry, and decreased depressibility of the soft palate. Neurologic signs such as seizures, behavioral changes, or cerebral dysfunction can be seen in cats with neoplasia or fungal infection due to extension of local disease. Regional lymph nodes are more likely to be enlarged in fungal infection or neoplasia than in CRS, and cytologic examination of aspirates from regional lymph nodes is recommended to assist in early diagnosis. Contributing dental disease or an oronasal fistula generally is not evident during a nonsedated examination.

For cats with unilateral nasal discharge and loss of nasal airflow, fungal infection and neoplasia should be high on the differential list. Cytologic analysis of nasal discharge is occasionally diagnostic for cryptococcosis by detection of a large (~20- to 30-μm) clear capsule surrounding a 3- to 8-μm organism (Figure 155-1). Cryptococcal antigen latex agglutination serologic testing should also be performed in cats with a loss of nasal airflow, since detection of circulating cryptococcal polysaccharide capsular antigen indicates infection. The assay has a high sensitivity (96% to 98%) and specificity (97% to 100%) when a pronase step is included in the method (pronase degrades antibodies that bind to the capsular antigen) (Malik et al, 1996; Trivedi et al, 2011). Fungal culture of a nasal swab also is indicated to isolate organisms for subsequent identification of species, antifungal susceptibility, and molecular subtype at a mycology reference laboratory. Nasal culture should not be used as a single diagnostic test for cryptococcosis, since it is possible for the nasal cavities of cats to be transiently colonized by cryptococcal organisms and not infected (Duncan et al, 2005).

Measurement of serum levels of galactomannan, a polysaccharide component of fungal cell walls, is a noninvasive test used in the early diagnosis of human

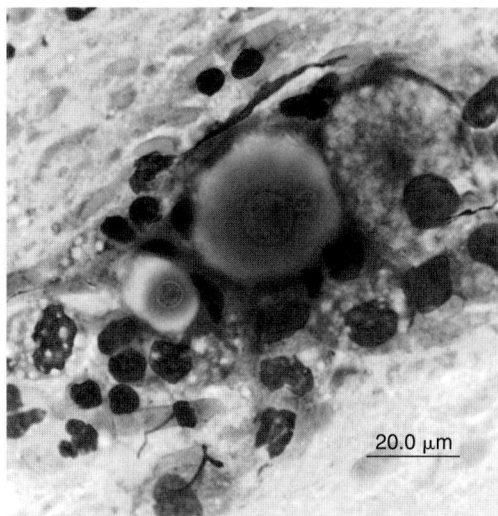

Figure 155-1 Smear from a nasopharyngeal cryptococcal granuloma treated with modified Wright-Giemsa (Diff-Quik) stain. The organisms, including a single budding yeast, are surrounded by a large polysaccharide capsule.

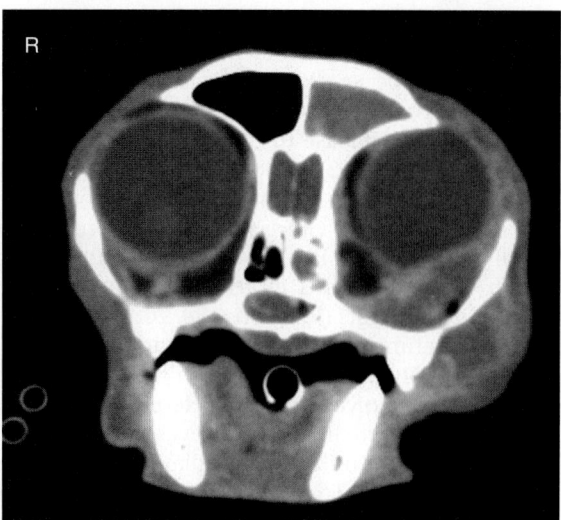

Figure 155-2 Transaxial contrast-enhanced computed tomographic scan for a cat with sino-orbital aspergillosis. There is a mass in the ventromedial orbit causing dorsolateral displacement of the globe as well as opacification of the left frontal sinus, left sphenoid sinus, and choanae. The mycotic granuloma in the orbit has spread to the paranasal soft tissues adjacent the maxilla. The pattern of contrast enhancement is heterogenous, with encapsulated areas of peripheral rim enhancement.

invasive aspergillosis (IA). It was evaluated recently for detecting upper respiratory tract (URT) aspergillosis in cats and was found to perform poorly, with a sensitivity of 23% and specificity of 78%. Immune-mediated clearance of galactomannan antigen is suspected to be a major reason for the poor sensitivity of this test in affected cats (Whitney et al, 2012). Antibodies against *Aspergillus* species were detected in the sera of four of nine cats with URT aspergillosis in several case reports, but the diagnostic usefulness of this serologic test has not been fully evaluated.

After laboratory testing (including tests for feline leukemia virus and feline immunodeficiency virus in cats with unknown viral or vaccination status), the first step in the diagnostic workup is to anesthetize the cat for skull radiography or preferably computed tomography. These images show variable degrees of turbinate lysis and increased fluid density within the nasal cavity in either rhinitis or neoplasia. The middle ear and sinuses are often fluid filled because of blocked drainage. Neoplasia and fungal infections usually have unilateral findings of a mass effect or soft tissue density. With invasive sino-orbital aspergillosis, an irregularly contrast-enhancing retrobulbar mass, paranasal soft tissue mass effect, and bony lysis generally are seen (Figure 155-2).

Rhinoscopy with biopsy and dental probing are performed after imaging to avoid creating artifacts on radiographs or CT. First, nasopharyngoscopy is accomplished by retroflexion of a flexible endoscope above the soft palate to rule out nasopharyngeal stenosis, foreign body, or a mass lesion. Neoplasia and fungal infections are often found in the choana and can be diagnosed with visualized sampling of the region for histopathology. Rhinoscopy of the rostral nasal cavity is best performed using a small (<2.8-mm) rigid telescope. Mucoid or purulent discharge is common in all causes of nasal discharge. Cats with CRS tend to have destructive rhinitis with loss of turbinates; in contrast, fungal infection or neoplasia

typically results in a mass lesion. Cats with aspergillosis can display a mass effect or occasionally have cavitated rhinitis and fungal plaques similar to those in dogs with the condition. Plaques or biopsy specimens from mass lesions should be submitted for fungal culture when infection is suspected. In patients with frontal sinus involvement and sinuses of adequate depth as assessed by CT, sinus trephination using a Jacob chuck and intramedullary pin (3.2 to 4 mm in diameter) enables endoscopic examination of the lateral compartment of the frontal sinuses and ready access to material for culture, histologic examination, and polymerase chain reaction (PCR) testing. Standard laboratory media such as Sabaraud's dextrose agar or cornmeal agar are adequate for isolation of most fungal pathogens of the upper respiratory tract. Differentiation of *A. fumigatus* from other species in the *A. fumigatus* complex often is not possible based on morphologic features alone but can be achieved using molecular techniques. A panfungal PCR procedure that amplifies the internal transcribed spacer 1 (ITS1) region of the ribosomal DNA gene cluster between the 18S and 5.8S ribosomal RNA genes can be performed using DNA extracted from formalin-fixed or fresh tissue biopsy specimens. Alternatively, using DNA extracted from fungal culture material, a panfungal PCR procedure that targets a larger region of the ribosomal DNA gene cluster including the ITS1, 5.8S gene, and ITS2 regions can be used and is more likely to yield reliable identification. These regions of the fungal genome are useful to amplify because they are multicopy (≥100 copies in the fungal genome) and they contain highly variable regions that facilitate identification of a diverse range of fungal genera from clinical specimens, including both filamentous fungi and yeasts. Comparative gene sequence analysis of an additional gene region such as the partial beta-tubulin or calmodulin genes may be necessary for definitive identification of some *Aspergillus* species. PCR products are sequenced and then compared with those in the National Institutes of Health GenBank database to obtain the identity of the fungus (Barrs et al, 2012).

Collecting nasal swab or biopsy specimens for bacterial culture in cats in which CRS is suspected is controversial. Potential pathogens are isolated from nasal samples from cats with chronic rhinitis more commonly than from those from healthy cats (Johnson et al, 2005), and culture results are sometimes helpful in guiding antibiotic therapy to control secondary bacterial rhinitis. It is unclear whether it is of clinical value to determine the type of inflammation present in CRS; however, histopathologic analysis is critical for ruling out neoplasia or fungal infection. In the cat with CRS, lymphoplasmacytic inflammation likely reflects the chronic nature of disease, whereas neutrophilic inflammation indicates an acute or bacterial component to the disease process. Eosinophilic infiltrates are relatively uncommon, but this finding might be considered suggestive of herpesvirus infection, as has been found in FHV-1–related facial dermatitis (Hargis et al, 1999). Since eosinophilic infiltrates can also occur in fungal rhinitis, special stains to detect fungal elements (e.g., periodic acid–Schiff or Gomori's methenamine silver) should be used.

After rhinoscopy, the oropharyngeal cavity is gently occluded with a moistened laparotomy pad and a copious flush is used to expel mucus and debris from the nasal cavity. Afterward, the cat is placed in dorsal recumbency and dental probing is performed to identify oronasal fistulae, palate defects, or deep periodontal pockets (>1 or 2 mm in depth) that could be responsible for dentally related nasal disease.

Treatment of Common Causes of Rhinitis

Chronic Rhinosinusitis

Antibiotics
Antibiotic therapy is usually prescribed in an attempt to control secondary bacterial rhinitis. Choice of antibiotics for the individual cat can be based on the results of culture of a deep nasal sample or on an understanding of potential pathogens that have been isolated previously from cats with rhinitis. These organisms include aerobes (*Pasteurella multocida, Escherichia coli, Corynebacterium ulcerans, Bordetella bronchiseptica, Streptococcus viridans, Pseudomonas aeruginosa, Actinomyces slackii*), anaerobes (*Peptostreptococcus anaerobius, Bacteroides fragilis, Bacteroides ureolyticus, Prevotella, Fusobacterium nucleatum*), and *Mycoplasma felis* (Johnson et al, 2005). Doxycycline (~50 mg per cat PO divided every 12 hours or given once daily) is a reasonable choice because it has efficacy against most bacteria involved, as well as *in vitro* efficacy against *Bordetella*. Doxycycline may help control clinical signs through antiinflammatory or immunomodulatory effects and is well tolerated by most cats, even when administered long term. The primary caution regarding the use of doxycycline hyclate preparations available in North America and Europe is esophageal stricture formation if

the pill lodges in the esophagus. Therefore the prescription label should call for administration of the pill with a small volume of water or food.

Other commonly used antibiotics are azithromycin, cephalexin, and amoxicillin/clavulanic acid. Azithromycin is an appealing option because it is available in liquid form and can be given once daily for 3 to 5 days at 5 mg/kg and then twice weekly since it accumulates in respiratory tissues. Penicillin-like drugs are helpful in many cats, although they lack efficacy against *Mycoplasma* species, which are cell wall–deficient organisms. These drugs are frequently associated with gastrointestinal adverse effects in cats. Fluoroquinolones generally are reserved for infections that are susceptible only to this class of antibiotic. Clindamycin can be effective in cases with extensive bony involvement because of its ability to penetrate bone. Since clindamycin administration has also been associated with esophagitis and stricture in cats it also should be administered with water or food (Beatty et al, 2006). Antibiotic treatment usually is continued for at least 3 to 6 weeks based on the assumption that turbinates are infected, but longer-term or intermittent therapy may be required.

Antiinflammatory Agents
Nasal inflammation can be partially ameliorated with piroxicam at 0.3 mg/kg PO daily or every other day. This drug is commercially available as a 10-mg tablet, and drug compounding is required. This nonsteroidal antiinflammatory agent causes subclinical gastric erosion, and caution is warranted in its use in older animals or in cats with renal insufficiency or gastrointestinal disease. Oral meloxicam is a tempting alternative to piroxicam because it is easier to dose and administer; however, currently it is licensed for long-term therapy only in Australia and Europe.

Glucocorticoids are sometimes advocated for treatment of cats with CRS, and in severely affected animals with inspissated mucus in the nasal cavity, administration of oral steroids may reduce mucus accumulation and promote appetite. Inhaled or topical steroids can be used, although it would seem wise to clear all mucus from the nasal cavity first so the drug can act locally on the mucosa. Antihistamine administration might temporarily improve clinical signs in some cats, although these drugs can also cause excessive drying of respiratory secretions. Nasal decongestants are rarely effective.

Antiviral Therapy
The role of FHV-1 in the induction or promotion of clinical signs in cats with CRS has not been clearly established; therefore specific antiviral therapy has not been recommended in cats with chronic disease. Dietary supplementation with lysine, an amino acid that competes with arginine and reduces FHV-1 replication *in vitro*, can be employed as trial therapy. The recommended dosage of lysine is 500 mg per cat PO twice daily; this dosage does not result in a drop in serum arginine levels. Lysine might be particularly indicated when intranuclear inclusions are detected or an eosinophilic inflammatory infiltrate is reported on histologic examination suggesting FHV-1 involvement. Anecdotal reports have suggested that

TABLE 155-1

Dosages of Antifungals Used in the Treatment of Fungal Rhinitis

Drug/Formulation	Dosage/Route of Administration	Indications for Therapy	Adverse Effects
Fluconazole 50-mg capsules 10- or 40-mg/ml oral suspension	2.5-10 mg/kg q12h PO or 50 mg per cat q12-24h	C	Gastrointestinal: inappetence Hepatotoxicity (rare)
Itraconazole 100-mg capsules 10-mg/ml oral suspension (Sporanox)	*Capsules:* 5 mg/kg q12h or 10 mg/kg q24h PO Administer with food *Oral suspension:* 1-1.5 mg/kg q24h PO	C, A	Gastrointestinal: anorexia, vomiting Hepatotoxicity: elevated liver enzyme levels, jaundice. Monitor ALP/ALT monthly. If hepatoxicity occurs, reduce dosage to 5 mg/kg q24h or 10 mg/kg q48h PO (capsules).
Posaconazole 40-mg/ml liquid (Noxafil)	5-7.5 mg/kg divided twice daily PO Administer with food	C, A	Hepatotoxicity: Unlikely to occur at 5 mg/kg divided twice daily PO
Voriconazole 50-mg tablets 40-mg/ml powder for oral suspension (Vfend)	5 mg/kg q24h PO	A	Neurologic problems: blindness, ataxia, stupor Consider use when other therapies have failed.
Terbinafine 250-mg tablets (Lamisil)	30 mg/kg q24h PO	A	Gastrointestinal: anorexia, vomiting, diarrhea
Flucytosine 250-mg capsules 75-mg/ml oral suspension	50 mg/kg q8h PO or 75 mg/kg q12h PO		Gastrointestinal: anorexia, vomiting, diarrhea
Amphotericin B deoxycholate 50-mg vial (Fungizone)	0.5 mg/kg of 5 mg/ml stock solution in 350 ml per cat of 0.45% NaCl + 2.5% dextrose SC two or three times weekly to a cumulative dose of 10-15 mg/kg	C, A	Nephrotoxicity: Monitor urea/creatinine every 2 wk. Discontinue for 2 to 3 wk if azotemic.
Liposomal amphotericin (AmBisome)	1-1.5 mg/kg IV q48h to a cumulative dose of 12-15 mg/kg Give as a 1-2 mg/ml solution in 5% dextrose by IV infusion over 1-2 hr	C, A	Nephrotoxicity: Azotemia can occur. Monitor urea/creatinine every 2-3 days during administration.

A, Aspergillosis; *ALP,* alkaline phosphatase; *ALT,* alanine aminotransferase; *C,* cryptococcosis; *PO,* orally.

famciclovir can be beneficial in controlling signs associated with CRS, and clinical studies are ongoing.

Adjunct Therapy and Prognosis

Vigorous flushing of the nasal cavity when the animal is anesthetized for diagnostic testing undoubtedly improves the clinical demeanor of cats with CRS. Cats can also benefit from intermittent airway humidification via steam inhalation, nebulizer treatment, or instillation of nasal saline drops. Oral *N*-acetylcysteine (150 to 250 mg per cat PO twice daily) can be helpful in reducing the viscosity of secretions and improving evacuation of the nasal cavity. It seems unlikely that cats with CRS can be cured given the abnormalities that often are found in nasal anatomy by the time diagnostic testing typically is performed or therapeutic intervention is sought. Owners should be aware that this disease may be controlled but rarely is cured, and a reasonable goal of therapy is to limit the severity and frequency of disease exacerbations.

Fungal Disease

Systemic Antifungal Therapy

Drugs used for treating fungal infections are listed in Table 155-1. Fluconazole is the recommended first-line therapy for treatment of cryptococcal rhinitis. Itraconazole is also effective but has more adverse effects, and longer courses of therapy may be required. When disease is severe or there is concurrent central nervous system involvement, combination therapy with amphotericin B, an azole, and flucytosine is recommended. Treatment should be continued until the cryptococcal antigen latex assay is zero, with follow-up antigen testing 1 month after therapy has been stopped and at subsequent recheck examinations, since relapse or reinfection can occur.

Systemic antifungal triazole drugs are recommended for the treatment of URT aspergillosis. Fluconazole should not be used because most species in the *A. fumigatus* complex are resistant. Posaconazole or itraconazole is recommended for first-line therapy. The pharmacologic characteristics of posaconazole have not been determined in cats, but it is well tolerated after oral administration (Barrs et al, 2012). Although isolates show *in vitro* susceptibility to voriconazole, this drug should not be used initially because of the reported high frequency of adverse neurologic events (Barrs et al, 2012; Quimby et al, 2010; Smith and Hoffman, 2010). In cases in which disease is confined to the nasal cavity (sinonasal aspergillosis) topical treatment is also recommended and should be discussed with a respiratory specialist. Some cases of sinonasal aspergillosis respond to topical therapy alone, but because of the propensity for orbital involvement from disease progression, systemic therapy is recommended in all cases. Correct identification of the fungal pathogen using the molecular methods described previously will help inform rational treatment selection. Sino-orbital aspergillosis in cats is most commonly caused by a single novel fungal species in the *A. fumigatus* complex (Barrs, unpublished data). *A. fumigatus* is the most common cause of sinonasal aspergillosis but has not been identified in sino-orbital infections. Infections due to *A. fumigatus* may be more likely to respond to topical antifungal therapies alone, although further research is required to support this assertion. For severe disease including orbital involvement, use of triazole antifungals in combination with amphotericin B and terbinafine may improve outcomes.

Adjunctive Therapy and Prognosis

Nasopharyngeal cryptococcal granulomas can be debulked surgically or endoscopically when upper airway obstruction is severe. In cases of sinonasal aspergillosis, fungal plaques should be débrided from the sinonasal cavity endoscopically followed by copious saline lavage prior to instillation of a 1% clotrimazole infusion in polyethylene glycol solution that is delivered intranasally or via sinus trephination. Adjunctive therapies in successfully treated cases of sino-orbital aspergillosis include orbital exenteration or débridement and lavage with a 1% solution of voriconazole (McClellan et al, 2006; Smith and Hoffman, 2010), although orbital débridement did not improve outcomes in one study (Barrs et al, 2012).

The prognosis for cryptococcal rhinitis with no central nervous system involvement and for sinonasal aspergillosis is generally good; however, long treatment courses of many months are often required. The prognosis for sino-orbital aspergillosis is poor. Recrudescent infection occurs in 15% to 20% of cases of cryptococcal infection in cats (O'Brien et al, 2006).

Nasal Neoplasia

The most common treatment for nasal neoplasia is radiation therapy, with survival times of 9 to 23 months. Nasal lymphoma is generally a B-cell lymphoma and is highly radioresponsive, with survival ranging from 4 to 55 months. Concurrent chemotherapy is often employed and improves outcome in some studies. An oncologist should be consulted to discuss treatment options.

Adverse effects of radiation therapy are predictable and expected. Early adverse effects include mucositis, conjunctivitis, and moist desquamation of skin. Late effects of radiation therapy such as bone necrosis, cataracts, and keratoconjunctivitis are generally irreversible, and treatment plans are designed to reduce the incidence of these delayed adverse effects. Stereotactic radiation holds promise for improved targeting of neoplastic tissue.

References and Suggested Reading

Barrs VR et al: Sinonasal and sino-orbital aspergillosis in 23 cats: aetiology, clinicopathologic features and treatment outcomes, *Vet J* 191(1):58, 2012. Epub March 8, 2011.

Beatty JA et al: Suspected clindamycin-associated injury in cats: five cases, *J Feline Med Surg* 8:412, 2006.

Duncan C et al: Sub-clinical infection and asymptomatic carriage of *Cryptococcus gattii* in dogs and cats during an outbreak of cryptococcosis, *Med Mycol* 43:511, 2005.

Hargis M et al: Ulcerative facial and nasal dermatitis and stomatitis in cats associated with feline herpesvirus 1, *Vet Dermatol* 10:267, 1999.

Johnson LR et al: Assessment of infectious organisms associated with chronic rhinosinusitis in cats, *J Am Vet Med Assoc* 227:579, 2005.

Malik R et al: A latex cryptococcal antigen agglutination test for diagnosis and monitoring of therapy for cryptococcosis, *Aust Vet J* 74:358, 1996.

McClellan GJ et al: Use of posaconazole in the management of invasive orbital aspergillosis in a cat, *J Am Anim Hosp Assoc* 42:302, 2006.

O'Brien CR et al: Long-term outcome of therapy for 59 cats and 11 dogs with cryptococcosis, *Aust Vet J* 84:384, 2006.

Quimby JM et al: Adverse neurologic events associated with voriconazole use in 3 cats, *J Vet Intern Med* 24:647, 2010.

Smith LN, Hoffman SB: A case series of unilateral orbital aspergillosis in three cats and treatment with voriconazole, *Vet Ophthalmol* 13:190, 2010.

Trivedi SR et al: Clinical features and epidemiology of cryptococcosis in cats and dogs in California, *J Am Vet Med Assoc* 239:357, 2011.

Whitney J et al: Serum galactomannan detection—evaluation of a new diagnostic test for invasive upper respiratory tract aspergillosis in cats, *Vet Microbiol*. Epub September 12, 2012.

CHAPTER 156

Brachycephalic Airway Obstruction Syndrome

CYRILL PONCET, *Arcueil, France*
VALÉRIE FREICHE, *Bordeaux, France*

Decades of genetic modification of brachycephalic breeds in the pursuit of ever flatter facial features have led to the progressive development of achondroplasia. This congenital and hereditary disorder leads to arrested elongation of nasal bones and results in relative hyperplasia of the soft tissues, with numerous deleterious consequences for the respiratory, gastrointestinal, and cutaneous systems. Since a close interaction has been established between respiratory and gastrointestinal disorders, the latter are considered an integral part of brachycephalic airway obstruction syndrome (BAOS).

In addition to stenotic nares and elongated soft palate, numerous other anomalies have been identified in these dogs. They may be congenital (primary) or acquired (secondary) (Table 156-1). The presence and severity of these anomalies vary from one dog to another and among the affected canine breeds. Although the clinical incidence of each entity may be expressed individually, each abnormality participates to a greater or lesser extent in an "engorgement" of the upper airways within a nondistensible cranial space.

A common pathophysiologic pathway seemingly can be identified for the respiratory and gastrointestinal anomalies of dogs with BAOS: gastroesophageal disorders and defective emptying of the upper gastrointestinal tract may aggravate the respiratory signs by encumbering the pharyngeal region and stimulating inflammation. Conversely, persistently increased respiratory effort promotes gastroesophageal reflux and other gastrointestinal conditions commonly described in these dogs. There is a clinical correlation between the severity of the respiratory disorders and the severity of gastrointestinal disorders that can be identified in the patient history.

Clinical Signs

The clinical presentation is dominated by respiratory signs, which are always present with inspiratory or mixed inspiratory-expiratory effort and noise. Intolerance of exercise, stress, and heat is characteristic. Snoring with stertor or stridor, coughing, and throat clearing are also reported. Episodes of cyanosis and syncope are commonly described in severely affected dogs. The progression of the clinical signs is notable, with gradual worsening over the months and with passing summers. Owners often consult a veterinarian during the dog's first summer after puppyhood or during an acute period of respiratory distress, although some owners consider these signs "normal" for the breed.

The prevalence of gastrointestinal disorders is significant in dogs with upper airway obstruction and can be the principal reason for consultation. A study of 73 cases (Poncet et al, 2005) showed a high incidence of concurrent gastrointestinal disorders in brachycephalic dogs brought for treatment primarily of respiratory disorders. The clinical signs most commonly described by the owners include vomiting (of gastric juices or food, indicative of gastric retention), regurgitation (sometimes linked to exertion, but very commonly occurring when the dog becomes excited), eructation, ptyalism and repeated swallowing, and ingestion of grass or other form of pica.

Diagnostic Approach

Various complementary examinations are required in the global management of obstructive airway syndrome. The purpose of these examinations is to determine an overall profile of the anomalies present, which is essential for planning treatment and determining prognosis. Cervical and thoracic radiographs are obtained to detect bronchopneumonia from food inhalation, bronchiectasis, pulmonary edema, tracheal hypoplasia, or deformation of the cardiac silhouette. Echocardiography is useful if heart disease is suspected. Computed tomography or magnetic resonance imaging can be helpful for modelling the soft palate and exploring the nasal cavities.

Endoscopy of the upper respiratory and gastrointestinal tracts provides a good overview of the lesions. Retrograde endoscopy of the nasopharynx enables documentation of choanal obstruction, notably via expansion of the ethmoidal turbinates. Antegrade rhinoscopy can be used to identify intranasal obstruction. Esophageal lesions commonly observed in brachycephalic dogs include esophageal deviation and distal esophageal erosions and inflammation secondary to chronic reflux. Other gastrointestinal findings include gastric fundal and antral inflammation (and notably follicular gastritis), gastric retention (evidenced by persistence of partially digested food despite prolonged consumption of a fluid-only diet), reduced pyloric diameter with hypertrophic mucosal folds, and gastroduodenal inflammation.

Endoscopy of the upper gastrointestinal tract enables visualization of gastrointestinal lesions and collection of gastric and duodenal biopsy samples; these are essential

TABLE 156-1

Soft Tissue Anomalies of the Upper Respiratory and Upper Gastrointestinal Tract Associated with Brachycephalic Airway Obstruction Syndrome

	Type of Anomaly	Origin	Prevalence	Clinical Significance*	Comments
Soft Tissue Respiratory Anomalies					
Nostrils	Stenotic nares	Primary	+++	+++	Alar cartilage important in stenotic nares
Nasal cavities	Distorted ethmoidal turbinates	Primary and secondary	++	Variable	Pug overrepresented
	Narrowing of cavities	Primary	+++	++	
Nasopharynx	Protrusion of ethmoidal turbinates	Primary	+	?	Pug overrepresented
	Pharyngeal soft tissue obstruction	Primary and secondary	++	+++	Dynamic obstruction that is difficult to interpret
Oropharynx	Elongation of soft palate	Primary	+++	+++	Variable according to breed
	Thickening of soft palate	Primary and secondary	+++	+++	Underdiagnosed, variable according to breed
	Macroglossa	Primary	++	+++	French and English bulldogs overrepresented
	Amygdalitis	Secondary	++	?	
	Superfluous soft tissues	Primary and secondary	+++	?	Increased with obesity
Larynx	Everted laryngeal ventricles	Secondary	+++	+	
	Collapse	Secondary	++	Variable	Variable severity, develops with age, pug overrepresented
Trachea	Tracheal hypoplasia	Primary	++	+	English bulldog overrepresented
Bronchi	Bronchial collapse	Secondary	+	?	Pug overrepresented, correlated with laryngeal collapse, no correlation with postsurgical outcome
Soft Tissue Gastrointestinal Anomalies					
Esophagus	Esophageal deviation	Primary	+	+	English bulldog overrepresented, may explain dribbling of saliva when excited
	Hiatal hernia	Secondary	+	+++	Often transient
	Cardial atony	Secondary	++	+++	Clinical sign markedly improved by airway surgery and medical treatment of gastrointestinal disorders
	Gastroesophageal reflux	Secondary	++	+++	Actively contributes to oropharyngeal inflammation
	Distal esophagitis	Secondary	++	+++	
Stomach	Gastric stasis	Primary	++	++	
	Pyloric mucosal hyperplasia	Primary and secondary	+++	++	
	Pyloric stenosis	Primary	++	++	Although a common finding, surgical modification of pylorus is rarely necessary
	Pyloric atony	Secondary	+	++	
	Duodenogastric reflux	Secondary	+	+	
	Diffuse inflammation	Secondary	+++	++	
	Punctiform inflammation	Secondary	++	++	Brachycephalics are predisposed to follicular gastritis
Duodenum	Diffuse inflammation	Secondary	++	+	White spicules, reflecting moderate local lymphangiectasia, are often found

*Clinical significance based on clinical retrospective study or personal observations.
+, Rare condition.
Prevalence: +, uncommon; ++, common; +++, frequent.
Clinical significance: +, minimal; ++, moderate; +++, important; ?, uncertain.

in dogs with gastrointestinal signs, because there is a poor correlation between the macroscopic and histologic appearance of the lesions. A prospective study of gastrointestinal lesions in 73 brachycephalic dogs (Poncet et al, 2005) revealed marked histologic lesions in 98% of cases in which biopsy samples were available. In this study a significant correlation was also established between the severity of the respiratory obstruction and the severity of gastrointestinal disorders.

Treatment

Early surgical treatment of BAOS facilitates surgery and optimizes surgical success by avoiding the development of secondary lesions such as eversion of the laryngeal ventricles, laryngeal collapse, and pharyngeal inflammation. In long-standing cases, emergency treatment may be required for acute respiratory distress using oxygen therapy, sedation, cooling, administration of steroidal antiinflammatories, and fluid therapy. Adjunctive therapy for gastrointestinal disease also improves outcomes.

Principles of Treatment

The objective of surgical treatment is to improve airflow (reduce resistance to flow and turbulence) from its entry (nares) up to its arrival (pulmonary alveoli). This principle is based on fluid mechanics and involves increasing the diameter of the areas that create significant airway resistance, including the nares, nasal cavities, soft palate, and larynx. Thus, the therapeutic approach to brachycephalic syndrome is above all surgical for the airway disease. In contrast, surgical correction of gastrointestinal abnormalities is rarely necessary, with the exception of sliding hiatal hernia or pyloric stenosis. However, medical treatment of gastrointestinal disease is an important adjunct in the overall management plan.

After complete exploration of all anatomic and functional anomalies, clearance of any obstructions to the upper airways should be planned. This often involves rhinoplasty and palatoplasty as first interventions. Advances in surgical techniques (notably enlarged palatoplasty and vestibuloplasty) should enable a significant reduction in the obstruction in these regions. Other surgical techniques can be used depending on the nature of the lesions observed (ventriculectomy, turbinectomy, and amygdalectomy, among others).

The medical treatment of gastrointestinal disorders should help to optimize the prognosis for these dogs, on both a gastrointestinal and a respiratory level. Treatment is dictated by the endoscopic appearance of the lesions and the severity of the histologic lesions. The most commonly used agents are acid-reducing drugs (omeprazole), gastrointestinal protectants (sucralfate, aluminium phosphate), and prokinetics (metoclopramide) in conjunction with corticosteroids (prednisolone) when gastroduodenal inflammation is marked. A medical treatment plan prescribed for a duration of 2 to 6 months led to improvement in more than 91% of cases in a study of 51 brachycephalic dogs monitored after surgical correction of respiratory abnormalities and medical treatment of gastrointestinal lesions (Poncet et al, 2006).

Specific Treatments for Respiratory Anomalies

A number of specific surgical procedures can be used in the management of BAOS. Some of the most common are summarized in the following sections. In some cases specialized equipment is necessary. Operators should obtain appropriate training before performing any of these procedures and should be comfortable with these surgical techniques. Ideally, these patients should be referred to a surgical specialist.

Rhinoplasty for Stenotic Nares

Rhinoplasty widens the opening of the nares and can be performed anytime after 5 months of age. A wide variety of surgical techniques have been described for the treatment of stenotic nares that vary in the orientation and location of the incision, but the necessity of this procedure in the management of BAOS is no longer disputed. It is important to concentrate the bulk of the surgical treatment on the alar cartilages, which seem to play a major role in the rostral obstruction of the nasal cavities. The cuneiform resection of the alar cartilages gives good results, both functionally (sufficient opening of the nares) and aesthetically (preservation of pigmentation).

Control of Cartilaginous Expansions of the Nasal Conchae

Cartilaginous expansions of the nasopharyngeal turbinates (conchae) can be identified in the nasopharynx of certain dogs. This phenomenon is encountered predominantly in the pug in our experience, and these protrusions present an additional source of obstruction of the nasal cavities. Laser-assisted turbinectomy is the only technique described to date that reduces resistance to airflow through the nasal cavities (Oechtering et al, 2007). A diode laser is used to excise obstructive mucosal folds and turbinates under videoscopic control. Although improvements in breathing have been noted, this technique is not widely available, and its use requires substantial time and expertise.

Palatoplasty for Elongated Soft Palate

Palatoplasty techniques have probably seen the greatest advances over the last few years. Hyperplasia of the soft palate (compressing the nasopharynx) associated with elongation should now be taken into account during palatoplasty at the same time that elongation is addressed. Several recent studies (Dunie-Mérigot et al, 2010; Findji and Dupré, 2009) have confirmed the clinical advantages of extending the resection to reduce both the length and thickness of the soft palate, and oropharyngeal function remains unaffected. A theoretical concern with excessive shortening of the soft palate is nasal regurgitation of liquid or food. The currently proposed technique is that of extended palatoplasty, which can be performed with a CO_2 laser (Figure 156-1).

Eversion of the Laryngeal Ventricles

In cases in which the cause of upper respiratory obstruction has been completely removed, eversion of the laryngeal ventricles can be reversible; this is why routine

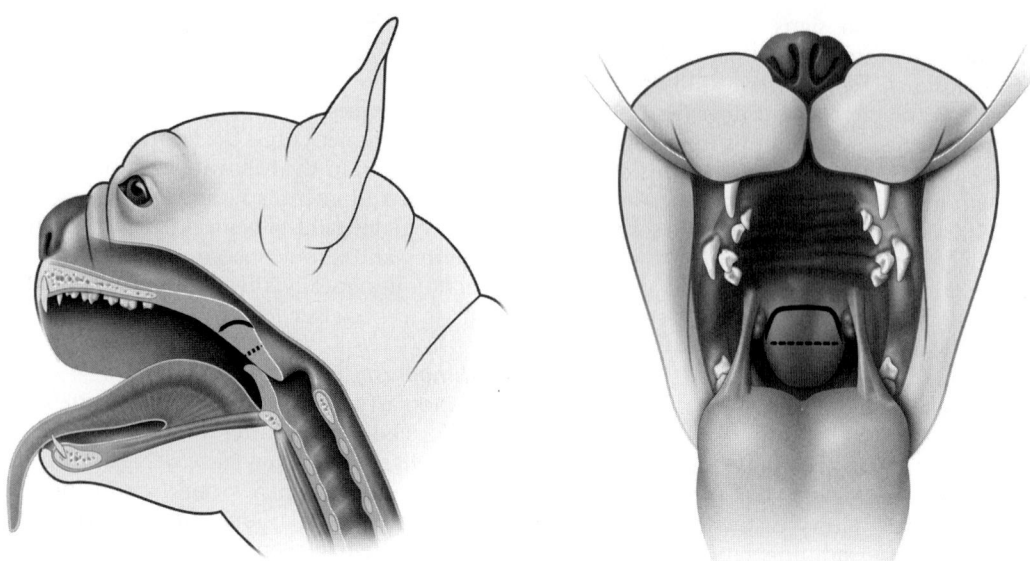

Figure 156-1 Diagram showing the lines of incision of the soft palate when performing a conventional (*solid line*) and extended (*dotted line*) palatoplasty. (After Dunie-Mérigot A, Bouvy B, Poncet C: Comparative use of CO_2 laser, diode laser and monopolar electrocautery for resection of the soft palate in dogs with brachycephalic airway obstructive syndrome, *Vet Rec* 167:700, 2010.)

ventriculectomy is a controversial recommendation in the management of BAOS. Although it plays a role in treating obstruction of the upper airways, ventriculectomy also may cause laryngeal edema and increase the risk of postanesthetic complications for the dog. We currently advise its use only in cases of significant eversion, ulceration, or formation of an inflammatory granuloma over these ventricles.

Management of Laryngeal Collapse

Laryngeal collapse is a respiratory obstruction caused by collapse of the arytenoid cartilages. Persistent negative pressure within the upper airways causes the cuneiform processes of the arytenoids to lose their rigidity and obstruct the laryngeal lumen. Obstruction is exacerbated by the presence of aggravating factors such as excitation, humidity, and exercise. Collapse of the cuneiform processes is known as *moderate* (grade 2 of 3) laryngeal collapse. In the event of collapse of the corniculate processes, which form the dorsal arch of the laryngeal orifice, the larynx is completely and critically obstructed (*severe*, grade 3 of 3). This situation represents a medical emergency.

Laryngeal collapse is a therapeutic challenge because no surgical solution enables effective reestablishment of the glottal opening, and removing upper airway obstruction through rhinoplasty and palatoplasty remains the priority. Lateralization of the arytenoid cartilage may be attempted in the event of moderate collapse; however, results are unpredictable. The significant flaccidity of the arytenoid cartilages in affected dogs often results in ineffective lateralization. An alternative may be to perform a partial excision of the arytenoid cartilages or a "consolidation" of the flaccid laryngeal structures using a laser technique. Cricoarytenoid lateralization combined with arytenoid laryngoplasty was recently reported to alleviate obstruction in dogs with laryngeal collapse (White, 2012).

A permanent tracheostomy can be envisaged as a last resort. The future lies in the development of precise new techniques for the surgical treatment of this serious disorder.

Management of Tracheal Hypoplasia

Tracheal hypoplasia is a congenital, static narrowing of the tracheal lumen, which may be associated with overlapping cartilaginous rings. It is particularly prevalent in the English bulldog. There is no surgical solution, but in the majority of cases, treatment of other causes of respiratory obstruction provides the dog with a satisfactory quality of life. None of the recent studies reports any modification in the prognosis for these dogs.

Prognosis

The period immediately after operation represents a critical time in these dogs, and swift action may be needed to restabilize the patient. Optimal conditions should be provided, including delayed extubation, constant monitoring, oxygenation via nasotracheal tube, avoidance of external pressure at the base of the tongue or neck, and preparation for reintubation or temporary tracheostomy if necessary.

The overall prognosis depends on the extent and severity of the lesions. Early treatment, a comprehensive diagnostic workup, and a logical approach to the management of observed lesions are important aspects of patient management. The surgical technique used, the experience of the operator, and the medical treatment of associated gastrointestinal disorders also are crucial aspects affecting the short- and medium-term prognosis in these dogs.

References and Suggested Reading

Brdecka DJ et al: Use of an electrothermal, feedback-controlled, bipolar sealing device for resection of the elongated portion of the soft palate in dogs with obstructive upper airway disease, *J Am Vet Med Assoc* 233:1265, 2008.

Dunie-Mérigot A, Bouvy B, Poncet C: Comparative use of CO_2 laser, diode laser and monopolar electrocautery for resection of the soft palate in dogs with brachycephalic airway obstructive syndrome, *Vet Rec* 167:700, 2010.

Findji L, Dupré G: Folded flap palatoplasty for treatment of elongated soft palate in 55 dogs, *Vet Med Austria* 95:56, 2009.

Ginn JA et al: Nasopharyngeal turbinates in brachycephalic dogs and cats, *J Am Anim Hosp Assoc* 44(5):243, 2008.

Grand JG, Bureau S: Structural characteristics of the soft palate and meatus nasopharyngeus in brachycephalic and non-brachycephalic dogs analysed by CT, *J Small Anim Pract* 52:232, 2011.

Oechtering GU et al: Laser-assisted turbinectomy (LATE)—treating brachycephalic airway distress at its intranasal origin, *Vet Surg* 36:E18, 2007.

Poncet C et al: Prevalence of gastro-intestinal tract lesions in 73 brachycephalic dogs with upper respiratory syndrome, *J Small Anim Pract* 46(6):273, 2005.

Poncet C et al: Long term results of upper respiratory syndrome surgery and gastrointestinal tract medical treatment in 51 brachycephalic dogs (2000-2003), *J Small Anim Pract* 47:1, 2006.

White RN: Surgical management of laryngeal collapse associated with brachycephalic airway obstruction syndrome in dogs, *J Small Anim Pract* 53:44, 2012. Epub November 28, 2011.

CHAPTER 157

Nasopharyngeal Disorders

SUSAN F. FOSTER, *Murdoch, Australia*
GERALDINE BRIONY HUNT, *Davis, California*

A variety of nasopharyngeal diseases are encountered in small animals. In cats, nasopharyngeal disease is most commonly caused by nasopharyngeal polyps, neoplasia, stenosis, foreign bodies, and cryptococcosis. In dogs, nasopharyngeal diseases include neoplasia, foreign bodies, nasal mites (*Pneumonyssoides caninum*), and congenital abnormalities. Clinical signs are similar regardless of cause, and a systematic approach to diagnosis is required to ensure that treatable diseases are recognized.

Clinical Signs of Nasopharyngeal Disease

Nasopharyngeal disease usually results in signs of upper airway obstruction, namely, inspiratory respiratory effort and stertor or snoring. In dogs, stertor is usually alleviated by open-mouth breathing. Cats are often unwilling or unable to breathe through the mouth and thus may exhibit severe respiratory distress. Pharyngeal discomfort, repeated attempts at swallowing, coughing, gagging, dysphagia, aerophagia, and changes in phonation also may occur. Animals with acute nasopharyngeal disease may paw at the nose and mouth or have facial discomfort and pruritus. Reverse sneezing is a specific nasopharyngeal sign in dogs. Sneezing is not typical of nasopharyngeal disease but may occur if the caudal nasal turbinates are irritated or if disease also affects the nasal cavity. Unless nasopharyngeal disease is accompanied by significant intranasal pathology, nasal discharge is usually mild or absent, because secretions from the nasopharynx tend to be swallowed. Purulent nasal discharge and fetid breath can be noted in animals with foreign bodies.

Signs of otitis media and vestibular disease can be seen when there is extension of disease from the nasopharynx into the tympanic bulla (or vice versa) or when the opening to the auditory (eustachian) tube is occluded. In one study, bullous effusion, considered most consistent with acute effusive disease, occurred in 34% of all cats with nasopharyngeal disease and 100% of cats with caudal nasopharyngeal disease (Detweiler et al, 2006). Thickening of the soft palate and reduced nasopharyngeal aperture have also been associated with the development of effusive otitis media in cavalier King Charles spaniels (Hayes et al, 2010). Conversely, expansile middle ear disease can cause nasopharyngeal obstruction. Horner's syndrome is commonly encountered in cats with involvement of the tympanic bullae. Deafness and signs of otic pain may occur, and there also may be signs of facial nerve dysfunction. Occasionally, the main presenting signs are neurologic, resulting from the spread of infection (such as cryptococcosis) or neoplasia, or signs may be related to the gastrointestinal tract (megaesophagus or hiatal hernia).

The speed of onset and severity of signs are variable and depend on the cause. Sudden onset of signs is suggestive of a foreign body, whereas gradual onset of stertor and attempted mouth breathing is more typical of a slow-growing nasopharyngeal mass.

Diagnosis of Nasopharyngeal Disease

Physical Examination

Mucous membrane color should be evaluated for cyanosis. Careful oral examination is required, and in quiet patients, palpation through the soft palate may reveal a nasopharyngeal mass. Unilateral or bilateral decreases in airflow are common. Enlargement of mandibular lymph nodes may be the first detectable finding in animals with nasopharyngeal neoplasia. Stertor, a snoring-type noise arising from the nasopharynx, should be differentiated from stridor (a high-pitched noise caused by disturbance of airflow through the larynx or trachea) before physical or chemical restraint is used. If possible, the effect of opening and closing the mouth on breathing and respiratory noise should be determined.

Diagnostic Imaging

The normal nasopharynx can be identified on plain lateral radiographs because of the presence of air dorsal to the soft palate. The hyoid apparatus and larynx define its caudal boundary. Space-occupying nasopharyngeal lesions are delineated by surrounding air, and radiopaque objects can be apparent; however, because of the complex anatomy of the region, and secretions within the nasopharynx, radiographic details may be obscured.

Computed tomography (CT) is increasingly used to assess the precise anatomic location of nasopharyngeal lesions and the involvement of other structures such as the middle ear, cribriform plate, brain, and bones of the skull. Use of a restraining device such as the VetMouse Trap allows CT to be performed in the conscious sedated small animal patient; however, assessment of the nasopharyngeal lumen and soft palate dimensions is reportedly more accurate with open-mouth positioning (Laurenson et al, 2011). CT is much quicker to perform than a full series of skull radiographs and is the preferred option if a mass is suspected.

Direct Visualization of the Nasopharynx

The oropharynx, laryngopharynx, and larynx are initially inspected before placement of a cuffed endotracheal tube sufficiently inflated to ensure a leakproof seal. The animal is best positioned in dorsal recumbency, with the maxilla held down firmly by tape applied over the upper canine teeth. Regional anesthesia of the nasopharynx with a topical anesthetic (2% lidocaine gel or lidocaine at 1 mg/kg) can decrease the plane of general anesthesia required to abolish reflexes resulting from mechanical stimulation of nasopharyngeal structures. Maxillary nerve blocks with 0.5% bupivacaine can also provide additional anesthesia. Rostral retraction of the caudal soft palate using a spay hook exposes the caudal nasopharynx. Using this method, the cranial nasopharynx and choanae also can be visualized in cats but not usually in dogs.

The most reliable method for evaluating the nasopharynx is nasopharyngeal endoscopy. A flexible endoscope is introduced into the pharynx and retroflexed above the soft palate or retroflexed before insertion and hooked over the soft palate. Rostral retraction of the retroflexed scope advances the scope (tip) toward the nose to allow visualization of the rostral nasopharynx. Lesions may not be apparent if they are obscured by mucus, blood, or pus. Vigorous saline flushing (via the endoscope or via the nostrils) usually helps with visualization.

Obtaining Diagnostic Samples from the Nasopharynx

Representative specimens for cytologic examination, histologic analysis, and microbial culture are required for definitive diagnosis. Fine-needle aspiration can be performed through the soft palate, and ultrasonographic guidance can aid in obtaining a representative sample. Blind Tru-Cut biopsy of lesions through the soft palate is also feasible, but there is a risk of hemorrhage if large blood vessels lateral to the nasopharynx are perforated. Ideally, biopsy tissue specimens are obtained by direct visualization via soft palate retraction, soft palate incision, or endoscopy. Endoscopic biopsy samples are small and may be superficial, yielding a diagnosis of nonspecific rhinitis rather than the true cause of disease. In some cases, a retroflexed endoscope can be used to visualize the nasopharynx while an independent biopsy forceps is advanced (antegrade) across the nasal cavity to the nasopharyngeal lesion.

When a mass is present, vigorous massage of the lesion through the soft palate often dislodges or fragments the mass, and anterograde flushing via the nares can be successful in dislodging part, or all, of it. The airways must be protected by gently occluding the laryngopharynx with packing material. In dogs, flushing is best achieved via catheters inserted into the ventral nasal meatuses; however, in cats, effective pressure can be generated by inserting the end of a 10-ml syringe directly into the naris and holding both nares closed with the fingers. Material dislodged from the nasal cavity or nasopharynx by flushing then collects on the packing material occluding the laryngopharynx. Anterograde passage of a catheter through the left and right ventral nasal meatuses is also helpful in dislodging foreign material and mucus. The advantages of a vigorous nasal flush technique over endoscopic biopsy are speed, cost, lack of need for any special equipment, immediate relief by debulking, dislodgment of foreign bodies, and usually better-sized biopsy samples; however, histopathologic analysis of nasal flush tissue can lead to inaccurate diagnoses.

Retrieval of canine nasal mites for diagnosis can be achieved with nasal flushing, although endoscopic visualization is preferable. Where permitted, flushing the nasal cavity with halothane can induce mites to migrate caudally into the nasopharynx where they can be easily retrieved and identified. It is conceivable that masking a dog with halothane or another inhalation anesthetic might have the same effect, but this has not been studied.

Adjunctive Tests for Diagnosis of Nasopharyngeal Disease

The results of cytologic analysis of squash-preparation specimens from nasopharyngeal masses in the cat showed good correlation with histologic findings in one study (De Lorenzi et al, 2008), although histopathologic analysis was recommended for differentiating lymphoma from lymphoid reaction. Cytologic examination and culture of nasal swabs may detect organisms such as *Cryptococcus* spp., but cats and dogs can have asymptomatic carriage of *Cryptococcus* spp. in the nasal cavity. Serologic testing is useful to differentiate asymptomatic carriage of *Cryptococcus* spp. from infection because animals with cryptococcosis should have a positive result on the latex cryptococcal antigen agglutination test.

Surgical Access to the Nasopharynx

When extraction of lesions such as inflammatory polyps, cryptococcal granulomas, or foreign bodies is not possible via palatine retraction, or better access is required to obtain diagnostic samples, the nasopharynx can be approached surgically via a longitudinal incision in the soft palate. In most cases, adequate access is obtained by maximally opening the jaws, placing a mouth gag, and having an assistant hold the endotracheal tube out of the way with a malleable retractor. Operating in this area requires some experience, and most cases are best managed by referral to a surgical specialist.

The soft palate is divided longitudinally from the caudal edge of the hard palate to within a centimeter of its caudal free edge. The caudal edge should be left intact to facilitate repair and support the incision during healing. Bleeding from the rich vascular plexuses within the soft palate should be anticipated but usually resolves spontaneously or with digital pressure. When extensive dissection is likely to be undertaken in dogs, blood loss may be ameliorated somewhat by temporary occlusion of the carotid arteries using Rummel tourniquets placed through a ventral midline cervical incision. This technique is not recommended for cats because it can result in permanent neurologic sequelae. In either species, if major blood loss is anticipated, contingency plans for replacement with whole blood or blood components should be made. The surgeon also should have a variety of hemostatic methods available, including sterile gauze for temporary packing of the nasal cavity or nasopharynx, and an implantable product such as Gelfoam. The soft palate incision can be continued rostrally as a mucoperiosteal incision and ventral rhinotomy if indicated, to provide excellent access to the ventral nasal cavity. Two- or three-layer repair of the soft palate with polydioxanone in a continuous suture pattern in the nasal mucosal and muscularis layers and in the oral mucosa provides excellent closure. Postoperative management is usually uncomplicated: animals display little evidence of pain and usually eat and drink within 24 hours of surgery unless systemic illness is present. Healing in this area is rapid and reliable, presumably due to the excellent blood supply. Soft food should be offered for 2 to 3 weeks after surgery and the incision examined at weekly intervals for signs of wound dehiscence.

Specific Nasopharyngeal Diseases and Their Treatment

Nasopharyngeal Mucus

Swelling of nasopharyngeal soft tissues is a common CT finding in cats with chronic upper respiratory tract disease. Mucosal hyperemia and swelling with multifocal lymphoid follicular hyperplasia and tenacious mucoid discharge are noted on retroflexed endoscopy. Feline mucus has a distinctive thick, ropey texture. Most cats cannot sneeze forcefully enough through narrowed nasal passages to clear this material, and nasopharyngeal obstruction can occur. Vigorous flushing with or without suction can provide immediate relief.

Nasopharyngeal Foreign Bodies

Foreign bodies include tablets, bones, stones, food, shrub and plant material (blades of grass are especially common in cats), trichobezoars (cats), needles, seaweed segments, and plastic. Nasopharyngeal foreign bodies can be dislodged by digital palpation or extracted under direct vision, endoscopically or surgically. Visualization and removal are facilitated by placing the animal in dorsal recumbency with head extension before retracting the soft palate. Foreign bodies may be coated with a thick layer of white to yellow mucopurulent material. It is often possible to dislodge foreign bodies caudally with a combination of anterograde flushing and passage of a urinary catheter. Alligator forceps also can be passed anterograde through the ventral nasal meatus and used to push the foreign body caudally for retrieval in the pharynx. Small stiff (Fogarty) embolectomy catheters with an inflatable balloon, passed via the nares and inflated at the choanae, can be useful to dislodge foreign bodies and push them into the pharynx. Surgery may be required to remove some foreign bodies such as fish bones or stones. After nonsurgical foreign body removal, the nasopharynx should be flushed with saline. If local ulceration is severe, broad-spectrum antibiotics with efficacy against anaerobes should be administered for 3 to 5 days.

Nasopharyngeal Parasites

The canine nasal mite *P. caninum,* reported in many countries (and probably worldwide), inhabits the nasal cavity, nasopharynx, and frontal sinus. Clinical signs of infestation include sneezing, reverse sneezing, and impaired olfaction. Diagnosis is established by direct observation of the mites in or around the external nares or endoscopic detection in the nasopharynx or nasal cavity. The diagnosis can be presumed when clinical signs resolve following miticidal treatment. Follicular hyperplasia in the nasopharynx should arouse suspicion even when mites are not visualized. Nasal mites can be effectively treated with milbemycin, ivermectin, or topical selamectin. The miticidal doses of selamectin, milbemycin, and ivermectin are higher than those required for heartworm prophylaxis. Milbemycin (0.5 to 1 mg/kg once weekly PO for 3 consecutive weeks) appears safe and effective. Topical selamectin (6 to 24 mg/kg every 2 weeks for three treatments) is also effective, but alopecia may develop at the higher dosages. Ivermectin has been effective at various doses (200 to 400 µg/kg SC or PO) and dosing frequencies (single dose or multiple doses at various intervals), although all doses are higher than the licensed dose and these dosages can have serious adverse effects in genetically predisposed, ivermectin-sensitive dogs such as collies.

It is advisable to supply a single antiinflammatory dose of prednisolone (0.5 mg/kg PO) either with the first miticidal treatment for prophylaxis or if signs worsen in severity after treatment. The transient increase in severity of signs that occurs in some dogs is presumed to be due to a host reaction to the dead and dying mites. Although this reaction is only transient, it can be distressing to both dogs and owners.

Cuterebra larvae are occasionally found in the feline pharynx, most commonly in the retropharyngeal tissues but also on the soft palate. The parasite may be seen through the "breathing hole" in the mucosal surface or may be found within a resected mass lesion. *Cuterebra* larvae are removed by excising the entire granuloma or by enlarging the breathing pore and grasping the parasite with forceps. Hypersensitivity reactions can occur if parasitic hemolymph escapes into the surrounding tissue, so care must be taken not to damage the larva during extraction.

Gapeworm (*Mammomonogamus ierei*) has been reported to be a common feline parasite in the Caribbean. The nematode attaches firmly to the mucosa of the nasopharynx causing inflammation and excessive mucus secretion. Respiratory distress, mucoid nasal discharge, sneezing, and respiratory noises are common. The diagnosis can be made through detection of a hookworm-type egg in a direct fecal smear from a cat with relevant clinical signs. Bronchoscopic removal of the adult worm might be required, and most parasiticides would likely be effective against the developmental stage.

Nasopharyngeal Cryptococcosis and Other Fungal Infections

In cats and dogs, the nasal cavity is usually the primary site of infection with *Cryptococcus* spp. If nasopharyngeal cryptococcomas are present, debulking by vigorous nasal flushing or surgery is recommended to alleviate upper airway obstruction and to hasten resolution. Cytologic examination, histopathologic analysis, and culture of retrieved material should be performed. Ideally, the isolate should be typed at a reference laboratory to establish whether it is *Cryptococcus neoformans* or *Cryptococcus gattii* and to determine drug susceptibility. This is especially important in places where *C. gattii* molecular types VGII and VGIII are endemic, such as northwestern North America, California, and Western Australia (Trivedi et al, 2011). Sequence analysis of polymerase chain reaction amplicons also may be necessary.

Fluconazole currently is regarded as the medical treatment of choice for localized nasopharyngeal cryptococcosis. Fluconazole is effective, has good penetration into the central nervous system (CNS), is well tolerated in the majority of cases, and is cheaper than itraconazole now that generic formulations are available. The dosage of fluconazole is 10 mg/kg q12h PO. Some cryptococcal isolates are resistant to fluconazole but susceptible to itraconazole or ketoconazole, both of which carry a greater risk of adverse effects including hepatotoxicity. Posaconazole is effective for treatment, although very costly.

Medical therapy should be continued until resolution of all clinical signs. Typically, this takes 3 to 12 months, although some cases require longer periods of treatment. Serum cryptococcal antigen titer should be monitored: a fourfold to fivefold reduction in titer suggests successful therapy, but cases ideally should be treated until the antigen titer declines to zero.

Other fungi reported to cause nasopharyngeal disease include *Aspergillus*, *Neosartorya* (sino-orbital aspergillosis), and *Trichosporon loubieri* (see Chapter 155).

Nasopharyngeal and Nasal Polyps

Nasopharyngeal polyps occur much more commonly in cats than in dogs. They arise from the mucosal lining of the nasopharynx, auditory tube, or middle ear. They are composed of fibrovascular connective tissue containing scattered lymphocytes, plasma cells, and macrophages and are covered by a stratified squamous or ciliated columnar epithelial layer that is often ulcerated. It has been proposed that nasopharyngeal polyps result from either congenital defects or chronic inflammatory middle ear disease caused by viral upper respiratory tract infection; however, an infectious cause has not yet been identified. Clinical signs can be respiratory, otic, or both. The external ear should be examined and CT considered to evaluate both compartments of the tympanic bulla.

Because of their caudal location in the nasopharynx, feline nasopharyngeal polyps are often amenable to removal by traction using grasping forceps with strong teeth. After intubation, the pharynx is packed with gauze. The cat is positioned in dorsal recumbency and its head is taped to the table or held manually. The soft palate is drawn rostrally to visualize the polyp. The polyp is grasped firmly across as much of its mass as possible, with care taken to ensure that pharyngeal mucosa is not included, and firm traction is applied. If grasping forceps with well-developed teeth are not available, artery forceps are preferred to conventional alligator forceps. The aim is to remove the polyp in its entirety, including its stalk. Removal of polyps piecemeal is likely to result in recurrence. Histopathologic examination is required to confirm the diagnosis of inflammatory polyp and eliminate the possibility of lymphosarcoma or cryptococcosis.

Owners should be warned that recurrence of the polyp is possible, and some surgeons have recommended ventral bulla osteotomy (VBO) for all cats. However, traction-avulsion is a good first option in cats with no radiographic evidence of bulla involvement, and because polyps do not always recur in cats with bulla involvement, traction-avulsion is probably a reasonable and practical first option for most cats. Anderson and others (2000) showed that cats with nasopharyngeal polyps were nearly four times more likely to be cured by traction alone than cats with aural polyps and that antiinflammatory doses of oral prednisolone following traction reduced the recurrence rate. VBO is indicated when polyps recur following traction, when there is evidence of a polyp in both the ear canal and the nasopharynx (MacPhail et al, 2007), when there is significant inflammatory disease extending beyond the tympanic bulla, and when the clinician is concerned that a neoplastic disease may be present. The nature of vascularized soft tissue within the bulla (polyp, otitis media, fibrous tissue following previous polyp extraction, neoplasia) cannot be determined using CT, and VBO may be required for collection of diagnostic samples. Samples for bacterial culture should be taken directly from the bulla if it is opened, because the microbial population may be different from that in the ear canal or nasopharynx. Owners should be informed that in deaf cats, VBO will not result in return of hearing and given that polyps can occur after VBO, total ear canal ablation may be preferable.

Horner's syndrome is common following VBO because of disruption of the sympathetic nerve fibers that are exposed along the promontory and ventromedial portion of the tympanic bulla. This usually resolves in 1 to 3 weeks. Facial nerve paralysis is also possible (but less likely) if the soft tissue dissection extends into the tissues ventral to the horizontal ear canal. Peripheral vestibular signs such as nystagmus, head tilt, and ataxia can occur as a result of aggressive curettage of the dorsomedial portion of the tympanic cavity and are temporary in most cases. Damage to the hypoglossal nerve is possible with aggressive dissection and retraction during the surgical approach. Likewise, damage to the retroarticular vein or internal carotid artery can result in major hemorrhage.

Inflammatory polyps of the nasal turbinates, previously termed *nasal polyps* but now thought to be feline mesenchymal hamartomas, arise in the nasal cavity and only occasionally extend into the nasopharynx (Greci et al, 2011). They usually occur in cats younger than 1 year of age and are possibly more common in Italy. They differ in gross appearance and histologic features from nasopharyngeal polyps. Per-endoscopic removal of the mass and visibly abnormal turbinates has been successful in some cats, although dorsal rhinotomy and turbinectomy may be required. Spontaneous resolution also has been reported.

In dogs, polyps usually arise from the caudal nasal turbinates, as a consequence of chronic rhinitis. They are usually situated rostrally in the nasopharynx, attached to the caudal nasal turbinates. This is also true of other forms of inflammatory granuloma. It may be possible to dislodge these by performing vigorous flushing or by grasping them endoscopically. In other cases, a ventral surgical approach to the nasopharynx can be combined with a ventral rhinotomy to obtain diagnostic samples and debulk the lesions.

Nasopharyngeal Turbinates

The finding of nasopharyngeal turbinates in brachycephalic dogs has been reported recently. These projections of the caudal nasal turbinates into the nasopharynx were present in 21% of brachycephalic dogs evaluated (Ginn et al, 2008) and appeared to cause obstruction of the choanae. The significance of nasopharyngeal turbinates and their possible contribution to the clinical signs associated with brachycephalic airway disease are yet to be determined; however, it seems advisable for clinicians evaluating brachycephalic dogs with upper airway obstruction to visualize the nasopharynx when possible.

Nasopharyngeal Stenosis

Nasopharyngeal stenosis can occur in cats and dogs as a result of chronic inflammation, infectious diseases, aspiration (Quimby and Lappin, 2010), or surgery or other trauma, or as a congenital abnormality (choanal atresia or soft palate dysgenesis). Regardless of cause, treatment aims are to establish patency of the choanae and nasopharynx and reduce the risk of stricture recurrence. Underlying conditions leading to the inflammation and mucosal ulceration must also be addressed to achieve long-term resolution of the nasopharyngeal obstruction.

Patency can be established by bougienage, dilation using artery forceps, stenting, or surgical excision of the obstructing tissue. It may be possible in some cases to restore the integrity of the nasopharyngeal mucosa by means of local flaps, but in most instances this is not feasible. The best results thus far have been achieved with balloon dilation of nasopharyngeal stenosis in dogs and cats. Multiple attempts at balloon dilation may be required before an acceptable long-term result is achieved, but it is worth persevering with this minimally invasive treatment before progressing to more aggressive options. Balloons of 10 to 15 mm in diameter are introduced orthograde through the ventral nasal meatus and inflated in stages until maximal dilatation of the stricture is achieved. Bradycardia, presumably mediated by the vagal nerve, can be encountered during the maneuver, and atropine administration should be considered before balloon inflation. Long-term control of clinical signs of nasopharyngeal disease is achieved in most patients; however, restenosis of variable severity can occur (Glaus et al, 2005).

Placement of balloon-expandable stents for primary treatment or for follow-up treatment of recurrent nasopharyngeal stenosis has also been accomplished (Berent et al, 2008). Complications included regrowth of the stricture through the stent and projection of the stent into the nasopharynx causing hairball entrapment and gagging.

Anecdotal experience with nasopharyngeal stenosis in dogs suggests that some stenoses are comprised of very dense (sometimes cartilaginous) tissue that may be resistant to dilation with regular valvuloplasty balloons, and for this reason some clinicians now use a specialized cutting balloon to make cuts in the fibrous tissue before balloon dilation. Positioning of the balloon or stent (or both) can be quick or time consuming depending on the accessibility and diameter of the stricture. In some patients, the nasopharynx is not patent, and a hole must be made with a stylet or biopsy punch. The goal is to position a guidewire across the stenosis by passing it either antegrade through the external nares or retrograde through a retroflexed endoscope. Once the guidewire is positioned, a cutting balloon or dilator can be passed to increase lumen diameter enough to receive a balloon catheter of appropriate diameter for the patient. The length of balloon is chosen and the balloon is positioned so as to avoid damaging normal turbinates within the nasal cavity.

Nasopharyngeal Cysts

Nasopharyngeal cysts arise as a result of caudal nasal turbinate disease (in dogs) or cystic malformation of structures adjacent to the nasopharynx, such as the thyroglossal duct or Rathke's cleft. In cystic Rathke's cleft, embryonic pituitary development proceeds abnormally and results in a progressively expansile cystic lesion within the sphenoid bone. Signs are often progressive, and owners may not seek veterinary attention until the patient reaches adulthood. Cystic Rathke's cleft may or may not be associated with pituitary dwarfism. Other types of developmental cysts have been encountered in dogs. A cystic or multilobulated appearance may also occur with cartilaginous and bony neoplasms of the skull, such as multilobular osteosarcoma, and advanced imaging and histopathologic analysis are important for diagnosis and surgical decision making. Cystic Rathke's cleft or other developmental bony cysts require complete excision or surgical débridement and debulking. Simple cysts of the nasal turbinates can be removed by traction or flushing, or may require surgical débridement.

Nasopharyngeal Neoplasia

Nasal tumors arise most commonly in the caudal one third of the nasal cavity, and nasopharyngeal involvement is common. Lymphosarcoma (lymphoma) is the most common nasopharyngeal tumor in cats. In a study of nasal and nasopharyngeal lymphoma, 10% of cats with lymphoma were found to have nasopharyngeal involvement only and 8% had both nasopharyngeal and nasal involvement (Little et al, 2007). Overall, the majority of tumors were classified as immunoblastic B-cell lymphomas; 60% of the masses with nasopharyngeal involvement only were B cell and 40% were T cell. Direct extension to the CNS has been reported, and multiorgan involvement was found in 67% of necropsied cats in one study (Little et al, 2007).

Nasopharyngeal lymphosarcoma is exceedingly rare in dogs, and there is little information about its treatment. Treatment usually involves multiagent chemotherapy protocols with prior surgical debulking only if respiratory signs are severe. Nonlymphoid nasal tumors that can involve the nasopharynx in dogs and cats include osteosarcoma, chondrosarcoma, fibrosarcoma, and carcinoma.

Olfactory neuroblastomas and oncocytomas with nasopharyngeal involvement or origin also have been reported in cats.

References and Suggested Reading

Anderson DM, Robinson RK, White RA: Management of inflammatory polyps in 37 cats, *Vet Rec* 147:684, 2000.

Berent AC et al: Use of a balloon expandable metallic stent for treatment of nasopharyngeal stenosis in dogs and cats: six cases (2005-2007), *J Am Vet Med Assoc* 233:1432, 2008.

De Lorenzi D, Bertoncello D, Bottero E: Squash-preparation cytology from nasopharyngeal masses in the cat: cytological results and histological correlations in 30 cases, *J Feline Med Surg* 10:55, 2008.

Detweiler DA et al: Computed tomographic evidence of bulla effusion in cats with sinonasal disease: 2001-2004, *J Vet Intern Med* 20:1080, 2006.

Ginn JA et al: Nasopharyngeal turbinates in brachycephalic dogs and cats, *J Am Anim Hosp Assoc* 44:243, 2008.

Glaus TM et al: Reproducible and long-lasting success of balloon dilation of nasopharyngeal stenosis in cats, *Vet Rec* 157:257, 2005.

Greci V et al: Inflammatory polyps of the nasal turbinates of cats: an argument for designation as feline mesenchymal nasal hamartoma, *J Feline Med Surg* 13:213, 2011.

Hayes GM, Friend EJ, Jeffery ND: Relationship between pharyngeal conformation and otitis media with effusion in Cavalier King Charles Spaniels, *Vet Rec* 167:55, 2010.

Laurenson MP et al: Computed tomography of the pharynx in a closed vs. open mouth position, *Vet Radiol Ultrasound* 52:357, 2011.

Little L, Patel R, Goldschmidt M: Nasal and nasopharyngeal lymphoma in cats: 50 cases (1989-2005), *Vet Pathol* 44:885, 2007.

MacPhail CM et al: Atypical manifestations of feline inflammatory polyps in three cats, *J Feline Med Surg* 9:219, 2007.

Quimby J, Lappin M: Feline focus: Update on upper respiratory diseases: condition-specific recommendations, *Compend Contin Educ Vet.* 32:E1, 2010.

Sfiligoi G, Théon AP, Kent MS: Response of nineteen cats with nasal lymphoma to radiation therapy and chemotherapy, *Vet Radiol Ultrasound* 48:388, 2007.

Trivedi SR et al: Clinical features and epidemiology of cryptococcosis in cats and dogs in California: 93 cases (1988-2010)., *J Am Vet Med Assoc* 239:357, 2011.

CHAPTER 158

Laryngeal Diseases

CATRIONA M. MACPHAIL, *Fort Collins, Colorado*
ERIC MONNET, *Fort Collins, Colorado*

The larynx is the collection of cartilages surrounding the rima glottis that is responsible for control of airflow during respiration. The four cartilages that constitute the larynx are the paired arytenoids and the unpaired epiglottis, cricoid, and thyroid cartilages. The cricoarytenoideus dorsalis muscle is solely responsible for opening the glottis. The muscle originates on the dorsolateral surface of the cricoid and inserts on the muscular process of the arytenoid cartilages. The recurrent laryngeal nerve innervates each of the intrinsic muscles of the larynx except the cricothyroid muscle.

The function of the larynx is to regulate airflow, protect the lower airway from aspiration during swallowing, and control phonation. Diseases most commonly affecting the larynx include laryngeal paralysis, laryngeal collapse, and laryngeal masses. Each of these conditions results in some degree of upper airway obstruction. Dogs and cats typically are brought to the veterinarian because of respiratory stridor, voice change, coughing, or gagging. Progression of clinical signs is highly variable.

Laryngeal Paralysis

Causes

Laryngeal paralysis is a common unilateral or bilateral respiratory disorder that primarily affects older (>9 years) large- and giant-breed dogs. However, a congenital form does occur in certain breeds such as Bouvier des Flandres, Siberian huskies, and bull terriers. A laryngeal paralysis-polyneuropathy complex has been described in dalmatians, rottweilers, and Pyrean mountain dogs. For the more frequently encountered acquired laryngeal paralysis, the Labrador retriever is the most common breed reported, but golden retrievers, Saint Bernards, Newfoundlands, and Irish setters are also overrepresented. Acquired laryngeal paralysis is caused by damage to the recurrent laryngeal nerve or intrinsic laryngeal muscles from polyneuropathy, polymyopathy, accidental or iatrogenic trauma, or intrathoracic or extrathoracic masses. In most dogs the cause remains undetermined, and these cases are traditionally classified as idiopathic. Recently, it was shown that many dogs develop systemic neurologic signs within 1 year following diagnosis of laryngeal paralysis, which is consistent with progressive generalized neuropathy (Stanley et al, 2010). Abnormalities in the results of electrodiagnostic tests and histopathologic analysis of nerve and muscle biopsy specimens reflecting generalized polyneuropathy have been documented in a small number of dogs with acquired laryngeal paralysis (Thieman et al, 2010).

Clinical Signs

In laryngeal paralysis, the arytenoid cartilages, and consequently the vocal folds, remain in a paramedian position during inspiration, creating upper airway obstruction. Dogs typically present with noisy inspiratory respiration and exercise intolerance. Early clinical signs include voice change and mild coughing and gagging. Severe airway obstruction results in respiratory distress, cyanosis, and collapse. Dogs may also have signs of dysphagia.

Progression of clinical signs is highly variable, and dogs may have clinical signs for several months to years before significant respiratory distress ensues. However, clinical signs are worsened by heavy exercise or increasing environmental temperature or humidity, which results in an acute exacerbation of a chronic condition. As respiratory rate increases, the mucosa covering the arytenoids obstructing airflow may become inflamed and edematous, which leads to further airway obstruction. A vicious cycle ensues that if unaddressed may become life threatening.

Diagnosis

Routine diagnostic evaluation for dogs thought to have laryngeal paralysis includes physical examination, neurologic examination, complete blood count, biochemical profile, urinalysis, thyroid function screening, thoracic radiographs, and laryngeal examination. Dogs with bilateral laryngeal paralysis are at risk of aspiration pneumonia both before and after surgery. Therefore thoracic radiographs are a necessary part of the diagnostic workup in dogs suspected to have laryngeal dysfunction. For dogs that present with dysphagia or vomiting, an esophagram should be obtained to rule out esophageal dysfunction or megaesophagus, which may not be apparent on plain thoracic radiographs. Severe progressive esophageal dysfunction has been reported in a set of dogs with idiopathic laryngeal paralysis and is likely reflects the proposed generalized progressive polyneuropathy (Stanley et al, 2010). Hypothyroidism may be found concurrently with laryngeal paralysis, although a direct causal link has yet to be established. Regardless, thyroid function screening is performed routinely in the workup for laryngeal paralysis. Thyroid supplementation should be instituted if indicated, although this does not seem to improve clinical signs associated with laryngeal paralysis.

Definitive diagnosis of laryngeal paralysis requires visual examination of the larynx. However, laryngoscopy can be confounding, and false-positive results are common because of the influence of anesthetic agents on laryngeal function. Laryngeal paralysis should not be diagnosed based solely on the lack of arytenoid movement; inflammation and swelling of the laryngeal cartilages also should be apparent. Diagnosis may additionally be confused by the presence of paradoxical movement of the arytenoids, resulting in a false-negative result. In this situation, the arytenoid cartilages move inward during inspiration because of negative intraglottic pressure that is created by breathing against an obstruction. The cartilages then passively return to their original position during the expiratory phase, which gives the impression of abduction. An assistant can state the phase of ventilation during laryngoscopy to help in distinguishing normal from abnormal motion.

Intravenous thiopental administered to effect is thought to be the best choice to allow assessment of laryngeal function. When a butorphanol-glycopyrrolate premedication is used, either thiopental or propofol allows excellent visualization of the larynx. The recent lack of availability of thiopental leaves propofol as the most appropriate induction agent for laryngeal examination in dogs. Doxapram HCl (1 mg/kg IV) has been advocated for routine use during laryngoscopy to increase respiratory rate and effort and improve intrinsic laryngeal motion, and should be administered if the diagnosis is in doubt. Some clinicians include doxapram administration as part of every laryngeal examination. Transnasal laryngoscopy, ultrasonography, and computed tomography (CT) all have been described as methods to diagnose laryngeal paralysis; however, none appears superior to traditional oral laryngeal examination under heavy sedation or light anesthesia.

Emergency Treatment

For dogs in acute respiratory distress, initial treatment is directed at improving ventilation, reducing laryngeal edema, and minimizing the animal's stress. A typical treatment regimen involves oxygen supplementation and administration of short-acting steroids (e.g., dexamethasone 0.2 to 1 mg/kg IV) and sedatives (e.g., acepromazine 0.02 mg/kg IV). Additional administration of buprenorphine (0.005 mg/kg IV) or butorphanol (0.25 mg/kg IV) also may be considered. These dogs are often also hyperthermic, and appropriate cooling procedures should also be instituted. If respiratory distress cannot be abated, intubation or a temporary tracheostomy should be considered. However, the use of a temporary tracheostomy tube in dogs with laryngeal paralysis has been shown to be a negative prognostic indicator following surgery, because dogs that received a temporary tracheostomy preoperatively were more likely to experience major complications.

Conservative Treatment

Often dogs are not severely affected clinically until they have bilateral laryngeal paresis or paralysis. Therefore dogs with unilateral laryngeal dysfunction are not surgical candidates. For dogs with bilateral laryngeal paralysis, the decision to recommend surgery is based on the quality of life of the dog, severity of clinical signs, and time of year. The goal of conservative management of dogs with laryngeal paralysis is to improve the quality of life through environmental changes, reduction of daily exercise, owner education, weight loss, and consideration of anti-inflammatory drugs to minimize laryngeal swelling. Unfortunately, this medical treatment path is insufficient for long-term management. For dogs that are diagnosed with concurrent hypothyroidism, thyroid supplementation should be instituted, but as noted earlier this rarely improves the clinical signs of laryngeal paralysis.

Surgical Treatment

Laryngeal paralysis is a surgical condition for significantly affected dogs. Numerous techniques have been described to treat laryngeal paralysis. Unilateral arytenoid lateralization is the current technique of choice for most surgeons, but various types of partial laryngectomy (bilateral vocal fold resection, partial arytenoidectomy) are also performed. Bilateral arytenoid lateralization is not recommended because it has been shown to result in unacceptable morbidity. Other techniques include castellated laryngofissure, reinnervation of the laryngeal musculature, and permanent tracheostomy. Castellated laryngofissure is performed rarely because of the technical difficulty of the procedure and inconsistent outcomes. Reinnervation does not provide immediate clinical relief, so it is therefore not a practical treatment option in dogs. Permanent tracheostomy is considered a salvage procedure for dogs most at risk of aspiration pneumonia, but it is associated with a high rate of major and minor complications and requires diligent postoperative and long-term care.

Several variations of unilateral arytenoid lateralization have been described. The most common technique involves suturing the cricoid cartilage to the muscular process of the arytenoid cartilage. This mimics the directional pull of the cricoarytenoid dorsalis muscle and rotates the arytenoid cartilage laterally. An alternative technique involves suture placement from the muscular process of the arytenoid cartilage to the caudodorsal aspect of the thyroid cartilage. This pulls the arytenoid cartilage laterally rather than rotating it and increases the area of the rima glottis to a lesser degree than the cricoarytenoid suture. However, differences in surgical technique and the degree of increase in surface area of the rima glottis do not appear to affect postoperative clinical signs and outcome. Increasing the surface area of the rima glottis beyond the edges of the epiglottis may put the animal at higher risk of aspiration. Limited lateral displacement of the arytenoid cartilage will significantly reduces airway resistance within the larynx and may decrease the risk of postoperative aspiration pneumonia (Greenberg et al, 2007). This is accomplished by minimizing the degree of dissection: separation of the cricothyroid articulation, transection of the sesamoid band connecting the paired arytenoid, and complete disarticulation of the cricoarytenoid joint are not necessary. A partial opening of the cricoarytenoid articulation allows accurate visualization of needle placement through the muscular process of the arytenoid but limits the degree of arytenoid cartilage abduction.

Partial laryngectomy encompasses various techniques for vocal cord excision and partial arytenoidectomy to increase the diameter of the glottis. Partial laryngectomy has been associated with complications, including laryngeal webbing, laryngeal scarring, and aspiration pneumonia. High complication rates have been reported by some. However, bilateral vocal fold resection alone resulted in fewer complications and better postoperative outcome than other partial laryngectomy techniques. This is thought to be to the result of better laryngeal protection during swallowing and decreased laryngeal irritation because the corniculate processes of the arytenoid cartilages are left intact. Bilateral vocal fold excision and thyroarytenoid lateralization performed through a ventral laryngotomy improves clinical signs and is associated with a low rate of aspiration pneumonia; however, recurrence of clinical signs is common, likely because of narrowing of the rima glottis (Schofield et al, 2007). Successful partial arytenoidectomy by photoablation of the left arytenoid cartilage tissue using a diode laser has been reported in a small set of dogs (Olivieri et al, 2009).

Prognosis

Aspiration pneumonia is the most common complication in dogs surgically treated for laryngeal paralysis. Although aspiration pneumonia is most likely in the first few weeks following surgery, it has been recognized that these dogs are at risk of this complication for the rest of their lives. Factors that have been found to be significantly associated with a higher risk of developing complications and a negative effect on long-term outcome include preoperative aspiration pneumonia, development of esophageal dysfunction, progression of generalized neurologic signs, temporary tracheostomy placement, and concurrent neoplastic disease. In the absence of surgical complications, unilateral arytenoid lateralization results in less respiratory distress and stridor and improved exercise tolerance. Owner satisfaction with this procedure has been reported as excellent, with the majority of owners believing that the quality of the dog's life was improved dramatically.

Laryngeal Paralysis in Cats

Laryngeal paralysis is an uncommon condition in cats. Clinical presentation is similar to that in dogs in that it occurs most often in middle-aged to older cats, and both unilateral and bilateral conditions have been reported. Cats with unilateral laryngeal paralysis can have significant clinical signs and require surgical intervention—unlike dogs, which rarely have clinical manifestations of the disorder. There may also be a prevalence of left-sided unilateral laryngeal paralysis in cats, which is similar to that reported in humans and horses.

The specific cause of laryngeal paralysis in cats is often unknown and it is deemed idiopathic, but several cases have been associated with trauma, neoplastic invasion, and iatrogenic damage (e.g., after thyroidectomy).

Neoplastic infiltration can lead to fixed laryngeal obstruction with both inspiratory and expiratory dyspnea and noise and should always be considered in the differential diagnosis of laryngeal paralysis in the cat.

Successful surgical treatment primarily using unilateral arytenoid lateralization has been reported in several small studies (Hardie et al, 2009; Thunberg and Lantz, 2010).

Laryngeal Collapse

Laryngeal collapse is a consequence of chronic upper airway obstruction, most often associated with brachycephalic airway syndrome (see Chapter 156). However, laryngeal collapse also may be associated with laryngeal paralysis, nasal and nasopharyngeal obstruction, or trauma. Chronic upper airway obstruction causes increased airway resistance and increased negative intraglottic luminal pressure. Over time this results in laryngeal collapse due to cartilage fatigue and degeneration. However, early onset of laryngeal collapse has been reported in brachycephalic dogs ranging in age from 4.5 to 6 months (Pink et al, 2006).

Diagnosis of laryngeal collapse requires oral laryngeal examination under heavy sedation or a light plane of general anesthesia without intubation. Functional, as well as structural, examination of the larynx should be performed. Recently, CT imaging and three-dimensional internal rendering was used in nine dogs with laryngeal collapse with no sedation or general anesthesia (Stadler et al, 2011).

The early stage of laryngeal collapse is still amenable to surgical treatment; however, options for treating advanced (grade 2 or 3) laryngeal collapse are limited (see Chapter 156).

Laryngeal Masses

Neoplasia

Tumors of the larynx are uncommon in the dog and cat. Numerous types of tumor have been reported in the dog, including rhabdomyosarcoma (oncocytoma), squamous cell carcinoma, adenocarcinoma, osteosarcoma, chondrosarcoma, fibrosarcoma, undifferentiated carcinoma, and mast cell tumor. Inflammatory nodules, especially those involving the vocal folds, should be considered in the differential diagnosis. Squamous cell carcinoma and lymphoma are the most common tumors of the larynx in the cat.

Small lesions may be resected by mucosal resection or partial laryngectomy through an oral approach or ventral laryngotomy. Aggressive surgical intervention involves complete laryngectomy with permanent tracheostomy but has been reported only in isolated cases. Radioresponsive tumors may be treated with radiation therapy. Otherwise most treatment is palliative, consisting of airflow bypass of the laryngeal area through a permanent tracheostomy. Prognosis for laryngeal tumors is guarded because most cases are quite advanced at the time of diagnosis. There are only isolated reports of management of canine and feline laryngeal tumors. Treatment of four cats with laryngeal squamous cell carcinoma with tube tracheostomy alone resulted in a median survival of only 3 days; chemotherapeutic treatment of five cats with laryngeal masses resulted in a median survival of 141 days (Jakubiak et al, 2005).

A recent study reported on the placement of permanent tracheostomies in five cats with laryngeal carcinoma (Guenther-Yenke and Rozanski, 2007). Survival at home ranged from 2 to 281 days with two cats dying from tracheostomy site occlusion and three cats euthanized because of disease progression.

Benign Growths

Inflammatory laryngeal disease is an uncommon non-neoplastic condition of the arytenoid cartilages of the larynx that has been reported in both dogs and cats. It can be granulomatous, lymphocytic-plasmacytic, or eosinophilic in nature, with multiple factors likely contributing to the development of the disease. Severe cases can result in laryngeal stenosis and significant upper airway obstruction. Biopsy of the mass is crucial to differentiate this disease from neoplasia, although it is still possible that inflammatory changes may represent a secondary response to underlying neoplasia. Treatment of inflammatory laryngeal disease is palliative and consists of debulking of the mass, steroid therapy, or permanent tracheostomy. Permanent tracheostomy has been associated with a higher mortality in cats with inflammatory laryngeal disease than in cats undergoing permanent tracheostomy for any other reason (Stepnik et al, 2009).

Benign laryngeal cysts also have been described in isolated feline cases. Cysts are typically epithelial in origin and stem from the ventral aspect of the larynx. Surgical removal is usually curative. Some cysts are very large and can significantly obstruct airflow.

References and Suggested Reading

Fasanella FJ et al: Brachycephalic airway obstructive syndrome in dogs: 90 cases (1991-2008), *J Am Vet Med Assoc* 237:1048, 2010.

Greenberg MJ, Bureau S, Monnet E: Effects of suture tension during unilateral cricoarytenoid lateralization on canine laryngeal resistance in vitro, *Vet Surg* 36:526, 2007.

Guenther-Yenke CL, Rozanski EA: Tracheostomy in cats: 23 cases (1998-2006), *J Feline Med Surg* 9:451, 2007.

Hardie RJ, Gunby J, Bjorling DE: Arytenoid lateralization for treatment of laryngeal paralysis in 10 cats, *Vet Surg* 38:445, 2009.

Jakubiak MJ et al: Laryngeal, laryngotracheal, and tracheal masses in cats: 27 cats (1998-2003), *J Am Anim Hosp Assoc* 41:310, 2005.

Olivieri M, Voghera SG, Fossum TW: Video-assisted left partial arytenoidectomy by diode laser photoablation for treatment of canine laryngeal paralysis, *Vet Surg* 38:439, 2009.

Pink JJ et al: Laryngeal collapse in seven brachycephalic puppies, *J Am Anim Hosp Assoc* 47:131, 2006.

Schofield DM, Norris J, Sadanaga KK: Bilateral thyroarytenoid cartilage lateralization and vocal fold excision with mucosoplasty for treatment of idiopathic laryngeal paralysis: 67 dogs (1998-2005), *Vet Surg* 36:519, 2007.

Stadler K et al: Computed tomographic imaging of dogs with primary laryngeal or tracheal airway obstruction, *Vet Radiol Ultrasound* 52:377, 2011.

Stanley BJ et al: Esophageal dysfunction in dogs with idiopathic laryngeal paralysis: a controlled cohort study, *Vet Surg* 39:139, 2010.

Stepnik MW et al: Outcome of permanent tracheostomy for treatment of upper airway obstruction in cats: 21 cases (1990-2007), *J Am Vet Med Assoc* 234:638, 2009.

Thieman KM et al: Histopathological confirmation of polyneuropathy in 11 dogs with laryngeal paralysis, *J Am Anim Hosp Assoc* 46:161, 2010.

Thunberg B, Lantz GC: Evaluations of unilateral arytenoid lateralization for the treatment of laryngeal paralysis in 14 cats, *J Am Anim Hosp Assoc* 46:418, 2010.

CHAPTER 159

Tracheal Collapse

BRIAN A. SCANSEN, *Columbus, Ohio*
CHICK WEISSE,* *New York, New York*

Tracheal collapse comprises a variety of conditions originally characterized as a degenerative disease of the cartilage rings in which hypocellularity and decreased glycosaminoglycan and calcium content lead to dynamic airway collapse during respiration. Other conditions include laxity of the dorsal tracheal membrane and malformed tracheal cartilage rings. Tracheal collapse is a disorder of predominantly small- and toy-breed dogs that can present with signs ranging from a mild, intermittent "honking" cough to severe respiratory distress from dynamic upper airway obstruction. Although more commonly seen in older patients, animals of all ages can be affected.

A careful history taking and physical examination are important to direct therapy and assist in determining prognosis. The history taking should be targeted to include any concurrent medical problems, the age of onset and duration of clinical signs, the progression of these signs, any factors that incite or worsen signs, the current frequency and severity of the signs, the effectiveness of any prior therapies in ameliorating cough or respiratory difficulty, and the occurrence of any episodes of cyanosis, syncope, or life-threatening respiratory distress. Further review of causes and diagnostic testing can be found in Chapter 144 of the previous edition of *Current Veterinary Therapy*.

General Treatment Considerations

Therapies are variable and depend on the severity of clinical signs, with some dogs requiring basic environmental modification and dietary therapy, others needing aggressive medical therapy, and the most severely affected requiring intervention. There is no definitive strategy that will work for all cases; for this reason, developing the final treatment strategy generally takes time and considerable trial and error with frequent client communication to achieve the most effective management. It is possible, however, to achieve a fair quality of life for most of these dogs as long as the appropriate expectation is explained to the client at the outset.

For those dogs with a primary history of cough, the most common complaint, environmental modification, weight loss, and medical therapy are the mainstays of therapy. Interventions such as intraluminal stenting or surgical prostheses should be reserved for dogs with

*Disclosure: Chick Weisse is a consultant for Infiniti Medical LLC and has been involved in the specifications chosen for the Vet Stent-Trachea and Delivery System.

life-threatening clinical signs or those for which medical therapy has failed. At what point such intervention is necessary is admittedly subjective. In most cases, after carefully evaluating a patient's history, response to therapy, and current clinical status, the veterinarian and owner can determine when the time has arrived to consider an intervention. An exception to this rule is the emergent, intubated patient for which attempts at extubation have failed. An owner's inability to administer medication is not a valid reason to perform one of these invasive procedures, because the majority of patients will still require medication following treatment. Placement of an intraluminal stent will initially stimulate the cough reflex; therefore, if the cough cannot be controlled medically, it is unlikely to improve with intervention. Furthermore, although intraluminal stenting and surgical prostheses can provide successful palliation for many dogs, both are associated with a moderate risk of complications. Therefore client education is critical, and the decision to proceed with tracheal intervention should be made only as a final option.

A detailed discussion of the diagnosis of tracheal collapse is beyond the scope of this chapter. In general the accepted diagnostic procedures include thoracic radiography, tracheal radiography, fluoroscopy, and endoscopy. Other primary or secondary respiratory disorders must be evaluated concurrently and addressed before more invasive therapies for tracheal collapse are implemented. For example, many dogs have concurrent bronchial collapse and others are affected by chronic bronchitis (see Chapter 160). Animals with concurrent cardiac or pulmonary disease often can benefit substantially from medical treatment of those conditions, so that more invasive tracheal collapse treatments can be avoided or postponed.

Clinical Syndromes of Tracheal Collapse

Conservative Therapy for Activity-Induced Cough

Many dogs with tracheal collapse have activity-induced coughing. Conservative therapy should be the first line of treatment for these patients. Weight loss, restricted exercise, and avoidance of secondhand smoke or inhaled irritants can reduce clinical signs. In addition, management of comorbidities such as cardiac disease or pulmonary disease can help reduce the incidence of respiratory crisis episodes. If the cough is infrequent, these modifications may be sufficient to control signs and avoid pharmacologic intervention or invasive procedures.

Medical therapy is critical to control signs in dogs with cough. Antitussive medications are the mainstay of therapy, with several options available. In the authors' opinion, hydrocodone-based cough suppressants (Hycodan, Tussigon) are the most effective antitussives in dogs. A common misconception is that if the cough is not controlled on a standard dosage of hydrocodone, typically considered 0.25 mg/kg PO q6-8h, then this medication has failed. However, the authors have found that most dogs with tracheal collapse require higher dosages, and it is the rare dog whose cough cannot at least be improved with hydrocodone. As noted earlier, client education is critical, and the authors instruct clients that a gradual escalation of hydrocodone therapy may be required, with the dose typically increasing in 0.25-mg/kg increments every 5 to 7 days based on the dog's response. The dose is gradually increased until either the cough is controlled or adverse effects of the hydrocodone manifest, usually excessive sedation or constipation. In the authors' experience, hydrocodone dosages of 0.5 to 1 mg/kg PO q6-8h are typically effective; a dosage greater than 1.5 mg/kg PO q6-8h is rarely necessary. For small dogs, a liquid suspension of hydrocodone (often formulated to 1 mg/ml) is easier to use than tablets and makes incremental dose adjustments more feasible. When medical therapy is first initiated, a tapering course of prednisone is also begun to suppress tracheal irritation and inflammation in hopes of breaking the cycle of coughing that has already been initiated. The authors prescribe prednisone at a starting dosage of 0.5 to 2 mg/kg/day PO with a taper over 2 to 3 weeks. For some dogs, the addition of maintenance therapy with inhalant corticosteroids is beneficial to minimize cough. Fluticasone is the authors' preferred inhaled corticosteroid, given at 110 µg/puff twice daily via a canine-specific spacing chamber and face mask.

The use of bronchodilators (e.g., theophylline, terbutaline) is often considered in dogs with tracheal collapse complicated by lower airway disease. In the authors' experience, these medications provide minimal palliation of respiratory signs and, given their sympathomimetic properties, may exacerbate excitability and anxiety in these dogs, thereby inducing more adverse respiratory events. However, because many anecdotal reports suggest benefit from these medications, the veterinarian may consider a 2- to 4-week trial of extended-release theophylline at a conservative dosage (5 to 10 mg/kg q12h PO) to assess for a positive clinical response in an individual dog. If no improvement is noted by the client while the animal is receiving theophylline, continued use is not advisable. This medication may be most beneficial in those dogs with bronchial collapse demonstrated as an expiratory push upon exhalation. Inhaled albuterol (given before the fluticasone) may help through local delivery and may theoretically assist in achieving better lower airway steroid penetration.

Although bacterial infections have not been demonstrated to be common in tracheal collapse, it is conceivable that chronic lower airway disease combined with chronic tracheal collapse and subsequent failure of the mucociliary apparatus may impart increased susceptibility to tracheal infection or colonization. For this reason, a course of antibiotics (e.g., doxycycline or azithromycin) is often prescribed by the authors as part of a multimodality treatment regimen in hopes of controlling clinical signs and avoiding intervention if possible.

The final medical strategy for the patient with tracheal collapse is sedation before known episodes of excitement that may precipitate respiratory distress. The mild sedative effects of hydrocodone provide some benefit to minimize respiratory distress, but stressful events such as travel, visitors to the home, and so on, can lead to decompensation. To avoid this, acepromazine (0.5 to 2 mg/kg PO) may be prescribed as needed, to be given 30 to 45 minutes before an event known to lead to excitement and worsened respiratory signs. More recently, the authors and others have found use of the serotonin modulator trazodone at a dosage of 5 mg/kg q12h PO beneficial to minimize anxiety and excitement in dogs with tracheal collapse.

Management of Respiratory Distress

Another common clinical sign affecting a large proportion of dogs with tracheal collapse is respiratory distress secondary to an inadequate airway. There is often minimal history of coughing in these dogs, but respiratory signs may be severe, including *cyanosis, syncope,* or *severe exercise intolerance.* Medical therapy as outlined earlier can be considered in these dogs but is rarely sufficient in controlling signs in the long term. These dogs are the appropriate candidates for intervention—whether intraluminal stenting or surgical ring prostheses—because no medical therapy can restore tracheal rigidity and airway patency.

Recently, there has been a trend away from the use of ring prostheses with a higher proportion of dogs treated by intraluminal stenting. Unfortunately, there are no prospective studies directly comparing these two treatment strategies. The placement of extraluminal support rings around the trachea through an open cervical approach was associated with an overall success rate of 75% to 85% in reducing clinical signs in 90 dogs according to one report (Buback et al, 1996). This procedure is not without complications, however, because 5% of animals died perioperatively, 11% developed laryngeal paralysis from the surgery, 19% required permanent tracheostomies (half within 24 hours), and approximately 23% died of respiratory problems, with a median survival of 25 months. In addition, only 11% of the dogs in this study had intrathoracic tracheal collapse (all dogs had extrathoracic tracheal collapse). The authors of the retrospective study advised against the use of this technique in patients with intrathoracic tracheal collapse, because the resulting morbidity was unacceptably high.

The combination of surgical risk and the inability of the ring procedure to treat intrathoracic collapse adequately led to the evaluation of human-intended intraluminal tracheal stents for the treatment of affected dogs. A number of stents have been previously evaluated in the canine trachea, including both balloon-expandable (Palmaz) stents, and self-expanding stents (stainless steel, laser-cut nickel-titanium [nitinol], and knitted nitinol). Clinical improvement has been reported in 75% to 90% of animals treated with intraluminal stainless steel, self-expanding stents (Moritz et al, 2004), and long-term improvement was noted in 10 of 12 dogs treated with nitinol self-expanding metallic stents (Sura and Krahwinkel, 2008). Immediate complications were typically minor; late complications included stent shortening, development of excessive inflammatory tissue, progressive tracheal collapse, and stent fracture.

Neither surgery nor stenting is a cure for tracheal collapse. However, when used appropriately in the proper patients, either intervention can significantly improve the patient's quality of life when medication alone is no longer adequate. Please see Chapter 145 of the previous edition of *Current Veterinary Therapy* for a complete description of the method for stent selection and the technique for placing intraluminal tracheal stents.

Management of Stent Complications

Given the increased use of intraluminal tracheal stents in dogs with tracheal collapse over the last decade, a discussion of the common postoperative complications and current treatment strategies for these complications is relevant to this chapter.

Improper Stent Position or Size

The best way to manage complications after stenting is to minimize their development. Many postoperative difficulties following tracheal stenting are related to improper selection of stent size, incorrect stent placement, or both. A complete description of stent selection and placement can be found in Chapter 145 of the previous edition of *Current Veterinary Therapy*, but a few additional comments are pertinent. The critical radiographic landmarks for stent placement are the cricoid cartilage cranially and the carina caudally. The cranial extent of the stent should be at least 3 to 5 mm caudal to the caudal margin of the cricoid cartilage. The cricoid cartilage represents a bony landmark of the larynx; therefore, if the stent extends to this level, it will be within the laryngeal apparatus and may lead to laryngospasm, cough, and laryngeal dysfunction (Figure 159-1, *A*). Likewise, the caudal extent of an intraluminal tracheal stent should be at least 3 to 5 mm cranial to the carina to avoid caging off a main-stem bronchus. In Figure 159-1, *B* the stent is positioned too far caudally, extending into the left caudal bronchus. Positioning of a stent this caudally should be avoided because it may lead to mucus entrapment, effectively closing off a large bronchus. To avoid these problems, the authors typically aim to achieve stent placement approximately 10 mm from the cricoid cartilage and 10 mm from the carina to provide a margin of safety.

Although the length should be chosen to span the area of collapse, it is the authors' experience that most dogs requiring a stent have diffuse disease throughout the trachea and do best with a stent that spans both the intrathoracic and extrathoracic trachea. When a short stent is placed for solely intrathoracic or extrathoracic collapse, it is not uncommon for the dog to be brought in for treatment later with signs referable to collapse of the nonstented portion of the trachea and to require a second stent procedure. Figure 159-1, *C* illustrates the

case of a dog with a stent placed initially for intrathoracic collapse that now shows severe extrathoracic collapse and requires a second stent placement.

The stent should be chosen in a diameter that is 10% to 20% larger than the maximal tracheal diameter as measured under positive pressure ventilation during fluoroscopy or radiography. Undersizing of the stent results in an increased risk of stent migration and dislodgement. An example of a stent that is undersized to the diameter of the trachea is seen in Figure 159-1, *D*. It should be kept in mind that the normal trachea is oval in cross section, often having a wider diameter in the left-to-right direction than the dorsal-to-ventral direction, and oversizing is important to maintain full apposition. Additionally, if the sides of the stent are not well apposed to the tracheal epithelium, mucus trapping between the stent and the tracheal wall, as shown in Figure 159-2, can lead to recurrent cough or infection.

Inflammatory Tissue

Among the more common complications following intraluminal tracheal stenting is the development of excessive inflammatory tissue within the tracheal lumen. It is unclear why this occurs in some locations (predominately at the cranial aspect of the stent) but not others. It may develop secondary to stent motion, and the authors suspect it is most likely to occur under conditions of persistent coughing. A tapering course of steroids after stenting and aggressive antitussive therapy is critical to reducing the risk of this complication. Many dogs require lifelong antitussive therapy after placement of a stent, and the client should be cautioned that any coughing postoperatively is potentially problematic. Scheduled radiographs should be taken after stenting at approximately 4 weeks, 3 months, and every 3 to 6 months thereafter to monitor for the development of any stent-related complications. Endoscopy may be considered to evaluate the tracheal lumen if there is a question about inflammatory tissue growth that is not clear on radiographs. The newer woven nitinol stents (Vet Stent-Trachea) appear less likely to induce inflammatory tissue in the authors' personal experience, but this has not been rigorously evaluated, and the authors have seen inflammatory tissue occur with many varieties of tracheal stents.

Presenting signs in an animal with excessive inflammatory tissue after stenting are typically similar to those of tracheal collapse and include stridulous breathing, exercise intolerance, cyanosis, and respiratory distress. Most cases of excessive inflammatory tissue can be treated medically, in the authors' experience. Prednisone is prescribed at a high starting dosage, typically 2 mg/kg/day for the first week, and then the dose is halved and gradually tapered over the next 6 to 8 weeks. A repeat radiograph obtained at the end of the first week of high-dose corticosteroid therapy should show improvement if not resolution of the soft tissue density (Figure 159-3). The authors often prescribe a broad-spectrum antibiotic for 10 to 14 days at the time the steroids are started. Transitioning the dog to inhaled fluticasone may allow a more rapid taper of the systemic steroid, although high doses of oral corticosteroids are required to induce regression of the

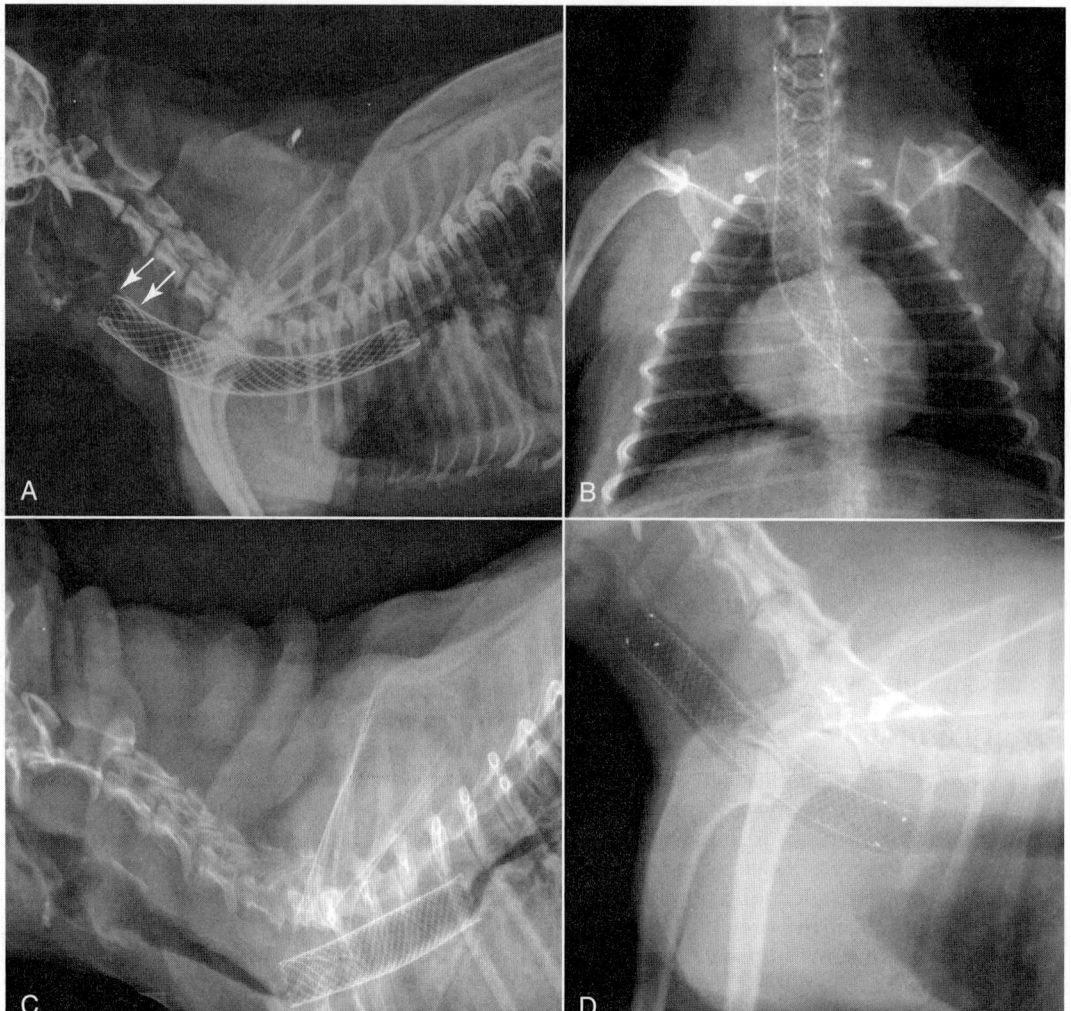

Figure 159-1 Radiographic images illustrating improper stent size and position. **A,** Placement of the stent too far cranial may leave the stent within the cricoid cartilage *(between arrows)* and disrupt laryngeal function. **B,** Placement of the stent too far caudal will engage a lobar bronchus and cage off the other bronchi because of mucus trapping. **C,** Use of a stent that is too short may result in persistent collapse cranial (or caudal) to the stented portion, seen as cervical collapse in this dog with an intrathoracic stent. **D,** A stent diameter that is undersized will not have appropriate apposition to the tracheal wall, which increases the risk of migration or mucus trapping.

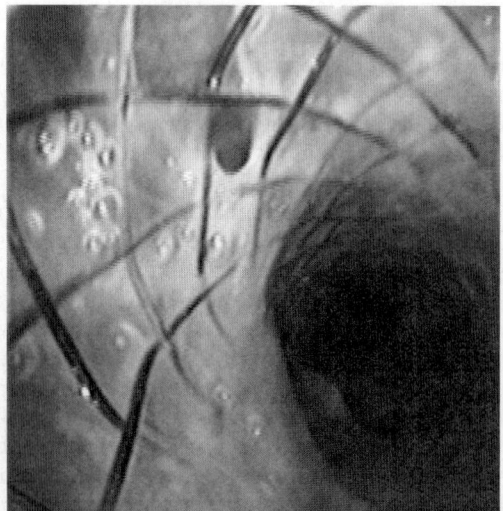

Figure 159-2 Tracheoscopic image of an undersized tracheal stent showing poor apposition to the tracheal endothelium and mucus trapping between the stent and tracheal wall.

tissue. In some cases excessive granulation tissue can be so severe as to nearly occlude the tracheal lumen (Figure 159-4). If clinical signs are perceived to be too severe for medical therapy, options include intubation and mechanical ventilation to give the steroids time to work or the placement of an additional stent at the site of tissue obstruction. Tissue regression with oral colchicine has also been reported and could be considered in refractory cases (Brown et al, 2008). In humans, endobronchial laser resection is used to resect granulation tissue, and this approach may be adopted in veterinary medicine in the future.

Stent Fracture

Although made of a durable metal, intraluminal stents are susceptible to excessive cycling, material fatigue, and fracture (Figures 159-5 and 159-6). If fracture occurs, the stent may lose all of its structural stability, and the dog's signs typically recur immediately. Clients should be

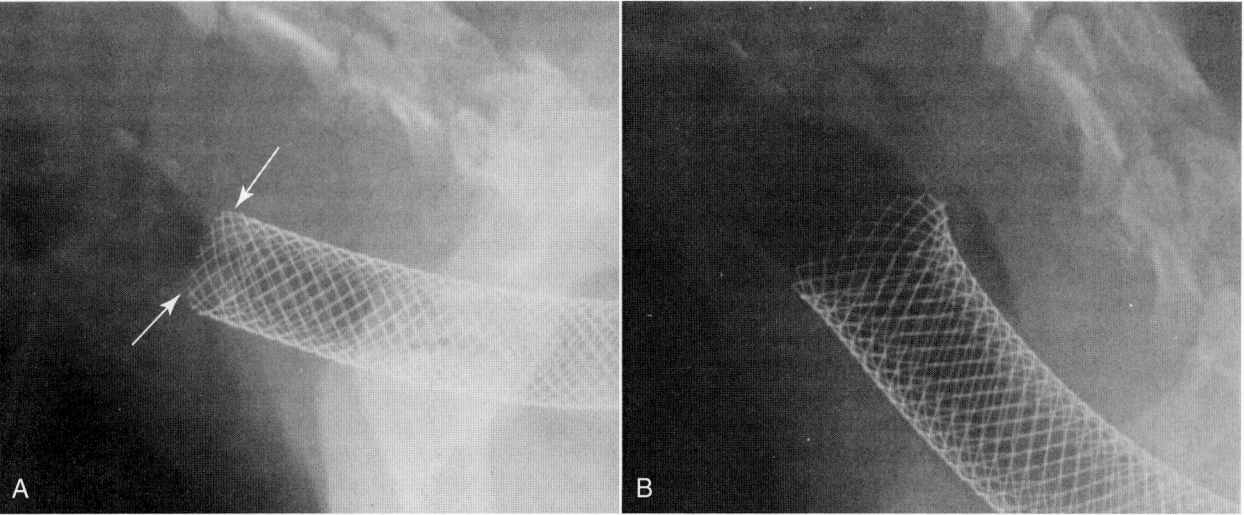

Figure 159-3 Radiographs of inflammatory tissue in a dog with an intraluminal tracheal stent. **A,** Soft tissue opacity is seen within the tracheal lumen *(arrows)* at the cranial aspect of the stent. **B,** After a course of prednisone, the inflammatory tissue has radiographically resolved.

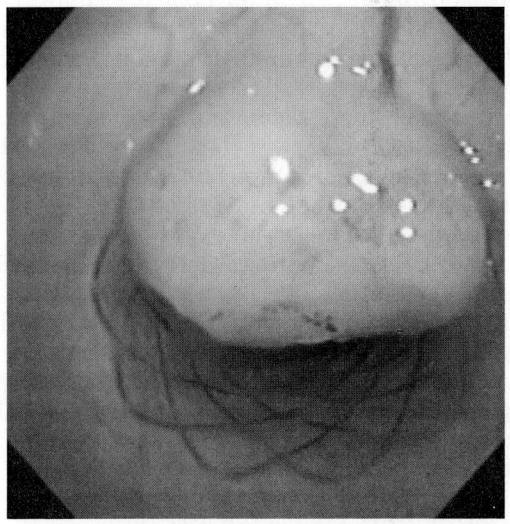

Figure 159-4 Tracheoscopic image for a cat with a tracheal stent showing severe inflammatory tissue reaction at the dorso-cranial aspect of the stent that nearly occludes the tracheal lumen.

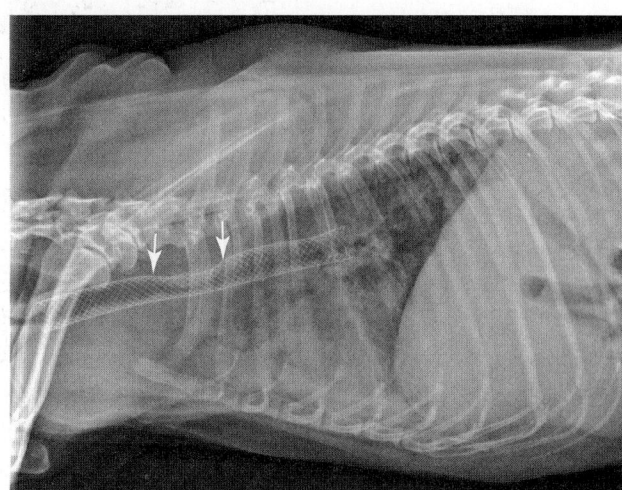

Figure 159-5 Lateral radiograph for a dog with fracture of a tracheal stent *(between arrows)* and concurrent pneumonia.

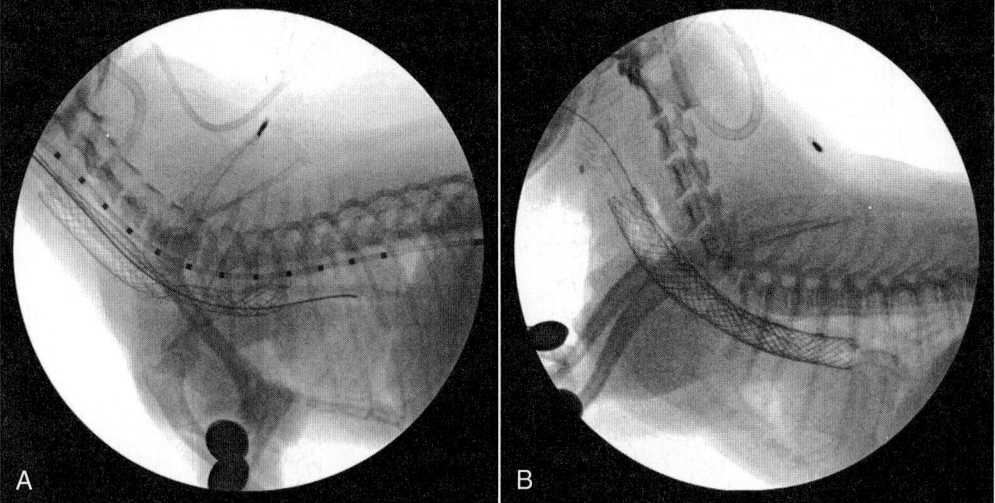

Figure 159-6 Fluoroscopic images taken during restenting of a fractured tracheal stent. A radiopaque guidewire is advanced through the lumen of the fractured stent **(A)** to guide delivery of the second stent and thereby restore an open tracheal lumen **(B).**

cautioned to seek veterinary care at once if sudden worsening of respiratory signs develops in an animal with a tracheal stent. Persistence of coughing after stenting leads to excessive forces on the stent and increases the risk of stent fracture; therefore the medical therapy described earlier, in particular antitussive medications, is critical. If stent fracture occurs, treatment involves restenting within the fractured stent. Evaluation of preliminary stent fracture data from one of the authors (C. Weisse) suggests that the long-term survival of a dog with a tracheal stent fracture is no different from that of dogs without fracture once the fracture is restented. The placement of a second stent into the trachea of a dog with a fractured stent is technically more challenging than the placement of the initial stent. It is important to confirm that the delivery system for the new stent is within the true lumen of the airway and the prior stent. Confirmation of this is best achieved by placing a wire into the tracheal lumen over which the new stent delivery system can be delivered and by evaluating orthogonal views before deployment of the new stent (see Figure 159-6).

Bronchial Collapse

Much debate remains concerning the use of intraluminal stents in dogs with bronchial collapse. Unfortunately, there are currently no data available to recommend or oppose the routine use of intraluminal stents in these dogs, and therefore, regrettably, one can offer only opinion. The questions raised are twofold:

1. *Should stents be placed within collapsing bronchi?* Stenting of collapsing bronchi currently is not routinely recommended by the authors. Placing stents into lobar bronchi will cage off other bronchi and consequently prevent drainage from the associated lobes. In addition, secondary and tertiary bronchi will continue to collapse, and therefore the benefit achieved from the bronchial stenting will likely be minimal, and temporary, compared with the risks.
2. *Should tracheal stents be placed in patients with large bronchial collapse?* Certain dogs will benefit from tracheal stenting, even with concurrent bronchial collapse. The dog should be carefully evaluated to determine the primary clinical signs. Tracheal collapse can lead to inspiratory-expiratory respiratory distress, persistent cough, or both. If obstructed breathing is the major clinical sign and tracheal collapse is present, a tracheal stent can help relieve the dynamic obstruction. In particular, those dogs with inspiratory dyspnea can benefit from stenting because the clinical signs are localized to the cervical trachea (which suggests minimal contribution of the bronchial collapse to the presenting signs). If the dog's primary problem is coughing, then it becomes difficult to determine if coughing is due to tracheal

collapse or bronchial collapse. For these dogs, the authors always warn the owner that continued coughing will likely be present because collapse of the large bronchi (as well as collapse of the smaller bronchi) will continue. In addition, in the authors' experience, continued intractable coughing will increase the risk of stent fracture and predispose to the formation of excessive inflammatory tissue. Persistent coughing must be treated aggressively to minimize the risk of these complications.

Pneumonia

Placement of an intraluminal tracheal stent impairs normal mucociliary clearance by the tracheal epithelium initially. However, chronic tracheal collapse likely alters normal ciliated tracheal epithelium, which is subsequently replaced with squamous metaplasia. Therefore tracheal stenting should prevent repeated collapse and might theoretically permit reestablishment of a normal mucociliary apparatus over time. This may not occur quickly, consistently, or throughout the entire tracheal lumen. The foreign material of a stent likely stimulates mucus production before epithelialization, and the mucus may not be mobilized adequately out of the upper airway. Prevention and surveillance are important to control and minimize the risk of pneumonia in dogs with tracheal stents. The authors prescribe a 7- to 10-day course of a broad-spectrum antibiotic (amoxicillin trihydrate/clavulanate potassium [Clavamox] 14 mg/kg q12h PO) at the time of tracheal stenting. Radiographic surveillance is then advised as described earlier to monitor for early evidence of interstitial or alveolar densities consistent with pneumonia. If such signs are noted, aggressive antibacterial therapy is advised for 4 to 6 weeks with regular radiographic monitoring. Antibiotic therapy should be continued for at least 1 week after radiographic resolution of the pneumonia.

References and Suggested Reading

Brown SA, Williams JE, Saylor DK: Endotracheal stent granulation stenosis resolution after colchicine therapy in a dog, *J Vet Intern Med* 22(4):1052, 2008.
Buback JL, Boothe HW, Hobson HP: Surgical treatment of tracheal collapse in dogs: 90 cases (1983-1993), *J Am Vet Med Assoc* 208(3):380, 1996.
Mittleman E et al: Fracture of an endoluminal nitinol stent used in the treatment of tracheal collapse in a dog, *J Am Vet Med Assoc* 225(8):1217, 2004.
Moritz A, Schneider M, Bauer N: Management of advanced tracheal collapse in dogs using intraluminal self-expanding biliary wallstents, *J Vet Intern Med* 18:31, 2004.
Radlinsky MG et al: Evaluation of the Palmaz stent in the trachea and mainstem bronchi of normal dogs, *Vet Surg* 26(2):99, 1997.
Sura PA, Krahwinkel DJ: Self-expanding nitinol stents for the treatment of tracheal collapse in dogs: 12 cases (2001-2004), *J Am Vet Med Assoc* 232(2):228, 2008.

CHAPTER 160

Chronic Bronchial Disorders in Dogs

LYNELLE R. JOHNSON, *Davis, California*

Chronic bronchial disorders in dogs most typically result in the clinical complaint of cough, with gradual development of exercise intolerance and labored respirations. The most common diagnoses include infectious bronchitis, chronic bronchitis (airway inflammation in the absence of a specific cause), and bronchomalacia (bronchial or airway collapse). Chronic, low-grade aspiration injury might also play a role in chronic cough syndrome. Airway collapse can occur as a sole entity or can accompany chronic or infectious bronchitis, perhaps because of weakening of cartilage or from effects of inflammatory mediators on cartilage or airway smooth muscle. Diagnosing the cause of cough typically requires the use of radiography, fluoroscopy, and bronchoscopy with cytologic examination and culture of samples from the airway. Although infectious bronchitis can respond to specific antimicrobial therapy, the remaining diseases generally require lifelong management.

Clinical Findings

Infectious bronchitis can be found in young and mature dogs, whereas the remaining bronchial disorders are diseases of middle-aged to older dogs. Both large- and small-breed dogs are affected, and a harsh cough is generally reported, although it can be moist or productive when copious respiratory secretions are produced. Gagging, retching, regurgitation, or voice change can suggest laryngeal dysfunction or gastroesophageal reflux disease and subsequent aspiration injury as a cause of cough. Paroxysms of coughing or a "goose-honk" cough are more often encountered in dogs with airway collapse. Dogs are systemically healthy, although in the later stages of disease, exercise intolerance or labored respirations can be reported and activity becomes limited by exercise-induced coughing. Severely affected animals can demonstrate cyanosis or collapse.

On physical examination, dogs with airway disease are often overweight. Some dogs are tachypneic or pant incessantly, whereas dogs severely affected by bronchitis or airway collapse may have prolonged expiration or an expiratory push. Thoracic auscultation can reveal coarse, diffuse crackles or expiratory wheezes, but findings may also be normal. Tracheal sensitivity is usually present because of nonspecific airway inflammation. Airway collapse should be suspected when a snapping sound is auscultated over the thoracic cage as intrathoracic airways collapse on expiration. In small breeds a murmur of mitral regurgitation is a common coincident finding in dogs with bronchitis or bronchomalacia. When present, hepatomegaly is likely caused by obesity.

Diagnosis

The diagnosis of chronic bronchitis is one of exclusion because airway infection (with *Mycoplasma, Bordetella,* parasites), bronchomalacia, or an airway foreign body can cause similar clinical signs. Therefore the diagnosis optimally is based on the history, clinical findings, thoracic radiographs, fluoroscopy, endoscopy, and airway sampling for bacterial culture and cytologic examination.

Clinicopathologic abnormalities typically are absent, even in dogs with infectious bronchitis. Thoracic radiography is an important part of the diagnostic workup, and a generalized increase in interstitial or bronchial infiltrates can be found in dogs with airway inflammation. However, radiography is relatively insensitive for chronic bronchitis, and in a case-controlled evaluation only increased thickness of airway walls and increased numbers of visible airway walls differentiated dogs with bronchitis from normal dogs (Mantis et al, 1998). Dogs with long-standing disease can develop irreversible bronchiectasis, which, when severe, will be visible radiographically (Figure 160-1). Normal-appearing chest radiographs are found relatively often in dogs with chronic bronchitis. Radiographs are also highly insensitive for documentation of airway collapse (Johnson and Pollard, 2010; Macready et al, 2007). Fluoroscopy might be considered the gold standard for identification of tracheal and bronchial collapse, although bronchoscopy is often required to document more subtle degrees of bronchomalacia or small airway collapse.

Collecting airway samples by tracheal wash or bronchoscopy is recommended to characterize the cellular infiltrate in the airway and to rule out infectious causes of cough. Bronchoscopy is particularly useful when typical radiographic findings of bronchitis are lacking or when bronchomalacia is suspected. Dogs with chronic bronchitis have airway hyperemia, the airway mucosa has a cobblestone or irregular appearance, and many have increased mucus lining the airway. In animals with long-standing bronchitis fibrous nodules can be seen protruding into the bronchial lumen. Bronchomalacia is characterized by a static circumferential narrowing of the bronchial lumen (Figure 160-2) or by dynamic changes in airway caliber during respiration.

Cytologically, chronic bronchitis is characterized by the presence of nondegenerate neutrophils. Some dogs

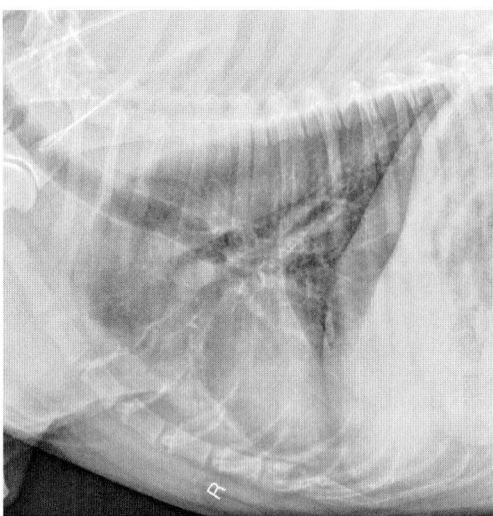

Figure 160-1 Right lateral radiograph for a 9-year-old male castrated chow-chow with a 5-year history of cough. The lobar bronchi to the left cranial lung lobe (both cranial and caudal segments) are obviously dilated with loss of normal tapering, airway walls are thickened, and a distal alveolar infiltrate is noted.

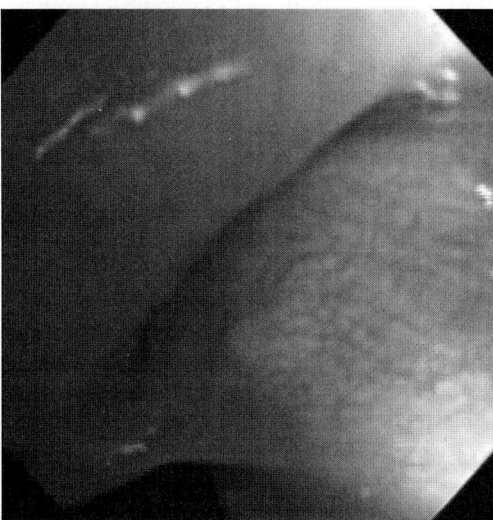

Figure 160-2 Bronchoscopic image demonstrating bronchomalacia, with 100% collapse of the left cranial lobar bronchus at the top of the image.

have a predominance of eosinophils in airway washings or mixed inflammation, and this might indicate parasitic bronchitis or a form of eosinophilic lung disease (see Chapter 163). Increased mucus is often present, and Curschmann's spirals (bronchial casts of airway mucus) are sometimes noted. Epithelial cells and squamous metaplasia can also be seen. Dogs with bronchomalacia can have normal findings on cytologic examination of bronchoalveolar lavage fluid, can have hypercellular lavage fluid, or can have cytologic evidence of concurrent bronchitis. Whether inflammation is a cause or a consequence of cough has not been determined.

Infectious bronchitis is characterized by the presence of septic suppurative inflammation. Organisms are generally recognizable on cytologic examination; however,

Mycoplasma spp. are uncommonly seen cytologically and may be isolated only through culture on specialized media or by polymerase chain reaction testing. Caution is warranted when interpreting results of airway specimen culture because the trachea and carina of dogs are not sterile and various species of commensal bacteria and oral flora can be found in tracheal wash or bronchoalveolar lavage samples despite careful attention to technique. True bacterial infections of the lower respiratory tract are characterized by quantitative cultures of bronchoalveolar lavage fluid yielding more than 1.7×10^3 colony-forming units/ml, lack of squamous cells or the oropharyngeal *Simonsiella* spp. on cytologic examination, and a variably increased percentage of neutrophils (Peeters et al, 2000).

Pulmonary function tests or advanced imaging can be performed to assess the severity of gas exchange or gas flow abnormalities. Arterial blood gas analysis generally shows only nonspecific, mild to moderate hypoxemia. Computed tomography is useful for detecting early signs of bronchiectasis.

Treatment of Bronchial Disorders

Antiinflammatory Agents

Clinical signs of chronic bronchitis are caused by airway inflammation, and treatment with glucocorticoids is successful in resolving clinical signs in the majority of dogs. Infectious diseases should be ruled out before the initiation of antiinflammatory treatment. When airway sampling is not possible, a trial of doxycycline (3 to 5 mg/kg q12h PO) is a reasonable therapeutic option.

Dosing of glucocorticoids should be tailored to the individual, with the severity of clinical signs, chronicity of disease, and general systemic health considered in decisions regarding treatment. Short-acting steroids such as prednisone or prednisolone are generally safe and effective in dogs with uncomplicated bronchitis. In the early stages of disease dogs often require dosages of glucocorticoids ranging from 0.5 to 1 mg/kg q12h PO for 5 to 10 days to induce remission of clinical signs. As clinical signs abate, the dosage should be decreased by half every 10 to 14 days; and, when possible, drugs should be administered on an alternate-day basis to allow normalization of the pituitary-adrenal axis. Long-term therapy (2 to 3 months) can be anticipated in most cases, although discontinuation of medication may be possible. If disease worsens in the early stages of treatment, a return to the higher dose of glucocorticoid that controlled clinical signs is generally required. It is important to note that some dogs with bronchomalacia may not have substantial airway inflammation, and steroid therapy will not be beneficial in these dogs.

Alternatively, treatment with inhaled steroids, bronchodilators, or antitussive agents can be added (see following paragraphs). Long-acting glucocorticoids such as dexamethasone, triamcinolone, and methylprednisolone acetate do not have a therapeutic advantage over prednisone and are associated with more severe derangements of the pituitary-adrenal axis. I have not used cytotoxic drugs or antihistamines in the treatment of chronic bronchitis.

To avoid systemic effects of glucocorticoids, inhaled medications can be considered in animals that tolerate administration via a face mask. Various types of steroids are available for inhalation in metered dose inhaler canisters. I generally start with fluticasone propionate (Flovent) 110 µg/puff or 220 µg/puff administered at 1 puff two to four times daily via spacing chamber and face mask. Spacing chambers are available through a variety of respiratory supply corporations or pharmacies. The AeroKat and AeroDawg spacers are supplied with two round face masks that fit most animals. Brachycephalic dogs can also be fit with face masks obtained from a local pharmacy because the shape of their face is similar to that of humans; for dolichocephalic breeds, anesthetic or cone-shaped face masks may be most effective but may require minor adaptation to fit snugly on the spacer. Drug delivery seems to be adequate when the dog has the nose and lips enclosed by the mask during actuation of the drug and breathes normally for 8 to 10 breaths (i.e., does not pant).

Bronchodilators

It is unlikely that bronchoconstriction plays a role in canine chronic bronchitis, and airway collapse affects primarily large airways, which are not the site of action for bronchodilators. However, bronchodilators often are clinically helpful in reducing signs in dogs with bronchitis or bronchomalacia or can allow a reduction in the dosage of glucocorticoid required to control signs. Both methylxanthine derivatives and β-agonists seem to act synergistically with glucocorticoids in the control of inflammatory lung disease. Bronchodilators may provide other beneficial effects by improving pulmonary perfusion, reducing respiratory effort, stimulating mucociliary clearance, and improving expiratory airflow. In dogs with bronchomalacia that lack airway inflammation or in dogs with chronic bronchitis that fail to respond adequately to glucocorticoids, a 2-week trial of a supplemental bronchodilator is a reasonable therapeutic option for improving expiration and reducing cough.

The two main classes of bronchodilators used in veterinary medicine are methylxanthine derivatives and β$_2$-agonists. Methylxanthine drugs were originally thought to act through phosphodiesterase inhibition, which causes smooth muscle relaxation through accumulation of cyclic adenosine monophosphate; however, it is likely that multiple mechanisms contribute to their action, such as adenosine antagonism or alterations in intracellular calcium handling. Theophylline also appears to have antiinflammatory effects, improves diaphragmatic strength, and may enhance mucociliary clearance. Generic forms of extended-release theophylline are recommended at 10 mg/kg q12h PO. For dogs with concurrent disease or dogs that may show drug sensitivity, a starting dosage of 5 mg/kg q12h PO should be considered initially with escalation of the dose as the dog will tolerate. Extended-release properties of most forms of theophylline are maintained when the pill is halved but not with quartering, which limits the size of dog that can be treated with the drug. Adverse effects of methylxanthines probably also are related to adenosine antagonism and include gastrointestinal upset, tachycardia, and hyperexcitability.

β$_2$-Agonists such as terbutaline and albuterol also have been used successfully in dogs with chronic bronchitis. Terbutaline is available through a wide number of pharmaceutical companies. Small dogs receive 0.625 to 1.25 mg q12h PO, medium-sized dogs are given 1.25 to 2.5 mg q12h PO, and larger dogs receive 2.5 to 5 mg q12h PO. Albuterol is available as a liquid and can be dosed at 50 µg/kg q8h PO. As with methylxanthines, β$_2$-agonists can result in excitability or tremors during initial therapy, but animals usually become accustomed to the drug. β$_2$-Agonists are widely available for inhaled therapy, but since bronchoconstriction is not a feature of canine bronchitis or bronchomalacia, these formulations are rarely used.

Antibiotics

When infection has been documented through appropriate culturing techniques and cytologic findings confirm infection, antibiotic treatment is warranted. Antibiotic choice should be based on culture and sensitivity results whenever possible, and the drug selected should have a broad spectrum of activity against bacteria commonly found in the lung, such as *Pasteurella* spp., *Staphylococcus* spp., *Streptococcus* spp., and various gram-negative organisms. The antibiotic chosen should be lipophilic to facilitate penetration of the airway and should be relatively free of adverse effects. When possible, I prefer doxycycline (3 to 5 mg/kg q12h PO) because this drug has all of the desired attributes and is relatively devoid of adverse effects. Owners should be instructed to supply water after administering the drug to propel the pill fully into the stomach and avoid the possibility of an esophageal stricture caused by delay in esophageal transit. Enrofloxacin (Baytril) is generally reserved for severe infection and true bacterial pneumonia. If enrofloxacin is needed, it is important to note that this drug inhibits metabolism of theophylline, and the concurrent use of the two agents results in toxic plasma levels of theophylline (Intorre et al, 1995). At least a 30% reduction in theophylline dosage is recommended when enrofloxacin is required to treat coincident infection. Length of antibiotic treatment depends on whether pneumonia is present or whether bronchial colonization and infection are suspected. True pneumonia generally requires 3 to 6 weeks of antibiotic therapy, whereas 7 to 10 days of treatment usually resolves signs related to bronchial colonization. If *Bordetella* is isolated from an airway wash, aerosolization with gentamicin (Gentocin) might be considered to reduce bacterial numbers in the airway. An ultrasonic nebulizer and face mask are used to administer 3 to 5 mg/kg of gentamicin once daily for 5 days.

Infection appears to play a predominant role in dogs with concurrent bronchiectasis. Bronchiectasis is defined as a dilatation of the lower airways; suppuration is usually present. It can occur as a sequela to uncontrolled airway inflammation or infection. Mucus trapping and obstruction of the airway are severe, and recurrent pneumonia is commonly encountered. Long-term antibiotic therapy is often required in these patients, and broad-spectrum antibiotics or combinations of antibiotics should be chosen because infection might involve various gram-negative bacteria (especially *Pseudomonas*) and anaerobes. Doxycycline, chloramphenicol (30 to 50 mg/kg q8h PO), trimethoprim/sulfamethoxazole (15 mg/kg q12h PO), or clindamycin (Antirobe, 11 mg/kg q12h PO) combined with enrofloxacin can be helpful in resolving long-standing pulmonary infection.

Antitussive Agents

The cough reflex is of major importance in the dog with bronchitis because it serves the essential function of clearing viscid secretions from the airway. Suppression of this reflex before resolution of inflammation can be deleterious, because mucus can become trapped in small airways. Prolonged contact between inflammatory mediators in the mucus and epithelial cells perpetuates airway inflammation. When clinical signs suggest that inflammation is resolving yet the cough persists, or when concurrent airway collapse is present, cough suppression is desirable, because chronic coughing can lead to repeated airway injury and syncopal events. Over-the-counter dextromethorphan-containing compounds might be useful in some animals.

When more potent suppression of a dry cough is required, narcotic agents should be prescribed. I prefer hydrocodone (Tussigon, 0.22 mg/kg q6-12h PO) or butorphanol (Torbutrol, 0.5 mg/kg q6-12h PO). These agents must be given at an interval that suppresses coughing without inducing excessive sedation or gastrointestinal effects. I generally start with a high dose given frequently and taper the dose and frequency of administration downward as cough resolves. This therapy seems to avoid induction of tolerance, which is important because long-term therapy can be required in some patients, particularly when tracheal or airway collapse is also present.

Mucolytic Therapy

Dogs with chronic bronchitis can benefit from saline nebulization to reduce the viscosity of airway secretions and improve clearance. An ultrasonic nebulizer that produces particles 2 to 5 μm in diameter is preferred for respiratory therapy because particles will penetrate deep into the airways. Sterile saline or water (without preservatives) is required for use in various types of nebulizers. Coupage of the chest or gentle exercise after nebulization facilitates clearance of secretions.

Oral N-acetylcysteine also may help thin respiratory secretions by breaking sulfur-sulfur bonds in mucus. It also has the purported benefit of acting as an antioxidant, and oxidant-antioxidant imbalance may be impaired in canine bronchial disorders as has been seen in other species. Empiric dosing of 200 to 600 mg (depending on the size of the dog) q12h PO has been associated with some clinical improvement, and adverse effects have not been noted to date.

Additional Therapy

Obesity worsens clinical signs in dogs with bronchial disease by decreasing thoracic wall compliance, increasing the work of breathing, and increasing abdominal pressure on the diaphragm. Improvements in exercise tolerance and arterial oxygenation can be seen with weight loss alone. Owners should be given reasonable goals for the dog's optimal weight and the time in which weight loss can be achieved. A 1% to 2% weight loss per week is desirable; therefore a dog with a body condition score of 8 out of 9 (30% overweight) could be anticipated to require 4 to 6 months to lose an appropriate amount of weight. This can be achieved by using a high-protein calorie-controlled diet and by providing gradually increasing amounts of exercise. Close monitoring of owner compliance and accomplishments in the weight-loss program seems to enhance overall success.

Animals with concurrent tracheal collapse or marked tracheal sensitivity benefit from having a harness instead of a collar. When stresses in the environment such as cigarette smoke, pollutants, heat, or humidity are encountered, the animal should be removed to a cool, clean area. Dogs that are suspected to have chronic aspiration injury caused by laryngeal dysfunction may benefit from altered feeding strategies, such as feeding upright or altering the consistency of the food.

Prognosis

Owners should be aware that many bronchial diseases are chronic and can be controlled but never cured. Providing reasonable expectations for the level of control possible improves owner satisfaction, because the majority of dogs have residual cough and exhibit clinical signs periodically throughout life. The presence of fibrosis and chronic inflammation on biopsy specimens or the presence of bronchiectasis or bronchomalacia indicates the irreversibility of airway disease. The goals of disease management are to control inflammation and thus limit clinical signs, to diagnose and treat infection when it occurs, and to prevent the development of debilitating sequelae such as bronchiectasis and cor pulmonale.

References and Suggested Reading

Adamama-Moraitou KK et al: Canine bronchomalacia: a clinico-pathological study of 18 cases diagnosed by endoscopy, Vet J 191(2):261, 2012. Epub December 21, 2010.

Hawkins EC et al: Demographic, clinical, and radiographic features of bronchiectasis in dogs: 316 cases (1988-2000), J Am Vet Med Assoc 223:1628, 2003.

Hawkins EC et al: Cellular composition of bronchial brushings obtained from healthy dogs and dogs with chronic cough and cytologic composition of bronchoalveolar lavage fluid obtained from dogs with chronic cough, Am J Vet Res 67:160, 2006.

Intorre L et al: Enrofloxacin-theophylline interaction: influence of enrofloxacin on theophylline steady-state pharmacokinetics in the beagle dog, J Vet Pharmacol Ther 18:352, 1995.

Johnson LR, Pollard RE: Tracheal collapse and bronchomalacia in dogs: 58 cases (2001-2008), J Vet Intern Med 24:298, 2010.

Macready DM, Johnson LR, Pollard RE: Fluoroscopic and radiographic evaluation of tracheal collapse in 62 dogs, J Am Vet Med Assoc 230:1870, 2007.

Mantis P, Lamb CR, Boswood A: Assessment of the accuracy of thoracic radiography in the diagnosis of canine chronic bronchitis, J Small Anim Pract 39:518, 1998.

Peeters DE et al: Quantitative bacterial cultures and cytological examination of bronchoalveolar lavage specimens in dogs, J Vet Intern Med 14:534, 2000.

CHAPTER 161

Chronic Bronchitis and Asthma in Cats

PHILIP PADRID, *Corrales, New Mexico*

For purposes of this chapter, the term *chronic bronchial disease* refers to a noninfectious airway inflammatory disorder in cats that occurs most commonly in two forms: chronic bronchitis and asthma. *Chronic bronchitis* is defined as an inflammatory disorder of the lower airways that causes a daily cough, for which other causes of cough (including heartworm disease, pneumonia, lungworms, idiopathic interstitial disease, and neoplasia) have been excluded. *Asthma* is more loosely defined as a disorder of the lower airways that causes airflow limitation, which may resolve spontaneously or in response to medical treatment. *Airflow limitation* is generally the result of some combination of airway inflammation, accumulated airway mucus, and, in typical asthma, airway smooth muscle contraction. Signs of asthma can be dramatic, including acute wheeze and respiratory distress. However, most commonly in cats the only sign of asthma-induced airflow limitation is a daily cough.

The definitive diagnosis of human asthma usually is based on both history and specific pulmonary function studies that require patient cooperation. Because both bronchitis and asthma in cats usually cause a daily cough as the only clinical sign, there are many times when it is not possible to distinguish bronchitis from asthma in the feline patient. Fortunately, the diagnosis, prognosis, and treatment options for both diseases overlap with great frequency.

Pathophysiology

The potential causes of bronchitis and asthma are numerous; however, the airways are capable of responding to noxious stimuli in a limited number of ways. Airway epithelium may hypertrophy, undergo metaplastic change, erode, or ulcerate. Airway goblet cells and submucosal glands may hypertrophy and produce excessive amounts of viscid mucus. Bronchial mucosa and submucosa, which are usually infiltrated with variable numbers and types of inflammatory cells, may become edematous. Bronchial smooth muscle may remain unaffected, become hypertrophied, or spasm. In almost all cases, the unifying and underlying problem is chronic inflammation, but the exact cause is undetermined.

The resulting clinical signs of wheeze, cough, and lethargy can be traced to limitation of airflow, excessive mucus secretions, airway edema, and airway narrowing from cellular infiltrates. In addition, cats with asthma may experience acute airway narrowing from bronchoconstriction. This has important clinical implications because the diameter of an airway has a profound effect on the velocity of airflow, pressure changes, and volume of air that can traverse that airway. A 50% reduction in airway luminal radius results in a sixteenfold increase in the static resistance to flow across that airway. The clinical implications are twofold: (1) relatively small amounts of mucus, edema, or bronchoconstriction can partially occlude airways and cause a dramatic fall in airflow; and (2) any therapy that increases airway diameter, even slightly, may dramatically improve clinical signs of airway obstruction.

Cough also may result from stimulation of mechanoreceptors located in inflamed and contracted airway smooth muscle, which seems fundamentally linked to inflammation. Although a number of different inflammatory cell types have been identified within asthmatic airways of cats, eosinophils represent the primary pathophysiologic effector cell in *allergic asthmatic* disease. Highly charged cationic proteins within eosinophil granules are released into airways and cause epithelial disruption and sloughing. In addition, these granular proteins can make airway smooth muscle more "twitchy" and prone to contraction after exposure to low levels of stimulation (airway hyperreactivity). In contrast, *chronic bronchitis* in the feline species is more commonly associated with a *neutrophilic* infiltrate, although this distinction requires more study (Cocayne et al, 2011).

Studies of Naturally Occurring Disease

Feline bronchial disease has been recognized for over a century. In 1906 Hill described cats with increased airway mucus, airway inflammation, labored breathing, and wheezing (Hill, 1906). In this monograph, airway reactivity was suggested ("ammoniacal odors [urine? in the barn?] excited the symptoms"). However, only in the last 15 years have veterinarians begun to study the disorder in earnest. Dye and associates (1996) identified pulmonary function abnormalities in cats with signs of chronic lower airway inflammation. Some of these cats had increased pulmonary resistance that resolved after treatment with terbutaline, a β_2-agonist, which indicated the presence of reversible bronchoconstriction. In addition, some of these cats experienced dramatic bronchoconstriction after exposure to low levels of methacholine, a drug with minimal effects on pulmonary function when used in equivalent doses in nonasthmatic cats. This was the first demonstration of *spontaneous,* naturally occurring airway hyperreactivity and reversible bronchoconstriction in a nonhuman species. In addition, histologic changes in airway specimens from asthmatic cats include epithelial erosion, goblet cell and submucosal gland hyperplasia and hypertrophy, and an increased mass of smooth muscle, which are features of human asthmatic airways. Additional reviews have demonstrated the variation in clinical findings, radiographic patterns, and responses to therapy in cats with bronchitis and asthma (Foster et al, 2004). This likely is a result of differences in the staging of these disorders and the confusion caused by other respiratory disorders such as pulmonary fibrosis and occult heartworm infection (Cohn et al, 2004).

Experimentally Induced Feline Asthma

Experimental models of feline asthma have been developed to elucidate the immunologic mechanisms and objectively determine responses to therapy. The first model of feline asthma involved antigen sensitization and long-term aerosol challenge with *Ascaris suum.* These cats developed persistent airway eosinophilia and hyperresponsiveness to nebulized acetylcholine along with typical morphologic changes observed in spontaneous bronchial disease of cats. These studies suggested mast cell–derived serotonin as a primary mediator contributing to airway smooth muscle contraction (Padrid et al, 1995). This mediator is absent in human, equine, and canine airways. According to this hypothesis, inhaled antigens promote mast cell degranulation, with the release of preformed serotonin precipitating the acute asthmatic attack through contraction of airway smooth muscle. The role of histamine is less certain given the variable effects of nebulized histamine, which range from bronchoconstriction to airway dilation. In clinical practice, antihistamine drugs do not demonstrate a beneficial effect in the treatment of cats with chronic bronchitis or asthma. Leemans and colleagues (2012) also have used the feline *A. suum* model of airway inflammation to demonstrate that inhaled fluticasone propionate was as effective as oral prednisolone in dampening eosinophilia in bronchoalveolar lavage (BAL) fluid and allergen-induced airway reactivity.

Reinero and colleagues (2005) developed an experimental feline model in which cats were sensitized and recurrently challenged with either Bermuda grass allergen (BGA) or house dust mites to mimic well-recognized antigenic triggers of human asthma. These cats showed enhanced production of allergen-specific immunoglobulin E (IgE); allergen-specific serum and BAL fluid IgG or IgA; airway hyperreactivity; airway eosinophilia; an acute helper T cell type 2 cytokine profile in peripheral blood mononuclear cells and BAL fluid cells; and histologic evidence of airway remodeling. This model has been particularly helpful in evaluating specific immunomodulating treatment strategies. For example, when cats sensitized and challenged with BGA were then treated with rush immunotherapy (high parenteral doses of BGA), eosinophil counts decreased significantly. Norris and associates. (2003) used CpG motifs (microbial oligodeoxynucleotide products that modulate activity in human and murine

lymphocytes) in cats with BGA-induced airway inflammation and hyperreactivity. This approach dampened the eosinophilic response normally seen in these antigen-sensitized and -challenged cats; however, the hyperactivity within airways was unaffected. More recently, this group has shown that allergen-specific immunotherapy (with or without a CpG adjuvant) can suppress BAL fluid eosinophilia and that irrelevant antigen can dampen the eosinophilic response (Reinero et al, 2009b). This latter finding is significant because the offending antigens that play a role in the pathogenesis of naturally occurring feline asthma have not been identified. Finally, IgE, nitric oxide, interleukin-4, interferon-γ, and tumor necrosis factor all have been identified and measured in BAL fluid or serum in this model, but none of the levels of these biomarkers has been elevated significantly enough to be recommended for diagnostic purposes in clinical practice (Delgado et al, 2010; Nafe et al, 2010).

Clinical Findings

Incidence and Prevalence

Currently there are no reliable data regarding the incidence and prevalence of asthma in cats. The prevalence of lower airway disease in the general adult cat population is estimated to be approximately 1%; prevalence in the Siamese breed may be 5% or higher as also suggested by an informal survey at a website (www.fritzthebrave.com) devoted to feline asthma (Hopper, n.d.).

Clinical Signs

Clinical signs are variable. Cats with *bronchitis* have a daily cough and may be absolutely free of signs between episodes of cough. Alternatively, they may be tachypneic at rest. This is different from dogs with chronic bronchitis, in which tachypnea is rare, and suggests that cats with chronic bronchitis should be treated aggressively early in the course of the disease. *Asthmatic* cats may cough, wheeze, and struggle to breath on a daily basis. In mild cases, signs may be limited to occasional and brief coughing. Some cats with asthma may be asymptomatic for weeks or months between occasional episodes of acute airway obstruction. Severely affected cats may have a persistent daily cough and experience repeated episodes of life-threatening acute bronchoconstriction.

As previously noted, in a cat with chronic coughing, it is difficult to distinguish chronic bronchitis from asthma as the underlying cause. Although these two disorders are frequently lumped together under the title of *chronic bronchial disease* or *lower airway disease,* different therapeutic approaches are needed and the disorders carry dissimilar prognoses. For example, asthmatic but not bronchitic cats may benefit from bronchodilator treatment.

Physical Examination Findings

There are no consistent physical examination findings on which to base a diagnosis of asthma. Importantly, cats with bronchitis or asthma may have normal physical examination findings at rest. When respiratory distress is evident, it occurs during expiration, which is a hallmark finding of both disorders in cats. Adventitious sounds including crackles often are heard. Wheezes are more characteristic of feline asthma.

Diagnostic Tests

Some cats with chronic cough have been exposed to cigarette smoke in the home, and these patients more commonly have chronic bronchitis. Aside from this distinction, the cat's historical signs do not allow the practitioner to distinguish between coughing cats with chronic bronchitis and coughing cats with asthma.

Reversible bronchoconstriction is one of the defining features of asthma and can be used to distinguish asthma from chronic bronchitis. However, demonstration of reversible bronchoconstriction via pulmonary function studies generally requires specific equipment and expertise. These tests are available in some veterinary university settings and occasionally in veterinary specialty hospitals (Rozanski and Hoffman, 2004). Otherwise, therapeutic response to a bronchodilator can point the practitioner toward a diagnosis of asthma. If a patient is wheezing during the physical examination, the author administers albuterol by inhalation (two puffs into a spacer held over the face for 7 to 10 breaths). Alternatively, terbutaline (0.01 mg/kg IM) can be administered and the patient reevaluated in 5 to 10 minutes. Resolution of wheezing implies reversible bronchoconstriction. With the exception of this maneuver, there are no practical tests that can be used for definitive diagnosis of asthma or bronchitis in cats. Therefore the author generally relies on clinical criteria, including the following:

- A history that includes one or more of these chronic persistent or intermittent clinical signs: acute wheeze, tachypnea, or respiratory distress, including labored, open-mouth breathing. These signs are usually relieved quickly with some combination of oxygen, bronchodilators, and corticosteroids. The diagnosis of chronic bronchitis requires the presence of a daily cough. But many cases of asthma also present with daily or intermittent chronic cough as the only problem.
- Findings on routine survey chest radiographs may be normal, and this result does not rule out asthma. However, frequently radiographs demonstrate diffuse prominent bronchial markings consistent with inflammatory airways ("doughnuts and tram lines"). Air trapping may be evidenced by hyperinflated airways. This is seen most prominently on the lateral view and can be appreciated by recognizing the position of the diaphragmatic crus at approximately the level of L1-L2. In the author's experience approximately 10% of radiographs in cats with bronchial disease have increased density within the right middle lung lobe associated. This may be associated with a mediastinal shift to the right. This is evidence of atelectasis. It is usually easier to see this pattern on a dorsoventral or ventrodorsal exposure because the right middle lung lobe

silhouettes with the cardiac silhouette on the lateral view. Atelectasis with or without bronchial stenosis most commonly occurs in the right middle lung lobe (Johnson and Vernau, 2011) because of mucus accumulation within the bronchus. This lobe is involved most commonly because its bronchus demonstrates a dorsoventral orientation and is more susceptible to gravitational influences.

- In more extreme cases, fluffy, ill-defined heavy interstitial infiltrates in multiple lung lobes may be appreciated. These changes may stem from multiple small areas of atelectasis associated with diffuse small mucus plugs. This presents a diagnostic challenge because this radiographic change is consistent with a number of disorders, including neoplasia and diffuse interstitial pneumonitis.
- Clinicopathologic evidence of airway inflammation is found, including the recovery of large numbers of eosinophils from tracheobronchial secretions in asthmatic airways and nonseptic neutrophils in bronchitic airways. Interestingly, until the 1980s it was generally assumed that eosinophils played only a beneficial role in the immune system by protecting against parasitic infection. However, within the last 30 years it has become clear that the presence of these cells in the wrong place at the wrong time can result in significant cellular and tissue damage. Therefore it is of great interest that eosinophils (often 20% to 25% of total count) can be recovered in large numbers from the tracheobronchial washings of many healthy cats (Padrid et al, 1991), and these cells appear to cause no damage to the local tissue environment. Their presence should not be assumed to indicate allergy or parasitism. Thus eosinophil counts can be somewhat confusing because of this normally high value. Similarly, alveolar macrophages are a normal cell within the lung parenchyma and are the most common cells recovered from BAL fluid obtained from healthy cats. These cells should not be interpreted as granulomatous or histiocytic inflammation when obtained in BAL fluid from bronchitic or asthmatic cats. These cells may also be resistant to eradication with corticosteroid therapy (Cocayne et al, 2011).

Cytologic specimens for evaluation of the airways can be obtained in the anesthetized cat by using a bronchoscope or by placing an endotracheal catheter (or cuffed small endotracheal tube) to lavage the bronchial tree and distal airways blindly. Both methods carry some risk, and critical studies comparing these two techniques have not been published. Both methods can yield samples for culture and evaluation of cellularity. However, for a number of reasons the author does not routinely collect tracheobronchial washings when considering the diagnosis of asthma or bronchitis in cats. These disorders usually can be diagnosed from a careful history taking, physical examination, interpretation of radiographs (with exclusion of other causes of respiratory signs), and observation of response to therapy. It is only when the clinical criteria for diagnosis are not fulfilled using these methods, and especially when the patient does not respond to standard treatment protocols, that the diagnosis is revisited and bronchoscopy or airway washings are considered. Although some clinicians do prefer to obtain and culture airway washings before initiation of long-term respiratory therapy, the points made previously about the normally high eosinophil and mononuclear cell counts obtained from feline airways must be considered when interpreting the cytologic findings or culture results.

Bronchoscopy

As suggested earlier, bronchoscopy is rarely required to make an accurate diagnosis of bronchitis or asthma in feline patients. Bronchoscopy in cats is not a trivial undertaking, and in cats with cough and respiratory compromise, it may be a life-threatening procedure. Instead, the previously described historical and physical examination findings and results of chest radiography are sufficient to make a *tentative* diagnosis. *Definitive* diagnosis usually can be made in these patients by a strongly positive response to therapy. In the author's experience the primary indication for bronchoscopy in these patients is the failure to observe an otherwise predictable cessation or minimization of clinical signs after 6 to 7 days of aggressive corticosteroid treatment.

Tracheobronchial Culture

The presence of a mixed population of aerobic bacteria in airways has been reported previously in cats with bronchial disease. However, neither the lower airway nor the lung parenchyma of healthy cats is sterile. Organisms usually considered as pathogens such as *Klebsiella* and *Pseudomonas* spp. can be recovered from healthy feline airways. Interestingly, one well-designed study showed that cats with signs of bronchial disease had fewer positive results on airway cultures than a cohort population of healthy cats (Dye et al, 1996). *Mycoplasma* may be an exception to this rule because it is not found in the lower airways of healthy cats. Also, *Mycoplasma* (and certain viruses) can degrade neutral endopeptidase, which is an enzyme responsible for biodegradation of substance P, a protein capable of causing bronchoconstriction and edema in the feline airway. *Mycoplasma* might then indirectly prolong the effects of substance P on airway smooth muscle. It is tempting to speculate that *Mycoplasma* or viruses such as herpes, which can remain dormant in feline airways, might be responsible for increasing the levels of substance P in cat airways and contribute to spontaneous bronchoconstriction.

Treatment

The primary signs of asthma include cough and wheeze, and these signs are frequently the result of some degree of airway smooth muscle contraction. It is tempting to treat coughing cats with suspected bronchial disease by using only bronchodilators to relax the airway smooth muscle contraction. Although this is a pivotal treatment when acute signs develop, both asthmatic and bronchitic

airways in cats show evidence of chronic, ongoing inflammation, whether the patient is showing clinical signs or not (Cocayne et al, 2011). Additionally, there is renewed concern about the risk of long-acting bronchodilator therapy (Reinero et al, 2009a). Therefore treatment strategies are most successful when directed toward *decreasing the underlying inflammatory component* of the disease in addition to addressing the acute clinical signs of cough, wheeze, and increased respiratory effort.

Long-Term Corticosteroids

The most effective long-term treatment of chronic noninfectious bronchial disease is systemically administered corticosteroids. This class of drugs is most likely to suppress airway inflammation. An important effect of steroids is to inhibit the synthesis of cytokine genes that are important in generating airway inflammation. The adverse effects of systemic corticosteroids given over long periods can be considerable. Fortunately, inhaled steroids are available that have minimal if any systemic adverse effects, and inhaled therapy has enhanced greatly our ability to treat patients with bronchial disease (see the section on aerosol delivery of steroids and bronchodilators later in the chapter).

For bronchitic or asthmatic cats with signs that occur more than once weekly, the author begins treatment with prednisolone (1 to 2 mg/kg q12h PO for 5 to 7 days). At this point, most cats with newly diagnosed disease have greatly diminished signs. If there is no response to this initial approach, then the original diagnosis is rethought. The dosage of steroids is then tapered slowly, over at least 2 to 3 months. This approach is much more effective than giving low doses of prednisolone for short periods and in response to acute flare-ups. Importantly, if a patient does not have a good response to oral corticosteroids, it is unlikely the patient will respond any better to an inhaled corticosteroid.

Some cats are managed effectively and safely by low-dose, alternate-day administration of corticosteroids. However, most cats with chronic bronchial disease continue to wheeze and cough when treated in this conservative manner. For patients that show a positive response to higher doses of consistently administered systemic corticosteroids, inhaled corticosteroid therapy should be encouraged as an alternative to reduce adverse effects (see later).

Cats with signs that occur less than once weekly (without medication) are generally not considered to have chronic severe active inflammatory airway disease. These patients may be treated safely with bronchodilators when needed.

Injectable Steroids

Parenteral administration of long-acting corticosteroids is limited to patients for which no other method of drug administration is feasible, such as intractable cats or those unable to be given pills. In such cases, injection of methylprednisolone (Depo-Medrol, 10 to 20 mg IM total dose) once every 4 to 8 weeks may be very effective. However, this therapy, if repeated over time, is likely to result in significant and serious adverse effects, including weight gain, diabetes mellitus, and reduced immunity as well as uncontrolled airway inflammation that could lead to airway remodeling and emphysematous lung disease. Precipitation of a congestive heart failure syndrome also has been observed. Therefore reposital corticosteroids represent the treatment of last resort.

Bronchodilators

The use of bronchodilators is based on the assumption that clinically significant bronchoconstriction is evident, which at times can be life threatening (Padrid, 2000). Bronchodilators can be beneficial to these patients. These drugs are classified generally as β-receptor agonists, methylxanthine derivatives, or anticholinergics. Drugs with preferential affinity for β_2-receptors provide more effective bronchodilation with fewer side effects. The two principal β_2-agonists currently marketed in preparations that can be readily and regularly used in small animals are terbutaline sulfate and albuterol sulfate.

Terbutaline Sulfate

Terbutaline is a selective β_2-receptor agonist that produces relaxation of the smooth muscle found principally in bronchial, vascular, and uterine tissues. Terbutaline is available as a tablet, elixir, and injectable preparation suitable for subcutaneous, intramuscular, or intravenous use. The dosage rate has been reported to range from 0.01 mg/kg given parenterally to up to 0.1 to 0.2 mg/kg every 8 hours given by mouth. The *major clinical indication* for terbutaline is treatment of the patient with acute respiratory difficulty when inhaled albuterol therapy is not possible. Terbutaline can be prescribed as a long-term oral treatment for bronchodilation when clients are not compliant with inhalant therapy.

The home use of a rapid-acting bronchodilator such as inhaled albuterol or injected terbutaline can preclude the need for a stressful emergency room visit. The author teaches clients to use an inhaler or to administer terbutaline to their asthmatic cats at a dose of 0.01 mg/kg SC or IM. An obvious beneficial response generally occurs within 15 to 30 minutes. This treatment may be repeated if a significant benefit is not observed after one dose. To determine if the drug has been absorbed and if a beneficial effect has occurred, heart rate and respiratory rate and effort are monitored. A respiratory rate or effort (or both) that declines by 50% or more suggests a beneficial effect.

At usual doses terbutaline has little effect on β_1-receptors; thus direct cardiostimulatory effects are unlikely. However, terbutaline always should be used with care in patients that may have increased sensitivity to adrenergic agents—in particular, cats with preexisting hypertrophic cardiomyopathy, diabetes mellitus, hyperthyroidism, hypertension, or seizure disorders. Use with various inhalation anesthetics may predispose the patient to ventricular arrhythmias.

Albuterol Sulfate

Albuterol is a selective β_2-receptor agonist with pharmacologic properties similar to those of terbutaline. Albuterol is available as a tablet and syrup and is contained in various inhalants. The author has used only the inhaled form of albuterol in feline patients. The inhaled formulation of albuterol comes as a single-strength 17-g metered dose inhaler (MDI) and delivers 90 µg per actuation of the device.

The pharmacokinetic profile of inhaled albuterol in cats has not been rigorously studied. When administered by inhalation to humans, albuterol produces significant bronchodilation within 15 minutes that lasts for 3 to 4 hours. It is also well absorbed orally and may have bronchodilatory effects for up to 8 hours. Anecdotal experience with this drug in clinical practice suggests a similar pharmacokinetic profile in cats. Albuterol undergoes extensive hepatic metabolism. Adverse effects occur rarely and include mild skeletal muscle tremors and restlessness, which generally subside after 2 to 3 days. Precautions should be taken similar to those noted earlier for terbutaline. Inhaled R,S-albuterol has been demonstrated to augment inflammation in cats with experimentally induced asthma (Reinero et al, 2009a).

Methylxanthines: Theophylline and Aminophylline

The methylxanthines relax smooth muscle, particularly bronchial smooth muscle. Although the author does not use this class of drugs to treat feline patients with asthma, methylxanthines are used frequently in the veterinary profession and thus are addressed briefly. Theophylline is considered a less potent bronchodilator than the β-agonists. It has been shown in other species to produce centrally mediated increased respiratory effort for any given alveolar partial pressure of carbon dioxide; to improve diaphragmatic contractility with reduced diaphragmatic fatigue; to mildly increase myocardial contractility and heart rate; and to increase central nervous system (CNS) activity, gastric acid secretion, and urine output. Not all of these effects have been demonstrated in cats. Interestingly, at therapeutic concentrations of theophylline, only adenosine receptor blockade has been demonstrated reliably. This has been suggested to explain the varied effects of theophylline.

Because of the relatively low therapeutic index and pharmacokinetic characteristics of theophylline, dosage rates should be based on lean body mass. The dosage depends on the preparation used. For standard preparations the recommended dosage for cats is 4 mg/kg every 8 to 12 hours. When sustained-release preparations are used a dosage of 15 to 19 mg/kg every 24 hours given at night should be considered.

Although theophylline can produce CNS stimulation and gastrointestinal disturbances, these effects most often are associated with excessive dosing and resolve with dosage adjustments. Seizures or cardiac arrhythmias may occur in severe toxicity. There are a number of drugs *known to interact with theophylline,* including enrofloxacin (Baytril). The effects of theophylline may be diminished by phenytoin and phenobarbital and enhanced by cimetidine, allopurinol, clindamycin, and lincomycin. The effects of theophylline and β-adrenergic blockers may be antagonized if they are administered concurrently. Theophylline increases the likelihood of arrhythmias induced by adrenergic agonists and halothane and the likelihood of seizures with ketamine.

Cyclosporine

In the experimental asthma model developed by the author and colleagues, we found that treatment with cyclosporin A (CsA) dramatically inhibited the pathologic changes in airway structure and function seen in cats not treated with CsA (Padrid et al, 1996). CsA is approved for use in cats to treat atopic dermatologic disease, and further studies using CsA to treat cats with asthma are needed.

Antibiotics

There is no objective evidence that bacterial infection plays a significant role in the cause or continuation of feline chronic bronchitis or asthma. Similarly, there is no objective evidence that antibiotic therapy has any effect on the duration or intensity of signs displayed by the cat with chronic bronchial disease. Despite a lack of such evidence, there are feline patients with chronic bronchial disease that occasionally have a flare-up, which responds quickly to antibiotic therapy. Because respiratory secretions are obtained very rarely for culture in this setting, it is unclear whether this represents true resolution of infection or coincidence. It is important to remember that the clinical signs of asthma in cats frequently wax and wane both in severity and in frequency of occurrence. Many anecdotal reports describe the therapeutic effect of antibiotics in controlling asthmatic signs, but these descriptions are consistent with the waxing and waning nature of the disease.

In the author's opinion, antibiotics are rarely indicated for cats with chronic bronchitis or asthma and are appropriate only when there is strong evidence of superimposed airway infection. This may be inferred from growth of a pure bacterial culture on a primary culture plate from material obtained from tracheobronchial secretions or by detection of intracellular bacteria on cytologic examination of suppurative material. Prophylactic or long-term therapy should be avoided unless there is documentation of a chronic airway infection, which is uncommon.

One possible exception to these statements involves *Mycoplasma* spp. *Mycoplasma* has been isolated from the airway of as many as 25% of cats with signs of lower airway disease, but it has not been cultured from the airway of healthy cats. For this reason, and because *Mycoplasma* infection has the potential to cause significant structural damage to airway epithelium, it may be prudent to treat any cat for which a culture of airway secretions is *Mycoplasma* positive with an appropriate antibiotic such as doxycycline or azithromycin.

Cyproheptadine

Cyproheptadine (Periactin) is marketed as an antihistamine; however, it has been used for years as an appetite stimulant for depressed or anorectic cats because of its antiserotonin properties. As mentioned earlier, serotonin is a primary mediator released from activated mast cells into feline airways and causes acute smooth muscle contraction (bronchoconstriction) in cats but not in humans. We have shown that the ability of cyproheptadine to block serotonin receptors in muscle cells is effective in preventing antigen-induced airway smooth muscle constriction in vitro. However, in clinical practice, this drug has *not* been effective in decreasing clinical signs and likely has limited value.

Antileukotrienes: Zafirlukast, Montelukast, and Zileuton

Leukotrienes belong to a family of inflammatory mediators that are derived from arachidonic acid and are known collectively as *eicosanoids*. The leukotrienes LTC_4, LTD_4, and LTE_4 collectively are known as the *cysteinyl leukotrienes* and play an important role in airway inflammation in people. These mediators produce mucus hypersecretion, increased vascular permeability, and mucosal edema; induce potent bronchoconstriction; and act as chemoattractants to inflammatory cells, particularly eosinophils and neutrophils.

The orally administered antileukotriene drugs are competitive, highly selective, and potent inhibitors of the production or function of LTC_4, LTD_4, and LTE_4. Specifically, zileuton (Zyflo) blocks leukotriene biosynthesis by inhibiting production of the 5-lipoxygenase enzyme, whereas both montelukast and zafirlukast block adhesion of leukotrienes to their common leukotriene receptor (cysteinyl leukotriene receptor 1). In humans leukotrienes inhibit asthmatic responses to allergen, aspirin, exercise, and cold, dry air.

There have been few investigations regarding the role of leukotrienes in feline airway disease. Although LTE_4 is found in increased concentrations in the urine of asthmatic humans, no such increase in urinary LTE_4 was found in cats with experimentally induced asthma (Padrid, 1995). In another experimental model of feline asthma, no increase in cysteinyl leukotrienes was found in either urine or BAL fluid after challenge exposure to sensitizing antigen (Norris et al, 2003). In addition, zafirlukast did not inhibit airway inflammation or airway hyperreactivity in this feline model (Norris Reinero et al, 2004). Although there is at least one claim of efficacy using zafirlukast (1 to 2 mg/kg twice daily) or montelukast (0.5 to 1 mg/kg once daily) for treatment of feline asthma (Mandelker and Padrid, 2000), there is no compelling evidence that drugs that affect leukotriene synthesis or receptor ligation play a significant role in the treatment of feline respiratory disease.

Aerosol Delivery of Steroids and Bronchodilators

Aerosol administration of the corticosteroid fluticasone and the bronchodilator albuterol rely on delivery of drug to the distal airways, which in turn depends on the size of the aerosol particles and various respiratory parameters such as tidal volume and inspiratory flow rate. Even in cooperative humans only approximately 10% to 30% of the inhaled dose enters the lungs; however, clinical benefit may be observed. Recent studies in cats have demonstrated that passive inhalation through a spacer-mask combination (AeroKat) is an effective method of delivering sufficient medication to be clinically effective (Kirschvink et al, 2006; Reinero et al, 2005).

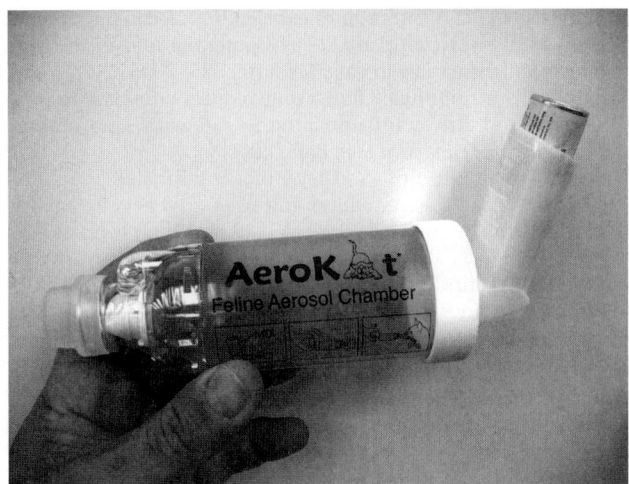

Figure 161-1 The AeroKat spacer is specifically made for the feline species. The metered dose inhaler fits snugly on one end, and the mask fits comfortably on the patient's nose. The Flow-Vu indicator is built into the front of the spacer to let the owner know when the patient takes a breath.

Drugs for inhalation typically come in a rectangular MDI or a round "Diskus" form. At the present time only the MDI form is practical for use in cats. Although the most effective means of using an MDI involves coordination between inhalation and actuation of the device, this is not reliable in animals.

The approach in cats involves use of a spacer device and a mask specifically designed for feline patients (Figure 161-1). A small, aerosol-holding chamber is attached to an MDI on one end and a face mask on the other. The mask is designed to cover the nose of the cat, and it can be helpful to acclimate the cat to the mask beforehand. The MDI supplies precise doses of the aerosol drug, and the holding chamber contains the aerosol so it can be inhaled when the patient inspires. The designers of the AeroKat spacer have shown that a holding chamber with a length of 11 cm and a diameter of 3.5 cm or larger delivered almost all of a therapeutically "ideal" aerosol (i.e., aerosol of equivalent aerodynamic diameter of ≤2.8 μm) produced by an MDI; and in some cases delivery was enhanced because of evaporation of large, suspended particles (Foley, n.d.). The choice of spacer is relevant because cats have a tidal volume of between 5 and 10 ml of inspired air per pound of body weight. Currently only the AeroKat brand spacers have been designed specifically based on the tidal volume characteristics of the cat. When these spacer devices are used, cats inhale the majority of drug propelled into the spacer by breathing *7 to 10 times* through the spacer-mask combination after actuation of the MDI. Owners can confirm normal inspiratory motions by noting movement of a Flow-Vu indicator at the terminal end of the spacing chamber.

When inhalation therapy is administered, the MDI is first shaken to open an internal valve within the canister, and then it is attached to the spacer. The mask attached to the other end of the spacer is placed snugly on the animal's nose or muzzle, and the MDI is pressed to release the medication into the spacer.

The use of inhaled medications to treat asthma and bronchitis is considered the standard of care in humans and now is recommended widely for cats with chronic bronchial disease. This approach avoids many of the adverse effects previously seen in patients treated with systemic medications.

Fluticasone Propionate

The most commonly used inhaled corticosteroid is fluticasone propionate (Flovent), a synthetic corticosteroid with an eighteenfold higher affinity for the corticosteroid receptor than dexamethasone. Binding of the steroid to this receptor results in a new molecular complex that leads to up- or down-regulation of the gene and its products. Like other corticosteroids, fluticasone acts to inhibit mast cells, eosinophils, lymphocytes, neutrophils, and macrophages involved in the generation and exacerbation of allergic airway inflammation by transcriptional regulation of these target genes. Preformed and newly secreted mediators, including histamine, eicosanoids, leukotrienes, and multiple cytokines, are inhibited as well.

Fluticasone is a large molecule and acts topically within the airway mucosa. Because there is poor absorption across gut epithelium, there is minimal oral systemic bioavailability. Plasma levels do not predict therapeutic effects. This explains the lack of systemic side effects; however, it also suggests that clinically effective absorption into the airway mucosa is delayed. Therefore optimal clinical effects may not occur for 1 to 2 weeks. For this reason, cats treated with fluticasone should first be stabilized with systemic corticosteroids if signs of asthma or bronchitis are evident at the time of diagnosis.

Fluticasone has been used to treat cats with bronchial asthma at least since 1993. Since then a number of manuscripts have demonstrated the clinical effectiveness of fluticasone for treatment of cats with allergic bronchitis and asthma (both naturally occurring and experimentally induced).

There have been no published controlled studies to determine the optimal dose or interval for use of fluticasone in cats; however, there are anecdotal reports that describe more than 500 small animal patients treated with fluticasone over a period covering 1995 through 2006. Dosage recommendations are based on these observations and recently published studies. Cohn and colleagues (2010) have shown in an experimental model of feline asthma that the lowest dose of fluticasone (44 μg) can suppress BAL fluid eosinophilia as effectively as the highest dose of fluticasone (220 μg). No pulmonary function results or clinical data were evaluated in this study. At this writing, the number of eosinophils in BAL fluid found in this model should not be used as a guide to determine the dose of fluticasone to be used in treating patients with naturally occurring bronchitis or asthma.

Fluticasone comes in three strengths: 44 μg, 110 μg, and 220 μg per actuation. The author has found that 44-μg dosing twice daily does not consistently result in acceptable clinical responses. For cats with mild to moderate disease, *110 μg given twice daily* frequently results in clinical responses equivalent to those achieved by administration of 5-mg oral doses of prednisone given twice daily. Cats with more serious disease may require

220 µg inhaled fluticasone twice daily. In the author's experience, administration of fluticasone more than twice daily has not resulted in clinical benefit.

Albuterol Sulfate

The pharmacology of albuterol, a selective β_2-adrenergic bronchodilator, has been described previously. This drug is available through different manufacturers and is commonly prescribed as Ventolin or Proventil. Albuterol comes in only a single uniform strength (90 µg per inhalation). Albuterol administration usually results in relaxation of airway smooth muscles within 1 to 5 minutes; thus the effect is almost immediate. This drug should be used in animals with documented or assumed bronchoconstriction. Signs that may indicate bronchoconstriction are wheezing, noisy lower airway breathing, a prolonged expiratory phase of ventilation, and coughing. Albuterol can be used once daily before administering fluticasone or as needed for acute coughing and wheezing. In emergency cases albuterol can be used every 30 minutes for up to 4 to 6 hours without serious side effects.

References and Suggested Reading

Cocayne CG, Reinero CR, DeClue AE: Subclinical airway inflammation despite high dose oral corticosteroid therapy in cats with lower airway disease, *J Feline Med Surg* 13:558, 2011.

Cohn LA et al: Identification and characterization of an idiopathic pulmonary fibrosis-like condition in cats, *J Vet Intern Med* 18(5):632, 2004.

Cohn LA et al: Effects of fluticasone propionate dosage in experimental model of feline asthma, *J Feline Med Surg* 2:91, 2010.

Delgado C et al: Feline-specific serum total IgE quantitation in normal, asthmatic and parasitized cats, *J Feline Med Surg* 12:991, 2010.

Dye JA et al: Bronchopulmonary disease in the cat: historical, physical, radiographic, clinicopathologic and pulmonary functional evaluation of 24 affected and 15 healthy cats, *J Vet Intern Med* 10:385, 1996.

Foley M: Personal communication. Trudell Medical International, London, Ontario, Canada.

Foster SF et al: Twenty-five cases of feline bronchial disease (1995-2000), *J Feline Med Surg* 6(3):181, 2004.

Hill JW: Diseases of the respiratory organs. In *The diseases of the cat*, New York, 1906, William R Jenkins, p 11.

Hopper K: Personal communication.

Johnson LR, Vernau W: Bronchoscopic findings in 48 cats with spontaneous lower respiratory tract disease (2002-2009), *J Vet Intern Med* 25:236, 2011.

Kirschvink N et al: Collection of exhaled breath condensate and analysis of hydrogen peroxide as a potential marker of lower airway inflammation in cats, *Vet J* 169:385, 2005.

Kirschvink N et al: Inhaled fluticasone reduces bronchial responsiveness and airway inflammation in cats with mild chronic bronchitis, *J Feline Med Surg* 8:45, 2006.

Leemans J et al: Effect of short-term oral and inhaled corticosteroids on airway inflammation and responsiveness in a feline acute asthma model, *Vet J* 192(1):41, 2012. Epub February 26, 2012.

Mandelker L, Padrid P: Experimental drug therapy for respiratory disorders in dogs and cats, *Vet Clin North Am Small Anim Pract* 30:1357, 2000.

Nafe LA et al: Evaluation of biomarkers in bronchoalveolar lavage fluid for discrimination between asthma and chronic bronchitis in cats, *Am J Vet Res* 15:583, 2010.

Norris CR et al: Concentrations of cysteinyl leukotrienes in urine and bronchoalveolar lavage fluid of cats with experimentally induced asthma, *Am J Vet Res* 64:1449, 2003.

Norris-Reinero C et al: An experimental model of allergic asthma in cats sensitized to house dust mite or Bermuda grass allergen, *Int Arch Allergy Immunol* 135:117, 2004.

Padrid PA et al: Cytologic, microbiologic, and biochemical analysis of bronchoalveolar lavage fluid obtained from 24 healthy cats, *Am J Vet Res* 52(8):1300, 1991.

Padrid PA: Personal observations, 1995.

Padrid PA: Feline asthma, *Vet Clin North Am Small Anim Pract* 30:1279, 2000.

Padrid PA et al: Cyproheptadine-induced attenuation of type-I immediate hypersensitivity reactions of airway smooth muscle from immune-sensitized cats, *Am J Vet Res* 56:109, 1995.

Padrid PA, Cozzi P, Leff AR: Cyclosporine A attenuates the development of chronic airway hyper-responsiveness and histological alterations in immune-sensitized cats, *Am J Respir Crit Care Med* 154:1812, 1996.

Rozanski EA, Hoffman AM: Lung mechanics using plethysmography and spirometry. In King LG, editor: *Respiratory disease in dogs and cats*, St Louis, 2004, Sanders, p 175.

Reinero CR et al: Effects of drug treatment on inflammation and hyperreactivity of airways and on immune variables in cats with experimentally induced asthma, *Am J Vet Res* 66:1121, 2005.

Reinero CR et al: Enantiomer-specific effects of albuterol on airway inflammation in healthy and asthmatic cats, *Int Arch Allergy Immunol* 150:43, 2009a.

Reinero CR et al: Immunomodulation with allergen specific immunotherapy in feline asthma. In *Proceedings of the XX Annual ACVIM Forum*, 2009b.

CHAPTER 162

Pneumonia

RITA M. HANEL, *Raleigh, North Carolina*
BERNIE HANSEN, *Raleigh, North Carolina*

Pneumonia can be categorized in several ways. In humans, it is most commonly classified by where or how it was acquired (community acquired, hospital acquired, ventilator associated, and aspiration); by the area of affected lung (lobar, bronchial, interstitial, alveolar, or any combination of these); by progression (acute, subacute, or chronic); or by the causative organism (bacterial, viral, fungal, protozoal, or parasitic). This chapter focuses primarily on bacterial pneumonia using the classification scheme that is based on *where* or *how* the infection was acquired. The use of this scheme may help guide diagnostic and therapeutic decisions for companion animals.

Community-Acquired Bacterial Pneumonia

Community-acquired pneumonia (CAP) is defined as pneumonia that develops in a patient that has not recently been hospitalized. The incidence of CAP in dogs and cats is unknown. Infection of the lung may occur by aspiration, inhalation, or hematogenous spread of virulent bacteria or opportunistic pathogens in immunosuppressed individuals. The different forms of CAP with distinguishing characteristics and pathogens are summarized in Table 162-1.

Aspiration (discussed in more detail later) and opportunistic organisms appear to be more common causes of infection than virulent bacteria in adult dogs and cats. Causes of immunosuppression that are associated with pneumonia in mature animals include preexistent disease (e.g., diabetes mellitus, hypothyroidism, neoplasia, or bronchiectasis) and therapeutic immunosuppression related to treatment of primary or acquired immunologic conditions (e.g., immune-mediated hemolytic anemia, lupus, or pemphigus). In a report of a case series describing bacterial pneumonia in 93 dogs, most affected animals were older than 5 years of age and 57% had concurrent medical problems that may have contributed to aspiration or immunosuppression (Jameson et al, 1995).

Bacterial cultures of specimens from the level of the carina yield oropharyngeal bacteria in up to 40% of healthy dogs and 75% of healthy cats (Box 162-1), and some of these organisms have been associated with pneumonia in dogs with aspiration injury or other causes of compromised immune function. Infection in young animals without concurrent illness is often associated with exposure to more virulent organisms, but a significant stressor (e.g., housing, transport, or environmental) may contribute to some degree of immune dysfunction and compromised resistance to infection.

Some pathogens causing CAP establish colonization with specialized virulence factors, regardless of the immune status of the patient. Some examples are extraintestinal pathogenic *Escherichia coli* and *Streptococcus equi* subsp. *zooepidemicus,* which have been responsible for hemorrhagic or necrotizing pneumonia in dogs and cats. Outbreaks of *S. equi* subsp. *zooepidemicus* also have been reported to cause fatal hemorrhagic pneumonia in dogs (Byun et al, 2009; Priestnall and Erles, 2010) and necrotizing suppurative pneumonia in cats (Blum et al, 2010). These organisms typically result in peracute to acute infections, the animals are profoundly ill with pyrexia and tachypnea, and mortality is high. Most affected animals had experienced a stressor, such as shipment or housing in a facility or shelter, that may have contributed to increased host susceptibility.

Another cause of CAP in both dogs and cats is infection with *Bordetella bronchiseptica.* This gram-negative aerobic coccobacillus has the capacity to colonize the airway as either a commensal or a pathogenic organism, and it frequently plays a role in canine infectious respiratory disease complex (see Chapter 153). The outcome of infection is difficult to predict and can range from mild subclinical disease to fatal pneumonia. *B. bronchiseptica* displays a myriad of virulence factors that influence the pathologic consequences of infection and may be affected by various environmental conditions. In a case series of puppies with CAP, *B. bronchiseptica* was isolated in 49% (32 out of 65) and predominantly gram-negative enteric bacteria were isolated in the rest, all of which were susceptible to most antimicrobials tested (Radhakrishnan et al, 2007).

Mycoplasma spp. are considered a normal inhabitant of the oropharynx of both dogs and cats, and they have been cultured from the lungs of many animals with pneumonia; however, most cases showed resolution of clinical disease without specific anti-*Mycoplasma* therapy (Jameson et al, 1995). This has led to speculation that these organisms may be an incidental contaminant or that they may have low pathogenicity on their own. However, *Mycoplasma* spp. also have been recovered as the sole pathogen from the airways of animals that subsequently responded to anti-*Mycoplasma* therapy. Several of those animals had findings consistent with bronchitis, asthma, or airway collapse, and whether *Mycoplasma* contributed to airway disease or was able to colonize as a downstream consequence of this disease is unknown. At present it seems likely that colonization of the lower respiratory tract by the organism does have clinical significance that warrants therapeutic consideration, especially in the cat.

TABLE 162-1

Community-Acquired Pneumonia (CAP) and Early-Onset Hospital-Acquired Pneumonia: Distinguishing Characteristics, Common Bacterial Isolates, and Antimicrobial Recommendations

Species	Distinguishing Characteristics	Common Bacterial Pathogens in Descending Order of Frequency	Antimicrobial Recommendations*/Comments
Dog	Acute to chronic adult-onset CAP, including aspiration pneumonia	Gram-negative enterics (*Escherichia coli*, *Klebsiella*, *Enterobacter*) *Pasteurella* *Streptococcus* *Staphylococcus* *Pseudomonas* Anaerobes *Mycoplasma*	Amoxicillin/clavulanate or Trimethoprim/sulfonamide or Enrofloxacin Consider combination with clindamycin or first-generation cephalosporin for broad-spectrum coverage.
Dog	Peracute to acute hemorrhagic CAP	Extraintestinal *E. coli* *Streptococcus equi* subsp. *zooepidemicus*	Enrofloxacin and first-generation cephalosporin
Dog	Young age (<1 yr) or recent environmental stressor	*Bordetella* Gram-negative enterics *Staphylococcus* *Pseudomonas* *Streptococcus* *Pasteurella*	Doxycycline or Amoxicillin/clavulanate
Cat	Acute to chronic adult-onset CAP	*Mycoplasma* *Pasteurella* *Bordetella* *Streptococcus* Gram-negative enterics	Doxycycline and amoxicillin/clavulanate or Doxycycline and a fluoroquinolone or Doxycycline and trimethoprim/sulfonamide
Cat	Peracute to acute necrotizing suppurative CAP	Extraintestinal *E. coli* *S. equi* subsp. *zooepidemicus*	Fluoroquinolone and first-generation cephalosporin
Cat	Young age (<1 yr) or environmental stressor	*Bordetella* *Pasteurella* *Mycoplasma* *Escherichia* *Streptococcus* If interstitial pattern is present, consider sepsis and hematogenous pneumonia (*E. coli*, *Streptococcus*, or *Pasteurella*)	Doxycycline or Azithromycin or Fluoroquinolone Consider blood culture with interstitial disease. Consider broad-spectrum therapy with systemic signs: Amoxicillin/clavulanate or Trimethoprim/sulfonamide

*Avoid fluoroquinolones in puppies. Use caution with trimethoprim/sulfonamide and monitor patients for ocular or hematologic abnormalities.

BOX 162-1

Bacterial Isolates from the Trachea of Healthy Animals

Canine	Feline
Gram Positive	
Staphylococcus	Staphylococcus
Streptococcus	Streptococcus
Corynebacterium	Corynebacterium
	Micrococcus
Gram Negative	
Pasteurella	Pasteurella
Klebsiella	Klebsiella
Bordetella	Escherichia
Escherichia coli	Pseudomonas
Enterobacter	Enterobacter
Pasteurella	Acinetobacter
Pseudomonas	Bordetella

Hematogenous acquisition of pneumonia is not well documented. Theoretically, hematogenous dissemination of bacteria can result in a diffuse interstitial pneumonia, given that the bloodstream is the portal of entry.

Hospital-Acquired Bacterial Pneumonia

Hospital-acquired pneumonia (HAP) is defined as pneumonia that occurs 48 hours or longer after admission and was not incubating at the time of admission (American Thoracic Society and Infectious Diseases Society of America, 2005). *HAP* can be used synonymously with *nosocomial pneumonia* and is the second most common nosocomial infection in humans in the United States. HAP in humans accounts for up to 25% of all intensive care unit (ICU) infections and more than 50% of antibiotics prescribed, and is associated with morbidity and mortality rates of 33% to 50%. Although the incidence in dogs and cats is unknown, in the authors' opinion HAP is a significant problem in veterinary referral hospitals and needs to be considered separately from CAP. In humans the length of time from admission to development of HAP has implications for therapy. Early-onset HAP, defined as HAP occurring within the first 4 days of hospitalization, typically carries a better prognosis because it is more likely to be caused by antibiotic-sensitive bacteria. Late-onset HAP, defined as HAP occurring after 5 days of hospitalization or longer, is more likely to be caused by multidrug-resistant (MDR) pathogens and is associated with increased morbidity and mortality.

In veterinary medicine, there are few studies that specifically address HAP. Nevertheless, veterinarians are finding similar patterns of MDR bacterial infections in our patients. One report described antimicrobial therapy and susceptibility patterns in isolates from various sources (urinary, respiratory, peritoneal) obtained from animals in a veterinary ICU (Black et al, 2009). MDR pathogens comprised 27% of isolates (19 out of 70) and were significantly more likely to be identified after 48 hours of hospitalization. Initial empiric antibiotic selection was appropriate in only 30% of animals that had received antibiotics in the month before culture submission. Antibiotics prescribed after submission of the sample but before final bacteriologic culture and susceptibility (minimal inhibitory concentration) results became available were appropriate only 75% of the time (Black et al, 2009). These findings underscore the importance of identifying antimicrobial susceptibility patterns in patients in the ICU. A 2010 case series (Epstein et al, 2010) compared airway microbial culture and susceptibility patterns in dogs and cats in the ICU that required positive pressure ventilation due to respiratory failure with findings in animals with respiratory infection that did not require intensive care during the same time period. Although the authors of that report did not specifically differentiate CAP from HAP, there was a clear distinction in severity of disease and level of care. In animals with respiratory failure gram-negative enteric organisms were more likely to be isolated, whereas in animals with respiratory infection gram-negative nonenteric and anaerobic organisms predominated. Fewer bacterial isolates from the respiratory failure group than from the respiratory infection group were susceptible to amoxicillin/clavulanate (35% versus 84%, respectively), enrofloxacin (33% versus 69%, respectively), and ticarcillin/clavulanate (47% versus 83%, respectively). The findings described in these reports suggest that the historical recommendation to prescribe therapy based on bacterial identification alone is likely inadequate in the setting of HAP. Animals with late-onset HAP or other risk factors for MDR pathogens (Box 162-2) should be treated with antibiotics that are more likely to be effective against MDR organisms (Table 162-2) while awaiting susceptibility results.

Aspiration Injury

Aspiration pneumonitis is a chemical injury caused by the inhalation of sterile gastric contents, whereas aspiration pneumonia is an infection caused by the inhalation of oropharyngeal or gastric contents that are contaminated by pathogenic bacteria. The incidences of both are

---

BOX 162-2

Risk Factors for Multidrug-Resistant Pathogens in Animals That Develop Pneumonia While Hospitalized

Antimicrobial therapy in the previous 90 days
Hospitalization within the previous 90 days
Current hospitalization for >48 hours
High incidence of antibiotic-resistant infections within the hospital

---

BOX 162-3

Risk Factors for Gastric Colonization

Small bowel obstruction or ileus
Gastroparesis
Enteral nutrition via feeding tube
Treatment with histamine antagonists or proton pump inhibitors

---

TABLE 162-2

Antimicrobial Recommendations for Patients with Late-Onset Hospital-Acquired Pneumonia or Patients at Risk of Infection with Multidrug-Resistant Pathogens

Species	Antimicrobial Recommendations
Dog	First-generation cephalosporin and second- or third-generation cephalosporin *or* Carbapenem *or* Amikacin and ticarcillin/clavulanate or amoxicillin/sulbactam
Cat	Same recommendations as for dogs; however, consider addition of enrofloxacin or doxycycline for treatment of *Mycoplasma* infection

NOTE: It is recommended that the practitioner consult an antibiogram, if available, and adjust therapy based on resistance patterns in his or her hospital.

---

unknown in veterinary medicine. The true incidence in humans also has been difficult to establish because there are no sensitive and specific markers for aspiration. If the patient does not have a reason for gastric colonization (Box 162-3) and has good oral hygiene, the initial aspiration event should be nearly sterile and acidic in nature, leading to a biphasic lung injury. The first phase, occurring in 1 to 2 hours, is secondary to direct injury of pulmonary parenchyma from acidic stomach contents. The second phase is typical of acute lung injury and develops as neutrophils infiltrate the alveoli as part of the postinjury inflammatory process. This host defense response,

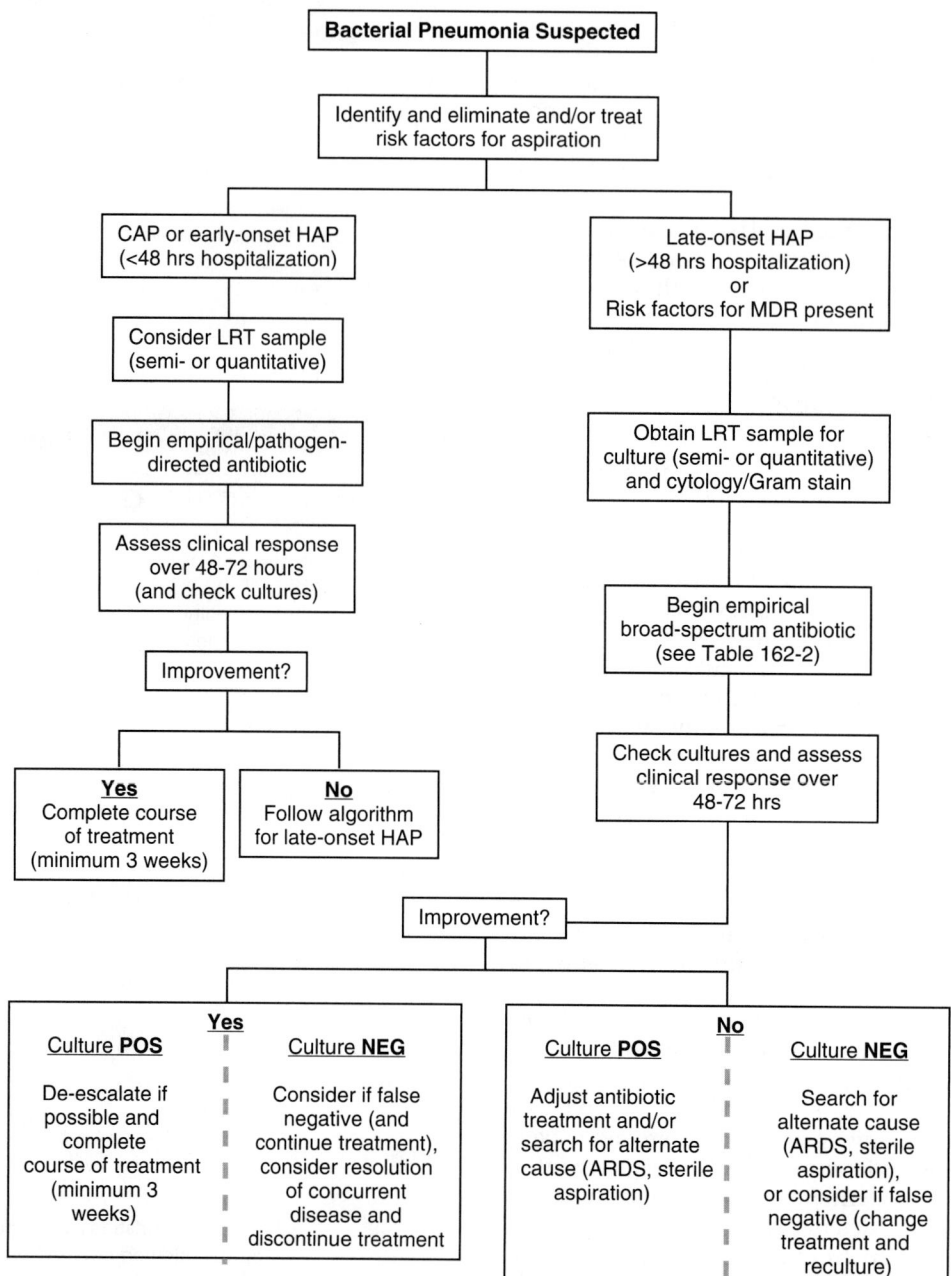

Figure 162-1 Algorithm for diagnosis and treatment of suspected bacterial pneumonia. *CAP,* Community-acquired pneumonia; *HAP,* hospital-acquired pneumonia; *LRT,* lower respiratory tract; *MDR,* multidrug resistant; *NEG,* negative; *POS,* positive; *Tx,* therapy.

which is essential to remove inhaled particulate matter, begins several hours after the event and can progress over the next 24 to 48 hours. This phase represents true pneumonitis that does not require initial antimicrobial therapy. In fact, administration of antibiotics may tend to select for more resistant organisms if a secondary infection is established. However, many animals do not have good oral hygiene, and many of the disease processes leading to the aspiration event are treated with therapies that contribute to gastric colonization, including proton pump inhibitors and enteral nutrition (see Box 162-3). Therefore treatment of aspiration injury in dogs and cats should follow the same recommendations as those for

treatment of uncomplicated CAP (see Table 162-1) unless the patient has risk factors for MDR organisms (see Box 162-2). In the latter case, the authors recommend following the therapeutic recommendations for late-onset HAP (Figure 162-1 and Table 162-2) and obtaining samples for culture and a cytologic specimen representative of the lower airway to guide therapy.

The diagnosis of aspiration pneumonia in veterinary medicine relies primarily on a high index of suspicion from clinical findings and the detection of characteristic infiltrates on thoracic radiographs. These are typically alveolar infiltrates in the right middle or cranial lung lobes with a heavier dependent distribution. Two recent case series identified risk factors for aspiration pneumonia in dogs that included esophageal disease, vomiting, neurologic disorders, laryngeal disease, and recent anesthesia (Kogan et al, 2008a; Tart et al, 2010). Both reports found survival rates in affected dogs of approximately 80%, which did not appear to be influenced by the underlying cause of aspiration. There was conflicting evidence regarding prognostic factors because one group found no association with radiographic severity (Kogan et al, 2008b), whereas the other reported the intuitively logical finding that dogs with only one affected lung lobe were more likely to survive (Tart et al, 2010). In the latter study microbial culture results were positive in 36 of 47 samples, with two or more organisms isolated in 21 of 36 cases. The four most frequently identified isolates were *E. coli* (39% of samples), *Mycoplasma* spp. (21%), *Pasteurella* spp. (19%), and *Staphylococcus* spp. (17%). All of the dogs in that series were treated with broad-spectrum antibiotics, and there was no apparent relationship between choice of antibiotic and survival. Although microbial culture was performed in fewer than 40% of dogs, the nearly 50% incidence of cultures yielding two or more genera of bacteria underscores the importance of using broad-spectrum antibiotic therapy for initial empiric treatment of these patients.

The ideal treatment for aspiration pneumonia is prevention, and four interventions should be considered for animals at risk: proper body positioning, enteral feeding, use of promotility agents, and gastric pH modification. There are numerous studies documenting an increased risk of aspiration in supine human patients. Although body positioning considerations in animals are different from those in humans, it seems prudent to consider elevation of the head or upper one third of the body in recumbent patients, especially those with neurologic disease or an inability to guard the airway. Excessive sedation should be avoided in any patient without a protected airway. Nasogastric tube feeding can promote the reflux of gastric contents. For this reason, nasoesophageal or gastric tube feeding is preferred. When administered frequently or given as a constant infusion, enteral nutrition can increase the pH of the gastric lumen and promote gastric colonization with bacteria, which warrants vigilance to prevent aspiration. Increased gastric residual volume often is cited as a risk factor contributing to aspiration, but there is little agreement regarding the volume required to put a patient at risk in human or veterinary medicine. However, increasing gastric residual volume in an animal at risk of aspiration should prompt the clinician to consider decreasing the rate, volume, or frequency of feeding. The use of prokinetic agents to prevent aspiration injury in humans is controversial, and none has been shown to decrease its incidence even when the agents are effective at reducing gastric residual volume. The potential for antacid therapy to increase the risk of aspiration pneumonia is also controversial. Modification of gastric pH is used frequently to treat or prevent gastroesophageal reflux disease despite the fact that this treatment may contribute to gastric colonization, primarily with gramnegative species. Two metaanalyses of clinical trials in humans published in the 1990s concluded that the incidence of pneumonia is reduced in patients treated with sucralfate compared to those treated with histamine antagonists or antacids. However, multiple studies performed since that time have not found the same effect. At present, there does not appear to be a compelling reason to use or to avoid antacid therapy in dogs or cats as a means of reducing the risk of pneumonia.

Diagnosis

The diagnosis of bacterial pneumonia is based primarily on information from the history, physical examination, and thoracic radiographs. Clinicopathologic findings can be supportive but are neither sensitive nor specific. Microbial culture results are usually confirmatory; however, the availability of culture results is delayed, and both falsepositives (recovery of normal flora; see Box 162-1) and false-negatives (failure to grow a pathogen contributing to the syndrome) can occur.

Clinical History

Signs of pneumonia include a productive cough, pyrexia, breathing difficulty, increased respiratory rate, nasal discharge, inappetence, lethargy, exercise intolerance, and altered mentation. In the setting of aspiration injury, pneumonia should be considered in patients with any of these signs and a history of gastrointestinal disease, neurologic disease, or recent anesthesia. Some dogs and cats may have only subtle or nonspecific signs early in the course of the disorder, and diagnosis may require a high index of suspicion. Historical findings that should prompt investigation include any of the risk factors listed in the discussion of aspiration injury, a recent environmental stressor such as shipping or boarding, a new pet in the household, or a history of chronic airway disease that may predispose the patient to bacterial infection (e.g., bronchiectasis).

Physical Examination

Physical examination findings may include pyrexia, increased respiratory rate, abnormal lung sounds, nasal discharge, or cough on tracheal palpation. In a review of lower respiratory tract infections in cats, tachypnea was the most common findings, followed by abnormal lung sounds (Foster et al, 2004). A recent case series of dogs with aspiration pneumonia reported increased, decreased, or adventitious lungs sounds in 68%, and increased body temperature, heart rate, or respiratory rate in fewer than 50% of cases (Kogan et al, 2008b). Regardless, signs may be subtle and any combination of the aforementioned historical and physical findings should prompt investigation.

Radiographic Findings

Radiographic findings in animals with bacterial pneumonia are variable, ranging from a diffuse bronchointerstitial pattern to a regional or focal alveolar pattern to complete consolidation. In cats, there is often a bronchiolar component, and changes can be patchy or diffuse. Both species also can have pulmonary nodules caused by abscessation or a diffuse interstitial to alveolar pattern caused by hematogenous pneumonia. Since any and all lung lobes can be affected, it is important to obtain both left and right lateral projections and a ventrodorsal exposure (or a dorsoventral view if the patient will not tolerate lying on its back). Finally, the absence of radiographic changes in peracute disease does not rule out a diagnosis of pneumonia because parenchymal changes are secondary to the ensuing inflammatory response.

Clinicopathologic Findings

Clinicopathologic findings are neither sensitive nor specific for the diagnosis of pneumonia. When abnormalities are present, the most common is a neutrophilia with or without a left shift. Hypoalbuminemia with or without hyperglobulinemia, consistent with an acute inflammatory response, is occasionally found. Hypoxemia or arterial hemoglobin desaturation may be identified on blood gas analysis or pulse oximetry, respectively, with a concurrent increase in the alveolar-arterial oxygen gradient. Identification of an inappropriately high venous or arterial partial pressure of carbon dioxide confirms developing respiratory failure. Hypoxemia is not specific to bacterial pneumonia because it occurs with ventilation-perfusion mismatch from any cause. However, abnormalities of gas exchange indicate the presence of severe lung dysfunction and should prompt aggressive diagnostic and therapeutic efforts.

Bacterial Identification

Ideally, a lower airway sample should be collected for culture and susceptibility testing in any animal with clinical findings consistent with serious infection. However, collection of a sample requires restraint, sedation, or general anesthesia, any of which can pose harm to an animal with significant respiratory compromise. Animals with minimal respiratory reserve capacity that are becoming exhausted may decompensate easily with restraint or heavy sedation and have a difficult or prolonged recovery. They may not tolerate the volume of saline that must be instilled in the airways for certain modes of sample collection. Animals that are in this fragile a condition often are in need of more aggressive supportive care such as mechanical ventilation and should be referred to a center capable of providing this level of care and obtaining airway specimens for culture in a more controlled situation. However, the majority of animals with bacterial pneumonia are not that ill, and other factors such as finances or owner compliance may have more influence on decisions about diagnosis and treatment. If the animal has never been treated for pneumonia, has a suspected CAP or early-onset HAP, and has none of the risk factors for MDR (see Box 162-2), then empiric pathogen-based therapy may be appropriate (see Table 162-1). However, if the history is consistent with late-onset HAP, risk factors for MDR are present, or previous therapy has failed, an airway sample should be obtained for culture and susceptibility testing, cytologic analysis, and Gram staining to guide therapy (see Figure 162-1 and Table 162-2).

There are several methods for obtaining a lower airway sample, including transtracheal wash, endotracheal wash, bronchoalveolar lavage, and guarded brush techniques. Although an in-depth description of these techniques is beyond the scope of this chapter, there are some relevant considerations when planning a diagnostic workup. A significant advantage of the transtracheal wash method over other techniques is that the procedure can be performed under local anesthesia with minimal or no sedation in dogs weighing more than about 5 kg. However, because the technique requires that saline be injected into and recovered from the distal trachea, multiple attempts may be required to obtain a sufficient sample, and recovered organisms may not be representative of the microbes in the pulmonary parenchyma. The endotracheal wash technique has the same limitations as transtracheal wash but requires sedation or anesthesia sufficient to allow intubation; furthermore, the patient is unlikely to cough, so that lavage fluid may simply pool away from the catheter tip. This technique is better for smaller patients or those with tracheal or skin diseases, in which the percutaneous transtracheal wash technique may be difficult or associated with additional risks. Bronchoalveolar lavage is typically performed through a bronchoscope and may be technically more challenging and expensive. It also must be performed under general anesthesia. However, the sample recovered is more representative of the distal airways and can be obtained from a specific lung lobe when the disease is not uniform in distribution. The guarded brush technique is simple, quick, and cheap if performed through an endotracheal tube without bronchoscopic guidance. The brush can be directed to the affected site when the technique is performed using a bronchoscope. Although the brush yields a small sample and does not reach the alveoli, it can be passed beyond the first bronchial division to obtain a sample from deeper in the lung than in the transtracheal wash method. The guarded brush technique does not require the instillation of fluid into the airway.

Whenever possible, a portion of the recovered sample should be reserved for cytologic analysis and Gram staining to help guide therapy while the results of culture are awaited. Because the sample-handling requirements for recovery of microorganisms may be somewhat specific to each laboratory, it is recommended to confirm these with laboratory personnel before obtaining samples to ensure that all the necessary items are collected and appropriately handled. In particular, anaerobic cultures can be time sensitive, and recovery of *Mycoplasma* spp. may require a separate media vial. Personnel should use proper hand-cleaning and gloving techniques and emphasize activities to prevent cross contamination of patients.

Treatment

Inpatient versus Outpatient Therapy
To minimize client expense and limit contamination of the hospital environment with potential pathogens from infected animals, it is always preferable to manage animals with infectious pneumonia as outpatients. However, some findings, such as the need for supplemental oxygen, an inability to tolerate oral medications or pill

administration, signs of shock or cardiovascular instability, or indicators of organ dysfunction (high blood urea nitrogen, creatinine, or bilirubin levels), indicate that hospitalization is necessary. If none of these conditions is present, hospitalization for intravenous antibiotic administration still should be considered in patients with leukopenia, recent exposure to immunosuppressive therapy, motility disorders, or questionable gastrointestinal absorption.

Antimicrobials: Selection, Timing, and Duration of Antibiotic Therapy

As previously mentioned, antibiotic choice should be guided in part by a determination of whether the infection is likely to be CAP, early-onset HAP, or late-onset HAP. Patients with risk factors for MDR infections (see Box 162-2) should be treated the same as those with late-onset HAP. Figure 162-1 provides a diagnostic and therapeutic algorithm for use in these patients, and Tables 162-1 and 162-2 outline recommended antimicrobials. In general, all patients should receive empiric therapy pending the results of diagnostic testing, with the anticipation of alterations in antimicrobial therapy when susceptibility results are available. In animals with CAP, this choice is frequently based on an understanding of which pathogen most likely will be isolated. In animals with late-onset HAP or factors contributing to MDR, therapy targeted for such infection is recommended, with refinement of the treatment regimen after interpretation of culture results. Antibiotic therapy should be initiated as early as possible, particularly in animals at risk of sepsis.

Therapy should be continued until resolution of disease, but it should be kept in mind that unnecessarily prolonged antimicrobial therapy can alter microbial populations and select for resistance in other airway bacteria. The most widely accepted standard is to continue treatment for 1 week after clinical resolution, which should occur within 4 to 6 weeks. Clinical response is determined by resolution of signs and abnormalities in physical examination findings or diagnostic test results. Resolution of radiographic abnormalities can lag behind clinical response, and such abnormalities may even worsen in the first 48 hours of therapy. In general, radiographic abnormalities should begin to resolve within 72 hours of therapy, and findings should be monitored until resolution is complete.

Supportive Therapy

Hospitalization for intravenous fluid therapy is recommended to maintain hydration in animals that are not eating and drinking. Fever, hyperventilation, panting, and mucus production contribute to free water loss, and maintaining normal mucociliary clearance and alveolar emptying via hydration is beneficial. Excessive administration of high-sodium replacement fluids can be detrimental if it contributes to pulmonary edema, so the type and volume of fluid administered should be calibrated to meet but not exceed patient metabolic needs.

Administration of bronchodilators is controversial. Lobar bronchoconstriction in response to regional hypoxia caused by infiltration protects gas exchange elsewhere, and pharmacologic bronchodilation could potentially worsen ventilation-perfusion inequality. However, bronchodilators may be beneficial in animals with generalized bronchoconstriction from global disease or in cats with concurrent asthma (see Chapter 151). Treatment with a direct-acting bronchodilator (e.g., terbutaline) may be particularly important in acute aspiration pneumonia in which gastric acid triggers bronchoconstriction. Infection with *Bordetella* theoretically has the potential to increase airway resistance, and a course of terbutaline might be beneficial in affected patients. Methylxanthines may impart additional benefit to dogs with impending respiratory failure by increasing the resistance of the diaphragm to fatigue.

Oxygen should be administered to patients with clinical signs of hypoxemia (e.g., increased respiratory rate or effort, lethargy), hemoglobin desaturation as measured by pulse oximetry, or arterial hypoxemia documented by blood gas analysis. During initial patient assessment this can be accomplished with oxygen flow-by or mask delivery. For prolonged administration, the easiest method is placement of a nasal or nasopharyngeal oxygen catheter. Alternatively, oxygen can be administered by hood or oxygen cage, which is preferred in cats and in brachycephalic breeds. Supplemental oxygen should be humidified and delivered at a rate of 50 to 100 ml/kg/min (via nasal catheter) or set to a fraction of inspired oxygen of 40% to 60% (in a cage or hood) depending on clinical response.

Nebulization and coupage should be considered for patients with alveolar disease or lung consolidation. For airway hydration, nebulization with 10 to 20 ml of saline over 10 to 20 minutes is delivered, followed by coupage. The nebulizer must be capable of forming droplets that are less than 5 µm in diameter to reach and hydrate the lower airways. Consequently, humidifiers and vaporizers cannot be used in lieu of a nebulizer. Coupage, or percussion of the thorax to aid in mobilization of secretions, is best performed in conjunction with other physical therapy; encouraging the patient to rise, walk, and cough also aides in alveolar clearance. Coupage should be avoided in animals with esophageal disease or vomiting disorders. Nebulized mucolytics such as acetylcysteine have limited value because they can be irritating to the epithelium and may cause reflex bronchoconstriction. Recumbent patients should be turned at least every 4 to 6 hours.

Reasons for Treatment Failure

Even with optimal therapy it may take up to 48 to 72 hours to observe clinical improvement. If the patient deteriorates during this time or there is a lack of improvement after 72 hours, culture and sensitivity testing must be performed or repeated (see Figure 162-1) and reasons for a lack of response must be identified. Possible reasons include inadequate or inappropriate antimicrobial therapy (e.g., infection with an MDR pathogen or *Mycoplasma* spp.), wrong diagnosis (e.g., cancer and not pneumonia), and complicating factors (e.g., lung abscessation, which may require surgical intervention). Another possibility is the presence of an unidentified concurrent illness causing an inflammatory response that is inhibiting resolution (e.g., catheter infection or pancreatitis). In these cases further diagnostic testing including a comprehensive serum chemistry panel should be performed, any intravenous catheters should be carefully inspected for evidence of infection, and other diagnostic tests such as abdominal ultrasonographic examination should be considered.

References and Suggested Reading

American Thoracic Society, Infectious Diseases Society of America: Guidelines for the management of adults with hospital-acquired, ventilator-associated, and healthcare-associated pneumonia, *Am J Respir Crit Care Med* 171:388, 2005.

Black DM, Rankin SC, King LG: Antimicrobial therapy and aerobic bacteriologic culture patterns in canine intensive care unit patients: 74 dogs (January-June 2006), *J Vet Emerg Crit Care* 19(5):489, 2009.

Blum S et al: Outbreak of *Streptococcus equi* subsp. zooepidemicus infections in cats, *Vet Microbiol* 144(1-2):236, 2010.

Byun JW et al: An outbreak of fatal hemorrhagic pneumonia caused by *Streptococcus equi* subsp. zooepidemicus in shelter dogs, *J Vet Sci* 10(3):269, 2009.

Epstein SE, Mellema MS, Hopper K: Airway microbial culture and susceptibility patterns in dogs and cats with respiratory disease of varying severity, *J Vet Emerg Crit Care* 20(6):587, 2010.

Foster SF et al: Twenty-five cases of feline bronchial disease (1995-2000), *J Feline Med Surg* 6(3):181, 2004.

Jameson PH et al: Comparison of clinical signs, diagnostic findings, organisms isolated, and clinical outcome in dogs with bacterial pneumonia: 93 cases (1986-1991), *J Am Vet Med Assoc* 206(2):206, 1995.

Kogan DA et al: Etiology and clinical outcome in dogs with aspiration pneumonia: 88 cases (2004-2006), *J Am Vet Med Assoc* 233:1748, 2008a.

Kogan DA et al: Clinical, clinicopathologic, and radiographic findings in dogs with aspiration pneumonia: 88 cases (2004-2006), *J Am Vet Med Assoc* 233:1742, 2008b.

Mandell LA et al: Infectious Diseases Society of America/American Thoracic Society consensus guidelines on the management of community-acquired pneumonia in adults, *Clin Infect Dis* 44:S27, 2007.

Marik PE: Aspiration pneumonitis and aspiration pneumonia, *N Engl J Med* 344(9):665, 2001.

Priestnall S, Erles K: *Streptococcus zooepidemicus:* an emerging canine pathogen, *Vet J* 188(2):142, 2011.

Priestnall SL et al: Characterization of pneumonia due to *Streptococcus equi* subsp. zooepidemicus in dogs, *Clin Vaccine Immunol* 17(11):1790, 2010.

Radhakrishnan A et al: Community-acquired infectious pneumonia in puppies: 65 cases (1993-2002), *J Am Vet Med Assoc* 230(10):1493, 2007.

Tart KM, Babski DM, Lee JA: Potential risks, prognostic indicators, and diagnostic and treatment modalities affecting survival in dogs with presumptive aspiration pneumonia: 125 cases (2005-2008), *J Vet Emerg Crit Care (San Antonio)* 20(3):319, 2010.

CHAPTER 163

Eosinophilic Pulmonary Diseases

CÉCILE CLERCX, *Liège, Belgium*
DOMINIQUE PEETERS, *Liège, Belgium*

Definition and Causes

Eosinophilic bronchopneumopathy (EBP) is a disease characterized by eosinophilic infiltration of the lung and bronchial mucosa. Several terms, including *pulmonary infiltration with eosinophils, pulmonary eosinophilia,* and *eosinophilic pneumonia* have been used in the literature to describe the same disease (Clercx et al, 2000). Possible causes include occult heartworm disease due to *Dirofilaria immitis,* migration of larvae of *Angiostrongylus vasorum* through pulmonary parenchyma, and infection with a parasite such as *Oslerus osleri, Filaroides hirthi, Crenosoma vulpis,* or *Paragonimus kellicotti.* Suspected but unconfirmed causes in dogs include allergic bronchopulmonary aspergillosis, chronic pulmonary infections caused by mycobacteria or fungi, drug reactions, and tumors (lymphoma and mast cell tumor). However, a specific cause is rarely identified even with extensive diagnostic workup, and most cases of EBP are considered to be idiopathic, although a hypersensitivity to aeroallergens is suspected.

Pathogenesis

In idiopathic EBP, a dominant helper T cell type 2 (T_H2) immune response is suspected, based on a selective increase in CD4+ T cells in bronchoalveolar lavage fluid (BALF) (Clercx et al, 2002) and increased levels of messenger RNA encoding for eotaxins, the strongest chemoattractants for eosinophils, in bronchial biopsy specimens from dogs with EBP (Peeters et al, 2006). The cause of these changes is unknown. A limited number of positive intradermal skin test reactions have been described in affected dogs; however, the relationship between positive intradermal skin test results and detection of aeroallergens responsible for EBP is still unclear. Lower airway and pulmonary destruction and remodeling observed in canine EBP may be connected to up-regulation of collagenolysis, related perhaps to increased activity of matrix metalloproteinase 8 (MMP-8), MMP-9, and MMP-13 (Rajamaki et al, 2002).

Signalment and Clinical Signs

Dogs affected with EBP are usually young adult dogs, although age at onset of disease varies greatly (up to 13 years). Females are more frequently affected than males. Siberian huskies and Alaskan malamutes appear to be predisposed, and although the disease also is frequently diagnosed in small breeds as well as in dogs of other large breeds, it is rarely encountered in miniature or giant breeds.

Harsh cough, followed by gagging and retching, is the most common clinical sign. Other frequent clinical signs are labored respirations, some degree of exercise intolerance, and nasal discharge. Auscultation findings may be normal, but increased bronchial sounds can be noted as well as wheezes or crackles.

Diagnosis

Diagnosis of EBP is usually suspected based on signalment, history, previous positive response to corticosteroids (and absence of or moderate response to other treatments), and clinical signs. Diagnosis must be confirmed before treatment is initiated and relies on identifying a combination of the frequently observed signs of peripheral eosinophilia, characteristic radiographic and bronchoscopic findings, and airway or tissue eosinophilic infiltration as demonstrated by cytologic analysis of BALF or histopathologic examination of bronchial biopsy specimens. Importantly, known causes of eosinophilic infiltration of the lower airways must be excluded and clinical response to corticosteroid therapy demonstrated.

Thoracic radiographs always show diffuse pulmonary lesions of variable intensity with a moderate to severe bronchointerstitial pattern. Peribronchial cuffing, marked thickening of the bronchial walls, alveolar infiltration, and bronchiectasis are other reported findings. Hematologic abnormalities include leukocytosis in up to half of cases, eosinophilia in up to 60%, neutrophilia in about 25%, and basophilia in up to 50% (Clercx et al, 2000). It is important to note that an absence of peripheral eosinophilia does *not* exclude a diagnosis of EBP. Serum biochemistry values are unremarkable.

Bronchoscopy allows observation of macroscopic findings typical of EBP, such as the presence of a moderate to large amount of yellow-green secretions (Figure 163-1), moderate to severe thickening of the bronchial mucosa with an irregular to polypoid aspect, bronchiectasis, and possibly bronchomalacia in chronic cases. Eosinophils constitute the predominant inflammatory cell type seen on BALF smear cytology or brush cytology. Secondary bacterial infection is uncommon but should be recognized and treated promptly before treatment with glucocorticoids is initiated. Histopathologic examination of perendoscopic mucosal bronchial biopsy specimens also can reveal eosinophilic infiltrates.

Occult heartworm disease can be ruled out using heartworm enzyme-linked immunosorbent assays. Fecal zinc sulphate centrifugation-flotation and Baermann's sedimentation test are advised to detect eggs or larvae from most pulmonary parasites. However, a negative result on fecal examination by either method is not conclusive, and therefore it is advised that the animal be treated for potential parasites using a course of an appropriate

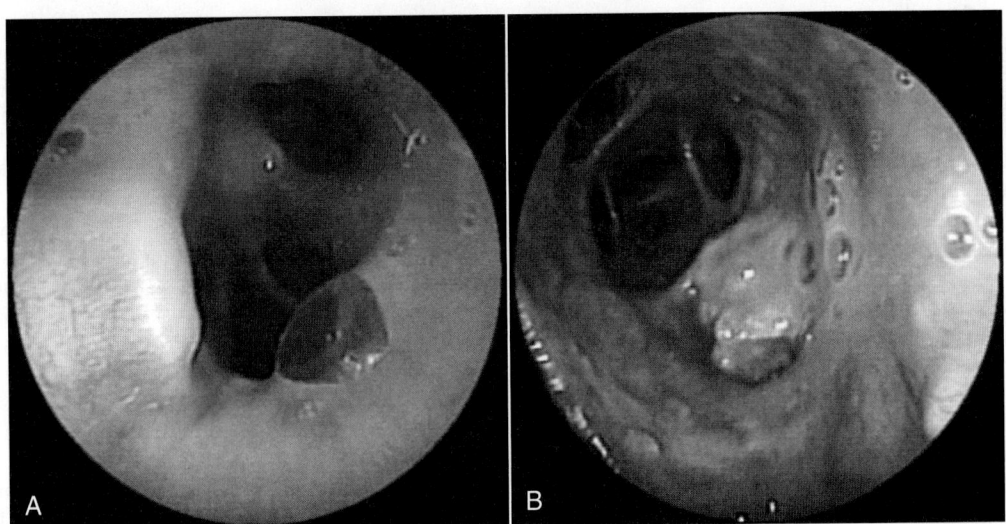

Figure 163-1 Endoscopic view of the bronchi of a 5-year-old female rottweiler with eosinophilic bronchopneumopathy showing a large amount of sticky yellow material **(A)** and bronchiectasis with the presence of almost solid material **(B)**.

antihelmintic (e.g., fenbendazole, thiabendazole, iver-mectin, or levamisole).

Pulmonary function tests are not widely used in veterinary medicine; however, noninvasive pulmonary function tests have been described that do not require patient cooperation and are suitable for clinical purposes, such as tidal breathing flow volume loops and barometric whole body plethysmography. Such tests, combined with a bronchoprovocation challenge, allow noninvasive measurement of airway reactivity in unrestrained, conscious, and spontaneously breathing animals, as well as noninvasive follow-up of the response to treatment. The authors have used barometric whole body plethysmography in some dogs with EBP to demonstrate a decrease in the H-Penh300 index, the concentration of histamine required to increase enhanced pause by 300% (an indirect assessment of airway reactivity), together with return to normal after treatment. Studies of large numbers of affected dogs have not yet been published.

Treatment

Excellent response to oral corticosteroid therapy is generally observed, although adverse effects are frequent. The treatment of choice for canine EBP is methylprednisolone, initiated at a dosage of 0.5 to 1 mg/kg every 12 hours PO during the first week, followed by the same dosage given on alternate days and then by a gradual decrease in dosage until maintenance levels are achieved (approximately 0.125 mg/kg every other day up to 0.5 mg/kg every other day in severe cases). Cough and respiratory difficulty improve within days. Cough totally disappears in most cases, but sometimes still occurs after exercise. Decreased exercise tolerance persists in some dogs, and nasal discharge is sometimes more refractory to steroid treatment. Radiographic and bronchoscopic abnormalities improve, although chronic lesions often persist. Blood eosinophilia and eosinophilic inflammation in BALF or bronchial biopsy samples improve or even resolve.

Response to steroids is often temporary. Within weeks or months after drug discontinuation, most dogs experience relapse, although a limited number do not. Neither time from onset of clinical signs until diagnosis nor age at the time of diagnosis seem to influence the response to treatment. The poorest responses to therapy occur in animals that are treated with repeated abrupt cessation of high doses of medication or with irregular parenteral administration of depository steroid injections.

In most cases, response to oral corticosteroid therapy is considered to be very satisfactory. However, despite a gradual decrease in dosage, some animals still require relatively high doses of glucocorticoids, and weight gain, polyuria, and polydipsia can become intolerable. In other animals, the use of glucocorticoids is contraindicated because of concurrent health problems such as heart failure, diabetes mellitus, or obesity, and alternate therapeutic agents should then be considered.

The use of inhaled medication appears to be promising for control of signs associated with EBP. A study published in 2006 has shown that inhaled corticosteroids can be used successfully for the management of chronic

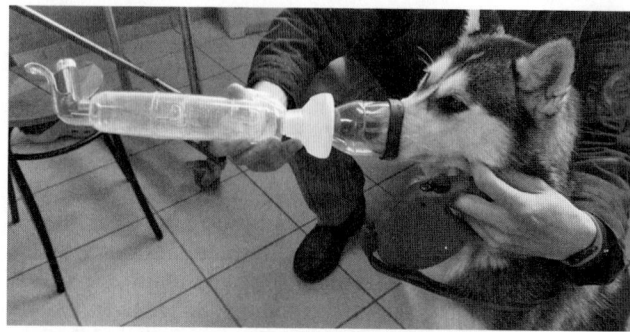

Figure 163-2 Treatment of a dog with eosinophilic bronchopneumopathy using inhaled fluticasone propionate administered twice daily through an aerosol chamber (pediatric model, commercially available) and nasal mask.

bronchitis and EBP in dogs (Bexfield et al, 2006). In the authors' experience, inhaled therapy with fluticasone propionate, administered at a dosage of 220 μg (and 110 μg in small breeds) twice daily through an aerosol chamber and nasal mask (AeroDawg) (Figure 163-2), is well tolerated by dogs. It results in excellent improvement in clinical signs and reduction in adverse effects in most cases with minimal endocrine or systemic immunologic effects (Cohn et al, 2008). In a small percentage of cases, clinical signs persist and combined oral and inhaled steroid therapy allows a reduction in the oral dosage. However, further prospective studies are warranted in larger numbers of animals to define optimum treatment protocols and investigate potential adverse effects.

In severe cases, treatment with a steroid can be initiated using a short-acting injection of steroid at the time the dog recovers from anesthesia (required for bronchoscopy and bronchoalveolar lavage), followed by oral or nebulized steroids. Injections of long-acting (repositol) steroids are not recommended because these drugs do not allow adequate long-term management.

Antibiotics are not required even when the initial high dose of steroids is used, unless significant secondary bacterial infection is documented by clinical signs (fever, lethargy), alveolar pattern on thoracic radiographs, and the presence of intracellular bacteria on cytologic examination of BALF. In these cases, administration of broad-spectrum antibiotics, such as amoxicillin/clavulanate, is advised during the first 2 to 4 weeks of treatment.

There is rarely a need for additional therapy such as bronchodilators or mucolytic agents because steroids are effective in rapidly reducing excess mucus and because active bronchoconstriction is not a common feature of eosinophilic pulmonary disease in dogs compared with cats.

As stated earlier, the role of aeroallergens in EBP is still unclear. Hyposensitization does not appear to be a treatment of choice, and dogs with EBP probably would require concomitant glucocorticoid therapy if such therapy were attempted. However, in rare cases hyposensitization has been used after positive results on an intradermal skin test and has led to clinical improvement (McKiernan, n.d.).

Cyclosporine, a cyclic oligopeptide macrolide that possesses immunomodulating properties, is a drug that has been used successfully in the treatment of canine atopic dermatitis. Although no clinical trials are available in canine EBP, the authors have successfully used oral cyclosporine (Atopica, 5 mg/kg q24h PO) to control clinical signs and decrease airway reactivity (as shown by barometric whole body plethysmography).

The recent advances in molecular biology that have enhanced the understanding of the mechanisms by which eosinophils are recruited to the lungs also have led to the discovery of potential new drug targets. New therapeutic strategies based on the use of immunomodulatory substances are being investigated in humans with bronchial asthma and in murine models of the disease. These strategies include (1) suppression of the effects of specific interleukins, like interleukin 5 or interleukin 13; (2) interference with CC chemokine receptor type 3 (the main receptor involved in the recruitment of eosinophils); and (3) the use of CpG oligodeoxynucleotides that modulate the inflammatory reaction toward a T_H1-type response. To the authors' knowledge, none of these novel therapies has been used in canine EBP. Given the remarkable efficacy of oral and inhaled corticosteroids in the treatment of EBP, potential future new therapies will need to be proven rigorously to be superior to corticosteroids before a change in standard practice is advised.

References and Suggested Reading

Bexfield NH et al: Management of 13 cases of canine respiratory disease using inhaled corticosteroids, *J Small Anim Pract* 47:377, 2006.

Clercx C et al: Eosinophilic bronchopneumopathy in dogs, *J Vet Intern Med* 14:282, 2000.

Clercx C et al: An immunologic investigation of canine eosinophilic bronchopneumopathy, *J Vet Intern Med* 16:229, 2002.

Cohn LA, DeClue AE, Reneiro CR: Endocrine and immunologic effects of inhaled fluticasone in healthy dogs, *J Vet Intern Med* 22:37, 2008.

McKiernan BC: Personal observation.

Peeters D et al: Real-time RT-PCR quantification of mRNA encoding cytokines, CC chemokines and CCR3 in bronchial biopsies from dogs with eosinophilic bronchopneumopathy, *Vet Immunol Immunopathol* 110:65, 2006.

Rajamaki MM et al: Clinical findings, bronchoalveolar lavage fluid cytology and matrix metalloproteinase-2 and -9 in canine pulmonary eosinophilia, *Vet J* 163:168, 2002.

CHAPTER 164

Pleural Effusion

DAVID HOLT, *Philadelphia, Pennsylvania*
LORI S. WADDELL, *Philadelphia, Pennsylvania*

Pleural effusion is a pathologic accumulation of fluid within the pleural space. The volume of the effusion may be scant and mainly of diagnostic significance or so large as to create a life-threatening situation. Pleural effusions are a common cause of respiratory distress in dogs and cats. These disorders call for an organized diagnostic approach and often demand prompt therapeutic measures. This chapter begins with an overview of pleural effusions in dogs and cats that considers the general causes, differential diagnosis, diagnostic approach, and initial treatment. Specific types of pleural effusions are considered next. Finally, the diagnostic and management approaches appropriate for patients with pyothorax or chylothorax are discussed.

Overview of Pleural Effusions in Dogs and Cats

A wide variety of diseases result in accumulation of fluid in the pleural space and cause respiratory compromise as expansion of the lungs is diminished. The underlying cause generally determines the prognosis and management. But first, the condition must be recognized in the patient and a sample of pleural fluid obtained for analysis. At that point, the pleural effusion can be classified into one of several primary *categories* (Table 164-1) based on the gross appearance, protein content, specific gravity, total nucleated cell count, and cytologic characteristics of the cells. Additionally, aerobic and anaerobic cultures may be indicated. Analysis of biochemical characteristics of the fluid, especially the triglyceride and cholesterol levels, is indicated if the effusion is suspected to be chylous (these values should be compared with serum levels). By identifying the type of effusion present, potential causes and the *differential diagnoses* for the effusion can be generated (Box 164-1).

In dogs, common disease processes that cause pleural effusions include pyothorax, pericardial effusion, cranial mediastinal mass, chylothorax, metastatic neoplasia in the pulmonary parenchyma, and dilated cardiomyopathy. In cats, the most common underlying diseases associated with pleural effusion are pyothorax, mediastinal

TABLE 164-1

Characterization of Pleural Effusions

Fluid Type	Total Protein	Total Nucleated Cell Count
Pure transudate	<2.5 mg/dl	<1500/μl
Modified transudate	2.5-7.5 mg/dl	1000-7000/μl
Exudate	>3.0 mg/dl	>7000/μl

BOX 164-1

Causes of Pleural Effusion

Transudates
Pure transudate
   Hypoalbuminemia
Modified transudate
   Heart disease
   Neoplasia
   Pericardial effusion
   Diaphragmatic hernia
   Systemic inflammatory
      response syndrome
      (SIRS)

Hemorrhagic Effusion
Trauma/iatrogenic
Coagulopathy
Neoplasia
Lung lobe torsion

Neoplastic Effusion
Lymphoma
Mesothelioma
Carcinoma
Sarcoma

Nonseptic Exudates
Feline infectious peritonitis
Neoplasia

Septic Exudates
Pyothorax

Chylous Effusion
Idiopathic
Neoplasia
Heart disease
Heartworm
Lung lobe torsion
Trauma

lymphoma, heart disease, and feline infectious peritonitis (FIP).

Bilateral pleural effusion is most common in dogs and cats because the mediastinum is functionally incomplete. Unilateral effusion may be encountered, is more common in cats than in dogs, and typically is associated with inflammatory processes. This point is clinically important because it is often assumed that drainage of one hemithorax also provides drainage of the other side, but this is not always the case.

Clinical Signs of Pleural Effusion

Respiratory signs caused by pleural effusion are all secondary to reduced lung expansion (and tidal volume), which initially results in rapid, shallow breathing. An asynchronous respiratory pattern also can be seen, and respiratory difficulty often is characterized by increased abdominal effort. Ultimately, the animal may exhibit an orthopneic position with the elbows abducted and neck extended to minimize resistance to breathing. If hypoxia

becomes severe, mucous membranes can become pale or even cyanotic.

Thoracic auscultation reveals that lung and heart sounds diminish ventrally but are often still present dorsally. The degree of respiratory compromise is generally proportional to both the volume of fluid within the pleural cavity and the rate of accumulation. Fluid that accumulates gradually may reach a larger volume before producing clinical signs. Once a certain volume is exceeded, critical respiratory compromise exists, and rapid decompensation can occur if the patient is not handled extremely cautiously. Other signs and physical examination findings, depending on the cause and associated clinical complications, may include coughing, pyrexia, depression, anorexia, weight loss, arrhythmias, murmurs, jugular venous distension, and ascites.

Diagnostic Tests in Patients with Pleural Effusion

Patients with pleural effusion usually are affected by a serious to life-threatening disease and should be assessed carefully. A typical workup includes a complete blood count and serum biochemical profile as well as other tests relevant to the clinical situation. These may include urinalysis, viral testing in cats (feline leukemia virus, feline immunodeficiency virus), and specific tests for infectious diseases when appropriate. Advanced evaluations such as flow cytometry or thoracoscopy may be required to identify an elusive neoplastic process.

Diagnostic imaging is a critical part of the evaluation. Thoracic radiography should be delayed until the patient's condition has been stabilized, usually after thoracocentesis. Additionally, the underlying cause of a pleural effusion may become obvious after thoracocentesis. Thoracic ultrasonography and computed tomography (CT) can be used to identify mass lesions in the pulmonary parenchyma or mediastinum when radiographs yield negative results. Echocardiography may be indicated to evaluate the heart and pericardial space. If metastatic or multicentric neoplasia is suspected, abdominal ultrasonographic examination of organs and regional lymph nodes should be considered.

Thoracocentesis and pleural fluid analysis are indicated when physical examination raises suspicion of a significant pleural effusion or when pleural fluid is identified following thoracic radiography. As mentioned previously, analysis of a fluid sample is pivotal to the differential diagnosis. The gross appearance of pleural effusions can vary, ranging from clear to opaque; from translucent to flocculent; and from straw colored to yellow, milky, sanguineous, or red. Effusions of different causes, including those due to chylothorax and pyothorax, can contain red blood cells that create a pink to red fluid coloration; the underlying cause cannot be determined without microscopic and biochemical evaluations. If the effusion is caused by a septic process, it is often thick and opaque and may be malodorous. Evaluation of fluid samples should include cell count, measurement of total protein level, cytologic examination, and culture. Cytologic evaluation should identify the predominant cell type as well as any inflammatory, reactive, or neoplastic cells. When neutrophils are present these should be inspected for degenerative or toxic changes as well as for intracellular and extracellular bacteria. Special stains may be needed to identify chylomicrons. Additional aspects of the diagnostic workup for pyothorax and chylothorax are considered later.

Initial Management of Pleural Effusion

Recognition of the patient in respiratory distress is essential. Oxygen supplementation should be provided while the physical examination is performed. Placement of an intravenous catheter is beneficial, if tolerated by the patient, to allow for sedation if needed (see later) and provide immediate vascular access if the patient experiences respiratory or cardiovascular arrest while being handled. If pleural effusion is strongly suspected based on auscultation of the chest, thoracocentesis should be performed for both diagnosis and stabilization. Thoracic radiography is not necessary and may pose a significant risk to the patient. If ultrasonography is available, a quick scan of the chest can confirm the presence and location of the effusion to facilitate thoracocentesis. Thoracocentesis helps stabilize the patient's condition and provides a sample of the fluid for diagnostic evaluation (see the following section on the thoracocentesis procedure).

Radiography or ultrasonography can be used after thoracocentesis to document successful evacuation of the pleural cavity. Radiographs may show an underlying cause that would have been obscured by the presence of fluid and collapse of the lung lobes before thoracocentesis. Ultrasonographic examination may reveal mass lesions or evidence of pericardial or cardiac disease.

If an animal remains in significant respiratory distress after successful aspiration of pleural fluid, concurrent heart or lung disease should be suspected (e.g., neoplasia, pulmonary contusions, pulmonary edema, or pneumonia). Fibrosing pleuritis or iatrogenic pneumothorax also should be considered.

The patient's cardiovascular system should be assessed to determine whether any treatment is necessary to stabilize cardiovascular parameters. This may include administration of a bolus of intravenous fluids if hypovolemic or septic shock is present, or administration of diuretics if the patient has volume overload from congestive heart failure.

Procedure for Thoracocentesis

Performing thoracocentesis is an essential skill because thoracocentesis can be both therapeutic and diagnostic for patients with pleural space disease. Equipment needed includes clippers, surgical scrub, large syringe (10 to 60 ml), three-way stopcock, extension tubing and needle or butterfly catheter, collection bowl, and tubes for samples, including one with ethylenediaminetetraacetic acid (EDTA) and one without anticoagulant. A short over-the-needle catheter can be used to reduce the risk of laceration of the lung or blood vessels, although these catheters can kink once the stylet is removed, which negates any benefits they may carry. Sedation that spares the cardiovascular system may be needed depending on

the stability of the patient's condition and the patient's temperament. A combination of an opioid and a benzodiazepine (e.g., butorphanol 0.1 to 0.3 mg/kg IV and diazepam 0.1 to 0.3 mg/kg) often is sufficient. Oxygen supplementation should be provided if the patient is in respiratory distress. With an assistant restraining the animal (preferably in sternal recumbency or standing), the appropriate rib space should be clipped and aseptically prepared. When pleural fluid is expected, use of the seventh or eighth intercostal space is recommended, at approximately the costochondral junction. Sterile gloves should be worn for insertion of the appropriately sized needle or butterfly catheter. For medium to large dogs a 1- or 1.5-inch needle may be required to penetrate the chest wall, whereas a $7/8$-inch butterfly needle is sufficient for most cats and small dogs. The needle tip should be placed just cranial to the rib to avoid intercostal blood vessels and nerves that are located caudally and should be inserted gently into the thorax perpendicular to the chest wall with the bevel of the needle pointing up while the hub of the needle and extension tubing are carefully observed for any signs of fluid. In cats with pleural effusion caused by heart failure, care must be taken to avoid puncturing a dilated left auricle, which often extends toward the left thoracic wall. Once the pleural space has been punctured, the needle can be directed ventrally so that the needle is almost parallel to the chest wall.

If a small amount of frank blood is suddenly and unexpectedly aspirated from the thorax, or if the lungs can be felt rubbing against the tip of the needle, the procedure should be stopped and the needle removed and replaced at a slightly different location. If a large amount of blood is withdrawn from the thorax, 1 to 2 ml should be placed in a red-topped tube to see if the blood clots. Blood from a hemothorax should not clot within the tube, whereas blood from the heart or a blood vessel will clot normally, provided there is no significant concurrent coagulopathy. If any other type of fluid is seen in the hub of the needle, aspiration should continue until no more fluid can be removed. If the patient will tolerate it, the needle can be directed ventrally while the patient is rolled slightly to the side on which thoracocentesis is being performed, and reaspirating from a more ventral location can facilitate removal of as much fluid as possible.

Complications of Thoracocentesis

Potential complications of thoracocentesis include iatrogenic pneumothorax from lung laceration, cardiac tamponade from cardiac laceration and bleeding, intrathoracic hemorrhage from laceration of blood vessels, and reexpansion pulmonary edema in situations of chronic pleural effusion. Severe pneumothorax after thoracocentesis is much more common in patients with severe chronic pulmonary disease or inflammatory pleural effusions. Acute death from the stress of restraint is also possible. Appropriate sedation may reduce these risks, but care should be taken to choose drugs with minimal respiratory suppression, as mentioned earlier. After thoracocentesis, the patient should be monitored for recurrence of respiratory distress, which might indicate return of fluid to the pleural space or development of an iatrogenic pneumothorax or hemothorax (less common).

Types of Pleural Effusions

Once a pleural effusion has been identified and sampled, the fluid typically is classified based on physical, cytologic, and chemical characteristics. Although there is some overlap among these categorizations, this organizational approach facilitates diagnosis.

Transudates

Transudates are the result of a disturbance in the overall balance of capillary hydrostatic pressure, intravascular colloid osmotic pressure, and vascular endothelial permeability, which are responsible for the formation of fluid in the pleural space and the rate of pleural fluid absorption. A decrease in absorption can occur secondary to inflammation of the pleura, obstruction of the pleural lymphatics with neoplasia or emboli, or lymphatic hypertension.

A pure transudate can be seen in severe hypoalbuminemia, which results in decreased intravascular oncotic pressure. Usually the albumin level must be less than 1.5 g/dl to result in pure transudate formation. Hypoalbuminemia may be caused by a protein-losing enteropathy or nephropathy, hepatic disease, or marked loss of inflammatory fluid through a wound or into a body cavity. Animals with hypoalbuminemia also may have ascites or peripheral edema.

Cardiac disease can affect the formation and absorption of fluid in the pleural space by increasing pulmonary and systemic capillary hydrostatic pressures. Systemic venous hypertension resulting from right-sided and bilateral congestive heart failure may result in accumulation of pleural transudate and is accompanied by other signs of cardiac disease. Cats can develop pleural effusion with right- or left-sided congestive heart failure. The fluid that is seen with heart disease typically is a modified transudate (slightly higher protein level than a pure transudate), but in some cats a chylous effusion is identified.

Lung lobe torsion or a diaphragmatic rupture can obstruct venous and lymphatic drainage, resulting in leakage of variable types of fluid through the organ capsule into the pleural space; one such fluid is a modified transudate, sometimes with a prominent number of red blood cells. Lung lobe torsion is not common in dogs, although Afghan hounds appear to be predisposed. Lung lobe torsion develops as a primary entity, particularly in deep-chested dogs, but also occurs as a consequence of pleural effusion in any breed. It is often difficult to determine whether pleural effusion or lung lobe torsion occurred first, and underlying causes for pleural effusion should be ruled out. Lung lobe torsion has been associated with trauma, chylothorax, pulmonary neoplasia, respiratory disease, and thoracic surgery. The right middle lung lobe followed by the right cranial lung lobe are most frequently affected. Radiography after pleural drainage usually reveals diffuse consolidation of a lung lobe, a vesicular gas pattern in the affected lung lobe, and possibly altered orientation or abrupt termination of the lobar bronchi. Lung lobe torsion requires immediate surgical treatment to remove the affected lung lobe.

Neoplasia can cause a modified transudate, particularly if it is not exfoliating into the effusion. Obstruction of lymphatic drainage is the most common way that neoplasia leads to this type of effusion. Systemic inflammatory response syndrome can cause a modified transudate pleural effusion due to increased endothelial permeability.

Hemorrhagic Effusions

A hemorrhagic effusion appears grossly bloody, does not clot, and has a packed cell volume and total protein level similar to those of peripheral blood. A major cause of hemorrhage into the pleural cavity is thoracic trauma resulting in fractured ribs or pulmonary parenchymal lacerations. A small amount of hemorrhage is common after thoracic surgery, but it can be marked if an intercostal vessel has been lacerated. An intrathoracic tumor or a coagulopathy (e.g., anticoagulant rodenticide toxicity) also can result in spontaneous hemorrhage into the pleural cavity.

Depending on the severity of blood loss, animals may require supportive treatment with fluid therapy and possibly a blood transfusion. Animals that have anticoagulant rodenticide toxicity also require treatment with vitamin K_1 (5 mg/kg SC initially, followed by 2.5 mg/kg q12h or 5 mg/kg q24h PO for 4 to 6 weeks) and active clotting factors from fresh whole blood or fresh frozen plasma (see Chapter 31). The coagulation profile should be reassessed within 1 to 3 days of therapy to confirm return to normal values. Maintenance of a normal coagulation profile after vitamin K_1 treatment has been discontinued for 2 to 3 days ensures that treatment has been adequate.

Neoplastic Effusions

Primary and metastatic thoracic neoplasia produces a variety of pleural effusions by a number of different mechanisms. These include inflammation of the pleura, hemorrhage into the space, and obstruction of lymphatic drainage. These effusions typically can be classified as a transudate, exudate, or hemorrhagic effusion. Cytologic examination reveals neoplastic cells in only approximately 50% of animals with a neoplastic pleural effusion; therefore absence of neoplastic cells on cytologic evaluation does *not* rule out neoplastic disease. Mediastinal lymphosarcoma may exfoliate lymphoblasts into pleural fluid. Mesothelioma (neoplasia of the pleura) usually is characterized by a severe pleural effusion and also may affect the pericardium, causing a pericardial effusion. It is particularly difficult to differentiate reactive from malignant mesothelial cells on cytologic examination (this usually requires analysis by a specialist in cytology). Biopsy of the pleura is indicated in these cases and can be performed via thoracoscopy or exploratory thoracotomy. A modified transudate may be seen in neoplasia, which makes diagnosis of the cause of effusion challenging. Advanced imaging of the chest including thoracic ultrasonography or CT can be helpful and should be done before surgical exploration is considered.

Nonseptic Exudates

Nonseptic exudates are characterized by high protein levels and high nucleated cell counts, without the presence of bacteria. A major cause of this type of effusion in cats is FIP, and both pleural and peritoneal effusions often occur in this condition. A diagnosis of FIP is strongly supported by the finding of a globulin concentration of more than 32% of the total protein concentration in the effusion. Positive results on immunocytochemical assay or polymerase chain reaction testing of thoracic fluid can contribute to the suspicion of FIP; however, the criteria for definitive diagnosis are controversial. If the albumin component is more than 48% or the albumin:globulin ratio of the effusion is more than 0.81, FIP is unlikely (Lappin, 1998). Serum hyperproteinemia, with or without hypoalbuminemia, is also a common finding. FIP also can cause a modified transudate pleural effusion.

Septic Exudates

Pyothorax is characterized by the accumulation of a septic purulent fluid within the pleural space. It has been described in both dogs and cats but is more common in cats. Bacteria typically are visualized cytologically both intracellularly and extracellularly in pleural fluid, and mixed populations of bacteria often are cultured from the fluid in cats and dogs. The causes, pathogenesis, and management of pyothorax are described in more detail later in this chapter.

Chylous Effusions

Chylothorax is the accumulation of lymphatic fluid in the pleural space that leaks from the thoracic duct system. Thoracic duct fluid has three main sources: lymph from the intestines (chyle), lymph of hepatic origin, and lymph from the hindquarters. The term *chyle* refers to lymphatic fluid drained from the intestines that has a high fat content, which gives chylous fluid its milky appearance. This fat is mainly in the form of chylomicrons, which are aggregates of triglycerides, phospholipid, lipoprotein, and cholesterol formed in the intestinal epithelial cells from fats that have been digested and absorbed. In addition to chylomicrons, thoracic duct lymph contains fluid and proteins similar in type and concentration to those of plasma. The thoracic duct system provides a major pathway for the return of fluid and protein from the interstitial space to the circulation. The proteins, including albumin and the various globulins, are important in the maintenance of normal colloid osmotic pressure and immune function and in the transport of protein-bound hormones and drugs. Thoracic duct lymph also contains electrolytes and trace minerals. The main cellular component of lymph is the small lymphocyte; however, chronic chylothorax can lead to a significant neutrophilic reaction, especially in cats. The causes, pathogenesis, and management of chylothorax are described in more detail at the end of this chapter.

Pyothorax

The cause of pyothorax in cats is most commonly bite wounds to the chest or environmental contamination from penetrating thoracic injuries. Other possibilities are rupture or perforation of the esophagus, trachea, or bronchi; migrating foreign bodies (grass awns) or lung parasites; bacterial pneumonia leading to lung abscesses and rupture; and iatrogenic contamination from thoracocentesis or thoracotomy. The most common bacterial isolates from cats with pyothorax are the anaerobes *Peptostreptococcus, Bacteroides, Fusobacterium,* and *Prevotella* and the aerobes *Pasteurella* and *Actinomyces* (Walker et al, 2000).

In dogs, reported causes of pyothorax include penetrating wounds to the chest, neck, or mediastinum; esophageal perforations; lung parasites; bacterial pneumonia with abscessation and rupture; hematogenous or lymphatic spread from other septic foci; spread from cervical or lumbar discospondylitis; neoplasia with secondary abscessation; iatrogenic contamination from thoracocentesis or thoracotomy; and migrating foreign bodies such as grass awns. The hunting and working breeds of dogs are overrepresented in most retrospective studies, and aspiration of grass awns and subsequent migration through the respiratory tract are thought to play an important role in the development of pyothorax in these breeds. The most common bacterial isolates from dogs with pyothorax are the anaerobes *Peptostreptococcus, Bacteroides, Fusobacterium,* and *Porphyromonas* and the aerobes *Actinomyces, Pasteurella, Escherichia coli,* and *Streptococcus* (Walker et al, 2000). These bacterial isolates are similar to those identified from cats, with the addition of the enteric *E. coli.*

Once bacterial infection enters the pleural cavity, the release of inflammatory mediators causes increased permeability of the endothelial lining of the pleural capillaries and impairment of lymphatic outflow. This results in accumulation of fluid, protein, and inflammatory cells in the pleural space. Increased protein concentration in the pleural fluid causes increased oncotic pressure, which favors additional fluid movement out of the capillaries and into the pleural space.

Clinical Signs and Physical Examination Findings

Clinical signs in a dog or cat with pyothorax often are delayed for weeks to months after the inciting incident. Penetrating thoracic injuries, such as bite wounds, often are healed by the time respiratory compromise develops, which makes diagnosis of the underlying cause difficult to impossible. Common clinical signs in cats include respiratory difficulty, depression, lethargy, pallor, anorexia, and pain. In dogs, exercise intolerance, labored respirations or panting, reluctance to lie down, anorexia, lethargy, and cough are common. Clinical presentation can vary widely, from mild respiratory signs to collapse from severe septic shock.

Physical examination findings usually include varying degrees of respiratory distress: increased respiratory effort, tachypnea, dull lung sounds ventrally with harsh sounds dorsally, and orthopnea all may be present. Signs of septic shock, such as hyperthermia or hypothermia, tachycardia (or, in cats, bradycardia), injected or pale mucous membranes, and bounding or weak pulses, may be present. Recent weight loss may be reported by the owner and a poor body condition may be noted. Additional findings include depression and dehydration.

Diagnostic Tests in Pyothorax

Cytologic evaluation of the pleural effusion should identify neutrophils as the predominant cell type, often with degenerative or toxic changes evident. In cases of chronic pyothorax, increased numbers of macrophages and plasma cells, and occasionally sulfur granules, may be seen in the fluid. Septic effusions often contain intracellular and extracellular bacteria (Walker et al, 2000); however, the absence of bacteria does not exclude pyothorax from the differential list, especially if the patient already has been treated with antibiotics. Therefore, when an inflammatory exudate is present, fluid should be submitted for aerobic and anaerobic culture and sensitivity testing.

In cases of septic effusion a marked leukocytosis usually is evident, with or without an increased number of band neutrophils and toxic changes. In severe cases, leukopenia and a degenerative left shift may be found. Anemia may be present owing to chronic disease. Serum chemistry values may be normal or show changes consistent with sepsis, including hypoalbuminemia, hypoglycemia, and increased alanine transaminase and total bilirubin levels; the latter two are consistent with cholestasis. Changes indicating dehydration and hemoconcentration are seen in some patients.

Initial Stabilization

Measures to stabilize the condition of a patient with pyothorax in respiratory distress should include oxygen supplementation, minimization of handling and stress, thoracocentesis, and intravenous catheter placement. Fluid therapy, including shock boluses, may be indicated depending on the patient's cardiovascular status at the time of presentation.

Broad-spectrum antimicrobials active against gram-positive, gram-negative, and anaerobic bacteria are administered until culture and sensitivity results are available. A broad-spectrum approach is appropriate due to the frequency with which dogs and cats are infected with a mixed population of aerobic, facultative, and anaerobic bacteria. Options for antimicrobial coverage include ampicillin (22 mg/kg IV q8h) and enrofloxacin (10 to 15 mg/kg IV q24h) in dogs and ticarcillin/clavulanate (50 mg/kg IV q6h) in cats. Antibiotics are administered intravenously while the patient is in critical condition but can be given orally once the patient's condition has been stabilized. Appropriate antibiotic therapy based on culture and sensitivity results should be continued for several months following discharge from the hospital. Fluid therapy should be continued at maintenance rates or more, depending on the amount of pleural effusion that is produced. Keeping the patient adequately hydrated is essential to maintain the effusion in a consistency that

permits easy aspiration via thoracocentesis or thoracostomy tubes.

Medical Management and Thoracostomy Tube Placement

Drainage of pleural effusion is one of the mainstays of therapy for patients with pyothorax. This can be accomplished by intermittent thoracocentesis or by placement of thoracostomy tubes, with either intermittent aspiration or continuous drainage. Thoracostomy tubes are preferred because they allow for more complete drainage of the thoracic cavity and eliminate the need for the potentially stressful restraint required for multiple thoracocenteses. Thoracostomy tubes are best placed with the patient under general anesthesia, so initial stabilization with fluid therapy and pleural drainage by thoracocentesis should precede anesthesia induction in what can be a very critically ill patient. Bilateral placement of thoracostomy tubes is indicated unless the patient has only unilateral effusion.

Lavage of the thoracic cavity with warm physiologic saline or another balanced electrolyte solutions has been recommended. A dose of 20 ml/kg instilled over 10 to 15 minutes every 6 to 24 hours can be used, but care must be taken to maintain strict aseptic technique so as not to introduce a nosocomial infection resistant to the antimicrobials that the patient is already receiving. Addition of antibiotics or other medications including chymotrypsin, streptokinase, and heparin has been recommended in various reports; however, none of these additives has been evaluated critically, and antibiotic therapy is most useful when administered intravenously. Lavage probably should be limited to those patients in which the pleural effusion is too thick to aspirate through the chest tube and performed at the time of thoracostomy tube placement. This reduces the risks of iatrogenic infection and of introduction of a large volume of fluid into the chest without the ability to retrieve it. The authors do not routinely perform lavage in these patients, and if lavage is used, they do not add any medications to the fluid.

The efficacy of therapy is assessed by decreasing volume of fluid production and by performing a cell count and cytologic examination on pleural fluid daily. Successful treatment is indicated by a reduction in cell count (particularly in neutrophil count) and an absence of intracellular bacteria. At the time that the thoracostomy tube is withdrawn, repeat bacterial culture of pleural effusion should be considered.

In cats, medical treatment that includes thoracostomy tube drainage, intravenous fluids, and intravenous antibiotic therapy usually is successful. If the cat is not responding to medical therapy, or if an obvious surgical lesion such as an abscessed lung lobe or foreign body is identified, surgical intervention is indicated. Failure of medical management can be defined as the inability to aspirate effusion through properly placed and functional thoracostomy tubes or the failure of the effusion to resolve over a reasonable period of time (usually a week). In one study of pyothorax, dogs were shown to have improved outcomes with surgical intervention (Rooney and Monnet, 2002). This probably relates to the more frequent association of pyothorax with foreign body disease in dogs, and the observation that surgery is often considered sooner in this species. However, some recent studies have shown excellent outcome in dogs without surgical intervention (Johnson and Martin, 2007) or failed to support the finding that surgical treatment is superior to medical management (Boothe et al, 2010).

Surgical Treatment

Surgical treatment of pyothorax requires a complete exploratory thoracotomy. Preoperative CT can be considered to define lung parenchymal abnormalities or foreign bodies. The goal of surgery is to identify and remove any necrotic tissue or foreign material and to allow for complete lavage of the thoracic cavity. Samples for aerobic and anaerobic culture are obtained at surgery. Options for surgical therapy include thoracoscopy, median sternotomy, and occasionally, lateral thoracotomy. Advantages of thoracotomy include the ability to perform full exploration of the thoracic cavity and remove of all exudate from the pleural space with lavage. Disadvantages include increased cost, longer hospital stay, and pain associated with the procedure.

Median sternotomy allows full evaluation of the right and left hemithoraces. The lungs, pericardium, trachea, mediastinum, pleural surfaces, and lymph nodes can be evaluated for signs of abscessation, bleeding, inflammation, or leakage of air. Adhesions of fibrous tissue need to be broken down to allow complete evaluation, especially when a possible foreign body is being sought. Any necrotic, abscessed, or severely inflamed tissue should be resected, including lung lobes, lymph nodes, mediastinum, and pericardium. A lateral thoracotomy is indicated only if the inflammatory process is limited to one hemithorax. Occasionally the origin of a unilateral pyothorax can be isolated to a single abscessed lung lobe or a foreign body, in which case a lateral thoracotomy may be preferred. Even with surgical exploration of the thoracic cavity, the underlying cause of pyothorax often is not identified. Thoracostomy tubes, either unilateral or bilateral as indicated, should be placed at the time of the surgery.

Postoperatively, these patients require intensive care and monitoring, especially for the first 24 to 48 hours after surgery. Septic shock and systemic inflammatory response syndrome can develop. Fluid therapy in the postoperative phase is very important and often consists of crystalloids, colloids, and blood products. Vasopressors may be needed to treat refractory hypotension once volume expansion has been accomplished. Respiratory, acid-base, and electrolyte abnormalities should be evaluated and treated, as needed. These patients are at high risk of the development of disseminated intravascular coagulation, and coagulation parameters must be monitored closely. A complete blood count and cytologic evaluation of pleural effusion should be performed daily.

Prognosis

A poor prognosis and frequent recurrence have been reported in cats and dogs with pyothorax. Many patients may be euthanized based on these reports and because of owners' financial constraints, which perpetuates the poor prognosis. For cats and dogs that receive aggressive and appropriate medical and surgical therapy, the survival rate is more than 50%, with a recurrence rate of less than 5% to 10% (Rooney and Monnet, 2002; Waddell et al, 2002). Many of the patients with pyothorax that do not survive either die naturally or are euthanized within the first 24 hours of presentation; the survival rate increases significantly for patients that are alive 24 hours after admission (Waddell et al, 2002).

Chylothorax

The accumulation of chyle within the pleural space usually indicates an abnormality of lymphatic drainage in the thoracic duct. Given the variable anatomy found in dogs and cats in both the number and location of lymphatic vessels, *thoracic duct system* is probably a more appropriate term for these structures. Chyle can be relatively irritating to pleural surfaces, especially in the cat, so that secondary inflammation and thickening of the parietal, visceral, and mediastinal pleura may develop.

Chyle is normally drained into the systemic venous system via the thoracic duct. In dogs, the thoracic duct system generally begins its course on the right side of the mediastinum dorsal to the aorta. In a study of 20 dogs (Birchard et al, 1982), only 1 dog had a single vessel in the caudal mediastinum, 5 dogs had two collateral vessels, and 14 dogs had three or more vessels. Most of the collateral vessels were in close relationship to one another. However, in some dogs, portions of the vessel system crossed the midline in widely distinct areas (over three vertebral spaces). In the cranial mediastinum, the thoracic duct system terminates as a single lymphatic vessel at the junction of the jugular and brachiocephalic veins with the cranial vena cava. Other dogs have multiple lymphatic vessels that send some terminal branches to mediastinal lymph nodes.

In the normal cat, the thoracic duct system consists of a single duct on the left side of the caudal mediastinum. In the middle of the mediastinum there are multiple ducts in a vast majority of cats. The thoracic duct system terminates at the jugulosubclavian angle, the left external jugular vein, or the brachiocephalic vein. These variations in anatomy have important implications for the surgical approach when thoracic duct ligation is considered.

Causes of Chylothorax

Chylothorax remains an enigmatic disease in many dogs and cats because of the difficulty in identifying a specific cause and defining an effective treatment. Congenital cases have been described, but these are rare. In the majority of dogs and cats, chylothorax is associated with dilation of lymphatic vessels (lymphangiectasia) and leakage from the thoracic duct lymphatic system. Experimentally, thoracic duct system lymphangiectasia and leakage can be produced by ligating the cranial vena cava close to the right atrium, so conditions that increase pressure in the cranial vena cava have the potential to cause chylothorax (Fossum and Birchard, 1986). Thoracic duct system lymphangiectasia and leakage also can occur secondary to physical obstruction caused by neoplasia. Hence chylothorax has been associated with heart disease (including congenital conditions, heart base tumors, and cardiomyopathies—especially in cats), mediastinal lymphosarcoma or thymoma, foreign body or fungal granulomas, heartworm disease, and cranial vena caval thrombosis. Chylothorax also can occur in association with more generalized lymphatic abnormalities such as intestinal lymphangiectasia and lymphangioleiomatosis. Previously many cases of chylothorax were thought to be traumatic in origin, with chylous fluid leaking from a ruptured thoracic duct system. However, many affected animals had no history of major trauma, and experimentally the thoracic duct system in normal dogs heals rapidly after deliberate transection (Hodges et al, 1993).

Recently the role of pericardial diseases in chylothorax has received attention. Restriction of the right atrium or right ventricle by a restrictive or effusive pericardial disease can increase pressure in the cranial vena cava and theoretically can contribute to development or maintenance of chylothorax. Although there are many dogs with significant pericardial effusions that have no associated chylothorax, pericardectomy is reported to be an effective treatment for chylothorax in many cases, perhaps because inflammatory pericarditis or mediastinitis—induced by a chylous effusion—increases systemic venous pressures and restricts lymphatic drainage.

Similarly, the cause-and-effect association between lung lobe torsion and chylothorax remains unclear. Some authors list lung lobe torsion as a potential cause of chylothorax. Although torsion of the right middle lung lobe could be argued to cause obstruction of or increased pressure in the thoracic duct system, it is equally possible that chylous effusion floats and mobilizes the right middle lung lobe, facilitating torsion. Regardless of these arguments, it is important for veterinarians to realize that these two conditions can occur simultaneously.

In many cases, search for a disease underlying chylothorax yields no definitive answer. These cases are then classified as idiopathic. In some of these "idiopathic" cases an identifiable underlying cause eventually may be revealed, such as microscopic neoplasia obstructing the thoracic duct system that is undetectable without a surgical or postmortem biopsy. In spite of these frustrations, the investigation for underlying causes is important when an animal's prognosis and treatment are being considered. Identification of an underlying cause, such as heart failure or cranial mediastinal lymphosarcoma, suggests that medical treatment may resolve the chylothorax without the need for surgery. In idiopathic cases, the clinician is left to treat the consequences of the disease (i.e., the chylous pleural effusion) rather than its root cause.

Clinical Signs and Physical Examination Findings

Chylothorax can affect any breed of dog or cat. However, Afghan hound and shiba inu dogs and Asian breeds of cats such as Himalayan and Siamese may be predisposed. Presentation to a veterinarian is usually precipitated by either respiratory abnormalities associated with chylous effusion or persistent coughing. Coughing may be due to airway compression by pleural effusion or may be caused by a disease process underlying the chylothorax, such as cardiomyopathy or thoracic neoplasia, or potentially pleural irritation. Other clinical signs include anorexia, lethargy, and weight loss.

Physical examination findings usually include an increased respiratory rate and variably muffled lung and heart sounds. Jugular venous pressure may be increased. Although this is not specific for heart failure, it does indicate a need to rule it out. Poor body condition may reflect debilitation associated with the loss of fats and proteins into the pleural space.

Thoracic radiographs should be taken unless positioning the animal causes worsening respiratory difficulty. In these instances, a thoracocentesis is performed before radiography as both a diagnostic and a therapeutic measure. Orthogonal lateral radiographs of the thorax provide better evaluation of right and left lung fields. Dorsoventral positioning is less stressful for the animal than ventrodorsal positioning. Radiographs often show only nonspecific signs of pleural effusion such as rounding of the lung margins, interlobar fissure lines, and separation of the lungs from the thoracic wall. Conditions underlying chylothorax may be visible on thoracic radiographs, depending on the severity of pleural effusion. Caudal displacement of the cardiac silhouette and widening of the cranial mediastinum may indicate a mediastinal mass. Enlargement of the cardiac silhouette may indicate pericardial effusion or cardiac disease. Marked consolidation of one lung lobe with a prominent, aberrantly located air bronchogram is suggestive of lung lobe torsion. Lung lobes that have a persistent shrunken, rounded appearance, even after removal of pleural effusion, may be affected by fibrosing pleuritis, in which scarring and contraction of the visceral pleura occurs in response to chronic pleural effusion.

Ultrasonography is another useful tool for evaluating the heart and mediastinum for diseases that can cause chylothorax. Echocardiography is especially important in cats because heart failure represents the second or third most common cause of chylothorax in this species in some centers. A moderate amount of fluid in the pleural space provides an acoustic window and allows optimal evaluation of thoracic structures with ultrasonography. In many instances, masses can be biopsied or aspirated with ultrasonographic guidance, providing material for a definitive diagnosis. Ultrasonography also can be used to evaluate the hilus of a suspected lung lobe torsion and the cranial vena cava for evidence of thrombosis, although this vessel is more difficult to assess along its entire length.

Thoracocentesis is performed to relieve respiratory distress and to obtain fluid for analysis. Fluid from thoracocentesis is placed in an EDTA tube. A fluid analysis (including cell count) is performed and fluid triglyceride levels are determined. Chylous effusions are generally opaque and either white or pink. Redder effusions should raise concern for lung lobe torsion. The specific gravity of chylous effusions ranges from 1.022 to 1.027 in dogs and from 1.019 to 1.050 in cats. Total protein concentrations range from 2.5 to 6.2 g/dl in dogs and 2.6 to 10 g/dl in cats. The total nucleated cell count is usually less than 10,000 white blood cells/µl in both species. Although the predominant cell is typically the small lymphocyte, secondary inflammation (especially in cats) can lead to a marked neutrophilic reaction that can be confused with an inflammatory pleuritis. Chylothorax is diagnosed by evaluation of pleural fluid triglyceride levels. In true chylothorax, the concentration of pleural fluid triglycerides is higher than that of serum triglycerides. In one study, all dogs with pleural fluid triglycerides at a concentration of more than 100 mg/dl had chylothorax (Waddle and Giger, 1990). This pleural fluid–serum concentration difference usually is marked (tenfold difference or greater) unless the affected animal is anorexic, in which case pleural triglyceride levels can drop toward those of serum levels.

Medical Management

Treatment should be aimed at any identifiable disease causing chylothorax. Successful management of the underlying disease may lead to resolution of the chylothorax, although this can take several months and intermittent thoracocentesis may be required. Experimentally, no diet has been shown to reduce the volume of chyle transported in the thoracic duct system, although a diet of homemade boiled tuna and rice resulted in lower thoracic duct fat content than either low- or high-fat commercial diets (Sikkema et al, 1993). Benzopyrones have been given to animals with chylothorax in the hope of improving macrophage function and increasing chyle reabsorption from the pleural space. Although chylous pleural effusion has resolved in some treated animals, it is not clear if this is due to the benzopyrone treatment or represents spontaneous resolution of the disease. The benzopyrone rutin has been administered to animals at dosages ranging from 50 to 100 mg/kg three times daily.

Supportive care of animals with chylothorax involves correcting dehydration and electrolyte imbalances. Nutritional support should be considered in anorexic, severely malnourished animals and can be provided by a nasoesophageal, esophageal, or gastric feeding tube. Enteral nutritional support is a two-edged sword because it will invariably increase the thoracic duct lymph flow, and this in turn may necessitate more frequent thoracocentesis or even chest tube placement.

Surgical Treatment

Surgery is indicated to obtain biopsy samples to confirm underlying disease, to remove nonlymphomatous mediastinal masses or torsed lung lobes, and to treat the majority of cases that are *idiopathic* and have not responded to conservative therapy. Anecdotally, many surgeons feel that fibrosing pleuritis is a contraindication to surgical treatment of chylothorax, and preoperative radiographs, ultrasonographic scans, or CT images should be evaluated carefully for signs of this condition. Given the wide range of surgical procedures described and the limited number of large studies evaluating these techniques, it is difficult to provide indications for selecting one technique over

another in individual cases. Surgery for chylothorax usually is a referral procedure and should be performed by individuals with the appropriate training and experience to achieve the best outcomes.

Thoracic duct ligation has been the mainstay of surgical chylothorax treatment for many years. After thoracic duct ligation, new lymphatic-to-venous anastomoses form in the abdominal cavity to transport lymph to the venous system while bypassing the thoracic duct system. Successful thoracic duct ligation can resolve chylothorax completely; however, in 20% to 50% of dogs and 50% to 80% of cats, either chylothorax or a serosanguineous pleural effusion persists after surgery (Birchard et al, 1988; Kerpsak et al, 1994). Reasons for failure of surgical treatment include failure to visualize and ligate branches of the thoracic duct system during surgery and persistence of the underlying disease.

Omentalization
Placing omentum in the thoracic cavity and removing the pericardium are additional procedures tried initially when thoracic duct ligation failed to resolve chylothorax. Both of these procedures are now used as primary surgical treatments for chylothorax, either in combination with each other or combined with thoracic duct ligation. The omentum has a substantial blood and lymphatic supply and classically has been used to help seal and repair intestinal surgical sites in dogs and cats. The omentum is thought either to act as a physiologic drain when placed into the thoracic cavity to treat chylothorax or to assist in sealing the leaking thoracic duct system. The physiologic drain theory is difficult to support logically because the omental lymphatics drain back into the thoracic duct system.

Pericardectomy
As mentioned in the section on causes of chylothorax, primary pericardial disease or pericardial (or mediastinal) thickening in response to chronic chylous effusion potentially elevates vena caval pressures and contributes to chylothorax in some cases. In one small series thoracic duct ligation and pericardiectomy resulted in an 80% positive response rate in cats with idiopathic chylothorax (Fossum et al, 2004). The authors have seen several canine cases in which a biopsy specimen from a thickened pericardium removed to treat persistent chylothorax revealed microscopic carcinoma.

Pleuroperitoneal Shunting
The technique of pleuroperitoneal shunting has been used to treat chylothorax when thoracic duct ligation has failed. In this technique, a commercially available shunt catheter is implanted, and the owner pumps pleural fluid into the peritoneal cavity. After surgery the pump chamber is pumped 100 to 200 times every 4 to 6 hours initially. Potential complications include dislodgment and flipping of the pump chamber, and obstruction of the pump chamber with fibrin.

Pleural Port Placement
An alternative procedure for drainage of chylous effusion that cannot be resolved with surgery is the placement of

a subcutaneous pleural port with an intrapleural tube that allows the veterinarian or the owner to aspirate fluid periodically from the pleural space using a Huber needle to access the subcutaneous port. These ports are used more commonly in patients requiring frequent anesthesia (e.g., for radiation therapy) but have been applied successfully to treat cats and dogs with recurrent pleural effusions (Brooks and Hardie, 2011).

References and Suggested Reading

Birchard SJ, Cantwell MD, Bright RM: Lymphangiography and ligation of the canine thoracic duct: a study in normal dogs and three dogs with chylothorax, *J Am Anim Hosp Assoc* 18:769, 1982.

Birchard SJ, Smeak DD, Fossum TW: Results of thoracic duct ligation in 15 dogs with chylothorax, *J Am Vet Med Assoc* 19:68, 1988.

Boothe HW et al: Evaluation of outcomes in dogs treated for pyothorax: 46 cases (1983-2001), *J Am Vet Med Assoc* 236:657, 2010.

Brooks AC, Hardie RJ: Use of the pleural port device for management of pleural effusion in six dogs and four cats, *Vet Surg* 40:935, 2011.

Fossum TW et al: Severe bilateral fibrosing pleuritis associated with chronic chylothorax in five cats and two dogs, *J Am Vet Med Assoc* 201:317, 1992.

Fossum TW et al: Thoracic duct ligation and pericardectomy for treatment of idiopathic chylothorax, *J Vet Intern Med* 18:307, 2004.

Fossum TW, Birchard SJ: Lymphangiographic evaluation of experimentally induced chylothorax after ligation of the cranial vena cava in dogs, *Am J Vet Res* 47:967, 1986.

Hodges CC, Fossum TW, Evering W: Evaluation of thoracic duct healing after experimental laceration and transection, *Vet Surg* 22:431, 1993.

Johnson MS, Martin MWS: Successful medical treatment of 15 dogs with pyothorax, *J Small Anim Pract* 48:12, 2007.

Kerpsak SJ, McLoughlin MA, Birchard SJ: Evaluation of mesenteric lymphangiography and thoracic duct ligation in cats with chylothorax: 19 cases (1987-1992), *J Am Vet Med Assoc* 205:711, 1994.

Lappin MR: Polysystemic viral diseases. In Nelson R, Couto G, editors: *Small animal internal medicine*, ed 2, St Louis, 1998, Mosby, p 1290.

Neath PJ, Brockman DJ, King LG: Lung lobe torsion in dogs: 22 cases (1981-1999), *J Am Vet Med Assoc* 217:1041, 2000.

Rooney MB, Monnet E: Medical and surgical treatment of pyothorax in dogs: 26 cases (1991-2001), *J Am Vet Med Assoc* 221:86, 2002.

Sikkema DA et al: Effect of dietary fat on triglyceride and fatty acid composition of thoracic duct lymph in dogs, *Vet Surg* 22:398, 1993.

Smeak DD et al: Treatment of chronic pleural effusion with pleuroperitoneal (Denver) shunts: 14 dogs (1985-1999), *J Am Vet Med Assoc* 219:1590, 2001.

Waddell LS, Brady CA, Drobatz KJ: Risk factors, prognostic indicators, and outcome of pyothorax in cats: 48 cases (1982-1999), *J Am Vet Med Assoc* 221:819, 2002.

Waddle JR, Giger U: Lipoprotein electrophoresis differentiation of chylous and nonchylous pleural effusions in dogs and cats and its correlation with pleural effusion triglyceride concentration, *Vet Clin Pathol* 19:80, 1990.

Walker AL, Jang SS, Hirsch DC: Bacteria associated with pyothorax of dogs and cats: 98 cases (1989-1998), *J Am Vet Med Assoc* 216:359, 2000.

CHAPTER **165**

Pneumothorax

ELIZABETH A. ROZANSKI, *North Grafton, Massachusetts*
ERIN MOONEY, *Melbourne, Australia*

Pneumothorax is defined as free air in the pleural space. Normal intrapleural pressure is approximately −5 cm H_2O, which means that, in the healthy dog or cat, intrapleural pressure is negative compared with the atmosphere. This negative intrathoracic pressure helps to maintain lung expansion and promote venous return. Normal intrapleural pressure varies depending on the phase of respiration, with inspiration associated with more negative pressure during spontaneous breathing. Pneumothorax develops when there is either leakage of air from damaged or diseased pulmonary parenchyma or external damage to the thoracic cavity resulting in the entrance of air into the chest cavity from the atmosphere.

Clinical signs of pneumothorax include a short and shallow ("restrictive") breathing pattern and absent lung sounds on thoracic auscultation. Diagnosis of pneumothorax may be confirmed with thoracic radiographs (Figure 165-1) or by a positive thoracocentesis. Computed tomography (CT) will also highlight pneumothorax (Figure 165-2). In emergency practice, limited ultrasonography of the thoracic cavity (thoracic focused assessment with sonography for trauma [T-FAST]) also has been used to detect pneumothorax in dogs and cats with suspected traumatic pneumothorax (Lisciandro, 2008). Pneumothorax can be characterized as traumatic, spontaneous, or iatrogenic, and as open or closed (Pawloski and Broaddus,

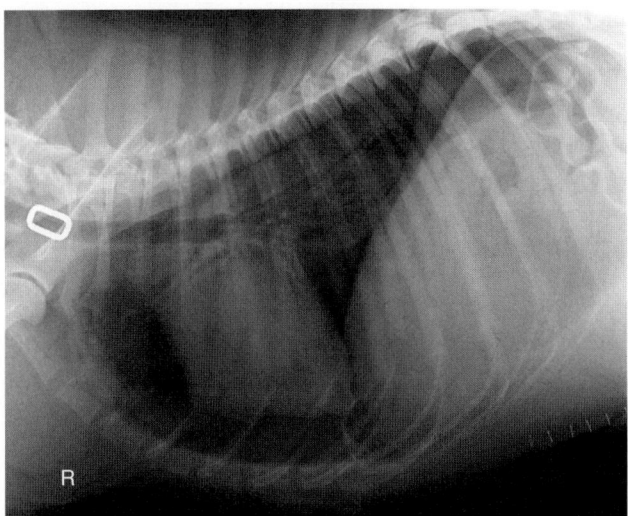

Figure 165-1 Lateral thoracic radiograph documenting pneumothorax in a dog. Note apparent "lifting" of the heart off of the sternum and retraction of the dorsal lung fields.

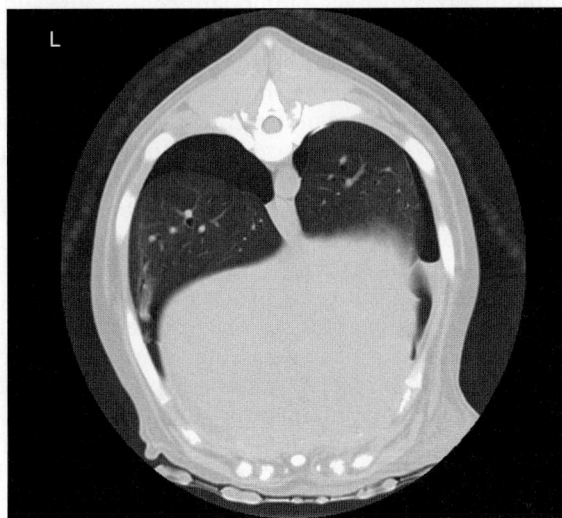

Figure 165-2 Computed tomographic image of spontaneous pneumothorax in a dog showing retraction of the lung from the rib cage on the left and pleural air accumulation.

2010). A tension pneumothorax can result from any type of pneumothorax, although it is usually closed. It is characterized by a barrel-shaped (hyperinflated) appearance to the chest cavity with limited thoracic motion despite vigorous movements of the head and neck in an attempt to ventilate, and by hypoxemia and cardiovascular collapse caused by continued entrapment of air within the pleural space due to lack of an escape pathway.

Therapeutic Options for Treatment of Pneumothorax

The recommendations for management of pneumothorax differ based on the cause. Simple supportive care is adequate in some cases, whereas other cases benefit from more aggressive medical or surgical therapy including placement of a thoracostomy (chest) tube. However, it is important to remember that clinically significant pneumothorax may develop even if a chest tube is in place, and if there is any doubt as to the patency of the chest tube, a new tube should be placed or needle thoracocentesis performed in a patient showing new or progressive respiratory distress.

Observation

Observation is appropriate for the animal with a small-volume pneumothorax of known cause detected radiographically that is not showing clinical signs or evidence of progression, because small volumes of air will be reabsorbed across the pleural space over a period of a few days to a week. However, ideally, animals with pneumothorax should be observed continuously for the first 24 to 36 hours.

Supplemental Oxygen

Oxygen therapy has been proposed as a method to hasten the resolution of pneumothorax. For animals breathing room air, the major component of pleural air is nitrogen gas (78%) and a much smaller proportion is oxygen (21%). Thus, if supplemental oxygen is provided to a patient, the relative partial pressure of nitrogen decreases in the surrounding tissues, and nitrogen is reabsorbed more quickly. Regardless, if pneumothorax is causing clinical signs, the clinician should evacuate the pleural space rather than relying solely on oxygen therapy.

Needle Thoracocentesis

Pneumothorax can be treated by evacuation using a syringe, extension set, and needle or butterfly catheter. Intravenous catheters also may be used in place of a needle and have the advantage of limiting the potential for iatrogenic trauma, but slightly more technical acumen is required to use them effectively. Needle thoracocentesis is a good first-line approach for most cases of pneumothorax. Recall that the mediastinum in small animals typically is not intact, and although bilateral chest tap may be performed, there is not a clinical concern regarding the volume of air withdrawn from each hemithorax. Caveats include the need to make sure the needle is long enough to reach the pleural space as well as the need to recognize that, if there is a large volume of intrapleural air, needle thoracocentesis may be insufficient to allow rapid recovery of ventilation. Classically, needle thoracocentesis for removal of air is performed more dorsally on the chest wall; however, in severe cases air can be retrieved from any location.

Small-Bore Chest Tube

A small-bore chest tube has been introduced in recent years as a modification of a jugular catheter (MILA chest tube). These catheters (14 gauge [6.3 Fr]) are placed readily using a modified Seldinger technique and can be secured easily in an awake patient. They are proving particularly popular in patients with moderately large-volume pneumothoraces, and their use appears to be more comfortable than placement of standard large-bore chest tubes or intermittent thoracocentesis. Small-bore chest tubes are less effective when continuous suction is required because generation of continuous negative pressure (–15 to –25 cm H_2O) appears to collapse the chest tube. Sterile red rubber feeding catheters also are recruited occasionally for use as chest tubes. These are an acceptable alternative, although they typically require general anesthesia or heavy sedation combined with local analgesia for placement because of the need to tunnel the catheter under the skin. A thoracic radiograph should be taken after placement of a small-bore chest tube to ensure adequate location in the thorax.

Large-Bore Chest Tube

Large-bore chest tubes (20 to 36 Fr) are placed when larger-volume pneumothoraces are present or when continuous suction is chosen as a therapeutic modality. Large-bore chest tubes typically are inserted under general anesthesia in all but the most severely compromised patients, although occasionally clinicians prefer placement using local anesthetics. As with small-bore chest tubes, thoracic radiographs should be obtained after placement of a large-bore chest tube to confirm proper positioning.

Heimlich Valves

Heimlich valves are one-way valve devices that attach to large-bore thoracostomy tubes. They are used very commonly in people and large animals such as horses. In cats and in dogs weighing less than 20 kg Heimlich valves are potentially less effective because of limited intrathoracic pressure changes. However, a recent report describes successful use of Heimlich valves in 34 dogs (Salci et al, 2009), and their use should be considered, particularly when continuous-suction units are not available. Each Heimlich valve costs approximately $30 USD. A potential problem with valves is that blood or other fluid sometimes can collect in the valve. This can lead to clogging and malfunction of the device. Patients with Heimlich values should be closely monitored.

Continuous-Suction Units

Continuous-suction units are used for treatment of large ongoing fluid or airway leaks and have the advantage of keeping the lung inflated, which assists in healing. Continuous-suction units require a source of continuous suction from a central or local suction device and provide negative pressure underwater seal set to the clinician's preference, typically –15 to –25 cm H_2O. The units are relatively expensive (approximately $120 USD).

Thoracotomy

In severe cases of ongoing pneumothorax or in cases of spontaneous pneumothorax in dogs, exploratory thoracotomy may be pursued to resect diseased lung and to explore the chest cavity for evidence of other pathologic processes. Although thoracotomy is considered the method of choice for spontaneous pneumothorax, there are issues associated with this treatment approach. These include the need for general anesthesia and positive pressure ventilation in an animal with an already damaged lung as well as difficulty in identifying the optimal site for the thoracotomy incision (relative to the putative pulmonary tear). Often a sternotomy is advocated to approach both lungs, but this procedure is best reserved for those with experience in thoracic surgery and the related complications.

Characteristics of Specific Causes of Pneumothorax

Traumatic pneumothorax results from injury to the chest. It may be further categorized as *open* when there is a wound connecting the chest cavity and the outside air, and as *closed* when air leak is from damaged lung parenchyma. Traumatic pneumothorax is considered the most common type of pneumothorax in dogs and probably also in cats. Management of traumatic pneumothorax depends on clinical signs. Many pets with traumatic pneumothorax also have pulmonary contusions, and it may be challenging to determine which specific cause of respiratory distress is contributing most to clinical signs. Dogs are thought to experience thoracic trauma more commonly than cats; the most frequent causes are impact by a car (e.g., road traffic accidents) and bite wounds. Identification of traumatic pneumothorax tends to occur in one of two ways. In the first the pet is brought in for treatment shortly after a traumatic event and is clearly very short of breath, with orthopnea and anxiety. In this case, rapid thoracocentesis with immediate resolution of pneumothorax is optimal both diagnostically and therapeutically. In the second case, in which emergent thoracocentesis is not performed, thoracic radiography or T-FAST is useful to document and quantify pneumothorax.

Thoracocentesis should not be undertaken if the pet is not showing signs of respiratory compromise, even in the presence of radiographically apparent pneumothorax. Pleural air will be rapidly reabsorbed, and needle thoracocentesis is not without risk, including hemorrhage or iatrogenic pneumothorax.

Chest tube placement is indicated in traumatic pneumothorax in animals that have severe signs at presentation and marked air leakage (e.g., >1 L with no end point reached) and in animals that have recurrent pneumothorax over the first 24 hours requiring more than three chest taps (the "three strikes" rule). The decision also should reflect the relative comfort level of the hospital staff with management and the clinician's comfort in placing the chest tube. Animals with chest tubes ideally should not be left unattended, and complications associated with placement, although uncommon, certainly are possible. Traumatic pneumothorax associated with blunt trauma (e.g., being hit by car) *rarely* requires surgical intervention to control the air leakage. Dogs or cats with penetrating chest trauma (e.g., bite wounds) may require surgical management to clean infected or devitalized tissues. Traumatized lung lobes will quickly seal and heal if the underlying parenchyma and pleura are normal because of the high tissue thromboplastin content of lung tissue (Osterud et al, 1986). The prognosis for traumatic pneumothorax is good.

Occasionally, dogs and cats with thoracic trauma have flail chest, which is defined as the presence of two or more fractures in three or more ribs. A flail segment is physiologically important because it moves paradoxically during ventilation and is invariably associated with a severe underlying pulmonary contusion. Historical references recommended surgical stabilization of a flail segment; however, more recent evidence suggests that this is not required, and analgesia and time are sufficient to allow adequate ventilation in most cases (Pettiford et al, 2007). However, if the thorax is undergoing exploration for treatment of another injury (e.g., bite wounds), or if severe instability is evident, the ribs can be stabilized surgically.

Spontaneous pneumothorax is pneumothorax that occurs without associated trauma. It is termed *primary* when there is no underlying lung disorder and *secondary* when it is due to lung disease. Spontaneous pneumothorax is most common in dogs, in which rupture of blebs, bullae, or the lesions of bullous emphysema results in primary spontaneous pneumothorax. Northern breeds such as huskies, deep-chested breeds, and possibly golden retrievers appear to be overrepresented among dogs with spontaneous pneumothorax. Clinical signs include restlessness, respiratory distress, and tachypnea. In affected dogs, it is important to distinguish spontaneous pneumothorax from pneumothorax due to an unobserved trauma because the approach to management of these two conditions is very different. Preoperative diagnostics should include three-view chest radiography and baseline laboratory testing. Other testing, such as echocardiography, abdominal ultrasonography, heartworm or lungworm testing, or CT is performed at the discretion of the attending clinician.

Spontaneous pneumothorax in dogs is considered a surgical disease, and prompt surgical intervention is associated with a higher cure rate and shorter duration of hospitalization (Puerto et al, 2002). In cats, it is less clear whether surgery should be pursued immediately because the incidence of spontaneous pneumothorax appears to be far lower in cats than in dogs (Mooney et al, 2012). Surgical exploration is typically via a median sternotomy to allow exploration of both hemithoraces. In some cases, even with an open surgical approach it has been difficult to identify the source of the air leak. In people, inhalation of sterile fluorescein occasionally has been used to try to document the lesion responsible for pleural leakage (Noppen et al, 2004), and this technique may have a role in management of spontaneous pneumothorax in dogs as well.

The usefulness of advanced imaging in the management of spontaneous pneumothorax is a point of controversy, with some clinicians strongly advocating preoperative CT scanning and others advising prompt surgical exploration via a median sternotomy (Au et al, 2006). The potential benefits of CT scanning include identification of a leaking bulla or bleb and exclusion of likely neoplastic disease. The potential disadvantages of CT include the possibility that the leaking site may not be apparent on CT scan because the lesion has ruptured,

the added costs, and additional anesthesia time required. The best answer is unknown, and in our practice, we do not perform CT routinely except when dogs have an atypical signalment or when there are concerns about neoplasia.

Secondary spontaneous pneumothorax can be seen in both dogs and cats and develops without trauma but is associated with preexisting lung disease. It has been reported in dogs secondary to neoplasia, pulmonary thromboembolism, and rarely pneumonia. In cats the most likely cause is thought to be asthma/airway disease or heartworm disease. Accumulation of small volumes of pleural air can be managed conservatively (medically); the presence of large volumes can require chest tube placement; and spontaneous pneumothorax associated with a mass lesion should be treated surgically. The prognosis for spontaneous pneumothorax treated surgically is good in dogs unless it is associated with a tumor. In cats the prognosis is less clear, but spontaneous pneumothorax appears more likely to be due to an underlying disease, and the prognosis reflects that condition.

Iatrogenic pneumothorax is pneumothorax associated with veterinary care. It may be created out of necessity—such as with a thoracotomy, in which case it is self-limiting—but it also may develop following thoracocentesis in a pet with a chronic effusion or in association with positive pressure ventilation. Pneumothorax arises in these pets because of damage to the pleural tissues covering the lung. In normal animals, the pleura are thin and will seal rapidly if punctured. However, if the pleura are thickened because of a chronic high-protein effusion (classically chylous effusion), there is a much greater chance of damage to the pleura that will not be self-sealing. Chronic effusions either can be identified clinically from the medical history or can be suspected if the lungs appear rounded on radiographs (Figure 165-3).

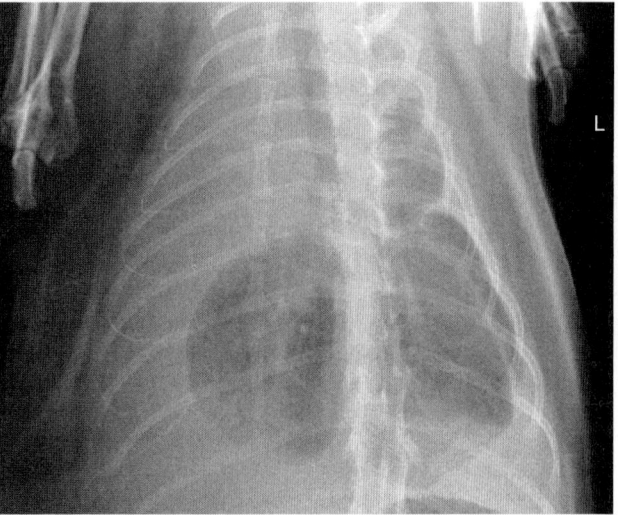

Figure 165-3 Thoracic radiograph showing chylous effusion in a cat. Note the rounded lung borders (most notably in the region of the right caudal lung lobe), which raise concern about the possibility of an iatrogenic pneumothorax following thoracocentesis.

Iatrogenic pneumothorax also is observed in dogs and cats being treated with intermittent positive pressure ventilation and particularly in dogs undergoing ventilation at high tidal volumes and/or high airway pressures. If possible, the plateau pressure should be kept at less than 35 cm H_2O, but the critical care veterinarian should always be vigilant for the possibility of pneumothorax and promptly intervene if desaturation occurs. Treatment of iatrogenic pneumothorax can be very challenging because the preexisting chronic effusion may make the surgical management unappealing for the client and risky for the patient, may limit the likelihood of successful resolution, and, in animals with ventilator-associated pneumothorax, may decrease the chances of successful therapy.

Autologous Blood Patching—
An Emerging Technique?

Blood patching or *pleurodesis* refers to the instillation of autologous fresh whole blood into the pleural space in an attempt to stop air leak from the pulmonary parenchyma. The mechanism by which this is successful is debated; most likely coagulated blood "plugs" the site of air leak rather than inducing a true pleurodesis (Rinaldi et al, 2009). This concept is supported by the rapid resolution of pneumothorax reported in many studies, typically with minimal to no complications. The major benefits are that the technique is painless, inexpensive, and easy to perform, and that the patient's blood is readily available.

The published literature on this topic in veterinary medicine currently is limited to one case report of the use of a blood patch in a 15-kg dog with persistent pneumothorax after surgery for chronic diaphragmatic hernia (Merbl et al, 2010). This dog had been managed with a thoracostomy tube and continuous suction for 4 days. Eighty milliliters of whole blood was instilled through the thoracostomy tube and the pneumothorax resolved immediately.

The most common complication of blood patching seen in humans is pyothorax. Iatrogenic tension pneumothorax due to blood clotting in the thoracostomy tube also is possible. To limit these complications, the blood always must be collected from the patient in a sterile fashion, the blood must be transferred immediately through the largest-bore thoracic catheter possible, and the catheter then must be flushed with sterile saline. Further investigation of blood patching in dogs and cats is warranted.

References and Suggested Reading

Au JJ et al: Use of computed tomography for evaluation of lung lesions associated with spontaneous pneumothorax in dogs: 12 cases (1999-2002), *J Am Vet Med Assoc* 228(5):733, 2006.

Lisciandro GR: Abdominal and thoracic focused assessment with sonography for trauma, triage, and monitoring in small animals, *J Vet Emerg Crit Care* 21(2):104, 2008.

Merbl Y et al: Resolution of persistent pneumothorax by use of blood pleurodesis in a dog after surgical correction of a diaphragmatic hernia, *J Am Vet Med Assoc* 237(3):299, 2010.

Mooney E et al: Spontaneous pneumothorax in 35 cats (2001-2010), *J Fel Med Surg* 14(6):384, 2012.

Noppen M et al: Fluorescein-enhanced autofluorescence thoracoscopy in primary pneumothorax, *Am J Respir Crit Care Med* 170(6):680, 2004.

Osterud B et al: Thromboplastin content in the vessels of different arteries and organs of rabbits, *Thromb Res* 42(3):323, 1986.

Pawloski DR, Broaddus KD: Pneumothorax: a review, *J Am Anim Hosp Assoc* 46:385, 2010.

Pettiford BL, Luketich JD, Landreneau RJ: The management of flail chest, *Thorac Surg Clin* 17:25, 2007.

Puerto DA et al: Surgical and nonsurgical management of and selected risk factors for spontaneous pneumothorax in dogs: 64 cases (1986-1999), *J Am Vet Med Assoc* 220(11):1670, 2002.

Rinaldi S, Felton T, Bentley A: Blood pleurodesis for the medical management of pneumothorax, *Thorax* 64:258, 2009.

Salci H, Bayram AS, Gorgul OS: Outcomes of Heimlich valve drainage in dogs, *Aust Vet J* 87:148, 2009.

CHAPTER 166

Pulmonary Thromboembolism

SUSAN G. HACKNER, *Stamford, Connecticut*

Pulmonary thromboembolism (PTE) occurs when thrombi that develop in the venous circulation dislodge and become trapped in the pulmonary vasculature. If the degree of obstruction overwhelms compensatory mechanisms, respiratory (and sometimes hemodynamic) compromise ensues. Although the clinical manifestations of PTE may be mild, a seemingly high proportion of patients exhibit significant morbidity or even experience acute death. The prevention and management of PTE is the focus of this chapter. Critical to this therapy is a basic understanding of antithrombotic drugs.

PTE is a common complication of medical illness and surgery in humans, accounting for significant morbidity and over 100,000 deaths annually in the United States. Although less common in small animals, PTE is nevertheless an important clinical entity, and prevalence is highest in certain patient populations. For example, the mortality of canine immune-mediated hemolytic anemia (IMHA) is reportedly 50% to 70%, and PTE may account for up to 60% to 80% of these deaths.

PTE results from an increased thrombotic tendency, termed *thrombophilia*. Thrombophilia arises from some combination of three major mechanisms, as described by Virchow's triad: endothelial injury, blood stasis, and prothrombotic alterations of the hemostatic system (hypercoagulability). The first feature is likely of greater importance in arterial thromboembolic pathophysiology and the latter in venous. Hypercoagulability results from platelet hyperaggregability, deficiencies of natural anticoagulants (antithrombin, protein C), or defective fibrinolysis.

The term *hypercoagulable state* refers to disorders in patients with underlying disease known to be associated with thrombophilia and an increased risk of thrombosis. In animals, these are acquired disorders, and the pathogenesis is generally multifactorial and complex. PTE in dogs is associated with IMHA, protein-losing nephropathy (PLN), neoplasia, necrotizing pancreatitis, hypercortisolism (hyperadrenocorticism and corticosteroid therapy), protein-losing enteropathy (PLE), cardiac disease (dirofilariasis, endocarditis, and cardiomyopathy), diabetes mellitus, sepsis, atherosclerosis, trauma, and major surgical procedures. In canine necropsy studies, 59% and 64% of dogs with PTE had more than one disorder potentially causing hypercoagulability, and many of these dogs also had thrombosis in nonpulmonary organs (LaRue et al, 1990; Johnson et al, 1999). PTE in cats is associated most commonly with neoplasia or cardiomyopathy; other infrequently reported conditions include necrotizing pancreatitis, IMHA, PLN, PLE, hypercortisolism, and

sepsis. In one study, 47% of cats had multiple potentially prothrombotic disease processes (Norris et al, 1999).

The pathophysiologic consequences of PTE and its diagnosis are reviewed in the previous edition of this textbook. This chapter focuses on treatment and prevention of PTE. Unfortunately, it is largely impossible to make evidence-based recommendations regarding the management of PTE in animals because of a lack of sufficient clinical trials in well-defined patient populations. As a result, one is forced to extrapolate from the human literature and leverage the limited information available from veterinary trials, case studies, and anecdotal reports. Thus the reader should be aware that clinical recommendations are based on limited evidence.

Antithrombotic Agents: General Principles

Antithrombotic agents are indicated to prevent thrombosis in patients considered at risk (primary thromboprophylaxis) or to prevent thrombus propagation and recurrence in patients that have experienced a thromboembolic event (secondary thromboprophylaxis). Antiplatelet drugs inhibit platelet aggregation and generally are indicated for the prevention of arterial thromboembolism (e.g., aortic, cerebrovascular), whereas anticoagulants are recommended for the prevention of venous thromboembolism (e.g., PTE). Consequently, in human patients, antiplatelet drugs are used for management of atherosclerosis and arterial thromboembolic risk, whereas anticoagulants are used when the risk of venous thromboembolism is high.

Thromboembolism in animals, however, is less clearly defined. Certainly thrombotic risk in IMHA is almost exclusively venous, whereas the risk with atherosclerosis is almost exclusively arterial. However, most hypercoagulable states in dogs are less predictable and can result in venous or arterial thrombosis. Consequently, the choice of anticoagulant versus antiplatelet drug for primary thromboprophylaxis in animals is less clear. Moreover, an adjunctive role for antiplatelet drugs in venous thromboprophylaxis now is apparent. Selection of antithrombotic therapy also involve issues such as overall thromboembolic risk, the route and anticipated duration of therapy, potential adverse effects (mainly bleeding), owner compliance, and cost.

Treatment of Pulmonary Thromboembolism

Initial treatment of the patient with PTE includes (1) respiratory and cardiovascular support, (2) prevention of thrombus propagation or recurrence (secondary thromboprophylaxis), and, infrequently, (3) thrombolysis. In the normal dog, thrombi begin to lyse spontaneously within hours. Even in patients with disturbed fibrinolysis, some degree of reorganization and lysis occur in the days following the event. If the patient can be supported through the compromise and further thrombosis can be prevented, survival is likely unless ischemic injury to tissues is severe or cannot be managed appropriately. In some cases, however, vascular compromise may be so extreme that thrombolysis is a consideration.

Respiratory and Cardiovascular Support

Oxygen supplementation is indicated when dyspnea is evident or when the arterial partial pressure of oxygen (PaO_2) decreases below 70 mm Hg. In addition to relieving hypoxemia, oxygen supplementation has been shown to dilate pulmonary vessels, reduce pulmonary hypertension, and improve right ventricular function. Perfusion should be optimized because hypoperfusion will further exacerbate already reduced tissue oxygen delivery. Moreover, correction of hypoperfusion reverses prothrombotic effects of vascular stasis and hypoxia-induced endothelial injury. Hyperbaric oxygen therapy has been suggested to have potential value to counteract pulmonary ischemic vasoconstriction, but data from controlled clinical trials still are needed.

Secondary Thromboprophylaxis

Anticoagulation using either intravenous unfractionated heparin (UFH) infusion or subcutaneous low-molecular-weight heparin (LMWH) is the mainstay of initial therapy. Intermittent subcutaneous UFH administration is not recommended for the initial treatment of PTE.

Unfractionated Heparin

The primary mechanism of action of heparin is the potentiation of antithrombin activity, leading to the inactivation of various coagulation factors, most notably thrombin (factor IIa) and factor Xa. The interaction of heparin with antithrombin is mediated by a unique pentasaccharide sequence. UFH is composed of mucopolysaccharides of varying molecular weights. The relative effect of heparin on factors II and X depends on molecular size, and chain lengths exceeding 18 saccharide units are required for the heparin-antithrombin complex to bind with and inhibit thrombin. In contrast, formation of such a large complex is not required for heparin's inhibition of factor Xa. UFH has a ratio of anti-Xa/anti-IIa activity of 1:1. Other effects of heparin include reduced blood viscosity, decreased platelet function, increased vascular permeability, enhanced release of tissue factor pathway inhibitor, and mildly enhanced fibrinolysis. These effects also contribute to the heparin-associated hemorrhagic risk.

The anticoagulant effects of a standard dose of UFH vary widely among patients. Bioavailability after subcutaneous administration is variable and often poor. The plasma clearance of UFH depends on a rapid, dose-related, saturable cellular mechanism and a slower, non–dose-related renal clearance. For this reason, the intensity and duration of effect increase disproportionately with increasing dose. Higher-molecular-weight species are cleared more rapidly than lower-molecular-weight species, which results in varied anticoagulant activity over time. Binding of UFH to plasma proteins, endothelial cells, and platelets contributes to the unpredictable response. Moreover, the concentration of UFH-binding proteins is increased in patients with inflammation, which results in heparin resistance and necessitates the use of higher doses to achieve effective anticoagulation. Because of the markedly variable pharmacokinetic profile of UFH, successful therapy requires monitoring of the anticoagulant response and titration of the dose to the individual patient (Hirsh and Raschke, 2004). It has been shown in human patients that, in the absence of such measures, many patients receive inadequate heparinization, which results in an increased incidence of recurrent thromboembolism.

Anticoagulant response to UFH traditionally is monitored using the partial thromboplastin time (PTT) because point-of-care testing enables practical dose titration. The therapeutic goal in human patients is a PTT of 1.5 to 2.5 times control or pretreatment values. Studies suggest that this goal results in supratherapeutic heparin concentrations in dogs, and a target PTT range of 1.5 to 2.0 times baseline has been suggested. A limitation in the use of the PTT to guide UFH therapy is that this measure is not correlated directly with anticoagulant activity and clinical efficacy, largely because the effect of UFH on PTT reflects primarily its factor IIa inhibition. A more accurate method for monitoring UFH effects is measurement of plasma anti-Xa activity, which has been correlated directly with plasma heparin concentration. However, results of this test are not commonly available for same-day dosage adjustments. It is unclear whether thromboelastography (TEG) will prove useful for guiding UFH therapy. A study in healthy dogs implied that TEG parameters are affected by even low plasma levels of heparin, and thus the test may be too responsive to identify adequate or excessive anticoagulation (Pittman et al, 2010; see Chapter 15).

In human patients, intravenous continuous-rate infusion of UFH using a heparin nomogram has been the traditional standard of care for acute PTE (Hyers et al, 2001). The author uses an extrapolation of this nomogram in dogs (Table 166-1). There are no reports of such an application in cats.

Subcutaneous UFH is not recommended for acute therapy because this route is unreliable in achieving therapeutic ranges rapidly. Even high dosages of UFH (300 U/kg q6h SC) and titration based on PTT or anti-Xa activity failed to result in therapeutic ranges within 48 hours in 10 of 18 dogs with IMHA (Breuhl et al, 2009). Therefore SC UFH should not be used in patients with IMHA suspected of having PTE unless other means of therapy are not feasible.

In cats, UFH at a dosage of 250 U/kg q8h SC commonly is recommended as part of the initial treatment regimen for arterial thromboembolism. A small study in healthy cats demonstrated anti-Xa activity within or above the target range at this dosage, but correlation with PTT results currently is unclear (Alwood et al, 2007).

TABLE **166-1**

Weight-Based Nomogram for the Intravenous Infusion of Heparin in Dogs

Heparin is administered in an intravenous bolus of 80-100 U/kg, followed by a continuous-rate infusion of 18 U/kg/hr.

Partial thromboplastin time (PTT) is evaluated 6 hr after initiation of therapy. Adjustments are as follows:

PTT	Dose Change (U/kg/hr)	Additional Action	Next PTT
<1.2 × mean normal	+4	Readminister bolus of 80 U/kg	6 hr
1.2 to 1.5 × mean normal	+2	Readminister bolus of 40 U/kg	6 hr
1.5 to 2.0 × mean normal	0	0	6 hr for first 24 hr, then daily
2.0 to 3.0 × mean normal	−2	0	6 hr
>3.0 × mean normal	−3	Stop infusion 1 hr	6 hr

Low-Molecular-Weight Heparin

LMWH is derived through depolymerization of UFH to yield smaller molecules. The smaller molecular size translates to higher anti-Xa:anti-IIa ratios (of 2:1 to 4:1). For this reason, anticoagulant effect cannot be monitored by PTT but is assessed by anti-Xa assay. However, favorable bioavailability with subcutaneous administration, a prolonged half-life, reduced plasma protein binding, dose-dependent renal clearance, and predictable antithrombotic responses enable weight-based, once- or twice-daily dosing in humans without the need for routine monitoring except in select populations (patients with renal failure, obese patients). Other advantages of LMWHs include their lesser effects on platelet function and vascular permeability compared with UFH, which possibly account for the fewer hemorrhagic effects noted at comparable antithrombotic dosages. The major disadvantage of LMWH therapy is the cost of the drug, which can be considerable when it is used in long-term situations.

Limited data are available regarding dosing protocols in dogs and cats, and the clinical efficacy or superiority (compared to UFH) of the LMWHs is not yet established. A number of studies in healthy animals have evaluated the pharmacokinetics of dalteparin (Fragmin) and enoxaparin (Lovenox), primarily with respect to anti-Xa activity. In canine studies, dalteparin administered at 150 U/kg SC achieved therapeutic ranges in healthy dogs (Mischke et al, 2001). Pharmacokinetic studies of dalteparin in cats show excellent bioavailability, with peak levels within 2 hours of administration (Alwood et al, 2007). Dalteparin at 100 U/kg SC did not result reliably in peak therapeutic anti-Xa activity, whereas a dose of

200 U/kg was supratherapeutic in some cats. Therefore a dose of 150 U/kg has been recommended, although it has not been investigated fully. A small study in healthy greyhound dogs indicated that enoxaparin at 0.8 mg/kg SC achieved target anti-Xa levels within 4 hours of administration (Lunsford et al, 2009). Enoxaparin at 1.0 mg/kg has been shown to result in appropriate anticoagulation in experiments in cats (Van De Wiele et al, 2010).

The preceding studies showed waning of anti-Xa activity below therapeutic range within 6 to 8 hours. As a result, investigators have recommended more frequent dosing intervals in dogs and cats (every 6 to 8 hours). However, these recommendations are controversial. The therapeutic target in human patients is peak anti-Xa activity of 0.5 to 1.0 U/ml measured at 4 hours; however, it is unlikely that this activity must be maintained, and the minimal effective anti-Xa activity in humans is undetermined. Also, in the feline venous stasis model of Van De Wiele and colleagues (2010), enoxaparin at 1 mg/kg q12h reliably resulted in a measurable antithrombotic effect that persisted well after anti-Xa levels had declined below target range. It is also worth noting that the applicability in other species of therapeutic anti-Xa activity established in humans has not been verified. This complexity underscores the need for clinical trials with outcome measures.

Based on current knowledge, the author uses a starting dosage of dalteparin 150 U/kg q8-12h SC or enoxaparin 1 mg/kg q12h SC in dogs and cats. Peak anti-Xa activity is monitored (4 hours after administration in dogs, and 2 hours after administration in cats) and the dose adjusted until an effective dose is established for that patient. The clinician should be aware that, until the efficacy of LMWH protocols is investigated in animals and dosing regimens are established that avoid the need for anti-Xa testing, initial therapy with LMWHs at the recommended dosages could result in inadequate heparinization.

Thrombolysis

Thrombolytic agents, such as tissue plasminogen activator (t-PA) and streptokinase, are plasminogen activators that augment fibrinolysis. t-PA offers advantages over other agents in that it is more clot specific and, in humans, has proved to be clinically superior in most studies.

The goal of thrombolytic therapy is to restore circulation rapidly in such a way that the procedure is clinically beneficial and the risks of therapy justifiable. The risk of systemic hemorrhage, however, is high. Therefore thrombolysis is reserved for patients with life-threatening thromboembolism that are unlikely to survive without rapid reperfusion and those with persistent thromboembolism that significantly affects organ or tissue function. In human PTE patients, thrombolysis is recommended only for those patients that are in hemodynamically unstable condition or have echocardiographic evidence of right ventricular dysfunction. Contraindications to thrombolysis include active internal bleeding, recent (within 2 to 3 weeks) surgery or organ biopsy, and gastrointestinal ulceration.

The role of thrombolytic agents in animals with PTE remains to be investigated, although a small number of reports describe the use of these agents for arterial thromboembolism. The successful use of t-PA has been reported in a dog with aortic thromboembolism (peripheral administration) and in a dog with vena caval thrombosis (administration at the site of the thrombus). Cats with arterial thromboembolism of recent onset (<6 hours) have been treated both successfully and unsuccessfully with t-PA (see Chapter 181). However, the risk of bleeding and of potentially fatal reperfusion hyperkalemia must be appreciated. Thrombolytic therapy carries an appreciable risk in a patient already in unstable condition, and referral to a specialty facility or consultation with a specialist is advised before such treatment is considered.

Maintenance Therapy

Once the patient's condition has stabilized, initial therapy is transitioned to maintenance thromboprophylaxis in preparation for hospital discharge. Antithrombotic options include LMWHs, intermittent SC UFH, warfarin, and possibly antiplatelet drugs (see later section on primary thromboprophylaxis).

Prevention of Pulmonary Thromboembolism

The mortality rate of animals with PTE is substantial, with some deaths occurring before the diagnosis can be confirmed and effective treatment implemented. Moreover, diagnosis is difficult, and treatment is not universally successful. This makes primary prophylaxis imperative in patients at risk of thromboembolism. Prevention should address all aspects of Virchow's triad. This includes (1) minimizing vascular stasis by maintaining adequate perfusion and mobility, (2) minimizing vascular injury by the appropriate placement and handling of venous catheters, and (3) altering the hemostatic system with antithrombotic drugs. Drugs are indicated when a significant risk of thromboembolism is likely.

Risk Assessment

Determination of thromboembolic risk in veterinary patients is exceedingly difficult. The prevalence of PTE in specific diseases is largely unknown, and there are few laboratory tools to confirm hypercoagulability in a given individual. Risk assessment is largely subjective. The extent of risk might be estimated by consideration of (1) thromboembolic history, (2) laboratory evidence of hypercoagulability, (3) underlying condition, (4) severity of disease, and (5) presence of concomitant prothrombotic conditions.

Undoubtedly the most convincing evidence of risk is a prior thromboembolic episode. Unless the underlying cause has been reversed, risk should be considered substantial, and thromboprophylaxis is indicated.

Laboratory assessment of hypercoagulability is extremely helpful; unfortunately, this is not achieved easily. Low antithrombin concentrations are correlated with risk of embolization, but this measure is useful only in conditions in which antithrombin deficiency is an important mechanism of hypercoagulability (e.g., PLN).

Similarly, hyperfibrinogenemia is prothrombotic but occurs only in a few inflammatory conditions. Of currently available tests, TEG demonstrates the greatest utility for the diagnosis of hypercoagulability in the individual patient (see Chapter 15). The predictive value of TEG in animals, however, has yet to be determined fully. Nevertheless, the presence of hypercoagulability indicates risk in the patient that should inform decisions regarding prophylaxis.

Hypercoagulable states are not equivalent with respect to risk. IMHA carries a high thromboembolic risk (see Chapter 60). Thromboembolism is a major cause of death in affected dogs, and venous thromboemboli are found on necropsy in up to 80% of dogs with IMHA. Risk also should be considered to be significant in patients with PLN, acute necrotizing pancreatitis, and sepsis. The author recommends thromboprophylaxis in each of these conditions.

Risk stratification of patients within certain hypercoagulable states appears to be affected by severity of disease and concomitant risk factors. Patient with severe necrotizing pancreatitis or severe IMHA are at greater risk compared with those with milder forms of these diseases. Risk factors also are cumulative. The patient with a hypercoagulable state may not develop thromboembolism unless it is precipitated by another hypercoagulable state or prothrombotic condition such as surgery, tissue damage, inflammation, hypoperfusion, catheterization, or immobility. For these reasons, PTE is relatively common in critically ill patients. The incidence of venous thromboembolism in human patients in the intensive care unit (ICU) ranges from 10% to 80%, and hypercoagulability was demonstrated in 11 of 27 dogs admitted to an ICU (Wagg et al, 2009). Patients with uncomplicated hyperadrenocorticism or diabetes mellitus appear to have a low incidence of PTE, and the need for prophylactic drugs in these patients is doubtful. Risk increases, however, when another thrombophilic condition occurs in these patients, such as surgery, pancreatitis, or PLN.

Primary Thromboprophylaxis

Anticoagulants
The choice of anticoagulant for PTE prophylaxis depends on the anticipated duration, route of administration, potential adverse effects, cost, and owner compliance. For short-term primary thromboprophylaxis (days to weeks), anticoagulant options are UFH or LMWH. UFH is inexpensive but, in the absence of close monitoring, effective anticoagulation cannot be predicted. LMWHs offer the advantage of less frequent monitoring and less frequent dosing but are considerably more expensive. For long-term thromboprophylaxis (months to years), warfarin can be prescribed, although the advantages of warfarin (oral dosing and low cost) are offset by fluctuating efficacy and a relatively high incidence of bleeding that demands close monitoring. Although LMWHs are an attractive option in animals, cost and route of administration are prohibitive for many owners. Antiplatelet drugs offer numerous theoretical and practical advantages. However, although some antithrombotic efficacy is assured, it is unclear whether the efficacy of antiplatelet

drugs is comparable to that of anticoagulants for venous thromboprophylaxis.

Subcutaneous UFH is indicated for short-term primary thromboprophylaxis. Traditionally, low-fixed-dose UFH (100 to 200 U/kg q8-12h SC) was used in dogs, but without any evidence of efficacy. In human patients, this regimen has been shown to result in a high rate of rethrombosis. In a retrospective study of dogs with IMHA, treatment with low-fixed-dose UFH did not have any positive effect on outcome. Effective anticoagulation is shown with higher doses of UFH. In healthy beagles, a UFH dosage of 250 U/kg q6h SC resulted in sustained therapeutic anti-factor Xa concentrations. Intuitively, one would expect higher dose requirements in patients with inflammatory disease. Indeed, in dogs with IMHA, a UFH dosage of 300 U/kg q6h SC resulted in target-range anti-Xa activity within 48 hours in only 8 of 18 dogs (Breuhl et al, 2009). Moreover, individual responses were extremely varied, which underscores the importance of aggressive and individualized dosage regimens.

Warfarin is used for long-term outpatient thromboprophylaxis. Warfarin is a vitamin K antagonist that alters the synthesis of vitamin K–dependent coagulation factors II, VII, IX, and X as well as the anticoagulant proteins C and S; the resulting factors have greatly reduced or absent activity. The anticoagulant effect of warfarin is not immediate because the newly synthesized inactive coagulation factors must first replace their functional counterparts. During the first 24 to 48 hours of therapy, only proteins with short half-lives, factor VII and protein C, are affected significantly, so that thromboembolic risk is potentiated in the initial days of therapy. For these reasons, heparin therapy should overlap warfarin therapy for at least the first 2 days and until therapeutic levels of warfarin are achieved.

Warfarin is initiated at a dosage of 0.05 to 0.1 mg/kg q24h PO in the dog and the cat. Therapy is monitored via prothrombin time (PT) or international normalization ratio (INR), and the dosage is adjusted to achieve a PT of 1.25 to 1.5 times baseline or an INR of 2.0 to 3.0. A therapeutic range generally is achieved within 5 to 7 days. Advantages of warfarin include oral administration, once-daily dosing, and affordability. However, numerous disadvantages outweigh these benefits. Therapeutic index is low, and pharmacokinetics are influenced by diet, comorbidity, and numerous other drugs. Because of the unpredictable pharmacokinetics and common occurrence of bleeding, strict owner compliance with instructions and close therapeutic drug monitoring are essential.

LMWHs can be used for both short- and long-term thromboprophylaxis. Onset of action is rapid, LMWHs are less associated with hemorrhage than warfarin, and, after the initial establishment of an effective dosage, LMWHs do not require ongoing monitoring (see earlier section on treatment). These benefits contribute to offsetting the costs of these drugs. As previously discussed, effective protocols for LMWH thromboprophylaxis have yet to be validated in small animals. Moreover, even in human patients, for whom therapeutic ranges have been established for secondary thromboprophylaxis, protocols for primary thromboprophylaxis are less clear, and recent trends are toward lower dosages for long-term prevention.

Until further data become available, the author uses the same dosages for primary and secondary prophylaxis.

Antiplatelet Drugs

Over and above the inability to predict venous versus arterial thromboembolism in most hypercoagulable states, there are other compelling reasons to consider a role for antiplatelet drugs in venous thromboprophylaxis. Platelet hyperaggregability has been demonstrated in numerous hypercoagulable states, including IMHA and neoplasia. Moreover, venous thrombi activate platelets, causing the release of agonists that promote bronchoconstriction, vasoconstriction, and pulmonary hypertension; antiplatelet drugs may ameliorate these effects.

Although antiplatelet drugs show efficacy as adjunctive agents for venous thromboprophylaxis in *humans* they are decidedly inferior to anticoagulants and are not recommended as sole therapy. There is clinical evidence of a beneficial effect of antiplatelet drugs in dogs as well. In a retrospective study of dogs with IMHA, improved survival was demonstrated in dogs that received ultra-low-dose aspirin (0.5 mg/kg q24h PO) (Wienkle et al, 2005). Although this effect was not shown to be directly related to thromboprophylaxis, the study did suggest a positive effect of aspirin on outcome. Based on the results of this study, together with the low cost, oral administration, and attractive safety profile of aspirin, ultra-low-dose aspirin has become standard therapy for primary thromboprophylaxis in canine IMHA, a condition associated primarily with venous thromboembolism. However, as in humans, appropriate anticoagulation might provide more benefit than aspirin in dogs at high risk of venous thromboembolism. A small retrospective study of dogs with IMHA showed better survival in dogs that received individually adjusted UFH therapy (7 of 8 dogs survived) than in those that received low-dose aspirin (10 of 25 dogs survived) (Orcutt et al, 2009). Larger prospective, controlled trials are needed to evaluate these antithrombotics, alone or in combination, in various subpopulations.

Aspirin irreversibly inhibits cyclooxygenase (COX) activity, preventing the formation of prostaglandins, including thromboxane A_2 (TXA_2) and prostacyclin (prostaglandin I_2). TXA_2 is produced by platelets, is largely a COX-1–derived product, and induces platelet aggregation. The antiplatelet effect of aspirin is almost immediate and is saturable. Prostacyclin, produced by vascular endothelial cells, is derived from both COX-1 and COX-2 activity and inhibits platelet aggregation. Aspirin is approximately fiftyfold more potent in inhibiting COX-1 than COX-2. Thus antiplatelet therapy with aspirin should use a low dose that inhibits TXA_2 production while sparing prostacyclin. This also limits the adverse gastrointestinal effects of aspirin, which are dose-related.

The ideal antiplatelet dosage of aspirin is unclear. A dosage of 0.5 to 1.0 mg/kg q24h PO generally is recommended. But in spite of the improved outcome demonstrated in Weinkle and colleagues' study of dogs with IMHA, other studies have suggested that even dosages of 1 mg/kg q24h do not reliably inhibit platelet aggregation in healthy dogs (Hoh et al, 2011).

In cats with aortic thromboembolism, there was no statistical difference in outcome or recurrence between the group treated with low-dose aspirin (5 mg per cat q72h PO) and the group treated with aspirin at the traditional dosage (81 mg per cat q72h PO), but significantly fewer cats in the low-dose therapy group experienced adverse effects (22% versus 4%) (Smith et al, 2003). This was a retrospective study encompassing a relatively small numbers of treated cats, however, so the results cannot be viewed as definitive without the accumulation of more data.

Clopidogrel (Plavix) is an alternative to aspirin that inhibits adenosine diphosphate–induced platelet aggregation. Clopidogrel is a prodrug, requiring hepatic metabolism to acquire antiplatelet activity. Onset of action is not immediate; platelet inhibition occurs by 2 days and reaches a steady state after 5 to 7 days. As with aspirin, the platelet defect persists for the life of the platelet.

In healthy dogs, a loading dosage of clopidogrel of 10 mg/kg q24h PO effectively inhibited platelet aggregation within 24 hours, and a subsequent daily dosage of 2 mg/kg q24h PO maintained adequate platelet inhibition (Mellett et al, 2011). This protocol, alone or in combination with low-dose aspirin, was safe and was associated with short-term survival similar to that with aspirin alone in a small group of dogs with IMHA. In cats, clopidogrel is effective *in vitro* in preventing platelet aggregation and was well tolerated when administered long term at 18.75 mg per cat q24h PO, although a small percentage of cats developed mild, self-limiting diarrhea (Hogan et al, 2004).

Duration of Thromboprophylaxis

Prophylaxis is continued until the risk of thromboembolism is considered sufficiently decreased. TEG evaluation might be useful in this regard because it allows global assessment of hypercoagulability. In the absence of TEG, the determination usually is subjective. In patients with short-term reversible causes of a thrombotic state, such as necrotizing pancreatitis or sepsis, thromboprophylaxis usually is discontinued at hospital discharge or within a week thereafter. In patients with IMHA, in which a more sustained, intermediate-term hypercoagulability is expected, the author continues prophylaxis until there is no evidence of ongoing hemolysis and corticosteroid therapy is discontinued or substantially reduced. Heparin therapy is tapered over several days because rebound thrombin generation and hypercoagulability can occur with abrupt cessation of either UFH or LMWH. The use of adjunctive antiplatelet therapy might attenuate this rebound effect. Indefinite thromboprophylaxis is recommended in patients with thromboembolism complicating malignancy or cardiac disease and in patients with ongoing and severe PLN.

References and Suggested Reading

Alwood AJ et al: Anticoagulant effects of low-molecular-weight heparins in healthy cats, *J Vet Intern Med* 21:378, 2007.

Breuhl EL et al: A prospective study of unfractionated heparin therapy in dogs with primary immune-mediated haemolytic anemia, *J Am Anim Hosp Assoc* 45:125, 2009.

Hirsh J, Raschke R: Heparin and low-molecular-weight-heparin: the seventh AACCP conference on antithrombotic and thrombolytic therapy, *Chest* 126:188S, 2004.

Hogan DF et al: Antiplatelet effects and pharmacodynamics of clopidogrel in cats, *J Am Vet Med Assoc* 225:1406, 2004.

Hoh CM et al: Evaluation of the effect of low-dose aspirin administration on urinary thromboxane metabolites in healthy dogs, *Am J Vet Res* 72:1038, 2011.

Hyers TM et al: Antithrombotic therapy for venous thromboembolic disease (sixth ACCP consensus conference on antithrombotic therapy), *Chest* 119:176S, 2001.

Johnson LR et al: Pulmonary thromboembolism in 29 dogs: 1985-1995, *J Vet Intern Med* 13:338, 1999.

LaRue MJ et al: Pulmonary thromboembolism in dogs: 47 cases (1986-1987), *J Am Vet Med Assoc* 197:1368, 1990.

Lunsford KV et al: Pharmacokinetics of subcutaneous low molecular weight heparin (enoxaparin) in dogs, *J Am Anim Hosp Assoc* 45:261, 2009.

Mellett AM, Nakamura RK, Bianco D: A prospective study of clopidogrel therapy in dogs with primary immune-mediated thrombocytopenia, *J Vet Intern Med* 25:71, 2011.

Mischke R et al: Amidolytic heparin activity and values for several hemostatic variables after repeated subcutaneous administration of high doses of a low molecular weight heparin in healthy dogs, *Am J Vet Res* 62:595, 2001.

Norris CR et al: Pulmonary thromboembolism in cats: 29 cases (1987-1997), *J Am Vet Med Assoc* 215:1650, 1999.

Orcutt ES et al: Comparison of individually monitored unfractionated heparin versus low-dose aspirin on survival of dogs with immune-mediated hemolytic anemia, *J Vet Intern Med* 23:692, 2009 (abstract).

Pittman JR, Koenig A, Brainard BM: The effect of unfractionated heparin on thromboelastographic analysis in healthy dogs, *J Vet Emerg Crit Care* 20:216, 2010.

Smith SA et al: Arterial thromboembolism in cats: acute crisis in 127 cases (1992-2001) and long-term management with low dose aspirin in 24 cats, *J Vet Intern Med* 17:73, 2003.

Thompson MF, Scott-Montcrief JC, Hogan DF: Thrombolytic therapy in dogs and cats, *J Vet Emerg Crit Care* 11:111, 2001.

Van De Wiele CM et al: Antithrombotic effect of enoxaparin in clinically healthy cats: a venous stasis model, *J Vet Intern Med* 24:185, 2010.

Wagg CR et al: Thromboelastography of dogs admitted to an intensive care unit, *Vet Clin Pathol* 28:453, 2009.

Weinkle TK et al: Evaluation of prognostic factors, survival rates, and treatment protocols for immune-mediated hemolytic anemia in dogs: 151 cases (1993-2002), *J Am Vet Med Assoc* 26:1869, 2005.

CHAPTER 167

Pulmonary Hypertension

MICHELE BORGARELLI, *Blacksburg, Virginia*

Definition and Classification

Pulmonary hypertension (PH) refers to elevations in pulmonary artery (PA) pressure. The PA pressure depends on flow across the pulmonary circulation (cardiac output) as well as resistance to flow with pressure. Resistance to PA flow can occur at the level of the pulmonary arteries and arterioles, within the alveolar capillary units, and at the levels of the pulmonary veins and left atrium. Thus disorders of the left side of the heart, diffuse diseases of the lung, and pulmonary arterial diseases can lead to PH.

The diagnosis of PH is confirmed by cardiac catheterization in human patients, but in veterinary medicine it is usually defined as an elevated systolic PA pressure as estimated noninvasively by Doppler echocardiography (Figure 167-1). Veterinary publications have used estimated systolic PA pressures of more than 31 mm Hg (up to 45 mm Hg) as indicators of PH. Despite publication of a number of clinical studies and reports, no consensus statements or prospective studies are available to definitively guide diagnosis or management of PH in dogs or cats. It should be noted that healthy dogs, as well as humans and other animal species, can reach much higher values of PA pressure while exercising, and this point certainly is relevant in animals with tachycardia that are undergoing Doppler echocardiographic examination.

PH is a well-recognized condition of dogs and has been described sporadically in cats. A variety of conditions and a spectrum of histopathologic lesions within the pulmonary vasculature lead to PH. Historically PH was classified as primary (idiopathic) or secondary depending on the presence or absence of identifiable causes; however, more recently PH has been classified in relation to pathophysiologic mechanisms, histologic lesions, and therapeutic options. In dogs primary PH is a relatively rare condition. Although specific diseases commonly associated with PH in animals differ from those in humans, similar classifications can be devised (Table 167-1). Analysis of data from different case series encompassing a total of 197 dogs with PH of varying causes showed that the most common identified reason for PH was left-sided heart failure (category 2, 50% of cases). Primary lung disease (category 3) represented the second most common reason for PH (24% of cases). Diseases affecting the pulmonary arteries (pulmonary arterial hypertension, or category 1) were responsible for 10% of cases. Chronic thrombotic or embolic disease (category 4) was the cause of 9% of cases, whereas category 5—a compilation of miscellaneous conditions—was last, accounting for 7% of cases.

The most commonly identified reasons for PH in each category were as follows: heartworm disease and congenital systemic-to-pulmonary shunts for category 1; myxomatous mitral valve disease (MMVD) and dilated cardiomyopathy for category 2; pulmonary interstitial fibrosis, chronic bronchial disease, and tracheal collapse for category 3; heartworm disease and pulmonary thromboembolism for category 4; and neoplasia for category 5 (Bach et al, 2006; Guglielmini et al, 2010; Johnson et al, 1999; Kellum and Stepien, 2007; Pyle et al, 2004).

Diagnosis and Clinical Presentation

Right-sided heart catheterization is considered the gold standard for diagnosis of PH. This technique provides accurate measurements of systolic, diastolic, and mean PA pressures and also can provide information about cardiac output and right ventricular function and filling pressures. However, in veterinary medicine right-sided heart catheterization rarely is performed in routine practice, and PH generally is diagnosed based on the presence of clinical and echocardiographic findings.

Clinical Signs

The presentation of dogs with PH is varied, and in general the severity of clinical signs relates to the severity of PH. Owners most commonly report cough, exercise intolerance, tachypnea or respiratory distress, and syncope. In dogs PH is one of the more common causes of sudden collapse or syncope and should always be considered in such cases, especially when these signs are associated with exertion. Physical examination findings may include tachypnea, abnormal respiratory sounds, ascites from right-sided heart failure, and cyanosis. A prominent jugular pulsation may be evident during careful examination.

Dogs with PH frequently have a systolic murmur; however, in most cases this is caused by mitral or tricuspid regurgitation due to MMVD. One possible exception to this generalization is cases in which a systolic murmur is detected with greatest intensity over the tricuspid valve area; some of these dogs will be found to have PH related to cor pulmonale. Dogs with PH might show other auscultatory findings, including increased intensity or abnormal splitting of the second heart sound, a soft ejection murmur into the PA, and rarely a soft diastolic murmur caused by pulmonic insufficiency.

Diagnostic Tests

Commonly performed diagnostic tests include thoracic imaging, echocardiography (see later), and diagnostic

Figure 167-1 Continuous wave spectral Doppler tracings of a regurgitant tricuspid jet *(left)* and pulmonary insufficiency jet *(right)* in a dog with pulmonary hypertension caused by chronic respiratory disease. The maximum right ventricular to right atrial velocity is 4.2 m/sec and the pressure gradient is 73 mmHg (see text), which suggests severely elevated pulmonary systolic pressure. The maximum pulmonary artery to right ventricular velocity is 2.4 m/sec and the pressure gradient is 23 mmHg, which suggests elevated pulmonary artery diastolic pressure.

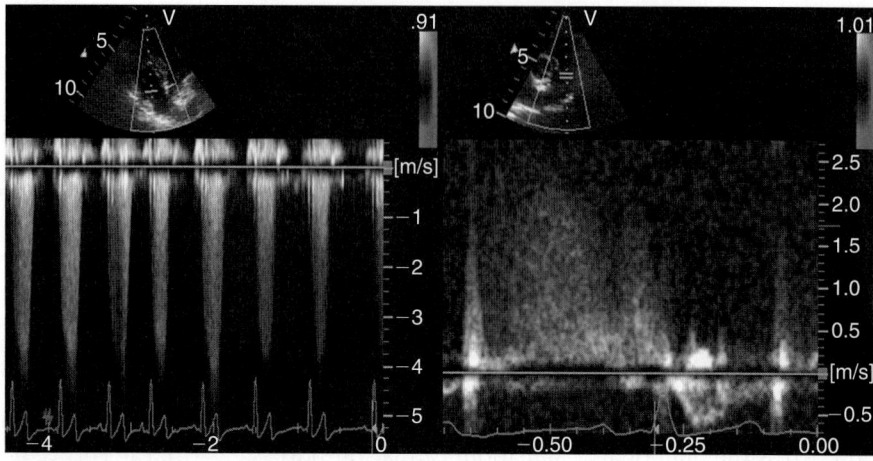

TABLE 167-1

Clinical Classification, Associated Diseases, and Histologic Lesions of Pulmonary Hypertension (PH) in Dogs

Category	Associated Diseases	Histologic Lesions
1. Pulmonary arterial hypertension	Idiopathic PH Familial PH Heartworm disease Congenital systemic-to-pulmonary shunts Collagen vascular disease Drugs or toxins Eisenmenger's syndrome	Pathologic lesions of distal pulmonary arteries Medial hypertrophy Intimal proliferative and fibrotic changes Adventitial thickening with moderate perivascular inflammatory infiltrates Complex lesions (plexiform, dilated lesions) Thrombotic lesions Pulmonary veins are unaffected
2. PH with left-sided heart disease	Myxomatous mitral valve disease Myocardial disease	Enlarged and thickened pulmonary veins Pulmonary capillary dilatation Interstitial edema Alveolar hemorrhage Lymphatic and lymph node enlargement
3. PH associated with lung disease and/or hypoxemia	Chronic obstructive pulmonary disease Interstitial lung disease Sleep-disordered breathing Alveolar hypoventilation disorders Long-term exposure to high altitude Developmental abnormalities	Medial hypertrophy and intimal obstructive proliferation of distal pulmonary arteries Variable degrees of destruction of the vascular bed in emphysematous or fibrotic areas also may be present

4. PH caused by chronic thrombotic or embolic disease	Thromboembolic obstruction of proximal or distal pulmonary arteries
	Nonthrombotic pulmonary embolism
	  Heartworm or other parasitic disease
	  Neoplasia
	  Foreign bodies (catheter, coil, Amplatz canine duct occluder)
		Thromboembolic obstruction:
		  Organized thrombi tightly attached to the pulmonary arterial medial intima
		  Complete occlusion of the lumen or different grades of stenosis
		  Lesions in nonoccluded areas that are histopathologically indistinguishable from those in category 1
		  Collateral vessels from the systemic circulation can grow and reperfuse the areas distal to complete obstruction

5. Miscellaneous	Compression of pulmonary vessels Lymphadenopathy Granulomatous disease Other: sarcoidosis, histiocytosis X, lymphangiomatosis	Different pathologic pictures seen

Adapted from Galiè et al: Guideline for the diagnosis and treatment of pulmonary hypertension, *Eur Respir J* 34:1219, 2009; and Henik RA: Pulmonary hypertension. In Bonagura JD, Twedt DC, editors: *Kirk's current veterinary therapy XIV,* St Louis, 2009, Saunders, p 697.

tests for pulmonary parenchymal diseases or vascular diseases. The latter may include arterial blood gas analysis, cytologic analysis and culture of respiratory secretions, fine-needle aspiration or biopsy of the lung, and routine hematologic testing. Tests for heartworm disease are usually indicated in cases of suspected PH. Diagnostic tests for coagulopathy, such a platelet count, D-dimer level, and thromboelastography (see Chapter 15) may be useful to exclude or support a diagnosis of pulmonary thromboembolism. Echocardiography is usually the diagnostic test of choice for PH and is discussed later.

Thoracic Imaging

The lungs, pulmonary vasculature, mediastinum, and pleural space can be evaluated by combinations of radiography, noncardiac ultrasonography, and computerized tomography. *Thoracic radiographs* are of great importance for assessing the type and severity of underlying thoracic disease but lack sensitivity for the diagnosis of PH. Enlarged and tortuous pulmonary arteries can be observed in more severe cases, particularly in dogs with heartworm disease, but these changes often are subtle and difficult to interpret. Right ventricular enlargement and dilatation of the main pulmonary artery is common in severe PH. Thoracic *computerized tomography* is probably more sensitive for diagnosis of some pulmonary parenchymal diseases and also can be useful for recognition of pulmonary vascular changes and pulmonary thromboembolism.

Electrocardiography

The electrocardiograph (ECG) is important for diagnosing underlying arrhythmias, but findings are not specific. The most commonly observed arrhythmias are pronounced sinus arrhythmia, isolated premature atrial or ventricular contractions, atrial fibrillation, and various degrees of atrioventricular block. Aside from pronounced respiratory sinus arrhythmia, most of these arrhythmias are identified in dogs with concomitant left-sided heart failure or are a consequence of the disease responsible for PH. ECG findings of P pulmonale or right ventricular hypertrophy occasionally can be seen in dogs with moderate to severe PH, but these are found inconsistently. Echocardiography is more sensitive for detection of mild to moderate right-sided heart enlargement and is discussed in the next section.

Doppler Echocardiography

The noninvasive gold standard for the diagnosis of PH in veterinary medicine is Doppler echocardiography (Figures 167-2 and 167-3; see Figure 167-1). This method also can establish the diagnosis of PH due to primary cardiac disease. It should be stressed that the diagnosis of PH in veterinary medicine is based on a combination of clinical and echocardiographic signs, and a single observation or variable cannot be relied upon.

Estimation of Pulmonary Artery Pressure. Provided a jet of tricuspid regurgitation (TR) or pulmonary insufficiency (PI) is present, the simplified Bernoulli equation (pressure gradient = $4 \times V^2$, where V [velocity] is measured in meters per second) can be used to detect and quantify PH. As long as the right ventricular outflow tract is not obstructed, systolic PA pressure and peak right ventricular

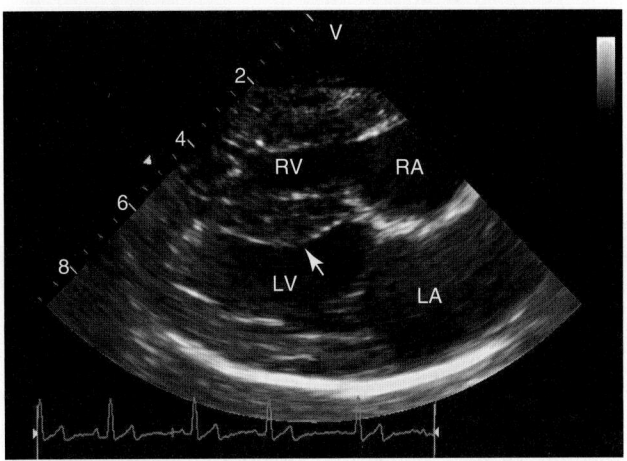

Figure 167-2 Right parasternal four-chamber long axis view in mid-diastole in a dog with severe pulmonary hypertension. A mixed concentric-eccentric hypertrophy pattern of the right ventricle is present. The interventricular septum *(arrow)* bows into the left ventricle, which decreases left ventricular size. *LA,* Left atrium; *LV,* left ventricle; *RA,* right atrium; *RV,* right ventricle.

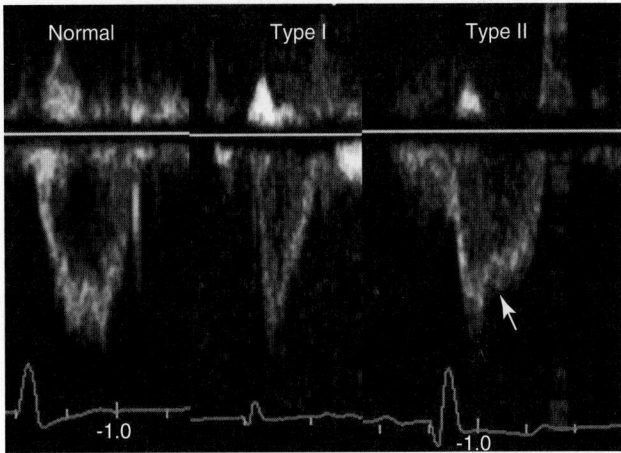

Figure 167-3 Pulsed spectral Doppler pulmonary flow traces for a normal dog and two dogs with pulmonary hypertension (type I and II). Pulmonary hypertension causes a rapid increase in velocity with a sharp peak and short acceleration time in the flow (type I). In more severe cases (type II) the deceleration phase can show a flow reversal, represented by a notch *(arrow)*.

systolic pressure are equivalent. Thus, when the peak velocity of the TR jet is faithfully recorded and inserted into the Bernoulli equation, peak PA pressure is known. Diastolic PA pressures can be estimated by examining the PI jet. Right atrial pressure and right ventricular diastolic pressures should be added to the calculated values for TR and PI, respectively; however, because these are often close to zero, most published studies in veterinary medicine use only the peak velocities and calculated pressure gradient to establish the diagnosis of PH (see Figure 167-1). There is no agreement on the pressure gradient that establishes the diagnosis of PH with optimal sensitivity and specificity; the values proposed by various authors range from 2.5 to 3.5 m/sec for TR and from 2 to

2.2 m/sec for PI. In general PH is considered mild if the gradient between right ventricular pressure and right atrial pressure is between 30 and 50 mm Hg, moderate if it is between 50 and 80 mm Hg, and severe if it is more than 80 mm Hg. PA pressure estimated by Doppler echocardiography acceptably correlates with PA pressure values measured by right-sided heart catheterization in human patients; however, this correlation decreases significantly in patients with less severe PH (Janda et al, 2011). Simultaneous Doppler echocardiography and catheterization studies have not been reported in dogs or cats.

Doppler echocardiography has several limitations in estimating PA pressure. First, a TR jet can be present in up to 80% of normal dogs, and some normal dogs have a TR velocity of about 3 m/sec (Schober and Baade, 2006). Second, TR peak velocity is affected by both right ventricular contractility and volume overload, and patients with severe PH commonly have right ventricular failure with impaired contractility and elevations of mean right atrial and right ventricular diastolic pressures. In these situations, using TR to estimate PA pressure can lead to a significant underestimation of the severity of PH. On the other hand, increased contractility or volume overload is associated with increased TR velocity and can lead to an overestimation of the severity of PH. As stated previously, TR and PI may not be present in all dogs with PH. Lastly, PA pressure may be underestimated if correct alignment with the TR or PI jets is not possible.

Pulmonary Artery Velocity Profile. Other echocardiographic findings can help in the diagnosis of PH. Pulmonary flow profiles are altered in the majority of dogs with PH (see Figure 167-3) (Johnson et al, 1999; Schober and Baade, 2006). In dogs a ratio of less than 0.31 between acceleration and deceleration time of pulmonary flow has a sensitivity and specificity of 73% and 87%, respectively, for predicting a systolic PA pressure of more than 45 mm Hg (Schober and Baade, 2006). Critically important is ensuring proper angulation of the ultrasound beam and proper placement of the pulsed wave cursor because technical errors can create a PH-like appearance of the PA profile even in healthy dogs.

Two-Dimensional Imaging. The diagnosis of PH can be supported by two-dimensional imaging, and in those cases in which TR or PI jets cannot be found, the two-dimensional echo may provide the best evidence for PH. Moderate to severe PH is usually associated with varying degrees of right ventricular enlargement and hypertrophy. Hypertrophy presents as concentric (thick walls with small lumen), eccentric (dilated chamber with normal wall thickness), or mixed patterns. In general concentric patterns are more common in congenital heart defects causing PH, whereas a mixed or eccentric pattern of right ventricular hypertrophy is more typical of acquired diseases with chronic elevations in PA pressure (see Figure 167-2). Severe cases of PH can exhibit flattening of the interventricular septum and paradoxical motion of the septum. Another common two-dimensional echocardiographic finding is dilatation of the main pulmonary artery and very often involvement of the main left and right branches of the PA. In normal dogs the ratio between the aortic root and pulmonary artery is about 1:1. In dogs with PH the ratio is less than 1.

Treatment

Goals of therapy include (1) treating the underlying process responsible for PH, (2) managing the consequences of PH such as right-sided heart failure, and (3) decreasing PA pressures. Knowing the cause and the underlying pathophysiologic mechanisms leading up to PH is helpful in determining the appropriate treatment. In humans several medications have been approved for the treatment of PH, including calcium channel blockers (CCBs), prostacyclin analogs, endothelin receptor antagonists, and phosphodiesterase 5 (PDE5) inhibitors. However, veterinary experience with most of these drugs is very limited. Furthermore, some of these medications require continuous infusions (e.g., epoprostenol) and are costly, which limits their use. Pimobendan has been proposed for the treatment of PH in dogs with category 2 disease (Atkinson et al, 2009), and there are a number of reports on the use of PDE5 inhibitors in veterinary medicine.

The gold standard for objectively monitoring response to therapy is right-sided heart catheterization. However, this is rarely done. Doppler echocardiography may not be sufficiently sensitive to evaluate the efficacy of treatment because in most cases only the pressure gradient is measured, and no estimates are made of pulmonary vascular resistance or PA flow. Pulmonary arterial vasodilation may reduce right ventricular afterload, increase cardiac output, and reduce clinical signs but produce little to no reduction in peak PA systolic pressures owing to improved pulmonary flow. In veterinary patients the clinical response to therapy is very important to gauge. These responses can include improved exercise capacity, reduced respiratory rate, and reduction or elimination of exertional collapse or syncope.

General Measures and Supportive Therapy for All Pulmonary Hypertension

The most common sign in patients with PH is exercise intolerance, and excessive physical activity should be avoided. In addition, traveling to an altitude above 1500 to 2000 m or flying without supplemental oxygen should be avoided because this can significantly worsen PH as a result of hypoxemia and reactive vasoconstriction.

Dogs that have right-sided heart failure require treatment with diuretics and positive inotropic agents such as pimobendan or digoxin. Diuretics should be used carefully in these patients because high-dose diuretics can reduce ventricular filling, induce low cardiac output, and promote the development of prerenal azotemia. An aldosterone antagonist (e.g., spironolactone) can be considered in these cases since secondary hyperaldosteronism often is present. We commonly use a combination of furosemide (1 mg/kg q12h PO), spironolactone (2 mg/kg q24h PO), and pimobendan (0.25 to 0.3 mg/kg q12h PO) in dogs with PH and right-sided heart failure.

Pulmonary Arterial Hypertension

The pathophysiology of category 1 pulmonary arterial hypertension (PAH) is multifactorial and involves

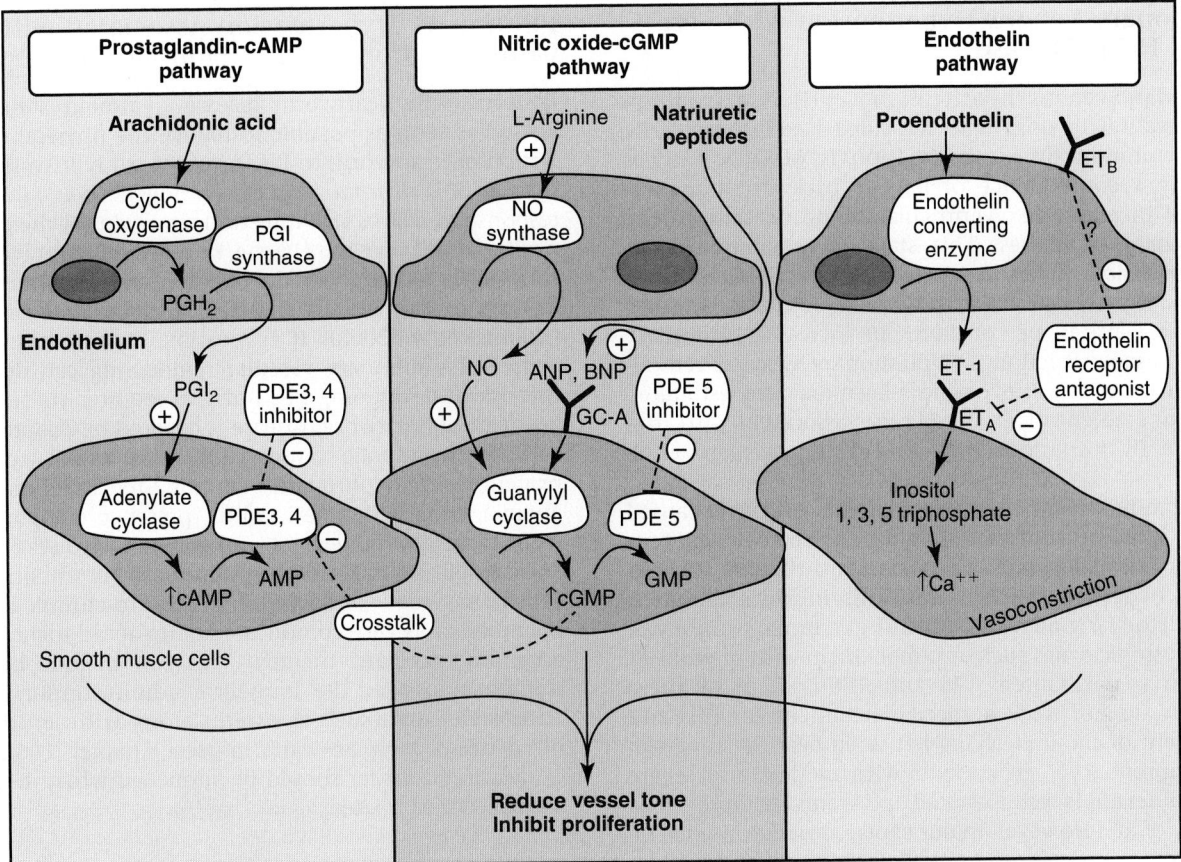

Figure 167-4 The three main mechanisms leading to development of pulmonary arterial hypertension and the site of action of possible medical treatment. *ANP,* Atrial natriuretic peptide; *BNP,* brain natriuretic peptide; *cAMP,* cyclic adenosine monophosphate; *NO,* nitric oxide; *PDE,* phosphodiesterase; *PGH2,* prostaglandin G/H synthase isoenzyme 2; *PGI,* prostacyclin. (From Hill NS: *Pulmonary hypertension therapy,* Armonk, NY, 2006, Summit Communications.)

vasoconstriction, remodeling of pulmonary arteries, inflammation, and thrombosis (Figure 167-4). Therefore treatment of PAH is specifically targeted to block these factors. CCBs such as diltiazem (0.5 mg/kg three times daily) and amlodipine (0.1 mg/kg twice daily) have been used to treat PAH because of their vasodilator effect on the pulmonary arterial tree. However, this effect is not specific for the lungs and CCBs can cause systemic hypotension, so systemic arterial blood pressure should be monitored closely. If CCBs are prescribed, they should be started at a low dose and titrated up slowly. Notably, only a small number of humans with primary PAH show a positive response to CCB treatment (Gailè et al, 2009), and responsiveness in dogs has not been reported.

PDE5 inhibitors are one of the approved treatments for PAH in humans. PDE5 inhibition reduces the degradation of cyclic guanosine monophosphate (cGMP), which results in increased intracellular cGMP, decreased intracellular calcium concentration, and vasodilation through the nitric oxide–cGMP pathway (see Figure 167-4). The pulmonary vasculature has a high concentration of PDE5, so the vasodilatory effects of these drugs are particularly evident in the lungs. Currently three PDE5 inhibitors are approved for use in human medicine: vardenafil, sildenafil, and tadalafil. All three medications

cause significant pulmonary vasodilation, with maximum effects observed after 40 to 45 minutes, 60 minutes, and 75 to 90 min, respectively (Gailè et al, 2009). In dogs sildenafil is the medication most commonly used for the treatment of PAH (Bach et al, 2006; Brown et al, 2010; Kellum and Stepien, 2007; Pyle et al, 2004). The current recommended starting dosage is 1 mg/kg every 8 hours PO, and dose varies between 0.5 and 5.6 mg/kg at dosing intervals of every 8 to 24 hours PO. Sildenafil is well tolerated by dogs, and systemic hypotension generally is not observed. Reported adverse effects are lethargy, clear nasal discharge, erect ears, and cutaneous flushing (Bach et al, 2006; Brown et al, 2010; Kellum and Stepien, 2007). In clinical studies sildenafil decreased PA pressure compared with baseline, increased exercise capacity, improved clinical scores, and improved the quality of life in some but not all of the treated dogs. Other reported positive effects of sildenafil include improved pulmonary gas exchange, increased myocardial contractility, reduced ventricular afterload, facilitated action of natriuretic peptide, and blunted adrenergic stimulation. Recently a small study in five dogs with congenital cardiovascular shunts and PAH showed that sildenafil improved the class of heart failure after 6 months of therapy (Nakamura et al, 2011).

Pulmonary Venous Hypertension with Left-Sided Heart Disease

Pulmonary venous hypertension (PVH) is a common complication in dogs with left-sided heart disease. The most common disease association is MMVD. PVH is initially a consequence of passive backward transmission of increased left ventricular filling pressure to the pulmonary capillaries. This stage is generally considered reversible if left ventricular dysfunction is treated successfully. However, if pulmonary venous pressure remains elevated or continues to increase, pulmonary artery vasoconstriction and pulmonary vascular remodeling can cause irreversible elevation. An estimated pressure gradient of 48 mm Hg was associated with irreversible PVH in dogs with MMVD (Chiavegato et al, 2009).

The initial treatment goal in patients with PVH caused by left-sided heart disease should be to decrease left ventricular filling pressures using standard therapy for left-sided congestive heart failure. This includes diuretics, vasodilators/angiotensin-converting enzyme inhibitors, and inotropic drugs such as pimobendan with or without digoxin (see Chapters 175 and 176). Many of these patients do not need a specific treatment for PH, and treatment of the underlying left-sided heart dysfunction can improve PVH. In patients with moderate to severe PVH, sildenafil is well tolerated and seems to improve the quality of life. However, in our experience response to the treatment is variable, and not all dogs improve after sildenafil is added to heart failure treatment. Acute pulmonary arterial vasodilation can increase left ventricular preload and filling pressure, causing pulmonary edema. Therefore, in patients with PVH, the starting dosage of sildenafil should be low (0.5 mg/kg q12h PO) and the dose should be titrated up slowly. Again, pimobendan (0.25 mg/kg q12h PO) has been proposed for the treatment of PVH in dogs with MMVD and is part of the standard of care for left-sided heart failure in these dogs. In a pilot study pimobendan was associated with a significant reduction of PA pressure but not with significant improvement in quality-of-life score (Atkinson et al, 2009).

Pulmonary Hypertension Associated with Lung Disease and/or Hypoxemia

The underlying lung disease associated with PH should be managed with appropriate treatment such as bronchodilators, antimicrobials, or steroids. Because hypoxia can contribute to the development of PH, severely affected patients benefit from oxygen administration. Although treatment can be complicated, in our experience long-term administration of oxygen is a feasible option for some owners and should be considered in dogs with PH due to a primary respiratory disease. Specific treatment aimed at decreasing PA pressure, including PDE5 inhibition, also should be considered in dogs with clinical signs due to PH and right-sided heart failure.

Pulmonary Hypertension Associated with Chronic Thrombotic or Embolic Disease

In dogs with heartworm disease treatment should be started as soon as possible to reduce the physical contribution of heartworm to PH. A recent study investigating the role of Wolbachia sp. in the pathogenesis and immune response to heartworm infection showed that the combination of doxycycline (10 mg/kg q24h PO) and ivermectin (6 μg/kg weekly PO) reduced perivascular inflammation in dogs experimentally infected with Dirofilaria immitis (Kramer et al, 2008). It is possible that reducing the degree of pulmonary vascular remodeling can decrease the risk of developing PH, but this requires study. Management of heartworm disease is covered in Chapter 184.

Thromboembolic causes of PH are associated with protein-losing nephropathy, immune-mediate hemolytic anemia, constrictive pericarditis, presence of right-sided heart catheters and devices, and systemic diseases that are poorly defined in terms of pulmonary thrombotic risk. The management of dogs with PH due to chronic thromboembolism is very complicated and should include lifelong anticoagulant therapy. This can include heparin initially and later the long-term administration of an antiplatelet drug such as aspirin along with antithrombotic drugs such as warfarin (see Chapter 166). Any underlying disorder should be addressed when it can be identified and treated.

Prognosis

PH generally is associated with a poor prognosis. In two case series survival time ranged from 1 day to 34 months. Moderate to severe PH has the worst prognosis, whereas mild to moderate PH may have a more favorable outcome (Pyle et al, 2004). The ability to treat the underlying condition can influence the outcome. Dogs with heartworm disease and PH have a better outcome if heartworm disease is treated successfully. Dogs with category 2 PH can survive longer if they respond well to treatment for their cardiac disease. The presence of right-sided heart failure generally is associated with a poor quality of life and short life expectancy. A small retrospective study reported that survival time in dogs with category 1 or 2 PH had survival times ranging between 8 and 734 days. After initiation of therapy, dogs that survived the first week had a 95% probability of survival at 3 months, 84% probability at 6 months, and 73% probability at 12 months (Kellum and Stepien, 2007).

References and Suggested Reading

Atkinson KJ et al: Evaluation of pimobendan and N-terminal pro-brain natriuretic peptide in the treatment of pulmonary hypertension secondary to degenerative mitral valve disease in dogs, J Vet Intern Med 23:1190, 2009.

Bach JF et al: Retrospective evaluation of sildenafil citrate as a therapy for pulmonary hypertension in dogs, J Vet Intern Med 20:1132, 2006.

Brown AJ, Davison E, Sleeper MM: Clinical efficacy of sildenafil in treatment of pulmonary arterial hypertension in dogs, J Vet Intern Med 24:850, 2010.

Chiavegato D et al: Pulmonary hypertension in dogs with mitral regurgitation attributable to myxomatous valve disease, *Vet Radiol Ultrasound* 50:253, 2009.

Galiè N et al: Guideline for the diagnosis and treatment of pulmonary hypertension, *Eur Respir J* 34:1219, 2009.

Guglielmini C et al: Serum cardiac troponin I concentration in dogs with precapillary and postcapillary pulmonary hypertension, *J Vet Intern Med* 24:145, 2010.

Janda S et al: Diagnostic accuracy of echocardiography for pulmonary hypertension: a systematic review and meta-analysis, *Heart* 97:612, 2011.

Johnson L, Boon J, Orton C: Clinical characteristics of 53 dogs with Doppler-derived evidence of pulmonary hypertension: 1992-1996, *J Vet Intern Med* 13:440, 1999.

Kellum HB, Stepien RL: Sildenafil citrate therapy in 22 dogs with pulmonary hypertension, *J Vet Intern Med* 21:1258, 2007.

Kramer L et al: *Wolbachia* and its influence on the pathology and immunology of *Dirofilaria immitis* infection, *Vet Parasitol* 158:191, 2008.

Nakamura K et al: Effects of sildenafil citrate on five dogs with Eisenmenger's syndrome, *J Small Anim Pract* 52:595, 2011.

Pyle RL, Abbott J, MacLean H: Pulmonary hypertension and cardiovascular sequelae in 54 dogs, *Int J Appl Vet Med* 2:99, 2004.

Schober K, Baade H: Doppler echocardiographic prediction of pulmonary hypertension in West Highland White Terriers with chronic pulmonary disease, *J Vet Intern Med* 20:912, 2006.

SECTION VIII

Cardiovascular Diseases

Chapter 168:	Nutritional Management of Heart Disease	720
Chapter 169:	Systemic Hypertension	726
Chapter 170:	Bradyarrhythmias	731
Chapter 171:	Supraventricular Tachyarrhythmias in Dogs	737
Chapter 172:	Ventricular Arrhythmias in Dogs	745
Chapter 173:	Feline Cardiac Arrhythmias	748
Chapter 174:	Congenital Heart Disease	756
Chapter 175:	Drugs for Treatment of Heart Failure in Dogs	762
Chapter 176:	Management of Heart Failure in Dogs	772
Chapter 177:	Chronic Valvular Heart Disease in Dogs	784
Chapter 178:	Dilated Cardiomyopathy in Dogs	795
Chapter 179:	Arrhythmogenic Right Ventricular Cardiomyopathy	801
Chapter 180:	Feline Myocardial Disease	804
Chapter 181:	Arterial Thromboembolism	811
Chapter 182:	Pericardial Effusion	816
Chapter 183:	Feline Heartworm Disease	824
Chapter 184:	Canine Heartworm Disease	831

The following web chapters can be found on the companion website at www.currentveterinarytherapy.com

Web Chapter 58:	Arrhythmogenic Right Ventricular Cardiomyopathy in Cats
Web Chapter 59:	Bradyarrhythmias and Cardiac Pacing
Web Chapter 60:	Cardioversion
Web Chapter 61:	Infective Endocarditis
Web Chapter 62:	Mitral Valve Dysplasia
Web Chapter 63:	Myocarditis
Web Chapter 64:	Patent Ductus Arteriosus
Web Chapter 65:	Pulmonic Stenosis
Web Chapter 66:	Subaortic Stenosis
Web Chapter 67:	Syncope
Web Chapter 68:	Tricuspid Valve Dysplasia
Web Chapter 69:	Ventricular Septal Defect

CHAPTER 168

Nutritional Management of Heart Disease

LISA M. FREEMAN, *North Grafton, Massachusetts*

General Nutritional Issues for Animals with Heart Disease

For many years the role of nutrition in the management of heart disease consisted primarily of feeding a low-sodium diet. We now know that severe sodium restriction is not necessary in all animals with heart disease. It also is becoming apparent that supplementation of certain nutrients, either to correct a deficiency or to provide pharmacologic effects, may have profound benefits in animals with heart disease. Research now is beginning to show that nutrition can modulate heart disease by slowing the progression, minimizing the number of medications required, improving quality of life, and in rare cases actually curing the disease. Therefore attention to diet at all stages of heart disease is critical for optimal care of the cardiac patient.

A single diet does not work for all animals with heart disease, and dietary modifications need to be individualized. Patients with heart disease vary in their clinical signs, laboratory parameters, and food preferences, all of which affect diet selection. For example, more severe sodium restriction would be required for a cat with congestive heart failure (CHF) than for a cat with asymptomatic heart disease. Animals with heart disease may be hyperkalemic, hypokalemic, or normokalemic, which influences the choice of diet. Concurrent diseases also alter diet choice and are present in many animals with heart disease (61% of dogs and 56% of cats) (Freeman et al, 2003; Torin et al, 2007).

Based on patient characteristics, one or more diets can be selected. Currently at least two commercial veterinary cardiac diets are available in the United States. The specific characteristics of each diet differ, but both are moderately to severely sodium restricted (i.e., 17 to 50 mg/100 kcal). One cardiac diet also includes supplemental taurine, carnitine, arginine, antioxidants, and omega-3 fatty acids.

In some cases a veterinary diet designed for another disease or an over-the-counter diet may have the nutritional properties desired for an individual patient. Having a number of choices is particularly beneficial for animals with severe CHF, a condition in which loss or change of appetite is common. I generally try to recommend multiple diets so the owner can determine which is most palatable to the pet.

In addition to the pet food selected, the owner also must receive careful instructions on treats and table food. In some cases animals may be eating an ideal pet food but are obtaining large amounts of sodium from treats. Over 90% of dogs and 30% of cats with heart disease received treats (Freeman et al, 2003; Torin et al, 2007). Examples of appropriate treats are given in Table 168-1. Including all sources of dietary sodium in the overall diet plan is important to achieve success with nutritional modifications.

Although a diet must be selected based on desired nutritional properties and palatability, it also is important to devise an overall dietary plan that includes an effective method for administering medications. Most dog owners (57%) and many cat owners (34%) use food for medication administration, and the most commonly used foods are high in sodium (e.g., cheese, hot dogs, lunch meats) (Freeman et al, 2003; Torin et al, 2007). Therefore examples of appropriate methods for administering medications should be provided (Box 168-1).

All dietary changes should be made gradually over a period of 3 to 5 days. However, major dietary changes should not be instituted while the patient is sick or hospitalized. Usually it is better to wait several days until the patient's condition has improved before initiating the change. Food aversions may develop and prevent adequate intake of the food over the long term. It also is important to instruct the owner to notify the veterinarian if the patient does not eat adequate amounts of the new food so that other options can be devised.

Nutritional Modifications Based on Severity of Disease

Asymptomatic Heart Disease

Over the years, recommendations for nutritional therapy for dogs and cats with asymptomatic heart disease have resembled a pendulum. Initially very-low-sodium diets were recommended when a heart murmur was first detected. Veterinarians then moved toward the approach that severe sodium restriction may not be ideal at this stage of disease because of early activation of the renin-angiotensin-aldosterone (RAA) system. This led to the idea that no nutritional modifications can or should be

TABLE 168-1

Examples of Low-Sodium Treats

Treat	Kilocalories* per Treat	Sodium* (mg/treat)
Dogs		
Iams original formula biscuits (small)	22	10
Hill's Prescription Diet Hypoallergenic Treats (canine)	17	9
Hill's Prescription Diet Treats (canine)	14	5
Hill's Science Diet Simple Essentials Treats Small & Toy Oral Care Adult Small Nugget	6	5
Hill's Science Diet Simple Essentials Treats Small & Toy Light Adult Small Biscuit with Real Chicken	3	3
Baby carrots	4	4
Alpo Healthy Snacks Variety Snaps with Real Meat	13	1
Apple (raw, one slice) or orange (one section)	10	0
Cats		
Purina Whisker Lickin's Crunch Lovers Tartar Control cat treats (all flavors)	3	4
Hill's Prescription Diet Hypoallergenic Treats (feline)	2	2

*Nutrient composition as of July, 2013.

BOX 168-1

Recommended Methods for Medication Administration

- Teach the owner to administer the pill to the animal without using foods.
- Use a pet piller or pet pill gun.
- Switch from pills to a compounded, flavored liquid medication. (NOTE: The pharmacokinetics may be altered.)
- Place pill fragments within an empty gelatin capsule.
- Place medications within low-sodium foods.
  - Meat or fish, home cooked, without salt (not lunch meats)
  - Fresh fruit (e.g., banana, orange, melon, berries)
  - Low-sodium canned pet food
  - Peanut butter (labeled as "no salt added")

made for animals with asymptomatic heart disease. Veterinarians are now swinging back toward the middle because new research is supporting the idea that dietary modification in early heart disease might be beneficial and the nutritional management of animals with asymptomatic heart disease should not be ignored.

One of the earliest and major compensatory responses in heart disease is activation of the RAA system, and sodium restriction can further elevate renin, angiotensin, and aldosterone concentrations. Thus severe sodium restriction in animals with early heart disease theoretically could be detrimental by triggering early and excessive activation of the RAA system. I recommend only mild sodium restriction in asymptomatic heart disease

(<100 mg/100 kcal for animals with International Small Animal Cardiac Health Council [ISACHC] class 1a or 1b heart disease; see Chapter 176). However, this is also an opportune time to begin talking to the owner about the animal's overall dietary patterns (e.g., the pet's food, treats, table food, and methods of administering medications), since it is generally much easier to institute dietary modifications when the animal is asymptomatic.

In addition to mild sodium restriction, another important goal is to achieve or maintain optimal body condition. Goals for body condition in animals with CHF may be different (see later), but in asymptomatic heart disease, veterinarians should assess the animal's body weight, body condition score, and muscle condition score at every visit as part of nutritional screening (which should be performed on every patient at every visit [World Small Animal Veterinary Association, 2011; World Small Animal Veterinary Association website]). If the animal is above the weight for an optimal body condition, a gradual and comprehensive weight-loss program should be instituted with careful monitoring.

Finally, there is the potential for benefit from nutritional modification in the asymptomatic animal. One study compared a moderately reduced-sodium cardiac diet that was enriched with omega-3 fatty acids, antioxidants, arginine, taurine, and carnitine with a placebo diet in dogs with asymptomatic chronic valvular disease (CVD) (Freeman et al, 2006). The cardiac diet increased circulating levels of key nutrients (e.g., antioxidants, omega-3 fatty acids) and also reduced cardiac size. This reduction in cardiac size did not appear to be an effect of sodium restriction. In addition, one retrospective study showed a significantly longer survival time in dogs with cardiac disease that were receiving omega-3 fatty acid supplementation (Slupe et al, 2008). Future prospective studies are needed to confirm such findings and to provide a better understanding of the role of nutritional modification in this early stage of disease.

Mild to Moderate Congestive Heart Failure

When CHF develops, additional nutritional concerns arise. Maintaining optimal body condition is of primary importance in the animal with CHF. Although obesity still can be present at this stage, animals with CHF more commonly begin to demonstrate weight loss. This weight loss, or cardiac cachexia, is unlike that seen in a healthy animal, which loses primarily fat. In an animal with CHF, the primary tissue lost is lean body mass. The term *cachexia* does not necessarily imply an emaciated, end-stage patient; there is a spectrum of severity of cachexia. In the early stages it can be very subtle and even may occur in obese animals (i.e., an animal may have excess fat stores but still lose lean body mass). Loss of lean body mass usually is noted first in the epaxial, gluteal, scapular, or temporal muscles. Cardiac cachexia can occur with any underlying cause of CHF (e.g., dilated cardiomyopathy [DCM], CVD, congenital heart diseases) but typically does not occur until CHF has developed (although it can occur in dogs with advanced CVD with severe left atrial enlargement). Cardiac cachexia is a common finding in animals with CHF and has deleterious effects on strength, immune function, and survival; thus it is important to recognize cachexia at an early stage and seize opportunities to manage it effectively.

The loss of lean body mass in cardiac cachexia is a multifactorial process caused by anorexia, increased energy requirements, and increased production of inflammatory cytokines such as tumor necrosis factor (TNF) and interleukin-1 (IL-1). These cytokines cause anorexia, increase energy requirements, and increase the catabolism of lean body mass. In addition, TNF and IL-1 also cause cardiac myocyte hypertrophy and fibrosis and have negative inotropic effects.

The nutritional management of cardiac cachexia consists primarily of providing adequate calories and protein and modulating cytokine production. One of the most important issues in managing anorexia (which is defined here to include either complete or partial loss of appetite) is to optimize medical therapy. An early sign of worsening CHF or the need for medication adjustment is a reduction in food intake in an animal that has previously been eating well. Medication adverse effects such as digoxin toxicity or azotemia secondary to angiotensin-converting enzyme (ACE) inhibitors or diuretic use also can cause anorexia. Providing a more palatable diet can help to improve appetite. This might involve switching from a dry food to a canned food, changing to a different brand, or feeding a balanced, cooked homemade diet formulated by a veterinary nutritionist. It also may be helpful to use flavor enhancers to increase food intake (e.g., yogurt, maple syrup, or applesauce in dogs; small amounts of home-cooked meats or fish in cats). Modulation of cytokine production also can be beneficial for managing cardiac cachexia. Supplementation of fish oil, which is high in omega-3 fatty acids, can decrease inflammatory cytokine production and improve cachexia (see later).

Unlike in the healthy animal or the asymptomatic person, dog, or cat with cardiac disease, obesity actually may be associated with a protective effect once CHF is present; this is known as the *obesity paradox* (Finn et al, 2010; Slupe et al, 2008). Although there are a number of hypothesized reasons for the obesity paradox, the benefit of obesity in CHF likely is due more to a *lack* of cachexia than to the obesity per se, given the adverse effects associated with cachexia.

Protein

As early as the 1960s, protein restriction was recommended for animals with CHF to reduce the metabolic load on the kidneys and liver. Restricting protein actually is detrimental because it can contribute to lean body mass loss and malnutrition. Animals with CHF should not be protein restricted unless they have concurrent advanced renal disease. Some diets designed for dogs with cardiac disease are very low in protein. Similarly, protein-restricted renal diets are sometimes recommended for animals with heart disease because these diets often (but not always) are moderately sodium restricted. Unless concurrent disease dictates otherwise, high-quality protein should be fed to meet minimum requirements for dogs (5.1 g/100 kcal) or cats (6.5 g/100 kcal). This should be a primary goal in animals with heart disease, particularly as CHF becomes more severe.

Another important issue with regard to protein is the still widespread misconception that dietary protein should be restricted in early renal disease. Some dogs receiving ACE inhibitors develop azotemia. Azotemia occurs more frequently when ACE inhibitors are used in conjunction with diuretics, but in a small number of dogs azotemia can develop from ACE inhibitors alone. When concurrent ACE inhibitor and diuretic use causes azotemia, reduction of the diuretic dose and/or temporary cessation of the ACE inhibitor is indicated. A protein-restricted diet is not recommended in this situation unless medication changes do not correct the problem and renal disease progresses.

Fat

In addition to serving as a source of calories and essential fatty acids, fat also can have significant effects on immune function, production of inflammatory mediators, and hemodynamics (Freeman, 2010). Most canine and feline diets contain primarily omega-6 fatty acids (e.g., linoleic acid, arachidonic acid). The omega-3 fatty acids eicosapentaenoic acid (EPA) and docosahexaenoic acid (DHA) normally are found in very low concentrations in the cell membrane compared with the omega-6 fatty acids, but their level can be increased by consumption of a food or supplement enriched in omega-3 fatty acids. The benefit of having a higher concentration of omega-3 fatty acids in cell membranes is that breakdown products of the omega-3 fatty acids (eicosanoids) are less potent inflammatory mediators than eicosanoids derived from omega-6 fatty acids. This decreases the production of cytokines and other inflammatory mediators. Fish oil also reduces the production of TNF and IL-1 and improves muscle mass. In some animals fish oil supplementation also improves appetite. Another potential benefit is that omega-3 fatty acids have antiarrhythmic effects.

Although an optimal dose of omega-3 fatty acids has not been determined, I currently recommend a daily dose of 40 mg/kg of EPA and 25 mg/kg of DHA for animals with anorexia or cachexia and also for most animals with CHF if there are no contraindications (e.g., dietary fat intolerance, coagulopathies) and it can be administered successfully (Freeman, 2010). Unless the diet is one of a few specially designed therapeutic diets, supplementation is necessary to achieve this omega-3 fatty acid dose. When a fish oil supplement is to be recommended, it is important to know the exact amount of EPA and DHA in a specific fish oil brand since supplements vary widely. However, the most common formulation of fish oil is 1-g capsules that contain approximately 180 mg of EPA and 120 mg of DHA. At this concentration fish oil can be administered at a dose of 1 capsule per 10 lb of body weight to achieve the recommended EPA and DHA dosages. Fish oil supplements always should contain vitamin E as an antioxidant, but other nutrients should not be included to avoid toxicities. Cod liver oil and flaxseed oil should not be used to provide omega-3 fatty acids to dogs and cats.

Sodium

Sodium restriction is one method, along with the use of diuretics and venous vasodilators, to treat excessive increases in preload in patients with CHF. In the 1960s, when few medications were available for treating animals with CHF, dietary sodium restriction was one of the few methods of reducing fluid accumulation. In this situation severe sodium restriction clearly was beneficial in reducing signs of congestion. However, with the current availability of newer and more effective medications, the role of severe sodium restriction in early CHF (ISACHC class 1 or 2) is no longer clear. I currently recommend moderate sodium restriction (i.e., <80 mg/100 kcal) for animals with ISACHC class 2 heart disease.

Most owners are unaware of the sodium content of pet and human foods and need very specific instructions regarding appropriate pet foods, acceptable low-salt treats, and methods for administering medications (Tufts HeartSmart website). Owners also should be counseled on specific foods to avoid, such as baby food; bread; canned vegetables (unless labeled "no salt added"); cheeses, including squirtable cheeses (unless specifically labeled "low sodium"); condiments (e.g., ketchup, soy sauce); lunch meats and cold cuts (e.g., ham, corned beef, salami, sausages, bacon, hot dogs); most pet foods and treats; pickled foods; pizza; processed foods (e.g., potato mixes, rice mixes, macaroni and cheese); snack foods (e.g., potato chips, packaged popcorn, crackers); and soups (unless homemade without salt). Mild to moderate reduction in dietary sodium can be achieved with a veterinary diet designed for animals with early cardiac disease or with certain over-the-counter diets designed for use in senior pets. If a diet designed for senior pets is used, it is very important to look at the characteristics of the individual product. There is no legal definition for a senior diet; thus the levels of calories, protein, sodium, and other nutrients

can vary dramatically among products from different companies. In a recent study of 37 over-the-counter senior diets for dogs, the sodium content ranged from 33 to 412 mg/100 kcal (Hutchinson et al, 2011).

Potassium and Magnesium

Potassium and magnesium are nutrients of concern in cardiac patients because depletion of these electrolytes can cause cardiac arrhythmias, decreased myocardial contractility, and muscle weakness and can potentiate the adverse effects of cardiac medications. Many of the medications used in animals with CHF, such as loop diuretics (e.g., furosemide) and thiazide diuretics (e.g., hydrochlorothiazide), can predispose a patient to hypokalemia. Inadequate dietary intake of potassium, which occurred in nearly half of dogs with heart disease in one study, also can predispose an animal to hypokalemia (Freeman et al, 2003). However, it is also important to note that the increased use of ACE inhibitors, which results in renal potassium sparing, also makes hyperkalemia a potential problem in animals with CHF. In addition, spironolactone, an aldosterone antagonist and potassium-sparing diuretic, is being used with greater frequency in dogs with heart disease and can cause hyperkalemia. Finally, some commercial pet foods are high in potassium, which can exacerbate hyperkalemia.

Magnesium plays a critical role in normal cardiovascular function, and many of the medications used to treat cardiac conditions, including digoxin and loop diuretics, are associated with magnesium depletion in people. Therefore animals with CHF have the potential to develop hypomagnesemia. Studies have reported variable prevalence rates of hypomagnesemia (from 2% to over 50%) in dogs with heart disease.

Serum potassium concentrations should be monitored routinely in CHF patients, particularly those receiving an ACE inhibitor or large doses of diuretics. Serum magnesium concentrations also should be measured, but clinicians should be aware that serum magnesium concentrations are a poor indicator of total body stores. Nonetheless, serial evaluations in an individual patient may be useful, especially in patients with arrhythmias or in those receiving high doses of diuretics. Diets vary greatly in their potassium content; thus, if hypokalemia or hyperkalemia is present, a diet with a higher or lower potassium content, respectively, should be selected. Similarly, diets high in magnesium may be beneficial in a hypomagnesemic animal.

Severe or Refractory Congestive Heart Failure

In severe CHF greater restriction of dietary sodium (<50 mg/100 kcal) may allow lower dosages of diuretics to be used to control clinical signs. Diets should be selected carefully to achieve this level of sodium restriction and to provide for other nutritional needs of the individual animal (e.g., protein). There also is a higher risk of potassium and magnesium abnormalities in severe CHF; thus monitoring of electrolytes is important.

At this stage of disease cardiac cachexia becomes more common; thus it is critical to maintain adequate calorie and protein intake. This can be a challenge since appetite in severe CHF is often cyclical, and owners should be warned that appetite might be highly variable. Another issue to consider is that anorexia in an animal that has been eating can be an early sign of worsening disease or the need for medication adjustment and should trigger a reevaluation. In addition to optimizing medical therapy, it can be helpful to offer multiple choices of appropriate pet foods, a nutritionally balanced homemade diet, or even single food items that can increase calorie intake without exacerbating the underlying disease. In this regard, home-cooked meat, low-sodium breakfast cereals, or energy bars can be very useful. Palatability enhancers also can be very helpful for pets with severe CHF, including cooked unsalted meat or fish for cats and cooked unsalted meat, yogurt, applesauce, or maple syrup for dogs. Encouraging the owner to try offering foods at different temperatures (e.g., warmed versus room temperature versus cold) may increase food intake in some animals. Omega-3 fatty acid supplementation also can be beneficial in some animals in which appetite is poor. Other tips that may increase food intake are providing smaller, more frequent meals; feeding the recommended diet(s) from the owner's plate; and putting the recommended diet(s) into a treat jar.

Special Situations

Feline Dilated Cardiomyopathy

The role of taurine deficiency in feline DCM has been well described, and there has been a dramatic decline in the incidence of the disease since the late 1980s. Most current cases of feline DCM appear to be independent of taurine status. Taurine deficiency still should be suspected whenever the diagnosis of feline DCM is made. A complete diet history should be obtained because cats that are eating a vegetarian, unbalanced homemade, or other unconventional diet are at higher risk of taurine deficiency. Even commercial vegetarian diets that include taurine in the ingredient list can be severely taurine deficient. Plasma and whole blood taurine levels should be analyzed, and treatment with taurine (125 to 250 mg q12h PO) should begin concurrent with medical therapy. If the cat is eating an unconventional diet, the owner also should be counseled to switch to a nutritionally balanced meat-based commercial cat food.

Canine Dilated Cardiomyopathy

Supplementation of certain nutrients, either in the diet or in the form of dietary supplements, is most often proposed for dogs with DCM. Advancing recommendations can be difficult because there is a paucity of published date but many unsubstantiated claims for dietary supplements that owners find when researching online. A discussion of the role of some of these nutrients in canine DCM follows.

Taurine
Unlike cats, dogs are thought to be able to synthesize adequate amounts of taurine endogenously, and taurine is not considered a requirement in canine diets. Although

breeds that typically develop DCM (e.g., Doberman pinscher, boxer) do not appear to have reduced taurine concentrations, taurine deficiency has been reported in some dogs of certain breeds affected with DCM. These include the American cocker spaniel, Newfoundland, and golden retriever. Perhaps taurine deficiency occurs more commonly in certain breeds because of higher requirements or breed-specific metabolic abnormalities. Diet also may play a role. As an example, lamb meal and rice as well as high-fiber or very-low-protein diets have been associated with taurine deficiency, although the exact role of diet is not yet known.

The benefits of taurine supplementation are far less certain in canine DCM than in feline DCM associated with dietary deficiency. Although several small studies have shown some improvements in clinical or echocardiographic parameters in taurine-deficient dogs given taurine supplements, the response is generally not as dramatic as is seen in cats with taurine deficiency–induced DCM (Kittleson et al, 1997). More research is needed. I currently recommend measuring plasma and whole blood taurine concentrations when dogs with DCM are at high risk of taurine deficiency (e.g., cocker spaniels, Newfoundlands, golden retrievers) and when DCM is encountered in dogs of an atypical breed (e.g., Welsh corgis or basset hounds). In addition, taurine concentrations should be measured in dogs with DCM eating lamb meal and rice–based diets, high-fiber diets, or diets that are highly protein restricted. Although the extent of benefit of supplementation is unclear, I recommend taurine supplementation until plasma and whole blood taurine concentrations for the patient are available. The optimal dose of taurine for correcting a deficiency has not been determined, but the dosage currently recommended is 500 to 1000 mg every 8 to 12 hours PO.

L-Carnitine
L-Carnitine plays an important role in long-chain fatty acid metabolism and energy production. Carnitine is in high concentrations in the myocardium, and carnitine deficiency syndromes can be associated with primary myocardial disease in humans. Carnitine deficiency was reported in a family of boxers in 1991. Since that time L-carnitine has been supplemented in some dogs with DCM, but no controlled prospective studies have been reported. Even if primary carnitine deficiency is not present, a secondary carnitine deficiency may develop in CHF, and carnitine supplementation may have benefits for myocardial energy metabolism. One limitation impacting the study of carnitine deficiency relates to the need to measure myocardial concentrations of L-carnitine to document a deficiency. Plasma concentrations are often normal, even in the face of myocardial deficiency.

L-Carnitine supplementation has few side effects, but it is expensive, and this may be a significant deterrent for some owners when efficacy is uncertain. I offer the option of L-carnitine supplementation to owners of dogs with DCM, especially boxers, but do not consider it essential. The minimal or optimal dose of L-carnitine necessary achieve repletion in a dog with low myocardial carnitine concentrations is unknown, but the dosage that has been recommended is 25 to 75 mg/kg every 8 to 12 hours PO.

Antioxidants

Although antioxidants have received a great deal of attention in the popular press in terms of preventing and treating cardiovascular diseases, most of the research in human cardiology has been on coronary artery disease. Antioxidants are produced endogenously but also can be supplied exogenously if there is an imbalance between the levels of oxidants produced and the antioxidant protection available. The major antioxidants include enzymatic antioxidants (e.g., superoxide dismutase, catalase, glutathione peroxidase) and oxidant quenchers (e.g., vitamin C, vitamin E, and β-carotene). Recent studies have shown that in dogs with CHF caused by either DCM or CVD, there is an imbalance between oxidant production and antioxidant protection. Supplemental antioxidants are now provided in many commercial veterinary diets, including at least one cardiac diet; however, the benefits of antioxidant supplementation in dogs and cats with CHF remain theoretical at this time.

Coenzyme Q₁₀

The roles of coenzyme Q_{10} in energy production and as an antioxidant have prompted some investigators to propose coenzyme Q_{10} deficiency as a possible cause of DCM. Coenzyme Q_{10} supplementation has been reported to be beneficial in human studies, but most of these have been poorly controlled and results are conflicting. The current recommended (but empiric) dosage in dogs is 30 mg every 12 hours PO, although up to 90 mg every 12 hours PO has been recommended for large dogs. The purported benefits of supplementation include correction of a deficiency, improved myocardial metabolic efficiency, and increased antioxidant protection. Controlled prospective studies are necessary to judge accurately the efficacy of this supplement.

Dietary Supplements: General Issues

In many cases the desired nutrient modifications can be achieved through diet alone. However, supplementation of certain nutrients may be desirable if they are not available in a particular diet or are not present in high enough levels in that diet to achieve the desired effect. The clinician and pet owner should understand that dietary supplements can be marketed without proof of safety, efficacy, or quality. Therefore careful consideration of the type, dose, and brand may be important to avoid toxicities or a complete lack of efficacy. Clearly more information is

needed to define the role of dietary supplements in heart disease.

Another important issue related to administration of dietary supplements is their usage in place of standard cardiac medications. Animals with severe CHF already may be receiving many pills each day, and it may not be clear to owners that it is more important to give the cardiac medications than the dietary supplements. In situations in which pill administration is becoming overwhelming for an owner, the veterinarian can assist the owner in determining which dietary supplements have the least potential benefits and might be discontinued.

References and Suggested Reading

Backus RC et al: Low plasma taurine concentration in Newfoundland dogs is associated with low plasma methionine and cyst(e)ine concentrations and low taurine synthesis, *J Nutr* 136:2525, 2006.

Finn E et al: The relationship between body weight, body condition, and survival in cats with heart failure, *J Vet Intern Med* 24:1369, 2010.

Freeman LM: Beneficial effects of omega-3 fatty acids in cardiovascular disease, *J Small Anim Pract* 51:462, 2010.

Freeman LM et al: Nutritional alterations and the effect of fish oil supplementation in dogs with heart failure, *J Vet Intern Med* 12:440, 1998.

Freeman LM et al: Dietary patterns in dogs with cardiac disease, *J Am Vet Med Assoc* 223:1301, 2003.

Freeman LM et al: Effects of dietary modification in dogs with early chronic valvular disease, *J Vet Intern Med* 20:1116, 2006.

Hutchinson D et al: Survey of opinions about nutritional requirements of senior dogs and analysis of nutrient profiles of commercially available diets for senior dogs, *Int J Vet Res Vet Med* 9:68, 2011.

Kittleson MD et al: Results of the multicenter spaniel trial (MUST): taurine- and carnitine-responsive dilated cardiomyopathy in American cocker spaniels with decreased plasma taurine concentration, *J Vet Intern Med* 11:204, 1997.

Slupe JL et al: The relationship between body weight, body condition, and survival in dogs with heart failure, *J Vet Intern Med* 22:561, 2008.

Torin DS et al: Dietary patterns of cats with cardiac disease, *J Am Vet Med Assoc* 230:862, 2007.

Tufts HeartSmart website for pet owners. Available at: www.tufts.edu/ret/heartsmart. Accessed July 24, 2013.

WSAVA Nutritional Assessment Guidelines Taskforce, Freeman L, et al: 2011 Nutritional assessment guidelines, *J Small Anim Pract* 52:385-396, 2011.

WSAVA Nutrition toolkit. Available at www.wsava.org/nutrition-toolkit. Accessed July 24, 2013.

CHAPTER 169

Systemic Hypertension

REBECCA L. STEPIEN, *Madison, Wisconsin*

Systemic hypertension (pathologic elevation of systemic blood pressure [BP]) is increasingly recognized as a cause of morbidity in pet cats and dogs. Systemic hypertension (HT) usually represents a complication of other systemic diseases in dogs and cats and therefore is classified as *secondary* hypertension. However, in some cases a causative disease is not apparent after careful investigation and the HT is deemed *primary* or *idiopathic*. Whether primary or secondary, persistent systemic HT indicates a failure of the body's physiologic adaptations to normalize BP in the setting of inappropriate elevation.

Overview of Systemic Hypertension in the Population

Persistent elevation of systolic BP to values higher than 160 mm Hg is associated with progressive renal injury in dogs, and the severity of renal injury has been correlated with the degree of elevation (Finco, 2004). Potential renal pathologic changes induced by systemic HT include both glomerular and tubulointerstitial changes with resulting ischemia, necrosis, atrophy, and exacerbation of proteinuria. These gradual and additive changes may be difficult to quantify in living animals with preexisting renal disease, but systolic HT (>160 mm Hg) at the time of presentation increases the odds of uremic crisis and death in dogs with renal disease (Jacob et al, 2003). Systolic BP higher than 180 mm Hg has been associated with ocular injury, including retinal or intraocular hemorrhage; retinal vascular tortuosity; and retinal detachments and retinal degeneration that may cause acute blindness, especially in cats. Neurologic abnormalities, most often intracranial—including seizures, mentation changes, and vestibular signs—have been noted in dogs and cats with HT and are more likely when systolic pressures exceed 180 mm Hg. Although variable cardiac hypertrophy has been documented in cats with naturally occurring HT (Chetboul et al, 2003; Henik et al, 2004; Nelson et al, 2002) and has been shown to regress with successful antihypertensive therapy (Snyder et al, 2001), the degree of hypertrophy has not been shown to correlate with severity of HT. In dogs with experimentally induced HT, hypertrophy and diastolic dysfunction without fibrosis occurred within 12 weeks (Douglas and Tallant, 1991). Although congestive heart failure caused by systemic HT appears to be rare in either species, hypertensive veterinary patients may exhibit signs of congestive heart failure or circulatory volume overload in response to excessive intravenous fluid administration. The onset, development, and clinical repercussions of cardiac changes resulting from sustained HT await further study in cats and dogs with naturally occurring systemic HT.

Systemic HT may be recognized when BP is measured as part of a diagnostic evaluation in animals known to have, or suspected of having, systemic diseases associated with the development of HT. Alternatively, elevated BP may be detected when clinical signs of HT-related target organ damage (typically retinal detachment or intracranial neurologic signs) lead to BP measurement (Box 169-1). Although periodic BP evaluation in healthy patients has been advocated by some authors, the moderate sensitivity (53% to 71%) and specificity (85% to 88%) of oscillometric and Doppler methods of detecting systolic BP higher than 160 mm Hg in conscious dogs increases the risk of false-positive and false-negative readings (Stepien et al, 2003). However, in cats these concerns may be modulated by the increased prevalence of diseases (chronic renal insufficiency and hyperthyroidism) associated with the development of systemic HT in older cats. Because these diseases may have an insidious onset, annual BP screening of apparently healthy older cats may be warranted.

Diagnosis of systemic HT as a complication of systemic disease requires an understanding of the diseases likely to produce systemic HT as a comorbid factor. The rate of HT in the general canine population is thought to be low, approximately 1% to 10% (Bodey and Michell, 1996; Remillard et al, 1991), and the prevalence of HT in the healthy feline population is unknown. In both species, systemic HT is more common in subpopulations affected by particular diseases (Table 169-1). Published prevalence rates are highly variable for many diseases based on the criteria used for diagnosis (i.e., the BP value used as a cutoff for normal), advances in the early recognition of some diseases, and variability in BP measurement techniques.

In cats, renal disease is the most likely cause of systemic HT. Renal disease is highly prevalent in the feline population, and HT occurs in approximately 20% to 30% of cats with this disease (Syme et al, 2002). In early studies as many as 86% of hyperthyroid cats had BP above the reference range, but recent evidence suggests that the prevalence rate of HT in hyperthyroid cats is much lower (≈10% to 30%), perhaps as a result of increased screening and earlier detection of hyperthyroidism (before hypertensive complications develop) (Williams et al, 2010). Many elderly cats have both chronic renal insufficiency and hyperthyroidism, which complicates analysis of the prevalence of HT in these diseases. The prevalence of HT in cats with diabetes mellitus is poorly documented, but BP screening in diabetic cats is warranted clinically,

BOX 169-1

Indications for Measurement of Blood Pressure in Dogs and Cats*

Both Species
- Intraocular hemorrhage
- Retinal hemorrhage or detachment
- Intracranial neurologic signs
- Renal disease
- Diabetes mellitus
- Primary hyperaldosteronism
- Left ventricular hypertrophy not associated with outflow obstruction
- Use of medications that may increase blood pressure
- Sudden decompensation of left-sided cardiac disease, especially in response to intravenous fluid administration

Dogs: Additional Indications
- Hyperadrenocorticism
- Pheochromocytoma

Cats: Additional Indications
- Hyperthyroidism
- Acromegaly
- Left ventricular hypertrophy
- Heart murmur
- Gallop rhythm

*For all cats, systemic hypertension should be excluded as a cause of left ventricular hypertrophy before a diagnosis of idiopathic hypertrophic cardiomyopathy is made.

especially if proteinuria is present. Other uncommon diseases associated with systemic HT in cats are acromegaly and primary hyperaldosteronism.

Numerous studies in dogs support chronic renal disease (especially glomerular disease), hyperadrenocorticism, and diabetes mellitus as the most common disorders associated with secondary systemic HT. Other uncommon endocrine diseases associated with HT in dogs are pheochromocytoma and primary hyperaldosteronism. The use of vasoactive medications such as phenylpropanolamine or corticosteroids may elevate BP primarily or additively with a causative disease. Healthy sight hounds may have resting BP values up to 15 mm Hg higher than other breeds of similar size (Bodey and Michell, 1996) and should be assessed accordingly.

Diagnosis of Systemic Hypertension

Studies of the ease of use, accuracy, and precision of various noninvasive BP measurement systems have been performed in normal and hypertensive dogs and cats. In general, Doppler methods using a forelimb (radial) cuff are recommended for use in cats. In dogs, oscillometric or Doppler methods with radial, metatarsal, or proximal tail cuffs are used. In all cases the patient should be calm and acclimated to the environment and position (sternal or lateral recumbency) before measurement, and BP measurement should precede or be separated by at least 30 minutes from stressful procedures (e.g., blood draw). The cuff width chosen should approximate 40% of the

TABLE 169-1

Conditions Associated with the Development of Systemic Hypertension in Dogs and Cats*

Condition	Estimated Prevalence of Systemic Hypertension (If Known) (%)	Comments
Dogs		
Renal disease	60-90	Animals with proteinuria may be at higher risk.
Hyperadrenocorticism	70-80	Animals with proteinuria may be at higher risk.
Diabetes mellitus	25-50	Only data for small numbers of patients have been analyzed.
Pheochromocytoma	Unknown	Systemic hypertension may be periodic with catecholamine surges.
Primary hyperaldosteronism	Unknown	
Acromegaly	Unknown	
Use of hypertension-inducing medications	Unknown	Phenylpropanolamine and corticosteroids are implicated most frequently.
Cats		
Renal disease	20-65	Early studies documented higher prevalence.
Hyperthyroidism	10-86	Early studies documented higher prevalence.
Diabetes mellitus	Unknown	One study suggested a low prevalence.
Primary hyperaldosteronism	Unknown	
Use of hypertension-inducing medications	Unknown	Corticosteroids are implicated most frequently.

*See text for references.

circumference of the limb at the point of placement, and the limb or tail should be positioned so that the cuff site is at the level of the heart during measurement. Typically six consecutive BP measurements with simultaneous heart rates are recorded. The first measurement and any obviously spurious measurements are discarded, and the remaining values are averaged for a representative reading. Careful training of specific practice personnel is recommended, and priority should be placed on measuring BP carefully and recording values consistently. Frequently cuff size is relatively too narrow to occlude the artery effectively, and measured pressure is higher than actual arterial pressure. The opposite occurs if the cuff is relatively too wide. When elevated BP is identified, some clinicians recommend remeasuring pressure in the opposite limb or an alternative site to exclude anatomic factors that may have an impact on arterial occlusion.

Measurements obtained from an initial session should be interpreted in conjunction with the patient's clinical signs or concurrent disease and the observed level of patient agitation at the time of measurement. Either isolated systolic HT or combined systolic and diastolic HT is identified in the majority of hypertensive dogs. For this reason, and because noninvasive measurement methods in current use most reliably deliver systolic BP measurements, decisions regarding diagnosis and therapy are usually based on systolic readings.

Studies of human hypertensive patients indicate a progressive increase in risk of target organ damage as BP increases above normal values. Although antihypertensive therapy is indicated in an individual patient as soon as target organ damage begins to occur, in veterinary patients the pressure at which an animal begins to sustain end-organ damage is usually unknown. Since recognizable injury to various organ systems has been documented when systolic BP exceeds 160 mm Hg over the long term, antihypertensive medications currently are recommended for patients in this group (Brown et al, 2007). It is likely that this current cutoff value will change as more information becomes available. Target organ injury most often is manifest as ocular injury (retinal hemorrhage, hyphema, retinal detachment), neurologic signs (intracranial signs of depression or obtundation), renal injury (proteinuria, decreased renal function), or cardiac remodeling (left ventricular concentric hypertrophy). Ocular injury is prevalent and easily detectable in hypertensive dogs and cats (LeBlanc et al, 2011; Maggio et al, 2000); for this reason, a complete ocular examination should be performed in any patient in which systemic HT is detected. (Similarly, identification of retinal lesions in a mature cat or dog with a murmur or gallop indicates the need to assess BP carefully).

If elevated BP is documented at a single session and no clinical signs of HT (ocular or neurologic) or obvious target organ injury is present, BP measurement should be repeated, preferably within a week. If elevated BP is confirmed, a detailed diagnostic evaluation should be initiated to search for a causative disease (Box 169-2). If a known causative disease is evident when elevated BP first is detected, therapy for HT can be started immediately in conjunction with optimal management of the underlying disorder. If systolic BP is between 160 and 180 mm Hg

---

BOX 169-2

Recommended Diagnostic Testing for Patients with Systemic Hypertension

Dogs
- Funduscopic examination
- Serum chemistry panel
- Urinalysis
- Urine protein screening
- Hyperadrenocorticism screening
  - Adrenocorticotropic hormone stimulation test
  - Dexamethasone suppression test
- Abdominal ultrasonography if indicated for additional renal and adrenal evaluation

Cats
- Funduscopic examination
- Serum chemistry panel
- Urinalysis
- Urine protein screening
- Thyroid screening if appropriate based on age
- Abdominal ultrasonography if indicated for additional renal and adrenal evaluation (if hyperaldosteronism is suspected)

---

and no clinical signs of HT are present, BP may be monitored until the diagnostic evaluation is complete. If BP remains elevated and causative disease is found, treatment of the underlying disease (e.g., hyperadrenocorticism) can be pursued concurrently with medical management of HT. If thorough diagnostic evaluation fails to reveal a causative disease, animals with consistently elevated BP should be treated with antihypertensive medications and monitored for development of systemic disease or complications.

Treatment of Systemic Hypertension

Multiple therapeutic options are available to treat the hypertensive veterinary patient. As is the case in humans, many animals need more than one medication to control HT adequately, and medication dosages may need to be modified over time. This is predictable based on the complex neurologic and endocrine control of the cardiovascular system. Mean arterial pressure is controlled by the interaction of systemic vascular resistance and cardiac output. In turn, cardiac output relies on the interaction of the heart rate and stroke volume, a value affected by preload (a reflection of blood volume), afterload, and contractile function. With intricate interplay of the sympathetic and parasympathetic nervous systems, endocrine control of blood volume, and vascular tone modulation through the renin-angiotensin-aldosterone and other systems, the cardiovascular system is capable of at least partially compensating for medication effects.

It is reasonable to assume that better control of BP may be possible if direct vasodilating medications (e.g., amlodipine besylate) are combined with medications that limit the ability of the compensatory mechanisms to adjust to medication-induced changes (e.g., angiotensin-converting enzyme [ACE] inhibitors). For many clinicians, the combination of amlodipine plus an ACE inhibitor represents typical therapy for feline HT. In addition, concern has been expressed regarding the possible detrimental effects of using calcium channel blockers as monotherapy. Calcium channel blockers such as amlodipine besylate cause preferential vasodilation of afferent renal arterioles and increase intraglomerular pressure in some circumstances. This afferent vasodilation, if combined with inadequate decreases in systemic BP, actually may promote glomerular damage (Brown et al, 1993; Jacob et al, 2003). In theory, combining the efferent arteriolar dilation associated with ACE inhibitors with the stronger antihypertensive effects of amlodipine or other dihydropyridine calcium channel blockers may provide optimal BP management while conferring some degree of renal protection against progressive injury. Finally, some conditions have recognized indications for specific medications (e.g., ACE inhibitors in proteinuric diseases, sympathetic nervous system blockade in symptomatic pheochromocytoma, aldosterone antagonists in hyperaldosteronism). In these cases, indicated medications should form the basis of therapy, with additional medications having different mechanisms of action added as needed. In nonemergent cases (systolic BP less than 200 mm Hg, no evidence of ocular or neurologic signs), at least 7 days should elapse before new antihypertensive medications are added.

Antihypertensive Therapy in Cats

Systemic HT in cats (idiopathic or secondary to renal insufficiency or diabetes mellitus) responds well to therapy with amlodipine besylate (0.625 to 1.25 mg/cat q24h, PO), and consistent administration typically results in long-term BP control (Elliott et al, 2001). In addition, early therapy with amlodipine in cats with blindness caused by retinal detachment may allow return of at least partial visual ability (Maggio et al, 2000). Transdermal administration of an amlodipine preparation has been studied in a small number of cats (n = 6), but although it was effective in maintaining some BP control, it did not reach the same blood concentrations as orally administered amlodipine (Helms, 2007). Transdermal administration of amlodipine is not recommended in animals with evidence of target organ damage. In cats with proteinuria, addition of an ACE inhibitor to amlodipine therapy may reduce renal protein loss, but an ACE inhibitor is very unlikely to control significant HT when used as a monotherapy. ACE inhibitors in common use in hypertensive cats are enalapril maleate (0.25 to 0.5 mg/kg q12-24h PO) and benazepril (0.25 to 0.5 mg/kg q24h PO). Benazepril may be preferred in cats with renal disease because it has some hepatic elimination compared with exclusively renal elimination for enalapril, but this potential benefit has not been subjected to clinical investigation. Cats with controlled HT should be reevaluated at regular intervals to assess BP and renal function.

Hypertensive cats with hyperthyroidism may benefit from amlodipine therapy with simultaneous β-blockade (e.g., atenolol 6.25 to 12.5 mg/cat q12h PO) to help control tachycardia and other cardiovascular effects of thyrotoxicosis. However, atenolol as a monotherapy is unlikely to control significant HT in cats. If medical or surgical resolution of the hyperthyroidism occurs, antihypertensive medications can be cautiously reduced or eliminated, and the BP rechecked. Nonetheless, some cats remain hypertensive after resolution of thyrotoxicosis and require long-term antihypertensive therapy, often because of concurrent renal disease (Williams et al, 2010).

Antihypertensive Therapy in Dogs

Canine HT typically is more challenging to control than feline HT. The reason for this disparity is unknown, but it makes dogs much more like humans, in whom the need for more than one antihypertensive medication to control BP is the norm. The effects of antihypertensive medications on BP are additive, but presumably so are the adverse effects. Ideal antihypertensive therapy would consist of optimal control of the causative disease paired with the minimal number of antihypertensive medications required to reduce BP to target systolic values of 140 to 150 mm Hg.

When specific abnormalities are identified (e.g., catecholamine excess in pheochromocytoma, excessive aldosterone secretion in primary hyperaldosteronism), targeted medical therapy such as α- and β-blockers or aldosterone antagonists (e.g., spironolactone 1 to 2 mg/kg q12h PO) is indicated. If systemic HT persists, addition of an ACE inhibitor or amlodipine may be beneficial.

In dogs with renal disease, hyperadrenocorticism, or diabetes mellitus, a standard progressive protocol can be used and results in control of systemic HT in the majority of cases. ACE inhibitors such as enalapril (0.5 mg/kg q12-24h PO) or benazepril (0.5 mg/kg q12-24h PO) are indicated to limit renal protein loss in dogs with proteinuria, and administration usually results in an approximately 10% decrease in systolic BP in these and other patients with renal insufficiency. If systemic HT is mild, this 10% decrease may be sufficient to decrease BP to within an acceptable range. Although twice-daily dosing of an ACE inhibitor may result in more rapid onset of effect than once-daily dosing, it is unclear whether twice-daily dosing is more effective for BP control at steady state. Current recommendations for therapy for both proteinuria and HT are to begin at once-daily dosing and increase to twice-daily dosing if inadequate response is noted.

The calcium channel blocker amlodipine besylate (0.2 to 0.4 mg/kg q24h PO) is a direct vasodilator useful in the management of systemic HT of any cause. Amlodipine appears to cause minimal reflex tachycardia, an adverse effect of some other direct vasodilators. As is the case with an ACE inhibitor, once-daily dosing is used and increased to maximal dosing as needed. Some animals require higher doses of amlodipine than typically recommended; animals receiving doses above the recommended range should be monitored closely for hypotension, changes in renal function, and other adverse effects. The long elimination half-life of amlodipine in dogs may require a 1-week follow-up to allow full evaluation of the antihypertensive effect.

Apparently refractory or difficult-to-manage systemic HT occurs occasionally in the canine population. In any case of apparently refractory HT, owner understanding of and compliance with the dosing schedule should be checked. Ideally BP should be measured approximately 12 hours after steady state is attained; measurement of BP several hours after dosing may underestimate medication effects. Additional diagnostics may be required to identify causative factors in animals with more than one predisposing condition (e.g., discovery of hyperadrenocorticism in a patient with diabetes). In cases of truly refractory HT, other medications (hydralazine, prazosin, spironolactone, diuretics) can be added to the patient's therapeutic plan. In general, addition of multiple medications based on theoretic benefit should be approached with caution, and all additional medications should be initiated at the low end of the dosing range with close BP and biochemical monitoring. There is a distinct shortage of clinical data supporting the safety and efficacy of multidrug regimens in the canine and feline hypertensive population. Additional medications may contribute to hypotension, dehydration with resultant renal dysfunction, and remote adverse effects such as inappetence, or they may complicate the therapeutic plan for the caregiver without evidence of advantage over simpler routines.

Hypertensive Emergencies in Dogs

Emergent hypertension with severe end-organ injury (active retinal detachment, intraocular bleeding, progressive central nervous system signs) should be treated in the hospital; immediate continuous intravenous infusion of sodium nitroprusside provides the most rapid and titratable method of lowering BP, but oral amlodipine and/or hydralazine may be used when sodium nitroprusside is not available. Oral hydralazine, with its relatively rapid onset, can be combined effectively with oral amlodipine, which has a slower onset, to decrease BP over several hours to a short-term target of a 25% decrease in systolic BP. It is reasonable to contact a specialist to discuss treatment in complicated or nonresponsive cases. Careful and consistent (at least hourly) monitoring of BP is required during initial therapy.

Prognosis

Few clinical studies are available that address the prognosis for survival of cats and dogs affected with HT as a primary problem or as a complication of systemic disease, but HT at diagnosis has been associated with a worse prognosis in dogs with chronic renal failure (Jacob et al, 2003) and in cats with hyperthyroidism (Williams et al, 2010). Prognosis likely varies based on the underlying disease, severity of hypertension, and presence and severity of clinical signs. Present therapeutic recommendations are aimed at ameliorating clinical signs and preventing progression of end-organ damage.

References and Suggested Reading

Bodey AR, Michell AR: Epidemiological study of blood pressure in domestic dogs, *J Small Anim Pract* 37:116, 1996.

Brown SA et al: Long-term effects of antihypertensive regimens on renal hemodynamics and proteinuria, *Kidney Int* 43:1210, 1993.

Brown S et al: Guidelines for the identification, evaluation, and management of systemic hypertension in dogs and cats, *J Vet Intern Med* 21:542, 2007.

Chetboul V et al: Spontaneous feline hypertension: clinical and echocardiographic abnormalities, and survival rate, *J Vet Intern Med* 17:89, 2003.

Douglas PS, Tallant B: Hypertrophy, fibrosis and diastolic dysfunction in early canine experimental hypertension, *J Am Coll Cardiol* 17:530, 1991.

Elliott J et al: Feline hypertension: clinical findings and response to antihypertensive treatment in 30 cases, *J Small Anim Pract* 42:122, 2001.

Finco DR: Association of systemic hypertension with renal injury in dogs with induced renal failure, *J Vet Intern Med* 18:289, 2004.

Helms SR: Treatment of feline hypertension with transdermal amlodipine: a pilot study, *J Am Anim Hosp Assoc* 43:149, 2007.

Henik RA, Stepien RL, Bortnowski HB: Spectrum of M-mode echocardiographic abnormalities in 75 cats with systemic hypertension, *J Am Anim Hosp Assoc* 40:359, 2004.

Jacob F et al: Association between initial systolic blood pressure and risk of developing a uremic crisis or of dying in dogs with chronic renal failure, *J Am Vet Med Assoc* 222:322, 2003.

LeBlanc NL, Stepien RL, Bentley EB: Ocular lesions associated with systemic hypertension in dogs: 65 cases (2005-2007), *J Am Vet Med Assoc* 238:915, 2011.

Maggio F et al: Ocular lesions associated with systemic hypertension in cats: 69 cases (1985-1998), *J Am Vet Med Assoc* 217:695, 2000.

Nelson OL et al: Echocardiographic and radiographic changes associated with systemic hypertension in cats, *J Vet Intern Med* 16:418, 2002.

Remillard RL, Ross JN, Eddy JB: Variance of indirect blood pressure measurements and prevalence of hypertension in clinically normal dogs, *Am J Vet Res* 52:561, 1991.

Snyder PS, Sadek D, Jones GL: Effect of amlodipine on echocardiographic variables in cats with systemic hypertension, *J Vet Intern Med* 15:52, 2001.

Stepien RL et al: Comparative diagnostic test characteristics of oscillometric and Doppler ultrasonographic methods in the detection of systolic hypertension in dogs, *J Vet Intern Med* 17:65, 2003.

Syme HM et al: Prevalence of systolic hypertension in cats with chronic renal failure at initial evaluation, *J Am Vet Med Assoc* 220:1799, 2002.

Williams TL et al: Survival and the development of azotemia after treatment of hyperthyroid cats, *J Vet Intern Med* 24:863, 2010.

CHAPTER 170

Bradyarrhythmias

BRUCE G. KORNREICH, *Ithaca, New York*
N. SYDNEY MOÏSE, *Ithaca, New York*

Bradyarrhythmias are defined as cardiac rhythms that result in heart rates that are lower than normal for an animal's signalment and activity. Based on 24-hour ambulatory electrocardiographic (ECG) recordings (Holter monitoring), the average heart rate for healthy dogs is 75 beats/min irrespective of size, whereas the average heart rate for healthy cats is approximately 165 beats/min. However, when rhythms are being evaluated with Holter monitoring in the home, it is equally important to know that a rate of 35 beats/min with sinus pauses of 3 seconds is quite common in a healthy sleeping dog. Importantly, these averages and lower limits may not be applicable to a nervous animal in a stressful environment such as a veterinary hospital. Most clinicians would investigate a heart rate that is persistently less than 140 beats/min in a hospitalized cat and less than 60 beats/min in a hospitalized dog, especially if the rate does not increase with stimulation. When a bradyarrhythmia is diagnosed either in the hospital or via 24-hour Holter monitoring, understanding the cause and significance of the rhythm, and determining optimal management, depends on knowing whether the mechanism is physiologic, iatrogenic, or pathologic.

Physiologic Bradyarrhythmias

Physiologic bradyarrhythmias are those that occur secondary to alteration of extracardiac factors, including body temperature, systemic blood pressure, intrathoracic pressure, intracranial pressure, ocular pressure, gastrointestinal distention, intraabdominal pressure, and pharyngeal or soft palate tension. These bradyarrhythmias are mediated primarily by increases in vagal tone or decreases in sympathetic tone.

A frequently observed physiologic bradyarrhythmia is the development of sinus bradycardia secondary to activation of the baroreceptor reflex. The baroreceptor reflex is an intrinsic physiologic response to an increase in systemic blood pressure that results in an elevation in cardiac vagal tone and a decrease in sympathetic tone (Figure 170-1). The baroreceptors responsible for this response are found primarily in the aortic arch and carotid sinus.

A second physiologic bradyarrhythmia is observed in animals that have brain injury or a disease that increases intracranial pressure and is part of the Cushing's response. Cushing's response is a reflex that occurs when the increased hydrostatic pressure of cerebrospinal fluid exceeds mean arterial pressure, which leads to compression of cerebral arterioles that decreases blood flow to the brain. Chemoreceptors in the medulla sense the ischemia-induced increase in carbon dioxide pressure and decrease in pH, resulting in reflex activation of the sympathetic nervous system and peripheral vasoconstriction. This vasoconstriction triggers peripheral baroreceptors to increase vagal tone, and bradycardia results.

Any abnormality in the distribution of the sensory afferent trigeminal nerve fibers can cause an elevation of cardiac vagal tone via activation of the vagal motor nucleus. Space-occupying or infiltrative lesions in the nasal cavity, as well as lesions in the eye or orbital region, may stimulate vagal afferent nerves, which travel via either the ophthalmic, maxillary, or mandibular nerves to the trigeminal ganglion and ultimately activate the vagal motor nucleus. The result of this activation is increased vagal tone and decreased heart rate.

Finally, animals experiencing moderate to severe hypothermia may demonstrate sinus bradycardia secondary to a hypothermia-induced decrease in sinoatrial (SA) node discharge rate.

In each of these examples, a regular or irregular sinus bradycardia is the observed rhythm, but physiologic slowing of atrioventricular (AV) node conduction also can be seen. Although elevated vagal tone is typically the mechanism for physiologic sinus bradycardia, treatment with parasympatholytic agents is not recommended if the animal's condition and blood pressure are stable; rather, treatment of the underlying problem (e.g., hypothermia, increased intracranial pressure) should be the primary goal. Treatment with atropine or glycopyrrolate may have a dose-dependent pharmacologic effect that is longer than desired. Although the atropine response test has been proposed as a diagnostic test to differentiate physiologic bradycardia from sinus node dysfunction (see the section on sick sinus syndrome later), caution is advised when administering parasympatholytic agents to dogs with potential sinus node dysfunction. The sinus node discharge rate in most dogs with diseased sinus nodes will still increase in response to parasympatholytic agents, which causes some dogs to develop tachycardias that overdrive suppress escape rhythms and can potentially precipitate an asystolic crisis.

Iatrogenic Bradyarrhythmias

Iatrogenic bradyarrhythmias most commonly result from the administration of drugs that decrease SA node discharge rate, AV node conduction, or both. Drugs that slow the heart rate generally are referred to as *negative chronotropes*. Drug-induced bradycardias most commonly occur in animals given medications for sedation or pain

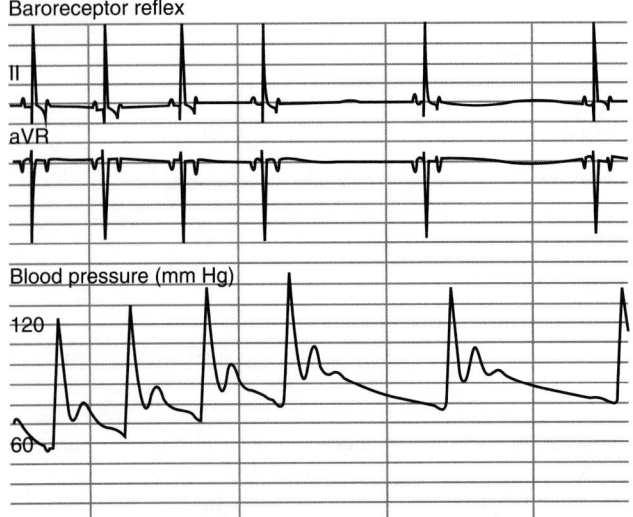

Figure 170-1 Baroreceptor reflex in an anesthetized dog. Lead II and aVR surface electrocardiograms are shown on top and the arterial blood pressure tracing is shown below. The increase in systemic pressure is associated with a decrease in sinus rate.

relief and in animals receiving medications used to treat tachyarrhythmias. Centrally acting opioids (e.g., morphine, hydromorphone, butorphanol, fentanyl) and α_2-agonists (e.g., dexmedetomidine and medetomidine) can cause a dose-dependent bradycardia. When overdose or adverse response to centrally acting opioids causes a physiologically unstable bradycardia, an opioid antagonist (e.g., naloxone) can be used to reverse the narcotic's effects. The bradycardic adverse effects of α_2-agonist overdose can be reversed with the α_2-antagonist atipamezole. Alternatively, anticholinergics such as glycopyrrolate or atropine may be used in either of these situations if symptomatic bradycardia is observed. It should be noted that hypothermia, as commonly occurs in an anesthetic setting, interferes with the effectiveness of anticholinergics in reversing bradycardia.

β-Adrenergic blockers and calcium channel blockers used to treat supraventricular arrhythmias decrease sinus rate and AV node conduction. The latter effect is the rationale for the use of these drugs in controlling the ventricular response rate in atrial fibrillation. Sustained-release diltiazem (2 to 4 mg/kg q12h PO) often is combined with a low dose of digoxin (0.003 mg/kg lean body weight q12h PO) to control ventricular response rate to atrial fibrillation. Digoxin decreases the ventricular rate via its presumed vagomimetic effect on AV node conduction. The authors have had success in controlling ventricular rate without excessive bradycardia using this combination, but the importance of careful monitoring by Holter recordings and serum digoxin concentrations is emphasized (these drugs should be dosed to achieve rate control with serum digoxin concentrations of 0.8 to 1.2 ng/dl and no adverse effects). Importantly, diltiazem's effect on ventricular rate when given either intravenously or orally is dose dependent, and high doses may induce bradycardia.

Ventricular tachycardia is often treated with sotalol, which has both potassium channel and β-adrenergic

blocking effects. The dosage of sotalol required to suppress ventricular arrhythmias (e.g., 2 to 3 mg/kg q12h PO) often decreases the sinus rate by 15% to 20% and may cause a marked increase in the number of pauses exceeding 2 seconds in duration during wakefulness. The duration of pauses during sleep may also be increased by sotalol, and pauses of 5 seconds' duration are not uncommon in dogs receiving this drug. The bradycardic effects of sotalol most often subside after 4 weeks of treatment, but if sotalol-induced bradycardia is excessive, careful reconsideration of the appropriateness of sotalol therapy and of dosage is recommended.

Finally, general anesthetics have a depressant effect on sinus node function, and in dogs with preexisting conduction system disease, general anesthesia may also suppress ventricular escape activity, leading to asystole. Breeds at risk of sick sinus syndrome (see later) should be monitored carefully during induction and maintenance of anesthesia.

Pathologic Bradyarrhythmias

Pathologic bradyarrhythmias are those nonphysiologic and noniatrogenic bradyarrhythmias that result in a heart rate that is too low to meet the metabolic and perfusion demands of the patient and that therefore result in clinical signs. The clinical signs most commonly observed in patients with pathologic bradyarrhythmias are lethargy, weakness, mental dullness, collapse, and syncope. Pathologic bradyarrhythmias can be categorized loosely into abnormalities of impulse initiation and abnormalities of impulse conduction. Abnormalities of impulse initiation primarily involve an inappropriately low or absent SA node discharge rate and include syndromes such as sick sinus syndrome and persistent atrial standstill. Abnormalities of impulse conduction most commonly consist of a failure of the AV conduction system (AV node, bundle of His, bilateral proximal bundle branches) to conduct a sufficient percentage of depolarizations of sinus origin to the ventricle; the results can include high-grade second-degree and third-degree atrioventricular block (AVB). Third-degree (complete) AVB and sick sinus syndrome are the most common bradyarrhythmias prompting pacemaker implantation in dogs.

Sinoatrial Node Abnormalities

Sick Sinus Syndrome (Sinus Node Dysfunction)
Sinus node dysfunction is a condition in which the SA node intermittently fails to discharge, and this dysfunction may lead to the clinical syndrome of sick sinus syndrome (SSS), in which animals display clinical signs of weakness, lethargy, collapse, or syncope that may or may not be exercise induced. The syncope seen in dogs with SSS is extremely variable with respect to frequency and duration of episodes, and although it is uncommon, dogs with SSS can die if not appropriately treated with pacemaker implantation. Even without a high risk of sudden death, frequent syncope negatively affects quality of life and may prompt unnecessary euthanasia if a client perceives the dog to be suffering.

Although the cause of SSS in dogs is still unclear, mutations in cardiac sodium channels (e.g., SCN5A), connexins, and α smooth muscle heavy-chain proteins; dysfunction of ryanodine receptor 2, which comprises the calcium clock in the SA node; and SA node fibrosis have been identified in people with this disease. SSS is seen most commonly in middle-aged or older small-breed dogs, and canine breeds that are predisposed to SSS include the miniature schnauzer, West Highland white terrier, dachshund, boxer, and cocker spaniel. These breed predispositions suggest a genetic component to the cause of canine SSS. Dogs with SSS may demonstrate sinus bradycardia or a sinus rhythm with periods of sinus arrest. Periods of sinus arrest may be interrupted by junctional or ventricular escape beats or rhythms. Importantly, the escape beats and rhythms in dogs with SSS often are inadequate and delayed, which suggests concurrent dysfunction of secondary (rescue) pacemaker sites in the more distal conduction system. Dogs with SSS also commonly demonstrate a sinus rhythm with intermittent bouts of supraventricular tachycardia that are characterized by positive or negative P waves (bradycardia-tachycardia syndrome) (Figure 170-2). AV conduction disturbances ranging from first- to second-degree AVB of varying severity have been observed, but the prevalence of coexisting AVB is not known. A prolongation of QT interval and sometimes prominent T waves are seen in some dogs with SSS. Abnormal findings may not be apparent on a baseline ECG in dogs with SSS, which highlights the importance of performing 24-hour Holter monitoring or capturing the cardiac rhythm during a clinical event on a loop recorder (event monitor) for definitive diagnosis in many cases. Even if a dog does not have a collapsing episode during the time that Holter monitoring is performed, findings such as a 6- to 7-second sinus pause may strongly suggest a diagnosis of SSS.

The definitive therapy for SSS patients is pacemaker implantation. The authors advise atrial pacing (e.g., AAI pacing mode) in dogs with SSS and no evidence of AV node disease to maintain AV synchrony. However, other veterinary cardiologists believe that the greater risk of lead dislodgement with atrial pacing, the typical geriatric age (and lower exercise capacity) of SSS dogs, the potential for diffuse conduction disease, and the fact that most dogs are not completely pacemaker dependent also support the use of ventricular pacing (e.g., VVIR pacing mode). In practical terms, both pacing modes are successful in preventing syncope and improving quality of life. Alternatively, dual-chamber pacing (e.g., DDD pacing mode) may be elected for SSS dogs, although the requirement for two leads in this mode may increase the risk of cranial vena cava thrombosis/obstruction in small dogs.

Some dogs with bradycardia-tachycardia syndrome associated with SSS may require pharmacologic management of the tachycardic component of their disease following pacemaker implantation. It is important that therapy for the tachycardia be withheld until pacing is performed to avoid life-threatening bradyarrhythmias and suppression of escape activity. Interestingly, some dogs with bradycardia-tachycardia syndrome experience a reduction in the occurrence of tachycardia following pacemaker implantation alone.

Persistent Atrial Standstill

Persistent atrial standstill (PAS) is a relatively rare bradyarrhythmia in which the atria fail to depolarize despite normal SA node discharge. PAS has been reported in both dogs and cats, although it is more commonly identified in dogs. The atria of affected animals usually are electrically and mechanically quiescent. PAS must be distinguished from the intermittent failure of atrial depolarization that may be observed in animals with hyperkalemia, digitalis toxicity, or hypothermia. PAS commonly is accompanied by a junctional or ventricular escape rhythm. Careful inspection of the ECG may indicate disorganized atrial activity (atrial fibrillation) or low-amplitude P waves that are not conducted to the ventricles.

The cause of PAS is the subject of debate, but proposed mechanisms in humans include infiltration of the atria by fibrosis, inflammatory cells, or amyloid; and mutation

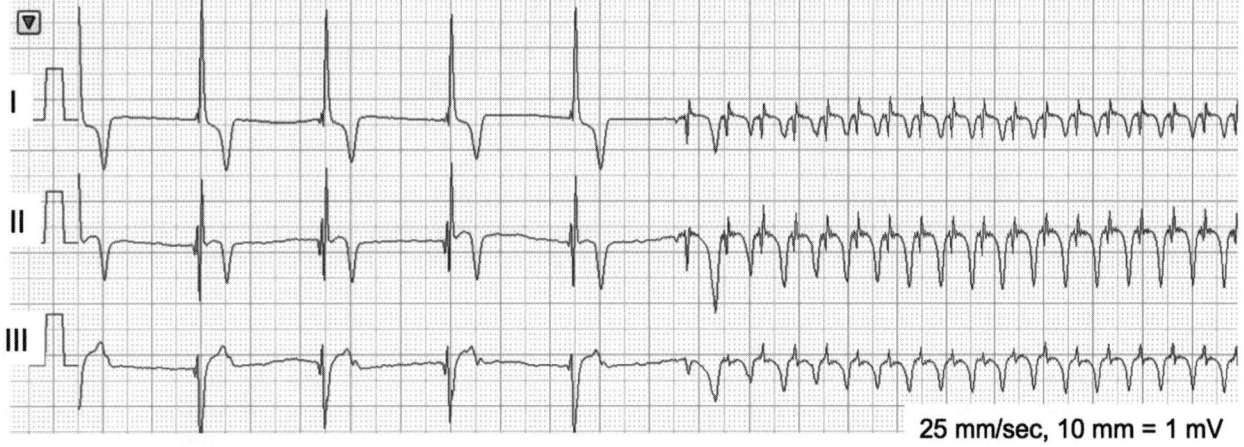

25 mm/sec, 10 mm = 1 mV

Figure 170-2 Lead I, II, and III surface electrocardiograms obtained from a 6-year-old female spayed miniature schnauzer with sick sinus syndrome. Note the initial sinus arrest with ventricular escape rhythm followed by supraventricular tachycardia initiated with negative P waves in leads I and II.

of the cardiac SCN5A sodium channel, connexin 40, or ryanodine receptor 2. At necropsy, the atria of affected animals often are grossly thinned and may appear translucent, but these findings likely represent the end stage of disease. Histologic evaluation often reveals atrial fibrosis with occasional fatty replacement of atrial myocardial cells and variable populations of chronic inflammatory cells within the atria. In rare cases, the ventricular myocardium may be infiltrated with inflammatory cells as well.

PAS can be persistent or intermittent, and it may occur as a familial disease in the English Springer spaniel, which suggests a genetic origin in this breed. PAS is diagnosed most commonly in young to middle-aged dogs. Clinical signs include lethargy, collapse, syncope that may not be related to exercise, and congestive heart failure, and are due to a combination of a loss of atrial contribution to ventricular preload and the effects of bradycardia on cardiac output. Imaging by radiography and echocardiography classically shows severe right atrial and right ventricular dilatation, but some cases show severe biatrial enlargement with marked enlargement of the left atrium and all cardiac chambers.

Definitive treatment for PAS is permanent pacemaker implantation, often combined with pharmacologic therapy to control clinical signs associated with congestive failure. Given the physical and electrical abnormality of the atria in affected individuals, ventricular demand pacing (VVIR mode) is the ideal therapy. Although pacemaker implantation may extend the life span of individuals with PAS, patients often succumb to progressive myocardial failure and congestive heart failure.

Atrioventricular Conduction Abnormalities

Second-Degree Atrioventricular Block

Second-degree AVB is defined as the intermittent failure of the AV conduction system to carry atrial depolarization to the ventricles. This failure of conduction can be characterized either by a gradual prolongation of AV conduction time (i.e., P-R interval) followed by a loss of AV conduction (Mobitz type I or Wenckebach block) or by a sudden loss of AV conduction without antecedent P-R interval prolongation (Mobitz type II block). Mobitz type I AVB most commonly occurs as a result of conduction disturbance in the compact AV node. Mobitz type II AVB most commonly is associated with conduction disturbance in the His-Purkinje system. Common patterns for Mobitz type II AVB include 2:1 conduction (every other P wave is conducted with a fixed P-R interval) and higher grades of block such as 3:1 or 4:1; the pattern also can vary. Mobitz type I AVB generally is viewed as a more transient and benign condition and more likely to be due to a drug effect (e.g., digoxin or an α_2-agonist) or other causes of high vagal tone. Both Mobitz type I and Mobitz type II may progress to third-degree AVB, although this is more common with Mobitz type II block, especially if conducted QRS complexes demonstrate a bundle branch block pattern (which suggests more diffuse His-Purkinje conduction disease). Second-degree AVB is characterized electrocardiographically by P waves with intermittent loss of subsequent QRS complexes. High-grade AVB has been

defined loosely as the absence of QRS complexes following P waves in consecutive cycles, and the more frequently block occurs, the more likely bradycardia will result in clinical signs (weakness, lethargy, collapse). A recent study identified the Afghan, Catahoula leopard dog, chow-chow, cocker spaniel, German wirehaired pointer, and Labrador retriever breeds as predisposed to high-grade second-degree AVB.

A variety of pathologic conditions can induce second-degree AVB, and these must be distinguished from physiologic and iatrogenic causes of AVB. Potential causes include infiltrative (e.g., neoplastic), ischemic, metabolic, degenerative, inflammatory, and traumatic diseases. Because some of these processes may be acute and induce myocardial cell injury, serum cardiac troponin I (cTnI) should be measured in any patient demonstrating second-degree AVB. In most cases a complete workup is done to evaluate the patient for concurrent cardiac and noncardiac diseases. Permanent pacemaker implantation is the definitive therapy in the vast majority of animals with second-degree AVB sufficient to cause clinical signs. This is discussed in more detail in Chapter 4 and Web Chapter 59.

Third-Degree Atrioventricular Block

Third-degree AV block is defined as a complete failure of conduction of atrial impulses into the ventricles. The level of block can be the AV node, the bundle of His, or both proximal bundle branches. This loss of sinus node pacing of the ventricles creates a reliance on an escape rhythm below the level of the block to maintain cardiac output. In most cases these are ventricular escape rhythms that originate in either ventricular myocardial or Purkinje cells and depolarize the ventricles through the slowly conducting myocardium. This results in wide-complex QRS complexes as well as abnormal and prolonged ventricular repolarization. Occasionally, junctional escape rhythms are observed in dogs with third-degree AVB. Patients with third-degree AVB often have accelerated atrial rates—essentially sinus tachycardia—in response to baroreceptor reflex–mediated elevation of sympathetic tone.

Third-degree AVB is characterized electrocardiographically by P waves and QRS complexes without any regular or consistent relationship; the atria are paced by the SA node at one rate, and the ventricles are paced by a spontaneous ventricular rhythm at substantially slower rates (Figure 170-3). Ventricular escape rates in younger healthy dogs often vary between 40 and 60 beats/min, whereas in many older dogs the ventricular escape rate is between 25 and 40 beats/min. Feline ventricular escape rates most commonly are in the range of 120 to 140 beats/min (and AVB may be overlooked during a cursory physical examination). Although the escape rhythms may have constant morphology and RR intervals, this is not always sustainable. In the authors' experience, the less regular the ventricular escape rhythm in dogs, the more likely it will become hemodynamically unstable. Despite preservation of myocardial systolic function in most cases, the associated bradycardia limits cardiac output sufficiently to lead to clinical signs of weakness, lethargy, or collapse, which often are not associated with exercise. The four-chamber dilatation induced by the prolonged diastolic filling

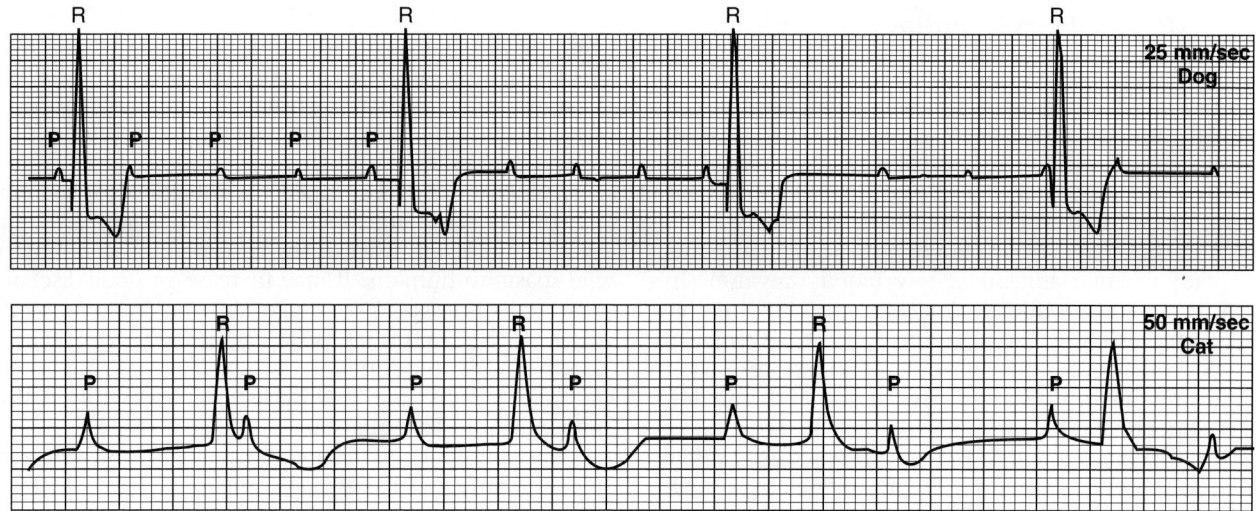

Figure 170-3 Lead II electrocardiograms obtained from a dog *(top)* and a cat *(bottom)* with third-degree atrioventricular block. Note the lack of association between P waves and QRS complexes and the ventricular escape rhythm in both cases.

periods and fluid retention in response to reduced cardiac output can lead to congestive heart failure, which commonly is right-sided unless there is concurrent cardiac disease (e.g., mitral regurgitation). Cats with third-degree AVB may not show any clinical signs, which may reflect their relatively sedentary lifestyles, and some survive for months to years with no apparent clinical progression of disease. Complete AVB can be extremely sporadic in some cats, with the rhythm changing suddenly from normal sinus rhythm to third-degree AVB. Failure to develop an escape rhythm or the loss of a previously stable escape rhythm can lead to clinical signs such as syncope (see Web Chapter 67). Unless the arrhythmia is detected, affected cats may be misdiagnosed as having a seizure disorder.

Causes of third-degree AVB involve the same processes implicated in second-degree AVB, as described earlier. Serum cTnI concentration should be measured in all animals with third-degree AVB. The authors have seen examples of third-degree AVB associated with elevated serum cTnI concentrations in both dogs and ferrets. In the authors' experience, third-degree AVB that is associated with elevated cTnI concentrations carries a less favorable long-term prognosis.

The treatment for symptomatic second-degree and third-degree AVB is permanent cardiac pacing (see Web Chapter 59). Since AV conduction is abnormal in animals with AVB, single-lead pacing from the atrium (AAI mode) is contraindicated. There are a number of potentially beneficial pacing lead configurations for these patients. One approach is transvenous placement of a special pacing lead that can sense native atrial depolarizations and pace the ventricle following a physiologically relevant period of time (VDD mode). Another approach is dual-chamber pacing (DDD mode) with two leads (one in the right atrium and one in the right ventricle). As in VDD pacing, the pacemaker is programmed to provide a physiologic AV interval to allow for appropriate ventricular filling and coronary perfusion. These two modes should provide

optimal pacing because the atrial sensor can respond to physiologic changes in the sinus node (as long as the dog is not in atrial fibrillation) and AV synchrony can be maintained. The third and simplest method involves a single transvenously placed ventricular lead with a pacemaker that is typically programmed to respond to activity or movement (VVIR mode). In our practice, we strive to pace in a mode that maintains AV synchrony whenever possible. Although there are some drawbacks to VVIR pacing in terms of loss of AV synchrony, and in spite of the fact that studies have demonstrated the benefits of pacing that maintains AV synchrony in human patients, many dogs and cats do very well with single-chamber ventricular pacing. Furthermore, rate responsiveness with activity can be demonstrated in these cases during pacemaker interrogation. Discussion of the pros and cons of different pacing systems for specific patients is beyond the scope of this chapter. Studies that evaluate both survival and exercise benefits of different pacing systems are lacking in veterinary patients.

The use of epicardial pacing systems has decreased dramatically, but these still may be applicable in certain cases. Cats, ferrets, and some toy-breed dogs may be good candidates if the transvenous pacing system is too large. Some patients undergo pacing during abdominal surgery (e.g., splenectomy), and a surgeon can readily place a left ventricular epicardial lead via the abdomen. These are subtleties best discussed with a cardiologist.

Particular care should be exercised in managing dogs with third-degree AVB and ventricular arrhythmias because these dogs are prone to develop ventricular fibrillation. Considering the use (heart rate) dependence of lidocaine, this drug is more likely to suppress rapid ventricular tachycardia than slower ventricular escape rhythms. Nevertheless, lidocaine should be administered very carefully in these cases, which are best referred to a cardiologist for temporary transvenous pacing to ensure ventricular activity while permitting more aggressive ventricular antiarrhythmic treatment.

Reflex-Mediated Bradycardias

Neurocardiogenic (reflex or vasovagal) syncope is a potential cause of fainting in dogs (see Web Chapter 67). Although the definitive mechanism for this type of syncope is the subject of some debate, it is characterized by reflex activation of the parasympathetic nervous system, suppression of the sympathetic nervous system, and the consequences of bradycardia and decreased peripheral vascular tone (i.e., low blood pressure). In humans, the predominant mechanism can involve cardiac depression, vasodilation, or both. Vasovagal syncope is believed to occur when stimulation of ventricular stretch receptors leads to activation of the medullary vasodepressor region of the brainstem. The reflex (described by Bezold and Jarisch) is mediated by cardiac C fibers, and in dogs it seems to be precipitated by sudden excitement or exercise. Hypotension leads to decreased cerebral perfusion with subsequent loss of consciousness. Vasovagal episodes may be triggered by a number of stimuli, including cough, defecation, and micturition, as well as excitement and sudden exertion.

The mechanism for vasovagal syncope observed in coughing (especially in small-breed brachycephalic breeds) may be multifactorial, associated with decreases in venous return, decreased ventricular preload, increased intracranial pressure, and decreased cerebral perfusion. Syncope might be explained by the combination of decreased preload (which briefly stimulates the sympathetic nervous system and predisposes to ventricular hypercontraction and activation of cardiac mechanoreceptors) and the other aforementioned factors.

In some breeds with severe ventricular arrhythmias (e.g., boxers), sinus arrest may follow a run of rapid ventricular tachycardia. This asystole, rather than the actual tachycardia, may be the cause of collapse, and in some of these animals suppression of the ventricular tachycardia eliminates the sinus arrest, possibly because the stimulus for the Bezold-Jarisch reflex (i.e., myocardial ischemia) is eliminated. However, it is important to remember that some boxers actually have primary sinus node dysfunction and require pacemaker implantation.

Other Treatments for Pathologic Bradycardias

The definitive therapy for the majority of pathologic bradyarrhythmias is permanent pacemaker implantation, as discussed earlier (see Web Chapter 59). In some cases of reflex-mediated bradycardias, eliminating or decreasing triggers such as cough or excitement may be a reasonable therapeutic goal, although some dogs with these syndromes ultimately may require pacemaker implantation. It should be understood, however, that if the predominant mechanism for syncope is vasodilation, pacing may not be effective (as has been shown in a number of human studies).

Palliative pharmacologic therapy may be attempted if the animal has comorbid medical conditions that preclude pacemaker implantation, if logistics preclude immediate pacemaker placement, or if the owner does not wish to pursue pacemaker implantation. Unfortunately, medical therapy rarely is effective. Pharmacologic therapy for bradyarrhythmias generally consists of treatment with either a parasympatholytic drug, an A_1 adenosine receptor antagonist, or a sympathomimetic drug (also see Web Chapter 67). In general, however, none of the drugs described in the following paragraphs is intended for long-term therapy.

Hyoscyamine is a competitive antagonist of the postganglionic cholinergic receptors in the SA and AV nodes that sometimes is used in the treatment of gastrointestinal spasm in humans. It may increase SA node discharge rate and improve AV node conduction in some pathologic bradyarrhythmias. A dosage of 0.003 to 0.006 mg/kg q8h PO is recommended in dogs. The most common adverse effects are mydriasis, decreased salivation, anorexia, and constipation.

Propantheline is another postganglionic cholinergic receptor antagonist that may increase SA node discharge rate and AV node conduction in animals with pathologic bradycardia. A dosage of 0.25 to 0.5 mg/kg q8-12h PO is recommended in dogs. The adverse effect profile of this drug is similar to that of hyoscyamine. Propantheline has become more difficult to procure in recent years, which has prompted more frequent use of other drugs to control bradycardia where indicated.

Some clinicians report success with oral administration of the parenteral formulation of atropine sulfate at a dosage of 0.04 mg/kg diluted 1:10 in a vehicle such a corn syrup to counteract the bitterness of the parenteral drug, although that authors have not used this therapeutic option in bradycardic animals.

Some sympathomimetic drugs commonly used to treat airway disease may be useful in the pharmacologic management of bradycardias. The methylxanthine theophylline, by competitive antagonism of A_1 adenosine receptors, may increase sinus node discharge rate and AV node conduction in animals with pathologic bradycardia. The recommended dosage is 10 mg/kg of the extended-release formulation q12h in dogs. The β_2 agonist terbutaline may also increase SA node discharge rate and improve AV node conduction via either a nonspecific effect on cardiac β_1-receptors or a baroreceptor-mediated increase in cardiac sympathetic tone secondary to a decrease in peripheral arterial pressures resulting from antagonism of vascular smooth muscle cell β_2 receptors. The recommended dosage is 0.14 mg/kg q8-12h PO in dogs and 0.1 to 0.2 mg/kg q12h PO in cats.

Parenteral administration of the nonselective β-adrenergic receptor agonist isoproterenol also may increase sinus rate and improve AV node conduction in hospitalized animals that are awaiting pacemaker implantation or that are being stabilized during an acute crisis. The recommended dosage in dogs is 0.04 to 0.08 µg/kg/min IV. Blood pressure and heart rhythm should be monitored carefully when either parasympatholytic or sympathomimetic drugs are administered because these agents may exacerbate the intermittent tachyarrhythmias that sometimes are observed in animals with pathologic bradycardias (e.g., bradycardia-tachycardia syndrome in SSS patients); this results in the suppression of escape rhythms and dangerously long periods of asystole. In addition, the elevation in sinus rate that may be observed when these agents are administered may exacerbate AV node block secondary to tachycardia-induced refractoriness of AV node tissue. Finally, drugs such as isoproterenol are pure β-agonists and also lead to vasodilation, which reduces diastolic blood pressure and potentially coronary perfusion.

References and Suggested Reading

Gladuli A et al: Poincare plots and tachograms reveal beat patterning in sick sinus syndrome with supraventricular tachycardia and varying AV nodal block, *J Vet Cardiol* 13:63, 2011.

Hanas S et al: Twenty four hour Holter monitoring of unsedated healthy cats in the home environment, *J Vet Cardiol* 11:17, 2009.

Lai SR: Atrioventricular muscular dystrophy in a 5 month old English springer spaniel, *Can Vet J* 50:1286, 2009.

Lamp AP, Meurs KM, Hamlin RL: Correlation of heart rate to body weight in apparently normal dogs, *J Vet Cardiol* 12:107, 2010.

Monfredi O et al: The anatomy and physiology of the sinoatrial node: a contemporary review, *Pacing Clin Electrophysiol* 33:1392, 2010.

Nikolaidou T et al: Structure-function relationship in the sinus and atrioventricular nodes, *Pediatr Cardiol* 33(6):890, 2012.

Wess G et al: Applications, complications, and outcomes of transvenous pacemaker implantation in 105 dogs (1997-2002), *J Vet Intern Med* 20:877, 2006.

CHAPTER **171**

Supraventricular Tachyarrhythmias in Dogs

ROMAIN PARIAUT, *Baton Rouge, Louisiana*
ROBERTO A. SANTILLI, *Varese, Italy*
N. SYDNEY MOÏSE, *Ithaca, New York*

Definition

Tachyarrhythmias are rapid rhythms, with rates typically above 180 to 200 beats/min in dogs, that appear out of proportion to the animal's level of activity or stress. This chapter outlines the diagnostic approach and management strategies for common and uncommon supraventricular tachyarrhythmias (SVTs) in dogs. Additional information regarding management of focal atrial tachycardias, atrial flutter, and atrial fibrillation can be found in Chapters 175, 176, and 178.

Tachyarrhythmia management is based on the discrimination between supraventricular and ventricular rhythms. SVTs have in common that their maintenance necessitates the participation of at least one cardiac structure situated above the ventricles. These structures include the sinus and atrioventricular (AV) nodes, the bundle of His, the atrial myocardium, the tributary veins such as the coronary sinus, the pulmonary veins or venae cavae, and on occasion accessory pathways. The main characteristic of SVTs on the surface electrocardiogram (ECG) is a narrow QRS complex (<70 ms in dogs), which indicates that electrical impulses, once they reach the ventricles, propagate within specialized muscular bundles of the His-Purkinje conduction system, similar to normal sinus beats. However, it is not unusual for SVTs to display broader QRS complexes as a result of an anatomic lesion or a rate-dependent prolongation of intraventricular conduction (e.g., bundle branch block).

Pathophysiology

The initiation of arrhythmias requires precipitating factors and a suitable substrate. Supraventricular structures such as vascular orifices opening into the atria (cranial and caudal vena cava, coronary sinus, pulmonary veins), muscular ridges (crista terminalis, eustachian ridge), and valve annuli create areas of block, slow conduction, and tissue boundaries that facilitate arrhythmia wave front propagation. Although myocyte depolarization is usually limited to the sinus and AV nodes, other supraventricular structures, in particular the crista terminalis and pulmonary veins, can become sources of focal ectopic activity. Ischemia, interstitial fibrosis, inflammation, and atrial chamber dilation also contribute the arrhythmogenic substrate. Additionally, autonomic influences and electrolyte abnormalities can contribute to the initiation and perpetuation of arrhythmias. It is therefore understandable that heart failure is frequently accompanied by SVTs.

Electrophysiologic mechanisms responsible for SVTs can be categorized into abnormalities of electrical impulse formation and abnormalities of impulse propagation. The first group of mechanisms encompasses abnormal automaticity in which myocytes depolarize spontaneously at a faster rate than sinus node cells and triggered activity in which spontaneous depolarization of cells is precipitated by repolarization abnormalities from the preceding action potential. Another mechanism known as *reentry* is the repetitive propagation of an impulse around an area of nonconducting tissue, such as a vein, a valve annulus, or a fibrotic region.

Classification

SVTs, currently diagnosed by electrophysiologic studies in dogs, can be classified according to the site of origin and the underlying arrhythmogenic mechanism. They include atrioventricular reciprocating tachycardia, focal atrial tachycardia, macro-reentrant atrial tachycardia or atrial flutter, focal junctional tachycardia, and atrial fibrillation. Although atrioventricular nodal reentrant tachycardia is a common cause of paroxysmal tachycardia in people, it has not been identified in dogs.

Atrioventricular reciprocating tachycardias (AVRTs) are macro-reentrant arrhythmias in which the electrical wave front moves along an anatomic circuit formed by the AV-His-Purkinje system, the ventricles, accessory pathways, and the atria. Accessory pathways are congenital muscular bundles that do not regress during the formation of the cardiac skeleton. These pathways represent an alternative route of AV or ventriculoatrial (VA) conduction besides the AV node. In the dog, accessory pathways are predominantly right-sided in the posteroseptal and right posterior area of the tricuspid annulus (in human nomenclature), rarely are multiple, and frequently present with unidirectional retrograde conduction (70% of cases) with no evidence of ventricular preexcitation during sinus rhythm. Two forms of AVRT have been described in human patients: orthodromic, in which the wave front descends from the atria to the ventricles along the AV node and returns to the atria along the accessory pathway, and antidromic, in which the wave front circles in the opposite direction. Only orthodromic AVRT and a preexcited form of atrial fibrillation have been described thus far in dogs.

Focal atrial tachycardias (FATs) correspond to the rhythmic atrial activation of a small area of atrial tissue (focus) from which wave fronts spread out centrifugally. In dogs, FATs are more commonly right sided (63% of cases) and automatic (78% of cases). It has been observed that FATs arising from the pulmonary veins trigger atrial fibrillation in 25% of the dogs examined.

Atrial flutter (AFL) is a macro-reentrant atrial tachycardia characterized by an organized atrial rhythm with a rate typically above 300 beats/min. The anatomic circuit of AFL includes the cavotricuspid isthmus, which is an area of the low posterior right atrium delimited by the caudal vena cava and the eustachian ridge posteriorly and the tricuspid valve annulus anteriorly. Based on the rotation pattern around the tricuspid valve annulus, two forms of cavotricuspid isthmus–dependent AFL have been identified: typical and reverse typical. During typical AFL the activation wave front turns counterclockwise around the tricuspid valve annulus when viewed from above, whereas during reverse typical AFL it turns clockwise.

Focal junctional tachycardia (FJT) is caused by an abnormally rapid discharge from the junctional region just posterior to the AV node and the bundle of His.

Atrial fibrillation (AF) is a rhythm disturbance characterized by uncoordinated atrial activations with consequent deterioration of atrial mechanical function and an irregular ventricular response rate.

Other features widely used in the human literature to characterize SVTs include their clinical presentation, duration, and mode of onset and termination. Accordingly, SVTs can be described as nonsustained (<30 seconds in duration), sustained >30 seconds in duration or causing syncope), incessant (lasting >12 hours a day), repetitive (runs of nonsustained tachycardia alternating with period of normal sinus rhythm), or paroxysmal (abrupt initiation and termination). A classification specific to AF differentiates it into paroxysmal (self-limiting and lasting <7 days), persistent (uninterrupted, but sinus rhythm can be restored with electrical or pharmacologic cardioversion), or permanent (sinus rhythm cannot be restored).

As suggested by the brief preceding discussion, SVTs are in many ways more complicated to classify and diagnose than ventricular tachycardias. Except in straightforward cases, such as persistent or permanent AF, the veterinarian should consider consultation or referral to a cardiologist because advanced methods of diagnosis and therapy might be necessary.

Clinical Manifestations and Evaluation

Common signs associated with SVT include weight loss, lethargy, exercise intolerance, excessive panting, and dyspnea. However, it is not uncommon for dogs to be asymptomatic. Owners of dogs with SVT may report seeing the dog's heart pounding in the chest during episodes of tachycardia. Episodic weakness and transient loss of consciousness are less common with SVT, unless the vasomotor reflex is inadequate. Additionally, SVTs may be recognized only at the time of physical examination in dogs with signs of congestive heart failure. In these situations, it is difficult to determine the contribution of the arrhythmia to the clinical signs and to the degree of myocardial dysfunction because an uncontrolled ventricular rate can lead to progressive myocardial failure independent of any underlying structural disease. This phenomenon is known as *tachycardiomyopathy*, and it is likely that a sustained rate above 250 beats/min will induce severe myocardial dysfunction within 3 to 4 weeks. It is noteworthy that, even when overt tachycardia-related myocardial failure is absent, atrial remodeling in the form of ion channel alteration, myocytolysis, glycogen accumulation, or contractility dysfunction occurs secondary to sustained SVT. This explains the tendency of some SVTs to resist antiarrhythmic therapy or to recur after conversion to sinus rhythm.

Cardiac auscultation is a useful diagnostic tool to calculate heart rate, detect occasional ectopic beats, and distinguish between paroxysmal and sustained arrhythmias. Whereas paroxysmal SVTs are usually regular, SVTs associated with variable AV conduction have an irregular rhythm. This occurs with AF, which is easily recognized on auscultation as a sustained and irregular tachycardia. Pulses may be weaker during bouts of tachycardia, and pulse deficits also may be recognized. However, some dogs with paroxysmal SVT are in sinus rhythm at the time of presentation.

Obtaining a 6- to 12-lead surface ECG is the initial step in identifying the arrhythmia. Further characterization of the SVT is obtained by ambulatory 24-hour ECG recordings (Holter monitoring). The information collected from the recording should include the number of episodes and their duration, the modes of arrhythmia onset and termination, and precise information about SVT cycle length and overall heart rate, especially when the animal is in a familiar environment. Evaluation of heart rate distribution over 24 hours in conjunction with an activity log completed by the owner during the period of recording is a source of valuable information on the circadian pattern of the arrhythmia and on the contribution of adrenergic tone to the initiation and rate of the arrhythmia.

Imaging also is part of the diagnostic workup. Dogs with clinical signs of congestive heart failure should be evaluated by thoracic radiography. An echocardiogram is indicated to identify structural cardiac disease and assess ventricular function.

Electrocardiographic Differential Diagnosis

In the last decade, detailed endocardial mapping has established the underlying arrhythmogenic mechanism and the site of origin of the most common SVTs in the dog. With this information as a guide, a stepwise approach to ECG interpretation can be used to diagnose SVTs (Figure 171-1). The duration of the QRS complex is the first parameter that should be assessed to distinguish SVTs from ventricular tachycardia. This step should be followed by determination of the ventricular rate, the regularity of the R-R interval, signs of atrial activation, the relationship between ventricular and atrial activation, presence of QRS complex alternans, ST-segment anomalies, and finally the AV conduction ratio during tachycardia. Signs of ventricular preexcitation, characterized by a consistent and short P-R interval, should be sought during periods of sinus rhythm.

SVTs are usually tachycardias with a narrow QRS complex (<70 ms) unless there is a functional bundle branch block (due to phase 3 aberrancy) or antegrade conduction into the ventricular myocardium along an accessory pathway (as with antidromic AVRT or preexcited AF).

Different ventricular rates during SVT have been reported: 190 to 300 beats/min for AVRT, 210 to 230 beats/min for FAT, 180 to 350 beats/min for AFL depending on the presence of AV conduction block, 130 to 260 beats/min for AF, and 120 to 200 beats/min for focal junctional tachycardia (FJT). Although the ventricular rate during FJT often is lower than 180 beats/min, it is usually considered a tachycardia because it arises from the junctional region where normal automaticity ranges from 40 to 60 per minute. Additionally, in an individual dog the rate may exceed the usual rates given here.

Tachycardias with a narrow QRS complex can be classified further into SVTs with a regular or irregular R-R interval. SVTs with a regular R-R interval include AVRT, FJT, and AFL with fixed AV conduction. SVTs with an irregular R-R interval include FAT, AFL with variable AV conduction, and AF. However, subtle beat-to-beat cycle length alternans of more than 20 ms has been reported in dogs with orthodromic AVRT. Automatic FAT also can present with regular R-R intervals during sudden periods of cycle-length irregularity caused by a warm-up and cooldown behavior of the automatic focus.

Atrial activation during SVT is represented on the ECG by P′ waves, flutter (F) waves, or fibrillation (f) waves. Often, because of the elevated rate, atrial waves are hidden in the previous ST segment or T wave. Sometimes these buried atrial waves can be located by comparing the morphology of the P-QRS-T complexes during sinus rhythm and during tachycardia. It is also helpful to pay particular attention to sections of slower heart rate that might occur with physiologic AV block or during a decrease in the rate of atrial activation.

P′ waves result from atrial activation that spreads from an ectopic focus (FAT), from the atrial insertion of an accessory pathway (AVRT), or from the AV node (FJT with 1:1 VA conduction). In dogs, the most common site of origin of FATs is the crista terminalis; such FATs are characterized by P′ waves with a superior-to-inferior (cranial-to-caudal in veterinary nomenclature) axis (−20 to +90 degrees). The second most common origin is the ostium of the coronary sinus, which gives rise to P′ waves with an inferior-to-superior (caudal-to-cranial) and right-to-left axis (−20 to −80 degrees). Less commonly, the focus lies in the left atrium with an atrial activation directed toward the right, with P′ waves that are negative in leads aVL and I. In addition, the P′-wave axis is deviated inferiorly (+90 to +180 degrees) when the impulse originates from the roof of the left atrium, and it is deviated superiorly (−180 to −100 degrees) when it starts from the floor of the atrium. When a P′ wave results from a retrograde activation starting from the atrial insertion of an accessory pathway or from the AV node, as in the case of FJT with 1:1 VA conduction, it is usually concentric, with an atrial vector directed inferior to superior (−100 to −80 degrees). The presence of positive P′ waves in lead aVR is diagnostic of orthodromic AVRT.

In the case of typical AFL, the F waves appear as a continuous and organized oscillation of the baseline with a rate above 300 beats/min, a saw-toothed morphology, and no isoelectric line between consecutive F waves. In the case of reverse typical AFL, the F-wave deflections are usually positive in the inferior leads (II, III, and aVF), and they can be separated by an isoelectric line. In contrast, atrial depolarizations during AF are characterized by low voltage and baseline oscillations of variable morphology (f waves) with a rate between 400 and 600 beats/min and with no isoelectric line between them.

If P′ waves are detected, the next step is to assess their relationship with the R wave. This is particularly useful in cases of FAT and orthodromic AVRT. The RP′ interval is considered short when it lasts less than 50% of the

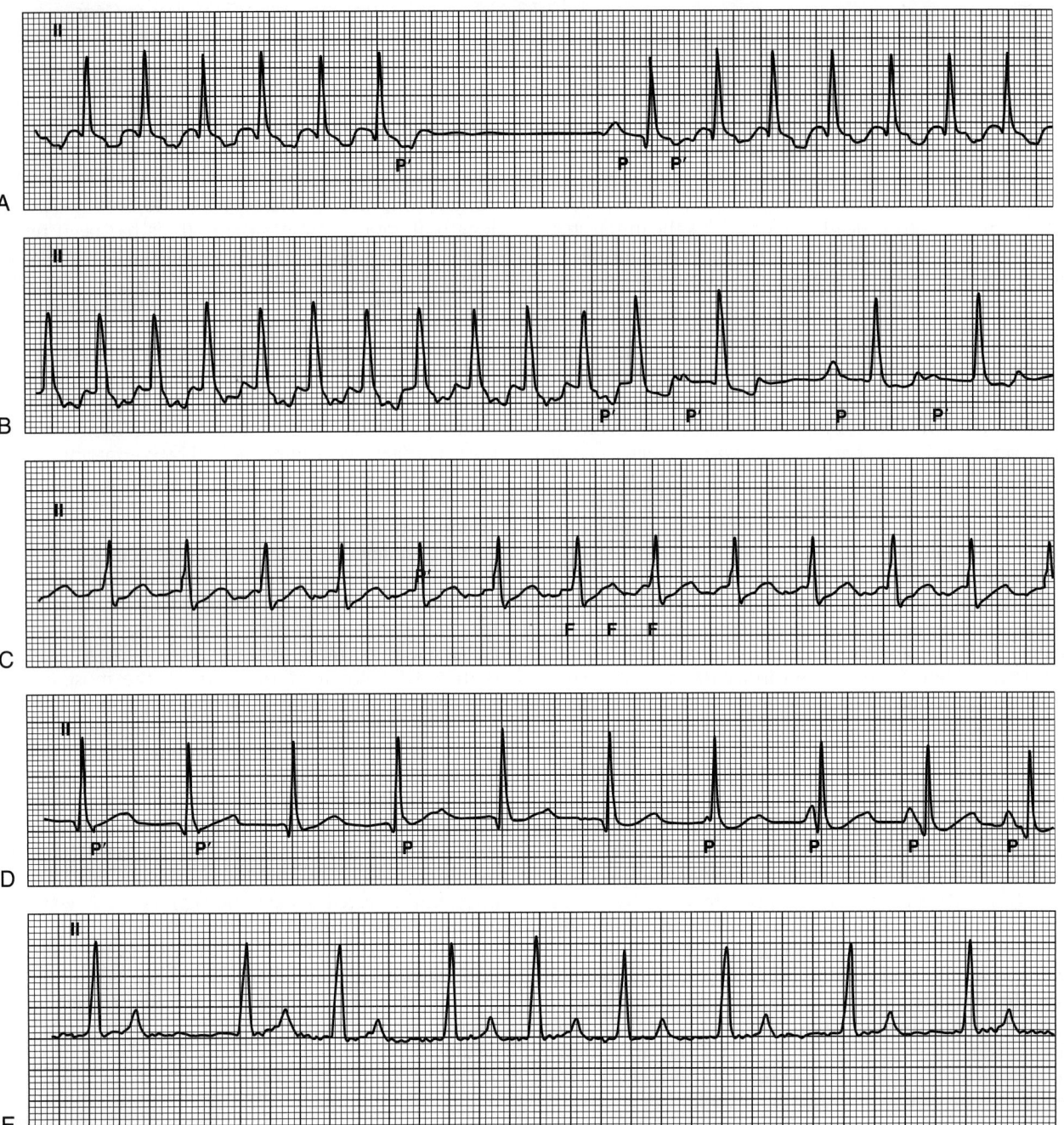

Figure 171-1 Surface electrocardiographic tracings of common supraventricular tachyarrhythmias. **A,** Orthodromic atrioventricular reciprocating tachycardia. The first part of the tracing shows a narrow-QRS tachycardia with a regular cycle length of 200 msec (300 beats/min); after the sixth beat the tachycardia stops suddenly and a sinus beat occurs (P); the tachycardia then restarts with the same cycle length. During the tachycardia a retrograde atrial activation is visible in the ST segment with an inferior-to-superior axis on the frontal plane (P') and a short RP' interval (shorter than 50% of the relative RR interval, RP':P'R = 0.57). The P'R interval after the sinus beats is longer; this indicates prolonged conduction along the AV node, which triggers the onset of tachycardia. **B,** Focal atrial tachycardia arising from the crista terminalis. The first part of the tracing shows a narrow-QRS-complex tachycardia with a regular cycle length of 200 msec (300 beats/min). After the twelfth beat a cycle-length irregularity occurs characterized by a longer RR interval in which the ectopic atrial activation (P') appears after the T wave; then a sinus beat occurs (P), followed by an ectopic beat. In the first part of the tracing, the P' is superimposed on the previous ST segment with a superior-to-inferior axis on the frontal plane and a RP':P'R of 0.8. After the twelfth beat, the depolarization rate of the ectopic focus decreases, which causes a longer RP'; AV conduction prolongation explains the longer P'R interval. **C,** Typical atrial flutter with a 2:1 conduction ratio. The tracing shows a narrow-QRS tachycardia with a regular cycle length of 240 msec (250 beats/min). Atrial activations (F) are continuous and regular with a saw-toothed appearance. Every other F wave is blocked in the AV node. **D,** Focal junctional tachycardia with 1:1 ventriculoatrial retrograde conduction progressing to isorhythmic atrioventricular dissociation. The first part of the tracing shows a narrow-QRS-complex tachycardia with a regular cycle length of 400 msec (150 beats/min). In all but the last beat the ventricular depolarization starts from the junctional area. The atria are depolarized in the first two beats in a retrograde manner along the AV node and appear as pseudo S waves (P'); then, starting from the third beat, the atria are depolarized by the sinus node at a progressively faster rate, which induces a shift of the P waves from the right to the left of the relative QRS complex with a secondary increase in the PQ interval (isorhythmic atrioventricular dissociation). As soon as the sinus rate is faster than the junctional rate, the ventricles are depolarized starting from the sinus node, and a sinus beat appears (last QRS complex). **E,** Atrial fibrillation. The tracing shows a narrow-QRS-complex tachycardia with an irregular cycle length and an average ventricular rate of 140 beats/min. Atrial activations are characterized by low voltage and oscillations of variable morphology (f waves). Lead II; paper speed, 50 mm/sec; calibration, 10 mm/mV.

respective R-R interval and long if it lasts longer than 50%. Orthodromic AVRTs have a RP':P'R ratio of less than 0.7, whereas FATs have a RP':P'R ratio of more than 0.7.

A pearl of ECG diagnosis is identification of QRS complex alternans. This is a beat-to-beat variation of the QRS amplitude of 0.1 mV in at least one lead. It is particularly common in orthodromic AVRT (86%) but also has been observed with FAT and AFL.

Deviation of the ST segment during tachycardia can be caused by the presence of a hidden P' wave or the heterogeneity of action potential duration in the ventricles during tachycardia. ST shift is present in almost 65% of dogs with orthodromic AVRT.

Assessment of AV conduction during tachycardia allows differentiation between orthodromic AVRT, which always presents with 1:1 conduction, and FAT, AFL, and AF, in which conduction can be associated with different degrees of AV block. FJT usually is characterized by isorhythmic AV dissociation alternating with periods of 1:1 VA conduction.

The presence of ventricular preexcitation during sinus rhythm proves the existence of an accessory pathway with antegrade conduction and suggests a risk of orthodromic AVRT. The term *ventricular preexcitation* describes the activation of part of the ventricular myocardium before the atrial wave front reaches the ventricular myocardium along the His-Purkinje system. Accessory pathways conduct bidirectionally in only 25% of dogs described in published reports, whereas 75% have orthodromic AVRT mediated by antegrade conduction over the AV node and only retrograde conduction (i.e., concealed conduction) across the accessory pathway. The ECG features of ventricular preexcitation in the dog include short PQ interval (<60 ms); presence of a delta wave on the upstroke of the QRS complex; wide QRS complex, commonly with a splintered appearance; ST deviation; and T-wave anomalies.

Clinical Management

Factors Associated with the Decision to Treat

Treatment is justified when SVTs cause clinical signs or impair ventricular performance. These outcomes usually are related directly to the rate and duration of the tachyarrhythmia. The timing of VA activation during the tachycardia also may be an important contributor to clinical signs. A short VA interval, which indicates that the atria and the ventricles are activated almost simultaneously, results in the contraction of the atria against closed AV valves, which leads to the elevation of intraatrial pressures with subsequent chamber enlargement and decreased cardiac output. In the absence of obvious clinical signs, treatment should be considered if tachycardia-induced cardiomyopathy is suspected. When SVTs are intermittent, relating the clinical signs to the arrhythmia may be challenging. In this situation, long-term recording of the cardiac rhythm with ambulatory 24-hour Holter recording, or preferably using a wearable or implantable loop event recorder, is indicated.

Rate Versus Rhythm Control

Heart rate control and heart rhythm control are the two general approaches taken when managing SVTs. The rate-control approach aims at slowing ventricular rate in response to rapid supraventricular impulses to alleviate clinical signs and prevent further deterioration of ventricular function. However, it does not terminate the arrhythmia. Rate control is based on increasing AV node filtering by prolonging the refractory period of the calcium-dependent AV nodal cells. This strategy is preferred when arrhythmia triggers cannot be eliminated and therefore the arrhythmia would likely recur soon after its termination, as is the case when heart failure is present.

For example, the rate-control strategy is the standard approach to AF in dogs and most commonly involves therapy with some combination of digoxin, diltiazem, and a β-blocker, depending on the clinical situation (see later and Chapters 176 and 178. Virtually all dogs with AF and heart failure require heart rate control. In contrast, in dogs with lone AF (AF without structural disease or heart failure), the need for pharmacologic control of the heart rate is best determined from the heart rate distribution obtained from a baseline 24-hour Holter recording because an ECG recorded at a single point of time may not be representative of overall control. The effect of therapy in both situations is best assessed using follow-up Holter recording about 2 weeks after treatment initiation. What constitutes adequate rate control in dogs with heart failure and in those with lone AF has not been precisely defined and may depend on the animal's underlying myocardial function. Usually, an average heart rate of 120 to 140 beats/min is considered adequate to observe clinical improvement. If the average heart rate is considered too high, drug dosages are increased by small increments with close monitoring of the animal's clinical status.

The rhythm-control strategy terminates the arrhythmia and restores sinus rhythm. This may be accomplished in some cases with drugs or in acute settings with direct-current electrical cardioversion (see Web Chapter 60). Although theoretically rhythm control represents the optimal approach, its implementation is hampered by the limited number of effective and safe options for terminating and maintaining sinus rhythm over the long term. Accordingly, rate control is often a more attractive alternative. Sometimes a drug is administered for rate control but converts the rhythm back to sinus rhythm. This is usually an after-the-fact indication that the AV node was a critical component of the arrhythmia mechanism, as is the case for AVRTs.

Pharmacologic Treatment

Antiarrhythmic drugs are the mainstay of SVT treatment (Table 171-1). However, antiarrhythmic drug administration should be preceded or accompanied by consideration of potential triggers for the arrhythmia. For example, electrolyte disturbances, hypoxemia, hypovolemia, and acidosis are potentially correctable causes of SVT. It also should be noted that hormones, in particular thyroid supplements, have also been linked to SVTs in dogs.

TABLE 171-1

Pharmacologic and Nonpharmacologic Management of Supraventricular Tachyarrhythmias

	ARRHYTHMIA CLASSIFICATION				ATRIAL FIBRILLATION (AF)		
	Focal Atrial Tachycardia	Focal Junctional Tachycardia	Atrioventricular Reciprocating Tachycardia	CTI-Dependent Atrial Flutter	Paroxysmal	Persistent	Permanent
Pharmacologic							
Class IA (Na blockers) Procainamide *Slow IV bolus: 5-15 mg/kg*	Conversion	—	Conversion	Conversion	—	—	—
Class IB (Na blockers) Lidocaine *Slow IV bolus (max. 4): 2 mg/kg*	—	—	Conversion	—	Conversion (vagally mediated AF)	—	—
Class II (β-blockers) Atenolol *Oral: 0.2-1 mg/kg q12-24h* Esmolol *Slow IV bolus: 0.2-0.5 mg/kg* Metoprolol *Oral: 0.2-0.8 mg/kg q12h (start with low end of dose range)*	Rate control	Conversion SR maintenance	Conversion SR maintenance	Rate control	Rate control	Rate control	Rate control ± digoxin
Class III (K blockers) Sotalol *Oral: 1-3 mg/kg q12h*	Conversion SR maintenance	—	Conversion SR maintenance	Conversion SR maintenance	—	—	—
Amiodarone *Oral: Loading dosage, 10-30 mg/kg q24h for 2-14 days; maintenance dosage, 6-15 mg/kg q24h*	Conversion SR maintenance	—	Conversion SR maintenance	Conversion SR maintenance	Conversion SR maintenance	Conversion Rate control	Rate control
Class IV (Ca blockers) Diltiazem *IV bolus: 0.1-0.4 mg/kg over 5 min; CRI: 1-4 µg/kg/min; Oral: 1-2 mg/kg q8h (standard) or 3-5 mg/kg q12h (extended release)*	Rate control	Conversion SR maintenance	Conversion SR maintenance	Rate control	Rate control	Rate control	Rate control ± digoxin
Cardiac glycoside Digoxin *Oral: 0.005 mg/kg q12h*	Rate control	—	—	Rate control	—	Rate control	Rate control
Radiofrequency ablation	SR maintenance	SR maintenance	SR maintenance	SR maintenance	SR maintenance	—	—
Direct-current cardioversion	Conversion	Conversion	Conversion	Conversion	Conversion	Conversion	—

CRI, Constant-rate infusion; *CTI,* cavotricuspid isthmus; *IV,* intravenous; *max.,* maximum; *SR,* sinus rhythm.

Antiarrhythmic drugs are indicated for immediate termination of arrhythmias in animals in hemodynamically unstable condition, for long-term rate-control management of SVTs, and for maintenance of sinus rhythm after initial cardioversion. Drug selection is based on the type of arrhythmia, the risk of adverse reactions, and the degree of cardiac dysfunction. Other factors to take into account are decreased oral medication absorption, drug metabolism and elimination in the presence of ascites, and the decreased hepatic and renal blood flow that accompany heart failure. Moreover, drug selection may depend on the level of certainty regarding the nature of the arrhythmia; for example, it may be challenging to determine the origin of a wide-complex tachycardia. Drugs used for rate-control management of SVTs, diltiazem in particular, may cause hemodynamic collapse if given in the presence of rapid ventricular tachycardia that would persist at a fast rate despite treatment.

Atrioventricular Node–Blocking Drugs

The nondihydropyridine calcium channel blocker diltiazem is widely used for the management of SVTs. A graded dose of diltiazem results in a decrease in ventricular response rate because of slower propagation of the action potential in the AV node. This decrease is accentuated at faster heart rates, a phenomenon known as the *use-dependent effect*. On occasion, diltiazem terminates SVTs if the arrhythmia mechanism depends on the AV node. Diltiazem can be administered by intravenous bolus and constant-rate infusion for short-term management of tachyarrhythmias. Oral formulations include standard and extended-release forms. When the drug is evaluated for long-term management of AF, a dosage of 3 to 5 mg/kg every 12 hours PO for the extended-release formulation usually achieves satisfactory rate control. Better rate control, especially during periods associated with high adrenergic tone, can be obtained by adding digoxin to the treatment regimen at a dosage of 0.0055 to 0.0075 mg/kg every 12 hours PO. Calcium channel blockers decrease ventricular contractility and may cause hypotension when used in animals with severely depressed cardiac function.

The range of indications for and adverse effects of β-blockers such as atenolol are very similar to those of calcium channel blockers. β-Blockers are indicated when adrenergic tone is thought to play an important role in the initiation and maintenance of the arrhythmia. They are frequently combined with other antiarrhythmic medications to improve control of the arrhythmia. Esmolol is a short-acting intravenous β-blocker that is rapidly metabolized by plasma esterases. It is used for rate control and termination of AV node–dependent SVTs. However, it may be less effective than intravenous diltiazem.

The occurrence of episodes of transient loss of consciousness in dogs treated with rate-control medications should raise the suspicion of drug-induced periods of sinus arrest or AV block as the cause of the syncope.

Sodium Channel Blockers

Sodium channel blockers include procainamide, flecainide, and lidocaine. These drugs are potentially effective for management of SVTs, but there are issues with each. Unfortunately, procainamide no longer is available in an oral formulation, and availability of the intravenous formulation is limited outside the United States. Lidocaine has been used successfully to treat some acute (vagally induced) SVTs, but its value is limited to those situations. Flecainide is used in human patients with AF, but its effectiveness and safety in dogs requires better delineation.

Procainamide has been used to manage reentrant arrhythmias and to slow conduction in accessory pathways displaying antegrade conduction. It also is indicated for short-term management of wide-complex tachycardias when discrimination between supraventricular and ventricular tachycardia is difficult because it also is very effective in terminating ventricular arrhythmias. For short-term management of a suspected orthodromic AVRT, procainamide at 2 mg/kg IV repeated four to six times or 8 to 12 mg/kg every 4 to 6 hours IM may be considered.

Although lidocaine is used extensively as the first-line therapy for immediate termination of ventricular tachycardia, its use for treatment of SVT has been reported only recently. It has been shown to terminate episodes of SVTs in the presence or absence of an accessory pathway. Lidocaine also has been used successfully to terminate recent-onset paroxysmal AF initiated by elevated vagal tone in large-breed dogs with normal cardiac function. One or two boluses of lidocaine restores sinus rhythm within 30 to 90 seconds but causes transient mild hypotension following the intravenous bolus.

Potassium Channel Blockers

Potassium channel blockers, including sotalol and amiodarone, are widely used in human patients with a variety of SVTs, but there is limited information about their effectiveness and safety in dogs. These drugs have been used empirically both to convert SVTs and to maintain control of sinus rhythm after successful conversion.

Sotalol combines potassium channel–blocking properties that prolong atrial and ventricular myocyte refractory periods with a mild β-blocking effect. Peak plasma concentration is reached 2 to 4 hours after oral administration. Sotalol has been used to terminate arrhythmias in patients in hemodynamically stable condition because it takes from a few hours to a few days for conversion to occur. However, because of its stronger effect on the refractory period at slower heart rates, a property known as the *reverse use-dependent effect*, sotalol may be more effective in preventing arrhythmia recurrence than in terminating SVTs. The negative inotropic effect of sotalol is modest compared with that of other β-blockers. Nonetheless, dogs with myocardial failure should be monitored closely while receiving sotalol.

Amiodarone shares properties of all four classes of antiarrhythmic drugs. The drug increases the refractory period in supraventricular tissues and slows AV conduction. Amiodarone has been used by some cardiologists for maintenance of sinus rhythm after electrocardioversion and for control of SVTs. Unfortunately, adverse effects are frequent and can be severe. Administered orally, amiodarone has been shown to cause hepatopathy, thyroid dysfunction, and gastrointestinal upset. When it is given intravenously, dogs frequently develop skin reaction, pruritus, and on occasion hypotension (although a new intravenous preparation may minimize some of these effects). Owing to these risks, the authors do not use amiodarone routinely to manage SVTs in dogs.

Nonpharmacologic Treatment

Synchronized direct-current cardioversion can be successful in terminating SVTs, including AF, and its use is detailed in Web Chapter 60. In most cases cardioversion is a referral procedure and is considered by the majority of cardiologists to be most feasible when treating either dogs with structurally normal hearts (e.g., lone AF) or those with drug-resistant tachyarrhythmias.

Radiofrequency catheter ablation (RFCA) has been used to treat SVTs in dogs and can be very effective but demands special equipment and training. Its application has been described for the treatment of orthodromic AVRT, FAT, and AFL. Radiofrequency current has a non-modulated sinusoidal waveform of a high frequency (0.3 to 30 kHz). For cardiac ablation, low frequencies (<10 kHz) are avoided to prevent stimulation of cardiac tissues. Once absorbed, radiofrequency energy is converted into heat, which warms the endocardium or epicardium and induces a coagulation necrosis with secondary loss of the electrophysiologic properties of the tissue. The range of temperatures used for RFCA is 50° to 90°C (122° to 194°F). Most electrophysiologic laboratories perform RFCA using a thermocouple-tipped, steerable 7 Fr catheter connected to a radiofrequency generator with temperature control.

In veterinary cardiology, accessory pathways are the most common target for ablation. To ablate an orthodromic AVRT circuit, the ablation catheter is placed at the atrial endocardial insertion of the accessory pathway around the tricuspid valve annulus or within the coronary sinus. Ablation procedures are guided by intracardiac recording: for bipolar recordings the shorter VA interval, or bypass tract potentials, are sought during

tachycardia or ventricular pacing, and for unipolar recordings a sharp, negative waveform is sought.

FATs arising from foci along the crista terminalis, right atrial appendage, triangle of Koch, pulmonary veins, and coronary sinus are the second indication for RFCA. To map automatic foci, either bipolar or unipolar recordings should be used. The goal of mapping is to identify the electrical epicenter of atrial activation, which is characterized by the earliest high-frequency, low-amplitude, and fragmented signal on a bipolar recording timed to the surface P' waves (this signal usually precedes the onset of P' waves with a mean interval of -39.9 ± 17.7 msec) and by a sharp, negative waveform on a unipolar recording.

RFCA is the treatment of choice for typical and reverse typical AFL. In these arrhythmias, the target of ablation is the cavotricuspid isthmus, where a linear lesion is created to obtain a bidirectional conduction block. The end point of ablation is demonstrated by the presence of a collision of waveforms while pacing the coronary sinus, with a superoinferior activation of the right free wall, a prolongation of isthmic conduction pacing either from the low right free wall or the coronary sinus, and a double potential at the site of linear ablation.

References and Suggested Reading

Gelzer AR et al: Combination therapy with digoxin and diltiazem controls ventricular rate in chronic atrial fibrillation in dogs better than digoxin or diltiazem monotherapy: a randomized crossover study in 18 dogs, *J Vet Intern Med* 23:499, 2009.

Pariaut R et al: Lidocaine converts acute vagally associated atrial fibrillation to sinus rhythm in German Shepherd dogs with inherited arrhythmias, *J Vet Intern Med* 22:1274, 2008.

Santilli RA et al: Utility of 12-lead electrocardiogram for differentiating paroxysmal supraventricular tachycardias in dogs, *J Vet Intern Med* 22:915, 2008.

Santilli RA et al: Electrophysiologic characteristics and topographic distribution of focal atrial tachycardias in dogs, *J Vet Intern Med* 24:539, 2010a.

Santilli RA et al: Radiofrequency catheter ablation of cavotricuspid isthmus as treatment of atrial flutter in two dogs, *J Vet Cardiol* 12:59, 2010b.

CHAPTER 172

Ventricular Arrhythmias in Dogs

MARK A. OYAMA, *Philadelphia, Pennsylvania*
CARYN A. REYNOLDS, *Baton Rouge, Louisiana*

Ventricular arrhythmias are encountered frequently in canine patients. The clinical setting ranges from single ventricular premature complexes in an asymptomatic dog to life-threatening ventricular tachycardia requiring immediate treatment. The decision whether to initiate antiarrhythmic therapy is contingent on clinical signs and the severity and underlying cause of the arrhythmia. Since ventricular arrhythmias in dogs can occur either as a consequence of primary cardiac disease or secondary to other systemic illness, successful management often requires a thorough diagnostic workup.

Diagnosis

Impulses originating from the ventricle are recognized by the presence of abnormally wide QRS complexes with large T waves typically displaying a polarity opposite that of the QRS complex. Because the impulse originates from an ectopic focus in the ventricle, it is not consistently associated with a preceding P wave. Ventricular premature complexes (VPCs) or ventricular tachycardia (VT) is seen on the electrocardiogram (ECG) as impulses originating from the ventricle and occurring at a faster heart rate than the sinus rate. Determining the most likely underlying cause of the rhythm disturbance has practical importance because it affects whether therapy is needed, whether there is a risk of sudden death, and whether any treatment is likely to be short-lived or lifelong.

The most malignant ventricular arrhythmias typically occur in dogs with significant underlying cardiac disease, such as cardiomyopathy, valvular heart disease, or myocarditis. These animals are more likely to have VT at rapid heart rates (>200 beats/min), which reduces cardiac output, causes clinical signs such as syncope or weakness, and has the potential to culminate in fatal ventricular fibrillation or asystole. Boxers and English bulldogs with arrhythmogenic right ventricular cardiomyopathy, Dobermans with dilated cardiomyopathy, and German shepherds with inherited ventricular arrhythmias are at particularly high risk of sudden death from ventricular arrhythmias. Malignant VT also may result from myocardial hypoxia in diseases that cause ventricular hypertrophy, such as subaortic stenosis or pulmonic stenosis.

Single VPCs and less malignant VT often are associated with noncardiac illness. Although the precise mechanism for these rhythm disturbances may not be known, the clinical associations are well established. For example, splenic masses and other abdominal neoplasms, gastric dilatation and volvulus, trauma, hypoxia, and systemic inflammatory states such as immune-mediated cytopenias or pancreatitis often are related to the incidental finding of ventricular arrhythmias. Ventricular rhythms at relatively slower heart rates (<150 beat/min) are unlikely to affect cardiac output, cause clinical signs, or result in sudden death, and therefore treatment usually is not necessary. These "slow VT" or accelerated idioventricular rhythms often occur at heart rates similar to the sinus rate and resolve without antiarrhythmic therapy once the underlying systemic illness has been resolved.

Diagnostic Approach

The clinical importance of ventricular arrhythmias depends on the underlying cause. In breeds with a high incidence of primary cardiac causes of arrhythmias (e.g., boxers and Doberman pinschers), single VPCs, although unlikely to be causing clinical signs, raise suspicion of underlying cardiomyopathy. In these animals, additional diagnostic tests, such as echocardiography, thoracic radiography, or 24-hour ambulatory ECG (Holter) monitoring, are performed routinely to corroborate the diagnosis, assess the risk of future congestive heart failure, and evaluate the need for antiarrhythmic therapy. In other breeds of dogs with less risk of underlying cardiomyopathy and in dogs with hearts of normal size and function, a search for noncardiac causes of ventricular arrhythmias is indicated, and further diagnostic testing might include complete blood count and blood chemistry studies, infectious disease titers, serum cardiac troponin I level, abdominal ultrasonography, and thoracic radiography. If intermittent arrhythmias are suspected, Holter monitoring generally is recommended to determine the presence and malignancy of any arrhythmias and their relationship to any clinical signs that might be noted.

Indications for Treatment

The efficacy of long-term antiarrhythmic therapy to prevent sudden death in dogs with ventricular arrhythmias is unknown. For this reason, antiarrhythmic therapy generally is reserved for arrhythmias that are rapid (>180 beats/min), sustained (lasting >30 seconds), or associated with clinical signs (e.g., syncope, weakness). In these instances, clinical signs can be improved in the majority of patients with antiarrhythmic therapy. Single VPCs or slower ventricular rhythms (<150 beats/min) are unlikely to cause clinical signs, and therapy typically is not indicated in these cases (Figure 172-1).

Treatment

Dogs that have sustained VT associated with clinical signs of hypotension, syncope, or cardiac shock should receive immediate treatment (Figure 172-2). Intravenous lidocaine at 2 mg/kg is the first-line drug of choice (Table 172-1). If the rhythm does not convert to sinus rhythm

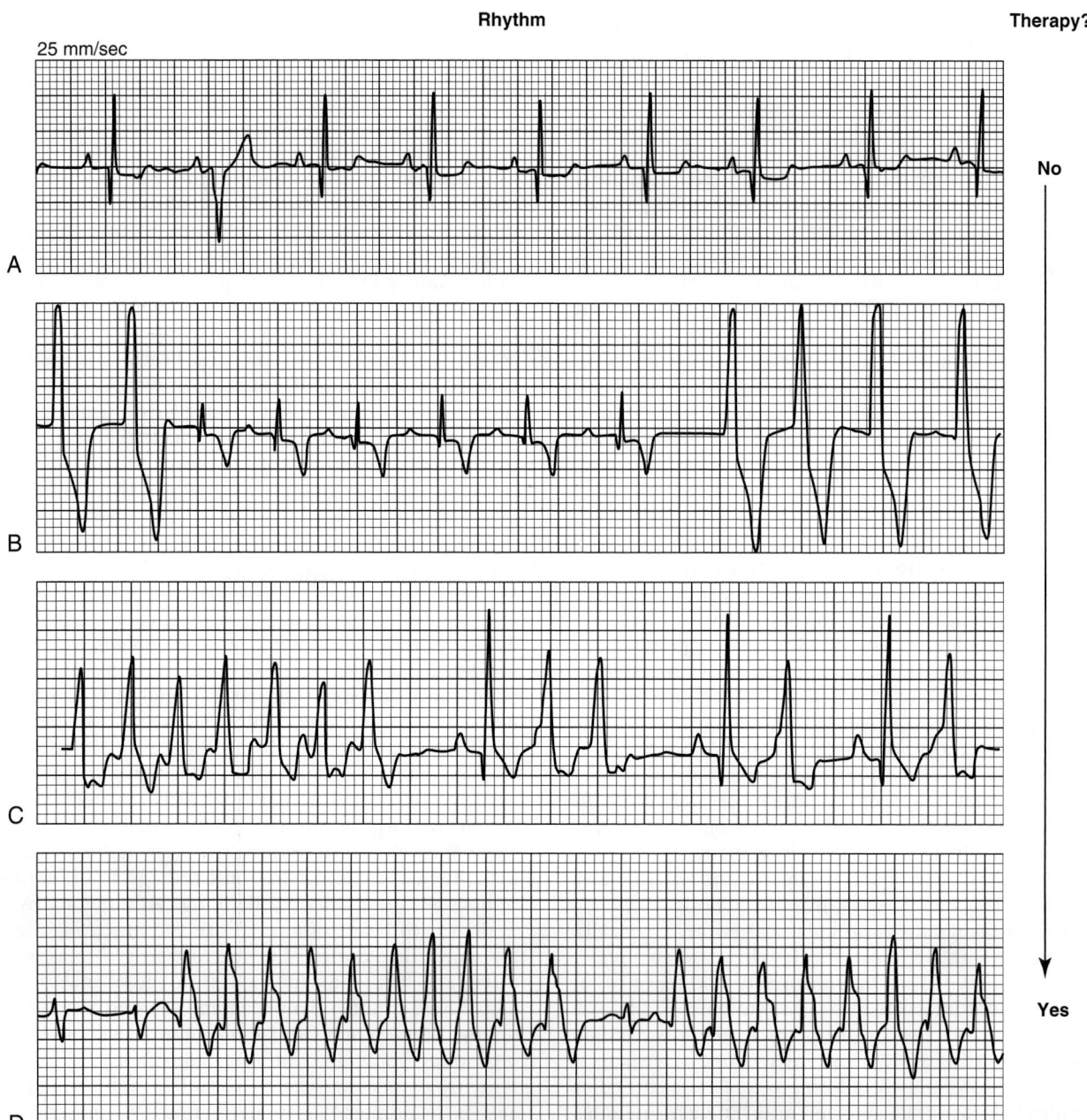

Rhythm   Therapy?

25 mm/sec

A

B

C

D

No

Yes

Figure 172-1 Examples of common ventricular arrhythmias and criteria for therapy. **A,** Sinus rhythm with a single ventricular premature complex, for which antiarrhythmic therapy typically is not indicated. **B,** A ventricular rhythm occurring at a rate similar to the sinus rate. When at relatively slow heart rates, ventricular arrhythmias usually do not cause clinical signs of hypotension and rarely require antiarrhythmic therapy. **C,** Nonsustained rapid ventricular rhythm that is most likely secondary to myocardial disease. Holter monitoring should be considered, and if clinical signs are present, long-term oral antiarrhythmic therapy probably is indicated. **D,** Rapid ventricular tachycardia. Clinical signs of weakness, collapse, or syncope are likely present and intravenous antiarrhythmic therapy is indicated.

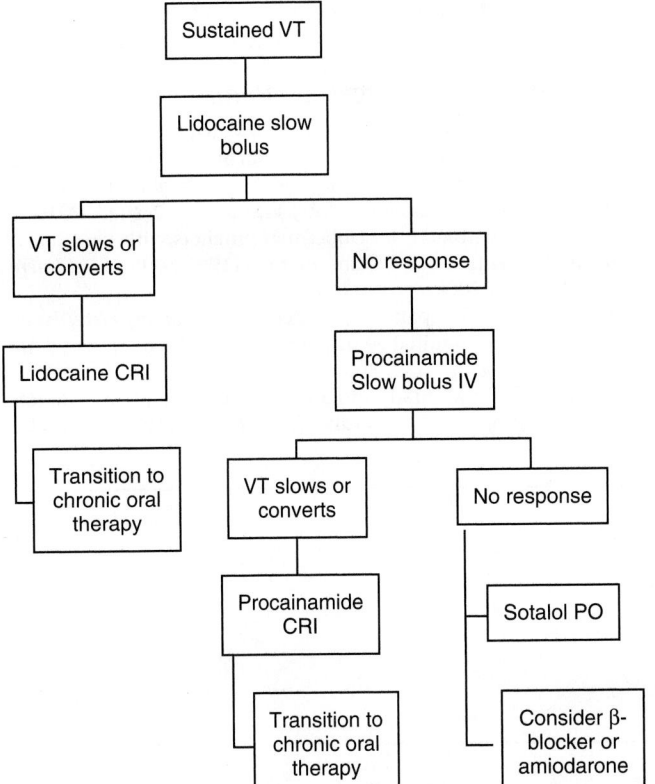

Figure 172-2 Flow diagram for treatment of severe, life-threatening ventricular tachycardia.

TABLE 172-1

Drugs Commonly Used for Treatment of Ventricular Arrhythmias

Drug	Canine Dosage
Lidocaine	2 mg/kg slow bolus IV (can repeat 2-3 times) 25-75 µg/kg/min continuous IV infusion
Procainamide	5-10 mg/kg slow bolus IV (can repeat if needed) 25-50 µg/kg/min continuous IV infusion
Sotalol	1-3 mg/kg q12h PO
Mexiletine	6-10 mg/kg q8h PO
Atenolol	0.5-1 mg/kg q12h PO
Amiodarone*	5 mg/kg slow bolus IV (over 10 min) Loading dosage of 10-30 mg/kg q24h PO for 2-14 days Maintenance dosage of 6-15 mg/kg q24h PO

IV, Intravenous; *PO*, by mouth.
*Nexterone brand of amiodarone does not contain polysorbate 80 or benzyl alcohol.

within 5 minutes following the first bolus, two or three additional boluses can be administered. The bolus should be given slowly, over about 1 minute, and the dog monitored for transient hypotension, vomiting, and seizures. If the rhythm converts to sinus or the VT slows, a continuous-rate infusion of lidocaine at 25 to 75 µg/kg/min should be instituted. If a dog fails to respond to

lidocaine, the authors often administer procainamide 5 to 10 mg/kg as a slow IV bolus (note that this drug has limited availability outside the United States). The authors generally do not exceed a total dose of 15 mg/kg of procainamide. Dogs should be monitored for hypotension and vomiting during administration of the bolus. Procainamide therapy also can be continued as a constant-rate infusion of 25 to 50 µg/kg/min in animals that show a response. If there is no response to either of these sodium channel–blocking drugs, a medication with potassium-blocking activity, such as amiodarone or sotalol, can be considered. The authors have only limited experience with administration of amiodarone as a slow IV bolus of 5 mg/kg over 10 minutes in the setting of ventricular arrhythmias. When amiodarone is administered intravenously, there is a risk of hypotension and anaphylaxis-like reactions, presumably from the polysorbate 80 or benzyl alcohol contained in most preparations, and careful monitoring is required. (Nexterone, a newer preparation of amiodarone, is now available and may be safer, but more experience is needed.) The authors often administer sotalol at 1 to 2 mg/kg PO to try to restore sinus rhythm in dogs with VT refractory to lidocaine and procainamide. In the authors' experience, many dogs show successful rhythm conversion within a few hours of oral sotalol administration.

When long-term oral therapy is necessary, Holter monitoring ideally is performed before antiarrhythmic medications are started to (1) establish ventricular arrhythmia as the cause of clinical signs; (2) assess the rate, duration, and frequency of the arrhythmia; and (3) serve as a basis of comparison with posttreatment Holter monitoring results to help assess efficacy of therapy. In instances when Holter monitoring is not possible, serial ECG examinations can be performed. In most cases, sotalol is the first-line oral drug of choice for long-term therapy because of its apparent efficacy and overall good tolerability. Sotalol most often is used in cases of dilated cardiomyopathy and arrhythmogenic right ventricular cardiomyopathy. However, due to its β-blocking activity and negative inotropic effect, dogs with severely decreased systolic function may not tolerate sotalol. Thus, if systolic function is poor (fractional shortening of <12% to 15%), sotalol can be initiated at a dose of 1 mg/kg, then increased to 2 mg/kg in 10 to 14 days while the dog is monitored for signs of low output or congestion. Alternatively, a drug without β-blocking properties such as mexiletine can be used. As do all antiarrhythmics, sotalol has the potential to worsen clinical signs or arrhythmias in some animals, and these effects can be identified by posttreatment Holter monitoring. Sotalol should not be chosen as an initial sole agent in dogs with conditions known to be aggravated by bradycardia, particularly German shepherds with inherited ventricular arrhythmias (Gelzer et al, 2010) and boxers with bradycardia-associated syncope (Thomason et al, 2008). Successful antiarrhythmic therapy is achieved when episodes of syncope or weakness are less frequent, runs of VT are eliminated, and the overall number of VPCs is reduced by more than 85% on Holter monitoring.

The authors' second drug of choice for long-term oral treatment of malignant ventricular arrhythmias is mexiletine, which is a sodium channel blocker similar to lidocaine. Mexiletine is often used in combination with sotalol because the reduction in the number of VPCs is greater than with monotherapy using either drug (Gelzer et al, 2010). The combination of mexiletine and atenolol also has been shown to be an effective therapy for VT in boxers (Meurs et al, 2002). In some dogs, decreased appetite, vomiting, or diarrhea is observed as an adverse effect of mexiletine; these signs often can be improved by administering the medication with food.

Oral amiodarone generally is reserved for VT refractory to other antiarrhythmics due to the high incidence of adverse effects, including hepatotoxicity, thyroid dysfunction, neutropenia, corneal microdeposits, and potentially pulmonary fibrosis. Hepatotoxicity is the most common adverse effect and, in one Doberman case series, was dose related and reversible (Kraus et al, 2009); monitoring of liver enzyme levels therefore is recommended.

References and Suggested Reading

Gelzer AR et al: Combination therapy with mexiletine and sotalol suppresses inherited ventricular arrhythmias in German shepherd dogs better than mexiletine or sotalol monotherapy: a randomized cross-over study, *J Vet Cardiol* 12(2):93, 2010.

Kraus MS et al: Toxicity in Doberman pinchers with ventricular arrhythmias treated with amiodarone (1996-2005), *J Vet Intern Med* 23(1):1, 2009.

Meurs KM et al: Comparison of the effects of four antiarrhythmic treatments for familial ventricular arrhythmias in Boxers, *J Am Vet Med Assoc* 221:522, 2002.

Thomason JD et al: Bradycardia-associated syncope in 7 Boxers with ventricular tachycardia (2002-2005), *J Vet Intern Med* 22(4):931, 2008.

CHAPTER **173**

Feline Cardiac Arrhythmias

ÉTIENNE CÔTÉ, *Prince Edward Island, Canada*

Like other species, cats may have cardiac arrhythmias that range in importance from harmless variations to life-threatening disorders. The decision-making process that determines the degree of concern and intervention warranted for a cat's arrhythmia—triage—should focus on at least five factors: (1) type of arrhythmia; (2) presence, type, and severity of structural heart disease; (3) reversible contributing factors; (4) presence or absence of syncope; and (5) heart rate during the arrhythmia.

The *type of arrhythmia* can be known only by analysis of an electrocardiogram (ECG), which may be obtained via standard ECG in the hospital or, for intermittent arrhythmias, via ambulatory ECG (Holter or event monitoring).

The *presence or absence of structural heart disease* is not suspected reliably from physical examination findings alone: depending on the criteria used, as few as 18% of cats with heart murmurs have evidence of left ventricular concentric hypertrophy on an echocardiogram (Paige et al, 2009; Wagner et al, 2010). The suspicion of structural heart disease may be increased or decreased by the results of thoracic radiography with or without N-terminal prohormone B-type natriuretic peptide testing (Côté et al, 2011b, 2011c; Ettinger, 2010; Fox et al, 2011), and confirmation requires echocardiography.

Reversible contributing factors to an arrhythmia are identified through routine laboratory tests. For example, hypokalemia, anemia, and hypoxemia can induce premature ventricular complexes and potentially render these refractory to antiarrhythmic treatment (Côté et al, 2011a). Such abnormalities may be identified or suspected via basic clinical testing (Figure 173-1).

The *presence or absence of syncope* is described by the owner; however, many owners cannot recognize the features of syncope. Since some cats produce subtle signs that could be explained either by syncope or by such nonsyncopal disorders as behavioral or metabolic disturbances, obtaining information during an episode can be enormously helpful. Owners may be instructed to record episodes on video at home for review by the veterinarian or to record an ECG during an episode via Holter or event monitoring. The information obtained is especially valuable when episodes are infrequent or ambiguous in their expression. It is also important to recognize that cats with syncope often are misdiagnosed with a seizure disorder because facial twitching and tonic-clonic motion are common signs of feline syncope. In feline medicine, it remains unresolved whether cats with clinical signs caused by bradyarrhythmias have cerebral hypoxia leading to an epileptic focus and true seizure activity or whether physical manifestations of syncope closely resemble seizure activity (Penning et al, 2009).

Finally, the *heart rate* generated during the arrhythmia may provide an indication that the cardiac output is too low because of inadequate diastolic filling time (tachycardias) or simply because of too few heartbeats per minute (bradycardias). Either extreme can produce similar signs of presyncope (transient ataxia and/or disorientation) or syncope, which emphasizes the need for an ECG diagnosis of the heart rhythm during such episodes for appropriate treatment selection and determination of an accurate prognosis.

Sinus Tachycardia

Normal sinus rhythm in the cat is evident when spontaneous automaticity in the sinoatrial node produces a heart rate of 110 to 180 beats/min. Each atrial depolarization leads to a ventricular depolarization. Therefore, on the ECG, each P wave is followed by a QRS complex at a fixed PR interval. The R-R interval is unchanging and thus the rate is constant, or if it changes, it does so gradually over a few heartbeats, not immediately from one beat to the next. These features are identical in *sinus tachycardia,* the equivalent of normal sinus rhythm but with a rate of more than 180 beats/min in cats (see Figure 173-1).

Treatment

Specific treatment to reduce the heart rate or suppress sinus tachycardia is virtually never appropriate and could be harmful, since sinus tachycardia generally arises as a physiologic response to such systemic stimuli as anxiety, pain, hyperthyroidism, hypovolemia, fever, congestive heart failure, or allergic airway disease (including status asthmaticus). Intervention for sinus tachycardia therefore centers on reducing or eliminating its inciting cause, not on altering the heart rate or rhythm. β-Blockade (e.g., atenolol 6.25 mg per cat q12-24h PO) may be initiated in profoundly hyperthyroid cats if a very rapid sinus tachycardia (e.g., >260/min) is present initially; this treatment is ended when euthyroidism is achieved.

Particularities in Cats

A number of key points can be made regarding sinus tachycardia in cats:

- Sinus tachycardia is the cardiac rhythm expected in essentially all cats in the clinical setting (Côté et al, 2011a) because of anxiety and arousal. A heart rate of less than 160 beats/min on physical examination during an appointment should trigger a suspicion of relative bradycardia. An ECG is then warranted to rule out a pathologic bradycardia like second- or third-degree atrioventricular (AV) block.
- QRS complexes in normal feline ECGs may be positive or negative because of the wide normal range of the mean electrical axis of the feline ventricles.
- QRS complexes in normal feline ECGs may be very small, and no minimum limit of normal has been recognized for the height of the R wave in the cat in lead II.

Premature Atrial Complexes, Atrial Tachycardia, and Atrial Fibrillation

It may seem paradoxical that diseased heart tissue tends to fire more than normal, not less. The paradox is clarified by contrasting normal and abnormal cardiac cells. Healthy cardiomyocytes maintain a stable, inactivated state until triggered to depolarize, like dominos in a tumbling series, by each heartbeat's advancing wave of normal electrical activity. Disruption of myocardial tissue interferes with this organized, sequential pattern of cardiac depolarization. In cats, myocyte stretch and myocardial interstitial fibrosis, in particular, are common atrial lesions that are associated with such disruptions (Boyden et al, 1984). These alterations render a cell less stable and more prone to depolarizing inappropriately. To continue the analogy, a single domino topples out in the periphery, creating a rogue heartbeat (ectopy) that propagates outward and commands the rhythm of the heart for that beat. A premature depolarization may not occur if it begins too prematurely, when the adjacent myocardium is refractory because all the dominos have tumbled and have not yet been prepared for the next tumble (i.e., have not yet repolarized).

This concept of premature depolarization applies to all chambers of the heart. In humans, these arrhythmias involve various substrates and mechanisms, like the origin of atrial fibrillation from the pulmonary venous-atrial junction, but these mechanisms have not been investigated *in vivo* in the cat. In the atria of cats, premature, spontaneous atrial depolarizations may occur singly (*premature atrial complexes* or PACs; synonyms include *atrial premature complexes, atrial premature contractions,* and *premature atrial depolarizations*), in a series of four or more from the same focus in the atrium (*atrial tachycardia* or AT), or as a series of chaotic, seemingly randomly generated atrial impulses (*atrial fibrillation* or AF) (see Figure 173-1). The ECG characteristics of these rhythms can be summarized as follows:

- *PACs:* Shorter R-R interval (i.e., the heartbeat occurs prematurely), with the P wave of the PAC (called *P'* or *P-prime*) often superimposed on the normal T wave of the preceding beat. The morphology of the QRS complex is identical or nearly identical to that of a normal sinus QRS complex. The next sinus beat generally occurs at an interval that is not in phase with the expected timing of normal sinus rhythm had the PAC not occurred. This creates a *noncompensatory pause* following the PAC, which suggests that the PAC penetrated and reset the sinoatrial nodal cycle.
- *AT:* As described for PACs, but consisting of four or more consecutive PACs. The QRS following the initial PAC of the sequence occasionally may be different in morphology owing to abnormal ventricular conduction (aberrancy).
- *AF:* Absence of P waves in all ECG leads. The morphology of the QRS complex is identical or nearly identical to that of the normal sinus QRS complex, often with subtle variation in the QRS complexes. Fine baseline undulations (atrial

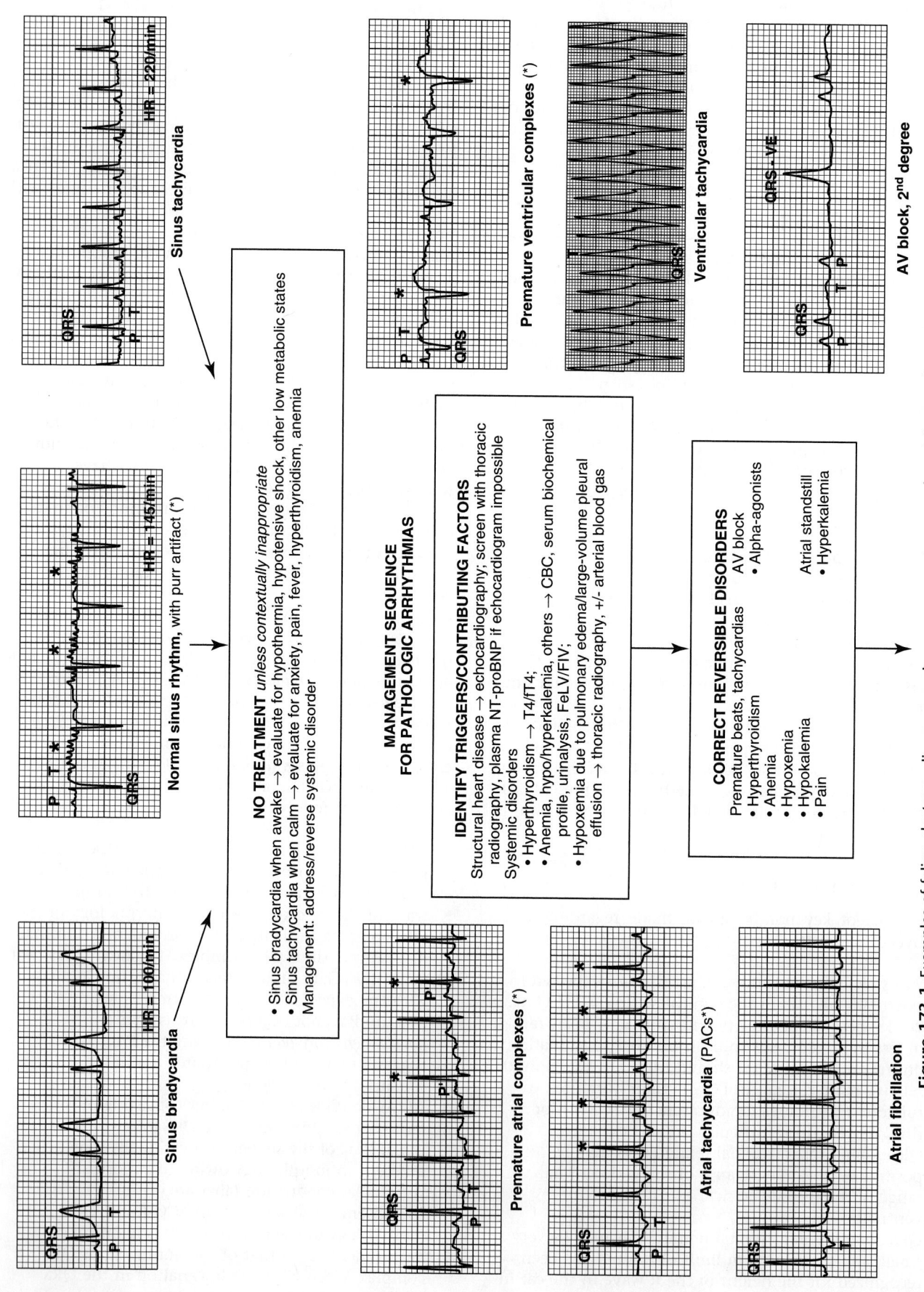

Figure 173-1 Examples of feline electrocardiograms and a management approach to feline cardiac arrhythmias.

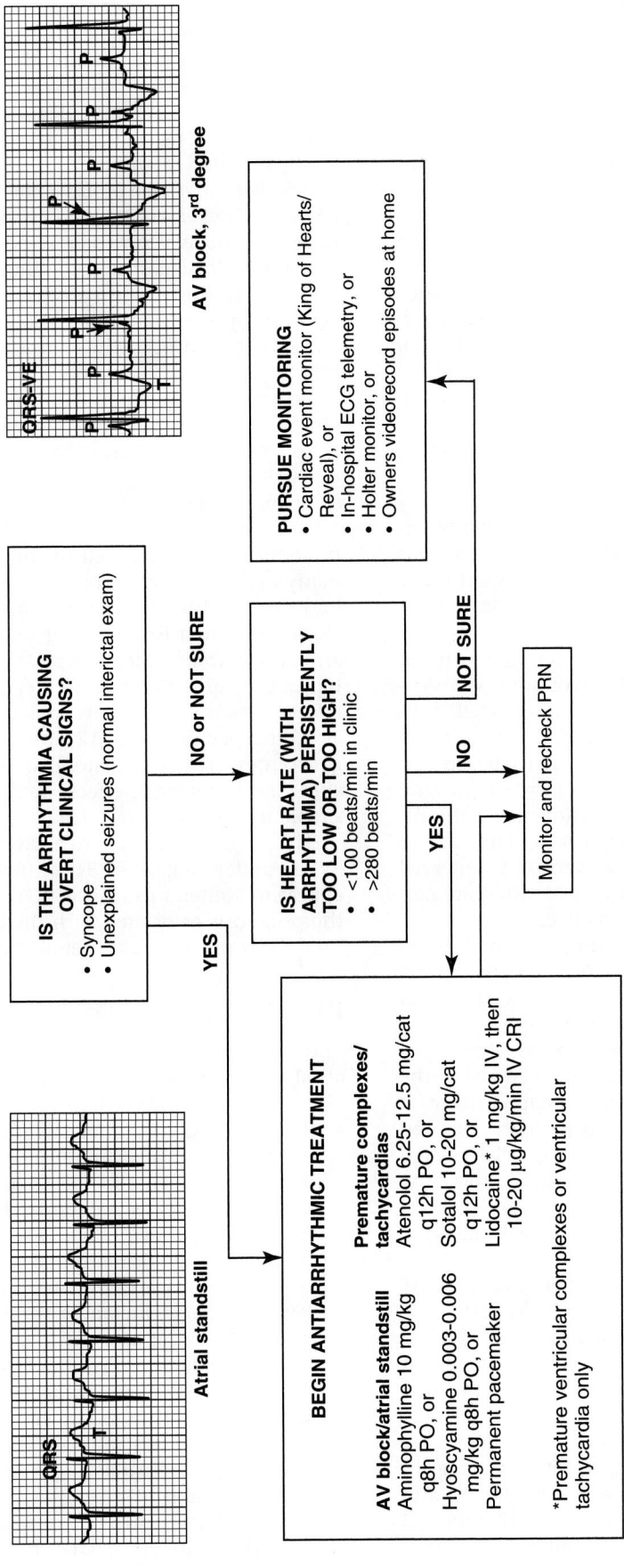

AV block, 3rd degree

Atrial standstill

IS THE ARRHYTHMIA CAUSING OVERT CLINICAL SIGNS?
- Syncope
- Unexplained seizures (normal interictal exam)

YES → **BEGIN ANTIARRHYTHMIC TREATMENT**

NO or NOT SURE → **IS HEART RATE (WITH ARRHYTHMIA) PERSISTENTLY TOO LOW OR TOO HIGH?**
- <100 beats/min in clinic
- >280 beats/min

NOT SURE → **PURSUE MONITORING**
- Cardiac event monitor (King of Hearts/Reveal), or
- In-hospital ECG telemetry, or
- Holter monitor, or
- Owners videorecord episodes at home

NO → **Monitor and recheck PRN**

YES → **BEGIN ANTIARRHYTHMIC TREATMENT**

BEGIN ANTIARRHYTHMIC TREATMENT

AV block/atrial standstill
Aminophylline 10 mg/kg q8h PO, or
Hyoscyamine 0.003-0.006 mg/kg q8h PO, or
Permanent pacemaker

Premature complexes/tachycardias
Atenolol 6.25-12.5 mg/cat q12h PO, or
Sotalol 10-20 mg/cat q12h PO, or
Lidocaine* 1 mg/kg IV, then 10-20 μg/kg/min IV CRI

*Premature ventricular complexes or ventricular tachycardia only

Legend: AF = atrial fibrillation; AV = atrioventricular; CBC = complete blood count; FeLV/FIV = feline leukemia virus/feline immunodeficiency virus; fT4 = free thyroxine by equilibrium dialysis; PRN = as needed; QRS-VE = ventricular escape; T4 = thyroxine. All tracings 25 mm/sec. Sinus bradycardia ECG courtesy of Dr. Cate Creighton, Atlantic Veterinary College.

Figure 173-1, cont'd

fibrillation waves) are seen. The rhythm is irregularly irregular; that is, the R-R interval has no discernible consistency or pattern through the ECG tracing.

Since PACs, AT, and AF are associated so commonly with underlying structural heart disease, their detection should trigger an investigation of underlying cardiac structure through thoracic radiography and echocardiography.

Treatment

Specific antiarrhythmic treatment of PACs (individual, pairs, or triplets) is not necessary. They are considered markers of structural or electrical atrial disease, and treatment consists of managing the underlying disorder, if warranted (e.g., treatment of congestive heart failure if it is present; anticoagulation if there is marked atrial enlargement; correction of hypokalemia).

Specific treatment of AT and of AF in cats is similar and considered necessary if the resulting heart rate is excessive and persistent. A healthy cat in a veterinary examination room may have a heart rate of 260 beats/min because of anxiety, but such a heart rate (from sinus tachycardia) normally would decrease after several hours of hospitalization or after the cat returned home. A cat with AT or AF whose heart rate remains consistently at or above 280 beats/min in the hospital, or certainly while at home, can be expected to have reduced diastolic ventricular filling because of the tachycardia, and targeted treatment is warranted. In addition to treating any predisposing condition, management of atrial tachyarrhythmias can include either controlling the heart rate by suppressing the ectopic focus or blocking conduction down the AV node, or actually converting the ectopic activity back to normal. Sometimes spontaneous conversion is observed regardless of drug therapy, but AT and AF often are persistent or permanent rhythm disturbances.

In most cases, initial therapy for the cat with AT or AF involves a β-blocker, typically atenolol 6.25 to 12.5 mg per cat every 12 to 24 hours PO. A logical approach in the cat whose AT or AF is not producing overt signs of hemodynamic compromise (e.g., syncope) is to prescribe atenolol 6.25 mg every 24 hours PO, administered in the evening and followed up with a daytime appointment. If reevaluation reveals AT or AF with a persistently elevated heart rate (e.g., >200 beats/min) despite β-blockade, then the therapy can be surmised either to be ineffective or to last less than 24 hours (the case in about three quarters of cats by anecdotal observation). In this case the atenolol dosage is increased to 6.25 mg per cat every 12 hours PO. If a subsequent recheck identifies persistence of AT or AF with a ventricular response of more than 200 beats/min, the atenolol dosage may be increased to up to 12.5 mg every 12 hours PO, but excessive suppression of the heart rate must be avoided, especially in cats with impaired systolic function or congestive heart failure (see later). A recheck appointment always is warranted when higher dosages of atenolol are prescribed, to identify sluggishness or dyspnea and to document the heart rate and rhythm by ECG. Sotalol 20 mg per cat every 12 hours PO can be used as an alternative to atenolol, particularly if ventricular arrhythmias also are present.

β-Blockers potentially are dangerous in some settings. Excessive bradycardia can induce congestive heart failure in cats previously in stable condition. Importantly, in cats with congestive heart failure, β-blockers should be prescribed only *after* the reduction or elimination of pulmonary edema or voluminous pleural effusion with injectable diuretics or thoracocentesis, respectively, to avoid worsening any fluid retention.

An alternative to β-blockers for AT or AF is the calcium channel blocker diltiazem. This drug can block the AV node to reduce ventricular response rate to AT or AF. As with β-blockers it is sometimes associated with suppression of the rhythm disturbance. However, in the author's opinion, the ability of oral calcium channel blockers to control the heart rate of cats with AT or AF is inferior to that of β-blockers.

Less commonly, when AT or AF with rapid ventricular rate is associated with an eccentrically hypertrophied or grossly dilated ventricle, such as that caused by ventricular septal defect or dilated cardiomyopathy, digoxin (0.01 mg/kg q48h PO) may be prescribed. This dosage typically corresponds to $\frac{1}{4}$ of a 0.125-mg tablet every 48 hours PO and is preferred to the pediatric elixir, which many cats dislike. A β-blocker, or alternatively diltiazem, may be added if rate control is insufficient with digoxin alone. Diltiazem is dosed at 1 mg/kg every 8 hours PO, although current tablet sizes make this more difficult, and typically $\frac{1}{4}$ of a 30-mg tablet per cat is given; extended-release versions also are available and typically are dosed at 15 mg per cat every 12 hours PO, although adverse gastrointestinal and hepatobiliary effects, and unpredictable pharmacokinetic effects, make these versions undesirable in the cat.

The prognosis for cats with PACs, AT, or AF is governed by the underlying cause. These three arrhythmias do not appear to confer a prognosis that is better or worse than the prognosis associated with the cat's underlying structural heart disease (Atkins et al, 2001).

Particularities in Cats

The following points are especially pertinent for cats with atrial arrhythmias:

- P waves on the ECGs of cats may be very small or isoelectric in one or more ECG leads. Therefore, to minimize misdiagnosis of AT or AF, ideally all 10 leads (6 limb leads, 4 chest leads) should be recorded and examined for P waves, and obtaining a high-quality tracing with minimal to no motion artifact or poor contact is essential.
- Several artifacts, including those caused by poor electrode contact and purring, are seen as fine baseline undulations on the ECG. These can appear identical to AF waves. Artifacts do not alter the underlying rhythm, however, and the unchanging R-R interval of normal sinus rhythm is the principal differentiator of artifact from AF (see Figure 173-1). This distinction may be difficult to make in AF causing higher ventricular response rates (e.g., heart rate >180 beats/min), when the variation in R-R interval may be very subtle.

- A *vagal maneuver,* such as carotid sinus massage, can help slow AV node transit time and reveal a more convincingly irregular R-R interval in AF when the heart rate is above 180 beats/min. To perform carotid sinus massage, place the cat in comfortable lateral recumbency, with the ECG electrodes connected and in good contact with the cat's skin (clear ECG tracing); have the ECG monitor printing; and then gently, comfortably squeeze the soft depression directly dorsal to the larynx bilaterally, using thumb and index finger, for 10 seconds—or less if a visible slowing of heart rate occurs. Stop if the cat shows resentment. A decrease of 10% or more in heart rate after the first several seconds of pressure is a typical response and allows the irregularity of the R-R interval to become more apparent in cases of AF. For a cat, the amount of pressure to be applied should be 2.5 to 3 kPa, or a force of 3 to 4 N (approximately the maximal digital force one could apply to a ripe grape without crushing it).
- Cats with AF almost always have atrial enlargement (90% to 100% of cases depending on the criteria used for defining atrial enlargement), but overt signs of heart failure need not be present; 22% of cats with AF were diagnosed with the arrhythmia as an incidental finding in one study (Côté et al, 2011a).
- Cats with AF may live 1 year or longer after the diagnosis of AF, as 33% did in one study (Côté et al, 2011a). Therefore, despite the extensive cardiac lesions often present when AF exists in cats, AF cannot be considered an indicator of a uniformly poor prognosis in the cat.

Ventricular Arrhythmias

Premature ventricular complexes (PVCs, VPCs) are spontaneous, unnecessary cardiac impulses generated by the ventricles. These may be caused by structural heart disease, notably the cardiomyopathies, or by systemic disturbances such as hyperthyroidism (Côté et al, 2011a). Many of the electrophysiologic features and hemodynamic consequences of ventricular arrhythmias are similar to those associated with arrhythmias affecting the atria as described earlier. Healthy cats have been reported to experience between 0 and 150 PVCs per day, usually fewer than 60 per day and often none in cats younger than 8 years of age (Côté et al, 2011a).

The ECG features of PVCs are indicated by the acronym itself: PVCs are premature, that is, the QRS complex of the PVC occurs sooner than a heartbeat would be expected given the background rhythm, producing a shorter R-R interval; and they are ventricular in origin, that is, they generate a QRS complex with a visibly different morphology than a normal sinus QRS complex. PVCs may occur singly or in clusters, and four or more consecutive PVCs are called *ventricular tachycardia* (VT) if the resulting rate is 240 beats/min or more in the cat; if it is less than 240 beats/min, the series of consecutive PVCs is more appropriately referred to as an *accelerated idioventricular rhythm.* The prognosis associated with PVCs in cats is not known to be different from the prognosis of the underlying disease.

Treatment

Antiarrhythmic treatment of ventricular arrhythmias in cats depends on the type of structural heart disease, the impact of the arrhythmia on the circulation, the safety of the antiarrhythmic medication, and practical factors including client and patient compliance. There are no formal guidelines for such treatment; the author's recommendations are shown in Figure 173-1. Broadly, PVCs, accelerated idioventricular rhythm, or VT, when associated with such overt signs as presyncope or syncope, should be treated with antiarrhythmic medications in essentially all cases. VT occurring at a persistently rapid heart rate (e.g., >280 beats/min) also justifies antiarrhythmic treatment, even in the absence of syncope. Contributing factors such as hyperthyroidism must be treated first or at least managed concurrently. The goal of treatment is not to normalize the ECG but to maintain a perfusing rhythm with the lowest risk of arrhythmia-induced complications such as hypotension or myocardial hypoperfusion. In practical terms, this is assessed by monitoring the heart rate (via ECG), pulse quality, and mentation. Cats that experience syncope or collapse and have sustained VT at a rate of 280 beats/min or more should receive intravenous antiarrhythmics beginning with lidocaine (see Figure 173-1), whereas cats that have evidence of adequate tissue perfusion (acceptable pulse quality, warm extremities) and are not experiencing syncope may be treated with oral medications, as shown in Figure 173-1. The selection of antiarrhythmic medication should be compatible with the underlying structural heart disease. For example, β-blockers such as atenolol or sotalol generally have better antitachycardia effects in cats than do calcium channel blockers and would be the preferred treatment for rapid but stable PVCs or VT in a cat with hypertrophic cardiomyopathy. Up-titration of antiarrhythmics is challenging because 24-hour Holter monitoring is necessary for complete assessment of the baseline and response during treatment with antiarrhythmic medication. However, this evaluation is performed very infrequently in cats, even though most indoor cats tolerate Holter monitors. Up-titration of β-blockers in cats with ventricular arrhythmias may be undertaken in the same way as described earlier for PACs, AT, and AF.

Particularities in Cats

The following issues are pertinent to management of ventricular arrhythmias in cats:

- On physical examination of cats with rapid heart rates, it is common for single PVCs to produce a hypodynamic beat that is inaudible to auscultation. Rather than detecting the premature beat, the examiner more often hears the pause that follows the PVC. Because of this, single PVCs in cats easily may be misinterpreted as second-degree AV block on auscultation because only the post-extrasystolic pause is noted, which gives the impression of a dropped beat. An ECG provides the correct diagnosis.
- In cats PVCs occur more commonly with structural heart disease and less often with systemic disease

compared with dogs: 102 of 106 cats (96%) with PVCs had underlying structural heart disease compared with 95 of 138 dogs (69%) in one study (Côté et al, 2011a).

Atrioventricular Block

A delay in the transmission of current from the atrial to the ventricular myocardium is referred to as *AV block* when it is caused by conduction delay in the AV node, bundle of His, or both bundle branches. The extent of AV block may be minimal to complete. When each impulse is delayed in its passage through the AV node but successfully reaches the ventricles, the diagnosis is *first-degree AV block*. When no impulses pass successfully through the AV node and depolarization of the ventricles relies on an escape rhythm, the ECG diagnosis is *complete* or *third-degree AV block*. Logically, then, when some impulses successfully pass to the ventricles but others do not, the diagnosis is *second-degree AV block*.

The ECG characteristics correspond to these designations. Prolongation of the PR interval by more than 0.09 seconds defines first-degree AV block in the cat, but this can be recognized only by examining an ECG. Second-degree AV block is characterized by an arrhythmia with some P waves associated with QRS complexes and other P waves not followed by QRS complexes (with or without junctional or ventricular escape complexes). When all P waves are unrelated to the QRS complexes the rhythm is third-degree AV block, and the ventricular rate often is slow in affected cats because junctional or ventricular escape beats prevent ventricular asystole. Cats with overt clinical signs due to complete AV block often demonstrate intermittent arrhythmia with periods of normal sinus rhythm (with or without first- or second-degree AV block) and then periods of complete AV block, sometimes with protracted absence of escape activity. This asystole can lead to periodic syncopal events (often misinterpreted as seizures when the hospital auscultation findings and ECG are normal). Some cases are discovered only fortuitously or when an ambulatory ECG event monitor (or other loop recorder) is attached to record periodic block and asystole.

Second-degree AV block is further characterized as Mobitz type I (progressive lengthening of the PR interval leading up to the blocked beat) or Mobitz type II (no lengthening of the PR interval forewarning a blocked P wave). Although sometimes Mobitz type I is thought to represent a vagally induced or physiologic phenomenon and Mobitz type II is considered a more ominous precursor to third-degree AV block, this notion is unsubstantiated in the cat, and no prognostic information can be derived from Mobitz classification in cats.

Treatment

The need for treatment depends on the hemodynamic impact of the AV block: whether the remaining ventricular activity provides a perfusing rhythm in the cat and can be expected to continue to do so. First-degree AV block, since it does not reduce the number of sinus impulses reaching the ventricles, is clinically silent and never requires treatment. Second- and third-degree AV block require treatment if they lead to insufficient cardiac output. This conclusion may be reached through consideration of clinical signs—whether the cat shows syncope, near syncope, or sluggishness associated with a slow heart rate (typically <100 beats/min)—or may be suspected based on the slow heart rate alone, since many cats are inactive by nature and the presence of sluggishness or lethargy may be difficult to identify. The treatment of choice for AV block causing overt clinical signs is implantation of a permanent cardiac pacemaker.

Medical therapy sometimes is attempted when pacemaker implantation is not possible. Treatment with oral anticholinergics (e.g., hyoscyamine 0.003 to 0.006 mg/kg q8h PO), methylxanthines (e.g., aminophylline regular formulation, not sustained-release, 10 mg/kg q8h PO), or the β-agonist terbutaline rarely is effective in the experience of most cardiologists; however, these agents have not been studied rigorously and can be tried as nonsurgical options in syncopal cats. Adjunctive medical therapy occasionally may be needed for the progressive volume overload observed in some cats with chronic bradycardias. These cats typically have enlarged hearts, small to moderate pleural effusions, and jugular venous distension. Such patients can be managed with low dosages of furosemide and an angiotensin-converting enzyme inhibitor to control volume retention. Follow-up examination is directed at rechecking any clinical signs, jugular venous pressure, thoracic radiographs, and renal function.

Particularities in Cats

The following points are pertinent to cats with AV block:

- The ventricular escape rhythm of cats often is faster than might be anticipated, frequently approaching or matching the rate expected for sinus rhythm, with a median of 120 beats/min reported by Kellum and Stepien (2006). For this reason, third-degree AV block is discovered as an incidental finding on ECGs in cats (23% of cases) more often than in other species.
- Third-degree AV block in the cat may be transient, with periods of complete AV block interspersed with periods of improved, or even normalized, conduction. This is in contrast to the dog, in which complete heart block is typically permanent.
- Many cats with third-degree AV block that do not receive a pacemaker do very well. Kellum and Stepien (2006) found that the median survival time for cats with complete AV block that did not receive a pacemaker was 386 days, and one cat survived for 5.7 years.
- There is a common association between third-degree AV block and hypertrophic cardiomyopathy in cats, likely due to fibrosis of proximal segments of the His-Purkinje system (Côté et al, 2011a). Clinical experience confirms this association and makes the long-term prognosis for pacemaker implantation a guarded one in such patients; resolving the bradycardia does not correct the underlying hypertrophic cardiomyopathy.

- Cats dislike the taste of atropine (profound hypersalivation results), so oral atropine compounded liquid usually is not a viable option for medical treatment of second- or third-degree AV block.
- Transvenous pacemaker implantation has been associated with pleural effusions and chylothorax in cats, perhaps related to obstruction of systemic venous return. For this reason, many cardiologists advocate an epicardial approach (via thoracotomy or laparotomy) for pacemaker implantation in the cat. Unfortunately, this treatment sometimes is associated with system failure owing to exit block, in which extensive fibrosis or migration around the epicardial electrodes leads to a failure to capture and pace the heart.

Atrial Standstill

The absence of any atrial electrical activity is referred to as *atrial standstill* or silent atrium. This rhythm disturbance may occur transiently, typically in the setting of hyperkalemia, or permanently, as with fibrosis or senescence of the atrial myocardium. In the cat, hyperkalemia is most commonly a result of urethral obstruction, reperfusion injury, or acute anuric kidney injury, whereas atrial myocardial degeneration almost always is associated with a form of myocardial disease (hypertrophic, dilated, restrictive/unclassified, or arrhythmogenic right ventricular cardiomyopathies).

The ECG characteristics are the absence of P waves in all leads and (usually) a regular (constant R-R interval) ventricular rhythm. In hyperkalemia the QRS complex eventually widens and the T waves tend to be large. It is uncertain whether such rhythms represent escape rhythms or sinoventricular rhythm with conduction abnormalities of the ventricles. Additionally, the ventricular rate in cats with hyperkalemia can vary from slow to fast. In persistent atrial standstill, a slow to normal heart rate is more typical. The differential diagnosis includes atrial fibrillation with fine or inapparent f waves and relatively regular ventricular rate response.

Treatment

Since there are two principal causes of atrial standstill, treatment options are straightforward. Hyperkalemia is managed medically as described in greater detail elsewhere in this volume. Given the high proportion of ionized hypocalcemia in cats with urethral obstruction in some reports, the best initial choice for treating hyperkalemia may be calcium gluconate (50 to 200 mg/kg, or 3 ml of 10% solution for a typical cat, given slowly IV over 5 to 15 minutes; treatment should stop if sudden bradycardia, new-onset PVCs, or shortened QT interval develops). This can be followed if necessary by potassium-lowering treatments such as sodium bicarbonate or insulin (with dextrose). In the absence of hyperkalemia,

atrial standstill is considered to be caused by atrial stretch–associated fibrosis by exclusion and therefore is not amenable to correction. The underlying condition—often congestive heart failure—is managed when possible. Implantation of a pacemaker may be considered in cases of persistent atrial standstill, but the prognosis typically remains guarded to poor because of the extent of structural heart disease usually present.

Particularities in Cats

The following are important points related to atrial standstill in cats:

- Given the very small size of some cats' P waves, "atrial standstill" may be misdiagnosed easily if normal P waves are isoelectric in the ECG lead under examination. Therefore a 10-lead ECG is indicated to identify atrial standstill by exclusion.
- Although the classic textbook appearance of the T wave in hyperkalemia is positive and tented, many hyperkalemic cats (perhaps the majority) exhibit large but negative T waves in lead II.
- Cats with hyperkalemia can exhibit normal to high heart rates and wide QRS complexes and T waves; this combination can mimic VT, and hyperkalemia must be ruled out when the ECG is suggestive of sustained VT in a cat.

References and Suggested Reading

Atkins CE et al: Prognosis in feline heartworm infection: comparison to other cardiovascular diseases. In *Proceedings of the American Heartworm Society Symposium*, Dallas, TX, 2001.

Boyden PA et al: Mechanisms for atrial arrhythmias associated with cardiomyopathy: a study of feline hearts with primary myocardial disease, *Circulation* 69:1036, 1984.

Côté E et al: Cardiac arrhythmias and other electrocardiographic abnormalities. In *Feline cardiology*, Ames, IA, 2011a, Wiley-Blackwell, p 213.

Côté E et al: Cardiac biomarkers. In *Feline cardiology*, Ames, IA, 2011b, Wiley-Blackwell, p 69.

Côté E et al: Radiography. In *Feline cardiology*, Ames, IA, 2011c, Wiley-Blackwell, p 37.

Ettinger SJ: The cat is not a dog: cardiac biomarkers. *Proceedings of the 27th Annual American College of Veterinary Internal Medicine Forum*, Anaheim, CA, June 11, 2010.

Fox PR et al: Multicenter evaluation of plasma N-terminal pro-brain natriuretic peptide (NT-proBNP) as a biochemical screening test for asymptomatic (occult) cardiomyopathy in cats, *J Vet Intern Med* 25:1010, 2011.

Kellum HB, Stepien RL: Third-degree atrioventricular block in 21 cats (1997-2004), *J Vet Intern Med* 20:97, 2006.

Paige CF et al: Prevalence of cardiomyopathy in apparently healthy cats, *J Am Vet Med Assoc* 234:1398, 2009.

Penning VA et al: Seizure-like episodes in 3 cats with intermittent high-grade atrioventricular dysfunction, *J Vet Intern Med* 23:200, 2009.

Wagner T et al: Comparison of auscultatory and echocardiographic findings in healthy adult cats, *J Vet Cardiol* 12:171, 2010.

CHAPTER 174

Congenital Heart Disease

BRIAN A. SCANSEN, *Columbus, Ohio*
RICHARD E. COBER, *Annapolis, Maryland*
JOHN D. BONAGURA, *Columbus, Ohio*

Congenital heart disease (CHD) is found in a small subset of dogs and cats brought in for veterinary care and is estimated to account for less than 10% of cardiac disease in these species. Acquired heart disease is encountered with greater frequency in general veterinary practice. However, the spectrum of CHD is broad and complex, which makes determining the diagnosis, treatment, and prognosis for these animals more challenging. In addition, some forms of CHD are curable, and therefore it is imperative that such lesions not be missed during pediatric general examination of these animals. A detailed overview of all forms of CHD is beyond the scope of this chapter; rather, the prevalence of certain defects is described and the typical diagnostic approach and treatment strategies are presented. The interested reader also is directed to other chapters within this section that detail some of the more common congenital malformations observed in dogs and cats.

Animals with complex or severe CHD may be brought for treatment within the first days to weeks of life because of failure to thrive, dyspnea, cyanosis, or syncope. In general this population is made up of species that routinely receive neonatal care—that is, valuable farm animals (calves, crias, foals) or purebred dogs and cats. It is likely that most puppies and kittens with severe cardiac malformations die early in life and before veterinary examination. The more common presentation for dogs and cats with CHD is that of an asymptomatic pet with an appointment for a wellness examination, deworming, and vaccination. Auscultation of these patients often provides the first and earliest clue that CHD may be present, and for this reason careful and thorough auscultation of all young animals is advised. Rarely, animals with CHD are identified later in life and often as a result of complications of their cardiovascular disorder (heart failure, syncope, or cyanosis) if it was not detected at an earlier age.

In the dog, persistent patency of the ductus arteriosus (see Web Chapter 64), pulmonary valve stenosis (see Web Chapter 65), and subaortic stenosis (see Web Chapter 66) are the most common forms of CHD. In the cat, ventricular septal defect (see Web Chapter 69) appears to be the most common form of CHD encountered. In both species, less commonly observed defects include atrial septal defect, mitral valve dysplasia (see Web Chapter 62), tricuspid valve dysplasia (see Web Chapter 68), atrioventricular septal defect, tetralogy of Fallot, vascular ring anomalies, and peritoneal-pericardial diaphragmatic hernia, among others.

Prevalence

The prevalence of CHD in the dog and cat is difficult to quantify due to a lack of routine perinatal care, occurrence of conditions that are not apparent on routine physical examination, and hospital biases in published reports. The work of Detweiler and Patterson in the Philadelphia area suggested a CHD prevalence rate of 0.56% among 4831 dogs surveyed in the mid-twentieth century (Detweiler and Patterson, 1965), whereas Buchanan found a rate of 0.67% for all dogs brought to the University of Pennsylvania between 1987 and 1989 (Buchanan, 1992). In a study of 1679 puppies aged 6 to 18 weeks at a pet store, murmurs were observed in 11, which suggests an incidence of CHD of 0.66% (Ruble and Hird, 1993). However, this may be an underestimation because it fails to include those puppies that died from CHD before the age of 6 weeks or those animals whose disease was silent to auscultation at that age. Conversely, this study may have overestimated the incidence of CHD because further testing was not performed to determine if the murmur was reflective of true CHD or simply functional or physiologic in origin. Additionally, the pet store population is likely biased toward purebred dogs, which are known to carry a higher proportion of hereditary defects than mixed-breed dogs.

Although the true prevalence of CHD in dogs and cats is unknown, data are available that indicate the relative incidence of specific malformations in each species. In an attempt to compile these data, several studies of CHD prevalence were analyzed and the data were combined (Tables 174-1 and 174-2). Ten applicable studies of CHD prevalence in dogs were found in the veterinary literature, comprising a sum of 4694 defects (see Table 174-1). When the defects were totaled, patent ductus arteriosus (PDA) (25.7%), subaortic stenosis (SAS) (23.5%), and pulmonary valve stenosis (PS) (22.1%) were found to be the most common and of nearly equal incidence, together comprising almost three fourths of all instances of CHD in the dog. Defects in the ventricular septum (8.8%) and atrial septum (1.9%) accounted for an additional 10.7% of cases, whereas dysplasias of the mitral valve (4.3%) and tricuspid valve (4.6%) were present in nearly equal frequency. The constellation of defects known as tetralogy of Fallot (ToF) accounted for 2.3% of defects, whereas more complex lesions not easily classified into the aforementioned categories made up 3.4% of CHD. Not all studies provided data on vascular ring anomalies, which may present with noncardiac signs and therefore likely are underrepresented in these data.

TABLE **174-1**

Congenital Heart Disease in Dogs

Defect	Number	Percentage
Patent ductus arteriosus (PDA)	1207	25.7
Subaortic stenosis (SAS)	1102	23.5
Pulmonary valve stenosis (PS)	1039	22.1
Ventricular septal defect (VSD)	413	8.8
Tricuspid valve dysplasia (TVD)	216	4.6
Mitral valve dysplasia (MVD)	204	4.3
Other defects	160	3.4
Persistent right aortic arch or other vascular ring anomaly (PRAA)	155	3.3
Tetralogy of Fallot (ToF)	110	2.3
Atrial septal defect (ASD)	89	1.9
Total	4694	100

Combined data from Patterson DF: Epidemiologic and genetic studies of congenital heart disease in the dog, *Circ Res* 23:171, 1968; Mulvihill JJ, Priester WA: Congenital heart disease in dogs: epidemiologic similarities to man, *Teratology* 7:73, 1973; Hunt GB, Church DB, Malik R: A retrospective analysis of congenital cardiac anomalies (1977-1989), *Aust Vet Pract* 20:70,1990; Buchanan JW. Causes and prevalence of cardiovascular disease. In Kirk RW, Bonagura JD, editors: *Current veterinary therapy XI: small animal practice,* Philadelphia, 1992, Saunders, p 647; Tidholm A: Retrospective study of congenital heart defects in 151 dogs, *J Small Anim Pract* 38:94, 1997; Kittleson MD: The approach to the patient with cardiac disease. In Kittleson MD, Kienle RD, editors: *Small animal cardiovascular medicine,* St Louis, 1998, Mosby, p 195; Buchanan JW: Prevalence of cardiovascular disorders. In Fox PR, Sisson DD, Moise NS, editors: *Textbook of canine and feline cardiology,* ed 2, Philadelphia, 1999, Saunders, p 458; Baumgartner C, Glaus TM: Congenital cardiac diseases in dogs: a retrospective analysis, *Schweiz Arch Tierheilkd* 145:527, 2003; Gregori T et al: Congenital heart defects in dogs: a double retrospective study on cases from University of Parma and University of Zaragoza, *Ann Fac Medic Vet di Parma* 28:79, 2008; Oliveira P et al: Retrospective review of congenital heart disease in 976 dogs, *J Vet Intern Med* 25:477, 2011.

TABLE **174-2**

Congenital Heart Disease in Cats

Defect	Number	Percentage
Ventricular septal defect (VSD)	80	18.4
Patent ductus arteriosus (PDA)	49	11.3
Tricuspid valve dysplasia (TVD)	47	10.8
Mitral valve dysplasia (MVD)	44	10.1
Atrioventricular septal defect (AVSD)	42	9.7
Aortic stenosis (AS)	31	7.1
Tetralogy of Fallot (ToF)	30	6.9
Atrial septal defect (ASD)	26	6.0
Persistent right aortic arch or other vascular ring anomaly (PRAA)	23	5.3
Endocardial fibroelastosis (EFE)	21	4.8
Pulmonary valve stenosis (PS)	17	3.9
Other defects	11	2.5
Double-outlet right ventricle (DORV)	7	1.6
Cor triatriatum sinister	7	1.6
Total	435	100

Combined data from Liu SK: Pathology of feline heart diseases, *Vet Clin North Am Small Anim Pract* 7:323, 1977; Harpster N, Zook B: The cardiovascular system. In Holzworth J, editor: *Diseases of the cat: medicine and surgery,* Philadelphia, 1987, Saunders, p 820; Hunt GB, Church DB, Malik R: A retrospective analysis of congenital cardiac anomalies (1977-1989), *Aust Vet Pract* 20:70, 1990; Kittleson MD: The approach to the patient with cardiac disease. In Kittleson MD, Kienle RD, editors: *Small animal cardiovascular medicine,* St Louis, 1998, Mosby, p 195; Michaelsson M, Ho SY: *Congenital heart malformations in mammals,* London, 2000, Imperial College Press.

Fewer data are available about CHD prevalence in the cat. Table 174-2 compiles CHD cases from five studies to provide cumulative data on 435 defects. Ventricular septal defect (VSD) appears to be the most common defect in the cat, comprising over 18% of cases. PDA is not considered a common defect in the cat, compared with the dog, but accounted for over 11% of defects tabulated in these studies. Mitral valve dysplasia (MVD) and tricuspid valve dysplasia (TVD) each accounted for an additional 10% of defects. Abnormalities of the atrioventricular septum (AVSDs; formerly known as *endocardial cushion defects* or *atrioventricular canal defects*) are not infrequent in the cat, comprising a tenth of the cases reported. However, not all studies clearly defined the location of tabulated atrial septal defects (ASDs) and VSDs, nor fully described the morphology of diagnoses of MVD and TVD—all of which may be forms of AVSD. For this reason, the proportion of at least partial AVSDs is likely higher than tabulated here. Earlier studies described a high proportion of endocardial fibroelastosis in kittens, particularly the Burmese and Siamese breeds, but this disease was not described in more

recent studies. Compared with dogs, abnormalities of the outflow tracts (PS and SAS) appear much less common in cats.

Diagnostic Testing

Screening for congenital cardiac disease typically begins with a thorough physical examination performed at the first general health examination. One of the most important aspects of the cardiac physical examination and one of the initial diagnostic tests for CHD is a thorough auscultation of the heart and great vessels. Auscultation is imperative for screening for CHD because the most common forms of CHD, as well as many complex CHDs, typically present with a systolic murmur (SAS, PS, VSD, MVD, and TVD) or continuous murmur (PDA). Auscultation in puppies and kittens should be performed in a quiet room and all valve areas should be evaluated, including the mitral valve area where the apical impulse is felt most strongly, the semilunar valve area (aortic and pulmonary valves) at the base of the left side of the heart (the ventral second to fourth intercostal spaces), the area of the great vessels just dorsal to the base of the left side of the heart, and the tricuspid valve area on the right chest wall. The left and right thoracic inlet and sternal borders also should be auscultated so as not to miss atypically radiating murmurs or very focal defects. In many cats and very small dogs, distinguishing separate valve areas is not possible because of the small chest size, and most murmurs in cats tend to be loudest adjacent to the sternal borders. The use of a pediatric stethoscope head can aid in the auscultation of very small animals.

Murmur location and intensity are useful in differentiating between types of CHD as well as in distinguishing an innocent or functional murmur from that caused by CHD. Left (mitral regurgitation) and right (tricuspid regurgitation) apical systolic murmurs commonly are due to defects of mitral valve dysplasia and tricuspid valve dysplasia, respectively. The murmur of a VSD typically is systolic at the right sternal border. Left basilar systolic murmurs can be more problematic, however, because they can indicate either an innocent murmur or a CHD such as SAS, PS, or ASD, especially when soft in intensity. Murmur intensity coupled with location can be helpful in discerning different types of CHD and differentiating CHD from an innocent or functional murmur. High-intensity murmurs (grade 3 out of 6 or louder) usually indicate the presence of significant CHD regardless of location and are an indication for more advanced diagnostic testing. However, less intense murmurs (grade 3 or lower) either may originate from a functional cause or may indicate CHD. In general, a soft left basilar systolic murmur heard in a young puppy or kitten that decreases in intensity over the first months of life or disappears by 6 months of age is more likely to be innocent. However, if the murmur persists at the same intensity or becomes louder as the animal ages, it is more likely to reflect CHD, and advanced diagnostic testing such as echocardiography should be recommended. A continuous murmur, a diastolic murmur, other cardiac signs (arrhythmia, cough, syncope), and a very loud murmur all likely indicate CHD, and further testing should be advised.

Other aspects of a cardiac physical examination are evaluations of the mucous membranes, jugular veins, and pulse quality. Mucous membranes should be assessed for evidence of cyanosis or prolonged capillary refill time, which may be indicative of a right-to-left intracardiac shunt or decreased cardiac output and reduced peripheral perfusion even in the absence of an obvious heart murmur. Variations in pulse quality also may be suggestive of CHD. Hypokinetic pulses commonly are detected in moderate to severe subaortic stenosis, whereas a hyperkinetic pulse quality is suggestive of a wide pulse pressure caused by PDA or severe aortic insufficiency. Jugular pulsation with or without distention can indicate tricuspid regurgitation or elevated right-sided pressures due to TVD, PS, or pulmonary hypertension from severe left-to-right shunting defects.

Although the physical examination is an important aspect of screening for the presence of CHD, it is difficult to make a definitive diagnosis from signalment and physical examination alone. Ancillary diagnostic tests, like thoracic radiography and electrocardiography (ECG), may be useful in narrowing the differential diagnostic list and determining disease severity but can also add cost to the initial evaluation without providing definitive diagnostic information.

Thoracic radiographs should be evaluated in a systematic manner and should include examination of orthogonal views, the cardiac silhouette, pulmonary vasculature, pulmonary parenchyma, and vena cava. Thoracic radiography is useful in diagnosing congestive heart failure (CHF) as well as in detecting cardiac changes due to moderate to severe CHD. However, radiographs have limited diagnostic capability in mild CHD because there may be minimal to no radiographic change. The radiographic diagnosis of left-sided CHF includes left-sided cardiomegaly, specifically left atrial enlargement; pulmonary venous distention; and interstitial to alveolar infiltrates in the perihilar to caudodorsal lung fields in dogs. Cats with CHF also have left atrial enlargement and venous congestion but may have a variety of pulmonary parenchymal changes such as a ventrally distributed interstitial pattern, patchy interstitial to alveolar infiltrates, and pleural effusion. Right-sided CHF has the radiographic signs of enlargement of the right side of the heart, caudal vena caval dilation, hepatomegaly, and varying degrees of either loss of abdominal detail from ascites or signs of pleural effusion.

Although the specific radiographic diagnosis of CHD is beyond the scope of this chapter, in general left atrial and ventricular enlargement are common secondary to mitral regurgitation (MVD) or left-to-right shunting defects (PDA, VSD). Conversely, left atrial enlargement without ventricular enlargement more likely is related to mitral valve stenosis. Left-to-right shunting defects, in addition to left-sided cardiomegaly, also have signs of overcirculation (dilatation) of both the pulmonary arteries and the pulmonary veins. Right atrial and ventricular enlargement may occur with tricuspid regurgitation (TVD), PS, ASD, or ToF. Rarely, left-to-right shunting defects may result in pulmonary vascular changes and secondary pulmonary hypertension, which also may cause radiographic evidence of enlargement of the right side of the heart. Isolated right atrial enlargement without right ventricular enlargement can be caused by tricuspid valve stenosis and TVD. SAS can show left ventricular enlargement in conjunction with dilation of the aortic root and ascending aorta, whereas PS results in dilation of the main pulmonary artery segment in addition to enlargement of the right side of the heart.

ECG may be beneficial in detecting cardiac changes related to CHD, although it is most useful for characterizing dysrhythmias heard on auscultation. Diseases affecting the right side of the heart such as PS, TVD, and ToF can show *P pulmonale* (tall P waves), indicating right atrial enlargement, or a right-axis deviation of the QRS complex, indicating right ventricular enlargement or right bundle branch block. Diseases affecting the left side of the heart can show *P mitrale* (wide P waves), indicating left atrial enlargement, or a tall or wide QRS complex, indicating left ventricular enlargement. CHDs that cause ventricular enlargement, such as PS and SAS, may provide a substrate for ventricular arrhythmias secondary to myocardial ischemia. However, ECG is a test that is more specific than sensitive because animals with significant CHD may have a normal ECG. ECG also is unlikely to be of use for definitive diagnosis of a CHD, although it is very useful for definitive diagnosis of dysrhythmias associated with CHD.

In recent years the use of cardiac biomarkers to screen animals for the presence of cardiovascular disease has gained in popularity. There have been limited studies looking at the usefulness of these tests in animals with CHD. The biomarkers receiving the most attention in veterinary cardiology are cardiac troponin I (cTnI) and B-type natriuretic peptide (BNP), especially the N-terminal (amino end) of the prohormone (NT-proBNP). The biomarker cTnI is a myocardial protein released in the setting of myocyte damage or death; for this reason, the level of cTnI is profoundly elevated in the setting of myocardial necrosis, and high-sensitivity assays also have found mild to modest elevations in conditions leading to cardiac remodeling. B-type natriuretic peptide is a hormone released by the myocardium in response to stretch, hypertrophy, or hypoxia; the N-terminal of the prohormone is more stable in serum and is therefore the preferred assay target.

There are few studies evaluating the use of cTnI as a biomarker in animals with CHD. A mild elevation (median, 0.20 ng/ml; range, 0.20 to 1.29) was shown in 30% of dogs with PS before balloon valvuloplasty (Saunders et al, 2009b). However, a study by a different group found normal cTnI values (≤0.05 ng/ml) in dogs with PDA and PS before intervention (Shih et al, 2009). Based on these limited data, cTnI level does not appear to be a reliable screening test for CHD in animals, although further studies are needed.

More data are available to suggest that NT-proBNP levels are elevated in dogs with CHD. A study by Saunders and colleagues (2009a) found median NT-proBNP values of 724 pmol/L (range, 50 to 3000) in dogs with PDA, 746 pmol/L (range, 278 to 3000) in dogs with PS, and 833 pmol/L (range, 388 to 2194) in dogs with ASD compared with 333 pmol/L (range, 161 to 826) in normal dogs. Also in 2009, Farace and colleagues found that NT-proBNP values in dogs with SAS were elevated and correlated with the severity of the stenosis: normal dogs had a mean NT-proBNP level of 361 pmol/L (range, 307 to 415), dogs with mild SAS had a level of 344 pmol/L (range, 239 to 448), dogs with moderate SAS showed a level of 1011 pmol/L (range, 86 to 1936), and those with severe SAS had a level of 2529 pmol/L (range, 1841 to 3217). Although NT-proBNP level does appear to have some usefulness in determining the presence or absence of CHD, it cannot distinguish the type of defect present. More comprehensive studies are needed to better define the value of NT-proBNP in screening young animals for the presence of CHD.

History, physical examination, thoracic radiography, ECG, and NT-proBNP level all are useful diagnostic tools for determining the presence of CHD but are less capable of providing a definitive diagnosis, assessing disease severity, or ruling out the presence of multiple or complex congenital lesions. In veterinary medicine, Doppler echocardiography is the noninvasive gold standard for definitive diagnosis of CHD. All animals in which CHD is suspected should undergo a detailed echocardiographic examination performed by a veterinarian trained in the diagnosis of CHD. Echocardiography allows identification of specific types of CHD and detection of concomitant defects, as well as assessment of disease severity and risk of complications, determination of the direction of cardiac shunting, estimation of intracardiac pressures, and assessment of the likelihood of CHF. Echocardiography is necessary for determining the need for therapy as well as for planning interventional or surgical therapies.

Medical Therapy

Medical therapy for CHD depends on what type of CHD is identified, how severe the disorder is, whether obvious clinical signs are present, and whether there are concomitant arrhythmias or CHF. Treatment of asymptomatic CHD depends on the specific underlying type and severity of CHD; therefore definitive diagnosis is essential. Mild, asymptomatic CHD may not require medical therapy if echocardiography suggests that the disease is unlikely to show significant progression, cause symptom development, or have an adverse impact on life expectancy. An example is mild PS in a full-grown dog with minimal cardiac remodeling—no therapy is needed in such a dog. Moderate to severe asymptomatic CHD, however, has a much greater probability of leading to symptoms, and therapy (medical, interventional, or surgical) is typically recommended.

In general, diseases with moderate to severe outflow tract obstruction causing concentric hypertrophy, such as SAS and PS, commonly are treated by the authors with β-blockers such as atenolol. Atenolol typically is given with an up-titration in dose over 4 to 8 weeks, starting at 0.2 to 0.5 mg/kg q12h PO and increasing to a target dose of 1 to 1.5 mg/kg q12h PO. Concentric hypertrophy leads to decreased myocardial perfusion, subendocardial ischemia, myocardial fibrosis, and development of dysrhythmias. β-Blockade reduces heart rate, decreases force of contraction, and prolongs diastolic filling, thereby enhancing myocardial perfusion. Such effects potentially reduce the risk of myocardial ischemia and the development of ventricular arrhythmias, although this has not been proven in controlled clinical trials. β-Blockers also act as nonspecific ventricular antiarrhythmic agents.

Whether asymptomatic diseases of volume overload, such as moderate to severe mitral or tricuspid regurgitation and left-to-right shunting defects like PDA, should be treated before CHF develops is controversial. However, the addition of angiotensin-converting enzyme (ACE) inhibitors such as enalapril at 0.5 mg/kg q12h PO is common if there is severe eccentric hypertrophy, impaired cardiac output, and atrial enlargement causing high risk of development of CHF and activation of the renin-angiotensin-aldosterone system.

Medical treatment of symptomatic CHD depends on the type of lesion and developing symptoms. Diseases of outflow tract obstruction (SAS, PS) commonly cause exercise intolerance and syncope related to reduced cardiac output, inappropriate baroreceptor activation, or ventricular arrhythmias. Syncope commonly is treated with exercise modification, antiarrhythmic agents, and β-blockers. Syncope is more likely to occur with high levels of intense activity because of the inability to increase cardiac output to match the level of exercise, possible inappropriate baroreceptor activation, and induction of arrhythmias by high sympathetic tone and myocardial ischemia. Modification of exercise level with avoidance of high-level intense or burst activity commonly reduces this symptom. β-Blockade potentially is beneficial in decreasing syncope because of a reduction in heart rate and force of contraction, the potential for increasing myocardial perfusion and reducing ischemia, and a decrease in sympathetic tone.

Diseases of left-sided volume overload commonly cause symptoms such as coughing before the onset of CHF because of severe left atrial enlargement and resultant left bronchial compression. Bronchial compression may be treated with ACE inhibitors and low-dose furosemide (1 mg/kg q12-24h PO) to decrease preload and left atrial pressure, which reduces bronchial compression and minimizes symptoms. Other therapies for bronchial compression include cough suppressants such as hydrocodone (0.5 mg/kg q8-12h PO) and bronchodilators such as extended-release formulations of theophylline (10 mg/kg q12h PO). Although cough suppressants may reduce the symptoms of bronchial compression, they also may mask early signs of CHF; therefore the animal's resting respiratory rate should be monitored carefully by the client (target respiratory rate is <30 to 35 breaths/min) so as not to miss symptoms of early CHF.

Pulmonary hypertension can develop in CHD secondary to left-to-right shunting lesions such as PDA, VSD, and ASD or secondary to chronic, severe elevations in left atrial pressure. Pulmonary hypertension therapy is instituted in response to the development of secondary symptoms such as severe exercise intolerance, syncope, right-sided CHF, and shunt reversal causing right-to-left shunting, hypoxemia, and polycythemia. Therapy is aimed at pulmonary vasodilation, most commonly using phosphodiesterase 5 inhibitors like sildenafil (usual dose is 2 mg/kg q8-12h PO).

Defects leading to pulmonary hypertension and shunt reversal (so-called Eisenmenger's physiology) cause cyanosis and secondary polycythemia (packed cell volume of >65%) and are treated with periodic phlebotomy or administration of chemotherapeutic agents causing reduction in red blood cell production, such as hydroxyurea. The aim of phlebotomy or hydroxyurea therapy for cyanotic heart disease is to achieve a packed cell volume of approximately 55% to 60% because this level of erythrocytosis provides increased oxygen-carrying capacity without excessive hyperviscosity.

Severe congenital cardiac disease due to either pressure or volume overload commonly leads to the development of left- or right-sided CHF. Left-sided CHF presents with coughing, tachypnea, and dyspnea secondary to pulmonary edema, whereas right-sided CHF presents with signs of jugular distention, hepatomegaly, ascites, or pleural effusion. CHF, regardless of cause, is treated with diuretics and ACE inhibitors. Furosemide is the diuretic of choice for both right- and left-sided CHF and is given at varying dosages, typically starting at 2 mg/kg q12h PO; the goal is to administer the lowest dose that controls clinical signs effectively, and usually the maximal oral dosage is up to 8 to 12 mg/kg/day. Right-sided CHF commonly requires higher doses of furosemide because of the potential for intestinal edema, which causes decreased gastrointestinal absorption. Other diuretics available for use in conjunction with furosemide are spironolactone and hydrochlorothiazide (see Chapter 175). ACE inhibitors always should be used in the treatment of chronic CHF to decrease the activation of the renin-angiotensin-aldosterone system associated with advanced heart failure and diuretic administration. Contraindications to ACE inhibition include the presence of systemic arterial hypotension or significant preexisting azotemia.

Pimobendan therapy has become the standard of care in the treatment of CHF secondary to acquired cardiac diseases such as dilated cardiomyopathy and chronic degenerative valve disease. Although no definitive data are available on the use of pimobendan in congenital cardiac disease, most cardiologists advocate its use in CHF caused by diseases of volume overload such as PDA or MVD. The use of pimobendan in the treatment of CHF secondary to diseases of pressure overload like SAS and PS is controversial as positive inotropes technically are contraindicated in diseases of outflow tract obstruction because of the resulting increase in pressure gradient, wall stress, and myocardial oxygen consumption. However, some cardiologists advocate the use of pimobendan in cases of SAS and PS when there is advanced CHF with myocardial failure and impaired systolic function, in order to improve control of CHF.

Surgical and Interventional Therapy

CHD can be palliated medically, as noted earlier, but also may be treated by minimally invasive (interventional) or traditional surgical techniques whenever possible. An accurate diagnosis of CHD is critical to guide therapy appropriately because some animals can live a normal life if treated early. For example, one study suggested that up to 60% of dogs with PDA will die within a year of diagnosis if the shunt is not closed, whereas those undergoing PDA closure before the onset of heart failure typically have a near-normal life span (Eyster et al, 1976). Likewise, balloon pulmonary valvuloplasty for PS can reduce the obstruction to right ventricular outflow and has been shown to prolong survival and improve quality of life for dogs with PS (Johnson and Martin, 2004).

The decision whether to operate or pursue transcatheter therapy depends on the expertise of the institution, the anatomy of the defect, and client preference. The treatment of CHD in children has trended toward interventional strategies because of reduced morbidity, shorter recovery times, and reduced costs compared with open surgical options. A similar trend has occurred in veterinary cardiology; for example, dogs with PS seldom have been treated using surgical techniques since the advent of balloon pulmonary valvuloplasty in the 1980s. Although the trend is toward transcatheter therapy, it is imperative that the adoption of a minimally invasive approach for a given condition be validated by scientific analysis proving noninferiority to traditional surgical techniques. Prospective comparison studies are sadly lacking in veterinary medicine, although retrospective data on PDA closure suggests comparable or improved outcomes using a transcatheter approach compared with surgery. Gordon and colleagues (2010) achieved complete PDA occlusion in 40 of 41 dogs treated using a transarterial canine-specific device with no perioperative mortality compared with a perioperative mortality of 2% to 8% during open PDA ligation reported in the surgical literature (Birchard et al, 1990; Eyster et al, 1976).

The CHD conditions for which there is currently a well-established surgical or interventional treatment option are PDA (see Web Chapter 64), vascular ring anomalies, and PS (see Web Chapter 65). Prior studies suggested that surgical or interventional therapy for SAS provided no survival advantage compared with medical therapy (Meurs et al, 2005; Orton et al, 2000). However, a new interventional approach using cutting and high-pressure balloon aortic valvuloplasty has shown early improvement in dogs with SAS by reducing the transvalvular gradient (Schmidt et al, 2010), although long-term results remain unknown. Dogs with VSD or ASD (see Web Chapter 69) have been treated successfully with both surgical and interventional techniques, and although they are costly, open surgical repair and newer transcatheter devices for closure of these defects may be considered. In cyanotic dogs with ToF, palliation can be achieved by surgical construction of a systemic-to-pulmonary anastomosis, typically a modified Blalock-Taussig shunt, which improves pulmonary blood flow and lessens central cyanosis. Open-heart repair of ToF also has been described in the dog. Atrioventricular valve dysplasia seldom is treated by surgical or interventional techniques; however, if a stenotic component is present, balloon valvuloplasty of the tricuspid or mitral valve may be considered. Case reports of open surgical mitral valve repair as well as valve replacement for mitral dysplasia are found in the veterinary literature. Newer transcatheter approaches to mitral valve repair are entering the human marketplace and may prove a viable option for animals in the future. Larger case series of tricuspid valve replacement have been reported recently (Arai et al, 2011; Brockman, 2010); results were fair, although the risk of valve failure secondary to thrombosis or inflammatory pannus remains a long-term concern in dogs.

References and Suggested Reading

Arai S et al: Bioprosthesis valve replacement in dogs with congenital tricuspid valve dysplasia: technique and outcome, *J Vet Cardiol* 13(2):91, 2011.

Birchard SJ, Bonagura JD, Fingland RB: Results of ligation of patent ductus arteriosus in dogs: 201 cases (1969-1988), *J Am Vet Med Assoc* 196(12):2011, 1990.

Brockman DJ: The RVC experience: tricuspid valve replacement and RVOT reconstruction. In *Proceedings of the ACVS Veterinary Symposium,* Seattle, WA, 2010.

Buchanan JW: Causes and prevalence of cardiovascular diseases. In Kirk RW, Bonagura JD, editors: *Current veterinary therapy XI: small animal practice,* Philadelphia, 1992, Saunders, p 647.

Detweiler DK, Patterson DF: The prevalence and types of cardiovascular disease in dogs, *Ann N Y Acad Sci* 127(1):481, 1965.

Eyster GE et al: Patent ductus arteriosus in the dog: characteristics of occurrence and results of surgery in one hundred consecutive cases, *J Am Vet Med Assoc* 168(5):435, 1976.

Farace G, et al: Correlation of N-terminal prohormone brain natriuretic peptide with left ventricular outflow tract in dogs with subaortic stenosis, *J Vet Intern Med* 23:2, 2009 (abstract).

Gordon SG et al: Transarterial ductal occlusion using the Amplatz® Canine Duct Occluder in 40 dogs, *J Vet Cardiol* 12(2):85, 2010.

Johnson MS, Martin M: Results of balloon valvuloplasty in 40 dogs with pulmonic stenosis, *J Small Anim Pract* 45(3):148, 2004.

Meurs KM, Lehmkuhl LB, Bonagura JD: Survival times in dogs with severe subvalvular aortic stenosis treated with balloon valvuloplasty or atenolol, *J Am Vet Med Assoc* 227(3):420, 2005.

Orton EC et al: Influence of open surgical correction on intermediate-term outcome in dogs with subvalvular aortic stenosis: 44 cases (1991-1998), *J Am Vet Med Assoc* 216(3):3, 2000.

Ruble RP, Hird DW: Congenital abnormalities in immature dogs from a pet store: 253 cases (1987-1988), *J Am Vet Med Assoc* 202(4):633, 1993.

Saunders AB et al: NT-proBNP concentrations in canine congenital heart disease, *J Vet Intern Med* 23:1, 2009a (abstract).

Saunders AB et al: Cardiac troponin I and C-reactive protein concentrations in dogs with severe pulmonic stenosis before and after balloon valvuloplasty, *J Vet Cardiol* 11(1):9, 2009b.

Schmidt M et al: Combined cutting balloon and high pressure balloon angioplasty in dogs with severe subaortic stenosis is effective at mid-term follow-up, *Catheter Cardiovasc Interv* 76(1):S10, 2010 (abstract).

Shih AC et al: Effect of routine cardiovascular catheterization on cardiac troponin I concentration in dogs, *J Vet Cardiol* 11:S87, 2009.

CHAPTER 175

Drugs for Treatment of Heart Failure in Dogs

JOHN D. BONAGURA, *Columbus, Ohio*
BRUCE W. KEENE, *Raleigh, North Carolina*

Therapy for canine heart failure (HF) requires careful orchestration of a multiple-drug treatment regimen. Cardiovascular drugs are potent in their relief of clinical signs and can be life prolonging, but these compounds also can injure the patient. In this chapter we consider the general classification, mechanism of action, indications, uses, and adverse effects of drugs used for treatment of canine HF. The coordinated use of these drugs and some of the clinical trial data indicating their benefit are discussed next in Chapter 176. The reader also is directed to the Appendix for a listing of alternative dosages. The dosages summarized in Table 175-1 focus exclusively on *dogs;* dosages for cats can be found in Chapters 173 and 180. One of the authors (BK) also has developed an on-line dosage calculator that veterinarians and veterinary technicians may find useful (see www.cardiologycarenetwork.com/network/dosage_calc.php).

The number of drugs capable of affecting heart and vascular functions is considerable (Box 175-1), and the pharmacologic effects of drugs used in treatment of HF can become confusing. Some treatments for congestive heart failure (CHF) affect ventricular pumping (inotropes), whereas others reduce venous pressures and ventricular preload (diuretics and venodilators), improving or preventing signs of congestion. Drugs with arterial vasodilator effects decrease blood pressure (BP), ventricular afterload, and mitral regurgitant volume, with the consequence of increasing forward stroke volume leaving the ventricle. Some agents demonstrate very rapid hemodynamic effects (e.g., intravenously administered diuretics, nitrovasodilators, and catecholamines). Others confer benefits by modulating the chronically activated neurohormonal, inflammatory, and profibrotic mediators of CHF (these include the "cardioprotective" drugs such as the angiotensin-converting enzyme [ACE] inhibitors, β-adrenergic blockers, and aldosterone receptor blockers).

The clinician should be mindful of the clinical pharmacology of these compounds (Brunton et al, 2010; Gordon and Kittleson, 2008; Opie and Gersh, 2013) and also appreciate that many drugs we use in veterinary practice are prescribed in an extralabel manner. For example, most of the vasodilator drugs and all of the antiarrhythmic drugs mentioned in this chapter are approved for human use and administered off label to dogs based on current standards of care. Although this chapter offers an overview of the important drugs used to manage HF in dogs, the reader is directed to

comprehensive textbooks in the reference list for a fuller recounting. The ABCD stages of HF are described fully in the next chapter, but for reference, stage C represents CHF that is manageable with standard four-drug therapy and dosages and stage D represents refractory CHF that requires additional therapies and higher dosages of the standard-treatment drugs. In this context, standard therapy for CHF in the dog is furosemide, an ACE inhibitor, pimobendan, and spironolactone.

Many HF drugs are available in generic formulations, which can help to control the cost of multiple-medication regimens such as the one just mentioned. However, proprietary formulations must be used in some countries based on applicable laws: this can create problems for some clients faced with high drug costs in the absence of any insurance reimbursement. Therefore the cost of drugs should be discussed with owners before prescribing and adjustments made as practical.

Diuretics

Diuretics are administered to cardiac patients in acute situations for mobilization of edema and in chronic HF to prevent ongoing sodium and water retention. Low dosages also may be useful (when combined with an ACE inhibitor) in the control of cough related to left bronchial compression when it occurs before the onset of overt CHF. When diuretics are prescribed for long-term use, dietary sodium intake should be restricted (see Chapter 168) and an ACE inhibitor and aldosterone receptor blocker (spironolactone) coadministered.

Furosemide and Torsemide

Furosemide and torsemide are potent diuretics that block the 2-chloride symporter in the thick loop of Henle and increase urinary losses of chloride, sodium, potassium, hydrogen ions, and water. Furosemide (also known as *frusemide*) is the most commonly used diuretic for management of CHF in dogs. Loop diuretics also block free-water clearance and increase the loss of magnesium ions. These agents are "high ceiling," demonstrating high potency in preventing renal sodium reabsorption with a strong dose-response relationship. There is far less experience with torsemide in veterinary medicine, but this drug is thought to have better oral bioavailability and a longer duration of action than furosemide. It is used increasingly in advanced CHF when furosemide seems to become less

BOX 175-1

General Classes of Cardiovascular Drugs Used in the Treatment of Canine Heart Failure

Diuretics
Diuretics acting on the loop of Henle: furosemide, torsemide
Aldosterone antagonists: spironolactone
Diuretics acting on the distal convoluted tubules:
    hydrochlorothiazide

Positive Inotropic Drugs
Cardiac glycosides: digoxin
Calcium sensitizers: pimobendan, levosimendan
Catecholamines: dobutamine, dopamine
Phosphodiesterase inhibitors: milrinone, pimobendan

Vasodilator Drugs
Angiotensin-converting enzyme inhibitors (see later)
Nitrovasodilators: nitroglycerine ointment, sodium nitroprusside
Calcium channel blockers: amlodipine
Phosphodiesterase (PDE) inhibitors: sildenafil (PDE 5),
    pimobendan (PDE 3), milrinone (PDE 3)
Other vasodilators: hydralazine

Angiotensin-Converting Enzyme Inhibitors
Enalapril, benazepril, imidapril, other "-prils"

β-Adrenergic Blockers
Second generation (cardioselective β_1-blocker): atenolol,
    metoprolol, bisoprolol, esmolol
Third generation (β_1-, β_2-, α_1-blockers, antioxidant): carvedilol

Antiarrhythmic Drugs
Sodium channel blockers (class I):
    Class IA: procainamide
    Class IB: lidocaine, mexiletine
    Class IC: flecainide
β-Adrenergic blockers (class II): sotalol, atenolol, carvedilol
Potassium channel blockers (class III): sotalol, amiodarone
Calcium channel blockers (class IV): diltiazem
Others: digoxin (increases vagal tone), omega-3 fatty acids

effective. Furosemide is effective when administered by intravenous, intramuscular, subcutaneous, and oral routes, and the relative onset of diuresis also follows this order from fastest to slowest. When used in dogs, torsemide is administered by mouth.

Furosemide is carried by renal blood flow to the proximal nephron and actively secreted into the plasma filtrate where it is carried to the loop of Henle. If renal blood flow is impaired because of severe CHF, plasma volume contraction, or the administration of a nonsteroidal antiinflammatory drug, the delivery of drug to the proximal nephron may be inadequate. Because of this possibility, a relatively high initial furosemide dose (such as 2 to 4 mg/kg IV) usually is administered to patients with severe CHF. When relative diuretic resistance is evident, a constant-rate IV infusion of furosemide can be initiated after the initial bolus. For a continuous IV infusion, 0.5 to 1 mg/kg/hr is administered using an accurate syringe pump for 3 to 12 hours. The patient is monitored closely for evidence of effective diuresis (by counting the respiratory rate, assessing respiratory effort, and checking for urination every 15 to 30 minutes; the bladder also can be palpated or imaged by ultrasonography if there is a question about urine formation). Once diuresis begins and the respiratory rate falls (to <40 to 45 breaths/min) the furosemide dosage is reduced to 2 mg/kg q6-12h IV, IM, or SC.

Oral maintenance dosages of furosemide can be initiated once the dog is in clinically stable condition and ready to be released from the hospital. The usual oral dosage is 2 to 4 mg/kg two times daily. The frequency can be increased to three times daily and the dosage up-titrated to as high as 12 mg/kg daily in refractory cases of CHF provided renal function and electrolyte status are monitored. When fluid retention becomes unresponsive to standard dosages of furosemide (stage D CHF), other diuretic options should be considered, including flexible subcutaneous dosing of furosemide or the addition of another diuretic such as torsemide or hydrochlorothiazide (see Chapter 176 for details). Torsemide ostensibly is more potent than furosemide in this setting and may be considered at approximately $\frac{1}{10}$ of the furosemide milligram dosage. It can be substituted for one or more daily doses of furosemide.

Adverse effects of loop diuretics include polydipsia, polyuria, reduction in BP, plasma volume depletion, (prerenal) azotemia, and depletion of electrolytes, especially chloride, potassium, and magnesium. Monotherapy with a loop diuretic activates the renin-angiotensin-aldosterone system; accordingly, long-term diuretic therapy should incorporate an ACE inhibitor (and optimally spironolactone) as part of the treatment plan. Clients should be instructed not to administer the drug at bedtime to avoid urinary accidents, and they should never restrict water (except in rare circumstances of profound hyponatremia). Mild azotemia is not a reason to discontinue diuretic therapy, but moderate to severe azotemia should prompt dosage reductions (see Chapter 176 for a detailed discussion of this issue). Potassium supplements are needed infrequently in dogs receiving combined therapy with furosemide, spironolactone, and enalapril because the latter two drugs "spare" potassium by reducing urinary losses. Ototoxicity and renal failure are potential adverse effects, especially when aminoglycosides are coadministered.

Spironolactone

Spironolactone is a synthetic, antiandrogenic, steroidal compound that blocks aldosterone receptors in the kidney, heart, and in other tissues (*eplerenone* is a related drug not sufficiently studied in veterinary medicine). Despite its classification as a diuretic, the urine-enhancing effects of spironolactone are weak to nonexistent in the dog, likely related to the locus of its antimineralocorticoid activity in the most distal segments of the renal tubule. The major reasons for prescribing spironolactone in heart disease relate to its potassium-sparing action and the potential for antifibrotic effects in the heart, kidneys, and other tissues. Drugs of this class (including eplerenone) also may normalize baroreceptor function, which has been shown to be depressed in canine CHF. There is some evidence—although it is not definitive—for a survival

TABLE 175-1

Drugs Used in the Treatment of Heart Failure and Arrhythmias in Dogs

Drug	Preparations	Commonly Used Dosages	Comments/Adverse Effects
Amiodarone	200, 400 mg tablets	8-12 mg/kg q24h PO for 7-10 days, then reduce to 4-6 mg/kg q24h PO	Long elimination half-life Hepatotoxicity is common Thyroid dysfunction, bone marrow suppression
Amlodipine	2.5, 5, 10 mg tablets	0.1-0.4 mg/kg q24h or divided BID PO	Slowly up-titrate dose in CHF Higher doses often needed in systemic hypertension caused by chronic kidney disease Hypotension
Atenolol	25, 50, 100 mg tablets	0.2-1 mg/kg q12h PO	Gradual up-titration required in CHF Dogs without CHF can tolerate higher doses Bradycardia, AV block, hypotension Depression of contractility, CHF
Benazepril	5, 10, 20, 40 mg tablets	0.25-0.5 mg/kg q12h PO	Start at lower range and increase to maximal dose with monitoring of renal function and BP Acute renal failure, azotemia, hyperkalemia
Carvedilol	3.125, 6.25, 12.5, 25 mg tablets	0.1-0.5 mg/kg q12h PO in DCM Up to 1.0 mg/kg q12h, PO in dog with normal LVSF	Gradual up-titration required in CHF Precipitation of HF possible, especially in DCM Dogs without CHF tolerate higher doses
Butorphanol	2 mg/ml or 10 mg/ml injectable 5, 10 mg tablets	0.1-0.5 mg/kg IM or IV Typical CHF dose is 0.2-0.25 mg/kg IM or IV 0.5-1.0 mg/kg orally as needed up to TID	Dose-dependent sedation Higher doses tolerated in dogs without CHF Respiratory depression
Digoxin	0.125, 0.25 mg tablets (preferred); 0.05 mg/ml and 0.15 mg/ml elixirs	0.0055 to 0.011 mg/kg q12h, PO	Begin at lower end of dosage range to limit toxicity Target trough serum levels of 0.8-1.2 ng/ml Renal failure delays elimination Anorexia, depression, vomiting, diarrhea Junctional tachycardia, AV block, PVCs/VT
Diltiazem	30, 60, 90, 120 mg tablets Sustained release: 60, 180, 240 mg 5 mg/ml injectable	0.5-2.5 mg/kg q8h PO (standard) 1-3.5 mg/kg q12h PO (sustained release) Total daily dosage: 2-7 mg/kg total 0.05-0.1 mg/kg IV over 5-10 minutes; can repeat up to 0.3 mg/kg cumulative dose for SVT	Gradual up-titration in CHF to target HR Dogs without CHF can tolerate higher doses Negative inotropy and vasodilation Use IV with caution, especially with DCM or decreased LVSF; monitor BP before each IV dose Hypotension, AV block, myocardial depression
Dobutamine	250 mg (20 ml) vial for injection Generic concentrations—variable	2.5-20 µg/kg/min CRI IV	Start at ~2.5 µg/kg/min and increase every 15-30 minutes to target systolic BP Tachycardia, premature complexes, seizures
Enalapril	1, 2.5, 5, 10 mg tablets	0.25-0.5 mg/kg q12h PO	Start at lower range and increase to maximal dose with monitoring of renal function and BP Acute renal failure, azotemia, hyperkalemia
Flecainide	50, 100, 100 mg	1-2 mg/kg q8 to 12h PO	Use with caution in CHF or DCM Proarrhythmia, VT, negative inotropy
Furosemide	Veterinary: 12.5 and 50 mg tablets Human generic: 20, 40, 80 mg tablets 1% furosemide syrup (10 mg/ml)	Acute CHF: 2 mg/kg IV; repeated in 30 min Acute CHF: 0.5-1 mg/kg/hour CRI IV CHF (stage C): 2-4 mg/kg q12h PO CHF (stage D): 3-4 mg/kg q8-12h PO	Dosage is increased in stepwise fashion in chronic CHF; use with ACE-inhibitor and spironolactone; restrict dietary sodium Polydipsia, polyuria, exacerbates incontinence Azotemia, renal failure, hypochloremia, hypokalemia, hypomagnesemia, hyponatremia
Hydralazine	10, 25, 50 mg tablets	Dosage range: 0.5-3 mg/kg q12h PO Initial dose: 0.5-1.0 mg/kg	Gradual up-titration required; monitor BP In CHF dogs initial dosage is lower In resistant hypertension higher dosages are used Hypotension, reflex tachycardia, anorexia

TABLE **175-1**

Drugs Used in the Treatment of Heart Failure and Arrhythmias in Dogs—cont'd

Drug	Preparations	Commonly Used Dosages	Comments/Adverse Effects
Hydrochlorothiazide	25, 50 mg tablets	1-4 mg/kg q12-24h PO Initial doses once daily or every other day	Used with furosemide/spironolactone Stage D CHF Start with low dose; recheck biochemical profile in 3 to 5 days Acute renal failure, profound electrolyte loss
Hydrocodone	5 mg tablets	0.25 mg/kg BID-QID	Adjust dosage as needed for cough; much higher dosages are tolerated chronically
Lidocaine	2% solution (20 mg/ml)	2 mg/kg IV bolus; may be repeated to 6 mg/kg over 10 min 25-75 µg/kg/min CRI IV	Used primarily to control ventricular ectopy; toxicity signs include anorexia, vomiting, tremors, seizures
Mexiletine	150, 200, 250 mg capsules	4-6 mg/kg q8h, PO	Can combine with sotalol or beta-blocker Anorexia, vomiting, tremors, seizures
Pimobendan	1.25, 5 mg chewable tablets, capsules	0.25-0.3 mg/kg q12h PO	Extralabel use TID in end-stage CHF Initial doses before feeding Minimal reported adverse effects
Procainamide	100 mg/ml, 10 ml vial 500 mg/ml, 2 ml vial Oral unavailable (can compound)	2-20 mg/kg, IV (see notes) 25-40 µg/kg/min CRI IV 10-20 mg/kg q4-6h, IM SC 10-20 mg/kg q8h PO (sustained release)	No acetylated metabolite (NAPA) in the dog IV: 2 mg/kg boluses every 2-3 minutes to a maximum of 20 mg/kg; monitor BP and ECG Depression of myocardial function, hypotension
Nitroglycerine 2% ointment	15 mg per inch (ointment) Transdermal patch 2.5, 5, 10 mg/24h	¼-¾ inch (~4-12 mg) q12h, cutaneously Giant breeds: 1 inch (15 mg) q12h, cutaneously	Delivered dose relates to surface area applied Rub off after 6 hours to allow nitrate-free interval Typically used for 24 to 48 hours in hospital Hypotension, headache?
Nitroprusside sodium	50 mg/2 ml vials Other generic formulations	0.5 to 5 µg/kg/min CRI IV	Dosed to achieve target systolic BP (see text) Read insert for dilution and delivery Light sensitive Hypotension, reflex tachycardia, cyanide toxicity
Sildenafil	25, 50, 100 mg tablets (proprietary) 20 mg tablets (generic) Compounded suspension	1-3 mg/kg q8-12h PO	Administer with L-arginine 250-500 mg q12h PO Start with lower end of dose; monitor BP Hypotension, abnormal behavior
Sotalol	80, 120, 240 mg tablets	1-2 mg/kg q12h PO	Potential for proarrhythmia Negative inotrope, can precipitate CHF AV block
Spironolactone	25, 50 mg tablets	1 mg/kg q12h PO or 2 mg/kg once daily PO	No significant diuretic effect Hyperkalemia
Torsemide	5, 10, 20 mg tablets	CHF (stage D): 0.25-0.4 mg/kg	See text for details; adverse effects per furosemide

AV, Atrioventricular; *BP,* systolic arterial blood pressure; *CHF,* congestive heart failure; *CRI,* constant rate infusion; *DCM,* dilated cardiomyopathy; *ECG,* electrocardiogram; *LVSF,* left ventricular systolic function; *PVCs,* premature ventricular complexes; *VT,* ventricular tachycardia.

benefit in canine HF when spironolactone is dosed at approximately 2 mg/kg daily PO. Based on the available tablet sizes, the daily dose can be administered in a single pill or divided into two daily doses. Some cardiologists also use this drug empirically for cardioprotection in cases of preclinical dilated cardiomyopathy (DCM) based on evidence from experimental models of myocardial disease.

When compared with humans, dogs appear to have minimal adverse effects from spironolactone. Breeders should be advised of potential effects on reproduction. Elevated serum potassium levels may be observed with spironolactone, especially in the setting of ACE inhibitor cotherapy, but this typically is mild and is ignored. Potassium supplements should not be given routinely to dogs receiving spironolactone unless hypokalemia is documented.

Hydrochlorothiazide

Hydrochlorothiazide (HCT) occasionally is used in combination with furosemide for the management of refractory stage D CHF, especially in dogs with intractable edema or effusions. This drug blocks the sodium-chloride symporter that is insensitive to loop diuretics, inhibiting sodium, chloride, and water reabsorption in the distal tubule and the connecting segment. Additionally, potassium and magnesium are lost in the urine. When used in combination with furosemide, HCT prevents some of the distal sodium reabsorption that escapes the effects of the loop diuretics (as part of a sequential nephron blockade). The usual dosage is 1 to 2 mg/kg once or twice daily PO, provided the drug is tolerated. To prevent rapid volume depletion and electrolyte disturbances, when HCT is added to furosemide, the authors recommend administering the drug once a day or every other day for the first week, starting at the lower end of the dosage range. Laboratory values should be checked within 7 days, or immediately if the dog becomes depressed or ill. If renal function and electrolyte levels remain stable, the frequency of dosing can be increased.

Adverse effects are similar to those described earlier for furosemide. When combination diuretic therapy is administered, profound azotemia, hypokalemia, hypochloremia, and hyponatremia can develop within a matter of days, regardless of cotreatment with spironolactone or an ACE inhibitor.

Angiotensin-Converting Enzyme Inhibitors and Other Vasodilators

Vasoconstriction is a feature of HF and is mediated by the interaction of calcium with myosin light-chain kinase within the smooth muscle cell. Calcium enters the cell by crossing L-type channels to release intracellular stores of calcium. Opening of the calcium channel is modulated by a number of receptors on the vascular smooth muscle, including the α-adrenergic receptor, the angiotensin II receptor, the endothelin receptor, and the vasopressin receptor, among others. Conversely, the generation of cyclic nucleotides by stimulation of vascular β_2-receptors, natriuretic peptide receptors, or muscarinic receptors leads to vasodilation by interfering with intracellular calcium dynamics.

The chronic activation of vasoconstricting systems observed in CHF is considered maladaptive, and ACE inhibitors are mainstays of CHF therapy. Additionally other vasodilator drugs may be useful in specific situations. For example, phosphodiesterase inhibitors such as pimobendan and sildenafil prevent the breakdown of cyclic adenosine monophosphate (cAMP) and cyclic guanosine monophosphate (cGMP), respectively, thereby potentiating the physiological vasodilator effect.

Drugs that induce venodilation can cause pooling of blood in systemic veins and reduce venous pressures and pulmonary congestion, while drugs that cause systemic arteriolar dilation lower arterial BP and potentially ventricular afterload. Mitral regurgitant volume usually is reduced by the lowering of diastolic BP; this is another potential benefit of ACE inhibitors and arterial vasodilators like sodium nitroprusside, amlodipine, pimobendan, and hydralazine.

Angiotensin-Converting Enzyme Inhibitors

The renin-angiotensin-aldosterone system (RAAS) is activated by the sympathetic nervous system, reduced renal perfusion, and impaired sodium delivery to the juxtaglomerular apparatus of the kidneys. The results of RAAS activation are direct vasoconstriction and augmented release of norepinephrine and vasopressin via central pathways; aldosterone release with resultant sodium and water retention; and activation of growth-promoting systems in tissues. The ACE inhibitors, including *benazepril, enalapril, imidapril, lisinopril, ramipril,* and *quinapril,* inhibit the RAAS by blocking the kininase (converting enzyme) that converts angiotensin I to the active peptide hormone angiotensin II. This leads to decreased plasma angiotensin II and as well as delayed degradation of vasodilating kinins, which have effects on both arteries and veins. The RAAS also can be blocked earlier in the pathway with renin inhibitors (e.g., aliskiren) or at the level of the angiotensin II receptor (e.g., losartan or valsartan); however, drugs in these classes have not been studied sufficiently in the treatment of canine CHF. Angiotensin II receptor blockers are currently under clinical investigation.

ACE inhibitors reduce serum aldosterone concentration and limit sodium retention and potassium loss in the urine. Additionally, ACE inhibitors protect cardiac muscle, renal tissues, and blood vessels from RAAS-induced injury while down-regulating the sympathetic nervous system. Vasodilation associated with ACE inhibition is not as dramatic as that observed with calcium channel blockers or intravenous nitrates so the overall effect on arterial BP is modest, especially in the treatment of dogs with systemic hypertension. The published dosage ranges for enalapril and benazepril vary considerably from as low as 0.25 mg/kg once or twice daily to as high as 0.5 mg/kg twice daily. The authors generally start with enalapril at approximately 0.25 mg/kg q12h PO and double the dosage to approximately 0.5 mg/kg q12h PO at the time of first reevaluation as long as arterial BP and renal function are acceptable (see Chapter 176).

The use of ACE inhibitors is considered a standard of care for management of established CHF in dogs caused by chronic valvular disease or DCM. They also are used more controversially for treatment of advanced, preclinical mitral valve disease and with greater acceptance for treatment of preclinical (occult) DCM. ACE inhibitors are appropriate treatments for dogs with systemic hypertension associated with chronic kidney disease, but as stated earlier, are less potent than amlodipine or the α-adrenergic blocker prazosin for control of moderate to severe hypertension.

The main *adverse effects* of ACE inhibitors and other vasodilator drugs are systemic hypotension (causing weakness or lethargy) and impairment of renal function. Glomerular filtration is augmented by angiotensin II constriction of the efferent arteriole of the glomerulus. Therefore the sudden blocking of the RAAS can induce acute renal failure by suddenly lowering pressure in the glomerular tuft, especially in dogs that have been volume depleted with furosemide. In most cases, this adverse effect is responsive to withdrawal of the ACE inhibitor, reduction of the diuretic dose, and judicious volume replacement with 0.45% saline with potassium chloride supplementation. Most of these dogs eventually can tolerate an ACE inhibitor, but slow up-titration of the dose is necessary once a stable diuretic dosage that controls CHF has been established. Hyperkalemia is a risk with all ACE inhibitors, especially when they are combined with spironolactone (but mild hyperkalemia is acceptable).

Other Vasodilators

A number of other vasodilator drugs are used for specific situations in canine HF. These include life-threatening pulmonary edema, systemic hypertension, and pulmonary hypertension. The vasodilators used most often in current veterinary practice are the ACE inhibitors, nitrovasodilators, amlodipine, and sildenafil. Pimobendan (discussed later) is an inodilator; that is, it is both an inotropic drug and a vasodilator.

Nitrovasodilators

Topically administered *2% nitroglycerine ointment* and intravenously administered *sodium nitroprusside* are hospital therapies used to treat life-threatening pulmonary edema. These drugs work by either increasing the formation of nitric oxide (NO) or stimulating formation of the second messenger of NO, cGMP, in arterioles and veins. Cyclic nucleotides inhibit the calcium-myosin light-chain kinase interaction in vascular smooth muscle, limiting vasoconstriction. Topically administered nitroglycerine is believed to dilate mainly systemic veins and venules, causing blood to pool away from the lungs. Sodium nitroprusside is a rapidly acting venous and arterial dilator, reduces pulmonary and systemic venous pressures, lowers systemic arterial BP, and effectively unloads the failing left ventricle. These drugs are used by the authors in conjunction with intravenous furosemide, inhaled oxygen, and butorphanol sedation when pulmonary edema is viewed as life threatening. Nitroglycerine ointment is simplest and safest to use but less potent. The decision to use sodium nitroprusside is made when a patient is unresponsive to simple diuresis, exhibits hemoptysis or expectorates frothy fluid, or has severe alveolar infiltrates on thoracic radiographs that create a "white-out" lung (Figure 175-1).

Clinical trial evidence demonstrating the efficacy of nitrates for managing CHF is lacking, but nitroglycerine ointment may be considered because of the simple delivery system and the potential benefits of pooling of blood away from the lungs. Many cardiologists view sodium nitroprusside as a lifesaving drug for dogs with fulminant pulmonary edema caused by mitral regurgitation with ruptured chordae tendineae. It also is a potential treatment for severe systemic hypertension in dogs, although it is rarely used for that purpose.

Dosages of these drugs are summarized in Table 175-1. Nitroglycerine usually is applied every 12 hours, but the ointment is wiped off approximately 6 hours after administration to provide a nitrate-free interval that allows for regeneration of NO responsiveness. Staff should wear gloves when applying the ointment and use the applicator paper for measuring and deciding on the area of coverage. Because the dose depends in part on the surface area over which the vehicle is applied, the often-used ear pinnae may not be an optimal site for dogs with cropped ears. Serial monitoring of arterial BP is essential when using nitroprusside; in fact, the infusion rate is determined by targeting a systolic BP of about 90 mm Hg and then maintaining that for 12 to 24 hours, until clinical signs are controlled. Sodium nitroprusside must be handled properly and protected from light (read the package insert). Metabolism leads to the release of cyanide,

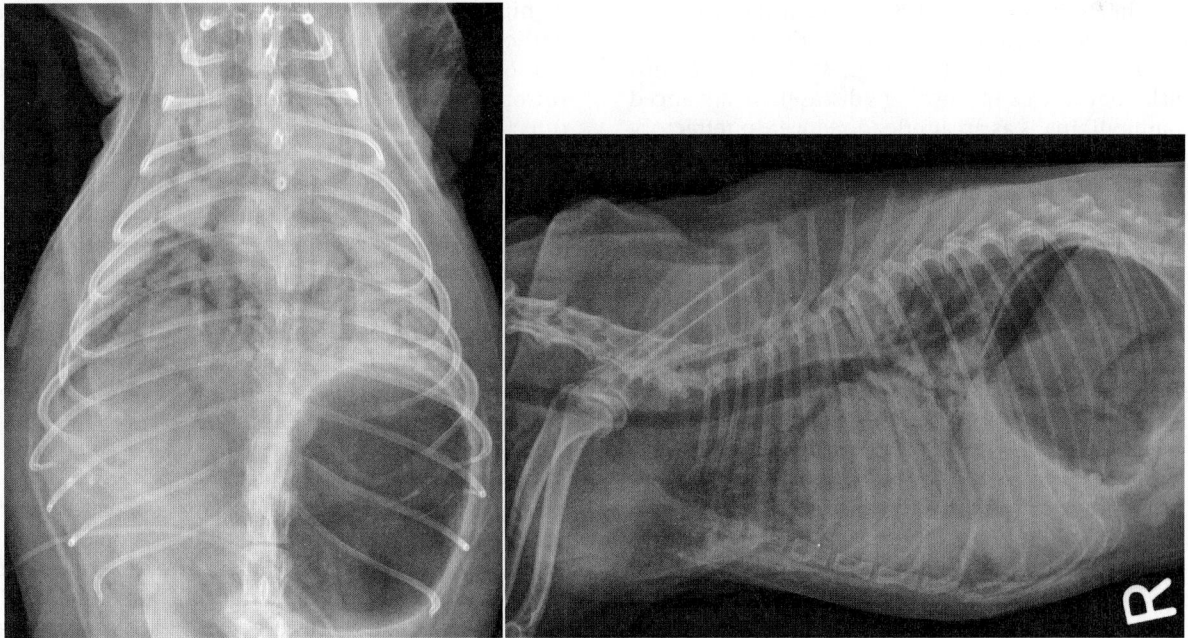

Figure 175-1 Severe alveolar pulmonary edema in a dog with ruptured mitral valve chordae tendineae. The infiltrates obscure the vascular structures and parts of the diaphragm and cardiac borders. There is marked aerophagia. The dog was successfully treated and released from the hospital.

which limits the use of nitroprusside to 24 hours or less in the authors' hospitals.

Hydralazine

Hydralazine is an orally administered compound with predominately arteriolar dilating effects. The mechanisms of action for hydralazine likely are multiple and are not completely understood but include the formation of NO with increases in cGMP within vascular smooth muscle. The clinical effect begins within 1 hour of dosing and reaches a peak in dogs within 3 hours (Gordon and Kittleson, 2008). Hydralazine reduces ventricular afterload and decreases mitral regurgitant volume, but it is not as rapid in onset, or as easy to control, as an infusion of sodium nitroprusside. It is no longer prescribed for long-term therapy and is used infrequently in the intensive care unit; however, some clinicians still find it a useful drug when treating severe left-sided CHF.

Amlodipine

The dihydropyridine calcium channel blockers, typified by amlodipine besylate in veterinary medicine, impede calcium entry across the L-type calcium channels in vascular smooth muscle. The resulting arterial vasodilation reduces systemic vascular resistance, decreases arterial BP, and presumably lowers left ventricular afterload. The effects of amlodipine on pulmonary arterioles are weaker and its use in pulmonary hypertension usually is limited by the development of systemic hypotension. The drug is very well absorbed from the gastrointestinal tract, protein binding is high, and elimination is by hepatic mechanisms. The elimination half-life is relatively long (about 30 hours in healthy dogs).

Because of its vascular selectivity, amlodipine is used mainly for control of *systemic hypertension,* often in combination with an ACE inhibitor. Because high BP impairs left-sided heart function in HF, the identification and control of hypertension is an important management point, especially for patients at highest risk (those with chronic kidney disease or Cushing's disease). An advanced use for amlodipine is as an afterload reducer in refractory (stage D) left-sided CHF. Lowering BP should improve forward stroke volume from the ventricle, especially in the setting of severe mitral regurgitation. Unlike diltiazem, amlodipine causes little direct depression of the sinus node or cardiac muscle, but reflex changes mediated by baroreceptors and the sympathetic nervous system may be observed if BP is sufficiently lowered.

The initial dosage of amlodipine for CHF patients is 0.05 to 0.1 mg/kg q12-24h PO; however, higher dosages (usually 0.2 to 0.4 mg/kg q12-24h PO) are needed to treat dogs with severe systemic hypertension. Accordingly, when amlodipine is used in the setting of CHF, the dose is up-titrated gradually with monitoring of BP and observation for clinical signs of hypotension. Again, with a long elimination half-life, it may take 3 to 7 days before dosage changes are fully evident.

Sildenafil

The phosphodiesterase 5 inhibitors such as sildenafil (Viagra, Revatio) and related compounds like tadalafil (Cialis) are reserved for treatment of severe, symptomatic *pulmonary hypertension.* These drugs demonstrate relatively selective pulmonary arterial vasodilation by preventing the degradation of the cGMP in pulmonary arteries and thereby lowering resistance to blood flow. There is considerable experience with its extralabel use in dogs for management of precapillary pulmonary hypertension (see Chapter 167), but no clinical trial data. Retrospective reports and clinical experience indicate that some dogs show significant response to sildenafil with a reduction in the number of collapsing episodes or syncopal attacks along with improved exercise capacity. Peak effect likely occurs within 2 to 3 hours after oral administration, and sildenafil optimally is administered three times daily to dogs. Because of increased pulmonary blood flow, pulmonary artery pressures may not change significantly. In cases of pulmonary hypertension associated with left-sided CHF, standard HF therapy should be administered first because lowering left atrial pressure will improve (postcapillary) pulmonary hypertension.

Long-term administration of sildenafil involves uptitration of the initial dosage (typically 1 to 2 mg/kg q12h PO) to up to 3 mg/kg q8-12h PO). The drug probably is metabolized by the canine liver, and other drugs with hepatic metabolism might interfere with sildenafil transformation.

Adverse Effects of Vasodilators

As for ACE inhibitors, the major adverse effects of vasodilators relate to a decrease in arterial BP. If systolic BP falls below 80 to 85 mm Hg the risk of depression, excessive sleeping, weakness, exertional collapse, or syncope is higher. Unlike ACE inhibitors, most vasodilators do not preferentially impact renal hemodynamics, but renal failure is still a potential concern. Particular caution must be exercised with sodium nitroprusside because this drug is highly potent and can induce severe hypotension without consistent and diligent monitoring of BP. The risk of cyanide toxicosis increases with the duration of nitroprusside treatment. The decrease in BP caused by direct vasodilators, including nitroprusside, amlodipine, and hydralazine, can induce reflex sympathetic and RAAS activation with sodium retention and potentially sinus tachycardia (especially nitroprusside and hydralazine). Sildenafil use has been associated with nonspecific signs including abnormal behavior within a few hours of administration (note that central nervous system and visual side effects are observed in people), but it is difficult to determine cause and effect without controlled clinical trials.

Inotropic Drugs

The positive inotropic drugs include catecholamines (dobutamine, dopamine), the glycoside digoxin, and the inodilators pimobendan, levosimendan, and milrinone. These drugs work by increasing the availability of calcium to the cardiomyocyte or by making the contractile apparatus more sensitive to cytosolic calcium. The result is an increase in ventricular stroke volume for any given level of cardiac filling and afterload. Atrial contractile function also may be enhanced. Indirect effects of these drugs can be important; for example, digoxin stimulates barorecep-tor activity and has neurotropic effects. Inodilators exhibit significant vasodilator effects in dogs, and dobutamine exerts dose-dependent effects on vascular tone.

Increasing contractile force is not always a positive. Positive inotropy can exert a negative effect on myocardial energetics (increasing oxygen demand); this often is observed with catecholamines. Inotropic drugs that increase calcium influx can impair relaxation if calcium uptake into the sarcoplasmic reticulum is not accelerated at the same time; this effect has been demonstrated in failing myocardium with digoxin. More importantly, increases in cytosolic calcium level often are associated with a less stable transmembrane electrical potential, afterdepolarizations, and subsequent ventricular ectopy.

Catecholamines

Catecholamines are used only in the hospital setting and are administered intravenously by constant-rate infusion. Dobutamine is a synthetic catecholamine with strong β_1-adrenergic and weaker β_2- and α_1-adrenergic effects. Contractility is enhanced by stimulation of the predominant β_1-receptors located within the myocardium; these generate higher intracellular concentrations of cAMP and increase opening of the L-type calcium channels. Heart rate increases at higher infusion rates. In healthy dogs myocardial lusitropy (relaxation) also is enhanced. The net effect of dobutamine is an increase in arterial BP caused mainly by increased cardiac output. The vascular effects are dose dependent. Within the dosage range typically used in dogs (see Table 175-1), dobutamine probably changes from being a weak vasodilator, to exerting a balanced vascular effect, to causing predominately vasoconstriction. For this reason it usually is preferred to dopamine or norepinephrine for treatment of cardiogenic shock because it is less likely to cause sinus tachycardia or profound vasoconstriction (see Chapter 3). Dobutamine is not difficult to monitor in the critical care setting. It typically increases stroke volume (as measured noninvasively by Doppler echocardiographic methods), increases arterial BP and the strength of the pulse, raises rectal temperature, and improves other indicators of tissue perfusion such as capillary refill time and mentation.

Accordingly, dobutamine—along with oxygen supplementation and furosemide treatment for pulmonary edema—is the initial inotrope of choice for stabilizing cardiogenic shock (defined here as a dog with CHF accompanied by a systolic BP of <80 mm Hg with hypothermia, impaired peripheral perfusion, and elevated blood lactate). Volume infusions should be avoided in patients with CHF; instead, the goal is an increase in cardiac output to fill the arterial tree more effectively.

Dobutamine is administered as a constant-rate infusion starting at 2.5 µg/kg/min and increasing by 1 to 2 µg/kg/min about every 30 minutes until systolic BP is 90 mm Hg. This end point generally is reached at an infusion of 5 to 10 µg/kg/min, although higher infusion rates may be needed. Once the systolic BP is stable (90 to 100 mm Hg), other drugs can be added. If the patient can swallow, pimobendan should be started as soon as the BP starts to increase. Pimobendan is a potent inotropic drug

but also a vasodilator, and in the authors' experience is not as effective as dobutamine for initial stabilization of cardiogenic shock caused by DCM. Additionally, the patient in stable condition can receive a nitrate, sodium nitroprusside, or an ACE inhibitor to unload the left ventricle depending on the degree of congestion and response to furosemide and oxygen. Heart rate should be monitored and increases above 140 beats/min avoided if possible. The presence of ventricular or atrial premature complexes indicates possible catecholamine toxicity, and the infusion rate should be lowered. An attempt usually is made to wean a patient in stable condition off dobutamine after 24 hours of therapy, but infusions may be needed for as long as 48 hours before this can be accomplished (with acceptance that further down-regulation of β-receptors is likely). The dobutamine infusion rate is reduced by 50% every 2 to 4 hours, and once the dosage has been lowered to approximately 2 µg/kg/min the infusion is discontinued. By that time the dog should be taking oral drugs for CHF, including pimobendan.

Pimobendan

Pimobendan (Vetmedin), a benzimidazole pyridazinone, is a potent, orally administered inotropic drug with arterial and venous vasodilator properties. It is classified as a calcium sensitizer with phosphodiesterase 3 (and possibly phosphodiesterase 5) inhibitory properties. The inotropic effect is attributed mostly to calcium sensitization as opposed to phosphodiesterase 3 activity, but myocardial relaxation might be enhanced by the phosphodiesterase effect. The drug is well absorbed, although the label indicates it should be given 1 hour before eating, especially at the onset of therapy. Effects usually are evident within 1 to 3 hours of dosing, and the duration of action is 8 to 12 hours. The drug is administered twice daily by mouth but can be dosed three times daily (in an extralabel manner) for dogs in stage D failure.

Pimobendan is useful for treatment of both acute and chronic HF in dogs. It can be initiated in hospital along with parenteral furosemide, oxygen, and a nitrate for acute treatment of CHF. When used long term pimobendan is combined with oral furosemide, an ACE inhibitor, and spironolactone; this four-drug therapy represents the current standard of care for management of canine CHF. Another potential indication is prevention of CHF in Doberman pinschers with well-defined preclinical DCM (as studied in the Pimobendan Randomized Occult DCM Trial to Evaluate Clinical Symptoms and Time to Heart Failure [PROTECT]; see Chapter 176). However, at this time clinicians should be cautious about generalizing the results of PROTECT to other breeds of dogs with preclinical DCM (a cardiologist should be consulted). The value of this drug in the treatment of advanced preclinical mitral valve disease is under study (Evaluating Pimobendan In Cardiomegaly [EPIC] trial), and at the time of this writing pimobendan is *not* recommended for small-breed dogs that have not developed CHF. Most cardiologists find pimobendan very effective in the treatment of low cardiac output or CHF associated with severe pulmonary hypertension, although the drug is not labeled for these uses. In dogs with atrial fibrillation pimobendan should be used in conjunction with digoxin (or another rate-control drug) because pimobendan does not slow atrio-ventricular (AV) node conduction.

Contraindications may include hypertrophic cardio-myopathy or disorders characterized by dynamic ventricular outflow obstruction. Adverse effects seemingly are uncommon with this drug, with rare cases of hypotension and gastrointestinal upset reported. Thus far pimobendan does not appear to aggravate ventricular arrhythmias, but vigilance still is advised considering the low number of dogs with ventricular ectopy studied in the clinical trials.

Digoxin

Digoxin has been used for hundreds of years to treat CHF and can be characterized as a weak to moderate positive inotrope that also slows heart rate by sensitizing baroreceptor function to alter autonomic tone to the cardiovascular system. The mechanism of inotropic action involves inhibition of the sodium-potassium pump, which increases intracellular sodium and activates a sodium-calcium exchanger; this in turn increases cytosolic calcium concentration. Baroreceptor function has been shown to be impaired in experimental canine HF, and digoxin partially corrects this insensitivity, leading to a baroreceptor-like response of increased vagal tone with withdrawal of sympathetic activity. Thus ventricular stroke volume increases and resting heart rate decreases under the influence of cardiac glycosides. In atrial fibrillation increased vagal tone slows AV node conduction and the resultant ventricular rate response to atrial fibrillation, especially at rest. These autonomic effects may help to suppress isolated atrial premature complexes, but conversely, enhanced vagal tone can predispose to atrial fibrillation. Comparatively speaking, the inotropic response to digoxin is far less than that achieved with catecholamines or pimobendan, and the AV node–blocking properties unfortunately become most evident at near-toxic blood levels.

The main indications for digoxin today are refractory CHF (stage D), CHF with *atrial fibrillation,* and CHF that cannot be treated with pimobendan (due to drug cost). There are no clinical trials demonstrating efficacy. Contraindications to its use include complex ventricular arrhythmias, bradyarrhythmia (sinus node dysfunction, AV block), and moderate to severe renal dysfunction because digoxin is eliminated by the kidneys. The oral tablet formulation is used most often, but there also is an alcohol-based elixir that has slightly greater bioavailability. There is some protein binding, but it probably is not clinically important in most cases. The elimination half-life is variable and highly dependent on glomerular filtration rate; an interval of 24 hours is a useful value to remember, which means that it will take about 3.5 to 5 days to achieve near steady-state blood levels. Elimination is affected by a number of drugs, and considering the infrequent use of digoxin today, the clinician is advised to consult a reference book to identify any noncardiac drug interactions. Targets for therapeutic concentrations used to be higher (1 to 2.5 ng/ml), but most cardiologists now aim for a trough level of 0.8 to 1.2 ng/ml to avoid

adverse effects, although higher serum concentrations may be tolerated. Values of more than 2.0 ng/ml at trough (8 to 12 hours after treatment) are more likely to cause anorexia or other adverse effects.

Central nervous system effects of digoxin likely account for the toxic signs of anorexia and vomiting. Other signs of toxicosis are depression, diarrhea, and cardiac arrhythmias (sinus node depression, AV node block, junctional tachycardia, premature ventricular complexes). These are best prevented by avoiding loading doses, starting treatment at the lower end of the dosing range (see Table 175-1), and monitoring serum digoxin concentrations.

Other Drugs Used in the Management of Canine Heart Failure

There are a number of other drugs that are potentially beneficial in the management of CHF. These include β-adrenergic blockers, antiarrhythmic drugs, oxygen (see Chapter 10), and drugs that treat concurrent respiratory disease such as cough suppressants and airway dilators (see Chapter 160).

β-Adrenergic Blockers

The pharmacologic effects of β-adrenergic blockade can be understood as reversal of the physiologic effects of β-stimulation. The sympathetic nervous system, acting on the β-receptor, increases (1) sinus node discharge rate (chronotropy), (2) speed of current conduction across the myocardium and conduction system (dromotropy), (3) myocardial contractility (inotropy), (4) rate of myocardial relaxation (lusitropy), and (5) excitability of subsidiary cardiac pacemakers (bathmotropy). Myocardial oxygen demand is increased by β-stimulation, and the diastolic time available for coronary artery and ventricular filling is abbreviated. The deleterious effects of long-term activation of sympathetic nervous activity on heart muscle (necrosis, apoptosis, fibrosis) also are relevant in patients with HF. The *β-blockers inhibit all of these effects.* The pharmacology of these drugs is diverse and beyond the scope of this chapter given the relative paucity of data regarding their efficacy in spontaneous canine HF. Of importance is selectivity (cardiac-selective β_1-blockade or nonselective β_1- and β_2-blockade); drug elimination (hepatic for most; renal for atenolol and sotalol; plasma esterases for esmolol); formulation (e.g., long-acting metoprolol); and additional properties of the so-called third-generation β-blockers (such as α-blocking and antioxidant properties for carvedilol).

The β-blockers carvedilol, metoprolol (long acting), bisoprolol, and atenolol sometimes are prescribed by veterinary cardiologists to protect the heart muscle in dogs with HF. The hope is that with long-term use, myocardium at risk will be protected from neurohormonal assault and demand ischemia; heart rate will be controlled; left ventricular ejection fraction will improve (as observed in human patients); and fatal cardiac arrhythmias will be suppressed. In studies in canine models, β-blockers are cardioprotective, but *this effect has not been proven* in clinical studies of dogs with DCM or chronic mitral regurgitation. This is a major difference from the situation in human patients, and the reasons for this discrepancy are unresolved. Thus, although dogs with preclinical HF usually tolerate β-blockade, the use of these drugs is empiric, and β-blockers *are not yet considered a standard of care* for management of chronic HF in dogs.

To be specific about the recommendations, the authors do not use β-blockers in the treatment of small-breed dogs with mitral valve disease except in some cases in which heart rhythm control is needed (see later). The authors do consider, on a case-by-case basis, introduction of a β-blocker (carvedilol, atenolol, or metoprolol) in dogs with clear evidence of impaired left ventricular systolic function on echocardiography, especially those with preclinical disease (i.e., not in CHF). The recommendation for those uncertain about using these drugs is to consult with a cardiologist before any treatment is started. β-Blockers *never should be used in uncontrolled CHF,* and *gradual up-titration of dose* is most appropriate when these drugs are prescribed to dogs with systolic ventricular dysfunction or following stabilization of CHF. Concurrent use of pimobendan seems to offset some of the negative inotropic effects of β-blockers in dogs with HF. Anticipated adverse effects of these drugs include weakness, hypotension, bradycardia, and worsening of edema or effusions.

Antiarrhythmic Drugs

The management of heart rhythm disturbances in dogs is discussed in more detail in Chapters 170, 171, 172, and 179, and in Web Chapters 59 and 60. The following comments are confined largely to the treatment of arrhythmias in dogs with CHF.

The most important arrhythmia to treat in CHF is atrial fibrillation. The authors generally aim for heart rate control because in their experience conversion to sinus rhythm is not sustained in most dogs with CHF, and the anesthetic risk associated with cardioversion is not negligible. The AV node can be partially blocked with the combination of digoxin (previously discussed) and the calcium channel blocker diltiazem. Some cardiologists use β-blockers to further decrease the ventricular rate response in dogs with atrial fibrillation. Carvedilol, low doses of atenolol, or other β-blockers may have a beneficial effect on the rate control.

Treatment of severe ventricular arrhythmias (complex premature ventricular complexes, ventricular tachycardia) in the setting of CHF is difficult because most drugs depress ventricular function and represent yet another pill for clients to administer. There also are adverse effects associated with most of these drugs. Some clients actually prefer that their dogs experience a sudden death rather than face the difficult spiral of worsening CHF and repeated considerations of euthanasia. Obviously clients should be carefully educated about the pros and cons of ventricular antiarrhythmic therapy. Many cardiologists do not try to suppress occasional premature ventricular complexes in the setting of CHF, even if they are multiform or distributed as couplets. Monomorphic ventricular tachycardia also may be left untreated if the heart rate is not too fast (<200 beats/min), the runs are brief, and there are no clinical signs such as collapse or syncope. The drugs that are used to manage ventricular arrhythmias are summarized in the following sections.

Class I Antiarrhythmic Drugs

The Vaughan Williams classification lists procainamide (class IA), lidocaine and mexiletine (class IB), and flecainide (class IC) as sodium channel blockers with other pharmacologic and electrophysiologic characteristics. *Procainamide* currently is unavailable as an oral drug except through compounding pharmacies. It is used to control ventricular tachycardia. Injectable forms are available for in-hospital use. Procainamide depresses heart function and BP. *Lidocaine* is used in hospital to control canine ventricular arrhythmias that are rapid or have a dangerous morphology. It is useful for short-term treatment and importantly does not depress heart function or heart rate significantly. A related compound for oral use, *mexiletine,* may be effective for long-term use if adverse effects are not an issue and the client can tolerate three-times-daily dosing. Elimination is hepatic, and metabolites may be active. Adverse effects of both drugs include anorexia, vomiting, tremors, and seizures.

The sodium channel blocker *flecainide* has not been studied sufficiently in dogs but can be administered at an initial dosage of 1 to 2 mg/kg q8-12h PO for ventricular arrhythmias. Unfortunately, it is more likely to be proarrhythmic in the setting of ventricular failure, and this limits or contraindicates its use in dogs with CHF until more data are obtained.

Class II Antiarrhythmic Drugs

Class II antiarrhythmic drugs are the β-blockers described previously. Additionally, the ultra-short-acting drug esmolol is available for intravenous use. However, esmolol is a significant negative inotrope and has limited applicability for arrhythmia treatment in the setting of CHF. The class III antiarrhythmic drug sotalol also has β-blocking properties (see later). β-Blockers work mainly by impairing calcium entry into cardiac cells and reducing the afterpotentials that can lead to premature complexes. AV node conduction and sinus node discharge rates also are depressed by β-blockade so that heart rate response in atrial fibrillation is reduced and resting and exercise heart rates are blunted. Depression of contractility is the major concern and limitation of this group of drugs.

Class III Antiarrhythmic Drugs

Class III antiarrhythmic drugs are potassium channel blockers that delay repolarization of heart muscle cells. *Sotalol* (1 to 2 mg/kg q12h PO) often is effective and is well tolerated except for its β-blocking properties, which can depress myocardial contractility and cardiac output. This drug is best avoided until CHF has been stabilized. It then can be used cautiously at the lower dosage. Combined therapy with mexiletine also is possible, but client compliance and enthusiasm for more pills may be low.

Amiodarone is a complex drug that sometimes is used for rhythm control after electrical or drug-induced cardioversion of atrial fibrillation. It also can be used for suppression of malignant ventricular arrhythmias and may be highly effective (dosage is 8 to 10 mg/kg once daily

PO for 2 weeks [some clinicians use it twice daily during the loading period], then 4 to 6 mg/kg once daily PO). However, owing to liver toxicity, liver enzyme levels and liver function (as well as thyroid function and complete blood count) must be followed. Dogs who become ill from amiodarone may take days to recover owing to the very long elimination half-life. However, considering the limited life span of many dogs with CHF and malignant arrhythmias, and the potential for once-daily dosing with this drug, amiodarone may be acceptable to some clinicians and clients for dogs with truly life-threatening ventricular tachycardia.

Class IV Antiarrhythmic Drugs

Class IV antiarrhythmic drugs are represented by *diltiazem,* a calcium channel blocker with widespread effects on specialized heart cells, cardiomyocytes, and vascular smooth muscle. Physiologically, calcium is responsible for sinoatrial node and AV node cell depolarizations, for contraction of cardiac muscle, and for contraction of vascular smooth muscle. In muscle cells calcium ions enter the long-lasting (L-type) channel to trigger further release from the sarcoplasmic reticulum. Calcium entry and its related effects are blocked by diltiazem (and verapamil). Although diltiazem directly depresses heart rate, reflex sympathetic activation from vasodilation and lowered BP

can maintain sinus node discharge. Direct effects on the AV node cells are leveraged for controlling heart rate in atrial fibrillation. The dosage usually is up-titrated quickly (starting at ~0.5 mg/kg PO and increased every 8 to 12 hours to as high as 2.5 mg/kg q8h PO for standard diltiazem; an alternative is long-acting diltiazem at a dosage of 0.5 to 3.5 mg/kg q12h). Hypotension and bradycardia are adverse effects of overdosage and are related to cardiac depression and vasodilation. The ultimate dose depends on response, with target in-hospital heart rates of less than 180 beats/min (optimally 120 to 140 beats/min) in atrial fibrillation. Ambulatory electrocardiographic (Holter) monitoring can be done to assess daily rate control objectively, aiming for an average ventricular rate of about 90 to 100/minute.

References and Suggested Reading

Brunton L, Chabner BA, Knollmann BC, editors: *Goodman and Gilman's the pharmacological basis of therapeutics,* ed 12, New York, 2010, McGraw-Hill, Section III: Modulation of cardiovascular function.

Gordon SG, Kittleson MD: Drugs used in the management of heart disease and cardiac arrhythmias. In Maddison JE, Page SW, Church DB, editors: *Small animal clinical pharmacology,* ed 2, St Louis, 2008, Saunders, p 380.

Opie LH, Gersh BJ: *Drugs for the heart,* ed 8, St Louis, 2013, Saunders.

CHAPTER 176

Management of Heart Failure in Dogs

BRUCE W. KEENE, *Raleigh, North Carolina*
JOHN D. BONAGURA, *Columbus, Ohio*

Heart failure (HF) is very common in dogs, and this section of *Current Veterinary Therapy* (and the accompanying digital version) offers a detailed consideration of the different congenital and acquired heart diseases responsible for this clinical syndrome. This chapter focuses on canine HF, beginning with an overview, describing methods for staging the severity of heart disease, and then discussing the authors' specific approaches for management of patients with chronic HF. The chapter concludes with a consideration of some special but relevant issues related to HF: namely, an approach to management of respiratory signs in dogs with heart disease, initial hospital treatment of acute congestive heart failure (CHF) and cardiogenic shock, and the

treatment of heart rhythm disturbances in the setting of HF.

Overview of Heart Failure

The term *heart failure* describes the situation in which the heart, despite normal to increased venous pressures, cannot maintain a cardiac output or arterial blood pressure (BP) sufficient to satisfy the perfusion demands of the tissues. From a pathophysiologic perspective the initial event in the syndrome of HF is arterial underfilling, triggered by systolic or diastolic dysfunction of the heart. Initially, inadequate tissue perfusion is apparent only during exercise; therefore early signs of HF may be subtle or go unrecognized. However, eventually venous pressures increase to support or augment cardiac filling. This situation contrasts sharply with most cases of shock, in which a reduced cardiac output is due mostly to decreased venous pressures and reduced cardiac filling. The elevated venous pressures associated with a failing heart increase capillary hydrostatic pressure and lead to more obvious clinical signs of CHF.

Physiologic control systems coordinate an array of vascular, neurologic, and endocrine responses involving the heart, blood vessels, kidney, lung, and central nervous system. These systems maintain blood volume, arterial and venous pressures, heart rate, cardiac output, and ventilation at levels sufficient to meet metabolic needs at rest, with exercise, and during other times of stress. HF triggers a cascade of these compensatory events, all focused on refilling the arterial tree and restoring BP toward normal. These physiologic controls predominately activate vasoconstrictor and sodium-retaining systems, attenuate vasodilator and natriuretic systems, and stimulate tissue mediators of inflammation. Prominent features of these compensations include (1) arterial and venous constriction mediated by the sympathetic, renin-angiotensin, vasopressin, and vascular endothelial systems; (2) redistribution of blood flow away from the skin, gut, kidneys, and skeletal muscle; (3) sodium and water retention mediated by altered renal blood flow; release of norepinephrine, aldosterone, and vasopressin; and inhibition of natriuretic hormones; (4) activation of inflammatory and growth-promoting systems that include fetal gene programs in the cardiac muscle cells and apoptosis.

If the cause of decreased cardiac output and arterial BP is rapidly reversible, activation of these systems is transient, and no permanent harm is apparent. However, when continually activated to support cardiac output and arterial BP, these compensations become maladaptive, persisting at the expense of structural and functional damage to blood vessels and cardiac muscle (hypertrophy, interstitial remodeling, and fibrosis), renal function, and skeletal muscle. These compensations also support the circulation, which makes many heart diseases difficult to diagnose until they have caused extensive cardiac remodeling and damage. However, the progression of heart disease and pump dysfunction triggers a spiral of increasing dependence on neurohormonal activity to maintain normal arterial BP and flow and eventually may lead to overt CHF. This is the stage most often managed by practicing veterinarians.

Clinical signs of CHF traditionally were classified as "forward" or "backward." So-called *forward HF* produces signs of low cardiac output and inadequate tissue perfusion that include weakness, lethargy, and prerenal azotemia. *Backward HF* identifies the inability of the heart to drain blood from the venous system. The resultant increases in venous pressures induce lung or tissue congestion or the development of body cavity effusions and also may impair renal and abdominal organ function. Clinical signs include tachypnea, dyspnea, and cough from pulmonary edema or pleural effusion. Additionally, jugular venous distention, hepatomegaly, and ascites are observed when the right side of the heart has failed. Metabolic disturbances in HF include weight loss, especially of muscle mass (cardiac cachexia), azotemia, and possibly insulin resistance. Although hemodynamic changes may explain the acutely life-threatening clinical signs of HF, morbidity and mortality in patients with chronic HF appear to be related strongly to the tissue effects of the accentuated neurohormonal and cytokine-mediated compensations that develop in response to the reduced output of the failing heart.

Most causes of canine HF cannot be reversed with the exceptions of pericardial effusions, some congenital heart defects, and sustained cardiac arrhythmias. Accordingly, drug therapy represents the major therapeutic method for treating HF in dogs. The treatment of acute HF is focused on identifying and correcting life-threatening hemodynamic derangements. The long-term treatment of HF is aimed at maintaining hemodynamic gains while modulating and blunting the maladaptive compensatory responses to protect tissues and prolong life while minimizing clinical signs.

Classifications of Heart Disease and Heart Failure

HF is not a specific disease but a clinical syndrome, precipitated by a definable cardiac lesion and characterized by hemodynamic, renal, neurohormonal, and proinflammatory abnormalities. Causes of heart disease can be classified anatomically, morphologically, etiologically, and by predominant pathophysiologic disturbances. Although these classifications are not always necessary, they do focus the clinician on the correct diagnosis and inform the prognosis and therapy. Additionally, the functional status of the *patient,* relative to the heart disease, helps to organize the optimal management approach (see the following section on functional classifications).

The *anatomic location* and *morphology* of the lesions that characterize the heart disease should be identified before a diagnosis of HF is accepted. The abnormalities can include structural heart lesions such as a thickened mitral valve as well as secondary responses evident in the cardiac chambers such as atrial or ventricular dilatation and hypertrophy. Anatomic and morphologic lesions, which often are verified in patients by echocardiography, can be classified simply by location and pathologic features.

For example, heart diseases can be described as *pericardial* diseases (idiopathic pericardial hemorrhage, pericarditis, and hemopericardium associated with hemangiosarcoma, chemodectoma, and mesothelioma), *myocardial* diseases (dilated cardiomyopathy [DCM], right ventricular cardiomyopathy, myocarditis), *valvular* diseases (congenital malformations, degenerative disease, infective endocarditis), intracardiac or extracardiac *shunts* (atrial septal defect, ventricular septal defect, patent ductus arteriosus), and *vascular* diseases (systemic hypertension, pulmonary hypertension, heartworm disease).

The *cause* of cardiac disease may be obvious or uncertain, and without doubt some disorders are primary or idiopathic; however, the underlying cause often can be identified. Etiologic categories include malformations, degeneration, metabolic and endocrine disorders, nutritional diseases, infections, immune-mediated diseases, ischemia, inherited/genetic diseases, tumors, trauma, and toxins.

Pathophysiologic disturbances of heart function usually are identified in patients with cardiac failure. These include *valvular regurgitation* (mitral and tricuspid valvular regurgitation), *valvular stenosis* (subaortic or pulmonic stenosis), intracardiac or extracardiac *shunting*, and heart *rhythm disturbances* (e.g., atrial fibrillation and ventricular tachycardia). Additionally, the basic mechanism by which the ventricle fails can be labeled as *systolic HF* or *diastolic HF*, although both abnormalities often are present to varying degrees. *Systolic dysfunction* indicates ineffective cardiac contraction because of myocardial or valvular dysfunction. Typical examples are DCM and chronic mitral regurgitation (MR). *Diastolic dysfunction* means that the heart cannot fill unless atrial or venous pressures are increased and suggests impaired myocardial relaxation, increased ventricular chamber stiffness, or both conditions. Examples include concentric hypertrophy associated with aortic stenosis or untreated systemic hypertension. Additionally, pericardial diseases compress or constrain the ventricles, also leading to diastolic HF. Finally, cardiac arrhythmias usually compromise both filling and pumping of the heart.

The clinician often classifies CHF as right-sided, left-sided, or biventricular. In some cases, right-sided CHF is a consequence of the pulmonary hypertension caused by severe left-sided heart disease. Most patients with HF experience clinical signs related to limited cardiac output, such as reduced exercise capacity. With *left-sided CHF* respiratory signs tend to dominate the clinical picture related to pulmonary congestion, with or without pleural effusion. *Right-sided CHF* in dogs is characterized by ascites (with or without pleural effusion). *Biventricular CHF* is most common in cases of left-sided heart disease complicated by either pulmonary hypertension or atrial fibrillation. Some dogs with DCM also have signs of biventricular HF. Finally, a small subset of dogs exhibit clinical signs of both forward and backward HF along with profound hypotension and biochemical markers of hypoperfusion (e.g., lactic acidosis). These cases are classified as *cardiogenic shock*.

These diagnostic categorizations are reviewed because the clinician's first step in treating cardiac failure involves identifying the underlying cardiac lesion(s) and the "heart disease" responsible for CHF. Therapy is predicated on these anatomic, morphologic, etiologic, and functional diagnoses. In the authors' experience, the most common mistake made when treating HF in practice is the use of "appropriate" HF therapy in a dog with clinical signs attributable to primary airway or lung disease. This error can be avoided by remembering that HF is not a disease but a consequence of a cardiac disorder that requires appropriate delineation.

Functional Classifications

The clinical signs of CHF are similar regardless of the underlying cardiac disease. Similarly, classification systems that grade the severity of HF or stage patients with heart disease are largely independent of anatomic or etiologic diagnoses.

A number of functional classifications of heart disease and heart failure have been applied to animals. These include the symptom-based classifications of the New York Heart Association (NYHA) and modifications of the scheme originally proposed by the International Small Animal Cardiac Health Council (ISACHC). The newer American College of Cardiology (ACC)/American Heart Association (AHA) classification scheme has been modified recently for dogs by an American College of Veterinary Internal Medicine (ACVIM) consensus panel. Each system provides a framework for discussing the clinical signs in patients with HF and a semiquantitative method for comparing these signs and, to some extent, estimating the need for various therapies.

Classifications Based on Clinical Signs
The first two systems assume that heart disease is *present* and that any functional impairment can be summarized as follows:

- **NYHA/ISACHC class I:** No clinical signs are evident at exercise or at rest.
  Notes: The modified ISACHC system subcategories include class IA (heart disease without cardiomegaly) and ISACHC class IB (heart disease with associated cardiomegaly).
- **NYHA/ISACHC class II:** There is mild functional limitation with clinical signs or limitations evident only with exercise or activity. There are no clinical signs at rest.
- **NYHA class III:** There is moderate functional impairment with clinical signs developing with mild exercise. The patient is comfortable only at rest.
  Note: There is no specific ISACHC classification comparable to NYHA class III.
- **NYHA class IV/ISACHC class III:** Severe functional limitations with clinical signs that are evident during exercise and at rest.
  Notes: ISACHC subclass IIIA indicates that home therapy for HF is possible; ISACHC subclass IIIB indicates that hospitalization is needed.

Although some animals with heart disease follow an orderly progression through functional classes, both the NYHA and ISACHC schemes allow an animal to move freely in both directions, for example, from class I to IV (or IIIB) following a dietary salt load, ruptured chordae tendineae, or hemodynamically significant arrhythmia, and then back from class IV to class II following successful medical management of CHF.

Modified ACC/AHA Classification
As an improvement on the clinical signs–based systems, the ACC and the AHA developed a staging system that emphasizes the progressive nature of most underlying diseases. This scheme was adapted for canine use in the report of the ACVIM consensus panel on the diagnosis and treatment of valvular heart disease (Atkins et al, 2009). This scheme can be summarized as follows:

- **Stage A:** Patients are at high risk of the development of HF but without apparent structural abnormality at the present time.

Examples: Cavalier King Charles spaniels, boxers, and Doberman pinschers, as well as other dogs belonging to breeds, families, or demographic groups known to be predisposed to heart disease.

- **Stage B:** Patients have a structural abnormality but have never demonstrated any (client-recognized) symptoms or clinical signs of HF. Stage **B1** includes dogs with normal heart size based on evaluation of radiographs (and, optimally, echocardiographic findings). Stage **B2** includes dogs with evidence of cardiomegaly and ventricular remodeling.

  Examples: An asymptomatic dog with a murmur of MR; an apparently healthy Doberman pinscher with systolic myocardial dysfunction and left ventricular dilatation on echocardiography.

- **Stage C:** Patients have a structural abnormality and current or previous clinical signs of HF.

  Examples: This stage includes all patients that have experienced an episode of clinical HF. Importantly, most dogs with cardiac disease remain in this stage despite improvement of their clinical signs with standard medical and dietary therapy for CHF.

- **Stage D:** Patients have clinical signs of CHF that are refractory to standard treatments.

  Examples: In human patients this stage includes those receiving standard dosages of diuretics, angiotensin-converting enzyme (ACE) inhibitors, β-blockers, and digoxin; in veterinary medicine, "standard therapy" for canine CHF (as discussed in detail later) includes usual dosages of furosemide, spironolactone, an ACE inhibitor, and pimobendan.

This staging emphasizes the progressive structural abnormalities that underlie the pathogenesis of HF. The system is meant to encourage a program of management and education that supports early detection and screening for heart disease and provides a loosely defined "stepped" plan of treatment intensification that may be applied as heart disease progresses. This staging system further departs from the NYHA and ISACHC functional classifications in that a patient can still progress suddenly from stage B to stage D but the entire path cannot be traveled in reverse.

This modified ACC/AHA staging system is more analogous to the standard clinical classification of cancer; that is, the screening and identification of patients that are known to be at risk of disease (stage A); the identification and treatment of patients with *in situ* disease (stage B); and the identification and treatment of patients with established (stage C) or widespread (stage D) disease. The main *limitation* of the ACC/AHA system is the categorization of dogs in which CHF first manifests as an acute condition requiring aggressive short-term treatment that may include hospital management and intravenous or other nonstandard therapies; such a patient would be classified as stage D, but the patient's condition actually may be stabilized back to stage C.

Management of Heart Failure in Dogs

Considering what we know regarding the origin, pathogenesis, progression, and response to therapy of the common acquired heart diseases of dogs (valvular heart disease and DCM), a practical therapeutic framework for managing HF in dogs should include diagnostic, treatment, and educational plans specific for each stage of heart disease and HF. Management plans should consider the natural history of the disease and carefully weigh what is known regarding the potential benefits and risks of each medication, and their combination, when used in a specific clinical setting. Using the ABCD classification just reviewed, a framework can be advanced for treatment of canine heart disease. Specific recommendations are offered in the following sections, with chronic MR and DCM used to illustrate the key issues. More details about cardiovascular drugs, including a table of common dosages, are provided in Chapter 175 and in the Appendix. The balance of the chapter offers specific management approaches to canine HF. Further details about degenerative valvular disease and canine cardiomyopathies can be found in other chapters in this section of the book.

Stage A: Dogs at Risk of Heart Disease

Stage A classification indicates that the dog is at risk of heart disease but currently has no clinical signs. Cavalier King Charles spaniels, dachshunds, and other small breeds at increased risk of development of chronic valvular heart disease should be screened by thorough cardiac auscultation. In otherwise healthy animals, the absence of a systolic click or the typical murmur of mitral valve regurgitation (a systolic murmur heard best over the left cardiac apex) adequately rules out significant degenerative valvular disease. Repeated annual screenings are indicated. If results of a screening examination are positive for valvular disease, then the classification is stage B. It should be emphasized that auscultation is an appropriate screening examination for degenerative valvular heart disease. However, if the clinician is interested in screening for preclinical DCM or arrhythmogenic right ventricular cardiomyopathy, different examinations (e.g., echocardiography or Holter ECG monitoring) are required.

Stage B: Asymptomatic Canine Heart Disease

Stage B is a "prefailure" state which indicates that cardiac disease is present in an otherwise asymptomatic dog. A typical case example is a mature small-breed dog in which a holosystolic murmur of MR is auscultated over the left apex. In this case the heart disease almost certainly is degenerative (myxomatous) valvular disease (i.e., endocardiosis). The workup should start with acquisition of high-quality lateral and dorsoventral (or ventrodorsal) thoracic radiographs. Objective quantitation of heart size using a vertebral heart size is useful at this stage because most dogs that develop clinical signs of CHF in the future will demonstrate a marked increase in heart size. In contrast, dogs coughing from primary airway or lung disease often exhibit little change in cardiac size compared with the previous examination. This approach not only provides a baseline for assessing progressive heart disease but also improves future differentiation of cardiac causes from primary respiratory causes of cough or dyspnea. Radiographs are especially helpful when an effort is made to obtain serial studies with similar positioning and exposure technique.

Depending on availability and client acceptance, a two-dimensional echocardiogram, optimally with Doppler studies, should be obtained to confirm the presence and severity of the valvular disease (presumably) responsible for the murmur. Echocardiography also is indicated in dogs younger than 6 years of age to rule out the possibility of congenital heart disease. Older dogs should be screened for systemic hypertension that might be caused by chronic kidney disease or Cushing's disease because high BP can worsen the severity of MR. Again, other clinical scenarios would suggest different diagnostic tests, especially for assessment of an asymptomatic dog at high risk of cardiomyopathy. In these patients, serial echocardiography and ECG have higher priorities in the cardiac workup.

Stage B1

To summarize: for dogs with MR and stage B degenerative valvular disease a workup should involve thoracic radiography, noninvasive BP measurement, and optimally Doppler echocardiography. If cardiac size is close to normal, repeat imaging would be recommended in about 1 year and *no therapy would be prescribed*. Diagnosis of stage B1 DCM is difficult since no remodeling would be evident at this stage, and there would have to be some reason for ordering an echocardiogram (e.g., a murmur, positive genetic test results, or a breeder's desire for a screening echocardiogram).

Stage B2

If either radiography or echocardiography reveals obvious cardiomegaly, the patient would be classified as having stage B2 disease. Treatment of dogs in this stage certainly is controversial, and therapeutic recommendations are different depending on whether the heart disease is chronic MR from valvular degeneration or preclinical DCM. Clients should be educated regarding the presence of significant heart disease and different treatment options discussed within the context of available evidence on prevention of CHF, quality of life, and long-term prognosis. Additionally, the cost of therapy and monitoring should be addressed. There are a number of therapeutic possibilities for dogs with stage B2 cardiac disease, and these are now considered.

ACE inhibitors such as enalapril and benazepril are controversial therapies at this stage in dogs with degenerative valvular disease. Two randomized, prospective, blinded clinical trials have yielded results considered negative and inconclusive. One study did show a possible benefit equivalent to an approximately 3-month extension of time before the onset of HF during a 3-year treatment period. Therefore the authors do not recommend an ACE inhibitor for dogs with MR and only mild cardiomegaly. The authors do start ACE inhibitor treatment in the following situations: (1) when moderate to severe cardiomegaly is present based on vertebral heart size obtained via echocardiography or radiography; (2) when a significant increment in cardiac size has been observed compared with the previous examination (e.g., an increase in

vertebral heart size of >0.5); or (3) when there is definitive evidence of systemic hypertension. This recommendation would be tempered in those countries in which low-cost generic ACE inhibitors cannot be prescribed to dogs because the cost : benefit ratio might be quite high in these locations.

In dogs with clearly documented preclinical DCM, the authors recommend a full dosage of enalapril (0.5 mg/kg q12h PO), benazepril, or other ACE inhibitor as cardioprotection based on the results of one open-label prospective study as well as experimental evidence of cardiac muscle protection conferred by this drug class. Similarly, the authors consider larger-breed dogs (>20 kg) with chronic MR to be at risk of progressive left ventricular myocardial dysfunction and treat these patients the same way those with DCM are treated; that is, an ACE inhibitor is prescribed for these patients when there is evidence of cardiac remodeling or impaired left ventricular systolic function.

β-Adrenergic blockers such as atenolol, bisoprolol, metoprolol, or carvedilol are even more controversial for treatment of stage B heart disease. Recently a multicenter prospective clinical trial of bisoprolol was stopped due to apparent lack of efficacy in delaying the onset of clinical HF. Accordingly, the authors *do not recommend use of a β-blocker* in small-breed dogs with stage B MR. Some evidence from studies of experimentally induced mitral valve disease in dogs suggests a potential cardioprotective benefit in larger-breed dogs (>20 kg) with MR. In the setting of significant left ventricular remodeling or impaired left ventricular systolic function in a large-breed dog with MR a β-blocker (carvedilol, metoprolol, or atenolol) can be considered, but such therapy is empiric. A similar approach is taken in dogs with preclinical (occult) DCM. Owing to the negative inotropic effects of this class of drugs, the clinician should appreciate the risk of precipitating CHF in dogs with impaired left ventricular systolic function.

Whether or not to use inotropic drugs still is unresolved. *Digoxin* is not recommended by the authors or by the ACVIM consensus panel at this stage of disease based on a lack of any clinical trial evidence. Similarly, *pimobendan* is not recommended for this stage of disease in smaller-breed dogs with MR. A clinical trial (Evaluating Pimobendan In Cardiomegaly [EPIC]) currently is under way in dogs with advanced stage B2 MR (with an end point of prevention of CHF), but results are not likely until after 2014. The use of pimobendan in preclinical DCM also is controversial, but a recent multicenter study of Doberman pinschers with preclinical DCM (Pimobendan Randomised Occult DCM Trial to Evaluate Clinical Symptoms and Time to Heart Failure [PROTECT]; Summerfield et al, 2012) did demonstrate a significant benefit for the primary end points of delaying the onset of CHF and all-cause mortality. Accordingly, in Doberman pinschers with well-defined DCM (including left ventricular dilatation) use of pimobendan can be justified. Whether this approach can be generalized to other breeds with preclinical DCM, however, cannot be determined from this study. Until there are further data for other breeds with preclinical DCM, the routine use of pimobendan to treat a lower than normal ejection fraction in a dog with no clinical signs cannot be advocated; accordingly, the authors suggest that a cardiologist be consulted in these cases.

Spironolactone is not recommended by the authors for stage B2 disease in dogs with MR until further studies are conducted. Because there are theoretical advantages to treatment with aldosterone receptor antagonists in preclinical stage B2 cardiomyopathy, some cardiologists prescribe spironolactone empirically, especially where it is available in a generic formulation.

Nutraceuticals have been discussed frequently for the early treatment of heart disease in dogs; however, there are no trial data to recommend taurine, L-carnitine, coenzyme Q_{10}, omega-3 fatty acid–containing fish oils, pomegranate extracts, hawthorn berry, or other holistic therapies except in very specific conditions of known dietary or metabolic deficiencies. None of these supplements is recommended by the authors for this stage of valvular heart disease. In cases of preclinical DCM the diet and the breed should be considered carefully because dietary or metabolic deficiencies of taurine and of L-carnitine have been reported on occasion. In addition, some special diets (vegan diets, exclusively lamb and rice diets) have been reported to be deficient in these micronutrients.

Sodium (salt)–restricted diets could be of potential benefit because there is evidence of abnormal sodium handling in animals with experimental valvular insufficiency before the onset of CHF. However, from a practical standpoint, sodium restriction is unlikely to be important at this stage of disease unless extremely high-sodium meals or treats are consumed by a dog on the verge of developing CHF. Some sodium-restricted diets (especially the renal diets) are relatively low in protein, and these may not be helpful to the cardiac patient. Many senior diets are controlled in sodium and include appropriate protein content for cardiac disease. See Chapter 168 for more details.

Stage C: Chronic Congestive Heart Failure

Stage C is hemodynamically significant heart disease and is characterized by obvious clinical signs of HF. Many dogs with chronic valvular heart disease and most dogs with DCM are diagnosed first at this stage, and with effective management these cases respond well to standard therapy as summarized later. Some patients progress to this stage slowly, begin to cough more often, but are otherwise well. Radiographic findings may be inconclusive, and these cases constitute a diagnostic dilemma (see the discussion of left bronchial compression later in the chapter in the section on respiratory signs). Other dogs develop significant, even life-threatening signs of CHF and require urgent care and stabilization (see the section on acute congestive heart failure later in the chapter).

The clinical signs of left-sided CHF are most common in stage C, and owners may notice respiratory distress or apparent dyspnea (shortness of breath, often associated with orthopnea or reluctance to lie down). Coughing is another common sign. There may be a history of exercise intolerance, lethargy, reduced appetite, and possibly weight loss. The heart rate often is elevated for a resting dog (>140 beats/min), as is the respiratory rate (>40 breaths/min). If the patient is not too anxious or distressed, confirmation of the diagnosis with thoracic radiography always is indicated.

In general, standard therapy for stage C patients involves controlling dietary sodium intake (see earlier) and prescribing four drugs: (1) *furosemide* for preload reduction (initial parenteral administration is followed by daily oral therapy); (2) *pimobendan* for inotropic and vasodilator effects; (3) an *ACE inhibitor* (enalapril, benazepril, or imidapril) to reduce ventricular load and mitigate neurohormonal activation; and (4) the aldosterone receptor blocker *spironolactone,* which exerts antifibrotic, weak diuretic, and potassium-sparing effects (Box 176-1). Common dosages for these agents are summarized in Chapter 175.

There are reasonably convincing clinical trial data for dogs in this stage supporting the use of ACE inhibitors and pimobendan (along with background therapy of furosemide with or without spironolactone); inconclusive trial data on monotherapy with spironolactone (the drug is approved in the European Union; a multicenter study is ongoing in North America); and no trial data for furosemide as monotherapy (but there is little doubt the drug is effective as a diuretic). Despite the overwhelming evidence of effectiveness in human patients with HF, there is no compelling proof that β-blockers are beneficial in canine CHF. If such treatment is contemplated, the drug should be initiated at a low dosage and only after clinical signs of CHF have been resolved for at least a week. The authors are most likely to add a β-blocker to standard HF therapy in cases of well-controlled DCM and use a slow up-titration of the dose. Dietary sodium intake should be discussed and clients warned about feeding treats or foods with high sodium content (see Chapter 168).

These patients remain in stage C even if clinical signs resolve completely with therapy. Long-term treatment of stage C heart disease will be needed for the life of the dog and encompasses three goals: (1) altering hemodynamics (cardiac output, arterial and venous pressures, vascular resistances) to permit a comfortable life and reasonable level of activity while minimizing signs of CHF; (2) prolonging life by reducing the ongoing damage to the heart muscle, blood vessels, kidneys, and other organs inflicted by neurohormonal systems and proinflammatory cytokines; and (3) minimizing the adverse effects of cardiac drugs on other organs, especially the kidneys. For most owners (and veterinarians) a good quality of life trumps longevity as the main treatment goal; however, both aims should be attainable with combination medical therapy and stepped increases in dietary sodium restriction. Two additional therapeutic goals are the prevention of drug-induced toxicosis and the avoidance of unplanned hospital visits because these two situations can lead to stressful and costly emergency examinations and may prompt euthanasia. Adverse effects of cardiovascular drugs are summarized in Chapter 175.

Follow-up Examinations

Long-term management of patients with stage C (and stage D) heart failure requires detailed client education about heart disease, treatments, and home monitoring

BOX 176-1

Management of Heart Failure in Dogs

Diuretics
Furosemide
Spironolactone
Torsemide[a]
Hydrochlorothiazide[a]

Inotropic Drugs
Pimobendan
Digoxin[b]
Dobutamine/dopamine[c]

**Angiotensin-Converting
Enzyme Inhibitors[d]**
Enalapril or benazepril
Imidapril

Dietary Management
**Controlled or restricted
  sodium intake**
Nutraceuticals (taurine,
  L-carnitine, L-arginine,
  omega-3 fatty acids)[e]
Potassium chloride
  supplementation[e]

Vasodilator Drugs
**Angiotensin-converting
  enzyme inhibitors**

Nitrovasodilators:
  nitroglycerine ointment,
  sodium nitroprusside[f]
Amlodipine[g]
Hydralazine
Sildenafil[h]

β-Adrenergic Blockers[i]
Carvedilol
Atenolol
Metoprolol

Antiarrhythmic Drugs[j]
Digoxin
Diltiazem
Lidocaine, mexiletine
Procainamide
Sotalol
Amiodarone

Other Agents
Sedatives (butorphanol)
Oxygen
Cough suppressants

Core therapies for stage C and D canine heart failure are indicated in **bold.**
[a]Used in stage D congestive heart failure (CHF) with caution; see text for details.
[b]Used for management of atrial fibrillation or end-stage CHF.
[c]Catecholamines used in the treatment of cardiogenic shock.
[d]The angiotensin-converting enzyme inhibitors are considered equivalent in efficacy, and choice depends on preference and country; enalapril or benazepril is most often chosen.
[e]See text for details; L-arginine is used in conjunction with phosphodiesterase 5 inhibitors such as sildenafil in treatment of pulmonary hypertension.
[f]Used in the hospital management of severe CHF; see text for details.
[g]Used for control of concurrent systemic hypertension or as a stage D treatment to further reduce afterload in the setting of severe mitral regurgitation.
[h]Sildenafil and related drugs are used specifically for management of documented pulmonary hypertension.
[i]The use of β-blockers in preclinical heart failure is controversial but may be beneficial; in overt CHF (stages C and D) these drugs must be used with great care and mainly are considered for dogs with well-controlled dilated cardiomyopathy, for further rate control in atrial fibrillation, or for control of ventricular arrhythmias (in the form of sotalol).
[j]Digoxin and diltiazem are used for rate control in atrial fibrillation; the others are potential treatments for life-threatening ventricular arrhythmias.

along with regularly scheduled follow-up examinations (Box 176-2), which are preferable to emergency department visits. The authors typically schedule reevaluations in about 1 week after initial diagnosis of CHF; 1 to 2 weeks after any significant change in diuretic dosing; at least every 3 months in patients in stable condition; and as dictated by clinical signs and circumstances. Although there are no recipes for these reexaminations, certain aspects of the history, physical examination, and laboratory evaluation are germane. Owners should report on

BOX 176-2

Canine Congestive Heart Failure: Follow-up Examinations

Medication Review
- Record the drug, tablet or formulation strength, current dose, and frequency of administration
- Calculate the total daily dose per body weight for each drug
- Address any compliance or drug administration issues
- Determine the need for refills
- Identify any signs of possible drug intoxication

Medical History and Quality of Life
- Appetite
  - Current diet and amount (assess sodium and protein contents)
  - Treats and supplements (assess sodium content)
- Activity and exercise capacity
- Attitude—interactions with family members and other pets
- Sleeping—ability to rest comfortably throughout the night
- Respiratory rate during sleep (review owner's log)
- Owner-recognized symptoms: coughing, difficult breathing, tiring, collapse or syncope
- Drinking and urinary habits

Physical Examination
- Body weight
- Hydration status
- Overall body condition score, evidence of cachexia
- Vital signs: temperature, pulse rate at rest, respiratory rate at rest
- Signs of congestive heart failure: elevated jugular venous pressure, hepatomegaly, ascites, abnormal findings on thoracic auscultation (pulmonary crackles or pleural fluid line)
- Heart rate and cardiac rhythm (assessed by auscultation)

Noninvasive Arterial Blood Pressure Measurement
- Identify hypotension (systolic blood pressure < 90 mm Hg)
- Identify elevated systolic blood pressure (>150-160 mm Hg)

Electrocardiography (if indicated)
- Record an electrocardiogram when an arrhythmia is detected during auscultation
- Record an electrocardiogram for accurate heart rate response if the patient has atrial fibrillation

Thoracic Radiography (as indicated)
- Review radiographs for control of pulmonary edema and effusions
- Consider other causes of respiratory signs (tracheal collapse, bronchial compression or collapse, bronchiectasis, pneumonia, pulmonary neoplasia)
- Compare current radiographs with prior studies

Clinical Laboratory Tests (as indicated)
- Packed cell volume/total solids (complete blood count if patient is acting sick)
- Renal function and electrolyte levels
- Serum concentrations of drugs (e.g., serum digoxin level)
- Advanced diagnostic testing (in select circumstances)
  - Specialized Doppler echocardiographic studies (to assess filling pressures, identify pulmonary hypertension)
  - Natriuretic peptide levels (to assist in prognosis, differential diagnosis of cough and tachypnea [?])

the dog's appetite, diet, and water consumption; activity and exercise capacity; interaction with people and other pets; respiratory rate during sleep; and any ongoing "symptoms" they have observed such as cough or restlessness at night. These simple quality-of-life indicators can provide reassurance to the caretaker that treatments are working and alert the clinician to developing complications. Respiratory rates at or below 30 breaths/min argue against radiographic evidence of pulmonary edema. Conversely, even when radiographic findings for pulmonary edema are equivocal, the sudden increase in resting respiratory rate or an average that exceeds 40 breaths/min is a cause for reexamination.

At the hospital the technician should carefully weigh the patient (specifically noting any changes) and obtain an accurate temperature, heart rate, and respiratory rate once the dog is calm. The clinician should auscultate the heart and lungs with attention to rate and rhythm (to detect arrhythmias), gallop sounds (indicating high venous pressures), lung crackles (suggesting pulmonary edema or chronic pulmonary fibrosis), and fluid lines (to detect pleural effusions). Attention to hydration status and jugular venous pressure as well as palpation of the abdomen for signs of right-sided CHF (hepatomegaly and ascites) also are important. Commonly performed blood tests are packed cell volume/total solids (to assess hydration), blood urea nitrogen (BUN) level, creatinine concentration, and serum electrolyte levels. Levels of natriuretic peptides (e.g., N-terminal prohormone B-type natriuretic peptide, B-type natriuretic peptide) are not measured routinely, but there is emerging evidence that their determination after treatment may be of prognostic value. Repeat radiographs of the thorax are often obtained, and in referral centers Doppler echocardiographic indices of cardiac filling and diastolic function might be analyzed. Doppler assessment of a tricuspid regurgitant jet can be used to identify and quantify pulmonary hypertension, and quantitation of a mitral regurgitant jet provides insight about systemic arterial BP. Although ECG is unnecessary for most patients, it is essential to characterize any heart rhythm or pulse disturbance evident during physical examination. ECG also is useful in dogs with atrial fibrillation to measure heart rate accurately.

When initial signs of CHF are severe enough to dictate hospitalization for diuresis, serum renal and electrolyte studies, thoracic radiography, and noninvasive BP measurement should be performed just before hospital release. Once home therapy begins, these studies should be repeated in about a week so the treatment response can be assessed and metabolic complications associated with HF and cardiac medications identified. The veterinarian should inquire about compliance with the drug regimen, review current therapy and potential adverse effects, and consider the potential to increase or decrease dosages. For example, the combination of diuretics and ACE inhibitors often reduces plasma volume, systemic arterial BP, and glomerular filtration rate. Generally, drug adjustments for BP, are unnecessary as long as systolic pressure is more than 90 mm Hg. But when mild or moderate azotemia (or an increase of 1.5 to 2 times baseline) is recorded, the furosemide dosage should be lowered by at least 25% provided the patient is "dry." Conversely, if clinical and radiographic signs of CHF are persistent, the dosage of furosemide or other heart medications should be increased, even in the setting of azotemia. Clinicians should develop the confidence to accept some degree of reduced glomerular filtration rate and "prerenal" azotemia to ensure that pulmonary edema is controlled. It helps to look at the patient: if the dog seems bright, is eating well, and is not exhibiting signs of uremia such as vomiting, it is likely the diuretic and ACE inhibitor dosages are tolerable. Fortunately, many patients show little or no change in renal function on the initial recheck, which provides the chance to optimize the ACE inhibitor dosage. As an example, the authors typically start enalapril therapy at a dosage of approximately 0.25 mg/kg q12h PO and then double the dose to approximately 0.5 mg/kg q12h at the first recheck. Ideally renal function should be reevaluated 1 to 2 weeks after any significant increase in diuretic or ACE inhibitor dosage.

Mild hypochloremia and metabolic alkalosis (elevated serum bicarbonate concentration) are anticipated complications of diuretic therapy and are ignored. These are to some degree indicators of loop diuretic efficacy. Initial diuresis often reduces serum potassium level, but in most cases, the value normalizes under the influence of ACE inhibitor and spironolactone therapy because each drug is potassium sparing. If moderate hypokalemia or profound hypochloremia becomes evident, and if the patient is free of edema, the diuretic dosage is reduced (~25% initially). In these cases potassium chloride supplements can be administered or salt substitute (KCl) sprinkled on the food, but these supplements can be unpalatable or lead to vomiting.

The development of moderate to severe azotemia (e.g., creatinine concentration of >3 mg/dl, BUN level of >60 mg/dl) in a dog that is still drinking is a serious concern (one should first ensure that the client is not withholding water to minimize urinary output). The presence of significant azotemia when standard diuretic and ACE inhibitor dosages are being administered suggests concurrent chronic kidney disease or a strong dependence on angiotensin II for maintenance of glomerular filtration. The latter situation is especially likely if the BUN and creatine concentrations increase suddenly with the introduction of an ACE inhibitor during the postdiuresis period. Clinical signs of acute renal failure can include anorexia, vomiting, and severe depression and may be misinterpreted as worsening HF. These patients are difficult to manage long term because of the competing goals of fluid management in CHF and in chronic kidney disease. Given that ACE inhibitors and spironolactone potentially are beneficial for both organs, these drugs should be continued, but lower dosages of ACE inhibitors may be needed and dosage titration should be more gradual. The short-term treatment of acute or severe azotemia involves 1 or 2 days of hospital stabilization with cautious intravenous fluid therapy (0.45% saline with KCl supplementation), temporary stoppage of the ACE inhibitor, and a lowering of the furosemide dosage. In some cases renal function test results actually return to the normal range.

Stage D: Refractory Congestive Heart Failure

Progression to stage D is defined somewhat arbitrarily as a need for treatment beyond the standard therapy and usual dosages of furosemide, pimobendan, ACE inhibitor, and spironolactone. The sudden development of severe, previously untreated CHF does reveal a limitation of this ABCD classification system, but staging (C or D) can await initial hospital management of HF (see the later section on acute congestive heart failure).

Treatment of refractory HF of any cause is a challenging and potentially frustrating endeavor for both the veterinarian and the client. A thorough search for factors commonly involved in the progression of HF should be undertaken. Some of these factors are listed in Box 176-3. Therapeutic principles involve maintenance of whatever cardioprotective regimens were tolerated in stage C, optimization of hemodynamics through the use of higher dosages of standard drugs, and addition of other vasodilators, inotropes, antiarrhythmic drugs, or experimental therapies as appropriate. Human patients with stage D disease sometimes are offered sophisticated electrical or mechanical circulatory aids, heart valve repair, and other interventions that would be helpful if the procedure could be performed with a high success rate and acceptable cost. However, thus far, surgical treatments have met with limited success and the cost still is too high. Many practitioners find consultation with a cardiologist helpful when navigating these options and managing patients in the final stages of heart disease.

The initial question to consider is whether the patient should be hospitalized or treated as an outpatient. This decision may require the collection of more data, such as performing complete serum biochemical testing, complete blood count, and urinalysis; obtaining thoracic radiographs (if tolerated) and fast or detailed thoracic and cardiac ultrasonographic studies; and of course performing a thorough physical examination. Sometimes the decision can be made simply, after observing the patient ventilate and assessing the work of breathing. At other times the patient just seems "sick," and an open mind may help the clinician identify a complicating or unrelated disease responsible for clinical signs.

Hospital-based therapies for patients with stage D heart disease may include oxygen administration, mechanical removal of effusions (thoracocentesis or abdominal paracentesis), and intravenous infusions of furosemide, dobutamine, sodium nitroprusside, or lidocaine, among other treatments. These are discussed in the following section.

BOX 176-3

Factors Exacerbating Clinical Signs of Congestive Heart Failure

Progression of Heart Disease
Progression of the primary cardiac disease
  Uninhibited neurohormonal activation
  Progressive degenerative changes
Complications of chronic valvular heart disease
  Ruptured chordae tendineae
  Secondary left or right ventricular myocardial dysfunction
  Tearing of the left atrium—cardiac tamponade or acquired atrial septal defect
  Intramural coronary artery disease—myocardial ischemia

Heart Rhythm Disturbances
Atrial fibrillation
Ventricular tachycardia or frequent ventricular premature complexes
Sustained or recurrent atrial or supraventricular tachycardias

Elevated Blood Pressure
Systemic hypertension
  Idiopathic
  Secondary: chronic kidney disease, Cushing's disease, other causes
  Drug related: vasoconstrictor drugs such as phenylpropanolamine
Pulmonary hypertension
  Secondary to left-sided heart failure (postcapillary)
  Pulmonary vascular reaction (precapillary)
  Secondary to widespread lung disease (pulmonary fibrosis)

Other Medical Disorders
Increased demands for cardiac output
  Hyperthyroidism (usually iatrogenic in dogs)

Anemia
Infections, especially those causing fever
Chronic kidney disease
Urinary sphincter incontinence (complicates tolerance of diuretic therapy)
Chronic respiratory diseases: tracheal collapse, bronchial collapse/bronchomalacia, chronic bronchitis, pulmonary fibrosis, respiratory infection

Medication Issues
Insufficient therapy or drug dosages for the stage of heart failure
Iatrogenic disease: inappropriate therapy or excessive drug dosages
Poor client adherence to the medication regimen
Addition of negative inotropic drugs: β-blockers, calcium channel blockers, antiarrhythmic drugs
Concurrent use of nonsteroidal antiinflammatory drugs (NSAIDs)

Dietary Issues
Poor or unpalatable diet (inadequate caloric intake)
Excessive dietary sodium intake in food or food treats
Low protein intake (e.g., renal diets)
Missing micronutrients (e.g., vegan diet, exclusively lamb and rice diet, poor formulation)

Other Issues
Excessive exercise for stage of heart failure
Environmental stress (heat, high humidity)
Inadequate patient follow-up

Home-based treatments for advanced CHF should start with optimizing the dosages of the standard four drugs and shortening the dosing interval of furosemide or pimobendan from twice to three times daily (an extra-label use for pimobendan). Diet should be reconsidered critically in patients with stage D disease, with calculated daily sodium intake compared with basic needs (about 12 mg/kg of sodium daily). Additionally, omega-3 fatty acids found in fish oils may help to prevent cardiac cachexia (see Chapter 168).

Another common strategy is to modify the diuretic regimen using one of three approaches. One involves the addition of parenteral doses of furosemide to the weekly treatment plan. Clients can be taught to administer a subcutaneous injection, starting at three times a week. A second strategy is to prescribe oral torsemide and substitute it for the midday dose (or all doses) of furosemide at about ⅛ to ¹⁄₁₀ of the furosemide dose. This loop diuretic is believed to have a higher absorption, better renal delivery, and more sustained duration of action. Other cardiologists prefer adding a third diuretic such as hydrochlorothiazide with a different mechanism of action. This creates a sequential nephron blockade, because thiazides work distally to the loop diuretics and proximally to aldosterone antagonists. Judicious initial dosages (1 mg/kg daily or every other day) are advised. Practitioners must exercise caution with all of these approaches and reassess the patient within 3 to 7 days, including monitoring of kidney function and serum levels of sodium, potassium, bicarbonate, and chloride.

Digoxin is a modest positive inotrope that sensitizes arterial baroreceptors and thereby increases vagal tone to the heart. Digoxin largely has been supplanted by pimobendan for treatment of CHF in dogs, but it can be considered in stage D failure. It also should be given (in addition to pimobendan) in the setting of atrial fibrillation complicating CHF. Relative contraindications to digitalis therapy include complex ventricular ectopy, moderate to severe azotemia, sinus node dysfunction, and preexisting atrioventricular block. These comorbidities, especially renal dysfunction, limit the use of digoxin in advanced CHF.

The clinician also should ensure that the patient is not hypertensive (as might occur with chronic kidney disease or Cushing's disease) and aggressively lower BP when necessary to the range of 90 to 120 mm Hg (systolic BP). This can be done by optimizing the ACE inhibitor dosage and adding the calcium channel blocker amlodipine starting at a conservative dose (0.1 mg/kg q24h PO) and up-titrating to effect. Even if BP is normal, cautiously reducing systolic pressure with the combination of an ACE inhibitor and amlodipine can reduce afterload, MR, and left atrial pressure in refractory left-sided CHF due to MR.

Chronic Right-Sided Congestive Heart Failure
When CHF leads to ascites or pleural effusions, the usual explanation is one of the following: MR complicated by pulmonary hypertension and tricuspid regurgitation; severe pulmonary hypertension (including dirofilariasis-associated pulmonary hypertension and idiopathic pulmonary hypertension); superimposition of atrial fibrillation on structural heart disease; DCM or right ventricular cardiomyopathy; pericardial disease; or unrecognized congenital right-sided heart disease (tricuspid valve malformation, pulmonary stenosis). In addition to the treatments mentioned earlier, other measures should be considered. It also is important to ensure that the CHF is not caused by pericardial effusion and cardiac tamponade (see Chapter 182) because the initial treatment for this condition is pericardiocentesis, not administration of cardiac drugs.

Ascites is associated with extreme sodium and water retention, and exercise and dietary sodium restrictions should be enforced; it may be useful to consult a veterinary nutritionist for dietary recommendations (see Chapter 168). *Thoracocentesis* should be performed in any dog with a large pleural effusion. *Abdominocentesis* is recommended in cases of tense ascites, and the effusion should be fully or partially drained (at least one half of the volume) to relieve pressure on the diaphragm and abdominal organs. Hepatomegaly should be distinguished from ascites before abdominocentesis (this can be more difficult than it sounds; a lateral abdominal radiograph or brief abdominal ultrasonographic examination offers assurance). Recurring body cavity effusions indicate that adjustments in medical therapy are needed. Some modification of diuretic therapies, as discussed earlier, should be carried out. Increasing the frequency of pimobendan administration from two to three times daily is another common strategy.

When Doppler echocardiography indicates the presence of moderate to severe pulmonary hypertension, a trial course of *sildenafil* (Viagra) or *tadalafil* (Cialis) is recommended along with supplementation with the amino acid L-arginine (250 mg q12h PO). Although clinical trial data are lacking, this class of phosphodiesterase inhibitors seems to help some dogs, especially in improving exercise tolerance and preventing exertional collapsing spells (see Chapters 167 and 175). Oxygen rarely is prescribed for home use but also can be considered, especially in smaller-breed dogs. When concurrent chronic bronchitis or major airway collapse leads to intractable coughing in dogs with CHF, symptomatic relief may be provided by a cough suppressant such as hydrocodone or courses of prednisone or inhaled fluticasone (see Chapters 159 and 160).

Prognosis in Chronic Congestive Heart Failure

The prognosis for stage C heart failure depends on the cause, the severity of disease, and the care provided. Many dogs in this stage survive for longer than 1 year after the first signs of CHF appear provided they receive the optimal veterinary and home care described earlier. Advancing a 6- to 12-month prognosis for CHF caused by chronic MR is reasonable as long as the dog's condition can be well stabilized initially. In general, the prognosis for CHF due to DCM is more guarded and more variable because of the severity of left ventricular dysfunction and the risk of sudden arrhythmic death (see Chapters 178 and 179). Human-related factors including the cost of care and clients' perceptions about heart disease in their dogs exert a profound influence on the overall outcome, which makes it difficult to establish specific prognoses for individual dogs. Clearly the attending veterinarian has a large role to play in advising the client, and this is likely to affect the prognosis. In human patients with CHF, referral to a cardiology specialist improves outcomes, and referral to a veterinary cardiologist may have the same impact. Thus specialty consultation should be considered, if only to verify that the diagnosis is correct and that an optimal treatment plan has been undertaken. Complicating factors, including concurrent renal failure, the development of atrial fibrillation or ventricular tachycardia, and severe comorbidities (e.g., diabetes mellitus or multicentric neoplasia), certainly worsen the outlook. Once CHF has progressed to severe failure (stage D), the outlook generally is guarded to poor (1 to 6 months' survival), but again, unexpected outcomes sometimes are achieved in dogs receiving meticulous medical management.

There are no randomized controlled clinical trials that prospectively evaluate prognostic criteria for the four-drug combination therapy described in this chapter. As indicated previously, randomized, multicenter studies of ACE inhibitors, pimobendan, furosemide, and spironolactone have been published. Most of these have suggested a benefit when drug treatments are combined.

Clients often want to understand the *causes of death* in chronic CHF. Although the causes are variable, the most common are (1) a sudden electrical event (asystole or ventricular fibrillation), (2) hypoxemia (from uncontrolled pulmonary edema, pleural effusion, or respiratory arrest), (3) multisystemic organ failure (especially in CHF complicated by renal failure), and, most important, (4) a client's desire for euthanasia based on a host of perceived medical and personal factors. Other causes of sudden death may include pulmonary embolism and myocardial infarction, but these are poorly characterized in dogs.

Special Situations in the Management of Canine Heart Failure

This section considers the treatment of dogs with heart disease and respiratory signs of ambiguous origin, the hospital management of life-threatening CHF, and the control of heart rhythm disturbances in the setting of HF.

Respiratory Signs in Stage B2 Heart Disease

Delineating the transition between stages B2 and C can be confusing even when a complete workup is performed. The onset of clinical signs in dogs with advanced valvular disease often is very gradual and usually is heralded by intermittent coughing. Although this can indicate pulmonary edema and CHF (stage C), the lungs may be radiographically clear and the coughing caused by *compression of the left main-stem bronchus* (between the descending aorta and dorsal left atrium). This feature of chronic MR in dogs is not synonymous with left-sided CHF but can be difficult to distinguish from signs of pulmonary edema. Even more confusing is the finding that levels of a biomarker for CHF—namely, N-terminal

prohormone B-type natriuretic peptide—sometimes are very high in these patients (>2500 pmol/L) despite clear lungs and normal respiratory rates. In symptom-based classification schemes, these dogs probably are classified as having CHF, but in the ABCD classification they probably are categorized as having stage B2 disease with airway complications.

The authors' approach to management of these dogs is to initiate treatment with enalapril or benazepril (0.25 mg/kg q12h for 1 to 2 weeks then 0.5 mg/kg q12h thereafter) along with low-dose furosemide (~1 to 2 mg/kg once daily PO) to contract the plasma volume. In most cases the cough improves if it is caused by bronchial compression (or early CHF). If the cough returns weeks or months later or if respiratory rate increases at home (to >40 breaths/min), then radiographs are repeated, the dog is reclassified as stage C, and standard four-drug therapy for CHF is initiated as described previously.

It should be emphasized that failure of the cough to respond to a low dose of a diuretic and a full dose of an ACE inhibitor should prompt reconsideration of the diagnosis; in particular, the clinician should rule out *chronic bronchitis, bronchomalacia,* and *other airway diseases* (including laryngeal disease and tracheal collapse), as well as pulmonary parenchymal disorders (pneumonia, neoplasia, heartworm disease). These patients ideally are evaluated by radiography and fluoroscopy or even by computerized tomography. It may be helpful to obtain a second opinion about the interpretation of the thoracic radiographs from a radiologist or cardiologist. If CHF is unlikely, appropriate respiratory diagnostic testing (e.g., bronchoscopy with cytologic analysis and culture of airway specimens) should be offered. When diagnostic testing is limited by client concerns, a trial course of doxycycline or prednisone may be instructive (and may relieve signs related to infection or noninfective bronchitis). Cough suppressants, especially codeine-derived agents, can be prescribed as a last resort for symptom relief.

Hospital Management of Acute Congestive Heart Failure—

Clinical signs of left-sided or biventricular CHF can be life-threatening. These dogs have respiratory distress and hypoxemia at presentation. A number of standard treatment approaches have proven useful for acute management of these patients. If the patient's condition is stable enough to allow minimal manipulation, placement of an intravenous catheter in a peripheral vein and attachment of ECG monitoring leads at the outset of therapy makes patient management and monitoring easier.

The combination of intravenous furosemide, oxygen, and a nitrovasodilator (topical nitroglycerine or sodium nitroprusside) closely followed by pimobendan represents the initial treatment plan and is applicable to most cases of CHF regardless of cause. Most dogs are distressed and sedation is beneficial; butorphanol is used most often (0.25 mg/kg IM, repeated in 30 to 60 minutes if needed). When this protocol is used, diuresis is initiated, oxygen saturation is increased, ventricular loading is reduced, the tendency toward pulmonary edema is decreased, myocardial contractility is supported, and anxiety is relieved. If the patient becomes heavily sedated, the torso is positioned in sternal recumbency, the neck is extended and the chin supported with a towel or soft pad, and nasal oxygen prongs (or cannula) are inserted to deliver oxygen. Thoracocentesis should be performed if moderate to large pleural effusions are clearly evident.

After administration of an initial IV bolus of 2 mg/kg furosemide, the dose, route, and frequency of the drug can be adjusted to the clinical response (respiratory rate, anxiety level, auscultation findings). In life-threatening or poorly responsive pulmonary edema a constant-rate infusion of furosemide along with aggressive afterload reduction with sodium nitroprusside also should be considered (see Chapter 175 for administration guidelines). This is especially useful when there is MR because the regurgitant volume will be decreased by load reduction. Less potent and less controllable alternatives to sodium nitroprusside are oral hydralazine or an ACE inhibitor.

Cardiogenic Shock

The findings of pulmonary edema or pleural effusion with severe hypotension (BP < 80 mm Hg), along with other indicators of low cardiac output (pallor, hypothermia, depression, elevated blood lactate) are highly suggestive of cardiogenic shock. Dogs with DCM (often Doberman pinschers) represent the typical case. Other potential causes of cardiogenic shock include myocardial infarction and pulmonary embolus as might occur following treatment for adult heartworms or after formation of a large pulmonary thrombus. Although initial treatment is generally the same as that discussed in the previous section (furosemide, oxygen, nitroglycerine, pimobendan), there are other therapeutic considerations. First, these hypotensive patients often are very depressed, so sedation is needed only infrequently. Second, the clinician should determine if centesis is necessary because dogs with cardiogenic shock can have both pulmonary edema and large cavity effusions. Third, volume infusion (i.e., fluid therapy) is *not* appropriate to raise BP because it will only worsen edema; furthermore, diuretics and venodilators can further depress BP, so other treatments are needed to stimulate cardiac output.

A catecholamine can be given to provide cardiac support by stimulating contractility, increasing cardiac output, and facilitating diuresis. Dobutamine (or dopamine) is administered as a constant-rate IV infusion starting at 2.5 µg/kg/min, and the infusion is increased by 1 to 2 µg/kg/min every 15 to 30 minutes until systolic BP is 90 mm Hg or higher (see Chapters 3 and 175). This end point generally is reached at an infusion rate of 5 to 10 µg/kg/min, although higher rates may be needed. Once the BP is stable, other vasoactive drugs, such as nitroprusside or an ACE inhibitor, can be added to unload the left ventricle. After 24 to 48 hours of dobutamine therapy, the dobutamine infusion rate is reduced by 50% every 2 to 4 hours, and once the dosage has been lowered to approximately 1 to 2 µg/kg/min, the infusion is discontinued. By that time the dog should be taking oral drugs, including the inodilator pimobendan, which can

be administered as cotherapy because it exerts a potent inotropic effect via a different cellular mechanism.

Arrhythmias in Congestive Heart Failure

In HF complicated by hemodynamically significant ventricular or supraventricular arrhythmias, antiarrhythmic drugs are needed, and referral to a critical care center with a cardiologist on staff generally is the best option if it is available and the owner is willing. Common arrhythmias in CHF are isolated atrial and ventricular premature complexes, atrial fibrillation, and ventricular tachycardia.

Atrial fibrillation can precipitate CHF in a canine patient in previously stable condition. This problem usually is managed with heart rate control as opposed to cardioversion (to normal rhythm; see Chapter 171). Rate control involves initiation of oral digoxin (0.005 to 0.0075 mg/kg q12h PO) followed within 24 hours by up-titration of oral diltiazem. Diltiazem is administered until a hospital heart rate of less than 180 beats/min is achieved (optimally a resting rate of 120 to 140 beats/min). Effective treatment of CHF also is useful because it allows for some withdrawal of sympathetic tone with attendant reduction of ventricular rate response.

Initial doses of 0.5 to 1 mg/kg PO of standard diltiazem can be increased with each sequential dose to a total daily dose of approximately 6 mg/kg (in two or three divided doses, depending on the formulation used). Rate response is best evaluated by 24-hour (Holter) ECG monitoring once a stable home dosage has been established. Average daily heart rates in the range of 90 to 110 beats/min are probably evidence of good control in a dog with CHF. Electrical cardioversion from atrial fibrillation to sinus rhythm has been used by some in managing this arrhythmia (see Web Chapter 60), but the authors' experience is that dogs with CHF usually revert back to atrial fibrillation in a short time, so the authors mainly recommend rate control in their practices.

Isolated premature ventricular complexes are not treated in CHF cases. However, sustained runs of rapid ventricular tachycardia require treatment to maintain BP and are managed initially with boluses of lidocaine (2-mg/kg IV boluses; 40- to 60-µg/kg/min IV infusion). Mexiletine (5 to 8 mg/kg q8h PO) is an oral alternative to lidocaine. Antiarrhythmic drugs are a problem in the setting of HF because they depress myocardial function. Lidocaine and mexiletine are the safest in this regard, but reduced hepatic blood flow could lead to drug accumulation and toxicity (tremors, vomiting, seizures). Ensuring that the patient is well oxygenated and that serum electrolyte values (especially potassium and magnesium) are normal also is important. Use of digoxin is *contraindicated* in this setting. When possible, a cardiologist should be consulted about management approaches and associated risks. It also is useful to gauge the client's expectations and concerns because some simply accept the risk of sudden cardiac death, especially if antiarrhythmic drug therapy is likely to exacerbate CHF or induce adverse effects such as anorexia, vomiting, or hepatic toxicity.

With regard to other hospital and long-term treatment options, injectable procainamide is available in some locales and can be effective in the hospital, but it is a negative inotropic drug and also may result in peripheral vasodilation, lowering BP. Since sotalol has β-blocking actions, it should be used with caution in the setting of CHF, although sometimes there are no other options, and the negative inotropic effect may be partly managed with concurrent administration of pimobendan. Initial dosages of sotalol should be conservative (~1 mg/kg q12h PO). Amiodarone is another consideration (see Chapter 175), but its use requires diligent monitoring for toxicity and it is not devoid of negative inotropic effects.

References and Suggested Reading

Atkins CE et al: Results of the veterinary enalapril trial to prove reduction in onset of heart failure in dogs chronically treated with enalapril alone for compensated, naturally occurring mitral valve insufficiency, *J Am Vet Med Assoc* 231(7):1061, 2007.

Atkins C et al: ACVIM consensus statement: guidelines for the diagnosis and treatment of canine chronic valvular heart disease, *J Vet Intern Med* 23:1142, 2009.

BENCH (BENazepril in Canine Heart disease) Study Group: The effect of benazepril on survival times and clinical signs of dogs with congestive heart failure: results of a multicenter, prospective, randomized, double-blinded, placebo-controlled, long-term clinical trial, *J Vet Cardiol* 1(1):7, 1999.

COVE Study Group: Controlled clinical evaluation of enalapril in dogs with heart failure: results of the Cooperative Veterinary Enalapril Study Group, *J Vet Intern Med* 9(4):243, 1995.

Häggström J et al: Effect of pimobendan or benazepril hydrochloride on survival times in dogs with congestive heart failure caused by naturally occurring myxomatous mitral valve disease: the QUEST study, *J Vet Intern Med* 22(5):1124, 2008.

Kvart C et al: Efficacy of enalapril for prevention of congestive heart failure in dogs with myxomatous valve disease and asymptomatic mitral regurgitation, *J Vet Intern Med* 16(1):80, 2002.

Summerfield NJ et al: Efficacy of pimobendan in the prevention of congestive heart failure or sudden death in Doberman Pinschers with preclinical dilated cardiomyopathy (the PROTECT Study), *J Vet Intern Med* 26(6):1337, 2012.

CHAPTER 177

Chronic Valvular Heart Disease in Dogs

JOHN E. RUSH, *North Grafton, Massachusetts*
SUZANNE M. CUNNINGHAM, *North Grafton, Massachusetts*

Chronic valvular heart disease (CVHD) is the most common acquired heart disease in dogs, with an overall cumulative incidence of more than 40%. CVHD often results in congestive heart failure (CHF). Cardiac disease is an important cause of morbidity and mortality in dogs, responsible for approximately 10% of all canine deaths and with a higher incidence in some breeds of dogs such as the cavalier King Charles spaniel. The mitral valve most commonly is affected in CVHD, but concurrent tricuspid valve disease often is noted. Most veterinarians are very familiar with CVHD; thus the goal of this chapter is to discuss and highlight some important concepts about this disorder, consider frequently discussed topics, and review recent developments in diagnosis and therapy.

Etiology, Pathology, and Pathophysiology

The cause of CVHD currently is unknown, although a genetic tendency to develop the disease has been proven in the cavalier King Charles spaniel and suspected in other breeds. As the field of canine cardiac genetics continues to develop, it is likely that specific genes causing or contributing to the development of CVHD will be identified. In addition, poorly defined environmental and epigenetic factors likely play a role in the rate of onset or severity of the disease.

Advanced myxomatous degeneration leads to grossly thickened and shortened valve leaflets with curled, nodular margins (Figure 177-1). Valvular hemorrhage and calcification may be seen. There is fibrosis of the valves, loss of collagen fibers, and an accumulation of acid-staining glycosaminoglycans within affected valves. Chordae tendineae often are affected and may become thickened, stretched, or ruptured, which allows portions of the diseased valve leaflets to bulge or prolapse into the atrial chamber. Electron microscopy has documented great variation in endothelial cell size and morphology of affected valves, with focal loss of the endothelial layer, collagen exposure, and activation of valvular interstitial cells. It is not clear which of these findings is a result of the disease and which might be a cause or contributor to

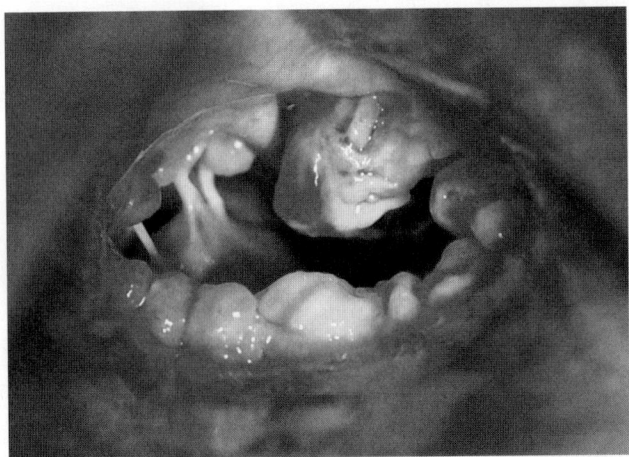

Figure 177-1 Gross pathologic image of the mitral valve from a dog with advanced chronic valvular heart disease. The left atrium has been opened allowing visualization of the atrial surface of the valve. Note the severely thickened, shortened leaflets and the retracted, nodular leaflet edges.

disease progression. CVHD historically has been considered a noninflammatory, myxomatous degeneration of the atrioventricular valve, but there is growing interest in the role that serotonin or other inflammatory mediators may play in accelerating the pathologic development of the disease. There is one report of elevated C-reactive protein concentrations in the serum of affected dogs, which suggests a possible role of low-grade systemic inflammation in the progression of the disease (Rush et al, 2006). Another study evaluating genomic expression patterns in the valves of dogs with CVHD confirmed activation of several pathways involved in cell signaling, inflammation, and extracellular matrix activation, with several inflammatory cytokines and serotonin–transforming growth factor-β pathways identified as contributory to the development of the degenerative process in the valve (Oyama and Chittur, 2006). Increased serum serotonin levels have been found in dogs with CVHD, and increased autocrine production of serotonin, as well as up-regulation of the serotonin receptor 5HT-R$_{2\beta}$, has been detected in affected valves. Increased serotonin signaling or decreased clearance can activate mitogenic pathways in valvular interstitial cells, resulting in their transformation to a more active myofibroblast phenotype. These activated interstitial cells are believed to play a role in pathologic valve remodeling via increased deposition of glycosaminoglycans, collagen turnover, and expression of transforming growth factor-β1 and other signaling molecules (Oyama and Levy, 2010). Further research into the role that serotonin pathways play in the pathogenesis of the valvular remodeling accompanying CVHD is ongoing.

In addition to valvular abnormalities, many dogs with CVHD have histopathologic lesions in the myocardium, including small foci of myocardial fibrosis and necrosis, as well as more widespread intramural coronary arteriosclerosis (Falk et al, 2006). The role that arteriosclerosis, myocardial fibrosis, and microinfarction resulting from occlusion of these arteriosclerotic lesions might play

in the progression toward ventricular dilation, systolic dysfunction, and CHF is not well understood at this time, but these lesions seem to offer possible alternative avenues for investigation as treatment or interventional opportunities.

Progressive valvular thickening leads to poor leaflet coaptation and worsening valvular regurgitation with progressive dilation and eccentric hypertrophy of the atria and ventricles. As the regurgitant fraction increases, forward cardiac output may diminish, and compensatory neurohumoral pathways are activated (e.g., adrenergic activation, enhanced renin-angiotensin-aldosterone system activity) in an attempt to restore blood pressure and maintain tissue perfusion. As long as the dilated left atrium remains sufficiently compliant to accept the regurgitant blood volume, CHF does not develop, although coughing may occur due to left main-stem bronchial compression. Increased left ventricular filling pressure eventually precipitates CHF as the volume of regurgitated blood becomes overwhelming; chordal rupture suddenly increases the regurgitant fraction; and the limits of left atrial or ventricular compliance are exceeded, or the left ventricular myocardium starts to fail. Atrial rhythm disturbances, including atrial fibrillation, also can contribute to cardiac dysfunction and precipitation of CHF. The onset of decompensated CHF typically is manifested by the development of pulmonary edema in mitral valve disease. Chronic left-sided heart failure often leads to postcapillary pulmonary hypertension (PHTN), which further strains the right side of the heart and leads to signs of right-sided CHF with accumulation of ascitic fluid and possibly pleural effusion. In some dogs, there is evidence of severe PHTN beyond that explained simply by elevated pulmonary venous pressures.

Clinical Evaluation of Dogs with Chronic Valvular Disease

CVHD is identified most commonly in middle-aged or older dogs of small to medium-sized breeds. Although primary valvular disease also occurs in large-breed dogs, dilated cardiomyopathy is a more common cause of CHF in these breeds than is CVHD. When large-breed dogs develop CVHD, concurrent myocardial failure, evidenced by global systolic dysfunction and inadequate left ventricular hypertrophy, often is noted relatively early in the disease. The incidence of CVHD is higher in male dogs than in females (1.5 : 1).

Clinical Presentations in Chronic Valvular Disease

Most dogs are first diagnosed with CVHD based on the finding of a cardiac murmur in the absence of any signs of cardiac decompensation. The period between first detection of a murmur and onset of clinical signs generally is years. As the disease advances, many dogs develop a cough as the first sign of CVHD, caused by either early CHF or left atrial enlargement leading to main-stem bronchial compression. Panting, dyspnea, exercise intolerance, weight loss, weakness, and syncope are additional causes for a visit to a veterinarian. Specific triggers that cause a sharp increase in fluid retention or decrease in cardiac performance may precipitate CHF. These include increased dietary intake of salty foods, vigorous exercise or exertion in the previous 48 hours, recent onset of a rapid tachyarrhythmia, overzealous fluid therapy, general anesthesia, and potentially glucocorticoid administration.

Evaluation of Asymptomatic Dogs with a Heart Murmur

Many dogs with CVHD have an audible murmur for years before the onset of cardiac decompensation and CHF (see Table 177-1 for the American College of Cardiology/American Heart Association [ACC/AHA] staging classification). An extra systolic sound known as a *midsystolic click* is often detected before the onset of this murmur and has been associated with mitral or tricuspid valve prolapse; this is a sign of early CVHD. With rare exceptions, clinically significant CVHD is accompanied by a holosystolic murmur of medium to loud intensity. Point of maximal murmur intensity is over the left apex with radiation dorsally and to the right in most cases. In most dogs the intensity of the murmur is correlated roughly with the severity of mitral regurgitation (MR) as long as arterial blood pressure is normal. Thus in dogs with soft murmurs of MR the volume of regurgitation is unlikely to result in clinical signs; however, once a loud murmur is present, one cannot readily predict the onset of CHF in a given dog.

TABLE 177-1

Modified ACC/AHA Classification Scheme

ACC/AHA Stage	Patient Population
Stage A	Patient at high risk of developing heart disease with no current identifiable structural cardiac abnormality (e.g., Cavalier King Charles spaniels with no cardiac murmur)
Stage B	Patients with structural cardiac disease but no past or present clinical signs of heart failure *Stage B1:* Asymptomatic patients with no echocardiographic or radiographic evidence of cardiac remodeling *Stage B2:* Asymptomatic patients with echocardiographic or radiographic evidence of cardiac enlargement
Stage C	Patients with past or present clinical signs of heart failure secondary to structural cardiac disease
Stage D	Patients with end-stage heart failure that are refractory to standard therapies (high-dose furosemide, ACE-I, and pimobendan)

Modified from Atkins C et al: ACVIM consensus statement: guidelines for the diagnosis and treatment of canine chronic valvular heart disease, *J Vet Intern Med* 23:1142, 2009; and Hunt SA et al: ACC/AHA guidelines for the evaluation and management of chronic heart failure in the adult: executive summary: a report of the American College of Cardiology/American Heart Association Task Force on Practice Guidelines (Committee to revise the 1995 Guidelines for the Evaluation and Management of Heart Failure). *J Am Coll Cardiol* 38:2101, 2001.

When a murmur is auscultated in a dog without clinical signs, baseline testing can be offered to the owner and often is helpful for comparison at subsequent examinations (see Table 177-2 for American College of Veterinary Internal Medicine [ACVIM] consensus recommendations on diagnostic testing). At a minimum the client should be clearly informed of the presence of the murmur and the fact that the disease ultimately may progress to CHF. Baseline testing ideally should include thoracic radiography to assess for cardiomegaly and optimally echocardiography to confirm the diagnosis and help assess cardiac size and function. A baseline B-type natriuretic peptide or N-terminal prohormone B-type natriuretic peptide (NT-proBNP) level also may be helpful in disease staging, and an NT-proBNP concentration above 1500 pmol/L indicates a higher chance of cardiac decompensation in the next 6 to 12 months. A blood pressure measurement is indicated to exclude systemic hypertension, which might accelerate progression of MR. If hypertension is identified, an underlying cause such as renal or adrenal disease should be sought. Baseline laboratory evaluation should include, at a minimum, assessment of hematocrit, total solids, serum creatinine level, and urinalysis. However, a complete blood count, full serum chemistry analysis, urinalysis, and possible urine protein:creatinine ratio are recommended in hypertensive animals or dogs with other signs of systemic disease.

Evaluation of Dogs with Signs of Cardiac Dysfunction

Once heart failure develops, a range of clinical presentations are possible, related to the degree and duration of valvular dysfunction. In an acute setting clinical signs usually are pulmonary or behavioral and may include cough, tachypnea, retching or gagging, nocturnal dyspnea, orthopnea or reluctance to settle down, and sometimes either excessive clinginess or social isolation. Less commonly, abdominal distention from ascites may be present, or the client may detect a "racing heart." Exertional collapse or syncope may be the initial sign of heart disease and can occur as a result of significant arrhythmias, secondary to low cardiac output, in association with a vasovagal reflex (neurocardiogenic) response, or following a coughing spell (tussive syncope). In our experience syncope can be seen at the time of the initial presentation of heart failure, and syncope in this setting likely has a reflex-mediated or vasovagal component. Moderate to severe PHTN also has been associated with syncope in dogs with CVHD. Some dogs exhibit decreased exercise tolerance and weight loss for weeks to months before the onset of CHF, but these are often overlooked and rarely are the cause of a trip to a veterinarian.

Physical Examination

Pulmonary auscultation may reveal loud bronchovesicular sounds that can progress to pulmonary crackles with the onset of alveolar edema. The latter may be particularly prominent over the hilar or caudal lung fields on inspiration. Hepatomegaly and ascites may be evident in dogs with right-sided CHF from advanced tricuspid

TABLE **177-2**

2009 ACVIM Consensus Recommendations for the Diagnosis and Treatment of Canine Chronic Valvular Heart Disease

Modified ACC/AHA Classification	Diagnosis	Treatment
Stage A	• Yearly auscultation of small-breed dogs at risk of CVHD • Yearly screening by a cardiologist for breeding animals or those at very high risk	• No drug therapy • No dietary therapy • Remove from breeding program those animals with early onset (<6-8 years of age) mitral regurgitation
Stage B	• Baseline thoracic radiographs • Blood pressure measurement • Echocardiography in large dogs; also consider in small dogs if radiographs and auscultation findings inconclusive • Baseline laboratory work (HCT, TS, serum creatinine, and UA at minimum)	*B1* • No drug or dietary therapy • Reevaluate via echocardiography or thoracic radiographs in 12 months *B2* • No consensus on use of ACE-I, β-blockers, or dietary modification

Stage C	• CHF diagnosis based on review of:
	  • Signalment and physical examination
	  • Thoracic radiographs
	  • Echocardiogram
	  • Basic labwork
	• Presence of a typical mitral murmur in a coughing dog is *not* sufficient to diagnose CHF
	• Obtain baseline CBC/Chem/UA
		Acute Therapy
		• Furosemide to effect
		  • 1-4 mg/kg repeated bolus dosing
		  • 1 mg/kg/min CRI after initial bolus for life-threatening CHF
		  • Free access to H₂O
		• Pimobendan: 0.25-0.3 mg/kg PO q12h
		• Oxygen supplementation
		• Remove effusions if contributing to respiratory distress
		• Sedation for anxious patients (e.g., butorphanol, buprenorphine, low-dose acepromazine)
		• Sodium nitroprusside CRI for ≤ 48 hr for life-threatening pulmonary edema
		Chronic Therapy
		• Titrate oral furosemide dosing to effect to maintain patient comfort (1-2 mg/kg PO q12h for mild CHF, up to 4-6 mg/kg PO q8h for severe CHF)
		  • Monitor renal values and electrolytes
		• Continue or start ACE-I (e.g., Enalapril 0.5 mg/kg q12h or equivalent dose of other ACE-I)
		  • Monitor creatinine and electrolytes after 3-7 days
		• Continue pimobendan–0.25-0.3 mg/kg PO q 12h
		• β-Blockers should *not* be started in the face of active CHF

Stage D	• Same diagnostic recommendations for Stage C, plus finding of failure to respond to standard therapies outlined for Stage C	*Acute Therapy*
		• See *Stage* C recommendations: continue ACE-I and pimobendan
		• Administer additional furosemide in absence of severe azotemia
		• Vigorous afterload reduction if tolerated
		  • Nitroprusside: start at 0.5-1 µg/kg/min
		  • Amlodipine: 0.05-0.1 mg/kg PO
		  • Hydralazine: 0.5-2 mg/kg PO
		  • Maintain systolic BP >85 mm Hg or MAP >60
		  • Measure serum creatinine before and after 24-72 hr
		• Consider mechanical ventilation
		Chronic Therapy
		• Up-titrate furosemide dose as needed to decrease signs of congestion, if use not limited by renal azotemia
		  • Monitor creatinine 12-48 hr after dose increases
		• Start or continue spironolactone (0.25-2.0 mg/kg PO q12-24h)
		• Avoid β-blockade in the presence of congestive signs

regurgitation (TR) or mitral disease with postcapillary PHTN. Jugular venous distention is commonly appreciated in dogs with ascites. Often the femoral pulses are easily palpated and prominent, even at the time of onset of CHF. Irregularities in pulse rate and strength may be noted in association with an arrhythmia. In animals with CHF the heart rate usually is elevated or in the upper-normal range, and sinus arrhythmia typically is absent, although this is variable. The ventricular apex beat is hyperdynamic and is progressively shifted caudally from the fifth intercostal space with increasing disease severity. If present, a precordial thrill also is palpable over the left apex. A louder murmur or more pronounced thrill on the right hemithorax typically indicates concurrent TR and PHTN. There may be a left ventricular heave or apical thrust. There may be other abnormalities since most CVHD patients are geriatric; therefore a complete physical examination is warranted.

Thoracic Radiography

Thoracic radiographs are *essential* to the management of CVHD. The earliest characteristic findings on thoracic radiographs are mild left ventricular enlargement and left atrial enlargement, which may be best noted as an auricular prominence on the dorsoventral view at the 2- to 3-o'clock position. Left atrial and left ventricular enlargement elevate the trachea and carina on the lateral radiographic projection, with a decrease in the angle between the trachea and the thoracic spine. The left main-stem bronchus may become elevated and compressed in cases of moderate to severe left atrial enlargement. There is straightening of the caudal cardiac border and loss of the caudal cardiac waist. Pulmonary venous dilation occurs; this finding may be best appreciated in the cranial lung fields in the lateral view. Distended pulmonary veins (and arteries in severe cases) also can be identified in the caudal lung fields on the dorsoventral or ventrodorsal projections. Early pulmonary edema is seen as a diffuse increase in interstitial density in the hilar or caudal lung fields, progressing to perihilar densities with air bronchograms corresponding to alveolar edema. Cardiogenic pulmonary edema appears to have a propensity for the right caudal lung fields in some dogs, and this finding may be noted on the dorsoventral view. With TR and right-sided or biventricular CHF, the cranial aspect of the trachea may be elevated, the caudal vena cava increases in size, and small-volume pleural effusion may be noted.

Not only is radiographic evaluation useful for monitoring cardiac chamber size and documenting CHF, but it also serves to guide therapy and exclude other disorders. Pneumonia can develop in an older dog with CVHD and CHF; thus, in a patient with new signs or a poor response to therapy, infection or another problem such as lung cancer should be considered. Chronic bronchitis also is common in many dogs with CVHD and occasionally can be recognized by the presence of severe bronchial patterns or bronchiectasis. The rate of increase in vertebral heart score has been shown to accelerate in the 6 to 12 months before the onset of CHF; thus sequential monitoring of radiographs may be helpful in predicting impending heart failure (Figure 177-2).

Electrocardiography

Electrocardiographic findings can include evidence of left ventricular hypertrophy, widened P waves of left atrial enlargement (P mitrale), and, infrequently, P pulmonale (P wave > 0.4 mV). P pulmonale is seen more frequently in dogs with concurrent respiratory disease. ST-segment slurring or depression, which may result from myocardial disease, ischemia, or hypoxia, is evident in some dogs

with left ventricular hypertrophy. Sinus rhythm or sinus tachycardia is typical of dogs with CVHD and CHF. Atrial arrhythmias, especially atrial premature depolarizations, are common. Atrial fibrillation develops in some dogs with marked atrial enlargement. On the other hand, ventricular arrhythmias are relatively uncommon in animals with compensated disease, and even in dogs with CHF ventricular ectopy is far less common than in animals with dilated cardiomyopathy.

Echocardiography

Echocardiography is valuable in assessing cardiac structure and function, although thoracic radiography is more useful in identifying CHF. Valvular thickening and valvular prolapse into the atria can be appreciated early in the course of disease (Figure 177-3, *A*). Rupture of a chorda tendinea leads to a flail mitral leaflet with chaotic valve motion and complete eversion of a tip of the leaflet into the left atrium in systole. With advancing disease the valve becomes progressively thickened, and left atrial and left ventricular enlargement are noted. With severe MR the left atrium enlarges disproportionately to the left ventricle.

Left ventricular systolic function can be difficult to assess accurately in dogs with CVHD and severe MR (Bonagura and Schober, 2009). Fractional shortening is normal or increased in the early stages of the disease and increases with increasing regurgitant fraction. With the onset of myocardial failure fractional shortening can move from hyperdynamic to the normal range and may even become decreased. The latter two findings are more often noted in large-breed dogs. The left ventricular free wall often develops a relatively reduced excursion compared with the septum (the opposite of the situation in normal dogs).

Although left atrial size is a better objective measure of severity of chronic MR, Doppler methods also can be used. The location and extent of the regurgitant jet can be mapped using color flow Doppler echocardiography as a crude indicator of disease severity (Figure 177-3, *B*). Additional Doppler methods such as semiquantitative assessment of the MR jet area in relation to the left atrial area or evaluation of the proximal isovelocity surface area may permit more accurate estimation of the regurgitant flow fraction using color Doppler methods. However, each of these methods is imperfect, especially when considered in isolation. Doppler studies of transmitral flow velocities and tissue Doppler imaging are used in the evaluation of systolic and diastolic function and prediction of left ventricular filling pressures; however, these are also confounded by the presence of volume overload. In general, a peak transmitral E-wave velocity of more than 1.2 m/sec in the setting of an enlarged left atrium is indicative of severe MR and considered a negative prognostic indicator (Borgarelli et al, 2008).

Frequently there is concurrent evidence of tricuspid valve disease. This can include tricuspid prolapse, valvular thickening, and Doppler imaging evidence of TR. High-velocity TR is a marker for PHTN, which can become severe in some dogs with CVHD. Pericardial effusion related to right-sided CHF or left atrial tear is observed

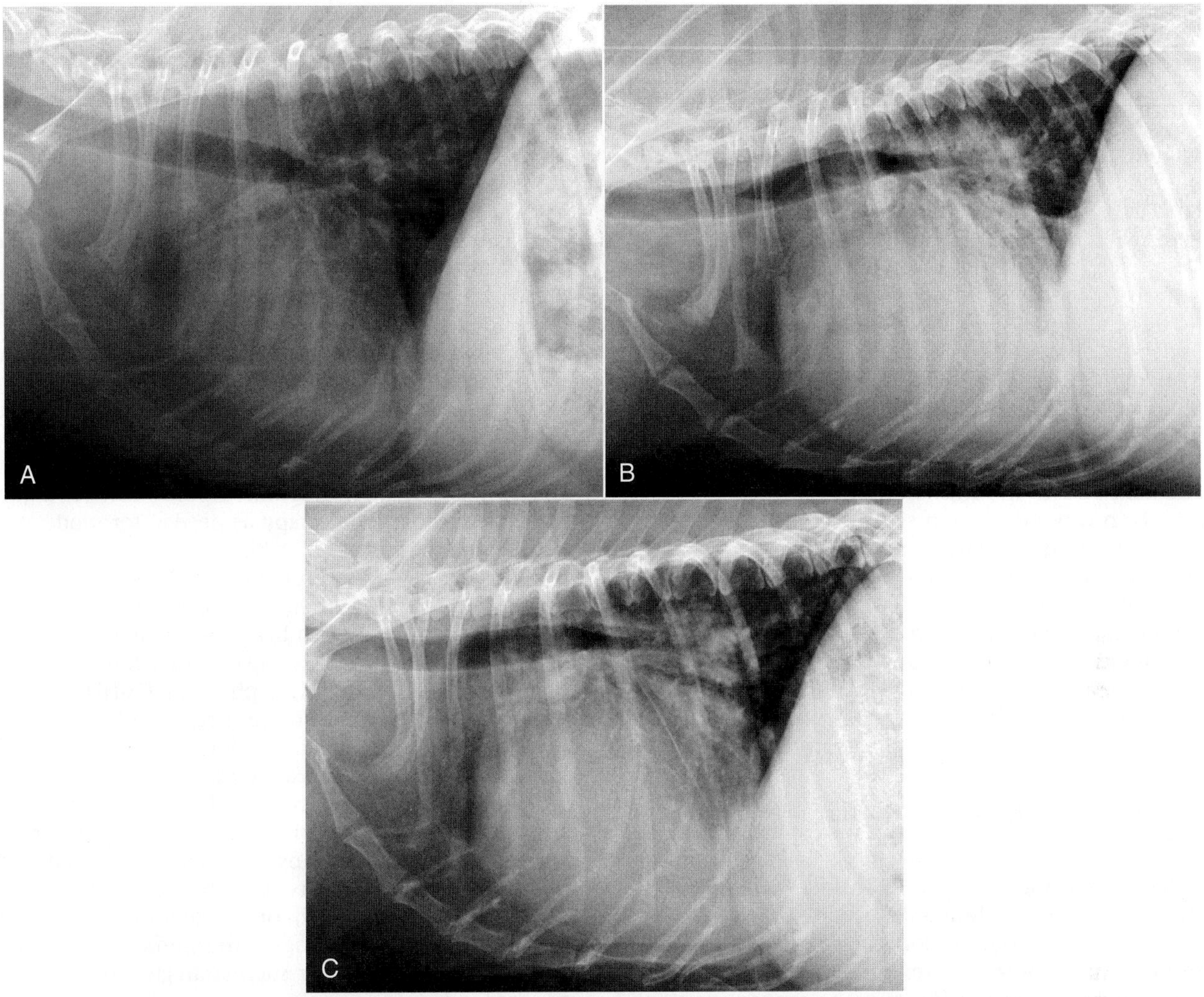

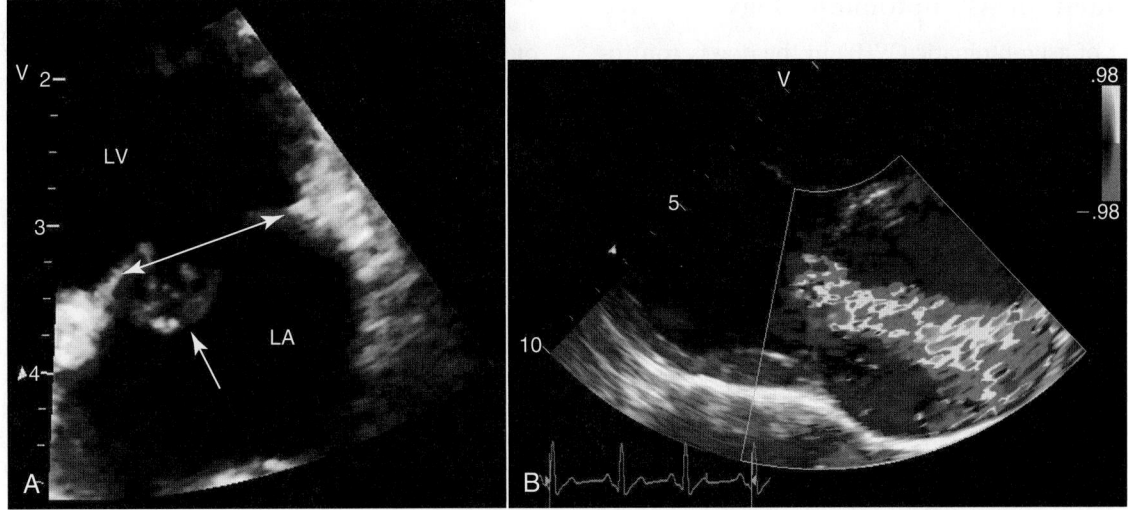

Figure 177-2 A to **C,** Serial thoracic radiographs taken from a dog with mitral and tricuspid chronic valvular heart disease. Note the progressive increase in cardiac size, elevation of the trachea, and compression of the left main-stem bronchus. Perihilar infiltrates and a pleural fissure line can be visualized in **C.**

Figure 177-3 A, 2D echocardiogram from a dog with severe mitral valve prolapse secondary to chronic valvular heart disease. The white arrow is pointing to the anterior mitral leaflet, which is bulging into the left atrium during systole. **B,** Color flow Doppler demonstrating a large jet of mitral insufficiency extending to the dorsal wall of the LA. *LA,* Left atrium; *LV,* left ventricle.

occasionally on echocardiography (see the later section on left atrial tear or splitting).

Biomarkers

Natriuretic peptides, including B-type natriuretic peptide (BNP) and atrial natriuretic peptide (ANP) and their N-terminal propeptide segments (NT-proBNP and NT-proANP), are released in response to ventricular and atrial stretch, and the levels of these peptides increase progressively with worsening disease severity and onset of CHF. Studies have documented that levels of these peptides are elevated in dogs with CVHD and CHF and increase progressively as the heart enlarges (Oyama et al, 2008). Natriuretic peptides hold great promise for early identification of patients at risk of developing CHF (e.g., NT-proBNP > 1500 pmol/L indicates higher risk of CHF in the next 6 to 12 months) and for confirmation of the diagnosis in those dogs with signs consistent with CHF. Natriuretic peptide levels also may offer some prognostic information as stand-alone tests or in conjunction with other clinical, imaging, or laboratory findings. It remains to be seen whether these hormones can be used to assist in treatment decisions or evaluate response to therapy. Commercial assays are currently available for canine BNP and NT-proBNP, and in-house (point-of-care) natriuretic peptide testing may become available in the near future.

Treatment of Chronic Valvular Heart Disease

The therapy for dogs with CVHD includes consideration of the patient with preclinical disease and the dog coughing from bronchial compression, the need for both short-term in-hospital and long-term at-home treatment plans for the dog with overt CHF, and the management of additional complications of this disorder. See Table 177-2 for ACVIM consensus recommendations on the treatment of CVHD at various stages of the disease.

Management of Asymptomatic Dogs

Treatment of asymptomatic CVHD in the dog is controversial. Although angiotensin-converting enzyme (ACE) inhibitors are useful in the treatment of overt CHF, the Scandinavian Veterinary Enalapril Project (SVEP) trial evaluating the use of the ACE inhibitor enalapril in asymptomatic cavalier King Charles spaniels failed to show a significant preventive benefit in terms of delaying onset of CHF (Kvart et al, 2002). However, the recently reported Veterinary Enalapril Trial to Prove Reduction in Onset of Heart Failure in Dogs (VETPROOF) suggested a possible modest long-term survival benefit for enalapril therapy in dogs with advanced mitral disease treated before the onset of CHF (Atkins et al, 2007). Clearly, more studies are needed before definitive recommendations can be made. In view of the results of these studies most cardiologists do not initiate therapy in small-breed dogs with chronic MR in the absence of significant cardiomegaly. Some clinicians initiate ACE inhibitor therapy in animals with preclinical disease when there is moderate to severe heart enlargement or when marked progressive

cardiac enlargement is observed on serial examinations. However, this therapy still is considered empiric, and there is no unanimity about such treatment.

Aside from the controversy noted previously, there may be some other reasons to consider ACE inhibition in CVHD. For example, in larger-breed dogs with MR, cardioprotective therapy with an ACE inhibitor with or without a β-blocker may be reasonable, especially when there is evidence of volume overload, because progressive left ventricular dilation and systolic dysfunction are more common in this patient group. A dog with left atrial enlargement that is coughing from presumed bronchial compression may benefit from ACE inhibitor therapy (or an ACE inhibitor and a low-dose diuretic, pimobendan, or cough suppressant). In dogs with CVHD and concurrent systemic hypertension the hypertension should be managed; ACE inhibitors generally are selected first in this particular setting, with amlodipine added for adjunctive antihypertensive therapy as needed for moderate to severe hypertension.

β-Blockers are dangerous to initiate in dogs with uncontrolled CHF, but there may be a role for these drugs in dogs with compensated heart failure or asymptomatic disease. There certainly is some enthusiasm for the use of β-blockers in the preclinical phase of CVHD based on extrapolation of results of research studies in canine models of volume overload. However, clinical studies documenting a clear clinical benefit in dogs with spontaneous CVHD are still ongoing, and evidence of benefit in this disease is lacking at the current time, with a recent study of bisoprolol failing to demonstrate favorable effects. When a β-blocker is prescribed, most cardiologists use carvedilol, bisoprolol, or metoprolol (see Chapter 175). Again, large-breed dogs with significant CVHD may be the best candidates for such strategies to protect the myocardium.

Severe dietary sodium restriction is not recommended in dogs with asymptomatic CVHD because of the potential for early activation of the renin-angiotensin-aldosterone system. However, client education on avoidance of high-sodium diets, treats, and table foods is important. One study evaluating the use of a novel diet for management of dogs with asymptomatic CVHD identified a reduction in cardiac size during the 4-week dietary trial, which demonstrates the impact of dietary sodium on plasma volume and cardiac size (Freeman et al, 2006). Studies that document a clear clinical benefit such as a delay in the onset of CHF or improved survival are lacking; thus firm dietary recommendations cannot be made at this time.

Management of Dogs with Congestive Heart Failure

Once CHF develops, many options are available for patient management (see Chapter 176 and Table 177-2). The patient with severe pulmonary edema requires aggressive diuresis. Oxygen administration and sedation (e.g., butorphanol 0.1 to 0.2 mg/kg IM as needed) are helpful supplements in treatment of hospitalized patients. Some clinicians use topical 2% nitroglycerin as a venodilator for dogs in the hospital setting, but efficacy data for this approach are lacking. Sodium nitroprusside is useful in cases of life-threatening pulmonary edema caused by ruptured chordae tendineae (see the section on chordae tendineae rupture later in the chapter). Once in stable condition, most dogs are treated with a combination of oral drugs in the home setting to prevent recurrence of CHF, minimize clinical signs, and prolong life.

Furosemide is the most commonly used diuretic, and the dose is titrated to effect (i.e., to control clinical signs resulting from fluid accumulation). In patients with severe pulmonary edema, intravenous boluses of 1 to 4 mg/kg of furosemide are indicated, and some clinicians transition from bolus dosing to a constant-rate infusion of furosemide at 0.5 to 2 mg/kg/hr for particularly severe or refractory cases. The dose of furosemide required to clear significant edema accumulations and cause the animal to be minimally symptomatic (the desired dose) is often close to that resulting in electrolyte disturbances, dehydration, and the development of prerenal azotemia. Dosages of furosemide can vary from 2 mg/kg/day in mild CHF to 4 to 6 mg/kg every 8 hours in advanced disease. Azotemia and electrolyte imbalance can result from the combined use of ACE inhibitors and diuretics; thus serial monitoring of the appropriate laboratory parameters is indicated. Baseline levels of blood urea nitrogen (BUN), creatinine, and serum electrolytes should be obtained, with rechecks of these values 3 to 7 days after starting these drugs and 3 to 7 days after any significant dosage adjustment, followed by routine evaluation every 3 to 6 months.

ACE inhibitors combined with diuretics may not be well tolerated in some dogs with preexisting renal disease; thus careful monitoring of clinical signs (appetite and activity) and more frequent assessment of electrolyte, BUN, and creatinine levels are advisable in these patients. The development of acute renal failure with the initiation of ACE inhibitor therapy should prompt reconsideration of this treatment because some dogs simply cannot tolerate the usual dosages of these drugs, especially when undergoing diuresis. Some of these dogs respond favorably to discontinuation of the ACE inhibitor and judicious volume expansion with 0.45% NaCl solution. Once the animal is in stable condition, acceptable renal values can be maintained in some dogs by using low-dose ACE inhibition combined with standard medical therapy.

Several clinical trials in dogs with CVHD and CHF have demonstrated the clinical benefits of ACE inhibitors in reducing clinical signs or delaying the time until clinical deterioration or death (Woodfield et al, 1995). Drugs such as enalapril, lisinopril, or benazepril can be initiated in the hospital or home setting. A full dosage of these drugs generally is considered to be 0.5 mg/kg every 12 hours PO, but many clinicians initiate therapy at one half that dosage and optimize to a full dosage at the time of first or subsequent follow-up. Measurement of blood pressure and renal function often is used to monitor treatment.

Pimobendan (Vetmedin), a calcium sensitizer and phosphodiesterase inhibitor, is an effective drug for management of CHF, and this drug is associated with minimal adverse effects. The positive inotropic and mixed vasodilator properties of pimobendan result in improved control of CHF and clinical signs of heart failure. Pimobendan does not appear to have significant proarrhythmic properties at commonly used clinical dosages. Several small clinical trials have documented that pimobendan combined with diuretic therapy is at least as effective as furosemide and ACE inhibitors and may have fewer adverse effects than many of the commonly used cardiovascular medications. The larger Quality of Life and Extension of Survival Time (QUEST) Trial demonstrated a distinct survival advantage to treatment with pimobendan and furosemide relative to treatment with benazepril and furosemide in dogs with CVHD (Haggstrom et al, 2008). However, no studies have evaluated the efficacy of combined therapy with pimobendan, furosemide, and an ACE inhibitor, the treatment approach advanced by the vast majority of cardiologists. Cardiologists hold some differing opinions on the role that pimobendan plays in the management of CHF in dogs with CVHD. Some believe that initial management of CHF should center on furosemide and pimobendan, whereas others opt for furosemide with an ACE inhibitor. In our practice, and in the ACVIM consensus statement, the initial treatment strategy for dogs with CVHD and well-defined CHF includes combined triple therapy with furosemide, pimobendan, and an ACE inhibitor (with or without spironolactone).

As cardiac disease progresses, additional medications will be required to control advancing CHF. This therapy may include a dose escalation of furosemide; administration of supplemental doses of furosemide by subcutaneous injection every 12 to 48 hours; addition of other diuretics to combat diuretic resistance; treatment with digoxin or antiarrhythmics as necessary; and various dietary manipulations. Diuretic resistance typically is defined as the need for dosages of furosemide in excess of 4 to 6 mg/kg/day to control congestive signs during long-term treatment of CHF (ACC/AHA stage D heart failure). In this situation the addition of spironolactone (1 to 2 mg/kg once or twice daily PO) or a combination of hydrochlorothiazide and spironolactone is recommended. If hydrochlorothiazide is prescribed, initial dosages should be conservative (0.5 to 1 mg/kg q12-24h PO) and renal function and electrolytes should be evaluated within 3 to 7 days. Another diuretic that may be added in severe CHF is the potent loop diuretic torsemide. Torsemide is approximately 10 times more potent than furosemide, has a longer half-life, and has ancillary aldosterone-antagonizing effects. The initial dose typically is one tenth of the furosemide dose that would be added. In addition to diuretic "stacking," careful investigation to identify other causes of fluid retention, such as high-sodium diets or treats or glucocorticoid therapy, is indicated in patients with apparent diuretic resistance. Nonsteroidal antiinflammatory drugs also have been implicated in the development of diuretic resistance in people, but this has not been documented in dogs with CVHD.

Digoxin still has some role in the management of CVHD, although it has largely been supplanted by newer drugs with fewer adverse effects. There is no consensus on the use of cardiac glycosides in dogs with CVHD; however, in cases of CHF with atrial fibrillation or CVHD with frequent or sustained supraventricular arrhythmias, digoxin should be considered. In addition, digoxin may be useful in the management of syncope in dogs with CVHD when no clear cause for collapse (e.g., arrhythmia or severe PHTN) can be established. Digoxin toxicosis leading to anorexia, depression, and gastrointestinal signs has the potential to contribute to a decision for euthanasia, and the narrow therapeutic window for digitalis glycosides predisposes to its occurrence. Serial monitoring of serum digoxin levels is advisable, with target serum concentrations 8 hours after dosing in the range of 0.8 to 1.2 mg/ml. The combination of digoxin and diltiazem has been shown to be more effective in controlling the ventricular response rate to atrial fibrillation than either agent used alone (see Chapter 171). Thus, for dogs with persistently rapid ventricular response rates, either extended-release diltiazem or a β-blocker may be required in addition to digoxin to reduce the heart rate to less than 160 beats/min during the recheck examination. Amiodarone also has been demonstrated to reduce the ventricular response rate to atrial fibrillation; however, in our practice this drug is not recommended as first-line therapy in this setting because of concerns about the potential for multiple organ toxicities and relative lack of efficacy for rate reduction or conversion to sinus rhythm.

β-Blockade has gained favor as a therapeutic modality for treatment of CHF in human patients, and several studies have documented the benefits that accrue from long-term treatment, although these effects often are not seen for several months. Reported benefits include up-regulation of previously down-regulated β-receptors, improved cardiac performance (increased stroke volume), and improved survival. These clinical benefits appear to have a sound theoretic basis, but there is no consensus among cardiologists about the use of β-blockers in dogs with CVHD, and in the ACVIM survey (and two surveys of cardiologists) β-blockers are not considered standard therapy. Carvedilol is tolerated by many dogs with naturally occurring CHF caused by both cardiomyopathy and CVHD when started at a low dose that is then slowly increased. Since β-blockers are negative inotropes, their most demonstrable effect when used in dogs with active CHF is likely to be a worsening of CHF. The negative inotropic and chronotropic effects of β-blockers can be harmful to dogs with active heart failure and those at the edge of compensation. If used at all, β-blockers are best administered to patients that are minimally symptomatic with early or mild heart failure and those with later stages of CHF in which the disease already is well controlled by a stable cardiac drug regimen (see Chapter 175 for more details). Carvedilol, metoprolol, bisoprolol, and atenolol all have been used for cardioprotection in dogs with CVHD, but carvedilol may have some advantages because of its concurrent α-blockade (which lowers vascular resistance), potent antioxidant effects, and more convenient dosing formulations. If metoprolol is used, the extended-release formulation is recommended for twice-daily administration. Addition of any β-blocker in a dog with advanced cardiac disease or congestive heart failure must be undertaken cautiously. Our recommendation is that a cardiologist should be consulted before initiating this form of treatment.

Moderate dietary sodium restriction also is important in the management of dogs with CVHD. The owners of asymptomatic dogs with CVHD and cardiac enlargement should be counseled to avoid feeding diets high in sodium as well as to avoid giving treats or table food (or any foods used to administer medications) high in sodium. For dogs with advanced disease but no signs of cardiac failure, the selected diet should have a sodium content of less than 100 mg/100 kcal of energy. Once CHF develops, additional sodium restriction is recommended (<80 mg/100 kcal). This does not necessarily require use of a commercial cardiac diet, and care should be taken to avoid diets designed for dogs with renal disease or cardiac diets that are excessively low in protein (e.g., many of the diets formulated for kidney disease) since these can contribute to loss of muscle mass and cardiac cachexia. As CHF progresses, stricter dietary sodium restriction may allow the use of lower dosages of diuretics to control clinical signs. A variety of other dietary considerations may be important in individual cases. Some diets are designed to contain or are supplemented with various levels of certain nutrients such as potassium, magnesium, taurine, L-carnitine, arginine, antioxidants, or omega-3 fatty acids (see Chapter 168).

Exercise restriction in cases of severe CHF is essential; however, controlled exercise in dogs with stable chronic heart failure often is well tolerated and improves quality-of-life scores. Repetitive or strenuous activities such as ball chasing and running should be restricted once advanced heart disease or serious arrhythmias develop.

Clinical Complications and Challenges

Cough in Dogs with Concurrent Chronic Valvular Disease and Respiratory Disease

The cause of a cough can be difficult to determine in dogs with concurrent cardiac and respiratory disease, and the presence of a typical mitral murmur in a coughing dog does *not* necessarily indicate CHF. Body condition can provide a clue inasmuch as dogs coughing from primary pulmonary disease often are overweight or have no history of weight loss, whereas weight loss or cardiac cachexia are more common with CHF.

Many dogs with tracheobronchial disease demonstrate tracheal sensitivity, a very productive cough, or a cough of long duration (often longer than 2 to 4 months). Auscultation frequently indicates only a soft murmur or no murmur at all, which argues strongly against a diagnosis of heart failure from CVHD. In contrast, most dogs with a cardiac cough have a loud murmur, some weight loss, and a cough of more recent onset. Sinus arrhythmia is more common in dogs with respiratory disease, whereas dogs with CHF often have normal sinus rhythm, sinus tachycardia, or atrial arrhythmias. Both CHF and respiratory diseases such as chronic bronchitis and pulmonary fibrosis can cause crackles and wheezes on auscultation; thus the presence of these auscultatory findings rarely is a helpful discriminating factor.

Radiography is critical in the differential diagnosis of coughing in the dog with CVHD, and when necessary, a second opinion should be sought regarding the images. A radiographic series that includes a vertebral heart score measured when the dog was asymptomatic offers useful baseline information. A stable heart size (vertebral heart score) in a coughing dog with chronic MR argues against the diagnosis of CHF. In most cases, the first onset of CHF is associated with significant increases in cardiac size over baseline. The radiographic findings of pulmonary edema with interstitial to alveolar infiltrates in the perihilar regions, pulmonary venous prominence, and an enlarged left atrium support a diagnosis of CHF, especially when these abnormalities improve following diuresis. Marked left atrial enlargement may compress the main-stem bronchi and lead to cough; this cough often improves with therapy for heart failure, presumably due to a decrease in the size of the left atrium.

Dogs with primary respiratory disease often have right-sided heart enlargement and a lack of left atrial enlargement on thoracic radiographs. Measurement of BNP or NT-proBNP concentrations in the coughing dog can be helpful in discriminating between cardiac and noncardiac causes. Although BNP level may be elevated to a modest degree by PHTN accompanying respiratory disease, a marked elevation in BNP level is more consistent with a diagnosis of heart failure.

In some cases, it may be difficult to decide whether the cause of coughing is cardiac, respiratory, or both. In those cases the response to a short clinical trial of furosemide or medications for primary airway diseases (see Chapter 151) may be instructive about the underlying cause of signs.

Rupture of the Chordae Tendineae

Acute rupture of a chorda tendinea may lead to catastrophic heart failure and may be appreciated clinically by a marked change in the murmur intensity and sudden onset of pulmonary edema. Acute CHF develops because the left atrium is unable to increase its compliance rapidly enough to accommodate the acute increase in regurgitant volume. Historically, chordal rupture has been associated with a grave prognosis. However, a recent review (Serres et al, 2007) concluded that survival time of affected dogs was longer than previously described, with 58% of affected and aggressively treated dogs surviving longer than 1 year after diagnosis. It should be noted that cardiologists do not always agree with the echocardiographic criteria used in this study for the diagnosis of ruptured chordae tendineae; nevertheless, these data suggest that not all chordal ruptures are lethal and that it is very reasonable to undertake therapy. In addition to aggressive diuresis, oxygen therapy, and sedation as required, the use of sodium nitroprusside infusion at a rate of 1 to 5 μg/kg/min for 24 to 48 hours can be successful in immediate afterload reduction and management of catastrophic heart failure and severe pulmonary edema in dogs with CVHD. Infusion of nitroprusside generally is started at a low dose of 0.5 to 1 μg /kg/min and up-titrated according to clinical response, or to a target systolic blood pressure of approximately 90 to 95 mm Hg. Once the nitroprusside infusion is discontinued, the blood pressure should be reevaluated and amlodipine added at a dose of approximately 0.1 to 0.2 mg/kg every 24 hours PO as needed for sustained afterload reduction.

Left Atrial Tear or Splitting

Left atrial tear can result from atrial stretch due to MR and endocardial damage caused by the constant impingement of the mitral regurgitant jet on the left atrial endocardium. The weakened endocardium can split, and at times a full-thickness atrial tear may develop, allowing hemorrhage into the pericardial sac. The resultant cardiac tamponade may be fatal. Alternatively, a tear in the interatrial septum instead may result in an acquired atrial septal defect.

Treatment of left atrial tear involves aggressive lowering of left atrial pressure through preload reduction and, if tolerated, afterload reduction. Pericardiocentesis rarely is indicated unless tamponade is imminently life threatening. The volume of blood in the pericardial sac identified by echocardiography may be relatively small, and great care should be used when tapping the pericardium, especially from the left side, because the dilated left auricle is punctured easily. In dogs that are not already receiving pimobendan, it has been our practice to delay the initiation of pimobendan therapy for at least several days after the diagnosis of left atrial tear.

Pulmonary Hypertension

PHTN is defined as a resting systolic pulmonary artery pressure of more than 25 mm Hg. PHTN may occur in isolation (idiopathic or primary PHTN), secondary to pulmonary thromboembolism or chronic respiratory disease, as a result of long-standing left-to-right shunting, or due to left-sided CHF. PHTN often leads to syncope and signs of right-sided CHF such as ascites or pleural effusion, especially if concurrent TR is present. PHTN most often is diagnosed by noninvasive continuous wave Doppler echocardiography with application of the Bernoulli equation to the tricuspid regurgitant jet velocity:

$$\text{Pulmonary artery pressure} = (\text{peak velocity})^2 \times 4 + \text{estimated right atrial pressure}$$

where velocity is in meters per second. Other echocardiographic indicators of significant PHTN include dilation of the main pulmonary artery and right heart chambers, septal flattening, midsystolic notching of pulmonary artery flow profiles, and a shortened pulmonary artery acceleration time in relation to ejection time. Tissue Doppler echocardiographic evaluation of the right ventricular free wall also may provide early evidence of PHTN. Moderate PHTN is common in advanced CVHD and can be well tolerated, but severe PHTN generally is associated with a poor prognosis. Pimobendan may reduce pulmonary artery pressures in selected cases, especially if the primary cause of PHTN is left-sided CHF. Sildenafil (Viagra, Revatio) and tadalafil (Cialis) have been described as therapeutic options in both humans and dogs with PHTN. We currently add sildenafil (1 to 2 mg/kg q8-12h PO) or tadalafil (1 mg/kg q24h PO) to the treatment regimen of dogs with CVHD and severe PHTN (estimated systolic pulmonary artery pressures of >75 mm Hg) and of dogs with moderate PHTN (estimated systolic pulmonary artery pressures between 50 and 75 mm Hg) and unresolved syncope or tachypnea following radiographic resolution of pulmonary edema. It is important to recall that concurrent sildenafil and nitrate therapy theoretically is contraindicated because of the potential for severe hypotension and cardiovascular collapse. Currently, the off-label use of these drugs is quite expensive in most countries.

Surgical Intervention in Chronic Valvular Disease

Surgical procedures have been developed to repair or replace the mitral valve in dogs with CVHD. Cardiopulmonary bypass is required for these procedures. Successful cardiopulmonary bypass requires a dedicated team of surgeons, perfusionists, anesthesiologists, cardiologists, and intensive care specialists, and strong veterinary technician support. The cost associated with surgery can be prohibitive ($8000 to $15,000). Once these techniques are mastered and refined for veterinary medicine, it seems probable that surgery or emerging catheter-based interventions (or hybrid procedures) to limit MR will become the preferred treatment for those that can afford the procedure.

References and Suggested Reading

Atkins CE et al: Results of the veterinary enalapril trial to prove reduction in onset of heart failure in dogs chronically treated with enalapril alone for compensated, naturally occurring mitral valve insufficiency, *J Am Vet Med Assoc* 231:1061, 2007.

Bonagura JD, Schober KE: Can ventricular function be assessed by echocardiography in chronic canine mitral valve disease? *J Small Anim Pract* 50:12, 2009.

Borgarelli M et al: Survival characteristics and prognostic variables of dogs with mitral regurgitation attributable to myxomatous valve disease, *J Vet Intern Med* 22:120, 2008.

Falk T et al: Arteriosclerotic changes in the myocardium, lung and kidney of dogs with chronic congestive heart failure and myxomatous mitral valve disease, *Cardiovasc Pathol* 15:185, 2006.

Freeman LM, Rush JE, Markwell PJ: Effects of dietary modification in dogs with early chronic valvular disease, *J Vet Intern Med* 20:1116, 2006.

Griffins LG, Orton EC, Boon JA: Evaluation of techniques and outcomes of mitral valve repair in dogs, *J Am Vet Med Assoc* 224:1941, 2004.

Haggstrom J et al: Effect of pimobendan or benazepril hydrochloride on survival times in dogs with congestive heart failure caused by naturally occurring myxomatous mitral valve disease: the QUEST study, *J Vet Intern Med* 22:1124, 2008.

Kvart C et al: Efficacy of enalapril for prevention of congestive heart failure in dogs with myxomatous valve disease and symptomatic mitral regurgitation, *J Vet Intern Med* 16:80, 2002.

Oyama MA et al: Clinical utility of serum N-terminal pro-B-type natriuretic peptide concentration for identifying cardiac disease in dogs and assessing disease severity, *J Am Vet Med Assoc* 232:1496, 2008.

Oyama MA, Chittur SV: Genomic expression patterns of mitral valve tissues from dogs with degenerative mitral valve disease, *Am J Vet Res* 67:1307, 2006.

Oyama MA, Levy RJ: Insights into serotonin signaling mechanisms associated with canine degenerative mitral valve disease, *J Vet Intern Med* 24:27, 2010.

Rush JE et al: C-reactive protein concentration in dogs with chronic valvular disease, *J Vet Intern Med* 20:635, 2006.

Serres R et al: Chordae tendineae rupture in dogs with degenerative mitral valve disease: prevalence, survival and prognostic factors (114 cases, 2001-2006), *J Vet Intern Med* 21:258, 2007.

Woodfield JA et al: Acute and short-term hemodynamic, echocardiographic, and clinical effects of enalapril maleate in dogs with naturally acquired heart failure: results of the invasive multicenter PROspective Veterinary Evaluation of Enalapril study, *J Vet Intern Med* 9:234, 1995.

CHAPTER 178

Dilated Cardiomyopathy in Dogs

AMARA H. ESTRADA, *Gainesville, Florida*
HERBERT W. MAISENBACHER III, *Gainesville, Florida*

Dilated cardiomyopathy (DCM) is a myocardial disease characterized by primary systolic dysfunction of the left ventricle with secondary eccentric hypertrophy and left atrial dilation. Left ventricular diastolic dysfunction is identified in some dogs. The right heart chambers are variably involved in this disease. DCM is the most common myocardial disease in dogs and the second or third most common cause of acquired canine heart disease in most surveys, after degenerative valvular disease and heartworm disease (where *Dirofilaria immitis* is endemic). Although DCM begins with an asymptomatic phase, also called a *preclinical* or *occult* phase, of variable duration, it is a progressive and usually fatal disease that leads to congestive heart failure (CHF), arrhythmias, and often sudden cardiac death.

Causes

Most cases of DCM in dogs are considered idiopathic; however, it is recognized in both human and veterinary medicine that one or more factors can trigger the DCM phenotype of myocardial failure with cardiac chamber enlargement. Potential causes include genetic, infectious, immune-mediated, toxic, nutritional, and metabolic processes. The term *dilated* cardiomyopathy usually is reserved for idiopathic or familial forms. When a specific cause is identified, the appropriate modifier should be used instead, as in *taurine-deficiency* cardiomyopathy or *doxorubicin-induced* cardiomyopathy.

Several predisposed dog breeds exhibit a familial inheritance pattern of DCM, and a genetic basis is strongly suspected in these breeds. In humans, 20% to 50% of patients with idiopathic DCM are affected by a familial form, and mutations in more than 20 genes have been established as causes or risk factors (Hare, 2011). Based on known gene mutations in humans and molecular studies in affected dogs, a number of candidate genes have been evaluated in canine breeds affected with familial DCM. Until recently, no genetic markers for canine DCM had been identified. However, in 2010, Meurs and colleagues reported a mutation in Doberman pinschers in the gene that encodes pyruvate dehydrogenase kinase 4, a mitochondrial protein that regulates glucose metabolism. Undoubtedly, other genetic abnormalities will be discovered in the future, and these hold promise for identifying dogs at risk and for reducing the overall incidence of DCM in the canine population by modifying breeding practices.

Nutritional deficiencies have been associated with a DCM phenotype in dogs (see Chapter 168), but taurine-deficiency cardiomyopathy in dogs is very uncommon, and a response to L-carnitine supplementation is considered rare. Although viral and autoimmune factors have been postulated to be important causes of DCM in humans, there is little evidence to support an infectious (viral or other pathogenic) or immune-mediated cause of DCM in the majority of dogs. Toxic cardiomyopathies may be induced by anthracycline chemotherapeutic agents such as doxorubicin and may occur with newer tyrosine kinase inhibitors (TKIs), although this has not been reported with toceranib (Palladia), the only TKI labeled for veterinary use. It also is possible for persistent tachyarrhythmias to induce myocardial failure and ventricular dilation (tachycardia-induced cardiomyopathy). This is an important disorder to recognize because it is usually reversible with restoration of a sinus rhythm or adequate heart rate control.

Diagnosis

Clinical Presentation

DCM typically is an adult-onset disease of large- and giant-breed dogs, with the greatest prevalence in Doberman pinschers, Irish wolfhounds, Great Danes, and Newfoundlands. Other breeds that may be overrepresented include Scottish deerhounds, dalmatians, German shepherds, Saint Bernards, Airedales, standard poodles, and Old English sheepdogs. The disease generally is rare in small- and medium-breed dogs with the exception of American and English cocker spaniels, and juvenile forms are recognized in Portuguese water dogs and the toy Manchester terrier. Although historically boxers have been listed among the breeds predisposed to DCM, they most likely share a unique and familial disease process more accurately classified as arrhythmogenic right ventricular cardiomyopathy (see Chapter 179). Most studies have demonstrated an increased prevalence in male dogs compared with females. Most cases are diagnosed in dogs aged 4 to 9 years, and the incidence increases with age. However, it may be diagnosed in dogs as young as 2 years (and infrequently in even younger dogs). The specific juvenile form of DCM affecting Portuguese water dogs typically develops within the first 6 months of life.

As noted earlier, DCM is characterized by a prolonged asymptomatic phase, referred to as *preclinical or occult* DCM, which may last for up to 2 to 4 years. Once clinical signs develop, the disease is referred to as *overt* DCM. Clinical manifestations are attributable to left ventricular dysfunction, heart rhythm disturbances, or both. Initial clinical signs can be subtle, such as exercise intolerance or weight loss, and may go unrecognized except in athletic or working dogs. Most commonly, DCM is recognized when clinical signs of CHF develop. Left-sided CHF signs usually predominate and include cough, tachypnea, and dyspnea; with right-sided or biventricular CHF, ascites and pleural effusion also may occur. Ventricular arrhythmias can cause syncope and even sudden death. These may precede any other signs, and sudden cardiac death is especially common in Doberman pinschers compared with other breeds.

There is an interest in identifying and often treating DCM in the preclinical or occult phase, and a number of screening programs have been suggested, especially for breeding animals. Both ambulatory electrocardiographic (ECG), or Holter, monitoring and echocardiographic methods have been used to identify early disease in animals at risk. Some suggest that members of predisposed breeds should be screened annually beginning at 2 years of age. Early work suggests that the cardiac biomarker N-terminal prohormone B-type natriuretic peptide (NT-proBNP) may have some ability to detect preclinical disease, but further studies are needed to define the precise usefulness of this screening modality (Wess et al, 2011). In general, the adult onset of the disease makes genetic counseling to promote breeding of unaffected animals a significant challenge.

Physical Examination

Cardiac auscultation may reveal a low-grade systolic left apical murmur caused by mitral regurgitation, an S_3 gallop caused by increased left ventricular filling pressure, or arrhythmias. Soft heart sounds sometimes are detected, related to impaired ventricular contractility even in the absence of overt effusions. Similarly, murmurs of mitral regurgitation often are softer than those encountered in primary degenerative valvular disease of dogs.

Weak femoral pulses from reduced ventricular ejection or pulse deficits associated with arrhythmias may be palpated. With left-sided CHF, increased bronchovesicular sounds or pulmonary crackles may be auscultated, but the lack of these does not rule out the presence of pulmonary edema. Ascites, hepatomegaly, jugular venous distension or pulsation, and muffled lung sounds caused by pleural effusion may be present with right-sided or biventricular CHF.

Echocardiography

Echocardiography is the test of choice for the diagnosis of DCM in both the occult and overt phases. The diagnosis is established by identifying primary left ventricular systolic dysfunction, often with evidence of cardiac remodeling. Comprehensive echocardiography with Doppler examination offers a combined assessment of disease severity, ventricular and secondary valvular dysfunction, and estimated ventricular filling pressures (indicating risk of CHF). Although echocardiography also is used as the main screening test for DCM, distinguishing between early DCM and systolic function at the lower end of normal variation is a challenge. Frequently, divergent results for left ventricular systolic function are obtained when different echocardiographic indices are used, and in these cases, serial examinations can be important for identifying progressive trends. Additionally, a normal echocardiogram does not rule out the future development of DCM; thus annual screening of dogs of predisposed breeds is recommended.

On two-dimensional or M-mode echocardiography, left ventricular, and sometimes right ventricular, chamber size is increased in both systole and diastole as assessed by left ventricular internal diameters at end systole and end diastole or by calculated end-systolic and end-diastolic left ventricular volumes. These measurements must be compared with established normal ranges based on body weight, for specific breeds when available, or indexed to body surface area. Recently, Wess and colleagues (2010) reported that in Doberman pinschers, an end-systolic and end-diastolic volume indexed to body surface area of more than 55 ml/m² and 95 ml/m², respectively, was superior to standard M-mode measurements for detection of occult DCM. Decreases in indices of left ventricular function, including fractional shortening and calculated ejection fraction, also are observed, but the diagnosis of DCM should not be based solely on a reduced fractional shortening or ejection fraction without assessment of the left ventricular chamber sizes in systole and diastole individually. Importantly, there is no single value for left ventricular shortening fraction that is both sensitive and specific for DCM in all breeds. Although the atria may be normal in size with occult DCM, the left atrium, and sometimes the right atrium, often is enlarged, and this is a consistent feature of overt DCM with CHF.

Doppler echocardiography often demonstrates a central jet of mitral regurgitation, which occurs because of mitral annular dilation and papillary muscle displacement. The mitral coaptation point often is displaced apically from the annulus in DCM (increased valve tenting). So-called secondary mitral regurgitation due to DCM sometimes can be differentiated from primary mitral valve degeneration with systolic dysfunction by imaging findings: a degenerative valve is typically thickened; one or both leaflets are likely to prolapse into the left atrium; and the jet of regurgitation typically is eccentric. Many dogs with DCM also develop Doppler imaging evidence of diastolic dysfunction, which may be demonstrated on transmitral flow. Experienced examiners generally look for evidence of impaired relaxation, indicating left ventricular dysfunction, but a restrictive transmitral filling pattern is more often associated with CHF. The latter finding is an important negative prognostic indicator. Recently several indices of ventricular filling pressure derived from Doppler and tissue Doppler imaging also have been shown to correlate with the presence and resolution of CHF in dogs with DCM (Schober et al, 2010,

2011). Other tissue Doppler imaging–derived indices such as tissue velocity, strain, and strain rate may be useful in assessing left ventricular systolic and diastolic function with perhaps more sensitivity than M-mode and two-dimensional indices, but there is not yet widespread acceptance of or data regarding these variables.

Electrocardiography

Although many dogs with DCM have ECG abnormalities such as evidence of left ventricular enlargement, left atrial enlargement, or left bundle branch block, the standard resting ECG is neither sensitive nor specific for DCM. The most useful application of ECG in DCM is diagnosis of arrhythmias. DCM often is associated with atrial fibrillation (AF), and this appears to be more common in giant-breed dogs. Giant-breed dogs, especially Irish wolfhounds, also can develop lone AF without any evidence of underlying structural heart disease. In some dogs lone AF progresses to overt DCM; thus annual screening of these dogs is recommended. The onset of AF may precipitate CHF signs because AF causes an abrupt reduction in cardiac output.

Ventricular arrhythmias, including ventricular premature complexes (VPCs or PVCs) and ventricular tachycardia (VT), also are common in dogs with DCM. Particularly malignant ventricular arrhythmias often are identified in Doberman pinschers, but dogs of other breeds also can demonstrate frequent or complicated ventricular ectopy. In dogs affected with syncope, VT is usually the cause, and degeneration of VT into ventricular fibrillation can lead to sudden death. Ventricular arrhythmias often precede the onset of echocardiographic changes in Doberman pinschers that develop DCM. Therefore 24-hour Holter monitoring is a good screening test in Doberman pinschers and is recommended annually with echocardiography. The occurrence of more than 50 to 100 VPCs in 24 hours or any couplets, triplets, or runs of VT are considered diagnostic for DCM in this breed. Although a recommendation for routine ambulatory ECG monitoring cannot be extended currently to all breeds as risk of DCM, it should be appreciated that breeds other than the Doberman pinscher (e.g., Great Danes) also may be at risk of malignant ventricular arrhythmias. Ventricular asystole also has been observed as a cause of syncope and sudden death in DCM.

Thoracic Radiography

Thoracic radiographs may demonstrate cardiomegaly with left ventricular and left atrial enlargement, and these changes are invariable in overt DCM. Radiographs are imperative for the diagnosis of left-sided CHF with pulmonary edema and also are useful in the differential diagnosis of respiratory signs or distress. Right-sided chamber enlargement and pleural effusion may be observed with right-sided or biventricular CHF.

Other Diagnostic Tests

A DCM phenotype has been reported in some cocker spaniels and also in breeds that are atypical of those affected by idiopathic-familial DCM. Taurine deficiency has been described in dogs fed vegetarian or off-brand diets, and in these cases, blood taurine levels should be evaluated because supplementation may dramatically improve left ventricular function and prognosis.

BNP is a hormone released from the ventricular myocardium in response to wall stress or hypertrophy, so that increased circulating levels are found in a multitude of heart diseases including overt and occult DCM. Commercial tests are now available for the prohormone of BNP (NT-proBNP) and for BNP in dogs. Special sample handling is required for these tests, and noncardiac diseases, including systemic hypertension and renal disease, can increase BNP concentrations in the blood. In mixed populations of dog breeds, especially in those with low risk of cardiac disease, concentrations of these biomarkers are not sufficiently sensitive or specific to be used as a screening test for asymptomatic cardiac disease. They are more useful for differentiating between cardiac and noncardiac disease (i.e., CHF or not) in dogs with respiratory signs. In a specific population of dogs at high risk of DCM, such as Doberman pinschers, NT-proBNP concentration may be useful as a screening test, but appropriate cutoffs must be established (Wess et al, 2011) and the test results should not be interpreted in isolation. A recent study suggests that BNP levels also may be useful to guide CHF therapy because levels decrease when pulmonary edema resolves, but more research is necessary to define this use (Schober et al, 2011). As a general point, therapy for DCM never should be based solely on the level of a circulating biomarker.

As indicated earlier, many cases of DCM are familial, and it is likely that genetic testing will become a prominent method for evaluating dogs at risk of this disease. Currently a test for the pyruvate dehydrogenase 4 gene mutation in Doberman pinschers is available that uses either a blood sample or a cheek swab (contact the North Carolina State University Veterinary Cardiac Genetics Laboratory). Initial results demonstrated that all affected dogs were either homozygous or heterozygous for the mutation, but some genetically positive dogs did not show any evidence of DCM at the time of testing (Meurs et al, 2010). This could reflect the delayed onset of the disease or reduced penetrance.

Treatment

Ideal therapy for DCM would target the underlying cause, but this rarely is possible. Current treatments are designed to delay progression of disease, control clinical signs, improve quality of life, and prolong survival. There are differing opinions regarding the ideal therapy for dogs with DCM, and unfortunately, there is little high-grade scientific evidence to support most treatment decisions for this disease. The ideal therapy likely varies depending on breed, stage of disease, and clinical signs; therefore treatment should be tailored to the individual patient.

Occult (Preclinical) Dilated Cardiomyopathy

Although there are no prospective studies evaluating the efficacy of angiotensin-converting enzyme (ACE) inhibitors in dogs with occult DCM, there is considerable evidence that ACE inhibitors delay progression of the disease in humans (Hare, 2011). Activation of the renin-angiotensin-aldosterone system has numerous deleterious effects on the failing heart, including vasoconstriction, fluid retention, increased sympathetic tone, and cardiac and vascular remodeling. Inhibiting the formation of angiotensin II with ACE inhibitors may block or attenuate these effects. A retrospective study in Doberman pinschers with occult DCM demonstrated that treatment with benazepril delayed the onset of overt DCM (O'Grady et al, 2009). It is likely that this benefit extends to all ACE inhibitors, and enalapril or benazepril (0.25 to 0.5 mg/kg q12h PO) is recommended for all dogs with occult DCM. One might argue in theory that the highest dose would be most likely to demonstrate beneficial results as a preventive treatment.

It is known that persistent sympathetic stimulation of the heart leads to β-receptor down-regulation, cardiac remodeling and fibrosis, myocyte death, and tachyarrhythmias, all of which may contribute to progressive myocardial dysfunction and ventricular dilation in DCM. β-Blockers can prevent these effects and have been demonstrated to reduce morbidity and mortality as well as improve myocardial function in humans with DCM (Hare, 2011). To date, there have been no studies evaluating the effect of β-blockers in dogs with occult DCM, and there is no consensus on the use of β-blockers in canine DCM. However, if there is a beneficial effect, it is most likely to be demonstrated when these drugs are administered in the occult phase of the disease. Therefore it is reasonable to discuss the potential benefits and risks of β-blocker therapy with owners and to emphasize that treatment in dogs with occult DCM can be based only on comparative (human) and laboratory model evidence at this time.

Carvedilol, a nonspecific β-blocker and α₁-blocker, and metoprolol, a selective β₁-blocker, demonstrate the most clearly defined benefits in humans and have been used in canine models of left ventricular dysfunction in laboratory settings. For DCM, β-blockers initially must be administered at very low dosages and gradually up-titrated over several months to a target or maximum tolerated dosage. It is emphasized that some patients cannot tolerate β-blockers even at low dosages, and administration can lead to decompensation and precipitate CHF. Carvedilol has been prescribed to dogs at a starting dosage of 0.05 to 0.1 mg/kg every 12 hours PO, with the dose gradually increased every 2 weeks to a maximum dosage of 0.5 to 1 mg/kg every 12 hours. During the up-titration phase, dogs must be monitored closely for the development of weakness, lethargy, or signs of CHF, and the dose must be reduced if any of these is noted.

With regard to positive inotropic drugs, it should be mentioned that in humans with DCM treatment with positive inotropic drugs has not improved, and sometimes has reduced, survival. Accordingly one should not necessarily treat low fractional shortening with an inotropic drug like digoxin or pimobendan in a dog without heart failure.

Very recently, however, a clinical trial of pimobendan (Vetmedin), a positive inotrope and balanced vasodilator, has been completed in Doberman pinschers with occult DCM (Summerfield et al, 2012). The results indicated a statistically significant improvement in time to onset of CHF and survival in dogs receiving pimobendan versus those given placebo. Onset of CHF or sudden death was delayed by an average of 9 months and death due to any all-cause mortality was delayed by an average of 5 months. Although the study was small and focused on only one breed, these results suggest possible benefit of the drug in preclinical DCM. Risk of sudden death was no different in the two groups. Unresolved issues associated with this study include the generalizability of these results to other breeds (in addition to the Doberman pinscher), the cost of therapy for the approximately 2 years needed to identify these benefits, and the value, if any, of cotherapy. In this study pimobendan was compared with placebo but not with cardioprotectant drugs like ACE inhibitors or β-blockers. Drugs in the latter two classes often are prescribed by cardiologists (empirically) for occult DCM.

Congestive Heart Failure

Since most clinical signs of DCM are due to CHF, most of the therapy for overt DCM is aimed at controlling CHF. For additional information on the treatment of CHF, including acute heart failure, see Chapter 176. The long-term management of CHF after initial stabilization has been accomplished is discussed here.

Clinical signs due to the presence of pulmonary edema, ascites, or pleural effusion necessitate treatment with diuretics to control ongoing fluid retention. Furosemide typically is the first-line diuretic treatment in CHF therapy and has a wide dosage range (1 to 5 mg/kg q8-12h PO). It should be administered at the lowest effective dose that controls clinical signs to avoid dehydration, azotemia, and electrolyte loss. However, as DCM progresses and CHF recurs, it will be necessary to increase the furosemide dose. Spironolactone (1 to 2 mg/kg q12-24h PO) is a potassium-sparing but weak diuretic that often is administered in addition to furosemide as CHF worsens. In humans, addition of low-dose spironolactone to standard heart failure therapy has been shown to improve survival modestly due to antagonism of systemic aldosterone effects, but this has not been demonstrated conclusively in dogs. Most North American cardiologists include spironolactone in their long-term therapy regimens for CHF according to recent surveys. Thiazide diuretics typically are used in addition to furosemide and spironolactone in cases of refractory CHF. However, this regimen may result in severe dehydration, azotemia, and electrolyte depletion, so the authors initially recommend low-dose hydrochlorothiazide (1 to 2 mg/kg q48-72h PO) with careful monitoring of relevant parameters. The use of other diuretics, such as the loop diuretic torsemide, requires more study before general recommendations can be advanced.

Blockade of the renin-angiotensin-aldosterone system is a cornerstone of CHF therapy, and there is good evidence from prospective, placebo-controlled trials of ACE inhibitors in dogs with DCM supporting an improvement in clinical signs and survival. These benefits are likely to occur with any ACE inhibitor, but experience in dogs is most extensive with enalapril and benazepril (0.25 to 0.5 mg/kg q12h PO). Especially when ACE inhibitors are administered in combination with diuretics, animals must be monitored for adverse effects of azotemia and hypotension.

Since the primary cardiac abnormality in DCM is systolic dysfunction, it is logical that positive inotropes would be beneficial in treating the disease. Pimobendan is a calcium sensitizer and phosphodiesterase 3 inhibitor and as such is both a positive inotrope and balanced vasodilator. Prospective, placebo-controlled studies of dogs with DCM and CHF given pimobendan in addition to the standard therapy of furosemide and ACE inhibitors have demonstrated an improvement in quality of life, time to treatment failure, and survival (O'Grady et al, 2008). Therefore pimobendan (0.2 to 0.3 mg/kg q12h PO) should be administered to dogs with DCM and CHF.

Digoxin is a weak positive inotrope with a narrow therapeutic range and has been largely supplanted by pimobendan, but it does have additional effects, including increasing vagal tone and improving baroreceptor function. There are no studies of the effectiveness of digoxin therapy in veterinary medicine, but human studies have shown beneficial effects and indicate that these effects may be observed with a lower incidence of toxicity when the drug is administered at lower dosages. The authors typically prescribe digoxin only when AF is present, but it may be considered as an additional treatment for CHF, especially in refractory disease. Of note, the two relative contraindications for digoxin are complex ventricular arrhythmias and azotemia, two conditions that are likely to occur in dogs with CHF.

Because of the beneficial effects discussed earlier, β-blockers are considered to be standard-of-care therapy for CHF in humans, but the issue is unresolved in dogs. If the decision is made to prescribe a β-blocker, therapy should be administered *only* after CHF has been stabilized completely. The use of carvedilol has been studied in a small group of dogs with DCM and stabilized CHF; no significant positive or negative effects were demonstrated (Oyama et al, 2007). As indicated earlier, if there is a beneficial effect of β-blockers in dogs with DCM, it is possible that it will not be observed in the overt phase because survival with CHF is short, and the effects of β-blockade are time dependent. Currently the authors do not recommend β-blocker therapy in dogs with DCM and CHF.

Arrhythmias

In dogs with DCM, AF further reduces cardiac output because of the reduction in ventricular filling from the loss of atrial contraction and the rapid ventricular rate. Therapeutic options include cardioversion to restore a sinus rhythm and the use of negative chronotropic drugs to slow the ventricular response rate. Techniques for electrical and pharmacologic cardioversion have been described (see Web Chapter 60), but in most dogs with CHF, heart rate control is the goal. It should be noted that dogs with CHF and sinus rhythm have a higher resting heart rate than healthy dogs (by about 30 beats/min), so an acceptable target heart rate range for dogs with AF and

CHF likely will be higher than that for a healthy dog. A practical target for rate control during clinical examination or in-hospital ECG is a rate of about 120 to 160 beats/min. In this regard, 24-hour Holter monitoring may be useful in the assessment of overall response in terms of average heart rate and peak heart rates that develop with exercise. The drugs used for heart rate control include digoxin, the calcium channel blocker diltiazem, and β-blockers. Although digoxin is the only positive inotrope in this group, it usually is insufficient as a single agent. The authors administer digoxin at a low dosage (0.002 to 0.003 mg/kg q12h PO) and monitor trough serum levels, accepting a therapeutic range of 0.8 to 1.5 ng/ml. In addition to digoxin, or in place of digoxin in dogs that exhibit gastrointestinal signs or have considerable ventricular arrhythmias, the authors administer diltiazem (0.5 to 2 mg/kg q8h PO for the standard formulation or 2 to 6 mg/kg q12h PO for the sustained-release formulation). An argument can be made for administering β-blockers given the potential beneficial effects, but these drugs need to be increased very gradually to a therapeutic dosage, and most often dogs with DCM and AF also have severe CHF.

Ventricular arrhythmias are common in dogs with DCM, especially Doberman pinschers, and may cause weakness, lethargy, syncope, or sudden death. Indications for therapy include clinical signs caused by hemodynamic compromise, VT, and potentially other malignant characteristics such as fast couplets or triplets (two or three VPCs) as well as the R-on-T phenomenon (closely coupled VPC on the previous T wave). Because of a lack of data there is no consensus on when or how to treat serious ventricular ectopy.

The goals of therapy may include the elimination of clinical signs, the control of VT or other malignant features, and the prevention of sudden death. The number of single VPCs does not serve as an indication for or a goal of treatment. Although often it is possible to control clinical signs, reduce the number or frequency of VPCs, and suppress runs of VT, there is no evidence that any antiarrhythmic therapy is protective against sudden death.

Several drugs are recommended for the long-term management of ventricular arrhythmias, but none has proven effects in dogs with DCM. Sotalol (1 to 2 mg/kg q12h PO), a potassium channel blocker and nonspecific β-blocker, is prescribed most frequently, and the authors recommend an up-titration from one quarter to one half of the desired dose over 2 to 4 weeks to avoid decompensation due to β-blockade. Mexiletine (5 to 8 mg/kg q8h PO) is a sodium channel blocker similar to lidocaine and often is more effective when combined with β-blockers, including sotalol. Gastrointestinal adverse effects usually can be avoided by administering with food. Three-times-daily administration is a problem for many clients. Amiodarone (10 mg/kg q12h for 2 weeks and then 5 mg/kg q24h PO) is a potent antiarrhythmic with effects in every antiarrhythmic class; however, its use often is limited by extensive adverse effects, including hepatotoxicity, neutropenia, and altered thyroid function, among others. Flecainide has not been studied sufficiently in this group of patients but has been used by some cardiologists.

Other Therapies

In addition to taurine supplementation for dogs found to be taurine deficient, several other nutritional recommendations, including moderate dietary sodium restriction and omega-3 fatty acid supplementation, may be advanced for dogs with DCM (see Chapter 168). Sufficient protein intake also is important because these dogs often exhibit cardiac cachexia.

Gene and stem cell therapy have the potential to revolutionize the treatment of DCM by improving or even curing the underlying abnormalities that lead to DCM (Sleeper et al, 2011). There appears to be great promise in these therapies in light of data from experimental animal models of cardiac dysfunction and the discovery of gene mutations in dogs with DCM. Although several investigators currently are exploring the potential of gene and stem cell therapies, to date none of these has been proven to be beneficial in clinical canine DCM.

Prognosis

Overall the long-term prognosis for dogs with DCM is guarded to poor; however, the prognosis is variable and depends on disease severity, breed, causes, concurrent diseases, and quality of veterinary and home-based management. Dogs with occult DCM may live for up to 2 to 4 years before developing any clinical signs. Once CHF develops, survival usually is limited to 6 to 12 months, although it has improved dramatically with the use of ACE inhibitors and pimobendan. Variables that have a negative impact on prognosis include young age at the onset of clinical signs, biventricular failure, AF, severely increased end-systolic volume index, and a restrictive transmitral flow pattern. Most of these predictors are logical and indicate that the heart is severely dilated, left ventricular function is severely impaired, and maladaptive neurohormonal responses are fully active. Most dogs with DCM die of CHF or are euthanized because of severe clinical signs, declining quality of life, or poor prognosis. Clients should be warned that sudden death also is common.

References and Suggested Reading

Hare JM: The dilated, restrictive, and infiltrative cardiomyopathies. In Bonow RO et al, editors: *Heart disease*, ed 9, Philadelphia, 2011, Saunders, p 1561.

Meurs KM et al: A splice site mutation in a gene encoding for a mitochondrial protein is associated with the development of dilated cardiomyopathy in the Doberman pinscher, *J Vet Intern Med* 24:693, 2010 (abstract).

O'Grady MR et al: Effect of pimobendan on case fatality rate in Doberman pinschers with congestive heart failure caused by dilated cardiomyopathy, *J Vet Intern Med* 22:897, 2008.

O'Grady MR et al: Efficacy of benazepril hydrochloride to delay the progression of occult dilated cardiomyopathy in Doberman pinschers, *J Vet Intern Med* 23:977, 2009.

Oyama MA et al: Carvedilol in dogs with dilated cardiomyopathy, *J Vet Intern Med* 21:1272, 2007.

Schober KE et al: Detection of congestive heart failure in dogs by Doppler echocardiography, *J Vet Intern Med* 24:1358, 2010.

Schober KE et al: Effects of treatment on respiratory rate, serum natriuretic peptide concentration, and Doppler echocardiographic indices of left ventricular filling pressure in dogs with congestive heart failure secondary to degenerative mitral valve disease and dilated cardiomyopathy, *J Am Vet Med Assoc* 239:468, 2011.

Sleeper M et al: Status of therapeutic gene transfer to treat cardiovascular disease in dogs and cats, *J Vet Cardiol* 13:131, 2011.

Summerfield NJ et al: Effect of pimobendan in the prevention of congestive heart failure or sudden death in Doberman pinschers with preclinical dilated cardiomyopathy (the PROTECT study), *J Vet Intern Med* 26:1337, 2012.

Wess G et al: Use of Simpson's method of disc to detect early echocardiographic changes in Doberman pinschers with dilated cardiomyopathy, *J Vet Intern Med* 24:1069, 2010.

Wess G et al: Evaluation of N-terminal pro-B-type natriuretic peptide as a diagnostic marker of various stages of cardiomyopathy in Doberman pinschers, *Am J Vet Res* 72:642, 2011.

CHAPTER 179

Arrhythmogenic Right Ventricular Cardiomyopathy

KATHRYN M. MEURS, *Raleigh, North Carolina*

The condition previously known as *boxer cardiomyopathy* is now more commonly referred to as *arrhythmogenic right ventricular cardiomyopathy* (ARVC). ARVC is a primary myocardial disease that typically presents in one of three forms: an asymptomatic form with ventricular premature complexes (VPCs); a symptomatic form with VPCs; and a form with ventricular dilation, myocardial dysfunction, and ventricular and supraventricular tachyarrhythmias. Affected dogs may live for years with the disease and remain asymptomatic, may experience sudden death, or may gradually progress to congestive heart failure. ARVC is an adult-onset familial disease that appears to be inherited in an autosomal-dominant fashion. It has variable penetrance and expressivity; that is, not all boxers with the disease have cardiomyopathy to the same degree or develop it at the same age, although the frequency of disease, as well as disease severity, increases with age in affected dogs.

A small percentage of boxers with myocardial disease brought for treatment for the first time have ventricular dilation and myocardial dysfunction without a history of ARVC. It is possible that these boxers have a separate myocardial disease that might be caused by an inherited carnitine deficiency, viral myocarditis, or some other myocardial insult that results in the development of a cardiomyopathic state.

Causes

In human beings, ARVC is an inherited disease most commonly associated with a genetic mutation in a gene that encodes for one of many desmosomal proteins. In the boxer dog, a deletion mutation has been identified in the 3′ untranslated region of striatin, a gene that encodes for a desmosomal protein. This mutation has approximately 70% penetrance in dogs with the deletion, which means that about 70% of dogs with the mutation eventually show the disease (30% do not). It should be remembered that in human beings there are numerous genetic causes for the disease, and this may be the situation in the boxer dog as well.

Diagnosis

Arrhythmogenic Right Ventricular Cardiomyopathy

A single diagnostic test for boxer ARVC is unavailable, and the diagnosis is best based on a combination of findings. Genetic evaluation for the deletion mutation can be performed. A test result that is positive for the mutation means that the dog is at increased risk of the disease and supports a diagnosis in dogs with clinical signs. However, a positive genetic test result does not mean that the dog absolutely will develop the disease since about 30% of dogs with the mutation show no signs of the disease (due to the variable penetrance described earlier). Similarly, if the test result is negative, it does not mean that the dog does not have ARVC since there may be more than one cause for the disease. Therefore genetic testing is a useful tool for screening dogs for a breeding program but is less helpful as a single diagnostic test. A family history of disease, the presence of a ventricular tachyarrhythmia, a history of syncope or exercise intolerance, and the exclusion of other systemic and cardiovascular diseases that could be responsible for the clinical presentation all are factors that support the diagnosis. Generally a thorough physical examination, electrocardiography (ECG), blood pressure measurement, and echocardiography should be performed when a diagnosis is suspected. In addition, ambulatory ECG (Holter) monitoring provides important information for both the initial treatment and long-term management of the case and should be performed whenever possible.

Physical examination findings may include the auscultation of premature beats with post-extrasystolic pauses, a persistent or paroxysmal tachyarrhythmia, or no abnormalities at all. It should be emphasized that many affected dogs have very intermittent bouts of the arrhythmia, and the absence of a tachyarrhythmia during examination does not rule out the diagnosis. In addition, since this is primarily an electrical disease, the majority of affected boxers do not have a heart murmur, although a left apical systolic murmur of mitral regurgitation may be identified in dogs that also have myocardial dysfunction and many boxers have a left basilar ejection murmur of uncertain cause.

The classic ECG findings of ARVC include the presence of upright VPCs with positive QRS complexes with a morphology resembling that of left bundle branch block on lead II (Harpster, 1991). However, in some affected dogs the morphology of the VPCs is different or, when the arrhythmia is intermittent, the ECG may not demonstrate any VPCs. It is important to note that normal ECG findings do not exclude a diagnosis of ARVC; if suspicion persists because of clinical signs (syncope, exercise intolerance), auscultation of an arrhythmia, or a family history of disease, 24-hour Holter monitoring and genetic testing is strongly suggested. Even if occasional VPCs are identified on an in-house ECG, Holter monitoring is generally recommended to allow better assessment of the overall frequency and complexity of the arrhythmia. In addition, a pretreatment Holter ECG recording provides useful baseline information when one attempts to determine treatment efficacy as well as to assess for potential proarrhythmic effects of treatment once it has started.

The results of Holter monitoring can be very useful in establishing a diagnosis of ARVC, particularly if the ECG findings are within normal limits. It is unusual for mature adult dogs to have ventricular ectopy. The median number of VPCs detected on the Holter readings from 600 mature asymptomatic boxers was 10 VPCs in 24 hours. Therefore the identification of frequent ventricular ectopy (>100 VPCs in 24 hours) in an adult boxer dog is strongly suggestive of a diagnosis of ARVC, particularly if there is significant complexity (couplets, triplets, bigeminy, or ventricular tachycardia) within the arrhythmia. However, in some cases a diagnosis of ARVC in a boxer is strongly suspected, based on the breed and a history of syncope, but the Holter monitor recording clearly does not show abnormalities. This may be explained by the significant day-to-day variability in the number of VPCs (up to 83%) in affected dogs. Alternatively, reflex-mediated syncope (e.g., vasovagal syncope, characterized by vasodilation and bradycardia) may be occurring. Reflex-mediated syncope has been observed in boxers and should be considered in a fainting boxer with no evidence of ventricular arrhythmias. In cases of uncertain cause, a second round of Holter monitoring or ambulatory ECG event monitoring may be performed to better determine the relationship of heart rhythm and syncope in a boxer dog.

Blood pressure measurement, echocardiography, and in certain cases splenic ultrasonography are recommended in cases of suspected ARVC. Although in the majority of cases the blood pressure, cardiac chamber sizes, and systolic ventricular function are within normal limits, an echocardiogram can rule out other, less common causes of ventricular ectopy (e.g., neoplasia). Likewise, splenic masses are a known cause of ventricular arrhythmias in dogs and should be considered in the diagnostic workup of ventricular arrhythmias, particularly in older dogs. Blood pressure measurement may offer insight into additional systemic diseases capable of causing syncope. In addition, echocardiography is necessary to identify the small percentage of dogs with ARVC that develop right and left ventricular enlargement and myocardial dysfunction.

Dilated Cardiomyopathy

A small percentage of boxers have a clinical presentation consistent with dilated cardiomyopathy. Affected dogs may experience syncope or show signs of left-sided heart failure, including coughing and tachypnea, or signs of biventricular failure, such as coughing, tachypnea, and ascites. Thoracic radiographs may demonstrate left-sided or biventricular enlargement, pulmonary edema, and pulmonary venous congestion. The echocardiogram may demonstrate left or biventricular enlargement associated with systolic dysfunction. The cause in these cases is unknown, although an association has been identified between homozygosity for the striatin deletion (two copies of the defective gene) and the development of the disease. Additionally, other causes of myocardial dysfunction, including L-carnitine deficiency and myocarditis (see Web Chapter 63), should be considered.

Screening

Given the inheritable nature of ARVC, there is significant interest on the part of breeders and enthusiasts of the boxer breed in the development of a screening program. Genetic testing plays an important role in the development of a screening program because dogs with the mutation are at increased risk of developing clinical signs. Dogs that are found to be heterozygous for the related mutation should be evaluated annually for signs of disease. Adult dogs that do not show signs of disease may exhibit a reduced genetic expression and, if they demonstrate other positive breed attributes, might be bred to mutation-negative dogs. Puppies of this mating should be screened for the mutation, and over a few generations, mutation-negative puppies may be selected to replace the mutation-positive parent and gradually decrease the number of mutation-positive dogs in the population. Boxers homozygous for the mutation probably should not be used for breeding. They appear to be at higher risk of having significant clinical disease, and since both copies of their gene have the mutation, they certainly will pass on the mutation to future offspring. Dogs negative for the mutation still should undergo clinical screening for ARVC (e.g., Holter monitoring) since there may be more than one genetic cause for ARVC in boxers (as in people). Given this possibility of multiple genetic causes for ARVC, a dog that is negative for the striatin mutation still could develop clinical findings of disease.

Multiple factors should be considered when making decisions about clinical screening results, including a family history of ARVC and results of repeated abnormal Holter monitor readings. Given the adult onset of the disease, many perform the first Holter monitoring at the age of 3 years and reevaluate on an annual basis. Holter monitor results should be evaluated for both the number of VPCs and the complexity of arrhythmia (e.g., singles, couplets, triplets, ventricular tachycardia). However, there still are many unanswered questions about ARVC and the relationship of the ventricular arrhythmia to the development of clinical signs. Some affected dogs can have thousands of VPCs and never develop clinical signs; others demonstrate severe clinical signs with a fairly low number of VPCs. We have not found the number of VPCs or the complexity of the arrhythmia to differ statistically in symptomatic (syncopal) dogs compared with asymptomatic affected dogs. In fact, the only factors that have been shown to correlate statistically with severe clinical signs (sudden death) are the presence of myocardial dysfunction (low fractional shortening) and the presence of homozygosity for the striatin mutation. Breeders should be encouraged strongly to screen for the disease but should be advised about the complexities of screening and counseled not to remove dogs completely from a breeding program because of a single abnormal Holter reading. Annual Holter monitoring is recommended strongly, and an emphasis should be placed on the results of multiple evaluations in an asymptomatic animal.

The results of 24-hour Holter monitoring in over 600 asymptomatic adult boxers yielded a median of 10 VPCs per 24 hours, with 25% and 75% confidence intervals of 2 and 110 VPCs, respectively. Based on this information we have developed the following initial classification system for screening asymptomatic dogs:

Grade 1. 0 to 50 single VPCs per 24 hours: within normal limits

Grade 2. 51 to 100 VPCs per 24 hours: indeterminate; suggest repeat testing in 6 to 12 months

Grade 3. 100 to 300 single VPCs per 24 hours: suspicious; consider keeping the dog out of the breeding program for 1 year and repeating the Holter study

Grade 4. 100 to 300 VPCs per 24 hours with increased complexity (frequent couplets, triplets, ventricular tachycardia) or 300 to 1000 single VPCs per 24 hours: the dog likely is affected

Grade 5. More than 1000 VPCs per 24 hours: the dog is affected; may consider treatment as discussed in the following paragraphs

These criteria are based on evaluation of the results of a single round of Holter monitoring in mature boxers with no history of syncope. Additional studies that evaluate long-term outcomes for boxers with arrhythmias of various grades are ongoing. This information is provided as a possible starting point for making screening recommendations. As indicated earlier, multiple criteria should be considered for each dog before any strict recommendations are advanced. The family history, evidence of any ongoing systemic disease that could be associated with ventricular arrhythmia, and results of repeated Holter studies are particularly important.

Treatment

In affected boxers, antiarrhythmic therapy has been shown to decrease the number of VPCs, the complexity (grade) of the arrhythmia, and the frequency of syncope. However, the ability of antiarrhythmic therapy to decrease the risk of sudden death has been neither proven nor disproven. In addition, ventricular antiarrhythmic agents can demonstrate significant proarrhythmic effects in some patients. Therefore the risks and benefits always should be assessed when treatment is considered.

For the asymptomatic dog the author generally recommends therapy to decrease the number and complexity of the arrhythmias if there are at least 1000 VPCs per 24 hours or if runs of ventricular tachycardia or evidence of the R-on-T phenomenon are identified. It should be remembered that some dogs with ARVC die suddenly without ever having any documented episodes of syncope. Thus the absence of a history of syncope does not imply a lack of risk, and a recent report has suggested that a history of syncope may not always increase the risk of sudden cardiac death. Ideally, boxers with syncope and

ventricular arrhythmias should be treated after results of 24-hour Holter monitoring are analyzed to quantify the pretreatment arrhythmia. If the syncope is frequent or if ventricular tachycardia is observed, a Holter monitoring evaluation may not be performed to avoid delay in initiating therapy. However, in these cases, the absence of pretreatment Holter monitoring recordings can make it difficult to assess fully the response to therapy. Therefore, whenever possible, a Holter monitoring evaluation should be performed first. If there is great concern about the risk of sudden death, the owner is advised to start therapy immediately after removing the monitoring electrodes (while awaiting the results).

A few therapeutic protocols appear to be effective in reducing the number of VPCs and the degree of complexity of the arrhythmia in boxer dogs with ARVC. One is sotalol (1.5 to 2.5 mg/kg q12h PO); a second is mexiletine (5 to 6 mg/kg q8h PO). In some hard-to-control cases, both sotalol and mexiletine, at the dosages given, can be administered. This combination can be quite effective and typically is well tolerated by affected dogs. In management of most cases of boxer ARVC, sotalol as a monotherapy generally is chosen first because of the ease of dosing twice a day, the low level of adverse effects, and the demonstrated reduction in the number of VPCs in most dogs. However, in some cases, sotalol does not suppress the arrhythmia sufficiently and the addition of mexiletine may be useful. Occasionally, mexiletine causes a loss of appetite or mild gastrointestinal upset, which may improve if the drug is given with a small meal. Failure of the combination of sotalol and mexiletine to work should prompt referral to or consultation with a cardiologist.

Despite their potential for beneficial antiarrhythmic effects, the aforementioned medications can exert proarrhythmic effects or may be insufficiently effective in some boxers with ARVC. Therefore a Holter ECG evaluation is recommended both before treatment and 2 to 3 weeks after treatment has been initiated. This evaluation can help determine the effect of treatment and confirm that the arrhythmia has not gotten worse. Significant day-to-day variability (up to an 83% change in daily VPC count) has been observed in affected boxers (Spier and Meurs, 2004). Therefore a positive therapeutic response is confirmed when at least an 80% reduction in VPC number along with a reduction in the complexity of the arrhythmia is observed on the posttreatment Holter recording. In contrast, an increase in symptoms after initiation of treatment or an increase of more than 80% in the number of VPCs per day may suggest a proarrhythmic effect.

References and Suggested Reading

Basso C et al: Arrhythmogenic right ventricular cardiomyopathy causing sudden death in boxer dogs: a new animal model of human disease, *Circulation* 109:1180, 2004.

Harpster N: Boxer cardiomyopathy, *Vet Clin North Am Small Anim Pract* 21:989, 1991.

Keene B: l-Carnitine supplementation in the therapy of dilated cardiomyopathy, *Vet Clin North Am Small Anim Pract* 21:1005, 1991.

Meurs KM et al: Familial ventricular arrhythmias in boxers, *J Vet Intern Med* 13:437, 1999.

Meurs KM et al: Comparison of in-hospital versus 24-hour ambu-
    latory electrocardiography for detection of ventricular prema-
    ture complexes in mature boxers, *J Am Vet Med Assoc* 218:222,
    2001.
Meurs KM et al: Comparison of the effects of four antiarrhythmic
    treatments for familial ventricular arrhythmias in boxers, *J Am
    Vet Med Assoc* 221:522, 2002.

Meurs KM et al: Genome-wide association identifies a mutation
    in the 3′ untranslated region of Striatin, a desmosomal gene,
    in a canine model of arrhythmogenic right ventricular cardio-
    myopathy, *Hum Genet* 128:315, 2010.
Spier AW, Meurs KM: Spontaneous variability in the frequency
    of ventricular arrhythmias in boxers with arrhythmogenic car-
    diomyopathy, *J Am Vet Med Assoc* 224:538, 2004.

CHAPTER **180**

Feline Myocardial Disease

VIRGINIA LUIS FUENTES, *Hatfield, Hertfordshire, United Kingdom*
KARSTEN ECKHARD SCHOBER, *Columbus, Ohio*

Definition of Myocardial Disease

Myocardial disease in cats is a heterogeneous group of
conditions, paralleling the spectrum of diseases that make
up human cardiomyopathy. Feline cardiomyopathies
originally were categorized according to morphology and
function, in line with the contemporary human classification. The main categories were hypertrophic, dilated,
restrictive, and unclassified cardiomyopathy, with the
later addition of arrhythmogenic right ventricular cardiomyopathy (ARVC). Human cardiomyopathies now are
divided into primary cardiomyopathies in which the
myocardial changes are the major abnormality (e.g.,
hypertrophic cardiomyopathy, or HCM) and secondary
cardiomyopathies in which a multiorgan systemic disease
(e.g., hyperthyroidism) affects the myocardium (Maron
et al, 2006). Primary cardiomyopathies are divided into
those with a genetic basis, those with an acquired cause,
and those involving a combination of genetic and
acquired factors (mixed). Hypertrophic cardiomyopathy
and ARVC are considered genetic in humans, whereas
dilated cardiomyopathy (DCM) and restrictive cardiomyopathy (RCM) are classed as mixed. There is evidence that
HCM can be genetic in cats: two separate mutations in
the cardiac myosin-binding protein C gene have been
identified in Maine coon and Ragdoll cats with HCM. A
deficiency in dietary taurine can result in a feline DCM
phenotype. Secondary cardiomyopathies found in cats
include myocardial disease related to hyperthyroidism,
systemic hypertension, and chronic anemia, which commonly affect cardiac chamber size and function.

Despite this classification, there is considerable overlap
among groups. Cats may progress from one phenotype to
another. Myocardial infarction can complicate HCM,
resulting in regional wall thinning and hypokinesis that
resembles a DCM phenotype. An end-stage form of HCM
also has been described in human and feline patients,
characterized by left ventricular hypertrophy with dilation and reduced systolic function. Left ventricular
remodeling in HCM with interstitial fibrosis and loss of
cardiac myocytes can result in a morphology that is closer
to RCM than to classic HCM, and chronic myocarditis
may mimic RCM or DCM. Even on a genetic level, some
sarcomeric mutations are associated with both DCM and
HCM phenotypes. In addition, abnormal mitral valve
morphology can be associated with dynamic outflow
tract obstruction and left ventricular hypertrophy, which
blurs the boundaries between congenital heart disease
and primary cardiomyopathy.

Diagnostic Approach

In addition to the difficulties in trying to assign a particular label to the cardiomyopathy in individual cats, feline
cardiac disease presents a number of other diagnostic
challenges.

Healthy cats may have innocent heart murmurs that
are not associated with any structural cardiac abnormality. The prevalence of murmurs in the healthy cat population is high, but as many as half of all feline murmurs
may be functional and not actually caused by structural
heart disease (Wagner et al, 2010). These low- to moderate-
intensity systolic murmurs often are associated with conditions characterized by increased sympathetic tone and
high cardiac output, such as stress, anemia, hyperthyroidism, and fever, with the murmur arising from the left
or the right ventricular outflow tract. Dynamic right
ventricular outflow tract obstruction can be normal in
cats. The best way to differentiate cats with functional
murmurs from those with heart disease is with echocardiography. Unfortunately, interpretation of echocardio-
grams in cats requires a high level of expertise, particularly

in distinguishing between normal cats and cats with mild structural cardiac changes. Thoracic radiography may be used to identify cardiomegaly in asymptomatic cats, but the sensitivity of this method is low, especially in cats with mild structural changes. Plasma biomarker assays such as those for N-terminal prohormone B-type natriuretic peptide (NT-proBNP) and high-sensitive cardiac troponin I are showing promise as screening tests for cardiomyopathy in this setting but always should be used in conjunction with other tests (Fox et al, 2011). It is relatively easy to screen for secondary cardiomyopathies by measuring blood pressure, thyroxine concentration, and hematologic parameters.

Noncardiac disease can cause respiratory distress that must be distinguished from congestive heart failure (CHF). Auscultation of a gallop sound in a cat with tachypnea is highly suggestive of CHF. Radiography can be helpful if cardiomegaly or venous engorgement is detected. If the cardiac silhouette is obscured or interpreted as normal, radiography is less useful as a discriminatory test because the distribution of pulmonary infiltrates with cardiogenic pulmonary edema is very variable in cats, and the presence of a pleural effusion is nonspecific. The careful positioning necessary for diagnostic radiography also can jeopardize patient safety when the cat is tachypneic. Although plasma NT-proBNP concentration may discriminate well between cardiac and noncardiac causes of respiratory distress in cats, it is not yet available as a cage-side test, and the delay in receiving results limits its usefulness.

Cats with myocardial disease may have no detectable abnormalities on physical examination. The extent of this problem is unclear, although a recent study evaluating 103 apparently normal cats found heart murmurs in only 5 of the 16 cats with echocardiographic evidence of cardiomyopathy (Paige et al, 2009). Additionally, it is common for cats brought for treatment of aortic thromboembolism (ATE) and advanced cardiomyopathy to have shown no signs of cardiac disease at previous examinations. Without preemptive screening, these at-risk cats likely will continue to be denied the opportunity for cardiac therapy.

Therapeutic Approach

Clearly it is never appropriate to treat a cat for heart disease based solely on the presence of an auscultatory abnormality such as a murmur or even a gallop sound or click. Most cats with heart disease have cardiomyopathy, but those with secondary cardiomyopathies must be identified because their treatment should be directed at the underlying disease. It is more important to determine symptomatic status than to try to categorize the cardiomyopathy phenotype because cats with clinical signs are managed differently from those without. Treatment decisions ideally should be evidence based, but relevant data mostly are lacking in feline heart disease. In the absence of valid evidence, management should focus on targeting cats at risk of recognized complications of cardiomyopathy. The most common sequelae of cardiomyopathy are CHF and ATE, although the incidence of sudden death is probably underestimated. When specific hemodynamic disturbances (e.g., systolic dysfunction) are identified, therapy should be tailored to the specific functional problem. Nevertheless, it is important to recognize that many cats with myocardial disease remain asymptomatic for long periods without any intervention (Payne et al, 2010), and any incremental benefit from therapy in these cats may not justify the additional expense, time, and stress. Management strategies are presented in the following sections according to risk stratification for stages of heart disease (Table 180-1).

Asymptomatic Cardiomyopathy (Low Risk)

Cats with occult cardiomyopathy exhibit a spectrum of risks, from those cats that will survive to old age and never experience any clinical signs associated with their heart disease to those at imminent risk of CHF or ATE. Cats at the low-risk end of this spectrum are likely to have a normal-sized left atrium (Payne et al, 2010) and may be difficult to differentiate from healthy cats if ventricular changes are subtle. Echocardiography is the most effective test for evaluating left atrial size in cats, although radiography can provide an approximate assessment in cats with moderate or severe atrial enlargement. Alternatively, plasma NT-proBNP concentrations may be used to provide an initial risk assessment to guide further testing (Fox et al, 2011).

It is difficult to justify therapy in cats with a normal-sized left atrium as a means of improving survival because most cats in this category do well without treatment, including cats with dynamic left ventricular outflow tract obstruction (DLVOTO), which typically is associated with systolic anterior motion of the mitral valve apparatus and mitral-septal contact. It is not known whether cats with DLVOTO experience the chest pain that some human HCM patients experience. Moreover, whether the well-known effect of moderate and severe DLVOTO on activity and exercise level in people also occurs in cats is largely undetermined. These are some potential reasons for treating feline DLVOTO in the absence of any demonstrated effect on survival (see the later section on DLVOTO).

Note that although cats with mild occult disease are unlikely to require treatment and often remain in stable condition for long periods, the risk remains that CHF will develop in response to interventions such as intravenous fluid therapy, anesthesia, or depot corticosteroid administration, or to periods of prolonged tachycardia associated with stress. Worryingly, cats in this category also may be at risk of sudden death (Payne et al, 2011).

Asymptomatic Cardiomyopathy (at Risk)

Cats at the high-risk end of the occult cardiomyopathy spectrum are likely to have left atrial enlargement. Such cats have an increased likelihood of developing CHF or ATE compared with those with no left atrial enlargement. Although results of a few short-term trials of therapy in asymptomatic cats have been published, no therapy has been reported to be unequivocally beneficial. However, enrollees frequently have included cats with normal-sized left atria, which minimizes the likely benefit of intervention over a short period.

TABLE **180-1**

Treatment Recommendations for Feline Myocardial Disease

	STAGE B			STAGE C		STAGE D	
	Asymptomatic HCM (Normal LA)	Asymptomatic HCM (Normal LA) + DLVOTO	Asymptomatic Other Cardiomyopathy (LA Enlargement)	Symptomatic (CHF)	Symptomatic (Acute Low-Output Signs)	Refractory CHF	Specific Indications
Atenolol	X	✓	X	X	X	X	DLVOTO with syncope
Diltiazem	?✓	X	X	X	X	X	Atrial fibrillation, supraventricular tachycardia
Furosemide	X	X	X	✓	X	✓	
ACE inhibitor	?✓	?✓	?✓	✓	X	✓	
Pimobendan	X	X	X	?✓ *(only if no DLVOTO)*	✓	✓ *(if no DLVOTO)*	Systolic dysfunction
Spironolactone	X	X	X	X	X	✓	
Aspirin ± clopidogrel	X	X	✓	✓	✓	✓	
Sotalol	?✓ *(if ventricular tachycardia)*	?✓ *(if ventricular tachycardia)*	?✓ *(if ventricular tachycardia)*	X	X	X	Ventricular arrhythmias *(if structural heart disease but normal systolic function)*

See text for details.

X, Not indicated; *✓,* used by the authors; *?,* greater degree of uncertainty; *ACE,* angiotensin-converting enzyme; *CHF,* congestive heart failure; *DLVOTO,* dynamic left ventricular outflow tract obstruction; *HCM,* hypertrophic cardiomyopathy; *LA,* left atrium.

Stage B, Heart disease without clinical signs; Stage C, heart failure treated with "standard methods" and dosages; Stage D, advanced or refractory heart failure.

Without experimental evidence to provide guidance, therapeutic decisions are based on extrapolation from human treatment protocols or knowledge of pathophysiology. This is the patient group about which there is the most controversy in terms of treatment decisions for feline cardiomyopathy. The theoretical goals of therapy in cats at high risk of decompensation might include improvement of hemodynamic function, reduction of left ventricular filling pressures, counteraction of neurohormonal activation, and modulation of platelet function. Treatments suggested include β-adrenergic antagonists (atenolol), calcium channel blockers (diltiazem), angiotensin-converting enzyme (ACE) inhibitors, and antiplatelet drugs (aspirin and clopidogrel).

β-Blockers reduce myocardial oxygen consumption, an effect that should reduce demand ischemia. This benefit, along with slowing of the heart rate and prolongation of diastolic filling, may have some overall benefit on diastolic function in HCM. Atenolol also reduces or eliminates dynamic outflow obstruction (see following paragraph). Anecdotal evidence suggests that relief of moderate and severe outflow tract obstruction may be associated with increased activity and exercise level in some cats that were previously classified as asymptomatic. Moreover, poor tolerance of tachycardia frequently

has been documented in people with HCM and has been proposed as a mechanism for the development of CHF in patients with occult HCM. Prevention of unwanted tachycardia therefore may be beneficial in some cats. The total daily dosage of atenolol is generally 1 to 4 mg/kg q12h PO. Liquid atenolol can be easier to dose than tablets in some cats, but in others the relatively small pill fractions can be hidden in food, treats, pill pockets, or gelatin capsules. Many clinicians dose atenolol to a heart rate effect (e.g., to achieve a rate of 120 to 160 beats/min during physical examination in a hospital setting). Doppler echocardiography can be used to confirm that the dose of atenolol is sufficient to control DLVOTO, and the associated murmur should decrease in intensity or disappear completely. Adverse effects of atenolol in asymptomatic cats can include excessive bradycardia and cardiac dilation.

The calcium channel blocker diltiazem has been said to improve left ventricular relaxation, although definitive evidence of this effect in cats is lacking. Diltiazem also slows heart rate, although less consistently than atenolol. Standard-release diltiazem is dosed at 7.5 mg per cat q8h PO, which is impractical for most cat owners. Extended-release preparations of diltiazem such as Dilacor XR permit once- or twice-daily dosing at 15 to 30 mg per cat q12-24h PO. These long-acting diltiazem compounds can achieve therapeutic plasma levels, but precise dosing guidelines for cats have not been reported. Adverse effects of diltiazem include salivation, anorexia, and weight loss.

Although ACE inhibitors have theoretic benefits in cardiomyopathy, there are no data supporting their use in asymptomatic cats. Well-controlled studies in asymptomatic Maine coon cats failed to show a benefit of 12 months of treatment with ramipril at 0.5 mg/kg q24h PO (MacDonald et al, 2006). Another randomized, controlled study (Taillefer and Di Fruscia, 2006) comparing the effects of benazepril (0.5 mg/kg q24h PO) and diltiazem CD (10 mg/kg q24h PO) in 21 cats with preclinical HCM did not identify any relevant difference between groups after 6 months, although a control group was not studied. However, some cardiologists do consider an ACE inhibitor for treatment of asymptomatic cats demonstrating moderate and severe left atrial enlargement.

Although severe left ventricular hypertrophy has been identified as an independent risk factor in people with HCM, and thus therapeutic targeting of left ventricular hypertrophy has been suggested, similar information is not available in feline HCM. Moreover, the mechanisms of hypertrophy may be so diverse in different forms of HCM that one common therapeutic strategy may not be capable of achieving the desired result. ACE inhibitors or angiotensin II receptor antagonists, spironolactone, diltiazem, and statins all have been used successfully in experimental HCM models. However, neither the ACE inhibitor regimen in the study cited previously nor 4 months of treatment with the aldosterone antagonist spironolactone (2 mg/kg q12h PO) showed any effect on estimates of left ventricular diastolic function or chamber dimensions in cats with preclinical HCM (MacDonald et al, 2006, 2008). In the spironolactone study, several cats developed skin lesions with chronic administration.

The specific risk of ATE in asymptomatic cats with HCM has not been reported. Most clinicians view left atrial enlargement as a likely risk factor for this complication, and many consider antithrombotic therapy appropriate in cats with HCM with this echocardiographic finding. This treatment is discussed in the following paragraphs and in Chapter 181. Evaluation of size, content, and flow velocity in the left auricle may contribute to the decision on whether to use antithrombotic treatment (Schober and Maerz, 2006).

Hypertrophic Cardiomyopathy with Dynamic Left Ventricular Outflow Tract Obstruction

In human HCM patients, DLVOTO is associated with increased risk of heart failure and death (Maron et al, 2003). Control of DLVOTO usually is initiated when patients become symptomatic (e.g., with syncope or exertional dyspnea), when DLVOTO is feared to be contributing to the development of left ventricular hypertrophy, or when DLVOTO is associated with more than mild mitral regurgitation, contributing to left atrial enlargement. In cats there is some controversy over the clinical significance of DLVOTO because several retrospective feline studies have shown an association between systolic anterior motion of the mitral valve and longer survival times (Fox et al, 1995; Payne et al, 2010; Rush et al, 2002). Often it is possible to control DLVOTO with β-blockers in cats, and anecdotal evidence suggests some clinical benefits on activity level following administration of β-blockers in cats with occult HCM. It is possible that symptomatic cats are more difficult to identify than symptomatic humans, particularly since human symptoms include signs such as chest pain and exercise intolerance. Cats with severe DLVOTO may be treated with atenolol and reexamined within the first month of treatment to confirm that DLVOTO has been controlled and that no adverse effects (e.g., bradycardia or an increase in left atrial size) have developed. Cats with CHF are less likely to demonstrate DLVOTO, but it is unclear whether any benefits of atenolol in this patient group are outweighed by its negative inotropic effects. β-Blockers should be used with great care (or not at all) in cats with DLVOTO and CHF.

Cardiomyopathy with Congestive Heart Failure

Myocardial disease should be high on the differential list for cats with respiratory distress. Physical examination findings that might arouse suspicion of myocardial disease with CHF include combinations of a systolic murmur, gallop sounds, or arrhythmias with tachypnea, pulmonary crackles, and jugular vein distention. Crackles are a helpful finding for parenchymal disease but are not always evident. Muffled breath sounds ventrally may suggest pleural effusion or lung consolidation. Soft heart sounds with normal breath sounds have been identified in cats with ventricular dysfunction, especially DCM. Sometimes no auscultatory abnormalities are present, although respiration generally is labored in inspiration and often in expiration. The differential diagnosis of CHF in cats includes other causes of respiratory distress, pulmonary infiltration, pleural effusion, and airway obstruction. Acute pulmonary infiltration with labored breathing and tachypnea can be associated with thoracic trauma, excessive infusion of crystalloid, noncardiogenic pulmonary edema (see Chapter 9), severe pulmonary infections, vasculitis, lung parasitism (see Web Chapter 57), or spontaneous heartworm death (see Chapter 183). The two most common types of pleural effusion identified in cats with CHF are modified transudates (with small lymphocytes on cytologic examination) and chylothorax related to obstruction of systemic venous and lymphatic return. The differential diagnosis of pleural effusion is extensive and is considered in Chapter 164. Feline asthma can be associated with acute dyspnea but is readily distinguished from CHF by physical examination and radiography (see Chapter 161). Uncommonly, cats with dyspnea are found to have major airway obstruction related to nasopharyngeal polyps (see Chapter 157), laryngeal paresis or neoplasia (see Chapter 158), or tracheal obstruction. Tachypnea in cats with ATE may be related to severe pain rather than CHF.

Imaging is critical to diagnosis. Radiography can be helpful for documenting pulmonary infiltrates or pleural effusion associated with CHF and excluding other causes of respiratory distress, although great care always should be taken when handling dyspneic cats. Sedation (butorphanol 0.1 mg/kg IM, repeated to a 0.3 mg/kg cumulative dose) may allow safer handling of stressed feline patients. These cats are very fragile, and thoracic ultrasonography with the cat in sternal recumbency may offer a safer option for identifying pleural effusions and perhaps the comet tail artifacts often related to pulmonary infiltration or edema.

Echocardiography is the only practical way of identifying the underlying structural and functional abnormality of the heart, and demonstration of left atrial enlargement can be extremely useful as a means of supporting a clinical suspicion of CHF and assessing the risk of thromboembolic complications. A full echocardiographic examination always can be delayed until the cat is in a more stable condition.

Short-term goals of therapy in cats with CHF include relieving life-threatening hypoxemia, lowering left ventricular filling pressure, and improving cardiac function. Improving hemodynamic function is particularly difficult in cats with diastolic heart failure as occurs in HCM.

Acute Congestive Heart Failure

Severely dyspneic cats must be handled with care, and stress should be avoided at all costs. Most cats benefit from low doses of butorphanol (0.1 mg/kg IM, repeated as needed) as sedation. Oxygen supplementation, diuresis, and venodilation all are appropriate treatments for any cat with left-sided heart failure. Pleural effusion must be drained if it causes respiratory distress, and this can be achieved using a 23-gauge butterfly cannula with the cat in sternal recumbency. Furosemide is the mainstay of treatment for cats with acute pulmonary edema. Doses should be lower than those used in dogs, but some cats still require aggressive diuresis, and intravenous furosemide should be titrated to effect. Doses of 1 to 2 mg/kg should be repeated q30-60min until respiratory rate is near normal. Renal function, electrolyte levels, and blood pressure must be monitored. A constant-rate infusion of furosemide also can be considered (see Chapter 175). Reduction of respiratory rate is the most vital monitoring variable indicating successful diuretic therapy. Although ACE inhibitors may have some favorable venodilating effects, caution should be used in administering these drugs to cats with hypotension, and they are best avoided until systemic arterial pressures have reached at least 100 mm Hg.

The severity of short-term clinical signs associated with CHF does not necessarily relate to prognosis. Cats that respond promptly to therapy may become asymptomatic and remain so for long periods. This is particularly true of cats in which CHF has been precipitated by some event, such as stress, intravenous fluid therapy, or general anesthesia.

Low-Output Heart Failure

Some cats have signs of low cardiac output, with or without CHF, which would be characterized by some as cardiogenic shock. These cats typically are hypothermic, bradycardic, and severely hypotensive (systolic blood pressure of <70 mm Hg). Although traditionally positive

inotropes are considered to be contraindicated in HCM because of the likelihood of an increase in myocardial oxygen consumption and aggravation of outflow obstruction, dobutamine appears to be very effective in improving cardiac output and clinical signs in cats with low cardiac output, irrespective of the type of underlying cardiomyopathy. Cats in a low-output state rarely exhibit DLVOTO. Dobutamine doses should be started at lower ranges than those used for dogs, with initial infusion rates of 1 to 2 µg/kg/min followed by cautious upward titration (up to 10 µg/kg/min, or even higher in very hypothermic, unresponsive cats) over several hours, depending on pressure response and heart rate and rhythm. The therapeutic targets are improvements in systolic blood pressure to higher than 100 mm Hg, increase in heart rate, and normalization of body temperature, at which point the infusion can be tapered and withdrawn over several hours. Some cats show signs of nausea or restlessness at relatively low dosages, and infusions exceeding 24 hours rarely are needed; the risk of seizures becomes higher after 24 hours of treatment.

Owing to its favorable pharmacokinetic properties and lack of adverse effects, pimobendan (0.25 mg/kg q12h PO; based on available preparations most often dosed at either 0.625 mg or 1.25 mg per cat q12h) also may be useful in cats with low-output failure that can tolerate oral medication. Although DLVOTO is a definite contraindication to the use of any positive inotrope, absence of a murmur makes DLVOTO unlikely. Warmth and supportive care are important, and in the rare cases in which low-output signs are present in the absence of CHF, it even may be necessary to consider cautious intravenous fluid therapy with low-sodium fluids such as 0.45% NaCl, particularly if levels of renal function indicators (blood urea nitrogen, creatinine) are elevated significantly.

Although the mortality rate for cats with low-output signs can be high, the rewards for aggressive short-term management can be good. For those cats that survive the initial 36 hours, the longer-term prognosis can be surprisingly good, especially for young cats.

Home Management of Congestive Heart Failure

Long-term goals of therapy for CHF include relief of symptoms through prevention of abnormal sodium and water retention, modulation of adverse neurohormonal activation, delay or reversal of myocardial changes, control of arrhythmias, and prevention of thromboembolism. The first two goals may be achievable with the use of oral furosemide and an ACE inhibitor alone in many cats. Furosemide should be titrated to effect (usually 1 to 3 mg/kg q8-24h PO) to achieve resolution of pulmonary edema and pleural effusion. Once congestive signs have resolved, the furosemide dose should be reduced as low as possible. Some cats experience an acute episode of pulmonary edema but, once in stable condition, show good compensation for long periods with minimal doses of furosemide (and furosemide may even be withdrawn in a few cats). In hypotensive cats ACE inhibitors should be introduced cautiously, at quarter or half dose. Such cats often tolerate the full dose of ACE inhibitor in the long term but are vulnerable to worsening hypotension and azotemia following initial administration. ACE inhibitors do not appear to have an adverse effect on dynamic left ventricular outflow tract obstruction and should counteract adverse renin-angiotensin system activation triggered by concurrent furosemide administration. There is not enough evidence to demonstrate superiority of one ACE inhibitor in cats over another. Specific presentations may require specific adjustments in therapy.

Hypertrophic Cardiomyopathy with Congestive Heart Failure and Dynamic Left Ventricular Outflow Tract Obstruction

Previously asymptomatic cats that have HCM with CHF and DLVOTO and *already are receiving* atenolol can be treated with furosemide and an ACE inhibitor as described earlier, in addition to the therapy they already are being given. In some cases congestive signs may be easier to control if the β-blocker is withdrawn or at least reduced by 50% in particular in animals that are hypotensive. Treatment with β-blockers *never should be started* while cats have any signs of CHF and probably is indicated only in cats with well-compensated HCM with DLVOTO.

Systolic Dysfunction

Taurine deficiency is uncommon now, and most cats with a DCM phenotype have normal plasma taurine concentrations. In cats with global systolic dysfunction, it still may be worth administering taurine (250 mg per cat q12h PO) until plasma taurine concentration results are available. A positive inotrope may be helpful, and pimobendan (0.625 to 1.25 mg per cat q12h PO or a dose of approximately 0.25 mg/kg q12h PO) appears to be better tolerated than digoxin in cats. Treatment for CHF is the same as for other cats with cardiomyopathy: furosemide to effect, and an ACE inhibitor. Antithrombotic treatment also should be considered.

Management of Recurrent or Refractory Congestive Heart Failure

Furosemide can be titrated up or down to effect, but some cats have recurrent or persistent congestive signs. In these cats higher doses of furosemide and an ACE inhibitor may be tried at the expense of progressive azotemia. Although mild elevations in serum blood urea nitrogen and creatinine levels are well tolerated, moderate to severe azotemia may result in clinical signs of uremia.

In a cat with progressive fluid accumulation it is reasonable to introduce spironolactone as an additional diuretic and neurohormonal modulator. Spironolactone appears to be tolerated reasonably well and can be given as ¼ of a 25-mg tablet *per cat* q24h. Development of dermal lesions or facial excoriation should be considered an adverse effect of spironolactone in cats, and this finding likely will require discontinuation of the medication. Cats that become truly refractory to furosemide tend to exhibit a lack of both beneficial and adverse effects of the drug. In these cases the dosage of furosemide and ACE inhibitors can be increased, or clients (if willing) can be given preloaded syringes with furosemide (1 mg/kg) that can be administered subcutaneously two or three times weekly in place of oral therapy.

An alternative is the addition of a thiazide diuretic such as hydrochlorothiazide (1 to 2 mg/kg q12-24h PO).

This should be started without subtracting any of the prior therapy. Thiazides should be added at the lowest end of the dosage range and titrated up to effect with careful monitoring of renal function and serum electrolyte levels. Extralabel use of pimobendan (0.625 to 1.25 mg per cat q12h PO) also is potentially beneficial for these cats. Additionally, many cats with CHF can tolerate between 0.25 and 0.5 mg/kg of enalapril or benazepril twice daily rather than once daily PO, and this may be another option to consider for progressive or unresponsive CHF. Periodic thoracocentesis or a brief hospitalization and parenteral diuresis may be needed to treat decompensation associated with marked dyspnea. The benefits of sodium-restricted diets in cats with chronic heart failure are undetermined.

There have been no prospective, multicenter, randomized trials of drug therapy in cats with CHF, and published data, although instructive, do not compare specific treatment approaches or correct for client perceptions that may prompt euthanasia. Perhaps surprisingly to some, survival of 1 year or longer is not uncommon for a cat following the first episode of CHF provided there is appropriate initial therapy, excellent owner compliance, and continuing veterinary support. Many cats can tolerate small to moderate amounts of pleural fluid as long as they are not stressed, and clients can be taught to monitor respiratory rate and depth, activity, appetite, and attitude as markers of quality of life and control of CHF. Ultimately, the combination of progressive CHF and advanced kidney failure tends to limit the success of these therapies. Other cases are complicated by ATE or sudden death.

Cardiomyopathy with Arrhythmias

Arrhythmias can complicate the whole spectrum of feline cardiomyopathy. Atrial and ventricular arrhythmias often are observed in restrictive or unclassified forms of cardiomyopathy. Supraventricular tachycardias have been recognized in young cats and can result in a tachycardia-mediated cardiomyopathy with a DCM phenotype. In management of supraventricular tachycardias, heart rate or rhythm control is essential and can be achieved with oral diltiazem, atenolol, or sometimes sotalol (10 mg per cat q12h PO) as described in more detail in Chapter 173. Great care should be taken because of the negative inotropic effects of sotalol and β-blockers, and these agents should not be used in cats with systolic dysfunction or uncontrolled CHF. Atrial fibrillation sometimes is found in cats with severe left atrial enlargement. If it is associated with excessively fast heart rates, diltiazem can be titrated to effect to control the ventricular response rate. Ventricular arrhythmias may be responsible for some cases of sudden death in cats with HCM or ARVC phenotypes, but ambulatory electrocardiographic monitoring is used less in cats than in dogs and most of these arrhythmias go undiagnosed. Sotalol has been used for control of ventricular arrhythmias in cats.

Arterial (Aortic) Thromboembolism

Cats with all forms of cardiomyopathy are at risk of ATE, and this is particularly true of cats in the more advanced stages of myocardial disease. Atrial dilatation and dysfunction, as discussed previously, are recognized risk factors for ATE. In some cats an episode of ATE is the first sign of myocardial disease. Typically these cats show sudden onset of signs of pain, vocalizing, and paresis when the aortic trifurcation is affected. Forelimbs also can be affected, sometimes with quick spontaneous recovery. Clinical signs may be more confusing with cerebral, mesenteric, renal, or coronary embolism.

Management of Acute Thromboembolism

Cats with thromboembolism are acutely distressed, and pain management is paramount. Fentanyl (3 to 5 µg/kg as a slow IV bolus followed by 2 to 5 µg/kg/hr as a constant-rate infusion) or methadone (0.6 mg/kg q4-6h as a slow IV infusion) are suitable analgesics. Cats that are normothermic, have only one limb affected, or have partial motor function have a better prognosis. This should be taken into consideration when advising the owner about euthanasia. Although the prognosis may be worse for cats with concurrent CHF, the resulting tachypnea can be difficult to differentiate from the effects of pain unless radiography is performed. Some cats die during the first 24 hours of sudden hyperkalemia associated with reperfusion. There is still controversy over the risk : benefit ratio of thrombolytic therapy, and most clinicians opt for prevention of thrombus extension. Aspirin, clopidogrel, unfractionated heparin (300 U/kg q8h SC initially, increase to 500 U/kg if necessary), and low-molecular-weight heparin all are used. However, if thromboembolism is detected within a few hours of the event, intravenous administration of tissue plasminogen activator (0.75-mg bolus followed by 2.5 mg as a constant-rate infusion over 30 minutes and then 1.75 mg as a constant-rate infusion over 1 hour to a total dosage of 5 mg/cat) may be beneficial provided no cardiac thrombus is detectable on echocardiography and the cat can be monitored closely by biochemical testing and electrocardiography for hyperkalemia. Although limb perfusion may be improved by thrombolytic therapy, there is an increased risk of reperfusion injury, which can be fatal. Supportive care is important, and confirmed signs of concurrent congestive disease should be treated as described earlier. Management and prevention of ATE are discussed in more detail in Chapter 181.

Prevention of Thromboembolism

There is no consensus on the optimal therapy for prevention of aortic thromboembolism. Aspirin has been used for many years with a relatively low rate of adverse effects. Its efficacy has not been established, and a low compounded dose (5 mg per cat q3d PO) does not appear to be any less effective than a higher dose (81 mg per cat q3d PO) based on retrospective analysis. Lower dosages do appear to have a lower rate of adverse effects such as anorexia and vomiting (often related to gastrointestinal irritation). Warfarin is associated with an unacceptable

rate of adverse effects and an impractically high level of monitoring requirements. Clopidogrel (Plavix, 18.75 mg per cat q24h PO) offers some hope as a new antithrombotic treatment and currently is under evaluation in the Feline Aortic Thromboembolism Clopidogrel versus Aspirin Trial (FATCAT). Preliminary analysis of the FATCAT trial data has demonstrated superiority of clopidogrel over aspirin (see Chapter 181). Clopidogrel can be combined with aspirin, although it probably is safest to use the lowest aspirin dosage possible in this situation (5 mg per cat q3d PO) and to have clients monitor appetite as a marker of gastrointestinal side effects. It is stressed that although each of these treatments hypothetically is beneficial and these drugs have been shown to alter clotting function in cats, there are no definitive, evidence-based guidelines for therapy or prevention of ATE in cats with cardiomyopathy.

References and Suggested Reading

Fox PR et al: Multicenter evaluation of plasma N-terminal pro-brain natriuretic peptide (NT-pro BNP) as a biochemical screening test for asymptomatic (occult) cardiomyopathy in cats, *J Vet Intern Med* 25:1010, 2011.

Fox PR, Liu SK, Maron BJ: Echocardiographic assessment of spontaneously occurring feline hypertrophic cardiomyopathy. An animal model of human disease, *Circulation* 92:2645, 1995.

MacDonald KA et al: The effect of ramipril on left ventricular mass, myocardial fibrosis, diastolic function, and plasma neurohormones in Maine Coon cats with familial hypertrophic cardiomyopathy without heart failure, *J Vet Intern Med* 20:1093, 2006.

MacDonald KA et al: Effect of spironolactone on diastolic function and left ventricular mass in Maine Coon cats with familial hypertrophic cardiomyopathy, *J Vet Intern Med* 22:335, 2008.

Maron BJ et al: American College of Cardiology/European Society of Cardiology clinical expert consensus document on hypertrophic cardiomyopathy, *J Am Coll Cardiol* 42:1687, 2003.

Maron BJ et al: Contemporary definitions and classification of the cardiomyopathies, *Circulation* 113:1807, 2006.

Paige CF et al: Prevalence of cardiomyopathy in apparently healthy cats, *J Am Vet Med Assoc* 234:1398, 2009.

Payne J et al: Population characteristics and survival in 127 referred cats with hypertrophic cardiomyopathy (1997 to 2005), *J Small Anim Pract* 51:540, 2010.

Payne JR et al: Risk factors for sudden death in feline hypertrophic cardiomyopathy, *J Vet Intern Med* 25:1479, 2011.

Rush JE et al: Population and survival characteristics of cats with hypertrophic cardiomyopathy: 260 cases (1990-1999), *J Am Vet Med Assoc* 220:202, 2002.

Schober KE, I Maerz: Assessment of left atrial appendage flow velocity and its relation to spontaneous echocardiographic contrast in 89 cats with myocardial disease, *J Vet Intern Med* 20:120, 2006.

Taillefer M, Di Fruscia R: Benazepril and subclinical feline hypertrophic cardiomyopathy: a prospective, blinded, controlled study, *Can Vet J* 47:437, 2006.

Wagner T et al: Comparison of auscultatory and echocardiographic findings in healthy adult cats, *J Vet Cardiol* 12:171, 2010.

CHAPTER 181

Arterial Thromboembolism

DANIEL F. HOGAN, *West Lafayette, Indiana*

Background

Arterial thromboembolism (ATE) is a sudden interruption of arterial blood flow caused by thrombotic material that is derived from a distant site. This obstruction leads to infarction of tissues served by that arterial bed. Localized arterial thrombosis is associated with abnormalities of the vascular endothelium or vascular wall and may stem from high-shear flow within a narrowed blood vessel. This condition seems relatively rare in dogs and cats. Conversely, ATE occurs commonly in small animals.

In some cases of ATE, the site of the originating thrombus is either known or reliably suspected. For example, cardiogenic embolism (CE) typically results from thrombi located within a dilated left atrium or auricle, whereas septic cardioemboli develop with valvular or mural endocarditis. However, in other cases, such as neoplasia, protein-losing nephropathy, hyperadrenocorticism, and immune-mediated hemolytic anemia, the thrombus source cannot be determined. It has been suggested that in some cases of ATE where a source of the arterial thrombus cannot be identified, systemic venous thrombi may be the source of the embolic material, causing paradoxical (right-to-left) ATE. In human patients paradoxical ATE often is associated with deep venous thrombosis in which thrombotic material crosses a congenital cardiac defect from the right to the left side of the circulation, often across a patent foramen ovale (PFO). Cryptogenic stroke (a stroke of uncertain origin) is three times more likely in human patients with a PFO, and human patients with a PFO are 34 times more likely to experience silent brain infarction. Paradoxic embolism has been reported in veterinary medicine and in one recent study (Hogan and Meltzer, 2011) evidence of right-to-left shunting at the atrial level was identified in approximately 50% of dogs with congenital heart disease using agitated saline contrast echocardiography. Such findings could explain the relatively high frequency of silent renal infarcts on abdominal ultrasonography in cats and dogs and the development of systemic ATE in veterinary patients with hypercoagulable disorders.

Pathogenesis

In the normal healthy state, there is an equilibrium between thrombus formation and thrombus dissolution, which prevents unregulated thrombus formation. Primary hemostasis occurs when platelets are exposed to subendothelial collagen. This leads to platelet adhesion and activation, with subsequent aggregation and release of proaggregating and vasoconstrictive substances. Platelet release products, in conjunction with circulating factors within the plasma, initiate the coagulation cascade. Fibrinolytic and antithrombotic mechanisms are activated simultaneously to break down the developing hemostatic plug, which prevents excessive thrombus formation. Pathologic thrombosis can result from any combination of impaired or overwhelmed antithrombotic mechanisms, increased function of prothrombotic mechanisms, or impaired fibrinolysis.

The development of pathologic thrombosis classically has been linked to Virchow's triad, which includes endothelial injury, blood stasis, and the presence of a hypercoagulable state, with each arm adding to the risk of thrombosis (cumulative thrombotic risk). Examples of endothelial injury are a dilated left atrium in a cat with hypertrophic cardiomyopathy, a damaged aortic valve in a dog with subaortic stenosis, and tumor invasion of the arterial tree. Blood stasis is associated with dilated or poorly contracting cardiac chambers, restricted blood flow from tumor growth, or sluggish venous flow. The hypercoagulability arm of the triad has been poorly defined in domestic animal species, although there are known clinical conditions associated with thrombosis in animals (see Chapter 166).

Known hypercoagulable states in humans include inherited abnormalities in the procoagulant factors IIa (thrombin), Va, and VIIIa as well as the antithrombotic proteins antithrombin (AT), protein C, and protein S. Additional hypercoagulable states include platelet hypersensitivity and increases in homocysteine, lipoprotein (a), plasminogen activator inhibitor, and thrombin-activatable fibrinolysis inhibitor. Suspected hypercoagulable states in dogs and cats include platelet hypersensitivity, decreased AT and protein C activity, and increased levels of in factors II, V, VII, VIII, IX, X, XII, and fibrinogen.

Early pathologic thrombus composition is classified as platelet rich but progressively becomes more fibrin rich as the thrombus continues to grow. As the thrombus ages, superficial portions can break off forming emboli that cause infarction in distant arterial beds. The clinical signs that result from the arterial infarction depend on the site and completeness of the arterial obstruction, the availability of arterial anastomoses and collateral circulation, and the metabolic demands of the tissues. Platelet-released vasoactive substances reduce the collateral flow around the site of obstruction and contribute to the clinical signs of ischemic neuromyopathy. This is similar to what is observed in humans with thrombotic stroke, cardiogenic embolism, and pulmonary embolism. In experimental feline models of aortic ATE, pretreatment with the antiserotonergic drug cyproheptadine and clopidogrel (which inhibits platelet activation and has a vasomodulating effect) maintains the collateral network and reduces the signs of ischemic neuromyopathy.

Clinical Signs

The type and severity of clinical signs relates to the location and completeness of the arterial obstruction. Organs often have a collateral network that can be recruited to provide blood flow around a site of arterial obstruction, but flow through these networks appears to be impaired with acute thrombotic infarction.

Renal infarction can present with renal pain and acute renal failure, whereas infarction of the cranial mesenteric artery can result in severe abdominal pain, vomiting, and diarrhea. Nonspecific signs of lethargy, anorexia, vomiting, and diarrhea have been reported with splenic infarction. The clinical signs of cerebrovascular accidents or stroke can be profound, depending on the neural location of the infarction and the territory served by the affected artery. Signs can include paresis, vestibular dysfunction, cranial nerve deficits, and seizures.

Infarction caused by obstruction of the distal aortic trifurcation (a saddle thromboembolus) accounts for the majority of ATE cases in dogs and cats and results in a loss of blood flow to the pelvic limbs, causing ischemic neuromyopathy. Paresis or paralysis of the pelvic limbs with absence of segmental reflexes, firm and painful pelvic limb musculature, and cold and pulseless limbs with cyanotic nail beds are typical features. These findings can be bilateral and symmetric, or unilateral and asymmetric, depending on the degree of infarction and blood flow through collateral vessels. The tail often is involved. Cats appear to be more severely affected with ischemic neuromyopathy than are dogs, which may be indicative of species differences in platelet function or preservation of the collateral circulation. The clinical signs of ischemic neuromyopathy are peracute in onset and can worsen, but usually remain stagnant or improve over the following several days to 3 weeks.

Infarction of the subclavian artery, typically the right subclavian, is the second most common site for ATE in cats and occasionally is seen in dogs. The clinical signs associated with infarction at this site are essentially identical to those for infarction of the aortic trifurcation, although the signs are confined to the affected forelimb.

Clinical Thrombotic Conditions

There are a number of clinical conditions in which thrombotic complications are commonly recognized, increase morbidity and mortality, may require acute treatment, and should initiate consideration for antithrombotic therapy. For this discussion, systemic ATE and pulmonary ATE are included in the pathologic process of ATE.

Immune-Mediated Hemolytic Anemia
Pulmonary embolism has been identified in 30% to 80% of dogs with immune-mediated hemolytic anemia (IMHA) at necropsy and often is speculated to be the cause of death. Altered hemostatic parameters, including prolonged coagulation times and increased levels of fibrinogen, D-dimers, and fibrin degradation products as well as reduced AT levels, have been noted. Oxidative stress and platelet hyperactivation appear to be associated with thrombosis in humans with IMHA. One study identified an eightfold increase in P-selectin expression in dogs with IMHA, which suggests that dogs with the disorder have an increase in circulating activated platelets (Weiss and Brazzell, 2006).

Hyperadrenocorticism
Pulmonary embolism appears to occur in up to 18% of dogs with hyperadrenocorticism, and increases in the procoagulant factors II, V, VII, IX, X, XII, and fibrinogen have been noted. There is a fourfold increase in pulmonary embolism in humans with hyperadrenocorticism, and as in dogs, elevations in procoagulant factors II, V, VII, IX, X, and XII have been identified.

Protein-Losing Nephropathy
Thromboembolic complications have been reported to occur in over 20% of dogs with protein-losing nephropathy. Reduced circulating AT levels are thought to result from loss through the damaged glomerular tuft; a correlation also has been noted between platelet hypersensitivity and hypoalbuminemia. This platelet hypersensitivity appears to resolve with increases in albumin concentration following therapy. The incidence of thromboembolic disease in humans with nephrotic syndrome is approximately 1% per year, and risk is related to the degree of proteinuria and hypoalbuminemia. In addition to loss of AT, other possible causes of hypercoagulability in humans include increased thrombin-activatable fibrinolysis inhibitor and reduced protein C activity.

Neoplasia
The reported frequency of neoplasia in dogs and cats with ATE ranges from 2.5% to 30%. Suspected causes include an unknown hypercoagulable state, paraneoplastic thrombocytosis, tumor embolization, and local tumor extension. Thrombosis is seen in up to 15% of human cancer patients, and there are a number of proposed causes for the hypercoagulable state, including the presence of a cysteine proteinase (cancer procoagulant factor), acquired protein C resistance, and increased P-selectin levels.

Cerebrovascular Accidents (Strokes)
Although representing fewer than approximately 2% of all neurologic cases in dogs, cerebrovascular accidents or strokes have become more widely identified clinically with the advent of advanced brain imaging. Apparent clinical associations include hypothyroidism, diabetes mellitus, hypertension, and suspected but undefined hypercoagulable states. Cavalier King Charles spaniels and greyhounds, breeds with known platelet abnormalities, appear to be overrepresented.

Cardiogenic Embolism
Thromboembolic complications associated with cardiac disease probably are the most common cause of ATE in

veterinary medicine, with cats affected far more commonly than dogs. The frequency of CE in cats with cardiac disease has been reported to be between 6% and 17%. Males are overrepresented, and breeds that appear to have an increased risk are Ragdoll, Birman, Tonkinese, and Abyssinian. Possible markers of hypercoagulability have been identified in cats with a previous history of CE and include platelet hypersensitivity as well as reductions in AT and protein C activity. Survival rates with an initial ATE event range from 33% to 39%. Survival is dramatically better with single-limb infarction than with bilateral infarction (68% to 93% versus 15% to 36%, respectively) and is negatively impacted by hypothermia, reduced heart rate, and absence of motor function. Reported median survival times range from 51 days to 443 days with recurrence rates of 17% to 75% over the first year (Laste and Harpster, 1995; Smith et al, 2003). A recent trial comparing clopidogrel with aspirin demonstrated significant improvement in survival with clopidogrel (Fat Cat trial, Hogan et al, 2013).

Clinical Management

Key elements in the acute management of ATE include preventing continued thrombus formation associated with the embolus, improving blood flow to the infarcted tissues, and managing pain.

Reduce Thrombus Formation

Unfractionated heparin (UFH) is a group of heterogeneous molecules with a mean molecular weight of approximately 15,000 D. Heparin molecules contain a pentasaccharide sequence that binds to AT, which facilitates the inhibition of factors IIa, Xa, IXa, and XIIa. Thrombin-catalyzed activation of factors V and VIII is inhibited as well. UFH also exhibits a mild antiplatelet effect in normal humans. Objective studies evaluating the bleeding risk with UFH therapy in dogs and cats are unavailable, but clinically relevant bleeding has been observed in both species. There is no documented report of heparin-induced thrombocytopenia in dogs or cats, although this severe condition has been reported in up to 10% of human patients receiving UFH. Ideally, coagulation testing including platelet count, prothrombin time (PT), and activated partial thromboplastin time (aPTT) should be performed before heparin therapy is begun. Adequate dosing of heparin in dogs and cats has been shown to be quite variable, and dosing requirements may change over time because of a decrease in AT levels. Dosing guidelines call for an initial dose of 250 to 375 IU/kg followed by 150 to 250 IU/kg q6-8h SC for cats, and an initial dose of 200 to 300 IU/kg IV followed by 200 to 250 IU/kg q6-8h SC for dogs. Constant-rate infusions also are used by some clinicians (see Chapter 166). Serial measurement of the aPTT can be used to monitor heparin therapy with a target of 1.5 to 2.0 times the baseline value.

The *low-molecular-weight heparins* (LMWHs) are smaller in molecular size than UFH and can be used in lieu of UFH. The cost of these agents is considerably more than that of UFH (approximately $3 to $5 per dose) and there is no clear indication of clinical benefit over UFH in the acute management period. Dalteparin (Fragmin) and enoxaparin (Lovenox) have been used in dogs and cats at 100 IU/kg q12h SC and 1.0 to 1.5 mg/kg q12h SC, respectively, during the acute management period.

Improvement of Blood Flow

Thrombolytic Therapy
Thrombolytic drugs have been used in dogs and cats to dissolve emboli and reestablish arterial blood flow. These should be administered as soon as possible after the embolic event, with many clinicians considering 6 hours a reasonable therapeutic window, although effective therapy has been documented as late as 18 hours after initial clinical signs of ATE. Severe and potentially fatal adverse effects can be associated with thrombolytic therapy; therefore caution should be exercised when considering these drugs. The sudden resumption of arterial flow to infarcted organs can result in the rapid development of life-threatening hyperkalemia and metabolic acidosis (reperfusion injury), and this is most likely to occur with complete aortic occlusion and severe infarction of rear limb muscles. The reported frequency of reperfusion injury following thrombolytic therapy in cats with CE is from 40% to 70% with reported survival rates from 0% to 43%, and some of these fatality rates are higher than those observed with more conservative therapy (heparin, pain management, time for reperfusion). Because of potential adverse effects and cost, the author considers thrombolytic therapy only in cases in which the loss of arterial flow makes survival unlikely.

Tissue plasminogen activator (t-PA) forms an intimate relationship with plasminogen within thrombi, resulting in a relative fibrin-specific conversion of plasminogen to plasmin. However, when t-PA is administered at clinical doses, a systemic proteolytic state and bleeding can be seen.

Although there is overall little experience with the use of human recombinant t-PA (Activase) in dogs and cats, it has been administered intravenously either as a constant-rate infusion in cats (0.25 to 1 mg/kg/hr IV for a total dose of 5 mg/kg) or multiple-bolus therapy in dogs (1 mg/kg IV). The success rate in two isolated case reports of dogs was variable. There is one reported clinical trial of t-PA therapy in six cats with CE that recorded a 50% survival rate. Perfusion was restored within 36 hours and motor function returned within 48 hours in 100% of surviving cats. Complications included minor hemorrhage from catheter sites (50%), fever (33%), and reperfusion injury (33%).

Urokinase, similar to streptokinase, is no longer commercially available, and is considered relatively fibrin specific. Urokinase has been administered to cats and dogs for treatment of ATE using a protocol of 4400 IU/kg IV as a loading dose given over 10 minutes followed by 4400 IU/kg/hr IV for 12 hours. There is one published study in cats (Whelan et al, 2005a), which reported a 42% survival rate; 30% regained pulses, 60% regained motor function, and 25% developed reperfusion injury. The published clinical experience in dogs (Whelan et al, 2005b) has been much less encouraging, with a mortality rate of 100% in treated dogs.

Improvement of Collateral Blood Flow

Increasing perfusion to the infarcted organ has been attempted by administering drugs that may potentially increase flow through the collateral arterial network. The use of vasodilators such as acepromazine has not been demonstrated to be effective and may have a negative clinical impact by inducing hypotension, which further reduces perfusion. The platelet-release products serotonin and thromboxane have been implicated as factors involved in loss of collateral circulation. Clopidogrel (Plavix) has been shown to reduce serotonin release from activated platelets in cats and improve collateral flow, with reduced clinical signs of ischemic neuromyopathy in a cat model of aortic thromboembolism. Maximal platelet inhibition is achieved within 72 hours at dosage of 1 to 4 mg/kg q24h PO in dogs and cats, but an oral loading dose of 10 mg/kg in dogs resulted in comparable effects within 90 minutes with no adverse effects. Daily administration of 1 to 2 mg/kg in cats (approximately 18.75 mg) is well tolerated and is not associated with adverse effects. Therefore the author administers a loading dose of 75 mg of clopidogrel PO upon presentation with ATE in an attempt to improve collateral flow and reduce thrombus formation.

Pain Management

ATE can result in severe pain that must be treated aggressively, especially within the initial 24 to 36 hours after the event when pain is most severe. Opiates generally are selected for this purpose. These include *butorphanol tartrate* (0.1 to 0.4 mg/kg q1-4h SC, IM, or IV for dogs and cats), *hydromorphone* (0.08 to 0.3 mg/kg q2-6h SC for dogs and cats), *buprenorphine hydrochloride* (0.005 to 0.02 mg/kg q6-12h SC, IM, or IV for dogs and cats), *oxymorphone hydrochloride* (0.05 to 0.2 mg/kg q1-3h SC, IM, or IV for dogs and cats), and *fentanyl citrate* (4 to 10 µg/kg IV bolus followed by 2 to 10 µg/kg/hr IV infusion for dogs and cats). The use of these drugs is discussed more fully in Chapter 12 of this book. In general, strong mu agonists (such as fentanyl or hydromorphone) provide the best analgesia, compared with partial (butorphanol) or mixed (buprenorphine) analgesics, and should be considered for initial therapy. Availability of specific opiates within the practice may influence the selection of drugs.

Prevention

Primary prevention of ATE is defined as preventing the first event in an animal at risk of ATE. Although primary prevention would be an ideal and logical goal, there is a poor understanding of thrombotic risk in dogs and cats. The greatest body of evidence relates to CE in cats. Cats appear to be at a greater risk of ATE if they have an increase in left atrial size or evidence of stagnant left atrial blood flow ("smoke") or diminished left auricular emptying as evidenced by echocardiography. Therefore prophylactic antithrombotic therapy should be considered in cats with these risk factors.

Secondary prevention is defined as preventing a recurrent ATE event, and the largest body of evidence again relates to CE in cats. However, these data are problematic because they are based on retrospective, non–placebo-controlled studies of individual antithrombotic agents. Thus there is no scientific basis for conclusions that any antithrombotic agent is effective, completely ineffective, or superior to another agent. Reported recurrence rates for cats receiving some antithrombotic drug range from 17% to 75%, with a 1-year recurrence rate of 25% to 50%.

Antithrombotic Drugs

Due to their direct effect on thrombus formation, antithrombotic agents have become a mainstay for primary and secondary prevention of ATE in dogs and cats. However, it should be emphasized that the goal of complete prevention of recurrent embolic events in animals with chronic diseases such as cardiac disease or nephrotic syndrome is unrealistic.

Antiplatelet Agents

Antiplatelet agents inhibit some aspect of platelet function and impair the formation of the initial platelet-rich thrombus. Some of these drugs also exhibit vasomodulating effects by reducing the release of or interfering with the activity of vasoactive substances released by platelets.

Aspirin irreversibly acetylates platelet cyclooxygenase, preventing the formation of thromboxane A_2, a potent proaggregating and vasoconstrictive molecule. Aspirin is considered a modest and indirect antiplatelet agent. The standard dosage in cats is 81 mg q72h PO, but adverse effects such as anorexia and vomiting have been reported in up to 22% of treated cats. A low-dose protocol of 5 mg q72h PO has been associated with reduced adverse effects. Reported recurrence rates of ATE in aspirin-treated cats range from 17% to 75%, regardless of aspirin dose. There has been very little published regarding the clinical use of aspirin for the prevention of thrombosis in dogs, but 0.5 mg/kg q24-12h PO generally is used, and one study reported an increased survival in dogs with IMHA.

Clopidogrel, which must undergo hepatic biotransformation to form the active metabolite, induces specific and irreversible antagonism of the adenosine diphosphate P2Y12 receptor along the platelet membrane and results in more potent platelet inhibition than aspirin. The vasomodulating effects of clopidogrel already have been mentioned. Unlike aspirin, clopidogrel is not associated with gastroduodenal ulceration. When dosed at 1 to 3 mg/kg q24h PO in cats and dogs, maximal antiplatelet effects are seen by 3 days of drug administration and are lost within 7 days after drug discontinuation. Because of the size of the commercially available tablet, the typical cat dosing protocol is 18.75 mg per cat q24h PO. There have been anecdotal reports of sporadic vomiting in cats receiving clopidogrel clinically. Administering clopidogrel in a gel capsule or with food appears to reduce this occurrence dramatically. Preliminary analysis of an ongoing trial indicated that clopidogrel confers a survival benefit over aspirin in cats that had previously survived a cardiogenic embolus (Hogan et al, 2013). Clopidogrel sometimes is combined with aspirin in human patients, but whether this combination might be effective in dogs and cats is unknown.

Anticoagulant Agents

Anticoagulant drugs inhibit the coagulation cascade by interfering with the formation of one or more active coagulation factors. Some of these drugs also exhibit relatively minor antiplatelet effects.

Warfarin inhibits the formation of the vitamin K–dependent coagulation factors II, VII, IX, and X as well as the anticoagulant proteins C and S. Numerous studies in humans have demonstrated superior efficacy of warfarin over antiplatelet drugs for primary and secondary prevention of CE in patients with atrial fibrillation. Warfarin therapy is adjusted by monitoring the international normalized ratio (INR), which normalizes an individual animal's PT for a given laboratory. The pharmacokinetics and pharmacodynamics of warfarin have been evaluated in dogs and cats, and wide interindividual and intraindividual variability have been noted. Published dosing protocols call for 0.06 to 0.09 mg/kg q24h PO for cats and 0.05 to 0.2 mg/kg q24h PO for dogs. Warfarin is not evenly distributed throughout the tablet, so it is best to have it compounded by a pharmacist if partial-pill dosing is required. Careful monitoring of the INR (with a target value of 2 to 3) or PT (with a target value of 1.3 to 1.6 times baseline) is required, and owners should be aware of this requirement for frequent blood draws and dosing adjustments. Warfarin dosing changes are often accomplished by changing the total weekly dose (as opposed to daily dose) in response to INR monitoring. Published CE recurrence rates for warfarin-treated cats in retrospective studies range from 42% to 53% with estimated mean survival times of 210 to 471 days. Bleeding is the most common complication and is seen in 13% to 20% of cats, with fatal hemorrhage reported in up to 13% of cats. Because of the difficulty in dosing accurately, wide variability in drug response, and requirement for diligent monitoring, warfarin rarely is used for prevention of ATE in cats. Warfarin is easier to administer to dogs, and there are small retrospective studies demonstrating practical clinical use in this species.

The *LMWHs* are smaller in molecular size than UFH but maintain the pentasaccharide sequence that binds to AT, so that they inhibit factor Xa but have a greatly reduced inhibition of factor IIa. Recommended dosing protocols are dalteparin 100 IU/kg q24-12h SC for cats and dogs and enoxaparin 1.0 to 1.5 mg/kg q24-12h SC for cats and dogs (see Chapter 166). Although some have advocated monitoring LMWH therapy by measuring anti–factor Xa activity, it has been shown that anti–factor Xa activity does not correlate with thrombus inhibition in cats, so monitoring is not indicated in the author's opinion. The ATE recurrence rate in cats treated with dalteparin is similar to that in cats given warfarin, but bleeding rarely is experienced. The major limiting factors for these drugs are that they must be administered by injection and are quite expensive.

Future Directions in Prevention

Most recently a number of drugs have been developed that selectively inhibit factor Xa (*Xa inhibitors*). These drugs are some of the first to have been proven to be at least as effective as warfarin for the prevention of CE in humans. They also are being used for the prevention of venous thromboembolism in humans. This group includes the drugs fondaparinux, rivaroxaban, and apixaban. Most of these drugs can be given orally and generally do not require monitoring. The development of a drug that is as efficacious as warfarin for ATE, can be given orally, and does not require clinical monitoring would be the greatest advancement in ATE prevention to date.

References and Suggested Reading

Hogan DF: Prevention and management of thromboembolism. In August JR, editor: *Consultations in feline internal medicine*, vol 5, St Louis, 2005, Saunders, p 331.

Hogan DF, Meltzer L: Frequency of right-to-left shunting in dogs with congenital cardiac disease undergoing interventional cardiovascular procedures. In *Proceedings of the 29th Annual ACVIM Forum*, 2011.

Hogan D et al: Analysis of feline arterial thromboembolism: clopidogrel vs. aspirin trial (Fat Cat) in *Proceedings of the American College of Veterinary Internal Medicine*, Seattle, June 2013 (abstract).

Laste NJ, Harpster NK: A retrospective study of 100 cases of feline distal aortic thromboembolism: 1977-1993, *J Am Anim Hosp Assoc* 31:492, 1995.

Smith SA et al: Arterial thromboembolism in cats: acute crisis in 127 cases (1992-2001) and long-term management with low-dose aspirin in 24 cases, *J Vet Intern Med* 17:73, 2003.

Weiss DJ, Brazzell JL: Detection of activated platelets in dogs with primary immune-mediated hemolytic anemia, *J Vet Intern Med* 20:682, 2006.

Whelan MF et al: Retrospective evaluation of urokinase in cats with arterial thromboembolism, *J Vet Emerg Crit Care* 15:S8, 2005a (abstract).

Whelan MF et al: Retrospective evaluation of urokinase use in dogs with thromboembolism (4 cases: 2003-2004), *J Vet Emerg Crit Care* 15:S8, 2005b (abstract).

Winter RL et al: Aortic thrombosis in dogs: presentation, therapy, and outcome in 26 cases, *J Vet Cardiol* 14:333, 2012.

CHAPTER 182

Pericardial Effusion

O. LYNNE NELSON, *Pullman, Washington*
WENDY A. WARE, *Ames, Iowa*

The double-layered pericardial sac surrounding the heart normally contains a small volume (≈0.25 ml/kg) of serous fluid between its outer fibrous layer (parietal pericardium) and inner serous membrane (visceral pericardium or epicardium). Excessive fluid accumulation (pericardial effusion) is the most common pericardial disorder in small animals. It occurs much more frequently in dogs than in cats.

Pathophysiology

Pericardial effusion disturbs cardiac function by impeding filling. Because the pericardium is relatively noncompliant, increases in pericardial fluid volume can increase intrapericardial pressure sharply. When intrapericardial pressure equals or exceeds normal cardiac filling pressure, cardiac filling is impaired. This condition is known as cardiac tamponade. The rate of pericardial fluid accumulation and the distensibility of the pericardial sac determine whether and how quickly cardiac tamponade develops. Rapid accumulation of a small volume (e.g., 50 to 100 ml) can raise intrapericardial pressure markedly because the pericardium can stretch only slowly. Fibrosis and pericardial thickening may further limit the compliance of this tissue. Pericardial fibrosis and inflammatory cell infiltrates are seen with idiopathic and neoplastic causes of effusion. Conversely, if effusion accumulates slowly, the pericardium may enlarge sufficiently to accommodate the increased volume at low pressure. As long as intrapericardial pressure is lower than normal venous pressures, cardiac filling and output are maintained and signs of tamponade are absent. Therefore large-volume pericardial effusion implies a gradual process.

The external cardiac compression that occurs with tamponade progressively limits filling, initially of the right side of the heart but subsequently of the left side as well. Systemic venous pressure increases while cardiac output falls. Diastolic pressures in all cardiac chambers and great veins eventually equilibrate. Neurohumoral compensatory mechanisms of heart failure become activated as cardiac output falls. External signs of systemic venous congestion and right-sided congestive heart failure (CHF) become especially prominent with time.

Cardiac tamponade exaggerates the variation in arterial blood pressure that occurs normally during the respiratory cycle. If the inspiratory fall in left heart output causes a 10 mm Hg or greater fluctuation in systolic arterial pressure, this is known as *pulsus paradoxus.* Although myocardial contractility is not affected directly by pericardial effusion, inadequate ventricular filling combined with reduced coronary perfusion during tamponade can lead to systolic and diastolic ventricular impairment. Low cardiac output, arterial hypotension, systemic venous congestion, and poor perfusion of the heart, as well as other organs, can lead ultimately to cardiogenic shock and death.

Presentation

Cardiac tamponade is relatively common in dogs but rare in cats. Clinical signs reflect the consequences of systemic venous congestion and poor cardiac output. Right-sided congestive signs usually predominate, especially abdominal enlargement (ascites). Tachypnea and weakness or syncope with exertion are common in the history. Lethargy, poor exercise tolerance, inappetence, cough, and other nonspecific signs can occur before obvious ascites develops. Loss of lean body mass (cachexia) is apparent in some chronic cases. Rapid pericardial fluid accumulation can cause acute tamponade, shock, and death. In such cases clinical signs of jugular venous distention, hypotension, and possibly pulmonary edema may be evident without pleural effusion, ascites, or radiographic cardiomegaly.

Physical examination findings typically include jugular venous distention or positive hepatojugular reflux, hepatomegaly, ascites, labored respiration, and weakened femoral pulses. Subcutaneous edema occasionally is evident. Greater attenuation of femoral pulse strength during inspiration is occasionally discernible in patients with pulsus paradoxus because of the phasic reductions in pulse (as well as mean arterial) pressure. This also may be detected with a Doppler flow system as expiratory "breakthrough" flow signals that are heard when the pressure within the blood pressure cuff is held just above the level of systolic pressure recorded during inspiration. High sympathetic tone associated with reduced cardiac output can lead to sinus tachycardia, mucous membrane pallor, and prolonged capillary refill time. Fever may accompany infective pericarditis, and affected patients may appear very ill.

The precordial impulse is palpably weak when pericardial fluid volume is large. Heart sounds become muffled (or distant) with moderate to large pericardial effusions. Lung sounds are muffled ventrally when pleural effusion is present. Although pericardial effusion does not cause a murmur, concurrent cardiac disease may do so. Large-volume pericardial effusions sometimes cause clinical signs by virtue of their size, even in the absence of overt tamponade. Lung or airway compression can provoke dyspnea or cough; esophageal compression can cause dysphagia or regurgitation.

Causes

Most pericardial effusions in dogs are serosanguineous or sanguineous (hemorrhagic) and are either neoplastic or idiopathic ("benign") in origin. Transudates, modified transudates, and exudates are found occasionally in both dogs and cats. Cardiac and heart-base neoplasia are common causes of pericardial effusion in the dog. Peritoneopericardial diaphragmatic hernia or (rarely) other congenital pericardial malformations including cysts may be associated with effusion in both species.

In cats pericardial effusion is identified most often in association with CHF (especially hypertrophic cardiomyopathy). Cardiac tamponade rarely develops in cats with CHF. Infection with feline infectious peritonitis virus is reported as an important cause of pericardial effusion in the older literature, but this origin seems less common today, at least in North America. Pericardial effusions caused by lymphoma, other systemic infections, and, rarely, renal failure also are reported in cats. Whereas cardiac tumors occur relatively frequently in dogs, these are rare in cats.

Hemorrhagic effusions tend to be dark red, with a packed cell volume of more than 7%, specific gravity of more than 1.015, and protein level of more than 3 g/dl. A hemorrhagic effusion with a packed cell volume similar to that of peripheral blood (hemopericardium) suggests active hemorrhage; considerations include acute tumor bleed, coagulopathy (e.g., rodenticide toxicity), and atrial tear. Besides red blood cells, reactive mesothelial, neoplastic, or other cells may be seen on cytologic examination. Pericardial fluid generally does not clot unless hemorrhage was very recent. Neoplastic hemorrhagic effusions are more common in older dogs, although middle-aged and even younger dogs sometimes are affected. Hemangiosarcoma (HSA) is by far the most common cause, followed by heart-base tumors and pericardial mesothelioma. HSA usually arises within the right side of the heart, especially the right auricular appendage. HSA appears to have an increased prevalence in certain breeds such as the German shepherd, golden retriever, Afghan hound, English setter, American cocker spaniel, Doberman pinscher, Labrador retriever, and miniature poodle but is observed in many breeds of dogs.

Chemodectoma or aortic body tumor (arising from chemoreceptor cells at the base of the aorta) is the most common heart-base tumor. Breeds with a predilection include boxers, Boston terriers, and bulldogs, but not all dogs with chemodectomas are of brachycephalic breeds. Other heart-base tumors include thyroid, parathyroid, lymphoid, or connective tissue neoplasms. Pericardial mesothelioma is confirmed occasionally in the dog and cat but represents a challenging diagnosis because discrete mass lesions are not always evident by echocardiography. Mesothelioma may mimic idiopathic pericardial effusion in dogs. Pericardial effusion secondary to metastatic tumors appears to be rare, although some necropsy reports indicate that metastatic cancer to the heart is underdiagnosed. Neoplastic pericardial effusion in cats most often is associated with lymphoma; various other cardiac tumors are involved rarely.

Idiopathic pericardial effusion is most common in medium to large dog breeds. Although dogs of any age can be affected, the median age appears to be about 6 to 7 years. The Saint Bernard dog is listed as predisposed in some reports. Mild pericardial inflammation with areas of hemorrhage and diffuse pericardial fibrosis have been described histologically. Less common causes of intrapericardial hemorrhage are left atrial rupture from severe chronic mitral regurgitation, coagulopathy, and penetrating trauma.

Transudative effusions usually are modified rather than pure transudates. Transudative effusions can occur with CHF, peritoneopericardial diaphragmatic hernia, hypoalbuminemia, pericardial cysts, or toxemias that increase vascular permeability (including uremia). Usually these conditions are associated with a small volume of pericardial effusion, and cardiac tamponade rarely develops. Effusions caused by cardiac lymphoma and rarely by heart-base masses also can appear as transudative rather than hemorrhagic.

Exudative pericardial effusions are rare in small animals. Exudates appear cloudy to opaque or serofibrinous to serosanguineous. They are characterized by a high nucleated cell count (well over 3000 cells/μl), high protein concentration (usually much higher than 3 g/dl), and high specific gravity (>1.015). Cytologic findings are related to the originating condition. Infectious causes usually are related to plant awn migration, bite wounds, or extension of infection in nearby structures. Various aerobic and anaerobic bacterial infections, actinomycosis, coccidioidomycosis, disseminated tuberculosis, and rarely systemic protozoal infections have been identified. Sterile exudative effusions have occurred with leptospirosis, canine distemper, uremia, and idiopathic pericardial effusion in dogs and with feline infectious peritonitis and toxoplasmosis in cats.

Diagnostic Evaluation

Blood Pressure Measurement

Arterial blood pressure should be measured in all cases of suspected pericardial disease. Hypotension (arterial systolic blood pressure of <90 mm Hg) generally is an indication of critical tamponade. As discussed previously, Doppler flow detectors may document respiratory variation in audible signal strength compatible with pulsus paradoxus.

Radiography

Thoracic radiography classically reveals a very round cardiac silhouette with large-volume pericardial effusion. The globoid cardiac shadow is especially apparent on the ventrodorsal or dorsoventral projection. However, smaller volumes of pericardial fluid often result in mild to moderate generalized cardiomegaly with still-evident chamber contours, which makes radiographic diagnosis of pericardial effusion less certain. Sometimes pleural effusion is present. Other radiographic findings commonly associated with pericardial effusion and tamponade are caudal vena cava distention, hepatomegaly, and ascites. Pulmonary vascular underperfusion or interstitial pulmonary edema also may be noted. A soft tissue mass effect may be evident in cases of heart-base tumor. The trachea may be deviated or appear displaced dorsally and to the right, distinctly separate from the heart base. Thoracic radiographs also are helpful to screen for other potentially associated lesions such as metastatic lung disease and lymphadenopathy.

Electrocardiography

Electrocardiography (ECG) is fairly insensitive for detecting pericardial effusion; in many cases the ECG tracing appears normal. However, ECG findings that can suggest pericardial effusion include diminished complex size (<1 mV in all leads in dogs), electrical alternans, and ST-segment elevation (from epicardial injury). Electrical alternans or alternating QRS complex height results from physical swinging of the heart within the pericardium in cases of large-volume pericardial effusion. It is often best appreciated when the ECG is recorded with the animal in a standing position. Sinus tachycardia is the most common cardiac rhythm associated with pericardial effusion, but atrial or ventricular tachyarrhythmias also may be noted. Atrial fibrillation can complicate chronic pericardial disease, especially in large-breed dogs.

Echocardiography

Echocardiography is a sensitive test for detecting even small volumes of pericardial effusion. In most cases the pericardial fluid is hypoechoic; thus pericardial effusion appears as an echo-free space between the epicardium and the intensely hyperechoic parietal pericardial interface. Because the pericardium adheres more tightly to the heart base and fluid initially collects ventrally, the apical and caudal left atrial regions are good places to screen for small amounts of pericardial effusion. Occasionally pleural effusion, a markedly enlarged left atrium and auricle, or a persistent left cranial vena cava with dilated coronary sinus can be confused with pericardial effusion. Performing a thorough scan from numerous positions differentiates these conditions. Particularly when scanning is done from the right parasternal window, the right ventricular free wall commonly appears hyperechoic because of the dramatic difference in density between the pericardial effusion and the epicardium. This should not be interpreted as a right ventricular abnormality or thickened epicardium.

Echocardiography is especially useful in determining the severity and impact of the effusion, which correlates with clinical severity. The echocardiographic correlate of clinical cardiac tamponade is seen as diastolic collapse of the right atrium and sometimes the right ventricle and is a direct reflection of intrapericardial relative to intracardiac pressures and diminished cardiac filling (Figure 182-1). Prolonged diastolic compression or inversion of the right atrial and ventricular chamber walls is especially

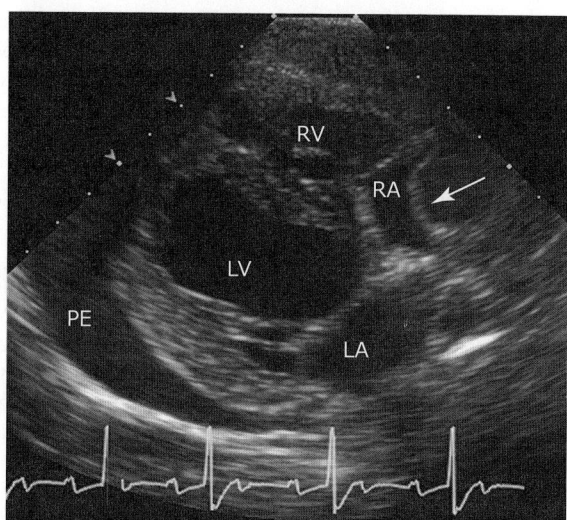

Figure 182-1 Image of a 10-year-old golden retriever with signs of cardiac tamponade (from mesothelioma). Arrow shows right atrial wall collapse associated with tamponade. (Right parasternal long axis image at onset of systole.) *LA,* Left atrium; *LV,* left ventricle; *PE,* pericardial effusion; *RA,* right atrium; *RV,* right ventricle.

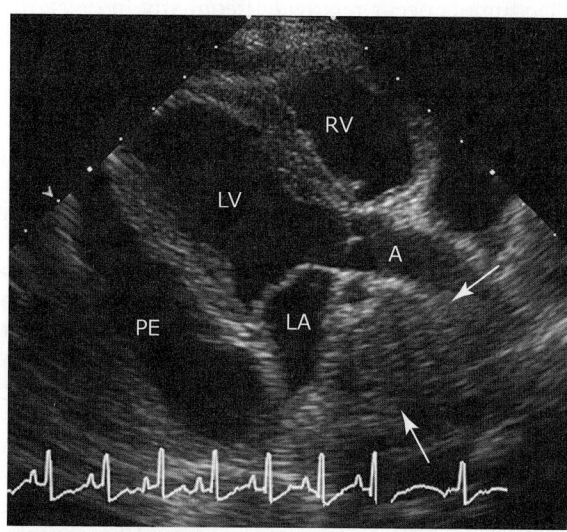

Figure 182-2 Image of a 10-year-old cocker spaniel with progressive cough, lethargy, and decreased appetite. Cardiac tamponade and a large heart-base mass *(arrows)* around the ascending aorta, extending dorsal to the left atrium, are present. The dog experienced arrest during pericardiocentesis; necropsy was denied. (Right parasternal long axis image.) *A,* Aorta; *LA,* left atrium; *LV,* left ventricle; *PE,* pericardial effusion; *RV,* right ventricle.

notable and usually an indication for immediate pericardiocentesis.

Echocardiography can establish the cause of pericardial effusion if cardiac or heart-base masses are identified (Figure 182-2) and can screen for concurrent conditions such as valvular disease, cardiomyopathy, or congenital abnormalities. Whenever possible, it is best to perform echocardiographic evaluation before pericardial fluid is removed. The presence of fluid generally improves

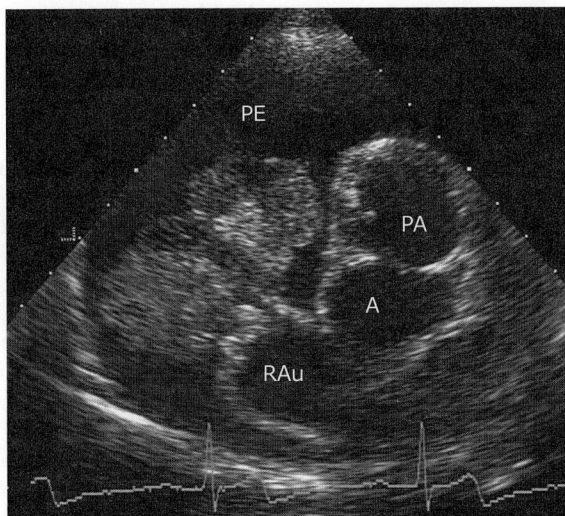

Figure 182-3 Image of a 10-year-old Keeshond that showed progressively increased respiratory effort over the past few months and recent lethargy. Large-volume pericardial effusion is noted, with an approximately 6-cm mass attached to the tip of the right auricle. (Left cranial short axis view with dorsal angulation.) *A,* Aorta; *PA,* main pulmonary artery; *PE,* pericardial effusion; *RAu,* right auricular appendage.

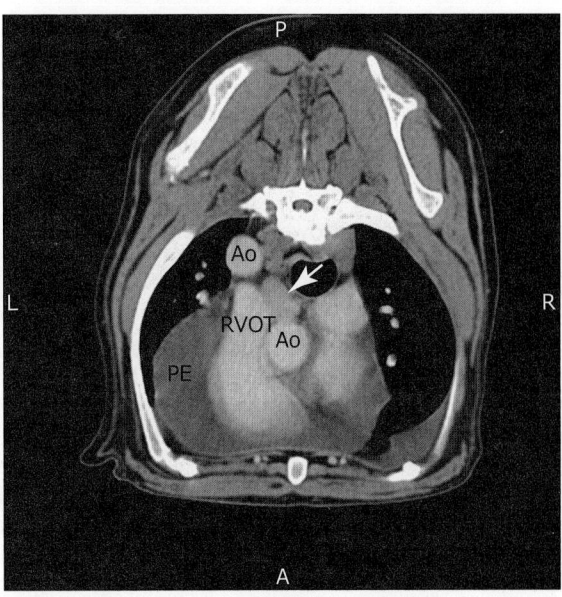

Figure 182-4 Contrast-enhanced computed tomographic image of a 12-year-old hunting dog with pericardial effusion. This study revealed a moderately enhancing soft tissue opacity *(arrow),* which in this case was an enlarged hilar lymph node (with a differential diagnosis of aortic body tumor). *Ao,* Aorta; *PE,* pericardial effusion; *RVOT,* right ventricular outflow tract.

visualization of the heart base and the location or point of adherence of any mass lesions. Thorough examination of the right atrium and auricle (especially from the left cranial long axis position), ascending aorta, and parietal pericardium is important to screen for neoplasia. In some cases the location of a lesion may narrow the list of differential diagnoses for the effusion; for example, masses of the right atrium or auricular appendage are consistent with a diagnosis of HSA (Figure 182-3). Transesophageal echocardiography can be especially useful in examination of the heart-base regions for suspected mass lesions and enlarged lymph nodes; however, this study requires anesthesia and equipment that is not widely available. The usefulness of transthoracic echocardiography for recognizing cardiac masses (as confirmed by surgery or necropsy) was evaluated in 107 dogs in a recent study and showed a sensitivity of 80%, a specificity of 100%, a positive predictive value of 100%, and a negative predictive value of 75% (MacDonald et al, 2009). These data suggest that the finding of a cardiac mass on echocardiography, if the imaging is performed by a trained and experienced sonographer, is a highly effective tool for discriminating the neoplastic origin of a pericardial effusion in a dog; however, not seeing a mass on the initial echocardiogram does not completely rule out a neoplastic cause.

Advanced Imaging Techniques

The major advantage of computed tomography (CT) and magnetic resonance imaging (MRI) techniques is the ability to view internal structures noninvasively with a high degree of resolution. Characterization of tissue (other than calcium content) with CT is more limited than with MRI, and injection of iodinated contrast agent frequently is needed to enhance visualization of tissues with different densities, such as tumors (Figure 182-4). Another limitation of CT is its use of ionizing radiation. Newer models of CT scanners with improved cardiac imaging capability can minimize motion artifacts produced by the beating heart. These provide the advantage of dramatically reduced image acquisition time and also may negate the need for general anesthesia in many cases.

Because MRI relies on the magnetic environment of the cellular nuclei, ionizing radiation is avoided. The information collected also is computer processed to form various two-dimensional images, and cine sequences that loop through the phases of the cardiac cycle can be obtained. With advances in software, many pulse sequences can be used for cardiac imaging. They generally are divided into dark (black) blood and bright (white) blood techniques. Vessels, cardiac chambers, and soft tissues of varying densities are distinguished more easily, and contrast enhancement is needed less often than with CT. Generally, image acquisition must be linked (gated) to a specific point in the cardiac cycle to avoid image blur. Despite its potential for increased tissue differentiation and image resolution, a recent small retrospective study (Boddy et al, 2011) concluded that MRI did not substantially improve the diagnosis of cardiac tumors compared with transthoracic echocardiography, although it did yield useful descriptive information regarding extent and anatomic location. The study also suggested that cardiac MRI requires extensive training and experience for tumor identification. Even so, MRI and CT imaging are potentially valuable tools for detecting and assessing cardiac mass lesions in veterinary patients.

Diagnostic Difficulties

The most difficult diagnosis involves the mature dog with a hemorrhagic effusion but no overt mass lesion or metastatic disease evident on cardiac, abdominal, and thoracic imaging. Careful serial imaging over 2 to 3 months may be required to identify HSA, chemodectoma, and mesothelioma as the tumor grows. Breeds at higher risk of HSA also should undergo careful examination of the spleen and liver.

Differentiating idiopathic hemorrhagic pericardial effusion from mesothelioma-related pericardial effusion is particularly challenging. Several studies have compared presenting clinical signs and diagnostic and histopathologic findings in cases ultimately diagnosed as either pericardial mesothelioma or idiopathic pericardial effusion. Unfortunately, clinical signs and results of noninvasive diagnostic tests are insufficient to differentiate idiopathic effusion from mesothelioma unless a discrete pericardial or intrapericardial mass is observed. Even the results of surgical pericardial biopsy can be misleading since both conditions lead to extensive pericardial fibrosis with a mixed inflammatory response incorporating large numbers of reactive mesothelial cells. One retrospective evaluation suggested that recurrence of pleural effusion within 120 days of pericardectomy increases the likelihood of a mesothelioma diagnosis (Stepien et al, 2000). Survival for longer than 120 days after pericardectomy without chemotherapeutic intervention was unusual in dogs in which mesothelioma ultimately was diagnosed.

Immunohistochemical staining of biopsy material may help determine the cause of pericardial effusion in questionable cases. Preliminary investigations (Church et al, 2005) have evaluated the staining patterns of cardiac HSA, chemodectoma, mesothelioma, and idiopathic pericardial effusion using antibodies specific for CD31, desmin, cytokeratin, vimentin, synaptophysin, chromogranin, and endothelin. In this study the antibody for CD31 was specific for HSA. Synaptophysin and chromogranin demonstrated high specificity but only moderate sensitivity for chemodectoma. Cytokeratin was specific for mesothelial tissue, and desmin occasionally differentiated mesothelioma from reactive mesothelial tissue. If the staining characteristics of cells obtained from pericardial fluid are similar, immunocytochemical staining could improve the diagnostic capability of pericardial fluid analysis. *Flow cytometry* methods also may have potential value for the isolation of neoplastic cells in fluid or blood.

Pericardial Fluid Analysis

Pericardial fluid is submitted routinely for cytologic analysis and culture. If an obvious mass is not identified by echocardiography, fluid analysis may take on a more important role in determining the next diagnostic and therapeutic steps. Standard laboratory and cytologic evaluation rarely is helpful in distinguishing neoplastic from benign hemorrhagic pericardial effusion, although it may identify suppurative, mycotic, or chylous effusions. In addition, mesothelial cells lining the pericardium can become very reactive and may exfoliate into the effusion. These cells are difficult to differentiate from neoplastic cells, particularly mesothelioma. Other cardiac-related tumors rarely exfoliate cells into the effusion, with the possible exception of lymphoma.

The therapeutic approach (and prognosis) for animals with pericardial effusion depend directly on the underlying cause of the effusion. Neoplasia-related effusion and idiopathic pericardial effusion are the most common types of pericardial effusion in the dog, but unfortunately fluid cytologic analysis does not differentiate these causes reliably. In addition, certain neoplastic disorders (e.g., HSA) are associated with notoriously short survival times. Biochemical analyses of pericardial fluid and serum have been examined as a way to distinguish between inflammatory, noninflammatory, and cancerous causes of pericardial effusion. Studies in dogs evaluating pericardial fluid pH have been conflicting. In general, the effusions of dogs with neoplastic causes of pericardial effusion have lower glucose levels, pH, bicarbonate levels, and chloride levels but higher lactate levels, hematocrit, and urea nitrogen levels than the effusions of dogs with nonneoplastic causes (de Laforcade et al, 2005). Although differences have been documented between neoplastic pericardial effusions and nonneoplastic effusions in various biochemical parameters, the clinical usefulness of these tests is hampered by the large degree of overlap between these groups.

Elevated plasma cardiac troponin I concentration also has been correlated with the presence of cardiac HSA rather than other causes of pericardial effusion; a value of more than 0.25 ng/ml was able to distinguish cardiac HSA as a cause of pericardial effusion with a sensitivity of 81% and a specificity of 100% in a small series of dogs (Chun et al, 2010). Further studies are needed to define the predictive value of cardiac troponin I in differentiating the cause of pericardial effusion in dogs.

Management

Myocardial systolic function is normal in most cases, and positive inotropic drugs are not warranted. Vasodilators and diuretics likewise have negligible effect on intrapericardial fluid volume and pressure and may serve only to lower systemic arterial pressure. Diuretics can worsen hypotension and may precipitate cardiogenic shock by decreasing the high preload needed to maintain even a minimal cardiac output during severe tamponade. Furthermore, the pericardium is avascular and minimally absorptive, so the greatest reduction in cardiac size actually may be related to reduced chamber filling, as opposed to reduced pericardial effusion. Accordingly, initial therapy for patients with pericardial effusion and tamponade must be directed at reducing intrapericardial pressure as soon as possible to enhance cardiac filling. Pericardiocentesis is therefore the treatment of choice, and it potentially provides some diagnostic information as well. Clinical signs of right-sided heart failure should resolve within days after effective pericardiocentesis.

Pericardiocentesis

Pericardiocentesis is the treatment of choice for initial stabilization of animals with cardiac tamponade.

Pericardial fluid analysis also is a part of the diagnostic process. Aspiration of even a small amount of fluid can markedly reduce intrapericardial pressure and improve clinical status. As indicated earlier, diuretic therapy without pericardiocentesis is not helpful for cardiac tamponade except when effusion is caused by CHF.

Pericardiocentesis is performed most routinely from the right side of the chest because the cardiac notch reduces the potential for lung injury and the major coronary vessels in the dog are located on the left. On a standard examination table the animal is securely restrained in sternal or left lateral recumbency. A radiographic wedge can be used to elevate the spine slightly. Sometimes pericardiocentesis can be done with the dog in the standing position, depending on the animal's temperament and the operator's approach. If an echocardiography table or other elevated table with an appropriately sized cutout is available, the animal can be placed in right lateral recumbency and tapped from underneath. Sedation seldom is required in dogs, but low doses of butorphanol (initially 0.1 to 0.2 mg/kg IM or IV) can be used if needed. Echocardiographic guidance may be used but is not often necessary. The ECG should be carefully monitored during the procedure. Needle-catheter contact with the epicardium often induces ventricular arrhythmias (usually with an upright configuration in lead II); this should prompt retraction of the device and may require administration of a lidocaine bolus at 2 mg/kg IV if persistent arrhythmias are noted. Dorsal puncture of the atrium, however, does not induce ventricular premature complexes.

An over-the-needle type of catheter is used most commonly for pericardiocentesis (Figure 182-5). Depending on the size of the animal, a 12- to 20-gauge, 2- to 6-inch catheter is selected. Extra side holes may be cut near the catheter tip using a sterile No. 11 blade or scissors to facilitate drainage of large-volume or flocculent fluid. Extension tubing is attached to the needle stylet, and a three-way stopcock is placed between the tubing and collection syringe. Box 182-1 summarizes the pericardiocentesis procedure.

The next therapeutic step after initial pericardiocentesis depends on the underlying cause of the effusion. In animals with infectious pericarditis, treatment depends on the organism identified by cytologic examination, culture, or possibly serologic testing. Most cases of infectious pericarditis benefit from surgical pericardectomy; this provides more effective drainage and helps avoid subsequent constrictive pericardial disease. Dogs with idiopathic pericarditis (culture negative) often are treated conservatively with one or more pericardiocentesis procedures (as needed). Some cardiologists empirically prescribe a course of broad-spectrum antibiotic therapy as well as antiinflammatory dosages of prednisone (e.g., 1 mg/kg/day, tapering off over 2 to 4 weeks) to dogs with idiopathic pericarditis; however, there are no prospective data indicating that such therapy is effective. Recovery appears to occur with this conservative approach in about 50% of cases. In animals with persistently recurrent effusions, surgical subtotal pericardectomy with pericardial biopsy is indicated and has yielded long median survival times. Removal of pericardium

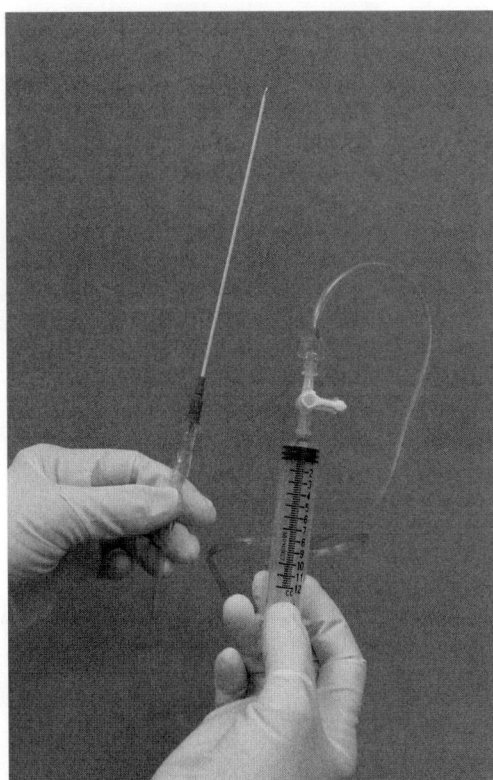

Figure 182-5 Common apparatus for pericardiocentesis procedure: a 16-gauge, 6-inch over-the-needle catheter connected to extension tubing and a three-way stopcock.

allows the fluid to drain onto the larger absorptive surface of the thoracic pleura.

Neoplastic pericardial effusion with tamponade also is treated initially by pericardiocentesis. Chemotherapy may be palliative in some cases of lymphosarcoma and more rarely in HSA and mesothelioma. Periodic pericardiocentesis can be done in some animals with neoplastic disease until the effusion becomes unmanageable. In some cases surgical approaches offer the best management options for neoplastic effusions.

Surgical Management

Pericardectomy is considered a definitive treatment for benign or idiopathic pericardial effusion and a palliative treatment for some malignant pericardial effusions. It is indicated when multiple pericardiocentesis procedures fail to resolve the effusion, when pericardial constrictive disease is suspected, and when exploration and biopsy are needed to rule out suspected neoplastic or infectious disease. Subtotal pericardectomy has been done most commonly, with removal of the pericardium below the phrenic nerves. However, thoracoscopic partial pericardectomy also may provide good results. The pericardium and biopsy samples obtained from any mass lesions should be submitted for histopathologic evaluation. Most neoplastic lesions are too extensive at the time of diagnosis to allow complete excision of the tumor; however, in rare cases a small discrete mass (e.g., at the tip of the right auricle) may be found that can be completely removed.

BOX 182-1

Step-by-Step Approach to Pericardiocentesis

1. Shave the hair over the right precordium (third to seventh rib spaces, sternum to costochondral junction). Prepare the area using an aseptic surgical scrub technique.
2. Attach an electrocardiographic monitor and noninvasive blood pressure monitor if available.
3. Identify the catheter insertion site by palpating the strongest precordial impulse and considering radiographic evaluation and echocardiographic guidance.
4. Provide local anesthesia, especially if large catheters are used.
   a. Generously infiltrate lidocaine (2%) from the insertion site into the underlying intercostal muscles and pleura.
   b. Make a small stab incision in the skin (No. 11 blade) if using a large catheter.
5. Insert the catheter with care to avoid the intercostal vessels just caudal to the ribs.
6. Once the needle penetrates the skin and after every increment of advancement, apply gentle negative pressure to the syringe and observe for fluid.
   a. Pleural fluid is typically straw colored.
   b. Pericardial fluid is typically dark and bloody; often this fluid is under positive pressure.
7. Subtle scratching of the needle tip on the pericardial surface may be noted or a loss of resistance may be felt as the needle enters the pericardial space. Usually this is not associated with ventricular arrhythmias.
8. If the needle contacts the epicardium, a marked scratching or pulsing sensation usually is felt. This often provokes ventricular arrhythmias. Retract the needle slightly.
9. When a catheter system is used, especially with smaller-volume pericardial effusions, advance the catheter, remove the needle, and attach extension tubing to the catheter.
10. After a small amount of fluid is obtained, take steps to differentiate bloody pericardial fluid from hemorrhage.
    a. Place a drop of fluid onto the table or into a clot tube and observe for clotting (pericardial effusion should not clot).
    b. Obtain a packed cell volume (PCV) measurement on the fluid and compare it with the PCV of peripheral blood.
11. Aspirate as much fluid as possible from the pericardial space. Submit samples for cytologic examination (and culture if indicated).
12. Verify the reduction of effusion and tamponade by echocardiography.

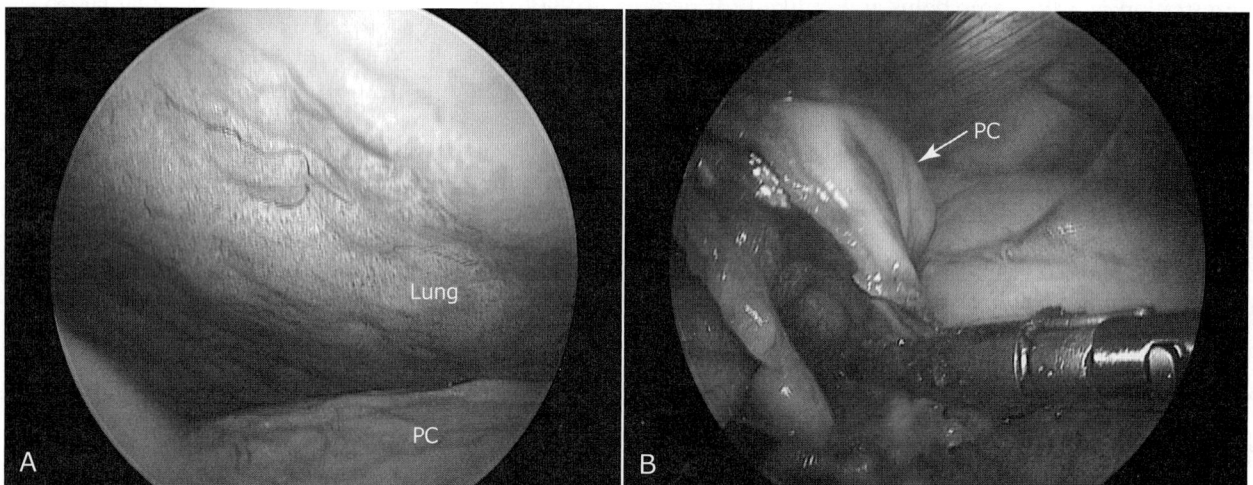

Figure 182-6 Thoracoscopic images of the same dog as in Figure 182-4. **A,** Insufflation of the thoracic cavity reveals good visualization of lung tissue and a thickened, opaque pericardium. **B,** A subtotal pericardectomy is performed; the fibrotic pericardium is retrieved with forceps after trimming *(arrow)*. Histologic analysis revealed chronic fibrosing pericarditis with bacterial colonies of *Corynebacterium* and *Staphylococcus* species (thought to be the result of a migrating foreign body). *PC,* Pericardium.

The prognosis for dogs with idiopathic pericardial effusion typically is very good after pericardectomy because the pleural space can readily absorb the relatively small amount of fluid and the risk of pericardial constriction is reduced markedly. Animals with neoplastic disease have a more variable prognosis. Cardiac HSA often has a rapidly progressive course, and metastases commonly are present at the time of diagnosis. Pericardectomy should be performed cautiously in animals with cardiac HSA because tumor rupture and bleeding into the chest cavity can have dire consequences. Chemotherapy may be considered, and there is some evidence that chemotherapy modestly prolongs survival in dogs with right atrial HSA that underwent surgical resection; in a series of 23 dogs, median survival was 175 days for dogs that received adjuvant chemotherapy versus 42 days for dogs that did not receive chemotherapy (Weisse et al, 2005).

Pericardectomy also helps alleviate cardiac tamponade in animals with pericardial mesothelioma; however, the procedure can facilitate metastatic dissemination throughout the thoracic cavity. Even so, animals may survive longer with pleural effusion than with pericardial effusion, and periodic thoracocentesis usually is easier to perform (or, alternatively, a pleural drainage port system can be placed that allows thoracocentesis to proceed without the repeated need for puncture of the thorax). Intracavitary chemotherapy has been attempted in thoracic mesothelioma, with limited success. Survival times after identification of pericardial effusion range from 3 to 10 months.

Chemodectoma tends to be slow growing and locally invasive, with a low rate of metastasis. Pericardectomy can prolong survival with good quality of life for many months and sometimes years in animals with chemodectoma and is a good option in many cases.

Thoracoscopic subtotal pericardectomy is gaining in popularity for the management of chronic pericardial effusion in veterinary patients. The procedure is feasible in dogs using bilateral lung ventilation; visualization of structures is quite good (Figure 182-6). The advantages of this technique over thoracotomy include lower morbidity and mortality, minimal recovery time, potential for decreased cost, and greater owner acceptance. Disadvantages include the need for specialized equipment and extensive clinician training. An alternative approach is to perform a "mini-thoracotomy" and use long surgical or laparoscopic instruments to remove a segment of pericardium via the small incisions. Yet another minimally invasive technique that may be useful for dogs with chemodectoma and idiopathic pericardial effusion when thoracoscopy is unavailable is percutaneous balloon pericardiotomy. This technique involves percutaneous transthoracic positioning of a balloon dilation catheter into the pericardium using fluoroscopic guidance and general anesthesia. Inflation of the balloon as it straddles the pericardium creates a small pericardial window, which allows for continued fluid drainage.

References and Suggested Reading

Aronsohn MG, Carpenter JL: Surgical treatment of idiopathic pericardial effusion in the dog: 25 cases (1978-1993), *J Am Anim Hosp Assoc* 35:521, 1999.

Boddy KN et al: Cardiac magnetic resonance in the differentiation of neoplastic and nonneoplastic pericardial effusion, *J Vet Intern Med* 25:1003, 2011.

Chun R et al: Comparison of plasma cardiac troponin I concentrations among dogs with cardiac hemangiosarcoma, noncardiac hemangiosarcoma, other neoplasms, and pericardial effusion of nonhemangiosarcoma origin, *J Am Vet Med Assoc* 237:806, 2010.

Church WM et al: Characterization of immunohistochemical staining patterns for cardiac hemangiosarcoma, idiopathic pericarditis, heart base chemodectomas, and pericardial mesothelioma, *J Vet Intern Med* 19:416, 2005.

Davidson BJ et al: Disease association and clinical assessment of feline pericardial effusion, *J Am Anim Hosp Assoc* 44:1, 2008.

De Laforcade AM et al: Biochemical analysis of pericardial fluid and whole blood in dogs with pericardial effusion, *J Vet Intern Med* 19:833, 2005.

Dupre GP, Corlouer JP, Bouvy B: Thoracoscopic pericardectomy performed without pulmonary exclusion in 9 dogs, *Vet Surg* 30:21, 2001.

Ehrhart N et al: Analysis of factors affecting survival in dogs with aortic body tumor, *Vet Surg* 31(1):44, 2002.

Fine DM, Tobias AH, Jacob KA: Use of pericardial fluid pH to distinguish between idiopathic and neoplastic effusions, *J Vet Intern Med* 17:525, 2003.

Hall DJ et al: Pericardial effusion in cats: a retrospective study of clinical findings and outcome in 146 cats, *J Vet Intern Med* 21:1002, 2007.

MacDonald KA, Cagney O, Magne ML: Echocardiographic and clinicopathologic characterization of pericardial effusion in dogs: 107 cases (1985-2006), *J Am Vet Med Assoc* 235:1456, 2009.

Mayhew KN et al: Thoracoscopic subphrenic pericardectomy using double-lumen endobronchial intubation for alternating one-lung ventilation, *Vet Surg* 38:961, 2009.

Monnet E: Interventional thoracoscopy in small animals, *Vet Clin North Am Small Anim Pract* 39:965, 2009.

Savitt MA et al: Physiology of cardiac tamponade and paradoxical pulse in conscious dogs, *Am J Physiol* 265:H1996, 1993.

Sidley JA et al: Percutaneous balloon pericardiotomy as a treatment for recurrent pericardial effusion in 6 dogs, *J Vet Intern Med* 16:541, 2002.

Stepien RL, Whitley NT, Dubielzig RR: Idiopathic or mesothelioma related pericardial effusion: clinical findings and survival in 17 dogs studied retrospectively, *J Small Anim Pract* 41(8):342, 2000.

Tobias AH: Pericardial diseases. In Ettinger SJ, Feldman EC, editors: *Textbook of veterinary internal medicine*, ed 7, St Louis, 2010, Elsevier, p 1342.

Ware WA, Hopper DL: Cardiac tumors in dogs: 1982-1995, *J Vet Intern Med* 13:95, 1999.

Weisse C et al: Survival times in dogs with right atrial hemangiosarcoma treated by means of surgical resection with or without adjuvant chemotherapy: 23 cases (1986-2000), *J Am Vet Med Assoc* 226:575, 2005.

CHAPTER 183

Feline Heartworm Disease

CLARKE E. ATKINS, *Raleigh, North Carolina*

Prevalence in the United States

Heartworm infection is less common in cats than in dogs, with the feline prevalence approximating 5% to 20% of the canine prevalence in a given geographic area (Ryan et al, 1996). The result has been a low index of suspicion for feline heartworm disease (FHWD), with consequent underdiagnosis. In addition, the diagnosis of FHWD often is obscured because (1) cats are frequently amicrofilaremic; (2) serologic tests (specifically, the enzyme-linked immunosorbent assay [ELISA] antigen and antibody tests) have lacked sensitivity or specificity in cats; (3) worm burdens are small; (4) aberrant sites are more common than in dogs; (5) clinical signs are often nonspecific and different from those seen in dogs; and (6) FHWD can be mistaken easily for feline bronchial disease (asthma) and clinical signs often improve with similar therapies. For these reasons, despite recent efforts at defining the scope of this problem in cats, the exact prevalence of FHWD is unknown and likely underestimated. Moreover, fewer than 5% of cats in the United States receive monthly heartworm preventive medication.

The greatest numbers of cases of feline heartworm infection (FHWI) have been reported from the southeastern United States, the Eastern Seaboard, the Gulf Coast, and the Mississippi River valley (Ryan and Newcomb, 1996). Prevalence studies have focused mainly on cats in shelters (Figure 183-1). Although the shelter population provides a very specific diagnosis by postmortem examination, such studies are not necessarily applicable to pet cats, even in the same geographic region. These studies have revealed a prevalence of FHWI ranging from 0% to 14% (see Figure 183-1). There are limited data for pet cats, but a study performed in cats brought to the teaching hospitals of North Carolina State University and Texas A&M University for evaluation of cardiorespiratory signs demonstrated a mature infection prevalence of 9% and an "exposure" rate of 26%; the latter figure is based on antibody titers (Atkins et al, 1998). Serologic surveys, performed primarily in asymptomatic cats, have found positive antibody test results in 5% to 33% of cats, even in areas where heartworm is not considered heavily endemic. Among cats exhibiting respiratory and gastrointestinal signs, positive antibody test results have been found in as many as 44% of cats (Robertson-Plough et al, 1998). The largest survey to date found a nationwide exposure rate of nearly 12% (Figure 183-2) in over 2000 largely asymptomatic cats from areas not considered to be highly endemic for heartworm infection (Miller et al, 1998). In this author's opinion, heartworm infection should be considered a risk for cats in any locale in which dogs are considered at risk.

Diagnosis

The diagnosis of FHWI or FHWD poses a unique and problematic set of issues. The clinical signs in cats often are different from those in dogs and the index of suspicion still is generally low. Furthermore, the diagnosis often is elusive because eosinophilia is transient or absent and most cats are amicrofilaremic. Radiography, although helpful, is neither adequately sensitive nor specific, requires expertise in interpretation, and is excessively expensive as a screening tool. Echocardiography shows promise in terms of specificity and sensitivity for mature infection, but is costly, requires special equipment and expertise, and is useless in cases of immature infection. Currently the most useful tests are the ELISA serologic tests, but these too are imperfect. The antigen test is very specific but is inadequately sensitive, missing 30% to 50% of natural infections (McCall et al, 1995). On the other hand, the laboratory feline antibody test is very sensitive for exposure (i.e., at least transient infection, with abortion of infection at larval or young adult stages), but its specificity is low for mature infection, which means that a positive test result does not necessarily indicate adult infection (McCall et al, 1995, 1998). In fact, the great majority of antibody-positive cats do not have mature FHWI. The two ELISA tests are often used in combination or in sequence. In the latter instance, the antibody test is done first; if results are positive, the antigen test is then performed. Unfortunately, cats with mature infections commonly are antibody positive and antigen negative; however, cats with positive results on antigen or microfilariae tests are presumed always to harbor adult infections.

Signalment, History, and Clinical Signs

Although no breeds of cats have been shown to be at increased risk of FHWI, most authors do suspect a male predisposition. This suspicion is based on the overall preponderance of males among cats diagnosed with FHWI (71%; Ryan et al, 1996) and the greater experimental infection rate in males than in females (McTier et al, 1993). However, the experience at North Carolina State University suggests that, although more males (61%) than females are diagnosed with FHWI, the male:female ratio is not significantly different from that of the general population of cats seen at a teaching hospital (53% male;

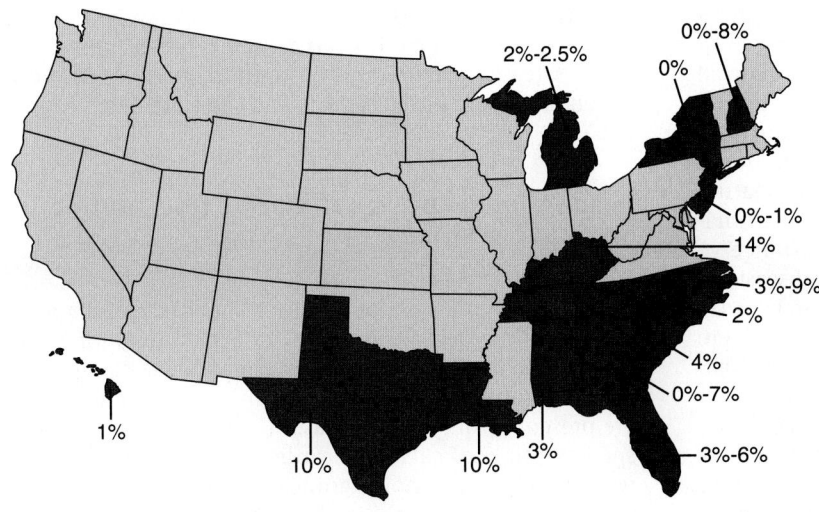

Figure 183-1 Prevalence of necropsy-proven heartworm infection in shelter cats. The shaded states are those in which such studies have been completed. One Michigan study, which showed a prevalence of 2%, was an antigen study.

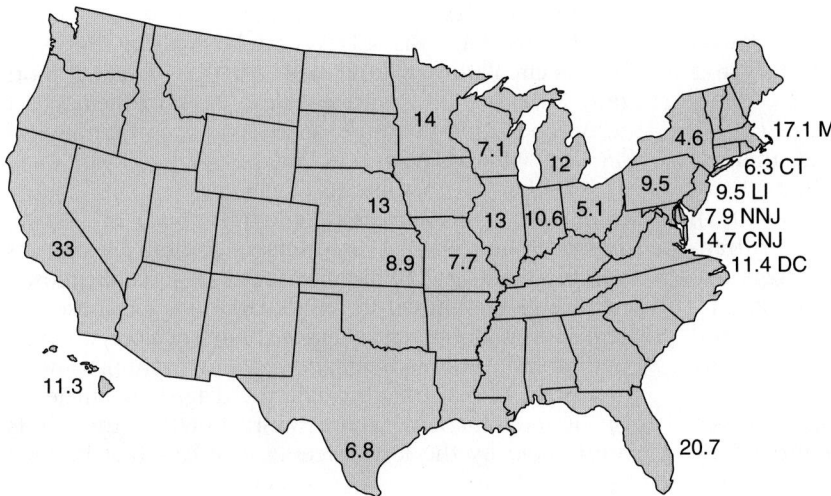

Figure 183-2 Prevalence of heartworm exposure (percent antibody positive) in over 2000 largely asymptomatic cats in 19 states (21 regions). *CNJ*, Central New Jersey; *LI*, Long Island, NY; *NNJ*, north New Jersey. (From Miller MW et al: Prevalence of exposure to *Dirofilaria immitis* in cats from multiple areas of the United States. In Soll MD, Knight DH, editors: *Proceedings of the Heartworm Symposium '98*, Batavia, IL, 1998, American Heartworm Society, p 161.)

Atkins et al, 2000). Indeed, the higher proportion of male cats with FHWI is comparable to that in the population of cats brought for treatment of cardiorespiratory signs (60% male; Atkins et al, 1997). The typical cat with FHWI is 4 to 6 years of age, but the age at presentation varies widely (range, <1 to 19 years). A history of outdoor exposure predicts a heightened risk of heartworm exposure (Miller et al, 1998). Nevertheless, over one fourth of heartworm-infected cats are reported by their owners to be housed *totally indoors* (Atkins et al, 2000). This may mean that indoor cats can be infected, that owners misinterpret the question when asked, or both. Although some have suggested a seasonal trend (August to December) for diagnosis of FHWD (Guerrero et al, 1992), other studies do not support this contention (Atkins et al, 2000).

Heartworm-infected cats are often asymptomatic and clinical manifestations, when present, may take either an acute (often cataclysmic) or a chronic (often waxing and waning) course. Acute or peracute presentation usually is caused by dead worm embolization, an anaphylaxis-like reaction, or migration of worms to the central nervous

system. Signs variably include salivation, tachycardia, shock, dyspnea, cough, hemoptysis, vomiting and diarrhea, syncope, dementia, ataxia, circling, head tilt, blindness, seizures, and death. Sudden death, with few or no premonitory signs, has been observed in approximately 10% to 23% of cases (Atkins et al, 2000; Ryan et al, 1996). Postmortem examination typically reveals pulmonary congestion and edema. Caval syndrome also has been recognized in cats.

Findings in chronic FHWD may include cough, dyspnea, anorexia, weight loss, lethargy, exercise intolerance, vomiting, and signs of right-sided heart failure. Cough is a relatively consistent finding (>50% of cases, compared with 15% in cats with cardiorespiratory signs but no FHWI). When cough is noted in cats from endemic areas, the suspicion of FHWD should increase. Likewise, dyspnea, although less specific than cough, is present in 40% to 60% of cases. The pulmonary response to *in situ* heartworms in cats includes type II pneumocyte hyperplasia and activation of pulmonary intravascular macrophages. The latter response, not recognized in dogs, may explain the asthma-like syndrome recognized in some cats, even after they have been cleared of *Dirofilaria immitis* (Dillon et al, 1996).

Recent research involving experimental and natural infections suggests that even infections that fail to mature can produce disease, affecting lung parenchyma, airways, and pulmonary arteries with inflammatory and proliferative lesions. It is believed that the death of immature final-stage heartworms in the lung incites the inflammatory and proliferative lesions. The exact importance of this so-called heartworm-associated respiratory disease, or HARD (Blagburn and Dillon, 2007), is unclear because experimental infections that produced these lesions were heavy. Nevertheless, Browne and colleagues in 2005 reported that 50% of shelter cats thought to have been exposed without a mature infection had characteristic proliferative and obstructive pulmonary arterial lesions. There is diagnostic importance to this finding because even transient heartworm infection can produce disease, with clinical signs of wheezing and coughing but negative findings on an antigen test and echocardiogram. However, the antibody test results and thoracic radiographic findings in such cases typically are positive. A comparison of HARD and mature heartworm disease is provided in Table 183-1 (Lee and Atkins, 2010). Somewhat speculatively, if one assumes that 20% of cats in Florida are antibody positive (see Figure 183-2), that 5% have adult infections (see Figure 183-1), and that 50% of cats with HARD show clinical signs (Browne et al, 2005), then 12.5% of the cats in Florida experience at least transient heartworm disease. Finally, it has been suggested, although not proven, that HARD may lead to inflammatory airway disease ("asthma") that persists well beyond the time at which young adult heartworm infections are cleared.

Physical examination is often unrewarding, although a murmur, a gallop, or diminished or adventitial lung sounds may be noted. In addition, cats may be thin or demonstrate dyspnea. If heart failure is present, elevated heart rate, jugular venous distention, pleural effusion (often chylous), and occasionally ascites are detected.

Hematologic and Microfilarial Tests and Serologic Testing

Hematologic Tests

Although the presence of eosinophilia or basophilia may increase the index of suspicion for FHWI, tests for these conditions are of limited value. Hematologic changes are transient (occurring at 4 to 7 months after infection) and are present in only 33% of cases (Dillon, 1984). In a prospective study of cats with cardiorespiratory signs, those with FHWD were not significantly more apt to have eosinophilia or basophilia than those not shown to be infected (Atkins et al, 1997).

Microfilarial Tests

A definitive diagnosis of FHWI can be made by the detection of circulating microfilariae using the modified Knott test, Millipore filter, direct smear, or microhematocrit techniques. One literature review indicated that 36% of 45 cats with FHWD were microfilaremic (Ryan et al, 1996), whereas other reports have indicated that no more than 20% of infected cats are microfilaremic (Atkins et al, 1997; Dillon, 1984). This discrepancy probably reflects the fact that at the time of early reports diagnostic methods were limited to microfilaria tests and postmortem examination. Increasing the volume of blood samples, performing multiple tests, and drawing evening samples are methods that may increase the diagnostic efficiency of the microfilaria-dependent tests; however, these tests are limited by the low percentage of cats that become

---

TABLE 183-1

Comparison of HARD (Heartworm-Associated Respiratory Disease or Immature Heartworm–Associated Respiratory Disease) and Chronic Heartworm Disease in Cats

	HARD	Chronic Heartworm Disease
Onset of clinical signs after infection	3 mo	>7-8 mo
Cause	Arrival and death of immature heartworms in pulmonary arteries	Presence, death, and deterioration of adult heartworms and pulmonary vascular, lung, and cardiac response to worms
Clinical signs	Dyspnea, coughing, wheezing	Dyspnea, coughing, hemoptysis, collapse, vomiting, neurologic signs, heart failure, sudden death
Serologic test results Antigen test Antibody test	 Negative Often positive	 Positive or negative Positive or negative
Microfilaremia	Absent	Occasionally present
Radiographic findings	Bronchointerstitial pattern	Variably, bronchointerstitial pattern, pulmonary artery enlargement, pulmonary hyperinflation; less commonly, pleural effusion and pulmonary consolidation
Echocardiographic findings	Normal (no heartworms discernible)	Heartworm(s) often found in pulmonary artery and/or right ventricle or atrium, possible pulmonary hypertension

From Lee A, Atkins C: Understanding feline heartworm infection: disease, diagnosis, and treatment, *Top Companion Anim Med* 25:224, 2010, with permission.

microfilaremic, the transient nature of microfilaremia, and the low numbers of microfilariae.

Antigen Tests

All heartworm antigen tests currently marketed for dogs can be used in cats. There is now one antigen test kit designed specifically for the cat (SNAP Feline Heartworm Antigen test). Although virtually 100% specific, ELISA antigen tests have been of somewhat limited use in cats because of their inability to detect all-male, immature, and low worm burden mature female infections (zero to one). In general, naturally infected cats have one to three worms (most often one worm, and almost always fewer than five worms). Importantly, since current tests detect antigens presumably produced in the reproductive tracts of mature female worms, these tests do not detect infections with immature worms (<7 months) or all-male infections. These factors may result in false-negative results, and their importance is underscored by a review of 108 cases of naturally occurring FHWD that identified single-worm infections in 53% and all-male infections in 18% (Ryan et al, 1996). Furthermore, as stated earlier, it is now clear that pulmonary abnormalities and presumably clinical signs may exist before worm maturation, at a time when cats are antigen negative (Blagburn and Dillon, 2007; Browne et al, 2005; Selcer et al, 1996). These limitations are demonstrated in two studies. First, in a study of six commercial ELISA antigen tests, positive test results were obtained 36% to 93% of the time from the sera of 31 known heartworm-positive cats harboring one to seven female worms (McTier et al, 1993). Although sensitivity increased with greater female worm burdens, no all-male heartworm infections were detected. Second, a commercial antigen test allowed detection of fewer than 40% of necropsy-proven natural infections (McCall et al, 1995).

Thus false-negative antigen test results occur frequently, depending on the test used, the maturity and gender of the worms, and the worm burden. Improvements in the sensitivity of ELISA antigen tests, however, probably have increased their efficiency in the diagnosis of infections containing at least one female worm. Although the specificity of antigen tests is well accepted, the risk of false-positive results nevertheless increases in low-prevalence areas. Therefore positive test results should be confirmed by a second test or supported by the presence of appropriate clinical findings (e.g., cough, radiographic lesions, echocardiographic signs).

Antibody Tests

The terminology used for antibody tests is confusing. A positive test result means that the cat has been exposed and that heartworm larvae have developed to the larva 4 (L4) stage. The infection may then be aborted at the early L5 (immature adult) stage or allowed to further mature. Because immature infections can produce disease (HARD), the positive antibody state indicates more than exposure but often does not indicate a mature infection.

Three "send-away" ELISA antibody tests designed specifically for the diagnosis of FHWI and one ELISA antibody test designed for in-house use (Solo Step FH) are available commercially. Published data on the send-away tests suggest higher specificity than has been found with previous antibody tests (McCall et al, 1998). Although less specific for mature infections than the antigen tests, the commercial ELISA antibody test is capable of detecting male-only and immature infections and has been shown to be useful in the identification of mature, developing, and aborted FHWI, even when antigen test results are negative (McCall et al, 1995). The antibody tests were shown to be 100% specific in determining cats to be heartworm negative before infection and detected 80% of experimental infections by 2 months, 97% to 100% by 3 months, and 100% by 4 months after infection (McCall et al, 1998). The antibody test was used to screen 215 random-source cats and detected seven of eight necropsy-proven cases (sensitivity of 88%) but at the same time gave false-positive results for 21 cats (90% specificity). The strength of this antibody test lies in its ability to *rule out **mature** infection* (>99% negative predictive value), but a positive test result clearly does not always indicate mature or current infection (positive predictive value of <25%). A negative antibody test result indicates either no infection or an early (<60- to 90-day) infection. A positive test result is thought to mean any of the following: (1) adult worms are present in the heart and/or pulmonary arteries; (2) a past infection has resolved but antibodies are still present; (3) precardiac late L4 or immature L5 infection exists; or (4) ectopic infection is present. Ideally a positive test result should be confirmed with an antigen test, echocardiography, or angiography and supported by the presence of appropriate clinical findings (e.g., cough, radiographic lesions). In addition to aiding in making a diagnosis of FHWI, the antibody test result may be useful as an indicator of exposure to heartworms, even in cats that never develop mature infection. Finally, the antibody test currently is the most logical single screening test for asymptomatic (and symptomatic) cats.

Imaging

Radiography

Radiographic findings of FHWD (Figure 183-3) include enlarged caudal pulmonary arteries, often with ill-defined margins; pulmonary parenchymal changes, including the presence of focal or diffuse infiltrates (interstitial, bronchointerstitial, or even alveolar); perivascular density; and occasionally atelectasis or pleural effusion. Pulmonary hyperinflation and enlargement of the right side of the heart also may be evident. Thoracic radiography has been suggested as an excellent screening test for FHWD. However, although it is often helpful, thoracic radiography is neither sensitive nor specific in making the diagnosis of FHWD. The single most sensitive radiographic sign—a left caudal pulmonary artery diameter greater than 1.6 times that of the ninth rib at the ninth intercostal space—can be identified in only 53% of cases (Schafer and Berry, 1995) and also may be noted in heartworm-free cats with heart failure. Likewise, pulmonary parenchymal changes are detectable radiographically in only approximately 50% of cases of natural FHWD (Schafer and Berry, 1995). Even though most cats with clinical signs have some radiographic abnormality, the findings are not specific for FHWD, are variable, and often are

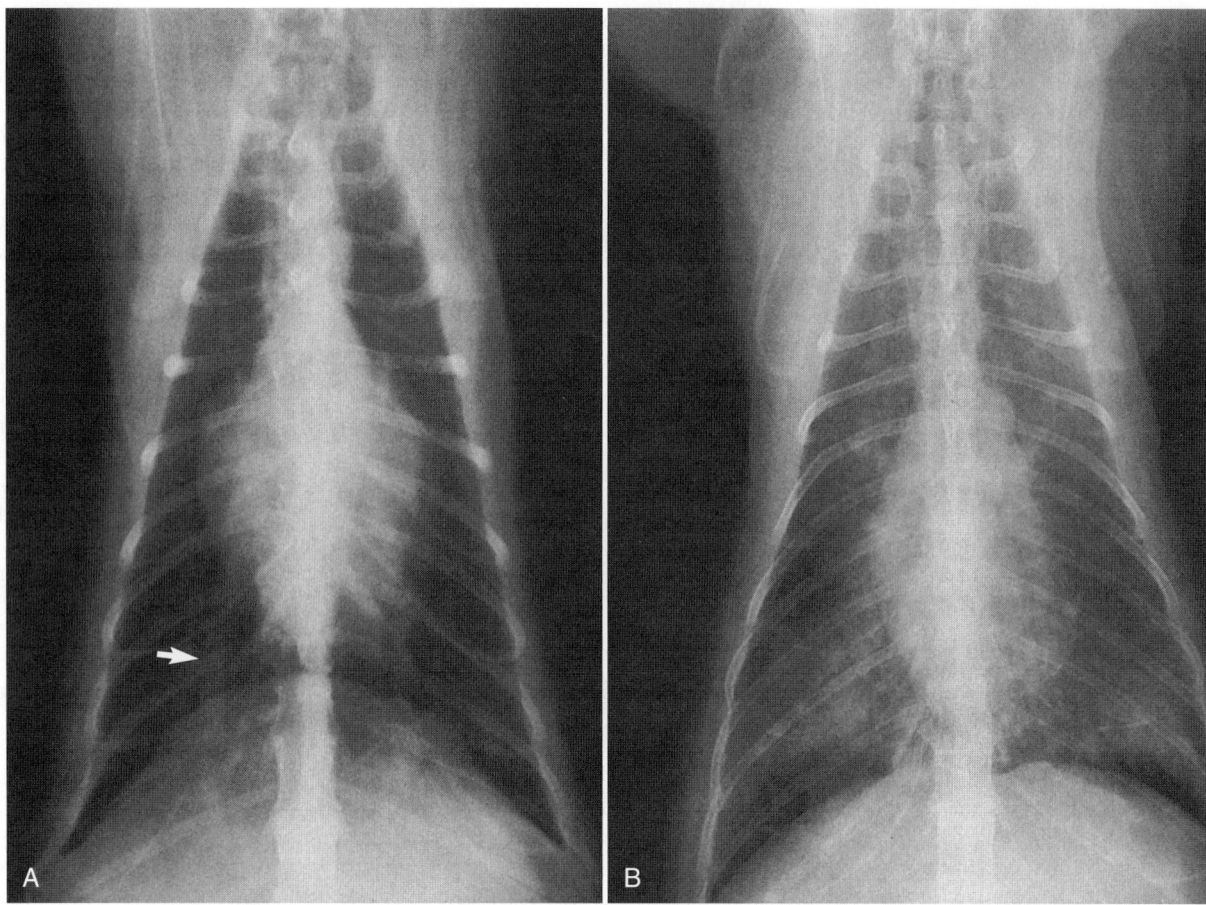

Figure 183-3 A, Thoracic radiograph of a cat with mild radiographic signs of heartworm disease. Note the right caudal pulmonary artery *(arrow)*. The arrow is located at the ninth intercostal space, the site for comparison of the ninth rib with the caudal lobar pulmonary artery (either right or left). The finding of a pulmonary artery that is 1.6 times or more the radiographically measured diameter of the ninth rib is suggestive of heartworm disease in the cat. **B,** Thoracic radiograph of a more severely affected cat. Note the alveolar infiltrate in caudal lung lobes. (From Schafer M, Berry CR: Cardiac and pulmonary artery mensuration in feline heartworm disease, *Vet Radiol Ultrasound* 36:499, 1995, with permission.)

transient (Selcer et al, 1996). Finally, false-positive radiographic abnormalities have been detected in experimentally exposed cats that ultimately resisted heartworm maturation and were heartworm-negative on postmortem examination (Blagburn and Dillon, 2007; Selcer et al, 1996). Pulmonary angiography can be used to make a definitive diagnosis by the demonstration of radiolucent intravascular "foreign bodies" and enlarged, tortuous, and blunted pulmonary arteries, but it is done infrequently.

Echocardiography

Echocardiography is more sensitive in cats than in dogs for the detection of heartworm infection. Typically a double-lined echodensity (Figure 183-4) is evident in the main pulmonary artery, one of its branches, the right ventricle, or occasionally at the right atrioventricular junction. FHWI was detected echocardiographically in 7 of 9 natural infections and 12 of 16 experimental infections (Atkins et al, 1997; Selcer et al, 1996). A thorough examination that allows clear visualization of the

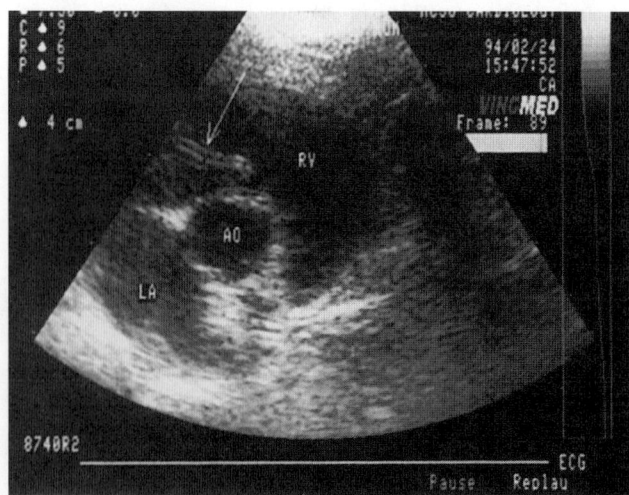

Figure 183-4 Two-dimensional echocardiogram for a cat with heartworm disease. A double-lined density (adult heartworm, indicated by arrow) is evident and is diagnostic for heartworm infection. *Ao,* Aorta; *LA,* left atrium; *RV,* right ventricle.

bifurcation of the pulmonary artery is essential. A retrospective review of data for a larger case series (DeFrancesco et al, 1998) revealed a lower sensitivity when worms were not specifically sought and particularly when studies were performed by noncardiologists. This observation underscores the need for a high index of suspicion, appropriate imaging equipment, and clinical expertise if this technique is to be of value in the diagnosis of FHWI. Although echocardiography can be a useful diagnostic tool, it cannot reliably determine worm numbers because of the coiling or serpentine posture of heartworms, which produces redundant shadows.

Prevention

Only 5% of cats in the United States receive heartworm-preventive medication. This is partly because owners and veterinarians question the need for heartworm prophylaxis in cats because they are not the natural host to *D. immitis* and because the incidence in cats is low. When a decision is being made about whether to institute prophylaxis, it is worth considering that the prevalence of FHWI in the southeastern United States and the Mississippi River valley approximates or even exceeds that of feline leukemia virus and feline immunodeficiency virus infections in the United States (Levy et al, 2006). Furthermore, a 1998 nationwide antibody survey in which over 2000 largely asymptomatic cats were tested revealed an exposure prevalence of nearly 12% (see Figure 183-2; Miller et al, 1998). Finally, the consequences of FHWD are potentially dire, with no clear therapeutic solutions. Therefore the author advocates preventive therapy in cats in endemic areas or, stated another way, in regions where heartworm preventives are advocated for dogs, they should be offered to cat owners as well.

Four heartworm preventives with Food and Drug Administration approval are marketed for use in cats in the United States (Table 183-2): ivermectin (Heartgard for cats), provided in a chewable formulation; milbemycin (Interceptor), a flavored tablet; selamectin (Revolution), a broad-spectrum topical parasiticide; and 10% imidacloprid/1% moxidectin (Advantage Multi for Cats), a broad-spectrum topical parasiticide. It is important to emphasize that four feline heartworm preventives are available, all highly effective with monthly administration and with varied spectra and methods of administration to meet the needs of most patients and clients.

As previously noted, cats rarely have microfilaremia, and when it is present, microfilariae occur in low numbers. Moreover, because rapid elimination of microfilariae is not seen with most monthly preventives, screening for FHWI before initiation of a preventive is not absolutely necessary. Although there is no reason to expect adverse reactions to prophylaxis in cats with existing FHWI, it still may be useful to know the heartworm status of a cat before institution of preventive therapy as a gauge of heartworm risk (both for that individual and for other animals) in the practice area. The current ELISA antigen tests are not adequately sensitive for this purpose and are not recommended unless the client is properly educated about their limitations. The ELISA antibody test (alone or with an antigen test) currently is more appropriate because of its higher sensitivity and ability to identify cats at risk (infected or exposed).

Based on the severity of FHWD, the lack of an effective and safe adulticidal therapy, and the difficulty in making a definitive diagnosis, the author advocates that clients in endemic areas be offered a heartworm preventive for their feline pets and that cats already infected with heartworms and their house mates receive preventive therapy.

Treatment

Since the vast majority of cats are amicrofilaremic, microfilaricidal therapy is unnecessary in this species. The use of arsenical adulticides is problematic. Thiacetarsamide is no longer available, and the data on the use of melarsomine in experimental (transplanted) FHWI are limited and contradictory. Although there is an abstract report in which one injection (2.5 mg/kg, one half the recommended canine dosage) of melarsomine was administered to experimentally infected cats without treatment-related mortality, the worm burdens after treatment were not significantly different from those in untreated control cats (Goodman et al, 1996). Diarrhea and heart murmurs were noted frequently in treated cats. A second study also reported in an abstract, which used either the standard canine protocol (2.5 mg/kg injected twice 24 hours apart) or a split-dosage regimen (one injection followed by two additional injections [2.5 mg/kg] 24 hours apart in 1 month), gave more favorable results (McLeroy et al, 1998). The standard treatment and split-dosage regimen resulted in a 79% and 86% reduction in worm burdens, respectively, and there were no adverse reactions.

TABLE **183-2**

Comparison of Macrolides Currently in Use in Cats for Heartworm Prevention and Parasite Control

Drug	Heartworm	Hookworm	Whipworm	Roundworm	Tapeworm	Flea/Eggs	Tick	*Sarcoptes*	Ear Mites
Ivermectin	+	+							
Milbemycin	+	+		+					
Selamectin	+	+		+		+/+			+
Imidacloprid/ moxidectin	+	+		+		+/−			+

Although promising, these unpublished data need to be interpreted with caution since the transplanted worms were young (<8 months old) and more susceptible, and the control cats experienced a 53% worm mortality (i.e., the average worm burden was reduced by 53% simply through the act of transplantation). In addition, the clinical experience in naturally infected cats generally has been unfavorable, with an unacceptable mortality. Because of the inherent risk, lack of clear benefit, and short life expectancy of heartworms in this species, the author does *not* advocate adulticidal therapy in cats. Surgical or catheter-based removal of heartworms has been successful and is attractive because it minimizes the risk of thromboemboli. Unfortunately, the mortality seen in the largest published case series was unacceptable (two of five cats; Venco et al, 1999). However, this procedure may hold promise for the future with the use of a less traumatic loop snare, which presumably can reduce anaphylaxis resulting from worm trauma. The author and colleagues have experienced success using this technique and have cured four cats of heart failure and chylothorax (Small et al, 2008).

Cats with FHWI should receive a monthly preventive and short-term corticosteroid therapy (prednisolone 1 to 2 mg/kg BID to q48h PO) to manage respiratory signs. If signs recur, alternate-day steroid therapy (at the lowest dosage that controls signs) can be continued indefinitely. For embolic or anaphylactic emergencies, oxygen, corticosteroids (dexamethasone 1 mg/kg IV or IM, or prednisolone sodium succinate 50 to 100 mg IV per cat), and bronchodilators (aminophylline 6.6 mg/kg q12h IM; theophylline, sustained-release formulation, 20 mg/kg (100 mg per cat) q24h PO; or terbutaline 0.01 mg/kg SC) may be administered. The use of bronchodilators in urgent situations is based on the ability of agents such as the xanthines (aminophylline and theophylline) to improve the function of fatigued respiratory muscles. In addition, the finding of hyperinflation of lung fields may indicate bronchoconstriction, a condition for which bronchodilation would be indicated. Nevertheless, the author does not use bronchodilators routinely in FHWD.

The use of aspirin has been questioned because vascular changes associated with FHWI consume platelets, increasing their turnover rate, and thereby effectively diminish the antithrombotic effects of the drug. Conventional dosages of aspirin did not prevent angiographically detected vascular lesions (Rawlings, 1990). Dosages of aspirin necessary to produce even limited benefit as assessed by histologic examination approached the toxic range. Despite this, because therapeutic options are limited, aspirin may be given and, at conventional dosages (40-80 mg per cat q72h PO), is well tolerated, generally harmless, inexpensive, and convenient; and because the quoted study used relatively insensitive estimates of platelet function and pulmonary arterial disease (and thus possibly missed subtle benefits), the author advocates aspirin for *asymptomatic* cats with FHWI. Aspirin is *not* prescribed concurrently with corticosteroid therapy. Management of other signs of FHWD is largely symptomatic.

There is some debate as to whether doxycycline should be administered to heartworm-infected animals to target the *Wolbachia* endosymbiont. Although reduced reaction to dying worms has been observed in dogs given doxycycline and ivermectin before adulticide therapy (Kramer et al, 2008), similar benefits have yet to be demonstrated in the cat. Consequently, the use of doxycycline in cats should be considered empiric, and this treatment cannot be generally recommended as an adjunctive therapy in cats at this time.

Prognosis

In the study of 50 cats with naturally acquired heartworm infection described earlier, at least 12 cats died of causes other than heartworm disease. Seven of these and two living cats were considered to have survived heartworm disease (i.e., lived ≥1000 days; Atkins et al, 2000). The median survival for all heartworm-infected cats living beyond the day of diagnosis was 1460 days (4 years; range, 2 to 4015 days), whereas the median survival of all cats (n = 48 with adequate follow-up) was 540 days (1.5 years; range, 0 to 4015 days). Survival of 11 cats treated with sodium thiacetarsamide (mean, 1669 days) was not significantly different from that of the 30 cats managed without adulticide (mean, 1107 days). Likewise, youth (≤3 years of age), presence of dyspnea, presence of cough, ELISA positivity for heartworm antigen, presence of identifiable worms on echocardiography, and gender of the cat did not appear to affect survival. Comparison of the prognosis for other cardiovascular diseases with that for FHWI reveals that survival in FHWI is roughly equivalent to that in hypertrophic cardiomyopathy (Atkins et al, 2003).

References and Suggested Reading

Atkins CE: Veterinary CE advisor: heartworm disease: an update, *Vet Med* 93(Suppl):12:2, 1998.

Atkins CE et al: Prevalence of heartworm infection in cats with signs of cardiorespiratory abnormalities, *J Vet Med Assoc* 212:517, 1997.

Atkins CE et al: Heartworm infection in cats: 50 cases (1985-1997), *J Vet Med Assoc* 217:355, 2000.

Atkins CE et al: Prognosis in feline heartworm infection: comparison to other cardiovascular disease. In Seward LR, Knight DH, editors: *Proceedings of the Heartworm Symposium '01*, Batavia, IL, 2003, American Heartworm Society, p 41.

Blagburn BL, Dillon AR: Feline heartworm disease: solving the puzzle, *Vet Med* 102(Suppl):7-14, 2007.

Browne LE et al: Pulmonary arterial disease in cats seropositive for *Dirofilaria immitis* but lacking adult heartworms in the heart and lungs, *Am J Vet Res* 66:1544, 2005.

DeFrancesco TC et al: Diagnostic utility of echocardiography in feline heartworm disease. In Soll MD, Knight DH, editors: *Proceedings of the American Heartworm Symposium '98*, Batavia, IL, 1998, American Heartworm Society.

Dillon AR: Feline dirofilariasis, *Vet Clin North Am* 114:1184, 1984.

Dillon AR, Warner AE, Molina RM: Pulmonary parenchymal changes in dogs and cats after experimental transplantation of dead *Dirofilaria immitis*. In Soll MD, Knight DH, editors: *Proceedings of the Heartworm Symposium '95*, Batavia, IL, 1996, American Heartworm Society, p 97.

Goodman DA et al: Evaluation of a single dose of melarsomine dihydrochloride for adulticidal activity against *Dirofilaria Immitis* in cats, *Proc Am Assoc Vet Parasitol* 41:64, 1996 (abstract).

Guerrero J et al: Prevalence of *Dirofilaria immitis* infection in cats from the southeastern United States. In Soll MD, editor: *Proceedings of the Heartworm Symposium '92*, Batavia, IL, 1992, American Heartworm Society, p 91.

Kramer L et al: Wolbachia and its influence on the pathology and immunology of *Dirofilaria immitis* infection, *Vet Parasitol* 158:191, 2008.

Lee A, Atkins C: Understanding feline heartworm infection: disease, diagnosis, and treatment, *Top Companion Anim Med* 25:224, 2010.

Levy JK et al: Seroprevalence of feline leukemia virus and immunodeficiency virus infection among cats in North America and risk factors for seropositivity, *J Vet Med Assoc* 228:371, 2006.

McCall JW et al: Utility of ELISA-based antibody test for detection of heartworm infection in cats. In Soll MD, Knight DH, editors: *Proceedings of the American Heartworm Symposium '95*, Batavia, IL, 1995, American Heartworm Society, p 127.

McCall JW et al: Evaluation of antigen and antibody tests for detection of heartworm infection in cats. In Soll MD, Knight DH, editors: *Proceedings of the American Heartworm Symposium '98*, Batavia, IL, 1998, American Heartworm Society, p 127.

McLeroy LW et al: Evaluation of melarsomine dihydrochloride (Immiticide) for adulticidal activity against *Dirofilaria immitis* in cats, *Proc Am Assoc Vet Parasitol* 43:67, 1998 (abstract).

McTier TL et al: Evaluation of ELISA-based adult heartworm antigen test kits using well-defined sera from experimentally and naturally infected cats. In *Proceedings of the 38th Annual Meeting of the American Association of Veterinary Parasitologists*, Minneapolis, 1993, p 37 (abstract).

Miller MW et al: Prevalence of exposure to *Dirofilaria immitis* in cats from multiple areas of the United States. In Soll MD, Knight DH, editors: *Proceedings of the Heartworm Symposium '98*, Batavia, IL, 1998, American Heartworm Society, p 161.

Rawlings CA: Pulmonary arteriography and hemodynamics during feline heartworm disease, *J Vet Intern Med* 4:285, 1990.

Robertson-Plough CK et al: Prevalence of feline heartworm infection among cats with respiratory and gastrointestinal signs: results of a multicenter study. In Soll MD, Knight DH, editors: *Proceedings of the Heartworm Symposium '98*, Batavia, IL, 1998, American Heartworm Society, p 127.

Ryan WG, Gross SJ, Soll MD: Diagnosis of feline heartworm infection. In Soll MD, Knight DH, editors: *Proceedings of the Heartworm Symposium '95*, Batavia, IL, 1996, American Heartworm Society, p 121.

Ryan WG, Newcomb KM: Prevalence of feline heartworm disease: a global review. In Soll MD, Knight DH, editors: *Proceedings of the Heartworm Symposium '95*, Batavia, IL, 1996, American Heartworm Society, p 79.

Schafer M, Berry CR: Cardiac and pulmonary artery mensuration in feline heartworm disease, *Vet Radiol Ultrasound* 36:499, 1995.

Selcer BA et al: Radiographic and 2-D echocardiographic findings in eighteen cats experimentally exposed to *D. immitis* via mosquito bites, *Vet Radiol Ultrasound* 37:37, 1996.

Small MT et al: Use of a nitinol gooseneck snare catheter for removal of adult *Dirofilaria immitis* in two cats, *J Am Vet Med Assoc* 233:1441, 2008.

Venco L et al: Surgical removal of heartworms in naturally infected cats. In Seward RL, Knight DH, editors: *Proceedings of the Heartworm Symposium '98*, Batavia, IL, 1999, American Heartworm Society, p 241.

CHAPTER 184

Canine Heartworm Disease

MATTHEW W. MILLER, *College Station, Texas*
SONYA G. GORDON, *College Station, Texas*

Despite the availability of numerous effective and safe preventive medications, heartworm disease (HWD) continues to be an important disorder affecting both dogs and cats. This chapter briefly reviews the life cycle of the parasite, diagnostic studies, and staging of disease and focuses on the treatment and prevention of canine dirofilariasis. Feline HWD is described in Chapter 183.

Diagnosis and Staging of Canine Heartworm Disease

Life Cycle of *Dirofilaria Immitis*

A basic knowledge of the life cycle of the heartworm parasite is imperative for understanding strategies for prevention, diagnosis, and therapy. The mosquito is a requisite intermediate host for transmission of this disease. The first-stage larvae (L1) or microfilariae are ingested by the female mosquito following a blood meal from an infected animal. The parasite molts twice within the mosquito, and these molts are required for the parasite to develop into the infective third stage (L3). The parasite maturation within the mosquito from L1 to L3 requires approximately 1 to 3 weeks depending on environmental conditions, most notably an ambient temperature of at least 14°C (57°F).

The L3 larvae are the infective stage of the parasite and are transmitted to a susceptible host through a bite from an infected mosquito. The third larval stage travels within the subcutaneous tissues of the host, molting to the fourth larval stage (L4) in approximately 1 to 2 weeks and becoming a young adult (L5) 30 to 60 days after initial inoculation. These young adults migrate and enter the systemic venous system where they are carried to the lungs approximately 100 days after infection. Under ideal conditions the infection may become patent (adult worms producing microfilariae) in 5 months. More often, however, this complete cycle requires in excess of 7 months.

Establishment of a Diagnosis

The American Heartworm Society (AHS; www.heartworm society.org) recommends the use of a test that detects adult heartworm antigen (Ag) as the primary screening test for HWD in dogs. A number of manufacturers supply heartworm Ag tests, and readers are referred to the excellent articles by Atkins (2003) and Courtney and Zeng (2001) for data about the relative sensitivity and specificity of these tests. Ag tests are substantially more sensitive than microfilarial concentration tests for detection of heartworm infection. In addition, the widespread use of macrocyclic lactone (ML) or macrolide preventive medications further decreases the sensitivity of the microfilarial tests for diagnosis by rendering the vast majority of infections amicrofilaremic (occult). In contrast, these drugs have no effect on the sensitivity of the Ag tests. Circulating Ag generally is undetectable until 6 to 7 months following infection, and this interval can be as long as 9 months after infection in dogs intermittently receiving MLs. As a general rule, weakly positive test results should be rechecked either by repeating the original test or preferably by submitting a sample for evaluation by a different Ag test at a reference laboratory. *False-positive* results occur infrequently and almost always are associated with technical errors. *False-negative* test results usually are the result of immature infections, infections with low numbers of female worms, or all-male infections. Although once thought uncommon, complexing of circulating Ag with specific or nonspecific host antibody may leave insufficient concentrations of free Ag for detection and subsequently lead to a false-negative test result.

Blood smear examination or use of a concentration test for the detection of circulating microfilariae is not recommended for routine screening of dogs, even when infection is suspected. The simultaneous use of both an adult heartworm Ag test and a concentration test for microfilariae has been advocated by some as the optimal screening protocol. However, addition of a concentration test probably increases the likelihood of diagnosis in a negligible percentage (≈1%) of cases, such as when a very low number of gravid females is present or when the circulating Ag is complexed to host antibody. Once a positive Ag test result is obtained, however, a concentration test should be performed to identify any circulating microfilariae. This information is important because it helps confirm the accuracy of the positive Ag test result and also may influence the preventive medication used in that patient.

Some preventive medications, most notably those containing the active ingredient milbemycin, are potent microfilaricides at the suggested preventive dosage and may be associated with substantial risk of a shocklike reaction when administered to dogs with a heavy burden of circulating microfilaria. The risk of a rapid microfilaria kill is much lower with ML preventives containing ivermectin, selamectin, or moxidectin. Dogs with severe microfilaremia optimally should be kept in the clinic when the first dose of any preventive medication is given. It also is prudent to recommend that the client observe a patient without microfilaremia for the entire day following administration of the first dose of preventive medication, regardless of which agent is used or what the concentration of circulating microfilariae.

Classification and Staging

It has been suggested that dogs with documented adult heartworm infection be classified, optimally based on radiographic findings and laboratory studies, before initiation of adulticidal therapy. In the vast majority of dogs with heartworm infection, the disease is diagnosed during routine wellness examinations. These dogs typically do not have demonstrable clinical signs nor do they commonly display radiographic or biochemical alterations associated with the infection. When HWD causes clinical signs, these generally are attributable to pulmonary parenchymal injury, pulmonary arterial injury, or cardiac dysfunction. Less frequently encountered clinical syndromes include severe glomerular disease, caval syndrome (see later), and disseminated intravascular coagulopathy.

There are a number of ways to classify patients with positive heartworm test results. One approach is related to the use of the Immiticide brand of melarsomine and is based on the U.S. Food and Drug Administration (FDA)–approved label. The drug package insert for Immiticide provides very detailed and specific information about this classification system, although there is some potential for overlapping of clinical and laboratory findings when this three-class system is used. Another method is to consider heartworm patients in terms of clinical syndromes or presentations, an approach that considers the aforementioned classification system but also provides additional perspective regarding treatment approaches. Dogs can be characterized clinically as follows:

- *Asymptomatic* or equivocal signs: Heartworm infection is documented, but there is no clear evidence of disease.
- *Respiratory signs* of HWD, including cough and tachypnea with exercise: These problems often are related to heartworm-induced pneumonitis; some but not all dogs also have evidence of pulmonary vascular disease.
- *Cor pulmonale,* radiographic evidence of significant pulmonary vascular disease: Typical clinical findings include limited exercise capacity and possibly exertional collapse or syncope; some but not all dogs have significant pulmonary parenchymal changes.
- *Congestive heart failure* (CHF): Right-sided heart failure is an advanced complication of severe pulmonary vascular disease, pulmonary hypertension, and subsequent cor pulmonale.

- *Caval syndrome*—an acute syndrome related to a large worm burden, severe pulmonary hypertension, and right ventricular dysfunction with tricuspid regurgitation: Hepatic congestion and intravascular hemolysis with hemoglobinuria are classic clinical signs.
- Heartworm infection or disease in a dog with *serious comorbid conditions:* Examples are malignant neoplasia, diabetes mellitus, and chronic renal failure.

Role of *Wolbachia*

Like all filarial nematodes that use an arthropod intermediate host and vector, *D. immitis* harbors obligate, intracellular, gram-negative bacteria belonging to the genus *Wolbachia* (Rickettsiales). Studies of non–*D. immitis* filariae demonstrated that treatment with tetracyclines during the first month of infection was lethal to some *Wolbachia*-harboring filariae but not to a filaria that did not harbor *Wolbachia*. In addition, treatment of *Wolbachia*-harboring filariae suppressed microfilaremia and made surviving microfilariae noninfectious. There is strong evidence to show that doxycycline at a dosage of 10 to 20 mg/kg/day PO in dogs substantially reduces the number of adult parasites and in some cases results in the gradual elimination of *D. immitis* when coadministered with ivermectin. In addition, with this combination of drugs there is loss of uterine content in adult female heartworms, microfilariae (L1 stage) are removed from the circulation, and although microfilariae still can molt within the mosquito from L2 to L3, these L3 organisms are rendered noninfectious. Ongoing studies suggest that doxycycline combined with ivermectin may be a feasible alternative adulticidal therapy for some dogs unable to be treated with melarsomine and may render the majority of dogs heartworm Ag negative after 36 to 45 weeks of therapy. However, it remains to be determined whether some combination of doxycycline and an ML can serve as a safe and effective alternative adulticidal option. Concerns with this approach include the potential for ongoing pulmonary and vascular injury during the relatively long period required to eliminate some infections as well as the possibility that not all infections will be completely resolved by this strategy.

It has been suggested that *Wolbachia* contributes to pulmonary and renal inflammation through its surface protein WSP, independently from its endotoxin component; however, the data supporting this supposition are not strong. Nevertheless, there is keen interest in studies to determine the role of *Wolbachia* in the pathogenesis of HWD, and there is hope that suppressing this symbiote with doxycycline before initiating adulticidal therapy may reduce the severity of lung and vascular injury after adulticide administration. Based on available data, the AHS suggests *pretreatment of animals with doxycycline for 30 days before adulticidal therapy* to reduce *Wolbachia* numbers. This preadulticide protocol offers the potential benefits of time to allow juvenile worms to mature fully to the susceptible adult stage and increased death of adult worms, higher levels of seroconversion, and reduction in the severity of clinical signs associated with the inevitable pulmonary embolization of dead and dying adult parasites. If there are shortages of doxycycline, minocycline can be substituted at a dose of 5 to 10 mg/kg q12h PO. There are no studies with minocycline in canine heartworm disease, but it has similar antibacterial activity.

Adulticidal Therapy for Canine Heartworm Disease

If necessary, steps should be taken to stabilize the condition of dogs with HWD before adulticidal therapy is begun. Dogs with *significant respiratory signs* and pulmonary infiltration generally are treated with supplemental oxygen therapy coupled with prednisone at 0.5 mg/kg once or twice daily PO for at least 7 to 14 days. Patients with eosinophilic pneumonitis often show a marked improvement in clinical signs. Dogs with *severe cor pulmonale* based on radiographic signs with or without evidence of CHF should be maintained on strict exercise restriction before, during, and after adulticidal treatment. The addition of a phosphodiesterase 5 inhibitor such as sildenafil (see Chapters 167 and 175) may help minimize the severity of clinical signs. Although other therapies, including aspirin and heparin, have been used empirically in dogs with severe cor pulmonale, there is no consensus on their use and we do not recommend these drugs. There is a clear risk of gastrointestinal bleeding with aspirin therapy, and this risk is extremely high when nonsteroidal antiinflammatory drugs are combined with corticosteroids.

When *right-sided CHF* is evident, adulticidal therapy typically is delayed for a number of weeks until CHF has been stabilized and resolved medically (see Chapter 176). In general, the management of CHF in HWD involves strict rest and administration of furosemide to effect, an angiotensin-converting enzyme inhibitor, a phosphodiesterase 5 inhibitor, and pimobendan.

Dogs with caval syndrome should be referred immediately to a hospital experienced in removing filarial parasites by minimally invasive catheter-based therapy. Melarsomine should *not* be given to dogs with caval syndrome. Patients with heartworm infection that have other serious systemic disorders generally are managed on a case-by-case basis.

Melarsomine Dihydrochloride Therapy

The only drug currently approved for adulticidal therapy of canine HWD is melarsomine dihydrochloride (Immiticide). Three specific dosing regimens are listed as approved protocols on the package insert. The most commonly employed regimens are the first two approaches.

Method 1 (two doses): Administration of two doses of melarsomine (2.5 mg/kg IM) with the second dose administered 24 hours after the first IM treatment.
Method 2 (three doses): An initial injection of melarsomine (2.5 mg/kg IM) followed approximately 1 month later by two injections as described previously for method 1. This method has been referred to as the *split-dose* approach and is discussed in more detail in the next section.
Method 3 (four doses): Two injections of melarsomine (2.5 mg/kg IM) separated by 24 hours (method 1 previously) and then repeated 4 months later.

Although this is the least frequently used protocol in clinical practice, the original data supporting FDA approval of this product demonstrated that this protocol was associated with the highest rate of seroconversion to negative Ag status of the three methods.

By definition, successful pharmacologic adulticidal therapy dictates that thromboembolic events will occur. The goal of adulticidal therapy is to eliminate all adult heartworms while minimizing the clinical manifestations of thromboembolic events. The severity of this complication can be diminished by restricting exercise after melarsomine administration and by using the split-dose regimen recommended for advanced HWD. A 4- to 6-week period of severe exercise restriction after each dose of adulticidal therapy is recommended. The method and degree of exercise restriction vary with the client's needs and the pet's inherent activity level but might include hospitalization, cage rest, sedation, housing in a restricted room of the house or garage, and only gentle leash walks. Nevertheless, some owners do not or cannot restrict exercise, which results in the occurrence or worsening of thromboembolic complications.

Split Versus Standard Dosing of Melarsomine

To minimize the chance of thromboembolic complications the use of a three-injection (split-dose) method of treatment can be supported for all dogs treated with melarsomine, regardless of the severity of disease. Studies have shown that dogs treated with the split-dose regimen (three doses in total) have a higher rate of seroconversion to a negative Ag status (89.7%) than patients treated with sodium thiacetarsamide (65.9%), which is no longer available, or the regimen of two doses (in total) of melarsomine (76.2%). In addition, in a study of experimental heartworm infection in dogs, the more effective adulticidal activity of three doses did not appear to increase the severity of clinically apparent pulmonary hypertension or thromboembolism. Perhaps more importantly, killing

adult worms in two increments and over a longer period seemingly diminishes the insult to the lung and pulmonary vasculature compared with the initial two-dose approach (method 1 described previously). This is especially critical in dogs with advanced cor pulmonale. After approximately 50% of the worms are killed with the first (single) dose, there is a 1-month interval for the lungs to heal before a second insult of dying worms begins. Furthermore, if there is a significant adverse reaction to the initial adulticidal injection, the second and third injections can be delayed (or even cancelled) until clinical signs have resolved and damaged tissue has healed (typically in 2 to 3 months). If such a delay is required, it is imperative to ensure that these patients continue to receive MLs to minimize the possibility of a new infection becoming established.

There are potential disadvantages to this split or two-step approach. First is the added cost of the third dose and attendant veterinary care. This cost may be balanced by a reduction in adverse reactions, which often require hospitalization and intensive therapy. Second, the total arsenic dose is increased, which may be a concern in a dog with significant renal disease. Finally, exercise restriction is a problem for some owners, and the split-dose regimen requires approximately 2 months of exercise restriction. Despite these drawbacks, we have found the approach to be generally well tolerated, and we advocate a split regimen. In dogs with significant renal disease, supportive fluid therapy may be appropriate to minimize the potential for renal injury.

Thus we strongly recommend a split-dose approach with a total of three injections for melarsomine administration and believe this provides the best management strategy for nearly all heartworm-infected dogs (Figure 184-1). There is evidence that this treatment regimen is safer and more effective than the two-dose regimen, which justifies the increased cost. The AHS also advocates this approach. Even if owners cannot afford the minimum set of tests for evaluation of general health and assessment of severity of HWD, they still may benefit

Figure 184-1 Our preferred approach to adulticidal therapy in all dogs with heartworm infection (HWI) includes three doses of melarsomine dihydrochloride (Immiticide). Macrocyclic lactone prophylaxis is begun at the time of diagnosis, if it is not already in use, and is continued according to product labeling 12 months of the year for the remainder of the patient's life. Doxycycline therapy at a dosage of 10 mg/kg/day should be initiated at the time of diagnosis. Minocycline may be substituted for doxycycline (see text). If microfilaremia is present, care should be taken to prevent or observe and treat adverse reactions, based on microfilarial numbers and the macrolide used. See text for complete description.

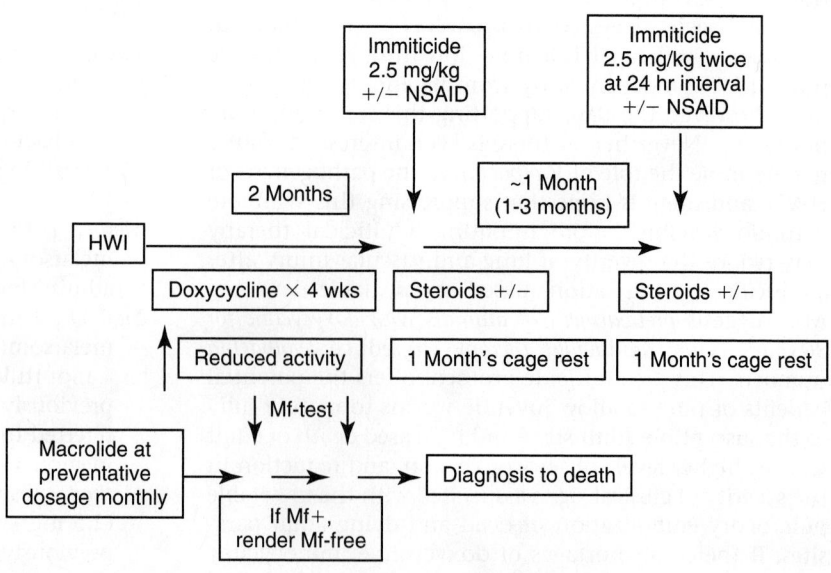

financially in the end from the use of a three-dose regimen because the likelihood of adverse reaction (and attendant costs) can be reduced by this approach.

Administration and Clinical Use of Melarsomine in Dogs

At the time of heartworm diagnosis by a positive Ag test result, we recommend compiling a database that includes the findings from a patient history and complete physical examination as well as the results of a microfilaria (concentration) test, serum chemistry panel, complete blood count, urinalysis, and thoracic radiography. In general, echocardiography is indicated in canine HWD only when there is a suspicion of caval syndrome or when the dog demonstrates clinical signs of severe cor pulmonale (e.g., exertional syncope or right-sided CHF).

We initiate doxycycline treatment at a dosage of 10 mg/kg/day and continue this therapy for 30 days. Based on currently available data this will most likely suppress *Wolbachia* numbers for 3 to 6 months (Bazzocchi et al, 2008). Administration of a macrolide preventive should be initiated *immediately* and continued according to label directions for the remainder of the patient's life (see Figure 184-1 and details later). These treatments will prevent further infection, begin to eliminate microfilariae (which removes the dog as a potential reservoir of infection), and destroy developing L4 larvae, a stage not susceptible to adulticidal therapy. The risk of an adverse reaction in microfilaria-negative dogs (dogs with occult infection) is very low with any preventive medication.

In *microfilaria-positive dogs* the first macrolide dose is administered in the hospital or at home with observation so that an adverse reaction can be recognized and treated promptly. Common clinical manifestations of rapid microfilarial death include hypotension, pale mucous membranes, tachycardia, and collapse. Dogs at high risk should be observed for the first 8 to 12 hours following administration of potentially microfilaricidal drugs. In our practice, we administer a corticosteroid (either dexamethasone 0.25 mg/kg IV *or* prednisolone 1 mg/kg PO) 1 hour before and sometimes 6 hours after administration of the first dose of preventive. Corticosteroids are used to reduce the potential for adverse reaction in patients with high microfilaria counts. It is important to emphasize that adverse reactions are unusual when macrolides are given at preventive dosages; however, the risk is probably greater for milbemycin oxime products than for those containing ivermectin, selamectin, or moxidectin as the active ingredients.

Depending on the time of year (and the geographic location), as long as 2 to 3 months might be allowed to lapse before adulticidal therapy is administered, although we most commonly initiate melarsomine therapy 1 month following diagnosis. Monthly macrolide administration ensures that the dog is at no further risk of infection and should prevent maturation of the majority of infections of shorter than 2 months' duration if the medication is continued indefinitely. Theoretically, an infection of longer than 4 months but less than 6 months cannot be halted from advancing with a monthly ML preventive, and the immaturity of the worms also renders them relatively resistant to melarsomine. Therefore the administration of preventives for 2 to 3 months before the first dose of melarsomine not only prevents new infections (or those of <60 days' duration) from maturing but also allows enough time for older larvae to mature to adulthood, which ensures their vulnerability to melarsomine therapy (see Figure 184-1).

The manufacturer's insert should be read carefully before the administration of melarsomine dihydrochloride. Melarsomine is administered by deep IM injection (2.5 mg/kg) into the lumbar musculature as described in the illustration accompanying the package insert. The injection needle is changed before injection, and care is taken to inject deep into the muscle and to record the injection site in the medical record. It is important to place the injection within the center of the epaxial muscle. Typically patients are hospitalized on the day of the injection. Some dogs seem to experience discomfort, depression, or nausea following injection; for this reason some clinicians administer butorphanol (0.3 to 0.4 mg/kg IM) before injection of melarsomine. Sedation also helps to ensure optimal injection technique. The need for exercise restriction for at least 1 month is emphasized, and sedatives or tranquilizers are dispensed if necessary. The owners are advised that they must return for a second series of two injections in approximately 1 month.

Owners also are advised regarding potential adverse reactions (fever, lethargy, inappetence, cough, dyspnea, and collapse) and are told to call if they have concerns. Since these signs often are predictable, related to pulmonary reaction to dead worms, some clinicians routinely dispense prednisolone (0.5 mg/kg daily) to be given at home when any of these clinical signs first is observed. Generally 5 to 7 days of therapy is sufficient to overcome pulmonary reactions to dead worms.

If serious systemic reaction results, the second stage of the adulticidal treatment may be delayed or even cancelled. However, even when severe reactions occur after adulticide administration, the entire treatment protocol generally is completed within 2 to 5 months. After a minimum interval of 1 month (1 to 2 months is typical) the melarsomine injection procedure is repeated; the injection site again is recorded. If significant local reaction was noted after the first injection, dexamethasone or oral nonsteroidal antiinflammatory drugs are administered to minimize pain at the injection site. Butorphanol also can be used as described previously. The following day (approximately 24 hours after the first injection) the process is repeated with injection into the *opposite* lumbar area. Client instructions are similar to those given previously, with reemphasis of the need for strict exercise restriction.

Heartworm Ag testing is repeated 6 months following the second series of injections; a positive test result indicates incomplete adulticidal efficacy. It is emphasized that, despite the proven effectiveness of melarsomine, not all worms are killed in every patient. Typically worm burden is reduced markedly, but if as few as one to three adult female worms remain, positive results on Ag tests are likely. Whether or not repeat adulticidal therapy is warranted under these circumstances is decided on a case-by-case basis, with input from the owners and perhaps from a specialist.

Monthly Preventives as Adulticides

Much has been written about the adulticidal properties of the monthly ML preventives. Some individuals have suggested that, because of their adulticidal properties, these drugs represent an alternative to melarsomine. The variable efficacy of the preventives is correlated with what frequently is called *reach-back*. This term is misleading because the property being described is simply a reflection of efficacy against older infections. Based on data published thus far, ivermectin has the highest efficacy against mature infections. McCall and colleagues (2001) reported that, when given monthly for longer than 24 months at the standard preventive dosage, ivermectin is 98% effective against 5-month-old worms and 95% effective against 7-month-old worms. Similar efficacy data for older infections have not been published. Despite these intriguing results, Rawlings and colleagues (2001) showed that dogs with preexisting 5.5- to 6.5-month-old infections administered the label dosages of either ivermectin or milbemycin developed radiographic changes and necropsy findings similar to those in dogs with infections of the same duration that remained untreated. These results reinforced the recommendations of the AHS that dogs be tested using an Ag test *before* preventive therapy is initiated and that *dogs found to be heartworm Ag positive receive treatment with an approved adulticide* and not simply be placed on a preventive medication.

Elimination of Circulating Microfilariae

Historically, elimination of circulating microfilariae has been attempted several months following adulticidal therapy as the second step in the treatment of a patent infection. The general recommendation now is that elimination of circulating microfilariae be accomplished as a secondary benefit of chemoprophylaxis, although some argue that rapid elimination of circulating microfilariae eliminates a potential disease reservoir more quickly. Despite this contention, the monthly ML preventives eliminate microfilariae and also that reservoir of infection; administration of these agents is initiated as soon as a positive diagnosis is established. As mentioned earlier, the concurrent use of doxycycline can facilitate elimination of circulating microfilariae. Even if microfilariae from dogs receiving doxycycline are ingested by a mosquito, these larvae are rendered noninfective by the previous doxycycline exposure. It sometimes is difficult to eliminate circulating microfilariae before completion of adulticidal therapy. However, even without adulticidal therapy, circulating microfilariae often are eliminated after several sequential months of treatment with an ML.

The ML drugs are the safest and most effective microfilaricidal drugs to date. However, none of these drugs is approved currently as a microfilaricide by the U.S. FDA. Use of the monthly preventives for this purpose is covered by the Animal Medicinal Drug Use Clarification Act of 1994, which allows licensed veterinarians extralabel use of certain drugs that have an established clinical application, provided a valid veterinarian-client-patient relationship has been established. Ensuring proper dose administration and providing appropriate aftercare when products are used in an extralabel application are the personal responsibilities of the dispensing veterinarian. The AHS has taken a firm stance against the once-common use of high-dose ivermectin for rapid elimination of microfilariae. The AHS also indicates in its guidelines that if rapid elimination of circulating microfilariae is deemed important, milbemycin oxime should be used since it is the most potent microfilaricide and produces the most rapid rate of microfilarial clearance. Additionally, clearance of circulating microfilariae can be accelerated by administering the monthly preventive dosage of any of the currently available macrolides every 2 weeks and in combination with doxycycline. Once the microfilariae are cleared, the standard dosage should be administered monthly. The potential for shocklike reaction, the need for clinical or client observation after ML treatment of a microfilaria-positive dog, and the potential value of pretreatment with corticosteroids for the first dose of an ML have been discussed previously in this chapter.

Heartworm Prevention in Dogs

Canine HWD is an almost completely preventable disease despite the fact that the dog is an exceptionally susceptible host. Administration of heartworm prophylaxis is suggested for all dogs living in endemic areas. Although year-round chemoprophylaxis may not be necessary in the northern half of the country, it is important to remember that successful seasonal prophylaxis depends on proper timing of heartworm *preventive* administration. When heartworm transmission potentially can occur over longer than 6 months, seasonal chemoprophylaxis may not be the most effective method of prevention. Additionally, there is ample evidence to suggest that although the vast majority of potential heartworm infections can be prevented by a single dose of an ML within 30 days of transmission of larvae, the efficacy of these products is enhanced further by administration of multiple sequential doses. Thus year-round preventive treatment should be considered to enhance compliance, and many of the available products also control other parasitic infections.

The currently available macrolides (ivermectin, milbemycin, moxidectin, and selamectin) all have been shown to have exceptional efficacy when administered appropriately at the recommended doses and dosing intervals. The ideal *preventive* medication is the product that best promotes client compliance and best fits other geographically determined needs for parasite control as well as the practicalities of practice management.

Product Switching

Occasionally the type of preventive medication used needs to be switched. Rarely does this result from intolerance of the product. More often it is related to perceived superiority, preference for administration route (topical versus oral), desire for additional antiparasitic activity, or practice management issues.

When product switching occurs, it may be important to establish a temporal line of evidence regarding the Ag status of the given animal so that, in the unlikely event of a prevention failure, the circumstances of the break can be ascertained. Although this may seem unnecessary, so-called lack-of-efficacy claims, when carefully investigated, most commonly have been found to be associated with a compliance issue, and this approach establishes the most likely cause. This practice also may be relevant in light of recent reports about ML resistance in parts of the southern United States.

We recommend obtaining a current Ag test result at the time of product switch. Any infection that is 6 months old or older would be expected to result in an Ag-positive status and therefore implicate the first product as responsible for prevention failure. If the Ag test result is negative, the new product is begun at the appropriate dosage, and a retesting schedule is established. Any infection that is 2 to 3 months old or younger almost certainly will be prevented from progressing by repeated monthly administration or a single injection of all the currently available preventives. On the other hand, a 4-month-old infection, although not identified by the initial Ag test, more likely will progress to become a mature infection. Seroconversion most likely will occur 6 to 9 months after infection, but it may take as long as 9 months because these dogs have been receiving at least intermittent ML treatments that are known to prolong parasite maturation and reduce or eliminate circulating microfilariae. Maturation at 6 to 9 months after infection would correspond to 2 to 5 months after the product switch occurred and the original Ag test was performed. Any new infection associated with exposure during that time would be too young to be detected by an Ag test.

Therefore repeating the Ag test 5 months after the product switch allows the veterinarian to determine if a prevention break occurred while the patient was receiving the initial product. Negative results on the Ag test at 5 months is very strong evidence that the initial product was effective. Seroconversion to a positive status 5 months or longer after product switching implicates the replacement product as the cause of the prevention break. We routinely repeat Ag testing 12 months after a product switch, and then that date becomes the annual testing date for that patient.

Concerns Regarding Resistance to the Macrocyclic Lactones

Initial concerns regarding perceived resistance to the MLs were voiced by practicing veterinarians in the Mississippi River Delta region based on observed prevention breaks and the subsequent inability to eliminate circulating microfilariae in certain patients. The number of affected dogs was relatively small, but the array of ML drugs used in these dogs coupled with the large doses and increased dosing frequency employed in an attempt to eliminate microfilariae prompted intense evaluation. Microfilariae from these dogs were collected and exposed to increasingly high levels of MLs *in vitro*. The motility of these microfilariae (low responders) was found to be minimally affected by this exposure compared with that of available laboratory and field strains. Genetic evaluation of these microfilariae showed a strong correlation between the GG-GG genotype of the P-glycoprotein and the low-responder phenotype. Furthermore, laboratory studies performed during the same time period as the aforementioned investigations documented imperfect protection following heavy experimental inoculation (100 infective L3 larvae) with the MP3 strain of *D. immitis* when a single dose of some ML drugs was given (Blagburn et al, 2011). It should be noted, however, that the MP3 strain is genetically very dissimilar to the low-responder field strain. Also, the dog from which the MP3 strain was isolated originated in an area of the country not reporting increased lack-of-efficacy claims. Additionally, administration of three sequential monthly doses of MLs was associated with 100% efficacy against the MP3 strain of *D. immitis* (Snyder et al, 2011). Finally, the low-responder microfilariae were passaged through mosquitoes and allowed to develop to the infective (L3) stage. When an established *in vitro* assay was used, these L3 larvae were found to have the same susceptibility to the MLs as available field and laboratory strains of *D. immitis* (Moorhead et al, 2011). Although the evolving body of data clearly documents that there is variability in susceptibility of different strains of *D. immitis* to the MLs, it is not clear that widespread resistance to the currently available preventive medications is developing.

References and Suggested Reading

Atkins CE: Comparison of results of three commercial heartworm antigen test kits in dogs with low heartworm burdens, *J Am Vet Med Assoc* 222(9):1221, 2003.

Bazzocchi C et al: Combined ivermectin and doxycycline treatment has microfilaricidal and adulticidal activity against *Dirofilaria immitis* in experimentally infected dogs, *J Parasitol* 38:1401, 2008.

Blagburn BL et al: Comparative efficacy of four commercially available heartworm preventive products against the MP3 laboratory strain of *Dirofilaria immitis*, *Vet Parasitol* 176:189, 2011.

Case JL et al: A clinical field trial of melarsomine dihydrochloride (RM340) in dogs with severe (class 3) heartworm disease. In Soll MD, Knight DH, editors: *Proceedings of the American Heartworm Symposium 1995*, Batavia, IL, 1995, American Heartworm Society, p 243.

Courtney CH, Zeng Q: Comparison of heartworm antigen test kit performance in dogs having low heartworm burdens, *Vet Parasitol* 96(4):317, 2001.

Kramer L et al: Is *Wolbachia* complicating the pathological effects of *Dirofilaria immitis* infections? *Vet Parasitol* 133(2-3):133, 2005.

McCall JW et al: Further evidence of clinical prophylactic, retro-active (reach-back) and adulticidal activity of monthly administrations of ivermectin (Heartgard Plus™) in dogs experimentally infected with heartworms. In Seward RL, editor: *Recent advances in heartworm disease: symposium*, Batavia, IL, 2001, American Heartworm Society, p 189.

Miller MW et al: Clinical efficacy of melarsomine dihydrochloride (RM340) and thiacetarsamide in dogs with moderate (class 2) heartworm disease. In Soll MD, Knight DH, editors: *Proceedings of the American Heartworm Symposium 1995*, Batavia, IL, 1995, American Heartworm Society, p 233.

Moorhead AD et al: In vitro bioassay for measuring anthelmintic susceptibility in *Dirofilaria immitis*. In *Proceedings of the American Association of Veterinary Parasitologists 56th Annual Meeting, 2011*, p 109 (abstract).

Rawlings CA et al: Disease response to trickle kill when ivermectin or milbemycin is started during *Dirofilaria immitis* infection in dogs. In Seward RL, Knight DH, editors: *Proceedings of the American Heartworm Symposium 2001*, Batavia, IL, 2001, American Heartworm Society, p 179.

Simón F et al: Immunopathology of *Dirofilaria immitis* infection, *Vet Res Commun* 1(2):161, 2007. Epub December 23, 2006.

Snyder DE et al: Ivermectin and milbemycin oxime in experimental adult heartworm *(Dirofilaria immitis)* infection of dogs, *J Vet Intern Med* 25:61, 2011.

SECTION IX

Urinary Diseases

Chapter 185: Applications of Ultrasound in Diagnosis and Management of Urinary Disease   840

Chapter 186: Recognition and Prevention of Hospital-Acquired Acute Kidney Injury   845

Chapter 187: Proteinuria/Albuminuria: Implications for Management   849

Chapter 188: Glomerular Disease and Nephrotic Syndrome   853

Chapter 189: Chronic Kidney Disease: International Renal Interest Society Staging and Management   857

Chapter 190: Use of Nonsteroidal Antiinflammatory Drugs in Kidney Disease   863

Chapter 191: Medical Management of Acute Kidney Injury   868

Chapter 192: Continuous Renal Replacement Therapy   871

Chapter 193: Surveillance for Asymptomatic and Hospital-Acquired Urinary Tract Infection   876

Chapter 194: Persistent *Escherichia coli* Urinary Tract Infection   880

Chapter 195: Interventional Strategies for Urinary Disease   884

Chapter 196: Medical Management of Nephroliths and Ureteroliths   892

Chapter 197: Calcium Oxalate Urolithiasis   897

Chapter 198: Canine Urate Urolithiasis   901

Chapter 199: Minilaparotomy-Assisted Cystoscopy for Urocystoliths   905

Chapter 200: Multimodal Environmental Enrichment for Domestic Cats   909

Chapter 201: Medical Management of Urinary Incontinence and Retention Disorders   915

Chapter 202: Mechanical Occluder Devices for Urinary Incontinence   919

Chapter 203: Top Ten Urinary Consult Questions   923

The following web chapters can be found on the companion website at www.currentveterinarytherapy.com

Web Chapter 70: Laser Lithotripsy for Uroliths

Web Chapter 71: Urinary Incontinence: Treatment with Injectable Bulking Agents

CHAPTER 185

Applications of Ultrasound in Diagnosis and Management of Urinary Disease

SILKE HECHT, *Knoxville, Tennessee*

Diagnostic imaging traditionally has played an important role in the workup of veterinary patients with disorders of the urinary system. With increases in technical quality and operator experience, ultrasonographic examinations and ultrasound-guided procedures have become invaluable tools and have partially replaced more conventional techniques such as survey radiography and radiographic contrast procedures. Ultrasound is useful for the diagnosis of various disorders of the kidneys, ureters, urinary bladder, and urethra; allows controlled needle placement for further diagnostic and therapeutic procedures; and helps in monitoring a patient's response to treatment.

Indications and Limitations

Ultrasound not only is indicated in patients with signs related to the urinary tract such as hematuria, stranguria, and increased frequency of urination but also is useful in the assessment of patients with nonspecific clinical signs such as abdominal pain or palpable abdominal masses. It is excellent for the evaluation of diffuse or focal renal parenchymal lesions, renal pelvis and ureteral dilation, intraluminal and mural lesions of the urinary bladder, and abnormalities of the intraabdominal part of the urethra. However, when one is deciding which imaging modality to choose for a patient with suspected urinary tract disease, the limitations of ultrasound need to be taken into consideration. In general, the diagnostic quality of abdominal ultrasound may be limited in large, deep-chested, and obese patients and may be affected significantly by the presence of a large amount of gas or ingesta within the gastrointestinal tract. Normal (nondistended) ureters and the intrapelvic part of the urethra typically are not visible when an ultrasonographic examination is performed and, depending on the indication, usually are better examined by means of an excretory urogram or a urethrogram, respectively. Ultrasound is inferior to survey radiography in the diagnosis of mineral opaque calculi in ureters and urethra, in the determination of the exact number of cystic calculi, and in the verification of the number of kidneys in the rare case of missing or supernumerary kidneys. Finally, contrast procedures such as excretory urography and cystourethrography are superior in the diagnosis of ureteral or urinary

bladder rupture, respectively; in the identification of the bladder in cases in which numerous large fluid-filled mass lesions are present in the caudal abdomen; and in the assessment of most urethral lesions.

Technique

The choice of transducer type and frequency is dictated in most instances by the equipment available in the examiner's practice. A microconvex, multifrequency transducer is desirable because it has a small contact area with the skin, allows the right kidney to be imaged through an intercostal approach without interference from overlying ribs, and provides the option of adjusting the transducer frequency during the examination. Curvilinear or linear transducers may be used if a microconvex transducer is not available. The transducer frequency should be chosen based on patient size and depth of the organs to be imaged. In large-breed dogs a frequency as low as 5 to 8 MHz may be needed to image the kidneys, whereas kidneys in small animals and the urinary bladder can be imaged with a higher frequency (8 to 12 MHz). As in the examination of other organ systems, the highest transducer frequency allowing evaluation of an organ should be chosen for each patient, and frequency may need to be adjusted separately for kidneys and urinary bladder.

The technique for the ultrasonographic evaluation of the urinary tract follows the same principles as that for a general abdominal examination. The animal is positioned in dorsal (or, depending on examiner preference, lateral) position, the abdomen is clipped, and ultrasonographic coupling gel is applied. The left kidney and urinary bladder usually are visualized easily using a ventral abdominal approach, as are dilated ureters and the proximal part of the urethra. The right kidney may be difficult to image because of its position in the craniodorsal abdomen immediately caudal to the liver, especially in large-breed and deep-chested dogs. In these cases use of a right dorsal intercostal approach, with the patient in left lateral recumbency, is beneficial to visualize the kidney and proximal right ureter. In male dogs the penile urethra can be scanned via a perineal and ventral approach.

The majority of the ultrasonographic examination is performed using routine grayscale B-mode ultrasound.

Color Doppler or power Doppler examination is helpful in assessing blood flow to an organ (e.g., in cases of suspected renal infarction) and in distinguishing vascular lesions such as bladder or renal neoplasms from nonvascularized lesions such as blood clots in the urinary bladder or renal cysts. Spectral Doppler ultrasonography and measurement of specific hemodynamic parameters such as resistive and pulsatility indices are not performed commonly in veterinary patients because of their low diagnostic yield in common urinary tract disorders.

If an ultrasound-guided interventional procedure is to be performed after the scan, all ultrasound gel should be cleaned off the abdomen. For simple procedures such as cystocentesis, thorough cleaning of the abdominal wall with alcohol is sufficient. When more invasive procedures such as renal biopsy are performed, surgical preparation of the abdominal wall is indicated. Cystocentesis and fine-needle aspiration of a kidney in a small patient can be accomplished using a 1.5-inch 22-gauge needle and syringe. However, aspiration of deeper structures necessitates the use of longer needles (e.g., 2.5-inch or 3.5-inch spinal needles). When long needles are used needle placement is more difficult to monitor with ultrasound. For these cases, and for biopsies utilizing larger bore sizes or extended procedures (such as drainage of large cysts), use of needle guides is strongly recommended. The guides consist of probe attachments and needle channels that direct the intraabdominal course of the needle in a predetermined direction and thus minimize the risk of injury to surrounding structures.

Normal Findings

Normal kidneys have an ovoid shape and are smoothly marginated. Generally, the size of the left and right kidney in the same animal should be similar. Because of the large variability in size between dogs of different breeds renal size traditionally has been evaluated with radiography rather than ultrasound. A normal range of 5.5 to 9.1 for kidney:aorta ratio has been proposed recently that allows objective assessment of renal size in a given dog. In cats, renal size is more consistent and should be approximately 3.0 to 4.5 cm in length. The renal cortex is hyperechoic to the strongly hypoechoic centrally located medulla (Figure 185-1), hypoechoic to the spleen, and isoechoic to hypoechoic to hepatic parenchyma. Many factors affect the echogenicity of the renal cortex, including normal variation, renal fat deposition, and transducer frequency so care must be taken not to overinterpret a mild generalized increase in renal cortical echogenicity as a pathologic change. The medulla is hypoechoic, and interlobar and arcuate vessels can be followed as anechoic tubular structures with hyperechoic walls crossing the renal medulla and branching at the level of the corticomedullary junction, respectively. When the kidney is investigated with color Doppler ultrasonography additional smaller branches (interlobular vessels) may be seen in the renal cortex. The renal pelvis may or may not be visible and should measure less than 2 mm wide in normal dogs and cats. Normal ureters usually are not visualized.

The urinary bladder is of variable size and filled with anechoic urine. A few echogenic speckles occasionally are

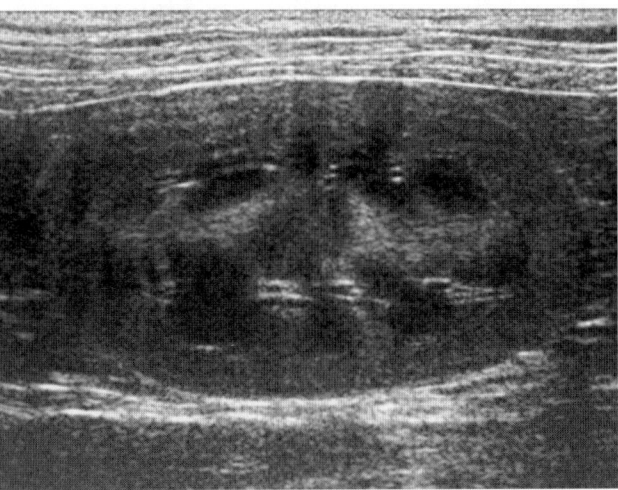

Figure 185-1 Sagittal ultrasonographic image of the normal left kidney in a cat. The medulla is hypoechoic compared with the surrounding cortex and the centrally located peripelvic fat.

observed within the urinary bladder in healthy animals and are thought to be the result of highly concentrated urine and excretion of normal substances. Given adequate (moderate) distention of the urinary bladder, wall thickness should be less than 2 mm in dogs and between 1.3 and 1.7 mm in cats. The healthy bladder wall is smoothly marginated. In some animals (especially in polyuric patients and animals receiving diuretics) ureteral "jetting" may be observed originating from the two small ureteral papillae located at the level of the trigone. The normal urethra typically is not visible in its entirety; the intraabdominal portion may be seen as a thin tubular structure extending caudally from the bladder neck toward the pelvic canal.

Congenital Disorders

Renal aplasia or agenesis is a rare diagnosis in dogs and cats and is characterized by absence of one kidney, often in association with an increase in the size of the contralateral kidney because of compensatory hypertrophy. Renal dysplasia is a congenital disease that has been reported in a variety of breeds. Affected animals typically are identified at a young age. Ultrasonographically the kidneys appear small and irregular, often with complete loss of the normal corticomedullary architecture (Figure 185-2). Ectopic kidneys occasionally are encountered, usually are incidental findings, and are characterized by an abnormal position. Supernumerary kidneys or failure of the kidneys to separate adequately from their common precursor (congenital renal fusion or horseshoe kidney) are very rare and poorly documented in the veterinary literature.

Ectopic ureters are a rather frequent congenital abnormality of the urinary tract and are defined as termination of one or both ureters in the urethra or reproductive system caudal to the level of the trigone. Ultrasound may be helpful in tracing dilated ureters past the level of their expected termination. However, the technique is neither sensitive nor specific for the diagnosis of ureteral ectopia, and excretory urography (with or without computed

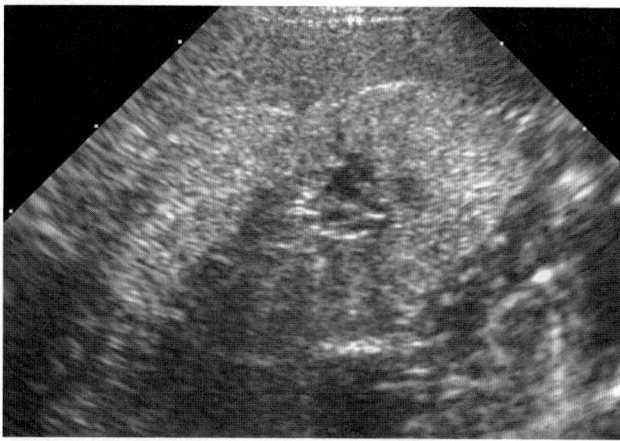

Figure 185-2 Renal dysplasia in a 2-year-old Australian shepherd. The kidney is small and has an irregular margin. Renal cortex and medulla are isoechoic, which results in complete loss of corticomedullary distinction. The ultrasonographic findings are similar to those observed in severe chronic degenerative renal disease ("end-stage kidneys").

tomography) and endoscopy therefore remain the modalities of choice to establish a diagnosis. Ultrasonographic diagnosis of a ureterocele as a focal dilation of the terminal ureter usually is straightforward. However, determination of the exact position of the ureterocele with respect to the bladder lumen (orthotopic versus ectopic) is difficult.

A pelvic bladder occasionally is diagnosed in animals with a presenting complaint of incontinence. The bladder is small and at least partially located within the pelvic canal. Because the degree of filling of the bladder and its position in normal animals are quite variable, this ultrasonographic diagnosis should be made only in association with supporting radiographic, endoscopic, and clinical findings and may not be the actual cause of incontinence. A urachal diverticulum is the result of a failure of the urachus to obliterate completely and appears as a focal rounded to triangular outpouching at the apex of the urinary bladder. The urine pool in this pouch can serve as a reservoir for bacteria, and affected animals often exhibit concurrent changes consistent with cystitis. Other congenital disorders of the bladder or urethra are extremely uncommon.

Acquired Disorders

Acquired disorders of the kidneys can result in changes in size and shape, alterations in overall echogenicity, focal or multifocal parenchymal lesions, abnormalities of the collecting system, and perinephric abnormalities. It is important to remember that there is variability in the size and echogenicity of the kidneys in normal animals and that a normal renal appearance on ultrasound does not rule out renal disease.

Changes in Renal Size

Differential diagnoses for diffusely enlarged kidneys include compensatory hypertrophy, acute inflammatory renal diseases (interstitial nephritis or glomerulonephritis), metabolic nephropathies, portosystemic shunt, toxic insult, and diffuse infiltrative neoplasia such as lymphosarcoma. A unilateral or bilateral decrease in renal size, usually associated with an irregular contour, indicates longstanding inflammatory or degenerative renal disease ("end-stage kidneys"). Small kidneys also may be seen in some congenital diseases such as renal dysplasia (see earlier).

Changes in Diffuse Renal Echogenicity

A diffuse increase in renal cortical echogenicity is a common finding and may be associated with a benign or incidental process such as fat deposition. Renal diseases that may result in increased renal cortical echogenicity include inflammation, metabolic disorders, toxic renal disease, and infiltrative neoplasia. Chronic degenerative renal changes also may result in an increased cortical echogenicity, typically in association with decreased corticomedullary distinction and a decrease in renal size.

Focal Parenchymal Lesions

Both focal and multifocal lesions are identified and characterized more easily than diffuse alterations in echogenicity. Depending on their size and position, lesions may be embedded completely within renal parenchyma, may distort the renal contour, or may result in complete loss of the normal renal architecture. Renal cysts typically appear as well-circumscribed, round, anechoic structures with distal sound-beam attenuation. Complex cysts may contain echogenic contents and are indistinguishable from other fluid-filled renal masses such as abscesses, hematomas, and cavitary tumors. Chronic renal infarcts are sharply marginated, hyperechoic, triangular or linear cortical lesions in perpendicular orientation to the renal capsule. Infarcts are often associated with a divot in the renal surface. Primary or metastatic renal neoplasms manifest as masses of variable size, shape, and echogenicity (Figure 185-3). Different tumor types cannot be distinguished ultrasonographically; biopsy or fine-needle aspiration is needed for a definitive diagnosis. Other focal lesions such as abscesses or hematomas are rare, have a variable but usually cavitary appearance, and commonly are associated with additional intrarenal or perirenal abnormalities (e.g., retroperitoneal effusion).

Collecting System Abnormalities

Abnormal dilation of the renal pelvis may be encountered secondary to an obstruction (hydronephrosis) or a nonobstructive process (e.g., pyelonephritis). Especially in mild cases, the diagnosis is best established from transverse ultrasound images, on which the dilated pelvis appears as a fluid-filled V-shaped structure in the center of the kidney. With increasing severity (typically secondary to an obstructive lesion) the size of the pelvis increases, and over time the surrounding renal parenchyma is reduced to a thin rim of tissue (Figure 185-4). Pelvic mineralization and nephroliths appear as sharply marginated, strongly hyperechoic structures with distal shadowing.

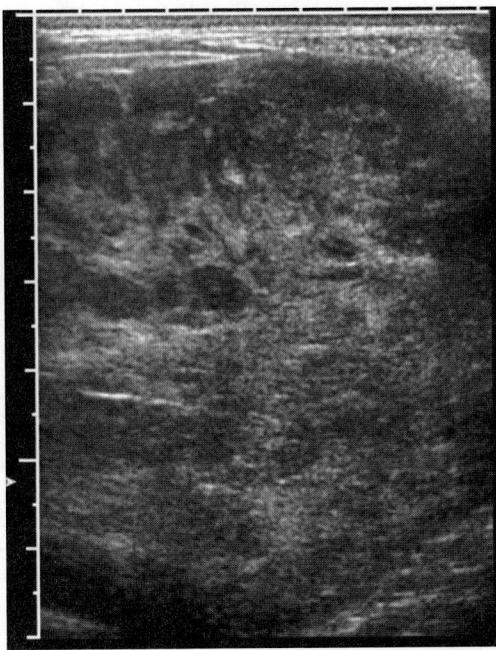

Figure 185-3 Large mixed-echogenic mass originating from the cranial pole of the right kidney in a 12-year-old bichon frise with complete disruption of normal renal architecture. Histologic diagnosis was renal carcinoma.

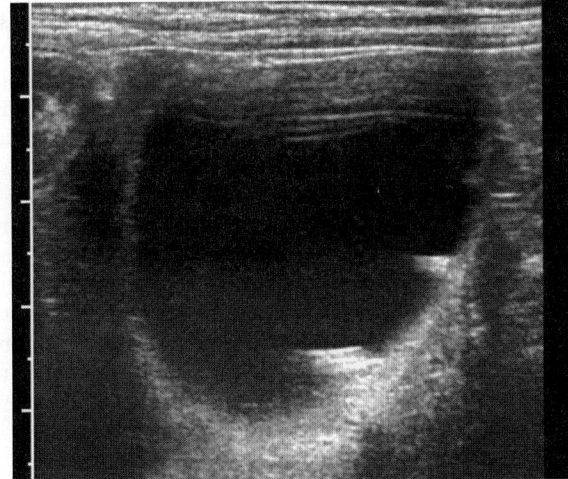

Figure 185-4 Severe hydronephrosis secondary to chronic ureteral obstruction in an 11-year-old Shih Tzu. The renal pelvis is severely distended with anechoic fluid, and the renal cortex is reduced to a very thin rim.

Other abnormalities of the renal collecting system (e.g., mass lesions) are rare.

Perinephric Abnormalities

Abnormalities occasionally encountered in the vicinity of the kidneys include encapsulated cystlike lesions in cases of perinephric pseudocysts or retroperitoneal effusion (e.g., transudate in acute inflammatory or toxic renal disease, or hemorrhage in renal neoplasia or trauma).

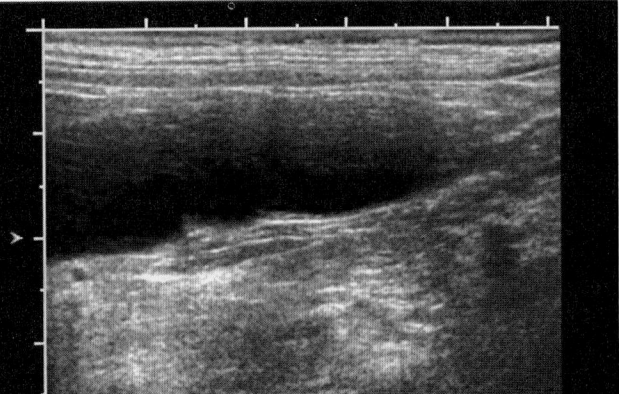

Figure 185-5 Severe hydroureter secondary to chronic obstruction in an 11-year-old Shih Tzu (same dog as in Figure 185-4). The ureter measures more than 1 cm wide on midsagittal image and could be traced from the hydronephrotic kidney to multiple calculi located within the distal ureter.

Ureteral Abnormalities

Acquired disorders of ureters can be subdivided into luminal and mural lesions. A dilation of the ureter (hydroureter) is observed in cases of obstructive uropathy, usually secondary to a bladder tumor or a ureterolith. The dilated ureter can be traced as a thin-walled anechoic tube of variable diameter from the level of the dilated renal pelvis to the obstructive lesion (Figure 185-5). Ureteroliths appear as intraluminal hyperechoic structures with distal shadowing that may be difficult to visualize unless they result in ureteral obstruction. Ureteral wall thickening and irregularity (e.g., secondary to ureteritis or ureteral neoplasia) are rare but readily identified during the ultrasonographic examination.

Urinary Bladder Abnormalities

Acquired disorders of the urinary bladder also can be subdivided into mural and intraluminal lesions. Generalized thickening and mucosal irregularity of the bladder wall are common indicators of cystitis (Figure 185-6). Focal bladder masses typically are indicative of neoplasia, although some inflammatory conditions (e.g., polypoid cystitis) can mimic neoplastic lesions. Transitional cell carcinoma is the most common bladder tumor and appears as irregular infiltrative masses of variable size (Figure 185-7). Although transitional cell carcinomas have a predilection for the trigone area, where they may result in ureteral or urethral obstruction, they can be found anywhere in the urinary bladder. Common intraluminal bladder abnormalities include echogenic urine (which indicates cellular contents; e.g., secondary to cystitis or hematuria), blood clots appearing as echogenic masslike lesions, and mineralized sediment or bladder calculi appearing as strongly hyperechoic structures with distal shadowing in the dependent portion of the urinary bladder (see Figure 185-6). It is important not to overinterpret small amounts of echogenic material in the urinary bladder.

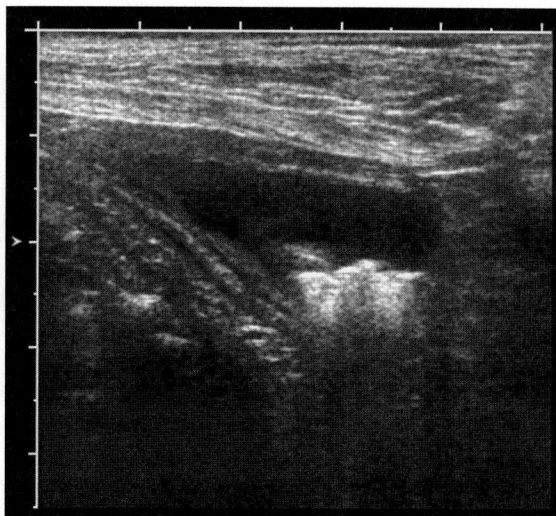

Figure 185-6 Cystitis and multiple bladder calculi in a dog. The urinary bladder wall shows moderate general thickening (5 mm), and multiple strongly hyperechoic structures with distal shadowing are noted in the dependent portion of the urinary bladder.

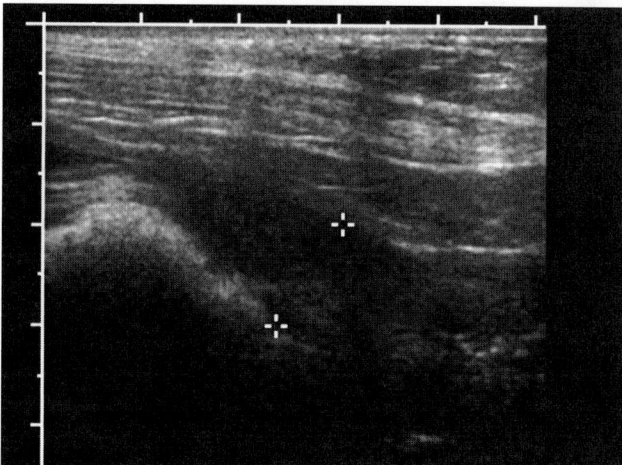

Figure 185-8 Urethral neoplasia in a 10-year-old female spayed border collie. The urethra *(between cursors)* is thickened, hypoechoic, and more conspicuous than in normal dogs. The diagnosis of transitional cell carcinoma was established by traumatic catheter aspiration/biopsy.

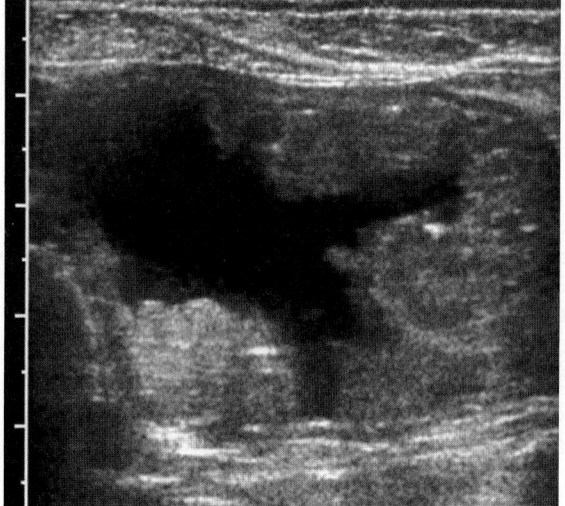

Figure 185-7 Bladder neoplasia (transitional cell carcinoma) in an 11-year-old beagle. Numerous irregularly marginated masses infiltrate the bladder wall.

Urethral Abnormalities

Acquired disorders of the urethra are similar to those described for the urinary bladder. Inflammatory or neoplastic disorders can result in thickening and mucosal irregularity of the urethral wall, which make the urethra more conspicuous (Figure 185-8). Urethral calculi appear as hyperechoic structures within the lumen and may or may not be associated with urethral obstruction. Urethral obstruction is characterized by distention of the bladder and urethra proximal to the inciting cause.

Ultrasound-Guided Procedures

A variety of ultrasound-guided procedures can aid in the diagnostic workup or treatment of urinary tract disorders.

Cystocentesis is a routine technique employed in small animal practice and in many cases does not require image guidance. However, in animals with a consistently small bladder, animals with pain, and obese animals, ultrasound allows controlled needle placement and increases safety. Ultrasound-guided sampling of contents within a dilated renal pelvis (pyelocentesis) commonly is performed in cases of suspected or therapy-resistant pyelonephritis. A modification of this technique (antegrade pyelography) can be used for the diagnosis and characterization of ureteral obstruction (see Chapter 195). A catheter is placed into the dilated renal pelvis under ultrasound guidance, positive contrast medium is injected, and flow of contrast medium is monitored by means of fluoroscopy or serial radiography. In cases of obstruction the renal pelvis and ureter proximal to the obstructive lesion will be dilated with contrast medium, whereas no contrast medium or only a small amount will be present in the ureter distal to the lesion.

Ultrasound-guided fine-needle aspiration or biopsy of renal parenchymal abnormalities is performed following established guidelines. Postprocedural hemorrhage is more common after renal biopsy than after biopsy of other organs, and the patient and the hematocrit should be closely monitored following the procedure so that appropriate treatment (transfusion) can be instituted if needed. Ultrasound-guided aspiration of bladder and urethral masses is considered contraindicated by some because of the risk of seeding of neoplastic cells along the needle tract. Alternatively, ultrasound can be used in these cases to monitor placement of a urinary catheter in the area of interest and to guide intraluminal traumatic catheterization (suction biopsy). In addition to assisting in these diagnostic procedures, ultrasound may be used in treatment in selected cases; for example, ultrasound may be used to guide drainage of cavitary lesions such as large renal cysts.

References and Suggested Reading

Adin CA et al: Antegrade pyelography for suspected ureteral obstruction in cats: 11 cases (1995-2001), *J Am Vet Med Assoc* 222(11):1576, 2003.

D'Anjou MA: Kidneys and ureters. In Penninck DG, d'Anjou MA, editors: *Atlas of small animal ultrasonography*, Ames, IA, 2008, Blackwell Publishing, p 339.

Hecht S: Nephropyelocentesis and antegrade pyelography. In Polzin DJ, Bartges J, editors: *Nephrology and urology of small animals*, Ames, IA, 2011, Wiley-Blackwell, p 43.

Hecht S, Henry GA: Ultrasound of the urinary tract. In Polzin DJ, Bartges J, editors: *Nephrology and urology of small animals*, Ames, IA, 2011, Wiley-Blackwell, p 128.

Kirberger RM, Stander N: Interventional procedures. In Gaschen L, Barr F, editors: *BSAVA manual of canine and feline ultrasonography*, Gloucester, UK, 2011, British Small Animal Veterinary Association, p 24.

Mareschal A et al: Ultrasonographic measurement of kidney-to-aorta ratio as a method of estimating renal size in dogs, *Vet Radiol Ultrasound* 48(5):434, 2007.

Nyland TG et al: Urinary tract. In Nyland TG, Mattoon JS, editors: *Small animal diagnostic ultrasound*, ed 2, Philadelphia, 2002, Saunders, p 158.

Stoneham AE et al: Retroperitoneal effusion in dogs and cats, *J Vet Emerg Crit Care* 14(S1):S1, 2004.

Sutherland-Smith J: Bladder and urethra. In Penninck DG, d'Anjou MA, editors: *Atlas of small animal ultrasonography*, Ames, IA, 2008, Blackwell Publishing, p 365.

Vaden SL et al: Renal biopsy: a retrospective study of methods and complications in 283 dogs and 65 cats, *J Vet Intern Med* 19(6):794, 2005.

CHAPTER 186

Recognition and Prevention of Hospital-Acquired Acute Kidney Injury

MARIE E. KERL, *Columbia, Missouri*
CATHY E. LANGSTON, *New York, New York*

There has been a shift in terminology in the human medical field within the last 10 years to establish a more concise and clinically relevant definition of acute renal failure (ARF). By the traditional definition, ARF is a rapid fall in glomerular filtration, which manifests clinically as an abrupt and sustained increase in the serum levels of urea and creatinine with an associated disruption of salt and water homeostasis. Since this definition cannot be quantified for clinical use, comparing incidence and outcome across clinical studies is challenging. To formulate guidelines to provide a more concise definition for ARF, physicians have proposed a definition of acute kidney injury (AKI) that includes reduction in kidney function within 48 hours defined by the occurrence of at least one of the following: (1) an absolute increase in serum creatinine concentration of at least 0.3 mg/dl (26.4 mmol/L), (2) an increase in serum creatinine concentration of more than 50% of baseline, or (3) oliguria of less than 0.5 ml/kg/hr for more than 6 hours.

Through the use of two similar classification schemes to stratify human patients with regard to severity of AKI—the Risk-Injury-Failure-Loss-End-stage disease (RIFLE) criteria and the Acute Kidney Injury Network (AKIN) criteria (Table 186-1)—multiple retrospective and prospective studies have proven a significant association between increasing severity of AKI and mortality, even with minimal increases in creatinine concentration that previously were not considered important.

In human medicine, AKI is recognized primarily as hospital acquired rather than community acquired. The term *hospital-acquired acute kidney injury* (HA-AKI) is used to identify this event. Veterinary patients have potential exposure to a wide variety of factors causing AKI, but people are less likely to be exposed to these factors in a community setting. In contrast, hospitalized people are more likely to be exposed to medications or diagnostic agents (e.g., radiocontrast agents) that predispose to AKI. Sepsis and the systemic inflammatory response also result

TABLE **186-1**

Comparison of Acute Kidney Injury Network (AKIN) and Risk-Injury-Failure-Loss-End stage disease (RIFLE) Criteria for Evaluating Hospital-Acquired Acute Kidney Injury

| | | CREATININE LEVEL | | | |
		Increase from Baseline	Absolute Increase	GFR Decrease	Urine Output
AKIN	Stage 1	≥150%-200%	≥0.3 mg/dl		<0.5 ml/kg/hr for ≥6 hr
	Stage 2	>200%-299%			<0.5 ml/kg/hr for ≥12 hr
	Stage 3	≥300%	≥4.0 mg/dl + acute increase of ≥0.5 mg/dl		<0.3 ml/kg/hr for ≥24 hr or anuria for ≥12 hr
RIFLE	Risk (R)	≥1.5-fold		≥25%	<0.5 ml/kg/hr for ≥6 hr
	Injury (I)	≥2.0-fold		≥50%	<0.5 ml/kg/hr for ≥12 hr
	Failure (F)	≥3.0-fold	≥4.0 mg/dl + acute increase of ≥0.5 mg/dl	≥75%	<0.3 ml/kg/hr for ≥24 hr or anuria for ≥12 hr

GFR, Glomerular filtration rate.

in multiorgan dysfunction in the severely ill. Aged adults often have reduced renal function compared with younger individuals.

Epidemiology and Etiology of Hospital-Acquired Acute Kidney Injury

Both AKI and HA-AKI have been investigated in the veterinary literature. In a retrospective review by Thoen and Kerl (2011) of data for 164 dogs admitted to the intensive care unit (ICU), 14.6% were noted to have developed AKI, as defined by an increase in creatinine concentration of at least 150% of baseline or an absolute increase of 0.3 mg/dl or more during the hospital stay. In another retrospective review (Harison et al, 2012), 15.2% to 19.3% of dogs for which at least two creatinine measurements were taken within a 2-, 3-, or 7-day period (n = 401, 477, and 646, respectively) developed AKI, as defined by an increase in serum creatinine concentration of 0.3 mg/dl or more. In both studies, only cases with serum creatinine levels of less than 1.6 mg/dl on the initial sample were included. There are no published prospective studies of the incidence of HA-AKI in dogs admitted to the ICU, but preliminary data suggest an incidence of around 10% to 17%. In cats, 20% to 21.3% of the at-risk population for which at least two creatinine measurements were taken within 2, 3, or 7 days (n = 128, 165, and 221, respectively) developed AKI, as defined by an increase in serum creatinine concentration of 0.3 mg/dl or more (Harison et al, 2012).

Commonly recognized risk factors for HA-AKI include preexisting renal disease, dehydration and volume depletion, decreased cardiac output, advanced age, fever, hypotension, hypertension, hypoalbuminemia, sepsis, electrolyte imbalances, acidosis, hyperviscosity syndromes, liver disease, administration of nephrotoxic drugs, administration of radiocontrast media, pancreatitis, diabetes mellitus, anesthesia, and surgery. Of 29 dogs that developed HA-AKI, most had been exposed to a nephrotoxicant (72%); were older than 7 years of age (69%); had chronic heart disease (41%), preexisting renal

disease (35%), a neoplastic condition (31%), or fever (28%); or had undergone anesthesia (14%) (Behrend et al, 1996). The nephrotoxicant drugs included aminoglycosides alone or in combination, cardiac drug combinations, cisplatin, and nonsteroidal antiinflammatory drugs. In contrast, almost 40% of 332 people who developed HA-AKI had experienced decreased renal perfusion (Nash et al, 2002). The causes of decreased renal perfusion included volume contraction, congestive heart failure, hypotension, cardiac arrest, inadequate blood pressure control, third-space losses, and arrhythmia. Other causes of HA-AKI were nephrotoxic medications, radiographic contrast media, postoperative status, and sepsis.

Biomarkers of Acute Kidney Injury

Early recognition of HA-AKI is clinically useful for case management decisions as well as for prognosis. Unfortunately, renal injury can occur before the development of azotemia and uremia. Current and future studies of serum and urine biomarkers may define the clinical utility of measuring substances that indicate early or ongoing damage to nephrons. Urine biomarkers are biochemical substances in the urine that provide an indication of glomerular or tubular cell dysfunction and death. For example, veterinarians can measure the level of albumin in the urine, and in the absence of inflammation elevations in albumin level compared with urine creatinine level indicate glomerular injury (see Chapter 188).

A number of urine protein and enzyme markers also can be used to identify and localize structural injury and dysfunction. An elevation of urine albumin level concurrently with an increase in the urine level of other high-molecular-weight proteins (HMWPs) such as immunoglobulin or transferrin confirm glomerular injury, and a high ratio of HMWPs to albumin in the sample can indicate more severe glomerular injury.

Low-molecular-weight proteins (LMWPs) are filtered freely by the glomerulus and under normal physiologic conditions should be reabsorbed completely by the proximal tubule; identification of LMWPs in the urine implies damage to the proximal tubular segments. One LMWP under investigation is urinary retinol-binding protein (URBP). In a recent study (Schaefer et al, 2011) dogs with naturally occurring systemic inflammatory response syndrome were found to have significantly increased urine protein:urine creatinine (UC) ratios, increased urine albumin to UC, and increased URBP to UC compared with healthy controls. The authors suggested that the presence of increased quantities of URBP could occur from direct tubular damage as an indication of AKI or from competition with other HMWPs for tubular binding sites. Further study is needed to determine the clinical significance of this urine biomarker.

In addition to measurement of proteins, renal injury can be detected by measurement of urine enzymes. The enzymes used commonly for this purpose are large (>80 kD) and therefore are expressed only in the urine from leakage of damaged tubular cells. Enzyme measurements often are more sensitive than protein measurements because (1) enzyme levels will become elevated in urine before the onset of overt dysfunction, (2) analysis of urine enzymes often is easier than analysis of proteins, and (3) the amount of enzyme leaked may be predictive of the degree and severity of ongoing injury. The most common enzymes studied in human patients are glutathione S-transferases and enzymes located within the proximal tubule and brush border. N-acetyl-β-D-glucosaminidase (NAG) and γ-glutamyl transpeptidase are renal proximal tubular cellular enzymes. These enzymes have been measured in urine of healthy dogs to determine reference ranges. Maddens and colleagues (2010) evaluated NAG as well as urine protein biomarkers in bitches with naturally occurring pyometra and found increases in the ratios of all urine biomarkers compared with UC at the time of surgical management for pyometra. At 6-month postsurgical follow-up, urine biomarker levels had decreased and were similar to urine biomarker quantities in age-matched control dogs. Evaluation of a panel of multiple proteins and enzymes most likely will provide greater diagnostic accuracy in identifying and localizing renal injury.

Outcome of Hospital-Acquired Acute Kidney Injury

The development of HA-AKI has a negative impact on outcome. Survival to hospital discharge was 38% for dogs with AKI in one study (Behrend et al, 1996). In another retrospective study, 46% of dogs with AKI survived to discharge, compared with 84% of dogs that did not develop AKI (Thoen and Kerl, 2011). Decrease in survival was significant with both mild and severe changes in creatinine concentration. In a third study (Harison et al, 2012), 30-day survival was 56% in dogs developing AKI within 2 days of hospitalization, compared with 75% in dogs not developing AKI; 90-day survival in these dogs was 43%, compared with 71% in those dogs not developing AKI. In this study, mild changes in measured creatinine concentration (serum creatinine level of <1.6 mg/dl despite a rise of ≥0.3 mg/dl) did not have a significant impact on survival at 30 days, but there was a significant impact on 90-day survival. In the same study, the 30-day

survival rate for cats with developing AKI within 2 days of hospitalization was 48%, compared with 85% survival in those not developing AKI. The survival difference was not significant for cats developing mild AKI, but it was significant for cats developing more severe AKI (serum creatinine level of >1.6 mg/dl and a rise of ≥0.3 mg/dl).

People with HA-AKI have a longer duration of hospitalization. There is no information on the impact of HA-AKI on duration of hospitalization in dogs or cats. Approximately half of dogs and cats who survive an episode of AKI develop chronic kidney disease as defined by a persistently elevated serum creatinine concentration.

Prevention of Hospital-Acquired Acute Kidney Injury

One of the main goals of fluid therapy in critically ill patients is to maintain adequate perfusion of all organ systems, and indeed, careful fluid therapy is the mainstay of preventing and treating AKI. Prerenal and ischemic acute tubular necrosis account for 30% to 75% of AKI in people.

Early goal-directed therapy (EGDT) for fluid resuscitation in septic shock decreases the incidence of AKI in people. With EGDT, the physiologic targets to achieve within 6 hours of diagnosis are mean arterial pressure of 65 mm Hg or more, central venous pressure between 8 and 12 mm Hg, improvement of blood lactate levels, central venous oxygen saturation of more than 70%, and urine output of 0.5 ml/kg/hr or more.

The optimal type of fluid to administer still is under debate. Information exists linking the use of hetastarch to AKI in humans with sepsis, but the situation is not clear in people with other disease processes. The effect of cumulative colloid dose, use of hyperoncotic versus isooncotic solutions, and molecular weight differences remains to be determined. There are no reports on the effect of hydroxyethyl starch (of any molecular weight) on the risk of HA-AKI in dogs or cats.

The evidence on early aggressive crystalloid resuscitation clearly indicates improvement in mortality and renal function in people with sepsis. Continuation of fluid therapy after the initial resuscitation period, especially to the point of overhydration, may be detrimental to renal function and outcome. Septic people with AKI had more fluid accumulation than those that did not develop AKI. Fluid accumulation is a predictor of mortality in patients with AKI. The risk of death is two to three times higher in patients with more than 10% weight gain. A study by Lin and colleagues (2006) found that, although more fluid was administered during the initial 6 hours in the group receiving EGDT than in the group receiving standard care, the total volume of fluid administered over 72 hours was the same in both groups despite a decrease in AKI in the EGDT group. In another study comparing a conservative fluid plan with a liberal fluid plan (which matched standard care), the group treated using the conservative fluid strategy had a cumulative balance of −136 ± 491 ml over 7 days, compared with 6992 ± 502 ml in the patients treated using the liberal fluid strategy (Widemann et al, 2006). There was no difference between groups in the development of AKI. Although no difference was seen in 60-day mortality in the two groups, the patients treated using the conservative fluid plan spent less time receiving mechanical ventilation and ICU care. In veterinary patients, for which assisted ventilation is costly and limited in availability, fluid overload can be life threatening and is considered an end point as clients decide whether to continue treatment. As noted by Prowle and colleagues (2010), no studies have demonstrated a worsening of renal function when restrictive fluid strategies are used.

Although the evidence is mounting that a positive fluid balance is associated with worse outcomes, a positive fluid balance also may be a marker of disease severity. Ill patients with poor or deteriorating renal function have limited ability to excrete sodium and water. Therefore these patients may have more capillary leakage and greater edema formation and may not be able to handle renal replacement therapy as well as less severely affected patients. Alternatively, fluid accumulation itself may impair renal function. Intraabdominal hypertension, caused by an increase in abdominal visceral edema, increases the risk of AKI. Positive fluid balance also may contribute to renal swelling and impair renal blood flow. Appropriate fluid therapy for established AKI, as well as other strategies for management, are detailed in Chapter 191.

Beyond timely and precise fluid management, other interventions for preventing AKI remain unproven. Initial reports suggested that tight glycemic control (avoidance of large glucose loads) could play a role in preventing AKI, but subsequent studies failed to find a protective effect and noted a higher incidence of hypoglycemic episodes.

Avoidance of nephrotoxic drugs, sustained hypotension, and other renal insults is prudent in patients at high risk.

References and Suggested Reading

Behrend E et al: Hospital-acquired acute renal failure in dogs: 29 cases (1983-1992), *J Am Vet Med Assoc* 208:537, 1996.

Brunker JD, Ponzio NM, Payton ME: Indices of urine N-acetyl-β-D-glucosaminidase and γ-glutamyl transpeptidase activities in clinically normal adult dogs, *Am J Vet Res* 70:297, 2009.

Dart AB et al: Hydroxyethyl starch (HES) versus other fluid therapies: effects on kidney function, *Cochrane Database Syst Rev* 1:CD007594, 2011.

Harison E et al: Acute kidney injury (AKI) as a predictor of mortality in dogs and cats, *J Vet Intern Med* 26:1093, 2012.

Lin SM et al: A modified goal-directed protocol improves clinical outcomes in intensive care unit patients with septic shock: a randomized controlled trial, *Shock* 26:551, 2006.

Maddens B et al: *Escherichia coli* pyometra induces transient glomerular and tubular dysfunction in dogs, *J Vet Intern Med* 24:1263, 2010.

Nash K, Hafeez A, Hou S: Hospital-acquired renal insufficiency, *Am J Kidney Dis* 39:930, 2002.

Nolan CR, Anderson RJ: Hospital-acquired acute renal failure, *J Am Soc Nephrol* 9:710, 1998.

Prowle JR et al: Fluid balance and acute kidney injury, *Nat Rev Nephrol* 6:107, 2010.

Schaefer H et al: Quantitative and qualitative urine protein excretion in dogs with severe inflammatory response syndrome, *J Vet Intern Med* 25:1292, 2011.

Thoen ME, Kerl ME: Characterization of acute kidney injury in hospitalized dogs and evaluation of a veterinary acute kidney injury staging system, *J Vet Emerg Crit Care* 21(6):648, 2011.

Wiedemann HP et al: Comparison of two fluid-management strategies in acute lung injury, *N Engl J Med* 354:2564, 2006.

CHAPTER 187

Proteinuria/Albuminuria: Implications for Management

GREGORY F. GRAUER, *Manhattan, Kansas*

*P*roteinuria is a general term that is used to describe the presence of excessive amounts of any type of protein in the urine. In most dogs and cats, in both health and disease, albumin is the primary urine protein. Proteinuria/albuminuria can arise from numerous causes (e.g., physiologic or benign; prerenal, renal, or postrenal). Therefore, when proteinuria is detected, localization of its source is a primary diagnostic objective. When renal proteinuria/albuminuria is suspected, the next diagnostic objectives are longitudinal monitoring and documentation of persistence followed by quantitation of the magnitude of proteinuria/albuminuria.

Proteinuria/albuminuria long has been established as a marker of kidney disease in dogs, but not long ago it was viewed to be primarily a marker of canine glomerular disease and likely not significant unless the urine protein/creatinine ratio was higher than 3.0 or it was associated with hypoalbuminemia. Today we recognize that proteinuria/albuminuria often is associated with chronic kidney disease (CKD) in both dogs and cats and that it can arise from both glomerular and tubular lesions. We also have recognized that even low-level proteinuria/albuminuria is a risk factor for CKD progression in both dogs and cats. For these reasons, detection, monitoring, and treatment of dogs and cats with renal proteinuria/albuminuria have received renewed interest.

Detection of Proteinuria

The dipstick colorimetric test is the most common screening test for proteinuria. This test is inexpensive, easy to use, and primarily measures albumin. However, sensitivity and specificity for albuminuria are relatively low with this method. False-negative results (decreased sensitivity) may occur with Bence Jones proteinuria, low urine concentrations of albumin, or dilute or acidic urine. The lower limit of detection for the conventional dipstick test is approximately 30 mg/dl. False-positive results also are common in both cats and dogs with dipstick testing but occur more frequently in cats. For example, when 599 canine and 347 feline urine samples were analyzed by both a conventional urine protein test strip method (Multistix Reagent Strips or Roche Chemstrip 9) and a canine or feline albumin-specific quantitative enzyme-linked immunosorbent assay (ELISA) (see later) there were disparate results. The sensitivity of conventional urine protein dipsticks for albuminuria in canine and feline urine (a trace positive reaction or greater) was 81% and

90%, respectively, but the specificity was only 48% and 11%, respectively (Lyon et al, 2010).

The sulfosalicylic acid (SSA) precipitation test is performed by mixing equal quantities of urine supernatant and 3% to 5% SSA in a glass test tube and grading the turbidity resulting from precipitation of protein on a 0 to 4+ scale. In addition to albumin, the SSA test can detect globulins and Bence Jones proteins to a greater extent than the dipstick test. False-positive results may occur if the urine contains radiographic contrast agents, penicillin, cephalosporins, sulfisoxazole, or thymol (a urine preservative), and for unknown reasons. The protein content also may be overestimated with the SSA test if uncentrifuged, turbid urine is analyzed. The reported sensitivity of the SSA test is approximately 5 mg/dl. Because of the relatively poor specificity of conventional dipstick analysis, many reference laboratories confirm a positive dipstick test result for proteinuria using the SSA test. The sensitivity of the SSA test for albuminuria in canine and feline urine (a trace positive reaction or greater) was found to be 73% and 58%, respectively, but the specificity was only 64% and 25%, respectively (Lyon et al, 2010).

Based on the study of canine urine mentioned earlier, if the urine dipstick or SSA result is 2+ or higher there is a high probability that the sample is positive for albumin. However, if the dipstick result is trace or 1+ positive, a turbidimetric SSA analysis should be performed to confirm the diagnosis of proteinuria. When both tests are performed simultaneously they should be interpreted in series to increase specificity (results of both tests should be positive for the sample to be considered positive for albuminuria), rather than in parallel fashion. If dipstick and SSA results both fall into the trace to 1+ range, positive results for albuminuria should be confirmed with a more specific assay such as the ELISA-based test.

For feline urine samples, both routine screening tests (dipstick and SSA) performed poorly and appear to be of minimal diagnostic value because of an unacceptably high number of false-positive results. For both dipstick and SSA tests, the positive and negative likelihood ratios were close to 1 and the positive and negative predictive values were close to 50%, which indicates that neither test provided useful information regarding albuminuria. Based on these data, urine albumin detection in the feline patient always should be performed with a higher-quality assay such as the species-specific ELISA. In cats with chronic kidney disease, the accuracy of the dipstick and SSA tests improves in comparison with the feline-specific albuminuria assay (Hanzlicek et al, 2012), presumably due to a higher magnitude or a higher percentage of albumin in the urine.

Proteinuria detected by these semiquantitative screening methods historically has been interpreted in light of the urine specific gravity and urine sediment. For example, a positive dipstick reading of trace or 1+ proteinuria in hypersthenuric urine often has been attributed to urine concentration rather than abnormal proteinuria. In addition, a positive dipstick reading for protein in the presence of hematuria or pyuria often has been attributed to urinary tract hemorrhage or inflammation. Although both variables must be taken into consideration, the conventional interpretation may not be correct. Given the limits of sensitivity of the conventional dipstick test, any positive result for protein, regardless of urine concentration, may indicate an abnormality (except in the case of false-positive results). Likewise, hematuria and pyuria have an inconsistent effect on urine protein/albumin concentrations; not all dogs with hematuria and pyuria have albuminuria. In patients with gross hematuria or microscopic pyuria, the source of the hemorrhage or inflammation should be diagnosed and treated before further assessment of the proteinuria/albuminuria.

Detection of Albuminuria

Albuminuria can be measured by point-of-care semiquantitative tests (e.g., the Heska E.R.D.-HealthScreen urine test) and quantitative immunoassays at reference laboratories. These tests are both sensitive and specific for canine and feline albumin. *Microalbuminuria* is defined as concentrations of albumin in the urine that are higher than normal (>1.0 mg/dl) but below the limit of detection using conventional urine dipstick tests (<30 mg/dl). Urine albumin concentrations can be adjusted for differences in urine concentration by dividing by urine creatinine concentrations. Alternatively, and more commonly, urine can be diluted to a standard specific gravity (1.010) before assay.

The use of microalbuminuria tests is indicated in the following circumstances:

1. When conventional screening tests for proteinuria produce equivocal or conflicting results or false-positive results are suspected.
2. When conventional screening tests for proteinuria give negative results in apparently healthy older dogs and cats and a more sensitive screening test is desired.
3. When conventional screening tests for proteinuria give negative results in apparently healthy young dogs and cats with a familial risk for developing proteinuric renal disease and a more sensitive screening test is desired.
4. When conventional screening tests for proteinuria give negative results in dogs and cats with chronic illnesses that are associated with proteinuric renal disease and a more sensitive screening test is desired.
5. Follow-up after a positive result on a previous microalbuminuria test to document persistence of the albuminuria.

Proper interpretation and follow-up of microalbuminuria testing is critical. Like other tests for proteinuria, microalbuminuria tests can be affected by lower urinary tract inflammation, and therefore assessment of patient history and urine sediment changes is important. A negative microalbuminuria result is a useful finding because it obviates any concern about albuminuria until the next testing interval. A positive test result is more complex to interpret and needs to be confirmed with follow-up testing approximately 7 to 10 days later. If the result of the second test is negative, the initial positive test result likely was caused by transient benign or physiologic albuminuria that is unlikely to have any long-term consequence for the patient. If results of follow-up tests continue to be positive, more frequent monitoring and further investigation is indicated. Monitoring can verify persistence as well as changes in the magnitude of the albuminuria. In the absence of postrenal inflammation and hemorrhage (see next section), increases in the magnitude of microalbuminuria likely are indicative of active, ongoing renal injury and should prompt further investigation to detect any infectious, inflammatory, or neoplastic disease that might be the underlying cause of the animal's renal disease.

Localization of the Source of the Proteinuria

When proteinuria is detected by screening tests, it is important to identify the source of the excess urine protein. Proteinuria may be caused by physiologic or pathologic conditions. Physiologic or benign proteinuria is often transient and abates when the underlying cause is corrected. Strenuous exercise, seizures, fever, exposure to extreme heat or cold, and stress are examples of conditions that may cause physiologic proteinuria. Decreased physical activity also may affect urine protein excretion in dogs; one study showed that urinary protein loss was higher in dogs confined to cages than in dogs with normal activity levels (McCaw et al, 1985).

Pathologic proteinuria may be caused by urinary or nonurinary abnormalities. Nonurinary disorders associated with proteinuria often involve the production of low-molecular-weight proteins (dysproteinemias) that are filtered by the glomeruli and subsequently overwhelm the reabsorptive capacity of the proximal tubule. An example of this "prerenal" proteinuria is the production of immunoglobulin light chains (Bence Jones proteins). Genital tract inflammation (e.g., prostatitis or metritis) also can result in pathologic nonurinary proteinuria. Obtaining urine samples via cystocentesis reduces the potential for urine contamination with protein from the lower urinary tract, although inflammatory exudate from the prostate may reflux into the bladder and cystocentesis is contraindicated in cases of suspected pyometra.

Pathologic urinary proteinuria may be renal or nonrenal in origin. Nonrenal proteinuria most frequently occurs in association with lower urinary tract inflammation or hemorrhage (also referred to as *postrenal proteinuria*). Changes observed in the urine sediment usually are compatible with the underlying inflammation (e.g., pyuria, hematuria, bacteriuria, and increased numbers of transitional epithelial cells). On the other hand, renal proteinuria is frequently caused by increased glomerular filtration of plasma proteins associated with intraglomerular hypertension, structural abnormalities of the glomerular capillary wall, or the presence of immune complexes or vascular inflammation in the glomerular capillaries. Renal proteinuria also may be caused by decreased reabsorption of filtered plasma proteins due to tubulointerstitial disease. Glomerular lesions usually result in proteinuria of higher magnitude than the proteinuria associated with tubulointerstitial lesions. Renal proteinuria may also be caused by inflammatory or infiltrative disorders of the kidney (e.g., neoplasia, pyelonephritis, and leptospirosis), which often are accompanied by an active urine sediment.

Monitoring of Renal Proteinuria/Albuminuria

Transient proteinuria/albuminuria is likely of little consequence and does not warrant treatment. On the other hand, persistent proteinuria/albuminuria for which prerenal and postrenal causes have been ruled out indicates the presence of renal disease. Persistent proteinuria/albuminuria can be defined as positive test results on three or more occasions on samples obtained two or more weeks apart. Because persistent proteinuria/albuminuria can be constant or increase or decrease in magnitude over time, monitoring should use quantitative methods to determine disease trends or response to treatment. Changes in the magnitude of proteinuria always should be interpreted in light of the patient's serum creatinine concentration since proteinuria may decrease in progressive renal disease as the number of functional nephrons decreases. Decreasing proteinuria in the face of a stable serum creatinine concentration suggests improving renal function, whereas decreasing proteinuria in the face of an increasing serum creatinine level suggests disease progression.

Quantitation of Proteinuria/Albuminuria

If the results of the screening tests show persistent proteinuria/albuminuria of suspected renal origin, urine protein excretion should be quantified. This helps to evaluate the severity of renal lesions and to assess the response to treatment or the progression of disease. Methods used to quantitate proteinuria include the urine protein/creatinine ratio (UP/C) and immunoassays for albuminuria that are expressed as either urine albumin/creatinine ratios or in milligrams per deciliter in urine samples that have been diluted to a standard urine specific gravity. Albumin levels of 30 mg/dl or more in urine diluted to a urine specific gravity of 1.010 usually result in UP/C ratios of 0.4 and 0.5 or more in cats and dogs, respectively. Most studies have shown that normal urine protein excretion in dogs and cats is 10 mg/kg or less per 24 hours and that normal UP/C ratios are 0.2 or less. UP/C values between 0.2 and 0.5 in dogs and between 0.2 and 0.4 in cats are considered borderline. Persistent proteinuria that results in a UP/C ratio of more than 0.4 and 0.5 in cats and dogs, respectively, for which prerenal and postrenal proteinuria

have been ruled out, is consistent with either glomerular or tubulointerstitial CKD. UP/C ratios above 2.0 are strongly suggestive of glomerular disease. It is possible that the definition of a normal UP/C ratio will continue to change with additional research. It is interesting to note that, although the UP/C ratio was a specific test for canine and feline albuminuria when compared with the species-specific quantitative albuminuria immunoassay, the cutoff value of 0.2 for UP/C ratio resulted in an unacceptable number of false-negative results. Therefore determination of the UP/C ratio is not recommended as a routine screening test for urine albumin level in dogs or cats, especially for low levels of albuminuria.

Based on longitudinal testing results in dogs with X-linked hereditary nephropathy, the UP/C ratio must change by at least 35% at high UP/C values (near 12) and by 80% at low UP/C values (near 0.5) for the difference between serial values to be significant. A single measurement was found to estimate the UP/C ratio reliably when the values were less than 4, but two or more determinations were necessary to estimate the UP/C ratio reliably when values were higher than 4. Studies have shown that making one UP/C determination after equal pooling of three urine samples produces results as valid as those derived by averaging the values from three samples (±20%) (LeVine et al, 2010).

Treatment of Renal Proteinuria

Once persistent renal proteinuria/albuminuria has been documented by monitoring, the appropriate treatment depends on the magnitude of the proteinuria and the health status of the patient (e.g., the presence or absence of azotemia or hypertension). In nonazotemic, persistently proteinuric patients, further investigation and appropriate treatment of potential concurrent infectious, inflammatory disorders, or neoplastic diseases is warranted. Neoplasia, infection, polyarthritis, hepatitis, hyperadrenocorticism, immune-mediated hemolytic anemia, and systemic hypertension are common concurrent medical problems in dogs with renal proteinuria/albuminuria. In cats, viral diseases, neoplasia, immune-mediated disease, polyarthritis, and systemic hypertension are some of the more common conditions associated with renal proteinuria/albuminuria. Unfortunately, in many cases an underlying disease is not identified or may be impossible to eliminate (e.g., neoplasia).

In cases of persistent proteinuria/albuminuria in which an underlying disorder cannot be identified or treated, the need for treatment depends on the magnitude of proteinuria. Proteinuria resulting in UP/C ratios of more than 1.0 to 2.0 in nonazotemic dogs and cats should be treated, whereas continued monitoring and patient investigation should be the primary focus in cases with proteinuria of lesser magnitude. In azotemic dogs and cats, treatment of proteinuria is generally recommended when the UP/C ratio is 0.5 and 0.4 or higher, respectively. Treatment recommendations usually include reduction of dietary protein (early renal disease diets), omega-3 fatty acid supplementation (found in most early renal disease diets), angiotensin-converting enzyme inhibitors (e.g., enalapril or benazepril 0.5 to 1.0 mg/kg q24h PO), and for higher-magnitude proteinuria low-dose aspirin for dogs (0.5 to 1.0 mg/kg q24h PO). Note, however, that it is difficult to separate the effects of individual treatments when they are used in combination.

Supportive Care

In addition to the treatments described earlier, supportive therapy is important in the management of proteinuric renal disease and should be aimed at decreasing hypertension, edema, and the tendency for thromboembolism to occur. Reduction of systemic hypertension may reduce intraglomerular hypertension, especially in dogs and cats with renal disease that has resulted in loss of renal blood flow autoregulation. Low-dose aspirin is administered easily on an outpatient basis and does not require extensive monitoring. Since fibrin accumulation within the glomerulus is a frequent consequence of proteinuric renal disease, low-dose aspirin treatment may serve a dual purpose. Finally, renal disease diets also should be recommended in an attempt to decrease glomerular hyperfiltration and proteinuria/albuminuria. See Chapters 188 and 189 for more information about management of significant glomerular disease and chronic kidney disease.

References and Suggested Reading

Burkholder WJ et al: Diet modulates proteinuria in heterozygous female dogs with x-linked hereditary nephropathy, *J Vet Intern Med* 18:165, 2004.

Cook AK, Cowgill LD: Clinical and pathological features of protein-losing glomerular disease in the dog: a review of 137 cases (1985-1992), *J Am Anim Hosp Assoc* 32:313, 1996.

Grauer GF et al: Effects of enalapril vs placebo as a treatment for canine idiopathic glomerulonephritis, *J Vet Intern Med* 14:526, 2000.

Grodecki KM et al: Treatment of X-linked hereditary nephritis in Samoyed dogs with angiotensin converting enzyme (ACE) inhibitor, *J Comp Pathol* 117:209, 1997.

Hanzlicek AS et al: Comparison of urine dipstick, sulfosalicylic acid, urine protein-to-creatinine ratio, and a feline-specific immunoassay for detection of albuminuria in cats with chronic kidney disease, *J Fel Med Surg* 14:882, 2012.

Jacob F et al: Evaluation of the association between initial proteinuria and morbidity or death in dogs with naturally occurring chronic renal failure, *J Am Vet Med Assoc* 226:393, 2005.

Lees GE et al: Assessment and management of proteinuria in dogs and cats; 2004 ACVIM Forum Consensus Statement (Small Animal), *J Vet Intern Med* 19:377, 2005.

LeVine DN et al: The use of pooled vs. serial urine samples to measure urine protein:creatinine ratios, *Vet Clin Pathol* 39:53, 2010.

Lyon SD et al: Comparison of dipstick, sulfosalicylic acid, urine protein creatinine ratio, and species-specific ELISA methodologies for detection of albumin in canine and feline urine samples, *J Am Vet Med Assoc* 236:874, 2010.

McCaw DL et al: Effect of collection time and exercise restriction on the prediction of urine protein excretion, using urine protein/creatinine ratio in dogs, *Am J Vet Res* 46:1665, 1985.

Nabity MB et al: Day-to-day variation of the urine protein:creatinine ratio in female dogs with stable glomerular proteinuria caused by X-linked hereditary nephropathy, *J Vet Intern Med* 21:425, 2007.

Syme HM et al: Survival of cats with naturally occurring chronic renal failure is related to severity of proteinuria, *J Vet Intern Med* 20:528, 2006.

CHAPTER 188

Glomerular Disease and Nephrotic Syndrome

SHELLY L. VADEN, *Raleigh, North Carolina*
BARRAK M. PRESSLER, *Columbus, Ohio*

The prevalence of glomerular disease in dogs with renal disease is unclear but is likely between 43% and 90%. Treatment of dogs and cats with glomerular disease is nonspecific; however, the standard of care for affected people often includes immunosuppressive drugs or inflammatory modulators based on disease histologic subtype. As the evaluation of renal biopsy specimens from dogs and cats increases, disease-specific protocols hopefully will be developed for the treatment of animals with glomerular disease. The purpose of this chapter is to review briefly the diagnosis and initial evaluation of dogs and cats with protein-losing nephropathies and to present a more detailed review of recommended specific and nonspecific management of glomerular diseases and nephrotic syndrome.

Diagnosis of Glomerular Disease

Clinical signs and physical examination findings in dogs and cats with glomerular disease are associated with the severity of the proteinuria, the stage of kidney disease, and perhaps the histologic subtype of glomerular disease. Most animals are asymptomatic or variably uremic at the time of initial diagnosis. Less common clinical signs include dyspnea, ascites, subcutaneous edema, and hyphema, which may develop secondary to extravascular fluid accumulation, thromboembolic disease, and hypertension.

Glomerular diseases frequently are associated with a specific set of clinicopathologic findings. Proteinuria (i.e., a urine protein/creatinine [UP/C] ratio >0.5) is the hallmark of glomerular injury. Certain glomerular disease histologic subtypes are associated with greater amounts of urine protein loss and higher UP/C ratios in people, but similar associations in dogs or cats with glomerular disease have been demonstrated inconsistently (Cook and Cowgill, 1996; Klosterman et al, 2011). Human patients with UP/C values of more than 2.0 to 3.5 or more than 300 to 350 mg/mmol are referred to as having *nephrotic-range proteinuria*. However, ranges of UP/C values noted in dogs with glomerular disease with and without nephrotic syndrome overlap so that identification of a similar clinically useful value has not been possible (Klosterman et al, 2011). If injury to renal tubules develops at a slower rate than does the glomerular injury, some renal concentrating ability may persist despite development of

azotemia. In a subset of dogs and cats with glomerular disease, hypoalbuminemia and proteinuria are accompanied by hypercholesterolemia and extravascular fluid accumulation, referred to as *nephrotic syndrome*.

Many cases of glomerular disease in dogs and cats are believed to be consequences of systemic inflammation. Animals with persistent glomerular proteinuria therefore should be evaluated thoroughly for concurrent neoplastic, infectious, or noninfectious inflammatory (NIN) disorders. Thorough physical examination should include careful evaluation of the oral cavity and skin as well as thoracic auscultation and abdominal palpation because commonly encountered conditions, including periodontal disease and atopy, should not be overlooked. Serologic testing for regional infectious diseases and antinuclear antibodies should be considered in patients when appropriate. Radiographic or ultrasonographic evaluation of the abdomen should include thorough assessment of all organs in addition to examination of the kidneys in order to detect concurrent disease processes, and thoracic radiography should be performed to evaluate for evidence of neoplastic disease.

Renal biopsy is required to determine the specific histologic subtype of glomerular disease. However, this test may not be indicated in every patient, and more study is needed to determine which patients may benefit from renal biopsy evaluation. Animals with International Renal Interest Society (IRIS) stage 1 or 2 (and possibly stage 3) chronic kidney disease that have UP/C values in or nearing the nephrotic range suggested in people likely will benefit most (see Chapter 189). Once collected, renal biopsy specimens should be divided appropriately and placed in fixatives suitable for evaluation with light, electron, and immunofluorescent microscopy. Although the findings of light microscopy may be highly suggestive of a particular glomerular disease, electron microscopy often is required for definitive characterization of histologic subtype, and immunofluorescent microscopy is needed to determine the specific nature of immune deposits.

Nonspecific Management of Glomerular Disease

Certain therapies are indicated in all dogs and cats with glomerular disease, regardless of the histologic diagnosis.

These nonspecific management recommendations can be divided into three major categories: (1) monitoring for and treatment of underlying NIN disorders, (2) reduction of proteinuria, and (3) management of uremia and other complications of renal failure.

Monitoring for and Treatment of Neoplastic, Infectious, or Noninfectious Inflammatory Disorders

NIN disorders responsible for glomerular disease may not be detected at first presentation. Because occult diseases may become overt months after initial diagnostic testing, continued observation and evaluation of any newly developed clinical signs or abnormal findings on physical examination are necessary. Identification and treatment of any underlying NIN disorder is perhaps the most important step in the management of dogs and cats with persistent proteinuria. Following treatment, animals should be evaluated for resolution of proteinuria, which may occur slowly over a period of months.

Reduction of Proteinuria

Intraglomerular hydrostatic pressure is a primary determinant of net protein movement across the glomerular filtration barrier. Angiotensin-converting enzyme (ACE) inhibitors, angiotensin II type 1 receptor blockers (ARBs), and aldosterone receptor antagonists inhibit the renin-angiotensin-aldosterone system (RAAS) and reduce glomerular capillary bed hydrostatic pressure, thus reducing proteinuria (Figure 188-1). Although the precise mechanisms by which these agents exert their beneficial effects have not been fully elucidated, it appears that reduction in proteinuria is greater than would be expected from their antihypertensive effects alone.

ACE inhibitors preferentially decrease efferent glomerular arteriolar resistance, which leads to decreased or normalized glomerular transcapillary hydrostatic pressure and also may preserve renal function by additional, less well-described mechanisms. Treatment of dogs with glomerular diseases with enalapril significantly reduces proteinuria and delays onset or progression of azotemia and

therefore is considered a standard of care (Grauer et al, 2000). ACE inhibitors are administered once or twice daily; if the magnitude of azotemia is relatively stable and there has been only partial or no reduction in proteinuria after 4 to 8 weeks, the dosage may be increased to the upper end of the recommended ranges (e.g., enalapril or benazepril 2 mg/kg PO per day). Although serum creatinine concentration should be monitored after therapy is begun, it is uncommon for dogs and cats to become azotemic or to experience severe worsening of preexisting azotemia (i.e., >30% increase from baseline) as a result of ACE inhibitor administration alone. Although differences exist in the elimination pharmacokinetics of enalapril and benazepril, there is no evidence that one ACE inhibitor is pharmacokinetically superior to others in either dogs or cats. In people, up-titration of doses of ACE inhibitors beyond current recommendations maximizes reduction of proteinuria and recently has been suggested to improve prognosis (Schjoedt et al, 2009); similar studies have not been performed yet in dogs or cats.

Although ARBs are used commonly in people with glomerular disease, their use in dogs still is being developed. Losartan is the most commonly used ARB. Even though dogs do not produce one of the major active metabolites, losartan does have anti-RAAS pharmacodynamic effects and anecdotally has an antiproteinuric effect in dogs with glomerular disease. In theory there may be an added benefit to combined therapy with an ACE inhibitor and an ARB because monotherapy with either drug class likely does not provide complete RAAS blockade. Studies in people have suggested that these drugs may have additive or synergistic effects in reducing proteinuria, although there have not been any equivalent studies in dogs (Linas, 2008). In addition, because the dose of each individual drug can be reduced during combined therapy, adverse effects in people may be reduced; however, elderly patients prescribed this combination have a higher risk of kidney failure and death.

Serum aldosterone concentrations increase over time (known as *aldosterone escape*) in people treated with maximal dosages of ACE inhibitors or ARBs, which may have adverse effects on the heart, systemic blood vessels, and glomeruli (Bakris, 2008). Aldosterone receptor antagonists reduce proteinuria and stabilize kidney function, acting in an additive fashion with ACE inhibitors and ARBs in people. Spironolactone (1.0 to 2.0 mg/kg q12h PO) is used most commonly in veterinary medicine; however, there are no published data examining its usefulness in the treatment of dogs or cats with glomerular disease. This drug likely would be most effective in animals with high serum aldosterone concentrations and persistent proteinuria despite treatment with an ACE inhibitor, ARB, or both. Anecdotal experience suggests that spironolactone is not very effective in reducing proteinuria in dogs with glomerular disease.

Hyperkalemia is a common adverse effect of RAAS inhibition in dogs with kidney disease. Thrombocytosis also is common in dogs with glomerular disease, and therefore pseudohyperkalemia should be excluded as a cause of increased serum potassium concentration before therapy is modified. True hyperkalemia can be managed by reducing the dosage of ACE inhibitor, ARB,

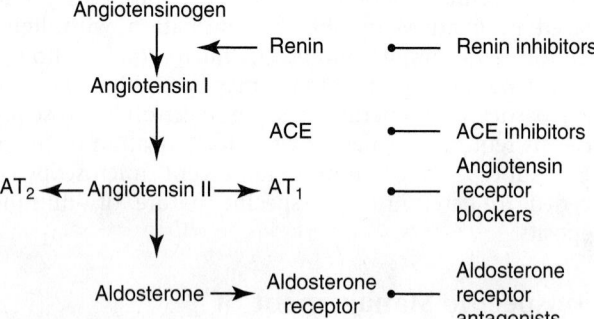

Figure 188-1 Renin-angiotensin-aldosterone system and the sites of action of inhibitors used to reduce the severity of proteinuria in human and veterinary medicine.

or spironolactone; feeding a reduced-potassium diet; or administering a gastrointestinal potassium binder (e.g., Kayexalate).

Treatment with antihypertensives often leads to a reduction in the magnitude of proteinuria in patients with high blood pressure. ACE inhibitors and ARBs are relatively weak antihypertensive agents and do not routinely reduce blood pressure by more than 10 to 15 mm Hg; additional antihypertensive agents (e.g., amlodipine) may be required if hypertension persists. Treatment with amlodipine alone also may result in reduction of proteinuria, but typically to a lesser degree than that seen with ACE inhibitor or ARB therapy. In addition, amlodipine may induce preferential dilation of the afferent glomerular arteriole, thereby increasing intraglomerular hydrostatic pressure, as well as RAAS activation in dogs and potentially also cats (Atkins et al, 2007). Some clinicians recommend that amlodipine not be administered to a dog or cat with chronic kidney disease without simultaneous administration of an ACE inhibitor.

Specific Management of Glomerular Disease Subtypes

Membranous Glomerulopathy

Membranous glomerulopathy (MG) results from the deposition of immune complexes on the subepithelial glomerular basement membrane surface, although immune complexes also may be found in the mesangium of dogs and cats with secondary MG. Deposition of subepithelial immune complexes results in podocyte injury and foot process effacement, with eventual thickening of the glomerular basement membrane. Because these immune complexes are located extravascularly, exposure to inflammatory mediators is limited, and a vigorous cellular immune response is uncommon. MG occurs in 10% to 45% of glomerular disease cases in dogs with glomerular disease and is the most common subtype of glomerular disease in cats.

The clinical course of idiopathic MG in people varies from spontaneous complete remission in 33% to 65% of patients to rapid progression to end-stage renal disease and dialysis dependence. The risk of progression in people correlates with the magnitude of proteinuria and the severity of renal functional impairment; patients with more severe proteinuria and azotemia show more rapid progression than less severely affected patients. MG appears to be progressive in most dogs and cats; however, the worsening of glomerular damage may be slow enough that many animals maintain good quality of life and relatively normal life spans. Following identification and treatment of potentially inciting disease processes and initiation of nonspecific management strategies, immunosuppressive therapy may be warranted in nonazotemic animals with idiopathic MG. Although immunosuppressive treatment protocols for MG in people have not been established clearly, some patients respond to corticosteroids combined with an alkylating agent. Beneficial effects have been shown most clearly in people

when methylprednisolone and chlorambucil are administered alternately every other day for 6 months. The best immunosuppressive protocol has not been established for dogs or cats with MG.

Amyloidosis

Amyloidosis accounts for approximately one fourth of cases of glomerular disease in dogs, whereas cats rarely develop glomerular amyloidosis. Reactive amyloidosis is the most common form of this disease in both dogs and cats, and older animals are affected more commonly. Except in the Chinese shar-pei, amyloid is deposited primarily in the glomerular mesangium, with eventual deposition in the subendothelial space. Proteinuria associated with glomerular amyloidosis may be massive, and dogs may be predisposed to development of thromboembolic complications (Segev et al, 2012). Chinese shar-pei dogs and Abyssinian cats have a familial form of reactive amyloidosis characterized by both glomerular and medullary amyloid deposition, with medullary deposits typically predominating.

Amyloid fibrils are relatively insoluble and resistant to proteolysis due to their β-pleated sheet configuration, so specific treatment is relatively ineffectual. Familial renal amyloidosis in shar-pei dogs and Abyssinian cats is analogous in some ways to familial Mediterranean fever in people, which results in cyclical fevers, renal amyloidosis, and pleuritis, peritonitis, and synovitis. Treatment with colchicine may prevent continued deposition of amyloid in human patients, which has led to the recommendation that colchicine be given to shar-pei dogs with renal amyloidosis, recurrent fevers, and probable polyarthritis. Colchicine (0.01 to 0.03 mg/kg q24h PO) anecdotally has led to remission of proteinuria in this breed, but there is no evidence to support the effectiveness of this drug once renal failure is present. Gastrointestinal upset is the primary adverse effect.

Administration of dimethyl sulfoxide (DMSO) to dogs with amyloidosis is controversial, and its use has been reported in only a limited number of dogs. Benefits likely are due to this drug's antiinflammatory effects, which lead to reduction of interstitial fibrosis and inflammation and, in some cases, improved renal function and reduced proteinuria. DMSO does not solubilize amyloid fibrils *in vivo*. Unfortunately, DMSO (90 mg/kg three times weekly PO or SC) has an unpleasant odor that may lead to poor owner compliance. To reduce injection site pain DMSO should be diluted 1:4 with sterile water before administration, although nausea and anorexia still may occur in some dogs.

Other Glomerular Disease Histologic Subtypes

Membranoproliferative glomerulonephritis (20% to 60% of glomerular disease cases in dogs; rare in cats), mesangioproliferative glomerulonephritis (2% to 16% of glomerular lesions in dogs), and focal segmental glomerulosclerosis have no recommended specific treatments at this time for either dogs or cats. However, it is reasonable to try controlled immunosuppressive therapy in animals with these histologic subtypes if there is documented evidence of active immune complex deposition via electron or immunofluorescent microscopic evaluation of a renal biopsy specimen. Minimal change disease, in which glomeruli are unremarkable on light microscopic evaluation but diffuse foot process effacement is observed on electron microscopy, is highly responsive to corticosteroid therapy in adult human patients but rarely has been described in dogs. No specific treatments beyond feeding a renal diet and administering ACE inhibitors are available for people or animals with hereditary nephritis, in which the unique lesions of irregular glomerular basement membrane splitting require electron microscopic evaluation of renal tissue for identification.

Treatment of Nephrotic Syndrome

Nephrotic syndrome resulting in fluid accumulation and edema is a consequence of severe proteinuria. The pathogenesis of nephrotic syndrome is unclear; rather than being due solely to low oncotic pressure, edema may be caused by a circulating "permeability factor" that increases net fluid extravasation from vascular beds and simultaneously widens glomerular endothelial pore size, resulting in proteinuria. Nonspecific management strategies for dogs or cats with glomerular disease should be implemented in animals with nephrotic syndrome, with aggressive inhibition of RAAS and lowering of the UP/C ratio.

Specific intervention to remove extravascular fluid is recommended only if patient quality of life is impaired or fluids have accumulated in a life-threatening location. Direct removal of ascitic fluid via peritoneocentesis should be limited to removing sufficient fluid to restore good quality of life (i.e., ability to eat and lie down comfortably) rather than attempting to remove all fluid; removal of large volumes of ascitic fluid may result in severe hypovolemia and electrolyte derangements, and worsened kidney injury. If antiproteinuric therapy is only partially successful at inhibiting fluid extravasation and patient discomfort is still apparent, then low-dose diuretic therapy can be instituted. Loop diuretics (e.g., furosemide) are effective for initial fluid mobilization, but use of spironolactone is preferred for maintenance therapy, if needed.

Use of intravenous colloids is not recommended in patients with nephrotic syndrome unless they require immediate increases in intravascular oncotic pressure to prevent or minimize life-threatening fluid accumulation. Patients with extravascular fluid accumulation that otherwise do not require hospitalization frequently experience worsening of their edema or ascites when intravenous colloids are administered. In these dogs and cats, there is likely rapid loss of colloidal molecules into the urine, and the remaining transfused high-sodium fluid increases vascular hydrostatic pressure, which promotes further fluid loss. When life-threatening pleural or pericardial effusion is present, or when ascitic fluid is accumulating at a sufficiently rapid rate that daily fluid removal is necessary, intravenous administration of plasma is preferred in small-breed dogs and administration of human albumin in larger patients.

Follow-up Evaluation

Successful management of dogs and cats with glomerular disease requires regular patient reevaluation. Urinalysis and measurement of the UP/C ratio, body weight, body condition score, systolic blood pressure, and serum albumin and creatinine concentrations should be performed monthly while modifications in the therapeutic plan are being made. However, evaluation every 3 to 6 months may be sufficient once clinical signs are stable and therapeutic changes become less necessary. Day-to-day UP/C variations of up to 50% in dogs and 90% in cats have been described, and therefore averaging results of two to four UP/C ratios measured over a 3- to 5-day period is ideal for estimating the severity of proteinuria in an individual patient. Alternatively, the UP/C can be measured in a sample made from combining equal aliquots from three samples collected over a 3- to 5-day period. Serial ratio measurements that increase or decrease by more than 50% in dogs or 90% in cats indicate a meaningful change in the magnitude of proteinuria.

Prognosis

Survival of dogs with glomerular disease is highly variable; many dogs are euthanized shortly after diagnosis, whereas others live several years and die of unrelated causes. Concurrent azotemia appears to be a negative prognostic indicator; median survival of nonazotemic nonnephrotic dogs with glomerular disease is 605 days, versus 45 days for azotemic nonnephrotic dogs with glomerular disease (Klosterman et al, 2011). Based on this recent finding, aggressive intervention is warranted in proteinuric nonazotemic dogs, with nonspecific medical management and potentially biopsy and specific therapy if indicated, because slowing the course of disease progression has important short- and long-term effects on mortality. Prognosis for cats with MG is unclear because few studies have included large numbers of animals, and the treatment options available have expanded since the publication of initial reports.

References and Suggested Reading

Atkins CE et al: The effect of amlodipine and the combination of amlodipine and enalapril on the renin-angiotensin-aldosterone system in the dog, *J Vet Pharmacol Ther* 30:394, 2007.

Bakris GL: Slowing nephropathy progression: focus on proteinuria reduction, *Clin J Am Soc Nephrol* 3:S3, 2008.

Cattran D: Management of membranous nephropathy: when and why for treatment, *J Am Soc Nephrol* 16:1188, 2005.

Cook AK, Cowgill LD: Clinical and pathological features of protein-losing glomerular disease in the dog: a review of 137 cases (1985-1992), *J Am Anim Hosp Assoc* 32:313, 1996.

Grauer GF et al: Effects of enalapril vs placebo as a treatment for canine idiopathic glomerulonephritis, *J Vet Intern Med* 14:526, 2000.

Klosterman ES et al: Association between nephrotic syndrome and signalment, clinicopathologic abnormalities, histologic diagnosis, and prognosis in dogs with glomerular disease, *J Vet Intern Med* 25:206, 2011.

Linas SL: Are two better than one? Angiotensin-converting enzyme inhibitors plus angiotensin receptor blockers for reducing blood pressure and proteinuria in kidney disease, *Clin J Am Soc Nephrol* 3:S17, 2008.

McAlister FA et al: The safety of combining angiotensin-converting enzyme inhibitors with angiotensin-receptor blockers in elderly patients: a population-based longitudinal analysis, *Can Med Assoc J* 183:E309, 2011.

Schjoedt KJ et al: Optimal dose of lisinopril for renoprotection in type 1 diabetic patients with diabetic nephropathy: a randomised crossover trial, *Diabetologia* 52:46, 2009.

Segev G et al: Renal amyloidosis in dogs: a retrospective study of 91 cases with comparison of the disease between Shar-pei and non Shar-pei dogs, *J Vet Intern Med* 26:259, 2012. Epub January 23, 2012.

CHAPTER **189**

Chronic Kidney Disease: International Renal Interest Society Staging and Management

JONATHAN ELLIOTT, *London, United Kingdom*
A.D.J. WATSON, *Sydney, Australia*

The International Renal Interest Society (IRIS) has developed a staging system for chronic kidney disease (CKD) in cats and dogs that aims to improve communication about diagnosis and management of this complex syndrome. The IRIS CKD Staging system is considered a work in progress, to be reviewed and modified at least annually as additional information becomes available; the most recent version can be accessed at www.iris-kidney.com. Since its inception, the staging system has gained increasing acceptance among veterinary nephrologists and clinicians. Publications have now appeared that use this approach to report accurately staged case series, together with treatments and outcomes that improve our overall understanding of the natural history of CKD in cats and dogs and help identify better approaches to management (Cortadellas et al, 2010; Hsu et al, 2011). Consistent and accurate use of IRIS staging of CKD should help individual practitioners provide prognostic information and identify the likely consequences that require monitoring and management at the different stages of dysfunction.

Diagnosis of Chronic Kidney Disease

When faced with an animal suspected of having CKD, practitioners should adopt a logical approach to diagnosis. The recommended minimum set of data to be obtained for such patients is shown in Box 189-1. The historical and physical abnormalities that led to this suspicion should be reviewed because these findings and other evidence may highlight specific problems that warrant further investigation to determine the type of kidney disease present. This review also may indicate whether an underlying cause is likely to be identified by further investigations and whether concomitant diseases should be suspected.

Laboratory evaluation should include appropriate blood biochemical tests, hematologic studies, and complete urinalysis. The results of these tests should confirm the clinical diagnosis but also may give indications of the causes and the possible presence of underlying diseases. Because kidney disease increases in prevalence as cats and dogs age, the practice of performing geriatric screening tests to detect kidney dysfunction has become more widespread. The IRIS minimum recommended geriatric screening tests for this purpose, together with a more ideal complete version, are presented in Box 189-2.

Selection of Cats and Dogs for Staging

It must be emphasized that the IRIS CKD Staging system is applicable only to cats and dogs with stable CKD—it is not appropriate for other disorders affecting kidney function in which blood creatinine concentrations can change dramatically over a short period of time. Therefore it is important to ensure that primary intrinsic kidney disease

BOX 189-1

Minimal Data Set for Patients Suspected of Having Kidney Disease

History
- Water intake
- Body weight
- Food intake
- Vomiting?

Physical Examination
- Body temperature
- Hydration status
- Body weight and body condition score
- Mucous membrane color
- Cardiac auscultation
- Kidney palpation
- Coat condition
- Oral examination
- Fundic examination
- Thyroid palpation (cat)
- Blood pressure

Laboratory
Obtain all samples before treatment initiation.

Hematology (at least):
- Hematocrit
- Reticulocyte count
- Total solids

Blood Biochemical Tests (at least):
- Creatinine
- Urea
- Phosphate
- Calcium and albumin
- Bicarbonate (or total carbon dioxide)
- Potassium
- In cats >10 yr of age, check alanine transaminase and screen for hyperthyroidism

Urinalysis* (at least):
- Cystocentesis preferred (record method)
- Dipstick testing of supernatant for pH, glucose, hemoglobin, protein
- Specific gravity by refractometry
- Sediment examination (centrifuge at least 3 ml of urine)

*If possible, urinalysis should include estimation of the ratio of urine protein to creatinine for both cats and dogs.

BOX 189-2

Geriatric Screening Tests (for Cats and Dogs Older than 6 Years)

Minimum
- Hematocrit
- Total solids
- Urinalysis
- Creatinine
- Urea

More Complete
- Complete hematologic studies
- Full biochemical panel
- Complete urinalysis

is present and that any prerenal and postrenal contributions to azotemia have been eliminated before CKD is staged in a patient. If the patient has acute kidney injury or decompensated chronic disease (also known as *acute on chronic disease*), it is possible that the condition will stabilize into CKD after 4 to 8 weeks of management, at which time IRIS CKD Staging can be considered.

Staging Based on Blood Creatinine Concentration

The primary indicator for IRIS staging of CKD is the concentration of creatinine in plasma or serum because currently this is the most useful and readily available test of kidney function in veterinary practice. The patient must be fasting and well hydrated at the time blood is sampled. The blood creatinine concentrations used to define IRIS CKD Stages 1 to 4 shown in Table 189-1 were reached by debate and consensus based on the clinical experiences of veterinary nephrologists and data derived from longitudinal studies. As noted previously, they and other elements of staging may be modified in the future as more knowledge is gained.

The IRIS board now proposes an "at-risk" stage of CKD to identify patients that, because of their history (e.g., exposure to nephrotoxic drugs), breed (in which familial kidney disease is common), or geographic location and lifestyle (e.g., residence in an area where leishmaniasis is very common) warrant close monitoring of kidney function. These patients differ from those with IRIS CKD Stage 1 in that they have no laboratory or physical abnormality at the time of examination. The first two numbered stages of the system reflect the fact that a large proportion of kidney tissue has to be damaged before a rise in blood creatinine concentration is detectable. Hence IRIS CKD Stage 1 and early Stage 2 encompass creatinine concentrations that are within or overlap the reference ranges for most laboratories.

It is likely that some animals with CKD pass through all four IRIS stages if their kidney disease progresses. But some animals remain in stable condition within one stage and die of another disease before kidney disease has a chance to progress. Affected animals may be brought to the veterinarian at any stage, depending on how observant the owner is and whether routine regular health screening is being practiced.

Substaging of Chronic Kidney Disease

Following staging, it is recommended that substaging be performed using the quantity of protein excreted in the urine and the systemic arterial blood pressure. Evaluation of these two variables is warranted because abnormalities in each can occur separately or together at any stage of CKD. Moreover, increases in both are known independent risk factors for progressive renal injury in human medicine that warrant specific treatment; the same is likely to be true in veterinary patients.

Proteinuria

Proteinuria is singled out for special attention because there is good evidence that it is a prognostic indicator in dogs and cats with CKD. For IRIS CKD substaging based on proteinuria to be used, the proteinuria must be of renal origin; therefore prerenal and postrenal causes of proteinuria have to be ruled out first. Because persistent proteinuria is considered more likely to be significant than transient proteinuria, substaging ideally requires proteinuria to be demonstrated in three or more urine

TABLE 189-1

IRIS CKD Staging Based on Blood Creatinine Concentration

Stage	Creatinine (mg/dl [μmol/L])*	Comments
At risk	As for Stage 1	History suggests the animal is at increased risk of developing CKD in the future because of a number of factors (e.g., exposure to nephrotoxic drugs, breed, high prevalence of infectious disease in the area, or old age).
1	<1.4 (125) dogs <1.6 (140) cats	Nonazotemic. Some other renal abnormality present (e.g., inadequate urinary concentrating ability without identifiable nonrenal cause, abnormal renal palpation or renal imaging findings, proteinuria of renal origin, abnormal renal biopsy results, increasing blood creatinine concentrations in samples collected serially).
2	1.4-2 (125-180) dogs 1.6-2.8 (140-250) cats	Mild renal azotemia (lower end of the range lies within reference ranges for many laboratories, but the insensitivity of creatinine concentration as a screening test means that animals with creatinine values close to the upper reference limit often have excretory failure). Clinical signs usually mild or absent.
3	2.1-5 (181-440) dogs 2.9-5 (251-440) cats	Moderate renal azotemia. Many extrarenal clinical signs may be present.
4	>5 (>440) dogs and cats	Severe renal azotemia. Many extrarenal clinical signs usually are present.

*Note that these blood creatinine concentrations apply to dogs of average size; for those of extreme size (e.g., miniature and giant breeds) these ranges may not be appropriate.
IRIS, International Renal Interest Society; *CKD,* chronic kidney disease.

TABLE 189-2

IRIS CKD Substaging by Urine Protein/Creatinine (UP/C) Ratio

UP/C Value*	Substage
<0.2 cats and dogs	Nonproteinuric (NP)
0.2-0.4 cats 0.2-0.5 dogs	Borderline proteinuric (BP)
>0.4 cats >0.5 dogs	Proteinuric (P)

*Calculated using mass units.
IRIS, International Renal Interest Society; *CKD,* chronic kidney disease.

samples over at least a 2-week period. It is important that urine sediment be examined microscopically on each occasion to rule out the presence of inflammation in the urinary tract (see Chapter 187). The three substages are nonproteinuric (NP), borderline proteinuric (BP), and proteinuric (P), based on the urine protein/creatinine (UP/C) ratio (determined using mass units), as shown in Table 189-2. Note that UP/C ratios classified as NP or BP may be categorized as microalbuminuric when other test methods are used. Because the significance of microalbuminuria in predicting future renal health is not understood at present, the current IRIS recommendation is to continue monitoring these patients for proteinuria using UP/C determinations. For animals found to have P or BP disease, the significance of the finding depends on the concurrent stage of CKD. Thus the P substage is more significant at Stage 3 than at Stage 1; this is because the filtered protein load presented to tubules reduces as the functioning nephron mass declines. Consequently, a

given level of proteinuria has higher significance as glomerular filtration rate (GFR) declines. Note that UP/C ratios at the BP or P level can indicate tubular or glomerular dysfunction, but once the UP/C ratio exceeds 2.0 it most likely indicates a primary glomerular problem. Response to any treatment given to reduce proteinuria (see later) should be monitored at appropriate intervals using the UP/C ratio.

Blood Pressure

Kidney disease can affect blood pressure regulation, leading to inappropriately high blood pressure. This in turn can be damaging to the kidneys and also can damage other organs such as the heart (left ventricular hypertrophy), the eye (hyphema, hypertensive chorioretinopathy), and the brain (dullness, lethargy, seizures), which may result in extrarenal signs and morbidity. Therefore IRIS recommends that arterial blood pressure be measured in all patients with CKD. There are several methods for blood pressure measurement and no agreed standard approach at present, but it is most important for practitioners to standardize the techniques they use. Patients should be examined for accompanying clinical signs of end-organ damage and acclimatized to the measurement conditions. Repeated measurements are required because prognosis and therapy depend on the reliability of this assessment. The final classification is based on measurements made during multiple patient visits to the clinic on separate days. However, making several determinations during the same visit is acceptable if they are separated by at least 30 to 120 minutes, which allows sufficient time for the animal to respond to the second measurement session as a separate event.

The persistence of risk should be judged based on multiple sequential blood pressure measurements made

TABLE 189-3

IRIS CKD Substaging by Arterial Pressure in Cats and Dogs* Based on Risk of Future Target-Organ Damage†

Systolic Pressure (mm Hg)	Diastolic Pressure (mm Hg)	Risk of Target-Organ Damage	Arterial Pressure (AP) Substage
<150	<95	None or minimal	AP0
150-159	95-99	Low	AP1
160-179	100-119	Moderate	AP2
≥180	≥120	High	AP3

*Although there are interbreed differences in blood pressure in dogs, only the difference for sight hounds (values 20 mm Hg higher for each category) necessitates separate categorization at present.
†If reliable measurements indicate different risk assessments when based separately on the patient's systolic and diastolic blood pressures, the patient's AP substage should be taken as the higher of the two assessments. If pressures are not measured, the substage assigned is *RND* (risk not determined).
IRIS, International Renal Interest Society; *CKD,* chronic kidney disease.

TABLE 189-4

Examples of IRIS CKD Staging and Substaging Before and After Treatment

Cat A

Before Treatment	*After Treatment*
Creatinine 3.0 mg/dl (260 µmol/L) UP/C ratio 0.3 Systolic blood pressure 200 mm Hg	*Creatinine 3.4 mg/dl (300 µmol/L) UP/C ratio 0.3 Systolic blood pressure 155 mm Hg*
IRIS CKD Stage 3-BP-AP3	*IRIS CKD Stage 3-BP-AP1(T)*

Dog B

Before Treatment	*After Treatment*
Creatinine 1.8 mg/dl (160 µmol/L) UP/C ratio 0.8 Systolic blood pressure 155 mm Hg	*Creatinine 1.9 mg/dl (170 µmol/L) UP/C ratio 0.4 Systolic blood pressure 155 mm Hg*
IRIS CKD Stage 2-P-AP1	*IRIS CKD Stage 2-BP-AP1(T)*

IRIS, International Renal Interest Society; *CKD,* chronic kidney disease; *UP/C,* urine protein/creatinine ratio.

over a 2-month period if the animal is at moderate risk, or over 1 to 2 weeks if the animal is at severe risk. However, if extrarenal target-organ damage already is present, demonstration of persistence is not necessary and treatment should begin immediately (see later).

Blood pressure–based substages are assigned according to what the arterial pressure measurement is and whether extrarenal target-organ damage is present or threatens. Table 189-3 defines pressure ranges associated with minimal, low, moderate, and high risk of target-organ damage; if pressure is not assessed, the designation applied is *RND* (risk not determined). Blood pressure–based substaging can be qualified by noting whether signs of complications (c) or no complications (nc) secondary to high blood pressure have been detected clinically (e.g., hypertensive chorioretinopathy). For example, in a patient with a systolic blood pressure of 165 mm Hg in which no complications were detected the arterial pressure (AP) substage would be AP2(nc), whereas in a patient with a systolic pressure of 170 mm Hg and evidence of hyphema the substage would be AP2(c).

Combining Stages and Substages

The following examples show how IRIS CKD stages and substages are combined to define CKD.

1. A nonproteinuric cat (UP/C ratio of 0.12) with a systolic blood pressure of 210 mm Hg, retinal detachment, and blood creatinine concentration of 2.0 mg/dl (176 µmol/L) would be classified as having IRIS CKD Stage 2-NP-AP3(c), where *NP* indicates absence of proteinuria and *AP3(c)* denotes arterial blood pressure associated with a high risk of target-organ damage and evidence of complications secondary to high blood pressure present at initial staging.

2. A dog with borderline proteinuria (UP/C value of 0.35) and blood creatinine concentration of 5.4 mg/dl (475 µmol/L) that did not undergo blood pressure assessment would be considered to have IRIS CKD Stage 4-BP-RND, where *BP* denotes borderline proteinuria and *RND* indicates that the risk of target-organ damage associated with arterial blood pressure was not determined.

3. A proteinuric dog (UP/C ratio of 0.7) with a systolic pressure of 120 mm Hg and blood creatinine concentration of 3.4 mg/dl (300 µmol/L) would be identified as having IRIS CKD Stage 3-P-AP0(nc), where *P* denotes proteinuria and *AP0(nc)* designates an arterial pressure status associated with minimal or no risk of target-organ damage accompanied by no evidence of hypertensive complications.

Revision of Staging and Substaging after Therapy

The stage and substages assigned to the patient's CKD should be revised appropriately as changes occur. For example, if antihypertensive (or antiproteinuric) therapy has been instituted, the CKD designation on reevaluation should reflect the current blood pressure (or UP/C ratio) rather than the original status, with an additional sign, *(T)*, after the relevant substage indicator to show that the current designation reflects treatment effects. Two examples are shown in Table 189-4.

Treatment and Monitoring

IRIS staging for CKD is not a "set and forget" process. It is necessary to monitor clinical progress at appropriate intervals, modify treatments according to the patient's response, and revise assigned stage and substages as changes occur. All treatments given are to be tailored to the individual patient. The following recommendations are useful starting points for the majority of animals at each stage. Specific dosages usually are not stipulated; standard dosages apply for starting therapy with most agents, but caution is advisable with drugs eliminated mainly by renal mechanisms.

General Management

The following are general basic guidelines to consider in the management of patients with CKD:

- Discontinue all potentially nephrotoxic drugs.
- Identify and treat any prerenal or postrenal abnormalities.
- Rule out any treatable condition within the urinary tract (e.g., renal urolithiasis, pyelonephritis).
- Rule out any treatable underlying disease outside the urinary system that can perpetuate renal damage (e.g., hyperthyroidism, hyperadrenocorticism, pyometra, infectious disease).
- Consider dietary manipulation. Changing to an established renal diet can help meet several aims of treatment and acts against hyperphosphatemia and hyperparathyroidism, proteinuria, hypertension, hypokalemia, and azotemia. It may be advantageous to do this early in the course of CKD (perhaps in late IRIS CKD Stage 2) before inappetence results from deteriorating function and uremia. Cats can be particularly difficult to transfer onto a renal diet, and a number of practical tips to facilitate this transition have been published (Roudebush et al, 2009).

Dehydration

At all stages of CKD, most patients have decreased urine concentrating ability, so it is important to correct clinical dehydration with isotonic, polyionic replacement fluids and to ensure that fresh drinking water is available at all times. Regular parenteral administration of such fluids may be needed to meet maintenance requirements if vomiting is present, especially at IRIS CKD Stages 3 and 4. If a feeding tube is in place, it can be used to administer fluids also.

Proteinuria

Note that the intervention points for proteinuria differ according to the IRIS CKD stage. At Stage 1 and early Stage 2 the number of filtering nephrons through which protein can be lost is high, so that borderline and low-level proteinuria (UP/C ratios of <2.0) are investigated and monitored closely. On the other hand, treatment is recommended at a lower UP/C ratio at IRIS CKD Stages 2 to 4.

Cats in IRIS CKD Stage 1 with a UP/C ratio of more than 1.0 should undergo investigation to identify the disease process leading to proteinuria (see steps 1 and 2 later) and should receive antiproteinuric treatment (steps 3, 4, and

5 later). Those with less marked proteinuria (UP/C ratio of 0.4 to 1.0) should be investigated and monitored (steps 1 and 4).

Cats with more advanced CKD (IRIS CKD Stages 2 to 4) and a UP/C ratio above 0.4 should undergo investigation to determine the disease process causing proteinuria (steps 1 and 2 later) and should receive antiproteinuric therapy (steps 3, 4, and 5). Those with borderline proteinuria (UP/C ratio of 0.2 to 0.4) require close monitoring (steps 1 and 4).

Dogs in IRIS CKD Stage 1 with a UP/C ratio of more than 2.0 should undergo investigation to identify the disease process leading to proteinuria (steps 1 and 2 later) and should receive antiproteinuric treatment (steps 3 and 5). If the UP/C ratio is 1.0 to 2.0, thorough investigation and close monitoring is warranted (steps 1, 2, and 4). In those with a UP/C ratio of 0.5 to 1.0 investigation and monitoring (steps 1 and 4) should be carried out.

Dogs with more advanced CKD (IRIS CKD Stages 2 to 4) and a UP/C ratio above 0.5 should undergo investigation to determine the disease process causing proteinuria (steps 1 and 2) and should receive antiproteinuric therapy (steps 3 and 5). Those with borderline proteinuria (UP/C ratio of 0.2 to 0.5) require close monitoring (steps 1 and 4).

The following is a stepwise approach for the evaluation and management of proteinuria (see also Chapter 187).

1. Look for any concurrent associated disease process that can be treated.
2. Consider kidney biopsy to identify the underlying disease (consult experts if unsure of indications for this).
3. Institute treatment with dietary protein reduction and angiotensin-converting enzyme (ACE) inhibitor therapy. Note that ACE inhibitor use is contraindicated if the patient is clinically dehydrated or showing signs of hypovolemia. Dehydration should be corrected before these drugs are used; otherwise GFR may drop precipitously.
4. Monitor response to treatment and progression of disease; a stable creatinine concentration with a decreasing UP/C ratio indicates a good response, but serial increases in creatinine concentrations or increases in UP/C ratios suggest that CKD is progressing. Therapy usually is lifelong unless the underlying disease resolves, in which case reducing drug dosage while monitoring UP/C ratio might be considered.
5. For dogs, institute low-dose acetylsalicylic acid therapy (1 to 5 mg/kg q24h PO) if serum albumin concentration is less than 2.0 g/dl (20 g/L). Although the risk of thromboembolism is probably similar in cats and dogs, it is difficult to achieve a selective antiplatelet effect in cats; in this species, administration of acetylsalicylic acid at 1 mg/kg q72h PO is suggested if serum albumin concentration is less than 2.0 g/dl (20 g/L).

Hypertension

The blood pressure required to prevent kidney disease progression is unknown, but the goal is to reduce systolic blood pressure to less than 160 mm Hg and to minimize the risk of extrarenal target-organ damage. If systolic pressure is persistently 160 mm Hg or above, treatment should be instituted; if target-organ damage is evident, the animal should be treated without requiring demonstration of the persistence of increased blood pressure.

Reducing blood pressure is a long-term aim in patients with CKD. A gradual and sustained reduction in blood pressure is the goal, and sudden or severe decreases leading to hypotension should be avoided; a systolic pressure of less than 120 mm Hg or clinical signs of weakness or tachycardia are suggestive of hypotension. A reduction in blood pressure may lead to small and persistent increases in blood creatinine concentration (increase of <0.5 mg/dl or <45 μmol/L). A marked increase suggests an adverse drug effect, whereas a progressively increasing creatinine concentration indicates progressive kidney damage. Serial monitoring is essential, with treatment adjustment as necessary. Once blood pressure has been stabilized, monitoring should be undertaken at least every 3 months.

For cats with hypertension, a logical stepwise approach to management is as follows:

1. Restrict dietary sodium. This can be done by introducing a commercial renal diet with low salt content. There is no evidence that this measure alone actually reduces blood pressure; if it is attempted, it should be done gradually and in conjunction with drug therapy because there is evidence that salt restriction enhances the efficacy of some antihypertensive agents, particularly those that interfere with the renin-angiotensin-aldosterone system.
2. Administer the calcium channel blocker (CCB) amlodipine (e.g., amlodipine 0.625 mg per cat q24h PO).
3. Increase the dosage of amlodipine to effect (see earlier), up to a maximum of 0.5 mg/kg q24h PO.
4. Add an ACE inhibitor to CCB treatment. If the patient has IRIS CKD Stage 3 or 4 and is in unstable condition or dehydrated, ensure that the patient is hydrated adequately before administration of the ACE inhibitor; otherwise GFR may drop precipitously.

For dogs with hypertension, the suggested stepwise approach is as follows:

1. Restrict dietary sodium, but see step 1 earlier for cats.
2. Start ACE inhibitor therapy at the standard dosage.
3. Double the dose of ACE inhibitor (this will improve antihypertensive efficacy in some patients).
4. Combine the ACE inhibitor with a CCB (e.g., amlodipine). Caution: see step 4 earlier for cats.
5. Add hydralazine to combined ACE inhibitor and CCB treatment.

Phosphate Intake

Renal secondary hyperparathyroidism develops early in the course of CKD, and many cats with IRIS CKD Stage 2 disease already have increased blood parathyroid hormone (PTH) concentrations even when blood phosphate concentrations remain within reference limits (Barber and Elliott, 1998).

There is evidence that reducing dietary phosphate intake in cats and dogs with CKD is beneficial. The goal is to maintain blood phosphate concentrations below 4.6 mg/dl but above 2.7 mg/dl (<1.5 mmol/L but >0.9 mmol/L). In practice, this target may be difficult to achieve in IRIS CKD Stages 3 and 4, for which more realistic goals would be less than 5.0 mg/dl and less than 6.0 mg/dl (<1.6 mmol/L and <1.9 mmol/L), respectively.

The following measures can be introduced sequentially in attempting to reduce blood phosphate concentrations.

1. Restrict phosphate intake by instituting an appropriate renal diet, ideally early in the course of CKD, before inappetence develops.
2. If blood phosphate concentration remains too high after dietary restriction, give an enteric phosphate binder (e.g., aluminium [aluminum] hydroxide, aluminium carbonate, calcium carbonate, calcium acetate, or lanthanum carbonate), starting at 30 to 60 mg/kg q24h PO divided (if fed twice daily) and mixed with the food. The dose required will vary with the phosphate intake and CKD stage. Treat to effect, although signs of toxicity may limit the upper possible dosage in the patient. Monitor blood calcium and phosphate concentrations every 4 to 6 weeks until they stabilize and then every 12 weeks. Microcytosis or generalized muscle weakness suggests aluminium toxicity if an aluminium-containing binder is used; switch to another form of phosphate binder should this occur. Hypercalcemia is to be avoided. Combinations of aluminium- and calcium-containing phosphate binders may be needed sometimes.
3. For dogs with IRIS CKD Stage 3 or 4 there is evidence that judicious use of calcitriol (1.5 to 3.5 ng/kg q24h PO) prolongs survival when phosphate is controlled and ionized calcium and PTH are monitored. However, beneficial effects of calcitriol have not been demonstrated yet for cats.

Metabolic Acidosis

If metabolic acidosis occurs (blood bicarbonate or total CO_2 of <16 mmol/L for cats or <18 mmol/L for dogs) once the patient's condition has been stabilized on the renal diet of choice, then supplementation with oral sodium bicarbonate or potassium citrate (if hypokalemic) should be initiated, with dosage adjusted to maintain blood bicarbonate or total CO_2 in the range of 16 to 24 mmol/L for cats and 18 to 24 mmol/L for dogs.

Anemia

Treatment for anemia should be considered if it is affecting the patient's quality of life; typically this occurs when the packed cell volume is less than 20% (0.20 L/L). Human recombinant erythropoietin is the most effective treatment but is not approved for veterinary use. Darbepoetin is preferable because it is less antigenic than epoetin alfa. The patient's hematocrit should be monitored to avoid erythrocytosis and to detect whether refractoriness to treatment is developing. Anabolic steroids are of no proven benefit and may be detrimental.

Vomiting, Nausea, and Inappetence

Vomiting, decreased appetite, or nausea should be treated with a histamine-2 receptor blocker (e.g., ranitidine) or proton-pump inhibitor (e.g., omeprazole) and an antiemetic (e.g., metoclopramide, maropitant, or ondansetron). However, further investigations are necessary to determine whether these drugs are useful for managing gastrointestinal disturbances in cats and dogs with CKD and uremia. Efforts to prevent protein-calorie malnutrition should be intensified. It may be necessary to consider placing a feeding tube (e.g., percutaneous gastrostomy or esophageal tube), which also can be used to administer fluids if necessary.

Hypokalemia

Cats (but not dogs) with CKD sometimes have reduced blood potassium concentrations. Commercial diets formulated for feline CKD patients often have increased potassium content, but additional potassium may be required. If so, potassium gluconate should be given orally to effect (typically 1 to 2 mmol/kg q24h PO).

Drug Therapy

Any drug that relies predominantly on renal function for clearance from the body should be used with caution in IRIS CKD Stages 3 and 4. It may be necessary either to adjust the dose of these drugs (depending on their therapeutic indices) to prevent accumulation or to avoid them completely.

References and Suggested Reading

Barber PJ, Elliott J: Feline chronic renal failure: calcium homeostasis in 80 cases diagnosed between 1992 and 1995, *J Small Anim Pract* 39:108, 1998.
Cortadellas O et al: Calcium and phosphorus homeostasis in dogs with spontaneous chronic kidney disease at different stages of severity, *J Vet Intern Med* 24:73, 2010.
Hsu V et al: Prevalence of IgG antibodies to *Encephalitozoon cuniculi* and *Toxoplasma gondii* in cats with and without chronic kidney disease from Virginia, *Vet Parasitol* 176:23, 2011.
Roudebush P et al: Therapies for feline chronic kidney disease. What is the evidence? *J Feline Med Surg* 11:195, 2009.

Website
International Renal Interest Society (IRIS): www.iris-kidney.com. In the Education section are recent items on diagnosis and staging of chronic kidney disease, including articles on hypertension by SA Brown and proteinuria by GF Grauer.

CHAPTER 190

Use of Nonsteroidal Antiinflammatory Drugs in Kidney Disease

SCOTT A. BROWN, *Athens, Georgia*

Nonsteroidal antiinflammatory drugs (NSAIDs) are the most commonly prescribed analgesic agents in veterinary medicine. Their analgesic, antiinflammatory, and antipyretic effects are attributed to reduction of prostaglandin synthesis caused by inhibition of cyclooxygenase (COX) enzymes. Unfortunately, gastrointestinal, hepatic, and renal toxicities have been associated with use of these agents. Other potential adverse effects appear to be less important (e.g., delayed bone and soft tissue healing) or have not been well studied (e.g., increased systemic arterial blood pressure) in dogs and cats. The effects of NSAIDs on the kidneys, particularly in animals with chronic kidney disease (CKD), deserve special attention largely because prostaglandins play a pivotal role in the maintenance of renal function. Furthermore, the effects of newer NSAIDs on the kidneys cannot be predicted from studies of their gastrointestinal effects.

Cyclooxygenase Isoenzymes

The COX-1 isoenzyme generally is thought of as the "housekeeping" isoform that mediates the formation of constitutive prostaglandins produced by many tissues.

When the presence of isoforms in the kidney was discovered, it was believed that the renal COX-1 isoenzyme was the constitutive form responsible for control of renal function and that COX-2 was the inducible form, being expressed primarily in the presence of renal inflammation associated with renal diseases. Although it still is generally accepted that COX-2 is the isoenzyme that contributes to renal inflammation, COX-2 is expressed constitutively in the kidney, is important in the control of renal blood flow and glomerular filtration rate, is up-regulated in volume depletion and in both inflammatory and noninflammatory forms of CKD, and contributes to the viability of renal tubular and interstitial cells (Cho et al, 2009; Radi, 2009). There is a third COX isoenzyme, a splice variant of COX-1, that is referred to variously as COX-1 variant or COX-3. Its role in renal function is not understood.

There are important differences between the distribution of these isoforms in human and in canine kidneys. The COX-1 isoenzyme is expressed constitutively in the canine collecting duct cells, medullary interstitial cells, endothelial cells, and smooth muscle cells of the preglomerular and postglomerular vessels. Critically, the COX-2 isoform has a wider constitutive distribution in the canine kidney and is present in the canine glomerulus, loop of Henle, macula densa, renal interstitial cells, and blood vessels. The distribution pattern is more extensive in canine kidneys than in human kidneys, and this has led to the assertion that dogs are more susceptible to nephrotoxicity from COX inhibition in general, and COX-2 inhibition in particular, than are people (Khan et al, 1998; Radi, 2009). Although isoenzyme distribution in the feline kidney is incompletely understood, a recent report has identified the presence of both isoenzymes in the feline kidney and suggested there is up-regulation of COX-2 in both canine and feline CKD (Yabuki et al, 2012).

Renal Effects of NSAIDs

NSAIDs in Normal Animals

Several inhibitors of COX enzymes have been used for management of postoperative pain and osteoarthritis in dogs and cats. These can be classified broadly into two categories: nonselective NSAIDs, which inhibit both COX-1 and COX-2 (e.g., aspirin and ibuprofen), and COX-2–selective NSAIDs, which preferentially inhibit COX-2 (e.g., carprofen, deracoxib, etodolac, firocoxib, and meloxicam). The selectivity of NSAIDs in the latter category varies, and all agents inhibit both isoenzymes to some extent.

In the kidney, prostaglandins have a variety of homeostatic effects, including a contribution to control of hemodynamic function (i.e., renal blood flow and glomerular filtration rate) and cytoprotective functions (e.g., sustaining interstitial and tubular cells in the medulla, which is a hypertonic, comparatively hypoxic environment). Although early proposals held that renal COX-1 was constitutive and was responsible for the maintenance of renal blood flow and glomerular filtration rate and that renal COX-2 was present only in renal disease or inflammation, both isoenzymes are constitutive and inducible in the kidney and both contribute to the control of renal blood flow, glomerular filtration rate, renin release, and cytoprotection. Although these roles are important in patients at risk (see later), neither preferential inhibition of COX-2 with selective NSAIDs nor inhibition of both isoenzymes with nonselective NSAIDs appears to have important effects on kidney function in normal dogs and cats (Goodman et al, 2009; Surdyk et al, 2011, 2012).

NSAID Nephrotoxicity

There are two general syndromes of NSAID nephrotoxicity (Table 190-1): acute hemodynamic insult (acute cortical nephrotoxicity) and chronic cytotoxic insult (chronic medullary cytotoxicity). Although either or both syndromes may occur in any particular patient, most reports to date in veterinary medicine implicate NSAIDs in what appears to be hemodynamically mediated acute cortical nephrotoxicity that manifests as classical acute kidney injury (Bacia et al, 1986; Poortinga and Hungerford, 1998). Most affected patients have one or more factors that place them at risk (see Table 190-1). Early clinical findings include the presence of renal tubular cells and casts in urine sediment, renal enzymuria, and proteinuria (microalbuminuria). Subsequently, there is a loss of renal concentrating ability and the development of electrolyte and acid-base disorders. Renal azotemia, with serum creatinine concentration proportional to the magnitude of renal damage, is a comparatively late finding. Although originally it was hoped that the newer generation of selective NSAIDs would pose less risk of nephrotoxicity, data to support this hypothesis are lacking. Inhibition of either or both COX isoenzymes can result in toxicity in animals at risk. In dogs, the deleterious renal hemodynamic effects of NSAIDs do not appear to differ between selective and nonselective NSAIDs (Surdyk et al, 2011, 2012).

The renal medulla is a harsh environment characterized by hypertonicity, comparatively low oxygen tension, and precarious blood flow. Chronic medullary cytotoxicity from NSAIDs is believed to occur as a result of renal tubular and interstitial cell death and disruption of medullary blood flow. Typically it is manifested as papillary necrosis, which initially is patchy and incomplete in other species. Although severe azotemia associated with papillary necrosis may occur, medullary cytotoxicity is difficult to identify because it usually is a gradual subclinical toxicity until its late stages and there are no known biomarkers to identify its presence early in the course of toxicity. Given the distribution of COX isoenzymes in the dog and cat kidneys, inhibition of either or both isoenzymes would be expected to enhance the likelihood of this toxicity, and evidence suggests that dogs are particularly susceptible. Although there have been studies of chronic medullary cytotoxicity in dogs (Sellers et al, 2004; Tsuchiya et al, 2005), the importance of this toxicity in cats is not known.

NSAIDs in Animals at Risk of Nephrotoxicity

Since NSAIDs have little effect on renal function in normal animals, the key to preventing nephrotoxicity lies in the identification and management of factors that

TABLE **190-1**

Syndromes of Renal Injury Associated with Nonsteroidal Antiinflammatory Drug (NSAID) Use*

	Acute Cortical Nephrotoxicity	Chronic Medullary Cytotoxicity
Risk factors	Extracellular fluid volume depletion, especially dehydration Systemic hypotension General anesthesia Dietary salt restriction Diuretic use Administration of antihypertensive agents that are not renal vasodilators Higher NSAID dosage Hypoalbuminemia Genetic factors?	Chronic dehydration Chronic hypotension or multiple acute bouts of hypotension Administration of antihypertensive agents that are not renal vasodilators Higher NSAID dosage Hypoalbuminemia Genetic factors?
Toxic effect	Loss of renoprotective effects of vasodilatory prostaglandins	Loss of cytoprotective effects of prostanoids
Primary effects of toxicity	Decreased renal blood flow and glomerular filtration rate	Necrosis of medullary interstitial and tubular cells (papillary necrosis)
Isoenzyme	Inhibition of COX-1 more important than inhibition of COX-2	Inhibition of COX-2 more important than inhibition of COX-1
Early clinical findings	Renal cells and casts in urine sediment, renal enzymuria, proteinuria, or microalbuminuria	None
Intermediate clinical findings	Serum electrolyte abnormalities, reduced urine concentrating ability	Renal enzymuria, decreased urine concentrating ability
Late clinical findings	Rising serum creatinine concentration	Serum electrolyte and acid-base abnormalities, rising serum creatinine concentration
Interspecies differences in susceptibility	Dogs more susceptible than people; cat susceptibility unknown	Dogs more susceptible than people; cat susceptibility unknown

*Limited clinical information is available for dogs and cats. Information is extrapolated from clinical reports of nephrotoxicity in veterinary medicine, laboratory studies in dogs and cats, and results of studies in other species.
COX, Cyclooxygenase.

place patients at risk (see Table 190-1). Renal function is particularly dependent on COX function in the preexisting conditions listed in Table 190-1 that otherwise would result in renal vasoconstriction, sometimes referred to as *high-renin states.* In these conditions, both COX isoenzymes produce vasodilatory prostaglandins that maintain renal blood flow and glomerular filtration rate. Prostaglandins also contribute to control of renal tubular handling of water and electrolytes and to opposition of the vasoconstrictive effects of angiotensin II. In this setting, the function of both COX-1 and COX-2 are essential for renoprotection.

Iatrogenic risk factors also place patients at risk of acute cortical nephrotoxicity. Antihypertensive agents that do not enhance renal perfusion are an important example because these agents may be used in geriatric patients in which CKD and painful conditions may coexist. In this regard, calcium channel blockers and agents that interfere with the renin-angiotensin system (e.g., converting enzyme inhibitors) are preferred over β-blockers or diuretic agents because the former agents produce renal vasodilatation.

Of additional concern are anecdotal reports of acute cortical nephrotoxicity in previously normal animals undergoing elective surgical procedures. Although hypotensive anesthesia by itself does not result predictably in nephrotoxicity (Boström et al, 2002; Goodman et al,

2009), some animals appear to be at higher risk, perhaps from comorbid effects of anesthetic agents that reduce medullary perfusion, postoperative dehydration, or other poorly understood factors. Since NSAIDs generally are highly protein bound, hypoalbuminemia would be expected to increase free drug concentration and place a patient at risk of nephrotoxicity. In people, there also are genetic factors that alter the metabolism of NSAIDs, placing specific individuals at risk (Blanco et al, 2008). Although the importance of genetic factors in dogs and cats is largely unknown, German shepherds may be more susceptible to NSAID nephrotoxicity (Poortinga and Hungerford, 1998).

Despite its importance in people and rodent models, comparatively little is known about the clinical significance of chronic medullary cytotoxicity in dogs and cats. However, conditions that lead to increased osmolality in the medullary interstitium or reduced medullary blood flow (e.g., dehydration or hypotension, especially if chronic) could be expected to place animals at risk of this form of NSAID nephrotoxicity (see Table 190-1).

NSAIDs in Animals with Chronic Kidney Disease

Because animals with acute kidney injury have inherently unstable renal function, NSAIDs should not be used in these patients. The judicious use of NSAIDs in patients with CKD can be appropriate. Studies in rodents (Cho et al, 2009) as well as a recent report on dogs and cats (Yabuki et al, 2012) indicate that expression of either or both isoenzymes is up-regulated in CKD. Although it is tempting to speculate that animals with CKD are at risk of NSAID toxicity, available studies do not support this contention. Results of laboratory studies of NSAID administration in otherwise healthy cats with induced CKD suggest that NSAIDs do not result in a substantial change in glomerular filtration rate (Surdyk et al, 2013). The findings of studies of a similar manipulation, supplementation of diet with omega-3 polyunsaturated fatty acids to blunt the effects of up-regulation of COX activity in azotemic dogs, are consistent with the proposal that, in the absence of risk factors, use of agents that interfere with prostaglandin production may be safe in animals with CKD (Brown et al, 2000). The increased cortical and medullary blood flow rates and reduced medullary fluid osmolality likely to be present in dogs and cats with spontaneous CKD in fact may be protective. In some rodent models, NSAIDs actually slow the rate of progression of CKD (Harding et al, 2003). A similar effect may be present in cats with CKD because one study demonstrated that meloxicam could be administered safely at low dosages (0.01 to 0.03 mg/kg q24h) to cats with CKD, and although cause and effect was not established, this NSAID use was associated with a slowing of the rate of progression of CKD in cats (Gowan et al, 2011).

Despite this evidence, clinicians should exercise caution when considering NSAID administration in animals with CKD; other approaches to pain management should be attempted before NSAIDs are used. First, animals with CKD have modest renal reserves, and any nephrotoxicity is likely to be clinically significant. Second, although NSAIDs generally are metabolized by the liver, metabolites are variously cleared by the kidney and gastrointestinal tract, and reduced renal function may slow clearance rates. Furthermore, hypoalbuminemia, as may be observed in animals with nephrotic syndrome or chronic malnutrition, increases the free (active) fraction of these highly protein-bound drugs.

Use of NSAIDs in Chronic Kidney Disease

Regardless of the indication for NSAID use, client education is critical. The U.S. Food and Drug Administration has provided Client Information Sheets (available at www.fda.gov), and these are intended to be distributed when NSAIDs are prescribed. Clients should participate in the decision to employ these agents, be cautioned as to possible adverse events, and be educated in how to identify these events. Clients also should be made aware that increased dosage heightens risk and that any suspected adverse effect of NSAID therapy mandates immediate discontinuation of the medication and evaluation by a veterinarian.

Short-Term NSAID Use

Given the plethora of alternative options for managing acute pain of less than 14 days' duration, it seems wise

to use alternatives to NSAIDs in an animal with CKD that has an acutely painful condition for which analgesics are appropriate. If an animal is well hydrated and other risk factors are absent or well managed, an NSAID may be used at the lowest dosage for which efficacy is expected and for as short a treatment duration as possible, generally less than 7 days. Baseline medical testing that should be performed before therapy includes a complete blood count, biochemical panel, complete urinalysis with sediment examination and quantification of proteinuria (i.e., ratio of urine protein to creatinine or microalbuminuria test), and urine culture. If the data obtained indicate previously unknown renal disease (e.g., urinary tract infection) or unstable renal function (e.g., serum creatinine concentration increased from previous values), use of NSAIDs is not appropriate.

Long-Term NSAID Use

It is well known that CKD and chronically painful conditions frequently coexist in veterinary patients, particularly in older dogs and cats. Evidence suggests that long-term use of NSAIDs in dogs and cats is relatively safe if risk factors are absent or well managed (Gowan et al, 2011; King et al, 2012; Narita et al, 2005; Raekallio et al, 2006; Roberts et al, 2009). On the basis of this available evidence, judicious use of NSAIDs for chronic pain management in an animal with CKD can be appropriate (Box 190-1) if the animal's quality of life in the absence of NSAID use is considered unacceptable by the owner and veterinarian and if alternative pain management approaches are ineffective.

Before long-term NSAID therapy is initiated, risk factors should be identified and managed. Some patients with CKD, such as animals who have experienced more than one unexplained bout of marked dehydration, are not suitable for long-term NSAID administration. Management of chronic dehydration (e.g., through the routine administration of fluids at home) should be instituted in affected CKD patients before NSAIDs are given. Baseline

---

BOX 190-1

Guidelines for Judicious Use of Nonsteroidal Antiinflammatory Drugs (NSAIDs) in Animals with Chronic Kidney Disease

- Use other pain management approaches first, such as weight loss, controlled exercise, physical therapy, and alternative analgesic agents.
- Avoid or manage factors that place animals at risk of nephrotoxicity (see Table 190-1).
- Use the lowest effective dosage, preferably intermittently.
- Select an NSAID with a low risk of gastrointestinal toxicity, generally a selective cyclooxygenase-2 inhibitor.
- Routinely screen the patient before and after each dosage adjustment.
- If evidence of toxicity is identified (see Table 190-1), permanently discontinue all use of NSAIDs.

medical testing before therapy includes a complete blood count, biochemical panel, complete urinalysis with sediment examination and quantification of proteinuria (i.e., ratio of urine protein to creatinine or microalbuminuria test), and urine culture. Although one study indicated that the use of meloxicam in cats with CKD was relatively safe (Gowan et al, 2011), comparable studies in dogs have not been done.

In terms of avoiding nephrotoxicity, there are no data to suggest that selective NSAIDs are safer than nonselective agents such as ibuprofen. However, the potential for gastrointestinal toxicity also must be considered; consequences of this more common adverse event also could lead to decompensation of CKD. Thus COX-2 selective agents are preferred when NSAIDs are indicated in CKD patients. Because CKD may alter drug pharmacokinetics and the potential for toxicity is related to dosage, the initial dosage should be subtherapeutic with upward adjustments made no more frequently than every 14 days until a minimal, acceptably effective dosage is reached. It also is preferable to use this minimal dosage intermittently, 7 to 10 days at a time, rather than continuously.

To determine whether adverse renal effects are present, evaluations should be made within 14 days of any dosage increase and before every dosage adjustment. Minimally, these should include measurement of serum creatinine, blood urea nitrogen, and electrolyte levels, and a complete urinalysis with sediment examination and quantification of proteinuria. Once a stable dosage has been identified, the patient should be evaluated similarly at 3-month intervals. If these data provide evidence of adverse effects on the kidney, NSAIDs should be discontinued immediately because an alternative pain management strategy is necessary. Changing to an alternate NSAID in the face of evidence of nephrotoxicity is not appropriate.

References and Suggested Reading

Bacia J et al: Ibuprofen toxicosis in a dog, *J Am Vet Med Assoc* 188:918, 1986.

Blanco G et al: Interaction of CYP2C8 and CYP2C9 genotypes modifies the risk for nonsteroidal anti-inflammatory drugs-related acute gastrointestinal bleeding, *Pharmacogenet Genomics* 18:37, 2008.

Boström IM et al: Effects of carprofen on renal function and results of serum biochemical and hematologic analyses in anesthetized dogs that had low blood pressure during anesthesia, *Am J Vet Res* 63:712, 2002.

Brown SA et al: Effect of dietary fatty acid supplementation in early renal insufficiency in dogs, *J Lab Clin Med* 135:275, 2000.

Cho KH et al: Niacin ameliorates oxidative stress, inflammation, proteinuria, and hypertension in rats with chronic renal failure, *Am J Physiol* 297:F106, 2009.

Goodman LA et al: Effects of meloxicam on plasma iohexol clearance as a marker of glomerular filtration rate in conscious, normal cats, *Am J Vet Res* 70:826, 2009.

Gowan R et al: Retrospective case control study of the effects of long-term dosing with meloxicam on renal function in aged cats with degenerative joint disease, *J Feline Med Surg* 13:752, 2011.

Harding P, Glass WF, Scherer SD: COX-2 inhibition potentiates the antiproteinuric effect of enalapril in uninephrectomized SHR, *Prostaglandins Leukot Essent Fatty Acids* 68:17, 2003.

Khan KNM et al: Interspecies differences in renal localization of cyclooxygenase isoforms: implications in nonsteroidal antiinflammatory drug-related nephrotoxicity, *Toxicol Pathol* 26:612, 1998.

King JN et al: Safety of oral robenacoxib in the cat, *J Vet Pharmacol Ther* 35(3):290, 2012. Epub July 8, 2011.

Narita T et al: Effects of long-term oral administration of ketoprofen in clinically healthy beagle dogs, *J Vet Med Sci* 67:847, 2005.

Poortinga EW, Hungerford LL: A case-control study of acute ibuprofen toxicity in dogs, *Prev Vet Med* 3:115, 1998.

Radi ZA: Pathophysiology of cyclooxygenase inhibition in animal models, *Toxicol Pathol* 37:34, 2009.

Raekallio MR et al: Evaluation of adverse effects of long-term orally administered carprofen in dogs, *J Am Vet Med Assoc* 228:876, 2006.

Roberts ES et al: Safety and tolerability of 3-week and 6-month dosing of Deramaxx (deracoxib) chewable tablets in dogs, *J Vet Pharmacol Ther* 32:329, 2009.

Sellers RS, Senese PB, Khan KN: Interspecies differences in the nephrotoxic response to cyclooxygenase inhibition, *Drug Chem Toxicol* 27:111, 2004.

Surdyk K, Sloan D, Brown SA: Evaluation of the renal effects of ibuprofen and carprofen in euvolemic and volume-depleted dogs, *Int J Appl Res Vet Med* 9:129, 2011.

Surdyk K, Sloan DL, Brown SA: Renal effects of carprofen and etodolac in euvolemic and volume-depleted dogs, *Am J Vet Res* 73:1485, 2012.

Surdyk K, Brown CA, Brown SA: Evaluation of glomerular filtration rate in cats with reduced renal mass and administered meloxicam and acetylsalicylic acid, *Am J Vet Res* 74(4):648, 2013.

Tsuchiya Y et al: Early pathophysiological features in canine renal papillary necrosis induced by nefiracetam, *Toxicol Pathol* 33:561, 2005.

Yabuki A et al: A comparative study of chronic kidney disease in dogs and cats: induction of cyclooxygenases, *Res Vet Sci* 93:892, 2012.

CHAPTER 191

Medical Management of Acute Kidney Injury

LINDA ROSS, *North Grafton, Massachusetts*

The term *acute kidney injury* (AKI) has replaced the historical term *acute renal failure* because it is believed to better describe the pathophysiologic changes and duration of the different phases of injury. It is defined as the rapid loss of nephron function (over hours to several days) resulting in azotemia; fluid, electrolyte, and acid-base abnormalities; and uremia. Many causes of AKI have been identified in dogs and cats. Although supportive therapy is similar in all cases, the prognosis and clinical outcome have been shown to vary depending on the cause (Vaden et al, 1997).

AKI can be divided into four pathophysiologic stages. The first, initiation, occurs during and immediately following the renal insult when pathologic damage to the kidneys is occurring. The second stage is extension during which ischemia, hypoxia, inflammation, and cellular injury continue, leading to cellular apoptosis or necrosis. The initiation and extension stages usually last less than 48 hours, and clinical and laboratory abnormalities may not be apparent during this time. The third stage, maintenance, is characterized by azotemia, uremia, or both and may last for days to weeks. Oliguria (<1 ml of urine per kilogram of body weight per hour) or anuria (no urine production) may occur during the maintenance stage. Urine production can be highly variable. The fourth stage is recovery, during which azotemia improves and renal tubules undergo repair. Marked polyuria may occur during this stage as a result of partial restoration of renal tubular function and osmotic diuresis of accumulated solutes. Renal function may return to normal, or the animal may be left with residual renal dysfunction. This stage also may last for weeks to months. Nonazotemic renal failure can occur and is characterized by abnormalities similar to those seen during the polyuric recovery stage of AKI. Treatment of AKI consists of treatment specific for the cause and supportive therapy based on the stage of AKI and the animal's fluid, electrolyte, and acid-base status. It is important to remember that the doses of drugs excreted primarily by the kidneys should be reduced or the dosing interval extended in proportion to the degree of azotemia.

Specific Therapy

Specific therapy to correct or eliminate the cause of AKI should be instituted if the cause is known or suspected. For example, in animals with known ethylene glycol ingestion vomiting should be induced if the ingestion occurred no more than 3 hours earlier, or drugs such as 4-methylpyrazole or ethanol should be given to prevent the metabolism of ethylene glycol to its toxic components. In geographic areas where leptospirosis occurs, all dogs with presumed AKI should receive an antibiotic effective against leptospires (penicillin, amoxicillin, or doxycycline). Empiric antibiotic therapy is indicated until pyelonephritis is ruled out by culture of urine or renal tissue.

Supportive Therapy

Fluid Therapy

Intravenous fluid therapy remains the mainstay of treatment for AKI. Frequent monitoring of the animal's hydration status, renal function, acid-base status, and electrolyte levels is necessary to determine appropriate intravenous fluid types and amounts. Placement of a catheter in the jugular vein allows monitoring of central venous pressure and more precise assessment of intravascular volume status. However, if hemodialysis is a treatment option, the jugular veins should not be used for intravenous catheters or even for venipuncture to obtain blood samples; rather, they should be preserved for placement of a central catheter for hemodialysis or other renal replacement therapy (see Chapter 192).

The initial volume of fluid to be administered should be calculated based on the animal's body weight and degree of hydration. Water deficits should be corrected within 4 to 6 hours to restore renal blood flow to normal as soon as possible. Maintenance fluid requirements (44 to 66 ml/kg/day) must be met and estimated fluid losses from vomiting or diarrhea replaced. Urine production should be monitored during the first few hours of fluid therapy. Placement of an indwelling urinary catheter is the most accurate method for such monitoring. However, the benefits of an indwelling catheter must be weighed against the risk of ascending infection and the need for sedation or anesthesia to place the catheter. The risk of infection can be reduced by scrupulous attention to sterile placement of the catheter, maintenance of a closed collection system, and daily cleansing of the visible portions of the catheter with disinfectant. Changing the urinary catheter every 2 to 3 days is recommended because the incidence of catheter-induced infections increases rapidly after 3 days when the same catheter is left in (Barsanti, 2010).

An isotonic, polyionic fluid such as lactated Ringer's solution or Plasma-Lyte A may be administered initially.

If hyperkalemia is present or suspected because of oliguria or anuria, use of a potassium-free fluid such as 0.9% sodium chloride is indicated. Following rehydration, the type of fluid should be adjusted based on the animal's fluid and electrolyte status. Polyionic fluids may contain too much sodium for maintenance, and half-strength lactated Ringer's solution or 0.45% sodium chloride in 2.5% dextrose may be used for long-term therapy.

Traditionally, intravenous fluids have been administered at as high a rate as the animal will tolerate without adverse signs, with the goal of maximizing glomerular filtration rate and renal blood flow and increasing elimination of metabolic waste products. However, an increase in fluid administration does not necessarily equate to increased urinary excretion of such substances. Recent studies in people have concluded that fluid overload is associated with adverse consequences and decreased survival; mortality decreased when fluid overload was corrected by dialysis (Bouchard et al, 2009). Although similar studies in clinical veterinary patients have not been reported, it would seem reasonable that avoiding fluid overload would be similarly beneficial, especially because dialysis is not readily available to many practices. One of the reasons for fluid overload is failure to adjust the fluid administration rate in the face of decreased urine production (see Chapter 186).

Management of Oliguria or Anuria

Once the animal has been hydrated, urine flow should increase rapidly to 2 to 5 ml/kg/hr, depending on the rate of intravenous fluid administration. If urine production is not sufficient, the clinician first should reassess the animal's circulating blood volume. Such assessment may include physical examination of hydration status, visual estimation of jugular venous pressure, measurement of packed cell volume and total solids, thoracic radiography to evaluate cardiac size and pulmonary vascular markings, and ultrasonographic imaging of the cardiac chambers and hepatic veins. Failure to restore circulating volume to normal is a common reason for decreased urine volume. If circulating blood volume is normal or increased, the rate of fluid administration should be slowed to prevent fluid overload. An indwelling urinary catheter should be placed if not already present. Calculation of inputs and outputs then can be used to provide appropriate quantities of intravenous fluids to match urine output. The maintenance fluid requirement (estimated at 22 ml/kg/day for insensible losses) is calculated for a short interval of time, typically 4 hours. The volume of urine produced during the previous time interval is added to the maintenance amount to obtain the volume of intravenous fluids to be administered over the next 4-hour period. This protocol helps maintain hydration while minimizing the risk of fluid overload.

Specific therapy to increase urine flow, consisting of administration of one or more diuretics, should be instituted next (Table 191-1). Furosemide can be administered as a bolus of 2 mg/kg IV, with escalation of doses to 4 to 6 mg/kg at hourly intervals if the initial dose fails to increase urine production. However, constant-rate infusion (CRI) has been shown to be more effective in

TABLE **191-1**

Drugs to Promote Urine Production in Animals with Oliguria or Anuria

Drug	Dosage
Furosemide	1.0 mg/kg IV bolus, followed by 1.0 mg/kg/hr CRI *or* 2 mg/kg IV bolus If effective, diuresis begins within 15-30 min Increase dosage to 4-6 mg/kg IV at hourly intervals if initial dose does not induce diuresis
Mannitol 20%	Contraindicated if animal has fluid overload, pulmonary edema, or congestive heart failure 0.5-1 g/kg IV bolus slowly, then 1-2 mg/kg/min CRI *or* Repeat bolus every 4-6 hr at a dose of 0.25-0.5 g/kg IV *or* 2 to 10 ml/min for the first 10 to 15 min IV, then 1 to 5 ml/min CRI for a total daily dose of 22 to 66 ml/kg; alternate with administration of a polyionic solution
Fenoldopam	0.8 µg/kg/min CRI

CRI, Constant-rate infusion; *IV,* intravenous.

producing diuresis than intermittent bolus doses (Adin et al, 2003). A loading dose of 1.0 mg/kg followed by a CRI at 1.0 mg/kg/hr is recommended. If furosemide administration fails to increase urine flow, osmotic diuresis can be attempted. Twenty percent mannitol can be given as a bolus dose of 0.5 to 1 g/kg of body weight over 15 to 20 minutes. If it is effective, urine flow will increase within 1 hour. Repeat bolus doses then can be administered every 4 to 6 hours, or mannitol can be administered as a CRI at 1 to 2 mg/kg/min. Mannitol may have additional beneficial effects in addition to its action as a diuretic. It inhibits renin release because of its hyperosmolar effect on tubular luminal filtrate. Mannitol also acts as a free-radical scavenger, blunting damaging increases in intramitochondrial calcium, and may result in a beneficial release of atrial natriuretic peptide. In actuality, mannitol is used infrequently because administration of a hypertonic solution is contraindicated in oliguric animals that are volume overloaded, and oliguria often is not recognized until overload already is present. Dopamine infusion traditionally has been recommended for oliguric or anuric animals. However, it is no longer considered to have a role in the prevention or treatment of AKI in people, based on several metaanalyses that failed to show a clinical benefit with regard to survival or need for dialysis (Friedrich et al, 2005; Kellum and Decker, 2001). There is little or no documentation of the efficacy of dopamine in dogs and cats with AKI, and its routine use to increase urine production in oliguric or anuric AKI cannot be justified.

In contrast, fenoldopam, a selective dopamine D1 receptor agonist, has been found to be renoprotective in people. A small number of studies in normal cats and dogs have suggested that fenoldopam administration may have beneficial effects on glomerular filtration rate and urine volume. Fenoldopam may be administered as a CRI of 0.8 µg/kg/min. Animals should be monitored for hypotension during administration (Bloom et al, 2012).

Management of Polyuria

Animals that recover from the oliguric or anuric phase of AKI, or those that have milder renal injury and do not develop azotemia, often have profound polyuria for days to weeks. These animals can develop electrolyte abnormalities, especially hyponatremia and hypokalemia, that need to be corrected with intravenous or sometimes oral therapy. Serum electrolyte levels should be monitored frequently and therapy adjusted until urine output decreases and renal function and serum electrolyte concentrations stabilize.

Correction of Acid-Base and Electrolyte Abnormalities

Metabolic acidosis occurs in AKI. Alkalinizing therapy is not recommended unless the blood pH is less than 7.2 or the serum bicarbonate level is less than 14 mEq/L after correction of fluid deficits because it can result in significant complications, including paradoxical cerebrospinal fluid acidosis, decreased ionized serum calcium concentration, and hypernatremia. If necessary, the bicarbonate deficit is calculated as follows:

$$\text{Body weight (in kg)} \times 0.3 \times (24 - \text{measured bicarbonate}) = \text{mEq bicarbonate deficit}$$

One quarter of the deficit is added as sodium bicarbonate to the intravenous fluids over 12 hours, and acid-base status is reassessed before further administration.

Moderate to severe life-threatening hyperkalemia may occur if the animal is oliguric or anuric. The first and most important step in therapy for hyperkalemia is to ensure urine production and excretion. Animals with severe hyperkalemia or those in which oliguria persists may benefit from additional specific therapy such as sodium bicarbonate, regular insulin, and glucose, or in life-threatening situations calcium gluconate. Hypokalemia may occur during the diuretic phase of AKI. Therapy consisting of intravenous or oral potassium chloride is indicated if the serum potassium concentration is below the normal range, although clinical signs not are usually apparent until it falls below 2.5 mEq/L.

Treatment of Other Uremic Signs

Vomiting

Vomiting can be a significant problem in animals with AKI. Drugs that inhibit gastric acid production are indicated because uremia results in hypergastrinemia. These drugs include histamine receptor antagonists such as famotidine (0.5 to 1 mg/kg q24h PO) and proton pump inhibitors such as omeprazole (0.7 mg/kg q24h PO) or pantoprazole (Protonix; 0.7 to 1.0 mg/kg q24h IV). Centrally acting antiemetics also may be necessary.

Metoclopramide, a dopamine antagonist, may be given as intermittent therapy at a dosage of 0.2 to 0.5 mg/kg q8h IV or as a CRI at 1 to 2 mg/kg q24h IV. Other centrally acting drugs are dolasetron (Anzemet; 0.6 mg/kg q24h PO or SC or diluted in compatible IV fluid and administered over 15 min IV) and ondansetron (Zofran; 0.1 to 0.2 mg/kg q8h SC or 0.5 mg/kg IV loading dose and then 0.5 mg/kg/hr CRI). The neurokinin-1 antagonist maropitant (Cerenia; 1 mg/kg q24h SC) is effective as a centrally and peripherally acting antiemetic in treating nausea and vomiting from renal failure. Phenothiazine-derivative antiemetics such as chlorpromazine (0.2 to 0.5 mg/kg q6-8h SC, IM, or IV) can be tried if vomiting persists despite other therapy. Adverse effects of phenothiazines include sedation and decreased blood pressure.

Hypertension

Arterial hypertension was found in 37% of dogs with AKI at the time of hospital admission in one study. This percentage increased to 81% during hospitalization, which was attributed to progressive disease, aggressive fluid therapy, oliguria or anuria, stress, and pain (Geigy et al, 2011). Treatment of hypertension includes reducing the rate of intravenous fluid administration, administering diuretics, and performing dialysis to remove excess fluid if the animal is oliguric or anuric. Pharmacologic treatment is limited because most antihypertensive drugs are available only in oral formulations, and the vomiting associated with AKI often precludes oral administration. If hypertension is severe, parenteral antihypertensives that can be used include nitroprusside (initial dose 1 to 2 µg/kg/min CRI IV; titrate up q5min to achieve desired blood pressure) and hydralazine (0.5 to 3 mg/kg q12h IV or 0.1 mg/kg loading dose IV and then 1.5 to 5 µg/kg/min CRI IV). Administration of both drugs requires close monitoring. Oral antihypertensives include amlodipine (dogs: 0.1 to 0.25 mg/kg q12-24h PO; cats: 0.625 to 1.25 mg per cat q24h PO) and angiotensin-converting enzyme (ACE) inhibitors such as enalapril (0.25 to 0.5 mg/kg q12-24h PO) and benazepril (Lotensin; 0.25 to 0.5 mg/kg q24h PO). Rectal administration of amlodipine dissolved in a small amount of saline has been reported to be effective (Geigy et al, 2011). ACE inhibitors have been associated with worsening of renal function in humans.

Nutritional Management

Nutritional support has been shown to be important for recovery from AKI. These animals are in a state of negative nutritional balance at a time when protein and energy are needed to support regeneration of damaged renal tissue. Enteral nutrition via an esophagostomy or gastrostomy tube can be used if the animal is not vomiting; otherwise parenteral nutrition is indicated.

Prognosis and Duration of Therapy

The prognosis for dogs and cats with AKI depends on the cause and the response to therapy. Those patients in which the cause is identified and treated early in the course of the disease (e.g., pyelonephritis and leptospirosis) have a relatively good prognosis. Animals with ethylene glycol toxicity that are already azotemic when diagnosed have been shown to have a poor to grave prognosis, even with therapy. Other factors that have been shown to confer a poor prognosis are severe azotemia (serum creatinine level of >10 mg/dl), lack of improvement or worsening of azotemia in spite of appropriate fluid and supportive therapy, and concurrent systemic disease such as pancreatitis or sepsis.

Supportive and specific treatment should be continued until one of the following occurs: (1) renal function returns to normal; (2) renal function improves and stabilizes, although not at normal levels, and the animal is doing well clinically; (3) renal function worsens, fails to improve, or does not improve sufficiently for the animal to be managed medically at home for the resulting renal insufficiency. In the first two cases fluid therapy can be tapered and other supportive medications adjusted in response to the animal's clinical signs. In the third case dialysis may be considered to support the animal for a longer period of time to see if renal function improves. If dialysis is not an option, euthanasia may be indicated at this point.

References and Suggested Reading

Adin DB et al: Intermittent bolus injection versus continuous infusion of furosemide in normal adult greyhound dogs, *J Vet Intern Med* 17:632, 2003.

Barsanti JA: Urinary tract catheterization and nosocomial infections in dogs and cats. In *Proceedings of the 29th Annual Internal Veterinary Medicine Forum*, 2010, p 445.

Bloom CA et al: Preliminary pharmacokinetics and cardiovascular effects of fenoldopam continuous rate infusion in six healthy dogs, *J Vet Pharmacol Ther* 35(3):224, 2012. Epub July 6, 2011.

Bouchard J et al: Fluid accumulation, survival, and recovery of kidney function in critically ill patients with acute kidney injury, *Kidney Int* 76:422, 2009.

Cowgill LD, Langston C: Acute kidney insufficiency. In Bartges J, Polzin DJ, editors: *Nephrology and urology of small animals*, Chichester, UK, 2011, Wiley-Blackwell, p 472.

Friedrich JO et al: Meta-analysis: low-dose dopamine increases urine output but does not prevent renal dysfunction or death, *Ann Intern Med* 142:510, 2005.

Geigy CA et al: Occurrence of systemic hypertension in dogs with acute kidney injury and treatment with amlodipine besylate, *J Small Anim Pract* 52:340, 2011.

Kellum JA, Decker JM: Use of dopamine in acute renal failure: a meta-analysis, *Crit Care Med* 29:1526, 2001.

Langston C: Managing fluid and electrolyte disorders in renal failure. In DiBartola SP, editor: *Fluid, electrolyte, and acid-base disorders in small animal practice*, ed 4, St Louis, 2012, Saunders, p 544.

Ross LA: Acute kidney injury, *Vet Clin North Am Small Anim Pract* 41:1, 2011.

Vaden SL, Levine J, Breitschwerdt EB: A retrospective case-control of acute renal failure in 99 dogs, *J Vet Intern Med* 11:58, 1997.

CHAPTER 192

Continuous Renal Replacement Therapy

MARK J. ACIERNO, *Baton Rouge, Louisiana*

Continuous renal replacement therapy (CRRT) is a relatively new blood purification modality that is rapidly gaining acceptance for the treatment of azotemia as well as acid-base, electrolyte, and fluid imbalances associated with acute kidney injury (AKI). As its name implies, CRRT is a continuous modality, and once a patient begins treatment, therapy continues until renal function returns or the patient is transitioned to intermittent dialysis. Potential advantages of CRRT over intermittent dialysis include better control of acid-base and electrolyte balance. CRRT also is appealing because it does not require a significant investment in water purification facilities and maintenance, as is the case with intermittent dialysis. This chapter provides a brief overview of the principles, methodology, and indications for CRRT in dogs and cats.

Principles and Mechanisms

All extracorporeal blood purification takes places within the dialyzer, where the patient's blood is divided and directed into thousands of strawlike semipermeable membranes. Traditional hemodialysis primarily is a *diffusive* modality in which the strawlike semipermeable membranes are bathed in dialysate solution. Substances that are in higher concentration in the blood, such as urea, diffuse across the membrane into the dialysate, whereas substances that are in higher concentration in the dialysate, such as bicarbonate, leave the dialysate and enter the blood. Movement of individual molecules in or out of the blood can be controlled by adjusting the concentration of a given substance in the dialysate.

CRRT uses diffusion as well as *convection* and *adhesion*. Convection exposes blood traveling through the straw-like semipermeable membranes to a positive transmembrane pressure. This forces fluid, called *ultrafiltrate*, out of the blood. Uremic toxins, electrolytes, and other small molecules are carried with the fluid and then discarded. A sterile balanced electrolyte solution is added to the blood to replace the ultrafiltrate. The primary advantage of convection is its ability to remove larger molecules from the blood than can diffusion; however, convection is technically challenging because the fluid removed must be replaced with accuracy or acid-base, electrolyte, and fluid imbalances can occur rapidly.

Adhesion is the tendency of molecules to adhere to the dialyzer's semipermeable membrane. For example, inflammatory cytokines can be removed by adhesion from the blood of septic patients receiving CRRT; however, it is not clear if this actually improves patient survival.

Continuous Renal Replacement Therapy Modalities

Although CRRT often is thought of as a single treatment modality, it actually combines the principles of diffusion, convection, and adhesion to provide four different therapies: slow continuous ultrafiltration, continuous venovenous hemofiltration, continuous venovenous hemodialysis, and continuous venovenous hemodiafiltration. Many CRRT systems also can perform *therapeutic plasma exchange,* which can be used in the treatment of autoimmune diseases and may be helpful in removing some protein-bound toxins.

Slow continuous ultrafiltration (SCUF) (Figure 192-1) is a purely convective modality in which a positive transmembrane pressure forces fluid (ultrafiltrate) out of the blood and the hemoconcentrated blood is returned to the patient. In human medicine, SCUF is used widely for the treatment of diuretic-resistant congestive heart failure. Its utility in veterinary medicine currently is under investigation.

Continuous venovenous hemofiltration (CVVH) (Figure 192-2) also is a purely convective modality; however, unlike SCUF, the ultrafiltrate is replaced with a sterile balanced electrolyte solution. The solution can be added to the blood before or after it passes through the dialyzer. In a postdialyzer configuration, a positive transmembrane pressure forces fluid out of the blood, which increases hemoconcentration. Before the patient's blood is returned, replacement fluids are added to restore it to physiologic packed cell volume. This is an extremely effective way to remove uremic toxins; however, as the blood becomes hemoconcentrated, there is a risk that the dialyzer will sludge and clot. This limits the amount of fluid that can be removed by CVVH to approximately 25% of blood

SCUF

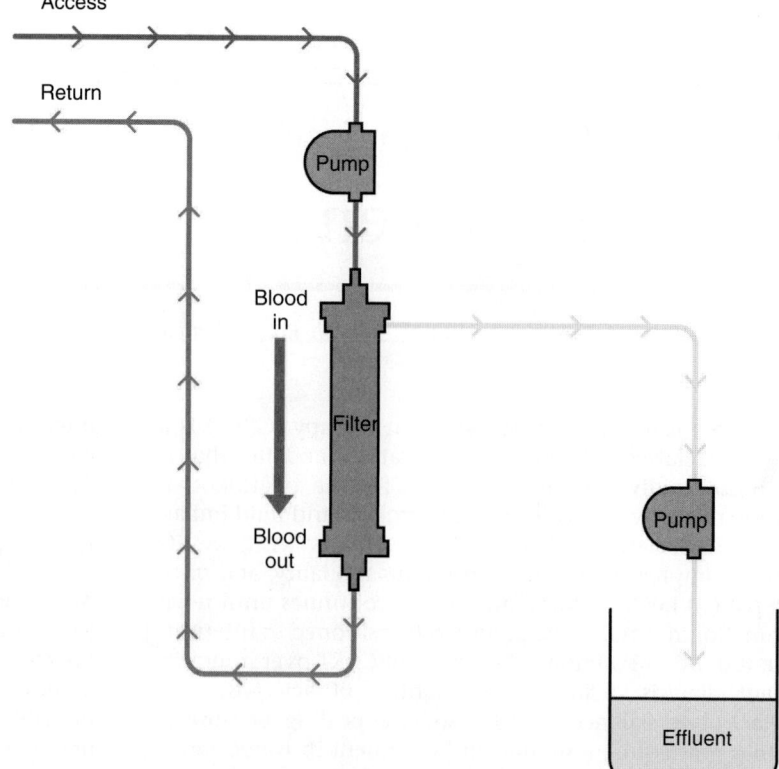

Figure 192-1 Slow continuous ultrafiltration (SCUF) is a purely convective modality that generates ultrafiltrate that is not replaced. (Used with permission, Veterinary Learning Systems.)

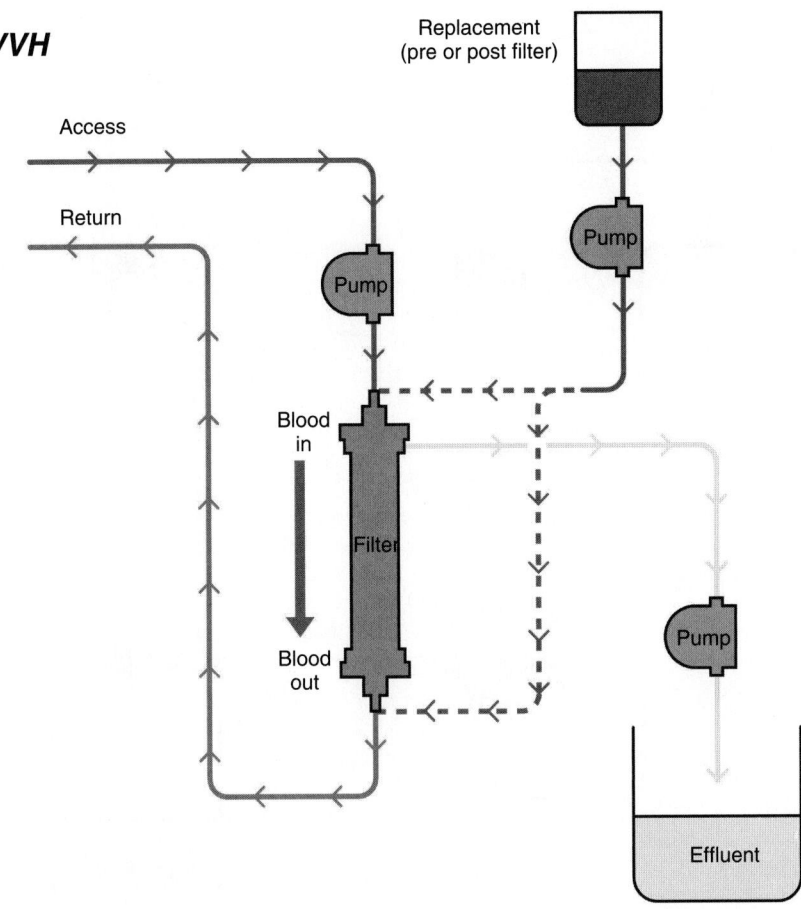

CVVH

Figure 192-2 Continuous venovenous hemofiltration (CVVH) is a convective modality that generates ultrafiltrate. Unlike in slow continuous ultrafiltration, the ultrafiltrate is replaced with a sterile balanced electrolyte solution. This fluid can be added before or after the blood passes through the dialyzer. (Used with permission, Veterinary Learning Systems.)

plasma volume. Alternatively, replacement fluids can be added to the blood before it passes through the dialyzer. The diluted blood then enters the dialyzer, where the excess fluid is removed by convection. Although this is less likely to result in dialyzer clotting, the prefilter arrangement is significantly less effective in removing uremic toxins.

Continuous venovenous hemodialysis (CVVHD) is a diffusive therapy that closely resembles intermittent hemodialysis (Figure 192-3). Blood enters the dialyzer, where it is divided into thousands of strawlike semipermeable membranes that are bathed in dialysate. Substances that are in high concentration in the blood leave the blood and enter the dialysate, whereas substances whose concentration is higher in the dialysate enter the blood.

Continuous venovenous hemodiafiltration (CVVHDF) combines the diffusive aspects of CVVHD with the convective aspects of CVVH (Figure 192-4). Blood flowing through the dialyzer's semipermeable membranes are bathed in dialysis solution and exposed to a positive transmembrane pressure so that both diffusion and ultrafiltration guides the movement of solutes.

It is not clear which modality is most effective for uremic animals. Convective modalities (CVVH, CVVHDF) have an advantage in the size of the molecules that they are capable of removing; however, the role that large molecules play in uremia and azotemia is unclear. Diffusion (CVVHD) is just as efficient in removing smaller

molecules such as urea and creatinine. In our hospital, we have been employing convective modalities (CVVH, CVVHDF) with good success.

Key Technical Considerations

Anticoagulation

Although CRRT circuits are made of highly biocompatible material, inadequate anticoagulation results in dialyzer clotting. This leads to a loss of patient blood, requires replacement of a costly dialyzer circuit, and represents time that the patient is not receiving treatment. Systemic heparinization and regional citrate infusion are the two most commonly employed CRRT anticoagulation techniques. Heparin is inexpensive, simple to monitor, and effective; however, under certain conditions, it can be associated with bleeding. Citrate can be added to blood as it leaves the patient, providing regional anticoagulation of the CRRT circuit. Calcium is then returned directly to the patient as a constant infusion. The primary advantage of citrate is that it anticoagulates only the CRRT circuit. Large studies in people have demonstrated that the use of citrate may be associated with fewer patient compilations and longer intervals between dialyzer failures; however, citrate anticoagulation in dogs and cats has been associated with significant alkalosis and hypocalcemia and thus necessitates significant acid-base and

CVVHD

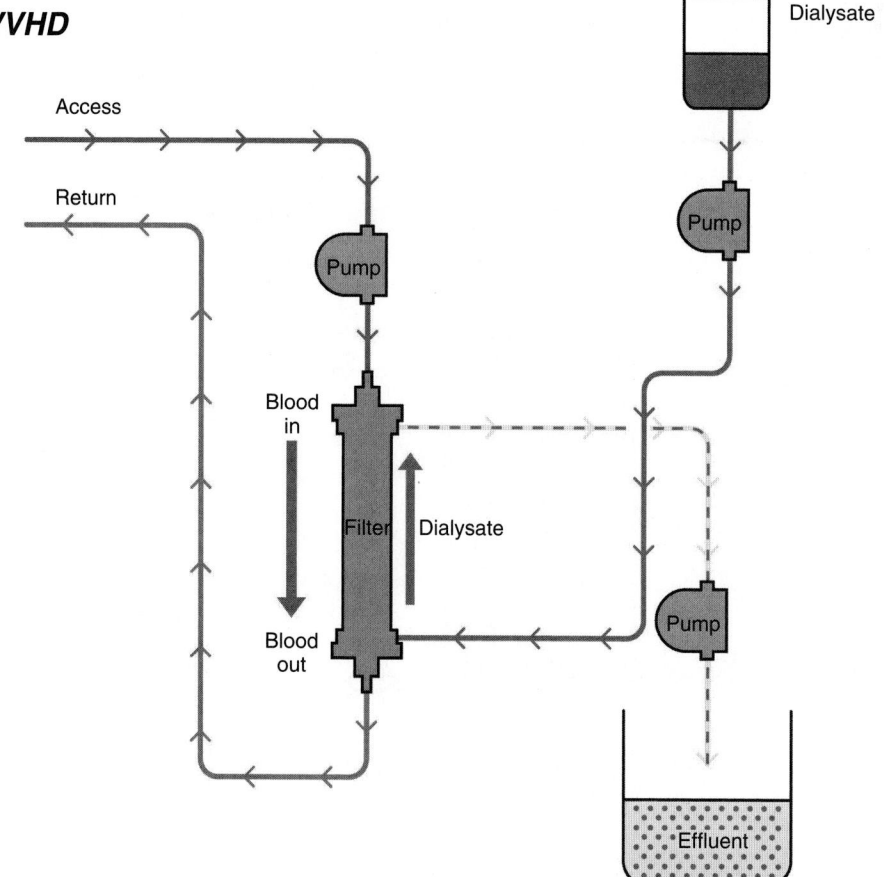

Figure 192-3 Continuous venovenous hemodialysis (CVVHD) is a diffusive therapy in which the movement of small molecules is guided by their relative concentrations in the dialysate. (Used with permission, Veterinary Learning Systems.)

CVVHDF

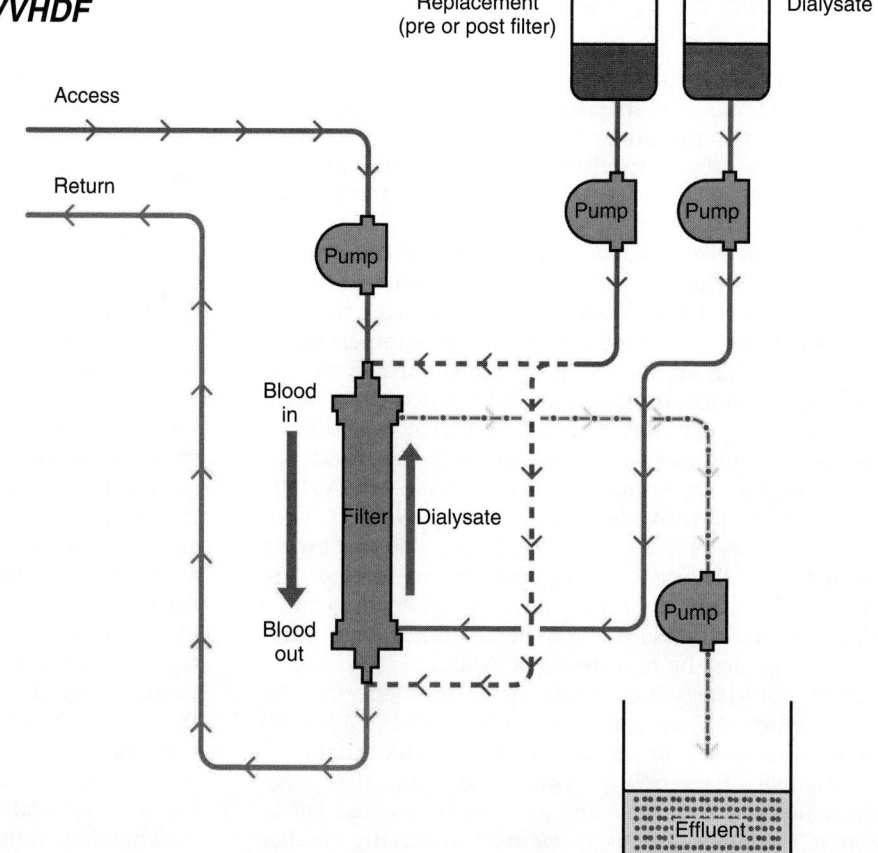

Figure 192-4 Continuous venovenous hemodiafiltration (CVVHDF) combines the diffusive aspects of continuous venovenous hemodialysis with the convective properties of continuous venovenous hemofiltration. Convection guides the movement of both large and small molecules, whereas diffusion is efficient in removing smaller molecules such as urea and creatinine. (Used with permission, Veterinary Learning Systems.)

electrolyte monitoring. Because of its lower cost, ease of use, and lower complication rate, most veterinary centers use heparin anticoagulation for both intermittent hemodialysis and CRRT.

Blood Access

In all but the smallest patients, a dual-lumen temporary dialysis catheter can be placed in the jugular vein using the Seldinger technique. Typically, a 13.5 Fr catheter is placed in large dogs, medium dogs get an 11.5 Fr catheter, whereas smaller dogs and cats receive a 7 Fr catheter. In the smallest patients we typically place a single-lumen 5 Fr dialysis catheter in each jugular vein.

Treatment Adequacy

Calculation of the CRRT prescription (blood flows, dialysate rates, convective rates) is based on formulas that take into account patient urea clearance. One such formula uses urea clearance per unit of time for a given volume of distribution and is known as Kt/V. Detailed information regarding these calculations can be found elsewhere (Acierno, 2011).

Indications

The most common indications for CRRT are the treatment of AKI in patients whose kidneys are expected to recover in a short period of time (days to weeks) and the stabilization of patients that will be transitioned to intermittent dialysis. We have successfully treated cases of AKI secondary to leptospirosis, tumor lysis syndrome, melamine toxicity, and heat stroke. Removal of drugs and toxins may be another indication for CRRT; however, intermittent dialysis may be more effective depending on the toxin's characteristics. Fluid removal in patients with congestive heart failure unresponsive to diuretics is a recognized use of CRRT in people, and CRRT may be useful in this setting in cats and dogs. Some important considerations before referring a case for CRRT are listed in Boxes 192-1 and 192-2. The most up-to-date listing of centers offering CRRT can be found on the Veterinary CRRT Web Page (www.vetcrrt.net).

References and Suggested Reading

Acierno MJ: Continuous renal replacement therapy, *Vet Clin North Am Small Anim Pract* 41(1):135, 2011.

Antoun TA, Palevsky PM: The clinical application of CRRT—current status: selection of modality of renal replacement therapy, *Semin Dial* 22(2):108, 2009.

Diehl SH, Seshadri R: Use of continuous renal replacement therapy for treatment of dogs and cats with acute or acute-on-chronic renal failure: 33 cases (2002-2006), *J Vet Emerg Crit Care* 18(4):370, 2008.

Langston CE: Hemodialysis. In Polzin D, Bartges J, editors: *Nephrology and urology of small animals*, Ames, IA, 2009, Wiley-Blackwell, p 255.

Martin A, Acierno MJ: Continuous renal replacement therapy in the treatment of acute kidney injury and electrolyte disturbances associated with acute tumor lysis syndrome, *J Vet Intern Med* 24(4):986, 2010.

CHAPTER 193

Surveillance for Asymptomatic and Hospital-Acquired Urinary Tract Infection

KATE S. KUKANICH, *Manhattan, Kansas*

Generally a patient develops a urinary tract infection (UTI) when microbial colonization leads to adherence, multiplication, and persistent invasion of the urinary tract. However, in some patients bacteria exist within the urinary tract without causing disease or clinical signs, and these patients are said to have bacterial colonization or bacteriuria. Long-term asymptomatic bacteriuria has been documented in human patients; it may result when organisms lack the virulence traits necessary to adhere and cause disease, and these organisms may protect the urinary tract by competing with pathogenic bacterial strains. Although specific diagnostic and therapeutic guidelines have been developed for asymptomatic bacteriuria in human beings, the role and significance of asymptomatic or subclinical bacteriuria is much less clear in veterinary medicine, and evidence-based guidelines are not yet available.

Pathophysiology

Host factors and bacterial factors both affect whether a microbial organism can persist and cause infection within the urinary tract. Numerous local and systemic components of the host immune system protect against infection, and alterations in these immune defenses can predispose to the development of UTI. Local immunity involves normal micturition (complete and regular voiding), physiologic and anatomic features (peristalsis, length of the urethra, ureterovesical valves), mucosal defense barriers (glycosaminoglycans, mucosal exfoliation, competition from normal distal flora), and antimicrobial properties of urine (urea, organic acids, Tamm-Horsfall proteins, hyperosmolality, and extreme pH), whereas systemic immunity can be humoral or cell mediated.

The majority of UTIs are caused by bacteria that ascend the urogenital tract, and bacteria may possess virulence traits that increase their ability to overcome local defenses and ascend, adhere, and cause disease. These virulence factors can include adhesins (fimbriae, pili), toxins (cytotoxic necrotizing factor, hemolysin), methods of avoiding the host immune system (capsular antigen), and ways to utilize host nutrients (aerobactin). In addition to bacteria, *Candida* can cause ascending UTI, especially in immunosuppressed patients. Hematogenous spread of bacterial and fungal organisms to the urinary tract occurs less frequently.

Risk Factors

Various studies have evaluated the risk and prevalence of UTI in veterinary patients with specific comorbidities or concurrent therapies. Although most authors consider a finding of more than 1000 colony-forming units (CFU)/ml in a quantitative culture of urine (collected by cystocentesis) to be significant, authors use a variety of definitions of UTI; specific definitions used in each study described here have been included when relevant.

Exogenous and Endogenous Steroids

It has long been believed that glucocorticoid therapy, by suppressing local and systemic immunity, may predispose to UTI. Two studies found positive urine culture results in 39% of dogs (Ihrke et al, 1985) and 18% of dogs (Torres et al, 2005) with chronic skin disorders that received long-term low-dose corticosteroids, compared with no positive urine culture results in dogs with chronic skin disorders that did not receive steroids. In these studies, no dogs had clinical signs of UTI. The type of steroid administered, frequency of administration, duration, and dosage of corticosteroid were not correlated with culture results. Dogs receiving short-term steroid therapy also may be affected because dogs administered dexamethasone in the 48 hours before hospital admission for surgical fixation of intervertebral disk disease were 11.4 times more likely to have a positive urine culture result (>5 CFU/ml) than dogs undergoing such surgery that had not received dexamethasone (Levine et al, 2008). For patients with intervertebral disk disease, this increased risk may be due to the immunosuppressive properties of dexamethasone in combination with altered neurologic function (inability to void completely). Of dogs with naturally occurring hyperadrenocorticism, 46% were found to have a UTI (>1000 CFU/ml), but clinical signs of UTI were rare (Forrester et al, 1999). UTI in these dogs may be caused by systemic immunosuppression, dilute urine causing local alterations in immunity, or concurrent disease. The antiinflammatory properties of glucocorticoids also may influence the development of clinical signs related to UTI and the presence of pyuria on urine sediment examination.

Diabetes Mellitus

Veterinary patients with diabetes mellitus have been considered at increased risk for UTI because of factors such as immunosuppression, inappropriate urine concentration, and glucosuria. In human patients, diabetic individuals with asymptomatic bacteriuria do not have an increased risk of developing symptomatic UTI or other diabetic complications requiring hospitalization; no similar data are available for companion animals. In canine studies, UTI (>1000 CFU/ml) was present in 24% to 37% of dogs with diabetes mellitus, but few patients had clinical signs specific for UTI (Forrester et al, 1999; McGuire et al, 2002). Cats with diabetes mellitus also may be at increased risk of subclinical UTI, with 12% to 13% of diabetic cats found to have bacterial growth in their urine; clinical signs were present in 14% to 44% of those with bacterial growth (Bailiff et al, 2006; Mayer-Roenne et al, 2007). Emphysematous cystitis, most often caused by gas production associated with *Escherichia coli* invasion of the urinary bladder wall, is a complication of UTI specifically recognized in diabetic veterinary patients as well.

Kidney Disease

Dogs and cats with chronic kidney disease (CKD) may have impaired systemic immunity (neutrophil dysfunction, reduced cell-mediated immunity) and local immune function (altered urine composition) that could lead to increased risk of UTI. In two studies bacterial growth in urine culture was identified in 22% to 30% of cats with CKD, with 23% of these cats showing clinical signs of lower urinary tract disease (Barber et al, 1999; Mayer-Roenne et al, 2007). Although female sex was associated with UTI in both studies, there was no association between UTI and age (>10 years) in either study, which suggests that young and middle-aged cats with CKD also are at risk of UTI.

Miscellaneous Systemic Conditions

Numerous other systemic illnesses may predispose dogs and cats to clinical or subclinical UTI. In one study, 12% of hyperthyroid cats had positive urine culture results, but no cats had clinical signs of a UTI (Mayer-Roenne et al, 2007). In dogs with parvoviral enteritis, 23% developed subclinical UTI (>1000 CFU/ml), suspected to be caused by fecal contamination of the urogenital tract combined with neutropenia (Koutinas et al, 1998). It is also commonly believed that veterinary patients receiving chemotherapy or nonsteroidal immunosuppressive therapy (e.g., cyclosporine) are at increased risk of UTI due to immunosuppression. Finally, morbidly obese dogs (>45% body fat) have been documented to have 7.5 times greater risk of asymptomatic UTI than dogs with less than 45% body fat (Lusby et al, 2011).

Local Urogenital Conditions

Any disorder that alters the uroepithelial surface (uroliths, neoplasia), micturition (obstruction, neurologic dysfunction, ectopic ureters), or the distal urogenital tract (juvenile vulva) may predispose to UTI by altering local immune defenses and potentially creating a nidus for infection. In these cases, it may be difficult to recognize clinical signs of a developing UTI because they may overlap with signs from the predisposing condition. Cats with feline lower urinary tract disease (FLUTD) are a common exception in terms of this risk factor (<3% UTI prevalence); risk of UTI increases in older cats with FLUTD (45% UTI prevalence in cats >10 yr), often as a comorbidity with CKD (Kruger et al, 1991). Cats with FLUTD that recently underwent catheterization or perineal urethrostomy and have clinical signs also have increased risk of bacteriuria and UTI (Griffin and Gregory, 1992).

Hospitalization

UTIs represent up to 40% of all hospital-acquired infections reported in human patients. High-risk patients include those with indwelling urinary catheters, those undergoing urogenital procedures, and those with debilitating diseases (Kalsi et al, 2003). In veterinary medicine, UTIs are among the most common hospital-acquired infections as well, with the causative bacteria originating from the patient's fecal flora or the hospital environment. In catheterized patients, bacterial ascension can occur from either within or around the catheter to the urinary bladder. Risk of UTI comes from catheter-induced damage to the uroepithelium, from the catheter itself (through introduction of bacteria and bypassing of urethral defenses), and from biofilm formation. Up to 45% of dogs with indwelling urinary catheters develop a UTI (>1000 CFU/ml), and the odds of UTI in a hospitalized dog with an indwelling catheter increase with age (by 20% for each advanced year), with duration of catheterization (by 27% per day), and with antimicrobial administration (by 454%) (Bubenik et al, 2007). Hospital-acquired UTIs also may occur in systemically immunosuppressed patients (e.g., patients with immune-mediated hemolytic anemia, chemotherapy patients), those with urogenital disease, and those with diarrhea.

Surveillance and Diagnosis

It is estimated that up to 14% of dogs will develop a UTI during their lifetime; however, the overall incidence of asymptomatic bacteriuria or UTI is not known. Nor is there a consensus in the veterinary literature on which patients should be screened for UTI or how frequently screening should occur. For a dog or cat with an identified risk factor, two considerations can be used to determine the clinical importance of screening: (1) Could clinical signs of UTI be present but overlooked in this individual patient? (2) What are the consequences of not promptly addressing a UTI in this patient? Clinical signs of UTI may not be recognized in veterinary patients as quickly as in human patients and may be overlooked because of an animal's stoic nature, environmental factors (e.g., outdoor dogs), or concurrent disease. Possible consequences, such as risk of bacterial ascension from the urinary bladder to cause development of pyelonephritis or sepsis, may be a concern for patients that are immunocompromised either locally or systemically, and these consequences and their incidence have not been thoroughly evaluated in veterinary medicine.

Therefore each case should be evaluated individually, with consideration of perceived risk factors for UTI and the potential consequences of untreated UTI, to determine if and when screening is necessary. Clients should be educated about the clinical signs of UTI so that their vigilance may detect signs early. Because of the increased risk and potential consequences of UTI for the upper urinary tract (e.g., pyelonephritis) in patients with CKD, it is recommended that urine culture be performed twice a year in dogs and cats with CKD. Although endocrine disorders may increase the risk of UTI, untreated UTI also may interfere with regulation of endocrine disorders. Similarly, a urine culture is recommended for all dogs newly diagnosed with diabetes or Cushing's syndrome, and culture should be repeated in cases of insulin resistance, diabetic ketoacidosis, or uncontrolled hyperadrenocorticism (Hess et al, 2000). For patients with uroliths or bladder neoplasia that are undergoing procedures, culture of the uroliths and bladder mucosa may be more sensitive than urine culture (Gatoria et al, 2006). There is no consensus on how frequently to culture urine in patients with transitional cell carcinoma, but a change in clinical signs may suggest infection. Ideally, in these patients urine should be collected by midstream free catch rather than cystocentesis to avoid disrupting and seeding neoplastic cells. For midstream samples, growth of an organism at more than 100,000 CFU/ml is considered significant.

There are no evidence-based guidelines for screening hospitalized veterinary patients for UTI. A recent consensus suggests that for patients with indwelling catheters and no clinical signs of UTI, a urine culture should be performed at the time of catheter removal only if that patient is considered at high risk of complications from an untreated UTI (Weese et al, 2011). If a patient with an indwelling catheter develops clinical signs of UTI (e.g., fever, hematuria) and has evidence of infection on urine sediment examination, urine should be submitted for culture and the catheter should be removed (ideally) or replaced before therapy. Similarly, urine culture should be considered for intensive care patients without indwelling urinary catheters when fever or sepsis of unknown cause occurs or when clinical signs of UTI are observed.

Surveillance Process

Urinalysis, including a sediment examination, is recommended in combination with urine culture when screening for UTI. Urine specific gravity and glucose concentration may provide information about concurrent disease. Urine sediment examinations may show evidence of pyuria and bacteriuria in veterinary patients with clinically significant UTIs; however, these findings are not always present, and their absence does not rule out a clinically important infection. When urine culture is performed, quantitative bacterial assessment should be requested to determine if a positive culture result on a specimen collected by cystocentesis likely reflects contamination (<100 CFU/ml) or significant growth (>1000 CFU/ml); for samples obtained via catheter, more than 10,000 CFU/ml is considered significant. Research currently is ongoing to determine whether analyzing urine for bacterial virulence factors and host mucosal response (cytokine production) may help to indicate pathogenicity and invasiveness and differentiate benign bacteriuria from clinically important UTI (Wood, 2011).

Treatment

The decision to treat a patient with an asymptomatic UTI should be made by weighing the potential risks of complications from an untreated UTI (e.g., pyelonephritis, urosepsis) against the potential risks of therapy, including adverse effects, cost, and potential development of subsequent antimicrobial resistance. Of course, proper identification and treatment of underlying diseases that increase the risk of UTI are the primary components of prevention and control of UTI.

The recommendation in human medicine is to treat adults with asymptomatic bacteriuria if they are pregnant, if they are undergoing urogenital surgical procedures that may cause mucosal bleeding, or if bacteriuria is persistent 48 hours after a urinary catheter is removed; specific treatment is not recommended in patients with other concurrent diseases such as diabetes mellitus (Nicolle et al, 2005). Similar specific guidelines are not available for veterinary patients. If significant bacteriuria (>1000 CFU/ml) is found incidentally in a clinically healthy animal, therapy may not be needed, although a repeat urine culture in 1 to 2 weeks should be considered. In patients with concurrent conditions that are considered at risk for bacterial ascension to the kidneys or systemic circulation, consensus suggests that treatment is warranted even when clinical signs are not appreciated (Weese et al, 2011). Until further studies are available, veterinary patients in this category may include patients receiving immunosuppressive therapy; those with hyperadrenocorticism, diabetes mellitus, and CKD; and others whose systemic and local defenses may be altered.

Despite increased risk of bacteriuria caused by indwelling urinary catheters, catheterized patients should not receive prophylactic antibiotic therapy while the catheter is indwelling. Therapy should be reserved for those patients with clinical signs of UTI and a quantitative urine culture showing more than 1000 CFU/ml and should be initiated after the urinary catheter is removed or replaced (Weese et al, 2011). A similar approach may be appropriate for patients with voiding dysfunction that is expected to resolve quickly (e.g., intervertebral disk disease, acute overdistention or obstruction). Selection of an antimicrobial agent for treatment of UTI should be based on results of culture and susceptibility testing and ideally should be targeted at all pathogenic bacteria identified. Guidelines for antimicrobial selection, dosage, and duration of treatment for simple, complicated, and multidrug-resistant UTIs are available elsewhere.

Prevention

Although prevention of bacteriuria and UTI may not always be possible, precautions should be taken in an attempt to minimize their impact in veterinary patients. Promptly diagnosing and treating conditions that may affect a patient's normal defenses are one way to minimize risk. In cases in which comorbidities continue, clients can be educated about the risk of UTI and can be the first line of surveillance for clinical signs. To minimize hospital-acquired UTIs, urinary catheters should be placed only when absolutely necessary and should be removed as soon as possible. Catheters should be placed using aseptic technique, with minimal trauma, and should be maintained as closed systems. Veterinary hospitals should stress hand hygiene for all employees, especially those in intensive care units coming in contact with immunosuppressed patients or those with urinary catheters. Making every effort to keep urinary catheters and the surrounding skin clean and free of fecal and environmental contamination also may help to reduce the risk of hospital-acquired UTIs.

References and Suggested Reading

Bailiff NL et al: Frequency and risk factors for urinary tract infection in cats with diabetes mellitus, *J Vet Intern Med* 20:850, 2006.

Barber PJ et al: Incidence and prevalence of bacterial urinary tract infections in cats with chronic renal failure, *J Vet Intern Med* 13:251, 1999.

Bubenik LJ et al: Frequency of urinary tract infection in catheterized dogs and comparison of bacterial culture and susceptibility testing results for catheterized and noncatheterized dogs with urinary tract infections, *J Am Vet Med Assoc* 231:893, 2007.

Forrester SD et al: Retrospective evaluation of urinary tract infection in 42 dogs with hyperadrenocorticism or diabetes mellitus or both, *J Vet Intern Med* 13:557, 1999.

Gatoria IS et al: Comparison of three techniques for the diagnosis of urinary tract infections in dogs with urolithiasis, *J Small Anim Pract* 47:727, 2006.

Griffin DW, Gregory CR: Prevalence of bacterial urinary tract infection after perineal urethrostomy in cats, *J Am Vet Med Assoc* 200:681, 1992.

Hess RS et al: Concurrent disorders in dogs with diabetes mellitus: 221 cases (1993-1998), *J Am Vet Med Assoc* 217:1166, 2000.

Ihrke PJ et al: Urinary tract infection associated with long-term corticosteroid administration in dogs with chronic skin diseases, *J Am Vet Med Assoc* 186:43, 1985.

Kalsi J et al: Hospital-acquired urinary tract infections, *Int J Clin Pract* 57:388, 2003.

Koutinas AF et al: Asymptomatic bacteriuria in puppies with canine parvovirus infection: a cohort study, *Vet Microbiol* 63:109, 1998.

Kruger JM et al: Clinical evaluation of cats with lower urinary tract disease, *J Am Vet Med Assoc* 199:211, 1991.

Levine JM et al: Adverse effects and outcome associated with dexamethasone administration in dogs with acute thoracolumbar intervertebral disc herniation: 161 cases (2000-2006), *J Am Vet Med Assoc* 232:411, 2008.

Lusby AL et al: Prevalence of asymptomatic bacterial urinary tract infections in morbidly obese dogs, *J Vet Intern Med* 25:717, 2011.

Mayer-Roenne B, Goldstein RE, Erb HN: Urinary tract infections in cats with hyperthyroidism, diabetes mellitus, and chronic kidney disease, *J Feline Med Surg* 9:124, 2007.

McGuire NC, Schulman R, Ridgway MD: Detection of occult urinary tract infections in dogs with diabetes mellitus, *J Am Anim Hosp Assoc* 38:541, 2002.

Nicolle LE et al: Infectious Disease Society of America guidelines for the diagnosis and treatment of asymptomatic bacteriuria in adults, *Clin Infect Dis* 40:643, 2005.

Torres SM et al: Frequency of urinary tract infection among dogs with pruritic disorders receiving long-term glucocorticoid therapy, *J Am Vet Med Assoc* 227:239, 2005.

Weese JS et al: Antimicrobial use guidelines for treatment of urinary tract disease in dogs and cats: Antimicrobial Guidelines Working Group of the International Society for Companion Animal Infectious Diseases, *Vet Med Int* 2011:263768, 2011. Epub June 27, 2011.

Wood MW: What is a pathogenic UTI? In *Proceedings*, ACVIM Forum 686-687, 2011.

CHAPTER 194

Persistent *Escherichia coli* Urinary Tract Infection

JULIE R. FISCHER, *San Diego, California*

Bacteria account for the majority of urinary tract infections (UTIs), and *Escherichia coli* strains are isolated from 35% to 50% of cultures. The urogenital tract hosts an extensive array of commensal bacteria that can appear in urine because of ascension or sample contamination during voiding or urethral catheterization. The presence of bacteria in urine *(bacteriuria)* therefore is not equivalent to UTI, which specifically implies colonization of the bladder (or ureters, kidneys, or proximal urethra).

UTI develops when bacterial virulence factors overcome host defense mechanisms, which permits adhesion of bacteria to urothelium or renal cells and enables persistence and proliferation. UTI occurs frequently in dogs, with a lifetime incidence around 14%. UTI is less prevalent in cats, particularly young cats; however, common geriatric feline diseases (e.g., chronic kidney disease, diabetes mellitus, hyperthyroidism) dramatically increase UTI prevalence. Up to 30% of cats with stable chronic kidney disease are found to have a UTI. Most UTIs caused by *E. coli* represent easily curable episodes of uncomplicated cystitis, but animals in which rapid, durable cure is not easily achieved require additional assessment and targeted management.

Uropathogenic *Escherichia coli*

Medically significant *E. coli* strains can be grouped into three major categories: commensal strains (chiefly from phylogenetic groups A and B1), intestinal pathogenic strains (chiefly from groups A, B1, and D), and extraintestinal pathogenic strains (chiefly from groups B2 and D). Spontaneously occurring bacterial UTI in dogs and cats, as in humans, most often is caused by a subset of extraintestinal pathogenic strains termed *uropathogenic E. coli* (UPEC), which possess genes for one or more virulence factors (e.g., adhesins, iron acquisition systems, toxins, host defense avoidance mechanisms) that specifically capacitate colonization of and persistence within the urinary tract. Until recently, UPEC strains generally either have expressed virulence factors *or* have demonstrated significant drug resistance; however, UPEC strains that demonstrate both virulence *and* resistance now have been documented in companion animal populations.

Traditionally, pathogenic *E. coli* was classified as strictly extracellular, but recently the capacity for UPEC to invade urothelial cells has been demonstrated. This intracellular presence permits establishment of potentially long-lived reservoirs of organisms shielded from both host immunologic defenses and antimicrobial exposure, and likely plays a major role in persistence and relapse of UTI caused by UPEC. Cell entry is facilitated by several independent virulence factors that permit increased contact with host cells and easier penetration of cell membranes. Pili (or fimbriae) are several different types of filamentous organelles critical for bacterial adhesion to host cells; the most prevalent pili in UPEC are called type 1 pili. In many UPEC strains, type 1 pili have a tip adhesin, FimH, that binds monomannose molecules. This specific binding affinity increases the strength and duration of interaction with urothelial cells and thus also increases resistance to clearance from the bladder. Other virulence factors lead to cell membrane disruption and increased host cell mobilization, and thus facilitate easier entry of the bound UPEC first into the more superficial urothelial cells and then into deeper cell layers as well. As mentioned earlier, capacity for intracellular residence, particularly in deeper cell layers, permits bacterial persistence in the face of both physiologic defense and clearance mechanisms and also antimicrobial pressure.

Definitions

Reinfection

A UTI is classified as a *reinfection* when, after one UTI is cured, another occurs due to a different isolate (although not necessarily a different bacterial species) and usually bespeaks an anatomic abnormality, physiologic dysfunction, or immunologic deficiency impairing host defenses against bacterial colonization (Box 194-1). Reinfection may occur shortly after an initial UTI is cured, or months may elapse between UTIs.

Relapse

The term *relapse* is applied when, following effective treatment of one UTI, another occurs that is caused by the same isolate. Relapse often indicates a persistent nidus or reservoir that shields bacteria from contact with antimicrobials present in the urine, then permits recolonization of the urinary tract once antimicrobial pressure is removed. These sites may be host tissues (e.g., renal parenchyma, prostate, thickened bladder wall, bladder mass) or foreign objects (e.g., uroliths, intraluminal suture material). Relapse also commonly occurs without an obvious nidus; as described earlier, UPEC can behave as an opportunistic intracellular pathogen, and creation of intracellular reservoirs of bacteria likely plays a lead role in the pathogenesis of relapse. Distinguishing between reinfection and relapse when the same bacterial species is isolated can be challenging; using antimicrobial susceptibility profiles to discriminate between the two has been shown to be unreliable. Genetic sequencing techniques such as pulsed-field gel electrophoresis are required for accurate assessment of clonality or differences between strains, but these assays are not widely available for routine clinical use.

Persistence

A *persistent* UTI is one in which appropriate therapy fails to clear infection; documentation requires a positive urine culture result during antimicrobial administration or within 1 week after termination of treatment. Persistence may be due to drug factors (e.g., inappropriate drug selection, inadequate dose or duration, noncompliance with administration), bacterial factors (e.g., acquisition of resistance, sequestration in tissues), or patient factors (e.g., inadequate drug absorption, uncorrected anatomic or physiologic urinary tract abnormality), but it is thought most often to result from impaired host defenses. Cure usually depends on identification and correction of the underlying issues.

Superinfection

Infection with a different isolate that occurs during therapy for the original infecting strain is termed *superinfection.* Superinfections occur most frequently when a cystostomy tube or urinary catheter is in place during antimicrobial therapy.

Multidrug Resistance

Although virulence factors mediate the pathogenicity of specific UPEC strains, they are not generally associated with the development of multidrug resistance (MDR), which is defined as lack of susceptibility to three or more classes of antibacterial drugs. Usually MDR UPEC strains produce *extended-spectrum β-lactamases,* enzymes whose substrates are later-generation β-lactam antimicrobials (e.g., third-generation cephalosporins). Multidrug resistance usually develops under pressure of antimicrobial use, which is a major predisposing factor. Many MDR *E. coli* isolates will respond to high-dose amoxicillin/clavulanic acid even when they appear resistant on susceptibility testing; thus the use of this protocol (Box 194-2) is rational before selection of higher-tier antimicrobials such as the carbapenems.

Therapeutic Approaches

Reinfection and Prophylactic Antimicrobial Therapy

An obvious reinfection in which bacterial isolates are different species or a strongly suspected diagnosis of reinfection mandates focus on identification and resolution or management of underlying patient-associated predisposing factors. Examples are treatment of incontinence, removal and prevention of uroliths, surgical correction of vulvar hooding, and control of hyperadrenocorticism. In a significant number of patients, no underlying cause of reinfection is found. Reinfections that occur months or longer apart are treated either as sequential uncomplicated episodes of cystitis (with 7 to 10 days of culture-based antimicrobial therapy in female dogs and castrated male dogs) or as complicated cystitis in the case of cats and intact male dogs (requiring 4 to 6 weeks of therapy). In intact male dogs a prostate-penetrating antimicrobial (e.g., trimethoprim/sulfa, chloramphenicol, enrofloxacin) should be used. For animals with reinfections in which an underlying predisposition is either unresolvable or unidentified, prophylactic antimicrobial therapy may be considered.

Prophylactic antimicrobial therapy is used to prevent reinfection in an animal documented to develop UTIs three or four times per year or more. As with suppressive therapy (discussed later), it is important first to treat to urine sterility with an appropriate antimicrobial based on results of susceptibility testing. Once sterility is documented, bedtime administration (to maximize bladder contact time) of 30% to 50% of the daily therapeutic dose is initiated. Ideally, urine is cultured monthly to prove ongoing sterility. Generally, a minimum of 6 months of therapy with documented sterility is recommended before therapy is stopped. Following discontinuation of antibiotics, culture should be performed in 1 week, and if results are negative, culture should be repeated monthly for 3 months, then every 2 to 3 months, out to 1 year. If at any point infection returns, standard antimicrobial therapy based on sensitivity results should be reinitiated, and the process begun again once the reinfection is cleared.

Relapse and Suppressive Antimicrobial Therapy

When relapsing UTI is documented or strongly suspected, search for a nidus or reservoir and screening tests for diseases that might impair host defenses should be undertaken. As discussed earlier the reservoir may well be intracellular populations of organisms that are shielded from antimicrobial, mechanical, and immunologic clearance; thus, with relapse, ongoing presence of the organism in the body is presumed. Suppressive therapy to reduce the risk of bacteremia is instituted using essentially the same protocol as prophylactic therapy, and as with prophylactic therapy, trial discontinuation of antimicrobials after a minimum of 6 months is rational if a similar post–antimicrobial therapy surveillance protocol is used.

Possible Alternative and Nonantimicrobial Therapies

The following strategies have been suggested for management of relapsing or MDR infections with UPEC. Except where stated, no evidential basis for use in companion animal UPEC-related UTI has been established.

Cranberry Extract/Proanthocyanidins

The proanthocyanidins present in cranberries have been shown to convey *in vitro* UPEC antiadhesin effects to urine when orally administered to humans, and a recent abstract described similar changes in the urine of dogs fed cranberry extract. Since bacterial adhesion is critical in the establishment of UTI, preventing adhesion will theoretically impede the infective process; however, no studies to date have demonstrated *in vivo* efficacy of cranberry extract for this purpose in dogs or cats.

Probiotics

As in humans, most UTIs in dogs are presumed to be ascending infections caused by spread of fecal flora from the rectum to the urogenital tract. In women, ingestion of *Lactobacillus* probiotics has been shown to decrease recurrence of UTI. The mechanism is thought to involve restoration of vaginal flora to normal predominance of *Lactobacillus* and creation of a rectal floral environment that is less hospitable to UPEC. In children of both sexes with vesicoureteral reflux, oral administration of *Lactobacillus* has been shown as effective as oral trimethoprim/sulfa for reduction of UTI recurrence over the course of a year. Probiotics are used extensively in companion animals in the management of gastrointestinal diseases but have not been evaluated for improvement of urogenital health and prevention of UTI. Given the promising results in humans, the relatively low cost of therapy, and preexisting veterinary use and availability, probiotics merit further investigation as a tool for prevention of UTI in dogs and cats.

Methenamine Hippurate

Methenamine hippurate is a urinary antiseptic used alone or as ancillary agent with an antimicrobial to help prevent recurrence of UTI. It also sometimes is used as an ancillary agent for treatment of an existing UTI. At acid pH (<6.5) methenamine dissociates into formaldehyde and ammonia; the formaldehyde is bactericidal. Methenamine may cause gastrointestinal upset and should not be used in patients with renal failure (or other causes of metabolic acidosis) since it is an acidifying agent. Urine pH must be less than 6.5 for efficacy, so coadministration of vitamin C, ammonium chloride, or d,l-methionine sometimes is needed. The manufacture of methenamine mandelate salt reportedly has been discontinued in the United States.

Polysulfated Glycosaminoglycans

The bladder urothelium is protected by a glycosaminoglycan layer that accounts in part for its capacity to tolerate constant contact with urine and also helps prevent bacterial adhesion. Pentosan polysulfate (Elmiron) has been used extensively in the treatment of interstitial cystitis in women and has been suggested as an ancillary therapy in cases of relapsing UTI as a mechanism for reestablishment of a normal protective glycosaminoglycan layer. Pentosan polysulfate has been used safely in the treatment of cats with idiopathic cystitis with anecdotal reports of amelioration of clinical signs and has been shown to restore the antiadhesive properties of a normal bladder when topically applied to mucin-deficient rabbit bladders *in vitro*.

No clinical studies in dogs or cats document this effect with oral administration or show improved resistance to relapse with its use; however, the principles are mechanistically sound and its use merits further exploration.

Fosfomycin

Fosfomycin tromethamine (Monurol) is a cell wall–active bactericidal drug with demonstrated effectiveness against UPEC and MDR *E. coli* strains; in humans it is administered as a one-time dose (or for up to 3 days) as treatment for *E. coli* UTI. Although its bactericidal mechanism is similar to that of the β-lactams, it is not inactivated by any class of β-lactamases, and when resistance to fosfomycin does occur, it generally is single-drug resistance rather than MDR. Initial pharmacokinetic studies in dogs show that serum concentrations of fosfomycin following oral dosing at 80 mg/kg exceed the 90% minimal inhibitory concentration for MDR UPEC for at least 12 hours after administration. Fosfomycin is less expensive than higher-tier options such as carbapenems and may prove a valuable oral agent for treatment of MDR *E. coli* UTI.

Induction of Asymptomatic Bacteriuria

Deliberate induction of asymptomatic bacteriuria with a specific *E. coli* strain (that cannot express primary adhesins but has superior biofilm-forming capacity) has been shown in murine models and in humans to successfully prevent establishment of a range of UPEC strains in the bladder. Attempts to durably colonize healthy dog bladders by inoculation with this *E. coli* strain have been unsuccessful, but induction of UTI, even with UPEC strains, can be difficult in a healthy bladder. Studies in affected dogs and cats whose bladders are susceptible to colonization would provide more meaningful insights into the potential clinical utility of this method of UTI prevention in veterinary patients.

Bacteriophages

A recent study examined the use of bacterial viruses *(bacteriophages)* to kill a wide variety of UPEC strains isolated from canine and feline urine and demonstrated that the majority of the UPEC isolates were susceptible to lysis by naturally occurring bacteriophages (Freitag et al, 2008; Nishikawa et al, 2008). *In vivo* mouse studies have shown this method to be protective against peritonitis and septicemia and effective against *E. coli* strains producing extended-spectrum β-lactamases, but no *in vivo* studies related to UTI have been performed.

References and Suggested Reading

Barsanti JA: Genitourinary infections. In Greene CE, editor: *Infectious diseases of the dog and cat*, ed 3, St Louis, 2006, Saunders, p 935.

Barsanti JA: Multidrug-resistant urinary tract infection. In Bonagura JD, Twedt DC, editors: *Kirk's current veterinary therapy XIV*, St Louis, 2009, Saunders, p 921.

Bartges JW, Pressler B: Urinary tract infections. In Ettinger SJ, Feldman EC, editors: *Textbook of veterinary internal medicine: diseases of the dog and cat*, ed 7, St Louis, 2010, Saunders, p 2036.

Freitag T et al: Naturally occurring bacteriophages lyse a large proportion of canine and feline uropathogenic *Escherichia coli* isolates in vitro, *Res Vet Sci* 85:1, 2008.

Gibson JS et al: Multidrug-resistant *E. coli* and *Enterobacter* extraintestinal infection in 37 dogs, *J Vet Intern Med* 22:844, 2008.

Labato MA: Uncomplicated urinary tract infection. In Bonagura JD, Twedt DC, editors: *Kirk's current veterinary therapy XIV*, St Louis, 2009, Saunders, p 918.

Nishikawa H et al: T-even-related bacteriophages as candidates for treatment of *Escherichia coli* urinary tract infections, *Arch Virol* 153:507, 2008.

Seguin MA et al: Persistent urinary tract infections and reinfections in 100 Dogs (1989-1999), *J Vet Intern Med* 17:622, 2003.

Thompson MF et al: Canine bacterial urinary tract infections: new developments in old pathogens, *Vet J* 190:22, 2011.

CHAPTER 195

Interventional Strategies for Urinary Disease

ALLYSON BERENT, *New York, New York*
CHICK WEISSE, *New York, New York*

Interventional endoscopy (IE) involves the use of endoscopic visualization with other contemporary imaging, such as fluoroscopy, ultrasonography, or both, to perform minimally invasive diagnostic and therapeutic procedures. Interventional radiology (IR) uses fluoroscopy, with or without ultrasonography, to guide access to vessels and various lumens for the delivery of specific materials (stents, chemotherapy agents, embolization particles) for diagnostic and therapeutic purposes. These modalities are being employed for numerous endourologic procedures in veterinary patients and have become very popular over the past 5 to 10 years.

This chapter briefly reviews the use of IR/IE in the management of various abnormalities of both the upper and lower urinary tracts of veterinary patients. The relatively high incidence of upper and lower urinary tract disease, combined with the invasiveness and morbidity associated with traditional surgical techniques, makes the use of minimally invasive procedures appealing. Such endourologic procedures are considered the standard of care in human medicine, a trend that is occurring in veterinary medicine as well. There are many advantages to IR/IE techniques compared with traditional therapies. As a minimally invasive alternative, IR/IE contributes to reduced perioperative morbidity and mortality, shorter anesthesia times, and shorter hospital stays. In addition, some procedures provide treatment or palliation for diseases for which previously there were no good therapeutic alternatives (e.g., ureteral stenting or a ureteral bypass device for ureterolithiasis or ureteral strictures and palliative stenting for malignant urethral or ureteral obstructions). The main disadvantages are that these procedures are technically challenging, require expensive specialized equipment, and are routinely available in only a small number of institutions around the world. Furthermore, appropriate training in IR/IE is essential and the learning curve can be steep.

Equipment

Most IR/IE procedures are performed in a clean angiography or endoscopy suite with fluoroscopy. A traditional fluoroscopic unit often is sufficient, but a C-arm unit has the advantage of mobility, permitting imaging in multiple tangential views. Occasionally, ultrasonography is useful to guide percutaneous needle access into vessels or other structures (e.g., renal pelvis, urinary bladder).

Various flexible and rigid endoscopes are used for IE procedures. Rigid cystoscopy is commonly performed in female animals for urethral, bladder, and ureteral access. Recommended endoscope diameters (at the tip) range from 1.9 to 4 mm, depending on the size of the patient. Flexible ureteroscopes are used for urethral and bladder access in male dogs (2.5 to 2.8 mm) and for ureteral access in animals large enough to accept such diameters (>15 kg). Rigid nephroscopes are needed (5.3 to 7.3 mm) for percutaneous nephrolithotomy (PCNL) procedures. Different types of intracorporeal lithotriptors and lasers are available for various IE procedures such as ultrasonic, electrohydraulic, pneumatic, shock wave, and holmium: yttrium-aluminum-garnet (holmium:YAG) lithotriptors, and the diode-type laser (see Web Chapter 70). In addition, an arsenal of catheters, wires, stents (both metallic [urethral] and polyurethane [ureteral]), and baskets are useful for the varied patient population in veterinary practice. A subcutaneous ureteral bypass (SUB) device is now more commonly used for the treatment of feline ureteral obstructions. This is a nephrostomy catheter and a cystostomy catheter that are attached subcutaneously to a shunting port that allows urine to drain directly from the kidney to the bladder, without the need to salvage the ureter.

Kidney and Ureter

Interventional Approach to Nephrolithiasis

The direct treatment of nephroliths is necessary only when they become problematic, which is the case less than 10% of the time in the authors' experience. Nephroliths are considered problematic when one of the following occurs: recurrent urinary tract infections (despite administration of appropriate antibiotic therapy for >8 to 12 weeks), pyelectasia or hydronephrosis, worsening renal function, pain and discomfort, or resulting intermittent ureteral obstruction. Traditional open surgical options to treat problematic nephroliths (e.g., nephrotomy, nephrectomy) are associated with frequent complications and high long-term morbidity. In a clinical study of dogs, approximately 43% had stone fragments remaining after surgery and 23% had procedure-related complications (Gookin et al, 1996). Additionally, 67% of dogs had evidence of renal azotemia that developed following nephrectomy. In a feline study of normal cats there was a 10% to 20% decrease in the glomerular filtration rate of the kidney in which a nephrotomy was performed (King et al, 2006). It is important to realize that in healthy animals the renal hypertrophic mechanisms are still functional, but in clinically affected dogs and cats this process already has been exhausted, which makes the change in renal function more dramatic. The use of less invasive approaches, such as extracorporeal shock wave lithotripsy (ESWL) (for stones of <1.5 to 2 cm) or PCNL (for stones of >1.5 to 2 cm), has been shown to be associated with preservation of renal function in humans. PCNL is highly effective in removing all stone fragments in the calices and does not require cutting of the nephrons. Instead, tissues are spread apart with the use of a balloon dilation kit to allow an endoscope and intracorporeal lithotriptor to remove the stone debris effectively.

Extracorporeal Shockwave Lithotripsy

ESWL is a minimally invasive alternative for the treatment of small calculi in the renal pelvis or ureters. ESWL uses external shock waves that pass through a water medium (either a wet or dry unit) and the soft tissue of the patient. The shock waves are directed under fluoroscopic guidance. The stone is shocked anywhere from 1000 to 3500 times at different energy levels for implosion and powdering of the stone. The debris is then permitted to traverse the ureter into the urinary bladder over a 2- to 12-week period. ESWL is believed to be very safe for the kidney, although subclinical intrarenal hemorrhage does occur. The severity of the damage is dose dependent. Studies have shown minimal to no decreases in glomerular filtration rate both short and long term after ESWL in patients with kidney stones. Availability of ESWL is limited, however. For stones of larger sizes (>1.5 to 2 cm), PCNL often is recommended in both humans and veterinary patients alike (see next section).

Percutaneous Nephrolithotomy

In humans, PCNL is considered the standard of care for nephroliths or proximal ureteroliths too large to be treated with ESWL or laser lithotripsy (>1.5 to 2 cm). PCNL also has been performed successfully in clinical veterinary patients. This procedure has been shown to have minimal or no negative effect on renal function in both children and adults with large stone burdens, solitary kidneys, or renal insufficiency. This minimally invasive endoscopic procedure allows access to the renal pelvis through a small sheath that is placed under fluoroscopic guidance (Figure 195-1). Once a tract is made into the renal pelvis, a nephroscope and intracorporeal lithotrite are used for stone fragmentation and removal. The aim is to minimize morbidity and preserve as much renal function as possible while removing all stone fragments to prevent the development of a ureteral obstruction and progressive renal insufficiency. The success rate of PCNL has been documented at 90% to 100% in both the adult and the pediatric human populations, and the authors have experienced the same in veterinary patients.

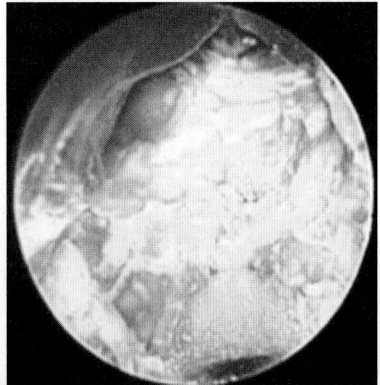

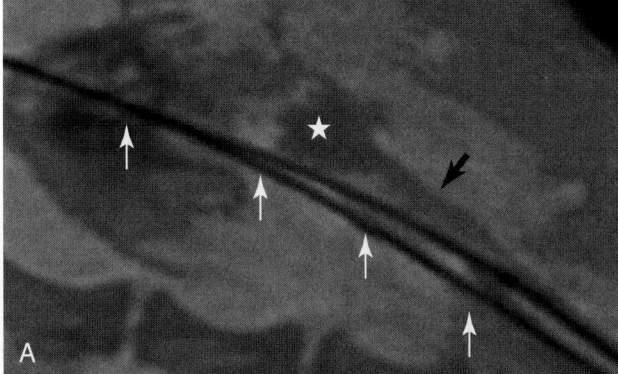

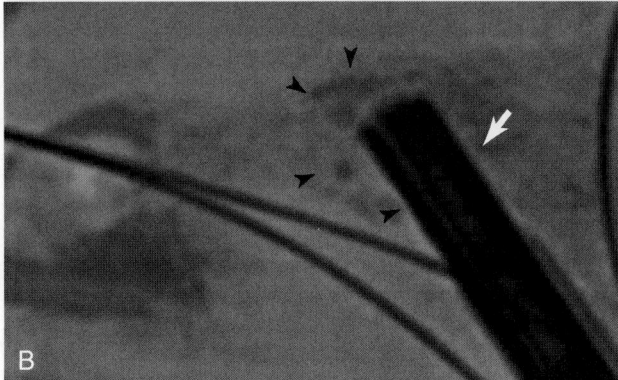

Figure 195-1 Dog with nephroliths undergoing percutaneous nephrolithotomy. The endoscopic image on the top shows the calcium oxalate nephrolith inside the renal pelvis during ultrasonic and electrohydraulic intracorporeal lithotripsy. **A,** Percutaneous access is obtained using ultrasonography and fluoroscopy. An 18-gauge catheter punctures the kidney onto the nephrolith *(asterisk)*. A guidewire *(white arrows)* is advanced down the ureter into the bladder and out the urethra for through-and-through access. A second wire is advanced down the ureter for placement of the renal access sheath *(black arrow)*. **B,** Nephroscope *(white arrow)* through the ureteral access sheath and multiple stone fragments are visualized *(black arrowheads)*.

Interventional Approach to Essential Renal Hematuria

Essential (idiopathic) renal hematuria is a rare condition in which a focal area of bleeding in the upper urinary tract results in long-term hematuria, iron deficiency anemia (if chronic) and the potential for clot formation, or blood calculi. In people, any hemangioma, angioma, or vascular malformation present may be visualized ureteroscopically and subsequently cauterized via ureteroscopy. Idiopathic renal hematuria is diagnosed most commonly in very young large-breed dogs and occurs bilaterally in 25% to 33% of affected patients. For unilateral disease, usually confirmed by cystoscopy, ureteronephrectomy was previously recommended to minimize blood loss. Currently, nephrectomy should be considered contraindicated because of the risk of progressive bilateral disease and the availability of kidney-sparing techniques.

Ureteroscopy

It is possible to perform ureteroscopy in dogs larger than approximately 15 kg for visualization of renal hemorrhage. This procedure is challenging to perform in dogs because the canine ureter typically is less than 2 mm in diameter and the smallest ureteroscope currently available is approximately 2.5 mm in diameter. Ureteral access is obtained via cystoscopy; a guidewire is advanced up the ureter into the renal pelvis and the endoscope is advanced over the guidewire under fluoroscopic and endoscopic guidance (Figure 195-2). The ureteral and renal pelvic mucosa are examined; if a bleeding lesion is identified, electrocautery can be applied endoscopically to stop the bleed.

Sclerotherapy

The use of silver nitrate and povidone-iodine as cauterizing agents is an alternative method for mitigating upper urinary tract bleeding. This can be done in any dog (male or female), regardless of size. Under cystoscopic and fluoroscopic guidance, the cauterizing agent is infused into the renal pelvis through a ureteral occlusion balloon catheter. In a recent study in which sclerotherapy was used for the treatment of IRH complete cessation of macroscopic hematuria occurred in 4 of 6 dogs within a median of 6 hours (range, postoperative to 7 days). Two additional dogs improved, one moderately and one substantially. None of the dogs required nephrectomy. Ureteroscopy for electrocautery has only been performed in a small number of patients, and this is typically reserved for patients that have failed sclerotherapy. There were no complications noted from the procedure when a stent was placed postinfusion.

Future Treatment Options for Chronic and Inflammatory Kidney Disease

Infusion of autologous mesenchymal stem cells, an adipose stromal component containing stem cells, currently is being investigated for the treatment of feline and canine renal diseases. With intravenous infusion,

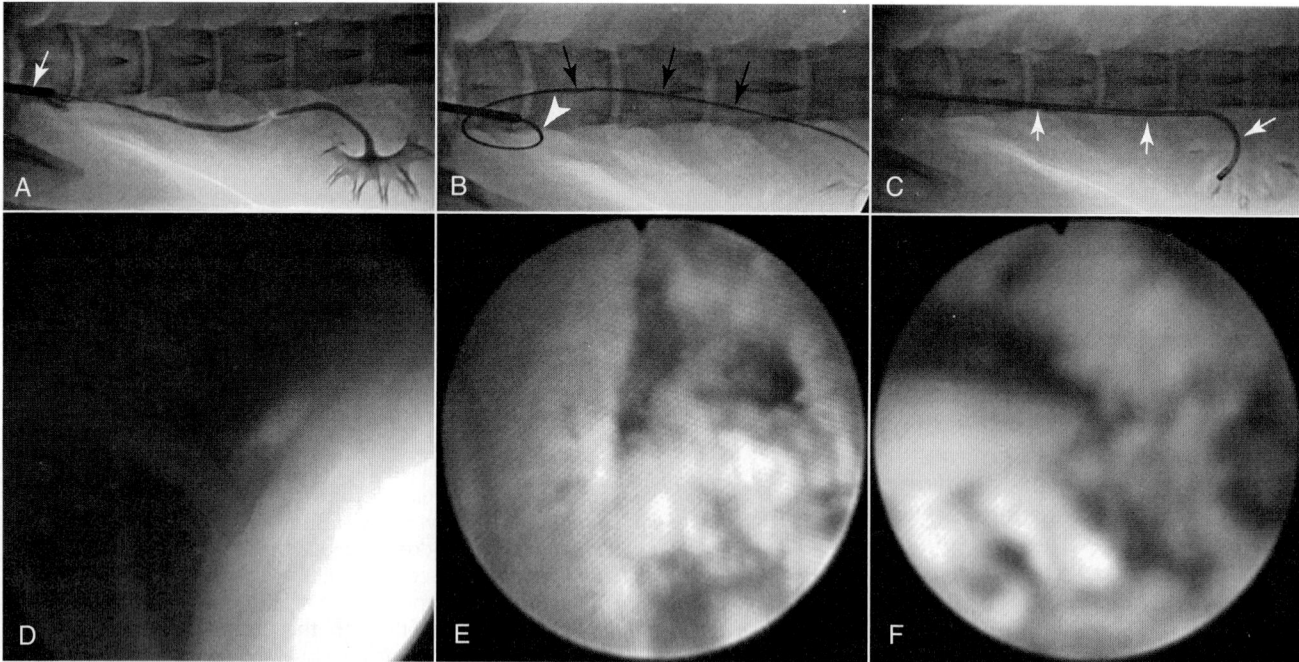

Figure 195-2 Female dog with idiopathic renal hematuria. Dorsoventral abdominal fluoroscopic image during ureteroscopy (caudal is left and cranial is right) and ureteroscopic images during cauterization. **A,** A cystoscope *(white arrow)* is used to identify the ureterovesicular junction, and a ureteral catheter is advanced up the most distal aspect of the ureter for retrograde ureteropyelography using a contrast agent (Iohexol). **B,** An angled-tipped hydrophilic 0.035-inch guidewire *(black arrows)* is advanced through the working channel into the ureteral opening, up the ureter, and into the renal pelvis. The J-hooked distal ureter is observed *(white arrowhead)*. **C,** The cystoscope is removed over the guidewire, and the flexible ureteroscope is advanced over the wire and into the renal pelvis *(white arrows)*. **D,** During cystoscopy the left ureterovesicular junction is seen to have jets of bloody urine identifying the side of bleeding. **E,** A lesion on the renal papilla inside the renal pelvis that is bleeding. **F,** An electrocautery probe *(blue)* is used through the flexible ureteroscope for cauterization.

first-pass extraction of the cells occurs in the lungs, which are the first capillary bed to encounter the cells. IR can facilitate direct delivery of the stem cells into the renal artery (via the femoral or carotid artery), where the glomeruli will be the first capillary bed to extract the cells. Randomized, placebo-controlled studies currently are under way to evaluate the safety and efficacy of this approach. The goals of stem cell therapy are to decrease the inflammatory reaction and fibrosis associated with both glomerulonephritis and interstitial nephritis through paracrine mechanisms. Tissue regeneration has not yet been proven, but studies are showing very promising results in various animal models. In the authors' practice over 95 treatments have been performed in both dogs and cats and it has proven safe. The efficacy to this point has been promising, although the studies are ongoing and the end points have not yet been met.

Interventional Approach to Ureteral Obstructions

Ureteral disorders can create significant management dilemmas in veterinary patients. The relatively common incidence of ureteral disease, combined with the morbidity associated with traditional surgical techniques, makes IR/IE options appealing.

Feline ureterolithiasis is the most common ureteral disorder. Other causes of ureteral obstruction are ureteral strictures, neoplasia, and dried solidified blood stones. The more that is learned about the pathophysiology of ureteral obstruction, the clearer it becomes that timely decompression of the renal pelvis is imperative so that renal function of the ipsilateral kidney is preserved and chronic progressive changes are avoided. Unfortunately, once medical management (e.g., intravenous fluid therapy, mannitol infusions, α-adrenergic blockade) fails to resolve the obstruction, management decisions become challenging because of the risk:benefit ratio of ureteral surgery. A retrospective study involving over 150 cats demonstrated a high rate of complications (>30%) and high mortality rates (18% to 38%) following surgery. Complications included continued obstruction from edema at the surgical site, urine leakage, recurrent obstruction from stones remaining in the renal pelvis, and ureteral stricture formation. Nevertheless, the survival rates were dramatically higher for cats that underwent surgery and had ureteroliths removed than for those treated with medical management alone (Kyles et al, 2005). Less-invasive, safer, and more effective alternatives certainly are desired, and interventional/endourologic options effectively have replaced open ureteral surgery in human medicine. The placement of a double-pigtail ureteral stent, nephrostomy tube, or ureteral bypass device could potentially circumvent the complications of surgery (e.g., leakage, stricture, and reobstruction), while quickly and efficiently stabilizing the patient, decreasing renal pelvic pressure, and stopping the cycle of pressure-induced nephron death. To date over 200 cats and 150 dogs have been treated in the authors' practice for ureteral obstructions with the following interventional therapies. These techniques can be applied for all causes of ureteral obstructions including tumors, strictures, and stones.

Percutaneous Nephrostomy

For rapid decompression, a temporary nephrostomy tube can be placed for urinary drainage (Figure 195-3). Because postrenal consequences are reduced, the patient's condition can be stabilized and intrinsic renal function can be assessed before ureteral surgery or other intervention is performed. IR assistance is useful in implementing percutaneous or surgically assisted techniques. Care should be taken to secure the tube adequately (nephropexy is recommended in cats) to avoid accidental dislodgement. Other complications include infection, hemorrhage, and leakage around the tube. The reason this option is no longer commonly used in the authors' practice is because it typically does require a second procedure for a definitive treatment, and the costs can be prohibitive. Now with the advent of the ureteral bypass device, nephrostomy tubes are rarely being used in our practice.

Ureteral Stenting

Ureteral stents are placed for a variety of disorders in both dogs and cats (Berent et al, 2011; Berent, Weisse, and Beal, 2011) and are used to (1) immediately divert urine from the renal pelvis into the urinary bladder while bypassing a ureteral obstruction, (2) encourage passive ureteral dilation (for urine flow, future placement of larger stents, or stone passage), (3) decrease surgical tension and prevent postoperative leakage or edema of the ureter during and after ureteral surgery (e.g., resection and anastomosis or proximal ureteral reimplantation), and (4) facilitate passage of fragments following ESWL for nephroliths. The use of IR/IE techniques has helped avoid traditional ureteral surgery, particularly in cases that are not considered good surgical candidates (Figure 195-4). For example, the number of stones found in the ureter and kidney in affected cats with nephroureterolithiasis appears to have increased recently (median of four stones per ureter in one study, with over 85% of cats having evidence of concurrent ipsilateral nephrolithiasis) (Berent et al, 2011).This stone burden makes a majority of the animals (nearly 60% to 80%) poor surgical candidates and a high risk for a future ureteral obstruction.

The most common type of ureteral stent is the double-pigtail stent, which lies entirely intracorporeally and can remain in place for years if necessary. Each loop of the pigtail is curled (one in the bladder and one in the renal pelvis), and the shaft of the stent travels through the entire ureteral lumen. This allows direct passage of urine from the kidney to the urinary bladder, around the stones or through a stricture. In dogs the stent typically is placed using cystoscopy and fluoroscopy to advance a guidewire into the vesicoureteral opening in a retrograde manner, with bypass of any obstruction. Successful retrograde placement is possible endoscopically in most dogs with obstruction but in only about 20% of cats. In feline patients stents are typically placed with surgical assistance in an antegrade manner, similar to the approach for a nephrostomy tube.

Ureteral stent placement requires careful patient selection, special training, and operator experience using wires, catheters, and stents. In a recent series of 75 cats (79 ureters), 95% of the cats had a significant improvement of their azotemia. The perioperative mortality rate was

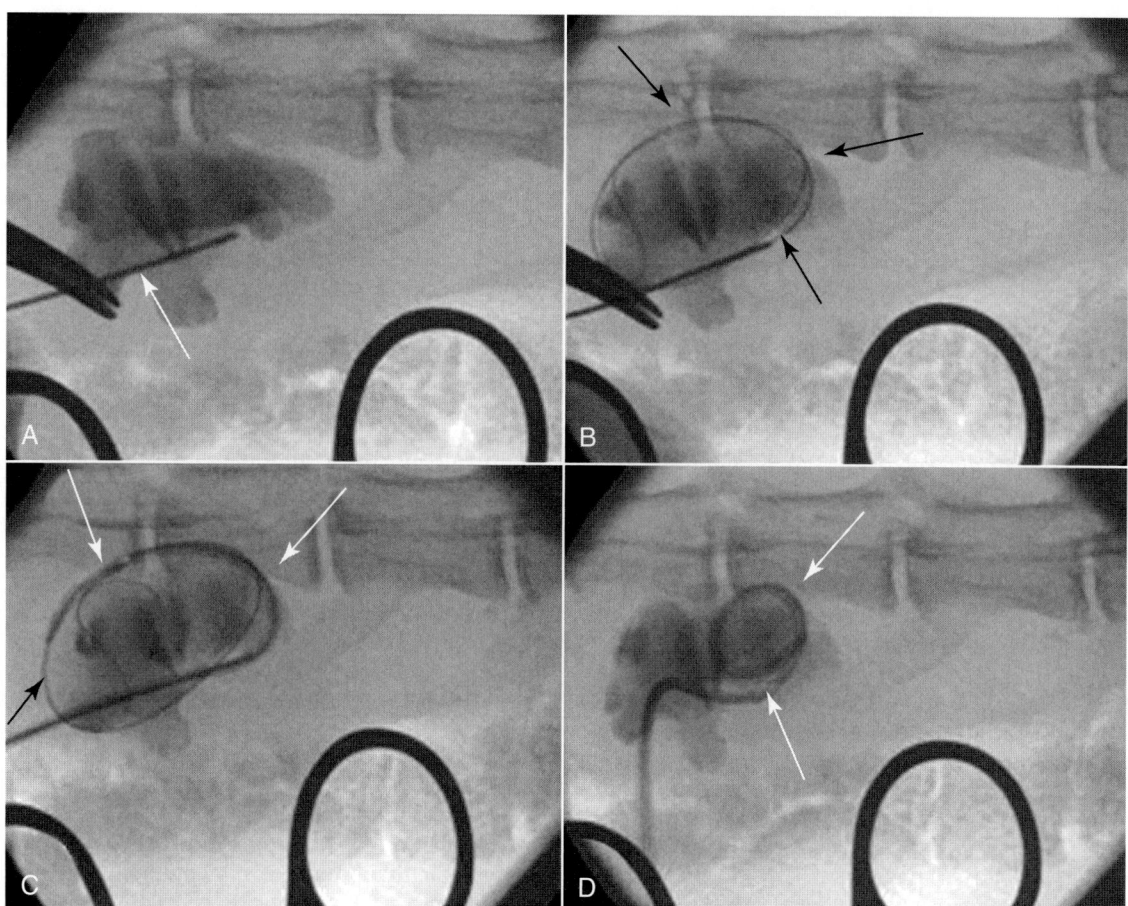

Figure 195-3 Placement of a percutaneous nephrostomy tube using the Seldinger technique under fluoroscopic guidance. **A,** Renal access is obtained using an 18-gauge renal access needle *(white arrow)* under ultrasonographic and fluoroscopic guidance. **B,** A 0.035-inch angled guide-wire *(black arrows)* is advanced through the needle and curled inside the renal pelvis. **C,** A locking-loop pigtail catheter is advanced over the guidewire *(black arrow)* until the entire loop is inside the renal pelvis *(white arrows)*. **D,** The guidewire is removed and the locking string is pulled to lock the catheter *(arrows)* in place.

7.5%, and no cat died because of surgical complications or associated with their ureteral obstruction. The rate of short-term complications (occurring within 1 month of stent placement) was 8%. Complications include stent misplacement, ureteral tear during stent placement, and urine leakage at a ureterotomy site that was performed concurrently. Urine leakage resolved following closed abdominal suction in all cases without the need for further intervention. The long-term complications (occurring after 1 month) were minor and included dysuria, stent migration, ureteral reaction to the stent, and occlusion around the stent (Berent et al, 2011). The most worrisome long-term complication of ureteral stenting is an occlusion of the stent. This is most commonly seen at the site of a stricture, which either was the primary obstructive lesion or developed after a ureterotomy was performed. This is most commonly seen 3 to 6 months after stent placement. The authors typically recommend placement of a SUB device (see next section) rather than a ureteral stent in cats with a known ureteral stricture. Overall, stenting is safe and effective in both dogs and cats, with very low perioperative complications; if a complication occurs

with the stent in the long term, it is usually minor, requiring an outpatient stent exchange or some medications to address dysuria. To date, the authors have placed stents successfully in over 250 dog or cat ureters for various clinical purposes, and outcomes have been excellent.

Subcutaneous Ureteral Bypass (SUB) Device Placement
Placement of a nephrostomy tube has been very useful in veterinary medicine when renal pelvic drainage is required (Figure 195-5). The biggest limitation of nephrostomy tubes is the external drainage apparatus, which requires hospitalization and intensive care management to prevent infection or dislodgement. The authors developed an indwelling nephrostomy device for veterinary patients using a combination locking-loop nephrostomy catheter and cystostomy catheter. This SUB device has a subcutaneous port that can be sampled and flushed as needed. In humans, a similar device has been shown to reduce the complications associated with externalized nephrostomy tubes and to improve patients' quality of life. The successful use of a SUB device in 23 cats and 2 dogs has been described recently (Berent, Weisse, and Bagley,

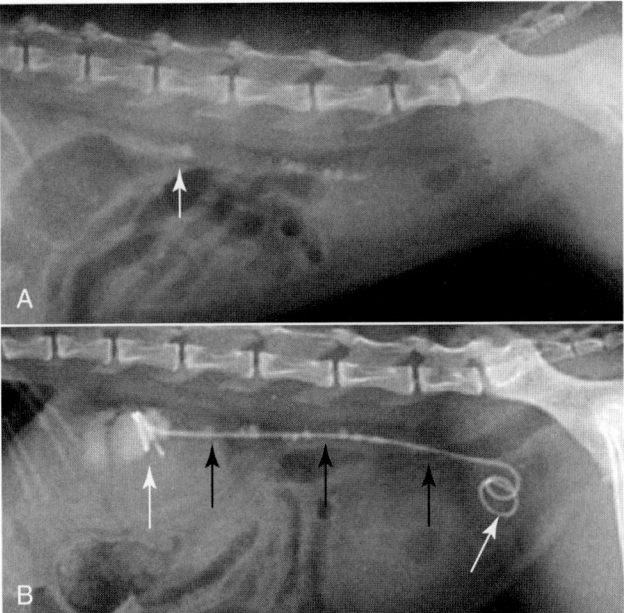

Figure 195-4 Radiograph of a feline patient before **(A)** and after **(B)** ureteral stent placement. Notice the numerous ureteroliths and nephroliths present *(arrow)*. The double-pigtail ureteral stent goes from the renal pelvis to the urinary bladder *(white arrows)* with the shaft travelling down the entire length of the ureter *(black arrows)*.

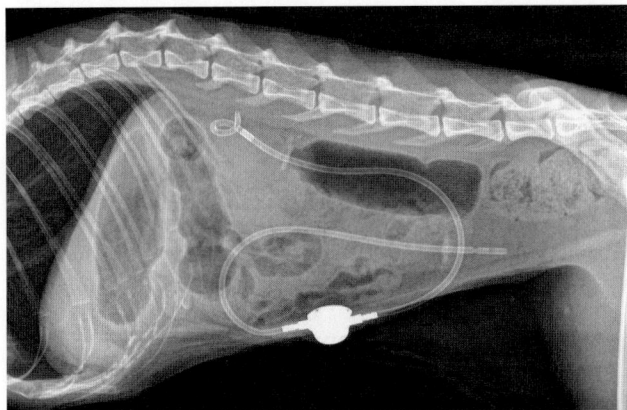

Figure 195-5 Lateral radiograph of a cat with a subcutaneous ureteral bypass device placed for a ureteral obstruction.

2011), and over 100 of these devices have been placed to date in our practice. Subcutaneous ureteral bypass is typically reserved for cases in which a ureteral stent cannot be placed or is contraindicated, such as those involving ureteral strictures or severe ureteritis. The perioperative, short-term, and long-term complication rate with the new commercially available product is very low (~5%). To prevent occlusion of the device regular flushing through the subcutaneous port is recommended (see Figure 196-5). At this time, the authors are performing this routinely for feline ureteral obstructions, of any cause, due to the lower rate of dysuria and reocclusion compared with feline ureteral stents. In dogs ureteral stenting is still considered ideal, and a SUB device is considered a salvage procedure.

Urinary Bladder and Urethra

Antegrade Urethral Catheterization

Transurethral catheterization is a simple and routine procedure and is used primarily to establish urinary drainage in patients with a urethral obstruction. Occasionally, standard retrograde catheterization can be difficult; for example, in very small female dogs or cats, females with obstructive tumors, or male cats with urethral tears or significant urethral trauma. With fluoroscopic guidance, percutaneous transvesicular catheterization can be performed in an antegrade manner. An 18-gauge catheter is advanced into the bladder to facilitate placement of a guidewire, which is passed through the urethra to the outside; then a small-diameter catheter is threaded over the guidewire. Minimally invasive antegrade catheterization can help to avoid the need for emergency surgical intervention in patients with obstruction and is especially valuable in managing urethral tears.

Urethral Stenting for Malignant Obstructions

Malignant obstructions of the urethra can cause severe dysuria and life-threatening azotemia in dogs. Transitional cell carcinoma affecting the bladder trigone, urethra, or prostate is encountered most commonly. Chemotherapy has been successful in slowing tumor growth in many cases; however, more aggressive debulking or diversion has been necessary to prolong good-quality life when obstruction occurs. Cystostomy tube drainage, transurethral resection or ablation, and surgical diversion have been described but are invasive procedures and often have poor outcomes. Placement of a self-expanding metallic stent using fluoroscopic guidance is fast, reliable, and safe in establishing urethral patency in both male and female dogs with malignant obstruction.

Using transurethral retrograde access, contrast cystourethrography is performed, and measurements of the normal urethral diameter and obstruction length are obtained (Figure 195-6). An appropriately sized self-expanding metallic stent is chosen to cross the entire obstruction. The stent is deployed under fluoroscopic guidance, and repeat contrast cystourethrography is performed to document restored urethral patency. Stent placement typically is performed as outpatient procedure.

The authors have found the procedure to be successful in 97% of attempts. The major adverse effect of urethral stent placement is moderate-to-severe urinary incontinence, which has been reported to occur in approximately 25% of both male and female dogs regardless of stent diameter or length. Overall, the median survival time after urethral stenting for carcinoma of the urinary tract was 78 days, but for dogs receiving adjunct chemotherapy it improved to 251 days (Blackburn et al, 2010). Urethral stenting also may be useful in patients with benign urethral strictures when traditional therapies have failed or when surgery is refused or not indicated. The authors have long-term experience with dogs and cats that underwent stenting for benign strictures, with some stents in place for over 5 years without complications. To

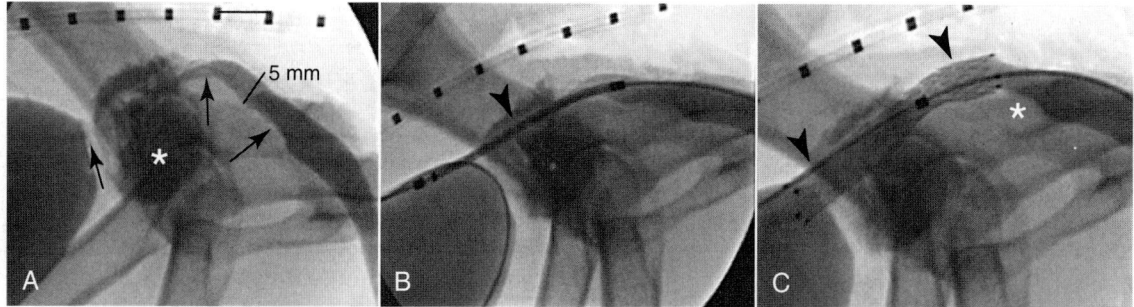

Figure 195-6 Fluoroscopic images of a dog with urethral and prostatic carcinoma before and after urethral stent placement (cranial is left and caudal is right). **A,** A urethrocystogram outlining the obstruction and tumor inside the urethra *(arrows)* and extravasation of contrast into the cystic prostate *(white asterisk).* The urethra is measured for appropriate stent placement *(lines)* using a colonic marker catheter to adjust for magnification. **B,** The self-expanding metallic stent (SEMS) *(arrowhead)* is advanced over the guidewire and situated across the obstructive lesion. **C,** The SEMS is deployed under fluoroscopic guidance to provide urethral patency. Some tumor is seen *(asterisk)* caudal to the stent and the obstruction is no longer present.

date over 150 urethral stents have been placed in the authors' practice.

Bladder and Urethral Stone Treatment

Numerous minimally invasive stone-retrieval techniques currently are available in veterinary medicine, including voiding urohydropropulsion, cystoscopic stone basketing, cystourethroscopically guided laser lithotripsy, and percutaneous cystolithotomy. Other chapters in this text discuss a majority of these in more detail.

Stone Basketing

Basket retrieval of bladder and urethral stones is performed routinely in both male and female dogs and female cats. This procedure is accomplished by transurethral cystourethroscopy. Stones of less than 5 mm in female dogs and 3 mm in male dogs and female cats routinely can be retrieved. This procedure typically is done on an outpatient basis.

Percutaneous Cystolithotomy

The newer minimally invasive technique termed *percutaneous cystolithotomy* (PCCL) (Runge et al, 2011) combines cystic and urethral stone retrieval for animals of any size, sex, or species, and stones of any size or number. This procedure is very easy to perform in both cats and dogs. An approximately 1-cm incision is made over the apex of the bladder appreciated during digital palpation. Then three stay sutures are placed to secure the bladder up to the incision so that a port can be placed at the apex. Antegrade cystoscopy (both rigid and flexible) then is performed, and a stone-retrieval basket is used for calculi removal. PCCL also allows for excellent visualization of the bladder, urethra, and ureterovesicular junction and assists in various interventions (upper and lower tract) when needed.

PCCL currently is the procedure of choice in the authors' practice for the retrieval of cystic or urethral calculi in cases that do not fit the criteria for other minimally invasive techniques. A similar technique is described in more detail in Chapter 199.

Intraarterial Chemotherapy for Lower Urinary Tract Neoplasia

Transitional cell carcinoma is the most common tumor of the canine urinary tract. Unfortunately, this disease often is diagnosed at an advanced stage, and a majority of animals are euthanized because of failure to control the local disease within the urinary tract. Current treatments include chemotherapy, radiation therapy, and surgical debulking, but none consistently produces durable remissions. Research suggests that these tumors can respond more favorably to higher concentrations of chemotherapy drugs or nonsteroidal antiinflammatory medications; however, both classes of drugs have significant deleterious adverse effects, which limits the systemic doses that can be administered. Recent advancements in IR now enable the administration of therapeutic agents directly into the arteries feeding the actual tumors via femoral or carotid arterial access (Figure 195-7). High regional drug concentrations can be achieved within the tumor without amplification of the systemic adverse effects. Studies confirm both higher levels of chemotherapy agents within the targeted tissues and improved tumor remissions in laboratory animals. Intraarterial delivery of carboplatin and meloxicam, as well as other agents, has been performed safely in dogs with carcinoma of the urinary tract. Investigation into intraarterial delivery of other chemotherapeutic agents currently is under way.

Cystoscopic-Guided Laser Ablation of Ectopic Ureters (CLA-EU)

Pharmacologic and endoscopic treatments for urethral sphincter mechanism incompetence are discussed in other chapters of this text and the accompanying electronic resources. Less commonly, incontinence is caused by congenital ectopic ureters, in which the ureteral orifice is positioned distal to the bladder trigone within the ureter, vagina, vestibule, or uterus. Over 95% of ectopic ureters traverse intramurally and exit into the urethra and are candidates for a minimally invasive IE procedure.

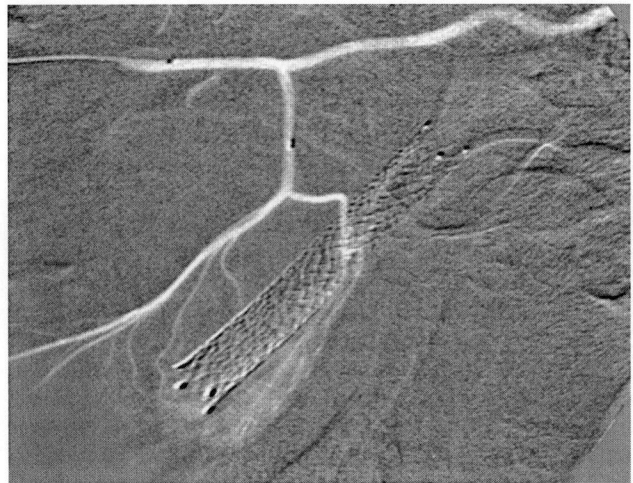

Figure 195-7 Fluoroscopic image of a dog with prostatic carcinoma during intraarterial chemotherapy delivery. Digital subtraction angiography is being used to view the caudal pudendal and prostatic arteries, which are feeding the caudal vesicle and urethral arteries. This patient also has a urethral stent in place.

Endoscopic repair of ectopic ureters has been performed over the past 5 to 7 years in male and female dogs and cats using fluoroscopy, cystoscopy, and a diode or holmium:YAG laser. The laser is applied to transect the medial side or the membrane of the ectopic ureter to separate the ureter from the normal trigone and urethra. The procedure can be performed on an outpatient basis at the same time as cystoscopic diagnosis of ectopic ureter(s) is made, which avoids the need for more than one anesthetic procedure for fixation. During the CLA-EU procedure various vaginal anomalies can be treated simultaneously as well (dual vagina, vaginal septum, persistent paramesonephric remnants). However, many affected dogs have concurrent urethral incompetence and require additional medication or procedures. A prospective study of CLA-EU in 30 female dogs was reported recently and showed an overall urinary continence rate of 77% after CLA-EU with the addition of medical management, collagen injections, or placement of a hydraulic occluder (Berent et al, 2012a). The success rate of the CLA-EU procedure alone in female and male dogs is 56%. The addition of a hydraulic occluder may increase the continence rate to nearly 90% (Figure 195-8).

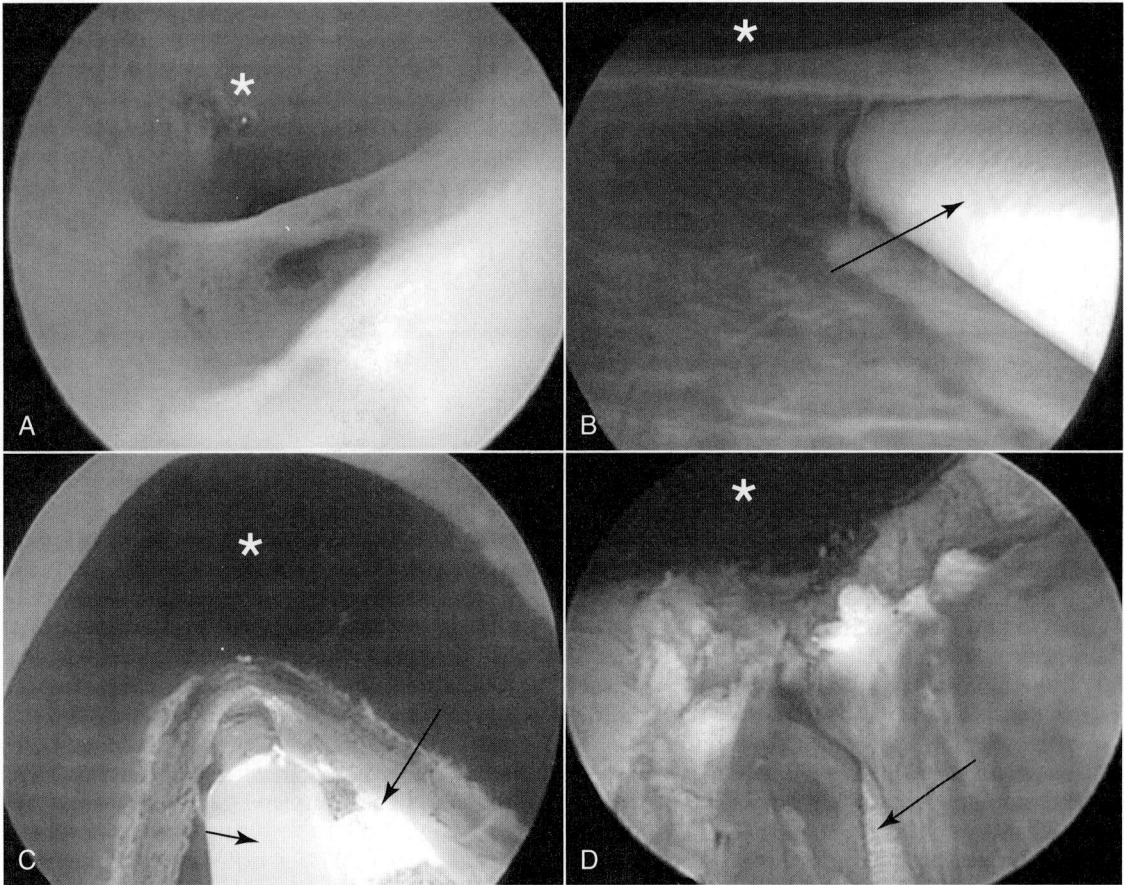

Figure 195-8 Endoscopic images of a female dog in dorsal recumbency during cystoscopically guided laser ablation of intramural ectopic ureters. **A,** The urethroscopic image shows the urethral lumen *(asterisk)* and the ectopic ureteral opening. **B,** A ureteral catheter *(black arrow)* is advanced into the ureteral lumen, and the urethral lumen is seen just ventral *(asterisk)*. **C,** A laser *(short arrow)* is used to ablate the common wall between the urethra *(asterisk)* and the ureter *(long arrow)* inside the urethral lumen. **D,** Once the laser ablation is complete the ureteral opening is successfully advanced to the level of the urinary bladder *(asterisk)*. A guidewire sits inside the ureteral lumen, and it is seen here to exit at the new ureteral orifice. Notice that there is no bleeding associated with this procedure.

References and Suggested Reading

Berent A: Ureteral obstructions in dogs and cats: a review of traditional and new interventional diagnostic and therapeutic options, *J Vet Emerg Crit Care* 21(2):86, 2011.

Berent A et al: Ureteral stenting for feline ureteral obstructions: 79 ureters with ureterolithiasis, 21st European College of Veterinary Internal Medicine—Companion Animals Congress, Sevilla, Spain. *J Vet Intern Med* 25(6):1506, 2011 (abstract).

Berent A et al: Prospective evaluation of cystoscopic guided laser ablation of intramural ectopic ureters in female dogs: 30 cases (2006-2009), *J Am Vet Med Assoc* 240:716, 2012a.

Berent A et al: Use of locking-loop pigtail nephrostomy catheters in dogs and cats: 20 cases (2004-2009), *J Am Vet Med Assoc* 241:348, 2012b.

Berent A, Weisse C, Bagley D: The use of a subcutaneous ureteral bypass device for ureteral obstructions in dogs and cats. American College of Veterinary Internal Medicine Forum, Denver, Colorado, *J Vet Intern Med* 25(3):632, 2011 (abstract).

Berent A, Weisse C, Beal M: Use of indwelling, double pigtail ureteral stents for the treatment of malignant ureteral

obstructions in dogs: 12 cases (2006-2009), *J Am Vet Med Assoc* 238(8):1017, 2011.

Blackburn A, Berent A, Weisse C: The use of self expanding urethral stents for the treatment of urothelial carcinoma: 42 dogs, American College of Veterinary Internal Medicine Forum, 2010, Anaheim, California, *J Vet Intern Med* 24(6):1577, 2010 (abstract).

Gookin JL et al: Unilateral nephrectomy in dogs with renal disease: 30 cases (1985-1994), *J Am Vet Med Assoc* 208:2020, 1996.

King MD et al: Effect of nephrotomy on renal function and morphology in normal cats, *Vet Surg* 35:749, 2006.

Kyles A et al: Management and outcome of cats with ureteral calculi: 153 cases (1984-2002), *J Am Vet Med Assoc* 226(6):937, 2005.

Runge J et al: Transvesicular percutaneous cystolithotomy for the removal of cystic calculi in dogs, *J Am Vet Med Assoc* 239:344, 2011.

Weisse C et al: Potential applications of interventional radiology in veterinary medicine, *J Am Vet Med Assoc* 233(10):1564, 2008.

CHAPTER **196**

Medical Management of Nephroliths and Ureteroliths

JESSICA E. MARKOVICH, *North Grafton, Massachusetts*
MARY ANNA LABATO, *North Grafton, Massachusetts*

Prevalence and Predisposition

Upper urinary tract uroliths currently represent approximately 3% of all uroliths submitted to the Minnesota Urolith Center (Albasan et al, 2009). Any of the uroliths typically identified in the lower urinary tract also can be found in the upper urinary tract; however, the prevalence of stone types does differ slightly. In cats, 70% to 98% of analyzed uroliths are calcium oxalate in composition, whereas the remaining 2% to 30% are calcium phosphate, magnesium ammonium phosphate (struvite), and dried solidified blood calculi (Osborne et al, 2009; Westropp et al, 2006). In dogs, there is nearly an equal distribution of calcium oxalate and struvite uroliths in submitted upper tract stones (Ling et al, 1998; Snyder et al, 2005).

Female dogs are more likely to form nephroliths than male dogs. Canine breeds at increased risk include the miniature schnauzer, Lhasa apso, Shih Tzu, and Yorkshire terrier. As with uroliths in the lower urinary tract, male dalmatians are more predisposed than females to the development of urate nephroliths. Cats differ from dogs

in that there is no gender predisposition to the development of renal calculi or ureteroliths, and domestic shorthairs and longhairs are the most commonly affected breeds. Both cats and dogs tend to be middle-aged or older at the time of initial presentation (mean age, 8 years) (Kyles et al, 2005a; Ling et al, 1998).

Diagnosis

Clinical signs associated with nephrolithiasis and ureterolithiasis may be completely absent or may include nonspecific signs such as vomiting, anorexia, weight loss, and lethargy. Abnormalities noted on physical examination may include pyrexia, pain on abdominal palpation, and enlarged or asymmetric kidneys (i.e., big kidney, little kidney). Clinicopathologic abnormalities may include hyperkalemia, hypercalcemia, hyperphosphatemia, azotemia, anemia, and a neutrophilic leukocytosis. Hematuria, pyuria, proteinuria, crystalluria, and bacteriuria all may be noted on routine urinalysis. Urine culture is an essential component of the diagnostic workup, and an estimated one third of cats and two thirds of dogs with ureterolithiasis have been found to have a concurrent bacterial infection.

Imaging

Radiography
Although a clinical suspicion may be present based on physical examination findings, definitive diagnosis is obtained via imaging. Abdominal radiography generally is the first-line diagnostic imaging modality used to evaluate the urinary tract for radiopaque uroliths. With radiography, the exact location and number of uroliths often can be determined, whereas these sometimes can be difficult to distinguish with other forms of imaging. On the other hand, radiography has the distinct limitation of being able to identify only radiopaque uroliths, and thus dried solidified blood calculi, mucus plugs, and radiolucent uroliths potentially can be missed. Furthermore, overlapping visceral organs occasionally can make diagnosis difficult; abdominal preparation with enemas is necessary if fecal material obscures the ureteral paths. The sensitivity of abdominal radiography for the diagnosis of ureteroliths was 81% in one feline study and 88% in one canine study (Kyles et al, 2005a; Snyder et al, 2005).

Ultrasonography
Parenchymal hyperechogenicity, perirenal effusion, and ureteral wall thickening may be observed on ultrasonographic examination. Although dried solidified blood calculi, mucus plugs, and radiolucent uroliths can be challenging to visualize via ultrasonography, renal pelvic and ureteral dilation would support a diagnosis of ureteral obstruction. Marked hydronephrosis or hydroureter may be noted with prolonged or complete obstruction. The sensitivity of abdominal ultrasonography was 77% for the detection of feline ureteroliths in one retrospective series, whereas in one canine study, sensitivity reached 100% (Kyles et al, 2005a; Snyder et al, 2005).

Abdominal ultrasonography and radiography are best used as complementary imaging modalities. When ultrasonography and radiography were evaluated in tandem, sensitivity for detection of uroliths was 90% in cats with ureteral obstruction (Kyles et al, 2005a). In dogs, ureteroliths and nephroliths were identified during ultrasonographic examination that were missed on abdominal radiographs (Snyder et al, 2005).

Other Modalities
When the location and degree of ureteral obstruction are difficult to document definitively, advanced techniques occasionally must be used to aid diagnosis and planning. One such technique is antegrade pyelography, in which a contrast agent is injected directly into the renal pelvis with ultrasonographic guidance, which minimizes systemic absorption. Fluoroscopy or serial radiography follows the flow toward the urinary bladder. Antegrade pyelography has a high specificity for ureteral obstruction; in a retrospective study of 11 cats with 18 obstructed kidneys, antegrade pyelography allowed correct identification of the anatomic location of the ureteral obstruction in 13 (72%) of the ureters (Adin et al, 2003). However, leakage of contrast material developed in 8 of 18 kidneys (44%) and prevented diagnostic interpretation in 5 of 18 studies (28%). Although highly useful, antegrade pyelography requires general anesthesia and a skilled sonographer. Hemorrhage also is a possible complication of the technique.

Treatment

Medical Management

Conservative Management of Nephroliths
Most nephroliths initially are managed conservatively and never require further intervention. The majority of nephroliths in dogs are asymptomatic. Nephroliths have not been associated with an increase in disease progression or poorer outcome in cats with concurrent kidney disease and nephrolithiasis compared with cats with chronic kidney disease alone (Ross et al, 2007).

Nephroliths can become damaging to renal function and patient comfort, however, when they contribute to recurrent urinary tract infection or obstruction. In 2006, Dalby and colleagues described seven cases of spontaneous retrograde movement of ureteroliths in two dogs and five cats. Based on this observational study, the authors theorized that some mobile nephroliths may contribute to continued kidney injury by intermittent obstruction of the ureter. The location of the nephrolith may influence the risk of obstruction; nephroliths that are located within the renal interstitium certainly pose less threat of intermittent obstruction than nephroliths located within the renal pelvis. Indications and options for intervention in cases of problematic nephroliths are discussed further in Chapter 195.

Management of Concurrent Urinary Tract Infection
In two studies of dogs with upper urinary tract urolithiasis, 65% to 70% of dogs had a concurrent urinary tract infection (Ling et al, 1998; Snyder et al, 2005). The most commonly observed bacteria were *Staphylococcus intermedius, Escherichia coli, Proteus mirabilis,* and *Streptococcus* spp, and infection was recognized more commonly in female than in male dogs. Cats with urolithiasis less commonly have an associated concurrent infection than do dogs, although approximately one third of cats have a bacterial infection (Ling et al, 1998). Antibiotic therapy should be guided by urine or urolith culture results and should be continued for a minimum of 4 to 6 weeks, with repeat urine cultures performed 1 to 2 weeks after the initiation of antibiotic therapy and 1 week after the completion of therapy (Weese et al, 2011). If the patient has concurrent azotemia, then the possibility of pyelonephritis should be considered and the duration of antibiotic therapy should be 6 to 8 weeks, with cultures performed every 2 weeks during therapy and 1 to 2 weeks after the termination of treatment. In dogs, in which 50% of nephroliths are struvite (infection-induced) uroliths, antibiotics may need to be administered for as long as 2 to 3 months before there is complete dissolution. Some dogs have had documented negative results on cultures of lower urinary tract specimens, but positive results on cultures of samples from the upper urinary

tract, particularly when the infection is associated with urolithiasis or antibiotics were administered before culture (Snyder et al, 2005).

Diuresis to Promote Ureterolith Passage
The ideal outcome of medical management of ureterolithiasis is that the urolith passes into the urinary bladder to be voided or removed. Medical dissolution of ureteroliths is not likely because ureteroliths are not bathed continuously in urine and most ureteroliths are composed of calcium oxalate and are not amendable to dissolution. The optimal time to allow for passage of ureteroliths by medical management is unknown, but the authors typically attempt medical management for a period of 2 to 3 days depending on the patient's clinical status and the owner's wishes. In one study of 52 cats with ureterolithiasis that underwent medical management, 7 cats (13.5%) responded with a significant decrease in serum creatinine concentration (Kyles et al, 2005b). Aggressive intravenous fluid therapy is recommended in an attempt to push the urolith along the ureter. Typically, the authors administer 80 to 120 ml/kg/day of crystalloids depending on the patient's cardiovascular status. Continued administration of fluids to patients with poor urine output can lead to overhydration, as can overzealous diuresis in an attempt to flush out stones. Careful monitoring of body weight, hydration status, and urine production are key in the management of obstructive ureteroliths.

Pharmacologic Agents
Pharmaceutical options to promote the movement of nephroliths and ureteroliths are limited, with few studies to validate their use in veterinary medicine. In human medicine, α_2-antagonists are considered the standard of care for ureteral dilation. Consequently, a number of α_2-antagonists have been investigated experimentally in dogs to evaluate their ureteral dilatory effects. The α_2-antagonists vary greatly in their selectivity, particularly in regard to ureteral dilatory effects. Phenoxybenzamine is a nonselective, noncompetitive antagonist, whereas the newer α_2-antagonists such as prazosin and tamsulosin all are variably selective. Possible adverse effects of all of the α_2-antagonists include hypotension, sedation, and occasionally urinary incontinence. The authors typically administer prazosin at a dosage of 0.25 to 0.50 mg q12-24h PO in cats and 1 mg/15 kg q12h PO in dogs. Blood pressure should be monitored, particularly in the first few days after initiation of therapy, because profound hypotension can occur in some animals.

A tricyclic antidepressant, amitriptyline, may be of assistance both by modulating the pain associated with the ureteral obstruction and by acting as a ureteral relaxant by causing the opening of voltage-gated potassium channels in smooth muscle. One report described the use of amitriptyline in cats with obstructed urethras and demonstrated in vitro relaxant effects on the porcine and human ureter (Achar et al, 2003). Recommended dosages of amitriptyline vary (1 to 2 mg/kg q24h PO); in cats, a starting dose of one 10-mg tablet per cat is recommended because of the extremely bitter taste of the medication when split or compounded into a liquid.

Glucagon is a hormone that is produced naturally by the pancreas and is known to have a variety of physiologic effects, including ureteral dilation and relief of pain associated with ureteral obstruction in people. One prospective study evaluating the intravenous administration of glucagon to cats with ureteral obstruction found that glucagon may promote urination in some cats; however, no long-term benefits were noted (Forman et al, 2004). Possible adverse effects of glucagon include significant functional gastrointestinal ileus with resultant diarrhea or vomiting, and respiratory effects such as tachypnea or dyspnea. Described intravenous dosages vary greatly and range from 0.05 to 0.1 mg per cat q6-24h. This medication should be administered with caution, and blood glucose and potassium levels should be monitored regularly with usage.

In addition to fluid diuresis, administration of diuretic agents, particularly osmotic diuretics such as mannitol, has been advocated but has not been evaluated prospectively or retrospectively in feline or canine patients with ureteral obstruction. The theory behind the use of diuretics is to increase the glomerular filtration rate and raise the intraureteral luminal pressure to push the ureterolith into the urinary bladder. These medications should be used concurrently with intravenous fluids so that the patient does not become systemically dehydrated or experience further kidney injury. At the authors' hospital, furosemide is used most frequently at a dosage of 0.5 to 1 mg/kg/hr after a 1- to 2-mg/kg initial bolus. Kidney function values and electrolyte levels should be monitored every 6 to 12 hours during the continuous administration of diuretics for ureteral obstruction.

Pain Management
Ureteral obstruction can be very painful, and use of opioid pain medications is recommended until the obstruction is resolved. Morphine specifically is not recommended, however, because in one in vitro canine ureteral study morphine was found to have spasmogenic effects that were not reversed by the administration of naloxone (Lennon et al, 1993). Meperidine, on the other hand, initially did cause ureteral spasms transiently, followed by complete inhibition of activity. The effects of meperidine also were not affected by naloxone (Lennon et al, 1993). The effects of other opioids on ureteral contraction have not been evaluated thus far in the canine or feline patient. Nonsteroidal antiinflammatory medications (NSAIDs) are not recommended at this time because of the potential for worsening kidney injury; however, NSAIDs currently are considered one of the first-line therapies in the treatment of renal colic in people (Yilmaz et al, 2009). Certain nonsteroidal agents—namely, diclofenac and indomethacin—were shown in one in vitro canine study to have spasmolytic effects on the canine ureter (Lennon et al, 1993). Further studies are indicated as to the role of NSAIDs in canine and feline ureterolithiasis.

The canine ureter has been shown to contain histamine receptors, both histamine-1 (H_1) and H_2 (Dodel et al, 1996). Interestingly, the two histamine receptors appear to demonstrate opposite but uneven clinical effects on the canine ureter in in vitro studies. The H_1 receptors demonstrate a contractile response, whereas the

H_2 receptors show a relaxant response and generally are activated after the stimulation of the H_1 response (Dodel et al, 1996). Chlorpheniramine, an H_1 receptor antagonist, has demonstrated spasmolytic effects and has been shown to directly inhibit the ureteral spasmogenic effects induced by morphine in an *in vitro* canine model (Lennon et al, 1993). In another *in vitro* canine study, the H_2 receptor antagonist cimetidine was found to significantly attenuate the relaxation effect of histamine in precontracted canine ureters (Dodel et al, 1996). These effects certainly are important considerations because it is not uncommon to administer an H_2-receptor antagonist to a patient with kidney disease, and this in fact may result in the inability of the body to provide relaxation of the ureter naturally. It appears wise to avoid administration of H_2-receptor antagonists in dogs with ureteral obstruction until further studies are performed to specifically elucidate the role of each H_2-receptor antagonist on the canine ureter. At this time, there are no similar studies analyzing the role of histamine in the feline ureter.

Other pharmacologic agents may help preserve kidney function during and immediately following ureteral obstruction. In experimental studies in dogs, angiotensin-converting enzyme (ACE) inhibitors have been shown to assist in the preservation of kidney function in animals with partial unilateral ureteral obstruction and to assist in recovery of renal function after the obstruction is eliminated (Soliman et al, 2009b). Similarly, the angiotensin receptor blocker losartan exhibited promising effects on the recovery of kidney function in dogs with experimentally induced unilateral partial chronic ureteral obstruction, presumably because of vasodilation and increased renal blood flow. Further studies of losartan have been performed in rats with complete ureteral obstruction, and losartan significantly decreased renal fibrosis, oxidative stress, and apoptosis (Soliman et al, 2009a). No studies have investigated the use of ACE inhibitors or angiotensin receptor blockers in cats with obstructive ureterolithiasis.

Advanced Supportive Modalities

Dialysis

The goals of hemodialysis or peritoneal dialysis in managing ureteral obstruction are multifactorial: (1) to reduce the degree of azotemia, hydration, or electrolyte derangements before induction of anesthesia for procedures or definitive treatment, (2) to provide time to treat infection, sepsis, or other concurrent abnormalities, and (3) to allow time to determine whether the ureteral calculus will pass on its own with medical management. Many of these patients have profound fluid overload, which renal replacement therapy also will normalize. Perioperative dialytic management is particularly beneficial in the patient in which kidney transplantation, ureteral surgery, or ureteral stent placement is planned.

Nephrostomy Tubes

Preoperative nephrostomy tube placement has goals similar to those of hemodialysis in terms of improving the stability of the patient's condition before surgery. A benefit of nephrostomy tubes over hemodialysis is the immediate decompression of the renal pelvis, which decreases the compressive damage to the renal parenchyma (see Chapter 195). Nephrostomy tubes can be lifesaving and can prevent further renal damage; however, in one study approximately half of cats in which nephrostomy tubes were placed experienced complications, which included urine leakage into the peritoneal cavity, poor drainage, and tube dislodgement (Kyles et al, 2005b). Unfortunately, decompression also may reduce the antegrade pressure on the obstructing material, minimizing other efforts to promote spontaneous passage.

Surgical and Interventional Therapies

If medical management has failed, the patient has many ureteroliths, or several levels of the urinary tract are affected, then a surgical or interventional procedure may be recommended. The type of surgery performed depends on the location of the ureterolith within the ureter, as well as the viability of the ureter and the preference of the surgeon. A ureteral stent may be placed during surgery after stone removal or, in dogs, occasionally may be placed with a cystoscope. Interventional stenting is discussed more extensively in Chapter 195.

Renal Transplantation

Renal transplantation has been considered a salvage procedure for cats with renal dysfunction due to urolithiasis. In one review of feline renal transplantation over a period of 8 years, approximately one fourth of all transplants were required because of confirmed or suspected calcium oxalate urolithiasis (Aronson et al, 2006). Furthermore, 60% of these cats continued to develop uroliths despite appropriate urolith prevention therapy. However, the recurrence of kidney and ureteral calculi did not cause these cats to have a lower mean survival time than cats that did not experience urolith recurrence.

Prevention

Dietary Therapy

Prevention and monitoring are essential in the long-term management of this dynamic disease. Except in cases of infection-induced struvite nephroliths, stone recurrence or growth is likely in all patients with nephroliths or ureteroliths. The saturation of stone-inducing minerals can be reduced with the use of therapeutic diets. As in all urinary diseases, diets that are high in water content are most beneficial for decreasing the recurrence of urolith formation. Canned diets allow the greatest percentage of water to be added to the diet; however, adding water to a dry diet also is possible. Urolith analysis is recommended to permit the most accurate recommendations to be made for dietary composition; however, a diet can be prescribed based on the most likely urolith type. Additionally, several feline diets currently are composed and marketed for the prevention of both magnesium ammonium phosphate and calcium oxalate urolithiasis and can be prescribed if the stone type is undetermined (see Chapter 197). Finally, underlying kidney disease is common in patients with nephroliths and ureteroliths (especially cats). In cats affected with both disorders, dietary management for renal disease often trumps the dietary considerations for urolithiasis. Patients with International Renal Interest Society stage 2 kidney disease or higher should be started on a diet that is restricted in protein, phosphorus, and sodium (see Chapter 189).

Monitoring and Recurrence

In one study, a second episode of ureterolithiasis was documented in 14 of 35 cats (40%) in which serial abdominal imaging was performed after medical or surgical management (Kyles et al, 2005b). In 12 of these 14 cats, nephroliths had been noted at the time of initial examination and had not been removed. Recurrence rates in dogs have not been reported.

Serum creatinine and electrolyte levels should be monitored at a frequency determined by the degree of azotemia and clinical progress of the patient. Monitoring including abdominal radiography or ultrasonography, urinalysis, urine culture, and blood chemistry studies should be repeated every 3 months for the first year and every 6 months thereafter, or sooner in the event that any changes in behavior or clinical signs are noted at home. Therapeutic targets include a urine specific gravity of less than 1.030 for cats and less than 1.020 for dogs, minimal crystalluria, stable or decreasing azotemia, stable or improving upper tract dilation, and lack of progression in urolith size and number.

References and Suggested Reading

Achar E et al: Amitriptyline eliminates calculi through urinary tract smooth muscle relaxation, *Kidney Int* 64:1356, 2003.

Adin CA et al: Antegrade pyelography for suspected ureteral obstruction in cats: 11 cases (1995-2001), *J Am Vet Med Assoc* 222:1576, 2003.

Albasan H et al: Rate and frequency of recurrence of uroliths after an initial ammonium urate, calcium oxalate, or struvite urolith in cats, *J Am Vet Med Assoc* 235(12):1450, 2009.

Aronson LR et al: Renal transplantation in cats with calcium oxalate urolithiasis: 19 cases (1997-2004), *J Am Vet Med Assoc* 228(5):743, 2006.

Dalby AM et al: Spontaneous retrograde movement of ureteroliths in two dogs and five cats, *J Am Vet Med Assoc* 229:1118, 2006.

Dodel RC, Hafner D, Borchard U: Characterization of histamine receptors in the ureter of the dog, *Eur J Pharmacol* 318(2-3):395, 1996.

Forman MA et al: Use of glucagon in the management of acute ureteral obstruction in 25 cats. In *Proceedings of the 22nd Annual ACVIM Forum*, 2004.

Kyles AE et al: Clinical, clinicopathologic, radiographic, and ultrasonographic abnormalities in cats with ureteral calculi: 163 cases (1984-2002), *J Am Vet Med Assoc* 226(6):932, 2005a.

Kyles AE et al: Management and outcome of cats with ureteral calculi: 153 cases (1984-2002), *J Am Vet Med Assoc* 226(6):937, 2005b.

Lennon GM et al: Pharmacological options for the treatment of acute ureteral colic: an *in vitro* experimental study, *Br J Urol* 71:401, 1993.

Ling GV et al: Renal calculi in dogs and cats: prevalence, mineral type, breed, age, and gender interrelationships (1981-1993), *J Vet Int Med* 12:11, 1998.

Osborne CA et al: Analysis of 451,891 canine uroliths, feline uroliths, and feline urethral plugs from 1981 to 2007: perspectives from the Minnesota Urolith Center, *Vet Clin North Am* 39(1):183, 2009.

Ross SJ, et al: A case-control study of the effects of nephrolithiasis in cats with chronic kidney disease, *J Am Vet Med Assoc* 230(12):1854, 2007.

Snyder DM et al: Diagnosis and surgical management of ureteral calculi in dogs: 16 cases (1990-2003), *N Z Vet J* 53(1):19, 2005.

Soliman SA et al: Recoverability of renal function after relief of chronic partial unilateral ureteral obstruction: study of the effect of angiotensin receptor blocker (losartan), *J Urol* 75:848, 2009a.

Soliman SA et al: Study of the effect of angiotensin converting enzyme inhibitor (enalapril) on renal function during and after relief of partial unilateral ureteral obstruction: a controlled canine study, *J Urol* 181(4 Suppl):662, 2009b (abstract).

Weese JS et al: Antimicrobial use guidelines for treatment of urinary tract disease in dogs and cats: Antimicrobial Guidelines Working Group of the International Society for Companion Animal Infectious Diseases, *Vet Med Int* 2011:263768, 2011.

Westropp JL et al: Dried solidified blood calculi in the urinary tract of cats, *J Vet Intern Med* 20:828, 2006.

Yilmaz E et al: Histamine 1 receptor antagonist in symptomatic treatment of renal colic accompanied by nausea: two birds with one stone? *Urology* 73(1):32, 2009.

CHAPTER 197

Calcium Oxalate Urolithiasis

BENJAMIN G. NOLAN, *Madison, Wisconsin*
MARY ANNA LABATO, *North Grafton, Massachusetts*

Calcium oxalate (CaOx) urolithiasis is a condition affecting dogs and cats that has become more common over the last several decades (Cannon et al, 2007; Low et al, 2010). A recent study examined the composition of uroliths submitted to the Minnesota Urolith Center between the years 1981 and 2007 (Osborne et al, 2008). During this time the percentage of CaOx stones in total submissions increased from 5% to 41% in dogs, whereas that in cats increased from 2% to 41%. Concurrently, the incidence of struvite uroliths decreased from 78% to 40% in dogs and from 78% to 49% in cats. It is thought that the primary factor causing this trend was dietary modifications made to address struvite urolithiasis. Overall, the pathophysiology of CaOx urolithiasis is complex, and much still remains to be understood. This chapter outlines what we know about CaOx urolithiasis and how this knowledge can be applied to design effective therapies for this disease.

Epidemiology

Dogs and cats affected with CaOx urolithiasis typically are middle-aged to older, male, and neutered. As in humans, obesity has been associated with a higher risk in dogs, but this has not yet been shown to be true for cats. Breeds of dogs most recently identified as having an increased risk of forming CaOx uroliths are the bichon frise, miniature schnauzer, Shih Tzu, Lhasa apso, Pomeranian, Cairn terrier, Yorkshire terrier, Maltese, and Keeshond. Cat breeds at higher risk include the Persian and Himalayan.

Pathophysiology

The physical chemistry governing crystal formation in urine is complex, and many variables must be considered. The two major factors that affect this process are supersaturation of urine with calculogenic materials (calcium and oxalate) and the balance between substances that promote and those that inhibit CaOx formation. When urine is supersaturated with calcium and oxalate, crystal formation is more likely to occur; one measure that reflects this state is the relative supersaturation of urine (RSS). This measure is used widely to assess the risk of CaOx formation in people and is finding use in veterinary medicine as well. In one study, the CaOx RSS of stone-forming dogs was found to be significantly higher than that of control dogs (Stevenson, Robertson et al, 2003).

To assess supersaturation of the urine with calculogenic materials, the relative importance of urinary water content, calcium concentration, and oxalate concentration have been examined. Water content is perhaps the single most important variable affecting CaOx formation. Increased water dilutes the urine and increases urine volume, thereby reducing CaOx RSS. Hyperoxaluria also plays a role. Urinary excretion of oxalate depends on dietary intake, intestinal absorption, renal tubular secretion, and the rate of endogenous synthesis. Intestinal absorption is influenced by factors that determine the amount of free oxalate in the gut lumen. Calcium and magnesium both can bind oxalate, creating complexes that are excreted instead of absorbed. Intestinal flora such as *Oxalobacter formigenes* and lactic acid bacteria can degrade oxalate and may play a role in the pathophysiology of this disease. Hyperoxaluria due to endogenous overproduction has been found to be a primary genetic condition in people caused by metabolic defects and exists in two forms (type I and type II). A few cases of primary hyperoxaluria also have been reported in cats and appear to be most similar to the type II variant in people (DeLorenzi et al, 2005).

Like oxalate excretion, urinary calcium excretion depends on dietary intake, intestinal absorption, and renal tubular excretion. Intestinal absorption of calcium is similar to that of oxalate in that calcium is poorly absorbed when it exists as a complex but is absorbed more readily when unbound. The appropriate level of calcium intake to minimize urinary CaOx RSS is thus intertwined with the amount of oxalate present, as well as the amount of other substances with which it may form complexes (e.g., phosphate). Hypercalciuria also can result from hypercalcemia, impaired tubular reabsorption of calcium (renal leak), and administration of certain drugs such as glucocorticoids or loop diuretics (e.g., furosemide).

Several substances have been identified as promoting or inhibiting CaOx formation in urine. Inhibitors include magnesium, citrate, and pyrophosphate, which form soluble complexes with calcium in the urine and prevent crystal formation with oxalate. Citrate also may lower the risk of CaOx formation by alkalinizing the urine. Proteins such as nephrocalcin and Tamm-Horsfall glycoprotein interfere with CaOx crystal formation and may play an additional role.

There most likely are many promoters of CaOx formation, but two that have been identified are uric acid and foreign material. Uric acid can block certain CaOx inhibitors, and a group of CaOx-forming miniature schnauzers was found to excrete significantly higher levels of uric acid than healthy controls (Lulich et al, 1991). The presence of foreign material such as intraluminal suture in the urinary tract can act as a nidus for crystal nucleation.

The urinary pH also has been evaluated for its role in CaOx formation, and there is controversy over its importance. The absolute solubility of CaOx in urine is affected marginally over a broad pH range, but there are several reasons why a low pH may promote CaOx formation: persistent aciduria is associated with low-grade metabolic acidosis, which induces calcium resorption from bone and can increase urinary calcium excretion; acidic urine may diminish the ability of citrate and pyrophosphate to act as CaOx inhibitors; and increased reabsorption of calcium from the distal tubule occurs when the urine is alkaline. Furthermore, feeding an acidifying diet has been identified as a risk factor for CaOx formation in cats and dogs. In dogs the risk was three times higher overall (Lekcharoensuk et al, 2002), whereas in cats the risk was three times higher when diets were fed producing a urinary pH of 5.99 to 6.15 compared with diets producing a pH of 6.5 to 6.9 (Lekcharoensuk et al, 2001). Studies also have evaluated the effect of pH specifically on CaOx RSS, but results so far have been conflicting.

Diagnostic Approach

The initial evaluation of a dog or cat with CaOx urolithiasis should include a thorough investigation for any underlying cause. A complete blood count, chemistry panel, urinalysis, and urine culture are considered a minimum database. If the total calcium concentration is elevated, the ionized calcium level should be measured, and if hypercalcemia is confirmed, measurement of parathyroid hormone, parathyroid hormone–related protein, and possibly serum vitamin D levels is recommended. Imaging should include both abdominal radiography and ultrasonography because in some cases stones may be missed when only one modality is used. This is especially the case for ureteroliths, which can cause severe illness. Ultrasonographic imaging also may reveal more detailed information about the urinary tract (e.g., ureteral obstruction, cystitis).

Treatment

Surgical and Interventional Management

There is no known protocol to dissolve CaOx uroliths at this time, and in many cases the only effective treatment is removal. Urolith removal can be achieved surgically, and less invasive methods are becoming increasingly available (see Chapters 195 and 199). Depending on the location of the urolith various techniques may be employed, such as lithotripsy (extracorporeal and intracorporeal), cystoscopic removal, or urohydropulsion. An obstructive stone also can be addressed by the placement of a stent, subcutaneous ureteral bypass device, or other interventional procedures.

Medical Management

Once CaOx urolithiasis is identified, preventive medical management of this problem still is of utmost importance

because this is a chronic disease. Dietary options and medications can be used to minimize the chance of stone recurrence or further growth. Additionally, regular monitoring of the patient is needed to evaluate response to therapy and to identify new stones that may form. In the case of a stone in the upper urinary tract (ureterolith, nephrolith), medical strategies are often instituted before surgery or other procedures (see also Chapter 196).

Diet

Perhaps the most important dietary modification that can be made is to increase water intake and urinary volume while decreasing urine specific gravity. Retrospective studies of cats (Lekcharoensuk et al, 2001) and dogs (Lekcharoensuk et al, 2002) with CaOx urolithiasis found a significantly lower risk of CaOx formation with higher dietary moisture content. Feeding a canned diet is the best way to increase water intake, but some dogs and cats will not eat canned food. In these cases, water or broth can be added to dry food, or broth can be added to the water supply. Water fountains also may be helpful to increase water intake in cats. Appropriate targets for specific gravity are less than 1.025 in cats and less than 1.020 in dogs; achieving dilute urine can be very difficult in cats.

Supplementation of sodium chloride has been investigated as a means of increasing water consumption but has been a point of controversy. Increased sodium consumption increases urinary calcium excretion and may increase the risk of CaOx urolithiasis. However, prospective studies have shown that increasing dietary sodium content significantly decreased the CaOx RSS in healthy and CaOx stone–forming dogs (Lulich et al, 2005; Stevenson, Hynds et al, 2003) as well as in healthy cats. The *total* daily urinary calcium excretion increased in these studies, but apparently the effect on CaOx RSS is offset by the increase in water intake and urine volume. These findings suggest a benefit to NaCl supplementation, but long-term studies still are needed. Sodium supplementation can be considered if there is an inadequate response to dietary therapy and the urine is not dilute, but patient selection must be done carefully. Short-term studies in cats have shown no adverse effects on kidney function or blood pressure, but caution is required when considering adding salt to the diets of dogs or cats with kidney disease or hypertension until longer-term studies are done. Additionally, high-sodium diets are contraindicated for animals with heart disease.

Higher dietary protein historically has been associated with an elevated risk of CaOx formation because it can promote acidosis and hypercalciuria. However, retrospective studies in dogs and cats have found a lower risk of CaOx formation with higher dietary protein (Lekcharoensuk et al, 2001, 2002). Overall, the exact amount and type of protein that is ideal has yet to be determined, but most diets designed to reduce CaOx urolithiasis have reduced protein levels.

The importance of the calcium and oxalate content of food was demonstrated by a study in healthy dogs (Stevenson, Hynds et al, 2003). In these dogs, urinary oxalate excretion and CaOx RSS increased when oxalate intake was increased, but *only* when the intake of calcium was low. The lowest CaOx RSS was found in dogs fed a diet that was lowest in both calcium and oxalate. If only calcium or only oxalate was decreased, the CaOx RSS increased. This emphasizes the need for a balanced amount of calcium and oxalate in the diet, but in all cases high calcium or oxalate content should be avoided. Examples of high-oxalate foods are leafy green vegetables and nuts. For a more complete list of foods with high oxalate content, see the Oxalosis and Hyperoxaluria Foundation website (www.ohf.org/diet.html).

Vitamin intake also can be important: hypercalciuria can result from excessive vitamin D intake because of enhanced intestinal absorption, and excessive vitamin C may promote hyperoxaluria, although this has yet to be proven in dogs and cats. A deficiency in vitamin B_6 (pyridoxine) also may play a role in urinary oxalate excretion. A study in healthy kittens showed that urinary oxalate excretion was higher in those fed a diet deficient in pyridoxine than in those fed a normal amount (Bai et al, 1989). Supplementation with vitamin B_6 (2 mg/kg q24-48h PO) thus can be considered as adjunct medical treatment.

Three studies have prospectively evaluated the effect of commercially available urinary diets on dogs and cats with CaOx urolithiasis. The diets evaluated were canned Royal Canin Canine SO Lower Urinary Tract Support, canned Hill's Prescription Diet Feline c/d-oxl, and canned Hill's Prescription Diet u/d. A fourth diet is available for cats (Purina Veterinary Diets UR Urinary St/Ox Feline Formula). Unpublished work indicates that feeding this diet to normal cats yielded urine that was metastable for CaOx, which suggests that it would be an appropriate option for cats with CaOx urolithiasis. However, published studies still are needed for a more complete evaluation.

In dogs fed canned Canine SO, the CaOx RSS was reduced significantly by 63% compared to that in dogs fed a maintenance diet (Stevenson et al, 2004). This group of dogs was followed for 12 months, during which time no recurrence of CaOx stones was noted.

In cats fed Prescription Diet Feline c/d-oxl, the activity product ratio (measure of CaOx supersaturation) was reduced significantly by 59% compared with that in the same group of cats fed a variety of dry maintenance diets (Lulich et al, 2004b). This diet is no longer available, but Hill's Prescription Diet c/d Multicare Feline has similar efficacy according to the manufacturer.

A third study evaluated the effect of feeding canned Prescription Diet u/d to dogs with CaOx urolithiasis (Lulich et al, 2001). Compared with dogs fed a maintenance diet, dogs fed Prescription Diet u/d had significantly lower urinary concentrations of both calcium and oxalate. Protein malnutrition is rare but possible during long-term feeding of Prescription Diet u/d; dogs fed this diet had a significantly lower serum albumin level than controls, although values remained in the normal range. The low protein levels make this diet contraindicated in dogs with dilated cardiomyopathy or in breeds that are predisposed to this disease. In recent years Hill's has supplemented Prescription Diet u/d with taurine and carnitine, but concerns still remain. In general, veterinary nutritionists recommend against using Prescription Diet

TABLE **197-1**

Target pH Values for Urinary Diets

Food	Target pH
Hill's Prescription Diet c/d Multicare Feline	6.2-6.4
Hill's Prescription Diet u/d Canine	7.1-7.7
Royal Canin Veterinary Diet Urinary SO Canine	5.5-6.0
Royal Canin Veterinary Diet Urinary SO Feline	6.0-6.3

u/d as a maintenance diet. Furthermore, this diet tends to be higher in fat and may not be the best choice for dogs with a history of pancreatitis or hyperlipidemia.

As mentioned earlier, acidifying diets have been associated with a higher risk of CaOx formation in both dogs and cats, but further studies have yielded conflicting results regarding the importance of daily urinary pH in CaOx prevention. Overall, it can be said that pH generally appears to be less important in controlling CaOx stone formation than in controlling formation of other stones such as struvite. Given the available information it seems prudent to avoid significant acidification of the urine. An appropriate initial target urine pH is approximately 7.0; however, with this in mind, the target urinary pH values achieved by feeding almost all of the diets listed in Table 197-1 are acidic. The only diet designed to produce a urinary pH of more than 7.0 is Hill's Prescription Diet u/d, with the others aiming for an acidic pH. This is because the goal of the Royal Canin Urinary SO formulation and Hill's Prescription Diet c/d Multicare is to prevent both CaOx *and* struvite uroliths. Since urine pH control is more important for dissolution and prevention in treating struvite stones than in treating CaOx stones, these diets target a lower pH as part of the strategy to prevent struvites. Despite causing a mildly acidic urine, all the listed diets are effective in producing urine with a low CaOx RSS. This apparent paradox exemplifies the complex nature of CaOx urolithiasis and the many factors must be considered in designing an appropriate diet. Of course, if CaOx uroliths continue to be a problem despite feeding an appropriate diet, alkalinization of the urine can be considered (see later) to potentially improve control.

Another important aspect of dietary treatment of CaOx urolithiasis is to control the types of treats, table food, and supplements given to dogs or cats. Owners often do not consider these things when dietary modifications are made, which can affect the efficacy of a diet adversely. Aside from being high in oxalate or calcium (see the previously referenced website for more details), certain treats or supplements can change the composition of urine by other mechanisms. Any discussion with owners concerning dietary recommendations thus should include a focus on this subject.

Medications
Pharmacologic agents can be added to the management plan for CaOx urolithiasis if dietary therapy alone is not effective in preventing stone growth or regrowth.

Potassium citrate has been used effectively in people as a urinary alkalinization agent, and it also may help due to the inhibitory action of citrate on CaOx formation. However, no study to date has shown a clear benefit to the use of citrate in dogs or cats. Furthermore, there is no evidence for hypocitraturia as a risk factor for CaOx formation in dogs or cats. One prospective study in healthy adult dogs was designed to evaluate the effect of supplemental potassium citrate on urinary parameters compared with controls (Stevenson et al, 2000). Overall, there was no significant difference in urinary pH, urinary citrate excretion, or CaOx RSS. However, when only the three miniature schnauzers in this group of dogs were considered, a significant decrease in CaOx RSS was observed. The dosage of potassium citrate used in this study was 75 mg/kg q12h PO, which is the currently recommended starting dose of this medication. Potassium citrate supplementation thus may be helpful in miniature schnauzers, but further studies are needed to confirm this and to determine if higher dosages would be more effective. If potassium citrate is used clinically for alkalinization, the starting dosage mentioned previously can be used and the dosage increased until a pH of approximately 7.0 is achieved. Serum potassium level should be monitored when this drug is used to avoid hyperkalemia.

Thiazide diuretics provide another medical option to reduce CaOx saturation. These drugs inhibit the sodium-chloride cotransporter in the distal tubule and by doing so stimulate calcium reabsorption and decrease urinary calcium excretion. The use of hydrochlorothiazide was evaluated in a group of dogs with a history of CaOx urolithiasis (Lulich et al, 2001). Urinary calcium excretion was significantly lower in dogs treated with the diuretic at a dosage of 2 mg/kg q12h PO. In a study of healthy cats treated with hydrochlorothiazide at a dosage of 1 mg/kg q12h PO, a significant decrease in urinary CaOx RSS was found (Hezel et al, 2007). Studies of the safety and effectiveness of long-term administration are lacking.

Monitoring

The probability of CaOx urolith recurrence varies among studies but in general is not uncommon. Two studies in cats have found differing results: resubmissions of uroliths were recorded from 7.1% of over 2000 affected cats within a 5-year period (mean resubmission time, 25 months) (Albasan et al, 2009), whereas 40% of a group of cats with ureteroliths exhibited recurrence within about a year (Kyles et al, 2005). Neither study group reflects the total population at risk. Two studies in dogs found CaOx stone recurrence rates of 57% at 2 years (Lulich et al, 2004a) and 36%, 42%, 48%, and 52% after years 1, 2, 3, and 6, respectively (Lulich et al, 1992). If new stones are identified before they become large, less invasive therapies such as voiding urohydropulsion may be used. The size of stone that can be expelled varies depending on breed and size, but in general bladder stones smaller than 5 mm in female cats, 1 mm in male cats, 10 to 15 mm in female dogs, and 1 to 3 mm in male dogs are amenable to urohydropulsion. Removal of larger uroliths requires a more invasive method. Radiography or ultrasonography

is recommended immediately following a removal procedure to verify that no stones remain, 4 weeks after the initial procedure, then at 3 and 6 months, and every 6 months thereafter.

Changes in diet or medical therapy designed to control CaOx formation also necessitate monitoring of urinalysis and blood work. Initially this testing is recommended 4 weeks after an intervention; it should then be repeated at 3 and 6 months, then every 6 months thereafter. The urine should be monitored for pH, specific gravity, and crystalluria. The timing of urine collection can affect interpretation. Urinary pH is not a constant and fluctuates during a 24-hour period. Various factors contribute, but in general pH is lowest through the night and highest during the day. In people, the greatest risk of CaOx crystallization was determined to be during the overnight period, and the same is thought to be true in dogs and cats. Thus it may be best to collect a urine sample in the morning before feeding. The urine specific gravity also is likely to be highest at this time, so two risk factors can be evaluated using the morning sample.

If potassium citrate is being administered, the urinary pH also can be measured after a meal to determine if it is having an alkalinizing effect. Measurement of pH can be done using a colorimetric reagent strip or a pH meter. However, pH values obtained using a colorimetric strip can vary by as much as 0.5 units on either side of the observed value. A pH meter is more accurate, and these are available in a benchtop model and a less expensive portable handheld meter. The pH values obtained by a handheld meter appear to correlate well with those obtained using the benchtop device. If a nephrolith or ureterolith is present, urine culture is recommended every 4 to 6 months. When either potassium citrate or thiazide diuretics are administered, serum or plasma electrolyte levels should be monitored at each re-evaluation. If a change in dosage is required, electrolyte levels should be checked again 2 weeks after the adjustment is made. For patients with concurrent conditions such as hypercalcemic disorders, hyperadrenocorticism, or urinary tract infection, additional parameters are monitored as well.

References and Suggested Reading

Albasan H, Osborne CA, Lulich JP: Rate and frequency of recurrence of uroliths after an initial ammonium urate, calcium oxalate, or struvite urolith in cats, *J Am Vet Med Assoc* 235:1450, 2009.

Bai SC et al: Vitamin B-6 requirement of growing kittens, *J Nutr* 19:1020, 1989.

Cannon AB et al: Evaluation of trends in urolith composition in cats: 5230 cases (1985-2004), *J Am Vet Med Assoc* 231:570, 2007.

DeLorenzi D, Bernardini M, Pumarola M: Primary hyperoxaluria (L-glyceric aciduria) in a cat, *J Feline Med Surg* 7:357, 2005.

Hezel A et al: Influence of hydrochlorothiazide on urinary calcium oxalate relative supersaturation in healthy young adult female domestic shorthaired cats, *Vet Ther* 8:247, 2007.

Kyles AE, Hardie EM, Wooden BG: Management and outcome of cats with ureteral calculi: 153 cases (1984-2002), *J Am Vet Med Assoc* 226:937, 2005.

Lekcharoensuk C et al: Association between dietary factors and calcium oxalate and magnesium ammonium phosphate urolithiasis in cats, *J Am Vet Med Assoc* 219:1228, 2001.

Lekcharoensuk C et al: Associations between dry dietary factors and canine calcium oxalate uroliths, *Am J Vet Res* 63:330, 2002.

Low WW et al: Evaluation of trends in urolith composition and characteristics of dogs with urolithiasis: 25,499 cases (1985-2006), *J Am Vet Med Assoc* 236:193, 2010.

Luckschander N et al: Dietary NaCl does not affect blood pressure in healthy cats, *J Vet Intern Med* 18:463, 2004.

Lulich JP et al: Evaluation of urine and serum metabolites in miniature schnauzers with calcium oxalate urolithiasis, *Am J Vet Res* 52:1583, 1991.

Lulich JP et al: Postsurgical recurrence of calcium oxalate uroliths in dogs. In *Proceedings of the 10th Annual ACVIM Forum*, 1992, p 802 (abstract).

Lulich JP et al: Effects of hydrochlorothiazide and diet in dogs with calcium oxalate urolithiasis, *J Am Vet Med Assoc* 218:1583, 2001.

Lulich JP et al: Biological behavior of calcium oxalate uroliths in Bichon Frise dogs. In *Proceedings of the 22nd Annual ACVIM Forum*, 2004a, p 861 (abstract)

Lulich JP et al: Effect of diet on urine composition of cats with calcium oxalate urolithiasis, *J Am Anim Hosp Assoc* 40:185, 2004b.

Lulich JP, Osborne CA, Sanderson SL: Effects of dietary supplementation with sodium chloride on urinary relative supersaturation with calcium oxalate in healthy dogs, *Am J Vet Res* 66:319, 2005.

Osborne CA et al: Analysis of 451,891 canine uroliths, feline uroliths, and feline urethral plugs from 1981-2007: perspectives from the Minnesota Urolith Center, *Vet Clin North Am Small Animal Pract* 39:183, 2008.

Stevenson AE et al: Effects of dietary potassium citrate supplementation on urine pH and urinary relative supersaturation of calcium oxalate and struvite in healthy dogs, *Am J Vet Res* 61:430, 2000.

Stevenson AE et al: Nutrient intake and urine composition in calcium oxalate stone-forming dogs: comparison with healthy dogs and impact of dietary modification, *Vet Ther* 5:218, 2004.

Stevenson AE, Hynds WK, Markwell PJ: The relative effects of supplemental dietary calcium and oxalate on urine composition and calcium oxalate relative supersaturation in healthy adult dogs, *Res Vet Sci* 75:33, 2003.

Stevenson AE, Robertson WG, Markwell P: Risk factor analysis and relative supersaturation as tools for identifying calcium oxalate stone-forming dogs, *J Small Anim Pract* 44:491, 2003.

CHAPTER **198**

Canine Urate Urolithiasis

JODY P. LULICH, *St. Paul, Minnesota*
CARL A. OSBORNE, *St. Paul, Minnesota*
HASAN ALBASAN, *St. Paul, Minnesota*

Between January 1, 2009, and December 31, 2010, the Minnesota Urolith Center received uroliths from 99,598 dogs. Purines made up 5.1% of uroliths submitted; of these, 84.5% were ammonium urate, 11.3% were other salts of urate, 2.5% were uric acid, and 1.7% were xanthine. Although purine uroliths were diagnosed in 111 breeds, dalmatians were the most common purine stone formers on every continent.

Uric acid is one of several biodegradation products of purine nucleotide biosynthesis and degradation. Purines are made up of three groups of compounds: (1) oxypurines (hypoxanthine, xanthine, uric acid, and allantoin), (2) aminopurines (adenine, guanine), and (3) methylpurines (caffeine, theophylline, and theobromine). In people, excess nucleotides are converted to xanthine and then uric acid via xanthine oxidase. In most dogs, excess uric acid is metabolized further to allantoin via the hepatic enzyme uricase. Allantoin is highly soluble in urine, whereas uric acid and xanthine are not.

Risk factors associated with urate lithogenesis in dogs include the following:

1. Increased renal excretion and urine concentration of uric acid
2. Increased renal excretion or renal production of ammonium ions
3. Increased microbial production of ammonium ions
4. Aciduria
5. Formation of highly concentrated urine
6. Presence of promoters or absence of inhibitors of urate urolith formation

Genetic factors also may be important. Hyperuricuria and urate urolithiasis have been linked to a mutation in a urate transporter that was identified recently in dalmatians, English bulldogs, and Black Russian terriers and sporadically in other breeds (Karmi et al, 2010).

To promote dissolution and prevention of urate uroliths, appropriate diets are prescribed to minimize the risk factors listed previously. In studies of normal dogs, consumption of high-protein foods was associated with greater urine uric acid excretion and increased urine saturation with uric acid, sodium urate, and ammonium urate, compared with consumption of low-protein foods. The same association was found in dalmatian dogs.

The following sections provide answers to questions essential for effective urate urolith management in dogs.

How Effective Is Medical Dissolution of Urate Uroliths?

Efficacy of medical dissolution depends on several key factors: the location of the uroliths, the treatments selected, owner compliance with the treatment regimen, any underlying disease(s), and disease severity. In an uncontrolled clinical trial, 25 dogs with naturally occurring urate urocystoliths (without hepatic portovascular anomalies) were prescribed canned Hill's Prescription Diet u/d and allopurinol (15 mg/kg q12h). Of these dogs, 36% experienced complete dissolution (median dissolution time, 3.5 months), 32% experienced partial dissolution, and 32% experienced no dissolution (Osborne et al, 2009). Aside from sporadic anecdotal reports, we are

not aware of the efficacy of other potentially litholytic diets (e.g., vegetarian diets, Royal Canin Veterinary Diet Urinary UC Low Purine, and other lower-protein diets formulated for dogs with renal failure, liver disease, or dermatologic disorders).

The role of a new selective xanthine oxidase inhibitor, febuxostat (Uloric), in safely promoting effective urolith dissolution also is unknown. Unlike allopurinol, febuxostat does not need to undergo hepatic transformation to more active metabolites. Therefore febuxostat would appear more suitable for dogs with portovascular shunts and urate urolithiasis; however, abnormal liver function test results were a frequent adverse event in humans taking the medication. Additional clinical studies are needed to evaluate the efficacy of contemporary diets and newer medications. Until such studies are completed, we recommend initially considering evidence-based medical dissolution therapies for dogs with asymptomatic or mildly symptomatic urate urocystoliths and nephroliths (Figure 198-1). More rapid urolith removal (surgery,

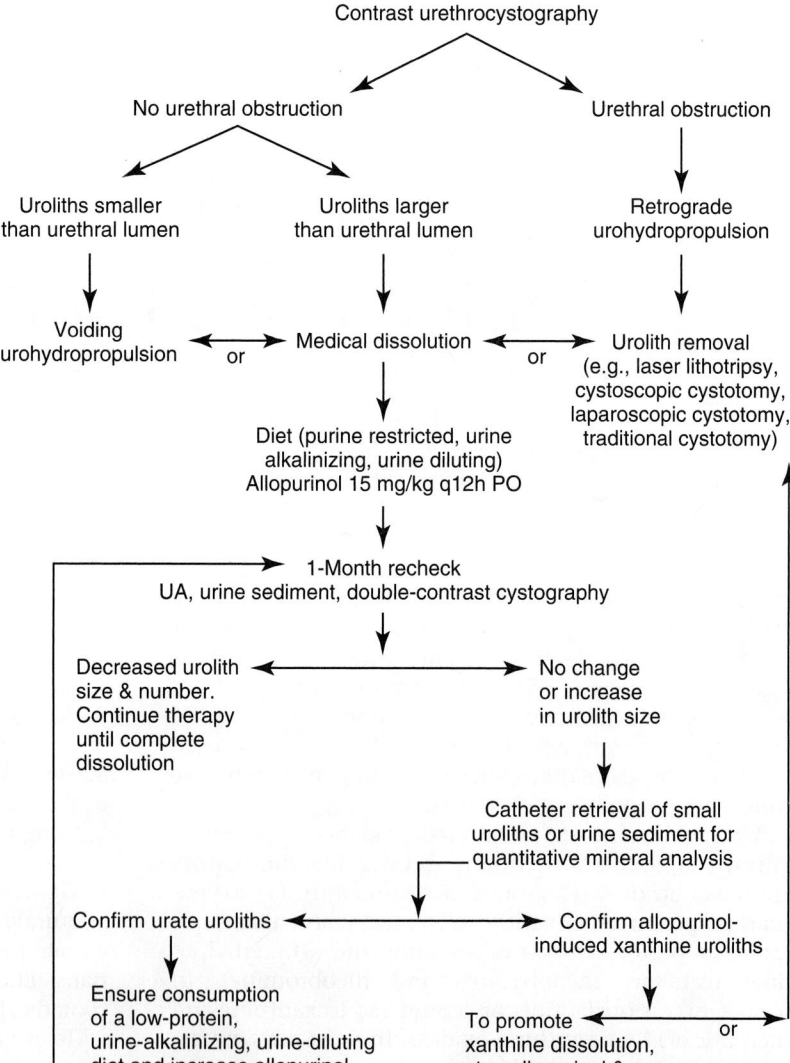

Figure 198-1 Managing urate uroliths in dogs.

lithotripsy, cystoscopically assisted cystotomy, or laparoscopic cystotomy) should be considered for dogs with urethroliths and clinically active disease (e.g., moderate to severe clinical signs or urinary obstruction).

How Should Medical Dissolution Be Monitored?

Frequent evaluations (monthly) are necessary to permit timely adjustments to therapy to improve dissolution and minimize adverse events. In addition to a defined history and physical examination, we use three tests to guide our assessment of progress.

Large Urine Sample

The night before the veterinary appointment, dog owners collect sufficient urine (200 to 500 ml by voiding midstream sampling) to allow quantitative evaluation of urine sediment. The urine can be refrigerated overnight and submitted to the clinic during the appointment. Absence of any visible sediment in a cooled urine sample is a good indication that therapy is balanced appropriately. For samples with visible sediment, the clinician should proceed as follows:

1. Decant the supernatant.
2. Place 10 ml of the remaining mixture in a 10- to 15-ml cone-tipped centrifuge tube. Centrifuge the sample to separate the sediment from the solution (alternatively, the sample can sit undisturbed to allow for separation by gravity).
3. Decant the supernatant again.
4. Repeat this process by adding additional urine to the centrifuge tube until sufficient sediment (i.e., 0.5- to 1-cm depth) is reclaimed.
5. Allow the sediment to air-dry for several days before submitting it for quantitative mineral analysis.

Unprocessed urine should not be submitted for quantitative mineral analysis.

Urinalysis of a Freshly Obtained and Rapidly Analyzed Urine Sample

Owners should be encouraged not to let their dog urinate 2 to 3 hours before the veterinary appointment so that a fresh sample can be collected and analyzed within 30 minutes. Ideally, urine specific gravity should be below 1.020 (the lower the better), pH should be above 7, and there should be no visible crystals. If crystals are observed, quantitative mineral analysis will be necessary to differentiate urate from xanthine precipitation in dogs receiving allopurinol. Urate crystalluria is an indication of insufficient dietary purine (protein) reduction, insufficient urine alkalization, insufficient urine dilution, insufficient allopurinol administration, or both. Xanthine crystalluria is an indication of excessive allopurinol administration in relation to insufficient dietary purine (protein) reduction, insufficient urine alkalization, or insufficient urine dilution.

Medical Imaging

It is difficult to monitor changes in urolith size and number by survey radiography because urate uroliths are marginally radiopaque. Therefore double-contrast cystography and ultrasonography often are used. Double-contrast cystography is superior to ultrasonography because (1) virtually all uroliths can be visualized, (2) urolith size, shape, and number can be assessed accurately, and (3) small uroliths often can be retrieved through the infusion catheter and can be submitted for quantitative mineral analysis. General anesthesia is not required to perform double-contrast cystography (however, local anesthesia and sedation improve patient comfort). Ultrasonography has the advantage of being noninvasive but is not a sensitive method of determining urolith size or number. In addition, urethroliths usually are missed by ultrasonography. When uroliths recur, the size and position of all uroliths should be assessed to determine if patients are candidates for voiding urohydropropulsion, basket retrieval, or retrograde urohydropropulsion. Therefore treatment planning should not be based on ultrasonography alone. Survey radiography and contrast urethrocystography are essential to ensure that the extent of disease is not underestimated.

Because the median urolith dissolution time is 3.5 months, medical imaging can be omitted during the first monthly evaluation but should be performed at all successive evaluations.

Is Urethral Surgery an Option for Urethroliths?

Because the surface of most urate uroliths is smooth, successful expulsion of urethroliths using retrograde urohydropropulsion should be anticipated in every patient after administration of sufficient anesthesia to relax the urethra properly. We recognize that for some patients, urethrotomy and urethrostomy may be required to avert the life-threatening consequences of complete urethral obstruction. However, urethrotomy is a common cause of urethral strictures, and urethrostomy is a common cause of recurrent urinary tract infections in male dogs. Avoidance of urethral surgery ensures that the integrity and function of the urinary tract will be preserved. Contemporary nonsurgical methods for removing urethroliths (e.g., retrograde urohydropropulsion and laser lithotripsy) are very successful and are becoming readily available at referral centers. Since surgery has no positive benefit for urolith prevention and can lead to urethral stricture, we recommend that urethral surgery be considered only as a salvage procedure when other approaches have been exhausted.

What Is the Appropriate Dosage of Allopurinol?

The dosage of allopurinol required to prevent urate urolith recurrence sufficiently without promoting xanthine urolith formation varies and is influenced by the severity of disease, the quantity of protein (i.e., purines) in the diet, urine pH, and urine volume. In a case series of 10 dogs with previous urate urolithiasis, allopurinol administration in excess of 9 to 38 mg/kg/day was associated with xanthine urolith formation (Ling, 1991). Xanthines form because allopurinol inhibits the breakdown of xanthine to uric acid and because xanthine is less soluble in urine than uric acid. Based on these observations, we recommend a dosage of 5 to 7 mg/kg/day to prevent urate uroliths safely. Because the dosage of allopurinol associated with urolith dissolution (10 to 15 mg/kg twice a day) is much higher, it is important to achieve decreased intake of dietary purine (i.e., protein), increased urine dilution, and increased urine pH before allopurinol is administered. Since allopurinol has a short half-life (2.5 hours) and requires hepatic transformation to its more effective, longer-lasting metabolite oxypurinol, an effective yet safe dosage has not been established for dogs with portovascular shunts (Ling et al, 1997).

Should Medical Treatment Be Considered to Manage Urate Crystalluria in Dogs without Uroliths?

Urate crystalluria in a fresh urine sample from an otherwise clinically healthy dog is an indication to look for an underlying cause (e.g., portovascular shunt, mutation in the SLC2A9 urate transporter, myeloproliferative cancers, tumor lysis syndrome). Medical imaging of the urinary tract should be performed in breeds at risk of urate urolithiasis (e.g., dalmatian, English bulldog, Russian terrier). In the absence of uroliths or a history of uroliths, therapy to prevent crystalluria usually is not warranted based on the following observations. There is no scientific evidence that urate crystalluria causes clinical signs. Although all dalmatians are assumed to be hyperuricosuric, few (less than 10%) form clinically recognizable urate uroliths. Clinical urolithiasis is primarily a disease of young adult (1- to 6-year-old) male dogs. Of the urate uroliths from almost 20,000 dalmatians that have been submitted to the Minnesota Urolith Center for quantitative analysis, fewer than 3% were from females and fewer than 20% were from dogs 8 years of age or older. Therefore these groups are not likely to form urate uroliths. In 2009 and 2010, urate uroliths from 457 Yorkshire terriers with presumed portovascular anomalies were analyzed; only 19% were from female dogs. Although the need for urolith prevention appears to be greater in males, we recommend that in all cases risk factors associated with urate urolith formation (e.g., high-protein/purine diets, urine acidification, aspirin therapy, water restriction) be eliminated, if possible.

How Quickly Will Urate Uroliths Recur?

Prospective studies addressing the issue of how quickly urate uroliths recur are limited. In one prospective crossover study, two diets (a canned maintenance food and a canned urolith-prevention food) were evaluated in six client-owned, male, urolith-forming dalmatians (age range, 2 to 5 years) (Lulich et al, 1997). Each diet was fed for 6 months. Dogs were randomly assigned as to which diet was fed first. To accurately assess urolith recurrence, dogs were evaluated monthly by double-contrast cystography. Uroliths that formed during the study were removed by voiding urohydropropulsion and submitted for quantitative analysis. When dogs were fed the canned maintenance diet (dry-matter protein content of 25%, chicken as the primary protein source), 87% of dalmatians developed recurrent urate uroliths within the 6-month period. Recurrent uroliths were small (<2 mm in diameter) and were not associated with clinical signs. These findings support the recommendation that following urate urolith removal, therapy to prevent urolith recurrence is needed. When the same dogs were fed the urolith-prevention diet (dry-matter protein content of 13%, egg as the primary protein source: Hill's Prescription Diet u/d), 50% of dogs developed recurrent urate uroliths within the 6-month period. Recurrent uroliths were small (<2 mm in diameter) and were not associated with clinical signs. These findings support the recommendation that therapeutic foods to prevent urolith recurrence are helpful; however, administration of xanthine oxidase inhibitors is also needed in most dogs to prevent urate urolith recurrence successfully. We are not aware of any other prospective studies evaluating only dietary efficacy using the clinically relevant end point of urolith recurrence.

Is a Vegetarian Diet Appropriate?

In general, vegetables have lower quantities of purines than meat-based foods. Vegetarian diets also have the advantage of minimizing urine acidity. However, the digestibility of vegetables and the biologic availability of vegetable proteins depend on the vegetables (or vegetable combinations) consumed and generally are lower than those of meat-based diets. Until vegetarian foods have been evaluated for their safety and efficacy, we recommend that these food sources be used cautiously with appropriate monitoring (e.g., for urate crystalluria, urolith recurrence, body weight, body condition).

If Dietary Protein Supplementation Is Desired, What Is an Appropriate Source?

Lower-protein diets, which equate to lower-purine diets, are recommended to minimize urate urolith recurrence in dogs. Commercially available diets for urolith prevention have undergone Association of American Feed Control Officials (AAFCO) feeding trials validating their nutritional completeness. However, in some situations (e.g., surgical recovery, increased physical activity, long-term feeding [for years]) additional protein may be needed. In these situations, we recommend protein sources with high biologic value and low purine content. A convenient, readily available source is pasteurized egg whites or eggs.

What Human Foods Are Low in Purines?

Dietary purines are present in most foods as constituents of nucleic acids and nucleotides. The end product of purine metabolism in most dogs with urate uroliths is most likely uric acid. Determining which foods are low in purines can be confusing because not only is uric acid

Foods Low in Purine and High in Purine

Permissible Low-Purine Foods
Eggs
Milk
Yogurt
Most fruits
Breads
Most vegetables (except those listed to avoid)

Higher-Purine Foods to Avoid
All meats and fish
Cauliflower
Broccoli
Brussels sprouts
Spinach
Cabbage
Soybeans and tofu
Sunflower seeds
Peanuts
Mushrooms

content important, but the quantity of uric acid precursors (adenine, guanine, hypoxanthine, xanthine) also must be measured. Box 198-1 provides a list of some foods with low uric acid content that can be fed in moderation to dogs with urate stones, along with a list of foods to avoid.

References and Suggested Reading

Karmi N et al: Validation of a urine test and characterization of the putative genetic mutation for hyperuricosuria in Bulldogs and Black Russian Terriers, *Am J Vet Res* 71:909, 2010.
Ling GV: Xanthine containing urinary calculi in dogs given allopurinol, *J Am Vet Med Assoc* 198:1935, 1991.
Ling GV et al: Pharmacokinetics of allopurinol in Dalmatian dogs, *J Vet Pharmacol Ther* 20:134, 1997.
Lulich JP et al: Effects of diets on urate urolith recurrence in Dalmatians, *J Vet Intern Med* 11:129, 1997.
Minnesota Urolith Center: Canine urate uroliths. Available at www.cvm.umn.edu/depts/minnesotaurolithcenter/recommendations/home.html. Accessed March 27, 2013.
Osborne CA et al: Paradigm changes in the role of nutrition for the management of canine and feline urolithiasis, *Vet Clin North Am Small Anim Pract* 39:127, 2009.

CHAPTER 199

Minilaparotomy-Assisted Cystoscopy for Urocystoliths

JOSEPH W. BARTGES, *Knoxville, Tennessee*
PATRICIA A. SURA, *Knoxville, Tennessee*
AMANDA CALLENS, *Knoxville, Tennessee*

Urocystolithiasis occurs commonly in dogs and cats. Although medical dissolution protocols are available for some types of uroliths (e.g., struvite, urate, and cystine), alternative methods of managing urocystoliths often are pursued because of failure of dissolution, inability to attempt dissolution, or lack of dissolution protocols (e.g., for calcium oxalate stones) (Bartges and Lane, 2003). Open cystotomy is the conventional means for removing urocystoliths; however, minimally invasive techniques such as transurethral cystoscopy and laser lithotripsy in female dogs and cats (Adams et al, 2008; Lulich et al, 2009) and laparoscopically or cystoscopically assisted cystotomy in male and female pets (Libermann et al, 2011; Rawlings et al, 2003; Runge et al, 2011) are becoming more commonplace. Minilaparotomy-assisted cystoscopic retrieval maximizes the advantages of both

and avoids the equipment and expertise required for laparoscopy. Rather than use a laparoscope to assist in urinary bladder identification and entry, which requires additional specialized equipment and establishment of pneumoperitoneum, minilaparotomy-assisted cystoscopy relies on the surgeon to isolate the apex of the urinary bladder and temporarily fasten it to the linea alba, which allows cystoscopy and stone removal to be performed through a small stab incision in the urinary bladder wall.

Indications

Indications for minimally invasive urocystolith retrieval are similar to those for open surgical cystotomy and include (1) medically nondissolvable urocystoliths (e.g., calcium oxalate or urate uroliths associated with portovascular anomalies), (2) client or patient factors that preclude medical dissolution, and (3) a need to remove the urocystoliths more rapidly than is possible with medical dissolution. Additionally, these minimally invasive procedures may be performed multiple times for a patient with recurrent urocystoliths; adhesions to the urinary bladder serosal surface appear to occur less commonly than with open cystotomy. Minilaparotomy-assisted cystoscopy typically is performed in male dogs and cats but can be performed in female dogs and cats when transurethral cystoscopy is not feasible. Minilaparotomy-assisted cystoscopy is most useful for patients with large stones that would require extended time to fragment with laser lithotripsy, for patients with large numbers of stones that would also make lithotripsy or open cystotomy time consuming, and for patients whose size precludes lithotripsy (see Web Chapter 70). In addition to allowing urolith retrieval, minilaparotomy-assisted cystoscopy also is useful for obtaining biopsy specimens of urinary bladder mucosa, evaluating whether hematuria is renal in origin by observing urine flow from ureteral orifices, and facilitating ureteral stent placement in certain circumstances. With the transvesicular placement of a rigid cystoscope, the proximal urethra, including the prostatic urethra in male dogs, may be examined in an antegrade fashion. Most of the remaining urethra can be visualized using an appropriately sized flexible endoscope.

Preprocedure

Before the procedure, a thorough history should be taken and a complete physical examination should be performed. Collection of a minimum data set including results of complete blood cell count, biochemical analysis, and urinalysis is indicated. Additional testing may include an aerobic bacteriologic culture of urine collected by cystocentesis, liver function testing if urate urocystoliths are suspected, and testing of adrenal function or calcium metabolism if calcium oxalate uroliths are likely. Abdominal survey radiography should be performed (Figure 199-1), but ultrasonographic examination or contrast studies also may be required to determine the locations of all uroliths and their impact on the urinary tract.

Procedure

The patient is placed under general anesthesia after appropriate premedication and is positioned in dorsal recumbency. If necessary, a urinary catheter is inserted in the urethra and urethroliths are retropulsed into the urinary bladder. Before final preparation of the abdominal wall, this urinary catheter is removed. The ventral abdominal wall is clipped, prepared, and draped as for standard laparotomy. The preputial sheath is flushed with 0.05% chlorhexidine solution for two minutes (Neihaus et al, 2011). A sterile urethral catheter then is inserted in male dogs and cats. The size of the catheter depends on the size of the patient: a 3.5 Fr catheter in a male cat, a 5 Fr to 10 Fr catheter in a male dog. Female dogs and cats usually do not require urinary catheterization to facilitate isolation of the bladder. The urinary bladder is distended with sterile fluid such as lactated Ringer's solution or normal saline so that the urinary bladder is palpable through the abdominal wall.

An incision is made through the skin on the ventral midline over the urinary bladder. In male dogs the incision is made just cranial to the preputial reflection or, if the urinary bladder is displaced caudally, it may be made in the right or left prepreputial area (Figure 199-2). The skin incision is 2 to 3 cm in length. The subcutaneous tissue is incised and the linea alba is identified. A stab incision is made through the linea alba and lengthened using Mayo scissors.

The urinary bladder is identified by digital palpation through the incision and is grasped with Babcock forceps or with needle and suture and brought to the incisional edges of the linea alba. Using 3-0 poliglecaprone 25 (Monocryl), the ventral surface of the urinary bladder near the apex is sutured to the right and left edges of the incision of the linea alba in a continuous pattern on each side. This temporary fixation stabilizes the urinary bladder to allow for manual and cystoscopic manipulation and minimizes leakage of urinary bladder contents into the abdominal cavity.

A stab incision is made into the urinary bladder using a No. 15 scalpel blade (Figure 199-3). A 2.7-mm

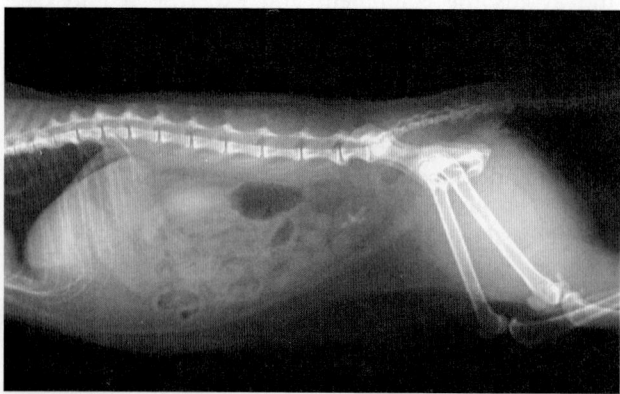
Figure 199-1 Lateral abdominal radiograph of an 11-year-old castrated male cat with multiple urocystoliths.

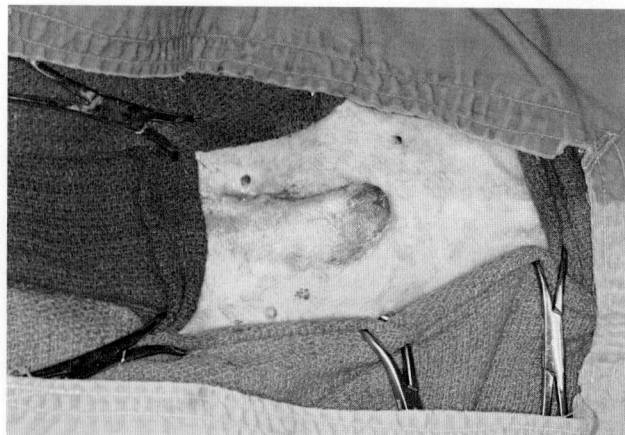
Figure 199-2 Final appearance of minilaparotomy-assisted cystotomy skin incision made in the right prepreputial area in a 6-year-old castrated male bichon frise.

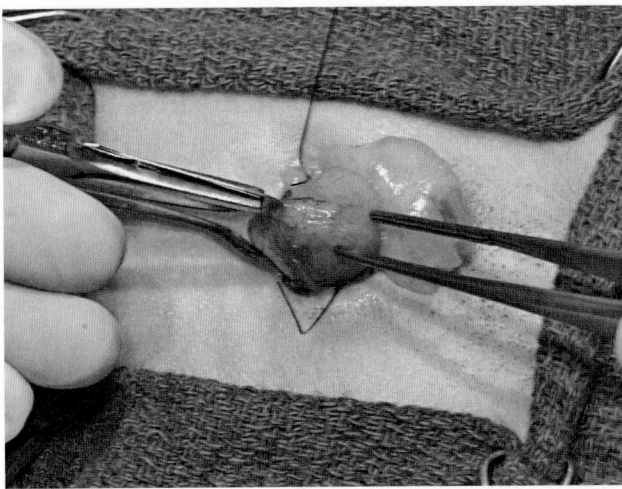

Figure 199-3 Stabilization of the urinary bladder to the lateral edges of the linear alba using 3-0 poliglecaprone 25 suture (Monocryl) and stab incision into the urinary bladder lumen with a No. 15 scalpel blade in the cat described in Figure 199-1. The initial approach was made on the ventral midline.

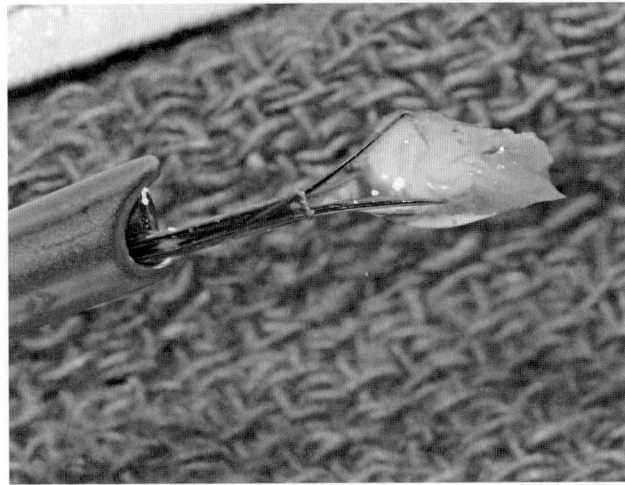

Figure 199-5 Retrieval of a urocystolith from the cat described in Figure 199-1.

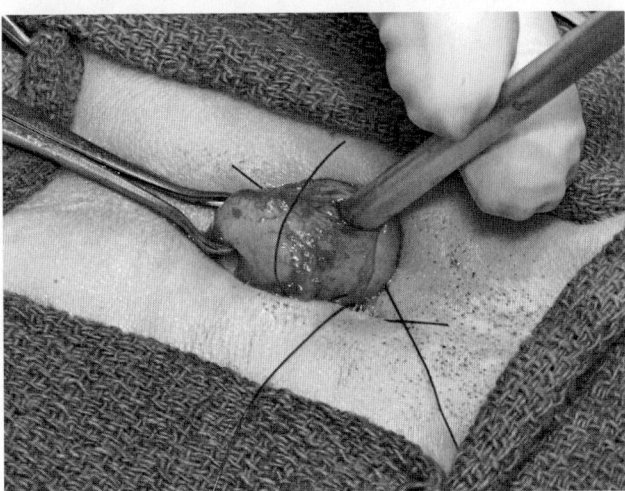

Figure 199-4 Insertion of a 2.7-mm, 30-degree, 15-cm rigid cystoscope and sheath through the stab incision in the ventral urinary bladder in the cat described in Figure 199-1.

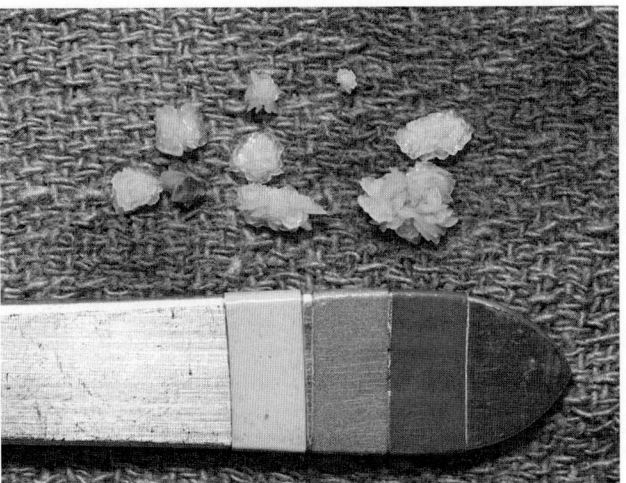

Figure 199-6 Urocystoliths removed via minilaparotomy-assisted cystotomy from the cat described in Figure 199-1.

cystoscope and sheath is inserted through the stab incision into the lumen of the urinary bladder (Figure 199-4). If desired, a threaded laparoscopic trocar can be inserted through the incision to maintain visualization, further prevent urine contamination, and minimize trauma associated with movement of the cystoscope. Sterile fluid (lactated Ringer's solution or 0.9% sodium chloride) is infused intermittently or continually through one port of the cystoscopy sheath to maintain bladder distention and visualization. Suction tubing or a syringe may be attached to the other port of the cystoscopy sheath and used to evacuate the urinary bladder as needed.

Uroliths are visualized and retrieved using cystoscopic graspers or baskets (Figures 199-5 and 199-6). Small uroliths can be retrieved by several methods. They can be aspirated with the fluid effluent through the cystoscope,

guided into the urethral catheter for aspiration, or directly retrieved using a biopsy instrument. Forceps retrieval is particularly useful for small uroliths or urolith fragments embedded in the urinary bladder mucosa (Figure 199-7). It may be necessary to enlarge the incision in the urinary bladder to facilitate removal of larger stones.

Once the uroliths are removed, the luminal surfaces of the urinary bladder and proximal urethra are inspected thoroughly. Biopsy is performed on lesions such as polyps or neoplastic masses through the operating port of the cystoscope. We routinely perform histopathologic examination and aerobic and anaerobic culture of tissue retrieved by biopsy. Ureteral orifices also are identified and urine is observed to flow through both ureters. For viewing of the trigone and proximal urethra, the urethral catheter is withdrawn to just inside the penile urethra and the catheter is flushed with sterile fluid while the trigone region is observed with the cystoscope. The urethral catheter then is slowly advanced back into the urinary bladder

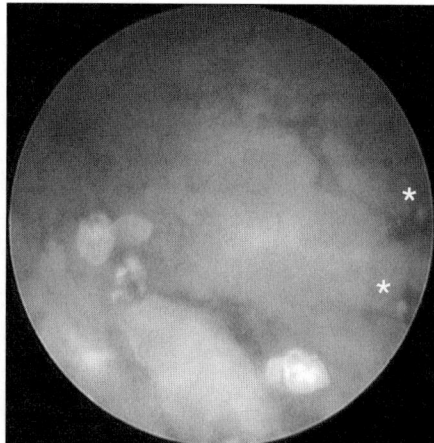

Figure 199-7 Intravesicular cystoscopic view of urocystoliths that are 1 to 2 mm in size and composed of calcium oxalate. The asterisks denote small (<1 mm) urocystoliths embedded in the urinary bladder mucosa. These were removed by aspiration.

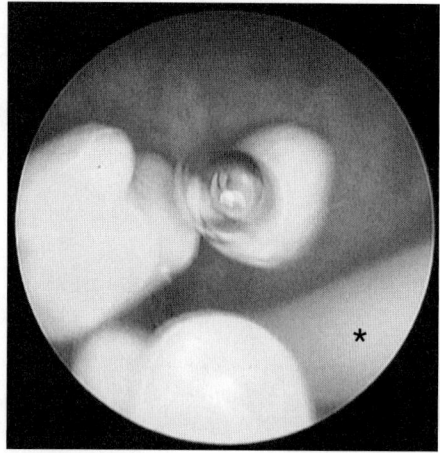

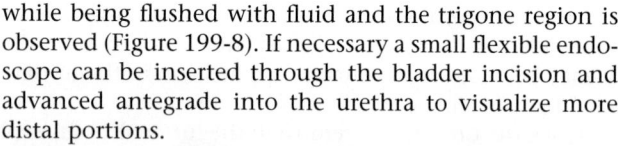

Figure 199-8 Intravesicular cystoscopic view of trigone region and small urate urocystoliths in a 4-year-old intact male English bulldog. The asterisk denotes a 8 Fr red rubber catheter that is visible entering the urinary bladder at the trigone.

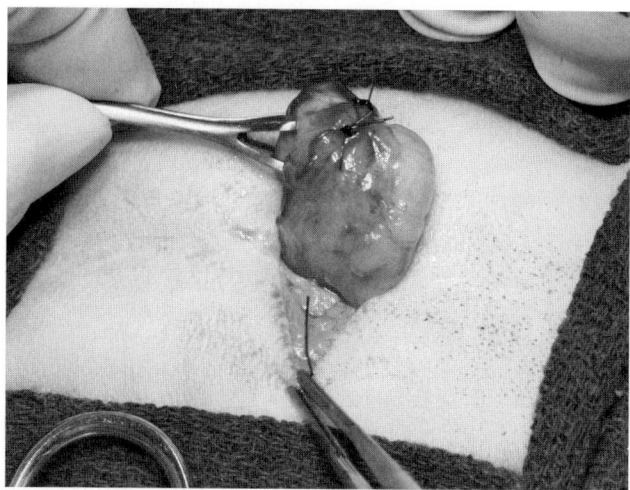

Figure 199-9 Closure of the urinary bladder stab incision with 3-0 poliglecaprone 25 suture (Monocryl) in the cat described in Figure 199-1.

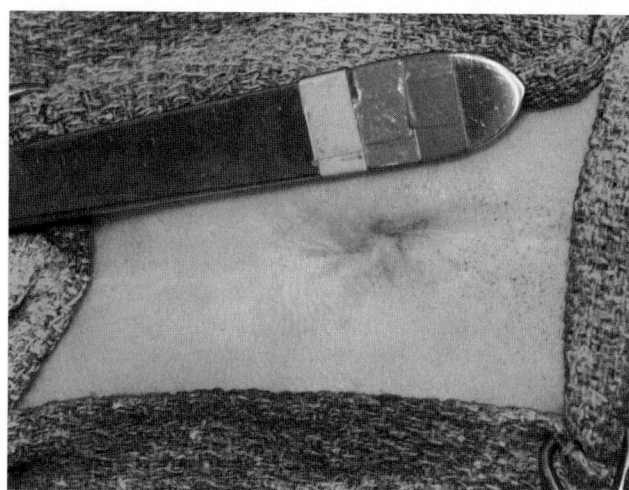

Figure 199-10 Final appearance of the minilaparotomy-assisted cystotomy skin incision in the cat described in Figure 199-1. An intradermal pattern of 3-0 poliglecaprone 25 suture (Monocryl) was used.

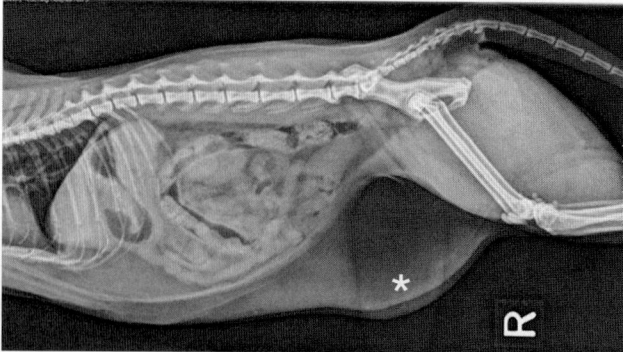

Figure 199-11 Lateral abdominal radiograph of the cat described in Figure 199-1 following minilaparotomy-assisted cystotomy for urocystolith removal. The asterisk denotes a wooden spoon applied to the lateral abdominal wall to isolate the urinary bladder by moving the intestines from overlying the urinary bladder.

while being flushed with fluid and the trigone region is observed (Figure 199-8). If necessary a small flexible endoscope can be inserted through the bladder incision and advanced antegrade into the urethra to visualize more distal portions.

The urinary bladder is closed in a simple continuous fashion. The suture is not allowed to extend into the urinary bladder lumen (Figure 199-9). The abdominal wall then is closed in a standard fashion (Figure 199-10). Lateral abdominal radiography is performed after the procedure to ensure removal of all urocystoliths (Figure 199-11). We routinely administer a single dose of ampicillin (22 mg/kg IV) and a postoperative dose of buprenorphine or hydromorphone. Meloxicam is administered for 3 days (0.1 mg/kg q24h PO) to dogs and buprenorphine is administered for 3 days (0.01 mg/kg q8-12h PO) to cats.

Outcome

In a recent report of the use of this technique in 27 cases procedural time ranged from 50 to 80 minutes. One patient had a residual urolith identified on radiographs that had to be retrieved in a second procedure. No major short- or long-term complications were reported (Adams et al, 2008). At our institution, we have performed over 150 cystoscopically assisted procedures. In three dogs, a single urocystolith remained in the bladder. The residual urocystolith was retrieved in a second procedure in one dog, whereas the urocystoliths passed during voiding in the other two dogs. Three dogs developed incisional infections. One case presumably was caused by licking of the surgical site and a second was thought to be due to extension of a urinary tract organism. The third dog underwent surgical exploration and excision of the abscessed site, which extended from the urinary bladder to the skin. A single dog sustained urinary bladder rupture during manipulation of the bladder with Babcock forceps; the damaged bladder wall was repaired after elongation of the abdominal incision. Only about 15% of the treated animals had macroscopic hematuria during recovery; most were discharged on the day of the procedure.

Minilaparotomy-assisted cystotomy appears to be an effective, safe, and efficient means for managing urocystoliths with a minimally invasive technique. Recovery time appears to be shorter than with conventional cystotomy.

References and Suggested Reading

Adams LG et al: Use of laser lithotripsy for fragmentation of uroliths in dogs: 73 cases (2005-2006), *J Am Vet Med Assoc* 232(11):1680, 2008.

Bartges JW, Lane IF: Medical management of urolithiasis. In Slater DH, editor: *Textbook of veterinary surgery*, Philadelphia, 2003, Saunders, p 1661.

Libermann SV et al: Extraction of urethral calculi by transabdominal cystoscopy and urethroscopy in nine dogs, *J Small Anim Pract* 52(4):190, 2011.

Lulich JP et al: Efficacy and safety of laser lithotripsy in fragmentation of urocystoliths and urethroliths for removal in dogs, *J Am Vet Med Assoc* 234(10):1279, 2009.

Neihaus SA et al: Presurgical antiseptic efficacy of chlorhexidine diacetate and povidone-iodine in the canine preputial cavity, *J Am Anim Hosp Assoc* 47(6): 406, 2011.

Rawlings CA et al: Use of laparoscopic-assisted cystoscopy for removal of urinary calculi in dogs, *J Am Vet Med Assoc* 222(6):759, 2003.

Runge JJ et al: Transvesicular percutaneous cystolithotomy for the retrieval of cystic and urethral calculi in dogs and cats: 27 cases (2006-2008), *J Am Vet Med Assoc* 239(3):344, 2011.

CHAPTER 200

Multimodal Environmental Enrichment for Domestic Cats

TRACI A. SHREYER, *Columbus, Ohio*
C.A. TONY BUFFINGTON, *Columbus, Ohio*

Enriched environments permit animals to perceive sufficient control and predictability so that they can engage in the widest range of general and species-typical activities possible for the situation. The goal of therapeutic environmental enrichment (EE) is to ensure that these conditions are present for all animals under our care. EE for all pets appears to be at least as important for long-term health and welfare as immunization and parasite prevention, and deserves at least as much attention during veterinary visits, when client attitudes and behaviors related to their cats are forming and most malleable. Multimodal efforts have proven particularly useful in cats with chronic, idiopathic lower urinary tract signs.

Applied to domestic cats, EE means providing opportunities to engage in important species-typical as well as general activities. The available conditions should promote expression of these normal behaviors. Appropriate EE provides preventive health care by maintaining an environment in which cats thrive; the result is sustained good health and positive interactions that the owner can enjoy. Owners confine most pet cats to spaces much smaller than their natural ranges; the smallest reported range is approximately 29,000 square feet (Liberg et al, 2000), more than 10 times the area of the average American home. Owners often keep cats indoors or allow access to small outdoor spaces that may contain perceived threats. Cats kept in these environments live akin to zoo animals, and, as with zoo animals, environmental quality can exert important effects on their health and welfare. Cats retain their drive to engage in species-typical behaviors regardless of environment. The motivations to explore, hunt, climb, scratch, and mark territory are not left at the door of the captive environments of house cats. Viewed from this perspective, EE is essentially husbandry, whose original meaning was "the administration and management of a household." Unfortunately, when owners are not educated that these behaviors are normal and are helped to provide opportunities for cats to engage in them, we risk depriving cats of appropriate outlets for their expression.

Additionally, an increasing number of cats are obtained as kittens from humane organizations. These animals are at increased risk of adverse experiences early in life, which can bias the activity of the central nervous system toward enhanced perception of threat (Buffington, 2009). Effective EE has been found to mitigate these changes in some studies of rodents, cats, and humans.

Although many indoor cats appear to survive perfectly well by accommodating to a wide range of surroundings, we advocate for environments that permit cats to thrive, rather than environments that meet minimum requirements for survival. Cats have a variety of unique behaviors and needs; we encourage owners to maximize their pet's health and welfare by providing a diverse, behaviorally enriched environment free from physical, psychologic, and social threats. Our current approach is to let clients choose the most appropriate intervention for their particular situation, after which we try to create and communicate a workable plan to implement changes. In our experience, the effectiveness of EE depends not only on the cat, but also on the housing situation, the client, and the quality and dedication of the veterinary team overseeing and supporting the client's efforts.

Assessing the Environment

Veterinary caregivers may consider the possibility of environmental influences on the health and welfare of any cat brought to the veterinarian for care of sickness behaviors in the absence of an identifiable medical cause. Sickness behaviors are a group of nonspecific behavioral and clinical signs including vomiting, diarrhea, voiding dysfunction, decreased food and water intake, fever, lethargy, somnolence, enhanced painlike behaviors, and decreased general activity, body care activities (grooming), and social interactions (Stella et al, 2011). Although these behaviors are well-documented responses to infection and a variety of structural disorders, they also can occur in response to adverse environmental events. Thus sickness behaviors can result both from peripheral (i.e., afferent) and central (i.e., efferent) pathways. The repeated observation that these behaviors largely resolve after exposure to an enriched environment provides additional evidence of a central nervous system disorder resulting in a chronic multisystem illness variably affecting other organs, as opposed to peripheral, organ-based problems (Buffington, 2011).

The health and welfare of pet cats also may be inferred from observation of their behaviors (Table 200-1) or the reports of clients. Pet cats enjoying good health and welfare typically engage in variable combinations of exploratory and interactive ("positive") behaviors. In contrast, cats suffering poor health or welfare tend not to engage in these behaviors but more commonly show "negative" behaviors suggestive of illness or threat. Negative behaviors may occur in response to threat, fear, or anxiety, or in response to pain or some structural disease process. The specific reason for the negative behavior can be difficult to determine; the field of assessment of the quality of life of companion animals is in its infancy and is sorely in need of well-validated and clinically useful instruments.

If the history or physical examination findings suggest that the environment may be adversely affecting the cat's health or welfare, the source of the problem may lie in either inanimate (physical) features, animate (human and other animal) features, or both. To improve the environment, we usually begin by ensuring an "environment of plenty": plenty of places to eat, drink, rest, and eliminate. We then can attempt to identify challenges or threats to the cat's perception of control and predictability that affect its interactions with other animals (including humans).

Space

General environmental needs for captive animals include enough safe space to provide opportunities for exploration, food acquisition and consumption, elimination, and resting. Regardless of the size of the cat's living space, it must provide a reasonable level of perceived controllability, consistency, and predictability. The smaller the space, the more attention must be paid to the cat's opportunities to move freely through the space in all three dimensions. Living space that keeps cats free from fear and distress and that provides a predictable daily routine over which the cat perceives it has some control is a basic feature of an enriched environment. Confined cats need unrestricted access to spaces that are safe from perceived threats, such as loud noises, dogs, other cats in the household, outdoor cats approaching the windows, and pursuit by small children. Cats seem to prefer soft resting surfaces such as pillows or fleece beds that are in warm areas, such as safely heated beds or sunny windows (the thermoneutral zone of unacclimated adult cats appears to lie between 30° and 38° C [86° and 100° F]). Owners of multicat households need to provide enough space to permit each cat to keep a social distance of 1 to 3 meters (horizontally as well as vertically) from other cats. Although some cats that are very comfortable with one another rest together and groom and rub (mark) each other, most cats use common resting, perching, and hiding locations at different times of the day. Hence owners of more than one cat need to provide safe, comfortable, and private locations for each cat to avoid creating competition for scarce resources.

Cats are prey as well as predators in nature, so climbing for observation and safe vantage is an important feline behavior. When this behavioral need is explained to owners, they usually enjoy providing acceptable opportunities for cats to climb, while protecting areas they do

TABLE 200-1

Observable Behaviors of Pet Cats

	Positive	Negative
Activity	• Moves around the home smoothly and confidently • Jumps normally • Relaxed body at rest • Seeks usual affection • Enjoys being petted or handled	• Reluctant to move, difficulty getting up from a lying position • Limps, cannot jump as high • Trembles or shakes • Seeks more affection • Avoids being held, picked up, handled, or petted • Restless • Gets up and lies down repetitively • Hides • Growls, hisses, bites, or scratches when approached
Daily habits	• Seeks social interaction • Usual eating, sleeping, and drinking • Usual litter box use	• Withdraws from social interaction • Changes in eating, sleeping, or drinking • Stops using the litter box • Urinates frequently
Facial expression	• Relaxed face • Calm gaze • Pupils normal for light conditions • Ears erect • Breathes quietly when at rest	• Grimaces, furrowed brow, vacant stare • Looks glazed, wide-eyed, or sleepy • Pupils enlarged • Ears flattened • Increased respiratory rate
Grooming	• Gentle, relaxed grooming of entire body	• Does not groom or grooms less, looks unkempt, overgrooms • Licks, bites, or scratches any particular areas of the body
Posture	• Generally lays on side in relaxed position • Carries body as usual	• Lays with feet tucked underneath • Arches back or tucks in abdomen
Vocalizing	• Happy meowing • Purring	• Decreased normal vocalizations • Plaintive meowing • Yowling • Hissing • Growling

Adapted from American Animal Hospital Association: How to tell if your cat is in pain. Available at http://secure.aahanet.org/eWeb/images/Trends/PDFs/CatHandout.pdf. Accessed March 22, 2013.

not want the cat to access. Then owners perceive the cat's climbing proclivity as natural rather than as an objectionable annoyance. Providing perching options throughout the house offers the cat both safety and a vantage point above people and other animals from which to view the surroundings. Examples of climbing structures include cat towers, window shelves, and wooden stepladders (which the cat also can scratch). Placing such structures near windows also permits the cat to safely survey the outdoor environment.

Food and Water

Although available commercial diets adequately meet the nutrient requirements of domestic cats, there is more to nutrition than nutrients. Hunting behavior and hedonic aspects of food (its look, feel in the mouth, taste, and smell) all contribute to the cat's feeding experience.

Providing food in ways that best mimic cats' natural preferences can provide additional enrichment. For example, owners can accommodate cats' natural predatory habits and increase their daily activity by offering food in puzzle toys, such as balls or other devices designed specifically for cats to release dry food or treats when

physically manipulated. Another option is a hollow toy that can be stuffed with frozen wet food, which requires cats to wait for the food to thaw and then work to remove the contents.

Play behaviors also may be part of prey-seeking behaviors in cats (although this relationship is controversial). Play behaviors appear similar to the natural predatory sequence of stalking, chasing, pouncing, and biting. Many cats enjoy playing with items they can pick up, toss in the air, and pounce upon. A safe way for owners to accommodate their cat's play drive is to use toys that permit a reasonable distance between the cat and the owner's body parts. Encouraging play and biting behaviors with hands and feet, on the other hand, may teach the cat that it is rewarding to stalk, pounce on, and bite the owner, which leads to play-related aggression problems. Examples of appropriate play objects are wand toys, battery-propelled toys that mimic prey, balls placed inside a box or bathtub, catnip-filled toys, and laser pointer games. Laser pointer use always should be followed by presentation of a treat or toy to reward the cat for the "hunt" and to avoid frustration.

Cats can display strong food preferences based on foods they encountered early in life, although these can be modified by later experience. Some cats also develop decreased preference for foods that have formed a large part of their diet in the past, the so-called monotony effect, and display preferences for novel foods. Food refusal is also a common feline response to environmental threat. The explanation for these seemingly contradictory food-related attitudes may lie in the role of the environment in food preference. In threatening environments, animals often avoid new foods, whereas in enriched environments they often prefer new foods.

Because cats evolved as solitary hunters of small prey, the provision of separate feeding containers out of sight of other cats' food facilitates "solitary" feeding and reduces the risk of conflict over resources. Food containers should be located in quiet areas, away from appliances that may begin operating unexpectedly and protected from interruption by other animals. Ideal placement permits the cat to eat without being disturbed. Cats with free access to food usually prefer to eat several small meals throughout the day as opposed to one or two large meals, and most will hunt for prey when given the option. Although free access to food may allow frequent feeding sessions, this feeding strategy removes the opportunity for expression of cats' natural predatory instincts that food puzzles provide, and may contribute to development of obesity and other health problems.

Cats also need adequate access to clean, fresh water and sometimes display preferences regarding its presentation. Some cats seem to prefer that their vibrissae do not touch the sides of containers during drinking, and some seem to enjoy drinking running water from faucets or fountains. Owners can be invited to investigate these preferences with their cats.

Litter Boxes

For cats, elimination consists of a sequence of behaviors that includes preelimination digging, elimination posturing, and postelimination digging and covering (Landsberg et al, 2003). Like food and water containers, litter boxes should be located in safe, quiet areas to ensure that the cat's access to or from the box cannot be blocked by another animal, and away from machinery that could come on unexpectedly and disrupt the normal elimination behavior sequence. Large (at least 1.5 times the length of the cat), open boxes, such as plastic storage containers, located away from food and water bowls provide safe places for cats to eliminate. Self-cleaning litter boxes offer increased cleanliness, although cats that find sound or movement aversive may avoid them. Covered litter boxes may trap odors and prevent the cat from having a safe vantage point for observing the approach of other animals during elimination, which makes them a less desirable option for many cats. In multicat households, owners should provide a box for each cat (or cat group) plus one additional box, with each box out of sight of all others. Most cats display a preference for unscented and finely particulate litter material, which makes clumping litter a desirable option. Plastic liners should be avoided if possible; many cats with intact claws find them aversive. Owners should be educated to provide enough litter so that the cat's feet do not come

into contact with the bottom of the box during digging, to scoop eliminations at least daily (adding more litter as needed), and to discard and replace the litter completely at least weekly, washing the box with mild, unscented soap and water before refilling.

Social Interactions

The social system of pet cats includes all animals that share their home space. Other animals may be perceived as threats (dogs, humans), competitors for resources (other cats), or prey (small birds, fish, and "pocket pets"). We advise owners to let the cat determine the timing and duration of contact with nonprey species to enhance the cat's perception of control of its environment. With regard to interactions with owners, some cats may prefer petting and grooming, whereas others seem to prefer play interactions. In single-cat homes, the human household members take on much of the social enrichment responsibility.

Cats interact with other cats in multicat households and shared outdoor spaces. Because cats do not appear to develop distinct linear dominance hierarchies or conflict resolution strategies with other cats to the extent that some other species do, they may attempt to circumvent antagonistic encounters by avoiding other cats or decreasing their activity. Related cats housed together in groups appear to spend more time interacting with each other than with unrelated cats. Cats housed together should be provided with their own separate food and water sources, litter boxes, and resting areas to avoid competition for resources and to permit cats to avoid unwanted interactions. For owners planning to acquire additional cats, published guidelines for introducing new cats into a home are available (Bohnenkamp, 1991).

Conflict among cats also can be manifested by the occurrence of sickness behaviors. Conflict can develop when cats perceive threats to their overall safety or competition for preferred resting or feeding areas in the home, from other animals in the home, or from outside cats. Conflict between cats can be open or silent. Signs of open conflict are easy to recognize; the cats may stalk each other, hiss, and turn sideways with legs straight and hair standing on end to make themselves look larger.* If neither cat backs down, the displays may increase to swatting, wrestling, and biting. In some cases, one or more of the confident cats in the home (sometimes referred to as "bully" cats) may begin to take control of both physical and social resources. This tends to become a problem as these cats reach the age of social maturity (2 to 5 years of age). The threatened or more fearful cats then begin to spend increasing amounts of time away from the family, staying in areas of the house that others do not use or interacting with family members only when the bullying cat is elsewhere. There may be open conflict between males, between females, or between males and females. Cats in conflict may never be "best friends," but in an enriched environment they usually can live together

---

*Illustrations of different cat postures are available at https://ckm.osu.edu/sitetool/sites/Indoorpetpublic/documents/hospital/indoorcat/Reading%20Cat%20Body%20Language.pdf.

without showing signs of conflict or conflict-related sickness behaviors. In severe cases, a behaviorist may be consulted for assistance in desensitizing and counterconditioning of cats in conflict so they can share the same spaces more comfortably if this is desired.

Body Care and Activity

Cats naturally engage in scratching, marking, and chewing behaviors. Owner frustration with these behaviors may be avoided by providing appealing, appropriate objects to cats as outlets for them. Scratching behavior maintains claw health and leaves both visual and pheromonal territorial marks. Objects such as sisal-covered posts or real bark-covered logs allow the cat to hook its claws into the material. Cats tend to scratch on prominent objects in areas where they spend much of their time. They also scratch more often when stretching after periods of rest or sleep. Hence placing scratching posts in frequently visited areas of the home, including near doorways and in proximity to preferred resting places, will increase their use.

Undesirable chewing can be avoided by offering a variety of cat-safe plants and grasses. Live planted greens and fresh catnip are two appealing options. An owner can rub the designated "cat plants" with tuna juice or wet cat food to encourage investigation and chewing, and keep other house plants in areas the cat cannot access. Applying commercially available bitter-tasting sprays or liquids also may make house plants less appealing. Toxic plants should be removed from the house or kept in a secure room that the cat cannot access. Other chewing options include moistened rawhide chews, dried fish, and beef or poultry jerky.

Making Changes

Usually a number of ways are available to provide EE to repair any identified deficits. There also are some strategies for minimizing the risk that cats will perceive changes in their environment as threats. First, the veterinarian should ensure that the owner agrees with the change and appreciates its value to the cat and the owner's relationship with it. Making suggestions that the owner does not want to or cannot implement only creates frustration, which may be perceived by the cat as a threat.

Increasing the client's perception of control by offering choices usually helps reduce the anxiety associated with change. We address this by "playing the waiter"—offering a number of possibilities and encouraging the owner to choose whichever is most appropriate for his or her unique situation. An example of helpful language is, "These approaches have worked for other clients. They might work for you, or stimulate your thinking about something that you can do in your home." This menu approach is a method that includes (1) avoiding unworkable solutions, which are met with "Yes, but..." by the client; (2) acknowledging and building on the client's greater understanding of the home environment; and (3) creating "buy-in" to enhance compliance.

Second, we recommend that whenever a change in a resource is made, the client offer the new resource adjacent to the familiar resource to permit the cat to display its preference for the new resource. If the new resource is preferred, it will be used; it not, it will be avoided. Imposing resources on a cat that it does not prefer to the familiar one may create an additional stressor in the cat's environment.

Third, we recommend that new resources be introduced at appropriate times. For example, we recommend that food puzzles be introduced at feeding, and at a time that the owner will be able to remain in the environment long enough to determine the effect of the change on the cat. We prefer that changes be offered or implemented on weekends when the owner usually has more time and fewer distractions, rather than just before leaving for work.

Fourth, if the change is intended to decrease a behavior, such as climbing on or scratching a piece of furniture, we advise owners to place an object acceptable for the cat to use adjacent to the one that owners want the cat to stop using. For example, if an owner decides to put foil or sticky tape on the arm of a couch a cat is scratching, a scratching post should be placed next to the couch and made as attractive to the cat as possible so the cat receives the message, "This new spot is so much better than that old one" rather than, "Get away!" Providing such alternatives can reduce frustration for both the owner and the cat simultaneously and promote healthier interactions between them.

Once clients understand the benefits of change and have agreed on a goal, a set of clear steps to achieve the goal can be crafted. We use a simple process for writing down plans called *SMARTR* plans to help ensure that goals are well defined, communicated clearly, and agreed upon by all involved in the change (Box 200-1). SMARTR plans are Specific, Measurable, Action oriented, Realistic, Time-driven/Timely, and Rewarded. More details about creation and implementation of SMARTR plans are available (Herron and Buffington, 2012).

The keys to successful implementation of EE goals are clarity on the objective(s) to be achieved, methods for recognizing when the goal is achieved, and willingness to change tactics to match changing situations by making other plans as necessary to achieve and maintain success.

BOX 200-1

Steps to Enhance the Success of SMARTR Plans

- Describe success in terms of observable changes in the cat's behavior by asking clients to create a diary to record the cat's behaviors in response to the recommendations.
- Write plans in positive, unequivocal terms.
- Be sure the goals are the client's goals.
- Advise that plans be posted in a prominent place, so that clients and others in the household can stay focused.
- Stay flexible; situations can and will change as life circumstances change. If a goal or a plan becomes unrealistic, change it to a more realistic one.

Follow-up

One of the crucial aspects of any successful treatment program is to follow the progress of the patient and provide coaching and support for the client's efforts. We tell clients what our follow-up schedule is and ask them to agree to a preferred method and time to be contacted. Our first contact with the client occurs within a week after initial recommendations are made, followed by repeat check-ins at approximately 3 to 6 weeks, 3 months, 6 months, and 1 year. Setting a schedule sends the message that we are committed to the program and allows us to monitor the patient's progress, to make adjustments as needed, and to continue to support and motivate the client at a frequency appropriate to conditions. It also helps to identify when the owner is becoming frustrated or having problems with the plan so that encouragement, modifications, or suggestions to help keep them on the plan can be offered.

Further information about EE for cats is available at http://indoorpet.osu.edu. The website is updated regularly as new information becomes available.

References and Suggested Reading

Bohnenkamp G: *From the cat's point of view*, San Francisco, 1991, Perfect Paws.

Buffington CAT: Idiopathic cystitis in domestic cats—beyond the lower urinary tract, *J Vet Intern Med* 25:784, 2011.

Buffington CAT: External and internal influences on disease risk in cats, *J Am Vet Med Assoc* 220:994, 2002.

Buffington CAT: Developmental influences on medically unexplained symptoms, *Psychother Psychosom* 78:139, 2009.

Buffington CAT et al: Clinical evaluation of multimodal environmental modification (MEMO) in the management of cats with idiopathic cystitis, *J Feline Med Surg* 8:261, 2006.

Ellis SL: Environmental enrichment: practical strategies for improving feline welfare, *J Feline Med Surg* 11:901, 2009.

Herron ME: Advances in understanding and treatment of feline inappropriate elimination, *Top Companion Anim Med* 25:195, 2010.

Herron ME, Buffington CAT: Feline focus: environmental enrichment for indoor cats: implementing enrichment, *Compend Contin Educ Pract Vet* 34:E1, 2012.

Landsberg GM, Hunthausen W, Ackerman L: Feline housesoiling. In Landsberg GM, Hunthausen W, Ackerman L, editors: *Handbook of behavior problems of the dog and cat*, ed 2, Philadelphia, 2003, Saunders, p 365.

Liberg O et al: Density, spatial organisation and reproductive tactics in the domestic cat and other felids. In Turner DC, Bateson P, editors: *The domestic cat: the biology of its behaviour*, ed 2, Cambridge, UK, 2000, Cambridge University Press, p 120.

Overall KL et al: Feline behavior guidelines from the American Association of Feline Practitioners, *J Am Vet Med Assoc* 227:70, 2005.

Stella JL, Lord LK, Buffington CAT: Sickness behaviors in response to unusual external events in healthy cats and cats with feline interstitial cystitis, *J Am Vet Med Assoc* 238:67, 2011.

Turner DC: The human-cat relationship. In Turner DC, Bateson P, editors: *The domestic cat: the biology of its behaviour*, ed 2, Cambridge, UK, 2000, Cambridge University Press, p 194.

CHAPTER 201

Medical Management of Urinary Incontinence and Retention Disorders

ANNICK HAMAIDE, *Liège, Belgium*

Micturition disorders can be divided into urinary incontinence and urinary retention. *Urinary incontinence* is defined as an involuntary escape of urine during the storage phase of the urinary cycle, whereas *urinary retention* is defined as a failure of the urine voiding phase of micturition, ultimately resulting in signs of overflow incontinence. An accurate characterization of the incontinence is warranted so that the appropriate pharmacologic treatment regimen can be chosen. This chapter reviews the mode of action of the pharmacologic agents available in veterinary medicine and gives an update on new agents and therapeutic approaches.

Urinary Incontinence

So that the most appropriate treatment can be provided, an accurate diagnosis of the cause of urinary incontinence should be made. Although urethral sphincter mechanism incompetence (USMI) is the most common cause of urinary incontinence in dogs, incontinence can be associated with low bladder capacity or detrusor instability. The goal of therapy in cases of urinary incontinence is improvement of urethral resistance, bladder capacity, or both. Two classes of drugs commonly are used to increase urethral resistance: sympathomimetic agents and estrogenic compounds. The use of additional agents with potential effects on both urethral and bladder functions can be contemplated in refractory cases. Recommended dosages are given in Table 201-1.

Sympathomimetic Agents

Phenylpropanolamine (PPA) is an indirect α-agonist amine producing a contraction of the bladder neck and proximal urethra by acting on the α-adrenergic receptors. PPA is very effective in the treatment of USMI, resulting in continence in 75% to 90% of the patients. PPA traditionally has been administered two or three times daily. However, recurrence of incontinence can be observed after prolonged administration. Urodynamic studies in beagle dogs have shown lack of modification of urethral resistance after 1 week of three-times-daily administrations of PPA, whereas significant increase in urethral resistance was observed clearly after 1 week of once-daily administration. In the author's experience, the administration of a single daily dose of PPA (1.5 mg/kg) in dogs

affected with USMI can achieve long-term continence in 90% of cases (Claeys et al, 2011). This administration regimen obviously is more convenient and less expensive for owners. Adverse effects of PPA include hypertension, restlessness, anxiety, and tachycardia. Therefore PPA should be administered cautiously to dogs with concurrent cardiovascular diseases or hypertension.

Ephedrine is a mixed-action sympathomimetic drug whose efficacy is slightly less predictable than that of PPA, with a complete response to treatment observed in about 75% of treated bitches. Adverse effects are those of sympathomimetic drugs. Experimental studies have shown that both PPA and ephedrine improved urethral function; however, bladder storage function also was improved after administration of ephedrine (Noël et al, 2012). This latter effect can be explained by stimulation of the β_3-adrenoreceptors present in the bladder dome. Therefore ephedrine potentially could be a useful drug in the treatment of refractory urinary incontinence with concurrent bladder dysfunction, but this hypothesis still needs to be confirmed in clinical cases.

Treatment with either ephedrine or PPA should be initiated at the recommended starting dosage, and then the dosage should be decreased progressively once the incontinence is controlled.

Pseudoephedrine is a stereoisomer of ephedrine that was shown to produce a lower increase in urethral resistance, a lower continence score, and more adverse effects in bitches with USMI compared with PPA (Byron et al, 2007). Pseudoephedrine generally is not recommended for the management of urinary incontinence.

Estrogenic Compounds

High-affinity estradiol receptors are located at the level of the proximal urethra, and estrogens are known to increase the number and the responsiveness of α-adrenergic receptors to sympathetic stimulation. Additional potential effects of estrogenic compounds include improvement of urethral vascularization, stimulation of collagen synthesis, and cellular proliferation leading to an increase in urethral wall thickness. Long-acting synthetic estrogen preparations are associated with bone marrow depletion and should no longer be used. *Estriol* is a short-acting natural estrogen compound with few adverse effects. It recently has received U.S. Food and Drug Administration

TABLE 201-1

Therapeutic Options for the Management of Urinary Incontinence

Agent	Recommended Dosage	Possible Adverse Effects
Phenylpropanolamine	Dog and cat: 1-1.5 mg/kg q8-12h PO or 1.5 mg/kg q24h PO	Restlessness, hypertension, tachycardia, anxiety
Ephedrine	Dog: 1-4 mg/kg q8-12h PO Cat: 2-4 mg per cat q8h or 2-4 mg/kg q6-12h	Restlessness, hypertension, tachycardia, anxiety, excitability
Pseudoephedrine	Dog: 0.2-0.4 mg/kg q8-12h PO	Restlessness, hypertension, tachycardia, anxiety, excitability
Estriol*	Dog: 0.5-2 mg per dog q24h PO	Vulvar swelling, attraction to males, metrorrhagia
Depot leuprolide	Dog: 1 mg/kg or 11-25 mg per dog	
Depot deslorelin	Dog: 5-10 mg per dog or Dog <30 kg: one 4.7-mg implant Dog >30 kg: one 9.4-mg implant	
Oxybutynin	Dog: 0.2 mg/kg q8-12h PO or Small dog: 0.75-1.25 mg per dog q8-12h PO Larger dog: 2.5-5 mg per dog q8-12h PO Cat: 0.5-1.25 mg per cat q8-12h	Diarrhea, constipation, urinary retention, hypersalivation, sedation, dry mouth, dry eyes, tachycardia, anorexia, vomiting, weakness, mydriasis
Propantheline bromide	Dog: 7.5-15 mg per dog q12h PO up to 30 mg per dog q8h or 0.2 mg/kg q6-8h PO Cat: 0.25-0.5 mg/kg q12-24h or 5-7.5 mg per cat every 3 days or 5-7.5 mg per cat q8h every 3 days	Dry mouth, dry eyes, urinary hesitancy, tachycardia, constipation
Imipramine	Dog: 5-20 mg per dog q12h PO Cat: 2.5-5 mg per cat q12h	Sedation, dry mouth, urinary retention, vomiting, constipation
Duloxetine†	Dog: 1 mg/kg q12h PO	

*Recommended dosages for other estrogenic compounds can be found in the previous edition of *Current Veterinary Therapy,* Chapter 207.
†Dosage is extrapolated from experimental studies in rabbits and cats and has not yet been investigated in dogs.
PO, Orally.

approval for use in veterinary medicine. Long-term administration is associated in rare cases with adverse effects such as pyometra or bone marrow suppression. Minor associated adverse effects include swelling of the vulva, attraction to males, and metrorrhagia. Success rate is lower with estrogen administration than with administration of sympathomimetic compounds, and complete continence is achieved in 65% of treated bitches (Mandigers and Nell, 2001). Estrogen administration can be chosen when the use of sympathomimetic agents is contraindicated, such as in dogs with concurrent cardiovascular disease or hypertension. Estrogen use is contraindicated in immature bitches with congenital USMI because of adverse effects associated with the negative feedback on the hypophysis. Estrogen administration also should be avoided in intact bitches and in male dogs.

Although the combination of estrogens and sympathomimetic agents has been advocated in cases of refractory incontinence to achieve a theoretical synergetic effect, the superiority of this combination still remains to be documented. Indeed, experimental urodynamic studies have failed to demonstrate a superior effect of this combination on urethral function compared with the effect of either estrogens or α-agonists alone (Hamaide et al, 2006). However, the combination still may be useful in individual dogs. If the drugs are used in combination, the dosage of each drug is identical to that used when the drug is given alone, and dosages of both medications also can be tapered over time.

Other Therapies

A role for gonadotrophins in the development of USMI has been suggested because ovariectomy induces a long-term increase in the levels of follicle-stimulating hormone and luteinizing hormone and a decrease in the expression of follicle-stimulating hormone and luteinizing hormone receptors in the lower urinary tract. Furthermore, the expression of gonadotropin-releasing hormone (GnRH) receptor messenger RNA is increased in the bladder after neutering. Therefore the role of *GnRH analogs* (leuprolide, deslorelin) as a treatment option also has been investigated. Long-term continence was achieved in 50% to 70% of incontinent bitches treated with deslorelin or leuprolide. No adverse effects were observed. However, the therapeutic effect of GnRH analogs typically is inferior to that of PPA, which should remain the first-line treatment. GnRH analogs represent an alternative when α-agonists are contraindicated (e.g., in animals with cardiovascular disease or hypertension). In some cases, the combined administration of PPA and a GnRH analog may restore continence. Interestingly, in spayed beagle dogs treatment with leuprolide did not demonstrably modify urethral function, but an increased bladder threshold volume was observed (Reichler et al, 2006a, 2006b). The improved continence observed with administration of GnRH analogs could be due to its effect on bladder function.

As previously mentioned, bladder overactivity can be a primary cause or concurrent cause of incontinence in dogs. Although the condition is rare in animals, the diagnosis is preferable to refractory USMI and can be made by cystometry. Clinical signs include nocturia, pollakiuria, urgency, and urinary incontinence. *Antimuscarinic* agents act on urinary bladder smooth muscle to improve storage and are used to treat bladder overactivity. Oxybutynin is used most commonly in dogs and cats. Propantheline bromide does not cross the blood-brain barrier and also has been used for the treatment of detrusor hyperreflexia. Emepronium bromide is an anticholinergic agent that has been shown to be effective in two bitches with detrusor instability and in one bitch with USMI (Holt, 1984). Tolterodine is a nonselective antimuscarinic agent acting on all muscarinic receptors and has fewer adverse effects than oxybutynin. Principal adverse effects in humans are sedation, vomiting, constipation, and urinary retention. In dogs, gastrointestinal upset and ptyalism can be encountered when higher dosages are used and usually resolve at lower dosages. The use of these agents must be avoided in animals with cardiac disease, arrhythmia, hypertension, hyperthyroidism, glaucoma, and obstructive uropathies (Lane, 2001). *Tricyclic antidepressants* (imipramine, amitriptyline, and duloxetine) are serotonin and norepinephrine reuptake inhibitors that may improve bladder storage by acting on both bladder and urethral smooth muscle through their anticholinergic, α-adrenergic, and β-adrenergic effects. Imipramine and amitriptyline are used in humans in the treatment of nocturnal enuresis, stress incontinence, and urge incontinence. The use of imipramine seldom is described in veterinary medicine. This agent could be an alternative for the treatment of urinary leakage or inappropriate voiding with a suspected behavioral origin (Lane, 2003). The main adverse effects of tricyclic antidepressants in humans are dry mouth, urine retention, constipation, nausea, and diarrhea.

Duloxetine is a serotonin and norepinephrine reuptake inhibitor used successfully in some women with stress incontinence. In dogs, results of experimental urodynamic studies are pending. Use of this class of drug has not yet been investigated in clinical cases.

Urinary Retention

Nonobstructive urinary retention is caused by urinary bladder atony, high urethral resistance, or both. The first therapeutic goal in cases of functional urinary retention is to decrease urethral resistance. Improvement of bladder contractility is considered once urethral resistance is decreased. Recommended dosages of various drugs for the management of urinary retention are given in Table 201-2.

Urethral Hypertonicity

Urethral resistance is maintained primarily by the urethral smooth and striated muscle. Other components of urethral tone include urethral vascularization, wall thickness, and urethral length and position. Management of urethral hypertonicity is aimed at the smooth or striated

TABLE **201-2**
Therapeutic Options for the Management of Urinary Retention

Agent	Recommended Dosage	Possible Adverse Effects
Phenoxybenzamine	Dog: 0.25 mg/kg q8-12h PO with total dose of 5-20 mg per dog Cat: 1.25-7.5 mg per cat q8-12h PO	Hypotension, hypertension, increased intraocular pressure, tachycardia, gastrointestinal upset, nasal congestion
Prazosin	Dog: 0.03 mg/kg q8h PO or 1 mg/15 kg q8-12h Cat: 0.25-0.5 mg per cat q12-24h PO	Hypotension at the first administration
Tamsulosin*	Dog: 0.1 mg/10 kg q24h or up to 1 mg per dog q24h PO	Hypotension
Diazepam	Dog: 2-10 mg per dog q8h PO Cat: 1-2.5 mg per cat q8h PO	Sedation, weakness, paradoxical excitement
Dantrolene	Dog: 1-5 mg/kg q8-12h PO Cat: 0.5-2 mg/kg q8h PO	Sedation, weakness, gastrointestinal upset
Bethanechol	Dog: 5-25 mg per dog q8h PO Cat: 1.25-5 mg per cat q8h PO	Vomiting, diarrhea, salivation, anorexia
Pyridostigmine*	Dog: 1 mg per dog q8h PO	
Cisapride	Dog: 0.5 mg/kg q8h PO Cat: 1.25-5 mg per cat q8-12h PO	Diarrhea

*Dosage and safety have not been investigated in veterinary medicine.
PO, Orally.

urethral musculature. It must be emphasized that the rationale for the use of the following agents is based on the results of experimental urodynamic studies in healthy dogs and cats or clinical results in humans. Investigation of the clinical and urodynamic effects of many of these agents in affected animals has not yet been reported.

Functional urethral outlet obstruction can be treated with *α-blocker agents* that act on the smooth muscle component of the urethral sphincter. Phenoxybenzamine is a nonselective, noncompetitive α-antagonist used in dogs and cats. It has been shown to decrease the urethral pressure in healthy female and male dogs as well as in cats. However, its effectiveness in dysuric dogs or in cats with urethrospasms is poorly documented. Adverse effects include hypotension, hypertension, miosis, increased intraocular pressure, tachycardia, gastrointestinal upset, and nasal congestion.

Prazosin is a selective $α_1$-antagonist, producing a selective and competitive inhibition of $α_1$-adrenergic receptors and reducing blood pressure and peripheral vascular resistance. The major adverse effect is hypotension. Prazosin appears to be an effective alternative to phenoxybenzamine in the treatment of detrusor-urethral dyssynergia or urethrospasms in cats, but pharmacokinetic and dose-response studies are needed to determine the optimal oral dosage protocol. Tamsulosin is a uroselective $α_1$-adrenoceptor antagonist used in men with prostatic hyperplasia. In healthy male dogs and in dogs with prostatic hyperplasia, it inhibits the prostatic intraurethral pressure in a dose-dependent manner without causing systemic hypotension. Tamsulosin could serve as an alternative to phenoxybenzamine or prazosin in refractory cases of detrusor-urethral dyssynergia.

Detrusor-urethral dyssynergia is associated with increased urethral striated muscle tone, which may or may not be accompanied by increased urethral smooth muscle tone. In cats, urethrospasms usually involve the striated part of the urethral sphincter. Therefore *somatic muscle relaxants* such as diazepam or dantrolene can be added. Diazepam depresses the central nervous system at a subcortical level and induces skeletal muscle relaxation and anticonvulsant effects. Possible adverse effects are sedation, weakness, and paradoxical excitement (Lane, 2001). Dantrolene is a direct striated muscle relaxant acting through inhibition of the excitation-contraction coupling mechanism by inhibiting calcium movement from the sarcoplasmic reticulum in muscle cells. Adverse effects include weakness, sedation, dizziness, headache, and gastrointestinal upset (Lane, 2001). Experimental urodynamic studies in healthy male cats showed no change in urethral pressure after administration of diazepam, whereas dantrolene induced a decrease in urethral pressure in the prostatic and penile portions of the urethra. Dantrolene may be more valuable for the pharmacologic management of urethral disorders in male cats but has had minimal application to date.

Bladder Atony

Detrusor atony in dogs and cats most commonly develops after acute or chronic bladder overdistention secondary to mechanical or functional urethral obstruction. Primary detrusor atony is rare but can develop with electrolyte disturbances, lesions of the pelvic nerves, lower motor neuron lesions, dysautonomia, hypoadrenocorticism, or administration of anticholinergic medications.

In cases of secondary bladder atony, α-blockers and possibly somatic muscle relaxants are administered first. When treatment is in place, and if some degree of bladder atony is suspected, other agents can be added to improve bladder contraction. These agents can be used alone in case of primary bladder atony.

Bethanechol is a parasympathomimetic agent most frequently used in the treatment of bladder atony in veterinary medicine. It has been shown to increase bladder contractility in a canine model. However, its clinical efficacy still is questionable. While response is awaited, it could be beneficial to place an indwelling urinary catheter for a few days to keep the bladder decompressed as the administration of bethanechol is started. Although the action of bethanechol is considered dose dependent, at a certain point a decreased response is observed after administration of much higher dosages. Adverse effects include vomiting, diarrhea, salivation, and anorexia.

Pharmacologic alternatives to parasympathomimetic agents include cholinesterase inhibitors, β-blocking agents, dopaminergic antagonists, prostaglandins, and prokinetic agents. *Cholinesterase inhibitors* such as pyridostigmine have been used to increase parasympathetic activity and can be administered in some refractory cases of detrusor-urethral dyssynergia. *Prokinetic agents* such as cisapride and metoclopramide also have been suggested to increase bladder contraction. In women, they decrease bladder capacity but do not seem to improve voiding function. However, the use of prokinetic agents for urinary retention in veterinary patients so far is anecdotal. If complete voiding still is not achieved even with medical treatment, intermittent urethral catheterization is needed, and an indwelling catheter or a cystostomy tube should be placed.

References and Suggested Reading

Byron J et al: Effect of phenylpropanolamine and pseudoephedrine on the urethral pressure profile and continence scores of incontinent female dogs, *J Vet Intern Med* 21:47, 2007.

Claeys S et al: Clinical evaluation of a single daily dose of phenylpropanolamine in the treatment of urethral sphincter mechanism incompetence in the bitch, *Can J Vet Res* 52:501, 2011.

Fischer JR, Lane IF: Incontinence and urine retention. In Brainbridge J, Elliott J, editors: *BSAVA: manual of canine and feline nephrology and urology*, ed 2, Gloucestershire, UK, 2007, British Small Animal Veterinary Association, p 26.

Hamaide A et al: Urodynamic and morphometric changes in the lower portion of the urogenital tract after administration of estriol alone and in combination with phenylpropanolamine in sexually intact and spayed dogs, *Am J Vet Res* 67:901, 2006.

Holt PE: Efficacy of emepronium bromide in the treatment of physiological incontinence in the bitch, *Vet Rec* 114:355, 1984.

Lane IF: Treatment of urinary disorders. In Boothe D, editor: *Small clinical pharmacology and therapeutics*, Philadelphia, 2001, Saunders, p 528.

Lane IF: Treating urinary incontinence, *Vet Med* 1:58, 2003.

Mandigers P, Nell T: Treatment of bitches with acquired urinary incontinence with oestriol, *Vet Rec* 22:764, 2001.

Noël S, Claeys S, Hamaide A: Acquired urinary incontinence in the bitch: update and perspectives from human medicine. Part 1: The bladder component, pathophysiology and medical treatment, *Vet J* 186:10, 2010a.

Noël S, Claeys S, Hamaide A: Acquired urinary incontinence in the bitch: update and perspectives from the human medicine. Part 2: The urethral component, pathophysiology and medical treatment, *Vet J* 186:18, 2010b.

Noël S, Massart L, Hamaide A: Urodynamic and haemodynamic effects of a single oral administration of ephedrine and phenylpropanolamine in continent female dogs, *Vet J* 192(1): 89, 2012. Epub June 28, 2011.

Reichler IM et al: Effect of long acting GnRH analogue or placebo on plasma LH/FSH, urethral pressure profiles and clinical signs of urinary incontinence due to sphincter mechanism incompetence in bitches, *Theriogenology* 66:1227, 2006a.

Reichler IM et al: Urodynamic parameters and plasma LH/FSH in spayed Beagle bitches before and 8 weeks after GnRH depot analogue treatment, *Theriogenology* 66(9):2127, 2006b.

CHAPTER 202

Mechanical Occluder Devices for Urinary Incontinence

CHRISTOPHER A. ADIN, *Columbus, Ohio*

Urinary incontinence is a common and serious problem in dogs. Acquired urethral sphincter mechanism incompetence (USMI) occurs in up to 20% of dogs after ovariohysterectomy, with ureteral ectopia, pelvic bladder, and other urogenital malformations contributing to the overall incidence of incontinence in dogs. Although urinary incontinence is not directly life threatening, the resultant house soiling is a major cause of euthanasia or abandonment of indoor pets. As a result, small animal practitioners often are pressured to provide effective options for the treatment of urinary incontinence that will produce a rapid and permanent resolution of clinical signs.

Therapeutic Options

Pharmacologic therapy is the standard of care for initial treatment of dogs with acquired urinary incontinence. Although treatment with α-agonists or estrogenic compounds (see Chapter 201) is effective in the majority of animals with acquired urinary incontinence, in approximately 20% of dogs with USMI the disorder is refractory to medical therapy. Male dogs with USMI and dogs with congenital malformations are far less likely to respond to drug therapy. Endoscopic or surgical procedures are considered as a means to improve control of urinary incontinence when the disorder shows no response to medical therapy or when clients feel that the lifelong administration of drugs is undesirable. Historically, endoscopic application of urethral bulking agents has provided a minimally invasive method for the treatment of USMI in female dogs (see Web Chapter 71). Although this procedure is effective in the majority of dogs (66% rate of complete continence; Byron et al, 2011), the durability of this effect is poor, with the mean duration of continence ranging from 5.2 to 16.4 months. In addition, the length of the male canine urethra makes endoscopic urethral bulking techniques impractical for use in male dogs. Because of the need for repeated injections over time and the limited availability of suitable bulking agents, many referral practices are actively seeking out other means of therapy for refractory incontinence.

Artificial Urethral Sphincter

The canine artificial urethral sphincter (AUS; Figure 202-1) is a modification of an inflatable silicone hydraulic vascular occluder that was intended for use in the temporary constriction of blood vessels in laboratory animals (Adin et al, 2004; Sereda et al, 2005). The device is similar in concept to an artificial urethral sphincter used in human beings with urinary incontinence (AMS 800), although that device requires manual deflation before each act of urination—a feature that prevented its direct application in dogs. Instead, the canine AUS is designed to produce a low level of static urethral compression, similar to the effect of urethral bulking agents. After the device was evaluated in cadavers, it was determined that these inflatable cuffs could be placed around the canine urethra through a caudal abdominal approach. Actuating tubing from the cuff is connected to a permanent subcutaneous injection port (Le Grande CompanionPort vascular access port) that is placed under the skin on the caudoventral abdomen. Incremental injections of fluid

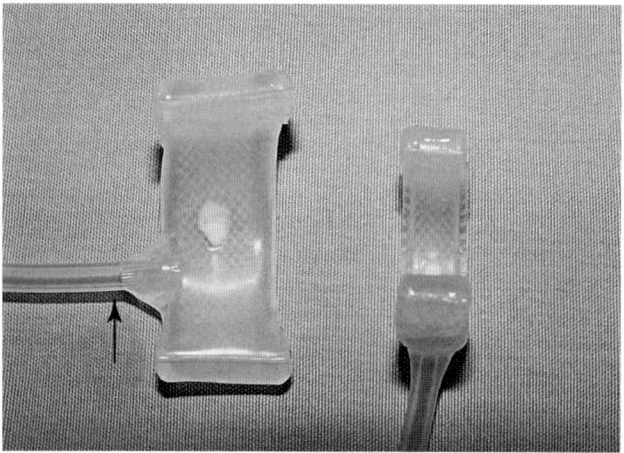

Figure 202-1 The silicone canine artificial urethral sphincter (AUS; DocXS Biomedical Products) at the left is a modification of a hydraulic vascular occluder *(right)*. The AUS cuff was widened to 1.4 cm to minimize atrophy of the urethra at an area of focal compression. The actuating tube *(arrow)*, used to inflate the device by injections into a subcutaneous port, was changed to a side-entry design to prevent kinking of the device on the urethra when the device is placed in the pelvic canal.

into the port created corresponding increases in urethral pressure in the cadaver study (Adin et al, 2004). Mechanical studies showed that devices that were inflated with sterile 0.9% NaCl remained inflated over a 5-month period of immersion in simulated body fluid (Sereda et al, 2006). Based on the success of these initial investigations and a subsequent pilot study in four client-owned dogs with refractory USMI (Rose et al, 2009), we now have performed the procedure in over 30 dogs with an expanding list of acquired and congenital causes of urinary incontinence.

Indications

In human beings, the AUS is used almost exclusively to treat men with urinary incontinence resulting from radical prostatectomy. Because of the severity of incontinence in affected men, significant urethral compression and a dynamic (deflatable) cuff are required to achieve continence and intermittent bladder emptying, respectively. In contrast, the canine AUS has been applied to treat the more commonly encountered female USMI—a condition that is more responsive to the mild, static increases in urethral pressure produced by this device. After experiencing initial success in treating female dogs with USMI, we now have expanded our criteria to include female dogs with pelvic bladder and urethral hypoplasia as well as those with continued incontinence after conventional or laser surgery for ureteral ectopia. Because of the extremely poor efficacy of alternative therapies, the canine AUS device has proven to be particularly useful in the treatment of male dogs with USMI.

Diagnostic Evaluation

Diagnostic screening of candidates for AUS implantation is similar to evaluation of any animal with urinary incontinence. Testing should include a complete blood count, serum biochemistry panel, urinalysis, and urine bacterial culture to rule out concurrent metabolic or infectious diseases that may be contributing to clinical signs of incontinence. Animals with a current urinary tract infection or with active pyoderma are treated with appropriate antibiotics to resolve any infection before implantation of a permanent implant such as the AUS is considered. Baseline urinary tract ultrasonography also is performed to screen for urolithiasis, ureteral dilation, renal parenchymal changes, or abnormalities in the bladder wall that may indicate preexisting urinary tract disease. In our practice, the medical history regarding the onset of incontinence is crucial in determining whether advanced imaging (computed tomographic excretory urography) or uroendoscopy are required to rule out concurrent anatomic abnormalities that should be corrected before AUS implantation is considered. A dog that has acquired USMI after gonadectomy is not subjected to advanced imaging, whereas an animal that has been leaking urine from birth is more likely to have concurrent ureteral ectopia, ureterocele, or other anomalies, and advanced imaging is recommended. Although urodynamic evaluation is a standard part of the screening of human patients with incontinence, it does not predict response to surgical therapy accurately and is not currently used as a standard screening test before AUS implantation.

Implant Selection

Canine AUS implants are sold based on the theoretical inside diameter of the closed cuff and are available in diameters ranging from 6 mm to 20 mm, with a cuff width of either 11 or 14 mm. Presterilized devices now are available and are sold with injection ports and optional filling catheters to prime the device with fluid before implantation. Guidelines in application of the human AUS suggest that the cuff circumference should approximate the circumference of the urethra, which allows placement of the uninflated device without any external compression of the urethra. Physicians keep an inventory of sizes and use a marked tape to measure the urethral circumference intraoperatively, selecting the appropriate device at that time. Companion animals have a much wider range of body sizes than the typical human patient populations, which makes sizing of the implants more challenging. Our approach has been to maintain a limited inventory that represents the most commonly applied sizes, with two of each of the following sizes kept in stock: 8 × 14 mm, 10 × 14 mm, 12 × 14 mm, and 14 × 14 mm. For animals that are outside the normal range of body sizes, additional small or large implants can be purchased and sterilized before the procedure is scheduled. Table 202-1 indicates the likely implant size given the animal's body weight based on our experience in performing the procedure. Fortunately, the Le Grande vascular access port that is used for fluid injection is compatible with the actuating tubing on all of the canine AUS devices, which allows a smaller stock of these items to be maintained. Veterinarians who are reluctant to keep an appropriate inventory of various-sized AUS implants are cautioned to

TABLE 202-1

General Guidelines for the Size of Artificial Urethral Sphincter Devices Based on the Body Weight of Female Dogs*

	BODY WEIGHT (KG)			
	<5 kg	5-25 kg	25-35 kg	30-40 kg
Device size (diameter × width)	6 × 11 mm	8 × 14 mm	10 × 14 mm	12 × 14 mm

*Intraoperative sizing of the device still is required. It is recommended that surgeons have available at least one size above the expected artificial sphincter diameter because it is safer to apply an oversized device and avoid risk of inadvertent urethral obstruction. See text for further details.

think carefully before performing the procedure because application of an inappropriately sized implant may result in failure of the procedure or iatrogenic obstruction of the urethra requiring revisional surgery.

Surgical Technique

Anesthetic technique is tailored to the individual animal because this caudal abdominal procedure does not carry a high degree of inherent perioperative risk or discomfort. Although AUS implantation is classified as a clean surgical procedure, standard antimicrobial prophylaxis is administered intravenously within 20 minutes of induction because a permanent synthetic device is being implanted. The ventral abdomen is shaved and aseptically prepared with the animal positioned in dorsal recumbency. A 5-cm caudal midline abdominal incision is made, extending to the pubis to allow maximal exposure of the abdominal urethra. The urinary bladder is exteriorized and stay sutures are placed at the apex to allow cranial retraction of the bladder, with exposure of several centimeters of the pelvic urethra. A 2-cm-wide section of the urethra is isolated by blunt dissection with Mixter right-angled forceps at least 3 cm caudal to the bladder neck to avoid constriction of the ureters at the trigone. In males, the device has been placed 1 cm caudal to the prostate, an area that can be exposed with careful cranial retraction of the bladder. The surgeon must avoid excessive manipulation of or trauma to the urethra and its blood supply, which could cause swelling and acute obstruction or delayed stricture formation. Once the urethra is dissected, the urethral circumference is estimated using a strand of suture and an AUS is selected that is slightly larger than the measured circumference to avoid inadvertent obstruction of the urethra. The selected AUS is primed with fluid by inserting a long catheter into the actuating tubing, with the air flushed from the device. A sterile vascular access port is inserted with a specially designed Huber point needle, which minimizes damage to the port, and the port is filled with sterile saline. The actuating tubing of the AUS then is connected to the injection port and the cuff is inflated five times to exercise the cuff membrane and to test for leakage (Figure 202-2). After leak testing, the AUS is closed to form a circle, and the volume required to fill the cuff is recorded. The deflated AUS then is passed around the urethra in the area of circumferential dissection and the cuff is closed around the urethra by tying a single strand of 2-0 polypropylene

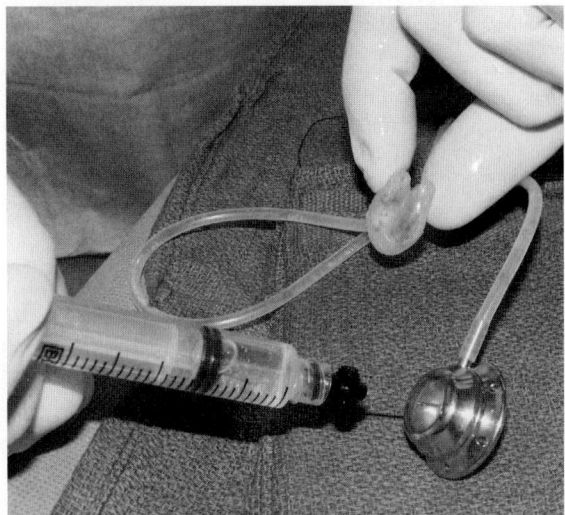

Figure 202-2 Before the implant is placed on the urethra, the device is primed with fluid and connected to a titanium vascular access port, and filling volume is recorded as the device is inflated using a specially designed Huber needle.

suture that has been threaded through the suture eyelets at the ends of the cuff (Figure 202-3). It is important to orient the cuff so that the actuating tubing is directed cranially (toward the bladder) so that the tube does not kink as the bladder retraction is released and the cuff moves into the pelvic canal. The port is disconnected temporarily while the infusion line is tunneled through the caudal abdominal wall, lateral to the rectus abdominus muscle and exiting through a separate skin incision just cranial to the flank fold on the caudolateral abdomen (Figure 202-4). The port is reattached to the actuating tubing and is sutured to the external rectus fascia using nonabsorbable sutures. The abdomen is closed routinely, and analgesia is provided using a nonsteroidal antiinflammatory drug and injectable opioid as needed. Animals are observed for the ability to urinate freely and produce a normal urine stream, then are discharged the day following surgery. We have not found it necessary to place urinary drainage catheters in the postoperative period.

Postoperative Adjustments

Animals are reevaluated at the time of suture removal, and urination behavior is assessed by direct observation

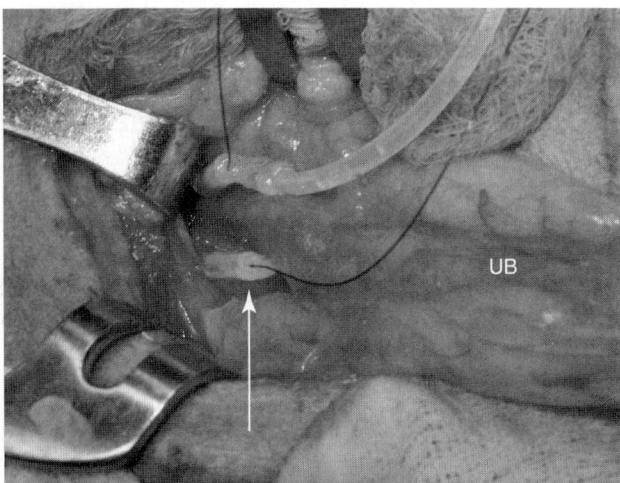

Figure 202-3 The artificial urethral sphincter (AUS) is placed around the urethra approximately 2 cm caudal to the urinary bladder (UB). The device then is closed around the urethra by placing nonabsorbable monofilament suture through the premade eyelets *(arrow)* and tying the suture into a secure knot.

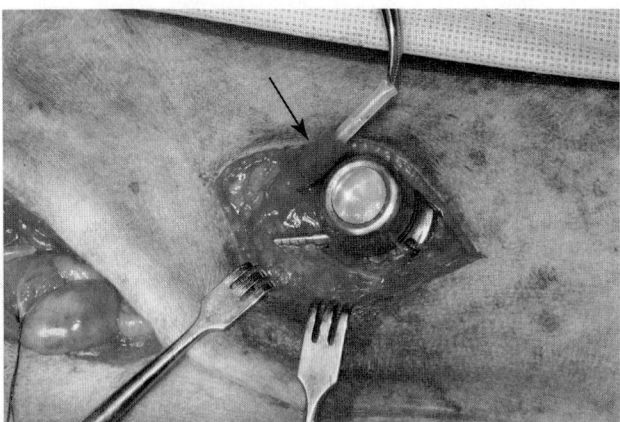

Figure 202-4 The titanium vascular access port is placed in a separate paramedian incision made just cranial to the flank fold. The actuating tubing is attached to the port and is secured to the port with a plastic boot *(arrow)* that improves the friction fit over the male connector on the port.

as well as by questioning of the pet owner. In our experience, more than 50% of dogs achieve an acceptable level of continence without any inflation of the AUS device, and these animals are discharged without need for further follow-up unless signs of incontinence or dysuria occur. In dogs that remain incontinent after implantation of the AUS, inflation is delayed until 6 weeks after surgery to allow for restoration of urethral blood supply and resolution of postoperative inflammation. Our initial report in cadavers suggested that infusion of 25% to 50% of the total fluid volume of the AUS would produce clinically relevant increases in urethral pressure; however, clinical experience has shown that injections of much smaller amounts of fluid can be effective. Thus, in animals with continued leakage at 6 weeks after surgery, volumes of 0.05 to 0.2 ml are injected once a week until signs resolve or until dogs begin to show evidence of stranguria due to excessive urethral compression. Injections are performed

using sterile 0.9% NaCl in a 1-ml (tuberculin) syringe with a 20- to 22-gauge Huber needle. The area of skin over the port is shaved and aseptically prepared. Sedation typically is not required in tractable animals. The injection is performed using sterile gloves; the subcutaneous port is stabilized with the left hand and the Huber needle is inserted through the skin and the thick membrane of the injection port until the needle contacts the titanium backing of the port. The priming fluid of the AUS system is aspirated to confirm that the needle is seated in the correct location. The priming volume and additional desired saline volume then are injected into the device before the needle and syringe are withdrawn. Before the dog is discharged, the animal is walked outside and urination behavior is observed directly by the clinician to confirm that an adequate urine stream is produced and that the bladder is emptied after urination. In animals that develop stranguria or incomplete bladder emptying, fluid should be withdrawn from the device using aseptic technique as described previously.

Outcome

Results of AUS implantation at our institution recently were summarized in a retrospective study involving 27 dogs with naturally occurring urinary incontinence (Reeves et al, 2013). Continence was scored using a visual analog scale with 1 representing constant leakage and 10 representing perfect continence. Before surgery, 25 of 27 dogs had incontinence refractory to medical management and 4 dogs had undergone failed urethral bulking procedures. Median continence score before surgery was 3. At a median of 12.5 months of follow-up, the median postoperative continence score had improved to 9. In 15 of 27 dogs injections were required to inflate the cuff after surgery. Median total volume of saline injected into the AUS was 0.3 ml. Two dogs developed unexplained stranguria and incomplete bladder emptying, requiring implant removal at 5 and 9 months after surgery. Minor complications included temporary worsening of incontinence, seroma formation over the port, and mild stranguria in the perioperative period. Overall, client satisfaction was high, with 24 of 27 owners describing themselves as either satisfied or very satisfied with the results of the procedure.

Although this study included only three male dogs, early experience with this technique was good. All three male dogs were restored to an acceptable level of continence, and no specific surgical or postoperative complications were associated with application of the device on the postprostatic urethra in this limited number of animals.

References and Suggested Reading

Aaron A et al: Urethral sphincter mechanism incompetence in male dogs: a retrospective analysis of 54 cases, *Vet Rec* 139:542, 1996.

Adin CA et al: Urodynamic effects of a percutaneously controlled static hydraulic urethral sphincter in canine cadavers, *Am J Vet Res* 65:283, 2004.

Arnold S et al: Urinary incontinence in spayed female dogs: frequency and breed disposition, *Schweiz Arch Tierheilkd* 131:259, 1989.

Arnold S et al: Treatment of urinary incontinence in bitches by endoscopic injection of glutaraldehyde cross-linked collagen, *J Small Anim Pract* 37:163, 1996.

Barth A et al: Evaluation of long-term effects of endoscopic injection of collagen into the urethral submucosa for treatment of urethral sphincter incompetence in female dogs: 40 cases (1993-2000), *J Am Vet Med Assoc* 226:73, 2005.

Byron JK et al: Retrospective evaluation of urethral bovine cross-linked collagen implantation for treatment of urinary incontinence in female dogs, *J Vet Intern Med* 25:980, 2011.

Holt PE, Moore AH: Canine ureteral ectopia: an analysis of 175 cases and comparison of surgical treatments, *Vet Rec* 136:345, 1995.

Reeves L et al: Outcome after placement of an artificial urethral sphincter in 27 dogs, *Vet Surg* 42(1):12, 2013.

Rose SA et al: Long-term efficacy of a percutaneously adjustable hydraulic urethral sphincter for treatment of urinary incontinence in four dogs, *Vet Surg* 38:747, 2009.

Sereda CW et al: Evaluation of a percutaneously controlled hydraulic occluder in a rat model of gradual venous occlusion, *Vet Surg* 34:35, 2005.

Sereda CW et al: Evaluation of manufacturing variability, diffusion of filling solutions, and long-term maintenance of occlusion in silicone hydraulic occluders, *Am J Vet Res* 67:1453, 2006.

CHAPTER 203

Top Ten Urinary Consult Questions

DIANNE I. MAWBY, *Knoxville, Tennessee*
AMANDA CALLENS, *Knoxville, Tennessee*
JOSEPH W. BARTGES, *Knoxville, Tennessee*

The scope of urologic problems in small animal veterinary practice is wide and encompasses upper and lower urinary tract problems as well as diagnostic, monitoring, and therapeutic challenges. Within this range of problems, 10 of the most common questions posed to specialists are summarized. The brief answers are designed to provide initial guidance for practitioners and often direct the reader to more specific information in this or previous editions of *Current Veterinary Therapy*.

1. Why Are Urine Culture Results Always Negative When I Send Specimens to the Diagnostic Laboratory?

The diagnostic plan for most patients with lower urinary tract signs includes urinalysis and urine culture. It can be frustrating to receive "false-negative" results when urinary tract infection (UTI) is suspected. False- and true-negatives can be related to procedural and biologic factors.

The timing of sample collection in relation to treatment selection is important. Samples should be collected before initiation of antimicrobial treatment in new cases whenever possible; if this is not possible, the diagnostic laboratory should be notified of current treatments.

Antimicrobial administration may inhibit bacterial growth in culture but may not be bactericidal *in vivo*. Additionally, anaerobic and mycoplasma organisms will not grow with standard aerobic methods.

Handling of the urine sample before transport may have adverse effects. Samples should be refrigerated and transported as soon as possible. Urine samples should not be transported in the same shipment with formalin-preserved biopsy samples. Duration and temperature of transport also may affect culture outcome. Bacteria must be alive at the time of inoculation in the laboratory for growth to occur, and long delays or high temperatures may affect bacterial viability.

Negative urine culture results, of course, often reflect a sterile sample accurately. Urine leukocyte indicators on some urine dipstick tests are not reliable for the detection of inflammatory cells in dog or cat urine, and "bacteria" are overestimated on urine sediment examination. Many artifacts mimic bacteria and even bacterial motion in urine examined microscopically. Sediment examination is enhanced by routine staining (clean Gram stain or new methylene blue) and review by qualified personnel.

Finally, not all lower urinary tract signs are caused by bacteria. Further evaluation for other causes (urolithiasis, neoplasia, idiopathic cystitis) should be pursued in patients with persistent signs and repeated negative culture results.

To overcome the procedural challenges, urine can be cultured initially at the clinic. A small incubator can be used for inoculated blood agar plates. If growth occurs, then these samples may be submitted for species identification and antimicrobial susceptibility testing. It is well worth the time and effort involved in setting up this initial culture in-house to ensure a more reliable outcome.

2. How Do I Treat Urinary Tract Infections That Keep Coming Back?

Sequential urine cultures are invaluable in sorting out recurrent bacterial UTIs. Repeated UTIs can be classified based on the species and pattern of bacteria observed. Recurrent signs caused by the same organism usually are due to a relapse of the original infection. Signs associated with a new infection usually are caused by a different organism. Granted, repeated *Escherichia coli* infections can be challenging to interpret since *E. coli* is a common infectious agent as well as a common persistent organism in some patients (see Chapter 194).

"Recurrent" infection also must be evaluated in relation to previous courses of treatment. In a relapse (same bacteria) questions target the effectiveness of the prior treatment plan: Was adequate treatment given to the patient including appropriate drug, dosage, and duration? Were urinalysis and culture results rechecked after treatment completion to ensure clearance of infection? Was it a simple or a complicated infection (especially prostatitis, pyelonephritis, or UTIs with concurrent disorders)?

When reinfections (different organisms) are detected, underlying predisposing causes must be considered. These include host defense problems such as anatomic abnormalities of the lower urinary tract (recessed vulva, vaginal urine pooling, and masses), urethral incompetence, neurologic impairment of micturition, and alteration in urine concentration and volume. Uroliths at any location in the urinary system also can act as a nidus for relapse or reinfection. Other underlying systemic predispositions include immunocompromise such as that associated with endocrine diseases (diabetes mellitus, hyperadrenocorticism) or corticosteroid therapy. Unfortunately, an underlying disorder cannot be detected in many cases.

Even when a distinct reason or underlying cause can be identified, management of recurrent UTIs still can be challenging. Underlying anatomic problems may be surgically corrected to solve the problem, and manageable systemic disorders can be addressed. Other predisposing disorders may or may not be able to be eliminated (e.g., poorly controlled endocrine disorders, irreversible neurologic impairment). These cases should be managed as a complicated UTI with long-term appropriate antimicrobial therapy. Pulse or low-dose daily antibiotic therapy or other prophylaxis can be considered once the initial infection is cleared.

Many of these recurrent infections involve *E. coli*, which first must adhere to the cell and may actually internalize. Oral therapies that may be used to prevent adhesion include cranberry extract and D-mannose. Cranberry extract contains proanthocyanidins that inhibit *E. coli* adhesion to epithelial cells. D-Mannose also may be an adhesion deterrent, but clinical studies of its efficacy are lacking.

3. How Do I Treat Highly Resistant Urinary Tract Infections?

Resistant UTIs usually occur in patients with unidentified or unmanageable underlying disease. Typically, many different classes of antimicrobials have been prescribed, and bacteria have become resistant. As with recurrent UTIs, an underlying disease or condition should be investigated and treated if possible.

The diagnostic laboratory can be of great help in maximizing effective antimicrobial choices. Laboratories report antibiotic susceptibility via agar disk diffusion (Kirby-Bauer method) or the antimicrobial dilution technique (minimum inhibitory [bacteriostatic] concentration, or MIC). In the MIC technique, each antibiotic is evaluated with respect to serum levels of the drug, but urinary concentrations may be significantly higher. Renally excreted antimicrobials may be effective even if the laboratory result reports intermediate susceptibility or resistance. Short-term use of injectable antimicrobials may be necessary to eliminate the infection. If aminoglycosides are used, urinalysis should be performed frequently to detect casts that indicate early renal tubular damage. In infections with susceptible organisms, antiseptic therapy with nitrofurantoin can be used, although potential adverse effects must be recognized. As discussed in the previous section, oral cranberry extract and D-mannose may be useful in management of some *E. coli* infections.

4. What Should I Do about Asymptomatic (Silent) Urinary Tract Infections?

A patient may not be showing clinical signs of lower urinary tract disease even with a culture positive for bacteria. First, urine contamination must be ruled out, and bacterial numbers should be evaluated. If one or two high-growth organisms are isolated from an appropriately handled cystocentesis urine sample, significant infection is likely. Patients with silent infections usually have an uncontrolled underlying disorder. In the course of frequent, deliberate urine cultures performed as part of a monitoring plan, infection may be discovered.

Initially, standard treatment approaches for complicated infections are pursued. Frustration arises when the infections can never be cleared, and resistance may occur. These patients still do not show clinical signs, but the concern is for ascending infection or possible struvite uroliths if bacteria are urease producers. In some cases, no treatment is successful in eliminating the organism. Inhibitory antimicrobial treatment (low-dose, once-daily administration) has been recommended to prevent complications; alternatively, all antimicrobial therapy may be discontinued and, with time, resistant bacteria may be replaced with other bacteria. The urine should be reevaluated and cultured after 1 to 2 months in hopes of finding treatable infection. In other cases, treatment is withheld unless clinical signs of infection or urosepsis occur. See Chapter 194 for more information.

5. How Do I Treat Canine Urinary Incontinence Not Responsive to Standard Therapy?

Incontinence in female dogs most commonly is associated with reproductive status and can occur months to years following ovariohysterectomy. Standard initial treatment for these spayed females is administration of reproductive hormones (e.g., estriol, conjugated estrogens, or diethylstilbestrol) or sympathomimetic drugs (phenylpropanolamine, phenylephrine, or pseudoephedrine). If these two classes of drugs are not effective alone, they can be combined to try to achieve continence. Antimuscarinic drugs also can be tried in refractory cases but are effective only in the rare dog with an element of bladder overactivity (see Chapter 201).

In dogs that are not responding to pharmacologic treatment, further diagnostic tests should be carried out. Urinalysis and urine culture always should be performed to evaluate for concentration and possible infections. A polyuric-polydipsic patient may be misdiagnosed as having primary incontinence if urinary accidents are occurring at night. Standard blood work including complete blood count and serum biochemistry testing should also be performed. Imaging of the bladder via radiology and ultrasonography can reveal anatomic abnormalities that may be contributing. Contrast urethral radiography can identify intraluminal or extraluminal problems in select cases. A urethral pressure profile is useful to determine the pressures at different locations in the urethra. Urethral endoscopy also can be useful to visualize the urethral and bladder mucosa and to rule out undetected ectopic ureters. If no other underlying problem is found, then urethral bulking or surgical placement of a percutaneously adjustable hydraulic urethral occluder are viable options (see Chapter 202).

6. Are There Any New Treatments for Feline Lower Urinary Tract Disease?

Feline lower urinary tract disease (FLUTD) encompasses many differential diagnoses that show similar clinical signs. It is important to rule out these diseases before making a diagnosis of feline idiopathic cystitis (FIC). Useful diagnostics tests, including imaging, urinalysis, urine culture, and basic blood work (complete blood count, serum biochemistry studies), should be completed, with priority given to urinalysis and survey radiography. If underlying disease is not found, then a presumptive diagnosis of FIC can be made. Triggers for episodes of FIC are not always known but may include stress and neurogenic stimuli. Therefore multimodal management to prevent recurrences includes stress reduction (environmental enrichment, use of facial pheromones; see also Chapter 200) and more traditional therapies of diet (moist food), increase in water intake, and analgesics.

Chronic cases are those in which cats continue to have clinical signs without remission or have frequent recurrences even after multimodal management. These cats should be provided with appropriate pain management to break the pain cycle using short-acting analgesics such as buprenorphine, butorphanol, or meloxicam. Pharmacologic treatment with amitriptyline may reduce recurrence through reduction of stress or via other pharmacologic effects. Use of feline facial pheromones may be beneficial in these cases by decreasing stress. Treatment with the oral glycosaminoglycan pentosan polysulfate (Elmiron), given long term (months to years), may reduce clinical signs in some cats, despite a lack of strong evidence. If this treatment is successful, therapy is lifelong. Use of other glycosaminoglycan drugs in these FIC patients also is anecdotal, and future studies are necessary. Each patient is unique, and trial therapies should be used to find the best management.

7. When Should I Consider Performing a Perineal Urethrostomy on a Cat?

Blockage of the urethra with a mucous or mucocrystalline plug in a male cat can be very frustrating in terms of both initial and long-term management. When the initial blockage is hard to resolve, urethral spasm can make recovery of voiding function difficult. The irritated urethra can spasm at any location, and the spasm can involve smooth or striated musculature. Recovery is prolonged and can involve multiple urinary catheter placements to overcome these spasms and pharmacologic therapy to help decrease urethral spasms.

After resolution of the initial blockage, management with diet, increased moisture intake, and multimodal environmental management may help prevent recurrence of urethral plugs. If several recurrences occur despite appropriate management, a perineal urethrostomy (PU) may be considered to prevent further blockage and the morbidity and expense incurred. For example, the authors are more likely to recommend that a PU be performed after a cat's third blockage. In other situations, a PU may be indicated as a salvage procedure when severe urethral trauma has occurred or for alleviation of blockage caused by a urethral stricture.

PU surgery is not innocuous. With loss of the distal urethra, normal barriers are lost; bacterial infection can occur and may ascend into the kidneys. The incidence of bacterial UTIs increases with PU surgery, and infection has been reported to occur in up to 50% of patients depending on the technique employed. PU is a delicate surgery, and if it is not done correctly, urethral leakage or stricture can occur. Finally, the cat still may experience episodes of nonobstructive lower urinary tract signs if medical management is not applied and continued.

8. When Should Nephroliths Specifically Be Treated?

The best treatment plan for a nephrolith depends on the type of nephrolith, the impact of the nephrolith on the patient, and the potential morbidity of available treatment options (see also Chapters 196, 197, and 198).

Nephroliths must be differentiated from renal mineralization and can vary in size from small to staghorn.

Nephroliths may be an incidental finding on survey radiographs or may be part of the primary problem. Mineral composition may be difficult to determine without removal and analysis. However, the most likely composition can be inferred from radiographic appearance, urinalysis (pH and crystalluria), presence of infections, and serum mineral levels (calcium).

In cats the most common nephroliths are calcium oxalate. Feline calcium oxalate nephroliths are best managed medically because surgical removal can cause renal damage; however, when proximal ureteral obstruction is present, surgery may be necessary. The goal is to prevent growth of the nephrolith because dissolution is not possible. Use of lithotripsy (extracorporeal) is not indicated because the feline kidney is unlikely to tolerate the shock wave dose required for complete fragmentation and ureteral passage of stone material. Medical management of cats includes evaluation for chronic kidney disease or hypercalcemia. Mild hypercalcemia, azotemia, and calcium oxalate nephrolithiasis commonly are seen together at presentation in feline patients. If idiopathic hypercalcemia is diagnosed, then therapy to decrease serum calcium concentration includes feeding a special diet, increasing fiber consumption, and possibly administering bisphosphonates. Nephroliths in a solitary functioning kidney (big kidney—little kidney syndrome) may pose additional concern but still usually are best managed with medical strategies.

Calcium oxalate nephroliths in dogs also should lead to investigation of underlying disease such as hypercalcemia or endocrinopathy (hyperadrenocorticism), although many breeds seem predisposed to this type of nephrolith. Treatment is similar to that in cats with the exception that extracorporeal lithotripsy may be used if conditions are suitable (in terms of nephrolith size and stability of the patient's condition). Surgical removal also may be indicated when a nephrolith is associated with infection, pain, or obstruction and renal pelvic dilation.

Suspected struvite nephroliths can be treated with dissolution diets and antimicrobial therapy (if infection induced). Ureteral obstruction is a possibility because the nephrolith becomes small enough to drop into the ureter; however, this appears to occur rarely in actual practice.

9. When Should I Worry about Crystalluria in an Asymptomatic Patient?

Crystalluria may be an indication of an underlying problem or may be insignificant. *In vivo*, crystals are formed in supersaturated urine. After collection of a urine sample, crystals can form or dissolve *in vitro* with changes in temperature, pH, evaporation, or technique of preparation. These changes can alter interpretation of results; therefore examination of recently acquired urine samples is preferred to determine crystal significance. The entire urinalysis findings should be reviewed to interpret crystals in relation to pH and specific gravity. Crystalluria often is not pathologic but may indicate a potential risk of urolith formation.

Magnesium ammonium phosphate (struvite) crystalluria is found in normal dogs and cats. However, these crystals also can occur with urinary bacterial infection via urease-induced production of ammonia. Therefore the presence of these crystals in dogs or pediatric cats plus other findings of the urinalysis such as pyuria or bacteriuria should prompt automatic culture of the urine sample. The detection of crystals in the presence of infection also should elicit further investigation for urolithiasis. Adult cats with struvite crystalluria usually do not have an underlying infection. Feline interstitial cystitis sometimes presents with overwhelming struvite crystalluria; struvite crystals remain the most common mineral component of urethral plugs.

Calcium oxalate crystalluria also can be a normal finding. The presence of significant quantities of crystals should prompt investigation for underlying disease such as hypercalcemia or ethylene glycol toxicity. Only 50% of animals with urolithiasis have crystalluria. If underlying disease or uroliths are not present in cases of persistent high-load crystalluria, then medical management with diet and oral potassium citrate may be necessary to decrease the risk of urolith formation (see also Chapter 197).

Urate crystals and especially ammonium urate crystals usually are not found in normal animals but can occur. Breed-specific urate crystalluria occurs in dalmatians and English bulldogs and puts them at risk of urolithiasis. Management depends on age, crystal load, and other individual factors. In other dog breeds and in cats, the presence of these crystals suggests underlying liver disease such as portovascular anomalies (shunts) and should prompt investigation of hepatic function (see also Chapter 198).

Cystine crystalluria is uncommon and usually indicates an underlying metabolic disorder, and the presence of crystals may lead to urolithiasis. These disorders are seen most commonly in a number of canine breeds, including English bulldogs, mastiffs, dachshunds, and others. The presence of these crystals should prompt further investigation.

Although crystalluria does not predict urolith formation, heavy crystalluria in a fresh urine sample indicates an increased risk of urolithiasis. Major changes in dietary composition are not necessarily indicated; however, increased water intake and increased surveillance are warranted. Uroliths that are detected early are small and may be removed by noninvasive means, followed by more aggressive management at that point.

10. When Should I Worry about Proteinuria in an Asymptomatic Dog or Cat?

Proteinuria detected on urine dipstick testing or by a screening microalbuminuria test may be an incidental finding but should not be ignored. The presence of protein should be confirmed using sulfosalicylic acid, and the source of the protein must be investigated. However, sulfosalicylic acid testing still may yield inaccurate results. Positive results occur with hemoglobinuria and myoglobinuria since these are composed of protein. For diagnosis of a true proteinuria caused by glomerular disease, urine sediment must not contain cells or bacteria. The first step is to evaluate urine sediment microscopically and to perform a urine culture. If there is inactive urine sediment and culture results are negative, then the urine protein/creatinine ratio (UP/C) should be determined to verify and quantitate the proteinuria.

Serial UP/C measurements are recommended to verify true persistent proteinuria. UP/C ratio is considered abnormal at a value of more than 0.5 in dogs and more than 0.4 in cats; however, most healthy dogs and cats have a UP/C ratio of less than 0.2.

When postrenal proteinuria is excluded, confirmed proteinuria usually is an indication of glomerular protein loss except in some tubular disorders such as Fanconi's syndrome. Glomerular disorders can be either primary or secondary, and proteinuria should be investigated. Secondary causes of glomerular disease include antigenic reactions; therefore a search must be made for an underlying antigenic stimulus such as heartworm disease or infection. Hypertension also can damage the glomerulus, which leads to proteinuria, and therefore systemic blood pressure should be measured. Cushing's disease or oral corticosteroid therapy in dogs causes a mild to moderate proteinuria that can resolve with treatment or cessation of therapy, respectively.

If an underlying cause cannot be found, renal biopsy should be considered. Since glomerulonephritis has different histopathologic forms, examination of a biopsy specimen helps with descriptive analysis as well as determination of future therapy (see also Chapters 187 and 188).

References and Suggested Reading

Bartges JW, Kirk CA: Interpreting and managing crystalluria. In Bonagura JD, Twedt DC, editors: *Kirk's current veterinary therapy XIV*, St Louis, 2009, Saunders, p 844.

Bartges J, Polzin DJ, editors: *Nephrology and urology of small animals*, Chichester, UK, 2011, Blackwell Publishing.

Forrester SD, Roudebush P: Evidence-based management of feline lower urinary tract disease, *Vet Clin Small Anim* 37:533, 2007.

Lane IF, Westropp JI: Urinary incontinence and micturition disorders: pharmacologic management. In Bonagura JD, Twedt DC, editors: *Kirk's current veterinary therapy XIV*, St Louis, 2009, Saunders, p 955.

Lees GE et al: Assessment and management of proteinuria in dogs and cats: 2004 ACVIM forum consensus statement (small animal), *J Vet Intern Med* 19:377, 2005.

Norris CR et al: Recurrent and persistent urinary tract infections in dogs: 383 cases (1969-1995), *J Am Anim Hosp Assoc* 36:484, 2000.

Osborne CA, Finco DR, editors: *Canine and feline nephrology and urology*, Philadelphia, 1995, Williams & Wilkins, p 136.

SECTION X

Reproductive Diseases

Chapter 204:   Breeding Management of the Bitch   930
Chapter 205:   Methods for Diagnosing Diseases of
               the Female Reproductive Tract   936
Chapter 206:   Endoscopic Transcervical Insemination   940
Chapter 207:   Pregnancy Diagnosis in Companion Animals   944
Chapter 208:   Dystocia Management   948
Chapter 209:   Postpartum Disorders in Companion Animals   957
Chapter 210:   Nutrition in the Bitch and Queen
               During Pregnancy and Lactation   961
Chapter 211:   Pyometra   967
Chapter 212:   Vulvar Discharge   969
Chapter 213:   Surgical Repair of Vaginal Anomalies in the Bitch   974
Chapter 214:   Early Age Neutering in Dogs and Cats   982
Chapter 215:   Estrus Suppression in the Bitch   984
Chapter 216:   Medical Termination of Pregnancy   989
Chapter 217:   Inherited Disorders of the Reproductive
               Tract in Dogs and Cats   993
Chapter 218:   Ovarian Remnant Syndrome in Small Animals   1000
Chapter 219:   Pregnancy Loss in the Bitch and Queen   1003
Chapter 220:   Benign Prostatic Hypertrophy and Prostatitis in Dogs   1012
Chapter 221:   Methods and Availability of Tests for
               Hereditary Disorders of Dogs and Cats   1015
Chapter 222:   Reproductive Oncology   1022
Chapter 223:   Reproductive Toxicology and Teratogens   1026
Chapter 224:   Acquired Nonneoplastic Disorders of the
               Male External Genitalia   1029

The following web chapters can be found on the companion website at www.currentveterinarytherapy.com

Web Chapter 72:   Aspermia/Oligospermia Caused by Retrograde
                  Ejaculation in Dogs
Web Chapter 73:   Priapism in Dogs

CHAPTER 204

Breeding Management of the Bitch

GARY C.W. ENGLAND, *Nottingham, England*
MARCO RUSSO, *Naples, Italy*

In the bitch the most significant problem with the management of breeding is the large variation that occurs in the time between the onset of proestrous behavior and the timing of ovulation. In addition, the behavior of the bitch and underlying endocrine events are correlated poorly. Often a misunderstanding of these two aspects of reproduction results in the owners choosing the wrong time to attempt to breed their bitches. Often mating occurs at a time remote from the fertilization period, resulting in a subsequent failure to achieve a pregnancy.

The aim of this chapter is to review methods available for the identification of the optimal time for breeding, which include observational assessments, measurement of circulating hormone concentrations, examination of exfoliated vaginal cells, vaginal endoscopy, and ovarian ultrasonography.

Unlike other domestic species, which are polyestrous, a nonpregnant bitch undergoes 57 days of luteal phase after estrus followed by a 5- to 6-month period of anestrus. The monoestrous nature of the bitch and the extended time until the return to proestrus highlight the importance of determining the timing of the period of greatest fertility.

Reproductive Physiology

The basic endocrinologic events in the bitch are not unlike those of other species in that a preovulatory surge of luteinizing hormone (LH) occurs approximately 2 days before ovulation. However, at the time of ovulation, oocytes are immature and cannot be fertilized immediately. Fertilization can occur only after extrusion of the first polar body and completion of the first meiotic division to form the secondary oocyte. Oocytes remain viable within the reproductive tract for 4 to 5 days after they have become fertilizable (i.e., they do not begin to undergo degeneration until 6 to 7 days after ovulation).

When compared with other species, this relative delay in the availability of oocytes for fertilization combined with their lengthened survival time has a significant impact on the onset and duration of the fertilization period of this species.

The Fertilization Period

For all species the fertilization period is the time when oocytes are available to be fertilized. In the bitch this period commences 2 days after ovulation and extends until approximately 5 days after ovulation (Figure 204-1). The fertilization period is the time of maximal fertility, which declines rapidly over the next few days because of degeneration of the oocytes and closure of the cervix, the latter of which prevents sperm from entering the reproductive tract.

Although the fertilization period is extremely important in the bitch, it is not the only period of time during which a breeding can result in pregnancy. Intrauterine insemination after closure of the cervix has resulted in pregnancies with a small litter size (presumably because of reduced fertilization rate in aging oocytes), whereas breeding before the fertilization period can result in pregnancy as long as the sperm survive until the fertilization period in the female reproductive tract.

The Fertile Period

The fertile period is the time during which a breeding could result in a conception. Therefore it includes the fertilization period, but it also precedes the fertilization period by several days because sperm can survive within the female reproductive tract (see Figure 204-1). In some stud dogs, sperm can survive for up to 7 days within the reproductive tract of some females. In this situation, the fertile period commences 5 days before ovulation (i.e., sperm surviving for 7 days fertilize oocytes 2 days after ovulation).

However, not every stud dog produces sperm able to survive such a protracted period of time within the female reproductive tract. Dogs with poor semen quality generally have reduced sperm survival, and this accounts largely for the poor fertility seen in these individuals. Sperm that have been preserved (chilled or frozen) also have a short survival time within the female reproductive tract. Therefore the potential fertile period is a feature of male fertility combined with female physiology.

The Optimal Time for Breeding

The period of peak fertility for natural breeding with fertile animals ranges from the day of ovulation until 4 days after ovulation (Table 204-1). The period of peak fertility commences before the true fertilization period because sperm are required to mature within the female reproductive tract; this process of capacitation may take approximately 6 hours or more. Litter size does not seem to depend on which of these days that bitches are mated. Breedings earlier or later commonly result in lower pregnancy rates and smaller litters. For the accurate prediction of the optimal time to breed, either the day of the onset of LH surge or ovulation should be identified. However, identifying these events can be challenging and imprecise.

Observational Assessments

Although in other domesticated species there are reasonable relationships between the time of ovulation and several aspects of the reproductive cycle, in the bitch this is not the case. The time of ovulation in relation to the onset of proestrus and the behavioral characteristics typical of estrus have a poor relationship with the fertilization period.

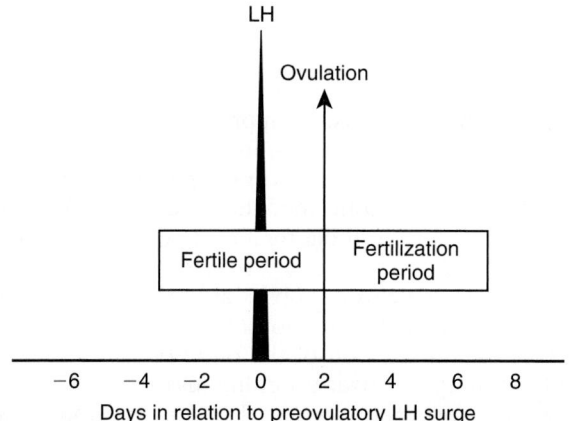

Figure 204-1 Schematic relationship among the fertilization period, fertile period, ovulation, and the luteinizing hormone surge.

The Number of Days from the Onset of Proestrus

Many breeders rely on counting the number of days from the onset of proestrus and believe that bitches ovulate a defined number of days from the onset of this event. This is not the case for all breeds (Figure 204-2). The duration of proestrus is variable among bitches (3 to 21 days). Although the "average bitch" may ovulate 12 days after the onset of proestrus, some bitches ovulate as early as day 5, and others as late as day 30 after the onset of proestrus.

The large variation in the time of ovulation (and therefore the fertilization period) explains most of the infertility that arises when bitches are bred on the twelfth and fourteenth day after the onset of proestrus, which is common breeding practice. Furthermore, the events of one estrus are not necessarily the same at the subsequent cycle; some bitches may vary in the day of ovulation by as much as 12 days from one cycle to the next (e.g., they ovulate on day 12 of one cycle and on day 24 of the next cycle).

The Onset of Estrous Behavior

In some species the onset of the behavioral signs of estrus (acceptance of mating) can be used to determine the optimal time for breeding. However, in the bitch there is often a poor correlation between endocrine events and behavioral events. Studies on laboratory-kept bitches suggest that the onset of standing estrus occurs, on average, at the same time as the onset of the LH surge (Concannon et al, 1977). Using these data, 3 or 4 days after the onset of standing estrus would be a suitable time for mating. However, as stated previously, in many other bitches the behavioral responses correlate poorly with the underlying hormonal events. This may be because bitches are housed away from the male and introduced only when the breeder considers the time to be correct, thus inhibiting natural courtship responses; or it simply may represent greater variation than was thought originally. A

TABLE **204-1**

Timing of Events in Relation to the Luteinizing Hormone Surge and Ovulation in the Bitch

Event	Days from Luteinizing Hormone Surge	Days from Ovulation
Period of potential fertility: the fertile period	3 days before LH surge until 7 days after LH surge	5 days before ovulation until 5 days after ovulation
Approximate time of oocyte maturation	4 or 5 days after LH surge	2 or 3 days after ovulation
Period of actual fertility: the fertilization period	4 or 5 days after LH surge until 7 days after LH surge	2 or 3 days after ovulation until 5 days after ovulation
Period of peak fertility	2 days after LH surge until 6 days after LH surge	The day of ovulation until 4 days after ovulation
Preferred breeding time using natural service or fresh semen insemination	2 days after LH surge until 6 days after LH surge	The day of ovulation until 4 days after ovulation
Preferred breeding time for males with poor quality semen or frozen-thawed semen insemination	5 to 6 days after LH surge	3 to 4 days after ovulation

Modified from England GCW, Concannon PW: *Determination of the optimal breeding time in the bitch: basic considerations,* accessed Sept 1, 2002, from www.ivis.org.
LH, Luteinizing hormone.

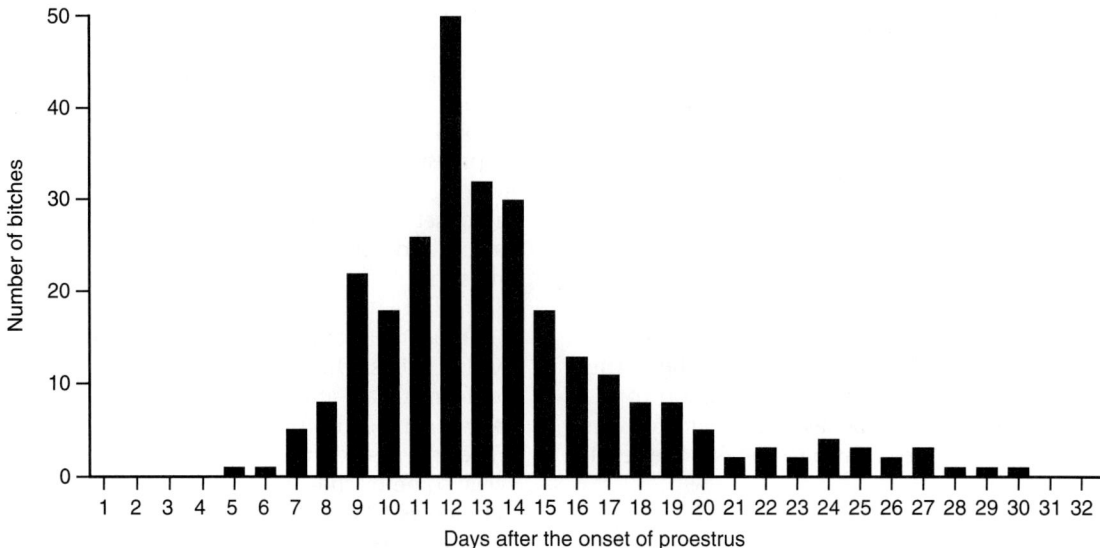

Figure 204-2 The relationship between day of ovulation and the onset of proestrus for normal fertile bitches.

further complication is that in some bitches the behavioral changes may be displayed poorly and therefore the onset of estrus may be indistinct.

It may be that, with regular examination using a standard stimulation (e.g., possibly with the use of a teaser male), the value of assessing estrous behavior could be improved. However, male dogs have been shown to demonstrate clear preferences for some females over others, thus making the interpretation of this criterion difficult to assess. When relying solely on the receptivity of the bitch, clinicians should plan breeding shortly after the onset of estrus and continue throughout the period of female receptivity.

Examination of the Caudal Reproductive Tract

Estrogen and progesterone have significant effects on the female reproductive tract. Although evaluation of changes within the uterine tubes and uterus is not possible, it is relatively simple to monitor changes of the vulva and vagina induced by fluctuations in hormonal concentration (as described below), thereby indirectly monitoring changes in these hormones.

The Onset of Vulvar Softening

One observational assessment that may be useful in establishing the optimal time for breeding is the change in the tone of the vulva that happens in most bitches. During proestrus the reproductive tract becomes edematous, and the vulva and perineal tissues become enlarged. In proestrus turgidity of the vulva increases in response to increasing concentrations of estrogen. At the time of the LH surge estrogen concentrations decline combined with a concomitant rise in progesterone. This results in a reduction in edema and a distinct softening of the vulva. Subjective examination of the vulva once or twice daily by gentle palpation easily demonstrates when this event has

occurred. Ovulation occurs approximately 2 days after softening of the vulva; therefore breeding should commence 3 days after observation of this event. However, recent work has not confirmed that changes in vulvar size or tone are valuable tools for breeding timing (Moxon et al, 2012).

In cases in which only observational assessments are available for the determination of the optimum time for breeding, a combination of the onset of standing estrus and the timing of vulvar softening may be used. Each of these events occurs on average 1 or 2 days before ovulation. Therefore, when no other tools are available for timing breeding, natural mating or fresh semen insemination breeding should be planned 2 or 3 days after vulvar softening and standing estrus has occurred. These assessments are not accurate enough for use with insemination of preserved semen, which frequently has a short life within the female reproductive tract. Not all bitches have vulvar edema occur during proestrus, and fertile breeding can occur in the absence of this symptom.

Exfoliative Vaginal Cytology

Collection, staining, and microscopic examination of exfoliated vaginal cells is a simple method for monitoring the stage of the estrous cycle, especially when examinations are performed serially. The increase in plasma estrogens during proestrus and estrus causes thickening of the vaginal wall predominantly by an increase in the number of epithelial cell layers, probably as a mechanism to protect the otherwise delicate mucosa at the time of mating. The mucosa changes from a cuboidal epithelium (in anestrus) through a transitional phase (during proestrus) into a stratified, keratinized squamous epithelium (during the fertile period). After the end of the fertilization period, as progesterone concentrations increase, there is rapid sloughing of the newly developed epithelium and an uncovering of a simple cuboidal epithelium similar to that observed during anestrus.

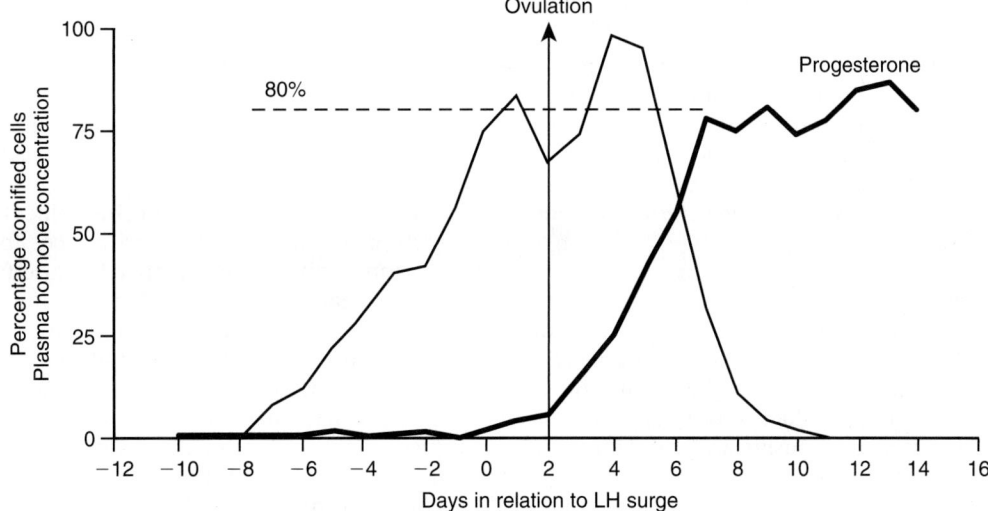

Figure 204-3 Schematic relationship among ovulation, plasma progesterone concentration, and the percentage of cornified epithelial cells.

Vaginal cells may be collected by aspiration of the vaginal cavity using a plastic catheter or by exfoliation using a saline-moistened cotton swab gently rolled over the surface of the vaginal mucosa. In the latter method, the swab must not be allowed to contact the vestibule mucosa or skin because collection of cells from these areas can give erroneous results. Swabs should be introduced and removed using a small speculum or guard.

Once collected, cells should be placed onto a glass microscope slide by lightly rolling the cotton swab or by application of the aspirated fluid, which is then spread into a thin film. Smears can be stained using either a modified Wright-Giemsa stain (e.g., Diff-Quik) or a modified trichrome stain. The former is readily available and has the advantage that sample preparation may take only minutes; the latter has the advantage of identification of cornified cells, but the staining technique is laborious.

During proestrus, as plasma estrogen concentrations increase, the surface epithelial cells alter in their shape, size, and staining character. They change from small, circular cells with little cytoplasm (parabasal cells) to larger, irregularly shaped, flat (squamous) nucleated cells (intermediate cells). Ultimately they become cornified squamous cells (superficial cells) and are characterized as having no nucleus or a faint and/or small pyknotic nuclear remnant. After the end of the fertilization period, the superficial cells disappear, and only small parabasal cells are found in the vaginal smear.

Polymorphonuclear leukocytes generally are present in small numbers in the anestrous vaginal smear but disappear from the smear during the fertile period because the thickened mucosa is a barrier to their migration to the surface. These polymorphonuclear leukocytes reappear, often in large numbers, at the end of the fertilization period as superficial epithelial cells are lost. The reappearance of these polymorphonuclear leukocytes is a result of a thinner mucosa and a chemotractant pool within the vaginal lumen.

The relative proportions of different types of epithelial cells can be used as broad markers of the endocrine environment. In general, the fertile period can be predicted approximately by calculating the percentage of epithelial cells that appear as cornified epithelial cells when using a modified Wright-Giemsa stain (Figure 204-3). Breeding should be attempted throughout the period when more than 90% of epithelial cells are cornified because in most bitches this coincides with the fertile period.

However, this varies widely among bitches, and in some cases the percentage of cornified cells reaches nearly 100% as early as 9 days before or as late as 2 days before ovulation. Conversely, in some cases, peak values of cornified cells may reach only 60% (England, 1992). Therefore changes in the vaginal cytology cannot be used accurately to time ovulation prospectively. Nevertheless, vaginal cytology permits monitoring of the normal progress of proestrus, and waiting for significant cornification allows avoidance of unnecessary testing, transportation, or breeding until the proestrous rise in estrogen is nearly complete.

As previously discussed, at the end of the fertilization period the cornified cell index of the vaginal smear declines rapidly, becoming dominated by small and medium-sized epithelial cells, cellular debris, bacteria, and polymorphonuclear leukocytes. This vaginal smear has been referred to as the onset of diestrus, and natural mating or vaginal insemination is rarely fertile when performed after this stage. In view of this, vaginal cytology is extremely valuable for demonstrating the end of the fertilization period, an event that is often unclear with use of endocrine testing.

Changes in Vaginal Fluid
Measurement of the electrical resistance of the vaginal fluid (vaginal wall) has been purported as useful for detecting the optimal time for breeding. This method is used to detect the optimal time of insemination in fox vixens. However, the authors recently used a commercial probe to measure electrical resistance daily in 48 bitches and found that only in two bitches were any useful trends

apparent. Similarly, the measurement of vaginal glucose concentration has failed to predict accurately the optimal time to breed. However, in a small number of bitches, crystallization of mucus collected from the anterior vagina has been found to develop after the peak in plasma estrogen concentration. Assessment of the mucus, which originates from cervical glandular tissue, may be useful in combination with vaginal cytology for determining the optimal mating time.

Vaginal Endoscopy
Vaginal endoscopy (vaginoscopy) is the examination of the luminal surface of the vaginal mucosa using a rigid endoscope. The principle underlying the technique is that endocrinologic changes influence the nature of the epithelium (as discussed previously) and therefore the appearance of the vaginal wall.

Vaginoscopic examination is well tolerated in most nonsedated bitches in proestrus or estrus. Examination normally is performed with the bitch standing. In most cases it can take as little as 2 minutes to make an evaluation of the stage of the cycle. The evaluation is based on assessment of the appearance of the vaginal wall (i.e., the mucosal fold contours and profiles and the color of the mucosa and of any fluid present) and the changes in this appearance at specific times of the estrous cycle.

During anestrus, the vaginal mucosa is relatively thin; therefore, when examined endoscopically, it appears flat and dry. Furthermore, it appears reddish because the submucosal vasculature is visible. At the onset of proestrus, the mucosa becomes thickened and edematous as a result of the increase in circulating estrogen concentrations. Therefore the mucosal folds appear greatly enlarged, thickened, edematous, and pink or whitish pink. Serosanguineous fluid can be observed within the lumen and may be seen to exit from the cervix. As proestrus progresses, the mucosal surface becomes progressively less pink and typically appears white because the thickened mucosa prevents the underlying capillaries that were visible during anestrus from being seen. In late proestrus or early estrus at approximately the same time as the LH surge, the folds shrink progressively, which is accompanied by further pallor. These effects are the result of an abrupt withdrawal of estrogen. Estrogen concentrations decline rapidly during and after the LH surge. Subsequently over the next several days, mucosal shrinkage is accompanied by gross wrinkling of the mucosal folds that now become angulated distinctly and are off-white to white.

The onset of the fertile period can be detected by observing the onset of mucosal shrinkage without excessive angulations, whereas gross shrinkage of entire mucosal folds with obvious angulation is characteristic of the fertilization period. Breeding is planned best approximately 4 days after the first detected mucosal shrinkage or at the onset of the period of obvious angulation of mucosal folds. The end of the fertilization period can be detected by observing sloughing of the vaginal epithelium (see section on Exfoliative Vaginal Cytology) and development of a variegated appearance to the color of the mucosal surface.

Observation of Follicular Dynamics Using Ultrasound

The ovaries of a bitch can be identified using real-time diagnostic B-mode ultrasound. Some bitches have a significant amount of fat within the ovarian bursa, which makes imaging difficult. However, with careful and repeated examination, monitoring follicular growth and detecting the time of ovulation are possible. In general, ovulation is difficult to identify because follicles do not collapse, changes in echogenicity are not always consistent, and new corpora lutea also have central fluid-filled cavities similar to those of the follicles.

Follicles appear as anechoic (black) structures that increase in size throughout proestrus and estrus to reach approximately 8 mm in diameter just before ovulation. Although difficult, it is possible to determine the time of ovulation using ultrasound. Usually the number of large anechoic follicles apparently decreases or they disappear completely because of an increase in echogenicity and/or a related apparent decrease in follicle size. The absence of anechoic structures may be detected best by repeated examination, during which it can persist for 1 to 2 days commencing approximately at the time of ovulation. It often is followed by the reappearance of anechoic structures in the ovaries, representing the early developing corpora lutea. Corpora lutea generally have thicker walls than preovulatory follicles and also contain central fluid. Cavitated corpora lutea are visible for several days to 2 weeks after ovulation. In clinical practice, using ovarian ultrasound to determine the fertilization period has little clinical application at the present time because of the difficulties in imaging the ovaries and the requirement for frequent examination.

Measurement of Plasma or Serum Hormone Concentrations

LH concentration surges significantly approximately 2 days before ovulation in the bitch; therefore detection of this event could be used to predict ovulation. In addition, another preovulatory event (follicular luteinization) cannot be dissociated temporally from the LH surge (Figure 204-4). This preovulatory luteinization results in a significant increase in circulating (plasma or serum) progesterone concentrations before ovulation, which can be detected by conventional assay methods.

Measurement of Plasma or Serum Luteinizing Hormone Concentration
The detection of a significant increase in plasma LH concentration is a reliable and accurate method for determining the time of ovulation and therefore the optimal time to breed. Most countries do not have a readily available commercial assay for canine LH, and measurement relies on radioimmunoassay techniques. As a result, this method is not used frequently outside of the United States because radioimmunoassays are expensive; furthermore, they result in a delay in obtaining the results because samples are assayed in batches. Another potential problem is the requirement to take regular (daily) blood samples because the duration of the LH surge is relatively short. However,

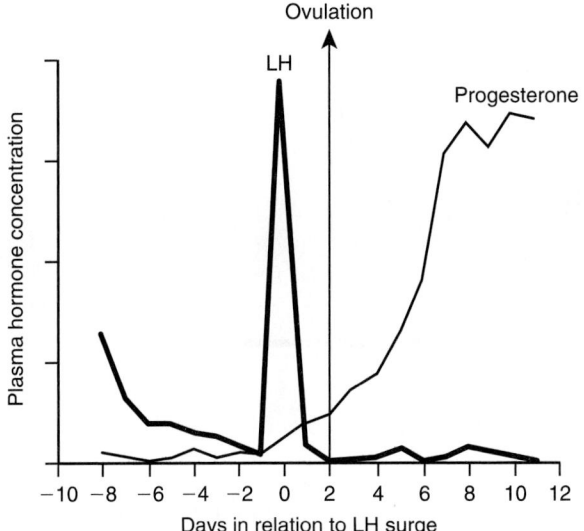

Figure 204-4 Schematic relationship among ovulation, the luteinizing hormone surge, and plasma progesterone concentration.

recently a quantitative enzyme-linked immunosorbent assay (ELISA) has been on the market for the measurement of canine LH. The method is simple and rapid and has been used successfully in the laboratory, although it has not been subjected to wide investigation. When these methods are used to detect the LH surge, breeding should commence 4 or 5 days after the surge has been identified because this coincides with the onset of the fertilization period.

Measurement of Plasma or Serum Progesterone Concentration

Luteinization of the follicle wall before ovulation results in circulating progesterone concentrations to increase rapidly from baseline approximately 2 days before ovulation at the same time as the onset of the LH surge. In fact, these two events (the rise in progesterone concentration and the onset of the LH surge) cannot be dissociated temporally. This distinct increase in circulating progesterone concentrations can be detected by serial monitoring. Progesterone concentrations continue to rise consistent with the occurrence of ovulation and then continue to rise throughout the first one third of diestrus. Because the initial rise in progesterone is progressive, collecting blood samples only every second or third day is necessary, unlike the daily sampling requirement when measuring LH concentrations. However, when the sampling interval is increased, the accuracy of determination of the day of the LH surge is decreased. Therefore, when semen is poor quality, it often is prudent to perform daily estimations close to the anticipated time of the LH surge.

Progesterone concentrations may be measured by radioimmunoassay, quantitative or qualitative ELISA, or immunochemiluminescence assay. Many veterinary and human diagnostic laboratories offer measurement of progesterone with reporting of results the same day. Several qualitative (or semi-quantitative) progesterone ELISA test kits have become available commercially for use in the veterinary practice. Results usually are available within 45 to 60 minutes of sample collection. The choice of assay method used is specific to each veterinary practice and is a balance of accuracy, speed of results, and the number of samples submitted (and therefore cost).

In general it is considered that progesterone concentrations are between 1.5 to 2.5 ng/ml (4.9 to 8.1 nmol/L) on the day of the LH surge; therefore breeding can be planned in relation to this event (i.e., 4 to 6 days later). Some reports suggest that breeding should commence 1 day after progesterone concentrations exceed 8 to 10 ng/ml (25 to 32 nmol/L), which typically are seen at the beginning of the fertilization period. Few data link absolute progesterone concentrations with the timing of the end of the fertilization period; this is detected best using vaginal cytology (see previous section).

References and Suggested Reading

Concannon P, Hansel W, Mcentee K: Changes in LH, progesterone and sexual behavior associated with preovulatory luteinization in the bitch, *Biol Reprod* 17:604, 1977.

England GCW: Vaginal cytology and cervicovaginal mucus arborisation in the breeding management of bitches, *J Small Anim Pract* 33:577, 1992.

England GCW, Allen WE: Crystallization patterns in anterior vaginal fluid from bitches in oestrus, *J Reprod Fertil* 86:335, 1989.

England GCW, Concannon PW: *Determination of the optimal breeding time in the bitch: basic considerations*, accessed Sept 1, 2002, from www.ivis.org.

England GCW, Yeager AE: Ultrasonographic appearance of the ovary and uterus of the bitch during oestrus, ovulation and early pregnancy, *J Reprod Fertil Suppl* 47:107, 1993.

Goodman M: Ovulation timing: concepts and controversies, *Vet Clin North Am Small Anim Pract* 31:219, 2001.

Hiemstra M et al: The reliability of vaginal cytology in determining the optimal mating time in the bitch, *Tijdschr Diergeneeskd* 126:685, 2001.

Jeffcoate IA, England GCW: Urinary LH, plasma LH and progesterone and their clinical correlates in the periovulatory period of domestic bitches, *J Reprod Fertil Suppl* 51:267, 1997.

Jeffcoate IA, Lindsay FEF: Ovulation detection and timing of insemination based on hormone concentrations, vaginal cytology and the endoscopic appearance of the vagina of domestic bitches, *J Reprod Fertil Suppl* 39:277, 1989.

Moxon R, Copley D, England GCW: Technical and financial evaluation of assays for progesterone in canine practice in the UK, *Vet Rec* 167:528, 2010.

Moxon R et al: Periovulatory changes in the endoscopic appearance of the reproductive tract and teasing behavior in the bitch, *Theriogenol* 78:1907, 2012.

van Klaveren NJ et al: The optimal mating time in the bitch based on the progesterone concentration in peripheral blood: a comparison of reliability between three ELISA test kits and a 125-iodine radioimmunoassay, *Tijdschr Diergeneeskd* 126:680, 2001.

CHAPTER 205

Methods for Diagnosing Diseases of the Female Reproductive Tract

HERNÁN J. MONTILLA, *Corvallis, Oregon*

Vaginoscopy

Clinical Uses

In the bitch, vaginoscopy is a valuable tool to evaluate reproductive anomalies and presence and severity of trauma, to determine the source of vulvar discharge, and to detect reproductive related causes of urinary incontinence and recurrent urinary tract infection (Lulich, 2006). In the normal estrous bitch, vaginoscopy can be used to stage the cycle when timing artificial insemination along with vaginal cytology and endocrine testing. During proestrus, the vaginal mucosal folds are edematous, moist, and pink. During estrus, the vaginal folds appear wavy with an almost serrated appearance (crenulated).

Technique

Preparation

Vaginoscopy can be performed with a vaginal speculum, otoscope, or pediatric proctoscope, but the lack of distention of the vaginal lumen can limit access to the cranial vagina. Endoscopic vaginoscopy can provide for better evaluation of the cranial vagina and cervix. This can be performed with a flexible or rigid endoscope or a cystoscope.

During the estrus phase most bitches allow for evaluation without sedation. In the anestrus animal or evaluation for a pathologic process, it is beneficial to use sedation or general anesthesia and perform the exam with the animal in dorsal recumbency.

Perivulvar hair should be clipped and the tail wrapped in long-haired dogs. The perivulvar region and perineum should be cleaned thoroughly with povidone-iodine or mild soap and water to minimize contamination. A lubricating agent is applied on the sides of the endoscope to pass it through the vulvar folds and into the vestibule with caution not to apply lubricant to the tip of the scope, which would obstruct the view.

Procedure

Initially the scope is passed with the tip acutely angled toward the spine of the dog to avoid the clitoris and clitoral fossa. Once inside, the vestibule can be distended with air or sterile, warm, isotonic fluid through a port on the scope. To prevent loss of fluid during vaginal distention, the thumb and first finger are used to lightly occlude the vulvar commissure around the tip of the scope. Room air can be used to insufflate the vaginal vault and vestibule. A vaginal cannula with an inflatable cuff could aid greatly in maintaining distention of the vaginal walls. A complete seal is not necessary and difficult to maintain; therefore a steady stream of fluid or air helps to maintain distention of the vaginal lumen. Insufflation with air is the best choice for sample collection for cytology or cultures, whereas distention with fluids could be useful to evaluate for structural and anatomic integrity of the different structures.

The vestibule should be examined when the scope is just past the vulvar commissure. Common lesions that may be found in the vestibule are anatomic and congenital anomalies, areas of hyperemia, lacerations, presence of discharge or blood, and foreign bodies. However, other than foreign material and mucosal pathologies, pathologies rarely are found in the vestibule. In some cases of urinary incontinence a vaginal termination of ectopic ureter can be identified. Next the vestibulovaginal junction and urethral os should be identified. This junction should be smooth and continuous with a symmetric opening. Asymmetry can be an indication of pathology. The vestibulovaginal opening should be dorsal to and wider than the urethral opening. A smaller or narrower vestibulovaginal opening should be considered a stricture. If the junction is divided into two or more openings, a diagnosis of vaginal septa or vaginal duplication may be made.

After the vestibule is evaluated, the scope is passed through the vestibulovaginal junction into the vagina. If discharge is present, the clinician should try to identify its origin. The wall of the vagina should be examined thoroughly for lesions and pathologies by rotating or changing the angle of the scope. The same technique should be used to evaluate the cranial vagina and the external cervical os. Care must be taken not to touch the vaginal fornix in the awake animal because this can be a sensitive area and pressure often results in discomfort.

Samples or biopsy may be obtained by several methods if any pathology is identified. A long 22- or 25-gauge needle can be passed through the biopsy channel of the scope to obtain fine-needle aspirates. Small biopsy forceps can be directed through the biopsy channel as well to collect a larger sample (Gunzel-Apel et al, 2001).

Vaginal Cytology

Clinical Uses

Vaginal cytology is a simple, quick, and economical tool commonly used to monitor hormonal influence on the canine vaginal epithelium. Vaginal cytology is most valuable as an estrogen bioassay in the bitch and queen. Vaginal cytology also can be used to identify an inflammatory pathology in the female reproductive tract (e.g., vaginitis, pyometra).

During the stages of anestrus, proestrus, and diestrus, the predominant cell type found on vaginal cytology is the round parabasal cell. Red blood cells, neutrophils, and bacteria also may be seen in low numbers. As proestrus progresses, the follicles produce more estradiol. In response to increased estradiol concentrations, there is hyperplasia of the vaginal epithelium. As the thickness of the vaginal epithelium increases, superficial cells move farther away from the blood supply of the basement membrane. These cells become nonviable anuclear cells. The highest number of these cornified superficial epithelial cells is found during estrus. A vaginal cytology sample taken during estrus should contain more than 80% cornified superficial epithelial cells. Red blood cells can be found in low numbers and neutrophils should not be present. At the onset of diestrus (6 to 7 days after ovulation in the bitch), vaginal cytology changes quickly from full cornification to 40% to 60% parabasal and intermediate cells. At this time neutrophils, parabasal cells with a neutrophils in the cytoplasm (metestrum cells), and parabasal cells with vacuoles in the cytoplasm (foam cells) may be seen.

Technique

The technique for obtaining vaginal cytology specimens is simple. The clinician's fingers can be used to open the vulvar folds, applying gentle traction caudally with the index and middle finger at the cranial aspect of the base of the vulva while applying gentle caudal ventral traction with the thumb at the ventral commissure of the vulva. A long cotton-tipped applicator (premoistened with saline to prevent friction) can be introduced through the vulva and vestibule into the vagina. When introducing the swab, the clinician should avoid picking up keratinized cells from the clitoral fossa on the ventral surface because these can be confused with superficial vaginal epithelial cells. The swab is passed dorsally and cranially to avoid the urethral papilla located ventrally caudal to the vestibule-vaginal junction. After the ischial arch is reached, the swab should be leveled and advanced cranially. The swab is rotated within the vagina a few times and then withdrawn. The swab is rolled onto a microscope slide in two to three nonoverlapping rows. After the smear is prepared, the slide is air dried and stained with a modified Wright-Giemsa stain (Diff-Quik). The stained slides should be evaluated at 40× magnification under the microscope.

Vaginal Culture

Clinical Uses

Vaginal cultures may help identify an overgrowth of a specific pathogen in the female reproductive tract. The vagina is not a sterile environment and cultured samples from healthy animals usually contain gram-positive and gram-negative bacteria, including but not limited to *E. coli*, *Staphylococcus* spp., *Streptococcus* spp., *Proteus* spp., *Pseudomonas* spp., *Mycoplasma* spp., and *Ureaplasma* spp. A positive vaginal culture does not always indicate vaginal or uterine infection. However, a pure culture (e.g., single organism) instead of a mixed culture may have more significance.

Technique

The technique for obtaining a vaginal culture is similar to obtaining vaginal cytology specimens. It is important to have the most adequate transport media for the suspected pathogen (e.g., Amies media for *Mycoplasma* spp. culture). Communication with the diagnostic lab for any specifics or particulars pertaining sample management, preparation, and shipment is beneficial. Often multiple types of transport media must be inoculated from the same sample collection. If cytology is to be performed also, a separate sample may be desired.

Transcervical Hysteroscopy

Clinical Uses

Hysteroscopy can be a sensitive tool for assessment of canine endometrial health along with endometrial cytology and culture. Endometrial lesions and cysts often can be diagnosed with this technique. In the postpartum bitch, a small endoscope may be passed directly through the cervix to visualize the endometrial surface. Dark-brown sites of implantation can be observed in the normal postpartum endometrium.

Technique

A 3- to 4-mm diameter laparoscope at least 10 to 20 cm in length, straight or with 30-degree view angle, and a port for insufflation can be used (Gerber and Nöthling, 2001). Introduction of the scope into the vagina uses the same technique described for vaginoscopy. Once the external cervical os is reached, the end of the scope can be used to stabilize the tissues so that the scope can be advanced through the cervix. In some cases, passing a catheter through the external cervical os before the scope may help to identify the best angle to proceed. When access through the cervix is not achieved readily, then the uterus can be exposed by means of a laparotomy. A small hysterotomy port or biopsy hole can be used for access to the uterine lumen with the endoscope. Insufflation can be achieved by passing air directly through a port on the scope, a blunt needle, or a catheter placed into the uterine lumen. The endometrial surface and uterotubal junctions should be visible and evaluated in all bitches. In some cases, uterine discharge and air escape through the cervix, reducing visibility. The cervix and caudal uterine body may not always be visualized in every patient.

Complications

Some complications reported from transcervical hysteroscopy include vaginal inflammation, vaginal tearing, and endometritis (Gerber and Nöthling, 2001). These side effects have a higher potential of occurring when instruments are forced and when samples are taken during anestrus (Root Kustritz, 2006).

Transcervical Uterine Cytology and Culture

Clinical Uses

Indications for collecting samples for uterine cytology and culture include a history of reproductive tract infection or infertility. The presence of pathologic discharge from the uterus identified on vaginoscopy warrants uterine cytology and culture. Different techniques have been described to collect samples adequate for endometrial cytology and bacterial cultures. Some of these techniques are less invasive but only possible in dogs (e.g., transcervically), and some are more invasive (e.g., via hysterotomy for endometrial biopsies or full-thickness uterine biopsies). Collection of adequate cell and tissue samples by laparotomy with or without hysterotomy have an increased potential for negative side effects because of inherited risks of anesthesia and surgery. Transcervical sample collection is less traumatic and successful for obtaining adequate samples for cytology and culture of endometrial surfaces.

Technique

For transcervical sample collection, the bitch can be sedated if necessary. The endoscope is passed as described for vaginoscopy. Once into the vagina, the scope is passed to the level of the external cervical os. Using the end of the endoscope to stabilize the external cervical os, a 4- to 7-Fr catheter can be passed through the biopsy port of the scope. To pass the catheter through the cervix, the catheter is rotated gently while advancing it. Once in the desired location, a small volume of sterile saline (several milliliters) is infused and aspirated (Watts, Wright, and Whithear, 1996).

Normal endometrial epithelial cells collected from this method have a degenerated appearance during late diestrus throughout anestrus. Bacteria normally can be found present during proestrus and estrus but should not be found during the other stages of the estrous cycle in normal bitches. Neutrophils are a common finding during proestrus, estrus, and diestrus, whereas lymphocytes and macrophages are more common during anestrus (Root Kustritz, 2006).

Uterine cytology specimens can be used for cultures as long as they are isolated and packaged for transport with minimal contamination or new samples should be collected. Growth of bacteria from specimens collected during proestrus and estrus is not uncommon because these can represent normal vaginal flora (Root Kustritz, 2006; Schultheiss et al, 1999; Watts et al, 1997; Watts, Wright, and Lee, 1998; Watts, Wright, and Whithear, 1996) that has ascended into the uterus during this stage of the estrous cycle. Growth of bacteria during other stages of the cycle is consistent with infection or contamination. Anaerobic bacteria and *Mycoplasma* spp. should not be grown from uterine cultures, even though *Mycoplasma* spp. have been isolated from the reproductive tract of normal bitches without any signs or evidence of pathology (Watts et al, 1996).

Radiography

Two radiographic techniques may aid in diagnosing reproductive pathologies in the reproductive tract: conventional (plain) radiography and radiography with positive or negative contrast. Positive contrast uses iodine or barium compounds, whereas negative contrast involves the use of air to delineate a cavity. Certain congenital anomalies require the use of these contrast techniques to identify them using radiography.

Conventional Radiography

Conventional radiography can be useful for diagnosing normal events during pregnancy in cats and dogs. The uterus usually is not seen until its diameter exceeds that of the small bowel. Applying gentle pressure at the level of the caudal abdomen with a paddle or spoon made of radiolucent material can help push the intestines cranially and improve visualization of the uterus, enhancing the appearance of its serosal margins. An enlarged uterus often can be seen by 35 days of gestation. Individual fetal swellings are difficult to identify. The pregnant uterus has no pathognomonic appearance at this stage of gestation and as a result, pyometra, mucometra, or pregnancy cannot be differentiated with radiography (see Figure 207-2). By 45 days of gestation, fetal bones begin to ossify. A fetal count can be determined by counting fetal skulls and spines. Fetal oversize also may be estimated. Fetal viability can be assessed roughly by evaluating the integrity of the fetal skeletons. If no information of litter size is available, it is sometimes beneficial to perform radiographs postpartum to confirm that no fetuses remain in the uterus after parturition apparently has been completed.

Conventional radiography also can be useful for diagnosing reproductive pathology. Normal ovaries should not be visible on abdominal radiographs. Ovaries visible by radiography suggest the presence of an ovarian mass, either cystic or neoplastic.

After ovariohysterectomy, a granuloma may develop in the uterine stump or at the site of ligation of an ovarian vessel when nonabsorbable ligature material is used. Granulomas may be seen as mass lesions on conventional radiographs. These granulomatous lesions involving the uterine stump also may involve the bladder or ureters, causing clinical signs similar to those of urinary tract infections.

Contrast Radiography

Retrograde vaginourethrography is a useful method for diagnosing pathologies such as ectopic ureters, vaginal masses, and strictures. In some cases, air may be adequate contrast. Urethrorectal and urethrovaginal fistulae have been described (Ralphs and Kramek, 2003) but are not encountered commonly. Positive contrast retrograde urethrography offers the best means of outlining these fistulae along with ruptures, stenosis, and neoplasia of the vagina.

With the patient under general anesthesia, a cuffed catheter (e.g., Foley catheter) or a standard catheter (e.g., polypropylene tom cat catheter, red rubber catheter, or large intravenous catheter) is inserted into the vestibule. Depending on the patient's size, a regular intravenous catheter may be needed. The catheter is inserted between the lips of the vulva and held in place by gently clamping the vulvar lips together. The cuff is inflated, and sufficient contrast medium is injected to distend the vagina. Iodinated contrast medium (1 ml/kg) is injected carefully to prevent vaginal trauma from overinflation. Lateral, ventrodorsal, and oblique radiographic views are obtained.

Ultrasonography

Clinical Uses

Ultrasonographic evaluation of the female reproductive tract can yield valuable information in regard to uterine and ovarian health as well as the events during pregnancy. Ultrasonographic examination is a sensitive test for detecting intrauterine fluid or exudate. However, ultrasonographic diagnosis of cystic endometrial hyperplasia (CEH) in bitches is not always possible because the variable degree of the lesions ranging from moderate to not identifiable. When found, CEH appears as many variable-size cysts in the uterus, irregular surface of the endometrium, hypertrophic or atrophic endometrium, with or without hyperechoic uterine content. Ultrasonography also can be used to examine ovaries for pathologic changes (e.g., cysts, neoplasia).

An estimation of gestational age can be made using ultrasonography (see Tables 207-1 and 207-2). Several fetal measurements are used to estimate gestational age (Kutzler et al, 2003). Crown-rump length (CRL) is the measurement from the most rostral point of the crown to the base of the tail. Body diameter (BD) is determined by taking the mean of two transverse measurements made at 90-degree angles at the level of the fetal liver and stomach. Biparietal diameter (BPD) can be measured after day 30 of gestation.

Technique

A wide range of ultrasonographic units are capable of providing two-dimensional, grayscale (B-mode), real-time ultrasound images of the reproductive tract in dogs and cats. A linear or curved-linear transducer with frequencies ranging from 5 to 12 MHz should be used. Ultrasonographic studies can be performed on individuals in dorsal recumbency with or without sedation, depending on the patient's demeanor and level of cooperation. A 35% to 45% alcohol solution or transmission gel is used as a coupling agent applied copiously to the ventral abdomen. In some cases it may be necessary to trim or shave the abdominal hair to improve contact between the face of the probe and the skin. The uterus may be located by starting the study with the transducer at the cranial edge of the pubic bone and scanning transversely between the urinary bladder and the colon. The uterus should appear as a continuous hypoechoic structure between a hyperechoic, crescent-shaped colon and an anechoic urinary bladder, or just at either side from this location. The uterus and cervix can be located best when under the influence of estradiol or progesterone. The cervix should be located just cranial to the trigone of the bladder. Uterine horns can be difficult to visualize unless enlarged from pregnancy, hormonal influence, or pathology. To visualize ovaries, the clinician should scan caudally and slightly lateral to the caudal poles of either kidney. Experience and training level of the operator along with the use of high-definition equipment can improve on the sensitivity and the diagnostic results allowing for the development of an adequate treatment plan.

References and Suggested Reading

Gerber D, Nöthling J: Hysteroscopy in bitches, *J Reprod Fertil* 57(suppl):415, 2001.

Gunzel-Apel A et al: Development of a technique for transcervical collection of uterine tissue in bitches, *J Reprod Fertil* 57 (suppl):61, 2001.

Kutzler M et al: Accuracy of canine parturition date prediction using fetal measurements obtained by ultrasonography, *Theriogenology* 60:1309, 2003.

Lulich J: Endoscopic vaginoscopy in the dog, *Theriogenology* 66: 588, 2006.

Ralphs S, Kramek B: Novel perineal approach for repair of a urethrorectal fistula in a bulldog, *Can Vet J* 44(10):822, 2003.

Root Kustritz M: Collection of tissue and culture samples from the canine reproductive tract, *Theriogenology* 66:567, 2006.

Schultheiss P et al: Normal bacterial flora in canine and feline uteri, *J Vet Diag Invest* 11:560, 1999.

Watts J et al: New techniques using transcervical uterine cannulation for the diagnosis of uterine disorders in bitches, *J Reprod Fertil* 51:283, 1997.

Watts J, Wright P, Lee C: Endometrial cytology of the normal bitch throughout the reproductive cycle, *J Small Anim Pract* 39:2, 1998.

Watts JR, Wright PJ, Whithear KC: Uterine, cervical and vaginal microflora of the normal bitch throughout the reproductive cycle, *J Small Anim Pract* 37:54, 1996.

CHAPTER 206

Endoscopic Transcervical Insemination

MARION S. WILSON, *Levin, New Zealand*
FIONA K. HOLLINSHEAD, *Matamata, New Zealand*

In many species frozen-thawed semen must be deposited into the uterus rather than the vagina to achieve good pregnancy rates and litter size. The options available to achieve intrauterine semen deposition are surgical or transcervical insemination (TCI). Many veterinarians choose to deposit semen surgically into the uterus of the bitch because the surgery is easy to perform. However, surgery is an invasive insemination technique and has risks associated with general anesthesia and surgery, which restrict the veterinarian to a single insemination. In a number of European countries the surgical insemination procedure is not permitted because it is considered ethically unacceptable. Furthermore, many owners and veterinarians prefer a noninvasive, nonsurgical option.

Dr. Marion Wilson developed the noninvasive TCI technique using a rigid endoscope specifically to deposit frozen-thawed semen into the uterus of the bitch (Wilson, 2001). Research of this technique resulted in identification of several features relating to the anatomy of the canine reproductive tract. These points are relevant to endoscopic TCI and are considered first, followed by a description of relevant procedures for TCI.

Anatomy

The cranial vagina (paracervix) is dominated by the dorsal median fold (DMF), which significantly reduces the vaginal lumen in the approach to the cervix. The restricted vaginal lumen limits the diameter of equipment that can be passed through the area. This feature, together with a particularly long vagina in the bitch, limits the number of endoscopes suitable for the technique. The DMF ends cranially at the vaginal portion of the cervix, which exists as a distinct tubercle (cervical tubercle). The paracervix is limited cranially by the fornix, which is a slitlike space cranioventral to the cervical tubercle. It appears as a blind end when viewed through the endoscope and is another important landmark. The cervix lies diagonally across the uterovaginal junction with the canal of the cervix directed craniodorsally from the vagina to the uterus. Consequently the external os is located ventrally in the cervical tubercle.

Equipment

The endoscope initially identified as meeting the criteria with regard to length and diameter was a rigid, extended length cystourethroscope (Table 206-1). An 8 Fr urinary catheter is used for insemination in the majority of bitches using this endoscope, although a 6 Fr gauge sometimes is required in small or maiden bitches. More recently, a longer (43 cm) and thinner (graduated 9.5 Fr to 13.5 Fr) rigid renourethroscope has been developed for the TCI procedure in bitches. A specially designed 70 cm × 5 Fr catheter (Minitube) with removable stylet is used for insemination of most bitches. Occasionally a 4 Fr catheter is required in small or toy breeds that can have a smaller os and cervical canal.

The longer, thinner endoscope has a number of advantages. First, the significantly narrower shaft greatly facilitates passage under the DMF, which is often a tight and narrow space. This feature is particularly beneficial in maiden bitches and certain individual bitches that can have a narrow vaginal canal. The longer endoscope has eliminated any limitations previously associated with insemination of large and giant breed bitches. However, despite the increased length of the new endoscope, it still can be used with relative ease in toy breeds. Finally, the renourethroscope is technically easier to use in regard to manipulation and catheterization of the os cervix compared with the cystourethroscope.

Furthermore, a "TCI Shunt System" (Minitube) has recently been developed to be used in combination with the renourethroscope for intrauterine insemination of bitches. This device consists of a shunt made of metal and a Foley catheter 55 mm or 105 mm in length. The shunt has multiple functions. Firstly the Foley component creates a tight seal in the vagina, thus eliminating air loss from the vaginal space during air insufflation. This allows the TCI endoscope to pass easily through the caudal vagina and under the dorsal median fold to the cervix. The shunt enhances stabilization of the TCI endoscope and fixation and catheterization of the cervical os. The Foley component also causes stretching of the vaginal wall, stimulating release of local oxytocin and resultant vaginal and uterine contractions, which facilitate sperm transport to the site of fertilization.

A specially designed platform is used to restrain the bitch in the standing position. The platform provides a tie point to the dog's collar and an abdominal support to restrict sideways movement and discourage any attempt to sit (Figure 206-1). A hydraulic chair together with a hydraulic table for the platform ensures the optimum position of the bitch relative to the operator during the

TABLE **206-1**			
Equipment for Transcervical Insemination			
Manufacturer	Catalog Number	Equipment	Specifications
Minitube	23700/1510	Renourethroscope	Length: 43 cm Diameter: 9.5 to 13.5 Fr instrument shaft with 8 Fr distal tip, no sheath Comments: Up to 5 Fr central channel, angled eyepiece with 6-degree telescope
ENDOWORLD	96182028E	Cystourethroscope (extended length)	Length: 29 cm Diameter: 3.5 mm, with sheath Comments: Straight eyepiece with 30-degree telescope
Minitube	17500	Insemination catheter	Length: 70 cm Diameter: 4 to 8 Fr Comments: Single or dual ports available

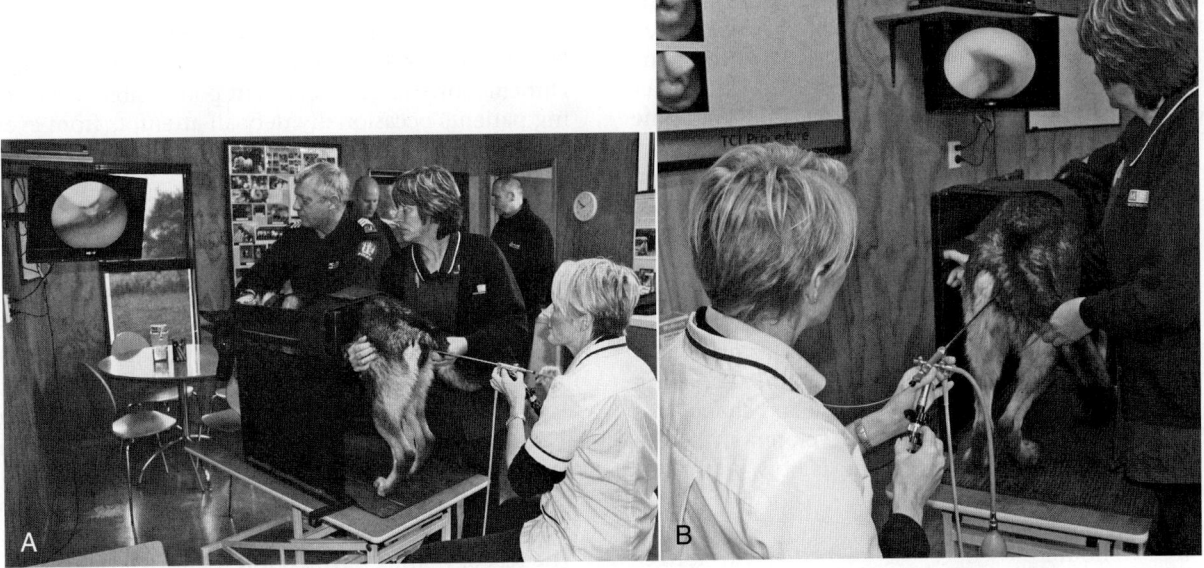

Figure 206-1 Table with abdominal support recommended for performing transcervical insemination (TCI) viewed from the side **(A)** and from behind **(B).** (Photos courtesy Dr. Marion Wilson and Fiona Hollinshead.)

procedure. This is important particularly when the endoscope is used without a camera. Bitches in estrus exhibiting standing behavior show excellent tolerance to the technique and sedation is rarely necessary.

Technique

The endoscope is introduced through the vulva and into the vestibule, taking care to avoid the clitoris and urethral orifice. It is advanced through the vaginal folds by observing the direction of the vaginal lumen. Air insufflation allows greater visualization of the vaginal lumen so that it can be "followed" easily to the cervix. Air insufflation is especially necessary for the renourethroscope because it does not have a sheath. In proestrus and early estrus, the rounded vaginal folds can make advancing the endoscope towards the cervix more difficult because the folds tend to fill the lumen. As estrus progresses, dehydration

and crenulation of the folds result in a less obstructive lumen. The DMF and crescentlike lumen of the cranial vagina represent important landmarks in locating the cervical os. At this point, the vaginal lumen can be narrow in some bitches, requiring manipulation of the endoscope to the widest space. This may result in the endoscope being pushed to one side of the DMF rather than continuing ventrally under the DMF. The ventral location of the cervical os means that it is not immediately obvious and the scope has to be directed under the cervical tubercle until the os, located in the center of a rosette of furrows, can be identified. The catheter is advanced into the cervical os by manipulation of the endoscope and catheter. The rigidity of the endoscope is used to move the cervical tubercle, line up the os, and change the angle of the canal.

Once the tip of the catheter is introduced into the cervical os, it is advanced steadily using a clockwise twisting motion to aid its passage through the cervical canal. The catheter should be passed through the cervix as far as it will go without force. Use of 5-cm marked graduations on the catheter is helpful in determining how far the catheter has advanced. The semen is inseminated slowly under continual observation to ensure that no significant backflow of semen into the vagina occurs. If this happens the catheter should be relocated, either further in or back slightly, and insemination started again.

Practical Considerations

The cost of the TCI equipment is a major consideration for general veterinary practice. Veterinarians must understand what they can expect from the technology, how easy the techniques are to learn, and what problems and results they can expect. Theoretically the technique is simple but takes time, patience, and mostly practice to perfect. The attachment of a video camera to the endoscope allows for direct training by an experienced operator. However, the skill can be learned without the assistance of others. Most operators find that the challenge of catheterizing the cervical os can be overcome confidently in a relatively short time. However, mastering the peculiarities of all breeds and sizes takes much longer.

Limiting Factors and Problems

For the technique to be adopted widely, it is essential that it can be applied successfully to all, or at least most, bitches. It is also important that the majority of bitches can be inseminated using the same endoscope. Looking at the vast array of breeds of various size and shape, this would seem unlikely, but with the development of the longer, thinner renourethroscope, this is now possible.

Vaginal Length

With the renourethroscope, the cervix is no longer beyond the reach of the equipment in large-breed bitches. Therefore vaginal length is no longer a limiting factor.

Paracervix Diameter

The amount of space available in the paracervix was a limiting factor initially identified when the technique was developed. In a small percentage of small or medium-size maiden bitches and some toy breeds (e.g., Chihuahua), the diameter of the paracervix was too narrow to advance the endoscope through this area. However, with the narrower and sheathless renourethroscope, this limitation mostly has been eliminated.

Cervical Os Identification

Theoretically, once the endoscope has passed through the paracervix, it should be possible to catheterize the cervix of all bitches. The ability to identify the cervical os comes from experience (i.e., appreciating what it looks like, where it is usually located, and how to search for it when it is not obvious). Some bitches have vaginal folds that can be mistaken for the cervical os, but in these instances, there is no opening for the catheter to pass through. Uterine fluid associated with estrus passing through the

cervix can facilitate the identification of the correct location.

Cervical Cannulation

Ensuring that the catheter advances once the tip is within the cervical os depends on application of appropriate pressure and at the correct angle to account for the angle of the cervical canal. Sometimes progress is limited by the diameter of the canal and a smaller-gauge catheter is necessary.

Visibility

Vaginal discharge can result in poor visibility, which can cause significant problems especially when learning this technique. Profuse vaginal discharge can be breed related and often is seen in bulldog bitches, in which pooling of estrous secretions occurs cranial to the pelvic brim.

Most of the problems encountered with TCI result from not fully understanding the anatomy of the female reproductive tract or not having developed the skill of manipulating the endoscope and catheter together. However, some bitches are more difficult to catheterize. Difficult entry angles, recurrent poor visibility, and fidgeting patients occasionally defy all attempts from even the most skilled operator.

Confidence in the Technique

Intrauterine Deposition

Visualization of the cervix eliminates any doubt that catheter placement and semen deposition is intrauterine. Continued viewing of the insemination process ensures that all of the semen is deposited in the uterus. A video camera allows the client and the operator to observe the intrauterine deposition of the semen. This is a particularly positive aspect of videoendoscope technology.

Safety

The risk of trauma or infection resulting from the insemination procedure is an important consideration. It is difficult to imagine that the soft TCI catheter could ever perforate the vaginal or uterine wall especially during estrus unless a pathologic condition preexisted. However, the paracervical area can be traumatized by the use of inappropriate force with the endoscope. If advancing the endoscope causes obvious discomfort to the bitch, the procedure should be stopped.

TCI could introduce infection to the uterine environment. The tip of the TCI catheter likely becomes contaminated with normal vaginal flora as the endoscope passes through the vagina despite air sufflation and therefore may introduce vaginal flora into the uterus. However, the semen deposited into the uterus is not "sterile." Furthermore, normal flora vaginal bacteria routinely are isolated from the uterus during proestrus and estrus, whether the bitch is inseminated artificially, naturally mated, or not bred during that heat. Estrus is a time when the cervix is open, thus allowing ascension of normal flora from the vagina into the uterus. This does not result in pathology because ascending normal flora from the vagina are cleared out of the uterus naturally before the onset of diestrus. Therefore a reasonable assumption is that any bacteria introduced into the uterus when advancing a catheter from the vagina during estrus are cleared naturally in bitches that do not have any existing predispositions to the development of endometritis. However, care must be taken to prevent introduction of potential primary pathogens (e.g., *Brucella canis*) or an overwhelming number of organisms resulting from inadequately cleaned instruments. The equipment should be cleaned and disinfected before each use.

Frozen Semen

The purpose of TCI is to facilitate the intrauterine deposition of semen that is a vital component for successful results when using frozen semen. Equally important to the site of insemination is the timing of insemination, semen quality, and the female's fertility. The success of endoscopic TCI, like any other artificial insemination method, relies upon optimizing all of these factors.

Other Transcervical Insemination Methods. TCI also can be performed using the *Norwegian* or *Scandinavian catheter*. The Norwegian method was described by Linde-Forsberg (1991). Briefly, this method uses a 10-mm outer protecting nylon sheath and 1- to 2-mm wide steel catheter with a 0.75- to 1-mm diameter tip. The catheter is produced in three lengths (20, 30, or 40 cm) to accommodate different size bitches. The technique requires palpation and fixation of the cervix through the abdominal wall. Manipulation of the cervix then enables catheterization with the metal catheter. Similar to the endoscopic TCI technique, this method also requires practice and patience. However, in contrast to endoscopic TCI, there is no visualization of the cervix or visual confirmation of intrauterine deposition of the semen. Because the cervix can be difficult to palpate and manipulate in giant breeds and nervous and overweight females, some bitches are unsuitable for using Norwegian catheters, which is another limiting factor with this method.

Expected Outcomes of Transcervical Insemination. Whelping rates after insemination of frozen-thawed semen using the Norwegian TCI technique range from 71% to 84% with experienced operators. Similar pregnancy and whelping rates have been reported after insemination with frozen-thawed semen using the endoscopic TCI technique. A recent retrospective study in 137 greyhound bitches reported a pregnancy rate of 89.9% after a single timed insemination of frozen-thawed semen using the endoscopic TCI technique (Linde-Forsberg, 1991). These results compare favorably with results from other trials using frozen semen and the surgical intrauterine insemination method, indicating no undesirable effects from TCI (Pretzer, Lillich, and Althouse, 2006). In fact, the intrauterine insemination technique used has a negligible effect on pregnancy rate, whereas the operator, timing of the insemination, semen quality and quantity, and female's fertility are the most important factors.

However, one advantage that transcervical intrauterine insemination has over intrauterine insemination via surgical laparotomy is the ability to perform repeat inseminations, which can increase pregnancy rates and litter size. TCI allows for multiple inseminations, whereas surgery does not. When the semen is of lower quality and possibly reduced longevity, repeat inseminations allow more semen to be inseminated over an extended period covering the "fertile period." Repeat inseminations are useful also when the bitch is difficult to time relative to phase of the estrous cycle.

Fresh or Chilled Semen

In any insemination, intrauterine deposit of semen allows reasonable expectations of better results than with vaginal deposition. This applies to chilled and fresh semen, particularly when semen quality is poor or low numbers of sperm are used. Using TCI for fresh and chilled inseminations not only results in excellent conception rates and litter sizes but also provides the opportunity to develop experience and expertise for many more situations.

Other Uses

Other than insemination, the renourethroscope can be used for a number of diagnostics and treatments.

Routine Vaginoscopy for Breeding Timing. The endoscope can be used for routine vaginoscopy to determine the progression through the estrous cycle, which can greatly assist the accurate timing of insemination.

Endometritis Diagnosis. With the longer renourethroscope, transcervical hysteroscopy has been used to study the intrauterine environment with respect to microbiology and cytology throughout the reproductive cycle of the bitch, providing valuable data into the pathogenesis of pyometra and the incidence of endometritis. Uterine biopsies and swabs can be collected in a minimally invasive manner with the renourethroscope and additional specialized equipment for collecting these samples. Endometrial histopathology, cytology, and culture with sensitivity can assist greatly in the workup of infertility cases.

When examinations are performed during anestrus and diestrus, the vaginal walls are thinner and more susceptible to trauma. Therefore extreme care must be taken in these situations. Bitches not in standing heat do not tolerate vaginal endoscopy well, thus sedation with acepromazine maleate (0.01 mg/kg IV) and butorphanol tartrate (0.2 mg/kg IV) usually is required in these cases. Sedation diminishes the dog's reaction to manipulation of the endoscope; therefore the operator should exercise extreme care. The uterus is likely to be more susceptible to infection during diestrus when under the influence of high progesterone concentrations. Not only are special care and aseptic technique crucial at this stage of the cycle but also removal of progesterone by induction of luteolysis with a either a progesterone receptor antagonist (aglepristone [Alizine] 10 mg/kg q24h twice SC) or increasing incremental doses of a prostaglandin $F_2\alpha$ (dinoprost tromethamine [Lutalyse] 10 to 50 µg/kg q8h SC) over 5 days is recommended after examination to prevent the development of a pyometra.

Pyometra Treatment. Treatment of open and closed pyometra using the renourethroscope has been described. The transcervical endoscopic catheterization technique (TECT) involves flushing the uterus to remove the pus and then instilling intrauterine cephazolin (22 mg/kg once) and prostaglandin $F_{2\alpha}$ (10 µg/kg once) to assist with uterine contractions and fluid evacuation. After TECT treatment, pyometra resolves after only 3 to 5 days compared with 5 to 10 days, which is the average time taken after medical management with luteolytic drugs and systemic antibiotics alone. Despite these promising preliminary results, the authors recommend that great care be taken with patient selection when considering the TECT treatment for pyometra. The possibility of uterine rupture or leakage of pus into the abdomen during flushing resulting in peritonitis is a potential adverse and fatal side effect.

References and Suggested Reading

Andersen K: Insemination with frozen dog semen based on a new insemination technique, *Zuchthygiene* 10:1, 1975.
Linde-Forsberg C: Achieving canine pregnancy by using frozen or chilled extended semen, *Vet Clin North Am Small Anim Pract* 21:467, 1991.
Lindsay FEF: The normal endoscopic appearance of the caudal reproductive tract of the cyclic and non-cyclic bitch: post uterine endoscopy, *J Small Anim Pract* 24:1, 1983.
Pretzer SD, Lillich RK, Althouse GC: Single, transcervical insemination using frozen-thawed semen in the greyhound: a case series study, *Theriogenology* 65:1029, 2006.
Verstegen J, Dhaliwal G, Verstegen-Onclin K: Mucometra, cystic endometrial hyperplasia and pyometra in the bitch: advances in treatment and assessment of future reproductive success, *Theriogenology* 70:364, 2008.
Watts JR, Wright PJ: Investigating uterine disease in the bitch: uterine cannulation for cytology, microbiology and hysteroscopy, *J Small Anim Pract* 36:201, 1995.
Wilson MS: Transcervical insemination techniques in the bitch, *Vet Clin North Am Small Anim Pract* 31:291, 2001.

CHAPTER 207
Pregnancy Diagnosis in Companion Animals

DANA R. BLEIFER, *Pasadena, California*
LEANA V. GALDJIAN, *Pasadena, California*
CINDY BAHR, *Woodland Hills, California*

Early pregnancy diagnosis in the bitch and queen is a valuable step in managing a prospective litter of puppies and kittens. Early and accurate pregnancy diagnosis and prepartum care are essential to ensure viable offspring. Pregnancy diagnosis may be performed using several different techniques. Abdominal palpation and transabdominal ultrasonography commonly are used to diagnose pregnancy. Another less commonly used method of pregnancy diagnosis is to detect the hormone relaxin through a blood test. Whichever technique is used to confirm pregnancy, one of the most important factors in the diagnosis of pregnancy is ruling out the differential diagnosis of a potential false pregnancy, mucometra, or pyometra.

Methods for Pregnancy Diagnosis

Abdominal Palpation

Abdominal palpation is used frequently because it does not require expensive equipment; however, the skill and experience of the practitioner can be a variable. The best time to perform palpation in bitches is between 25 and 35 days after the luteinizing hormone (LH) surge. For queens, palpation is recommended between day 21 and 25 after breeding, at which time the fetal vesicles are approximately 2.5 cm in diameter (Johnston, Root Kustritz, and Olson, 2001b). During this time, amnionic vesicles can be palpated within the uterus, usually with the patient in a standing position. This technique is most successful in dams that are not overweight or overly tense. If the first examination reveals no palpable vesicles, then the procedure should be repeated 1 week later. A disadvantage of this technique is that a fluid-filled uterus can be misinterpreted as pregnancy in some cases, especially in a saccular form of pyometra. Any bitch or queen with palpable swelling in the uterus also should be checked for vaginal discharge, and the owner should be asked general health questions regarding polyuria, polydipsia, vomiting, lethargy, or unusual interest by males, which can be symptoms of pyometra.

Abdominal Ultrasonography

Another method of diagnosing pregnancy is with real-time (B-mode) ultrasonography. Ultrasound is the application of sound waves to the abdomen that reflect off of different tissues to create an image on the monitor. This technique is one of the preferred methods for determining pregnancy. Ultrasonography can be performed with the patient in dorsal recumbency or standing position. The advantages of ultrasonography include the identification of amnionic vesicles (as early as 21 days after LH surge for bitches and as early as 16 to 25 days after breeding for queens), embryonic/fetal structures, and fetal heartbeat (as early as 25 days after LH surge). An accurate fetal count usually can be achieved in bitches between 30 and 37 days from LH surge (Figure 207-1) and in queens from day 28 to 35 from breeding. With experience and training, gestational age can be determined quantitatively (Table 207-1) as well as qualitatively (Table 207-2). The main disadvantage of ultrasonography is the cost of the equipment and experience necessary for an accurate interpretation.

Abdominal Radiography

Abdominal radiography can be used in pregnancy diagnosis. However, in early gestation, it is not possible to differentiate between pregnancy and a nonpregnant fluid-filled uterus (e.g., mucometra, pyometra) (Figure 207-2). In addition, radiography before organogenesis is completed (before 45 days after LH surge) is potentially hazardous to embryos. Mineralization of the canine fetal skeleton occurs at approximately 45 days after the LH surge. For queens, radiographic identification of calcification of fetal bones may occur as early as 38 to 40 days after breeding (Johnston, Root Kustritz, and

Olson, 2001b). Therefore abdominal radiographs should be taken a few days after these minimum gestational ages to ensure adequate skeletal calcification to make a diagnosis of pregnancy. Similar to ultrasonography, radiography can be used to determine gestational age quantitatively and qualitatively (Table 207-3). Abdominal

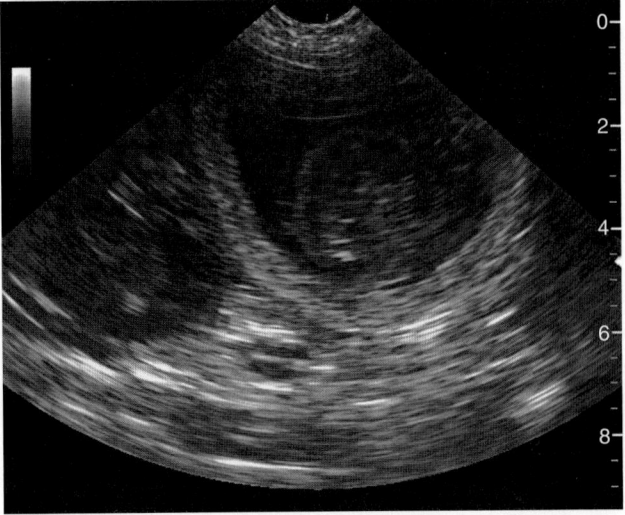

Figure 207-1 Transabdominal ultrasonography performed on a bitch 33 to 35 days after breeding (37 days after LH surge). Two fetuses can be identified readily in this view.

TABLE **207-1**

Using Transabdominal Ultrasonography, Days Before Parturition Determined Quantitatively in Queens and Small to Medium-Size Bitches by Applying Gestational Sac Diameter, Crown-Rump Length, Body Diameter, and Biparietal Diameter Measurements into Formulas

Stage of Gestation	Parameter	Species	Breed	Days Before Parturition Formula
Early pregnancy	GSD	Bitch	Small breed	(GSD in mm − 82.13) ÷ 1.8
			Medium-size breed	(GSD in mm − 68.88) ÷ 1.53
				$45.34 - (6.27 \times$ GSD in cm)
				$45 - (6 \times$ GSD in cm)
	CRL	Bitch	Small breed	$38 - (3 \times$ CRL in cm)
			Medium-size breed	$40.36 - (4.54 \times$ CRL in cm$) + (0.24 \times$ CRL^2 in cm)
Late pregnancy	BD	Queen		$43.5 - (10.9 \times$ BD in cm)
				$61 - (11 \times$ BD in cm $+ 21)$
		Bitch	Medium-size breed	$36 - (7 \times$ BD in cm)
				$42.11 - (12.75 \times$ BD in cm$) + (1.17 \times$ BD^2 in cm)
	BPD	Queen		$61.2 - (24.6 \times$ BPD in cm)
				$61 - (25 \times$ BPD in cm $+ 3)$
		Bitch	Small breed	(BPD in mm − 25.11) ÷ 0.61
			Medium-size breed	(BPD in mm − 29.18) ÷ 0.7
				$43.92 - (14.88 \times$ BPD in cm$) + (0.11 \times$ BPD^2 in cm)
				$45 - (15 \times$ BPD in cm)
	BD and BPD	Bitch	Medium-size breed	$35 - (6 \times$ BPD in cm$) - (3 \times$ BD)
				$34.27 - (5.89 \times$ BPD in cm$) - (2.77 \times$ BD in cm)

Data from Davidson AP, Baker TW: Reproductive ultrasound of the bitch and queen, *Top Companion Anim Med* 24:55, 2009; Michel E et al: Prediction of parturition date in the bitch and queen, *Reprod Dom Anim* 46:926, 2011.
BD, Body diameter; *BPD,* biparietal diameter; *CRL,* crown rump length; *GSD,* gestational sac diameter.

TABLE 207-2

Using Transabdominal Ultrasonography, Days Before Parturition as Determined Qualitatively in Queens and Bitches by Identifying Changes in Embryonic Structures

Appearance of Embryonic Structures	Species	Days Before Parturition
Gestational sac (spherical anechoic structure with thin and hyperechoic borders)	Queen	54-55
	Bitch	45
Embryo protrudes into gestational sac	Queen	48-50
	Bitch	40-42
Fetal heartbeat	Queen	47-49
	Bitch	40-42
Limb buds	Queen	46-48
	Bitch	30-32
Fetal movement	Queen	37
	Bitch	29-31
Spherical anechoic urinary bladder at the caudal pole of fetus	Queen	33-36
	Bitch	26-30
Spherical anechoic stomach caudal to liver	Queen	35-36
	Bitch	26-29
Lungs hyperechoic to liver	Queen	33-36
	Bitch	23-27
Intestines with intestinal layers	Queen	9-13
	Bitch	2-8

Data from Johnston SD, Root Kustritz MV, Olson PNS: Canine pregnancy. In Johnston SD, Root Kustritz MV, Olson PNS, editors: *Canine and feline theriogenology*, Philadelphia, 2001, WB Saunders, p 66; Johnston SD, Root Kustritz MV, Olson PNS: Feline pregnancy. In Johnston SD, Root Kustritz MV, Olson PNS, editors: *Canine and feline theriogenology*, Philadelphia, 2001, WB Saunders, p 414; Michel E et al: Prediction of parturition date in the bitch and queen, *Reprod Dom Anim* 46:926, 2011.

TABLE 207-3

Using Radiography, Days Before Parturition Determined Quantitatively in Queens and Bitches by Identifying Mineralization of Fetal Structures

Mineralization of Fetal Structures	Species	Days Before Parturition
Skull and spinal column mineralized	Queen	21-29
	Bitch	19-22
Scapula, humerus, and femur mineralized	Queen	17-24
	Bitch	14-19
Radius and tibia mineralized	Queen	15-22
	Bitch	12-15
Pelvis mineralized	Queen	8-20
	Bitch	8-12
Digits mineralized	Queen	0-11
	Bitch	1-10
Teeth mineralized	Queen	1-6
	Bitch	2-7

Data from Haney DR et al: Use of fetal skeletal mineralization for prediction of parturition date in cats, *J Am Vet Med Assoc* 223:1614, 2003; Johnston SD, Root Kustritz MV, Olson PNS: Canine pregnancy. In Johnston SD, Root Kustritz MV, Olson PNS, editors: *Canine and feline theriogenology*, Philadelphia, 2001, WB Saunders, p 66; Johnston SD, Root Kustritz MV, Olson PNS: Feline pregnancy. In Johnston SD, Root Kustritz MV, Olson PNS, editors: *Canine and feline theriogenology*, Philadelphia, 2001, WB Saunders, p 414; Michel E et al: Prediction of parturition date in the bitch and queen, *Reprod Dom Anim* 46:926, 2011.

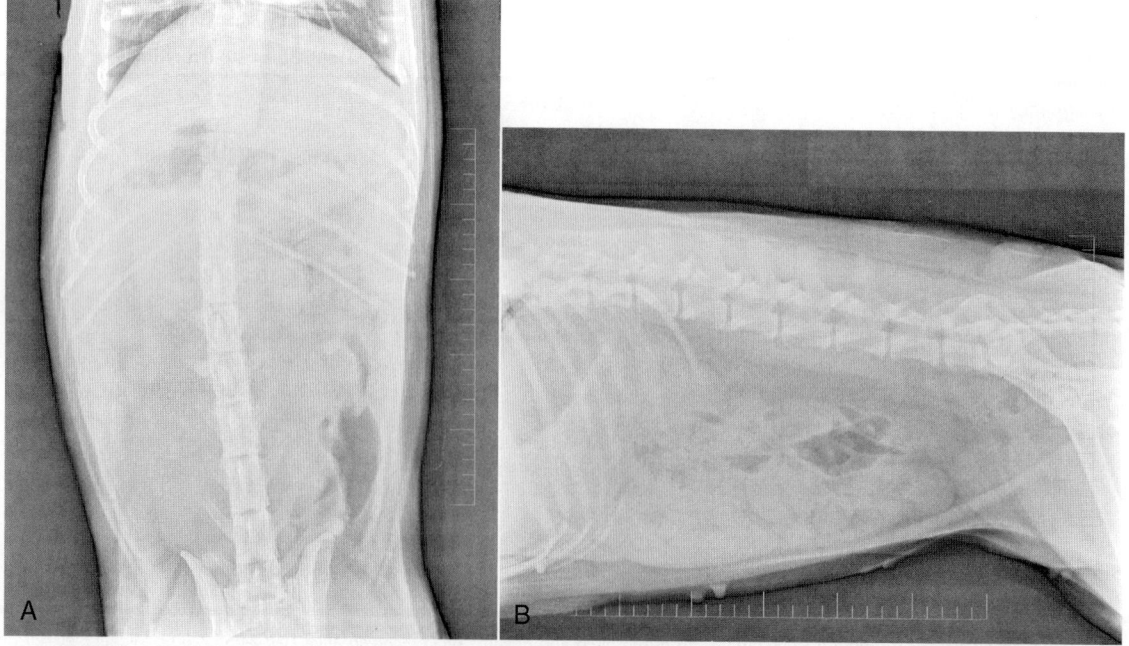

Figure 207-2 Ventrodorsal **(A)** and lateral **(B)** radiographs taken from an inappetent bitch 35 days after breeding (40 days after LH surge). The uterus is enlarged with a fluid density. It is not possible to make a diagnosis of pregnancy or pyometra based upon radiography alone at this stage of gestation.

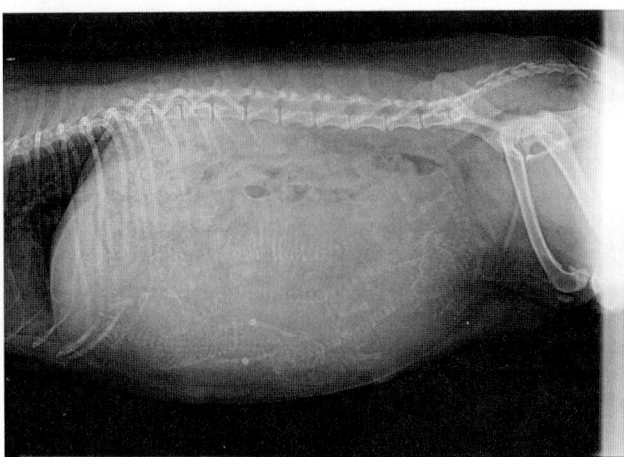

Figure 207-3 Lateral radiograph taken from a bitch 53 days after breeding (57 days after LH surge). Five fetuses are identified readily in this view.

radiography performed during the last week of pregnancy can provide an accurate fetal count (except in the case of very large litters) (Figure 207-3). This information can be helpful when discussing parturition management with the client.

Relaxin

A less common method of pregnancy diagnosis is to measure circulating relaxin concentrations. An in-house enzyme-linked immunosorbent assay (ELISA) is commercially available in the United States (Witness Relaxin Canine Pregnancy Test Kit). According to the manufacturer's instructions, canine and feline pregnancy can be diagnosed with this method as early as 20 days after the LH surge. A negative result detected between 20 and 28 days after the LH surge should be rechecked at 31 days, when hormone levels peak. The breed and body weight of the dam and litter size (e.g., placental number) may influence circulating relaxin concentrations. The authors recommend that this method be followed up with an ultrasound to evaluate fetal development and litter size.

Pregnancy Differential Diagnoses

Overt False Pregnancy

In examination of a bitch that may be pregnant, a few differentials should be considered. Overt false pregnancy, also called *pseudopregnancy* or *pseudocyesis*, is a common condition in intact bitches. Clinical signs of overt false pregnancy are not associated with an endocrine abnormality, but they are related to elevated circulating prolactin concentrations. As progesterone concentrations decrease in the second half of diestrus, prolactin concentrations increase. Although progesterone concentrations in bitches with overt false pregnancy are not different than in pregnant bitches, bitches experiencing overt false pregnancy may overly produce prolactin or may have an increased sensitivity to the hormone (Gobello, de la Sota, and Goya, 2001b).

When a bitch or a queen shows signs of overt pseudopregnancy, a definitive diagnosis should be confirmed by the methods described above. Clinical signs of overt pseudopregnancy vary but can include mammary gland enlargement (with or without lactation), behavioral changes (e.g., nesting, nursing a "litter" of toys, nervousness, aggression, dullness), and milky vulvar discharge. Mastitis may occur in some cases because of lactation. Clinical signs usually manifest 6 to 12 weeks after estrus and may last from weeks to months. Cases that manifest only behavioral changes may be difficult to identify, but a recurrent cyclic pattern may indicate pseudopregnancy. Treatment is not always indicated and depends upon type and severity of clinical signs. An 8-day food restriction has been shown to hasten involution of overt pseudopregnancy symptoms in bitches (Hermo et al, 2009).

Pyometra and Mucometra/Hydrometra

Pyometra and mucometra/hydrometra are diseases of the uterus that can be life threatening. These should be ruled out when examining a bitch or a queen for pregnancy if the clinical signs include lethargy, poor appetite, fever, or vulvar discharge. Occasionally, pyometra can occur simultaneously with pregnancy. Patient history, physical exam, vaginal cytology, serum chemistry with a complete blood cell count, and transabdominal ultrasonography to examine the uterus may be used to differentiate these conditions. Ultrasound can identify the presence of fluid in the uterus. In a pregnant uterus, the fluid-filled areas should be uniform in size with visible structures within the fluid-filled sac. With pyometra and mucometra/hydrometra, the fluid-filled areas are often different sizes with no apparent structure within the fluid. If any vulvar discharge is noted, the presence of numerous neutrophils (with or without toxic change) on a vaginal cytology should increase the suspicion of pyometra. In cases of pyometra, an immature neutrophilia may be present. Depending on the severity of symptoms, the clinician should determine the treatment (medical and/or surgical). Complete ovariohysterectomy is the recommended treatment for closed-cervix pyometra for dogs that are not intended to be bred. Seriously ill animals should be stabilized prior to surgery with IV fluids and antimicrobial therapy (e.g., enrofloxacin 5 mg/kg q24h PO if tolerated by patient). Medical treatment with prostaglandins can sometimes be used on young, healthy bitches with open-cervix pyometra. Any signs of suspected pyometra or mucometra/hydrometra should be monitored closely and broad-spectrum systemic antimicrobial therapy (e.g., amoxicillin/clavulanic acid [Clavamox] 13.75 mg/kg q12h PO) should be initiated immediately.

Complications During Pregnancy

In cases in which complications are suspected, fetal viability can be assessed by monitoring fetal heart rate (normal between 180 and 220 bpm) by ultrasonography. If the pregnancy is not near term, the fetuses may not survive premature delivery because of inadequate surfactant production until 62 days after the LH surge (in bitches) (Ruaux, 2011). If the fetuses are less than 62 days of gestation (relative to the LH surge), medical intervention may be appropriate to maintain the pregnancy and achieve a viable litter. The authors have had puppies delivered at 60 days after the LH surge survive to weaning. Serial progesterone measurements and CBCs should be performed to determine a treatment plan. Altrenogest (0.2 ml/10 lb q24h PO [Regu-Mate]) or progesterone in oil (2 mg/kg q72h IM) should be administered if serum progesterone concentrations drop below 5.0 ng/ml and the dam is less than 61 days after LH surge. Altrenogest cannot be detected by serial progesterone monitoring, whereas injectable progesterone in oil can. If premature labor is present, terbutaline sulfate (0.03 mg/kg q8h PO or by continuous IV infusion to effect) should be administered to decrease uterine contractions. Terbutaline should be discontinued 48 hours prior to whelping or 24 hours prior to cesarean section. Altrenogest should be discontinued 24 hours before whelping or cesarean section, whereas progesterone in oil should be discontinued 72 hours before whelping or cesarean section. Broad-spectrum systemic antimicrobial therapy (e.g., amoxicillin/clavulanic acid [Clavamox] 13.75 mg/kg q12h PO) should be prescribed if the dam has leukocytosis on CBC or if nonviable puppies were detected by abdominal ultrasonography. Viable fetuses within the stressed pregnancy should be monitored serially every other day by transabdominal ultrasonography.

References and Suggested Reading

Davidson AP, Baker TW: Reproductive ultrasound of the bitch and queen, *Top Companion Anim Med* 24:55, 2009.

DiGangi BA et al: Use of a commercially available relaxin test for detection of pregnancy in cats, *J Am Vet Med Assoc* 237:1267, 2010.

Gobello C, de la Sota RL, Goya RG: A review of canine pseudo-cyesis, *Reprod Domest Anim* 36:283, 2001a.

Gobello C, de la Sota RL, Goya RG: Study of the change of prolactin and progesterone during dopaminergic agonist treatments in pseudopregnant bitches, *Animal Reprod Sci* 66:257, 2001b.

Haney DR et al: Use of fetal skeletal mineralization for prediction of parturition date in cats, *J Am Vet Med Assoc* 223:1614, 2003.

Hermo G et al: Effect of short-term restricted food intake on canine pseudopregnancy, *Reprod Domest Anim* 44:631, 2009.

Johnston SD, Root Kustritz MV, Olson PNS: Canine pregnancy. In Johnston SD, Root Kustritz MV, Olson PNS, editors: *Canine and feline theriogenology*, Philadelphia, 2001a, WB Saunders, p 66.

Johnston SD, Root Kustritz MV, Olson PNS: Feline pregnancy. In Johnston SD, Root Kustritz MV, Olson PNS, editors: *Canine and feline theriogenology*, Philadelphia, 2001b, WB Saunders, p 414.

Michel E et al: Prediction of parturition date in the bitch and queen, *Reprod Dom Anim* 46:926, 2011.

Ruaux C: The respiratory system. In Peterson ME, Kutzler MA, editors: *Small animal pediatrics*, St Louis, 2011, Elsevier Saunders, p 328.

CHAPTER 208

Dystocia Management

AUTUMN P. DAVIDSON, *Davis, California*

Although many dogs and cats deliver in the home or kennel/cattery setting without difficulty, requests for veterinary participation in the field of veterinary obstetrics have become more common. The increased financial and emotional value of stud dogs and toms, brood bitches and queens, and their offspring to the dog and cat fancier makes the preventable loss of even one neonate undesirable. Breeding colonies in academic, scientific, and industrial facilities must maximize neonatal survival for financial and ethical reasons.

Veterinary involvement in obstetrics has several goals: to increase neonatal viability (minimizing offspring born dead from the difficulties in the birth process), to minimize morbidity and mortality in the dam, and to contribute to better survival rates of neonates during the first week of life. Neonatal survival is related directly to the quality of labor. Optimal management of parturition requires an understanding of normal labor and delivery in the bitch and queen, as well as the clinical ability to detect and treat abnormalities in the delivery process.

Dystocia is defined as difficulty in the normal vaginal delivery of a neonate from the uterus. Dystocia must be detected in a timely fashion for medical or surgical intervention to improve outcome. In addition, the cause of dystocia must be identified for the most appropriate therapeutic decisions to be made.

Normal Gestation in the Bitch

Clinicians commonly are asked to ascertain if a bitch is at term pregnancy and ready chronologically to deliver a litter and even to intervene if labor has not begun when anticipated. Because there are no well-documented, predictable, and safe labor induction protocols for the bitch, this generally means a cesarean section.

Prolonged gestation is a form of dystocia. Normal gestation in the bitch is 56 to 58 days from the first day of diestrus (detected by serial vaginal cytologies, defined as the first day that cytology returns to 50% or fewer cornified/superficial cells) or 64 to 66 days from the initial rise in progesterone from baseline (generally between 1.0 and 2.5 ng/ml), which equates to the day of the luteinizing hormone (LH) surge, or 58 to 72 days from the first instance that the bitch permitted breeding. Predicting gestational length without any prior ovulation timing is difficult because of the disparity between estrual behavior and the actual time of conception in the bitch and the length of time semen can remain viable in the bitch reproductive tract, often up to more than 7 days. As a result, breeding and conception dates do not correlate closely enough to permit highly accurate prediction of whelping dates. In addition, clinical signs of term pregnancy are not specific: the radiographic appearance of fetal skeletal mineralization varies at term; fetal size varies with breed and litter size, making ultrasonographic gestational aging imprecise; and the characteristic drop in body temperature preceding stage I labor (typically less than 100° F) varies and may not be detected in all bitches.

Breed, parity, and litter size also can influence gestational length. Astute dog owners and clinicians may be able to detect subtle signs of impending delivery, such as relaxation of the perineum, mammary engorgement, or a change in the appearance of the gravid abdomen, but these are not sensitive or specific. The inability to manage clinically prematurity in the canine (primarily because of lack of surfactant) effectively makes excessively early delivery undesirable. Unfortunately an overly conservative (delayed) approach resulting in intrauterine fetal death also is undesirable.

Bitches typically enter stage I labor within 24 hours of a decline in serum progesterone to below 2.0 ng/ml, which occurs in conjunction with elevated circulating prostaglandins and is associated commonly with a transient drop in body temperature usually to less than 100° F. Monitoring serial progesterone levels for gestational length is problematic because in-house kits enabling rapid results are inherently less accurate between 2 and 5 ng/ml. Commercial laboratories offering quantitative progesterone by chemiluminescence enzyme immunoassay typically have a 12- to 24-hour turnaround time, which is not rapid enough to enable decisions about an immediate indication for obstetric intervention. Progesterone levels can drop precipitously over an 8- to 12-hour period; thus results are helpful in supporting the decision to perform an elective cesarean section only if the level drops below 2.0 ng/ml. Some bitches experience a typical drop in progesterone level but still do not have normal labor. Clearly it is beneficial to obtain information about ovulation timing, minimally by determining the onset of cytologic diestrus, for accurately evaluating gestational length at term. The clinician should avoid electively delivering puppies younger than 62 gestational days (days from the LH surge), unless an indication of impending fetal demise or maternal morbidity is present. Doppler or ultrasonographic fetal heart rate monitoring may be helpful; if fetal heart rates are consistently less than 150 beats/min, fetal stress is likely.

Normal Gestation in the Queen

The queen is an induced ovulator. Typical feline gestation length is 61 to 63 days from the date of effective coital contact inducing the LH surge. Prediction of gestational age is facilitated by housing the queen with a tom for only short periods during behavioral estrus (2 to 4 days).

Normal Labor and Delivery

Stage I labor in the bitch and queen normally lasts from 12 to 24 hours, during which time the uterus has myometrial contractions of increasing frequency and strength associated with cervical dilation. No abdominal effort (visible tenesmus) is evident during stage I labor. Bitches and queens may exhibit changes in disposition and behavior, becoming reclusive and restless and nesting intermittently, often refusing to eat, and sometimes vomiting. Panting and trembling may occur. Vaginal discharge typically is clear and watery.

Normal stage II labor is defined to begin when external abdominal efforts can be seen accompanying myometrial contractions to culminate in the delivery of a neonate. Presentation of the fetus at the cervix triggers the Ferguson reflex, promoting the release of endogenous oxytocin from the hypothalamus. Typically these efforts should not last longer than 1 to 2 hours between fetuses, although this varies greatly. The entire delivery can take between 1 and more than 24 hours; however, normal labor outcome is associated with shorter total delivery time and intervals between neonates. Vaginal discharge can be clear, serous to hemorrhagic, or reddish brown in queens or green (uteroverdin) in bitches. Typically dams continue to nest between deliveries and may nurse and groom neonates intermittently. Anorexia, panting, and trembling are common.

Stage III labor is defined as the delivery of the placenta. Dams typically vacillate between labor stages II and III until the delivery is complete. During normal labor all fetuses and placentae are delivered vaginally, although they may not be delivered together in every instance. Occasionally placentae are delivered hours after delivery of all of the offspring is complete. Dams typically consume placentae, making client counts potentially inaccurate.

Detecting Abnormalities in Canine and Feline Labor

The standard approach to labor management in companion animals has involved subjective monitoring of the dam's behavior, rectal temperature (in bitches), progression of labor, and the physical condition of the neonates. Little accurate, timely, and evidence-based information is made available to the clinician concerning actual uterine activity or prepartum fetal viability with this methodology. Telephone consultations between the veterinarian and breeder or kennel manager usually entail interpretation of indirect information such as time between

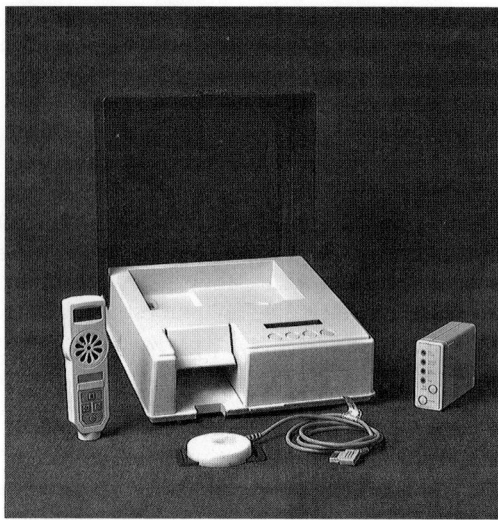

Figure 208-1 Veterinary obstetrical monitoring equipment consists of a tocodynamometer (sensor, recorder, and modem, *right*) and hand-held Doppler unit (*left*).

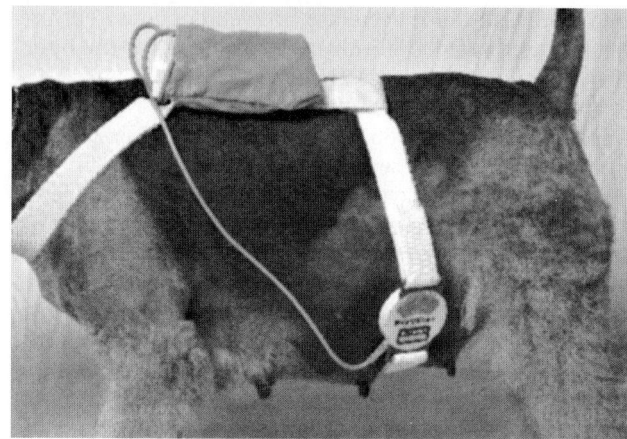

Figure 208-2 A monitoring session showing a pregnant Airedale bitch with tocodynamometer sensor in place. The sensor is placed over a lightly clipped area of the gravid lateral abdomen.

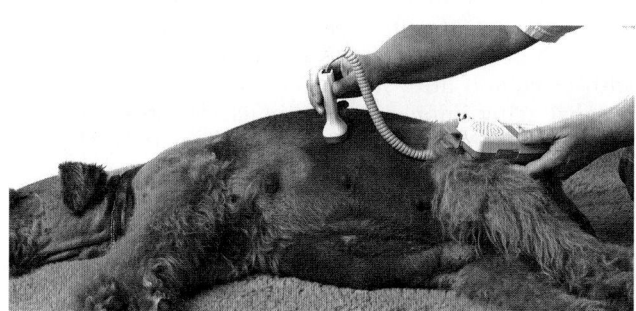

Figure 208-3 Evaluating fetal heart rate with a handheld Doppler. Fetal heart rates can be detected audibly or read from the unit.

deliveries, color of vaginal discharge, presence and nature of externally visible tenesmus, and occurrence of stillborn offspring. Although generally acceptable (associated with a favorable outcome) for the uneventful delivery in a young, healthy dam, parturition associated with fetal and maternal morbidity and mortality is familiar to most clinicians in reproductive practice. For these cases, improved diagnostic tools are desirable, such as those used in human obstetrics. Clinical information about the onset, duration, and progression of the stages of labor, frequency and strength of myometrial contractions, progression of delivery of fetuses into the uterine body and vagina for birth, and physical status of the fetuses is helpful for obstetric decision making. Evaluating the metabolic status of dams presented for dystocia is important if hypocalcemia or hypoglycemia is suspected but neither commonly is detected.

Recently a system for monitoring labor and fetal viability in the bitch or queen has become available commercially (Veterinary Perinatal Services, Inc.). This system is intended for use by veterinarians in the clinical setting when evaluating a bitch or queen in labor or by dog or cat fanciers or kennel or cattery managers with veterinary supervision in the home or kennel/cattery setting. The Veterinary Perinatal Service (VPS) design is based on labor monitoring systems used routinely in human obstetrics. The uterine monitoring system consists of a tocodynamometer (sensor), a recorder, and a modem (Figure 208-1). The uterine sensor detects changes in intrauterine and intraamniotic pressures. The sensor is strapped over a lightly clipped area of the dam's caudolateral abdomen using an elasticized strap. The sensor's recorder is worn in a small backpack placed over the caudal shoulder area in medium and large bitches or adjacent to this area in smaller bitches or queens (Figure 208-2). Dams should be at rest in the nesting box, cage, or a crate during the monitoring sessions. The monitoring equipment is well tolerated. Subsequent to each recording

session, data are transferred from the recorder to the service center using a modem with the telephone.

Fetal heart rate assessments can be performed easily with either real-time ultrasound or a handheld Doppler unit. Normal fetal heart rates generally range above 220 beats/min. Normal canine and feline fetuses at term have heart rates at least twice the maternal rate. Fetal distress is evident by persistent fetal bradycardia of 120 to 150 beats/min. In a model of impaired oxygen delivery, heart rates in fetal dogs were recorded during hypoxic episodes; they showed that decelerations were an early sign of fetal hypoxia.

Fetal heart rate monitoring, performed with either a real-time ultrasound scanhead (5 to 7.5 MHz) or a handheld Doppler unit, is best used with dams in lateral recumbency, using acoustic coupling gel (Figure 208-3). Visualization of the fetal cardiac valve motion enables estimation of the heart rate with real-time ultrasound. Directing the handheld Doppler perpendicularly over a fetus results in a characteristic amplification of the fetal heart sounds, distinct from maternal arterial, digestive, or cardiac sounds, enabling audible determination of fetal heart rates. The presence of fetal distress is reflected by sustained deceleration of the heart rates. Decelerations associated with uterine contractions suggest mismatch between the size of the fetus and the birth canal or fetal malposition or malposture. Malpresentation is generally not a problem in canine or feline deliveries because approximately 50% are delivered in caudal longitudinal presentation. Transient accelerations occur with normal fetal movement.

The Prepartum Visit

Dog or cat fanciers or kennel/cattery personnel can perform labor and fetal monitoring with veterinary guidance by telephone after previous demonstration of equipment in the clinic or on site. Ideally such demonstration should take place during a prepartum office visit or house call. After performing a physical examination of the gravid dam (including palpation/evaluation of the mammary glands and a digital vaginal examination for strictures in bitches), the clinician reviews labor management with the client or kennel/cattery personnel, including the use of monitoring equipment and administration of any medications, as well as delivery equipment and neonatal resuscitation. Light clipping of the hair coat over the gravid area of the lateral flanks allows proper contact later of the uterine sensor and fetal Doppler. In addition, proper technique for the subcutaneous administration of injectable drugs is taught during the prepartum consult. Calcium gluconate, 10% solution with 0.465 mEq Ca^{2+}, and oxytocin, 10 USP units/ml can be dispensed in predrawn syringes for later use on veterinary orders.

Specific orders (Figure 208-4) are written for each dam by the attending veterinarian concerning the indication, frequency of administration, and dosage of medications (calcium gluconate and oxytocin) and faxed to VPS. A copy is retained for the medical record. An abdominal radiograph may be obtained at the prepartum visit to best estimate litter and relative fetal size.

Clinical Labor Monitoring

Use of this monitoring equipment in a veterinary clinical setting is dictated by the presentation or referral of dams for labor evaluation and is helpful in making immediate assessment of the quality of labor and fetal viability. Minimal monitoring of uterine activity for 30 minutes is advised. Fetal heart rate monitoring can be performed immediately after uterine monitoring while uterine data are being sent via modem and generally takes 5 to 10 minutes, depending on the number of fetuses and skill of the operator.

For labor evaluation during parturition in the home or kennel/cattery setting, uterine and fetal monitoring should be initiated at least 1 week before the first predicted parturition date and generally are performed twice daily for 1 hour at each episode approximately 12 hours apart. This permits prospective identification of normal prelabor myometrial activity and the onset and duration of stages I and II of labor (Figures 208-5 and 208-6). Owners should attempt to identify a heartbeat for each fetus with the Doppler unit at each monitoring session. Obstetric personnel (licensed human obstetric nurses) are available 24 hours a day at the VPS central office to receive and interpret uterine contractile recordings and

subsequently communicate such findings by telephone to the attending veterinary clinician. Once a dam enters stage I labor, the subsequent frequency of uterine and fetal monitoring is based on the recommendation of such obstetric personnel and the attending veterinarian evaluating the progression of labor and neonatal condition. Obstetric personnel generally consult by telephone with the veterinary clinician continuously during actual labor monitoring.

Therapeutic Intervention in Dystocia

The diagnosis of dystocia can be made objectively if uterine contractility is determined to be inappropriate (generally infrequent, weak myometrial contractions) for the stage of labor (Figure 208-7) or if excessive fetal stress as determined by fetal heart rate monitoring is resulting from labor. Subjectively the diagnosis of dystocia can be made if stage I labor is not initiated at term, if stage I labor is longer than 24 hours without progression to stage II, if stage II labor does not produce a vaginal delivery within 1 to 2 hours, if fetal or maternal stress is excessive, if moribund or stillborn neonates are resulting, or if stage II labor does not result in the completion of deliveries in a timely manner (within 6 to 12 hours).

Dystocia results from maternal factors, fetal factors, or a combination of both. Maternal factors include uterine inertia, fluid abnormalities, and pelvic canal anomalies. Uterine inertia (i.e., failure of the myometrium to contract in an effective manner) can be primary or secondary. Primary uterine inertia is multifactorial, with genetic, mechanical, hormonal, and physical components. Dams exhibiting primary inertia fail to proceed into an effective labor pattern, and cesarean section is indicated. Dams exhibiting secondary inertia fail to complete expulsion of all fetuses because of exhaustion of the uterine muscle. Medical management may be successful. Clinically secondary uterine inertia is the most common maternal cause of dystocia. Abnormalities of fetal/placental fluids include hydrops, an excessive accumulation of allantoic fluid associated with each fetus, causing the fetal unit to be markedly oversized. Underproduction of uterine fluid surrounding the amniotic membranes occurs rarely, resulting in dystocia caused by a lack of lubricating fluids. Disorders of the birth canal contributing to dystocia include pelvic abnormalities, such as narrowing from a healed fracture or congenital disorders, and vaginovulvar abnormalities, such as strictures. In dogs, successful natural breedings can occur despite the presence of septate (dorsoventral) bands in the vaginal vault. Unfortunately, subsequent vaginal delivery of fetuses usually is impaired. The veterinarian should detect septate bands and strictures in bitches at the time of the soundness examination before breeding and revise them if possible. Annular (circular) strictures often are detected at the time of breeding because they can interfere with the ability to attain a natural tie. These may be resected with some difficulty before breeding; however, recurrence is common, and artificial insemination and elective cesarean delivery are actually less problematic. Dams with unusually small vulvar openings may require a partial episiotomy to deliver offspring vaginally.

WhelpWise™ Veterinary Orders
Please circle all that apply

Client _____ Client Phone _____ Due Date _____

Animal Name _____ Breed _____ Wt._____

1. Initiate the WhelpWise™ service. Instruct client in use of equipment. Encourage client to monitor uterine contractions twice daily, preferably 10 to 12 hours apart. At the onset of an active labor pattern, client and WhelpWise staff will determine the frequency and duration of subsequent monitor sessions.

    Notify DVM of onset of labor: **YES   NO**   After hours: **YES   NO**

2. In the presence of inertia as documented by the external uterine contraction monitor, begin labor augmentation per protocol. **YES   NO   Notify DVM before beginning medications: YES   NO**

3. All medication doses are based on the uterine contraction pattern, and used to treat inertia only. **Medication will not be given in the presence of a strong, regular contraction pattern**

    Oxytocin: _____ to _____**UNITS** administered **SC or IM** every _____minutes to maintain an adequate uterine contraction pattern. (Usual dose 0.25–2.5 U/bitch or queen)

    10% Calcium gluconate solution _____ ml, **subcutaneously** every _____ hrs. **(Usual dose 1.0 ml/10 lb or /4.5 kg BW)**

    Post partum oxytocin? _____, **dose?** _____ after deliveries are complete.

4. Encourage client to monitor the fetal heart rates a minimum of once a day prior to labor, and every 1-2 hours or more frequently during active labor. Notify me if decelerations or repeated absence of fetal heart rates is noted. Recommend that the client assess the fetal heart rates prior to administration of any medication.

5. If the case being monitored is a planned cesarean section, notify DVM at the onset of labor. Yes   No

6. Notify me of the details of labor monitoring and outcome at the conclusion of service by_____ phone _____fax

Other Instructions:

_____

_____

_____

Signature _____

Veterinarian _____   phone _____

Backup Veterinarian _____ phone _____

Clinic Name: _____   **Address** _____

Clinic Phone _____   **Fax** _____

Veterinary Perinatal Specialties Inc.   9111 W. 38ᵗʰ Ave. Wheat Ridge, CO 80033
1-888-281-4867,   (303) 423-3429   Fax: (303) 423-8242

Figure 208-4 Veterinary orders form. The supervising veterinarian determines whether medications (calcium gluconate and oxytocin) may be given by an owner and if so, under which circumstances and at what dosage. This form is faxed to Veterinary Perinatal Services when home monitoring is initiated. (Courtesy Veterinary Perinatal Specialties, Inc., Wheat Ridge, CO.)

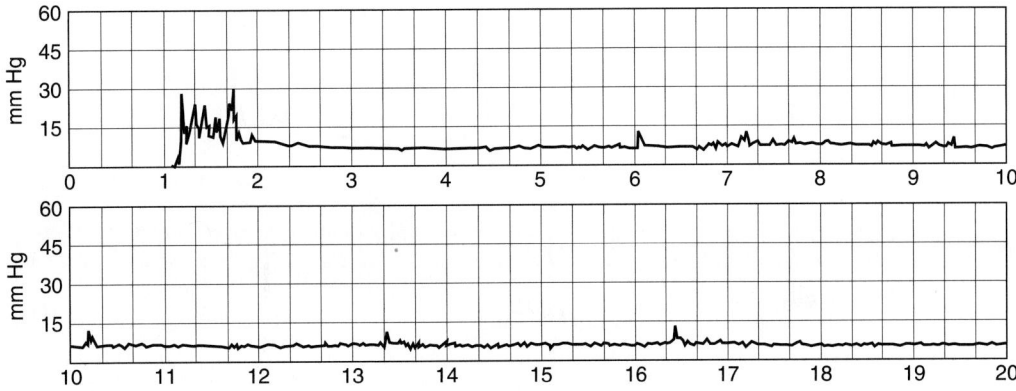

Figure 208-5 Normal uterine baseline recording (prelabor), no contractions evident. X-axis represents time in minutes; Y-axis strength of contraction in millimeters of mercury.

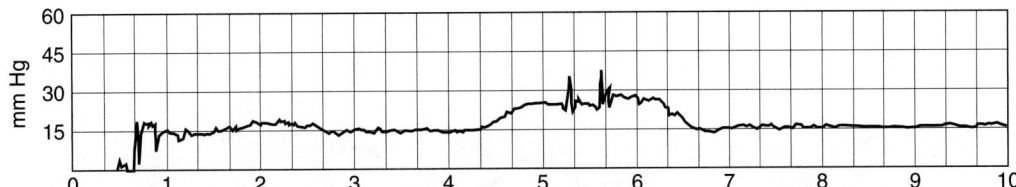

Figure 208-6 Normal myometrial contraction, prelabor. Note excursion off baseline during contraction with return to baseline.

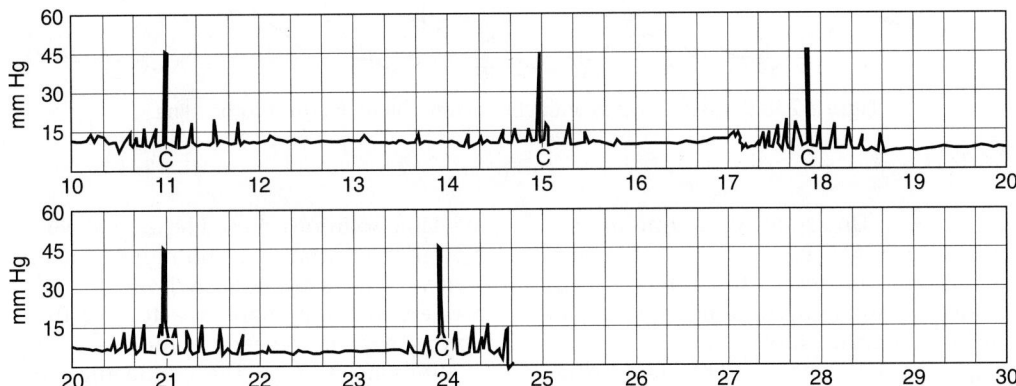

Figure 208-7 Uterine inertia: abdominal efforts (seen as vertical spikes "c") with no myometrial contractions evident.

Fetal causes of dystocia include fetal oversize; fetal anomalies; and abnormal fetal position, presentation, or posture. Fetal oversize can occur with prolonged gestation in abnormally small litters and is the most common fetal cause of dystocia. Fetal anomalies such as anasarca and hydrocephalus (abnormalities of body fluid distribution) can cause a mismatch between the size of the birth canal and the fetus. Because craniad (head first) and caudad (breech) presentation are normal in dogs and cats, only a transverse (sideways) presentation is associated with dystocia and is rare. Fetuses normally are positioned with the fetal spine adjacent to the dorsal surface of the uterus. Malpositioning (fetal spine adjacent to ventral surface of uterus rather than the maternal dorsum) can cause dystocia. Abnormalities of posture, the normal being fully extended forelimbs (as if diving), are the second most frequent fetal cause of dystocia. Malpositioning of the head (elevated), forelimbs, or hind limbs of the canine or feline fetus is not corrected readily with the use of forceps, traction, or digital manipulation because of the limitations of the size of the birth canal.

The use of uterine and fetal monitors allows the veterinary clinician to detect and monitor labor and manage dystocia medically or surgically with insight. Clinical use of the monitoring equipment should dictate subsequent medical or surgical intervention. In the home or kennel setting, the administration of medications is initiated as indicated by monitoring information and only with authorization from the attending veterinary clinician. Continued monitoring permits evaluation of the response

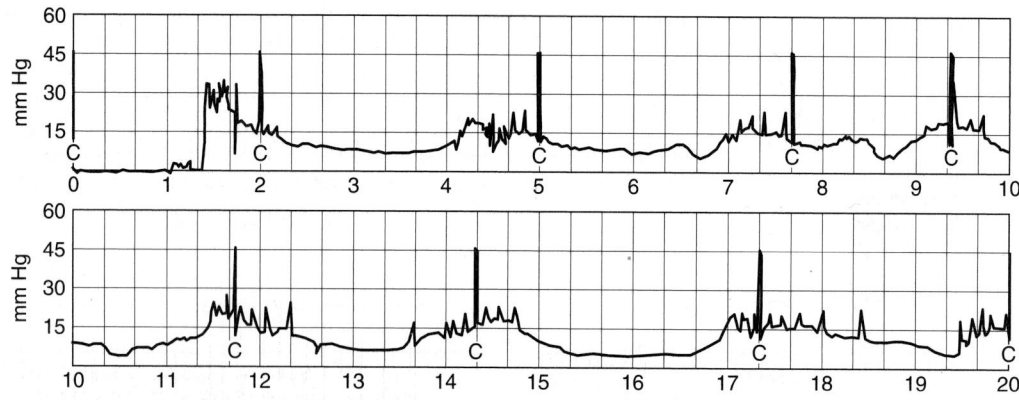

Figure 208-8 Inertia as seen in Figure 208-7 treated with 1 unit of oxytocin subcutaneously; normal contraction pattern evident.

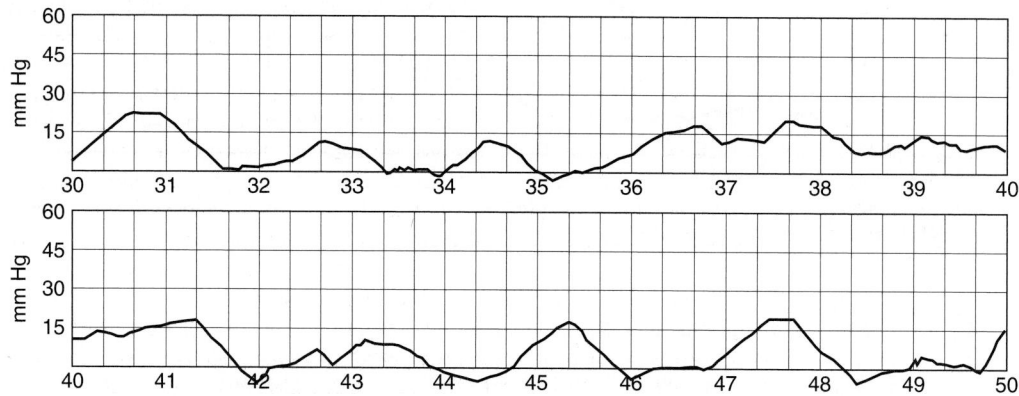

Figure 208-9 Uterine hypercontractility; note minimal return to baseline.

to therapy (Figure 208-8). Unresponsive uterine inertia, obstructive dystocia, aberrant uterine contractile patterns, or progressive fetal distress without response to home medical management are indications for return to the veterinary facility for cesarean section.

Medical management revolves around the administration of calcium gluconate and oxytocin, based on the results of monitoring. Drugs are given only after 8 to 12 hours of an established contraction pattern (stage I labor) as detected by the uterine monitor and only if inertia is detected when stage II labor is anticipated. Premature administration of drugs results in suboptimal response; for this reason prelabor monitoring permitting recognition of the onset of labor is ideal.

Generally the administration of calcium increases the strength of myometrial activity, and oxytocin increases the frequency of myometrial contractions. Despite normocalcemia, the administration of calcium gluconate can result in improved myometrial tone. A 10% solution of calcium gluconate can be given when ineffective, weak uterine contractions are detected. Calcium gluconate 10% (0.465 mEq/ml) is dosed at 1 ml/4.5 kg of body weight (bitch or queen), generally every 4 to 6 hours. Subcutaneous administration of calcium gluconate avoids the potential for cardiac irritability associated with intravenous administration. More concentrated commercially

available solutions should be diluted with sterile water to a final concentration of no more than 11.5%.

Oxytocin is administered when uterine contractions are less frequent than expected for the stage of labor. Oxytocin given too early or too late during whelping has a minimal effect on the contractile pattern. The most effective time for dosing is when uterine inertia begins to develop, before the complete cessation of uterine contractility occurs. High doses of oxytocin saturate the receptor sites and make it ineffective as a uterotonic. Substantially lower-than-traditional doses of oxytocin are now known to be effective for improving the quality of myometrial contractions. Oxytocin is commercially available at a concentration of 10 units/ml, permitting accurate small dosing. Refrigeration is not required. An initial dose of 0.25 to 0.5 units per bitch or 0.25 to 0.5 unit per queen administered subcutaneously is advised. Subsequent doses range from 0.5 to 2 units per bitch or queen. Higher doses of oxytocin or intravenous boluses can cause tetanic, ineffective uterine contractions that compromise fetal oxygen supply during placental compression. If fetal stress is evident (persistent bradycardia) and response to medications poor, surgical intervention is indicated. Uterine hyperstimulation with elevated baseline levels of contractility compromising placental blood supply (Figure 208-9) or a uterine obstructive pattern also

TABLE 208-1

Author's Protocol for Cesarean Section Anesthesia

Preanesthesia	Anesthesia Induction	Anesthesia Maintenance	Postoperative Analgesia
Preoxygenate by face mask	Propofol 6 mg/kg IV to effect	Isoflurane or sevoflurane	Bupivacaine local block up to 2 mg/kg
Glycopyrrolate 0.01-0.02 mg/kg SC			Hydromorphone 0.05-0.1 mg/kg IV as needed

negates further use of calcium gluconate or oxytocin. Use of intrapartum monitoring has been demonstrated to lead practitioners to perform cesarean section earlier in some cases of dystocia, decreasing offspring mortality and dam morbidity in these cases.

A written summary concerning the labor pattern and response to medical intervention can ultimately be incorporated into the dam's medical record for reference in future breedings. The monitoring equipment can be leased for constant use in a busy reproductive practice for a monthly fee. Alternatively, the equipment may be leased and shipped directly to the veterinary client for use during with an individual dog during labor. Practitioner and client acceptance of the equipment once familiarity is established is generally good.

Surgical intervention (cesarean section) is indicated if a bitch or queen fails to respond to in-hospital medical management, or if fetal distress is apparent despite adequate to increased uterine contractility (suggesting mismatch of maternal birth canal to fetal size, or fetal malposition or malposture incompatible with vaginal delivery), or if aberrant contractile patterns are noted by uterine monitoring. Well-orchestrated cesarean sections result when anesthetic and neonatal resuscitative protocols already are established and coordinated, and the preoperative preparation of the dam optimized.

Clinicians should always remember that the dam may be debilitated and require careful anesthetic management, there may be little time for routine preanesthetic preparation, and the dam may have been fed recently. Minimally, the hematocrit, total solids, serum calcium, and glucose levels should be evaluated preoperatively. Intravenous fluid support at an operative rate minimally is indicated (10 ml/kg/hr).

For premedication, atropine is best not given routinely, because it crosses the placenta and blocks the normal, adaptive bradycardic response of the fetus to hypoxia and causes relaxation of the lower esophageal sphincter, making maternal aspiration more likely. However, the use of an anticholinergic is indicated for the dam because of the anticipated vagal stimulation during manipulation of the gravid uterus. Glycopyrrolate (0.01 to 0.02 mg/kg SC) does not cross the placenta and is preferred. Most dams are tractable and do not need preanesthetic tranquilization, which has a depressant effect on the fetuses. Phenothiazine tranquilizers are transported rapidly across the placenta and are depressants. α_2-Adrenoceptor agonists such as dexmedetomidine and xylazine are contraindicated because of their severe cardiorespiratory depressant

effects. Similarly, the respiratory depressant effect of opioids makes them unpopular before removal of the fetuses. If tranquilization is necessary with an intractable dam, narcotic sedatives are preferable because their effects can be reversed (naloxone 1 to 10 µg/kg IV or IM) during neonatal resuscitation. Metoclopramide (0.10 to 0.20 mg/kg) can be administered subcutaneously or intramuscularly before the induction of anesthesia to reduce the risk of vomiting; metoclopramide also promotes the release of prolactin and facilitates lactation.

Preoxygenation by mask (5 to 10 minutes) always is indicated. Initial preparation of the abdomen (clipping and first scrubbing) can be undertaken during this time. For induction of anesthesia, dissociative agents such as ketamine and the barbiturates are best avoided because they produce profound depression of the fetuses. Propofol (6 mg/kg to effect IV) appears to be most useful. Its redistribution is rapid, therefore it has a limited effect upon the fetuses after delivery. Mask induction actually produces more maternal and fetal hypoxemia than propofol induction. For maintenance of anesthesia, volatile agents are preferable, especially those with low partition coefficients such as isoflurane and sevoflurane. These agents show rapid uptake and elimination by the animal, and it may have a better cardiovascular margin of safety than the more soluble agents such as halothane. Nitrous oxide may be used to reduce the dose of other anesthetic agents, it is transferred rapidly across the placenta, and, although it has minimal effects upon the fetus in utero, it may result in a significant diffusion hypoxia after delivery. Using a local anesthetic (bupivacaine 2 mg/kg) line block in the skin and subcutaneous tissues before incising permits a more rapid entry to the abdomen while the dam is making transition from propofol induction to inhalant maintenance and helps with postoperative discomfort (Table 208-1).

Operative speed is important because surgical delay and prolonged anesthetic time are associated with fetal asphyxia and depression. However, care should be taken during incision of the linea alba to ensure that the gravid uterus is not also incised. Ideally the uterus should be exteriorized and packed off with moistened laparotomy sponges to prevent abdominal contamination with uterine fluid. This process should be undertaken carefully to ensure that the uterus and its broad ligament do not tear; it may be easier in some cases to exteriorize one horn at a time. The uterus should be penetrated in a relatively avascular area, and it is best to elevate the uterine wall from the fetus and to extend the incision with scissors to ensure that the fetus is not lacerated. The fetuses may be brought to the incision by gently "milking" them along the uterus, although in some cases or in large dams it may be necessary to make more than one incision. As the fetal fluid is released it is best to remove this by suction and then to clamp the umbilicus (twice, incising between clamps) before passing the fetus to an assistant for immediate resuscitation. After each fetus is removed, the associated placenta should be detached by gentle traction, but the placentas may be left *in situ* if they are attached firmly and their removal causes significant hemorrhage. Placentas can be passed spontaneously postoperatively, or managed medically. The uterine horns, the uterine body, and the vagina must be inspected thoroughly to ensure that all fetuses have been removed. Finally, after closure the uterus, its broad ligament and the vascular supply should be inspected carefully to ensure that any previously unnoticed tears have been identified before closure of the abdomen. Ovariohysterectomy at the time of cesarean section is again the option of the surgeon and owner but results in longer anesthetic time for the dam, delayed nursing for the neonates, and increased loss of blood in the dam, so should be postponed if reasonable. Some believe that estrogen acts in a permissive fashion for prolactin receptors in the mammary glands, making ovary removal at cesarean section undesirable. If uterine viability is questionable, an ovariohysterectomy should be performed. In the normal dam the uterus begins to involute shortly after removal of the fetuses. However, if this is not the case, oxytocin may be administered (0.25 to 1.0 units per dam) to facilitate involution and arrest any hemorrhage; this also promotes milk letdown.

Postsurgical discomfort should be acknowledged in the dam. Once the fetuses are removed, narcotic analgesia can be administered parenterally to the dam. Postoperatively, nonsteroidal antiinflammatories are not advisable because of their uncertain metabolism by the nursing neonates with immature renal and hepatic metabolism. Narcotic analgesia is preferable. Oral narcotics (e.g., Tramadol, 10 mg/kg q24h) in divided doses provide excellent postoperative analgesia for nursing dams with minimal sedation of the neonates. In all cases, clients should be advised to monitor closely dams postoperatively until normal maternal behavior emerges. After cesarean section, dams can be clumsy and inattentive to the neonates and even can become aggressive because the normal mechanisms of maternal bonding have been bypassed. Nursing should be supervised and neonatal care ensured.

References and Suggested Reading

Darvelid AW, Linde-Forsberg C: Dystocia in the bitch: a retrospective study of 182 cases, *J Small Anim Pract* 35:402, 1994.

Davidson AP: Primary uterine inertia in four Labrador bitches, *J Am Anim Hosp Assoc* 47:83, 2011.

Davidson AP: Problems during and after parturition. In England G, von Heimendahl A, editors: *BSAVA manual of canine and feline reproduction and neonatology*, ed 2, Gloucester, 2010, BSAVA, p 121.

Davidson AP: Uterine and fetal monitoring in the bitch, *Vet Clin North Am Small Anim Pract* 31:305, 2001.

England GC: Ultrasonographic assessment of abnormal pregnancy, *Vet Clin North Am Small Anim Pract* 28:849, 1998.

Gaudet DA, Kitchell BE: Canine dystocia, *Compend Contin Educ Small Anim Pract* 7:1406, 1985.

Jackson PGG: Cesarean section. In Jackson PGG, editor: *Handbook of veterinary obstetrics*, Cambridge, 2004, Elsevier, p 173.

Johnston SD et al: Prenatal indicators of puppy viability at term, *Compend Contin Educ Small Anim Pract* 5:1013, 1983.

Münnich A, Küchenmeister U: Dystocia in numbers—evidence-based parameters for intervention in the dog: causes for dystocia and treatment recommendations, *Reprod Domest Anim* 44(suppl 2):141, 2009.

Wallace MS: Management of parturition and problems of the periparturient period of dogs and cats, *Semin Vet Med Surg (Small Anim)* 9:28, 1994.

CHAPTER 209

Postpartum Disorders in Companion Animals

MICHELLE ANNE KUTZLER, *Corvallis, Oregon*

The interval from parturition to weaning, the post-partum period, is typically 6 to 8 weeks in dogs and cats. During the postpartum period, endometrial remodeling at the placental sites occurs, which is histologically complete by 12 weeks after delivery. Postpartum vaginal discharge of lochia, initially dark green in dogs, may persist for 3 to 6 weeks, over which time the discharge changes to reddish brown before it subsides completely. Abnormal events arising during the postpartum period are described in the following paragraphs with a summary of recommended therapies at the end of this chapter (Table 209-1).

Hemorrhage

Scant bleeding after parturition is normal; however, excessive bleeding may indicate uterine or vaginal parturient trauma or may be evidence of an underlying coagulopathy. Vaginoscopy may be useful to identify the source of bleeding (e.g., uterine or vaginal). Intravenous fluid support and blood transfusions may be needed to stabilize the patient, depending on the overall condition of the animal and the total amount of blood lost. When correcting blood volume deficits, clinicians should consider that the normal hematocrit in most bitches and queens at term is 30%, as a result of a hemodilution that occurs during gestation. Although oxytocin (0.1 to 0.2 units/kg, not to exceed 10 units q2-3h SC) may reduce the diameter of the uterine lumen, its efficacy for the treatment of acute postpartum hemorrhage has not been evaluated critically, and ovariohysterectomy often is indicated.

Subinvolution of Placental Sites

Subinvolution of the placental sites (SIPS) involves a delay in the normal process of cytotrophoblast apoptosis (placental degeneration) and endometrial reconstruction. Although the exact etiopathogenesis is unclear, cytotrophoblasts persist within the endometrium instead of degenerating after parturition, preventing endometrial blood vessels from developing thromboses, resulting in persistent endometrial bleeding. Trophoblasts also may invade the myometrium and on rare occasions may penetrate through the serosa, resulting in peritonitis.

SIPS generally occurs in primiparous bitches younger than 2½ years old, with an incidence of 10% to 20% in postpartum bitches. SIPS has never been reported in queens, which is curious given the similarity between the canine and feline placenta. The only clinical sign of SIPS is persistent hemorrhagic (with or without clots) to serosanguineous discharge for more than 6 weeks after delivery. However, SIPS may occur in the absence of any vaginal discharge. A presumptive diagnosis of SIPS is made based upon the clinical history. Bitches with SIPS are afebrile and otherwise healthy, which differentiates SIPS from metritis; however, abnormalities within the bladder or vagina also should be ruled out. Abdominal palpation may identify discrete, firm spheroid enlargements within the uterine horns (approximately 2.5 cm in diameter). Abdominal ultrasonography may identify increased fluid in the uterine horn lumen with prominent placental attachment sites. Identification of multinucleated, basophilic staining trophoblasts with highly vacuolated cytoplasm on cytologic examination of the discharge or histologic examination of a uterine biopsy provides a definitive diagnosis. A cystocentesis with urinanalysis and vaginoscopic examination should rule out the urinary tract and vagina as the source of the discharge.

The clinical management of SIPS must be based on the individual patient and client. Most cases of SIPS are self-limiting, which is fortunate because medical treatment has not proven to be effective. Administration of antibiotics, progestins, or oxytocin does not decrease the duration, amount, or character of the vaginal discharge. Bitches intended for future breeding should be monitored cautiously until the discharge resolves spontaneously. Monitoring includes deliberate daily observation of the bitch's general appearance by the owner and weekly vaginal cytologic examinations and complete blood cell counts to confirm the absence of metritis or anemia. However, in cases of uterine rupture or severe hemorrhage or if the patient is no longer a valuable breeding animal, ovariohysterectomy is recommended. Normal fertility has been reported in bitches after recovery from SIPS.

Uterine Prolapse

Uterine prolapse is relatively uncommon in the queen and bitch but has been reported in the literature more frequently in queens than bitches. Uterine prolapse can occur during or within a few hours after parturition, involving either one or both uterine horns. Dystocia, delivery of large litters, placental retention, advanced maternal age, and excessive relaxation of the pelvic and perineal region are considered predisposing factors.

TABLE 209-1

Recommended Therapies for Postpartum Disorders in Companion Animals

Drug	Dosage	Indications	Side Effects	Additional Information
Acepromazine	0.5-2 mg/kg SC	Agalactia	Bradycardia, hypotension	
Cabergoline	5 μg/kg q24h PO for 5 days	Adjunctive therapy for treating mastitis or puerperal tetany to suppress lactation	None observed at this dosage	
Calcium carbonate	100 mg/kg q24h PO	To prevent recurrence of puerperal tetany	May cause gastrointestinal irritation and constipation	
Calcium gluconate (10%)	0.22-0.44 ml/kg IV (slowly)	Puerperal tetany	Bradycardia and other arrhythmias	Should be administered in conjunction with careful cardiac monitoring
Cefadroxil	22 mg/kg q12h PO	Susceptible bacterial infections in lactating bitches and queens	May cause gastrointestinal effects in susceptible animals	Has not been observed to affect nursing offspring
Oxytocin	0.1-0.2 units/kg, not to exceed 10 units q2-3h SC	Postpartum hemorrhage, secondary agalactia	Uterine cramping and abdominal discomfort	Milk will let down within 2 minutes of injection
Prostaglandin $F_{2\alpha}$ (Lutalyse)	25-50 μg/kg q4-6h SC	Metritis	Hypersalivation, purring (cats only), vomiting, diarrhea, abdominal discomfort	At this low dose, side effects are minimal to nonexistent

Examination reveals a firm soft tissue mass protruding from the vagina, which should be differentiated from a vaginal prolapse or neoplasia by palpation of the cervix and clinical appearance. Patients with a uterine prolapse quickly can develop hypotensive or hemorrhagic shock, especially if the ovarian or uterine vessels have been ruptured. While stabilizing the patient, the clinician should cover prolapsed tissues with warm, saline-moistened towels or gauze. After gentle cleaning and copiously lubricating the tissue, manual reduction, with or without an episiotomy, under epidural or general anesthesia should be attempted. Manual reduction may be accomplished with a gloved finger, test tube, or syringe case. Systemic antibiotics are warranted because the risk of metritis after a uterine prolapse is high. Cefadroxil (22 mg/kg q12h PO) is recommended because it has broad-spectrum antibacterial activity and has not been observed to affect nursing puppies or kittens. If the uterine tissue is not viable or the dam is no longer intended for breeding, manual reduction should be followed by an ovariohysterectomy. If the uterus cannot be reduced manually, the urethra should be catheterized, and the uterus may be amputated externally. The amputation procedure involves individual ligation of the uterine arteries, transection, and oversewing of the transected uterine body. A laparotomy should follow amputation to complete the ovariohysterectomy.

Septic Metritis

Septic metritis is an acute ascending bacterial infection of the uterus (usually caused by *Escherichia coli*), typically at the sites of placental attachment, occurring in the immediate postpartum period. Obstetric manipulations during dystocia, abortion, retained fetal or placental tissue, and uterine prolapse are predisposing factors. Clinical signs include rectal temperature higher than 39.5°C (>103°F), dehydration and anorexia, depression, disinterest in offspring, agalactia, and malodorous sanguineous vaginal discharge. Abdominal palpation may reveal a doughy, enlarged, and painful uterus. Vaginal cytology reveals large numbers of degenerative neutrophils, bacteria, and debris. Clinical pathology often shows elevated total solids (secondary to dehydration) with immature leukocytosis; however, leukopenia can occur in severely ill patients. Ultrasonography or hysteroscopy may aid in identifying an underlying cause. Evaluation of the uterine lumen postpartum for retained placentas or mummified fetuses is accomplished best with ultrasound. Although not diagnostic for metritis, guarded cranial vaginal cultures with sensitivity may be helpful in determining appropriate antibiotic therapy.

Removal of offspring from the dam and administration of intravenous fluids and broad-spectrum antibiotics are necessary for treatment of septicemia. Amikacin (5 to 10 mg/kg q12h IV) with cephalothin (22 mg/kg q8h IV) is recommended; however, antibiotics alone may be ineffective in treating postpartum metritis. Uterine evacuation using prostaglandin $F_{2\alpha}$ tromethamine (Lutalyse) at a dosage of 25 to 50 μg/kg q4-6h SC results in a clinical cure with minimal side effects (e.g., emesis, hypersalivation, diarrhea, purring [queens]). If the patient is no longer needed for breeding, ovariohysterectomy is recommended when the patient is stable for general anesthesia. Bitches and queens recovering from acute postpartum metritis have retained their fertility and have demonstrated this by normal subsequent whelpings without future postpartum complications.

Agalactia

Agalactia can present as either complete failure of mammary gland development (primary) or failure of milk to let down (secondary). Debilitating maternal illness, dehydration, malnutrition, and endocrine imbalances are predisposing factors. In addition, extremely stressed dams may have elevated epinephrine concentrations, leading to decreased pituitary release of oxytocin. Acepromazine (0.5 to 2 mg/kg SC) promotes prolactin secretion, which may increase pituitary oxytocin release. Oxytocin administered either parenterally (0.1 to 0.2 units/kg, not to exceed 10 units q2-3h SC) or intranasally using a nebulizing spray (Syntocinon) into one nostril (q2-3h) results in milk letdown within 2 minutes. In addition, efforts should be made to correct the underlying maternal condition. Neonates should be offered supplemental feedings or reared as orphans if the condition persists.

Septic Mastitis

Acute septic mastitis, an ascending bacterial infection involving one or more of the mammary glands, can occur secondary to unsanitary housing or galactostasis. Clinical signs include rectal temperature higher than 39.5°C (>103°F); dehydration and anorexia; depression; disinterest in offspring and agalactia; and painful, firm, and reddened mammary glands. Expressed mammary secretions tend to be sticky, chunky, and discolored (either purulent or blood tinged). Clinical pathology reveals a leukocytosis with marked immature neutrophilia. Cytologic examination of the mammary secretions may reveal bacteria, white blood cells, and erythrocytes. A Gram stain performed on mammary secretions improves antibiotic selection. Bacterial culture of mammary secretions typically yields *Staphylococcus* spp., *Streptococcus* spp., and *E. coli* as causal organisms. Milk white blood cell counts have been recommended in the past for diagnosing mastitis, but this test has not been reliable because cell counts tend to differ between individual animals as well as within glands from the same animal.

Until culture and sensitivity results are obtained, cefadroxil (22 mg/kg q12h PO) is recommended because it has broad-spectrum antibacterial activity and has not been observed to affect nursing offspring. Neonates should be allowed to nurse because nursing may speed resolution of the disease. However, if many glands are affected or the mother is severely ill, the offspring should be hand raised. If the neonates are weaned, cabergoline (Dostinex) (5 μg/kg q24h PO for 5 days) should be used to stop lactation and prevent further bacterial extension. Warm compresses can be applied two to three times a day along with milking out the affected glands. Ultrasound of a mastitic mammary gland can be helpful in identifying fluid pocket development (abscessation) that warrants surgical intervention and in monitoring response to therapy (Figure 209-1). In cases of abscessation or gangrenous mastitis (Figure 209-2), surgical drainage and removal of the affected mammary gland may be necessary. In these cases a clear line of demarcation separates the healthy tissue from the gangrenous tissue.

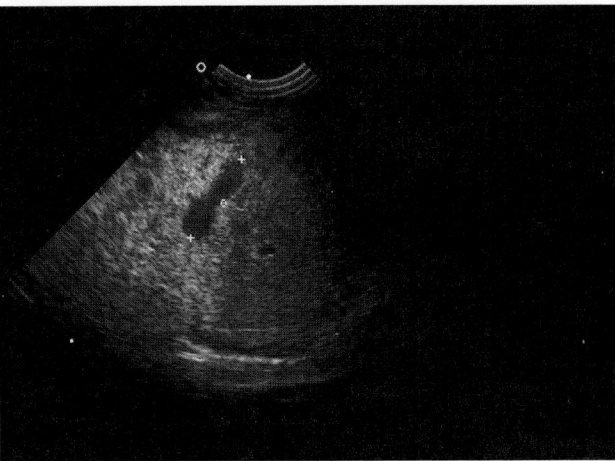

Figure 209-1 Acute septic mastitis. *Cursors* indicate a hypoechoic fluid accumulation suggesting abscessation. (Reprinted with permission from Davidson AP, Baker TW: Reproductive ultrasound of the bitch and queen, *Top Companion Anim Med* 24:55, 2009.)

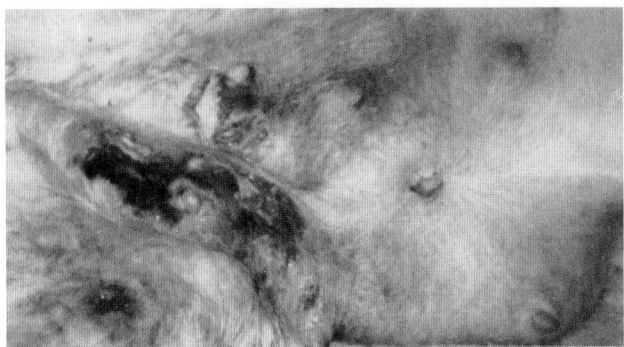

Figure 209-2 This 5-year-old yellow Labrador retriever bitch was 2 weeks postpartum when the owner first noticed swelling in her left hind leg (note presence of dermatitis in the medial thigh). When examined in left lateral recumbency, both pairs of mammary glands (caudal abdominal and inguinal) are swollen and erythematous. In addition, the overlying skin is necrotic in multiple areas with evidence of abscessation.

Puerperal Tetany

Puerperal tetany, also known as postpartum hypocalcemia or eclampsia, generally develops less than 28 days after delivery but can occur during late pregnancy or during parturition. In the dog, puerperal tetany occurs most commonly in small-breed bitches, less frequently in medium-sized bitches, and rarely in large-breed bitches. Puerperal tetany has been reported in queens (pre- and postpartum) but occurs at a much lower incidence than in bitches. Other than breed, predisposing factors in dogs include young age, large litter size in relation to body weight, and diet during pregnancy. Diets high in calcium, animal protein (egg or meat), or containing cereals with phytates (a compound that binds ionized calcium making it biologically unavailable), may predispose to puerperal tetany.

Puerperal tetany occurs with an acute decrease in ionized calcium concentration. A reduction in calcium concentrations increases membrane permeability in nerve cells to sodium ions, causing increased frequency of spontaneous nervous activity noticeable as muscle fasciculations. Clinical signs are related not only to the absolute decrease in ionized calcium concentrations but also to the rate and progression of its decline. The onset of clinical signs is usually rapid, and the progression of signs is predictable. Early clinical signs include restlessness, whining, panting, salivation, anorexia, vomiting, and behavioral changes. As the signs progress, muscle fasciculations, stiffness, ataxia, tonic-clonic muscle spasms, hyperthermia, tachycardia, seizures, and death may ensue. Ionized serum calcium concentrations less than 0.6 to 0.8 mmol/L are definitive for diagnosing puerperal tetany. If ionized calcium quantification is not available, total serum calcium measurements can be used, with concentrations less than 1.625 mmol/L highly indicative of puerperal tetany. Ionized calcium concentrations are typically 30% to 50% of total calcium concentrations; however, alkalosis resulting from hypersalivation may increase the protein-bound calcium fraction, resulting in a lower net decrease in ionized calcium levels. In addition to measuring calcium levels, a full serum chemistry evaluation is necessary because hypoglycemia and other electrolyte disturbances may develop concurrently with puerperal tetany.

Treatment for puerperal tetany is aimed at returning ionized calcium concentrations to normal values. This is achieved by slow intravenous administration of 10% calcium gluconate (0.22 to 0.44 ml/kg) in combination with careful cardiac auscultation or electrocardiography. The development of bradycardia and other arrhythmias during intravenous calcium administration is indicative of too rapid replacement. Full recovery or clinical cure occurs within minutes of the intravenous treatment. Judicious administration of intravenous fluids and anticonvulsants (diazepam 1 to 5 mg once IV) is indicated for treatment of hyperthermia and seizures. The offspring should be removed from the dam and hand fed a milk supplement for at least 12 to 24 hours to prevent a relapse. If the litter is older than 4 weeks old, they can be weaned. Lactation can be terminated using cabergoline (Dostinex) (5 µg/kg q24h for 5 days PO). Oral supplementation with calcium carbonate (100 mg/kg q24h) and vitamin D (10,000 to 25,000 units q24h) also is recommended to prevent a relapse. Bitches and queens may suffer from a puerperal tetany at the next parturition. However, dams should not be supplemented with calcium during pregnancy because this increases the likelihood of developing puerperal tetany rather than preventing its recurrence.

References and Suggested Reading

Biddle D, Macintire DK: Obstetrical emergencies, *Clin Tech Small Anim Pract* 15:88, 2000.

Burstyn U: Management of mastitis and abscessation of mammary glands secondary to fibroadenomatous hyperplasia in a primiparturient cat, *J Am Vet Med Assoc* 236:326, 2010.

Davidson AP, Baker TW: Reproductive ultrasound of the bitch and queen, *Top Companion Anim Med* 24:55, 2009.

Dickie MB, Arbeiter K: Diagnosis and therapy of the subinvolution of placental sites in the bitch, *J Reprod Fertil Suppl* 47:471, 1993.

Drobatz KJ, Casey KK: Eclampsia in dogs: 31 cases (1995-1998), *J Am Vet Med Assoc* 217:216, 2000.

Grundy SA, Davidson AP: Acute metritis secondary to retained fetal membranes and a retained nonviable fetus, *J Am Vet Med Assoc* 224:844, 2004.

Sontas HB et al: Full recovery of subinvolution of placental sites in an American Staffordshire terrier bitch, *J Small Anim Pract* 52:42, 2011.

Vaughan L, McGuckin S: Uterine prolapse in a cat, *Vet Rec* 132:568, 1993.

Ververidis HN et al: Experimental staphylococcal mastitis in bitches: clinical, bacteriological, cytological, haematological and pathological features, *Vet Microbiol* 124:95, 2007.

Wiebe VJ, Howard JP: Pharmacologic advances in canine and feline reproduction, *Top Companion Anim Med* 24:71, 2009.

CHAPTER 210

Nutrition in the Bitch and Queen During Pregnancy and Lactation

DAVID A. DZANIS, *Santa Clarita, California*

Gestation and lactation place some of the most rigorous nutritional demands on the dam, especially when compared with the adult, nonreproducing animal. A dietary deficiency or excess in one or more nutrients during this life stage can have profound effects on the ability of the dam to conceive, deliver, and raise a healthy litter.

Successful nutritional management of the dam during pregnancy and lactation takes more than just recommending a particular brand of pet food. Instead, considering the nutrient needs of the individual animal, assessing the qualities of the ration in meeting those needs, and feeding the ration in an appropriate manner are critical elements. The American College of Veterinary Nutrition (ACVN) has developed a graphic representation to help demonstrate these basic principles (Figure 210-1).

Determining Nutrient Requirements

Energy

The nutrient of greatest increased demand during pregnancy and especially lactation is energy. Because daily caloric need of a given individual also is influenced greatly by body size, breed, age, activity, and environmental conditions, perhaps the best means of expressing energy needs for pregnancy and lactation is as a proportion of the normal energy requirements of the same animal at maintenance. However, to do that requires knowledge of the dam's energy needs at maintenance.

A number of equations are used to determine maintenance energy requirements of the dog, but perhaps the most widely accepted equation provided by the National Research Council (NRC, 2006) is for metabolizable energy (ME) in kilocalories per day:

$$\text{ME (kcal/day)} = 130 \times \text{Body weight (kg)}^{0.75}$$

Although some equations do not rely on an exponent and thus are easier to calculate, determination of metabolic body weight by this method best accounts for the great diversity in adult body size in dogs. The constant in the formula (130) was determined in dogs under laboratory conditions; thus it assumes the dog to be at a moderate activity level and in environmentally favorable conditions during most of the day. Actual maintenance requirements of a given individual may vary up to 30% either way. A mostly indoor, sedentary house pet requires less to maintain body weight than an outdoor, kenneled dog. Breed and body size are also factors. For example, the equation coefficient may vary from 94 for a large pet dog to 175 for a highly active pet Border collie.

For cats, the equations recommended by NRC (2006) for estimating maintenance energy requirements are similar in format to the dog equation. Cats have less of a range of adult body sizes and are less apt to be highly active or exposed to extreme environmental conditions compared with dogs. Therefore variability in caloric requirements between individuals may be narrower. However, differences in requirements are seen with increasing body condition score (BCS); overweight cats require fewer calories per kilogram (kg) to maintain body weight. To account for this difference, ME can be calculated by two equations, one for "lean" (BCS ≤5 on a scale of 1 to 9) and one for "overweight" (BCS >5):

$$\text{Lean cats: ME (kcal/day)} = 100 \times \text{Body weight (kg)}^{0.67}$$

$$\text{Overweight cats: ME (kcal/day)} = 130 \times \text{Body weight (kg)}^{0.4}$$

Because of the potentially large variation in caloric requirements, especially in dogs, perhaps a more practical means of determining needs of an individual is simply to monitor the amount of a given food (and number of calories that amount of food delivers) required to keep the animal in optimum body condition during prebreeding. During gestation and lactation the amount of the same food then can be adjusted by the appropriate proportion. If a more calorie-dense food is fed during these periods, the proportional increase would be modified relative to the calorie content of the old and new diets.

In the bitch the energy requirements for early and midgestation are approximately the same as those for maintenance (Figure 210-2). Although the fetuses are developing rapidly, they remain relatively small. Only in the last few weeks of gestation are additional calories needed for growth of the fetuses and maternal tissues. Depending on the number of fetuses, total weight gain by the time of parturition should be around 15% to 25%. At this time the bitch likely is consuming approximately

150% of her normal maintenance needs. Expressed differently, the increase in energy requirements above maintenance from the fourth week after mating until parturition is approximately 26 kcal of ME per kilogram of body weight per day.

Unlike in the bitch, increase in body weight and therefore caloric requirements of the gestating queen between mating and parturition are linear; that is, weight gain is steady and consistent throughout gestation. The weight gain in the queen during early pregnancy is not associated with fetal growth but apparently serves as an energy reserve to support later demands for lactation. Depending on the number of kittens, the mean body weight gain at the end of gestation is usually around 40% over premating body weight.

In the bitch, dramatic increases in energy needs are seen after the first week of lactation, even though the dam may be approaching or even falling below her prebreeding body weight after delivery. This effect is tempered somewhat in queens; she remains above prebreeding weight at parturition but then uses the fat stored during early pregnancy for lactation. Still, increased energy is needed in bitches and queens to meet the monumental nutritional demands of milk production for the ever-growing offspring. For both species, the calorie requirement of a given individual depends on the amount of milk production, which in turn is correlated with the number of offspring. In bitches with litters of one to four neonates, milk production can be estimated at 1% of the bitch's body weight per pup, which increases the bitch's energy requirement by 24 kcal of ME per kilogram of body weight per day for each puppy in the litter. For litters larger than four, milk production and caloric needs per additional pup are approximately half of these values, and the increase in milk yield as litters exceed eight pups is negligible. Put more simply, in a bitch during peak lactation (4 weeks after parturition) with a moderate-to-large litter, energy needs could be three or even up to four times the normal maintenance requirements. As the offspring are weaned and milk production declines, the calorie needs for lactation drop, and more energy can be directed toward reestablishing normal body weight.

The increase in caloric requirements for the queen may not be as dramatic as in the bitch, because the queen still is using energy she stored during early gestation and continues to lose weight during lactation. In the lactating queen, NRC (2006) recommends energy requirements in

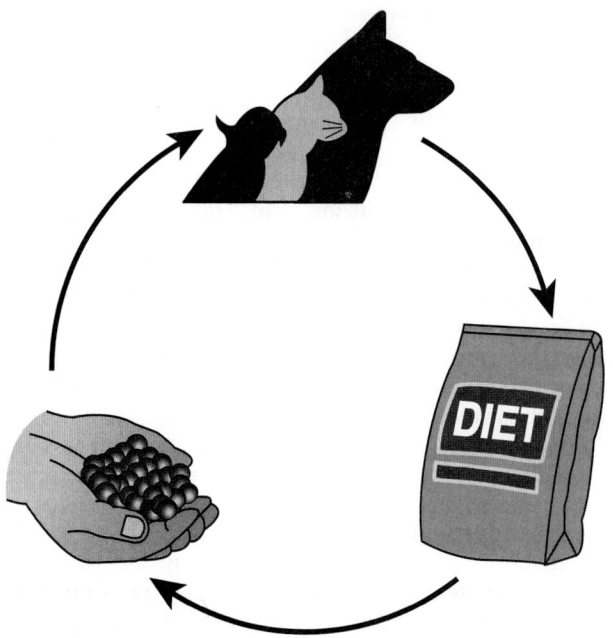

Figure 210-1 The American College of Veterinary Nutrition Iterative Process of Nutritional Assessment requires consideration of the animal, the ration, and the feeding management. (Courtesy American College of Veterinary Nutrition.)

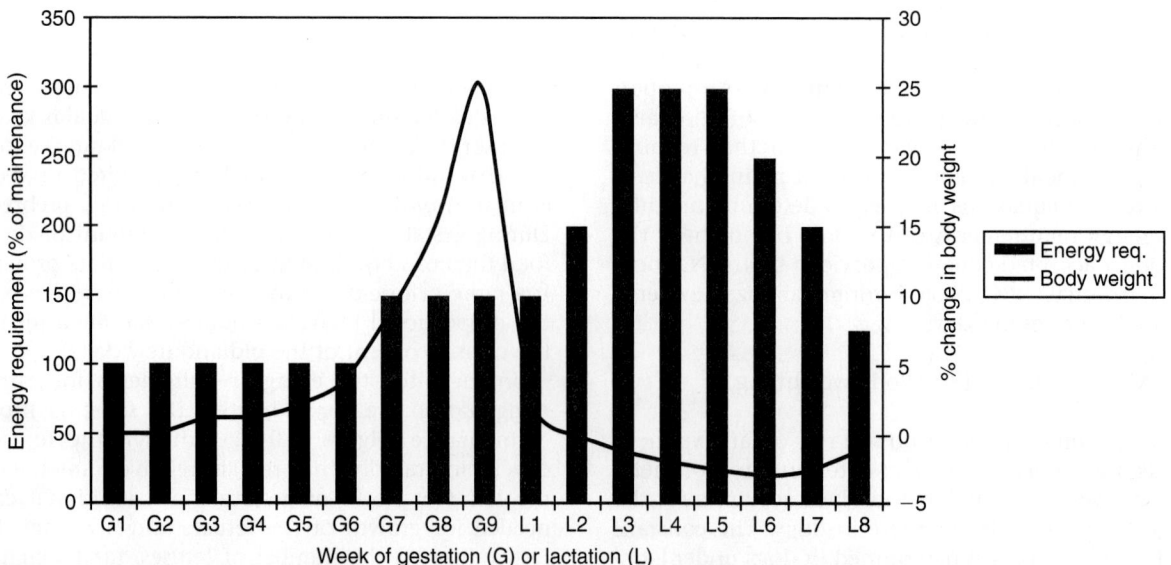

Figure 210-2 Energy needs and expected body weight changes of the bitch during gestation and lactation. (Modified from Case LP et al: *Canine and feline nutrition*, ed 3, St Louis, 2010, Mosby.)

kilocalories (kcal) per day above maintenance by the following equation:

$$ME\ (kcal/day) = maintenance + [K \times L \times Body\ weight\ (kg)]$$

Where K = 18, if number of kittens in litter less than 3,

K = 60, if number of kittens in litter 3 or 4, and

K = 70, if number of kittens in litter greater than 4,

And where L = 0.9 at first or second weeks of lactation,

L = 1.2 at third and fourth weeks of lactation,

L = 1.1 at fifth week of lactation,

L = 1.0 at sixth week of lactation, and

L = 0.8 at seventh week of lactation

For example, a 4-kg queen with three kittens in peak lactation (fourth week) would require 288 kcal per day above the 253 kcal/day required for maintenance. As a rule of thumb, an energy need 2 to 2.5 times the maintenance requirement is expected during lactation.

Other Essential Nutrients

In addition to calories, the needs for most other essential nutrients (e.g., amino acids, minerals, vitamins) increase during this life stage. For example, more protein, calcium, and phosphorus are needed for proper growth and bone development of the puppies and kittens. The Association of American Feed Control Officials (AAFCO) Dog and Cat Food Nutrient Profiles indicate for which nutrients are increased dietary needs above maintenance of the reproducing bitch or queen. For example, increased intake of dietary salt above maintenance needs is indicated to support normal milk production in the bitch, whereas the dietary levels of vitamins A and D are higher for reproducing queens versus cats at adult maintenance. Although many of the nutrient requirements in the AAFCO profiles appear the same for all life stages, absence of an established difference in the profiles between growth and reproduction versus maintenance reflects the lack of data showing a decreased need in the adult at maintenance (especially for many of the trace minerals and vitamins). Furthermore, although the amount in the diet may appear to remain the same, the actual daily intake of a given nutrient is higher in the gestating/lactating bitch or queen because of increased food intake.

Fatty Acids

One recommendation by the NRC not incorporated into the AAFCO Dog or Cat Food Nutrient Profiles is for dietary omega-3 fatty acids, specifically of α-linolenic acid (ALA) and eicosapentaenoic acid (EPA) and docosahexaenoic acid (DHA) in combination. Although no apparent developmental abnormalities caused by omega-3 fatty acid deficiencies have been reported for any commercial pet food, DHA, and to a lesser extent its precursors ALA and EPA, appear to be important in normal nervous tissue development of puppies and kittens. Notwithstanding inclusion of fish oil or other sources of DHA in foods intended for postweaned puppies to improve "trainability," only recently has there been evidence of effect on brain development or learning by this stage in either the puppy's or the kitten's life (Zicker et al, 2012). However, improvement in retinal function in young dogs was seen when the dams were fed omega-3 fatty acids during gestation and lactation, perhaps by transfer *in utero* but more likely via the milk during the early neonatal period (Bauer et al, 2006). Regardless, inclusion of omega-3 fatty acids in the diet of the gestating/lactating bitch and queen is prudent. The NRC recommended allowance for foods for dogs in gestation and lactation for ALA is 0.08% dry matter or 0.2 g/1000 kcal ME and for EPA and DHA in combination is 0.05% dry matter or 0.13 g/1000 kcal ME. The NRC also recommends these fatty acids for gestating/lactating queens but at lower amounts (ALA = 0.02% dry matter, 0.05 g/1000 kcal ME; EPA/DHA = 0.01% dry matter or 0.025 g/1000 kcal ME). Revisions to the AAFCO Dog and Cat Food Nutrient Profiles are expected by 2014, including anticipated similar minimum requirements for these fatty acids in foods intended for growth and reproduction.

Nutritional Disorders During Pregnancy and Lactation

Eclampsia

The presence of eclampsia, a condition characterized by periparturient hypocalcemia in both species (more commonly in the bitch, especially during early lactation), may be thought to imply that dietary calcium requirements of late gestation have not been met and that further supplementation is indicated. Although definitive studies on the prevention of this condition in companion animals are lacking, a lesson may be drawn from what is known about milk fever, a similar condition in dairy cows. Contrary to intuition, the calcium needs of the growing fetus are relatively low, and a high dietary calcium intake during gestation initiates responses to suppress calcium intestinal absorption and bone and kidney resorption in the mother. Then, when lactation ensues, the dramatic loss of calcium into the milk cannot be countered by normal metabolic responses, and the animal cannot maintain normocalcemia regardless of dietary intake of calcium at that stage. On the other hand, a low calcium intake in cattle helps ensure that bone calcium remains relatively mobile and responsive to the sudden demands of lactation. The syndromes in companion animals and cows are different. Data are lacking to indicate that a low-calcium diet in late gestation is an effective preventive in dogs and cats. However, calcium supplementation beyond that already provided in a balanced diet (which is already increased compared with diets intended for maintenance) may be imprudent at best.

Hypoglycemia

Although infrequent in the dog and not well documented in the cat, periparturient hypoglycemia can occur, usually in the last weeks of gestation. Although carbohydrates are not recognized as essential nutrients in either species, the diet of the gestating/lactating dam should provide at least 20% of its energy content from carbohydrates to mitigate the risk of periparturient hypoglycemia, to ensure ample glucose for the developing fetuses, and to help maintain lactose levels in the milk. Historically, most pet foods (and all dry or semi-moist foods) contained an ample source of carbohydrates, with the exception of some exclusive canned and frozen pet food products (e.g., "all beef"). However, considering the increased popularity for feeding pets "low-carb" diets in recent years, the clinician should assess the food for adequate carbohydrate content regardless of form.

Dehydration

Finally, adequate water intake should not be overlooked, especially during periods of heavy demand such as at peak lactation. Lack of adequate intake could hurt the dam and the offspring from decreased milk production. Although data are lacking on the minimum water requirement of gestating/lactating bitches and queens, it is presumed to be proportional to energy intake (1 ml water per 1 kcal ME consumed for dogs, 0.6 ml water per 1 kcal ME consumed for cats). Clean, fresh water should be made available at all times, and dams must be monitored for signs of dehydration and/or decreased milk production.

Choosing the Appropriate Food

An abundance of high-quality, nutritionally "complete and balanced" commercial foods are available for feeding bitches and queens in gestation and lactation. The flavor, form (dry vs. canned), and presence or absence of a particular ingredient are not as important as the product's substantiation of nutritional adequacy. To ensure that the product is suitable to be fed as the sole source of nutrition, the information panel on the label should bear either of the following: "(Product Name) is formulated to meet the nutritional levels established by the AAFCO Dog (or Cat) Food Nutrient Profiles," or "Animal feeding tests following AAFCO procedures substantiate that (Product Name) provides complete and balanced nutrition." If it bears the statement that it is intended "for intermittent or supplemental feeding only," includes reference to AAFCO in a manner other than either of the previous statements, refers to an organization other than AAFCO, or contains no reference to nutritional adequacy, the product should not be presumed to be nutritionally sufficient.

The first AAFCO nutritional substantiation method requires that the product contain adequate but not excessive quantities of all recognized essential nutrients compared with the AAFCO Profiles, such as amino acids, calcium, and vitamin A. These levels were established using the results of scientific studies demonstrating adequacy of a given nutrient and then adding adjustment factors to allow for differences in bioavailability of nutrients in commonly used ingredients. For the feeding trial method, a specified number of bitches or queens must be fed the product as the sole source of nutrition (except water) from breeding through peak lactation (4 and 6 weeks after parturition, for dogs and cats, respectively). Performance is judged on acceptable maintenance of body weight compared with prebreeding, normal hematologic and serum biochemical values, and lack of any other clinical or pathologic sign of nutritional deficiency or excess. In addition, litter size, survivability, and weight of the puppies or kittens at the end of the trial must compare favorably to animals fed a ration previously shown to be complete and balanced nutritionally.

The profile method and the feeding trial method have their advantages and disadvantages, and neither is perfect. Overall the feeding trial method is the preferred choice of substantiation. However, under current AAFCO Model Pet Food Regulations for a "product family," a pet food deemed to be "nutritionally similar" to a tested product can bear a statement suggesting completion of animal feeding tests, even though the food actually never underwent the feeding trial. This is particularly troublesome because products substantiated under the product family criteria share the disadvantages of the profile and the feeding trial methods and therefore offer the least assurance of nutritional adequacy. Some product family member labels may bear a statement that accurately reflects the fact that the product is "nutritionally similar" to a tested product, but because of a provision in the regulations most circumvent this statement. Instead, most product family members bear the same statement allowed on the tested "lead member" products. Thus the veterinarian or pet owner may not know whether the particular food was tested solely on the basis of labeling.

The good news is that the majority of products bearing the "animal feeding tests" label statements also are formulated to meet the AAFCO Profiles but simply do not allude to that fact on the label. On the other hand, a product bearing the AAFCO Profile statement most probably has not been subject to a feeding trial. Because each method has its pros and cons the best assurance of nutritional adequacy is if the product meets *both* criteria. The manufacturer's representative for any specific product should be able to attest to and document its product family status and whether the feeding-tested product also meets the AAFCO Profiles.

Another component of the nutritional adequacy statement is the food's suitability for the intended life stage. Few if any labels bear reference to nutritional adequacy for female reproduction. Instead, most cite suitability for "all life stages," which includes the rigorous demands of gestation and lactation. Not all intended uses of the product may be evident from the front panel designation. Many of the higher-end "adult" foods may in fact be suitable for all life stages, as would be indicated on the information panel. This is meant to distinguish the product from the manufacturer's "puppy" or "kitten" product, which is generally a bit higher in nutrient density than the adult formula. Regardless, both have been held up to the same nutritional criteria, and, although relatively more of the adult formula may have to be fed compared with the growth formula, both should perform as expected. In some cases the all-life stage, "adult" formula may be more appropriate for the dam with a propensity for excessive weight gain.

Clients who prefer to offer a raw or other home-formulated food rather than a commercial food should realize that a given recipe from books, Internet websites, or elsewhere is not obligated to meet regulatory requirements to be "complete and balanced." Although testimonials or other assurances of the suitability of a given home formulation may abound, clients should seek the advice of a board-certified veterinary nutritionist or other professional sufficiently trained to evaluate scientifically the nutritional content of the proposed diet. Furthermore, recipes in which ingredients are not cooked may present an increased risk of harboring potentially pathogenic organisms. To mitigate the possible risk to animal and human health, appropriate handling and sanitary measures must be followed.

Feeding Management

Feeding management of the reproducing bitch or queen should begin well before breeding. Difficulties in conception, parturition, and successful rearing of healthy offspring may occur in a dam that is either underconditioned or overweight. Strategies to bring the dam to optimum weight should begin many months before expected breeding. By the time of mating, the bitch or queen should be at a stable, if not ascending, plane of nutrition. By no means should success be assumed if the animal is on a weight loss regimen at the time of breeding.

Under AAFCO Model Pet Food Regulations, feeding directions are required on all "complete and balanced" product labels, although the ranges of recommended feeding amounts are often too broad to be useful. Also, foods meeting the "all life stage" nutritional criteria but designated just for adult use generally do not have directions for the pregnant or lactating dam. A preferred method to determine amounts to be fed is to calculate the energy needs of the animal as described previously and then compare them to the calorie content of the diet. Voluntary calorie content label statements are allowed; however, except as required for "lite" or "less calories" products intended for weight loss, these statements rarely appear on the label. If stated, the energy content must be expressed in terms of kilocalories per kilogram of food as fed. More consumer-friendly units (e.g., kilocalories per cup or can) also may be given. If the latter information is not provided, measuring the number of cups in a known weight of food such as a 20-pound bag usually gives a more accurate estimate than trying to weigh precisely a single cup of product.

In 2005 the ACVN proposed an amendment to the AAFCO regulations to require calorie content statements on all dog and cat food labels and to require these statements in terms of kilocalories of ME per kilogram and kilocalories of ME per cup or can. The amendment was adopted by AAFCO in January 2013, and the revised regulations will appear in the 2014 Official Publication. However, there will be a grace period for enforcement. Although the length of time to allow for complete compliance has yet to be decided, it is possible that some products may not bear the required calorie content statement until 2017. Until that time, alternative methods of determining calorie content may be necessary. If the label calorie content information is absent or incomplete, the manufacturer's representative may be able to provide that information. Alternatively, calorie content can be estimated from the guaranteed analysis values using the following formula:

$$ME \text{ (kcal/kg as fed)} = [(3.5 \times CP) + (8.5 \times CF) + (3.5 \times NFE)] \times 10$$

where CP = percentage of crude protein, CF = percentage of crude fat, and NFE = percentage of nitrogen-free extract (carbohydrate), which is 100 minus the sum of percentages for crude protein, crude fat, crude fiber, moisture, and ash (AAFCO, 2013). This formula tends to overestimate the true calorie content of high-fiber or poor-quality foods and underestimate that of very digestible products. However, the equation tends to be more predictive of true caloric content for cat foods than for dog foods, not because of a species difference but probably because of less variability in crude fiber and NFE content between cat foods.

A reportedly more accurate, albeit more complicated, calculation of ME for dog foods has been suggested by the NRC (2006):

$$Gross \text{ energy (GE)} = (5.7 \times CP) + (9.4 \times CF) + [4.1 \times (NFE + \% \text{ crude fiber})]$$

$$Percentage \text{ energy digestibility (PED)} = 91.2 - [1.43 \times (\% \text{ Crude fiber/proportion dry matter})]$$

$$Digestible \text{ energy (DE)} = GE \times PED/100$$

$$ME = [DE - (1.04 \times CP)] \times 10$$

A similar equation also exists for cat foods but with different values used to estimate energy digestibility and energy loss from metabolism.

An example of estimation of ME for a dog food using both methods on the same guaranteed analysis values is found in Figure 210-3. The NRC method does yield a higher estimate for this relatively higher-fat, lower-fiber example. As an alternative to using the NRC method, substitution of the coefficients for CP, CF, and NFE with the values 4, 9, and 4, respectively, in the previous AAFCO formula may yield more accurate results when estimating the calorie content of a higher-quality or homemade diet for either a cat or dog. Regardless, the AAFCO formula is still a good means of comparing energy content among products. Because this formula calculates energy on an as-fed basis, further conversion to dry matter (i.e., the derived value divided by the proportion of the nonmoisture component of the diet) is necessary to compare among products of different moisture contents such as a dry versus a canned or semi-moist product.

Regardless of feeding directions or previous estimates of energy needs, an individual animal may vary greatly in its true requirements. Therefore careful monitoring of body weight and body condition score, with adjustment

Guaranteed analysis:
    Crude protein 28%
    Crude fat   16%
    Crude fiber   3%
    Moisture   10%
    Ash   5%
                   62% Nitrogen-free extract (NFE) = 100% − 62% = 38%

Proportion dry matter = (100% − 10%)/100% = 0.9

AAFCO Method

28 × 3.5 = 98
16 × 8.5 = 136
38 × 3.5 = 133
     Total   367

Calorie content = 367 × 10 = 3670 kcal ME/kg as fed
                = 3670/0.9 = 4078 kcal ME/kg dry matter

NRC Method

28 × 5.7 = 159.6
16 × 9.4 = 150.4
41 × 4.1 = 168.1
     Total   478.1

91.2 − (1.43 × 3/0.9) = 86.4
478.1 × 86.4/100 = 413
413 − (1.04 × 28) = 384

Calorie content = 384 × 10 = 3840 kcal ME/kg as fed
                = 3840/0.9 = 4267 kcal ME/kg dry matter

Figure 210-3 Example of estimating calorie content in a dog food from label guaranteed analysis values using Association of American Feed Control Officials and National Research Council formulas.

in intake as needed to maintain optimum condition, is warranted.

In the bitch, no change in food, feeding amount, or frequency usually is indicated the first two thirds of gestation. A temporary drop in voluntary food consumption may be observed during estrus and again in midgestation, but this is normal and does not indicate a need for adjusting the feeding management as long as body weight and condition are acceptable. Beginning about 3 weeks before expected whelping, a gradual increase in nutrient intake should be initiated. This can be done simply by increasing the amount of food offered or by switching to a more calorie-dense food. The frequency of feeding may have to be increased to accommodate the increased intake. By time of parturition, a calorie intake approximately 50% above prebreeding needs should be anticipated.

In the queen, an increase in feeding amounts should begin immediately after mating. At this stage, free-choice feeding usually is indicated if not already the norm. If the recommended energy allowance of 25% to 50% above maintenance needs is not met by increased consumption, a change to a more calorie-dense food is prudent. As with the bitch, some fluctuation in appetite during gestation may be observed but generally does not indicate a problem as long as body weight continues to increase.

As the dam enters peak lactation, caloric requirements may double or more for queens and triple or more for bitches. If not already switched during gestation, switching the diet to a more energy-dense product generally is indicated. Offering food free choice may be necessary for the bitch to be able to consume adequate quantities throughout the day. Some degree of weight loss compared with prebreeding may be anticipated; however, if body weight drops more than a few percent below weight at maintenance, a more calorie-dense food should be offered. As the offspring are weaned and the dam regains any lost weight, the amounts offered can be cut back slowly so that she is near normal food intake and body weight by the time milk production has ceased.

Assuming that the appropriate food is selected as discussed previously, no dietary supplementation should be necessary. At best supplements may do no harm, but injudicious use may create nutrient excesses. The example of calcium is given earlier. However, even something as simple as added fat to increase total caloric intake may be detrimental if it suppresses intake of the mainstay diet because it decreases intake of all other essential nutrients.

References and Suggested Reading

Association of American Feed Control Officials: *Official publication*, Oxford, Ind, 2013, AAFCO.

Bauer JE et al: Retinal functions of young dogs are improved and maternal plasma phospholipids are altered with diets containing long-chain n-3 polyunsaturated fatty acids during gestation, lactation, and after weaning, *J Nutr* 136(suppl):1991S, 2006.

Case LP et al: *Canine and feline nutrition*, ed 3, St Louis, 2010, Mosby.

Debraekeleer J, Gross KL, Zicker SC: *Feeding reproducing dogs*. In Hand MS, editor: *Small animal clinical nutrition*, ed 5, Topeka, Kan, 2010, Mark Morris Institute, p 281.

Dzanis DA: Ensuring nutritional adequacy. In Kvamme JL, Phillips TD, editors: *Petfood technology*, Mt. Morris, Ill, 2003, Watt Publishing, p 62.

National Research Council: *Nutrient requirements of dogs and cats*, Washington, DC, 2006, National Academies Press.

Zicker SC et al: Evaluation of cognitive learning, memory, psychomotor, immunologic, and retinal functions in healthy puppies fed foods fortified with docosahexaenoic acid–rich fish oil from 8 to 52 weeks of age, *J Am Vet Med Assoc* 241:583, 2012.

CHAPTER 211

Pyometra

FRANCES O. SMITH, *Burnsville, Minnesota*

Pyometra is a disease of the uterus, literally meaning *pus in the uterus*. Similar clinical entities include mucometra and hydrometra. Pyometra typically occurs in the estrogen-primed uterus during the period of progesterone dominance (diestrus) or thereafter (anestrus). It most commonly is diagnosed in an intact bitch from 4 weeks to 4 months after an estrous cycle. Pyometra is not as common in the queen as in the bitch because the queen is an induced ovulatory and thus does not experience repetitive estrogen and progesterone influences on the uterus. Many studies highlight an increased incidence of pyometra in nulliparous bitches and in bitches over 4 years of age. The queen has an increased incidence of pyometra with increasing age. In addition, African lions have been shown to have an increased risk of developing pyometra.

Pregnancy has a sparing effect on the uterus. In one study of multiple breeds, previous pregnancy had a protective effect on the incidence of pyometra in the rottweiler, collie, and Labrador retriever but was not protective for the golden retriever. Thus protective factors and risk factor may vary between breeds. There is no correlation between clinical signs of false pregnancy and pyometra in the bitch.

Pathogenesis

In one colony of beagles the incidence of pyometra was 15.2% of bitches older than 4 years of age, with the average age of onset 9.36 ± 0.35 years (Fukuda, 2001). In a population of insured dogs in Sweden in which routine ovariohysterectomy is disallowed, the crude 12-month incidence of pyometra over the 2-year period from 1995 through 1996 was approximately 2% in bitches under 10 years of age (Egenvall et al, 2001). A recent publication involving Swedish bitches lists the incidence of pyometra of bitches under 10 years of age at 25% (Hagman et al, 2011).

The pathogenesis of pyometra in the bitch involves estrogen stimulation followed by prolonged periods of progesterone dominance. Progesterone results in endometrial proliferation, glandular secretions, and decreased myometrial contractions. Leukocyte inhibition in the progesterone-primed uterus tends to support bacterial growth. These effects are cumulative with each estrous cycle, exacerbating the uterine pathology. Cystic endometrial hyperplasia (CEH) pyometra has four stages. Stage one is uncomplicated CEH. Stage two is CEH with endometrial infiltration of plasma cells. Stage three is CEH with acute endometritis. Finally, Stage four is CEH with chronic endometritis.

Estrogen therapy is associated with an increased risk of pyometra in bitches from 1 to 4 years of age. Use of estrogens (estradiol cypionate) for mismating in diestrous bitches is particularly dangerous and has resulted in approximately a 25% occurrence rate of pyometra. Furthermore, use of estrogens in the bitch has a potential for idiosyncratic, non–dose-related bone marrow suppression. The one (and only) time this author used estradiol cypionate for mismating in an 18-month-old golden retriever resulted in an open cervix pyometra. In queens, the administration of medroxyprogesterone acetate for estrus suppression increases the risk for development of pyometra.

Risk for pyometra is increased in several breeds, including the golden retriever, miniature schnauzer, Irish terrier, Saint Bernard, Airedale terrier, cavalier King Charles spaniel, rough collie, rottweiler, and Bernese mountain dog.

Clinical Findings

The medical history of a female dog with pyometra can be nonspecific. The queen may have nonspecific illness and a vaginal discharge. In older bitches the client may not recognize an estrous cycle and assume that the bitch has experienced "menopause." The client also may mistake a serosanguineous vaginal discharge associated with pyometra with that of a normal estrus. Vaginal cytology helps to differentiate the prevailing hormonal events at the time of initial examination. Clinical history of bitches and queens with pyometra often includes depression, inappetence, polydipsia, polyuria, lethargy, and abdominal enlargement with or without vaginal discharge. Pyometra always should be in the differential diagnosis of a sick, intact bitch or queen.

Bitches and queens with pyometra typically are afebrile. An elevated white blood count is typical, and hyperproteinemia and hyperglobulinemia also are common. An acute phase protein α-1-acid glycoprotein is elevated in the bitch with pyometra; however, this test is not readily available in clinical practice. Prerenal azotemia accompanies dehydration, but urine-concentrating ability may be impaired. Bitches with pyometra that have urine protein creatinine ratio (UPC) greater than 1.0 or high ratios of urinary biomarkers may have clinically significant renal lesions and should receive follow-up monitoring of renal function after the resolution of the pyometra. Cystocentesis is associated with the risk of perforation of the fluid-filled uterus and possible spillage of uterine contents into the abdomen. The most common organism isolated from the uterus or vaginal discharge of a bitch with pyometra is *Escherichia coli*. Culture and sensitivity of the vaginal discharge or of intrauterine fluid at the time of ovariohysterectomy should be performed to guide antibiotic therapy.

The vaginal discharge in the CEH/pyometra complex may be purulent, sanguinopurulent (the color and consistency of tomato soup), mucoid, or frankly hemorrhagic. Vaginal discharge of any description should alert the clinician to include pyometra in the differential diagnosis. Other causes of vaginal discharge include vaginitis, estrus, immune-mediated thrombocytopenia (bloody discharge), anticoagulant toxicity, metritis, and subinvolution of placental sites.

Diagnosis is accomplished best with ultrasonography and/or radiography. The classic radiographic finding is a fluid-filled, tubular organ between the descending colon and the bladder that presents a sausage-like appearance. The uterus is visualized best with a lateral abdominal radiograph. A fluid-filled organ can be identified ultrasonographically, and the uterine wall thickness and proliferative changes also can be noted.

Therapy

The preferred treatment for any aged or ill bitch or for a bitch or queen with closed cervix pyometra is complete ovariohysterectomy. Medical treatment of bitches with closed cervix pyometra may result in uterine rupture or in seepage of uterine contents into the abdomen. This author does not advocate the use of medical management for any bitch with a closed cervix pyometra. Surgical uterine drainage and lavage with a 5% povidone-iodine in saline solution via transcervical catheterization was successful in the treatment of eight bitches with pyometra. All eight bitches conceived and whelped after treatment (DeCramer, 2010). Bitches that are seriously ill should be stabilized medically with appropriate intravenous fluid therapy and broad-spectrum antibiotics before surgery. The clinician should be prepared to deal with bacteremia and endotoxemia. Disseminated intravascular coagulation is an infrequent but possible complication of pyometra.

Young bitches or queens with breeding value and an open cervix, normal organ function, together with a compliant and reasonable owner, may be treated with prostaglandins. Prostaglandins increase myometrial contractility, encourage cervical relaxation, allow expulsion of the uterine contents, and with repeated doses result in lysis of the corpus luteum. Serum progesterone should be measured before treatment with prostaglandins.

The most frequently administered drug is prostaglandin $F_2\alpha$ ($PGF_2\alpha$) at a dosage of 250 µg/kg q12h SC until the uterus reduces to near normal in size, which typically takes 3 to 5 days. Therapy that requires a longer treatment period or a recurrence of fluid in the uterus signals a negative prognosis for prostaglandin treatment success. In 20

queens treated for open cervix pyometra with $PGF_2\alpha$, 90% responded to therapy and subsequently delivered a normal litter (Johnston, Kustritz, and Olson, 2001). A vaginal culture should be obtained before treatment, and appropriate antibiotics administered for 3 to 4 weeks after therapy. Many other protocols have been published, starting with doses of $PGF_2\alpha$ as low as 50 µg/kg and gradually increasing to 250 µg/kg over the treatment period to decrease the side effects of panting, nausea, salivation, vomiting, and diarrhea—all of which are commonly seen 15 to 45 minutes after each injection. The side effects decrease in severity with each dose. One study described the use of $PGF_2\alpha$ (150 µg/kg) in 17 bitches with pyometra administered by infusing 0.3 ml/10 kg of body weight into the vaginal canal one or two times daily for 4 to 12 days (Gabor, Siver, and Szenci, 1999). Bitches received intramuscular antibiotics and the intravaginal infusion. Treatment was effective in 86.6% of these bitches. It has been reported that cloprostenol, a $PGF_2\alpha$ analog, has been used successfully for treatment of open cervix pyometra. However, this author does not use cloprostenol because it is far more potent and has great potential for accidental overdosage. Also, progesterone receptor blockers (e.g., mifepristone and aglepristone) have been used to treat open cervix pyometra in Europe. Aglepristone treatment was most effective in bitches under 5 years of age. These antiprogestins are not commercially available in the United States. Prostaglandins are not approved for small animal use in the United States; thus an informed consent form, including risks of treatment, should be obtained before therapy. In this author's opinion, prostaglandins should *never* be dispensed for client administration because of the narrow safety index and the potential for triggering asthmatic events and pregnancy loss in humans.

Bitches treated with prostaglandins may have their interestrous interval shortened slightly. The bitch should have a vaginal culture, be treated with appropriate antibiotics, and be bred to a fertile male at her next estrous cycle. Success results in conception rates of 50% to 65%. Fertility in bitches after pyometra therapy is decreased when compared with normal bitches. Failure to conceive or failure to be bred results in a high incidence of recurrence of pyometra, with recurrence rates as high as 77%. This author has observed pyometra in subsequent generations of chow-chows and English setters of young age, suggesting a possible familial tendency toward early development of CEH in these animals.

References and Suggested Reading

Bowen RA et al: Efficacy and toxicity of estrogens commonly used to terminate canine pregnancy, *J Am Vet Med Assoc* 186:783, 1985.

De Cramer KG: Surgical uterine drainage and lavage as treatment for canine pyometra, *J S Afr Vet Assoc* 81:172, 2012.

Egenvall A et al: Breed risk of pyometra in insured dogs in Sweden, *J Vet Intern Med* 15:530, 2001.

Fukuda S: Incidence of pyometra in colony-raised beagle dogs, *Exp Anim* 50:325, 2001.

Gabor G, Siver L, Szenci O: Intravaginal prostaglandin F2 alpha for the treatment of metritis and pyometra in the bitch, *Acta Vet Hung* 47:103, 1999.

Hagman R: Serum α-1-acid glycoprotein concentrations in 26 dogs with pyometra, *Vet Clin Pathol* 40:52, 2011.

Hagman R et al: A breed-matched case-control study of potential risk-factor for canine pyometra, *Theriogenology* 75(7):1251, 2011.

Johnston SD, Kustritz MV, Olson PNS: Disorders of the canine uterus and uterine tubes (oviducts). In Johnston SD, Kustritz MVR, Olson PNS, editors: *Canine and feline theriogenology,* Philadelphia, 2001, WB Saunders, p 206-469.

Jurka P et al: Age-related pregnancy results and further examination of bitches after aglepristone treatment of pyometra, *Reprod Domest Anim* 45:525, 2010.

Maddens B et al: Evaluation of kidney injury in dogs with pyometra based on proteinuria, renal histomorphology and urinary biomarkers, *J Vet Intern Med* 25:1075, 2011.

Troxel MT et al: Severe hematometra in a dog with cystic endometrial hyperplasia/pyometra complex, *J Am Anim Hosp Assoc* 38(1):85, 2002.

CHAPTER 212

Vulvar Discharge

RICHARD WHEELER, *Fort Collins, Colorado*

*V*aginal discharge, more accurately described as *vulvar discharge*, is a common presentation of intact or spayed bitches. Too often it is diagnosed erroneously as *vaginitis,* when in fact it is a symptom of an underlying problem of the urogenital system. The discharge actually may originate from the perivulvar region, vulva, vestibule, cervix, uterus, urethra, or urinary bladder with or without involvement of the vagina. Vulvar discharge in queens is uncommon and usually has a uterine cause (e.g., pyometra). Inappropriate use of antibiotics (overuse or insufficient duration) and failure to address the inciting cause are the most common reasons for treatment failure.

Clinical Signs

Presenting complaints include vulvar discharge, vulvar licking, vulvar swelling and hyperemia, clitoral hypertrophy, "scooting," pollakiuria, or recurrent urinary tract infections. Vulvar discharge may be mucoid, mucopurulent, purulent, or hemorrhagic. Purulent discharge may be suppurative (indicating irritation or infection) or lymphocytic (indicating allergic or immune mediated). Vaginal cytology rarely determines the etiology of the inflammation but confirms the presence of neutrophils. Degenerate neutrophils with swollen nuclei and intracellular bacteria indicate a septic component, whereas neutrophils with hypersegmented nuclei suggest a noninfectious, reactive component. A speculum or vaginoscopic exam is necessary to determine if the purulent discharge is confined to the vestibule or extends from the vagina. In spayed or nonestrous bitches, vaginal examination may require heavy sedation or anesthesia.

Etiology

Uterine Causes

In intact bitches, normal vulvar discharge originates from the uterus. It may be estral bleeding, cervical mucus during late gestation, fetal fluids at parturition, or lochia for up to 4 weeks after parturition. All other vulvar discharges in intact female dogs and all vulvar discharges in spayed females are abnormal. Pathologic uterine causes of vulvar discharges in intact and spayed bitches are summarized in Table 212-1. Involvement of the uterus must be ruled out when working up the complaint of vulvar discharge. Further insight into uterine diseases is beyond the scope of this chapter.

Lower Reproductive Tract Causes

The causes of vulvar discharges (not originating from the uterus) are similar in intact or spayed dogs and can be categorized broadly as causing *vaginitis* (inflammation of the vaginal vault from the vaginovestibular junction to the cervix), *vestibulitis* (inflammation of the vestibule from the vulvar mucosal margin to the vaginovestibular junction), and *perivulvar dermatitis* (inflammation of the skin around the vulva). These three entities may occur independently or one may incite either or both of the other two conditions. Also, a bacterial component may or may not be present. Proper treatment relies on elucidating and resolving the inciting condition.

Vaginitis

Vaginitis is inflammation, and commonly infection, of the mucosa cranial to the vaginovestibular junction

Pathologic Uterine Causes of Vulvar Discharges in Intact Bitches and Spayed Bitches with a Uterine Stump

Intact	Spayed
Subinvolution of placental site (SIPS)	Stump pyometra-ovarian remnant syndrome
Pyometra	Suture reaction (granulomatous)
Metritis	Infection (e.g., *Brucella canis*, enterics)
Ovarian diseases resulting in persistent estrus	Neoplasia
Uterine neoplasia	

Aerobic Bacteria Isolated from the Vagina of Healthy Dogs

Aeromonas	*Alcaligenes faecalis*
Bacillus spp.	*Bacteroides* spp.
*Chlamydia psittaci**	*Corynebacterium* spp.
*Clostridium perfringens**	*Escherichia coli**
*Enterococcus**	*Enterobacter* spp.*
Flavobacterium	*Lactobacillus*
Haemophilus spp.	*Klebsiella* spp.*
Micrococcus	*Moraxella*
Neisseria	*Pasteurella* spp.
Proteus spp.*	*Plesiomonas*
Pseudomonas spp.	*Staphylococcus aureus**
*Staphylococcus intermedius**	*Staphylococcus pseudintermedius*
Streptococcus spp. (β-hemolytic)*	*Streptococcus* spp. (α-hemolytic)
*Streptococcus pyogenes**	

*Bacteria isolated from dogs with vulvar discharge.

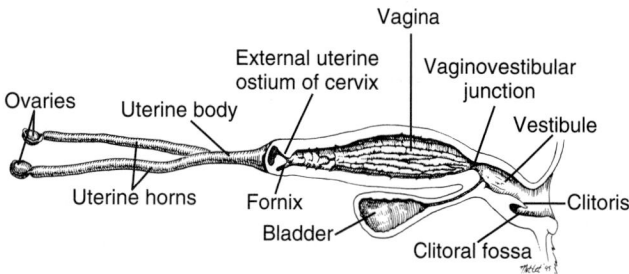

Figure 212-1 The canine female reproductive tract comprises ovaries, uterus, cervix, vagina, vaginovestibular junction, vestibule, vulva, and clitoris. (Used with permission from Johnston SD, Root Kustritz MV, Olson PNS: Sexual differentiation and normal anatomy of the bitch. In Johnston SD. Root Kustritz MV, Olson PNS, editors: *Canine and feline theriogenology,* Philadelphia, 2001, WB Saunders, p 1 [Figure 1-5A on page 6].)

(Figure 212-1) and is most often the symptom of an underlying problem. It often presents as purulent or mucopurulent vulvar discharge, and it must be differentiated from vestibulitis, pyometra, and other diseases that present as vulvar discharge. Direct visualization of the vaginal canal by speculum or vaginoscope helps to elucidate whether the discharge is originating from the vestibule, vagina, or cranial to the cervix. Cytologic examination and culture of a guarded swab passed cranial to the vestibule may implicate vaginal involvement. Finally, a vaginal biopsy definitively indicates the presence or absence of inflammation in the vagina. Vaginitis often is categorized into juvenile (puppy) vaginitis or adult-onset vaginitis.

Juvenile (Puppy) Vaginitis. Juvenile vaginitis commonly is seen in bitches between 6 weeks and 1 year of age. It develops as the bitch establishes a symbiotic relationship with her endogenous bacteria and naïve vagina. Puppy vaginitis may persist for months without detrimental effects on the puppy. In fact, juvenile vaginitis usually poses greater distress to the owner than to the puppy. Cytologic evaluation of the discharge usually demonstrates mature, hypersegmented, nondegenerate neutrophils; culture often results in no significant growth (that is, either no growth or low-level, mixed populations of normal vaginal flora [Table 212-2]).

Owners often request antibiotic treatment; however, conservative treatment usually is advised. Antibiotic therapy may predispose to opportunistic bacterial overgrowth in the absence of normal bacterial flora and development of antibiotic resistant strains of bacteria. If puppy vaginitis persists for more than 2 months or becomes excessive, irritating, or problematic, antibiotic therapy may be initiated based on culture and sensitivity results. However, discharge commonly returns when antibiotics are discontinued.

Conflicting opinions exist whether to spay affected bitches before the first estrus. The rationale for waiting until after the first estrus is that the influence of estradiol on the vaginal mucosa increases vascular circulation and local immune function, thereby clearing up the vaginitis. No clear evidence supports or disparages this theory.

Adult-Onset Vaginitis. Adult-onset vaginitis in the dog is often idiopathic. Common etiologies for vaginitis in adults include primary infections (*Brucella canis* or canine herpesvirus), infection secondary to a foreign body, urinary incontinence or urine pooling, ascending infections from vestibulitis, tumors or masses of the vagina, and abnormal development of the vagina such as strictures or vaginal bands.

Vestibulitis

Vestibulitis, or inflammation of the vestibule, involves the region from the vulvar mucosal junction to the

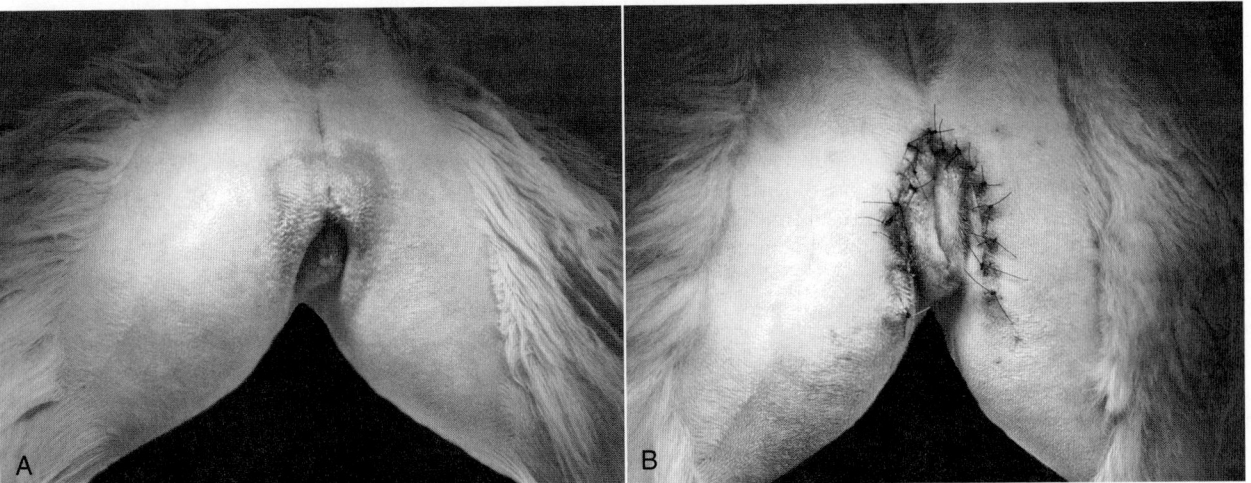

Figure 212-2 A hooded vulva predisposes the bitch to vestibulitis, perivulvar dermatitis, and vulvar discharge. The dorsal vulvar fold envelops more than one third of the lateral folds of the vulva **(A)**, which is surgically resolved with vulvoplasty **(B)**.

vaginovestibular junction (see Figure 212-1). Vestibulitis is perhaps the most common cause of purulent vulvar discharge and vulvar licking. It frequently occurs as a primary condition without involving the vagina or perivulvar region. Conformational abnormalities of the vulva (such as inverted vulvar folds, hooded vulva, clitoral hypertrophy, or ectopic hairs) and perineum (excessive perivulvar fat folds), or urinary incontinence (possibly subclinical) may induce mucosal irritation and subsequent vulvar discharge.

Perivulvar Dermatitis

Perivulvar dermatitis is inflammation of the skin around the vulva. Perivulvar dermatitis is caused commonly by allergies. *Atopy* commonly induces a histamine response associated with the perivulvar region as well as the axilla, interdigital spaces, and auricula. However, allergies do not appear to be associated with primary vestibulitis or vaginitis. Perivulvar dermatitis also may result from the same conformational defects and urinary incontinence that cause vestibulitis. The ensuing perivulvar irritation caused by any of these conditions induces chronic vulvar licking, which further maintains a moist environment, aggravates the condition, and often induces a swollen, erythematous vulva. Trapped or persistent moisture leads to secondary bacterial or yeast infections of the perivulvar skin, vestibule, or vagina. Yeasts isolated from the vagina and perineum of dogs include *Candida* spp., *Rhodotorula* spp., and *Malassezia pachydermatis*. These yeasts appear to be commensal organisms of the vagina and are not involved in causing vaginitis or vestibulitis. Chronic licking of the perivulvar region may result in development of a secondary vestibulitis or ascending vaginitis. Conversely, vestibulitis or vaginitis may initiate chronic licking that then results in secondary perivulvar dermatitis. Treatment of perivulvar dermatitis requires resolving the inciting cause and long-term antibiotics (4 to 6 weeks) to resolve completely the associated dermatitis to avoid reoccurrence.

Predisposing Factors

Conformational or Functional

Hooded Vulva

Hooded vulva (Figure 212-2), also called "juvenile vulva," is a conformational defect in which the dorsal fold of the vulva envelops and covers more than one third of the lateral vulvar folds. The overhanging skin traps moisture and predisposes the bitch to perivulvar dermatitis and vestibulitis. The entrapped hair also causes chronic irritation of the vulvar mucosa, contributing to vestibulitis. Clinically, it presents with vulvar discharge and vulvar licking. It is treated successfully by vulvoplasty (see Chapter 213).

Vestibulovaginal Stenosis

Narrowing of the reproductive tract at the level of the vaginovestibular junction is conformationally and functionally normal (see Figure 212-1). This narrowing prevents or limits ascending infection and retrograde movement of urine or foreign bodies into the vaginal vault. In maiden bitches, this is the location of the hymen, which may or may not be intact. The vaginovestibular junction is significantly narrow in bitches spayed before their first estrus (early [juvenile] spaying) because the reproductive tract has not matured; this should not be confused with vaginal stenosis. Vestibulovaginal stenosis is defined as when the ratio between the maximum vaginal lumen diameter and the diameter of the vaginal lumen at the level of the vaginovestibular junction is less than 0.33 as measured by retrograde vaginourethrography. A follow-up study showed no significance to narrowing of the vagina until the ratio approached less than 0.20 (Crawford and Adams, 2002). Strictures commonly are diagnosed as the cause of vaginitis; however, they are most likely incidental findings to which a diagnosis is attributed (Wang et al, 2006a; Wang et al, 2006b). Surgical correction of these strictures has not been shown to significantly affect resolution of vaginitis.

Vestibulovaginal Bands

Vestibulovaginal bands are vertical bands at the level of the vaginovestibular junction. They are remnants of embryonic development, in which fusion of the cranial and caudal vagina is incomplete. Although they often are implicated in causing vaginitis, they are likely incidental findings because many normal bitches are diagnosed with similar bands and no history of vaginitis. Surgical correction of vertical bands has not been shown to significantly resolve vaginitis.

Clitoral Hypertrophy

Clitoral hypertrophy occurs as a primary condition in pseudohermaphrodites and as a result of fetal masculinization from *in utero* exposure to exogenous progestins or testosterone. Clitoral hypertrophy also can develop from postnatal exposure to exogenous androgens (e.g., testosterone, mibolerone) or exogenous estrogens (e.g., diethylstilbestrol, topical human estrogen replacements). Chronic irritation and masturbation also can result in enlargement of the clitoris. Chronic exposure of the enlarged clitoris can result in desiccation, inflammation, and excoriation as well as ascending infection of the vestibule and vagina. If the inciting cause for clitoral hypertrophy cannot be determined and eliminated, clitoridectomy may be curative.

Neoplasia

The most common neoplasms affecting the vestibule and vagina are fibromas, polyps, leiomyomas, and transmissible venereal tumors. These have been covered in more detail in Chapter 222.

Foreign Body

Incidence of vaginal foreign bodies as the cause of vaginitis and vulvar discharge has been documented, but it is rare. Vaginoscopy is the diagnostic tool of choice. The most common foreign bodies are iatrogenic or fetal remains from prior pregnancies.

Infectious

Viral

Canine Herpesvirus. Canine herpesvirus infection can cause vesicular lesions on the vaginal or vestibular mucosa surface and may result in a secondary bacterial infection and subsequent vulvar discharge. Canine herpesvirus infection usually is self-limiting and does not require treatment.

Bacterial

Culture of suppurative vulvar discharge or a vaginal swab usually results in mixed growth of normal vaginal bacteria (see Table 212-2). Growth of a single type of bacteria may indicate bacterial overgrowth of a more virulent or opportunistic strain of bacteria, indicating an upset to normal bacterial flora. Culture rarely implicates a single bacterial agent and rarely elucidates the cause of vulvar discharge.

Brucella canis. *Brucella canis* is the only primary bacterial pathogen of the canine urogenital tract. It is an intracellular, gram-negative coccobacillus that localizes in the reproductive tract, eye, and spinal column. The incidence of *B. canis* is increasing in the United States in recent years because of the increased relocation of stray and abandoned dogs and increased breeding and use of shipped semen. *B. canis* rarely causes a primary vaginitis but should be considered in cases of chronic vulvar discharge because infection of the uterus or uterine stump by *B. canis* is possible.

Screening for *B. canis* is done routinely by a rapid card agglutination test or tube agglutination test. Both tests detect antibodies to *Brucella* spp. with a high sensitivity but low specificity. 2-Mercaptoethanol may be added to improve specificity and therefore rule out false-positive tests. Confirmation of all positive tests is recommended by agar gel immunodiffusion. The greatest limitation to serologic testing is the delay of seroconversion, which may take up to 12 weeks after exposure to be detectable. Chronically infected animals may have titers too low to detect (after 1 to 5 years), resulting in false negatives (e.g., negative test on a truly infected animal). Culture is the definitive positive diagnostic test; however, if the affected animal is not bacteremic at the time of sampling or if the bacteria go undetected because of low concentrations or overgrowth by other bacteria, false negatives can occur. Recent advances in ELISA and PCR technologies may make rapid detection of a very low concentration of *B. canis* possible and appear promising in the future diagnosis of *B. canis*. Serology and culture should be used in conjunction to identify reliably infected animals; testing should be repeated at multiple time points if indicated.

Recommended treatment of animals infected with *B. canis* is euthanasia to prevent the spread of *B. canis* to other dogs or people. (*B. canis* is zoonotic but is not contracted as easily as *B. abortus* or *B. ovis*.) The zoonotic potential of *B. canis* is becoming especially relevant with the increase in immune-compromised persons living with pets. Neuter (spay or castration) and long-term antibiotics can be attempted as treatment. However, the potential for transmission (although low) remains relevant because *B. canis* is not eliminated completely from the site of infection because antibiotic penetration into the cells is difficult. Antibiotic protocols include doxycycline (10 mg/kg q12h PO) in conjunction with rifampin (20 mg/kg q12h PO) for a minimum of 30 days; or enrofloxacin (5 mg/kg q12h PO) alone for a minimum of 30 days. However, owners who choose treatment over euthanasia should be warned of the potential for recurrence and transmission (to humans and other dogs). The dog should be isolated from all other dogs for the rest of its life and rechecked every 6 months by blood or vaginal swab culture for recrudescence and retreated if indicated.

Mycoplasma Species. *Mycoplasma* spp. are gram-negative, intracellular bacteria with no cell wall. They can be diagnosed easily and routinely in culture, but special requests using special media are necessary. Some *Mycoplasma* spp. do not grow well in culture and may go undetected. *Mycoplasma* is a commensal isolate from the canine vagina (23% to 73% normal dogs) and is considered normal bacterial flora (Box 212-1). The incidence of *Mycoplasma* isolation increases after antibiotic therapy. In addition to the reproductive tract, species of *Mycoplasma* have been isolated from the respiratory tract, oral cavity,

BOX 212-1

Isolates within the *Mycoplasma* Family (Mycoplasmataceae) from Healthy Dogs

Mycoplasma arginine
*Mycoplasma bovigenitalium**
Mycoplasma canis†‡*
Mycoplasma cynos‡*
Mycoplasma felis
*Mycoplasma feliminutum**
*Mycoplasma gateae**
Mycoplasma haemocanis
Mycoplasma edwardii†*
Mycoplasma molare†‡*
Mycoplasma maculosum†*
Mycoplasma opalescens†
Mycoplasma spumans†*
Ureaplasma canigenitalium†‖*
Acholeplasma laidlawii§‖*

*Isolated from canine genital tract.
†Canine specific.
‡Sialidase secreting.
§Specific to canine genital tract.
‖Belonging to the same class of "Mollicutes" and genetically isolated with the same DNA primers used for *Mycoplasma* species.

and auricular canal. *Mycoplasma canis* is the species most commonly isolated from the vagina.

Some disease conditions (e.g., canine infectious respiratory disease, also known as kennel cough) may be caused by *Mycoplasma* synergistically working with other infectious agents. *Mycoplasma* has a known synergistic relation in inducing infertility and abortion in ruminants, but no distinct correlation has been made in dogs. Although it is suspected in cases of canine infertility, pregnancy loss, and chronic vaginitis, experimental infections with *M. canis* have failed to fulfill satisfactorily Koch's postulates in reliably inducing disease. Further investigation is necessary to determine if specific *Mycoplasma* spp. are associated with infertility or abortion in bitches. Sialidase is a known virulence factor of bacteria and has been found in certain strains of *Mycoplasma* spp. in dogs. It functions by increasing microbial colonization and facilitating tissue invasion by inducing molecular damage to cell walls and extra cellular matrix. Sialidase-producing *Mycoplasma* spp. may be more virulent and someday may be shown to affect fertility adversely. Antibiotic treatment (e.g., doxycycline [5 mg/kg q12h PO] or enrofloxacin [5 to 10 mg/kg q12h PO]) often is used empirically as a treatment against *Mycoplasma* spp. for chronic vaginitis or infertility.

Treatment

Successful treatment of vulvar discharge is aimed at resolving the inciting cause. Many cases of adult-onset vaginitis and most cases of juvenile-onset vaginitis resolve with no specific treatment. Oral supplementation of probiotics has been shown to help maintain or establish healthy bacterial flora in the gut, and extrapolation to the vagina has been suggested. Some species of *Lactobacillus*

and *Enterococcus* alter the vaginal pH and may inhibit pathologic overgrowth of bacteria. Orally administered probiotic bacteria do transfer to the urogenital tract by fecal-oral transfer; but no benefit in treating or preventing vaginitis has been shown.

Treatment with antibiotics is discouraged unless an inciting cause has been diagnosed and treated or if perivulvar dermatitis is present. If antibiotics are used, their selection should rely on culture and sensitivity results. Numerous studies have isolated antibiotic-resistant bacteria, including methicillin-resistant *Staphylococcus pseudintermedius* from the canine vagina. Some veterinarians have been advocates of dilute Betadine solution or chlorhexidine solution lavage of the vagina in lieu of antibiotics. No evidence suggests that this facilitates a cure, and it has been implicated in delayed healing, supposedly from chronic irritation either from the retention of fluid or abrasion from the delivery device. In addition, dilute vinegar lavages or commercially available human vaginal douches are not indicated because canine vestibulitis and vaginitis have not been shown to be caused by yeasts.

Corticosteroid therapy in conjunction with antibiotics seems beneficial when allergies or immune stimulation appears to be related to the cause. This is the case with perivulvar dermatitis or when lymphocytes are present on cytologic evaluation of the vulvar discharge.

Some cases of vulvar discharge respond well to estrogen therapy. Estrogen increases the thickness of the vaginal mucosa (increasing resistance to bacteria) and increases blood supply to the vagina (improving immune function). Estrogen supplementation is most appropriate when urinary incontinence is present because it is probably the effect of diethylstilbestrol on urethral sphincter tone, which facilitates healing.

References and Suggested Reading

Brito EHS et al: The anatomical distribution and antimicrobial susceptibility of yeast species isolated from healthy dogs, *Vet J* 182:320, 2009.

Crawford JT, Adams WM: Influence of vestibulovaginal stenosis, pelvic bladder, and recessed vulva on response to treatment for clinical signs of lower urinary tract disease in dogs: 38 cases (1990-1999), *J Am Vet Med Assoc* 221:995, 2002.

Johnston SD, Root Kustritz MV, Olson PNS: Sexual differentiation and normal anatomy of the bitch. In Johnston SD, Root Kustritz MV, Olson PNS, editors: *Canine and feline theriogenology*, Philadelphia, 2001, WB Saunders, p 1.

Keid LB et al: Comparison of agar gel immunodiffusion test, rapid slide agglutination test, microbiological culture and PCR for the diagnosis of canine brucellosis, *Res Vet Sci* 86:22, 2009.

Makloski CL: Canine brucellosis management, *Vet Clin North Am Small Anim Prac* 41:1209, 2011.

May M, Brown DR: Secreted sialidase activity of canine mycoplasmas, *Vet Microbiol* 137:380, 2009.

Rota A et al: Isolation of methicillin-resistant *Staphylococcus pseudintermedius* from breeding dogs, *Theriogenology* 75:115, 2011.

Wang KY et al: Vestibular, vaginal, and urethral relations in spayed dogs with and without lower urinary tract signs, *J Vet Intern Med* 20:1065, 2006a.

Wang KY et al: Vestibular, vaginal and urethral relationships in spayed and intact normal dogs, *Theriogenology* 66:726, 2006b.

Wanke MM, Delpino MV, Baldi PC: Use of enrofloxacin in the treatment of canine brucellosis in a dog kennel (clinical trial), *Theriogenology* 66:1573, 2006.

CHAPTER 213

Surgical Repair of Vaginal Anomalies in the Bitch

ROBERTO E. NOVO, *Vancouver, Washington*

A number of developmental and acquired conditions affect the canine vagina and vulva. Congenital conditions, which affect primarily younger dogs, include rectovaginal fistula; vulvar/vaginal hypoplasia; anovulvar cleft; clitoral enlargement; and vaginal septa, bands, or stenosis. Acquired conditions generally affect older dogs and include vaginal neoplasia and vaginal prolapse. Some acquired conditions such as vaginal hyperplasia and perivulvar dermatitis can affect younger dogs. Invariably congenital and acquired abnormalities overlap somewhat because some acquired anatomic problems may develop secondary to congenital abnormalities within the reproductive tract. Surgery to correct these abnormalities often corrects the presenting clinical signs. These procedures may be as simple as digital breakdown of a thin vaginal band or more complex (e.g., complete vaginal ablation).

Surgical Approaches to the Canine Vagina

Most surgical procedures of the vagina (and vestibule) can be approached via a perineal or caudal episiotomy. More involved procedures may require a ventral approach, which may necessitate a combined abdominal approach with or without a pubic osteotomy. With either surgical approach, strong consideration should be given to management of postoperative pain. The use of a fentanyl patch or epidural analgesia should be considered before surgery. An appropriately sized fentanyl patch (4 µg/kg/hr in dogs) should be applied the day before surgery. Alternatively, an epidural with the use of preservative-free morphine (0.1 mg/kg), bupivacaine (0.5 to 1 mg/kg), or a combination of both can be administered before or immediately after surgery. If epidural analgesia is elected, the surgeon should review the various techniques and dosing guidelines described in the veterinary literature.

Caudal Approach with Episiotomy

When performing an episiotomy, the surgeon should place the animal in sternal recumbency with the pelvic limbs hanging over the end of the table. The edges of the table should be well padded to avoid trauma to the limbs. The table is tilted so that the animal's head is down about 30 degrees and the vulva is at a comfortable working height. This head-down position may make ventilation of the patient more difficult, requiring assisted manual or mechanical ventilation to maintain adequate

oxygenation and anesthetic plane. These patients are also at increased risk of gastric reflux/regurgitation and subsequent aspiration. These animals must be fasted at least 12 hours before surgery and receive H_2 blockers to decrease gastric acidity. A loading dose of metoclopramide (1 mg/kg IV), followed by a constant rate infusion (1 mg/kg/hr) during anesthesia also may reduce the incidence of gastroesophageal reflux. In addition, a cuffed endotracheal tube should be used, and the pharynx should be evaluated and suctioned at the end of the procedure. A purse-string suture is placed around the anus to prevent fecal contamination of the surgical field. A piece of surgical tape marked "purse string" should be placed on the patient's head to remind the surgeon and anesthetist to remove the sutures once the procedure is finished. The vestibule and caudal vagina is flushed with dilute povidone-iodine solution as part of the surgical scrub. Three to four flushes of a 1:10 dilution of povidone-iodine with sterile water should be used to minimize vaginal mucosal irritation.

An incision along the median raphe is made from the level of the caudodorsal aspect of the horizontal vaginal canal, descending to the dorsal commissure of the vulvar cleft. The incision is continued along the same plane of the skin incision through the vaginal musculature and mucosal layers. Placement of a flat instrument (e.g., scalpel handle) in the vestibule can be used to stabilize the tissues while the incision is made through the dorsal vestibular mucosa. Alternatively, Metzenbaum scissors can be used to cut the mucosal layer. Cautery, vessel ligation or compression of the vestibular wall using two Doyen bowel clamps (positioning one on each side with one blade in the vestibular lumen and one on the skin surface) can be used for hemostasis (Figure 213-1). Hemorrhage often is associated with surgery to this region because of the increased vascularity to the vaginal tissues. Exposure is maintained with the use of self-retaining retractors (i.e., Gelpi, Weitlander, or ring retractors) or stay sutures. A urinary catheter should be placed if there is potential for tissue manipulation around the urethra and urethral tubercle.

Closure of the episiotomy is performed in four layers: mucosa, muscular tissue, subcutaneous tissue, and skin. A simple interrupted or continuous pattern of 3-0 monofilament absorbable suture is used for the mucosa. The muscular and subcutaneous tissues can be closed together or separately, depending on the size of the animal, using a simple continuous pattern of 3-0 or 4-0 absorbable suture. The skin edges can be closed with sutures (simple interrupted or cruciates) or surgical staples.

Perineal Approach with Episiotomy

In some cases, the episiotomy can be modified by limiting the approach to the perineum. This approach allows access to the vestibulovaginal region without incising into the dorsal aspect of the vestibule, therefore limiting

the intraoperative hemorrhage and minimizing postoperative pain. It can be used for resection and anastomosis of vestibulovaginal stenosis and to access pedunculated masses of the vagina or vestibule. This approach also can be combined with a ventral abdominal approach for vaginal ablation.

An incision along the median raphe is made from the level of the caudodorsal aspect of the horizontal vaginal canal, descending to the dorsal commissure of the vulvar cleft. Digital palpation during the approach facilitates identification of the vagina and helps identify the location of interest (Figure 213-2, *A*). The incision is continued along the same plane of the skin incision until the muscular wall of the vagina/vestibule is reached. Cautery vessel ligation should be used for hemostasis. Exposure is maintained with the use of self-retaining retractors. Blunt dissection can be performed around the vagina as needed (Figure 213-2, *B*). Careful dissection along the ventral aspect of the vagina is necessary to avoid trauma to the urethra. A urinary catheter should be placed if there is potential for tissue manipulation around the urethra and urethral tubercle.

Closure of the perineum is performed in two layers: subcutaneous tissues and skin. The subcutaneous tissues can be closed together or separately, depending on the size of the animal, using a simple continuous pattern of 3-0 or 4-0 absorbable suture. The skin edges can be closed with sutures (simple interrupted or cruciates) or surgical staples.

Ventral Approach

Fortunately, the ventral approach to the canine vagina is not used often because it requires a pelvic osteotomy. The ventral approach often is used for vaginal ablations.

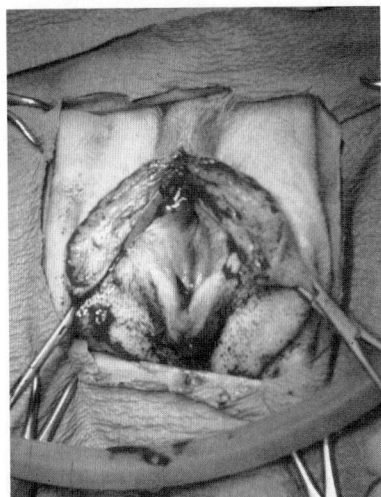

Figure 213-1 An episiotomy over the dorsal aspect of the vulva allows access to the lumen of the vestibule/vagina. Two Doyen bowel clamps are placed on the edges of the incision (positioning one on each side with one blade in the vestibular lumen and one on the skin surface to control hemorrhage and allow visualization).

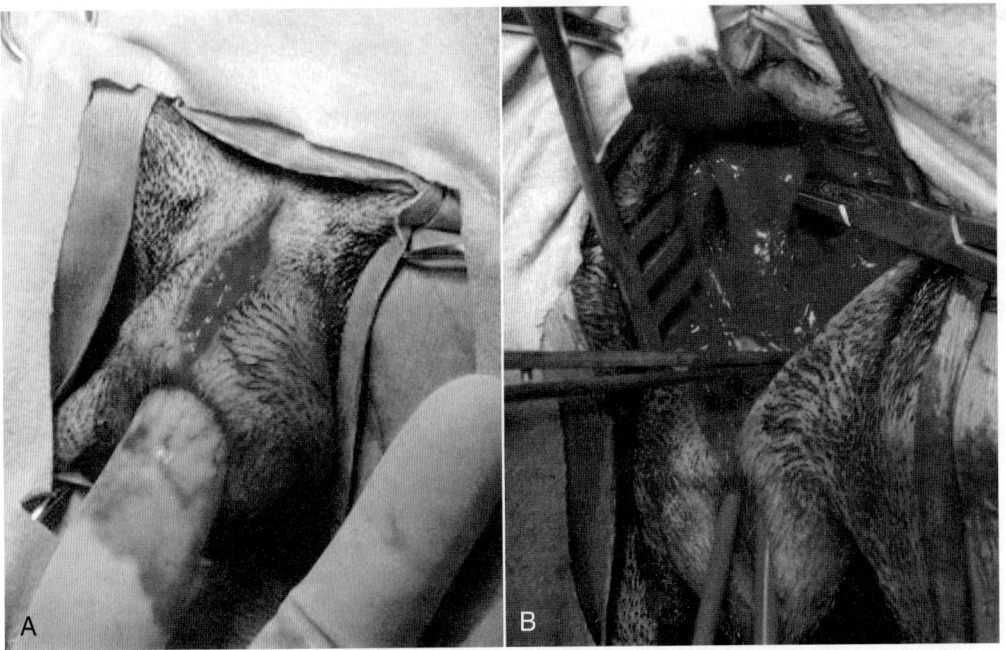

Figure 213-2 Perineal approach to the vestibule/vagina. **A,** Digital palpation of the vestibule with an incision along the median raphe. **B,** Continued dissection along the midline to the vagina and careful dissection circumferentially around the vagina using right-angled forceps. A red rubber catheter is placed in the urethra for identification and protection during dissection.

However, surgery through an abdominal or caudal/perineal approach often is possible to avoid the need for a pelvic osteotomy (see next section). The urethra should be catheterized to aid in identification and prevent iatrogenic trauma.

A standard ventral midline approach is performed in the caudal abdomen up to the cranial pelvic rim. The urinary bladder can be manipulated aside to provide access to the vagina. The pelvic osteotomy is performed to increase the exposure to the vagina and urethra. The incision is extended caudally over the midline of the pubic symphysis. The adductor muscles are elevated laterally with periosteal elevators to expose the pubic and ischial rami. A partial or complete pelvic osteotomy can be performed, depending on the location and amount of exposure needed. A partial pelvic osteotomy involves osteotomies through the pubic rami and across the pubic symphysis at the level of the obturator foramen. A complete pelvic osteotomy through both pubic rami and ischial rami gives the greatest exposure. Once the surgeon has determined the location of the osteotomy, holes are predrilled on either side of the osteotomy site. It is much easier to drill these holes before performing the osteotomy, especially if using a hand chuck and pin. The osteotomy is performed with Gigli wire, rotating burr, sagittal saw, or bone cutters. The internal obturator muscle is elevated off the pubic symphysis on one side of the pelvis and hinged on the contralateral internal obturator muscle to expose the pelvic canal.

Alternatively an osteotomy through the pubic symphysis, separating the hemipelvis, can be performed. The flexibility of the pelvis allows the placement of retractors to separate the hemipelvis, giving exposure to the pelvic canal. Holes can be predrilled on either side of the pubic symphysis. Self-retaining retractors (i.e., Finochietto retractors) facilitate exposure (Figure 213-3). Care must be taken not to put excessive stress on the hemipelvis, which can create a fracture or sacroiliac luxation (especially in young dogs or cats). Closure of this approach begins with reduction of the pelvic floor, using 18- to 20-gauge cerclage wire. The predrilled holes allow for rapid and accurate alignment of the pubic and ischial rami. The obturator and adductor muscle fascia from either side is sutured to its contralateral partner along the midline. Closure of the linea, subcutaneous tissue, and skin is performed routinely. Because of the osteotomy, activity should be restricted for 4 months after surgery. In small patients the pubic symphysis does not have to be replaced. Closure of the obturator and adductor muscles along the midline provides adequate support of the pelvic floor.

Combined Abdominal and Caudal/Perineal Approach

In most cases, the cranial aspect of the vagina can be accessed through a caudal abdominal approach combined with a caudal or perineal approach, avoiding the need for a pubic osteotomy. This approach can be used for vaginal ablation secondary to a vaginal neoplasia and can be combined with an ovariohysterectomy if the patient is intact.

Once the caudal abdomen is approached via a routine midline laparotomy, the bladder can be retroflexed to allow exposure to the vagina and associated structures. Fascial and peritoneal attachments between the vagina and rectum are bluntly dissected free. Similarly, dissection of attachments between the vagina and the urethra is performed, avoiding any disruption of the craniolateral aspect of the urethra and the periurethral tissues and avoiding damage to the ureters and urethral innervations. The cranial and caudal branches of the vaginal artery and vein are ligated. Once the vagina is dissected free, a stay suture can be placed through all layers of the vagina and the loop of the suture pushed caudally or passed into the vaginal lumen. The laparotomy is closed routinely.

The intraluminal stay suture then can be grasped via a caudal approach with episiotomy; the extraluminal stay suture can be grasped via a perineal approach. Once the stay suture is identified, it is retracted caudally, withdrawing the cranial vagina into the perineal site, allowing for complete resection of the vagina.

Congenital Abnormalities

Anovulvar Cleft

A cleft or trough is located between the ventral anus and dorsal vulva. This rare defect occurs as a result of inappropriate fusion of the urogenital folds and can be observed in sexually normal female dogs or dogs with intersex disorders. The vestibular floor and clitoris are exposed, resulting in fecal contamination and hyperemia. Correction of this defect with a perineoplasty reduces infection and abrasion of the exposed mucous membranes and provides a more cosmetic appearance.

An H-shaped or inverted V-shaped incision is made along the mucocutaneous junction of the anovulvar cleft. The vestibular mucosal margin and skin edge must be separated. Interrupted sutures of an absorbable suture are used to close the vestibular mucosa and submucosa. This is followed by subcutaneous and skin sutures. Because of the proximity of the incision to the anus, the incision may become infected. The area must be kept clean until sutures are removed. Prophylactic antibiotics may be used, but they are not necessary. An Elizabethan

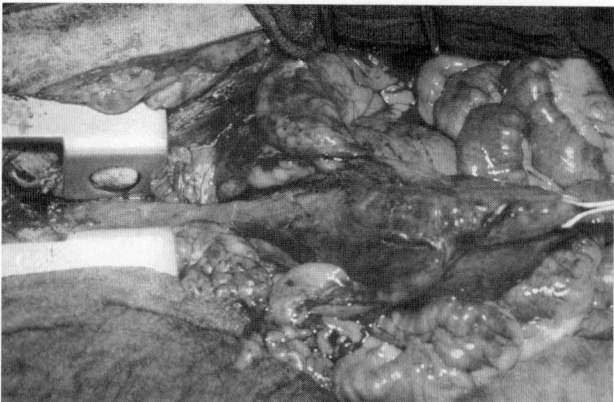

Figure 213-3 A ventral approach to the female urogenital system via a pubic symphysis osteotomy. Finochietto retractors increase exposure and allow for visualization of the structures within the pelvic canal.

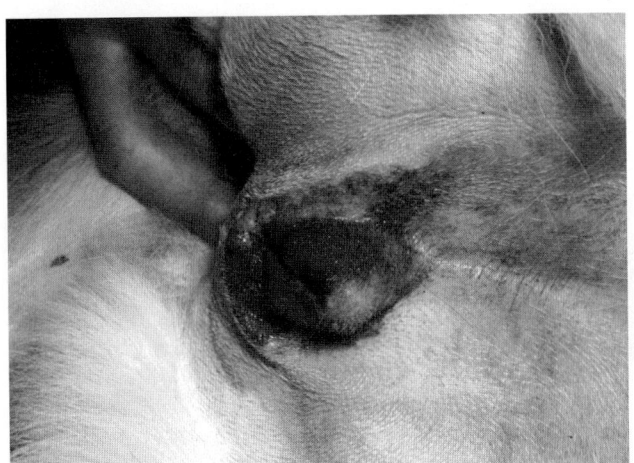

Figure 213-4 Dog with vulvar excoriations secondary to self-mutilation associated with perivulvar fold dermatitis.

collar is recommended to prevent self-mutilation to the incision.

Vulvar Hypoplasia

Vulvar hypoplasia occurs frequently in spayed female dogs. The vulva is small and recessed into the perineal skin folds. This condition is also referred to as a *juvenile/infantile vulva*. Dogs with juvenile vulva often have perivulvar moist dermatitis (Figure 213-4), which is aggravated by retention of urine and/or feces within the folds of skin. A similar condition occurs in obese dogs when the redundant perineal skin covers the vulvar cleft. Recurrent vaginitis and urinary tract infections are common in these patients. Surgical removal of the perivulvar folds and antibiotic management help to alleviate clinical signs. In obese patients weight reduction may help alleviate the perivulvar dermatitis. However, before surgery is recommended, medical management should be instituted to decrease the inflammatory and infectious process around the vulva. The affected area is cleansed gently with a benzoyl peroxide shampoo and a mild topical astringent. The use of oral antibiotics and topical antibiotic-steroid cream also can be recommended. Once the inflammatory reaction has subsided, an episioplasty can be performed.

An episioplasty is performed to remove the excess perivulvar skinfolds and the underlying subcutaneous fat. Before surgery the perivulvar skin is plicated to determine how much skin should be removed. The goal is to remove enough skin so that the vulva is no longer recessed without creating excessive tension on the incision site. A crescent-shaped skin incision is made around the vulva, starting lateral to the ventral vulvar commissure, extending laterally and dorsally to a point about 1 cm dorsal to the dorsal vulvar commissure, and then extending ventrolaterally to the contralateral side. A second crescent-shaped incision begins and ends at the same points as the first incision; however, this incision extends wider than the first (Figure 213-5). The perivulvar skin between the incisions is excised with Metzenbaum scissors. If uncertain about how much skin to remove, the surgeon should consider starting the second incision with a narrow arch

and, if the vulva is still recessed, creating a wider incision to remove more skin. This prevents unnecessary tension on the incision line.

Excessive subcutaneous fat dorsal to the vulva is removed. This is critical in obese animals. Hemorrhage is controlled with cautery and ligation. The subcutaneous tissues are closed using absorbable suture in a simple interrupted pattern. The first subcutaneous suture should be placed at the dorsal midpoint, followed by additional sutures at the midpoints of the remaining defect. The skin is closed with simple interrupted nonabsorbable sutures. Again skin sutures are placed at 12, 9, and 3 o'clock positions to ensure a cosmetic closure.

Rectovaginal and Rectovestibular Fistula

This fistula is an abnormal communication between the rectum and the dorsal aspect of the vagina or vestibule. Affected dogs often have atresia ani or an imperforate anus. The dogs present because of passage of soft feces through the vulva. Severity of clinical signs varies with size of the fistula, type of diet, and presence of atresia ani. Dogs with atresia ani may have megacolon as a complicating factor. Vaginography or a barium sulfate enema can be used to demonstrate the location and size of the fistula.

Repair of this defect is twofold, involving restoration of the vaginal/vestibular lumen followed by restoration of the rectal lumen and anal orifice. Surgery is performed via a perineal approach. An incision is made between the anus (or region of the anus) and the dorsal vulvar cleft, along the median raphe. The subcutaneous tissues are dissected bluntly until the fistula is identified. A red rubber catheter placed within the fistula may aid in identification. The communications with the rectum and vagina/vestibule are ligated and resected. The rectal mucosa should be oversewn to ensure a tight seal. If the fistula is short and wide, ligation may not be possible. The stoma should be resected and then closed primarily with absorbable simple interrupted sutures. Again the defects should be oversewn. The subcutaneous tissues and skin should be closed routinely.

In the event of anal atresia, surgery must be performed to recreate a stoma between the rectum and anus (if present). The degree of anal abnormalities may vary from an imperforate anus in which a membrane remains at the level of the anus to complete anal atresia, in which the anus and associated anal muscles are absent. Patients with an imperforate anus require opening of the anal canal. This can be performed by breaking down the membrane digitally, by blunt dissection, or by surgical resection of the membrane. Dogs with an imperforate anus must be evaluated carefully with a barium contrast study to differentiate the disorder from anal atresia, which may clinically appear the same. Dogs with an imperforate anus generally have normal anal function and tone.

If anal atresia is present, evidence of an anus is minimal to nonexistent, and on contrast radiography of the colon a section of rectum caudal to the fistula is absent. A rectal pull-through procedure is performed, creating a new anal orifice. Because the anal musculature and innervation are absent, these animals have fecal incontinence. Muscle

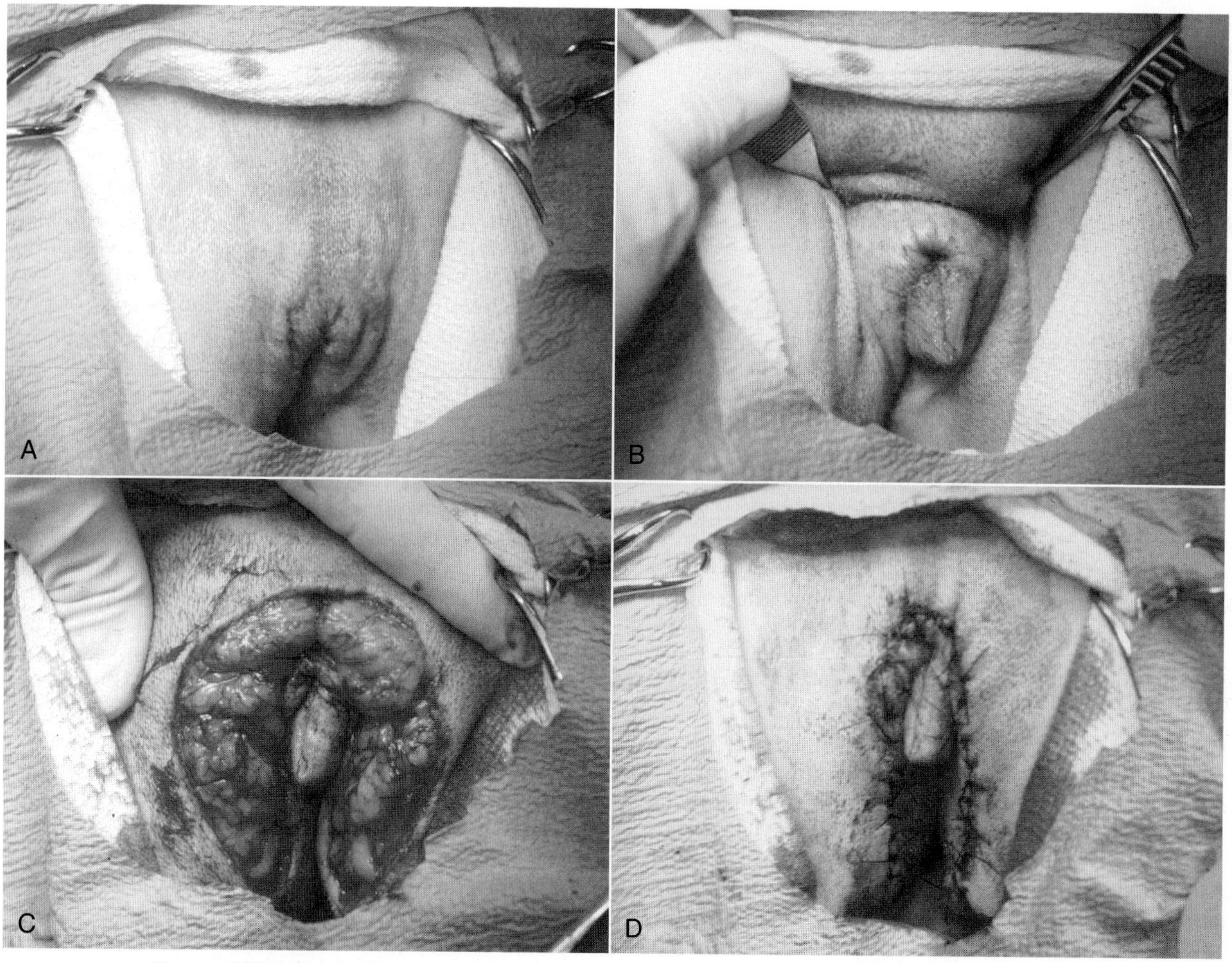

Figure 213-5 Episioplasty for correction of a recessed juvenile vulva or for redundant perivulvar skin. **A,** Appearance of a dog with a recessed vulva. Note that the vulva is not visible under the redundant skin folds. **B,** The redundant skin is retracted to visualize the vulva. The excess skin is plicated to determine the amount of skin that will have to be excised. **C,** Two crescent-shaped skin incisions are made around the vulva. **D,** The subcutaneous tissue and skin are closed with multiple simple interrupted sutures.

flaps can be attempted to increase tone to the new opening; however, results have been inconsistent.

Clitoral Hypertrophy

Clitoral hypertrophy may occur in dogs with intersex disorders, dogs receiving anabolic steroids, or dogs with hyperadrenocorticism; however, this condition also may be found in normal females. Some dogs with chronic vaginitis may present with clitoral hypertrophy caused by excessive vulvar licking. The clitoris often protrudes through the vulvar cleft (Figure 213-6). These dogs generally are presented by an owner for cosmetic reasons, clitoral irritation and vestibular inflammation, or mutilation of the protruded clitoris. Treatment of hyperadrenocorticism or termination of steroid administration may cause resolution of clitoral hypertrophy. In cases in which the clitoris is protruding through the vulvar cleft, amputation of the clitoris is recommended. Clitoral amputation is performed by simple submucosal dissection. Dogs with

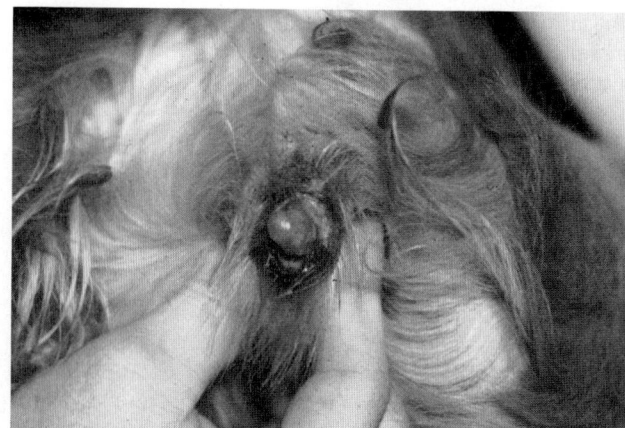

Figure 213-6 Dog with clitoral hypertrophy. The end of the enlarged clitoris is extruded between the vulvar cleft.

intersex disorders may have significant bleeding during the dissection because of the presence of erectile tissue. Performing an episiotomy may improve visualization and assist with hemostasis.

Vaginal Band, Septum, and Stenosis

A number of vaginal and vestibular congenital abnormalities occur as a result of imperfect joining of the genital folds, genital swellings, or müllerian ducts. These conditions may be incidental findings on a physical examination, or occasionally they cause a variety of clinical presentations. Bitches with stenosis or bands may present with clinical signs of chronic vaginitis, which may be associated with urine pooling in the anterior portion of the vagina. Other bitches may present for artificial insemination after unsuccessful attempts at natural breeding. The female and/or male may demonstrate pain when attempting to breed. Vaginal bands also are associated frequently with dogs having ectopic ureters. A digital vaginal examination may be most informative because visual inspection with speculums or otoscopes may bypass the abnormality. A vaginogram may be necessary to determine the extent and severity of the abnormality.

A persistent or imperforate hymen can be corrected with digital breakdown of the membrane. Vaginal bands or septa that cannot be corrected digitally may require an episiotomy and surgical resection (Figure 213-7). Depending on the extent of the mucosal defect remaining after surgical removal of the band or septa, the defect can be left to heal by second intention or surgically closed using an absorbable suture in a simple continuous manner.

Vestibulovaginal stenosis is diagnosed as a palpable submucosal fibrous ring at the level of a persistent hymen. Vaginal stenosis is a region of vaginal hypoplasia, in which the lumen over a given area is narrower than the rest of the vagina or vestibule. Bitches with stenosis of

the vestibulovaginal junction that exhibit clinical signs tend to respond poorly to digital and surgical attempts at dilation. If surgery is indicated, a vaginogram should be performed to determine the extent of the affected region and to determine the vestibulovaginal ratio. The vestibulovaginal junction should be larger than a third of the diameter of the vagina. The measurement guideline that has been used is the vestibulovaginal ratio, which is calculated by dividing the height of the vestibulovaginal junction by the maximum height of the vagina on a lateral vaginourethrogram (Figure 213-8). A ratio of less than 0.20 is considered severe stenosis; 0.20 to 0.25 moderate stenosis; 0.26 to 0.35 mild stenosis; and more than 0.35 anatomically normal.

Three surgical techniques have been recommended for correction of these defects: T-vaginoplasty, stenosis

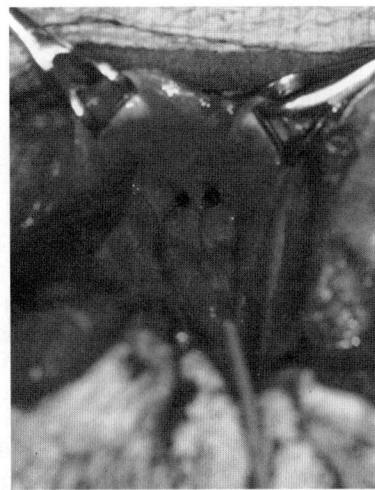

Figure 213-7 Episiotomy performed for visualization of a vaginal band. A urinary catheter identifies the urethral opening at the base of the vestibulovaginal junction.

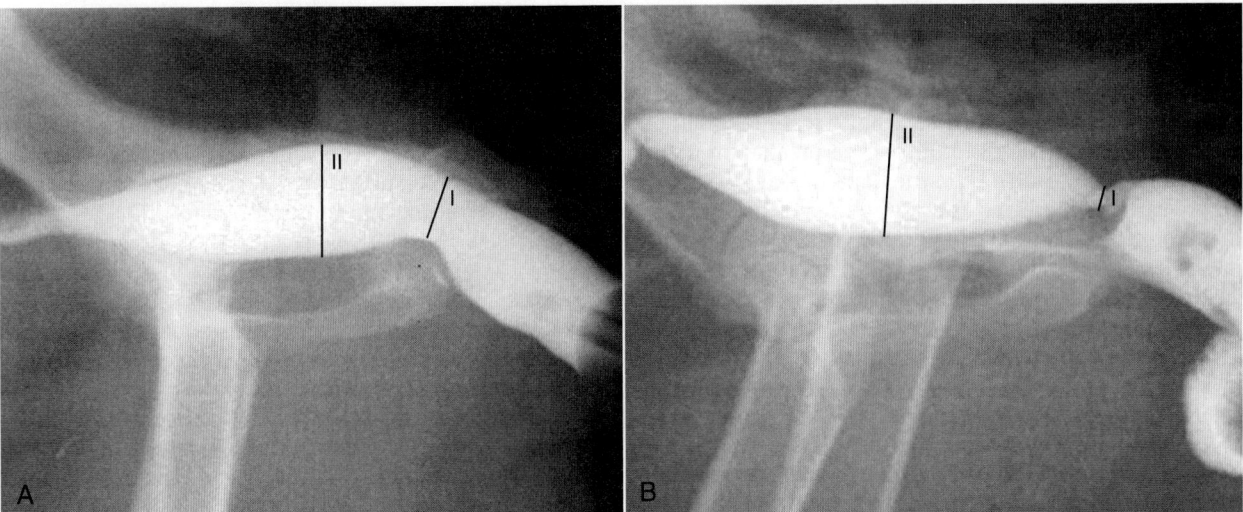

Figure 213-8 A positive contrast vaginourethrogram. The height of the vestibulovaginal junction (I) and the maximum height of the vagina (II) are measured on lateral vaginourethrographic views to calculate the vestibulovaginal ratio (I divided by II). **A,** Normal vaginogram. **B,** Patient with vestibulovaginal stenosis.

resection, and partial/complete vaginectomy. Resection of the stricture/stenosis has a better outcome than the T-vaginoplasty for complete resolution of clinical signs; however, the procedure is more difficult technically and therefore can have higher surgical complications. The T-vaginoplasty has been shown to resolve clinical signs in some dogs. Surgical recommendations vary with severity of the stenosis. Severe stenosis most likely would respond to resection and anastomosis, whereas the milder stenosis probably would respond to a less invasive T-vaginoplasty.

The T-vaginoplasty is performed via a standard caudal approach with episiotomy or perineal approach. A longitudinal incision is made on the dorsal aspect of the vaginal stenosis, followed by a T-shaped closure to increase the vaginal diameter. However, this procedure has met with variable results. Bitches with submucosal fibrous rings may not require full-thickness incisions. These annular stenoses located at the vestibulovaginal junction require only resection of the fibrous tissue through a mucosal incision. The fibrous ring is resected, and the remaining mucosal defect is closed so that none of the deeper vaginal tissues are exposed. In spayed bitches only the ventral 180 degrees of the stenosis is removed in mild cases to allow adequate drainage of vaginal fluids. Positive postoperative results have been reported on the few cases in which complete resection and anastomosis of the defect were performed.

This technique is technically more difficult because it requires a 360-degree dissection of the stenosis. A standard caudal with episiotomy or perineal approach provides the surgeon with adequate visualization of the defect. Full-thickness excision of vaginal stenosis is recommended for moderate to severe stenosis, as determined by the vestibulovaginal ratio and clinical signs. Two circumferential incisions are made cranial and caudal to the defect. Catheterization and protection of the urethra are critical when performing a vaginal resection and anastomosis. Ligation and cautery of superficial and muscular vessels are mandatory. The remaining defect can be closed once the stenosis is resected, using absorbable suture in a simple interrupted pattern.

A complete vaginectomy is the final option for correction of vaginal stenosis in bitches that are not intended for breeding. Results with this technique seem favorable. A standard caudal with episiotomy or perineal approach, combined with a caudal midline laparotomy may be used. The vagina is resected anterior to the urethral tubercle, making sure that the entire stenotic vagina is removed. A Parker-Kerr oversew or other inverting suture patterns are used to close the vagina.

Acquired Abnormalities

Vaginal Prolapse

Vaginal prolapse includes two different disease processes. One process involves prolapse of edematous mucosa on the floor of the vaginal vault. This disease also is referred to as *vaginal edema* and previously was referred to as *vaginal hyperplasia*. The second process involves a true prolapse of the vagina, in which the prolapse is circumferential and often includes the cervix. These dogs have *true vaginal prolapse*. For ease of discussion, the terms *vaginal edema* and *true vaginal prolapse* are used when discussing the two disease processes.

Vaginal Edema and Hyperplasia

Young, intact bitches in proestrus or estrus frequently are reported with this condition. Large and brachycephalic breeds are overrepresented. Normally during the follicular phase of the estrous cycle the vaginal and vestibular mucosa become thickened and edematous. Occasionally an exaggerated response occurs, resulting in excessive edema. The submucosal tissue edema and redundant mucosa at the floor of the vagina just cranial to the urethral tubercle can protrude through the vulvar labia as a fleshy red mass (Figure 213-9). The exposed tissue is prone to trauma, desiccation, and self-mutilation. The urethra is not exteriorized and can be catheterized at the base of the edematous tissue. The location of the urethral tubercle helps distinguish vaginal edema from vaginal prolapse, in which the urethral opening may be exteriorized with the prolapsed vagina.

Conservative management consists of protection of the exteriorized portion of the mass with lubricants and prevention of self-mutilation with an Elizabethan collar. Vaginal edema is seen most commonly during the first estrous period and regresses spontaneously during the luteal phase. However, recurrence is common during subsequent estrous cycles. Owners should be cautioned that the edematous tissue also may recur at parturition, resulting in dystocia. Hormonal therapy with megestrol acetate (2 mg/kg q24h PO for 7 days) or gonadotropin-releasing hormone (2.2 μg/kg IM) also may be attempted. Owners should be advised of specific side effects of hormonal therapy.

Ovariohysterectomy is curative and should be considered to prevent recurrence. Surgical resection of the mass should be considered if the bitch is intended for breeding or if the tissues are traumatized. A standard caudal approach with episiotomy is performed to expose the base of the edematous tissue. The mass is lifted off of the vestibular floor, and the urethra catheterized to prevent iatrogenic trauma. A transverse elliptical incision is made around the base, and the redundant vaginal tissue is amputated. The vaginal mucosal defect is closed with absorbable suture in a simple continuous pattern, carefully avoiding the urethral orifice.

True Vaginal Prolapse

True vaginal prolapse occurs less frequently than vaginal edema and can be either partial or complete. In a complete true vaginal prolapse, the cervix is exteriorized. In both cases the vaginal tissues demonstrate a doughnut-shaped eversion. This is differentiated from vaginal edema in that there is circumferential involvement of the vaginal mucosa and the urethral tubercle. Brachycephalic breeds in normal estrus are predisposed to vaginal prolapse.

No treatment may be necessary in cases with mild prolapse because spontaneous regression occurs during diestrus. More severe prolapses may require protection of

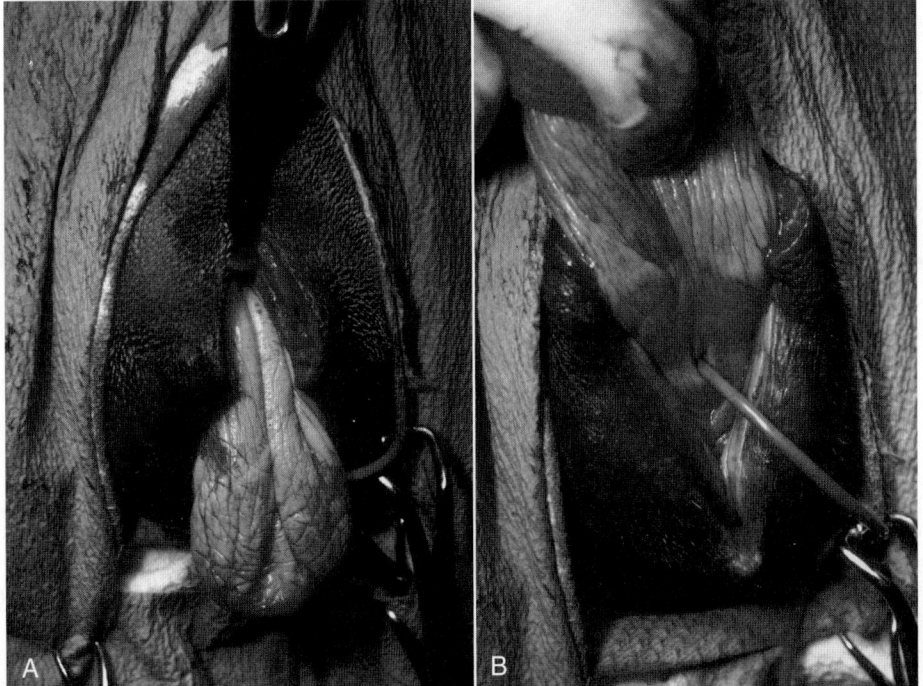

Figure 213-9 Hyperplasia of the vaginal floor. **A,** An episiotomy is performed to expose the base of the hyperplastic tissue. **B,** The pedunculated hyperplastic tissue is elevated, exposing the urethral opening. A urinary catheter is inserted to maintain visual recognition and protection of the urethra during resection of the hyperplastic tissue.

exposed tissues. General anesthesia is required if attempting to replace the prolapsed mucosa. The everted tissue is cleaned with a dilute antiseptic solution or saline. If the edema is severe, manual compression or application of 50% dextrose solution to the mucosal surface may decrease its size, therefore facilitating reduction. A lubricated plastic syringe can be used to reduce the tissues. An episiotomy may be necessary to provide better exposure for reduction. Reduction also can be assisted by traction on the uterus via a ventral abdominal approach. Once the vagina is reduced, reprolapse can be minimized by suturing the uterine body or the broad ligament to the abdominal wall. A urinary catheter should be maintained until the vaginal swelling resolves.

Dogs with long-standing prolapses may have secondary necrosis, infection, or hemorrhage of the prolapsed tissues. These dogs should be evaluated and treated as necessary for hypotension and/or sepsis. Surgical resection of the devitalized tissues is indicated in these patients to prevent further sepsis and self-mutilation. An episiotomy helps with exposure and placement of a urinary catheter. A stepwise full-thickness circumferential incision is made in the vaginal wall. A section of 1 to 2 cm of the outer mucosal layer is incised, followed by resection of the inner noninverted mucosal layer. Horizontal mattress sutures are used to close the incision edges. Hemorrhage can be significant and should be controlled with cautery and ligation. This is continued circumferentially in small sections until the entire prolapsed tissue is resected.

References and Suggested Reading

Crawford JT, Adams WM: Influence of vestibulovaginal stenosis, pelvic bladder, and recessed vulva on response to treatment for clinical signs of lower urinary tract disease in dogs: 38 cases (1990-1999), *J Am Vet Med Assoc* 221:995, 2002.

Hammel SP, Bjorling DE: Results of vulvoplasty for treatment of recessed vulva in dogs, *J Am Anim Hosp Assoc* 38:79, 2002.

Hedlund CS: Surgery of the female reproductive tract. In Fossum TW et al, editor: *Small animal surgery*, ed 3, St Louis, 2007, Mosby, p 729.

Kieves NR, Novo RE, Martin RB: Vaginal resection and anastomosis for treatment of vestibulovaginal stenosis in 4 dogs with recurrent urinary tract infections, *J Am Vet Med Assoc* 239:972, 2011.

Mathews KG: Surgery of the canine vagina and vulva, *Vet Clin North Am Small Anim Pract* 31: 271-290, 2001.

Pettit GD: Vagina and vulva: surgical treatment of vaginal and vulvar masses. In Bojrab MJ, Ellison GW, Slocum B, editors: *Current techniques in small animal surgery*, ed 4, Baltimore, 1998, Lippincott, Williams & Wilkins, p 503.

Rahal SC et al: Rectovaginal fistula with anal atresia in 5 dogs, *Can Vet J* 48:827, 2007.

Wang KY et al: Vestibular, vaginal and urethral relations in spayed dogs with and without lower urinary tract signs, *J Vet Intern Med* 20:1065, 2006.

Wang KY et al: Vestibular, vaginal and urethral relationships in spayed and intact normal dogs, *Theriogenology* 66:726, 2006.

Wykes PM, Olson PN: Vagina, vestibule, and vulva. In Slatter D, editor: *Textbook of small animal surgery*, ed 3, Philadelphia, 2002, WB Saunders, p 1502.

CHAPTER **214**

Early Age Neutering in Dogs and Cats

MICHELLE ANNE KUTZLER, *Corvallis, Oregon*

Pet overpopulation in the United States is an ongoing problem. Surgical removal of the gonads (gonadectomy) in dogs and cats has long been a basis of population control and part of routine veterinary health maintenance programs for animals not intended for breeding. In the United States, neutering is the most common surgical procedure performed in dogs and cats younger than 1 year of age. However, the optimal age to neuter female and male dogs and cats is not defined by the veterinary literature. For the purposes of this chapter, the term *neutering* is used to describe ovariohysterectomy (spay) and orchidectomy (castration).

Although these elective surgical procedures traditionally are delayed until the patient is 6 to 7 months old (but still before puberty), mandatory preadoption neutering as early as 6 to 14 weeks of age occurs in many animal shelters throughout the United States. Recently, the Society for Theriogenology (SFT) and the American College of Theriogenologists (ACT) developed a consensus statement opposing mandatory neutering programs, stating that "the pet overpopulation problem that exists in the United States [compared to other developed countries] is due to cultural differences on the importance of pets, the responsibility of pet owners, and the ability of the government and national agencies to properly educate the public." Early age castration is forbidden in Germany under the Law for Prevention of Cruelty to Animals (Tierschutzgesetz) (Günzel-Apel, 1998).

Many veterinarians and pet owners are starting to ask, "What are the long-term effects of early age gonadectomy?" Several long-term effects must be taken into consideration. The focus of this chapter is to compare the benefits (Table 214-1) and concerns (Table 214-2) between early age and traditional age neutering of dogs and cats as well as briefly illustrate some technical differences when performing early age neutering. For the purposes of this chapter, early age neutering is defined as neutering between the ages of 6 to 23 weeks (before 6 months), and traditional age neutering is defined as neutering after 24 weeks (6 months) of age. Regardless of whether it is performed at an early or a traditional age, most elective neutering in female dogs and cats occurs prepubertally because puberty typically occurs after 8 months of age in male and female dogs and cats. Benefits and concerns of early age neutering are discussed.

Benefits

Short-term advantages of early age neutering include a quicker recovery and shorter surgery time for the patient (Howe, 1997). Fewer surgical complications are reported when patients are neutered before 12 weeks of age compared with after 24 weeks of age (Howe, 1997). In addition, long-term benefits are associated with early age neutering. In cats, up to 70.5% of litters from owned cats are unplanned (Murray et al, 2009), and neutering these animals before adoption completely eliminates the possibility of unplanned offspring stemming from poor owner compliance of neutering at the traditional age. With respect to the health effects, cats neutered before 23 weeks of age had a decreased incidence of asthma, gingivitis, and abscesses (Spain, Scarlett, and Houpt, 2004a). Moreover, cats neutered at an early age had decreased incidence of sexual behavior, urine spraying, and aggression toward veterinarians compared with cats neutered at the traditional age (Spain, Scarlett, and Houpt, 2004a). Some investigators have found that early age neutering in dogs decreases separation anxiety, escaping behavior, and inappropriate elimination when frightened (Spain, Scarlett, and Houpt, 2004b) compared with traditional age neutering. However, the influence of the age at neutering on behavior in dogs is controversial: some investigators have found no behavioral differences between early age and traditional age neutered dogs (Howe et al, 2001).

Concerns

Behavioral

Some investigators have reported increased noise phobia and sexual behavior in dogs neutered before 23 weeks of age compared with traditional age neutered dogs. Cats neutered before 23 weeks of age had a higher incidence of shyness compared with traditional age neutered cats.

Immunologic

Dogs neutered before 24 weeks of age are more likely to contract an infectious disease later in life compared with dogs neutered after 24 weeks of age (Howe et al, 2001).

TABLE **214-1**

Summary of Long-Term Health Risks Decreased with Early Age Neutering Compared with Traditional Age Neutering

System	Species Affected	Health Risks
Behavioral	Feline	Aggression towards veterinarians
		Sexual behavior
		Urine spraying
	Canine	Escaping behavior
		Inappropriate elimination when frightened
		Separation anxiety
Immunologic	Feline	Abscesses
		Asthma
		Gingivitis

TABLE **214-2**

Summary of Long-Term Health Risks Increased with Early Age Neutering Compared with Traditional Age Neutering

System	Species Affected	Health Risks
Behavioral	Canine	Noise phobias
	Feline	Shyness
Immunologic	Canine	Contraction of an infectious disease
Musculoskeletal	Canine, feline	Growth plate closure delay
	Canine	Cranial cruciate ligament rupture
	Canine	Hip dysplasia
Urogenital	Canine	Cystitis
	Canine	Paraphimosis
	Canine	Perivulvar dermatitis
	Canine	Preputial hypoplasia
	Canine	Urinary incontinence
	Canine	Vaginitis
	Feline	Phimosis

Musculoskeletal

Dog neutered at 7 weeks of age have a greater delay in radius and ulna growth plate closure compared with dogs neutered at 7 months of age, resulting in longer bone length in dogs neutered at 7 weeks of age (Howe et al, 2001; Salmeri et al, 1991). The effect of increased physeal growth is believed to be responsible for the increased incidence of hip dysplasia and cranial cruciate ligament rupture (Duerr et al, 2007) reported in early age neutered dogs compared with those neutered at the traditional age. Because of these increases risks, the SFT and ACT recommend that neutering should be postponed until after

puberty for potential canine athletes. Increased physeal growth also has been reported in cats neutered at an early age.

Urogenital

Early age neutering results in an increased rate of cystitis and urinary incontinence in dogs compared with traditional age neutering (Spain et al, 2004b; Stöcklin-Gautschi et al, 2001). The risk of urinary incontinence is greatest in dogs spayed before 3 months of age. In addition incidence of perivulvar dermatitis and vaginitis is increased in bitches neutered at an early age compared with those neutered at the traditional age. Early age neutering in male dogs permanently arrests the normal development of the balanopreputial fold, resulting in preputial hypoplasia and an increased incidence of paraphimosis. Neutering male cats at 7 weeks of age causes a phimosis by permanently preventing complete penile extrusion, which complicates urinary catheter placement and management of feline urologic syndrome.

Surgical Technique

Many physiologic differences between young and older patients must be considered before surgery. Younger dogs and cats do not have the ability to concentrate urine and have a greater fluid requirement relative to body mass than older patients. In addition, hepatic glycogen is minimal and declines rapidly during fasting, resulting in hypoglycemia. For these reasons, water and food restriction before surgery should not exceed 1 hour and 4 to 8 hours, respectively.

Early age ovariohysterectomy is performed in a similar manner to the procedure in older patients with a few exceptions. The ventral midline abdominal incision should be made in the middle third of the distance between the umbilicus and pubis rather than the cranial third used for older dogs. Inside the abdominal cavity, kittens and puppies less than 16 to 20 weeks old normally have a substantial amount of clear fluid in the peritoneal cavity. The reproductive tracts from puppies and kittens are small, lack vasculature, and lack adipose tissue. Tissues in general are more delicate in puppies and kittens and therefore require gentle handling. In 6- to 14-week-old male kittens, it also has been suggested not to use castration techniques in which the spermatic cord is tied onto itself or the vas deferens and spermatic artery are tied together because the spermatic artery is allegedly too small and fragile (Goeree, 1998). Soft, nonirritating suture materials, such as polyglactin 910, are recommended for a suture material for spermatic cord and pedicle ligation. Multifilament or coated nonabsorbable suture materials should be avoided. Polydioxanone suture also should be avoided for ligation because it has been reported to cause calcinosis circumscripta in two young dogs (Kirby et al, 1989).

References and Suggested Reading

Duerr FM et al: Risk factors for excessive tibial plateau angle in large-breed dogs with cranial cruciate ligament disease, *J Am Vet Med Assoc* 231(11):1688, 2007.

Goeree G: Pediatric neuters can be technically challenging, *Can Vet J* 39:244, 1998.

Günzel-Apel AR: Early castration of dogs and cats from the point of view of animal welfare, *Dtsch Tierarztl Wochenschr* 105(3):95, 1998.

Howe LM: Short-term results and complications of prepubertal gonadectomy in cats and dogs, *J Am Vet Med Assoc* 211:57, 1997.

Howe LM et al: Long-term outcome of gonadectomy performed at an early age or traditional age in dogs, *J Am Vet Med Assoc* 218:217, 2001.

Kirby BM et al: Calcinosis circumscripta associated with polydioxanone suture in two dogs, *Vet Surg* 18:216, 1989.

Murray JK et al: Survey of the characteristics of cats owned by households in the UK and factors affecting their neutering status, *Vet Rec* 164:137, 2009.

Salmeri KR et al: Gonadectomy in immature dogs: effects on skeletal, physical, and behavioral development, *J Am Vet Med Assoc* 198:1193, 1991.

Society for Theriogenology, American College of Theriogenologists: Basis for position on mandatory spay-neuter in the canine and feline, accessed December 31, 2011, from http://therio.org/associations/2746/files/Basis%20for%20Position%20on%20Mandatory%20Spay%20SFT%20ACT%20FINAL.pdf.

Spain CV, Scarlett JM, Houpt KA: Long-term risks and benefits of early-age gonadectomy in cats, *J Am Vet Med Assoc* 224:372, 2004a.

Spain CV, Scarlett JM, Houpt KA: Long-term risks and benefits of early-age gonadectomy in dogs, *J Am Vet Med Assoc* 224:380, 2004b.

Stöcklin-Gautschi NM et al: The relationship of urinary incontinence to early spaying in bitches, *J Reprod Fertil Suppl* 57:233, 2001.

CHAPTER 215

Estrus Suppression in the Bitch

PATRICK W. CONCANNON, *Ithaca, New York*

The use of estrous cycle suppressing hormone therapy should be proposed only for animals intended for breeding within 1 to 3 years of initiating treatment. Animals not intended for breeding are best managed by surgical sterilization. In North America, no new methods or products for estrus prevention or suppression in dogs and cats have been introduced in the last three decades. The oral progestin megestrol acetate (Ovaban) remains the only drug marketed for suppression of ovarian cycles in dogs. The only indication is for use in adult dogs. In Europe and some Latin American countries, other progestins are marketed for estrus suppression in small animals, including proligestone and medroxyprogesterone acetate (MPA). These progestins often are marketed with an indication for use in prepubertal dogs and adults. Drugs marketed for human use sometimes are administered as contraceptive treatments in small animals by or at the request of owners; practitioners should be aware of these and their possible application and side effects. In North America these include depot MPA and various anabolic androgens, including testosterone and mibolerone. Mibolerone, previously marketed as a brand-name dog contraceptive, was withdrawn from the market after its labeling as a regulated anabolic steroid but remains in use in a generic oral liquid formulation available from compounding pharmacies. Annual or semiannual administration of gonadotropin-releasing hormone (GnRH) agonist implants that down-regulate pituitary secretion of gonadotropic hormones also can be used to suppress ovarian cycles in bitches. Such implants containing deslorelin (Suprelorin) are marketed for suppression of testis function in dogs in Europe, Scandinavia, Australia, and New Zealand. The extent of off-label use for estrus suppression in females is not known. Such application has been demonstrated safe and effective but with the side effect of inducing estrus in adult bitches treated during anestrus and in young bitches in the late prepubertal period. These implants are also marketed for treatment of adrenocortical disease in ferrets in the United States but extralabel use in other species is prohibited. Practitioners should be aware of all possible modalities of contraception previously available to animals they are treating and the potential side effects particularly of gonadal steroids.

Steroid Contraceptive Mechanism of Action

Progestins

When progestins are given by serial administration or depot injection to bitches, the result is an artificial luteal phase that mimics many of the effects of the progesterone secreted during the 2-month luteal phase that normally follows ovulation in the ovarian cycle. Mechanisms include an antigonadotropic action potentially resulting in lowered luteinizing hormone (LH) and follicle-stimulating hormone (FSH) pulsatile secretion and plasma concentrations; an antiestrogen action achieved by reducing the concentrations of intracellular estrogen receptors in many tissues, including those regulating gonadotropin secretion; and progestational actions on the reproductive tract occurring out of the normal sequence of the ovarian cycle, resulting in altered endometrial growth and secretion, altered cervical secretion, reduced sperm transport, and altered uterine-tube motility. In addition, progestins can have an antiovulatory effect by preventing a preovulatory surge release of gonadotropins (LH and FSH) from the pituitary, the normal stimulus for ovulation, if administered before a large rise in estrogen. However, administration at or immediately after the follicular phase peak in estrogen can facilitate and advance the preovulatory LH surge and ovulation. When administered beginning several days or more before the peak in estrogen would have occurred, progestins typically prevent the LH surge, possibly by interfering with hypothalamic and pituitary responses to estrogen.

However, none of these actions provides an explanation of how the typical clinical administration of a progestin during anestrus causes an apparent prolongation of anestrus and prevents and delays the occurrence of a new ovarian follicular phase or an associated proestrus. Long-term progestin administration in bitches does not lower the systemic concentrations of LH below those typically observed during most of normal anestrus and actually may result in a small increase in basal LH (Colon et al, 1993), perhaps by acting as an antiestrogen and partially interfering with the normal negative feedback effects of estrogen.

During normal ovarian cycles, elevated progesterone reduces GnRH pulsatility, and thus reduces LH and FSH pulsatility. As a result, the luteal phase prevents any increase in gonadotropin pulsatility that would stimulate the next follicular phase. Contraceptive progestin treatment has the same effect. The progestin prevents any increase in gonadotropin pulsatility sufficient to initiate another estrus cycle. Why the effect lasts 1 to several months after withdrawal of progestin is not understood, but it is similar to what is observed after luteolysis during the normal ovarian cycle. In dogs, proestrus does not occur until after many weeks or months of an obligate anestrus after the end of the 7- to 10-week luteal phase and the decline in progesterone concentrations to nearly undetectable levels. A contraceptive progestin treatment mimics a luteal phase and postpones and reestablishes the onset of anestrus.

Androgens

The estrous cycle postponing effects of androgens, like those of progestins, appear to involve primarily a negative feedback effect at the level of the hypothalamus and possibly the pituitary. The contraceptive and other effects of androgens in females may be the same as in males by binding to androgen receptors or may involve cross-talk with other steroid receptors. Androgen receptors have been observed in estrogen target tissues, and androgen binding can result in reduced responsiveness to estrogen. The duration of effect after hormone withdrawal may vary among androgens. Androgen therapy including testosterone reportedly is followed often by rapid return to estrus within a few weeks after withdrawal (England, 1998), although some androgen therapy such as mibolerone typically has required 2 to 3 months for return to estrus, with a range of 1 to 7 months, as with progestins. In addition, termination of long-term androgen use in bitches, especially with testosterone, can result in a prolonged or even permanent anestrus, as observed in some racing greyhound bitches.

Side Effects of Contraceptive Steroids

Progestin side effects can occur from excessive dosing, prolonged exposure to lower doses, or an idiosyncratic sensitivity and responsiveness of some bitches to a particular regimen. These side effects have included uterine hyperstimulation, development of mammary tumors, diabetes mellitus, gallbladder disease, growth hormone hypersecretion, and acromegaly. Stimulation of the endometrium can result in mucometra, cystic endometrial hyperplasia, and eventually pyometra. Uterine effects may be more pronounced when progestin is administered during or after stimulation by endogenous estrogen during proestrus or estrus. Insulin resistance occurs possibly as a direct effect of the progestin but also is related to increased serum growth hormone in some bitches. Progestin-induced growth hormone secretion can result in signs of acromegaly of varying severity and appears to mimic luteal phase induction of signs of acromegaly reported in some older intact bitches. Progestin-induced increased serum growth hormone concentrations appear to result from hypersecretion of growth hormone by mammary tissue, although pituitary growth hormone activity increases as well. Reduced adrenal size and reduced concentrations of cortisol also have been observed with high doses of progestin.

Side effects of androgens include increased muscle mass and strength, aggression, and clitoral hypertrophy. Anal gland inspissation and excessive lacrimation have been noted with at least one androgen, mibolerone. Androgens and progestins can result in masculinization of female fetuses if administered to pregnant bitches.

Progestin Products and Applications

Megestrol Acetate Tablets

Megestrol acetate is marketed in North America as Ovaban tablets for the prevention and postponement of proestrus and estrus in anestrus bitches and for the curtailment of proestrus and prevention of ovulation and estrus in early proestrus bitches. Ovaban is marketed in bottles of 5- or 20-mg tablets for oral administration. The generic drug tablets are available in those sizes and others from compounding pharmacies. The recommended dosage is

0.55 mg/kg/day (or 0.25 mg/lb/day) for 32 days in anestrus bitches. Higher dosages of 2.2 mg/kg/day (or 1 mg/lb/day) for 8 days are given to bitches already in early proestrus. The indication is for use in adult bitches for up to two successive cycles. In some countries, including the United Kingdom, megestrol acetate is used in pubertal dogs as well as adults. Diabetes mellitus, mammary tumors, uterine disease, and liver disease are contraindications to the use of megestrol acetate. Bitches with an unknown or ill-defined reproductive history should be confirmed to be in anestrus by vaginal cytology and progesterone assay before treatment. Administration during pregnancy can result in masculinization of female fetuses. Treatment should not be repeated beyond two successive estrous cycles without allowing an intervening normal cycle.

Administration during anestrus should be initiated 1 to 2 weeks or more before the next expected proestrus. If initiated too late in anestrus, a spontaneous proestrus may occur and require changing to the higher, proestrus-regimen dosing. If treatment is started immediately before the onset of proestrus, the subsequent proestrus may occur a few weeks after withdrawal. If megestrol acetate is initiated too early in anestrus, there may be no apparent postponement of the next cycle. The next proestrus typically occurs 4 to 6 months after treatment, with a range of 1 to 7 months. The advantages of the oral formulation are ease of administration and administration by the owner; concerns include compliance by the owner and potential for underdosing or overdosing. The bitch's body weight should be determined with exactitude, and the precise number of tablets or partial tablets of a specific formulation to be administered each day should be provided with written instructions.

Administration of megestrol acetate in early proestrus should begin within 3 days of proestrus onset. Client education regarding the signs of early proestrus is important. A bitch with a normal proestrus usually lasting less than 4 days or longer than 20 days is reportedly not a good candidate for megestrol acetate treatment during proestrus. Early proestrus status can be confirmed by vaginal cytology showing less than 50% superficial cells, increasing rather than decreasing vulval turgidity, and serum progesterone concentrations less than 0.5 ng/ml. Proestrus treatment with megestrol acetate should be combined with isolation of the bitch from males for 3 to 8 days and until the end of serosanguineous discharge, following the recommendation of the manufacturer. The suppression of proestrus symptoms occurs by 3 to 8 days after initiation of treatment. The subsequent proestrus is expected in 4 to 6 months but ranged from 1 to 7 months in clinical trials. Administration too late in proestrus can likely result in induction of ovulation, failure to prevent ovulation, or the occurrence of estrus.

Megestrol acetate is currently the only cycle preventive or estrus preventive marketed for dogs in the United States and is approved for use in two successive cycles. In the United Kingdom similar dosages of megestrol acetate (Ovarid) are recommended, including 0.55 mg/kg/day for 40 days in anestrus, or 2 mg/kg/day for 8 days in early proestrus. However, for the bitch in pubertal proestrus, or with a history of pseudopregnancy, or housed with other

bitches and susceptible to pheromone effects, the recommendation has been to use a dose of 2 mg/kg for 4 days and then 0.55 mg/kg for 16 days. The onset of proestrus must be determined accurately for use in proestrus, especially in pubertal bitches. The treatment of bitches in anestrus also includes the option to continue treating with lower doses of 0.2 mg/kg twice weekly for up to 4 months after the initial 40 days of treatment but then allowing a normal estrus to occur before retreating. The 40-day regimen also can be followed with an early proestrus treatment at the next estrous cycle.

In other countries, generic megestrol acetate is marketed under many brand names for use in dogs and/or cats in tablets of various content (5, 10, or 20 mg), sometimes of a single content (10 mg). The 10-mg tablets can make it difficult to dose accurately smaller animals. The drug should be administered according to the manufacturer's recommendation, unless assuming that a lower dose or shorter period of treatment will be effective is reasonable based on recommendations of other manufacturers or review articles. Side effects in dogs most frequently mentioned by manufacturers include increased appetite and weight gain, decreased aggression, increased docility, and mammary enlargement. Megestrol acetate tablets also are marketed as a human product (Megace).

Megestrol acetate at the higher proestrus dose also has been proposed and used to prevent the induction of proestrus at the onset of a treatment with a GnRH-agonist subcutaneous implant administered for long-term estrus suppression (see below).

Medroxyprogesterone Acetate Injections

A depot injectable formulation of MPA (dMPA) was marketed as a female dog contraceptive (Promone) in North America several decades ago but removed from the market because of a high incidence of uterine disease (namely, pyometra). However, dMPA marketed as a human contraceptive (Depo Provera) has been administered to bitches. Several dMPA products are marketed for veterinary use in Europe and other locales under various trade names (Promone-E, Perlutex Injection, Supprestal, Vetoquinol) with an indication for prevention of estrous cycles in bitches during anestrus. Various regimens for dosage and injection intervals have been recommended. They include 2.5 to 3 mg/kg every 5 months and 50 mg/bitch every 6 months. Side effects appear to be dose dependent, and dosing on a body weight basis would be more appropriate. Side effects of dMPA in high-dose toxicity tests or with long-term treatment with lower doses include cystic endometrial hyperplasia, pyometra, acromegaly, gallbladder calculi and mucosal hyperplasia, and mammary tumors (Concannon et al, 1980). The mammary tumors, although sometimes large, were mostly benign, but adenocarcinomas have been observed. Development of diabetes also has been reported. Injectable dosages near the minimal effective dose (e.g., 2 mg/kg every 3 months, 2.5 mg/kg every 5 months) are clinically more appropriate than higher doses. If used in dogs, depot MPA should be administered only during confirmed anestrus. Administration during mid-proestrus, late-proestrus, or early estrus can result in ovulation, in pregnancy, and in possibly failure of parturition, in pyometra, or in pseudopregnancy. Directions to use dosages much greater than those mentioned previously are likely inappropriate, although anecdotal evidence suggests that the same progestin from different manufacturers may have different biopotencies per unit of product weight.

Proligestone Injections

Proligestone is available as a depot injectable progestin in Europe (Delvosteron, Covinan) and other locations, with indications for estrus prevention in female dogs, cats, and ferrets. It is not marketed in North America. Dosages of 10 to 33 mg/kg vary inversely with body weight. For example, for bitches that are 20 kg the dose is 17.5 mg/kg but for those over 60 kg the dose is 10 mg/kg. The manufacturer's recommended dosing frequency for bitches is at 0, 3, and 7 months of treatment and subsequently at 5-month intervals. It also is indicated during proestrus to prevent ovulation and estrus. Both published reports (Selman et al, 1995) and anecdotal evidence have suggested that uterine disease, including pyometra, mammary tumors, and acromegaly, are side effects of proligestone, as with other progestins, and that administration is initiated best during anestrus with an appreciation of potential occurrences of side effects similar to those observed with other progestins.

Other Progestin Formulations

Oral formulations of MPA are marketed as human drugs in the United States and elsewhere (Provera, Farlutal) and as veterinary drugs in many countries (Perlutex Vet Tablets). A suggested dosing regimen in dogs is reported to be 10 mg/bitch for 4 days and then 5 mg/bitch for 12 days, doubling the doses for bitches weighing over 15 kg (England, 1998). As with any drug, dosing on a body-weight basis would be more appropriate.

Contraceptive Steroid Implants

Subcutaneous silastic implants that release a progestin have been used experimentally, especially for the contraception of exotic carnivores in zoos. Such implants can have a functional life of up to several years. Contraceptive steroids that have been incorporated into such implants have included progesterone, melengestrol acetate, megestrol acetate, and levonorgestrel. Uterine side effects have been reported. None are marketed commercially. Silastic implants formulated to steadily release natural progesterone in low doses were reported to have contraceptive efficacy without side effects over a 4-year treatment period, with treatment initiated during anestrus in all cases. However, plans for commercial development have not been reported.

Androgen Products

Natural androgens, including testosterone, and synthetic androgens are by definition all masculinizing and anabolic steroids, and effects are dose dependent. None are marketed with an indication for prevention of ovarian cycles in small animals in the United States, and none can be considered to be recommended or appropriate. Several are marketed in Europe and elsewhere with such indications.

Mibolerone

The androgen mibolerone, an androgen receptor-specific steroid previously was marketed in the United States for cycle prevention in dogs. The liquid oral formulation (Cheque drops) was recommended at a dosage of 30, 60, 120 or 180 µg/day continuously for up to 2 years, with the dose depending on body weight (<12, 12 to 22, 23 to 45, or >45 kg, respectively) and all Alsatians or Alsatian-derived bitches receiving the highest dosage. Withdrawal from market likely was related to abuse by athletes and listing as an anabolic steroid controlled substance in several states. Mibolerone has anabolic effects on skeletal muscle and is sometimes encountered as a contraceptive used in working and racing bitches.

Mibolerone liquid (100 µg/ml) for oral administration is available from some veterinary compounding pharmacies. Considerations include confirmation of anestrus status before treatment initiation, potential masculinization of fetuses in pregnant bitches, possible increased incidence in ovarian fibromas with long-term use, clitoral hypertrophy, and potential for anal gland inspissation with overdosage. Another extralabel use of mibolerone is to postpone estrus briefly (i.e., for 3 to 6 months) in bitches with a history of abnormally short estrous cycles.

Testosterone

Testosterone in various chemical states and formulations and several other androgens are marketed as anabolic steroids for use in human geriatric, surgical, and anemia patients, among others, and are also subject to abuse. Testosterone particularly has been used by animal owners to effect estrous cycle prevention and contraception in dogs used in sporting events, including sled dogs and racing greyhounds. In greyhounds, weekly oral administration of 25 mg of methyl testosterone for up to 5 years also has been used. Masculinizing and anabolic side effects are common. Permanent or prolonged anestrus may be a complication after treatment. The extent to which anabolic steroids are used in sporting dogs is not known. Androgen use should be considered as a possible complication in racing bitches with clitoral hypertrophy or anal gland inspissation.

In Europe, available androgen products used for pet contraception include methyl testosterone and mesterolone tablets for oral administration and injectable solutions of testosterone propionate, testosterone phenylpropionate, and mixtures of testosterone esters. The most common use of androgens as an estrous cycle preventive administered during anestrus is the depot injection of mixed testosterone esters (25 mg/kg), typically every 4 to 6 weeks, often supplemented with oral dosages of methyl testosterone at 0.25 to 0.50 mg/kg (England, 1998).

Gonadotropin-Releasing Hormone Agonists and Antagonists

Gonadotropin-Releasing Hormone Agonist Implants

GnRH agonist (deslorelin)-releasing biodegradable, lipophilic-matrix implants that result in the down-regulation of LH and FSH secretion and suppression of gonadal function in male dogs (Suprelorin) currently are marketed in Australia, New Zealand, and more than a dozen European countries for use in male dogs only. The implants have been marketed as 6-month implants (SL-6, containing 4.7 mg) and more recently also as 12-month implants (cSL-12, containing 9.4 mg; Suprelorin-12). The implants (2 mm × 12 mm and 2 mm × 25 mm, respectively) come preloaded in an insertion device. The recommended site of implant placement is subcutaneously between the shoulder blades. Use in female dogs remains extralabel and unapproved. Implants are also available on an experimental basis for use in zoo animals. The 4.7-mg implant is also marketed as an Indexed Product in North America as "Suprelorin F" for treatment of adrenal hyperplasia in ferrets. However, extralabel use in other species is forbidden by the Food and Drug Administration (FDA). Suprelorin 9.4 mg is also marketed in European countries both for adrenal suppression and for reproduction suppression in ferrets.

A GnRH agonist like deslorelin in the circulation binds to GnRH receptors on the pituitary cells and, after an initial transient phase of stimulation of LH and FSH release, the agonist down-regulates gonadotrope cell GnRH-receptors and chronically prevents release of gonadotropins in the amounts and patterns needed to support normal gonadal function. Experimental and extralabel use of implants of deslorelin and other GnRH agonists in bitches have demonstrated efficacy and safety as a female contraceptive despite the potential problem of initial induction of a fertile estrus and ovaries subsequently are maintained in an anestrous-like state.

Continuous treatment with down-regulating (i.e., desensitizing) doses of a GnRH agonist initiated in young (3½ to 5 months) prepubertal bitches has been shown to be 100% effective in suppressing ovarian cycles throughout treatments of 1 year and longer. It is without any obvious side effects and allows for a return to a normal puberty (albeit at an adult age) and fertility following implant removal (Rubion et al, 2006). In adult bitches and in prepubertal bitches 7 months of age or older, the same treatment is equally effective long term and likewise reversible, except that typically an initial ovarian-stimulation response results in a proestrus and fertile estrus during the first 2 weeks after treatment onset. The induced estrous cycle involves increased estrogen secretion in response to the initial stimulation of LH and FSH release and can result in a spontaneous ovulation-inducing LH surge and fertile ovulation. However, pregnancies that result from breeding at the induced estrus typically fail to proceed much beyond implantation because of abnormal luteal function that occurs during continued GnRH agonist administration and gonadotropin suppression. The same technology, with discontinuation of treatment following estrus induction and mating in adult bitches, has been used experimentally to synchronize pregnancies and treat prolonged anestrus in research dogs (Concannon et al, 1993; Walter et al, 2011).

A nonbiodegradable (silastic-agonist matrix) implant releasing the GnRH agonist azaglynafarelin (Gonazon CR) initially was proposed for marketing as a pet contraceptive in Europe. However, the drug is being marketed as a spawning-regulation product for the fish farming industry and is unlikely to be promoted for use in small animals. Interestingly, Gonazon-induced suppression of puberty in bitches and the resulting delay in puberty onset to 18 months of age and older had no effect on growth or body weight measured at 22 months of age when compared with untreated control bitches (Rubion et al, 2006). The investigators speculate that perhaps weight gains sometimes associated with surgical spaying are less likely to occur with the GnRH-agonist mode of contraception.

The undesirable GnRH agonist side effect of estrus induction in adult bitches is typically not seen when bitches are treated during early or mid-metestrus (diestrus) and when progesterone is above 5 ng/ml. Some reports suggest that the estrus induction effect can be suppressed or inhibited by pretreatment with megestrol acetate at 2 mg/kg but not 1 mg/kg daily for 2 weeks (but not 1 week) before and 1 week after initiation of agonist treatment. The progestin blunts the LH response to deslorelin (Sung et al, 2006). Megestrol for 4 days before implant prevented estrus (but not proestrus) induction in most but not all bitches (Corrada et al, 2006). Prolonged estrus and follicular cysts following administration of a deslorelin implant has been reported in a mature bitch.

Gonadotropin-Releasing Hormone Agonist versus Antagonist

A single injection of a GnRH antagonist (acyline) in early proestrus can transiently block GnRH-dependent gonadotropin secretion, suppress proestrus, and delay the occurrence of estrus for 2 to 5 weeks (Valiente et al, 2009). Furthermore, it may be useful for acute management of estrous cycles in bitches in which planned breeding is preferably delayed without using a more prolonged or unpredictable contraceptive regime.

The Future of Small Animal Contraception

As reviewed earlier (in the previous edition of *Current Veterinary Therapy*; Kutzler and Wood, 2006), several alternative technologies are currently being tested, including immunization against GnRH, GnRH-multimers, LH receptor, or ovarian zona pellucida or other oocyte proteins, and the administration of GnRH (or other reproductive hormones or hormone analogs) conjugated to cytotoxins and thus targeting the destruction of pituitary gonadotroph cells (or other reproductive cell types) as cells required for normal cycles and/or fertility. No marketable method has resulted to date. GonaCon, a USDA research-developed, GnRH-mollusk blue protein conjugate vaccine is approved for use in multiple wild and feral animal species in the United States and is being studied coadministered with rabies vaccine to feral dogs. Similar testing has involved the vaccination of feral dogs with a biosynthetic rabies virus protein into which two copies of GnRH-peptide sequence are incorporated.

References and Suggested Reading

Colon J et al: Effects of contraceptive doses of the progestagen megestrol acetate on luteinizing hormone and follicle-stimulating hormone secretion in female dogs, *J Reprod Fertil Suppl* 47:519, 1993.

Concannon P: Reproductive endocrinology, contraception and pregnancy termination in dogs. In Ettinger S, Feldman E, editors: *Textbook of veterinary internal medicine*, Philadelphia, 1995a, Saunders, p 1625.

Concannon P et al: Growth hormone, prolactin, and cortisol in dogs developing mammary nodules and an acromegaly-like appearance during treatment with medroxyprogesterone acetate, *Endocrinology* 106:1173, 1980.

Concannon PW: Contraception in the dog. In Raw ME, Parkinson TJ, editors: *The veterinary annual*, Oxford, UK, 1995b, Blackwell Scientific, p 177.

Concannon PW: Reproductive cycles of the domestic bitch, *Anim Reprod Sci* 124:200, 2011.

Concannon PW et al: Synchronous delayed oestrus in beagle bitches given infusions of gonadotrophin-releasing hormone superagonist following withdrawal of progesterone implants, *J Reprod Fertil Suppl* 47:522, 1993.

Corrada Y et al: Short-term progestin treatments prevent estrous induction by a GnRH agonist implant in anestrous bitches, *Theriogenology* 65:366, 2006.

England G: Pharmacological control of reproduction in the bitch. In Simpson G, England GE, Harvey MJ, editors: *Manual of small animal reproduction and neonatology*, Birmingham, UK, 1998, British Small Animal Association, p 197.

Kutzler M, Wood A: Non-surgical methods of contraception and sterilization, *Theriogenology* 66:514, 2006.

Romagnoli S, Concannon P: Clinical use of progestins in bitches and queens: a review. In Concannon P, England G, Verstegen J, Linde-Forspurg C, editors: *Recent advances in small animal reproduction*, (ePub:International Veterinary Information Service), 2003, accessed June 27, 2013 from www.ivis.org.

Rubion S et al: Treatment with a subcutaneous GnRH agonist containing controlled release device reversibly prevents puberty in bitches, *Theriogenology* 66:1651, 2006.

Selman PJ et al: Comparison of the histological changes in the dog after treatment with the progestins medroxyprogesterone acetate and proligestone, *Vet Q* 17:128, 1995.

Sung M, Armour AF, Wright PJ: The influence of exogenous progestin on the occurrence of proestrous or estrous signs, plasma concentrations of luteinizing hormone and estradiol in deslorelin (GnRH agonist) treated anestrous bitches, *Theriogenology* 66:1513, 2006.

Valiente C et al: Interruption of the canine estrous cycle with a low and a high dose of the GnRH antagonist, acyline, *Theriogenology* 71:408, 2009.

Walter B et al: Estrus induction in Beagle bitches with the GnRH-agonist implant containing 4.7 mg Deslorelin, *Theriogenology* 75:1125, 2011.

CHAPTER 216

Medical Termination of Pregnancy

BRUCE E. EILTS, *Townsville, Australia*

A perfect pregnancy termination drug could be given at any stage of estrus or pregnancy, would be 100% effective, would cause no vaginal discharge, would have no side effects, would not impair future fertility, would be readily available, and would be inexpensive. Unfortunately such a drug does not exist. In cases in which the patient is not a valuable breeding animal, the client should be counseled that the best option is to terminate the pregnancy and to prevent future pregnancies surgical sterilization is recommended. Drugs available for pregnancy termination are discussed under the general categories of those used after pregnancy is confirmed and those used before pregnancy is confirmed. A comprehensive list of drugs to terminate pregnancy commonly available in the United States is discussed.

Drugs Used After Confirmed Pregnancy

If the bitch mated or is thought to have mated, a pregnancy diagnosis should be performed before proceeding to terminate the pregnancy. Even though conception rates in controlled breeding situations resulted in a pregnancy rate of about 90% when only a single mating was allowed on any day of estrus (up to the last 2 days of estrus) (Holst and Phemister, 1974), only 38% of bitches presented for mismate actually may be pregnant (Feldman et al, 1993). A pregnancy examination should be performed at least 30 to 40 days after the last possible breeding to minimize false-negative diagnoses caused by errors in calculating the gestation duration from a mating that occurred early in estrus. Therapy is instituted only if a bitch is pregnant. Drugs that terminate pregnancy can cause premature luteal demise by acting as a direct luteolytic, inhibiting prolactin secretion, or blocking the progesterone receptors or unknown mechanisms.

Prostaglandins

Protocols

Prostaglandin $F_{2\alpha}$ ($PGF_{2\alpha}$) induces lysis of the corpora lutea. In dogs, the natural $PGF_{2\alpha}$ (Lutalyse) given at a dosage of 0.1 to 0.25 mg/kg q8-12h SC is effective at terminating pregnancy after pregnancy confirmation. One protocol reported to have few side effects is administration of $PGF_{2\alpha}$ at 0.1 mg/kg q8h SC for 2 days and then 0.2 mg/kg q8h SC until abortion is complete (Feldman et al, 1993). Abortion usually is complete within 9 days, but some dams still have live fetuses after 9 days. It is extremely important to continue the treatments until abortion is complete. In queens, natural $PGF_{2\alpha}$ is most effective after 40 days of gestation. Beginning at 45 days of gestation, $PGF_{2\alpha}$ (0.2 mg/kg q12h SC first day, 0.5 mg/kg q12h SC for up to 5 days) caused abortion in 75% of queens.

Synthetic $PGF_{2\alpha}$ analogs are more potent and have fewer side effects than natural $PGF_{2\alpha}$. Cloprostenol (Estrumate) at a dosage of 1 to 2.5 µg/kg q24h SC for 4 to 5 days was 100% effective at inducing abortion (Verstegen, 2000). Once-per-day treatments with synthetic $PGF_{2\alpha}$ analogs provide an advantage over the three-times-per-day treatments required with natural $PGF_{2\alpha}$. Hospitalization or frequency of injections adds greatly to client cost when using $PGF_{2\alpha}$ as an abortifacient.

To shorten the treatment period required to induce abortion with $PGF_{2\alpha}$, $PGF_{2\alpha}$ (0.1 mg/kg q8h SC for 2 days and then 0.2 mg/kg q8h SC to effect) can be combined with PGE_1 (misoprostol, Cytotec) at a dosage of 1 to 3 µg/kg q24h deposited into the cranial vaginal vault. The mean time to complete abortion using this combination was 2 days shorter compared with $PGF_{2\alpha}$ alone (5 days vs. 7 days, respectively) (Davidson et al, 1997). Similar results have been reported using PGE_1 with the synthetic $PGF_{2\alpha}$, alfaprostenol (Agaoglu et al, 2011).

Adverse Effects

Adverse effects of natural $PGF_{2\alpha}$ are more common in dogs than cats and include vomiting, diarrhea, and possibly circulatory collapse. The adverse effects usually subside within 20 minutes, but the bitch should be monitored carefully during this time. To minimize caloric loss, bitches should be fed at least 1 hour after treatment. Minimal to no adverse effects are observed when using $PGF_{2\alpha}$ analogs at a 1 µg/kg q24h SC dosage.

Drugs used to decrease the adverse effects of natural $PGF_{2\alpha}$ include a combination of atropine sulfate (0.025 mg/kg), prifinium bromide (0.1 ml/kg), and metopimazine (0.5 mg/kg) SC 15 minutes before $PGF_{2\alpha}$ administration. Lower doses of natural $PGF_{2\alpha}$ also decrease adverse effects.

Complete pregnancy termination 5 days after starting treatment with minimal adverse effects (tachypnea lasting less than 15 minutes) was reported after administration of natural $PGF_{2\alpha}$ at a dose of 0.012 mg/kg q6h SC at 30 days of gestation (Len et al, 2011). Clients must be able to administer safely multiple injections to their animals, or the animals must be hospitalized. The safety and efficacy of this protocol makes it the author's primary choice as an abortifacient in the bitch.

Prolactin Inhibitors

Dopaminergic drugs are prolactin inhibitors. Commercially available prolactin inhibitors include bromocriptine, cabergoline, and metergoline. Bromocriptine (Parlodel) administered at a dosage of 62.5 µg/kg q12h PO to dogs at 43 to 45 days after ovulation resulted in only 50% of bitches aborting; side effects included emesis and loose stools (Wichtel et al, 1990). Because the dosage is so low and the tablets contain so much active drug the bromocriptine tablets can be crushed and dissolved in water to ease dosing. Cabergoline at a dose of 1.65 µg/kg q24h SC for 5 to 6 days at 25 to 40 days after the first mating resulted in abortion for 100% of bitches greater than 40 days of gestation but only for 25% and 67% at 25 days and 30 days of gestation, respectively. Side effects were minimal, and bitches that aborted became pregnant after treatment. In the United States, cabergoline is available in a 0.5-mg tablet. When given at a dose of 160 µg PO to a 32-kg German shepherd dog after 40 days of gestation, it resulted in abortion after 7 days with no side effects (Arbeiter and Flatscher, 1996). Although cabergoline is not expensive for each dose, it may be difficult to administer because of the amount of drug per tablet (0.5 mg) is considerably higher than the dose for a 10-kg dog (0.05 mg). Metergoline (0.6 mg/kg q12h PO starting after the onset of cytologic diestrus and continued to effect) induced abortion in 89% of bitches with no side effects (Nöthling et al, 2003). Cabergoline (5 to 15 µg/kg q24h PO) administered to feral cats 36 to 40 days of pregnancy for 4 to 9 days caused abortion in 100% of queens (Jochle and Jochle 1993).

Prolactin Inhibitors in Combination with Prostaglandin $F_{2\alpha}$ Analogs

Combining prolactin inhibitors with $PGF_{2\alpha}$ increases the efficacy of pregnancy termination and reduces the side effects of treatment. Cloprostenol (1 or 2.5 µg/kg SC once) in combination with cabergoline (1.65 µg/kg q24h SC for 5 days) from midgestation induced abortion with no adverse side effects (Onclin et al, 1995). After an average of 9 days, cabergoline (5 µg/kg q24h PO) 1 hour after cloprostenol (1 µg/kg q48h SC) caused fetal death with no side effects when started at 25 days of gestation peak (Onclin and Verstegen, 1996). Treatment with cabergoline (5 µg/kg q24h PO) for 10 days combined with either one dose (2.5 µg/kg SC) or two doses (1 µg/kg SC repeated 4 days later) of cloprostenol at the start of the treatment was successful at inducing pregnancy termination. Similarly, bromocriptine (30 µg/kg q8h PO) for 10 days with either one dose (2.5 µg/kg SC) or two doses (1 µg/kg SC repeated 4 days later) of cloprostenol at the start of the treatment was successful at inducing pregnancy termination (Onclin and Verstegen, 1999). All bitches in the aforementioned study became pregnant during the subsequent estrous cycle, which occurred sooner than normally anticipated. As with $PGF_{2\alpha}$ alone, using PGE_1 with the cabergoline combined with a synthetic $PGF_{2\alpha}$ decreased the time to abortion compared with those not receiving PGE_1. Oral cabergoline (5 µg/kg q24h PO) combined with cloprostenol (5 µg/kg q48h SC) starting at the thirtieth day after coitus caused abortion in 100% of queens after an average of 9 days of treatments.

Progesterone Receptor Blockers

The progesterone receptor blocker mifepristone (Mifeprex), more commonly known as RU486 or RU38486 for its use in preventing human pregnancies, administered at a dosage of 2.5 mg/kg q12h PO for $4\frac{1}{2}$ days starting at day 32 of gestation resulted in no side effects and 100% abortion in bitches with pregnancy loss occurring 3 days after treatment initiation (Concannon et al, 1990). Doses as low as 8.3 mg/kg and up to 20 mg/kg q24h PO for one or two treatments resulted in abortion within 2 to 11 days at days 35 to 39 of pregnancy (Linde-Forsberg et al, 1992). In the United States, mifepristone is available only in a 200-mg tablet.

Aglepristone (Alizine) is another progesterone receptor blocker that is commercially available in several European countries but not in the United States. Two doses of aglepristone (9.9 mg/kg q24h SC) caused uncomplicated abortions within 14 days in 94.4% of bitches after 26 days of pregnancy (Fieni et al, 2003) Side effects included slight depression, transitory anorexia, and mammary gland congestion. Similar to $PGF_{2\alpha}$ alone, administration of PGE_1 (200 to 400 µg q24h) intravaginally in combination with aglepristone reduced the time to abortion when compared with aglepristone alone. In cats, aglepristone (10 mg/kg q24h SC) administered twice caused abortion in 5 ± 2 days in 100% of queens (Favre et al, 2007).

Unknown Mechanisms

Although the mechanism of action is not completely known, dexamethasone was effective at terminating pregnancy from midgestation after a $10\frac{1}{2}$-day dosage schedule (Table 216-1). Pregnancies lasting less than 40 days generally had no fetuses expelled with mild vaginal discharge seen in about 34% of the bitches (Wanke et al, 1997; Zone et al, 1995). Pregnancy loss generally was complete 10 to 23 days after the treatment started. The main side effects of dexamethasone treatment included anorexia, polydipsia, and polyuria. The side effects usually begin around 2 to 3 days after treatment is initiated, are most pronounced 4 to 5 days later, and then subside 3 to 4 days after the termination of treatment. Successful pregnancies were obtained in 90% of bitches bred during the first estrus after treatment. In the author's experience, dexamethasone (0.2 mg/kg q12h PO) until pregnancy termination has occurred (with no tapering of the dose) has similar results with no greater side effects. The advantages of dexamethasone treatment for pregnancy termination

TABLE **216-1**

Dosing Schedule for Canine Pregnancy Termination with Dexamethasone

Treatment Days	Dexamethasone Dose or Dosage
Days 1 to 7	0.2 mg/kg q12h PO
Day 8 (AM)	0.16 mg/kg PO
Day 8 (PM)	0.12 mg/kg PO
Day 9 (AM)	0.08 mg/kg PO
Day 9 (PM)	0.04 mg/kg PO
Day 10 (AM)	0.02 mg/kg PO

over the previously mentioned drugs include that it eliminates most of the side effects reported with other pregnancy termination drugs, avoids the requirement for hospitalization or office visits for injections, is inexpensive, is readily available, can be administered easily by clients, is effective, and has few side effects. However, this author is aware of anecdotal reports of prolonged treatment times, treatment failures, and even patient death associated with dexamethasone pregnancy termination. The author is unaware of its effect on pregnancy termination in the queen.

Several other drugs have been used to terminate pregnancy in the bitch, including tamoxifen citrate (Noladex), which acts as an estrogen; epostane, which inhibits steroid synthesis by inhibition of 3β-hydroxysteroid dehydrogenase; and Δ5-4 isomerase and isoquinolones L-12717 (Lotifren). These are either not efficacious or not available in the United States.

Drugs Used Before Confirmed Pregnancy

During Diestrus

Before pregnancy confirmation, prolactin inhibitors are ineffective at terminating pregnancy because of their mechanism of action (as discussed above). Although $PGF_{2\alpha}$ can be used to terminate pregnancy before pregnancy confirmation, the dosage required to induce luteolysis at this stage of diestrus approaches the LD_{50}. Progesterone receptor blockers should be effective at this stage of gestation in dogs and cats, but controlled studies to demonstrate their efficacy before pregnancy confirmation have not been performed.

During Estrus

The only drugs available to terminate pregnancy during estrus are the estrogens, which act by blocking embryo transit in the oviducts. The use of estrogens for mismate management is cited in many texts and by many academicians as being unsafe to the extent of being malpractice; however, little published data substantiate these statements. Estrogens should be used only during estrus because their use during diestrus significantly increases the chance of inducing a pyometra. A vaginal cytology examination having 90% to 100% cornified cells shows that the bitch is truly in estrus, whereas if the cells are not cornified, the bitch is not in estrus. Side effects such as prolonged estrus, pyometra, and aplastic anemia (pancytopenia) are possible; therefore it should be documented that the bitch actually was bred based on owner observation of a mating or laboratory identification or the presence of sperm cells in a vaginal swab. Sperm cells can be identified in 100% of bitches mated within 24 hours and 75% of bitches mated within 48 hours by placing the tip of the vaginal cytology swab into a tube containing 0.5 ml saline for 10 minutes, squeezing the swab dry into a tube and centrifuging the fluid at 2000 × g for 10 minutes, and finally staining the sediment.

Estradiol cypionate (ECP, Depo-Estradiol) was shown to have 100% efficacy and no side effects during the study period when administered at a dose of 44 µg/kg intramuscularly one time during estrus; however, a 25% (¼) incidence of pyometra was seen when administered during diestrus (Bowen et al, 1985). Although the drug marketed as ECP is no longer available, estradiol cypionate can still be obtained from compounding pharmacies. Estradiol benzoate (oestradiol benzoate) at a dosage of 0.01 mg/kg IM at 3 and 5 days (and occasionally 7 days) after mating in 358 bitches resulted in only 4.5% (16/358) of the bitches actually whelping; in none of the bitches was bone marrow aplasia reported. The 7.3% incidence of pyometra reported was not different from the normal prevalence reported as 2% to 10%. Although a more recent study showed a statistically higher incidence of pyometra associated with estradiol benzoate pregnancy termination treatment (8.7% in estradiol benzoate–treated bitches compared with 1.3% in untreated bitches) (Whitehead, 2008). Administration of diethyl stilbestrol is not effective at terminating pregnancy (Bowen et al, 1985).

In queens, ECP (250 µg/cat IM) administered 6 days after coitus retarded uterine tubal embryo transport and development. Administration of ECP (125 to 250 µg/cat IM) 40 hours after coitus has been suggested to be an effective mismating regimen in queens; however, no data are available on its actual efficacy (Heron and Sis, 1974).

This author does not encourage estrogen use for routine pregnancy termination because alternative treatments are available once the bitch is diagnosed pregnant. However, the use of estrogens for pregnancy termination is not condemned unconditionally as malpractice.

References and Suggested Reading

Agaoglu AR et al: The intravaginal application of misoprostol improves induction of abortion with aglepristone, *Theriogenology* 76:74, 2011.

Arbeiter K, Flatscher C: Induction of abortion in the bitch using cabergoline (Galastop), *Kleintierprax* 41:747, 1996.

Bowen RA et al: Efficacy and toxicity of estrogens commonly used to terminate canine pregnancy, *Amer Vet Med Assn* 186:783, 1985.

Cetin Y et al: Intravaginal application of misoprostol improves pregnancy termination with cabergoline and alfaprostol in dogs, *Berl Munch Tierarztl Wochenschr* 123:236, 2010.

Concannon PW, Yeager A, Frank D: Termination of pregnancy and induction of premature luteolysis by the antiprogestagen, mifepristone, in dogs, *J Reprod Fertil* 88:99, 1990.

Davidson AP, Nelson RW, Feldman EC: Induction of abortion in 9 bitches with intravaginal misoprostol and parenteral PGF2α, *J Vet Intern Med* 11:123, 1997.

Favre RN et al: Induction of abortion in queens by administration of aglepristone (Alizine): preliminary results, *Theriogenology* 68:499, 2007.

Feldman EC et al: Prostaglandin induction of abortion in pregnant bitches after misalliance, *J Amer Vet Med Assn* 202:1855, 1993.

Fieni F et al: Clinical use of anti-progestins in the bitch, *Int Vet Inform Serv*, accessed October 30, 2011, from http://www.ivis .org/advances/Concannon/fieni/ivis.pdf.

Heron MA, Sis RF: Ovum transport in the cat and the effect of estrogen administration, *Amer J Vet Res* 35:1277, 1974.

Holst PA, Phemister RD: Onset of diestrus in the Beagle bitch: definition and significance, *Amer J Vet Res* 35:401, 1974.

Jochle W, Jochle M: Reproduction in a feral cat population and its control with a prolactin inhibitor, cabergoline, *J Reprod Fertil Suppl* 47:419, 1993.

Len JA et al: Low dose prostaglandin F$_{2a}$ for luteal regression in the bitch, *Clin Theriogenol* 2:362, 2011.

Linde-Forsberg C, Kindahl H, Madej A: Termination of mid-term pregnancy in the dog with oral RU 486, *Small Anim Pract* 33:331, 1992.

Nöthling J et al: Abortifacient and endocrine effects of metergoline in beagle bitches during the second half of gestation, *Theriogenology* 59:1929, 2003.

Onclin K, Silva LDM, Verstegen JP: Termination of unwanted pregnancy in dogs with the dopamine agonist, cabergoline, in combination with a synthetic analog of PGF2Alpha, either cloprostenol or alphaprostol, *Theriogenology* 43:813, 1995.

Onclin K, Verstegen JP: Comparisons of different combinations of analogues of PGF2à and dopamine agonists for the termination of pregnancy in dogs, *Vet Rec* 144:416, 1999.

Onclin K, Verstegen JP: Practical use of a combination of a dopamine agonist and a synthetic prostaglandin analogue to terminate unwanted pregnancy in dogs, *Small Anim Pract* 37:211, 1996.

Sutton DJ, Geary MR, Bergman JGHE: Prevention of pregnancy in bitches following unwanted mating: a clinical- trial using low-dose estradiol benzoate, *J Reprod Fertil Supp* 51:239, 1997.

Verstegen JP: Overview of mismating for the bitch. In Bonagura JD, editor: *Current veterinary therapy: small animal practice*, ed 13, Philadelphia, 2000, WB Saunders, p 947.

Wanke M et al: Clinical use of dexamethasone for termination of unwanted pregnancy in dogs, *J Reprod Fertil Supp* 51:233, 1997.

Whitehead M: Risk of pyometra in bitches treated for mismating with low doses of oestradiol benzoate, *Vet Rec* 162:746, 2008.

Wichtel JJ et al: Comparison of the effects of PGF2a and bromocryptine in pregnant beagle bitches, *Theriogenology* 33:829, 1990.

Zone M et al: Termination of pregnancy in dogs by oral administration of dexamethasone, *Theriogenology* 43:487, 1995.

CHAPTER 217

Inherited Disorders of the Reproductive Tract in Dogs and Cats

VICKI N. MEYERS-WALLEN, *Ithaca, New York*

Normal Sexual Development

Normal sexual development depends on successful completion of three consecutive steps: (1) establishment of chromosomal sex, (2) development of gonadal sex, and (3) development of phenotypic sex. *Chromosomal sex*, which corresponds to genetic sex in normal animals, is established at fertilization. The zygote receives either two X chromosomes or an X and a Y chromosome and maintains this chromosomal constitution in all cells by mitotic division. Morphology of early XX and XY embryos is sexually indifferent. Both have a genital ridge, from which the testis or ovary develops. They also have müllerian and wolffian ducts, a urogenital sinus, a genital tubercle, and genital swellings, from which the internal and external genitalia will arise (Figure 217-1). Differentiation of the genital ridge into a testis or an ovary defines gonadal sex and marks the end of the sexually indifferent stage. Although several genes are necessary for normal development through the sexually indifferent stage, genes that determine gonadal sex have a pivotal role in sexual development.

Gonadal sex typically is determined by sex chromosome constitution: presence of the Y chromosome results in testis development, whereas its absence results in ovarian development. The sex-determining region Y gene, *SRY*, is located normally on the Y chromosome, and the SRY protein is the signal for initiating testis differentiation in the genital ridge (Jakob and Lovell-Badge, 2011). In the absence of the Y chromosome and *SRY*, the genital ridge normally becomes an ovary. However, ovarian induction is not a passive process: testis-promoting and ovary-promoting signaling pathways are responsible for gonadal sex determination (Quinn and Koopman, 2012).

Phenotypic sex is controlled normally by gonadal sex. If the genital ridges are removed from XX or XY embryos before gonadal differentiation occurs, a female phenotype develops, indicating that the embryo is programmed to develop as a female and must be diverted from this pathway to develop as a male. The critical diverting step is testis development. The testis secretes two substances that act within embryonic critical periods to induce masculinization: (1) müllerian-inhibiting substance/antimüllerian hormone (MIS/AMH), which causes the müllerian ducts to regress, and (2) testosterone, which stimulates formation of the vasa deferentia and epididymides from the wolffian ducts (see Figure 217-1). In the external genitalia, testosterone is converted to dihydrotestosterone (DHT) by the enzyme 5α-reductase. Dihydrotestosterone stimulates formation of the prostate and male urethra, penis, and scrotum from the urogenital sinus, genital tubercle, and genital swellings, respectively (see Figure 217-1). Descent of the testes into the scrotum completes the male external genitalia, but the genetic and hormonal control of this process is incompletely understood. Testosterone and insulin-like 3 factor (*INSL3*), both secreted by Leydig cells, are required for testis descent, as are their receptors, but other unknown factors also likely are involved. In the absence of testicular secretions, female genitalia develop (see Figure 217-1).

Diagnosis of Disorders of Sexual Development

For the purpose of pursuing a diagnosis, it is useful to identify the initial step at which development differs from normal, either at the level of chromosomal sex, gonadal sex, or phenotypic sex (Table 217-1). A more precise diagnosis defines the disorder according to its etiology, preferably by the specific gene mutation responsible for the defect. To eliminate older, confusing terms such as pseudohermaphrodite and facilitate incorporation of molecular diagnoses, a new nomenclature has been established (Pasterski, Prentice, and Hughes, 2010). With this terminology, intersex individuals are described as having a disorder of sexual development (DSD), a non-specific term. All DSDs are categorized initially by karyotype, with *sex chromosome DSD* including all errors at the level of chromosomal sex. Errors occurring at the level of gonadal sex or phenotypic sex now are divided according to karyotype, either *XX DSD* or *XY DSD* (see Table 217-1).

Regardless of the nomenclature used, the diagnostic plan for any DSD includes a karyotype (dog 78,XX or 78,XY; cat 38,XX or 38,XY). The presence or absence of the *SRY* gene in dogs and cats can be tested by polymerase chain reaction (PCR). Gonadal sex is determined by histology and may require serial gonadal sections for identification of ovotestes. A concise description of the

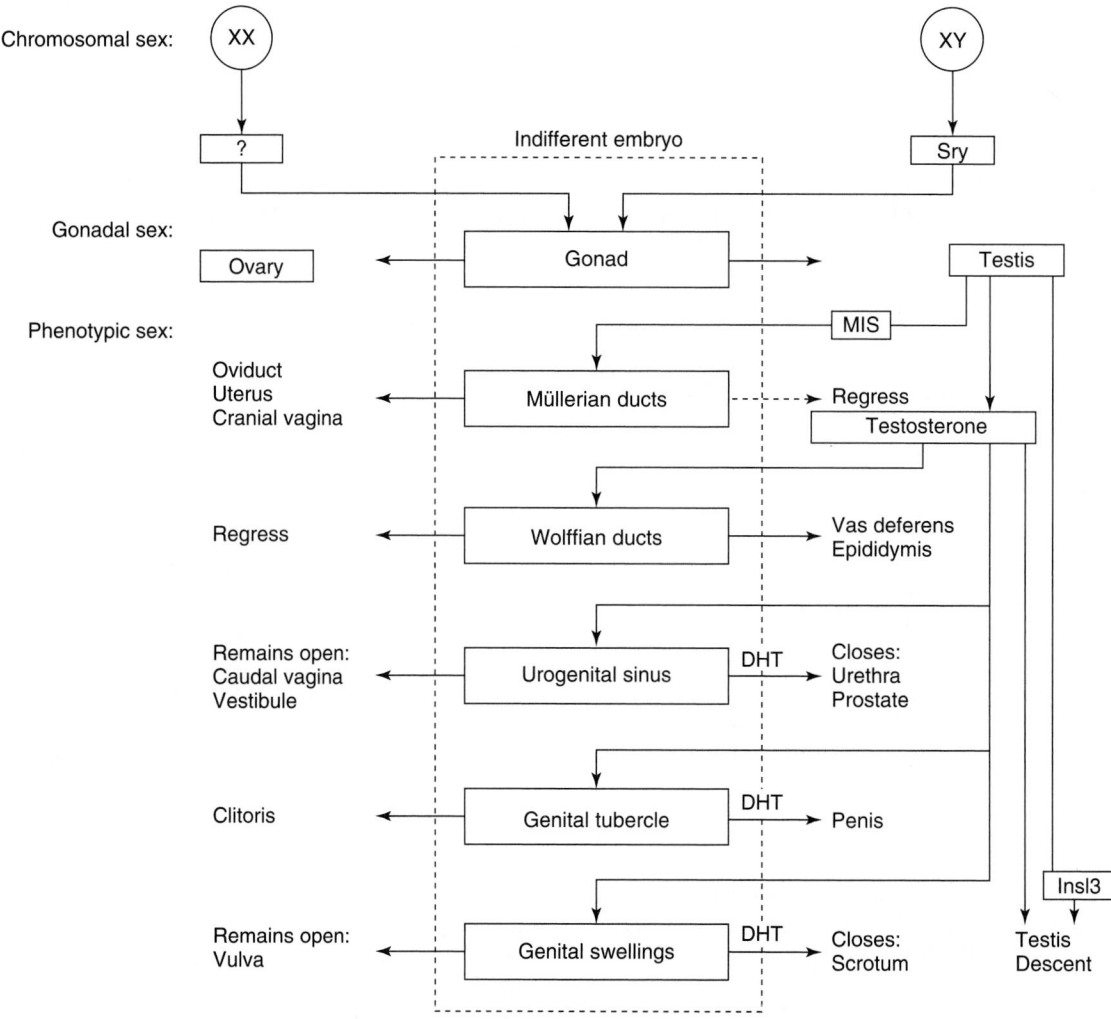

Figure 217-1 Major steps in normal sexual development. (Modified with permission from: Meyers-Wallen VN, Patterson DF: Disorders of sexual development in the dog. In Morrow DA, editor: *Current therapy in theriogenology*, ed 2, Philadelphia, 1986, WB Saunders, p 567.)

internal and external genitalia is necessary to define phenotypic sex. Assays of peripheral hormones may be helpful but are not a substitute for gonadal histology. Gonadotropin-releasing hormone (GnRH) or human chorionic gonadotropin (hCG) stimulation tests, rather than single peripheral samples, are necessary in many cases, particularly those in which peripheral androgen concentrations are of concern.

Sex Chromosome Disorders of Sexual Development

Many disorders of sexual differentiation have been reported, in which the primary cause was an abnormality in the number or structure of the sex chromosomes. To summarize, animals with abnormalities in sex chromosome number, such as those with XXY and XO syndromes and their variants, generally have underdeveloped genitalia and are sterile but are unambiguously male or female in phenotype (see Table 217-1). However, some XXX dogs have exhibited estrous cycles, and pregnancy was reported in an XXX variant cat. The gonadal sex of

chimeras and mosaics depends on the distribution of XX and XY cells within the genital ridge. Phenotypic sex then is determined by the presence and amount of functional testicular tissue in the gonad. Sex chromosome DSDs usually are caused by errors in chromosome segregation or by fusion of zygotes. Therefore familial aggregation of affected individuals is not expected.

XX Disorders of Sexual Development

All animals with XX disorders of sexual development (XX DSDs) have a female karyotype and are separated according to whether the primary defect occurs at or below the level of the gonad (see Table 217-1).

Disorders of Gonadal Development
For those individuals with the primary defect occurring at the level of the gonad, these animals develop testicular tissue (ovotestis or testis) despite having a normal female karyotype. This has been reported in dogs but not in cats. Such animals previously were termed sex-reversed because the chromosomal sex and the gonadal sex of the

TABLE 217-1

Main Features of Selected Disorders of Sexual Development Reported in Dogs or Cats

	Karyotype	Gonads	Müllerian Duct Derivatives	Wolffian Duct Derivatives	External Genitalia	Diagnosis
Abnormality of Chromosomal Sex	XO	Streak gonad	Uterus, uterine tubes, vagina	None	Female	Sex chromosome DSD
	XXX	Ovary ± hypoplastic	Uterus, uterine tubes, vagina	None	Female	Sex chromosome DSD
	XXY	Testis	None	Epididymis, vas deferens	Male	Sex chromosome DSD
	XX/XY	Ovary or ovotestis or testis	Varies with amount of functional testis	Varies with amount of functional testis	Female ± ambiguous or male	Sex chromosome DSD
Abnormality of Gonadal Sex	XX	Ovotestis	Uterus ± uterine tube	Epididymis (±)	Female or enlarged clitoris	XX DSD, ovotesticular
	XX	Testis	Uterus	Epididymis ± vas deferens	Cryptorchid, hypospadias, displaced prepuce	XX DSD, testicular
	XY	Testis lacking germ cells	Uterus (±)	Epididymis (±)	Ambiguous	XY DSD, testicular dysgenesis (partial)
	XY	Ovotestis	Uterus, uterine tube	Epididymis ± vas deferens	Male	XY DSD, ovotesticular
Abnormality of Phenotypic Sex	XX	Ovary	Uterus, uterine tube	None	Ambiguous or Male	XX DSD, androgen excess
	XX	Ovary	Uterus: unicornuate, hypoplastic or segmental aplastic (+ renal agenesis or ectopy)	None	Female	XX DSD, müllerian agenesis, or hypoplasia
	XY	Testis	None	None or epididymis	Female or ambiguous	XY DSD, androgen insensitivity syndromes
	XY	Testis	Uterus, uterine tube, cranial vagina	Epididymis, vas deferens	Male	XY DSD, persistent müllerian duct syndrome
	XY	Testis	None	Epididymis, vas deferens	Male with hypospadias only	XY DSD, isolated hypospadias
	XY	Testis	None	Epididymis, vas deferens	Male with cryptorchidism only	XY DSD, isolated cryptorchidism

individual disagree. Affected dogs have at least one ovo-testis (ovotesticular XX DSD) or bilateral testes (testicular XX DSD) and previously were called XX true hermaphrodites or XX males, respectively. Both phenotypes can appear in the same family. Phenotypic masculinization depends on the amount of testicular tissue in the affected individual. Thus those with ovotestes may have normal female external genitalia, an enlarged clitoris with an os clitoris that resembles a penis, or any phenotype in between. Those with bilateral testes generally have a cau-dally displaced prepuce and a penis with hypospadias and are bilaterally cryptorchid. This DSD has been reported as a familial trait in at least 28 canine breeds and two mixed breeds (Box 217-1). In the American cocker spaniel, this DSD is inherited as an autosomal-recessive trait, but the mode of inheritance has not been determined in all breeds. The Y-linked *SRY* gene is absent in all affected dogs reported, ruling out translocation as the cause.

BOX 217-1

Canine Breeds in Which Testicular or Ovotesticular XX DSD Has Been Reported

American cocker spaniel	German shepherd dog
Afghan hound	German shorthaired pointer
American pit bull terrier	Golden retriever
American Staffordshire terrier	Jack Russell terrier
Australian shepherd	Kerry blue terrier
Basset hound	Norwegian elkhound
Bernese mountain dog	Podenco dog
Beagle	Pug
Border collie	Soft-coated wheaten terrier
Brussels griffon	Tibetan terrier
Doberman pinscher	Vizsla
English cocker spaniel	Walker hound
French bulldog	Weimaraner
German pinscher	Wheaten terrier

Diagnosis depends on confirmation of a 78,XX karyotype and histology demonstrating at least one ovotestis or testis. To define the etiology more precisely and aid in genetic counseling, the diagnostic workup should include a molecular test for *SRY*. Whereas elevation in peripheral testosterone concentrations in response to GnRH or hCG stimulation strongly suggests that testicular tissue is present, it is not diagnostic. The inability to provoke testosterone elevation by a stimulation test does rule out the diagnosis. In addition to dogs, ovotesticular or testicular XX DSD in which the individuals are *SRY* negative has been reported in several mammals. Mutations that cause *SOX9* or *SOX3* overexpression or reduce *RSPO1* expression have been identified in affected humans and mice (Jakob and Lovell-Badge, 2011).

This form of canine XX DSD has been studied most extensively in a pedigree derived from the American cocker spaniel, in which an autosomal-recessive mode of inheritance was identified through experimental matings (Meyers-Wallen, 2012). A genome-wide linkage analysis in this model pedigree identified linkage to CFA29. A candidate gene has not been identified, and *SOX9, RSPO1,* and *SOX3* are not located in this region. The causative mutation is likely to be the same in American and English cocker spaniels because they share recent common ancestry. It is unclear whether the same gene locus is responsible in other breeds.

Treatment is limited to surgical removal of the gonads and uterus and, if the dog is uncomfortable, excision of the enlarged clitoris and os clitoris. Although all dogs with testicular XX DSD and most with ovotesticular XX DSD are sterile, some of the latter have exhibited estrous cycles and reproduced as females. Nevertheless, the mating of affected dogs of any breed is discouraged strongly because it will increase the frequency of the causative mutation within the breed and lead to production of more affected dogs. Similarly, parents of affected dogs should not be bred. As the causative mutation is unknown, a laboratory test to detect carriers and affected dogs is not available.

Androgen Excess
These animals have a female karyotype and bilateral ovaries but develop ambiguous genitalia in response to androgen exposure during development (see Table 217-1). They are categorized according to the androgen source, either fetal or maternal. These are errors of phenotypic sex, formerly categorized as female pseudohermaphroditism.

Fetal Origin. Although adrenal enzyme defects (adrenogenital syndromes) are a common cause of fetal androgen excess in humans, they are apparently rare in dogs and cats. Steroid precursors accumulate at the enzyme block and are shunted to the androgen synthesis pathway. Excess adrenal androgen production from 11 beta-hydroxylase deficiency has been reported in a 38,XX calico cat that presented with male external genitalia, but the testes were not palpable. Internal genitalia consisted of ovaries, bicornuate uterus, and uterine tubes. Clinical signs included polydipsia, polyuria, and inappropriate urination. After ovariohysterectomy, penile spines persisted and peripheral testosterone concentrations were in the normal range of an intact male. Subsequent

to prednisone treatment, testosterone concentrations decreased and clinical signs ceased. This DSD has not been reported in dogs.

Maternal Origin. Canine cases of androgen excess have been 78,XX individuals with bilateral ovaries, a complete uterus, and phenotypic masculinization ranging from mild clitoral enlargement to nearly normal male external genitalia and a prostate gland internally. An iatrogenic cause was known in some cases: either an androgen (testosterone, mibolerone) or a progestagen had been administered to the pregnant dam. Presenting signs were related to bleeding at the onset of proestrus, urinary incontinence, or uterine infection. Feline cases have not been reported.

Diagnosis of XX DSD, androgen excess depends on confirmation of a female karyotype, bilateral ovaries, and evidence of androgen-dependent masculinization. Before gonadectomy, the diagnostic workup could include tests for endogenous androgen production. Elevation of serum testosterone in response to GnRH or hCG would suggest testicular androgen production, which along with a female karyotype would suggest a diagnosis of ovotesticular or testicular XX DSD (above). Gonadal histology is necessary for distinguishing the difference. Abnormal elevation of serum androgens in response to adrenocorticotropic hormone (ACTH) stimulation would suggest adrenal androgen production and androgen excess of fetal origin, as in adrenogenital syndromes (above). If no evidence of endogenous androgen production is found, historical confirmation of exogenous androgen exposure to the pregnant dam should be sought.

Ovariohysterectomy, with gonadal histopathology, is recommended. However, when urinary abnormalities are present, contrast studies are recommended before surgery to determine whether additional surgical treatment is necessary. Because the most common cause in dogs is iatrogenic androgen administration prevention is achieved by avoidance of steroid administration, such as androgens or progestagens, during gestation. Because the canine internal and external genitalia normally develop between gestational days 34 and 46, counting from the serum luteinizing hormone (LH) peak of the dam, it is prudent to avoid steroid administration particularly during this period.

Müllerian Agenesis or Hypoplasia
Müllerian duct aplasia or hypoplasia in humans is associated strongly with renal agenesis or ectopy and cervicothoracic somite dysplasia: if one component is identified, the other anomalies should be investigated. This syndrome in humans is referred to as MURCS (müllerian duct aplasia, unilateral renal agenesis, and cervicothoracic somite anomalies). A survey of cats and dogs undergoing elective ovariohysterectomy identified several cases of unicornuate uterus, unilateral uterine segmental aplasia, and uterine horn hypoplasia. In 29.4% of cats and 50% of dogs with uterine abnormalities in which the kidneys were also evaluated, ipsilateral renal agenesis was present (McIntyre et al, 2010). This suggests that further study, including a karyotype and evaluation of the cervical spine and thoracic skeleton, is needed in such cases to determine whether there is a feline or canine counterpart of MURCS.

XY Disorders of Sexual Development

All animals with XY disorders of sexual development (XY DSDs) have a male karyotype and are separated according to whether the primary defect occurs at the level of the testis, the androgen-dependent tissues, or the remaining genitalia (see Table 217-1).

Disorders of Gonadal Development

Partial Testicular Dysgenesis. These animals have defects in testis induction or early differentiation, which affects masculinization that is dependent upon testicular hormones. This has been reported rarely in dogs and has not been reported in cats (Meyers-Wallen, 2012).

An *SRY*-positive 78,XY poodle presented with ambiguous external genitalia, consisting of an enlarged clitoris protruding from the vulva. The undescended testes contained seminiferous tubules lined by Sertoli cells, but germ cells were absent. The testes were attached to the horns of a bicornuate uterus, in which the endometrial glands were small in size and number. Because androgen and MIS-dependent masculinization were incomplete in this case, the diagnosis is likely XY DSD partial testicular dysgenesis. The molecular cause is unknown.

Another case was an *SRY*-positive 78,XY Labrador retriever that presented with an enlarged clitoris protruding from the vulva. One testis was located near the vulva, whereas the other was in the abdomen. Both testes contained Leydig cells and seminiferous tubules lacking spermatogenesis. Incompletely developed epididymides were adjacent to each testis, but vasa deferentia were absent. No müllerian duct derivatives were identified. Because partial androgen-dependent masculinization and complete müllerian duct regression were confirmed, this case could be either XY DSD partial testicular dysgenesis or an XY DSD of androgen synthesis or action (below). The molecular cause is unknown.

Ovotestes. These animals have a male karyotype but develop ovotestes. They now are classified as ovotesticular XY DSD but were classified formerly as XY sex reversal (XY true hermaphrodite). One cat has been reported, which was a 1-year-old mixed breed, phenotypic male presented as bilaterally cryptorchid (Schlafer et al, 2011). The karyotype was 38,XY and the *SRY* sequence was the same as a normal male control. Ovotestes, located at the caudal pole of the kidneys, were composed primarily of testis, with a thin rim of ovarian tissue in the cortex. Epididymides were adjacent to each gonad, but vasa deferentia were found adjacent only to the cranial uterine horns. There was complete failure of müllerian duct regression; a bicornuate uterus, uterine tubes, and fimbria were present. The causative mutation is unknown.

Disorders in Androgen Synthesis or Action

These animals have a normal male karyotype, testes, and normal müllerian duct regression. However, genitalia that require androgens for masculinization fail to develop normally because of defects in androgen production, 5α-reductase, or the androgen receptor.

Complete Androgen Insensitivity Syndrome. Complete androgen insensitivity syndrome (CAIS) disorders are caused by androgen receptor (AR) defects and formerly were called androgen resistance syndromes or testicular feminization. One affected 38,XY cat has been reported (Meyers-Wallen et al, 1989). The external genitalia were unambiguously female at 6 months of age when presented for routine ovariohysterectomy. Bilateral abdominal testes were present, but there were no epididymides or vasa deferentia. The uterus was absent, which is expected in such cases because MIS production and response is unaffected. High-affinity binding of DHT was virtually undetectable in cultured genital fibroblasts, confirming receptor malfunction.

Partial Androgen Insensitivity Syndrome. One case of canine partial androgen insensitivity syndrome (PAIS) was reported in a 78,XY mixed-breed dog (Peter et al, 1993). It was phenotypically female at 6 months of age, but scrotal-like swellings containing testes later were identified on each side of the vulva, which opened into a blind vaginal pouch. Peripheral testosterone and DHT concentrations were normal after hCG stimulation. Epididymides were present adjacent to the testes, indicating that T-dependent masculinization was unimpaired during embryonic development. High-affinity binding of DHT was undetectable in cultured genital fibroblasts. These data suggest that DHT binding was abnormal but testosterone binding was not. Testosterone and DHT bind to the same androgen receptor, which is encoded by a single gene. Nevertheless, there is pharmacologic evidence that the androgen receptor can exhibit different binding affinity preference for DHT relative to testosterone in adult canine tissues. Therefore an AR mutation could affect DHT-dependent masculinization but not testosterone-dependent masculinization, as the findings in this case would suggest.

Diagnosis of CAIS or PAIS is dependent on confirmation of a normal male karyotype, bilateral testes, and abnormal androgen binding in androgen-responsive tissues. GnRH/hCG stimulation tests in the intact animal confirm that peripheral androgens are present, providing further evidence for androgen insensitivity. It is now possible to diagnose these defects at the level of the canine or feline AR gene. Castration is recommended for affected dogs and cats. Prevention is limited to genetic counseling regarding the X-linked inheritance of this disorder. Because carrier females are fertile, 50% of their male offspring are affected, whereas 50% of the female offspring are carriers, on average. However, 50% of the male offspring will not receive the X chromosome bearing the AR mutation, will have normal genitalia, and can be used in a breeding program.

Other Causes

This category includes persistent müllerian duct syndrome, isolated hypospadias, and isolated cryptorchidism (see Table 217-1).

Persistent Müllerian Duct Syndrome. Persistent müllerian duct syndrome (PMDS) has been reported in the miniature schnauzer in several continents, the basset hound in Europe, and a mixed-breed dog; it also may occur in the Persian cat (Meyers-Wallen, 2012). Affected miniature schnauzers are XY males with bilateral testes and normal androgen-dependent masculinization of the internal and external genitalia. However, because of a

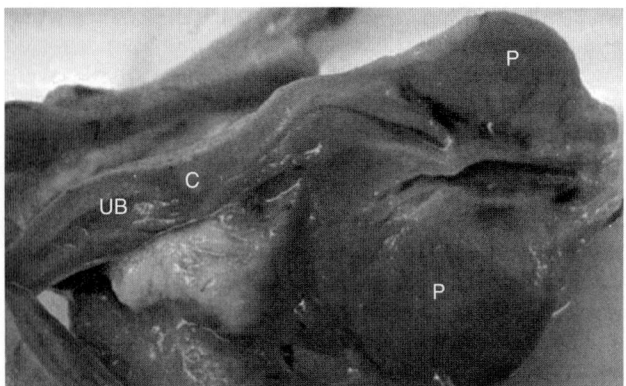

Figure 217-2 Caudal reproductive tract of a dog with persistent müllerian duct syndrome (PMDS). This fixed specimen is bisected longitudinally to show the uterine body (UB), the cervix (C), and the cranial vagina entering the craniodorsal aspect of the prostate gland (P). Note the thin separation between the vagina and prostatic urethra. In some PMDS dogs there is a small diameter connection here between the vagina and the urethra. (Reprinted with permission from Wu X et al: A single base pair mutation encoding a premature stop codon in the MIS type II receptor is responsible for canine persistent müllerian duct syndrome, *J Androl* 30:46, 2009.)

defect in the MIS receptor, they also have bilateral uterine tubes, a complete uterus with cervix, and the cranial portion of the vagina, which terminates within the craniodorsal aspect of the prostate gland (Figure 217-2). Approximately 50% of PMDS dogs have unilateral or bilateral cryptorchidism, whereas the remainder have bilateral descended testes and are fertile. Although PMDS rarely is detected by physical examination alone, PMDS dogs are diagnosed most frequently when clinical signs arise related to pyometra, urinary tract infection, prostate infection, or neoplasia in cryptorchid testes. The dilated uterus and cranial vagina can be misdiagnosed as a large prostatic abscess.

Diagnosis of PMDS depends on confirmation of a normal male karyotype, bilateral testes, and the presence of all müllerian duct derivatives (see Table 217-1). However, diagnosis in the miniature schnauzer can be obtained by DNA testing. In this breed, a mutation in the MIS type 2 receptor (*MISRII/AMhR2*) eliminates receptor function (Wu et al, 2009). PMDS dogs are homozygous for this mutation, which appears to be widely distributed in this breed. Treatment is limited to castration and hysterectomy, taking care to remove the cervix and cranial vagina at the craniodorsal aspect of the prostate gland (see Figure 217-2). In some cases, a small-diameter communication between the cranial vagina and the prostatic urethra is present and should be ligated since it could allow ascending infection into the uterus. In the miniature schnauzer, PMDS is inherited as a sex-limited, autosomal-recessive trait; only homozygous males express the affected phenotype. A mutation test is commercially available (Pujar and Meyers-Wallen, 2009). Members of this breed should be tested before entering a breeding program to identify noncarriers, affected males, carrier males, and carrier females. Affected dogs and homozygous females should be removed from the breeding

population because they will transmit the mutation to all of their offspring, producing only carriers or affected dogs. Furthermore, to prevent production of affected dogs, male or female carriers should be bred only to noncarriers or be removed from the breeding population.

Isolated Hypospadias. Hypospadias is an abnormality in location of the urinary orifice caused by incomplete masculinization of the urogenital sinus during formation of the male urethra. As a result, the urethral opening may be located anywhere along the embryologic course of the urogenital sinus to the genital tubercle. Because hypospadias can occur in association with other defects, such as testicular or ovotesticular XX DSDs, these should be included in the differential diagnosis, particularly when cryptorchidism, scrotal abnormalities, anorectal defects, or a uterus is present. However, isolated hypospadias refers to hypospadias not associated with other DSDs.

Isolated hypospadias has been reported as a familial defect in some dog breeds, particularly in the Boston terrier. Rare reports in cats include the domestic shorthair and two cases in the Himalayan breed. The diagnostic plan includes karyotype, gonadal histology, and ruling out association with other DSD. Surgical correction of mild hypospadias is usually unnecessary because hypospadias usually does not cause urinary difficulties. However, cosmetic repair may be indicated for severe hypospadias. Although affected animals with mild hypospadias may be able to breed normally, affected dogs should be removed from the breeding program to prevent further dissemination of familial hypospadias.

Isolated Cryptorchidism. Cryptorchidism is associated with other DSDs, such as testicular XX DSD and PMDS above, but also can appear as the only defect of the reproductive system, which is isolated cryptorchidism (see Table 217-1).

Feline cryptorchidism has been reported infrequently and appears to be uncommon. Hospital surveys of male cats admitted for neutering reported that 1.3% to 1.7% were affected; most are unilateral cryptorchid (Meyers-Wallen, 2012). In contrast, isolated cryptorchidism is the most common disorder of the reproductive tract reported in dogs, ranging from 6.8% of males presented for neutering to 1.4% of dogs at 6 to 12 months of age.

A diagnosis of canine cryptorchidism is warranted if either testis is not palpable within the scrotum at 8 weeks of age because the testes normally descend by 10 days after birth. Although canine testis descent later than 10 days is known anecdotally to most veterinarians, the frequency of delayed descent is unknown. In one study, pups with cryptorchidism were examined every 2 weeks from 6 to 14 weeks of age, then again at 6 and 12 months of age. They observed that 24.6% of cryptorchid testes descended by 6 months of age, with the majority descending by 14 weeks of age (Dunn et al, 1968). Testis descent after 6 months of age was not observed in any case monitored. Evidence in humans and mice shows that delayed testis descent is a variation of cryptorchidism rather than a variation of normal. For example, delayed testis descent is observed in men with heterozygous *INSL3* mutations (Tomboc et al, 2002).

Dogs with bilateral cryptorchidism are sterile, whereas those with unilateral cryptorchidism can be fertile.

However, the recommended treatment for both is bilateral castration. First, the risk of Sertoli cell tumor is increased in cryptorchid testes. Second, isolated cryptorchidism is clearly a familial trait in several breeds and is likely to be inherited in dogs, as it is in other mammals. Although mutations in *INSL3* and its receptor have been identified to cause isolated cryptorchidism in mice and humans, such mutations have not been identified in cryptorchid dogs. Furthermore, mutations in those genes account for a small number of human cases (1.4%), indicating that additional genes are likely to play a role in cryptorchidism.

Although the genetic cause presently is unknown, it is being pursued. Inheritance of isolated cryptorchidism as a sex-limited recessive trait is consistent with available data, but it may be a polygenic trait that is genetically heterogeneous between breeds. Using this model, the first recommendation is that affected dogs be removed from the breeding population. The second is that both the father and mother of affected dogs should be considered carriers. Therefore removing carrier parents and affected males from the breeding population is probably the minimum program that should be pursued in dogs. As some full siblings of the affected dog are also carriers, it also may be necessary to remove these from the breeding program, but there is no practical way at present to determine which are carriers. Although medical regimens have been suggested to induce testicular descent in cryptorchid dogs, no published reports confirm that these are more successful than no treatment, in which 24.6% of cryptorchid testes could descend by 6 months of age. Furthermore, even if delayed testis descent occurs, the genes responsible for cryptorchidism remain unchanged and are transmitted to the offspring. Therefore cryptorchid dogs and those with late testicular descent should be removed from the breeding program to reduce the frequency of the causative mutations in the population.

References and Suggested Reading

Dunn ML, Foster WJ, Goddard KM: Cryptorchidism in dogs: a clinical survey, *J Am Anim Hosp Assoc* 4:180, 1968.

Jakob S, Lovell-Badge R: Sex determination and the control of *Sox9* expression in mammals, *FEBS J* 278:1002, 2011.

McIntyre RL et al: Developmental uterine anomalies in cats and dogs undergoing elective ovariohysterectomy, *J Am Vet Med Assoc* 237:542, 2010.

Meyers-Wallen VN: Gonadal and sex differentiation abnormalities of dogs and cats, *Sexual Development* 6:46, 2012.

Meyers-Wallen VN et al: Testicular feminization in a cat, *J Am Vet Med Assoc* 195:631, 1989.

Pasterski V, Prentice P, Hughes IA: Impact of the consensus statement and the new DSD classification system, *Best Pract Res Clin Endocrinol Metab* 24:18, 2010.

Peter AT, Markwelder D, Asem EK: Phenotypic feminization in a genetic male dog caused by nonfunctional androgen receptors, *Theriogenology* 40:1093, 1993.

Pujar S, Meyers-Wallen VN: A molecular diagnostic test for persistent Müllerian duct syndrome in miniature schnauzer dogs, *Sex Devel* 3:326, 2009.

Quinn A, Koopman P: The molecular genetics of sex determination and sex reversal in mammals, *Semin Reprod Med* 30(5):351, 2012.

Schlafer DH et al: A case of *SRY*-positive 38,XY true hermaphroditism (XY Sex Reversal) in a cat, *Vet Pathol* 48:822, 2011.

Tomboc M et al: Insulin-like 3/Relaxin-like factor gene mutations are associated with cryptorchidism, *Clin Endocr Metab* 85:4013, 2002.

Wu X et al: A single base pair mutation encoding a premature stop codon in the MIS type II receptor is responsible for canine persistent Müllerian duct syndrome, *J Androl* 30:46, 2009.

CHAPTER 218

Ovarian Remnant Syndrome in Small Animals

CARLOS M. GRADIL, *Amherst, Massachusetts*
ROBERT J. MCCARTHY, *North Grafton, Massachusetts*

Ovarian remnant syndrome (ORS) is a reported complication after ovariohysterectomy (OHE), a common surgical procedure to prevent estrus, pregnancy, and pyometra and to decrease the incidence of tumors. Failure to remove all ovarian tissue may result in the continued secretion of reproductive hormones with overt signs of proestrus or estrus, uterine stump pyometra, or neoplasia of the ovary, mammary gland, and/or the vagina. Dogs with ORS have a higher rate (23.8%) of neoplasms (e.g., sex-cord stromal tumors in the residual ovarian tissue) than the reported incidence of 6.25% in sexually intact female dogs.

Recognizing bitches with ORS can be challenging, depending on the phase of the reproductive cycle. Most dogs with ORS are presented with periodic or continuous symptoms of vulvar swelling, serosanguineous vaginal discharge, and attractiveness to male dogs. The actual interval from OHE to the time of examination and diagnosis of ORS is highly variable and is attributed partially to failure of owners to recognize clinical signs of proestrus or estrus. The interval between OHE and diagnosis of ORS in animals with neoplasm is significantly longer than in animals without neoplasms.

Potential Causes for Ovarian Remnant Syndrome

Because remnant ovarian tissue is found in typical anatomic locations and is not considered ectopic tissue in dogs, surgical error is suspected as the cause of ORS. In dogs, location of remnant ovarian tissue is found more frequently in the region of the right ovarian pedicle, probably because the more cranial position of the right ovary and difficulty in exposure and removal of the right ovary during OHE. However, Miller (1995) found remnant ovarian tissue to be distributed equally between the right and left side.

Differences between dogs and cats provide further support for surgical error as the cause of ORS and may account for more dogs than cats being affected. Dogs have more adipose tissue surrounding the ovaries that can obscure exposure. The suspensory ligament of the ovary in dogs is more difficult to rupture to achieve adequate exposure, compared with cats. In addition, dogs typically have a deeper abdominal cavity, which makes it more challenging to exteriorize each ovary (Figure 218-1).

Other possible causes of ORS that have been proposed include the revascularization and autotransplantation of free-floating ovarian tissue that becomes separated from the ovary at the time of OHE or surgical inexperience (e.g., veterinarian with <5 years of experience that can lead to surgical errors). However, experience of the surgeon was not identified as a factor in some studies. Proper exposure of the ovary and appropriate placement of hemostats before placement of ligatures should ensure complete removal of ovarian tissue and prevent ORS.

Ectopic ovarian tissue (i.e., supernumerary ovaries or accessory ovarian tissue) has not been reported in dogs. However, accessory ovarian tissue located within the proper ligament of the ovary has been reported in cats, cows, and women. This tissue may be separated partially or completely from the ovary by connective tissue; therefore it may be difficult to distinguish from residual tissue because of improper placement of hemostats at the time of OHE.

Preexisting intraabdominal abnormalities (e.g., endometriosis, pelvic inflammatory disease, and previous abdominal surgery) that obscure identification of the ovaries at the time of surgical removal have not been reported in domestic animals.

Signalment and Medical History

No breed predilection is apparent in the incidence of ORS. Age of animals at the time of OHE can be categorized as those that undergo OHE before puberty (<4 months old), as a juvenile (5 to 12 months old), or as an adult (>12 months old). No correlation has been shown between occurrence of ORS and age of the dog at OHE. The interval between OHE and diagnosis of ORS could be years.

Clinical Signs

Differential clinical signs should include vaginitis, stump pyometra, neoplasia, trauma, exogenous therapy, or coagulopathies. If at the time of OHE a functional corpus luteum is present, overt false pregnancy may occur after surgery but subsides in less than 4 weeks without treatment.

Clinical signs of ORS are consistent with the influence of estrogen. Clinical signs related to the functional remnant ovarian tissue include signs of proestrus and estrus with vulvar swelling and serosanguineous vaginal discharge and, in some cases, pyometra. Some dogs may show only behavioral signs of estrus. Dogs that do not show signs of proestrus or estrus but may have mammary

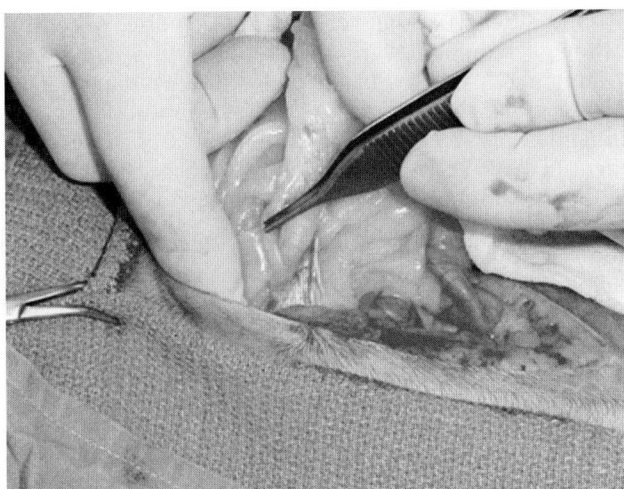

Figure 218-1 Canine ovarian tissue *in situ*. Dogs typically have a deeper abdominal cavity, which makes it more challenging to exteriorize each ovary during OHE. (Photo courtesy Dr. Robert J. McCarthy, Tufts Cummings School of Veterinary Medicine, North Grafton, MA.)

gland enlargement may have a progesterone concentration consistent with luteal activity. Clinical signs may not be recognized in some animals for several years after OHE. Once cyclic estrus returns, dogs with ORS may have an extended interestrus interval (e.g., 8 to 9 months). Animals with neoplasms have a significantly longer interval (8 years) between OHE and diagnosis of ORS, compared with the interval between OHE and diagnosis of ORS for animals without neoplasms (1 year).

Affected queens may show normal estrus and may allow copulation but do not become pregnant if bred. The time interval from OHE to return to estrus could be days to years. Then estrus recurs at normal interval.

Diagnostic Tests

Besides clinical signs, to confirm the presence of remnant ovarian tissue before laparotomy/laparoscopy, diagnostic tests to consider should include vaginoscopy and vaginal cytologic examination, hormonal assays, and ultrasonography.

Vaginoscopy and Vaginal Cytologic Examination

Observation of mating behavior, vaginoscopy, and vaginal cornification (anuclear squames, superficial cells) can confirm the effect of estrogens.

Hormonal Assays

Hormonal assays should evaluate the basal plasma estrogen and progesterone levels, plasma concentrations of luteinizing hormone (LH), estradiol-17β or progesterone before and after administration of gonadotropin-releasing hormone (GnRH), or to detect adrenal gland disease, which also may result in high concentrations of sex hormones.

Gonadotropins

In dogs with remnant ovarian tissue, changes in the pituitary-ovarian axis are noticeable. The concentrations of circulating gonadotropins are significantly higher in ovariectomized bitches than in bitches in anestrus because of the loss of negative feedback of ovarian hormones after ovariectomy. However, despite the fact that plasma gonadotropin concentrations may suggest the presence of ovarian tissue, the pulsatile secretion of gonadotropins can cause overlapping of their plasma concentrations between ovariectomized bitches and bitches in anestrus. Thus a single high LH concentration does not confirm spayed status because sexually intact dogs can have brief episodic surges in serum LH concentrations throughout the estrous cycle. Dogs with high (>1 ng/ml) LH concentrations on 2 separate days are consistent with the presence of remnant ovarian tissue and help eliminate false positives resulting from pulsatile secretion of gonadotropins.

Among bitches with remnant ovarian tissue, basal plasma LH concentration is higher in those in which the interval between ovariectomy and the appearance of estrus is more than 3 years. The LH response to GnRH stimulation is lower in bitches with remnant ovarian tissue than in ovariectomized bitches or those in anestrus.

In bitches with granulosa cell tumor (GCT), the pituitary-ovarian axis is affected and is characterized by relatively high plasma LH concentrations in GCT-ORS bitches and a subnormal LH response to GnRH stimulation in GCT bitches compared with those in anestrus and ovariectomized bitches. The relatively high proportion of dogs with remnant ovarian tissue in GCT bitches may point to a pathogenic role for elevated gonadotropin secretion in the pathogenesis of GCT.

Estrogen and Progesterone

When there is behavioral evidence of an increased plasma estradiol, estrus may be confirmed by vaginal cytology; checking the progesterone concentration 2 to 3 weeks later verifies luteinization or ovulation.

In cases of no behavioral or clinical evidence of an increased plasma estradiol concentration, recognition of bitches with remnant ovarian tissue is challenging. The production of estradiol and of progesterone decreases markedly after ovariectomy, but basal plasma concentrations of both hormones in anestrous and ovariectomized bitches overlap.

A preoperative diagnosis of ORS can be attained by the use of hormone stimulation tests. Stimulation of the pituitary-ovarian axis with GnRH may help to distinguish between ovariectomized bitches and those in anestrus, because administering GnRH causes a significant rise in plasma estradiol concentration only if ovarian tissue is present.

In dogs and cats with behavioral estrus, stimulation of ovulation and luteinization can be induced with GnRH (Table 218-1).

Elevated Estrogen. Diagnosis of ORS during the follicular phase should show an elevated plasma concentration of estradiol, produced by granulosa cells in developing ovarian follicles. Estradiol concentration of more than

Gonadotropic-Releasing Hormone and Human Chorionic Gonadotropin Stimulation Protocol

Dogs	50 µg GnRH IM or 400 IU hCG IV or 500 IU IM and 500 IU IV	2-3 weeks later	P4 >2 ng/ml
Cats	25 µg GnRH IM	2-3 weeks later	P4 >2 ng/ml

hCG, Human chorionic gonadotropin; *GnRH,* gonadotropin-releasing hormone; *P4,* progesterone.

20 pg/ml is consistent with follicular activity for bitches and queens. For animals with suspected adrenal gland disease, an ACTH stimulation test or low-dose dexamethasone suppression test should be performed. However, adrenal diseases associated with high estrogens are less common than ORS as a cause of vaginal cornification in spayed bitches.

Elevated Progesterone. During the late follicular phase, ovulation, and the luteal phase, the plasma concentration of progesterone (secreted by partially luteinized granulosa cells before ovulation and by mature luteal cells after ovulation) is increased, providing evidence for remnant ovarian tissue. Progesterone concentration more than 2 ng/ml is consistent with luteal activity for bitches and queens.

Antimüllerian Hormone. Antimüllerian hormone (AMH) is produced by the fetal testes in mammals. It inhibits müllerian (paramesonephric) duct development in the male embryo. However, following the development of the müllerian ducts into the oviduct, uterus, and upper vagina in female mammals, the ovaries produce AMH, which can be measured in the peripheral circulation. The ovaries appear to be the sole source of AMH in the circulation. A commercially available human-based assay is available for measurement of AMH concentration in dogs and cats.

Ultrasonographic Examination

Ultrasonography (US) may be helpful as an adjunct diagnostic test in animals with or without signs consistent with proestrus or estrus, or with mammary gland enlargement. The success or failure of being able to identify ovarian tissue by use of US may be related to the expertise of the ultrasonographer, stage of the estrous cycle of the animal at the time of examination, and size of the remnant ovarian tissue. Clinical signs of proestrus or estrus or its absence do not appear to affect the ability to identify correctly remnant ovarian tissue at the time of US exam.

US examinations may present as acoustic enhancement, echogenic fluid, hyperechoic septations, and anechoic follicles. Some US features of remnant ovarian tissue may resemble simple cysts or cysts with multiple septations. These cystlike structures also can have a rim of presumed ovarian tissue with arterial and venous blood flow.

One differential diagnosis for a false-positive identification of remnant ovarian tissue during US is a suture granuloma at the site of ligation of the ovarian pedicle. Suture material can cause a localized immunologic and inflammatory reaction. Suture granulomas have been identified by US as clearly defined hypoechoic lesions with or without double or single hyperechoic lines within the lesion. Suture granulomas frequently involve nonabsorbable suture material; however, suture granulomas involving absorbable suture also have been reported, as well as granulomas involving metallic surgical staples. Although most suture granulomas would be expected to develop and resolve within a short period after surgery, suture granulomas have been identified in humans for months and possibly years.

Remnant ovarian tissue detected during US and found subsequently during surgery should be confirmed histologically.

Laparotomy

Exploratory laparotomy for suspected remnant ovarian tissue, if present, will be most likely in the region of the right or left ovarian pedicles, and bilaterally in the region of both ovarian pedicles in a small number of animals. Statistically, it would be expected that remnant ovarian tissue would have an equal chance of being found on the right or the left side (50% for each side). However, the presence of remnant ovarian tissue in the region of the right ovarian pedicle is significantly higher than the expected 50%.

Histologic Examination

Histologic examination performed on suspected remnant ovarian tissue excised from suspected ORS may confirm ovarian tissue (Figure 218-2). Histopathologic findings include differentiated ovarian tissue singly, or a combination of ovarian follicles or follicular cysts, corpora lutea, ovarian neoplasms, adenomatous hyperplasia, and paraovarian cysts.

Uterine remnants excised and evaluated histologically may be enlarged and may show evidence of cystic endometrial hyperplasia. Microbial culture of uterine remnants may yield bacteria (e.g., *Escherichia coli, Enterococcus* spp.), which indicates a uterine stump pyometra. Some dogs may have neoplasms of the reproductive system, including the ovaries, mammary glands, and vagina. Ovarian tumors may include sex-cord stromal or granulosa cell tumors, cystadenoma, mammary gland tumor, adenoma, vaginal tumors, and leiomyoma.

Treatment

The preferred treatment for ORS is surgical removal of remnant ovarian tissue. To facilitate visualization of the ovarian remnant surgery should be performed when the animal is in proestrus, estrus, or diestrus because of follicles or corpora lutea in the ovarian tissue and prominence of ovarian blood vessels. Surgical removal of remnant ovarian tissue results in resolution of clinical signs of estrus or proestrus.

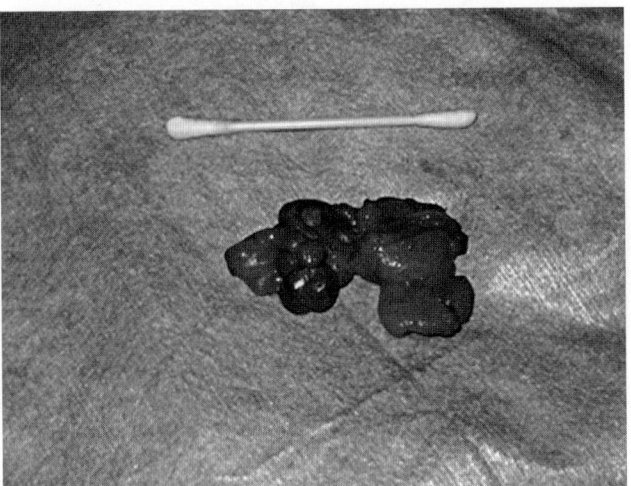

Figure 218-2 Excised ovarian tissue from a mixed breed dog spayed at 4½ years of age. Six months after ovariohysterectomy, the bitch displayed proestrous clinical signs (vaginal bleeding, attractive to males, licking vulva) but otherwise was clinically normal. Vaginoscopy was performed and revealed edematous vaginal folds and brownish-yellow watery discharge. The serum progesterone concentration was 3.2 ng/ml. Eight months later, she was again in heat, which was confirmed by exfoliative vaginal cytology (70% superficial, cornified epithelial cells). After the end of estrus, a laparotomy was performed and ovarian tissue was removed. (Photo courtesy Dr. Tuire Tamminen, Faculty of Veterinary Medicine, University of Helsinki, Finland.)

References and Suggested Reading

Ball R et al: Ovarian remnant syndrome in dogs and cats: 21 cases (2000-2007), *J Am Vet Med Assoc* 236:548, 2010.

Beijerink NJ et al: Basal and GnRH-induced secretion of FSH and LH in anestrous versus ovariectomized bitches, *Theriogenology* 67:1039, 2007.

DeNardo GA et al: Ovarian remnant syndrome: revascularization of free-floating ovarian tissue in the feline abdominal cavity, *J Am Anim Hosp Assoc* 37:290, 2001.

Fleischer AC et al: Sonographic features of ovarian remnants, *J Ultrasound Med* 17:551, 1998.

Jeffcoate IA: Gonadotrophin-releasing hormone challenge to test for the presence of ovaries in the bitch, *J Reprod Fertil Suppl* 47:536, 1993.

Löfstedt RM, Vanleeuwen JA: Evaluation of a commercially available luteinizing hormone test for its ability to distinguish between ovariectomized and sexually intact bitches, *J Am Vet Med Assoc* 220:1331, 2002.

Magtibay PM, Magrina JF: Ovarian remnant syndrome, *Clin Obstet Gynecol* 49:526, 2006.

Miller DM: Ovarian remnant syndrome in dogs and cats: 46 cases (1988-1992), *J Vet Diagn Invest* 7:572, 1995.

Okkens AC, Dieleman SJ, v d Gaag I: Gynaecological complications following ovariohysterectomy in dogs, due to: (1) partial removal of the ovaries. (2) inflammation of the uterocervical stump [in Dutch], *Tijdschr Diergeneeskd* 106:1142, 1981.

Place NJ et al: Measurement of serum anti-Müllerian hormone concentration in female dogs and cats before and after ovariohysterectomy, *J Vet Diagn Invest* 23:524, 2011.

Wallace MS: The ovarian remnant syndrome in the bitch and queen, *Vet Clin North Am Small Anim Pract* 21:501, 1991.

CHAPTER **219**

Pregnancy Loss in the Bitch and Queen

LINDA K. KAUFFMAN, *Ames, Iowa*
CLAUDIA J. BALDWIN, *Ames, Iowa*

Conception rates in a normal bitch can exceed 95% with the proper breeding management. Breeding of a fertile queen and tom should result in attainment of pregnancy 70% of the time. The exact number of bitches and queens that undergo embryonic and fetal loss is difficult to determine if pregnancy is suspected but not confirmed before the loss occurs. Methods for pregnancy diagnosis are discussed in Chapter 207. Making a diagnosis of pregnancy loss is also difficult because females may consume the fetuses and show few clinical signs. Pregnancy loss during the second half of gestation often is associated with a hemorrhagic vulvar discharge.

Some females that experience fetal death in late gestation do not abort but retain their dead fetuses. Mummification results when fetal death occurs under sterile autolytic conditions. This includes absorption of the placental and fetal fluids and does not occur in the first half of gestation because fetal bone mineralization does not begin until day 40 to 45 of gestation (England, 2006). Mummification can occur in the presence of other live fetuses while maintaining the pregnancy until birth of the live fetuses or all the fetuses can be mummified and be retained past the whelping or queening date. Actual incidence of mummification in the bitch and queen is unknown but it is thought to be low. Retained dead fetuses that are not mummified can become macerated and emphysematous; these require surgical removal. These females may be systemically ill and have a foul vulvar discharge.

Historical Findings of Pregnancy Loss

A bitch or queen with the complaint of pregnancy loss or conception failure requires the clinician to obtain a complete medical history to assess the individual female and the colony. Dietary records as well as details about how the female is housed, housing practices of the breeding facility (pregnant vs. nonpregnant vs. neonates), and isolation protocols should be discussed in depth. Vaccine history, deworming history, serologic testing for heartworm disease, *Brucella canis* testing status (bitches only), feline leukemia virus (FeLV) and feline immunodeficiency virus (FIV) (queens), and any other important medical history of the female in question as well as other animals at the facility should be reviewed carefully. Breeding dates, type of breeding management used, stud or tom used and his breeding history (breeding soundness results if any), and the relationship of the stud to the female are important factors for review. Past reproductive history of the female, her relatives, and the rest of the colony are important to evaluate. All medications, supplements, holistic therapies, and preventives (flea, tick, heartworm, gastrointestinal anthelmintics) prescribed or used must be recorded.

Specific history related to pregnancy loss may be variable. There may be no additional history other than a bitch or queen that fails to produce offspring at the time of expected end of gestation. Other findings related to pregnancy loss may include decreased appetite, weight loss, vomiting, diarrhea, or simply a decrease in abdominal size. If the owners have witnessed the abortion, they should be instructed to collect materials carefully, wearing gloves and placing material in plastic bags or containers, and refrigerate at 1.7° to 3.3° C (35° to 38° F). They should be questioned about fetal material delivered, viability of fetuses at the time of delivery, and placental passage. Owners may have noticed only a vulvar discharge (mucoid, greenish, or serosanguineous) and nothing more at the time of pregnancy loss. In rare cases, a client may bring in a female that has delivered one or more stillborn or mummified fetuses.

Clinicopathologic Findings of Pregnancy Loss

To determine if a reproduction problem exists, a complete physical examination of the bitch or queen using observation, auscultation, and palpation should be performed. A closer examination of the reproductive system should include vaginal inspection (in bitches) via a speculum or via vaginoscopy to look for discharge or the presence of a fetus, whereas careful vaginal inspection via rectal palpation and digital vulvovaginal inspection and vaginoscopy should be performed in the queen. Abdominal palpation, radiographs, or ultrasonography may be used to confirm pregnancy loss. Confirmation of early embryonic loss in the bitch before implantation is not possible

currently in clinical practice, but pregnancy loss after day 21 of gestation may result in a positive relaxin test that persists up to a week after complete pregnancy loss has occurred. Early in gestation, anechoic gestational sacs are visible via ultrasound imaging. In the queen, uterine segmental swellings associated with gestational sacs, fetal poles, heartbeat, and fetal membranes may be seen as early as days 11, 15, 16, and 21, respectively, using ultrasound imaging (Davidson, Nyland, and Tsutsui, 1986). If the gestational sacs fail to develop embryonic structures over time, this confirms pregnancy loss. Later in gestation, fetal death can be confirmed by the absence of a heartbeat and fetal movement during the last 7 to 14 days of pregnancy, which can be confirmed by ultrasound if necessary. Radiographic imaging also can be used to look for signs of fetal death, assess presence and location of remaining fetuses, and estimate the stage of gestation and size of the remaining fetuses. A final form of pregnancy loss is the stillborn. This is well recognized and much easier to confirm. Stillbirths may represent an average of 13% of total kitten births. The mammary glands should be examined for stage of development and presence of colostrum or milk. The primiparous queen tends to develop earlier than the multiparous queen, which can be confusing to the cat owner, making the client concerned about pregnancy loss or undetected abortion. Any fetal, placental, or neonatal materials available should be inspected closely and handled aseptically to allow for further diagnostics (e.g., bacterial culture, virus isolation, karyotyping). Any abnormalities should be noted and investigated.

Diagnostic testing may be indicated to assess the general health of the bitch and queen. Repeating a careful history of the individual bitch and queen and the population, health maintenance practices, and housing may be helpful. Abnormalities in hematology, serum biochemistries, and urinalysis may reflect specific underlying disease. The bitch and queen normally develop a dilutional normochromic, normocytic anemia during gestation with a significant decrease in the percentage packed cell volume. Serum protein concentrations also decrease. These changes are at their greatest by 8 weeks' gestation and quickly return to normal after parturition. *Brucella canis* status of the bitch and the breeding facility is indicated if not yet performed and reassessed if the breeding facility is not closed. Canine herpesvirus titer may provide useful information if elevated. Reassessment of FeLV and FIV status is useful in the queen.

Diagnosis of Disorders Associated with Pregnancy Loss

Differential diagnoses for pregnancy loss in the bitch and queen are numerous, but some owners have a hard time discerning normal pregnancy events from an abortive event. The history, physical examination findings, and imaging should be able to confirm the current pregnancy status. Occasionally, a late gestation bitch or queen may have a mucoid vulvar discharge. Cytology of this discharge may reveal numerous nondegenerate neutrophils with minimal bacteria present; this can be a normal finding. If the clinician suspects a normal pregnancy, the owner should be instructed to isolate the bitch or queen and monitor for signs of labor (e.g., temperature drop [bitch], nesting behavior, straining). If the bitch or queen is presented already in stage II of parturition, noted by active straining and passage of term offspring, then the clinician must determine if normal delivery can occur or if a problem requires assistance. If the bitch or queen has presented with one or more stillborn full-term fetuses, then it is necessary to determine if they are a result of dystocia and if the remaining fetuses require assistance (cesarean section). Owners must be counseled about their diagnostic options and potential outcomes in the following instances:

1. No evidence of pregnancy after breeding
2. Uterine changes suggesting disease
3. Mummified fetuses found
4. Resorbed fetuses or placentation sites in an otherwise healthy bitch or queen

First and foremost, optimal breeding management should be discussed at length with the owner. The owner should be advised to confirm the pregnancy after the next breeding so that it can be monitored closely. Older bitches and queens may benefit from additional diagnostic testing (e.g., complete blood count, serum biochemistries, urinalysis, thyroid levels [T_4/TSH] in the bitch) along with ultrasonographic imaging of the reproductive tract.

A single differential diagnostic plan cannot be followed when working through a case of pregnancy loss in the bitch or queen. Pregnancy loss can be caused by maternal disorders that result in the death of developing embryos or fetuses. This may be caused by disease of a single organ system or be multisystemic. Pregnancy loss also can be caused by fetal disorders that cannot be attributed solely to the bitch or queen (Table 219-1).

Maternal Disorders

Maternal causes of pregnancy loss include obvious and subtle disorders. A careful history and physical examination should help identify underlying diseases (e.g., renal, cardiac, endocrine, respiratory). Cardiac disease should be suspected in females with murmurs or irregular rhythms or poor perfusion or pulse quality. Endocrine disease should be suspected in females with signs of polyuria, polydipsia, weight loss, or weight gain. Diagnostic blood work should be performed as a screening tool if underlying disease is suspected. Parasite load should be assessed by fecal floatation, fecal PCR, or antigen testing when available; testing for heartworm should be repeated in endemic areas. Cats should be reassessed for FeLV or FIV status. In addition, knowledge of the genetic or medical conditions that some breeds are predisposed to is helpful when working with these types of cases. Other congenital or developmental diseases not associated with breed may compromise pregnancy maintenance as well. Treatment of these conditions depends on the specific disease identified.

Primary uterine disease that is inflammatory or infectious may be responsible for pregnancy loss or may mimic pregnancy in some cases (Figure 219-1). Cystic endometrial hyperplasia, pyometra, and metritis are types of

TABLE **219-1**

Causes of Pregnancy Loss

Condition	Species
Inflammatory	
Cystic endometrial hyperplasia	Bitch and queen
Pyometra	Bitch and queen
Metritis	Bitch and queen
Infectious	
Bacterial	
Staphylococcus spp.	Bitch and queen*
Streptococcus spp.	Bitch only
Escherichia coli	Bitch and queen
Mycoplasma spp.	Bitch and queen†
Coxiella burnetii	Queen only
Brucella spp.	Bitch only
Campylobacter spp.	Bitch and queen*
Group G *Streptococcus*	Bitch and queen‡
Leptospira spp.	Bitch only
Salmonella spp.	Bitch and queen*
Viruses	
Canine herpesvirus (CHV)	Bitch only
Canine parvovirus (type 1)	Bitch only
Canine distemper virus (CDV)	Bitch only
Feline panleukopenia (FPLV)	Queen only
Feline leukemia virus (FeLV)	Queen only
Feline herpesvirus-1 (FHV-1)	Queen only
Feline immunodeficiency virus (FIV)	Queen only

*Uncommon.
†Experimental in cats.
‡Reported to cause toxic shock and neonatal sepsis in cats.

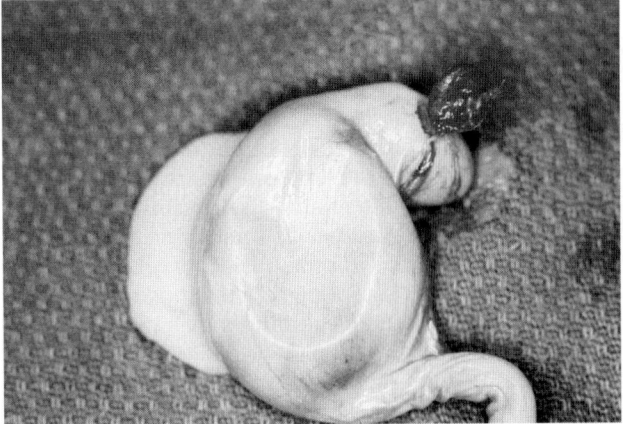

Figure 219-1 Photograph of segmental pyometra in a queen that could have been mistaken for normal segmental swelling of the uterus because of pregnancy. Ovarian pedicle is located in the upper right of the photograph.

inflammatory lesions that can be found in the uterus and may be related to early embryonic death. The lesions may be segmental, likely associated with sites of fetal resorption, or the lesions may be more diffuse, involving one horn or the entire uterus. The bitch or queen may show no clinical signs of disease even when the pathology in the uterus is sufficient enough to prohibit implantation and support of the pregnancy. In other cases abdominal distention may be a notable sign. When the cervix is open, a purulent to serosanguineous vulvar discharge may be present. Cytology of the discharge would reveal an abundance of degenerate neutrophils with intracellular bacteria, suggestive of a septic condition.

Numerous bacteria, including normal vaginal flora (e.g., *Staphylococcus* spp., *Streptococcus* spp., *Escherichia coli*, *Mycoplasma* spp., and in the queen *Coxiella burnetii*) and pathogens (e.g., *Brucella* spp., *Campylobacter* spp., group G *Streptococcus, Leptospira* spp., and *Salmonella* spp.), have been associated with pregnancy loss in the bitch or queen (Pretzer, 2008). More severe clinical signs such as fever, anorexia, dehydration, collapse, and shock can be seen in the bitch and queen when these bacteria cause pregnancy loss. Viral agents are the most commonly reported infectious causes of abortion in queens and include feline panleukopenia (FPLV), FeLV, FIV, and feline herpesvirus-1 (FHV-1). Some of these agents are thought to produce abortion because of the maternal illness and fever in the (FHV-1) infected queen, whereas others, such as FeLV, FIV, and FPLV, cause placental lesions, early embryonic death, and viremia in the fetus (Verstegen, Dhaliwal, and Verstegen-Onclin, 2008). Viral agents involved in pregnancy loss in the bitch include canine herpesvirus (CHV), canine parvovirus (CPV type 1), and canine distemper virus (CDV). Hematologic and biochemistry abnormalities associated with pregnancy loss can include leukopenia or leukocytosis along with a varying degree of azotemia as well as other abnormalities (see Table 219-1).

Ultrasonographic examination of the uterus should assist in diagnosis of pregnancy loss. Segmental areas of inflammation may not compromise the pregnancy but can be a reason for concern. Metritis or pyometra, with or without pregnancy, requires medical or surgical treatment (see Chapter 211). Dystocia must be considered as a cause of pregnancy loss in the bitch and queen (see Chapter 208). Other causes of pregnancy loss include uterine displacement, torsion, and uterine rupture, although these conditions do not occur often. Uterine torsion can occur when one or both horns twist along the long axis or around the opposite horn, or the entire uterine body can rotate around itself. Clinical signs can vary depending on the type of torsion that occurs and range from almost no symptoms to those consistent with an acute abdomen. Severe uterine torsions can obstruct blood supply to the uterus, leading to possible rupture of uterine vessels, shock, and fetal or maternal death. Diagnosis is based on clinical signs, diagnostic imaging, and exploratory surgery. Treatment includes hysterotomy to remove the fetuses and correct the torsion or ovariohysterectomy if the uterus is not salvageable. Uterine rupture can follow a uterine torsion or trauma, although this condition is rare. If fetal circulation is not compromised,

this condition may go undiagnosed until dystocia results because of the fetuses failing to enter the birth canal. Fetuses expelled into the peritoneal cavity may die immediately and be resorbed (if before fetal bone mineralization has occurred) or become retained fetal mummies. Maternal peritonitis secondary to the uterine rupture is a possible sequel. Treatment includes surgical correction of the uterine rupture, removal of any retained fetuses, and correction of the uterine torsion, if needed.

Failure to maintain the pregnancy may result from insufficient production of progesterone (hypoluteoidism/ inadequate luteal phase). Progesterone concentrations greater than 1.5 to 2 ng/ml are thought to be required for pregnancy maintenance. This condition could be suspected in a bitch or queen that suffers from repeated pregnancy loss once infectious and other causes of pregnancy loss have been ruled out, although not definitively documented in the queen (Verstegen, Dhaliwal, and Verstegen-Onclin, 2008). Confirmation requires serial progesterone testing. It has been suggested that giving these bitches supplemental progestogen (type and dose remain a source of debate) after day 40 of gestation until 1 week before anticipated whelping date can prevent pregnancy loss. Owners must be warned that progestogen supplementation can cause masculinization of female offspring (pseudohermaphrodism) (Johnson, Root Kustritz, and Olson, 2001) and male offspring that become cryptorchid (England et al, 2006). In addition a decrease in progesterone concentration can be a normal response to terminate an abnormal pregnancy for either maternal (e.g., placentitis, intrauterine infections) or fetal (e.g., primary abnormality, infection) reasons. Pharmaceutic maintenance of an abnormal pregnancy could result in pyometra, dystocia, and even septicemia of the bitch, so caution is important when offering this option to clients.

Maternal Polysystemic Disorders: The DAMNITT Approach

The development of differential diagnoses often is approached best in a systematic way. The DAMNITT (Degenerative, Allergic, Metabolic, Neoplastic, Iatrogenic, Toxic, Traumatic) scheme has been used for many years in medicine to categorize causative diagnoses as Degenerative, developmental; Allergic, autoimmune (immunemediated); Metabolic; Neoplastic, nutritional; Iatrogenic, ischemic, idiopathic, infectious/noninfectious, inflammatory, or immune-mediated; Toxic; or Traumatic puts this diagnostic approach to use when considering potential causes of pregnancy loss in the bitch and queen.

Developmental/Genetic. More than 400 genetic diseases have been reported in dogs that have survived gestation, so it is presumed when these defects are more severe, resorption or abortion occurs. Inbreeding lines of dogs and cats also can play a part in neonatal mortality; mixedbreed dogs have a higher reproductive performance than purebred dogs (Johnson, Root Kustritz, and Olson, 2001). Genetic defects are seen with close inbreeding in the cat and may be responsible for 15% of infertility or pregnancy loss or in abortion of domestic animals, including cats. Owners should be advised about the availability of genetic counseling before the start of breeding so that they are less likely to make choices that produce high-risk

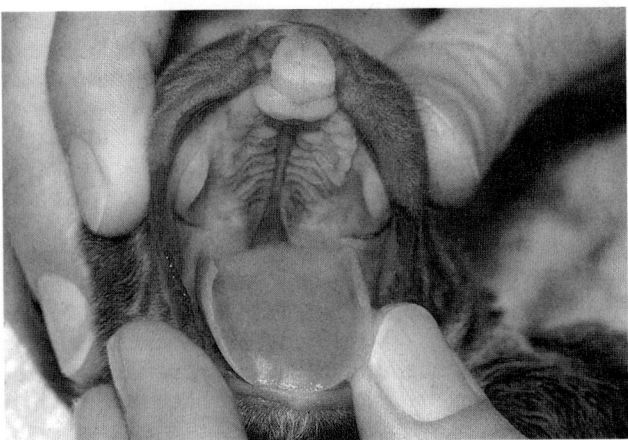

Figure 219-2 Photograph of a full-term puppy with cleft palate, which is a developmental defect. (Photo courtesy Dr. Lawrence Evans.)

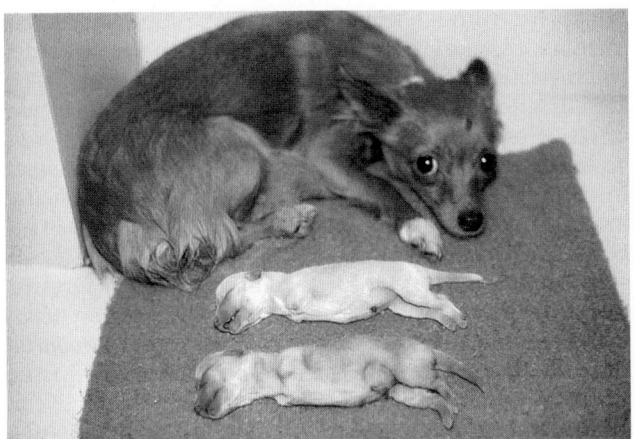

Figure 219-3 Photograph of two full-term puppies both affected with thoracic ectromelia, another type of developmental defect. (Photo courtesy Dr. Lawrence Evans.)

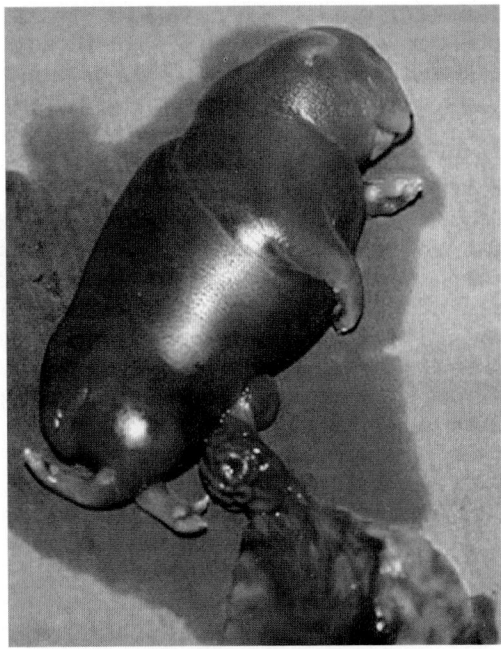

Figure 219-4 Photograph of a kitten delivered vaginally near term. This kitten was affected by *Hydrops fetalis* or anasarca.

Diabetes mellitus, hypothyroidism (bitches), hyperthyroidism (queens), adrenal insufficiency, and hyperadrenocorticism are diseases that can affect fertility and embryonic and fetal development. Owners of females diagnosed with these diseases should be advised of the risk of infertility and pregnancy loss plus the potential of maternal loss in severe cases (e.g., DKA with diabetes mellitus) if they choose to breed this female.

Neoplastic. Neoplastic disease that may occur in a breeding female certainly could lead to pregnancy loss. Neoplasia causes dysfunction of the organs involved and promotes metabolic changes and possibly fever; all of which can compromise the pregnancy, resulting in resorption or abortion. Affected bitches and queens must be identified so that treatment can be implemented, which normally means they are no longer part of a breeding program.

Nutritional. Proper nutrition is important to reproductive health (see Chapter 210). Nutritional lack or excess can play a role in reproductive disturbance. In addition, oversupplementing of vitamins, minerals, or nutraceuticals may alter the developmental process of pregnancy (Verstegen, Dhaliwal, and Verstegen-Onclin, 2008). Assessing the body condition score of a bitch and queen before breeding along with knowledge of her normal activity level is important prebreeding information because an overweight, sedentary female may be more difficult to impregnate. While taking the history from an owner, the clinician should use care in questioning about the diet. Many "natural foods" are marketed as premium line but may not provide needed nutrition for adult canines, much less the nutrition needed for gestating or lactating dams. "Raw diets" may be another area of contention with some owners because of veterinary concerns about *Salmonella* and *E. coli* infections.

pregnancies or offspring with genetic abnormalities. Conditions such as cleft palate, thoracic ectromelia, and anasarca are examples of such developmental defects (Figures 219-2 through 219-4).

Autoimmune. Although immune factors are considered a contributing factor to human abortions, the role of immunologic factors in early embryonic death and abortion in companion animals remains unknown at this time. A female with underlying immune disease (e.g., immune-mediated thrombocytopenia or multisystemic polyarthropathy) most likely should not be considered for breeding stock because of the potential for high-risk pregnancy and possible pregnancy loss. Owners should be advised of these considerations when making choices regarding whether to breed a female.

Metabolic. Metabolic disorders can occur in any breed and at any age. Effects of these disorders, if severe and widespread, can threaten the bitch's or queen's ability to reproduce or maintain a pregnancy. A thorough history and complete physical examination are helpful in diagnosis along with the appropriate diagnostic tests.

Education of the owner about appropriate dietary intake for a breeding female is an ongoing process. Taurine-deficient rations (<200 ppm of diet), fed to queens for at least 6 months before breeding, resulted in decreased reproductive performance including resorption, abortion, and stillbirths. These effects persisted after feeding a diet with normal amounts of taurine for 6 months (Sturman, 1991). Effects on the queens and the liveborn kittens also were apparent in these and similar studies.

Inflammatory/Infectious. A number of infectious agents have been identified in pregnancy loss in the bitch and queen. This section summarizes them into the following categories: bacteria, viral, parasites, and other. Each agent is reviewed briefly; transmission, diagnosis, and treatment also are described.

Bacteria

Brucella canis *(canine only).* This intracellular bacterium is the causative agent of a sexually transmitted disease whose hallmark sign is abortion in the bitch at 7 to 9 weeks' gestation along with prolonged vaginal discharge postabortion. It also can cause embryonic death, testicular atrophy, epididymitis, and infertility (stud or bitch). Generalized lymphadenitis, diskospondylitis, and anterior uveitis also can be seen in the stud or bitch, or no clinical signs may be noted. Stillborn or weak pups have been delivered by infected bitches. The main mode of transmission is through ingestion of infected aborted material (fetal or placental) and vaginal discharge of infected bitches. Venereal transmission also has been documented mainly from infected male to female but occasionally from infected female to male. Urine, saliva, semen, mammary secretions, and nasal secretions may contain organisms and also serve as potential fluids for transmission. Definitive diagnosis is made by isolation of the organism via culture, but isolation of this organism can be difficult at times. Current diagnostic testing involves serologic testing relying on antibody production to *B. canis,* which normally takes 6 to 8 weeks to occur. The rapid slide agglutination test (RSAT) is used by most veterinarians as a screening test for *B. canis,* but false-positive results are common because of cross-reaction with antibodies produced against mucoid *Pseudomonas* or *Staphylococcus* species, other *Brucella* species, and *Bordetella bronchiseptica.* Positive RSAT results should be confirmed with either 2-mercaptoethanol (2-ME) RSAT testing or an agar gel immunodiffusion (AGID) test performed at Cornell Diagnostic Laboratory.

More recently quantitative polymerase chain reaction (qPCR) testing has been looked at as a way to identify bacterial DNA in a bitch in the absence of antibodies (recently infected, chronic disease). Antibiotic therapy usually is unsuccessful as treatment for this disease because the bacteria is intracellular and recrudescence of the disease common. Spaying and neutering infected dogs decrease spread of disease, but this disease has the potential for zoonosis in immunocompromised individuals. A case of brucellosis regardless of species is reportable to the state veterinarian in most states. Some states have mandated euthanasia of confirmed infected dogs as a way to try to eradicate the disease from their states.

Other Brucella *species.* Brucella abortus, Brucella suis, and *Brucella melitensis* have been implicated in canine abortion, although the role of these species causing abortion is not large. Known exposure to infected livestock is a key part of the history associated with these cases. Transmission is usually by ingestion of infected fetal or placental material. Diagnosis is not through traditional *B. canis* RSAT testing. Instead specific screening for each organism is needed to confirm the cause of the abortion was due to one of these organisms.

Campylobacter *species.* This bacterium has been associated with pregnancy loss in the bitch and queen, placentitis leading to abortion, and gastrointestinal signs in adults. There is zoonotic potential when dealing with this bacterium, and diagnosis is usually through isolation of the organism from infected tissue (placenta, fetus, vaginal swab). Several antibiotics can be used to treat this bacterium, but eradication of the organism from a kennel or cattery may not be possible, and reinfection with subsequent pregnancy loss can occur.

Leptospirosis (canine only). Leptospira serovar *bratislava* has been linked to canine abortions and infertility. Transmission is through the urine, penetration of mucous membranes, or abraded skin. There is zoonotic potential when dealing with this organism, and diagnosis is by identification of the organism in infected tissue (placenta or fetus) or urine. Elevated serum titers also can be suggestive of disease with paired serum titers most desired. Initial treatment during the leptospiremic phase usually includes a penicillin derivative and supportive care. This is followed by a tetracycline (doxycycline) for the leptospiruric phase. Vaccines are available for certain serovars with little cross-protection between serovars.

Salmonella *species.* Strains of this bacterium (*Salmonella panama*) have been implicated in pregnancy loss in the bitch and queen. This organism is not normal flora of the vaginal tract but can be shed in some feces intermittently. Transmission can be from fomites or by consuming contaminated water or food. Airborne transmission occasionally may occur as well. *Salmonella* spp. can survive outside of a host for relatively long periods of time. This bacterium has zoonotic potential, especially in immunocompromised people. Diagnosis is through isolation of the organism from infected tissue (placenta or fetus). Selective antibiotic treatment should be restricted to animals with moderate to severe clinical signs because treatment can promote a carrier state and may promote bacteria resistance.

Escherichia coli. This is the most common bacteria isolated from the canine and feline vagina, commonly cultured from bitches and queens with metritis and pyometra. Sometimes it is associated with pregnancy loss (Johnson, Root Kustritz, and Olson, 2001). This bacterium is known to produce endotoxins that can cause further damage to the bitch and to the fetuses. These bacteria have zoonotic potential, and diagnosis is through isolation of the organism from infected tissue (e.g., uterus, vaginal tract, placenta, or fetus). If a metritis occurs during a pregnancy and the fetuses are found to be alive via ultrasound, then antibiotic therapy could be attempted to try to save the pregnancy. Careful, daily ultrasound monitoring of the pregnancy would be needed to see if the therapy works; if not, most likely the pregnancy will be lost.

Coxiella burnetii. *Coxiella burnetii*, a bacterium known to cause Q fever, has been documented as a cause of abortion in the cat. The cat may not show any signs of disease other than abortion. Infection may occur by tick bites or by ingestion or inhalation. This disease is also important because of the public health aspects. There are numerous reports of people contracting Q fever after exposure to queens during abortion or parturition. Aerosols or fomites are believed to be the route of infection. Diagnostic tests include antibody tests on serum measured by complement fixation, enzyme-linked immunosorbent assay (ELISA), or fluorescent antibody.

Canine viruses

Canine herpesvirus (canine only). Canine herpesvirus (CHV) is considered ubiquitous in the kennel environment, and most dogs are exposed at some point in their lifetime, resulting in a mild or inapparent respiratory or genital tract disease. This virus is linked to early embryonic death, mummification, abortion, premature birth, and stillbirths when a naïve bitch is exposed to the virus during breeding or some time during her pregnancy. Canine herpesvirus also has been linked to neonatal death (e.g., fading puppy syndrome). Transmission is primarily through saliva and nasal mucus (licking) or via aerosolization (coughing). *In utero* and venereal transmissions are also common. A definitive diagnosis is made by virus isolation and the presence of intranuclear inclusion bodies within infected tissue of the fetus. An elevated CHV titer of greater than 1:16 is suggestive of an active infection. Pregnancy loss in the bitch from CHV should be self-limiting after she develops immunity. Subsequent litters should not be affected, although she can still shed the virus at the time of whelping leading to neonatal infection. Treatment of this virus is generally unrewarding. A vaccine is available in Europe.

Canine parvovirus (type 1) (canine only). This virus has been proposed to cause to early pregnancy loss in the bitch. However, this virus is part of a combination vaccine commonly used in the United States, so most dogs are protected.

Canine distemper virus (canine only). Canine distemper virus (CDV) can cross the placenta to cause abortion and congenital infection in newborn pups. Abortion occurs because of the systemic illness from the virus or it can occur from a direct infection of the placenta or fetuses. Diagnosis can be through finding viral antigens in the bitch or in the aborted material. Lesions suggestive of CDV may be noted on the fetuses at necropsy. This virus is also part of a combination vaccine commonly used in the United States, so most dogs are protected.

Feline viruses. A number of viral agents have been incriminated in pregnancy loss in the queen. Additional infectious agents are being recognized, through traditional and newfound diagnostic techniques, which also may play a part. Those most clearly documented are presented below.

Feline panleukopenia. Feline panleukopenia is a viral disease caused by a parvovirus. *In utero* infection is possible. Infection early in gestation may result in resorptions, mummified fetuses, or abortions. Infection later in gestation additionally may produce kittens with neural

tissue injury (primarily cerebellar hypoplasia). This finding may be helpful when attempting to make a definitive diagnosis. Although queens may exhibit fever, depression, vomiting, and diarrhea, some queens do not exhibit any clinical signs. Many diagnostic tests for this are available to clinical practices. Methods include serum virus neutralization, hemagglutination, fluorescent antibody detection in tissues, and others. ELISA testing of feces is available commercially.

Feline leukemia virus. Feline leukemia virus (FeLV) infection in cats also has been identified as a cause of pregnancy loss in the queen. All breeding queens should be tested for the infection by ELISA and retested before introduction into the colony. Unfortunately, overt signs of infection in the queen may not be shown before pregnancy loss. The virus can be transmitted placentally. Losses seen include resorption and abortion usually in late gestation. Metritis at the placentation site and bacterial endometritis may be found. Those kittens surviving may demonstrate infection later in life. Testing and retesting of queens by ELISA or IFA may be helpful in confirmation of this disease. Other diagnostic options to identify this virus include fetal and reproductive tract tissue evaluated by IFA or PCR (Verstegen, Dhaliwal, and Verstegen-Onclin, 2008).

Feline immunodeficiency virus. Feline immunodeficiency virus (FIV) also is recognized as a cause of pregnancy loss. Breeding queens should be tested before introduction to the colony and retested. Losses are seen as arrested fetal development, abortion, and stillbirths. The queen may be infected before breeding. Alternatively, the virus can be introduced to a naïve queen by an infected male via semen, although this is less common. Recently, it has been shown that shedding of virus in semen of cats can occur during the acute phase of infection before demonstration of clinical signs or detection of disease by ELISA. The virus then can spread to the fetus and reproductive tract. Placental immunopathology has been documented in experimentally infected cats. In that study, litter sizes were smaller in queens infected with the virus than with controls, and the fetal death rate was much higher (60%) in infected queens compared with controls (3.2%) (Weaver et al, 2005). Clinical signs in the queen vary depending on the stage of infection. There may be no outward signs of illness, except during the acute phase or the terminal phase. Diagnostic evaluation of the breeding pair should include FIV-specific antibody detection by ELISA, before breeding, although prior vaccination or maternal antibodies can be detected by this method and create false positives. Diagnostic accuracy by use of PCR has been investigated and is clearly not 100% sensitive and specific (Sellon and Hartmann, 2012).

Upper respiratory pathogens. The upper respiratory pathogens shown to interfere with reproductive performance include feline herpesvirus (FHV-1) and feline calicivirus. Vaccination to protect against these pathogens should be done routinely; however, many cats are virus carriers or are infected chronically and shed virus intermittently. Studies infecting pregnant queens with FHV-1 by intranasal and intravenous routes resulted in fetal death and abortion. The queens displayed severe upper respiratory signs when infected intranasally and mild signs when infected by intravenous route. Uterine, placental, and fetal pathology, along with virus detection, occurred in queens infected by the intravenous route but not by the intranasal route. This suggests that the pregnancy loss seen via intranasal infection, as would occur naturally in a colony, is due to the clinical illness in the queen (Hoover and Griesemer, 1971). Calicivirus has been identified from a dead fetus that was harvested surgically. Three other kittens in the litter also died but the virus was not identified in them. The queen was in the acute phase of calicivirus infection (van Vuuren et al, 1999). This suggests calicivirus also must be considered in the differential diagnosis of pregnancy loss. Clinical signs associated with upper respiratory disease may be acute or chronic. Colony history and health of kittens in the colony should be explored because the queen may not have obvious signs of disease when pregnancy loss occurs. Diagnostic testing for these pathogens has included virus isolation (VI), indirect fluorescent antibody (FA), and polymerase chain reactions (PCR). Hopefully, advancement of diagnostic techniques will make these organisms easier to identify.

Feline infectious peritonitis. Feline infectious peritonitis (FIPV) is a disease caused by a mutation of the feline enteric corona virus (FECV). FECV is common in high-volume populations and easily spread. Heritability to mutation and thus susceptibility of FIPV can be high in some breeds and catteries. FIPV as a major cause of pregnancy loss is now questioned, however (Verstegen, Dhaliwal, and Verstegen-Onclin, 2008). The mutated virus is not thought to be spread horizontally. To avoid problems with FIPV, lineage should be studied carefully, common ancestors removed from the breeding population, persistent fecal shedders of FECV culled, population density minimized, and exposure to fecal material decreased. Colonies with reproductive failure, abortion, and dead fetuses at birth should assess titers to FECV in affected queens. Development of this fatal disease also can be seen in nonpurebred littermates based on the authors' observations. Definitive diagnosis of FIP is difficult and should be based on histology and PCR. Virus detection by FA and immunocytochemistry also may be available. PCR techniques also have been applied but are not sensitive nor specific enough.

Parasites

Toxoplasma gondii. This protozoan organism can infect the dog and cat and cause abortion because of systemic illness in the bitch. Transmission is through congenital infection, ingestion of infected tissues, and ingestion of oocyte-infected food or water. Transplacental transmission is thought to be less common in the dog than small ruminants. Prevention is by avoiding contaminated food, including raw meat. This pathogen also can cause pregnancy loss in the queen. Infection induced in pregnant queens can cause placentitis and result in infection in the fetus. Stillborns have been documented. The presence of tachyzoites in stillborn tissues is diagnostic. Clinical signs of toxoplasmosis in the queen are variable. A tentative diagnosis may be made with compatible clinical signs and careful interpretation of serologic titers (IgG and IgM).

Other

Mycoplasma and ureaplasma. Both of these organisms are part of the normal mucosal flora of the nasopharyngeal and reproductive tracts of dogs, but they have been associated with reproductive diseases in the dog. Poor conception, early embryonic death, fetal resorption, abortion, stillborn weak pups, and neonatal deaths have been linked to these organisms (Feldman and Nelson, 1996). Diagnosis is through specialized culture of the organism from infected tissue (placenta or fetal) or uterine or preputial discharge. Antibiotic treatment can be attempted, but avoidance of contaminated breeding dogs and less stressful conditions helps as well. Reinfection is common after treatment because these organisms are ubiquitous in the environment.

Other infectious agents certainly can threaten pregnancy, especially when they endanger the life of the queen or bitch. However, predictions, in the authors' experience, are not always accurate. An example of this is a multiparous queen that presented with symptomatic pulmonary blastomycoses and was treated with itraconazole. Any intervention to end the pregnancy was considered too dangerous. Despite the poor prognosis, the queen delivered a live healthy singlet kitten several days after release from the hospital.

Toxicity

Some drugs are known to be embryotoxic or teratogenic or to cause abortion (see Chapter 223). Use of these drugs sometimes requires weighing the benefits against the risks to the bitch or queen, to the pregnancy, and to the fetuses. The critical timing for embryotoxicity in the bitch and queen is from 6 to 20 days after the LH surge (Johnson, Root Kustritz, and Olson, 2001). Tetracyclines are known to cause bone and teeth malformations in the fetus along with potentially causing toxicity in the female. Quinolones have been associated with articular cartilage defect in the canine fetus. Aminoglycosides easily cross the placenta and have been associated with incidence of cranial nerve VIII toxicity or nephrotoxicity. Antifungal drugs are known to be toxic and teratogenic. Administration of griseofulvin is known for the ability to produce defects (head, brain, palate, skeleton) in the developing fetus. Steroids such as dexamethasone and prednisone carry the risk of cleft palate and other congenital malformations. These drugs also may induce premature labor, causing abortion and fetal death. Before using any drug in a pregnant female, the clinician should have an in-depth discussion with the owner about the need and reason for use of the drug along with the potential side effects of the drug on the bitch or queen, the pregnancy, and the fetuses. Owners must be aware of the pros and cons of the medication being prescribed to their female and agree to these risks (if any) before medication is dispensed.

Trauma and Stress

Physical trauma can threaten gestation. Severe trauma (e.g., being hit by a car) can produce abortion, though this may be due to the blunt physical trauma, physiologic stress caused by the event, or a combination of the two. Environmental stress caused by poor housing conditions or exposure to environmental toxins (paint fumes, smoke fumes, poor ventilation) also could lead to pregnancy loss. An in-depth health history, including information on housing conditions or a breeding facility visit, may be necessary to get a clear picture of the environmental stress a breeding female is under to help determine if that played a role in the pregnancy loss.

Fetal Disorders

Fetal defects can occur secondary to exposure to certain pathogens or substances during a critical time of development. The magnitude of the defect dictates whether fetal death will occur. Usually the entire litter is affected in these cases and the cause of the disorder may never be identified. Fetal lesions also can be related to chromosomal defects. Lethal gene combinations have been known to occur in some canine and feline breeds when bred for certain physical characteristics. Karyotyping and other forms of genetic testing are available to investigate cases of pregnancy loss related to fetal defects if an owner wishes to pursue these options. Inborn errors of metabolism also may cause pregnancy loss. Urine submission to a genetics laboratory also may be useful for confirmation.

Therapy and Management

Owner counseling concerning breed screening for inherited or prevalent diseases before breeding is highly recommended to help select the best bitches and queens for breeding. Maternal health should be assessed and a reproductive exam should be performed before the female comes into estrus. Instruction regarding appropriate preventive medicine (e.g., vaccination, deworming, other pathogen preventives [e.g., tick and flea control]) and dietary and housing should be offered. Appropriate diagnostic testing is recommended if abnormalities are noted, and treatment or therapy instituted if needed. Owner education on all infectious disease that may affect health of the bitch or queen is necessary, and testing should be performed when possible. In the bitch, *Brucella canis* testing should be performed; this is a known pathogen that affects reproductive status and can be zoonotic. Mandatory tests for cats include an ELISA for FeLV and FIV.

Isolation of a pregnant female, especially one with a high-risk pregnancy, is recommended to help decrease the chance of exposure to infectious agents. This typically is done around mid-gestation, at the time of pregnancy diagnosis. Sometimes hospitalization of the female is necessary for closer monitoring of the pregnancy, but the cost of that additional extra stress must be weighed against the advantages of better monitoring of her pregnancy. In most cases of an ongoing or threatened abortion, it is unlikely that medical management will stop the abortion.

Assessment of the bitch or queen at the time of presentation determines how the case must be handled. General supportive care (e.g., intravenous fluids, thermoregulation, supplemental nutrition) should be offered if it is needed. If any specific diseases have been diagnosed at this time, then implementation of treatment or therapy should be initiated. The attending veterinarian always should discuss potential side effects of any treatment on the gestating fetuses (if still present). The owner then must decide whether to treat the bitch or queen at this time and risk effects to the litter or not treat at this time and risk effects to her health. If a recently diagnosed condition involving the bitch or queen threatens her overall health, medical pregnancy termination can be considered as long as it can be done safely.

Pregnant females with a history of pregnancy loss may benefit from serial ultrasound exams to follow the pregnancy closely, especially if a cause for the pregnancy loss has not been identified. Serial measurements of progesterone concentrations during gestation are also advisable, monitoring for decreases below 2 ng/ml signaling impending parturition. When a genetic defect is suspected, the owner can try using a different stud or tom not closely related to the last. Other owners try to repeat the breeding to determine if the pregnancy loss is repeatable or not. With genetic testing, females and studs can be screened for breed-specific genetic diseases so that affected and carrier states are known before breeding, and good breeding stock can be selected.

References and Suggested Reading

Davidson AP, Nyland TG, Tsutsui T: Pregnancy diagnosis with ultrasound in the domestic cat, *Vet Radiol* 27:109, 1986.

England GCW: Pregnancy diagnosis, abnormalities of pregnancy and pregnancy termination. In Simpson GM, England GCW, Harvey M, editors: *Manual of small animal reproduction and neonatology*, United Kingdom, 2006, British Small Animal Veterinary Association, p 113.

Feldman EC, Nelson RW: Periparturient diseases. In Feldman EC, Nelson RW, editors: *Canine and feline endocrinology and reproduction*, ed 2, Philadelphia, 1996, WB Saunders, p 572.

Hoover EA, Griesemer RA: Experimental feline herpesvirus infection in the pregnant cat, *Am J Path* 65:173, 1971.

Johnson SD, Root Kustritz MV, Olson PNS: Canine pregnancy. In Johnson SD, Root Kustritz MV, Olson PNS, editors: *Canine and feline theriogenology*, Philadelphia, 2001, WB Saunders, p 66.

Pretzer SD: Bacterial and protozoal causes of pregnancy loss in the bitch and queen, *Theriogenology* 70(3):320, 2008.

Sellon RK, Hartmann K: Feline immunodeficiency virus infection. In Green CE, editor: *Infectious diseases of the dog and cat*, ed 4, St Louis, 2012, Elsevier Saunders, p 136.

Sturman JA: Dietary taurine and feline reproduction and development, *J Nutr* 121:S166, 1991.

Van Vuuren M et al: Characterization of a potentially abortigenic strain of the feline calicivirus isolated from a domestic cat, *Vet Record* 144:636, 1999.

Verstegen J, Dhaliwal G, Verstegen-Onclin K: Canine and feline pregnancy loss due to viral and non-infectious causes: a review, *Theriogenology* 70(3):304, 2008.

Weaver CC et al: Placental immunopathology and pregnancy failure in the FIV-infected cat, *Placenta* 26:138, 2005.

CHAPTER 220

Benign Prostatic Hypertrophy and Prostatitis in Dogs

KAITKANOKE SIRINARUMITR, *Bangkok, Thailand*

The prostate is the major accessory sex gland in the male dog. It is an encapsulated, bilobed, and bilaterally symmetric ovoid gland located caudal to the bladder and circling the proximal urethra. The canine prostate is composed of glandular acini and stromal components. Prostatic fluid is secreted from the glandular acini and excreted through the prostatic duct and prostatic urethra during ejaculation. In intact male dogs, the prostate continues to grow from birth to approximately 2 years of age. After 2 years of age, the gland is maintained with no further normal growth. The Doberman pinscher and the German shepherd are breeds most frequently identified with prostatic diseases. A retrospective study on 36 dogs with prostatitis found that the percentage of dog breeds with prostatitis was 42% in small breeds (less than 10 kg), 33% in medium breeds (10 to 25 kg), and 25% in large breeds (25 to 40 kg) (Limmanont and Sirinarumitr, 2009).

Benign Prostatic Hypertrophy

Benign prostatic hypertrophy (BPH) is a spontaneous and age-related condition in men and intact dogs. More than 80% of intact dogs older than 5 years of age have either gross or microscopic evidence of BPH. The prostate gland of dogs with BPH is enlarged symmetrically and of moderately firm texture when examined by rectal palpation. Dogs with BPH are predisposed to prostatic cysts, infection, and prostatic abscessation, and the enlarged prostate may compress the descending colon or rectum. In dogs older than 5 years of age, the overall rate of cell growth, which is modulated by estrogen and dihydrotestosterone (DHT), outpaces the rate of cell death, which is modulated by apoptosis, leading to a gradual increase in prostate size.

Pathogenesis of Benign Prostatic Hypertrophy

The pathogenesis of BPH is not known completely. Testosterone, DHT, estradiol, and some growth factors such as epidermal growth factor, transforming growth factor, keratinocyte growth factor, and basic growth factor are involved in prostatic growth. DHT, a form of testosterone metabolized by 5α-reductase enzyme, is a major hormone involved in prostatic enlargement; it enhances growth of stromal and glandular components. The uptake of DHT by prostatic cells is stimulated by estradiol. Prostatic DHT concentration in dogs with BPH was reported to be approximately two to four times greater than in normal intact male dogs. However, plasma and prostatic testosterone concentration of dogs with BPH were in the normal range.

Diagnosis of Benign Prostatic Hypertrophy

The diagnosis of BPH is based on clinical signs and a detection of prostate enlargement without any other prostatic diseases. Some affected dogs may be diagnosed after blood contamination is found in semen during routine breeding soundness examination without any other clinical signs. In the dog BPH may be suspected based on clinical signs including constipation, sanguineous discharge dripping from the tip of the penis, blood in the urine or semen, and difficult urination. Straining to defecate may result in perineal hernias. Scottish terriers may have more severe clinical signs of BPH than in other breeds. Digital rectal examination reveals a symmetrically large, smooth surface and firm prostate with no sign of pain during examination. A dog with BPH and a large intraprostatic cyst may have an asymmetric prostatic lobe. The complete blood count in dogs with BPH is usually normal.

Prostatic enlargement is diagnosed radiographically when the prostatic diameter on the lateral radiograph exceeds 70% of the distance between the sacral promontory and the pubis. Ultrasonographically the prostate gland usually is enlarged symmetrically with parenchyma that is homogeneous in echogenicity and either with or without cavitating cystic lesions. A prostatic cyst is usually visible as a discrete, hypoechoic lesion within the parenchyma. The volume of prostatic tissue (cm³) can be calculated using the following formula:

$$[1/2.6\,(L \times W \times D)] + 1.8$$

where L = the greatest craniocaudal length, W = the transverse dimension, and D = the dorsoventral length of the prostate measured in centimeters (Kamolpatana, Johnston, and Johnston, 2000). Prostatic volume in the dog with BPH is usually greater than 10 ml, which is generally 2 to 6.5 times greater than that of normal dogs of similar weight.

Prostatic fluid collected by ejaculation, prostatic massage, or prostatic aspiration (ultrasound guided) in the dog with BPH should yield less than 10^4 colony-forming units (CFUs) of aerobic bacteria per milliliter and no anaerobic bacteria, *Mycoplasma* spp., or *Ureaplasma* spp. Normal seminal fluid sediment cytology lacks inflammatory cells containing less than 3 white blood cells (WBC)/hpf. Sometimes diagnosis of squamous metaplasia of the prostate is possible if the seminal fluid has an abundance of squamous cells in the sediment cytology.

Medical Treatment of Benign Prostatic Hypertrophy

The treatment objectives in dogs with BPH are to decrease the size of the prostate gland and to alleviate signs related to BPH. Castration is a permanent BPH treatment and is recommended for most dogs with BPH. Medical management using hormone therapy is an alternative to castration for BPH in cases in which the risk of anesthesia or surgery is high. However, hormone therapy is only a temporary treatment for BPH. For breeding dogs, medical treatment is necessary.

Finasteride (Proscar) 5-mg tablet, at a dosage of 0.1 to 0.5 mg/kg (or 1 tablet/dog weighing between 1 and 50 kg) q24h PO is recommended for medical BPH treatment in dogs. Finasteride is a 5α-reductase inhibitor that blocks production of DHT from testosterone. The prostate in dogs with BPH treated with finasteride involutes by programmed cell death (apoptosis) rather than necrosis; thus no inflammatory process is associated. Finasteride significantly decreases prostatic volume and serum DHT concentration by 40% to 50% but does not affect adversely semen quality, libido, or serum testosterone in dogs with BPH. The only effect of finasteride on semen quality is a decrease in semen volume. Clinical signs related to BPH, such as constipation or blood in the semen, abate within 1 to 4 weeks after the onset of finasteride treatment. No adverse effects have been reported using finasteride. During and after finasteride treatment, dogs with BPH have bred bitches successfully that subsequently underwent normal pregnancy, gestation duration, and litter size. Dogs with BPH should receive finasteride treatment for 1 to 4 months. Prostate size and clinical signs are decreased significantly at the end of 1 month of treatment in most dogs. About 45% of treated dogs showed recurrence of BPH clinical signs within 4 months after cessation of treatment with finasteride using a dose of 0.1 to 0.5 mg/kg for 4 months. Finasteride had no adverse effect on complete blood count or serum biochemistry during and after the 4 months of therapy. Deslorelin (Suprelorin), a synthetic gonadotropin-releasing hormone (GnRH) analog, has been used for BPH treatment in dogs (Limmanont, Phawaphutanont, and Sirinarumitr, 2011). Suprelorin is available as a 4.7 or 9.4 mg deslorelin acetate for subcutaneous implantation and can last for 6 months or 12 months, respectively. Prostatic size and seminal fluid volume are decreased during the 6-month treatment period after administration of 4.7 mg of deslorelin. Within 4 months of deslorelin implantation, anejaculation (inability to ejaculate) was reported in all treated dogs. After 4 months from hormone cessation (10 months after implant administration), all treated dogs still had anejaculation, no recurrence of BPH clinical signs, and small prostatic sizes. No skin reaction at the implantation site (between the shoulder blades) was detectable, and there were no adverse effects on complete blood or serum biochemistry during and after the 4 months of treatment. However, deslorelin implantation for BPH treatment is not recommended for stud dogs because of the actions of decrease in testicular sizes and testosterone levels, resulting in poor semen quality and anejaculation. It is unknown how long normal testicular function remains impaired after deslorelin treatment in male dogs.

Other medical treatments used to reduce prostatic size in BPH dogs include diethylstilbestrol (0.2 to 1 mg/dog q48-72h for 3 to 4 weeks PO), medroxyprogesterone acetate (3 mg/kg [with a minimum dose of 50 mg] SC given at least 4 weeks apart), megestrol acetate (0.55 mg/kg q24h PO for up to 4 weeks), and flutamide (5 mg/kg q24h PO). The potential side effects of estrogen treatment in dogs include bone marrow suppression with resultant anemia, thrombocytopenia, or pancytopenia. Repeated estrogen treatments may incite growth of fibromuscular stroma and induce squamous metaplasia of the prostate. Adverse effects of medroxyprogesterone acetate treatment in dogs include increased appetite, hypothyroidism, diabetes mellitus, testicular degeneration, and decreased serum concentration of testosterone. Flutamide significantly decreased prostate size within 10 days of treatment. Libido and sperm production were unchanged in male dogs treated with flutamide for 1 year; however, a course of flutamide treatment is prohibitively expensive.

Prostatitis

Canine prostatitis is one of the most important prostatic disorders commonly seen in sexually intact male dogs more than 5 years old. The disease can be either acute or chronic. Prostatitis usually is caused by ascending infection of normal (aerobic) urethral bacteria into the hypertrophied gland. Bacterial prostatitis may progress and develop into prostatic abscessation. Prostatitis is predisposed with prostatic diseases such as BPH, prostatic cyst, prostatic neoplasia, or altered prostatic secretions, and with urinary tract infection or altered urine flow. Bacteria isolated from prostatic fluid are generally similar to bacteria associated with urinary tract infection. *Escherichia coli*, the most common organism, is found in 70% of dogs with prostatitis, followed by (in order of prevalence) *Staphylococcus* spp., *Streptococcus* spp., *Klebsiella* spp., *Proteus* spp., *Mycoplasma* spp., *Pseudomonas* spp., *Enterobacter* spp., *Pasteurella* spp., and *Haemophilus* spp. Infection with anaerobic bacteria or fungi also has been reported. One retrospective study of seminal fluid cultures in dogs with prostatitis found 50% had *Staphylococcus* spp., followed by *Pseudomonas* spp. (16%), *Streptococcus* spp. (8%), and *E. coli* (8%). The results of urine culture from these same prostatitis dogs identified *Staphylococcus* spp. (27%), *E. coli* (27%), and *Streptococcus* spp. (18%), which suggests urine cultures do not always correlate with seminal fluid cultures (Limmanont and Sirinarumitr, 2009).

Clinical Signs

Acute Prostatitis

Clinical signs in dogs with acute prostatitis include fever, pain, depression, straining to urinate or defecate, a "stiff-legged" gait, hematuria, and pollakiuria. There may be edema of the scrotum, prepuce, or hind limb. Dogs with acute prostatitis usually show signs of pain during digital rectal examination of the prostate. The prostate is generally symmetric to palpation. Asymmetric enlargement of a lobe may be found in prostatitis abscessation. The gland may have a fluctuant swelling or be firm on rectal examination. Dogs with prostatic abscessation may show signs of septicemia.

Chronic Prostatitis

Dogs with chronic prostatitis may be infertile and have signs of poor semen quality, such as a decrease in progressive sperm motility, although morphologically normal sperm may be evident. If prostatic contraction is painful, dogs may show decreased libido. Chronic prostatitis dogs may show signs of lower urinary tract disease. Prostatic character on digital rectal examination is symmetric, and some dogs may show signs of pain during rectal examination. One study found that 45% of dogs with prostatitis had signs of constipation, followed by hematuria (35%), stranguria (15%), pyuria (5%), and abdominal pain (5%) (Limmanont and Sirinarumitr, 2009).

Diagnosis of Prostatitis

Prostatitis should be suspected on the basis of a history of previous illness related to prostatic disease, clinical signs, results of complete general physical examination, and digital rectal examination of the prostate. Laboratory findings often are variable. A complete blood count in dogs with acute prostatitis usually shows a leukocytosis, whereas dogs having chronic prostatitis may have normal white blood cell counts. The urinalysis results may contain blood, bacteria, or leukocytes. When prostatitis is suspected, a quantitative urine culture (CFUs/ml) should be performed. Quantitative culture of prostatic fluid usually contains bacteria greater than 10,000 CFUs/ml with the exception of *Brucella canis*.

Imaging of the prostate is essential in suspected cases of prostatitis. Routine abdominal radiographs or retrograde urethrocystography may be performed. However, ultrasonography is preferred over radiography for diagnosis of prostatic disease. Ultrasonographically, prostatitis parenchyma is usually heteroechogenic and prostatic abscesses are visible as discrete hypoechoic or anechoic lesions with or without distant enhancement. Unfortunately prostatic abscesses cannot be differentiated from cysts solely using ultrasonography. Prostatic volume measurement by ultrasonography should be performed as described above.

Prostatic fluid also should be collected by ejaculation, prostatic massage, or prostatic aspiration (using ultrasound guidance), and generally the fluid contains significant numbers of inflammatory cells. Inflammatory cells in prostatic fluid sediment is graded as mild (1 to 3 WBC/hpf), mild to moderate (4 to 6 WBC/hpf), moderate (7 to 10 WBC/hpf), and severe (>10 WBC/hpf).

Treatment of Prostatitis

Treatment strategies for canine prostatitis center on an appropriate antimicrobial therapy with other supportive treatments. Antimicrobial therapy is based upon the result of bacterial culture and sensitivity from prostatic fluid collected by ejaculation, prostatic massage, or prostatic aspiration. If the prostatic fluid culture cannot be performed, the antibiotic selection then is based on the results of antibiotic sensitivity from the urine culture. The antimicrobial drug diffusion into the prostatic fluid may be enhanced by treatments to decrease prostatomegaly caused by BPH and should be combined with antibiotic therapy. Finasteride, deslorelin, or castration is appropriate.

Antimicrobial drugs for prostatitis treatment should have high lipid solubility, low protein binding in plasma, and low pK_a, allowing diffusion of the nonionized form of the drug across the lipid prostatic membrane. Antimicrobial drugs that are highly lipid soluble include trimethoprim-sulfa, chloramphenicol, and the fluoroquinolones. These drugs are effective against susceptible aerobic bacterial infections. Fluoroquinolones (e.g., enrofloxacin, ciprofloxacin) are also effective against *Mycoplasma* spp. infection. Chloramphenicol is effective against anaerobic infections; however, chloramphenicol is used infrequently in companion animal practice. One retrospective study of canine prostatitis found that 58% of bacteria cultured from prostatitic fluid were susceptible to amoxicillin-clavulanate and doxycycline.

Treatment with a specific antimicrobial drug should be continued for at least 4 to 6 weeks. Before and 1 week after antimicrobial therapy is withdrawn, a complete blood count, blood chemistry profiles, quantitative bacterial prostatic fluid and urine culture, grading inflammatory cells in the prostatic fluid sediment, and comparison measurement of prostatic or abscess size by ultrasonography should be evaluated. If the selected antibiotic is appropriate, clinical signs will resolve and prostatic abscessation will be reduced in size or resolve. The number of CFUs/ml from prostatic bacterial culture, numbers of inflammatory cells on prostatic fluid sediment, and total white blood cell count will be decreased. Prostatic fluid and or urine also should be recultured 7 to 10 days after cessation of treatment and again at 30 days once antibiotic treatment is concluded to ensure resolution of the bacterial infection. Some dogs with prostatitis may require antimicrobial therapy for up to 8 to 24 weeks. Adverse effects associated with long-term antibiotic therapy should be considered when treating cases requiring prolonged antibiotic therapy.

Treatment of Prostatic Abscesses

In the author's opinion, some large prostatic abscesses or cysts may be aspirated using ultrasound guidance to obtain prostatic fluid for bacterial culture and cytology as well as to decompress the abscess or cyst to reduce abdominal pressure and pain. However, the dog should be under heavy sedation or general anesthesia during aspiration. The clinician should begin treatment with an appropriate antimicrobial drug immediately if it is an abscess. Long-term antimicrobial therapy (up to 4 months) with finasteride treatment may be necessary to achieve medical resolution. Prostatic ultrasonography and complete blood counts should be performed every 3 to 4 weeks to monitor resolution of an abscess. Treatment should continue until the abscess is no longer visible ultrasonographically.

After resolution of the prostatic abscess castration, finasteride treatment or deslorelin implantation should be used to further decrease prostate size and likelihood of recurrence. If the prostatic abscessation or cysts remain enlarged after antimicrobial and finasteride treatment, surgical drainage should be performed. The author prefers to combine prostate omentalization with castratión in cases unresponsive to medical management. After surgery dogs should be evaluated at least every 2 months and selective antimicrobial drug therapy continued for at least 4 to 6 weeks.

References and Suggested Reading

Freitag T et al: Surgical management of common canine prostatic conditions, *Compend Contin Educ Vet* 29:656, 660, 662, 2007.

Johnston SD et al: Prostatic disorders in the dog, *Anim Reprod Sci* 60:405, 2000.

Johnston SD, Root Kustritz MVR, Olson PNS: Disorders of the canine prostate. In *Canine and feline theriogenology*, Philadelphia, 2001, WB Saunders, p 337.

Kamolpatana K et al: Effect of finasteride on serum concentrations of dihydrotestosterone and testosterone in three clinically normal sexually intact adult male dogs, *Am J Vet Res* 59:762, 1998.

Kamolpatana K, Johnston GR, Johnston SD: Determination of canine prostatic volume using transabdominal ultrasonography, *Vet Radiol Ultrasound* 41:73, 2000.

Limmanont C, Phawaphutanont J, Sirinarumitr K: Adverse effects of 5alpha-reductase inhibitor and GnRH-agonist and disease recurrence after cessation of treatment in dogs with benign prostatic prostatic hypertrophy: a clinical trial. The 36th World Small Animal Veterinary Association World Congress, Jeju, Korea, Oct 14-17, 2011, p 130.

Limmanont C, Sirinarumitr K: A retrospective study of canine prostatitis. The 15th Veterinary Practitioner Association of Thailand Regional Congress, Bangkok, Thailand, April 26-29, 2009, p 258.

Sirinarumitr K et al: Effects of finasteride on size of the prostate gland and semen quality in dogs with prostatic hypertrophy, *J Am Vet Med Assoc* 218:1275, 2001.

Sirinarumitr K et al: Finasteride-induced prostatic involution by apoptosis in dogs with benign prostatic hypertrophy, *Am J Vet Res* 63:495, 2002.

Weichselbaum RE et al: Imaging the reproductive tract in the male dog. In Kirk RW, Bonagura JD, editors: *Kirk's current veterinary therapy XII (small animal practice)*, Philadelphia, 1995, WB Saunders, p 1052.

CHAPTER **221**

Methods and Availability of Tests for Hereditary Disorders of Dogs and Cats

EDWARD E. (NED) PATTERSON, *St. Paul, Minnesota*

The study of the biochemical and physiologic bases of canine and feline heritable disorders over the last 10 to 20 years has identified mutations responsible for a number of diseases. The progress of the canine genome maps and the recent publication of the canine genome sequence, coupled with comparative data from human genome research, have led to the recent discovery of the molecular basis of additional canine inherited disorders. More than 570 inherited diseases and traits in dogs and more than 290 in cats are recognized, but in many the biochemical or molecular basis is not yet identified. More than 80 polymerase chain reaction (PCR) DNA tests are associated with canine diseases and more than 10 DNA tests are available for cats. With additional research and emerging technologies, the number of available tests will grow exponentially in the near future. A working knowledge of the basic methods and availability of such tests will be an increasingly important part of the knowledge base of the small animal veterinarian. Biochemical, direct mutation, and genetic marker tests are the three major categories of inherited disease diagnostic tests.

Scientific Basis of the Tests

The basis, methods, techniques, and quality control of inherited disease testing are not standardized for small animals. In addition, animal genetic testing laboratories and companies have no oversight or accreditation. Regulations and guidelines for small animal genetic testing are needed. Until these are enacted, veterinarians submitting samples for canine genetic disease testing must evaluate each test individually to determine its accuracy and reliability. A basic knowledge of the methods of the test and an evidence-based approach to its evaluation are important to guide decisions about when to use a specific test. Criteria for molecular genetic testing should be similar to those for any diagnostic medical test. Within a reasonable amount of time after development, the data and results of the test should be published in a peer-reviewed scientific journal. Ideally the test should be verified independently by an outside group. Any test, evidence, and data without the scrutiny of a peer review should be used cautiously or evaluated critically. For some of the currently available tests, only patent information is available; this information can be reviewed through the U.S. patent website (www.uspto.gov/main/patents.htm). In some cases companies offering tests are awaiting resolution of intellectual property issues.

Biochemical Tests

Biochemical tests for inherited disorders in dogs and cats have been available for many years. They continue to play an important role in diagnosis of inherited disorders in which the chromosomal location or gene for the defect has not been identified. Most biochemical tests require only a simple blood or urine sample. Biochemical tests are also necessary to help evaluate newly developed molecular genetic tests, especially those lacking documentation or presenting controversy. Examples of some of the currently available biochemical tests include those for mucopolysaccharidosis, Fanconi syndrome, erythrocyte osmotic fragility, methylmalonic aciduria, cystinuria, urinary acids, urinary amino acids, urinary carbohydrates, urinary glycosaminoglycans, urinary oligosaccharides, cobalamin malabsorption, hypersarcosinemia, and other inborn errors of metabolism performed at the University of Pennsylvania School of Veterinary Medicine (PennGen) (Table 221-1). Factor assay tests for von Willebrand's

disease and other inherited coagulopathies are performed at a number of veterinary diagnostic laboratories. In many cases biochemical tests are the best estimate of the genetic status of an individual (i.e., affected, carrier, or clear). However, test results can fall into overlapping categories, causing potential problems with classification and definition.

Deoxyribonucleic Acid–Based Tests

Many genetic markers do not code for messenger ribonucleic acid or proteins (noncoding markers). These markers are interspersed throughout all chromosomes, and many noncoding markers are near every gene. The markers tend to be variable among individuals because changes in the nucleotides do not have any known functional effect. Many of the markers used in past canine genetic studies and marker tests are repeats of nucleotides (e.g., CA repeated 10 to 30 times). Restriction enzymes cut DNA at specific, short sequences. The resulting different lengths of DNA can be detected on a gel because the fragments migrate in an electrical field in inverse proportion to their size. The varying lengths of the marker are called different alleles, just as various blood types represent different alleles of a coding gene. Single nucleotide polymorphisms (SNPs), such as a C or T at the exact same chromosomal location (locus), are another type of genetic marker. Canine SNP arrays that can genotype thousands of SNP markers for one individual have been available for a number of years. Currently, most canine genetic disease research looks for association of SNP markers with the disease of interest for particular breed or a group of related breeds. A SNP array has just been developed and now is available for feline research.

A genetic marker can be associated strongly or linked with a disease gene if it is close to a gene and the marker has more than one allele. The farther a marker is from a gene on the same chromosome, the more likely recombination is to have occurred during meiosis. The percentage of time a marker and gene have recombination between them is termed the *recombination fraction*. For a marker to be potentially useful as a screening genetic test, a recombination fraction of 5% or less typically is required.

TABLE 221-1

Some Laboratories and Companies Offering Canine and Feline Genetic Testing in the United States and United Kingdom

Name	Phone	Website
Animal Health Trust (AHT) (United Kingdom)	44-(0)1638-555621	www.aht.org.uk
DDC Animal DNA Testing	800-625-0874	http://www.vetdnacenter.com/
OptiGen LLC (Ithaca, NY)	607-257-0301	www.optigen.com
Orthopedic Foundation for Animals (OFA) (Columbia, MO)	573-442-0418	www.offa.org/dnatesting/
PennGen (University of Pennsylvania)	215-898-3375	www.vet.upenn.edu/penngen
Veterinary Genetics Laboratory (University of California, Davis)	530-752-2211	www.vgl.ucdavis.edu
VetGen LLC (Ann Arbor, MI)	800-483-8436	www.vetgen.com

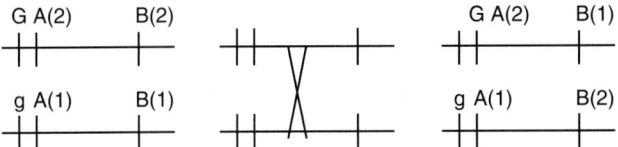

Figure 221-1 Genetic linkage of a marker A and gene G and recombination between G and marker B. The left portion shows two homologous chromosomes with gene G and markers A and B. G refers to the normal gene allele and g refers to the mutated gene allele. A(2) is marker A allele 2, and A(1) is marker a allele 1. The left side shows the A(1) and B(1) marker alleles linked with the mutation g. The middle shows a recombination event during meiosis, and the right side shows that marker A, which is close to the gene, still has allele A(1) linked with the mutation g. However, marker B now has changed to allele B(2) linked with mutation g as a result of the recombination event. A marker must be close to the gene with a low recombination frequency and with specific population dynamics of the alleles to be a reliable screening test.

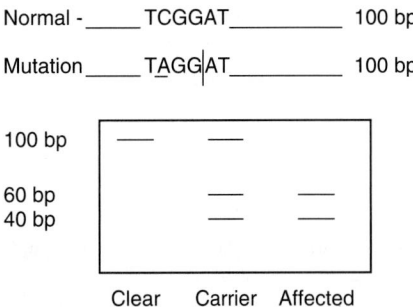

Figure 221-2 Gel electrophoresis results for a hypothetic direct mutation test for a recessive disease. The normal and mutation polymerase chain reaction sequence products are both 100 base pairs (bp) long. They differ in a C to A substitution in the second nucleotide shown. A restriction enzyme cuts the mutation sequence between the G and A into a 60- and a 40-base pair fragment but does not cut the normal product. The fragments are size separated and visualized on a gel. The results unequivocally categorize individuals into clear, carrier, or affected for this one specific mutation. This does not test for other mutations in the same gene. Laboratories always should run positive and negative controls for all molecular genetic tests.

Figure 221-1 illustrates marker and gene linkage and recombination. A marker allele is linked to a disease; this is probably the most difficult concept pertaining to an understanding of published chromosomal locations of causative genes and molecular genetic disease testing.

Direct mutation tests detect DNA sequence differences in the specific causative gene. A genetic marker test detects a marker allele linked to a mutation in a nearby, unknown gene. For either type of molecular genetic test only a small DNA sample obtained from a special cheek swab kit or an ethylenediaminetetraacetic acid (EDTA) whole-blood sample is needed. Instructions for the type of sample are found easily on the laboratory website or via phone contact. These tests can be performed at any age after weaning and are done only once in a lifetime. Laboratories always should run positive and negative controls for all molecular genetic tests to ensure accuracy and reliability. A list of the major canine and feline molecular genetic testing laboratories can be found in Table 221-1. This is not an inclusive list because new laboratories are established frequently.

Direct Mutation Tests

The testing procedure for a direct mutation test is straightforward and relatively simple. Depending on the exact mutation, there are several different detection methods. For many of the tests the specific DNA in the area of the specific known mutation is PCR amplified and then cut with a restriction enzyme that differentially cuts or does not cut the normal and mutated sequences. The restriction enzyme products then are separated by size on a gel, and the different-sized products can be categorized into normal, heterozygous (carrier for a recessive disease or affected for a dominant disease), and homozygous-affected categories. A hypothetic example that illustrates direct mutation testing with a restriction enzyme for a recessive disease is given in Figure 221-2. Currently, using automated fluorescent SNP detection methods is common to find the normal and mutant allele for direct mutation testing. Each specific direct mutation test checks for only

one mutation in the gene. Table 221-2 contains a list of some of the direct mutation tests currently available for dogs.

Once a causative mutation for an inherited disorder has been well documented, a direct mutation test can be nearly 100% accurate if the disease in the breed has been passed on by a popular breeding animal. Many genetic diseases in the dog and cat are recessive because of this founder effect. In humans with recessive diseases, affected individuals often are compound heterozygotes (i.e., they have two different mutations of the same gene causing the disease). On the other hand, affected dogs and cats often have two identical copies of the same mutation passed on from the founding individual through both their sire and dam lines. If the founder effect is strong within a breed for a particular disease and no other similar forms of the disease are caused by a different mutation in the same gene or other genes, a direct mutation test is highly accurate. However, clinicians always must consider the possibility of a new *(de novo)* mutation occurring in the same gene or a similar gene and the possibility of heterogeneity of an identical-appearing disorder caused by a different mutation in the same gene or a mutation in a different gene. Among breeds the specific mutations are sometimes exactly the same, as in some instances of type I von Willebrand's disease, in which the exact same mutation is shared by a number of breeds. In other instances the mutations are breed specific as with the three different mutations for narcolepsy in the hypocretin receptor gene of Doberman pinschers, Labrador retrievers, and dachshunds.

Genetic Marker Tests

A genetic marker test is based on linkage and/or association between a genetic marker allele and a disease. There are two major ways to prove these associations. The first

TABLE **221-2**

Some of the Common Direct Mutation Tests for Canine Inherited Disorders

Disease	Breed(s)	Inheritance	Laboratory	Basis
Arrhythmogenic right ventricular cardiomyopathy	Boxer	Variable penetrance?	North Carolina State	Patent pending
Canine leukocyte adhesion deficiency	Irish setter	AR	OptiGen	PBL
		AR	AHT	PBL
Canine multifocal retinopathy	Bullmastiff	AR?	OptiGen	NDY
	Coton de tulear	AR?	OptiGen	NDY
	Great Pyrenees	AR?	OptiGen	NDY
Cataracts	Staffordshire bull terrier	AR	AHT	NDY
Centronuclear myopathy	Labrador retriever	AR	Alfort, France	PBL
Ceroid lipofuscinosis	American bulldog	AR	U of MO	PBL
	Border collie	AR	AHT	PBL
	Dachshund	AR	U of MO	PBL
	English setter	AR	U of MO	PBL
Cobalamin malabsorption (methylmalonic aciduria)	Australian shepherd	AR	PennGenn	PBL
	Giant schnauzer	AR	PennGenn	PBL
Collie eye anomaly	Australian shepherd	AR	OptiGen	Patent pending
	Border collie	AR	OptiGen	Patent pending
	Rough collie	AR	OptiGen	Patent pending
	Shetland sheepdog	AR	OptiGen	Patent pending
	Smooth collie	AR	OptiGen	Patent pending
Cone degeneration	German shorthaired pointer	AR	OptiGen	NDY
Congenital stationary night blindness	Briard	AR	OptiGen	PBL
		AR	AHT	PBL
Copper toxicosis	Bedlington terrier	AR	AHT	PBL
		AR	VetGen	PBL
Cystinuria	Newfoundland	AR	Penn	PBL
		AR	OptiGen	PBL
		AR	VetGen	PBL
Degenerative myelopathy	>15 breeds	AR(P)?	OFA	PBL
Dilated cardiomyopathy	Doberman pinscher	AR?	NCSU	Patent Pending
Exercise induced collapse (DNM1)*	Labrador retriever and 5 other breeds	AR	U of MN*	PBL
Familial nephropathy (hereditary nephritis)	English cocker spaniel	AR	OptiGen	PBL
Factor VII deficiency	Beagle	AR	Penn	PBL
	Scottish deerhound	AR	Penn	PBL
Factor XI deficiency	Kerry blue terrier	AD(P)?	Penn	NDY
Fucosidosis	English springer spaniel	AR	Penn	PBL
		ARAHT	PBL	
Glanzmann's thrombasthenia (I)	Great Pyrenees	AR	Auburn	PBL
	Otter hound	AR	Auburn	PBL
Hemophilia B	German wirehaired pointer	XL	Cornell	PBL
Hyperuricosuria (SLC2A9)	Dalmatian and 11 other breeds	AR	UC Davis	PBL
Hyperparathyroidism	Keeshond	AD	Cornell	NDY
Hypothyroidism (congenital)	Rat and toy fox terrier	AR	MSU	PBL
Ivermectin toxicity	Australian shepherd	AR	Wash State	PBL
	Collie	AR	Wash State	PBL
	Longhaired whippet	AR	Wash State	PBL
	Old English sheepdog	AR	Wash State	PBL
	Shetland sheepdog	AR	Wash State	PBL
L-2-hydroxyl glutaric aciduria	Staffordshire bull terriers	AR	AHT	PBL
Mucopolysaccharidosis IIIB	Schipperke	AR	Penn	PBL

TABLE **221-2**

Some of the Common Direct Mutation Tests for Canine Inherited Disorders—cont'd

Disease	Breed(s)	Inheritance	Laboratory	Basis
Mucopolysaccharidosis VI	Miniature pinscher	AR	Penn	PBL
Mucopolysaccharidosis VII	German shepherd	AR	Penn	PBL
Myotonia congenita	Miniature schnauzer	AR	Penn	PBL
		AR	OptiGen	PBL
Narcolepsy	Dachshund	AR	OptiGen	PBL
	Doberman pinscher	AR	OptiGen	PBL
	Labrador retriever	AR	OptiGen	PBL
Neuronal ceroid lipofuscinosis	American bulldog	AR	OFA	PBL
	Dachshund	AR	U of MO	PBL
	English setter	AR	U of MO	PBL
	Tibetian terrier	AR	OFA	PBL
Neonatal encephalopathy	Standard poodle	AR	U of MO, OFA	PBL
Phosphofructokinase deficiency	American cocker spaniel	AR	OptiGen	PBL
		AR	Penn	PBL
		AR	VetGen	PBL
	English springer spaniel	AR	OptiGen	PBL
		AR	Penn	PBL
		AR	VetGen	PBL
		AR	AHT	PBL
Progressive retinal atrophy (PRA) type A	Miniature schnauzer	AD(P)	OptiGen	NDY
Progressive retinal atrophy (dominant)	Bullmastiff	AD	OptiGen	PBL
	Old English mastiff	AD	OptiGen	PBL
Progressive retinal atrophy (X-linked)	Siberian husky	XL	OptiGen	PBL
	Samoyed	XL	OptiGen	PBL
Progressive retinal atrophy (Rcd3)	Cardigan Welsh corgi	AR	OptiGen	PBL
Pyruvate kinase deficiency	Basenji	AR	OptiGen	PBL
		AR	Penn	PBL
		AR	Vetgen	PBL
		AR	AHT	PBL
	Beagle	AR	Penn	PBL
	Cairn terrier	AR	Penn	PBL
	Dachshund	AR	Penn	PBL
	Eskimo	AR	Penn	PBL
	West Highland white terrier	AR	Penn	PBL
		AR	AHT	PBL
Rod cone dysplasia-1 (Rcd1)	Irish setter	AR	OptiGen	PBL
		AR	VetGen	PBL
		AR	AHT	PBL
Rod cone dysplasia-1 (Rcd1a)	Sloughi	AR	OptiGen	PBL
		AR	AHT	PBL
Rod cone dysplasia-3 (form of PRA)	Cardigan Welsh terrier	AR	OptiGen	PBL
Progressive rod cone degeneration (PRCD)	American Eskimo	AR	OptiGen	Patent
	Australian cattle dog	AR	OptiGen	Patent
	Australian shepherd	AR	OptiGen	Patent
	Chesapeake Bay retriever	AR	OptiGen	Patent
	Chinese crested	AR	OptiGen	Patent
	English cocker spaniel	AR	OptiGen	Patent
	Labrador retriever	AR	OptiGen	Patent
	Nova Scotia duck tolling retriever.	AR	OptiGen	Patent
	Miniature and toy poodle	AR	OptiGen	Patent
	Portuguese water Dog	AR	OptiGen	Patent
Severe combined immunodeficiency	Bassett hound	XL	Penn	PBL
	West Highland white terrier	XL	Penn	PBL
	Cardigan Welsh corgi	XL	Penn	PBL

Continued

TABLE 221-2

Some of the Common Direct Mutation Tests for Canine Inherited Disorders—cont'd

Disease	Breed(s)	Inheritance	Laboratory	Basis
von Willebrand's disease type I	Bernese mountain dog	AR?	VetGen	Patent
	Doberman pinscher	AR?	VetGen	Patent
	German pinscher	AR?	VetGen	Patent
	Kerry blue terrier	AR?	VetGen	Patent
	Manchester terrier	AR?	VetGen	Patent
	Papillon	AR?	VetGen	Patent
	Pembroke Welsh corgi	AR?	VetGen	Patent
	Poodle (all varieties)	AR?	VetGen	Patent
von Willebrand's disease type II	German shorthaired pointer	AR	VetGen	PBL
von Willebrand's disease type III	Scottish terrier	AR	VetGen	PBL
	Shetland sheepdog	AR	VetGen	Patent

AD, Autosomal-dominant; *AD(P),* autosomal-dominant with partial penetrance; *AR,* autosomal-recessive; *NDY,* no published data yet; *Patent,* patent that can be viewed on U.S. patent website; *PBL,* peer-reviewed publication; *Un,* unknown; *XL,* X-linked–recessive. Direct mutation tests can be virtually 100% accurate if there is a strong founder effect within the breed, but another mutation in the same gene or a different gene causing the disease is always a possibility in some percentage of the cases.
*The author has a patent for the exercise induced collapse genetic test and receives a portion of the royalties for the genetic testing. (All information in this table is deemed reliable at the time of writing, but the author does not guarantee its accuracy or completeness; consult the individual laboratory for full details.)

is a family linkage study, in which marker alleles are tracked through generations of affected families in a breed to determine if the marker allele cosegregates with the disease. Statistically significant linkage found through a significant log of odds score of 3 or greater is direct evidence of the causative mutation residing on the chromosomal segment containing the marker. Association between a marker allele and a disease also is shown by a marker association study, which is done by testing markers on a group of affected individuals versus a matched group of normal control individuals. A statistically significant association by chi square or other similar statistical analysis can identify chromosomal regions that potentially contain the causative gene for an inherited disorder. This type of association of a marker allele and disease is termed *linkage disequilibrium.* It indicates that one allele of a marker is associated with a disease far more often than would be expected if the marker allele frequencies were in Hardy-Weinberg equilibrium. Statistical association in marker studies is not necessarily direct evidence that a gene is in a chromosomal segment close to the marker. Confounding variables and false positives caused by familial relationships of the dogs always are possible. A hypothetic example of a genetic marker test done on a family is illustrated in Figure 221-3.

Genetic marker tests are never 100% accurate for all individuals in a breed; therefore they should be considered screening tests only. As previously discussed, depending on population dynamics and other factors, a direct mutation test can sometimes be close to 100% accurate and therefore is considered the definitive test. The accuracy of the genetic marker test depends on linkage disequilibrium, the recombination fraction between the marker and the gene, and the population dynamics of the breed. One specific allele of the marker most often is associated with the mutation because of a popular founding individual. However, often a few individuals have the

same specific allele but do not have the mutation because of a previous recombination event between the marker and the gene. This false association also can be caused by population dynamics in which some family lines always hold the same specific marker allele yet not associated with the mutated gene. The sensitivity, specificity, positive predictive value, and a negative predictive value can be calculated from sufficient data for a genetic marker test. Currently available genetic marker tests for canine inherited disorders are listed in Table 221-3. Some of the current major genetic testing laboratories are listed in Table 221-1 and the Canine Health Foundations keeps an updated online list of many of the laboratories (http://www.akcchf.org/canine-health/health-testing/laboratory).

Genetic marker tests are often temporary screening tests because once a genetic marker is documented, the nearby causative genetic mutation is likely to be identified by positional cloning. An example of this is copper toxicosis in Bedlington terriers, for which a linked marker and corresponding marker test were identified in 1997. The genetic linkage test was verified in a larger population shortly thereafter, and a number of years later the putative mutation was identified.

Future Test Development, Other Services, and Updated Test Lists

The field of veterinary molecular genetics is evolving at a fast pace; therefore the list of available tests and services also is changing rapidly. Individual results for a direct mutation test generally have a straightforward interpretation. If direct mutation test results are used in a breeding program or if results of a genetic marker test are used for breeding decisions, a veterinary geneticist should be consulted for genetic counseling. Many of the listed laboratories (see Table 222-1) and some other laboratories offer

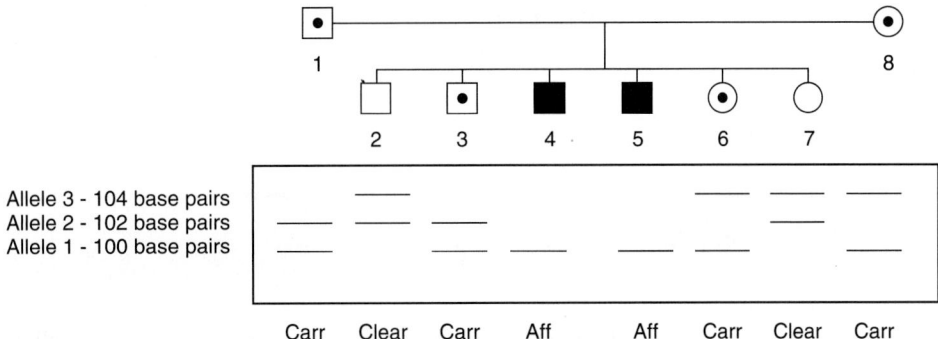

Figure 221-3 Gel electrophoresis results for a hypothetic genetic marker test in a family. Marker A has three alleles that vary in size by two base pairs in size of a dinucleotide marker repeat such as CA. The marker is linked closely to the gene defect, with allele 1 usually associated with the disease allele and alleles 2 and 3 usually associated with the normal gene allele. The alleles from each individual can be separated and visualized on a gel by electrophoresis. Squares are males and circles are females. Individuals 1 and 8 are the parents and are both carriers. Individuals 4 and 5 are affected and have two copies of the 1 allele (only one band is visualized because the alleles from each parent are the same size). The status indicated below each set of gel band for each individual is the most likely genetic status for a hypothetic recessive disease (Clear = likely clear, Carr = likely carrier, Aff = likely affected). Genetic marker tests are never 100% accurate because of recombination events and/or population dynamics, but they can be good screening tests if there is a low recombination frequency and a strong founder effect. Eventually the actual mutation should be identified and a direct gene test developed. Laboratories always should run positive and negative controls for all molecular genetic tests.

TABLE 221-3

Genetic Marker Tests for Canine Inherited Disorders

Disease	Breed(s)	Inheritance	Laboratory	Basis
Copper toxicosis	Bedlington terrier	*AR*	Vetgen	*PBL*
Dilated cardiomyopathy (juvenile)	Portuguese water dog	*AR?*	PennGen	*NDY*

AR, Autosomal-recessive; *NDY,* no published data yet; *PBL,* peer-reviewed publication. Refer to Table 221-1 for complete laboratory details. Genetic linkage tests are never 100% accurate and should be used as screening test only until the mutation is identified.

additional services such as individual DNA identification, parentage testing, DNA storage, coat color genetic testing, and/or karyotyping.

The principles and details outlined here apply equally well to testing for inherited disorders of cats. Updated lists of the available tests for dogs and cats can be found at the website for the World Small Animal Veterinary Association (WSAVA) Genetic Database (http://research.vet .upenn.edu/DNAGeneticsTestingLaboratorySearch/tabid /7620/Default.aspx).

References and Suggested Reading

Hungs M et al: Identification and functional analysis of mutations in the hypocretin (orexin) genes of narcoleptic canines, *Genome Res* 11(4):531, 2001.

Lee YJ et al: Diagnosis of feline polycystic kidney disease by a combination of ultrasonographic examination and PKD1 gene analysis, *Vet Rec* 167:614, 2010.

Lindblad-Toh K et al: Genome sequence, comparative analysis and haplotype structure of the domestic dog, *Nature* 438(7069):803, 2005.

Lyons LA: Feline genetics: clinical applications and genetic testing, *Top Companion Anim Med* 25:203, 2010.

Mellersh C: DNA testing and domestic dogs, *Mamm Genome* 2011. DOI 10.1007/s00335-011-9365-z.

Metallinos DL: Canine molecular genetic testing, *Vet Clin North Am Small Anim Pract* 31:421, 2001.

Ostrander EA, Galibert F, Patterson D: Canine genetics comes of age, *Trends Genet* 16:117, 2000.

Patterson DF: Companion animal medicine in the age of medical genetics, *J Vet Intern Med* 14:1, 2000.

Shelton GD: Routine and specialized laboratory testing for the diagnosis of neuromuscular diseases in dogs and cats, *Vet Clin Pathol* 39:278, 2010.

van de Sluis B et al: Identification of a new copper metabolism gene by positional cloning in a purebred dog population, *Hum Mol Genet* 11:165, 2002.

CHAPTER 222

Reproductive Oncology

SHAY BRACHA, *Corvallis, Oregon*

Reproductive tumors in the dog and cat are rare in comparison to other cancers because of the common practice of castration and ovariohysterectomy. However, some reproductive tumors have increased incidences in recent decades. Most reproductive tumors are benign and usually are an incidental finding. Therefore local clinical signs typically are seen in these patients, whereas systemic clinical signs may be present in cases of hormone-producing tumors. Treatments and prognosis vary according to the tumor type and invasiveness; however, through the use of surgery, chemotherapy, and radiation therapy, many types of reproductive tumors can be managed more easily.

Testicular Tumors

Testicular tumors are among the most common malignancies in intact male dogs, whereas they are extremely rare in cats. Most of these tumors are undiagnosed and detected as a primarily incidental finding on either physical exam or abdominal ultrasound. In recent decades according to one study, incidences in intact dogs are increased. The prevalence of testicular tumors in the same study was 27%; interstitial cell tumors and seminomas are the most common, followed by Sertoli cell tumor. Although interstitial cell tumors and seminomas do not exhibit prominent clinical signs, Sertoli cell tumors are more likely to be detected because of the manifestation of obvious symptoms associated with hyperestrogenism. In the last decades, only a limited number of cases have been reported in the cat and included seminomas, interstitial cell tumors, teratomas, and Sertoli cell tumors.

Many dogs present with bilateral tumors and occasionally have more than one tumor type. Intact older dogs and dogs of certain breeds such as boxers, German shepherds, and Afghan hounds present an increased risk for testicular tumors. Cryptorchidism significantly increases the risk for tumor manifestation in the dog, particularly for Sertoli cell tumor and seminomas. Cryptorchidism seems to increase the potential of a malignant testis in cats as well. Although studies in people showed an increased risk of testicular cancer after an exposure to environmental factors such as pesticides and radiation, it has yet to be determined in the dog. A possible association to chemical exposure was assumed in dogs that served in Vietnam.

Testicular tumors can be classified into several categories by tissue of origin, such as germinal epithelium of the seminiferous tubules, sex cord stroma, mixed tumors, and tumors of different origin. Germinal epithelium cells give rise to seminoma, teratoma, embryonal carcinoma, and yolk sac carcinoma. Sertoli cell tumors as well as Leydig cell tumors arise from the sex cord stroma, and a mixed characters group of germ cell and sex-cord stromal tumors. Tumors of different origin, such as adenocarcinomas, sarcomas, and gonadoblastomas, rarely have been reported.

The World Health Organization classification of seminomas in the dog labels the tumor histologic morphology as either intratubular (invasive or noninvasive) or diffuse. Further classification of classical seminoma and spermatocytic seminoma can be done and relates to the origin of the tumor cell. Spermatocytic seminomas originate from well-differentiated mature spermatocytes and therefore present a more benign nature in people. Classical seminomas, on the other hand, originate from undifferentiated gonocytes and therefore have a more malignant course. Immunohistochemistry can further differentiate between the two seminoma types. Classical seminomas typically stain positive to placental alkaline phosphatase and periodic acid stain, whereas spermatocytic seminomas are periodic acid stain negative. A recent study found that the expression of CKIT receptor is a sensitive marker for canine seminomas, whereas OCT 3/4, which is a sensitive marker in human seminomas, did not show the same sensitivity in the dog. The same study suggests that because CD30 was not expressed in seminomas it may be a good marker for distinguishing embryonal carcinoma from seminoma.

Interstitial cell tumors are the least common to metastasize, and seminomas and Sertoli cell tumors rarely metastasize in the dog. Tumors that originate in a cryptorchid testicle show a higher metastatic risk in the dog. The most common sites of metastasis are the sublumbar lymph nodes, but metastasis to any organ is possible, including lungs, spleen, kidneys, skin, and central nervous system. In people, the rate of metastasis is much higher than in the dog, in which the incidence is less than 15%.

A common finding of testicular tumors is a palpable mass on the affected testicle or, in the case of a cryptorchid dog, in the inguinal area. These may be accompanied with atrophy of the scrotum and the other testicle. Systemic clinical signs are not common, and when present, usually are associated with Sertoli cell tumor and hyperestrogenism. Estrogen myelotoxicity may have fatal consequences and should be considered as a potentially life-threatening condition in dogs with testicular tumors. Clinical signs associated with myelotoxicity and pancytopenia may include hemorrhage, petechiation, lethargy, decreased appetite, ataxia, and fever. Other clinical signs associated with hyperestrogenism include feminization, symmetric bilateral alopecia, hyperpigmentation, atrophied scrotum and penis, and metaplasia of the prostate. Although feminization was not reported in cats with testicular tumors, masculine behavior was observed in two cases and in one case was attributed to a potential increase in serum testosterone levels. Testosterone production may result in a perianal hernia in the dog, as well as hyperplasia of the prostate and of the perianal glands.

Although a histologic sample is needed for a definitive diagnosis, a fine-needle aspirate has a relatively high sensitivity and high specificity. Generally, aspirates are performed with ultrasound guidance and typically are reserved for owners who resent castration. A thorough physical exam including rectal palpation should be performed. A complete blood count (CBC) may reveal hematologic abnormalities associated with estrogen myelotoxicity, such as pancytopenia. In addition, plasma levels of estradiol-17β should be measured in dogs with feminization signs. However, clinical signs of feminization may exist in the absence of increased levels of estradiol-17β. Complete staging also should include an abdominal ultrasound and thoracic radiographs.

The majority of dogs present with local disease and the preferred treatment is castration with en bloc scrotal ablation. Prevalence of metastasis in cats is increased; however, the number of reported cases is limited. For dogs with estrogen myelotoxicity, the prognosis is guarded even with intensive supportive treatment of broad-spectrum antibiotics and blood transfusions. Recovery of such an insult to the bone marrow may take several weeks to months. Bleomycin sulfate (Blenoxane) and cisplatin (Platinol-AQ) were reported for the treatment of metastatic disease but had mixed results. Cisplatin typically is administered at a dose of 60 mg/m² IV over 20 minutes, generally every 3 weeks. However, an intravenous saline diuresis should be performed 4 hours before and 2 hours after the administration of cisplatin at a rate of 20 ml/kg/hr. Although reports on radiation treatment are limited, it proved to be effective in the management of testicular tumors.

Penile and Preputial Tumors

Penile and preputial tumors in dogs are rare and no reports exist in the cat. Multiple forms of skin cancer can affect the prepuce and penis; however, transmissible venereal tumor (dogs only) and squamous cell carcinoma are the most common. Transmissible venereal tumors are more common in younger dogs in tropical climate weather, whereas squamous cell carcinoma is more common in lightly pigmented dogs with history of exposure to solar radiation. Mast cell tumors have been reported on the prepuce and may involve the penis. Other tumors of the prepuce and penis include benign masses such as papilloma, hemangioma, fibroma, and sebaceous adenoma. Malignant tumors include lymphoma, hemangiosarcoma, and fibrosarcoma.

Preputial and penile tumors are usually visible and palpable. Clinical signs may include paraphimosis, pineal prolapse, hematuria, hemorrhagic discharge from the prepuce or penis, and dysuria resulting from obstruction. Diagnosis can be determined with fine-needle aspirates or impression smears. A histologic sample should be obtained for definite diagnosis. Further staging requires a CBC, blood chemistry panel, and urinalysis. Because of the potential metastasis of some of the tumors, such as hemangiosarcoma, mast cell tumor, squamous cell carcinoma, and fibrosarcoma, thoracic radiographs and an abdominal ultrasound are warranted. Although transmissible venereal tumors have a low risk to metastasize, such incidences were reported in up to 15% of the cases in one study and therefore complete staging is recommended.

Surgical excision is the preferred treatment for most penile and preputial tumors, excluding transmissible venereal tumors, that typically show complete response with chemotherapy treatment. The extent of surgery and postsurgical therapy should be determined by the type of tumor.

Vincristine (Oncovin or Vincasar PFS) is a common effective treatment for transmissible venereal tumors administered at a dosage of 0.5 to 0.70 mg/m² IV once a week. Treatment with doxorubicin hydrochloride (Adriamycin) may be attempted in cases of resistance to vincristine. Transmissible venereal tumors are also sensitive to radiation, and in some cases a cure was reported with a single treatment of 1000 cGy. In one study, the entire cohort of 18 dogs achieved complete remission when 1 to 3 fractions of 1000 cGy were delivered.

Scrotal Tumors

As in other locations of the dog's skin, mast cell tumors are the most common on the scrotum. The aggressiveness of mast cell tumors in the inguinal area is debated. However, to date, survival seems to be equivalent for patients with the same grade disease regardless of the tumor location on the skin. Other possible tumors of the scrotum include squamous cell carcinoma, sweat gland carcinoma, hemangioma, myxoma, plasmacytoma, and melanoma. Scrotal tumors in the cat have not been reported.

In most circumstances, scrotal tumors are obvious and easy to palpate. Squamous cell carcinomas usually have a nodular confined appearance and are more common in older dogs with lightly pigmented skin. Myxosarcoma may present as a nodular mass without defined borders, whereas mast cell tumors may present as a confined mass or more diffusive. Edema, bruising, and ulceration may be associated with mast cell tumors. Needle aspirates, impression smears, or tissue biopsies for a definite diagnosis should be obtained and ideally accompanied with complete staging. In cases of potential mast cell tumors, an injection of diphenhydramine hydrochloride (Benadryl) 20 minutes before the procedure may prevent possible complications associated with cell degranulation. The typical dose of diphenhydramine hydrochloride is 2 mg/kg SC or IM.

Surgical excision of the scrotum usually is curative. In the case of metastatic disease, chemotherapy may be necessary depending on the type of tumor.

Prostatic Cancer

The prevalence of prostate cancer increases with the age of the dog. An epidemiologic study based on the

Veterinary Medical Data Base demonstrated an increased risk of prostate cancer in castrated male dogs. This study examined data from more than three decades and revealed a higher chance of metastatic disease in castrated males in comparison to those intact. Regardless of castration status, mixed-breed dogs and certain breeds such as Doberman pinschers, Shetland sheepdogs, Scottish terriers, beagles, German shorthaired pointers, Airedale terriers, and Norwegian elkhounds were reported to have a higher prevalence for prostate cancer. Prostatic tumors in the cat have not been reported.

Dogs with prostate cancer often present with difficulties to defecate, hematuria, stranguria, and incontinence. The few reports in cats demonstrated similar clinical presentation. Metastasis to sublumbar lymph nodes and lungs are common. As in humans, skeletal metastasis is common as well, and younger dogs have an even increased risk for skeletal involvement. Neurologic deficits attributed to musculoskeletal disease were reported in about a third of dogs with prostate cancer. According to one study, the most common skeletal sites of metastasis were the lumbar vertebra, the pelvis, and the femur.

A rectal examination may reveal enlarged prostate and sublumbar lymph nodes. Lameness and/or pain on spinal palpation may be evident in the case of skeletal involvement. Complete staging includes a CBC, blood chemistry, urinalysis, and urine culture. Thoracic radiographs and abdominal ultrasound may reveal metastatic disease to lymph nodes or other visceral organs. Fine-needle aspirates and biopsies ideally should be obtained with ultrasound guidance.

Estrogen has a significant role in the differentiation of epithelial and stromal cells in the prostate. Expression of estrogen receptors was examined with immunohistochemistry (IHC) and IHC labeling in normal, hyperplastic, and neoplastic tissues. A marked nuclear expression was demonstrated in the normal and hyperplastic cells. However, neoplastic cells showed a reduced expression that was related to the cells' poor differentiation. Immunohistochemistry staining for cytokeratin 7 can differentiate between tumors of epithelial origin or urothelium origin. Cytokeratin 7 stains positive in masses of urothelium origin and negative in prostate epithelium origin. A study of prostate carcinoma proteomics showed a significant overexpression of cytokeratin 7, GRP78, and endoplasmin when compared with the profile of normal prostate and normal urinary bladder. Protein profiling may help in the near future to develop a deeper understanding of prostate cancer type and origin and potential therapeutic targets.

In one study a histological examination of prostatic cancer showed that about half of the tumors had a mixed morphology and about a third of the tumors were considered to be adenocarcinomas. The rest of the tumors were classified as squamous cell carcinomas and urothelial carcinomas. A more recent study indicated that canine prostate cancer can be classified as adenocarcinoma or poorly differentiated. The same study further classified prostatic adenocarcinoma and found that intraalveolar is the most common subtype in castrated dogs, whereas intact dogs had the small acinar type. Surgical methods that can be used are the total prostatectomy and subtotal intracapsular prostatectomy. Total prostatectomy can be attempted but may result in serious postsurgical complications such as uncontrolled bleeding, sepsis, and acute renal failure. Less severe complications are urinary incontinence and urethral damage. Dogs that had subtotal intracapsular prostatectomy had fewer complications and longer survival times when compared with dogs that had total prostatectomy. In most instances, a prostatectomy is not performed because of the potential high morbidity involved with these procedures and the lack of evidence that it prolongs survival. In an advanced stage disease a partial or a complete obstruction of the urethra may take place. Possible palliative treatments include urethral stenting and tube cystostomy.

Reports are limited regarding the treatments with chemotherapy. Prostate cancer in humans and dogs express COX-2. Although COX-2 could not be linked directly to disease progression in prostate cancer of the dog, treatment with nonsteroidal antiinflammatory drugs (NSAIDs) still may be valuable. The NSAID piroxicam (Feldene), with a dosage of 0.3 mg/kg q24h PO in a combination with mitoxantrone hydrochloride (Novantrone) at 5.0 mg/m^2 IV once every 3 weeks, have proven to be effective in the treatment of transitional cell carcinoma and may be effective when the prostate is involved. Other potential treatments for metastatic disease may include carboplatin (Paraplatin) 300 mg/m^2 IV once every 3 weeks and doxorubicin hydrochloride 30 mg/m^2 IV once every 3 weeks. In humans, docetaxel is used commonly for the treatment of castration-resistant prostate cancer. Treatment with photodynamic therapy includes the administration of a photosensitizer (e.g., 5 aminolevulinic acid), a laser light source, and oxygen. Photodynamic therapy in dogs with prostatic cancer has had limited use; however, this therapeutic model may prove a good method for local disease control.

Ovarian Tumors

Ovarian tumors are seldom seen in dogs, most probably because of the common practice of ovariohysterectomy. The prevalence of ovarian tumors is less than 1.2% in dogs, whereas in humans the incidence rate is 12.8 per 100,000 per year. Several breeds such as boxers, German shepherds, Yorkshire terriers, pointers, and bulldogs have a higher risk. Most affected dogs are older, except in the cases of granulosa cell tumors and teratomas, which are seen more commonly in younger dogs. According to one report the left ovary seems to be affected more frequently; however, not all studies support this observation.

Classification is by the tissue of origin, including germ cell tumors, epithelial tumors, sex-cord stromal tumors, and mesenchymal tumors. Epithelial cell tumors typically are more common in older females and account for 40% to 50% of ovarian tumors. Epithelial tumors include papillary adenomas, cystadenoma, papillary adenocarcinomas, and undifferentiated carcinomas; of which papillary adenoma is the most common. Sex cord stromal tumors reported in the dog include thecomas, Sertoli-Leydig cell tumors (benign), and granulosa cell tumors (responsible for up to 50% of all ovarian tumors in the dog). Germ cell tumors account for a small percentage of the ovarian tumors and include dysgerminoma tumors and teratomas. Mesenchymal tumors are rare and may include hemangioma, hemangiosarcoma, and leiomyoma. Sex cord tumors, germ cell tumors, and epithelial tumors have been reported in the cat. However, epithelial tumors are diagnosed much more often in the dog than in the cat. Cats most commonly have malignant granulosa cell tumors.

Production of hormones may be associated with sex cord stromal tumors. These tumors are known to secrete inhibin, estrogen, progesterone, and, in some cases, testosterone. Production of estrogen may result in a pyometra, vaginal discharge, symmetric alopecia, polyuria, polydipsia, and abnormal estrous behavior. Estrogen myelotoxicity may result in severe anemia and sepsis, in which case the dog may become pyretic and lethargic. The production of progesterone can induce mammary hyperplasia. In the case of testosterone, behavioral changes (e.g., aggression) may be observed. Pulmonary metastasis or pleural effusion may cause coughing and dyspnea. A mass effect or ascites may result in a distended abdomen in dogs.

In the dog about 30% of ovarian masses metastasize and hence a physical examination and complete staging are necessary for evaluation of the disease stage. A cytologic or histologic sample should be obtained for the determination of the nature of the tumor. Complete staging should follow any diagnosis of ovarian tumor. Cats may present with advanced disease because of the likelihood of malignant tumors. Breathing difficulties may point to lung metastasis or pleural effusion. Thoracic radiographs may show pulmonary metastasis or pleural fluid associated with carcinomatosis. Abdominal distention may be the result of a mass-occupying effect or malignant ascites. Abdominal ultrasound may reveal masses with or without free fluid. Scanning of the abdomen also may display bilateral ovary involvement, which can be associated with papillary adenomas and adenocarcinomas. Needle aspirates of ovarian tumors showed an accuracy of 94.7%; however, a histologic sample is warranted for a definitive diagnosis. Aspiration of free abdominal fluid that can accompany ovarian carcinomas may reveal malignant cells on cytologic evaluation.

Ovariohysterectomy should follow a complete staging and is the treatment of choice for cases in which the tumors are confined to the ovaries. However, surgery should be reconsidered in the presence of metastatic disease. Chemotherapy can be considered specifically for metastatic disease. Systemic chemotherapy may be attempted, such as carboplatin (Paraplatin) 250 mg IV (for cats) or 300 mg/m^2 IV (for dogs) once every 3 weeks; doxorubicin hydrochloride 30 mg/m^2 IV (cats and dogs) once every 3 weeks; or mitoxantrone hydrochloride 5.0 to 5.5 mg/m^2 IV (for cats) or 5.0 mg/m^2 IV (for dogs) once every 3 weeks.

The use of NSAIDs may be effective in the case of metastatic carcinoma; however, dosages should be calculated carefully when combined with other chemotherapies (e.g., carboplatin) to minimize the risk toward renal and gastrointestinal toxicities. Draining of pleural and abdominal effusion may provide a temporary relief for patients, but usually the procedure has a short-lived outcome. Intracavitary chemotherapy with carboplatin or mitoxantrone may yield temporary control in cases of carcinomatosis with abdominal or thoracic effusion. Immense supportive care should take place in the cases of dogs with myelotoxicity, which may include blood transfusions and broad-spectrum antibiotics.

The prognosis is excellent for dogs with benign disease and fair for dogs with malignant tumors confined to the ovaries. However, metastatic disease presents a rather guarded prognosis even with chemotherapeutic treatment. Dogs with myelotoxicity may have a long recovery course that can take several weeks to months after the elimination of the myelotoxic insult.

Uterine Tumors

Canine Uterine Tumors

Uterine tumors are more likely to be diagnosed in older dogs and account for only 0.4% of all tumors. Two main uterine tumors are reported in the dog: the leiomyoma (benign) and leiomyosarcoma (malignant). Although not common in the dog, epithelial origin tumors are the most frequent uterine cancer in cats. Other tumors reported in the cat include müllerian tumor, hemangiosarcoma, fibroma, fibrosarcoma, leiomyoma, and leiomyosarcoma. In the dog, leiomyomas are diagnosed more commonly and usually are an incidental finding. In contrast, leiomyosarcomas are less commonly diagnosed and account for only 10% of uterine tumors. German shepherds may be predisposed to uterine leiomyomas because of a mutation on the BHD gene, which is inherited in an autosomal dominant manner. Along with the formation of uterine leiomyomas, German shepherds with a mutated BHD gene also may show multifocal renal cystadenocarcinomas and nodular dermatofibrosis. To date, no other breeds have been reported to have a predisposition to uterine tumors.

Physical examination, CBC, and blood chemistry are part of a basic workup. Abdominal ultrasound and thoracic radiographs are desirable for complete staging, especially in the case of leiomyosarcoma. Ovariohysterectomy is the treatment of choice for both types of tumors in dogs, with excellent prognosis for leiomyoma and good prognosis for leiomyosarcoma, considering there is no evidence of metastasis at time of diagnosis. Uterine and cervical carcinomas and adenocarcinomas were reported as a rare event in the dog. On one report, three of five dogs were described to have multiple tumors in the uterus and cervix accompanied with advanced metastasis. Common metastatic sites were the kidneys and lungs.

Feline Uterine Tumors

Uterine neoplasia is rare in cats, making up 0.29% of all feline neoplasms. Uterine tumors are found more commonly in older, intact female cats between 4 and 16 years of age. Only one case of uterine adenocarcinoma has been reported in an ovariohysterectomized cat. Types of uterine tumors reported in the cat include leiomyoma, adenocarcinoma, leiomyosarcoma, adenoma, lymphosarcoma. squamous cell carcinoma, mixed müllerian tumor, mixed mesodermal tumor, paramesonephric carcinosarcoma, endothelioma, hemangioma, fibroadenoma, cystadenoma, and submucosal fibroma. Leiomyoma and adenocarcinoma are the most common in cats. Concurrent mammary adenocarcinoma may occur with uterine adenocarcinoma. The clinical signs of uterine tumors in cats vary but can include abdominal distention, weight loss, anorexia, pain, vaginal bleeding, and infertility.

As with the dog, physical examination, CBC, and blood chemistry are part of the basic workup. Abdominal ultrasound and thoracic radiographs are desirable for complete staging, especially in the case of adenocarcinoma. Ovariohysterectomy is the preferred treatment for all uterine tumors in cats provided there is no evidence of metastasis at time of diagnosis. In the cat, carcinomas and adenocarcinomas frequently metastasize and hence carry a guarded prognosis.

References and Suggested Reading

Bryan JN et al: A population study of neutering status as a risk factor for canine prostate cancer, *Prostate* 67:1174, 2007.

Fan TM, Lorimier LP: Tumors of the male reproductive system. In Withrow SJ, Vail DM, editors: *Withrow and Macewen's small animal clinical oncology*, ed 4, St Louis, 2007, Saunders Elsevier, p 637.

Grieco V et al: Canine testicular tumours: a study on 232 dogs, *J Comp Pathol* 138:86, 2008.

Klein MK: Tumors of the female reproductive system. In Withrow SJ, Vail DM, editors: *Withrow and Macewen's small animal clinical oncology*, ed 4, St Louis, 2007, Saunders Elsevier, p 610.

LeRoy B et al: Protein expression profiling of normal and neoplastic canine prostate and bladder tissue, *Vet Comp Oncol* 5:119, 2007.

Masserdotti C et al: Cytologic features of testicular tumours in dog, *J Vet Med A Physiol Pathol Clin Med* 52:339, 2005.

Patnaik AK, Greenlee PG: Canine ovarian neoplasms: a clinicopathologic study of 71 cases, including histology of 12 granulosa cell tumors, *Vet Pathol* 24:509, 1987.

Taylor KH: Female reproductive tumors. In Henry CJ, Higginbotham ML, editors: *Cancer management in small animal practice*. St Louis, 2010, Saunders, p 268.

Taylor KH: Male reproductive tumors. In Henry CJ, Higginbotham ML, editors: *Cancer management in small animal practice*, St Louis, 2010, Saunders Elsevier, p 282.

Yu CH et al: Comparative immunohistochemical characterization of canine seminomas and Sertoli cell tumors, *J Vet Sci* 10:1, 2009.

CHAPTER **223**

Reproductive Toxicology and Teratogens

MICHAEL E. PETERSON, *Albany, Oregon*

Reproductive Toxicity

Sexually intact dogs and cats constitute a small percentage of patients in the average veterinary practice. Clinical focus on reproduction in small companion animals is a relatively new field, limited to breeding primarily purebred dogs and cats. Clients concerned about a reproductive disorder in their animals generally seek reproductive workups when the animals fail to conceive. Early ultrasonographic or hormonal diagnosis of pregnancy (within the first half of gestation) is of greatest benefit when dams fail to produce offspring from a breeding. The ability to distinguish between the failure to conceive and failure to carry a pregnancy to term defines the problem and correctly directs the workup between the dam, the sire, and the breeding management.

The differential diagnosis of a reproductive toxicity usually does not result until a specific problem is identified as the source of the infertility. At this point, the effect of exposure is apparent (e.g., ovulation failure as in the case of methanol exposure), but the underlying cause may never be known. In addition, some toxic effects may not become apparent until the next generation, as is the case of male offspring with decreased testosterone levels and low sperm counts whose dams were exposed to lindane while pregnant or lactating. Specific treatments for reproductive toxicities are limited to a number of conditions. For example, recovery of spermatogenesis after cyclophosphamide exposure may be improved with GnRH treatment.

Reproductive problems in kennels or catteries in which multiple animals are housed are presented less commonly but are easier to work up with an epidemiologic approach. Diagnosing reproductive intoxications depends on a thorough history, physical examination, and appropriate laboratory testing. The history should include family reproductive history as well as past and current feeding and husbandry practices (Box 223-1). Industrial hygienists may be useful in site visits because these professionals are experienced in assessing sick building syndrome and workplace exposures to toxins. Assessing any exposure requires more than finding a suspect xenobiotic (Box 223-2). The Environmental Protection Agency (EPA)

BOX 223-1

Patient History Questions to Identify a Potential Case of Reproductive Toxicity

Family Reproductive History
- Have the sire and dam both produced offspring and if so, how long ago?
- Did either parent receive any drug therapy in the days to months before conception?

Feeding
- Have there been any feed changes?
- What feed supplements are used and how much?

Housing
- How are the animals housed?
- Are the animals in a rural or urban setting?
- What is used for pest control (both rodents and insects)?

Cleaning
- What disinfectants are used?
- Are any fungicides or herbicides used?
- Have any new shampoos been used?

BOX 223-2

A Partial List of Potential Reproductive Toxins

Acrylonitrile	Manganese and its
Aniline	compounds
Arsenic and its compounds	Mercury and its compounds
Benzene	(Inorganic)
Benzo(a)pyrene	Methyl n-butyl ketone
Beryllium	Methyl chloroform
Boric acid (Boron)	Methyl ethyl ketone (MEK)
Cadmium and its compounds	Nitrogen dioxide
Carbon monoxide	Ozone
Chlordecone (Kepone)	Platinum and its compounds
Chloroform	Polybrominated biphenyls
Chloroprene	(PBB) and polychlorinated
Dibromochloropropane	biphenyls (PCB)
(DBCP)	Selenium and its compounds
Dichlorobenzene	Styrene
1,1-Dichloroethane	Tellurium and its compounds
Dichloromethane	Tetrachloroethylene
Dioxane	Thallium and its compounds
Epichlorohydrin	Toluene and
Ethylene dibromide	toluene-2,4-diisocyanate
Ethylene dichloride	o-Toluidine
Ethylene oxide	Trichloroethylene
Fluorocarbons	Vinyl chloride
Formaldehyde	Vinylidene chloride
Formamides	Xylene
Lead (organic)	

---

currently is assessing 87,000 compounds for their impact on the endocrine system. Issues relative to the total dose received, route of exposure, and length of exposure to a possible reproductive toxicant or teratogen are important in determining if the cause is sufficient to result in the particular disorder diagnosed. The level, timing, and nature of the exposure are paramount in assessing the possible reproductive risk to either the male or female breeding animal. It is not enough to determine exposure alone. In the case of the bitch or queen, was exposure preconception or postconception?

Target Sites

Hypothalamus

The hypothalamus produces gonadotropin-releasing hormone (GnRH), which is responsible for initiation of estrus and ovulation. The correct timing, amount, and frequency of GnRH release is controlled by positive and negative feedback responses. The primary action of GnRH is to induce the anterior pituitary gland to synthesize, store, and secrete gonadotropins (follicle-stimulating hormone [FSH] and luteinizing hormone [LH]).

The hypothalamus responds to exposure to catecholamines, dopamine, serotonin, GABA, and endorphins by increasing or decreasing release of GnRH. These exposures can have significant negative reproductive effects.

Anterior Pituitary

The anterior pituitary is responsible for synthesis and release of FSH, LH, prolactin, growth hormone (GH), thyroid-stimulating hormone (TSH), and adrenocorticotropic hormone (ACTH). In the female, the primary function of FSH, LH, and prolactin is to control ovarian cyclicity, follicular recruitment/maturation, ovulation, and luteinization. In the male, the main function of FSH on testicular Sertoli cells is to stimulate spermatogenesis, whereas the primary function of LH on testicular Leydig cells is to stimulate steroidogenesis. Prolactin has synergistic action with LH in males. Generally these processes are controlled with positive or negative feedback from the gonads as well as by stimulation from hypothalamic GnRH.

Gonads

Ovaries. The ovary is responsible for follicular development and maintenance of proper hormonal environment for correct growth and maturation of the oocyte. This process relies on endocrine stimulation and feedback. The ovary contains all the primordial eggs at birth, so any toxin exposure potentially affects all of the female's eggs. Primordial follicle damage may take years to identify and may manifest as a decrease in reproductive lifespan. Environmental toxin exposure during estrus may damage preovulatory follicles, resulting in decreased litter size.

Testes. Testosterone produced by Leydig cells stimulates testicular Sertoli cells to induce spermatogenesis. It also regulates the hypothalamus and anterior pituitary to inhibit release of GnRH, LH, and FSH. Inhibin and estradiol are produced by the Sertoli cells, which also act to inhibit FSH secretion.

The high rate of division of spermatic germ cells makes them particularly susceptible to toxic xenobiotics and environmental insults. The more primitive the germ cell affected by the toxin, the longer the effects will last on future spermatogenesis.

Diagnosis

Stud or tom fertility workup is easier: sperm can be evaluated relative to count, motility, and morphology. Semen quality may be more reflective of xenobiotic exposures occurring during spermatogenesis 80 or more days previously. Any particular defect directs the clinician to specific locations or events in the male reproductive tract, helping to define the source of the problem. For example, abnormal motility usually is indicative of morphologic abnormalities of the midpiece or tail. Monthly serial semen collections over a span of 1 year can be used to monitor progress in returning to normal. Chromosomal testing can be performed. The endocrine axis can be evaluated by hormone-stimulating test. No response or poor response in serum testosterone levels after hormonal stimulation testing is an indicator for testicular biopsy to evaluate the spermatogenic germ cell population.

Treatment

There are no general treatments for exposure to reproductive toxins. Patients should be treated with the same techniques employed for other potential toxic exposures. Once a diagnosis of toxicity is made, the patient should be removed from the source of the exposure and decontaminated if warranted. Any specific antidote (e.g., chelator for heavy metal intoxication) should be used. The patient then should be monitored for evidence of recovery and return to normal reproductive health. Serial testing of induced hormonal responses can be used to aid in the monitoring process. The prognosis always is guarded until the patient returns to normal reproductive health and function.

Endocrine Disruption

Discussions about endocrine disruption often are clouded with political implications; therefore a precise definition is necessary. Common sources of endocrine disruptors are pesticides, herbicides, plasticizers, and other industrial and agricultural waste products. In veterinary medicine, the most common source of endocrine disruptors is synthetic rather than natural and is generally from an environmental exposure. Endocrine disruptors may cause hormonal signal interference by disrupting communication between cells, organs, or animals. Endocrine disruptors bind to steroid hormone receptors (estrogenic, androgenic, and progestogenic). These compounds may have either inhibitory or stimulatory actions. Endocrine disruptors are capable of interfering with hormonal signaling, thereby inducing reproductive failure.

Teratogens

Teratogenesis is defined as developmental defects induced by toxic exposures between conception and birth. Typically these defects are associated with embryonic or fetal death; morphologic, functional, and/or neurobehavioral anomalies; decreased birth weight; and decreased growth rates. Teratogenic defects occur not only because of exposure to a toxicant but also because this exposure happened at a specific time or developmental stage. Genetic damage may occur, inducing a variety of defects that can result in the loss of the pregnancy or birth of offspring with abnormalities. A particularly high-risk period for canine and feline fetuses is the first two thirds (approximately 40 days) of the pregnancy during organogenesis.

Reproductive intoxicants and teratogens induce adverse effects on the physiologic processes, associated behaviors, and anatomic structures involved in normal reproduction and development. These xenobiotics usually act by inducing cellular dysregulation and alterations in normal cellular maintenance. Often the normal defensive mechanisms of the body allow the affected processes to be repaired.

References and Suggested Reading

Ellington JE, Wilker CE: Reproductive toxicology of the male companion animal. In Peterson ME, Talcott TA, editors: *Small animal toxicology*, ed 2, St Louis, 2006, Elsevier, p 500.

Evans T: Reproductive toxicity and endocrine disruption. In Gupta RC, editor: *Veterinary toxicology—basic and clinical principles*, New York, 2007, Academic Press.

Wilker CE, Ellington JE: Reproductive toxicology of the female companion animal. In Peterson ME, Talcott TA, editors: *Small animal toxicology*, ed 2, St Louis, 2006, Elsevier, p 475.

CHAPTER 224

Acquired Nonneoplastic Disorders of the Male External Genitalia

MICHELLE ANNE KUTZLER, *Corvallis, Oregon*

The subject of disorders of the male external genitalia is too vast to cover thoroughly in this concise chapter. Neoplastic disorders of the male genitalia are discussed in Chapter 222 in this text. Therefore the focus of this chapter is on acquired conditions affecting the male external genitalia. Congenital disorders (e.g., cryptorchidism, persistent frenulum, hypospadias) are not included.

Penis and Prepuce

Paraphimosis and Phimosis

Paraphimosis is the inability to withdraw completely the penis into the prepuce. Paraphimosis is the opposite of phimosis, which is the inability to extrude the penis from the prepuce. Paraphimosis occurs 14 times more frequently than phimosis. It is seen most commonly in young, intact male dogs (boxers and poodles are overrepresented in case reports), is uncommon in castrated male dogs, and is rare in cats. Although still uncommon, phimosis is reported in the literature more frequently in cats than dogs.

The causes of paraphimosis are summarized in Box 224-1. The cranial preputial muscles normally draw the prepuce cranially about 1 cm in front of the tip of the penis. If the preputial musculature cannot retract effectively the penis into the prepuce because of muscular or neurologic deficits, then the prepuce may end at the tip of the penis or be shorter than the penis, allowing the tip of the penis to remain exposed continuously. About 30% of paraphimosis cases are idiopathic (Papazoglou, 2001). Like paraphimosis, phimosis can have a number of developmental or acquired causes. The acquired causes of phimosis are summarized in Box 224-1.

Paraphimosis
The diagnosis of paraphimosis typically is made by visual inspection of the penis protruding from the prepuce. The entire length of the penis and prepuce should be examined to determine if any other urogenital abnormalities exist. Chronic protrusion of the penis causes the penile mucosa to become dry, congested, erythematous, inflamed, edematous, ischemic, excoriated, and painful, which may lead to self-mutilation. Evidence or history of trauma or concurrent stranguria indicates the need for radiographs of the penis to determine if the os penis has been fractured.

The treatment goal is to replace the penis in the prepuce as soon as possible and prevent recurrence of the problem. Penile size (edema and inflammation) can be reduced using cold compression bandages, massage with topical hyperosmotic solutions, and systemic antiinflammatory therapy. Urine production should be monitored closely. If in doubt about urethral patency and/or bladder integrity, the clinician should place a urinary catheter. General anesthesia facilitates replacing the penis into the prepuce by reducing preputial muscle contraction. Before attempting manual replacement of the penis, the clinician should clip the hair around the preputial opening (in the dog) or pluck this hair (in the cat) and apply copious amounts of lubricant to the penile mucosa. If the penis cannot be replaced manually, surgery is required. If a preputiotomy is performed, the tissues should be closed carefully to the original state. Penile and preputial surgical repair requires a thorough understanding of normal anatomy and basic reconstruction principles. Castration often is performed in conjunction with surgical correction of paraphimosis, but castration alone is not successful in correcting paraphimosis.

If the penis will not stay within the prepuce after replacement, additional surgery is needed. These techniques include a purse-string suture at the preputial orifice, preputial orifice narrowing, preputial lengthening (preputioplasty), cranial preputial advancement, preputial muscle myorrhaphy, and phallopexy. Phallopexy is the author's preferred method for penile retention, which is a technique of creating a permanent adhesion between the dorsal surface of the penis and the preputial mucosa (Somerville and Anderson, 2001). If the penis cannot be returned to the prepuce or if it has been severely damaged, a complete or subtotal penile amputation with concurrent urethrostomy should be performed (Pavletic and O'Bell, 2007). The prognosis is good to guarded for resolution of paraphimosis, depending on the severity and duration of clinical signs. The owner must be informed that erection and ejaculation in the animal may be impaired after paraphimosis.

Phimosis
Common owner complaints for a patient with phimosis is that their pet may lick its prepuce excessively, may

Acquired Causes of Paraphimosis and Phimosis

Paraphimosis
Ineffective preputial musculature that cannot effectively retract the penis into the prepuce
Neurologic deficits in dogs with posterior paresis (e.g., from intervertebral disk disease)
Trauma (e.g., from os penis fracture)
Constriction of preputial hair around the penis
Hypoplastic prepuce resulting from early age castration
Too large of preputial orifice
Priapism
Idiopathic

Phimosis
Excessively thick penis from a penile tumor (which may be palpable through the preputial skin)
Too small of preputial orifice (stenotic, fibrotic, or scarred) from excessive licking, previous wound, etc.
Balanoposthitis
Penis that is adhered to the preputial mucosa from trauma, chronic balanoposthitis, etc.

dribble urine from the preputial opening after urination, may suffer from an offensive or hemorrhagic preputial discharge, or may have a fluid-distended prepuce, stranguria, and pollakiuria. The diagnosis is often obvious once attempts are made to extend the penis for examination. In cases in which urine is voided into the preputial cavity, a secondary balanoposthitis may be evident as inflammation (reddening, swelling, and ulceration) of the tissues at the preputial opening. A bacterial culture and sensitivity must be submitted before treating balanoposthitis. Fluid (usually retained urine) may be palpable inside the preputial cavity; this also should be cultured. Other than direct examination, the diagnosis can be made using contrast radiography or ultrasonography. Contrast radiography is accomplished by filling the preputial cavity with saline and then taking radiographs of the penis and prepuce. Ultrasonographic examination largely can achieve the same results as contrast radiography. Ultrasonography allows for the detection of adhesions between the penis and preputial mucosa that were not detected by palpation through the preputial skin (Payan-Carreira and Bessa, 2008).

Symptomatic cases of phimosis require surgical correction. Antimicrobial therapy targeted with sensitivity testing should be initiated 48 to 72 hours before surgery. The simplest corrective surgery involves widening an excessively narrow preputial opening. This can be accomplished by making a longitudinal, full-thickness incision through the dorsal aspect of the preputial ring. Making an incision through the ventral aspect of the preputial opening should be avoided because this results in the persistent exposure of the tip of the penis. In cases in which adhesions are present between the penile and preputial mucosa, the preputial cavity must be exposed through a ventral longitudinal incision in the middle of the prepuce. This allows adhesions to be broken by blunt and sharp dissection. Once separated, the penile and preputial mucosal defects should be closed with absorbable suture material. Leaving the defects open may result in

the formation of new adhesions and a recurrence of the problem.

The prognosis for most phimosis cases that have been subjected to corrective surgery is good to excellent with appropriate postsurgical care to prevent self-trauma.

Balanoposthitis

Balanoposthitis is an inflammation of the penis and the prepuce. In puppies, balanoposthitis can occur as a primary condition, similar to juvenile-onset vaginitis in the bitch. However, in most cases, balanoposthitis occurs as a sequela of another condition. In the cat, a case of balanoposthitis has been reported to occur secondary to chronic prostatitis, cystitis, and pyelonephritis (Pointer and Murray, 2011). Balanoposthitis may result after phallopexy if this procedure is performed too far caudally in the prepuce. Balanoposthitis occurs secondary to phimosis, especially if urine is accumulating within the prepuce, which can lead to urine scalding and eventually infection because of overgrowth of resident bacteria. Balanoposthitis may cause ulceration of the preputial and penile mucosa that over time leads to adhesion formation, creating a vicious cycle until corrected.

Trauma

Injury to the prepuce and penis may occur from blunt force trauma (e.g., vehicular accidents); bite wounds; breeding; or self-mutilation (e.g., secondary to separation anxiety) (Ghaffari et al, 2007). The degree of trauma varies widely from superficial lacerations of the prepuce to penile amputation. The need for surgical intervention depends on the existence of or potential for urethral obstruction or uncontrolled hemorrhage.

Lacerations of the Prepuce and Penis

Although lacerations of the external prepuce are readily apparent, injuries to the penis may be less obvious. Small volumes of blood may drip slowly and continuously from the preputial orifice, or large amounts may be released intermittently as the preputial cavity fills and overflows. Hemorrhage from a lacerated penis may be exacerbated by penile erection, particularly when wounds are deep and penetrate the cavernous spaces. Minor injuries to the penis (e.g., punctures) should be managed as open wounds, treated with topical and systemic antimicrobials, and allowed to heal by second intention. For lacerations demonstrating significant hemorrhage, surgical debridement, ligation of compromised vasculature, and a double layer closure of the tunica albuginea and penile mucosa using absorbable suture must be performed. In cases in which urethral integrity may be compromised, placement of an indwelling urinary catheter for the first several days after repair may reduce self-trauma and deter stricture formation.

Traumatic Penile Amputation

Traumatic penile truncation or amputation has been reported in the dog. The injury site should be cleaned and débrided, and a new urethral opening fashioned through apposition of the urethral mucosa to the penile mucosa using an indwelling urinary catheter as a guide. In cases in which a large proportion of the penis has been lost or in which the os penis is exposed, partial penile amputation with preputial urethrostomy or complete penile amputation with scrotal or perineal urethrostomy are indicated.

Fracture of the Os Penis
The function of the os penis is to stiffen the penis to assist in intromission. It has a lower mineral density than long bones (e.g., radius), which may be a mechanism designed to decrease the stiffness and thus reduce the risk of fracture during copulation (Sharir et al, 2011).

Males suffering from an acute fracture of the os penis may present with concurrent preputial or penile laceration, penile deviation, hemorrhagic preputial discharge, and/or dysuria. However, chronic os penis fractures tend to present with histories of hematuria and/or dysuria for months to years, possibly after a traumatic event. Urinary obstruction is associated with callus formation resulting from healing fracture. Although clinical signs of hematuria and/or dysuria in the presence of penile deviation, crepitus, and pain on palpation of the penis are suggestive of a fracture of the os penis, radiography confirms the diagnosis. The feline os penis can be visualized on radiographs (especially computed versus analog) and should not be mistaken for a pathologic finding (e.g., urolithiasis or dystrophic mineralization) (Piola et al, 2011). Urinary catheter placement before radiography or retrograde contrast urethrography aids in determining the degree of urethral canal impingement.

Fractures of the os penis are most often simple and may be managed conservatively with placement of an indwelling urinary catheter to impart stability during healing. The catheter is positioned proximal to the fracture site and left in place for 5 to 7 days, during which time systemic antimicrobial and antiinflammatory medications are administered. Fractures of the os penis may be reduced openly and stabilized through internal fixation using a titanium or stainless steel finger plate. Progressive dysuria with or without hematuria is the hallmark of urinary outflow compromise secondary to bone callus formation in healing os penis fractures. Surgical callus removal may be accomplished through resection of the lateral wall of the urethral groove of the os penis (partial ostectomy), complete removal of the os penis (total ostectomy), or penile amputation and urethrostomy, depending upon the size and location of the callus. Penile amputation generally is favored by surgeons over total ostectomy of the os penis because removal of the os penis in its entirety is technically challenging, may precipitate profuse hemorrhage, and may injure the urethra, resulting in stricture formation and urinary obstruction. As mentioned previously, penile and preputial surgical repair requires a thorough understanding of normal anatomy and basic reconstruction principles.

Scrotum

Lesions of the scrotum and the scrotal contents are not uncommon in intact males. Clinical problems involving the scrotum typically present as the presence of fluid in the scrotum, pain and discomfort with or without discoloration of the scrotum, or changes in size, shape, or consistency of the scrotal contents. Scrotal dermatitis may accompany any of the above signs. Pyoderma, dermatophytes, keratinization defects, immune-mediated skin disease, or food allergy can result in scrotal lesions. A common client complaint is that the patient repeatedly is licking his scrotum. Episodic scrotal mutilation has been reported.

Trauma

Lacerations of the scrotum may be caused by blunt force trauma (e.g., vehicular accidents) and bite wounds. Most scrotal injuries should be treated as open wounds with the goal to minimize inflammation and resulting pressure necrosis. Systemic antibiotics should be administered in all cases of scrotal trauma.

Hernia

When a scrotal hernia occurs, abdominal contents move through the inguinal canal into the vaginal process within the scrotum. Scrotal hernias can cause acute onset of severe pain and swelling. Strangulation of the abdominal contents within the hernia is a surgical emergency. Severe damage to the scrotal wall and testes often requires surgical removal of the affected tissue (e.g., unilateral or bilateral orchidectomy). Ultrasound and nuclear imaging are valuable tools in identification of a scrotal hernia. Ultrasonographic examination of a scrotal hernia reveals a normal-appearing testis amid fluid and portions of omentum. Nuclear imaging is useful in ruling out a concurrent testicular torsion.

Dermatitis

Scrotal skin is thinner than most of the skin on the body with few hair follicles and is irritated readily. Temperature extremes, insect bites, allergic eruption, and trauma may result in rapid progression from a minor scrape to a lesion resembling pyotraumatic dermatitis. The affected area rapidly becomes firm, thickened, warm to the touch, and exquisitely painful. Treatment must be aggressive to avoid injury to the testicles. Topical therapy is usually successful and includes corticosteroids, antihistamines, and judicious use of tranquilizers (to prevent self-trauma).

The scrotum is also exquisitely sensitive to contact dermatitis from a large range of substances and chemical irritants. The diagnosis of contact dermatitis is made by results of avoidance and/or provocation testing or patch testing. Avoidance testing is against floor detergents, bleach, cement, laundry detergent, and plastic. Once an etiologic agent is identified, treatment is straightforward, consisting of agent avoidance.

Testes

Trauma

Testicles are not traumatized commonly in dogs and cats because of their mobile nature within the scrotum.

Clinical signs of testicular trauma include pain and swelling of the affected testicle with possible corresponding hind limb lameness. In more severe cases scrotal swelling and bruising may be seen. Severe blunt trauma may result in local hemorrhage and rupture of the tunica albuginea, the fibrous covering of the testis. Sperm granulomas are possible sequelae of testicular rupture. Diagnosis of testicular trauma is by careful physical examination. Rupture of the tunica albuginea may be difficult to detect because of local swelling. Severe testicular trauma may require unilateral or bilateral castration. Castration should be delayed until the extent of testicular damage is evaluated completely using ultrasonography.

References and Suggested Reading

May LR, Hauptman JG: Phimosis in cats: 10 cases (2000-2008), *J Am Anim Hosp Assoc* 45:277, 2009.

Ghaffari MS et al: Penile self-mutilation as an unusual sign of a separation-related problem in a crossbreed dog, *J Small Anim Pract* 48:651, 2007.

Papazoglou LG: Idiopathic chronic penile protrusion in the dog: a report of six cases, *J Small Anim Pract* 42:510, 2001.

Pavletic MM, O'Bell SA: Subtotal penile amputation and preputial urethrostomy in a dog, *J Am Vet Med Assoc* 230:375, 2007.

Payan-Carreira R, Bessa AC: Application of B-mode ultrasonography in the assessment of the dog penis, *Anim Reprod Sci* 106:174, 2008.

Piola V et al: Radiographic characterization of the os penis in the cat, *Vet Radiol Ultrasound* 52:270, 2011.

Pointer E, Murray L: Chronic prostatitis, cystitis, pyelonephritis, and balanoposthitis in a cat, *J Am Anim Hosp Assoc* 47:258, 2011.

Sharir A et al: The canine baculum: the structure and mechanical properties of an unusual bone, *J Struct Biol* 175:451, 2011.

Somerville ME, Anderson SM: Phallopexy for treatment of paraphimosis in the dog, *J Am Anim Hosp Assoc* 37:397, 2001.

Trenti D et al: Suspected contact scrotal dermatitis in the dog: a retrospective study of 13 cases (1987 to 2003), *J Small Anim Pract* 52:295, 2011.

SECTION XI

Neurologic Diseases

Chapter 225: Congenital Hydrocephalus 1034

Chapter 226: Intracranial Arachnoid Cysts in Dogs 1038

Chapter 227: Treatment of Intracranial Tumors 1039

Chapter 228: Metabolic Brain Disorders 1047

Chapter 229: New Maintenance Anticonvulsant Therapies for Dogs and Cats 1054

Chapter 230: Treatment of Cluster Seizures and Status Epilepticus 1058

Chapter 231: Treatment of Noninfectious Inflammatory Diseases of the Central Nervous System 1063

Chapter 232: Peripheral and Central Vestibular Disorders in Dogs and Cats 1066

Chapter 233: Canine Intervertebral Disk Herniation 1070

Chapter 234: Canine Degenerative Myelopathy 1075

Chapter 235: Diagnosis and Treatment of Atlantoaxial Subluxation 1082

Chapter 236: Diagnosis and Treatment of Cervical Spondylomyelopathy 1090

Chapter 237: Craniocervical Junction Abnormalities in Dogs 1098

Chapter 238: Diagnosis and Treatment of Degenerative Lumbosacral Stenosis 1105

Chapter 239: Treatment of Autoimmune Myasthenia Gravis 1109

Chapter 240: Treatment of Myopathies and Neuropathies 1113

Chapter 241: Vascular Disease of the Central Nervous System 1119

The following web chapters can be found on the companion website at www.currentveterinarytherapy.com

Web Chapter 74: Physical Therapy and Rehabilitation of Neurologic Patients

CHAPTER 225

Congenital Hydrocephalus

WILLIAM B. THOMAS, *Knoxville, Tennessee*

Causes

Hydrocephalus is active distention of the ventricular system of the brain caused by obstruction of the flow of cerebrospinal fluid (CSF) from its point of production to its point of absorption (Rekate, 2009). CSF is produced at a constant rate by the choroid plexuses of the lateral, third, and fourth ventricles; the ependymal lining of the ventricular system; and blood vessels in the subarachnoid space. The CSF circulates through the ventricular system into the subarachnoid space, where it is absorbed by arachnoid villi. Obstruction can be caused by developmental abnormalities or acquired lesions such as neoplasia or inflammatory lesions.

A number of conditions such as infarction and necrosis can result in decreased volume of brain parenchyma that leaves a vacant space filled passively with CSF. Although this situation previously was referred to as *hydrocephalus ex vacuo,* it does not cause active distention of the ventricles and therefore is not classified as hydrocephalus.

Early hydrocephalus initially damages the ependymal lining of the ventricles. This allows water and larger molecules to leak into the adjacent white matter, causing periventricular edema. Further enlargement of the ventricles compresses the white matter, which leads to demyelination and axonal degeneration. The septum pellucidum separating the lateral ventricles can become fenestrated or completely destroyed, so that one single, large ventricle is created (Figure 225-1). In some cases, the cerebral cortex is preserved. In more severe cases, the cortex becomes thin, with neuronal vacuolation and loss of neurons. This affects the prognosis after surgical shunting. If the cortex is preserved, shunting results in reexpansion of the white matter and regeneration of remaining axons. However, if the cortex is damaged, the neuronal damage persists even after shunting. With severe obstruction to CSF flow, the volume of CSF can increase so fast that it causes an increase in intracranial pressure, which leads to further brain damage and impairs blood flow to the brain.

Clinical Features

Based on the age of onset, hydrocephalus can be classified broadly as pediatric or acquired. Pediatric hydrocephalus is caused by developmental abnormalities, and clinical signs often are noticed by several months of age. Toy and brachycephalic dogs are at increased risk, including the Maltese terrier, Yorkshire terrier, English bulldog, Chihuahua, Lhasa apso, Pomeranian, toy poodle, cairn terrier, Boston terrier, pug, and Pekingese. The most commonly identified cause in these breeds is stenosis of the mesencephalic aqueduct associated with fusion of the rostral colliculi. In many cases, however, an obvious site of obstruction is not apparent. These cases may be due to obstruction at the level of the subarachnoid space or arachnoid villi, which is difficult to detect. Another possibility is the occurrence of intraventricular obstruction during a critical stage of development with later resolution of the obstructive lesion so that only the ventricular enlargement remains. Pediatric hydrocephalus also may be associated with other malformations such as meningomyelocele, Chiari's malformation, Dandy-Walker syndrome, and cerebellar hypoplasia. Many toy and brachycephalic dogs have enlarged ventricles with no apparent neurologic dysfunction. Hydrocephalus is seen sporadically in kittens, and although a genetic basis has been suggested in the Siamese, this has not been confirmed with genetic studies.

Clinical signs of pediatric hydrocephalus include an enlarged, dome-shaped head with persistent fontanelles and open cranial sutures. However, not all patients with a persistent fontanelle have hydrocephalus, and not all patients with pediatric hydrocephalus have a persistent fontanelle. Enlargement of the calvaria can be assessed subjectively by noticing whether the most lateral aspect of the parietal bone extends laterally beyond the level of the zygomatic arch. There may be ventral or ventrolateral strabismus due to either malformation of the orbit or brainstem dysfunction.

Affected patients often are unthrifty and smaller than normal. Common neurologic deficits include abnormal behavior and cognitive dysfunction, such as inability to become house trained. Visual deficits include unilateral or bilateral blindness with normal pupillary function. (One should remember that the menace response may not develop until at least 4 weeks of age in normal puppies and kittens.) Ataxia, seizures, circling, and vestibular dysfunction also are possible.

The clinical course is variable and difficult to predict. Neurologic deficits can progress over time, remain static, or even improve after 1 to 2 years of age. The condition of affected patients often is fragile and can worsen later in life coincident with other diseases. Patients with very large lateral ventricles and a thin cerebral cortex are at risk of intracranial hemorrhage from relatively trivial head trauma that results in tearing of bridging veins. This can result in chronic subclinical hematomas or sudden neurologic deterioration due to intracranial bleeding.

Acquired hydrocephalus can develop at any age and can be caused by neoplasia, head trauma, and meningoencephalitis. Neurologic deficits are similar to those in

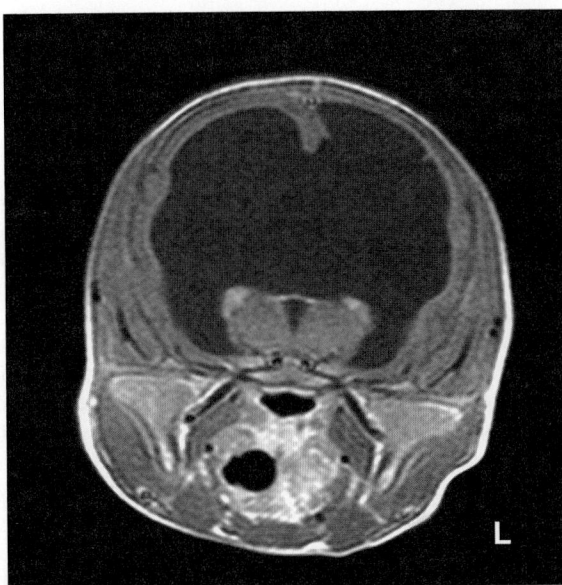

Figure 225-1 MRI of a golden retriever puppy with pediatric hydrocephalus. The septum pellucidum separating the lateral ventricles is completely destroyed, giving rise to one single large ventricle.

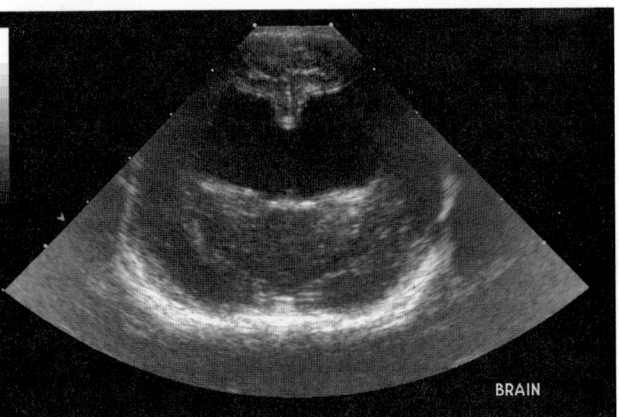

Figure 225-2 Transverse ultrasound performed through the fontanelle. The lateral ventricles are evident as a single large anechoic structure.

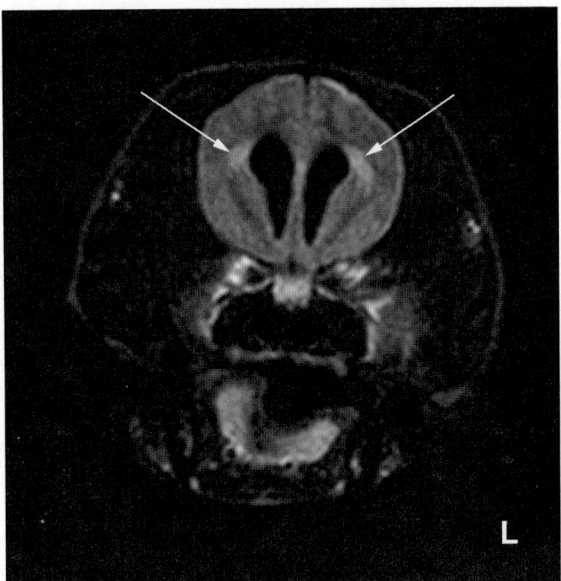

Figure 225-3 Transverse T2-weighted fluid-attenuated inversion recovery (FLAIR) MRI. The lateral ventricles are seen as hypointense (dark) structures. Periventricular edema is evident as hyperintensity (bright) regions *(arrows)* adjacent to the ventricles.

young animals, but if hydrocephalus develops after the cranial sutures have closed, malformation of the skull does not develop. Clinical signs also may reflect the underlying cause of the hydrocephalus.

Diagnosis

Diagnosis is based on the clinical features and brain imaging to assess ventricular size and identify any specific causes. Ventricular size usually is assessed subjectively by noting the progressively greater proportion of the intracranial volume occupied by the lateral, third, or fourth ventricles. However, there is poor correlation between clinical signs and ventricular size. Also, symmetric or asymmetric enlargement of the lateral ventricles is relatively common in normal animals. Therefore diagnosis of hydrocephalus is based on clinical features, not just ventricular size.

In pediatric patients with persistent fontanelles, ultrasonography allows easy detection of obviously enlarged ventricles. Normal-sized ventricles appear as paired, slit-like anechoic structures just ventral to the longitudinal fissure on either side of the midline. Enlarged ventricles are seen easily as paired anechoic regions. With marked ventricular enlargement, the septum pellucidum that normally separates the lateral ventricles is absent and the ventricles appear as a single, large anechoic structure (Figure 225-2).

Computed tomography (CT) and magnetic resonance imaging (MRI) enable accurate determination of ventricular size, extent of cortical atrophy, and the presence of any focal lesions that may account for the hydrocephalus. Imaging also is useful for monitoring patients after surgical placement of ventriculoperitoneal shunts. Obstructing masses such as tumors, granulomas, and cysts may be

identified. MRI is more sensitive than CT in demonstrating small focal lesions, especially those in the caudal fossa.

Periventricular edema may be identified on CT as blurring or loss of the normally sharp ventricular margins. On MRI, this edema is best appreciated on T2-weighted images as increased intensity compared with normal white matter. Heavily T2-weighted FLAIR (fluid-attenuated inversion recovery) sequences are useful in detecting subtle periventricular lesions (Figure 225-3). Periventricular edema usually is associated with acute hydrocephalus and increased intraventricular pressure, rather than chronic, relatively compensated hydrocephalus with normal intraventricular pressure.

It is critical to differentiate between hydrocephalus and ventricular enlargement secondary to brain atrophy. Atrophy is characterized by widening of the cerebral sulci and subarachnoid space. On the other hand, effacement of sulci, periventricular edema, and rounding of the frontal portion of the lateral ventricles and ventral displacement of the third ventricle suggest hydrocephalus with increased intraventricular pressure.

Analysis of CSF is helpful in cases of suspected meningoencephalitis. CT or MRI is performed first to identify any shifting of brain tissue, such as caudal cerebellar herniation, or other abnormalities that may increase the risk of CSF collection from the cerebellomedullary cistern. In some cases, it may be safer to collect CSF from an enlarged lateral ventricle through a persistent fontanelle.

Treatment

Medical Therapy

Medical therapy is used when surgery is not an option or is not indicated and for short-term management of acute deterioration. Several medications have been shown to decrease CSF production and may provide temporary relief of clinical signs. Acetazolamide (10 mg/kg q8h PO) is a carbonic anhydrase inhibitor that decreases CSF production. Furosemide (1 mg/kg q24h PO) inhibits CSF formation to a lesser degree by partial inhibition of carbonic anhydrase. The proton pump blocker omeprazole (0.5 mg/kg q24h PO) decreases CSF production in normal dogs (Javaheri et al, 1997). Glucocorticoids also are commonly used to treat hydrocephalus in veterinary patients. One protocol is prednisone given at a dosage of 0.25 to 0.5 mg/kg q12h PO until signs improve, followed by a dose reduction at weekly intervals until 0.1 mg/kg q48h PO is reached.

Removal of CSF sometimes is performed to provide temporary relief and to help predict which patients will benefit from surgical shunting. In pediatric patients with a fontanelle, an enlarged lateral ventricle can be punctured with a 25-gauge needle inserted at the lateral aspect of the fontanelle, with care taken to avoid the sagittal sinus on the midline. Ultrasonography is helpful in determining the depth of the center of the ventricle; optimally this procedure should be performed by a specialist with experience in the technique. Approximately 2 ml of CSF can be removed safely in most patients.

Ventriculoperitoneal Shunt

Definitive treatment is insertion of a shunt to divert CSF from the ventricular system to another body cavity, typically the peritoneal space. The presence of enlarged ventricles alone does not indicate the need for surgery. The key findings in recommending surgery are progressive neurologic deficits, progressive enlargement of the ventricles on repeated imaging, or image features indicating increased intraventricular pressure, such as periventricular edema.

A variety of shunt systems designed for human patients are available and have been used in dogs and cats. All of the shunt manufacturers make pediatric or low-profile versions designed for small infants, and these work well in small dogs and cats. Several trials in human pediatric patients failed to demonstrate any difference in outcome among various systems (Kestle et al, 2000; Pollack et al, 1999).

A shunt consists of three components: a ventricular catheter that is inserted into the ventricle, a valve, and a peritoneal catheter placed in the abdomen. Most valves are differential pressure valves that open when the pressure across the valve exceeds a certain threshold and close when the pressure drops below that level. The most common design is a diaphragm valve, in which a silicone membrane is deflected in response to pressure to allow the flow of CSF. Some shunts employ a slit valve consisting of one or more slits in the distal tubing that open and close at certain pressures. Valves are available in low-, medium-, and high-pressure versions, which roughly correlate with pressures of 5, 10, and 15 cm H_2O.

Several manufacturers provide externally adjustable valves that enable the clinician to regulate the opening pressure after the shunt is implanted using a device that emits a magnetic field. An advantage of this type of valve is that the function of the shunt can be adjusted noninvasively based on the individual patient's clinical response without the need for surgery to change the valve. Because these valves contain ferromagnetic material, they create an artifact on MRI scans. Another disadvantage is the additional cost of the shunt and the programming device compared with that of nonadjustable valves.

Surgical Technique

Surgical technique is similar for all ventriculoperitoneal shunts, although details vary slightly based on the specific system. Aseptic technique and meticulous hemostasis are critical to minimize the chance of shunt infection and obstruction. The site of the incision over the skull is determined using preoperative brain imaging so that the catheter tip is placed in the center of the occipital horn or frontal horn, caudal or rostral to the choroid plexus. The abdominal incision is located 2 to 3 cm caudal to the last rib, about halfway between the lumbar spine and the ventral aspect of the abdomen. The patient is measured to determine the proper shunt length so that approximately one third to one half the shunt is placed in the abdomen. The patient is clipped and prepared from the head to the side of the abdomen. The skin and subcutaneous tissues are incised over the skull and abdomen. A subcutaneous tunnel is created connecting the two incisions, and the catheter is pulled from the cranial incision through subcutaneous tissues to the abdominal incision. The ventricular catheter is placed into the ventricle through a burr hole in the skull and secured with sutures placed through one or two small holes in the bone. Securely anchoring the catheter to the skull is important to prevent dislodgement of the catheter. The abdominal muscles and peritoneum are incised to allow the distal end of the shunt to be placed into the peritoneal cavity. The shunt tubing is secured to the abdominal wall using nonabsorbable suture tied to an anchoring clip or tied in a finger-trap fashion to the tubing and the abdominal muscle is apposed with absorbable suture. The

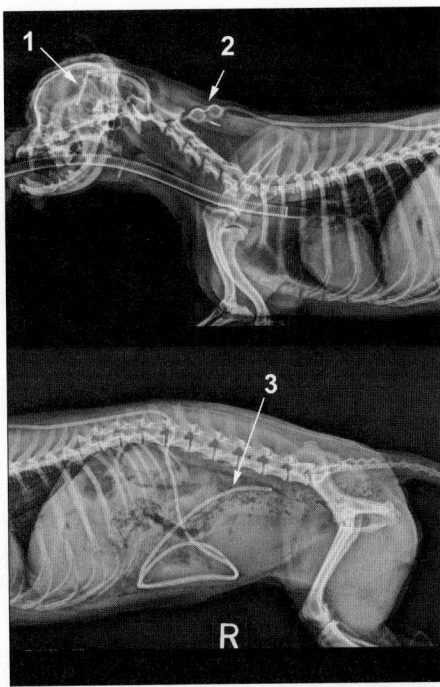

Figure 225-4 Radiographs after insertion of a ventriculoperitoneal shunt. 1, Ventricular catheter. 2, Valve. 3, Peritoneal catheter.

subcutaneous and skin incisions are closed routinely. A postoperative radiograph is obtained to document adequate shunt placement (Figure 225-4).

Complications

Ventriculoperitoneal shunting is prone to several complications. Most common is obstruction of flow through an intact shunt as a result of scarring or ingrowth of the choroid plexus at the ventricular catheter tip, valve occlusion by blood or proteinaceous debris, or scarring or adhesions around the peritoneal tubing. Lower-pressure valves are more prone to obstruction by proximal occlusion because they allow slightly more drainage of CSF and smaller ventricles (Robinson et al, 2002). Distal slit valves are more prone to obstruction with omentum or debris than are valve of other designs (Cozzens et al, 1997). Therefore the author generally uses medium- or high-pressure valves and avoids slit-valve designs. Obstruction can occur at any time after implantation and is accompanied by recurrence of signs of hydrocephalus. Shunt obstruction is suspected in any patient that initially improves after surgery and then develops lethargy, ataxia, or abnormal behavior. An imaging finding of ventricles that are larger than on a previous scan is a strong indication of obstruction.

Other postoperative complications are migration of an intact shunt, fracture or disconnection of shunt components, and infection. These adverse events usually require replacement of the shunt. Securely anchoring the shunt at the skull and the abdomen decreases the risk of migration. Infection is manifested as wound infection, fever, or obstruction. Cytologic analysis and culture of CSF collected percutaneously from the shunt reservoir is helpful in the diagnosis of shunt infection. The infection may resolve after 4 weeks of antibiotic therapy guided by culture and sensitivity testing; obstruction or persistent infection indicates the need to replace the shunt. Perioperative antibiotic administration and meticulous aseptic technique are important to decrease the risk of infection. Antibiotic-impregnated shunts are available and decrease the risk of infection in human patients, but veterinary trials are lacking.

Prognosis

Some patients can be managed successfully with medication, especially when the hydrocephalus is not progressive. But in many cases medical therapy provides only temporary benefit. Approximately 85% of dogs treated with shunting have long-term improvement. Fifteen percent of patients require shunt revision, usually due to shunt obstruction, fracture, or migration (de Stefani et al, 2011; Shihab et al, 2011).

References and Suggested Reading

Cozzens JW, Chandler JP: Increased risk of distal ventriculoperitoneal shunt obstruction associated with slit valves or distal slits in the peritoneal catheter, *J Neurosurg* 87:682, 1997.

De Stefani A et al: Surgical technique, postoperative complications and outcome in 14 dogs treated for hydrocephalus by ventriculoperitoneal shunting, *Vet Surg* 40:183, 2011.

Javaheri S et al: Different effects of omeprazole and Sch 28080 on canine cerebrospinal fluid production, *Brain Res* 754:321, 1997.

Kestle J et al: Long-term follow-up data from the Shunt Design Trial, *Pediatr Neurosurg* 33:230, 2000.

Klimo P Jr et al: Antibiotic-impregnated shunt systems versus standard shunt systems: a meta- and cost-savings analysis, *J Neurosurg Pediatr* 8:600, 2011.

Pollack IF, Albright AL, Adelson PD: A randomized, controlled study of a programmable shunt valve versus a conventional valve for patients with hydrocephalus. Hakim-Medos Investigator Group, *Neurosurgery* 45:1399, 1999.

Rekate HL: A contemporary definition and classification of hydrocephalus, *Semin Pediatr Neurol* 16:9, 2009.

Robinson S, Kaufman BA, Park TS: Outcome analysis of initial neonatal shunts: does the valve make a difference? *Pediatr Neurosurg* 37:287, 2002.

Shihab N et al: Treatment of hydrocephalus with ventriculoperitoneal shunting in twelve dogs, *Vet Surg* 40:477, 2011.

CHAPTER 226

Intracranial Arachnoid Cysts in Dogs

CURTIS W. DEWEY, *Ithaca, New York*

Intracranial arachnoid cyst (IAC), also termed *intraarachnoid cyst* and *quadrigeminal cyst,* is a developmental brain disorder in which cerebrospinal fluid (CSF) is believed to accumulate within a split of the arachnoid membrane during embryogenesis. The developing neural tube is surrounded by a loose layer of mesenchymal tissue called the *perimedullary mesh;* this tissue eventually becomes the pia and arachnoid layers of the meninges. In normal development, pulsatile CSF flow from the choroid plexuses is thought to divide the perimedullary mesh into pia and arachnoid layers, effectively creating the subarachnoid space. It is postulated that some aberration of CSF flow from the choroid plexuses during this stage of development forces a separation within the forming arachnoid layer that eventually leads to the creation of an IAC. The intraarachnoid location of IACs has been demonstrated via light and electron microscopy in people.

The mechanisms by which an IAC continues to expand with fluid are unknown, but several theories have been proposed. Fluid may be secreted by the arachnoid cells lining the cyst cavity. There is evidence that cells lining the IAC may have secretory capacity. There also may be fluid movement into the cyst via an osmotic pressure gradient. Considering that the fluid within the IAC is nearly identical to CSF, this latter theory is unlikely. In addition, there have been documented cases in people in which the IAC and the subarachnoid space communicate via small slits. These slits act as one-way valves, diverting CSF into the cyst during systole but preventing return to the subarachnoid space during diastole.

Although IAC has been reported to occur in several locations in humans, all reported canine cases have been in the caudal fossa. Because IAC typically is associated with the quadrigeminal cistern in dogs, these accumulations of fluid often are called *quadrigeminal cysts* in this species. Also termed *intracranial intraarachnoid cyst,* IAC accounts for 1% of all intracranial masses in people and has been sporadically reported in dogs. IAC often is an incidental finding in humans; it has been suggested recently that this also may be the case in dogs.

Clinical Findings

In the veterinary literature, there have been nine clinical reports of IAC in dogs, with a total of 53 cases described. The IAC was suspected to be an incidental finding in approximately one third to over one half of the reported cases. The likelihood of clinical signs probably relates to the extent to which the cyst compresses the occipital lobe. The vast majority of reported IAC cases in dogs have involved small breeds, with a predominance of brachycephalic dogs. The breeds and numbers reported to date include the Shih Tzu (12), Maltese (4), pug (4), cavalier King Charles spaniel (4), Yorkshire terrier (4), Lhasa apso (4), Chihuahua (3), Staffordshire bull terrier (3), bulldog (3), Pekingese (2), West Highland white terrier (2), and one each of bichon frise, Pomeranian, cairn terrier, Jack Russell terrier, terrier mix, beagle, miniature schnauzer, and German shorthaired pointer.

There is a wide range in age at the time of clinical presentation (2 months to 10 years), with an approximate average age of 4 years. The most common clinical signs are attributed to forebrain dysfunction (including seizure activity), central vestibular (cerebellovestibular) disease, or both. Dogs also may be brought in with a primary complaint of neck pain.

Diagnosis of IAC typically is made via computed tomography or (preferably) magnetic resonance imaging (Figure 226-1). IACs also can be visualized using ultrasound imaging (via the foramen magnum, a temporal window, or a persistent bregmatic fontanelle), especially in younger dogs. The characteristic appearance of IAC is that of a large, well-demarcated fluid-filled structure that is isointense with the CSF spaces and is located between the caudal cerebrum and rostral cerebellum. Because IAC may be an incidental finding, it is important to rule out concurrent inflammatory disease (i.e., by CSF examination). In the author's opinion, it is often difficult or impossible to discern whether IAC in the presence of another brain disorder is purely an incidental finding. Since the presence of a large fluid-filled structure within the cranial vault likely decreases intracranial compliance, some IACs may contribute to clinical signs rather than being simply an incidental finding. Because this disorder is believed to represent a developmental abnormality of the intracranial ventricular CSF system, it may occur concurrently with other fluid abnormalities (including congenital hydrocephalus). The cyst may or may not communicate with the remainder of the ventricular system. When one is faced with evidence of IAC and another disease (e.g., granulomatous meningoencephalitis) in the same patient, obtaining an optimal response to treatment may entail treating both conditions.

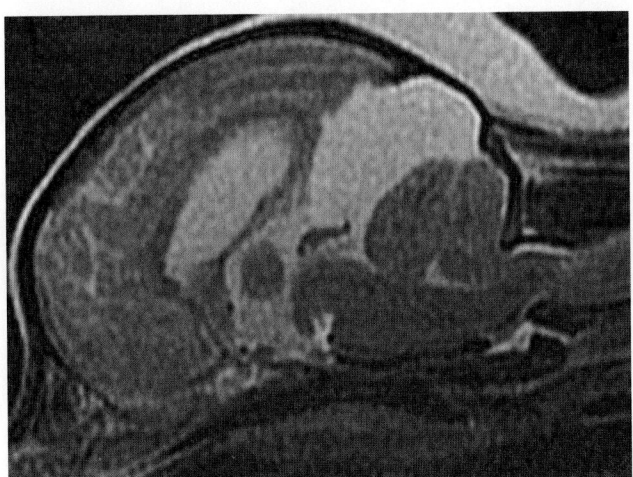

Figure 226-1 Sagittal T2-weighted brain image of a dog with a large intracranial arachnoid cyst.

Treatment

Medical treatment for IAC is identical to that described for congenital hydrocephalus; namely, corticosteroids, diuretics, and anticonvulsants if indicated. Dogs with IAC tend to respond initially to medical therapy, but the response often is temporary. Surgical management of IAC in people typically is achieved via either cyst fenestration or cystoperitoneal shunt placement. Both procedures have been reported in dogs with IAC.

Five cases have been reported in which IAC was considered the primary disease and was treated by fenestration. In three cases reimaging was performed after surgery; two of the three dogs had evidence of cyst persistence on magnetic resonance imaging. However, only one of these two dogs required reoperation. The author has reported successful cystoperitoneal shunting in four dogs with IAC. The success rate for surgical management of IAC appears to be high in humans and dogs, and whether fenestration or cystoperitoneal shunting is the preferred procedure remains controversial in both species.

References and Suggested Reading

Dewey CW et al: Craniotomy with cystoperitoneal shunting for treatment of intracranial arachnoid cysts in dogs, *Vet Surg* 36:416, 2007.

Dewey CW et al: Intracranial arachnoid cysts in dogs, *Compend Contin Educ Vet* 31(4):160, 2009.

Duque C et al: Intracranial arachnoid cysts: are they clinically significant? *J Vet Intern Med* 19:772, 2005.

Matiasek LA et al: Clinical and magnetic resonance imaging characteristics of quadrigeminal cysts in dogs, *J Vet Intern Med* 21:1021, 2007.

Vernau KM et al: Magnetic resonance imaging and computed tomography characteristics of intracranial arachnoid cysts in 6 dogs, *Vet Radiol Ultrasound* 38:171, 1997.

Vernau KM et al: Intracranial arachnoid cysts with intracystic hemorrhage in two dogs, *Vet Radiol Ultrasound* 43:449, 2002.

CHAPTER 227

Treatment of Intracranial Tumors

ERIN N. WARREN, *Knoxville, Tennessee*
JILL NARAK, *Knoxville, Tennessee*
TODD W. AXLUND, *Akron, Ohio*
ANNETTE N. SMITH, *Auburn, Alabama*

Intracranial tumors cause a devastating clinical picture, with signs that may include seizures, behavioral changes, proprioceptive deficits, altered mentation, vestibular disease, and other cranial nerve abnormalities. Clinical signs are caused in part by destruction of normal brain tissue by the neoplasm, but patients also deteriorate due to secondary lesions. These include peritumoral edema and hemorrhage that lead to increased intracranial pressure and potentially brain herniation.

Intracranial neoplasia affecting dogs and cats can arise from primary or secondary sources. Primary tumors originate from intracranial structures and include meningioma, glial tumors, neuroepithelial tumors, neural tumors, pituitary gland tumors, pineal gland tumors, and germ cell tumors. Secondary tumors arise from extracranial structures and include extension of nasal or skull tumors and metastatic neoplasia.

All intracranial tumors carry a poor prognosis; however, often it is difficult to discuss prognosis because treatment sometimes is initiated without a definitive diagnosis. Definitive treatment relies on an accurate histopathologic tumor diagnosis, although correlations between tumor appearance on magnetic resonance imaging (MRI) and histopathologic diagnoses have been reported (Kraft et al,

1997; Snyder et al, 2006). The patient's prognosis is related to tumor biologic behavior, as well as severity and progression of clinical signs. Without treatment intracranial tumors offer a grave prognosis.

Definitive Therapies

Definitive treatments include surgical excision, irradiation, and chemotherapy. These therapies aim to reduce or eradicate the tumor mass and decrease its secondary effects, such as peritumoral edema, hemorrhage, and intracranial hypertension.

Surgical Excision

Surgical Approaches and Considerations

Surgical removal of an intracranial tumor achieves many treatment goals. There is decompression and reduction of intracranial pressure. Moreover, a histopathologic diagnosis can be obtained, which allows for accurate prognostication and additional treatment planning in the case of subtotal resection. Surgical approaches include rostrotentorial, caudotentorial, transfrontal, and suboccipital craniotomies or craniectomies, and combinations of these approaches may be used. The tumor size, degree of invasiveness, and location determine whether or not surgical removal is a viable option; these also guide the neurosurgical approach. Intraaxial tumors, which are located within the brain parenchyma, are more difficult to remove than extraaxial tumors. In addition, approaches to the caudal fossa are difficult and seldom attempted because of the possibility of inducing iatrogenic trauma to the brainstem, which can result in severe clinical signs. However, one recent case report describes a novel basiooccipital surgical approach to relieve compression of the caudal brainstem and cranial cervical spinal cord caused by a meningioma in a canine patient (Barreau et al, 2010).

In most cases the goal of surgery is removal of the entire mass. Tumor removal can be achieved using a combination of sharp and blunt dissection, or an ultrasonic aspirator can be used. Adequate dissection can be difficult because many tumors are not well delineated from normal tissue, and adjacent normal brain tissue may be compromised because of peritumoral edema or hemorrhage. Endoscopy has been used to assist in removal of residual intracranial tumor after a debulking procedure (Klopp et al, 2009). This is particularly useful when removing a tumor from the olfactory and frontal regions of the brain as well as the cerebellum. In these procedures, an endoscope increases the visibility of regions that otherwise receive inadequate exposure in routine surgical approaches.

The dura mater must be incised or removed to obtain adequate visualization of the underlying brain structures. The defect can be closed using a graft (synthetic or fascial), or it may be left open. In dogs and cats cerebrospinal fluid (CSF) typically does not cause complications when leaked into the surrounding tissues (Niebauer et al, 1991). To protect the underlying brain, the skull defect generally is replaced when using a transfrontal or radical rostrotentorial approach; replacement is not necessary when other approaches are used.

To assess the completeness of resection, the neurosurgeon can check the gross surgical margins intraoperatively using a sterile ultrasonographic technique or after surgery using advanced brain imaging (most commonly computed tomography [CT] or MRI). However, in certain instances it may be difficult to distinguish between residual tumor and inflammation secondary to the surgical procedure itself via MRI. If it is indicated, the surgeon can reoperate immediately to remove more tumor tissue or address life-threatening postoperative hemorrhage or cerebral swelling. Microscopic surgical margins can be assessed intraoperatively by histopathologic analysis using cryosectioned biopsy samples.

A tissue diagnosis also may be obtained using the less-invasive CT- or MRI-guided biopsy; stereotactic or freehand image-guided biopsy may be performed. Both techniques may induce iatrogenic hemorrhage, and a craniotomy may have to be performed to manage hemostasis.

Anesthetic Considerations

Intracranial tumor patients typically are older animals, and concurrent disease may be present. Preanesthetic screening, including complete blood count (CBC), serum biochemistry profile, urinalysis, thoracic radiography, and abdominal ultrasonography, is indicated both to ensure the general health of the patient and to identify potential metastatic or other systemic disease, which could change the management approach.

In addition, these patients often have elevated intracranial pressure; thus the anesthetist should take measures to avoid or reduce intracranial hypertension, including maintaining normotension (systolic blood pressure of 110 to 160 mm Hg or mean arterial pressure of 80 to 110 mm Hg), eucarbia (35 to 45 mm Hg), and analgesia. Inhalant anesthetics increase cerebral blood flow (see Chapter 13), which can lead to or potentiate intracranial hypertension; injectable agents such as propofol and fentanyl can be used to decrease the requirement of inhalant anesthetics. Diuretics and glucocorticoids may be given to decrease brain edema (Table 227-1). Intracranial surgery can be associated with intraoperative hemorrhage; thus one should be prepared for a blood transfusion. After surgery the patient should be allowed to recover gradually from anesthesia. It is critically important to avoid excitement on recovery, and additional sedation may be required. Analgesia should be continued and titrated to the patient's needs.

Intraoperative and Postoperative Considerations

Intraoperative complications include hemorrhage, hypotension, intracranial hypertension, and air embolism. Postoperative infection may be of concern after transfrontal craniotomy because the approach involves incision through the contaminated frontal sinus. However, postoperative infection is not a typical complication after intracranial surgery, possibly because of the routine use of perioperative antibiotics (see Table 227-1). Intracranial hypertension is a concern following surgery, and patient positioning can aid in maintaining intracranial pressure within the normal range. Intracranial pressure can be measured directly, or it can be monitored indirectly by

TABLE 227-1

Medications Used in the Treatment of Intracranial Tumors

Drug	Dosage	Use/Indication
Carmustine	50 mg/ml q6wk IV (over 15-20 min)	Nitrosourea chemotherapeutic agent; may be used to treat meningioma and glioma
Cefazolin	22 mg/kg q90min IV	Perioperative antibiotic
Cytarabine (cytosine arabinoside)	20-100 mg/m^2 q1wk intrathecally; 50 mg/m^2 SC for 2 days. Repeat every 3 weeks	Chemotherapeutic agent used to treat CNS lymphoma
Diazepam and midazolam	0.5 mg/kg as needed IV; or 2 mg/kg as needed per rectum	Anticonvulsant used in emergency management of status epilepticus or cluster seizures
Dimenhydrinate	Dog: 25-50 mg q8-24h PO Cat: 12.5 mg q8-24h PO	Antihistamine used as antiemetic in vestibular disease
Hydroxyurea	Dog: 50 mg/kg once daily, 3 days per week PO Cat: 25 mg/kg once daily, 3 days per week PO	Chemotherapeutic agent; may be used to treat meningioma
Levetiracetam	20 mg/kg q8h PO 20-60 mg/kg IV for status epilepticus	Anticonvulsant
Lomustine	Dog: 60-90 mg/m^2 q3-6wk PO Cat: 50-60 mg/m^2 q6wk PO	Nitrosourea chemotherapeutic agent; may be used to treat meningioma and glioma
Mannitol	0.5-1 g/kg q4h or as needed IV	Osmotic diuretic used to decrease brain edema and lower intracranial pressure
Meclizine	25 mg/dog and 12.5 mg/cat q24h PO	Antihistamine used as antiemetic in vestibular disease
Methylprednisolone sodium succinate	30 mg/kg once IV; or 100 mg/kg given over 24 hr IV	Glucocorticoid used to decrease peritumoral brain edema and lower intracranial pressure
7.5% NaCl	5-20 ml/kg as needed IV	Osmotic diuretic used to decrease brain edema and lower intracranial pressure
Phenobarbital	Loading dosage: 5 mg/kg as needed IV (up to 20 mg/kg total) Maintenance dosage: 2-8 mg/kg q12h PO (Adjust dose by monitoring blood concentrations)	Anticonvulsant
Potassium bromide	Loading dosage: 200 mg/kg per day every 3-5 days Maintenance dosage: 30-40 mg/kg q24h PO	Anticonvulsant
Prednisone	0.5-1 mg/kg q12h PO	Glucocorticoid used for supportive treatment of intracranial tumors
Zonisamide	10 mg/kg q12h PO	Anticonvulsant

CNS, Central nervous system; IV, intravenously; PO, orally.

observing for changes associated with intracranial hypertension, including Cushing's response (systemic hypertension with reflex bradycardia) and changes in pupil size and symmetry. The patient's head should be elevated (approximately 30 degrees), jugular occlusion should be avoided (e.g., no jugular venipuncture or neck leads), and pain and excitement should be prevented. If necessary, diuretics with or without glucocorticoids can be continued in the postoperative period. If the patient is recumbent, urinary catheterization may be necessary. Care should be taken to keep the patient clean and dry, and appropriate bedding with frequent rotation or placement in a sling to prevent the formation of decubital ulcers is required. To avoid aspiration pneumonia the patient should be given nothing by mouth for 24 hours postoperatively. Nutritional and intravenous fluid support is indicated in a patient who cannot maintain adequate nutrition orally.

Meningioma

Meningiomas usually are easily accessible to the neurosurgeon since they are often extraaxial masses. However, meningiomas located along the brainstem and those located on the falx cerebri, tentorium cerebelli, or along the lateral ventricles may be more difficult to access.

Surgical removal of feline meningiomas may be curative since the entire mass often can be removed in total. Accordingly, surgical excision is the treatment of choice for feline meningiomas. Troxel and associates (2003) reported that cats treated by surgical removal of meningiomas had a significantly longer survival time than cats treated by any other modality (Table 227-2). Niebauer and colleagues (1991) reported that 50% of cats were alive 2 years after surgery.

Canine meningiomas are more difficult to remove totally. Histologically these tumors tend to be more aggressive and invasive in dogs than in cats. Thus surgical

TABLE 227-2

Comparison of Median Survival Times in Dogs and Cats with Intracranial Tumors Treated with Surgical Excision and/or Irradiation

Study	Tumor Type	Number of Patients	Treatment	Results/Median Survival Time (Days)
Troxel et al	Meningioma	34 cats	Surgical excision	685
Greco et al	Meningioma	17 dogs	Surgical excision	1254
Axlund et al	Meningioma	14 dogs	Surgical excision	210
	Meningioma	12 dogs	Surgical excision followed by irradiation	495
Brearley et al	Extraaxial tumor	41 dogs	Irradiation	347
	Intraaxial tumor	34 dogs	Irradiation	282
	Pituitary tumor	8 dogs	Irradiation	147
Turrel et al	Meningioma	2 dogs	Irradiation	322
	Undifferentiated sarcoma	1 dog		
	Astrocytoma	1 dog		
Heidner et al	Meningioma	9 dogs	Irradiation (some dogs + hyperthermia, some dogs + surgery)	137
	Other tumor types	8 dogs		
	Unknown tumor types	8 dogs		
Evans et al	Meningioma	4 dogs	Irradiation	9 dogs (39 Gy): 1545
	Lymphoma	1 dog		dogs (45 Gy): 519
	Pituitary adenoma	1 dog		
	Metastatic anaplastic carcinoma	1 dog		
	Oligodendroglioma	1 dog		
	Granulomatous meningoencephalitis	1 dog		
	Unknown tumor type	5 dogs		
Iwamoto et al	Meningioma	18 dogs	Irradiation	Clinical improvement and decrease in tumor size
	Glioma	6 dogs		
	Pituitary tumor (presumed)	1 dog		
LaRue et al	Unknown tumor type	65 dogs	Irradiation (some dogs + surgery)	405
Spugnini et al	Meningioma	21 dogs	Irradiation	250
	Glioma	4 dogs		
	Choroid plexus tumor	3 dogs		
Kent et al	Pituitary tumor	19 dogs	Irradiation	1405
Mayer et al	Pituitary tumor	8 cats	Irradiation	522
Bley et al	Extraaxial tumor	22 dogs	Irradiation	1174
	Intraaxial tumor	13 dogs		
	Pituitary	13 dogs		

removal often leaves behind microscopic disease, and further treatment with follow-up radiation therapy or chemotherapy is necessary. Greco and colleagues (2006) reported that histopathologic tumor subtype influenced prognosis: transitional and meningothelial meningiomas were associated with higher median survival times than fibroblastic, anaplastic, and psammomatous meningiomas. Théon and associates (2000) found that a high tumor proliferative index, noted on immunohistochemical analysis of histologic tumor sections, was a significant prognostic indicator for tumor progression in dogs with meningioma.

Glioma

Surgical removal of gliomas can be helpful for debulking and histopathologic confirmation of the diagnosis of glioma. However, gliomas are invasive tumors, and it is difficult to obtain clean margins. These tumors typically are highly vascular, and because of their deep location, surgical resection may damage normal brain parenchyma. Tumor location also may make visualization difficult during surgery. Intraoperative ultrasonography may help to delineate tumor margins. For these reasons surgical removal of gliomas usually is followed by radiation therapy.

Other Neoplasms

Pituitary microadenomas may be amenable to surgical removal, but macroadenomas typically are too large for excision. Radiation therapy is the treatment of choice for those tumors, although the prognosis is worse if neurologic signs are present. The ratio of pituitary height to brain area is used to discriminate between pituitary microadenoma and macroadenoma and to determine the feasibility of surgical removal. Traditionally a macroadenoma may be defined as a pituitary gland that is greater than 1 cm in height, although Meij and associates (1998) describe that in veterinary medicine a pituitary tumor is classified as a macroadenoma when the ratio of pituitary height to brain area is more than 0.31. Techniques described for pituitary microadenoma removal include use of the transsphenoidal and transcranial approaches.

Neuroepithelial tumors such as choroid plexus papillomas and ependymomas may be removed surgically; however, they often are situated in difficult locations within the ventricular system. As a result, obstructive hydrocephalus may occur and exacerbate clinical signs. To relieve hydrocephalus, a viable palliative option is the placement of a ventriculoperitoneal shunt. This procedure may be combined with tumor removal in selected cases.

Radiation Therapy

Radiation therapy may be used as adjunct treatment to surgical excision. In fact, it may be most effective when combined with surgical tumor removal (Table 227-3). Radiation therapy also can be used as sole therapy for intracranial tumors. Because of the potential morbidity associated with surgical removal of brainstem masses, the use of radiation as sole therapy is the treatment of choice for tumors in those locations. The use of radiation as sole

therapy is justified if a qualified surgeon is not available; however, radiation therapy typically requires referral to a specialty center. Megavoltage radiation is recommended, but orthovoltage also has been used. Radiation oncologists base treatment planning on the known or suspected tumor type and location, keeping in mind the acute and late adverse effects that may be induced by radiation therapy.

The goal of radiation therapy is to deliver a tumoricidal dose of radiation while sparing normal brain tissue. High doses of radiation improve control of brain tumors but put the patient at risk of radiation-induced brain necrosis; thus the risk:benefit ratio needs to be considered for each patient. Radiation-induced brain damage is the result of focal necrosis and local hemorrhage. Fractionation is a strategy used to avoid radiation-induced brain necrosis. This approach relies on the ability of normal tissue to repair itself between doses of radiation. Tumor cells have lost this ability for repair; thus the radiation doses are lethal to the tumor mass. Typical fractionation schedules call for three to five anesthetic episodes per week, which can be stressful to the typical geriatric brain tumor patient. Ideally, to avoid radiation-induced brain necrosis, treatments are delivered in fractions of less than 300 cGy to reach a total dose of 45 to 50 Gy.

Therapy may fail as a result of tumor recurrence or radiation-induced brain necrosis. Advanced imaging cannot distinguish between these processes, and both

---

TABLE **227-3**

Comparison of Treatment Results in Dogs with Intracranial Tumors Treated Using Various Chemotherapy Protocols

Study	Protocol	Tumor Type	Number of Patients	Survival Time
Couto et al	Cyclophosphamide, vincristine, cytosine arabinoside, prednisone, chlorambucil	CNS lymphoma	2 dogs	1 dog: 63 days 1 dog: complete remission after 90 days
Cook et al	BCNU 50 mg/m² IV q4-6wk	Glioma	3 dogs	9-11 mo
		1 benign vascular tumor and 1 unidentified tumor	2 dogs	>12 mo
		Meningioma	Unknown	4-6 mo
		Pituitary tumor	Unknown	Little to no response
Dimski et al	BCNU 50 mg/m² IV q6wk + Phenobarbital + Oxacillin + Prednisone	Astrocytoma	1 dog	7 mo
Jeffery et al	CCNU 60-80 mg/m² PO q4wk	Glioblastoma multiforme	1 dog	4 mo
		Meningioma	1 dog	11 mo
Tamura et al	Hydroxyurea 30 mg/kg 3 times per wk PO × 5 mo then increased to 45 mg/kg 3 times per wk × 2 mo then discontinued + Dexamethasone	Meningioma	1 dog	14 mo
Jung et al	Lomustine 60 mg/m² PO × q6wk + Prednisone 1 mg/kg BID PO	Meningioma	1 dog	13 mo

Adapted from Van Meervenne SAE et al: Therapy of brain tumors in dogs and cats, *Vlaams Diergen Tijds* 76:165, 2007.
BCNU, Carmustine; *BID,* twice daily; *CCNU,* lomustine; *CNS,* central nervous system; *IV,* intravenously; *PO,* orally.

conditions present with similar clinical signs. It can be difficult to know if a patient is deteriorating as a result of tumor progression or brain necrosis. A severe and rapid neurologic decline may be the result of radiation-induced brain necrosis, whereas a slowly progressive decline in neurologic status may represent tumor regrowth (Brearley et al, 1999). Ultimately, this differentiation can be made only at postmortem examination. Brain is a late-responding tissue; thus these radiation adverse effects may not be noted until months to years after treatment, and Spugnini and associates (2000) reported that only 5% to 20% of veterinary patients with brain tumors survive to be at risk of these effects. Another late adverse effect to consider is new tumor growth induced by radiation, as noted in one report by Théon and colleagues (2000).

Acute adverse effects of radiation therapy in the brain can be seen weeks to months after therapy and include transient demyelination, which usually responds to anti-inflammatory dosages of corticosteroids (see Table 227-1). Other acute adverse effects of radiation therapy depend on the normal tissues included in the treatment portal. These may include keratoconjunctivitis, corneal ulcers, mucositis, otitis externa, and dermatitis. Although these effects are not life threatening, they may cause debilitation in the short or long term and require management.

Stereotactic radiosurgery is a technique that allows for the precise delivery of radiation to the tumor while sparing adjacent normal brain tissue. Fewer anesthetic episodes are required because a sufficient dose of radiation is delivered to the tumor at once or over a few treatment sessions, whereas only a fraction is delivered to normal brain tissue. This technique can be used to treat tumors of relatively small diameter and requires referral to an adequately equipped specialty center. Other techniques such as boron neutron capture therapy and brachytherapy have been attempted to deliver a precise dose of radiation to the tumor tissue.

Chemotherapy

Chemotherapy has been largely ineffective in the treatment of brain tumors, but certain therapeutic agents deserve consideration (see Table 227-3). The blood-brain barrier is impermeable to large hydrophilic compounds. Consequently most drugs are unable to penetrate the blood-brain barrier and exert tumoricidal effects. However, in the face of significant lesions, the blood-brain barrier may not be completely impenetrable, and some drugs may gain limited access to the tumor.

Agents that increase the permeability of the blood-brain barrier (e.g., mannitol) may be given to enhance the effectiveness of a chemotherapeutic agent; however, this technique may increase the toxic effects of the drug, so the approach generally is not advised. To achieve maximum delivery into the central nervous system (CNS), agents can be injected directly into the subarachnoid space (intrathecal injection). Alternatively, intratumoral injections of chemotherapeutic agents have been used in humans and may deliver a precise dose of the drug directly into the tumor; however, this technique is limited by the invasiveness of the procedure.

Certain tumors are considered to be relatively chemo-responsive, including CNS lymphoma, medulloblastoma, and oligodendroglioma, but chemotherapy may be considered for any patient with an intracranial tumor. In particular, lymphoma of the CNS is considered a nonsurgical disease and is treated with systemic and sometimes intrathecal chemotherapy. Chemotherapy is also used to treat metastatic brain neoplasia; the protocol used depends on the primary tumor. Surgical debulking and radiation therapy may not be advised for metastatic brain neoplasia because of the poor prognosis; however, these modalities can be offered as palliative therapy. Standard protocols for chemotherapy for the treatment of intracranial tumors have not yet been developed, but certain chemotherapeutic agents are discussed here.

Nitrosoureas
Nitrosoureas are highly lipophilic and obtain rapid passage across the blood-brain barrier. Lomustine (CeeNU) and carmustine (BiCNU) are used as adjunct therapy for brain tumors (see Table 227-1). These agents have been used to treat glioma and meningioma with varying degrees of success. Adverse effects of the nitrosoureas include myelosuppression; thus CBCs should be monitored weekly, beginning after the first week of treatment. Maximum myelosuppression may not occur until 4 to 6 weeks after treatment, and the effects (neutropenia and thrombocytopenia) may be cumulative. If the patient becomes neutropenic with a count of less than 1000×10^3 neutrophils/μl but otherwise appears to be healthy, administration of broad-spectrum oral antibiotics may be advised; if the patient is neutropenic with less than 1000×10^3 neutrophils/μl and displays signs of sepsis or systemic illness (lethargy, vomiting, diarrhea, or fever), the patient should be hospitalized and given broad-spectrum intravenous antibiotics with monitoring for progression of sepsis. Lomustine also can cause hepatotoxicity and nephrotoxicity; thus it is important to monitor the results of serial serum biochemical tests. Prophylactic administration of Denamarin (S-adenosylmethionine and silybin) has been used to prevent liver toxicity (Skorupski et al, 2011). If evidence of toxicity is present, hepatic and renal function tests and/or abdominal ultrasonography should be performed.

Hydroxyurea
Hydroxyurea is a chemotherapeutic agent that also crosses the blood-brain barrier and may be useful in the treatment of intracranial tumors (see Table 227-1). Hydroxyurea has shown promise in treating humans with unresectable or recurrent meningioma, but there is no evidence demonstrating its efficacy in dogs or cats. The most serious adverse effect of hydroxyurea is myelosuppression; serial CBCs should be monitored.

Cytarabine
Intrathecal delivery of cytarabine (cytosine arabinoside, Cytosar) has been used in the treatment of CNS lymphoma when malignant cells are found in the CSF. Cytosine arabinoside may be delivered intrathecally (see Table 227-1). The chemotherapy is continued until 1 week beyond a finding of no atypical lymphocytes on CSF tap; three to six

treatments usually are necessary. Intrathecal delivery of chemotherapy requires general anesthesia and the technical expertise to perform a CSF tap. Systemic chemotherapy is recommended in conjunction with intrathecal chemotherapy. An oncologist or neurologist should be consulted regarding protocols. Response to treatment usually occurs in weeks to months.

Other Chemotherapeutic Drugs

The combination of procarbazine, lomustine, and vincristine has been used to treat certain types of human glioma. Temozolomide is an alkylating agent that also has been used with varying success in humans with glioma. Methotrexate has been used intrathecally to treat humans with CNS lymphoma. Studies are needed in veterinary medicine to address the efficacy and safety of these drugs.

Supportive Therapies

Supportive therapy is aimed at seizure control and reduction in intracranial pressure and is often instituted regardless of whether or not definitive treatments are undertaken. When used in combination with definitive therapy such as surgery or radiation, these treatments aid in reducing the patient's clinical signs in the short term during the wait for definitive treatments to take effect. Supportive therapies can be used as the sole means of treatment, but owners should be made aware that the patient's prognosis is poor; these therapies treat only the symptoms of the intracranial tumor and do not affect the tumor itself. The usefulness of supportive therapies as the sole means of treatment is short-lived because eventually the tumor mass enlarges and exacerbates the patient's clinical signs. However, supportive care can extend a patient's life in the short term and temporarily alleviate clinical signs associated with the intracranial tumor.

Treatment of Acute Intracranial Hypertension

Intracranial hypertension can develop because of the presence of the brain tumor or because of secondary complications such as edema and hemorrhage. Left untreated, intracranial hypertension can cause brain herniation and death. Intravenous fluid support is implemented to maintain normotension and support blood flow to the brain since cerebral perfusion pressure relies on adequate mean arterial blood pressure. Methylprednisolone sodium succinate (Solu-Medrol) is a glucocorticoid effective in decreasing peritumoral edema (see Table 227-1). Diuretics also may be given to decrease brain edema. Mannitol and hypertonic saline are osmotic diuretics effective in decreasing intracranial pressure (see Table 227-1). It is important to monitor the patient's hydration status when using diuretics since therapy can lead to hypovolemia and hypotension, which can exacerbate cerebral ischemia caused by hypoxia.

Anticonvulsants

Phenobarbital and potassium bromide are the typical first-line anticonvulsants used in veterinary patients, but recently other drugs such as levetiracetam and zonisamide have become popular (see Table 227-1). Serum phenobarbital concentrations should be measured 2 weeks after maintenance therapy is initiated; the therapeutic range is 15 to 45 μg/ml when phenobarbital is used as monotherapy. High levels of phenobarbital may be associated with hepatotoxicity. Increased alkaline phosphatase levels may be noted in the serum biochemistry profile, although this is associated with hepatic enzyme induction rather than hepatotoxicity. Bone marrow hypoplasia is an uncommon adverse effect of phenobarbital therapy. Additional adverse effects are polydipsia and polyuria, polyphagia, sedation, ataxia, and paraparesis. These adverse effects often resolve within 1 to 2 weeks of therapy initiation. In patients receiving phenobarbital, serial serum biochemistry profiles should be measured and serum phenobarbital concentration should be monitored regularly to aid in dose adjustments if needed.

Potassium bromide may be used as monotherapy to suppress seizures or it may be added to phenobarbital therapy in refractory cases. Because it takes a long time to reach steady state, patients usually are given a loading dose for 5 days, followed by a maintenance dosage. Serum concentrations of potassium bromide should be measured in 3 weeks, and the dosage adjusted accordingly. Adverse effects of potassium bromide are similar to those of phenobarbital. Potassium bromide is not known to cause hepatotoxicity, although it may be associated with pancreatitis. Potassium bromide is not recommended for use in cats because it has been linked with the development of inflammatory pneumonitis. It is important to keep the salt content of the patient's diet consistent during bromide therapy since increased dietary chloride can reduce the serum levels of bromide and affect seizure control.

The appearance of cluster seizures or status epilepticus is an emergency, and treatment includes the administration of diazepam (Valium) or midazolam (Versed). Phenobarbital may be given as a loading dose (see Table 227-1). If these anticonvulsants cannot control the patient's seizures, anesthetics such as pentobarbital, propofol, and inhalant anesthetics should be considered, with recognition that the patient may require ventilatory support.

Corticosteroids

Glucocorticoids may be given to reduce peritumoral edema and decrease CSF production. An antiinflammatory dosage of prednisone is recommended (see Table 227-1). This dosage can be adjusted based on the patient's response to therapy.

Antihistamines

Meclizine and dimenhydrinate are antihistamines with antiemetic effects that are useful to alleviate nausea in patients with vestibular disease (see Table 227-1).

Emerging Therapies

Emerging molecular therapies such as immunotherapy, gene therapy, and oncolytic viral therapy have been used with varying success in humans, and these approaches represent future directions for research in veterinary patients. Both gene therapy and vaccination have been tested for treatment of malignant gliomas in dogs and have shown promising results as an adjunctive therapy to surgery or radiation. Gene therapy is the insertion, alteration, or deletion of genes within an individual's cells to treat disease. Vaccination, on the other hand, is the administration of antigenic material to stimulate the immune system of an individual to develop adaptive immunity to a disease. One recent study (Xiong et al, 2010) demonstrated the usefulness of an adenoviral vector for delivery of genes encoding an immunostimulatory cytokine (human soluble fms-like tyrosine kinase 3 ligand, or hsFlt3L) to leukocytes in a peripheral canine blood culture. The study showed that this therapy triggers an antitumor immune response which leads to increased production of antigen-presenting cells (dendritic cells) demonstrating antitumor activity (phagocytic activity, increased secretion of antitumor cytokines).

Vaccination against tumor cells also has been used in conjunction with gene therapy and surgery to improve outcomes in dogs with malignant gliomas. In one canine case study (Pluhar et al, 2010), a dog with spontaneous glioma was treated using a combination of surgery, gene transfer, and vaccination. In this study, an adenovirus vector was used to deliver the gene for intratumoral interferon-γ into the brain resection cavity following debulking surgery for the glioma. Interferon-γ has been shown to increase recruitment of lymphocytes to brain tumor sites in murine models but has extended survival times only modestly when used as a single agent. The vaccine used in this study consisted of a glioma cell lysate with a potent vaccine adjuvant that promotes signaling through toll-like receptor 9 in dendritic cells and B cells to induce an adaptive, antitumor immune response. The adjunctive use of these treatment modalities resulted in complete resolution of clinical signs in the dog and tumor-free survival for at least 450 days following surgery.

Nonthermal irreversible electroporation (N-TIRE) is a promising new modality for treatment of intracranial tumors. N-TIRE is a novel, minimally invasive technique that involves placing electrodes in or around a targeted area and delivering a series of short, intense electrical pulses that destabilizes the cellular membranes within tissues and leads to increased membrane permeability. This increased membrane permeability ultimately leads to cell death due to loss of cell homeostasis and thus ablation of tumor cells within the treated area. One advantage of N-TIRE over other focal ablation techniques is that the electrical pulses do not cause the thermal damage associated with resistive heating; therefore major blood vessels, extracellular matrix, and other surrounding tissue structures are spared.

References and Suggested Reading

Axlund TW, McGlasson ML, Smith AN: Surgery alone or in combination with radiation therapy for treatment of intracranial meningiomas in dogs: 31 cases (1989-2002), *J Am Vet Med Assoc* 221:1597, 2002.

Barreau P et al: Canine meningioma: a case report of a rare subtype and novel atlanto basioccipital surgical approach, *Vet Comp Orthop Traumatol* 23(5):372, 2010.

Bley CR et al: Irradiation of brain tumors in dogs with neurologic disease, *J Vet Intern Med* 19(6):849, 2005.

Brearley MJ et al: Hypofractionated radiation therapy of brain masses in dogs: a retrospective analysis of survival of 83 cases (1991-1996), *J Vet Intern Med* 13:408, 1999.

Couto CG et al: Central nervous system lymphosarcoma in the dog, *J Am Vet Med Assoc* 184(7):809, 1984.

Dimski DS et al: Carmustine-induced partial remission of an astrocytoma in a dog, *J Am Anim Hosp Assoc* 26:179, 1990.

Evans SM et al: Radiation therapy of canine brain masses, *J Vet Intern Med* 7(4):216, 1993.

Greco JJ et al: Evaluation of intracranial meningioma resection with a surgical aspirator in dogs: 17 cases (1996-2004), *J Am Vet Med Assoc* 229:394, 2006.

Heidner GL et al: Analysis of survival in a retrospective study of 86 dogs with brain tumors, *J Vet Intern Med* 5(4):219, 1991.

Iwamoto KS et al: Diagnosis and treatment of spontaneous canine brain tumors with a CT scanner, *Radiother Oncol* 26(1):76, 1993.

Jeffery N et al: Brain tumours in the dog: treatment of 10 cases and review of recent literature, *J Small Anim Pract* 34:367, 1993.

Jung DI et al: Long-term chemotherapy with lomustine of intracranial meningioma occurring in a miniature schnauzer, *J Vet Med Sci* 68(4):383, 2006.

Kent MS et al: Survival, neurologic response, and prognostic factors in dogs with pituitary masses treated with radiation therapy and untreated dogs, *J Vet Intern Med* 21(5):1027, 2007.

Klopp LS, Ridgway M: Use of an endoscope in minimally invasive lesion biopsy and removal within the skull and cranial vault in two dogs and one cat, *J Am Vet Med Assoc* 234(12):1573, 2009.

Kraft SL et al: Retrospective review of 50 canine intracranial tumors evaluated by magnetic resonance imaging, *J Vet Intern Med* 11:218, 1997.

LaRue SM et al: Recent advances in radiation oncology, *Comp Contin Educ Pract* 16:795, 1993.

Mayer MN et al: Outcomes of pituitary tumor irradiation in cats, *J Vet Intern Med* 20(5):1151, 2006.

Meij BP et al: Results of transsphenoidal hypophysectomy in 52 dogs with pituitary-dependent hyperadrenocorticism, *Vet Surg* 27:246, 1998.

Nakaichi M et al: Primary brain tumors in two dogs treated by surgical resection in combination with postoperative radiation therapy, *J Vet Med Sci* 58(8):773, 1996.

Niebauer GW, Dayrell-Hart BL, Speciale J: Evaluation of craniotomy in dogs and cats, *J Am Vet Med Assoc* 198:89, 1991.

Pluhar GE et al: Anti-tumor immune response correlates with neurological symptoms in a dog with spontaneous astrocytoma treated by gene and vaccine therapy, *Vaccine* 28(19):3371, 2010.

Skorupski KA et al: Prospective randomized clinical trial assessing the efficacy of Denamarin for prevention of CCNU-induced hepatopathy in tumor-bearing dogs, *J Vet Intern Med* 25:838, 2011.

Snyder JM et al: Canine intracranial primary neoplasia: 173 cases (1986-2003), *J Vet Intern Med* 20:669, 2006.

Spugnini EP et al: Primary irradiation of canine intracranial masses, *Vet Radiol Ultrasound* 41:377, 2000.

Tamura S et al: A canine case of skull base meningioma treated with hydroxyurea, *J Vet Med Sci* 69(12):1313, 2007.

Théon AP et al: Influence of tumor cell proliferation and sex-hormone receptors on effectiveness of radiation therapy for dogs with incompletely resected meningiomas, *J Am Vet Med Assoc* 216:701, 2000.

Troxel MT et al: Feline intracranial neoplasia: retrospective review of 160 cases (1985-2001), *J Vet Intern Med* 17:850, 2003.

Turrel JM et al: Radiotherapy of brain tumors in dogs, *J Am Vet Med Assoc* 184(1):82, 1984.

Van Meervenne SAE et al: Therapy of brain tumors in dogs and cats, *Vlaams Diergen Tijds* 76:165, 2007.

Xiong W et al: Human Flt3L generates dendritic cells from canine peripheral blood precursors: implications for a dog glioma clinical trial, *PLoS One* 5(6):e11074, 2010.

CHAPTER 228

Metabolic Brain Disorders

CRISTIAN FALZONE, *Zugliano, Italy*

Metabolic disorders affecting the brain are relatively common, and clinical signs can range from subtle to severe. This chapter considers selected primary disorders of the brain associated with disturbances of energy metabolism including mitochondrial encephalopathies, inborn errors of metabolism, and methylmalonic aciduria and malonic aciduria.

Energy Metabolism in the Brain

Although the brain represents only 2% of the body weight, it performs many vital functions, even during sleep. Constant high energy production is needed, and any metabolic disorder potentially can have dramatic effects on brain function. Almost all the energy produced and used by the brain is derived from the metabolism of glucose, which is mostly oxidized to CO_2 and H_2O, with concurrent production of high-energy compounds (see later). Approximately 25% of total body glucose and 20% of total body oxygen consumption (at rest) occurs in the brain. Because glucose is produced or stored only minimally in the brain, the majority must be delivered via the arterial blood flow, with the brain receiving about 15% of the cardiac output. Brain energy metabolism therefore represents an equilibrium between blood flow, glucose utilization, and oxygen consumption.

Cerebral blood flow (CBF), glucose metabolism, and oxygen consumption are closely related. CBF is influenced and regulated by a number of factors, including arterial blood pressure, intracranial pressure, venous outflow, blood viscosity, arterial partial pressures of carbon dioxide ($PaCO_2$) and oxygen (PaO_2), collateral flow, vasoreactivity and the status of cerebral autoregulation. Chemical mediators such as K^+, Ca^{2+}, H^+, and adenosine also may play a role in regulation of CBF. However, cerebral metabolism is the major determinant of regional blood flow. The distribution of capillaries is organized functionally throughout the central nervous system (CNS); hence capillary density may provide an anatomic indicator of oxidative and glucose metabolism. Areas with the greatest capillary density are most commonly located in the gray matter, but regional heterogeneity can be identified. CBF increases with increased neuronal activity. Hemodynamically, CBF is determined by the ratio of cerebral perfusion pressure to cerebral vascular resistance, where cerebral perfusion pressure is the difference between mean arterial blood pressure (MABP) and intracranial pressure (ICP).

High-energy phosphates, predominantly adenosine triphosphate (ATP), are the most important energy source for the brain. ATP is produced almost entirely by oxidative metabolism of glucose. Glucose is derived from the diet and is transported into the brain by transmembrane proteins known as *glucose transporters*. There glucose undergoes metabolic degradation via glycolysis or the Krebs cycle (tricarboxylic acid cycle); these processes generate 2 and 36 molecules of ATP, respectively. Glycolysis also leads to the production of pyruvate, which can follow three different pathways: (1) it can be metabolized to ethanol (alcoholic fermentation); (2) it can be reduced to lactate (lactic fermentation); or (3) it can be transferred to the mitochondria, where it is used in the tricarboxylic acid cycle. Most of the energy obtained from the tricarboxylic acid cycle is captured by the oxidized form of nicotinamide adenine dinucleotide and flavin adenine dinucleotide, and later converted to ATP via an electron transport chain in mitochondria, known as *oxidative phosphorylation*.

Most of the ATP (~65%) is used to maintain energy-dependent ion transport—in particular, the Na^+,K^+-ATPase pump—which represents the main energy-consuming process in neural cells. The remaining energy is used for axonal transport and for the synthesis of neurotransmitters, proteins, lipids, and glycogen. Despite that only small quantities of neurotransmitters are stored in the brain, neurotransmitter synthesis actually can account for about 5% of the energy consumption, and it takes place almost entirely in the glial cells. Although brain energy metabolism often is considered to reflect predominantly neuronal energy metabolism, it is now clear that other cell types—namely, neuroglial and vascular endothelial cells—not only consume energy but also can play an active role in the flux of energy substrates to neurons. Glial cells, which make up almost 50% of the brain volume, have a much lower metabolic rate than neurons and account for less than 10% of total cerebral metabolism. Among the glial cells, astrocytes seem mainly to contribute to brain energy metabolism. Moreover, other energy substrates such as lactate and pyruvate can be released by astrocytes, and they can potentially be used to a lesser degree to support the metabolism of neurons.

Brain function and tissue integrity also are highly dependent on a continuous supply of oxygen. Changes in local brain energy metabolism now can be studied in humans using functional magnetic resonance imaging (MRI) and positron emission tomography (PET). These studies can monitor alterations in the relationships between blood flow, glucose utilization, and oxygen consumption during activation of specific brain areas.

In addition to oxygen supply, clearance of carbon dioxide also is very important. Minimal changes in $PaCO_2$ can have a marked impact on cerebral blood flow by changing the hydrogen ion concentration and then modulating extracellular pH. This can modify the cerebrovascular resistance and blood flow. Of importance to clinicians, hypercapnia relaxes vascular smooth muscles, whereas hypocapnia produces vasoconstriction and reduces flow.

Disruption of blood flow, glucose utilization, oxygen supply, and clearance of metabolites all potentially can lead to metabolic encephalopathy. Metabolic encephalopathies can be divided into either primary or secondary, depending on whether the encephalopathy is due to a local metabolic disorder or a systemic disease, respectively. Systemic diseases that can cause a secondary metabolic encephalopathy, including those associated with hepatic, renal, and cardiovascular diseases as well as hypoglycemia, electrolyte disorders, and acid-base disturbances, are beyond the scope of this chapter. The focus here is on those brain diseases that are caused primarily by abnormal cellular metabolism or abnormal function of the mitochondrial respiratory chain.

Primary Metabolic Brain Diseases

Primary metabolic brain disorders are the direct result of a defect in cellular metabolism, caused by deficiencies of either mitochondrial respiratory chain enzymes or, less commonly, cytosolic enzymes. This group of diseases usually is referred to as *mitochondrial encephalopathy*. In addition, encephalopathies due to an abnormal metabolism of organic and amino acids are discussed briefly at the end of the chapter.

Mitochondrial Encephalopathies

Mitochondria are organelles located in the cytoplasm of almost all mammalian cells and they are inherited maternally. Because several important biochemical functions take place in mitochondria, such as the tricarboxylic acid cycle and oxidative phosphorylation as described earlier, defects in the respiratory chain complexes can lead to different metabolic disorders. Most of these defects are heritable and are the result of either a nuclear DNA or a mitochondrial DNA mutation (with mitochondrial DNA being of maternal inheritance). The clinical expression of a mitochondrial DNA mutation is heterogeneous. Tissues with high metabolic demand such as brain, heart, and muscle are more prone to develop dysfunction. Although pure neurologic syndromes involving either the central nervous system (CNS) or peripheral nervous system (PNS) are possible, multisystemic disorders are not uncommon. Different syndromes can be associated with the same mutation, and a single syndrome can be associated with different mutations.

In humans, many mitochondrial encephalopathies, myelopathies, and myopathies have been reported. Recently, several inherited myopathies, mitochondrial encephalopathies, and encephalomyelopathies have been reported in dogs.

Clinical Signs

In humans with mitochondrial encephalopathy, severity can vary from acute life-threatening disease to a subacute progressive degenerative disorder. Progression may be unrelenting with rapid deterioration over hours, episodic with intermittent decompensations and asymptomatic intervals, or insidious with slow degeneration over decades. The presenting clinical signs of these neurometabolic diseases often are very non specific and are caused by progressive destruction of motor, mental, and perceptual functions potentially associated with seizures and with earlier death, often before adulthood.

As in people, relatively nonspecific, progressive or episodic, classically life-threatening signs of CNS dysfunction related to neurometabolic diseases have been reported in isolated cases or families of dogs (Table 228-1). Since the neurons have the highest metabolic demand of the different brain cells, the cerebral cortex is the most susceptible to energy metabolism disorders. Thus the overwhelming majority of animals with metabolic encephalopathies initially experience neurologic signs referable to forebrain dysfunction; these signs then can progress to more generalized brain involvement (brainstem or cerebellar signs may develop later on) and eventually death. The neurologic signs usually develop in the first year of life; however, the age of onset may vary from as young as 4 months to 6 years or older. Clinical signs usually are compatible with a generalized bilateral and symmetric encephalopathy or a multifocal CNS disease (e.g., cerebrum and cerebellum, or cerebrum and spinal cord).

Clinical signs generally correlate well with the location of structural lesions observed on gross and microscopic examination of the CNS. However, the abnormalities also may reflect a functional disturbance of neuronal

TABLE 228-1

Clinical Signs and Imaging Findings in Dogs with Mitochondrial Encephalopathy

Breed	Clinical Signs	Imaging Findings
Alaskan husky	Ataxia, seizures, behavioral abnormalities, blindness, facial hypalgesia and difficulty in prehension of food	MRI: Bilateral lesions in center of brainstem, extending from midthalamus to medulla; to a lesser degree, lesions in putamen, caudate nucleus, and claustrum. Lesions were hyperintense with T2 weighting and isointense/hypointense nonenhancing with T1 weighting.
Yorkshire terrier	Behavioral changes with or without seizures, visual deficits, generalized ataxia	Well-circumscribed, noncontiguous, bilateral, oblique areas within basal nuclei, midthalamus and brainstem that appeared hypodense on CT and on MRI images; hyperintense with T2 weighting and hypointense nonenhancing with T1 weighting.
Jack Russell terrier	Ataxia/hypermetria, fine head tremor, bilateral blindness and deafness	Imaging not performed.
English springer spaniel	Ataxia/hypermetria, visual deficits, positional nystagmus, delayed postural reactions in all four limbs	Imaging not performed.
Shih Tzu	Progressive bilateral brachial plexus/caudal cervical spinal cord disorder; later, brain signs (behavioral changes such as aggressiveness and vocalization)	MRI: Two well-demarcated, intraaxial lesions into cervical spinal cord, caudal colliculi, vestibular nuclei, medulla of cerebellum; hyperintense with T2 weighting and FLAIR, and hypointense nonenhancing with T1 weighting.
Australian cattle dog	Seizures, followed by progressive ataxia and tetraparesis	MRI: Multiple ovoid, bilaterally symmetric, T2 hyperintense, T1 isointense/hypointense nonenhancing lesions on interposital nuclei, vestibular nuclei, pontine nuclei, and caudal colliculi.
Shetland sheepdog and Australian cattle dog	Seizures, followed by depressed mental status, hypermetric gait, intention head and neck tremor, and eventually inability to walk with extensor spasticity of all four limbs	CT: Diffuse hypomyelination (i.e., hypodense areas) and dilated lateral and fourth ventricles.

CT, Computed tomography; FLAIR, fluid attenuated inversion recovery; MRI, magnetic resonance imaging.

populations not visible by light microscopy, and this is relatively common in metabolic disorders. In cases of forebrain localization, mental obtundation, blindness, and behavioral changes with or without seizures have been reported most commonly. Brainstem-cerebellar signs such as generalized ataxia, dysmetria, and a wide-based stance also have been reported with a relatively high frequency. A combination of these signs is seen with a diffuse or multifocal problem.

Encephalopathies proved or suspected to be due to a mitochondrial disorder have been reported sporadically in Alaskan huskies, Yorkshire terriers, Jack Russell terriers, springer spaniels, Shih Tzus, Australian cattle dogs, and Shetland sheepdogs. However, other dogs previously reported to have vacuolar or spongiform encephalopathy of idiopathic origin currently are suspected to have an underlying mitochondrial dysfunction. The encephalopathy described in the Alaskan husky shares many similarities with that reported in the Yorkshire terrier, springer spaniel, and, to a lesser degree, the Jack Russell terrier and resembles subacute necrotizing encephalomyelopathy, or Leigh's syndrome, in humans. This syndrome includes a heterogeneous group of heritable neurodegenerative diseases. Currently, most of the diseases reported are known

to be caused by diverse defects of the mitochondrial respiratory chain.

In dogs with changes similar to those in Leigh's syndrome, the clinical signs usually include ataxia (mostly cerebellar-quality ataxia), seizures, behavioral abnormalities (including obtundation and propulsive pacing), and visual deficits. Moreover, the neurologic examination commonly reveals delayed postural reactions and some other cerebellovestibular signs like nystagmus and head tremor. Varying degrees of tetraparesis, facial hypalgesia, and difficulty in prehending food also have been reported in Alaskan huskies.

In Australian cattle dogs, after an initial presentation of psychomotor seizures (episodes of running in circles, vocalizing, and urinating), usually progressive fatigue and thoracic limb stiffness, and eventually spastic tetraparesis occur over a 6- to 12-month period (Harkin et al, 1999; Brenner et al, 1997b). In one dog, the thoracic limb stiffness was exacerbated while the dog was placed in lateral recumbency; the thoracic limbs were in fact rigidly extended in a tetanic posture with persistent contraction of extensor muscles (Harkin et al, 1999). In the single Shih Tzu recently reported in which a mitochondrial CNS disease was suspected, the signs initially were compatible with a progressive bilateral brachial plexus–caudal cervical spinal cord disorder that mostly spared the back legs; only later did the dog develop concurrent brain signs consisting of behavioral changes such as aggressiveness and vocalization (Kent et al, 2009). In the Shetland sheepdogs the clinical signs were intermittent, present from puppyhood, and composed mainly of seizures. As the disease progressed, depressed mental status, hypermetric gait, and intention head and neck tremor developed, and ultimately these dogs became unable to walk, with extensor spasticity of all four limbs (Wood et al, 2001).

Diagnostic Tests

Results of urinalysis and routine blood tests, including a serum biochemistry profile, usually are within normal limits. In humans with Leigh's syndrome serum lactate and pyruvate levels can be elevated. Lactate and pyruvate levels were elevated in the cerebrospinal fluid (CSF) of the affected Australian cattle dogs, and in one of them, mild CSF pleocytosis and increase in protein content were detected (Brenner et al, 1997b). The remaining dogs had normal CSF findings.

Advanced imaging such as computed tomography (CT) and MRI has been performed in a small number of canine cases, and as with humans, lesions associated with the diagnosis seem to be evident using magnetic resonance imaging. Some of the key features identified in dogs are summarized in Table 228-1. When CT examination was performed (Yorkshire terriers and Alaskan husky), changes were the same in distribution as those reported on MRI scans, and they were compatible with bilateral and symmetric cavitary lesions. In Shetland sheepdogs, in which the major histopathologic finding is the spongy degeneration of the white matter of the cerebrum and spinal cord (see next section), CT changes compatible with diffuse hypomyelination (i.e., hypodense areas) and dilated lateral and fourth ventricles were reported. However, MRI or CT findings reported in dogs with mitochondrial encephalomyelopathy are not pathognomonic and may be encountered to varying degrees in other brain diseases, including nutritional disorders (e.g., thiamine deficiency), toxicosis, and degenerative diseases (e.g., spongy degeneration of the CNS).

Pathologic Findings

The definitive diagnosis of Leigh's syndrome in people is based on gross and histopathologic demonstration of characteristic lesions in the brain and spinal cord. Lesions usually are bilateral and symmetric and show a tendency to be noncontiguous. Characteristic features of acute lesions are loosening and spongiosis of the neuropil followed by necrosis. There is capillary proliferation, macrophage infiltration, gliosis, and occasional perivascular cuffs. An important feature is the relative preservation of neurons. Findings may vary in different regions in the same individual: although some areas may have end-stage lesions, others may show florid changes. The destructive process is episodic, and total tissue damage is cumulative. These lesions in humans with Leigh's syndrome bear a considerable resemblance in their distribution and quality to those observed in the dog, the characteristics of which

are summarized in Table 228-2. There are differences between the canine and human disorders mainly in the topography of the lesions; the thalamus is the most severely affected region in dogs, whereas it is involved in fewer than half of Leigh's syndrome cases. In the single springer spaniel with mitochondrial encephalopathy reported, no gross abnormalities were noted. Microscopically, the lesions were bilateral and symmetric throughout the brain and spinal cord. Other findings identified in affected canine breeds are summarized in Table 228-2. Interestingly, the histopathologic changes in Shetland sheepdogs delineated a leukodystrophy or leukoencephalomyelopathy resembling human Canavan's disease, but amino acid and organic acid metabolism abnormalities were not detected. Diminished aspartoacylase enzyme activity in tissue and excessive N-acetylasparticaciduria, which are the hallmark abnormalities in Canavan's disease, were not found in the affected dogs.

The relative sparing of the neurons in all these forms except for the generalized involvement of astrocytes indicates an active role for the latter cells in brain metabolism, and this is further supported by histochemical studies that showed an abundance of enzymes in astrocytes that take part in different metabolic pathways. Astrocytic compromise is presumed to be diffuse throughout the neuraxis, whereas the multifocal involvement is believed to reflect regional variations in neuronal metabolism. Increased neuronal activity presumably increases the workload of adjacent astrocytes. Thus lesion topography as seen on histologic and MRI examinations may reflect glial sensitivity to the metabolic disturbance as well as regional neuronal functional activity.

Ultrastructurally, mitochondrial abnormalities of either morphology or number in neuronal cells and more commonly astrocytes have been reported in Australian cattle dogs, Yorkshire terriers, English springer spaniels, Jack Russell terriers, and Shih Tzus (see Table 228-2). The lack of mitochondrial structural abnormalities cannot rule out the diagnosis of mitochondrial disease, and such abnormalities are identified in only a small percentage of people with mitochondrial disorders. In Yorkshire terriers an abnormal mitochondrial respiratory chain activity has been demonstrated. Moreover, in two families of dogs with the spongiform leukoencephalomyelopathy (Australian cattle dogs and Shetland sheepdogs) a maternally inherited missense mutation in mitochondrial DNA was identified that was related to respiratory chain dysfunction, but no overt changes in the mitochondria were apparent. The disorder in dogs initially was thought to resemble Canavan's disease in people; however, these canine findings are more similar to a mitochondrial disorder known as *Kearns-Sayre syndrome*, in which the major pathologic finding is the spongy change of the white matter caused by the splitting of the myelin sheath, as is reported in the affected dogs.

Treatment and Prognosis

Treatments for mitochondrial encephalopathies in human patients have been unrewarding despite major advances in the understanding of mitochondrial diseases. Pharmacologic therapies have been reported to be of some isolated benefit, but for the vast majority of patients, the

TABLE 228-2

Pathologic Changes and Related Mitochondrial Abnormalities in Dogs with Mitochondrial Encephalopathy

Breed	Pathologic Changes	Mitochondrial Abnormality
Alaskan husky	Bilateral and symmetric V-shaped cavitated foci in thalamus and basal nuclei, and sometimes extending into caudal brainstem. Microscopic lesions: varying degree of neuronal loss, spongiosis, gliosis, and cavitation. Minor multifocal lesions at base of sulci in cerebral cortex and in ventral vermis of cerebellum.	Not reported.
Yorkshire terrier	Changes similar to those reported in Alaskan husky.	Increased number of dysmorphic mitochondria. Abnormal mitochondrial respiratory chain activity.
Jack Russell terrier	Bilateral, symmetric neuronal degeneration and mineralization in cochlear and cerebellar nuclei, dorsal areas of medulla oblongata, vestibulocochlear nerve, and plexus choroideus, and within granule cell layer of ventral cerebellar hemispheres.	Mitochondria that were increased in number and enlarged.
English springer spaniel	Astrogliosis, mild focal spongiosis, and mild neuronal, mostly Purkinje cell, loss. Diffuse neuropil spongiosis in brain and spinal cord.	Giant and bizarre mitochondria within neuronal perikarya and axons.
Shih Tzu	Spongiosis of neuropil with reactive astrocytes in cervical spinal cord, caudal colliculi, and vestibular and cerebellar nuclei (polioencephalomyelopathy).	Mitochondria that were increased in number and swollen, mainly in astrocytes.
Australian cattle dog	Bilateral and symmetric foci of malacia in nuclei of cerebellum, caudal colliculi, lateral vestibular nuclei, lateral cuneate nuclei, lateral reticular nuclei, and gray matter of spinal cord associated with cervical and lumbosacral intumescences. Minor lesions in interpositial nucleus and spinal nuclei of trigeminal nerve (polioencephalomyelopathy).	Marked mitochondrial accumulation and swelling in astrocytes.
Shetland sheepdog and Australian cattle dog	Spongiosis of white matter in cerebellar medulla and folia, in cerebral white matter, and in dorsal funiculi of spinal cord. Purkinje cells were slightly swollen.	Missense mutation in mitochondrial DNA but no changes in morphology or number.

current emphasis primarily is supportive. In many situations, supportive care for mitochondrial disease is no different from that for any other progressive illness. Reports of treatment efficacy thus far primarily are anecdotal or are based on small clinical trials using surrogate (as opposed to major clinical) end points.

Dietary change and supplementation with various quantities of B vitamins, vitamin E, and other ergogenic aids such as coenzyme Q_{10} (CoQ_{10}) have been used. CoQ_{10} is an essential component of the respiratory chain, and in a few well-documented cases of isolated CoQ_{10} deficiency its use has been highly effective. However, results were inconclusive in the only published double-blind, multicenter study of CoQ_{10} supplementation in humans with mitochondrial myopathies (Bresolin et al, 1990). Riboflavin and thiamine (B_2 and B_1 vitamins, respectively) are cofactors in respiratory chain complexes or enzymes. However, their therapeutic effects seem minimal at best. L-Carnitine often is used in conjunction with CoQ_{10} in patients with respiratory chain disease. Although only a minority of human patients with respiratory chain defects have a secondary carnitine deficiency, many individuals have reported an improvement in symptoms with L-carnitine treatment. However, the precise mechanism of benefit remains obscure. Corticosteroids also have been

TABLE 228-3

Recommended Dosages of Supplements in Canine Mitochondrial Myopathies

Supplement	Dosage
L-Carnitine	50 mg/kg q12h PO
Coenzyme Q_{10}	100 mg q24h PO
Riboflavin	100 mg q24h PO

PO, Orally.

used in patients with MELAS (mitochondrial myopathy, encephalopathy, lactic acidosis, and strokelike episodes) and other mitochondrial encephalomyopathies, but again there have been conflicting results. Thus far, reported canine cases have not been treated systematically, and all dogs have died or have been euthanized. Empiric therapy can be considered (Table 228-3). The inadequacy of these current biochemical therapeutic strategies has led to the consideration of gene therapy, which is still investigational.

Encephalomyelopathy and Organic Acidopathies

Inborn errors of metabolism, distinct from mitochondrial encephalopathies, rarely are reported in the veterinary medical literature. Several inherited diseases in people that involve abnormal metabolism of organic and amino acids leading to neurologic dysfunction have been reported in dogs, including L-2-Hydroxyglutaricaciduria, methylmalonic aciduria, and malonic aciduria with progressive encephalopathy or encephalomyelopathy. Hexanoylglycineaciduria, similar to medium-chain acyl-coenzyme A dehydrogenase deficiency in humans, was reported recently in a 2-month-old cavalier King Charles spaniel with refractory seizures that seemed to respond positively to levetiracetam therapy (Platt et al, 2007).

L-2-Hydroxyglutaricaciduria

L-2-Hydroxyglutaricaciduria is the best characterized of the inborn errors of metabolism associated with encephalomyelopathy, and it is attributed to a mutation in the canine homolog of the L-2-hydroxyglutarate dehydrogenase (L2HGDH) gene. Although the specific metabolism of L-2-hydroxyglutaric acid and its physiologic and pathologic role are unknown, it is thought that a link may exist between L-2-hydroxyglutaric acid and lysine catabolism or oxidative stress from L-2-hydroxyglutaric acid buildup in the brain, and possibly interference with creatine kinase activity in the cerebellum.

Clinical Signs

In humans the clinical signs usually start during childhood and are characterized by progressive psychomotor delay with intellectual impairment, ataxia, and occasionally seizures. In dogs the disease first was reported in Staffordshire bull terriers and subsequently in a West Highland white terrier and a Yorkshire terrier. Although the development of clinical signs generally is thought to be insidious and progressive, cases also have been reported with acute manifestations, especially in dogs with seizures. Signs usually occur within the first few years of life. Forebrain signs are common clinical findings in affected dogs, with behavioral changes, visual deficits, tonic-clonic seizures, and postural reaction deficits. Generalized ataxia, hypermetria, and head-neck tremors also have been documented as a result of cerebellar involvement.

Diagnostic Tests and Pathologic Findings

Results of laboratory studies (including hematologic testing, biochemistry studies, and urinalysis) are normal in affected dogs. As in humans, MRI can reveal typical changes in dogs. Specific MRI characteristics of human L-2-hydroxyglutaricaciduria consist of prominent hyperintensities of the subcortical white matter tracts and hyperintensities in the gray matter regions of the basal ganglia and dentate nucleus with T2-weighted imaging. The areas of hyperintensity on T2-weighted images often correlate with regions of non-enhancing hypointensity on T1-weighted images. The cerebellum is prominently involved in most cases. In dogs, as in the mitochondrial encephalopathies previously described, T2-weighted MRI reveals bilaterally symmetric and hyperintense lesions. These generally involve the cerebral and cerebellar cortices, thalamus, dorsal portion of the brainstem, and basal and cerebellar nuclei. The same areas are isointense to hypointense on T1-weighted images, with no evidence of contrast enhancement after intravenous injection of gadolinium.

Results of routine CSF analysis are unremarkable. In humans, the diagnosis of the disorder is based on urinary organic acid screening with demonstration of a high concentration of L-2-hydroxyglutaric acid, which, however, also is consistently high in the CSF and plasma. High levels of L-2-hydroxyglutaric acid have been detected consistently in the CSF, plasma, and urine of affected dogs by means of gas chromatography and mass spectroscopy. The reported urine concentration ranges from 2223 mmol/mol of creatinine to 3922 mmol/mol creatinine. High levels of methylmalonic acid, lysine, or arginine also have occasionally been reported, although their significance is unknown.

Since L-2-hydroxyglutaricaciduria is inherited in both people and dogs as an autosomal-recessive disease, diagnosis may be confirmed through DNA testing for the mutation of the gene encoding L2HGDH.

In one Staffordshire bull terrier a histopathologic examination of brain tissue was performed (Abramson et al, 2003). No gross lesions were identified in the brain. Microscopy of the brain mainly revealed clear or empty vacuoles in the gray matter astrocytes around neurons and blood vessels; changes extended into the adjacent white matter, with vacuoles found in astrocytes and myelin sheaths. Most of these changes were compatible with cytotoxic edema mainly affecting the gray matter (polioencephalopathy), although differences between gray and white matter lesions in dogs and those in humans were identified.

Treatment and Prognosis

Currently there is no known treatment for L-2-hydroxyglutaricaciduria, and as previously described for mitochondrial encephalopathy, metabolic disorders may require dietary manipulation to compensate for altered metabolic pathways. Thus supportive treatment and antioxidant diet supplementation with L-carnitine, CoQ_{10}, and riboflavin have been attempted. The long-term prognosis is guarded. In dogs with seizure activity, phenobarbital has controlled clinical signs adequately. Cobalamin supplementation has been implemented in cases of concurrent methylmalonicaciduria, with uncertain results (see later). As with mitochondrial encephalopathies, gene therapy represents a possible future treatment option.

Methylmalonic Aciduria and Malonic Aciduria

A progressive encephalomyelopathy has been reported in a 12-week-old Labrador retriever with a variety of forebrain and brainstem signs (Podell et al, 1996). Clinical findings included stiffness and ataxia that progressed to tetraparesis, nystagmus, decreased menace response, anisocoria, ventrolateral strabismus, diminished gag reflex, and apparent dysphonia. Significant biochemical abnormalities included methylmalonic aciduria and malonic aciduria, mild lactic aciduria, and pyruvic aciduria. Disordered cobalamin metabolism was suspected, although serum cobalamin levels were normal. The condition was considered an inborn error of metabolism resulting in abnormal organic acid accumulation with similarities to methylmalonicacidemia in neonatal humans (an autosomal-recessive disorder). Many human patients respond to large doses of vitamin B_{12}, but cobalamin-unresponsive cases also have been reported. Results of B_{12} therapy are controversial.

In the reported case, an 8-week-course of L-carnitine (1000 mg/day), vitamin B_{12} (0.5 mg/day), and a protein-restricted diet resulted in marked improvement in the organic acid values in this dog. However, clinical improvement was not observed, which prompted euthanasia. At necropsy, enlargement of the lateral, third, and fourth ventricles of the brain and white and gray matter atrophy were grossly visible. Syringohydromyelia extended from the cervical to the lumbar intumescence.

Malonic aciduria without elevated serum levels of methylmalonic acid has been reported in a family of Maltese dogs with signs of episodic seizures and stupor, along with hypoglycemia, acidosis, and ketonuria (O'Brien et al. 1999). Interestingly, treatment with frequent feedings of a low-fat diet high in medium-chain triglycerides resulted in normalization of clinical signs and a resolution of the malonic aciduria in one dog.

References and Suggested Reading

Abramson CJ et al: L-2-hydroglutaric aciduria in Staffordshire bull terriers, *J Vet Intern Med* 17(4):551, 2003.

Baiker K et al: Leigh-like subacute necrotising encephalopathy in Yorkshire Terriers: neuropathological characterisation, respiratory chain activities and mitochondrial DNA, *Acta Neuropathol* 118(5):697, 2009.

Brenner O et al: A canine encephalomyelopathy with morphological abnormalities in mitochondria, *Acta Neuropathol* 94(4):390, 1997a.

Brenner O et al: Hereditary polioencephalomyelopathy of the Australian cattle dog, *Acta Neuropathol* 94(1):54, 1997b.

Brenner O et al: Alaskan Husky encephalopathy—a canine neurodegenerative disorder resembling subacute necrotizing encephalomyelopathy (Leigh syndrome), *Acta Neuropathol* 100(1):50, 2000.

Bresolin N et al: Ubidecarenone in the treatment of mitochondrial myopathies: a multi-center, double blind trial, *J Neurol Sci* 100:70, 1990.

Garosi LS et al: L-2-hydroxyglutaric aciduria in a West Highland white terrier, *Vet Rec* 156(5):145, 2005.

Gruber AD et al: Mitochondriopathy with regional encephalic mineralization in a Jack Russell Terrier, *Vet Pathol* 39(6):732, 2002.

Harkin KR et al: Magnetic resonance imaging of the brain of a dog with hereditary polioencephalomyelopathy, *J Am Vet Med Assoc* 214(9):1342, 1999.

Kent M et al: Clinicopathologic and magnetic resonance imaging characteristics associated with polioencephalomyelopathy in a Shih Tzu, *J Am Vet Med Assoc* 235(5):551, 2009.

Li FY et al: Canine spongiform leukoencephalomyelopathy is associated with a missense mutation in cytochrome b, *Neurobiol Dis* 21(1):35, 2006.

Magistretti PJ et al: Brain energy metabolism: an integrated cellular perspective. In Bloom FE, Kupfer DJ, editors: *Psychopharmacology: the fourth generation of progress*, New York, 1995, Raven, p 657.

Mariani CL et al: Magnetic resonance imaging of spongy degeneration of the central nervous system in a Labrador retriever, *Vet Radiol Ultrasound* 42(4):285, 2001.

O'Brien DP et al: Malonic aciduria in Maltese dogs: normal methylmalonic acid concentration and malonyl-CoA decarboxylase activity in fibroblasts, *J Inherit Metab Dis* 22(8):883, 1999.

Penderis J et al: L-2-hydroxyglutaric aciduria: characterisation of the molecular defect in a spontaneous canine model, *J Med Genet* 44(5):334, 2007.

Platt S et al: Refractory seizures associated with an organic aciduria in a dog, *J Am Anim Hosp Assoc* 43(3):163, 2007.

Podell M et al: Methylmalonic and malonic aciduria in a dog with progressive encephalomyelopathy, *Metab Brain Dis* 11:239, 1996.

Rosenberg RN et al: Mitochondrial disorders. In Rosenberg et al, editors: *The molecular and genetic basis of neurological disease*, ed 2, Boston, 1998, Butterworth-Heinemann, p 35.

Sanchez-Masian DF et al: L-2-hydroxyglutaric aciduria in two female Yorkshire terriers, *J Am Anim Hosp Assoc* 48:5, 2012.

Taylor RW et al: Treatment of mitochondrial disease, *J Bioenerg Biomembr* 29(2):195, 1997.

Wakshlag JJ et al: Subacute necrotising encephalopathy in an Alaskan husky, *J Small Anim Pract* 40(12):585, 1999.

Wood SL, Patterson JS: Shetland Sheepdog leukodystrophy, *J Vet Intern Med* 15(5):486, 2001.

Zauner A, Muizelaar JP: Brain metabolism and cerebral blood flow. In Reilly P, Bullock R, editors: *Head injury*, London, 1997, Chapman & Hall, p 89.

CHAPTER 229

New Maintenance Anticonvulsant Therapies for Dogs and Cats

CURTIS W. DEWEY, *Ithaca, New York*

Over the last 15 years the paradigm for treating dogs and cats with seizure disorders has changed, coincident with the introduction of several new anticonvulsant drugs. Although phenobarbital (dogs and cats) and bromide (dogs) remain valuable first-choice anticonvulsant drug options for pets with seizure disorders, a number of alternative drugs can be used as either adjunctive treatment (i.e., for refractory seizures) or sole therapy. The major impediments to widespread use of these newer anticonvulsant drugs have been principally higher cost compared with phenobarbital and bromide and clinical unfamiliarity with their usage. Since several of these drugs (gabapentin, zonisamide, levetiracetam) are now available in generic forms, cost is now less of a concern. Information is available concerning several newer anticonvulsant drugs for canine use. Unfortunately, much of the information regarding new anticonvulsant therapy for cats remains largely anecdotal, and the majority of clinical trials are neither randomized nor placebo controlled. This chapter provides information on some of these newer anticonvulsant drugs with recommendations based on published literature and my own clinical experience. Additionally, the next generation of some of these compounds is discussed briefly.

Gabapentin

Gabapentin, a structural analog of γ-aminobutyric acid (GABA), probably exerts its antiseizure effects via inhibition of voltage-gated calcium channels in the brain. Gabapentin is well absorbed in both dogs and people, with peak serum concentrations occurring within 1 to 3 hours after ingestion. In dogs 30% to 40% of the orally administered dose of gabapentin undergoes hepatic metabolism to N-methyl-gabapentin. Although gabapentin undergoes some hepatic metabolism in dogs, there is no appreciable induction of hepatic microsomal enzymes in this species. The half-life of elimination for gabapentin in dogs is between 3 and 4 hours. Because of its short half-life in dogs, gabapentin probably needs to be administered at least every 8 hours and possibly every 6 hours to maintain serum gabapentin concentrations within the therapeutic range. The potential need for dosing every 6 hours can make it difficult for some pet owners to administer gabapentin consistently.

The recommended *daily* dosage range of gabapentin for dogs is 25 to 60 mg/kg of body weight in *divided doses* q6-8h. I recommend an initial dosage regimen of 10 mg/kg of body weight q8h. The suspected therapeutic plasma concentration for dogs is 4 to 16 mg/L. Gabapentin concentrations seldom are measured in dogs.

The efficacy of gabapentin therapy in dogs has been evaluated in some small studies. In one prospective study evaluating gabapentin as an add-on treatment for dogs with refractory seizure activity, no significant decrease in overall seizure activity was seen over a 4-month evaluation period. Despite this, 3 of 17 dogs became seizure free, and 4 others experienced a reduction of 50% or more in seizure frequency during the evaluation period. In a similar study evaluating 11 dogs, an overall significant reduction in seizure frequency was found, and 6 dogs experienced a reduction of 50% or more in seizure frequency. Sedation and pelvic limb ataxia were the only reported adverse effects in these two studies. In my experience gabapentin occasionally is helpful as an anticonvulsant drug in dogs. In humans gabapentin appears to be much more effective in the treatment of focal seizure disorders than in the treatment of generalized seizures.

Long-term canine toxicity trials for gabapentin have not been reported. However, the drug seems to be very well tolerated in this species, usually with few to no adverse effects. Sedation does not appear to be a major problem. However, I have had many clients report that their dog experienced mild sedation or mild polyphagia and weight gain in association with gabapentin use.

Only anecdotal information is available regarding gabapentin use in cats. A dosage of 5 to 10 mg/kg of body weight q8-12h PO has been suggested but is not based on any published data. The elimination half-life of gabapentin in cats (approximately 3 hours) is similar to that in dogs, which suggests that a lower dose or longer dosing interval for this species is not necessary.

A new gabapentin analog, pregabalin, has been approved recently for human use. Pregabalin has a greater affinity for the $\alpha_2\delta$-subunit of voltage-gated calcium channels than gabapentin and purportedly is more effective in people than its predecessor as both an anticonvulsant and a pain-relieving drug. The elimination half-life of pregabalin is approximately 7 hours in dogs and 11 hours in cats. In a small, prospective clinical trial involving epileptic dogs, administration of pregabalin (as an add-on therapy) was associated with an overall reduction in seizures of 57%. The response rate in this study was 78%, and the responding dogs had a mean 64% reduction in seizures. The main adverse effect of pregabalin appears to be sedation. The target dosage for canine epilepsy is about 3 to 4 mg/kg q12h. However, the starting dosage should be 2 mg/kg q12h for at least the first week to avoid severe sedation. I suspect the dosage range for cats (based on pharmacokinetic data) to be about half that for dogs (i.e., 1 to 2 mg/kg q12h).

Felbamate

Felbamate is a dicarbamate drug that has demonstrated efficacy in the treatment of both focal (partial) and generalized seizures in experimental animal studies and human clinical trials. Proposed mechanisms of action include blocking of N-methyl-d-aspartate (NMDA)–mediated neuronal excitation, potentiation of GABA-mediated neuronal inhibition, and inhibition of voltage-sensitive neuronal sodium and calcium channels. Felbamate also may offer some protection to neurons from hypoxic-ischemic damage.

Approximately 70% of the orally administered dose of felbamate in dogs is excreted in the urine unchanged; the remainder undergoes hepatic metabolism. The half-life of felbamate in adult dogs typically is between 5 and 6 hours (range, 4 to 8 hours). Felbamate is well absorbed after oral administration in adult dogs, but bioavailability in puppies may be only 30% that in adults. The half-life of elimination also has been shown to be much shorter in puppies than in adult dogs (approximately 2.5 hours). For adult dogs I recommend an initial felbamate dosage regimen of 15 mg/kg of body weight q8h. Felbamate has a wide margin of safety in dogs, with serious toxic effects usually not apparent below a daily dose of 300 mg/kg of body weight per day. If the initial dose of felbamate is ineffective, the dose is increased by 15-mg/kg increments every 2 weeks until efficacy is achieved, unacceptable adverse effects are evident, or the cost of the drug becomes prohibitive. The therapeutic range for serum felbamate concentration in dogs is believed to be similar to that in people (20 to 100 μg/ml). Typically serum felbamate assays are costly. In addition, the wide therapeutic range and low toxicity potential of felbamate make routine serum drug monitoring of questionable clinical value. I do not routinely check felbamate levels in dogs.

The limited published material regarding clinical efficacy of felbamate is similar to my experience with the drug. In one report of refractory epilepsy in dogs, 12 of 16 patients experienced a reduction of seizure frequency following initiation of felbamate therapy. In another report of six dogs with suspected focal seizure activity, all dogs experienced a substantial reduction in seizure frequency when felbamate was used as the sole anticonvulsant drug; two of these dogs became seizure free.

I have used felbamate extensively in the treatment of dogs with seizure disorders. Felbamate appears to be very effective both as an add-on therapy and as a sole anticonvulsant agent for patients with focal and generalized seizures. Because of its lack of sedative effects, felbamate is particularly useful as monotherapy in dogs exhibiting obtunded mental status as a result of their underlying neurologic disease (e.g., brain tumor, cerebral infarct). I have found adverse effects from felbamate to be very infrequent, especially when it is used as the sole anticonvulsant drug. Hepatic dysfunction associated with felbamate use tends to resolve following discontinuation of the drug. In dogs with evidence of preexisting hepatic disease, felbamate should be avoided. Because of the potential for hepatoxicity, it is recommended that serum biochemistry analysis be performed every 6 months in dogs receiving felbamate, especially if the drug is given concurrently with phenobarbital. It also may be advisable to evaluate complete blood counts every few months in the unlikely event that a blood dyscrasia develops.

Adverse effects are observed infrequently with felbamate use in dogs. Unlike other anticonvulsants, felbamate does not cause sedation. Because felbamate does undergo some hepatic metabolism, liver dysfunction is a potential adverse effect. In one study 4 of 12 dogs receiving felbamate as an add-on therapy developed liver disease; however, each of these dogs was also receiving high doses of phenobarbital. In humans felbamate has been shown to increase serum phenobarbital concentrations in some patients receiving combination therapy. It is unclear whether felbamate, phenobarbital, or the combination of the two drugs is responsible for the reported hepatotoxicity in dogs. In humans serious hepatotoxicity rarely is associated with felbamate use and usually occurs in patients concurrently receiving other anticonvulsant drugs. Aplastic anemia (caused by bone marrow suppression) has been reported to occur in people receiving felbamate at a rate of 10 per 100,000 patients; this uncommon and severe adverse effect also usually is encountered in patients receiving combination anticonvulsant drug therapy. Fortunately this does not appear to occur in dogs. However, in one report reversible bone marrow suppression was suspected in two dogs receiving felbamate; one dog developed mild thrombocytopenia, the other mild leukopenia. Both of these abnormalities resolved following discontinuation of the drug. One patient in this report developed bilateral keratoconjunctivitis sicca; it is unknown whether this was related to felbamate use, although I have encountered several patients given felbamate that developed keratoconjunctivitis sicca. Generalized tremor activity in small-breed dogs receiving high dosages of felbamate also has been reported as a rarely encountered adverse effect.

To my knowledge there is no clinical information regarding the use of felbamate in cats. Because of the potential for felbamate-associated hepatotoxicity and blood dyscrasias in dogs, felbamate is not likely to become a viable anticonvulsant option for cats.

Because of the problems of hepatoxicity and blood dyscrasias occasionally associated with felbamate use in people, a new derivative of the drug—fluorofelbamate— has been developed and is undergoing clinical trials for human use. In experimental animal epilepsy models fluorofelbamate has been shown to have equal or superior anticonvulsant potency compared with felbamate. A reactive aldehyde intermediate that is formed from felbamate metabolism has been linked to the hepatic and hematologic adverse effects of this drug. This toxic intermediate is not produced from metabolism of fluorofelbamate.

Levetiracetam

Levetiracetam is a new piracetam anticonvulsant drug that has demonstrated efficacy in the treatment of focal and generalized seizure disorders in people as well as in several experimental animal models. Although generally recommended as an add-on anticonvulsant drug, levetiracetam has been used successfully as monotherapy in people. In humans with refractory epilepsy, levetiracetam has manifested antiseizure effects within the first day of treatment. The mechanism of action of the anticonvulsant effects of levetiracetam is not entirely clear but appears to be related to its binding with a specific synaptic vesicle protein (SV2A) in the brain. Unlike other anticonvulsant drugs, levetiracetam does not appear to have a direct effect on common neurotransmitter pathways (e.g., GABA, NMDA) or ion channels (e.g., sodium, T-type calcium). Levetiracetam has demonstrated neuroprotective properties and may ameliorate seizure-induced brain damage. Levetiracetam also has been reported to have an "antikindling" effect, which may diminish the likelihood of increasing seizure frequency over time. Orally administered levetiracetam is approximately 100% bioavailable in dogs, with a serum half-life of 3 to 4 hours. In dogs approximately 70% to 90% of the administered dose of levetiracetam is excreted unchanged in the urine; the remainder is hydrolyzed in the serum and other organs. The effective serum levetiracetam concentration in people is 5 to 45 µg/ml. Because there is no clear relationship between serum drug concentration and efficacy for levetiracetam, and because the drug has an extremely high margin of safety, routine therapeutic drug monitoring is not typically recommended for this drug in humans.

In one small, uncontrolled clinical study, oral levetiracetam was found to decrease seizure frequency by over 50% in epileptic dogs when used as an add-on therapy. Subsequent to that report, however, levetiracetam was shown to be ineffective as an add-on antiseizure drug in a placebo-controlled clinical trial. There was also one report suggesting that levetiracetam shows a distinct "honeymoon" effect in dogs, working fairly well initially, then fading in efficacy over time. There is evidence that levetiracetam metabolism is accelerated over time in dogs concurrently receiving phenobarbital. This phenomenon may explain at least partially the apparent failure of levetiracetam as an add-on antiseizure drug. In the placebo-controlled levetiracetam study, it was found that 38% of dogs had levetiracetam plasma drug concentrations below the level considered to be the lower limit of the therapeutic range for the drug. In terms of cost, levetiracetam is more expensive than zonisamide but less expensive than felbamate.

Based on recent evidence, it may be that the recommended levetiracetam dosage of 20 mg/kg three times daily may be too low for dogs, especially for those patients concurrently receiving phenobarbital therapy.

Long-term toxicity data for levetiracetam in dogs confirm that the drug is extremely safe. In one study dogs were administered levetiracetam at dosages of up to 1200 mg/kg/day PO for 1 year. One of eight dogs receiving 300 mg/kg/day developed a stiff, unsteady gait. Other adverse effects (salivation, vomiting) were seen only in dogs receiving 1200 mg/kg/day. There were no treatment-related mortalities or histopathologic abnormalities.

My colleagues and I have prospectively investigated the use of oral levetiracetam as an add-on anticonvulsant therapy for cats with epilepsy refractory to phenobarbital. Levetiracetam appears to be very well tolerated in this species, usually with no apparent adverse effects. The half-life of elimination is approximately 3 hours after oral administration. A dosage of 20 mg/kg q8h PO typically achieves a serum drug level within the therapeutic range reported for people. Two of twelve cats experienced transient inappetence and lethargy that resolved without dose adjustment within 2 weeks. Although there is some degree of variability among cats, the mean reduction of seizure frequency in cats receiving levetiracetam as an add-on drug is approximately 68%; this was found to be statistically significant when compared with seizure frequency before initiation of levetiracetam therapy. In addition, 7 of 10 cats evaluated for seizure frequency reduction showed a response (i.e., reduction of seizure frequency of 50% or more), with a mean reduction of seizures of 92%. I consider levetiracetam to be the preferred add-on anticonvulsant drug for cats receiving phenobarbital because of lack of serious adverse effects and evidence of efficacy.

Intravenous administration of levetiracetam has shown promise as a treatment for experimental status epilepticus in a rat model. In this study intravenous levetiracetam and diazepam appeared to potentiate the anticonvulsant effect of one another. Intravenous levetiracetam seems well tolerated in dogs, even at doses as high as 400 mg/kg of body weight. The pharmacokinetics of intravenous levetiracetam has been investigated in dogs. In my practice I have had success using intravenous levetiracetam for years as an emergency seizure drug. There is recent clinical evidence supporting the efficacy of intravenous levetiracetam for treating canine seizures in an emergency situation (e.g., status epilepticus and cluster seizures).

Since the discovery of levetiracetam's unique binding site in the brain, two related anticonvulsant drugs—brivaracetam and seletracetam—have been developed that have higher affinity than levetiracetam for the SV2A receptor. These drugs have been demonstrated to have better anticonvulsant activity than levetiracetam in experimental animal seizure models and currently are being evaluated in human clinical epilepsy trials.

Zonisamide

Zonisamide is a sulfonamide-based anticonvulsant drug recently approved for human use; it has demonstrated efficacy in the treatment of both focal and generalized seizures in people with minimal adverse effects. Suspected anticonvulsant mechanisms of action include blockage of T-type calcium and voltage-gated sodium channels in the brain, facilitation of dopaminergic and serotonergic neurotransmission in the central nervous system, scavenging of free radical species, enhancement of the actions of GABA in the brain, inhibition of glutamate-mediated neuronal excitation in the brain, and inhibition of carbonic anhydrase activity. Zonisamide is metabolized primarily by hepatic microsomal enzymes, and the elimination half-life in dogs is approximately 15 to 20 hours. The elimination half-life of zonisamide in cats is substantially longer (approximately 33 hours). In humans it has been shown that the elimination half-life of zonisamide is dramatically shorter in patients who are already receiving drugs that stimulate hepatic microsomal enzymes than in patients who are not receiving such drugs. A similar phenomenon appears to occur in dogs. When zonisamide is used as an add-on therapy for dogs already receiving drugs requiring hepatic metabolism (e.g., phenobarbital), I recommend an initial zonisamide dosage of 10 mg/kg of body weight q12h PO. This dosage regimen has been shown to maintain canine serum zonisamide concentrations within the therapeutic range reported for people (10 to 40 µg/ml) when used as an add-on therapy. For dogs not concurrently receiving drugs that induce hepatic microsomal enzymes, it is recommended that zonisamide be started at a dosage of 5 mg/kg of body weight q12h. I generally check trough serum zonisamide concentrations after approximately 1 week of zonisamide treatment. Zonisamide has a high margin of safety in dogs. In one study minimal adverse effects occurred in beagles administered zonisamide at dosages of up to 75 mg/kg of body weight per day for 1 year. However, there is some potential for hepatotoxicity with zonisamide use in dogs; routine blood monitoring (every 6 months) therefore is recommended.

In one study zonisamide was found to decrease seizure frequency by at least 50% in 7 of 12 dogs with refractory idiopathic epilepsy. In this responding group the mean reduction in seizure frequency was 81.3%. In six of the seven responding dogs phenobarbital dose was able to be reduced by an average of 92.2%. Mild adverse effects (e.g., transient sedation, ataxia, vomiting) occurred in six dogs (50%); none of the adverse effects was considered severe enough to require discontinuing zonisamide therapy. In another similarly designed study, 9 of 11 dogs with refractory epilepsy treated with zonisamide showed a response, with a median seizure reduction of 92.9%; transient ataxia and sedation occurred in six dogs.

Zonisamide has been shown to be very effective as a sole anticonvulsant drug in people. I have used zonisamide as the sole anticonvulsant drug in a large number of dogs. Zonisamide appears to be effective as anticonvulsant monotherapy, with few to no apparent adverse effects in dogs.

My colleagues and I have successfully treated a number of epileptic cats with zonisamide as a sole drug or as an add-on to phenobarbital therapy. In some cats, once-daily dosing is possible, presumably due to the long elimination half-life in this species. The recommended starting dosage is either 5 mg/kg twice daily or 10 mg once daily in cats. The main adverse effect of zonisamide use in cats is anorexia; the occurrence of this adverse effect has necessitated discontinuation of zonisamide for resolution. Further data are needed regarding the use of zonisamide in cats.

References and Suggested Reading

Bailey KS et al: Levetiracetam as an adjunct to phenobarbital treatment in cats with suspected idiopathic epilepsy, *J Am Vet Med Assoc* 232:867, 2008.

Bialer M: New antiepileptic drugs that are second generation to existing antiepileptic drugs, *Expert Opin Investig Drugs* 15:637, 2006.

Dewey CW: Anticonvulsant therapy in dogs and cats, *Vet Clin Small Anim* 36:1107, 2006.

Dewey CW et al: Zonisamide therapy for refractory idiopathic epilepsy in dogs, *J Am Anim Hosp Assoc* 40:285, 2004.

Dewey CW et al: Pharmacokinetics of single-dose intravenous levetiracetam administration in normal dogs, *J Vet Emerg Crit Care* 18:153, 2008.

Dewey CW et al: Pregabalin as an adjunct to phenobarbital, potassium bromide, or a combination of phenobarbital and potassium bromide for treatment of dogs with suspected idiopathic epilepsy, *J Am Vet Med Assoc* 235:1442, 2009.

Govendir M, Perkins M, Malik R: Improving seizure control in dogs with refractory epilepsy using gabapentin as an adjunctive agent, *Aust Vet J* 83:602, 2005.

Hardy BT et al: Double-masked, placebo-controlled study of intravenous levetiracetam for the treatment of status epilepticus and acute repetitive seizures in dogs, *J Vet Intern Med* 26:334, 2012.

Hasegawa D et al: Pharmacokinetics and toxicity of zonisamide in cats, *J Feline Med Surg* 10:418, 2008.

Mazarati AM, Sofia RD, Wasterlain CG: Anticonvulsant and antiepileptogenic effects of fluorofelbamate in experimental status epilepticus, *Seizure* 11:423, 2002.

Moore SA et al: The pharmacokinetics of levetiracetam in healthy dogs concurrently receiving phenobarbital, *J Vet Pharmacol Ther* 34:31, 2010.

Munana K et al: Evaluation of levetiracetam as adjunctive treatment for refractory canine epilepsy: a randomized, placebo-controlled, crossover trial, *J Vet Intern Med* 26:341, 2012.

Ramael S et al: Levetiracetam intravenous infusion: a randomized, placebo-controlled safety and pharmacokinetic study, *Epilepsia* 47:1128, 2006.

Salazar V et al: Pharmacokinetics of single-dose oral pregabalin administration in normal dogs, *Vet Anaesth Analg* 36:574, 2009.

Sia KT et al: Pharmacokinetics of gabapentin in cats, *Am J Vet Res* 71:817, 2010.

Vartanian MG et al: Activity profile of pregabalin in rodent models of epilepsy and ataxia, *Epilepsy Res* 68:189, 2006.

Volk HA et al: The efficacy and tolerability of levetiracetam in pharmacoresistant epileptic dogs, *Vet J* 176:310, 2008.

Von Klopman T et al: Prospective study of zonisamide therapy for refractory idiopathic epilepsy in dogs, *J Small Anim Pract* 48:134, 2007.

CHAPTER 230

Treatment of Cluster Seizures and Status Epilepticus

DANIEL J. FLETCHER, *Ithaca, New York*

Acute-onset seizures are common presenting complaints in veterinary emergency practice. They are caused by focal groups of abnormal neurons that initiate and then propagate bursts of aberrant activity. These episodes generally are short-lived, but prolonged seizure activity or repeated seizures can be life threatening and must be treated aggressively. Treatment of cluster seizures or status epilepticus should focus on rapid treatment of the seizures, identification and treatment of systemic sequelae such as hypoperfusion, hyperthermia, and deficits in ventilation and oxygenation, and in-patient therapy targeted at achieving a 24-hour seizure-free interval. Additional workup to identify the underlying cause of the seizures should be initiated once the patient's condition has been stabilized. Finally, an anticonvulsant treatment plan tailored to the needs of the patient and client must be devised. This chapter considers these aspects of diagnosis and therapy.

Pathophysiology

A seizure is initiated by a high-frequency burst of action potentials within a local, hypersynchronized population of neurons. When a large enough population of neurons is involved, a characteristic spike can be seen in the electroencephalogram (EEG). Within this population, individual neurons experience a sequence of events that includes the following: (1) an intracellular influx of calcium and sodium, leading to a high-frequency burst of action potentials at approximately 700 to 1000/sec; (2) a phase during which the cell remains depolarized; and finally (3) rapid influx of chloride or efflux of potassium mediated by γ-aminobutyric acid (GABA) receptors, which leads to rapid repolarization and hyperpolarization. Although the cause commonly is forebrain disease, other areas of the brain, including the thalamus, subcortical nuclei, and brainstem, can participate in the genesis and propagation of seizures.

Individual, infrequent, and short-duration seizures may not require therapy, but severe, acute seizures are life-threatening emergencies, and aggressive therapy is warranted. Cluster seizures and status epilepticus are the two most life-threatening types of seizures. A cluster of seizures is defined clinically as more than one seizure within a 24-hour period, between which the patient returns to normal mentation and activity. Status epilepticus is seizure activity that continues unabated for longer than 5 minutes or multiple seizures between which the

patient does not return to normal mentation. With these types of severe seizures, direct neuronal damage is common and predisposes the patient to more frequent and severe seizures in the future. In addition, systemic sequelae such as traumatic injury to other parts of the body, hyperthermia leading to disseminated intravascular coagulation (DIC), aspiration pneumonia, and noncardiogenic pulmonary edema are common, so that close monitoring and intensive supportive care are required even after the seizures have been controlled. Aggressive management of cluster seizures and status epilepticus is essential, and both intracranial and extracranial priorities must be addressed.

Differential Diagnoses and Diagnostic Workup

Both extracranial and intracranial diseases may cause seizures. Determining the definitive cause of an individual patient's seizures can require an extensive diagnostic workup, but development of the best treatment plan and accurate estimation of prognosis depends upon an accurate diagnosis.

Extracranial Causes of Seizure

Metabolic disturbances and systemic disease can lead to alterations in the electrophysiology of the brain, causing paroxysmal neuronal discharges and seizures. In general, these types of diseases are likely to cause widespread disturbances affecting both hemispheres. Therefore generalized seizures are more common than focal seizures.

Endogenous toxins accumulating because of hepatic or renal disease can lead to seizures. Metabolic disturbances such as hypoglycemia, hyperlipidemia, hypocalcemia, and hypermagnesemia as well as endocrine diseases such as hypothyroidism and hyperosmolar nonketotic diabetes mellitus also can lead to seizures. Many toxicoses, including bromethalin, theobromine, caffeine, lead, or organophosphate poisoning, can result in seizures.

Initial diagnostic testing should include a complete blood count to rule out systemic inflammation or infection and platelet disorders, as well as a chemistry panel and urinalysis to rule out electrolyte and glucose derangements and to assess renal and hepatic function. Taking a thorough history to rule out potential toxin exposure also is essential. For patients in which there is a high index of suspicion of extracranial disease, further diagnostic studies including abdominal ultrasonography or specific organ function testing may be warranted.

Intracranial Causes of Seizure

Once extracranial causes of seizure are ruled out, the many primary intracranial causes of seizure must be considered. In patients with localizing neurologic deficits (e.g., cranial nerve dysfunction or lateralized proprioceptive deficits), intracranial disease is more likely than extracranial disease. A classification scheme such as DAMNIT-V can be helpful for organizing this large list of disorders. See Table 230-1 for a compilation of differential diagnoses using the DAMNIT-V scheme. Definitive diagnosis of intracranial causes of seizure commonly requires advanced imaging such as magnetic resonance imaging or computed tomography and cerebrospinal fluid analysis, which usually cannot be done until the patient is in stable condition and seizures are controlled. Basic historical and signalment data can be useful in ranking the relative likelihood of each of the differential diagnoses. In dogs younger than 6 months of age, infectious or anomalous diseases are most common. In dogs between 6 months and 6 years of age, idiopathic epilepsy is most common, and in dogs older than 6 years of age, neoplasia is most likely. In younger cats, infectious and anomalous diseases are most common. In outdoor cats, parasitic diseases like cuterebriasis should be considered, and in

TABLE 230-1

Differential Diagnosis of Acute-Onset Seizures (DAMNIT-V Scheme)

D	Degenerative	Storage diseases
A	Anomalous	Hydrocephalus, lissencephaly
M	Metabolic	Extracranial diseases: hepatic, renal
N	Neoplasia	Primary: meningioma, glioma, astrocytoma Metastatic: lymphoma, hemangiosarcoma, carcinomas, etc.
I	Infectious	Viral: rabies, distemper, feline infectious peritonitis Bacterial: inoculation via wounds or hematogenous spread Fungal: cryptococcosis Protozoal: toxoplasmosis (dog and cat), neosporosis (dog) Rickettsial: Rocky Mountain spotted fever (*Rickettsia rickettsii* infection) Parasitic: cuterebriasis, visceral larva migrans
	Inflammatory	Granulomatous meningoencephalomyelitis, steroid-responsive meningitis/arteritis, necrotizing encephalitis (Yorkshire terrier, pug)
	Idiopathic	Epilepsy
T	Trauma	Traumatic brain injury
	Toxin	Bromethalin, theobromine, caffeine, lead, organophosphate poisoning
V	Vascular	Thromboembolic disease, intracranial hemorrhage

catteries and multicat households, feline infectious peritonitis becomes more likely.

Treatment

Treatment includes emergent anticonvulsant therapy and extracranial stabilization. A number of anticonvulsant drugs are effective in the acute setting, but careful patient monitoring is important. The management of extracranial complications and support of other organ systems is also of vital importance.

Emergent Anticonvulsant Therapy

It is vital that seizure activity be stopped as soon as possible to prevent continued injury to the brain and to reduce the potential for systemic sequelae. The goal of emergent anticonvulsant therapy is to stop all seizure activity immediately and to prevent all additional seizures for a 24-hour period. It should be recommended strongly to the owner of any patient with cluster seizures or status epilepticus that the animal be admitted to the hospital for a minimum of 24 hours for intravenous anticonvulsant therapy. If the patient has additional seizures within the first 24 hours of therapy, the 24 hour time period should be restarted.

Benzodiazepines

Intravenous diazepam (0.5 to 1.0 mg/kg) or midazolam (0.066 to 0.22 mg/kg) should be considered first-line therapy for patients with severe, acute seizures. These drugs are GABA agonists and cause hyperpolarization of neurons via influx of chloride ions, which results in cessation of seizure activity. They generally are effective and safe when given intravenously in dogs and cats, and have a low likelihood of significant adverse effects, although a small number of cats have been reported to develop fatal acute hepatic necrosis when administered diazepam orally. For patients in whom intravenous access is not readily available, diazepam at a dose of 1 to 2 mg/kg can be administered rectally and is absorbed rapidly. To ensure adequate retention of the drug when administered rectally, it should be injected through a red rubber catheter passed into the colon and flushed with saline or air. Intramuscular midazolam has also recently been shown to be as effective and safe as intravenous benzodiazepines for status epilepticus in people and may be considered an alternative to rectal diazepam in patients without IV access. If the patient responds to benzodiazepine therapy but shows rapid recrudescence, an intravenous constant-rate infusion should be considered. Diazepam at 0.5 to 2.0 mg/kg/hr often is effective, but the drug should be protected from light and drawn up from a glass vial freshly every 6 hours because of its capacity to bind to plastic.

Barbiturates

For those patients with seizures refractory to benzodiazepine therapy, barbiturates (pentobarbital, phenobarbital) sometimes can be effective. Phenobarbital is the barbiturate of choice for treating seizures. It is a highly effective anticonvulsant (2 to 6 mg/kg IV) but can take 15 to 20 minutes to show an effect. If an effect is not noted within 15 to 30 minutes, the dose may be repeated to raise blood levels to the therapeutic range more rapidly (to a maximum loading dose of 16 mg/kg within the first 24 hours); however, care must be taken to avoid overdose, which can cause hypoventilation or apnea. Close monitoring of ventilation via arterial or venous blood gas measurement or end-tidal capnography is recommended. Pentobarbital (2 to 15 mg/kg IV) can terminate the physical manifestations of seizure activity effectively within several minutes, but it generally is not considered to be an effective anticonvulsant, and its ability to stop seizure activity in the brain is questionable.

Propofol

Propofol is a rapidly acting injectable anesthetic that is a centrally acting GABA agonist. It may be administered to effect via slow intravenous injection at a dose of 1 to 6 mg/kg and has been shown to be effective at stopping seizure activity (cluster seizures and status epilepticus) in human and veterinary medicine. If the initial bolus dose is effective but seizures recur, a constant-rate infusion at 0.1 to 0.6 mg/kg/min may be instituted. Apnea, vasodilation, and cardiovascular depression are important adverse effects to consider, and it is the author's opinion that any animal receiving a propofol infusion should be intubated to protect the airway. Ventilation should be closely monitored to detect hypoventilation. Patients that persistently hypoventilate while receiving propofol may need to undergo mechanical ventilation.

Levetiracetam

Levetiracetam (Keppra) is a piracetam anticonvulsant that has shown efficacy for treatment of seizures in people and experimental animals. This drug exerts its anticonvulsant effect via several mechanisms, including stabilization of presynaptic vesicles by V2 receptor activation, which reduces the release of excitatory neurotransmitters. It does not appear to act via the more common neurotransmitter receptors or ion channels. It has a high bioavailability in dogs and is excreted unchanged in the urine without any significant hepatic metabolism. It has no sedative adverse effects. Intravenous administration is well tolerated in dogs, even at very high doses of 400 mg/kg (published oral dose is 20 mg/kg q8h PO). It is available in an intravenous formulation (also administered at 20 mg/kg IV as a bolus). Because of its high therapeutic index, intravenous administration may be repeated frequently in patients with cluster seizures or status epilepticus. There are limited but encouraging data suggesting that this drug also is effective in cats, both as monotherapy and as part of a multidrug anticonvulsant therapeutic regimen.

Extracranial Stabilization

Rapid identification and treatment of life-threatening extracranial sequelae of seizures is essential for successful case management and good patient outcome. Rapid primary assessment to identify cardiovascular or respiratory dysfunction and adequacy of systemic perfusion is crucial.

Hyperthermia

Sustained seizure activity produces a large amount of heat, overwhelming the body's cooling mechanisms and resulting in severely elevated body temperature. Body temperature should be measured as soon after presentation as possible. Any patient with a core body temperature higher than 40.6° C (105° F) should be cooled actively. Administering room temperature intravenous fluids, wetting the fur, cooling with fans, and placing the animal directly on a metal surface are recommended. Core body temperature should be rechecked frequently, preferably with the use of an indwelling rectal temperature probe. Active cooling should be discontinued when the temperature drops to 39.4° C (103° F) to reduce the risk of hypothermia. The use of ice packs or ice baths is not recommended because these can lead to peripheral vasoconstriction, which decreases radiant, convective, and conductive heat loss through the skin. The application of alcohol to the foot pads also is discouraged because the effectiveness of evaporative cooling over such a small surface area is questionable and the flammability of the alcohol puts the patient at risk, especially if electrical defibrillation is required should the patient experience cardiopulmonary arrest.

Hyperthermia can lead to many systemic sequelae, including DIC, hypoglycemia, acid-base disturbances, hypotension, pulmonary edema, and multiorgan failure. Meticulous serial monitoring of the patient after cooling is recommended and should include blood pressure measurement, assessment of oxygenation and ventilation status, and daily platelet counts to identify early signs of DIC.

Perfusion

Hypotension and poor perfusion are common in patients with cluster seizures and status epilepticus because of vasodilation secondary to hyperthermia or neurogenic shock and hypovolemia from fluid loss. Aggressive fluid therapy using isotonic crystalloids, hypertonic crystalloids, or synthetic colloids (see Chapter 2) should be initiated early in the course of treatment to normalize blood pressure. In patients with persistent, inappropriate vasodilation that remain hypotensive in the face of adequate volume resuscitation, pressor therapy (e.g., norepinephrine, or vasopressin) should be considered (Chapters 3 and 4), but only if hypovolemia has been addressed adequately first. Clinical signs of persistent vasodilation include hyperemic oral mucous membranes, fast capillary refill times (<1.5 sec), and bounding pulses. Patients with poor blood pressure and evidence of peripheral vasoconstriction (pale oral mucous membranes and capillary refill time of >2 sec) are unlikely to benefit from vasoconstrictors, and these drugs should be avoided. Recommended fluid resuscitation and vasopressor dosages are listed in Table 230-2.

Ventilation

The partial pressure of CO_2 in the arterial blood ($PaCO_2$) is a potent regulator of cerebrovascular tone. Normocapnia ($PaCO_2 > 35$ mm Hg and < 45 mm Hg) is essential for the maintenance of cerebral perfusion and prevention of cerebral hyperemia, which can cause increased

TABLE 230-2

Recommendations for Fluid Resuscitation in the Seizure Patient

Indication	Drug	Dosage	Comments
Fluid Resuscitation for Hypovolemia			
Dehydrated patients	Isotonic crystalloids (0.9% saline, lactated Ringer's, Normosol-R, Plasma-Lyte A)	20-30 ml/kg over 15 min; may be repeated	Generally safe, effective, and inexpensive. Repeat doses may be administered until resuscitation end points are achieved.
Euhydrated patients	Synthetic colloids (hetastarch, dextran 70, pentastarch)	5-10 ml/kg over 15 min; may be repeated	Volume expansion effects much greater than volume administered. Particularly useful in hypoproteinemic patients. May exacerbate coagulopathies or platelet disorders.
	Hypertonic saline (7%) + synthetic colloid	3-5 ml/kg over 15 min; may be repeated	Contraindicated in hyponatremic patients. Monitor serum sodium concentrations with repeat dosing. If using 23.4% solution, dilute 1 part hypertonic saline with 2 parts colloid.
	Hypertonic saline (7%-7.8%)	3-5 ml/kg over 15 min; may be repeated	Contraindicated in hyponatremic patients. Monitor serum sodium concentrations with repeat dosing. If using 23.4% solution, dilute 1 part hypertonic saline with 2 parts 0.9% saline or sterile water.
Vasopressor Therapy			
Vasodilation and hypotension in the face of adequate volume resuscitation	Norepinephrine	1-10 µg/kg/min	Potent vasoconstrictor with primarily α_1 effects. Start at 1 µg/kg/min and titrate up by 1 µg/kg/min q15 min until desired blood pressure is reached.
	Vasopressin	1-4 mU/kg/min	Very potent vasoconstrictor via V1 receptors. Start at 1 mU/kg/min and titrate up by 0.5 mU/kg/min until desired blood pressure reached.

intracranial pressure (ICP). Many anticonvulsants (e.g., benzodiazepines, barbiturates, propofol) can lead to sedation and hypoventilation, which requires intubation or tracheostomy and mechanical ventilation. Patients receiving constant-rate infusions of propofol should be intubated using a sterile endotracheal tube with an inflated cuff to reduce the risk of aspiration pneumonia because these patients often fail to protect the airway. The tube should be suctioned using sterile technique as needed. Acid-base disturbances and hyperthermia can lead to hyperventilation, which causes cerebral vasoconstriction and decreased delivery of oxygen and nutrients to the brain. These conditions should be treated aggressively to minimize effects on cerebral blood flow. Serial monitoring of ventilation is recommended for all patients during hospitalization. Arterial blood gas analysis is the preferred method, but the partial pressure of CO_2 (PCO_2) in venous blood never should be lower than that in arterial blood and can be used to monitor for hypoventilation. End-tidal CO_2 monitoring is useful in intubated patients for continuous monitoring of ventilation status.

Oxygenation

The brain has a high basal metabolic rate and is intolerant of deficits in oxygen and nutrient delivery. Supplemental oxygen should be provided to all patients with status epilepticus or cluster seizures via mask, oxygen cage, nasal catheter, or intubation. In cases of severe edema or pneumonia, mechanical ventilation may be required to address hypoxemia. Serial monitoring of oxygenation using pulse oximetry measurements or arterial blood gas analysis is recommended for all patients with status epilepticus or cluster seizures because of the risk of noncardiogenic pulmonary edema and aspiration pneumonia. Thoracic radiographs should be obtained after stabilization for any patient with persistent hypoxemia (pulse oximetry O_2 saturation < 95% on room air or PaO_2 < 80 mm Hg on room air). Oxygen-carrying capacity of the blood is determined primarily by the amount of hemoglobin present. Packed red blood cell or whole blood transfusion should be considered in anemic patients, especially if the anemia is acute.

Intracranial Stabilization

A number of treatments and physical modifications can be used to provide intracranial stabilization.

Mannitol

Because of accumulations of intracellular sodium and calcium and increased cerebral vascular permeability, cerebral edema is common during and after severe acute seizures. Mannitol is a highly effective therapy for patients with increased ICP and has been shown to reduce cerebral edema, increase cerebral perfusion pressure and cerebral blood flow, and improve neurologic outcome in patients with cerebral edema. It has a rapid onset of action, with clinical improvement occurring within minutes of

TABLE 230-3

Drugs and Dosages for Treatment of Increased Intracranial Pressure (ICP) in the Seizure Patient

Indication	Drug	Dosage	Notes
Increased ICP in normotensive or hypertensive patients	Mannitol 25%	0.5-1.0 g/kg IV over 15 min; may be repeated	Can lead to severe dehydration. Treat with crystalloids to prevent dehydration and hypovolemia. Closely monitor fluid input and output.
	Hypertonic saline (7%)	3-5 ml/kg over 15 min; may be repeated	Dilute 1 part 23.4% hypertonic saline with 2 parts sterile water or normal saline. Do not use in hyponatremic or hypernatremic patients because may cause rapid changes in serum sodium concentrations. Monitor serum sodium levels.
Increased ICP in hypovolemic/ hypotensive patients	Hypertonic saline (7%) + dextran or hetastarch	Dogs: 4 ml/kg over 15 min Cats: 2 ml/kg over 15 min May be repeated	Dilute 1 part 23.4% hypertonic saline with 2 parts hetastarch or dextran 70. Do not use in hyponatremic patients because may cause rapid changes in serum sodium concentrations. Monitor serum sodium levels.
	Hypertonic saline (7%)	2-4 ml/kg over 15 min; may be repeated	Dilute 1 part 23.4% hypertonic saline with 2 parts sterile water or normal saline. *Do not* administer undiluted 23.4% hypertonic saline. Do not use in hyponatremic patients because may cause rapid changes in serum sodium concentrations. Monitor serum sodium levels.

administration, and these effects can last as long as 1.5 to 6 hours. Mannitol boluses of 0.5 to 1.0 g/kg IV over 15 to 20 minutes have been recommended for treatment of increased ICP in dogs and cats (see Table 230-3 for dosing and indications). The diuretic effect of mannitol can be profound and can cause severe volume depletion and rebound hypotension. Therefore treatment must be followed by administration of isotonic crystalloid solutions or colloids to maintain intravascular volume.

Hypertonic Saline
Hypertonic saline (HTS) is a hyperosmotic solution that may be used as an alternative to mannitol in patients with cerebral edema at a dose of 4 ml/kg over 15 to 20 minutes in dogs and 2 ml/kg in cats (see Table 230-3 for dosing and indications). Because sodium does not freely cross an intact blood-brain barrier, HTS has osmotic effects similar to those of mannitol. Other beneficial effects of HTS include improved hemodynamic status via volume expansion and positive inotropic effects, as well as beneficial vasoregulatory and immunomodulatory effects. Rebound hypotension is uncommon with HTS administration because, unlike mannitol, sodium is reabsorbed actively in the kidneys, especially in hypovolemic patients. This makes it preferable to mannitol for treating patients with increased ICP and systemic hypotension due to hypovolemia. In euvolemic patients with evidence of elevated ICP, either mannitol or HTS may be a useful treatment option. If one drug is not having the desired clinical effect, treatment with the other may be successful.

Body Positioning
Facilitating venous drainage from the brain also can reduce ICP and maintain cerebral perfusion to the injured brain. Placing the patient on a slant board at a 15- to 30-degree angle has been shown to optimize venous drainage while maintaining cerebral blood flow. Placing pillows or towels under the head should be avoided because bending the neck may result in occlusion of the jugular vein, which negates the beneficial effect of head elevation.

Minimization of Cerebral Metabolic Rate
The injured brain is at risk of ischemic damage due to decreased delivery of oxygen caused by elevated ICP as well as increased metabolic demand. Drugs that increase cerebral metabolism, including nitrous oxide and ketamine, should be avoided in these patients.

Corticosteroids
Although treatment with corticosteroids has been shown to be beneficial in patients with brain tumors because it reduces peritumor vasogenic edema, there is no evidence to support the use of these drugs in patients with seizure disorders due to any other cause. Recent data from a large human clinical trial showed that in patients with brain injury caused by trauma, the use of high-dose corticosteroids in the acute setting resulted in worse outcomes than with placebo. Given the similarity between the neuronal damage resulting from trauma and that caused by seizures, the use of corticosteroids in most patients with status epilepticus or cluster seizures is not recommended.

Prognosis

The prognosis for dogs and cats experiencing status epilepticus and cluster seizures has not been well studied but likely depends strongly on the underlying cause of the seizures. Animals with idiopathic epilepsy generally have a fair chance of enjoying a reasonable quality of life but are likely to require lifelong anticonvulsant therapy and are at risk of escalation of disease with every cluster of seizures or episode of status epilepticus. Patients with evidence of DIC due to hyperthermia at presentation have a guarded prognosis, are at risk of multiorgan failure, and often require intensive therapy, including administration of blood products and prolonged hospitalization. With rapid, targeted therapy, many patients with these disorders can be managed effectively long term, depending on the underlying cause of the seizures.

References and Suggested Reading

Dewey CW: Anticonvulsant therapy in dogs and cats, *Vet Clin North Am Small Anim Pract* 36(5):1107, 2006.

Dewey CW: *A practical guide to canine and feline neurology*, Ames, IA, 2009, Iowa State Press.

Lorenz MD, Coates J, Kent M: *Handbook of veterinary neurology*, ed 5, Philadelphia, 2010, Saunders.

Platt SR, McDonnell JJ: Status epilepticus: clinical features and pathophysiology, *Compend Contin Educ Pract Vet* 22(7):660, 2000.

CHAPTER 231

Treatment of Noninfectious Inflammatory Diseases of the Central Nervous System

LAUREN R. TALARICO, *Fairfax, Virginia*

Noninfectious inflammatory diseases commonly affect the central nervous system (CNS) of small animal patients. These diseases primarily cause inflammation of the brain parenchyma (encephalitis) or meninges (meningoencephalitis).

Overview

Among the subtypes of inflammatory CNS disease are granulomatous meningoencephalitis, necrotizing meningoencephalitis, necrotizing leukoencephalitis, and eosinophilic meningoencephalitis, referred to as *GME, NME, NLE,* and *EME*, respectively. GME has been reported to affect the spinal cord and cause a subsequent meningomyelitis. Steroid-responsive meningitis-arteritis (SRMA) is another suspected autoimmune disorder that affects primarily the spinal cord; this disorder is not considered here. As a group, these diseases often are referred to as *meningoencephalitis of unknown cause* because antemortem diagnosis is difficult to achieve in most cases. Given the increasing availability of less invasive stereotactic brain biopsy instruments guided by magnetic resonance imaging (MRI) or computed tomography (CT), we anticipate that definitive diagnoses will become more attainable in the near future.

The disorders NME and NLE sometimes are referred to as *pug dog encephalitis* and *Yorkshire terrier encephalitis*, respectively. It is important to realize that dogs of many other breeds can develop NME and NLE and that these disorders are not exclusive to pug and Yorkshire terrier breeds. The author also has diagnosed GME in pug dogs and Yorkshire terriers and therefore advises against using this breed-specific terminology. Furthermore, the majority of the literature contains reports of noninfectious meningoencephalitis (NIME) in small-breed dogs; however, the author has definitively diagnosed GME in several large-breed retriever dogs.

To date, a definitive cause of granulomatous, necrotizing, and eosinophilic meningoencephalitides has not been established. Genetic, infectious, and autoimmune causes have been proposed. A recent study by Barber et al (2010) evaluating the results of polymerase chain reaction testing of brain tissue and cerebrospinal fluid (CSF) demonstrated that *Ehrlichia, Anaplasma, Rickettsia,* and *Borrelia* are unlikely to be associated with NIME; however, the role of *Bartonella* still is uncertain. It is the author's belief that GME, NME, NLE, and EME are autoimmune in origin, and this constitutes the basis for our therapeutic approach. An underlying genetic predisposition for these diseases also may play a role.

Clinical Signs

The majority of NIME cases are small-breed dogs between 2 and 6 years of age brought in because of peracute- or acute-onset multifocal neurologic signs. Patients with noninfectious CNS inflammatory diseases rarely have extraneural signs, and results of routine blood work usually are unremarkable. The specific deficits found on the neurologic examination reflect the location of the lesion within the brain, meninges, and spinal cord. Typically multiple areas of the brain are affected. Animals with forebrain involvement can have seizures and show behavioral or mentation changes, circling, pacing, head pressing, and central blindness with normal pupillary light reflexes. Signs referable to brainstem involvement can include severe mental depression varying from obtundation to coma; mydriasis; hemiparesis or hemiplegia; tetraparesis or tetraplegia; decreased palpebral, corneal, and gag reflexes; facial and trigeminal paralysis; and central vestibular signs. Cerebellar signs, including intention tremors, titubation, hypermetria or dysmetria, and absent menace response with normal vision often are encountered. Head pain with or without neck pain is likely secondary to inflammation of the meninges. Animals with head pain back away when the examiner attempts to pet the head, and their eyes often appear squinted.

Clinical signs typically are progressive, but the rate of progression varies. It is important to realize that the severity of a patient's clinical signs at presentation is not correlated with survival time or achievement of disease remission.

Diagnosis

NIME is a histopathologic diagnosis, and a definitive antemortem diagnosis is not often achieved. With the advent of minimally invasive stereotactic MRI- or CT-guided brain biopsy tools at veterinary referral centers and veterinary colleges, definitive antemortem diagnoses are becoming more frequent. Nevertheless, the majority of cases are diagnosed presumptively based on a combination of signalment, clinical signs, MRI, and spinal fluid analysis (CSF tap). Infectious encephalitis, congenital malformations, storage diseases, toxin exposure, and neoplasia are differential diagnoses for multifocal neurologic signs with peracute onset in a young adult animal. A minimum data set consisting of results of a complete blood count, chemistry panel, urinalysis, and thoracic radiographs often is within normal limits.

MRI and CSF analysis provide the most helpful information for making a presumptive diagnosis. MRI typically reveals multifocal infiltrative lesions within the brain parenchyma that are hyperintense on T2-weighted and FLAIR (fluid-attenuation inversion recovery) images and hypointense to isointense compared with the surrounding parenchyma on T1-weighted sequences. Contrast enhancement is variable. The meninges also can be hyperintense on T2-weighted and T1-weighted postcontrast sequences. The lesion and associated edema often are space occupying, causing compression of the surrounding brain parenchyma and a midline shift. In extreme cases,

subfalcine and/or transtentorial herniation of the caudal cerebellum through the foramen magnum will occur.

GME tends to have a predilection for the white matter and typically affects both the brainstem and forebrain. There is a focal form of GME that produces a solitary space-occupying mass lesion which can closely resemble a neoplastic process. The majority of NME cases are supratentorial in distribution, predominately affecting both the gray and white matter of the forebrain. NLE is characterized by defacement of the white matter of both the brainstem and cerebral cortex. Additionally, the necrotizing encephalitides (NME and NLE) can be associated with visible areas of necrosis within the brain parenchyma in addition to inflammatory lesions as described earlier. Occasionally the MRI findings are normal and the diagnosis is based solely on the results of CSF analysis.

CNS inflammation is best documented by CSF analysis, consisting of cytologic examination and protein evaluation. GME, NME, and NLE are characterized by mononuclear cell pleocytosis (elevated lymphocytes and monocytes) and elevated protein level. These CSF findings are nonspecific because they cannot discriminate between autoimmune, neoplastic, viral, and protozoal CNS infections. EME is characterized by eosinophilic pleocytosis and elevated protein level. Differential diagnoses for eosinophilic pleocytosis are parasitic, protozoal, autoimmune, and neoplastic diseases. Cell counts and protein level can be quite variable, ranging from zero to several thousand cells per microliter and zero to several hundred grams per deciliter, respectively. The magnitude of the pleocytosis or protein level in the CSF is not prognostic. Occasionally the CSF tap findings can be normal, especially if the patient recently received corticosteroids. It is possible that animals with normal imaging findings but CSF results consistent with NIME are being seen early in the disease process before the formation of brain lesions.

Treatment

A standardized treatment regimen for NIME has yet to be determined, and the mainstay of treatment is aggressive immunosuppression. At the Cornell University Hospital for Animals, we treat GME, NME, NLE, and EME with a similar protocol which is based on the presumption that these diseases are autoimmune in origin. The combination of immunosuppressive agents used and the timing of their administration is individualized for each patient. It is important that a presumptive diagnosis be made (see earlier) before therapy is initiated. In addition to the diagnostic studies listed previously, we recommend routine infectious disease testing for toxoplasmosis, neosporosis, cryptococcosis, rickettsial diseases, and canine distemper to ensure that the underlying disease truly is noninfectious. In severe cases in which the animal's clinical status is declining rapidly, aggressive immunosuppression must be implemented before the results of infectious disease testing are available.

Corticosteroids

Initial therapy consists of immunosuppressive dosages of prednisone (1 to 2 mg/kg twice daily PO) for a minimum of 3 to 4 months. If the patient's mental status precludes the use of oral medications, an equivalent dose of dexamethasone can be given intravenously. In addition to having immunomodulatory properties, corticosteroids decrease perilesional edema and ideally improve neurologic signs. Treatment of NIME with corticosteroid monotherapy generally results in a guarded to poor prognosis, and relapses are common. In a study by Munana and Luttgen (1998), the mean survival time for 30 dogs with histopathologically confirmed GME treated with prednisone monotherapy was 14 days (range, 1 to >1215 days). These results may be biased toward the most severe cases because postmortem histopathologic confirmation of GME was an inclusion criterion. The dose of prednisone used in this study also was variable (0.25 mg/kg to 2 mg/kg twice daily), which possibly accounted for the variable survival times. A recent study reporting survival data for dogs treated with corticosteroid monotherapy noted a survival time of 357 days when the drug was administered at 1 to 2 mg/kg twice daily and tapered over a 3-month period.

Several unwanted side effects including polyuria, polydipsia, polyphagia, weight gain, liver and gastrointestinal damage, pancreatitis, and iatrogenic endocrinopathies can result from long-term steroid therapy. In an effort to maintain the patient's quality of life and owner compliance, the author typically uses a multimodal drug protocol (see later). The goal is to induce a clinical remission as soon as possible and to taper the dose of corticosteroids slowly to the lowest effective dose to minimize unwanted drug-related side effects. In the author's experience, most NIME patients require prolonged low-dose corticosteroid therapy to maintain remission.

Other Immunosuppressive Therapies

The reported overall median survival time ranges from 240 to 590 days for dogs treated with corticosteroids plus any other immunosuppressive drug combination (cyclosporine, lomustine, procarbazine, mycophenolate, cytarabine arabinoside, or leflunomide) compared with 28 to 357 days for those treated with corticosteroids alone.

At the Cornell University Hospital for Animals, NIME cases are treated using an aggressive multimodal immunosuppressive drug regimen. Our initial therapeutic protocol consists of immunosuppressive doses of prednisone (1 mg/kg twice daily PO), cyclosporine (4 mg/kg twice daily PO), and cytarabine (200 to 600 mg/m^2 as a constant-rate infusion over 24 hours). While infectious disease titers are awaited, doxycycline (10 mg/kg once daily PO) and clindamycin (10 mg/kg twice daily PO) also are administered. Patients that do not experience clinical remission within the first 48 to 72 hours of treatment according to this protocol are given additional immunosuppressive medications, including procarbazine, azathioprine, leflunomide, or some combination of these.

Cytarabine (cytosine arabinoside) is a chemotherapeutic agent. At the recommended dosages, it has immunosuppressive properties and can cross the blood-brain barrier, which makes it useful in the treatment of suspected autoimmune meningoencephalitis. Cytarabine exerts its effects on actively dividing cells by causing premature strand breaks and inhibition of repair. Commonly reported adverse effects include leukopenia and mild gastrointestinal upset. At the author's institution we administer this medication as a constant-rate infusion over 24 or 48 hours based on the clinical severity of the patient's neurologic signs. Previous reports have described giving this medication as four subcutaneous injections 12 hours apart over a 48-hour period. Our decision to administer this drug as a constant-rate infusion is based on the requirement for prolonged exposure to cytarabine to maintain minimum cytotoxic concentrations in the CNS. A complete blood count is performed 10 to 14 days after the first administration of the drug. If results are normal, continued monitoring of the leukocyte count is done every 4 to 6 months.

We administer cytarabine initially at 3-week intervals. Cytarabine regimens are individualized for each patient, and the interval between treatments is extended gradually over several months based on serial neurologic examinations. The cytarabine treatment intervals are increased until 8-week intervals are achieved. If the patient has not shown any indication of disease relapse after three rounds of cytarabine treatment at 8-week intervals, our group performs a repeat spinal tap to determine if the CNS inflammation has subsided. If the CSF results are normal, cytarabine treatments are discontinued.

Signs that a patient may be coming out of remission can be subtle and include inappetence, lethargy, depression, increased seizure frequency, or recurrence of initial neurologic signs. When an animal comes out of remission, we recommend increasing the prednisone dosage to 1 to 2 mg/kg twice daily PO, administering cytarabine as a constant-rate infusion (400 to 600 mg/m^2) over 24 hours, and instituting treatment with another immunosuppressive agent such as procarbazine, azathioprine, lomustine, or leflunomide.

Other Treatments

In addition to receiving immunosuppressive therapy, patients with seizures should be treated concurrently with anticonvulsant medications. Most NIME patients have mental obtundation, stupor, or coma as part of their underlying disease process. We recommend the use of anticonvulsants with minimal sedative side effects, including zonisamide (5 to 10 mg/kg twice daily PO) or levetiracetam (20 mg/kg three times daily PO or IV). If the patient's seizures are not adequately controlled, phenobarbital (2 to 4 mg/kg twice daily PO) is administered.

Patients with severe mental obtundation, stupor, or coma also should be treated with intravenous mannitol as needed (1 g/kg repeated as necessary). Fluid resuscitation and other supportive therapies such as oxygen administration also must be instituted on a case-by-case basis.

Prognosis

Historically, the prognosis for NIME has been considered to be guarded to poor. Clinical remission is achieved in the majority of the cases seen at the Cornell University Hospital for Animals within the first 24 to 36 hours of treatment. Relapses are uncommon at our institution, but do occur, and we counsel owners thoroughly to ensure that they are able to recognize subtle signs of a potential relapse. The average survival time for patients with NIME treated at the Cornell University Hospital for Animals is 2 to 3 years. With the advent of minimally invasive stereotactic brain biopsy equipment, it is our hope that definitive antemortem diagnoses will be achieved and more accurate data on survival times obtained.

References and Suggested Reading

Barber RM et al: Evaluation of brain tissue or cerebrospinal fluid with broadly reactive polymerase chain reaction for Ehrlichia, Anaplasma, spotted fever group *Rickettsia, Bartonella,* and *Borrelia* species in canine neurological diseases (109 cases), *J Vet Intern Med* 24:2, 2010.

Flegel T et al: Magnetic resonance imaging findings in histologically confirmed pug dog encephalitis, *Vet Radiol Ultrasound* 49:5, 2008.

Granger N, Smith PM, Jeffery ND: Clinical findings and treatment of non-infectious meningoencephalomyelitis in dogs: a systematic review of 457 published cases from 1962 to 2008, *Vet J* 184:3, 2010.

Munana KR, Luttgen PJ: Prognostic factors for dogs with granulomatous meningoencephalomyelitis: 42 cases (1982-1996), *J Am Vet Med Assoc* 212:12, 1998.

Scott-Moncrieff JC et al: Plasma and cerebrospinal fluid pharmacokinetics of cytosine arabinoside in dogs, *Cancer Chemother Pharmacol* 29:13, 1991.

Talarico LR, Schatzberg SJ: Idiopathic granulomatous and necrotizing inflammatory disorders of the canine central nervous system: a review and future perspectives, *J Small Anim Pract* 51:3, 2010.

CHAPTER **232**

Peripheral and Central Vestibular Disorders in Dogs and Cats

STARR CAMERON, *Ithaca, New York*
CURTIS W. DEWEY, *Ithaca, New York*

The vestibular system maintains the body's posture and balance. The vestibular system coordinates and communicates the position of the head in relation to the body and the body in relation to the ground. Vestibular disease is one of the more common presentations of an animal with neurologic disease, and it also can be one of the most terrifying for the owner to witness. This chapter reviews pertinent anatomy of the vestibular system, clinical signs of dysfunction, and some of the more common disease processes affecting the peripheral and central vestibular systems.

Vestibular Anatomy

A basic understanding of the neuroanatomy of the vestibular system is very helpful in neurolocalization, which aids in distinguishing the differential diagnoses and thus in selecting the diagnostic tests and treatments required.

Peripheral Vestibular System

The peripheral vestibular system is located within the inner ear and consists of receptors and the vestibular portion of cranial nerve VIII (vestibulocochlear nerve). The bony labyrinth, which is located in the petrous temporal bone, consists of the semicircular canals, vestibule, and cochlea and is filled with perilymph. The membranous labyrinth, filled with endolymph, is located within the bony labyrinth and is composed of the semicircular ducts, utricle, saccule, and cochlear duct. The semicircular ducts are located within the semicircular canals, the utricle and saccule are located within the vestibule, and the cochlear duct is located within the cochlea. The crista ampullaris is located in the semicircular ducts and responds to acceleration, deceleration, and rotation. Hair cells in the crista ampullaris respond to displacement of the endolymph. The dendrites of cranial nerve VIII synapse on these hair cells and are stimulated when they deflect.

Maculae are receptors located in the utricle and saccule that respond to linear movement. The surface is covered by hair cells that trigger an action potential in cranial nerve VIII when they are deflected. The receptors provide continual tonic input to cranial nerve VII, which functions to maintain normal posture of the head and body.

Central Vestibular System

The central vestibular system consists of the vestibular nuclei located in the medulla and the projections to the spinal cord, brainstem, and cerebellum. Spinal cord projections from the vestibular nuclei exert facilitatory and inhibitory effects on ipsilateral extensors and flexors, respectively. These projections also inhibit contralateral extensors. Brainstem projections relay information to the motor neurons of cranial nerves III, IV, and VI (oculomotor, trochlear, and abducens nerves, respectively) via the medial longitudinal fasciculus. These projections are responsible for normal eye position and physiologic nystagmus. Other brainstem projections are directed to the vomiting center within the reticular formation. Cerebellar projections travel via the caudal cerebellar peduncle to the vestibulocerebellum to maintain coordination.

Clinical Signs of Vestibular Disease

Nystagmus can be physiologic or pathologic and usually has a fast and a slow phase. Physiologic, or naturally occurring, nystagmus can be elicited during the neurologic examination by testing the vestibuloocular reflex, as by moving the head in a lateral or medial direction. Physiologic nystagmus requires coordination between the vestibular system and cranial nerves III, IV, and VI and the medial longitudinal fasciculus. Some animals, such as the Siamese cat, have resting nystagmus, which is considered normal for the breed.

Pathologic nystagmus is the jerking eye movements seen with physiologic nystagmus but it occurs when the head is at rest. Pathologic nystagmus can occur when the animal is in a normal position, termed *resting nystagmus,* or when the animal is put in an unusual position such as on its back, termed *positional nystagmus.* Traditionally, the nystagmus is characterized by the direction of the fast phase, and in most cases this movement is away from the lesion. For example, nystagmus in which the fast phase is toward the left and the slow phase is toward the right is termed *fast phase left* and is suggestive of a left-sided lesion in most cases. This terminology can be confusing, and a way to help remember the direction is the mnemonic that the nystagmus is "running away" from the lesion.

Strabismus is an abnormal eye position. Strabismus may be spontaneous (occurring at rest) or positional. In vestibular disease strabismus is either ventral or ventrolateral and occurs on the same (ipsilateral) side as the lesion.

Ataxia describes an uncoordinated gait. Vestibular ataxia is characterized by turning, rolling, falling, or circling to the side of the lesion. Usually it is very asymmetric and generally the circles are very tight circles. Some animals may be unwilling to walk and some have a broad-based stance.

A head tilt often is present in vestibular disease and usually is toward the side of the lesion. Head tilts can range from very mild to quite severe. For reasons unknown, a head tilt often persists long term or indefinitely after resolution of the other clinical signs of vestibular disease.

Peripheral Vestibular Disease

Peripheral vestibular disease is characterized by any combination of vestibular ataxia, head tilt, strabismus, and nystagmus. With peripheral disease the nystagmus can be in any direction, but vertical nystagmus is extremely rare in peripheral disease and should be considered central in origin. Many believe that nystagmus associated with peripheral disease should not change in character or direction, but nothing definitive has been published regarding this finding. Nystagmus can be spontaneous,or positional.

It is important not to misinterpret vestibular ataxia as proprioceptive deficits. Animals with peripheral vestibular disease often have quite dramatic clinical signs, and examining them thoroughly can be challenging. It is important to support the animal's weight during proprioception to prevent orthopedic disease or weakness from interfering with the ability of the animal to replace the paw to a normal position.

Bilateral vestibular disease can be confused easily with a more central condition because the clinical signs often are symmetric. Animals with bilateral vestibular disease tend to walk low to the ground in a crouched position and often fall to both sides. Lateral head excursions are common with bilateral vestibular disease. A head tilt and vestibuloocular reflex often are absent.

Central Vestibular Disease

Central vestibular disease has several hallmark features that can distinguish it from peripheral vestibular disease (Table 232-1). Central lesions may be accompanied by a change in mentation; for example, the animal may be overly dull or obtunded. If abnormalities in other cranial nerves, besides cranial nerves VII and VIII, are found on neurologic examination, then a central lesion should be considered. Proprioceptive deficits often are present with central lesions and are characterized by decreased placing or hopping on the side ipsilateral to the lesion. Any form of nystagmus, including vertical or changing nystagmus,

TABLE **232-1**

Clinical Signs of Peripheral versus Central Vestibular Disease

Neurologic Sign	Peripheral	Central
Head tilt	Yes	Yes
Strabismus	Yes	Yes
Nystagmus	Yes	Yes
Horizontal	Yes	Yes
Rotary	Yes	Yes
Vertical	No	Yes
Cranial nerve deficits (other than in cranial nerves VII or VIII)	No	Possible
Change in mentation	No	Possible
Proprioceptive deficits	No	Possible

may be present with central lesions. The other signs listed for peripheral vestibular disease, such as ataxia, head tilt, and strabismus, also can be seen with central lesions.

Paradoxic vestibular disease is the term used to describe the situation in which head tilt is contralateral to the lesion. Paradoxic vestibular disease always is a central lesion and occurs due to early disinhibition of the vestibular nuclei. All clinical signs seen with conventional central lesions may be observed with paradoxic vestibular disease. The proprioceptive deficits are always on the side of the lesion. For instance, a dog with a right-sided head tilt and left-sided proprioceptive deficits would have a left-sided central paradoxic lesion.

Causes of Vestibular Disease

The cause of the vestibular disease is a consideration in terms of both prognosis and therapy. Furthermore, different diagnostic tests may be appropriate based on the location-determined differential diagnosis for the lesion.

Peripheral Vestibular Disease

Otitis media/interna is the most common infectious cause of peripheral vestibular disease and accounts for up to 50% of canine peripheral vestibular disease cases. With otitis media/interna, cranial nerve VII, the facial nerve, also may be affected. Bilateral otitis media/interna can cause signs of bilateral vestibular disease. An otoscopic examination should be performed in every animal that has peripheral vestibular signs at presentation (see Chapter 108). Animals with chronic ear disease often have a stenotic or inflamed external ear canal, which can make examining the ear difficult or impossible. In addition, the presence of an intact tympanic membrane does not exclude otitis media/interna as a differential diagnosis. Bulla radiography, computed tomography (CT), or magnetic resonance imaging (MRI) can be used to investigate the internal ear structures further if otitis media interna is suspected. A myringotomy can be performed to collect samples for cytologic analysis and culture so that appropriate treatment can be initiated. Treatment should include cleaning the ears with solutions that are not ototoxic as well as administering systemic antibiotics for 6 to 8 weeks. Ideally the antibiotics should be chosen based on culture and sensitivity testing of a sample obtained by myringotomy. However, if a myringotomy is not possible, then broad-spectrum antibiotics should be used. If the animal shows no response to medical treatment, then a surgical procedure such as a bulla osteotomy or total ear canal ablation should be considered.

Ototoxicity has been reported with aminoglycoside antibiotics, erythromycin, furosemide, chemotherapy agents containing platinum, and certain ear-cleaning solutions. Vestibular signs may resolve if the medication is removed promptly. Deafness frequently accompanies vestibular signs and often is permanent.

Idiopathic (geriatric, old dog) vestibular disease is one of the most common causes of peripheral vestibular signs. If an animal is exhibiting clinical signs suggesting a central lesion, then the disorder cannot be idiopathic vestibular disease. Idiopathic vestibular disease also has been reported in cats but much less commonly than in dogs. Cats may be any age at presentation, whereas dogs tend to be older. Vestibular signs may be mild or quite severe, and the onset usually is acute. Clinical signs may take 2 to 3 weeks to resolve completely, but signs of improvement often are seen within 48 to 72 hours. Although many theories have been proposed regarding the origin of the disorder, no definitive cause has yet been found.

Congenital vestibular disease is uncommon but has been reported in Doberman pinschers, English cocker spaniels, Akitas, beagles, and German shepherd dogs. Siamese, Tonkanese, and Burmese cats also are known to be affected. Animals are young at presentation and may show bilateral vestibular signs. No definitive abnormality has been identified as the underlying cause, and there is no treatment for congenital vestibular disease.

Hypothyroidism can cause vestibular signs as well as affect cranial nerve VII, the facial nerve. Other clinical signs of hypothyroidism also may be present. It is important to measure thyroid function in an animal with peripheral vestibular signs when other causes of vestibular dysfunction have been ruled out. Clinical signs should resolve once the animal is receiving appropriate thyroid hormone supplementation.

Neoplasia such as ceruminous gland adenocarcinoma, squamous cell carcinoma, fibrosarcoma, chondrosarcoma, osteosarcoma, and lymphoma may affect the middle or inner ear. In addition, peripheral nerve sheath tumors can affect or compress cranial nerve VIII. Some tumors may be visible on otoscopic examination; however, CT or MRI may be needed. Depending on tumor location and extent of invasion, it may be possible to biopsy or even excise some tumors.

Inflammatory polyps may cause peripheral vestibular signs in addition to upper respiratory tract or pharyngeal disease. Polyps are much more common in cats than in dogs and usually cause unilateral signs. Polyps may be visualized with an oral or otoscopic examination. Removal of the polyp usually is possible. Recurrence has been noted with oral removal of the polyp as well as with bulla osteotomy and total ear canal ablation.

Finally, trauma to the petrous temporal bone is very rare but is possible, and can result in peripheral vestibular signs.

Central Vestibular Disease

Metronidazole toxicity has been shown to cause central vestibular signs in both dogs and cats and usually is associated with very high dosages of the drug (>60 mg/kg/day), although toxicity also can be seen with long-term use of lower dosages. Asking about metronidazole use always should be included as part of the history taking for an animal with central vestibular signs. Stopping the metronidazole treatment usually leads to resolution of clinical vestibular signs within 1 to 2 weeks, with an average of approximately 11 days. However, recently it was shown that administering diazepam at an initial IV bolus of 0.4 mg/kg, followed by 0.4 mg/kg PO q8h for 3 days, shortened the duration of clinical signs to a median of 38 hours.

Thiamine deficiency has been correlated with central vestibular signs in both dogs and cats and causes areas of necrosis and hemorrhage. Deficiency most commonly occurs when animals are fed cooked diets or diets that contain thiaminase. In cats the vestibular nuclei often are affected, which produces central vestibular signs. If the deficiency is diagnosed and treated early, animals may recover with appropriate thiamine supplementation.

Inflammatory disease, such as granulomatous meningoencephalomyelitis (GME), may cause vestibular signs, depending on the area of the brain affected (see Chapter 231). GME usually is seen in young to middle-aged small-breed dogs, but dogs of any breed or age may be affected. A diagnosis of GME usually is obtained by MRI and cerebrospinal fluid (CSF) analysis, along with negative results on infectious disease titers. GME is a very aggressive disease and should be treated aggressively with immunosuppressive medications. The prognosis is quite variable, and the severity of clinical signs at presentation does not correlate with short- or long-term prognosis.

Infectious organisms may enter the central nervous system and cause central vestibular signs. Viral infections include canine distemper and feline infectious peritonitis. There are no available treatments for either of these diseases, and prognosis is grave. Neosporosis, toxoplasmosis, cryptococcosis, coccidioidomycosis, blastomycosis, prototothecosis, Rocky Mountain spotted fever, and ehrlichiosis are other infections that may affect the vestibular system. In addition, infection from otitis media interna can extend into the brain if severe.

Neoplasia can compress or infiltrate any area of the vestibular system. Meningiomas, choroid plexus carcinomas, gliomas, adenocarcinomas, squamous cell carcinomas, and lymphomas all have been reported to cause central vestibular signs. Intracranial arachnoid cysts are nonneoplastic but space-occupying masses that may compress the cerebellum or brainstem and cause central vestibular signs. Depending on the location and tumor type, a combination of surgery, chemotherapy, and radiation therapy may be used for palliation or potential cure.

Vascular events such as infarcts or transient ischemic attacks (TIAs) are diagnosed with increasing frequency. The possibility of a vascular event should be considered in an animal with central or paradoxic vestibular signs. Both infarcts and TIAs can cause abrupt vestibular signs, and the signs of TIAs often improve within 24 hours. Diagnostic testing such as serum biochemistry studies, complete blood count, thyroid panel, and blood pressure measurement should be undertaken to investigate the cause of the infarct or TIA. If an underlying disease process is not found and properly treated, the animal is at greater risk of having another infarct or TIA.

Hypothyroidism has been reported to cause central vestibular signs as well as peripheral vestibular signs. Therefore a thyroid panel should be included as part of a workup for central vestibular disease. The pathophysiology is thought to be related to infarction from atherosclerosis secondary to hypothyroidism. Dogs usually recover with appropriate hormone supplementation.

Paradoxic vestibular disease occurs with lesions in the cerebellum or medulla. Signs of paradoxic vestibular disease usually are caused by a vascular or space-occupying lesion, such as a neoplasm or intracranial arachnoid cyst. However, vascular events also may cause paradoxic vestibular signs.

Diagnostic Tests

A thorough history taking and physical and neurologic examinations are important for localizing the disease to the vestibular system as well as for differentiating peripheral from central vestibular causes (see earlier section on clinical signs). A history of ear infections, topical ear treatments, consumption of a thiamine-deficient diet, or metronidazole ingestion could provide direction for further diagnostic testing and treatments. Physical examination findings consistent with an ear infection, clinical signs of hypothyroidism, or indications of an underlying coagulopathy could be suggestive of the underlying cause of the vestibular signs. As discussed previously, mentation changes, proprioceptive deficits, cranial nerve abnormalities (apart from those in cranial nerve VII or VIII), and the presence of vertical nystagmus are signs indicative of a central lesion.

A workup for peripheral vestibular disease in a dog should include an otoscopic examination, complete blood count, biochemistry studies, urinalysis, thyroid panel, and blood pressure measurement. Clinical signs indicative of a central lesion warrant further investigation in addition to the diagnostic tests listed previously, such as MRI and CSF analysis. An MRI scan may show neoplasia, evidence of an inflammatory brain disease, or an intracranial arachnoid cyst. CSF analysis may help support the diagnosis of a vascular event or inflammatory disease. In addition, in cases in which an infectious cause is suspected, titers may be performed specifically on the CSF or blood. Routinely, titers are ordered for *Neospora, Toxoplasma, Rickettsia rickettsii*, distemper virus (dogs only), *Cryptococcus, Anaplasma*, and *Ehrlichia* when an infectious cause is strongly suspected.

Treatment and Prognosis

The treatment and prognosis for vestibular disease depends completely on the underlying cause. Idiopathic vestibular disease often has the most dramatic presentation, yet it carries a very good prognosis. Animals with central vestibular disease may have had the intracranial lesion longer and therefore have learned to compensate for their disease, and they often have the most subtle signs at presentation. Benign and sinister causes can be cited for both peripheral and central vestibular disease. Therefore no animal should be condemned to a poor prognosis without identification of the underlying lesion or, in the case of idiopathic vestibular disease, the passage of time.

References and Suggested Reading

Bischoff MG, Kneller SK: Diagnostic imaging of the canine and feline ear, *Vet Clin North Am Small Anim Pract* 34(2):437, 2004.

Caylor KB, Cassimatis MK: Metronidazole neurotoxicosis in two cats, *J Am Anim Hosp Assoc* 37(3):258, 2001.

Cherubini GB et al: Rostral cerebellar arterial infarct in two cats, *J Feline Med Surg* 9(3):246, 2007.

De Lahunta A: *Veterinary neuroanatomy and clinical neurology*, ed 3, St Louis, 2009, Elsevier.

Dewey CW: *A practical guide to canine and feline neurology*, ed 2, Ames, IA, 2008, Wiley-Blackwell.

Evans J et al: Diazepam as a treatment for metronidazole toxicosis in dogs: a retrospective study of 21 cases, *J Vet Intern Med* 17(3):304, 2003.

Garosi LS et al: Thiamine deficiency in a dog: clinical, clinicopathologic, and magnetic resonance imaging findings, *J Vet Intern Med* 17(5):719, 2003.

Garosi LS et al: Neurological manifestations of ear disease in dogs and cats, *Vet Clin North Am Small Anim Pract* 42(6):1143, 2012.

Higgins MA, Rossmeisl JH Jr, Panciera DL: Hypothyroid-associated central vestibular disease in 10 dogs: 1999-2005, *J Vet Intern Med* 20(6):1363, 2006.

Kent M, Platt SR, Schatzberg SJ: The neurology of balance: function and dysfunction of the vestibular system in dogs and cats, *Vet J* 185(3):247, 2010.

Marks SL et al: Reversible encephalopathy secondary to thiamine deficiency in 3 cats ingesting commercial diets, *J Vet Intern Med* 25(4):949, 2011.

Negrin A et al: Clinical signs, magnetic resonance imaging findings and outcome in 77 cats with vestibular disease: a retrospective study, *J Feline Med Surg* 12(4):291, 2010.

Pickrell JA, Oehme FW, Cash WC: Ototoxicity in dogs and cats, *Semin Vet Med Surg (Small Anim)* 8(1):42, 1993.

Rossmeisl JH Jr: Vestibular disease in dogs and cats, *Vet Clin North Am Small Anim Pract* 40(1):81, 2010.

Rossmeisl JH Jr et al: Survival time following hospital discharge in dogs with palliatively treated brain tumors, *J Vet Med Assoc* 242(2):193, 2013.

Troxel MT, Drobatz KJ, Vite CH: Signs of neurologic dysfunction in dogs with central versus peripheral vestibular disease, *J Am Vet Med Assoc* 227(4):570, 2005.

CHAPTER 233

Canine Intervertebral Disk Herniation

JONATHAN M. LEVINE, *College Station, Texas*

Intervertebral disk herniation (IVDH) is the most common cause of spinal cord injury (SCI) in the dog, accounting for 2.3% of admissions to academic veterinary centers (Priester, 1976). The clinical signs associated with IVDH are numerous and reflect a combination of primary (biomechanical) injury to surrounding neuroparenchyma and secondary (biochemical) mechanisms. A basic understanding of the epidemiology and pathophysiology of this disease process is essential in making diagnostic and treatment recommendations.

Pathophysiology of Intervertebral Disk Disease

The intervertebral disk has three anatomic zones: the anulus fibrosus, nucleus pulposus, and cartilaginous end plate. The anulus fibrosus arises from mesenchymal cells and consists of overlapping lamellae, which are predominantly composed of type I collagen. These lamellae attach to the cartilaginous end plate and are capable of parallel motion during biomechanical loading. In some species, the outermost portions of the anulus are supplied by minute blood vessels and innervated by small, penetrating nerve fibers. The nucleus pulposus is centrally located, bounded by the anulus fibrosus, and contains an abundance of extracellular matrix. It arises from remnant notochordal and chondrocyte-like cells. These cell populations are responsible for the synthesis and maintenance of proteoglycans that bind extracellular water. The cartilaginous end plate serves as a connection between the bony end plate and anulus fibrosus. The hyaline cartilage that composes this structure has pores, which are essential in providing nutrition and removing waste materials from the largely avascular nucleus and anulus.

Intervertebral Disk Degeneration

Disk degeneration has been defined as structural failure of the intervertebral disk associated with abnormal or accelerated changes seen in aging (Adams and Roughley, 2006). Both mechanical and biochemical factors are responsible for disk degeneration. Mechanical degeneration results from chronic vertebral column loading, which leads to anular tearing with subsequent histologic changes in the nucleus and cartilaginous end plate. Biochemical degeneration results from either failure of nutrient delivery or premature senescence of remnant notochordal cells.

In veterinary medicine, disk degeneration traditionally is classified as chondroid or fibroid. This scheme probably is a vast oversimplification of complex, inherently interwoven processes. Chondroid metaplasia is primarily biochemical and is identified most commonly in young chondrodystrophoid dogs. Specifically, early notochordal cell senescence within the nucleus pulposus results in loss of proteoglycans, shifts in proteoglycan ratios, disk dehydration, and nuclear mineralization (Cappello et al, 2006). Fibroid metaplasia is identified frequently in older large-breed dogs and is believed to be principally the result of mechanical influences. The affected nucleus contains abundant fibrous tissue, has shifts in proteoglycan ratios, and is dehydrated; nuclear mineralization also has been recognized. A recent large-scale study suggested that disk degeneration in dogs and disk degeneration in humans bear critical similarities with reference to gross morphological changes, reductions in nuclear glycosaminoglycans, and increases in matrix metalloproteinases; histologic differences in degenerative patterns were not detected between chondrodystrophoid and nonchondrodystrophoid dogs (Bergknut et al, 2012).

It is important to note that disk degeneration may not result in clinically detectable signs. Clinical neurologic disease is believed to occur only when IVDH is present. Some individuals use the expression *intervertebral disk disease* as an umbrella term to refer to disk degeneration, subclinical IVDH, and clinical IVDH.

Intervertebral Disk Herniation

Intervertebral disk herniation is synonymous with the term *intervertebral disk prolapse* and refers to abnormal focal displacement of the intervertebral disk. Most frequently, displacement is dorsal or dorsolateral and impacts structures within the vertebral canal or intervertebral foramen. In dogs IVDH most often occurs in the setting of a previously degenerated disk. Traumatic IVDH has been reported and occurs when a supraphysiologic load is applied to the vertebral column. In such a case, it is possible for nondegenerate intervertebral disks to herniate. Disk herniation is classified as disk extrusion (Hansen's type I disk herniation) or disk protrusion (Hansen's type II disk herniation). Many investigators have ceased using Hansen's terminology because these eponyms are specific to veterinary medicine and do not reflect pathologic mechanisms.

Disk extrusion is defined as rupture of the anulus fibrosus with displacement of the nucleus pulposus into the vertebral canal or intervertebral foramen. In dogs disk extrusion typically is an acute event and is associated with chondroid metaplasia. Disk extrusion can be subclassified as nondispersed, dispersed, sequestered, and noncompressive. Nondispersed disk extrusion is contiguous with the intervertebral disk space and extruded material does not extend significantly over vertebral bodies. Dispersed disk extrusion is more extensive and implies that herniated material extends beyond the limits of the vertebral articulation. Disk sequestration occurs when extruded material is no longer contiguous with the anulus fibrosus. Noncompressive disk extrusion results in minimal displacement of nervous system tissues, even in the setting of significant clinical signs.

Disk protrusion is defined as rupture of the inner layers of the anulus fibrosus, partial displacement of the nucleus into the disrupted anulus, and annular hypertrophy. It is associated most frequently with fibroid metaplasia and may result in slowly progressive clinical signs. Spatial relationships with spondylosis deformans may exist. *Disk bulge* is reported uncommonly in veterinary medicine and is technically not a form of IVDH (Fardon and Milette, 2001). It is defined as symmetric hypertrophy of the anulus fibrosus over greater than 50% of the disk circumference without nuclear displacement.

Spinal Cord Injury and Pathologic Features

Mechanisms of nervous system injury typically are described as *primary* and *secondary*. Primary injury refers to the initial mechanical insult delivered to tissues. Subcategories of primary injury may include compression, contusion, concussion, laceration, and traction. Secondary injuries occur following primary events and are biochemical in nature. Inflammation (innate and adaptive), oxidative stress, excitotoxicity, and vascular injury are just a few of the often overlapping processes involved in secondary injury.

Dogs with acute SCI resulting from IVDH typically have significant spinal cord compression and contusion. The pathologic lesions seen with IVDH involve white and gray matter (Smith and Jeffery, 2006). White matter involvement may predominate and usually is most obvious in the dorsolateral, lateral, and ventral portions of the spinal cord. Intraparenchymal hemorrhage, axonal fragmentation, and demyelination typically occur in combination. In some cases wedge-shaped, infarctlike lesions are located within the white matter. Within the gray matter, ischemic neuronal necrosis, hemorrhage, and neuronal chromatolysis have been recognized.

Limited data are available concerning the pathologic alterations seen with chronic SCI resulting from IVDH, especially in the setting of disk protrusion. At the site of compression there is typically axonal loss and demyelination in all white matter funiculi. Cranial and caudal to the compression, stereotypical loss of white matter tracts reflecting wallerian-like degeneration has been described.

Epidemiology and Clinical Signs

Dogs with IVDH typically are young to middle-aged males of chondrodystrophoid breeds. Dachshunds have been reported to represent 48% to 72% of affected animals and may have a lifetime incidence of IVDH that approaches 20% (Levine et al, 2011). In one study, 83.6% of dogs with IVDH had compression located in the thoracolumbar vertebral column, whereas 16.4% had lesions in the cervical vertebral column (Gage, 1975).

The clinical signs associated with IVDH are variable. In the cervical vertebral column, IVDH may result in hyperesthesia, root signature, tetraparesis, and general proprioceptive ataxia in all limbs. Severely affected dogs may be tetraplegic and require mechanical ventilation.

Many dogs with cervical IVDH have hyperesthesia as their only clinical sign, perhaps because the ratio of vertebral canal diameter to spinal cord diameter is larger in the cervical region than in other vertebral column locations.

In dogs with thoracolumbar IVDH either the T3 to L3 or L4 to S3 spinal cord can be involved. Animals may have hyperesthesia, paraparesis or paraplegia, pelvic limb general proprioceptive ataxia, urinary voiding disability, fecal incontinence, and loss of pelvic limb nociception. Animals with acute IVDH localized to T3 to L3 may have Schiff-Sherrington syndrome. In some instances of acute IVDH, spinal shock can occur. Spinal shock results from interruption of corticospinal tracts and is manifest as a transient loss of pelvic limb spinal reflexes in the setting of an upper motor neuron lesion (Smith and Jeffery, 2005). About 5% to 10% of dogs with IVDH that lack pelvic limb deep nociception develop ascending-descending myelomalacia. The clinical signs of myelomalacia may include severe hyperesthesia, loss of pelvic limb reflexes in the setting of a compression located in the T3 to L3 vertebral column, anal dilation, flaccid bladder paralysis, and cranial migration of the cutaneous trunci reflex. In some instances myelomalacia may result in thoracic limb paresis and ventilatory compromise due to involvement of the cervical spinal cord.

Spinal Cord Injury Scores

Recently several groups have advocated the routine use of physical examination–based SCI scores in dogs with IVDH and other myelopathies. Examples of currently validated systems are the modified Frankel score, Texas Spinal Cord Injury Score, and 14-point gait score (Table 233-1) (Levine et al, 2011). These systems allow for objective, reliable measurement of clinical facets of SCI, such as nociception and gait. Scoring systems enhance medical record keeping, facilitate clinician communication, and provide objective functional milestones during recovery.

Diagnosis

Radiographic features of IVDH include disk space narrowing, disk space wedging, increased articular process overlap, and the presence of mineralized material in the vertebral canal. The diagnostic accuracy of radiography has been reported as 35% for cervical IVDH and 51% to 61% for thoracolumbar IVDH (Lamb et al, 2002; Somerville et al, 2001). Radiography is still viewed as a reasonable screening test because it is easy to perform, highly specific for vertebral fracture and luxation, has a high sensitivity for detecting diskospondylitis, and may permit the detection of osseous neoplasia.

TABLE 233-1

Comparison of Validated Ordinal Physical Assessment–Based Spinal Cord Injury Scales Commonly Used in Dogs

MFS*	TSCIS–Gait* (Individual Limb)†	14-Point Motor Score‡
0 = No motor function or deep nociception caudal to lesion site.	**0** = No limb movement.	**0** = No motor function or deep nociception caudal to lesion site.
1 = No motor function and no superficial nociception caudal to lesion site; deep nociception preserved.	**0** = No limb movement.	**1** = No motor function caudal to lesion site, but deep nociception preserved.
2 = No motor function caudal to lesion site, but deep and superficial nociception preserved.	**0** = No limb movement.	**1** = No motor function caudal to lesion site, but deep nociception preserved.
3 = Nonambulatory status with paresis and general proprioceptive ataxia.	**1** = Limb protraction with no ground clearance. **2** = Limb protraction with inconsistent ground clearance. **3** = Limb protraction with consistent ground clearance.	**3** = Non–weight-bearing protraction in at least one joint. **5** = Non–weight-bearing protraction with more than one joint involved >50% of the time.
4 = Ambulatory with paresis and ataxia.	**4** = Ambulatory, consistent ground clearance, moderate paresis-ataxia (falls occasionally). **5** = Ambulatory, consistent ground clearance, mild paresis-ataxia (does not fall).	**7** = Weight-bearing protraction 10%-50% of the time. **10** = Weight-bearing protraction 100% of the time with reduced strength. Mistakes 50%-90% of the time.
5 = Normal gait. Spinal hyperesthesia and hyperreflexia may be present.	**6** = Normal gait.	**14** = Normal gait.

*From Levine GJ et al: Description and repeatability of a newly developed spinal cord injury scale for dogs, *Prev Vet Med* 89:121, 2009.
†Only the gait component of the TSCIS is displayed. The TSCIS gait component scores each limb individually on a scale of 0 to 6.
‡From Olby NJ et al: Development of a functional scoring system in dogs with acute spinal cord injuries, *Am J Vet Res* 62:1624, 2001.
MFS, Modified Frankel scale; *TSCIS*, Texas Spinal Cord Injury Scale (gait component).

Myelography can be used to detect IVDH, with a reported accuracy in identifying surgical thoracolumbar lesions that ranges from 83.6% to 98% (Israel et al, 2009). The ability of myelography to detect diseases that may mimic IVDH, especially those that primarily involve spinal cord parenchyma, may be inferior to that of more modern modalities. Myelography has been associated with adverse events related to contrast delivery, such as seizures, myelopathy, cardiac arrhythmia, hemorrhage, and death. For these reasons, and because standard myelography is a two-dimensional technique, many clinics use other imaging modalities to detect IVDH.

Like myelography, computed tomography (CT) is used commonly to identify IVDH. Recent studies suggest that the accuracy of CT in detecting surgical thoracolumbar lesions ranges from 81.8% to 100% (Hecht et al, 2009; Israel et al, 2009). Imaging findings associated with IVDH include visible spinal cord compression, loss of epidural fat opacity surrounding the compressed spinal cord, the presence of mineral-dense material within the epidural space, and the presence of extradural material with a density consistent with hemorrhage. Like myelography, CT is believed to be a poor means of identifying intraparenchymal spinal cord diseases that can clinically resemble IVDH.

At many centers, magnetic resonance imaging (MRI) is used as the first-line technique for imaging the vertebral column. Like CT, MRI produces multiplanar images, can be performed quickly with a high-field magnet, and is noninvasive. It has a distinct advantage over CT in that it provides superior soft tissue contrast, which enhances imaging of the spinal cord, epidural space, and intervertebral disk. Unlike other modalities, MRI allows for the classification of disk degeneration and disk herniation subtypes. Additionally, in dogs with thoracolumbar IVDH the degree of hyperintensity within the spinal cord on T2 weighting has been shown to correlate with initial injury severity and functional recovery (Levine et al, 2009). MRI also is the best means to detect intraparenchymal diseases that mimic IVDH, such as myelitis, fibrocartilaginous embolism, and syringohydromyelia.

Treatment

Treatment of IVDH can involve nonsurgical and surgical methods. The optimal approach depends on the clinical evaluation and situation. Often combinations of therapeutic modalities are needed.

Nonsurgical Treatment

Medical treatment alone typically is selected for animals with acute mild clinical signs referable to IVDH (e.g., hyperesthesia with or without ambulatory ataxia and paresis). The hallmarks of medical therapy are analgesia, cage rest, and physical rehabilitation. Limited data are available regarding the best type of medical treatment. In one large retrospective study (Levine et al, 2007), dogs with presumptive IVDH that received medical treatment with glucocorticoids had poorer outcomes than dogs receiving other treatments, even after correction for duration and severity of injury in the analysis. Severe SCI

and chronic SCI both were negatively associated with outcome. In this same report, 14.4% of medically treated dogs with thoracolumbar IVDH experienced treatment failure (e.g., required euthanasia or surgery) and 30.9% had signs of clinical recurrence. Dogs with cervical IVDH had outcomes similar to those of dogs with thoracolumbar lesions. Our current medical treatment protocol consists of 2 to 4 weeks of cage rest and analgesia with nonsteroidal antiinflammatory drugs and opioids, with or without additional drugs for neuropathic pain. Physical rehabilitation is also a component of nonsurgical treatment.

Surgical Treatment

Surgical treatment is recommended for dogs with moderate to severe clinical signs (e.g., nonambulatory status or marked ambulatory ataxia and paresis), dogs with chronic clinical signs, and those that show no response to nonsurgical treatment. The goal of surgical therapy is to decompress the spinal cord or nerve roots. In dogs with cervical disk herniation this is typically accomplished via a ventral slot procedure. Dorsal laminectomy has been used in the cervical vertebral column, especially in cases of multilevel disk protrusion or disk protrusion associated with cervical spondylomyelopathy. Dorsal laminectomy has the disadvantage of not permitting direct removal of herniated disk material in most instances. Recently cervical hemilaminectomy has been described and may provide access to lateralized compressive lesions. In the thoracolumbar vertebral column, hemilaminectomy, pediculectomy, mini-hemilaminectomy, partial lateral corpectomy, and dorsal laminectomy all have been used to gain access to the vertebral canal.

For IVDH involving the cervical vertebral column, limited data are available regarding outcomes and clinical recurrence following surgery. Most studies suggest significant clinical improvement in more than 90% of dogs following decompression. In one report, 10% of dogs with cervical IVDH had recurrence of clinical signs following surgery (Cherrone et al, 2004). In dogs with thoracolumbar IVDH, pelvic limb deep nociception is the most important physical examination–based predictor of functional outcome. Among animals with intact pelvic limb deep nociception at admission, voluntary ambulation occurred in 86% to 96% following surgery (Levine et al, 2011). Dogs lacking pelvic limb deep nociception before surgery have a 43% to 62% chance of voluntary ambulation following surgery (Levine et al, 2011). In paraplegic dogs with intact deep nociception before surgery the median time to regain ambulation following surgical decompression is 9 days (Ferreira et al, 2002). Dogs lacking pelvic limb deep nociception have a mean time to ambulation of 7.5 weeks (Olby et al, 2003).

Recently biomarkers and MRI findings have been studied as outcome predictors in dogs with surgically treated thoracolumbar IVDH. For example, dogs with a cerebrospinal fluid myelin basic protein concentration of 3 ng/ml or more had 0.09 times the odds of long-term ambulation compared with dogs with a cerebrospinal fluid myelin basic protein concentration of less than 3 ng/ml (Levine et al, 2011). Cerebrospinal fluid creatine kinase concentration and matrix metalloproteinase 9 expression also are related to long-term ambulatory status. Two reports have shown that the length of a hyperintense area within the spinal cord on T2-weighted sagittal images is associated with initial severity of SCI and functional outcome. Data suggest that the biomarkers and MRI signal changes studied appear independent of the Modified Frankel Score, which may permit their use in combination with traditional physical examination–based measures of SCI severity to determine long-term ambulatory outcome.

Clinical recurrence has been identified in 12.7% to 20.2% of dogs with surgically treated thoracolumbar IVDH (Brisson et al, 2011). Episodes of reported recurrence may be mild or severe, requiring surgical intervention. Early recurrence often occurs at the surgical site, whereas later recurrence occurs at vertebral articulations adjacent to surgical sites. Results of a small, nonblinded, prospective study suggested that fenestration at the site of surgically treated IVDH reduces herniation of additional disk material in the early postoperative period (Forterre et al, 2008). A large, nonblinded, prospective study found that the rate of recurrence was lower in dogs with multisite fenestration (7.5%) than in those with single-site fenestration (17.9%); no dogs with IVDH that did not receive fenestration were studied (Brisson et al, 2011).

Glucocorticoids

Glucocorticoids, including methylprednisolone sodium succinate (MPSS), dexamethasone, and prednisone, have been used in the medical treatment of IVDH. Administration of glucocorticoids to dogs with IVDH can have two purposes: (1) neuroprotection in the setting of acute, severe SCI, and (2) modulation of inflammatory mediators in the setting of chronic IVDH-associated compression.

Glucocorticoid therapy has been studied in animal models and in humans with SCI for decades. In humans with traumatic myelopathies, only MPSS has been associated with improved outcomes. The benefits realized with MPSS administration likely relate to the antioxidant properties of the drug when it is administered at high dosages. In humans with SCI, MPSS must be administered within 8 hours of SCI, and effects on motor function have been reported as modest. Currently, the use of MPSS in humans with traumatic SCI is contentious due to variable outcome data. The only completed study on treatment with high-dose MPSS in dogs with thoracolumbar IVDH was retrospective and did not show an association with better outcomes. Currently a multicenter prospective clinical trial is under way to study the effects of MPSS in dogs with acute, severe IVDH-associated SCI. The use of glucocorticoids such as dexamethasone is strongly *discouraged* as a treatment for acute SCI resulting from IVDH because positive effects on outcome have not been detected. Dexamethasone administration increases the risk of urinary tract infection and gastrointestinal signs in dogs with thoracolumbar IVDH.

Limited data are available on the use of glucocorticoids in dogs with mild or chronic myelopathy associated with IVDH. A multicenter retrospective study suggested that, in dogs with presumptive IVDH, glucocorticoid therapy was negatively associated with improved functional outcome (Levine et al, 2007). Because this patient population was heterogeneous with respect to SCI severity, it is challenging to understand the implication of this result for mildly affected animals. A recent retrospective study in dogs with lumbosacral disk protrusion suggested a benefit for epidural administration of glucocorticoids (Janssens et al, 2009).

At many clinical centers, glucocorticoids are no longer administered to dogs suspected of having IVDH-mediated SCI. The reasons for this include the current lack of evidence to support an association with better outcomes, reported adverse events, and the recognition that dogs suspected of having IVDH can have other causes of SCI (e.g., myelitis) with divergent pathologic mechanisms.

Novel Therapies

The use of neuroprotective agents (those that mitigate acute secondary injury) and treatments to facilitate spinal cord regeneration or plasticity currently are under investigation in dogs with thoracolumbar IVDH. Polyethylene glycol (PEG) is a surfactant that physiologically and anatomically fuses spinal cord axons in SCI models. In 2004 an open-label phase I-II study (Laverty et al, 2004) examined the use of PEG in dogs lacking deep nociception because of thoracolumbar IVDH and compared outcomes with those for historical controls. The drug appeared to be safe, and in 17 of 19 dogs recovery of pelvic limb nociception occurred within 2 days of PEG administration. The open-label design of this study and the use of historical controls have led some to question the effects of PEG in dogs with IVDH. A phase III clinical trial is currently under way in dogs with IVDH that will provide valuable data regarding the efficacy of PEG administration.

Olfactory ensheathing cells (OECs) promote axonal growth and remyelination in SCI models. In dogs with thoracolumbar SCI lacking deep nociception, data from a phase I trial (Jeffery et al, 2005) suggest that OECs can be harvested safely and delivered via myelotomy. Spinal walking was observed in a subset of treated dogs. Recently, a blinded, randomized phase II investigation suggested that OECs improve motor function in dogs with chronic, complete SCI; in this population, there was no improvement in limb nociception, suggesting the possibility that OECs modulate the central pattern generator but do not result in repair of long tracts (Granger et al, 2012).

References and Suggested Reading

Adams MA, Roughley PJ: What is intervertebral disk degeneration, and what causes it? *Spine* 31:2151, 2006.

Brisson BA et al: Comparison of the effect of single-site and multiple-site disk fenestration on the rate of recurrence of thoracolumbar intervertebral disk herniation in dogs, *J Am Vet Med Assoc* 238:1593, 2011.

Bergknut N et al: The dog as an animal model for intervertebral disc degeneration? *Spine* 37:351, 2012.

Cappello R et al: Notochordal cells produce and assemble extracellular matrix in a distinct manner, which may be responsible for the maintenance of healthy nucleus pulposus, *Spine* 31:873, 2006.

Cherrone KL et al: A retrospective comparison of cervical intervertebral disk disease in nonchondrodystrophic large dogs versus small dogs, *J Am Anim Hosp Assoc* 40:316, 2004.

Fardon DF, Milette PC: Nomenclature and classification of lumbar disc pathology. Recommendations of the combined task forces of the North American Spine Society, American Society of Spine Radiology, and American Society of Neuroradiology, *Spine* 26:E93, 2001.

Ferreira AJ, Correia JH, Jaggy A: Thoracolumbar disc disease in 71 paraplegic dogs: influence of rate of onset and duration of clinical signs on treatment results, *J Small Anim Pract* 43:158, 2002.

Forterre F et al: Influence of intervertebral disc fenestration at the herniation site in association with hemilaminectomy on recurrence in chondrodystrophic dogs with thoracolumbar disc disease: a prospective MRI study, *Vet Surg* 37:399, 2008.

Gage ED: Incidence of clinical disc disease in the dog, *J Am Anim Hosp Assoc* 11:135, 1975.

Granger N et al: Autologous olfactory mucosal cell transplants in clinical spinal cord injury: a randomized double-blinded trial in a canine translational model, *Brain* 135:3227, 2012.

Hecht S et al: Myelography vs. computed tomography in the evaluation of acute intervertebral disk extrusion in chondrodystrophic dogs, *Vet Radiol Ultrasound* 50:353, 2009.

Israel SK et al: The relative sensitivity of computed tomography and myelography for identification of thoracolumbar disk herniations in dogs, *Vet Radiol Ultrasound* 50:247, 2009.

Janssens L, Beosier Y, Daems R: Lumbosacral degenerative stenosis in the dog. The results of epidural infiltration with methylprednisolone acetate: a retrospective study, *Vet Comp Orthop Traumatol* 22:486, 2009.

Jeffery ND, Lakatos A, Franklin RJM: Autologous olfactory glial cell transplantation is reliable and safe in naturally occurring canine spinal cord injury, *J Neurotrauma* 22:1282, 2005.

Lamb CR et al: Accuracy of survey radiographic diagnosis of intervertebral disc protrusion in dogs, *Vet Radiol Ultrasound* 43:222, 2002.

Laverty PH et al: A preliminary study of intravenous surfactants in paraplegic dogs: polymer therapy in canine clinical SCI, *J Neurotrauma* 21:1767, 2004.

Levine JM et al: Evaluation of the success of medical management for presumptive thoracolumbar intervertebral disk herniation in dogs, *Vet Surg* 36:481, 2007.

Levine JM et al: Magnetic resonance imaging in dogs with neurologic impairment due to acute thoracic and lumbar intervertebral disk herniation, *J Vet Intern Med* 23:1220, 2009.

Levine JM et al: Naturally occurring disk herniation in dogs: an opportunity for pre-clinical spinal cord injury research, *J Neurotrauma* 28:675, 2011.

Olby N et al: Long-term functional outcome of dogs with severe injuries of the thoracolumbar spinal cord: 87 cases (1996-2001), *J Am Vet Med Assoc* 222:762, 2003.

Priester WA: Canine intervertebral disk disease—occurrence by age, breed, and sex among 8,117 cases, *Theriogenology* 6:293, 1976.

Smith PM, Jeffery ND: Spinal shock—comparative aspects and clinical relevance, *J Vet Intern Med* 19:788, 2005.

Smith PM, Jeffery ND: Histological and ultrastructural analysis of white matter damage after naturally-occurring spinal cord injury, *Brain Pathol* 16:99, 2006.

Somerville ME et al: Accuracy of localization of cervical intervertebral disk extrusion or protrusion using survey radiography in dogs, *J Am Anim Hosp Assoc* 37:563, 2001.

CHAPTER 234

Canine Degenerative Myelopathy

JOAN R. COATES, *Columbia, Missouri*
SHINICHI KANAZONO, *Columbia, Missouri*

Canine degenerative myelopathy (DM) was first described as an insidious, progressive general proprioceptive ataxia and upper motor neuron (UMN) spastic paresis of the pelvic limbs ultimately leading to paraplegia and necessitating euthanasia (Averill, 1973). Although most of the dogs in the initial reports were German shepherd dogs, other breeds were represented (Averill, 1973; Braund and Vandevelde, 1978; Griffiths and Duncan, 1975). DM is now recognized as a common problem in a number of breeds, with an overall prevalence of 0.19% (Coates et al, 2007; Coates and Wininger, 2010). Additionally, the clinical spectrum of DM has been broadened to encompass both the UMN and lower motor neuron (LMN) systems. Discovery of a missense mutation in the superoxide dismutase 1 gene (*SOD1*) provided further understanding that this canine disease may share pathogenic mechanisms with some forms of human amyotrophic lateral sclerosis (ALS, or Lou Gehrig's disease) (Awano et al, 2009).

Pathophysiology

Since it was first described by Averill (1973), canine DM, because of its histopathologic features, was termed a *nonspecific degeneration of spinal cord tissue of undetermined cause.* Awano and colleagues (2009) identified a c.118G>A transition of glutamate to lysine in *SOD1* that predicted an E40K missense mutation underlying canine DM. In this initial study there was a highly significant association between homozygosity for the *SOD1:c.118A* allele and the DM phenotype in Pembroke Welsh corgis and also in four other dog breeds: boxer, Chesapeake Bay retriever, German shepherd dog, and Rhodesian ridgeback. SOD1 is a ubiquitous intracellular protein functioning as a free radical scavenger. Mutations in *SOD1* are known to cause some forms of familial ALS in humans. ALS, the most common adult motor neuron disease, is characterized by loss of motor neurons causing stiffness and slowing of muscle movements, difficulty speaking and swallowing, muscle atrophy, and severe weakness. The Greek word *amyotrophy* means "muscles without nourishment." *Lateral* is the location within the spinal cord of axonal disease, and *sclerosis* refers to replacement of diseased axons by sclerotic or "scar" tissue. In addition, Awano and associates (2009) demonstrated that, as in ALS, cytoplasmic aggregates that bind anti-SOD1 antibodies were present in the spinal cords of dogs with DM that were homozygotic for *SOD1:c.118A*. The aggregates are thought to form because amino acid substitutions force SOD1 to assume an unstable conformation. It is unclear if the aggregates cause or contribute to the neurodegeneration or are a by-product of other neurodegenerative processes. No similar SOD1 antigen–containing aggregates are found in healthy dogs lacking known *SOD1* mutations.

Not all *SOD1:c.118A* homozygotes develop clinical signs; therefore DM appears to be an incompletely penetrant autosomal-recessive disease, whereas most human *SOD1* mutations are autosomal dominant. Thus homozygosity for the E40K mutation is a *major risk factor* for canine DM. We have detected the DM-associated *SOD1:c.118A* allele in over 100 different dog breeds. The mutant allele appears to be very common in some breeds. It remains to be seen whether or not homozygosity for the mutation puts dogs of all of these different genetic backgrounds at risk of developing DM. Recently another mutation in *SOD1* has been discovered in a DM-affected Bernese mountain dog (Wininger et al, 2011). This finding serves as a reminder that direct DNA tests can indicate the presence or absence of disease-causing alleles but cannot be used to rule out a diagnosis because other sequence variants in the same gene or in a different gene might produce a similar disease phenotype.

Clinical Spectrum

Subsequent to the discovery of the *SOD1* mutation underlying canine DM, the clinical spectrum became more clearly defined with identification of the stages of disease progression (Table 234-1). Dogs with DM follow a predictive pattern of clinical signs that begins with UMN pelvic limb paresis and general proprioceptive ataxia, progresses to LMN paraparesis, and then spreads to involve the thoracic limbs and brainstem. The earliest clinical signs appear when dogs are at least 8 years or older, and the mean age of onset is 9 years. There is no sex predilection.

TABLE 234-1

Neurologic Signs in Dogs with Degenerative Myelopathy Based on Disease Progression

Time from Onset of Signs (Months)	Neurologic Signs
6 to 12	**Upper motor neuron paraparesis and general proprioceptive ataxia** Progressive general proprioceptive ataxia Asymmetric spastic paraparesis Intact spinal reflexes (patellar reflex may be decreased)
9 to 18	**Nonambulatory paraparesis to paraplegia** Mild to moderate loss of muscle mass in pelvic limbs Reduced to absent spinal reflexes in pelvic limbs ± Urinary and fecal incontinence
14 to 24	**Lower motor neuron paraplegia to thoracic limb paresis** Signs of thoracic limb paresis Flaccid paraplegia Severe loss of muscle mass in pelvic limbs Urinary and fecal incontinence
>24-36	**Lower motor neuron tetraplegia and brainstem signs** Flaccid tetraplegia Difficulty with swallowing and tongue movements Reduced to absent cutaneous trunci reflex Generalized and severe loss of muscle mass Urinary and fecal incontinence

NOTE: Shading represents the disease stages at which lower motor neuron signs are present.

The clinical course of DM can vary after the presumptive diagnosis is made; the mean disease duration is 6 to 12 months in larger dog breeds, at which point dogs become nonambulatory paraparetics. Pet owners usually elect euthanasia when their dogs can no longer support weight with their pelvic limbs. Dogs of smaller breeds can be cared for by the pet owner over a longer time; for example, the median disease duration in the Pembroke Welsh corgi was 19 months (Coates et al, 2007). DM-affected Pembroke Welsh corgis often have signs of thoracic limb paresis at the time of euthanasia.

Early Disease (Upper Motor Neuron Signs)

The earliest clinical signs of DM are general proprioceptive ataxia and mild spastic paresis in the pelvic limbs. Worn nails and the appearance of asymmetric pelvic limb lameness can be seen on physical examination. Asymmetry of signs at disease onset is reported frequently. At disease onset, spinal reflex abnormalities are consistent with UMN paresis localized in the T3 to L3 spinal cord segments. Patellar reflexes may be normal or exaggerated to clonic; however, hyporeflexia of the patellar reflex also has been described in dogs at a similar disease stage (Griffiths and Duncan, 1975). Involvement of the dorsal roots of the femoral nerve may inhibit sensory impulses from stretch receptors located in the quadriceps muscle. Flexor (withdrawal) reflexes also may be normal or show crossed extension (suggestive of chronic UMN dysfunction). Often within 6 to 12 months from the time of disease onset, dogs progress to nonambulatory paraparesis.

Late Disease (Lower Motor Neuron Signs)

If the DM-affected dog is not euthanized early, clinical signs will progress to LMN paraplegia and ascend to affect the thoracic limbs within 18 to 24 months. LMN signs emerge as hyporeflexia of the patellar and withdrawal reflexes, flaccid paralysis, and widespread muscle atrophy beginning in the pelvic limbs as the dogs become nonambulatory (Awano et al, 2009; Matthews and de Lahunta, 1985). The paresis becomes more symmetric and progresses to flaccid tetraplegia in dogs with advanced disease. Widespread and severe loss of muscle mass occurs in the axial and appendicular musculature. Most previous reports attributed loss of muscle mass to disuse, but flaccidity in dogs with protracted disease suggests denervation. Cranial nerve signs include difficulty swallowing and inability to bark. Urinary and fecal continence usually are spared until the latter disease stage of LMN paraplegia.

Differential Diagnoses

The diagnosis of DM in the early disease stage can be challenging because the clinical presentation can mimic that of other acquired spinal cord diseases. These disorders differ in anatomic distribution, clinical signs, and age of onset. Older dogs often have concurrent orthopedic and neurologic disease that can confound the interpretation of the neurologic findings. Paw replacement (proprioceptive positioning) is a very useful test that distinguishes between orthopedic and neurologic diseases because it does not require weight bearing. Animals with orthopedic disease do not have paw replacement deficits. Disorders that often mimic and coexist with DM include degenerative lumbosacral syndrome, intervertebral disk disease, spinal cord neoplasia, and degenerative joint diseases such as hip dysplasia or cruciate ligament disease. The Pembroke Welsh corgi is a chondrodystrophic breed and prone to Hansen type I intervertebral disk herniation. Hansen type II intervertebral disk herniation can be an incidental or clinically significant finding and is more common in older dogs of the large nonchondrodystrophic breeds. Pelvic limb dysfunction can present before thoracic limb paresis in cervical spinal cord disease (e.g., caudal cervical spondylomyelopathy) and in generalized neuromuscular diseases such as neuropathy, neuromuscular junction disorders, and myopathy.

Diagnostic Approach

Accurate antemortem diagnosis is based on recognition of the pattern of progression of clinical signs supported by inclusionary and exclusionary diagnostic testing.

Neurodiagnostic Testing

A careful neurologic examination is fundamental to developing a diagnostic approach. Lack of paraspinal hyperesthesia is a key clinical feature of DM that distinguishes it from other compressive myelopathies. As in a patient with a "definite" diagnosis of ALS, in a DM-affected dog neurologic signs progress from UMN to LMN signs, spread to two or more spinal regions, and eventually involve the brainstem (bulbar signs). An antemortem diagnosis of canine DM is based on ruling out other spinal cord–compressive diseases.

Neurodiagnostic techniques for evaluation of spinal cord disease include cerebrospinal fluid (CSF) analysis, spinal cord imaging, and electrodiagnostic testing. A presumptive diagnosis of DM often is made based on lack of clinically relevant compressive myelopathy as determined by magnetic resonance imaging (MRI). If MRI is unavailable, computed tomography/myelography can also be used. MRI is especially useful for identifying early intramedullary spinal cord neoplasia and providing evidence of extradural compressive myelopathy. Imaging often reveals disk protrusions, which can confound the diagnosis of DM. The clinician must be guided by clinical experience to evaluate for rapidity of disease progression, presence of paraspinal hyperesthesia, and amount of spinal cord compression to account for the severity of the myelopathy. CSF analysis can help to rule out meningitis and myelitis.

Electrodiagnostic testing is useful for detecting evidence of neuromuscular disease. Early in the progression of DM when UMN signs predominate, no spontaneous activity is detected by electromyography (EMG) and nerve conduction velocities are within normal limits. Later in the disease course with the emergence of LMN signs, EMG reveals multifocal spontaneous activity in the distal appendicular musculature. Fibrillation potentials and positive sharp waves are the more common waveforms recorded. Recordings of compound muscle action potentials (M waves) from stimulation of the tibial and ulnar nerves have been found to show temporal dispersion and decreases in amplitudes (Awano et al, 2009). The proximal and distal motor nerve conduction velocities have been found to be decreased when compared with the normal reference range. These findings provide evidence of motor axonopathy and demyelination in the late disease stage of DM.

A DNA test based on the *SOD1* mutation is commercially available. Dogs homozygous for the mutation are at risk of developing DM and will contribute one chromosome with the mutant allele to all of their offspring. Heterozygous dogs are DM carriers and are less likely to develop clinical DM, but they can pass on a chromosome with the mutant allele to half of their offspring. Dogs homozygous for the nonmutated (normal) allele are unlikely to develop DM and will provide all of their offspring with a protective normal allele. A test result showing that the dog is at risk can support a presumptive diagnosis of DM in the setting of typical clinical signs and normal findings on neuroimaging and CSF analysis. The *SOD1* DNA test is of potential use to dog breeders wishing to reduce the incidence of DM in the breed or line.

Neuropathologic Features

Because a variety of common acquired compressive spinal cord diseases can mimic DM by compromising the UMN pathways, a definitive diagnosis of DM can be accomplished only at postmortem examination. The pathologic features of DM include axonal degeneration with secondary demyelination and astroglial proliferation (sclerosis) in all spinal cord funiculi but consistently most severe in the dorsal portion of the lateral funiculus and in the dorsal columns of the middle to lower thoracic region (March et al, 2009). Absence of neuronal cell body degeneration or loss in the ventral horn of the spinal cord is not a prominent histopathologic finding. Histopathologic studies of tissue from dogs in late disease stage with LMN signs have documented denervation atrophy in muscle, nerve fiber loss with axonal degeneration, and secondary myelin loss in myelinated fibers of peripheral nerves (Awano et al, 2009; Shelton et al, 2012). Similarly, in ALS patients and DM-affected dogs, muscle biopsy specimens show evidence of reinnervation in the early disease stages (Shelton et al, 2012). Based on clinical signs and pathologic findings, DM is now considered a multisystem disease involving central and peripheral axons that has similarities to UMN-onset ALS.

Management Overview

The long-term prognosis of DM is poor. In the face of the inevitable gradual progression of DM regardless of the use of various therapeutic modalities, it is important to realize the emotional support a pet owner can provide to maintain quality of life for the pet. As a DM-affected dog progresses through the disease stages, the pet owner encounters the challenges of at-home management and provision of appropriate daily care for the pet. Ultimately, the pet owner will need to make a decision for humane euthanasia, often with the assistance of the veterinarian.

Pharmacotherapy

Pharmacotherapies for canine DM, including drugs and nutritional supplements, have been empiric, with a lack of evidence-based approaches for determining efficacy. The antiprotease agent ε-aminocaproic acid has been advocated for long-term management of DM (Clemmons, 1989). However, a recent study that evaluated combined therapy with ε-aminocaproic acid, N-acetylcysteine, and vitamins B, C, and E found no beneficial effects (Polizopoulou et al, 2008). Treatment with parenteral cobalamin or oral tocopherol did not affect neurologic progression in a study of DM-affected dogs; furthermore, serum concentrations of α-tocopherol in DM-affected German shepherd dogs were not significantly different from the concentrations in normal dogs (Fechner et al, 2003; Johnston et al, 2001; Williams et al, 1985).

ALS has no known cure, and effective treatments have remained elusive. The only drug currently approved by the U.S. Food and Drug Administration for use in treating humans with ALS is riluzole (Rilutek), an anti-excitotoxic agent that inhibits release of glutamate, and this drug has shown only marginal benefits in slowing disease progression (Bensimon et al, 1994; Miller et al, 2007). There has been no report of the use of riluzole in DM-affected dogs. Explanations for the negative results of other treatments for ALS include heterogeneity in disease susceptibility and pathogenic mechanisms, and defective design of clinical trials (Beghi et al, 2011). The pattern of clinical progression of canine DM is relatively uniform within breeds and among breeds. This may facilitate the establishment of longitudinal measures of disease progression for determining the efficacy of therapeutic approaches.

Physiotherapy

Physical rehabilitation is an evolving area in veterinary medicine. Goals for rehabilitation of the neurologic patient include maintaining joint function and range of motion, improving balance and proprioception, preserving or increasing muscle strength, and improving overall functioning (Millis, 2009). Physiotherapy and implementation of the principles of physical rehabilitation may improve quality of life and retard deterioration of function in DM-affected dogs (Millis, 2009; Sherman and Olby, 2004). Rehabilitation of dogs with neurologic disease has focused primarily on recovery after a disease insult. These protocols involve a combination of active and passive exercise, functional activities, and therapeutic modalities (Drum, 2010; Olby et al, 2005; Shealy et al, 2004). In veterinary medicine no formal evidence-based guidelines have been published for physiotherapy for animals with neuromuscular disease. Moreover, physiotherapy regimens and the efficacy of such regimens for management of neurodegenerative disorders in animals remain to be determined. The rationale for physiotherapy in the management of canine DM will continue to evolve as we gain further understanding of DM and its resemblance to ALS.

The role of exercise in people with ALS has been controversial, and it is possible that excessive exercise or strengthening exercises might induce overwork damage. The pattern of ALS onset and progression is highly variable, which has limited advancement in understanding whether exercise has beneficial effects in ALS management. Much of the current evidence for the neuroprotective potential of exercise in ALS comes from studies in rodent ALS models (McCrate and Kaspar, 2008). Transgenic ALS mice that engaged in moderate exercise showed slower disease progression, improved function, and longer survival than sedentary animals living in cages (Kaspar et al, 2005; Kierkinezos et al, 2003). However, high-resistance strengthening exercises do not have any benefit over moderate-resistance programs and can accelerate neurologic deterioration (Mahoney et al, 2004). Further beneficial effects of extensive exercise in the mouse ALS model were shown when exercises were alternated with periods of rest and were performed regularly (Kierkinezos et al, 2003; Liebetanz et al, 2004).

In human ALS, strength training in conjunction with aerobic training was considered more likely to be beneficial than to be deleterious in patients with ALS provided the exercise is individualized, monitored, and involves progressive resistance (Bello-Haas et al, 2007; Drory et al,

2001). A recent review assigned a level II evidence rating (likely to be effective) for muscle strengthening in ALS (Chen et al, 2008). For humans with ALS recommendations are for exercises that do not cause fatigue and that focus on maintaining mobility. Additionally, focused exercise programs can have positive psychologic effects on a patient's coping strategies. The efficacy of therapeutic interventions is related to the timing of interventions as well as the motivation and persistence of the patient and support from family members (Hallum, 2007).

To date, no prospective studies have established whether exercise has a beneficial effect in DM-affected dogs. Kathmann and colleagues (2006) reported survival data for 22 DM-affected dogs that received varying degrees of physiotherapy. Dogs that received intensive physiotherapy had significantly longer survival times (mean, 255 days) than dogs that received moderate physiotherapy (mean, 130 days) or no physiotherapy (mean, 55 days). The physiotherapy regimen consisted of active and passive exercises that did not take into account disease stage or UMN-LMN signs. Although study limitations included lack of randomization and definitive diagnosis, small group size, and bias from owner perceptions, the results warrant further investigation into the efficacy of physiotherapy in DM-affected dogs.

Physiotherapy Considerations

Two major factors must be considered when planning and implementing an activity or exercise program for patients with ALS and should be taken into account in cases of degenerative myelopathy: slowing of disuse muscle atrophy and minimizing of overuse injury (Figure 234-1).

Disuse Muscle Atrophy. Disuse muscle atrophy occurs with UMN weakness. Type I muscle fibers involving the postural muscles and those crossing one joint are most vulnerable to disuse atrophy. Disuse muscle weakness lowers muscle force production and reduces muscle endurance. Furthermore, disuse atrophy in combination with pathologic weakness and spasticity of specific muscle groups contributes to loss of coordination and lower efficiency of movements (Ropper and Samuels, 2009). Exercise recommendations for ALS patients suggest that progressive resistive exercises begin in the early stage of

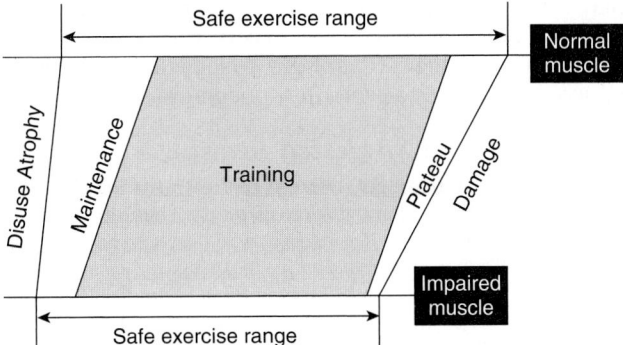

Figure 234-1 Exercise window for normal and damaged or denervated muscles. (Adapted from Maloney FP, Burks JS, Ringel SP, editors: *Interdisciplinary rehabilitation of multiple sclerosis and neuromuscular disorders,* New York, 1985, JB Lippincott. In Umphred DA, editor: *Neurological rehabilitation,* ed 5, St Louis, 2007, Elsevier.)

the neuromuscular disorder because strength training in patients with less than 10% of normal function generally was not effective (Milner-Brown and Miller, 1998). It is important to try to differentiate between muscle weakness from disuse and muscle weakness from overwork. Diagnosis of overwork weakness is based on a decrease in strength and endurance that can reasonably be related to specific overuse and by failure to regain strength with specific exercise (Bennett and Knowlton, 1958). Muscles weak from disuse will respond favorably to specific graduated exercise by showing increased strength.

Exercise-Induced Damage. In ALS patients fatigue occurs more easily in damaged or denervated muscle during anaerobic and aerobic exercise because of motor inefficiency caused by weakness (Sanjak et al, 2001). Loss of LMN innervations results in secondary compensatory axonal sprouting and a larger muscle mass innervated by a smaller pool of motor neurons. These macro motor units may be susceptible to failure due to dropout and defective neuromuscular transmission along the reinnervated nerve sprouts. In experimentally neurectomized muscles of rats, vigorous exercise caused further muscle damage if fewer than one third of motor units were functional (Reitsma, 1969). If more than one third of the motor units remained intact, exercise promoted hypertrophy of the functioning myofibers. Thus the extent of strengthening is proportional to the number of intact motor units. Importantly, exercise at a level to elicit a training effect in normal muscle may actually cause overwork damage in weakened, denervated muscle (Bennett and Knowlton, 1958; Tam et al, 2001). In concert with physiotherapy in ALS patients, high-resistance strengthening should be limited and strengthening exercises should emphasize concentric (muscle-shortening) rather than eccentric (muscle-lengthening) muscle contractions (Hallum, 2007). Thus when a physiotherapy program is being designed for animals with neuromuscular disease it is important that one "first do no harm."

Exercise Interventions Suggested for Canine Degenerative Myelopathy

When UMN signs predominate in DM-affected dogs, physiotherapy is directed at retarding further deconditioning and disuse muscle atrophy, and relieving spasticity. Spasticity, a hallmark clinical sign of UMN paresis, is a velocity-dependent increase in the resistance of muscles to a passive stretch stimulus. Spasticity is characterized by an increase in tonic stretch reflexes with an increase in resistance against quick and strong flexion force but a normal or lesser increase in resistance against slow and gradual flexion force (Ropper and Samuels, 2009). Spasticity in ALS patients contributes to worsening muscle dysfunction. A randomized controlled trial assessed the effect of moderate exercise on spasticity in ALS patients (Drory et al, 2001; reviewed in Ashworth et al, 2006). Although the study was too small to determine whether exercise was useful, the patients who performed the exercises had significantly less spasticity.

Active exercises are recommended for DM-affected dogs while spinal reflexes and at least some voluntary movements remain intact. Active exercises improve muscle mass and strength, neuromuscular balance, and coordination (Olby et al, 2005). Exercises that involve repetitive range-of-motion activity also serve to decrease spasticity (Katz, 1988). Such therapies include sit-to-stand and standing exercises, weight shifting, and ambulation exercises. Hydrotherapy such as walking on an underwater treadmill allows support of the dog's body weight through buoyancy effects, and the water provides resistance to movement for muscle strengthening. Dynamic balance exercises using balance balls or rolls or a balance board can improve proprioception. Other proprioceptive exercises include standing or walking on an uneven surface (e.g., air mattress, sand, and cushion) or weaving through obstacles or over obstacles. Balance exercises and coordination activities also strengthen core muscles of the trunk and reduce the exaggerated tone in antigravity muscles of the limbs. Moreover, ongoing or maintenance exercise programs serve to decrease muscle stiffness and slow immobility. If a DM-affected dog shows evidence of significant, persistent weakness after an exercise regimen is instituted or has persistent fatigue the day after exercise, the therapist will need to adjust the exercise program to prevent damage from excessive overwork and fatigue.

Passive range-of-motion (PROM) exercise is performed before active exercises and in neurologic patients who lack voluntary movement or strength. Regularly performing PROM exercise maintains joint health, retards contracture, enhances mobility of soft tissues and circulation, and reduces pain and spasticity (Millis et al, 2004; Olby et al, 2005). Before PROM exercise, the limbs should be warmed and massaged using stroking and pressure techniques. The therapist should gently grasp the limb, and the motion should be slow and steady. During flexion and extension of the limb, the joints are positioned into flexion to the point of resistance, and then extended in the same manner. The limb also is manipulated in a "bicycling" manner to simulate a normal gait pattern. PROM exercise is recommended at all stages of progression of DM. Extreme stretching exercises should be performed with caution in denervated muscle to prevent further muscle damage.

Once LMN paresis develops, as indicated by severe muscle atrophy, flaccidity, and absence of spinal reflexes, preservation of muscle mass becomes difficult. In DM-affected dogs development of neurogenic atrophy confounds the interpretation of disuse atrophy. Neuromuscular electrical stimulation (NMES) may attenuate muscle atrophy in the presence of LMN signs by helping to maintain potential functional capacity of the muscle fibers. As does active exercise, NMES may improve the timing or recruitment of muscles so that the muscles exert more force in a useful and coordinated manner. Continuous NMES was found to have positive effects on reinnervation and the sprouting process in denervated muscles of experimentally neurectomized dogs (Williams, 1996). Its use is considered contraindicated in cases of extreme muscle weakness, however, because of the risk of further muscle damage. In ALS patients, a rule of thumb is that NMES should no longer be performed when the patient no longer has voluntary muscle movements (Hallum, 2007).

It is important to establish outcome measures specific to DM to document prospectively the effects of active and passive exercise in DM-affected dogs. Another consideration is the effect of age on the neuromuscular system of dogs. Muscle mass declines with age, presumably because of myofiber loss and atrophy. A comparison study of aged dogs revealed little age-related variation in the diameter of type I myofibers, but the diameter of type IIA fibers was decreased uniformly in dogs 7 years and older (Braund et al, 1982).

Other Supportive Care

When the DM-affected dog becomes recumbent, supportive care that addresses psychologic and physical well-being is especially important. Assistive devices include a broad array of equipment to help caregivers with ambulation of their pets, to protect the extremities, and to improve quality of life for pets and their owners (Millis, 2009; Millis et al, 2004). In dogs with loss of proprioceptive placement, protective boots shield the dorsum of the paws and prevent wearing of the nails. The boots should be fitted properly and have properties that promote hygiene, water resistance and durability. Slings are available commercially for use as the dog becomes paraparetic. The sling should have a soft lining and be fitted properly to prevent chaffing. In dogs that are unable to ambulate without support, two- or four-wheel carts are available commercially. These assistive devices can provide independence for the DM-affected dog. However, the pet owner must monitor for fatigue in the thoracic limbs and ensure that the cart fits appropriately as the disease progresses.

It is important to prevent or minimize the secondary consequences of DM, such as contracture, decubitus ulcers, and pneumonia. Bedding should be supportive enough to distribute the dog's weight evenly, especially over bony prominences, to prevent decubital ulcers. The skin should be assessed twice daily for redness or other evidence of ulceration. Absorbent materials (lamb's wool, diaper pads) should overlay supportive materials (air, foam mattresses). If the dog is unable to reposition itself into a sternal position, rotation should be performed every 4 to 6 hours. Cleanliness is critical to prevent fecal and urine scalding because incontinence develops when the dog becomes nonambulatory. Hydrotherapy also can play a role in increasing circulation in the limb vasculature and preventing decubitus ulcers. In the late disease stage when the dog is tetraplegic, dysphagia will develop, which predisposes to aspiration pneumonia.

References and Suggested Reading

Ashworth NL, Satkunam LE, Deforge D: Treatment for spasticity in amyotrophic lateral sclerosis/motor neuron disease, *Cochrane Database Syst Rev* 1:CD004156, 2006.

Averill DR: Degenerative myelopathy in the aging German Shepherd dog: clinical and pathologic findings, *J Am Vet Med Assoc* 162(12):1045, 1973.

Awano T et al: Genome-wide association analysis reveals a *SOD1* mutation in canine degenerative myelopathy that resembles amyotrophic lateral sclerosis, *Proc Natl Acad Sci U S A* 106:2794, 2009.

Beghi E et al: The epidemiology and treatment of ALS: focus on the heterogeneity of the disease and critical appraisal of therapeutic trials, *Amyotroph Lateral Scler* 12:1, 2011.

Bello-Haas VD et al: A randomized controlled trial of resistance exercise in individuals with ALS, *Neurology* 68:2003, 2007.

Bennett RL, Knowlton GC: Overwork weakness in partially denervated skeletal muscle, *Clin Orthop* 12:711, 1958.

Bensimon G, Lacomblez L, Meininger V: A control trial of riluzole, ALS/Riluzole Study Group, *N Engl J Med* 330:585, 1994.

Boillée S, Vande Velde C, Cleveland DW: ALS: a disease of motor neurons and their nonneuronal neighbors, *Neuron* 52(1):39, 2006.

Braund KG, McGuire JA, Lincoln CE: Observations on normal skeletal muscle of mature dogs: a cytochemical, histochemical and morphometric study, *Vet Pathol* 19:577, 1982.

Braund KG, Vandevelde M: German Shepherd dog myelopathy— a morphologic and morphometric study, *Am J Vet Res* 39(8):1309, 1978.

Chen A, Montes J, Mitsumoto H: The role of exercise in amyotrophic lateral sclerosis, *Phys Med Rehabil Clin N Am* 19:545, 2008.

Clemmons RM: Degenerative myelopathy. In Kirk RW, editor: *Current veterinary therapy X: small animal practice*, Philadelphia, 1989, Saunders, p 830.

Coates JR et al: Clinical characterization of a familial degenerative myelopathy in Pembroke Welsh Corgi dogs, *J Vet Intern Med* 21:1323, 2007.

Coates JR, Wininger FA: Canine degenerative myelopathy, *Vet Clin North Am Small Anim Pract* 40:929, 2010.

Drory VE et al: The value of muscle exercise in patients with amyotrophic lateral sclerosis, *J Neurol Sci* 191:133, 2001.

Drum MG: Physical rehabilitation of the canine neurologic patient, *Vet Clin North Am Small Anim Pract* 40:181, 2010.

Fechner H et al: Molecular genetic and expression analysis of alpha-tocopherol transfer protein mRNA in German Shepherd dogs with degenerative myelopathy, *Berl Munch Tierarztl Wochenschr* 11:631, 2003.

Griffiths IR, Duncan ID: Chronic degenerative radiculomyelopathy in the dog, *J Small Anim Pract* 16(8):461, 1975.

Hallum A: Neuromuscular disease. In Umphred DA, editor: *Neurological rehabilitation*, ed 5, St Louis, 2007, Mosby, p 475.

Johnston PEJ et al: Central nervous system pathology in 25 dogs with chronic degenerative radiculomyelopathy, *Vet Rec* 146(22):629, 2000.

Johnston PEJ et al: Serum alpha tocopherol concentrations in German shepherd dogs with chronic degenerative radiculomyelopathy, *Vet Rec* 148:403, 2001.

Kaspar BK et al: Synergy of insulin-like growth factor-1 and exercise in amyotrophic lateral sclerosis, *Ann Neurol* 57:649, 2005.

Kathmann I et al: Daily controlled physiotherapy increases survival time in dogs with suspected degenerative myelopathy, *J Vet Intern Med* 20:927, 2006.

Katz RT: Management of spasticity, *Am J Phys Med Rehabil* 67:108, 1988.

Kierkinezos IG et al: Regular exercise is beneficial to a mouse model of amyotrophic lateral sclerosis, *Ann Neurol* 53:804, 2003.

Liebetanz D et al: Extensive exercise is not harmful in amyotrophic lateral sclerosis, *Eur J Neurosci* 20:3115, 2004.

Mahoney DJ et al: Effects of high-intensity endurance exercise training in the G93A mouse model of amyotrophic lateral sclerosis, *Muscle Nerve* 29:656, 2004.

March PA et al: Degenerative myelopathy in 18 Pembroke Welsh Corgi dogs, *Vet Pathol* 46:241, 2009.

Matthews NS, de Lahunta A: Degenerative myelopathy in an adult miniature poodle, *J Am Vet Med Assoc* 186(11):1213, 1985.

McCrate ME, Kaspar BK: Physical activity and neuroprotection in amyotrophic lateral sclerosis, *Neuromolecular Med* 10:108, 2008.

Miller RG et al: Riluzole for amyotrophic lateral sclerosis (ALS/ motor neuron disease [MND]), *Cochrane Database Syst Rev* CDOO1447, 2007.

Millis DL: Physical therapy and rehabilitation of neurologic patients. In Bonagura JD, Twedt DC, editors: *Kirk's current veterinary therapy XIV*, St Louis, 2009, Saunders, p 1131.

Millis DL, Levine D, Taylor RA: *Canine rehabilitation and physical therapy*, Philadelphia, 2004, Saunders.

Milner-Brown HS, Miller RG: Muscle strengthening through high-resistance weight training in patients with neuromuscular disorders, *Arch Phys Med Rehabil* 69:14, 1998.

Olby N, Halling KB, Glick TR: Rehabilitation for the neurologic patient, *Vet Clin North Am Small Anim Pract* 35:1389, 2005.

Polizopoulou ZS et al: Evaluation of a proposed therapeutic protocol in 12 dogs with tentative degenerative myelopathy, *Acta Vet Hung* 56(3):293, 2008.

Reitsma W: Skeletal muscle hypertrophy after heavy exercise in rats with surgically reduced muscle function, *Am J Phys Med* 48:237, 1969.

Ropper AH, Samuels MA: *Adams and Victor's principles of neurology*, ed 9, New York, 2009, McGraw-Hill.

Sanjak M et al: Quantitative assessment of motor fatigue in amyotrophic lateral sclerosis, *J Neurol Sci* 191:55, 2001.

Shealy P, Thomas WB, Immel L: Neurologic conditions and physical rehabilitation of the neurologic patient. In Millis DL, Levine D, Taylor RA, editors: *Canine rehabilitation and physical therapy*, Philadelphia, 2004, Saunders, p 388.

Shelton GD et al: Degenerative myelopathy associated with a missense mutation in the superoxide dismutase 1 (SOD1) gene progresses to peripheral neuropathy in Pembroke Welsh Corgis and Boxers, *J Neurol Sci* 318:55, 2012.

Sherman J, Olby NJ: Nursing and rehabilitation of the neurological patient. In Platt SR, Olby NJ, editors: *BSAVA manual of canine and feline neurology*, ed 3, Gloucester, UK, 2004, British Small Animal Veterinary Association, p 394.

Tam SL et al: Increased neuromuscular activity reduces sprouting in partially denervated muscles, *J Neurosci* 21:654, 2001.

Williams DA, Prymak C, Baughan J: Tocopherol (vitamin E) status in canine degenerative myelopathy. In *Proceedings of the 3rd ACVIM Forum*, 1985, p 154.

Williams HB: The value of continuous electrical muscle stimulation using a completely implantable system in the preservation of muscle function following motor nerve injury and repair: an experimental study, *Microsurgery* 17:589, 1996.

Wininger FA et al: Degenerative myelopathy in a Bernese mountain dog with a novel SOD1 missense mutation, *J Vet Intern Med* 25:1166, 2011.

CHAPTER 235

Diagnosis and Treatment of Atlantoaxial Subluxation

BEVERLY K. STURGES, *Davis, California*

Atlantoaxial (AA) instability with subluxation of C2 relative to C1 is a frequent cause of cervical pain as well as myelopathy in toy and miniature breeds of dogs. Congenital vertebral malformations along with abnormality or absence of ligamentous structures lead to contusion or compression of the cervical spinal cord and caudal brainstem. AA instability also occurs infrequently in large breeds of dogs and usually is secondary to traumatic injury of the cervical vertebral column. Because AA instability is a potentially life-threatening disease, it is important to recognize when it *may* be present so that the patient is handled appropriately. This will prevent exacerbation of the clinical signs until a definitive diagnosis is made and appropriate treatment is instituted.

General Considerations: Anatomy and Physiology

The atlas (C1) and axis (C2) form a pivotal joint that allows free movement of the head about the longitudinal axis of the spine. Most rotational head movement centers around the dens, a bony process projecting rostrally from the body of the axis. The dens is held in place on the ventral aspect of C1, within the vertebral canal, by several ligaments (Figures 235-1 and 235-2):

1. The *apical and alar ligaments* leave the apex of the dens and attach to the ventral aspect of the foramen magnum and the skull medial to the occipital condyles.
2. The *transverse atlantal ligament* is a strong ligament that runs transversely in the vertebral canal, crossing dorsally over the dens. This ligament is particularly important to AA joint stability since it holds the dens firmly against the ventral aspect of the atlas.
3. The *dorsal atlantoaxial membrane* is a fibrous extension of the joint capsule running between the arch of the atlas and the spinous process of the axis. It adds support limiting the amount of dorsoventral movement between C1 and C2.

The atlas articulates rostrally with the occipital condyles of the skull and forms a joint of which the main movements are flexion and extension of the head, the "yes" joint. Caudally, the atlas articulates with the axis allowing lateral and rotational movement of the head, the "no" joint. Working together, these two joints allow free motion of the head in all directions. The large nuchal ligament that attaches the spinous process of C2 to those of T1 and T2 functions in suspension of the head, forming a fulcrum at the AA joint (see Figures 235-1 and 235-2).

Pathophysiology

Instability of the AA region allows excessive flexion of the C1-2 joint that may result in subluxation of C2 relative to C1 and injury to the spinal cord (Figure 235-3). This usually occurs secondary to congenital or developmental abnormalities of the bones or ligaments of the AA joint, traumatic injury to the joint, or a combination of both (Figure 235-4). In many instances the abnormalities present are associated with the dens and include agenesis or hypoplasia of the dens, dorsal angulation of the dens, and fracture or avulsion of the dens from the axis. Absence or rupture of associated AA ligaments often contributes to the instability caused by congenital anomalies in the region. All of these findings are common in toy and miniature breeds of dogs. Traumatic rupture of the AA ligaments without associated anomalies of the AA joint is possible but usually occurs as a result of major traumatic injury to the cervical vertebral column. This is the most common cause of AA instability in large-breed dogs. Recently there have been reports (Owen et al, 2008; Warren-Smith et al, 2009) of larger-breed dogs with absence or incomplete ossification of the atlas (Figure 235-5). Associated AA subluxation in most of these dogs suggests another predisposing factor to AA instability. This was further investigated in another study characterizing the morphology of the atlas on computed tomography (CT) in various classes of dog breed (Parry et al, 2010). Dogs with ossification abnormalities involving the atlas were significantly more likely to have associated AA subluxation, although the underlying pathophysiology behind these findings is not known. AA subluxation rarely is seen in cats. Only a handful of cases have been reported, and all of them have been associated with congenital occipitoatlantoaxial malformations or malformations of the dens (C2).

Regardless of the underlying cause, dorsal displacement of the cranial portion of the body of the axis into the vertebral canal causes compression, edema, and inflammation of the spinal cord that may extend cranially into the caudal brainstem. In addition, intraaxial hemorrhage into the central nervous system parenchyma also may contribute to the clinical signs (Kent et al, 2010). Cervical pain, myelopathy of varying degrees, and possible caudal brainstem signs may occur.

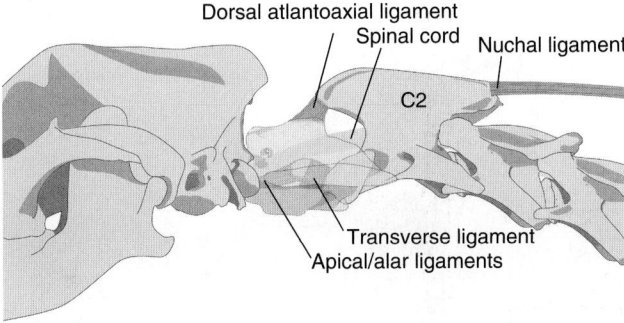

Figure 235-1 Normal atlantoaxial (AA) joint, lateral view. Note the relationships of the ligamentous and bony structures of the AA joint that allow normal head movement without injury to neural structures.

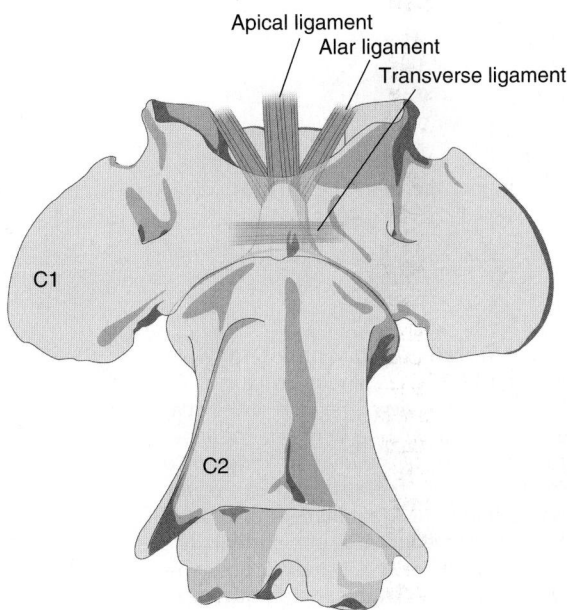

Figure 235-2 Normal atlantoaxial joint, ventrodorsal view. The apical and alar ligaments attach the dens to the occipital bones of the skull, whereas the transverse ligament crosses over the dens, maintaining it in place on the floor of the vertebral canal.

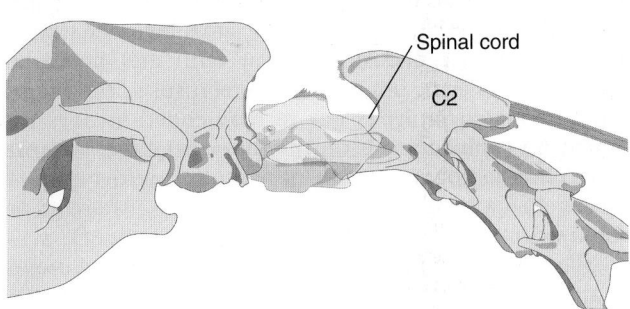

Figure 235-3 Atlantoaxial subluxation, lateral view. Subluxation of the axis (C2) relative to the atlas (C1) causes traumatic injury and compression of the cranial spinal cord. Associated hemorrhage and edema may extend rostrally to affect brainstem function.

Diagnosis

Clinical Presentation

Malformations of the AA joint occur most frequently in toy and miniature breeds of dogs, especially Chihuahuas, Yorkshire terriers, toy and miniature poodles, Pomeranians, Japanese chin, Maltese dogs, and others. Clinical signs of a C1 to C5 myelopathy or cervical pain occur and may be acute or chronic in onset and progressive, nonprogressive, or intermittent. Often the signs occur secondary to mild "trauma" such as jumping off the bed or roughhousing with other dogs. Although clinical signs typically are reported in the first year of life, it is not uncommon for dogs older than a year, including middle-aged or older animals, to begin showing clinical signs. Severity of signs varies from mild cervical pain to profound cervical pain to tetraparesis, respiratory paralysis, and caudal brainstem signs (e.g., hypoventilation, obtundation, vestibular signs). Traumatic AA instability, with or without an underlying congenital malformation, usually is the cause of AA subluxation in larger-breed dogs (>10 kg).

Occasionally dogs with AA instability have a history of seizurelike signs or episodes that occur intermittently. Owners often describe an associated transient apnea and paresis. The episodes may be related to a mild trauma, such as jumping out of a car or going down the stairs. These clinical signs may occur more commonly with malformations of the dens, specifically agenesis or dorsal angulation of the dens.

Differential diagnoses for dogs with suspected AA instability or subluxation include intervertebral disk disease, cervical trauma or spinal fracture, infectious or inflammatory disease (e.g., granulomatous meningoencephalitis), other craniospinal anomalies (e.g., syringomyelia, Chiari-like malformation), and neoplasia (of the cervical spine or brain). Since the history, signalment, and clinical signs of AA instability may be indistinguishable from those of other differential diagnoses, it is important to take appropriate precautions in any animal that may have vertebral instability at the AA joint.

Radiography

Plain cervical radiography provides the diagnosis in most instances. Because it is essential that positioning be accurate when the AA region of the cervical spine is evaluated, general anesthesia is necessary. It is easy to misdiagnose AA subluxation when positioning is imperfect or when the beam is not centered on C1-2. Care must be taken when manipulating an animal suspected of having AA instability during intubation, handling under anesthesia, and radiography since flexion of the animal's neck may result in further spinal cord compression. Placing a soft, padded bandage on the patient before inducing anesthesia, with the head positioned in mild extension, provides support and comfort for the animal and serves as a safeguard to keep the AA joint in extension.

On radiographs the body of the axis is displaced dorsally and cranially into the vertebral canal on neutral lateral projections. The distance between the dorsal arch

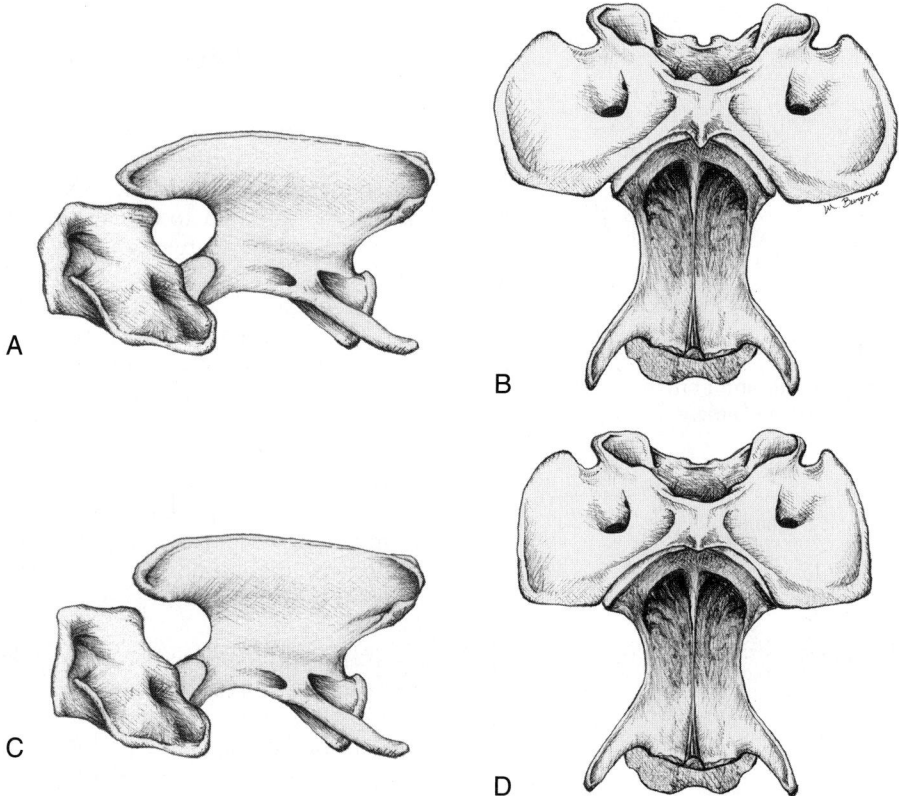

Figure 235-4 Comparison of C1 and C2 vertebrae. **A** and **B,** Lateral and ventrodorsal views illustrating the normal shape and relationship of C1 relative to C2. The spinous process of C2 typically spans the caudal third of the dorsal arch of C1 on the lateral view. The arch of the atlas is thicker than in toy or miniature breeds, with a layer of trabecular bone between the inner and outer layers of cortical bone, and the transverse process (wings) of the atlas are longer and thicker. **C,** Lateral view showing typical vertebral deformities seen in the atlas and axis of toy and miniature breeds. The spinous process of C2 often is foreshortened and minimally associated with the dorsal arch of C1. Dorsal atlantoaxial ligaments likely are reduced or nonexistent. The intervertebral foramen is comparatively large, and the vertebral arches of C1 and C2 are comparatively small and misshapen. **D,** Ventrodorsal view showing typical vertebral deformities seen in toy and miniature breeds. The wings of the atlas are very thin and often much smaller comparatively than in normal dogs. The articulation between C1 and C2 is widened and often malformed; there is much less bony mass in the body of C1 and C2. Significantly, these changes are accompanied by hypoplasia, agenesis, and abnormal angulation of the dens.

of the atlas and spinous process of the axis is increased (Figure 235-6, *A*). If the findings are not clearly diagnostic, the head should be extended gently to demonstrate further reduction of the subluxation (Figure 235-6, *B*). As a last resort, the head may be flexed gently to demonstrate abnormal movement at C1-2 and exacerbation of the subluxation. Abnormalities of the dens may be seen clearly on oblique lateral views, in which the wings of the atlas are not superimposed on the dens, or on ventrodorsal views.

Advanced Imaging

Myelography, CT imaging, or both modalities may be required to confirm that subluxation is present and to provide further delineation of regional problems when multiple congenital anomalies are present (Figure 235-7).

Such imaging also may be useful to rule out other differential diagnoses within the same neuroanatomic region (e.g., disk disease). Lumbar puncture should be done since cisternal puncture for cerebrospinal fluid sampling or myelography is not recommended in dogs for which AA subluxation is on the differential list. In most cases plain radiography with or without myelography or CT-myelography is sufficient to diagnose AA instability or subluxation.

Magnetic resonance imaging (MRI) may be very useful in the diagnosis of AA subluxation, especially in patients with clinical signs of brain or brainstem disease as well as cervical pain and myelopathy. The extent of central nervous system parenchymal injury to the cervical cord or caudal brainstem is best visualized with MRI (Figure 235-8). Typically a region of hyperintensity is visible in the cranial cervical spinal cord or caudal brainstem on

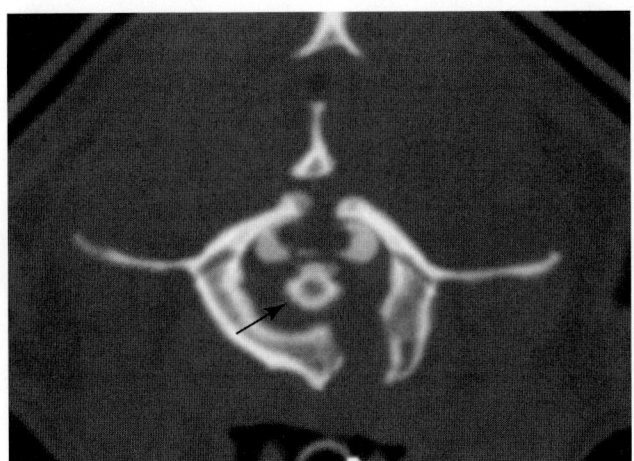

Figure 235-5 Transverse computed tomographic–myelographic image showing incomplete ossification of C1 in a 10-year-old Brittany spaniel with chronic cervical pain and tetraparesis. There is discontinuity of the dorsal arch as well as the body/ventral arch of C1. The dens is causing marked compression and dorsal displacement of the spinal cord within the vertebral canal. (Courtesy Dr. Robert Bergman.)

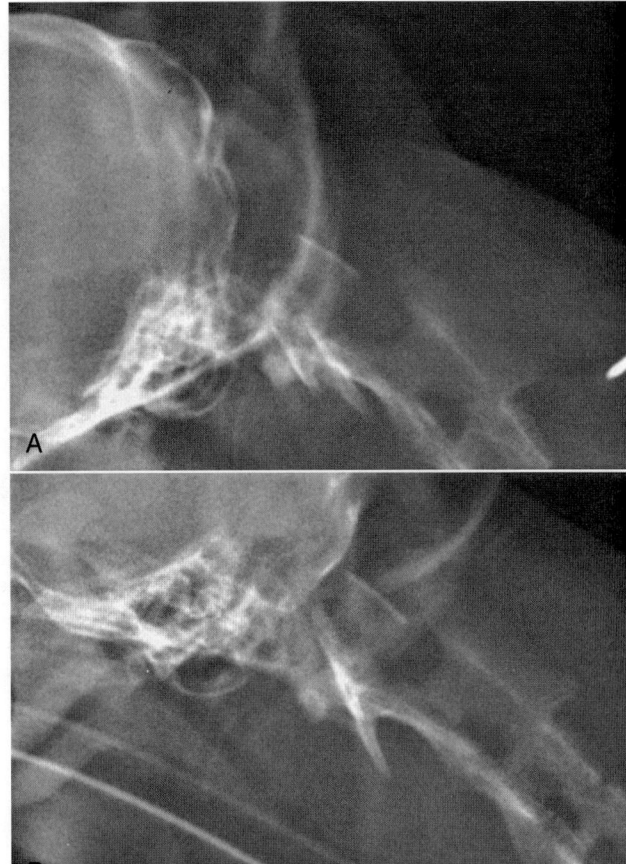

Figure 235-6 Plain lateral radiographs of a 0.75-kg 5-month-old Yorkshire terrier with acute-onset nonambulatory tetraparesis. **A,** The head is in a neutral position, and increased space can be seen between the arch of C1 and the spinous process of C2. This dog had several congenital abnormalities, including agenesis of the dens, an associated lack of normal atlantoaxial (AA) ligaments, and block vertebrae from C2 to C4. **B,** The head is now positioned in extension, which relieves compression on the spinal cord and allows C1 and C2 to assume a more normal relationship. This confirms that AA instability is present without the need to risk further spinal cord injury by flexing the head.

T2-weighted images. In addition, MRI is useful for ruling out the presence of concurrent diseases with clinical signs localizing to the same region and for identifying underlying disease that may influence long-term prognosis. For example, cavalier King Charles spaniels should be evaluated for the presence of a Chiari-like malformation and syringomyelia as well as AA instability when signs of cervical pain and myelopathy are present. Collection of cerebrospinal fluid is recommended in cases in which the diagnosis is not straightforward on imaging, especially in breeds of dogs typically prone to inflammatory disease of the brain (e.g., granulomatous meningoencephalitis).

Treatment

Animals with cervical pain only or minimal neurologic deficits may respond well to splinting of the head and neck in mild extension and strict cage rest for at least 6 weeks. However, the clinical signs may not completely resolve or may worsen, and recrudescence often occurs when the splint is removed. Surgical decompression and stabilization is indicated in animals with moderate to severe neurologic deficits or intense pain, and in those showing no response to nonsurgical treatment. Surgery also is recommended in animals in which angulation of the dens results in spinal cord injury. Animals younger than 6 months of age are best treated conservatively, if possible, to allow for more complete mineralization of bone and closure of vertebral physes before surgical stabilization is attempted. Certainly conservative treatment should be attempted in situations in which financial constraints do not allow surgical repair to be done.

Nonsurgical Treatment

Cage confinement, immobilization of the AA region, and possibly nonsteroidal antiinflammatory therapy often results in clinical improvement. Splinting allows for formation of fibrous tissues and some healing of ligamentous structures to restabilize the AA joint. Ideally the splint should extend from the mandible to the sternum incorporating the head in mild extension in an attempt to immobilize the AA joint as much as possible. Casting materials, thermoplast, or malleable metals may be used to form the splint, which then should be well padded before it is applied to the patient. Many patients do not tolerate this degree of immobilization well. Toy breeds, especially immature animals, may even have a hard time eating, walking, and supporting the cranial half of the body. Instead of a splint, a shorter, softer supportive bandage may be used that incorporates the head (including the caudal aspect of the mandible) down to the caudal cervical region. This is tolerable to the patient, keeps the head in mild extension, is easily supported, and appears to be effective, especially in very small dogs (Figure 235-9). Animals with splints and bandages of any kind

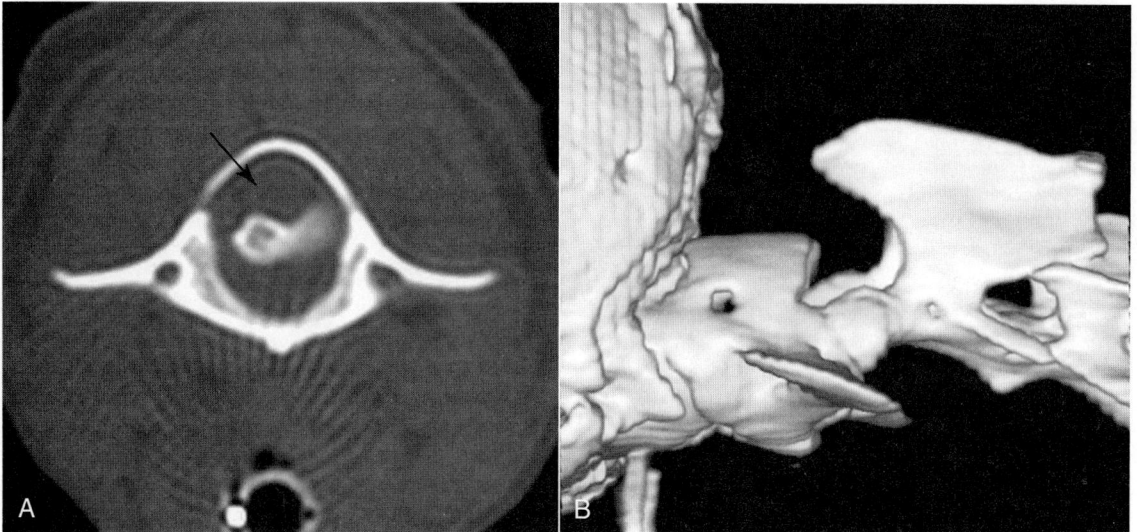

Figure 235-7 Computed tomographic images of a 3-year-old Yorkshire terrier with acute-onset cervical pain and ataxia. Although initially the dog was treated conservatively, clinical signs did not resolve. **A,** A transverse image through C1 shows the dens luxated into the vertebral canal and compressing the spinal cord *(arrow)*. **B,** A three-dimensional reconstruction confirms the abnormal position of C1 relative to C2.

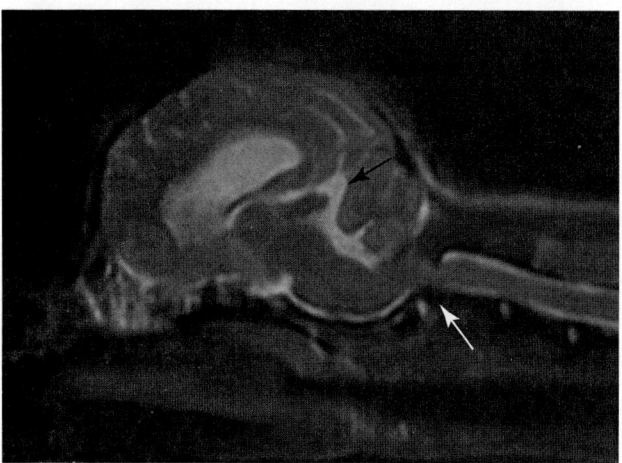

Figure 235-8 Midsagittal magnetic resonance image of a 15-month-old Chihuahua with acute onset of cervical pain, ataxia, and tetraparesis. Several abnormalities are noted in this dog. Ventriculomegaly is present along with a small quadrigeminal cyst *(black arrow)*. Mild crowding of the caudal fossa, occipital bone dysplasia, and dorsal atlantoaxial ligament hypertrophy also can be seen along with a dens that is subluxated into the vertebral canal *(white arrow)*. Hyperintensity in the spinal cord dorsal to the dens is consistent with edema, inflammation, or hemorrhage. The neurologic status of this dog returned to normal following surgical stabilization of C1-2.

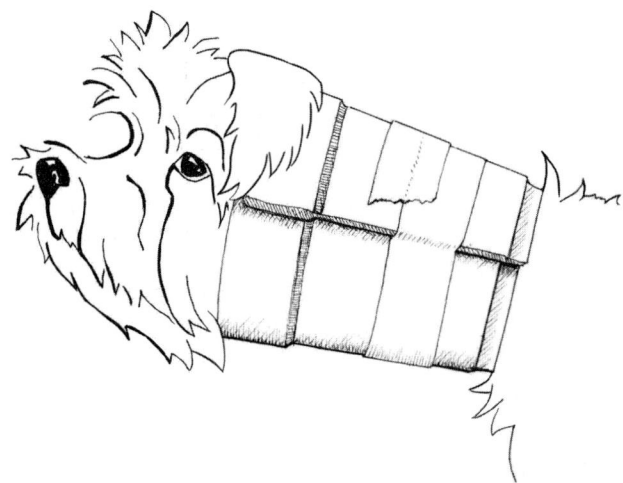

Figure 235-9 Removable supportive bandage for atlantoaxial (AA) instability in toy breed dogs. A small Styrofoam cup is cut from top to bottom and the base of the cup is removed. The cup is gently wrapped around the dog's neck, with the lip of the cup situated at the level of the temporomandibular joint and the base of the cup ending in the midcervical region. The cup is gently tightened and secured by overlapping the cut sides and taping in place. This provides comfortable support while limiting ventroflexion at the C1-C2 joint. Ear and jaw movements are not hindered and the bandage can be easily removed and replaced as needed.

should be checked regularly for any signs of complication, including otitis, facial and corneal excoriations, and dermatitis. Bandages typically are left on for a period of 4 to 8 weeks and then removed. The animal is allowed a gradual return to normal activity. If clinical signs of AA instability return, nonsurgical treatment may be reinstituted; however, surgical repair is strongly recommended at this point. Clients often become distraught with repeated episodes of pain or myelopathy and usually are

amenable to more definitive treatment with surgery after the first episode.

Surgical Treatment

Surgery is indicated for most dogs and cats with clinical signs of AA subluxation. Stabilization of the joint usually results in immediate relief of pain and improved neurologic status, even in the most severely affected animals.

Stabilization of the AA joint reduces the lateral and rotational mobility of the patient's head, although usually this is well tolerated physically by the animal. The "domino" effect, which frequently is of concern with fusion of vertebrae in the caudal cervical spine, does not appear to be a problem with stabilization of C1-2. Many surgical techniques for AA stabilization have been described in the veterinary literature that use either a dorsal or a ventral approach to the C1-2 joint. The following paragraphs briefly describe the procedures currently in common use.

Dorsal-Approach Surgical Techniques

Dorsal repairs of the AA joint were the earliest techniques described for immobilization (McCarthy et al, 1995). However, since fusion of the joint is not achieved, they are palliative procedures only and usually are not recommended as the first choice for treatment of AA subluxation. In most circumstances dorsal repairs have been replaced by ventral fusion techniques. Dorsal methods that are currently used include the following (Figure 235-10).

The *dorsal wiring-suturing technique* still is the most common dorsal method in use. The approach is technically easy, but correct placement of the wire or suture may

be difficult, and the procedure may be associated with several potential complications: (1) the spinal cord may be injured further during wire placement; (2) disruption of the internal vertebral venous sinus may lead to hemorrhage or hematoma formation within the vertebral canal, which exacerbates clinical signs; and (3) the wire or suture may cut through the lamina of C1, especially in soft, immature bones. Use of a splint or bandage is recommended for 6 weeks after surgery to immobilize the AA joint until scar tissue forms.

The *Kishigami atlantoaxial tension band repair* is an older technique. Recently the band has become available commercially, and its use in toy breeds for AA joint repair has been reported (Pujol et al, 2010).

Ventral-Approach Surgical Techniques

Ventral fixation of the AA joint generally is preferred since the ventral approach provides direct access to the C1-2 joint. This allows the surgeon to reduce the subluxation and decompress the spinal cord, perform an odontectomy if indicated, and promote arthrodesis between C1 and C2 by removing the articular cartilage and placing a bone graft. However, ventral approaches are technically more difficult, and complications may occur because (1) bones usually are very small, often malformed, and

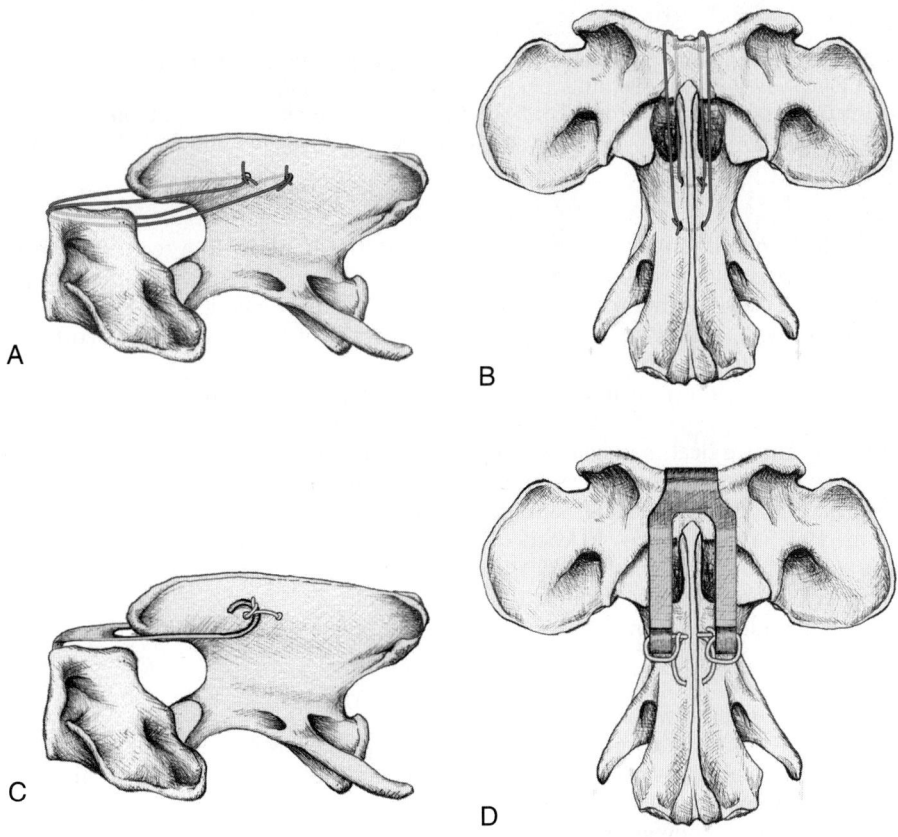

Figure 235-10 Dorsal surgical atlantoaxial (AA) repair techniques currently used to maintain C1-2 in reduction. **A,** Dorsal wiring technique using wire or suture. **B,** Kishigami band. Dorsal repairs do not provide the immobilization that ventral repairs do and are not recommended as the first choice for treatment of AA instability.

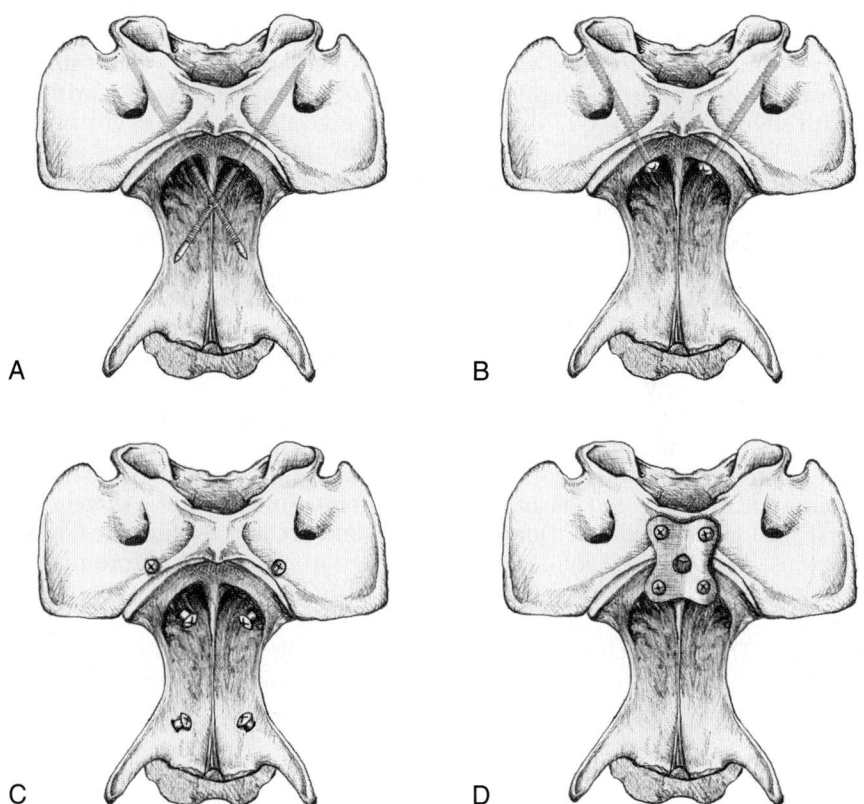

Figure 235-11 Ventral surgical stabilization techniques currently used to immobilize the atlantoaxial joint, ventrodorsal view. In addition to the implant, cancellous bone grafts are placed intraarticularly to promote arthrodesis at C1-2. **A,** Transarticular pins (with or without polymethyl methacrylate [PMMA]). **B,** Transarticular lag screws. **C,** Screw anchors and PMMA. **D,** Butterfly locking plate.

easily fractured during reduction and implant placement; (2) vertebral movement or incorrect positioning of the implant during placement can cause further injury to the spinal cord and possible paralysis, ventilatory failure, or death; and (3) trauma can occur to vital soft tissue structures in the area (e.g., vagosympathetic trunk, carotid artery, trachea, brainstem).

Many ventral techniques for surgical management of AA instability in dogs have been reported (Dickomeit et al, 2011; McCarthy et al, 1995; Platt et al, 2004; Sanders et al, 2004; Schulz et al, 1997; Sharp, 2005). In each of these procedures, the patient is positioned in dorsal recumbency with the neck in extension. Stabilization techniques in current use include the following (Figures 235-11 and 235-12):

- Transarticular pins, wires, or screws (with or without polymethyl methacrylate [PMMA]). A combination of pins, screws, and bone cement is used to immobilize the joint, and bony fusion at the site is promoted by the placement of a bone graft into the AA joint.
- Screw anchors and PMMA. Small screws are placed in the lateral masses of C1 and bony masses of C2, and sometimes of C3. These are then incorporated into PMMA.

- Butterfly plate. In a technique recently reported for use in small dogs (Dickomeit et al, 2011), a small (1.5-mm) locking plate is applied to the ventral aspect of C1-2 using monocortical screws.

Postoperative care usually is minimal, with pain medications needed for the first 24 to 36 hours and nonsteroidal antiinflammatory drugs used to treat associated inflammation as needed. Improvement in the neurologic status and pain score of the patient usually is seen immediately following surgery. Restriction of activity or cage confinement is recommended for the first 4 to 6 weeks.

Prognosis

The prognosis for animals with AA subluxation varies depending on the chronicity and severity of the spinal cord injury that occurs. Generally speaking, the long-term outcome is very good to excellent for animals treated surgically that have clinical signs of pain or mild to moderate neurologic deficits. Animals with severe tetraparesis or tetraplegia and respiratory distress, especially those with a long history of difficulties, have a guarded prognosis for good recovery of neurologic function (Beaver

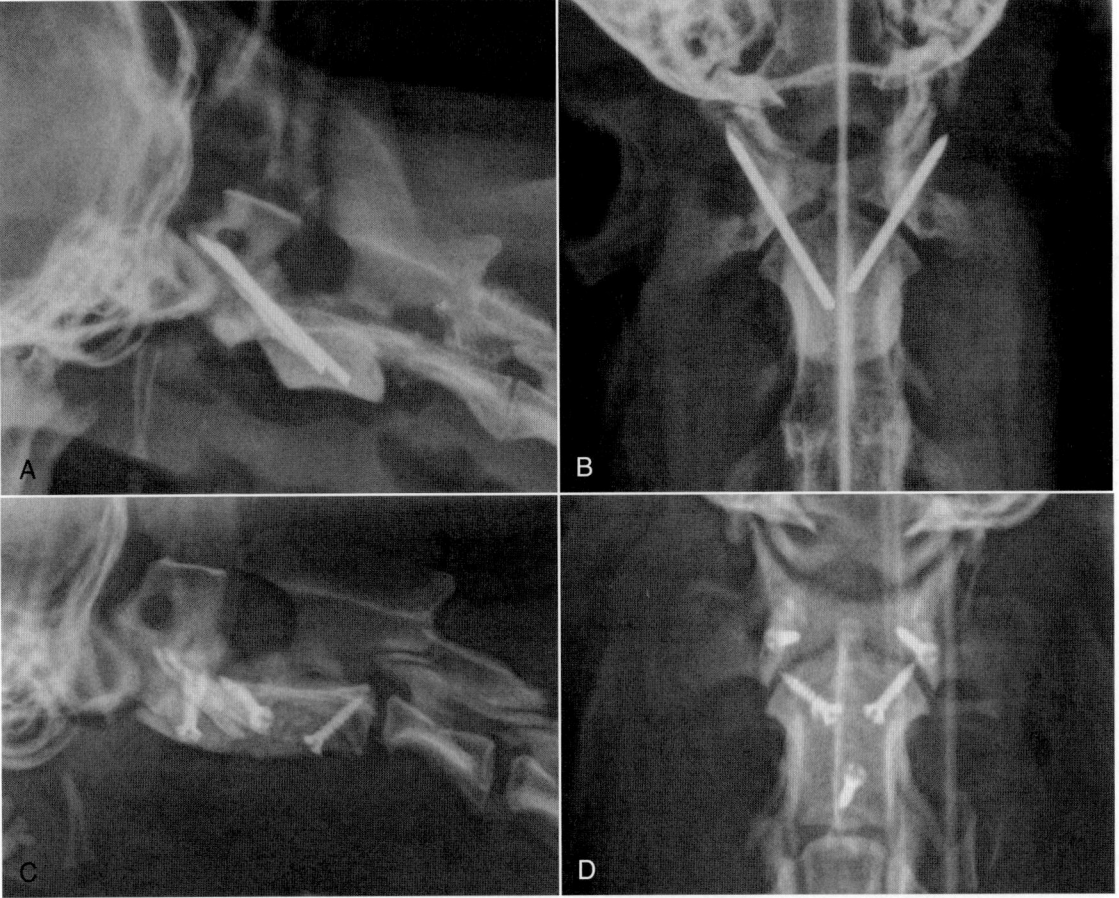

Figure 235-12 Common methods used to stabilize atlantoaxial subluxation. **A** and **B,** Postoperative lateral and ventrodorsal radiographs showing positive-profile threaded transarticular acrylic interface pins embedded in polymethyl methacrylate (PMMA). Note the block vertebrae present at C2, C3, and C4 in this dog. **C** and **D,** Titanium screw anchors in C1 and C2 embedded in PMMA. (**C** and **D** courtesy Dr. Andy Hopkins.)

et al, 2000; Knipe et al, 2002). Recently reported success rates for ventral surgical techniques vary from 79% to 92% for a good to excellent outcome (Beaver et al, 2000; Knipe et al, 2002; Platt et al, 2004; Sanders et al, 2004; Schulz et al, 1997); no one method proved superior to the others with respect to long-term survival. The experience and comfort level of the surgeon in performing surgery in the AA region is likely one of most important influences on the overall outcome for patients with AA disease. In practice, the patient almost always is referred to a surgical specialist for this procedure.

A recent study examining long-term outcomes in dogs treated nonsurgically found that dogs that had an acute onset of clinical signs and no history of signs of AA instability had a good outcome about 60% of the time, regardless of the severity of the neurologic signs at presentation (Havig et al, 2005). Dogs treated nonsurgically that had shown clinical signs for longer than 30 days were significantly more likely to have a poor final outcome. It should be noted that the presence of pain perception is of little prognostic value in animals with AA subluxation since compression severe enough to cause loss of deep pain at this level of the spinal cord usually results in respiratory paralysis and death.

References and Suggested Reading

Beaver DP et al: Risk factors affecting the outcome of surgery for atlantoaxial subluxation in dogs: 46 cases (1978-1998), *J Am Vet Med Assoc* 216:7, 2000.

Dickomeit M et al: Use of a 1.5mm butterfly locking plate for stabilization of atlantoaxial pathology in three toy breed dogs, *Vet Comp Orthop Traumatol* 24:246, 2011.

Havig ME et al: Evaluation of nonsurgical treatment of atlantoaxial subluxation in dogs: 19 cases (1992-2001), *J Am Vet Med Assoc* 222:2, 2005.

Kent M et al: Intraaxial spinal cord hemorrhage secondary to atlantoaxial subluxation in a dog, *J Am Anim Hosp Assoc* 46:132, 2010.

Knipe MF et al: Atlantoaxial instability in 17 dogs. 20th Annual ACVIM Forum Proceedings, Dallas, TX, *J Vet Intern Med*, 2002.

McCarthy RJ, Lewis DD, Hosgood G: Atlantoaxial subluxation in dogs, *Compend Contin Educ* 17:2, 1995.

Owen MC, Davis SH, Worth AJ: Imaging diagnosis—traumatic myelopathy in a dog with incomplete ossification of the neural arch of the atlas, *Vet Radiol Ultrasound* 49:570, 2008.

Parry AT et al: Computed tomography variations in morphology of the canine atlas in dogs with and without atlantoaxial subluxation, *Vet Radiol Ultrasound* 51(6):596, 2010.

Platt SR, Chambers JN, Cross A: A modified ventral fixation for surgical management of atlantoaxial subluxation in 19 dogs, *Vet Surg* 33:349, 2004.

Pujol E et al: Use of the Kishigami atlantoaxial tension band in eight toy breed dogs with atlantoaxial subluxation, *Vet Surg* 39:35, 2010.

Sanders SG et al: Outcomes and complications associated with ventral screws, pins, and polymethyl methacrylate for atlantoaxial instability in 12 dogs, *J Am Anim Hosp Assoc* 40:204, 2004.

Schulz KS, Waldron DR, Fahie M: Application of ventral pins and polymethylmethacrylate for the management of

atlantoaxial instability: results in nine dogs, *Vet Surg* 26:317, 1997.

Sharp NJH: Atlantoaxial subluxation. In Sharp NJH, Wheeler SJ, editors: *Small animal spinal disorders: diagnosis and surgery*, ed 2, St Louis, 2005, Mosby, p 161.

Warren-Smith CMR et al: Incomplete ossification of the atlas in dogs with cervical signs, *Vet Radiol Ultrasound* 50:235, 2009.

CHAPTER 236

Diagnosis and Treatment of Cervical Spondylomyelopathy

RONALDO CASIMIRO DA COSTA, *Columbus, Ohio*

Cervical spondylomyelopathy (CSM) is a very common disease of the cervical spine of large- and giant-breed dogs. CSM is characterized by dynamic and static compressions of the cervical spinal cord, nerve roots, or both leading to variable degrees of neurologic deficits and neck pain. CSM certainly is a controversial disease! Few other diseases in veterinary medicine have been called by 15 different names, with *wobbler syndrome, cervical vertebral instability, cervical malformation/malarticulation syndrome,* and *disk-associated wobbler syndrome* some of the more commonly used. Furthermore, few other disorders have been the target of 27 different proposed surgical treatments. This diversity reflects in part the lack of understanding regarding mechanisms of CSM.

Although the disease can affect essentially all canine breeds, two account for approximately 60% to 70% of all cases: the Doberman pinscher and the Great Dane. These breeds also illustrate the two distinct forms of the disease: disk-associated CSM (primarily affecting Dobermans) and the osseous form of CSM (affecting Great Danes).

Causes and Pathophysiology

The cause of CSM remains unresolved. Proposed causes include genetic, congenital, body conformation, and nutritional factors, with the latter two playing a less significant role. Based on current evidence CSM appears to be congenital. The genetic contribution to the development of the disease remains unclear, although recent evidence in Dobermans suggests that CSM is inherited as an autosomal dominant trait with variable penetrance in this breed.

The pathophysiology of CSM involves both static and dynamic factors. The key static factor is vertebral canal stenosis. It may be an absolute vertebral canal stenosis, which causes direct spinal cord compression and neurologic signs, or a relative vertebral stenosis, which by itself does not lead to myelopathic signs but predisposes the patient to development of myelopathy. Despite some degree of overlap, the spinal cord compressions can be divided into osseous compression and disk-associated compression based on pathophysiology.

Disk-associated compression typically is seen in middle-aged large-breed dogs (mostly Dobermans). It is caused by intervertebral protrusion with or without hypertrophy of the dorsal longitudinal ligament or ligamentum flavum (Figure 236-1). Three factors act in combination to explain the pathophysiology of disk-associated CSM: (1) relative vertebral canal stenosis, (2) more pronounced torsion in the caudal cervical spine leading to intervertebral disk degeneration, and (3) protrusion of larger-volume disks into the caudal cervical spine. Affected dogs apparently are born with a congenital vertebral canal stenosis that predisposes them to the development of clinical signs.

The vast majority of disk-associated spinal cord compressions are located in the caudal cervical spine, affecting the disks at C5-6 and C6-7. The biomechanical features of the caudal cervical spine explain the high incidence of lesions there. This region experiences three times more axial rotation or torsion than the cranial cervical spine, and torsion (more than axial compression) is the main biomechanical force leading to intervertebral disk degeneration in nonchondrodystrophic dogs. Additionally, a study found that Dobermans with CSM have larger

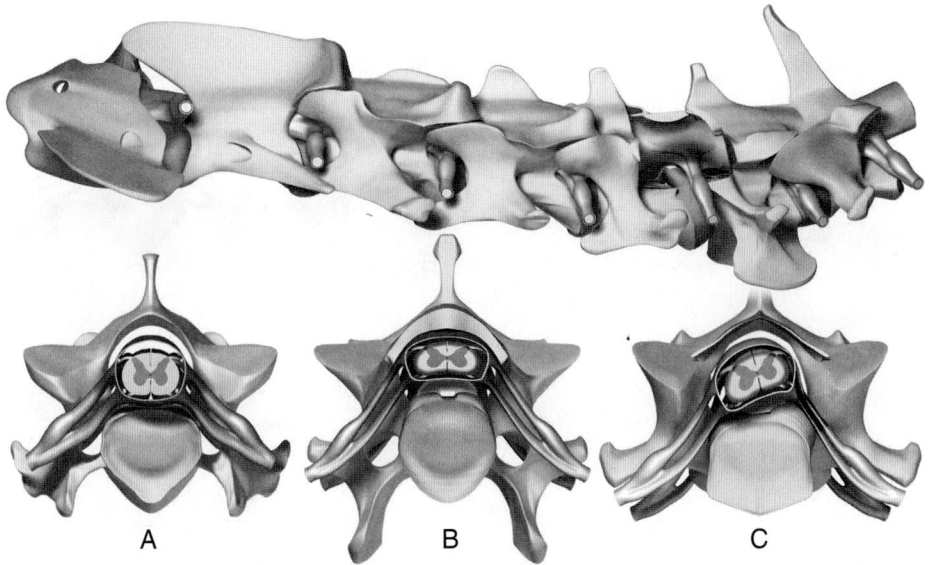

Figure 236-1 Disk-associated cervical spondylomyelopathy. *Top:* Ventral spinal cord compression and nerve root compression at C5-6 caused by intervertebral disk protrusion. Dorsally, hypertrophy of the ligamentum flavum causes mild spinal cord compression. **A,** Transverse section at the level of the C4-5 disk region showing normal spinal cord and vertebral canal. **B,** Ventral compression at the C5-6 region caused by intervertebral disk protrusion and hypertrophy of the dorsal longitudinal ligament and ligamentum flavum (leading to mild dorsal compression). **C,** Asymmetric intervertebral disk protrusion at C6-7 causing spinal cord and nerve root compression.

intervertebral disks than clinically normal Dobermans (da Costa et al, 2006b). This would cause a larger volume of disk protrusion into the vertebral canal. Since dogs with CSM have a narrow vertebral canal, the combination of a stenotic vertebral canal and protrusion of disks with larger volumes ultimately leads to clinical disease.

The pathophysiology of osseous or bony CSM is different. Osseous CSM is seen predominantly in young adult giant-breed dogs, especially in Great Danes. Although a hereditary basis still is unproven, a familial predisposition has been identified. Giant breeds usually have severe absolute vertebral canal stenosis secondary to proliferation of the vertebral arch (dorsally), articular facets (dorsolaterally), or articular facets and pedicles (laterally) (Figure 236-2). The cause of the compression appears to be a combination of vertebral malformation and osteoarthritic-osteoarthrotic changes at the level of the articular facets. Even though most giant-breed dogs have osseous compression, occasionally these compressions are complicated by disk protrusion, especially in older dogs. Ligamentous compression (by the ligamentum flavum) may be involved in the pathophysiology of the disease in giant- and large-breed dogs, but pure ligamentous compression as the single source of compression appears uncommon.

Critical to understanding the development of clinical signs in CSM-affected large-breed dogs is the concept of the dynamic lesion. Dynamic spinal cord compressions are present in both disk-associated and osseous forms of CSM. A dynamic lesion is one that worsens or improves with changes in the position of the cervical

spine. Continuous flexion and extension of the cervical spine can lead to spinal cord elongation causing axial strain and stress within the spinal cord, and this has been proposed as a key mechanism of spinal cord injury in cervical spondylotic myelopathy in humans. This is very different from instability, which has been defined as loss of the ability of the cervical spine to maintain its normal pattern of displacement under physiologic loads and thereby prevent damage to the spinal cord or nerve roots. Instability has not yet been proven in dogs with CSM, and it appears that with the severe disk and osseous degenerative changes, a restricted rather than an excessive motion occurs at the affected sites.

The most common location of compressive lesions in both large- and giant-breed dogs is at C5-6 and C6-7. The lesion is located at one of these sites in 90% of affected large-breed dogs. In giant-breed dogs, the C4-5 site also is commonly affected. Approximately 50% of large-breed dogs have a single site of spinal cord compression, and 50% have two or more sites of similar severity. In giant-breed dogs approximately 20% of dogs have a single site of compression, whereas 80% have multiple compressive lesions. A computed tomographic (CT)–myelographic study identified lesions affecting the T1-T2 and T2 regions in 14% of giant-breed dogs and the C7-T1 region in 22% of all dogs (da Costa et al, 2012). These lesions were not the primary site of compression but were part of the multiple compressions seen in giant-breed dogs. For this reason, it is important to include the cranial thoracic region in imaging studies of dogs suspected of having CSM.

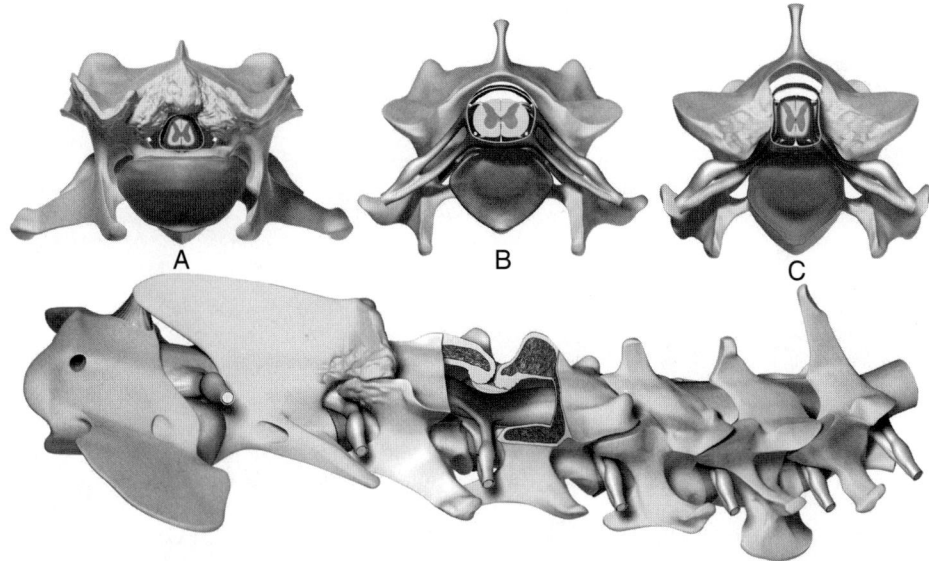

Figure 236-2 Osseous cervical spondylomyelopathy. **A,** Severe dorsolateral spinal cord compression at C2-3 caused by osseous malformation and osteoarthritic changes. **B,** Normal C3-4 disk region. **C,** Bilateral compression at C4-5 caused by osteoarthritic changes and medial proliferation of the facets resulting in absolute vertebral canal stenosis and foraminal stenosis, which lead to spinal cord and nerve root compression, respectively. *Bottom:* Dorsal spinal cord compression at C3-4 caused by lamina malformation and hypertrophy of the ligamentum flavum. Osteoarthritic changes also are shown at C2-3.

Diagnosis

As indicated earlier, CSM is primarily a disease of large- and giant-breed dogs. It is seen occasionally in small-breed dogs, but it is unclear whether small dogs also have vertebral canal stenosis. The majority of large-breed dogs (weimaraners, dalmatians) and Dobermans with CSM are older than 3 years of age at presentation (mean age, ~7 years). Great Danes and giant breeds (Mastiffs, rottweilers, Bernese and Swiss mountain dogs) with CSM usually are seen at a younger age. The mean age of giant-breed dogs with CSM is 3.8 years, and the disease may be seen in dogs just a few months old.

History and Clinical Signs

A history of chronic progressive signs persisting for several weeks to months is typical. Acute presentations usually are associated with neck pain. Neck pain or cervical hyperesthesia is a common historical finding but is not the typical reason for presentation. Neck pain is part of the clinical findings in approximately 65% to 70% of Dobermans and in 40% to 50% of dogs of other breeds, but it is the chief complaint in only 5% to 10% of dogs with CSM. Forceful manipulations of the cervical spine are unnecessary to document the presence of neck pain and can lead to severe neurologic decompensation. Careful assessment of posture and evaluation of voluntary range of motion (side to side, ventrally and dorsally) using a food treat is recommended to assess for cervical pain. Deep palpation of the transverse processes also can assist in the identification of neck pain.

Gait evaluation is the most important component of the examination in dogs suspected of having CSM because it reliably identifies proprioceptive ataxia, even in the absence of conscious proprioceptive deficits. Proprioceptive ataxia is seen in most dogs with CSM. Dogs with lesions in the cranial or midcervical spine tend to have ataxia affecting all four limbs more uniformly. However, affected dogs typically have obvious pelvic limb ataxia with milder abnormalities in the thoracic limbs. In some cases, the thoracic limb ataxia or weakness may be very mild in comparison with the pelvic limb signs, so that the thoracic limb abnormalities go unnoticed. The thoracic limb gait can appear short-strided or spastic with a pseudohypermetric ("floating") appearance. Occasionally thoracic limb lameness can be seen, which suggests nerve root entrapment. The pelvic limb gait often is wide based (abducted) and markedly incoordinated. The stride length of the pelvic limbs is increased, which causes the swaying movements of the hind end that are typical of the disease. Scuffing of the pelvic or thoracic limb toes and nails also can be seen. Postural reaction deficits (proprioceptive positioning deficits) are seen in most dogs with CSM but may not be evident in those with a history of long-standing signs despite the presence of proprioceptive ataxia. The reason for this discrepancy is that different tracts carry the pathways for conscious and unconscious proprioception. Approximately 10% of dogs with CSM have nonambulatory tetraparesis at initial presentation.

Evaluation of the spinal reflexes in dogs with CSM indicates a lesion located at either the C1 to C5 spinal cord segments (normal to increased spinal reflexes in all four limbs, with neurologic signs as described earlier) or C6 to C8 spinal cord segments. A C6 to C8 myelopathy is typical because the osseous and disk lesions are concentrated in the C5-6 and C6-7 intervertebral regions. In these cases, the gait is affected in all four limbs but more severely in the pelvic limbs. Evaluation of the spinal reflexes in the thoracic limbs shows a decreased flexor (withdrawal) reflex indicating involvement of the musculocutaneous nerve from the C6 to C8 spinal cord segments, with normal to increased extensor tone suggesting an upper motor neuron lesion and release of the radial nerve from spinal cord segments C7, C8, and T1, mostly C8 and T1. The pelvic limb reflexes are normal to increased.

Radiography

Survey radiographs can be used only as a screening test to rule out other differential diagnoses for cervical myelopathies, such as osseous neoplasia, trauma, vertebral osteomyelitis, and diskospondylitis. Radiographic findings in disk-associated CSM are primarily changes in the shape of the vertebral body (which assumes a triangular shape in severe cases), narrowing of the intervertebral disk space, and vertebral canal stenosis. Osteoarthritic, sclerotic changes of the articular facets are the radiographic hallmarks in giant-breed dogs with osseous compressions and can be seen on lateral and ventrodorsal projections. Some of the radiographic findings seen in dogs with CSM (e.g., vertebral tipping) also are seen in normal dogs. Studies in Doberman pinschers indicate that approximately 20% to 25% of clinically normal dogs have radiographic changes comparable to those seen in dogs with CSM.

Myelography

Myelography is no longer the method of choice to diagnose CSM. It can be used if CT and magnetic resonance imaging (MRI) are unavailable. Lateral and ventrodorsal views should be obtained. Oblique views also should be considered to increase diagnostic accuracy. Stress myelographic views also can be obtained, primarily in large-breed dogs. Because of the risk of severe neurologic decompensation after myelography with the animal in extension and flexion positions, only traction views are recommended. Myelograms obtained in these positions can, in theory, assist in differentiating a static from a dynamic lesion, but this distinction is highly subjective and no clear guidelines for testing and interpretation have been established. For some clinicians, a dynamic lesion is one that improves with traction, whereas others consider a lesion dynamic when it reduces completely. When traction is to be performed, the recommendation is to use a cervical harness and approximately 20% of the dog's weight for traction. Postmyelographic seizures occur in 25% of dogs with CSM. The risk of seizure can be minimized by restricting the total volume of contrast medium and using lumbar injections. Because of all of these issues, other imaging modalities are preferred.

Computed Tomography

CT is a rapid technique that allows visualization of transverse sections of the cervical spine. It must be combined with myelography to identify the exact location of the compressive lesion. It provides superior visualization of the direction and severity of the spinal cord compression compared with myelography as well as identification of spinal cord atrophy. Atrophy is identified on CT myelography as a widening of the subarachnoid space surrounding the spinal cord, with the cord assuming a triangular shape. Spinal cord atrophy may be a negative prognostic indicator in dogs with CSM. Plain CT can be performed with sedation only, which may be useful in cases in which general anesthesia is contraindicated or for long-term follow-up of osseous compressive lesions.

Magnetic Resonance Imaging

MRI is the gold standard test for evaluation of dogs suspected of having CSM. The main advantage of MRI is that it also detects signal changes in the spinal cord and thus allows assessment of the spinal cord parenchyma. These parenchymal signal changes are seen in approximately 50% of dogs with CSM and allow precise identification of the site most severely affected. A study compared myelography and MRI in the diagnosis of CSM and concluded that MRI was more accurate in predicting the site, severity, and nature of spinal cord compression (da Costa et al, 2006b).

The presence of spinal cord signal changes—namely, hyperintensity on T2-weighted images—is associated with the degree of severity of clinical signs, degree of severity of spinal cord compression, and chronicity of signs. Hyperintensity on T2-weighted images does not appear to correlate with prognosis in dogs, but preliminary evidence suggests that the combination of hyperintensity on T2-weighted images and hypointensity on T1-weighted images may be associated with a worse prognosis. Current evidence in humans suggests that multilevel hyperintensity on T2-weighted images and hypointensity on T1-weighted images are associated with a poorer prognosis.

In some cases, the degree of spinal compression is minimal relative to the severity of clinical signs. Dynamic spinal cord compressions are assumed in such cases. Testing for dynamic compression using traction MRI can be performed, and guidelines for testing have been published.

Additional Diagnostic Tests

Many large-breed dogs have concurrent medical conditions that potentially can increase anesthetic or surgical risk, or affect long-term prognosis. For this reason other studies beyond routine clinical laboratory tests should be performed in assembling a minimum data set. Tests of thyroid function usually are indicated because hypothyroidism is very common in Doberman pinschers and has been identified in a high percentage of dogs in association with CSM. Hypothyroidism can interfere with neurologic function and recovery from anesthesia. An understanding of the risks of hemorrhage related to von Willebrand status is necessary because a 73% prevalence of von Willebrand disease has been found in Doberman pinschers. Finally, assessment of heart rhythm (with a 5-minute electrocardiogram or Holter electrocardiography) as well as cardiac size and function (by echocardiography) is recommended before surgical treatment. General anesthesia can worsen cardiac function and lead to decompensation in dogs with occult dilated cardiomyopathy.

Treatment

Conservative (Medical) Treatment

Traditionally, medical treatment for CSM was considered a temporary measure to alleviate clinical signs. Without surgery, it was thought, the disease would be progressive and euthanasia would have to be contemplated. The only evidence to support these views came from a study conducted over 30 years ago involving mainly Great Danes that essentially received no treatment (Denny et al, 1977). Medical management of CSM was revisited recently in two studies (da Costa et al, 2008; De Decker et al, 2009). One study compared the outcomes of dogs treated medically and surgically and found that 54% of dogs treated medically improved and 27% showed no change in long-term follow-up. By comparison, surgical treatment led to improvement in 81% of dogs. These results show that, although surgery offers the best chances of improvement, medical management is an acceptable alternative. The fact that approximately 80% of dogs can experience improvement or maintenance of neurologic status with medical management makes this approach preferable to many owners because of financial constraints or concerns about anesthetic and surgical risks, especially in Doberman pinschers, a breed with high incidence of dilated cardiomyopathy. The author also prefers to initiate medical management to evaluate the improvement obtained and to give owners the opportunity to decide on surgery. The response to medical management (corticosteroids and exercise restriction) can be used indirectly to assess the degree of reversibility of spinal cord lesions.

The most important component of medical management is *exercise restriction* to minimize those high-impact activities that might exacerbate the dynamic component of spinal cord compression. Dogs can be walked on leash, but unsupervised exercise is strongly discouraged. A body harness should be worn instead of a neck collar.

Corticosteroids appear to benefit dogs with CSM, and antiinflammatory dosages of prednisone often are used (0.5 to 1.0 mg/kg q12-24h PO), with the dosage progressively tapered over the course of 2 to 3 weeks. In some patients dexamethasone appears to elicit a better response, and it can be used for more severely affected patients or as a rescue therapy for dogs with sudden deterioration. Only low dosages of dexamethasone should be used, never more than 0.25 mg/kg q24h PO because no incremental therapeutic benefit is gained by higher dosages and the risk of adverse effects is higher. The severe complications that have been reported with dexamethasone use were seen mainly when high dosages were used (1 to 2 mg/kg/day). The author prescribes dexamethasone at an initial dosage of 0.2 to 0.25 mg/kg q24h PO (to a maximum dose of 8 mg per dog) for 1 to 3 days, depending on the severity of clinical signs, and then continues treatment at a dosage of 0.1 mg/kg q24h. Corticosteroids, particularly dexamethasone, improve neurologic function in chronic spinal cord compression predominantly by decreasing vasogenic edema. Other proposed mechanisms include protection from glutamate toxicity and reduction of neuronal and oligodendroglial apoptosis.

Despite the potential benefits associated with corticosteroid therapy, the use of corticosteroids, particularly for long periods, can be associated with important adverse effects. Because of the possibility of gastrointestinal complications, omeprazole (0.7 mg/kg q24h) or famotidine (0.5 mg/kg q12-24h) often is used in conjunction with corticosteroid therapy. Nonsteroidal antiinflammatory drugs (NSAIDs) can be used in place of corticosteroids if neck pain appears to be a major component of the syndrome or if the adverse effects of the corticosteroids cannot be tolerated. Although many NSAIDs can be used effectively, the author often prescribes meloxicam (0.2 mg/kg initially, followed by 0.1 mg/kg q24h). Regardless of the NSAID used, *corticosteroids and NSAIDs never should be used in combination!*

One reason for the success of medical management is the slow progression of spinal changes associated with the disease. This has been documented in Dobermans and currently is under investigation in Great Danes. Surviving demyelinated axons also may remyelinate with treatment. Remyelination has been shown in the spinal cords of horses and humans with cervical myelopathy treated medically.

As previously mentioned, some dogs with CSM have concurrent hypothyroidism (8 out of 12 dogs in a study—da Costa et al, 2006a). Hypothyroid dogs with CSM may show remarkable improvement in strength and energy when thyroid supplementation is started. In these cases improvement usually is noticeable within a week. Hypothyroidism obviously should be treated before surgery for CSM is performed. Dogs with occult dilated cardiomyopathy can develop heart rhythm disturbances or congestive heart failure if excessive dosages of thyroid hormone are prescribed; accordingly, thyroxine levels should be measured after initiation of treatment. The general approach to diagnosis and treatment of CSM is outlined in Figure 236-3.

Surgical Treatment

Surgery is generally assumed to represent the treatment of choice for most dogs with CSM. Because most affected dogs have spinal cord compression, decompressing the spinal cord in theory provides the definitive treatment. However, the decision to recommend surgical treatment should be based on several considerations, including severity of neurologic signs, degree of pain, type and severity of compressive lesions, response to medical management, short- and long-term expectations of the owner, and presence of concurrent neurologic conditions, orthopedic problems, or other diseases such as dilated cardiomyopathy that could affect the long-term outcome.

Selection of a specific surgical technique can be complicated, and the following discussion provides an overview as well as the author's perspective on current surgical methods. Direct decompressive techniques include dorsal laminectomy, dorsal laminoplasty, ventral slot technique, inverted cone slot technique, and hemilaminectomy. Indirect decompressive techniques typically are grouped

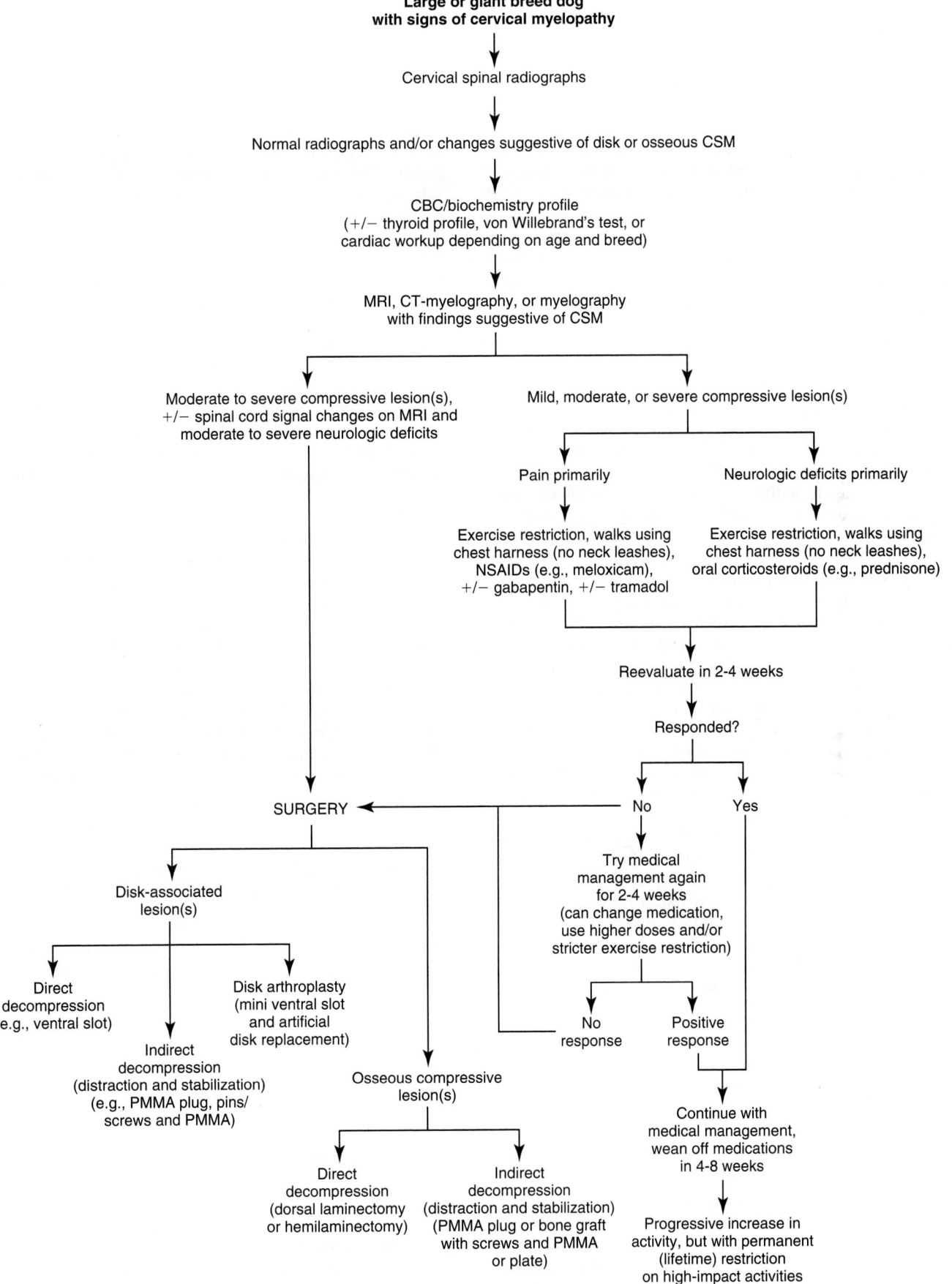

Figure 236-3 Algorithm illustrating the diagnostic and therapeutic approach for dogs suspected of having cervical spondylomyelopathy.

into the distraction-stabilization category, and procedures have been reported that use bone grafts of several types, pins (smooth, threaded) or screws and polymethyl methacrylate, interbody screws, washers, metallic spacers, metallic plates, plastic plates, Kirschner-wire spacer, Harrington rods, interbody polymethyl methacrylate plug, and fusion cage. All of these techniques have been combined with diskectomy or with partial or complete ventral slot procedures. Intervertebral disk fenestration also has been performed, and more recently motion-preserving techniques using disk arthroplasty or artificial disk replacement have been proposed. In general, because the source and direction of compression can be divided broadly into disk associated and osseous, general treatment recommendations can be focused on management of these types of compression.

It also is important to consider that a significant proportion of dogs show a worsening of CSM approximately 2 to 3 years after surgery; therefore, whenever possible, the surgical technique should allow long-term postoperative imaging using MRI. All metallic implants except those made of titanium cause significant artifacts that preclude the use of MRI. Polymethyl methacrylate and titanium implants (screws, plate, or artificial disk) produce minimal or no artifacts, which allows postoperative MRI.

Disk-Associated Compressions

Disk-associated CSM is the most common form of CSM and the one for which the largest number of corrective surgical techniques have been proposed. These surgical techniques have been based on the identification of static or dynamic lesions by stress or traction myelography, but as previously discussed, such determinations are highly subjective. Nevertheless, the outcomes for most of these techniques are similar and generally positive. Ventral static compressions usually are treated with the traditional ventral slot or inverted cone slot procedure. Dynamic compressions can be treated with distraction-stabilization techniques, and a polymethyl methacrylate plug or pins or screws combined with polymethyl methacrylate commonly are used. Multiple compressive sites can be treated with distraction-stabilization techniques, with the most common methods involving distraction with a polymethyl methacrylate plug. Dorsal laminectomy is an alternative for treatment of multiple ventral compressions. A newer approach is disk arthroplasty, which has the theoretical advantage of maintaining intervertebral mobility while allowing direct spinal cord decompression.

Osseous Compressions

Typically, osseous compressions are thought to be primarily static, and for this reason direct decompression of the affected sites is recommended. Commonly this is achieved by dorsal laminectomy, but cervical hemilaminectomy also can be used. Another way to treat osseous lesions is by distraction-stabilization of the affected segments ventrally. Stabilization and fusion of the affected segments does not decompress the affected sites directly but eliminates the dynamic component of the spinal cord compression. It also may allow regression of the osseous and

ligamentous lesions over time. The technique used in these cases is the polymethyl methacrylate plug.

Pure Ligamentous Compressions

Ligamentous hypertrophy usually occurs in combination with either disk-associated or osseous compressions. Pure ligamentous compression (hypertrophy of the ligamentum flavum) currently is an uncommon presentation. Surgical treatment can be achieved either by decompressing the affected sites (dorsal laminectomy) or by using the polymethyl methacrylate plug technique.

Surgical Complications

Surgical treatment can lead to several complications, including death. Hypotension and hemorrhage may be responsible for a large proportion of the cases of intraoperative and perioperative complications. Aggressive monitoring and maintenance of appropriate arterial blood pressure transoperatively is essential to minimize complications. When instrumentation is used, penetration of the vertebral canal or transverse foramina with implants as well as implant failure also can be observed, with an incidence ranging from 7.5% to 30% (Platt and da Costa, 2011).

"Domino" lesion, or *adjacent-segment disease*, is a late postoperative complication that occurs in approximately 20% of dogs following surgical treatment of CSM, predominantly when distraction-stabilization techniques are used. It typically occurs in the second or third year after surgery. The use of ventral slot techniques reportedly decreases the risk of domino lesion. The domino effect may occur secondary to bony fusion. Typically domino lesion affects only one disk region, either cranial or caudal to the operated area. Motion-preserving techniques such as disk arthroplasty appear to decrease the incidence of adjacent-segment disease in people. It remains to be seen if the same effect will be observed in dogs.

Natural History and Prognosis

Ideally the *natural history* of a disease should be understood so that treatment recommendations and prognosis can be based on this knowledge. Unfortunately, the natural history of CSM has not been defined. It appears that the disease progresses slowly in many dogs with disk-associated CSM. The same may be true for giant-breed dogs with osseous compressions. Current evidence suggests that the progressive course of the disease is limited mostly to the lesions seen at the time of initial diagnosis. Follow-up imaging studies of dogs with both disk-associated and osseous CSM have demonstrated that the compressive lesions progress slowly. It is uncommon to see the appearance of additional lesions in dogs treated conservatively (da Costa and Parent, 2007; De Decker et al, 2012).

When *prognosis* is discussed with clients, it is useful to understand that the outcome of surgical treatment of disk-associated CSM is very successful, with approximately 80% (range, 70% to 90%) of dogs improving after surgery. No one surgical technique stands as clearly superior, even for dogs with disk-associated CSM. Intervertebral disk fenestration is not recommended because the reported success rate has been only 33%. In contrast to older studies, recent reports on medical management indicate an improvement rate of approximately 50% (range, 45% to 54%) (da Costa et al, 2008; De Decker et al, 2009). Given that surgery more consistently leads to clinical improvement, it always should be considered in the treatment of dogs with CSM.

Surgery does not alter the long-term survival of dogs with CSM, however. The survival time of 76 dogs with CSM (33 dogs treated surgically and 43 dogs treated medically) was reported recently (da Costa et al, 2008). The median survival time was identical (36 months) regardless of whether the dogs were treated medically or surgically. This finding indicates that CSM continues to progress independently of the method of treatment and that the clinical deterioration seen months to years after treatment may not be due solely to failure of the surgery or development of adjacent-segment disease. Presumably, other mechanisms such as ischemia, apoptosis, or other molecular changes within the spinal cord are operative, and these represent future targets for therapy.

References and Suggested Reading

Adamo PF: Cervical arthroplasty in two dogs with disk-associated caudal cervical spondylomyelopathy, *J Am Vet Med Assoc* 239(6):808, 2011.

Burbidge HM: *Caudal cervical malformation in the Doberman pinscher, doctoral thesis,* New Zealand, 1999, Massey University, p 121.

da Costa RC: Pathogenesis of cervical spondylomyelopathy: lessons from recent years. In *Proceedings of the 25th Annual ACVIM Forum,* 2007, p 318.

da Costa RC: Cervical spondylomyelopathy (wobbler syndrome), *Vet Clin North Am Small Anim Pract* 40(5):881, 2010.

da Costa RC et al: Comparison of magnetic resonance imaging and myelography in the diagnosis of cervical spondylomyelopathy in Doberman pinscher dogs—18 cases, *Vet Radiol Ultrasound* 47(6):523, 2006a.

da Costa RC et al: Morphologic and morphometric magnetic resonance imaging features of Doberman pinscher dogs with and without clinical signs of cervical spondylomyelopathy, *Am J Vet Res* 67(9):1601, 2006b.

da Costa RC et al: Outcome of medical and surgical treatment in dogs with cervical spondylomyelopathy—104 cases, *J Am Vet Med Assoc* 233(8):1284, 2008.

da Costa RC, Echandi R, Beauchamp D: Computed tomography myelographic findings in dogs with cervical spondylomyelopathy, *Vet Radiol Ultrasound* 53(1):64, 2012.

da Costa RC, Parent J: One-year clinical and magnetic resonance imaging follow-up of Doberman pinscher dogs with cervical spondylomyelopathy treated medically or surgically, *J Am Vet Med Assoc* 231(2):243, 2007.

Denny HR, Gibbs C, Gaskell CJ: Cervical spondylopathy in the dog: a review of thirty-five cases, *J Small Anim Pract* 18(2):117, 1977.

De Decker S et al: Clinical evaluation of 51 dogs treated conservatively for disc-associated wobbler syndrome, *J Small Anim Pract* 50(3):136, 2009.

De Decker S et al: Evolution of clinical signs and predictors of outcome after conservative medical treatment for disk-associated cervical spondylomyelopathy in dogs, *J Am Vet Med Assoc* 240(7):848, 2012.

Jeffery ND, McKee WM: Surgery for disc-associated wobbler syndrome in the dog—an examination of the controversy, *J Small Anim Pract* 42(12):574, 2001.

Johnson JA et al: Kinematic motion patterns of the cranial and caudal canine cervical spine, *Vet Surg* 40(6):720, 2011.

Platt SR, da Costa RC: Cervical spine. In Tobias KM, Johnston SA, editors: *Veterinary surgery: small animal,* ed 1, Philadelphia, 2011, Saunders, p 410.

Sharp NJH, Wheeler SJ: Cervical spondylomyelopathy. In Sharp NJH, Wheeler SJ, editors: *Small animal spinal disorders: diagnosis and surgery,* ed 2, St Louis, 2005, Mosby, p 211.

Craniocervical Junction Abnormalities in Dogs

CURTIS W. DEWEY, *Ithaca, New York*
DOMINIC J. MARINO, *Plainview, New York*
CATHERINE A. LOUGHIN, *Plainview, New York*

Craniocervical junction abnormality (CJA) is a term that encompasses a number of developmental anatomic aberrations at the region of the caudal occiput and first two cervical vertebrae. Chiari-like malformation (CM) appears to be the most common CJA encountered in dogs, and there has been a tremendous amount of clinical investigation into this disorder in recent years. Other abnormalities in this region include atlantooccipital overlap (AOO), dorsal constriction at C1 and C2, and atlantoaxial instability. Atlantoaxial instability is discussed in detail in Chapter 235 and is not covered here.

CJAs in small-breed dogs increasingly are being recognized as common and challenging disorders. In particular, CM, the canine analog of human Chiari type I malformation, has emerged in recent years as the possible cause of major health problems in several small-breed dogs, most notably the cavalier King Charles spaniel. The term *craniocervical junction abnormality,* as used in human medicine, serves as an umbrella term for a variety of malformations that occur in the craniocervical region. The craniocervical junction refers to the occipital bone (primarily the supraoccipital component) that forms the boundaries of the foramen magnum, the atlas (C1), and the axis (C2). In veterinary medicine, the term *Chiari-like malformation* has been used widely to describe constrictive disorders at the cervicomedullary junction that are apparent on magnetic resonance imaging (MRI). Numerous abnormalities of the craniocervical junction in dogs are presumed to be heritable malformations; all have been associated with the secondary development of syringomyelia (SM). SM refers to the accumulation of fluid within the spinal cord parenchyma. The fluid cavity itself is called a *syrinx.* The term *hydromyelia* specifically describes fluid accumulation only within the central canal, and hydromyelia is considered a possible precursor to SM. Although the signalment features for some of the more newly reported disorders have not been defined clearly, all of the disorders tend to affect young small-breed dogs. The nomenclature used for these disorders often is confusing and generally assumes that these are all distinctly separate disorders. Included among these diseases is CM, also termed *caudal occipital malformation syndrome* or *COMS,* and occipital hypoplasia. Recently it has been found that many dogs have abnormalities in the craniocervical junction region that do not conform to traditional veterinary nomenclature. These include AOO and dorsal constriction at the C1-C2 vertebral junction. Both of these abnormalities may represent the canine analog of human basilar invagination. Finally, it has become apparent that some dogs with suspected "classic" atlantoaxial instability have other concurrent abnormalities at the craniocervical junction. Because the occipital region of the skull and the first two cervical vertebrae develop together embryologically, it makes inherent sense that multiple developmental disorders, as well as combinations of these disorders, should occur in this anatomic region in veterinary patients, as they do in humans. For these reasons, we place all of these disorders under the general heading of CJAs. It has been reported that, especially for purposes of surgical planning, developing an optimal description of a craniocervical junction disorder for an individual patient often depends on a combination of MRI and computed tomographic (CT) images.

Pathophysiology and Clinical Features

Chiari-like malformation, as noted earlier, is thought to be the canine analog of Chiari type I malformation in people. As in the human disorder, the cranial cavity is too small to accommodate the contents of the caudal fossa (cerebellum and brainstem), which results in overcrowding of the cerebellomedullary region of the brain (Figure 237-1). On MRI, the abnormality of the supraoccipital bone that causes an indentation of the caudal cerebellum often is visible. In addition, an impingement of the dorsal subarachnoid space typically occurs at the level of the cervicomedullary junction. Herniation of the caudal aspect of the cerebellum through the foramen magnum also is commonly appreciated (Figure 237-2). Most of these dogs also have cervical SM, evident on MRI (Figure 237-3). CM generally has been considered a congenital malformation of the caudal occipital region of the skull, leading to overcrowding of the caudal fossa and compression of the cervicomedullary junction at the level of the foramen magnum. However, the anatomic abnormalities associated with CM are far more complicated than simply a malformed skull in the caudal-most aspect of the occipital bone region causing a physical constriction near the foramen magnum. It is now apparent that the malformations of CM are not limited only to the caudal part of the

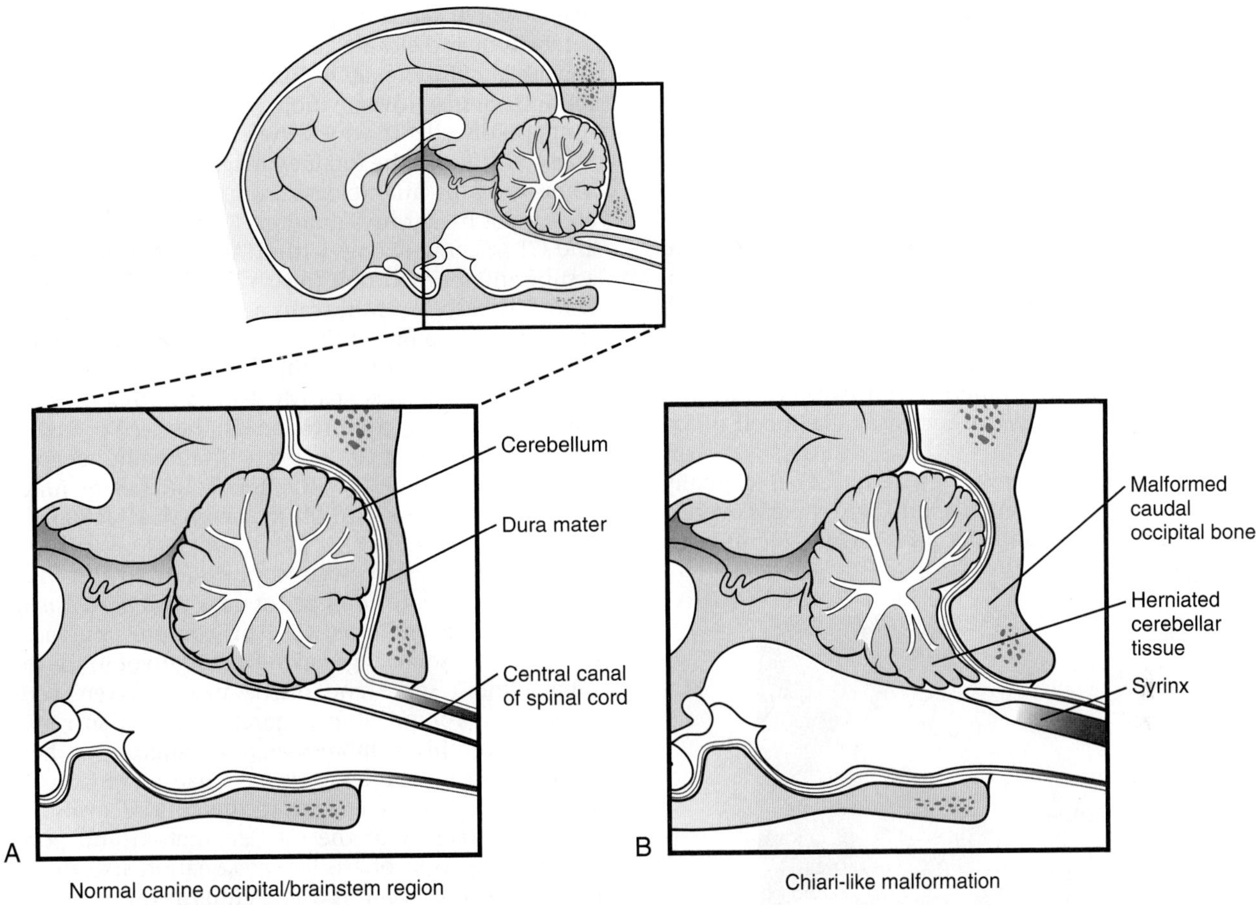

Cerebellum

Dura mater

Central canal
of spinal cord

Malformed
caudal
occipital bone

Herniated
cerebellar
tissue

Syrinx

A Normal canine occipital/brainstem region

B Chiari-like malformation

Figure 237-1 A, Schematic illustration of the normal shape of the caudal occipital region. **B,** Typical shape of this region in a dog with Chiari-like malformation. (From Dewey CW: Surgery of the brain. In Fossum TW, editor: *Small animal surgery,* ed 4, St Louis, 2013, Mosby, p 1438.)

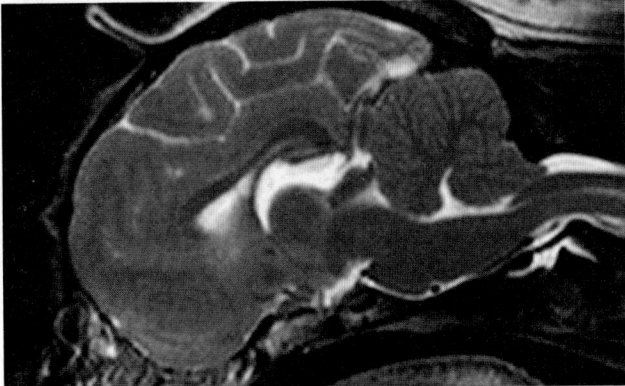

Figure 237-2 Midsagittal T2-weighted magnetic resonance image of a dog with Chiari-like malformation showing cerebellar herniation through the foramen magnum.

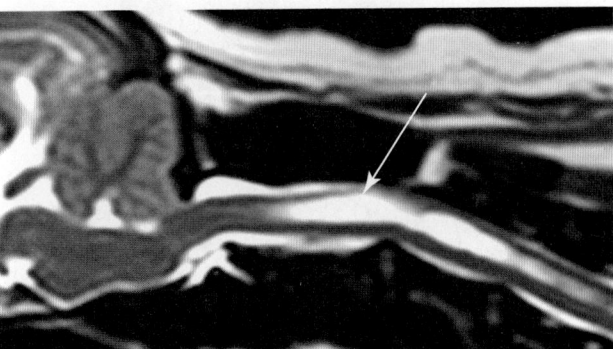

Figure 237-3 T2-weighted sagittal cervical magnetic resonance image of a dog with Chiari-like malformation showing syringomyelia.

skull. In addition, there is convincing evidence in Cavalier King Charles spaniels that there is a mismatch between the volume available in the caudal fossa region (also referred to as the *caudal cranial fossa*) and the parenchyma (cerebellum and brainstem) that resides within this volume; in other words, there is too much brain parenchyma in too small a space in the caudal fossa of Cavalier

King Charles spaniels (compared with other small-breed dogs and Labrador retrievers). This mismatch between parenchyma and available volume also has been demonstrated in the cranial fossa (rostral and middle fossae) of Cavalier King Charles spaniels. Increased ventricular size, increased relative parenchymal volume in the caudal fossa (as a percentage of total brain parenchymal volume), and increased relative cerebellar volume all have been associated with increased likelihood of the presence of SM in the cavalier King Charles spaniel breed. Increased syrinx width also has been associated with increased ventricular size and relative caudal fossa parenchymal volume in this breed. There is some evidence in the cavalier King Charles spaniel breed that the caudal fossa volume itself often is too small compared with other dog breeds. Other anatomic abnormalities of the skull reported in dogs with SM include minute or absent frontal sinuses and abnormally small jugular foramen volumes. With regard to this latter abnormality, it is hypothesized that the constricted venous drainage from the brain caused by small jugular foramina leads to intracranial venous hypertension and increased intracranial pressure; this would lead to an increased pressure differential between cranial and spinal compartments and an increased likelihood of SM development.

In *atlantooccipital overlap,* the atlas (C1) is cranially displaced into the foramen magnum, and there is overlap of the occipital bone and the atlas (Figure 237-4). This

displacement tends to compress the caudal aspect of the cerebellum and elevate and compress the caudal medulla (medullary kinking). AOO likely is a form of basilar invagination. Basilar invagination is a human craniocervical junction disorder in which the atlas or axis (C2), or both, telescope toward the foramen magnum. It is possible that some cases of atlantoaxial instability in dogs are also analogs of basilar invagination. Based on combined MRI and CT imaging of dogs with CJAs, there is evidence that a substantial proportion (nearly 30%) of dogs diagnosed with CM based on MRI scans actually may have AOO as the main anatomic abnormality causing compression at the cervicomedullary junction. Bone is poorly visualized by MRI, but CT images clearly delineate what bony structures are causing compression at the cervicomedullary junction. In short, it is likely that many dogs with constrictive disorders at the cervicomedullary junction that are diagnosed via MRI as having CM actually may have AOO.

Similar to the AOO seen in small- and toy-breed dogs, we have seen a large number of dogs with *dorsal compression at the level of C1 and C2.* This compression varies in severity, with some dogs having a mild divot in the dorsal subarachnoid space and others having severe cervical spinal cord compression (Figure 237-5). At surgery, the majority of this compressive mass appears to be soft tissue, although several cases have had an obvious bony component. We believe that this disorder also may involve instability at the C1-C2 junction and possibly represents a form of basilar invagination like the AOO problem. It can occur as a sole entity or in combination with CM or atlantoaxial instability.

Syringomyelia most often is discussed in the context of CM as a causative disorder. However, SM can occur secondary to any CJA or to any disorder that disturbs normal laminar CSF flow in the subarachnoid space of the vertebral canal. Multiple mechanisms have been proposed for the formation of SM, all of which are based on the pressure differential between cranial and spinal compartments created by constriction at the cervicomedullary junction. We have found that of dogs that undergo MRI of their entire spine (not just the cervical region), most have syrinxes in the thoracic and lumbar spinal cord

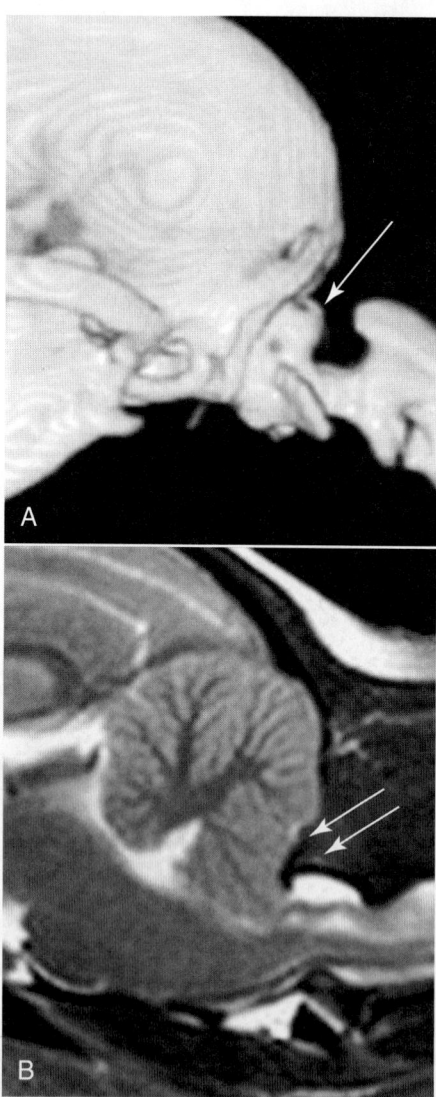

Figure 237-4 Midsagittal T2-weighted magnetic resonance image **(A)** and three-dimensional reconstructed computed tomographic image **(B)** of a dog with atlantooccipital overlap malformation.

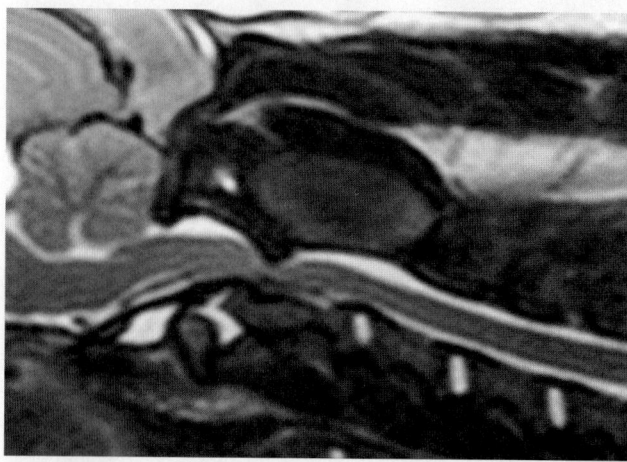

Figure 237-5 Sagittal T2-weighted magnetic resonance image of a dog with a severely compressive dorsal lesion at C1 and C2.

regions in addition to the cervical region. In a recent review of our unpublished MRI data for over 350 dogs, we found that syrinx formation begins in the cervical region and sequentially progresses to the thoracic region and finally to the lumbar region without skipping over a region. In one study of 49 Cavalier King Charles spaniels, 76% of the dogs had syrinxes in thoracic or lumbar regions or both, in addition to cervical SM (Loderstedt et al, 2011).

CM typically is encountered in small-breed dogs, with the cavalier King Charles spaniel being the most commonly affected. Other breeds affected by this disorder are the Brussels griffon, miniature poodle, Yorkshire terrier, Maltese, Chihuahua, bichon frise, Staffordshire terrier, pug, Shih Tzu, miniature dachshund, miniature pinscher, French bulldog, Pekingese, and Boston terrier. The typical age range at presentation appears to have changed over time, with many dogs developing clinical signs within the first year of life. In general, although the age range at clinical presentation is broad, CM is identified in most dogs by the time they are 4 years old. Dogs that are brought to the veterinarian at younger than 2 years of age often have more severe clinical signs than older dogs. In recent years, we have seen an increasing number of younger patients (<1 year of age); whether this trend reflects increasing severity of the disorder with subsequent generations, increased awareness within the veterinary community and the general public and hence earlier diagnosis, or a combination of these factors is unknown. Although AOO and dorsal C1-C2 compression are not as well characterized as CM, dogs with these disorders also tend to be young small-breed dogs, similar to the noncavalier King Charles spaniel CM population. In our experience, the very small breeds (e.g., Yorkshire terrier, Chihuahua) tend to be diagnosed more frequently with AOO than with CM.

Clinical signs of CM and related disorders are variable, but the most consistent clinical features are cervical pain and apparent pruritus of the head, neck, and shoulder regions. Clinical signs of CM with SM include neck pain, back pain, vestibular dysfunction, cervical myelopathy, incessant scratching activity, lameness, diminished hearing, and scoliosis. Cervical myelopathy (with associated neck pain) and cerebellovestibular dysfunction (e.g., strabismus, decreased menace response with normal vision, head tilt, nystagmus) are encountered most commonly. In most cases, cerebellovestibular dysfunction is revealed during a neurologic examination and has not necessarily been observed by the pet owner. Many dogs with CM have decreased to absent menace responses with normal vision as well as varying degrees of positional ventrolateral strabismus. An unusual and distinctive feature of the scratching activity associated with CM in dogs is that these patients typically do not make contact with the skin while scratching at the head and shoulder regions, so-called phantom scratching or air guitar. Scratching often occurs on only one side. Facial rubbing (pawing at the face or rubbing against objects) also is encountered in some dogs and is considered to be a manifestation of pain or paresthesia. Spinal hyperpathia (typically cervical), scratching activity, and scoliosis all are generally believed to be related to interference of the

syrinx cavity with ascending sensory pathways in the spinal cord. Scratching activity and neck discomfort often are exacerbated by abrupt weather changes, stress, or excitement, and by physical contact with the neck and shoulder region. The presence of both pain and scoliosis is correlated with syrinx width in cavalier King Charles spaniels with SM secondary to CM. Some of the neck pain may be related directly to constriction at the cervicomedullary junction or comorbid CJA. Occasionally dogs with CM and cervical SM have a specific variant of cervical myelopathy called *central cord syndrome.*

In these cases the outwardly expanding syrinx in the cervicothoracic intumescence causes damage to the lower motor neurons of the thoracic limbs within the regional gray matter; this leads to lower motor neuron paresis of the thoracic limbs while sparing the more peripherally located white matter tracts (upper motor neurons to the pelvic limbs). Damage to the regional white matter would cause general proprioceptive and upper motor neuron paresis in the pelvic limbs. The result is thoracic limb paresis (lower motor neuron in nature) that is notably worse than pelvic limb paresis. In some dogs with this syndrome, the pelvic limbs may appear normal.

Clinical signs in dogs with AOO typically are neck pain and varying degrees of ataxia of all four limbs. Similar clinical signs have been noted in dogs with dorsal compressive lesions at C1 and C2. It is important to realize that, especially in the cavalier King Charles spaniel breed, conditions other than CM-SM may account for some or all of the clinical signs identified. Recently it has been reported that more than 40% of cavalier King Charles spaniels with CM-SM are asymptomatic for the disorder, according to the dogs' owners (Couturier et al, 2008); however, in a recent unpublished pilot study we found that 41% of 227 dogs demonstrated clinical signs that went unrecognized by their owners. Idiopathic epilepsy also is a prevalent disorder in the cavalier King Charles spaniel breed.

Seizures have been reported to occur in 10% to 12% of humans with Chiari type I malformation; in the authors' experience, seizure activity is an infrequent occurrence in dogs with CM, and it is not possible to distinguish whether this seizure activity is due to CM or represents concurrent idiopathic epilepsy.

Congenital deafness also is well described in the cavalier King Charles spaniel breed. The severity and rate of progression of CM in dogs are variable, ranging from absence of symptoms (i.e., evidence of CM is found when imaging is performed for some other reason) to extreme pain and debilitation with rapid worsening over a short period. In addition, some dogs with CM have other unrelated concurrent disorders (e.g., disk extrusion, inflammatory brain disease) that could explain observed clinical signs. In such situations, it may be difficult to discern whether CM is the main problem, a contributory condition, or an incidental finding. An enigmatic ear problem seen in the cavalier King Charles spaniel breed called *primary secretory otitis media* also has been described. Clinical signs of primary secretory otitis media include apparent pain around the head and neck area, scratching of the head and neck, facial paralysis, and head tilt. Finally, other CJAs can occur concurrently with or be mistaken for CM. In the authors' opinion, determination of a complete and accurate diagnosis, including identification of all types of CJA, is essential for development of an effective treatment plan for dogs with suspected CM.

Diagnosis

The diagnosis of CM and similar disorders (like AOO) can be made only by MRI, which also is the preferred imaging modality for diagnosing SM. On MRI, the malformation is best visualized on a midsagittal view (preferably T2 weighted), which includes the caudal fossa and the cranial cervical spinal cord. Consistent findings on MRI indicative of CM are attenuation or obliteration of the dorsal subarachnoid space at the cervicomedullary junction and rostral displacement of the caudal cerebellum by the occipital bone. Other common MRI findings in CM include SM (usually at the C2 level caudally), herniation of the caudal cerebellum through the foramen magnum, and a kinked appearance of the caudal medulla. In one study of cavalier King Charles spaniels, it was found that using a flexed head position during MRI was more likely to exacerbate the degree of cerebellar herniation than using an extended head position (Upchurch et al, 2011). Phase-contrast MRI (cine MRI) often is used to measure cerebrospinal fluid flow in humans with Chiari type I malformation and recently has been evaluated for use in dogs with CM. It was found that cerebrospinal fluid flow velocity and flow pattern are useful predictors of CM-SM in cavalier King Charles spaniels. Occasionally dogs with MRI findings consistent with CM have evidence of other congenital disorders such as intracranial arachnoid (quadrigeminal) cyst, malformation-malarticulation of the C1 or C2 vertebra, and hydrocephalus. In the authors' opinion, most small-breed dogs normally have large lateral ventricles as a breed characteristic (ventriculomegaly) and are not truly hydrocephalic. In the absence of concurrent disease processes, cerebrospinal fluid analysis usually produces normal results; occasionally a mild mononuclear pleocytosis is apparent, however.

Medical Therapy

Medical therapy for dogs with CJAs generally falls into three categories: (1) analgesic drugs (implies relief of dysesthesia-paresthesia as well), (2) drugs that decrease cerebrospinal fluid production, and (3) corticosteroid therapy. Anecdotally, the most useful drug available for relief of scratching activity associated with SM has been gabapentin (10 mg/kg body weight q8h PO). It has been shown that neuropathic pain is accentuated over time because of up-regulation of the α2δ-1 subunit of voltage-gated calcium channels in dorsal root ganglion neurons and dorsal horn nociceptive neurons of the spinal cord. Gabapentin and the newer gabapentin analog pregabalin are believed to exert their antinociceptive effects by selectively binding to the α2δ-1 subunit and inhibiting calcium influx in these neurons. Adverse effects of gabapentin are minimal and usually are restricted to mild sedation, pelvic limb ataxia, and weight gain. Our recent experience with pregabalin (2 to 4 mg/kg q12h) suggests that it is a more effective drug in relieving pain and scratching

activity in dogs with CM-SM. Because the elimination half-life of pregabalin is nearly twice as long as that of gabapentin, twice-daily dosing is possible. It is important to start at the low end of the dosage range to avoid the adverse effects of sedation and ataxia. Orally administered opiate drugs sometimes are helpful in alleviating neck and head pain in dogs with CM-SM. We have had success using oral tramadol (2 to 4 mg/kg q8-12h), especially when it is administered in conjunction with either gabapentin or pregabalin.

Several drugs aimed at decreasing cerebrospinal fluid production have been used in dogs with CM-SM in an effort to diminish cerebrospinal fluid pulse pressure. All information regarding efficacy of these drugs is anecdotal. They include omeprazole (a proton pump inhibitor), acetazolamide (a carbonic anhydrase inhibitor), and furosemide (a loop diuretic). Omeprazole, a proton pump inhibitor, has been shown (in an experimental study) to decrease cerebrospinal fluid production by 26% when administered intrathecally in dogs (Javaheri et al, 1997). The oral dosage for dogs is 10 mg q24h for dogs weighing less than 20 kg and 20 mg q24h for dogs weighing more than 20 kg. Acetazolamide is a carbonic anhydrase inhibitor that is used to treat glaucoma, epileptic seizures, idiopathic intracranial hypertension, altitude sickness, and cystinuria and also is classified as a diuretic. Medically it may be used to treat conditions of moderate to severe metabolic or respiratory alkalosis. It does this by interfering with bicarbonate resorption in the kidneys, which reacidifies the blood (and thus alkalinizes the urine). Acetazolamide also is used to decrease the production of cerebrospinal fluid in idiopathic intracranial hypertension. Furosemide is a loop diuretic that acts on the distal tubules by abolishing the corticomedullary osmotic gradient and blocking negative as well as positive free water clearance. Its action is independent of any inhibitory effect on carbonic anhydrase or aldosterone. Because of the large NaCl absorptive capacity of the loop of Henle, diuresis is not limited by the development of acidosis, as it is with the carbonic anhydrase inhibitors. When treatment decisions are made, the potential adverse effects of long-term corticosteroid or diuretic therapy should be considered, along with the questionable efficacy of this therapy. Depletion of electrolytes (especially potassium) and dehydration are concerns when diuretics are used for prolonged periods, particularly when they are combined with corticosteroids.

Corticosteroids often are used in the medical management of CM-SM and other CJAs in dogs. Potential benefits include antiinflammatory effects, decreased cerebrospinal fluid production, and decreased expression of substance P (a nociceptive neurotransmitter) in spinal cord dorsal horn neurons. An initial antiinflammatory dosage of 0.5 mg/kg q12h PO often is effective in controlling clinical signs. This dose should be tapered, if at all possible, to an every-other-day schedule within the first month of therapy.

In most cases of CM-SM, medical therapy diminishes the severity of clinical signs, but resolution is unlikely. It is the authors' opinion that in most cases medical therapy should be viewed as a temporary treatment bridge until more definitive therapy such as surgical decompression with cranioplasty to restore normal cerebrospinal fluid flow can be performed.

Most dogs with CJAs respond favorably to medical therapy, although in many cases this response is temporary. In one group of 10 dogs with CM treated medically, 5 dogs were euthanized within 2 years because of disease progression and diminished responsiveness to therapy (Dewey et al, 2004). In another study, 36% of dogs with CM treated medically were euthanized because of the clinical signs of the disease at a mean of 1.7 years from the time of diagnosis (Rusbridge, 2007b). In one longer-term study evaluating the response to nonsurgical management, 48 cavalier King Charles spaniels with CM (with or without SM) were followed prospectively for a mean of 39 months; despite the fact that the majority (75%) of these dogs continued to deteriorate clinically over time (25% remained in static condition or improved), 75% of the total (36 dogs) were still alive at the end of the study period (Plessas et al, 2012). The response of dogs with AOO and C1-C2 dorsal compression to medical therapy has been similar to that of dogs with CM, although this statement is based on our anecdotal observations.

Surgical Therapy

We consider CJAs to be surgical disorders for the most part, although some can be managed medically long term. One of the difficulties in deciding which patients should receive nonsurgical therapy and which should receive surgical treatment for a CJA is our inability to predict accurately which patients will respond favorably to either approach over the long term. In people with symptomatic Chiari type I malformations, surgical therapy is considered the treatment of choice, with foramen magnum decompression being the preferred surgical procedure. Adjunctive surgical procedures occasionally are performed in people who have had a suboptimal response to foramen magnum decompression; such procedures usually involve placement of a shunt to divert SM fluid from the spinal cord region to another location for absorption (e.g., pleural or peritoneal cavity, subarachnoid space). Although a high degree of success has been achieved in surgical management of Chiari type I malformation in people, the reoperative rate varies from 8% to 30% for foramen magnum decompression; the most common problem necessitating reoperation is excessive scar tissue formation at the foramen magnum decompression site, which causes compression at the cervicomedullary junction that effectively re-creates the original disease state.

In our opinion, based on more than 300 operated cases, the preferred surgical procedure for treatment of CM in dogs is foramen magnum decompression with cranioplasty using titanium mesh and polymethyl methacrylate (PMMA). This procedure involves a suboccipital craniotomy and partial (at least 75% removal) or complete dorsal laminectomy of C1 and subsequent placement of a titanium mesh–PMMA plate on titanium screw anchor posts inserted around the circumference of the occipital bone defect (Figure 237-6). Proper plate

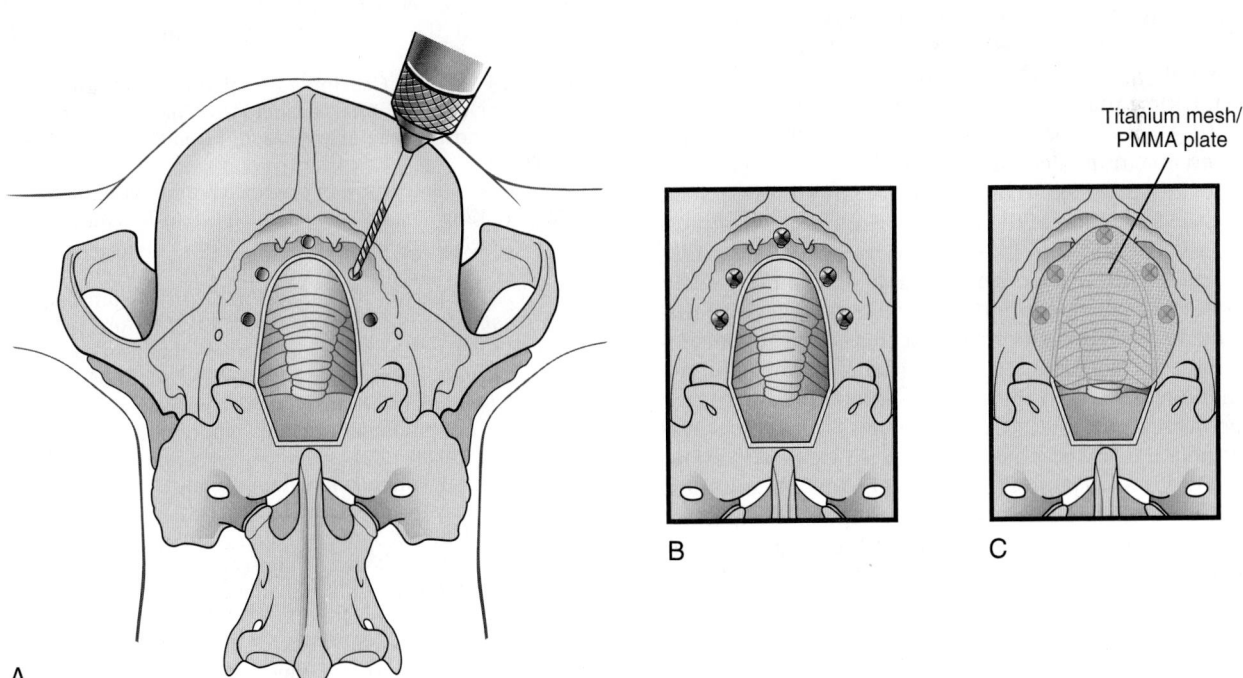

Figure 237-6 A, Schematic illustration depicting the typical pattern of guide hole placement for titanium screws in a cranioplasty procedure accompanying foramen magnum decompression. **B,** Schematic illustration showing placement of self-tapping titanium screws in guide holes. **C,** Schematic illustration depicting placement of a titanium mesh and polymethyl methacrylate (PMMA) plate to the foramen magnum decompression site. (From Dewey CW: Surgery of the brain. In Fossum TW, editor: *Small animal surgery,* ed 4, St Louis, 2013, Mosby, p 1438.)

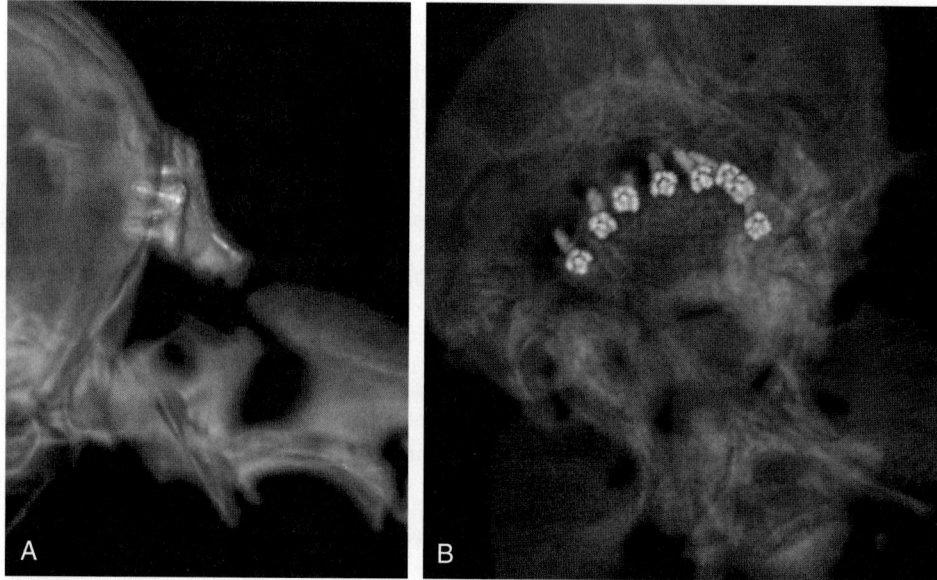

Figure 237-7 Lateral **(A)** and caudal **(B)** three-dimensional reconstructed computed tomographic postoperative views of a dog's skull following foramen magnum decompression with cranioplasty for Chiari-like malformation. (From Dewey CW: Surgery of the brain. In Fossum TW, editor: *Small animal surgery,* ed 4, St Louis, 2013, Mosby, p 1438.)

application is confirmed via radiography or (preferably) CT (Figure 237-7). The rate of short-term surgical success (sustained improvement in neurologic status or pain and scratching relief) with foramen magnum decompression in dogs with CM is approximately 80%, whether or not adjunctive cranioplasty is performed. One report found an inverse relationship between the length of time clinical signs were present before surgical intervention and the extent of postoperative improvement (Dewey et al, 2005). Unfortunately, a disease relapse rate ranging from 25% to 47% has been reported in cases treated with foramen magnum decompression alone; most of these relapses are suspected to be due to excessive postoperative scar tissue formation at the foramen magnum decompression site. We and our colleagues developed the cranioplasty procedure (based on a similar procedure used in human foramen magnum decompression surgery) to discourage excessive postoperative scar tissue from recompressing the operative site. Our initial report suggested a dramatic reduction in the rate of reoperation due to scar tissue formation after the cranioplasty procedure was instituted, but this was based on only 21 cases with about a 1-year follow-up period (Dewey et al, 2007). In our most recent unpublished analysis of more than 300 cases of foramen magnum decompression with cranioplasty, the reoperative rate was less than 1%. Syringosubarachnoid shunting has been evaluated retrospectively in a small cohort of 11 dogs with CM-SM; 9 dogs were judged to show neurologic improvement at 6-month follow-up, and 7 dogs were still alive a mean of 2.6 years after surgery.

References and Suggested Reading

Carrera I et al: Use of magnetic resonance imaging for morphometric analysis of the caudal cranial fossa in Cavalier King Charles spaniels, *Am J Vet Res* 70:340, 2009.

Cerda-Gonzalez S et al: Characteristics of cerebrospinal fluid flow in Cavalier King Charles Spaniels analyzed using phase velocity cine magnetic resonance imaging, *Vet Radiol Ultrasound* 50(5):467, 2009a.

Cerda-Gonzalez S et al: Imaging features of atlanto-occipital overlapping in dogs, *Vet Radiol Ultrasound* 50(3):264, 2009b.

Cerda-Gonzalez S et al: Congenital diseases of the craniocervical junction in the dog, *Vet Clin North Am Small Anim Pract* 40(1):121, 2010.

Couturier J, Rault D, Cauzinille L: Chiari-like malformation and syringomyelia in normal cavalier King Charles spaniels: a multiple diagnostic imaging approach, *J Small Anim Pract* 49:438, 2008.

Cross H et al: Comparison of cerebral cranium volumes between Cavalier King Charles spaniels with Chiari-like malformation, small breed dogs and Labradors, *J Small Anim Pract* 50:399, 2009.

Dewey CW: Surgery of the cervical spine. In Fossum TW, editor: *Small animal surgery,* ed 4, St Louis, 2013, Mosby, p 1467.

Dewey CW et al: Caudal occipital malformation syndrome in dogs, *Compend Contin Educ Pract Vet* 26:886, 2004.

Dewey CW et al: Foramen magnum decompression for treatment of caudal occipital malformation syndrome in dogs, *J Am Vet Med Assoc* 227(8):1270, 2005.

Dewey CW et al: Foramen magnum decompression with cranioplasty for treatment of caudal occipital malformation syndrome in dogs, *Vet Surg* 36(5):406, 2007.

Driver CJ et al: Morphometric assessment of cranial volumes in age-matched Cavalier King Charles spaniels with and without syringomyelia, *Vet Rec* 167(25):978, 2010.

Javaheri S et al: Different effects of omeprazole and Sch 28080 on canine cerebrospinal fluid production, *Brain Research* 754:321, 1997.

Loderstedt S et al: Distribution of syringomyelia along the entire spinal cord in clinically affected Cavalier King Charles spaniels, *Vet J* 190:359, 2011.

Marino DJ et al: Morphometric features of the craniocervical junction region in dogs with suspected Chiari-like malformation based on combined MR and CT imaging: 274 cases (2007-2010), *Am J Vet Res* 73:105, 2012.

Motta L et al: Syringosubarachnoid shunt as a management for syringohydromyelia in dogs, *J Small Anim Pract* 53:205, 2012.

Parker JE et al: Prevalence of asymptomatic syringomyelia in Cavalier King Charles spaniels, *Vet Rec* 168(25):667, 2011.

Plessas IN et al: Long-term outcome of Cavalier King Charles spaniel dogs with clinical signs associated with Chiari-like malformation and syringomyelia, *Vet Rec* 171(20):501, 2012.

Rusbridge C: Neurological diseases of the Cavalier King Charles spaniel, *J Small Anim Pract* 46(6):265, 2005.

Rusbridge C: Chiari-like malformation with syringomyelia in the Cavalier King Charles spaniel: long-term outcome after surgical management, *Vet Surg* 36(5):396, 2007a.

Rusbridge C: Pilot study: Chiari-like malformation with syringomyelia in the cavalier King Charles spaniel; long term follow up after conservative management, PhD thesis, Utrecht, The Netherlands, 2007b, p 138.

Rusbridge C et al: Syringomyelia in Cavalier King Charles spaniels: the relationship between syrinx dimensions and pain, *J Small Anim Pract* 48:432, 2007.

Rusbridge C et al: Chiari-like malformation in the Griffon Bruxellois, *J Small Anim Pract* 50(8):386, 2009.

Schmidt MJ et al: Volume reduction of the jugular foramina in Cavalier King Charles spaniels with syringomyelia, *BMC Vet Res* 8:158, 2012.

Shaw TA et al: Increase in cerebellar volume in Cavalier King Charles spaniels with Chiari-like malformation and its role in the development of syringomyelia, *PLoS One* 7:1, 2012.

Upchurch JJ et al: Influence of head positioning on the assessment of Chiari-like malformation in Cavalier King Charles spaniels, *Vet Record* 169:277, 2011

CHAPTER 238

Diagnosis and Treatment of Degenerative Lumbosacral Stenosis

CATHERINE A. LOUGHIN, *Plainview, New York*

Degenerative lumbosacral stenosis is a common radiculopathy in dogs and is noted most frequently in large working dogs. The most commonly affected breed is the German shepherd, but the disease also is encountered in other large breeds such as the Labrador retriever, golden retriever, and Doberman pinscher, and sometimes in smaller dogs. Males are more commonly affected than females, with reported ratios ranging from 1.3:1 to 5:1.

The lumbosacral region is bordered dorsally by the vertebral lamina, the articular facets, and the interarcuate ligament; ventrally by the dorsal longitudinal ligament, the annulus fibrosus, and the vertebral bodies of L7 and S1; and laterally by pedicles of the vertebral body. The intervertebral disk is attached to the cartilaginous end plates via strong collagen fibers called *Sharpey's fibers*. The vascular system in the region is made up of a vertebral venous plexus and paired lumbar arteries. The spinal cord ends in the sixth lumbar region and terminates into the seventh lumbar, the sacral, and the caudal nerve roots. The L7 nerve roots pass over the intervertebral disk space and exit through the intervertebral foramen between the L7 and S1 vertebral bodies.

Stenosis involves the narrowing of the vertebral canal or intervertebral foramina in the lumbosacral region. Pathophysiologically the disease involves soft tissue and bony abnormalities that compress the nerve roots. Disk degeneration is evident in many cases. Causes of this degeneration may be related to lumbosacral instability, Hansen's type II disk disease, or facet joint tropism (asymmetry of the left and right facet angles). Other causes of compression are diskospondylosis, osteophytosis, subluxation, hypertrophy of the interarcuate ligament, proliferation of the joint capsule, synovial cyst formation, and proliferation of the dorsal longitudinal ligament.

Diagnosis

Clinical signs of lumbosacral stenosis can be difficult to differentiate from those of other neurologic and orthopedic diseases. Signs include lumbosacral pain, hind limb paresis, urinary or fecal incontinence, pelvic limb lameness, muscle atrophy, dysesthesia, tail paresis, hyperesthesia or pruritus, and anal hyporeflexia. Owners often report that the dog has difficulty sitting, jumping, or climbing. To differentiate lumbosacral stenosis from other diseases such as canine hip dysplasia and degenerative myelopathy, diagnostic imaging becomes imperative.

The *physical examination* can help localize the cause to the lumbosacral region. Any changes in anal tone or tail function are an indicator of caudal nerve dysfunction. Decreased or absent hock flexion and a hyperreflexive patellar reflex can be indicators of sciatic dysfunction. Pain can be elicited directly by palpating over the lumbosacral region or by lifting the tail dorsally. Pelvic limb weakness can be evident on gait analysis and by observation of wearing of the nails on digits 3 and 4 of the hind limb paws. The findings of a comprehensive physical examination also can help guide the selection of optimal tests to arrive at the diagnosis and provide overall assessment of the dog.

Standard two-view *radiographs* are useful to assess bone changes in the lumbosacral region. Radiographs can reveal stenosis, diskospondylitis, osseous neoplasia, diskospondylosis, osteochondrosis, fracture, subluxation, and transitional vertebrae. Positional views, such as the extended and flexed views, can help determine whether movement of the lumbosacral region is normal and whether compression is present. In extension, the sacrum can displace ventrally and the vertebral canal is at its narrowest diameter. In flexion, the vertebral canal should be at its greatest diameter, but the diameter is decreased in dogs with lumbosacral stenosis.

Contrast studies can provide additional information beyond survey radiographs. Myelography is the least helpful of the contrast studies available. The dural sac termination site is variable in each dog. For myelography to provide diagnostic findings in cases of lumbosacral stenosis, the dural sac must extend into the sacrum. Diskography and epidurography provide better diagnostic information. Epidurography is used to evaluate neural compression (Figure 238-1). Diskographic abnormalities that confirm lumbosacral disease are intradiskal accumulation of the contrast agent, focal extravasation of contrast into the canal, and the presence of contrast within the disk. Transosseous and intravenous venography involve injection of a contrast agent into the vertebral venous sinus system to evaluate spinal cord compression indirectly.

Computed tomography (CT) provides cross-sectional images without the superimposition noted on radiographs. Dogs with lumbosacral disease have characteristic changes on CT images such as loss of epidural fat, dorsal bulging of the intervertebral disk, spondylosis, thecal sac displacement, narrowed foramen, narrowed central canal, thickened articular facets or joint capsule, articular process subluxation, and osteophytosis. Reformatting can create dorsal and sagittal images, and three-dimensional reconstruction also can make diagnosis of lumbosacral stenosis more visible.

Magnetic resonance imaging (MRI) provides the best soft tissue resolution, allows images to be acquired in multiple planes without degradation, and can detect disk degeneration earlier (Figure 238-2). Other advantages of MRI over CT are excellent visualization of the nerve roots, intervertebral disks, and ligaments and lack of exposure to ionizing radiation. MRI tends to be the most sensitive method for diagnosis of lumbosacral stenosis, but with

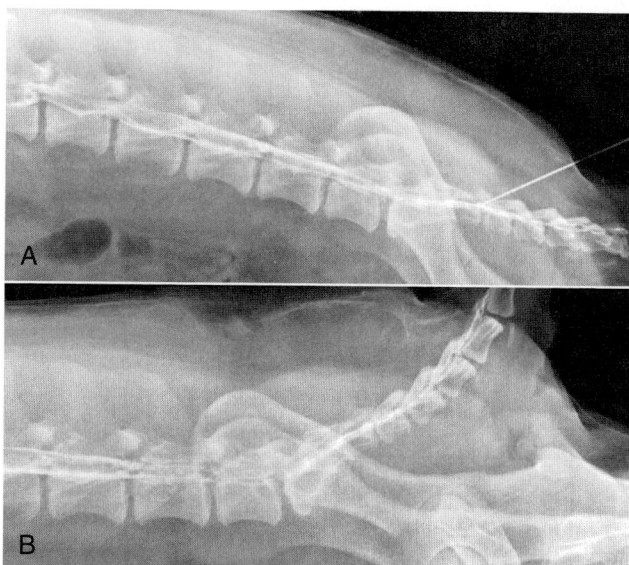

Figure 238-1 A, Lateral epidurogram for a 7-year-old neutered male Labrador retriever brought in because of back pain. He was diagnosed with a lumbosacral herniated disk. With the tail flexed there is minimal attenuation of contrast at the lumbosacral disk space. **B,** Epidurogram for the same dog with the tail extended. Note the bulge of the lumbosacral disk and attenuation of contrast.

excellent resolution also comes the potential for overdiagnosis. It is best to correlate imaging findings with the results of clinical assessment.

Other diagnostic modalities to consider are electromyography and medical thermal imaging. Electromyographic abnormalities of the pelvic limb, tail, and perineal musculature may be useful in confirming lumbosacral stenosis. Medical thermal imaging has been used to diagnose intervertebral disk disease in chondrodystrophic dogs, equids, and humans (Figure 238-3). Further studies may reveal the possibility of screening for lumbosacral disease in suspected cases.

Treatment

Treatment of lumbosacral stenosis is based on history, clinical signs, and the owner's ability to care for the dog. Dogs that are fully ambulatory with mild pain and dogs that demonstrate some neurologic deficits but are unable to receive decompressive surgery (because of client or other health issues) may be candidates for medical management. Dogs with more significant pain, weakness, urinary or fecal incontinence, or lack of response to medical management and working dogs are candidates for surgical decompression.

Medical Management

Medical management of lumbosacral stenosis consists of the traditional rest and treatment with antiinflammatory agents, but physical therapy, acupuncture, and administration of supplements (e.g., glucosamine, omega-3 fatty acids, vitamin B, and antioxidants) have been shown to be helpful in managing these cases. Acute signs of pain

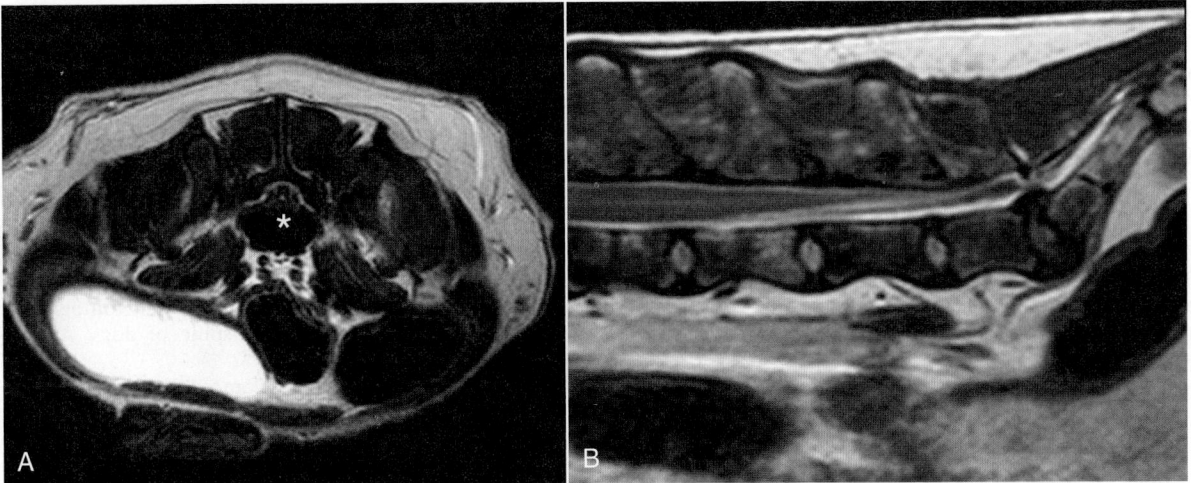

Figure 238-2 A, Axial T2-weighted magnetic resonance image of a 3-year-old neutered male French bulldog that became nonambulatory in the hind limbs and was diagnosed with a herniated lumbosacral disk. Note the compression of the nerve roots above the extruded disk *(asterisk).* **B,** Midsagittal T2-weighted MRI of the same dog. Note the compressive lumbosacral disk in the lumbar region.

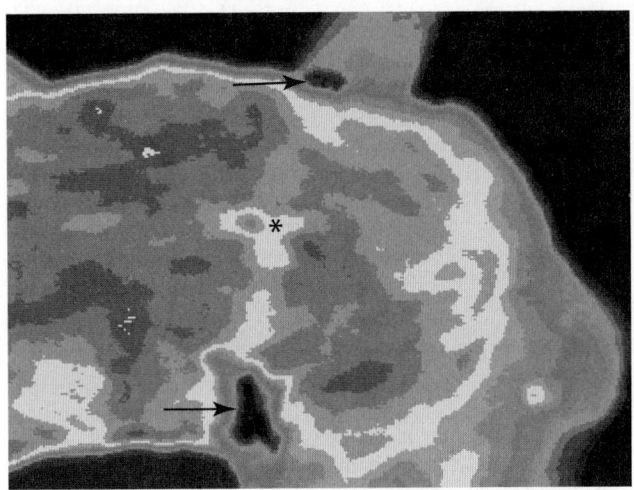

Figure 238-3 Medical infrared image of the dorsal lumbosacral region of an 11-year-old spayed female mixed-breed dog with a confirmed lumbosacral disk herniation on magnetic resonance imaging. The arrows indicate clips denoting the lumbosacral region as confirmed on radiographs. In the center of the image is a "cold" region indicating the area of the compressive disk *(asterisk).* This pattern is consistent with the findings on medical infrared imaging in humans with chronic disk disease.

and weakness are most commonly treated with corticosteroids and a pain medication (e.g., tramadol [Ultram]). For long-term treatment, a nonsteroidal antiinflammatory drug (NSAID) may be more beneficial, especially in animals with known or suspected osteoarthritis. Additionally, gabapentin (Neurontin) or tramadol, as well as supplements, can be used concurrently with a NSAID for long-term pain relief. In addition to medication, specific exercise programs can be prescribed that are tailored to the dog's condition to combat weakness and decrease the pain caused by stenosis. Physical therapy and acupuncture have been used in humans for years to treat pain and improve mobility. As more studies are performed in veterinary medicine, we may find that these modalities are underused and not only may provide more options for treatment but also may improve on the current medical and surgical outcomes.

Surgical Management

Surgical decompression can be accomplished with dorsal laminectomy, partial diskectomy, foraminotomy, and facetectomy. Dogs with lumbosacral instability also may require distraction and fusion of the joint. Dorsal laminectomy is the most commonly used procedure, and results of several studies indicate improvement in clinical signs after surgical intervention (De Risio et al, 2001; Jones, Banfield, and Ward, 2000; Lin et al, 2003; Suwankong et al, 2007; van Klaveren et al, 2005). Younger dogs and those with mild clinical signs before surgery have the best outcomes. As age and severity of signs increase, the prognosis worsens (Linn et al., 2003). Overall recovery rates vary, but recent studies report improvement in 73% to 79% of surgical cases (De Risio et al, 2001; Linn et al, 2003; Suwankong et al, 2007). Improvement has been confirmed by canine studies using force plate analysis (Suwankong et al, 2007; van Klaveren et al, 2005). Within 6 months of surgical decompression, normal propulsive forces were noted in the pelvic limbs. During this period owners also reported improvement in their dog's clinical signs.

Experimental treatment options such as lumbar sympathectomy have been shown to improve blood flow to the pelvic limbs and cauda equina. It is suspected that this type of procedure will not only improve blood flow but also improve function in the limbs and decrease pain. Further evaluation is needed to assess the usefulness of these procedures in dogs with intermittent clinical signs secondary to lumbosacral stenosis. Minimally invasive neurosurgical techniques also have been evaluated in humans, but less so in dogs. Endoscopically assisted foraminotomy has been evaluated and has been shown to improve visualization during the decompression procedure. As minimally invasive techniques become more readily available, more procedures for lumbosacral decompression may be developed.

Achievement of successful outcomes in dogs with lumbosacral stenosis often requires a combination of surgical decompression, medical management, and physical therapy. A thorough evaluation of the dog's history, signs, disease progression, and diagnostic test results—as well as the owner's expectations—can help direct development of an appropriate treatment plan. Although surgical decompression tends to be the treatment of choice of many surgeons, other factors, including the owner's desire for surgery and the dog's other health conditions, may render the dog an unacceptable surgical candidate. With advances in medicine and more frequent use of supplements, physical therapy, and acupuncture, a viable treatment protocol can be developed for the majority of cases. These same therapies also may be used postoperatively to reduce pain and improve ambulation.

References and Suggested Reading

Adams WH et al: Magnetic resonance imaging of the caudal lumbar and lumbosacral spine in 13 dogs (1990-1993), *Vet Radiol Ultrasound* 36(1):3, 1995.

Axlund TW, Hudson JA: Computed tomography of the normal lumbosacral intervertebral disc in 22 dogs, *Vet Radiol Ultrasound* 44(6):630, 2003.

Barthez PY, Morgan JP, Lipsitz D: Discography and epidurography for evaluation of the lumbosacral junction in dogs with cauda equina syndrome, *Vet Radiol Ultrasound* 35(3):152, 1994.

Breit S, Kunzel W: Breed specific osteological features of the canine lumbosacral junction, *Ann Anat* 183:151, 2001.

De Haan JJ, Shelton SB, Ackerman N: Magnetic resonance imaging in the diagnosis of degenerative lumbosacral stenosis in four dogs, *Vet Surg* 22:1, 1993.

De Risio L et al: Predictors of outcome after dorsal decompressive laminectomy for degenerative lumbosacral stenosis in dogs: 69 cases (1987-1997), *J Am Vet Med Assoc* 219:624, 2001.

Dhupa S, Glickman NW, Waters DJ: Functional outcome in dogs after surgical treatment of caudal lumbar intervertebral disk herniation, *J Am Anim Hosp Assoc* 35:323, 1999.

Feeney DA et al: Computed tomography of the normal canine lumbosacral spine: a morphologic perspective, *Vet Radiol Ultrasound* 37(6):399, 1996.

Gruenenfelder FI et al: Evaluation of the anatomic effect of physical therapy exercises for mobilization of lumbar spinal nerves and the dura mater in dogs, *Am J Vet Res* 67:1773, 2006.

Hankin EJ et al: Transarticular facet screw stabilization and dorsal laminectomy in 26 dogs with degenerative lumbosacral stenosis with instability, *Vet Surg* 41:611, 2012.

Jones JC et al: Comparison between computed tomographic and surgical findings in nine large-breed dogs with lumbosacral stenosis, *Vet Radiol Ultrasound* 37(4):247, 1996.

Jones JC et al: Use of computed tomographic densitometry to quantify contrast enhancement of compressive soft tissues in the canine lumbosacral vertebral canal, *Am J Vet Res* 63:733, 2002.

Jones JC et al: Effects of body position and clinical signs on L7-S1 intervertebral foraminal area and lumbosacral angle in dogs with lumbosacral disease as measured via computed tomography, *Am J Vet Res* 69:1446, 2008.

Jones JC, Banfield CM, Ward DL: Association between postoperative outcome and results of magnetic resonance imaging and computed tomography in working dogs with degenerative lumbosacral stenosis, *J Am Vet Med Assoc* 216:1769, 2000.

Jones JC, Inzana KD: Subclinical CT abnormalities in the lumbosacral spine of older large-breed dogs, *Vet Radiol Ultrasound* 41(1):19, 2000.

Jones JC, Wilson ME, Bartels JE: A review of high resolution computed tomography and a proposed technique for regional examination of the canine lumbosacral spine, *Vet Radiol Ultrasound* 35(5):339, 1994.

Jones JC, Wright JC, Bartels JE: Computed tomographic morphometry of the lumbosacral spine of dogs, *Am J Vet Res* 56(9):1125, 1995.

Karkkainen M, Punto LU, Tulamo RM: Magnetic resonance imaging of canine degenerative lumbar spine diseases, *Vet Radiol Ultrasound* 34(6):399, 1993.

Linn LL et al: Lumbosacral stenosis in 29 military working dogs: epidemiologic findings and outcome after surgical intervention (1990-1999), *Vet Surg* 32:21, 2003.

Mayhew PD et al: Association of cauda equina compression on magnetic resonance images and clinical signs in dogs with degenerative lumbosacral stenosis, *J Am Anim Hosp Assoc* 38:555, 2002.

Morgan JP et al: Lumbosacral transitional vertebrae as a predisposing cause of cauda equina syndrome in German Shepherd Dogs: 161 cases (1987-1990), *J Am Vet Med Assoc* 202(11):1877, 1993.

Onda A et al: Lumbar sympathectomy increases blood flow in a dog model of chronic cauda equina compression, *J Spinal Disord Tech* 17(6):522, 2004.

Pochaczevsky R et al: Liquid crystal thermography of the spine and extremities, *J Neurosurg* 56:386, 1982.

Ramirez O, Thrall DE: A review of imaging techniques for canine cauda equina syndrome, *Vet Radiol Ultrasound* 39(4):283, 1998.

Roberts RE, Selcer BA: Myelography and epidurography, *Vet Clin North Am Small Anim Pract* 23(2):307, 1993.

Scharf G et al: The lumbosacral junction in working German Shepherd Dogs—neurological and radiological evaluation, *J Vet Med* 51:27, 2004.

Seiler G et al: Staging of lumbar intervertebral disc degeneration in nonchondrodystrophic dogs using low-field magnetic resonance imaging, *Vet Radiol Ultrasound* 44(2):179, 2003.

Sharp NJH, Wheeler SJ: Lumbosacral disease. In Sharp NJH, Wheeler SJ, editors: *Small animal spinal disorders: diagnosis and surgery*, ed 2, St Louis, 2005, Mosby, p 181.

Shealy P, Thomas WB, Immel L: Neurologic conditions and physical rehabilitation of the neurologic patient. In Millis DL, Levine D, Taylor RA, editors: *Canine rehabilitation and physical therapy*, St Louis, 2004, Saunders, p 388.

Smolders LA et al: Pedicle screw-rod fixation of the canine lumbosacral junction, *Vet Surg* 41:720, 2012.

Steffen F et al: A follow-up study of neurologic and radiographic findings in working German Shepherd Dogs with and without degenerative lumbosacral stenosis, *J Am Vet Med Assoc* 231:1529, 2007.

Suwankong N et al: Agreement between computed tomography, magnetic resonance imaging, and surgical findings in dogs with degenerative lumbosacral stenosis, *J Am Vet Med Assoc* 229(12):1924, 2006.

Suwankong N et al: Assessment of decompressive surgery in dogs with degenerative lumbosacral stenosis using force plate analysis and questionnaires, *Vet Surg* 36(5):423, 2007.

Van Klaveren NJ et al: Force plate analysis before and after dorsal decompression for treatment of degenerative lumbosacral stenosis in dogs, *Vet Surg* 34(5):450, 2005.

Wood BC et al: Endoscopic-assisted lumbosacral foraminotomy in the dog, *Vet Surg* 33(3):221, 2004.

CHAPTER 239

Treatment of Autoimmune Myasthenia Gravis

G. DIANE SHELTON, *La Jolla, California*

The name *myasthenia gravis* (MG) originally was given to a human disease that was frequently fatal. As recently as 40 years ago, 25% of human MG patients died of the disease. Canine MG also has been associated with a high death rate and, according to many older textbooks of veterinary medicine, a poor prognosis for recovery. We now know that, with early recognition of the disease, a correct diagnosis, and appropriate treatment, the prognosis for a relatively normal quality of life and life span is favorable in both human and canine patients with MG.

Canine MG is the most common neuromuscular disease diagnosed in my laboratory. Feline autoimmune MG occurs much less frequently but is associated with a higher incidence of a cranial mediastinal mass (25.7%) than canine MG (3.4%).

Diagnosis of Myasthenia Gravis

The spectrum of clinical presentations in both cats and dogs is broad and variable; thus autoimmune MG should be high on the list of differential diagnoses for any dog or cat with focal or generalized neuromuscular weakness, acquired megaesophagus, or dysphagia. In-depth discussions of the diversity of clinical presentations in canine and feline MG can be found in the literature (Dewey et al, 1997; Shelton, 2002; Shelton, Ho, and Kass, 2000; Shelton and Lindstrom, 2001; Shelton, Schule, and Kass, 1997). The onset of clinical signs commonly is acute, occurring only a few days to a few weeks before presentation. Because of the propensity of dogs with MG to develop aspiration pneumonia, autoimmune MG is one disease in which a delay in obtaining a diagnosis or assumption of the wrong diagnosis can result in a fatal outcome.

When MG is suspected, ideally a serum sample should be collected for acetylcholine receptor (AChR) antibody testing and the diagnosis confirmed before initiation of therapy. The gold standard for the diagnosis of autoimmune MG continues to be the demonstration of autoantibodies against muscle AChRs by immunoprecipitation radioimmunoassay. The assay is specific and sensitive and documents an autoimmune response against muscle AChRs. Although seronegative MG occurs in approximately 2% of dogs with generalized MG, false-positive results are rare.

The edrophonium chloride challenge test (Tensilon or Enlon, 0.1 to 0.2 mg/kg in dogs and 0.25 to 0.5 mg total dose in cats IV) also should be performed since dramatic positive test results give a presumptive diagnosis of MG and allow initiation of therapy before serologic confirmation. A negative edrophonium chloride challenge result does not rule out a diagnosis of MG. In addition, a subjective improvement in muscle strength may be found in other neuromuscular diseases; thus, unless the response is dramatic, the edrophonium chloride challenge test should not be used alone to confirm a diagnosis.

Treatment of Focal and Generalized Myasthenia Gravis

No single treatment regimen is ideal for all cases of MG. Choices must be made among the therapeutic options, with the goal of obtaining the best result while keeping the risks and adverse effects as low as possible. Each case needs an individualized treatment plan, which may have to be changed from time to time depending on the stage of the disease and response to treatments. Relative to discussion of available treatments, autoimmune MG can be divided into focal (group 1), generalized (group 2), acute fulminating (group 3), and paraneoplastic (group 4) forms. Unlike humans with MG, in whom treatment is usually lifelong, dogs with MG routinely experience spontaneous remission if they survive the initial month following onset of clinical signs and do not have a thymoma (Shelton and Lindstrom, 2001).

Supportive Care

General supportive care and dedicated owners are integral parts of treatment for all groups of MG patients. The owners should be advised that treatment for MG may be as short as a few months or may need to be continued for several months to a couple of years, depending on the severity of disease.

Differentiation of vomiting from regurgitation and recognition of esophageal dilation or pharyngeal weakness are critical. Aspiration pneumonia should be treated aggressively (see Chapter 162). In cases of acute fulminating MG, referral of patients to centers with intensive care facilities is optimal. As for any dog with esophageal dilation, altered feeding procedures, including elevation of food and water or placement of a gastrostomy tube, should be used to facilitate adequate hydration, nutrition, and drug delivery. If there is a delay in recognition of megaesophagus, inadequate nutrition and poor hydration may occur, which could worsen the clinical status of the animal. Nutritional support can be expected to decrease morbidity and improve immune status.

Cholinesterase Inhibitors

Cholinesterase inhibitors are the cornerstone of treatment for MG and are advised for all patient groups. These drugs result in improved muscle strength by decreasing the hydrolysis of acetylcholine (ACh) at the neuromuscular junction. This allows a greater number of ACh molecules to bind to and activate AChRs on the postsynaptic membrane, prolongs the action of ACh, and enhances neuromuscular transmission. Cholinesterase inhibitors do not treat the underlying aberrant immune response and thus do not modify the course of the disease, but they do control the clinical signs. In canine nonthymomatous MG, this is not a problem since the natural course of the disease is to go into remission in the absence of immunosuppression. If an optimal response to therapy is obtained and normal limb muscle strength returns and regurgitation decreases or resolves, supportive care and management of megaesophagus, anticholinesterase therapy, and time may be all that is required.

Pyridostigmine bromide (Mestinon, 1 to 3 mg/kg q8-12h PO) and neostigmine bromide (Prostigmin, 2 mg/kg/day PO administered in divided doses to effect) are the most commonly used cholinesterase inhibitors; the former is preferred in most clinical situations because of its longer duration of action and fewer cholinergic adverse effects. The dosage must be adjusted individually for each animal, depending on the response to the drug and tolerance of the adverse effects.

Pyridostigmine bromide is available in syrup, tablet, and time-release forms. The syrup form may be optimal for dosing in smaller breeds of dogs but should be diluted 50:50 in water before use because gastric irritation may result if it is given straight. In animals in critical condition in which oral dosing is not possible, constant-rate infusion of pyridostigmine bromide (0.01 to 0.03 mg/kg/hr) may be used until oral feedings are resumed or a feeding tube is placed. For dosing in cats, pyridostigmine bromide (0.1 to 0.25 mg/kg IV q24h) has been recommended.

Adverse effects of cholinesterase inhibitors result from excessive cholinergic stimulation following the accumulation of ACh at muscarinic receptors of smooth muscle, autonomic glands, the central nervous system, and nicotinic receptors of skeletal muscle. Bradycardia, which results from excessive vagal activity, is seen almost exclusively after parenteral injections of ACh inhibitors. Gastrointestinal adverse effects may occur after administration by any route and include nausea, vomiting, abdominal cramping, loose stools, or overt diarrhea. Increased bronchial and oral secretions may be a problem if dysphagia is present. Adverse effects may be reduced by administering small doses of atropine or having the animal take medication after meals when feasible.

Overtreatment with cholinesterase inhibitors can result in excessive accumulation of ACh at the neuromuscular junction, with worsening of weakness as a result of depolarization or desensitization of the postsynaptic membrane. Any increase in anticholinesterase

medication that does not produce clear-cut improvement in muscle strength should be reversed promptly.

Corticosteroids

If myasthenic animals cannot be managed successfully with supportive care and cholinesterase inhibitors alone, corticosteroids may be added carefully. Corticosteroids have been shown to be of benefit in human MG and may improve the long-term prognosis in some cases of canine MG. However, the adverse effects may be life threatening. Glucocorticoids result in polydipsia and polyphagia in an animal that may have difficulty swallowing or is regurgitating. In addition, there is an increased susceptibility to infection. Increased weakness often occurs early in the course of steroid treatment, requiring hospitalization and sometimes intensive medical care with respiratory support. To prevent the initial steroid-induced weakness, low-dose prednisone therapy has been recommended in mild and moderately affected human patients with MG. I have also recommended a similar therapeutic approach for myasthenic dogs in groups 1 and 2. The use of anti-inflammatory dosages (0.5 mg/kg q24h PO), not immunosuppressive dosages, of corticosteroids is suggested. Relative contraindications for corticosteroid therapy include severe obesity, diabetes mellitus, uncontrolled hypertension, gastrointestinal ulcerations, and ongoing infections or aspiration pneumonia.

Although myasthenic cats can be treated successfully with anticholinesterase drugs, it is my impression that cats generally respond better to corticosteroid therapy. Exacerbation of muscle weakness and other unwanted adverse effects of high-dose corticosteroids may not occur as frequently in myasthenic cats as in myasthenic dogs.

Immunosuppressive Drugs

The use of other immunosuppressive drugs in canine and feline MG has not been studied adequately, and there are only a few case reports suggesting effectiveness. Clearly, controlled clinical trials are warranted. Since most cases of canine or feline MG can be managed successfully with anticholinesterase drugs alone or in combination with prednisone, most of these immunosuppressive drugs should be reserved for severe, nonresponsive forms of MG. Disadvantages of these agents are the time it takes for improvement to begin, the adverse effects, the expense, and the need for long-term administration.

Azathioprine

Azathioprine is the most frequently used immunosuppressive agent in MG after prednisone. Adverse effects are related to gastrointestinal and myelosuppressive toxicity. A complete blood cell count should be performed 7 to 10 days after initiation of therapy and monthly thereafter. Azathioprine may be used as an alternative to prednisone when the latter drug is relatively contraindicated and when a less rapid response to therapy is acceptable. Azathioprine also may be used for its "steroid-sparing" effects in patients that have developed unacceptable adverse responses to prednisone, when it has not been possible to reduce the dosage of prednisone to acceptable levels, or when the response to prednisone has not been satisfactory. The recommended dosage of azathioprine is 1.1 to 2.2 mg/kg q24-48h PO. Since azathioprine can result in neuromuscular blockade in cats, its use is not recommended in feline patients.

Cyclophosphamide

Cyclophosphamide can cause severe leukopenia, specifically neutropenia, and routine complete blood counts should be performed every 7 to 10 days after administration. Gastrointestinal disturbances also can occur. Sterile hemorrhagic cystitis is another serious adverse effect of cyclophosphamide and can occur not only with prolonged administration but after a single dose. This drug has not been evaluated in treatment of canine MG, and given the serious adverse effects, the risks do not outweigh the benefits.

Cyclosporine

Cyclosporine has been used to treat a variety of immune-mediated diseases in the dog but has not been evaluated specifically for the treatment of MG. In human MG cyclosporine is used in patients who are candidates for immunosuppression but who cannot take or who have not responded satisfactorily to azathioprine. It has been used as the primary immunosuppressant in human MG as well as combined with prednisone, which permits use of lower corticosteroid doses. The maximum response usually is seen within 3 to 4 months. Suggested dosage range for canine immune-mediated diseases is 5 to 10 mg/kg/day PO divided into two doses. Adverse effects include vomiting, diarrhea, weight loss, gingival hyperplasia, and involuntary shaking. Although the drug can be nephrotoxic in humans, dogs seem relatively resistant to this adverse effect.

Mycophenolate Mofetil

Mycophenolate mofetil (MMF) has been used widely in human medicine and recently in veterinary medicine for the treatment of MG. Although clinical studies have not documented a long-term benefit of MMF over other drugs, it may be useful as a rescue agent in the treatment of severe generalized MG or as an initial treatment to control clinical signs in the first months of disease. At a dosage of 20 mg/kg PO q12h gastrointestinal signs may be observed, including vomiting, diarrhea, and anorexia, which are dosage related. For this reason, in patients with MG a 50% reduction in MMF dosage should be made once significant improvement or resolution of clinical signs is noted.

Thymectomy

Most human neurologists recommend thymectomy for MG patients, although no controlled clinical trial has proven this treatment to be of significant benefit. In human patients there is a high incidence of thymic hyperplasia, but in my experience thymic hyperplasia is identified only rarely in canine or feline myasthenic patients. In canine and feline MG thymectomy should be reserved for animals with confirmed MG that also have a cranial mediastinal mass (group 4, paraneoplastic MG). In my opinion all animals with a cranial mediastinal mass should be tested for MG before surgical removal of the mass. Weakness may become apparent clinically after the surgery, and knowing the antibody status before surgery should aid in therapeutic management. If a cranial mediastinal mass can be removed completely, the AChR antibody titer should return to the reference range, and clinical signs of MG should resolve. If the mass cannot be removed completely, the antibody titer will remain positive, and treatment for MG will need to be continued. Specific treatments are similar to those for group 2 MG (preceding paragraphs) or group 3 MG (following paragraphs).

Treatment of Acute Fulminating Myasthenia Gravis

Management of acute, severe generalized MG (group 3, acute fulminating MG) can be difficult and ideally should be performed in intensive care facilities. In humans expensive short-term treatment modalities such as plasma exchange (plasmapheresis) and intravenous immunoglobulin commonly are used; however, because of the expense and technical difficulty of performing these therapies, they are not often used in veterinary medicine.

Ventilatory support and placement of a feeding tube usually are required. Respiratory failure, caused either by ventilatory failure due to weakness of the intercostal muscles or diaphragm or by severe aspiration pneumonia, may be the most common cause of death in dogs with acute fulminating myasthenic crisis. If possible, specimens should be obtained from the respiratory tract by tracheal wash and cultured, and broad-spectrum intravenous antibiotics should be instituted immediately. Aminoglycosides and ampicillin should be avoided because of possible detrimental effects on neuromuscular transmission.

For animals in critical condition in which oral medication is not possible, a constant-rate infusion of pyridostigmine bromide (0.01 to 0.03 mg/kg/hr) may be used until oral feedings are resumed. Alternatively, anticholinesterase therapy can be administered through a feeding tube.

Myasthenic crisis may be precipitated by concurrent infection or high daily doses of prednisone. Corticosteroids should be avoided initially in patients with overwhelming aspiration pneumonia. Once an infection has been controlled, corticosteroids or other immunosuppressive agents such as azathioprine, cyclosporine, or MMF can be added to the regimen if necessary (see earlier section). High-dose intravenous methylprednisolone sodium succinate therapy may be of benefit in severe cases of MG without causing a worsening of muscle weakness. In one study of 15 human patients, 2 g of methylprednisolone sodium succinate was given intravenously every 5 days for a total of 15 days. Satisfactory improvement without exacerbation of muscle weakness occurred in 10 of 15 patients.

Monitoring the Course of Autoimmune Myasthenia Gravis

Although a positive AChR antibody titer is diagnostic of autoimmune MG, there is a poor correlation between the severity of the disease and the antibody concentration. However, in the absence of immunosuppressive therapy, determination of serial AChR antibody titers in an individual animal is a good indicator of disease status and should help determine duration of treatment. As long as the AChR antibody titer remains positive, treatment should be continued. In my laboratory there has been an excellent correlation between resolution of clinical signs, including megaesophagus, and return of AChR antibody titers to within the reference range. Monitoring of the AChR antibody titer also is suggested in paraneoplastic MG since it gives a good indication of whether a cranial mediastinal mass has been removed completely. In most cases of canine autoimmune MG, once remission has occurred, recurrence of MG is rare. A therapeutically induced decrease in AChR antibody titer and absence of clinical signs while the dog is receiving immunosuppressive therapy should not be misinterpreted as a remission. In these cases clinical signs can return once the dosage of immunosuppressive drug is decreased. The natural course of autoimmune MG in cats has not been determined, although it is my impression that spontaneous remissions are not as common as in dogs.

With an accurate diagnosis and early treatment, autoimmune MG is a treatable disease. Since there is a genetic predisposition to autoimmune diseases, including MG, it is recommended that myasthenic animals not be bred. Myasthenic female dogs and cats should be spayed as soon as possible after MG is under control because heat cycles and pregnancy can exacerbate active MG. Finally, vaccination during active MG should be avoided because general immune stimulation can result in exacerbations of weakness and elevations of the AChR antibody titer. Whether or not vaccinations can trigger MG is still an unresolved question.

References and Suggested Reading

Abelson AL et al: Use of mycophenolate mofetil as a rescue agent in the treatment of severe generalized myasthenia gravis in three dogs, *J Vet Emerg Crit Care* 19:369, 2009.

Arsura E et al: High-dose intravenous methylprednisolone in myasthenia gravis, *Arch Neurol* 42:1149, 1985.

Dewey CW et al: Clinical forms of acquired myasthenia gravis in dogs: 25 cases (1988-1995), *J Vet Intern Med* 11:50, 1997.

Dewey CW et al: Mycophenolate mofetil treatment in dogs with serologically diagnosed acquired myasthenia gravis: 27 cases (1999-2000), *J Am Vet Med Assoc* 236:664, 2010.

Ducoté JM, Dewey CW, Coates JR: Clinical forms of acquired myasthenia gravis in cats, *Compend Contin Educ Pract Vet* 21:440, 1999.

Foy DS et al: Cholinergic crisis after neostigmine administration in a dog with acquired focal myasthenia gravis, *J Vet Emerg Crit Care* 21:547, 2011.

Khorzad R et al: Myasthenia gravis in dogs with an emphasis on treatment and critical care management, *J Vet Emerg Crit Care* 21:193, 2011.

King LG, Vite CH: Acute fulminating myasthenia gravis in five dogs, *J Am Vet Med Assoc* 212:830, 1998.

Shelton GD: Myasthenia gravis and disorders of neuromuscular transmission, *Vet Clin North Am Small Anim Pract* 32:189, 2002.

Shelton GD et al: Acquired myasthenia gravis: selective involvement of esophageal, pharyngeal, and facial muscles, *J Vet Intern Med* 4:281, 1990.

Shelton GD, Ho M, Kass PH: Risk factors for acquired myasthenia gravis in cats: 105 cases (1986-1998), *J Am Vet Med Assoc* 216:55, 2000.

Shelton GD, Lindstrom JM: Spontaneous remission in canine myasthenia gravis: implications for assessing human MG therapies, *Neurology* 57:2139, 2001.

Shelton GD, Schule A, Kass PH: Risk factors for acquired myasthenia gravis in dogs: 1154 cases (1991-1995), *J Am Vet Med Assoc* 211:1428, 1997.

CHAPTER 240

Treatment of Myopathies and Neuropathies

G. DIANE SHELTON, *La Jolla, California*

Neuromuscular diseases can be difficult diagnostic challenges with only a limited number of available therapeutic options. However, the most common diseases affecting muscle and peripheral nerve are treatable if a correct diagnosis is reached before irreversible pathologic changes occur. For other neuromuscular diseases, particularly the inherited myopathies and neuropathies, no therapeutic options currently are available. The old dictum "To help, or at least to do no harm" (Hippocrates) is particularly true for this group of diseases. Beginning a trial of corticosteroid treatment before performing at least the minimum necessary diagnostic tests can delay or impair the ability to reach a correct diagnosis, delay initiation of specific therapies, and possibly result in irreversible contractures or even death of the animal. Further, glucocorticoid treatment results in a polydipsic and polyphagic animal with an increased susceptibility to infection.

The first important step is to achieve accurate neuroanatomic localization. Neuromuscular diseases are disorders of the motor unit and as such affect neuronal cell bodies in the ventral gray matter (ventral horn) of the spinal cord (motor neuron disease), peripheral nerve (neuropathies), neuromuscular junction (disorders of neuromuscular transmission), and muscle (myopathies). A careful neurologic examination is critical. If the wrong anatomic localization is made, an incorrect diagnostic pathway will be chosen and valuable time wasted. An incorrect diagnosis can lead to inappropriate treatments that may result in severe debilitation or be life threatening.

Once clinical signs have been localized to the neuromuscular system, specific laboratory testing should be performed to reach an accurate diagnosis. Testing to collect a minimum data set for neuromuscular diseases should include a complete blood cell count, serum chemistry profile including creatine kinase (CK) activity and electrolyte concentrations, thyroid screen, urinalysis, and, in most cases, acetylcholine receptor antibody titer to test for myasthenia gravis. Electrodiagnostic testing, including electromyography and measurement of sensory and motor nerve conduction velocity, provides important information regarding the distribution and nature of the disorder but requires specialized equipment and expertise. Cerebrospinal fluid analysis may be beneficial in disorders of nerve roots such as acute polyradiculoneuritis and protozoal diseases. A definitive diagnosis ultimately requires histopathologic evaluation of appropriately collected and processed muscle and peripheral nerve biopsy specimens. Although a specific diagnosis may not be reached in all cases, information regarding the underlying pathologic process can guide empiric therapy.

Treatment of the most common inflammatory myopathies (masticatory muscle myositis, polymyositis, infectious myositis) and noninflammatory myopathies (endocrine and exogenous corticosteroid induced), the less common noninflammatory myopathies (inherited myopathies), and the neuropathies are described in this chapter. Specific treatments for the various clinical forms of myasthenia gravis are covered in Chapter 239.

Treatment of Inflammatory Myopathies

The inflammatory myopathies, including the immune-mediated forms (masticatory muscle myositis, polymyositis, extraocular myositis, and dermatomyositis) and those associated with infectious diseases (particularly infections with the protozoal organisms *Toxoplasma gondii*, *Neospora caninum*, and *Hepatozoon americanum*) are relatively common in dogs. Myositis associated with neoplasia as a paraneoplastic or preneoplastic process occurs less commonly. Inflammatory myopathies occur rarely in cats as a paraneoplastic syndrome (thymoma) or associated with feline immunodeficiency virus (FIV) or feline leukemia virus (FeLV) infection. In my experience, purely immune-mediated inflammatory myopathies are uncommon in cats. Following a histologic diagnosis of an inflammatory myopathy, infectious diseases should be ruled out by serologic testing, and screening for neoplasia should be initiated. If results are negative, an immune-mediated cause is likely.

Masticatory Muscle Myositis

Masticatory muscle myositis (MMM) is the most common inflammatory myopathy occurring in dogs and occurs in rare cases in cats. In MMM clinical signs are restricted to the muscles of mastication without involvement of the limb muscles or other muscle groups. MMM has been recognized in most breeds of dogs and can begin as early as 3 months of age. Although MMM is a bilateral disease, clinical signs can appear unilateral, with one side affected more markedly than the other. A particularly severe, breed-associated form of MMM has been identified recently in young cavalier King Charles spaniels. In the acute form of MMM, pain and swelling of the masticatory muscles and trismus are common clinical findings. Typically the jaws cannot be opened, even under anesthesia. The cause of this inability to the open the jaw in the acute stage has not been identified, and fibrosis is not obvious in muscle biopsy specimens. In the chronic stage there is atrophy of the masticatory muscles with or without jaw pain or immobility. In end-stage MMM, atrophy is severe, and the jaw may not open more than a couple of centimeters. In muscle biopsy specimens in end-stage disease, there is severe loss of muscle mass and replacement with fibrous tissue. MMM is very responsive to corticosteroid therapy in the acute stages and moderately so in the chronic stages. Once end-stage MMM is present, typically there is only minimal, if any, response to corticosteroids.

Because of the propensity for fibrosis, an early and accurate diagnosis is critical to achieve a positive clinical outcome. The serum CK activity usually is normal or only mildly elevated. Although a serologic assay currently is available for the diagnosis of MMM (through demonstration of antibodies to type IIM fibers by either immunohistochemical analysis or enzyme-linked immunosorbent assay), a biopsy of the temporalis muscle also is recommended to determine severity of the disease and long-term prognosis. Previous receipt of corticosteroid therapy at immunosuppressive dosages for longer than 7 to 10 days can lower antibody titers and produce negative results. In addition, animals with chronic, end-stage MMM can test negative for antibodies against type IIM fibers because most fibers of this type have been destroyed, which removes the antigenic stimulus. If a biopsy specimen is collected, care must be taken to ensure that the correct muscle is sampled. A common mistake is to biopsy the frontalis and not the temporalis muscle. The frontalis muscle lies directly under the skin and is not part of the masticatory muscle group. A biopsy specimen from the frontalis muscle will not be diagnostic. Instructions for collection of an appropriate temporalis muscle biopsy specimen are given in a 2004 review of MMM by Melmed and colleagues (2004).

Following confirmation of the diagnosis of MMM, immunosuppressive therapy with prednisone should be initiated at 1 to 2 mg/kg q12h PO. Treatment should be continued until the level of CK activity (if elevated) has returned to the reference range, jaw mobility has returned to normal, and clinically evident jaw pain has resolved. Prednisone dosage then should be gradually decreased to the lowest alternate-day dose that keeps the dog free of clinical signs and continued for a period of at least 4 to 6 months. Relapses are common if treatment is stopped too soon. The most frequent causes of a poor clinical outcome are a delay in initiating appropriate treatment, inappropriate dosages of corticosteroids, and treatment for too short a period of time. If prednisone is poorly tolerated, other immunosuppressive drugs such as azathioprine may be added to reduce the glucocorticoid dosages. There are no controlled clinical trials examining the efficacy of any therapeutic regimens in the treatment of canine inflammatory myopathies; thus recommendations for the use of other agents, including cyclosporine, mycophenolate mofetil, and intravenous immunoglobulin, cannot be given.

In end-stage MMM, fibrosis may be severe, and the jaw may open only a few centimeters, if that. In these cases resolution of clinical signs with corticosteroid therapy should not be expected. Maintenance of hydration and adequate nutrition may be problematic, and dogs may have generalized muscle wasting from malnourishment related to the lack of food intake. Under no circumstances should the jaw be opened forcibly, even under sedation or anesthesia, because a jaw fracture may result. Surgical procedures such as mandibular symphysiotomy or partial mandibulectomy or hemimandibulectomy may allow tongue movement for lapping food and water. These procedures are best performed by a surgical specialist. The position of the tongue should be noted under anesthesia to avoid inadvertent protrusion and swelling from venous congestion.

Polymyositis

Polymyositis (PM) is an immune-mediated inflammatory myopathy that can affect all muscle groups, including the masticatory muscles, the limb muscles, and the esophageal, pharyngeal, and laryngeal muscles. PM can occur alone or as part of a generalized autoimmune disorder such as systemic lupus erythematosus. The serum CK activity may be normal or mildly to moderately elevated, depending on the degree of muscle damage and the distribution of cellular infiltrates. The IIM antibody titer yields negative results in most cases, even with clinical involvement of the masticatory muscles. Clinical signs may include a stiff, stilted gait; muscle atrophy; variable myalgia; regurgitation and dysphagia; and contractures in chronic PM.

The diagnosis of PM is confirmed by muscle biopsy findings. Biopsy specimens should be collected from more than one muscle since cellular infiltrates can have a patchy distribution and may be missed on individual biopsy specimens. The large proximal limb muscles such as the vastus lateralis or biceps femoris of the pelvic limb and the triceps muscle of the thoracic limb are suggested as biopsy sites. Once a diagnosis of an inflammatory disorder has been histologically confirmed and infectious agents have been ruled out, immunosuppressive therapy should be initiated as for MMM. The serum CK activity should be monitored, and the animal should be observed for resolution of clinical signs. Because cardiac muscle also may be involved, testing for cardiac troponin I is warranted. Periodic screening for an underlying neoplasia also is suggested, particularly in the boxer breed. Breed-associated PM has been described in vizsla and Newfoundland dogs.

Extraocular Muscle Myositis

A focal, presumed immune-mediated inflammatory myopathy, extraocular myositis, selectively affects the extraocular muscles while sparing the masticatory and limb muscles. The clinical presentation is that of a bilateral exophthalmos in the acute stage or a restrictive strabismus in the chronic stage. The serum CK concentration is normal, and results of IIM antibody testing are negative. A presumptive diagnosis of extraocular myositis can be made by clinical presentation, a negative result on the IIM antibody test, and demonstration of swollen extraocular muscles by orbital ultrasonography or magnetic resonance imaging. In the acute stage resolution of clinical signs with immunosuppressive dosages of corticosteroids can be rapid. In chronic stages of extraocular myositis with fibrosis of the extraocular muscles, a favorable response to immunosuppression should not be expected. Restrictive strabismus may result when treatment is inappropriate or delayed.

Dermatomyositis

Canine dermatomyositis is a familial, immune-mediated inflammatory disease of striated muscle, skin, and microvasculature found in young collies, Shetland sheepdogs (shelties), and collie-crossbred dogs, but it can occur rarely in other breeds. In familial dermatomyositis the clinical diagnosis is based on the findings of classic skin changes and myositis in a collie or sheltie. The onset of clinical signs typically occurs within the first 6 months of life. Clinical signs of myositis develop after the dermatitis and approximately correlate in severity with the degree of dermatitis. Serum CK activity is only mildly elevated. A specific diagnosis is made by examination of skin and muscle biopsy specimens. Unlike in PM, in dermatomyositis the temporalis and distal limb muscles (such as the cranial tibial muscle) are affected more markedly. Treatment involves immunosuppression as in MMM and PM as well as symptomatic relief of skin lesions, including avoidance of sunlight, treatment of underlying pyoderma, and administration of vitamin E (400 U q24h PO).

Inflammatory Myopathies Secondary to Infectious Agents

In my laboratory the most common cause of infectious myositis in dogs is the protozoal organism *N. caninum*. Young dogs infected with *N. caninum* can show clinical signs of rigid pelvic limb hyperextension, muscle atrophy resulting from myositis, and concurrent polyradiculoneuritis. In older dogs infection can cause either an inflammatory or a necrotizing myopathy.

Infection with *T. gondii* is considered more common in cats, with clinical signs predominantly related to the central nervous system, respiratory system, and gastrointestinal system. Although parasitic cysts may be identified in muscle biopsy specimens from cats with neuromuscular diseases, an inflammatory myopathy with cellular reactions around the cysts is a rare finding. A presumptive diagnosis can be based on positive results on immunoglobulin G or immunoglobulin M antibody titers, but a definitive diagnosis requires demonstration of the organism within muscle or other tissue by immunohistochemical or molecular methods. A combination treatment of clindamycin (10 mg/kg q8h PO) and trimethoprim/sulfa (15 mg/kg q12h PO) for 4 weeks has been suggested for canine neosporosis. Clindamycin (25 to 50 mg/kg PO q8-12h) is the treatment of choice for feline toxoplasmosis.

Infection with other protozoal organisms, including *H. americanum* in the southern region of the United States

and *Leishmania infantum* in the Mediterranean area, may cause myositis in dogs. *Trypanosoma cruzi* may affect the myocardium and skeletal muscle of dogs in the temperate to tropical regions of the world. Severe myositis recently has been associated with infection with *Sarcocystis* spp. in dogs. Although bacterial and rickettsial infectious diseases are common in dogs and cats, reports of an associated myositis are infrequent. Virus-related inflammatory myopathies are well documented in people, with retroviruses and enteroviruses most commonly implicated. Inflammatory myopathies and neuropathies have been identified in my laboratory in FeLV- and FIV-infected cats. For more in-depth discussions of infectious causes of neuromuscular diseases and appropriate antimicrobial agents, references by Podell (2002) and Kent (2004) are suggested.

Treatment of Noninflammatory Myopathies

The largest group of treatable noninflammatory myopathies encountered in clinical practice consists of those associated with endocrine disorders such as hypothyroidism, hyperthyroidism, and Cushing's syndrome secondary to long-term corticosteroid therapy (so-called steroid myopathy) or with electrolyte abnormalities in metabolic disorders. The presence of weakness, stiffness, reluctance to move, muscle wasting, and myalgia may be the first indications of an underlying endocrine disorder in the absence of classic clinical signs.

Hypothyroid Myopathy

Among human patients newly diagnosed with hypothyroidism, as many as 38% have clinical muscular weakness, and 80% have complaints suggestive of muscle dysfunction. The incidence of myopathic signs in canine hypothyroidism is not known but may be similar. The serum CK activity may be normal or mildly elevated. A diagnosis of hypothyroidism can be strongly suspected from histochemical evaluation of a muscle biopsy specimen and confirmed with laboratory testing, including measurement of endogenous canine thyroid-stimulating hormone and serum free thyroxine levels by dialysis. The prognosis for recovery in hypothyroid myopathy is excellent, and resolution is rapid once the dog is restored to a euthyroid state.

Hyperthyroid Myopathy

Muscle weakness and tremors may occur in feline hyperthyroidism. The serum CK activity may be markedly elevated, but muscle biopsy specimens usually show normal findings. Resolution of clinical weakness rapidly follows correction of electrolyte abnormalities and return to a euthyroid state. An adverse effect of the antithyroid drug methimazole is the development of muscle weakness approximately 2 to 4 months after initiation of therapy, with a positive result on an acetylcholine receptor antibody titer diagnostic of acquired myasthenia gravis. Clinical signs of myasthenia resolve and the acetylcholine receptor antibody titer returns to the normal range after cessation of the drug.

Cushing's Myopathy and Myotonia

Muscle wasting, weakness, gait abnormalities, and in some cases myotonia may be found in older dogs with Cushing's syndrome. Muscle stiffness and lameness may be an early clinical indicator of an underlying endocrinopathy. Laboratory testing can confirm hyperadrenocorticism, and type II fiber atrophy and excessive lipid accumulation commonly are found on histochemical examination of muscle biopsy specimens, consistent with this disease. Although it has not been studied thoroughly, peripheral neuropathy also may be associated with Cushing's syndrome. If myotonia is absent, clinical signs of myopathic weakness should resolve following specific treatment. Muscle rigidity associated with myotonia is not as responsive to therapy, and deficits can persist.

Steroid Myopathy

Profound muscle weakness and atrophy can occur following long-term exogenous corticosteroid therapy in dogs. The masticatory muscles usually are the most severely affected; however, weakness and atrophy may affect the whole body musculature. As in myopathy associated with Cushing's syndrome, prominent atrophy of type II fibers is a classic histologic change in muscle biopsy specimens. The fluorinated corticosteroids such as triamcinolone, betamethasone, and dexamethasone have been reported to have the most myopathic potential; thus conversion to a nonfluorinated steroid preparation with alternate-day treatment is recommended. Addition of another immunosuppressive agent that would allow the dosage of corticosteroids to be lowered also is suggested. Improvement usually follows but can take several weeks. Nutritional supplements also may be of benefit (see the section on nutritional supplements at the end of this chapter).

Myopathies Associated with Electrolyte Abnormalities

Dramatic muscle weakness, including inability to raise the head, and markedly elevated serum CK activity may occur with electrolyte abnormalities, particularly in cats. Hypokalemia may be associated with renal failure, excessive potassium loss (from diuretics or intrinsic renal disease), thyrotoxicosis, or hyperaldosteronemia (Conn's-like syndrome), and can be a breed-associated condition in Burmese kittens. Muscle biopsy findings typically are normal, and the diagnosis is made by routine laboratory testing. Affected cats usually demonstrate substantial improvement in muscle strength within 2 to 3 days after oral potassium supplementation is initiated. Hypernatremic polymyopathy also has been reported in cats. Muscle weakness associated with hyperkalemia and hyponatremia in canine Addison's disease also is reversible and readily responds to treatment of the underlying condition.

Myopathies Associated with Inherited Diseases

Most of the inherited myopathies, including the muscular dystrophies (Shelton and Engvall, 2002) and other degenerative muscle diseases, occur in purebred dogs and cats younger than 1 year of age. In some cases gait abnormalities and small stature may be first noticed at the time of ambulation. The breed of an affected animal is one of the most useful distinguishing diagnostic criteria for inherited diseases (Compendium of Inherited Diseases, see Fyfe, 2002). For the majority of these diseases there is no cure, and treatment options are mainly supportive. An accurate pathologic diagnosis is of particular importance to breeding programs because the goal is development of reliable molecular testing procedures for identification of carrier animals. Obtaining a specific diagnosis of these diseases also is important because inherited diseases constitute a significant proportion of diseases that cause poor quality of life or death in all breeds of dogs and cats.

Treatment of Peripheral Neuropathies

Peripheral neuropathy continues to be a challenging area with regard to recognition, diagnosis, and therapy. Most often the cause of a peripheral neuropathy remains elusive despite extensive biochemical, toxicologic, electrophysiologic, histochemical, histopathologic, and electron microscopic studies of muscle and nerve biopsy specimens. This is partly because of the limited number of ways in which peripheral nerves react to disease. Even though a specific cause may not be identified, evaluation of peripheral nerve biopsy samples in plastic sections can provide valuable information regarding disease severity and presence or absence of regeneration.

Neuropathies Associated with Endocrine Diseases

Neuropathies associated with endocrine diseases are relatively common, and treatment is based on the primary endocrinopathy. Diabetes mellitus can cause both a sensory and a motor neuropathy in cats, with clinical signs of a plantigrade, and in some cases palmigrade, stance. Resolution of clinical signs usually follows adequate glycemic control; however, residual deficits may occur in cats with chronic, poorly controlled disease. Weakness and muscle atrophy consistent with neuropathy also may occur in diabetic dogs, although most cases are complicated by hypothyroidism or Cushing's syndrome. Hypothyroidism in dogs may be associated with peripheral neuropathy, although the mechanisms are poorly understood. Following hormone replacement, gradual improvement in neurologic signs should result; however, this may take several months. Neuropathy also is a rare complication of pancreatic beta-cell (adeno)carcinoma. Although clinical signs of neuropathy may improve following surgical intervention, the prognosis for complete remission from an insulinoma and the accompanying peripheral neuropathy is poor.

Nutritional and Toxic Polyneuropathies

Although polyneuropathies with nutritional or toxic causes are not common or well documented in veterinary medicine, they may be treatable; thus the owner should be questioned carefully about diet, dietary supplements, and any previous drug therapies. Review of the health history and a thorough physical examination also should be performed to identify any underlying gastrointestinal disease that could impair absorption. Although not fully documented in the veterinary literature, vitamin B_1 deficiency and toxic neuropathies associated with metronidazole and nitrofurantoin treatments are described in the human literature. In an experimental study (Dickinson et al, 2004), it was demonstrated that long-term dietary restriction of phenylalanine and tyrosine in cats may result in a predominantly sensory neuropathy.

Neuropathies and Neoplastic Disorders

Lymphoma is the most common tumor of nonneural origin that affects the peripheral nervous system. Particularly in cats, neoplastic cells can infiltrate the nerve and nerve roots, which results in clinical signs of polyneuropathy in addition to signs of multicentric lymphoma. The diagnosis is confirmed by electrodiagnostic testing and demonstration of neoplastic cells within a peripheral nerve biopsy specimen. Chemotherapy should be aimed at treating the underlying neoplasia. Chemotherapeutic drugs such as vincristine and cisplatin used in the treatment of lymphoma and solid tumors, respectively, may themselves cause peripheral neuropathy. Malignant peripheral nerve sheath tumors are the most common primary nerve tumor affecting the peripheral nervous system. Although surgical excision and amputation have been described, the prognosis is poor because recurrence is common with extension into the vertebral canal or thorax.

Inflammatory and Immune-Mediated Neuropathies

Organisms such as *T. gondii* and *N. caninum* can cause inflammatory and degenerative changes in peripheral nerves and nerve roots, as well as in muscle. Diagnosis and treatment are as described previously. Acute canine polyradiculoneuritis (coonhound paralysis) is one of the most commonly recognized canine peripheral neuropathies, characterized by lymphocytic radiculitis and demyelination of the ventral, and less commonly dorsal, nerve roots. Ascending tetraparesis or tetraplegia occurring over 1 to 2 days is characteristic of this disease. Treatment is supportive and includes physical therapy and bladder evacuation. Corticosteroids should not be given to dogs with acute canine polyradiculoneuritis because these drugs do not improve clinical signs or shorten the course of the disease and may in fact exacerbate the disorder and reduce survival rate.

The term *chronic (relapsing) demyelinating polyradiculoneuritis* refers to a group of chronic progressive or relapsing motor and sensory peripheral neuropathies that are associated with inflammatory changes in the spinal nerve roots as well as in the cranial nerves and more peripheral regions of appendicular nerves. An autoimmune attack against peripheral nerve myelin is suspected. A definitive diagnosis of the pathologic nature of the neuropathy and its severity and distribution is achieved by electrophysiologic evaluation and muscle and peripheral nerve biopsy. Because of the suspected immune-mediated nature of

this group of neuropathies, immunosuppression with prednisone (1 to 1.5 mg/kg PO q12h) has been recommended. Even with therapy, the long-term prognosis is guarded since relapses are common and the disease progresses over months to years.

Cellular infiltrates may invade the most distal intramuscular nerve branches and be evident in muscle biopsy specimens, particularly in cats. Young Bengal cats are predisposed to a relapsing polyneuropathy associated with demyelination and remyelination. The prognosis for recovery is good, although relapses can occur. Corticosteroids have been used in Bengal cats that recovered from polyneuropathy; however, recovery can occur in the absence of steroid treatment. It is possible that steroid treatment may result in a more rapid recovery, but further investigations are required. A similar relapsing form of polyneuropathy also has been identified in other purebred and mixed-breed cats.

Chronic Axonal Degeneration

Chronic, slowly progressive idiopathic axonal degeneration affects middle-aged to older large-breed dogs. Clinical presentation is that of progressive paraparesis or tetraparesis. Laryngeal paralysis may be an early clinical sign of a generalized peripheral neuropathy. A typical scenario is onset of peripheral weakness several months after laryngeal tie-back surgery, but weakness and atrophy of the distal limb muscles may be present at the time of surgery.

All diagnostic evaluations (biochemical, endocrine, or metabolic screening, as well as radiography and ultrasonography) yield normal results. Diagnosis is based on electrodiagnostic testing and muscle and peripheral nerve biopsy. Peripheral nerve biopsy is of particular importance in these cases because the extent of nerve fiber loss or endoneurial fibrosis and the presence or absence of regeneration are important in determining the course of the disease and long-term prognosis. At this time no therapeutic options are available that have been proven to be successful. Physical therapy and nutritional supplements are suggested in later sections.

Early-onset peripheral neuropathies associated with axonal degeneration and demyelination also occur in young pure-bred dogs, and many have been shown to have a genetic basis. Notably, genetic tests currently are available for early-onset polyneuropathy in Leonberger and St. Bernard breeds, for sensory ataxic neuropathy in golden retrievers, for polyneuropathy in greyhound show dogs, and for inherited polyneuropathy in Alaskan malamutes.

Adjunctive Therapy in Neuromuscular Diseases

Unless indicated by the presence of obvious cellular infiltrates within muscle and peripheral nerve biopsy specimens or signs of inflammation in cerebrospinal fluid, trials of treatment with glucocorticoids in the absence of a specific diagnosis can do more harm than good. Corticosteroids are catabolic and thus can lead to a decrease in muscle mass and exacerbate weakness. Suggested supportive therapies for myopathies or neuropathies without a specific underlying cause are physical therapy and nutritional supplementation.

Physical Therapy

Inactivity can diminish muscle mass further in cases of neuromuscular diseases, and weakness may be aggravated by contractures. Mild exercise may prevent some of the atrophy induced by glucocorticoid treatments or hyperadrenocorticism; thus walking should be encouraged. Passive range-of-motion exercises positively influence reinnervation and the sprouting process in denervated muscle and may be of therapeutic value.

Nutritional Supplements

Nutritional supplements may be beneficial when a specific diagnosis is not identified and may be used in conjunction with corticosteroids in inflammatory myopathies or neuropathies to counteract the adverse effects of additional drug-induced muscle atrophy and weakness. Although controlled studies have not yet been performed, various vitamins and nutritional supplements have been advocated for patients with neuromuscular diseases. The goal is to increase muscle mass and strength by the use of anabolic agents, exercise, and physical therapy rather than exacerbate muscle weakness and atrophy by inactivity and harmful drugs.

I recommend oral supplementation with L-carnitine (100 mg/kg q24h), coenzyme Q_{10} (4 mg/kg q24h), and B complex vitamins. This therapy should not be harmful and may help improve muscle strength. Several different muscle diseases are associated with low muscle carnitine concentrations, and dramatic improvement may result in some cases. The owners should be informed that in most instances this is not a cure, but, most important, it cannot be harmful. The metabolic benefits of L-carnitine include transportation of fatty acids into the mitochondria for energy generation and promotion of the urinary excretion of abnormal metabolites. Coenzyme Q_{10} functions as a cofactor in several enzyme systems related to energy conversion (electron transport) and is a vital catalyst for energy production at the cellular level. It also is a free radical scavenger. For degenerative peripheral nerve diseases, acetyl-L-carnitine may be more beneficial than the L-carnitine form. Clearly, controlled clinical trials are necessary to document the efficacy of these treatments for neuromuscular diseases.

References and Suggested Reading

Bensfield AC et al: Recurrent demyelination and remyelination in 37 young Bengal cats with polyneuropathy, *J Vet Intern Med* 25:882, 2011.

Cuddon P: Electrophysiology in neuromuscular disease, *Vet Clin North Am Small Anim Pract* 32:31, 2002.

Dickinson PJ et al: Assessment of the neurologic effects of dietary deficiencies of phenylalanine and tyrosine in cats, *Am J Vet Res* 65:671, 2004.

Dickinson PJ, LeCouteur RA: Muscle and nerve biopsy, *Vet Clin North Am Small Anim Pract* 32:63, 2002.

Evans J, Levesque D, Shelton GD: Canine inflammatory myopathies: a clinicopathologic review of 200 cases, *J Vet Intern Med* 18:679, 2004.

Fyfe JC: Molecular diagnosis of inherited neuromuscular disease, *Vet Clin North Am Small Anim Pract* 32:287, 2002.

Glass EN, Kent M: The clinical examination for neuromuscular disease, *Vet Clin North Am Small Anim Pract* 32:1, 2002.

Haley AC et al: Breed-specific polymyositis in Hungarian Vizsla dogs, *J Vet Intern Med* 25:393, 2011.

Kent M: Therapeutic options for neuromuscular diseases, *Vet Clin North Am Small Anim Pract* 34:1525, 2004.

Melmed C et al: Masticatory muscle myositis: pathogenesis, diagnosis, and treatment, *Compend Contin Educ Pract Vet* 26:590, 2004.

Nanai B et al: Life threatening complication associated with anesthesia in a dog with masticatory muscle myositis, *Vet Surg* 38:645, 2009.

Neravanda D et al: Lymphoma-associated polymyositis in dogs, *J Vet Intern Med* 23:1293, 2009.

Platt SR: Neuromuscular complications in endocrine and metabolic disorders, *Vet Clin North Am Small Anim Pract* 32:125, 2002.

Podell M: Inflammatory myopathies, *Vet Clin North Am Small Anim Pract* 32:147, 2002.

Shelton GD, Engvall E: Muscular dystrophies and other inherited myopathies, *Vet Clin North Am Small Anim Pract* 32:103, 2002.

Sykes JE et al: Severe myositis associated with *Sarcocystis* spp. infection in 2 dogs, *J Vet Intern Med* 25:1277, 2011.

Warman S et al: Dilatation of the right atrium in a dog with polymyositis and myocarditis, *J Small Anim Pract* 49:302, 2008.

CHAPTER 241

Vascular Disease of the Central Nervous System

LAURENT S. GAROSI, *Higham Gobion, England*
SIMON R. PLATT, *Athens, Georgia*

There has been a good deal of confusion in the veterinary literature regarding the terms *cerebrovascular disease, cerebrovascular accident,* and *stroke. Cerebrovascular disease* refers to any abnormality of the brain caused by a pathologic process compromising the blood supply. Pathologic processes that may result in cerebrovascular disease include occlusion of the lumen by a thrombus or embolus, rupture of a blood vessel wall, a lesion or altered permeability of the vessel wall, and increased viscosity or other changes in the quality of the blood. This chapter considers vascular disorders of the brain (stroke) and of the spinal cord (ischemic myelopathy).

Cerebrovascular Accident (or Stroke)

Stroke or cerebrovascular accident (CVA) is the most common clinical presentation of cerebrovascular disease and is defined as a sudden onset of nonprogressive focal brain signs secondary to cerebrovascular disease. By convention these signs must persist for longer than 24 hours to qualify for the diagnosis of stroke, which usually is associated with permanent damage to the brain. If the clinical signs resolve within 24 hours, the episode is called a *transient ischemic attack.* From a pathologic point of view, a CVA falls into one of two broad categories: (1) ischemia with or without infarction secondary to obstructed blood vessels, and (2) hemorrhage caused by rupture of the blood vessel wall.

Ischemic Stroke

With limited stores the brain relies on a permanent supply of glucose and oxygen to maintain ionic pump function (see Chapter 228). When perfusion pressure falls to critical levels, ischemia develops, progressing to infarction if hypoperfusion persists long enough. An infarct is an area of compromised or necrotic brain parenchyma caused by a focal occlusion of one or more blood vessels. It may be caused either by vascular obstruction that develops within the affected vessels (thrombosis) or by obstruction by material that originates from another vascular bed and travels to the brain (thromboembolism).

Depending on the size of vessel involved, infarcts can be the consequence of small-vessel disease (e.g., disease of a superficial or deep perforating artery), which gives rise to a lacunar infarct, or large-vessel disease (disease of a major artery of the brain or its main branches), which gives rise to a territorial infarct. Two distinct regions can be distinguished in ischemic stroke: the core, in which ischemia is severe and infarction develops rapidly; and the penumbra, which surrounds the core and demonstrates a less severe reduction of cerebral blood flow (CBF), so that longer durations of ischemic stress can be tolerated. The relative volume of pathologic effects within these two regions changes as the infarct evolves. The factors favoring evolution of the penumbra to irreversible brain injury are multiple and complex. The time window after which the penumbra is no longer viable depends on the degree of reduction in blood flow, the region of the brain involved, and the individual. In the penumbra neurons are still viable but at risk of becoming irreversibly injured. Penumbra tissue has the potential for recovery and therefore is the target of interventional therapy in acute ischemic stroke.

Ischemic strokes have been reported infrequently in veterinary publications compared with the human medical literature. Most reports have been based on postmortem results in dogs that either died or were euthanized as a result of the severity of the ischemic stroke or the suspected underlying cause of the stroke. This retrospective reporting may affect the prevalence and type of underlying causes identified in canine CVA because only the most severe cases are likely to be reported. In a similar vein, dogs in which infarction occurred secondary to a disease with a poor prognosis also would die or be euthanized.

Suspected underlying causes identified in histopathologically confirmed cases included septic thromboemboli, atherosclerosis associated with primary hypothyroidism and with hypertriglyceridemia in miniature schnauzers, aberrant parasitic migration (*Cuterebra* spp.) or parasitic emboli (*Dirofilaria immitis*), embolic metastatic tumor cells, intravascular lymphoma, embolism with an aortic or cardiac source, and fibrocartilaginous embolism. In our study (Garosi, 2005) using magnetic resonance imaging (MRI), a concurrent medical condition was detected in just over 50% of dogs affected by brain infarcts. Hypertension was documented in 30% of dogs. In these dogs chronic kidney disease and hyperadrenocorticism were the most commonly suspected underlying causes of the hypertension. No underlying cause could be identified antemortem in nearly half of the dogs. An infarct of unknown origin is called *cryptogenic.* No age, sex, or breed predisposition was identified. However, cavalier King Charles spaniels and greyhounds appeared overrepresented.

Reports of ischemic strokes in cats are limited. A concurrent medical condition is found more frequently in cats than in dogs. Concurrent conditions identified include *Cuterebra* parasitic migration, heartworm migration, intracranial telangiectasia, cardiovascular disease, hyperthyroidism, liver disease, and neoplasia elsewhere in the body.

Hemorrhagic Stroke

In hemorrhagic stroke blood leaks from the vessel directly into the brain, forming a hematoma within the brain parenchyma, or into the subarachnoid space. The mass of clotted blood causes physical disruption of the tissue and pressure on the surrounding brain. This alters central nervous system volume-pressure relationships with the possibility of increasing intracranial pressure (ICP) and decreasing CBF. In contrast to the high incidence observed in humans, intracerebral hemorrhage resulting from spontaneous rupture of vessels is considered rare in dogs. Secondary hemorrhage in dogs has been associated with rupture of congenital vascular abnormalities, primary and secondary brain tumors, inflammatory disease of the arteries and veins, intravascular lymphoma, brain infarction (hemorrhagic infarction), or impaired coagulation. Nontraumatic subarachnoid hemorrhage has been reported in dogs but remains very rare. This is in contrast to human patients, in whom aneurysmal rupture of blood vessels is the most common underlying cause of hemorrhagic stroke. Intraparenchymal hemorrhage in cats has been associated with primary or secondary hypertension, intracranial neoplasia, cerebral amyloid angiopathy, and feline infectious peritonitis.

Clinical Presentation of Stroke

In all forms of stroke the denominative feature is the temporal profile of neurologic events. The abruptness with which the neurologic deficits develop is highly suggestive that the disorder is vascular. This is followed by an arrest and then regression of the neurologic deficit in all except fatal strokes. Worsening of edema (associated with the secondary injury phenomenon) can result in progression of neurologic signs for a short period of 24 to 72 hours. Intracranial hemorrhage can be an exception to this description, presenting with a more progressive onset over a very short period of time. Clinical signs usually regress after 24 to 72 hours; this is attributable to diminution of the mass effect caused by hemorrhage with subsequent reorganization or to edema resorption. Neurologic deficits usually refer to a focal anatomic diagnosis and depend on the neurolocalization of the vascular insult (telencephalon, thalamus, midbrain, pons, medulla, cerebellum). Infarction of an individual brain region is associated with specific clinical signs that reflect the loss of function of that specific region. With hemorrhagic stroke the total clinical picture is different because the hemorrhage usually involves the territory of more than one artery, and pressure effects cause secondary signs.

Neurologic signs are related largely to increasing ICP, which gives rise to nonspecific signs of forebrain or brainstem disease. Fundus examination is important and may reveal findings such as tortuous vessels (suggestive of systemic hypertension), hemorrhage (suggestive of coagulopathy or systemic hypertension), or papilledema (suggestive of elevated ICP).

Imaging studies of the brain (computed tomography [CT], conventional and functional MRI) are necessary to confirm the suspicion of stroke, define the vascular territory involved and the extent of the lesion, and distinguish between ischemic and hemorrhagic stroke (Figure 241-1). Imaging studies also are necessary to rule out other causes of neurologic deficit such as tumor, head trauma, and encephalitis. (See References and Suggested Reading for more details.)

Ancillary diagnostic tests in ischemic stroke should focus on evaluating the animal for systemic hypertension (and underlying causes; see Chapter 169), endocrine disease (hyperadrenocorticism, hypothyroidism, hyperthyroidism, diabetes mellitus), kidney disease (especially protein-losing nephropathy), heart disease (a much greater risk factor in cats with cardiomyopathy), and metastatic disease. In cases of ischemic stroke, D-dimer assays and antithrombin III evaluation should be included routinely in the screening tests to identify thromboembolic disease as a possible cause of ischemic stroke. A D-dimer assay is considered to be a more useful test for detecting thromboembolic disease in dogs than traditional tests currently in use (platelet count and clotting times). In cases of hemorrhagic stroke, diagnostic tests should be targeted at screening the animal for a coagulation disorder (and underlying causes), hypertension (and underlying causes), and metastatic disease (particularly hemangiosarcoma).

Treatment and Prognosis of Stroke

Once the diagnosis of a stroke has been made, any potential underlying disease should be identified and treated accordingly. Generally treatment of these patients aims to provide supportive care, maintain adequate tissue oxygenation, and manage neurologic and nonneurologic complications. Nursing management of a recumbent dog is vital to the success of more specific therapies. Such management includes prevention of decubital ulceration, aspiration pneumonia, and urine scald, in addition to physical therapy and provision of enteral nutrition. More specific therapies are aimed at preventing further neurologic deterioration.

Treatment of Ischemic Stroke
Treatment of an ischemic stroke revolves around three principles: monitoring and correcting basic physiologic variables (e.g., oxygen level, fluid balance, blood pressure, body temperature), inhibiting the biochemical and metabolic cascades subsequent to ischemia to prevent neuronal death (the concept of neuroprotection), and restoring or improving CBF by thrombolytic therapy if a thrombus is present. The potentially salvageable portion of the ischemic zone (ischemic penumbra) is the presumed therapeutic target for both thrombolytic and neuroprotective

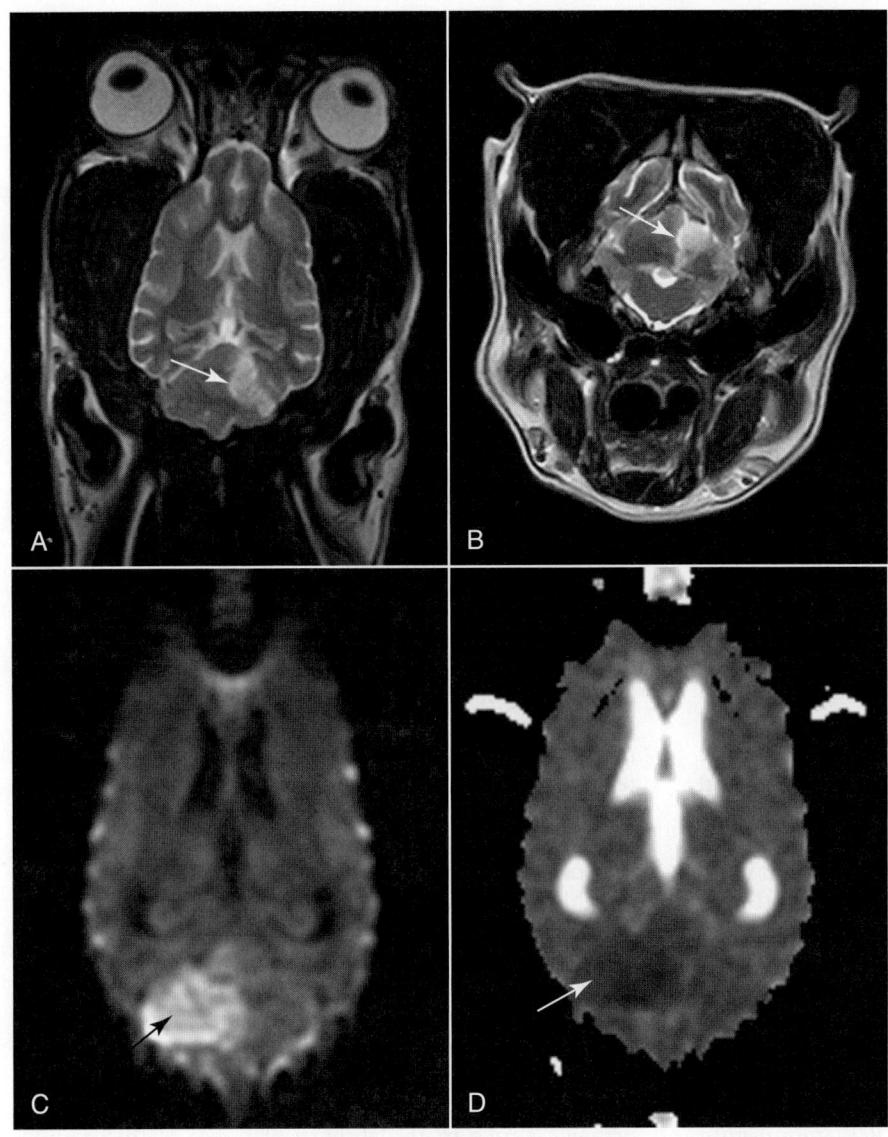

Figure 241-1 A and **B,** Dorsal and transverse T2-weighted magnetic resonance images of the brain showing a cerebellar territorial infarct *(arrow)* in the vascular territory of the rostral cerebellar artery. The sharp demarcation, lack of mass effect, and gray matter involvement are typical of an infarct. **C,** Diffusion-weighted image of a large ischemic cerebellar infarct *(arrow)* in a different dog than shown in **A** and **B. D,** Corresponding apparent diffusion coefficient map of the infarct *(arrow).* The nature of the lesion is confirmed because of the hyperintensity and hypointensity of the lesion, respectively. (**A** and **B** courtesy Dr. Cristian Falzone.)

stroke therapy. The time period during which injury may be reversible is called the *therapeutic window.* It is estimated that this "window of opportunity" is *approximately 6 hours* before irreversible neurologic damage occurs. Fortunately, the vast majority of ischemic stroke patients have no major difficulty maintaining the airway, breathing efforts, or circulatory competence early in the clinical course.

There is some controversy surrounding the management of hypertension in the setting of an ongoing acute ischemic stroke. Although hypertension is a potential risk factor for a CVA, it also can develop as a physiologic response to a stroke to ensure adequate cerebral perfusion pressure (CPP) in the penumbra of the infarct. Elevated blood pressure can persist for up to 72 hours after the onset of injury. Maintenance of systemic arterial blood pressure within the physiologic range is essential, and aggressive lowering of blood pressure should be avoided during the acute stages unless the patient is at a high risk of end-stage organ damage (systolic blood pressure remains >180 mm Hg). In such cases hypertension often can be controlled with an angiotensin-converting enzyme inhibitor such as enalapril (0.25 to 0.5 mg/kg twice daily PO) or benazepril (0.25 to 0.5 mg/kg twice daily PO) with or without a calcium channel blocker such as amlodipine (0.1 to 0.25 mg/kg once daily PO). Amlodipine is more effective in severe hypertension.

There is no evidence that glucocorticoid treatment provides any beneficial neuroprotection in stroke. Not only is there lack of proven benefit in veterinary stroke patients, the use of glucocorticoids may increase the risk of gastrointestinal complications and infection. Treatment strategies considered for ischemic stroke in humans that use other neuroprotective agents (*N*-methyl-d-aspartate antagonists, calcium channel blockers, sodium channel modulators) or antiplatelet and thrombolytic therapy remain to be evaluated clinically in dogs. Although these neuroprotective agents have resulted in a dramatic decrease in the size of stroke lesion in experimental animal models, they either have failed to prove their efficacy in clinical trials or are awaiting further investigation.

At the time of this writing, there are no definitive data in humans or animals to confirm a significant improvement in clinical outcome in patients with acute ischemic stroke treated with unfractionated heparin as anticoagulant therapy. Despite conflicting results regarding the efficacy of intravenous recombinant tissue plasminogen activator, it sometimes is used in human ischemic stroke patients if it can be given within the first 3 hours. This critical time window makes the use of thrombolytic treatment largely unrealistic in veterinary practice. Furthermore, this type of treatment carries a significant risk of intracranial hemorrhage following treatment. Antiplatelet therapy with low-dose aspirin (0.5 mg/kg once daily PO) or clopidogrel (2 to 4 mg/kg once daily PO) can be used prophylactically to prevent clot formation when a cardiac embolic source has been proven.

Treatment of Hemorrhagic Stroke

The medical management of dogs with intracranial hemorrhage commonly includes stabilization of the patient's condition (airway protection, monitoring and correction of vital signs); assessment and monitoring of neurologic status; determination and treatment of potential underlying causes of the hemorrhage; and assessment of the need for specific treatment measures, including management of increased ICP. The risk of neurologic deterioration and cardiovascular instability is highest during the first 24 hours after the onset of an intracranial hemorrhage as the space-occupying lesion slowly expands and cerebral vasogenic edema develops. Therefore careful monitoring, including assessment of vital parameters (e.g., oxygen levels, fluid balance, blood pressure, body temperature) and neurologic status, is essential during this initial period.

Unfortunately, clinical signs of raised ICP often are delayed, inconsistent, and nonspecific. The size of an intracranial hematoma can be difficult to estimate from the neurologic examination alone. ICP monitoring systems are used frequently in human hospitals, but these systems are largely unavailable in veterinary hospitals. As a hematoma develops initially, ICP may be maintained at a constant value as a result of a system of compensation. Within the closed space of the skull a change in the volume of one intracranial constituent (brain tissue, arterial blood, venous blood, or cerebrospinal fluid [CSF]) is balanced by a compensatory change in another incompressible constituent. This is the Monroe-Kellie doctrine, which explains why some animals with large intracranial bleeds develop substantial increases in ICP at the time of herniation. The exhaustion of the compensating mechanisms for an intracranial space–occupying lesion implies that any further increase in the volume of the hematoma will produce a massive rise in ICP, and clinically this can be associated with herniation.

Owing to mechanical autoregulation, CBF remains constant, even though CPP may vary between 40 and 120 mm Hg. The normal autoregulation of CBF may be impaired following a CVA, so that blood flow to damaged regions becomes directly dependent on systemic blood pressure. In such cases the animal may be unable to compensate for reductions in mean arterial blood pressure, which causes decreased CPP in the presence of increased ICP. This possibility emphasizes the importance of maintaining systemic blood pressure. In these circumstances systemic hypotension can result in inadequate perfusion of the brain, which leads to cerebral ischemic and secondary neuronal injury.

If decreased CPP is present, correction of tissue perfusion is an important stabilizing therapy in patients with hemorrhagic stroke. The primary goal of fluid therapy is rapid restoration of blood pressure, so that CPP is maintained above 70 mm Hg. Hypovolemia should be recognized and treated with volume expansion using artificial colloids or hypertonic saline (7.5%) to achieve rapid restoration of blood volume and pressure while limiting the volume of fluid administered (see Chapters 1 and 2). Central venous pressure monitoring can be useful as an aid in assessing the effectiveness of volume resuscitation, provided cardiac function is otherwise normal. The use of glucose-containing solutions is discouraged since hyperglycemia has been shown to correlate with poor outcome in human stroke patients. For this reason, blood glucose level should be monitored from the time of presentation.

Moderate levels of hypertension should not be treated because systemic hypertension may be secondary to the intense reflex sympathetic response to intracranial hypertension, which is a compensatory mechanism to maintain cerebral perfusion. In ischemic stroke, attempts to lower and normalize the blood pressure should be reserved for animals at high risk of end-stage organ damage (systolic blood pressure that remains >180 mm Hg) or animals with severe ocular manifestations of hypertension such as retinal detachment or intraocular hemorrhage. Treatment recommendations for lowering blood pressure are detailed in the preceding section on treatment of ischemic stroke.

There is no evidence in humans to support the routine use of oxygen supplementation for the treatment of hemorrhagic stroke in the absence of hypoxia. In a rapidly deteriorating animal hyperventilation can be used temporarily to reduce ICP. The aim of hyperventilation is to reduce cerebral blood volume and hence ICP by causing a hypocapnic vasoconstriction. However, excessive hyperventilation can be accompanied by a reduction in global CBF, which may drop below ischemic thresholds; therefore it is not a recommended therapy unless the arterial carbon dioxide pressure can be monitored closely with capnography or arterial blood gas analysis.

Mannitol has been used traditionally to treat intracranial hypertension associated with pathologic conditions such as head trauma, brain tumor, or encephalitis. There is insubstantial evidence to suggest that mannitol exacerbates intracranial hemorrhage; therefore osmotic diuretics are used routinely in the control of ICP in human patients with known intracranial hemorrhage. Mannitol therapy (0.25 to 2.0 g/kg IV over 10 to 20 minutes up to q4-8h) may be initiated to treat suspected elevated ICP secondary to hemorrhagic stroke. The main effect of mannitol is to enhance CBF by reducing blood viscosity. Surgical evacuation of the hematoma can be performed in dogs that have large hematomas (mostly subarachnoid) and a deteriorating neurologic status.

Prognosis

The prognosis for ischemic or hemorrhagic stroke depends overall on the initial severity of the neurologic deficit, the initial response to supportive care, and the severity of the underlying cause if one has been identified. Fortunately, in most cases of ischemic stroke recovery occurs within several weeks with only supportive care. In the authors' retrospective study of 33 dogs with MRI or necropsy evidence of brain infarction (Garosi 2005), there was no association between the region of the brain involved (telencephalon, thalamus-midbrain, cerebellum), the type of infarction (territorial or lacunar), and the outcome. However, dogs with a concurrent medical condition had a significantly shorter survival time than those with no identifiable medical condition. Dogs with a concurrent medical condition also were significantly more likely to show recurrent neurologic signs caused by subsequent infarcts.

Ischemic Myelopathy

Ischemic myelopathy is a vascular disease of the spinal cord most commonly caused by embolization of spinal cord blood vessels, but it also can be due to vessel thrombosis and vascular spasm, which often are secondary to trauma. Sudden reduction of blood flow to an area of the spinal cord causes ischemic necrosis resulting in clinical signs that can be peracute (<6 hours) or acute (6 to 24 hours), with distribution and severity referable to the site and extent of the lesion. Because the emboli most commonly documented to be responsible are fibrocartilaginous, this condition usually is called *fibrocartilaginous embolism* (FCE) or *fibrocartilaginous embolic myelopathy*.

Pathophysiology of Ischemic Myelopathy

Spinal cord arteries are functional end arteries, and their occlusion leads to ischemia of the area which they supply. The arterial blood supply to the lumbar spinal cord is illustrated in Figure 241-2. The most common cause of ischemic necrosis of the spinal cord is embolization of spinal arteries by fibrocartilage. The embolized fibrocartilage has a structure similar to that of the intervertebral disk nucleus pulposus; however, the mechanism of entry of this material into the vasculature is not completely understood. Direct penetration of nucleus pulposus fragments into the spinal cord vessels or into the vertebral vessels often has been proposed; however, arterial walls are naturally very tough and resistant to such damage, and venous damage would result in hemorrhage that has not been described. Other possible causes of the presence of fibrocartilage in vessels are the existence of embryonic remnant vessels within the nucleus pulposus (which is normally avascular in adults) and neovascularization of a degenerated intervertebral disk, either of which would allow entrance of the material into the vasculature.

Ischemic myelopathy also may result from obstruction of the intrinsic spinal blood vessels by material other than fibrocartilage, such as thrombi or bacterial, parasitic, neoplastic, or fat emboli. Preexisting medical conditions associated with CVAs in dogs and cats, including cardiomyopathy, hypothyroidism, hyperthyroidism,

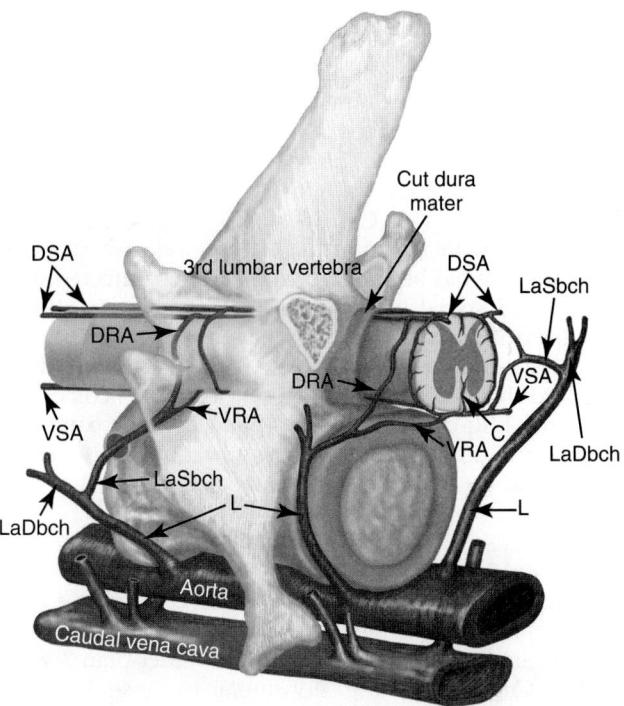

Figure 241-2 Diagrammatic representation of the arterial supply to the lumbar spinal cord. *C,* Central artery; *DRA,* dorsal radicular artery; *DSA,* dorsal spinal artery (paired); *L,* lumbar artery; *LaDbch,* lumbar artery, dorsal branch; *LaSbch,* lumbar artery, spinal branch; *VRA,* ventral radicular artery; *VSA,* ventral spinal artery. (Reproduced with permission from De Risio L, Platt SR: Fibrocartilaginous embolic myelopathy in small animals, *Vet Clin North Am Small Anim Pract* 40[5]:859, 2010.)

hyperadrenocorticism, chronic renal failure, and hypertension, should be considered as potential causes of ischemic myelopathy.

The ischemic injury caused by the arterial obstruction initiates a series of biochemical and metabolic events that result in neuronal and glial cell death. The gray matter, because of its greater metabolic demand, is affected more severely than the white matter.

Clinical Presentation of Ischemic Myelopathy

Ischemic myelopathy has been reported most commonly in large- and giant-breed dogs and only occasionally occurs in small-breed dogs (particularly miniature schnauzers). Approximately 80% of dogs with an antemortem diagnosis or histologic confirmation of ischemic myelopathy suspected to be caused by fibrocartilaginous emboli weigh more than 20 kg. The median age at diagnosis in dogs is 5 to 6 years in most studies and ranges from 2 months to 12 years.

Classically, the disease is characterized by a peracute onset of nonprogressive, nonpainful, often asymmetric spinal cord signs. Up to 80% of dogs are physically active (walking, running, or playing) and up to 50% of dogs exhibit a manifestation of pain (e.g., vocalization) at the time of onset only. Gradual improvement or stabilization of signs usually begins after the first 24 hours, depending on the extent and severity of the ischemic injury.

The degree of neurologic dysfunction resulting from the ischemia depends on its location and the severity of the injury; clinical signs are asymmetric in 53% to 86% of dogs. The most commonly affected spinal cord segments in dogs have been L4 to S3 (44% to 50%), T3 to L3 (27% to 42%), and C6 to T2 (30% to 33%). Commonly, neurologic deficits refer to the affected spinal cord segment (e.g., C1 to C5, C6 to T2, T3 to L3, or L4 to S3). In the acute stages of the disease, a decreased withdrawal reflex has been observed in severely affected dogs with T3-L3 spinal cord ischemia observable on MRI. It has been suggested that this may represent a form of spinal shock in these patients. Notably, most of these dogs exhibit a cutaneous trunci reflex "cutoff" consistent with the MRI-detected lesion. Spinal column palpation of affected dogs within the first few hours after onset can reveal focal mild to moderate discomfort, but this rapidly resolves.

Ischemic Myelopathy in Cats

Ischemic myelopathy seems to be less common in cats. The majority of cats reported with ischemic myelopathy have been domestic shorthairs and are older than 7 years of age. Clinical signs are very similar to those described in dogs; however, clinical deterioration has been observed for up to 5 days in a few cats with histologically confirmed lesions. Additionally, there rarely is a history of activity at the onset of disease, and spinal pain has not been reported. Severe ischemic lesions of the cord may be seen in cats with a history of trauma in the absence of evident structural changes in the spinal column. It is suspected that these lesions may relate to acute vasospasm of abdominal arteries supplying the spinal cord. In the absence of trauma, the most commonly affected spinal cord segments are C6 to T2, but any spinal cord segment can be involved.

Fibrocartilaginous Embolic Myelopathy versus Acute Disk Disease

In the differential diagnosis of FCE, another disorder that results in peracute onset of nonprogressive and often asymmetric spinal cord dysfunction must be considered—namely, *acute noncompressive nucleus pulposus extrusion* or *traumatic intervertebral disk extrusion*. In this disorder, nondegenerate nucleus pulposus extrusion causes spinal cord contusion with minimal or no spinal cord compression. Pain on palpation of the spinal column has been reported in up to 57% of dogs with acute noncompressive nucleus pulposus extrusion and usually persists for longer than 24 hours, which helps to differentiate this disease from FCE. Otherwise, accurate MRI interpretation is necessary to discriminate a nucleus extrusion from a suspected FCE. The MRI features of acute noncompressive nucleus pulposus extrusion include the presence of a focal intramedullary hyperintensity overlying a narrowed intervertebral disk and reduced volume and signal intensity of the nucleus pulposus on T2-weighted images. Extraneous material or signal change within the epidural space dorsal to the affected disk with absent or minimal spinal cord compression is noted in these cases.

Diagnosis of Ischemic Myelopathy

The definitive diagnosis of ischemic myelopathy, and specifically of FCE, requires histologic examination of the spinal cord. The clinical diagnosis is based on the typical clinical presentation and exclusion of other causes of peracute-acute focal myelopathy (by means of diagnostic imaging and CSF analysis). Spinal imaging is necessary to rule out other causes of spinal cord dysfunction and to suggest ischemic myelopathy.

Myelography

Myelography can be important for the exclusion of other causes of peracute-acute focal myelopathies, especially those that cause spinal cord compression, such as intervertebral disk extrusion. Myelographic findings can be normal or can reveal an intramedullary pattern suggestive of focal spinal cord swelling in the acute stage of FCE. This has been observed in 26% to 47% of dogs with FCE. Focal myelitis, intramedullary neoplasia, intraparenchymal hemorrhage, and acute noncompressive nucleus pulposus extrusion also can result in an intramedullary myelographic pattern, however.

Computed Tomography

CT also can help to rule out other causes of peracute-acute myelopathy. CT-myelography may reveal an intramedullary pattern in the acute stage of an ischemic myelopathy.

Magnetic Resonance Imaging

MRI is the diagnostic imaging modality of choice for the antemortem diagnosis of ischemic myelopathy. In addition to excluding other causes, it allows visualization of intraparenchymal signal intensity changes suggestive of ischemic infarction. A focal, relatively sharply demarcated, and often asymmetric lesion predominantly involving the gray matter is seen most commonly in affected cases. The lesion often is hyperintense to normal spinal cord gray matter on T2-weighted images and isointense or hypointense to normal spinal cord gray matter on T1-weighted images (Figure 241-3). However, MRI scans obtained within the first 24 to 72 hours may appear normal, and repeated MRI may be necessary. Various degrees of lesion enhancement following contrast administration occasionally can be seen within a week of onset of the myelopathy. The severity of neurologic dysfunction at the time of initial examination has been associated with the extent of the ischemic lesions affecting the spinal cord on MRI; dogs that are ambulatory on presentation are more likely to have normal MRI findings than nonambulatory dogs.

As with CVAs, the use of diffusion-weighted MRI increases the sensitivity and specificity for diagnosis of spinal cord infarction in the early stage of the disorder. Diffusion-weighted MRI has shown increasing intramedullary hyperintensity from 1 to 24 hours after embolization in experimental dogs with spinal cord infarction.

Cerebrospinal Fluid Analysis

CSF abnormalities (mainly an elevated protein concentration) have been reported in up to 46% of dogs with a

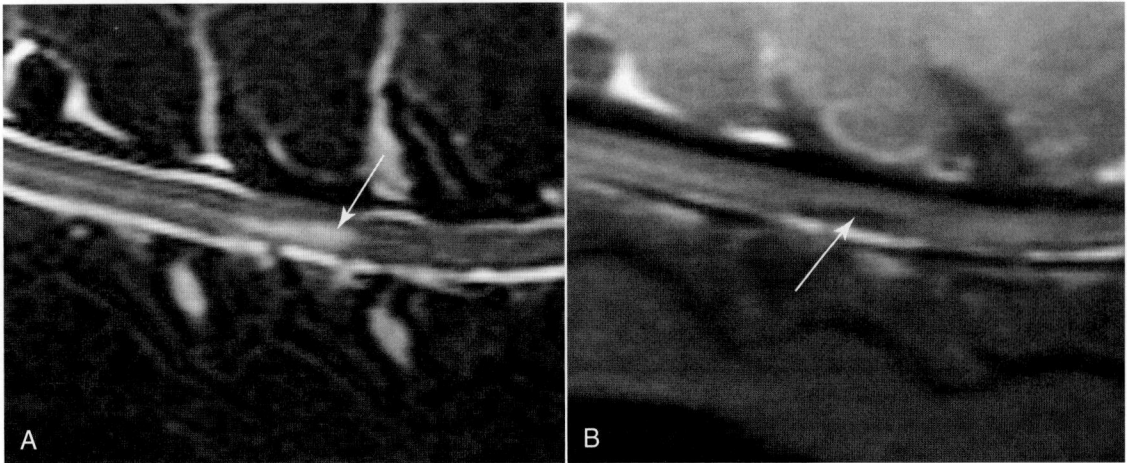

Figure 241-3 Sagittal T2-weighted **(A)** and T1-weighted/FLAIR (fluid-attenuated inversion recovery) **(B)** magnetic resonance images of the spinal cord demonstrating a well-defined hyperintensity and hypointensity, respectively *(arrows)*, in the parenchyma over the body of the sixth cervical vertebra.

histologic diagnosis of FCE and in up to 75% of dogs with an antemortem diagnosis of FCE. Other documented abnormalities include xanthochromia and mild to moderate pleocytosis (7 to 84 white blood cells/μl).

Histologic Examination

Fibrocartilaginous material in spinal vessels within or near an area of focal myelomalacia is evident when ischemic myelopathy is due to FCE. The distribution of the lesion frequently is asymmetric and the gray matter generally is more severely affected than the white matter, with lesion margins being well delineated from normal tissue. Infarcted areas usually are ischemic but sometimes may be accompanied by hemorrhage.

Treatment of Ischemic Myelopathy

Treatment of ischemic myelopathy can be similar to that described for patients with ischemic stroke. At this time there are no commercial pharmacologic therapies that have been proven to improve the outcome for spinal cord ischemia. Nursing care and physical therapy play an essential role in the management of patients, promoting recovery and helping prevent complications. Physical therapy can stimulate neuronal plasticity and therefore improve functional recovery; in addition, it can minimize disuse- and immobilization-related complications such as muscle atrophy and joint contractures. Nursing care includes provision of adequate bedding and regular patient turning, the prevention of decubital ulcers and urine scalding, bladder and bowel management, care of the respiratory system, and adequate nutrition.

Prognosis of Ischemic Myelopathy

The prognosis for recovery in patients with ischemic myelopathy depends on the severity and extent of the ischemic injury. Rates of recovery to the level of a functional pet with fecal and urinary continence vary from 58% to 84%. Loss of nociception, lower motor neuron

signs, severe neurologic signs at the time of initial examination, and lack of improvement within the first 14 days are considered negative prognostic indicators for an acceptable recovery. The extent of the ischemic intraparenchymal lesion on MRI also is associated with patient outcome. Dogs with a ratio of lesion length to vertebral length (C6 for cervical lesions and L2 for thoracolumbar lesions) of more than 2.0 or a percent cross-sectional lesion area of 67% or more (based on the cross-sectional area of the largest intramedullary hyperintensity on a transverse T2-weighted image as a percentage of the area of the spinal cord at the same level) are significantly more likely to have an unsuccessful outcome than dogs with lower values of these variables. However, the presence of CSF abnormalities (increased protein concentration with or without pleocytosis) does not seem to show a consistent association with patient prognosis.

Time intervals between the onset of neurologic signs and the recovery of voluntary motor activity, unassisted ambulation, and maximal recovery have been reported as 6 days (range, 2.5 to 15 days), 11 days (range, 4 to 136 days), and 3.75 months (range, 1 to 12 months), respectively.

References and Suggested Reading

Cerebrovascular Disease

Garosi LS et al: Results of diagnostic investigations and long-term outcome of 33 dogs with brain infarction (2000-2004), *J Vet Intern Med* 19:725, 2005.

Garosi LS et al: Clinical and topographical magnetic resonance characteristics of suspected brain infarctions in 40 dogs, *J Vet Intern Med* 20:311, 2006.

Garosi LS, McConnell JF: Brain infarct in dog and human: a comparative review, *J Small Anim Pract* 46:521, 2005.

Hillock SM et al: Vascular encephalopathies in dogs: diagnosis, treatment, and prognosis, *Compend Contin Educ Pract Vet* 28:208, 2006.

McConnell JF, Garosi LS, Platt SR: MRI findings of presumed cerebellar cerebrovascular accident in twelve dogs, *Vet Radiol Ultrasound* 46:1, 2005.

Platt SR, Garosi LS: Canine cerebrovascular disease: do dogs have strokes? *J Am Anim Hosp Assoc* 39:337, 2003.

Ischemic Myelopathy

Abramson CJ et al: Magnetic resonance imaging appearance of suspected ischemic myelopathy in dogs, *Vet Radiol Ultrasound* 46:225, 2005.

Cauzinille L, Kornegay JN: Fibrocartilaginous embolism of the spinal cord in dogs: review of 36 histologically confirmed cases and retrospective study of 26 suspected cases, *J Vet Intern Med* 10:241, 1996.

De Risio L et al: Magnetic resonance imaging findings and clinical associations in 52 dogs with suspected ischemic myelopathy, *J Vet Intern Med* 21:1290, 2007.

De Risio L et al: Association of clinical and magnetic resonance imaging findings with outcome in 50 dogs with suspected ischemic myelopathy, *J Am Vet Med Assoc* 233:129, 2008.

De Risio L et al: Association of clinical and magnetic resonance imaging findings with outcome in 42 dogs with presumptive acute non-compressive nucleus pulposus extrusion, *J Am Vet Med Assoc* 234:495, 2009.

Gandini G et al: Fibrocartilaginous embolism in 75 dogs: clinical findings and factors influencing the recovery rate, *J Small Anim Pract* 44:76, 2003.

Smith PM, Jeffery ND: Spinal shock—comparative aspects and clinical relevance, *J Vet Intern Med* 19:788, 2005.

SECTION XII

Ophthalmologic Diseases

Chapter 242: Pearls of the Ophthalmic Examination   1128
Chapter 243: Evaluation of Blindness   1134
Chapter 244: Canine Conjunctivitis   1138
Chapter 245: Tear Film Disorders in Dogs   1143
Chapter 246: Corneal Ulcers   1148
Chapter 247: Canine Nonulcerative Corneal Disease   1152
Chapter 248: Feline Corneal Disease   1156
Chapter 249: Canine Uveitis   1162
Chapter 250: Feline Uveitis   1166
Chapter 251: Canine Glaucoma   1170
Chapter 252: Feline Glaucoma   1177
Chapter 253: Disorders of the Lens   1181
Chapter 254: Canine Retinopathies   1188
Chapter 255: Feline Retinopathies   1193
Chapter 256: Orbital Disease   1197
Chapter 257: Canine Ocular Neoplasia   1201
Chapter 258: Feline Ocular Neoplasia   1207

The following web chapters can be found on the companion website at www.currentveterinarytherapy.com

Web Chapter 75: Diseases of the Eyelids and Periocular Skin
Web Chapter 76: Canine Retinal Detachment
Web Chapter 77: Epiphora
Web Chapter 78: Ocular Emergencies
Web Chapter 79: Tear Film Disorders of Cats
Web Chapter 80: Anisocoria and Abnormalities of the Pupillary Light Reflex: The Neuro-ophthalmic Examination

CHAPTER 242

Pearls of the Ophthalmic Examination

DAVID J. MAGGS, *Davis, California*

Although signalment and historical data often provide essential clues to ocular diagnoses, ready visualization of almost all parts of the eye means that nothing can replace a complete examination. Fortunately a thorough ophthalmic examination is performed with just five requirements, five skills, and minimal equipment.

There are five essential requirements for a thorough ophthalmic examination:

1. Patient and veterinarian at eye level with each other
2. Dim ambient light
3. A bright and focal light source
4. A source of magnification
5. An orderly and complete approach

To minimize the extent to which the eyelids and orbital structures obscure the ocular structures, the patient should always be placed at eye level with the examining veterinarian. This is usually achieved simply by placing the patient on the examination table, which also limits patient movement. Having an assistant rather than the owner restrain the pet further reduces movement and is especially important when a detailed examination with magnification is performed. Since many structures within the normal eye are transparent, they are best examined in a darkened room using a very focal light source. This combination maximizes reflections, which are useful for examining ocular surfaces. Dim ambient light also facilitates examination of the darker interior structures of the globe. Many ocular abnormalities are small and will be missed without a source of magnification and a bright light source. This combination can best be achieved in practice by using a magnifying head loupe (e.g., Optivisor) and Finnoff (Welch Allyn) transilluminator. A readily available alternative is the otoscope used without the plastic cone. This provides a focal light source and approximately 2× to 3× magnification, but does not permit the direction of illumination and examination to be varied independently of one another. Slit-lamp biomicroscopes are used by ophthalmologists and some general practitioners and maximize the combination of magnification and a focal light source. By focusing the light to a narrow slit, an optical section provides microscopic detail of transparent ocular media such as the tear film, cornea, aqueous, lens, vitreous, and (to a lesser extent) conjunctiva.

The ophthalmic examination should be carried out in a repeatable and sequential manner to ensure that nothing is overlooked. A prepared examination sheet reminds the practitioner to perform all necessary tests in the correct sequence and permits lesions to be drawn. The examination begins by observing the patient from a distance for behavioral evidence of vision loss. The patient's head and periocular tissues should then be more closely examined for facial symmetry, globe position and movement, periocular discharge, and overt ocular abnormalities. Brief but complete testing of the cranial nerves involved in normal ocular function follows. This should include tests of the menace response, palpebral reflex, direct and consensual pupillary light reflexes, and dazzle reflex. More detailed examination of each eye is then performed. Examining the unaffected eye before the affected eye in animals with unilateral disease ensures that the normal eye is not forgotten and provides information on each patient's normal ocular appearance.

Mastering the following five skills ensures that the essential findings from the anterior and posterior segments of the eye are not missed:

1. Retroillumination
2. Transillumination (or focal illumination)
3. Tonometry (measurement of intraocular pressure [IOP])
4. Assessment of aqueous flare
5. Fundic examination

Retroillumination is a simple but extremely useful technique for assessment of pupils and all parts of the transparent ocular media (tear film, cornea, aqueous, lens, and vitreous). A focal light source such as a Finnoff transilluminator is held close to the examiner's eye and directed over the bridge of the patient's nose from at least arm's length (Figure 242-1, *A*). Alternatively, the direct ophthalmoscope can be held against the examiner's eye (as for the fundic examination) but about arm's length from the patient. Either technique elicits the fundic reflection, which is usually gold or green in tapetal animals or red in nontapetal individuals (Figure 242-1, *B*). Because the examination is done at arm's length, each eye can be illuminated equally, and the fundic reflex can be used to assess and compare equality of pupil size and shape. In addition, opacities in any of the clear ocular media (e.g., corneal blood vessels, cataracts, vitreous debris) obstruct the fundic reflection and are noted as black "shadows" against the fundic reflection. These opacities should be noted for subsequent and more detailed examination, with retroillumination repeated from close to the patient following pupil dilation. They should also be examined using transillumination and a source of magnification.

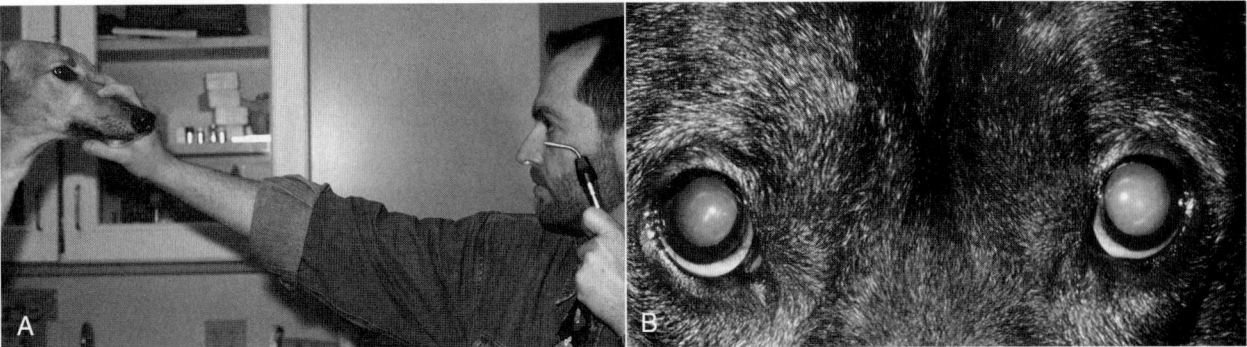

Figure 242-1 Retroillumination. **A,** A Finnoff transilluminator is held close to the examiner's eye and directed over the bridge of the patient's nose from at least arm's length. The reflection from the animal's fundus is used to judge pupil size and the clarity of the ocular media. **B,** This patient has nuclear sclerosis visible as a subtle ring inside the pupil. (From Maggs DJ et al: *Slater's fundamentals of veterinary ophthalmology,* ed 5, 2013, St Louis, Saunders.)

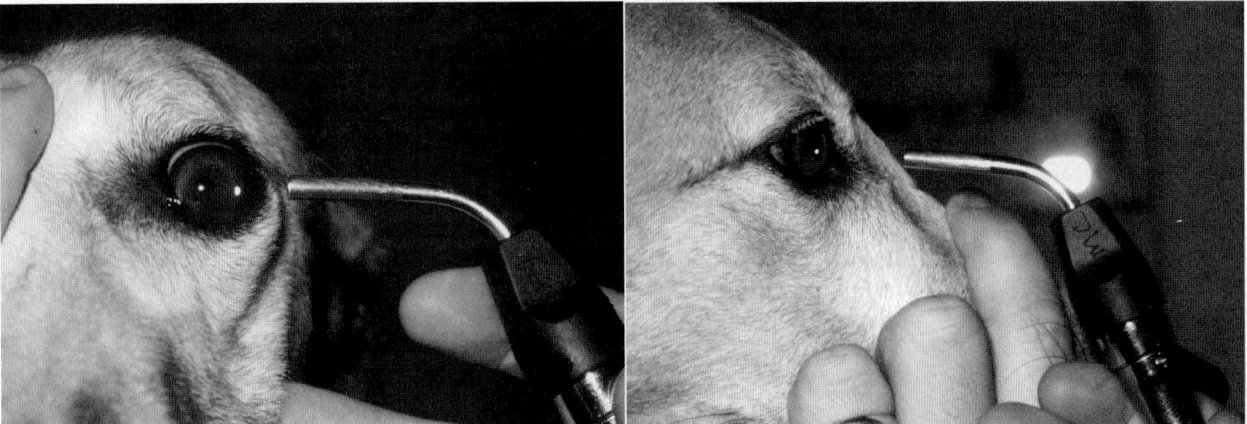

Figure 242-2 Transillumination. A focal light source is directed at the eye from many angles while the examiner simultaneously varies the viewing angle. Varying the viewing and lighting angles relative to each other permits the examiner to use parallax, reflections, perspective, and shadows to gain valuable information regarding lesion depth.

Retroillumination is particularly useful for differentiating nuclear sclerosis from cataract.

Transillumination (sometimes called *focal illumination*) is then used to sequentially examine all ocular structures in front of and including the lens (the "anterior segment"). A focal light source should be directed at the eye from many angles while the examiner simultaneously varies the viewing angle (Figure 242-2). Varying the viewing and lighting angles relative to each other permits the examiner to use parallax, reflections, perspective, and shadows to gain valuable information regarding lesion depth. This technique is particularly useful for examining the anterior chamber since changes within this chamber can be more easily differentiated from corneal, iridal, or lenticular changes when viewed transversely. In cats the corneal curvature and anterior chamber depth are so great that limited visualization of the iridocorneal angle is also possible.

The importance of a sequential anterior segment examination cannot be overstated. An obvious method is to begin at the front and progress to the back of the eye while simultaneously moving from peripheral to axial. This ensures that the eyelids (including periocular skin, eyelid margin, and cilia), conjunctiva (third eyelid, bulbar, and palpebral conjunctival surfaces, as well as nasolacrimal puncta), sclera, cornea (including the limbus and tear film), anterior chamber, iris, pupil, and lens are examined completely. Anterior segment examination should be initiated before dilation so that the iris face is easily examined; however, complete examination of the lens requires full dilation. The complete anterior segment should be examined using transillumination and a source of magnification such as the Optivisor, the otoscope head, or a slit-lamp biomicroscope. Following pupil dilation, retroillumination can be repeated from close to the patient and with a source of magnification so that lesions in the clear ocular media can be both backlit and magnified without the pupil constricting. The otoscope head is particularly useful for this because the examiner can alter the viewing angle until the lesion is either backlit by the tapetal reflection dorsally or viewed against the dull nontapetal area of the fundus ventrally while illuminated from in front.

In both cases the otoscope head is moved in or out from the eye until the lesion is in crisp focus and under full magnification against the chosen background.

Tonometry is the estimation of IOP and is essential for differentiating between the two major vision-threatening conditions in which red eye is the hallmark feature: uveitis and glaucoma (see Chapters 251 and 252). Digital tonometry, in which the IOP is crudely assessed by compressing the globe against the orbital rim, is completely unreliable. The Schiøtz tonometer is reliable but awkward to use and requires conversion tables to convert the scale reading to the standard unit of IOP (millimeters of mercury). The availability of easily used and reasonably priced tonometers such as the Tono-Pen and TonoVet has made estimation of IOP easier in all species, particularly cats. Unlike the Schiøtz tonometer, the Tono-Pen and TonoVet estimate IOP directly and do not require any conversion. They can also be held horizontally and therefore allow recordings to be performed with the patient's head held in a normal, relaxed position. Finally, they each have a small probe that permits measurement of IOP in even the smallest feline and pediatric canine eyes.

The Tono-Pen comes with an excellent instructional video and manual; however, the following tips may help the veterinarian achieve optimal results. The tonometer should be periodically calibrated according to the manufacturer's directions. A drop of topical anesthetic is applied to the cornea. A disposable cover is placed over the Tono-Pen tip, and the pen is turned on with firm, somewhat protracted pressure on the large black button about one third down the shaft. Correct patient restraint is essential. The patient should be lightly restrained so as to not artificially raise IOP. In particular, direct pressure on the jugular veins by the holder or by a collar should be avoided. Similarly, no pressure should be exerted on the globe itself via the eyelids. This is best achieved by having an assistant (not the owner) restrain the patient's head, holding the angle of the mandible and the occiput. The Tono-Pen is then held in the dominant hand, and the patient's eyelids are gently parted using the nondominant hand so that pressure is applied to the underlying orbital rim, not the globe. The hand holding the Tono-Pen should then be rested onto the hand holding the eyelids or onto the patient's head itself. Very small, rapid movements of the Tono-Pen away from and back toward the cornea such that the cornea is very lightly "blotted" with the Tono-Pen tip enhance the reliability and reproducibility of the readings while reducing the number of readings necessary. Particular attention should be paid to the "approach angle" of the Tono-Pen tip to the cornea. The flat surface of the tip should be exactly parallel to the corneal surface. This is best achieved by viewing the interface between the cornea and the tip from the side. Said another way, the Tono-Pen itself should approach the globe as close to perpendicular to the corneal surface as possible. Therefore, because of corneal curvature, the approach angle must be changed dramatically if any area other than the central cornea is used or if the patient redirects its gaze from straight ahead.

Each time the cornea is appropriately "blotted" with the probe, an electronic tone advises the operator that a reading has been obtained. When a suitable number of readings have been obtained, a longer tone of a different pitch sounds, and no further readings can be obtained without restarting the Tono-Pen using the black button. The number of readings required to achieve an average varies, depending on how disparate the readings are from each other and from the normal physiologic range. A small digital screen displays the IOP in mm Hg and provides an estimate of the "reliability" (coefficient of variance) of the result. This appears as a small bar located above one of four percentage readings. This bar should be above the 5% mark, or tonometry should be repeated for that eye. Estimates of IOP with the Tono-Pen are highly correlated with manometric pressure; however, this tonometer tends to overestimate pressure at lower IOPs and underestimate IOPs at higher pressures.

The TonoVet tonometer uses the mechanical principle called rebound tonometry to estimate IOP. A small probe is ejected at a fixed distance from the cornea and the motion of the probe is measured as it rebounds from the cornea and returns to the instrument. Since this technique is affected to some degree by ocular surface tension, it must be performed before application of any topical medications, including topical anesthetic, and it is unclear what effect reduced tear film might have on IOP readings obtained from patients with dry eye or other corneal pathologies. Tono-Pen applanation tonometers are probably less susceptible to erroneous readings attributable to these variables than rebound tonometers. The TonoVet has been calibrated for normal dogs, cats, and horses; thus the correct software must be selected before IOP recordings begin. Because of this species-specific calibration in normal animals, the rebound tonometer tends to estimate IOP very close to true pressure measurements as determined with a manometer.

Across large populations, normal canine and feline IOP is reported as approximately 10 to 20 mm Hg (using any tonometer). However, variation is noted between individuals, technique, tonometer, and time of day. Therefore comparison of IOP between right and left eyes is critical to interpretation of results. A good rule of thumb is that IOP should not vary between eyes of the same patient by more than 20%. Because IOP measured by the Schiøtz tonometer, Tono-Pen, and TonoVet can differ, it is important to record which tonometer was used.

Aqueous flare is a pathognomonic sign of uveitis and is the result of breakdown of the blood-aqueous barrier, with subsequent leakage of plasma proteins into the anterior chamber where, with special technique, they can be seen. Aqueous flare is best detected using a very focal, intense light source in a totally darkened room. The passage taken by the beam of light is viewed from an angle. In the normal eye a focal reflection is seen where the light strikes the cornea. The beam is then invisible as it traverses the almost protein- and cell-free aqueous humor in the anterior chamber. Because of the presence of lens proteins, the light beam becomes visible again as a focal reflection on the anterior lens capsule and then as a diffuse beam through the body of the normal lens. If uveitis has allowed leakage of serum proteins into the anterior chamber, these proteins will cause a scattering of the light as it passes through the aqueous humor (Figure 242-3). This is called *aqueous flare* and is seen as a beam

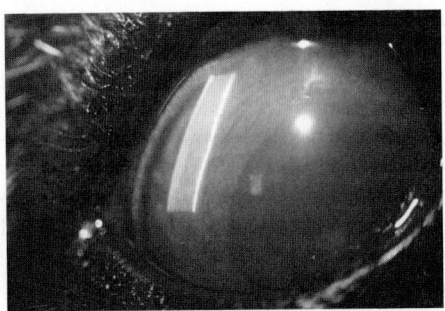

Figure 242-3 Aqueous flare is present in this dog with anterior uveitis. A very focal, intense beam of light is directed across the anterior chamber and viewed transversely with magnification in a totally darkened room. Leakage of serum proteins into the anterior chamber causes scattering of the light as the beam passes through the aqueous humor between the cornea and iris.

of light traversing the anterior chamber and joining the focal reflections on the corneal surface and the anterior lens capsule or iris. A slit lamp provides ideal conditions for detecting aqueous flare; however, the beam produced by the smallest circular aperture on the direct ophthalmoscope, at brightest illumination, in a completely darkened room, held as closely as possible to the cornea, and viewed transversely with some form of magnification also provides excellent results. The slit beam on the direct ophthalmoscope is not as intense as the small circular aperture and does not provide as many "edges" of light along which flare can be most readily appreciated. Aqueous flare is best seen against a black "backdrop," which in the eye is the pupil. Therefore assessment of flare is sometimes easier after complete pupil dilation. Combined assessment of IOP and aqueous flare should be performed whenever glaucoma or uveitis is suspected because of the frequency with which these conditions coexist.

Fundic examination is probably the greatest challenge in the ophthalmic examination. Fortunately, anterior segment abnormalities tend to outnumber fundic abnormalities in general practice. However, fundic examination is critical in the assessment of animals presenting with visual disturbance, pupil abnormalities, anterior uveitis, or systemic disease. Traditionally there have been two methods for viewing the fundus: direct and indirect ophthalmoscopy. Recently Welch Allyn and Keeler both introduced new ophthalmoscopes (the Panoptic and the Wide-Angle Twin Mag, respectively) that combine some of the best features of direct and indirect ophthalmoscopy. Regardless of which method is used, thorough fundic evaluation requires full pupil dilation. This is best achieved by examining the patient at least 15 minutes after topical application of a single drop of tropicamide.

The Direct Ophthalmoscope

The direct ophthalmoscope hangs on the walls of most veterinary examination rooms the world over and yet is not the best method for examining the fundus. It is used by turning the lens power to "0," selecting the largest circle of light that it emits, turning the light to the

minimum brightness that will permit examination but not distress the patient, turning the room lights off or to a dim setting, and resting the brow rest of the ophthalmoscope against the operator's brow. Ideally the operator's right eye should be used for examining the patient's right eye and vice versa, although some operators have trouble using their nondominant eye. While an assistant holds the animal's head steady, the examiner should hold the animal's eyes open and begin viewing at arm's length from the patient and move around until a bright tapetal reflection is obtained (as for retroillumination). The examiner should then slowly approach the animal, while always aiming at the tapetal reflection of the eye to be examined. Good focus in a normal patient should be reached within just a few centimeters of the eye. Therefore it is sometimes useful to extend a finger of the hand holding the ophthalmoscope and rest that finger against the patient's cheek.

Direct ophthalmoscopy provides a highly magnified, upright image of a very small region of the patient's fundus. In compliant human patients this instrument can then be used to slowly and sequentially examine the whole fundus in minute detail. However, in veterinary patients this small field of view frequently means that areas of the fundus, particularly peripherally, are never examined and that one area of the retina cannot be compared readily with another region.

The Indirect Ophthalmoscope

Because of the large field of view achieved with indirect ophthalmoscopy, this is the preferred method for examining the dog or cat fundus. This larger field of view permits the examiner to compare regions of the fundus against each other so that focal areas of subtle pathology may be detected by comparison with neighboring normal areas. It also makes a complete examination of the whole fundus more likely and easier than when performed with direct ophthalmoscopy. One perceived downfall is that the image is less magnified; however, this can be countered by moving closer to the patient while performing indirect ophthalmoscopy or by a subsequent (more magnified) examination of any "suspect" areas using the direct ophthalmoscope. Another difficulty for beginning ophthalmoscopists is that indirect ophthalmoscopy produces an inverted view. This makes navigation around the fundus and correct anatomic localization of lesions a little more difficult at first, but this disadvantage can be readily overcome with practice. In order of decreasing magnification, the Volk 20 D, 2.2 Pan Retinal, or 30 D indirect lens may be used for examining the dog and cat fundus.

Monocular Indirect Ophthalmoscopes

Monocular indirect ophthalmoscopes fit existing battery handsets commonly found in veterinary practices, are reasonably easily mastered, and produce a view of the fundus with many of the best features of those produced using direct and indirect ophthalmoscopy. The image is upright and moderately magnified and includes more of the fundus than is visible with the direct ophthalmoscope but less than that with indirect ophthalmoscopy.

Other Common Diagnostic Techniques in Veterinary Ophthalmology

Unlike assessment of other less accessible organs, visual examination of the eyes frequently provides all the clues necessary to reach a clinical diagnosis. However, ancillary tests can provide valuable information in specific disease conditions.

The *Schirmer tear test (STT)* records basal and reflex tearing as number of millimeters of wetting of a strip of absorbent paper placed in the lateral aspect of the ventral conjunctival fornix for 1 minute. The lateral aspect of the fornix is used to ensure that the strip lightly irritates the cornea and produces reflex tearing. If the strip is placed more medially, it may be prevented from contacting the cornea by the third eyelid, leading to erroneously low STT results. The STT should be performed before application of any topical solutions, particularly anesthetic or parasympatholytic (pupil-dilating) drops. General anesthesia and sedation also depress normal tearing for at least 48 hours. Normal STT values for dogs are well established; an STT reading of 15 mm or more in 60 seconds is considered normal. Wetting of less than 15 mm in 60 seconds is abnormal and is usually associated with evidence of keratoconjunctivitis. The range of reported STT values in normal cats (3 to 32 mm) is much wider and more difficult to interpret than in dogs and readings lower than the reported mean (17 mm in 60 seconds) can frequently be recorded in completely normal cats. This is probably because of autonomic control of tear secretion and short-term alterations in tear flow as a result of stress in the examination room. Feline STT values should still be recorded, compared between left and right eyes, and interpreted in conjunction with clinical signs.

Application of fluorescein dye to the cornea can yield a large amount of information. A strip impregnated with fluorescein is moistened with 1 to 2 drops of sterile ocular irrigation solution ("eye wash"). The strip is then lightly and briefly touched on the bulbar conjunctiva. Care should be taken not to touch the strip onto the cornea because this will cause fluorescein to be retained in the absence of ulceration. An absolute minimum amount of dye should be applied to reduce the need for flushing, which animals appear to find irritating; however, if excess dye is applied, it should be rinsed from the corneal surface. This simple, water-soluble dye has great affinity for the hydrophilic corneal stroma but is not absorbed by epithelial cells or Descemet's membrane. Therefore its most common use is identification and characterization of corneal ulcers. Excitement of the fluorescent dye with a cobalt blue light assists with identification of minor lesions. However, care must be taken not to overinterpret the normal pooling of dye, especially on roughened but not eroded epithelial surfaces. This risk can be reduced by ensuring that excessive dye is not applied or that it is adequately rinsed from the cornea, preventing the fluorescein strip from touching the cornea, and recalling that small, "scuffed" areas of corneal epithelium are occasionally seen following the STT.

Passage of fluorescein dye down the nasolacrimal duct is referred to as the *Jones test* and is used to assess functional and anatomic patency of the nasolacrimal apparatus. *Seidel's test* also uses fluorescein stain. This test is used to assess integrity of the cornea following suspected penetrating trauma or ulceration and to guide decisions regarding management of such wounds. In Seidel's test, an abundance of fluorescein is applied to the cornea, but is not rinsed from the cornea. Using a cobalt blue light source and magnification, the eye is examined for small rivulets in the fluorescein dye pooled on the corneal surface. These represent areas where the precorneal film of fluorescein is disrupted by aqueous humor egressing through a corneal perforation.

Rose bengal stain is retained by devitalized corneal or conjunctival epithelial cells. Even changes in the amount or quality of some normal tear film components such as mucin and albumin can cause otherwise viable epithelial cells to retain rose bengal stain. Therefore its clinical use is detection of subtle epithelial abnormalities as seen in keratoconjunctivitis sicca ("dry eye") or the dendritic ulcers that are pathognomonic for canine and feline herpesvirus keratitis. Rose bengal and fluorescein stains may affect results of culture, cytology, and possibly polymerase chain reaction (PCR). Therefore these stains should not be applied before collection of microbiologic samples. Rose bengal is also epitheliotoxic and may cause discomfort in some animals; therefore it should be reserved for cases in which it may provide useful additional information. For this reason some now prefer lissamine green in place of rose bengal stain.

Retropulsion of the globe is a simple but useful method for investigating orbital disease. It is performed by applying gentle digital pressure to both globes in a posterior direction through closed lids. The resistance to retropulsion and the resilience with which the globes "spring" back against the retropulsive force are subjectively assessed. Retropulsion of each globe in a variety of directions may further localize orbital masses or outline smaller masses that would be missed by direct caudal retropulsion only.

Cannulation of the nasolacrimal puncta and gentle flushing with saline can be readily performed in most conscious dogs following application of a topical ophthalmic anesthetic. However, it is particularly challenging in cats without sedation or general anesthesia. A ¾-inch, 22- or 24-gauge Teflon intravenous catheter without the stylet is easy to use and usually well tolerated; however, more rigid, specialized metal cannulae are also available. The inferior or superior punctum is identified and cannulated. Gentle injection of saline through one punctum should elicit flow from the other in the same eye without any resistance. Following assessment of patency between the superior and inferior puncta, gentle digital obstruction of the noncannulated punctum should cause passage of the solution through the nasolacrimal duct and out the ipsilateral nostril. Frequently in cats and brachycephalic dogs, the nasolacrimal ducts open caudally enough in the nose that flush solutions are not evident at the external nares but exit into the nasopharynx and then the oral cavity, causing licking or swallowing. Inclusion of a small amount of fluorescein in the flush solution and observation of the nares and oral cavity with a cobalt blue light source may assist with confirmation of patency. However, fluorescein should be avoided if culture or cytologic examination of nasolacrimal fluid is intended.

Samples for cytologic or histologic examination can be harvested relatively easily from ocular and periocular tissues, sometimes without sedation. Scraping or aspirate samples from the eyelid are collected using the same procedures as elsewhere on skin; however, particular care is taken not to damage the eyelid margin and to direct the instruments used away from the globe. Scrapings from the cornea or conjunctiva are performed following several applications of topical anesthesia and using either a Kimura platinum spatula, a commercially available cytology brush, or the dull, handle-end of a scalpel blade. Cytology specimens are spread gently onto glass slides and stained with Diff-Quik and/or Gram stains. Conjunctival "snip biopsies" can usually be harvested following application of topical anesthetic and without sedation. A small section of conjunctiva is gently "tented up" with fine forceps and resected with small tenotomy scissors. Minimal and careful handling is essential to avoid artifactitious disruption of this delicate tissue before histologic interpretation. Corneal biopsies are usually obtained by lamellar keratectomy and require general anesthesia, magnification, and sometimes neuromuscular blockade and therefore are more commonly performed by those with specialty training.

Imaging techniques for the globe and orbit are useful for diagnosis of orbital disease, and when opacity of the ocular media (cornea, lens, aqueous humor, or vitreous) prohibits detailed examination of intraocular structures. Ultrasonographic assessment has proved particularly useful. A 12 to 20 MHz probe is optimal but lower frequency probes often produce useful images. Examination of a conscious patient following application of topical anesthetic is preferred since sedation tends to cause ventral rolling of the eyeball and enophthalmos, which make obtaining adequate images difficult. Transcorneal or transpalpebral approaches are used most commonly; however, a temporal approach has been described for retrobulbar examination. Sterile, water-soluble coupling gel (preferably from single-use containers and without preservatives) is applied to the cornea or lids, and the probe is applied with gentle pressure sufficient to ensure a clear image. Eyes in which corneal perforation has occurred or is imminent should not undergo ultrasonography.

Radiographic assessment is particularly useful for identification of radiopaque foreign bodies, particularly gunshot injuries, and can also be used to diagnose orbital fractures or to detect bony involvement when invasive tumors are suspected. However, computed tomography scans provide a more sensitive method and permit three-dimensional reconstruction to better facilitate surgical planning. Magnetic resonance imaging also can provide valuable information regarding the extent and character of orbital disease.

Gonioscopy is the examination of the iridocorneal angle (ICA). In dogs a small plastic corneal lens is required. In cats (because of their large corneas and degree of corneal curvature) magnification and a focal light source (i.e., an otoscope head) permit some assessment of this area; however, this should be supplemented with a gonioscopic lens before a final assessment is made. The clinician should focus initially on the iris and then follow it out peripherally until the ICA and pectinate ligament come into view. The pectinate ligament is composed of numerous long and relatively straight filaments with large spaces between them. These filaments are usually pigmented to about the same degree as the iris. Examination of the ICA provides essential information for diagnosis and prognosis of glaucoma and uveitis. Although this technique is learned relatively easily, familiarity with angle anatomy and interpretation of abnormal findings require practice.

Anterior chamber, vitreous, and subretinal aspirates are sometimes used in the assessment of uveitis or intraocular masses if less invasive techniques have not yielded a diagnosis. Samples gathered in this fashion can be examined serologically or cytologically or submitted for PCR or culture and sensitivity testing. Due to the risk of irreversible globe damage during these procedures, they are best performed by ophthalmologists.

The *electroretinogram* is a measure of retinal electrical activity in response to stimulation with light. It is a routine part of assessment of patients before cataract surgery and may also be used to assist in the neuroanatomic localization of blindness resulting from retinal, optic nerve, or central neurologic disease. The specialized equipment and knowledge of the technique needed limit this study to specialist ophthalmology practices.

CHAPTER 243

Evaluation of Blindness

ANNE J. GEMENSKY METZLER, *Columbus, Ohio*

valuation of a patient brought to the veterinarian because of vision deficits or blindness can be a diagnostic challenge. Both ocular and neurologic causes must be considered. As with central nervous system disease, localization of an ophthalmologic lesion is imperative to formulate the differential diagnoses, diagnostic approach, and therapeutic plan, and to advance a prognosis. This chapter, in conjunction with Web Chapter 80 on the neuro-ophthalmic examination, provides a blueprint for the assessment of a blind patient.

Obtaining a Thorough History

The client should be questioned to ascertain the onset, duration, and character of the blindness. Answers to the following questions should be obtained to the extent possible: (1) Did the blindness occur fairly rapidly over hours or days or was the onset more gradual, occurring over weeks to years? (2) Was the onset of vision loss obvious or more insidious? (3) In what type of environment was the blindness first noticed? (4) What is the duration of the visual impairment or loss? (5) Has the vision loss been intermittent, waxing and waning, or constant since first noticed? (6) Has there been any difference in visual function in bright light compared with dim light or darkness? (7) Does the pet seem to be more impaired centrally or peripherally or on one side (right or left) more than the other? Although some clients are better observers than others, their responses to each of these questions offer valuable clues about the cause of vision loss.

It is useful to ask the client to describe the behavior of the pet that makes the client feel the pet has vision difficulties to help in discerning whether an ophthalmic problem is the source of the behavioral changes causing concern. In some situations, it is not apparent to the client that his or her pet is blind until the pet is taken to an unfamiliar environment. The client also should be questioned about the pet's general health, current and past administration of medications, and awareness of any genetically related pets that have been diagnosed with ophthalmic disorders.

Assessing the Patient

Once the history has been obtained, the pet's behavior and confidence navigating around the clinic and examination room should be assessed. Additional methods of assessing vision include menace response testing, cotton ball tracking, visual placing, maze testing, evaluation of the pupillary light reflexes (PLRs), and assessment of dazzle responses (see Chapter 242). Electroretinography,

although it does not directly assess vision, also may be useful for assessing retinal function. It is important to evaluate the vision in each eye independently as well as to assess the visual fields of each eye. Visual fields are assessed by covering one eye and checking menace responses in the other by advancing a fist toward the tested eye from both the nasal and the temporal sides of the globe. Baseline pupil symmetry, the presence or absence of anisocoria, and the PLRs should be evaluated in both a brightly lit and a dimly lit room and the findings recorded.

Any abnormality of the PLRs should be characterized (ranging from a mild decrease to complete absence) and qualified as an afferent or efferent deficit. Afferent PLR deficits are associated with vision deficits. The pupillomotor fibers split off from the optic tract just before the lateral geniculate nucleus; therefore lesions involving the Edinger-Westphal nucleus (the parasympathetic nucleus of cranial nerve III) and the efferent arm of the PLR pathway are not associated with loss of vision (Figure 243-1). Lesions that involve the visual pathway from the lateral geniculate nucleus to the optic striations in the visual cortex do not cause abnormalities of the PLR or anisocoria (Figure 243-2).

Localizing Blindness

After the neuro-ophthalmic assessment is conducted, a complete ophthalmic examination, including evaluation of the anterior and posterior segments, is performed to determine whether the blindness is of ocular or neurologic origin. There are four main ways that blindness can be produced: (1) opacification of the ocular media; (2) failure of the neural retina or optic nerve to process and transmit an image; (3) failure of the extraocular portion of the optic nerve, the optic chiasm, or optic tracts to transmit an image; and (4) failure of the visual cortex of the brain to process an image.

The cornea, anterior chamber, lens, and vitreous must be examined carefully to detect opacification of the ocular media. Ideally this examination should follow pharmacologic pupillary dilation and should employ a focal bright light source such as a transilluminator as well as some type of magnifying device. Types of corneal opacification that may impair vision include severe edema, vascularization, cellular and noncellular infiltrates, pigment, and fibrosis. In the anterior chamber, severe aqueous flare, fibrin, hyphema, and hypopyon may decrease vision, as can dense or extensive cataracts. Posterior segment lesions such as the presence of vitreal inflammatory cells and vitreal degeneration with consolidation and asteroid hyalosis are additional causes. It is stressed that although

1134

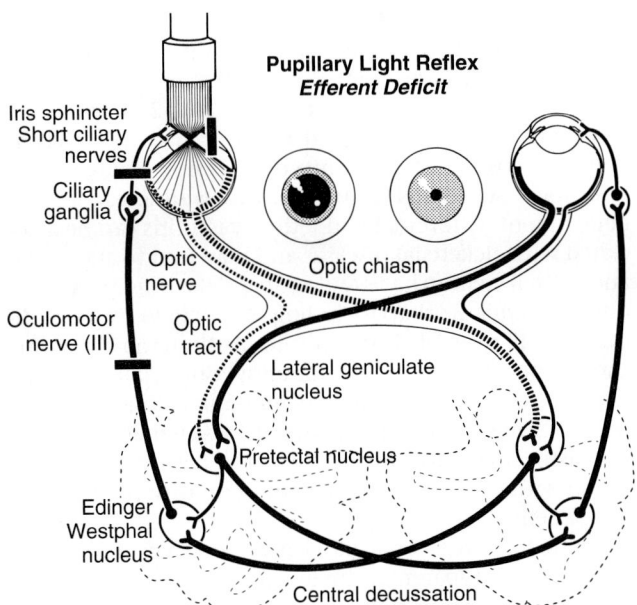

Figure 243-1 Diagram of an efferent pupillary light reflex deficit. Vision is not affected.

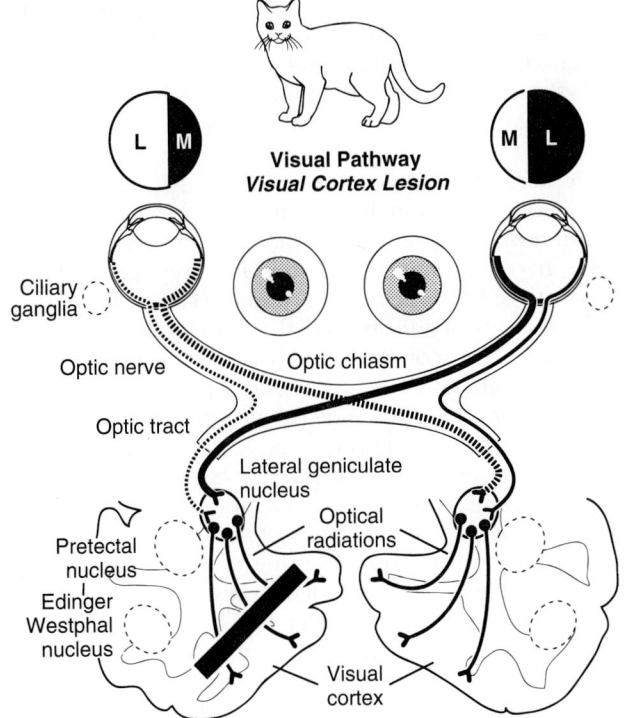

Figure 243-2 Diagram of a lesion involving the lateral geniculate nucleus, optic radiations, or the visual cortex. Loss of the ipsilateral nasal visual field and the contralateral lateral visual field occurs, whereas the pupillary light reflex is normal.

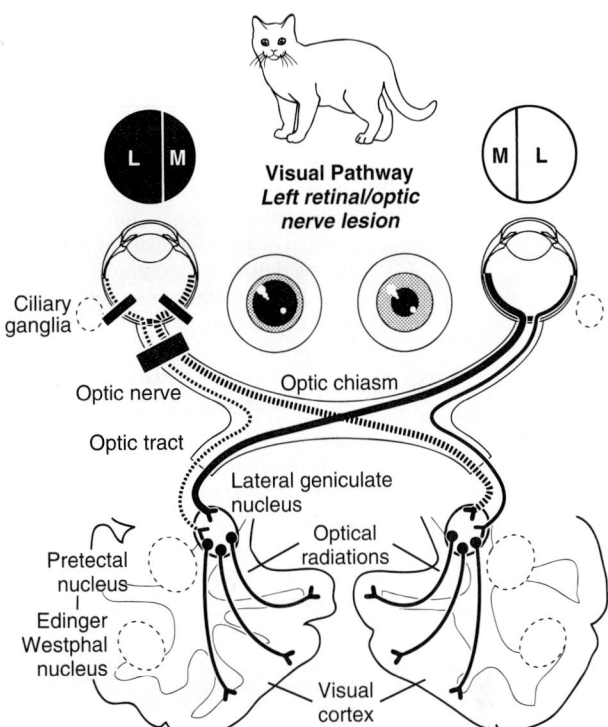

Figure 243-3 Diagram of a retinal or optic nerve lesion causing an afferent pupillary light reflex deficit.

opacity of the ocular media can alter light transmission sufficiently to cause blindness, the PLR and dazzle response should be present provided that the light source is bright and the neural pathways are intact.

Next the menace response, PLR, and dazzle response can be assessed further to localize the neuro-ophthalmic source. If the menace response is absent, the ability to blink should be tested using the palpebral reflex and vision loss should confirmed by another method such as cotton ball tracking or maze testing. If the menace response is absent and the PLR and dazzle responses are abnormal or absent, then the lesion involves the retina, optic nerve, optic chiasm, or optic tracts. If the PLR and dazzle responses are normal despite the presence of vision loss, then central blindness is most likely. Central blindness results from one or more lesions of the lateral geniculate nucleus, optic radiations, or visual cortex of the cerebrum.

Identifying and Treating the Cause of Blindness

Table 243-1 lists causes of blindness organized by the site of the lesion along the neuro-ophthalmic pathway.

Retinal and Optic Nerve Disorders

Lesions involving the retina or optic nerve cause blindness along with a decreased or absent PLR (Figure 243-3). Retinal or optic nerve diseases causing vision loss typically are associated with ophthalmoscopic changes such as tapetal hyperreflectivity, retinal vessel attenuation, retinal detachment, optic nerve pallor, or myelin loss.

Retinal Disorders
Retinal disorders often are diagnosed by signalment, history, and the presence of ophthalmic lesions. Electroretinography may be indicated to confirm and characterize the retinal dysfunction. Retinal degenerative disorders

TABLE 243-1

Causes of Blindness

Site of Lesion	Potential Causes

Retina	Progressive retinal atrophy
	Senile retinal degeneration
	Sudden acquired retinal degeneration
	Retinal dysplasia (geographic or
	  retinal nonattachment forms)
	Retinal detachment
	Glaucoma
	Chorioretinitis secondary to systemic
	  infectious/inflammatory disease

Optic nerve	Glaucoma Optic nerve hypoplasia Optic nerve coloboma Traumatic optic nerve avulsion Systemic mycosis Feline infectious peritonitis Granulomatous meningoencephalitis Meningioma
Retrobulbar optic nerve	Compressive orbital neoplasia or abscess/cellulitis
Optic chiasm	Pituitary tumor Traumatic optic nerve avulsion
Optic tract	Neoplasia Central nervous system infectious/ inflammatory disease Granulomatous meningoencephalitis
Lateral geniculate nucleus, optic radiations, visual cortex	Hydrocephalus Lissencephaly Hepatoencephalopathy Systemic mycosis Canine distemper viral encephalitis Granulomatous meningoencephalitis Neoplasia Ivermectin toxicity Traumatic edema or hemorrhage Hypoxia Cerebral edema secondary to seizure Vascular infarct Lead poisoning Congenital metabolic storage disease

such as progressive retinal atrophy or other inherited disorders, senile retinal degeneration, and sudden acquired retinal degeneration should be considered (see Chapter 254). DNA testing currently is available for many inherited retinal diseases. Retinal detachment (see Web Chapter 76) due to systemic hypertension or other causes; chorioretinitis related to systemic infectious, inflammatory, or neoplastic diseases; ivermectin toxicosis; and glaucoma also must be included in the differential diagnosis for blindness with an afferent PLR deficit. Systemic hypertension (see Chapter 169) is the most common cause of retinal detachment and blindness in the cat. In the dog systemic hypertension more commonly causes petechial hemorrhages than bullous retinal detachment, but detachment can occur with severe or sudden-onset hypertension as is seen in acute renal failure.

Hypertensive retinopathy has a fair to good prognosis for return of vision in cats and dogs with prompt diagnosis and institution of antihypertensive therapy.

Chorioretinitis (see Chapters 249 and 250) is associated with toxoplasmosis and systemic mycoses such as cryptococcosis and blastomycosis. Lesions range from multifocal subretinal granulomas to widespread retinal detachment. Choroidal and retinal vasculitis can be associated with rickettsial diseases and may lead to subretinal and retinal hemorrhage and retinal detachment. A thorough systemic workup including serologic testing is indicated for all cases of chorioretinitis. Antimicrobial therapy should be directed at the primary cause, although in many infectious cases, antiinflammatory dosages of systemic corticosteroids may help decrease the inflammation associated with the infection and improve or restore vision without causing significant immunosuppression in the patient.

Ivermectin toxicosis may cause mydriasis and vision loss without apparent changes in the fundus. However, multifocal punctate to vermiform gray lesions in the non-tapetal fundus also have been described. Supportive care is indicated because these patients usually have significant concurrent neurologic dysfunction. Vision typically returns days to weeks after the ingestion of ivermectin. In a case of severe toxicosis in a Border collie, intravenous lipid emulsion was used to bind ivermectin, and this treatment led to rapid improvement in clinical signs and shorter hospital stay (see Chapter 24 and Web Chapter 34).

Optic Nerve Disorders

The optic nerve can be affected by vision-threatening conditions such as glaucoma (see Chapters 251 and 252), optic nerve coloboma, optic nerve hypoplasia, optic nerve avulsion, optic neuritis, and infectious, neoplastic, and inflammatory disorders of the central nervous system. An optic nerve coloboma such as occurs in collie eye anomaly is characterized by a focal depression within the optic disc or a substantial defect encompassing the entire optic disc and surrounding sclera. Blindness occurs in severe cases. A congenitally hypoplastic optic nerve is small in diameter, relatively dark, and slightly depressed. Optic nerve hypoplasia causes blindness and absence of the PLR and dazzle response due to a complete lack of retinal ganglion cells and their axons. Hypoplasia is differentiated from micropapilla (an optic disc of small diameter that is composed of normal axons) mainly by the lighter color of the disc and the presence of vision in micropapilla. Optic nerve avulsion occurs most frequently because of globe proptosis (see Chapter 256) or head trauma. Vision may return after treatment with systemic corticosteroids with minor stretching of the optic nerve, but more commonly, blindness is irreversible.

Optic neuritis can be recognized by hyperemia, elevation, swelling, and sometimes hemorrhage of the optic disc. Peripapillary subretinal edema or exudates commonly are seen in conjunction with changes in the disc. Optic neuritis may be a primary immune-mediated disorder or a clinical manifestation of granulomatous meningoencephalitis. After systemic infectious diseases are ruled out by physical examination and serologic testing, immunosuppressive dosages of corticosteroids may be prescribed to control the inflammation. These should be tapered as soon as possible to the lowest effective dose that controls the disease. Azathioprine may be started in conjunction with corticosteroid treatment to maintain control as the corticosteroid is slowly tapered and discontinued. Prognosis is guarded to fair for a response to treatment, depending on the chronicity of the disease and the level of destruction of optic nerve axons.

Lesions involving the retrobulbar optic nerve (see Figure 243-3), optic chiasm, or optic tracts cause blindness with a decrease or absence of the PLRs. Retrobulbar optic neuritis can cause vision loss without any ophthalmoscopic abnormalities. Advanced imaging with magnetic resonance imaging (MRI) or computed tomography (CT) is more sensitive than orbital ultrasonography in evaluating the optic nerve and usually precedes collection of cerebrospinal fluid. Retrobulbar tumors can compress the optic nerve, which results in loss of vision (see Chapters 257 and 258) and are usually manifested as exophthalmia. Fundic examination may reveal scleral indentation with large or rigid masses. CT or MRI is useful in evaluating the origin and extent of orbital masses as well as in guiding collection of the aspirates or biopsy samples needed for definitive diagnosis. Primary tumors without bony extension may be treated effectively by exenteration of the orbit with or without adjunctive radiation.

Optic Chiasm Lesions

Pituitary tumors are the primary cause of blindness associated with an optic chiasm lesion. The chiasm contains the medial 75% of the optic nerve fibers from each eye, so that a lesion results in a decreased to absent PLR when the light is directed toward the medial and central retina along with loss of 75% of the peripheral to central visual fields (Figure 243-4). The lateral fibers continue to the ipsilateral side without decussating; hence the medial 25% of the visual field is retained. However, abnormalities often are not apparent to the client until the mass expands to include the adjacent nondecussating fibers. In this situation, pupils are dilated, the PLRs are significantly decreased or absent, and vision is severely diminished or lost (Figure 243-5). Some pituitary tumors are responsive to radiation therapy.

Optic Tract Lesions

Optic tract lesions result in a static anisocoria in which the contralateral pupil always remains more dilated regardless of which eye is illuminated. This is explained by the fact that the affected optic tract contains 75% of the optic fibers from the contralateral eye. Accordingly, a hemianopsia (partial visual field loss) occurs in which the ipsilateral nasal visual field and the contralateral temporal visual field are lost (Figure 243-6). In other words, with a left optic tract lesion, the right side of the visual field is lost from both eyes. Optic tract lesions are uncommon and usually are associated with neoplasia.

Central or Cortical Blindness

Lesions of the lateral geniculate nucleus, optic radiations, and visual cortex cause a central blindness, whereas the

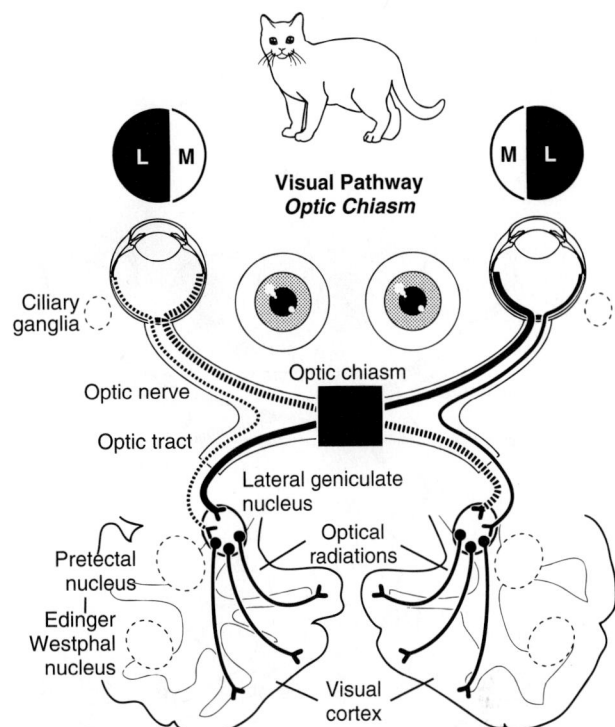

Figure 243-4 Diagram of an optic chiasm lesion illustrating the abnormalities of the pupillary light reflex and loss of the lateral visual field of both eyes.

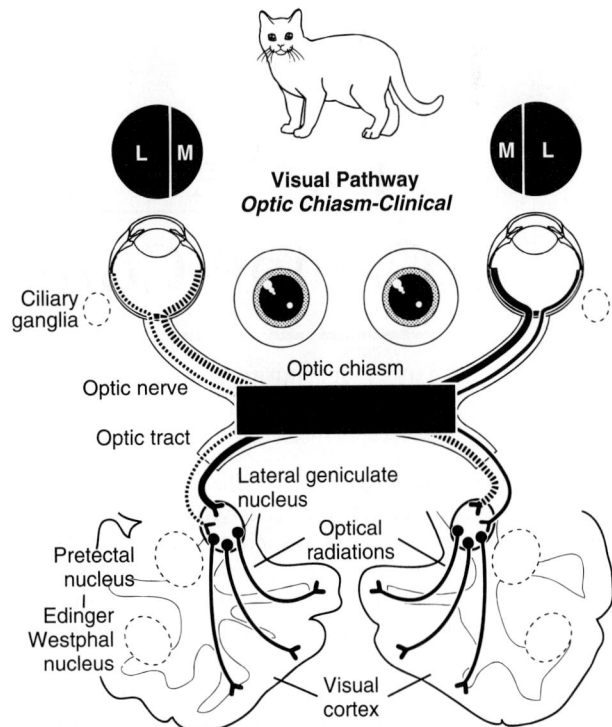

Figure 243-5 Diagram of an extensive optic chiasm lesion that also affects the adjacent nondecussating optic nerve fibers illustrating complete loss of the pupillary light reflex and vision in both eyes.

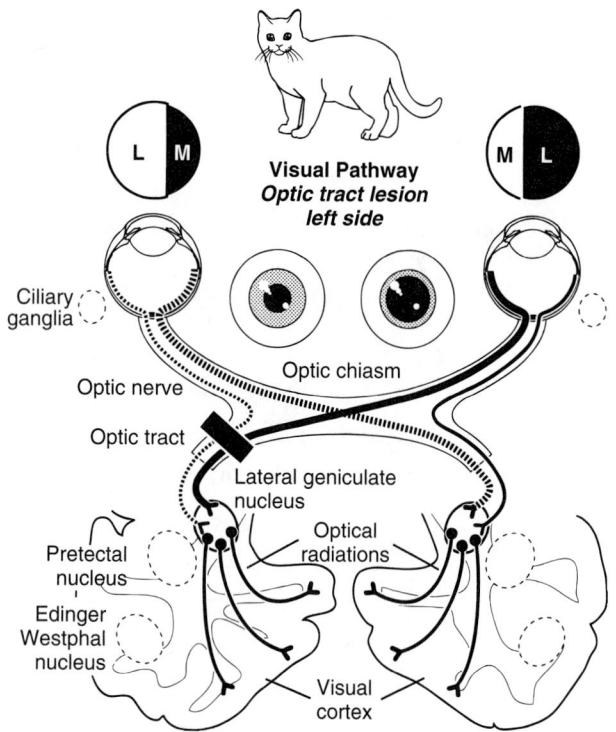

Visual Pathway
Optic tract lesion left side

Ciliary ganglia

Optic nerve

Optic tract

Optic chiasm

Lateral geniculate nucleus

Pretectal nucleus

Optical radiations

Edinger Westphal nucleus

Visual cortex

Figure 243-6 Diagram of an optic tract lesion showing the resulting pupillary light reflex abnormality and the loss of the ipsilateral nasal visual field and the contralateral lateral visual field.

PLRs remain unaffected (see Figure 243-2). Possible causes include central nervous system neoplastic and inflammatory diseases such as meningioma, granulomatous meningoencephalitis, and cryptococcosis. Other causes to consider are cerebral edema due to seizures, brain hypoxia, hepatoencephalopathy, and head trauma. The diagnostic workup may entail MRI or CT, cerebrospinal fluid tap, and serologic testing. Again, therapy is directed at the primary cause. Postictal blindness and blindness occurring after hypoxia or general anesthesia usually is transient and resolves within a few hours to a few weeks without treatment. Clients should be encouraged to demonstrate patience in these situations, especially if return of the pet to the home is not precluded by other serious medical issues.

References and Suggested Reading

Bley CR et al: Irradiation of brain tumors in dogs with neurologic disease, *J Vet Intern Med* 19(6):849, 2005.

Clarke DL et al: Use of intravenous lipid emulsion to treat ivermectin toxicosis in a Border Collie, *J Am Vet Med Assoc* 239(10):1328, 2011.

Kenny PJ et al: Retinopathy associated with ivermectin toxicosis in two dogs, *J Am Vet Med Assoc* 233(2):279, 2008.

Shamir MH, Ofri R: Comparative neuro-ophthalmology. In Gelatt KN, editor: *Veterinary ophthalmology*, ed 4, Oxford, UK, 2007, Blackwell Publishing, p 1406.

Theon AP, Feldman EC: Megavoltage irradiation of pituitary macrotumors in dogs with neurologic signs, *J Am Vet Med Assoc* 213(2):225, 1998.

CHAPTER 244

Canine Conjunctivitis

ERIC C. LEDBETTER, *Ithaca, New York*

Conjunctivitis is a common disorder in dogs. The causes of canine conjunctivitis are numerous, including primary conjunctival diseases and other extraocular, intraocular, and systemic conditions that lead to secondary conjunctivitis. Clinical manifestations of conjunctivitis frequently are nonspecific and may be similar in spite of diverse causes. Furthermore, severe ocular diseases and potentially life-threatening systemic conditions can present initially as conjunctivitis. Failure to consider both local and systemic causes of conjunctivitis can have dire consequences for ocular and systemic health; therefore a methodical clinical approach to conjunctivitis should be followed.

Essential Anatomy and Physiology

The conjunctiva is the mucous membrane covering the posterior aspect of the eyelids, palpebral and bulbar surfaces of the nictitans membrane, and anterior portion of the globe. The conjunctiva is composed of nonkeratinized, stratified epithelium, and the underlying connective tissue is referred to as the *substantia propria*. Mucin-producing goblet cells are present in the conjunctival epithelium, and the substantia propria contains vessels, nerves, and lymphoid tissue. The rich vascular supply, loose arrangement of the substantia propria, and resident lymphoid tissue contribute to the conjunctiva's ability to respond rapidly, and often dramatically, to insults.

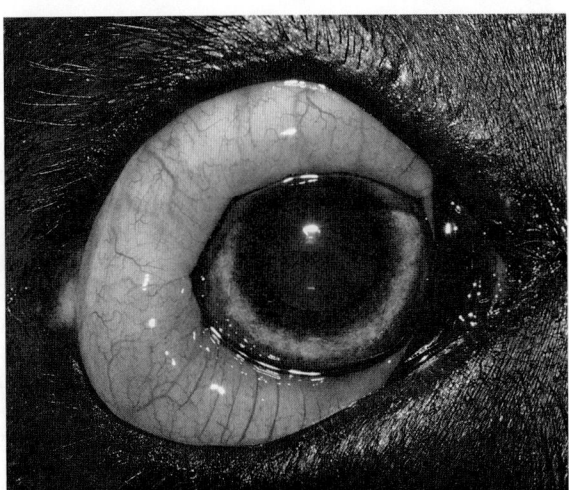

Figure 244-1 Allergic conjunctivitis in a dog with marked chemosis that occurred immediately following a Hymenoptera (honeybee) sting.

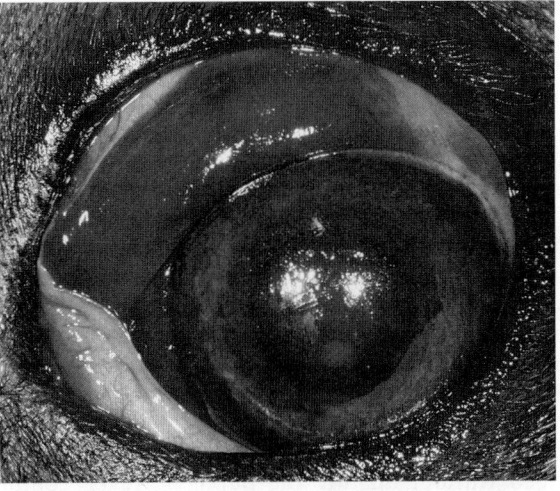

Figure 244-2 Conjunctivitis and subconjunctival hemorrhage in a dog resulting from blunt ocular trauma.

Clinical Signs

Conjunctivitis invariably is associated with some combination of the following clinical signs: ocular discharge, chemosis, hyperemia, discomfort, pruritus, tissue proliferation, ulceration, and hemorrhage. Ocular discharge may be characterized by serous, mucoid, mucopurulent, or serosanguineous fluids. Epiphora, overflow of serous tears, results from excessive production or inadequate nasolacrimal drainage. Chemosis appears as conjunctival swelling and is the clinical manifestation of conjunctival edema caused by increased vascular permeability and fluid extravasation (Figure 244-1). Hyperemia is a red conjunctival discoloration ("red eye") and is a clinically observable manifestation of vasodilation and increased blood flow. Ocular discomfort and pruritus most commonly manifest as blepharospasm and periocular rubbing.

Tissue proliferation is divided into two distinct types: lymphatic and epithelial. Lymphatic proliferation frequently is termed *follicular conjunctivitis* and appears as small, round, semitransparent, elevated lesions representing lymphocytic aggregates. The occasional occurrence of conjunctival lymphatic follicles on the posterior aspect of the nictitans membrane is normal; however, increased numbers of follicles or their presence in other anatomic locations is pathologic. Epithelial hyperplasia or keratinization results in irregular, opaque, pink to red, elevated lesions of variable size. Both lymphatic and epithelial conjunctival tissue proliferation are indicative of chronic inflammation but are otherwise nonspecific clinical findings.

Ulceration of the conjunctival epithelium may occur with any severe conjunctivitis but is most common in conjunctivitis of viral or traumatic origin. Conjunctival ulcers appear as flat, irregular, pale or pink regions on the conjunctival surface that retain fluorescein stain and are surrounded by a hyperemic border. Hemorrhage may occur in the conjunctival epithelium or subconjunctival space. Both intraconjunctival and subconjunctival hemorrhages appear as bright or dark red regions of variable shape and size (Figure 244-2). Conjunctival hemorrhage is frequently detected in dogs with traumatic or viral conjunctivitis but also can be a manifestation of systemic disease, including coagulopathy, hypertension, hyperviscosity, platelet disorders, and vasculitis.

Clinical Evaluation

The clinical approach to canine conjunctivitis is similar to the approach to any nonspecific ocular lesion that can have various causes, including investigation of both primary and secondary causes of conjunctival inflammation. A thorough history taking, physical examination, and ocular examination are performed to identify the specific cause when possible or to narrow the differential diagnosis and exclude more serious causes of conjunctivitis such as systemic or intraocular disease. Historical details to collect include the onset and duration of clinical signs, presence and nature of ocular discharge, changes in vision, presence of pain or pruritus, and known concurrent systemic and ocular diseases. All ocular and systemic drug treatments should be identified, including over-the-counter medications and medications administered by the client on his or her own accord. It is beneficial to request that clients not clean ocular discharge from the dog before the evaluation. A complete physical examination is performed on all dogs with conjunctivitis, including evaluation of body temperature, thoracic auscultation, oral cavity examination, and regional lymph node palpation.

A complete ophthalmic examination always is indicated for dogs with conjunctivitis, including Schirmer tear tests, ocular surface fluorescein staining, and tonometry (see Chapter 242). This simple examination strategy maximizes the chances of correctly identifying the cause of the conjunctivitis and prevents missing more serious ocular diseases that initially may resemble primary conjunctivitis. These include ulcerative keratitis, uveitis, and glaucoma. Examination should begin with a general evaluation of facial conformation and the size, position, and symmetry of the globe, orbits, eyelids, and pupils. The general evaluation is most productive when performed at a distance from the dog's head and with minimal restraint. Palpation of the periocular facial regions and adnexa is performed and menace responses, palpebral reflexes, pupillary light reflexes, ocular motility, and globe retropulsion are assessed.

Detailed examination of the adnexa, ocular surface, and intraocular structures is then performed with magnification and a bright focal light source. Eyelid conformation is assessed and the eyelid margins and conjunctiva are methodically examined to detect foreign bodies, cilia abnormalities, and other lesions. The bulbar surface of the nictitans membrane is examined for foreign material or the presence of abundant lymphoid follicles. Examination of the anterior segment of the globe may be performed without dilating the pupil; however, complete evaluation of the lens and posterior segment can be accomplished only with pharmacologic mydriasis.

Causes and Management of Canine Conjunctivitis

As indicated earlier, the causes of conjunctivitis include primary conjunctival diseases, secondary manifestations of other ocular diseases, and secondary manifestations of systemic diseases. Primary causes of conjunctivitis are those in which the disease process is limited to the conjunctiva and include allergic, frictional irritant, immune-mediated, infectious, and traumatic conditions.

Primary Conjunctival Diseases

Allergic Conjunctivitis

Conjunctivitis associated with allergic conditions occurs frequently in the dog and can be divided into three general types: atopic conjunctivitis, drug reaction conjunctivitis, and conjunctivitis caused by insect envenomation. Atopic conjunctivitis often is accompanied by atopic dermatitis but can occur alone. Dogs frequently show mild and seasonal hyperemia, chemosis, epiphora, and ocular pruritus. Conjunctival follicle formation occurs in chronic cases. Atopic conjunctivitis generally is a diagnosis of exclusion; however, atopic dermatitis and seasonality are suggestive of this cause. Allergen immunotherapy and allergen avoidance are definitive treatments for atopic conjunctivitis but may be impractical for some dogs. The use of topical ophthalmic corticosteroids applied two or three times daily for short durations (1 to 2 weeks) as needed for flare-ups generally is effective in controlling clinical signs. Dogs with recurrent episodes, a protracted clinical course, or contraindications to topical corticosteroids benefit from long-term or lifelong topical ocular cyclosporine therapy (0.2% to 2% solution or ointment, applied twice daily). Continual cyclosporine therapy generally reduces or eliminates the need for pulse therapy with topical corticosteroids.

Drug reaction conjunctivitis is a hypersensitivity reaction that often results in severe clinical signs. Concurrent blepharitis, often with dermal ulceration, frequently is present. Conjunctivitis may develop at any time during drug use and with any medication. Ophthalmic medications containing neomycin and carbonic anhydrase inhibitors are among the most common causes of allergic conjunctivitis in dogs. Treatment consists of discontinuing all ophthalmic medications for 1 to 2 weeks (when possible) and slowly reintroducing medications individually until the offending pharmaceutical is identified. Topical corticosteroid therapy can assist in relieving clinical signs, but a medication that is unlikely to be associated with this type of reaction should be chosen (e.g., prednisolone acetate 1% solution).

Insect bites and stings anywhere on the body—not just on periocular tissues—may result in dramatic conjunctivitis. This form of conjunctivitis typically has a rapid onset and is characterized by severe bilateral chemosis with the conspicuous absence of other acute clinical signs of conjunctivitis (see Figure 244-1). Therapy consists of a single dose of systemic corticosteroid and possibly an antihistamine followed by several days of topical corticosteroid administration. Rapid resolution of the chemosis is typical.

Frictional Irritant Conjunctivitis

Endogenous and exogenous irritants may result in conjunctivitis. These irritants include conjunctival foreign bodies (Figure 244-3), dermoids, and abnormalities of the eyelids such as masses, entropion, and ectropion. Additional causes are abnormal cilia (distichiasis and ectopic cilia) and periocular facial hair (trichiasis). Diagnosis of frictional irritant conjunctivitis is made by identifying one or more of these conditions during ocular examination. Definitive treatment involves removal of the irritant (e.g., surgical dermoid excision, surgical entropion correction, cryoepilation of abnormal cilia, foreign body removal), along with prevention of opportunistic bacterial infection with a topical ophthalmic antimicrobial.

Immune-Mediated Conjunctivitis

Despite the terms ascribed to these conditions, the conjunctiva is the actual focus of clinically apparent disease in both diffuse episcleritis and nodular granulomatous

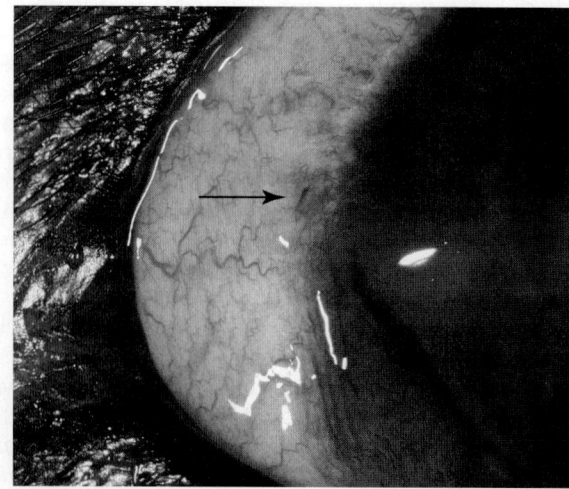

Figure 244-3 Frictional irritant conjunctivitis in a dog resulting from a conjunctival foreign body (thorn embedded in the conjunctiva indicated by the arrow).

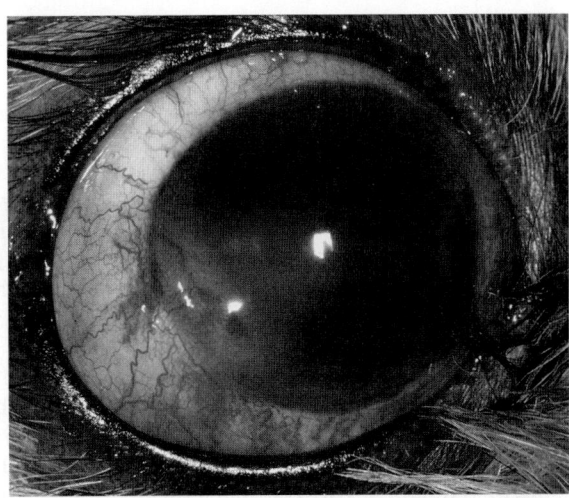

Figure 244-4 Nodular granulomatous episcleritis in a dog with a distinct, smooth-surfaced mass in the temporal bulbar conjunctiva and adjacent peripheral keratitis.

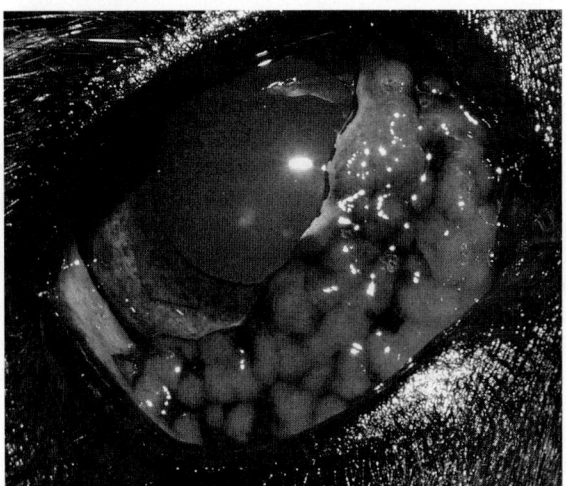

Figure 244-5 Atypical pannus (plasmoma) in a German shepherd dog with conjunctival hyperemia, thickening, multifocal follicle formation, and depigmentation of the nictitating membrane.

episcleritis. These conditions are characterized by granulomatous inflammation of the conjunctival substantia propria and episclera with variable infiltration by lymphocytes, plasma cells, histiocytes, and fibroblasts. Both conditions present with conjunctival hyperemia and thickening. Peripheral keratitis adjacent to the conjunctival lesions is common. Lesions may be unilateral or bilateral. The collie and American cocker spaniel breeds are predisposed, but episcleritis can be observed in any breed. Nodular granulomatous episcleritis is associated with formation of one or more distinct, proliferative, firm, smooth-surfaced masses (Figure 244-4). Diffuse episcleritis is likely a diffuse form of the same disease and is clinically similar, but without nodule formation.

Diagnosis usually is made solely from clinical appearance; however, conjunctival biopsy can provide confirmatory findings. Clinical signs in most dogs can be controlled with topical therapy only, and options include topical corticosteroids, cyclosporine, and tacrolimus (see Chapter 59). Topical corticosteroids provide rapid improvement in clinical signs but are associated with greater potential for adverse effects. Cyclosporine and tacrolimus have favorable adverse effect profiles, even with long-term use, but take longer to improve and resolve clinical signs. Combining a topical corticosteroid (three or four times daily) and cyclosporine (twice daily) is very effective, results in rapid clinical improvement, and allows the slow tapering and eventual discontinuation of the corticosteroid over several months. Once the condition is controlled, most dogs can be managed long term (lifelong therapy generally is required) with cyclosporine alone; however, short courses of corticosteroids may be required to control flare-ups. For severe cases or those refractory to topical treatment alone, a single subconjunctival corticosteroid injection within or adjacent to the lesions is helpful. For dogs that cannot or will not tolerate topical therapy, the combination of oral niacinamide and tetracycline is used. For dogs with body weights of more than 10 kg, 500 mg of both medications is administered three times daily; for dogs with body weights

of less than 10 kg, 250 mg of both medications is administered three times daily. Following resolution of clinical signs, administration frequency is reduced gradually to once daily over several months to provide long-term control. The potential adverse effects of these drugs should be appreciated, and referral to an ophthalmologist is recommended to confirm the diagnosis before embarking on alternative therapies.

Atypical pannus or plasmoma is an alternative presentation of pannus (i.e., chronic superficial keratitis) in which the primary clinical focus of lesions is the conjunctiva as opposed to the cornea. Atypical pannus is characterized by a lymphoplasmacytic infiltrate with concurrent fibrovascular proliferation and pigmentation. There are strong breed predilections for atypical pannus, including the German shepherd, greyhound, and Belgian sheepdog. Atypical pannus presents clinically as a bilateral hyperemic thickening of the nictitans conjunctiva associated with multifocal follicle formation and varying degrees of depigmentation and pigmentation. Atypical pannus has the clinical appearance of cobblestone granulation tissue (Figure 244-5). Treatment of atypical pannus is similar to treatment of diffuse episcleritis and nodular granulomatous episcleritis.

Infectious Conjunctivitis

Conjunctivitis may result from bacterial, viral, or parasitic infection. Unlike in many other species, bacterial infection is not a known cause of primary conjunctivitis in dogs. However, secondary bacterial conjunctivitis occurs commonly, exacerbates clinical lesions, and complicates the management of conjunctivitis associated with other causes in dogs. Development of bacterial conjunctivitis in dogs requires anatomic, physiologic, or immunologic compromise of the ocular surface. Resolution of bacterial conjunctivitis requires that the underlying cause be identified and corrected. Common underlying conditions in dogs with bacterial conjunctivitis include keratoconjunctivitis sicca, entropion, ectropion, euryblepharon, lagophthalmos, facial nerve dysfunction, distichiasis, ectopic cilia, trichiasis, and conjunctival foreign bodies. Concurrent treatment of the opportunistic bacterial infection hastens resolution. *Staphylococcus* and *Streptococcus* spp. are the most frequent isolates, and neomycin/polymyxin/bacitracin (or gramicidin), erythromycin, and tobramycin (administered three or four times daily until clinical signs resolve) are good empiric choices for topical therapy. Recurrent bacterial conjunctivitis is highly suggestive of a persistent and unresolved primary ocular abnormality and should prompt referral to a specialist.

Primary conjunctivitis may result from direct viral infection of the conjunctival epithelium, including infection with canine herpesvirus 1 (CHV-1) and canine adenovirus 2. Conjunctivitis also may be a prominent feature of various other systemic viral infections (e.g., canine distemper, canine influenza), but these dogs have concurrent systemic illness. Of the viruses causing primary conjunctivitis in dogs, CHV-1 is observed clinically the most frequently.

Conjunctivitis may occur from either primary or recurrent CHV-1 infection and can present as unilateral or bilateral disease. CHV-1 conjunctivitis often occurs in dogs with immunomodulating systemic conditions and in those receiving immunosuppressive therapeutics. Although the clinical features of CHV-1 conjunctivitis may be nonspecific and indistinguishable from those of other types of primary conjunctivitis (i.e., blepharospasm, conjunctival hyperemia, chemosis, ocular discharge), conjunctival ulceration and petechiae frequently are present with CHV-1 infection. Although they are not specific to CHV-1 infection, these clinical findings are uncommon in conjunctivitis due to most other causes (Figure 244-6). Definitive diagnosis of CHV-1 conjunctivitis is made by virus isolation or polymerase chain reaction analysis of conjunctival swabs. These assays should be considered when physical and ophthalmic examinations have failed to identify any other potential causes or when recent historical factors suggest possible exposure to dogs shedding the virus (e.g., hospitalization, kennels) or immunosuppression.

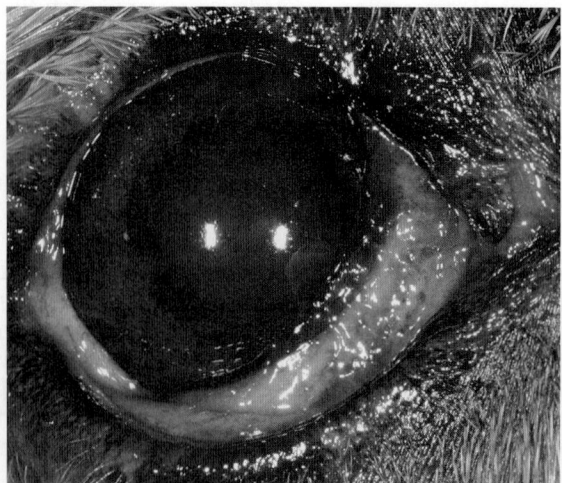

Figure 244-6 Canine herpesvirus 1 conjunctivitis in a dog associated with multifocal conjunctival epithelial ulceration and conjunctival petechiae.

In otherwise healthy dogs, CHV-1 conjunctivitis typically is self-limiting. Antiviral treatment shortens the duration of clinical disease and prevents development of more severe ocular or systemic sequelae in immunosuppressed dogs. In addition to nonspecific treatments to prevent secondary bacterial infection, antiviral therapy with 0.1% idoxuridine, 1% trifluridine, or 0.5% cidofovir ophthalmic solution can be used. Idoxuridine and trifluridine are administered six to eight times daily for the first 48 hours and then four times daily until active clinical signs resolve. Cidofovir is reportedly effective with twice-daily administration.

Parasitic conjunctivitis may result from infection with *Thelazia* or *Onchocerca*. Both parasites have a geographically restricted range. *Thelazia* spp. are nematodes transmitted by flies that reside in the conjunctival fornix and nasolacrimal duct. Diagnosis is made by identifying thin, white, motile, 1.0- to 1.5-cm-long parasites on the ocular surface. Therapy for *Thelazia* conjunctivitis includes manual parasite removal or use of antiparasitic agents, such as topical ophthalmic application of ivermectin or moxidectin or dermal application of imidacloprid and moxidectin. *Onchocerca* spp. are filaria that produce conjunctivitis associated with single or multiple bulbar conjunctival nodules. Diagnosis is by histopathologic demonstration of the parasites, typically with surrounding eosinophilic or granulomatous inflammation. Surgical excision of the nodules is the treatment of choice.

Traumatic Conjunctivitis

Blunt or penetrating trauma can produce conjunctivitis. Both forms may be self-inflicted in dogs with other painful or pruritic ocular diseases. Conjunctival trauma often is associated initially with dramatic chemosis and subconjunctival hemorrhage (see Figure 244-2). It is imperative to exclude the presence of other ocular injuries and foreign bodies, but this can be difficult on initial presentation if severe chemosis precludes performing a complete ocular examination. Ocular and orbital ultrasonography can be used in these situations or reexamination can be attempted following symptomatic therapy. Treatment includes application of cold compresses and a topical ophthalmic antimicrobial to prevent opportunistic bacterial infection. Systemic nonsteroidal antiinflammatory treatment hastens improvement in clinical signs. For penetrating or full-thickness wounds, a course of a systemic antimicrobial (e.g., cephalexin or amoxicillin/clavulanic acid) is indicated to prevent orbital infection. The extensive conjunctival vascular supply that results in dramatic conjunctivitis following trauma typically permits rapid resolution of clinical signs. Small conjunctival lacerations do not require surgical closure because the conjunctiva heals spontaneously and rapidly; however, foreign material should be removed by irrigation.

Secondary Manifestation of Other Ocular Diseases

Because of anatomic proximity, shared blood supply, and extensive vascular and lymphoid tissue, the conjunctiva may be secondarily affected by other ocular diseases.

Conjunctivitis is a frequent manifestation of a variety of potentially serious extraocular and intraocular diseases, including blepharitis, ulcerative keratitis, keratoconjunctivitis sicca, uveitis, glaucoma, and orbital disease. In these conditions, conjunctivitis develops from an active extension of inflammation or passively from increased regional blood flow or decreased venous drainage. Failure to exclude other ocular conditions as the cause of conjunctivitis in the dog is a common error and is avoided by performing a complete ocular examination. When conjunctivitis is a secondary manifestation, therapy should be directed toward the primary ocular condition.

Secondary Manifestation of Systemic Diseases

Because the conjunctiva is relatively accessible and observable, systemic diseases may first manifest in a detectable manner as conjunctivitis. The extensive vascular and lymphoid tissues within the conjunctiva also render it susceptible to generalized vascular and lymphatic diseases. A number of serious and potentially life-threatening systemic diseases can be associated with conjunctivitis. These include infectious diseases such as (in alphabetical order) anaplasmosis, borreliosis, botulism, canine distemper, canine influenza, ehrlichiosis, leishmaniasis, leptospirosis, listeriosis, protothecosis, Rocky Mountain spotted fever, systemic mycosis, and toxoplasmosis. Neoplastic disorders including lymphoma, multiple myeloma, and systemic histiocytosis can involve the conjunctival tissues. Vascular diseases and hematologic disorders, including coagulopathies and thrombocytopenia, hyperviscosity syndromes, plasminogen deficiency, polycythemia, and systemic hypertension, are additional systemic causes of conjunctivitis. The listed systemic conditions are especially likely to present as conjunctivitis, with or without additional ocular abnormalities. In the majority of dogs, historical and physical examination findings suggest a systemic disease process.

References and Suggested Reading

Bianciardi P, Otranto D: Treatment of dog thelaziasis caused by *Thelazia callipaeda* (Spiruda, Thelaziidae) using a topical formulation of imidacloprid 10% and moxidectin 2.5%, *Vet Parasitol* 129:89, 2005.

Gonzalez Alonso-Alegre EM, Rodriguez Alvaro A, Rollan Landeras E: Comparison of cyclosporin A and dexamethasone in the treatment of canine nictitans plasmacytic conjunctivitis, *Vet Rec* 144:696, 1999.

Hurn S, McCowam C, Turner A: Oral doxycycline, niacinamide and prednisolone used to treat bilateral nodular granulomatous conjunctivitis of the third eyelid in an Australian Kelpie dog, *Vet Ophthalmol* 8:349, 2005.

Ledbetter EC, Hornbuckle WE, Dubovi EJ: Virologic survey of dogs with naturally acquired idiopathic conjunctivitis, *J Am Vet Med Assoc* 235:954, 2009.

Lourenço-Martins AM et al: Allergic conjunctivitis and conjunctival provocation tests in atopic dogs, *Vet Ophthalmol* 14:248, 2011.

Peňa MA, Leiva M: Canine conjunctivitis and blepharitis, *Vet Clin North Am Small Anim Pract* 38:233, 2008.

CHAPTER 245

Tear Film Disorders in Dogs

ELIZABETH A. GIULIANO, *Columbia, Missouri*

Canine patients frequently are brought to the veterinary practitioner with chronic keratitis or conjunctivitis as a result of a tear film disorder. Keratoconjunctivitis sicca (KCS) is characterized by ocular discomfort, ocular discharge, redness, and corneal opacities that may lead to blindness. KCS results primarily from deficiency of aqueous tears, the fluid comprising approximately 95% of the total tear volume, and therefore sometimes is referred to as a *quantitative tear deficiency*. Deficiencies of the other primary tear components (mucin and lipid) have been referred to as *qualitative tear deficiencies*. This chapter focuses on *quantitative* tear film deficiencies in dogs.

Anatomy and Physiology

The precorneal tear film (PTF) is crucial for the maintenance of ocular surface health and clear vision. Its functions include serving as the primary oxygen source for the avascular cornea, lubricating between the eyelids and ocular surface, providing protective antimicrobial proteins, and removing debris and exfoliated cells. The PTF classically is described as a superimposition of three layers consisting of lipid, aqueous, and mucin components, including the innermost layer of glycocalyx extending from the superficial layer of the ocular surface epithelia.

The lipid layer is secreted by the meibomian glands and provides a thin, oily component to the PTF that retards evaporation and promotes a stable, even spread of tears over the cornea. Meibomian glands are highly developed in the dog; 20 to 40 glands per eyelid typically are present in the dog's tarsal plate and form linear aggregates of secretory acini. The aqueous component of the PTF provides the avascular cornea with glucose, electrolytes, oxygen, and water. In dogs, aqueous tears are secreted by orbital and third eyelid lacrimal glands and consist of water, inorganic salts, proteins, glucose, urea, and surface-active polymers composed primarily of glycoproteins. Mucus, the third component to the PTF, is produced primarily by conjunctival goblet cells and is composed of mucin, immunoglobulins, urea, glycoproteins, salts, glucose, leukocytes, cellular debris, and enzymes. The mucous layer helps to provide a smooth refractive surface over the cornea, lubricates the cornea and conjunctiva, anchors the aqueous tear film to the corneal epithelium thus decreasing shear forces, inhibits bacterial adherence, and prevents desiccation. The health and function of the PTF depends not only on the production of normal secretory components but also on eyelid integrity, normal ocular motility, and an intact blink mechanism.

Deficiency of aqueous tears (i.e., quantitative tear deficiency) may result in inflammation, metaplasia, and necrosis of surface cells by several mechanisms. Tear deficiency results in hypertonicity and dehydration of the conjunctiva and cornea, hypoxia of corneal epithelium and subepithelial corneal stroma, increased susceptibility to ocular infections, frictional irritation by the eyelids and third eyelid, and accumulation of potentially toxic tissue metabolites such as lactic acid, desquamated cells, denatured mucus, and other microscopic debris. Qualitative tear film deficiencies are characterized by more rapid tear film breakup due to an abnormality in either the lipid or mucin component of the PTF and subsequent tear film instability.

Causes

A decrease in lacrimal secretions may result from a single disease process or a combination of conditions affecting the orbital and third eyelid glands. Immune-mediated KCS appears to constitute the largest group of clinical cases in dogs. Infectious causes of lacrimal adenitis include canine distemper and bacterial blepharoconjunctivitis caused by chronic staphylococcal infection. Congenital acinar hypoplasia is a breed-related cause (e.g., in Yorkshire and Bedlington terriers). Drug-induced KCS may occur in dogs treated with either systemic sulfonamides or repeated topical administration of atropine. Preanesthetic and anesthetic agents are known to reduce tear secretion, and anesthetic events lasting longer than 2 hours have a more prolonged effect on Schirmer's tear test values than those lasting less than 2 hours. Removal of the third eyelid gland remains an important iatrogenic cause of dry eye in dogs. Decreased aqueous tear production may develop in association with systemic metabolic diseases such as hypothyroidism, diabetes mellitus, and Cushing's disease. Other causes include uncorrected third eyelid gland prolapse, traumatic and inflammatory orbital diseases, loss of parasympathetic innervation to the lacrimal glands (cranial nerve VII), and loss of sensory innervation to the ocular surface (cranial nerve V).

Clinical Signs

Clinical signs are nonspecific in the early stages of KCS (i.e., red, inflamed eyes with intermittent mucoid or mucopurulent discharge); therefore the disease often is misdiagnosed as an ocular allergy or primary bacterial conjunctivitis. As the KCS becomes subacute or chronic, the ocular surface develops a lackluster appearance, the conjunctiva appears more hyperemic, and tenacious mucopurulent ocular discharge is observed. As the disease progresses, keratitis develops, characterized by corneal vascularization, pigmentation, and fibrosis, with or without ulceration. Blepharitis with periocular dermatitis often appears simultaneously with accumulation of exudates along the eyelids. Ocular discomfort intensifies, and affected eyes are often partially squinted or completely closed.

Diagnosis

Tear film abnormalities are diagnosed based on the presence of typical clinical signs, positive results on ocular staining with vital stains, and a finding of quantitative or qualitative tear deficiency. Rose bengal stain detects devitalized cells and subtle epithelial defects on either conjunctival or corneal surfaces. Fluorescein stain is used primarily to detect concurrent corneal ulceration but also may be used to evaluate tear breakup, or the ability of the corneal surface to retain a homogeneous tear covering. Schirmer's tear test (STT) remains the standard for quantifying aqueous tear production. In any dog with a red, irritated eye, ocular discharge, or corneal disease of undetermined cause STTs should be performed.

STTs may be done either without topical anesthetic (STT I) or with topical anesthetic (SST II). Testing without anesthetic measures the ability of the eye to produce reflex tears in addition to basal secretions and is performed most commonly. STT I readings in dogs generally are interpreted as follows: 15 mm/min or more is considered normal production; 11 to 14 mm/min indicates early or subclinical KCS; 6 to 10 mm/min is classified as moderate or mild KCS; and 5 mm/min or less indicates severe KCS. Repetition of STT measurements is advised in dogs that are stressed by examination or receive medical therapy for ulcerative corneal disease because sympathetic stimulation caused by stress or current topical treatments (specifically atropine administration) may reduce tear secretions. Evaluation of patients with KCS also should include examination for possible associated systemic disease conditions (e.g., hypothyroidism), assessment of eyelid function and blink reflexes, and culture and cytologic analysis in selected cases. Secondary bacterial conjunctivitis is common in canine KCS cases and resistant microorganisms may develop if previous treatment has included a number of different antibiotic preparations.

Treatment

Medical Therapy

Medical therapy is the mainstay of canine KCS management. The specific treatment regimen is tailored to the individual patient and is influenced by the client's ability to comply with the recommended treatment schedule. Depending on the severity of KCS, medical treatment generally consists of some combination of the following: (1) tear stimulation, (2) tear replacement, (3) topical antimicrobial drugs, (4) mucinolytic therapy, and (5) antiinflammatory agents.

Lacrimostimulants

Lacrimostimulants, drugs administered to promote tear secretion, include two broad categories of therapeutic agents: cholinergics and immunomodulators such as cyclosporine.

Cholinergic Agents

The lacrimal gland is innervated both sympathetically and parasympathetically. In KCS cases resulting from parasympathetic denervation of the lacrimal gland, cholinergic drugs sometimes have been used successfully to stimulate tearing. Ophthalmic pilocarpine solution may be administered either topically or orally as a tear stimulant. Its effectiveness depends on the presence of some functional lacrimal gland, and thus its use generally is unrewarding in cases of absolute KCS. For oral administration a 1% to 2% ophthalmic solution is applied to the food. A safe initial oral dosage is one drop of 2% topical pilocarpine per 10 kg body weight in food twice daily. The dose may be increased gradually by one-drop increments until signs of systemic reaction develop, (i.e., salivation, vomiting, bradycardia, or diarrhea) and is then lowered to the previously tolerated dose. Concurrent administration of other parasympathomimetic agents (e.g., organophosphates or carbamate antiparasitic agents) should be avoided to prevent potentiation of adverse effects. Alternatively, topical dilute pilocarpine has been applied directly to the eyes with variable success. Concentrations of 0.125% or 0.25% can be applied after being diluted as follows: add 1 ml of 2% solution to 15 ml of artificial tears to make a 0.125% solution, or add 2 ml of 2% solution to 14 ml of artificial tears to make a 0.25% solution. Topical pilocarpine, even when diluted, may cause conjunctival hyperemia, miosis, and sufficient irritation to necessitate discontinuing topical treatments. The route of pilocarpine administration may be determined by the individual patient's tolerance for one method over the other.

Immunomodulators

An immune-mediated cause is presumed for most cases of canine KCS. Cyclosporine A (CsA), a derivative of the fungus *Tolypocladium inflatum,* and tacrolimus (formally FK-506), a macrolide antibiotic produced by *Streptomyces tsukubaensis,* are both T-cell activation inhibitors initially developed for their systemic uses in preventing graft rejection after organ transplantation. Although CsA and tacrolimus are structurally nonhomologous, the mechanism of action is similar for both drugs, with T-cell proliferation and activation altered by the inhibition of interleukin-2 (IL-2) gene expression in CD4$^+$ helper T lymphocytes. IL-2 transcription blockage leads to impaired proliferation of helper T and cytotoxic T cells. Both immunomodulating and tear-stimulating properties appear to account for the dramatic responses observed in many affected dogs after topical application. At present, topical CsA or tacrolimus represents the *primary treatment* for canine KCS.

To stimulate tear production, topical CsA usually is recommended first, with application every 12 hours to affected eyes. However, in severe cases treatment intervals can be reduced to every 8 hours. Several weeks of continuous treatment usually is needed before substantial increases in tear production are observed. In cases in which CsA treatment has been administered every 12 hours for 3 weeks or longer and the STT values remain at or below 10 mm/min, the topical frequency may be increased to every 8 hours or higher topical concentrations of CsA may be prescribed. The most accurate assessment of response to CsA is obtained when tear production is measured 3 hours after topical administration. When CsA administration every 12 hours restores tears to physiologic levels (STT reading of ≥15 mm/min) therapy often may be reduced to a once-daily maintenance regimen. In cases unresponsive to topical CsA therapy, tacrolimus is prescribed and applied topically every 12 hours. Tacrolimus has been estimated to be 10 to 100 times more potent than CsA *in vitro.* Formulations of 0.02% to 0.03% tacrolimus in aqueous or oil-based suspensions, as well as ointment formulations, are available through various compounding pharmacies in the United States. Some ophthalmologists prefer to use tacrolimus instead of CsA as their first-line drug of choice when treating dogs with KCS.

Tear Substitutes (Lacrimomimetics)

Tear substitutes contain ingredients to replace deficiencies in one or more of the three primary tear components (aqueous elements, mucin, lipid). Many ophthalmic solutions and ointments are available commercially for tear-replacement therapy (Table 245-1), and new products frequently emerge. Selection of a particular agent is influenced by the nature of the deficiency, availability, cost, clinician preference, patient compatibility, and owner acceptance. Aqueous tear-replacement agents initially are applied to affected eyes four to six times daily and generally are used concurrently with other topical therapeutic agents. Although more frequent applications (i.e., every 1 or 2 hours) often are desirable, this treatment frequency rarely is possible or practical for the pet owner. Despite these limitations, the use of lacrimomimetics is warranted in the treatment of qualitative tear film abnormalities and as an adjunct to lacrimostimulant therapy for quantitative tear film deficiencies.

Methylcellulose products are virtually inert, water soluble, viscous, semisynthetic cellulose colloids. Because cellulose derivatives are nonirritating to the eye, do not significantly delay corneal wound healing, and are compatible with most drugs, they commonly are used as aqueous tear substitutes and aqueous vehicles for other

TABLE 245-1

Tear Substitutes*

Product	Viscosity Agent/ Concentration	Preservative	Product	Viscosity Agent/ Concentration	Preservative
Polyvinyl Alcohol Solutions			Refresh	PVA 1.4%, povidone 0.6%	None
Akwa Tears	PVA 1.4%	BAC, EDTA	Refresh Tears Plus	PVA 1.4%, povidone 0.6%	Chlorobutanol
Artificial tears	PVA 1.4%	BAC, EDTA	Tears Naturale	HPMC 0.3%, DEX 0.1%	BAC, EDTA
Liquifilm Tears	PVA 1.4%	Chlorobutanol	Tears Naturale II	HPMC 0.3%, DEX-70 0.1%	POLYQUAD
Teargen	PVA	BAC, EDTA	Tears Naturale Free	HPMC 0.3%, DEX 0.1%	None
Cellulose-Based Solutions			Tears Renewed	HPMC 0.3%, DEX-70 0.1%	BAC, EDTA
Celluvisc	CMC 1%	None	**Viscoelastic Products**		
Comfort Tears	HEC	BAC, EDTA	Hylashield	Hylan 0.15%	None
GenTeal	HPMC 0.3%	None	Hylashield Nite	Hylan 0.4%	None
Isopto Tears Plain	HPMC 0.5%	BAC, EDTA	I-Drop	Hyaluronate 0.3%	None
Murocel	MC 1%	Methylparaben Propylparaben	**Glycerin Products**		
Nature's Tears	HPMC 0.4%	BAC, EDTA	Eye-Lube-A	Glycerin 0.25%	BAC, EDTA
Refresh Plus	CMC 0.5%	None	**Ointments**		
Refresh Tears	CMC 0.5%	None	Akwa Tears ointment	White petrolatum, MO	None
Teargen II	HPMC 4 mg	BAC, EDTA	Duratears Naturale	White petrolatum, lanolin, MO	None
Polymer Combinations			Hypo Tears	White petrolatum 85%, MO 15%	None
Aqua Site	PEG-400 0.2%, DEX 0.1%	EDTA	Moisture Eyes PM	White petrolatum 80%, MO 20%	None
Bion Tears	DEX 0.1%, HPMC 0.3%	None	Puralube	White petrolatum, MO	None
Hypo Tears	PVA 1%, PEG-400	BAC, EDTA	Refresh Lacri-Lube	Mineral Oil 42.5%, white petrolatum 56.8%	Chlorobutanol
Hypo Tears PF	PVA 1%, PEG-400	EDTA			
Lubri-Tears	HPMC 0.5%, DEX 0.1%	BAC, EDTA	Refresh P.M.	White petrolatum 56.8%, lanolin, MO 41.5%	None
Optixcare	Carbomer, sorbitol	EDTA, cetrimide			
Murine Eye Lubricant	PVA 0.5%, povidone 0.6%	BAC, EDTA	Tears Renewed	White petrolatum, MO	None
Nature's Tears	HPMC 0.4%	BAC, EDTA			
OcuCoat	DEX-70 0.1%, HPMC 0.8%	BAC			

From Giuliano EA: *Veterinary ophthalmology*, ed 5, Hoboken, NJ, Wiley-Blackwell (in press). Table compiled courtesy of Cynthia K. Gause, RPh.
*Percentage composition given when this information is available.
BAC, Benzalkonium chloride; *CMC*, carboxymethyl cellulose; *DEX*, dextran; *EDTA*, ethylenediaminetetraacetic acid; *GEL*, gelatin; *HEC*, hydroxyethyl cellulose; *HPMC*, hydroxypropyl methylcellulose; *MC*, methylcellulose; *MO*, mineral oil; *PEG*, polyethylene glycol; *POLYQUAD*, polyquaternium-1; *PSB*, polysorbate 80; *PVA*, polyvinyl alcohol.

ophthalmic preparations. Polyvinyl alcohol (PVA) is a hydrophilic resin that is less viscous than methylcellulose but has good corneal adhesive properties. Usually provided as a 1.4% solution, PVA is the primary ingredient in a number of artificial-tear products. One PVA-based product (Hypo Tears) is formulated as a hypotonic fluid to counter the hypertonic tears of patients with KCS.

Viscous lubricants enhance ocular surface wettability and have extended contact time with the ocular surface. Linear polymers such as dextran and polyvinylpyrrolidone (povidone) have mucinomimetic properties. Polymers have been combined with buffered solutions of substituted cellulose esters to form preparations for

treating deficiencies of both the aqueous and mucin components of the preocular tear film. Solutions containing linear polymers remain on the eye for longer periods than solutions without these derivatives.

Viscoelastic substances with mucinomimetic properties include sodium hyaluronate, chondroitin sulfate, and 1% to 2% methylcellulose preparations. A hyaluronic acid–derivative viscoelastic tear supplement is available commercially in North America (Hylashield) as a 0.15% or 0.40% drop. Anecdotal reports indicate that this product has been useful in managing KCS in dogs with suspected ocular mucin deficiency. Chondroitin sulfate, which is a glycosaminoglycan polymer made of disaccharide units, is slightly less viscous than sodium hyaluronate. One percent methylcellulose (Celluvisc) is more viscous than methylcellulose at the usual concentration of 0.5% and may serve as a less expensive substitute for sodium hyaluronate or chondroitin sulfate.

Lanolin, petrolatum, and mineral oil commonly are used as bases for ophthalmic lubricating ointments. These ingredients mimic the function of naturally occurring meibomian lipids by preventing evaporation and thus preserving existing tears. Duration of lubrication usually is of greater concern than transient blurring of vision in animals, and ointments are used extensively in veterinary patients. Nonmedicated ophthalmic ointments containing one or more of these ingredients are used to lubricate and protect the eyes when corneal exposure is a problem, such as during general anesthesia or in cases of eyelid paresis or eyelid swelling.

Ointment vehicles also prolong corneal and conjunctival contact for therapeutics such as corticosteroids and antibiotics. Antibiotic ointments may be more economical than and as effective as lubricants, with the additional advantage of having antibacterial effects. Although ophthalmic ointments remain on the eye longer than drops, they can be more difficult for some owners to apply. Warming the tube of ointment under hot water for 10 to 15 seconds (with the ointment cap firmly sealed) immediately before ointment instillation facilitates application.

Preservatives (e.g., benzalkonium chloride, chlorobutanol, methyl parathimerosal) often are used in lacrimomimetic formulations to maintain stability of solutions in multiple-dose bottles and to prolong shelf life. If a tear replacement containing preservative is recommended, topical application should be limited to six or fewer applications per day to avoid epithelial toxicity. Preservative-free tear solutions should be used when more frequent application is indicated or when a preservative causes irritation. Preservative-free products are more expensive and typically are dispensed in single-dose vials that can be cumbersome for an owner to use.

Antibacterials
Antibiotics with broad-spectrum activity, such as triple antibiotic ointment or solution, commonly are administered to control the secondary bacterial infections that often occur with inadequate wetting of the ocular surface. Initial frequency of treatment is usually three to four times daily. This is reduced to twice daily as mucopurulent discharge decreases, and the antibiotic eventually is discontinued once signs of infection have abated. In cases of persistent mucopurulent discharge, bacterial culture and sensitivity testing should be performed.

Mucinolytic and Anticollagenase Agents
Good ocular hygiene, including the frequent cleansing of ocular discharge, is essential to minimize accumulation of degradative enzymes that contribute to ocular surface inflammation and ulceration. A 5% to 10% solution of acetylcysteine may be applied topically two to four times daily to facilitate removal of the copious exudates and mucoid debris that accompany KCS. In addition, acetylcysteine's anticollagenase properties may aid in preventing enzymatic degradation of surface tissues and be useful in the treatment of corneal ulceration. The author advocates the use of preservative-free saline solution to rinse the ocular surface at least twice daily in dogs with moderate to severe KCS.

Antiinflammatory Agents
Antiinflammatory therapy can be a valuable adjunct to other medical therapy in improving clinical signs in cases of KCS. Topical corticosteroids commonly are administered to minimize conjunctivitis, alleviate discomfort, and reduce corneal opacities associated with chronic keratitis. Triple antibiotic ointment in combination with hydrocortisone is beneficial to many dogs with KCS. However, topical corticosteroids are contraindicated if the cornea retains fluorescein stain, and their use can complicate the healing of a corneal ulcer. Long-term administration of topical corticosteroids also can cause local immunosuppression and predispose the eye to secondary infections.

Besides their marked lacrimostimulant effects, topical CsA and tacrolimus have beneficial antiinflammatory properties such as reducing corneal vascularization. In contrast to corticosteroids, these drugs appear safe to use in the presence of corneal ulceration and also may be beneficial in reducing corneal pigmentation in animals with chronic pigmentary keratitis associated with KCS.

Surgical Therapy

Surgical procedures may be indicated in the management of selected cases of KCS, and these are best performed by an ophthalmologist. The most common procedures are parotid duct transposition, which allows saliva to substitute for tears, and permanent partial tarsorrhaphy, which reduces exposure and enhances blinking. Occlusion of the nasolacrimal puncta is used by some as a tear-conserving procedure and works by blocking tear drainage. Replacement of the third eye gland (versus gland removal) is regarded as a preventive surgical procedure for canine KCS. Descriptions of surgical procedures are beyond the scope of this textbook.

References and Suggested Reading

Berdoulay A, English RV, Nadelstein B: Effect of topical 0.02% tacrolimus aqueous suspension on tear production in dogs with keratoconjunctivitis sicca, *Vet Ophthalmol* 8:225, 2005.

Carter R, Colitz CMH: The causes, diagnosis, and treatment of canine keratoconjunctivitis sicca, *Vet Med* 97:683, 2002.

Gelatt KN et al: Effect of lacrimal punctal occlusion on tear production and tear fluorescein dilution in normal dogs, *Vet Ophthalmol* 9:23, 2006.

Hendrix DVH et al: An investigation comparing the efficacy of topical ocular application of tacrolimus and cyclosporine in dogs, *Vet Med Int* 2011:487592, 2011.

Moore CP: Qualitative tear film disease, *Vet Clin North Am Small Anim Pract* 20:565, 1990.

Plummer CE et al: Intranictitans tacking for replacement of prolapsed gland of the third eyelid in dogs, *Vet Ophthalmol* 11:228, 2008.

Sanchez RF et al: Canine keratoconjunctivitis sicca: disease trends in a review of 229 cases, *J Small Anim Pract* 48:211, 2007.

CHAPTER 246

Corneal Ulcers

AMBER LABELLE, *Urbana, Illinois*

Corneal Anatomy

The cornea and sclera make up the tough and protective fibrous tunic of the eye. The cornea is composed of five layers: precorneal tear film, epithelium with basement membrane, stroma, Descemet's membrane, and endothelium (Figure 246-1). The cornea can be described as a "fat-water-fat" sandwich; the epithelium and endothelium–Descemet's membrane are hydrophobic, whereas the collagenous stroma is hydrophilic.

The epithelium of the cornea is protected and nourished by the precorneal tear film, which consists of three layers: (1) a mucus layer produced by the goblet cells of the conjunctiva, (2) an aqueous layer produced by the orbital lacrimal gland and gland of the third eyelid, and (3) a lipid layer produced by the meibomian glands. Functions of the tear film include lubrication of the ocular surface, provision of oxygen and nutrients for the anterior cornea, removal of waste products, immunoprotection (via endogenous components, including immunoglobulin A and lysozyme), and maintenance of optical transparency. A normal, healthy tear film is critical for the maintenance of corneal health.

The corneal epithelium is approximately six to eight cell layers thick, with the deepest layer being comprised of columnar basal cells. The epithelium is nonkeratinized and firmly attached to the underlying stroma by hemidesmosomes. The epithelium has an important function as a physical barrier to prevent the seepage of the precorneal tear film into the cornea. It also acts as a barrier to microorganisms, preserving the integrity of all other ocular structures.

Stroma represents approximately 90% of the corneal thickness. It is composed of well-organized, parallel layers of collagen fibrils, glycosaminoglycans, and a relatively low number of keratocytes. The bulk of the stroma is comprised of water, which makes this corneal layer highly hydrophilic. The precise anatomic arrangement of the collagen fibrils allows light to pass through the cornea without scatter.

Descemet's membrane is the basement membrane (10 to 15 μm thick) of the corneal endothelium. It is highly hydrophobic and gets thicker with age. The endothelium is a single layer of hexagonal cells lining the inner surface of the cornea. The endothelial cell layer is very active metabolically and plays the major role in maintaining corneal transparency. Adenosine triphosphate–dependent pumps on the endothelial cells help to transport water actively out of the corneal stroma to maintain its relatively dehydrated state.

Physiology of Corneal Transparency

Corneal transparency is maintained by the following five mechanisms:

1. The corneal epithelium contains no pigment.
2. The cornea is avascular.
3. The corneal epithelium is nonkeratinized.
4. The stromal collagen lamellae have a precise anatomic arrangement.
5. The corneal stroma is relatively dehydrated.

Loss of corneal transparency results from a disruption of one of these normal physiologic mechanisms. Corneal ulceration results in corneal stromal edema due to loss of the hydrophobic epithelial barrier. Corneal vascularization or pigmentation may develop with chronic corneal ulceration. Keratinization typically is observed at a microscopic level in patients with keratoconjunctivitis sicca (KCS), but it usually is not associated with corneal ulceration. Alterations in the regular arrangement of the stromal lamellae lead to loss of transparency. Scar formation following injury of the stroma results in opacity due to misalignment of the collagen fibers.

Corneal Wound Healing

Wounds that involve the corneal epithelium heal differently than wounds that involve the stroma. Epithelium is mitotically active and quick to repair superficial wounds. Epithelial cells at the edges of the ulcerated area release their attachments to neighboring cells, migrate to cover the wound, undergo mitosis to rebuild the normal epithelial thickness, and then reestablish their connection to the underlying basement membrane. Epithelium migrates at a rate of approximately 1 mm/day from both sides of the ulcer bed. Stromal wounds are much slower to heal. For a wound involving stroma to resolve, epithelium must slide over the defect and keratocytes must be activated into a fibroblast phenotype, migrate to the wound bed, remodel the injured collagen, and synthesize new collagen. This process takes weeks to months to complete. Corneal fibrosis typically results from wounds involving the stroma because newly synthesized collagen does not have the precise anatomic orientation of mature collagen. If epithelialization precedes stromal remodeling, a corneal facet can occur. A facet is an area of thin stroma covered by intact epithelium. It is important to differentiate a healed facet from a descemetocele by carefully observing the fluorescein staining pattern of the lesion. A facet does not retain fluorescein dye, whereas a

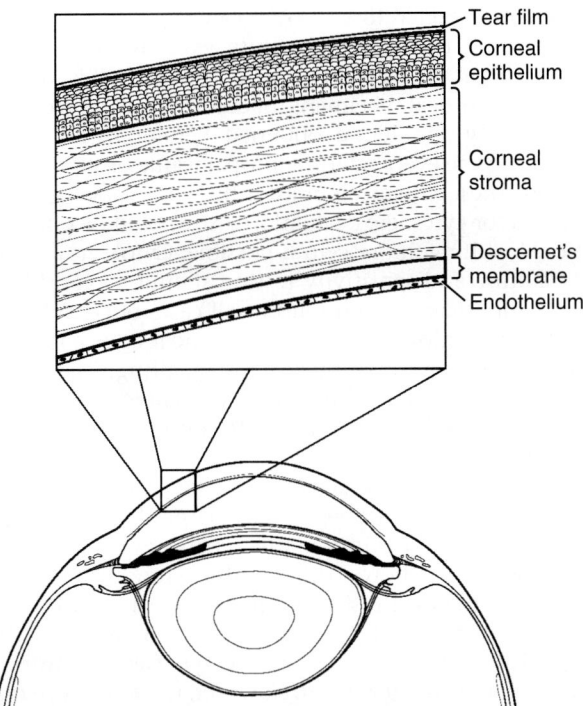

Figure 246-1 Diagram of equine cornea. Enlarged inset demonstrates relative proportions of corneal epithelium, stroma, and Descemet's membrane/endothelium. (From Gilger B: *Equine ophthalmology,* ed 2, St Louis, 2011, Saunders.)

descemetocele likely shows fluorescein retention in the wall but not in the base of the ulceration.

Diagnosis of Corneal Ulceration

A corneal erosion, also called an *abrasion,* is a loss of several layers of corneal epithelium without exposure of the underlying stroma. Ulceration occurs when there is full-thickness loss of the epithelial barrier and the underlying stroma is exposed. The diagnosis can be confirmed by the application of fluorescein sodium solution to the corneal surface. Sterile fluorescein paper strips are used, and after the application of one or two drops of eyewash or saline solution the strip is touched gently to the conjunctiva. Excess fluorescein should be rinsed from the ocular surface to prevent false-positive results. True fluorescein staining cannot be removed from the ocular surface by irrigation. The water-soluble fluorescein molecule normally is repelled by the hydrophobic corneal epithelium. When epithelium has been removed, as in the case of an ulcer, the hydrophilic stroma is revealed and fluorescein binds readily to the tissue, which results in a "positive" fluorescein retention or staining result. Descemet's membrane is hydrophobic, so if all the stroma has been lost (as in a descemetocele), the bottom of the ulcer will not show any fluorescein retention (but the exposed stroma in the walls of the ulcer will).

All corneal ulcers can be categorized as simple ulcers or complicated ulcers. Simple ulcers will heal with supportive care. Complicated ulcers require recognition and correction of the complicating factor before they will heal.

Simple Corneal Ulcers

Simple ulcers are defined by the following criteria:

1. *Superficial.* Only epithelium has been lost, with no loss of stroma.
2. *No evidence of infection.* Infection in the cornea usually appears as stromal infiltrate, which is caused by inflammatory cells migrating within the cornea that give it a yellow, white, or tan appearance.
3. *Healing in an appropriate amount of time.* Epithelium is very mitotically active, and even an ulcer that encompasses 90% of the corneal surface (provided it involves loss of epithelium and no loss of stroma) can be expected to be healed in 7 to 10 days. Ulcers usually take about 1 day to heal for every 1 mm of width.
4. *No complicating factors.* No underlying cause for the ulcer can be identified that would need to be corrected.

The cause of most simple ulcers is likely trauma. However, if the clinician identifies a cause (such as entropion) then the ulcer is no longer simple—it is complicated!

Treatment of Simple Ulcers

A topical antibiotic ointment or drop should be used every 6 to 8 hours until the corneal surface is negative for fluorescein staining, which indicates that reepithelialization has occurred. The purpose of topical antibiotics in treatment of a simple ulcer is to keep the wound from becoming infected. Systemic antibiotics do *not* achieve effective levels in the cornea, and topical medications are needed. A broad-spectrum antibiotic is most desirable. Triple antibiotic preparations (neomycin/polymyxin/ bacitracin or gramicidin) are ideal for their spectrum of coverage. Aminoglycosides should not be used alone because of their lack of efficacy against gram-positive organisms. Gram-positive bacteria constitute a significant proportion of the canine ocular flora and are likely opportunistic pathogens.

Atropine 1% solution or ointment should be administered every 12 to 24 hours. An axonal reflex mediated by cranial nerve V causes reflex uveitis, including spasm of the ciliary body musculature and miosis. Atropine induces cycloplegia, or paralysis of the ciliary body, which alleviates the pain caused by spasm of the ciliary body. Mydriasis is an additional effect of atropine and may make the patient more sensitive to light. In most cases, once-daily administration or a one-time administration of atropine during the first examination is sufficient to induce cycloplegia and mydriasis. Atropine administration is contraindicated in patients with or predisposed to glaucoma. A systemic nonsteroidal antiinflammatory (NSAID) or an opioid such as tramadol can be used for 3 to 5 days to provide additional analgesia. An Elizabethan collar may be necessary to prevent self-trauma but is unnecessary in most cases.

The average simple ulcer should be healed in less than a week, and in most cases within 3 to 4 days. Any prolonged healing should prompt complete and thorough reexamination and possibly referral to an ophthalmologist for a second opinion. Brachycephalic patients are more likely to experience complications in their wound healing than nonbrachycephalic breeds. A recheck 24 to 48 hours after initial diagnosis is warranted in these patients to ensure that the ulcer is healing as expected.

Complicated Corneal Ulcers

Complicated ulcers are defined by the following criteria:

1. *Increasing depth or stromal loss.* Whenever an ulcer involves loss of both epithelium and stroma, its healing process becomes more complicated. Although epithelium is highly mitotically active, stroma is composed of collagen fibers with few keratocytes. When the stroma is wounded, the process of activating keratocytes into fibroblasts that synthesize and replace the collagen is lengthy and prolongs the course of wound healing. Wounds that involve loss of stroma are slower to heal and are more likely to develop secondary complications like infection or malacia. An ulcer that has lost all stroma down to the level of Descemet's membrane is termed a *descemetocele.* In such a case, only a single layer of endothelium and its basement membrane remain, and complete rupture of the cornea is imminent.
2. *Infection or a melting appearance.* Infection is visible in the cornea as a yellow, white, or tan cellular infiltrate within the stroma. Infected ulcers also tend to be more painful because of the greater involvement of the stroma. The presence of infection can be confirmed by cytologic analysis and culture and sensitivity testing. Keratomalacia, or melting of the cornea, is the dissolving of the stromal collagen due to the action of collagenase and protease enzymes. There are two major sources of collagenase and protease: infectious organisms (bacteria, fungi) and white blood cells (especially neutrophils). Corneal melting can lead to corneal perforation if not treated appropriately.
3. *Failure to heal in an appropriate amount of time.* As indicated previously, any corneal ulcer that has not healed within 7 days should be considered a complicated ulcer and prompt reevaluation for complicating factors.
4. *Presence of complicating factors.* Complicating factors consist of a variety of causes of corneal ulceration that must be addressed before corneal wound healing can occur. Examples include KCS, entropion, eyelid tumors, lagophthalmos or inability to blink, ectopic cilia, glaucoma, corneal denervation or cranial nerve V deficit, and systemic immunocompromise (e.g., diabetes mellitus, Cushing's disease). If these underlying factors are not addressed, the ulcer will not heal. Once the complicating factor is resolved, the ulcer should heal within a reasonable time frame.

Diagnosis of Complicated Ulcers

A complete ophthalmic examination is key to making the correct diagnosis of complicated ulcer. Note that in cases of extreme stromal loss (>90%), caution should be taken in handling the patient because excessive restraint or struggling on the part of the patient may result in corneal rupture. If corneal specimens for culture are to be acquired, they ideally should be obtained before instilling any drops into the eye, including proparacaine or fluorescein, because these chemicals may inhibit microbial growth. Samples for cytologic evaluation also should be obtained before instilling fluorescein if possible. Cytologic analysis and culture and sensitivity testing should be considered mandatory diagnostic studies in all cases of complicated corneal ulceration, particularly chronic lesions and those showing stromal loss, infection, or melting. The results of cytologic evaluation guide initial choice of therapy, and culture and sensitivity results confirm or alter those choices.

If there is extreme stromal loss, avoiding Schirmer's tear test (STT) or tonometry may be prudent to prevent corneal rupture. It is important to perform these tests on the opposite eye, however, since the fellow eye may hold the key to the diagnosis. In a patient with KCS, the STT results may be within the normal range in an eye with a corneal ulcer because the patient hypersecretes tears in response to ocular irritation; however, the fellow eye may have an abnormally low STT value, revealing the diagnosis of KCS.

Treatment of Complicated Ulcers

The most important principle in treating complicated ulcers is to recognize the complicating factor and address it.

Treating Complicated Ulcers with Stromal Loss, Infection, and Melting

If there is more than a 50% stromal loss, the ideal treatment is surgical stabilization, such as a conjunctival graft. In these cases, the cornea is at risk of rupture with subsequent loss of vision from retinal detachment or chronic uveitis and cataract formation. These patients should be referred to a veterinary ophthalmologist for evaluation. If referral is not an option, the lesion should be managed as an infected or melting ulcer. Use of an Elizabethan collar to prevent self-trauma is important. In the case of corneal laceration with iris prolapse, referral should be strongly encouraged.

Results of the cytologic evaluation should guide initial antibiotic choices in the case of a deep melting or infected ulcer. If a mixed population of bacteria is observed, a fluoroquinolone such as ofloxacin 0.3% or levofloxacin 0.5% solution is recommended for broad-spectrum and potent coverage. An aminoglycoside such as gentamicin 0.3% or tobramycin 0.3% solution may be added if gram-negative bacteria or rods are observed. A cephalosporin or triple antibiotic may be added if gram-positive bacteria are noted. A triple antibiotic alone is not recommended because it has poor ability to penetrate into the cornea and anterior chamber. Antibiotic therapy should begin with administration every 2 to 4 hours and then decrease as the infection becomes controlled. Fungal keratitis is very rare in small animal patients. Since sensitivity to antifungal agents varies widely with geographic region, consultation with a local ophthalmologist who has experience with effective treatments in your region may be helpful. For example, in central Illinois, voriconazole 1% solution is the most common first-line antifungal agent.

Keratomalacia (melting) must be addressed with anticollagenase and antiprotease therapy. Autologous serum (serum harvested from the patient) is a highly effective anticollagenase-antiprotease. Serum can be obtained by collecting whole blood in a red-topped tube, centrifuging the clotted blood, and drawing the serum into a sterile eye dropper vial for dispensing. Serum should be stored aseptically in the refrigerator and replaced every 5 days. Ethylenediaminetetraacetic acid (EDTA), topical tetracyclines, systemic tetracyclines, and N-acetylcysteine are other anticollagenases-antiproteases that can be used in addition to autologous serum. An EDTA solution can be compounded in the clinic by filling a purple-topped (EDTA) blood collection vial half full with sterile 0.9% saline. The resultant EDTA solution can be administered directly to the corneal surface. Topical oxytetracycline/polymyxin B ointment (Terramycin) is a convenient way to administer tetracycline to the ocular surface. Alternatively, doxycycline 5 mg/kg q12h PO can be used. The frequency of administration of topical anticollagenases depends on the severity of the disease, with administration every 1 to 2 hours recommended for the most severely affected patients.

Most patients with deep infected or melting ulcers have significant concurrent uveitis. This uveitis is best addressed by administering systemic antiinflammatories such as oral NSAIDs or an antiinflammatory dose of oral corticosteroids. Topical atropine will relieve any accompanying ciliary body muscle spasm and also produce mydriasis, which prevents posterior synechiae. The use of topical corticosteroids is *contra*indicated for any corneal ulcer. The use of topical NSAIDs is controversial, and the author does not recommend their use in patients with complicated corneal ulcers.

Treating Complicated Ulcers with Slow Healing
As noted earlier, if a corneal ulcer is not healed within 7 days, it should be considered complicated. It is important then to consider why the ulcer is not healing and to look for evidence of stromal loss, infection or melting, or other complicating factors. If these all have been ruled out, then the ulcer may be indolent.

Treating Complicated Ulcers with Complicating Factors
Careful ophthalmic examination will reveal the presence of any complicating factors. It is imperative that these factors be corrected for the ulcer to heal. The treatment varies with the complicating factor and may include eyelid tacking to correct spastic entropion, medical therapy for dry eye, or surgical removal of an eyelid tumor that is abrading the cornea.

Treatment of the complicated ulcer can be rigorous. Medications may need to be administered very frequently, and multiple medications usually are required. Frequent recheck examinations may be needed in the case of the infected or melting ulcer. Adopting a systematic approach

to identifying factors that make an ulcer simple or complicated helps the clinician to create a logical and effective treatment plan.

Indolent Corneal Ulcers
Indolent ulcers represent a unique type of complicated corneal ulcer. They usually are diagnosed in older dogs and boxers. The classic clinical appearance is that of a superficial ulcer with nonadherent flaps of corneal epithelium at the margin of the ulcer. Fluorescein uptake may be observed beneath the ulcer edges. Superficial vascularization may or may not be present, and ocular pain is likewise variable. Most indolent ulcers are not associated with a significant degree of uveitis. An indolent ulcer is diagnosed based on the clinical characteristics as well as by exclusion of all other possible causes of corneal ulceration. Cytologic evaluation is recommended in all cases of suspected indolent ulcer and typically demonstrates abundant corneal epithelium with few or no inflammatory cells and no infectious organisms.

Treatment of Indolent Ulcers
Indolent ulcers in dogs are caused by a defect in the cell-cell adhesion molecules called *hemidesmosomes* that anchor epithelial cells to their underlying basement membrane and stroma. Treatment of an indolent ulcer requires disruption of that basement membrane to stimulate normal cell adhesion. These techniques, collectively called *anterior stromal puncture,* include such well-described methods as grid keratotomy and multiple punctate keratotomy. When anterior stromal puncture techniques fail, superficial keratectomy performed by a veterinary ophthalmologist may be curative, and referral is recommended in such cases. Several methods are summarized briefly in the following sections to explain the general approach to managing indolent ulcers, but the operator should be experienced before performing these procedures, and other textbooks detailing ophthalmologic procedures should be consulted.

Grid Keratotomy
Grid keratotomy is performed under gentle manual restraint and with topical anesthesia (proparacaine). The corneal surface may be prepared further by instilling dilute povidone-iodine solution. The nonadherent corneal epithelium then is gently débrided using a dry cotton-tipped applicator. All nonadherent epithelium must be removed for the grid keratotomy to be successful. A 25-gauge needle then is used to make fine lines in the anterior stroma by moving from normal cornea, across the ulcer bed, and then back into normal cornea on the other side of the ulcer. The entire surface area of the ulcer should be covered. Lines should be placed approximately 1 mm apart.

Therapy after grid keratotomy should be as for a simple ulcer with a recheck examination in approximately 2 weeks to ensure healing. Oxytetracycline/polymyxin B is the antibiotic of choice based on *in vitro* and clinical evidence of improved rates of epithelial migration and healing with tetracycline therapy. Oral doxycycline may be used if a topical tetracycline is not available. If the grid keratotomy does not produce resolution of the ulcer, then the practitioner should reconsider the possibility that the ulcer may not be indolent (some other factor is keeping it from healing) and refer for further evaluation.

Multiple Punctate Keratotomy

Preparation and postprocedure care for multiple punctate keratotomy are identical to those for grid keratotomy. To perform multiple punctate keratotomy, a 22-gauge needle is used to make superficial punctures in the anterior stroma. This procedure generally is more challenging for the inexperienced practitioner and is not recommended.

Diamond Burr Débridement

A new technique for treatment of the indolent ulcer has been reported recently. The diamond burr (AlgerBrush) is a handheld instrument with a round, textured ball tip that functions similarly to a Dremel tool. After a topical anesthetic is applied, the rotating burr tip is moved in smooth, circular strokes over the ulcer until all nonadherent epithelium has been removed. The instrument simultaneously creates microabrasions in the epithelial basement membrane that contribute to improved epithelial adhesion. Advantages of the diamond burr débridement technique over traditional anterior stromal puncture techniques include minimal postprocedure scarring; the simplicity of performing the procedure, which obviates the need for advanced surgical training; the low ulcer recurrence rate after treatment; and low cost. Treatment after débridement is similar to that for other anterior stromal puncture techniques. Preliminary work suggests that this technique is safe and efficacious for treatment of indolent ulcers in the dog; however, peer-reviewed studies comparing diamond burr débridement with anterior stromal puncture techniques are necessary.

References and Suggested Reading

Bentley E: Spontaneous chronic corneal epithelial defects in dogs: a review, *J Am Anim Hosp Assoc* 41:158, 2005.

Chandler HL et al: In vivo effects of adjunctive tetracycline treatment on refractory corneal ulcers in dogs, *J Am Vet Med Assoc* 237:378, 2010.

Garcia da Silva E et al: Histologic evaluation of the immediate effects of diamond burr debridement in experimental superficial corneal wounds in dogs, *Vet Ophthalmol* 14:285, 2011.

Gosling AA et al: Management of spontaneous chronic corneal epithelial defects (SCCEDs) in dogs with diamond burr debridement and placement of a bandage contact lens, *Vet Ophthalmol* 16(2):83, 2013.

Massa KL et al: Usefulness of aerobic microbial culture and cytologic evaluation of corneal specimens in the diagnosis of infectious ulcerative keratitis in animals, *J Am Vet Med Assoc* 215:1671, 1999.

Ollivier FJ et al: Proteinases of the cornea and preocular tear film, *Vet Ophthalmol* 10:199, 2007.

CHAPTER **247**

Canine Nonulcerative Corneal Disease

MARGI GILMOUR, *Stillwater, Oklahoma*

When a corneal lesion is identified the practitioner first should determine if the disease is ulcerative or nonulcerative. Nonulcerative corneal disease usually is not painful, whereas ulcerative corneal disease is painful and is associated with blepharospasm. It is very important to distinguish a primary nonulcerative keratitis from a keratitis secondary to a healed or healing corneal ulcer. For example, the treatment for the former condition often is a topical steroid, but steroids are contraindicated in the presence of a corneal ulcer.

Additionally, the practitioner always should consider the position and function of the eyelids, as well as the quality and quantity of the tear film, whenever corneal disease is diagnosed. The cornea depends on the eyelids, tear film, and aqueous humor for maintaining its health. The tear film and aqueous humor supply nutrients to the avascular cornea, and the eyelids are responsible not only for protection but for proper distribution and restructuring of the tear film. Accordingly, the diagnostic evaluation for nonulcerative keratitis always should include a Schirmer tear test as well as fluorescein staining of the cornea.

Nonulcerative corneal disease can be inflammatory in origin, and this keratitis can be acute or chronic. Inflammatory disease is indicated by the presence of active corneal vascularization. Active vessels can be distinguished from chronic vessels by their multiple branching pattern. Superficial vessels have treelike branching, whereas deep stromal vessels are compacted with bushlike branching or a paintbrush appearance. Granulation tissue and corneal edema are additional signs of active keratitis. The finding of corneal pigmentation, or melanosis, is an indication of chronic corneal disease or corneal irritation.

Congenital Disorders

Dermoid

A corneal dermoid is a choristoma—normal tissue (skin) in an abnormal location (cornea). Corneal dermoids usually are located on the lateral aspect of the cornea. Dermoids are nonpainful; however, they usually contain hair follicles, and the hair from the dermoid may cause irritation of the adjacent normal cornea. The thickened tissue itself interferes with normal tear film spread over the cornea. Keratectomy is the treatment of choice and is curative. Keratectomy should be performed using appropriate microsurgical technique and instrumentation to allow complete excision and is best performed by an ophthalmologist.

Neonatal Dystrophy

Congenital or neonatal corneal dystrophy is a light, gray to white corneal opacity in a patchy or lacy pattern. It may be detected in neonatal puppies and is considered an incidental finding. The opacities usually resolve by 10 weeks of age. There is no associated keratitis and the condition is nonpainful. No treatment is needed.

Noninflammatory Disorders

Epithelial Inclusion Cyst

Corneal inclusion cysts are uncommon and occur when there has been injury to the epithelium. The epithelial cells form an epithelium-lined cyst that accumulates white, yellow, or tan material. The cyst is well circumscribed with normal surrounding cornea. It protrudes from the surface of the cornea and extends into the corneal stroma. Keratectomy is curative.

Lipid Keratopathy

Corneal lipid deposits appear as gray to white, refractile or glitterlike opacities in the superficial stroma. They can be bilateral or unilateral and usually do not significantly enlarge but can become denser over time. Vision rarely is affected, and the lesions are not painful. Causes of these deposits include genetic dystrophy, hyperlipidemia, and lipid degeneration in association with corneal injury, scar, or active keratitis. The long-term topical use of corticosteroids is another association. Diagnostic testing should include measurement of fasting serum cholesterol and triglyceride concentrations, particularly when the opacity is perilimbal. There is no specific treatment for the lipid deposits other than treating any existing hyperlipidemia.

If the patient is receiving topical steroid medications, substitution of a topical nonsteroidal medication should be considered when possible.

Calcium-Related Degenerative Keratopathy

Calcium deposits in the epithelial and subepithelial cornea are seen most frequently in geriatric dogs, although dogs of all ages can be affected. The deposits are white, refractile, spicule opacities like an etching in glass. They are nonpainful and not associated with keratitis; however, it is not uncommon for a corneal ulcer to develop adjacent to an area of dense calcium deposits. Superficial vascularization may be seen in or surrounding the area of calcium deposition. Topical ethylenediaminetetraacetic acid (EDTA) 1% has been recommended for treatment in an attempt to chelate the calcium deposits, but even with long-term use, efficacy is variable. Calcium deposits in association with a deep corneal ulcer or descemetocele can be treated successfully with keratectomy and conjunctival pedicle graft.

Superficial Punctate Keratitis

Superficial punctate keratitis manifests as focal or multifocal, punctate, epithelial corneal opacities. The surface of the cornea may have an "orange peel" irregularity in the area of the opacities. Usually the opacities do not stain with fluorescein, but occasionally they can retain a dot of stain in the center. In some dogs the condition is associated with mild to moderate blepharospasm. Rarely there is associated superficial vascularization. The disorder appears to be familial in the sheltie and dachshund breeds. Clinical signs usually are controlled well with topical cyclosporine 1% administered every 12 hours. Lifelong treatment usually is needed.

Endothelial Dystrophy

The endothelium is a single cell layer on the inner surface of the cornea responsible for keeping the cornea dehydrated and transparent. When it is affected by disease the result is diffuse corneal edema. Endothelial dystrophy is a bilateral genetic or age-related loss of endothelial cells. The condition is nonpainful, and usually there is no associated keratitis. Vision loss is rare even with significant edema. With severe corneal edema epithelial bullae can develop on the surface of the cornea. Rupture of the bullae results in painful epithelial ulcers. Hypertonic sodium chloride 5% ointment can be used every 6 to 12 hours to help reduce the severity of edema and lessen the risk of bullae formation. Very severe cases can be referred to an ophthalmologist for thermokeratoplasty or a Gunderson flap procedure.

Florida Spots

Florida spots are a unique condition of unknown etiology seen in dogs living in tropical and subtropical climates. The underlying cause has not been identified definitively. The lesions are round, focal or multifocal, white-gray homogeneous opacities, sometimes overlapping, located in the superficial stroma. There is no associated keratitis. The condition is nonpainful and does not progress to affect vision. No successful treatment has been reported.

Inflammatory Disorders

Chronic Superficial Keratitis

Formerly called *pannus* or *German Shepherd pannus,* chronic superficial keratitis (CSK) is considered an immune-mediated disease targeting the superficial corneal tissue. Greyhounds, German shepherds, German shepherd mixes, and related breeds such as the Belgian Malinois, Belgian shepherd, and Belgian Tervuren are predisposed. CSK presents as bilateral, nonpainful, nonulcerative keratitis starting in the lower lateral quadrant of the cornea and steadily progresses to affect the entire cornea. Factors contributing to the severity of the disease include age (young dogs tend to have a more severe form that is less responsive to treatment) and ultraviolet light exposure (greater exposure is associated with more severe disease). Early clinical signs include hyperemic bulbar conjunctiva, corneal edema, and corneal neovascularization, followed by white cellular infiltrate, granulation tissue, and pigmentation (melanosis). As the vascularization and cellular infiltrate progress, vision decreases, and vision loss eventually occurs without treatment.

CSK can be controlled medically, and even severely affected dogs can regain vision; however, it cannot be cured, and lifelong treatment is required. Overall prognosis is good as long as maintenance therapy is continued. Treatment includes topical steroids, cyclosporine 1% or 2% or tacrolimus 0.02% or 0.03%, and in severe cases subconjunctival steroid injection. Initial therapy should be aggressive to attain control of the disease and resolve the active inflammation, then medication is tapered slowly to the lowest frequency needed to maintain remission. Topical steroids have a stronger antiinflammatory action than cyclosporine or tacrolimus and are best for controlling the initial, active keratitis. Prednisolone 1% or dexamethasone 0.1% should be used every 4 to 6 hours initially, then gradually tapered over several months once the cellular infiltrate, granulation tissue, and blood vessels are gone. Cyclosporine or tacrolimus can be started with the topical steroid, or added later, to help reduce the frequency of topical steroid administration required to maintain remission. Cyclosporine and tacrolimus also may help break up pigment with long-term use. A maintenance frequency of prednisolone or dexamethasone every 24 to 48 hours and/or cyclosporine or tacrolimus every 12 to 24 hours usually can be achieved. In patients with severe disease and those with a weak response to initial topical therapy, a subconjunctival steroid injection can be given to augment the topical therapy. Triamcinolone (Kenalog) 40 mg/ml can be used for subconjunctival injection by administering 0.1 ml (4 mg) beneath the bulbar conjunctiva.

Pigmentary Keratitis in the Pug

Pigmentary keratitis in the pug begins as a triangular area of pigmentation extending from the medial limbus toward the center of the cornea. The severity of the disease can vary from mild with minimal progression of the pigment and no effect on vision, to severe with pigment eventually covering the entire cornea and resulting in vision loss. The disease likely has multiple causes, including increased corneal exposure from exophthalmic conformation and macropalpebral fissures, both of which affect tear film spread; increased number of melanocytes in the limbal and perilimbal tissue; and lower medial entropion causing chronic irritation of the conjunctiva and cornea by hair. A complicating factor can be keratoconjunctivitis sicca because the pug is a predisposed breed. Treatment depends on the degree and progression of pigmentation. Because pigment is difficult to clear once deposited, prevention is ideal. Surgical alteration of conformation, such as medial entropion correction or permanent medial and lateral tarsorrhaphies, may be beneficial. These procedures resolve any medial entropion and also narrow the palpebral fissure to lessen exposure and improve tear film spread. Cyclosporine 1% or 2% or tacrolimus 0.02% or 0.03% can break up corneal pigment with long-term use in some dogs. This pigment-inhibitory effect of these drugs, in addition to their ability to increase basal tear production, makes cyclosporine and tacrolimus beneficial in the treatment of pigmentary keratitis. Topical dexamethasone or prednisolone can be used with cyclosporine or tacrolimus if corneal vascularization is present.

Disorders Secondary to Tear Film Deficiency

The cornea is avascular and must rely on the tear film to provide nutrition to the superficial layers. With long-term lack of nutrition, vascularization and edema occur initially, followed by fibrosis and pigmentation. The tear film is composed of three dynamic layers—the inner mucin layer, the middle aqueous layer, and the outer lipid layer. The mucin layer smooths the corneal epithelium and is hydrophilic, which allows prolonged contact between the cornea and the aqueous layer. The aqueous layer is the largest layer and the primary source of nutrition for the corneal cells, providing oxygen, glucose, electrolytes, and water.

Keratoconjunctivitis Sicca

Keratoconjunctivitis sicca (KCS) refers to inadequate production of the aqueous component of the tear film. It can result in an ulcerative or nonulcerative keratitis and present either unilaterally or bilaterally. Common clinical signs are blepharospasm; hyperemic conjunctiva; a thick, tenacious mucoid discharge that adheres to the eyelids and cornea; and various stages of keratitis, including neovascularization, edema, fibrosis, and pigmentation. Vision can be lost due to severe corneal pigmentation and fibrosis. Causes include immune-mediated inflammation of the lacrimal glands, neurogenic KCS caused by damage to the parasympathetic fibers that travel with the facial nerve and innervate the lacrimal glands, drug toxicity (sulfonamides and the nonsteroidal antiinflammatory drug etodolac), excision of the nictitans lacrimal gland, canine distemper virus infection, and congenital lacrimal gland hypoplasia in toy breeds, particularly the Chihuahua and Yorkshire terrier.

KCS can be diagnosed definitively by performing a Schirmer tear test. The tear strip should be placed carefully in the central to lateral lower conjunctival fornix. For accurate results the tear strip should be resting between the lower eyelid and cornea and not between the lower eyelid and nictitans. The strip should be read as soon as it is removed from the eye. The normal value is 15 mm or more in 60 seconds. Treatment is recommended when clinical signs are present, even if the results of the Schirmer tear test are normal or decreased by only a few millimeters, since response is always better when treatment is started earlier rather than later in the disease.

Treatment depends on the cause, but regardless of cause, cyclosporine often is used topically because it has been shown to increase tear production independently of its immunomodulatory effect. It is also a very safe drug to use, has antiinflammatory properties, and can inhibit pigment migration—all of which are beneficial regardless of the cause of KCS. Immune-mediated KCS usually is treated successfully with topical cyclosporine 0.2%, 1%, or 2% every 8 to 12 hours or topical tacrolimus 0.02% or 0.03% every 8 to 12 hours. Neurogenic KCS may respond to either oral pilocarpine 1% or 2%, or topical pilocarpine 0.1% or 0.2%, every 8 to 12 hours. In severe cases of KCS that are not responsive to medical therapy parotid duct transposition surgery can be performed to maintain vision and comfort. Once the underlying cause is controlled medically or surgically, the keratitis should be specifically addressed and resolved to avoid corneal scarring and pigmentation. Topical dexamethasone 0.1% and prednisolone 1% have stronger antiinflammatory action than cyclosporine or tacrolimus and can improve or resolve corneal neovascularization, edema, cellular infiltrates, and granulation tissue much more quickly. Topical steroids should be used cautiously in extremely dry eyes because such eyes may be more prone to ulceration, secondary infection, or complicated healing. The frequency of treatment can be tapered as the active keratitis is controlled. KCS of any cause except that due to trauma and transient damage to the facial nerve and parasympathetic branches requires lifelong treatment and routine monitoring of tear production and keratitis.

Mucin Deficiency

Mucin deficiency is less common than KCS. It is diagnosed by measuring tear breakup time. Undiluted fluorescein stain is instilled into the eye to stain the tear film. From a closed position, the eyelids are opened and held open while timing commences and the fluorescein-stained tear film is observed with a cobalt blue light. As soon as the tear film starts to break up on the surface of the cornea, indicated by the formation of dark patches in the green tear film, timing stops. A tear breakup time of less than 15 seconds is indicative of a deficient mucin layer. A deficient mucin layer leads to less contact time between the aqueous portion of the tear film and the cornea, which affects the nutrition of the cornea. Clinical

signs are not as severe as in KCS and usually manifest as a mild, chronic nonulcerative keratitis characterized by mild conjunctival hyperemia, superficial corneal vascularization, and corneal haze. Schirmer tear test values are usually normal. Dogs with mucin deficiency often benefit from topical application of cyclosporine or tacrolimus every 12 hours. Mucinomimetic artificial tear products such as Refresh Liquigel and Refresh Celluvisc or Systane Ultra and Systane Gel Drops also may be beneficial.

Disorders Secondary to Eyelid Abnormalities

Cilia Abnormalities

Constant irritation from cilia can cause chronic nonulcerative keratitis. Distichia, in which cilia arise from the meibomian glands and exit out the eyelid margin, can cause nonulcerative keratitis if the cilia are long or thick. Various forms of trichiasis, hairs arising from an anatomically correct location but touching the eye, also can result in nonulcerative keratitis manifested by mild vascularization, edema, and pigmentation. Common types of trichiasis include lower medial entropion in the pug and other brachycephalic breeds; medial canthal and caruncle trichiasis, especially in the Shih Tzu; and nasal fold hairs touching the cornea in the Pekingese. In distichia the cilia are removed by cryoepilation or electrocautery. Medial canthal trichiasis is treated surgically with medial canthoplasty or cryoepilation of caruncle hair follicles. Lower medial entropion is treated with surgical correction of the eyelid position. Nasal fold trichiasis is treated with nasal fold excision.

Entropion and Ectropion

Abnormal eyelid position can lead to compromised corneal health. Entropion can result in nonulcerative keratitis due to chronic hair irritation. Ectropion can result in nonulcerative keratitis due to increased exposure of the cornea and poor tear film spread. The degree of edema, vascularization, and pigmentation depend on both the severity and the duration of the entropion or ectropion.

Lagophthalmos and Macropalpebral Fissure

Inability to completely close the eyelids over the cornea (lagophthalmos) caused by facial nerve paralysis, exophthalmia, or buphthalmia, and incomplete blinks in dogs such as brachycephalic breeds with macropalpebral fissures (oversized eyelid apertures) result in poor tear film spread across the cornea. Without the normal tear film distribution and restructuring of the trilayer anatomy that occurs with a normal blink, corneal nutrition is impaired, which leads to nonulcerative keratitis, especially in the most exposed area of the cornea. Treatment approaches include surgical narrowing of the palpebral fissure, administration of cyclosporine or tacrolimus to increase basal tear production, and routine application of longer-lasting artificial tear gels and ointments.

Neoplasia

Corneal neoplasia is uncommon in dogs. Epibulbar melanocytoma and hemangioma-hemangiosarcoma frequently arise at the limbus and may secondarily affect the cornea. Corneal squamous cell carcinoma is rare in the dog compared with other species. Dogs with chronic keratitis and dogs receiving long-term cyclosporine therapy may be predisposed, but a direct causal link has not been established. Corneal squamous cell carcinoma presents as a unilateral raised, irregular, proliferative mass that is pink or red and must be differentiated from granulation tissue. Biopsy findings should provide a definitive diagnosis. Treatment is complete excision by keratectomy. The metastatic potential appears to be low and the prognosis good with excision.

References and Suggested Reading

Andrew SE: Immune-mediated canine and feline keratitis, *Vet Clin North Am Small Anim Pract* 38:269, 2008.

Gilger BC, Bentley E, Ollivier FJ: Diseases and surgery of the canine cornea and sclera. In Gelatt KN, editor: *Veterinary ophthalmology*, ed 4, Ames, IA, 2007, Blackwell Publishing, p 690.

Maggs DJ: Cornea and sclera. In Maggs DJ, Miller PE, Ofri R, editors: *Slatter's fundamentals of veterinary ophthalmology*, ed 4, St Louis, 2008, Saunders, p 175.

Sanchez RF et al: Canine keratoconjunctivitis sicca: disease trends in a review of 229 cases, *J Small Anim Pract* 48:211, 2007.

Williams DL: Immunopathogenesis of keratoconjunctivitis sicca in the dog, *Vet Clin North Am Small Anim Pract* 38:251, 2008.

CHAPTER 248

Feline Corneal Disease

CHERYL L. CULLEN, *New Brunswick, Canada*

The cornea is the transparent anterior aspect of the outer fibrous layer of the globe. The cornea is composed of five layers: a precorneal tear film over the outer stratified squamous epithelium, epithelial basement membrane, middle stroma, Descemet's membrane, and inner endothelium. The main functions of the cornea are to contain the intraocular contents and to aid in the refraction and transmission of light due to its curvature and transparency, respectively. The transparency of the cornea is maintained by a number of anatomic features: a lack of blood vessels, lymphatics, or pigmentation; a nonkeratinized surface epithelium maintained by the moisture of the preocular tear film; a unique lattice organization of small-diameter stromal collagen fibrils; and a functioning inner endothelial layer to maintain its relative state of dehydration. It is noteworthy that the feline cornea is only 0.5 mm thick at its periphery and 0.6 mm thick centrally. The cornea is rich in sensory nerve supply derived from the ophthalmic branch of the trigeminal nerve (cranial nerve V). A functional tear film; an intact and healthy corneal epithelium, stroma, endothelium, and nerve supply; and lack of corneal infiltrate are crucial for the overall health and functioning of the cornea. The unique necessity for the cornea to maintain transparency often is compromised because many corneal disorders lead to corneal opacification and impaired vision.

Cats are affected by a variety of nonulcerative and ulcerative corneal diseases. Feline herpesvirus type 1 is known to play a role in many forms of feline keratopathies, including dendritic corneal ulcers, eosinophilic keratitis, and corneal sequestra. Fortunately, many feline corneal diseases are responsive to medical or surgical therapies. The identification of appropriate treatments depends on the clinician's first establishing an accurate diagnosis. This chapter focuses on the diagnostic approach to feline corneal disease, describes both general and distinguishing clinical characteristics of the most common disorders, and provides an overview of currently available medical and surgical therapies.

Clinical Signs

There are a number of clinical signs associated with corneal disease in the cat. These signs generally are not specific for a type of disease. The most common findings are summarized in Box 248-1.

Feline Herpesvirus 1 Keratoconjunctivitis

Clinical Presentation and Diagnosis

Feline herpesvirus 1 (FHV-1) is a ubiquitous DNA α-herpesvirus that infects and causes necrosis of the epithelial surfaces of the respiratory tract and conjunctiva and, to a lesser extent, the corneal epithelium. Infection with FHV-1 generally causes a self-limiting primary

BOX 248-1

Clinical Signs of Feline Corneal Disease

Ocular discharge (serous, mucoid, mucopurulent, serosanguineous, crusty, dark brown or black)
Blepharospasm
Conjunctival or episcleral injection
Chemosis (conjunctival edema)
Corneal opacification due to the following:
   Edema (hazy gray in appearance)
   White blood cell infiltration (white to yellowish in appearance)
   Lipid (crystalline white in appearance)
   Scarring or fibrosis (dull white in appearance)
Corneal vascularization (superficial branching or straighter deep blood vessels)
Secondary reflex uveitis (miotic or constricted pupil; conjunctival hyperemia; aqueous flare; inflammatory cells in anterior chamber; fibrin in anterior chamber)
Raised pink to white chalky plaques from medial or lateral limbus (most consistent with proliferative eosinophilic keratitis)
Amber to black region of cornea (most consistent with corneal sequestrum)

TABLE 248-1

Corneal Diseases Associated with Feline Herpesvirus 1 Infection and Their Characteristic Clinical Signs

Corneal Disease	Characteristic Clinical Signs
Corneal ulceration	Positive staining with fluorescein ± rose bengal showing linear to dendritic or geographic appearance
Stromal keratitis	Vascularization and white to yellow ± gray opacification of deeper corneal stroma
Symblepharon	Adhesions of conjunctiva to cornea or itself
Keratoconjunctivitis sicca	Dry, nonlustrous corneal surface with Schirmer tear test values typically <5 mm/min from globe with signs of ocular irritation, including conjunctival injection ± corneal ulceration
Eosinophilic keratitis	Raised pink to white chalky plaques from medial or lateral limbus and corneal vascularization
Corneal sequestrum	Amber to black region of central to paracentral cornea ± corneal vascularization

disease. Primary FHV-1 disease is characterized by malaise, pyrexia, inappetence, sneezing or coughing, and nasal as well as ocular discharge. The virus is spread from cat to cat by direct contact, fomites, or aerosolization of the virus. Studies have estimated that over 90% of cats are seropositive for the virus. Approximately 80% of FHV-1–affected cats develop a lifelong latent infection (FHV-1 carriers), and of these cats, approximately 45% develop periodic reactivation of the virus and either asymptomatically shed FHV-1 or have clinical disease.

Many feline ocular diseases are caused directly by or associated with FHV-1, including most commonly conjunctivitis and ulcerative keratitis. FHV-1 produces disease via at least two mechanisms: (1) cytolytic infection during active viral replication resulting in cell rupture such as occurs during primary FHV-1 infection or following viral reactivation from latency, and (2) immune-mediated inflammation. Clinical ophthalmic manifestations of FHV-1 cytolytic infection are numerous and include conjunctivitis characterized by hyperemia, blepharospasm, chemosis, and ocular discharge. Conjunctivitis, unilateral or bilateral, is the most common FHV-1–related ocular disorder in adult cats without active respiratory disease, although some cats have concurrent sneezing or other mild signs of respiratory tract infection. Keratoconjunctivitis sicca (KCS) has been reported in cats with FHV-1–related conjunctivitis as well. FHV-1 is the sole documented viral cause of keratitis in cats; therefore every case of feline ulcerative and nonulcerative keratitis should be considered to be associated with FHV-1 unless proven otherwise. Dendritic or geographic corneal ulcers are a common manifestation of FHV-1 infection. If both the cornea and conjunctiva are ulcerated because of the cytolytic effects of FHV-1, corneal stroma and conjunctival substantia propria become exposed, which facilitates adhesion formation between these tissues (i.e., symblepharon). Neonatal ophthalmia may be caused by FHV-1 infection, either from maternal transmission to the kitten or infection shortly after birth.

Clinical disease caused by the immunopathologic mechanism of FHV-1 is an uncommon response to the viral infection. Stromal keratitis results from an immune-mediated response to viral antigen and is probably the most serious ocular manifestation of FHV-1 infection. Subconjunctival administration of dexamethasone has predisposed experimentally infected cats to develop stromal keratitis. Stromal keratitis, often secondary to chronic ulceration, is characterized by ocular discomfort, deep corneal vascularization, edema, and cellular infiltrates and can lead to significant corneal opacification and fibrosis. Table 248-1 provides a list of the corneal diseases in which FHV-1 infection plays a role and their characteristic clinical signs.

The frequency with which cats are vaccinated against FHV-1 as well as the number of clinically healthy cats that carry and shed FHV-1 make serologic and virus isolation detection methods unhelpful in the diagnosis of FHV-1 keratoconjunctivitis. Therefore, despite the wide availability of diagnostic tests such as virus isolation and fluorescent antibody tests, these are considered relatively insensitive in cats with chronic or recurrent ocular disease. Modern techniques that identify viral DNA, such as the polymerase chain reaction (PCR) assay, are more sensitive for diagnosis. However, several recent studies evaluating the use of PCR for the detection of FHV-1 in feline ocular samples have revealed that a high percentage of cats without clinical signs of ocular disease have detectable levels of FHV-1 DNA in their conjunctiva and corneas. Thus the diagnosis of FHV-1 keratoconjunctivitis typically is made based on detection of characteristic clinical signs such as dendritic corneal ulcers or scars or the finding of symblepharon along with a history of upper respiratory tract disease or a positive response to antiviral therapy.

Treatment

Owners of affected cats should be informed that the treatment of FHV-1 keratoconjunctivitis can be challenging and expensive and that recurrences of FHV-1–related ocular diseases are common. In general, cases of FHV-1 conjunctivitis are self-limiting and resolve within 7 to 14 days. Treatment of acute conjunctivitis involves the use of topical antibiotics such as tetracycline or erythromycin ointment three times daily or chloramphenicol ointment or solution three times daily or four times daily, respectively, for 10 to 14 days to prevent or treat secondary infections caused by *Chlamydophila* spp., *Mycoplasma* spp., or opportunistic bacterial flora. In cases of chronic conjunctivitis, topical or oral antiviral therapy and oral supplementation with l-lysine as described later generally are recommended. It is also prudent to consider tear supplementation in cats affected with FHV-1 conjunctivitis because recent studies have documented accelerated tear film breakup times in some affected cats.

FHV-1–related ulcerative and stromal keratitis typically require antiviral therapy. No antiviral agent has been developed specifically for cats. The following are topical antivirals with activity against FHV-1, listed in order of decreasing *in vitro* efficacy: (1) trifluridine, (2) idoxuridine < ganciclovir, (3) cidofovir < penciclovir, (4) vidarabine, (5) bromovinyldeoxyuridine, (6) acyclovir. It is of particular importance to note that these antiviral agents are virostatic and must be applied at least four to six times daily. The one exception is cidofovir, which accumulates in tissue and, when used clinically in cats at the 0.5% concentration, may be administered only twice daily for 14 days. Some of the medications listed (including topical trifluridine, idoxuridine, and vidarabine) have been widely tested and used in cats with FHV-1 infection, whereas the clinical efficacy and safety of the other agents remain unknown. Many cats experience irritation from topical antiviral drugs or do not readily tolerate the frequency of administration of these medications. Recent studies have evaluated the effectiveness and safety of the oral antiviral famciclovir in cats. Oral administration of famciclovir at 90 mg/kg q8h for 21 days improved outcomes with regard to not only ophthalmic variables but also systemic, clinicopathologic, virologic, and histologic variables in cats experimentally infected with FHV-1 (Thomasy et al, 2011). Famciclovir, a prodrug to penciclovir, has been used in client-owned cats with FHV-1–associated ocular disease at widely variable doses and frequencies (25 to 90 mg/kg q8-24h). There is evidence that dosages of 40 to 90 mg/kg q8h PO are safe and warranted based on pharmacokinetic data in cats; however, the pharmacokinetics of this drug are complex, and further studies are needed to determine dose rates and frequency.

Treatment of cats with FHV-1–induced corneal ulcers should include not only an antiviral medication but additional therapy when appropriate. For example, in cases of indolent or superficial refractory corneal ulcers, corneal débridement is indicated to reduce the number of viral particles, both to hasten healing and to help prevent development of stromal keratitis or sequestration. Cats should *not* undergo grid-striate or punctuate keratotomy to promote healing of a corneal ulcer (see Chapter 246) because this could seat virus particles within the stroma and predispose to stromal keratitis or corneal sequestration.

Treatment for KCS in cats with FHV-1 infection should commence with a topical viscous (gel) tear supplement three or four times daily in addition to antimicrobial therapy as described earlier. In KCS cases that are refractory to this form of symptomatic treatment, topical 0.2% cyclosporine ointment in addition to antiviral therapy may be used. Clients should be made aware of the possibility that the clinical signs of FHV-1 keratoconjunctivitis may worsen with administration of cyclosporine. Therefore increased ocular discomfort or corneal opacification following commencement of topical cyclosporine therapy warrants prompt reexamination of the cat's eyes. In general, if an immunosuppressive agent such as cyclosporine is used to treat FHV-1–related ocular disease, an antiviral medication should be used concurrently. Recombinant interferon has been used in cats with herpesvirus-related ocular disease, although studies that document its effectiveness have been limited to those involving experimental FHV-1 infection and *in vitro* investigations.

Lysine, in conjunction with low arginine levels, has been documented to be effective in reducing FHV-1 synthesis *in vitro* by antagonizing the availability of arginine, an essential amino acid used in viral synthesis. Clinical studies reveal that oral lysine is safe and reduces both the severity of conjunctivitis in cats with primary FHV-1 infection and the ocular viral shedding rate in cats with latent FHV-1 infection. However, recent studies evaluating the effectiveness of lysine supplementation in cats housed in animal shelters documented an increased severity of FHV-1 disease or increased detection of FHV-1 DNA. Despite these varying results, there are no studies evaluating the effectiveness of lysine use in client-owned cats with FHV-1 infection. Lysine administration is recommended for cats during active FHV-1 disease and as a long-term prophylactic treatment in cats with recurrent episodes of FHV-1 activity. Recommended dosages are one 500-mg bolus PO q12h in adults and one 250-mg bolus PO q12h in kittens (not as a dietary supplement). Lysine is now available as a powder, paste, or chewable treat for cats. For a review of antiviral therapy for FHV-1 infection, the reader is referred to Maggs (2010).

Eosinophilic Keratitis

Clinical Presentation and Diagnosis

Eosinophilic keratitis (EK), also known as *proliferative keratoconjunctivitis,* is a chronic, progressive disease of the feline cornea. Early clinical manifestations include superficial corneal vascularization perilimbally that progresses

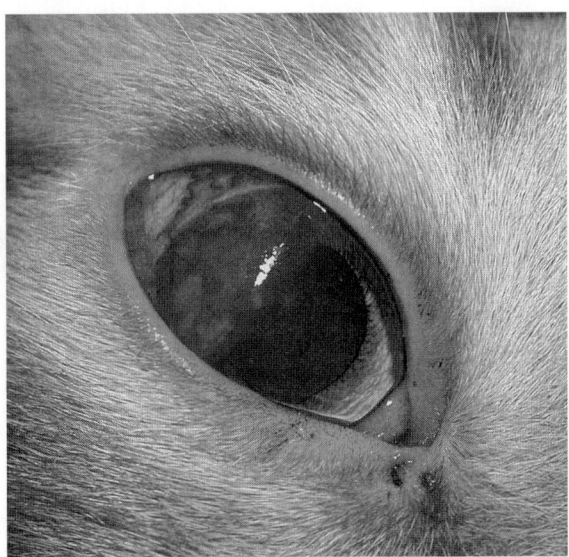

Figure 248-1 Right eye of a domestic shorthair cat with eosinophilic keratitis. Note the raised pink and white vascularized corneal plaque commencing at the lateral limbus.

to raised, vascularized, irregularly shaped plaques that are pink to chalky white and that typically start at the medial or lateral limbus (Figure 248-1). These corneal plaques are variably covered by epithelium and may or may not retain fluorescein stain. Most cases of EK are unilateral, although this ocular condition may be bilateral. Various ages and breeds can be affected with EK; however, young to middle-aged adult mixed-breed cats appear overrepresented. The characteristic corneal plaque is highly suggestive of EK; however, definitive diagnosis is established by cytologic sampling of the lesion using topical anesthesia (0.5% proparacaine or 1% tetracaine) and a sterile Dacron-tipped applicator or the handle end of a No. 15 Bard-Parker scalpel blade to scrape the lesion. The diagnosis of EK is confirmed by identification of as few as one eosinophil or mast cell. The cause and pathogenesis of EK have yet to be elucidated. However, the corneal scrapings of some cats with EK have tested positive for FHV-1 DNA via PCR and a corneal ulcer may be present prior to the development of EK, which suggests that FHV-1 may play a role in its pathogenesis.

Treatment

Topical corticosteroid treatment generally is effective for resolution of lesions and control of EK. Prednisolone acetate 1% ophthalmic suspension or dexamethasone 0.1% solution or ointment may be administered two to four times daily, depending on lesion severity, and slowly tapered in frequency (every 2 to 6 weeks) to the lowest effective dose. Additional treatment options include topical cyclosporine (0.2% ointment or 1.5% solution) usually applied two or three times daily. A recent study examining the use of topical cyclosporine 1.5% for treatment of EK demonstrated improvement in the treated eyes in 31 of 35 cats (88.6%), whereas in 4 cats (22.6%) the EK failed to respond to topical cyclosporine (Spiess et al, 2009). Although therapy can be discontinued

following resolution of the lesions, recurrences of EK are common. Long-term, often lifelong, therapy with a topical corticosteroid or cyclosporine at the lowest effective dose therefore is recommended. In some cases subconjunctival triamcinolone (4 mg) or oral megestrol acetate (5 mg/day initially tapered to 2.5 to 5 mg once weekly) has been used to treat EK. The inability to immediately cease the exposure to a corticosteroid following subconjunctival injection and the risk of serious systemic complications such as development of diabetes mellitus associated with megestrol acetate use indicate that these therapies should be used judiciously.

Corneal Sequestrum

Clinical Presentation and Diagnosis

Corneal sequestration is a common disorder in cats, particularly in the Persian and Himalayan breeds. The cause remains undetermined, but sequestra appear to develop in association with multiple factors, including chronic corneal disease caused by infection with FHV-1, chronic corneal irritation as occurs with entropion, corneal exposure due to lagophthalmos, and tear film deficiencies, among others. The condition is characterized by an area of corneal degeneration varying from an amber or dilute-tea color (Figure 248-2, *A*) to a dark brown or black discoloration (Figure 248-2, *B*). The lesions range in size from pinpoint sequestra to those occupying more than half the cornea. Corneal vascularization may be intense or absent, and ocular pain ranges from absent to severe. Corneal sequestration has been noted to occur after topical corticosteroid use in cats experimentally infected with FHV-1 as well as in naturally infected cats. In a study by Cullen and colleagues (2005), three of nine corneal sequestra keratectomy specimens tested positive for the presence of *Toxoplasma gondii* DNA, which indicates a possible role for this organism in corneal sequestration; however, the parasite was not detected ultrastructurally in the specimens. Corneal sequestra are diagnosed by their characteristic clinical appearance. Cats, unlike dogs, rarely develop corneal pigmentation in response to keratitis; for this reason, any degree of brown opacity of a feline cornea is considered nearly pathognomonic for corneal sequestration. Interestingly, tear porphyrins once were felt to be one possible cause of the amber to black discoloration of corneal sequestra, but a recent study by Newkirk and associates (2011) documented the absence of porphyrins in keratectomy samples from 18 corneal sequestra.

Treatment

In general, surgery to remove the corneal sequestrum via lamellar keratectomy with or without placement of a graft is considered the best treatment for affected globes. Surgery allows excision of the necrotic cornea, and if the remaining corneal lesion is deep (>50% of stromal depth), a graft is placed for tectonic support. Various forms of corneal grafting have been employed for affected eyes, including the use of amniotic membrane grafts and heterologous corneal grafts (canine donor cornea to avoid

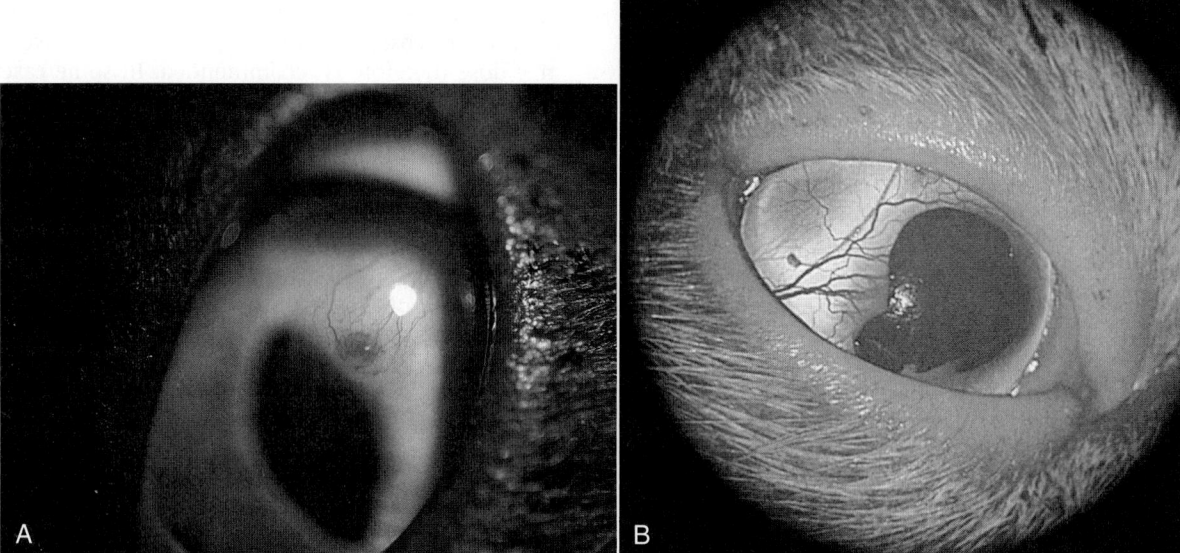

Figure 248-2 A, Right eye of a Devon rex cat demonstrating a small focal tea-colored area consistent with a corneal sequestrum within the dorsomedial cornea surrounded by superficial corneal vascularization and edema. **B,** Right eye of a Persian cat demonstrating a large paracentrally located black corneal sequestrum with overlying corneal ulceration and corneal vascularization.

the risk of spreading infectious organisms such as FHV-1 and feline leukemia virus), autogenous corneal grafts (feline donor cornea), and conjunctival island and pedicle grafts as well as corneoconjunctival transposition, among others. The choice of grafting method depends, in part, on availability of the material or tissue as well as on the size and location of the corneal sequestrum. Recurrences of corneal sequestra can arise, even after surgical therapy, and this is likely caused by some of the contributing factors that cannot be altered, including breed predisposition and FHV-1 infection. It is the author's experience that conjunctival pedicle flap placement without transection of the blood supply to the flap results in a reduced rate of recurrence.

Medical management of corneal sequestra is also an option; however, medical treatment alone usually results in greater morbidity for the affected globe and the cat. Sloughing or extrusion of the necrotic portion of cornea can require months to years, and over this time the cornea may ulcerate, which causes acute or chronic ocular pain as well as increased corneal opacification. In some cases the cornea may perforate following natural extrusion of the corneal sequestrum because the sequestrum may extend to the depth of Descemet's membrane.

The author recommends a number of strategies. Medical therapy is aimed initially at preventing secondary infections by using broad-spectrum topical antibiotics (solutions four times daily and ointments three times daily) during periods of corneal ulceration. Alternating between different topical antibiotics on a monthly basis may help prevent changing the conjunctival microflora. The second therapeutic goal is controlling ocular discomfort by using a topical nonsteroidal antiinflammatory agent such as diclofenac 0.1% ophthalmic solution once

or twice daily. Tear supplementation (e.g., application of a viscous tear gel from two to four times daily) is prescribed if a concurrent quantitative or qualitative tear film deficiency is detected. Lastly, in cases in which FHV-1 infection is suspected, a topical or systemic antiviral agent can be used in the short term (2 to 3 weeks at a time). Topical antiviral agents can be epitheliotoxic and should not be used for protracted periods.

Owners of affected cats should be made aware that in the long term the cost of medical management for a globe with corneal sequestration can be higher than the cost of surgery because medical therapy involves not only the medications for the eye but also periodic ocular reexaminations to monitor the status of the corneal sequestrum. Many cats with corneal sequestra develop superficial corneal ulcers overlying the portion of necrotic cornea that may not retain fluorescein stain. This lack of fluorescein dye uptake is due to the nonhydrophilic nature of necrotic corneal stroma along with masking by the dark coloration of many sequestra. A concurrent corneal ulcer should be suspected if the affected globe shows signs of ocular discomfort such as blepharospasm.

Surgical Indications and Options for Corneal Disease

A discussion of surgical treatments for feline corneal disease is beyond the scope of this textbook, and most of these procedures should be performed by a veterinary ophthalmologist. Table 248-2 summarizes a few of the available options so that practitioners can be familiar with some of the more advanced treatment methods available for management of feline corneal diseases.

TABLE 248-2

Surgical Indications and Options in Corneal Disease

Corneal Disease	Indications for Surgery	Surgical Option(s)
Corneal ulceration	Corneal ulcer that is >50% stromal depth; visible corneal crater or defect; ulcer down to level of Descemet's membrane (i.e., clear in center of ulcer bed) Chronic refractory superficial corneal ulcer with lips of nonadherent epithelium (indolent corneal ulcer)	Keratectomy to remove unhealthy portions of cornea associated with ulcer and some form of grafting procedure (e.g., conjunctival pedicle flap) to fill remaining corneal defect for tectonic support. Corneal débridement to remove unhealthy corneal epithelium; grid-striate or punctuate keratotomy should not be performed in cats because it could predispose to feline herpesvirus 1–related stromal keratitis or corneal sequestrum.
Stromal keratitis	Advanced generalized corneal opacification, blindness, and chronic ocular pain; poor response to medical therapy	Enucleation of severely compromised globes.
Keratoconjunctivitis sicca (KCS)	Schirmer tear test values remain consistently low or zero and medical therapies have failed to control not only the KCS but also the cat's symptoms	Parotid salivary duct transposition; rarely performed in cats compared with dogs.
Eosinophilic keratitis	Nonsurgical ocular disease unless a complex corneal ulcer develops (see corneal ulceration above)	Not applicable unless complex corneal ulcer develops (see corneal ulceration above)
Corneal sequestrum	Shorten healing time and decrease ocular discomfort	Keratectomy ± grafting procedure

References and Suggested Reading

Cullen CL et al: Ultrastructural findings in feline corneal sequestra, *Vet Ophthalmol* 8:295, 2005.

Dean E, Meunier V: Feline eosinophilic keratoconjunctivitis: a retrospective study of 45 cases (56 eyes), *J Feline Med Surg*, Jan. 15 Epub, 2013.

Gould D: Feline herpesvirus-1: ocular manifestations, diagnosis and treatment options, *J Feline Med Surg* 13:333, 2011.

Lim CC, Cullen CL: Schirmer tear test values and tear film break-up times in cats with conjunctivitis, *Vet Ophthalmol* 8:305, 2005.

Maggs DJ: Antiviral therapy for feline herpesvirus infections, *Vet Clin North Am Small Anim Pract* 40:1055, 2010.

Maggs DJ, Nasisse MP, Kass PH: Efficacy of oral supplementation with L-lysine in cats latently infected with feline herpesvirus, *Am J Vet Res* 64:37, 2003.

Newkirk KM, Hendrix DVH, Keller RL: Porphyrins are not present in feline ocular tissues or corneal sequestra, *Vet Ophthalmol* 14:2, 2011.

Sandmeyer LS, Keller CB, Bienzle D: Effects of interferon-alpha on cytopathic changes and titers for feline herpesvirus-1 in primary cultures of feline corneal epithelial cells, *Am J Vet Res* 66:210, 2005.

Spiess AK, Sapienza JS, Mayordomo A: Treatment of proliferative feline eosinophilic keratitis with topical 1.5% cyclosporine: 35 cases, *Vet Ophthalmol* 12:132, 2009.

Thomasy SM et al: Evaluation of orally administered famciclovir in cats experimentally infected with feline herpesvirus type-1, *Am J Vet Res* 72:85, 2011.

Townsend WM et al: Heterologous penetrating keratoplasty for treatment of a corneal sequestrum in a cat, *Vet Ophthalmol* 11:273, 2008.

CHAPTER 249

Canine Uveitis

ALEXANDRA VAN DER WOERDT, *New York, New York*

Uveitis is defined as inflammation of the vascular uveal tract within the eye. *Anterior uveitis* is inflammation of the iris and ciliary body. *Chorioretinitis* is inflammation of the choroid and the adjacent retina. Isolated *choroiditis* without involvement of the retina is rare. *Panuveitis* refers to inflammation that affects the entire uveal tract. Anterior uveitis and chorioretinitis are common ocular diseases in dogs and often are present at the same time. There are numerous causes of uveitis in dogs, and they include both systemic diseases and localized ocular diseases. Proper diagnosis and investigation of possible underlying diseases is important for the management of both the eye and the dog. This chapter provides a brief description of uveal anatomy and physiology, followed by a discussion of clinical signs, differential diagnoses, and treatment of uveitis in dogs.

Anatomy and Physiology

The uvea consists of the iris, ciliary body, and choroid. The uvea has many functions, including production of aqueous humor, regulation of the amount of light that enters the eye through constriction and dilation of the pupil, and supply of nutrients and oxygen to the nonvascularized or poorly vascularized portions of the eye. The uvea also is responsible for maintenance of the blood-aqueous barrier that protects the eye from toxins, infectious organisms, and exuberant inflammation. Inflammation starts either within the eye itself or in reaction to a disease process elsewhere in the body. Microorganisms or damaged tissue release inflammatory mediators such as histamine, serotonin, prostaglandins, and leukotrienes, which result in vasodilation and increased vascular permeability. This leads to breakdown of the blood-aqueous barrier. These inflammatory mediators also cause leukocyte activation and migration. Antigens are transported through the bloodstream to the spleen or other lymphoid tissues, which results in activation of T and B lymphocytes. These activated T and B lymphocytes are transported back to the eye through the bloodstream to the uveal tract. Uveitis resolves when inhibitory cytokines eliminate the inflammatory response and the initial offending antigen is removed. Chronic inflammation may occur when the initial offending antigen cannot be removed or the inflammatory response is not adequately suppressed.

Diagnosis

Clinical signs of anterior uveitis include blepharospasm, conjunctival hyperemia, corneal edema, aqueous flare,

hypopyon, swelling of the iris, rubeosis iridis (neovascularization of the iris in chronic uveitis), decreased intraocular pressure (IOP), decrease or loss of vision, and miosis. Table 249-1 lists the differential diagnoses for the various clinical signs associated with anterior uveitis. Blepharospasm is a sign of ocular pain associated with spasm of the ciliary body musculature and intraocular inflammation. Conjunctival hyperemia is a nonspecific sign associated with many ocular diseases and cannot be used to rule in or rule out uveitis. Corneal edema is caused by temporary malfunction of the endothelial cells resulting in decreased removal of fluid from the cornea. Breakdown of the blood-aqueous barrier results in the leakage of protein and inflammatory cells into the aqueous humor. The anterior chamber is best evaluated for the presence of aqueous flare by illumination using a bright pinpoint or slit-beam light source held in close proximity to the cornea in a dark room. A normal eye shows a white light beam on the cornea, no light reflection from the aqueous humor, and a white light beam on the iris-lens. An eye with uveitis has increased protein and cells in the aqueous humor, which can be seen as light reflecting between the beam on the cornea and the beam on the iris-lens. Severe breakdown of the blood-aqueous barrier may result in the presence of white blood cells in the anterior chamber, a condition called *hypopyon*. These often settle at the bottom of the anterior chamber. It is important to remember that the presence of hypopyon does not necessarily indicate intraocular infection but is pathognomonic for intraocular inflammation. Inflammation of the iris and ciliary body causes a decrease in IOP because of a decrease in the production of aqueous humor and an increase in the removal of aqueous humor through the inflamed iris. Miosis results from elevated levels of prostaglandins in the aqueous humor that stimulate contraction of the iris sphincter muscle. Blepharospasm, corneal edema, aqueous flare, and miosis all may contribute to a decrease in vision.

Chorioretinitis often causes a decrease in, or loss of, vision. Secretion of fluid between the choroid and the retina may result in focal or complete (serous) retinal detachment. Focal areas of chorioretinitis are visible within the retina as hyporeflective lesions that often are round and may have a different color from the surrounding tapetal and nontapetal areas.

Causes

Uveitis can have numerous causes in the dog. Uveitis can be divided into two main types: uveitis associated with systemic disease and uveitis secondary to other ocular

TABLE 249-1

Clinical Signs of Anterior Uveitis with Common Differential Diagnoses

Clinical Sign	Differential Diagnoses	Diagnostic Tests and Other Clinical Signs to Help Differentiate Diagnoses
Blepharospasm	Corneal ulceration Glaucoma Lens luxation Blepharitis Entropion	Thorough ophthalmic examination Measurement of IOP
Conjunctival hyperemia	Glaucoma Conjunctivitis 　Allergic 　Keratoconjunctivitis sicca Corneal ulceration	Schirmer tear test Measurement of IOP Fluorescein staining
Corneal edema	Corneal ulceration Glaucoma Anterior lens luxation Endothelial cell degeneration	Fluorescein staining Measurement of IOP Evaluation of lens position
Aqueous flare	Lipid-laden aqueous humor	Biochemistry profile with evaluation of cholesterol and total lipids
Hypopyon	Focal area of depigmentation in iris	Comfortable eye with no other signs of inflammation
Iris swelling	Normal iris crypts Major arterial circle visible at base of iris Neoplastic infiltration	No other signs of inflammation present with normal iris crypts
Rubeosis iridis	Major arterial circle may appear as a red vessel at base of iris in eyes with a light-colored iris	Circular, irregular vessel at base of iris
Miosis	Neurologic disease Use of miotic agents (i.e., latanoprost, pilocarpine)	
Low intraocular pressure	Advanced age	Absence of other clinical signs of uveitis in an older dog
Decreased or loss of vision	Severe corneal disease Cataract Lens luxation Retinal degeneration Sudden acquired retinal degeneration Optic neuritis Retinal detachment	Mydriasis usually present in the following: 　Retinal degeneration 　Sudden acquired retinal degeneration 　Optic neuritis 　Retinal detachment Difficult to evaluate intraocular details in severe corneal disease

IOP, Intraocular pressure.

diseases. Box 249-1 lists the most common causes of uveitis in dogs. In one large retrospective study (Massa et al, 2002), an underlying cause was unidentified in approximately 60% of cases of canine uveitis, which led to a default diagnosis of immune-mediated uveitis/uveitis of unknown cause in the majority of cases. It is important to prepare clients for this possibility because even a thorough workup may not reveal the cause of uveitis. Nevertheless, a complete workup is critically important to rule out any underlying neoplastic or infectious disease. A thorough physical examination, including careful palpation of regional lymph nodes, is indicated for all patients with uveitis. Obtaining a travel history is important because uveitis may indicate the presence of a disease not typically seen in the dog's home area. A complete blood count, serum biochemistry profile, and urinalysis are recommended as part of a systematic workup. Submission of blood for serologic testing for specific diseases should be guided by results of the physical examination and

knowledge of diseases specific to the geographic location or travel history. Aspiration of the anterior chamber or vitreous cavity to collect samples for cytologic analysis or culture is an additional diagnostic technique that can help establish a diagnosis, but such procedures usually are done under general anesthesia and often are best performed by a veterinary ophthalmologist.

Numerous infectious diseases can cause anterior uveitis in dogs. Patients typically show clinical signs of systemic disease in addition to ocular disease; however, a lack of systemic signs does not rule out systemic illness. Ocular lesions are most often bilateral but can be unilateral. Bacterial infections include leptospirosis, brucellosis, and the various tick-borne diseases. Brucellosis usually is manifested as a reproductive disease in intact male dogs, although it also can cause endophthalmitis, chorioretinitis, and hyphema. Uveitis is relatively uncommon in leptospirosis. Conversely, inflammation of the anterior and posterior segments of the eye is common in tick-borne

BOX 249-1

Causes of Uveitis in Dogs

Ocular Diseases
- Ulcerative keratitis
- Lens protein leakage
- Ocular neoplasia
- Pigmentary uveitis (golden retrievers)
- Immune-mediated disease (idiopathic)
- Trauma to the globe (blunt or penetrating)
- Scleritis

Systemic Diseases

Infectious

Bacterial
- Leptospirosis
- Brucellosis
- Lyme disease
- Ehrlichiosis
- Rocky Mountain spotted fever
- Bacteremia or septicemia (e.g., endocarditis, pyometra)

Viral
- Canine adenovirus 1 infection

Mycotic
- Blastomycosis
- Histoplasmosis
- Cryptococcosis
- Aspergillosis
- Coccidiomycosis

Parasitic
- Dirofilariasis
- Aberrant nematode larval migration

Protozoan
- Leishmaniasis
- Toxoplasmosis (rare in dogs)

Algal
- *Prototheca* infection

Immune Mediated
- Uveodermatologic syndrome
- Reaction to vaccine against canine adenovirus 1 or 2
- Idiopathic

Miscellaneous
- Hyperlipidemia
- Hypertension
- Hyperviscosity
- Metastatic neoplasia

---

diseases. Hemorrhage, such as hyphema and retinal hemorrhage, as well as retinal detachment may be present. Any disease associated with bacteremia, such as pyometra, can cause a secondary uveitis. Blastomycosis, histoplasmosis, coccidiomycosis, and cryptococcosis are the systemic fungal diseases most commonly associated with ocular inflammation, and uveitis, chorioretinitis, endophthalmitis, and optic neuritis can be evident. The inflammation often is severe. Cryptococcosis induces less ocular inflammation because the thick capsule of the *Cryptococcus* organism shields antigens from the immune system. Less common causes of canine uveitis are aberrant migration of parasitic larvae, toxoplasmosis, and infection with *Prototheca* or *Leishmania* spp.

Immune-mediated disease may be associated with uveitis. Uveodermatologic syndrome (or Vogt-Koyanagi-Harada–like syndrome) is a disease mediated by an immune response against pigmented tissues in the eye and the skin. Clinical signs include anterior uveitis, chorioretinitis, retinal detachment, poliosis, and vitiligo of

the mucocutaneous junctions of the head, nasal planum, scrotum, and footpads. Ulceration of the skin may occur as well. Predisposed breeds include the Akita, chow-chow, Siberian husky, and Samoyed. "Blue eye" or immune-mediated uveitis is associated with a type III hypersensitivity reaction to canine adenovirus (CAV) infection. Uveitis and endotheliitis of the cornea as a reaction to CAV-1 or CAV-2 vaccination is rare with modern vaccines but still can be observed sporadically. Clinical signs include an acute onset of severe corneal edema within a few days after vaccination.

Miscellaneous systemic diseases associated with uveitis include hyperlipidemia, hypertension, hyperviscosity syndromes, and metastatic neoplasia. Patients with uveitis and hyperlipidemia may be brought for evaluation of acute onset of a very cloudy appearance to the eye. The eye is often comfortable, and the anterior chamber appears to be filled with "milk-white" aqueous humor. The condition can arise suddenly but also can resolve very quickly. Breakdown of the blood-aqueous barrier is required for lipid to enter the anterior chamber. Hyperlipidemia also can be visible in the retinal vessels as lipemia retinalis, which gives the retinal vessels a light-red appearance. The anterior uveitis associated with systemic hypertension or hyperviscosity syndromes usually is mild and far less significant than the changes seen in the fundus. Retinal changes include retinal edema; supraretinal, subretinal, or intraretinal hemorrhage; hyphema; tortuous vessels; and retinal detachment. Metastatic neoplasia can manifest itself as discrete nodules in the iris, focal infiltrative lesions in the retina and choroid, or a diffuse infiltration of the iris or choroid.

Primary ocular causes of uveitis can be unilateral or bilateral. Corneal ulceration can cause significant reflex uveitis, especially if secondary bacterial infection is present. The degree of inflammation may be mild in a superficial corneal ulcer but can be quite pronounced with hypopyon in a deep, infected corneal ulcer.

Blunt or penetrating trauma to the eye can induce reflex uveitis but would likely be associated with other signs, including hyphema, corneal ulceration or laceration, scleral laceration, lens luxation, vitreous hemorrhage, and retinal detachment.

Lens-induced uveitis occurs when proteins from a cataract leak through an intact lens capsule into the aqueous humor (phacolytic uveitis). This is most common with hypermature cataracts and may be seen with any cataract larger than an incipient size (>10% of the lens volume). Phacoclastic uveitis is caused by acute rupture of the lens capsule and the release of lens proteins into the aqueous humor. Phacoclastic uveitis typically occurs 2 to 14 days after lens capsule rupture. The sudden exposure of the eye to large quantities of lens protein causes a severe inflammatory reaction that may be blinding. When rupture of the lens capsule is suspected, immediate referral to an ophthalmologist for lensectomy is indicated to optimize the chances of preserving vision.

Intraocular neoplasia is more likely to be associated with uveitis when it is secondary to ocular metastasis or multicentric neoplasia. Primary intraocular neoplasia rarely is associated with inflammation in the early stages of tumor development.

Pigmentary uveitis is a potentially blinding disease in golden retrievers. Clinically, iris cysts are one of the first abnormalities noted. Other clinical signs are fine streaking of pigment on the anterior lens capsule and darkening of the iris. A proteinaceous exudate may be present in the anterior chamber as the diseases progresses. The posterior segment remains unaffected unless secondary glaucoma develops. Complications including cataract formation and glaucoma are common. The eye often is comfortable until late in the disease, when secondary glaucoma makes the globe painful.

Complications

Ocular complications are common in anterior uveitis, especially if the inflammation is not adequately treated or if the disease becomes chronic or recurrent. Common complications are anterior and posterior synechiae, cataract formation, lens luxation, glaucoma, and blindness. Chronic inflammation is one of several ocular diseases in which preiridal fibrovascular membranes form on the anterior surface of the iris. These membranes are composed of fibrous and vascular components, and their presence predisposes the eye to the development of hyphema, entropion or ectropion uveae, and synechiae. These membranes also can lead to occlusion of the iridocorneal angle resulting in glaucoma.

Treatment

Treatment of uveitis has several components: addressing the underlying disease if possible; suppressing the inflammation; dilating the pupil; and controlling the discomfort associated with uveitis. Treatment of the underlying disease, if possible, is the most important aspect of managing uveitis. Topical symptomatic therapy for the eyes should be started at the same time as treatment for the underlying disease. Suppression of the inflammation is accomplished using topical corticosteroids, systemic corticosteroids, or nonsteroidal antiinflammatory medications (NSAIDs) (Table 249-2). Prednisolone acetate 1% solution and dexamethasone 0.1% solution are potent topical antiinflammatory medications with good intraocular penetration. Hydrocortisone is not recommended for the treatment of uveitis because of its poor intraocular penetration. The frequency of topical steroid use is determined by the severity of the uveitis and can range from once daily to hourly; however, in most cases, administration is every 4 to 8 hours and the time between doses is increased as inflammation subsides. Topical steroids should not be used when corneal ulceration is present. Topical medications are ineffective in treating inflammation of the posterior segment because a topically administered drop does not penetrate the eye past the lens. Oral corticosteroids can be used to treat inflammation of the posterior segment and also can be administered if severe anterior uveitis is present. Caution should be used in dosing oral corticosteroids when an infectious cause of chorioretinitis is suspected. Dosing should remain in the antiinflammatory range (0.5 to 1.0 mg/kg/day) and should not extend into the immunosuppressive range. Oral azathioprine (2.2 mg/kg q24h) may be useful in the long-term management of chronic uveitis. Uveodermatologic

TABLE **249-2**

Antiinflammatory Medications for Treatment of Uveitis

Oral Medications	Topical Medications
Steroidal Medications	**Steroidal Medications**
Prednisolone 0.5-2.2 mg/kg q12-24h Prednisone 0.5-2.2 mg/kg q12-24h	Prednisolone acetate 1% suspension, see text Dexamethasone 0.1% solution, see text Dexamethasone 0.05% ointment, see text
Nonsteroidal Antiinflammatory Drugs	**Nonsteroidal Antiinflammatory Drugs**
Carprofen 2.2 mg/kg q12-24h Deracoxib 1-2 mg/kg q24h Meloxicam 0.2 mg/kg first day, then 0.1 mg/kg once daily Tepoxalin 10 mg/kg q24h	Flurbiprofen 0.03% q6-12h Diclofenac 0.1% q6-12h Suprofen 1% q6-12h Ketorolac 0.4% q6-12h Nepafenac 0.1% q8h

syndrome, for example, often is treated with a combination of oral corticosteroids and azathioprine. Topical NSAIDs are recommended to treat uveitis when a concurrent corneal ulcer is present. Many topical NSAIDs are available, and several of the newer medications (e.g., nepafenac 0.1%) are potent antiinflammatory medications. They should be used with caution in animals at risk of the development of glaucoma because some NSAIDs may potentiate elevation of IOP. Of the oral NSAIDs available, oral tepoxalin has been suggested to be superior to other NSAIDs in suppressing experimentally induced uveitis.

Mydriatics such as atropine 1% solution are used to relieve the pain associated with ciliary body spasm and to induce mydriasis to prevent posterior synechiae from occluding the pupil. The use of tropicamide 1% solution is not recommended because this mydriatic has only weak cycloplegic properties and therefore is ineffective in relieving ciliary body spasm. Careful monitoring of the IOP is indicated when the various mydriatic agents are used. Severe uveitis can be very resistant to mydriatic agents. It may take multiple applications of atropine per day to dilate a pupil in the setting of uveitis. Once the pupil is dilated, the frequency of application can be reduced to the minimal frequency needed to maintain mydriasis.

When treating a patient with uveitis, it is important to reevaluate the patient regularly and decrease medications only when the clinical picture is improved. For example, reduced blepharospasm, mydriasis maintained with minimal application of atropine, decreased aqueous flare, and resolution of hypopyon are indicative of resolving disease. When antiinflammatory medications are tapered, it is recommended that treatment continue for several weeks past the clinical resolution of inflammation because microscopic inflammation may be present even when gross evidence is lacking. Monitoring IOP is a useful way to detect subclinical or ongoing inflammation. IOP is expected to normalize when uveitis has been adequately controlled.

Treatment of Uveitis in Combination with Other Ocular Diseases

Uveitis and Corneal Ulceration

Topical corticosteroids delay healing of a corneal ulceration and should be avoided if an ulcer is present. Topical NSAIDs and oral corticosteroids can be used to treat uveitis accompanied by a corneal ulcer.

Uveitis and Glaucoma

Normal IOP is between 10 and 20 mm Hg. IOP typically is low in cases of uveitis. Secondary glaucoma should be suspected if the IOP is normal in an eye with uveitis. Mydriatics are contraindicated in eyes with glaucoma or those at risk of glaucoma. Miotic agents such as prostaglandin analogs commonly are used in the treatment of glaucoma but should be avoided in eyes with uveitis. Concurrent uveitis and glaucoma are best treated with a combination of antiinflammatory medications and antiglaucoma medications that do not affect pupil size.

Carbonic anhydrase inhibitors are the safest antiglaucoma medication for use in a patient with uveitis and secondary glaucoma (see Chapter 251).

References and Suggested Reading

Gilmour MA, Lehenbauer TW: Comparison of tepoxalin, carprofen, and meloxicam for reducing intraocular inflammation in dogs, *Am J Vet Res* 70(7):902, 2009.

Johnson DA, Maggs DJ, Kass PH: Evaluation of risk factors for development of secondary glaucoma in dogs: 156 cases (1999-2004), *J Am Vet Med Assoc* 229(8):1270, 2006.

Massa K et al: Causes of uveitis in dogs: 102 cases (1989-2000), *Vet Ophthalmol* 5(2):93, 2002.

Sapienza JS, Simo FJ, Prades-Sapienza A: Golden retriever uveitis: 75 cases (1994-1999), *Vet Ophthalmol* 3(4):241, 2000.

Sigle KJ et al: Unilateral uveitis in a dog with uveodermatologic syndrome, *J Am Vet Med Assoc* 228(4):543, 2006.

Townsend WM: Canine and feline uveitis, *Vet Clin North Am Small Anim Pract* 38(2):323, 2008.

Zarfoss MK et al: Canine pre-iridal fibrovascular membranes: morphologic and immunohistochemical investigations, *Vet Ophthalmol* 13(1):361, 2010.

CHAPTER 250

Feline Uveitis

CYNTHIA C. POWELL, *Fort Collins, Colorado*

Uveitis is a painful, vision-threatening disease common in cats. Previous reports suggest that 40% to 70% of feline uveitis cases are associated with a systemic illness. A thorough workup to eliminate infectious causes is imperative because treatment of idiopathic uveitis is directed toward immunosuppression. Owners should be prepared for a potentially expensive diagnostic workup in which a definitive diagnosis is not identified. Some causes of uveitis in cats are different from those identified in the dog (see Chapter 249).

The uveal tract is comprised of the iris, ciliary body, and choroid. Anterior uveitis or iridocyclitis is inflammation of the iris and ciliary body. Posterior uveitis is more commonly referred to as *chorioretinitis* since the choroid and retina are affected concurrently in many cases. Anterior uveitis and chorioretinitis can occur separately or together.

Clinical Manifestations

Intraocular inflammation is initiated by tissue injury from trauma, infectious agents, or other antigen challenge. The tissue factors released from the damaged tissue and microorganisms result in vasodilation and changes in the vascular permeability of the intraocular vasculature. Inflammatory mediators cause leukocyte activation and migration. With moderate or severe anterior uveitis, increases in protein concentrations and inflammatory cells numbers lead to opacity of the normally transparent aqueous humor, also called *aqueous flare.* Hyphema, fibrin clots, and keratic precipitates (inflammatory cell and protein aggregates on the corneal endothelium) also may be observed. Conjunctival and scleral injection, photophobia, blepharospasm, enophthalmos, and epiphora are common with anterior uveitis but often are not present with chorioretinitis unless anterior uveitis also is present. Other ocular signs of anterior uveitis are corneal edema, miosis, edema and color changes in the iris, anterior and posterior synechia, and iris bombé. Decreased intraocular pressure (IOP) frequently is observed as a consequence of decreased aqueous humor formation. Normal feline IOP is reported as approximately 10 to 20 mm Hg. Ocular hypotony should resolve as the intraocular inflammation is controlled.

BOX 250-1

Causes of Uveitis in Cats

Exogenous
Trauma
- Secondary bacterial infection
- Sterile inflammation

Ocular Surgery
- Secondary bacterial infection
- Sterile inflammation

Keratitis
- Ulceration
- Infection

Endogenous
Infection
Bacterial
- *Ehrlichia* sp.
- *Bartonella* spp.
- Bacteremia or septicemia (e.g., pyometra, abscess)
Viral
- Feline leukemia virus
- Feline coronavirus (feline infectious peritonitis)
- Feline immunodeficiency virus
Mycotic
- *Cryptococcus neoformans*
- *Blastomyces dermatitidis*
- *Histoplasma capsulatum*
- *Coccidioides immitis*
- *Candida albicans*
Protozoal/parasitic
- *Toxoplasma gondii*
- *Leishmania* sp.
- Insect larvae (ophthalmomyiasis)

Neoplasia
Primary
- Diffuse iris melanoma
- Ciliary body adenoma
- Ciliary body adenocarcinoma
Metastatic
- Lymphosarcoma
- Others

Immune-Mediated Disorders
Lens Induced
- Cataract
- Lens subluxation/luxation
- Lens perforation or rupture
Idiopathic

Miscellaneous Causes of Blood-Eye Barrier Disruption
- Hyperviscosity syndrome
- Hypertension

Normal IOP in an actively inflamed eye raises the suspicion of concurrent glaucoma. Trends in IOP should be monitored closely throughout treatment.

Inflammatory cells sometimes accumulate in the anterior vitreous, obscuring the retina from direct visualization. This is referred to as *pars planitis* or *intermediate uveitis*. In the choroid and retina, exudates of protein and inflammatory cells accumulate within and beneath the retina and cause retinal and subretinal edema, hemorrhage, and retinal detachment. Since the retina and subretinal space are immediately anterior to the tapetum, tapetal reflectivity is decreased or obscured by areas of active chorioretinitis.

Diagnosis

Causes of feline uveitis generally are subdivided into the categories of trauma, infection, immune-mediated disease, and neoplasia (Box 250-1). Some causes can be identified by history (trauma) or ocular examination (trauma, lens disorders, neoplasia). Correlating infectious disease with uveitis is more challenging. Infectious causes generally cannot be differentiated by ocular findings alone, so the history, physical examination findings, and results of a complete blood count, urinalysis, and serum biochemical panel should be used to guide further diagnostic testing such as serologic studies, aqueous or vitreous humor analysis, radiography, ocular ultrasonography, and histopathologic evaluation. Ocular fluids can be used for cytologic analysis, culture and sensitivity testing, polymerase chain reaction (PCR) assay, and determination of antibody content.

Infectious Diseases Associated with Feline Uveitis

Toxoplasmosis

Infection with *Toxoplasma gondii* occurs primarily by ingestion of tissue cysts in prey animals. Chorioretinitis is the most common ocular manifestation of toxoplasmosis in systemically ill cats; however, the majority of infected cats do not become systemically ill. Cats with positive results on tests for *T. gondii* infection often exhibit anterior uveitis but are otherwise clinically normal. Evidence suggests that *T. gondii*–related anterior uveitis is immune mediated. Definitive diagnosis of ocular toxoplasmosis is difficult due to the high percentage of cats with serum titers showing positivity for *T. gondii*. The presence of serum immunoglobulin M, a rising serum immunoglobulin G level, and antibody production in the aqueous humor all support a diagnosis of ocular toxoplasmosis.

All sick cats that test positive for *T. gondii* should be treated with anti-*Toxoplasma* drugs. *T. gondii*-positive cat with uveitis, but no other clinical signs of infection by *T. gondii*, should be treated with anti-*Toxoplasma* drugs when other causes have been ruled out, especially if the uveitis responds poorly to antiinflammatory therapy alone. Clindamycin hydrochloride is recommended at 10 to 25 mg/kg q12h for 14 to 21 days.

Feline Infectious Peritonitis

Ocular disease (anterior and posterior uveitis) associated with feline infectious peritonitis (FIP) is most common in the dry, noneffusive form of FIP and usually is accompanied by signs of systemic disease. Rarely ocular signs may be the sole presenting complaint. FIP typically occurs in cats younger than 3 years of age. Currently available tests cannot distinguish antibodies against feline enteric coronavirus from those against FIP-inducing coronavirus; however, in a young cat with ocular disease, the findings of a coronavirus antibody titer of more than 1:1600, lymphopenia, and hypergammaglobulinemia are highly suggestive of FIP infection. Once clinical signs occur, the prognosis for FIP is grave. Cats with less severe disease may live for several months with therapy.

Immunosuppressive and antiinflammatory drugs may be used for palliative therapy. Several protocols have been described, but there is no consensus on optimal treatment of systemic disease. Ocular inflammation should be treated with topical and systemic glucocorticoids and with cycloplegics, depending on the location and severity of the inflammation (see treatment section).

Feline Leukemia Virus Infection/ Lymphosarcoma

Ocular disease occurs infrequently with feline leukemia virus (FeLV) infection except in association with lymphosarcoma or secondary infection associated with chronic immunosuppression. Fewer than 2% of cats with clinical FeLV infection have ocular disease. Ocular lymphosarcoma can be nodular or diffuse. When diffuse, ocular lymphosarcoma has an appearance to similar that of uveitis due to other causes. Isolated ocular lymphosarcoma is rare, and the diagnosis most frequently is confirmed after identification of multicentric neoplasia. FeLV status is useful for prognosis but not diagnosis, since only approximately 19% of cats with ocular lymphosarcoma test positive for FeLV. Anterior chamber/centesis with gentle iris vacuuming to obtain cells for cytologic evaluation occasionally demonstrates neoplastic cells. Treatment is by combination chemotherapy and empiric therapy for anterior uveitis when present.

Feline Immunodeficiency Virus Infection

Uveitis commonly is observed in cats with clinically apparent feline immunodeficiency virus (FIV) infection. The pathophysiology of disease includes direct viral invasion, opportunistic infection (57% of cats are coinfected with *T. gondii*), and initiation of secondary immune responses (e.g., immune complex formation). Diagnosis is supported by serum antibody testing with enzyme-linked immunosorbent assay (ELISA), immunofluorescence assay (IFA), or Western blot. These tests cannot differentiate antibodies induced by vaccination, which makes accurate diagnosis challenging. Ocular signs include anterior uveitis, pars planitis, and glaucoma. Pars planitis appears as white punctate infiltrates concentrated in the peripheral anterior vitreous. Ocular lymphosarcoma also has been associated with FIV infection. Treatment of FIV infection should be aimed at management of secondary infections when identified. Although use of topical corticosteroids to treat anterior uveitis is likely safe in cases of FIV infection, systemic corticosteroids should be used with caution since their effect on viral replication is unknown.

Systemic Mycoses

Granulomatous chorioretinitis with or without anterior uveitis can occur with cryptococcosis, histoplasmosis, blastomycosis, and coccidioidomycosis in cats. Cryptococcosis is the most common systemic mycosis in cats. Diagnosis is by demonstration of the organism on cytologic analysis of skin lesions, nasal exudate, or lymph node or bone marrow samples, or cytologic evaluation of subretinal or vitreous exudates. Serum antigen titers or ELISA test results for *Cryptococcus* are useful for diagnosis and monitoring of response to therapy.

Systemic therapy with fluconazole is considered ideal for ocular disease since it has fewer adverse effects and penetrates ocular tissues well. Treatment should continue for at least 1 month after clinical signs resolve and the *Cryptococcus* titer has dropped by at least two orders of magnitude. When present, anterior uveitis should be treated with a topical corticosteroid and atropine. Antiinflammatory dosages of oral corticosteroids along with antifungal therapy may be necessary to control inflammation associated with posterior segment infection. Eyes with secondary glaucoma or severe posterior segment involvement that are not responsive to antifungal medications require enucleation.

Bartonellosis

Infection with *Bartonella* spp. is common in cats, although clinical disease is less frequent. A recent study (Fontenelle et al, 2008) showed that healthy cats were more likely to be seropositive for *Bartonella* than cats with uveitis. After other causes have been ruled out, cats with uveitis unresponsive to traditional therapy should be tested for *Bartonella* infection, especially if there is a history of flea infestation. Diagnosis is by PCR testing, culture of whole blood, or IFA or ELISA antibody testing of serum. Oral doxycycline at a dosage of 10 mg/kg q12h for 2 to 4 weeks or oral enrofloxacin at a dosage of 5 mg/kg q24h or divided q12h can be used for treatment.

General Principles of Treatment

The primary goals in the treatment of uveitis are to stop inflammation, prevent or control complications caused by inflammation, and relieve pain. Specific therapy for uveitis must address any underlying cause of inflammation, including corneal ulceration or infectious disease. Nonspecific treatments include decreasing the ocular inflammatory response with antiinflammatory drugs, inducing mydriasis to prevent synechia formation, and paralyzing the ciliary body (cycloplegia) to decrease pain (Table 250-1). Therapy for glaucoma should be instituted when elevations in IOP are identified.

Ocular inflammation is treated primarily with topical or systemic glucocorticoids. Anterior uveitis is treated with topical administration of drugs unless contraindicated by concurrent corneal ulceration. The frequency of administration depends on the severity of inflammation.

TABLE 250-1

Drugs Commonly Used for Treatment of Uveitis

Topical Drugs	Dosing Schedule
Glucocorticoids	
Prednisolone acetate (1% suspension)	q2-12h
Dexamethasone (0.1% solution, 0.05% ointment)	q2-12h
NSAIDs	
Flurbiprofen (0.3% solution)	q6-12h
Ketorolac (0.5% solution)	q6-12h
Diclofenac (0.1% solution)	q6-12h
Mydriatic/Cycloplegic Drugs (Parasympatholytics)	
Atropine sulfate (0.5% and 1% solution and ointment)	q8-24h
Tropicamide (0.5% and 1% solution)	q8-24h
Mydriatic Drugs (Sympathomimetics)	
Phenylephrine hydrochloride (2.5% solution)	q8-12h Used in conjunction with parasympatholytic

Oral Drugs	Dosing Schedule
Corticosteroids	
Prednisolone (5-mg tablet) Prednisone (5- and 20-mg tablets)	0.5-2.2 mg/kg q12-24h (higher dosages for initial treatment of severe inflammation) 0.5-2.2 mg/kg q12-24h (higher dosages for initial treatment of severe inflammation)
NSAIDs	
Meloxicam	0.2 mg/kg PO in food then 0.1 mg/kg in food q24h × 2 days, then 0.025 mg/kg 2-3 times per wk
Acetylsalicylic acid (80-mg tablet)	3-10 mg/kg q48-72h
Ketoprofen (12.5-mg tablet)	≤2 mg/kg initially then ≤1 mg/kg q24h

NSAIDs, Nonsteroidal antiinflammatory drugs.

Mild inflammation requires topical antiinflammatory therapy every 8 to 12 hours and severe inflammation may require treatment as frequently as every 1 to 2 hours. When topical administration is impossible, oral or parenteral dosing may be necessary. If systemic infection is confirmed or suspected, immunosuppressive dosages of oral corticosteroids should be avoided, and antiinflammatory dosages should be used with caution. Topical drug administration is not adequate for chorioretinitis owing to the limited intraocular penetration of topically administered ophthalmic medications; systemic administration is needed to achieve therapeutic levels. Little is known about the effectiveness of nonsteroidal antiinflammatory drugs (NSAIDs) in the treatment of feline uveitis, and caution should be used in their administration.

The use of systemic NSAIDs in cats has been associated with potentially serious adverse effects, including bone marrow suppression, gastrointestinal ulceration, hemorrhage, vomiting, and diarrhea. Aspirin, ketoprofen, and meloxicam can be used systemically with careful attention to dosage and possible adverse effects. Topical application of NSAIDs may complicate bacterial or viral corneal infections and is not recommended in cases of uveitis with concurrent corneal ulceration.

As ocular inflammation subsides, antiinflammatory treatment should be tapered. The rate of reduction depends on both the duration and severity of inflammation. With acute mild inflammation drugs can be discontinued over a period of 1 to 2 weeks. Chronic or severe inflammation dictates a much slower taper, potentially over several months. Some cats with chronic inflammation require maintenance antiinflammatory therapy. The dosage should be decreased to the lowest possible to maintain control of inflammation.

Parasympatholytics such as atropine relieve ocular pain by relaxing the ciliary body musculature (cycloplegia). Atropine also induces mydriasis, which decreases the chance of posterior synechia. Atropine is more effective than tropicamide in the presence of uveitis because it has greater cycloplegic effects. Atropine carries a bitter taste, and cats often salivate profusely when atropine ophthalmic solutions are administered topically since they readily drain down the nasolacrimal duct. Atropine ointment generally is better tolerated. Judicious use of parasympatholytics is recommended since long-term dilation of the pupil can obstruct aqueous humor outflow. Parasympatholytic drugs also may be associated with transient decreases in tear production. Sympathomimetics, such as phenylephrine 2.5%, can be used in conjunction with parasympatholytics if severe, poorly responsive miosis is encountered.

Prognosis

The prognosis for the feline eye with anterior uveitis is influenced by a number of factors. Inflammation that can be brought under control quickly may leave behind no evidence of prior uveitis. Chronic inflammation has significant sequelae that can result in visual impairment or complete blindness. Iris inflammation and swelling, inflammatory cells and debris, and iris bombé secondary to posterior synechiae each can contribute to obstruction of the iridocorneal angle resulting in acute glaucoma. Chronic uveitis can stimulate the growth of a fibrovascular membrane across the iris, pupil, and iridocorneal angle, which also can lead to secondary glaucoma. Other sequelae of chronic anterior uveitis are cataract formation and extension of inflammation to the retina.

Permanent visual impairment is more likely to occur with chorioretinitis. Diffuse inflammation can cause generalized retinal degeneration and blindness. Focal inflammation leads to focal areas of retinal degeneration with little effect on visual function. The likelihood of visual impairment as a consequence of uveitis depends on the severity and chronicity of the inflammation, which in turn depends on the cause, the rapidity with which the diagnosis is made, and the response to appropriate therapy.

References and Suggested Reading

Brightman AH, Ogilvie GK, Tompkins M: Ocular disease in FeLV-positive cats: 11 cases (1981-1986), *J Am Vet Med Assoc* 198(6):1049, 1991.

Davidson MG et al: Feline anterior uveitis: a study of 53 cases, *J Am Anim Hosp Assoc* 27(1):77, 1991.

English RV et al: Intraocular disease associated with feline immunodeficiency virus infection in cats, *J Am Vet Med Assoc* 196(7):1116, 1990.

Fontenelle JP et al: Prevalence of serum antibodies against *Bartonella* species in the serum of cats with or without uveitis, *J Fel Med Surg* 10:41, 2008.

Giuilano EA: Nonsteroidal anti-inflammatory drugs in veterinary ophthalmology, *Vet Clin North Am Small Anim Pract* 34(3):707, 2004.

Lappin MR, Black JC: Bartonella spp. infection as a possible cause of uveitis in a cat, *J Am Vet Med Assoc* 214(8):1205, 1999.

Maggs D: Feline uveitis an "intraocular lymphadenopathy", *J Fel Med Surg* 11:167, 2009.

Powell CC, Lappin MR: Causes of feline uveitis, *Compend Contin Educ Pract Vet* 23(2):128, 2001.

CHAPTER **251**

Canine Glaucoma

JOHN S. SAPIENZA, *Plainview, New York*

Glaucoma is a common cause of blindness in dogs, with an incidence of 0.5% using the Veterinary Medical Data Base (VMDB). Glaucoma generally is characterized by the death of the retinal ganglionic cells leading to rapid loss of vision. The definition of glaucoma has evolved over the years to become more than simply elevated intraocular pressure (IOP). The retinal ganglionic cells, the cells that lead to the formation of the optic nerve, are exquisitely sensitive to changes in IOP, vascular abnormalities, and movement of the posterior scleral lamina cribrosa. The normal IOP in dogs can vary, but a general guideline for a normal range of IOP is between 15 and 25 mm Hg. Glaucoma usually is associated with an IOP much higher than these published numbers, and elevated IOP is a major risk factor for further optic nerve damage and subsequent blindness.

The main goals of management for the general practitioner are to diagnose the presence of glaucoma accurately, to distinguish primary from secondary causes of glaucoma, and to assess the potential for return or maintenance of vision or relief of ocular pain. Acute glaucoma truly is an ophthalmic emergency. This chapter provides practicing veterinarians with a framework for understanding the causes, diagnosis, and treatment of glaucoma in the dog.

Causes and Pathogenesis

Glaucoma can arise from both primary and secondary causes that are associated with increased IOP, which damages primarily the inner retina and the retinal ganglionic cells. Primary glaucoma has been observed in many breeds (Box 251-1) and is defined as an increase in IOP in the absence of concurrent ocular disease. It demonstrates a strong genetic basis with bilateral ocular involvement. Both primary open-angle and primary angle-closure glaucoma are identified in dogs. Primary angle-closure glaucoma is eight times more common than primary open-angle glaucoma in dogs. There is also a more than twofold higher frequency of primary angle-closure glaucoma in female dogs than in males. Secondary glaucoma occurs two times more frequently than primary canine glaucoma and may be related to disorders of the lens (cataract, intumescence, lens rupture or trauma, lens-induced uveitis), uveitis (see Chapter 249), hyphema, intraocular neoplasia, iridociliary cysts, misdirection of the vitreous, chronic retinal detachments, intraocular pigment dispersion or melanosis, and trauma.

A balance exists between aqueous humor production and aqueous outflow to maintain the normal shape and function of the eye. Aqueous humor is produced by the nonpigmented epithelium of the ciliary body through both active ionic transport and hydrostatic and colloidal diffusion of fluid. Carbonic anhydrase catalyzes the combination of carbon dioxide and water to form carbonic acid and is the key enzyme in the active production of aqueous humor. The IOP remains constant because of the equilibrium between aqueous production and aqueous outflow. This has importance for therapy because reduction in the production or increase in the outflow of aqueous humor can be accomplished medically with a number of oral and topical pharmaceuticals.

Two outlets for drainage of the aqueous humor are available: the conventional outflow through the iridocorneal angle and the unconventional outflow through the uveoscleral route. After production at the ciliary body, the

BOX 251-1

Breeds Predisposed to Glaucoma

Afghan hound	Great Dane
Akita	Maltese
Alaskan malamute	Manchester terrier
Bassett hound	Miniature pinscher
Beagle	Norfolk terrier
Border collie	Norwegian elkhound
Boston terrier	Pembroke Welsh corgi
Bouvier des Flanders	Poodle
Cairn terrier	Saluki
Cardigan Welsh corgi	Samoyed
Chihuahua	Scottish terrier
Chinese shar-pei	Sealyham terrier
Chow-chow	Shih Tzu
Cocker spaniel (English and	Shiba inu
American)	Siberian husky
Dachshund	Skye terrier
Dalmatian	Welsh springer spaniel
Dandie Dinmont terrier	Welsh terrier
English springer spaniel	West Highland white terrier
Fox terrier (smooth haired)	Whippet
Giant schnauzer	Wire fox terrier

aqueous fluid migrates into the posterior chamber (between the iris and the anterior portion of the lens), through the pupil, and into the anterior chamber, with the vast majority of fluid leaving through the iridocorneal angle into the trabecular meshwork. The conventional outflow is pressure sensitive and comprises 85% of the aqueous outflow in dogs. The uveoscleral outflow allows aqueous to drain through the iris stroma, ciliary body, and choroid into the posterior venous circulation and is independent of the IOP. Glaucoma occurs because of an obstruction to the outflow of aqueous. Overproduction of aqueous humor by the ciliary body does not occur.

Clinical Signs and Diagnosis

Clinical signs of glaucoma differ for acute and chronic glaucoma (Table 251-1). However, the IOP should be evaluated in all cases of a red eye with a dilated pupil.

Commonly observed ocular signs of acute glaucoma in dogs include a red eye caused by episcleral injection, squinting, diffuse corneal edema, a fixed or dilated pupil, and loss of vision to complete blindness (Figure 251-1). Fundus evaluation may demonstrate a swollen or edematous optic nerve head with or without peripapillary retinal edema or separation.

Clinical signs that may be observed in patients with chronic glaucoma include a red eye, corneal edema, corneal striae (caused by fractures in Descemet's membrane), a normal to enlarged globe (the latter called *buphthalmos*), a midsized to dilated pupil, a subluxated to completely luxated lens, degeneration of the optic nerve head with or without cupping, and tapetal hyperreflectivity (Figures 251-2 and 251-3).

The diagnosis of glaucoma usually is entertained based on the classic clinical signs (red eye, corneal edema, dilated pupil, loss of vision), breed predisposition (in cases of primary glaucoma), ophthalmoscopic findings, and measurement of IOP. Gonioscopic evaluation, high-frequency ocular ultrasonography, and occasionally advanced radiologic imaging may be useful in understanding the cause and differential diagnoses. Tonometry, the measurement of the IOP, can be performed with various tonometers such as by use of an indentation instrument (Schiøtz tonometer), by applanation (Tono-Pen), and by the rebound process (TonoVet) as discussed in Chapter 242. There should not be a difference of more than 2 to 4 mm Hg between the two eyes. Gonioscopy is a procedure usually performed by a veterinary ophthalmologist in which a special lens is used to view the iridocorneal angle to classify glaucoma based on the degree of angle opening (normal, narrowed, closed, and dysplastic). High-frequency ultrasonography (35 to 50 MHz) can be

TABLE 251-1

Clinical Signs Observed in Acute and Chronic Glaucoma in Dogs

Structure or Feature	Acute Glaucoma	Chronic Glaucoma
Intraocular pressure	Usually elevated	Usually elevated May be low to normal (due to ciliary body atrophy)
Conjunctiva	Episcleral injection	Episcleral injection
Cornea	Edema	± Edema ± Descemet's striae
Globe size	Normal	Normal to enlarged (buphthalmos)
Pupil size	Dilated	Midsized to dilated
Lens	Normal position	Normal, subluxated, luxated
Optic nerve	Normal or swollen optic nerve head	Atrophied and/or cupped
Retina	Normal or peripapillary retinal elevation/edema	Tapetal hyperreflectivity, retinal vessel attenuation, choroidal infarcts

used to evaluate the iridocorneal angle and ciliary cleft as well as the relationship between the iris and the anterior lens capsule.

Fundus examination is extremely important to evaluate for optic nerve damage and retinal changes. Both direct and indirect ophthalmoscopy should be employed. The PanOptic Ophthalmoscope is highly recommended to the general practitioner because of its ease of use. This instrument allows thorough fundus evaluation, particularly for the examiner who is uncomfortable performing posterior segment evaluations. With this ophthalmoscope, the optic nerve and peripapillary region can be assessed readily for glaucomatous alterations.

Treatment

The treatment goals depend on whether the glaucoma is primary or secondary, whether it is acute or chronic, and whether saving vision is an attainable goal. The optimal cases for referral to a veterinary ophthalmologist are those

in which glaucoma has been diagnosed rapidly in the early stage of disease. If the IOP remains elevated for as few as 24 to 48 hours, irreversible blindness may ensue. As stated earlier, acute glaucoma is a true ophthalmic emergency and requires immediate attention from a veterinary ophthalmologist.

The three main therapeutic goals are maintenance of vision, control of the IOP, and maintenance of the health of the retinal ganglionic cells. Additional therapeutic considerations in subacute glaucoma are the potential to preserve vision and relief of ocular pain when vision has already been lost. Once glaucoma is diagnosed, medical therapy is instituted to lower the IOP rapidly. This includes the use of hyperosmotic agents (mannitol or glycerol), oral and topical carbonic anhydrase inhibitors, topical miotic agents, β-blockers, and prostaglandin analogs as well as neuroprotective agents (Table 251-2). Often multiple medications are required.

Medical Treatment

Hyperosmotic agents—namely, mannitol and glycerol—are used to decrease the IOP rapidly in an acute glaucoma crisis (Box 251-2). These agents work by dehydrating the vitreous and thus decrease the intraocular volume. Mannitol typically is dosed at 1 to 2 g/kg IV administered over 30 minutes. The patient must be fasted and water must be withheld for at least 3 hours after mannitol treatment. The IOP should be evaluated 1 hour after therapy, and if it still is elevated (and the low end of the dose range was used initially), an additional mannitol treatment can be administered at one-half the original dosage. Mannitol can remain effective for 6 to 10 hours but is not the sole therapy for acute glaucoma. Glycerol is not recommended for use in diabetic dogs because blood glucose level will increase and the insulin requirements will be altered. Osmotic diuretics also should be avoided in dehydrated

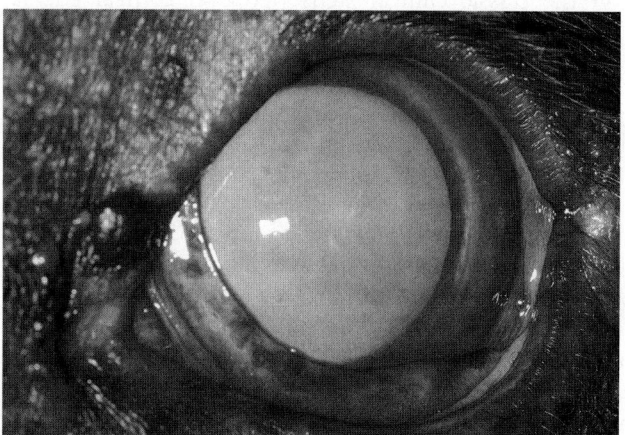

Figure 251-1 Acute glaucoma in a 9-year-old basset hound with an intraocular pressure of 45 mm Hg. Note the episcleral injection, diffuse corneal edema, and dilated pupil. (Courtesy Dr. Anne Gemensky Metzler.)

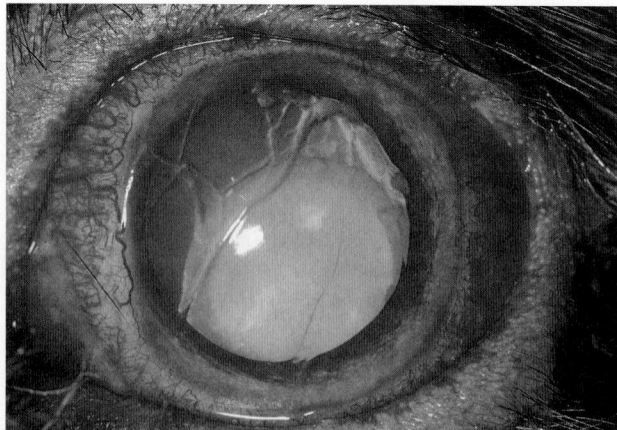

Figure 251-2 Chronic glaucoma in a 10-year-old cocker spaniel. Note the buphthalmos, severe episcleral injection, diffuse corneal edema, dilated pupil, and posteriorly subluxated and cataractous lens in this blind eye. The mucoid discharge is secondary to corneal exposure and keratoconjunctivitis sicca. (Courtesy Dr. Anne Gemensky Metzler.)

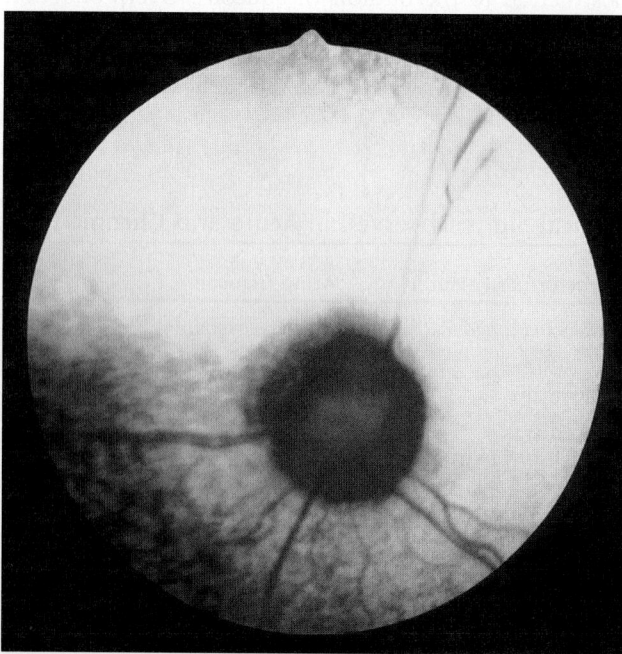

Figure 251-3 Fundus of a canine eye demonstrating a cupped and atrophic optic nerve secondary to chronic glaucoma. (Courtesy Dr. David Wilkie.)

patients as well as those with congestive heart failure, systemic hypertension, or significant renal disease. During mannitol administration adjunctive topical and oral medications should be started. In some patients with marked aqueous flare, the IOP may not be reduced effectively with hyperosmotic agents.

Prostaglandin drugs such as latanoprost, travoprost, and bimatoprost have changed glaucoma therapy markedly for canine patients. These agents work by increasing the uveoscleral outflow and can significantly reduce the IOP in dogs. Prostaglandin analogs can be used in acute glaucoma therapy instead of mannitol and also for long-term maintenance in chronic glaucoma. Prostaglandin analogs cause a marked miosis in canine patients, which can eliminate the pupillary blockade in some acute cases and often results in rapid resolution of the glaucoma with just one drop of drug. Prostaglandin agents are contraindicated in cases of anterior uveitis and anterior lens luxation. Clinically, prostaglandin agents can be used in conjunction with topical carbonic anhydrase inhibitors (CAIs) and also β-blockers but are not recommended for concurrent use with topical miotic drugs. A generic form of latanoprost is commercially available.

Topical and oral CAIs decrease the production of aqueous humor. Topical dorzolamide and brinzolamide commonly are prescribed in small animal practice. Dorzolamide is well tolerated by most dogs. Brinzolamide has been shown to reduce IOP significantly in dogs with glaucoma. A dorzolamide-timolol combination also is commercially available, and the recommended twice-daily administration may improve client compliance. Oral and topical CAIs commonly are used for long-term management of chronic glaucoma. Methazolamide and acetazolamide are available commercially, but the latter

---

BOX 251-2

Medications Commonly Prescribed for Treatment of Acute and Chronic Glaucoma in Dogs

Hyperosmotics (Mainly Used for Acute Glaucoma)
Mannitol 20% solution 0.5-1.5 g/kg IV slowly
Glycerol or glycerin 50% and 75% solutions 1-2 ml/kg q8h PO of a 40 mg/ml liquid emulsion

Carbonic Anhydrase Inhibitors*
Methazolamide (Neptazane) 2-3 mg/kg q8-12h PO
Acetazolamide (Diamox) 4-8 mg/kg q8-12h PO (not generally recommended due to systemic adverse effects)
Dorzolamide 2% (Trusopt) q8h topically
Brinzolamide 1% (Azopt) q8h topically

Prostaglandin Analogs
Latanoprost 0.005% (Xalatan) q12-24h
Bimatoprost 0.03% (Lumigan) q12-24h
Travoprost 0.004% (Travatan) q12-24h

Miotics
Pilocarpine 1-2% q6h
Demecarium bromide 0.25% q12h (available from a compounding pharmacy)

β-Blockers*
Timolol 0.5% (Timoptic) q12h
Metipranolol 0.3% (OptiPranolol) q12h
Betaxolol 0.5% (Betoptic) q12h

Neuroprotective Agents
Amlodipine (Norvasc) 0.125-0.4 mg/kg/day PO

*Also suitable for prophylactic therapy in eye with normal intraocular pressure.
IV, Intravenous; *PO*, orally.

TABLE 251-2

Medical Options for Treatment of Acute Glaucoma with and without Uveitis

No Uveitis	Uveitis
Consider mannitol therapy (1-2 g/kg IV slowly) or 1 drop of a prostaglandin analog (e.g., latanoprost or travoprost).	Avoid topical prostaglandin analog and miotic agents. Attempt IV mannitol therapy. Start concurrent topical and oral CAIs.
Evaluate IOP in 30-60 min.	Evaluate IOP in 30-60 min.
If IOP < 35 mm Hg, continue medical therapy with topical and oral CAIs and prostaglandin ± β-blocker, sympathomimetic agent, and neuroprotective agent. Provide early referral to veterinary ophthalmologist.	If IOP < 35 mm Hg, continue medical therapy with topical corticosteroid and topical and oral CAIs ± prostaglandin, β-blocker, sympathomimetic agent, and neuroprotective agent. Provide early referral to veterinary ophthalmologist.
If IOP > 35 mm Hg, may repeat mannitol (see text).	If IOP > 35 mm Hg, may repeat mannitol (see text).
If IOP < 35 mm Hg, follow above recommendations.	If IOP < 35 mm Hg, follow above recommendations.
If IOP > 35 mm Hg, refer immediately to specialist.	If IOP > 35 mm Hg, refer immediately to specialist.

CAIs, Carbonic anhydrase inhibitors; *IOP*, intraocular pressure; *IV*, intravenous.

is associated with more adverse effects and generally is not recommended for use in dogs. Dichlorphenamide is no longer available commercially but can be obtained from a compounding pharmacy. Adverse effects of CAIs caused by the systemic effects of the medications include polyuria and polydipsia, metabolic acidosis (with associated panting), vomiting, diarrhea, anorexia, rare blood dyscrasias, nephrolithiasis, and skin eruptions. Because potassium excretion is increased with the use of oral CAIs, supplementation with oral potassium is advised to avoid the potential sequelae of hypokalemia.

Miotic agents such as pilocarpine and demecarium bromide cause constriction of the pupil and opening of the iridocorneal angle, which increases the outflow of aqueous humor through the trabecular meshwork. These drugs are used much less often today because of their adverse effects (stinging, exacerbation of uveitis), availability of newer, improved topical medications, and difficulty in obtaining some of these miotics. Pilocarpine and demecarium bromide are direct and indirect parasympathomimetic agents, respectively. The frequency of use is every 6 to 8 hours for pilocarpine and twice daily for demecarium bromide. These miotics should *never* be used in patients with secondary glaucoma associated with uveitis or an anterior lens luxation because they can exacerbate the uveitis and cause entrapment of an anteriorly luxated lens. Also, miotic agents are ineffective if the IOP is more than 50 mm Hg. In terms of prevention, demecarium bromide 0.25% has been shown to delay the onset of primary glaucoma significantly in predisposed eyes.

β-Blockers such as timolol were long a mainstay in human ophthalmology but have been replaced by more effective topical medications. β-Blockers decrease the production of aqueous humor and can be added to other glaucoma medications in dogs, but their effectiveness as a sole agent is very limited. In contrast to the miotic agents, β-blockers do not cause breakdown of the blood-aqueous barrier. As noted earlier, combinations of timolol and the topical CAI dorzolamide are available. With regard to prevention of glaucoma in predisposed eyes, topical betaxolol 0.5% administered twice daily has been shown to lengthen the time to development of glaucoma. β-Blockers are absorbed systemically and therefore should be used with great caution in dogs with obstructive pulmonary disease, heart failure, or cardiac conduction system disease such as sick sinus syndrome.

Sympathomimetic agents reduce IOP by decreasing the production and increasing the outflow of aqueous humor. Many of the sympathomimetic drugs have been discontinued. An epinephrine prodrug called *dipivefrin hydrochloride* was available as Propine but now has been removed from the market. Compounding pharmacies still supply this medication. Dipivefrin is not a highly effective medication as a sole agent but may have an additive effect when combined with other drugs.

Neuroprotective pharmaceuticals have been used to minimize optic nerve damage associated with glaucoma, but their usage is controversial. Drugs such as amlodipine (a calcium channel blocker) and memantine (an N-methyl-d-aspartate inhibitor) have been used empirically in treatment of canine glaucoma, but efficacy data are lacking.

The author uses amlodipine in all visual glaucoma cases at a dosage of 0.125 to 0.4 mg/kg/day PO. Blood pressure should be monitored.

An important component of therapy in cases of primary glaucoma is prophylactic treatment of the contralateral eye, even if IOP in that eye is normal, because there is a strong likelihood that this eye also will develop glaucoma within a year's time. Either a topical CAI such as dorzolamide or a β-blocker such as timolol is a suitable choice for prophylactic therapy and may be administered every 8 to 12 hours. Clients should be advised of the importance of prophylactic treatment and careful monitoring of the "good" eye to ensure the best chance for long-term retention of vision.

Intraocular Pressure Monitoring

Once glaucoma has been diagnosed and a therapeutic regimen established, the IOP should be monitored every 1 to 3 months to ensure adequate control in the affected eye as well as to monitor for the onset of glaucoma in the contralateral eye (in cases of primary glaucoma). Ideally, IOP should not exceed 18 to 20 mm Hg when the patient is receiving prophylactic glaucoma medications. Clients should be well educated on the clinical signs of glaucoma (red eye plus blue eye plus dilated pupil with or without vision loss) and advised that the IOP should be measured immediately if a pressure spike is suspected. When the IOP is not controlled adequately with medical therapy, surgical options should be considered.

Surgical Options

The exact surgical procedure chosen depends on the surgeon's expertise, available equipment, and goals for the patient. The most important issue related to selection of surgical therapy is whether the salvage of *vision* or the relief of *pain* is the primary goal. Other considerations are the animal's breed, age, underlying metabolic or cardiac disorders, and globe size as well as the client's expectations and financial constraints. The surgical therapy for secondary glaucoma must target the underlying disease process. For example, if there is an anteriorly luxated lens in a visual eye, then an intracapsular lens extraction is advised. If intraocular neoplasia is present, enucleation and ocular biopsy is recommended after a thorough evaluation for metastatic disease.

Surgery has significant limitations in terms of outcomes. One must be mindful that glaucoma arguably is the most difficult disorder for an ophthalmologist to treat. Treatment failures are more frequent than surgical successes. However, in an appropriately diagnosed and treated case of early glaucoma, retention of vision may be an attainable goal. A dedicated client and an early diagnosis are imperative for success.

Visual Eyes

For visual eyes (or for those with a hope of retaining vision), the ophthalmologist usually performs a ciliodestructive procedure (selective damage to the ciliary body) or a fistulizing procedure (creation of an alternative outflow pathway). Combination ciliodestructive and alternative pathway procedures also are commonly advocated. Ciliodestructive procedures can entail the use of lasers, cryotherapy (freezing), diathermy (heat), and ultrasonic waves; laser and cryotherapy procedures most commonly are used. The laser treatment causes a decrease in aqueous production due to destruction of the pigmented cells of the ciliary body epithelium. Poorly pigmented animals (such as albinotic, subalbinotic, or blue iris patients) may respond in a less favorable fashion to laser cyclophotocoagulation than dogs with a brown iris. Previous reports of the use of diode transscleral cyclophotocoagulation demonstrated adequate IOP control in 92% of cases and an average decrease in IOP of 58% in treated eyes over a 12-month follow-up period (Hardman and Stanley, 2001). Vision was retained in 37% to 50% of the potentially visual eyes in previous reports. Complications noted with laser cycloablation include uveitis, hyphema, cataract formation, early posttreatment spikes of high IOP, recurrence of glaucoma, retinal detachment, corneal ulcer, and dyscoria. A combination technique using a glaucoma drainage implant (gonioimplant) and photocoagulation can provide immediate relief of IOP elevation in a recently laser-treated eye.

Freezing the area of the ciliary body (cyclocryotherapy) with either liquid nitrogen or nitrous oxide also is associated with cyclodestruction. The cryotherapy procedure is said to be more painful than the laser procedure in people, but in experienced hands, cryotherapy has been reported to be successful in dogs. Cryotherapy may be more effective than laser procedures in poorly pigmented eyes. Complications associated with cyclocryotherapy include an immediate IOP elevation, cataract formation, retinal detachment, ocular pain, and recurrence of glaucoma.

A relatively new procedure for cyclophotocoagulation in veterinary medicine is the diode endolaser, an endoscopically guided laser that can cause selective destruction of the ciliary body. This endoscopic cyclophotocoagulation (ECP) procedure has been used in human medicine since 1992. Complete visualization and treatment of the intended target tissue of the ciliary processes are possible with the endolaser, which allows a more precise laser placement and lower energy usage with ECP compared with the blind transscleral laser approach. Collateral damage to the lens, iris, and retina thus can be avoided. Several veterinary ophthalmologists are combining this ECP procedure with lens removal (phacoemulsification of the normal lens or cataract) to allow better access to the ciliary sulcus and ciliary processes as well as to avoid future cataract formation if the lens is left *in situ*. There are no published data on the results of the ECP procedure, but preliminary findings appear promising.

To minimize the postoperative IOP elevation associated with any laser treatment, prior or concurrent placement of a gonioimplant also has been advocated in cases of acute canine glaucoma with the hope of preserving vision. Results presented by Bras et al (2005) for 112 canine patients with primary glaucoma treated with ECP demonstrated control of IOP in 91% of cases and preservation of vision in 70% of cases. Lutz and Sapienza (2008) presented promising results in pseudophakic or aphakic dogs with secondary glaucoma, with control of IOP in 100% of cases at 2 months after ECP surgery and

maintenance or recovery of vision in 67% of cases. At present ECP (with or without a gonioimplant procedure) is considered the new wave of therapy for primary glaucoma in dogs.

Fistulizing procedures are surgeries that create an alternate pathway for aqueous outflow. Recently the use of gonioimplants or glaucoma shunts from the anterior chamber has gained popularity in small animal ophthalmology. Many types of glaucoma shunts are used, and these generally are placed in the anterior chamber to move aqueous humor to the subconjunctival space or frontal sinus. Suprachoroidal shunts, implants that direct the flow of aqueous humor into the supraciliary space (mimicking the uveoscleral outflow), also have been described, but their long-term success has not been demonstrated to date. Short-term complications with these gonioimplants include postoperative anterior uveitis, progression of glaucoma, and fibrin occlusion of the implanted anterior chamber tube. Long-term complications of glaucoma shunt placement include tube migration, fibrous capsule formation around the reservoir base, contact of the anterior chamber tube with the corneal endothelium, and recurrence of glaucoma.

The author has described and advocated a combined procedure of cyclodestruction with a contact diode laser and placement of an Ahmed glaucoma valve into the anterior chamber. In a study in which 51 dogs with primary glaucoma were treated using the combined procedure of laser diode cyclophotocoagulation and Ahmed glaucoma implant placement, a return or maintenance of vision occurred in 82% of operated eyes in the immediate short term, and long-term IOP control was achieved in 76% of cases. At 1 year after surgery, 41% of the eyes were still visual (Sapienza and van der Woerdt, 2005).

Paracentesis, or insertion of a needle into the anterior chamber to relieve pressure rapidly, is considered to be a poor technique as the sole therapy for primary glaucoma. The rapid decrease in IOP may induce a disastrous intraocular hemorrhage; in addition, there is the potential for intraocular damage to the iris or lens. Thus, as a primary way to treat glaucoma, paracentesis is *never* advised.

Painful Blind Eyes

For blind and painful eyes, salvage procedures are available to reduce the pain of a blind glaucomatous eye. The choice of procedure depends on a number of factors, including the size of the globe, the type of glaucoma (primary versus secondary), the presence of concurrent ocular diseases, cost, the dog's age and ability to undergo general anesthesia safely, and surgical preference. Choices include evisceration with intrascleral prosthesis (ISP) implantation, enucleation, intravitreal chemical injection, laser treatment, and cryocycloablation.

As a general rule, for irreversibly blind canine eyes with primary glaucoma, the author usually prefers to perform evisceration with implantation of an ISP. Tissues should be submitted for ocular histopathologic evaluation. ISP implantation is a procedure in which the intraocular contents are removed and a silicone sphere inserted through a scleral incision. The ISP procedure should be avoided in cases of severe corneal disease, intraocular infection (endophthalmitis), or neoplasia. ISP surgery is relatively

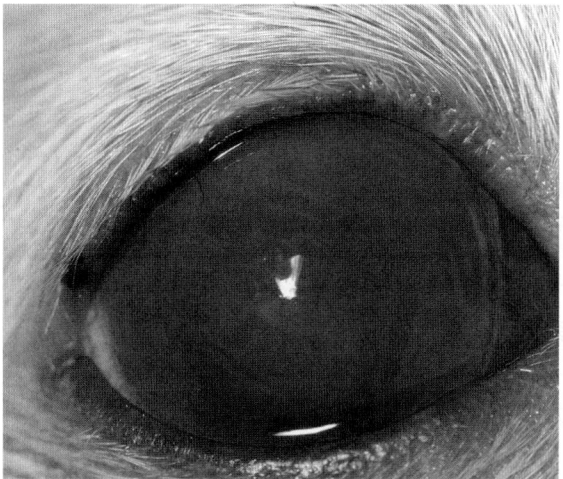

Figure 251-4 Cosmetic postoperative appearance of an intrascleral silicone prosthesis placed in a 6-year-old Maltese with blinding glaucoma. Note the subtle wrinkling of the corneal endothelium. (Courtesy Dr. Anne Gemensky Metzler.)

BOX 251-3

Available Surgical Options for Visual and Blind Eyes in Dogs

Surgical Options for a Visual Eye
Laser cyclophotocoagulation
Cyclocryotherapy
Endoscopic cyclophotocoagulation (with or without lens removal)
Gonioimplant placement
Frontal glaucoma shunt placement
Combination of laser therapy or cyclocryotherapy plus glaucoma shunt placement

Surgical Options for a Blind Eye in a Dog with Chronic Glaucoma
Evisceration with placement of an intrascleral prosthesis
Enucleation
Laser therapy (transscleral or endoscopic)
Cryotherapy
Intravitreal gentamicin or cidofovir injection

rapid and typically associated with few complications. Bilateral ISP surgery can be performed in dogs that have lost vision in both eyes because of chronic glaucoma. In most cases a very cosmetic result is achieved with a gray to black color of the eye (Figure 251-4). Possible complications associated with ISP surgery include corneal ulcer formation due to poor blinking ability, extrusion of the implant, infection, placement of an inadequately sized implant, development of keratoconjunctivitis sicca, unrecognized intraocular neoplasia, and inadequate evisceration of the intraocular contents.

Enucleation, or eye removal, is a technique preferred by many ophthalmologists in glaucoma cases. Ocular pain is relieved, and tissue is readily available for histopathologic analysis. Many owners, however, may be resistant to the idea of a one-eyed pet. Postoperative bleeding, cyst formation (due to inadequate removal of any epithelial or glandular tissue), and a sunken orbital pocket are potential complications associated with enucleation.

Intraocular injections of a toxic chemical to destroy the ciliary body also can be performed in a blind eye. Injections of gentamicin (or, less commonly, cidofovir) are used. The advantage of this technique is that the procedure is rapid, can be performed under sedation or deep topical or peribulbar anesthesia, and results in effective destruction of the ciliary body. The eye must be blinded already before this procedure is performed because this toxic intraocular injection will surely result in blindness due to retinal toxicity. The disadvantages of gentamicin injections are the relatively uncertain cosmesis of the globe, frequent development of a shrunken globe (phthisis bulbi), potential recurrence of glaucoma, and possibility of injection into an eye with an undiagnosed intraocular tumor.

Thus the choices for glaucoma therapy are numerous and are determined by the treatment goals, the equipment available, the surgeon's training, and surgeon and owner preferences (Box 251-3).

References and Suggested Reading

Bras TD et al: Diode endolaser cyclophotocoagulation in canine and feline glaucoma, *Vet Ophthalmol* 8(6):449, 2005.

Cook CS et al: Diode laser transscleral cyclophotocoagulation for the treatment of glaucoma in dogs: results of six and twelve month follow-up, *Vet Comp Ophthalmol* 7:148, 1997.

Cullen CL: Cullen frontal sinus valved glaucoma shunt: preliminary findings in dogs with primary glaucoma, *Vet Ophthalmol* 7:311, 2004.

Gelatt KN, Brooks DE, Källberg ME: The canine glaucomas. In Gelatt KN, editor: *Veterinary ophthalmology*, ed 4, Ames, IA, 2007, Blackwell Publishing, p 753.

Hardman C, Stanley RG: Diode laser transscleral cyclophotocoagulation for the treatment of primary glaucoma in 18 dogs: a retrospective study, *Vet Ophthalmol* 4:209, 2001.

Johnsen DA, Maggs DJ, Kass PH: Evaluation of risk factors for development of secondary glaucoma in dogs: 156 cases (1999-2004), *J Am Vet Med Assoc* 229:1270, 2006.

Lutz EL, Sapienza JS: Diode endoscopic cyclophotocoagulation in pseudophakic and aphakic dogs with secondary glaucoma, *Vet Ophthalmol* 11(6):423, 2008.

Reinstein SL, Rankin AJ, Allbaugh R: Canine glaucoma: medical and surgical options, *Compend Contin Educ Vet* 31:454, 2009.

Sapienza JS, van der Woerdt A: Combined transscleral diode laser cyclophotocoagulation and Ahmed gonioimplantation in dogs with primary glaucoma: 51 cases (1996-2004), *Vet Ophthalmol* 8:121, 2005.

Westermeyer HD, Hendrix DV, Ward DA: Long-term evaluation of Ahmed gonioimplants in dogs with primary glaucoma: nine cases (2000-2008), *J Am Vet Med Assoc* 238:610, 2011.

CHAPTER 252

Feline Glaucoma

AMY J. RANKIN, *Manhattan, Kansas*

Glaucoma is one of the most frustrating conditions to treat in veterinary ophthalmology. In most cases, despite intensive therapy, the disease process continues and eventually leads to loss of vision. Glaucoma is a group of diseases that have an abnormally elevated intraocular pressure (IOP) as a common feature. The elevated IOP may cause irreversible damage to the retina and optic nerve and lead to blindness. Clinical symptoms in cats often are subtle, and many cats are not brought for treatment until late in the course of the disease when the eye is already permanently blind.

The normal IOP range in cats has been reported to be between 15 and 25 mm Hg (mean, ~20 mm Hg). IOP is generated by aqueous humor production and outflow, which normally are in equilibrium. The elevated IOP in glaucoma is due to reduced outflow of aqueous humor rather than overproduction of aqueous humor. Glaucoma can be categorized as congenital, primary, or secondary.

Congenital glaucoma is very uncommon in cats. It is due to abnormalities in the aqueous humor outflow pathway and generally occurs in very young patients (<6 months of age). Most kittens with congenital glaucoma have an acute onset of buphthalmia (enlarged globe) and corneal edema (Figure 252-1). Congenital glaucoma can be either unilateral or bilateral and may occur along with other ocular abnormalities.

In cats primary glaucoma also is very rare. Primary glaucoma is not associated with any other ocular disease and in veterinary medicine is classified as open, narrow, or closed angle, depending on the appearance of the drainage angle. It has been reported in certain breeds including Burmese, Persian, European shorthair, and Siamese. The increased incidence of primary glaucoma in purebred cats likely is due to inbreeding. Pectinate ligament dysplasia is another form of primary glaucoma that has been reported in a group of related Siamese cats. Primary glaucoma is a bilateral, heritable condition in dogs, and although the mode of inheritance has not been established in cats, breeding of cats with primary glaucoma is not recommended.

Secondary glaucoma occurs when another disease condition causes a decrease in the outflow of aqueous humor from the eye. In cats secondary glaucoma is the most common form of glaucoma. Several conditions can cause an increase in IOP, including uveitis, hyphema, intraocular neoplasia, and aqueous misdirection. The two most common causes of secondary glaucoma in cats are chronic uveitis (intraocular inflammation) and neoplasia.

Uveitis is one of the most common and clinically important ophthalmic disorders in domestic cats (see Chapter 250). Uveitis in cats has been associated with trauma, primary or metastatic neoplasia, abnormalities of the lens, infectious agents, and idiopathic causes. In a retrospective histopathologic study of 158 eviscerated or enucleated feline globes, idiopathic lymphocytic-plasmacytic uveitis was found to be the most common type of uveitis (Peiffer and Wilcock, 1991). Infectious agents that have been associated with feline uveitis include *Toxoplasma gondii*, feline immunodeficiency virus, feline leukemia virus, feline infectious peritonitis virus, and fungi causing systemic infections (*Blastomyces dermatitidis*, *Cryptococcus neoformans*, and *Histoplasma capsulatum*).

Although it is important to establish a cause for uveitis, standard diagnostic studies such as cytologic analysis of aqueous humor and serologic testing often are unsuccessful, and the majority of cases are classified as idiopathic. This may be related to the sensitivity and specificity of the tests as well as the stage of the disease process when the cat shows signs of uveitis. In general a complete blood count (CBC), chemistry panel, urinalysis, feline leukemia virus assay, feline immunodeficiency virus assay, and possibly feline infectious peritonitis tests should be performed in cats with intraocular inflammation. Other diagnostic tests can be performed depending on the geographic location of the cat and the general health of the patient. Treatment of uveitis is aimed at decreasing intraocular inflammation and relieving signs of discomfort. Antiinflammatory medications in addition to a specific antimicrobial agent when an infectious cause has been identified are recommended for treatment of uveitis. In general, topical antiinflammatory medications, such as prednisolone acetate 1% suspension every 6 to 12 hours, are recommended to treat anterior uveitis (depending on the severity of the inflammation). Topical nonsteroidal antiinflammatory drugs, such as flurbiprofen 0.03% and diclofenac 0.1%, may increase IOP and should be avoided in feline patients with an elevated IOP.

Intraocular neoplasia is the second most common cause of secondary glaucoma in cats. Although any primary or metastatic intraocular tumor may lead to the development of increased IOP, diffuse iris melanoma is the most common tumor to cause secondary glaucoma in cats. This tumor generally starts as a small focal area of iris hyperpigmentation. These tumors progress slowly, over the course of several months to even years. As the tumor progresses, infiltration of the iridocorneal angle with neoplastic cells leads to the development of glaucoma. In a study evaluating the survival rate of cats in which enucleation was performed to treat diffuse iris melanoma, cats with secondary glaucoma due to the tumor had shorter survival times than cats with diffuse

1177

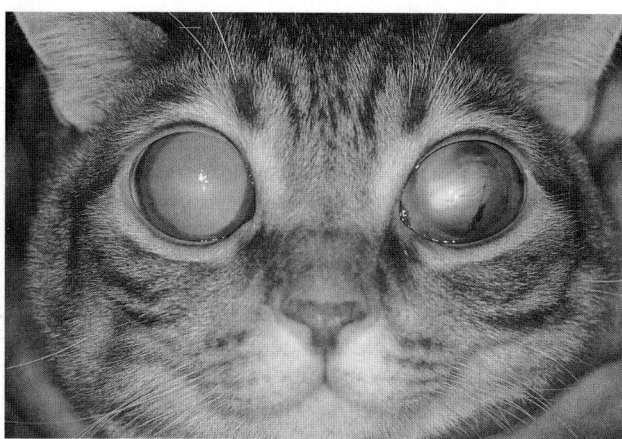

Figure 252-1 Bilateral congenital glaucoma and buphthalmia in a 3-year-old male castrated domestic shorthair. (Courtesy Kansas State University Veterinary Ophthalmology Service.)

iris melanomas that did not have secondary glaucoma. Lymphosarcoma is the second most common intraocular tumor to cause secondary glaucoma in cats. Typically it manifests as pinkish-whitish nodular lesions on the iris.

Hyphema (blood in the anterior chamber) is another cause of secondary glaucoma, which results from obstruction of the iridocorneal angle with blood. Hyphema can be caused by numerous disorders, such as trauma, coagulopathies, infectious diseases, and neoplasia, but in older cats systemic hypertension probably is the most common cause. In cats with systemic hypertension (systolic blood pressure of ≥160 mm Hg) a CBC, chemistry panel, urinalysis, and thyroxine level measurement should be performed to rule out chronic kidney disease or hyperthyroidism as the cause of systemic hypertension.

Aqueous misdirection, also known as *malignant glaucoma,* is another form of glaucoma that has been described in cats. In this condition the aqueous humor is misdirected into the vitreal space and the lens and iris are shifted anteriorly, which occludes the iridocorneal angle. Cats with aqueous misdirection may show mydriasis (dilated pupil), decreased pupillary light reflexes, decreased menace response, an abnormally shallow anterior chamber, elevated IOP, and glaucomatous changes in the optic nerve head. In a study of 32 cats with aqueous misdirection, the mean age at the time of diagnosis was found to be approximately 12 years, and female cats were affected significantly more often than males. This condition has been reported to occur more often unilaterally, but it can also occur bilaterally. Medical treatment of aqueous misdirection includes the use of topical carbonic anhydrase inhibitors such as dorzolamide 2% every 8 to 12 hours to reduce the production of aqueous humor. Drugs that cause miosis (constriction of the pupil) such as prostaglandin analogs, pilocarpine, and timolol should not be used to treat aqueous misdirection syndrome because these medications may exacerbate glaucoma by increasing contact between the iris and the lens and further decreasing the outflow of aqueous humor through the pupil. If the IOP cannot be controlled sufficiently with medical therapy, referral to an ophthalmologist for a lensectomy and anterior vitrectomy may be indicated.

Ideally the IOP should be less than 25 mm Hg to prevent the discomfort associated with elevated IOP and also to prevent damage to the retina and optic nerve, which could lead to loss of vision. With early detection and medical intervention many cats with this condition can remain comfortable and visual.

Clinical signs of glaucoma in cats usually are subtle, and most cats are not brought for treatment until late in the course of disease. Owners may notice mydriasis, a cloudy eye (corneal edema), or buphthalmos. In most cases of feline glaucoma conjunctival hyperemia is absent to minimal. On examination of the fundus retinal degeneration may be present, which is characterized by tapetal hyperreflectivity and vascular attenuation. Optic nerve cupping is difficult to appreciate in cats due to the lack of myelin on the optic nerve head. An optic nerve that is atrophied appears darker than a normal optic nerve.

Two commonly used instruments to measure IOP are the Tono-Pen and the TonoVet tonometers (see Chapter 242). The Tono-Pen is an applanation tonometer and estimates IOP by flattening the surface of the cornea. A topical anesthetic such as ophthalmic proparacaine must be used to obtain readings with this instrument. The instrument is held perpendicular to the corneal surface and is tapped lightly on the central portion of the cornea. Brief beeps indicate when an individual reading has been recorded, and a longer tone indicates that the mean of those IOP readings has been calculated. The mean IOP is displayed along with the coefficient of variation obtained from the readings (i.e., 5%, 10%, 20%, or >20%, calculated as standard deviation/mean). The Tono-Pen is very accurate in the normal range of IOPs but tends to overestimate IOP in the low range and underestimate IOP in the high range. Ideally readings with a coefficient of variation of 5% or less should be recorded as the IOP for that patient.

The TonoVet measures the rebound action of a magnetic probe as it contacts the corneal surface and bounces back. One of the advantages of the TonoVet tonometer is that it does not require the use of a topical anesthetic. The instrument should be held upright while taking measurements. The mean IOP reading obtained with the rebound tonometer (TonoVet) has been found to be 2 to 3 mm Hg higher than that measured with the applanation tonometer (Tono-Pen VET) in cats. Although a difference of 2 to 3 mm Hg is not clinically significant, it highlights the importance of using the same tonometer for follow-up examinations in the same patient.

IOP can be elevated artificially in cats without any ophthalmic abnormalities, which indicates that a single abnormal IOP measurement in the absence of other ophthalmic abnormalities may be insufficient for a diagnosis of glaucoma in cats. Artificially high IOP readings can occur in fractious or nervous cats. Excessive pressure on the globe, eyelids, or neck also can increase IOP readings artificially. Cats that have IOP readings of 25 mm Hg or more or a difference in IOP between the two eyes of 12 mm Hg or more but that do not show any ophthalmic abnormalities or changes in the optic nerve head may have a falsely high IOP. Tonometry should be repeated in these cats within a few weeks, and if the elevation in IOP persists, referral to an ophthalmologist for a more thorough examination may be warranted before antiglaucoma therapy is initiated.

Because secondary glaucoma is much more common than primary glaucoma it is important to diagnose the cause of glaucoma (e.g., uveitis or neoplasia) and address the underlying issue. In cases of uveitis, topical antiinflammatory therapy and specific antimicrobial agents when an infectious cause has been identified are recommended (see Chapter 250). Antiglaucoma medications can be used at the same time as topical antiinflammatories. In cases of intraocular neoplasia, enucleation and histopathologic examination of the eye is recommended. If an intraocular tumor is suspected, thoracic and abdominal radiography and abdominal ultrasonography should be discussed with the owner before surgery is undertaken to remove the eye.

The goals of glaucoma therapy are to preserve vision and alleviate discomfort. The therapeutic plan depends on the cause of the glaucoma and the patient's visual status.

Medical Treatment

Hyperosmotic Agents

The administration of hyperosmotic agents is indicated only in the treatment of acute glaucoma. Since the majority of cats have chronic glaucoma these medications very rarely are indicated. Mannitol can be administered over a 20- to 30-minute period at a dosage of 1 g/kg IV. Water or fluids should be withheld for 4 hours and then slowly reintroduced. Mannitol should not be administered to cats with heart failure, known cardiomyopathy, or renal impairment.

Carbonic Anhydrase Inhibitors

Systemic and topical carbonic anhydrase inhibitors (CAIs) are available. CAIs work by decreasing the production of aqueous humor. The administration of oral CAIs can be associated with anorexia, gastrointestinal disturbances, increased respiratory rate secondary to metabolic acidosis, hypokalemia, blood dyscrasias, and neurologic abnormalities. Cats appear to be more susceptible to the adverse effects of oral CAIs than other species, and oral CAIs should *not* be used in cats.

Because of the adverse effects associated with systemic CAIs topical formulations have been developed. The topical ophthalmic CAIs currently available commercially are dorzolamide hydrochloride 2% solution (Trusopt and generic) and brinzolamide 1% suspension (Azopt). Experimental evaluation of the use of dorzolamide 2% in normal cats showed a significant decrease in IOP compared with pretreatment values (Rainbow and Dziezyc, 2003; Dietrich et al, 2007; Rankin et al, 2011); however, the magnitude of effect of dorzolamide on IOP in normotensive cats may not be an accurate representation of the effect of this medication in cats with glaucoma. Dogs with glaucoma typically have a greater decrease in IOP than normotensive dogs when treated with topical and systemic CAIs. Cats with glaucoma are likely to have a

more dramatic response to topical CAIs than normal cats, so the practitioner should not be dissuaded from the use of this important class of medications. A recent study demonstrated a dramatic decrease in IOP in cats with primary congenital glaucoma that were treated three times daily with topical dorzolamide 2% solution (Sigle et al, 2011). The most common adverse effect with the use of topical CAIs is irritation after instillation, which is more common with dorzolamide than with brinzolamide. A solution of dorzolamide 2% and timolol 0.5% is commercially available but does not appear to lower IOP more than dorzolamide alone three times daily in cats. Also, because of the possible absorption of the medication and the small body size of cats, a β-blocker should be used with caution. Topical carbonic anhydrase inhibitors should be administered every 8 to 12 hours.

β-Blockers

Betaxolol is a selective β_1-antagonist and timolol is a nonselective β-antagonist. Both of these medications are available in 0.25% and 0.5% ophthalmic solutions. Topical administration of timolol 0.5% to normotensive cats causes a significant (22%) decrease in IOP. A significant miosis also is observed. After topical application of an ophthalmic medication, a portion of the medication is absorbed systemically through the conjunctiva or the nasal or oral mucosa after the medication passes through the nasolacrimal system. Although serum levels of drugs that are applied topically to the eye generally are low, there can be systemic side effects. β-Blockers may cause undesirable cardiac effects, including bradycardia, syncope, or reduced myocardial contractility. In addition to adverse cardiac effects, blockade of β_2-receptors by nonselective β-blockers could theoretically lead to respiratory complications, and these drugs should not be used in cats with a history of asthma. Because of the small body size of cats, topical β-blockers should be used with caution in cats, and the 0.25% ophthalmic solution should be administered every 12 to 24 hours.

α-Agonists

Apraclonidine is an α_2-agonist. Although it causes a significant decrease in IOP in normotensive cats, it should not be used because of the severe adverse effects associated with its administration, including decreased heart rate and vomiting.

Cholinergic Agents

Topical pilocarpine 2%, a direct-acting parasympathomimetic agent, has been reported to decrease IOP in normotensive cats. Parasympathomimetic medications are contraindicated in cases of uveitis because they may increase the permeability of the blood-aqueous barrier. Pilocarpine may be very irritating topically and also has the potential for serious systemic adverse effects, and should not be used in cats to treat glaucoma. Demecarium bromide is an indirect-acting parasympathomimetic that is available from compounding pharmacies in 0.125% and 0.25% solutions. Topically applied demecarium bromide can reach systemic concentrations high enough to result in toxicosis (diarrhea, salivation, and vomiting) and also should be avoided in cats.

Prostaglandin Analogs

Prostaglandin analogs are the newest antiglaucoma medications available. They are believed to lower IOP primarily by increasing uveoscleral outflow of aqueous humor via their action on iris and ciliary body musculature. In addition, there is evidence to suggest that prostaglandin analogs also have an effect on the conventional outflow pathway and decrease the production of aqueous humor. Topical application of prostaglandins decreases IOP in cats, but unfortunately the commercially available prostaglandin analogs, including latanoprost, bimatoprost, and unoprostone, do not consistently reduce IOP in cats. Although these medications cause significant miosis, they do not consistently decrease IOP and therefore are not recommended for the treatment of feline glaucoma.

Surgical Treatment

If medical therapy can no longer control the IOP, surgery may be indicated. In visual eyes, cyclocryotherapy and cyclophotocoagulation are options to decrease the production of aqueous humor. Cyclocryotherapy uses either nitrous oxide or liquid nitrogen applied to the sclera to cause cryonecrosis of the ciliary body. Complications associated with cyclocryotherapy include inflammation inside the eye, retinal detachment, and cataract formation.

Cyclophotocoagulation is destruction of the ciliary body using either a diode or neodymium:yttrium-aluminum-garnet (Nd:YAG) laser and generally is considered to be associated with fewer complications than cyclocryotherapy. The laser energy can be delivered to the eye either through the sclera (transscleral cyclophotocoagulation) or through an intraocular endolaser that applies the laser energy directly to the ciliary body. Complications include postoperative increases in IOP, corneal ulcers, cataract, hyphema, and retinal detachment.

Endoscopic cyclophotocoagulation offers a fairly high rate of success in IOP control and vision preservation.

In permanently blind eyes with glaucoma, a palliative surgical procedure is recommended to alleviate pain. In general, discomfort is not associated with an IOP of less than 25 mm Hg. Enucleation is recommended for painful blind eyes. If an intraocular tumor or uveitis is suspected, the globe should be submitted to a veterinary pathologist for histopathologic evaluation. Placement of an orbital prosthesis is not recommended in cats because of the high complication rate (40%) seen in this species. Evisceration and placement of an intraocular prosthesis is another option for cats that do not have an intraocular tumor or intraocular infection, but cats are more likely than dogs to have complications associated with the prosthesis. Chemical ablation of the ciliary body epithelium with an intravitreal injection of gentamicin is not recommended in cats because of the potential for inducing an intraocular sarcoma.

References and Suggested Reading

Czederpiltz JMC et al: Putative aqueous humor misdirection syndrome as a cause of glaucoma in cats: 32 cases (1997-2003), *J Am Vet Med Assoc* 227(9):1434, 2005.

Dietrich UM et al: Effects of topical 2% dorzolamide hydrochloride alone and in combination with 0.5% timolol maleate on intraocular pressure in normal feline eyes, *Vet Ophthalmol* 10(Suppl 1):95, 2007.

Peiffer R, Wilcock B: Histopathologic study of uveitis in cats: 139 cases, *J Am Vet Med Assoc* 198:135, 1991.

Powell CC, Lappin MR: Causes of feline uveitis, *Comp Contin Ed Pract Vet* 23(2):128, 2001a.

Powell CC, Lappin MR: Diagnosis and treatment of feline uveitis, *Comp Contin Ed Pract Vet* 23(3):258, 2001b.

Rainbow M, Dziezyc J: Effects of twice daily application of 2% dorzolamide on intraocular pressure in normal cats, *Vet Ophthalmol* 6:147, 2003.

Rankin A, Crumley W, Allbaugh R: Effects of ocular administration of ophthalmic 2% dorzolamide hydrochloride solution on aqueous humor flow rate and intraocular pressure in clinically normal cats, *Am J Vet Res* 73:1074, 2011.

Sigle K et al: The effect of dorzolamide 2% on circadian intraocular pressure in cats with primary congenital glaucoma, *Vet Ophthalmol* 14:48, 2011.

CHAPTER 253

Disorders of the Lens

DAVID A. WILKIE, *Columbus, Ohio*

The crystalline lens is an avascular, transparent, biconvex structure that serves, along with the cornea, to refract and focus an image on the retina. During embryogenesis, lens development is supported anteriorly by the pupillary membrane vasculature and posteriorly by the hyaloid vasculature. Abnormalities of these vascular structures may be associated with congenital lens malformations or cataracts.

The lens is supported by zonular fibers that originate at the ciliary body and insert at the lens equator. The zonules facilitate accommodation, which is controlled by the musculature of the ciliary body. Loss of zonular attachment results in lens instability and lens luxation.

The lens is divided into nuclear, cortical, and capsular regions. The lens nucleus is located centrally and is formed during embryogenesis. Abnormalities of the nucleus typically are congenital, but not all congenital lens abnormalities involve the nucleus. The lens cortex surrounds the nucleus and can be divided into anterior, posterior, and equatorial regions. The lens epithelial cells are located just under the anterior lens capsule. The epithelial cells undergo migration and replication and, at the lens equator, elongate anteriorly and posteriorly to form new lens cortical fibers, are displaced centrally, and join other lens fibers anteriorly and posteriorly at the regions known as the lens sutures. It is the regular arrangement of lens fibers that allows transparency. Changes in lens fiber arrangement or composition result in an opacity, termed a *cataract*. Insults to the lens epithelium may result in cell death, posterior cell migration, or epithelial-mesenchymal cell transformation, all of which contribute to cataractogenesis.

New lens fibers are added throughout life, but the lens is restricted in the size to which it can grow. As a result, rather than increase in size, the lens increases in density and the central lens becomes compressed. This results in lenticular sclerosis, a zone of change in transparency between the central and peripheral lens. Clinically this becomes apparent at the age of 6 years in most dogs and cats and increases with age (Figure 253-1).

The lens is surrounded by a capsule comprised of the basement membrane of the lens epithelial cells. The anterior lens capsule (50 to 75 μm) is thicker than the posterior capsule (5 μm). The capsule is a semipermeable membrane allowing nutritional substances and metabolic waste materials to pass while serving to isolate the antigenic lens protein. In hypermature cataracts, lens proteins can break down, leak across the capsule, and result in lens-induced uveitis. With traumatic or spontaneous rupture of the lens capsule, lens proteins enter the anterior chamber in large quantity, resulting in phacoclastic uveitis.

As an avascular structure, the lens relies on the aqueous humor for nutrition and waste removal. Abnormalities of the aqueous humor, as seen in uveitis, may alter lens metabolism and result in cataract formation. Abnormalities or changes of the lens include lenticular sclerosis, congenital malformations, cataract, lens instability, and trauma to the lens and its capsule.

Congenital Lens Anomalies

Congenital abnormalities of the lens may be solitary or part of multiple ocular anomalies and include variations in lens shape, size, location, or transparency. They may be inherited or result from toxic, infectious, nutritional, or other insults during embryogenesis. The most common congenital lenticular abnormalities are microphakia, lens coloboma, spherophakia, posterior lenticonus, cataract, and ectopia lentis. These may be associated with microphthalmia, persistent pupillary membranes, persistent hyaloid, persistent tunica vasculosa lentis, anterior segment dysgenesis, retinal dysplasia, retinal detachment, or other ocular malformations.

When a congenital ocular abnormality is present, a complete dilated ophthalmic examination of both eyes should be performed. If no obvious cause is apparent, the abnormality should be presumed to be inherited, and affected animals should not be used for breeding. In addition, parents and littermates should be examined whenever possible. Follow-up examination of affected animals should be performed to monitor for progression of cataract or glaucoma. When significant cataracts are present, surgical removal may be an option, but placement of an intraocular lens may be difficult or impossible in cases of microphakic lenses or microphthalmic eyes. Additionally, these eyes are at increased risk of postoperative glaucoma and retinal detachment compared with the eyes of routine cataract patients.

Cataract

A *cataract* is defined as an opacity of the lens or its capsule regardless of size. Cataracts are classified by age of onset, location, severity, and cause (Table 253-1). Cataracts may be congenital (present at birth), juvenile (appearing at <2 years of age), adult (appearing at 2 to 6 years of age), or senile (appearing at >6 years of age). Cataract locations are described as nuclear, cortical (anterior, posterior, equatorial), capsular, and axial versus peripheral. With respect

TABLE 253-1

Classification of Cataracts

Age of onset	Congenital (present at birth)
	Developmental
	    Juvenile (<2 yr)
	    Adult (2-6 yr)
	    Senile (>6 yr)

Severity	Incipient Immature Mature Hypermature Morgagnian
Cause	Inherited Associated with other congenital ocular abnormalities Metabolic disease—diabetes mellitus Trauma Retinal degeneration Inflammatory disease—uveitis Toxins or drugs Radiation Electric shock
Location	Capsular—anterior, posterior Cortical—anterior, posterior, equatorial Nuclear Equatorial vs. axial

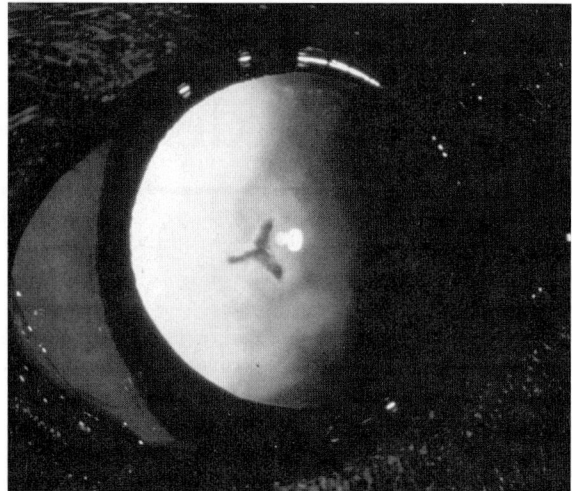

Figure 253-2 Incipient axial posterior cortical cataract involving the posterior suture in a 2-year-old Labrador retriever.

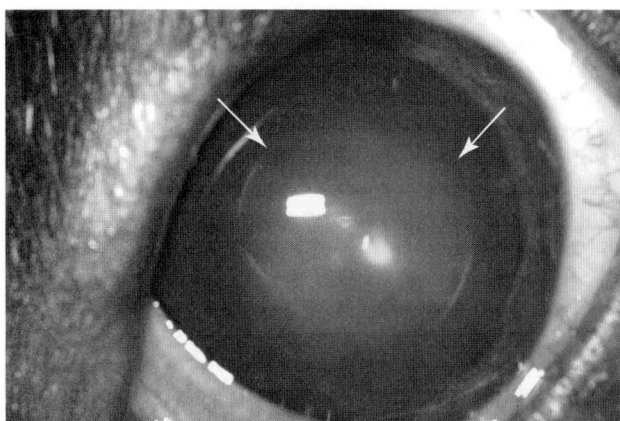

Figure 253-1 Lenticular sclerosis *(arrows)* of the axial lens in an 11-year-old Labrador retriever.

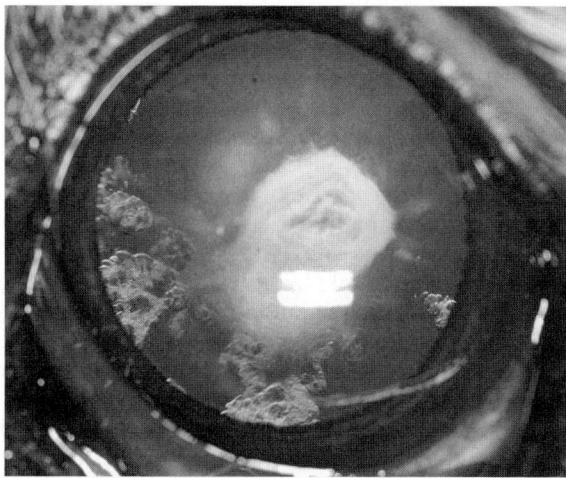

Figure 253-3 Immature cataract involving the posterior, anterior, and equatorial cortex in a 2-year-old golden retriever. The equatorial involvement shows cortical vacuoles suggestive of more recent and rapid cataract progression.

to severity and the amount of lens affected by a cataract, the terms used are *incipient* (does not affect vision significantly; Figure 253-2), *immature* (interferes with vision but does not completely prevent it; Figure 253-3), *mature* (obscures an image entirely; Figure 253-4), and *hypermature* (liquefactive degeneration of the lens proteins has occurred). Liquefaction of lens protein results in lens-induced uveitis that may lead to globe hypotony, iris hyperpigmentation, aqueous flare, miosis, synechia, keratic precipitates, lens instability, secondary glaucoma, vitreous degeneration, or retinal detachment (Figure 253-5). Hypermature cataracts are characterized clinically by irregularity of the lens surface, a deeper anterior chamber,

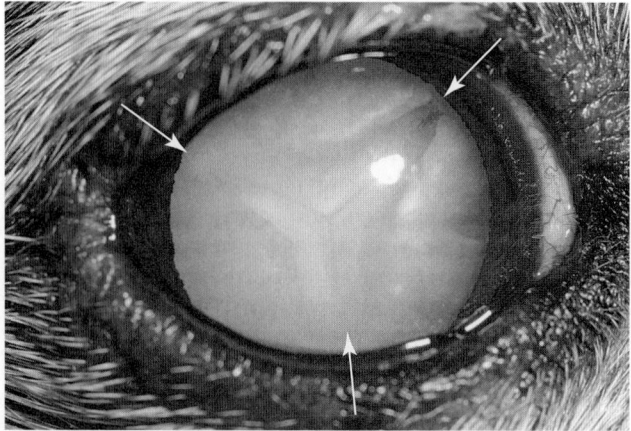

Figure 253-4 Mature intumescent (swollen) cataract with suture clefting *(arrows)* secondary to diabetes mellitus.

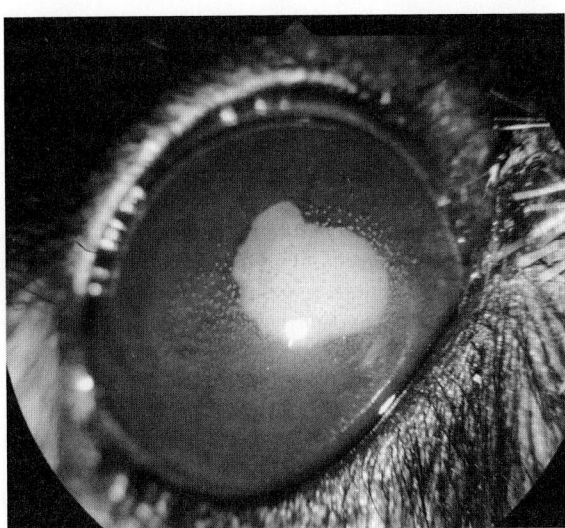

Figure 253-5 Hypermature cataract with secondary lens-induced uveitis. The uveitis has resulted in posterior synechia, dyscoria, and keratitic precipitates.

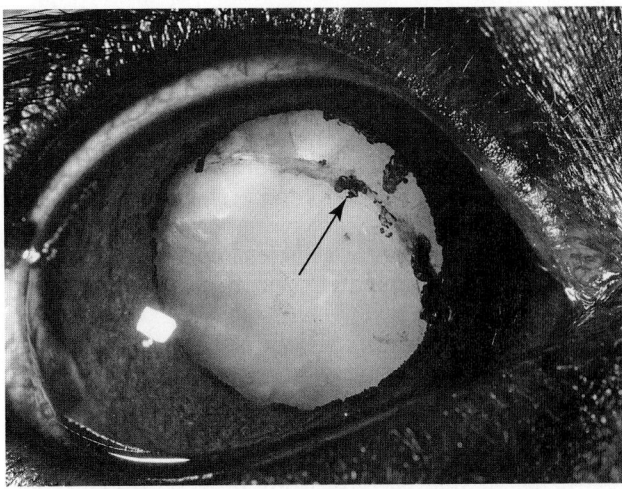

Figure 253-7 Spontaneous lens capsule rupture secondary to diabetes mellitus. The lens capsule has ruptured equatorially with retraction of the anterior lens capsule *(arrow)* and exposure of the lens cortex.

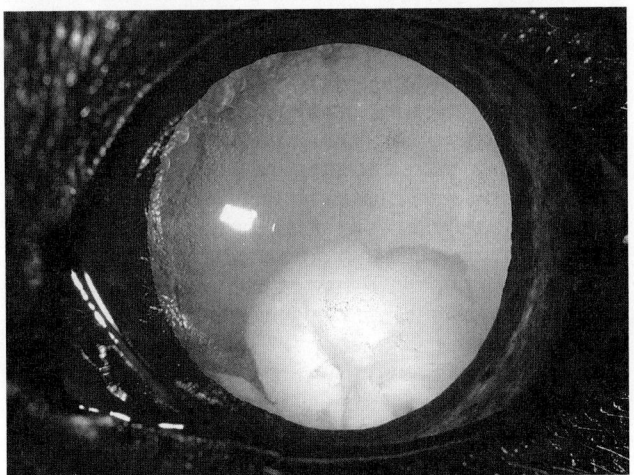

Figure 253-6 Hypermature morgagnian cataract. Because the majority of the cataractous lens cortex has been resorbed, the remaining lens nucleus has settled ventrally in the capsular bag.

capsule wrinkling, and mineralization. Hypermature cataracts occasionally may undergo substantial or complete resorption in which the cortex liquefies and the nucleus shifts and are then termed *morgagnian* cataracts (Figure 253-6). In some of these cases, the patient may regain vision as the cataract resorbs, although retinal detachment often occurs during rapid resorption.

Most canine cataracts are inherited or caused by diabetes mellitus. Inherited cataracts are seen in most breeds of dogs and in mixed-breed dogs. Inherited cataracts may be congenital or acquired and vary by breed in age of onset, location, severity, and progression. Affected animals should not be used for breeding regardless of the severity of the cataract. Metabolic causes of cataracts include diabetes mellitus and, less commonly, hypocalcemia. In dogs affected with diabetes mellitus, 50% will develop cataracts within 170 days of diagnosis of diabetes and 80%

will have cataracts by 470 days. Diabetic cataracts begin with vacuoles or "bubbles" in the equator of the lens that progress, often rapidly, to swelling and rupture of lens fibers with subsequent complete opacification and clefting of the lens fibers at the suture junctions due to fluid accumulation (see Figure 253-4). Diabetic cataracts result when the enzyme aldose reductase catalyzes the reduction of glucose to sorbitol. The intracellular accumulation of sorbitol in the lens leads to an osmotic shift and swelling and disruption of lens fibers. Due to rapid and dramatic swelling of the lens, subsequent spontaneous lens capsule rupture has been described in dogs with diabetes mellitus as well as in nondiabetic dogs with rapidly progressive cataracts (Figure 253-7). Spontaneous lens capsule rupture is both a medical and a surgical emergency, with phacoclastic uveitis expected within days of the rupture. Additional causes of cataracts in dogs include trauma, uveitis, retinal degeneration, nutritional deficiencies, electrical shock, and radiation. Feline cataracts most commonly occur secondary to anterior uveitis. Inherited cataracts have been described in cats, but cataracts secondary to diabetes are not typically seen in the cat.

The treatment of cataracts depends on the impact of the lesion on vision, the overall health and age of the patient, the presence of concurrent ocular abnormalities, and the owner's wishes and financial status. Cataracts that are incipient should be monitored for progression and generally do not require any additional treatment. Cataracts that are progressive, immature, mature, or hypermature should be considered as potential surgical candidates. With the introduction of intraocular lens implants, cataract surgery also can be offered in cases of unilateral cataract to restore binocular emmetropia. There is no medical treatment for cataracts that has any clinical benefit for vision restoration. Veterinarians and dog owners should not fall prey to the various holistic and dietary supplemental treatments sold to "cure" cataracts. Although proper nutrition may play a role in cataract prevention, once a cataract has occurred, the change in lens protein is irreversible. Hypermature cataracts are associated with an increased risk not only of lens-induced uveitis but also of secondary glaucoma, retinal detachment, lens capsular wrinkling and opacification, and lens instability. Therefore careful monitoring and prompt referral of patients with cataracts are imperative to ensure the best postoperative results and prognosis. For patients unable to be referred, the veterinarian should consider long-term monitoring for glaucoma and uveitis and use of a topical antiinflammatory drug to decrease secondary complications.

Lens-Induced Uveitis

Lens-induced or phacolytic uveitis (LIU) commonly is seen in dogs with cataracts, with one study suggesting a prevalence as high as 71% (Paulsen et al, 1985). It has been suggested that all stages of cataract are accompanied by some degree of LIU. Clinical signs of LIU include low intraocular pressure, conjunctival hyperemia and episcleral injection, aqueous flare, iris hyperpigmentation, ectropion uveae, keratic precipitates, delayed or incomplete pharmacologic mydriasis, and synechia. Although early retrospective studies suggested that preexisting LIU significantly reduced the long-term success of cataract surgery, this does not appear to be as significant with current surgical techniques. However, prompt recognition and treatment of LIU is imperative to ensure the best long-term prognosis for vision and ocular health. In general, pretreatment with topical or systemic antiinflammatory therapy (Table 253-2) for a period of a few days to weeks followed by phacoemulsification is the most appropriate means to manage LIU and avoid long-term sequelae. The consequences of uncontrolled LIU include secondary glaucoma, synechia, corneal edema, retinal detachment, lens luxation, vitreous degeneration, and phthisis bulbi.

TABLE 253-2

Antiinflammatory Treatment Options for Lens-Induced Uveitis before Cataract Surgery

Route of Administration	Drug Class	Drug and Dosage
Topical	Corticosteroid	Prednisolone acetate 1% q6-12h
		Dexamethasone 0.1% q6-12h
	NSAIDs	Diclofenac 0.1% q6-12h
		Ketorolac 0.4% q6-12h
		Flurbiprofen 0.03% q6-12h
		Nepafenac 0.1% q12h
	Mydriatic	Atropine 1% q12-24h
Oral	Corticosteroid	Prednisone 0.5 mg/kg q12h PO
	NSAIDs	Carprofen 2.2 mg/kg q12h PO
		Meloxicam 0.2 mg/kg once PO, then 0.1 mg/kg q24h PO

NSAIDs, Nonsteroidal antiinflammatory drugs; *PO,* orally.

Cataract Surgery

Cataract surgery has changed dramatically in recent years with regard to surgical technique, ocular pharmacology, and the availability of antiinflammatory agents, viscoelastic agents, and phacoemulsification; the most recent advancement is intraocular lens (IOL) implantation for dogs and cats. Despite these dramatic changes, cataract surgery remains a procedure for which a successful outcome depends on meticulous attention to detail, surgeon skill and experience, appropriate patient selection, and diligent postoperative treatment and monitoring.

Cataract surgery is considered to be an elective procedure since many animals adapt well to vision loss. It must be remembered, however, that if the owner elects not to perform cataract surgery, the patient still must be monitored long term for lens-induced complications such as LIU, secondary glaucoma, retinal detachment, and lens luxation. Younger animals with cataracts that do not undergo surgery may experience spontaneous resorption of the cataract and regain aphakic vision if the retina does not detach during resorption. In a study of 44 dogs with cataracts, eyes that received no medical or surgical treatment had a much greater risk of a poor outcome such as chronic ocular pain, secondary glaucoma, lens luxation, or enucleation or globe evisceration compared with eyes that were treated with antiinflammatory agents and those in which phacoemulsification was performed (Lim et al, 2011). Surgical outcome was better for immature cataracts than for mature and hypermature cataracts. Recent studies have suggested that dogs with significant cataracts that remain unoperated have a 20% risk of developing glaucoma in at least one eye, whereas the glaucoma risk following cataract surgery is 7% to 9% (Gelatt and MacKay, 2004). The conclusions are that early surgical intervention is associated with the highest success rate and that animals that do not undergo phacoemulsification should be managed with a topical antiinflammatory medication and monitored for the development of secondary glaucoma. If surgery is not performed, topical nonsteroidal antiinflammatories or a topical corticosteroid should be administered every 12 to 24 hours for life (or until the cataract has completely resorbed), and an ophthalmic examination should be performed every 6 to 9 months.

Before cataract surgery is undertaken a complete ophthalmic examination is required (see Chapter 242). In addition, ocular ultrasonography and electroretinography are performed to ensure that there are no abnormalities of the posterior segment, including vitreous degeneration, retinal detachment, or retinal degeneration. If LIU is present, it should be treated and controlled before surgery. The intraocular pressure should be measured to rule out early secondary glaucoma. A complete physical examination as well as a complete blood count, serum chemistry panel, and urinalysis are indicated to ensure that the animal is healthy enough to undergo general anesthesia.

Cataract surgery requires extensive equipment and training to become proficient and is considered a referral procedure. Clients with affected animals who are considering surgery should be referred early in the disease course to allow the veterinary ophthalmologist to visualize the posterior segment before the cataract becomes mature. Early surgical intervention before the cataract becomes hypermature and LIU begins results in a more favorable outcome. Rapidly progressive cataracts in dogs with diabetes mellitus can be considered somewhat of an emergency, and such patients should be referred promptly because these cataracts can result in severe LIU and spontaneous lens capsule rupture.

The success rate of cataract surgery in restoring long-term vision when performed using phacoemulsification and IOL implantation generally is considered to be 85% to 90%. Certain breeds of dogs are at increased risk of specific postoperative complications. Specifically, these complications include retinal detachment in the bichon frise and Shih Tzu, postoperative intraocular hypertension and glaucoma in the Labrador retriever and Boston terrier, and glaucoma in those breeds with a risk of primary glaucoma such as the American cocker spaniel and miniature poodle.

The current accepted standard of care for cataract surgery in small animals is phacoemulsification and IOL implantation. Phacoemulsification is carried out under general anesthesia and is performed through a small incision with minimal tissue trauma and restoration of emmetropia through implantation of an IOL specifically designed for the canine or feline eye (Figure 253-8). Without placement of an IOL, the eye is left 14 diopters hyperopic (far-sighted), and vision is significantly abnormal. Before surgery, topical mydriatics and topical and systemic antiinflammatories and antibiotics are used according to surgeon preference. If cataracts are bilateral, most surgeons choose to operate on both eyes during a single procedure. This minimizes cost, requires only one anesthesia induction, simplifies the postoperative management, and avoids leaving a cataract that may result in LIU and its associated complications.

Exercise restriction and use of an Elizabethan collar are required for the first 10 to 14 days following surgery.

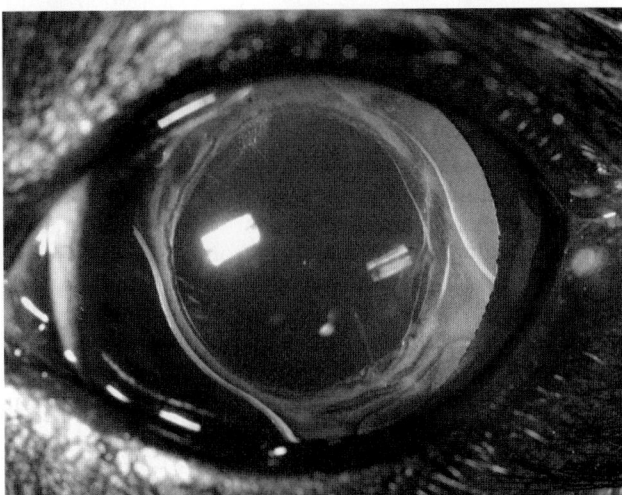

Figure 253-8 Acrivet 60V acrylic intraocular lens seen in the lens capsule. Fibrosis of the edge of the anterior lens capsule opening is noted, but the lens optic and visual axis remain clear.

Topical and systemic antiinflammatories and antibiotics are prescribed according to surgeon preference. Medications are gradually tapered and may be discontinued, and the period between follow-up examinations is extended. After the immediate postoperative period of 4 to 6 months, it generally is recommended that annual or semiannual ophthalmic examinations be performed by a veterinary ophthalmologist. These examinations are to monitor for uveitis, retinal detachment, secondary glaucoma, keratoconjunctivitis sicca, and other complications that may affect the long-term success of cataract surgery. Early diagnosis of these complications, should they occur, can result in successful medical or surgical management and vision preservation. Postoperative medications are adjusted on an individual animal basis, but some animals require some level of lifelong topical antiinflammatory therapy. This is especially true for dogs with diabetes mellitus.

The most common long-term complication of cataract surgery and IOL implantation in veterinary ophthalmology is posterior capsule opacification. Currently this occurs with varying severity in 100% of canine and feline patients. It results when residual lens epithelial cells undergo epithelial-mesenchymal transformation, migrate, and proliferate on the anterior and posterior lens capsule. It is more severe in young animals and may occur even before cataract surgery in cases of hypermature cataracts. Fortunately, it is rarely of clinical significance with respect to the animal's ability to navigate and function normally following surgery. Methods to limit or decrease posterior capsule opacification through IOL design, surgical technique, and pharmacologic intervention are currently under investigation.

When seeing a cataract patient after surgery, the primary care veterinarian should include evaluation of menace and pupillary light responses, measurement of tear production and intraocular pressure, and examination of the anterior and posterior segments of the eye as part of an annual wellness examination.

Lens Instability

Lens instability can occur as a primary abnormality or develop secondary to hypermature cataract, chronic LIU, trauma, or glaucoma. Primary lens luxation (PLL) is breed associated and is considered common in as many as 8 to 10 terrier breeds and the Australian cattle dog, border collie, and shar-pei. Primary lens instability typically appears between the ages of 2 and 6 years and, although often asymmetric at presentation, typically is a bilateral disease. The mode of inheritance is autosomal recessive, and a genetic test is commercially available for the canine PLL mutation. DNA results suggest that in some breeds, such as the miniature bull terrier in the United Kingdom, up to 40% of breed members may be carriers.

Unstable lenses may remain in the posterior chamber or may luxate into the anterior or vitreous chambers. Lens instability or lens subluxation may be recognized by the presence of an aphakic crescent (Figure 253-9), lens trembling (phacodonesis), iris trembling (iridodonesis), corneal edema, vitreous in the anterior chamber, and visualization of the lens in the anterior (Figure 253-10) or

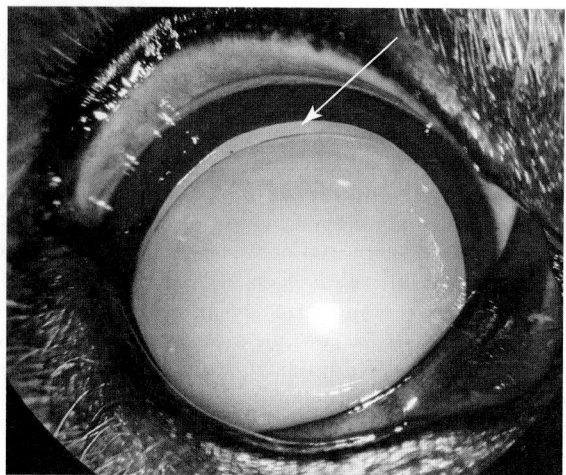

Figure 253-9 Mature cataract in a subluxated lens. The lens is unstable and has shifted ventrally, which results in an aphakic crescent *(arrow)*.

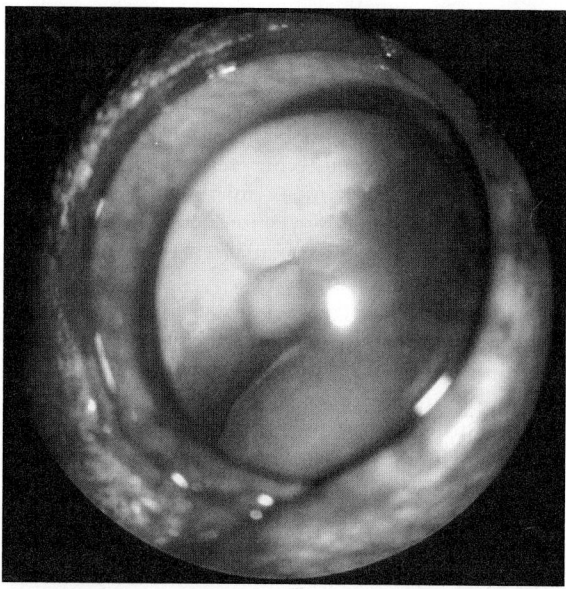

Figure 253-11 A complete posterior lens luxation of a cataractous lens in a canine eye.

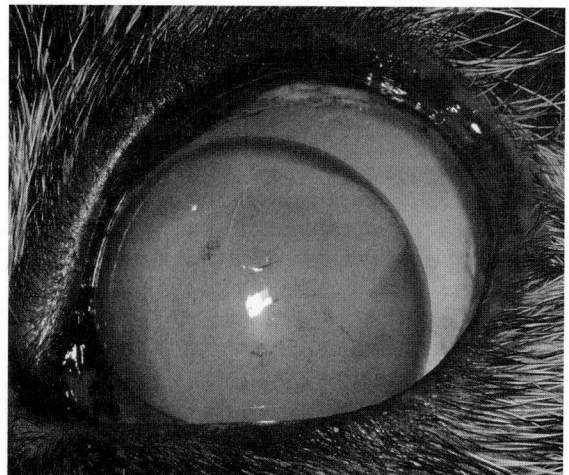

Figure 253-10 Complete anterior lens luxation in a feline eye.

vitreous chamber (Figure 253-11) A dog with an anteriorly luxated lens may be brought to the veterinarian because of acute onset of corneal edema and blepharospasm. If the corneal edema is not severe, the lens may be visualized in the anterior chamber by viewing the globe from the lateral side. Initial assessment and management consists of measurement of the intraocular pressure, assessment of vision status, and determination of the location of the lens. If the lens is located anteriorly, the use of topical miotic agents is contraindicated, and prompt referral is the most appropriate treatment. If the intraocular pressure is elevated and the lens is anterior, topical and oral carbonic anhydrase inhibitors and systemic osmotic agents such as mannitol may be used to lower intraocular pressure (see Chapter 251).

If the lens is located posterior to the iris and is unstable or luxated, topical miotic agents may be used to trap the lens and avoid anterior luxation. Topical miotic agents

include the prostaglandin analogs (latanoprost [Xalatan], travoprost [Travatan], bimatoprost [Lumigan]), which induce potent miosis and can be used every 12 hours indefinitely, and the parasympathomimetic drugs (demecarium bromide 0.125% and pilocarpine 2%). The miotic agents also serve to lower intraocular pressure and so have the advantage of managing both the lens instability and possible secondary glaucoma. In the author's opinion, topical latanoprost 0.005% every 12 hours is the most effective topical therapy for a posterior lens luxation. Referral of an animal with posterior lens luxation to a veterinary ophthalmologist is advised. If the lens instability is considered to be primary, examination of the contralateral eye is essential because it is also at risk.

There is considerable diversity of opinion among veterinary ophthalmologists regarding when unstable lenses should be removed. The most conservative approach is to use topical miotic agents to prevent anterior luxation and to perform surgery only when the lens luxates anteriorly. Once the lens has luxated completely, removal often requires an intracapsular surgical technique (intracapsular lens extraction) that uses a 160-degree incision and can be associated with significant postoperative complications (glaucoma, retinal detachment). Recent studies have revealed that the prognosis for vision after intracapsular lens extraction is poor if glaucoma is present at the time of surgery. The mechanisms by which unstable lenses cause glaucoma have not been identified, but some believe glaucoma begins early in the course of lens instability and then rapidly becomes irreversible. As a result, some advocate that unstable lenses be removed as soon as the instability is detected. DNA testing for PLL combined with early surgical intervention for unstable lenses should be considered in an effort to improve long-term outcomes.

The technique for removal of an anteriorly luxated or unstable lens depends on the degree of instability, the equipment available, the health of the vitreous, and surgeon preference. In general, if the lens is stable enough to allow phacoemulsification, this should be the preferred method of extraction. This method allows the use of small-incision techniques and has been shown to produce significantly better outcomes than intracapsular lens extraction. In addition, after phacoemulsification, implantation of an IOL into the capsular bag may be possible in some cases. For lens instability of more than 160 degrees or complete lens luxation, a sulcus-sutured IOL may be placed in selected cases to restore emmetropia. With the concurrent use of endoscopic cyclophotocoagulation, the incidence of postoperative glaucoma may be reduced.

Trauma

Ocular trauma can be divided into sharp and blunt. Blunt trauma typically results in an explosive type of rupture of the fibrous tunic, and the globe usually is not visual or able to be salvaged. Sharp trauma, such as puncture with a cat claw, results in laceration of the fibrous tunic and, if penetrating, may involve the lens and its capsule. After laceration of the lens capsule, a cataract will occur. Phacoclastic uveitis may develop if the lens capsule laceration is large enough so that sufficient exposure of lens proteins occurs. When a rupture of the lens capsule is suspected or diagnosed, prompt referral for corneal repair and lens removal is indicated. Systemic and topical nonsteroidal antiinflammatories and antibiotics should be prescribed until surgery can be performed. Although small lens capsule lacerations may seal themselves, which results in a focal cataract without phacoclastic uveitis, this is the exception and referral still is indicated.

References and Suggested Reading

Beam S, Correa MT, Davidson MG: A retrospective-cohort study on the development of cataracts in dogs with diabetes mellitus: 200 cases, *Vet Ophthalmol* 2:169, 1999.

Binder DR, Herring IP, Gerhard T: Outcomes of nonsurgical management and efficacy of demecarium bromide treatment for primary lens instability in dogs: 34 cases (1990-2004), *J Am Vet Med Assoc* 231:89, 2007.

Biros DJ et al: Development of glaucoma after cataract surgery in dogs: 220 cases (1987-1998), *J Am Vet Med Assoc* 216:1780, 2000.

Bras ID et al: Posterior capsular opacification in diabetic and nondiabetic canine patients following cataract surgery, *Vet Ophthalmol* 9:317, 2006.

Gould D et al: ADAMTS17 mutation associated with primary lens luxation is widespread among breeds, *Vet Ophthalmol* 14:378, 2011.

Gelatt KN, MacKay EO: Secondary glaucoma in the dog in North America, *Vet Ophthalmol* 7:245, 2004.

Gelatt KN, Wilkie DA: Surgical procedures of the lens and cataract. In Gelatt KN, Gelatt JP, editors: *Veterinary ophthalmic surgery*, St Louis, 2011, Saunders, p 305.

Lim CC et al: Cataracts in 44 dogs (77 eyes): a comparison of outcomes for no treatment, topical medical management, or phacoemulsification with intraocular lens implantation, *Can Vet J* 52:283, 2011.

Paulson ME et al: The effect of lens induced uveitis on the success of extracapsular cataract extraction: a retrospective study of 65 lens removals in the dog, *J Am Anim Hosp Assoc* 22:49, 1985.

Sigle KJ, Nasisse MP: Long-term complications after phacoemulsification for cataract removal in dogs: 172 cases (1995-2002), *J Am Vet Med Assoc* 228:74, 2005.

Wilkie DA et al: Canine cataracts, diabetes mellitus and spontaneous lens capsule rupture: a retrospective study of 18 dogs, *Vet Ophthalmol* 9:328, 2006.

Wilkie DA, Colitz CMH: Surgery of the canine lens. In Gelatt KN, editor: *Veterinary ophthalmology*, ed 4, Ames, IA, 2007, Blackwell Publishing, p 888.

CHAPTER 254

Canine Retinopathies

SIMON M. PETERSEN-JONES, *East Lansing, Michigan*

Retinopathies in dogs may be identified because of a loss of vision or an altered external appearance of the eyes. Many cases are detected only during a careful ophthalmoscopic examination (Figure 254-1) as part of a general physical examination or at a screening clinic (e.g., a Canine Eye Registration Foundation examination). This chapter considers hereditary and acquired diseases of the canine retina.

Hereditary Retinal Dystrophies

Retinal Dysplasia

Retinal dysplasia is a group of conditions that involve abnormal development of the retina. Retinal dysplasia is classified by both cause and severity. Categorized by cause, retinal dysplasias include acquired lesions, which may result from insults such as *in utero* infection or irradiation, and hereditary lesions. *Complete* or *total* retinal dysplasia is the most severe form and is characterized by blindness due to detachment or congenital nonattachment of the retina. Concurrent congenital abnormalities such as microphthalmos and cataract may be present. Nonocular congenital anomalies, such as skeletal dwarfism, also may be observed with complete or total retinal dysplasia. An example is oculoskeletal dysplasia, also referred to as *dwarfism with retinal dysplasia*. In the Labrador retriever and Samoyed breeds the causal gene mutations for dwarfism with retinal dysplasia have been identified.

A less severe retinal dysplasia known as *geographic retinal dysplasia* is seen in many breeds of dog (see Figure 254-1, *C*). The tapetal retina dorsal to the optic nerve head is affected most frequently. Affected regions may be focally detached or there may be regions of retinal thinning with subsequent pigmentation, which produces an appearance similar to that of a chorioretinal scar. Unless the geographic lesions are very extensive or a complete retinal detachment develops, vision is not noticeably affected.

A third form of retinal dysplasia is known as *multifocal retinal dysplasia*. In this form the lesions may appear as circular dots, linear streaks, or V- or Y-shaped streaks, most commonly in the tapetal fundus. Typically there is a duplication of the photoreceptor layer within the lesions, which also are called *rosettes* because of their appearance in histologic sections. The lesions usually have a different color from the surrounding normal fundus and may appear hyporeflective (due to thickening of abnormal retinal tissue). The affected retina also may degenerate, which leaves a hyperreflective spot or streak. Multifocal retinal dysplasia typically does not have any detectable effect on vision.

Canine Multifocal Retinopathy

Canine multifocal retinopathy (cmr) is an autosomal-recessive condition caused by mutations in the canine *BEST1* gene *(cBEST1)*. Three different mutations have been identified in *cBEST1* in different breeds of dog causing cmr1, cmr2, and cmr3. Mastiff breeds are affected with cmr1, the Coton de Tulear breed with cmr2, and the Lapponian herder with cmr3. Dogs affected with cmr develop multiple small bullous retinal detachments that have tan-colored subretinal fluid. These first develop in young dogs and then may remain unchanged for years. The cmr3 form may have a somewhat later onset than cmr1 and cmr2, with lesions developing at about 1 year of age. Histologically, the lesions show focal loss of photoreceptors, and the underlying retinal pigment epithelium is abnormal. Currently there is no treatment for the condition, although gene therapy is being investigated experimentally. Genetic tests for cmr1, cmr2, and cmr3 have been developed.

Progressive Retinal Atrophy

Progressive retinal atrophy (PRA) is a group of conditions that have a similar clinical presentation, although the age of onset and rate of progression can vary considerably by breed. The majority of forms are inherited in an autosomal-recessive fashion, although dominant and X-linked PRAs have been identified. There are forms of PRA that are breed specific (the causal mutation has been identified in only a single breed), others that occur only in closely related breeds, and one important form that is caused by a mutation in the progressive rod-cone degeneration gene *(PRCD)* that occurs in many different breeds. In attempts to categorize the different forms, PRA has been divided into categories based on age of onset and the pathologic changes that occur in the retina of affected dogs. Thus there are early, middle-aged, and late-onset forms and forms with descriptive names such as *rod dysplasia, rod-cone dysplasia* (types 1, 2, and 3), *early retinal degeneration,* and *progressive rod-cone degeneration.* Advances in molecular genetics have allowed the underlying gene mutation of several forms to be identified. This allows classification on a molecular basis so that the disorder is described as PRA due to a particular mutation in a certain gene (Table 254-1).

Classically, PRA results in an initial deterioration of vision in dim light followed by a progressive loss of

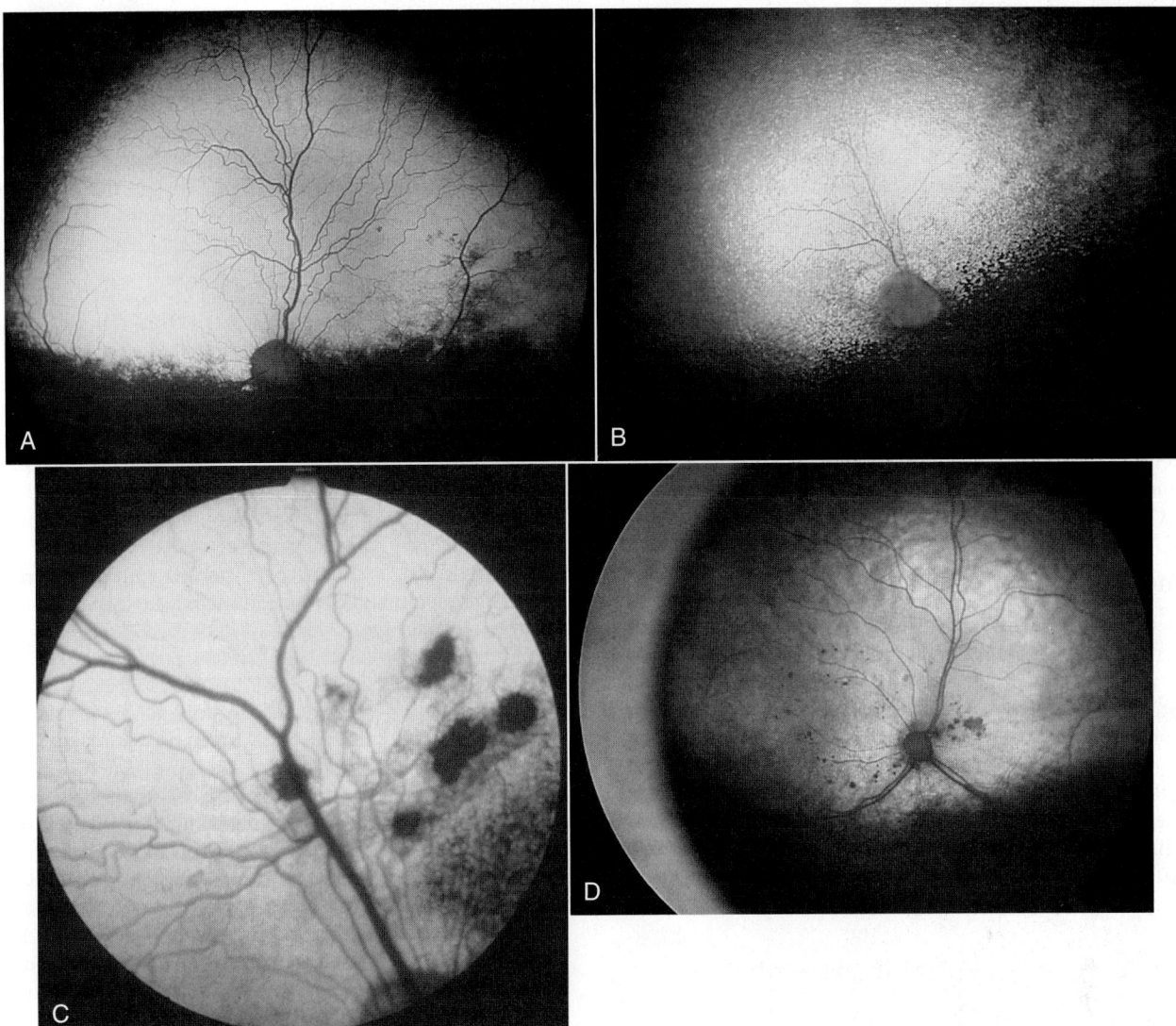

Figure 254-1 A, Wide-angle view of a fundus of a normal adult dog. **B,** Wide-angle view of a fundus of a Cardigan Welsh corgi with progressive retinal atrophy. The tapetal fundus is hyper-reflective due to retinal thinning and the retinal vasculature is attenuated. **C,** Fundus of a springer spaniel with geographic retinal dysplasia lesions. The lesions have an altered tapetal color and the larger ones have a pigmented center. **D,** Wide-angle view of a fundus of an elderly cat with hypertensive retinopathy. There are multiple spots of hemorrhage in the central retina. Some tapetal hyperreflectivity is present due to retinal thinning.

TABLE **254-1**

Examples of the Different Classifications for Four Forms of Progressive Retinal Atrophy (PRA)

Breed	Classification by Inheritance	Classification by Age of Onset	Classification by Pathologic Features	Classification by Genetic Mutation
Irish setter	Autosomal-recessive PRA	Early-onset PRA	Rod-cone dysplasia type 1 (RCD1)	Rod cyclic GMP phosphodiesterase β subunit (PDE6B)
Collie	Autosomal-recessive PRA	Early-onset PRA	Rod-cone dysplasia type 2 (RCD2)	Retinal degeneration 3 (RD3)
Cardigan Welsh corgi	Autosomal-recessive PRA	Early-onset PRA	Rod-cone dysplasia type 3 (RCD3)	Rod cyclic GMP phosphodiesterase α subunit (PDE6A)
Poodle, Labrador retriever, cocker spaniel, plus many other breeds	Autosomal-recessive PRA	Mid- to late-onset PRA	Progressive rod-cone degeneration (PRCD)	Progressive rod-cone degeneration (PRCD)

GMP, Guanosine monophosphate.

daytime vision and ultimate blindness. Owners also may notice that the pupils are unusually dilated and there may be increased "eye shine" due to a combination of the pupillary dilation and increased tapetal reflectivity. Cataract formation commonly accompanies PRA and may be the initial presenting complaint. Ophthalmoscopic signs of PRA include progressive development of a generalized hyperreflectivity of the tapetal fundus, which is a result of retinal thinning (see Figure 254-1, *B*). Retinal vasculature becomes progressively attenuated, and atrophy involving the optic nerve head also develops. Pigmentary changes (patchy increase and decrease in pigmentation) in the nontapetal fundus also may become apparent. Electroretinography, a diagnostic method used to measure the retinal electrical response to light stimulation, can be used for the early diagnosis of many forms of PRA and also for assessment of retinal function when ophthalmoscopic examination is not possible because of cataract. DNA tests now are available for many breeds.

Cone-Rod Dystrophy

The term *cone-rod dystrophy* (CRD) is used for retinal degenerative conditions in which the cone photoreceptors are affected earlier or more severely than the rod photoreceptors. This is in contrast to "classical" PRA in which rods are affected initially or more severely in the early stages of the condition compared with cones. The ophthalmoscopic changes in CRD may be very similar to those in PRA (tapetal hyperreflectivity, retinal vascular attenuation, optic nerve atrophy). Electroretinography is useful in differentiating the two conditions. DNA testing is available for many breeds.

Retinal Pigment Epithelial Dystrophy

Retinal pigment epithelial dystrophy (RPED) originally was called *central progressive retinal atrophy*. The condition is characterized by the accumulation of light brown pigment spots across the tapetal fundus. Experimental vitamin E deficiency and vitamin E deficiency caused by very poor diet have been described in dogs and result in a retinal dystrophy that appears very similar to RPED, which has led to speculation that RPED may be associated with vitamin E deficiency. Anecdotal evidence from the United Kingdom indicates that the incidence of RPED decreased dramatically when owners improved the quality of the diet that typically was fed. This direct and indirect evidence suggests that systemic or local abnormalities in vitamin E metabolism or transport may play a role in the development of some forms of RPED.

Congenital Stationary Night Blindness/ Retinal Dystrophy of Briards

Congenital stationary night blindness (retinal dystrophy of briards) is an autosomal-recessive trait of the briard. Affected dogs have markedly reduced visual sensitivity so that when the light level is reduced from full room light they become effectively blind. Although the condition initially was considered a stationary (nonprogressive) night blindness, in fact daytime vision also is affected to

a variable extent and the condition does progress slowly over several years, which makes the name a misnomer. The condition is caused by a mutation in the *RPE65* gene. A mutation in the same gene in humans is responsible for an important cause of blindness called *Leber's congenital amaurosis type II*. The *RPE65* gene product is expressed in the retinal pigment epithelium of the eye and is an important enzyme in the retinoid (visual) cycle. RPE65 deficiency is associated with very slow degeneration of the photoreceptors in affected dogs.

Achromatopsia

Achromatopsia (also *day blindness* or *hemeralopia*) is a term used to describe conditions that result in a lack of, or loss of, cone function. Affected dogs have visual impairment in bright light with restoration of normal vision in dim lighting conditions. Pupil size in bright light varies from pinpoint to normal to mydriatic. Achromatopsia in the Alaskan malamute and German shorthaired pointer have been shown to be caused by different mutations in the *CNGB3* gene, which is inherited in an autosomal-recessive fashion.

Treatment of Hereditary Retinal Dystrophies

Currently there are no proven therapies for retinal dystrophy that are in common clinical use. Dogs have proven to be important models for several human retinopathies, and significant developments have occurred through the study of canine patients. In applied veterinary medicine, the focus currently is on DNA-based testing for disease-causing gene mutations and selective breeding to eliminate those conditions. In the future, some of the novel treatment approaches developed in natural or experimental dog models of human retinopathy may become available to treat canine veterinary patients.

Treatments Applicable before Complete Photoreceptor Loss

Dietary Supplementation

Large clinical trials of dietary supplementation in human patients with retinal dystrophies such as retinitis pigmentosa have shown some positive effects of supplementation. The effects of dietary supplementation on retinal dystrophies in companion animals have not been the subject of well-designed clinical trials. Despite this lack of scientific proof, dietary supplements are being marketed for this use. There is a real need for carefully controlled large clinical trials examining dietary supplementation as a way of slowing retinal degeneration in conditions such as PRA. This paucity of hard evidence to support dietary supplementation in dogs with retinal dystrophies makes it impossible to give advice based on anything more than anecdotal evidence. Supplementation therefore should be advised with care and excessive supplementation of fat-soluble vitamins avoided so as not to risk toxicity effects.

Although RPED has strong similarities to vitamin E deficiency and vitamin E supplementation in affected dogs may seem a logical approach, clinical trials to investigate such supplementation as a method of treatment have not been reported. There is anecdotal evidence that ensuring that at-risk dogs receive a diet adequate in vitamin E and antioxidants reduces the incidence of RPED. The results from the clinical trials of human patients with retinitis pigmentosa mentioned earlier showed that vitamin E supplementation actually had a deleterious effect, which suggests that supplementation is not without risk.

Disease-Specific Gene Therapy

Recent advances in gene therapy have given scientists and practitioners alike a glimpse of the future possibilities of this novel treatment modality. Gene supplementation therapy in the *RPE65*-mutant briard dog has provided spectacular restoration and subsequent maintenance of visual function. One important feature of the retinal dystrophy in the dog with *RPE65* mutation is that although the visual deficits are present from the time of retinal maturation, the retinal cells degenerate only very slowly. This disconnect between function and structure provides a large window of opportunity to correct the genetic defect while photoreceptors remain and thus to restore vision. Modified adeno-associated viruses used to introduce a normal copy of the *RPE65* gene were injected into the subretinal space (between the photoreceptors and retinal pigment epithelial cells) and delivered the normal gene to the retinal pigment epithelium, which allowed restoration of visual function. These studies in *RPE65*-mutant dogs led to human clinical trials of similar gene therapy. Unfortunately, humans appear to have fewer surviving photoreceptors, so the success of gene therapy in the human trials to date has not been as spectacular as it is in dogs.

Unfortunately, the situation in many other retinal dystrophies is not as favorable for gene supplementation therapy. The loss of vision in a number of retinal dystrophies is the result of the death of photoreceptors, with vision deteriorating as the number of remaining functional photoreceptors dwindles. For gene supplementation to be successful, it would need to be applied before too many photoreceptors are lost. This would require the early identification of animals that are destined to go blind because of a retinal dystrophy and then provision of treatment early in the disease process. Because there are many different genes that can lead to a retinal dystrophy when mutated, this approach also would require the construction of a new therapeutic viral vector for each gene. Each unique construct would be able to treat only disease resulting from a mutation of that gene.

Further complicating successful gene therapy is the variation in the genetics of each dystrophy. Most of the conditions that would be amenable to gene supplementation therapy are recessively inherited and are caused by a lack of normal gene product. Carrier animals with only one functional copy of the gene instead of two have a reduced amount of the gene product, but this is still enough to allow for retinal function. Dominantly inherited retinal dystrophies result when having only one functional copy of the gene is not sufficient for normal function or when the mutated gene product is produced but has a deleterious effect. Simple gene supplementation therapy is unlikely to be successful in these cases.

Generic Gene Therapy

In gene supplementation therapy (adding a normal copy of a mutated gene) each gene therapy vector is suitable for use in only a small number of patients because the vector is specific to the particular breed mutation. A more generic treatment that could slow or prevent vision loss in a wide range of retinal dystrophies would be more attractive, particularly for commercialization. Research looking at factors to prevent photoreceptor cell death, including the introduction of therapeutic genes expressing growth factors, cell survival factors, and antiapoptosis factors, is under way.

Growth Factors

Therapy involving the delivery of growth factors to the retina has been developed and is being tested in human clinical trials. One approach that has been investigated extensively is the use of intravitreal implants of encapsulated cells altered to produce a particular therapeutic protein, such as ciliary neurotrophic factor. The therapeutic protein is produced by the modified cells in the device, leaks from the capsule, and reaches the retina following diffusion across the vitreous. This approach has been shown to preserve photoreceptors in many different animal models, including models with severe forms of PRA.

Treatments Applicable after Photoreceptors Have Died

Once retinal degeneration has advanced to the stage that the photoreceptor cells have died, therapeutic approaches that introduce a new copy of the defective gene or proteins that stop or slow down photoreceptor loss are no longer effective, and a different therapeutic approach is required. Three main approaches currently are being investigated: transplantation of retinal progenitor cells that can develop into replacement photoreceptors, introduction of light-sensitive channel proteins into the remaining cells of the inner retina, and implantation of an electrical microarray to act as an artificial retina.

Transplantation

Injection of progenitor photoreceptors into eyes with photoreceptor degeneration currently is being investigated in animal models. The most promising results so far have come from injection of progenitor cells rather than stem cells. These progenitor cells have been manipulated to commit them to becoming photoreceptors before they are injected into the subretinal space.

Introduction of Light-Responsive Channel Proteins

Another approach to restoration of vision involves the use of gene therapy to introduce a light-responsive channel protein into the cell membranes of remaining inner retinal neurons. Inner retinal neurons are still present in retinal dystrophies long after the photoreceptors have degenerated. The channel proteins allow these remaining neurons to create a difference in electrical potential across their membranes upon light stimulation. This results in the transmission of a neurologic message to the brain for conscious perception. This approach already has been shown to restore some light-driven responses in mice blinded because of retinal dystrophies.

Artificial Retina

An electrical microchip can be implanted into the eye and used to stimulate the remaining inner retinal neurons that it contacts. A camera is then used to send information to the microchip, creating a pattern of stimulation on the retina that is subsequently processed in the visual centers of the brain. This approach currently is being evaluated in human clinical trials.

Acquired Retinal Dystrophies

Diabetic Retinopathy

Diabetic retinopathy in humans is a very important problem, with proliferative retinal neovascularization and resultant hemorrhage developing in some patients and potentially causing vision loss. Diabetic dogs do develop retinal vascular changes and retinal hemorrhage, and microaneurysms are observed in some animals. A retrospective study of 52 diabetic dogs recorded retinal hemorrhages or microaneurysms in 21%, whereas in control animals the incidence was 0.6% (Landry et al, 2004). Fortunately, therapeutic intervention beyond adequate regulation of the diabetes generally is not necessary to control diabetic retinopathy in canine patients.

Hypertensive Retinopathy

Systemic hypertension can result in retinal changes ranging from arteriolar constriction and dilation (aneurysms) to retinal edema, retinal detachment, and retinal and preretinal hemorrhage (see Figure 254-1, *D*). The more severe changes may be vision threatening. Systemic blood pressure always should be measured when these signs are observed funduscopically. Control of the systemic blood pressure is key in the stabilization of the retinal changes (see Chapter 169). Prompt reduction of hypertension and maintenance of normal blood pressure can allow a detached retina to reattach and potentially restore vision.

Sudden Acquired Retinal Degeneration Syndrome

Sudden acquired retinal degeneration syndrome (SARDS) is a unique canine retinopathy that results in the sudden onset of vision loss. Typically, middle-aged dogs are affected. There may be a history of polydipsia and polyphagia. On examination the dogs are blind, but the pupillary light reflexes may be normal, delayed, or absent in association with mydriasis. Fundus examination reveals no retinal abnormalities. The main differential diagnosis for blindness with no apparent cause detectable on ophthalmoscopic examination is central blindness. An electroretinogram allows differentiation between SARDS and central blindness. In SARDS no electrical responses can be recorded from the retina in response to light stimulation, whereas in the initial stages central causes of blindness do not have a major effect on the electroretinogram. The cause of SARDS is not understood, and there does not appear to be an effective treatment.

Senile Retinal Degeneration

It is recognized that vision deteriorates with age. In elderly animals retinal thinning may become apparent; it is particularly evident in the peripheral retina and on ophthalmoscopic examination can be seen most readily as hyperreflectivity of the peripheral tapetal region.

References and Suggested Reading

Acland GM et al: Gene therapy restores vision in a canine model of childhood blindness, *Nat Genet* 28:92, 2001.

Gearhart PM, Gearhart CC, Petersen-Jones SM: A novel method for objective vision testing in canine models of inherited retinal disease, *Invest Ophthalmol Vis Sci* 49:3568, 2008.

Guziewicz KE et al: Bestrophin gene mutations cause canine multifocal retinopathy: a novel animal model for best disease, *Invest Ophthalmol Vis Sci* 48:1959, 2007.

Hurn SD, Hardman C, Stanley RG: Day-blindness in three dogs: clinical and electroretinographic findings, *Vet Ophthalmol* 6:127, 2003.

Komaromy AM et al: Gene therapy rescues cone function in congenital achromatopsia, *Hum Mol Genet* 19:2581, 2010.

Landry MP, Herring IP, Panciera DL: Funduscopic findings following cataract extraction by means of phacoemulsification in diabetic dogs: 52 cases (1993-2003), *J Am Vet Med Assoc* 225:709, 2004.

McLellan GJ et al: Clinical and pathological observations in English cocker spaniels with primary metabolic vitamin E deficiency and retinal pigment epithelial dystrophy, *Vet Rec* 153:287, 2003.

Tao W et al: Encapsulated cell-based delivery of CNTF reduces photoreceptor degeneration in animal models of retinitis pigmentosa, *Invest Ophthalmol Vis Sci* 43:3292, 2002.

Wrigstad A, Narfström K, Nilsson SE: Slowly progressive changes of the retina and retinal pigment epithelium in Briard dogs with hereditary retinal dystrophy. A morphological study, *Doc Ophthalmol* 87:337, 1994.

Zangerl B et al: Identical mutation in a novel retinal gene causes progressive rod-cone degeneration in dogs and retinitis pigmentosa in humans, *Genomics* 88:551, 2006.

Zangerl B et al: Assessment of canine BEST1 variations identifies new mutations and establishes an independent bestrophinopathy model (cmr3), *Mol Vis* 16:2791, 2010.

CHAPTER 255

Feline Retinopathies

KATHERN E. MYRNA, *Athens, Georgia*

Examination of the feline retina is an important part of a thorough systemic evaluation. Any cat with a pupillary abnormality, a presenting complaint of vision loss, a systemic illness of unknown origin, or a cardiac abnormality should undergo a complete retinal examination. Proper retinal evaluation can help the practitioner to focus the diagnostic search as well as monitor response to therapy. This chapter reviews the most common causes of retinal lesions in the feline and presents a diagnostic approach to retinal changes. Figure 255-1 provides a diagnostic algorithm for feline retinal disease.

The biggest obstacle to understanding retinal disease is the difficulty inherent in fundic examination. The fundus is defined as the visible structures in the posterior half of the eye and includes five overlapping layers of tissue with varying degrees of transparency. The fundus is composed of the sclera, the choroid, the tapetum, the retinal pigmented epithelium, and the neurovascular retina. The posterior blood-eye barrier is formed by the nonfenestrated capillaries of the neurovascular retina and the tight junctions between retinal pigmented epithelium cells, and acts to prevent substances in the bloodstream from entering the eye. Pathologic conditions result in a breakdown of this barrier, which can allow offending substances, including inflammatory cells, infectious organisms, or blood, to collect within and under the retina. These alterations in the layers of the fundus result in the characteristic changes in the appearance of the retina.

The first key to effective fundic evaluation is an understanding of the normal retinal appearance. Performing routine retinal examinations and using an ophthalmic atlas will help to establish a thorough recognition of normal variation. When retinal disease is detected, it is first important to differentiate active from inactive disease. When cells or fluid sit between the retina and the tapetum the tapetal reflection is blocked, which leads to a murky or blurry image. Thus active retinal lesions often are hyporeflective and fuzzy with irregular borders. Atrophy of the retina results in vascular attenuation and retinal thinning, which allows greater tapetal reflection. Thus inactive lesions are hyperreflective with sharp margins. Inactive lesions also may be associated with pigment clumping, leading to foci of hyperpigmentation within or adjacent to a hyperreflective lesion.

Hypertensive Retinopathy

Hypertensive retinopathy is perhaps the most common and clinically important retinopathy in the cat. It should be considered in all cases of acute blindness in older cats.

Hypertensive retinopathy has been used as a broad term to include both hypertensive retinopathy and choroidopathy. The retinal arteries autoregulate in response to increased systemic blood pressure. This results in vasoconstriction, which in turn leads to hypertrophy of the smooth muscle layer of the arteriole and ultimately to focal necrosis and rupture of the vessel. These focal ruptures produce multifocal areas of retinal edema or hemorrhage. As more vessel damage occurs, serum and blood continue to leak, which leads to complete retinal detachment and blindness. Additionally, the choroid does not autoregulate, and as the blood pressure increases, there is a substantial degree of choriocapillaris serum leakage resulting in serum collection beneath the retina and exudative retinal detachment.

The incidence of ocular signs in hypertensive cats is about 40% to 60%, and ocular signs are the most common form of target organ dysfunction associated with systemic hypertension. Hypertensive retinopathy is identified most often in cats older than 10 years of age with systolic blood pressures greater than 168 mm Hg when measured by an oscillometric technique (Sansom et al, 2004). The presence of ocular changes is an indication to start antihypertensive therapy even if blood pressure measurements do not consistently meet the criteria for hypertension.

Diagnosis

Clinical signs of hypertensive retinopathy can be unilateral but are typically bilateral. Presenting complaints include blindness, vision loss, or progressively dilated pupils. Hypertensive retinopathy also may have a subclinical presentation, noted only during routine examination of the fundus or during examination of cats with high blood pressure or those evaluated for a gallop sound or heart murmur. Serous retinal detachment often can be diagnosed with a penlight from arm's distance. Retroillumination of the eye is achieved by holding a light at arm's length from the patient. A normal eye should show bright yellow-green tapetal reflection in the pupil, although a blue eye may have a red pupil due to a lack of tapetum. Retinal detachment results in a dampening of that reflection caused by the presence of fluid between the retina and the tapetum. The proximity of the retina to the lens also sometimes allows the retinal vessels to be seen directly through the pupil. Retinal examination is difficult with retinal detachment, and the entire fundus may seem blurry. Focal areas of detachment are blurry and hyporeflective and are sometimes associated with hemorrhage beneath, within, or above the retina. Hyphema or vitreal hemorrhage also may be observed.

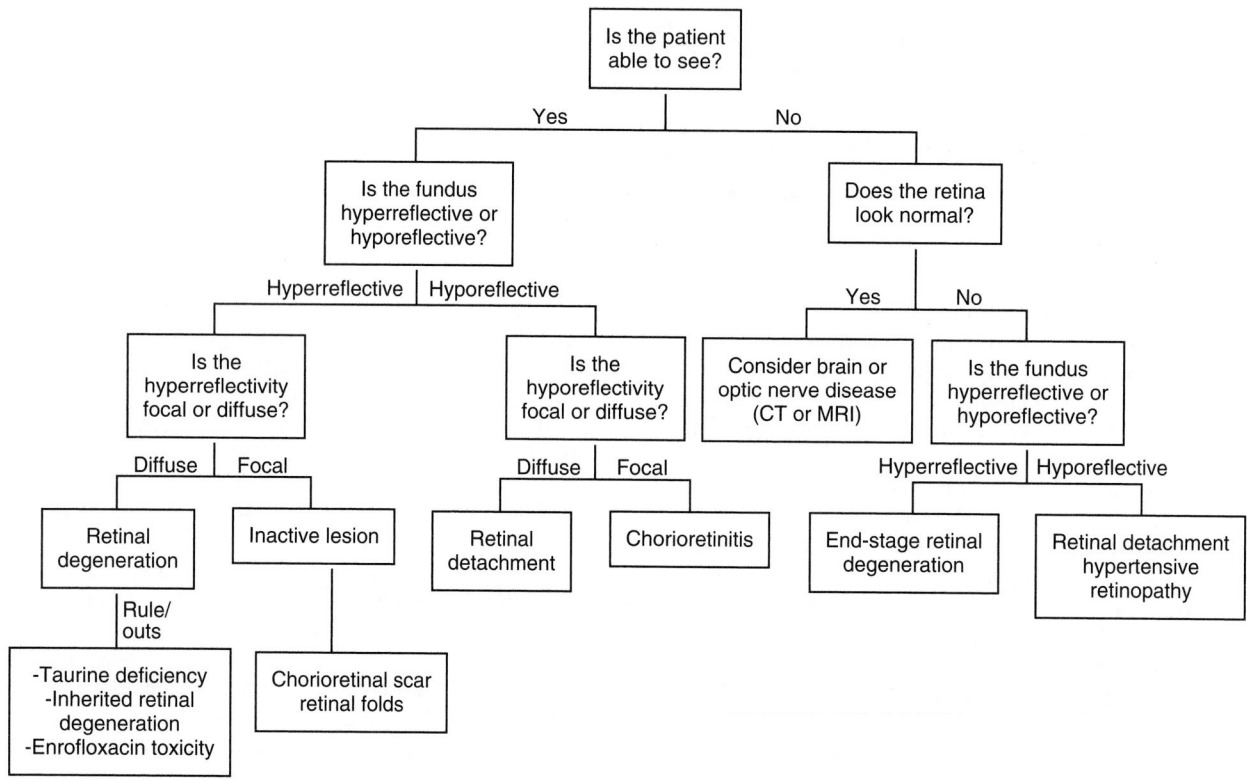

Figure 255-1 Diagnostic algorithm for the evaluation of feline retinopathies.

Treatment and Prognosis

Treatment of hypertensive retinopathy is focused solely on control of the systemic hypertension. No topical medications are indicated to treat the ocular component. Amlodipine has been demonstrated to be particularly effective in the resolution of systemic hypertension and hypertensive retinopathy (Maggio et al, 2000). Current recommendations for the treatment of systemic hypertension can be found in Chapter 169, but cats with hypertensive retinopathy should be evaluated for underlying systemic disease, including renal failure, hyperthyroidism, and the more uncommon condition of hyperaldosteronism (Conn's syndrome).

The prognosis for vision varies depending on the duration of the retinal detachment, with experimental models showing a return to function if the retina has been detached for 2 weeks or less. Unfortunately, because of cats' ability to adjust to vision loss, the retina typically is detached long before the patient is seen by a clinician. Although resolution of the hypertension usually results in reattachment of the retina, continued retinal degeneration is likely to occur. Thus some cats who are visual at presentation or regain vision immediately after treatment may continue to go blind despite adequate control of blood pressure.

Retinal Degeneration

The term *retinal degeneration* is a broad description for all disease states that result in progressive atrophy of the retina. There are nutritional, toxic, and inherited causes of retinal degeneration that can be challenging to differentiate. The clinical signs of retinal degeneration include progressive vision loss, dilated pupils, and a poor or incomplete pupillary light reflex. Fundic examination reveals diffuse bilateral retinal vascular attenuation and tapetal hyperreflectivity. Unfortunately, there is no way to differentiate the cause of retinal degeneration based on its appearance once the disease has progressed to clinical blindness. Thus all possible causes should be considered.

Taurine Retinopathy

Taurine is an essential amino acid for the cat and must be ingested in the diet to maintain health. Since the description of taurine deficiency and its associated retinopathy in 1975, commercial diets routinely have been supplemented with taurine. This has greatly decreased the incidence of the disease; however, deficiencies can be found in strays, patients fed homemade or canine-only diets, and occasionally in patients with seemingly appropriate diets.

Diagnosis

Taurine deficiency manifests initially as a pathognomonic lesion in the area centralis of the retina (see Figure 255-1). The area centralis is located superior and lateral to the optic disc and is characterized by a high concentration of photoreceptors. The taurine deficiency causes a focal retinal atrophy and a football-shaped area of hyperreflectivity. This proceeds to a band of hyperreflectivity extending across the visual streak. The retinal degeneration will progress to complete retinal atrophy without dietary modification. The presence of bilateral oval lesions or diffuse retinal degeneration is an indication to assess whole blood taurine levels. If the patient is found to have a taurine deficiency, a cardiac workup is recommended because the deficiency also is associated with dilated cardiomyopathy.

Treatment and Prognosis

If diagnosed early, taurine deficiency retinal degeneration can be halted but not reversed by restoring normal levels of taurine. Owners should be counseled to feed a commercial diet or to supplement their homemade diets with proper levels of taurine. Cats also can be given 125 to 250 mg of taurine twice daily PO. Although the precise time to retinal response is unknown, it can take 2 to 3 months before cardiac response is seen, and it is likely that retinal effects follow a similar timeline.

Enrofloxacin Toxic Retinopathy

Enrofloxacin toxicity first was identified in the mid-1990s when the dosing recommendations for cats were altered. After individual reports of rapid vision loss after systemic enrofloxacin administration, the toxicity was discovered to be dose related. Signs of retinal damage can be found in cats administered 25 mg/kg or more, with 50-mg/kg dosing resulting in retinal changes within days (Ford et al, 2007). The mechanism of toxicity is proposed to be a defect in a drug transporter gene that leads to accumulations of photoreactive fluoroquinolones; these subsequently generate toxic free radicals when exposed to light, which leads to photoreceptor cell death.

Diagnosis

Diagnosis is based on the presence of typical ocular signs combined with a history of high-dose enrofloxacin administration. The first clinical sign is the presence of dilated pupils, which is usually seen within several days of the enrofloxacin administration. Initially, increased granularity is appreciated in the area centralis, dorsotemporal to the optic disc. As in taurine deficiency retinopathy, this lesion progresses to include the horizontal visual streak. Eventually, vascular attenuation and diffuse tapetal hyperreflectivity characteristic of end-stage retinal degeneration are observed.

Treatment and Prognosis

At this time there is no treatment for enrofloxacin toxicity, and its resultant blindness is irreversible. However, early identification of the toxicity and discontinuation of the drug can preserve some vision. Although the toxicity is dose related, there are reported risk factors. These include rapid intravenous infusion of the drug, prolonged administration of the drug, and increased age of the patient. Given the severity of the retinal damage, enrofloxacin should be reserved for treatment of severe diseases, and dosages never should exceed 5 mg/kg q24h PO. Additional caution should be exercised when administering the drug intravenously and when choosing treatment for older cats. Although the toxicity is best understood for enrofloxacin, all fluoroquinolones hold the potential to cause retinal toxicity. Current studies have demonstrated higher safety thresholds with more recent generations of the drug including the recently released pradofloxacin.

Inherited Retinal Degeneration

The incidence of heritable retinal degeneration is significantly lower in cats than in dogs (see Chapter 254), and such disorders fall under the broad designation of *progressive retinal atrophy* (PRA). Abyssinian and Somali cats with PRA have been studied extensively, and two forms of the disease have been identified. The early-onset form is inherited as an autosomal-dominant trait and results in vision loss by 7 weeks of age. The late-onset PRA is an autosomal-recessive trait and results in vision loss by 3 to 5 years of age. The genetic basis for these degenerative disorders is known, and genetic testing is available. The single-nucleotide mutation in the *CEP290* gene discovered in Abyssinians with late-onset PRA (*rdAc*) also has been found in many other breeds. Siamese cats show a significantly increased incidence of this mutation, which may account for the anecdotal reports of PRA in Siamese and Siamese crossbreeds (Menotti-Raymond et al, 2010). An early-onset PRA has been reported in a domestic short-haired cat and a Persian cat, although the prevalence of this disease appears to be low. This disease entity (*Rdy*) is associated with a single base deletion in the CRX gene. Genetic testing is available for the early-onset PRA affecting Abyssinians and Somali cats (*Rdy* genotype) and the late-onset form (*rdAc* genotype) from the University of California at Davis.

Diagnosis

Diagnosis of inherited PRA in the cat is based on a combination of compatible clinical signs and signalment. The presence of bilaterally symmetric retinal vascular attenuation and diffuse hyperreflectivity in a 3- to 7-year-old cat of the appropriate breed should raise the index of suspicion for an inherited PRA. A diagnosis can be made by ruling out all other causes of retinal degeneration, including enrofloxacin toxicity and taurine deficiency, as well as testing for the *rdAc* genotype.

Treatment and Prognosis

There is no therapy to slow or reverse PRA. The rate of retinal degeneration is variable. Abyssinians and Somalis with early-onset PRA will lose vision by 7 weeks of age, and those with the late-onset form will be blind by 3 to 5 years of age. Although the inheritance is not understood in all breeds, it is prudent to recommend against breeding any cat with a suspected PRA. Blind cats generally have a high quality of life, although they should be confined inside to minimize the chance of accidents.

Chorioretinitis

Chorioretinitis is a term for inflammation that originates in the choroid and spreads to the adjacent retina. Chorioretinitis occurs with a breakdown of the blood-eye barrier and the introduction of infectious organisms, inflammatory cells, or exudate into the subretinal space or the retina itself. Because many disease processes can disrupt the blood-eye barrier, the causes of chorioretinitis are quite varied, and infection with any hematogenously disseminated pathogen could potentially result in chorioretinitis.

Diagnosis

Chorioretinitis is characterized by multifocal areas of active retinal inflammation. These areas have poorly defined or fuzzy borders and decreased reflectivity. Depending on the cellular makeup of the lesions, they can have a gray, white, yellow, or tan appearance. Severe chorioretinitis can result in complete retinal detachment. Once chorioretinitis has been identified, the focus should be on determination of the underlying cause. Potential causes of chorioretinitis in the cat are similar to the causes of uveitis (Chapter 250) and include systemic mycoses (cryptococcosis, blastomycosis, histoplasmosis, coccidiomycosis, systemic aspergillosis), feline infectious peritonitis (typically the dry form), and toxoplasmosis, as well as primary choroidal neoplasia. This list is not exhaustive but includes the most likely causes of chorioretinitis in the cat. Diagnostic workup should include a full physical examination, routine blood work, and urinalysis. Further diagnostic tests such as infectious disease titers, examination of lymph node aspirates, and imaging should be guided by the history and geographic location as well as the presence of concurrent clinical signs.

Treatment and Prognosis

Treatment is focused on the underlying cause of the chorioretinal lesions. Prognosis is good if the underlying disease can be identified and treated. However, chorioretinitis is more likely to result in permanent vision loss than other forms of intraocular inflammation. After resolution of the inflammation, the areas will atrophy, which results in focal areas of hyperreflectivity with pigment clumping.

Inactive Retinal Lesions

The last category of retinal change is that of inactive disease. This includes both chorioretinal scars and the congenital defect retinal dysplasia. All inactive retinal lesions are characterized by hyperreflectivity, and many are associated with clumps of pigment. Retinal dysplasia has a characteristic appearance of multifocal, linear, curving lesions with a central line of pigment surrounded by hyperreflectivity. In cats neonatal infection with panleukopenia or feline leukemia virus is a known cause of retinal dysplasia. Because these lesions are inactive and nonprogressive, no treatment is needed. Chorioretinal scars typically are circular rather than vermiform and are less regular in size. The impact of many chorioretinal scars on vision is unknown, but in this author's experience, a clinical visual defect never has been detected with these lesions.

References and Suggested Reading

Ford MM et al: Ocular and systemic manifestations after oral administration of a high dose of enrofloxacin in cats, *Am J Vet Res* 68:190, 2007.

Maggio F et al: Ocular lesions associated with systemic hypertension in cats: 69 cases (1985-1998), *J Am Vet Med Assoc* 217:695, 2000.

Menotti-Raymond M et al: Widespread retinal degenerative disease mutation (rdAc) discovered among a large number of popular cat breeds, *Vet J* 186:32, 2010.

Sansom J, Rogers K, Wood JL: Blood pressure assessment in healthy cats and cats with hypertensive retinopathy, *Am J Vet Res* 65:245, 2004.

Stepien R: Feline systemic hypertension diagnosis and management, *J Feline Med Surg* 13:35, 2011.

CHAPTER 256

Orbital Disease

RALPH E. HAMOR, *Urbana-Champaign, Illinois*

Orbital disease in dogs and cats can be caused by a variety of pathologic processes. Accurate assessment of the patient is essential for the selection of appropriate diagnostic studies and therapy. Orbital disease generally can be divided into those processes that lead to *exophthalmos* (protrusion of a normal-sized globe from the orbit) due to space-occupying disease, *enophthalmos* (recession of the globe within the orbit) due to decreased orbital contents, or *strabismus* (deviation of the globe within the orbit) (Box 256-1). The diagnostic challenge lies in the fact that clinical signs of orbital disease are evident only indirectly and involve changes in a wide variety of orbital tissues and surrounding structures.

Orbital Anatomy

Dogs and cats have an incomplete bony orbit. The orbit consists of the frontal, lacrimal, zygomatic, sphenoid, maxillary, and palatine bones. The lateral orbital wall is completed by a collagenous orbital ligament that attaches the frontal process of the zygomatic bone to the zygomatic process of the frontal bone. The masseter muscle completes the orbit posterolaterally, whereas the zygomatic salivary gland and medial pterygoid muscle fill the floor of the orbit. Most of the extraocular muscles arise from the posterior and medial aspect of the orbit to form a cone as they attach to the anterior aspect of the globe. The lacrimal gland is located dorsolaterally beneath the frontal bone in the lacrimal fossa. The frontal sinus is located dorsal to the orbit, and the maxillary sinus is rostral and ventral to the orbit. The ventral floor of the orbit is directly adjacent to the oral cavity as well as the roots of the upper premolar and molar teeth. The orbital cavity also contains the second, third, and fourth cranial nerves; the ophthalmic branch of the fifth cranial nerve; the sixth cranial nerve; numerous arteries and veins; and smooth muscle, and is surrounded by periorbital tissue. The orbit is most shallow and directed more laterally in brachycephalic breeds and is most deep and directed more medially in dolichocephalic breeds, with the orbit in mesaticephalic breeds lying somewhere in between.

Clinical Signs of Orbital Disease

Pathologic processes affecting the orbit involve one or more of three anatomic compartments: (1) within the extraocular muscle cone, (2) outside the cone but inside the periorbital tissue, and (3) inside the orbit but outside the periorbital tissue. Orbital disorders are characterized by clinical signs that alter the function, appearance, or position of the globe, eyelids, or ocular adnexal structures.

The orbit is a confined space with little capacity for its contents to expand. Primary and secondary clinical signs of orbital disease are the hallmark of orbital disorders. *Primary clinical signs* include exophthalmos, enophthalmos, and strabismus. *Secondary clinical signs* include chemosis, swelling of the eyelids and periorbital tissue, elevation of the third eyelid, pain upon opening the mouth, lagophthalmos (incomplete eyelid closure), exposure keratitis, visual impairment, abnormal pupillary light reflexes, scleral indentation, mild to moderate increase in intraocular pressure (only with extreme exophthalmos), and facial asymmetry.

One of the challenges in the diagnosis of orbital disease is the accurate interpretation of clinical signs. It is crucial for the clinician to differentiate buphthalmos (enlargement of the globe) from exophthalmos. Exophthalmos is a clinical sign of orbital disease, whereas buphthalmos is secondary to chronic glaucoma. Measuring the horizontal corneal diameter (from limbus to limbus) may be useful in differentiating buphthalmos from exophthalmos. The horizontal corneal diameters of the two globes should differ by 1 mm or less. Ultrasonography also can be used to measure the axial globe length. When assessing axial globe length, the operator should ensure that the ultrasound probe is positioned in the center of the globe so that the image is captured through the thickest section of the lens.

Diagnostic Approach

A thorough history taking and physical examination are prerequisites for the diagnostic workup of orbital disease. When orbital disease is suspected, initial examination should include palpation of the eye and periocular structures, retropulsion of the globe, and careful examination of the oral cavity. The sizes of the palpebral fissures should be compared, the orbit should be palpated, the position of the eyelids and third eyelid should be observed, the location and mobility of the globe within the orbit should be assessed, and the presence of any ocular discharge should be noted. The globe generally can be retropulsed if there are no space-occupying lesions in the orbit. *Retropulsion* of the globe is performed through closed eyelids by placing an index finger on the upper eyelid of each eye and gently pressing or pushing the globe caudally within the orbit. Brachycephalic breeds may have quite shallow orbits, and the amplitude of retropulsion may be decreased even in normal orbits.

Orbital Diseases Causing Exophthalmos, Enophthalmos, and Strabismus

Exophthalmos
Abscess (bacterial, fungal)
Cellulitis
Neoplasia
Zygomatic mucocele
Varix or vascular anomaly
Hemorrhage secondary to trauma
Coagulopathy
Masticatory myositis
Extraocular polymyositis
Relative exophthalmos
     (brachycephalic breeds)
Proptosis
Craniomandibular osteopathy

Enophthalmos
Relative enophthalmos (dolichocephalic breeds)
Phthisis bulbi
Microphthalmia
Pain
Horner's syndrome
Chronic inflammation
Atrophy of orbital tissues
Starvation or dehydration
Orbital fracture

Strabismus
Neoplasia
Proptosis
Relative strabismus (brachycephalic breeds)
Masticatory myositis
Zygomatic mucocele
Lacrimal cyst
Hydrocephalus
Orbital fracture

Digital pressure should never be used to assess intraocular pressure. Exophthalmic globes feel "hard" because of the resistance to retropulsion secondary to a space-occupying lesion within the orbit. When an exophthalmic globe is diagnosed incorrectly as glaucomatous because the globe feels hard, an incorrect differential diagnostic list and therapeutic plan will be formulated. In general, exophthalmic globes have normal intraocular pressure until the globe is quite exophthalmic, which causes the globe to be pressed against the eyelid margin. In these cases, the globe generally is not buphthalmic and does not have other clinical signs consistent with chronic glaucoma, including diffuse corneal edema, a dilated and unresponsive pupil, lens subluxation, retinal atrophy, and optic nerve cupping.

Once orbital disease is suspected, the most important clinical diagnostic test is to check for the presence or absence of resistance to opening the mouth. Pain upon opening or attempting to open the mouth as the coronoid process of the mandible impinges on the orbital tissues is indicative of retrobulbar inflammation. This test should be executed slowly, carefully, and gently because patients with orbital inflammation can have significant pain. A thorough oral examination should be performed. Sedation or general anesthesia may be necessary. Lack of pain upon opening the mouth more often is consistent with orbital neoplasia. Orbital neoplasia generally causes less orbital inflammation for a similar degree of exophthalmos. Some orbital neoplastic diseases may produce significant orbital inflammation, and some cases of orbital inflammation may not cause pain when the mouth is opened; however, evidence of pain on opening the mouth is more common in orbital inflammatory disease. Inappetence may be reported by the owner in association with oral pain.

Exophthalmos

Orbital Cellulitis or Abscess

The causes of orbital cellulitis include trauma, penetrating foreign body, extension of tooth root abscess or sinonasal disease, and hematogenous dissemination of infection or neoplasia. In some cases, an underlying cause may not be identifiable. The canine and feline orbit lacks a bony floor, which leaves it vulnerable to penetrating injury or puncture if the patient chews a bone or a stick. Foreign bodies often are implicated as the cause of orbital cellulitis but rarely are identified definitively. The onset of clinical signs generally is rapid. These signs may include exophthalmos, fever, pain upon opening the mouth, and chemosis. A soft, fluctuant swelling or hyperemia may be present caudal to the last molar. Tooth root abscesses of the fourth premolar can erupt through the skin causing a draining tract ventral to the orbit.

Diagnostic evaluation for orbital cellulitis or abscess should include a complete physical examination, a complete blood count, and a thorough oral examination. Dental radiography may be indicated to rule out dental disease. Skull radiographs may demonstrate radiodense foreign bodies, show evidence of extension of inflammation from adjacent sinuses, or reveal orbital fractures. Orbital ultrasonography may demonstrate diffuse hyperechogenicity posterior to the globe or a discrete hypoechoic mass. Ultrasonography of the fellow normal orbit may be useful for comparison and aid in the identification of subtle lesions. Advanced imaging (including magnetic resonance imaging [MRI] and computed tomography [CT]) provides the most detailed and accurate images of the orbit and retrobulbar tissue. CT generally is considered to be the imaging modality of choice for orbital disease. Fine-needle aspirates for cytologic evaluation or culture and sensitivity testing may be obtained from the retrobulbar space through the conjunctiva, skin, or oral cavity. Ultrasonographic or CT guidance may be useful to improve localization when aspiration is performed.

Treatment of Orbital Cellulitis or Abscess

Therapy consists of establishing surgical drainage under general anesthesia, performing local irrigation, and administering systemic antibiotics. Before any of these procedures is performed, the operator should ensure that the cuff of the endotracheal tube is well inflated to prevent aspiration of any exudates. The mucosa should be incised behind the last upper molar using a No. 10 or No. 15 Bard-Parker scalpel blade and a closed blunt mosquito hemostat should be inserted to enlarge the opening. The closed hemostat then should be opened gently to create a tract to allow drainage. Purulent material may not be immediately evident after establishment of a drainage tract. Samples should be procured for aerobic and aerobic culture and sensitivity testing if purulent material is obtained. The tract then may be flushed gently with dilute 1:10 povidone-iodine solution.

Systemic antibiotics should be administered after drainage has been established. Mixed aerobic and anaerobic bacterial infections occur most commonly in the dog and cat, and cephalosporins, extended-spectrum penicillins, potentiated penicillins, and carbapenems are recommended for initial antimicrobial treatment of orbital abscesses in dogs and cats (Wang et al, 2009). Administration of systemic nonsteroidal antiinflammatories and analgesics, including oral opioids such as tramadol hydrochloride, also is recommended until clinical signs resolve. Antiinflammatory dosages of oral corticosteroids may also be effective; however, immunosuppressive dosages should be avoided.

The patient should be evaluated carefully for the ability to completely close the lids over the globe. Many patients with exophthalmos develop secondary exposure keratitis from lagophthalmos. Corneal ulceration may occur in lagophthalmic patients. All patients with exophthalmos should be evaluated carefully for the presence of a corneal ulceration. Topical lubricating ointments should be applied every 2 to 6 hours to prevent desiccation of the ocular surface. A temporary tarsorrhaphy may be necessary if the exophthalmos is severe or prolonged.

Orbital Neoplasia

Orbital neoplasia is an important cause of exophthalmos in canine and feline patients (see Chapters 257 and 258). The clinical signs are similar to those of orbital cellulitis, but the onset of signs generally is less acute. Pain upon opening the mouth is not observed frequently, and fever or leukocytosis usually is absent. The most common clinical sign is slowly progressive unilateral exophthalmos. Patients with orbital neoplasia also are much more likely to have strabismus, which may assist in localization of the orbital mass. A patient with a tumor in the ventronasal aspect of the orbit often has dorsotemporal strabismus because the mass shifts the normal position of the globe away from the location of the orbital mass. As in orbital cellulitis, the intraocular pressure of the globe usually is within the normal range unless the exophthalmos is so severe that the eyelids are compressing the globe.

Diagnostic evaluation for orbital neoplasia should include a complete physical examination and systemic staging (complete blood work, three-view thoracic radiography, and abdominal ultrasonography). An oral examination also is warranted because in rare cases orbital neoplasia erodes or invades the ventral floor of the orbit. Orbital ultrasonography may be helpful, but more advanced imaging (MRI or CT) provides the most diagnostically useful information. Fine-needle aspiration or

biopsy is useful in establishing a diagnosis. In some cases, surgical orbital exploration may be necessary to obtain tissue for histopathologic analysis. Orbital exploration is best performed by a surgeon familiar with orbital anatomy and vasculature.

Masticatory Muscle Myositis

Masticatory muscle myositis is a canine autoimmune inflammatory disease. It commonly occurs in German shepherds, golden retrievers, and weimaraner dogs. This condition involves the muscles of mastication (masseter, temporalis, and sometimes pterygoid). Clinical signs include exophthalmos, blepharedema, protrusion of the third eyelid, and pain upon opening the mouth. Upon palpation, the involved masticatory muscles typically are hard and painful. Episodes of inflammation may last 10 to 21 days and commonly recur. Persistently affected dogs may be unable to open the mouth (trismus) and demonstrate atrophy or fibrosis of the temporalis and masseter muscles.

Diagnosis generally is made by observation of characteristic clinical signs and is confirmed by histopathologic evaluation. Peripheral eosinophilia is present inconsistently. Autoantibodies against type IIM myofibers have been identified in affected dogs (also see Chapter 240). Biopsy of the temporalis muscle demonstrates eosinophilic infiltration and type IIM myofiber antigen-antibody complexes. The mainstay of treatment is systemic corticosteroids (immunosuppressive dosage initially, with the dosage then slowly tapered over 4 to 6 weeks). Oral azathioprine also may be used for long-term therapy. During episodes of inflammation, patients can be encouraged to eat by providing frequent soft meals.

Extraocular Polymyositis

Extraocular polymyositis is an autoimmune inflammatory disease that is confined to the extraocular muscles. The syndrome is described most commonly in young large-breed dogs; golden retrievers are overrepresented. Clinical signs include acute-onset bilateral exophthalmos and mild chemosis. Because the exophthalmos is directly along the visual axis, affected animals have 360 degrees of scleral exposure. In rare cases, massive swelling of the extraocular muscles may compress the optic nerve and cause a visual deficit.

Diagnosis is made primarily by observation of the characteristic clinical signs. Findings of advanced imaging (MRI or CT) and biopsy of the extraocular muscles, which reveals infiltration of the muscle by lymphocytes and histiocytes, are supportive of the diagnosis. Treatment is similar to that for masticatory muscle myositis.

Cystic Orbital Disease

Exophthalmos may occur secondary to zygomatic or lacrimal mucoceles. Zygomatic mucocele is most common and may occur spontaneously or secondary to trauma. Mucoceles generally are nonpainful and may cause protrusion of the oral mucous membrane behind the last upper molar or protrusion of a mass beneath the conjunctiva in the inferior temporal or nasal conjunctival fornix. Ultrasonography may reveal a cystic mass in the orbit. Aspiration of the cyst generally reveals thick, stringy, clear to straw-colored fluid that forms mucoid strands when placed between the thumb and forefinger. Advanced imaging of the orbit may be useful. Treatment is generally surgical removal, but some patients respond to systemic broad-spectrum antibiotics and antiinflammatory agents.

Enophthalmos

Enophthalmos occurs when the globe becomes displaced posteriorly within the orbit. The globe may be normal sized or smaller than normal. Causes of enophthalmos in a normal-sized globe include age-related loss of periorbital and orbital muscle mass and fat leading to symmetric enophthalmos. Horner's syndrome causes enophthalmos secondary to loss of sympathetic innervation of the orbit (see Web Chapter 80). Enophthalmos also may occur when the globe is retracted actively by the retractor bulbi muscle. This is observed most commonly in patients with a painful ocular surface or intraocular disease. Microphthalmos is a unilateral or bilateral congenital lesion in which the globe is smaller than normal. Microphthalmos must be differentiated from phthisis bulbi (shrinking of a previously normal-sized globe), which occurs secondary to chronic and severe uveitis.

In addition to enophthalmos, clinical signs may include passive elevation of the third eyelid and secondary entropion of the lower lateral eyelid. Identification of the cause of enophthalmos is the most important component of treating enophthalmos. Age-related orbital tissue atrophy does not need treatment, but enophthalmos may be a clinical sign of serious intraocular disease that needs accurate identification and intervention.

Trauma

Traumatic lesions of the orbit include proptosis and fracture. Proptosis is discussed in Web Chapter 78.

Orbital fractures usually are caused by some traumatic event and may be associated with proptosis of the globe, especially in nonbrachycephalic breeds. Diagnosis of orbital fractures frequently can be made by palpation. Small nondisplaced fractures may be difficult to see radiographically. CT may be useful in such cases. Clinical signs include pain, periorbital swelling and contusions, crepitus, facial asymmetry, exophthalmos or enophthalmos, and corneal disease. Careful assessment of globe motility is indicated because bony fragments may lead to entrapment of extraocular muscles. A helpful maneuver to perform, when possible, is to move the head side to side as well as up and down while following the movement of both globes. The globes should move together and symmetrically. In a sedated or anesthetized patient, motility of the globe can be assessed by gently grasping the sclera with toothed forceps. The normal globe can be used for comparison. Visual prognosis is poor when extraocular muscles are entrapped in fractured bone.

Bony fragments can be removed, especially if they are protruding into the orbit. Large displaced fractures can be repaired or removed surgically. Consultation with an experienced orthopedic or ophthalmic surgeon is recommended. Although the patient may heal with some facial asymmetry and enophthalmos, most patients retain vision. It is not uncommon for the zygomatic arch to be fractured completely with significant head trauma. Complete removal or reconstruction may be necessary.

References and Suggested Reading

Allgower I et al: Extraocular muscle myositis and restrictive strabismus in 10 dogs, *Vet Ophthalmol* 3:21, 2000.

Armour MD et al: A review of orbital and intracranial magnetic resonance imaging in 79 canine and 13 feline patients (2004-2010), *Vet Ophthalmol* 14:215, 2011.

Miller PE: Orbit. In Maggs DJ, Miller PE, Ofri R, editors: *Slatter's fundamentals of veterinary ophthalmology*, ed 4, St Louis, 2008, Saunders, p 352.

Ramsey DT et al: Comparative value of diagnostic imaging techniques in a cat with exophthalmos, *Vet Comp Ophthalmol* 4:198, 1994.

Ramsey DT et al: Ophthalmic manifestations and complications of dental disease in dogs and cats, *J Am Anim Hosp Assoc* 32:215, 1996.

Wang AL, Ledbetter EC, Kern TJ: Orbital abscess bacterial isolates in *in vitro* antimicrobial susceptibility patterns in dogs and cats, *Vet Ophthalmol* 12:91, 2009.

CHAPTER 257

Canine Ocular Neoplasia

SANDRA M. NGUYEN, *Sydney, Australia*
AMBER LABELLE, *Urbana-Champaign, Illinois*

Ocular neoplasia is relatively uncommon compared with neoplasia affecting other body systems; however, it is the second most common cause of enucleation. Early detection of ophthalmic neoplasia is important for optimal treatment outcome. Ophthalmic disease, particularly uveitis, can be the first sign of systemic neoplasia, and multicentric neoplasia can involve the eye, which makes an ocular examination desirable in all canine oncology patients. These relationships emphasize the importance of a complete physical examination in all cases of canine uveitis. Additionally, owners may be less willing to pursue oncologic treatment in blind pets, which underscores the importance of early detection and aggressive treatment of ocular neoplasia.

General Diagnostic Approach

In general, a working diagnosis should be made based on ophthalmic and physical examination findings and results of fine-needle aspiration (FNA) or biopsy. Appropriate staging tests can be selected based on these results. For orbital tumors, computed tomography (CT) and magnetic resonance imaging (MRI) are very helpful in determining the local extent of disease and planning surgical and radiation treatment. For tumors involving the globe, ocular ultrasonography is useful for identifying and localizing masses obscured by corneal, aqueous, or lens opacity and for those located in the posterior segment. Ocular ultrasonography also is useful for guiding FNA, and high-resolution ultrasonography can be used to assess the extent of tumors in the cornea, sclera, and iris. Thoracic radiography and lymph node aspiration should be performed to detect metastatic disease, with recognition that the overall metastatic rate for most malignant ocular neoplasms is low. The eye also may be a site of metastatic or multicentric neoplasia (as in the case of lymphoma), so the initial diagnosis will influence the subsequent diagnostic and treatment decisions.

For eyelid lesions, which typically are benign, early diagnosis is the key to complete resolution without the need for complicated surgical reconstruction. One third of the eyelid margin length can be excised without impairing eyelid function. As for other skin lesions, cytologic analysis, examination of skin scrapings, and FNA are straightforward diagnostic procedures for periocular masses. The eye must be protected or retropulsed whenever a needle or blade is directed toward the globe, so chemical restraint often is indicated to prevent ocular trauma during the procedure.

For conjunctival lesions, most diagnostic procedures can be performed using topical anesthesia (proparacaine hydrochloride 0.5% solution) and gentle manual restraint. A sample of a conjunctival lesion for cytologic analysis can be obtained with the blunt end of a scalpel blade, a cytobrush, or a Kimura spatula. Biopsy of the conjunctiva also can be performed using topical anesthesia. The conjunctiva adjacent to the lesion should be grasped using small, toothed forceps and gently elevated, and then the lesion should be snipped free with small scissors. The sample then can be gently spread onto a tongue depressor for fixation. Alternatively, the sample can be placed directly into a histopathologic tissue cassette. Closure of conjunctival defects smaller than 4 mm in diameter is unnecessary. Although biopsy may be more invasive, it provides more information than cytologic analysis alone and may prove essential to obtaining a diagnosis. Subconjunctival or episcleral masses most often are inflammatory, but differentiating these from a neoplastic mass can be a diagnostic challenge. Biopsy of an episcleral mass may warrant referral to an ophthalmologist to avoid inadvertent penetration of the globe.

Examination of the third eyelid also can be performed with topical anesthesia. Nontoothed forceps may be used to grasp the leading margin and elevate the third eyelid, which allows the palpebral and bulbar surfaces to be visualized and palpated directly. Biopsy of the third eyelid conjunctiva may be performed as described earlier. For larger lesions for which excisional biopsy or removal of the entire third eyelid may be warranted, general anesthesia may be required. Because the development of keratoconjunctivitis sicca is a possible complication of complete third eyelid excision, it is important to ensure that informed consent is obtained before this procedure is performed.

Aqueous paracentesis is performed infrequently on visual eyes because it requires general anesthesia; carries a (low) risk of bacterial endophthalmitis, profuse iridal hemorrhage, or retinal detachment; and reliably induces transient uveitis. Aqueous humor cytologic evaluation is most sensitive for the diagnosis of lymphoma, if the diagnosis cannot be made by sampling other tissues. Vitreocentesis is most useful in cases of exudative or solid posterior segment masses in blind globes. For blind eyes, aqueous humor cytologic analysis or vitreal aspirate examination may yield a diagnosis before enucleation that may improve surgical planning, but enucleation is preferred in nonvisual eyes affected with neoplasia.

For orbital masses, FNA, collection of culture specimens, and Tru-Cut biopsy can be performed through the conjunctiva, periocular skin, or oral cavity behind the last molar. Tru-Cut biopsy is best performed under sedation or anesthesia in conjunction with ultrasonography or CT to avoid damage to the globe. Plain radiographs are useful mostly for identifying dental or nasal disease or osteolysis; CT or MRI is far superior for evaluating the soft tissues of the orbit and globe as well as for assessing involvement of orbital bone and sinuses. Orbital mucoceles and abscesses tend to have a more cavitary appearance than orbital tumors on ultrasonographic, CT, or MRI scans.

Signalment, history, and examination findings help further with differential diagnoses. For instance, dental disease and neoplasia are more common causes of orbital disease in older patients. Abscesses tend to arise more quickly and to elicit more pain than tumors. Application of topical lubricants or performance of a temporary tarsorrhaphy often is needed in cases of severe exophthalmos to protect the cornea while a definitive diagnosis is being made and therapy is implemented.

Histopathologic diagnosis of ophthalmic neoplasia can be complicated by the idiosyncrasies of ophthalmic anatomy and tumor physiology, species differences, the mount of inflammation present within a tumor, the orientation of the tissue, and the experience of the veterinary pathologist. Submitting a detailed history as well as drawings and photographs of the lesion *in situ*, inking the margins of adnexal tumors, and marking the scleral location of intraocular tumors with suture after enucleation are recommended to assist the pathologist in making the most accurate and informative diagnosis. When an enucleated globe is submitted for histopathologic analysis, fixation in a volume of formalin 10 times that of the globe is optimal for adequate fixation of intraocular tissue. A 25-gauge needle may be used to inject approximately 0.5 ml of formalin through the sclera posterior to the equator of the globe to improve fixation of the intraocular structures.

Primary Ocular Neoplasia

Adnexa and Conjunctiva

The most common canine eyelid neoplasms are *meibomian gland adenoma* and *epithelioma* (Figure 257-1) These tumors are benign but locally expansive, arising from the sebaceous glands and glandular epithelium, respectively. They typically occur in older dogs, have an irregularly textured to cobblestone surface, and can be seen protruding from the meibomian gland orifice as a pink, gray, or black mass at the eyelid margin. If the tumor remains within the meibomian gland it may cause obstruction of the gland orifice, resulting in accumulation of the glandular lipid secretions within the duct. When rupture of the gland ensues, marked granulomatous inflammation may develop in response to the release of inflammatory lipid products into the surrounding tissues. This secondary inflammation may give a small meibomian gland adenoma a falsely large appearance and can be quite uncomfortable for the patient. Meibomian gland adenomas and epitheliomas also can cause significant corneal irritation, and although these rarely are a direct cause of

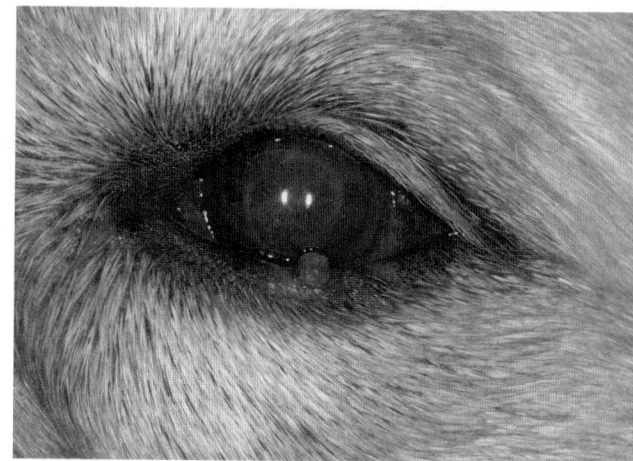

Figure 257-1 Meibomian gland adenoma in the lower central and upper lateral eyelid of a mixed-breed dog.

corneal ulceration, they may prevent epithelialization and delay corneal wound healing when an ulcer is present.

Squamous papillomas, which arise from the eyelids and periocular skin, have a clinical appearance and behavior similar to those of tumors of meibomian gland origin and also are frequent in older dogs. Squamous papillomas in younger dogs are more likely of viral origin and usually regress spontaneously without any treatment. Benign eyelid melanomas also are common in older dogs and typically are broad-based pigmented masses adjacent to but not usually involving the eyelid margin. Pedunculated forms rarely occur.

Surgical resection is the treatment of choice for most canine eyelid tumors. Surgical options include full-thickness eyelid resection, carbon dioxide laser ablation, and surgical debulking with cryoablation. When full-thickness eyelid resection is performed, it is imperative to achieve perfect reapposition of the eyelid margin to ensure normal eyelid function and long-term corneal health. Surgical debulking with cryoablation is an alternative to full-thickness eyelid resection that does not require general anesthesia in most patients. It can be performed under sedation (e.g., dexmedetomidine 375 to 500 $\mu g/m^2$ IV and butorphanol 0.1 mg/kg IV) and local anesthesia (0.5 ml of lidocaine 2% infiltrated into the base of the neoplasm). After an open-closed chalazion clamp is placed over the eyelid and tumor, small scissors are used to excise all neoplastic tissue visibly extruding from the meibomian gland orifice. Gentle digital pressure may be applied to the palpebral conjunctiva to extrude any glandular contents. If the tumor can be visualized through the palpebral conjunctiva, a No. 15 Bard-Parker scalpel blade can be used to sharply excise the overlying conjunctiva to the level of the tumor, which allows débridement with a 3- or 4-mm curette or sharp excision using Stevens tenotomy scissors. It is important not to incise the eyelid margin using this debulking approach and to ensure that any incisions extend only through the palpebral conjunctiva. After the majority of the tumor material has been removed, cryoablation can be performed using liquid nitrogen in a dispensing canister with a flat probe attached (Figure 257-2). The size of the ice ball generated provides

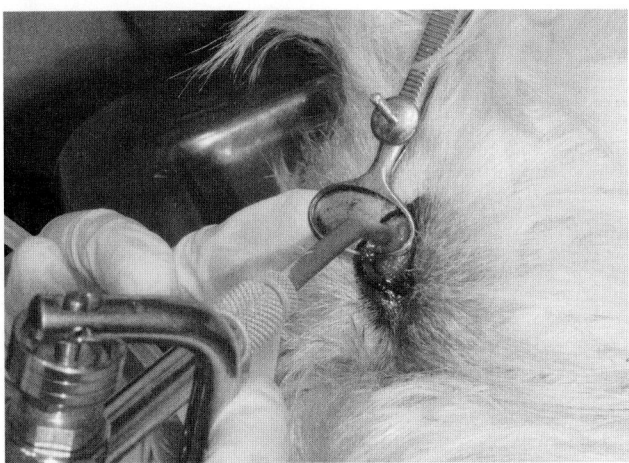

Figure 257-2 Intraoperative photograph demonstrating the use of an open-closed chalazion clamp to isolate a meibomian gland adenoma of the upper eyelid. A cryoprobe has been applied directly to the palpebral conjunctiva overlying the base of the tumor.

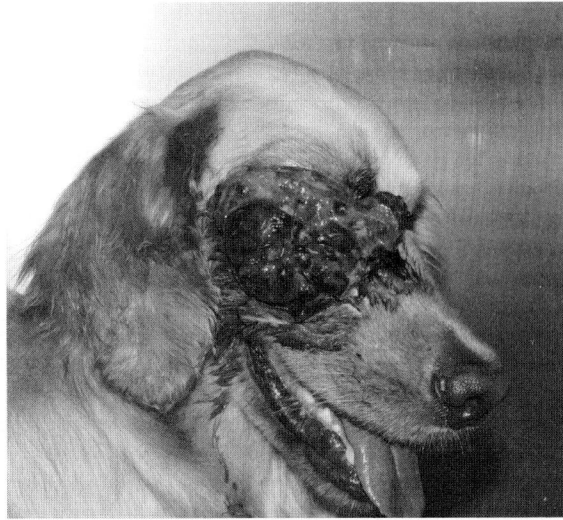

Figure 257-3 Biologically high-grade, histologically low-grade fibrosarcoma arising from the lower lid of a young golden retriever. The tumor has caused significant deviation of the globe and subsequent corneal rupture.

an estimate of the depth of cryopenetration. Use of two complete freeze-thaw cycles is recommended. The size of the tip selected for the cryoablation unit should approximate the size of the base of the tumor. Postoperatively, patients should be treated for 5 to 7 days with a broad-spectrum ophthalmic antibiotic ointment. Swelling and epidermal depigmentation occur commonly at the site of cryoablation, but repigmentation may be expected within weeks to months. In rare cases depigmentation remains at the eyelid margin, which may be a concern in patients for which cosmesis is important.

Histiocytomas appear as firm, well-circumscribed, pink or red, raised cutaneous masses that may involve the periocular skin in young dogs. Spontaneous regression occurs within 6 weeks in most cases. FNA usually is sufficient to confirm the diagnosis. If spontaneous regression does not occur, complete surgical excision is recommended.

Mesenchymal hamartomas are an infrequently reported benign tumor of the canine eyelid for which complete surgical excision is expected to be curative.

Primary *malignant neoplasms* of the canine adnexa include melanoma, adenocarcinoma, mast cell tumor, histiocytic sarcoma, hemangiosarcoma, basal cell carcinoma, squamous cell carcinoma, lymphoma, and fibrosarcoma (Figure 257-3). The majority of these tumors are locally invasive, and complete surgical excision is required to achieve a good outcome. It is also important to evaluate the patient and stage the tumor to ensure that the tumor is indeed primary and to assess for the presence of metastasis or multicentric disease, particularly with lymphoma, mast cell tumor, and histiocytic sarcoma. Cytologic or histopathologic evaluation is recommended before definitive surgery to confirm the diagnosis and assist in surgical planning. Enucleation is necessary in cases of very large eyelid tumors when achievement of adequate surgical margins makes surgical resection and repair impossible.

Neoplasia of the third eyelid is uncommon. Reported neoplasms include adenoma, adenocarcinoma, squamous cell carcinoma, mast cell tumor, melanoma, lymphoma, hemangioma, hemangiosarcoma, plasmacytoma, and papilloma. Clinical signs of third eyelid disease include elevation of the third eyelid, enophthalmos or exophthalmos, deviation of the globe, and a visible mass effect within the body of the nictitans. Conjunctivitis may occur as a secondary finding. It is important to differentiate third eyelid neoplasia from a glandular cyst or prolapsed gland of the third eyelid (also known as *cherry eye*). Removal of the third eyelid generally is not recommended because of the contributions the gland makes to the aqueous portion of the tear film; however, surgical resection may be curative for neoplasia of the third eyelid, and the subsequent keratoconjunctivitis sicca can be managed medically in most cases. Adenocarcinoma is the most frequently reported neoplasm of the third eyelid; local recurrence or metastasis is uncommon because complete surgical resection is expected to be curative. If the tumor extends into the orbit, exenteration may be necessary to achieve complete excision. Advanced diagnostic imaging, such as CT or MRI, may be useful in surgical planning when the tumor extends to the base of the nictitans or when orbital involvement is suspected.

Because of the intimate anatomic relationship of the eyelid and conjunctiva, primary conjunctival neoplasia can be quite difficult to differentiate from eyelid neoplasia. Determining the tissue of origin is particularly important for conjunctival melanoma, which has a significantly higher rate of local recurrence and potential to metastasize than melanoma of the periocular skin. Other reported neoplasms of the conjunctiva include squamous cell carcinoma, mast cell tumor, hemangioma, hemangiosarcoma, papilloma, lymphoma, and histiocytic sarcoma. Neoplastic conjunctival masses must be differentiated from nonneoplastic diseases such as episcleritis, parasitic granuloma, cysts, and subconjunctival fat prolapse. Most conjunctival neoplasms are amenable to surgical excision, potentially followed by cryoablation or beta irradiation of the margins. Conjunctival melanomas may have a higher rate of recurrence, and wide surgical excision is indicated for these neoplasms. Enucleation or exenteration may be required in some cases. Papillomas, which are found more frequently in young dogs, may regress spontaneously.

Sclera, Limbus, and Cornea

Neoplasia of the canine cornea and sclera are uncommon. Theoretically, all types of epithelial neoplasms could arise from their surfaces; however, squamous cell carcinoma and limbal melanoma are the most common and clinically important tumors. *Squamous cell carcinoma* may affect the conjunctiva, limbus, corneal surface, or some combination thereof. Chronic keratitis is a risk factor for the development of squamous cell carcinoma. Some authors have proposed that the long-term use of immunomodulatory agents such as cyclosporine or tacrolimus may be a risk factor for the development of squamous cell carcinoma; however, controlled studies are lacking. Squamous cell carcinoma appears clinically as a pink, raised mass with an irregular or ulcerated surface, and in younger dogs, it should be differentiated from a viral papilloma, which may have a similar appearance. Cytologic analysis may be useful for distinguishing the two neoplasms. Keratectomy is curative in most cases, and adjunctive treatment with beta irradiation, carbon dioxide laser ablation, or cryoablation may decrease the incidence of local recurrence.

Limbal melanomas are recognized easily by their clinical appearance as a black, smooth, circular mass at the limbus. They may invade into the cornea, iridocorneal angle, and anterior chamber. The German shepherd and Labrador retriever are predisposed. In young dogs the tumor may grow rapidly and invasively; surgical intervention is indicated in these cases. In older dogs, the tumors tend to grow very slowly and may not require treatment, although diligent monitoring with careful sequential measurements is indicated. Limbal melanomas must be differentiated from anterior uveal melanomas because uveal melanomas have a greater potential for destruction of intraocular tissues and vision loss, and therefore necessitate earlier intervention and possibly enucleation. Potential surgical interventions include full-thickness resection with grafting procedures to restore the integrity of the sclera and limbus and debulking followed by cryoablation, photoablation, or beta irradiation. Referral to an ophthalmologist is indicated in cases of limbal melanoma or squamous cell carcinoma.

Uvea

Uveal *melanoma* or *melanocytoma* is the most common intraocular neoplasm in the dog and must be differentiated from a uveal cyst. Uveal cysts arise from the posterior pigmented iris epithelium, tend to be round and translucent, and may be free floating within the anterior chamber or connected to the pupillary margin by a thin stalk. A neoplastic lesion also must be differentiated from

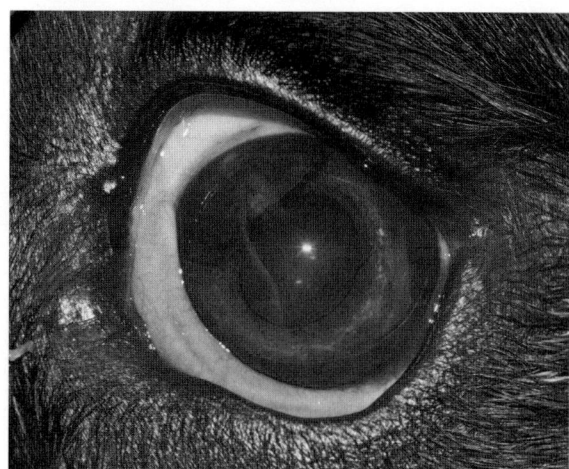

Figure 257-4 Melanocytoma located between the 9 o'clock and 12 o'clock positions in the iris of a Bernese mountain dog. The mass is causing dyscoria.

an iris nevus, which is the equivalent to a freckle on the skin; an iris nevus is a pigmented, flat, benign, and inactive lesion that is not expected to undergo neoplastic transformation. Anterior uveal melanoma and melanocytoma vary in clinical appearance from dark brown or black, flat or slightly raised lesions on the face of the iris, to large masses expanding or effacing the iris, to partially hidden but expansile masses of the ciliary body (Figure 257-4). Anterior uveal melanocytic neoplasms typically are locally invasive and expansive and may lead to intraocular inflammation, secondary glaucoma, and retinal detachment. These long-term complications frequently necessitate enucleation. When a slightly raised, well-circumscribed pigmented mass is present on the anterior surface of the iris, diode or neodymium:yttrium-aluminum-garnet (Nd-YAG) laser may be effective in arresting the growth of the lesion and eliminate the need for enucleation. Surgical resection by sector iridectomy may be a curative therapy for smaller lesions but is accompanied by significant risk of complications, including intraocular hemorrhage, endophthalmitis, and retinal detachment. Posterior uveal (choroidal) melanoma and melanocytoma are less common and necessitate enucleation in the majority of cases.

Most uveal melanocytic neoplasms in the dog are benign with no potential for metastasis, which makes recommending enucleation challenging for a visual and comfortable globe. Unfortunately, it is nearly impossible to differentiate a benign from a malignant tumor clinically, and histopathologic evaluation is essential for confirming the diagnosis. Referral to a veterinary ophthalmologist is warranted to determine treatment options and prognosis in individual cases. For melanomas that are expected to be biologically aggressive based on presentation and histopathologic features, the canine melanoma vaccine may be used after local control of the tumor is achieved, although peer-reviewed studies documenting its efficacy in this location are lacking.

Iridociliary adenoma is the second most common primary intraocular tumor in the dog (Figure 257-5). These tumors appear pink to pink-red and are seen as

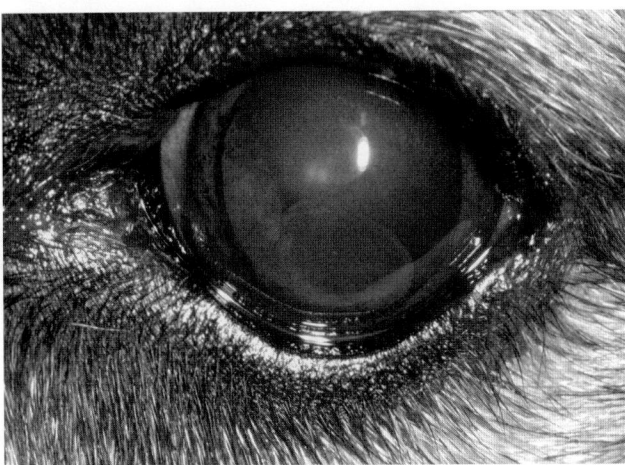

Figure 257-5 Ciliary body adenoma visible in the pupil of a mixed-breed dog. The mass has a significant cystic component and appears translucent at its most temporal aspect.

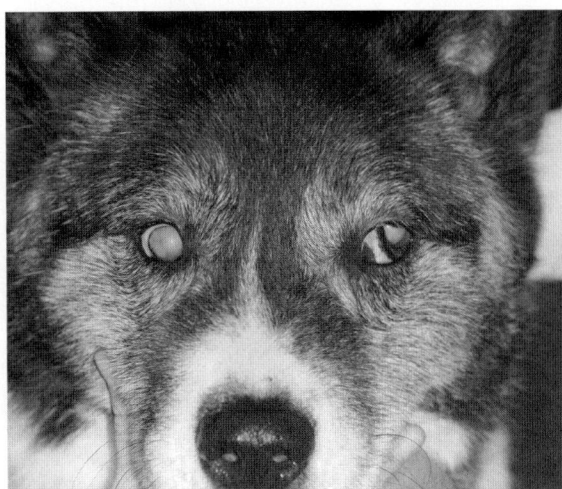

Figure 257-6 Enophthalmos, strabismus, and elevation of the nictitating membrane in a dog with an orbital mass.

well-circumscribed masses through the pupil and behind the iris. They arise from the ciliary body but may also involve the iris. Occasionally, iridociliary adenomas may appear pigmented, which makes them difficult to differentiate from an intraocular melanocytic neoplasm. In the early stages, iridociliary tumors are not associated with intraocular inflammation. As they increase in size, secondary intraocular disease such as uveitis, secondary glaucoma, hyphema, and retinal detachment are common. These secondary complications are the most likely reasons for enucleation. Surgical resection can be attempted and is most likely to be successful early in the disease process. Transscleral laser ablation may be effective in shrinking or slowing the growth of iridociliary neoplasms. Referral to an ophthalmologist is recommended for these surgical interventions. Iridociliary adenocarcinomas are less common and rarely metastasize. It is difficult to differentiate an iridociliary adenoma from an adenocarcinoma based on clinical presentation.

Spindle cell tumor of blue-eyed dogs is a mesenchymal neoplasm found in dogs with a blue or heterochromic iris. The tumor appears as an expansile mass within the iris leaflet and can extend into the ciliary body. Melanocytoma, melanoma, iridociliary epithelial neoplasia, and metastatic neoplasia are differential diagnoses for tumors with this clinical appearance. Enucleation and histopathologic analysis are required for definitive diagnosis. The tumor is considered benign, and metastasis is very rarely reported. Immunohistochemically, the tumor appears similar to a schwannoma; however, the cell type of origin has not been elucidated. Because it is difficult to distinguish this tumor clinically from metastatic neoplasia, enucleation is indicated.

Retina, Optic Nerve, and Orbit

The retina is an extremely uncommon site of primary neoplasia. *Gliomas*, which are further subcategorized into astrocytomas, oligodendrogliomas, ependymomas, and oligoastrocytomas, are the only reported primary retinal neoplasms. The optic nerve frequently is involved.

Clinically the tumor appears as a pink or pink-white mass protruding into the vitreous cavity from the optic nerve or retina, and often it is associated with vision loss and mydriasis. Intraocular hemorrhage frequently is seen with these tumors, which makes intraocular visualization difficult. Ocular ultrasonography is invaluable in these cases. Although such tumors rarely metastasize, local extension from the optic nerve toward the brain is common. When such extension is present, the prognosis is significantly poorer. Radiation therapy is likely to be an effective adjunctive treatment for a glioma patient after enucleation with incomplete excision, although the efficacy of this modality for tumors in this location is not well documented in the literature. *Medulloepitheliomas*, although uncommon in the dog, can present as pink masses in the anterior chamber or can arise from the retina. These tumors are congenital and originate from neuroectodermal tissue. Enucleation is recommended.

Meningioma is the most common tumor of the canine optic nerve. Meningiomas are divided into two categories: intraocular and retrobulbar-orbital. The intraocular form has a clinical appearance similar to that of gliomas and typically is visible on fundic examination. Exophthalmos, mydriasis, and vision loss are more common with the orbital form of meningioma. This tumor can arise from the central nervous system (CNS) with secondary extension along the optic nerve or may originate from the retrobulbar optic nerve sheath and extend both into the globe and toward the CNS. Surgical resection may be curative; however, local recurrence with extension into the CNS is common, although metastasis is rare. Radiation is likely to be an effective adjunctive therapy.

Although primary orbital neoplasia has a low frequency in the canine population, it is one of the most common diseases of the canine orbit (Figure 257-6). All orbital tissues may give rise to neoplasia. Reported tumors include osteosarcoma, fibrosarcoma, squamous cell carcinoma, chondrosarcoma, and meningioma. Advanced imaging, including MRI and CT, is important for assessing local disease in these patients and aids in surgical planning. Exenteration most often is the treatment of choice;

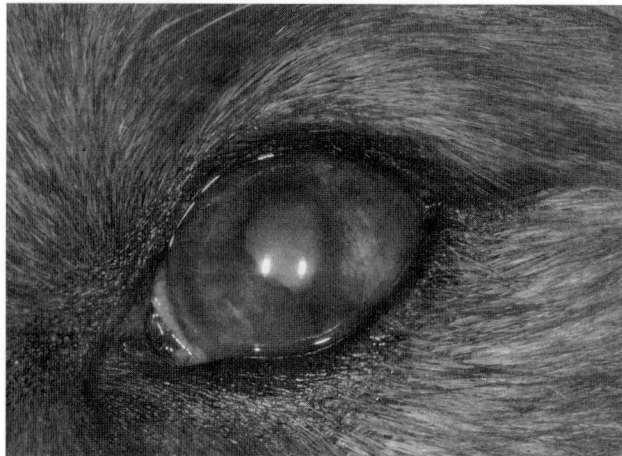

Figure 257-7 Iris bombé, dyscoria, and diffuse infiltration in the iris of an older golden retriever with multicentric lymphoma.

however, achieving complete excision of the tumor can be challenging in some cases. Follow-up radiation usually is indicated to ensure adequate local control.

Secondary Ocular Neoplasia

Secondary canine neoplasms more commonly involve the intraocular structures than the ocular surface. Although any neoplasm can metastasize to the eye and periocular tissues, certain tumor types are overrepresented. Lymphoma is the most common secondary ocular neoplasm (Figure 257-7). Sudden onset of blindness or hyphema may be the first clinical sign noted in a dog with lymphoma. Involvement of the highly vascular uveal tract often is associated with uveitis. Gross masses within the iris may be present concurrently with uveitis.

In addition to systemic chemotherapy for lymphoma, topical antiinflammatory therapy is warranted whenever uveitis is present. Topical ophthalmic steroid preparations such as prednisolone acetate 1% suspension should be administered every 4 to 8 hours until signs of uveitis are controlled. Topical ophthalmic atropine 1% solution may be useful in managing the pain associated with ciliary body muscle spasm that accompanies uveitis as well as preventing posterior synechia. Secondary glaucoma is an occasional complication and unfortunately is difficult to treat in isolation; achieving a systemic remission often manages the ocular component of disease. In some cases secondary glaucoma may be controlled with the judicious use of topical carbonic anhydrase inhibitor/β-blocker combinations. Topical prostaglandin analog therapy should be avoided if possible in cases of secondary

glaucoma associated with uveitis because of the potential for formation of posterior synechiae and exacerbation of the uveitis. A complete ophthalmic examination should be a regular component of reevaluation in a patient with lymphoma because ocular signs may be the first evidence that the disease is coming out of remission.

Ocular lesions also may be observed in dogs with multiple myeloma. Retinal hemorrhages, increased retinal vascular caliber and vascular tortuosity, retinal detachment, anterior uveitis, iridal hemorrhages, and secondary glaucoma may be evident. Hyperviscosity syndrome likely plays a role in the etiopathogenesis of these clinical signs. Prognosis for vision can be good with systemic therapy if remission is achieved.

Tumor extension from the oral, nasal, or sinus cavity into the retrobulbar space can cause exophthalmos, increased resistance to retropulsion of the globe, and ocular or nasal discharges. Squamous cell carcinoma is most commonly implicated, although primary nasal adenocarcinoma also commonly causes retrobulbar or orbital disease. Advanced imaging can confirm the suspected secondary involvement and help define the primary tumor.

Any hematogenously disseminating tumor can produce metastasis within the globe or orbit; however, with the exception of lymphoma, ocular involvement is not a common feature of any single neoplasm.

References and Suggested Reading

Boroffka SA et al: Assessment of ultrasonography and computed tomography for the evaluation of unilateral orbital disease in dogs, *J Am Vet Med Assoc* 230:671, 2007.

Dreyfus J, Schobert CS, Dubielzig RR: Superficial corneal squamous cell carcinoma occurring in dogs with chronic keratitis, *Vet Ophthalmol* 14:161, 2011.

Fife M et al: Canine conjunctival mast cell tumors: a retrospective study, *Vet Ophthalmol* 14:153, 2011.

Giuliano EA et al: A matched observational study of canine survival with primary intraocular melanocytic neoplasia, *Vet Ophthalmol* 2:185, 1999.

Kern TJ: Orbital neoplasia in 23 dogs, *J Am Vet Med Assoc* 186:489, 1985.

Krohne SG et al: Prevalence of ocular involvement in dogs with multicentric lymphoma: prospective evaluation of 94 cases, *Vet Comp Ophthalmol* 4:127, 1994.

Naranjo C, Schobert C, Dubielzig R: Canine ocular gliomas: a retrospective study, *Vet Ophthalmol* 11:356, 2008.

Pirie CG et al: Canine conjunctival hemangioma and hemangiosarcoma: a retrospective evaluation of 108 cases (1989-2004), *Vet Ophthalmol* 9:215, 2006.

Roberts SM, Severin GA, Lavach JD: Prevalence and treatment of palpebral neoplasms in the dog: 200 cases (1975-1983), *J Am Vet Med Assoc* 189:1355, 1986.

Zarfoss MK et al: Uveal spindle cell tumor of blue-eyed dogs: an immunohistochemical study, *Vet Pathol* 44:276, 2007.

CHAPTER 258

Feline Ocular Neoplasia

SANDRA M. NGUYEN, *Sydney, Australia*
AMBER LABELLE, *Urbana-Champaign, Illinois*

Ocular neoplasia is less common in the cat than in the dog, but the proportion of primary tumors that are malignant is much higher. For appropriate therapeutic intervention, it is important to distinguish primary tumors from secondary neoplasms. Staging of disease also is important, and the concepts applicable to the cat are discussed in the chapter on canine ocular neoplasia (see Chapter 257) in this section. Treatment of many ocular neoplasms is surgical, and complications of surgery, including scarring, can lead to a number of problems of the globe or adnexa. Thus optimal surgical outcomes are most likely when the procedure is performed by a specialist in ophthalmic surgery. Additionally, other treatments may involve advanced oncologic therapies that can be obtained only by referral.

Primary Ocular Neoplasia

Adnexa

Feline eyelid neoplasms are less common and more likely to be malignant than similar neoplasms in dogs. Virtually any epidermal or dermal tumor may affect the eyelid. The most commonly reported neoplasm is squamous cell carcinoma. Other tumors include fibrosarcoma, adenocarcinoma or adenoma, mast cell tumor, basal cell tumor, fibroma, papilloma, hemangiosarcoma, and melanoma. Large eyelid tumors require extensive reconstructive surgery after resection, which may deter owners from pursuing treatment. Because malignant eyelid tumors can result in death or euthanasia of the cat, it is best to examine and treat these tumors early in the course of disease.

Squamous cell carcinomas may appear as ulcerated or proliferative, pink, cobblestone masses. They are more common in older cats with lightly pigmented (pink) eyelid margins. Exposure to ultraviolet light is a significant risk factor for the development of squamous cell carcinoma. Squamous cell carcinoma is locally invasive and tends to metastasize late in the course of disease. The treatment of choice is complete surgical excision, although this may be challenging with large or multifocal lesions. Adjunctive therapies, including beta irradiation (using a strontium 90 probe) or cryotherapy can successfully induce remission in some patients with small tumors. If complete surgical excision is unattainable and adjunctive therapies are not available, enucleation or exenteration may be necessary. Piroxicam 0.3 mg/kg q48h PO is an empirical treatment for some cats with squamous cell carcinoma, but the patient must be closely monitored for nephrotoxicity and gastrointestinal ulceration as well as for efficacy.

Feline periocular peripheral *nerve sheath tumor* appears clinically as a firm intradermal mass with little to no alopecia or surface ulceration. Surgical resection with wide margins is recommended, and reconstructive surgery may be required to maintain eyelid function. Enucleation, with creation of rotational flaps to cover the orbital wound, may be necessary to prevent recurrence.

Apocrine gland hidrocystomas are an unusual type of benign neoplasia seen most commonly in aged brachycephalic cats. The clinical appearance is that of multiple 2- to 8-mm smooth, round, darkly pigmented masses that contain a brown serous fluid. Although the masses are benign, their rupture may be associated with ocular discomfort. Surgical excision alone is associated with recurrence. Topical application of trichloroacetic acid and cryoablation have been reported to be more effective therapies in preventing reappearance.

Neoplasia uncommonly affects the feline *nictitans.* Clinical signs include elevation of the nictitans, mass effect with deviation of the globe, conjunctivitis, and enophthalmos or exophthalmos. The most commonly reported tumor is squamous cell carcinoma, which may be a local extension from an eyelid or palpebral conjunctival lesion. Other reported tumors include adenocarcinoma, mast cell tumor, hemangiosarcoma, fibrosarcoma, lymphoma, and melanoma. Care must be taken to differentiate prolapse of the gland of the nictitans (also called *cherry eye*), a relatively uncommon condition in cats except for the Burmese and Bombay breeds, from neoplasia of the nictitans. Surgical excision is indicated for most neoplasms, with exenteration necessary when adequate surgical margins cannot be achieved with the globe *in situ.*

Cornea and Conjunctiva

Primary corneal neoplasia is uncommon in the cat. The limbus is the most frequently affected region of the cornea. Limbal or epibulbar melanoma is the most commonly recognized tumor of the feline limbus. *Limbal melanomas* arise from the pigmented melanocytes of the limbus and sclera. The clinical appearance is that of a black, smooth, well-circumscribed mass that may be observed to invade the cornea and sclera. Gonioscopy is useful to detect extension into the iridocorneal angle, and high-resolution (35- to 50-MHz) ultrasonography may be necessary to determine the extent of intraocular involvement. Because limbal melanomas in cats generally are benign and nonpainful, monitoring alone is indicated in most cases. If progression is noted, treatment options include surgical debulking and adjunctive treatment of the tumor bed (diode laser ablation, cryoablation, beta irradiation) or full-thickness surgical excision with grafting to restore scleral integrity. Digital photographs and detailed measurements are useful for detecting subtle changes in size and shape. Although distant metastasis of limbal melanoma has been reported, it is rare.

Other *primary corneal tumors* include squamous cell carcinoma, hemangiosarcoma, fibrous histiocytoma, and lymphoma. All would be expected to arise at the limbus and usually involve corneal neovascularization. Careful clinical examination and diagnostic cytologic examination or biopsy are required to differentiate these uncommon corneal neoplasms from the more common feline corneal diseases of eosinophilic keratitis or feline herpesvirus 1–associated keratoconjunctivitis. Keratectomy with adjunctive radiation therapy or cryotherapy is indicated for these primary corneal neoplasms.

Unlike limbal melanomas, *conjunctival melanomas* are more likely to be malignant and are associated with a higher rate of metastasis. Golden to brown granular pigmentation of the temporal bulbar conjunctiva, palpebral conjunctiva, and eyelid margin is a common ocular finding in cats with an orange coat and must not be confused with a conjunctival melanoma. Conjunctival melanomas typically are dark brown or black and raised. The palpebral, bulbar, or nictitans conjunctiva may be affected. Although excision and adjunctive treatment, including irradiation or cryoablation, may be effective in treating local disease, widespread metastasis still may result within weeks to months. Local recurrence may follow simple excision.

Primary *conjunctival hemangiomas* and *hemangiosarcomas* are diagnosed rarely. Their biologic behavior is locally aggressive with rare metastasis. Complete excision is recommended. A single report of B-cell lymphoma with the clinical manifestation of palpebral conjunctival masses suggests that the conjunctiva may be primarily involved in rare cases of lymphoma.

Uvea

Feline diffuse iris melanoma (FDIM) is a clinical syndrome that encompasses a spectrum of iris lesions. A nevus is a focal, flat, benign, pigmented iris lesion that remains unchanged over the course of a patient's life and is unassociated with other intraocular disease (Figure 258-1). FDIM must be differentiated from an iris nevus as well as from diffuse iris hyperpigmentation resulting from chronic uveitis. An FDIM lesion can be distinguished from a nevus by its typically darker pigmentation (dark brown to black), raised surface with loss of normal iris architecture, and "velvety" appearance (Figures 258-2 and 258-3). The tumors are more likely to be associated with secondary uveal or pupillary changes, pigment dispersion into the aqueous humor, and secondary glaucoma. Magnification is helpful when scrutinizing the iris surface and differentiating a benign nevus from lesions of FDIM. Frequently the diagnosis is not straightforward, and referral to an ophthalmologist may be helpful. Gonioscopy may

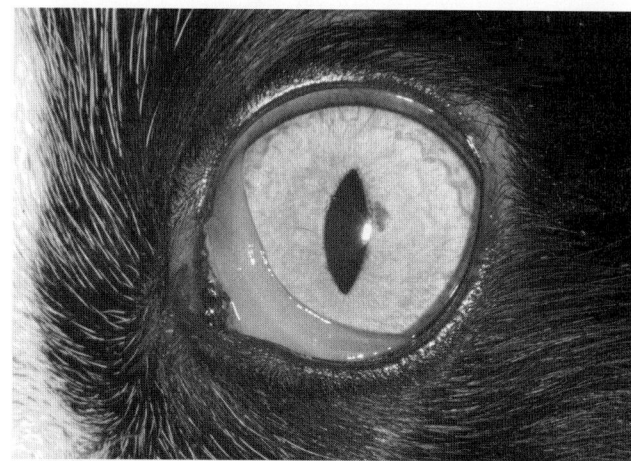

Figure 258-1 Benign iris nevus located temporal to the pupillary margin in a young domestic shorthair cat.

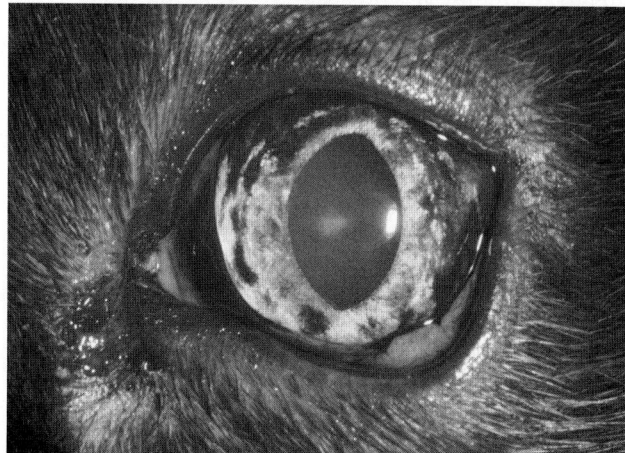

Figure 258-2 Darkly pigmented multifocal iris lesions consistent with feline diffuse iris melanoma.

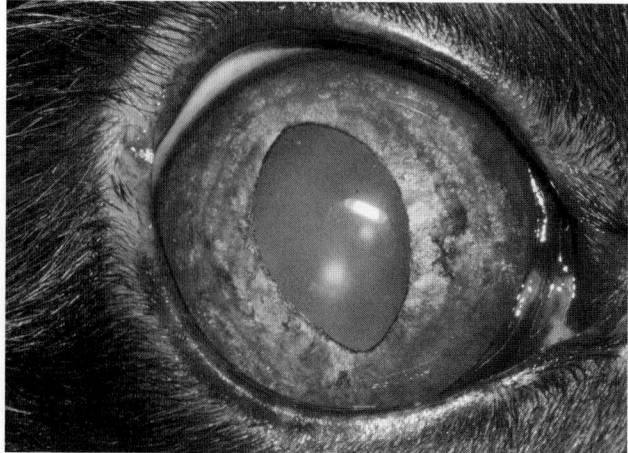

Figure 258-3 Diffuse iris thickening with loss of normal architecture and velvety pigmentation of the iris consistent with feline diffuse iris melanoma.

be useful to examine the iridocorneal angle for the presence of pigment. Determining when a pigmented iridal lesion has undergone malignant transformation to a neoplasm is a major clinical challenge. A focal pigmented lesion associated with some dyscoria but no significant uveitis or secondary glaucoma presents a significant dilemma to the clinician.

Once clinical changes suggestive of malignancy (dyscoria, uveitis, pigment dispersion, or glaucoma) are documented, complete staging (based on results of local lymph node aspiration, thoracic radiography, and abdominal ultrasonography) followed by enucleation is recommended. Alternatives to enucleation include laser (neodymium:yttrium-aluminum-garnet [Nd:YAG] or diode) ablation of iridal lesions and, rarely, surgical excision of FDIM, but to date there is little documentation on the long-term benefit of these treatments. Although enucleation does provide tissue for histopathologic interpretation, iris biopsy has not proven useful clinically for making treatment decisions. Histopathologic features such as iris stromal invasion and a high mitotic rate may be poor prognostic indicators. When metastasis occurs, regional lymph nodes, lung, liver, and spleen are affected most frequently. Uveal melanomas in cats rarely may arise in the choroid. These lesions carry a poorer prognosis because their posterior location means detection occurs relatively late in the disease process. Early enucleation, particularly when performed before the development of secondary glaucoma, is the best-known treatment strategy for survival.

Feline posttraumatic sarcoma (FPTS) is a poorly understood neoplasm unique to the cat. Trauma to the eye is hypothesized to result in liberation of lens epithelium from the lens capsule. The cells subsequently undergo neoplastic transformation and give rise to several types of neoplasms, including fibrosarcoma, anaplastic sarcoma, osteosarcoma, and a round cell variant of FPTS. The time between trauma and onset of clinically apparent neoplasia is widely variable, ranging from months to years. Any patient with traumatic lens capsule rupture, penetrating corneal trauma, chronic lens-induced uveitis, or a penetrating scleral wound should be considered at risk for future development of FPTS. The neoplasm typically lines the globe and may cause its expansion, which may be particularly noticeable to owners in cases in which the globe has undergone phthisis bulbi (decrease in globe size associated with chronic inflammation) and subsequently begins to expand to "normal" size. The tumor will extend up the optic nerve and can invade the brain, so that early detection and enucleation are critical for a successful outcome. Enucleation of blind chronically inflamed or previously traumatized feline eyes should be considered to prevent the development of FPTS.

Tumors of the feline ciliary body include *iridociliary adenoma* and *iridociliary adenocarcinoma*. The tumor appears clinically as a pink or white mass protruding from the region of the ciliary body and often is visible within the pupil. The tumor may be pigmented in rare cases. Dyscoria may result from impingement of large masses on the pupillary margin. If the mass is associated with uveitis or secondary glaucoma, enucleation is recommended. Small lesions may be surgically resectable. Metastasis is reported infrequently.

Optic Nerve and Orbit

Primary neoplasia of the feline optic nerve is uncommon; however, orbital neoplasms may involve the optic nerve secondarily. Clinical signs of orbital disease in cats include exophthalmos, decreased eye movements, increased resistance to retropulsion, strabismus, pain on opening of the mouth, elevation of the nictitans, enophthalmos, ocular discharge, conjunctival hyperemia, mydriasis, and blindness. Reported primary orbital tumors include fibrosarcoma, hemangioma, carcinoma, plasmacytoma, retrobulbar teratoma, meningioma, melanoma, and osteosarcoma. Careful clinical examination and advanced imaging, including computed tomography or magnetic resonance imaging, with ultrasonically guided fine-needle aspiration or biopsy is indicated.

Feline *restrictive orbital myofibroblastic sarcoma* is a newly recognized feline orbital neoplasm. It is most often bilateral with infiltration of the orbital and periocular connective tissue. Clinical signs include inability to blink, restriction of globe movement, and exposure keratitis. Involvement of the oral cavity (gingivitis and gingival infiltration) is common. Middle-aged cats are affected most often. Attempts at treatment, including oral immunosuppressive therapy, local antiinflammatory therapy, and radiation therapy, generally have been unsuccessful. Enucleation may be palliative in some cases but has not been demonstrated to prevent involvement of the fellow eye.

Secondary Ocular Neoplasia

The uveal tract is the most common site of metastatic neoplasia (Figure 258-4). Its vascular nature makes the uvea a logical site for hematogenous metastasis. *Lymphoma* is the most frequently recognized feline uveal tumor to involve the eye. Lymphoma may appear as a discrete mass in the iris or may be associated with

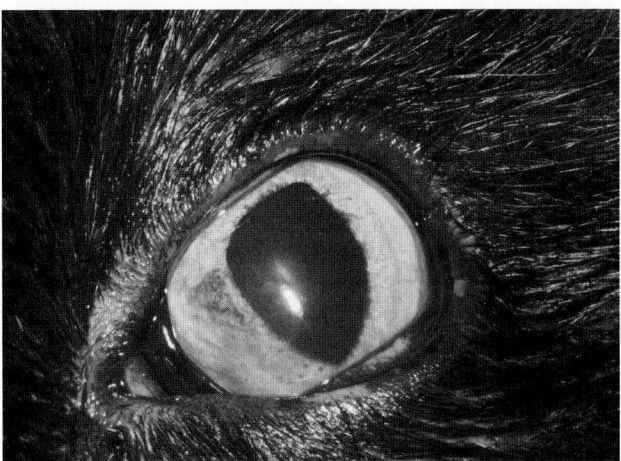

Figure 258-4 Focal mass in the nasal iris associated with uveitis, rubeosis iridis, keratic precipitates, and dyscoria in a domestic shorthair cat with a metastatic intraocular carcinoma.

generalized uveitis, iritis, rubeosis iridis, miosis, aqueous flare, keratic precipitates, and secondary glaucoma. Choroidal lesions may include intraretinal hemorrhage, retinal detachment, and subretinal masses. Uveitis may be the first clinical sign of lymphoma, which underscores the importance of performing a complete physical examination and systemic workup in all feline patients with uveitis. Aqueous paracentesis may be useful for collecting neoplastic cells to make a definitive diagnosis when sampling of other organs is not feasible. Topical steroids (dexamethasone 0.1% or prednisolone acetate 1% solution q6-12h) are most effective in controlling inflammation. Adding a topical nonsteroidal antiinflammatory drug (flurbiprofen 0.03% or diclofenac 0.1% solution) may increase the antiinflammatory effect in severe cases. Topical atropine 1% solution q12-24h can alleviate painful ciliary body muscle spasm and decrease the formation of posterior synechiae by causing mydriasis. Systemic chemotherapy in conjunction with local treatment of uveitis is most effective in treating the ocular manifestations of lymphoma.

Primary *bronchogenic carcinoma* is associated with a syndrome of angioinvasive pulmonary carcinoma in which tumor cells invade and cause infarction in the choroidal vasculature, which results in ischemic chorioretinopathy. The clinical manifestations include vision loss, wedge-shaped black or tan lesions of the tapetal fundus associated with tapetal necrosis, multifocal serous retinal exudate, and retinal vascular attenuation. Patients are invariably blind and may be affected unilaterally or bilaterally. The distal extremities of these patients similarly are affected by infarcted lesions. Successful treatment has not been reported.

The feline orbit is affected more commonly by secondary neoplasms than by primary neoplasms. Extension of neoplasia from nearby anatomic structures such as the oral and nasal cavity often is implicated in orbital disease, including squamous cell carcinoma, adenocarcinoma,

and lymphoma. The conjunctiva and third eyelid also may become involved in a secondary orbital neoplasm. Advanced imaging such as computerized tomography is invaluable in cases of orbital neoplasia for distinguishing a primary from a secondary lesion; this permits image-guided aspiration or biopsy and more accurate assessment of prognosis. Unfortunately, visual and comfortable globes may need to be sacrificed via exenteration when orbital access is essential for treatment. In some cases of nasal lymphoma, radiation therapy or chemotherapy may be globe sparing.

References and Suggested Reading

Bell CM, Schwarz T, Dubielzig RR: Diagnostic features of feline restrictive orbital myofibroblastic sarcoma, *Vet Pathol* 48:742, 2011.

Cantaloube B, Raymond-Letron I, Regnier A: Multiple eyelid apocrine hidrocystomas in two Persian cats, *Vet Ophthalmol* 7:121, 2004.

Cassotis NJ et al: Angioinvasive pulmonary carcinoma with posterior segment metastasis in four cats, *Vet Ophthalmol* 2:125, 1999.

Gilger BC et al: Orbital neoplasms in cats: 21 cases (1974-1990), *J Am Vet Med Assoc* 201:1083, 1992.

Hoffman A et al: Feline periocular peripheral nerve sheath tumor: a case series, *Vet Ophthalmol* 8:153, 2005.

Holt E et al: Extranodal conjunctival Hodgkin's-like lymphoma in a cat, *Vet Ophthalmol* 9:141, 2006.

Newkirk KM, Rohrbach BW: A retrospective study of eyelid tumors from 43 cats, *Vet Pathol* 46:916, 2009.

Pirie CG, Dubielzig RR: Feline conjunctival hemangioma and hemangiosarcoma: a retrospective evaluation of eight cases (1993-2004), *Vet Ophthalmol* 9:227, 2006.

Schobert CS, Labelle P, Dubielzig RR: Feline conjunctival melanoma: histopathological characteristics and clinical outcomes, *Vet Ophthalmol* 13:43, 2010.

Zeiss CJ, Johnson EM, Dubielzig RR: Feline intraocular tumors may arise from transformation of lens epithelium, *Vet Pathol* 40:355, 2003.

Chapter 259:	Infectious Agent Differentials for Medical Problems	1212
Chapter 260:	Rational Empiric Antimicrobial Therapy	1219
Chapter 261:	Infectious Causes of Polyarthritis in Dogs	1224
Chapter 262:	Immunotherapy for Infectious Diseases	1229
Chapter 263:	Systemic Antifungal Therapy	1234
Chapter 264:	Infectious Diseases Associated with Raw Meat Diets	1239
Chapter 265:	Pet-Associated Illness	1244
Chapter 266:	Vaccine-Associated Adverse Effects in Dogs	1249
Chapter 267:	Update on Vaccine-Associated Adverse Effects in Cats	1252
Chapter 268:	Treatment of Canine Babesiosis	1257
Chapter 269:	Canine Bartonellosis	1261
Chapter 270:	Feline Bartonellosis	1267
Chapter 271:	Borreliosis	1271
Chapter 272:	Management of Feline Retrovirus-Infected Cats	1275
Chapter 273:	*Hepatozoon americanum* Infections	1283
Chapter 274:	Leptospirosis	1286
Chapter 275:	*Neospora caninum*	1290
Chapter 276:	Canine and Feline Monocytotropic Ehrlichiosis	1292
Chapter 277:	Toxoplasmosis	1295
Chapter 278:	Rational Use of Glucocorticoids in Infectious Disease	1299
Chapter 279:	Feline Infectious Peritonitis Virus Infections	1303

The following web chapters can be found on the companion website at www.currentveterinarytherapy.com

Web Chapter 81:	American Leishmaniasis
Web Chapter 82:	Canine and Feline Hemotropic Mycoplasmosis
Web Chapter 83:	Canine Brucellosis
Web Chapter 84:	Feline Cytauxzoonosis
Web Chapter 85:	Pneumocystosis
Web Chapter 86:	Pythiosis and Lagenidiosis

CHAPTER 259

Infectious Agent Differentials for Medical Problems

MICHAEL R. LAPPIN, *Fort Collins, Colorado*

For most clinical problems or syndromes recognized in small animal practice, there are several infectious agents that may be the cause. Bacterial, fungal, parasitic, rickettsial, and viral agents frequently are encountered in small animal practice. Common infectious agents and the clinical problems with which they are associated are summarized in Tables 259-1 to 259-4. Recognizing the infectious agents that are most commonly associated with medical problems or syndromes allows the veterinary clinician first to rank the list of differential diagnoses using the signalment, history, and clinical examination findings. Diagnostic assays to aid in the diagnosis of small animal infectious diseases are plentiful and relatively inexpensive. However, starting with a syndromic approach allows the differential list to be narrowed and subsequently aids in selection of the optimal diagnostic assays for further evaluation of the case or choice of the most logical empiric therapeutic trials. In this chapter, the bacterial, fungal, parasitic, rickettsial, and viral agents associated with common medical problems are discussed briefly.

Common Medical Problems

Azotemia

A number of infectious agents are associated with renal azotemia. Pyelonephritis caused by aerobic bacteria is thought to be the most common. Acute pyelonephritis resulting in azotemia often is accompanied by signs of fever and renal discomfort on physical examination. However, chronic pyelonephritis can have an insidious onset, and clinical findings are less clear. Most, but not all, patients with clinical illness associated with pyelonephritis have systemic manifestations of disease that would trigger the clinician to perform a complete blood cell count, serum biochemical studies, and urinalysis. All dogs and cats with azotemia, with or without pyuria or bacteriuria on urinalysis, should be assumed to have pyelonephritis; aerobic urine culture and antimicrobial susceptibility testing should be performed, and the patient should be treated accordingly while culture results are awaited (Weese et al, 2011). It is now recognized that *Leptospira* spp. infections are present throughout the United States and many other countries, and so serologic testing for the organism with or without polymerase chain reaction (PCR) testing of urine is indicated for all dogs with renal azotemia (Sykes et al, 2011). In areas endemic for *Borrelia burgdorferi* (northeastern United States, upper midwestern United States, and some areas

of northern California), renal azotemia can develop secondary to Lyme nephropathy. Appropriate diagnostic assays and treatments for *B. burgdorferi* are indicated in these cases (Littman et al, 2006). Infectious agents associated with induction of vasculitis also can cause azotemia; acute *Ehrlichia canis* and *Rickettsia rickettsii* infections are notable examples that should be considered on the differential list for dogs with an appropriate history and other characteristic clinical or laboratory findings.

Ataxia, Seizures, and Other Central Nervous System Signs

Canine distemper virus infection still is one of the most common causes of central nervous system (CNS) disease in young, inadequately vaccinated dogs. Chronic CNS disease also can occur in some dogs. Most dogs with CNS distemper had previous signs of gastrointestinal or respiratory disease. Chorioretinitis or chorea myoclonus may be noted on physical examination. Rabies is the other significant viral cause of CNS disease and always should be considered in dogs and cats with CNS disease, particularly if the vaccination history is poor or unknown. Both aerobic and anaerobic bacteria have been documented as causes of CNS infections. Infectious agents associated with induction of vasculitis, including *Bartonella* spp., *E. canis*, and *R. rickettsii*, can cause diffuse meningoencephalitis and should be on the differential list for dogs with appropriate clinical histories. The systemic fungal agents *Blastomyces dermatitidis*, *Coccidioides immitis*, *Cryptococcus* spp., and *Histoplasma capsulatum* should be considered as causes of CNS infections in dogs or cats in endemic areas. *Toxoplasma gondii* infection is a differential diagnosis in kittens or puppies that may have been infected transplacentally, those that are immunocompromised, and those that could be exposed to the organism in prey species or uncooked meat. *Neospora caninum* neuromuscular infections generally develop in puppies after transplacental transmission and are characterized by ascending paralysis. Puppies with neosporosis more commonly are rural dogs, and there is often a history of similar problems in previous litters because repeated transplacental transmission can occur.

Cardiac Murmur or Arrhythmias

Valvular murmurs related to infectious agents often are accompanied by fever and other multisystemic signs of disease. Agents commonly isolated from the blood of

TABLE 259-1

Common Bacterial Agents Infecting Small Animals and Associated Primary Clinical Findings

Agent	Common Problems and Syndromes
Anaerobes (including *Actinomyces* and *Nocardia*)	Abscesses, stomatitis, rarely pneumonia
Bacterial endocarditis (multiple bacteria)	Fever, cardiac murmur
Bartonella henselae	Fever, uveitis, hyperglobulinemia, lymphadenopathy, myocarditis, endocarditis
Bartonella vinsonii subsp. *berkhoffii* (dogs)	Fever, epistaxis (vasculitis), endocarditis, thrombocytopenia, hemolytic anemia, polyarthritis, pyogranulomatous inflammation
Borrelia burgdorferi (dogs)	Lameness (polyarthritis), proteinuria with azotemia
Bordetella bronchiseptica	Sneezing or coughing
Brucella canis (dogs)	Reproductive failure, orchitis, uveitis, hyperglobulinemia; zoonotic
Campylobacter spp.	Mixed bowel diarrhea with or without vomiting
Chlamydia felis (cats)	Conjunctivitis; potentially sneezing and nasal discharge
Clostridium perfringens	Large bowel diarrhea, polycythemia, occasionally vomiting
Discospondylitis (multiple bacteria)	Fever, lameness, pain at the site of infection
Helicobacter spp.	Vomiting, nausea, weight loss, no diarrhea
Leptospira spp.	Fever, vomiting (nephritis, hepatitis), thrombocytopenia
Mycoplasma spp.	Sneezing or coughing (upper respiratory tract disease in cats and canine infectious respiratory disease complex in dogs), lameness (polyarthritis), reproductive failure
Mycoplasma haemominutum (cats)	Pale mucous membranes from hemolytic anemia
Mycoplasma haemofelis (cats)	Pale mucous membranes from hemolytic anemia
Mycoplasma turicensis (cats)	Pale mucous membranes from hemolytic anemia
Mycoplasma haemocanis (dogs)	Subclinical infection except in immunosuppressed dogs and then pale mucous membranes from hemolytic anemia may occur
Mycoplasma hematoparvum (dogs)	Subclinical infections except in immunosuppressed dogs, which can develop pale mucous membranes from hemolytic anemia
Salmonella spp.	Mixed bowel diarrhea with or without vomiting
Streptococcus equi var. *zooepidemicus* (dogs)	Cough
Staphylococcus pseudintermedius	Pyoderma
Yersinia pestis	Fever, lymphadenopathy, rarely cough or dyspnea

bacteremic animals include aerobic and anaerobic bacteria: *Staphylococcus, Streptococcus, Enterococcus, Corynebacterium, Escherichia coli, Salmonella, Klebsiella, Enterobacter, Pseudomonas, Proteus, Pasteurella, Clostridium, Fusobacterium,* and *Bacteroides.* Many of these affected animals have an apparent primary site of infection, which commonly is the skin, urogenital system, or mouth, and the animal may have clinical findings related to those sites of infection. Recently, a number of *Bartonella* spp., including *Bartonella vinsonii* subsp. *berkhoffii* (dogs), *Bartonella henselae* (dogs and cats), *Bartonella koehlerae* (dogs and cats), and *Bartonella quintana* (dogs and cats), have been found to be associated with bacterial endocarditis (Breitschwerdt et al, 2010). *Bartonella* spp. infection should be on the differential list for dogs or cats with suspected valvular endocarditis, particularly if there is a history of exposure to fleas or ticks. The diagnostic procedures and treatment regimens for *Bartonella* spp. are different from those for other bacteria causing valvular endocarditis, so it is important that these agents be identified (Breitschwerdt

et al, 2010) (see Chapters 269 and 270). Ventricular arrhythmias can be associated with infections caused by *Trypanosoma cruzi, T. gondii, N. caninum,* and the bacterial or rickettsial agents that induce vasculitis.

Diarrhea

Diarrhea is characterized by increased frequency of defecation, increased fluid content of the stool, or increased volume of stool. Markedly increased frequency of defecation, small-volume stools, tenesmus, urgency, hematochezia, and passage of mucus are consistent with large bowel diarrhea. Slight increase in the frequency of defecation, large-volume stools, melena, steatorrhea, and multisystemic clinical signs are more consistent with small bowel diarrhea. Mixed bowel diarrhea shows a combination of characteristics or clinical signs. Some dogs with gastrointestinal infections have vomiting concurrently with diarrhea or have vomiting alone. For example, infections involving *Helicobacter* spp. and some nematodes

TABLE 259-2

Common Fungal and Rickettsial Agents Infecting Small Animals and Associated Primary Clinical Findings

Agent	Common Problems and Syndromes
Fungal	
Aspergillus spp.	Sneezing, mucopurulent nasal discharge, epistaxis, multisystemic signs in German shepherd dogs
Blastomyces dermatitidis	Dyspnea, cough, weight loss, uveitis, multisystemic signs; rarely urogenital
Coccidioides immitis	Dyspnea, cough, lameness (osteomyelitis), multisystemic signs
Cryptococcus neoformans	Rhinitis, chorioretinitis, multisystemic signs
Histoplasma capsulatum	Large bowel diarrhea, weight loss, aplastic anemia in cats, dyspnea, multisystemic signs
Sporothrix schenckii	Draining tracts, zoonotic skin disease communicable to people
Rickettsial	
Anaplasma phagocytophilum	Fever, lameness (polyarthritis), thrombocytopenia
Anaplasma platys (dogs)	Fever, thrombocytopenia, uveitis
Coxiella burnetii	Stillbirth or abortion in cats; zoonotic respiratory disease communicable to people
Ehrlichia canis	Fever, nonregenerative anemia, thrombocytopenia, neutropenia, hyperglobulinemia, central nervous system inflammation
Ehrlichia ewingii (dogs)	Fever, lameness (polyarthritis), thrombocytopenia
Neorickettsia helminthoeca (dogs)	Mixed bowel diarrhea with or without vomiting
Neorickettsia risticii (dogs)	Fever, cytopenias in dogs
Rickettsia rickettsii	Fever, epistaxis (vasculitis), thrombocytopenia, multisystemic signs

TABLE 259-3

Common Parasitic Agents Infecting Small Animals and Associated Primary Clinical Findings

Agent	Type	Common Problems and Syndromes
Aelurostrongylus abstrusus (cats)	Lungworm	Coughing or dyspnea from bronchitis
Ancylostoma caninum (dogs)	Hookworm	Diarrhea with blood, pale mucous membranes
Ancylostoma tubaeforme (cats)	Hookworm	Diarrhea with blood, pale mucous membranes
Babesia vogeli (dogs)	Piroplasm	Pale mucous membranes and weakness from hemolytic anemia in dogs
Babesia gibsoni (dogs)	Piroplasm	Pale mucous membranes and weakness from hemolytic anemia in dogs
Babesia conradae (dogs)	Piroplasm	Pale mucous membranes and weakness from hemolytic anemia in dogs
Baylisascaris procyonis (dogs)	Roundworm	Subclinical in dogs; zoonotic
Cryptosporidium spp.	Coccidian	Small bowel diarrhea and weight loss
Cytauxzoon felis (cats)	Piroplasm	Pale mucous membranes and weakness from hemolytic anemia in cats
Dipylidium caninum	Cestode	Subclinical or unthrifty
Dirofilaria immitis	Heartworm	Coughing or dyspnea from bronchitis or emboli, proteinuria
Echinococcus granulosa (dogs)	Cestode	Subclinical or unthrifty; zoonotic
Echinococcus multilocularis	Cestode	Subclinical or unthrifty; zoonotic
Oslerus osleri (dogs)	Nematode	Coughing or dyspnea from worms in trachea
Giardia spp.	Flagellate	Small bowel diarrhea and weight loss
Hepatozoon americanum (dogs)	Coccidian	Lameness due to muscle inflammation and periosteal bone inflammation
Isospora spp.	Coccidian	Large bowel diarrhea or subclinical
Leishmania spp.	Flagellate	Skin disease, weight loss, multisystemic signs, Walker hounds
Ollulanus tricuspis (cats)	Nematode	Vomiting in cats
Neospora caninum (dogs)	Coccidian	Abortion, stillbirth, ascending neuromuscular disease

TABLE 259-3

Common Parasitic Agents Infecting Small Animals and Associated Primary Clinical Findings—cont'd

Agent	Type	Common Problems and Syndromes
Paragonimus kellicotti	Fluke	Cough
Physaloptera canis	Nematode	Vomiting
Pneumonyssoides caninum (dogs)	Mite	Serous nasal discharge and sneezing
Strongyloides stercoralis	Nematode	Mixed bowel diarrhea
Toxocara canis (dogs)	Roundworm	Vomiting, abdominal distention, failure to thrive
Toxocara cati (cats)	Roundworm	Vomiting, abdominal distention, failure to thrive
Toxascaris leonina	Roundworm	Vomiting, abdominal distention, failure to thrive
Trichuris vulpis (dogs)	Whipworm	Large bowel diarrhea, occasional vomiting
Taenia spp.	Cestode	Subclinical or unthrifty
Toxoplasma gondii	Coccidian	Fever, uveitis, lameness (muscle pain)
Tritrichomonas foetus	Flagellate	Large bowel diarrhea
Trypanosoma cruzi (dogs)	Flagellate	Ventricular arrhythmias, myocarditis

TABLE 259-4

Common Viral Agents Infecting Small Animals and Associated Primary Clinical Findings

Agent	Common Problems and Syndromes
Canine adenovirus 1	Vomiting, icterus, diarrhea (canine infectious hepatitis)
Canine adenovirus 2	Sneezing, nasal discharge, cough (part of CIRDC)
Canine coronavirus	Small bowel diarrhea in puppies
Canine distemper virus	Vomiting, diarrhea, sneezing, coughing, seizures, chorea, myoclonus, posterior uveitis
Canine herpesvirus	Vomiting, diarrhea, abdominal distention in fading puppies, possibly cough as part of CIRDC
Canine influenza virus	Cough, sneezing, nasal discharge (part of CIRDC)
Canine parvovirus	Vomiting, neutropenia, bloody diarrhea
Canine respiratory coronavirus	Cough, sneezing, nasal discharge (potentially part of CIRDC)
Feline calicivirus	Sneezing, stomatitis, vasculitis (virulent systemic strains)
Feline coronaviruses	Small bowel diarrhea, fever, uveitis, hyperglobulinemia, failure to thrive, central nervous system disease
Feline immunodeficiency virus	Fever, weight loss, multisystemic signs with involvement of most body systems
Feline herpesvirus 1	Sneezing, nasal discharge, keratitis, conjunctivitis, rarely stomatitis
Feline leukemia virus	Multisystemic signs due to immunodeficiency and secondary invaders, cytopenias, aplastic anemia, lymphoma
Feline panleukopenia virus	Vomiting, bloody diarrhea, neutropenia
Canine parainfluenza virus	Cough, sneezing, nasal discharge (part of CIRDC)
Rabies virus	Neurologic signs; zoonotic

CIRDC, Canine infectious respiratory disease complex.

(Physaloptera, Ollulanus, Toxocara spp.) commonly cause vomiting and no diarrhea. Bacterial, fungal, parasitic, rickettsial, and viral infections usually are associated with diarrhea and vomiting in dogs and cats around the world. The causative agents are summarized in Tables 259-1 through 259-4. The American College of Veterinary Internal Medicine consensus statement on enteropathogenic bacteria (Marks et al, 2011; www.acvim.org) and the Companion Animal Parasite Council (www.capcvet.org) are excellent sources of further information on many of the common enteric agents. Regurgitation related to infection usually is associated only with granulomas caused by Spirocerca lupi, which can develop in some parasitized dogs in endemic areas.

Dyspnea from Pleural Effusions

The most common causes of dyspnea from pleural effusions are effusive feline infectious peritonitis (FIP) and pyothorax. Effusions in cats with FIP are sterile, are colorless to straw colored, may contain fibrin strands, and may clot when exposed to air. Protein concentration on fluid analysis commonly ranges from 3.5 g/dl to 12 g/dl. Mixed inflammatory cell populations of lymphocytes, macrophages, and neutrophils occur most commonly; nondegenerate neutrophils predominate in most cases, but in some cats macrophages are the primary cell type observed. If the albumin:globulin ratio of the effusion is more than 0.8, FIP is unlikely. If the albumin:globulin ratio of the effusion is less than 0.4, FIP is the likely cause. Reverse transcriptase PCR testing can be used to amplify coronavirus RNA from effusions, and positive results support the diagnosis of FIP.

Cytologic examination of infection-related effusions from dogs or cats generally reveals signs of suppurative inflammation with degenerative and nondegenerative neutrophils. If bacteria are seen, mixed bacterial morphologic forms may be noted. The bacteria commonly isolated from pleural effusions of cats with pyothorax include *Fusobacterium*, *Prevotella*, *Porphyromonas*, *Bacteroides*, *Peptostreptococcus*, *Clostridium*, *Actinomyces*, and *Filifactor villosus*. *Pasteurella* spp., *Streptococcus* spp., and *Mycoplasma* spp. also have been isolated. *Staphylococcus* spp., gram-negative bacteria other than *Pasteurella*, and organisms such as *Nocardia* spp. and *Rhodococcus equi* have been isolated less frequently. Cats with pyothorax often have a history of cat fights or feline upper respiratory tract disease (URTD). Aerobic and anaerobic bacterial cultures of pleural effusions from dogs often reveal mixed anaerobes: *Prevotella* spp., *Peptostreptococcus* spp., *Propionibacterium acnes*, *Clostridium* spp., *Bacteroides* spp., *Fusobacterium* spp., and Enterobacteriaceae, especially *E. coli* and *Klebsiella pneumonia*. However, many other bacteria have been cultured, including *Streptococcus canis*, *Staphylococcus* spp., *Enterococcus* spp., *Corynebacterium* spp., *Bacillus* spp., *Arcanobacterium pyogenes*, *Pasteurella* spp., *Acinetobacter* spp., *Capnocytophaga* spp., *Enterobacter* spp., *Stenotrophomonas maltophilia*, *Aeromonas hydrophila*, *Achromobacter xylosoxidans*, *Serratia marcescens*, *Pseudomonas* spp., *Actinomyces* spp., *Nocardia* spp., and *Streptomyces* spp. (Boothe et al, 2010). Pyothorax in dogs commonly results from bite wound inoculation, migrating plant foreign bodies, or trauma.

Epistaxis

Dogs and cats with bleeding from the nares generally have local diseases of the nasal cavity or sinuses, coagulopathies, vasculitis, or hypertension. *Aspergillus* spp., *Cryptococcus* spp., *Penicillium* spp., and *Sporothrix schenckii* are the fungal agents most commonly associated with epistaxis from local disease. These animals usually have a history of a chronic progressive condition and have concurrent mucopurulent disease. The infectious agents associated with thrombocytopenia rarely induce thrombocytopenia of a magnitude great enough to produce spontaneous bleeding unless vasculitis is present concurrently.

Bartonella spp., *E. canis*, and *R. rickettsii* are the infectious agents most commonly associated with vasculitis that can induce epistaxis acutely and often without other discharges. The rhinitis caused by bacterial and viral agents generally is associated with mucopurulent nasal discharges, and blood is noted only rarely.

Gingivostomatitis

Secondary bacterial infections of the mouth are common when normal colonizing bacteria overgrow secondary to another primary cause of disease such as plaque or calculus formation. In cats, feline calicivirus is the viral agent that has been implicated most frequently in both acute and chronic cases of gingivostomatitis and was estimated to be the cause of approximately one half of the cases of caudal stomatitis in one study (Dowers et al, 2010). Feline herpesvirus 1 also may be associated with caudal stomatitis syndrome in some cats (approximately 10%). There is conflicting evidence in support of a relationship between *Bartonella* spp. exposure and gingivostomatitis in cats with the majority of published papers failing to find evidence of involvement, and the syndrome never has been reported in cats experimentally infected with *B. henselae* or *B. clarridgeiae*. Performing diagnostic tests for infectious agents did not aid in the diagnosis of gingivostomatitis in one study (Quimby et al, 2008).

Lameness

Infections associated with polyarthritis, osteomyelitis, discospondylitis, and polymyositis can cause an animal to be brought to the veterinarian for evaluation of lameness. The signalment, physical examination findings, and history can help rank the differential diagnoses. Many of the organisms causing infectious polyarthritis in dogs or cats are vector borne, and so the animal's location or travel history can be instrumental in formulation of a differential list (see Chapter 261). Classic examples are *Anaplasma phagocytophilum* and *B. burgdorferi* infections, which are found primarily in the Northeast, upper Midwest, and northern California in the United States because of the distribution of the tick vector (*Ixodes* spp.). *Bartonella* spp., *E. canis*, *Ehrlichia ewingii*, and *R. rickettsii* also are isolated more commonly in areas with heavy exposure to appropriate vectors (see Chapter 276).

The most common causes of infectious polymyositis in dogs are *T. gondii*, *N. caninum*, and *Hepatozoon canis*. *T. gondii* infection is most common in dogs or cats fed uncooked meat or allowed to hunt. Other multisystemic signs of disease such as fever, uveitis, and dyspnea due to pulmonary infections may be seen. Myositis associated with neosporosis usually occurs in puppies that live in a rural environment after transplacental infection from the dam. Repeated transplacental infection can occur from the same dam, so there may be historical evidence of the problem. Dogs also can become infected by ingesting infected bovine placentas. *Amblyomma maculatum* (the Gulf Coast tick) is the vector for *Hepatozoon americanum*, which explains the geographical distribution of infection with this parasite. Clinical manifestations of disease are most common in puppies. Reactive signs in the periosteum next to inflamed muscles are characteristic radiographic findings in *H. americanum* infection.

Osteomyelitis can be caused by any bacterium. Most infections are due to direct inoculation or hematogenous spread, and so there may be other physical examination or historical findings that suggest a cause. Infection with *Bartonella* spp. recently has been linked to osteomyelitis, and these animals frequently have a history of exposure to fleas or ticks. *Brucella canis* is one of the predominant bacterial causes of discospondylitis, and affected dogs may have a breeding history or came from crowded environments like pet stores or puppy mills. *Staphylococcus* spp. and *Streptococcus* spp. infections also are commonly associated with discospondylitis in dogs, and this may explain why many affected dogs respond to empiric cephalosporin antibiotic therapy. All of the systemic fungal agents have been associated with osteomyelitis, but infection with *C. immitis* in dogs residing in the southwestern United States is most common.

Pale Mucous Membranes

Pale mucous membranes result from decreased perfusion or anemia. Any chronic infectious disease can induce anemia of chronic disease. *E. canis* (dogs), *E. canis*–like organism (cats), and feline leukemia virus (FeLV) are the infectious agents most commonly associated with aplastic anemia. Occasionally, *H. capsulatum* will induce aplastic anemia in cats from bone marrow infection. Regenerative anemia due to blood loss can result from a number of infectious diseases, particularly hookworm infection of the gastrointestinal tract and infections leading to blood loss from vasculitis or thrombocytopenia (see earlier section on epistaxis). The tick-borne infectious agents most commonly associated with hemolytic anemia are *Babesia vogeli*, *Babesia gibsoni*, and *Babesia conradae* in dogs and *Cytauxzoon felis* in cats. Other clinical findings or risk factors can raise or lower the position of these agents on the differential list. For example, *B. vogeli* infections are common in greyhounds and other dogs exposed to *Rhipicephalus sanguineous*, *B. gibsoni* infections are common in American pit bull terriers and other dogs exposed to pit bulls, *B. conradae* infections are most common in California, and *C. felis* infections are most common in outdoor cats in areas with *Amblyomma americanum* ticks. Infection with *B. vinsonii* subsp. *berkhoffii* should be a differential diagnosis for hemolytic anemia in dogs exposed to fleas. However, *B. henselae* infection does not appear to cause hemolytic anemia in cats.

Pollakiuria

The majority of dogs with pollakiuria have bacterial urinary tract infections, whereas in cats with this clinical sign, the urine usually is sterile on bacterial culture. Approximately 75% of the bacterial urinary tract infections in dogs are caused by gram-negative organisms; *E. coli*, *Proteus*, *Klebsiella*, *Pseudomonas*, and *Enterobacter* infections are common. Similar organisms are cultured from dogs with prostatitis or prostatic abscesses. In cats that previously have been catheterized, *E. coli* is the most common cause of bacterial urinary tract infection;

Staphylococcus and *Streptococcus* organisms commonly are cultured after urethrostomy. *Mycoplasma* and *Ureaplasma* infections have been documented in small proportions of dogs with pollakiuria. Infection with fungal agents like *Blastomyces* (in dogs in endemic areas) or *Candida* (in animals previously treated with antibiotics) is associated with pollakiuria in rare cases. Guidelines are available to direct the use of antimicrobials in the treatment of urinary tract infections (Weese et al, 2011).

Sneezing or Coughing

There are multiple infectious causes of sneezing or coughing in dogs and cats. The most common viral causes of feline URTD are feline herpesvirus 1 and feline calicivirus. Feline herpesvirus 1 infection is most likely if ocular inflammation (conjunctivitis or keratitis) occurs concurrently with sneezing and nasal discharges. Feline calicivirus infection is most likely if stomatitis occurs concurrently. *Bordetella bronchiseptica* can be a primary pathogen in some cats and usually is associated only with respiratory disease (rhinitis, bronchitis, or pneumonia). *Chlamydia felis* is associated primarily with conjunctivitis in cattery cats. *Mycoplasma* spp. are normal commensal organisms but can be associated with rhinitis, conjunctivitis, bronchitis, or pneumonia. Each of these agents can be grown or amplified by molecular assays in samples from normal cats, and modified live vaccine administration can influence the results of these tests. Thus proving the primary cause of disease can be difficult because results of PCR panels designed to detect multiple pathogens have poor positive predictive value and do not accurately aid in the development of a treatment plan. *Staphylococcus* spp., *Streptococcus* spp., *Pasteurella* spp., *E. coli*, and anaerobes are commensal bacteria that can cause secondary infections in association with rhinitis, bronchitis, or pneumonia. Other infectious or parasitic agents that are less commonly associated with URTD in cats are *Cryptococcus* spp., *Sporothrix* spp., *Aspergillus* spp., and *Cuterebra*. These agents should be ruled out if routine treatments do not resolve the signs of URTD.

Canine infectious respiratory disease complex (CIRDC) can be caused by a number of viral and bacterial pathogens. Canine adenovirus type 2, canine distemper virus, canine respiratory coronavirus, canine herpesvirus, canine influenza virus, and canine parainfluenza virus are detected most commonly in countries that have studied the syndrome. Bacteria that may be involved as primary pathogens in CIRDC include *B. bronchiseptica*, *Streptococcus equi* subsp. *zooepidemicus*, and *Mycoplasma* spp. *Mycoplasma cynos* was the species most commonly isolated in cases with clinical signs according to one report in the United Kingdom (Chalker et al, 2004). However, *M. cynos* infection was not associated with clinical signs of disease in a study in the United States (Lappin unpublished data, 2013). Thus the role of *Mycoplasma* spp. as primary causes of respiratory tract disease in dogs and cats still is unclear. As with the organisms associated with URTD in cats, all of the agents associated with CIRDC can be grown or amplified by molecular assays in specimens from normal dogs, and modified live vaccine administration can influence the results of some assays. Thus proving the primary cause of disease can be difficult, and results of PCR panels designed to detect multiple pathogens have poor positive predictive value.

Bronchitis in dogs and cats often is manifested by coughing and is associated with many different causes, including inhaled irritants, bacteria, viruses, respiratory parasites, and allergies. The bacteria and viruses associated with feline URTD and CIRDC also can result in bronchitis with cough. The respiratory parasitic conditions most commonly associated with coughing in the United States are pulmonary migration of *Toxocara* spp. in puppies and kittens and *Aelurostrongylus abstrusus* infections in cats (see Table 259-1). The presence of *Oslerus osleri,* the tracheal nodular worm, is associated with formation of nodules, tracheitis, and resultant cough in some affected dogs, and the lesions may be noted as soft tissue densities on thoracic radiographs.

Primary bacterial pneumonia in dogs and cats is uncommon but can occur after infection with *B. bronchiseptica, Mycoplasma* spp., *S. equi, S. canis,* and *Yersinia pestis* (primarily in cats). These agents generally cause infection after inhalation and so have alveolar radiographic patterns. In one study of 65 puppies younger than 1 year of age with pneumonia in the United States, 49% were infected with *B. bronchiseptica* (Radhakrishnan et al, 2007). *Y. pestis* infection is most common in outdoor cats in the western United States, and infected cats often have a history of hunting. If a primary bacterial pathogen is not identified in dogs or cats with bacterial pneumonia, other conditions like viral infections, aspiration, or immune deficiency are likely to be involved and should be considered during the diagnostic evaluation. Organisms commonly isolated from the lower respiratory tract include *E. coli, Pasteurella* spp., β-hemolytic *Streptococcus* spp., *B. bronchiseptica,* nonhemolytic *Streptococcus/Enterococcus* spp. group, *Mycoplasma* spp., coagulase-positive *Staphylococcus* spp., and *Pseudomonas* spp.

The most common causes of fungal pneumonia are *B. dermatitidis, C. immitis, Cryptococcus* spp., and *H. capsulatum.* These organisms are distributed geographically and usually show interstitial patterns radiographically. *Toxoplasma gondii* and *Neospora caninum* infections are the other major causes of interstitial pneumonia in dogs and cats and should be considered if other known risk factors are present. The infectious agents causing interstitial pulmonary disease are less likely to induce cough than are agents causing alveolar pulmonary disease or bronchitis.

Stillbirth or Abortion

B. canis infection causes a number of clinical syndromes in dogs, including epididymitis, orchitis, endometritis, stillbirth, abortion, discospondylitis, uveitis, and hyperglobulinemia. Because this agent is a significant zoonotic, brucellosis always should be included on appropriate differential lists. *Coxiella burnetii* is the cause of Q fever in people and can be associated with abortion in cats. Thus care should be taken (mask and gloves should be used) when caring for aborting cats. *Mycoplasma* spp. are suspected to be causes of reproductive failure in dogs and cats, but because these agents are also normal commensal agents in the genital region, it is difficult to document cause and effect. Exposure to *T. gondii* or *N. caninum in utero* can lead to abortion or stillbirth. These agents are found most commonly in dogs (*N. caninum* or *T. gondii*) or cats (*T. gondii*) allowed to hunt or fed raw meat. Exposure to canine herpesvirus or feline herpesvirus 1 during parturition can result in neonatal death (fading puppies or kittens, respectively). *In utero* transmission of FeLV but not of feline infectious peritonitis virus can result in stillbirth or neonatal death.

Uveitis

Any chronic infection can be associated with anterior uveitis from immune complex deposition in the choroid. In dogs, the systemic fungal agents (*B. dermatitidis, C. immitis, Cryptococcus* spp., *H. capsulatum*), *T. gondii,* and agents that induce vasculitis (*Bartonella* spp., *E. canis, R. rickettsii*) are associated with anterior or posterior uveitis. In cats, FeLV-related lymphoma and infection with feline immunodeficiency virus, FIP, *T. gondii, B. henselae,* or the systemic mycoses are associated most commonly with anterior or posterior uveitis.

References and Suggested Reading

Boothe HW et al: Evaluation of outcomes in dogs treated for pyothorax: 46 cases (1983-2001), *J Am Vet Med Assoc* 236:657, 2010.

Breitschwerdt EB et al: Bartonellosis: an emerging infectious disease of zoonotic importance to animals and human beings, *J Vet Emerg Crit Care* 20:8, 2010.

Chalker VJ et al: Mycoplasmas associated with canine infectious respiratory disease, *Microbiology* 150:3491, 2004.

Dowers KL, Hawley JR, Brewer MM: Association of *Bartonella* spp., feline calicivirus, and feline herpesvirus 1 infection with gingivostomatitis in cats, *J Feline Med Surg* 12:314, 2010.

Littman MP et al: ACVIM small animal consensus statement on Lyme disease in dogs: diagnosis, treatment, and prevention, *J Vet Intern Med* 20:422, 2006.

Marks SL et al: Enteropathogenic bacteria in dogs and cats: diagnosis, epidemiology, treatment, and control, *J Vet Intern Med* 25:1195, 2011.

National Association of State Public Health Veterinarians: Compendium of animal rabies prevention and control, 2011, *MMWR Recomm Rep* 60(RR-6):1, 2011.

Neer TM et al: Consensus statement on ehrlichial disease of small animals from the infectious disease study group of the ACVIM. American College of Veterinary Internal Medicine, *J Vet Intern Med* 16:309, 2002.

Quimby JM et al: Evaluation of the association of *Bartonella* species, feline herpesvirus 1, feline calicivirus, feline leukemia virus and feline immunodeficiency virus with chronic feline gingivostomatitis, *J Feline Med Surg* 10:66, 2008.

Radhakrishnan A et al: Community-acquired infectious pneumonia in puppies: 65 cases (1993-2002), *J Am Vet Med Assoc* 230:1493, 2007.

Sykes JE et al: Association between *Bartonella* species infection and disease in pet cats as determined using serology and culture, *J Feline Med Surg* 12:631, 2010.

Sykes JE et al: 2010 ACVIM small animal consensus statement on leptospirosis: diagnosis, epidemiology, treatment, and prevention, *J Vet Intern Med* 25:1, 2011.

Weese JS et al: Antimicrobial use guidelines for treatment of urinary tract disease in dogs and cats: Antimicrobial Guidelines Working Group of the International Society for Companion Animal Infectious Diseases, *J Vet Intern Med* 2011:263768, 2011.

CHAPTER 260

Rational Empiric Antimicrobial Therapy

PATRICIA M. DOWLING, *Saskatoon, Canada*

Concerns regarding bacterial resistance to antimicrobials are increasing the awareness of their rational use in human and veterinary medicine. Empiric antimicrobial therapy requires matching the likely pathogens with the antimicrobial drugs that should be effective against them (Table 260-1). A successful empiric antimicrobial dosage regimen depends on both a measure of drug exposure (pharmacokinetics [PK]) and a measure of the potency of the drug against the infecting organism (pharmacodynamics [PD]). New information is emerging rapidly regarding the PK:PD relationships that determine antimicrobial efficacy in both human and veterinary patients (McKellar et al, 2004). The PK parameters used in drug dosage design are the area under the plasma concentration versus time curve (AUC) from 0 to 24 hours, the maximum plasma concentration (Cmax), and the time the antimicrobial concentration exceeds a defined PD threshold (T). The most commonly used PD parameter is the bacterial minimum inhibitory concentration (MIC). In relating the PK and PD parameters to clinical efficacy, antimicrobial drug action is classified as either concentration dependent or time dependent.

Concentration-Dependent Antimicrobials

For antimicrobials whose efficacy is concentration dependent, high plasma concentrations relative to the MIC of the pathogen (Cmax:MIC) and the area under the plasma concentration–time curve that is above the bacterial MIC during the dosing interval (area under the inhibitory curve, $AUC_{0\text{-}24\,hr}$:MIC) are the major determinants of clinical efficacy (Figure 260-1). These drugs also have prolonged postantibiotic effects, which allows once-daily dosing with maintenance of maximum clinical efficacy. For fluoroquinolones (enrofloxacin, orbifloxacin, pradofloxacin, marbofloxacin), clinical efficacy is associated with achieving either an $AUC_{0\text{-}24\,hr}$:MIC of more than 125 or a Cmax:MIC of more than 10. For aminoglycosides (gentamicin, amikacin), achieving a Cmax:MIC of more than 10 is considered optimal for efficacy. Other antimicrobials that appear to have concentration-dependent activity are metronidazole (Cmax:MIC > 10 to 25) and azithromycin ($AUC_{0\text{-}24\,hr}$:MIC > 25). These PK:PD targets are met when antimicrobials are administered at label dosages for the pathogens indicated on the label. For extralabel pathogens with high MIC values, such as *Pseudomonas aeruginosa,* achieving the optimum PK:PD ratios systemically may be impossible with label or even higher than label dosages. In such cases, underdosing is ineffective and merely contributes to antimicrobial resistance.

Time-Dependent Antimicrobials

For antimicrobials whose efficacy is time dependent, the time during which the antimicrobial concentration exceeds the MIC of the pathogen (T > MIC) determines clinical efficacy (Figure 260-2). How much above the MIC and for what percentage of the dosing interval concentrations should be above the MIC still is being debated and likely is specific for individual bacteria-drug combinations. Typically, exceeding the MIC by one to five multiples for between 40% and 100% of the dosing interval is appropriate for time-dependent antimicrobial agents. The time that the concentration exceeds MIC should be closer to 100% for bacteriostatic antimicrobials and for patients that are immunosuppressed. Therefore these drugs typically require frequent dosing or constant-rate infusions for appropriate therapy. An exception is cefovecin; this third-generation cephalosporin maintains concentrations above the target MIC for 7 days because of its high degree of protein binding. In sequestered infections, penetration of the antimicrobial to the site of infection may require high plasma concentrations to achieve a sufficient concentration gradient. In such cases, the $AUC_{0\text{-}24\,hr}$:MIC or Cmax:MIC, or both, also may be important in determining the efficacy of an otherwise time-dependent antimicrobial. The penicillins, cephalosporins, most macrolides and lincosamides, tetracyclines, chloramphenicol, and potentiated sulfonamides are considered time-dependent antimicrobials.

Urinary Tract Infections

Bacterial urinary tract infection (UTI) results when normal skin and gastrointestinal tract flora ascend the urinary tract and overcome the normal urinary tract defenses that prevent colonization. Large retrospective studies have documented the most common species of uropathogens in dogs and cats, with *Escherichia coli* being the single most common isolate in both acute and recurrent UTIs (Ball et al, 2008). Gram staining and determination of pH of a urine sample help direct empiric antimicrobial therapy. If the urine is persistently alkaline, a urease-producing pathogen such as *Staphylococcus* spp. should be suspected if Gram-positive cocci are seen, and *Proteus* if Gram-negative rods are seen. If the urine is acidic,

TABLE 260-1

Suggested Empiric Antimicrobial Therapy by Site of Infection Based on the Likely Pathogens and Their Antimicrobial Susceptibility

Site of Infection	First-Choice Antimicrobials
Urinary tract	Amoxicillin Cephalexin or cefadroxil Nitrofurantoin Tetracycline or doxycycline
Pyoderma	Cephalexin or cefadroxil Amoxicillin/clavulanic acid Cloxacillin, dicloxacillin, or oxacillin Clindamycin, lincomycin, or erythromycin
Upper respiratory tract	Amoxicillin/clavulanic acid Cephalexin or cefadroxil Azithromycin Doxycycline
Lower respiratory tract	Amoxicillin/clavulanic acid ± fluoroquinolone* or aminoglycoside† Cephalosporin ± fluoroquinolone* or aminoglycoside† Clindamycin ± fluoroquinolone* Chloramphenicol Tetracycline or doxycycline Azithromycin
Musculoskeletal: surgical prophylaxis	Potassium penicillin G Cefazolin
Musculoskeletal: septic arthritis, tenosynovitis, osteomyelitis	Cephalosporins Clindamycin Amoxicillin/clavulanic acid Fluoroquinolones* Aminoglycosides†
Septicemia/bacteremia	Cefazolin Cefazolin or penicillin + enrofloxacin Cefazolin or penicillin + aminoglycoside† Cefoxitin

*Fluoroquinolones include enrofloxacin, orbifloxacin, marbofloxacin, and pradofloxacin, but only enrofloxacin is available in an injectable formulation.
†Aminoglycosides include amikacin and gentamicin. In orthopedic infections, these drugs can be used in local therapy to avoid toxicity.

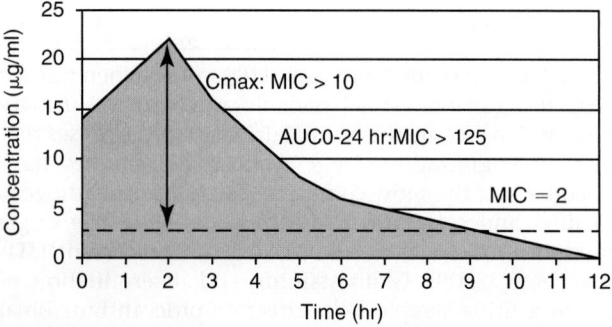

Figure 260-1 For concentration-dependent antimicrobials, the ratio of maximum plasma concentration (Cmax) to minimum inhibitory concentration (MIC) and the ratio of area under the curve to MIC are the major determinants of clinical efficacy.

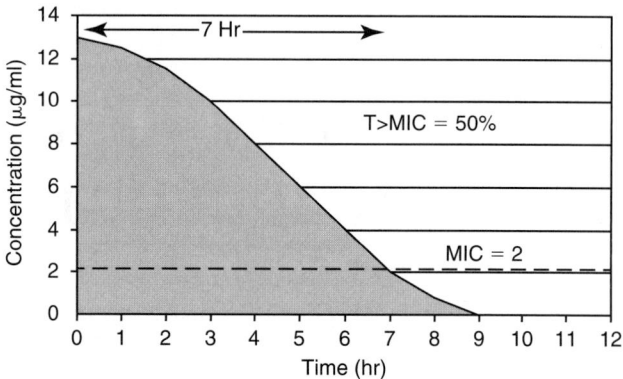

Figure 260-2 For time-dependent antimicrobials, the time during which the antimicrobial concentration exceeds the minimum inhibitory concentration for the pathogen determines clinical efficacy.

the most likely pathogens are *E. coli* if Gram-negative rods are seen, and *Enterococcus* spp. or *Streptococcus canis* if Gram-positive cocci are seen. Initial treatment of uncomplicated UTIs is straightforward because most antimicrobials undergo renal elimination to a great extent, so urine concentrations may be up to 100 times peak plasma concentrations. All of the first-choice treatments are time-dependent antimicrobials, so frequent dosing is important for efficacy. Amoxicillin has excellent activity against staphylococci, streptococci, enterococci, and *Proteus* and can achieve high enough urinary concentrations to be effective against *E. coli* and *Klebsiella* if dosed frequently. Therefore amoxicillin every 8 hours is the most rational empiric therapy for bacterial UTI while culture and susceptibility results are pending. Amoxicillin/clavulanic acid has excellent bactericidal activity against β-lactamase–producing staphylococci, *E. coli,* and *Klebsiella.* However, clavulanic acid undergoes some hepatic metabolism and excretion, so the efficacy of amoxicillin/clavulanic acid may be due primarily to the high concentrations of amoxicillin achieved in urine; therefore it is not preferred over amoxicillin for first-line therapy.

First-generation cephalosporins, such as cephalexin or cefadroxil, have greater stability to β-lactamases than penicillins and therefore have greater activity against staphylococci and Gram-negative bacteria. They have excellent activity against staphylococci, streptococci, *E. coli, Proteus,* and *Klebsiella. Pseudomonas,* enterococci, and *Enterobacter* are resistant, and the use of cephalosporins predisposes patients to nosocomial enterococcal infections. Thus cephalexin and cefadroxil are suitable empiric alternatives to amoxicillin, as long as enterococcal infection has been ruled out by the Gram stain results and urine pH. Nitrofurantoin is an old antimicrobial approved only for treatment of UTIs in people because therapeutic concentrations are not attained in plasma or tissues. It is also a good first-line treatment for UTIs caused by *E. coli,* enterococci, staphylococci, *Klebsiella,* and *Enterobacter.* Bacterial resistance to nitrofurantoin usually does not convey resistance to other antimicrobial classes, so this old antimicrobial is increasingly recommended as a first-line treatment in women. Similarly, recommendations for its use in veterinary medicine are increasing, but good

PK : PD studies have not been carried out in dogs and cats, and its adverse effects profile in dogs and cats is not well documented.

Tetracyclines are broad-spectrum antimicrobials that can be used empirically for the treatment of UTIs, but because of plasmid-mediated resistance, staphylococci, enterococci, *Enterobacter, E. coli, Klebsiella,* and *Proteus* have variable susceptibility. However, the tetracyclines are excreted unchanged in the urine, so high urinary concentrations may result in therapeutic efficacy despite susceptibility test results that indicate resistance. Doxycycline is a very lipid-soluble tetracycline that is better tolerated in cats and achieves therapeutic concentrations in the prostatic and renal tissues. Because of biliary elimination, it was thought initially not to be useful for treatment of uncomplicated UTIs, but effective concentrations for treatment of the most common pathogens are achieved in the urine of dogs and cats. Combinations of trimethoprim or ormetoprim with a sulfonamide are synergistic and bactericidal against staphylococci, streptococci, *E. coli,* and *Proteus.* Activity against *Klebsiella* is variable, and *Enterococcus* spp. and *Pseudomonas* are resistant. Although their spectrum of activity makes the potentiated sulfonamides rational first-line treatment choices, they are associated with a number of adverse effects that discourage more frequent selection. Enrofloxacin, orbifloxacin, and marbofloxacin are all fluoroquinolones approved for treatment of UTIs in dogs and some are approved for cats, but all are used in cats. All fluoroquinolones have excellent activity against staphylococci and Gram-negative bacteria but have variable activity against streptococci and enterococci. The therapeutic advantage of these drugs is their Gram-negative antimicrobial activity and excellent penetration into the prostate gland and activity in infected tissues. Their concentration-dependent killing allows for client-convenient once-daily dosing. However, it is inappropriate to use these important antimicrobials for empiric treatment of uncomplicated UTIs. Their use should be reserved for complicated UTIs, such as cases of pyelonephritis that involve Gram-negative bacteria, and for UTIs in intact male dogs in which prostatic involvement is likely.

Pyoderma

Pyoderma is a common primary bacterial skin disease of dogs caused by *Staphylococcus pseudintermedius,* whereas pyoderma occurs in cats only secondary to a primary pathologic problem (e.g., flea allergy). *S. pseudintermedius* is part of normal skin flora and colonizes the upper respiratory tract, the oral cavity, the anal region, and the external ear canal of dogs. Most canine staphylococci produce slime that allows the bacteria to adhere to cells, and contain protein A, which activates the complement cascade and incites inflammation. *E. coli, Proteus* spp., and *Pseudomonas* spp. can colonize the skin transiently and occasionally may become involved in pyoderma secondary to the staphylococcal infection. Treatment of the primary staphylococcal infection usually is sufficient to resolve these secondary infections.

Effective treatment of pyoderma requires systemically administered antimicrobials and topically applied antibacterial agents, along with specific treatment of any underlying causes (e.g., atopy). Appropriate empiric antimicrobials must be resistant to β-lactamase produced by staphylococci. Historically, *S. pseudintermedius* isolates did not demonstrate significant antimicrobial resistance because they did not readily retain antimicrobial resistance plasmids. However, methicillin-resistant *S. pseudintermedius* (MRSP) infections in dogs and cats have become increasingly common since 2006 and present a significant therapeutic challenge. MRSP can contain a wide range of different antimicrobial resistance genes, which makes these organisms resistant not only to all β-lactam antibiotics but also to other classes of antimicrobial drugs, including the fluoroquinolones. Two major clonal MRSP lineages have disseminated in Europe and North America. Isolates originating in North America often are susceptible to chloramphenicol, whereas isolates in Europe often are resistant. There are reports of MRSP isolates resistant to all approved veterinary antimicrobials, which has resulted in pressure to use "last-resort" antimicrobials approved for human use, such as linezolid.

Amoxicillin/clavulanic acid and first-generation cephalosporins, such as cephalexin or cefadroxil, are the usual empiric treatment choices for staphylococcal pyoderma, and dosing every 12 hours achieves a concentration above the MIC for 40% to 50% of the dosing interval. Cefpodoxime proxetil and cefovecin, third-generation cephalosporins, are attractive for use because of their client-convenient dosing schedules but should be reserved for more serious skin infections than superficial pyoderma. The antistaphylococcal penicillins (cloxacillin, dicloxacillin, and oxacillin) are excellent first choices for treatment of pyoderma, but because of a limited spectrum of activity these human-approved drugs usually are not on stock in a veterinary clinic, although they can be prescribed easily from a pharmacy. Because of poor oral bioavailability and rapid renal elimination, they must be dosed every 6 hours, which makes client compliance difficult. The macrolides and lincosamides are reasonable empiric choices for treatment of pyoderma, but recurrent infections are likely to be resistant. Erythromycin is associated with a high incidence of gastrointestinal upset in dogs. This can be avoided by using enteric-coated tablets, administering with food, prescribing antiemetics for the first 2 or 3 days of therapy, and initiating therapy with a lower dose. This treatment regimen is too complicated and inconvenient for most clients, and most clinicians prefer to use antimicrobials that do not routinely induce vomiting. Lincomycin has the same activity as erythromycin and does not cause gastrointestinal upset. Clindamycin typically is very active against *Staphylococcus* spp. and anaerobic bacteria. Trimethoprim or ormetoprim combined with a sulfonamide is effective in most cases of superficial pyoderma, but the risks of adverse effects such as keratoconjunctivitis sicca and multisystemic drug reactions limit their use. Enrofloxacin, marbofloxacin, and orbifloxacin are first choices only for antimicrobial treatment of deep pyoderma. Pradofloxacin is specifically approved for skin infections in cats. Fluoroquinolones have ideal pharmacokinetic properties; they accumulate in leukocytes and retain activity in necrotic and purulent debris. Since they are concentration-dependent killers, high-dose once-daily administration is ideal and increases client compliance with the treatment regimen. The fluoroquinolones initially have excellent activity against *S. pseudintermedius, Pseudomonas,* and *Proteus,* but MRSP frequently also is resistant to fluoroquinolones and *Pseudomonas* readily becomes resistant if the underlying pathologic condition is not addressed.

Respiratory Tract Infections

Upper Respiratory Tract

Primary bacterial disease of the upper respiratory tract is uncommon, but almost all dogs and cats with a mucopurulent or purulent nasal discharge have some bacterial component to their disease. *Bordetella bronchiseptica* can cause primary upper respiratory tract (URT) infections in dogs, whereas *B. bronchiseptica, Mycoplasma,* and *Chlamydophila felis* cause primary URT infections in cats. Most cases of rhinitis are secondary to other diseases, and because of the variety of normal flora found in the nasal passages, culture and susceptibility test results are difficult to interpret. Treating the bacterial infection without correcting the underlying cause is very unrewarding and encourages emergence of antimicrobial-resistant pathogens such as *P. aeruginosa.* Empiric therapy for URT infections in dogs and cats includes amoxicillin, amoxicillin/clavulanic acid, cephalexin or cefadroxil, or drugs with efficacy against *Mycoplasma* and *C. felis,* such as doxycycline or azithromycin. Doxycycline is considered the most effective therapy, but clinical signs of chlamydiosis improve with any of these drugs; yet cats frequently continue to have positive results on polymerase chain reaction or immunofluorescent antibody testing. In children, doxycycline is the least likely of the tetracyclines to cause dental damage, and there are no published reports of dental abnormalities from the use of doxycycline in puppies and kittens. However, oral administration of doxycycline to cats has been associated with esophagitis in some cats that can lead to stricture, so administration of tablets or capsules should be followed with consumption of food or water to ensure passage into the stomach. Fluoroquinolones should be reserved for resistant infections, preferably on the basis of culture and susceptibility testing. Enrofloxacin and orbifloxacin should be used carefully in cats because of the potential for retinal damage; marbofloxacin and pradofloxacin are not associated with such retinal toxicity. Tetracycline, chloramphenicol, or erythromycin ophthalmic ointments can be used to treat concurrent conjunctivitis. For chronic URT infection in dogs or cats, drugs that penetrate bone and target anaerobic bacteria, such as clindamycin, amoxicillin/clavulanic acid, or cephalexin or cefadroxil, should be chosen.

Lower Respiratory Tract

Bacterial pneumonia in dogs and cats usually is secondary to some pathologic process that disrupts normal pulmonary defense mechanisms. Treatment depends on the specific cause and the clinical status of the patient. In dogs with community-acquired bacterial infections,

the likely causative pathogens are *B. bronchiseptica, Mycoplasma* spp., *Streptococcus zooepidemicus, Pasteurella* spp., and *E. coli.* In cats, the pathogens are similar with the addition of *C. felis.* In previously ill animals or animals with hospital-acquired illness, *E. coli, Klebsiella, Pasteurella,* streptococci, staphylococci, anaerobes, *B. bronchiseptica, Pseudomonas,* and *Mycoplasma* frequently are involved, and more than one bacterial pathogen commonly is isolated. The unpredictable antimicrobial susceptibility of *E. coli* and other Gram-negative bacteria makes it difficult to choose antimicrobial therapy without susceptibility testing. In the critically ill patient a broad-spectrum parenteral antimicrobial regimen should be started as soon as possible until definitive culture results are obtained. Gram-negative rods frequently are susceptible to potentiated sulfonamides, gentamicin, chloramphenicol, third-generation cephalosporins (e.g., cefpodoxime proxetil), and the fluoroquinolones (enrofloxacin, orbifloxacin, marbofloxacin, pradofloxacin). *B. bronchiseptica* typically is susceptible to amoxicillin/clavulanic acid, tetracyclines, or azithromycin, but some isolates are resistant to the fluoroquinolones. Gram-positive cocci frequently are susceptible to amoxicillin/clavulanic acid, chloramphenicol, cephalosporins, or azithromycin. Aminoglycosides or enrofloxacin can be administered concurrently with parenteral formulations of penicillins or cephalosporins for broad-spectrum treatment of seriously ill patients. Clindamycin or metronidazole provides activity against β-lactamase–producing *Bacteroides fragilis.*

Musculoskeletal Infections

Prophylactic Antimicrobials

Veterinary surgeons routinely administer prophylactic antimicrobials to surgical patients undergoing orthopedic procedures, but there is little evidence from clinical trials to demonstrate the efficacy of this practice. In human patients undergoing clean bone surgery, antimicrobials are administered intravenously from 30 minutes before skin incision to no longer than 24 hours after the operation. Cefazolin typically is the prophylactic antimicrobial of choice in small animal practice. However, in the only published veterinary trial of prophylactic antimicrobial therapy in dogs undergoing elective orthopedic surgery, prophylaxis decreased the postoperative infection rate, but potassium penicillin G was as effective as cefazolin (Whittem et al, 1999). Prophylactic antimicrobial therapy should be followed by close observation and treatment with appropriate antibiotics and surgery if postoperative infection is diagnosed.

Septic Arthritis, Tenosynovitis, Osteomyelitis

Because of the variety of pathogens involved in musculoskeletal infections, appropriate samples must be submitted for culture and susceptibility testing. Aggressive empiric antimicrobial therapy must be initiated as soon as there is sufficient evidence of infection because of the devastating consequences of bone, joint, or tendon sheath infections. While culture results are awaited, initial antimicrobial selection can be based on the clinical case characteristics. In adult dogs and cats, septic arthritis and tenosynovitis commonly result from wounds or iatrogenic contamination with bacteria. In wounds, a variety of Gram-positive and Gram-negative bacteria typically are present, whereas *Staphylococcus aureus* and *S. pseudintermedius* are the usual isolates from iatrogenic infections, with methicillin-resistant *S. aureus* (MRSA) and MRSP increasingly reported in veterinary cases. Osteomyelitis in dogs and cats most commonly is caused by *S. pseudintermedius*. Polymicrobial infections are common in small animals, and organisms may include mixtures of streptococci, enterococci, Enterobacteriaceae (*E. coli, Klebsiella, Pseudomonas*), and anaerobic bacteria. Cat fight abscesses typically are caused by *Pasteurella multocida* and anaerobes. *Pseudomonas* often colonizes devitalized tissues, such as those occurring with big dog–little dog degloving injuries. For most bone and joint infections caused by β-lactamase–producing staphylococci, cephalosporins (cefazolin, cephalexin, cefpodoxime proxetil), clindamycin, and amoxicillin/clavulanic acid are effective. In treating MRSA or MRSP infections in dogs and cats, clindamycin may be selected for empiric therapy because of its antimicrobial activity and good tissue distribution. However, an inducible form of clindamycin resistance may be present in canine MRSA isolates. These staphylococcal strains appear susceptible on routine antimicrobial susceptibility testing, but resistance is induced during clindamycin treatment, resulting in treatment failure. On a Kirby-Bauer plate, strains with this inducible resistance are difficult to detect because they appear erythromycin resistant and clindamycin sensitive *in vitro*. However, if the clindamycin disk is placed next to the erythromycin disk, inducible resistance is detected by the presence of a D-shaped zone of inhibition around the clindamycin disk. Therefore it is recommended that the D-test be performed for all erythromycin-resistant isolates that initially test as susceptible to clindamycin. Clindamycin and metronidazole are effective for musculoskeletal infections caused by anaerobic bacteria. The aminoglycosides (amikacin, gentamicin) and fluoroquinolones (enrofloxacin, orbifloxacin, marbofloxacin, pradofloxacin) typically have good activity against staphylococci and excellent activity against Gram-negative pathogens. The excellent broad-spectrum antimicrobial activity and good safety profiles of the fluoroquinolones and the availability of injectable (enrofloxacin) and oral formulations make them popular choices for treatment of musculoskeletal infections. Although amikacin usually has good activity against *Pseudomonas*, it has poor activity against streptococci compared with gentamicin. Because nephrotoxicity and ototoxicity are related to duration of treatment, the aminoglycosides often are reserved for treatment of musculoskeletal infections by local delivery techniques. The newer human macrolide antimicrobials (azithromycin, clarithromycin) also may be effective for musculoskeletal infections and have good safety profiles in dogs and cats.

Septicemia/Bacteremia

Septicemia is common in critically ill canine and feline patients, and the majority that are septicemic have blood cultures positive for bacteria. In dogs, Gram-negative bacteria (especially *E. coli*) are most common, followed by Gram-positive cocci and anaerobes. Polymicrobial infections also are common and usually involve Gram-negative enterics and anaerobes. Bacteria cultured from cats are primarily Gram-negative enterics or anaerobes. Therefore it is common to use intravenous cephalosporins or β-lactam/aminoglycoside or β-lactam/enrofloxacin combinations for initial treatment of septic dogs and cats. The concentration-dependent drugs are administered once daily, but the time-dependent β-lactam drugs either must be administered by constant-rate infusion or must be given at least every 6 hours. Cefoxitin is a second-generation cephalosporin with good activity against anaerobes and Gram-negative enterics that can be used to treat septic dogs and cats. Imipenem, meropenem, and vancomycin occasionally are used to treat resistant infections in severely ill dogs and cats, but because of their importance in human medicine their use should not be routine in veterinary patients.

References and Suggested Reading

Ball KR et al: Antimicrobial resistance and prevalence of canine uropathogens at the Western College of Veterinary Medicine Veterinary Teaching Hospital, 2002-2007, *Can Vet J* 49:985, 2008.

Faires MC et al: Inducible clindamycin-resistance in methicillin-resistant *Staphylococcus aureus* and methicillin-resistant *Staphylococcus pseudintermedius* isolates from dogs and cats, *Vet Microbiol* 139:419, 2009.

Giguere S et al: *Antimicrobial therapy in veterinary medicine*, ed 4, Ames, IA, 2006, Iowa State University Press.

McKellar QA, Sanchez Bruni SF, Jones DG: Pharmacokinetic/pharmacodynamic relationships of antimicrobial drugs used in veterinary medicine, *J Vet Pharmacol Ther* 27:503, 2004.

Weese JS et al: Antimicrobial use guidelines for treatment of urinary tract disease in dogs and cats: Antimicrobial Guidelines Working Group of the International Society for Companion Animal Infectious Diseases, *Vet Med Int* 2011:263768, 2011.

Whittem TL et al: Effect of perioperative prophylactic antimicrobial treatment in dogs undergoing elective orthopedic surgery, *J Am Vet Med Assoc* 215:212, 1999.

CHAPTER 261

Infectious Causes of Polyarthritis in Dogs

RICHARD E. GOLDSTEIN, *New York, New York*

MICHAEL R. LAPPIN, *Fort Collins, Colorado*

Dogs with lameness and pain usually have disease of the muscles, joints, bone, or meninges, or have referred pain from parenchymal organs such as the prostate. The site of pain or lameness usually can be determined on careful physical examination. Some, but not all, dogs with polyarthritis have swollen, hot, painful joints. Since many causes of polyarthritis involve immune complex deposition (see discussion later), the small joints often are affected. Discomfort frequently is most evident in the carpi. Dogs with polyarthritis usually are reluctant to move, and when they ambulate the gait often is described as "walking on eggshells" because they do not want to flex the small joints.

There are three primary clinical groupings of polyarthritis based on joint fluid cytologic analysis: mononuclear polyarthritis (primary osteoarthritis and rarely primary immune disease); septic, suppurative polyarthritis (the organism causing disease is present in the joint); and nonseptic, suppurative polyarthritis (organisms are not demonstrated). Dogs with nonseptic, suppurative polyarthritis usually have either a primary immune disease (idiopathic polyarthritis or systemic lupus erythematosus [SLE]), an infectious disease, or a secondary immune reaction to noninfectious antigens. Polyarthritis also can be classified by whether the syndrome is erosive or nonerosive.

Hypersensitivity reactions are an amplification of the host's normal defense mechanisms. These reactions are most common with infectious disease agents that cause chronic infection and persist within the body. Primary immune-mediated diseases like SLE and neoplasia also can induce hypersensitivity reactions. Immunologic hypersensitivity reactions often contribute greatly to the overall extent of pathogenic changes, particularly when the organisms involved are of relatively low virulence such as the systemic fungal agents and *Bartonella* spp. Type III (immune complex) hypersensitivity reactions are thought to be involved in a number of primary immune or infectious causes of polyarthritis. These reactions develop as immune complexes (antibody and specific antigen) form and are deposited in or on tissues, which leads to secondary inflammation. Alternatively, free antigen can bind to membranes and subsequently react with circulating antibody. After the immune complex is deposited, complement is fixed, which leads to an inflammatory reaction. Neutrophils and platelets are attracted to the area and release lysosomal enzymes and vasoactive substances, respectively, that lead to increased vascular permeability. Synovial membranes commonly are affected in type III hypersensitivity reactions.

Differential Diagnosis

Dogs with septic joints generally are systemically ill and have swollen, hot, red, and painful joints. Synovial fluid cytologic examination reveals increased numbers of nondegenerative neutrophils, degenerative neutrophils, and macrophages; bacteria, fungi, or protozoans may or may not be observed. In dogs, bacterial arthritis generally involves only one joint, and often there is a portal of entry such as a laceration or bite wound.

In most dogs with nonseptic, suppurative polyarthritis the clinical signs include intermittent fever, general malaise, anorexia, joint pain, and stiffness. However, some affected dogs can have normal findings on joint palpation. It is important to remember that the infectious causes of nonerosive, nonseptic, suppurative polyarthritis often are clinically indistinguishable from primary immune causes.

A number of vector-borne or non–vector-borne infectious agents causing polyarthritis are relatively common in the United States and include *Anaplasma phagocytophilum* (dogs or cats), *Bartonella* spp. (dogs), *Borrelia burgdorferi* (dogs), *Ehrlichia canis* (dogs or cats), *Mycoplasma* spp. (dogs or cats), and *Rickettsia rickettsii* (dogs). Since these organisms generally are not seen in the joints, the joint fluid usually is classified cytologically as nonseptic. Secondary immune-mediated, suppurative, nonerosive polyarthritis commonly occurs due to infectious diseases that do not directly involve the joints but cause inflammation from type III hypersensitivity. Examples are brucellosis, ehrlichiosis, bacterial endocarditis, chronic otitis externa, pyometra, actinomycosis, coccidioidomycosis, and leishmaniasis. Nonerosive, nonseptic, suppurative, polyarthritis also is believed to occur as a manifestation of vaccine reactions, although this is not well documented in dogs. It occurs most frequently with modified live calicivirus vaccination of kittens.

There may be other historical data and clinical signs associated with infectious causes of nonerosive, nonseptic, suppurative polyarthritis that vary with the infectious agent. For example, *R. rickettsii* replicates in endothelial cells, which leads to severe inflammation in multiple tissues, and so most clinically affected dogs are extremely ill. *R. rickettsii* infection (Rocky Mountain spotted fever) has only an acute stage; this finding, combined with the fact that tick vectors are not active in the winter, make this a seasonal syndrome (spring through fall). Most cases of *R. rickettsii* infection are reported in the midwestern and southeastern United States. In contrast, *Ehrlichia ewingii* is not seasonal, clinical signs other than polyarthritis are minimal, and infection occurs mostly in dogs living in states harboring the Lone Star tick, *Amblyomma americanum*. Another classic finding is that polyarthritis associated with *A. phagocytophilum* or *B. burgdorferi* infection occurs almost exclusively in dogs that have visited areas endemic for the deer tick, *Ixodes* spp. Finally, *A. phagocytophilum*, *E. ewingii*, and *R. rickettsia* primarily are associated only with acute disease, which leaves *Bartonella* spp., *B. burgdorferi*, *E. canis*, and *Mycoplasma* spp. as the most likely infectious agent differentials if polyarthritis has been present long term.

Diagnostic Plan

When polyarthritis is suspected, the initial diagnostic plan generally includes radiography of the affected joints to determine whether osteoarthritis or erosive changes are present and a complete blood cell count, serum biochemical testing, and urinalysis to evaluate for possible causes or sites of inflammation. Arthrocentesis usually is performed to determine whether the joint fluid is septic or nonseptic and whether the predominant cells are mononuclear cells, degenerative neutrophils, or nondegenerative neutrophils.

If bacteria are seen, synovial fluid should be cultured for aerobes, anaerobes, and *Mycoplasma* spp. In all dogs in which the predominant cells are neutrophils, urine also should be cultured regardless of whether the neutrophils are degenerative or nondegenerative, even if bacteria are not seen. Transport media and specific culture media are required for successful culture of *Mycoplasma* spp. Thoracic and abdominal radiography or ultrasonography should be considered for dogs with nonerosive, nonseptic, suppurative polyarthritis to evaluate for occult infectious or neoplastic antigen sources. Urine and blood cultures should be considered. Protein:creatinine ratio should be determined if proteinuria without hemorrhage or inflammation is detected on initial urinalysis. Echocardiography can be performed to evaluate heart valves for changes associated with bacterial endocarditis. In some dogs with valvular endocarditis murmurs may not be auscultated.

The decision to perform tests for primary immune diseases depends on the individual case. It has been shown that positive results on tests for antinuclear antibodies and rheumatoid factors do not correlate with the presence of primary immune-mediated diseases (Smith et al, 2004). However, because most dogs with SLE are antinuclear antibody positive, a negative test result may rule out this syndrome as a cause of the polyarthritis.

The signalment, risk of vector exposure, vector disease control history, travel history, and clinical findings should be used to rank the differential list. The clinician then can select tests for individual infectious disease agents to complete the diagnostic workup. Several laboratories now offer panels of infectious agent serologic tests or polymerase chain reaction (PCR) assays that amplify the DNA

of infectious disease agents. However, the results of these assays can be positive in healthy dogs as well as in dogs with polyarthritis, so positive test results do not always correlate with illness. See the later sections on each individual agent for a discussion of currently available diagnostic tests.

Treatment

Animals with septic polyarthritis should be treated with antibiotics that kill aerobes, anaerobes, and gram-positive and gram-negative organisms until culture results return. The combination of a quinolone with a penicillin or a cephalosporin is a logical first choice. Quinolones often are effective against gram-negative bacteria as well as *Bartonella* spp., L-form bacteria, *Mycoplasma*, and *R. rickettsii*. Penicillin derivatives are effective against gram-positive bacteria, anaerobic bacteria, and *B. burgdorferi*.

Animals with nonseptic, suppurative polyarthritis often are administered doxycycline (5 to 10 mg/kg q12-24h PO) while the workup is completed. Doxycycline generally is effective for management of infections with *A. phagocytophilum*, *B. burgdorferi*, *Ehrlichia* spp., *Mycoplasma* spp., and *R. rickettsii*. However, *Bartonella* spp. infections of dogs rarely respond to doxycycline alone, and so this agent should stay on the differential list for dogs with polyarthritis in which a doxycycline trial fails (see the section on *Bartonella*). An additional benefit of doxycycline is that it has antiinflammatory properties and may lessen discomfort in some affected dogs nonspecifically. If doxycycline is unavailable or not tolerated, alternative options do exist such as minocycline (at the same dose as doxycycline), penicillins, or cephalosporins for *B. burgdorferi*; minocycline or imidocarb for *E. canis*; and so forth. Because the inflammation usually is neutrophilic, low-dose prednisone administered at 1 mg/kg q12-24h PO initially may give dramatic improvement in clinical signs of disease. However, excessive doses can activate some infectious agents such as *B. burgdorferi*. If the syndrome turns out to be a primary immune-mediated disorder, increased doses of prednisone with or without other immunosuppressive drugs may be required.

Specific Infectious Agents

Anaplasma phagocytophilum

Anaplasma phagocytophilum, a gram-negative, obligate, intracellular bacterium in the order Rickettsiales, is the cause of canine granulocytotropic anaplasmosis. This organism was previously thought to be an *Ehrlichia* sp. and was described in different reports as *Ehrlichia equi*, *Ehrlichia phagocytophila*, and the agent causing human granulocytic ehrlichiosis.

Like *B. burgdorferi*, *A. phagocytophilum* is vectored by *Ixodes* spp. Thus areas around the world that are considered endemic for Lyme disease in dogs or people also are endemic for *A. phagocytophilum*. Cats also can develop acute clinical signs of disease after exposure to infected ticks. Definitive hosts are thought to be small rodents and the white-tailed deer. The transmission from the tick occurs during the blood meal. The transition into the tick salivary glands and eventual infection of the dog is thought to require at least 24 hours of feeding. Coinfection of dogs with *A. phagocytophilum* together with other organisms like *B. burgdorferi* is thought to play a role in the pathogenic potential. It also is known that some *A. phagocytophilum* strains are more pathogenic than others, which partially explains the high prevalence of seropositive healthy dogs.

Dogs experimentally exposed to *A. phagocytophilum*–infected ticks either develop subclinical infections or demonstrate vague clinical signs of illness including fever, lethargy, malaise, anorexia, and general muscle pain resulting in reluctance to move. Some dogs exhibit joint pain and lameness resulting from inflammatory polyarthritis. These signs are remarkably similar to those of acute Lyme disease, and because of the very high prevalence of coinfection it often is impossible to determine which agent is causing the disease. Although the organism is known to persist in the blood and synovial fluid of experimentally inoculated dogs, associations with chronic polyarthritis or other inflammatory diseases are unclear. Other clinical findings are gastrointestinal signs such as vomiting, diarrhea, or both, or respiratory signs such as coughing and labored breathing. Central nervous system disease (meningitis) also can occur, resulting in seizure activity, ataxia, or neurologic deficits.

Dogs infected with *A. phagocytophilum* are more likely than those infected with *B. burgdorferi* to have laboratory abnormalities, with mild to moderate thrombocytopenia being noted most commonly. Morulae may be seen within the cytoplasm of circulating neutrophils or those in synovial fluid. It has been shown that some acutely infected dogs have positive results on PCR analysis of blood samples before detectable levels of serum antibodies appear, so seronegative dogs should be evaluated by PCR testing of blood or both tests should be run simultaneously. One experimental study found that diagnostic sensitivity was not increased by performing PCR analysis of synovial fluid in addition to testing the blood.

Although dose optimization studies have not been performed, administration of doxycycline at 5 to 10 mg/kg q12-24h PO generally leads to rapid resolution of clinical signs of disease (Neer et al, 2002). Experimentally infected dogs treated with doxycycline at 10 mg/kg q24h PO for 28 days tested negative for *A. phagocytophilum* DNA in blood during and after treatment (Moroff et al, 2011). However, immunosuppressive therapy was not given in an attempt to reactivate infection. Although penicillins and some cephalosporins are effective for the treatment of clinical borreliosis, they are not effective for anaplasmosis. Thus doxycycline always should be considered the drug of choice for dogs with nonseptic polyarthritis, especially in areas with *Ixodes* ticks. The prognosis for acute disease appears to be good. However, tick control should be maintained because reinfection can occur and *A. phagocytophilum* is a significant zoonotic agent.

Bartonella Species

Bartonella vinsonii subsp. *berkhoffii* initially was isolated from a dog with endocarditis in North Carolina (Breitschwerdt et al, 1995). Since that time, additional *Bartonella* species have been isolated from dogs or have had DNA amplified from blood or tissues, including *B. henselae, B. clarridgeiae, B. koehlerae, B. washoensis, B. quintana, B. rochalimae,* and *B. elizabethae* (see Chapter 270). Although each of these organisms potentially can induce illness in dogs, most have been infected with *B. vinsonii* subsp. *berkhoffii, B. henselae,* or *B. clarridgeiae*. Each of these agents is associated with fleas, and so *Bartonella* spp. should be high on the differential list for dogs with nonerosive, nonseptic polyarthritis that also have current or previous flea infestations. Coinfection with other agents, such as *Anaplasma* spp. or *Ehrlichia* spp., may play a role in the pathogenesis of clinical canine bartonellosis. For example, in one study of valvular endocarditis, all dogs with *Bartonella* spp.–associated disease also were seropositive for *A. phagocytophilum* (MacDonald et al, 2004).

Clinical findings or syndromes most frequently attributed to *Bartonella* spp. infections in dogs are endocarditis, fever, arrhythmias, hepatitis, granulomatous lymphadenitis, cutaneous vasculitis, rhinitis, polyarthritis, meningoencephalitis, thrombocytopenia, eosinophilia, monocytosis, immune-mediated hemolytic anemia, epistaxis, idiopathic cavitary effusions, and uveitis. *B. henselae* and *B. vinsonii* subsp. *berkhoffii* seem to be the most likely species to be associated with clinical disease, and both should be on the differential list for dogs with polyarthritis.

Serum antibodies can be detected in both healthy and clinically ill dogs, so the presence of antibodies does not always correlate with illness. In addition, approximately 50% of dogs with clinical bartonellosis are seronegative, and so serum antibody testing never should be used as the sole diagnostic method in suspect cases. *Bartonella* spp. can be difficult to grow or amplify from dogs because the agents frequently are present in low numbers. Thus the combination of serologic testing with culture and PCR assay of blood often is needed to confirm infection (Duncan et al, 2007; Galaxy Diagnostics, 2013). For some dogs, samples must be tested repeatedly to prove the presence of the organism. It also is unclear whether there is benefit in performing PCR testing and culture of synovial fluid in addition to blood. If test results are positive in a clinically ill dog and no other explanation for the illness is obvious, treatment is indicated.

Doxycycline treatment alone has failed in dogs with suspected bartonellosis; thus failure to respond to this drug should not exclude the diagnosis. Dual therapy is thought by some veterinarians to be more effective than monotherapy, but more information is needed. Doxycycline at 5 mg/kg q12h PO combined with a veterinary fluoroquinolone such as enrofloxacin at 5 to 10 mg/kg q24h PO is recommended. Rifampin in combination with another antibiotic may be required in resistant cases. Amikacin administered at 20 mg/kg q24h IV commonly is recommended for the treatment of endocarditis but requires monitoring for potential renal toxicity. No matter which drug is used, a minimum of 4 to 6 weeks of treatment usually is recommended. Flea and tick control also should be maintained to avoid reinfection and to lessen the risk of zoonotic transfer of disease.

Borrelia burgdorferi

Lyme disease (Lyme borreliosis), caused by *Borrelia burgdorferi* and transmitted by *Ixodes* spp. ticks, is reviewed in Chapter 271. *Ixodes* spp. are found mainly in the Northeast, the Upper Midwest, and some parts of northern California in the United States. Lyme disease should be included in the differential list for dogs with acute or chronic polyarthritis that live or have visited those areas, particularly if strict tick control has not been maintained.

Evidence suggests that about 5% to 10% of dogs that are exposed to *B. burgdorferi* will develop clinical disease within 2 to 5 months of infection. Why some dogs but not others develop polyarthritis is not completely understood. Experimental studies have shown that the number of infected ticks that feed is critical, and the age and immune status of the animal also seem to be important. Humans with certain haplotypes of the major histocompatibility complex are prone to more severe clinical manifestations of the disease, and there may be a genetic link in dogs as well.

In experimentally infected dogs, overt clinical illness begins 2 to 5 months after tick exposure and consists of fever, inappetence, lethargy, lymphadenopathy, and episodic shifting limb lameness related to polyarthritis. Arthritis starts first in the joint that is closest to the tick bite. It has been shown that the release of proinflammatory cytokines and especially interleukin-8 plays an important role in the pathogenesis of acute and possibly more chronic progressive arthritis in dogs. Synovial fluid analysis findings are typical for a suppurative polyarthritis, with leukocyte counts ranging from 2000 to 100,000 nucleated cells/µl; however, the organism generally is not seen cytologically. PCR assay to detect *B. burgdorferi* DNA in blood is not indicated because the organism migrates in connective tissue. However, if clinical signs of disease are present, PCR testing can be used to detect *B. burgdorferi* DNA in joint fluid and samples of synovium. PCR assays cannot distinguish between live and dead organisms, but *B. burgdorferi* DNA was cleared within 3 weeks of injection in experimental animals. Research has shown that small DNA fragments of *B. burgdorferi* can persist in synovial membranes after treatment, and these fragments can be amplified by PCR. Although the sensitivity of PCR is high, the sample must contain *B. burgdorferi* DNA to yield positive results. A negative PCR result therefore never excludes the presence of the organism elsewhere in the body. As discussed in Chapter 271, multiple serologic assays are available, but positive results alone do not correlate with Lyme polyarthritis because of the high exposure rates in endemic areas.

The antibiotics that are most effective for treating *B. burgdorferi* infection are the tetracyclines, ampicillin or amoxicillin, some third-generation intravenous cephalosporins, and erythromycin and its derivatives; current protocols are reviewed in Chapter 271. Improvement in polyarthritis often occurs within 24 to 48 hours of initiation of antimicrobial therapy in acute cases. The greatest success is achieved in the initial phases of clinical illness. Research suggests that the organism is difficult to eliminate from animals with established infection and that relapses occur despite seemingly adequate treatment regimens. Most treatment is instituted for a minimum of 30 days. However, on the basis of research studies, clearance of the organism after 30 days of treatment is questionable. Relapse can occur and PCR results can become positive after discontinuation of antimicrobials. Also, inflammatory changes that occur in various tissues, such as the joints, may become self-perpetuating. Intraarticular persistence of *B. burgdorferi* may stimulate chronic immune and inflammatory processes. Dogs with more chronic borreliosis are less likely to show improvement or to have relapses, even if treatment is continued for weeks to months. Nonsteroidal antiinflammatory drugs may be helpful for pain relief during episodes of recurrent *B. burgdorferi*–associated arthritis. Immunosuppressive doses of glucocorticoids definitely should be avoided because immunosuppression may potentiate infection exacerbation. Tick-exposed dogs that had recovered from clinical signs of Lyme disease and were treated with oral prednisolone for a 2-week period 16 months after the original exposure again demonstrated lameness and polyarthritis.

Administration of *B. burgdorferi* vaccines before exposure can lessen the likelihood of development of polyarthritis. Whether vaccination potentiates polyarthritis in previously exposed dogs is unclear. Tick control should be maintained in endemic areas to help prevent infection or reinfection.

Ehrlichia canis

Canine monocytotropic ehrlichiosis caused by *Ehrlichia canis* is reviewed in Chapter 276. Because this agent is vectored by the brown dog tick (*Rhipicephalus sanguineus*), it has a worldwide distribution and should be on the differential list for all dogs with clinical manifestations of polyarthritis. In addition, *R. sanguineus* lives within homes and kennels and feeds year round, so ehrlichiosis should be considered a year-round differential. *Anaplasma platys*, *Babesia* spp., *Hepatozoon canis*, and *R. rickettsii* are other agents transmitted by this tick, and the presence of coinfections may potentiate *E. canis*–associated disease.

Although most exposed dogs never develop clinical illness, polyarthritis can occur in either the acute or chronic phases of disease. In the acute phase, polyarthritis may relate to vasculitis, and in the chronic phase it may relate to immune complex disease. Polyarthritis rarely is the only manifestation of disease in dogs with monocytotropic ehrlichiosis. As discussed in Chapter 276, dogs in the acute phase can be seronegative by immunofluorescence assay or point-of-care diagnostic assays (Neer et al, 2002). Thus PCR testing of blood should be considered in these cases; very little has been published concerning synovial fluid cytologic findings or PCR assay results in dogs with monocytotropic ehrlichiosis. Dogs with chronic ehrlichiosis usually are seropositive, but the presence of serum antibodies does not always correlate with disease. Unlike in canine granulocytotropic ehrlichiosis (caused by *E. ewingii*), morulae rarely are detected in blood or synovial fluid. Doxycycline generally is the drug of first choice for treatment, and current protocols are reviewed in Chapter 276. There currently is no licensed vaccine, so strict tick control should be maintained to lessen the likelihood of infection or reinfection.

Ehrlichia ewingii

Canine granulocytotropic ehrlichiosis caused by *Ehrlichia ewingii* is documented most commonly in dogs and human beings that reside in the central region as well as the southern and southeastern United States. For example, in a recent study by Beall et al (2012) seroreactivity to *E. ewingii* was highest in the central region (14.6%) followed by the southeast region (5.9%). The geographic distribution relates to that of the vector, *A. americanum* (Lone Star tick). The incubation period after tick exposure is approximately 13 days, so some clinically affected dogs are seronegative when initially screened. To date, only acute clinical signs of disease have been detected, and these generally are less severe than those caused by *E. canis* infection. Concurrent disease or infections may play a significant role in the pathogenesis of *E. ewingii* infection.

Nonspecific signs of *E. ewingii* infection include fever, lethargy, anorexia, depression, and signs consistent with polyarthritis, such as stiffness. Other clinical signs are vomiting, diarrhea, and peripheral edema and neurologic signs such as ataxia, paresis, and vestibular disease. As in infection with *A. phagocytophilum* and *R. rickettsii*, acute disease seems to be most common; thus *E. ewingii* infection should be highest on the list of differential diagnoses from spring through autumn when *A. americanum* is most active.

Suppurative polyarthritis is common with *E. ewingii* infection, and morulae of *E. ewingii* can be detected inconsistently in neutrophils and eosinophils from peripheral blood and in neutrophils from synovial fluid. Other clinicopathologic findings include mild to moderate thrombocytopenia as described for acute *E. canis* or *A. phagocytophilum* infections. Antibodies can be detected by several methods, but since they can be detected in healthy as well as diseased dogs, the presence of *E. ewingii*–specific antibodies cannot be used alone to diagnose clinical granulocytotropic ehrlichiosis. Some dogs with acute disease have negative test results on presentation, so antibody testing during convalescence is required. PCR assays for amplification of *E. ewingii* DNA in blood currently are available, and test results are likely to be positive before seroconversion. Whether there is clinical utility in performing PCR testing of synovial fluid in addition to blood is unknown.

Supportive care should be provided as indicated. The treatment protocols discussed for *A. phagocytophilum* and *E. canis* infections generally are effective. Reinfection probably can occur and the agent also infects humans, so strict tick control should be maintained.

References and Suggested Reading

Battersby IA et al: Retrospective study of fever in dogs: laboratory testing, diagnoses and influence of prior treatment, *J Small Anim Pract* 47:370, 2006.

Beall MJ et al: Seroprevalence of *Ehrlichia canis*, *Ehrlichia chaffeensis* and *Ehrlichia ewingii* in dogs in North America, *Parasit Vectors* 8(5):29, 2012.

Berg RI et al: Effect of repeated arthrocentesis on cytologic analysis of synovial fluid in dogs, *J Vet Intern Med* 23:814, 2009.

Breitschwerdt EB et al: Endocarditis in a dog due to infection with a novel *Bartonella* subspecies, *J Clin Microbiol* 33:154, 1995.

Clements DN et al: Type I immune-mediated polyarthritis in dogs: 39 cases (1997-2002), *J Am Vet Med Assoc* 224:1323, 2004.

Colopy SA, Baker TA, Muir P: Efficacy of leflunomide for treatment of immune-mediated polyarthritis in dogs: 14 cases (2006-2008), *J Am Vet Med Assoc* 236:312, 2010.

Duncan AW et al: A combined approach for the enhanced detection and isolation of *Bartonella* species in dog blood samples: pre-enrichment liquid culture followed by PCR and subculture onto agar plates, *J Microbiol Methods* 69:273, 2007.

Foley J et al: Association between polyarthritis and thrombocytopenia and increased prevalence of vector borne pathogens in Californian dogs, *Vet Rec* 160:159, 2007.

Galaxy Diagnostics: The most effective test for active Bartonella infection, 2013. Available at www.galaxydx.com. Accessed June 29, 2013.

Goodman RA et al: Molecular identification of *Ehrlichia ewingii* infection in dogs: 15 cases (1997-2001), *J Am Vet Med Assoc* 222:1102, 2003.

Goodman RA, Breitschwerdt EB: Clinicopathologic findings in dogs seroreactive to *Bartonella henselae* antigens, *Am J Vet Res* 66:2060, 2005.

Hegemann N et al: Cytokine profile in canine immune-mediated polyarthritis and osteoarthritis, *Vet Comp Orthop Traumatol* 18:67, 2005.

Johnson KC, Mackin A: Canine immune-mediated polyarthritis. Part 1: Pathophysiology, *J Am Anim Hosp Assoc* 48:12, 2012a.

Johnson KC, Mackin A: Canine immune-mediated polyarthritis. Part 2: Diagnosis and treatment, *J Am Anim Hosp Assoc* 48:71, 2012b.

Littman MP et al: ACVIM small animal consensus statement on lyme disease in dogs: diagnosis, treatment, and prevention, *J Vet Intern Med* 20:422, 2006.

MacDonald KA et al: A prospective study of canine infective endocarditis in northern California (1999-2001): emergence of *Bartonella* as a prevalent etiologic agent, *J Vet Intern Med* 18:56, 2004.

Moroff S et al: Detection of antibodies against *Anaplasma phagocytophilum* in experimentally infected dogs using an automated fluorescence based system (Accuplex4™ BioCD). In *Proceedings of the 29th Annual ACVIM Forum*, June 2011.

Neer TM et al: Consensus statement of ehrlichial disease of small animals from the infectious disease study group of the ACVIM, *J Vet Intern Med* 16:309, 2002.

Rondeau MP et al: Suppurative, nonseptic polyarthropathy in dogs, *J Vet Intern Med* 19:654, 2005.

Smith BE et al: Antinuclear antibodies can be detected in dog sera reactive to *Bartonella vinsonii* subsp. *berkhoffii*, *Ehrlichia canis*, or *Leishmania infantum* antigens, *J Vet Intern Med* 18:47, 2004.

Stull JW et al: Canine immune-mediated polyarthritis: clinical and laboratory findings in 83 cases in western Canada (1991-2001), *Can Vet J* 49:1195, 2008.

CHAPTER **262**

Immunotherapy for Infectious Diseases

STEVEN DOW, *Fort Collins, Colorado*
JESSICA M. QUIMBY, *Fort Collins, Colorado*

Role of Immune-Stimulatory and Immunosuppressive Therapy

Some infections in dogs and cats cannot be treated effectively with antimicrobial drugs alone. Often these are chronic infections, typically in sites that may not be fully accessible so that effective antimicrobial drug concentrations can be reached. These difficult-to-treat infections include chronic viral infections in cats (e.g., feline herpesvirus 1, feline calicivirus, feline coronavirus, feline immunodeficiency virus infections) as well as chronic infections in dogs caused by certain intracellular pathogens (e.g., *Toxoplasma gondii, Mycobacterium* spp, *Ehrlichia canis, Coccidioides immitis,* canine papilloma virus). For these infections, active immunotherapy can be an effective alternative or adjunct to conventional antimicrobial therapy.

At the other extreme, there are some infections in which the immune response to infection elicits such a marked inflammatory response that inflammation actually causes more injury to the host than the pathogen itself. Examples of these infections include acute rickettsial infections (e.g., *E. canis* and *Rickettsia rickettsii* infection), hemoplasma infections (e.g., *Mycoplasma haemofelis, Candidatus Mycoplasma haemominutum*), and some bacterial pneumonias and meningitides. For these infections, brief immunosuppression with glucocorticoids can reduce host inflammatory responses and thereby ameliorate the damage caused by unchecked inflammation, while at the same time not interfering with the overall effectiveness of treatment with conventional antimicrobial drugs (see Chapter 278).

Principles of Immune-Stimulatory Therapy

The primary goal of active immunotherapy for treatment of most infections is to induce repeated production of large amounts of both type I interferons, or IFNs (IFN-α, IFN-β) and type II IFNs (IFN-γ). Depending on the site and distribution of infection, the immune-stimulatory drug is administered either locally (e.g., intranasally) or systemically. Strong IFN responses, particularly those that include type I IFNs, can suppress replication and increase intracellular killing of most pathogens, including viral, bacterial, and fungal pathogens. In addition, repeated activation of innate immune responses can lead to the generation of pathogen-specific T-cell responses.

Key Role of Type I Interferons in Antiviral Immunity

Type I IFNs, which actually consist of a family of closely related isoforms of IFN-α plus a single isoform of IFN-β, play a key role in early immune responses to viral infections and infections with certain bacterial pathogens. IFN-α is produced by all nucleated cells in the body in response to viral entry and replication and represents one of the primary immune defenses against viral pathogens (Seo and Hahm, 2010). For example, IFN-α suppresses viral replication in the host cell and augments cellular immunity, especially natural killer (NK) cell activity and CD8 T-cell responses. After chronic infection has become established, type I IFNs remain important, but IFN-γ responses become much more important as mediators of effector T-cell antiviral activity, including both CD4 T-cell and CD8 T-cell activity.

Major Role of Interferon-γ in Antibacterial and Antifungal Immunity

IFN-γ plays a key role in regulating both early and late immunity to bacterial and fungal pathogens, and the importance of IFN-γ has been established clearly in a number of different animal models (Seder et al, 1999). Unlike the production of type I IFNs, the production of IFN-γ is restricted to only a few cell types in the body, primarily NK cells and T lymphocytes. Early after infection, IFN-γ is produced primarily by NK cells, whereas later in the course of infection, IFN-γ production is restricted to antigen-specific CD4+ and CD8+ T cells. Production of IFN-γ by T lymphocytes is largely responsible for maintaining sustained immune control of bacteria, fungal, and viral infections. IFN-γ has numerous immune effects, including direct suppression of intracellular replication as well as induction of effective intracellular killing mechanisms by macrophages and neutrophils.

Effective Immune Therapeutics and Balanced Interferon Production

Both type I and type II IFNs are important for controlling persistent infections by viruses, fungi, and bacteria. Therefore the most effective immunotherapeutics are those that produce balanced induction of both type I and type II IFN responses. For example, Zylexis, a veterinary immune stimulant produced from inactivated parapoxviral particles, has been shown potently to induce IFN production (Fachinger et al, 2000). Type I IFN and type II IFNs exert critical and nonredundant activities against intracellular pathogens. However, although most currently licensed veterinary immune therapeutics can elicit some IFN-γ production, few are strong inducers of IFN-α production, with the possible exception of Zylexis. Thus there is still a need for veterinary immune therapeutics capable of potently activating both IFN-α and IFN-γ production *in vivo*.

Importance of Sustained Interferon Production

Effective immunotherapeutics should induce sustained immune activation and IFN production, which may require the administration of relatively long-acting immune stimulants (e.g., live bacille Calmette-Guérin) or repeated administration of shorter-acting immune activators (e.g., Toll-like receptor 3 [TLR-3] or TLR-9 agonists; see Table 262-1). For example, effective intracellular killing of persistent intracellular pathogens often requires prolonged exposure to activating concentrations of IFNs because effective pathogen elimination typically takes time to develop. This principle is one of the primary drawbacks to the use of recombinant cytokines, such as human recombinant IFN-α (Roferon-A, others), for treatment of persistent viral infections in cats. Frequent and repeated dosing also means that there is a higher likelihood of development of neutralizing antibodies against human recombinant cytokines such as IFN-α (Zeidner et al, 1990). The use of recombinant feline IFN omega (currently available only in Europe) avoids the issue of neutralizing antibodies, but long-term, frequent treatment still is required, and optimal daily dosing regimens have not been established for most pathogens.

Cytokine Induction Profiles of Currently Available Immune Therapeutics

Currently little published information is available allowing direct comparison of the ability of commercially available immune stimulants to induce production of cytokines (and especially IFN-γ). However, several general trends can be discerned from experimental studies of different classes of immune therapeutics. Immune therapeutics based on nucleic acids (or inactivated viral particles) appear to be the most effective inducers of both type I and type II IFN responses. For example, Zylexis was shown to induce IFN-γ production by porcine peripheral blood mononuclear cells, most likely by activation of the TLR-3 pathway (Fachinger et al, 2000). Likewise, an immune stimulant comprised of cationic liposomes and noncoding plasmid DNA (a TLR-9 agonist) has been shown by us and others to induce high levels of IFN-α and IFN-γ production in mice, cats, and dogs (Kamstock et al, 2006; Veir et al, 2006).

In contrast, immune stimulants based on purified or enriched bacterial or fungal extracts tend to induce high levels of tumor necrosis factor-α (TNF-α) production, but lower amounts of IFN-γ and little or no IFN-α production. For example, killed *Propionibacterium acnes* (ImmunoRegulin) has been reported to induce TNF-α production by bovine leukocytes. Likewise, *Staphylococcus* phage lysate (SPL) has been reported to activate innate immunity. Cell wall extracts of *Aloe vera* (Acemannan Immunostimulant), which are rich in polysaccharides, are reported to induce TNF-α production by macrophages *in vitro* (Zhang and Tizard, 1996).

TABLE 262-1

Immunotherapeutics for Use in Infectious Diseases

Drug	Mechanism of Action	Indications	Dosage	Adverse Effects
Killed *Propionibacterium* (ImmunoRegulin)	Activation of innate immunity	Chronic staphylococcal pyoderma	0.03-0.06 ml/kg IV as needed	Fever, injection site reactions
Staphylococcus phage lysate (SPL)	Activation of innate immunity	Chronic staphylococcal pyoderma, bacterial infection	0.5-1.5 ml twice to once weekly SC	Local or systemic vaccine reactions
Cationic liposomes with Toll-like receptor ligands	Activation of innate immunity	Chronic viral or fungal infections	1-2 ml SC or IP as needed	Lethargy and fever
Human recombinant interferon alfa (Roferon-A, others)	Activation of innate and adaptive immunity	Feline viral infections	1 million units/kg IV or SC injection daily for 5 consecutive days	Anemia, hepatotoxicity
Feline interferon omega (Virbagen Omega)	Direct antiviral activity	Feline viral infections	1 million units/kg every other day to weekly SC	Anemia, lethargy, fever
Inactivated parapoxvirus (Zylexis)	Activation of innate immunity	Viral or fungal infections	Not published for dogs or cats	Fever, cutaneous reactions

IL, Intralesionally; *IV,* intravenously; *IP,* intraperitoneally; *SC,* subcutaneously.

Potential Adverse Effects of Immune Stimulants

Strong activation of the immune system has the potential to cause harmful adverse effects, in addition to enhancing pathogen immunity. The primary adverse effect is overstimulation of innate immunity with excessive production of proinflammatory cytokines such as TNF-α, interleukin-6 (IL-6), and IL-1β, which can cause fever and hypotension. Overstimulation of innate immunity is more likely to occur when immune stimulants are administered systemically than following subcutaneous or mucosal administration.

In the case of recombinant cytokines, overdosing is a more substantial risk, particularly with potent cytokines such as IFN-α or IL-2. However, to date, significant adverse effects from overdosing of recombinant cytokines have not been reported in veterinary medicine, although adverse effects from intravenous administration of human recombinant IL-2 have been noted in dogs with cancer. Administering xenogeneic recombinant cytokines (e.g., human recombinant IFN-α) to animals also introduces the risk of development of broadly cross-reactive neutralizing antibodies. Thus in theory treatment of a cat or dog with human recombinant IFN-α can induce antibodies that not only neutralize the foreign human IFN but may also neutralize the animal's own endogenous IFN-α, although this adverse effect has not been specifically documented in companion animals.

Immunotherapy for Persistent Infections in Dogs

There are several chronic infections in dogs that may benefit from active immunotherapy, although in most cases clinical trials have not been completed. For example, animals with persistent infections with rickettsial agents or fungal organisms in the bone marrow or lymphoid tissues may benefit from activation of innate immunity with nonspecific immunotherapy. Chronic bacterial infections are relatively rare in dogs, although persistent infections with atypical mycobacteria (e.g., *Mycobacterium avium* spp.) have been reported. More commonly, dogs with acquired deficiencies in adaptive immunity (e.g., animals being treated with glucocorticoids or cyclosporine), or those with immunoglobulin deficiency, may develop persistent or recurrent infections with common bacterial agents such as *Staphylococcus* or *Streptococcus* and may benefit from immunotherapy.

Although chronic viral infections are uncommon in dogs, papillomatosis due to chronic infection with canine papillomavirus is an exception and appears to be increasing in prevalence. In part, the increase in canine papillomatosis may be iatrogenic, driven by the increasing use of potent T-cell immunosuppressants such as cyclosporine, which is believed to result in reactivation of viral replication at mucous membrane surfaces (Lange and Favrot, 2011). Although still relatively rare, papillomatosis can be a devastating disease in older animals because of interference with eating and swallowing (Figure 262-1). A number of strategies have been evaluated in the past for treatment of papillomatosis in dogs, although few have been consistently effective. We recently have observed a high response rate in dogs with persistent papillomatosis treated with a liposome-based immunotherapeutic (cationic liposome-DNA complexes, or CLDCs) (see Figure 262-1). The CLDC immune therapeutic has been widely evaluated in rodent models as well as in dogs with cancer and cats with chronic upper respiratory virus infection and is noteworthy because of its strong induction of both

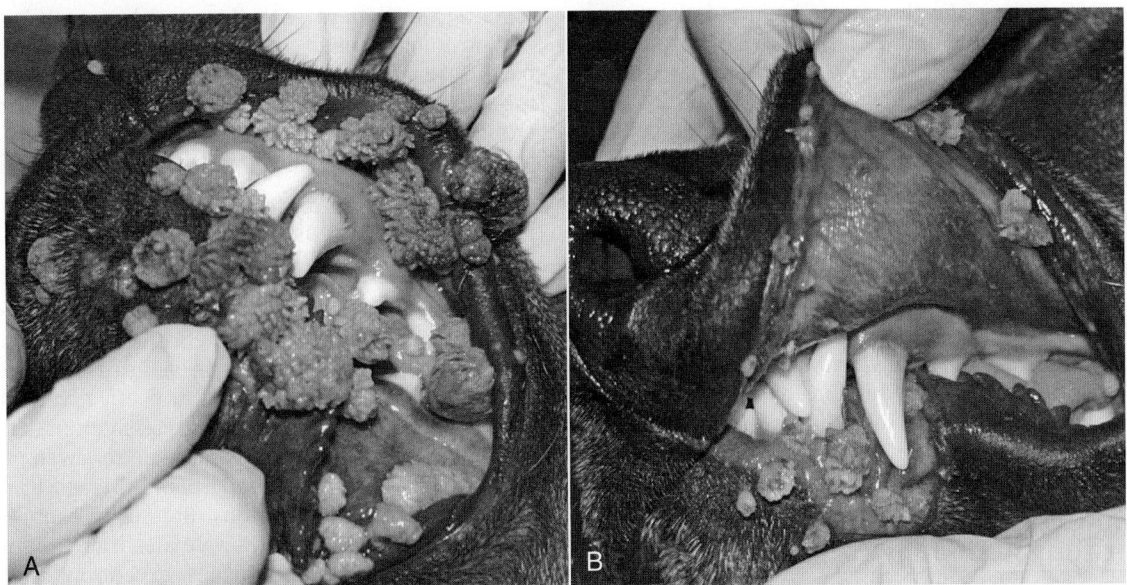

Figure 262-1 Oral papillomatosis lesions and response to nonspecific immunotherapy. **A,** A 9-month-old Rhodesian ridgeback dog with chronic, unresponsive oral papillomatosis of 5 months' duration. The dog was treated with weekly injections of cationic liposome-DNA complex (CLDC) immunotherapy. **B,** The oral lesions following 4 weeks of treatment.

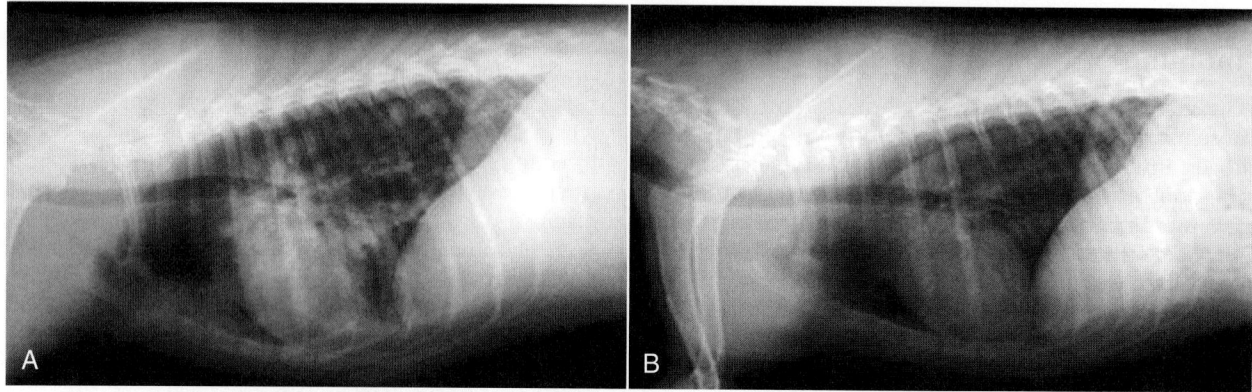

Figure 262-2 Response to immunotherapy in a dog with primary immune deficiency and disseminated toxoplasmosis. A 3-year-old Border collie developed progressive, disseminated toxoplasmosis that was unresponsive to clindamycin, azithromycin, and trimethoprim/sulfonamide therapy. **A,** Thoracic radiographs revealing marked pulmonary infiltrates associated with disseminated *Toxoplasma gondii* infection. Immunotherapy with weekly injections of cationic liposome-DNA complex (CLDC) was instituted, followed by injections every other week for 3 months. **B,** Thoracic radiographs taken after 2 months of CLDC treatment in conjunction with clindamycin treatment revealing complete resolution of the pulmonary parenchymal changes.

type I and II IFNs. Immunotherapy with CLDC also has shown activity in cats and dogs with chronic *Cryptococcus neoformans* infections and in animals with disseminated toxoplasmosis (Figure 262-2).

Immunotherapy for Persistent Viral Infections in Cats

Cats suffer disproportionately from persistent viral infections, especially chronic upper respiratory tract and oral mucosal infections with feline herpesvirus 1 and feline calicivirus (Veir et al, 2008). For these patients, recurrent infections are common and treatment is frustrating and often requires combinations of antibiotic therapy, appetite stimulants, and antiviral agents such as lysine or famciclovir. Cats persistently infected with pathogenic feline coronaviruses that induce feline infectious peritonitis also currently lack effective treatment options. However, the key role played by cellular immunity in controlling coronavirus replication suggests that an active immune-stimulatory therapeutic that could augment cellular immunity (i.e., T-cell immunity) should be effective in suppressing viral replication and reducing immune sequelae. It was reported in one study that treatment with feline IFN omega reduced clinical signs and improved survival in cats with feline immunodeficiency virus and feline leukemia virus infections (de Mari et al, 2004). Treatment with feline IFN omega and glucocorticoids also resulted in disease remission and prolonged survival in one third of treated cats with feline infectious peritonitis in a small study (Ishida et al, 2004).

Immunotherapy to Augment Antimicrobial and Antifungal Therapy

Immunotherapy also may be used to amplify the effectiveness of conventional antimicrobial therapy. For example, we reported recently that IFN-γ immunotherapy markedly enhanced the effectiveness of antibiotic therapy

against the intracellular bacterial pathogen *Burkholderia* (Propst et al, 2010). It also has been noted that the effectiveness of antibiotic therapy against *Mycobacterium tuberculosis* was enhanced *in vitro* by combining IFN-γ therapy with antimycobacterial drugs. In addition, the effectiveness of vancomycin therapy against infection with *Enterococcus* sp. was enhanced by IFN-γ treatment *in vitro*. IFN-γ immunotherapy also has been reported to increase the effectiveness of antifungal therapy against *Cryptococcus neoformans* in a mouse model of infection (Lutz et al, 2000).

The use of immunoantimicrobial therapy for treatment of chronic fungal infections may have clinical utility. For example, we observed that cats and dogs with chronic *Cryptococcus* infection that failed to respond to sustained treatment with fluconazole responded rapidly when the immune therapeutic CLDC was added to fluconazole treatment. There is preclinical data from rodent models to support the use of combined immunoantimicrobial therapy for treatment of selected chronic fungal infections.

Immunosuppressive Therapy in the Management of Infectious Diseases?

There are also examples of infections in which brief immunosuppression and reduction of inflammation can generate important benefits. In veterinary medicine few studies have addressed either the effectiveness or the safety of combined immunosuppressive and antimicrobial therapy. However, there has been renewed interest in the role of short-term glucocorticoid therapy in the management of certain infectious diseases in humans. In an interesting metaanalysis (McGee and Hirschmann, 2008) it was determined that, with few exceptions, administration of glucocorticoids to humans with infections either was clearly beneficial or had no effect on patient outcomes. In only two situations did glucocorticoid administration worsen clinical disease: prolonged glucocorticoid administration for chronic viral hepatitis and for cerebral malaria. Based on these findings, it was concluded that a brief course of modest doses of glucocorticoids could be beneficial for many infectious diseases, while not interfering with resolution of infection.

What are the lessons for veterinary medicine? For years, it has been dogma that glucocorticoids never should be administered to patients with infections. However, it may be time now to reexamine the use of glucocorticoids for the management of certain infections. Although there are few published data to guide recommendations for veterinary patients, the following examples describe situations in which brief, low-dose glucocorticoid therapy may benefit patients and improve overall treatment outcomes, as suggested in a recent review (see also Chapter 278).

Glucocorticoid therapy is nearly always likely to be beneficial in the management of bacterial meningitis in dogs or cats, where even short-term inflammation can cause significant collateral damage to the central nervous system. Glucocorticoids also have been recommended to suppress the inflammation that develops following initiation of antifungal therapy in dogs with disseminated *Blastomyces* or *Histoplasma* infection. In one study, brief glucocorticoid therapy reduced coughing while not worsening the underlying infection in animals with fungal infection. Although not yet examined in a properly controlled clinical trial, it also has been recommended that a brief antiinflammatory course of glucocorticoids (e.g., 0.5 mg/kg q24h PO for 3 to 5 days) in dogs with acute tracheobronchitis can reduce the severity of clinical signs, while not altering the disease course.

Similarly, the brief use of glucocorticoids has been recommended for dogs with acute infections with *E. canis* or *R. rickettsii*, primarily to reduce the immunologic sequelae of red blood cell and platelet destruction. For cats with infections with hemoplasmas, glucocorticoid therapy may be especially beneficial in reducing the immune-mediated destruction of red blood cells. Although currently not supported by well-designed clinical trials, the use of glucocorticoids to ameliorate pulmonary inflammation in animals with acute bacterial pneumonia (e.g., following inhalational pneumonia) also has been proposed. Clearly, additional, carefully controlled clinical studies are warranted before these recommendations can be more widely adopted.

Summary and Recommendations

Immune therapy is an attractive and currently underutilized treatment option for primary management of persistent infections in dogs and cats. Recent studies suggest that immunotherapy also may be a way to increase the effectiveness of conventional antimicrobial therapy for certain chronic infections, especially fungal and bacterial infections. It is also important to understand that in some infections short-term suppression of host immunity actually may be more beneficial than stimulation of immunity.

References and Suggested Reading

de Mari K et al: Therapeutic effects of recombinant feline interferon-omega on feline leukemia virus (FeLV)-infected and FeLV/feline immunodeficiency virus (FIV)-coinfected symptomatic cats, *J Vet Intern Med* 18:477, 2004.

Fachinger V et al: Poxvirus-induced immunostimulating effects on porcine leukocytes, *J Virol* 74:7943, 2000.

Ishida T et al: Use of recombinant feline interferon and glucocorticoid in the treatment of feline infectious peritonitis, *J Feline Med Surg* 6:107, 2004.

Kamstock D et al: Liposome-DNA complexes infused intravenously inhibit tumor angiogenesis and elicit antitumor activity in dogs with soft tissue sarcoma, *Cancer Gene Ther* 13:306, 2006.

Lange CE, Favrot C: Canine papillomaviruses, *Vet Clin North Am Small Anim Pract* 41:1183, 2011.

Lutz JE, Clemons KV, Stevens DA: Enhancement of antifungal chemotherapy by interferon-gamma in experimental systemic cryptococcosis, *J Antimicrob Chemother* 46:437, 2000.

McGee S, Hirschmann J: Use of corticosteroids in treating infectious diseases, *Arch Intern Med* 168:1034, 2008.

Propst KL et al: Immunotherapy markedly increases the effectiveness of antimicrobial therapy for treatment of *Burkholderia pseudomallei* infection, *Antimicrob Agents Chemother* 54:1785, 2010.

Seder RA, Gazzinelli RT: Cytokines are critical in linking the innate and adaptive immune responses to bacterial, fungal, and parasitic infection, *Adv Intern Med* 44:353, 1999.

Seo YJ, Hahm B: Type I interferon modulates the battle of host immune system against viruses, *Adv Appl Microbiol* 73:83, 2010.

Veir JK et al: Prevalence of selected infectious organisms and comparison of two anatomic sampling sites in shelter cats with upper respiratory tract disease, *J Feline Med Surg* 10:551, 2008.

Veir JK, Lappin MR, Dow SW: Evaluation of a novel immunotherapy for treatment of chronic rhinitis in cats, *J Feline Med Surg* 8:400, 2006.

Zeidner NS et al: Alpha interferon (2b) in combination with zidovudine for the treatment of presymptomatic feline leukemia virus-induced immunodeficiency syndrome, *Antimicrob Agents Chemother* 34:1749, 1990.

Zhang L, Tizard IR: Activation of a mouse macrophage cell line by acemannan: the major carbohydrate fraction from *Aloe vera* gel, *Immunopharmacology* 35:119, 1996.

CHAPTER 263

Systemic Antifungal Therapy

JANE E. SYKES, *Davis, California*
AMY M. GROOTERS, *Baton Rouge, Louisiana*
JOSEPH TABOADA, *Baton Rouge, Louisiana*

Over the past three decades, immunocompromise associated with human immunodeficiency virus infection and transplantation medicine has resulted in the emergence of opportunistic fungi as increasingly important causes of morbidity and mortality in human patients. The subsequent demand for safer and more effective antifungal therapies has led to the development of new pharmacologic agents that selectively target components unique to fungi (such as the cell wall), as well as the reformulation of drugs with good efficacy but a narrow therapeutic window (such as amphotericin B) in ways that make them less toxic. In addition, new drugs with a broader spectrum of activity have been developed in classes of drugs (such as the azoles) that traditionally have been valuable for the treatment of fungal infections in veterinary patients. Consequently, veterinarians recently have gained access to a number of new antifungal drugs with high efficacy and low toxicity that, despite being limited in use in some patients because of high cost, hold significant promise for the treatment of mycotic infections in small animal patients. The purpose of this chapter is to provide indications, initial drug protocol recommendations, and information concerning potential toxicities for the antifungal drugs most frequently prescribed to dogs and cats (Table 263-1). For amphotericin products, the drug generally is dosed repeatedly to a cumulative drug target as described. For the other antifungal drugs, duration of therapy varies with the fungal species and clinical manifestations in the individual case. However, the duration of therapy is generally weeks to months.

Amphotericin B

Amphotericin B, a polyene antibiotic, traditionally has been the treatment of choice for invasive fungal infections in human and veterinary patients because it is highly active against a wide range of fungal organisms. Because it is absorbed poorly from the gastrointestinal tract, amphotericin B must be given parenterally. Following intravenous administration, amphotericin B is highly protein bound and then is redistributed quickly to tissues. It acts by binding to ergosterol in the fungal cell membrane; this compromises membrane stability and alters permeability, which leads quickly to leakage of cell contents and cell death. Although amphotericin B has greater affinity for fungal ergosterol than for mammalian cholesterol, its clinical usefulness has been hampered by dose-limiting nephrotoxicity, which may be mediated by direct renal epithelial cytotoxicity as well as renal vasoconstriction. As a result, when the original formulation of amphotericin B (amphotericin B deoxycholate [Fungizone]) is used for the treatment of systemic mycoses in dogs and cats, nephrotoxicity may occur before an effective cumulative dose can be administered. However, the development of novel delivery systems for amphotericin B in the early 1990s resulted in three newer (albeit more expensive) formulations with reduced nephrotoxicity and improved organ-specific drug delivery: amphotericin B lipid complex (Abelcet), amphotericin B colloidal dispersion (Amphotec), and liposomal amphotericin B (AmBisome).

Amphotericin B is used for the initial treatment of rapidly progressive or severe systemic mycoses (for which oral azoles are not likely to act quickly enough) or treatment of systemic mycoses that fail to respond to azole therapy, and provides a less expensive alternative to parenteral azole therapy in the treatment of fungal disease of the gastrointestinal tract when frequent vomiting precludes the use of oral medications. Amphotericin B has been used successfully in both human and veterinary patients for the treatment of blastomycosis, histoplasmosis, cryptococcosis, coccidioidomycosis, aspergillosis, hyalohyphomycosis, phaeohyphomycosis, sporotrichosis, zygomycosis, disseminated candidiasis, and rarely pythiosis.

Amphotericin B Deoxycholate

Amphotericin B deoxycholate typically is administered as a series of intravenous infusions. Dogs receive 0.5 to 1 mg/kg IV three times weekly to a cumulative dose of 4 to 8 mg/kg or until azotemia develops; cats receive 0.25 mg/kg IV three times weekly to a cumulative dose of 4 to 6 mg/kg. Each dose should be diluted in 5% dextrose and administered to a well-hydrated patient over 10 minutes to 5 hours. Sodium loading and longer infusion times may reduce nephrotoxicity and diminish infusion-related adverse effects, such as trembling, pyrexia, and nausea. Infusion-related adverse effects also may be lessened by pretreatment with diphenhydramine (0.5 mg/kg IV or PO), aspirin (10 mg/kg PO) or other nonsteroidal antiinflammatory drugs, or a physiologic dose of a glucocorticoid. Not all animals experience infusion-related adverse effects, so nonsteroidal antiinflammatory drugs and glucocorticoids should be only administered if such adverse effects are likely based on previous observations. Additionally, tolerance to infusion-related adverse effects

TABLE **263-1**

Drugs Used for Systemic Antifungal Therapy in Dogs and Cats

Drug*	Dosage	Formulations
Amphotericin B deoxycholate	0.5-1 mg/kg IV infusion three times weekly to a cumulative dose of 4-8 mg/kg (dogs) 0.25 mg/kg IV infusion three times weekly to a cumulative dose of 4-6 mg/kg (cats)	50-mg vial (reconstitute with 10 ml sterile water, then dilute to 0.1 mg/ml with 5% dextrose for IV infusion)
Amphotericin B lipid complex	1-3 mg/kg IV infusion three times weekly to a cumulative dose of 12-36 mg/kg (dogs) 1 mg/kg IV infusion three times weekly to a cumulative dose of 12 mg/kg (cats)	100-mg vial (dilute to 1 mg/ml in 5% dextrose for IV infusion); although each 100-mg vial is labeled for single use only, the doses for each treatment can be aliquoted into sterile vials and used for up to 1 wk after the 100-mg vial is opened
Itraconazole	5-10 mg/kg/day PO (dogs) 5 mg/kg q12h PO (25 or 50 mg per cat)	100-mg capsule 10-mg/ml oral solution
Fluconazole	5-10 mg/kg/day PO or IV (dogs) 50-100 mg per cat per day PO (cats)	50-mg, 100-mg, 150-mg, 200-mg oral tablets; 150-mg oral capsule 10-mg/ml, 40-mg/ml powder for oral suspension 100 ml or 200 ml of 2-mg/ml solution for IV infusion
Voriconazole	4 mg/kg q12h PO or IV (dogs) Do not use in cats	50-mg, 200-mg oral tablets 40-mg/ml powder for oral suspension 200-mg vial (reconstitute with sterile water to 10 mg/ml for IV infusion)
Posaconazole	5 mg/kg q24h PO (dogs and cats)	40-mg/ml powder for oral suspension
Ketoconazole	10-15 mg/kg q12h PO (dogs) 5-10 mg/kg q24h PO (cats)	200-mg oral tablet
Caspofungin	1 mg/kg IV infusion q24h (dogs)	50-mg, 70-mg vials (dilute in 0.9% saline for IV infusion)
Flucytosine	50 mg/kg q6-8h PO (cats) Do not use in dogs	250-mg, 500-mg oral capsules
Terbinafine	10-30 mg/kg q24h PO (dogs and cats)	250-mg oral tablets

*For amphotericin products, the drug generally is dosed repeatedly to a cumulative drug target as described. For the other antifungal drugs, duration of therapy will vary by the fungal agent and clinical manifestations in the individual case. However, the duration of therapy generally is weeks to months.

often occurs over time, which reduces the need for pretreatment with antiinflammatory drugs. Saline diuresis before administration of amphotericin B may decrease its effect on renal blood flow and should be considered in patients with preexisting renal disease or those at high risk of nephrotoxicity. Other adverse effects reported in humans treated with amphotericin B include hypokalemia, distal renal tubular acidosis, hypomagnesemia, anemia, and nephrogenic diabetes insipidus.

Serum levels of blood urea nitrogen (BUN) and creatinine should be measured before each infusion. If azotemia develops, infusions should be discontinued until it has resolved. Amphotericin B–induced azotemia usually is reversible, but it may take weeks to months for BUN and creatinine levels to return to baseline. Permanent renal damage is more likely to occur in patients with underlying renal disease and in those that are receiving other nephrotoxic drugs concurrently.

A protocol for subcutaneous administration of amphotericin B was developed with the intent of decreasing nephrotoxicity and avoiding the need for prolonged vascular access, and its use for the treatment of cryptococcosis was described by Malik and colleagues (1996) in three dogs and three cats. Amphotericin B deoxycholate (0.5 to 0.8 mg/kg) was diluted in 400 ml (for cats) or 500 ml (for dogs) of 0.45% NaCl/2.5% dextrose and administered subcutaneously two to three times per week

to a cumulative dose of 8 to 26 mg/kg. Although this protocol was successful in the six patients described, sterile abscesses caused by local tissue irritation occurred at concentrations higher than 20 mg/L, which is unavoidable in very large dogs. In addition, sterile abscesses often are seen even in smaller dogs for which more dilute concentrations are attainable. Despite this significant adverse affect, this protocol provides an alternative for antifungal therapy when financial limitations preclude the use of triazoles or amphotericin B lipid complex.

Amphotericin B Lipid Complex

Of the three newer formulations of amphotericin B designed to be less nephrotoxic, amphotericin B lipid complex (ABLC) has been the most extensively used and evaluated in veterinary patients. In dog studies, it is 8 to 10 times less nephrotoxic than amphotericin B deoxycholate, due in part to the fact that binding of amphotericin B to phospholipids decreases its ability to interact with cholesterol in the mammalian cell membrane and facilitates its selective transfer to ergosterol in fungal membranes. The efficacy of ABLC is increased by uptake of the lipid-complex drug by cells of the reticuloendothelial system, followed by liberation of amphotericin B from its lipid complex by lipases released from inflammatory cells at the site of infection.

For administration, ABLC is diluted in 5% dextrose to a concentration of 1 mg/ml and infused over a 1- to 4-hour period. Dogs receive 1 to 3 mg/kg IV three times weekly to a cumulative dose of 12 to 36 mg/kg; cats receive 1 mg/kg IV three times weekly to a cumulative dose of 12 mg/kg. The authors typically start with a dose at the lower end of the range and then increase the dose in subsequent infusions to the higher end of the range if the dose is well tolerated; this allows a reasonable cumulative dose to be administered within a 3-week period. Saline diuresis does not appear to be necessary before administration of ABLC but may be beneficial in animals with preexisting renal disease. As with amphotericin B deoxycholate, BUN and creatinine levels should be closely monitored, and infusion-related adverse effects may be diminished by pretreatment with antihistamines, aspirin, or glucocorticoids. Other adverse effects of amphotericin B such as hypokalemia, distal renal tubular acidosis, and nephrogenic diabetes insipidus rarely occur with these less nephrotoxic formulations.

Azoles

The azoles are an essential class of antifungal agents that block ergosterol biosynthesis by inhibiting lanosterol 14α-demethylase, a cytochrome P-450 enzyme that allows conversion of lanosterol to ergosterol. This disrupts fungal cell membrane function by causing depletion of ergosterol and accumulation of lanosterol and other 14-methylated sterols. Azoles are classified based on the number of nitrogen atoms contained in the azole ring: imidazoles (ketoconazole, clotrimazole, miconazole) contain two nitrogen atoms, whereas triazoles (itraconazole, fluconazole, voriconazole, posaconazole) contain three. Because of their more potent inhibitory effects on mammalian cytochrome P-450 enzymes, imidazoles such as ketoconazole tend to cause more adverse effects than triazoles. In addition, several azoles interfere with the activity of hepatic microsomal enzymes, which can lead to increased blood concentrations of concurrently administered drugs, such as cyclosporine and digoxin. In general, the triazoles play a major role in the treatment of systemic mycoses in human and veterinary patients because they provide an alternative to intravenous amphotericin B, which allows endemic mycoses such as blastomycosis and histoplasmosis to be treated with oral medication on an outpatient basis. Imidazoles such as ketoconazole have been largely replaced by the triazoles for treatment of systemic fungal infection because the triazoles have fewer adverse effects and better efficacy. Nevertheless, several imidazoles still are used in topical preparations.

Itraconazole

Itraconazole (Sporanox) is a triazole released in the early 1990s that has become the initial treatment of choice in dogs and cats for most systemic mycoses that are not immediately life threatening. Itraconazole is a weak base that requires an acid environment for maximal gastrointestinal absorption. Therefore its oral bioavailability is increased when it is given with food or cola beverages and decreased when it is given with antacids. Itraconazole is highly protein bound, but because of its lipophilicity, it distributes well to most tissues. However, it does not cross the blood-brain, blood-prostate, or blood-ocular barriers well, and its concentration in cerebrospinal fluid (CSF) and urine is low. Despite this fact, itraconazole often is used successfully for the treatment of fungal infections of the central nervous system (CNS) and eye, perhaps because inflammation-mediated compromise of these barriers allows more of the drug to move across them into infected tissues.

In dogs and cats, itraconazole typically is used to treat systemic fungal infections at a dosage of 5 to 10 mg/kg/day PO (either once daily or 10 mg/kg divided twice daily). It is available as both an oral capsule (100 mg) and an oral solution (10 mg/ml), the latter of which has improved gastrointestinal absorption. Itraconazole is notorious for its erratic oral bioavailability, especially when generic preparations are used. For this reason, substitution with generic itraconazole is not recommended because it may not result in therapeutic plasma concentrations, especially when the generic powder is compounded. If therapeutic drug monitoring can be performed, the recommended trough concentration target is between 0.25 and 0.5 µg/ml.

Adverse effects associated with itraconazole often are dose dependent and include gastrointestinal signs, hepatotoxicity, and cutaneous vasculitis. When gastrointestinal adverse effects occur, dividing the daily dose into two treatments, administered 12 hours apart, may be beneficial. Liver enzyme levels should be monitored every 4 weeks during itraconazole therapy, or sooner if inappetence or vomiting occurs. Increased transaminase activity is common but is not an indication to discontinue therapy unless it is accompanied by anorexia, vomiting, abdominal pain, or hyperbilirubinemia. Cutaneous vasculitis manifested as an ulcerative dermatitis most often is observed at dosages higher than 10 mg/kg/day. Therefore the development of ulcerative skin lesions in an animal receiving high-dose itraconazole should prompt biopsy of the lesion rather than an assumption that the lesion is caused by the underlying fungal infection. Lesions typically resolve when the dose of itraconazole is reduced.

Fluconazole

Fluconazole (Diflucan) is a triazole that traditionally has been used for the treatment of cryptococcosis and candidiasis. Because it crosses the blood-brain, blood-prostate, and blood-ocular barriers well, it often is chosen for the treatment of fungal infections of the eye or brain. Fluconazole is highly water soluble and minimally protein bound, achieving high concentrations in urine. It is not affected by gastric pH, and its oral bioavailability generally is consistent and is not affected by food or antacids. In general, fluconazole is more active against yeasts than molds. Therefore fluconazole is most often indicated in dogs and cats for the treatment of cryptococcosis and candidiasis or for ocular and CNS infections, whereas itraconazole or other triazoles are more likely to be effective for systemic mold infections such as aspergillosis and hyalohyphomycosis. The recent availability of fluconazole in an inexpensive generic formulation has expanded its use to include diseases such as blastomycosis and histoplasmosis that traditionally have been treated successfully with itraconazole. Results of a recent investigation failed to show that fluconazole was noninferior to itraconazole for the treatment of blastomycosis and did show that dogs treated with fluconazole were treated longer than dogs receiving itraconazole (Mazepa et al, 2011). A higher mortality in the fluconazole-treated dogs appeared to be limited to the first 2 weeks of therapy, which may indicate that there is a difference in early efficacy. However, clinicians who commonly treat blastomycosis have not observed a clinically significant difference between itraconazole and fluconazole, and often choose fluconazole as initial therapy for the treatment of this disease because of its much lower cost, even when longer treatment times are required.

Fluconazole is available as tablets of various strengths, an oral suspension, and an injectable formulation. Cats typically receive 50 mg per cat per day, which can be increased to 100 mg per cat divided twice daily if needed. Dogs typically receive 5 to 10 mg/kg q24h PO. Fluconazole generally is well tolerated, occasionally causing moderate subclinical increases in transaminase activity.

Voriconazole

Voriconazole (Vfend) is a fluconazole derivative with greater potency and a broader spectrum of activity than fluconazole. In human patients, it is currently the drug of choice for treatment of invasive aspergillosis. It also is used to treat other invasive and refractory mycoses such as those caused by *Scedosporium* spp. (*Pseudallescheria* spp.) and *Paecilomyces* spp. It is at least as active as itraconazole against veterinary isolates of *Cryptococcus* spp., *Candida* spp., and *Aspergillus fumigatus*. It is not active against *Sporothrix schenckii* and zygomycetes.

Voriconazole is available as a tablet, oral suspension, and an intravenous solution. Like fluconazole, it has excellent oral bioavailability, but its absorption is reduced in the presence of fatty food. Voriconazole is poorly water soluble and moderately protein bound. It is metabolized extensively by hepatic cytochrome P-450 enzymes and eliminated into bile. Of all the triazoles, it also is the most potent inhibitor of P-450 enzymes, and it can even induce its own metabolism over time. It has good penetration of the CNS, and although it is expensive, it has been used with some success to treat systemic aspergillosis in dogs and CNS coccidioidomycosis. If therapeutic drug monitoring can be performed, the recommended targets are a trough concentration of between 2 and 5.5 mg/L and a peak concentration of less than 5.5 mg/L to minimize toxicity.

Adverse effects have not yet been well documented in dogs, but the authors have observed decreased appetite, increased serum liver enzyme activities, and in uncommon cases CNS signs, including ataxia and staring or "star gazing". Tachypnea and marked pyrexia after intravenous infusion was observed in one dog. Cats are highly sensitive to the adverse effects of voriconazole and develop inappetence; CNS signs such as ataxia, pelvic limb paresis, mydriasis, apparent blindness, decreased pupillary light responses, and a decreased menace response; cardiac arrhythmias; and hypokalemia. As a result, the use of voriconazole in cats currently is not recommended. Among the adverse effects of voriconazole in humans are reversible visual effects including photophobia and blurred vision, hallucinations, peripheral neuropathies, and photosensitization, as well as the same toxicities seen with other triazoles.

Posaconazole

Posaconazole (Noxafil) is an itraconazole analog that has demonstrated good activity in the treatment of several refractory deep mold infections in dogs and cats, including infections with *Aspergillus* spp. and *Mucor* spp. in cats and systemic infections with *Aspergillus* spp. in dogs. Its spectrum of activity is similar to that of voriconazole, with the addition of zygomycetes. Posaconazole is available as an oral suspension. Because of variable absorption in different individuals, therapeutic drug monitoring is recommended in human patients, with target peak concentrations of more than 1.48 mg/L. As with itraconazole, in humans its absorption is promoted by the concurrent presence of fatty food and gastric acidity. Absorption also is improved when the total daily dose is divided into two to four doses. Posaconazole is highly protein bound (>95%) and undergoes hepatic metabolism, with some inhibition of P-450 enzymes. Most administered posaconazole is eliminated in the feces. Data on CSF concentrations of posaconazole are not yet available. Adverse effects appear to be less common in cats than with voriconazole.

Ketoconazole

Ketoconazole largely has been replaced by itraconazole for treatment of many mycoses because of the greater toxicity and lower efficacy of ketoconazole compared with triazole antifungal drugs. Because of its low cost, it continues to be used in veterinary medicine when the cost of other antifungal drugs is prohibitive for the client, and it remains effective for the treatment of *Malassezia* spp. dermatitis, feline nasal and cutaneous cryptococcosis, and long-term treatment of coccidioidomycosis. The dosage is 10 to 15 mg/kg PO q12h for dogs and 5 to 10 mg/kg PO q12h for cats. The absorption of ketoconazole is improved when the drug is administered with food and inhibited by concurrent use of antacids. Ketoconazole is highly protein bound and is metabolized extensively by the liver, with inactive products being excreted in bile and, to a lesser extent, in urine. It has poor penetration of the CNS and generally is ineffective for treatment of CNS mycoses.

Vomiting, anorexia, lethargy, and diarrhea are relatively common adverse effects of treatment with ketoconazole. Administration of ketoconazole with food may help to reduce gastrointestinal adverse effects. Liver enzyme activities should be monitored monthly during treatment and earlier if gastrointestinal signs occur. It is common to see mild increases in the activity of serum transaminases during treatment, which do not warrant discontinuation of the drug. Less commonly, ketoconazole causes a hepatopathy, which may be accompanied by anorexia, vomiting, lethargy, increased activities of serum alanine transaminase and alkaline phosphatase, and hyperbilirubinemia. The drug should be discontinued if this occurs. Pruritus and cutaneous erythema have been reported in fewer than 1% of dogs treated with ketoconazole. Lightening of the hair coat color and cataract formation also rarely have been associated with ketoconazole administration in dogs.

Ketoconazole is a potent inhibitor of mammalian cytochrome P-450 enzymes and efflux transporter proteins such as P-glycoprotein. It inhibits testosterone and cortisol synthesis in mammals. Ketoconazole also can interfere with P-glycoprotein transport of ivermectin, which predisposes dogs to ivermectin toxicity. Inhibition of adrenal steroid synthesis can cause transient infertility during treatment of intact male animals and in rare cases clinical signs of hypoadrenocorticism.

Echinocandins

Echinocandins represent a new class of lipopeptide antifungal agents that target the cell wall rather than the cell membrane. Specifically, they inhibit the formation of $(1,3)$-β-d-glucans in the fungal cell wall. The prototype drug is caspofungin acetate (Cancidas). Other drugs in this class are micafungin and anidulafungin. Their use in dogs and cats has been limited by their high cost and need for once-daily intravenous infusion. Caspofungin was used successfully to induce remission in a dog with disseminated aspergillosis (1 mg/kg diluted in 250 ml 0.9% NaCl administered IV over 1 hour q24h). Synergism has been reported when echinocandins are used in combination with other antifungal drugs. The echinocandins are not active against *Cryptococcus* spp., which possess little glucan synthase. In human patients, caspofungin is approved for treatment of refractory invasive aspergillosis.

In human patients, caspofungin is extensively protein bound and is metabolized slowly by the liver, with some renal excretion. It has limited ability to penetrate the CNS and eye. Adverse effects noted in humans include fever, phlebitis, and elevated alanine transaminase levels (<20% of patients). The proper dose and the extent to which adverse effects occur in dogs and cats are unknown.

5-Flucytosine

Flucytosine is a fluorinated pyrimidine related to fluorouracil. Its use is limited to treatment of *Cryptococcus* and *Candida* infections in cats. These fungi deaminate flucytosine to 5-fluorouracil, which interferes with DNA replication and protein synthesis. Mammalian cells cannot convert flucytosine into 5-fluorouracil, so toxicity to mammalian cells is limited. Marked drug resistance arises during treatment (secondary drug resistance), and so flucytosine always must be used in combination with other drugs, most commonly amphotericin B, with which it has synergistic activity.

Flucytosine is absorbed rapidly and well from the gastrointestinal tract, and penetration of the CSF and aqueous humor is excellent. Because about 80% of the dose is

excreted unchanged in the urine, high urinary concentrations can be achieved. For the same reason, flucytosine toxicity is greatly increased in cats with renal failure, so the drug should be avoided in these animals. Because amphotericin B can cause impaired renal function, careful monitoring for toxicity is indicated when flucytosine is used in conjunction with amphotericin B. The use of flucytosine in animals has been limited mostly by its relatively high cost, especially when combined with costly treatment with amphotericin B.

The most common adverse effects of flucytosine therapy are myelosuppression and gastrointestinal signs. The complete blood count should be monitored during treatment. Administration of flucytosine to dogs frequently is followed by the development of a severe (but reversible) drug eruption within 2 to 3 weeks of starting treatment.

Terbinafine

Terbinafine (Lamisil) is a synthetic allylamine that inhibits ergosterol biosynthesis by interfering with squalene epoxidase; this results in ergosterol deficiency and squalene accumulation that disrupts fungal cell membrane function. It is highly lipophilic and keratinophilic, which leads to high concentrations in skin, hair, and nails. It is commonly used for the treatment of dermatophytosis and onychomycosis in human and veterinary patients. Although terbinafine does not have good efficacy for the treatment of systemic fungal infections when administered alone, it has been used with some success in combination with triazole or echinocandin therapy. Adverse effects are uncommon and usually limited to gastrointestinal signs, with hepatotoxicity in rare cases.

References and Suggested Reading

Evans N et al: Focal pulmonary granuloma caused by *Cladophialophora bantiana* in a domestic short haired cat, *Med Mycol* 49:194, 2011.

Foy DS, Trepanier LA: Antifungal treatment of small animal veterinary patients, *Vet Clin North Am Small Anim Pract* 40:1171, 2010.

Malik R et al: Combination chemotherapy of canine and feline cryptococcosis using subcutaneously administered amphotericin B, *Aust Vet J* 73:124, 1996.

Mazepa AS, Trepanier LA, Foy DS: Retrospective comparison of the efficacy of fluconazole or itraconazole for the treatment of systemic blastomycosis in dogs, *J Vet Intern Med* 25:440, 2011.

McLellan GJ et al: Use of posaconazole in the management of invasive orbital aspergillosis in a cat, *J Am Anim Hosp Assoc* 42:302, 2006.

Mehta AK, Langston AA: Use of posaconazole in the treatment of invasive fungal infections, *Expert Rev Hematol* 2:619, 2009.

Murphy KF et al: Successful treatment of intra-abdominal *Exophiala dermatitidis* infection in a dog, *Vet Rec* 168:217, 2011.

O'Brien CR et al: Long-term outcome of therapy for 59 cats and 11 dogs with cryptococcosis, *Aust Vet J* 84:384, 2006.

Quimby JM et al: Adverse neurologic events associated with voriconazole use in 3 cats, *J Vet Intern Med* 24:647, 2010.

Roffey SJ et al: The disposition of voriconazole in mouse, rat, rabbit, guinea pig, dog, and human, *Drug Metab Dispos* 31:731, 2003.

Schultz RM et al: Clinicopathologic and diagnostic imaging characteristics of systemic aspergillosis in 30 dogs, *J Vet Intern Med* 22:851, 2008.

CHAPTER 264

Infectious Diseases Associated with Raw Meat Diets

RACHEL A. STROHMEYER, *Kingston, Washington*

Over recent years, the commercial pet food industry has been under intense scrutiny. In 1999 and 2005 fungal toxins were found in some commercially available dry dog foods and were responsible for numerous pet illnesses and deaths. In March 2007, 91 commercial canned pet foods manufactured by several prominent companies in North America were recalled and later implicated in the deaths of potentially thousands of dogs and cats in the United States. Although no definitive cause was ever proven, it is suspected that melamine from wheat gluten in these foods was the source of the 2007 deaths. Although some owners always have opted to feed homemade or alternative diets, the new concerns over the safety and nutritional content of commercially available canine and feline diets and a greater interest in "natural and holistic" options has created an increased trend toward feeding homemade diets, many of these consisting at least partially of raw meat. This trend raises many concerns not only for the companion animals being fed these diets but also for the humans feeding and preparing the food and for family members being exposed to the food, bowls, and feces of these animals.

Why Feed Raw?

For years high-performance dogs such as racing greyhounds and sled dogs have been fed diets consisting mainly of raw meat because it is an inexpensive high-protein source. The trend toward feeding raw is gaining popularity in the companion animal world. The BARF (biologically appropriate raw food) diet has many supporters, including dog and cat breeders and pet owners who laud the "miraculous" health benefits of feeding raw. Many health claims are made regarding why feeding pets a raw diet is superior to feeding commercial diets. Some of these include potentiation of immune responses; lack of dental, skin, and gastrointestinal disease; lack of anal gland and allergy problems; and longer life expectancy. There also are claims that feeding raw helps animals maintain their ideal weight and that the animals have healthier coats. It is widely thought by those that feed their pets raw diets that a raw diet provides better nutrition because the cooking process breaks down vital nutrients. One of the strongest arguments in favor of feeding raw meat is the claim that wild canines and felines have always eaten raw and it is the natural way.

It should be noted, however, that the health benefit claims of feeding raw have never been scientifically substantiated.

Why Not Raw?

Proponents touting the benefits of feeding raw in general have not factored domestication into the recommendation process. The role of companion animals has changed significantly over the last 20 years. Pets are sleeping in their owners' beds, licking their owners' faces, eating off their owners' plates, walking on kitchen counters, and sitting on kitchen tables. Not to mention that these pets are urinating and defecating where people spend a significant amount of time, including private yards and public parks. There are certain health risks to the companion animals being fed a raw diet, but more importantly there are significant potential health risks to the pet owners, their families, and the general public. Because pets are playing a more significant role in people's lives there is a significantly greater risk of exposure to zoonotic diseases potentially associated with feeding a raw food diet than in previous times.

In the United States there are approximately 78.2 million pet dogs and 39% of households own at least one dogs; there are approximately 86.4 million pet cats and 33% of households have at least one cat. In general it is estimated that at least 50% of households in the United States have at least one companion animal. In addition, it has been estimated that at least 10 million people, or 3.6% of the United States population, can be considered immunocompromised, defined as being positive for human immunodeficiency virus or acquired immunodeficiency syndrome, being an organ transplant recipient, or being a cancer patient (Kahn, 2008). The number of immunocompromised people is even higher if those taking immunosuppressive drugs or those with suboptimal immune systems such as the elderly, pregnant women, infants, and children are included. It is estimated that 30% to 40% of immunocompromised people in the United States have at least one companion animal. It is highly recommended that immunocompromised people and households in which an immunocompromised person lives not feed raw diets to their companion animals (Kaplan et al, 2009).

Sources of Raw Meat for Companion Animal Diets

There are three main sources of raw meat fed to companion animals: meat obtained directly from facilities processing human food; meat from animals that have died from means other than slaughter (what is considered

"4D" meat—down, dead, dying, or diseased animals); and meat originally offered but no longer considered suitable for human consumption. Because the latter two sources could contain significantly more bacterial contamination, the U.S. Food and Drug Administration (FDA) recommends that only sources of animal tissue that come from U.S. Department of Agriculture (USDA)–inspected facilities and have passed USDA inspection for human consumption be used for manufacturing foods that contain raw meat or other raw animal tissues for consumption by dogs, cats, and other companion or pet animals (U.S. FDA, 2004). Aside from this, there are few or no regulations for commercial raw meat diets for companion animals, and many of the diets have not passed Association of American Feed Control Officials (AAFCO) feeding trials.

Infectious Organisms in Raw Meat

Many zoonotic bacteria and parasites potentially are associated with raw protein diets (Box 264-1). The purpose of this chapter is to provide the general practitioner with information concerning the most common agents associated with raw meat diets to use as a resource in helping educate clients who either are feeding or are considering feeding raw protein diets to their pets. It is important to note that there are many factors that affect microbial contamination of raw meat, including factors associated with the specific microbial contaminant, species of animal used to produce the product, degree of processing, number of times the product has been handled, facility where the product is produced, and sampling methods.

Bacteria

Campylobacter spp. are gram-negative flagellated spirochetes that have been linked to numerous food-borne illnesses in humans. Although there are many serovars of *Campylobacter*, *Campylobacter jejuni* is most commonly implicated in food-borne illness. The internal body temperature of avians is ideal for this bacterium to live and proliferate, and so consumption of raw or undercooked poultry products appears to be the most common path of transmission. The CDC reports that in 2005 *Campylobacter* spp. was present on 47% of raw chicken breasts tested through the FDA-NARMS (National Antimicrobial Resistance Monitoring System) Retail Food program.

Some serovars of *Campylobacter* are pathogenic, and a small number of bacteria can be responsible for causing significant illness in humans. Animals consuming raw poultry are at risk of *Campylobacter* infection. One serotyping study showed that *Campylobacter* spp. isolated from dogs with diarrhea also were isolated from poultry carcasses the dogs had been fed (Remillard, 2005). Although some dogs and cats exposed to *Campylobacter* spp. develop gastrointestinal disease, others remain healthy but become colonized and shed the organism in their feces, thus serving as a source of potential human exposure.

A common gram-positive commensal bacterium inhabiting the gastrointestinal tract of many animals is *Enterococcus faecalis*. It is a common contaminant of raw meat. A 2001-2002 study in Iowa of retail meat found 29% of samples to be contaminated with *E. faecalis* (Hayes et al, 2003). Although this bacterium seems to cause mostly incidental disease in companion animals, it is a bacterium that can exhibit extreme antibiotic resistance and is a growing concern for nosocomial infections in the humans. After ingesting the organism, animals can shed the resistant organism in their feces, contaminating the environment with antibiotic-resistant bacteria.

Escherichia spp. are facultative anaerobic gram-negative rod bacteria that populate the gastrointestinal tract of most species. These organisms are spread fecally and orally and can result in subclinical infection or significant gastrointestinal or systemic disease, including death, depending on both host and bacteria characteristics. *Escherichia coli* contamination is common in raw meat. In the 2010 Retail Meat Report presented by NARMS, of meat considered fit for human consumption, *E. coli* contamination rates were 67.6%, 83.1%, 43.2%, and 82.1% for ground beef, chicken breast, pork chop, and ground turkey samples, respectively (on average from 2002 to 2010). One veterinary study found 53% of commercially available raw meat diets consisting of beef, lamb, chicken, or turkey to be contaminated with non–type specific *E. coli* (Strohmeyer et al, 2006).

Methicillin-resistant *Staphylococcus aureus* (MRSA) has emerged as a great concern for human medical doctors, and this "superbug" is beginning to become more of a problem in veterinary medicine. Although most people associate this organism with hospitals and shopping cart handles, a common source is raw meat. MRSA has been cultured from numerous raw meat samples that were sold for human consumption. For example, a study published in June 2011 found that 65 (22.5%) of 289 beef, chicken, and turkey samples from grocery stores in Detroit, Michigan, were positive for *S. aureus* on culture (Bhargava et al, 2011). Of these 65 positive samples, six were positive for MRSA. A similar study in Baton Rouge, Louisiana, that tested 120 raw pork and beef products from grocery stores found 45.6% of pork and 20% of beef samples to be contaminated with *S. aureus*. Of these samples, five pork and one beef sample were positive for MRSA (Shuaihua et al, 2009). Other studies worldwide show similar results. In these other studies, raw pork samples have shown the highest numbers of MRSA isolates on culture. *S. aureus* is different from other potential food-borne pathogens because it colonizes the skin, not the intestinal tract.

BOX 264-1

Pathogens Potentially Associated with Raw Meat Diets Fed to Companion Animals

Bacteria	Parasites
Campylobacter spp.	*Cryptosporidium* spp.
Enterococcus spp.	*Echinococcus* spp.
Escherichia spp.	*Giardia lamblia*
Staphylococcus aureus	*Neospora caninum*
Salmonella spp.	*Toxocara* spp.
	Toxoplasma gondii

Pyoderma and skin allergies are common illnesses of companion animals. The question has been raised, If a companion animal has an underlying skin disorder and is fed a raw diet contaminated with MRSA, is this animal more susceptible to developing a MRSA infection (from the environment or from licking or chewing itself)? More research needs to be done, but this could prove to be a significant human and animal issue.

Salmonella spp. are gram-negative rod bacteria that are one of the most common pathogens associated with food-borne illness in humans and animals. Infected hosts with subclinical disease can be carriers and shed the bacteria in normal feces. *Salmonella* spp. enter through the digestive tract and can survive for weeks outside of the living body. It is estimated that at least 1% of human *Salmonella* infections in the United States are associated with contact with companion animals, and because the diagnosis of salmonellosis commonly is missed, this percentage may be much higher (Finley et al, 2006). As recently as the fourth quarter of 2011, the USDA Food Safety and Inspection Service reported that 1.7% to 49.9% of poultry carcasses and ground poultry products intended for human consumption tested positive for *Salmonella* spp. According to the CDC approximately 0.05% of eggs (1 in 20,000) sold in the shell are contaminated with *Salmonella* spp. Although the percentage of *Salmonella*-infected eggs is small, it still amounts to approximately 2.3 million contaminated eggs per year. It also is estimated that approximately 2% of the beef sold in the United States for human consumption is contaminated with *Salmonella* spp. According to the USDA Food Safety and Inspection Service fourth quarter report in 2011, 7.5% of ground beef samples tested positive for *Salmonella* spp. Information on food-borne disease in companion animals for the most part is lacking, but because *Salmonella* spp. are such common and potentially serious pathogens, there is considerable information pertaining to raw pet food contamination with this bacterium. For example, one study of commercially available raw meats for canines in the United States showed 5.9% to be contaminated with *Salmonella enterica* (Strohmeyer et al, 2006). In two studies of dogs fed raw meat diets in Canada, 3 of 10 dogs consuming a homemade diet and 5 of 7 dogs consuming a commercially available diet shed *Salmonella* spp. (Finley et al, 2006). *Salmonella* spp. have been implicated in disease and death in racing greyhounds, and one study found that 75% of 4D meat samples at one greyhound breeding facility and 93% of fecal samples from dogs at the same facility tested positive for *Salmonella* spp. (Morley et al, 2006). Finally, two cats in a single household died of salmonellosis that was linked to the raw meat diet being fed (Stiver et al, 2003).

Parasites

Cryptosporidium spp. are obligate single-celled protozoan parasites that infect the intestinal tract of their host, usually causing significant gastrointestinal issues. The infective stage is the oocyst, which is shed in the feces of the host and is immediately infectious. Hosts can shed over a million oocysts in one bowel movement, and infection with as few as 10 oocysts can cause clinical disease. The most common source of *Cryptosporidium* spp. infection is contaminated water, but raw meat and vegetables also can serve as a source of infection. Data from the CDC's Foodborne Diseases Active Surveillance Network (FoodNet) for 2007 reported cases of *Cryptosporidium* spp. infection to be on the rise, with children under 4 years old at the greatest risk. *Cryptosporidium parvum* and *Cryptosporidium hominis* usually are associated with disease in people. The host-adapted strains in dogs and cats, *Cryptosporidium canis* and *Cryptosporidium felis,* generally are not causes of disease in humans. However, meat used for pet consumption could be contaminated with *C. parvum,* and it is known that cats can harbor this zoonotic strain, shedding oocysts for months after infection (Scorza et al, 2005).

Echinococcus spp. are cyclophyllidean tapeworms in the family Taeniidae. Predators including dogs become infected with these tapeworm parasites by eating tissue from an infected intermediate host and serve as the final host. The parasites remain in the predator's gastrointestinal system shedding eggs into the environment, and the eggs then are eaten by an intermediate host. Sheep, goat, and swine are the most common, but small rodents, and sometimes humans, can also serve as intermediate hosts, depending on the species of *Echinococcus.* In 2002 a study of red foxes in Nebraska showed that 37.5% were infected with *Echinococcus multilocularis* and in Idaho 62% of wolves were found to have the parasite (Storandt et al, 2002). Echinococcosis in humans can be severe, with the manifestations (hydatid disease) depending on the *Echinococcus* sp. ingested. Although there is little information on how many cases of echinococcosis occur in the United States every year, it is thought that the majority of these cases are caused by passage of the parasite from pet dogs to humans. Thus feeding raw meat containing this parasite to dogs could increase risk of human exposure.

Giardia lamblia is a protozoan (flagellate) that colonizes the small intestine of infected hosts. The organism currently is classified genetically into different assemblages; assemblages A and B are those generally associated with human infection but are less common than the host-adapted assemblages C, D, and F in dogs and cats (Scorza et al, 2012). Human giardiasis generally is acquired by ingestion of water contaminated with these assemblages and can result in significant gastrointestinal disease, particularly in immunocompromised people and pets. It is thought that "the greatest risk of zoonotic transmission appears to be from companion animals such as dogs and cats" (Thompson, 2004). Food animal species commonly are infected with *Giardia* spp; one study estimated that 17.7% of sheep and 10.4% of cattle have *Giardia* spp. infection. Prevalence of *Giardia* spp. infection in sheep and cattle appears to decrease with age. The Animal and Plant Health Inspection Service's (APHIS) National Animal Health Monitoring System showed that as many as 45.9% of calves without diarrhea carried *Giardia* spp. Meat can become contaminated with *Giardia* spp. during the slaughter process, and so feeding raw meat could lead to amplification of zoonotic assemblages in the human environment.

Neospora caninum is a coccidian parasite that is shed in feces as oocysts after primary infection of dogs. Cattle are the most common food animal species that serve as intermediate hosts and develop tissue infection. Thus ingestion of raw beef by dogs perpetuates the life cycle. The consequences of *N. caninum* infection of humans have not been fully detailed, but infection may be common. In one study, 69 (6.7%) of 1029 people tested were seropositive (Tranas et al, 1999).

Toxocara canis and *Toxocara cati* are nematodes that account for 10,000 clinical cases of visceral larva migrans or ocular larva migrans (toxocariasis) in the U.S. human population each year. Cattle, pigs, sheep, and rabbits all can serve as paratenic hosts. Eating raw tissues from these animals has the potential to infect dogs or cats, which then contaminate the human environment with eggs that larvate over time and are infectious to humans.

Cats are the only definitive host of the coccidian *Toxoplasma gondii* and as such pass oocysts in feces for a period of time after primary infection. After a 1- to 3-day sporulation period, *T. gondii* oocysts are infectious and can survive in the environment for months. Many species, including humans, are intermediate hosts for *T. gondii* and develop tissue infections that can be associated with clinical signs of disease, particularly if the host is immunocompromised. *T. gondii* tissue cysts are found most frequently in pork, venison, and lamb but also have been found in tissues from free-ranging chickens. Humans are thought to be infected most commonly by ingestion of tissue cysts in undercooked meat, but ingestion of sporulated oocysts also can induce toxoplasmosis. Thus it is incredibly dangerous to feed felines raw meat, particularly if there are immunocompromised family members and the feline feces are not discarded daily. Dogs cannot magnify the infection but have been shown to pass *T. gondii* oocysts in feces after ingestion of infected cat feces.

Organizations Taking a Stand

With the increased prevalence of feeding raw, several prominent animal organization are taking a stand against feeding raw diets to companion animals. The American Animal Hospital Association (AAHA) issued a Raw Protein Diet Position Statement in August 2012: "Feeding a raw protein diet no longer concerns only each individual pet, but has become a larger community health issue; for this reason, AAHA can no longer support or advocate the feeding of raw protein diets to pets" (www.aahanet.org/Library/Raw_Food_Diet.aspx). The American Association of Feline Practitioners (AAFP) and the National Association of State Public Health Veterinarians (NASPHV) both endorsed AAHA's statement.

The American Veterinary Medical Association (AVMA) issued its "Raw or Undercooked Animal-Source Protein in Dog and Cat Diets" policy in August 2012 (www.avma.org). This policy states that "AVMA discourages the feeding to cats and dogs of any animal source protein that has not first been subjected to a process to eliminate pathogens because of the risk of illness to cats and dogs as well as humans."

The FDA issued the following statement in May 2004 and later revised in November of the same year: "FDA does not believe raw meat foods for animals are consistent with the goal of protecting the public from

significant health risks, particularly when such products are brought into the home and/or used to feed domestic pets."

The *Companion Animal Parasite Council* (www.capcvet.org) posted an alert regarding the concerns with feeding raw diets to pets. Listed were the parasites with which animals potentially could become infected after eating raw meat. Besides basic parasite control and fecal checks, feeding cooked food and fresh water were listed as ways of decreasing a pet's overall risk of exposure to zoonotic pathogens that might be transferred to humans.

The *Pet Partners program* (formerly the Delta Society) is a national organization that trains and screens owners and their pets. The pets are used for animal-assisted therapy and work in hospitals, nursing homes, hospices, schools, and other locations. As of June 30, 2010, the board of directors voted to "preclude animals eating raw protein foods from participating in Pet Partners' Therapy Animal Program." The animals have to be off the raw protein food for a minimum of 4 weeks before being allowed back into the programs.

Client Still Insist on Feeding Raw?

Even with education about the potential dangers of feeding companion animals raw meat diets, some clients still are going to insist on feeding raw protein diets. Thus veterinarians should be prepared to educate these clients as well as possible about how to minimize the risk of food-borne illness for owners.

Clients should be encouraged to purchase food that has a decreased chance of contamination, such as food that has undergone irradiation. In general, ground meat has undergone more processing and therefore has a greater likelihood of contamination. Discouraging the feeding of preground meat may decrease the potential for handling of infectious contaminants. Clients also should be aware of the source of the raw meat they are purchasing; meat for human consumption has a lower chance of contamination than meat from other sources.

Clients need to be educated about proper handling and ways to minimize cross contamination. Freezing may inactivate some infectious agents (*T. gondii*, *Giardia* spp.) but does not inactivate others (most bacteria). Freeze drying also is not uniformly effective. One way to reduce the potential for diet-associated infections is to thaw the food in the refrigerator and not at room temperature, at which the bacteria have a greater chance to proliferate. Owners should be educated about avoiding cross contamination from utensils, cutting boards, dishes, and dishcloths. Water bowls should be cleaned and water changed regularly because of probable salivary contamination.

The optimal way to lessen the likelihood of infecting dogs or cats with the agents described is to cook the protein source. *Salmonella* spp. are killed when heated at 55°C (131°F) for 1 hour or at 60°C (140°F) for a half-hour. Poultry should reach an internal temperature of 74°C (165°F) to kill *Campylobacter* spp., and *T. gondii* is killed when whole cuts of meat are heated to 63°C (145°F), ground meat to 71°C (160°F), and poultry to 74°C (165°F).

According to the Companion Animal Parasite Council, all animals, not just those fed raw protein diets, should be receiving parasite preventives monthly and should be evaluated for enteric parasites through bi-yearly fecal checks. These recommendations are even more vital for those animals fed a raw diet because of their greater chance of exposure to some of the common zoonotic parasites.

The CDC website (www.cdc.gov) is an excellent resource and has useful information on how to minimize the risk of food-borne illness for humans.

References and Suggested Reading

Animal and Plant Health Inspection Services Web site: *Cryptosporidium* and *Giardia* in beef calves, National Animal Health Monitoring System. Available at http://www.aphis.usda.gov/animal_health/nahms/beefcowcalf/downloads/chapa/CHAPA_is_Crypto.pdf. Accessed April 7, 2013.

Bhargava K et al: Methicillin-resistant *Staphylococcus aureus* in retail meat, Detroit, Michigan, USA, *Emerg Infect Dis*, June 2011 (letter). Available at wwwnc.cdc.gov/eid/article/17/6/10-1905_article.htm. Accessed September 29, 2011.

Centers for Disease Control and Prevention, 2012.

Companion Animal Parasite Council: Veterinarian council issues pet food alert. Available at www.capcvet.org/downloads/RawFoodWarning.pdf. Accessed August 4, 2011.

Finley R, Reid-Smith R, Weese JS: Human health implications of *Salmonella*-contaminated natural pet treats and raw pet food, *Clin Infect Dis* 42:686, 2006.

Hayes JR et al: Prevalence and antimicrobial resistance of *Enterococcus* species isolated from retail meats, *Appl Environ Microbiol* 69:7153, 2003.

Jackson CR et al: Prevalence, species distribution and antimicrobial resistance of enterococci isolated from dogs and cats in the United States, *J Appl Microbiol* 107:1269, 2009.

Kahn LH: The growing number of immunocompromised, 2008, Bulletin of the Atomic Scientists Web site. Available at: http://www.thebulletin.org/web-edition/columnists/laura-h-kahn/the-growing-number-of-immunocompromised. Accessed April 7, 2013.

Kaplan JE et al: Guidelines for prevention and treatment of opportunistic infections in HIV-infected adults and adolescents, *MMWR Recomm Rep* 58(RR04):1, 2009.

Lefebvre SL et al: Evaluation of the risks of shedding *Salmonellae* and other potential pathogens by therapy dogs fed raw diets in Ontario and Alberta, *Zoonoses Public Health* 55:470, 2008.

LeJeune JT, Hancock DD: Public health concerns associated with feeding raw meat diets to dogs, *J Am Vet Med Assoc* 219:1221, 2001.

Lucio-Forster A et al: Minimal zoonotic risk of cryptosporidiosis from pet dogs and cats, *Trends Parasitol* 26:174, 2010.

Morley PS, Strohmeyer RA, Tankson JD: Evaluation of the association between feeding raw meat and *Salmonella enterica* infections at a Greyhound breeding facility, *J Am Vet Med Assoc* 228:1524, 2006.

Pet Partners: Raw protein diet policy. Available at www.petpartners.org/Page.aspx?pid=638. Accessed August 4, 2011.

Remillard R: NAVC clinician's brief, November 2005. Available at: www.hilltopanimalhospital.com/raw%20meat%20diets.htm.

Scorza AV et al: Detection of *Cryptosporidium spp* in feces of cats and dogs in the United States by PCR assay and IFA (abstract), *J Vet Intern Med* 19:437, 2005.

Scorza AV et al: Comparisons of mammalian *Giardia duodenalis* assemblages based on the β-giardin, glutamate dehydrogenase and triose phosphate isomerase genes, *Vet Parasitol* 189 (2-4):182, 2012. Epub May 8, 2012.

Scorza AV, Brewer MM, Lappin MR: Polymerase chain reaction for the detection of *Cryptosporidium* spp in cat feces, *J Parasitol* 89:423, 2003.

Shuaihua P, Feifei H, Beilei G: Isolation and characterization of methicillin-resistant *Staphylococcus aureus* strains from Louisiana retail meats, *Appl Environ Microbiol* 75:265, 2009.

Stiver SL et al: Septicemic salmonellosis in two cats fed a raw-meat diet, *J Am Anim Hosp Assoc* 39:53, 2003.

Storandt ST et al: Distribution and prevalence of *Echinococcus multilocularis* in wild predators in Nebraska, Kansas, and Wyoming, *J Parasitol* 88:420, 2002.

Strohmeyer RA et al: Evaluation of bacterial and protozoal contamination of commercially available raw meat diets for dogs, *J Am Vet Med Assoc* 228:537, 2006.

Thompson RC: The zoonotic significance and molecular epidemiology of *Giardia* and giardiasis, *Vet Parasitol* 126:15, 2004.

Tranas J et al: Serological evidence of human infection with the protozoan *Neospora caninum*, *Clin Diagn Lab Immunol* 6:765, 1999.

US Food and Drug Administration, Center for Veterinary Medicine: Guidance for industry: manufacture and labeling of raw meat foods for companion and captive noncompanion carnivores and omnivores, revised November 9, 2004. Available at www.fda.gov/.../guidancecomplianceenforcement/guidanceforindustr. Accessed August 4, 2011.

CHAPTER 265

Pet-Associated Illness

ANDREA WANG, *Athens, Georgia*
CRAIG E. GREENE, *Athens, Georgia*

In the broadest terms, zoonoses are infectious or parasitic diseases that are common to both animals and humans. True zoonoses are those that are transmitted to people directly from animals, their secretions, or shared fomites or vectors. This chapter addresses zoonoses associated with companion cats and dogs.

In the United States, more than 60% of households own pets (Bingham et al, 2010; Glaser et al, 2012; Oehler et al, 2009), with an estimated 78.2 million owned dogs and 88 million owned cats. The attachment between people and their pets cannot be underestimated. Dog owners spend an average of $248 per year on veterinary visits, whereas cat owners spend slightly less, at $219 per year. Companion animals have become an integral part of many families. Cohabitation with companion animals provides humans physiologic and emotional benefits that are multifaceted and that have been recognized for years. The benefits to owners of having companion animals include decreased blood pressure, decreased cholesterol and triglyceride levels, decreased anxiety and depression, and increased physical activity and socialization (Barker and Wolen, 2008; Parslow and Jorm 2003).

According to the World Health Organization, there are over 200 zoonotic diseases, with approximately 40 true zoonoses associated with dogs and cats. Among public health professionals, veterinarians are uniquely prepared to educate clients regarding the risks of pet-associated illnesses and to provide treatment and prevention methods (Chomel and Marano, 2009; Glaser et al, 2012). Veterinarians generally receive more training in the zoonotic diseases than most physicians except human infectious disease specialists. Surprisingly, surveys have shown that veterinarians and physicians rarely communicate about zoonotic disease; however, physicians believe veterinarians should be involved in the prevention of zoonotic diseases.

There are several major routes of transmission for infectious diseases to move from animals to humans, and these provide the sections for this chapter. These include transmission by percutaneous contact through a scratch, bite, or skin wound; transmission by inhalation or ingestion of infectious bodily secretions or excretions; transmission by aerosolized infectious particles; transmission by contact with contaminated feces or urine; transmission by direct or indirect mucosal contact; transmission by ingestion of infected or infested tissue; and transmission by shared vectors (Table 265-1). Additional information on individual organisms can be obtained from the Centers for Disease Control and Prevention (CDC) website at www.cdc.gov as well as in the book chapters listed in Table 265-1.

Recommendations by Route of Transmission

Bite and Salivary Spread

Dog and cat bites are the most common source of zoonoses and account for approximately 1% of emergency room visits annually (Oehler et al, 2009). More than 130 pathogens have been isolated from cat and dog bite wounds (Freshwater, 2008; Talan et al, 1999). Immunocompromised individuals are at particular risk of developing systemic infections from bite wound injuries.

Rabies, a progressive viral encephalitis that can affect any mammal, is almost universally fatal in humans and is a serious public health concern (National Association of State Public Health Veterinarians [NASPHV] and CDC, 2011). Humans are infected through a bite from a rabid animal or by contamination of mucous membranes or open wounds with infected saliva or nervous tissue. Clinical signs in affected mammals can include any neurologic signs and invariably progress to rapid onset of neurologic dysfunction and death. Rabies in humans can be prevented by eliminating contact with wildlife, by providing exposed persons with post-exposure rabies prophylaxis, and by vaccinating persons considered at high risk (e.g., veterinary professionals). Cats and dogs should be vaccinated according to current recommendations of the NASPHV (NASPHV and CDC, 2011). The recommendation for disposition of dogs and cats that are suspected of having rabies is covered in the NASPHV rabies compendium (Brown et al, 2011; NASPHV, 2011).

Pasteurella organisms are facultative anaerobic, gramnegative coccobacilli. Pasteurellosis in humans most commonly is caused by bite or scratch wounds from a cat or dog. Although 20% to 30% of dog bite wounds are contaminated with *Pasteurella* organisms, the contamination rate is reported to be up to 80% for cat bite wounds (Freshwater, 2008; Greene and Goldstein, 2012). Pasteurellosis also can be transmitted through animal kissing, sharing of saliva, licking, and aerosolized mucous secretions (Chomel and Sun, 2011). Prophylactic antimicrobial treatment is indicated for cat and dog bite wounds because of the likelihood of infections transmitted through bite wounds. Routine bite wound culture and susceptibility testing is indicated to characterize the

TABLE 265-1

Zoonoses Contracted from Companion Animals by Route of Transmission

Zoonosis	Kirk's Current Veterinary Therapy XII, XIII: Page XIV, XV: Chapter	Infectious Diseases* Chapter
Bite and Salivary Spread		51
• Bartonellosis	XIV: 270, XV: 269, 270	52
• Blastomycosis	XIV: 277	57
• Bordetellosis	XIV: 147	6, 14, 100
• Capnocytophagosis		51
• Helicobacteriosis	XIV: 113, XV: 124	37
• Mycoplasmosis	XIV: 271	31, 32
• Pasteurellosis		35, 51
• Rabies	XIII: 294	20
• Tularemia	XIII: 296	46
Scratch or Close Physical Contact		
• Bartonellosis	XIV: 270, XV: 269, 270	52
• Capnocytophagosis		51
• Cheyletiellosis	XIV: 86	
• Dermatophytosis	XIII: 577, XIV: 105	56
• Pasteurellosis		35, 51
• Staphylococcosis/MRSA infection	XIV: 102	34
• Sporotrichosis		61
• Trypanosomiasis (Chagas' disease)	XIV: 177	72
• Tularemia	XIII: 296	46
Respiratory Particle Spread		
• Bordetellosis	XIV: 147, 279	6, 14, 100
• Coxiellosis	XII: 288	46
• *Rhodococcus* infection		33
• Tularemia	XIII: 296	46
• Yersiniosis (plague)		45
Fecal Contamination		
• Ancylostomiasis	XII: 711	
• Campylobacteriosis	XIII: 626	37
• Cestodiasis	XIII: 1237	
• Cryptosporidiosis	XII: 272, 728	81
• Giardiasis	XII: 716, XIV: 279, XV: 129	77
• Helicobacteriosis	XIV: 113, XV: 124	37
• Salmonellosis	XII: 1123	37
• Toxoplasmosis	XV: 277	79
• Toxocariasis	XII: 711	
• Yersiniosis (enteric)	XIII: 626	37
Urogenital Spread		
• Leptospirosis	XV: 274	42
• Coxiellosis	XII: 288	46
• Brucellosis	XV: Web Ch. 83	38
Ingestion of Infected Meat		
• Cestodiasis/cysticercosis	XIII: 1237	
• Toxoplasmosis	XV: 277	79
• Tularemia		46
Vector Transmission		24
• Babesiosis	XIV: 283, XV: 271	76
• Bartonellosis	XIV: 270, XV: 269, 270	52
• Borreliosis	XV: 271	43
• Dipylidiasis		
• Dirofilariasis	XV: 183, 184,	
• Ehrlichiosis		26
• Leishmaniasis		73
• *Rickettsia* infection (Rocky Mountain spotted fever)	XV: 276	27
• Trypanosomiasis (Chagas' disease)		72
• Yersiniosis (plague)		45

MRSA, Methicillin-resistant *Staphylococcus aureus*.
*Greene CE, editor: *Infectious diseases of the dog and cat*, ed 4, St Louis, 2012, Elsevier.

population and antimicrobial susceptibility of common oral bacteria of cats and dogs.

Pet owners often are unaware of the potential for development of life-threatening diseases secondary to animal bite wounds. Any individual, particularly if immunocompromised (Box 265-1), should seek professional medical treatment immediately after sustaining bite wounds from an animal. Treatment of bite wounds may include wound management, deep culture, radiography, débridement, antimicrobial therapy, and rabies prophylaxis if applicable. Prevention of bite wounds includes facilitating early recognition of behaviors of both the human and pet that lead to bites, educating families in the awareness and assessment of risk factors, and advocating behavioral training to benefit pets and owners alike (de Keuster and Overall, 2011).

Scratch or Close Physical Contact

Up to 62% of pet owners allow their animals to sleep on their beds (Chomel and Sun, 2011). Zoonotic infections acquired by close contact with a pet usually are uncommon; however, severe cases of illness have been reported. Unlike infections from bite wounds, transmission of disease from a scratch or close physical contact often is overlooked due to the constant and common nature of incurring minor scratches, kissing a pet, being licked by a pet, and sharing beds with pets. For instance, zoonotic transmission of *Bartonella henselae* (cat-scratch disease) occurs by close contact with cats infested by the cat flea *Ctenocephalides felis felis*. However, only 30% of reported cases of cat-scratch disease involve a history of a cat scratch. Immunocompromised individuals (see Box 265-1) should be discouraged from sharing their beds with their pets, playing roughly with their pets, and regularly kissing their pets to decrease risk of transmission. Routine hand washing as recommended by the CDC (2013) should be performed after contact with pets. In the veterinary setting, developing habits of frequent hand washing and using personal protective gear can aid in the prevention of disease transmission. The presence of pets in the house should be brought to the attention of physicians if any unusual or prolonged human illness is present.

Aerosolized Infectious Particles

Infections transmitted through the respiratory tract of animals are rare. However, pneumonia is the most common disease manifestation when spread by this route and can be severely debilitating or life threatening.

Bordetella bronchiseptica is a commensal bacterium of the dog and cat respiratory tract. Although bordetellosis is common in dogs and cats because of the pathogenic potential of *B. bronchiseptica,* the bacterium is not commonly transmitted to people. Routine vaccination is recommended for dogs to decrease the incidence and severity of canine bordetellosis. Areas where animal density is high, such as dog parks, shows, kennels, and sporting meets, should be avoided to prevent transmission of *Bordetella,* particularly when households include immunocompromised individuals (see Box 265-1).

Q fever, caused by *Coxiella burnetii,* is a risk for individuals handling placentas. Prevention is through proper use of personal protective equipment, including protective masks, eyewear, gloves, and barrier garments, when handling reproductive tissues.

Yersinia pestis usually is transmitted to humans from rodent fleas. However, infected cats can transmit the organism directly by aerosolization, causing the deadly form of disease, pneumonic plague.

Tularemia is caused by *Francisella tularensis,* an endemic and highly infectious bacterium found in lagomorphs and rodents. Humans are infected by bites from ticks, flies, or mosquitoes, or from infected cats via scratches, bites, or aerosols.

Fecal Contamination

Enteric organisms posing zoonotic risk may be directly infectious or may shed eggs, oocysts, or cysts, which are immediately infectious or subsequently become infectious in the environment. Many of these can be identified in the feces of the infected host. Although a number of these organisms can be shared between pets and humans, diseases are transmitted more commonly between humans. This is the case for human giardiasis, cryptosporidiosis, campylobacteriosis, and helicobacteriosis. On the other hand, canine and feline roundworms, hookworms, and *Toxoplasma gondii* pose significant risks to humans, and infections with these organisms are among the most commonly reported zoonoses. Each of these agents requires a period of time in the environment before becoming infectious.

Cutaneous larva migrans is a superficial skin disease of humans caused by hookworm larvae. Adult hookworms live in the small intestine of cats and dogs and shed eggs in feces and into the environment, where they hatch and develop into first-, second-, then the infective third-stage larvae (L_3) within 2 to 9 days. Dogs and cats become infected with hookworms via ingestion of L_3 from a contaminated environment, larval penetration of the skin, or ingestion of other vertebrate or invertebrate hosts with infective larvae in their tissues. Immature and adult worms migrate and attach to the mucosa of the small intestine, digest the tissue, inject anticoagulants, and suck blood. Humans are considered accidental hosts when their skin makes contact with larvae, and aberrant migration through the dermis causes dermatitis characterized by cellulitis, erythema, and edema secondary to hypersensitivity. Abdominal pain also has been reported in some people who ingest larvated eggs. The Companion Animal Parasite Council (CAPC, 2011) has recommended treatment and prevention protocols for canine and feline ectoparasites and endoparasites.

Toxocariasis most commonly is caused by the roundworms *Toxocara canis* and *Toxocara cati,* which normally are carried by their definitive hosts, the dog and cat, respectively. *Toxocara* spp. infect humans as accidental hosts through human ingestion of contaminated soil, consumption of raw or undercooked meat from infected paratenic hosts, or indirect contamination of food. Dogs and cats are infected by ingesting paratenic hosts or via the transmammary route while nursing. Eggs shed via dog and cat feces become embryonated and infective in the environment within 3 weeks to several months. An estimated 5.3% of dogs and 5.5% of cats are shedding *Toxocara* eggs in the United States. Americans have an average seroprevalence of 13.9%, with a majority of infected individuals being asymptomatic. However, toxocariasis may cause serious disease in humans by aberrant migration, including ocular larva migrans, visceral larva migrans, and neural toxocariasis. Although most infections are undetected, clinical signs may include fever, nonspecific generalized symptoms, coughing and wheezing, cognitive dysfunction, seizures, and even death.

T. gondii is an obligate intracellular two-host coccidian parasite that infects animals globally, including mammals, birds, reptiles, and amphibians. Domestic and wild felids are the only definitive host of *T. gondii,* and no other host sheds oocysts. Three to 10 days after a naïve cat ingests bradyzoite cysts in paratenic host tissue, it becomes infected and sheds oocysts through the gastrointestinal tract for only 7 to 10 days. The prevalence of oocyst shedding is low in cats (1%) because of the short duration of shedding following acute infection. Oocysts need to be exposed to moisture and air for 1 to 5 days before they become infectious. For this reason, daily cleaning of the litter box is an effective way of preventing toxoplasmosis in humans. Disease caused by *T. gondii* is secondary to rapidly dividing tachyzoites and the development of *T. gondii* granulomas with ensuing necrosis and inflammation. Seroprevalence is 25% to 50% in people in temperate regions and 30% in dogs and cats. Seroprevalence rates increase toward equatorial regions. Although infection in people usually causes mild and transient symptoms, toxoplasmosis is an important zoonosis because of the possibility of acute infection, placentitis, and transplacental transmission in seronegative pregnant women. Immunocompromised individuals may develop severe disease or a reactivation of previously encysted bradyzoites.

Cyclophyllidean tapeworm infections are shared between humans and pets and can be life threatening.

Zoonotic species include *Dipylidium caninum, Taenia* spp., *Echinococcus* spp., and *Mesocestoides* spp. Dogs and cats become infected by ingesting intermediate or paratenic hosts such as fleas, lice, rodents, and ruminants containing larval cestodes. Eggs released from proglottids shed in the feces of the definitive hosts are ingested by the intermediate or paratenic hosts. Mature adult cestodes live in the gastrointestinal tract and frequently do not cause clinical disease. Humans are infected after ingesting eggs shed by definitive hosts or by consuming undercooked or raw meat of intermediate hosts. *Taenia* and *Echinococcus* eggs are immediately infectious when passed and can cause serious cyst-forming disease in people, which serve as intermediate hosts. Humans are the definitive hosts of *Dipylidium caninum,* and infection can occur by ingestion of fleas or proglottids shed in feces. Stringent adherence to flea and lice control measures is required to remove the paratenic host and prevent *D. caninum* infection in dogs and cats. Prevention of predation and scavenging activity will limit the opportunity for dogs and cats to acquire infection with *Taenia* spp. or *Echinococcus* spp. via ingestion of cysts in intermediate hosts. In areas where *Echinococcus granulosus* and *Echinococcus multilocularis* are present, routine monthly deworming of dogs with praziquantel is recommended. The prevention of cestode infection in humans, cats, and dogs can be achieved by following cesticidal and ectoparasite control guidelines as recommended by the CAPC (2011).

Animal feces should be removed from the environment daily, with the feces bagged and trashed, burned, or flushed down a toilet. Aggressive decontamination measures are necessary to eradicate resistant stages such as oocysts or eggs. These measures include application of heat (boiling water, steam, propane gun, fire), removal of contaminated substrate (5 to 6 inches of soil), or entombment of eggs under concrete or asphalt. Children's sandboxes should be covered when not in use. Metal or concrete surfaces should be decontaminated with bleach or ammonia solutions, whereas soil and gravel should be decontaminated with heat or a desiccant such as sodium borate to remove hookworm larvae.

Urogenital Spread

Infection with organisms spread by urogenital contact can be prevented by avoiding direct contact with animal urine, reproductive organs, and urogenital secretions. *Brucella canis, C. burnetii,* and leptospires are the most common organisms spread in this manner (see Table 265-1). Wearing protective clothing and gear when handling these infectious materials is important.

Leptospirosis is caused by motile obligate aerobic bacterial spirochetes of the genus *Leptospira.* Pathogenic serovars of leptospires persist by infecting maintenance hosts, which typically do not manifest clinical signs. The organism is transmitted to incidental hosts (including humans) by direct or indirect contact of mucosae or damaged skin with urine or contaminated fomites, respectively. Although most human infections are associated with environmental exposure to contaminated water, the zoonotic potential of canine leptospirosis should be considered significant. Gloves, disposable gowns, and face protection should be worn while handling animals suspected of infection and while cleaning cages. A urinary catheter may be placed in the patient to control urine handling and cleaning until bacteriuria is eliminated. Shedding is terminated within 24 hours of initiation of antimicrobial therapy. Vaccines containing antigens of organisms in serogroups canicola, pomona, icterohaemorrhagiae, and grippotyphosa are recommended in dogs at risk of exposure and may lessen shedding of leptospires if the vaccinated dog contacts the agent.

Ingestion of Infected Meat

Ingestion of undercooked meat is the main route of transmission of *T. gondii* to humans. Transmission of zoonotic disease by ingestion of infected meat with cysts of tapeworms and *T. gondii* can be prevented by thoroughly cooking meat to an internal temperature of 71° C (160° F). Rodents, rabbits, and hares can have tularemia, and care should be taken to avoid direct contact with, aerosolization of, or ingestion of undercooked meat. In general, animal meat of unknown origin or undercooked meat should not be fed to household pets.

Vector Transmission

Vector-borne zoonotic diseases are transmitted indirectly to humans by ticks, mosquitoes, flies, lice, and mites. Wildlife species, rather than cats and dogs, serve as reservoirs for the majority of these diseases. Vector-borne diseases can be prevented by practicing ectoparasite control for people and pets. Tick-borne disease transmission often requires a period of attachment of the tick to its host. Routine and thorough inspection and removal of ticks from people and pets after exposure can prevent transmission effectively. The CAPC guidelines (2011) recommend vaccination against *Borrelia burgdorferi* for at-risk dogs in endemic areas.

Human cutaneous dirofilariasis is a rare infection caused by filarial worms of the genus *Dirofilaria*, which includes various species that naturally infect cats and dogs, including the heartworm *Dirofilaria immitis*. Microfilariae are carried by dogs, cats, and raccoons, and transmission to humans occurs by infected mosquito bites. Humans are dead-end hosts, and symptoms are related to aberrant migration in subcutaneous and ocular tissue. Pesticides or growth regulators approved by the Environmental Protection Agency can be applied to the premises to kill environmental stages of mosquitoes, fleas, and ticks. Animals in regions with endemic parasitic disease should be tested annually for vector-transmitted pathogens.

Preventive Measures for Pets

Compared with the incidence of all human infectious or parasitic diseases, the incidence of true zoonoses from dogs or cats is low. However, veterinarians are in the unique position of having been alerted to specific zoonoses through veterinary training and often serve as the first line in recognizing these diseases. Therefore veterinarians need to be aware of potential zoonotic agents to be able to identity, treat, and prevent the infecting animals, and also to educate clients and the general population on the risks. Household pets should be kept free of ectoparasites, routinely dewormed, and regularly examined by a veterinarian. The following information gives recommendations and sources for preventing zoonotic infections in dogs and cats.

The CAPC (2011) provides guidelines for veterinarians and owners for the prevention of infection with endoparasites and ectoparasites, many of which can carry or are themselves the cause of zoonotic diseases. CAPC recommendations include lifelong, year-round treatment with broad-spectrum heartworm anthelmintics that have activity against parasites with zoonotic potential. The targeted endoparasites include various species of roundworms, hookworms, whipworms, tapeworms, and heartworms. The targeted ectoparasites include various species of fleas, ticks, mites, and mosquitoes. Many commercially available formulations contain combinations of endoparasiticides and ectoparasiticides (CAPC, 2011).

Heartworm testing and a fecal flotation and smear analysis should be conducted at least yearly as disease surveillance in cats and dogs. Puppies and their dams should be treated with anthelmintics when puppies are 2, 4, 6, and 8 weeks of age and then should receive preventive therapy monthly. Kittens should receive biweekly treatment starting at 3 weeks of age and should begin monthly preventive therapy at 9 weeks of age.

Environmental control is an integral component of parasite prevention and control because of the many resistant environmental stages (eggs, larvae, oocysts, cysts, oocytes) of various enteric zoonotic organisms. Parasitized animals should be treated aggressively to prevent environmental contamination and monitored by fecal examination to confirm treatment efficacy. Predation behavior should be eliminated in household pets to prevent ingestion of infected paratenic hosts.

Preventive Measures for People

Individuals with altered immune systems may be particularly susceptible to all diseases, including zoonotic diseases. Groups of people with conditions that may put them in an immunocompromised state are listed in Box 265-1. Veterinarians should be particularly vigilant in identifying these individuals and counseling them in zoonosis prevention. Additional steps veterinarians can take to increase awareness of zoonotic diseases are engaging in frequent discussions with clients, physicians, and public health agencies; providing educational brochures on common zoonotic diseases to clients; and attending or providing continuing education on zoonoses.

Hand washing is the most important preventive step for reducing disease transmission. Hands always should be washed immediately after contact with animals and soil, after cleaning up feces or urine, and before eating or drinking. Soap is the best agent for hand washing. If soap is not available, alcohol-based hand sanitizers with at least 60% alcohol can be used to reduce the number of infectious agents on hands. The CDC (2013) has posted recommendations for proper hand-washing techniques.

The prevention of zoonotic diseases is the most effective way to eradicate them. Vigilance on the veterinarian's part can increase awareness in veterinary professionals, medical professionals, and clients alike.

References and Suggested Reading

Barker SB, Wolen AR: The benefits of human-companion animal interaction: a review, *J Vet Med Educ* 35:487, 2008.

Bingham GM, Budke CM, Slater MR: Knowledge and perceptions of dog-associated zoonoses: Brazos County, Texas, USA, *Prev Vet Med* 93:211, 2010.

Brown CM et al: Compendium of animal rabies prevention and control, 2011, *J Am Vet Med Assoc* 239:609, 2011.

Centers for Disease Control and Prevention: Handwashing: clean hands save lives, updated January 11, 2013. Available at www.cdc.gov/handwashing/. Accessed [April 4, 2013].

Chomel BB, Marano N: Essential veterinary education in emerging infections, modes of introduction of exotic animals, zoonotic diseases, bioterrorism, implications for human and animal health and disease manifestation, *Rev Sci Tech* 28:559, 2009.

Chomel BB, Sun B: Zoonoses in the bedroom, *Emerg Infect Dis* 17:167, 2011.

Companion Animal Parasite Council: CAPC general guidelines, updated May 2011. Available at www.capcvet.org/recommendations/. Accessed [April 4, 2013].

de Keuster T, Overall KL: Preventing dog bite injuries: the need for a collaborative approach, *Vet Rec* 169:341, 2011.

Freshwater A: Why your housecat's trite little bite could cause you quite a fright: a study of domestic felines on the occurrence and antibiotic susceptibility of *Pasteurella multocida*, *Zoonoses Public Health* 55:507, 2008.

Glaser CA, Powers EL, Greene CE: Zoonotic infections of medical importance in immunocompromised humans. In Greene CE, editor: *Infectious diseases of the dog and cat*, St Louis, 2012, Elsevier.

Greene CE, Goldstein EJC: Bite wound infections. In Greene CE, editor: *Infectious diseases of the dog and cat*, St Louis, 2012, Elsevier.

Humane Society of the United States: U.S. pet ownership statistics, August 12, 2011. Available at www.humanesociety.org/issues/pet_overpopulation/facts/pet_ownership_statistics.html. Accessed October 31, 2011.

National Association of State Public Health Veterinarians: NASPHV compendia and recommendations, 2011. Available at www.nasphv.org/documentsCompendia.html. Accessed [April 10, 2013].

National Association of State Public Health Veterinarians, Centers for Disease Control and Prevention: Compendium of measures to prevent disease associated with animals in public settings, 2011: National Association of State Public Health Veterinarians, Inc., *MMWR Recomm Rep* 60(RR-4):1, 2011. Available at www.ncbi.nlm.nih.gov/pubmed/21546893. Accessed October 31, 2011.

Oehler RL et al: Bite-related and septic syndromes caused by cats and dogs, *Lancet Infect Dis* 9:439, 2009.

Parslow RA, Jorm AF: Pet ownership and risk factors for cardiovascular disease: another look, *Med J Aust* 179:466, 2003.

Talan DA et al: Bacteriologic analysis of infected dog and cat bites. Emergency Medicine Animal Bite Infection Study Group, *N Engl J Med* 340:85, 1999.

World Health Organization: Zoonoses and veterinary public health, 2011. Available at www.who.int/zoonoses/en. Accessed October 31, 2011.

CHAPTER 266

Vaccine-Associated Adverse Effects in Dogs

GEORGE E. MOORE, *West Lafayette, Indiana*

Vaccines are a vital component of veterinary medicine, dramatically reducing the incidence, morbidity, and mortality of infectious diseases. Increasing use of vaccines is desirable, at least theoretically, to protect our patients against infectious pathogens. As immunologic stimulants, however, vaccines can produce undesirable side effects. The risk and occurrence of vaccine-associated adverse events, as well as concerns of disease risk, client costs, and vaccine protocol adjustments, limit the automatic addition of newly available vaccines into practice protocols. Public media attention on adverse events potentially associated with human vaccines has heightened owner awareness of vaccine risk, often decreasing their acceptance of vaccines as an important prophylactic measure against disease. Expanding our knowledge of these risks and our communication to owners regarding these risks will improve the acceptability of recommended protocols (Welborn et al, 2011).

Innate Immune Responses

Innate immunity provides rapid nonspecific, non–memory-associated response to tissue damage and foreign pathogens. These stimuli lead to activation and secretion of cytokines and chemokines as part of an inflammatory response that can help establish adaptive immunity. Vaccine components that can stimulate innate immunity include nucleic acids, peptides, carbohydrates, toxins, lipids, adjuvants, and other molecules. These can induce localized reactions within minutes or hours after vaccination with hallmark signs of inflammation including pain, erythema, and swelling. Pain at the time of vaccine injection also may be caused by vaccine components or biologic properties such as pH and osmolality. Various vaccine components can serve as immune stimulants, and greater antigen exposure (volume of vaccine per kilogram of body weight) increases the risk of a localized innate reaction. Mitigation or prevention of clinically apparent innate responses is common in human medicine through administration of nonsteroidal antiinflammatory drugs (NSAIDs). Prevaccination administration of NSAIDs to small animal patients is not routinely recommended because of the potential for drug-associated adverse events in young pets, inadequate timing in relation to onset of action, limited impact on immediate hypersensitivity reactions, or lack of acceptable over-the-counter products for administration by owners. Prevaccine administration of NSAIDs by veterinarians may be indicated for selected canine patients with a history of localized postvaccinal reactions.

Hypersensitivity Reactions

Immediate

Immediate (type I) hypersensitivity reaction is the most common serious adverse event following vaccination in dogs. This reaction is mediated by immunoglobulin E (IgE), the principal cellular component is the mast cell or basophil, and the reaction is amplified or modified by eosinophils, neutrophils, and platelets. The precise mechanism by which some patients are more prone to type I hypersensitivity is not clear. It has been shown in people that some individuals preferentially produce more type 2 helper T cells that secrete interleukin-4 (IL-4), IL-5, and IL-13, which favor IgE activation. IgE produced preferentially in response to certain antigens or allergens links with the allergen at receptors on mass cells and basophils to trigger mass cell degranulation. Mediators of immediate hypersensitivity include preformed agents such as histamine, tryptase, and kininogenase, and newly generated mediators such as leukotrienes and prostaglandins. These mediators increase vascular dilation and permeability and cause smooth muscle contraction.

Antigens within vaccines that can cause type I hypersensitivity reactions include foreign proteins such as residual culture media proteins, additives, preservatives, and possibly adjuvants. Protein of bovine origin from fetal calf serum has been incriminated as an IgE allergen causing hypersensitivity reactions in some dogs (Ohmori et al, 2005). Different vaccines, even with the same label antigen (e.g., *Leptospira*), may contain differing quantities of foreign proteins after the vaccine manufacturing process. Thus practitioners may observe different reaction rates when using the same antigen vaccines from different manufacturers. Continued vaccine quality improvements, however, have reduced hypersensitivity reaction rates for many vaccines in the last decade.

A dose-response relationship has been observed between the number of vaccines administered at one time and the likelihood of an immediate hypersensitivity reaction (Moore et al, 2005). This relationship derives from the increased risk associated with individual vaccines in smaller dogs (i.e., <10 kg) as well as the increase in risk as additional vaccines are given at one time to any dog. It is therefore prudent to limit the number of parenterally administered vaccines administered at one time, particularly to smaller dogs or dogs at high risk. Increased risk has been demonstrated for some small breeds such as dachshunds, pugs, miniature pinschers, Boston terriers, and Chihuahuas, and selected large breed dogs such as boxers and weimaraners. This increased risk most likely represents genetic predisposition to rapid mast cell degranulation in the face of low quantities of antigen. The optimal separation time between administration of different vaccines is not known, but a 2-week interval is considered reasonable.

Clinical signs of type I hypersensitivity commonly are noted in the skin and vascular systems and include facial or periorbital edema, wheals, urticaria, pruritus, hypotensive shock, or collapse. Vomiting with or without diarrhea and respiratory distress are noted less commonly. Treatment of immediate hypersensitivity reactions should be tailored to the severity of the clinical signs. Treatment may include the H_1 antihistamine diphenhydramine to block histamine receptors, rapidly soluble glucocorticoids to block arachidonic pathways, and intravenous crystalloid fluids to counteract hypotensive shock. Epinephrine and oxygen therapy are not often necessary but are indicated for cyanosis and respiratory distress. In patients with documented immediate hypersensitivity reactions to previous vaccinations, prevaccination administration of diphenhydramine (2 to 3 mg/kg IM) may prevent recurrence of type I reactions; untreated dogs may or may not demonstrate adverse effects after subsequent vaccinations.

Autoimmune

Vaccine-induced autoimmune hemolytic anemia (IMHA) or thrombocytopenia (ITP) can be a concern to practitioners because of the potentially life-threatening severity of these disorders. Because these diseases are immune mediated, vaccination through immune stimulation may be a possible inciting cause. Nevertheless, a cause-and-effect association with veterinary vaccines has not been established for IMHA or ITP in dogs (Huang et al, 2012), and retrospective studies have been severely limited or have produced conflicting results. Disease onset occurring within a month of vaccination may be a random occurrence, and critical predisposing factors are not known.

Vaccination of dogs previously diagnosed with IMHA or ITP is a more pragmatic issue. Vaccination should not be considered until the disease is in remission and administration of immunosuppressive drugs has been reduced. In dogs with controlled disease, titer testing may be prudent to evaluate the patient's immune protection for some vaccine antigens. If protective immunity cannot be determined or is not evident through testing, vaccination is indicated, but the number of vaccines given should be limited to minimize excessive immune stimulation.

Vasculitis

Ischemic dermatopathy and cutaneous vasculitis have been reported weeks or months after vaccination, most notably at sites of rabies vaccination. In case series reports, poodles appeared to be affected more commonly and vaccines from more than one manufacturer were associated with the lesion, which suggests a genetic predisposition. Lesions typically manifest as focal alopecia, although multifocal cutaneous disease involving pinnal margins, periocular regions, and footpads has also been reported. Because of a reduced number of blood vessels and lymphocytic cuffing around vessels, an ischemic vasculopathy appears to be the hallmark lesion. Treatment with pentoxifylline, a methylxanthine derivative used for vasculopathy in people, generally is recommended. Although the optimal dosage of pentoxifylline for this syndrome is not known, 15 mg/kg q8h PO commonly is administered. Through an increase in erythrocyte flexibility and reduction in erythrocyte fragmentation, vascular permeability and tissue perfusion are believed to be improved. Improvement in clinical signs may take days to weeks, however, and may or may not be treatment related.

Hypertrophic Osteodystrophy

Hypertrophic osteodystrophy of the metaphyseal region of long bones, often the distal radius and ulna, has been noted in young dogs within 2 weeks of vaccination. Large-breed dogs such as weimaraners, Great Danes, Irish setters, and German shepherds have been reported to be at increased risk of this disease. Because the disease most commonly is reported in young dogs of vaccination age, the cause-and-effect association is unclear. Clinical signs include lameness, metaphyseal swelling, fever, and lymphadenopathy with leukocytosis. Although lameness, joint swelling, and radiographic bony changes have prompted the use of NSAIDs for their antiinflammatory and analgesic properties, glucocorticoids may provide a superior response to NSAIDs and are the recommended treatment (Safra et al, 2013). High-dose pulse therapy with prednisolone at an initial dosage of 2 to 4 mg/kg q24h PO tapered to a physiologic dose within a week can produce dramatic improvement in affected patients.

Systemic Illness

Systemic illness is an uncommon adverse effect of vaccines but may occur as a self-limiting infection with modified live vaccines. Treatment with antiinflammatory, antipyretic, or even antibiotic drugs seldom is indicated but may be considered if opportunistic secondary infections also are present. Because systemic illness is associated with actual infection, discernment of the cause may be challenging if it involves pathogens that may be part of a disease complex—as, for example, with respiratory disease following administration of *Bordetella bronchiseptica* live vaccine.

Modified live virus vaccines given during pregnancy may result in fetal disease or reproductive disorders in the dam. These vaccines, if administered to very young puppies, also may produce neonatal infections. Administration of vaccine to gravid bitches is not recommended unless the vaccine is specified by the manufacturer as safe for use in pregnant animals.

Inadvertent parenteral administration of a live vaccine approved only for topical (e.g., intranasal) use also may lead to systemic illness. Subcutaneous administration of an intranasal *B. bronchiseptica*–canine influenza vaccine has been reported to cause fever, injection site cellulitis, leukocytosis, icterus, and diffuse hepatocellular necrosis in a dog (Toshach et al, 1997).

Vaccine Failure

Regrettably, no vaccine will stimulate a protective immune response in 100% of the patients receiving it. Furthermore, not all vaccines are licensed for prevention of disease; some vaccines may only reduce the severity of clinical illness. The acceptable vaccine efficacy for some biologics may be less than 90%, which indicates that some vaccinated animals may remain unprotected. Herd immunity may limit the occurrence of disease in these individuals. Factors that can cause vaccine failure may be related to the vaccine itself, the patient receiving the vaccine, or human error. The most common cause of vaccine failure in young animals is interference from maternal-derived antibodies. It is recommended that the last dose of modified live virus vaccine (e.g., canine distemper virus or canine parvovirus) given to a puppy not be administered before 14 weeks of age. Failure of killed vaccines can occur if the required second dose is not administered at a proper interval to stimulate adequate immunity and an anamnestic response. Practitioners should ensure that manufacturers' instructions are followed for proper administration and maximum patient protection.

Reporting of Adverse Effects

Adverse events may simply be chance instances of infection or disease occurring around the time of vaccination, not causally associated with administration of vaccine. Nevertheless, veterinarians should report vaccine-associated adverse events to the specific product manufacturer or to the U.S. Department of Agriculture (USDA) Center for Veterinary Biologics (http://aphis.usda.gov/animal_health/vet_biologics/vb_adverse_event.shtml). Manufacturers are required to submit adverse events summaries regularly to the USDA, which has regulatory oversight for animal vaccines. Adverse event reporting by veterinarians is critical for manufacturer awareness of product safety and better documentation of the incidence of frequently occurring and uncommon adverse effects observed after administration of a vaccine.

References and Suggested Reading

Day MJ: Vaccine side effects: fact and fiction, *Vet Microbiol* 117:51, 2006.

Huang AA et al: Idiopathic immune-mediated thrombocytopenia and recent vaccination in dogs, *J Vet Intern Med* 26:142, 2012.

Iwasaki A, Medzhitov R: Regulation of adaptive immunity by the innate immune system, *Science* 327:291, 2010.

Kang SM, Compans RW: Host responses from innate to adaptive immunity after vaccination: molecular and cellular events, *Mol Cells* 27:5, 2009.

Moore GE et al: Adverse events diagnosed within three days of vaccine administration in dogs, *J Am Vet Med Assoc* 227:1102, 2005.

Moore GE, HogenEsch H: Adverse vaccinal events in dogs and cats, *Vet Clin North Am Small Anim Pract* 40:393, 2010.

Ohmori K et al: IgE reactivity to vaccine components in dogs that developed immediate-type allergic reactions after vaccination, *Vet Immunol Immunopathol* 104:249, 2005.

Safra N et al: Clinical manifestations, response to treatment, and clinical outcome for Weimaraners with hypertrophic osteodystrophy: 53 cases (2009-2011), *J Am Vet Med Assoc* 242:1260, 2013.

Toshach K, Jackson MW, Dubielzig RR: Hepatocellular necrosis associated with the subcutaneous injection of an intranasal *Bordetella bronchiseptica*-canine parainfluenza vaccine, *J Am Anim Hosp Assoc* 33(2):126, 1997.

Welborn LV et al: 2011 AAHA canine vaccination guidelines, *J Am Anim Hosp Assoc* 47:1, 2011.

CHAPTER **267**

Update on Vaccine-Associated Adverse Effects in Cats

DENNIS W. MACY, *Fort Collins, Colorado*
MICHAEL R. LAPPIN, *Fort Collins, Colorado*

Adverse reactions potentially can occur after the administration of any vaccine. Reactions can be local or systemic and can vary considerably in severity and time to develop after vaccination. However, adverse reactions to vaccination, including failure to confer immunity, are relatively uncommon in dogs and cats. For example, in a study of more than 1.2 million dogs, the overall rate of adverse reactions was 38.2 out of 10,000 dogs that had been administered vaccines within the previous 3 days (Moore et al, 2005). In a study of 496,189 cats, the overall rate of adverse reactions was 51.6 out of 10,000 cats that had been administered vaccines within the previous 30 days (Moore et al, 2007). Vaccine-associated adverse effects can vary for each vaccine type and vaccine antigen and are discussed individually in most guideline committee reports (Richards et al, 2006; Welborn et al, 2011).

Vaccine-associated adverse events that occur over the long term and have a low incidence are more difficult to study; injection site sarcomas and potential immune-mediated sequelae associated with vaccination are two examples. The objective of this chapter is to provide updates on injection site sarcomas and vaccination-associated autoantibodies in cats.

Vaccine-Associated Sarcoma

It has been more than 20 years since Dr. Mattie Hendrick, a veterinary pathologist at the University of Pennsylvania, and her co-authors published an article titled "Postvaccinal Sarcomas in the Cat: Epidemiology and Electron Probe Microanalytical Identification of Aluminum" in *Cancer Research* (1992), which was the first manuscript to suggest a linked between vaccination and sarcoma development. Dr. Hendrick initially brought her concerns to the forefront in 1991 in a letter to the editor of the Journal of the American Veterinary Association, in which she suggested that a rise in sarcomas at vaccines sites might have been associated with the recent enactment of a state law in Pennsylvania requiring the rabies vaccination of cats. During the same period as the study (1985), the introduction of the first feline leukemia virus (FeLV) vaccine, which contained aluminum adjuvant, and the switch from a modified live rabies vaccine to an adjuvanted killed rabies vaccine occurred. Since then, many of Dr. Hendrick's observations and the studies and findings of other researchers have matured and solidified our understanding of the cause, the risk factors, and the incidence of vaccine-associated sarcoma (VAS) in cats. It also has become clear that sarcomas can develop locally after other medical events, including other injections and rarely microchip placement. Thus the global term currently used is feline injection site sarcoma. Although our understanding of this condition still is incomplete, this chapter presents an overview of the current information concerning the pathogenesis and clinical management of VAS.

Sarcoma Development

The association between sites of vaccine administration and subsequent development of high-grade sarcomas and other mesenchymal tumors in cats has been well documented and accepted by the veterinary community. The association between previous vaccination and tumor at vaccination sites in cats has been observed worldwide and has a reported prevalence ranging from 1 in 1000 to 1 in 10,000 in cats. It has been estimated that up to 22,000 new cases of VAS occur annually. Vaccination site tumors also have been reported in dogs, horses, and ferrets but far less frequently. The time from vaccination to tumor development may be as short as 3 months, with 93% of tumors developing within 4 years. Sarcoma development also has been reported sporadically at the site of injection or implantation of other substances, including lufeneron, cisplatin, long-acting penicillin, long-acting glucocorticoid preparations, meloxicam, and foreign material such as suture and microchips.

Tumor genesis associated with chronic inflammation is well documented in a variety of species and potentially correlates with the amount of inflammation and the degree of fibrous proliferation in response to the foreign materials in some cats. The observed chronic inflammation after the administration of adjuvant containing rabies and FeLV fits this model. A 2002 report from the United Kingdom found that injection site sarcomas were five times more likely to develop in cats that were administered aluminum-adjuvanted FeLV vaccines than nonadjuvanted vaccines. Further supporting the role of adjuvanted vaccines in the development of sarcoma was a recent study by Shaw and colleagues (2009). In that study, the change in the location of VASs from 1990 to 2006 was studied. In 1996, there was a recommendation to change the site of administration of the most frequently adjuvanted vaccines rabies and leukemia vaccines from the intrascapular space to the rear legs. In the time since this recommendation was made, a drop in sarcomas developing in the intrascapular space was noted and more than a doubling of sarcomas reported in the rear legs was observed.

The initial reports identified only FeLV and rabies vaccines as being associated with an increased risk of sarcoma development at site of vaccination. However, an additional study in Canada (Lester et al, 1996) suggested a role for other adjuvanted killed virus vaccines, including vaccines against panleukopenia and respiratory viruses, because sarcomas were noted in cats that had not received FeLV vaccination, and the incidence of sarcoma in the population decreased after a switch was made to modified live virus vaccines. Although tumors have been reported to develop subsequent to the administration of nonadjuvanted vaccines, this is thought to be less common and

may be associated with other factors such as trauma. Trauma associated with the injection process, including muscle tearing or the introduction of hair into the subcutaneous tissues at the time of injection, can result in inflammation. Although vaccines commonly contain aluminum hydroxide in suspension as an adjuvant, postvaccinal inflammation and sarcoma development also occur with vaccines using a soluble adjuvant (carbopol). It is clear that not all substances carry the same risk, and reports of sarcoma initiation following insulin administration in cats are lacking. It is thought that the risk of tumor development may relate to the reactive nature of the vaccine components or other injectable substances as well as the qualitative nature of the local inflammatory response and the various oxidative products generated by the cellular response. This is in addition to the magnitude of the fibrous response to the vaccine and its components.

Dr. Elizabeth McNiel (2001) at the University of Minnesota investigated the role of free radical damage associated with feline vaccines in producing mutations that may stimulate oncogenesis and found that cell cultures exposed to adjuvant-containing vaccines developed mutations that increased as vaccine concentration increased, whereas no mutations were found after exposure to nonadjuvanted vaccines. She further found that the mutations could be blocked by addition of a free radical scavenger. In 1999 the World Health Organization International Agency for Research on Cancer acknowledged the evidence for the potential carcinogenicity of feline adjuvanted vaccine.

Although not all veterinarians are convinced of the role of inflammation in the pathogenesis of VASs, chronic inflammation is a well-known tumor promoter in a variety of species. Cats are uniquely sensitive in this regard and frequently develop mesenchymal tumors secondary to chronic inflammation associated with ocular injury, more so than any other species. Species genetic susceptibility to foreign body inflammation–induced tumor genesis is not unique to the cat; it also has been studied in mice, and some strains are known to be resistant to foreign body sarcoma development, whereas other strains can be highly susceptible. Other potential causes such as viruses have been studied. Research appears to rule out the potential role of viral agents, including feline immunodeficiency virus, FELV, papillomavirus, and polyomavirus, as a cause of this disease in cats.

Injection site sarcomas also have been reported at sites at which only nonadjuvanted vaccines (including vectored vaccines) have been administered (Srivastav et al, 2012). These vaccines do not induce significant local inflammatory reactions, and the findings suggest that factors related to development of injection site sarcomas are more complex than inflammation alone. Genetic factors often are considered when cancers such as VAS occur in younger animals. Cats are more susceptible to oxidative injury (e.g., Heinz body formation from acetaminophen toxicity) than other species. This characteristic may be important in tumor initiation. At the University of Minnesota, Dr. Sagarika Kanjilal and her colleagues studied the role of genetic predisposition in the development of VAS. Normal p53 is up-regulated in the presence of DNA damage and suppresses tumor cell growth. Alterations in p53 were found in some cats with VAS. Mutations in p53 have been associated with initiation and progression of tumors in a variety of species. However, this link was not substantiated in a follow-up study (Mucha et al, 2012). Further studies are needed evaluating the genetic links to injection site sarcomas in cats.

Histologic Features

Tumors that arise at sites of previous vaccination are similar to those that arise from areas of chronic inflammation in other species and are mesenchymal in origin, with osteosarcoma, chondrosarcoma, fibrosarcoma, malignant histiocytoma, giant cell tumor, rhabdomyosarcoma, and leiomyosarcoma being reported. However, fibrosarcomas make up 80% of the tumors observed at sites of vaccination. This observation suggests a local pluripotential mesenchymal cell as the target for the malignant transformation.

In addition to recent immunohistologic and ultrastructural descriptions of VAS, good microscopic descriptions have provided pathologists with a better capability to identify these lesions. The characteristics of intratumoral lymphoplasmacytic inflammation, giant cells, intracellular basophilic material, and myofibroblastic differentiation have helped diagnostic pathologists in identifying these lesions. Of clinical significance, and a potential reason for frequent surgical failure in the management of VAS, is the finding that histologically normal-looking cells up to 5 cm from the tumor have up-regulated p53 indicating DNA damage, a potentially premalignant state, and risk of later treatment failure, a phenomenon known as field carcinogenesis.

Clinical Management

VASs typically are diagnosed in younger cats than are sarcomas at nonvaccination sites and usually appear within 4 years of vaccination, although some have been reported up to 10 years after vaccination. Postvaccination lumps are very common, especially after the administration of rabies and FeLV vaccines, which commonly are adjuvanted. The majority of these lumps take a benign course and resolve within 3 months. The task force guidelines can help the veterinarian in the management of these lumps. If a lump develops at the vaccine site or within 5 cm of the vaccine site, the veterinarian should follow the "3-2-1" rule. A biopsy of the mass should be done if the mass persists for longer than *3* months, is larger than *2* cm in diameter, or is increasing in size *1* month after injection. The degree of inflammation associated with these tumors makes cytologic evaluation unreliable; thus a core biopsy sample should be obtained. Simple lumpectomy is not recommended because if the lump is proven to be tumor, wider surgical margins are required to ensure that both tumor and premalignant tissues are excised. Tumor size and histopathologic type are prognostic indicators. Cats with malignant fibrous histiocytomas live half as long as those with fibrosarcomas (290 days versus 645 days, respectively). Cats with tumors smaller than 2 cm live longer than those with

tumors 2 to 5 cm, which in turn have longer survival than those with tumors larger than 5 cm; mean survival times are 643, 558, and 394 days, respectively. Most vaccine-associated tumors have short doubling times, with 86% of recurrences developing within 6 months. Clinical staging is recommended before surgery. Three-view chest radiography is standard care, but contrast-enhanced computed tomography, when available, can improve surgical planning and is superior to routine radiographic evaluation in detecting pulmonary metastasis. The most common site of metastasis is the lungs, followed by the lymph nodes and other internal organs. The rate of clinically detectable metastasis at the time of diagnosis is 5%, and overall reported rates of metastasis are 0% to 28%.

Surgical management generally is inadequate as the sole modality of treatment, with 30% to 70% local recurrence depending on tumor margins, but is considered the most important component in multimodality treatment regimen. Surgery should be aggressive and should include all recognizable tumor as well as margins of 3 to 5 cm and two muscle planes deep. A recent series in which tumor margins were 5 cm or larger laterally and two fascial planes deep reported a recurrence rate of only a 19%. Even with the usual aggressive surgical intervention (3 cm margins) and histopathologic reports indicating no tumor cells observed at the surgical margins there is a 50% recurrence rate. Infiltrative surgical margins are associated with a 10 times greater risk of recurrence compared with noninfiltrative margins. The recommendation to administer rabies and FeLV vaccines in the rear legs is based in part on the better survival rates in patients that develop sarcoma on the rear legs and then undergo amputation. Radiation therapy alone can be palliative but is seldom curative, although in a number of studies it has been shown to prolong survival significantly in patients when combined with surgery. Chemotherapy has been shown to have limited value in the management of VAS. Drugs with activity against vaccine-associated tumors, including carboplatin, vincristine, mitoxantrone, doxorubicin, and cyclophosphamide alone or in combination, have reported to lead to a 50% reduction in tumor size but with limited durability of response. The use of chemotherapy in the adjuvant setting with surgery or surgery and radiation has shown mixed results, with some studies indicating increased survival but others failing to show improved survival. Hendrick found expression of platelet-derived growth factor (PDGF) on fibroblasts in VAS, whereas non–vaccine-associated tumors failed to express PDGF, which suggests a biologic basis for the use of tyrosine kinase inhibitors in the management of these tumors. Tyrosine kinase inhibitors administered to block PDGF receptor signaling have been observed to show some activity against VAS in a limited number of cases.

The prognosis for VAS varies by the treatment modality. Based on an average of reported studies, the disease-free intervals for marginal resection and wide surgical resection are 79 days and 325 days, respectively. Approximate survival times also vary for marginal resection (9 months), wide excision (16 months), wide excision plus radiation therapy (650 days), and wide excision plus radiation therapy and chemotherapy (700 days).

Prevention

Given the high cost of treatment and relatively poor prognosis of VAS, prevention is highly desirable. The clear association between vaccination and tumor development in cats is well accepted; thus recommended vaccine protocols with less frequent administrations are desired and should be used if appropriate for each individual cat based on an annual risk assessment. The use of vaccines and other injectable products that produce less or no inflammation at the injection site is recommended when possible. Subcutaneous or intramuscular administration of substances should be avoided in cats previously proven to have developed an injection site sarcoma because a genetic predisposition to this syndrome is suspected.

Vaccine-Associated Autoantibodies

Feline viruses like feline herpesvirus 1, feline calicivirus, and feline panleukopenia virus usually are propagated on cell lines when being produced for use in vaccines (e.g., feline viral rhinotracheitis, calicivirus, panleukopenia [FVRCP] vaccine) or in immunodiagnostic assays (Lappin et al, 2005). During virus purification it is difficult to remove all of the cell-line proteins. As a consequence, if the viral preparation is used for vaccine production, the immunized cats are exposed and have immune responses not only to the viruses within the vaccine but also to any potential remnants of the cell line used to propagate the virus.

This issue first was studied in cats vaccinated with three FVRCP vaccines grown on the Crandell-Rees feline kidney (CRFK) cell line (Lappin et al, 2005). Although isolated from a kidney, the cell line has characteristics of a fibroblast. The objectives of the study were to determine whether cats inoculated with FVRCP vaccines grown on the CRFK cell line would develop antibodies against CRFK lysates or feline renal cell (FRC) lysates, whether cats hypersensitized with CRFK lysates would develop antibodies against CRFK cell lysates or FRC lysates, and whether FVRCP vaccination or hypersensitization with CRFK cell lysates would induce clinical pathologic or histopathologic abnormalities over a 56-week period.

Three FVRCP vaccines for subcutaneous administration and one FVRCP vaccine for intranasal/intraocular administration were used to vaccinate kittens three times as per the American Association of Feline Practitioners vaccine panel report and then to give booster injections 50 weeks later. Other cats were hyperinoculated (11 doses) with three different concentrations of CRFK lysates that were comparable to those concentrations found in the FVRCP vaccines studied, with the last dose administered at week 50. Renal biopsy specimens were collected from all kittens before they entered the study and at week 56. The kittens that were hyperinoculated were considered the positive control groups. Although the intranasal vaccine contains CRFK protein contaminants, mucosal immune responses generally do not develop against inactivated antigens, and so cats inoculated with this vaccine were considered the negative control group.

Complete blood cell counts, serum biochemical studies, urinalysis, microalbuminuria assays (some samples), and enzyme-linked immunosorbent assays (ELISAs) to detect antibodies against CRFK lysate or FRC lysate were performed on samples collected at intervals during the study. Renal biopsy specimens were assessed for abnormalities independently by two pathologists. None of the cats was positive for antibodies against CRFK lysate or FRC lysate before inoculation. All six cats administered CRFK lysate alone tested positive on the CRFK ELISA on multiple sample dates. Neither of the cats receiving intranasal/intraocular vaccination had samples that reached the positive cutoff value on the CRFK ELISA. Five of the six cats administered a parenteral vaccine had positive results on the CRFK ELISA at least once during the study. All six cats administered CRFK lysate tested positive on multiple sample dates on the FRC ELISA. All six cats administered a parenteral vaccine tested positive on multiple sample dates on the FRC ELISA. Neither of the cats administered the intranasal/intraocular vaccine had positive results on the FRC ELISA. Significant abnormalities in the results of the complete blood count, serum biochemical testing, urinalysis, microalbuminuria assay, and histopathologic analysis were not detected during the study. It was concluded that parenteral administration of vaccines grown on the CRFK cell line and subcutaneous inoculation of CRFK lysate alone induced CRFK antibodies and FRC antibodies in most cats in this study. However, the clinical pathologic and histopathologic results suggested that even hypersensitization with CRFK proteins was not associated with detectable renal dysfunction, renal inflammatory disease, or glomerular disease in the 56-week study period (Lappin et al, 2005).

In the preceding study, renal biopsy specimens were collected 6 weeks after the last vaccination or CRFK hyperinoculation; thus it is possible that inflammation of renal tissues occurred but was transient and resolved by the time of biopsy. In a second study, it was hypothesized that interstitial nephritis would be detected in cats that were hyperinoculated with CRFK lysates, received a booster with CRFK lysates, and then underwent biopsy 2 weeks after the booster (Lappin et al, 2006). The CRFK-hyperinoculated cats from the first study and the cats vaccinated with the intranasal/intraocular FVRCP vaccine (negative control group) were retained and housed for an additional 1 year with no manipulations. The same CRFK lysate dose or vaccine as used in the first study was administered to the same cats in the previous study and a renal biopsy specimen was obtained 2 weeks later. Mild to moderate interstitial nephritis was documented in three of six cats hyperinoculated with CRFK lysates, but not in cats vaccinated with the intranasal FVRCP vaccine. None of these three cats had significant inflammation in the renal biopsy specimens collected 6 weeks after the booster, 1 year previously. These data show that cats hyperinoculated with CRFK lysates develop significant interstitial nephritis, but the duration of inflammation may be brief. However, it is important to emphasize that the cats in the study were inoculated multiple times with CRFK lysates over the first year of the study. Whether such inflammation occurs after parenteral administration of CRFK-contaminated FVRCP vaccines using routine vaccination protocols remains to be proven.

The first study to determine whether anti-CRFK antibodies were induced in vaccinated cats was considered a pilot study and so included only two cats per group (Lappin et al, 2005). A larger study then was performed with five groups of cats (one receiving intranasal vaccine and four receiving parenteral vaccines) to gather further data on different levels of CRFK responses and to determine the immunodominant antigens contained in the lysates (Whittemore et al, 2010). It was shown that FVRCP vaccines administered parenterally induced a statistically greater magnitude of antibody response to CRFK proteins than the intranasal FVRCP vaccine, which confirmed the findings of the first study (Lappin et al, 2005). There were three immunodominant antigens in the CRFK lysates that were recognized by CRFK-hyperinoculated cats and cats vaccinated with FVRCP vaccines parenterally (Whittemore et al, 2010). Antibodies against two of the three antigens (α-enolase and annexin A2) have been associated with autoimmune disorders in people, including interstitial nephritis. Both of these antigens are in all mammalian cell lines and so are not specific to vaccines prepared from viruses propagated on CRFK cells.

In subsequent research, it was demonstrated that azotemic cats older than 10 years of age are more likely to have antienolase antibodies than normal cats and that cats, like people, show spontaneous production of antienolase antibodies as well as production of antienolase antibodies after vaccination with antigens grown on cell lines. Further data are being gathered to determine whether vaccines administered at longer intervals or vaccines not derived from viruses grown on cell lines are less likely to be associated with azotemia or renal inflammation than cell line–derived parenteral vaccines administered at annual intervals.

As discussed in the introduction to this chapter, vaccine-associated adverse effects generally are rare and therefore are difficult to predict in individual cats or to study in small groups of cats. Thus the best way to avoid potential vaccine-associated adverse effects is to administer only vaccines that currently are indicated, at the longest interval currently accepted. National and international vaccine panel reports like those of the American Association of Feline Practitioners and the International Society of Feline Medicine, the guidelines of the European Advisory Board on Cat Diseases, and guidelines from the World Small Animal Veterinary Association are excellent sources of guidance in tailoring optimal vaccine protocols for individual cats and are published in their respective websites.

References and Suggested Reading

Hershey AE et al: Aberrant p53 expression in feline vaccine associated sarcomas and correlation with prognosis, *Vet Pathol* 42:805, 2005.

Lappin MR et al: Use of serologic tests to predict resistance to feline herpesvirus 1, feline calicivirus, and feline parvovirus infection in cats, *J Am Vet Med Assoc* 220:38, 2002.

Lappin MR et al: Investigation of the induction of antibodies against Crandell Rees feline kidney cell lysates and feline renal cell lysates after parenteral administration of vaccines against feline viral rhinotracheitis, calicivirus, and panleukopenia in cats, *Am J Vet Res* 66:506, 2005.

Lappin MR et al: Interstitial nephritis in cats inoculated with Crandell Rees feline kidney cell lysates, *J Feline Med Surg* 8:353, 2006.

Lester S, Clemett T, Burt A: Vaccine site-associated sarcomas in cats: clinical experience and a laboratory review (1982-1993), *J Am Anim Hosp Assoc* 32(2):91, 1996.

McNiel E: Vaccine-associated sarcomas in cats: a unique cancer model, *Clin Orthop Relat Res* 382:21, 2001.

Moore GE et al: Adverse events diagnosed within 3 days of vaccine administration in pet dogs, *J Am Vet Med Assoc* 227:1102, 2005.

Moore GE et al: Adverse events after vaccine administration in cats: 2,560 cases (2002-2005), *J Am Vet Med Assoc* 231:94, 2007.

Mucha D et al: Lack of association between p53 SNP and FISS in a cat population from Germany, *Vet Comp Oncol*. Epub August 9, 2012. doi:10.1111/j.1476-5829.2012.00344.x.

Richards JR et al: The 2006 American Association of Feline Practitioners feline vaccine advisory panel report, *J Am Vet Med Assoc* 229:1405, 2006.

Shaw SC et al: Temporal changes in characteristics of injection site sarcomas in cats: 392 cases (1990-2006), *J Am Vet Med Assoc* 234:376, 2009.

Srivastav A et al: Comparative vaccine-specific and other injectable-specific risks of injection-site sarcomas in cats, *J Am Vet Med Assoc* 241:595, 2012.

Vaccine-Associated Feline Sarcoma Task Force: The current understanding and management of vaccine associated sarcomas in cats, *J Am Vet Med Assoc* 226:1821, 2005.

Welborn LV et al: 2011 AAHA canine vaccination guidelines, *J Am Anim Hosp Assoc* 47(5):1, 2011.

Whittemore JC et al: Antibodies against Crandell Rees feline kidney (CRFK) cell line antigens, α-enolase, and annexin A2 in vaccinated and CRFK hyperinoculated cats, *J Vet Intern Med* 24:306, 2010.

CHAPTER 268

Treatment of Canine Babesiosis

ADAM J. BIRKENHEUER, *Raleigh, North Carolina*

Babesiosis typically is characterized by thrombocytopenia, hemolytic anemia, and splenomegaly. Canine babesiosis is an important disease worldwide and can be caused by many different species of *Babesia* (Table 268-1). Molecular characterization of the parasite is critical for selecting the treatment with the best efficacy and lowest cost. Serologic testing for antibodies against *Babesia* spp. can be useful in cases in which parasitemia is below the limit of detection for molecular assays but because of cross-reactivity cannot always be used to predict accurately which species are causing infection. Serologic studies and polymerase chain reaction (PCR) testing should be considered complementary assays and should be used together to maximize the chances of making a definitive or presumptive diagnosis of babesiosis. Empirical therapy should be started immediately in critical cases in which there is a high index of suspicion of babesiosis while results of molecular diagnostic tests are pending. The following responses to frequently asked questions regarding the treatment of babesiosis are based on the literature and the author's experience.

Frequently Asked Questions

What Should I Expect When Treating *Babesia gibsoni* Infections?

After the discovery of *Babesia gibsoni* about a century ago every treatment that was used against it failed to clear infection. Then in 2004 the use of atovaquone and azithromycin was first described (Birkenheuer et al, 2004). Atovaquone and azithromycin combination therapy is the treatment of choice for *B. gibsoni* infection in dogs in North America in the author's opinion. Despite this improvement in treatment, this combination therapy seems to be "*Babesia*-static," not "*Babesia*-cidal," and requires that the dog have an intact functional immune system for maximum efficacy. It is typical for clinical signs and hematologic abnormalities to begin improving within 1 week of starting treatment. In the United States where reinfection via tick vectors is unlikely, this treatment is associated with parasite clearance or reduction of parasite burden below the limit of detection in 80% to 85% of cases. This treatment appears to be very safe, and no adverse effects have been reported in dogs. Unfortunately, it can be expensive, with a single 750-ml bottle of atovaquone costing $700 to $1200 at the time this chapter was published. Although this bottle contains enough drug to treat three 20-kg dogs, many pharmacies require purchase of the entire bottle. Several compounding pharmacies will sell it by the dose.

Is There a Less Expensive Form of Atovaquone?

There are two commercially available forms of atovaquone in the United States. A single-drug formulation (Mepron) is widely available and is the formulation the author recommends. A less expensive formulation (Malarone) in which atovaquone is combined with a second antiprotozoal drug, proguanil hydrochloride, also is widely available but has not been evaluated specifically for the treatment of *B. gibsoni*. In addition, in the author's experience administration of the atovaquone/proguanil combination is associated with severe vomiting in some dogs. Since parasite resistance can be selected for or develop rapidly, there is concern about an increased chance of resistance if the drugs are not well absorbed because of vomiting.

Do I Have to Use Atovaquone and Azithromycin Together for Treatment of *Babesia gibsoni?*

Atovaquone and azithromycin must be used in combination. Each drug alone has some antiprotozoal activity, but together they have been shown to work synergistically *in vivo* and can clear *Babesia* infections. Since resistance can be selected for or develop quickly it is recommended that these drugs be administered only in combination. The author is concerned about selection of resistant parasites and usually does not administer azithromycin while waiting for the atovaquone to arrive. Instead, other treatments such as administration of imidocarb dipropionate and supportive care are used to assist in stabilizing the patient's condition. Atovaquone is a hydroxynaphthoquinone that acts as a ubiquinone (coenzyme Q_{10}) analog. By binding to cytochrome *b*, atovaquone blocks the action of ubiquinone, and the mitochondrial electron transport chain is disrupted. Once the electron transport chain is disrupted, the mitochondrial membrane potential is collapsed, which inhibits most mitochondrial functions such as pyrimidine biosynthesis. Because of differences in the structure of cytochrome *b*, atovaquone does not affect mammalian mitochondrial functions. The exact mechanism of action of azithromycin against protozoa is not known but is speculated to involve inhibition of mitochondrial 70S–like ribosomal function.

What If the Owner Cannot Afford Atovaquone and Azithromycin?

The author often treats *B. gibsoni*–infected dogs with imidocarb dipropionate at the labeled dose and frequency.

TABLE **268-1**

Recommended Treatment Options for Canine Babesiosis Based on Infecting Species

Babesia Species	Treatment of Choice	Notes
Babesia gibsoni	Atovaquone (13.3 mg/kg q8h PO) and azithromycin (10 mg/kg q24h PO) given simultaneously for 10 days	Atovaquone should be given with a fatty meal to maximize absorption. The author's preference is Mepron over Malarone because of anecdotal experience of Malarone's causing severe adverse effects (vomiting). This dose and frequency are likely to eradicate or reduce parasitemia below detection limit of polymerase chain reaction testing in some dogs.
Babesia (canis) vogeli	Imidocarb dipropionate (6.6 mg/kg IM or SC, repeat in 14 days)	This dose and frequency are likely to eradicate parasites. Pretreatment with atropine or glycopyrrolate minimizes cholinergic adverse effects.
Babesia (canis) canis	Imidocarb dipropionate (2 mg/kg IM or SC once for premunition; 6.6 mg/kg IM or SC, repeat in 14 days, for sterilization)	This dose and frequency are likely to induce premunition but not eradicate the parasites. Pretreatment with atropine or glycopyrrolate minimizes cholinergic adverse effects.
Babesia (canis) rossi	Diminazene aceturate (3.5 mg/kg IM once; or imidocarb dipropionate 6.6 mg/kg IM or SC, repeat in 14 days)	This dose and frequency are likely to eradicate parasites. Pretreatment with atropine or glycopyrrolate minimizes cholinergic adverse effects.
Babesia sp. (Coco)	Imidocarb dipropionate (6.6 mg/kg IM or SC, repeat in 14 days)	There are not enough data to determine whether or not parasitemia is cleared consistently. Pretreatment with atropine or glycopyrrolate minimizes cholinergic adverse effects. Atovaquone and azithromycin should be considered if treatment fails to clear infection.
Babesia conradae	Atovaquone (13.3 mg/kg q8h PO) and azithromycin (10 mg/kg q24h PO) given simultaneously for 10 days	This dose and frequency are likely to eradicate or reduce parasitemia below the limit of detection in some dogs.
Babesia microti–like sp.	Optimal treatment unknown	

IM, Intramuscularly; *PO,* orally; *SC,* subcutaneously.

These dogs usually go into a state of premunition. Premunition is referred to as *immunity of infection,* and dogs can remain in this state without overt clinical signs for months to years. The owners then are instructed to save money to treat the dog at a later date with atovaquone and azithromycin. The author has waited as long as a year before treating with atovaquone and azithromycin.

Isn't Imidocarb Dipropionate Ineffective against *Babesia gibsoni*?

The use of imidocarb dipropionate for the treatment of *B. gibsoni* is an area in which there appears to be some confusion. There is a belief that imidocarb is not effective at all against *B. gibsoni*. This idea seems to have originated from a Japanese study that incorrectly states in the abstract (written in both English and Japanese) that imidocarb did not reduce mortality in experimentally infected dogs. However, the actual data in the article (written only in Japanese) demonstrate that none of the imidocarb-treated dogs died. Although imidocarb is unable to eradicate the parasite and definitely should not be considered the treatment of choice for *B. gibsoni* infection, the author has used it to induce a clinical remission in numerous cases.

What about the Clindamycin-Doxycycline-Metronidazole Combination for Treatment of *Babesia gibsoni* Infections?

In an uncontrolled trial, treatment with a combination of clindamycin (25 mg/kg q12h PO), doxycycline (5 mg/kg q12h PO), and metronidazole (15 mg/kg q12h PO) was associated with parasite clearance or reduction of *B. gibsoni* burden below the PCR limit of detection in three of four dogs after the dogs had been treated with diminazene aceturate (Suzuki et al, 2007). The three dogs from which the parasite could no longer be amplified were treated for approximately 90 days. The remaining dog was treated for 206 days. Ideally a randomized trial comparing the efficacy of this combination with the efficacy of atovaquone and azithromycin should be performed. Decreased cost commonly is cited as a reason to choose this combination. However, the cost of treatment of a 20-kg dog at the author's institution was $356 for a 10-day course of atovaquone and azithromycin and $325 for a 90-day course of clindamycin, doxycycline, and metronidazole.

How Should I Follow Up after Treatment of *Babesia gibsoni* Infections?

Follow-up after treatment for infection with any species of *Babesia* is similar and includes monitoring for resolution of clinical signs with complete blood counts, serum biochemical studies, urinalysis, measurement of urine protein:creatinine ratios, and so on. The author also usually recommends that two or three consecutive PCR tests be performed 2 to 4 weeks apart starting 60 days or longer after treatment. The wait is this long to make sure that antiprotozoal drugs (particularly azithromycin) have had adequate time to be cleared from the patient and to minimize the detection of dead or dying piroplasms in red blood cells that have not been cleared from circulation.

What Do I Do If Atovaquone and Azithromycin Treatment Fails in a *Babesia gibsoni*–Infected Dog?

Dogs that remain infected after treatment with atovaquone and azithromycin (as assessed by PCR performed ≥60 days after treatment) are unlikely to respond to additional treatment with atovaquone and azithromycin alone. These dogs are assumed to be infected with *B. gibsoni* organisms that have mutations in their cytochrome *b* genes leading to atovaquone resistance. Mutations can be confirmed by PCR assay and DNA sequencing. In the author's experience dogs in which atovaquone and azithromycin therapy fails often have been receiving immunosuppressive drugs for weeks to months before treatment or have undergone splenectomy before treatment. Atovaquone-resistant *B. gibsoni* organisms can be notoriously difficult to clear from infected dogs.

If the dog was being treated with immunosuppressive drugs, the author stops these before retreatment. In some cases, treatment with imidocarb dipropionate (every 1 to 2 weeks) is needed to maintain clinical remission during the corticosteroid weaning process. In animals in which atovaquone and azithromycin therapy was ineffective, the author uses a combination of clindamycin (25 mg/kg q12h PO), doxycycline (5 mg/kg q12h PO), and metronidazole (15 mg/kg q12h PO) given daily for 3 months because this combination was associated with parasite clearance in three of four dogs in an uncontrolled trial (Suzuki et al, 2007). Since using antiparasitic drugs with different mechanisms may increase efficacy, the author often combines this with imidocarb at the labeled dose, route, and frequency; an artemisinin derivative; and repeat treatment with atovaquone and azithromycin. Antiemetics often are administered during therapy to reduce nausea. In the author's experience most dogs treated with this protocol will remain in clinical remission with persistent parasitemia, and occasional dogs will persistently test negative for the presence of *B. gibsoni* by PCR assay after treatment. Some dogs with persistent infection after these treatments (particularly those that have undergone splenectomy) may need to receive some therapy indefinitely (usually a combination of clindamycin, doxycycline, and metronidazole) because their clinical signs often reappear shortly after treatment is stopped.

What Should I Expect When Treating *Babesia canis* Infections?

Imidocarb dipropionate is very effective against *Babesia (canis) vogeli*, *Babesia (canis) canis*, and *Babesia (canis) rossi.*

Imidocarb can be used against these species for treatment of dogs with acute babesiosis, for treatment of carriers with subclinical disease, or as chemoprophylaxis to prevent infection. It generally is accepted that imidocarb eradicates *B. (canis) vogeli*, *B. (canis) canis*, and *B. (canis) rossi* infections. The labeled dose of imidocarb is 6.6 mg/kg IM or SC with a repeat dose in 14 days. Several studies have demonstrated clinical efficacy (evidence of parasite clearance was not consistently evaluated and frequently molecular techniques were not used) against *B. (canis) canis* and *B. (canis) rossi* at lower doses. In Europe the typical recommended dose of imidocarb for the treatment of *B. (canis) canis* is 2 to 3 mg/kg; however, this strategy is aimed at inducing a state of premunition, not parasite clearance.

What about Other Diamidine Derivatives for the Treatment of *Babesia canis* Infections?

Some drugs in the diamidine derivative class of drugs are imidocarb dipropionate, phenamidine isethionate, pentamidine isethionate, diminazene aceturate, and diminazene diaceturate. These drugs are believed to interfere with parasite replication and function by binding to the minor groove in adenine-thymine–rich DNA sequences. Only one drug in this class, imidocarb dipropionate, has been approved by the Food and Drug Administration. Several formulations of diminazene are available outside the United States and appear to be equally effective for the treatment of *B. (canis) vogeli*, *B. (canis) canis*, and *B. (canis) rossi.* The chemoprophylactic utility of diminazene in dogs is not well characterized. Diminazene is considered more effective against *B. gibsoni* than imidocarb; however, diminazene alone still fails to eradicate *B. gibsoni* from infected dogs.

Do Any Other Antibiotics Work against *Babesia* Species Infections?

Clindamycin Hydrochloride
Clindamycin hydrochloride at high dosages (25 mg/kg q12h PO for 14 days) has been demonstrated to reduce morbidity and mortality in dogs with experimental *B. gibsoni* infections. It is important to note that this treatment did not eradicate infection. The exact mechanism by which clindamycin works against *Babesia* spp. is unknown. Less is known about the efficacy of clindamycin for the treatment of infection with other *Babesia* spp. in dogs, but it is likely the drug would have efficacy similar to that seen in treatment of *B. gibsoni.*

Tetracyclines
Tetracycline antibiotics have modest anti-*Babesia* activity *in vitro* and *in vivo*. Although these antibiotics are not recommended as single-agent treatments for babesiosis, their activity is important to note because many cases of canine babesiosis are suspected to be resistant rickettsial infections based on the reduction of clinical signs with tetracycline therapy and recurrence once the treatment is discontinued. However, coinfections with *Babesia* spp. and rickettsial agents can occur.

Trimethoprim/Sulfadiazine

Trimethoprim/sulfadiazine administered at a dosage of 30 mg/kg q12h PO for 7 days has been shown to reduce morbidity and mortality in dogs with *B. gibsoni* infections. The mechanism is presumed to interfere with protozoal folate production. This widely available treatment may be useful while more specific antiprotozoal treatments are awaited.

What Is Artemisia?

Artemisinin (*qinghaosu* in Chinese) is a chemical present in a type of Asian wormwood (*Artemisia annua* Linnaeus) that was found to have significant antimalarial activity. The exact mechanism by which artemisinin and its derivatives exert their antiparasitic effect remains unclear. The leading theories regarding the mechanism of artemisinin include inhibition of a calcium-dependent adenosine triphosphatase pump (PfATP6) and the production of reactive oxygen species after activation by an iron source such as hemoglobin. Artemisinins demonstrate activity against *B. gibsoni in vitro*. There are no clinical trials or reports of the use of artemisinins for the treatment of canine babesiosis. Parenteral administration of artemisinin derivatives in dogs has been associated with neurologic adverse effects. Adverse effects are not seen with oral administration. The author has anecdotal experience with the use of artemether (3.5 mg/kg q12h PO on the first day, then q24h PO for 5 days) in a handful of cases. This agent always has been given in combination with other antiprotozoal drugs. In these cases no adverse effects were noted. Clinical trials investigating the use of artemisinins alone or in combination with other antiprotozoal drugs are indicated.

Since the Hemolytic Anemia and Thrombocytopenia Associated with Babesiosis Are Immune Mediated, Should I Use Immunosuppressive Drugs?

It is the author's experience that, although hemolytic anemia and thrombocytopenia are immune-mediated pathologic processes, immunosuppressive therapy almost never is needed to ameliorate clinical signs of babesiosis. It is also the author's impression that treatments for babesiosis may be more *Babesia*-static than *Babesia*-cidal, and so having a fully functional immune system may improve outcome. In dogs that have been immunosuppressed before treatment with antiprotozoal drugs, parasitemia seems to fail to clear more frequently.

References and Suggested Reading

Birkenheuer AJ, Levy MG, Brietschwerdt EB: Efficacy of combined atovaquone and azithromycin for therapy of chronic *Babesia gibsoni* (Asian genotype) infections in dogs, *J Vet Intern Med* 18(4):494, 2004.

Bourdoiseau G: Canine babesiosis in France, *Vet Parasitol* 138 (1-2):118, 2006.

Di Cicco MF et al: Re-emergence of *Babesia conradae* and effective treatment of infected dogs with atovaquone and azithromycin, *Vet Parasitol* 187(1-2):23, 2012. Epub January 8, 2012.

Suzuki K et al: A possible treatment strategy and clinical factors to estimate the treatment response in *Babesia gibsoni* infection, *J Vet Med Sci* 69(5):563, 2007.

Takahashi K: Action of several antiprotozoal compounds against *Babesia gibsoni* infection in dogs, *J Jpn Vet Med Assoc* 37(4):203, 1984.

CHAPTER 269

Canine Bartonellosis

PEDRO PAULO VISSOTTO DE PAIVA DINIZ, *Pomona, California*

Currently the genus *Bartonella* comprises at least 30 species and subspecies of fastidious gram-negative bacteria. They are transmitted by hematophagous arthropods and capable of infecting and causing a chronic and persistent intraerythrocytic bacteremia in a wide variety of terrestrial and marine hosts. The identification of *Bartonella* DNA from a 4000-year-old human tooth and from 800-year-old cats demonstrates that these organisms have coevolved over the centuries with mammalian hosts. Overall, *Bartonella* spp. are not species specific, but selected bacterial species have adapted to specific mammalian hosts, such as *B. henselae* and *B. clarridgeiae* to cats; *B. vinsonii* subsp. *berkhoffii* and *B. rochalimae* to domestic dogs and wild canids; *B. bovis* to cattle; *B. washoensis* to ground squirrels; and *B. quintana* to humans. Consequently, these adapted species generally cause limited clinical manifestations in their preferred hosts, in spite of persistent bacteremia. Pathologic effects are more common in immunosuppressed hosts or when *Bartonella* spp. infect a non-adapted accidental host, resulting in a wide variety of clinical manifestations. However, the low levels of bacteremia and frequent lack of specific antibody response in immunocompetent cats, dogs, and human patients make the diagnosis a challenge (Boulouis et al, 2005; Breitschwerdt et al, 2010).

In recent decades, the evolution of laboratory diagnostic techniques has facilitated the identification of several *Bartonella* spp. infecting dogs, eight of them capable of infecting humans as well. Although the role of dogs as reservoirs for human infection has not been defined, dog infection may be an important epidemiologic sentinel for human exposure because both share the same environment. Bartonellosis is an emerging infectious disease in human patients, with veterinarians and other professionals in frequent animal contact considered at-risk groups (Maggi et al, 2011).

Bartonella Species in Dogs

Eleven species, subspecies, or species candidatus of *Bartonella* have been reported from dogs (Table 269-1): *B. bovis*, *B. clarridgeiae*, *B. elizabethae*, *B. henselae*, *B. koehlerae*, *B. quintana*, *B. rochalimae*, *B. vinsonii* subsp. *berkhoffii*, *Candidatus* B. merieuxii, *Candidatus* B. volans, and *Candidatus* B. washoensis. Worldwide, the two most frequent species in dogs are *B. henselae* and *B. vinsonii* subsp. *berkhoffii*. Dogs are considered the primary host of *B. vinsonii* subsp. *berkhoffii*, and they also may be reservoirs for *B. rochalimae*.

B. vinsonii subsp. *berkhoffii* has been identified as an important cause of endocarditis in dogs and also has been associated with myocarditis and anterior uveitis. Historically, this species was considered the most frequent species infecting dogs. Four genotypes of *B. vinsonii* subsp. *berkhoffii* have been described, based upon analysis of blood samples from coyotes, dogs, foxes, and humans. All four genotypes have been reported in dogs with endocarditis and a range of other clinical manifestations, but genotypes I, III, and IV are found infrequently. Antigenic differences among genotypes may explain negative serology titers in some infected dogs (Breitschwerdt et al, 2010; Maggi et al, 2006).

Cats are frequently infected with *B. henselae*. Recent data also suggest that *B. henselae* is the most frequent cause of bartonellosis in dogs, also detected in dogs coinfected with other *Bartonella* spp. In dogs, *B. henselae* has been associated with endocarditis, polyarthritis, idiopathic effusions, pyogranulomatous lymphadenitis, epistaxis, and hepatitis, but the pathogenicity of this organism has not been clearly established. In humans, *B. henselae* is the causative agent of cat-scratch disease (CSD), generally presented as self-limiting regional lymphadenopathy with fever and malaise. *B. henselae* infection in humans can be associated with retinitis, glomerulonephritis, endocarditis, granulomatous hepatitis, hemolytic anemia, and osteomyelitis. *B. henselae* demonstrates large genetic variability with several genotypes and strains of *B. henselae* described worldwide. It is unknown if dogs are predisposed to develop disease when infected with certain genotypes, but human infection frequently is caused by selected genotypes.

B. rochalimae was first isolated in 2007 from an American woman who became severely ill two weeks after returning to the United States from Peru, where she experienced multiple insect bites. Infection with *B. rochalimae* also was found in a dog with endocarditis in San Francisco, California, in a sick dog from Greece, and in 7.3% of 205 asymptomatic dogs in Peru (Diniz et al, 2012). The epidemiology of this organism is still limited, but gray foxes and raccoons may be the natural reservoir in California and red foxes in Europe and Israel (Henn et al, 2009). In addition, an experimental infection of two dogs, five cats, and six guinea pigs with *B. rochalimae* demonstrated that only dogs became highly bacteremic without any disease expression, suggesting that dogs could be the natural reservoir for this species (Chomel et al, 2009a).

Other species of *Bartonella* were described infecting dogs (see Table 269-1). The most common disease manifestation reported in these cases included endocarditis, followed by hepatic disease, weight loss, and, in one case, sudden death. Recently, 37% of 97 stray dogs in Iraq were

TABLE 269-1

Species of *Bartonella* Detected in Dogs, Other Accidental Mammalian Hosts, and Reported Syndromes in Humans

Species	Primary Host	Accidental Hosts	Disease in Humans
B. bovis	Cattle	Dog, cat, deer, elk	Not reported in humans
B. clarridgeiae	Cat	Human, dog	Endocarditis
B. elizabethae	Rat	Human, dog	Endocarditis
B. henselae	Cat	Human, dog, horse, rat, sea turtle, porpoise, beluga, wild felid	Cat-scratch disease, bacillary angiomatosis, bacillary peliosis, relapsing fever, meningitis, encephalitis, neuroretinitis, endocarditis, epithelioid hemangioendothelioma
B. koehlerae	Cat	Human, dog	Sensory neuropathy, epithelioid hemangioendothelioma
B. quintana	Human	Human, dog, cat, monkey	Trench fever, endocarditis, bacillary angiomatosis, bacillary peliosis, chronic lymphadenomegaly
B. rochalimae	Gray and red fox, raccoon	Human, dog, coyote	Carrion-like disease (fever, anemia, splenomegaly, and insomnia)
B. vinsonii berkhoffii	Dog, coyote	Human, cat, fox, sea turtle	Neurologic disease
Candidatus B. merieuxii	Dog (?)	Not reported	Not reported in humans
Candidatus B. volans	Squirrel	Dog, sea otter	Joint pain, mental confusion, seizures, encephalopathy
Candidatus B. washoensis	Squirrel	Human, dog, chipmunk	Myocarditis

found to be infected with a new species named *Candidatus* Bartonella merieuxii; however, its pathogenicity for dogs is still unknown (Chomel et al, 2012).

Epidemiology

Bartonella spp. have been found in all continents except Antarctica. Unlike in cats, the prevalence of *Bartonella* spp. in dogs is generally low. The epidemiology of these organisms is diverse in tropical areas, but low prevalence has been detected in dogs in subtropical regions. In Thailand, exposure to *B. vinsonii* subsp. *berkhoffii*, determined by antibody detection, was reported in 39% (19/49) of sick dogs. Similarly, 38% of 147 dogs from Morocco were seropositive for *B. vinsonii* subsp. *berkhoffii*. In contrast, seroprevalence of 10% or less for *B. henselae* or *B. vinsonii* subsp. *berkhoffii* was reported from southeastern Brazil, Granada, Hawaii, the United Kingdom, Israel, Taiwan, and Japan. Bacteremia, documented by PCR amplification of *Bartonella* DNA, was reported in 16.7% (9/54) of healthy dogs in Korea, 11.6% (7/60) of healthy dogs in southern Italy, 6.3% (5/80) of dogs in Algeria, 1.4% (1/73) of dogs in Grenada, and 1% (2/198) of sick dogs in Brazil. In the United States, a study involving 663 dogs from 11 states located in the northeastern, midwestern, or southern United States detected 61 bacteremic dogs (9.2%) infected with one species and 9 dogs (1.4%) coinfected with more than one species of *Bartonella* (Breitschwerdt et al, 2010; Chomel et al, 2010).

Transmission and Risk Factors

Several arthropod vectors including biting flies, fleas, keds, lice, sandflies, and ticks have been implicated in the transmission of *Bartonella* spp. among mammals. The mode of transmission in dogs is not well established, but epidemiologic evidence supports the role of ticks and fleas. *Bartonella* DNA was detected in *Ixodes* spp. and *Rhipicephalus sanguineus* (brown dog tick) collected in North America, Europe, and Asia. Transmission of the bacterial pathogen from fleas occurs through inoculation of contaminated flea feces into the skin via a scratch or bite. Consequently, heavy flea exposure, heavy tick exposure, cattle exposure, and a rural environment are risk factors for *Bartonella* spp. infection (Chomel et al, 2010).

Pathogenesis

Once *Bartonella* spp. gain access to the bloodstream, they infect a primary niche outside of circulating blood, possibly vascular endothelial cells or CD34+ progenitor cells in the bone marrow. This approach provides a potentially unique strategy for immediate access to erythrocytes, ideal for bacterial persistence within the circulatory system. *Bartonella* spp. also can infect dendritic cells, microglial cells, monocytes, and macrophages. Cell invasion by *Bartonella* spp. is mediated by two groups of virulence factors: adhesins and the type IV secretion system (T4SS). Adhesins mediate adhesion to the extracellular matrix of mammalian host cells, whereas the T4SS is capable of transporting DNA and effector proteins to the target host cell. *Bartonella* adhesin A (BadA) mediates bacterial adherence to endothelial cells and extracellular matrix proteins and triggers the induction of angiogenic gene programming. The VirB/VirD4 T4SS is responsible for inhibition of host cell apoptosis, bacterial persistence in erythrocytes, and endothelial sprouting. The Trw T4SS system of *Bartonella* spp. mediates host-specific adherence to erythrocytes. *In vitro*, the peak invasion of canine erythrocytes by *B. vinsonii* subsp. *berkhoffii* occurs after 48 hours postinoculation (PI). *In vivo,* approximately on day five PI, large numbers of bacteria are released into the bloodstream, where they bind to and invade mature erythrocytes. Bacteria then replicate in a membrane-bound compartment until reaching a critical number. For the remaining life span of the erythrocytes, the intracellular bacteria remain in a nondividing state. Continuous replication of the pathogen in the primary niche causes erythrocyte infection waves at approximately 5-day intervals, causing persistent bacteremia to facilitate the acquisition of the organism by the vector. Experimental infection of dogs with *B. vinsonii* subsp. *berkhoffii* induced immunosuppression, characterized by sustained suppression of peripheral blood CD8+ lymphocytes. Immunosuppression caused by *Bartonella* infection may predispose the host to opportunistic infections, including infection by other pathogens transmitted by the same vector; however, this hypothesis has not yet been proven (Franz and Kempf, 2011).

Clinical Presentation

The cyclic shedding of *Bartonella* spp. from the primary niche into the bloodstream facilitates the distribution of the organisms throughout the body, with consequent involvement of numerous cell types, many organ systems, and a wide range of disease manifestations (Box 269-1) and diagnoses (Box 269-2). Lesions may occur in the heart, liver, lymph nodes, joints, eye, nasal cavity, CNS, skin, and subcutaneous tissue. Unfortunately, clinical signs of *Bartonella* infection in dogs cannot be discriminated from other tick-borne infections, with the most frequent signs fever (40%), lethargy (40%), weight loss (34%), anorexia (32%), and lymphadenopathy (30%). Weight loss was significantly associated with *Bartonella* spp. infection in dogs when compared with sick dogs

suspected of other vector-borne diseases (Perez et al, 2013). Endocarditis is a common clinical finding in *Bartonella*-infected dogs. Endocarditis is documented more frequently in large-breed dogs with a predisposition for aortic valve involvement; however, 20% of cases involve the mitral valve or multiple valves. Endocarditis resulting from *B. vinsonii* subsp. *berkhoffii* infection is the most commonly reported; however, endocarditis resulting from *B. clarridgeiae, B. henselae, B. koehlerae, B. quintana, B. rochalimae,* or *B. washoensis* infection was reported in a limited number of dogs. The clinical abnormalities commonly reported in dogs with endocarditis resulting from *Bartonella* spp. are murmurs (89%), fever (72%), leukocytosis (78%), hypoalbuminemia (67%), thrombocytopenia (56%), elevated liver enzymes (56%), lameness (43%), azotemia (33%), respiratory abnormalities (28%), and weakness and collapse (17%) (Breitschwerdt et al, 2010; Chomel et al, 2009b).

Granulomatous inflammation, systemically or in a single tissue, has been reported in dogs infected with *B. vinsonii* subsp. *berkhoffii* or *B. henselae.* Several organ systems can be affected, including liver, lung, heart, spleen, lymph nodes, eyes, endocardium, mediastinum, omentum, kidneys, and/or salivary glands. Signs associated with granulomatous inflammation vary according to the organ system involved; however, syncope, exercise intolerance, apathy, and generalized weakness predominate. Neurologic signs also have been reported in

---

BOX 269-1

Summary of Clinical and Laboratory Abnormalities in Dogs Infected with *Bartonella* Species

Clinical Signs	Laboratory Abnormalities
Anorexia	Elevated liver enzymes
Ascites	Eosinophilia
Cardiac arrhythmias	Hemoglobinuria
Diarrhea	Hyperbilirubinemia
Epistaxis	Hyperglobulinemia
Fever	Hypoglobulinemia
Heart murmur	Leukocytosis
Lameness	Monocytosis
Lethargy	Neutrophilia
Lymphadenopathy	Nonregenerative anemia
Neurologic signs	Proteinuria
Ocular signs	Spherocytosis
Respiratory signs	Thrombocytopenia
Skin lesions	
Splenomegaly	
Weight loss	

BOX 269-2

Reported Diagnoses in Dogs Infected with *Bartonella* Species*

Cardiac	**Hepatic**
Endocarditis	Peliosis hepatis
Myocarditis	Granulomatous hepatitis
Polyarthritis	
	Nasal
Ocular	Granulomatous rhinitis
Anterior uveitis	
Chorioretinitis	**Splenic**
	Fibrohistiocytic nodules
Systemic	Hemangiosarcoma
Immune-mediated hemolytic anemia	Lymphoid nodular hyperplasia
Immune-mediated thrombocytopenia	**Dermal**
Polyarthritis	Dermatitis
Systemic pyogranulomatous inflammation	Granulomatous inflammation
	Hemangiopericytoma
	Lymphadenitis
Central Nervous System	Panniculitis
Meningitis	
Meningoencephalitis (neutrophilic or granulomatous)	**Miscellaneous**
	Hyperviscosity syndrome
	Idiopathic effusions
Myelopathy	Sialometaplasia

*Whether *Bartonella* spp. infection induced each of these clinical abnormalities, in particular the neoplasms, currently is unknown.

dogs infected with *Bartonella* spp. These organisms may affect any topographic portion of the nervous system; therefore clinical manifestation may vary. In immunocompetent humans, *B. vinsonii* subsp. *berkhoffii* and *B. koehlerae* have been associated with neurologic and neurocognitive abnormalities, including headaches, insomnia, depression, anxiety, mood swings, memory loss, incoordination, muscle spasms, seizures, hallucinations, and decreased peripheral vision. Improvement of neurologic signs in humans and animals has been documented after antibiotic therapy (Breitschwerdt et al, 2010; Mellor et al, 2006).

Recently, *B. vinsonii* subsp. *berkhoffii* and *B. henselae* have been detected from transudates, modified transudates, or chylous effusions from dogs with cavitary effusions and from a dog with a massively enlarged seroma. Vascular endothelial infection may contribute to increased vascular permeability and aberrant fluid accumulation. In one study, two out of five patients treated for bartonellosis demonstrated improvement after antibiotic therapy (Cherry et al, 2009; Diniz et al, 2009).

B. henselae and *B. vinsonii* subsp. *berkhoffii* also have been detected from canine synovial fluid. Dogs seroreactive to *Bartonella* spp. have three times the odds for presenting arthritis-related lameness than seronegative dogs. Moreover, lameness and neutrophilic polyarthritis are frequently diagnosed in dogs infected with *Bartonella* spp. (Henn et al, 2005).

Diagnosis

The diagnosis of canine bartonellosis in dogs is a great challenge for the clinician and requires documentation of a combination of compatible clinical signs and pathologic abnormalities, serologic testing, microbiologic identification of the organism (culture, PCR, and DNA sequencing), and diagnostic efforts to rule out other infectious and noninfectious diseases.

Clinical Laboratory Assays

Hematologic and biochemical abnormalities frequently reported in dogs infected with *Bartonella* spp. are provided in Box 269-1. Because of the diversity of affected tissues and organ systems, an array of laboratory abnormalities may occur, but no abnormality is pathognomonic for *Bartonella* spp. infection. Symptoms frequently reported from dogs seropositive or bacteremic with *Bartonella* spp. are anemia (33% to 38% of dogs), thrombocytopenia (34% to 50%), leukocytosis (36% to 50%), neutrophilia (23% to 50%), monocytosis (33%), eosinophilia (29%), increased alanine aminotransferase (ALT) (18%) and alkaline phosphatase (ALP) (33% to 38%), proteinuria (63%), and neutrophilic polyarthitis. Hypoproteinemia was significantly associated with *Bartonella* spp. infection in dogs when compared with sick dogs suspected of other vector-borne diseases (Perez et al, 2013). Anemia generally is regenerative, and a positive Coombs' test is frequently documented because of immune-mediated hemolytic anemia (IMHA). Antinuclear antibodies also may be present, which may result in a misdiagnosis of systemic lupus erythematosus (SLE).

Blood smear examination for detection of intraerythrocytic organisms is not useful for the diagnosis of canine bartonellosis.

DNA Amplification Assays

Different from cats, which usually sustain high levels of bacteremia (10^5 to 10^6 organisms/ul of blood), asymptomatic or sick dogs generally maintain very low levels (<1 to 10 organisms/ul of blood), which can be below the limit of PCR detection. Therefore the practicality of PCR for documenting *Bartonella* spp. infection in canine blood and other diagnostic sample sources, as currently offered at some universities or commercial diagnostic laboratories, is limited fundamentally by the number of organisms in circulation. Therefore *negative PCR or culture results should never be used to rule out* Bartonella *spp. infection in dogs*. Higher concentrations of these pathogens may be detected in targeted tissues, such as affected cardiac valves, synovial fluid, effusions, lymph nodes, or granulomatous lesions, and also should be tested by PCR or culture. However, the presence of *Bartonella* DNA in lymph nodes is not confirmatory for canine bartonellosis, as demonstrated in a study in healthy golden retrievers, in which 18% of dogs harbored the organism in their lymph nodes (Duncan et al, 2008). Immunosuppression with corticosteroid therapy also increases the odds of *Bartonella* spp. detection; however, it predisposes the patient to a more severe disease manifestation, especially endocarditis.

Antibody Detection Assays

The detection of antibodies against *Bartonella* spp. provides strong clinical evidence of prior exposure to these organisms. However, only one third to one half of infected dogs mount a detectable antibody response at the time of initial testing (Breitschwerdt et al, 2010). Therefore, similar to PCR assays, *negative results of serologic tests do not rule out* Bartonella *spp. infection in dogs*. Detection of *Bartonella* spp. antibodies by enzyme-linked immunosorbent assay (ELISA) or immunofluorescent antibody assay (IFA) has substantial diagnostic limitations. The patient's antibody response to an infecting strain or genotype may not be detectable when using a different genotype in the assay, causing false-negative results. Commercial laboratories do not offer serology panels discriminating the four genotypes of *B. vinsonii* subsp. *berkhoffii*, although one university laboratory recently has developed specific IFA assays for genotype I, II, and III* currently available only for research purposes. Because approximately only one in three seropositive dogs is bacteremic for these organisms, diagnostic efforts based on culture or PCR assays should be made to confirm active infection. Progressive decrease in antibody titers during antibiotic therapy is associated with positive therapeutic response, with no antibodies detected as early as 3 to 6 months following therapy. Therefore monitoring antibody titers after therapy may

---

*Vector Borne Disease Diagnostic Laboratory, North Carolina State University, College of Veterinary Medicine, Raleigh, NC. http://www.cvm.ncsu.edu/vhc/csds/ticklab.html.

be useful to determining the therapeutic elimination of *Bartonella* spp., but should be used in conjunction with PCR and/or culture methods (Breitschwerdt et al, 2010).

Culture Assays

Several culture techniques have been reported for the isolation of *Bartonella* spp. However, success rates in isolating these organisms from dog blood or other clinical specimens vary greatly because of the low bacteremia level in the host. Most of the successful canine isolates are obtained from tissue samples, such as cardiac valves or biopsies for granulomatous lesions. *Bartonella* spp. are fastidious and slow-growing organisms, requiring several weeks to more than a month for their isolation.

Combined Approach: Enrichment Culture and DNA Amplification (Enrichment PCR)

A new diagnostic platform (enrichment PCR), which uses a novel liquid media coupled with highly sensitive and specific PCR, has enhanced considerably the ability to detect and or isolate *Bartonella* spp. from dogs, humans, and other hosts (Duncan, Maggi, and Breitschwerdt, 2007). This combined approach uses a chemically modified insect-based cell media (*Bartonella* α-Proteobacteria Growth Medium, BAPGM) to improve organism growth before subculture isolation on solid blood-agar media. This approach offers two different environments (insect cell media and mammalian blood cells) to support *Bartonella* growth, which has shortened the processing time for results and has broadened the spectrum of species detected. PCR testing combined with DNA sequencing for *Bartonella* spp. identification is used at three different steps of the BAPGM diagnostic platform: from the original sample (blood or tissue); after BAPGM liquid culture enhancement; and when plate isolates are obtained. Currently, this is one of the most successful diagnostic techniques available, detecting 55% more dogs infected with *Bartonella* spp. than a single PCR assay from blood or tissue (Perez et al, 2013). However, similar to serology and PCR assays, *negative results do not rule out infection* because of the cyclic shedding of *Bartonella* spp. from the primary niches into the bloodstream The enrichment PCR diagnostic platform is offered by a private laboratory in the United States.*

Microscopy

Bartonella spp. are small, slightly pleomorphic organisms with bacillary morphology. They cannot be visualized on tissue samples stained with hematoxylin-eosin. Modified silver stains (e.g., Warthin-Starry stain or Dieterle's stain) are required for visualization of the *Bartonella* spp. Nevertheless, these special stains are not specific for *Bartonella* spp., and other bacterial genera including *Leptospira, Borrelia, Pseudomonas, Streptococcus, Staphylococcus, Enterococcus, Corynebacterium,* and some fungi also are visualized using these staining methods. Immunohistochemistry and fluorescent *in situ* hybridization (FISH) have been

described for specific identification of *Bartonella* spp. in tissue samples; however, these techniques are not yet available through commercial diagnostic laboratories in the United States.

Treatment

Because of the frequent challenges in diagnosing canine bartonellosis associated with the lack of large clinical therapeutic trials, optimal treatment of *Bartonella* spp. infection in dogs remains controversial. Therefore, the optimal course of therapy for dogs is unknown, and current recommendations are extrapolated from the human literature and from nonrandomized, non–placebo-controlled reports from dogs. Long-term antibiotic therapy is required to eliminate *Bartonella* spp. infection in dogs, and once an effective treatment is initiated, weeks to months of therapy should be expected. Historically, azithromycin for 6 weeks has proven effective for most but not all dogs. Doxycycline for 4 to 6 weeks as monotherapy or combined with azithromycin has achieved variable degrees of disease remission. Unfortunately, failure to eliminate *Bartonella* spp. infection, despite multiple courses of azithromycin or doxycycline, has been documented. Therefore *monotherapy with azithromycin or doxycycline is no longer recommended because of treatment failure and the risk of rapid development of antimicrobial resistance.* If there are shortages of doxycycline, minocycline may be substituted at a dose of 5 to 10 mg/kg q12h PO (dogs) and 10 mg/kg q24h PO (cats).

A multidrug therapy for eradicating *Bartonella* spp. infection in dogs has not been established. One current, yet unproven, recommendation for treatment is based on combining an antibiotic that achieves high intracellular concentrations with another antibiotic that maintains high plasma concentrations. Suggested antibiotic combinations are provided in Table 269-2. In clinically stable dogs, the second antibiotic should be started 5 to 7 days after the first antibiotic is introduced to decrease the risk of Jarisch-Herxheimer reaction. This reaction is characterized by lethargy, vomiting, and signs resembling bacterial sepsis, caused by rapid death of bacteria and release of endotoxins with consequent increase of inflammatory cytokines in the bloodstream. Once present, this reaction lasts for few days. Empirically, corticosteroids at antiinflammatory doses have been used to alleviate these signs. Clinicians should differentiate this reaction from an adverse drug event to avoid interruption of antibiotic therapy.

In one study, *B. henselae* isolates from cats and humans were more susceptible *in vitro* to pradofloxacin (a third-generation fluoroquinolone) than azithromycin and enrofloxacin (Biswas et al, 2010). However, the effectiveness of pradofloxacin as monotherapy or combined with other antibiotics in dogs naturally infected with *Bartonella* spp. is currently unknown. Unpublished data suggest the combination of doxycycline with a fluoroquinolone is effective in cats with resistant bartonellosis; this protocol also may be effective in dogs, although *in vivo* data is needed. Pradofloxacin suspension is approved for use in cats in the United States (7.5 mg/kg PO once daily). Once daily use is approved in Europe for dogs and cats (tablets: 3 mg/kg PO; suspension: 5 mg/kg PO).

---

*Galaxy Laboratories, Research Triangle Park, NC, USA. http://www.galaxydx.com.

TABLE 269-2

Recommended Antibiotic Dosages for Canine Bartonellosis

Drug	Dose	Interval (hours)	Route	Duration (weeks)
Doxycycline[¶] with enrofloxacin*	5-10 mg/kg 5 mg/kg	12 12	PO PO	4-6 4-6
Azithromycin with rifampin[‡]	5-10 mg/kg 5 mg/kg	24 24	PO PO	6[†] 6
Doxycycline[¶] with rifampin[‡]	5-10 mg/kg 5 mg/kg	12 24	PO PO	4-6 4-6
Doxycycline[¶] with amikacin	5-10 mg/kg 15-20 mg/kg	12 24	PO IV/IM/SC	4-6 See notes[§]

*Other fluoroquinolones might be considered, but experimental or clinical data is not available. See text for details.

[†]Initially given every 24 hours for 7 days, followed by every other day for an additional 5 weeks.

[‡]It should only be used in combination with other antibiotics because of the risk of the development of antibiotic resistance.

[§]It should only be used during inpatient treatment because it requires parenteral administration and renal function monitoring. This is the protocol currently recommended for endocarditis.

[¶]If doxycycline is not available, minocycline may be substituted (see text).

In dogs with acute or life-threatening infections (endocarditis, myocarditis, meningoencephalitis, among others), concurrent use of a fluoroquinolone or doxycycline with an aminoglycoside (amikacin) is recommended during the initial management of the patient, followed by combined antibiotic therapy for at least 6 weeks. Amikacin should be administered parenterally while monitoring evidence of kidney injury during therapy (e.g., urinalysis and azotemia). Therapeutic elimination of the organism can be monitored by following serum antibody titers if initially present; many dogs that experience resolution of the disease manifestations no longer have detectable antibodies within 6 months after treatment. Culture and PCR assay results also can be followed, but the very low bacteremic levels and the failure to seroconvert make it unclear whether long-term antibiotic therapy clears the organism or if the organisms remain in a subclinical "latent" form (Breitschwerdt et al, 2010).

Transmission to Humans

The two recent reports of a possible iatrogenic transmission by needle stick of B. vinsonii subsp. berkhoffii and B. henselae to two veterinarians who experienced chronic fatigue and frequent headaches or chronic undulant fever, persistent back pain, and lymphadenopathy emphasizes the zoonotic importance of this organism, especially for veterinarians and other individuals with increased animal or arthropod contact. A recent study on 192 humans, predominantly from the United States, with extensive arthropod exposure or frequent animal contact

detected that approximately half of them were seroreactive and one in four was bacteremic for Bartonella spp. The most common clinical signs and symptoms reported by the patient population included fatigue (79%), sleeplessness (64%), muscle pain (63%), joint pain (64%), chronic fatigue (63%), irritability (60%), and headaches (62%) (Maggi et al, 2011). Therefore individuals from high-risk groups should take precautions to avoid arthropod bites, contact with arthropod feces, bites and scratches from animals, and direct contact with bodily fluids from sick animals (Breitschwerdt et al, 2010). In addition, veterinarians play a major role in educating and advising the local community of the zoonotic risk of Bartonella spp. as well as infections with other vectorborne pathogens. Despite the fact that Bartonella DNA was detected in dog saliva, it is unclear if dog bites and scratches can transmit Bartonella spp. to humans or if dogs serve as a reservoir host for human infection. Dogs infected with Bartonella spp. may represent an epidemiologic sentinel for human exposure to a common vector; therefore tick and flea control is crucial to reduce or prevent transmission of Bartonella spp. to pets and potentially their owners.

References and Suggested Reading

Biswas S et al: Comparative activity of pradofloxacin, enrofloxacin, and azithromycin against Bartonella henselae isolates collected from cats and a human, J Clin Microbiol 48(2):617, 2010.

Boulouis HJ et al: Factors associated with the rapid emergence of zoonotic Bartonella infections, Vet Res 36(3):383, 2005.

Breitschwerdt EB et al: Bartonellosis: an emerging infectious disease of zoonotic importance to animals and human beings, J Vet Emerg Crit Care 20(1):8, 2010.

Cherry NA et al: Isolation or molecular detection of Bartonella henselae and Bartonella vinsonii subsp. berkhoffii from dogs with idiopathic cavitary effusions, JVIM 23(1):186, 2009.

Chomel BB et al: Dogs are more permissive than cats or guinea pigs to experimental infection with a human isolate of Bartonella rochalimae, Vet Res 40(4):27, 2009a.

Chomel BB et al: Bartonella endocarditis: a pathology shared by animal reservoirs and patients, Ann NY Acad Sci 1166:120, 2009b.

Chomel BB, Kasten RW: Bartonellosis, an increasingly recognized zoonosis, J Appl Microbiol 109(3):743, 2010.

Chomel BB et al: Candidatus Bartonella merieuxii, a potential new zoonotic Bartonella species in canids from Iraq, PLoS Negl Trop Dis 6(9):e1843, 2012.

Diniz PPVP et al: Co-isolation of Bartonella henselae and Bartonella vinsonii subsp. berkhoffii from blood, joint and subcutaneous seroma fluids from two naturally infected dogs, Vet Microbiol 138(3-4):368, 2009.

Diniz PPVP et al: Bartonella rochalimae in dogs in Peru. In Proceedings of the seventh International Conference on Bartonella as Animal and Human Pathogen, 2012, 21.

Duncan AW, Maggi RG, Breitschwerdt EB: A combined approach for the enhanced detection and isolation of Bartonella species in dog blood samples: pre-enrichment liquid culture followed by PCR and subculture onto agar plates, J Microbiol Methods 69(2):273, 2007.

Duncan AW et al: Bartonella DNA in the blood and lymph nodes of Golden Retrievers with lymphoma and in healthy controls, JVIM 22(1):89, 2008.

Franz B, Kempf VA: Adhesion and host cell modulation: critical pathogenicity determinants of Bartonella henselae, Parasit Vectors 4:54, 2011.

Henn JB et al: Seroprevalence of antibodies against Bartonella species and evaluation of risk factors and clinical signs associated with seropositivity in dogs, *Am J Vet Res* 66(4):688, 2005.

Henn JB et al: Bartonella rochalimae in raccoons, coyotes, and red foxes, *Emerg Infect Dis* 15(12):1984, 2009.

Maggi RG et al: A Bartonella vinsonii berkhoffii typing scheme based upon 16S-23S ITS and Pap31 sequences from dog, coyote, gray fox, and human isolates, *Mol Cell Probe* 20(2):128, 2006.

Maggi RG et al: *Bartonella* spp. bacteremia in high-risk immunocompetent patients, *Diagn Microbiol Infect Dis* 71(4):430, 2011.

Mellor PJ et al: Alpha1-proteinase inhibitor deficiency and *Bartonella* infection in association with panniculitis, polyarthritis, and meningitis in a dog, *J Vet Intern Med* 20(4):1023, 2006.

Perez C et al: An unmatched case controlled study of clinicopathologic abnormalities in dogs with *Bartonella* infection, *J Vet Intern Med*, in press, 2013.

CHAPTER 270

Feline Bartonellosis

LYNN F. GUPTILL, *West Lafayette, Indiana*

*B*artonella spp. are fastidious, vector-transmitted, gram-negative bacteria in the α-2 Proteobacteria family Bartonellaceae. At least 24 named *Bartonella* spp. are highly adapted to and likely evolved with mammalian reservoir hosts, in which long-term, apparently asymptomatic bacteremia occurs (Breitschwerdt et al, 2010; Guptill, 2010a). Since the first report of feline *B. henselae* infection in 1992, natural infection of cats with five *Bartonella* spp. (*B. henselae, B. clarridgeiae, B. koehlerae, B. quintana,* and *B. bovis* [formerly *B. weissii*]) has been reported. Feline infections with species other than *B. henselae* or *B. clarridgeiae* are uncommon (Chomel and Kasten, 2010). Approximately 14 *Bartonella* spp. are considered zoonotic; all five of the *Bartonella* spp. identified in cats are zoonotic.

The primary zoonotic *Bartonella* sp. associated with cats is *B. henselae,* which causes long-term bacteremia in healthy cats. It has been detected by polymerase chain reaction (PCR) in tissues of numerous other mammalian species, some of which are dogs, seals, whales, horses, and wild felids (Breitschwerdt et al, 2010). Domestic cats are considered the primary mammalian reservoir and vector for human infections with *B. henselae.*

B. henselae causes or has been associated with cat-scratch disease (CSD), bacillary angiomatosis, bacillary peliosis, relapsing fever with bacteremia, meningitis, encephalitis, neuroretinitis, endocarditis, and many additional conditions in humans (Chomel and Kasten, 2010). *B. clarridgeiae* was associated serologically with a CSD-like condition in two people (Breitschwerdt et al, 2010). *B. koehlerae,* isolated from several healthy cats, has been associated with human and canine endocarditis (Ohad et al, 2010) but did not cause clinical signs in cats inoculated experimentally. Although *B. quintana* has been identified in cats, it has not been established that it is transmitted zoonotically by cats. Humans are the reservoir host for *B. quintana,* which caused trench fever in World War I and also causes endocarditis, bacillary angiomatosis, bacillary peliosis, and chronic lymphadenomegaly in people (Chomel et al, 2006; Kaiser et al, 2011). This chapter focuses on *B. henselae,* the feline-associated *Bartonella* spp. for which the most information is known.

Epidemiology and Pathogenesis

Exposure of cats to *Bartonella* spp. is common worldwide. *B. henselae* bacteremia occurs in approximately 5% to 40% of cats in the United States on average, with higher prevalence in warmer, more humid regions with high flea prevalence. In some cat colonies, *Bartonella* seroprevalence reaches 90% or more. Most cats with *Bartonella* bacteremia are infected with *B. henselae*; between 10% and 31% of cats surveyed with *Bartonella* bacteremia were infected with *B. clarridgeiae. B. koehlerae* and *B. bovis* were detected in only a few cats. *Bartonella* spp. also were identified in wild felids in North America, Brazil, and Africa (Chomel et al, 2009b; Guptill, 2010a). Coinfection of cats with multiple *B. henselae* genetic types and with *B. henselae* and *B. clarridgeiae* is reported. There are regional differences in prevalence of infection of cats with different types of *B. henselae,* and there is remarkable molecular diversity among *B. henselae* isolates (Chomel et al, 2009b). Genomic variation in *B. henselae* during the course of infection in cats likely enhances the ability of *B. henselae* to persist in cats for prolonged periods. Genetics also may be a factor in the pathogenicity of various *Bartonella* spp. isolates.

Bartonella henselae is transmitted naturally among cats by cat fleas (*Ctenocephalides felis felis*). The primary mode of transmission is via intradermal exposure to flea feces;

it does not appear that transmission occurs via flea saliva. Ticks may have a role in transmission, and *Bartonella* spp. also have been detected in biting flies, lice, and other arthropods (Tsai et al, 2011). Transmission among cats does not appear to occur normally transplacentally or directly through grooming or sharing of food dishes and litter boxes when fleas are absent. Feline bacteremia with *B. henselae* is chronic and recurrent. Experimentally infected cats had relapses of bacteremia occurring at irregular intervals of between 1 and 4½ months. Persistent natural relapsing bacteremia in cats because of reinfection of cats with different strains of *B. henselae* over time also is reported (Breitschwerdt et al, 2010; Guptill, 2010a).

Cats have robust cellular and humoral immune responses to *Bartonella* spp. infections, and immunosuppression by *Bartonella* spp. infection has not been documented. Cell-mediated immunity appears important in reducing the level of bacteremia in experimentally infected cats. Cats maintained normal CD4 and CD8 lymphocyte numbers and ratios in one experimental study, whereas in another study some experimentally infected cats had transiently decreased CD4 lymphocyte numbers (Guptill, 2010a). Prior infection with *Bartonella* spp. does not appear to confer broad-based immunity to reinfection; most cats are susceptible to infection with *Bartonella* strains and species to which they have not been exposed previously (Breitschwerdt et al, 2010; Guptill, 2010a).

Bartonella spp. are generally intracellular bacteria, and *B. henselae* has been detected within erythrocytes of naturally infected cats. *Bartonella* spp. also may be located intracellularly in vascular endothelial cells of infected cats as has been suggested for rats infected with *B. tribocorum*. Extracellular *B. henselae* also are detected in blood and other tissues of infected cats (Chomel et al, 2009a; Guptill, 2010).

Clinical Findings

Experimental Studies

Most cats experimentally infected with *Bartonella* spp. exhibited no clinical signs. Clinical signs that did occur were, with some notable exceptions, generally mild, and varied with the strain of *B. henselae* used for inoculation (Guptill, 2010b). Cats developed induration or abscess at intradermal inoculation sites between approximately 2 and 21 days after inoculation. Other transient clinical findings included generalized or localized peripheral lymphadenomegaly that persisted for approximately 6 weeks after inoculation. Fever (>103° F; 39.4° C) occurred during the first 48 to 96 hours after inoculation and again for 24 to 48 hours at approximately 2 weeks after inoculation. Some cats were lethargic and anorexic when febrile. Mild neurologic signs (e.g., nystagmus, transient whole body tremors, decreased or exaggerated responses to external stimuli, mild behavior changes), and epaxial muscle pain also were reported in some cats. In one study, three of six cats infected by exposure to *C. felis* developed fever and one cat was euthanized because of severe cardiac disease. Reproductive failure occurred in some cats. There were no reported clinical signs in cats experimentally

infected with *B. koehlerae* or the proposed species *B. rochalimae* (Breitschwerdt et al, 2010; Guptill, 2010a; Chomel and Kasten, 2010).

Complete blood counts, serum biochemical tests, and urine analysis were normal in most experimentally infected cats. A few cats had transient mild anemia early in the course of infection, and some had persistent eosinophilia. Mature neutrophilia occurred in some cats during periods of skin inflammation. Cats had hyperplasia of lymphoid organs, small foci of lymphocytic, pyogranulomatous, or neutrophilic inflammation in multiple tissues (lung, liver, spleen, kidney, heart), and small foci of necrosis in the liver or spleen (Breitschwerdt et al, 2010; Guptill, 2010a).

Natural Infection

Clinical signs are not reported commonly in naturally infected cats. There were no clinical signs reported in 65 naturally infected cats in one study. *Bartonella* infection has been associated with uveitis in some cats (Breitschwerdt et al, 2010; Guptill, 2010b). *Bartonella* spp. were associated with endocarditis in two naturally infected cats (Chomel et al, 2009). Whether members of the genus *Bartonella* contribute to previously described instances of argyrophilic bacteria in lymph nodes of cats with persistent lymphadenomegaly is unknown. *Bartonella* DNA was not found in tissues of 14 cats with plasmacytic pododermatitis, or 26 cats with peliosis hepatis, and immunohistochemical staining was negative for *Bartonella* spp. in these cats (Guptill, 2010).

A potential causative role of *Bartonella* spp. in chronic diseases of cats has been proposed because *Bartonella* bacteremia in cats often is prolonged, and systemic inflammation is documented in infected cats. Contribution of *Bartonella* infections to development of chronic illnesses of cats has not been verified. Associations have been reported between seropositive status and gingivitis, stomatitis, lymphadenomegaly, unspecified urinary tract disorders, and hyperglobulinemia (Breitschwerdt et al, 2010; Chomel et al, 2006; Guptill, 2010b). However, the use of serology for establishing *Bartonella* spp. infection appears to be limited, and conclusions drawn from studies that rely solely on serologic methods for diagnosis of *Bartonella* spp. infection should be interpreted with caution.

Clinical conditions proposed as attributable to feline bartonellosis also may result from other causes, and determining which cats have clinical signs attributable to *Bartonella* spp. infection is difficult. Case-control studies evaluating naturally infected cats have failed to prove association of *Bartonella* spp. with anemia, gingivostomatitis, neurologic conditions, high serum trypsin-like immunoreactivity, inflammatory polyps, chronic rhinosinusitis, or uveitis (Guptill, 2010b; Stiles, 2011). In some of these studies, animals seropositive for *Bartonella* spp. were less likely to be affected by the clinical condition studied than were serologically negative animals. The prevalence of *Bartonella* DNA in the blood of febrile cats was almost statistically significantly greater (P = 0.057) than the prevalence of *Bartonella* DNA in the blood of afebrile cats (Breitschwerdt et al, 2010; Guptill, 2010b).

Because *Bartonella* spp. exposure is common in the domestic cat population, additional extensive, carefully controlled epidemiologic investigations are needed to determine whether particular clinical conditions truly are associated with *B. henselae* infections in cats. Veterinarians also must consider the likelihood that some clinical conditions have multiple causes, particularly in cats with exposure to arthropod vectors.

Diagnosis

Determining which sick cats are most likely to be ill because of *Bartonella* spp. infection is challenging. Because bartonellosis is zoonotic, veterinarians may be asked to test healthy cats belonging to clients with *Bartonella*-related illnesses, or to screen healthy cats under consideration as pets for immunocompromised people (see Public Health below).

Cytology

Detecting *B. henselae* in erythrocytes of infected cats is not effective using conventional staining methods. Intraerythrocytic and extracellular Bartonellae have been detected using immunocytochemical and immunohistochemical methods.

Serology

Serologic testing alone is problematic in that false-positive test results seem common regardless of the assay used. Serology probably is used best in conjunction with blood culture or polymerase chain reaction (PCR) testing. Serum IgG antibodies persist in experimentally infected animals for prolonged periods; how long antibodies persist after clearance of an infection is unknown. It remains difficult to document clearance of *Bartonella* spp. infection because of the relapsing nature of feline bacteremia and relative insensitivity of culture and molecular methods to detect low levels of bacteremia. False-negative results appear less common; 5% to 12% of cats with *B. henselae* bacteremia were seronegative (Breitschwerdt et al, 2010; Guptill, 2010b).

Immunofluorescent antibody (IFA), enzyme immunoassay (EIA), and Western blot tests are available. Infections with some strains or species of *Bartonella* may be missed using any serologic method, depending on the antigen preparations used. Positive predictive values of IFA and EIA tests for anti-*B. henselae* serum IgG antibodies for bacteremia in cats are 39% to 46%. The utility of a negative serologic test is greater; negative predictive values for these tests in cats are 89% to 97% (Breitschwerdt et al, 2010; Guptill, 2010a). The diagnostic accuracy of Western blot immunoassays has not been investigated as extensively.

Bacterial Isolation

A positive blood culture or culture of other tissue provides definitive diagnosis of active *Bartonella* spp. infection but does not indicate that *Bartonella* spp. are the cause of clinical disease. Because of the relapsing nature of feline *Bartonella* bacteremia, a single blood culture can be insensitive for bacteremia, and multiple blood cultures may be necessary. Combination of enriched culture and molecular detection may be the best method for diagnosing feline *Bartonella* spp. infections (Breitschwerdt et al, 2010).

Blood for culture should be obtained using sterile technique, and the blood is placed in ethylenediamine tetraacetic acid (EDTA)–containing tubes or lysis centrifugation blood culture tubes (Isolator tubes). Blood collected into EDTA tubes should be chilled or frozen for transport to the laboratory. Blood should be sent to laboratories familiar with *Bartonella* culture. Because enriched media are used for *Bartonella* culture, strict sterile technique when collecting blood samples is important. Even a small amount of contamination may result in overgrowth with less fastidious bacteria, or conversely, residual flea excrement at the site of venipuncture may result in a positive *Bartonella* culture using enriched media.

Nucleic Acid Amplification

Standard PCR testing for *Bartonella* DNA in blood may be no more sensitive than blood culture for detecting active *Bartonella* spp. infection, and detecting DNA does not equate always to detecting living organisms. Depending on the assay, real-time PCR may improve diagnostic sensitivity. The primer pairs used have a marked influence on the sensitivity of PCR assays. An advantage of PCR testing is that results are available more quickly than those of blood culture. The products of PCR reactions may be sequenced, making rapid identification of *Bartonella* spp. and strains possible. Samples for PCR testing should be obtained using strict sterile technique, and care must be taken in collection and processing to avoid sample contamination (and false positive results) or DNA degradation (and false negative results). For culture and PCR testing, individual laboratories should be contacted for collection and submission guidelines.

Coinfection

Cats may be coinfected with multiple pathogens; for example, cats may be coinfected with other vector-borne pathogens such as hemotrophic *Mycoplasma* spp. or rickettsial pathogens. Cats also may be coinfected with feline leukemia virus (FeLV) or feline immunodeficiency virus (FIV) and other *Bartonella* spp. Such coinfections make attributing clinical signs of disease to infection with a particular organism difficult and also have important implications for therapy.

Treatment

Treatment of feline *Bartonella* spp. infections remains challenging and controversial. Documenting clearance of feline *Bartonella* spp. infections through antibiotic treatment is difficult because of the relapsing nature of the bacteremia and persistence of serum antibodies. Treatment of *Bartonella* spp. infections appears to require long-term (at least 4 to 6 weeks) antibiotic administration. No regimen of antibiotic treatment has been proven effective for definitively eliminating *Bartonella* spp. infections in cats. Doxycycline and enrofloxacin have been shown to have mixed efficacy for treating experimentally infected cats. Doses reported as effective vary. When doxycycline (tablets) is used, precautions to avoid esophageal strictures are necessary. Because enrofloxacin causes retinal degeneration and blindness in some cats when administered at more than 5 mg/kg q24h, use of a higher dose is contraindicated. Results of a recent study showed good *in vitro* efficacy of pradofloxacin against *B. henselae*. However, another report documented naturally occurring fluoroquinolone resistance in *Bartonella* isolates, and it was recommended that fluoroquinolones not be used to treat *Bartonella*-related clinical conditions in humans (Biswas and Rolain, 2010). Antibiotics tested in experimental studies (erythromycin, amoxicillin, amoxicillin/ clavulanic acid, tetracycline hydrochloride) decreased the level of bacteremia in treated cats. Antibiotic treatment could not be deemed successful compared with no treatment because untreated cats became blood culture negative after the same length of time as did cats that were treated (Guptill, 2010b). Rifampin in combination with doxycycline has been recommended, but data regarding efficacy of this combination in cats have not been published. Rifampin should not be used alone because resistance develops rapidly (Biswas and Rolain, 2010).

Azithromycin has been used widely to treat feline *Bartonella* spp. infections, but no data from controlled feline studies support this practice. Macrolide-resistant strains of *Bartonella* spp. are reported, and concern was stated in one publication that a resistant *Bartonella* strain may have arisen as a result of animals exposed to macrolide antibiotics (Biswas et al, 2006; Guptill, 2010b). Recent *in vitro* data suggest that azithromycin's efficacy against *Bartonella* spp. may be limited, and resistance to azithromycin was induced *in vitro* (Biswas and Rolain, 2010). In addition, azithromycin appears to have important immunomodulatory and antiinflammatory properties in addition to its broad antimicrobial spectrum. It is therefore difficult to determine whether reports of beneficial effects from azithromycin treatment of cats are a result of anti-*Bartonella* activity or instead are a result of azithromycin's other properties, of the antimicrobial action of azithromycin on other bacteria, or of a combination of all of these. Taken together, the data suggest that azithromycin is not the best first choice for treating feline bartonellosis.

Antibiotic resistance in *Bartonella* spp. is an important consideration. Resistance to azithromycin was induced easily *in vitro* after only two passages. Resistance was induced to enrofloxacin and pradofloxacin after five *in vitro* passages. Gentamicin resistance was induced in *B. henselae* only after nine *in vitro* passages. Aminoglycosides may be the only class of antibiotic bactericidal for *Bartonella* spp. Investigators were unable to induce resistance *in vitro* to doxycycline or amoxicillin. They recommended that humans with *Bartonella*-related endocarditis be treated with doxycycline for 6 weeks plus gentamicin for 14 days (Biswas and Rolain, 2010). People with *Bartonella* spp. infections causing bacillary angiomatosis or peliosis, or endocarditis, are treated with a variety of antibiotics.

Erythromycin has been recommended for bacillary angiomatosis because of its antibiotic and antiangiogenic properties (Biswas and Rolain, 2010).

Because of the uncertainty of antibiotic efficacy and the concern that routine treatment for asymptomatic feline *Bartonella* spp. infections may induce resistant strains, treatment is recommended only for cats showing clinical signs of disease. Given recent findings regarding resistance, and data from experimental infections documenting some efficacy of doxycycline treatment, the preferred antibiotic for treating ill cats may be doxycycline. Additional controlled studies are needed to assess antibiotic treatment protocols for feline *Bartonella* spp. infections.

Client education is essential. The uncertainty of treatment efficacy and the importance of flea control and other means of preventing transmission must be emphasized. In addition, the likelihood that cats may be reinfected readily with *Bartonella* spp. after exposure to infected fleas, even after treatment, must be made clear to owners.

Prevention

Prevention of *Bartonella* spp. infections is accomplished best by avoiding exposure to fleas and other arthropod vectors. Because *B. henselae* and *B. clarridgeiae* have been transmitted through inoculation of infected cat blood, any cat that tests positive for *Bartonella* spp. via serology, culture, or PCR should not be used as a blood donor. No vaccine is available to prevent *Bartonella* spp. infection in cats.

Public Health

Bartonella spp. cause many clinical syndromes in humans, some of which include CSD (typical and atypical forms, including encephalopathies in children and other neurologic abnormalities), bacillary angiomatosis, parenchymal bacillary peliosis, relapsing fever with bacteremia, endocarditis, optic neuritis, pulmonary, hepatic, or splenic granulomas, and osteomyelitis (Kaiser et al, 2011). Immunocompetent individuals may have more localized infections, whereas infections that occur in immunocompromised individuals are more often systemic and can be fatal. Veterinarians, veterinary staff, groomers, and others with extensive companion animal contact are at a greater risk for *Bartonella* spp. exposure than are members of the general public (Breitschwerdt et al, 2010). Veterinary staff should receive specific training regarding the zoonotic potential of *Bartonella* spp. and potential modes of transmission.

Transmission of *B. henselae* from cats to humans probably occurs through contamination of cat scratches with flea excrement. Transmission may occur through cat bites if cat blood or flea excrement contaminates the bite site or the cat's saliva. Ticks are considered possible vectors for transmission of some *Bartonella* spp. infections, although their role in transmission remains undefined. Some persons with *Bartonella* spp. infections have reported exposure to dogs and not cats, and others report no animal contact at all (Breitschwerdt et al, 2010).

The 2009 *Guidelines for Preventing Opportunistic Infections Among HIV-Infected Adults and Adolescents* (Kaplan et al, 2009) recommend the following when acquiring a new cat: adopt a cat over 1 year of age that is in good health, avoid rough play with cats, maintain flea control, wash any cat-associated wounds promptly, and do not allow cats to lick wounds or cuts. The guidelines note no evidence of any benefit to cat owners from routine culture or serologic testing of healthy cats for *Bartonella* spp. There is no evidence that declawing cats decreases the probability of transmission of *B. henselae* from cats to humans. Control of fleas and other potential arthropod vectors is essential for interrupting transmission.

References and Suggested Reading

Biswas S, Rolain JM: *Bartonella* infection: treatment and drug resistance, *Future Microbiol* 5:171, 2010.

Biswas S, Raoult D, Rolain J-M: Molecular characterization of resistance to macrolides in *Bartonella henselae*, *Antimicrob Agents Chemother* 50:3192, 2006.

Boulouis H-J et al: Factors associated with the rapid emergence of zoonotic *Bartonella* infections, *Vet Res* 36:383, 2005.

Breitschwerdt EB et al: Bartonellosis: an emerging infectious disease of zoonotic importance to animals and human beings, *J Vet Emerg Crit Care* 20:8, 2010.

Brunt J et al: American Association of Feline Practitioners 2006 Panel report on diagnosis, treatment, and prevention of *Bartonella* spp. infections, *J Feline Med Surg* 8:213, 2006.

Chomel BB et al: *Bartonella* spp. in pets and effect on human health, *Emerg Infect Dis* 12:389, 2006.

Chomel BB et al: *Bartonella* endocarditis: a pathology shared by animal reservoirs and patients, *Ann N Y Acad Sci* 1166:120, 2009a.

Chomel BB et al: Ecological fitness and strategies of adaptation of *Bartonella* species to their hosts and vectors, *Vet Res* 40:29, 2009b.

Chomel BB, Kasten RW: Bartonellosis, an increasingly recognized zoonosis, *J Appl Microbiol* 109:743, 2010.

Guptill L: Bartonellosis, *Vet Microbiol* 140:347, 2010a.

Guptill L: Feline bartonellosis, *Vet Clin North Am Small Anim Pract* 40:1073, 2010b.

Kaiser PO et al: *Bartonella* spp: Throwing light on uncommon human infections, *Int J Med Microbiol* 301:7, 2011.

Kaplan JK et al: Guidelines for prevention and treatment of opportunistic infections in HIV-infected adults and adolescents: recommendations from CDC, the National Institutes of Health, and the HIV Medicine Association of the Infectious Diseases Society of America, *MMWR Recomm Rep* 58(RR-4):1, 2009.

Ohad DG et al: Molecular detection of *Bartonella henselae* and *Bartonella koehlerae* from aortic valves of Boxer dogs with infective endocarditis, *Vet Microbiol* 141:182, 2010.

Stiles J: Bartonellosis in cats: a role in uveitis? *Vet Ophthalmol* 14(Suppl 1):9, 2011.

Tsai YL et al: *Bartonella* species and their ectoparasites: selective host adaptation or strain selection between the vector and the mammalian host? *Comp Immunol Microbiol Infect Dis* 34(4):299, 2011.

CHAPTER **271**

Borreliosis

MERYL P. LITTMAN, *Philadelphia, Pennsylvania*

Lyme disease (Lyme borreliosis) in dogs is caused by a unicellular microaerophilic gram-negative motile spirochete, *Borrelia burgdorferi*, generally transmitted via *Ixodes* tick bites. In the United States, 95% of human Lyme disease is reported in just 12 endemic states: New Jersey, Pennsylvania, Wisconsin, New York, Massachusetts, Connecticut, Minnesota, Maryland, Virginia, New Hampshire, Delaware, and Maine. After 2 to 4 days of tick attachment, down-regulation of the spirochete's expression of OspA (the organism's outer surface protein, which attaches it to the tick's midgut) allows its passage into the new host. Migrating interstitially, this extracellular organism lives near collagen and fibroblasts, usually causing little if any inflammation in most hosts. Antigenic variation allows new antigens to be expressed over time by the spirochete in carriers, thereby evading the host's immune system. *Borrelia* spp. of the relapsing fever group may also cause illness in dogs.

The most common form of canine Lyme disease is the subclinical (asymptomatic) carrier. In endemic areas, up to 70% to 90% of healthy dogs are seropositive. In field studies, 95% of seropositive dogs had no signs of Lyme disease by history or at 20-month follow-up. Less than 5% of seropositive dogs show signs of *Lyme arthritis* (lameness ± fever/inappetence), which is self-limiting or quickly responsive to antibiotics. The least common but most serious form is *Lyme nephritis*, seen mostly in Labrador and golden retrievers. The incidence is unknown but thought to be very low (less than 1% to 2%) because proteinuria is uncommon even among seropositive retrievers. Other human manifestations (e.g., rash or cardiac or neurologic signs) are not well documented in dogs.

The experimental model for inducing Lyme disease in dogs (beagles) showed a self-limiting arthritis in puppies; adults became seropositive but remained subclinical. Puppies age 6 to 12 weeks of age exposed to endemic *Ixodes* ticks showed a 4-day self-limiting illness after a 2- to 5-month incubation, with fever, anorexia, and lameness or joint swelling or lymphadenopathy in the leg closest to where ticks fed. One to six similar self-limiting episodes several weeks apart in the same or different leg may follow because of migration of spirochetes expressing new antigens. Older pups (13 to 26 weeks) showed milder and fewer signs as well as number of days and episodes involved. Cultures and polymerase chain reaction (PCR) testing of skin biopsies from where ticks fed more than 1 year earlier showed that dogs remain subclinical carriers if not treated with antibiotics, and 10% to 15% of treated dogs were still not cleared. None developed Lyme nephritis, so the factors related to onset, progression, treatment, or prevention are unknown. Approximately 35% to 45% of these tick-exposed experimental dogs were coinfected with *Anaplasma phagocytophilum*, and a few were coinfected with *Babesia microti*.

Lyme nephritis (LN) was described first in seropositive dogs with protein-losing nephropathy (PLN) and a unique combination of renal histopathologic changes, including immune-mediated (usually membranoproliferative) glomerulonephritis (IMGN), diffuse tubular necrosis and regeneration, and lymphoplasmacytic interstitial nephritis. Affected dogs were younger than other dogs with PLN (5.6 ± 2.6 years vs. 7.1 ± 3.6 years), and almost half were Labrador or golden retrievers (Shetland sheepdogs also were overrepresented). Less than 30% of the dogs had a history of lameness. Most clinical findings were due to renal failure with primary glomerular disease (proteinuria, hypoalbuminemia, hypercholesterolemia, ascites or effusions, thromboembolic events, hypertension) and secondary tubular involvement (glycosuria sometimes, eventually isosthenuria). Mild to moderate thrombocytopenia also sometimes was seen, possibly because of consumption related to the hypercoagulability of PLN or because of coinfections. Studies show LN is a sterile nephritis, caused by immune-complex deposition rather than renal invasion of spirochetes. Affected dogs have on average higher levels of circulating *B. burgdorferi*–specific immune complexes than unaffected seropositive dogs, although the level is not predictive because many unaffected dogs also have high levels. The entity LN probably occurs during the chronic or carrier phase when antibody levels are high, although signs may appear as acute, chronic, mild, moderate, or severe. Some dogs progress rapidly and become oliguric or anuric soon after presenting with vomiting. One study showed positive staining of *B. burgdorferi*–specific immune complexes in 84% of renal cortical biopsies from suspect cases using immunohistochemistry (IHC) and rabbit antibodies directed against *B. burgdorferi* antigens p83, p34 (OspB), p31 (OspA), and lower molecular weight *B. burgdorferi* antigens. Other studies found involvement of *B. burgdorferi* antigens p39, p41 (flagellin), p22, and p31 (OspA). Whether there are immune-complex deposits not specific to *B. burgdorferi* in these cases is unknown. Without an inducible experimental model, it is unknown if there are

specific *Borrelia* spp. strains that trigger LN. A genetic predisposition may involve immune dysregulation or a structural or functional glomerulopathy. Most seropositive dogs (even seropositive retrievers) are not affected with LN and are not proteinuric.

Renal biopsies were described in severely affected dogs either at necropsy or end-stage disease. Without an experimental model for LN the appearance of the lesion and the clinical progression during earlier stages is unknown. There may be a time when occult proteinuria exists with milder glomerular changes, when intervention may be most helpful, before azotemia and/or tubular damage occurs.

Diagnostic Tests

Positive serology, supportive clinical signs, consideration of differentials, and response to therapy are clues, but Lyme disease easily is overdiagnosed because *B. burgdorferi* antibodies are common in healthy dogs, clinical signs are not pathognomonic, and response to therapy may be coincidental. In addition, no test predicts which seropositive dogs will become ill.

Serology

The organism does not circulate in blood and is found rarely in fluids or tissues, so antigen assays (e.g., culture or PCR assays) are not as useful. Measurement of serum antibodies against *B. burgdorferi* antigens is the test most widely used to aid in the diagnosis of Lyme disease.

The magnitude of any *B. burgdorferi* antibody titer does not predict illness because many dogs with subclinical infections also have high titers. The most commonly used test for natural exposure is the C6 peptide antibody test (SNAP-4DxPlus, SNAP-3Dx, Lyme C6Quant) against part of the VlsE antigen, which is not expressed in ticks, *in vitro*, or in any of the *B. burgdorferi* vaccines. Antibodies against the C6 peptide reach detectable levels 3 to 5 weeks after infection, well before clinical signs are recognized in experimentally infected dogs. A Lyme C6Quant level more than 30 confirms exposure but does not prove the organism is the cause of the clinical signs. Comparisons of pretreatment and 6-month posttreatment C6Quant levels may be helpful (if a dog is treated); a 50% decline or more may indicate decreased antigenic load and possible clearance, even if the qualitative SNAP test is still positive. In addition, the new baseline quantitative value may be useful for future comparison if clinical signs suggestive of Lyme disease recur. It currently is unclear whether the failure to achieve a decreased C6Quant level after treatment can be used as a prognostic indicator.

Whole-cell immunofluorescent antibody (IFA) and enzyme-linked immunosorbent assay (ELISA) antibody tests are available but do not differentiate antibodies induced by vaccination from those induced by natural exposure and may cross-react with other spirochetal antigens. Determination of IgM titers independent of IgG titers is not needed because dogs are not ill until after seroconversion to IgG, and IgM peaks can reoccur in carriers because of antigenic variation. Western immunoblot immunoassays may be useful to distinguish vaccinated from exposed dogs if a sole antibody band at p31 is seen after giving a subunit ospA vaccination. Otherwise banding patterns may not differentiate clearly antibodies induced by administration of *B. burgdorferi* bacterin vaccines from natural exposure antibodies. This is because *B. burgdorferi* carriers may recognize similar *B. burgdorferi* antigens found in dogs administered bacterins as the organism shows the host its antigenic repertoire, including antigens usually expressed in ticks, *in vitro*, or in bacterins. Some laboratories (e.g., New York State Diagnostic Laboratory and Antech Laboratories) are reporting serologic responses against multiple *B. burgdorferi* antigens; common targets include OspA, OspC, and OspF. OspA antibodies rise and fall after vaccination, but the protective titer level is unknown. OspA is not seen as commonly after natural exposure, although antigenic variation during the chronic phase may allow a nonvaccinated host to have anti-OspA antibodies. OspA expression is down-regulated during tick feeding, but a few OspA molecules may slip in, thus OspA antibodies may be seen transiently soon after infection. In contrast, OspC expression is up-regulated during tick feeding; OspC antibodies generally are detectable 2 to 3 weeks after infection and wane at 3 to 5 months (possibly before signs of illness). Because of reexposure, finding these "early antibodies" are a clue when the dog was last infected but not necessarily when it was first infected. The Nobivac Lyme vaccine may induce OspC antibodies, mimicking natural exposure antibodies. OspF antibodies generally are detectable 6 to 8 weeks after infection and persist; it is unknown whether posttreatment levels of OspF antibodies decline as C6 peptide antibodies do (whole-cell IFA and ELISA antibodies do not decline as much). More information is needed to determine optimal serologic assays.

Test for Proteinuria

All dogs with proteinuria localized as coming from the kidney should be tested for *B. burgdorferi* antibodies. If *B. burgdorferi* serology is used as part of a wellness evaluation, all seropositive dogs should be screened and monitored for proteinuria by urinalysis, microalbuminuria testing, or urine protein/creatinine ratio (UPC). However, if a seropositive dog has proteinuria, it may have LN or it may have proteinuria from another cause and just be seropositive coincidentally.

Differential Diagnosis

If the *B. burgdorferi* seroprevalence in an area is 40% in healthy dogs, then 40% of dogs with disk disease, cancer, genetic disease, or other diseases may be seropositive. Lyme disease is overdiagnosed in *B. burgdorferi* endemic areas because serologic testing is readily available. Owners and veterinarians may accept this trendy diagnosis, foregoing the expense of further diagnostic workup. Dogs may appear to respond to antibiotic treatment because of inadvertent treatment of coinfections, coincidental improvement, or because doxycycline has antiarthritic and antiinflammatory properties.

Borrelia burgdorferi seropositivity is a marker for exposure to wildlife and other tick-borne diseases (TBD) that may cause arthritis, fever, inappetence, lymphadenopathy, or proteinuria, such as anaplasmosis, ehrlichiosis, Rocky Mountain spotted fever (RMSF), babesiosis, and bartonellosis. Coinfections may increase the risk for illness. Joint tap cytology in cases with Lyme arthritis shows nonspecific nonseptic suppurative inflammation. Signs of Lyme arthritis may be mimicked by other TBDs; immune-mediated, septic, or rheumatoid arthritis; degenerative joint disease; intervertebral disk disease; trauma; panosteitis; osteomyelitis; polymyositis; neoplasia; or any reason for inability to rise (e.g., cardiopulmonary, metabolic, or neurologic disease). Glomerular proteinuria may be due to other TBDs, glomerulosclerosis, amyloidosis, or immune-mediated, microangiopathic, genetic, chronic inflammatory, or neoplastic disease. Diagnostic workup for PLN includes complete blood count, biochemical profile, urinalysis, urine culture, UPC, blood pressure measurements, a search for TBDs, neoplasia (chest radiographs and abdominal ultrasound), possible screening for immune diseases, genetic tests for PLN, and possible aspirates of lymph node or bone marrow, depending on other findings. If a dog with PLN is a candidate for the procedure, renal cortical biopsy is recommended to check for IMGN or other subtypes of PLN and to see if immunosuppressive therapy is warranted. Biopsies are most helpful when taken in early disease states, before end-stage damage or fibrosis obscures lesions. The International Veterinary Renal Pathology Service (IVRPS, a joint collaboration between Texas A&M and the Ohio State University) distributes kits and tubes with transit media. The date for the procedure must be coordinated with the IVRPS so that submitted biopsies are handled properly after overnight shipment on ice for immunofluorescence (IF), transmission electron microscopy (TEM), and thin-section (3 micron) light microscopy (LM). Special elution studies and immunohistochemistry (IHC) tests for *B. burgdorferi*–specific immune complexes are not routinely available. Samples of DNA (cheek swabs, 2 ml refrigerated whole blood in EDTA, or a sample of frozen tissue) from seropositive suspects of breeds at risk are requested for future genetic studies by this author.

Treatment and Monitoring

No evidence suggests that treatment of dogs with subclinical *B. burgdorferi* infection is warranted. Because overtreatment of dogs with antibiotics may cause side effects and promote environmental bacterial resistance, treatment is not recommended for all healthy, nonproteinuric dogs. However, because circulating immune complexes decline with treatment, treatment of seropositive retrievers may prevent LN. Doxycycline (5 to 10 mg/kg q12h PO) is the preferred antibiotic to treat clinically ill dogs because doxycycline also may treat coinfections and has antiinflammatory properties. Minocycline, amoxicillin, erythromycin, azithromycin, cefovecin, and ceftriaxone are alternative antimicrobial agents. One month of antibiotics is standard treatment for dogs with Lyme arthritis, but because not all dogs are cleared of infection after 1 month, longer treatment is preferred for dogs with LN until a 6-month follow-up C6Quant level is below 30 or wanes to below 50% of the pretreatment value. With antibiotics and good tick control, in the author's experience, the C6Quant generally wanes. If it did not and was still very high, it may be associated with ongoing infection, high circulating immune complexes, and continuing risk for glomerular deposition; therefore aggressive long-term antimicrobial therapy seems warranted. In the author's experience, dogs with pretreatment C6Quant values below 100 may not wane as much with treatment, possibly because of immune memory; therefore longer-term antimicrobials may not be warranted for those cases.

In addition to antibiotics, standard therapy for PLN should be used. To decrease proteinuria by inhibiting the renin-angiotensin-aldosterone system (RAA), dilating efferent and afferent arterioles at the glomerulus to decrease glomerular filtration pressure, an angiotensin-converting enzyme inhibitor (ACEI such as enalapril or benazepril) is first choice, starting at 0.5 to 1 mg/kg q24h PO, and increasing by 0.5 mg/kg q24h depending on response, up to 2 mg/kg q24h PO. Spironolactone, an aldosterone receptor antagonist with diuretic properties, may be added if necessary at 1 to 2 mg/kg q12h PO. Care must be taken to monitor serum potassium, because any RAA inhibitor is likely to cause hyperkalemia. If hypertension exists despite adequate antiproteinuric effects with RAA inhibition, a calcium-channel blocker antihypertensive is helpful (e.g., amlodipine 0.1 to 0.2 mg/kg q24h PO). A low antithrombotic dose of aspirin (1 to 2 mg/kg q24h PO) is recommended, especially for dogs with hypoalbuminemia. Other standard treatments for PLN include modified low-protein low-phosphorus diet, omega-3 fatty acid supplement, and the following as necessary: phosphate binder, antiemetics, antacids, appetite stimulants, and supportive and symptomatic treatment as for other renal failure cases. Dogs with PLN without anorexia or vomiting or with serum creatinine below 3.0 mg/dl may respond to antibiotics and standard PLN therapy without immunosuppressive drug administration. In more severely and dehydrated affected dogs, intravenous crystalloids and colloids are often necessary, and these have a poorer prognosis, in the author's experience.

Validation studies are needed to show which protocol is best for biopsy-confirmed cases of IMGN in general and LN in particular. If dogs respond to a therapy protocol with or without immunosuppression, it is difficult to know whether LN was occurring because renal biopsies may not have been done with TEM and IF and IHC to prove IMGN or Lyme-specific immune complex deposition in glomeruli. Anecdotal evidence supports the use of immunosuppressive therapy for biopsy-confirmed cases of IMGN or to use blindly for suspects that are deteriorating rapidly and if renal biopsy is contraindicated because of thrombocytopenia, unregulated hypertension, or owner constraints. Glucocorticoids are not usually first choice because of their side effects, including increased risk for thromboembolic events, gastric ulceration, and hypertension, for which PLN cases are already prone. But if IMGN is biopsy-confirmed, or if the case is rapidly deteriorating, glucocorticoids may be administered alone or in combination with other immunosuppressive drugs. Agents used include mycophenolate (CellCept 10 to 20 mg/kg q12h IV or PO long term), pulse therapy with glucocorticoids (e.g., methylprednisolone sodium succinate [Solu-Medrol] 2 mg/kg q24h IV for 2 days or prednisolone 1 to 2 mg/kg q24h PO, pulse or with taper), cyclophosphamide (Cytoxan 200 to 250 mg/m^2 q2-3wk IV or 50 mg/m^2 4 days/wk PO q2-3wk), azathioprine (Imuran 2 mg/kg q24h PO for 2 weeks, then 2 mg/kg q48h PO), or chlorambucil (Leukeran 0.2 mg/kg q24-48h PO). Although in one study cyclosporine failed to help dogs with nonspecific PLN, more study is warranted with more cases and with in-depth characterization of PLN subtype, as is obtained with biopsies sent to the IVRPS. Such a study may be able to show whether cyclosporine may be indicated for certain subsets of PLN, such as IMGN or LN.

Reexamination and monitoring of blood pressure measurement, UPC, packed cell volume (PCV), serum albumin, creatinine, blood urea nitrogen (BUN), phosphorus, Na/K, and bicarbonate is recommended every 7 to 14 days after discharge in moderately severe cases or every 30 days for several months in milder cases to see the trend for stability or progression and to reassess the management protocol. Daily variation of UPC can be as high as 80% at low UPC values and 35% at high UPC values, thus averaging three urine samples taken over 3 days by mixing equal aliquots of urine and submitting it as one sample is helpful. Based on progress, reconsider the protocol medications, diets, doses, and recommendations for frequency of rechecks.

Prevention

Tick control is vital in *B. burgdorferi* endemic areas because of coinfections. *Borrelia* and *Babesia* spp. may require 2 to 4 days of tick attachment to induce infection, which allows most acaricides adequate time. However, other organisms such as *Anaplasma*, *Bartonella*, *Ehrlichia*, *Mycoplasma*, and *Rickettsia* spp. may be transmitted after shorter periods of tick attachment. Thus the use of compounds such as amitraz or permethrin, which prevent attachment of *Ixodes* and other ticks, should be considered.

Borrelia burgdorferi vaccination is controversial because excellent tick control is needed in endemic areas to prevent other tick-borne diseases. Furthermore, most exposed dogs have subclinical infections or have self-limiting illness or illness that is quickly responsive to relatively safe and inexpensive antibiotics. Also the duration of immunity and efficacy for *B. burgdorferi* vaccines is lower, and postvaccine events are seen more frequently than with other vaccines. There are also concerns about possible immune-mediated sequelae from *B. burgdorferi* antigen-antibody complexes, especially in genetically predisposed dogs because the pathogenesis of the most serious form of Lyme disease is immune-mediated. Elevated levels of *B. burgdorferi*–specific circulating immune complexes occur for weeks to months after vaccination, and longer in already naturally seropositive or boostered dogs. Without an experimental induction model, it is unknown if vaccination prevents, sensitizes, or aggravates

LN. If the deposition of immune-complexes in LN occurs slowly over weeks to months, the presentation of sick dogs may not be related temporally to vaccination and an association may go unrecognized. Up to 30% of LN suspects had been vaccinated in Dambach's study; six dogs had been vaccinated with Lyme bacterin 2 weeks to 15 months before presentation, but it is unknown if vaccination was merely nonprotective, coincidental, or whether vaccinal immune complexes may be deposited independently or alongside natural exposure complexes.

References and Suggested Reading

Chou J et al: Detection of *Borrelia burgdorferi* DNA in tissues from dogs with presumptive Lyme borreliosis, *J Am Vet Med Assoc* 229:1260, 2006.

Dambach DM et al: Morphologic, immunohistochemical, and ultrastructural characterization of a distinctive renal lesion in dogs putatively associated with *Borrelia burgdorferi* infection: 49 cases (1987-1992), *Vet Pathol* 34:85, 1997.

Goldstein RE: Lyme disease. In Ettinger SJ, Feldman EC, editors: *Textbook of veterinary internal medicine*, ed 7, St Louis, 2010, Saunders Elsevier, p 868.

Goldstein RE et al: Microalbuminuria and comparison of serologic testing for exposure to *Borrelia burgdorferi* in nonclinical Labrador and Golden Retrievers, *J Vet Diagn Invest* 19:294, 2007.

Littman MP: Protein-losing nephropathy in small animals, *Vet Clin North Am Small Anim Pract* 41(1):31, 2011.

Littman MP et al: ACVIM Small Animal Consensus Statement on Lyme disease in dogs: diagnosis, treatment, and prevention, *J Vet Intern Med* 20(2):422, 2006.

Littman MP: Canine borreliosis. In Macintire DK, Breitschwerdt EB, editors: Emerging and re-emerging infectious diseases, *Vet Clin North Am Small Anim* 33(4):827, 2003.

Littman MP: A matter of opinion: should we treat asymptomatic, nonproteinuric Lyme-seropositive dogs with antibiotics? *Clinician's Brief* 9:13, 2011.

Littman MP: Lyme nephritis, *J Vet Emerg Crit Care* 23:163, 2013.

Slade DJ, Nolan TJ, Littman MP: Clinicopathologic findings in dogs with protein-losing nephropathy and anti-*Borrelia burgdorferi* antibodies, *J Vet Intern Med* 22(3):784, 2008.

CHAPTER 272

Management of Feline Retrovirus-Infected Cats

KATRIN HARTMANN, *Munich, Germany*

In domestic cats, three retroviruses have been identified: feline immunodeficiency virus (FIV), feline leukemia virus (FeLV), and feline foamy virus (FeFV). All three are global and widespread but differ in their potential to cause disease. FeFV (previously known as feline syncytium-forming virus, FeSFV), a spumavirus, is not associated with disease; thus routine testing is not performed.

FIV, a lentivirus that shares many properties with human immunodeficiency virus (HIV), can cause an acquired immune deficiency syndrome in cats leading to increased risk for opportunistic infections, neurologic diseases, and tumors. In most naturally infected cats, FIV infection does not cause a severe clinical syndrome, and with proper care FIV-infected cats can live many years. Many in fact die at an older age from causes completely unrelated to their FIV infection. In a study of naturally FIV-infected cats, the rate of progression was variable, with death occurring in about 18% of infected cats within the first 2 years of observation (about 5 years after the estimated time of infection). An additional 18% developed clinical signs, but more than 50% remained clinically asymptomatic during the 2 years of observation. FIV infection has little impact on a cat population and does not reduce the number of cats in a household. Thus overall survival time is not necessarily shorter than in uninfected cats, and quality of life is usually fairly high over an extended period of time.

FeLV, an oncornavirus, is the most pathogenic of the three viruses. Historically, it was considered to account for more disease-related deaths and clinical syndromes than any other single infectious agent in cats. More recently, prevalence and consequently the importance of FeLV as a pathogen in cats have been decreasing, mainly because of testing and eradication programs and the use of FeLV vaccines. The death rate of persistently viremic cats in multicat households is approximately 50% in 2 years and 80% in 3 years but is lower in cats kept strictly indoors in single-cat households. Despite the fact that persistent FeLV viremia is associated with a decrease in life expectancy, many owners elect to provide treatment for the clinical syndromes that accompany infection. With proper care, many FeLV-infected cats kept only indoors may live for many years with good quality of life.

Therefore a decision for treatment or for euthanasia of a cat should never be based solely on the presence of a retrovirus infection. FIV- and FeLV-infected cats are subject to the same diseases that befall cats free of those infections, and illness in a given cat may not be related to the retrovirus infection. However, in all cats, healthy or sick, FIV and FeLV status should be known because these infections affect health status and long-term patient management.

Management of Retrovirus-Infected Multicat Households

When a cat in a multicat household is diagnosed with a retrovirus infection, all cats in that household should be tested to determine their infection status. If positive and negative cats are identified within the same household, the owner must be informed of the potential danger to uninfected cats and told that the best method of preventing spread of infection is to isolate the infected individuals and prevent them from interacting with housemates. However, despite this admonition, the overall risk of transmission between these cats is not high for either infection. FIV transmission in households with a stable social cat environment is rare because FIV is transmitted mainly through biting and fighting; if no fights occur, FIV is not likely to be transmitted. Long-term studies of households with FIV-infected cats have shown that a few additional cats may become FIV-positive over time, but in some households no transmission occurred over many years. All cats in these households should be neutered, and new cats should not be introduced into the household because this may lead to fights and to increased risk for transmission, even between cats that have lived together peacefully for a long time. The benefit of FIV vaccination of FIV-negative cats living with a FIV-positive cat is controversial. The vaccine currently available has not been tested under these conditions. Usually the FIV subtype of the infected cat is unknown, and cross-protection by the vaccine against some FIV subtypes (e.g., the frequently found subtype B) is uncertain. Because the vaccine contains whole virus cats respond to vaccination by producing antibodies indistinguishable from those present during natural infection. Therefore vaccinated cats are antibody positive, and assessment of their true infection status can be difficult. Before vaccination is considered, ideally the veterinarian should ensure that the virus in the infected cat can be detected by polymerase chain reaction (PCR) (which is possible in only 50% to 90% of cases). Only if the virus strain of the infected cat is detectable by PCR is it possible to identify later another cat in the household that may become infected despite vaccination.

If an FeLV-infected cat has lived for some time in an otherwise FeLV-negative household, the other cats that have been in contact with the FeLV-shedding cat already will have been infected. Thus these cats most likely are immune to new infection, and an owner may elect to keep all of the cats together. However, studies in cluster households have shown that eventually other cats in these households may become FeLV viremic. This is most likely the result of reactivation of a long-persisting latent infection, but the risk of new infections cannot be excluded totally as virus-neutralizing antibodies may not persist for life. The risk of becoming viremic in adult FeLV antigen-negative cats is approximately 10% to 15% if they live with an FeLV-shedding cat for several months. If owners refuse to separate housemates, the uninfected cats should be administered FeLV vaccination to enhance their natural level of immunity. However, owners should be informed that vaccination may not provide sufficient levels of protection in these environments of high viral exposure.

Management of Individual Retrovirus-Infected Cats

The most important life-prolonging advice the veterinarian can give to owners of retrovirus-infected cats is to keep the cats strictly indoors. This avoids spread to other cats in the neighborhood and prevents exposure of the immunosuppressed, retrovirus-infected cat to infectious agents carried by other animals. In FIV-infected cats, secondary infections cause clinical signs and may lead to progression of the FIV infection. This is probably not the case in FeLV infection, in which the retroviral infection is more pathogenic and progresses relatively independently of cofactors.

"Routine vaccination" of retrovirus-infected cats is subject to much discussion. Although there is no scientific proof that retrovirus-infected cats are at increased risk from modified-life virus (MLV) vaccines, inactivated vaccines are recommended out of concern that MLV vaccines given to immunosuppressed animals may regain pathogenicity. FIV-infected cats are susceptible to secondary infection and while in an early stage of infection are able to mount appropriate levels of protective antibodies after vaccination; thus regular vaccination would seem indicated. However, it is the author's opinion that vaccines should not be given to FIV-infected cats if strictly kept indoors because immunosuppression and immune stimulation can lead to progression of FIV infection by altering the balance between the immune system and the virus. Stimulation of FIV-infected lymphocytes is known to promote virus production *in vitro*. *In vivo* vaccination of chronically FIV-infected cats with a synthetic peptide was associated with a decrease in the CD4/CD8 ratio. Thus the potential tradeoff to protection from infection with vaccination is progression of FIV infection secondary to increased virus production. If FIV-infected cats are kept strictly indoors, the risk of secondary infections may be lower than the possible adverse effects of vaccination. In some countries or states legal requirements for rabies vaccination may supersede these issues.

In contrast, FeLV-infected cats should be administered routine vaccinations. Studies investigating the immune response to rabies vaccination demonstrated that FeLV-infected cats may not be able to mount adequate immune responses. Therefore protection in an FeLV-infected cat after vaccination is not comparable with that in a healthy cat, and more frequent vaccinations than usually recommended must be considered (e.g., every 6 months), especially in cats allowed to go outside.

Retrovirus-infected cats should have routine health care visits at least semiannually to promptly detect changes in health status. A complete blood count (CBC), biochemistry profile, and urinalysis should be performed at least annually (CBC every 6 months in FeLV-infected cats to detect anemia or other cytopenias associated with FeLV infection). Intact male and female retrovirus-infected cats should be neutered to reduce stress associated with estrus and mating behavior and the desire to roam outside the house and interact aggressively. Surgery generally is well tolerated by asymptomatic retrovirus-infected cats, but perioperative antibiotic administration should be used for all surgeries and dental procedures. Because both viruses live for only minutes outside of the host and are susceptible to all disinfectants (including common soap) simple precautions and routine cleaning procedures prevent transmission in the hospital. Retrovirus-infected cats can be housed in the same ward as other hospitalized patients but in individual cages. They may be immunosuppressed and should be kept away from cats with other infectious diseases and therefore not be placed in a "contagious disease ward" with cats suffering from infections such as respiratory viruses.

If retrovirus-infected cats are sick, prompt and accurate identification of the secondary illness is essential. Treatment recommendations for specific situations are given in Boxes 272-1 and 272-2. Often the clinical signs of retrovirus-infected cats are not caused by the retrovirus infection and so intensive diagnostic testing for secondary diseases should proceed early in the course of illness to allow for appropriate therapeutic intervention. Many cats with a retrovirus infection respond as well as uninfected cats to appropriate medications, although a longer or more aggressive course of therapy (e.g., antibiotics) may be needed. Glucocorticoids or other immunosuppressive as well as bone marrow–suppressive drugs should be avoided. Griseofulvin has been shown to cause bone marrow suppression in FIV-infected cats and should not be used.

Recombinant human granulocyte colony-stimulation factor (rHuG-CSF, filgrastim) is contraindicated in FIV-infected cats. It increases neutrophil counts, but treatment can lead to a significant increase in virus load. Until data in FeLV-infected cats are available, rHuG-CSF therapy also cannot be recommended. In contrast, recombinant human erythropoietin (rHuEPO) can be administered safely to retrovirus-infected cats and may be effective in cats with nonregenerative anemia and those with neutropenia. Recombinant human insulin-like growth factor-1 (rHuIGF-1) is also safe and can induce thymic growth and stimulate T cell function. It may be considered in young FIV-infected cats, but no field studies so far show its effect in naturally FIV-infected cats. Its usefulness in FeLV infection is also unknown.

Antiviral Chemotherapy

Most antivirals used in cats (Table 272-1) are licensed for humans and are intended specifically for treatment of HIV infection. Some can be used to treat FIV infection because most enzymes of FIV and HIV have similar sensitivities to various inhibitors. However, few controlled

---

BOX 272-1

Suggested Treatment Recommendations for FIV-Infected Cats

Treatment with or without Clinical Signs
If no clinical signs are present:
- No treatment is recommended.
- Cats should be kept strictly indoors and should not be vaccinated.

If clinical signs are present:
- First any underlying diseases should be identified (FIV itself alone usually is not responsible for the clinical signs).
- Underlying diseases should be treated.

Treatment of FIV-Infected Cats with Stomatitis
- Glucocorticoids should be avoided.
- Treatment with AZT (5 to 10 mg/kg PO q12h) and antibiotics should be tried.
- If concurrent feline calicivirus infection is present, local oromucosal treatment with feline IFN-ω (0.1 IU/kg q24h) can be tried.
- In addition, lactoferrin should be applied topically (40 mg/kg q24h) to the oral mucosa.
- If this does not lead to improvement, removal of all teeth (usually in two sessions; total removal of all tooth roots has to be confirmed by x-rays) is recommended.

Treatment of FIV-Infected Cats with Neurologic Signs
- Any underlying disease causing the neurologic signs has to be identified.
- Underlying diseases should be treated.
- If no underlying disease is identified (and the neurologic signs are assumed to be caused by FIV directly), treatment with AZT (5 to 10 mg/kg PO q12h) should be initiated.

Treatment of FIV-Infected Cats with Recurring Infections
- Recurring infections should be treated aggressively (e.g., long-term antibiotics).
- Virus load should be determined by quantitative RNA qPCR.
- CD4+ and CD8+ cell counts and CD4/CD8 rations should be measured.
- If virus load is high and CD4+ cell counts are low, treatment with antivirals (e.g., plerixafor [0.5 mg/kg SC q12h] or AZT [5 to 10 mg/kg PO q12h]) should be considered.

---

studies have been performed to support their use in cats. Nucleoside analogs are usually less effective against FeLV when compared with FIV because FeLV is not related as closely to HIV.

Zidovudine (azidothymidine, AZT) is a nucleoside analog (thymidine derivative) that blocks the reverse transcriptase of retroviruses. AZT can inhibit FIV replication *in vitro* and *in vivo*, reduce plasma virus load, improve the immunologic and clinical status of FIV-infected cats, increase quality of life, and prolong life expectancy. In a placebo-controlled trial, AZT improved stomatitis in naturally infected cats. It should be used at a dosage of 5 to 10 mg/kg PO or SC q12h. The higher dose should be used

Suggested Treatment Recommendations for FeLV-Infected Cats

Treatment with or without Clinical Signs

If no clinical signs are present:
- No treatment is recommended.
- Cats should be kept strictly indoors.

If clinical signs are present:
- First any underlying diseases should be identified. (FeLV itself alone may not be responsible for the clinical signs [e.g., secondary infections may be present].)
- Underlying diseases should be treated.

Treatment of FeLV-Infected Cats with Lymphoma
- Multidrug chemotherapeutic protocols should be used (e.g., COP protocol, including cyclophosphamide, vincristine, and prednisone).
- Owners should be informed about the more guarded prognosis.

Treatment of FeLV-Infected Cats with Anemia
- Blood transfusions are recommended if anemia is severe.
- Erythropoietin (100 IU/kg SC q48h) treatment can be tried.
- If there is no effect, glucocorticoid treatment can be considered (because anemia in FeLV-infected cats may have an immune-mediated origin, and some cats may respond).

Treatment of FeLV-Infected Cats with Neurologic Signs
- Underlying diseases causing the neurologic signs should be identified (e.g., lymphoma).
- Underlying diseases should be treated.
- If no underlying disease is identified (and the neurologic signs are assumed to be caused by FeLV directly), treatment with AZT (5 mg/kg PO q12h) can be considered.

Treatment of FeLV-Infected Cats with Recurring Infections
- Recurring infections should be treated aggressively (e.g., long-term antibiotics).
- Immunomodulator treatment can be considered in addition (e.g., feline IFN-ω [10^6 IU/kg SC once a week] or SPA [10 μg/kg IP 2×/week]).

carefully because side effects can develop. For subcutaneous injection, the lyophilized product should be diluted in isotonic NaCl solution to prevent local irritation. For oral application, syrup or gelatin capsules (with dosage individualized for the cat) can be used. During treatment, a CBC should be performed regularly (weekly for the first month) because nonregenerative anemia is a common side effect, especially if the higher dosage is used. If blood values are stable after the first month, a monthly check is sufficient. Cats with bone marrow suppression should not be treated with AZT. Studies in which FIV-infected cats were treated for 2 years showed that AZT is well tolerated. Some cats may develop a mild decrease of hematocrit initially in the first 3 weeks that resolves even if treatment is continued. If hematocrit drops below 20%, discontinuation is recommended, and anemia usually

resolves within a few days. Unfortunately, as in HIV, AZT-resistant mutants of FIV can arise as early as 6 months after initiation of treatment. AZT is also effective against FeLV in vitro. When treated less than 1 week after experimental inoculation, cats were protected from FeLV bone marrow infection and persistent viremia. However, in a study with naturally FeLV-infected cats, 6 weeks of treatment with AZT did not lead to a statistically significant improvement of clinical, laboratory, immunologic, or virologic parameters. In general, the therapeutic efficacy of AZT in FeLV-infected cats seems to be less promising than in cats infected with FIV. It should be used only at low dosage (5 mg/kg PO or SC q12h) in FeLV-infected cats because of its bone marrow–suppressive effects.

Stavudine (2'-3'-didehydro-2'-3'-dideoxythymidine, D4T) is a thymidine-based nucleoside analog and is active against FIV in vitro. No in vivo data in FIV-infected cats are published, and D4T activity against FeLV is unknown.

Didanosine (2',3'-dideoxyinosine, ddI), an inosine analog, is also active against FIV in vitro. In one experimental study, FIV replication was suppressed significantly in animals treated with ddI, but treatment was associated with the development of antiretroviral toxic neuropathy. ddI is also active against FeLV in vitro, but efficacy in vivo is unknown.

Zalcitabine (2'-3'-dideoxycytidine, ddC) is an analog 2'-desoxycytidine. In vitro, antiviral efficacy has been demonstrated against FIV, but in vivo data are missing. It is effective against FeLV in vitro and has been used in experimental studies. It has a short half-life and therefore was administered via controlled-release subcutaneous implants that inhibited de novo FeLV replication and delayed onset of viremia; however, when therapy was stopped, an equivalent incidence and level of viremia as before treatment were reestablished rapidly. In a study using continuous IV infusion for 28 days, ddC was extremely toxic, causing death in 8 of 10 cats.

Lamivudine (2',3'-dideoxy-3'-thiacytidine, 3TC) is an analog of cytidine and often is combined with AZT in HIV-infected patients. 3TC is active against FIV in vitro, and combination of AZT and 3TC had synergistic anti-FIV activities in primary peripheral blood mononuclear cell cultures. One in vivo study was performed in experimentally FIV-infected cats in which a high-dose AZT/3TC combination protected some cats when the treatment was started before experimental infection. However, AZT/3TC treatment had no anti-FIV activity in chronically infected cats. Severe side effects, which included fever, anorexia, and marked hematologic changes, were observed in some of the cats. Data on the anti-FeLV activity of 3TC are not available.

Suramin, a sulfated naphthylamine, has been used primarily as an antiparasitic drug. It is also effective against several viruses through inhibition of reverse transcriptase. However, it is associated with severe side effects, including nausea and anaphylactic shock (during administration), peripheral neuritis, agranulocytosis, hemolytic anemia, and destruction of the adrenal cortex. No reliable studies show efficacy against FIV. Suramin was used to treat FeLV-infected cats, although only a limited number of cats were studied. FeLV-related anemia improved in these cats, and serum viral infectivity ceased transiently.

TABLE 272-1

Antiviral Drugs Used for Retrovirus-Infected Cats (Including EBM Grades for Judgment of the Available Efficacy Data)

Drug	Infection	Efficacy In Vitro	Controlled Study In Vivo	Efficacy In Vivo	Comments	EBM Level (1-4)
Nucleoside Analog Reverse Transcriptase Inhibitors						
Zidovudine (AZT)	FIV	Yes	Yes	Yes	Effective in some cats (e.g., with stomatitis, neurologic disorders)	1
	FeLV	Yes	Yes	No	Not very effective	1
Stavudin (D4T)	FIV	Yes	No	n.d.	Possibly effective, but no data in cats available	4
	FeLV	n.d.	No	n.d.	Possibly effective, but no data in cats available	4
Didanosine (ddI)	FIV	Yes	Yes	Yes	Effective in one experimental study, but neurologic side effects	2
	FeLV	Yes	No	n.d.	Possibly effective, but no data in cats available	4
Zalcitabine (ddC)	FIV	Yes	No	n.d.	Possibly effective, but no data in cats available	4
	FeLV	Yes	Yes	No	Not very effective	2
Lamivudine (3TC)	FIV	Yes	Yes	No	Not very effective, toxic in high dosages	2
	FeLV	No	No	n.d.	Possibly effective, but toxic	4
Nonnucleoside Reverse Transcriptase Inhibitors						
Suramin	FIV	No	No	n.d.	Possibly effective, but too toxic	4
	FeLV	No	No	n.d.	Possibly effective, but too toxic	2
Nucleotide Synthesis Inhibitors						
Foscarnet	FIV	Yes	No	n.d.	Effective in vitro, but too toxic	4
	FeLV	Yes	No	n.d.	Effective in vitro, but too toxic	4
Ribavirin	FIV	Yes	No	n.d.	Possibly effective, but too toxic in cats	4
	FeLV	Yes	No	n.d.	Possibly effective, but too toxic in cats	4
Receptor Homologs/ Antagonists						
Plerixafor	FIV	Yes	Yes	Yes	Some effect in a study in privately-owned cats, thus can be considered	1
	FeLV	n.d.	No	n.d.	Very likely ineffective	4

FeLV, Feline leukemia virus; *FIV*, feline immunodeficiency virus; *n.d.*, not determined.
EBM, evidence-based medicine:
EBM level 1 = confirmed by at least one placebo-controlled double-blind field study
EBM level 2 = shown in a controlled experimental study
EBM level 3 = supported by case series
EBM level 4 = only based on expert opinion

However, because these studies were not controlled, results must be interpreted carefully, and the severe side effects limit its use in cat patients.

Foscarnet is a pyrophosphate analog that reversibly inhibits virus-specific enzymes. It has a wide spectrum of activity against DNA and RNA viruses. *In vitro*, foscarnet has activity against FIV and FeLV, but no reliable data exist on its *in vivo* efficacy in cats, and its use in cats is limited because of toxicity. It is nephrotoxic and myelosuppressive and chelates cations such as calcium, so hypocalcemia, hypomagnesemia, and hypokalemia may develop. Foscarnet is also toxic to epithelial cells and mucous membranes, leading to severe gastrointestinal side effects and ulceration of genital epithelium.

Ribavirin has marked *in vitro* antiviral activity against a variety of feline and canine viruses, including FIV and FeLV. *In vivo*, however, therapeutic concentrations are not achieved because of toxicity, and cats are extremely sensitive to its side effects.

Plerixafor is a bicyclam that is not on the market as anti-HIV drug but is available and clinically used in humans for stem cell mobilization. Bicyclams bind selectively to the chemokine receptor CXCR4. CXCR4 is an important coreceptor in FIV infection and thus bicyclam derivatives inhibit FIV infection through selective blockage of the chemokine receptor CXCR4. Plerixafor is effective against FIV *in vitro*. Its efficacy also was confirmed in a placebo-controlled double-blind trial that investigated 40 naturally FIV-infected cats. Treatment of FIV-infected cats with plerixafor (0.5 mg/kg SC q12h for 6 weeks) caused a significant decrease in the provirus load but also a decrease in serum magnesium levels without clinical consequences.

Immune Modulator Therapy

Immune modulators or interferon inducers are used widely in retrovirus-infected cats (Table 272-2). These agents may benefit infected animals by restoring compromised immune function, thereby allowing the patient to control viral burden and recover from the disease. Some case reports suggest dramatic clinical improvement with these drugs, but when investigated in placebo-controlled

TABLE 272-2

Immune Modulators Used for Retrovirus-Infected Cats (Including Evidence-Based Medicine Grades for Judgment of the Available Efficacy Data)

Drug	Infection	Efficacy *In Vitro*	Controlled Study *In Vivo*	Efficacy *In Vivo*	Comments	EBM Level (1-4)
Interferons						
Human interferon-α (human IFN-α) SC high dose	FIV	Yes	No	n.d.	Likely ineffective	4
	FeLV	Yes	Yes	No	Ineffective	1
Human interferon-α (human IFN-α) PO low dose	FIV	Yes	Yes	Yes	Some effect (most likely more on secondary infections)	1
	FeLV	Yes	Yes	No	Ineffective	1
Feline interferon-ω (feline IFN-ω)	FIV	Yes	Yes	No	Ineffective	1
	FeLV	Yes	Yes	Yes	Some effect (most likely more on secondary infections)	1
Cytokines and Growth Factors						
Filgrastim (G-CSF)	FIV	n.d.	Yes	No	Contraindicated (may increase virus replication)	3
	FeLV	n.d.	Yes	No	Likely contraindicated	3
Sargramostin (GM-CSF)	FIV	n.d.	Yes	No	Contraindicated (may increase virus replication)	2
	FeLV	n.d.	No	n.d.	Likely contraindicated (may increase virus replication)	2
Erythropoietin (EPO)	FIV	n.d.	Yes	Yes	Weakly effective in cats with anemia and neutropenia	2
	FeLV	n.d.	No	n.d.	Possibly effective in cats with anemia and neutropenia	
Insulin-like growth factor-1 (IGF-1)	FIV	n.d.	Yes	Yes	Possibly effective in young cats	2
	FeLV	n.d.	No	n.d.	Likely ineffective	4
Interferon and Other Cytokine Inducers						
Staphylococcus protein A (SPA)	FIV	n.d.	No	n.d.	Likely contraindicated	4
	FeLV	n.d.	Yes	Yes	Weakly effective	1
Propionibacterium acnes	FIV	n.d.	No	n.d.	Likely contraindicated	4
	FeLV	n.d.	No	n.d.	Likely ineffective	3
Bacille Calmette-Guérin (BCG)	FIV	n.d.	No	n.d.	Likely contraindicated	4
	FeLV	n.d.	Yes	No	Ineffective	2
Serratia marcescens (S. marcescens)	FIV	n.d.	No	n.d.	Likely contraindicated	4
	FeLV	n.d.	Yes	No	Ineffective	2

TABLE **272-2**

Immune Modulators Used for Retrovirus-Infected Cats (Including Evidence-Based Medicine Grades for Judgment of the Available Efficacy Data)—cont'd

Drug	Infection	Efficacy *In Vitro*	Controlled Study *In Vivo*	Efficacy *In Vivo*	Comments	EBM Level (1-4)
Pind-avi/Pind-orf	FIV	n.d.	No	n.d.	Likely contraindicated	4
	FeLV	n.d.	Yes	No	Ineffective	1
Polyinosinic:poly-cytidylic acid (poly I:C)	FIV	n.d.	No	n.d.	Likely contraindicated	4
	FeLV	n.d.	No	n.d.	Likely ineffective	4
Acemannan	FIV	n.d.	No	n.d.	Likely contraindicated	3
	FeLV	n.d.	No	n.d.	Possibly weakly effective	3
Other Drugs with Immunomodulatory Activity						
Levamisole	FIV	n.d.	No	n.d.	Likely contraindicated	4
	FeLV	n.d.	No	n.d.	Likely ineffective	3
Diethylcarbamazine Citrate (DEC)	FIV	n.d.	No	n.d.	Likely contraindicated	4
	FeLV	n.d.	Yes	No	Ineffective	2
Lactoferrin	FIV	n.d.	No	n.d.	Possibly effective in cat with stomatitis	3
	FeLV	n.d.	No	n.d.	Possibly effective in cat with stomatitis	4
Nosodes	FIV	n.d.	No	n.d.	Likely contraindicated	4
	FeLV	n.d.	No	n.d.	Very likely ineffective	4

FeLV, Feline leukemia virus; *FIV,* feline immunodeficiency virus; *n.d.,* not determined.
EBM, evidence-based medicine:
EBM level 1 = confirmed by at least one placebo-controlled double-blind field study
EBM level 2 = shown in a controlled experimental study
EBM level 3 = supported by case series
EBM level 4 = only based on expert opinion

studies, these results cannot be reproduced. Most of these reports in the veterinary literature do not fulfill criteria of evidence-based studies and are difficult to interpret because of vague diagnostic criteria, lack of clinical staging or follow-up, small numbers of cats studied, absence of a placebo-treated control group, the natural variability of the course of disease, and the fact that additional supportive treatments were administered. In FIV infection, a nonspecific stimulation of the immune system may be contraindicated because it may lead to an increase in virus replication caused by activation of latently infected lymphocytes and macrophages.

Human interferon-α (human IFN-α) has immunomodulatory effects but also acts as a true antiviral compound by inducing a general antiviral state of cells that protects them against virus replication. Two common treatment regimens are used in cats: subcutaneous injection of high-dose IFN-α (10^4 to 10^6 IU/kg q24h) or oral application of a low-dose treatment (1 to 50 IU/kg q24h). Measurable serum levels can be obtained when given subcutaneously, but using this regimen human IFN-α becomes ineffective after 3 to 7 weeks because of development of neutralizing antibodies. Human IFN-α given by mouth is not absorbed but is destroyed in the gastrointestinal tract; no measurable serum levels develop. The only way PO interferons may have an effect is by stimulation of the local lymphoid tissue in the oral cavity. In murine studies it was

shown that subcutaneous administration of IFN-α had an antiviral effect, whereas PO administration only caused immune modulation. Human IFN-α is active against FIV *in vitro*. Low-dose human IFN-α (50 IU/cat PO) used in ill, naturally FIV-infected cats caused a significant difference in the survival rate after 18 months and in the clinical condition of the cats, but there was no difference in virus load, suggesting that the improvement was rather the result of treatment of opportunistic infections. This study would support the use of low-dose oral human IFN-α in FIV-infected cats, whereas on the other hand, nonspecific immune stimulation may be contraindicated in FIV infection. Human IFN-α inhibits FeLV replication *in vitro* and has been used in several studies in FeLV-infected cats. Treatment with high dosages of human IFN-α (1.6×10^4 and 1.6×10^6 IU/kg SC) in experimentally FeLV-infected cats resulted in significant decreases in circulating FeLV p27 antigen. In a study in naturally FeLV-infected cats, high-dose human IFN-α (1×10^5 IU/kg SC q24h for 6 weeks), however, did not lead to a statistically significant improvement of clinical, laboratory, immunologic, or virologic parameters. Low-dose human IFN-α (0.5 IU/cat PO or 5 IU/cat PO) did not lead to a difference in the development of viremia in an experimental placebo-controlled study when treatment started directly after challenge, although treated cats had significantly fewer clinical signs and longer survival times (with a better response using 0.5 IU/cat). In a placebo-controlled study in naturally FeLV-infected cats that were treated with low-dose human IFN-α (30 IU/cat PO q24h); however, there were no statistically significant differences in FeLV status, survival time, clinical or hematologic parameters, or subjective improvement in the owners' impression of clinical signs.

Feline interferon-ω (feline IFN-ω) is licensed for use in veterinary medicine in some European countries and Japan. Interferons are species specific; therefore feline IFN-ω can be used parenterally or orally for prolonged periods without antibody development. No side effects have been reported in cats. Feline IFN-ω is active against FIV *in vitro,* but only one study has been performed in field cats, and the study did not show significant changes in survival rate when compared with a placebo group. Feline IFN-ω also inhibits FeLV replication *in vitro.* In a placebo-controlled field study, 48 cats with FeLV infection were treated with feline IFN-ω (10^6 IU/kg SC q24h on 5 consecutive days repeated 3 times with several weeks between treatments). A significant difference was found in the survival time of treated versus untreated cats. However, no virologic parameters were measured during the study to support the hypothesis that the interferon actually had an anti-FeLV effect rather than an inhibition of secondary infections, and further studies are needed.

Staphylococcus protein A (SPA), a bacterial polypeptide purified from cell walls of *Staphylococcus aureus,* can bind to the Fc portion of certain immunoglobulin G subclasses and thus exhibits immunomodulatory effects. The efficacy of SPA against FIV is unknown. A variety of SPA treatment protocols have been used in FeLV-infected cats. In some studies, a high rate of tumor remission and conversion to FeLV-negative status was observed; in others, responses were less dramatic and short lived. However, in an experimental study that included kittens with experimental FeLV infection, SPA treatment neither reversed anemia nor improved humoral immune function. In a placebo-controlled study, treatment of ill client-owned FeLV-infected cats with SPA did not cause a statistically significant difference in FeLV status, survival time, or clinical and hematologic parameters when compared with a placebo-treated control group, but it did result in significant improvement in the owners' subjective impression of the health of their pets.

Propionibacterium acnes, formerly *Corynebacterium parvum,* is a killed bacterial product that stimulates macrophages and the release of various cytokines and interferons and enhances T cell and natural killer cell activity. Its efficacy against FIV is unknown. It has been used in FeLV-infected cats, but no prospective studies have been performed. Anecdotal reports note that about 50% of the treated cats improved.

Bacille Calmette-Guérin (BCG) is a cell wall extract of *Mycobacterium bovis* that was originally developed as a "vaccine" against tuberculosis in humans. Its efficacy against FIV is unknown. BCG treatment was not able to prevent tumor development or increase survival rate in kittens experimentally infected with feline sarcoma virus (FeSV), a recombinant virus that can develop *de novo* in a cat infected with FeLV.

Serratia (S.) marcescens preparations contain DNA and membrane components of the bacterium *S. marcescens* that stimulates feline bone marrow–derived macrophages to release IL-1, IL-6, and tumor necrosis factor. Its efficacy against FIV is unknown. In a study in FeLV-infected cats, treatment with BESM failed to prevent or reverse viremia but induced marrow stimulation through cytokine release leading to neutrophilia and fever.

Pind-avi (parapox virus avis) and pind-orf (parapox virus ovis) are inactivated poxviruses that belong to the so-called paramunity inducers. Their suggested mode of action is primarily induction of interferons and activation of natural killer cells. They have not been used against FIV. These compounds caused a sensation in Germany when it was published that their administration resulted in a cure of 80% to 100% of FeLV-infected cats, even those in moribund condition. Paramunity inducers quickly became the most commonly used treatment for FeLV infection in Europe. However, two placebo-controlled, double-blind trials (including 120 and 30 cats, respectively) using the same treatment protocol in naturally FeLV-infected cats under controlled conditions failed to reproduce these striking results. There were no significant differences between the cats treated with paramunity inducers and placebo-treated cats in the number of cats that terminated viremia or in any clinical, laboratory, immunologic, or virologic variable investigated.

Polyinosinic:polycytidylic acid (poly I:C) is a chemical IFN inducer used to treat cats and dogs; however, its efficacy against FIV or FeLV is unknown.

Acemannan, a water-soluble, long-chain complex carbohydrate polymer derived from the aloe vera plant, is thought to be taken up by macrophages, stimulating them to release cytokines, which in turn stimulate cell-mediated immune responses, including cytotoxicity. In an uncontrolled trial, 50 cats with natural FeLV infection were treated with acemannan. After 12 weeks 71% of the cats were alive, all remained FeLV antigen–positive, and no significant change was noted in their clinical signs or hematologic parameters. There was no control group; thus assessment of the survival rate is not possible.

Levamisole is a broad-spectrum anthelmintic drug that nonspecifically stimulates cell-mediated immunity. Levamisole has been given to FIV- and to FeLV-infected cats, but its effect never has been substantiated by controlled studies, and its use remains investigational. Toxicity of levamisole is relatively high, including hypersalivation, vomiting, diarrhea, and CNS signs.

Diethylcarbamazine citrate (N,N-diethyl-4-methyl-1-piperazine carboxamide dihydrogen citrate, DEC) also is an antiparasitic agent with some immunomodulatory effects. It has not been investigated in FIV-infected cats. In one controlled study, kittens were infected experimentally with a lymphoma-causing strain of FeLV, and although viremia still occurred, development of lymphoma was inhibited.

Lactoferrin is a mammalian iron-binding glycoprotein with antibacterial, antifungal, antiprotozoal, and antiviral properties. Antiviral activity may occur as a result of interaction with the viral receptors on the cell surface or by direct neutralization or inhibition of the viral particle. Lactoferrin is produced by mucosal epithelial cells of many mammalian species and is present mainly in secretions such as tears, milk, saliva, or seminal or vaginal fluids. Side effects are not described. Lactoferrin had some effect in cats with stomatitis, and it may be an option for treatment of FIV- and FeLV-related stomatitis.

Nosodes are homeopathic preparations of tissues from animals with the disease for which they are intended to prevent. Clinical trials involving nosodes to prevent infectious diseases have not been controlled, and information about their usefulness against FIV and FeLV and about their toxicity is not available.

References and Suggested Reading

Hartmann K: Antiviral and immunomodulatory chemotherapy. In Greene CE, editor: *Infectious diseases of the dog and cat*, St Louis, 2012, Elsevier Saunders, p 10.

Hartmann K: Feline leukemia virus infection. In Greene CE, editor: *Infectious diseases of the dog and cat*, St Louis, 2012, Elsevier Saunders, p 108.

Hosie MJ et al: Feline immunodeficiency. ABCD guidelines on prevention and management, *J Feline Med Surg* 11:575, 2009.

Levy JK et al: 2008 American Association of Feline Practitioners' feline retrovirus management guidelines, *J Feline Med Surg* 10:300, 2008.

Lutz H et al: Feline leukaemia. ABCD guidelines on prevention and management, *J Feline Med Surg* 11:565, 2009.

Sellon RK, Hartmann K: Feline immunodeficiency virus infection. In Greene CE, editor: *Infectious diseases of the dog and cat*, St Louis, 2012, Elsevier Saunders, p 106.

CHAPTER 273

Hepatozoon americanum Infections

KELLY E. ALLEN, *Stillwater, Oklahoma*
EILEEN MCGOEY JOHNSON, *Stillwater, Oklahoma*
SUSAN E. LITTLE, *Stillwater, Oklahoma*

Hepatozoon americanum is a tick-borne parasite infecting domestic dogs and coyotes in the United States and is the causative agent of American canine hepatozoonosis (ACH), a painful, debilitating, and often fatal clinical syndrome. ACH is considered an emerging disease, and recent molecular data obtained from clinically suspicious dogs presented to veterinarians throughout the United States in 2006 to 2008 indicate that the disease is no longer limited to south-central and southeastern states (Li et al, 2008). Thus veterinarians all over the United States, regardless of location, must recognize clinical signs of ACH. Although the disease is incurable, ACH can be well managed with drug therapy in many patients, especially if treatment begins soon after initial presentation of clinical signs (Macintire et al, 2001).

Pathogenesis

The accepted primary route of *H. americanum* transmission to domestic dogs and wild canids is ingestion of *Amblyomma maculatum* (Gulf Coast tick) that contain sporulated *H. americanum* oocysts. The ingestion of infected ticks is thought to be a result of grooming or inadvertent ingestion of infected ticks infesting prey or scavenged animals. In addition to the conventional route, recent experiments have confirmed transmission of *H. americanum* to domestic dogs via their consumption of cystozoites contained in tissues harvested from experimentally infected paratenic hosts (Johnson et al, 2009). Predator-prey relationships are important in the lifecycles of many *Hepatozoon* spp. and likely are involved in *H. americanum* transmission cycles.

H. americanum zoites are liberated within the canine alimentary tract and disperse by an unknown route to other tissues, particularly striated muscle, to undergo merogony. Several weeks after experimental infection, meronts of *H. americanum* can be observed within leukocytes situated between individual muscle fibers in stained histologic preparations of muscle biopsy samples. Meront-containing leukocytes are encysted within host cell–derived concentric layers of mucopolysaccharide, which resemble the layers of an onion. The characteristic lesions thus are termed "onion skin" cysts (Figure 273-1). Meronts increase in size as they mature and eventually rupture host cells to release merozoites, which then penetrate cyst

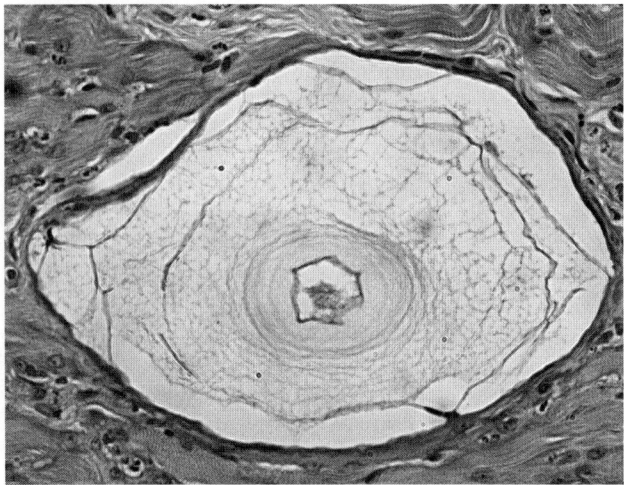

Figure 273-1 Onion skin cyst in the skeletal muscle of a dog infected with *H. americanum.*

walls and result in localized inflammatory reactions that often progress to pyogranulomata. Liberated merozoites invade new host leukocytes to form additional meronts or develop into gamonts, the sexually differentiated, peripherally circulating stages of parasite that are infective to feeding larval and nymphal *A. maculatum* (Panciera and Ewing, 2003).

Clinical Manifestations

Clinical Signs

ACH is diagnosed most often in dogs in rural areas, especially if kenneled outdoors or allowed to roam, that are not maintained diligently with acaricidal compounds and that prey on other animals. Clinical signs are a result of parasite merogonic cycles within tissues and associated inflammatory reactions and are seen as soon as 3 to 5 weeks after exposure in experimentally infected dogs (Panciera and Ewing, 2003). Dogs often are presented with fever (102.7° F to 105.6° F) that does not resolve with antibiotic treatment, a stiff and painful gait, lameness, ataxia, generalized weakness, reluctance to move, lethargy, and depression. Despite obvious discomfort, dogs often continue to eat and drink, but sometimes only when food and water are placed directly in front of them. However, weight loss still may be noted, which is a result of increased inflammatory processes, and marked muscle atrophy is not uncommon (Little et al, 2009; Medici and Heseltine, 2008; Panciera and Ewing, 2003; Potter and Macintire, 2010; Vincent-Johnson, 2003). A consistent feature of the syndrome is a copious mucopurulent ocular discharge. In addition, uveitis, retinal scarring, hyperpigmentation, and papilledema may be evident upon ophthalmic exam (Medici and Heseltine, 2008; Potter and Macintire, 2010). Although some dogs continue to decline after initial onset of clinical signs, other patients endure a waxing and waning course of disease, with obvious clinical signs spontaneously abating only to recur a few months later. The cyclic presentation and resolution of apparent illness is ascribed to interims of active and arrested parasite merogony, respectively (Macintire et al, 2001; Potter and Macintire, 2010).

Laboratory Findings

Complete blood count analyses are often valuable in the detection of *H. americanum* infections. Neutrophilic leukocytosis, with counts commonly ranging between 20,000 and 200,000 cells/ml, is a hallmark finding of ACH and often is observed before or coinciding with onset of clinical signs (Potter and Macintire, 2010; Vincent-Johnson, 2003). In general, a mature neutrophilia is present, but a left shift may be noted. Laboratory abnormalities may include mild normocytic normochromic nonregenerative anemia, and in cases of concurrent infections with rickettsial species, thrombocytopenia (Medici and Heseltine, 2008; Potter and Macintire, 2010).

Serum biochemical abnormalities commonly include a mild increase in alkaline phosphatase activity (AP), hypoalbuminemia, and hyperglobulinemia. In addition, hypoglycemia may be present, which is an artifact of the increased metabolism of glucose by abnormally high levels of leukocytes (Panciera and Ewing, 2003; Vincent-Johnson, 2003). Blood urea nitrogen (BUN) levels may be lowered, and in combination with the decreased levels of albumin and glucose and increased AP, the suspicion of liver failure may arise. However, fasting and postprandial bile acids are typically within normal ranges (Vincent-Johnson, 2003). In cases of chronic infections, complications of glomerulopathy and renal failure may result, with urinalyses possibly revealing proteinuria and elevations in urine protein-creatinine ratios (Medici and Heseltine, 2008; Panciera and Ewing, 2003; Potter and Macintire, 2010; Vincent-Johnson, 2003).

In dogs with ACH, periosteal bone proliferation occurs, particularly of the long bones. The osseous lesions are likely painful upon palpation, and the mechanisms behind their formation are not clear. On radiographs the lesions appear similar to those observed in cases of hypertrophic osteopathy (Panciera and Ewing, 2003; Vincent-Johnson, 2003).

Diagnosis

The history of tick exposure or predatory behaviors, clinical signs, neutrophilic leukocytosis, and radiographic evidence of periosteal bone proliferation should alert veterinarians to the possible diagnosis of ACH. Parasite gamonts, pale-blue staining ellipsoidal bodies (8.2 × 3.9 μm) with faintly staining nuclei, found within the cytoplasm of host leukocytes (Figure 273-2), are scant to absent on blood smears because parasitemia is often less than 0.1%. However, when rare gamonts are detected, they are considered confirmatory for *H. americanum* infection (Medici and Heseltine, 2008; Potter and Macintire, 2010). If numerous gamonts are observed on blood smears, *Hepatozoon canis*, which is now thought to be present in North America, is the more likely etiologic agent responsible for infection (Baneth, 2011; Li et al, 2008; Little et al, 2009). Gamonts of *H. americanum* have been observed on blood smears from experimentally infected dogs as soon as 5 weeks after exposure (Johnson et al, 2009).

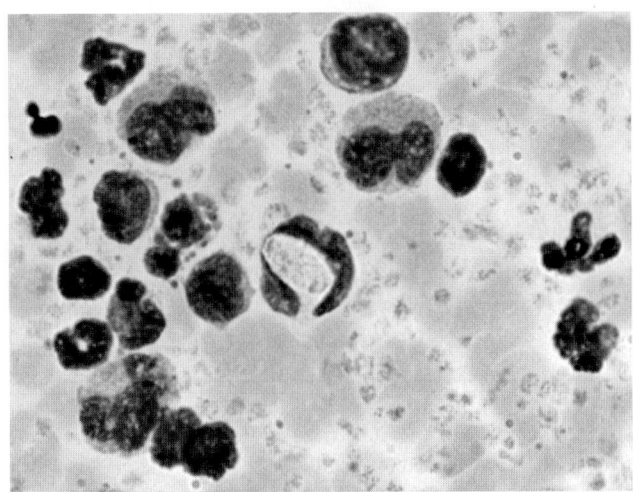

Figure 273-2 Gamont of *H. americanum* within a leukocyte on a peripheral blood smear.

Merogony of *H. americanum* occurs predominantly in striated muscle tissue; therefore muscle biopsy (2 × 2 cm), typically of the biceps femoris or semitendinosus muscle, is considered the most reliable and sensitive method for achieving a definitive diagnosis of ACH. Microscopic examination of histologic preparations of muscle biopsy usually reveals the presence of onion skin cysts and pyogranulomata, which are pathognomonic for *H. americanum* infection. Several areas of muscle tissue may have to be sampled to increase the likelihood of parasite detection (Medici and Heseltine, 2008; Potter and Macintire, 2010; Vincent-Johnson, 2003).

Real-time PCR assays for the detection of *Hepatozoon* spp. DNA in whole-blood samples in EDTA are available commercially through Auburn University's Molecular Diagnostics Laboratory (Auburn, Alabama) and through IDEXX Laboratories (Westbrook, Maine). The PCR specifically detects *Hepatozoon* spp. 18S rDNA present in whole blood and can differentiate *H. americanum* and *H. canis* infections (Li et al, 2008). Although very sensitive, some *H. americanum* infections are missed because of extremely low levels of circulating parasites, especially in dogs with chronic infections. A negative whole-blood PCR result in a dog presented with classic clinical signs should not preclude a diagnosis of ACH; histologic examination of muscle biopsy often reveals the organisms in these cases.

Treatment

In prostrate patients, conditions such as dehydration, anorexia, and hypoglycemia must be corrected (Potter and Macintire, 2010). Nonsteroidal antiinflammatory drugs (NSAIDs) should be administered to alleviate pain (Allen et al, 2010; Medici and Heseltine, 2008); many infected dogs regain function and maintain health while on NSAID therapy.

No known curative treatments exist for *H. americanum* infections. All drugs experimentally evaluated have failed to eliminate encysted parasite stages (Allen et al, 2010; Macintire et al, 2001; Potter and Macintire, 2010). However, the currently recommended treatment regimen of initial 14-day parasiticidal triple therapy with trimethoprim-sulfadiazine (15 mg/kg PO q12h), clindamycin (10 mg/kg PO q8h), and pyrimethamine (1 mg/kg PO q24h), followed by long-term administration of decoquinate (10 to 20 mg/kg PO q12h), affords affected dogs a better quality of life and extends life expectancy (Allen et al, 2010; Macintire et al, 2001). Ponazuril (10 mg/kg PO q12h) given for 14 days, also followed by long-term decoquinate therapy, may be administered as an alternative to TCP treatment (Allen et al, 2010).

Although TCP administration often results in a marked clinical improvement, the triple therapy does not have an enduring effect. Long-term follow-up decoquinate administration decreases the frequency of relapse, which often occurs within 2 to 6 months after initial onset of clinical signs and administration of TCP without supplemental decoquinate treatment (Macintire et al, 2001). Obtain the decoquinate 6% (27.2 gram/lb) powder. Decoquinate powder (Deccox) is available in bulk as a feed additive and can be mixed into wet food at a dose of 0.5 to 1 tsp/10 kg of body weight (10 to 20 mg/kg q12h PO). Decoquinate is not associated with any known side effects and can be administered long term without sequelae (Macintire et al, 2001; Medici and Heseltine, 2008). Infected animals should be maintained on the coccidiostat for 2 years (Macintire et al, 2001). Although some researchers contend that patients should be tested every 3 to 6 months by PCR, stop treatment when parasitemia can no longer be detected by the assay, and resume treatment when a positive PCR status is again determined (Medici and Heseltine, 2008; Potter and Macintire, 2010), withholding parasiticide treatment may allow exacerbation or recrudescence of clinical disease.

A study conducted at Oklahoma State University determined that after ponazuril treatment, administration of decoquinate to an experimentally, chronically infected dog successfully blocked transmission of *H. americanum* to feeding *A. maculatum* while the dog was on the coccidiostat. Before treatment, the infected dog had been able to infect ticks consistently throughout course of disease, regardless of clinical state, and in fact was maintained as a reservoir of parasite. Although data from this study are limited, they do indicate that maintaining infected dogs on decoquinate after TCP treatment may reduce the risk of *H. americanum* transmission to other dogs by preventing the infection of susceptible ticks in the environment.

Prognosis

ACH is a lifelong disease, and patients therefore should be monitored with that consideration. Acutely ill ACH patients receiving TCP, decoquinate, and NSAIDs often respond positively to treatment, especially if it is begun soon after the initial onset of clinical signs. Prognosis is more guarded in animals that have had chronic illness before treatment. If clinical relapse is observed, repetition of TCP and decoquinate treatment is recommended.

References and Suggested Reading

Allen KE et al: Treatment of *Hepatozoon americanum* infections: review of the literature and experimental evaluation of efficacy, *Vet Ther* 11:E1, 2010.

Baneth G: Perspectives on canine and feline hepatozoonosis, *Vet Parasitol* 181:3, 2011.

Johnson EM et al: Experimental transmission of *Hepatozoon americanum* to New Zealand White rabbits *(Oryctolagus cuniculus)* and infectivity of cystozoites for a dog, *Vet Parasitol* 164:162, 2009.

Li Y et al: Diagnosis of canine *Hepatozoon* spp. infection by quantitative PCR, *Vet Parasitol* 157:50, 2008.

Little SE et al: New developments in canine hepatozoonosis in North America: a review, *Parasit Vectors* 2:S5, 2009.

Macintire DK et al: Treatment of dogs infected with *Hepatozoon americanum*: 53 cases (1989-1998), *J Am Vet Med Assoc* 218:77, 2001.

Medici EM, Heseltine J: American canine hepatozoonosis, *Compend Contin Educ Vet* 30:E1, 2008.

Panciera RJ, Ewing SA: American canine hepatozoonosis, *Anim Health Res Rev* 4:27, 2003.

Potter TM, Macintire DK: *Hepatozoon americanum*: an emerging disease in the south-central/southeastern United States, *J Vet Emerg Crit Care* 20:70, 2010.

Vincent-Johnson NA: American canine hepatozoonosis, *Vet Clin North Am Small Anim Pract* 33:905, 2003.

CHAPTER 274

Leptospirosis

KATHARINE F. LUNN, *Raleigh, North Carolina*

Leptospirosis is a zoonotic bacterial disease of worldwide importance in human and veterinary medicine. Disease is caused by serovars of the pathogenic species *Leptospira interrogans* sensu lato. Infection is maintained in nature by mammalian reservoir hosts infected endemically with host-adapted strains. Examples of reservoir hosts include the vole and raccoon (both carrying serovar *grippotyphosa*), and the rat (serovar *icterohaemorrhagiae* and serovar *bratislava*). These hosts serve as a source of infection for incidental hosts, such as humans and dogs, through excretion of organisms in the urine. Survival of leptospires is optimum in warm and wet environments with stagnant or slow-moving water. Transmission to incidental hosts may be direct or indirect, through exposure to contaminated water, soil, food, or bedding.

Case reports and serologic surveys have demonstrated clinical and subclinical leptospirosis in dogs from many locations in North America. Because leptospirosis typically is contracted through indirect contact with the urine of wild animal hosts, it often has been assumed that working dogs, large-breed dogs, or dogs with an outdoor rural lifestyle are more likely to develop the disease. However, many clinicians, including this author, routinely diagnose leptospirosis in small-breed dogs and dogs that rarely leave the house and backyard. In support of this, it recently was shown that dogs in regions of the midwestern United States are at higher risk for leptospirosis if they live in urban areas (Raghavan et al, 2011). Thus any dog should be considered to be at risk, regardless of breed or lifestyle. The manifestations of leptospirosis in dogs range from peracute disease to subclinical infection and include sudden death, renal failure, hepatic failure, vasculitis, and uveitis. Because leptospires have zoonotic potential, veterinarians must maintain a high index of suspicion for this infection, particularly in those cases that do not have typical clinical signs. Feline leptospirosis rarely is recognized as a clinical entity; however, cats can be infected experimentally with the organisms and can seroconvert and shed leptospires in the urine. This chapter focuses on the clinical manifestations, diagnosis, and treatment of leptospirosis in dogs. There have been few new developments in the prevention of canine leptospirosis. Vaccination was discussed in the previous edition of this text (see Chapter 269 in the previous edition of *Current Veterinary Therapy*), in the 2011 American Animal Hospital Association Vaccine Guidelines (www.aahanet.org), and in the 2010 American College of Veterinary Internal Medicine Small Animal Consensus Statement on Leptospirosis: Diagnosis, Epidemiology, Treatment, and Prevention (Sykes et al, 2011).

Clinical Findings

Common Manifestations

Acute renal failure has been the most common presentation for canine leptospirosis in recent years. Affected animals can present with lethargy, anorexia, vomiting, abdominal pain, and a history of polyuria, oliguria, or anuria. Dogs that survive acute renal failure may return to normal or progress to chronic renal failure. Leptospirosis also should be considered in any dog with previously diagnosed chronic renal disease that develops "acute-on-chronic" renal failure.

Acute renal failure results from interstitial nephritis, renal swelling, and vasculitis, leading to decreased renal perfusion and decreased glomerular filtration rate (GFR). The leptospiral organisms also penetrate and colonize renal tubular cells. In humans the acute renal failure of leptospirosis is often nonoliguric and can be associated with hyponatremia and hypokalemia. These electrolyte changes also have been noted in canine leptospirosis, along with the expected changes of azotemia, hyperphosphatemia, and acidosis of renal failure. The hypokalemia of acute renal failure in leptospirosis has been attributed to decreased proximal tubular reabsorption of sodium leading to increased distal tubular sodium delivery with associated increased distal potassium secretion. These abnormalities may be caused by a Na^+/K^+ ATPase inhibitor associated with leptospiral endotoxin.

Polyuria and polydipsia (PU/PD) in the absence of azotemia is a less common manifestation of the renal effects of leptospirosis. PU/PD could result from a decrease in GFR sufficient to cause loss of renal concentrating ability without azotemia. However, this PU/PD also may be a form of nephrogenic diabetes insipidus. In guinea pigs experimentally infected with leptospirosis, the inner medullary collecting ducts of the renal tubules appear to be resistant to the effects of vasopressin.

Acute liver disease can accompany acute renal failure in dogs with leptospirosis, or it can occur alone. Affected dogs may be icteric, and serum biochemistry analysis reveals increased bilirubin and alkaline phosphatase (ALP) activity. Alanine aminotransferase (ALT) activity typically is less markedly increased than ALP activity. In humans and dogs, the icterus of acute leptospirosis appears to be associated with minimal histopathologic changes in the liver, suggesting that it is due to "cholestasis of sepsis" rather than hepatocellular damage.

Muscle pain, stiffness, weakness, trembling, or reluctance to move can be seen in dogs with leptospirosis and are attributed to vasculitis, myositis, or nephritis. Myalgia commonly is reported in human leptospirosis and is associated with the septicemic phase of the disease.

Uncommon Manifestations

Petechial hemorrhages, epistaxis, melena, and hematemesis occasionally are seen in dogs with leptospirosis. These findings most likely are due to vasculitis. Affected dogs also may be thrombocytopenic; however, platelet counts are rarely low enough to be responsible for spontaneous bleeding. The causes and mechanisms of bleeding disorders in leptospirosis are poorly understood, but they have been suggested to be associated with endothelial cell damage.

Pulmonary hemorrhage is one of the most common clinical signs in outbreaks of human leptospirosis. Reticulonodular pulmonary opacities have been described in the thoracic radiographs of dogs with leptospirosis and attributed to pulmonary hemorrhage (Baumann and Fluckiger, 2001). These changes may be diffuse or involve predominantly the caudodorsal lung fields. This was previously believed to be a rare finding in canine leptospirosis; however, clinical or radiographic signs of pulmonary disease have been noted in several dogs with leptospirosis, and recent case series suggest that pulmonary disease may be more common than suspected, at least in Europe (Baumann and Fluckiger, 2001; Klopfleisch et al, 2010; Kohn et al, 2010).

Uveitis is an uncommon manifestation of leptospirosis in dogs, although it may be underrecognized. Although uveitis is associated infrequently with experimental canine leptospirosis and has been reported only rarely in the literature (Townsend, Stiles, and Krohne, 2006), this author has observed it. Uveitis also has been reported in human patients with leptospirosis. In most human cases, uveitis occurs as a late complication after apparent recovery from leptospirosis and is likely immune-mediated. However, leptospirosis also can cause uveitis in the acute phase of the disease, in humans and animals, possibly associated with the vasculitis caused by the organism. In the horse, there is a well-known association between leptospirosis, uveitis, and periodic ophthalmia.

Additional clinical signs in dogs with leptospirosis may include vomiting, diarrhea, weight loss, fever, hypothermia, oculonasal discharge, lymphadenopathy, effusions, and edema.

Clinical Laboratory Findings

CBC changes may include neutrophilia, lymphopenia, monocytosis, anemia (resulting from blood loss), and thrombocytopenia. Serum chemistry may reveal increases in blood urea nitrogen, creatinine, phosphorus, bilirubin, lipase, amylase, and activities of ALP, ALT, aspartate aminotransferase (AST), and creatine kinase (CK). Electrolyte changes can include hyponatremia, hypochloremia and hypokalemia, or hyperkalemia. Metabolic acidosis may be present. Coagulation abnormalities may include increased fibrin degradation products and prolonged prothrombin time (PT) or activated partial thromboplastin time (aPTT). Urinalysis may reveal hyposthenuria, isosthenuria, or hypersthenuria, depending on the degree of renal involvement. Proteinuria, glucosuria, cylindruria, hematuria, and pyuria may be detected, reflecting renal tubular damage. Leptospirosis also could be potentially associated with renal tubular acidosis.

Diagnosis

Leptospirosis can be diagnosed by finding the organism or by detecting an immune response to the organism. However, as with other infectious diseases, neither finding the organism nor detecting an antibody response necessarily equates to clinical disease. For example, subclinically infected dogs can shed leptospires in the urine, and dogs can have circulating antibodies to leptospires as a result of vaccination or exposure. Thus the results of diagnostic testing always should be interpreted in light of the clinical signs and vaccination history. One of the difficulties associated with the evaluation of diagnostic tests for leptospirosis is the fact that there is no readily accessible "gold standard" test for *antemortem* diagnosis in the dog. For most patients, the diagnosis is based on a combination of clinical signs, clinicopathologic findings, and microscopic agglutination test (MAT) titers, sometimes combined with polymerase chain reaction (PCR) or other methods of organism detection.

The MAT still is considered to be the reference method for diagnosis of leptospirosis. In this test dilutions of a patient's serum are incubated with suspensions of live leptospires. The suspensions then are examined by dark-field microscopy for evidence of agglutination. The end-point is the highest dilution of the patient's serum at which 50% agglutination occurs. The MAT is available at many diagnostic laboratories, and each laboratory maintains cultures of serovars that are locally common or expected to cause disease in the animal species of interest. Laboratories that participate in the International Leptospirosis Society testing proficiency program should be used whenever possible. Most veterinary laboratories offer the MAT for serovars *canicola, icterohaemorrhagiae, pomona, grippotyphosa, hardjo,* and *bratislava. Autumnalis* and other serovars may be available upon request. Although the laboratories report results for the serovars tested, the MAT is a serogroup-specific assay.

The advantages of the MAT are that the test is widely available, has been used for many years, and is relatively inexpensive. Furthermore, a wealth of data is available from use of the assay in humans and animals. Disadvantages include the safety concerns associated with laboratory maintenance of live cultures of leptospires, the subjective nature of the interpretation of the end point of the test, the risk of cross-contamination of live cultures, and the significant occurrence of cross-reactions between different serogroups. The MAT also may give either false-positive or false-negative results in the diagnosis of leptospirosis, as discussed below. In a patient with consistent clinical signs and clinicopathologic abnormalities, a single MAT titer of 1:800 or greater often is considered to be diagnostic for leptospirosis. However, titers of this magnitude develop transiently in some dogs after vaccination with currently available products. If leptospirosis is suspected and the initial titer is not confirmatory, a convalescent titer should be performed. A fourfold (or greater) change (usually a rise) in titer between paired sera is regarded as confirming the diagnosis. The timing of the convalescent titer likely depends on the interval between the onset of clinical signs and presentation of the patient. This author has observed seroconversion within 8 days in patients that were clinically ill but seronegative at the time of the first MAT. Thus it may not be necessary to wait for the recommended 2 to 4 weeks.

The sensitivity of an initial titer of at least 1:800 (for any serogroup) for the diagnosis of leptospirosis ranges from 22% to 67%, depending on the laboratory used (Miller et al, 2008). This finding confirms that a single negative or low MAT titer cannot be used to rule out leptospirosis in the early stages of disease. The specificity of the MAT ranges from 69% to 100%, depending on the cutoff titers and laboratory used (Miller et al, 2008). Seroprevalence studies in healthy dogs also demonstrate that the detection of antibodies by the MAT does not correlate necessarily with clinical disease. In Michigan almost 25% of healthy dogs tested had evidence of exposure to leptospires (Stokes et al, 2007). The author also has surveyed healthy unvaccinated dogs in Wisconsin and found a

seroprevalence of 11%. Finally, when tested in specific-pathogen-free dogs, the MAT appears to have an extremely low false-positive rate.

The available evidence suggests that the MAT cannot be used reliably to predict the infecting serovar in a patient with leptospirosis. In a large study of culture-proven leptospirosis in human patients, it was found that the predominant serogroup (based on MAT results) predicted less than 50% of the serovars isolated (Levett, 2003). In human and veterinary medicine it is well recognized that patients with leptospirosis have high MAT titers to more than one serogroup. These cross-reactions are attributed to the presence of several common antigens among leptospires. In veterinary medicine it has been assumed that the serovar with the highest MAT titer represents the infecting serogroup. However, it was reported recently that in dogs with leptospirosis the identity of the serogroup with the highest titer varies between laboratories (Miller et al, 2011). This finding implies that the results of a single MAT from a single laboratory cannot predict accurately the infecting serogroup in a patient with leptospirosis.

In the human literature, "paradoxic" immune responses are well documented in leptospirosis; in this phenomenon the highest MAT titer is detected to a serogroup unrelated to the infecting strain. This is most common in the acute stages of leptospirosis, whereas convalescent MAT titers appear to reflect more accurately the infecting serogroup. This is attributed to the presence of common antigens between different leptospiral serovars, the fact that the MAT detects IgG and IgM antibodies, and the different rates of decline of cross-reacting titers. When MAT titers are followed, it was shown that the identity of the serogroup with the highest MAT titer can change in some dogs (Miller et al, 2011).

Vaccination of dogs with commercially available leptospirosis vaccines produces detectable MAT titers; however they appear to persist for a relatively short time. MAT titers were studied in puppies and adult dogs after giving a commercial subunit vaccine against *L. interrogans* serovar *pomona*/*L. kirschneri* serovar *grippotyphosa* (Barr et al, 2005). Titers to serovar *grippotyphosa* were 1:400 or less, most titers to serovar *pomona* were 1:800 or less, and titers to serovar *autumnalis* were as high as 1:12,800. All serovar *pomona* and serovar *grippotyphosa* titers were less than 1:100 by 16 weeks postvaccination, but low serovar *autumnalis* titers still were present at this time. High MAT titers to serovar *autumnalis* and serovar *bratislava* also were detected in some dogs after vaccination with a subunit vaccine against serovars *canicola, icterohaemorrhagiae, pomona,* and *grippotyphosa* (Miller et al, 2011). After administration of inactivated whole-cell bacterin vaccines against serovars *canicola* and *icterohaemorrhagiae,* high MAT titers are detected for up to 10 to 12 weeks postvaccination and usually decrease to less than 1:100 by 16 weeks. Some dogs may develop titers as high as 1:3200 after vaccination, and these titers can persist for 6 months or longer.

Although the results of MAT may not be used reliably to determine the identity of the infecting serogroup, the results of the test can be used to confirm a diagnosis of leptospirosis. In the presence of appropriate clinical signs and clinicopathologic findings, a single high MAT titer, or fourfold change in titer in paired samples, provides strong evidence in support of the diagnosis of leptospirosis. However, there is a need for tests that can be used much earlier in the course of infection. Point-of-care assays have been developed that detect serum IgM antibodies (Abdoel et al, 2011). These appear promising, although they have not been widely evaluated or adopted in veterinary medicine. Tests that detect the presence of the organism also can be used to diagnose leptospirosis in the early stages of infection. Culture of leptospires is not a useful test for clinicians because it requires special media, it is available at few laboratories, and the organisms are extremely slow growing. However isolation of leptospires from clinical cases is necessary and important for researchers in this field to further our understanding of the epidemiology and prevention of leptospirosis. PCR assays for the diagnosis of leptospirosis are becoming more widely available, although validation of these assays unfortunately is reported rarely in the literature. These tests are most likely to be useful when performed on blood samples within the first 10 days of infection and subsequently on urine samples. Recent vaccination does not appear to interfere with the use of PCR assays for the diagnosis of acute leptospirosis in dogs (Midence et al, 2012). False-negative results may occur when the number of organisms in the blood or urine is low, or when leptospiruria is absent or intermittent. PCR assays are generally specific for pathogenic leptospires but do not identify the infecting serovar.

Treatment

Appropriate supportive and nonspecific therapy should be provided to patients with acute renal failure, hepatic disease, uveitis, and other manifestations of leptospirosis. A dearth of literature is available to guide antibiotic choices for the treatment of canine leptospirosis. Current recommendations are to treat with a 2- to 3-week course of doxycycline (5 mg/kg q12h PO) to eliminate the leptospiremic and renal carrier phase of infection. In clinically ill patients that cannot tolerate oral medications, penicillin G (25,000 to 40,000 U/kg q12h IV) or ampicillin (25 mg/kg q8h IV) can be used to eliminate the leptospiremic phase, followed by a course of doxycycline to resolve leptospiruria. No published studies document the duration of shedding of leptospires in canine urine after antibiotic therapy.

References and Suggested Reading

Abdoel TH et al: Rapid test for the serodiagnosis of acute canine leptospirosis, *Vet Microbiol* 150:211, 2011.

Barr SC et al: Serologic response of dogs given a commercial vaccine against *Leptospira interrogans* serovar pomona and *Leptospira kirschneri* serovar grippotyphosa, *Am J Vet Res* 66:1780, 2005.

Baumann D, Fluckiger M: Radiographic findings in the thorax of dogs with leptospiral infection, *Vet Radiol Ultrasound* 42:305, 2001.

Greene CE et al: Leptospirosis. In Greene CE, editor: *Infectious diseases of the dog and cat*, ed 4, St Louis, 2012, Elsevier Saunders, p 431.

Harkin KR: Leptospirosis. In Bonagura JD, Twedt DC, editors: *Kirk's current veterinary therapy XIV*, St Louis, 2009, Saunders Elsevier, p 1237.

Klopfleisch R et al: An emerging pulmonary haemorrhagic syndrome in dogs: similar to the human leptospiral pulmonary haemorrhagic syndrome? *Vet Med Int* 2010, doi:10.4061/2010/928541.

Kohn B et al: Pulmonary abnormalities in dogs with leptospirosis, *J Vet Intern Med* 21:1277, 2010.

Levett PN: Leptospirosis, *Clin Microbiol Rev* 14:296, 2001.

Levett PN: Usefulness of serologic analysis as a predictor of the infecting serovar in patients with severe leptospirosis, *Clin Infect Dis* 36:447, 2003.

Midence JN et al: Effects of recent Leptospira vaccination on whole blood real-time PCR testing in healthy client-owned dogs, *J Vet Intern Med* 26:149, 2012.

Miller MD et al: Sensitivity and specificity of the microscopic agglutination test for the diagnosis of leptospirosis in dogs, *J Vet Intern Med* 22:787, 2008.

Miller MD et al: Variability in results of the microscopic agglutination test in dogs with clinical leptospirosis and dogs vaccinated against leptospirosis, *J Vet Intern Med* 25:426, 2011.

Raghavan R et al: Evaluations of land cover risk factors for canine leptospirosis: 94 cases (2002-2009), *Prev Vet Med* 101:214, 2011.

Stokes JE et al: Prevalence of serum antibodies against six *Leptospira* serovars in healthy dogs, *J Am Vet Med Assoc* 230:1657, 2007.

Sykes JE et al: 2010 ACVIM small animal consensus statement on leptospirosis: diagnosis, epidemiology, treatment, and prevention, *J Vet Intern Med* 25:1, 2011.

Townsend WM, Stiles J, Krohne SG: Leptospirosis and panuveitis in a dog, *Vet Ophthalmol* 9:169, 2006.

CHAPTER 275

Neospora caninum

JEANNE E. FICOCIELLO, *South Weymouth, Massachusetts*

Neospora caninum is a protozoal agent in the phylum Apicomplexa. The domestic dog and coyotes are definitive hosts, and herbivores, including deer and cattle, are considered intermediate hosts. Encephalomyelitis and myositis develop in experimentally infected kittens, and seropositive, naturally exposed cats have been detected, but clinical disease in naturally infected cats has not been reported (Bresciani et al, 2007). After the sexual phase is completed in the dog's gastrointestinal tract, infected dogs pass unsporulated oocysts in feces. After sporulation, the oocysts are infectious to definitive and intermediate hosts. However, in one study, dogs fed sporulated oocysts became infected and seroconverted but did not shed oocysts (Bandini et al, 2011). Dogs also become infected by ingesting bradyzoites in tissue cysts from intermediate hosts, including bovine placentas, or any meat from deer or cattle. The organism also has been detected in the tissues of free-ranging chickens. Transplacental infection also is common in dogs and can occur repeatedly once a bitch is infected.

Neospora caninum seroprevalence rates have varied from 0% to 100% depending on the country and lifestyle of the dog. Infections are found throughout the world, with prevalence rates higher in feral dogs than in domestic dogs. Furthermore, dogs that eat raw meat also have higher seroprevalence rates than do dogs fed commercial diets. However, because of the short duration of the shedding period, oocysts rarely are reported in fecal surveys. In one study of 24,677 dog samples, oocysts consistent with N. caninum were detected in only 0.3% of the samples (Barutzki and Schaper, 2011).

Clinical Findings

Clinical signs of neosporosis vary depending on the age of the animal at the time of infection. Dogs that are infected *in utero* or at a very young age (usually younger than 16 weeks) usually have ascending paralysis and rigidity of affected muscles (particularly the pelvic limbs). Stillbirth and neonatal death are also common. Clinical signs can be seen in puppies as young as 3 weeks of age and can progress to include dysphagia and megaesophagus. Young affected dogs often remain bright and alert because intracranial infection is rare. These puppies can survive for months if provided supportive care, although they often are paralyzed. Young dogs often succumb to the disease, even with attempted therapy.

Older dogs (usually older than 6 months) that become infected with N. caninum usually do so via the ingestion of infected, often raw, bovine or deer meat or aborted bovine fetuses. These dogs may be infected chronically yet show few to no clinical signs of illness. Neosporosis may become apparent only when the animals become spontaneously immunosuppressed or after immunosuppressive drug administration. At that time, affected dogs may show signs of dysfunction in any organ system; however, musculoskeletal, cardiopulmonary, and central nervous system abnormalities are most common. Clinical signs may include, but are not limited to, hyperesthesia, lower motor neuron signs, seizures, altered mental status, fever, arrhythmias, pyogranulomatous dermatitis, and dyspnea. Cerebral ataxia and atrophy recently are recognized clinical syndromes associated with neosporosis.

Diagnosis

Until the late 1990s, N. caninum often was misdiagnosed as *Toxoplasma gondii* via light microscopic examination of infected tissues. N. caninum oocysts are morphologically similar to those of T. gondii. With the advent of other diagnostic modalities, the two organisms can be distinguished readily.

Abnormalities detected on serum biochemical panels blood work may vary among affected dogs but often include increased activities of the liver enzymes, including aspartate transaminase (AST). Creatine kinase (CK) activity also may be elevated, although a normal CK does not exclude the possibility of neosporosis. Dogs with central nervous system neosporosis often have cerebral spinal fluid abnormalities that include elevated protein concentrations and mild, mixed pleocytosis (10 to 50 cells/µl) consisting of monocytes, lymphocytes, neutrophils, and occasionally tachyzoites.

Exposure to N. caninum can be documented serologically with indirect fluorescent antibody assay titer results of at least 1:50. Many dogs with clinical neosporosis have titers of 1:800 or greater. Because clinical signs of toxoplasmosis and neosporosis can be similar, dogs with suspected infection should be screened for antibodies against both organisms; if both titers are positive, the highest titer is likely the infective agent. If tissue biopsies are obtained, tachyzoites or bradyzoites can be detected by light microscopy with immunohistochemical stains or polymerase chain reaction assay used to distinguish N. caninum from T. gondii.

Therapy

None of the drugs used to treat neosporosis eliminate tissue infection; therefore the primary goals of treatment are survival and reduction of progressive disease. Although the prognosis for many dogs with neosporosis is grave, some have survived after treatment with trimethoprim-sulfadiazine combined with pyrimethamine; sequential treatment with clindamycin hydrochloride, trimethoprim-sulfadiazine, and pyrimethamine; or clindamycin alone. Administration of trimethoprim-sulfadiazine (15 mg/kg q12h PO) with pyrimethamine (1 mg/kg q24h PO) for 4 weeks or clindamycin (10 mg/kg q8h PO) for 4 weeks has been recommended for the treatment of canine neosporosis by some authors. If improvement is noted, treatment should be continued. Clindamycin induced significant clinical improvement after 18 weeks of administration to a 7-week-old Irish wolfhound with *N. caninum*–associated myositis (Crookshanks et al, 2007). Administration of clindamycin alone for 6 months (75 mg/puppy at 9 weeks of age q12h PO [dose doubled at 13 weeks]) lessened clinical signs of disease in naturally infected beagle puppies but did not eliminate the infection (Dubey et al, 2007). Four of six dogs with cerebellar disease associated with *N. caninum* infection treated with different combinations of clindamycin, trimethoprim, sulfadiazine, and pyrimethamine had a positive response (Garosi et al, 2010). Treatment of clinically affected dogs should be initiated before the development of extensor rigidity, if possible.

Prevention

There is no *N. caninum* vaccine; therefore avoiding infection is the primary means of prevention. Dogs should be fed processed food and never be fed raw beef or venison. Dogs living on farms should not have access to bovine tissues and aborted fetuses. Because infected bitches can transmit the organism to multiple litters those that have whelped infected puppies should not be bred in the future.

Zoonotic Considerations

Antibodies against *N. caninum* have been detected in the serum of people, but the organism has not been linked to abortion in women. However, meat to be eaten by immune-suppressed people or pregnant women should be cooked to medium well.

References and Suggested Reading

Bandini LA et al: Experimental infection of dogs (*Canis familiaris*) with sporulated oocysts of *Neospora caninum*, *Vet Parasitol* 176:151, 2011.

Barutzki D, Schaper R: Results of parasitological examinations of faecal samples from cats and dogs in Germany between 2003 and 2010, *Parasitol Res* 109(Suppl 1):S45, 2011.

Bresciani KD et al: Antibodies to *Neospora caninum* and *Toxoplasma gondii* in domestic cats from Brazil, *Parasitol Res* 100(2):281, 2007.

Cavalcante GT et al: Shedding of *Neospora caninum* oocysts by dogs fed different tissues from naturally infected cattle, *Vet Parasitol* 179:220, 2011.

Crookshanks JL et al: Treatment of canine pediatric *Neospora caninum* myositis following immunohistochemical identification of tachyzoites in muscle biopsies, *Can Vet J* 48:506, 2007.

Dubey JP et al: Neosporosis in beagle dogs: clinical signs, diagnosis, treatment, isolation and genetic characterization of *Neospora caninum*, *Vet Parasitol* 149(3-4):158, 2007.

Dubey JP, Schares G: Neosporosis in animals—the last five years, *Vet Parasitol* 180:90, 2011.

Galgut BI et al: Detection of *Neospora caninum* tachyzoites in cerebrospinal fluid of a dog following prednisone and cyclosporine therapy, *Vet Clin Pathol* 39:386, 2010.

Garosi L et al: Necrotizing cerebellitis and cerebellar atrophy caused by *Neospora caninum* infection: magnetic resonance imaging and clinicopathologic findings in seven dogs, *J Vet Intern Med* 24:571, 2010.

Ishigaki K et al: Detection of *Nesopora caninum*-specific DNA from cerebrospinal fluid by polymerase chain reaction in a dog with confirmed neosporosis, *J Vet Med Sci* 74(8):1051, 2012.

Meseck EK et al: Use of a multiplex polymerase chain reaction to rapidly differentiate *Neospora caninum* from *Toxoplasma gondii* in an adult dog with necrotizing myocarditis and myocardial infarct, *J Vet Diagn Invest* 2005;17:565.

Silva DA et al: Evaluation of serological tests for the diagnosis of *Neospora caninum* infection in dogs: optimization of cut off titers and inhibition studies of cross-reactivity with *Toxoplasma gondii*, *Vet Parasitol* 143:234, 2007.

Tranas J et al: Serological evidence of human infection with the protozoan *Neospora caninum*, *Clin Diagn Lab Immunol* 6:765, 1999.

CHAPTER 276

Canine and Feline Monocytotropic Ehrlichiosis

SUSAN M. EDDLESTONE, *Mandeville, Louisiana*

Canine Monocytic Ehrlichiosis

Cause

Canine monocytic ehrlichiosis (CME) is an important tick-borne disease of dogs caused by the rickettsial organism *Ehrlichia canis*. It is transmitted by the Ixodidae tick *Rhipicephalus sanguineus*, the "brown dog tick," found throughout the United States with noted prevalence in the southeastern, midwestern, and northeastern states. Other identified tick-borne rickettsial organisms that can infect the dog and cause similar clinical disease are *Ehrlichia ewingii, Anaplasma phagocytophilum, Neorickettsia risticii, Anaplasma platys,* and *Ehrlichia chaffeensis. E. chaffeensis,* the causative agent of human monocytotropic ehrlichiosis, can cause a milder form of disease in naturally infected dogs.

The known tick vectors for *E. chaffeensis* are *Amblyomma americanum* and *Dermacentor variabilis,* and *E. chaffeensis* also must be considered as a cause of canine ehrlichiosis. Distribution of infected ticks that carry *E. chaffeensis* has been reported in the south-central, southeastern, mid-Atlantic states, and California. In a large serosurvey conducted in the United States, antibodies to *Ehrlichia* spp. possibly induced by exposure to either *E. canis* or *E. chaffeensis* were more common in the southern states (Bowman et al, 2009).

Clinical Findings

Clinical signs of CME ehrlichiosis are multisystemic and can be mild to severe depending on the stage of disease. The German shepherd is considered particularly sensitive and susceptible to the severe form of CME. The varied presentations may be categorized into one of three stages: acute, subacute, and severe chronic. Most reports of the acute form of clinical disease are within 10 days postinfection or postexposure to ticks. The acute stage in most dogs is mild and may go undetected by the owner because only mild elevations in temperature, lethargy, and weight loss may occur. Overt signs of bleeding can occur and usually are due to thrombocytopenia or thrombocytopathia; petechiae, ecchymoses, and epistaxis are most common. Other clinical signs are uveitis, polymyositis, polyarthritis, and central nervous system signs, which may include seizures, ataxia, vestibular deficits, and cerebellar dysfunction. The granulocytic *Ehrlichia* spp. (*E. ewingii; A. phagocytophilum* [previously *E. equi*]) most commonly have been associated with polyarthritis. Recently a report of a German shepherd dog with severe acute hepatitis was determined to be associated with *E. canis* infection (Mylonakis et al, 2010). Apparently, many dogs exposed to *E. canis* seroconvert but never show clinical signs. It is unknown why they maintain high antibody titers. Do they truly clear the organism or harbor the organism and not show clinical signs for months to years? Reinfection in endemic areas is always possible, so it is difficult to distinguish from latency. The presence of coinfections with other tick-borne diseases such as *A. platys* or *Bartonella* spp. can make the clinical signs vary and difficult to attribute to a single specific agent; response to treatment may be less than expected than with just CME because of altered immune defenses.

Laboratory Findings

Clinicopathologic abnormalities most characteristic for CME are thrombocytopenia and mild regenerative anemia. However, infected dogs may have normal platelet counts. Dogs in the severe chronic phase of the disease, months to years after infection, may develop pancytopenia as a result of hypoplasia of all bone marrow precursor cells. Granular lymphocytosis, which may be confused with well-differentiated lymphocytic leukemia, has been reported. Hyperglobulinemia is reported in approximately one third of cases and is usually a polyclonal gammopathy, but monoclonal gammopathies have been reported in dogs and cats. Hypoalbuminemia and proteinuria have been found in all stages of the disease and may be asymptomatic. A common presentation of CME is the subclinical stage usually found incidentally with mild to moderate thrombocytopenia with the platelet count usually not below 60,000 ($\times 10^3/\mu l$), and the infected dog usually is not bleeding. Diagnosis of the disease at this stage and appropriate treatment are imperative so that the more severe, chronic phase does not occur. The chronic phase occurs when the bone marrow has been infected for weeks to months with irreversible bone marrow damage ensuing. The chronic stage often is not responsive to treatment and dogs either die or are euthanized because of poor quality of life.

Diagnostic Evaluation

Serologic test results can be of benefit in the diagnosis of CME in dogs. Serum antibodies can be detected by use of the indirect fluorescent antibody (IFA) assay; different point-of-care kits also are available commercially in some countries. In the IFA assay, it can take 7 to 28 days for a dog to become seropositive after initial infection. Clinical signs of CME may be present before the development of serum antibodies, and therefore the *E. canis* serum antibodies can be negative in acutely infected dogs. Repeat serologic testing in 2 to 3 weeks may show seroconversion and should be performed on dogs suspected of having CME. An *E. canis* IFA titer of more than 1:10 but less than 1:80 is considered suspect and should be repeated in 2 to 3 weeks. One point-of-care assay used to detect *E. canis* antibodies is calibrated to be positive at an IFA titer of approximately 1:100 or more (SNAP 4DX Plus). There is cross-reactivity between *E. canis* and other *Ehrlichia* spp. in some currently available antibody assays.

Positive *E. canis* antibody titers do not distinguish exposure from active infections. In endemic areas there are seropositive dogs exposed to the organism that either have cleared the organism naturally or may be infected currently. Serum antibody titers do not correlate with the duration of infection or the severity of disease. Apparently clinically ill or apparently healthy dogs with a positive antibody titer are not infected necessarily with *E. canis* and need further diagnostic investigation. Methods to document current infection include blood culture, cytologic demonstration of morulae, and amplification of *E. canis* DNA from blood or tissues by polymerase chain reaction (PCR). Blood culture for *E. canis* takes up to 8 weeks to become positive, is expensive and not widely available, and therefore is considered a research tool. Morulae are clusters of *E. canis* organisms found within mononuclear cells that stain purple on hematoxylin-eosin (H&E) blood smears. Detection of morulae confirms current infection; however, the sensitivity is low because morulae of CME are found rarely because they are present in the acute stage of the disease when most patients are infected subclinically. Because of these limitations, further evaluation of dogs for current CME infection generally is done by PCR assay, and positive test results confirm active infection. In general, *E. canis* DNA can be amplified from blood of experimentally infected dogs as soon as 4 to 10 days after the initial infection. PCR blood testing is specific for active infection and can detect infection earlier than IFA titers. However, healthy dogs also can be PCR positive, so this test also fails to prove definitely that the laboratory and clinical abnormities are related to CME. Not all commercial diagnostic laboratories are the same, and PCR assay results can be limited by quality controls used, which can result in false-positive and false-negative results.

The clinical diagnosis of CME usually is based on the combination of characteristic clinical signs, clinicopathologic abnormalities consistent with CME, a positive *E. canis* antibody titer, or a positive *E. canis* PCR assay on blood or tissue. Patients meeting these criteria should be treated for the infection. Whether to treat apparently healthy, seropositive dogs with no laboratory abnormalities is controversial. The pros and cons are discussed in the ACVIM Consensus Statement on Ehrlichial Disease of Small Animals from the Infectious Disease Study Group of the ACVIM (Neer et al, 2002). In one study using client-owned dogs, the authors concluded that serology alone should not be used to make a treatment decision (Hegarty et al, 2009).

Treatment Considerations

Standard treatment for *E. canis* was agreed on in the ACVIM Consensus Statement on Ehrlichial Disease of Small Animals in 2002: doxycycline 5 mg/kg q12h (or 10 mg/kg q24h) PO for 28 days. Clinical improvement generally is recognized within the first 24 to 48 hours after beginning treatment. Platelets increase during this time and are usually normal within 14 days of treatment. Chloramphenicol, 15 to 25 mg/kg q8h PO, IV, or SC for 28 days is also effective against *E. canis* infection and often is used in puppies to prevent the possibility of discolored teeth with the use of tetracycline drugs (although discolored teeth have never been proven to occur with doxycycline) and in those dogs resistant to doxycycline. It should be avoided in pancytopenic patients in the chronic stage of infection. Imidocarb dipropionate has been used for more than 20 years for the treatment of *Ehrlichia* spp. infections in dogs and still is used currently around the world today to treat effectively different strains and species of ehrlichia. In one recent study, imidocarb dipropionate has been proven ineffective in clinical improvement or clearing experimentally induced infection of the Louisiana strain of *E. canis* in dogs (Eddlestone et al, 2006).

Short-term immunosuppressive corticosteroids (prednisone 2 mg/kg q24h PO for 2 to 7 days) may be helpful in dogs with severe thrombocytopenia or those with neurologic signs resulting from the immune-mediated component elicited against the platelet and the deleterious effects of inflammation on CNS tissue. Use of prednisone at this dose does not inhibit organism clearance. Other supportive therapies that may be indicated are intravenous fluids, whole blood or packed RBCs, and platelet-rich plasma transfusions. Growth colony-stimulating factor products have not been assessed adequately in the chronic stage of CME to allow for definitive recommendations for the treatment of pancytopenia.

Posttreatment Monitoring

Monitoring of the patient posttreatment is important because some patients have persistent or latent infections. Serology may become negative within 6 to 9 months, but titers remain high in some patients for up to 34 months posttreatment. Thrombocyte counts usually normalize and hyperglobulinemia usually resolves in dogs after treatment. However, latent infections are a concern because research indicates that some apparently healthy dogs with or without treatment can maintain high *E. canis* IFA antibody titers and can have positive PCR assay results for months.

Performance of *E. canis* PCR assay on blood is considered to be more sensitive than serology for documenting organism clearance and should be performed 2 weeks after treatment. If *E. canis* DNA is amplified at that time, doxycycline should be administered for an additional 4 weeks with the PCR assay repeated on blood 2 weeks posttreatment. If the PCR assay is still positive after two cycles of treatment, another antiehrlichial drug protocol should be considered. If PCR results are negative, the test should be rechecked in 2 months; if still negative, clearance of the organism is likely. However, sequestration of the organism in other tissues such as spleen and bone marrow is possible. Reinfection is possible in dogs after an effective treatment and recovery from a previous infection, so tick control is imperative.

Prevention

Tick prevention is extremely important to prevent CME in endemic areas and in patients that are diagnosed and have recovered. Use of tick-repellant products and tick-control programs in kennels, as well as the isolation of dogs from ticks during the tick season in endemic regions are used in combination to attempt to prevent CME. Although no single product can protect against ticks with 100% efficacy, products currently used to best protect dogs from tick infestation are fipronil topical application, with an amitraz-impregnated collar, and imidacloprid and permethrin topical applications. In a recent study, administration of imidacloprid 10% and permethrin 50% to young dogs lessened incidence of *E. canis* infections by 94.6% (Otranto et al, 2010). Vaccines against CME are under investigation but not yet available commercially. Client education about tick prevention and regular patient screening for *E. canis* antibody titers in endemic areas are the best ways currently to prevent CME, which can be potentially a life-threatening disease.

Feline Monocytotropic Ehrlichiosis

Feline monocytotropic ehrlichiosis (FME) is not a well-described clinical disease in cats. *Ehrlichia* spp. infections of cats have been documented in Canada, Colorado, North Carolina, and several European countries based on characteristic morulae, serologic evidence, or amplification of *Ehrlichia* spp. DNA from blood or tissues.

At this time, any cat that has clinical signs and clinicopathologic abnormalities similar to CME or signs of autoimmune disease should be suspect for FME and an extensive search for a cause performed. Cats suspected to have FME have had fever, anorexia, lethargy, myalgia, dyspnea, and enlarged lymph nodes. Clinicopathologic

abnormalities reported include anemia, thrombocytopenia, leukopenia, and pancytopenia. Morulae are found rarely in the mononuclear cells on blood smears or lymph node aspirates. Validated serologic assays are not available currently, and some cats have been PCR positive, serum antibody assay negative. Thus performance of *E. canis* PCR assays on blood is considered optimal by some at this time. Treatment with doxycycline at the recommended dosage and duration for canines with CME is recommended for cats (5 mg/kg q12h PO for 28 days) suspected to be infected with *Ehrlichia* spp.

References and Suggested Reading

Bouloy RP et al: Clinical ehrlichiosis in a cat, *J Am Vet Med Assoc* 204(9):1475, 1994.

Bowman D et al: Prevalence and geographic distribution of *Dirofilaria immitis, Borrelia burgdorferi, Ehrlichia canis,* and *Anaplasma phagocytophilum* in dogs in the United States: results of a national clinic-based serologic survey, *Vet Parasitol* 160:138, 2009.

Breitschwerdt EB et al: Molecular evidence supporting *Ehrlichia canis*–like infection in cats, *J Vet Intern Med* 16:642, 2002.

Dawson JE, Ewing SA: Susceptibility of dogs to infection with *Ehrlichia chaffeensis,* causative agent of human ehrlichiosis, *Am J Vet Res* 538:1322, 1992.

Eddlestone SM et al: Failure of imidocarb dipropionate to clear experimentally induced *Ehrlichia canis* infection in dogs, *J Vet Intern Med* 20:840, 2006.

Harrus S et al: Amplification of ehrlichial DNA from dogs 34 months after infection with *Ehrlichia canis, J Clin Microbiol* 36:73, 1998.

Harrus S et al: Therapeutic effect of doxycycline in experimental subclinical canine monocytic ehrlichiosis: evaluation of a 6-week course, *J Clin Microbiol* 36:2140, 1998.

Hegarty BC et al: Clinical relevance of annual screening using a commercial enzyme-linked immunosorbent assay (SNAP 3Dx) for canine ehrlichiosis, *J Am Anim Hosp Assoc* 45:118-124, 2009.

Mylonakis ME et al: Severe heptatitis associated with acute *Ehrlichia canis* infection in a dog, *J Vet Intern Med* 24:633, 2010.

Neer TM et al: ACVIM Consensus Statement "Consensus Statement on Ehrlichial Disease of Small Animals from the Infectious Disease Study Group of the ACVIM, *J Vet Intern Med* 16:309, 2002.

Otranto D et al: Prevention of endemic canine vector-borne diseases using imidacloprid 10% and permethrin 50% in young dogs: a longitudinal field study, *Vet Parasitol* 172:323, 2010.

CHAPTER 277

Toxoplasmosis

MICHAEL R. LAPPIN, *Fort Collins, Colorado*

Familiarity with *Toxoplasma gondii* is important for all small animal practitioners because of pet ownership issues, as well as the occasional association of *T. gondii* with clinical illness in cats and dogs. The life cycle, diagnosis, treatment, and prevention of feline and canine toxoplasmosis has been reviewed extensively over the years (Dubey et al, 2009; Lappin, 2010). In addition, the American Association of Feline Practitioners and the Centers for Disease Control and Prevention have provided information concerning cat ownership as it relates to *T. gondii* and other infectious agents (Brown et al, 2003; Kaplan et al, 2009). This chapter emphasizes some of the most important points about this disease and provides recently published information concerning the zoonotic and clinical considerations for this protozoan.

Agent and Epidemiology

T. gondii is one of the most prevalent parasites infecting warm-blooded vertebrates; one survey of clinically ill cats in the United States showed an overall seroprevalence rate of 31.6% (Vollaire, Radecki, and Lappin, 2005). Approximately 20% of dogs in the United States are seropositive for *T. gondii* antibodies. Only cats complete the coccidian life cycle and pass environmentally resistant oocysts in feces. Dogs do not produce *T. gondii* oocysts like cats but can transmit oocysts mechanically after ingesting feline feces. *Sporozoites* develop in oocysts after 1 to 5 days of exposure to oxygen and appropriate environmental temperature and humidity. Thus, to lessen the potential of exposure to *T. gondii* for veterinary staff members in the laboratory, fresh feces should be used for fecal flotation, or the feces should be stored refrigerated until examined. *Tachyzoites* are the rapidly dividing stage of the organism; they disseminate in blood or lymph during active infection and replicate rapidly intracellularly until the cell is destroyed. Tachyzoites can be detected in blood, aspirates, and effusions in some dogs or cats with disseminated disease. *Bradyzoites* are the slowly dividing, persistent tissue stage that form in the extraintestinal tissues of infected hosts as immune responses attenuate tachyzoite replication. Bradyzoites form readily in the central nervous system (CNS), muscles, and visceral organs. *T. gondii* bradyzoites can be the source of reactivated acute infection (e.g., during immune suppression by feline immunodeficiency virus [FIV] or high-dose cyclosporine therapy), or they may be associated with some chronic disease manifestations (e.g., uveitis). Infection of warm-blooded vertebrates occurs after ingestion of any of these three life stages of the organism or transplacentally. In addition, it appears that cats can be infected lactationally, dogs can be infected by venereal contact, and repeated infections can occur in seropositive animals. Cats infected by ingesting *T. gondii* bradyzoites during carnivorous feeding shed oocysts in feces from 3 to 21 days. Fewer numbers of oocysts are shed for longer time periods if sporulated oocysts are ingested. Sporulated oocysts can survive in the environment for months to years and are resistant to most disinfectants. For dogs, cats, and humans it is believed that bradyzoites persist in tissues for the life of the host, regardless of whether drugs with presumed *T. gondii* activity are administered. Thus serum antibody titers are unlikely to decrease after treatment.

Clinical Features of Feline Infection

Approximately 10% to 20% of cats inoculated experimentally with *T. gondii* tissue cysts develop self-limiting small bowel diarrhea for 1 to 2 weeks; local replication of the organism during the intestinal phase of infection is presumed the cause. However, detection of *T. gondii* oocysts in feces rarely is reported in studies of client-owned cats with diarrhea, in part because of the short oocyst shedding period. Although *T. gondii* enteroepithelial stages were found in intestinal tissues from two cats with inflammatory bowel disease that responded to anti–*T. gondii* drugs, in the author's experience chronic gastrointestinal disease in cats from toxoplasmosis is uncommon.

Fatal toxoplasmosis can develop during acute dissemination and intracellular replication of tachyzoites; hepatic, pulmonary, CNS, and pancreatic tissues commonly are involved (Dubey et al, 2009). Transplacentally or lactationally infected kittens develop the most severe signs of extraintestinal toxoplasmosis and generally die of pulmonary or hepatic disease. Common clinical findings in cats with disseminated toxoplasmosis include depression, anorexia, fever followed by hypothermia, peritoneal effusion, icterus, and dyspnea. If a host with chronic toxoplasmosis is immunosuppressed, bradyzoites in tissue cysts can replicate rapidly and disseminate again as tachyzoites; this is common in humans with acquired immune deficiency syndrome (AIDS). Disseminated toxoplasmosis has been documented in cats concurrently infected with feline leukemia virus (FeLV), FIV, and feline infectious peritonitis virus. Commonly used clinical doses of glucocorticoids do not appear to predispose to activated toxoplasmosis. However, administration of cyclosporine to cats or dogs with renal transplantations or dermatologic disease has been associated with fatal disseminated toxoplasmosis (Barrs, Martin, and Beatty, 2006; Bernstein et al, 1999). Cats started on cyclosporine before exposure to *T. gondii* are most likely to develop significant illness, particularly if the trough blood level is higher than the normal range. Administration of cyclosporine at 7.5 mg/kg PO daily for 42 days failed to reactivate *T. gondii* in one experimental model performed by the author.

Chronic toxoplasmosis with vague and recurrent clinical signs of disease apparently occurs in some cats. *T. gondii* infection should be on the differential diagnoses list for cats with anterior or posterior uveitis, fever, muscle hyperesthesia, weight loss, anorexia, seizures, ataxia, icterus, diarrhea, or pancreatitis.

Based on results of *T. gondii*–specific aqueous humor antibody and polymerase chain reaction (PCR) studies, toxoplasmosis appears to be one of the most common infectious causes of uveitis in cats. It is unknown why the majority of cats infected with *T. gondii* are affected subclinically and other cats develop clinical signs of disease. Similar to what is reported in humans, kittens infected with *T. gondii* transplacentally or lactationally commonly develop ocular disease. Immune complex formation and deposition in tissues and delayed hypersensitivity reactions may be involved in chronic clinical toxoplasmosis. Because none of the anti-*Toxoplasma* drugs totally clear the body of the organism, recurrence of disease is common. This fact should be made clear to owners in discharge instructions, and the communication noted in the medical record.

Clinical Features of Canine Infection

Before 1988 many dogs diagnosed with toxoplasmosis based on histologic evaluation truly were infected with *Neospora caninum*. However, *T. gondii* infection frequently occurs in dogs and rarely can be associated with clinical disease. The most common syndromes associated with disseminated toxoplasmosis in dogs have involved the respiratory, gastrointestinal, or neuromuscular systems, resulting in fever, vomiting, diarrhea, dyspnea, and icterus. Disseminated toxoplasmosis is most common in immunosuppressed dogs, such as those with canine distemper virus infection or those receiving cyclosporine to prevent rejection of a renal transplant.

Neurologic signs depend on the location of the primary lesions and include ataxia, seizures, tremors, cranial nerve deficits, paresis, and paralysis. Dogs with myositis exhibit weakness, stiff gait, or muscle wasting. Rapid progression to tetraparesis and paralysis with lower motor neuron dysfunction can occur. Myocardial infection resulting in ventricular arrhythmias occurs in some infected dogs. Retinitis, anterior uveitis, iridocyclitis, nodular conjunctivitis, and optic neuritis occur in some dogs with toxoplasmosis but for unknown reasons seem to be less common than in the cat.

Clinical Diagnosis

Cats and dogs with clinical toxoplasmosis can have a variety of clinicopathologic and radiographic abnormalities, but none of the findings alone can be used to document the disease. Nonregenerative anemia, neutrophilic leukocytosis, lymphocytosis, monocytosis, neutropenia, eosinophilia, proteinuria, bilirubinuria, and increases in serum globulins and bilirubin concentration can be seen. In addition, increased activities of creatine kinase, alanine aminotransferase, alkaline phosphatase, and lipase occur in some affected animals. Pulmonary toxoplasmosis most commonly causes diffuse interstitial-to-patchy alveolar patterns or pleural effusion. Cerebrospinal fluid (CSF) protein concentrations and cell counts are often higher than normal; the predominant white blood cells in CSF are small mononuclear cells and neutrophils. The detection of these abnormalities should direct the clinician to perform additional, more specific *T. gondii* tests, particularly if in cases of a high likelihood of exposure to sporulated oocysts or uncooked meat or historical or other evidence of immunodeficiency.

The antemortem definitive diagnosis of toxoplasmosis can be made if the organism or its DNA is demonstrated; this is most likely to be achieved in cats or dogs with acute disseminated disease. Tachyzoites or bradyzoites have been detected in tissues, effusions, bronchoalveolar lavage fluids, aqueous humor, or CSF. Detection of *T. gondii* organisms is unlikely in cats or dogs with chronic disease manifestations. *T. gondii* DNA can be amplified from tissues and fluids; thus PCR detection is considered more sensitive and specific than cytologic or histopathologic detection of the organism. Multiple laboratories offer PCR assays that can amplify DNA of *T. gondii* and *N. caninum* (dogs); these assays should be considered if *T. gondii* or *N. caninum* is suspected but is not documented cytologically. Tissues, fluids, or aspirates for *T. gondii* PCR testing can be maintained frozen until assayed because the DNA is stable. *T. gondii* PCR assays seem to be less sensitive if performed on formalin-fixed samples; thus use of fresh tissue is preferred. Immunohistochemistry also can be performed on tissues to document the presence of *T. gondii* and to differentiate *T. gondii* from *N. caninum*.

Detection of 10×12 μm diameter oocysts in feces in cats with diarrhea suggests toxoplasmosis but is not definitive because *Besnoitia* and *Hammondia* spp. infections of cats produce morphologically similar oocysts. In these cases *T. gondii* serology should be performed, and, if the primary infection is *T. gondii*, seroconversion should be documented within 2 to 3 weeks. In dogs *N. caninum* oocysts are morphologically similar to *T. gondii* oocysts. These dogs can be screened for *N. caninum* and *T. gondii* antibodies in 2 to 3 weeks to determine the organism that was associated with the infection. Alternately, results of *T. gondii* and *N. caninum* PCR assays can be used to differentiate if a sample containing microbial DNA is available.

T. gondii antibodies can be detected in serum by a variety of different methods. Serum antibody assay results can be positive in healthy animals as well as those with clinical signs of toxoplasmosis; thus to make an antemortem diagnosis of clinical toxoplasmosis is impossible based on results of these tests alone. Of the serum tests, IgM titers correlate best with clinical toxoplasmosis because this antibody class is detected rarely in serum of healthy animals; thus many laboratories offer IgM and IgG test results separately. The antemortem diagnosis of clinical toxoplasmosis can be based tentatively on the combination of (1) clinical signs of disease referable to toxoplasmosis; (2) demonstration of antibodies in serum, which documents exposure to *T. gondii*; (3) demonstration of an IgM titer of more than 1:64 or a fourfold or greater increase in IgG titer, which suggests recent or active infection; (4) exclusion of other common causes of the clinical syndrome; and (5) positive response to appropriate treatment. In dogs neosporosis and toxoplasmosis appear clinically similar; thus the author frequently combines *T. gondii* and *N. caninum* serologic tests in his diagnostic workup of suspect patients.

T. gondii antigens or DNA can be detected in the blood of healthy or clinically ill cats and dogs; the source of the organism is likely bradyzoites from tissue cysts (Lee et al, 2008). The combination of *T. gondii*–specific antibody detection in aqueous humor or CSF and organism DNA amplification by PCR is the most accurate way to diagnose ocular or CNS toxoplasmosis in cats (Powell et al, 2010). CNS toxoplasmosis and neosporosis can appear clinically similar in dogs; thus the author frequently combines PCR testing for both organisms on CSF samples from dogs with inflammatory CNS disease.

Therapy

Supportive care should be instituted as needed. The author has used clindamycin hydrochloride administered at 10 to 12 mg/kg q 12h PO for 4 weeks or trimethoprim-sulfonamide combination administered at 15 mg/kg q12h PO for 4 weeks most frequently for the treatment of clinical feline or canine toxoplasmosis. These two drugs also can be used in combination. Trimethoprim sulfonamides are likely to penetrate an intact blood-brain barrier better than clindamycin and thus should be considered for CNS toxoplasmosis, particularly if the response to clindamycin is poor in the first 7 days of therapy. Azithromycin administered at 10.0 mg/kg q12h PO has been used successfully in a limited number of cats and dogs, but the optimal interval or duration of this expensive drug is unknown. Recently a case of azithromycin-resistant, clindamycin-responsive pulmonic toxoplasmosis in a dog was documented (Lappin MR, unpublished data). As with bacteria, different *T. gondii* isolates likely have different antimicrobial susceptibilities; thus, if the first drug attempted fails, an alternate drug should be attempted if the organism is still high on the differential list. Pyrimethamine combined with sulfa drugs is effective for the treatment of human toxoplasmosis but commonly results in toxicity in cats; thus the author never uses the drug for this purpose. Ponazuril has been used experimentally in *T. gondii*–infected rodents and there is evidence that ponazuril may be effective in kittens at a dose of 50 mg/kg once PO or 20 mg/kg per day × 2 days PO. More evidence for the use of this drug in cats is needed. However, ponazuril was administered at 20 mg/kg q24h PO for 28 days and was apparently successful in the treatment of a dog with suppurative keratitis and necrotizing conjunctivitis (Swinger et al, 2009).

Cats or dogs with systemic clinical signs of toxoplasmosis combined with uveitis should be treated with anti-*Toxoplasma* drugs in combination with topical, oral, or parenteral corticosteroids to avoid secondary glaucoma and lens luxations. Prednisolone acetate (1% solution) applied topically to the eye three to four times daily is generally sufficient. *T. gondii*–seropositive cats or dogs with uveitis that are otherwise normal can be treated with topical glucocorticoids alone unless uveitis is recurrent or persistent or if fever is present. Cases with concurrent systemic illness or recurrent uveitis should be administered a drug with anti-*T. gondii* activity.

Clinical signs not involving the eyes or the CNS usually begin to resolve within the first 2 to 3 days of clindamycin or trimethoprim-sulfonamide administration; ocular and CNS toxoplasmosis respond more slowly to therapy. If fever or muscle hyperesthesia is not lessening after 3 days of treatment, other causes should be considered, or an alternate anti-*Toxoplasma* drug prescribed. Recurrence of clinical signs may be more common in cats or dogs treated for less than 4 weeks. In cases of pulmonary toxoplasmosis, total resolution of radiographic abnormalities may not occur for several weeks. The prognosis is usually poor for cats or dogs with hepatic or pulmonary disease resulting from organism replication, particularly in those that are immunocompromised.

It currently is unknown whether benefit is gained from testing cats or dogs for *T. gondii* infection and treating the seropositive animals before administering cyclosporine therapy for other clinical diseases. If cyclosporine is to be used, it seems prudent to use the lowest dose possible to attempt to avoid exposure to *T. gondii* by restricting hunting activity and feeding processed foods and to measure blood concentrations to make sure the individual animal is not above the therapeutic range.

Zoonotic Aspects and Prevention

Primary infection of mothers with *T. gondii* during gestation can lead to clinical toxoplasmosis in the fetus; stillbirth, CNS disease, and ocular disease are common clinical manifestations. Primary infection in immunocompetent individuals results in self-limiting fever, malaise, and lymphadenopathy. As T-helper cell counts decline, approximately 10% of humans with AIDS develop toxoplasmic encephalitis from activation of bradyzoites in tissue cysts. *T. gondii* is known to alter behavior of prey species, which may benefit the organism by allowing the feline definitive host to ingest the parasite more easily and continue the life cycle. A number of papers suggest that chronic *T. gondii* infection of humans may result in a variety of CNS diseases, including behavior changes and schizophrenia (Arias et al, 2012). However, because *T. gondii* infection can be acquired in several ways, there is no reason to relinquish a personal cat for this concern.

Humans most commonly acquire toxoplasmosis by ingesting sporulated oocysts or tissue cysts or transplacentally. To prevent toxoplasmosis, humans should avoid eating undercooked meats or ingesting sporulated oocysts. Recently, *T. gondii* has been documented in free-ranging chickens and filter feeders such as oysters. Although owning a pet cat has been associated epidemiologically with acquiring toxoplasmosis in some studies, the majority of work suggests that touching individual cats is probably not a common way to acquire toxoplasmosis for the following reasons: (1) cats generally shed oocysts only for days to several weeks after primary inoculation; (2) repeat oocyst shedding is rare, even in cats receiving

BOX 277-1

Guidelines for Cat Owners to Avoid Acquiring Toxoplasmosis

- Wash hands after handling cats, especially if you are pregnant or immunocompromised.
- Remove fecal material from the home environment daily.
- If possible, do not have immunocompromised humans clean the litter box. If immunocompromised humans must clean the litter box, they should wear gloves and wash hands thoroughly when finished.
- Use litter box liners and periodically clean the litter box with scalding water and detergent.
- Wear gloves when gardening and wash hands thoroughly when finished.
- Cover children's sandboxes when not in use to lessen fecal contamination by outdoor cats.
- Feed cats only cooked or commercially processed food.
- Control potential transport hosts such as flies and cockroaches that may bring the organism into the home.
- Filter or boil water from sources in the environment.
- Housing cats indoors may lessen their exposure.
- Cook meat for human consumption to 80°C (176°F) for 15 minutes minimum (medium well).
- Wear gloves when handling meat and wash hands thoroughly with soap and water when finished.

glucocorticoids or cyclosporine or in those infected with FIV or FeLV; (3) cats with toxoplasmosis inoculated with tissue cysts 16 months after primary inoculation did not shed oocysts; (4) cats are fastidious and usually do not allow feces to remain on their skin for time periods long enough to lead to oocyst sporulation (the organism was not isolated from the fur of cats shedding millions of oocysts 7 days previously); (5) increased risk of acquired toxoplasmosis was not associated with cat ownership in studies of veterinary health care providers or humans with AIDS. However, because some cats repeat oocyst shedding when exposed a second time, feces always should be handled carefully. The feces should be collected daily until the oocyst shedding period is complete; administration of clindamycin (25 to 50 mg/kg divided q12h PO) or sulfonamides (100 mg/kg divided q12h PO) can reduce levels of oocyst shedding.

Because humans are not infected commonly with *T. gondii* from contact with individual cats, testing healthy cats for toxoplasmosis is not recommended (Kaplan et al, 2009). Fecal examination is an adequate procedure to determine when cats are shedding oocysts actively but cannot predict when a cat has shed oocysts in the past. No serologic assay accurately predicts when a cat shed *T. gondii* oocysts in the past, and most cats shedding oocysts are seronegative. Most seropositive cats have completed the oocyst shedding period and are unlikely to repeat shedding; most seronegative cats would shed the organism if infected. If owners are concerned that they may have acquired toxoplasmosis, they should seek medical evaluation. Common sense practices also should be followed (Box 277-1).

References and Suggested Reading

Arias I et al: Infectious agents associated with schizophrenia: a meta-analysis, *Schizophr Res* 136:128, 2012.

Barrs VR, Martin P, Beatty JA: Antemortem diagnosis and treatment of toxoplasmosis in two cats on cyclosporine therapy, *Aust Vet J* 84:30, 2006.

Bernstein L et al: Acute toxoplasmosis following renal transplantation in three cats and a dog, *J Am Vet Med Assoc* 215:1123, 1999.

Brown RR et al: Feline zoonoses guidelines from the American Association of Feline Practitioners, *Compend Contin Educ Pract Vet* 25:936, 2003.

Dabritz HA, Conrad PA: Cats and *Toxoplasma*: implications for public health, *Zoonoses Public Health* 57:34, 2010.

Dubey JP et al: Toxoplasmosis and other intestinal coccidial infections in cats and dogs, *Vet Clin North Am Small Anim Pract* 39:1009, 2009.

Holt N et al: Seroprevalence of various infectious agents in dogs with suspected acute canine polyradiculoneuritis, *J Vet Intern Med* 25:261, 2011.

Kaplan JE et al: Guidelines for prevention and treatment of opportunistic infections in HIV-infected adults and adolescents. Recommendations from CDC, the National Institutes of Health, and the HIV Medicine Association of the Infectious Diseases Society of America, *MMWR Recomm Rep* 58(RR04):1, 2009.

Langoni H et al: Detection and molecular analysis of *Toxoplasma gondii* and *Neospora caninum* from dogs with neurological disorders, *Rev Soc Bras Med Trop* 45:365, 2012.

Lappin MR: Update on the diagnosis and management of *Toxoplasma gondii* infection in cats, *Top Companion Anim Med* 25:136, 2010.

Lee JY et al: Nested PCR-based detection of *Toxoplasma gondii* in German shepherd dogs and stray cats in South Korea, *Res Vet Sci* 85:125, 2008.

Malmasi A et al: Prevention of shedding and re-shedding of *Toxoplasma gondii* oocysts in experimentally infected cats treated with oral clindamycin: a preliminary study, *Zoonoses Public Health* 56:102, 2009.

Mitchell SM et al: Prevention of recrudescent toxoplasmic encephalitis using ponazuril in an immunodeficient mouse model, *J Eukaryot Microbiol* 53:S164, 2006.

Powell CC et al: *Bartonella* species, feline herpesvirus-1, and *Toxoplasma gondii* PCR assay results from blood and aqueous humor samples from 104 cats with naturally occurring endogenous uveitis, *J Feline Med Surg* 12;923, 2010.

Swinger RL et al: Keratoconjunctivitis associated with *Toxoplasma gondii* in a dog , *Vet Ophthalmol* 12:56, 2009.

Vollaire MR, Radecki SV, Lappin MR: Seroprevalence of *Toxoplasma gondii* antibodies in clinically ill cats of the United States, *Am J Vet Res* 66:874, 2005.

CHAPTER 278

Rational Use of Glucocorticoids in Infectious Disease

ADAM MORDECAI, *Buffalo Grove, Illinois*
RANCE K. SELLON, *Pullman, Washington*

Evidence supporting the use of glucocorticoids for treatment of infections in small animal patients is based on anecdotal or retrospective reports. Few prospective controlled studies have evaluated critically the benefits or consequences of glucocorticoid use in this setting. Despite the fact that little scientific evidence supports their use, glucocorticoids frequently are suggested for patients with infectious disease. Frequently cited reasons for administration of glucocorticoids in treating infectious disease include suppression of harmful inflammatory or immune responses and suppression of presumed secondary immune-mediated processes. The aim of this chapter is to review the use of glucocorticoids in infectious disease situations and to offer guidelines for their use. This chapter does not address specifically the use of glucocorticoids, either topical or systemic, in patients with ocular infections or ocular manifestations of infectious disease, although they are used frequently.

Mechanism of Action

The mechanisms by which glucocorticoids mediate antiinflammatory activity are not understood completely. Glucocorticoids diffuse across the plasma membrane and bind to specific glucocorticoid receptors in the cytoplasm. The steroid-receptor complex then exerts a variety of effects. The complex can inactivate proinflammatory transcription factors and increase the production of proteins that inhibit cytokine production. Glucocorticoids also can mediate their actions through nontranscriptional means such as decreasing the half-life of messenger ribonucleic acid for inflammatory cytokines. Glucocorticoids attenuate inflammation by inducing lipocortin-1, which directly inhibits phospholipase A_2, an enzyme responsible for production of inflammatory prostaglandins, leukotrienes, and eicosanoids. Through these and other mechanisms, inflammation and immune function can be altered or suppressed by glucocorticoids.

Even at physiologic concentrations, glucocorticoids are immunomodulatory, leading to a shift in cytokine production from a proinflammatory to an antiinflammatory pattern. Pharmacologic doses are immunosuppressive and inhibit cellular and humoral responses (Sternberg, 2001); however, the cellular response is thought to be most compromised. Poor cellular immune responses could enhance the pathogenic potential of some infectious organisms, prevent cell-mediated clearance of organisms, and perpetuate inflammation secondary to persistence of organisms and activation of other inflammatory pathways. Glucocorticoids commonly are thought to decrease phagocytic and oxidative functions of phagocytic cells in a dose-dependent manner, thereby compromising the ability to kill ingested organisms. These general properties support the use of glucocorticoids in patients with infectious disease and raise concerns about the potential side effects and complications associated with their use.

Glucocorticoids in Humans with Infectious Disease

A survey of the human literature on the use of glucocorticoids as adjunctive treatment for infectious disease puts into perspective many of the uncertainties in veterinary medicine. Conclusions regarding the benefits of glucocorticoids given to humans with infectious disease vary depending on the infectious agent studied, the age of the patient group studied, the dose and/or duration of glucocorticoid therapy, the parameters assessed (e.g., immunologic or infectious agent parameters such as cytokine levels or quantity of infectious agent detected), the presence of other infectious agents, and by extension, perhaps, of other concurrent diseases. Many human studies either involve small numbers of patients or lack appropriate controls. One helpful review (McGee and Hirschmann, 2008) of published randomized, double-blinded studies comparing corticosteroids with placebo in the treatment of human infectious diseases categorized the role of glucocorticoids as either improving survival with some infections (e.g., bacterial meningitis, pneumocystis pneumonia), reducing long-term disability (e.g., bacterial arthritis), improving symptoms (herpes zoster, many others), providing no or uncertain benefit, or causing harm (viral hepatitis, cerebral malaria). The range of outcomes described in people indicates that no "one size fits all" approach is appropriate for the use of glucocorticoids in small animals with infectious diseases and suggests that blanket avoidance of glucocorticoids in patients with infectious disease is not clinically appropriate.

Glucocorticoids in Small Animals with Infectious Disease

Respiratory Infections

Clinicians have proposed that antiinflammatory doses of glucocorticoids for 5 to 7 days may be effective in ameliorating cough associated with uncomplicated infectious tracheobronchitis but do not shorten significantly the clinical course of disease. It is recognized commonly that after initial administration of antifungal agents to patients with fungal pneumonia (i.e., blastomycosis and histoplasmosis) respiratory signs can worsen presumably as a consequence of heightened inflammation associated with fungal death. Glucocorticoids are thought to prevent treatment-induced inflammation from occurring. In people who develop hypoxemia or respiratory distress after initiation of antifungal therapy for histoplasmosis, or who develop other inflammatory complications of the infection, treatment with glucocorticoids is recommended (Wheat et al, 2007). However, the evidence to support this recommendation is primarily physician experience and isolated reports instead of prospective, controlled clinical studies. A preliminary report of dogs with severe respiratory blastomycosis treated with either nonsteroidal antiinflammatory drugs (NSAIDs) or glucocorticoids, in addition to antifungal therapy, found no difference in clinical outcomes between the two treatment groups (Munks et al, 2011). A group of dogs treated with only antifungal drugs was not described, so it is difficult to know if antiinflammatory therapy had a positive impact on the clinical course of affected dogs. In a retrospective study of chronic histoplasmosis in dogs (Schulman, McKiernan, and Schaeffer, 1999), clinical signs of coughing from airway obstruction associated with hilar lymphadenomegaly resolved more quickly with administration of immunosuppressive dosages (2 to 4 mg/kg q24h) of prednisone alone or prednisone and antifungal drugs compared with those in dogs treated with antifungal chemotherapy alone (less than 3 weeks compared with approximately 9 weeks). In this study the glucocorticoid-treated dogs did not show evidence of dissemination of disease.

Central Nervous System Infections

In central nervous system (CNS) infections, inflammatory mediators and toxic factors produced by the immune system may be more responsible for CNS damage than the primary pathogen. Treatment of bacterial organisms can result in lysis and release of inflammatory cell wall components, including lipopolysaccharides and outer membrane vesicles. No controlled studies address the use of glucocorticoids in dogs or cats with infectious meningitis. However, anecdotal experience, case reports, and the human literature suggest a potential benefit, but not all human studies ascribe advantages in reduction of mortality and neurologic sequelae to glucocorticoid therapy.

At the authors' institution patients suspected to have CNS infection based on cerebral spinal fluid (CSF) pleocytosis, elevated CSF protein content, and/or consistent magnetic resonance imaging findings are treated with a broad-spectrum antimicrobial and antiinflammatory protocol (trimethoprim-sulfonamide 15 mg/kg q12h PO; clindamycin 12.5 mg/kg q12h PO; prednisone 0.5 mg/kg q12h PO) while awaiting more definitive results, including bacterial culture and titers or polymerase chain reaction results for viral and protozoal organisms. Diagnostic testing always should be performed before any treatment because it may affect CSF analysis and culture results. In addition, glucocorticoids may attenuate the increased blood-brain barrier permeability that results from inflammation, thereby theoretically reducing antimicrobial penetration into the CSF. Clinical studies in small animals with bacterial meningitis that address antibiotic penetration in the face of glucocorticoids are lacking, and long-term consequences of glucocorticoid therapy for infectious meningitis have not been established.

Disseminated and Miscellaneous Infections

Glucocorticoids are used frequently in conjunction with antimicrobials for hemolytic anemia or thrombocytopenia while awaiting results to differentiate a primary immune-mediated hemolytic process from hemolytic disease secondary to an infectious organism such as *Babesia* spp., the hemoplasmas, or rickettsial agents. Immune-mediated destruction may contribute to anemia or thrombocytopenia with these infections, and the addition of glucocorticoids has the potential to decrease immunologically mediated cell destruction. However, no controlled studies demonstrate proof of efficacy. In one study, dogs with experimentally induced *Rickettsia rickettsii* (Rocky Mountain spotted fever, RMSF) infection and treated with doxycycline and immunosuppressive doses of glucocorticoids did not have more severe clinical disease compared with dogs treated with doxycycline alone (Breitschwerdt et al, 1997). Although no adverse clinical effects were observed in these experimentally infected dogs, the authors were careful to state that their results were not an endorsement of routine glucocorticoid use in dogs with RMSF. Instead, they supported the notion that short courses of immunosuppressive doses of glucocorticoids are unlikely to harm an *R. rickettsii*–infected dog when clinical circumstances dictate a need to initiate antibiotics and glucocorticoids before a definitive diagnosis of RMSF is established. Treatment of other systemic infections with glucocorticoids, including the hemotropic *Mycoplasma* spp. of dogs and cats (hemoplasmas) or *Babesia* spp. in dogs has no support in controlled clinical studies, although glucocorticoids are used commonly in the treatment of patients infected with these organisms.

Of the many canine and feline infectious diseases, treatment of cats with feline infectious peritonitis (FIP) with glucocorticoids would be a logical application of the drugs, given the key role that immunopathology plays in the clinical disease. Glucocorticoids often are recommended for FIP despite an absence of any controlled clinical studies demonstrating benefits of such therapy (see Chapter 279). One study has suggested the benefit of concurrent use of recombinant feline interferon and glucocorticoid administration to cats with FIP, but the report included no controls, and the diagnosis of FIP was not confirmed in all cases (Ishida et al, 2004).

TABLE **278-1**

Glucocorticoid Dosing Recommendations (mg/kg/day) with Relative Glucocorticoid Potency of Formulations

Glucocorticoid	Physiologic Replacement	Antiinflammatory	Immune Suppression	Potency Relative to Hydrocortisone
Hydrocortisone	0.5 to 1.0	2.5 to 5	Not used	1
Prednisone	0.1 to 0.2	0.5 to 1	2 to 4 (dog); 4 to 8 (cat)	5
Dexamethasone	0.02 to 0.04	0.1 to 0.2	0.4 to 0.8	25

Juvenile cellulitis (puppy strangles) is a syndrome of facial swelling, lymphadenopathy, deep pyoderma of the head and face, fever, polyarthritis, anorexia, and depression. The disease is seen most often in young dogs and is attributed to immune-mediated responses to bacterial antigens. Affected patients usually respond to antimicrobials and immunosuppressive doses of glucocorticoids, and available literature provides reasonable (although not case-controlled) evidence for the use of immunosuppressive doses of glucocorticoids in the management of this disease. The disease may recur if corticosteroid therapy is tapered too quickly; thus a slower tapering protocol may be required.

Sepsis/Systemic Inflammatory Response Syndrome, Acute Respiratory Distress Syndrome, and Relative Adrenal Insufficiency

Systemic inflammatory response syndrome (SIRS) is a term used to describe the clinical consequences of severe systemic inflammation. Severe systemic inflammation can result in secondary conditions such as disseminated intravascular coagulopathy, acute respiratory distress syndrome (ARDS), and multiple organ dysfunction syndrome. Dysregulated systemic inflammation is a major contributor to the morbidity and mortality in sepsis and ARDS. Relative adrenal insufficiency (RAI) is defined as a usually transient lack of response to endogenous or exogenous adrenocorticotropic hormone (ACTH) and occurs in patients with widespread systemic inflammation (see Chapters 16 and 41). Suspicion of RAI often is based on poor systemic pressures despite appropriate hydration (central venous pressures ranging between 5 and 10 cm of water) and vasopressor (dobutamine, norepinephrine) dependency. RAI occurs with relative frequency in human septic SIRS patients and has been described recently in septic dogs (Burkitt et al, 2007). Human studies have demonstrated that a short course of glucocorticoids at physiologic doses improves clinical outcomes in patients with sepsis. Future studies likely will show similar benefits for dogs with sepsis and RAI.

Considerations for Glucocorticoid Use

Prednisone and prednisolone are ideal glucocorticoids for use in patients with infectious disease because of their short duration of activity (12 to 36 hours). Prednisolone sodium succinate (Solu-Delta-Cortef) or methylprednisolone sodium succinate (Solu-Medrol) are parenteral formulations that may be used if patients are unable to take oral formulations. Dexamethasone would be an additional alternative for these patients, but its activity is approximately 48 hours, making it perhaps a less ideal first choice. Given its long storage life and because it is relatively inexpensive compared with other glucocorticoids, practitioners may elect to use dexamethasone. Depot formulations such as methylprednisolone acetate (Depo-Medrol) are not recommended because of their long duration of activity.

Dosage

Systematic evaluation of glucocorticoid dosages in small animal infectious disease patients has not been performed. Typical therapeutic ranges (Table 278-1) to achieve either antiinflammatory or immunosuppressive effects have been suggested. Ideally therapy with glucocorticoids should be initiated at the lowest doses needed to obtain the desired clinical response. Clinicians should be aware of the relative potencies of the commonly used glucocorticoids (see Table 278-1) when selecting a glucocorticoid and dose.

Duration of Glucocorticoid Treatment

If the correct underlying cause has been identified and antiinfective treatment is effective, clinical improvement usually occurs within days. The authors recommend that concurrent glucocorticoid therapy should last only as long as needed to achieve and maintain the desired clinical response: in some patients that period may be days, in others weeks. The decision to stop glucocorticoid therapy depends on the patient's clinical status, clinician preference, and potential for clinical relapse or deterioration.

Common belief holds that glucocorticoid tapering is needed to prevent signs of iatrogenic hypoadrenocorticism. The authors believe that tapering is suited better to identify early relapse or recurrence of the syndrome requiring glucocorticoid therapy. If the need arises to acutely stop glucocorticoids, theoretically a clinician should be able to reduce immediately the amount to a physiologic dose given daily or every other day and prevent clinical signs associated with iatrogenic hypoadrenocorticism. The authors' argument is based on the fact that dogs with glucocorticoid deficiency from spontaneous hypoadrenocorticism fare well with prednisone given at physiologic or slightly higher doses (0.1 to 0.2 mg/kg/day). If the reduction in dose is well tolerated, a brief period of alternate-day therapy should allow return of normal adrenal function. The time period for return of normal adrenal function depends on many variables, including dose, formulation, duration of therapy, and variation in patient response preventing any absolute recommendations. In general, longer durations of therapy with higher doses or use of formulations with greater duration of activity may require a longer period of alternate day, or alternate day followed by every third day therapy, for return of normal adrenal function. Periodic testing in the form of drug cessation trials or ACTH stimulation may be required if iatrogenic hypoadrenocorticism is suspected. A period of dose reduction of glucocorticoids also should be considered when treating patients concurrently with glucocorticoids and ketoconazole for systemic fungal infections because ketoconazole impairs adrenal glucocorticoid synthesis and could lead to transient iatrogenic hypoadrenocorticism.

Adverse Effects of Glucocorticoids with Infectious Disease

Apart from the usual side effects of glucocorticoids, virtually no information is available regarding small animal patients that addresses adverse effects of glucocorticoids when given concurrently with antiinfective therapy for a specific infection. The potential for immunosuppression and exacerbation of existing infection or development of additional infections is a valid concern, yet it seldom seems to be recognized clinically. Perhaps it is more important that the clinician not be lulled into a false sense of security regarding apparent positive responses in patients with infections also treated with glucocorticoids. A patient could improve initially because of antiinflammatory properties and yet worsen with time because of decreased immunologic clearance of infectious organisms and progressive infection, particularly if antiinfective therapy is ineffective. Theoretically, supraphysiologic doses of glucocorticoids could inhibit the inflammation necessary for wound repair and could retard healing. When adverse effects are suspected secondary to immunosuppression (worsening of disease), rapid reduction of glucocorticoid doses as suggested previously may be required.

The causative agents of some infections such as endocarditis may be hard to confirm despite appropriate testing (i.e., blood cultures, urine cultures). Treatment with glucocorticoids may increase the chance of recovery of organisms such as *Bartonella* spp. (Dr. Ed Breitschwerdt, personal communication), but glucocorticoids are not advised for that specific intent.

Guidelines for Use of Glucocorticoids with Infections

The authors believe that some patients with infections benefit from treatment with antiinflammatory or occasionally higher doses of glucocorticoids. The authors suspect that this view is held by many other clinicians despite the absence of rigorous evaluation of glucocorticoid use in small animal infections. When using glucocorticoids in patients with infectious disease, whenever possible the authors try to adhere to the following guidelines:

- Diagnostic studies to identify the specific cause of infection should be completed before the administration of glucocorticoids.
- Glucocorticoid treatment should be implemented after or at the same time as antiinfective therapy.
- The decision to administer glucocorticoids to patients with an infection should be made on a case-by-case basis that weighs the patient's clinical status and relative benefits against the potential risks of complications and adverse effects.
- Glucocorticoid administration should not form a blanket approach to treatment of a given infectious agent.
- Doses of glucocorticoids should be appropriate for the goal of therapy (e.g., antiinflammatory, immunosuppressive, or physiologic replacement for patients with RAI).
- Administration of glucocorticoids with short or intermediate duration of activity (e.g., prednisone) is preferred to glucocorticoids with longer durations of antiinflammatory or immunosuppressive activity; depot forms of glucocorticoids are not advised.
- Glucocorticoids should be administered at the lowest dosages and for no longer than needed to achieve and maintain desired clinical responses.
- Patients treated with glucocorticoids should be assessed regularly and carefully for complications of therapy, particularly progressive infection. Because glucocorticoid administration can attenuate the very patient responses that alert clinicians to the existence of problems (e.g., fever, pain) that could otherwise suggest clinical deterioration in patients not receiving glucocorticoids, enhanced attention is warranted.
- In some patients receiving glucocorticoids concurrently with antiinfective therapy (e.g., those with systemic fungal infections), the duration of the antiinfective treatment period may have to be extended.
- Owners should be advised of the potential risks associated with a treatment approach (glucocorticoids for infection) that lacks support of appropriately performed clinical studies.

In summary, evidence in human medicine supports the administration of glucocorticoids to improve outcomes in some patients with infectious disease. Because the evidence in veterinary medicine is primarily anecdotal, definitive studies (randomized, blinded and placebo-controlled) that examine the benefits or complications of glucocorticoid use in veterinary patients with infections are needed to better characterize the indications and contraindications to the administration of these drugs. Until such studies are available, glucocorticoids should not be avoided absolutely in dogs or cats with infectious diseases but should be used judiciously on a case-by-case basis and with appropriate attention to the patient.

References and Suggested Reading

Breitschwerdt EB et al: Prednisolone at anti-inflammatory or immunosuppressive dosages in conjunction with doxycycline does not potentiate the severity of *Rickettsia rickettsii* infection in dogs, *Antimicrob Agents Chemother* 41:141, 1997.

Burkitt JM et al: Relative adrenal insufficiency in dogs with sepsis, *J Vet Intern Med* 21:226, 2007.

Ishida T et al: Use of recombinant feline interferon and glucocorticoid in the treatment of feline infectious peritonitis, *J Feline Med Surg* 6:107, 2004.

McGee S, Hirschmann J: Use of corticosteroids in treating infectious diseases, *Arch Intern Med* 168:1034, 2008.

Minneci PC et al: Meta-analysis: the effect of steroids on survival and shock during sepsis depends on the dose, *Ann Intern Med* 141:47, 2004.

Munks MJ et al: The use of anti-inflammatory therapy as adjunctive treatment in dogs with blastomycosis (abstract ID-1), *J Vet Intern Med* 25:705, 2011.

Schulman RL, McKiernan BC, Schaeffer DJ: Use of corticosteroids for treating dogs with airway obstruction secondary to hilar lymphadenopathy caused by chronic histoplasmosis: 16 cases, (1979-1997), *J Am Vet Med Assoc* 214:1345, 1999.

Simmons CP et al: The clinical benefit of adjunctive dexamethasone in tuberculous meningitis is not associated with measurable attenuation of peripheral or local immune responses, *J Immunol* 175:579, 2005.

Sternberg EM: Neuroendocrine regulation of autoimmune/inflammatory disease, *J Endocrinol* 169:429, 2001.

Wheat JL et al: Clinical practice guidelines for the management of patients with histoplasmosis: 2007 update by the Infectious Diseases Society of America, *Clin Infect Dis* 45:807, 2007.

White SD et al: Juvenile cellulitis in dogs: 15 cases (1979-1988), *J Am Vet Med Assoc* 195:1609, 1989.

CHAPTER 279

Feline Infectious Peritonitis Virus Infections

MICHAEL R. LAPPIN, *Fort Collins, Colorado*

Coronaviruses causing disease in cats include feline infectious peritonitis virus (FIPV) and feline enteric coronavirus (FECV). Enteric infection generally results in mild gastrointestinal signs; systemic infection can induce a clinical syndrome with diverse manifestations commonly referred to as feline infectious peritonitis (FIP) (Pedersen, 2009). FIP-inducing strains may arise from enteric strains by mutation (called the "*in vivo* mutation transition hypothesis"), or distinctive benign and pathogenic strains may circulate in a population with the pathogenic strains inducing disease in exposed cats with the appropriate predisposition (called the "circulating virulent-avirulent FCoV hypothesis") (O'Brien et al, 2012).

The effusive form of disease generally is believed to develop in cats with poor cell-mediated immune responses, and the noneffusive form develops in cats with partial cell-mediated immunity. The effusive form of disease is an immune complex vasculitis characterized by leakage of protein-rich fluid into the pleural space, the peritoneal cavity, the pericardial space, and the subcapsular space of the kidneys. In the noneffusive form pyogranulomatous or granulomatous lesions develop in multiple tissues, particularly the eyes, brain, kidneys, omentum, and liver. Some affected cats have characteristics of both forms of FIP.

Clinical Features

Enteric Coronavirus

Enteric replication of coronaviruses may result in fever, vomiting, and mucoid diarrhea in some kittens. However, most kittens have subclinical infections. Unfortunately, making an antemortem diagnosis of enteric coronavirus-associated illness is impossible with currently available assays. For example, a recent study failed to show an association between fecal scores and the presence of coronavirus RNA in feces (Gingrich et al, 2010).

Feline Infectious Peritonitis

Fulminant effusive FIP can occur in cats of any age but generally is recognized in cats younger than 5 years; most cases are younger than 1 year. Anorexia, weight loss, and general malaise are common presenting complaints.

Icterus, ocular inflammation, abdominal distention, dyspnea, or CNS abnormalities occasionally are noted by the owner. In cats with effusive disease, abdominal distention is common and a fluid wave often can be balloted. Pleural effusion can result in dyspnea and a restrictive breathing pattern (shallow and rapid) as well as muffled heart and lung sounds. Male cats sometimes have scrotal enlargement from fluid accumulation.

Fever and weight loss are common with the effusive and noneffusive forms of the disease. Pale mucous membranes or petechiae are noted in some cats. FIP is one of the most common causes of icterus in cats younger than 2 years; liver size can be normal or enlarged, and the margins are usually irregular. Occasionally masses (pyogranulomas or lymphadenopathy) can be palpated in the omentum, mesentery, or intestines. A solitary ileocecocolic or colonic mass, resulting in obstruction leading to vomiting and diarrhea, occurs in some cats. Kidneys can be small (chronic disease) or large (acute disease or subcapsular effusion); renal margins are usually irregular. Anterior uveitis and chorioretinitis occur most frequently with the noneffusive form of the disease and can be its only manifestation. Pyogranulomatous disease can develop anywhere in the CNS, leading to a variety of neurologic signs that include seizures, posterior paresis, and nystagmus. Seizures secondary to FIP are a poor prognostic indicator (Timmann et al, 2008).

Diagnosis

Enteric Coronavirus

As discussed, no assay is available to determine whether enteric coronaviruses are associated with diarrhea in cats. Cats with coronavirus RNA in feces should be evaluated for other causes of diarrhea.

Feline Infectious Peritonitis

Diagnostic tests for diagnosis of FIP have been reviewed (Giori et al, 2011; Hartmann et al, 2003). Cats with effusion disease are usually easy to confirm because the fluid is fairly characteristic. The fluid is sterile, appears colorless to straw colored, may contain fibrin strands, and may clot when exposed to air. The protein concentration on fluid analysis commonly ranges from 3.5 g/dl to 12 g/dl and is generally higher than that associated with other diseases. Mixed inflammatory cell populations of lymphocytes, macrophages, and neutrophils occur most commonly; neutrophils predominate in most cases, but in some cats macrophages are the primary cell type seen. In some cats the coronavirus antibody titers are greater in the effusion than in serum. Measurement of protein concentrations in effusions and calculation of the albumin/globulin ratio can aid in the diagnosis of effusive FIP. In one study an albumin/globulin ratio of 0.5 had a positive predictive value of 89%, and an albumin/globulin ratio of 1.0 had a negative predictive value of 91% (Hartmann et al, 2003). Coronavirus antigens commonly are detected by direct immunofluorescence in the effusions of cats with FIP but not in the effusions of cats with other diseases. In addition, viral RNA can be amplified detected by reverse transcriptase polymerase chain reaction (RT-PCR) in effusions and is unlikely to be in effusions from other causes.

Multiple hematologic, serum biochemical, urinalysis, diagnostic imaging, and CSF abnormalities develop in cats with noneffusive FIP. Several authors have assessed the predictive values of individual and combinations of tests (Giori et al, 2011; Hartmann et al, 2003). Other than histopathology, the positive predictive values of tests used to aid in the diagnosis of FIP are less than 100%, including the amplification of mRNA from blood. A presumptive diagnosis of noneffusive FIP usually is based on the combination of clinical and clinicopathologic findings and excluding other causes of the presenting clinical syndromes. Definitive diagnosis can be made by documenting appropriate histopathologic findings and coronavirus in tissues with immunohistochemistry.

Treatment

Because an antemortem diagnosis of FIP is difficult to make, assessment of studies reporting successful treatment is virtually impossible. A small percentage of cats have spontaneous remission, adding to the confusion concerning therapeutic response. Focal masses associated with FIP pyogranulomas associated with intestinal obstruction should be removed surgically. A number of protocols with at least some theoretic or proven clinical value that have been used in cats with effusive and noneffusive FIP are presented in the following sections and in Table 270-1 (Addie et al, 2009; Hartmann and Ritz, 2008).

Enteric Coronavirus

Supportive care is indicated for kittens with nonspecific diarrhea that may be related to enteric coronavirus. Lessening stress by increasing enrichment, feeding a controlled amount of a high-quality diet, and treating other concurrent diseases such as gastrointestinal parasites is likely to be beneficial for treatment of cats with enteric coronavirus and diarrhea. In one study, administration of the probiotic *Enterococcus faecium* (FortiFlora) to shelter cats greatly reduced the prevalence rate of nonspecific diarrhea present for 2 days or longer (Bybee, Scorza, and Lappin, 2011).

Feline Infectious Peritonitis

Supportive care, including correction of electrolyte and fluid balance abnormalities, should be provided to all cats with effusive or noneffusive FIP as needed. Lessening stress, improving enrichment, and treating concurrent disease syndromes as discussed for enteric coronavirus infections also are indicated.

Optimal treatment of FIP theoretically includes drugs to inhibit FIPV. *In vitro* inhibition of FIPV replication has been demonstrated with a number of drugs, including ribavirin, human interferon-α, feline interferon-omega, adenine arabinoside, amphotericin B, and cyclosporine (CsA). CsA inhibits replication of feline coronaviruses *in vitro*, but it is currently unknown whether this drug could be used as a treatment of FIP (Tanaka et al, 2012). The potent T lymphocyte inhibitory properties of CsA also could lead potentially to worsening of FIP. One potential future FIP treatment modality is the use of small interfering RNA (siRNA). siRNA can be synthesized to target different regions of the coronavirus genome to inhibit viral replication in vitro (McDonagh, Sheehy, and Norris, 2011). To date no uniformly successful antiviral treatment has been developed, and the drugs typically have potentially serious adverse effects and therefore are not recommended. High doses of human interferon-α or feline interferon-omega are likely to have anti-FIPV effects and have been attempted in the treatment of some cats with FIP given variable responses (Table 279-1).

Clinical manifestations of FIP are generally secondary to immune-mediated reactions against the virus. Thus modulation of the inflammatory reaction is the principal form of palliative therapy. Drugs used most frequently for this purpose include aspirin, prednisolone, dexamethasone, and chlorambucil (see Table 279-1). Some clinicians have administered glucocorticoids into the thoracic or peritoneal cavities as an attempt to lessen local inflammation. Administration of glucocorticoids may lessen clinical signs associated with ocular or CNS inflammation. However, optimal protocols have not been developed. Low-dose human interferon-α administered orally is believed to regulate cytokine cascades and has improved clinical abnormalities in cats with FIV (Pedretti et al, 2006). However, if immune stimulation also occurs, immune-mediated manifestations of FIP could be exacerbated (see Table 279-1).

The use of prednisolone and feline interferon-omega recently has been promoted for the treatment of effusive and noneffusive FIP (Ishida et al, 2004). In that study, four cats with effusive disease believed to be from FIP virus had prolonged remission. However, the results should be viewed cautiously because the cases were atypical (older cats), the diagnosis of FIP was not confirmed, no control group was used and, if a treatment response occurred, whether it was from the prednisolone or interferon-omega was impossible to determine because both drugs were

TABLE **279-1**

Drug Protocols Attempted for the Treatment of Feline Infectious Peritonitis

Drug/Compound	Likely Mechanism	Protocol	Comments
Chlorambucil	Immune suppression	1 to 2 mg/cat 3 times per week PO	Used in concert with glucocorticoids for noneffusive FIP; controlled studies are lacking
Dexamethasone	Antiinflammatory	1 mg/kg, intrathoracic or intraperitoneal	Used in some cats with effusive FIP; controlled studies are lacking
Feline interferon-omega	Antiviral?	*Effusive:* 1 million units/kg q48h SC, reducing to once weekly if remission occurs *Noneffusive:* 50,000 units per cat q24h PO until globulins, hematocrit, lymphocyte count, and clinical signs return to normal	Controlled studies are lacking; reported responses are variable
Human interferon-alpha: PO low dose	Immune modulation	50 U/cat q24h PO, indefinitely	If immune stimulation occurs, FIP associated disease could be worsened
Human interferon-alpha: high dose	Antiviral?	10,000 U/kg, q24h SC, optimal duration unknown	One clinical trial showed no effect on cats with FIP
Ozagrel hydrochloride	Thromboxane synthesis inhibitor aimed at treating the inflammatory response	5 to 10 mg/kg q12h PO, variable duration	Used in two cases with potential beneficial effect but was combined with prednisolone
Pentoxifylline	Decreases vasculitis?	10 to 15 mg/kg q12h PO, optimal duration unknown, or approximately one-quarter tablet (100 mg) per cat q12h PO	Some veterinarians in practice have tried this treatment, but there are no published studies or case reports for FIP in cats
Prednisolone	Antiinflammatory	1-2 mg/kg per day initially (may be divided into q12h), and taper to 0.5-1.0 mg/kg q48h PO	Although used as the preferred antiinflammatory drug in both effusive and noneffusive FIP, controlled studies are lacking
Salicylic acid (aspirin)	Antiinflammatory	5 mg/kg q24h PO	Controlled studies lacking; avoid use with high doses of glucocorticoids

FIP, Feline infectious peritonitis.

administered to all cats. In another study, administration of interferon-omega was ineffective for the treatment of FIP (Ritz, Egberink, and Hartmann, 2007).

The drugs pentoxifylline and propentofylline are used to treat vasculitis (see Table 279-1). As the manifestations of effusive form of FIP relate to vasculitis, some clinicians have used these drugs and reported successes anecdotally. However, when propentofylline was evaluated in a placebo-controlled study of naturally infected cats with effusive disease, the protocol assessed did not improve the quality of life or lessen the effusion (Fischer et al, 2011). Ozagrel hydrochloride, a thromboxane A_2 synthase inhibitor, was administered to one cat each at 5 mg/kg or 10 mg/kg q12h PO with positive responses noted (Watari et al, 1998). However, both cats also were treated with glucocorticoids.

Polyprenyl immunostimulant is believed to modify the immune response through its action on toll-like receptors. Th-1 cytokines are believed to be up-regulated, directing the immune response toward a cell-mediated immune response, which could aid in the destruction of virus-infected cells (Legendre and Bartges, 2009). Safety has been evaluated in a large number of cats and polyprenyl immunostimulant appears to be safe in cats at 10× dosing. Although the drug is reported ineffective for effusive FIP, three cats with noneffusive disease may have had a positive therapeutic effect (Legendre and Bartges, 2009). Additional data are being collected.

Antibiotics do not have primary antiviral effects but some, such as doxycycline and azithromycin, may have immune modulation effects. Antibiotics may be indicated for the treatment of secondary bacterial infection in cats with FIP. Other supportive care treatments, such as anabolic steroids (stanozolol 1 mg q12h PO) and ascorbic acid (125 mg q12h PO) also have been recommended for the treatment of FIP. Other drugs with theoretic benefit were reviewed previously (Addie and Ishida, 2008).

Most cats with systemic clinical signs of FIP die or require euthanasia within days to months of diagnosis. The effusive form of disease carries a grave prognosis. Depending on the organ system involved and the severity of polysystemic clinical signs, cats with noneffusive disease have variable survival times. Cats with only ocular FIP may respond to antiinflammatory treatment or enucleation of the affected eye(s) and seem to have a better prognosis than cats with systemic FIP.

References and Suggested Reading

Addie D et al: Feline infectious peritonitis. ABCD guidelines on prevention and management, *J Feline Med Surg* 11:594, 2009.

Addie DD, Ishida T: Feline infectious peritonitis: therapy and prevention. In Bonagura J, Twedt D, editors: *Current veterinary therapy XIV*, St Louis, 2008, Elsevier, p 1295.

Bybee SN, Scorza AV, Lappin MR: Effect of the probiotic *Enterococcus faecium* SF68 on presence of diarrhea in cats and dogs housed in an animal shelter, *Vet Intern Med* 25:856, 2011.

Fischer Y et al: Randomized, placebo controlled study of the effect of propentofylline on survival time and quality of life of cats with feline infectious peritonitis, *J Vet Intern Med* 25:1270, 2011.

Gingrich EN et al: Common enteric pathogens in cats before and after placement in an animal shelter, *J Vet Intern Med* 24:766, 2010. (Abstract).

Giori L et al: Performances of different diagnostic tests for feline infectious peritonitis in challenging clinical cases, *J Small Anim Pract* 52:152, 2011.

Hartmann K et al: Comparison of different tests to diagnose feline infectious peritonitis, *J Vet Intern Med* 17:781, 2003.

Hartmann K, Ritz S: Treatment of cats with feline infectious peritonitis, *Vet Immunol Immunopathol* 123:172, 2008.

Ishida T et al: Use of recombinant feline interferon and glucocorticoid in the treatment of feline infectious peritonitis, *J Feline Med Surg* 6:107, 2004.

Legendre AM, Bartges JW: Effect of polyprenyl immunostimulant on the survival times of three cats with the dry form of feline infectious peritonitis, *J Feline Med Surg* 11:624, 2009.

McDonagh P, Sheehy PA, Norris JM: In vitro inhibition of feline coronavirus replication by small interfering RNAs, *Vet Microbiol* 150:220, 2011.

O'Brien SJ et al: Emerging viruses in the Felidae: shifting paradigms, *Viruses* 4:236, 2012.

Pedersen NC: A review of feline infectious peritonitis virus infection: 1963-2008, *J Feline Med Surg* 11:225, 2009.

Pedretti E et al: Low-dose interferon-alpha treatment for feline immunodeficiency virus infection, *Vet Immunol Immunopathol* 109:245, 2006.

Ritz S, Egberink H, Hartmann K: Effect of feline interferon-omega on the survival time and quality of life of cats with feline infectious peritonitis, *J Vet Intern Med* 21:1193, 2007.

Tanaka Y et al: Suppression of feline coronavirus replication in vitro by cyclosporin A, *Vet Res* 43:41, 2012.

Timmann D et al: Retrospective analysis of seizures associated with feline infectious peritonitis in cats, *J Feline Med Surg* 10:9, 2008.

Watari T et al: Effects of a thromboxane synthetase inhibitor on feline infectious peritonitis in cats, *J Vet Med Sci* 60:657, 1998.

APPENDIX I

Table of Common Drugs: Approximate Dosages

MARK G. PAPICH, *Raleigh, North Carolina*

Drug Name	Other Names	Formulations Available	Dosage
Acepromazine	PromAce and many generic brands	5-, 10-, and 25-mg tablets and 10-mg/ml injection	Dog: 0.02-0.1 mg/kg IM, SC, IV; 0.56-2.25 mg/kg PO q6-8h Cat: 0.02-0.1 mg/kg IM, SC, IV; or 1-2 mg/kg PO q8-12h
Acetaminophen	Tylenol and many generic brands	120-, 160-, 325-, and 500-mg tablets	Dog: 15 mg/kg PO q8hr Cat: Not recommended
Acetaminophen with codeine	Tylenol with codeine and many generic brands	Oral solution and tablets. Many forms (e.g., 300 mg acetaminophen plus either 15, 30, or 60 mg codeine)	Follow dosing recommendations for codeine
Acetazolamide	Diamox	125- and 250-mg tablets	5-10 mg/kg PO q8-12h (glaucoma) 4-8 mg/kg PO q8-12h (other diuretic uses)
Acetylcysteine	Mucomyst	20% solution	Antidote: 140 mg/kg (loading dose) then 70 mg/kg IV or PO q4h for five doses Eye: 2% solution topically q2h
Acetylsalicylic acid	*See* Aspirin		
ACTH	*See* Corticotropin		
Activated charcoal	*See* Charcoal, activated		
Adequan	*See* Polysulfated glycosaminoglycan (PSGAG)		
Albendazole	Valbazen	113.6-mg/ml suspension and 300-mg/ml paste	25-50 mg/kg PO q12hr for 3 days For *Giardia* use 25 mg/kg q12h for 2 days
Albuterol	Proventil or Ventolin	2-, 4-, and 5-mg tablets; 2 mg/5 ml syrup	20-50 µg/kg q6-8h; up to maximum of 100 µg/kg q6-8h PO
Allopurinol	Lopurin, Zyloprim	100- and 300-mg tablets	10 mg/kg q8h, then reduce to 10 mg/kg q24h
Aluminum carbonate gel	Basalgel	Capsule (equivalent to 500 mg aluminum hydroxide)	10-30 mg/kg PO q8h (with meals)
Aluminum hydroxide gel	Amphojel	64-mg/ml oral suspension; 600-mg tablet	10-30 mg/kg PO q8h (with meals)
Amikacin	Amiglyde-V (veterinary) and Amikin (human)	50- and 250-mg/ml injection	Dog: 15-30 mg/kg IV, SC, IM q24h Cat: 10-14 mg/kg IV, SC, IM q24h
Aminopentamide	Centrine	0.2-mg tablet; 0.5-mg/ml injection	Dog: 0.01-0.03 mg/kg IM, SC, PO q8-12h Cat: 0.1 mg/cat IM, SC, PO q8-12h
Aminophylline	Many (generic) (Theophylline is preferred for oral therapy)	100- and 200-mg tablets; 25-mg/ml injection	Dog: 10 mg/kg PO, IM, IV q8h Cat: 6.6 mg/kg PO q12h
Amiodarone	Cordarone	200-mg tablets; 50-mg/ml injection	Dog: Start with 15-mg/kg loading dose, then 10 mg/kg/day thereafter

Continued

Drug Name	Other Names	Formulations Available	Dosage
Amitraz	Mitaban	10.6-ml concentrated dip (19.9%)	10.6 ml per 7.5 L water (0.025% solution). Apply three to six topical treatments q2wk. For refractory cases, this dose has been exceeded to produce increased efficacy. Doses that have been used include 0.025%, 0.05%, and 0.1% concentration applied twice per week and 0.125% solution applied to one-half body every day for 4 weeks to 5 months.
Amitriptyline	Elavil	10-, 25-, 50-, 75-, 100-, and 150-mg tablets; 10-mg/ml injection	Dog: 1-2 mg/kg PO q12-24h (range: 0.25-4 mg/kg q12-24h) Cat: 2-4 mg/cat/day PO; for cystitis: 2 mg/kg/day (2.5-7.5 mg/cat/day)
Amlodipine besylate	Norvasc	2.5-, 5-, and 10-mg tablets	Dog: 2.5 mg/dog or 0.1 mg/kg PO once daily Cat: 0.625 mg/cat/day PO initially and increase if needed to 1.25 mg/cat/day (average is 0.18 mg/kg)
Ammonium chloride	Generic	Available as crystals	Dog: 100 mg/kg PO q12hr Cat: 800 mg/cat (approximately ⅓ to ¼ tsp) mixed with food daily
Amoxicillin trihydrate	Amoxi-Tabs, Amoxi-drops, Amoxil, and others	50-, 100-, 200-, and 400-mg tablets; 50-mg/ml oral suspension	6.6-20 mg/kg PO q8-12h
Amoxicillin/clavulanic acid	Clavamox	62.5-, 125-, 250-, and 375-mg tablets; 62.5-mg/ml suspension	Dog: 12.5-25 mg/kg PO q12h, or q8h for gram-negative infections Cat: 62.5 mg/cat PO q12h; or q8h for gram-negative infections
Amphotericin B	Fungizone	50-mg injectable vial	0.5 mg/kg IV (slow infusion) q48h, to a cumulative dose of 4-8 mg/kg
Amphotericin B (Liposomal)	Amphotec, Abelcet, AmBisome		Dog: 2-3 mg/kg IV 3 times/wk for 9-12 treatments for a cumulative dose of 24-27 mg/kg Cat: 1 mg/kg IV 3 times/wk for 12 treatments
Ampicillin	Omnipen, Principen, others	250-, and 500-mg capsules; 125-, 250-, and 500-mg vials of ampicillin sodium	10-20 mg/kg IV, IM, SC q6-8h (ampicillin sodium) 20-40 mg/kg PO q8h
Ampicillin + sulbactam	Unasyn	1.5- and 3- gm vials in 2:1 combination for injection	10-20 mg/kg IV, IM q8h
Ampicillin trihydrate	Polyflex	10- and 25-mg vials for injection	Dog: 10-50 mg/kg SC, IM q24hr Cat: 10-20 mg/kg SC, IM q24hr
Amprolium	Amprol, Corid	9.6% (9.6 gm/dl) oral solution; soluble powder	1.25 gm of 20% amprolium powder to daily feed, or 30 ml of 9.6% amprolium solution to 3.8 L of drinking water for 7 days
Apomorphine hydrochloride	Generic	6-mg tablet	0.03-0.05 mg/kg IV or IM; 0.1 mg/kg, SC; or instill 0.25 mg in conjunctiva of eye (dissolve 6-mg tablet in 1-2 ml of saline)
Ascorbic acid	Vitamin C	Various forms	100-500 mg/animal/day (diet supplement) or 100 mg/animal q8h (urine acidification)
L-Asparaginase	Elspar	10,000 U per vial for injection	400 U/kg IV, IP, IM weekly; or 10,000 U/m² weekly for 3 wk

Drug Name	Other Names	Formulations Available	Dosage
Aspirin	Many generic and brand names (Bufferin, Ascriptin)	81-mg and 325-mg tablets	Dog: Mild analgesia: 10 mg/kg q12h Antiinflammatory: 20-25 mg/kg q12h Antiplatelet: 5-10 mg/kg q24-48h Cat: 81 mg per cat q48h PO
Atenolol	Tenormin	25-, 50-, and 100-mg tablets; 25-mg/ml oral suspension; and 0.5-mg/ml ampule for injection	Dog: 6.25-12.5 mg/dog q12h (or 0.25-1.0 mg/kg q12-24h) PO Cat: 6.25-12.5 mg/cat q12h (approximately 3 mg/kg) PO
Atipamezole	Antisedan	5-mg/ml injection	Inject same volume as used for medetomidine
Atracurium	Tracrium	10-mg/ml injection	0.2 mg/kg IV initially, then 0.15 mg/kg q30min (or IV infusion at 4-9 µg/kg/min)
Atropine	Many generic brands	400-, 500-, and 540-µg/ml injection; 15-mg/ml injection	0.02-0.04 mg/kg IV, IM, SC q6-8h 0.2-0.5 mg/kg (as needed) for organophosphate and carbamate toxicosis
Auranofin (triethylphosphine gold)	Ridaura	3-mg capsule	0.1-0.2 mg/kg PO q12h
Aurothioglucose	Solganol	50-mg/ml injection	Dog <10 kg: 1 mg IM first wk, 2 mg IM second wk, 1 mg/kg/wk maintenance Cat: 0.5-1 mg/cat IM q7days
Azathioprine	Imuran	50-mg tablet; 10-mg/ml for injection	Dog: 2 mg/kg PO q24h initially then 0.5-1 mg/kg q48h Cat (use cautiously): 0.3 mg/kg PO q48hr
Azithromycin	Zithromax	250-mg capsule; and 250- and 600-mg tablets; 20-mg/ml oral suspension	Dog: 10 mg/kg PO q48h or 3.3 mg/kg once daily Cat: 5-10 mg/kg PO every other day
AZT (azidothymidine)	See Zidovudine		
BAL	See Dimercaprol		
Benazepril	Lotensin	5-, 10-, 20-, and 40-mg tablets	Dog: 0.25-0.5 mg/kg PO q24h Cat: 0.5-1 mg/kg q24h PO or 2.5 mg/cat/day up to a maximum of 5 mg/cat/day
Betamethasone	Celestone	600-µg (0.6-mg) tablet; 3-mg/ml sodium phosphate injection	0.1-0.2 mg/kg PO q12-24h
Bethanechol	Urecholine	5-, 10-, 25-, and 50-mg tablets; 5-mg/ml injection	Dog: 5-15 mg/dog PO q8h Cat: 1.25-5 mg/cat PO q8h
Bisacodyl	Dulcolax	5-mg tablet	5 mg/animal PO q8-24h
Bismuth subsalicylate	Pepto Bismol	Oral suspension: 262 mg/15 ml or 525 mg/ml in extra-strength formulation; 262-mg tablet	1-3 ml/kg/day (in divided doses) PO
Bleomycin	Blenoxane	15-U vials for injection	10 U/m² IV or SC for 3 days, then 10 U/m² weekly (maximum cumulative dose 200 U/m²)
Bromide	See Potassium bromide		
Budesonide	Entocort	3-mg capsule	Dog, cat: 0.125 mg/kg q6-8h PO; dose interval may be increased to q12h when condition improves
Bunamidine hydrochloride	Scolaban	400-mg tablet	20-50 mg/kg PO

Continued

Drug Name	Other Names	Formulations Available	Dosage
Bupivacaine	Marcaine and generic	2.5- and 5-mg/ml solution injection	1 ml of 0.5% solution per 10 cm for an epidural
Buprenorphine	Temgesic (Vetergesic in the U.K.)	0.3-mg/ml solution	Dog: 0.006-0.02 mg/kg IV, IM, SC q4-8h Cat: 0.005-0.01 mg/kg IV, IM q4-8h Buccal administration in cats: 0.01-0.02 mg/kg q12h
Buspirone	BuSpar	5- and 10-mg tablets	Dog: 2.5-10 mg/dog PO q12-24h; or 1 mg/kg q12h PO Cat: 2.5-5 mg/cat PO q24h (may be increased to 5-7.5 mg/cat twice daily for some cats)
Busulfan	Myleran	2-mg tablet	3-4 mg/m² PO q24h
Butorphanol	Torbutrol Torbugesic	1-, 5-, and 10-mg tablets; 0.5- or 10-mg/ml injection	Dog: Antitussive: 0.055 mg/kg SC q6-12h or 0.55 mg/kg PO Preanesthetic: 0.2-0.4 mg/kg IV, IM, SC (with acepromazine) Analgesic: 0.2-0.4 mg/kg IV, IM, SC q2-4h or 0.55-1.1 mg/kg PO q6-12h Cat: Analgesic: 0.2-0.8 mg/kg IV, SC q2-6h, or 1.5 mg/kg PO q4-8h
Calcitriol	Rocaltrol, Calcijex	Available as injection (Calcijex) and capsules (Rocaltrol): 0.25- and 0.5-µg capsules; 1- or 2-µg/ml injection	Dog: 2.5 ng/kg once daily Cat: 0.25 µg/cat every other day; or 0.01-0.04 µg/kg/day, or 2.5 ng/kg PO once daily for hyperparathyroidism
Calcium carbonate	Many brands available: Titralac, Tums, generic	Many tablets or oral suspension (e.g., 650-mg tablet contains 260 mg calcium ion)	For phosphate binder: 60-100 mg/kg/day in divided doses PO For calcium supplementation: 70-180 mg/kg/day added to food
Calcium chloride	Generic	10% (100 mg/ml) solution	0.1-0.3 ml/kg IV (slowly)
Calcium citrate	Citracal (OTC)	950-mg tablet (contains 200 mg calcium ion)	Dog: 20 mg/kg/day added to food Cat: 10-30 mg/kg PO q8h (with meals)
Calcium disodium EDTA	See Edetate calcium disodium		
Calcium gluconate	Kalcinate and generic	10% (100 mg/ml) injection	0.5-1.5 ml/kg IV (slowly)
Calcium lactate	Generic	OTC tablet	Dog: 0.5 gm/dog/day PO (in divided doses) Cat: 0.2-0.5 gm/cat/day PO (in divided doses)
Captopril	Capoten	25-mg tablet	Dog: 0.5-2 mg/kg PO q8-12h Cat: 3.12-6.25 mg/cat PO q8h
Carbenicillin	Geopen, Pyopen	1-, 2-, 5-, 10-, and 30-gm vials for injection	40-50 mg/kg and up to 100 mg/kg IV, IM, SC q6-8h
Carbenicillin indanyl sodium	Geocillin	500-mg tablet	10 mg/kg PO q8h
Carbimazole	Neo-mercazole	Available in Europe	Cat: 5 mg/cat PO q8h (induction), followed by 5 mg/cat PO q12h
Carboplatin	Paraplatin	50- and 150-mg vial for injection	Dog: 300 mg/m² IV q3-4wk Cat: 200 mg/m² IV q4wk
Carprofen	Rimadyl (Zinecarp in the U.K.) Novox (generic)	25-, 75-, and 100-mg tablets 50 mg/ml solution	Dog: 2.2 mg/kg PO q12h; or 4.4 mg/kg once daily PO; 2.2 mg/kg q12h or 4.4 mg/kg once daily SC Cat: doses not available
Carvedilol	Coreg	3.125-, 6.25-, 12.5-, and 25-mg tablets	Dog: 0.2 to 0.4 mg/kg q12h PO; titrate dose up to 1.5 mg/kg q12h PO if needed
Cascara sagrada	Many brands (e.g., Nature's Remedy)	100- and 325-mg tablets	Dog: 1-5 mg/kg day PO Cat: 1-2 mg/cat/day

Drug Name	Other Names	Formulations Available	Dosage
Castor oil	Generic	Oral liquid (100%)	Dog: 8-30 ml/day PO Cat: 4-10 ml/day PO
Cefadroxil	Cefa-Tabs, Cefa-Drops	50-mg/ml oral suspension; 50-, 100-, 200-, and 1000-mg tablets	Dog: 22-30 mg/kg PO q12h Cat: 22 mg/kg PO q24h
Cefazolin sodium	Ancef, Kefzol, and generic	50 and 100 mg/50 ml for injection	20-35 mg/kg IV, IM q8h For perisurgical use: 22 mg/kg q2hr during surgery
Cefixime	Suprax	20-mg/ml oral suspension and 200- and 400-mg tablets	10 mg/kg PO q12h For cystitis: 5 mg/kg PO q12-24h
Cefotaxime	Claforan	500-mg and 1-, 2-, and 10-gm vials for injection	Dog: 50 mg/kg IV, IM, SC q12h Cat: 20-80 mg/kg IV, IM q6h
Cefovecin	Convenia	80 mg/ml injection	Dog, cat: 8 mg/kg SC once every 14 days
Cefoxitin sodium	Mefoxin, generic	1-, 2-, and 10-gm vials for injection	30 mg/kg IV q6-8h
Cefpodoxime proxetil	Simplicef, generic	100- and 200-mg tablets; 10- or 20-mg/ml human label suspension	Dog: 5-10 mg/kg PO once daily Cat: Dose not established
Ceftazidime	Fortaz, Ceptaz, Tazicef, generic	0.5-, 1-, 2- and 6-gm vials reconstituted to 280 mg/ml	30 mg/kg IV, IM q6h
Ceftiofur	Naxcel (ceftiofur sodium); Excenel (ceftiofur HCl)	50-mg/ml injection	2.2-4.4 mg/kg SC q24h (for urinary tract infections)
Cephalexin	Keflex, Rilexine, generic forms	150, 300, and 600 mg chewable tablets for dogs; 250- and 500-mg capsules; 250- and 500-mg tablets; 100-mg/ml or 125- and 250-mg/5-ml oral suspension	10-30 mg/kg PO q6-12h; for pyoderma, 22-35 mg/kg PO q12h
Cetirizine	Zyrtec	1-mg/ml oral syrup; 5- and 10-mg tablets	Dog: 5-10 mg/dog q12h PO, up to a dose of 2 mg/kg q12h PO Cat: 5 mg/cat PO q24h
Charcoal, activated	ActaChar, Charcodote, Toxiban, generic	Oral suspension	1-4 gm/kg PO (granules) 6-12 ml/kg (suspension)
Chlorambucil	Leukeran	2-mg tablet	Dog: 2-6 mg/m^{2}or 0.1-0.2 mg/kg PO q24h initially, then q48h Cat: 0.1-0.2 mg/kg q24h initially, then q48h PO
Chloramphenicol	Chloromycetin, generic forms	250-mg capsule; and 100-, 250-, and 500-mg tablets	Dog: 40-50 mg/kg PO q8h Cat: 12.5-20 mg/kg PO q12h
Chlorothiazide	Diuril	250- and 500-mg tablets; 50-mg/ml oral suspension and injection	20-40 mg/kg PO q12h or IV
Chlorpheniramine maleate	Chlor-Trimeton, Phenetron, and others	4- and 8-mg tablets	Dog: 4-8 mg/dog PO q12h (up to a maximum of 0.5 mg/kg q12h) Cat: 2 mg/cat PO q12h
Chlorpromazine	Thorazine	25-mg/ml injection solution	Dog: 0.5 mg/kg IM, SC q6-8h (before cancer chemotherapy administer 2 mg/kg SC q3h) Cat: 0.2-0.4 mg/kg q6-8h IM, SC
Chorionic gonadotropin	See Gonadotropin		
Cimetidine	Tagamet (OTC and prescription)	100-, 150-, 200-, and 300-mg tablets and 60-mg/ml injection	10 mg/kg IV, IM, PO q6-8h (in renal failure administer 2.5-5 mg/kg IV, PO q12h)
Ciprofloxacin	Cipro and generic	250-, 500-, and 750-mg tablets; 2-mg/ml injection	Dog: 25-30 mg/kg, PO, once daily; 15 mg/kg IV (slowly), q24h Cat: 10 mg/kg, q12h, PO; 10 mg/kg IV (slowly) q12h

Continued

Drug Name	Other Names	Formulations Available	Dosage
Cisapride	Must be compounded		Dog: 0.1-0.5 mg/kg PO q8-12h (doses as high as 0.5-1.0 mg/kg have been used in some dogs) Cat: 2.5-5 mg/cat PO q8-12h (as high as 1 mg/kg q8h has been administered to cats)
Cisplatin	Platinol	1-mg/ml injection; 50-mg vials	Dog: 60-70 mg/m^2 q3-4wk (administer fluid for diuresis with therapy) Cat: Do not use in cats
Clavamox	See Amoxicillin-clavulanic acid combination		
Clemastine	Tavist, Contac 12-hr allergy, and generic	1.34-mg tablet (OTC); 2.64-mg tablet (Rx); 0.134-mg/ml syrup	Dog: 0.05-0.1 mg/kg PO q12h
Clindamycin	Antirobe, Cleocin, and generic	Oral liquid 25-mg/ml; 25-, 75-, 150-, and 300-mg capsule; and 150-mg/ml injection (Cleocin)	Dog: 11-33 mg/kg q12h PO; for oral and soft tissue infection: 5.5-33 mg/kg q12h PO Cat: 11-33 mg/kg q24h PO for skin and anaerobic infections Toxoplasmosis: 12.5-25 mg/kg PO q12h for 4 wk
Clofazimine	Lamprene	50- and 100-mg capsules	Cat: 1 mg/kg PO up to a maximum of 4 mg/kg/day
Clomipramine	Anafranil (human label); Clomicalm (veterinary label)	10-, 25-, and 50-mg tablets (human) 5-, 20-, and 80-mg tablets (veterinary)	Dog: 1-2 mg/kg PO q12h up to a maximum of 3 mg/kg PO q12h Cat: 1-5 mg/cat PO q12-24h
Clonazepam	Klonopin	0.5-, 1-, and 2-mg tablets	Dog: 0.5 mg/kg PO q8-12h Cat: 0.1-0.2 mg/kg q12-24h PO
Clopidogrel	Plavix	75-mg tablets	Dog: give oral loading dose of 2-4 mg/kg, PO, followed by 1 mg/kg q24h, PO Cat: 19 mg per cat (¼ tablet) q24h PO
Clorazepate	Tranxene	3.75-, 7.5-, 11.25-, 15-, and 22.5-mg tablets	Dog: 2 mg/kg PO q12h Cat: 0.2-0.4 mg/kg q12-24h PO (up to 0.5-2 mg/kg)
Cloxacillin	Cloxapen, Orbenin, Tegopen	250- and 500-mg capsules; 25-mg/ml oral solution	20-40 mg/kg PO q8h
Codeine	Generic	15-, 30-, and 60-mg tablets; 5-mg/ml syrup; 3-mg/ml oral solution	Analgesia: 0.5-1 mg/kg PO q4-6h Antitussive: 0.1-0.3 mg/kg PO q4-6h
Colchicine	Generic	500- and 600-µg tablets; 500-µg/ml ampule injection	0.01-0.03 mg/kg PO q24h
Colony-stimulating factor	Sargramostim (Leukine) and Filgrastim (Neupogen)	300 µg/ml (Neupogen) and 250 or 500 µg/ml (Leukine)	Leukine: 0.25 mg/m^2 q12h SC or IV infusion Neupogen: 0.005 mg/kg (5 µg/kg) q24h SC for 2 wk
Corticotropin (ACTH)	Acthar	Gel 80 U/ml	Response test: Collect pre-ACTH sample and inject 2.2 IU/kg IM; collect post-ACTH sample in 2 hr in dogs and at 1 and 2 hr in cats
Cosequin	See Glucosamine chondroitin sulfate		
Cosyntropin	Cortrosyn	250 µg per vial (can be stored in freezer for 6 months)	Response test: Dog: Collect pre-ACTH sample and inject 5 µg/kg IV or IM and collect sample at 30 and 60 min Cat: 0.125 mg IV or IM and collect sample at 30 min and 60 min after IV administration and 30 and 60 min after IM administration

Drug Name	Other Names	Formulations Available	Dosage
Cyanocobalamin (vitamin B$_{12}$)	Many	100-µg/ml injection	Dog: 100-200 µg/day PO Cat: 50-100 µg/day PO
Cyclophosphamide	Cytoxan, Neosar	25-mg/ml injection; 25- and 50-mg tablets	Dog: Anticancer: 50 mg/m^2 PO once daily 4 days/wk or 150-300 mg/m^2 IV and repeat in 21 days Immunosuppressive therapy: 50 mg/m^2 (approx. 2.2 mg/kg) PO q48h or 2.2 mg/kg once daily for 4 days/wk Cat: 6.25-12.5 mg/cat once daily 4 days/wk
Cyclosporine (cyclosporin A)	Atopica, Neoral, Optimmune (ophthalmic)	Atopica: 10-, 25-, 50-, and 100-mg capsules; Atopica oral solution: 100 mg/mL Neoral: 25-mg and 100-mg microemulsion capsules; 100-mg/ml oral solution (for microemulsion) Optimmune: 0.2% ointment	Dog: 3-7 mg/kg/day; for atopic dermatitis some dogs are controlled with q48h dosing Cat: 5 mg/kg PO q24h; or 7.5 mg/kg of Atopica oral solution
Cyproheptadine	Periactin	4-mg tablet; 2-mg/5-ml syrup	Antihistamine: 1.1 mg/kg PO q8-12h Appetite stimulant: 2 mg/cat PO
Cytarabine (cytosine arabinoside)	Cytosar-U	100-mg vial	Dog (lymphoma): 100 mg/m^2 IV, SC once daily or 50 mg/m^2 twice daily for 4 days; Meningoencephalitis: 200 mg per square meter, IV infused over 8 hours, repeated twice in 48 hours Cat: 100 mg/m^2 once daily for 2 days
Dacarbazine	DTIC	200-mg vial for injection	200 mg/m^2 IV for 5 days q3wk; or 800-1000 mg/m^2 IV q3wk
Dalteparin	Fragmin	16 mg/0.2 ml; 32 mg/0.2 ml in prefilled syringes or 64 mg/ml multidose vials for injection	Dog: 100-150 units/kg q8h SC Cat: 180 units/kg q6h SC
Danazol	Danocrine	50-, 100-, and 200-mg capsules	5-10 mg/kg PO q12h
Dantrolene	Dantrium	100-mg capsule and 0.33-mg/ml injection	For prevention of malignant hyperthermia: 2-3 mg/kg IV For muscle relaxation: Dog: 1-5 mg/kg PO q8h Cat: 0.5-2 mg/kg PO q12h
Dapsone	Generic	25- and 100-mg tablets	Dog: 1.1 mg/kg PO q8-12h Cat: Do not use
Darbazine (prochlorperazine + isopropamide)	Darbazine	No. 1, 2, and 3 capsules	Dog, cat: 0.14-0.2 ml/kg SC q12h Dog 2-7 kg: 1-#1 capsule PO q12h Dog 7-14 kg: 1-#2 capsule PO q12h Dog >14 kg: 1-#3 capsule PO q12h
Deferoxamine	Desferal	500-mg vial for injection	10 mg/kg IV, IM q2h for two doses; then 10 mg/kg q8h for 24 hr
Deprenyl (l-deprenyl)	*See* Selegiline (Anipryl)		
Deracoxib	Deramaxx	25-, 100-mg tablets	Dog: 3-4 mg/kg q24h PO for 7 days; or 1-2 mg/kg q24h PO for long-term use Cat: 1 mg/kg PO, one-time dose
Desmopressin acetate	DDAVP	100-µg/ml injection and desmopressin acetate nasal solution (0.01% metered spray); 0.1- and 0.2-mg tablets	Diabetes insipidus: 2-4 drops (2 µg) q12-24h intranasally or in eye Animal oral dose: 0.05-0.1 mg/dog q12h PO initially, then increase to 0.1-0.2 mg/dog q12h as needed von Willebrand's disease treatment: 1 µg/kg (0.01 ml/kg) SC, IV, diluted in 20 ml of saline administered over 10 min
Desoxycorticosterone pivalate	Percorten-V, DOCP, or DOCA pivalate	25 mg/ml injection	1.5-2.2 mg/kg IM q25 days

Continued

Drug Name	Other Names	Formulations Available	Dosage
Dexamethasone (dexamethasone solution and dexamethasone sodium phosphate)	Azium solution in polyethylene glycol. Sodium phosphate forms include Dexaject SP, Dexavet, and Dexasone. Tablets include Decadron and generic	Azium solution, 2 mg/ml. Sodium phosphate forms are 3.33 mg/ml; 0.25-, 0.5-, 0.75-, 1-, 1.5-, 2-, 4-, and 6-mg tablets	Antiinflammatory: 0.07-0.15 mg/kg IV, IM, PO q12-24h Dexamethasone suppression test: Dog: 0.01 mg/kg IV Cat: 0.1 mg/kg IV Collect sample at 0, 4, and 8 hr
Dexmedetomidine	Dexdomitor	0.5-mg/ml injectable solution	Dog: Sedative and analgesic: 375 mg/m^2 IV or 500 mg/m^2 IM Dog: Preanesthetic: 125 mg/m^2 IM Cat: Sedative and analgesic: 40 µg/kg IM
Dextran	Dextran 70 Gentran-70	Injectable solution: 250, 500, and 1000 ml	10-20 ml/kg IV to effect
Dextromethorphan	Benylin and others	Available in syrup, capsule, and tablet; many OTC products	0.5-2 mg/kg PO q6-8h has been reported, but effective dose not established
Dextrose solution 5%	D5W	Fluid solution for IV administration	40-50 ml/kg IV q24h
Diazepam	Valium and generic	2- and 5-mg tablets; 5-mg/ml solution for injection	Preanesthetic: 0.5 mg/kg IV Status epilepticus: 0.5 mg/kg IV, 1.0 mg/kg rectal; repeat if necessary Appetite stimulant (cat): 0.2 mg/kg IV
Dichlorophen	Vermiplex (See Toluene)		
Dichlorvos	Task	10- and 25-mg tablets	Dog: 26.4-33 mg/kg PO Cat: 11 mg/kg PO
Dicloxacillin	Dynapen	125-, 250-, and 500-mg capsules; 12.5-mg/ml oral suspension	25 mg/kg IM q6h Oral doses not absorbed
Diethylcarbamazine (DEC)	Caricide, Filaribits	Chewable tablets; 50-, 60-, 180-, 200-, and 400-mg tablets	Heartworm prophylaxis: 6.6 mg/kg PO q24h
Diethylstilbestrol (DES)	DES, generic (no longer manufactured in U.S.)	1- and 5-mg tablet; 50-mg/ml injection	Dog: 0.1-1.0 mg/dog PO q24h Cat: 0.05-0.1 mg/cat PO q24h
Digoxin	Lanoxin, Cardoxin	0.0625-, 0.125-, 0.25-mg tablets; 0.05- and 0.15-mg/ml elixir	Dog: <20 kg body weight: 0.01 mg/kg q12h; >20 kg use 0.22 mg/m^2 PO q12h (subtract 10% for elixir) Dog: (rapid digitalization): 0.0055-0.011 mg/kg IV q1h to effect Cat: 0.008-0.01 mg/kg PO q48h (approximately $\frac{1}{4}$ of a 0.125-mg tablet/cat)
Dihydrotachysterol (vitamin D)	Hytakerol, DHT	0.125-mg tablet; 0.5-mg/ml oral liquid	0.01 mg/kg/day PO; for acute treatment administer 0.02 mg/kg initially, then 0.01-0.02 mg/kg PO q24-48h thereafter
Diltiazem	Cardizem, Dilacor	30-, 60-, 90-, and 120-mg tablets; 50-mg/ml injection	Dog: 0.5-1.5 mg/kg PO q8h, 0.25 mg/kg over 2 min IV (repeat if necessary) Cat: 1.75-2.4 mg/kg PO q8h For Dilacor XR or Cardizem CD dose is 10 mg/kg PO once daily
Dimenhydrinate	Dramamine (Gravol in Canada)	50-mg tablets; 50-mg/ml injection	Dog: 4-8 mg/kg PO, IM, IV q8h Cat: 12.5 mg/cat IV, IM, PO q8h
Dimercaprol (BAL)	BAL in oil	Injection must be prepared by compounding	Dog and cat: 4 mg/kg IM, q4h
Dinoprost tromethamine	See Prostaglandin F$_{2\alpha}$ 5-mg/ml injection		
Dioctyl calcium sulfosuccinate	See Docusate calcium		
Dioctyl sodium sulfosuccinate	See Docusate sodium		

Drug Name	Other Names	Formulations Available	Dosage
Diphenhydramine	Benadryl	Available OTC: 2.5-mg/ml elixir; 25- and 50-mg capsules and tablets; 50-mg/ml injection	Dog: 25-50 mg/dog IV, IM, PO q8h Cat: 2-4 mg/kg q6-8h PO or 1 mg/kg IM, IV q6-8h
Diphenoxylate	Lomotil	2.5 mg	Dog: 0.1-0.2 mg/kg PO q8-12h Cat: 0.05-0.1 mg/kg PO q12h
Diphenylhydantoin	*See* Phenytoin		
Diphosphonate disodium etidronate	*See* Etidronate disodium		
Dipyridamole	Persantine	25-, 50-, 75-mg tablets; 5-mg/ml injection	4-10 mg/kg PO q24h
Dirlotapide	Slentrol	5-mg/ml oral oil-based solution	Dog: Start with 0.01 ml/kg/day PO Monthly adjustments to dose should be done on the basis of animal's weight loss. Do not exceed 0.2 ml/kg/day. Cat: Do not administer to cats
Disopyramide	Norpace (Rhythmodan in Canada)	100- and 150-mg capsules (10-mg/ml injection in Canada only)	6-15 mg/kg PO q8h
Dithiazanine iodide	Dizan	10-, 50-, 100-, and 200-mg tablets	Heartworm: 6.6-11 mg/kg PO q24h for 7-10 days For other parasites: 22 mg/kg PO
Divalproex sodium	*See* Valproic acid		
Dobutamine	Dobutrex	250-mg/20-ml vial for injection (12.5 mg/ml)	Dog: 5-20 μg/kg/min IV infusion Cat: 2 μg/kg/min IV infusion
Docusate calcium	Surfak, Doxidan	60-mg tablet (and many others)	Dog: 50-100 mg/dog PO q12-24h Cat: 50 mg/cat PO q12-24h
Docusate sodium	Colace, Doxan, Doss, many OTC brands	50-, and 100-mg capsules; 10-mg/ml liquid	Dog: 50-200 mg/dog PO q8-12h Cat: 50 mg/cat PO q12-24h
Dolasetron mesylate	Anzemet	50-, 100-mg tablets; 20-mg/ml injection	Dog, cat: Prevention of nausea and vomiting: 0.6 mg/kg IV or PO q24h Treating vomiting and nausea: 1.0 mg/kg PO or IV once daily
Domperidone	Motilium	Not available in U.S.	2-5 mg/animal PO
Dopamine	Intropin	40-, 80-, or 160-mg/ml	Dog, cat: 2-10 μg/kg/min IV infusion
Doxapram	Dopram, Respiram	20-mg/ml injection	5-10 mg/kg IV Neonate: 1-5 mg SC, sublingual, or via umbilical vein
Doxorubicin	Adriamycin	2-mg/ml injection	30 mg/m^2 IV q21days or >20 kg use 30 mg/m^2 and <20 kg use 1 mg/kg Cat: 20 mg/m^2 or approximately 1-1.25 mg/kg IV q3wk
Doxycycline hyclate or Doxycycline monohydrate	Vibramycin and generic forms	10-mg/ml oral suspension; 100-mg injection vial; 50- or 100-mg tablets or capsules	Dogs and cats: 3-5 mg/kg PO, IV q12h or 10 mg/kg PO q24h For *Rickettsia* in dogs: 5 mg/kg q12h
Edetate calcium disodium (CaNa$_2$EDTA)	Calcium disodium versenate	20-mg/ml injection	25 mg/kg SC, IM, IV q6h for 2-5 days
Edrophonium	Tensilon and others	10-mg/ml injection	Dog: 0.11-0.22 mg/kg IV Cat: 0.25-0.5 mg/cat (total dose) IV
Enalapril	Enacard, Vasotec	2.5-, 5-, 10-, and 20-mg tablets	Dog: 0.5 mg/kg PO q12-24h Cat: 0.25-0.5 mg/kg PO q12-24h
Enflurane	Ethrane	Available as solution for inhalation	Induction: 2%-3% Maintenance: 1.5%-3%

Continued

Drug Name	Other Names	Formulations Available	Dosage
Enilconazole	Imaverol, Clina-Farm-EC	10% or 13.8% emulsion	Nasal aspergillosis: 10 mg/kg q12h instilled into nasal sinus for 14 days (10% solution diluted 50/50 with water) Dermatophytes: Dilute 10% solution to 0.2% and wash lesion with solution four times at 3- to 4-day intervals
Enoxaparin	Lovenox	30 mg/0.3 ml, 40 mg/0.4 ml, 60 mg/0.6 ml, 80 mg/0.8 ml, and 100 mg/1 ml in prefilled syringes for injection	Dog: 0.8 mg/kg SC q6h Cat: 1.25 mg/kg SC q6h
Enrofloxacin	Baytril	68-, 22.7-, and 5.7-mg tablets. Taste Tabs are 22.7 and 68 mg; 22.7-mg/ml injection	Dog: 5-20 mg/kg/day PO, IM Cat: 5 mg/kg/day PO (do not exceed dose)
Ephedrine	Many, generic	25- and 50-mg/ml injection	Vasopressor: 0.75 mg/kg IM, SC; repeat as needed
Epinephrine	Adrenaline and generic forms	1-mg/ml (1:1,000) injection solution	Cardiac arrest: 10-20 µg/kg IV or 200 µg/kg intratracheal (may be diluted in saline before administration) Anaphylactic shock: 2.5-5 µg/kg IV or 50 µg/kg intratracheal (may be diluted in saline)
Epoetin alpha (erythropoietin) (r-HuEPO)	Epogen, epoetin alfa (r-HuEPO)	2000-U/ml injection	Doses range from 35 or 50 U/kg three times/wk to 400 U/kg/wk IV, SC (adjust dose to hematocrit of 0.30-0.34) Cat: Start with 100 units/kg three times/wk and adjust dose based on hematocrit
Epsiprantel	Cestex	Coated tablet	Dog: 5.5 mg/kg PO Cat: 2.75 mg/kg PO
Ergocalciferol (vitamin D_2)	Calciferol, Drisdol	400-U tablet (OTC); 50,000-U tablet (1.25 mg); 500,000-U/ml (12.5 mg/ml) injection	500-2000 U/kg/day PO
Erythromycin	Many brands and generic	250- or 500-mg capsule or tablet	Antibacterial dose: 10-20 mg/kg PO q8-12h Prokinetic dose: 0.5-1.0 mg/kg PO q8h
Esmolol	Brevibloc	10-mg/ml injection	500 µg/kg IV, which may be given as 0.05-0.1 mg/kg slowly every 5 min or 50-200 µg/kg/min infusion
Estradiol cypionate (ECP)	ECP, Depo-Estradiol, generic	2-mg/ml injection	Dog: 22-44 µg/kg IM (total dose not to exceed 1.0 mg) Cat: 250 µg/cat IM between 40 hr and 5 days of mating
Etidronate disodium	Didronel	200- and 400-mg tablets; 50-mg/ml injection	Dog: 5 mg/kg/day PO Cat: 10 mg/kg/day PO
Etodolac	EtoGesic, veterinary; Lodine, human	150- and 300-mg tablets	Dog: 10-15 mg/kg PO once daily Cat: Dose not established
Etretinate	Tegison	10- and 25-mg capsules	Dog: 1 mg/kg PO, with food/day or for <15 kg 10 mg/dog PO q24h; >15 kg 10 mg/dog PO q12h Cat: 2 mg/kg/day
Famotidine	Pepcid	10-mg tablet; 10-mg/ml injection	Dog: 0.1-0.2 mg/kg IM, SC, PO, IV q12h; or 0.5 mg/kg PO q24h, or 0.5 mg/kg IM, SC, PO, IV q24h Cat: 0.2-0.25 mg/kg IM, IV, SC, PO q12-24h
Felbamate	Felbatol	400- and 600-mg tablets; 120-mg/ml oral flavored suspension	Dog: Start with 15 mg/kg PO q8h and increase gradually to maximum of 65 mg/kg q8h
Fenbendazole	Panacur, Safe-Guard	Panacur granules 22.2% (222 mg/gm); 100-mg/ml liquid	50 mg/kg/day PO for 3 days

Drug Name	Other Names	Formulations Available	Dosage
Fentanyl	Sublimaze, generic	50-µg/ml injection	0.02-0.04 mg/kg IV, IM, SC q2h or 0.01 mg/kg IV, IM, SC (with acetylpromazine or diazepam) For analgesia: 0.01 mg/kg IV, IM, SC q2h
Fentanyl transdermal	Duragesic	25-, 50-, 75-, and 100-µg/hr patch	Dog: 10-20 kg, 50-µg/hr patch q72h Cat: 25-µg patch every 118 hr
Ferrous sulfate	Many OTC brands	Many	Dog: 100-300 mg/dog PO q24h Cat: 50-100 mg/cat PO q24h
Finasteride	Proscar	5-mg tablets	Dog (BPH): 5-mg tablet/dog PO q24h
Firocoxib	Previcox	57- or 227-mg tablets	Dog: 5 mg/kg PO, once daily Cat: 1.5 mg/kg, once; long-term safety in cats has not been determined
Florfenicol	Nuflor	300 mg/ml (cattle)	Dog: 20 mg/kg q6h PO, IM Cat: 22 mg/kg q12h IM, PO
Fluconazole	Diflucan	50-, 100-, 150-, and 200-mg tablets; 10- or 40-mg/ml oral suspension; 2-mg/ml IV injection	Dog: 10-12 mg/kg day PO For *Malassezia* 5 mg/kg q12h PO Cat: 50 mg/cat PO q12h or 50 mg/cat/day PO
Flucytosine	Ancobon	250-mg capsule; 75-mg/ml oral suspension	Cats: 25-50 mg/kg PO q6-8h (up to a maximal dose of 100 mg/kg PO q12h) Dogs: Do not use in dogs
Fludrocortisone	Florinef	100-µg (0.1 mg) tablet	Dog: 0.2-0.8 mg/dog or 0.02 mg/kg PO q24h (13-23 µg/kg) Cat: 0.1-0.2 mg/cat PO q24h
Flumazenil	Romazicon	100-µg/ml (0.1 mg/ml) injection	0.2 mg (total dose) IV as needed
Flumethasone	Flucort	0.5-mg/ml injection	Dog, cat: Antiinflammatory: 0.15-0.3 mg/kg IV, IM, SC q12-24h
Flunixin meglumine	Banamine	250-mg packet granules; 10- and 50-mg/ml injection	1.1 mg/kg IV, IM, SC once or 1.1 mg/kg/day PO 3 days/wk Ophthalmic: 0.5 mg/kg IV once
5-Fluorouracil	Fluorouracil	50-mg/ml vial	Dog: 150 mg/m² IV once/week Cat: Do not use
Fluoxetine	Prozac, Reconcile	8-, 16-, 32-, and 64-mg chewable tablets for dogs. Human formulation is 10- and 20-mg capsules and 4-mg/ml oral solution	Dog: 1-2 mg/kg/day PO q24h Cat: 0.5-4 mg/cat PO q24h
Follicle-stimulating hormone (FSM)	*See* Urofollitropin		
Fomepizole	4-Methylpyrazole, Antizole, and Antizol-vet	5% solution	Dog: 20 mg/kg initially IV, then 15 mg/kg at 12- and 24-hr intervals, then 5 mg/kg at 36 hr; repeat q12h if necessary
Furazolidone	Furoxone	100-mg tablet	4 mg/kg PO q12h for 7-10 days
Furosemide	Lasix, generic	12.5-, 20-, and 50-mg tablets; 10-mg/ml oral solution; 50-mg/ml injection	Dog: 2-6 mg/kg IV, IM, SC, PO q8-12h (or as needed) Cat: 1-4 mg/kg IV, IM, SC, PO q8-24h
Gabapentin	Neurontin	100-, 300-, 400-mg capsules; 100-, 300-, 400-, 600-, 800-mg scored tablets; 50-mg/ml oral solution	Dog, cat: Anticonvulsant dose: 2.5-10 mg/kg q8-12h PO For analgesia: 10-15 mg/kg q8h PO
Gemfibrozil	Lopid	300-mg capsules; 600-mg tablets	7.5 mg/kg PO q12h
Gentamicin	Gentocin	50- and 100-mg/ml solution for injection	Dog: 9-14 mg/kg IV, IM, SC q24h Cat: 5-8 mg/kg IV, IM, SC q24h
Glipizide	Glucotrol	5- and 10-mg tablets	Dog: Not recommended Cat: 2.5-7.5 mg/cat PO q12h. Usual dose is 2.5 mg/cat initially, then increase to 5 mg/cat q12h

Continued

Drug Name	Other Names	Formulations Available	Dosage
Glucosamine chondroitin sulfate	Cosequin and others	Regular (RS) and double-strength (DS) capsules	Dog: 1-2 RS capsules/day (2-4 capsules of DS for large dogs) Cat: 1 RS capsule/day
Glyburide	Diabeta, Micronase, Glynase	1.25-, 2.5-, and 5-mg tablets	0.2 mg/kg/day PO; or 0.625 mg/cat
Glycerin	Generic	Oral solution	1-2 ml/kg, up to PO q8h
Glycopyrrolate	Robinul-V	0.2-mg/ml injection	0.005-0.01 mg/kg IV, IM, SC
Gold sodium thiomalate	Myochrysine	10-, 25-, and 50-mg/ml injection	1-5 mg IM on first wk, then 2-10 mg IM on second wk, then 1 mg/kg once/wk IM maintenance
Gold therapy	See Aurothioglucose, Gold sodium thiomalate, or Auranofin		
GoLYTELY	See Polyethylene glycol electrolyte solution		
Gonadorelin (GnRH, LHRH)	Factrel	50-µg/ml injection	Dog: 50-100 µg/dog/day IM q24-48h Cat: 25 µg/cat IM once
Gonadotropin, chorionic (HCG)	Profasi, Pregnyl, generic, A.P.L.	Injection sizes of 5,000, 10,000, and 20,000 U	Dog: 22 U/kg IM q24-48h or 44 U IM once Cat: 250 U/cat IM once
Gonadotropin-releasing hormone	See Gonadorelin		
Granisetron	Kytril	1-mg/ml injection; 1-mg tablet	0.01 mg/kg (10 µg/kg) IV
Griseofulvin (microsize)	Fulvicin U/F	125-, 250-, and 500-mg tablets; 25-mg/ml oral suspension; 125-mg/ml oral syrup	50 mg/kg PO q24h (up to a maximum dose of 110-132 mg/kg/day in divided treatments)
Griseofulvin (ultramicrosize)	Fulvicin P/G, GrisPEG	100-, 125-, 165-, 250-, and 330-mg tablets	30 mg/kg/day in divided treatments PO
Growth hormone (hGH, somatrem, somatropin)	Protropin, Humatrope, Nutropin	5- and 10-mg/vial	0.1 U/kg SC, IM three times/wk for 4-6 wk (Usual human pediatric dose is 0.18-0.3 mg/kg/wk)
Guaifenesin	Glyceryl guaiacolate, Guaiphenesin, Mucinex	Tablets: 100-, 200-mg; 600-mg extended-release tablets Oral solution: 20 mg/ml or 40 mg/ml	Dog, cat: Expectorant: 3-5 mg/kg q8h PO Dog: Anesthetic adjunct: 2.2 ml/kg/hr of a 5% solution IV
Halothane	Fluothane	250-ml bottle	Induction: 3% Maintenance: 0.5%-1.5%
Hemoglobin glutamer	Oxyglobin	13-gm/dl in 125-ml single-dose bags	Dog: One-time dose of 10-30 ml/kg IV at a rate not to exceed 10 ml/kg/hr Cat: One-time dose of 3-5 ml/kg slowly IV
Heparin sodium	Liquaemin (US); Hepalean (Canada)	1,000- and 10,000-U/ml injection	100-200 units/kg IV loading dose; then 100-300 units/kg SC q6-8h Low-dose prophylaxis (dog and cat): 70 U/kg SC q8-12h
Hetastarch	Hydroxyethyl starch (HES)	Injectable solution	Dog: 10-20 ml/kg/day IV Cat: 5-10 ml/kg/day IV
Hycodan	See Hydrocodone bitartrate		
Hydralazine	Apresoline	10-mg tablet; 20-mg/ml injection	Dog: 0.5 mg/kg (initial dose); titrate to 0.5-2 mg/kg PO q12h Cat: 2.5 mg/cat PO q12-24h
Hydrochlorothiazide	HydroDIURIL and generic	10- and 100-mg/ml oral solution and 25-, 50-, and 100-mg tablets	2-4 mg/kg PO q12h
Hydrocodone bitartrate	Hycodan	5-mg tablet; 1-mg/ml syrup	Dog: 0.22 mg/kg PO q4-8h Cat: No dose available

Drug Name	Other Names	Formulations Available	Dosage
Hydrocortisone	Cortef and generic	5-, 10-, 20-mg tablets	Replacement therapy: 1-2 mg/kg PO q12h Antiinflammatory: 2.5-5 mg/kg PO q12h
Hydrocortisone sodium succinate	Solu-Cortef	Various size vials for injection	Shock: 50-150 mg/kg IV Antiinflammatory: 5 mg/kg IV q12h
Hydromorphone	Dilaudid, Hydrostat, and generic	1-, 2-, 4-, 10-mg/ml injection Oral forms are available, but there is no assurance of oral absorption in dogs.	Dog: 0.22 mg/kg IM or SC. Repeat every 4-6 hr, or as needed for pain treatment Cat: 0.1-0.2 mg/kg IM or SC, q2-6hr, or as needed, or 0.05-0.1 mg/kg IV, q2-6hr
Hydroxyethyl starch (HES)	HES, Hetastarch	Injection	10-20 ml/kg IV to effect
Hydroxyurea	Hydrea	500-mg capsule	Dog: 50 mg/kg PO once daily, 3 days/wk Cat: 25 mg/kg PO once daily, 3 days/wk
Hydroxyzine	Atarax	10-, 25-, and 50-mg tablets; 2-mg/ml oral solution	Dog: 2 mg/kg q12h PO, IV, IM Cat: Safe dose not established
Imipenem	Primaxin	250- or 500-mg vials for injection	3-10 mg/kg q6-8h IV, SC, or IM; usually 5 mg/kg q6-8h IM, IV, or SC q6-8h
Imipramine	Tofranil	10-, 25-, and 50-mg tablets	Dog: 2-4 mg/kg PO q12-24h Cat: 0.5-1.0 mg/kg q12-24h PO
Indomethacin	Indocin	Safe dose has not been established	
Insulin, regular crystalline		100-U/ml injection	Ketoacidosis: animals <3 kg, 1 U/animal initially, then 1 U/animal q1h; animals 3-10 kg, 2 U/animal initially, then 1 U/animal q1h; animals >10 kg, 0.25 U/kg initially, then 0.1 U/kg IM q1h
Insulin, NPH isophane, Ultralente, or PZI		100-U/ml injection	Dog: Start with 0.75 U/kg q12h, SC and adjust dose with monitoring Cat: PZI or Ultralente initial dose 0.5-1.0 U/kg SC, usually twice/day
Interferon (interferon alpha, HuIFN-alpha)	Roferon	5- and 10-million U/vial	Dog: 2.5 million U/kg IV once daily for 3 days Cat: 1 million U/kg IV once daily for 5 consecutive days at 0, 14, and 60 days
Iodide	See Potassium iodide		
Ipecac syrup	Ipecac	Oral solution: 30-ml bottle	Dog: 3-6 ml/dog PO Cat: 2-6 ml/cat PO
Ipodate	Cholecystographic agent	50-mg capsules	Cat: 15 mg/kg q12h PO (usually 50 mg/cat q12h)
Iron	See Ferrous sulfate		
Isoflurane	AErrane	100-ml bottle	Induction: 5% Maintenance: 1.5%-2.5%
Isoproterenol	Isuprel	0.2-mg/ml ampules for injection	10 µg/kg IM, SC q6h; or dilute 1 mg in 500 ml of 5% dextrose or Ringer's solution and infuse IV 0.5-1 ml/min (1-2 µg/min) or to effect
Isosorbide dinitrate	Isordil, Isorbid, Sorbitrate	2.5-, 5-, 10-, 20-, 30-, and 40-mg tablets; 40-mg capsules	2.5-5 mg/animal PO q12h (or 0.22-1.1 mg/kg PO q12h)
Isosorbide mononitrate	Monoket	10- and 20-mg tablets	5 mg/dog PO two dose/day 7 hr apart
Isotretinoin	Accutane	10-, 20-, and 40-mg capsules	Dog: 1-3 mg/kg/day (up to a maximum recommended dose of 3-4 mg/kg/day PO) Cat: Dose not established

Continued

Drug Name	Other Names	Formulations Available	Dosage
Itraconazole	Sporanox and generic	100-mg capsules; 10-mg/ml oral solution	Dog: 2.5 mg/kg PO q12h or 5 mg/kg PO q24h For dermatophytes: 3 mg/kg/day PO for 15 days For *Malassezia*: 5 mg/kg q24h PO for 2 days, repeated each wk for 3 wk Cat: 1.5-3.0 mg/kg, up to 5 mg/kg PO for 15 days
Ivermectin	Heartgard, Ivomec, Eqvalan liquid	1% (10 mg/ml) injectable solution; 10-mg/ml oral solution; 18.7-mg/ml oral paste; 68-, 136-, and 272-μg tablets	Heartworm preventative: Dog: 6 μg/kg PO q30 days Cat: 24 μg/kg PO q30 days Microfilaricide: 50 μg/kg PO 2 wk after adulticide therapy Ectoparasite therapy (dog and cat): 200-300 μg/kg IM, SC, PO Endoparasites (dog and cat): 200-400 μg/kg SC, PO weekly Demodex therapy: Start with 100 μg/kg, then, increase to 600 μg/kg/day PO for 60-120 days
Kanamycin	Kantrim	200- and 500-mg/ml injection	10 mg/kg IV, IM, SC q6-8h; or 20 mg/kg q24h IV, IM, SC
Kaopectate (kaolin + pectin)	Kaopectate	Oral suspension 12 oz	1-2 ml/kg PO q2-6h
Ketamine	Ketalar, Ketavet, Vetalar	100-mg/ml injection solution	Dog: 5.5-22 mg/kg IV, IM (recommend adjunctive sedative or tranquilizer treatment) Cat: 2-25 mg/kg IV, IM (recommend adjunctive sedative or tranquilizer treatment)
Ketoconazole	Nizoral	200-mg tablet; 100-mg/ml oral suspension (only available in Canada)	Dog: 10-15 mg/kg PO q8-12h For *Malassezia canis* infection use 5 mg/kg PO q24h Hyperadrenocorticism: 15 mg/kg PO q12h Cat: 5-10 mg/kg PO q8-12h
Ketoprofen	Orudis-KT (human OTC tablet); Ketofen (veterinary injection)	12.5-mg tablet (OTC); 100-mg/ml injection	Dog, cat: 1 mg/kg PO q24h for up to 5 days or 2.0 mg/kg IV, IM, SC for one dose
Ketorolac tromethamine	Toradol	10-mg tablet; 15- and 30-mg/ml injection in 10% alcohol	Dog: 0.5 mg/kg PO, IM, IV q12h for not more than two doses
L-Dopa	*See* Levodopa		
Lactated Ringer's solution	Generic	250-, 500-, and 1,000-ml bags	Maintenance: 55-65 ml/kg/day IV For severe dehydration 50 ml/kg/hr IV or for shock 90 ml/kg IV (dogs) and 60-70 ml/kg IV (cats)
Lactulose	Chronulac, generic	10 gm/15 ml	Constipation: 1 ml/4.5 kg PO q8h (to effect) Hepatic encephalopathy: Dog: 0.5 ml/kg PO q8h Cat: 2.5-5 ml/cat PO q8h
Leucovorin (folinic acid)	Wellcovorin and generic	5-, 10-, 15-, and 25-mg tablets; 3- and 5-mg/ml injection	With methotrexate administration: 3 mg/m^2 IV, IM, PO Antidote for pyrimethamine toxicosis: 1 mg/kg PO q24h

Drug Name	Other Names	Formulations Available	Dosage
Levamisole	Levasole, Tamisol, Ergamisol	0.184-gm bolus; 11.7 gm/13-gm packet; 50-mg tablet (Ergamisol)	Dog (hookworms): 5-8 mg/kg PO once (up to 10 mg/kg PO for 2 days) Microfilaricide: 10 mg/kg PO q24h for 6-10 days Immunostimulant: 0.5-2 mg/kg PO three times/wk Cat: 4.4 mg/kg once PO For lungworms: 20-40 mg/kg PO q48h for five treatments
Levetiracetam	Keppra	250-, 500-, 750-mg tablets	Dog: Start with 20 mg/kg q8h PO; increase gradually as necessary Cat: 30 mg/kg q12h PO
Levodopa (L-dopa)	Larodopa, L-dopa	100-, 250-, and 500-mg tablets or capsules	Hepatic encephalopathy: 6.8 mg/kg initially then 1.4 mg/kg q6h
Levothyroxine sodium (T$_4$)	Soloxine, Thyro-Tabs, Synthroid	0.1- to 0.8-mg tablets (in 0.1-mg increments)	Dog: 18-22 μg/kg PO q12h (adjust dose via monitoring) Cat: 10-20 μg/kg/day PO (adjust dose via monitoring)
Lidocaine	Xylocaine and generic brands	5-, 10-, 15-, and 20-mg/ml injection	Antiarrhythmic: Dog: 2-4 mg/kg IV (to a maximum dose of 8 mg/kg over 10-min period); 25-75 μg/kg/min IV infusion; 6 mg/kg IM q1.5hr Cat: 0.25-0.75 mg/kg IV slowly; or 10-40 μg/kg/min infusion For epidural (dog and cat): 4.4 mg/kg of 2% solution
Lincomycin	Lincocin	100-, 200-, and 500-mg tablets	Dog and cat: 15-25 mg/kg PO q12h For canine pyoderma: Doses as low as 10 mg/kg q12h have been used
Linezolid	Zyvox	400- and 600-mg tablets; 20-mg/ml oral suspension; 2-mg/ml injection	Dog, cat: 10 mg/kg q8-12h PO, IV
Liothyronine (T$_3$)	Cytomel	60-μg tablet	4.4 μg/kg PO q8h For T$_3$ suppression test (cats): Collect presample for T$_4$ and T$_3$; administer 25 μg q8h for seven doses, then collect post samples for T$_3$ and T$_4$ after last dose
Lisinopril	Prinivil, Zestril	2.5-, 5-, 10-, 20-, and 40-mg tablets	Dog: 0.5 mg/kg PO q24h Cat: No dose established
Lithium carbonate	Lithotabs	150-, 300-, and 600-mg capsules; 300-mg tablet; 300-mg/5 ml syrup	Dog: 10 mg/kg PO q12h Cat: Not recommended
Lomotil	*See* Diphenoxylate		
Lomustine	CCNU, CeeNU	10-, 40-, 100-mg capsules	Dog: 70-90 mg/m², every 4 wk PO For brain tumors: Use 60-90 mg/m² q6-8wk PO Cat: 50-60 mg/m² PO q3-6wk or 10 mg/cat PO every 3 wk
Loperamide	Imodium and generic	2-mg tablet; 0.2-mg/ml oral liquid	Dog: 0.1 mg/kg PO q8-12h Cat: 0.08-0.16 mg/kg PO q12h
Lufenuron	Program	45-, 90-, 135-, 204.9-, and 409.8-mg tablets; 135- and 270-mg suspension per unit pack	Dog: 10 mg/kg PO q30 days Cat: 30 mg/kg PO q30 days, 10 mg/kg SC q6mo
Lufenuron + milbemycin oxime	Sentinel tablets and Flavor Tabs	Milbemycin/lufenuron ratio is as follows: 2.3/46-mg tablets; 5.75/115-11.5/230-, and 23/460-mg Flavor Tabs	Administer 1 tablet q30 days; each tablet formulated for size of dog
Luteinizing hormone	*See* Gonadorelin		

Continued

Drug Name	Other Names	Formulations Available	Dosage
L-LYSINE	Enisyl-F	250-mg/ml paste	Paste formulation: 1-2 ml/cat, PO, to adult cats (approximately 400 mg/cat) and 1 ml/cat, PO, for kittens
Magnesium citrate	Citroma, Citro-Nesia (Citro-Mag in Canada)	Oral solution	2-4 ml/kg PO
Magnesium hydroxide	Milk of Magnesia	Oral liquid	Antacid: 5-10 ml/kg PO q4-6h Cathartic: Dog: 15-50 PO ml/kg Cat: 2-6 ml/cat PO q24h
Magnesium sulfate	Epsom salts	Crystals, many generic preparations	Dog: 8-25 gm/dog PO q24h; for treating arrhythmias: 0.15-0.3 mEq/kg slowly IV over 5-15 min followed by 0.75-1.0 mEq/kg/day; fluid supplementation: 0.75-1.0 mEq/kg/day Cat: 2-5 gm/cat PO q24h
Mannitol	Osmitrol	5%-25% solution for injection	Diuretic: 1 gm/kg of 5%-25% solution IV to maintain urine flow Glaucoma or central nervous system edema: 0.25-2 gm/kg of 15%-25% solution IV over 30-60 min (repeat in 6 hr if necessary)
Marbofloxacin	Marbocyl, Zeniquim	25-, 50-, 100-, and 200-mg tablets	Dog, cat: 2.75-5.55 mg/kg PO q24h
Maropitant	Cerenia	10-mg/ml injection; 16-, 24-, 60-, 160-mg tablets	Dog: 1 mg/kg SC once daily for up to 5 days; 2 mg/kg PO once daily for up to 5 days For motion sickness: 8 mg/kg PO once daily for up to 2 days Cat: 1 mg/kg PO, SC, or IV once daily (same dose for all indications)
MCT oil	MCT oil (many sources)	Oral liquid	1-2 ml/kg/day in food
Mebendazole	Telmintic	Each gram of powder contains 40 mg	22 mg/kg (with food) q24h for 3 days
Meclizine	Antivert, generic	12.5-, 25-, and 50-mg tablets	Dog: 25 mg PO q24h (for motion sickness, administer 1 hr before traveling) Cat: 12.5 mg PO q24h
Meclofenamic acid (meclofenamate sodium)	Arquel, Meclomen	50- and 100-mg capsules	Dog: 1 mg/kg/day PO for up to 5 days Cat: Not recommended
Medium-chain triglycerides	See MCT oil		
Medroxyprogesterone acetate	Depo-Provera (injection); Provera (tablets)	150- and 400-mg/ml suspension injection; 2.5-, 5-, and 10-mg tablets	1.1-2.2 mg/kg IM q7days; for behavioral use 10-20 mg/kg SC; for prostate 3-5 mg/kg SC, IM every 3-4 weeks
Megestrol acetate	Ovaban	5-mg tablet	Dog: Proestrus: 2 mg/kg PO q24h for 8 days Anestrus: 0.5 mg/kg PO q24h for 30 days Behavior: 2-4 mg/kg q24h for 8 days (reduce dose for maintenance) Cat: Dermatologic therapy or urine spraying: 2.5-5 mg/cat PO q24h for 1 wk, then reduce to 5 mg once or twice/wk Suppress estrus: 5 mg/cat/day for 3 days, then 2.5-5 mg once/wk for 10 wk
Melarsomine	Immiticide	25-mg/ml injection; after reconstitution retains potency for 24 hr	Administer via deep IM injection. Class 1-2 dogs: 2.5 mg/kg/day for 2 consecutive days Class 3 dogs: 2.5 mg/kg once, then in 1 month two additional doses 24 hr apart

Drug Name	Other Names	Formulations Available	Dosage
Meloxicam	Metacam (veterinary); Mobic (human)	Veterinary: 1.5-mg/ml oral suspension and 5-mg/ml injection Human: 7.5-mg tablets	Dog: 0.2 mg/kg initially PO, then 0.1 mg/kg q24h PO thereafter; injection 0.1 mg/kg IV or SC Cat: 0.3 mg/kg SC one-time injection; 0.05 mg/kg q24-48h PO for chronic use
Melphalan	Alkeran	2-mg tablet	1.5 mg/m^2 (or 0.1-0.2 mg/kg) PO q24h for 7-10 days (repeat every 3 wk)
Meperidine	Demerol	50- and 100-mg tablets; 10-mg/ml syrup; 25-, 50-, 75-, and 100-mg/ml injection	Dog: 5-10 mg/kg IV, IM as often as q2-3h (or as needed) Cat: 3-5 mg/kg IV, IM q2-4h (or as needed)
Mepivacaine	Carbocaine-V	2% (20 mg/ml) injection	Variable dose for local infiltration. For epidural: 0.5 ml of 2% solution q30sec until reflexes are absent
6-Mercaptopurine	Purinethol	50-mg tablet	Dog: 50 mg/m^2 PO q24h Cat: Do not use
Meropenem	Merrem	500 mg in 20-ml vial, or 1-gm vial in 30-ml vial for injection	Dogs, cats: 8.5 mg/kg SC q12h up to 12 mg/kg SC q12h or 24 mg/kg IV q12h
Mesalamine	Asacol, Mesasal, Pentasa	400-mg tablet; 250-mg capsule	Veterinary dose has not been established, the usual human oral dose is 400-500 mg q6-8h (also see Sulfasalazine, Olsalazine)
Metaproterenol	Alupent, Metaprel	10- and 20-mg tablets; 5-mg/ml syrup; inhalers	0.325-0.65 mg/kg PO q4-6h
Methadone	Methadose and generic	2-mg/ml oral solution; 10- and 20-mg/ml solution for injection; 5-, 10-, 40-mg tablets	Dog: 0.5-2.2 mg/kg IV, SC, IM, or 0.5-1.0 mg/kg IV q3-4h for analgesia Cat: 0.2-0.5 mg/kg SC or IM, or 0.05-0.1 mg/kg up to 0.2 mg/kg IV q3-4h for analgesia
Methazolamide	Neptazane	25- and 50-mg tablets	2-3 mg/kg PO q8-12h
Methenamine hippurate	Hiprex, Urex	1-gm tablet	Dog: 500 mg/dog PO q12h Cat: 250 mg/cat PO q12h
Methenamine mandelate	Mandelamine and generic	1-gm tablet; granules for oral solution; 50- and 100-mg/ml oral suspension	10-20 mg/kg PO q8-12h
Methimazole	Tapazole (human brand); Felimazole (veterinary brand)	5- and 10-mg tablets	Cat: 1.25 mg to 2.5 mg per cat, q12h, PO then adjust by monitoring T$_4$ 1.25 mg to 2.5 mg methimazole is administered twice daily
DL-Methionine	See Racemethionine		
Methocarbamol	Robaxin-V	500- and 750-mg tablets; 100-mg/ml injection	44 mg/kg PO q8h on the first day then 22-44 mg/kg PO q8h
Methohexital	Brevital	0.5-, 2.5-, and 5-gm vials for injection	3-6 mg/kg IV (give slowly to effect)
Methotrexate	MTX, Mexate, Folex, Rheumatrex, generic	2.5-mg tablet; 2.5- or 25-mg/ml injection	2.5-5 mg/m^2 PO q48h (dose depends on specific protocol) or Dog: 0.3-0.5 mg/kg IV once/wk Cat: 0.8 mg/kg IV q2-3wk
Methoxamine	Vasoxyl	20-mg/ml injection	200-250 µg/kg IM or 40-80 µg/kg IV
Methoxyflurane	Metofane	4-oz bottle for inhalation	Induction: 3% Maintenance: 0.5%-1.5%
Methylene Blue 0.1%	Generic, also called New Methylene Blue	1% solution (10 mg/ml)	1.5 mg/kg IV, slowly
Methylprednisolone	Medrol	1-, 2-, 4-, 8-, 18-, and 32-mg tablets	0.22-0.44 mg/kg PO q12-24h

Continued

Drug Name	Other Names	Formulations Available	Dosage
Methylprednisolone acetate	Depo-Medrol	20- or 40-mg/ml suspension for injection	Dog: 1 mg/kg (or 20-40 mg/dog) IM q1-3wk Cat: 10-20 mg/cat IM q1-3wk
Methylprednisolone sodium succinate	Solu-Medrol	1- and 2-gm and 125- and 500-mg vials for injection	For emergency use: 30 mg/kg IV and repeat at 15 mg/kg IV in 2-6 hr
4-Methylpyrazole (fomepizole)	Antizole, Antizol-Vet (Fomepizole)	5% solution	See Fomepizol for dose
Methyltestosterone	Android, generic	10- and 25-mg tablets	Dog: 5-25 mg/dog PO q24-48h Cat: 2.5-5 mg/cat PO q24-48h
Metoclopramide	Reglan, Clopra, and others	5- and 10-mg tablets; 1-mg/ml oral solution; 5-mg/ml injection	0.2-0.5 mg/kg IV, IM, PO q6-8h or IV loading dose at 0.4 mg/kg followed by 0.3 mg/kg/hr IV
Metoprolol tartrate	Lopressor	50- and 100-mg tablets; 1-mg/ml injection	Dog: 5-50 mg/dog (0.5-1.0 mg/kg) PO q8h Cat: 2-15 mg/cat PO q8h
Metronidazole and metronidazole benzoate	Flagyl and generic	250- and 500-mg tablets; 50-mg/ml suspension; 5-mg/ml injection; the benzoate form is not available commercially and must be obtained from a compounding pharmacist	For anaerobes: Dog: 15 mg/kg PO q12h or 12 mg/kg q8h Cat: 10-25 mg/kg PO q24h For Giardia: Dog: 12-15 mg/kg PO q12h for 8 days Cat: 17 mg/kg (or approximately ⅓ of a 250 mg tablet per cat) q24h for 8 days
Mexiletine	Mexitil	150-, 200-, and 250-mg capsules	Dog: 5-8 mg/kg PO q8-12h (usually in combination with solatol, or beta-blocker) Cat: Do not use
Mibolerone	Cheque-drops	55-µg/ml oral solution	Dog: 0.45-11.3 kg, 30 µg; 11.8-22.7 kg, 60 µg; 23-45.3 kg, 120 µg; >45.8 kg, 180 µg; or approximately 2.6-5 µg/kg/day PO Cat: Safe dose not established
Midazolam	Versed	5-mg/ml injection	Dog: 0.1-0.25 mg/kg IV, IM (or 0.1-0.3 mg/kg/hr IV infusion) Cat: 0.05 mg/kg IV; or 0.3-0.6 mg/kg IV (combine with 3 mg/kg ketamine)
Milbemycin oxime	Interceptor and Interceptor Flavor Tabs	23-, 11.5-, 5.75-, and 2.3-mg tablets	Dog: Microfilaricide; 0.5 mg/kg; Demodex: 2 mg/kg PO q24h for 60-120 days Heartworm prevention: 0.5 mg/kg PO q30 days Cat: 2 mg/kg q30 days PO
Milk of Magnesia	See Magnesium hydroxide		
Mineral oil	Generic	Oral liquid	Dog: 10-50 ml/dog PO q12h Cat: 10-25 ml/cat PO q12h
Minocycline hydrochloride	Minocin	50-, 75-, and 100-mg tablets or capsules; 10-mg/ml oral suspension	Dog: 5-10 mg/kg, PO, q12h Cat: 8.8 mg/kg, PO, once daily, or 50 mg per cat PO, once daily
Misoprostol	Cytotec	0.1-mg (100 µg), 0.2-mg (200 µg) tablets	Dog: 2-5 µg/kg PO q6-8h; for atopic dermatitis 5 µg/kg q8h PO Cat: Dose not established
Mithramycin	See Plicamycin (Mithracin)		
Mitotane (o,p'-DDD)	Lysodren	500-mg tablet	Dog: For pituitary-dependent hypercorticism: 50 mg/kg/day (in divided doses) PO for 5-10 days, then 50-70 mg/kg/wk PO For adrenal tumor: 50-75 mg/kg day for 10 days, then 75-100 mg/kg/wk PO
Mitoxantrone	Novantrone	2-mg/ml injection	Dog: 6 mg/m² IV q21 days Cat: 6.5 mg/m² IV q21 days

Drug Name	Other Names	Formulations Available	Dosage
Morphine	Generic	1- and 15-mg/ml injection; 30- and 60-mg delayed-release tablets	Dog: 0.1-1 mg/kg IV, IM, SC (dose is escalated as needed for pain relief) q4-6hr Dog: 0.5 mg/kg q2hr IV, IM, or CRI 0.2 mg/kg followed by 0.1 mg/kg/hr IV Epidural: 0.1 mg/kg Cat: 0.1 mg/kg q3-6h IM, SC (or as needed)
Moxidectin	Cydectin	Injection	Dog: Heartworm prevention: 3 µg/kg Endoparasites: 25-300 µg/kg Demodex: 400 µg/kg/day up to 500 µg/kg/day for 21-22 wk
Moxifloxacin	Avelox	400-mg tablet	10 mg/kg q24h PO
Myochrysine	*See* Gold sodium thiomalate		
Mycophenolate	Cell Cept	250-mg capsule	Dog: 10-20 mg/kg q8h PO Cat: 10 mg/kg q12h, PO
Naloxone	Narcan	20- or 400-µg/ml injection	0.01-0.04 mg/kg IV, IM, SC as needed to reverse opiate
Naltrexone	Trexan	50-mg tablet	For behavior problems: 2.2 mg/kg PO q12h
Nandrolone decanoate	Deca-Durabolin	Nandrolone decanoate injection: 50-, 100-, and 200-mg/ml	Dog: 1-1.5 mg/kg/wk IM Cat: 1 mg/cat/wk IM
Naproxen	Naprosyn, Naxen, Aleve (naproxen sodium)	220-mg tablet (OTC); 25-mg/ml suspension liquid; 250-, 375-, and 500-mg tablets (Rx)	Dog: 5 mg initially, then 2 mg/kg q48h Cat: Not recommended
Neomycin	Biosal	500-mg bolus; 200-mg/ml oral liquid	10-20 mg/kg PO q6-12h
Neostigmine bromide and neostigmine methylsulfate	Prostigmin; Stiglyn	15-mg tablet (neostigmine bromide); 0.25- and 0.5-mg/ml injection (neostigmine methylsulfate)	2 mg/kg/day PO (in divided doses, to effect) Injection: Antimyasthenic: 10 µg/kg IM, SC, as needed Antidote for nondepolarizing neuromuscular block: 40 µg/kg IM, SC Diagnostic aid for myasthenia gravis: 40 µg/kg IM or 20 µg/kg IV
Nitenpyram	Capstar	11.4- or 57-mg tablet	1 mg/kg PO daily as needed to kill fleas
Nitrates	*See* Nitroglycerin, Isosorbide dinitrate, or Nitroprusside		
Nitrofurantoin	Macrodantin, Furalan, Furatoin, Furadantin, or generic	Macrodantin and generic 25-, 50-, and 100-mg capsules; Furalan, Furatoin, and generic 50- and 100-mg tablets; Furadantin 5-mg/ml oral suspension	10 mg/kg/day divided into four daily treatments, then 1 mg/kg PO at night
Nitroglycerin ointment	Nitrol, Nitro-Bid, Nitrostat	0.5-, 0.8-, 1-, 5-, and 10-mg/ml injection; 2% ointment; transdermal systems (0.2 mg/hr patch)	Dog: 4-12 mg (up to 15 mg) topically q12h Cat: 2-4 mg topically q12h (or ¼ inch of ointment per cat)
Nitroprusside	Nitropress	50-mg vial for injection	1-5, up to a maximum of 10 µg/kg/min IV infusion. Start with 2 mcg/kg/min and increase gradually until desired blood pressure is attained. At doses >10 mcg/kg/min seizures are more likely.
Nizatidine	Axid	150- and 300-mg capsules	Dog: 5 mg/kg PO q24h
o,p'-DDD	*See* Mitotane (Lysodren)		

Continued

Drug Name	Other Names	Formulations Available	Dosage
Olsalazine	Dipentum	500-mg tablet	Dose not established (usual human dose is 500 mg or 5-10 mg/kg PO twice daily)
Omeprazole	Prilosec (formerly Losec), Gastrogard (equine paste)	20-mg capsule	Dog: 20 mg/dog PO once daily (or 0.7 mg/kg q24h) Cat: 0.5-0.7 mg/kg q24h PO
Ondansetron	Zofran	4- and 8-mg tablets; 2-mg/ml injection	0.5-1.0 mg/kg IV, PO 30 minutes before administration of cancer drugs
Orbifloxacin	Orbax	5.7-, 22.7-, and 68-mg tablets, and 30 mg/mL oral suspension	Dogs and cats (tablets): 2.5-7.5 mg/kg PO once daily; cats: 7.5 mg/kg once daily (oral suspension)
Ormetoprim	See Primor (ormetoprim-sulfadimethoxine)		
Oxacillin	Prostaphlin and generic	250- and 500-mg capsules; 50-mg/ml oral solution	22-40 mg/kg PO q8h
Oxazepam	Serax	15-mg tablet	Cat: Appetite stimulant: 2.5 mg/cat PO
Oxtriphylline	Choledyl-SA	400- and 600-mg tablet (oral solutions and syrup available in Canada but not U.S.)	Dog: 47 mg/kg (equivalent to 30 mg/kg theophylline) PO q12h
Oxybutynin chloride	Ditropan	5-mg tablet	Dog: 5 mg/dog PO q6-8h
Oxymetholone	Anadrol	50-mg tablet	1-5 mg/kg/day PO
Oxymorphone	Numorphan	1.5- and 1-mg/ml injection	Dog: Analgesia: 0.1-0.2 mg/kg IV, SC, IM (as needed), redose with 0.05-0.1 mg/kg q1-2h Cat: 0.03 mg/kg bolus, followed by 0.02 mg/kg q2h Preanesthetic: 0.025-0.05 mg/kg IM, SC
Oxytetracycline	Terramycin	250-mg tablets; 100- and 200-mg/ml injection	7.5-10 mg/kg IV q12h; 20 mg/kg PO q12h
Oxytocin	Pitocin and Syntocinon (nasal solution) and generic	10- and 20-U/ml injection; 40-U/ml nasal solution	Dog: 5-20 U/dog SC, IM (repeat every 30 min for primary inertia) Cat: 2.5-3 U/cat SC, IM (repeat every 30 min)
2-PAM	See Pralidoxime chloride		
Pamidronate	Aredia	30-, 60-, 90-mg vials for injection	Dog: 2 mg/kg IV, SC For treatment of cholecalciferol toxicosis: 1.3-2 mg/kg for two treatments
Pancreatic enzyme	See Pancrelipase		
Pancrelipase	Viokase	16,800 U of lipase, 70,000 U of protease, and 70,000 U of amylase per 0.7 gm; also capsules and tablets	Mix 2 tsp powder with food per 20 kg body weight or 1-3 tsp/0.45 kg of food 20 min before feeding
Pancuronium bromide	Pavulon	1- and 2-mg/ml injection	0.1 mg/kg IV or start with 0.01 mg/kg and additional 0.01-mg/kg doses every 30 min
Pantoprazole	Protonix	40-mg tablets, 0.4-mg/ml vials for injection	Dog, cat: 0.5 mg/kg q24h IV or 0.5-1 mg/kg IV infusion over 24 hr
Paregoric	Corrective mixture	2 mg morphine per 5 ml of paregoric	0.05-0.06 mg/kg PO q12h
Paroxetine	Paxil	10-, 20-, 30-, and 40-mg tablets	Cat: 1/8 to 1/4 of a 10-mg tablet daily PO
D-Penicillamine	Cuprimine, Depen	125- and 250-mg capsules and 250-mg tablets	10-15 mg/kg PO q12h
Penicillin G benzathine	Benza-pen and other names	150,000 U/ml, combined with 150,000 U/ml of procaine penicillin G	24,000 U/kg IM q48h
Penicillin G potassium; penicillin G sodium	Many brands	5- to 20-million unit vials	20,000-40,000 U/kg IV, IM q6-8h
Penicillin G procaine	Generic	300,000 U/ml suspension	20,000-40,000 U/kg IM q12-24h
Penicillin V	Pen-Vee	250- and 500-mg tablets	10 mg/kg PO q8h

Drug Name	Other Names	Formulations Available	Dosage
Pentobarbital	Nembutal and generic	50 mg/ml	25-30 mg/kg IV to effect; or 2-15 mg/kg IV to effect, followed by 0.2-1.0 mg/kg/hr IV
Pentoxifylline	Trental	400-mg tablet	Dog: For use in canine dermatology and for vasculitis, 10 mg/kg PO q12h and up to 15 mg/kg q8h Cat: ¼ of 400-mg tab PO q8-12h
Pepto Bismol	*See* Bismuth subsalicylate		
Phenobarbital	Luminal and generic	15-, 30-, 60-, and 100-mg tablets; 30-, 60-, 65-, and 130-mg/ml injection; 4-mg/ml oral elixir solution	Dog: 2-8 mg/kg PO q12h Cat: 2-4 mg/kg PO q12h Dog and cat: Adjust dose by monitoring plasma concentration Status epilepticus: Administer in increments of 10-20 mg/kg IV (to effect)
Phenoxybenzamine	Dibenzyline	10-mg capsule	Dog: 0.25 mg/kg PO q8-12h or 0.5 mg/kg q24h Cat: 2.5 mg/cat q8-12h or 0.5 mg/cat PO q12h (in cats, doses as high as 0.5 mg/kg IV have been used to relax urethral smooth muscle)
Phentolamine	Regitine (Rogitine in Canada)	5-mg vial for injection	0.02-0.1 mg/kg IV
Phenylbutazone	Butazolidin and generic	100-, 200-, 400-mg and 1-gm tablets; 200-mg/ml injection	Dog: 15-22 mg/kg PO, IV q8-12h (44 mg/kg/day) (800 mg/dog maximum) Cat: 6-8 mg/kg IV, PO q12h
Phenylephrine	Neo-Synephrine	10-mg/ml injection; 1% nasal solution	0.01 mg/kg IV q15min 0.1 mg/kg IM, SC q15min
Phenylpropanolamine	PPA, Propalin, Proin PPA	25-, 50-, and 75-mg tablets and 25-mg/ml liquid	Dog: 1 mg/kg q12h PO and increase to 1.5-2.0 mg/kg as needed q8h PO
Phenytoin	Dilantin	30- and 125-mg/ml oral suspension; 30- and 100-mg capsules; 50-mg/ml injection	Antiepileptic dog: 20-35 mg/kg q8h Antiarrhythmic: 30 mg/kg PO q8h or 10 mg/kg IV over 5 min
Physostigmine	Antilirium	1-mg/ml injection	0.02 mg/kg IV q12h
Phytomenadione	*See* Vitamin K₁		
Phytonadione	*See* Vitamin K₁		
Pimobendan	Vetmedin	2.5- and 5-mg capsules (Europe and Canada); 1.25-, 2.5-, 5-mg chewable tablets (US)	Dog: 0.05 mg/kg/day in divided treatments q12h Cat: 0.25 mg/kg q12h, PO; 1.25 mg per cat q12h also has been used
Piperacillin	Pipracil	2-, 3-, 4-, and 40-gm vials for injection	40 mg/kg IV or IM q6h
Piperazine	Many	860-mg powder; 140-mg capsule, 170-, 340-, and 800-mg/ml oral solution	44-66 mg/kg PO administered once
Piroxicam	Feldene and generic	10-mg capsule	Dog: 0.3 mg/kg PO q48h Cat: 0.3 mg/kg q24h PO
Pitressin (ADH)	*See* Vasopressin, Desmopressin acetate		
Plicamycin (old name is mithramycin)	Mithracin	2.5-mg injection	Dog: Antineoplastic: 25-30 µg/kg day IV (slow infusion) for 8-10 days Antihypercalcemic: 25 µg/kg/day IV (slow infusion) over 4 hr Cat: Not recommended
Polyethylene glycol electrolyte solution	GoLYTELY	Oral solution	25 ml/kg PO repeat in 2-4 hr PO

Continued

Drug Name	Other Names	Formulations Available	Dosage
Polysulfated glycosaminoglycan (PSGAG)	Adequan Canine	100-mg/ml injection in 5-ml vial (for horses vials are 250 mg/ml)	4.4 mg/kg IM twice weekly for up to 4 wk
Potassium bromide (KBr)	No commercial formulation	Usually prepared as oral solution Must be compounded	Dog and cat: 30-40 mg/kg PO q24h If administered without phenobarbital, higher doses of up to 40-50 mg/kg may be needed. Adjust doses by monitoring plasma concentrations. Loading doses of 600-800 mg/kg divided over 3-4 days have been administered.
Potassium chloride (KCI)	Generic	Various concentrations for injection (usually 2 mEq/ml); oral suspension and oral solution	0.5 mEq potassium/kg/day; or supplement 10-40 mEq/500 ml of fluids, depending on serum potassium
Potassium citrate	Generic, Urocit-K	5-mEq tablet; some forms are in combination with potassium chloride	0.5 mEq/kg/day PO
Potassium gluconate	Kaon, Tumil-K, generic	2-mEq tablet; 500-mg tablet; Kaon elixir is 20-mg/15-ml elixir	Dog: 0.5 mEq/kg PO q12-24h Cat: 2-8 mEq/day PO divided twice daily
Potassium iodide			Cat: 30-100 mg/cat daily (in single or divided doses) for 10-14 days
Pralidoxime chloride (2-PAM)	2-PAM, Protopam Chloride	50-mg/ml injection	20 mg/kg q8-12h (initial dose) IV slow or IM
Praziquantel	Droncit	23- and 34-mg tablets; 56.8-mg/ml injection	Dog (PO): <6.8 kg, 7.5 mg/kg, once; >6.8 kg, 5 mg/kg, once (IM, SC): <2.3 kg, 7.5 mg/kg, once; 2.7-4.5 kg, 6.3 mg/kg, once; >5 kg, 5 mg/kg, once Cat (PO): <1.8 kg, 6.3 mg/kg, once; >1.8 kg, 5 mg/kg, once (for *Paragonimus* use 25 mg/kg q8h for 2-3 days) (IM, SC): 5 mg/kg
Prazosin	Minipress	1-, 2-, and 5-mg capsules	0.5- and 2-mg/dog or cat (1 mg/15 kg) PO q8-12h
Prednisolone	Delta-Cortef and many others	5- and 20-mg tablets	Dog (cat often requires two times dog dose) Antiinflammatory: 0.5-1 mg/kg IV, IM, PO q12-24h initially, then taper to q48h Immunosuppressive: 2.2-4.4 mg/kg/day IV, IM, PO initially, then taper to 2-4 mg/kg q48h Replacement therapy: 0.2-0.3 mg/kg/day PO
Prednisolone sodium succinate	Solu-Delta-Cortef	100- and 200-mg vials for injection (10 and 50 mg/ml)	Shock: 15-30 mg/kg IV (repeat in 4-6 hr) Central nervous system trauma: 15-30 mg/kg IV, taper to 1-2 mg/kg q12h
Prednisone	Deltasone and generic; Meticorten for injection	1-, 2.5-, 5-, 10-, 20-, 25-, and 50-mg tablets; 1-mg/ml syrup (Liquid Pred in 5% alcohol) and 1-mg/ml oral solution (in 5% alcohol); 10- and 40-mg/ml prednisone suspension for injection	Same as prednisolone, except that prednisone is not recommended for cats
Primidone	Mylepsin, Neurosyn (Mysoline in Canada)	50- and 250-mg tablets	8-10 mg/kg PO q8-12h as initial dose, then is adjusted via monitoring to 10-15 mg/kg q8h
Primor (ormetoprim + sulfadimethoxine)	Primor	Combination tablet (ormetoprim + sulfadimethoxine)	27 mg/kg on first day, followed by 13.5 mg/kg PO q24h
Procainamide	Pronestyl, generic	250-, 375-, 500-mg tablets or capsules; 100- and 500-mg/ml injection	Dog: 10-30 mg/kg PO q6h (to a maximum dose of 40 mg/kg), 8-20 mg/kg IV IM; 25-50 µg/kg/min IV infusion Cat: 3-8 mg/kg IM, PO q6-8h

Drug Name	Other Names	Formulations Available	Dosage
Prochlorperazine	Compazine	5-, 10-, and 25-mg tablets (prochlorperazine maleate); 5-mg/ml injection (prochlorperazine edisylate)	0.1-0.5 mg/kg IM, SC q6-8h
Progesterone, repositol	*See* Medroxyprogesterone acetate		
Promethazine	Phenergan	6.25- and 25-mg/5-ml syrup; 12.5-, 25-, 50-mg tablets; 25- and 50-mg/ml injection	0.2-0.4 mg/kg IV, IM PO q6-8h (up to a maximum dose of 1 mg/kg)
Propantheline bromide	Pro-Banthine	7.5- and 15-mg tablet	0.25-0.5 mg/kg PO q8-12h
Propiomazine	Tranvet	5-, 10-mg/ml injection or 20-mg tablet	1.1-4.4 mg/kg q12-24h PO or 0.1-1.1 mg/kg IM, IV (range of dose depends on degree of sedation needed)
Propofol	Rapinovet and PropoFlo (veterinary); Diprivan (human)	1% (10 mg/ml) injection in 20-ml ampules	6.6 mg/kg IV slowly over 60 seconds; constant-rate IV infusions have been used at 5 mg/kg slowly IV, followed by 100-400 µg/kg/min IV
Propranolol	Inderal	10-, 20-, 40-, 60-, 80-, and 90-mg tablets; 1-mg/ml injection; 4- and 8-mg/ml oral solution	Dog: 20-60 µg/kg over 5-10 min IV; 0.2-1 mg/kg PO q8h (titrate dose to effect) Cat: 0.4-1.2 mg/kg (2.5-5 mg/cat) PO q8h
Propylthiouracil (PTU)	Generic, Propyl-Thyracil	50- and 100-mg tablets	11 mg/kg PO q12h
Prostaglandin F2 alpha (dinoprost)	Lutalyse	5-mg/ml solution for injection	Pyometra: Dog: 0.1-0.2 mg/kg SC once daily for 5 days Cat: 0.1-0.25 mg/kg SC once daily for 5 days Abortion: Dog: 0.025-0.05 mg (25-50 µg)/kg IM q12h Cat: 0.5-1 mg/kg IM for two injections
Pseudoephedrine	Sudafed and many others (some formulations have been discontinued)	30- and 60-mg tablets; 120-mg capsule; 6-mg/ml syrup	0.2-0.4 mg/kg (or 15-60 mg/dog) PO q8-12h
Psyllium	Metamucil and others	Available as powder	1 tsp/5-10 kg (added to each meal)
Pyrantel pamoate	Nemex, Strongid	180-mg/ml paste and 50-mg/ml suspension	Dog: 5 mg/kg PO once and repeat in 7-10 days Cat: 20 mg/kg PO once
Pyridostigmine bromide	Mestinon, Regonol	12-mg/ml oral syrup; 60-mg tablet; 5-mg/ml injection	Dog: Antimyasthenic: 0.02-0.04 mg/kg IV q2h or 0.5-3 mg/kg PO q8-12h, or CRI of 0.01-0.03 mg/kg/hr Antidote (nondepolarizing muscle relaxant): 0.15-0.3 mg/kg IM, IV Cat: 0.1-0.25 mg/kg q24h, PO
Pyrimethamine	Daraprim, ReBalance (Equine)	25-mg tablet Equine formulation (ReBalance) contains 250 mg sulfadiazine and 12.5 mg pyrimethamine per ml	Dog: 1 mg/kg PO q24h for 14-21 days (5 days for *Neospora caninum*) Cat: 0.5-1 mg/kg PO q24h for 14-28 days
Quinidine gluconate	Quinaglute, Duraquin	324-mg tablets; 80-mg/ml injection	Dog: 6-20 mg/kg IM q6h; 6-20 mg/kg PO q6-8h (of base)
Quinidine sulfate	Cin-Quin, Quinora	100-, 200-, and 300-mg tablets; 200- and 300-mg capsules; 20-mg/ml injection	Dog: 6-20 mg/kg PO q6-8h (of base); 5-10 mg/kg IV
Quinidine polygalacturonate	Cardioquin	275-mg tablet	Dog: 6-20 mg/kg PO q6h (of base) (275 mg quinidine polygalacturonate = 167 mg quinidine base)
Racemethionine (DL-methionine)	Uroeze, MethioForm, and generic. Human forms include Pedameth, Uracid, and generic	500-mg tablets and powders added to animal's food; 75-mg/5 ml pediatric oral solution; 200-mg capsule	Dog: 150-300 mg/kg/day PO Cat: 1-1.5 gm/cat PO (added to food each day)

Continued

Drug Name	Other Names	Formulations Available	Dosage
Ranitidine	Zantac	75-, 150-, and 300-mg tablets; 150- and 300-mg capsules; 25-mg/ml injection	Dog: 2 mg/kg IV, PO q8h Cat: 2.5 mg/kg IV q12h, 3.5 mg/kg PO q12h
Retinoids	See Isotretinoin (Accutane), Retinol (Aquasol-A), or Etretinate (Tegison)		
Retinol	See Vitamin A (Aquasol-A)		
Riboflavin (vitamin B₂)	See Vitamin B₂		
Rifampin	Rifadin	150- and 300-mg capsules	Dog: 5 mg/kg q12h, PO
Ringer's solution	Generic	250-, 500-, and 1000-ml bags for infusion	55-65 ml/kg/day IV, SC, or IP; 50 ml/kg/hr IV for severe dehydration
Ronidazole	No formulation available; must be compounded	There are no commercial formulations. However, compounding pharmacies have prepared formulations for cats.	Dog: Dose not established Cat: 30 mg/kg/day PO for 2 wk. Dose of 30 mg/kg per day may be divided into twice daily treatments
Salicylate	See Aspirin, acetylsalicylic acid		
Selegiline (deprenyl)	Anipryl (also known as deprenyl, and l-deprenyl); human dose form is Eldepryl	2-, 5-, 10-, 15-, and 30-mg tablets	Dog: Begin with 1 mg/kg PO q24h; if there is no response within 2 months, increase dose to maximum of 2 mg/kg PO q24h Cat: 0.25-0.5 mg/kg q12-24h PO
Senna	Senokot	Granules in concentrate, or syrup	Dog: Syrup; 5-10 ml/dog q24h; granules: ½ to 1 tsp/dog q24h PO with food Cat: Syrup: 5 ml/cat q24h; granules: ½ teaspoon/cat q24h (with food)
Septra (sulfamethoxazole + trimethoprim)	See Trimethoprim/ sulfonamides		
Sildenafil	Viagra	25-, 50-, 100-mg tablets	Dog: 0.5-1 mg/kg q12h PO; higher dose of 2-3 mg/kg q8h may be needed in some cases Cat: 1 mg/kg q8h, PO
Silymarin	Silybin, Marin, "milk thistle"	Silymarin tablets are widely available OTC. Commercial veterinary formulations (Marin) also contain zinc and vitamin E in a phosphatidylcholine complex in tablets for dogs and cats.	30 mg/kg/day PO
Sodium bicarbonate (NaHCO₃)	Generic, Baking Soda, Soda Mint	325-, 520-, and 650-mg tablets; injection of various strengths (4.2% to 8.4%), and 1 mEq/ml	Acidosis: 0.5-1 mEq/kg IV Renal failure: 10 mg/kg PO q8-12h Alkalization of urine: 50 mg/kg PO q8-12h (1 tsp is approximately 2 gm)
Sodium bromide	No commercial form	Must be compounded	Same as potassium bromide, except dose is 15% lower (30 mg/kg potassium bromide is equivalent to 25 mg/kg sodium bromide)
Sodium chloride 0.9%	Generic	500- and 1,000-ml infusion	15-30 ml/kg/hr IV
Sodium chloride 7.5%	Generic	Infusion	2-8 ml/kg IV
Sodium thiomalate	See Gold sodium thiomalate		
Somatrem, Somatropin	See Growth hormone		
Sotalol	Betapace	80-, 160-, 240-mg tablets	Dog: 1-2 mg/kg PO q12h (one can start with 40 mg/dog q12h, then increase to 80 mg if no response) Cat: 1-2 mg/kg PO q12h
Spironolactone	Aldactone	25-, 50-, and 100-mg tablets	Dog: 2-4 mg/kg/day (or 1-2 mg/kg PO q12h) Cat: Questionable efficacy, may produce skin lesions

Drug Name	Other Names	Formulations Available	Dosage
Stanozolol	Winstrol-V	50-mg/ml injection; 2-mg tablet	Dog: 2 mg/dog (or range of 1-4 mg/dog) PO q12h; 25-50 mg/dog/wk IM Cat: 1 mg/cat PO q12h; 25 mg/cat/wk IM
Succimer	Chemet	100-mg capsule	Dog: 10 mg/kg PO q8h for 5 days, then 10 mg/kg PO q12h for 2 more wk Cat: 10 mg/kg q8h for 2 wk
Sucralfate	Carafate (Sulcrate in Canada)	1-gm tablet; 200-mg/ml oral suspension	Dog: 0.5-1 gm/dog PO q8-12h Cat: 0.25 gm/cat PO q8-12h
Sufentanil citrate	Sufenta	50-μg/ml injection	2 μg/kg IV, up to a maximum dose of 5 μg/kg
Sulfadiazine	Generic, combined with trimethoprim in Tribrissen	500-mg tablet; trimethoprim-sulfadiazine 30-, 120-, 240-, 480-, and 960-mg tablets	100 mg/kg IV, PO (loading dose), followed by 50 mg/kg IV, PO q12h (see also Trimethoprim)
Sulfadimethoxine	Albon, Bactrovet, and generic	125-, 250-, and 500-mg tablets; 400-mg/ml injection; 50-mg/ml suspension	55 mg/kg PO (loading dose), followed by 27.5 mg/kg PO q12h (see also Primor)
Sulfamethoxazole	Gantanol	50-mg tablet	100 mg/kg PO (loading dose), followed by 50 mg/kg PO q12h (see also Bactrim, Septra)
Sulfasalazine (sulfapyridine + mesalamine)	Azulfidine (Salazopyrin in Canada)	500-mg tablet	Dog: 10-30 mg/kg PO q8-12h (see also Mesalamine, Olsalazine) Cat: 20 mg/kg q12hr PO
Sulfisoxazole	Gantrisin	500-mg tablet; 500-mg/5 ml syrup	50 mg/kg PO q8h (urinary tract infections)
Tamoxifen	Nolvadex	10- and 20-mg tablets (tamoxifen citrate)	Veterinary dose not established; 10 mg PO q12h is human dose
Taurine	Generic	Available in powder	Dog: 500 mg PO q12hr Cat: 250 mg/cat PO q12hr
Telazol	See Tiletamine-Zolazepam		
Terbinafine	Lamisil	125-, 250-mg tablets	Dog: Malassezia dermatitis: 30 mg/kg/day PO Cat: Dermatophytosis: 30-40 mg/kg PO q24h
Terbutaline	Brethine, Bricanyl	2.5- and 5-mg tablets; 1-mg/ml injection	Dog: 1.25-5 mg/dog PO q8h Cat: 0.1-0.2 mg/kg PO q12h (or 0.625 mg/cat, ¼ of 2.5-mg tablet) For acute treatment in cats: 5-10 μg/kg q4h SC or IM
Testosterone cypionate ester	Andro-Cyp, Andronate, Depo-Testosterone and other forms	100- and 200-mg/ml injection	1-2 mg/kg IM q2-4wk (see also Methyltestosterone)
Testosterone propionate ester	Testex (Malogen in Canada)	100-mg/ml injection	0.5-1 mg/kg 2-3 times/wk IM
Tetracycline	Panmycin	250- and 500-mg capsules; 100-mg/ml suspension	15-20 mg/kg PO q8h; or 4.4-11 mg/kg IV, IM q8h
Thenium closylate	Canopar	500-mg tablet	Dog: >4.5 kg: 500 mg PO once, repeat in 2-3 wk 2.5-4.5 kg: 250 mg q12h for 1 day, repeat in 2-3 wk
Theophylline	Many brands and generic	100-, 125-, 200-, 250-, and 300-mg tablets; 27-mg/5 ml oral solution or elixir; injection in 5% dextrose	Dog: 9 mg/kg PO q6-8h Cat: 4 mg/kg PO q8-12h

Continued

Drug Name	Other Names	Formulations Available	Dosage
Theophylline extended-release	Inwood labs extended release	100-, 200-, 300-, and 400-mg tablets or 125-, 200-, 300-mg capsules	Dog: 10 mg/kg q12h PO of extended-release tablet or capsule Cat: 20 mg/kg q24-48h PO extended-release tablet or 25 mg/kg q24-48h PO extended-release capsule
Thiamine (vitamin B$_1$)	Bewon and others	250-µg/5 ml elixir; tablets of various size from 5 mg to 500 mg; 100- and 500-mg/ml injection	Dog: 10-100 mg/dog/day PO or 12.5-50 mg/dog IM or SC/day Cat: 5-30 mg/cat/day PO (up to a maximum dose of 50 mg/cat/day) or 12.5-25 mg/cat IM or SC/day
Thioguanine (6-TG)	Generic	40-mg tablet	40 mg/m^2 PO q24h Cat: 25 mg/m^2 PO q24hr for 1-5 days, then repeat every 30 days
Thiomalate sodium	See Gold sodium thiomalate		
Thiopental sodium	Pentothal	Various size vials from 250 mg to 10 gm (mix to desired concentration)	Dog: 10-25 mg/kg IV (to effect) Cat: 5-10 mg/kg IV (to effect)
Thiotepa	Generic	15-mg injection (usually in solution of 10 mg/ml)	0.2-0.5 mg/m^2 weekly, or daily for 5-10 days IM, intracavitary, or intratumor
Thyroid hormone	See Levothyroxine sodium (T$_4$), or Liothyronine		
Thyrotropin, thyroid-stimulating hormone (TSH)	Thytropar, Thyrogen	10-U vial; old forms difficult to obtain; Thyrogen is 1000 µg/vial	Dog: Collect baseline sample, followed by 0.1 U/kg IV (maximum dose is 5 U); collect post-TSH sample at 6 hr Cat: Collect baseline sample, followed by 2.5 U/cat IM and collect a post-TSH sample at 8-12 hr
Ticarcillin	Ticar, Ticillin	Vials containing 1, 3, 6, 20, and 30 gm	33-50 mg/kg IV, IM q4-6h
Ticarcillin + clavulanate	Timentin	3-gm/vial for injection	Dose according to rate for ticarcillin
Tiletamine + zolazepam	Telazol, Zoletil	50 mg of each component per milliliter	Dog: 6.6-10 mg/kg IM (short term) or 10-13 mg/kg IM (longer procedure) Cat: 10-12 mg/kg IM (minor procedure) or 14-16 mg/kg IM (for surgery)
Tobramycin	Nebcin	40-mg/ml injection	Dog: 9-14 mg/kg IM, IV, SC q24h Cat: 5-8 mg/kg IM, SC, IV q24h
Tocainide	Tonocard	400- and 600-mg tablets	Dog: 15-20 mg/kg PO q8h Cat: No dose established
Toluene	Vermiplex		267 mg/kg PO (of toluene), repeat in 2-4 wk
Tramadol hydrochloride	Ultram and generic	Tramadol immediate-release tablets are available in 50-mg tablets	Dog: 5 mg/kg PO q6-8h Cat: Start with 2 mg/kg q12h PO and increase gradually to 4 mg/kg q8-12h. Cats are more prone to adverse reactions
Trandolapril	Mavik	1-, 2-, and 4-mg tablets	Not established for dogs; human dose is 1 mg/person/day to start, then increase to 2-4 mg/day
Triamcinolone	Vetalog, Trimtabs, Aristocort, generic	Veterinary (Vetalog) 0.5- and 1.5-mg tablets. Human form: 1-, 2-, 4-, 8-, and 16-mg tablets; 10-mg/ml injection	Antiinflammatory: 0.5-1 mg/kg PO q12-24h, then taper dose to 0.5-1 PO mg/kg q48h (however, manufacturer recommends doses of 0.11 to 0.22 mg/kg/day)
Triamcinolone acetonide	Vetalog	2- or 6-mg/ml suspension injection	0.1-0.2 mg/kg IM, SC, repeat in 7-10 days Intralesional: 1.2-1.8 mg, or 1 mg for every cm diameter of tumor q2wk

Drug Name	Other Names	Formulations Available	Dosage
Triamterene	Dyrenium	50- and 100-mg capsules	1-2 mg/kg PO q12h
Tribrissen	See Trimethoprim-sulfadimethoxine combination		
Trientine hydrochloride	Syprine	250-mg capsule	10-15 mg/kg PO q12h
Trifluoperazine	Stelazine	10-mg/ml oral solution; 1-, 2-, 5-, and 10-mg tablets; 2-mg/ml injection	0.03 mg/kg IM q12h
Triflupromazine	Vesprin	10- and 20-mg/ml injection	0.1-0.3 mg/kg IM, q8-12h
Tri-iodothyronine	See Liothyronine		
Trilostane	Vetoryl	10-, 30-, 60-, and 120-mg capsules; no formulations approved in U.S.; must be imported	Dog: 3-6 mg/kg q24h, PO (adjust dose with cortisol measurements) Cat: 6 mg/kg q24h, PO and gradually increase as needed to 10 mg/kg q24h, PO
Trimeprazine tartrate	Temaril (Panectyl in Canada)	2.5-mg/5 ml syrup; 2.5-mg tablet	0.5 mg/kg PO q12h
Trimethobenzamide	Tigan and others	100-mg/ml injection; 100- and 250-mg capsules	Dog: 3 mg/kg IM, PO q8h Cat: Not recommended
Trimethoprim + sulfonamides (sulfadiazine or sulfamethoxazole)	Tribrissen and others	30-, 120-, 240-, 480-, and 960-mg tablets with trimethoprim to sulfa ratio 1:5	15 mg/kg PO q12h, or 30 mg/kg PO q12-24h For Toxoplasma: 30 mg/kg PO q12h
Tripelennamine citrate and Tripelennamine hydrochloride	Pelamine, PBZ	25- and 50-mg tablets; 5 mg/mL oral liquid elixir and 20-mg/ml injection (citrate); Tripelennamine hydrochloride is a 25 mg/mL injection	1 mg/kg PO q12h, or 0.25 mL per 5 kg of tripelennamine hydrochloride
TSH (thyroid-stimulating hormone)	See Thyrotropin		
Tylosin	Tylocine, Tylan, Tylosin tartrate	Available as soluble powder 2.2 gm tylosin per tsp (tablets for dogs in Canada)	Dog, cat: 7-15 mg/kg PO q12-24h Dog: For colitis: 10-20 mg/kg q8h with food initially, then increase interval to q12-24h
Urofollitropin (FSH)	Metrodin	75 U/vial for injection	75 U/day IM for 7 days
Ursodiol (ursodeoxycholate)	Actigall	300-mg capsule, 250-mg tablets	10-15 mg/kg PO q24h
Valproic acid, divalproex	Depakene (valproic acid); Depakote (divalproex)	125-, 250-, and 500-mg tablets (Depakote); 250-mg capsule; 50-mg/ml syrup (Depakene)	Dog: 60-200 mg/kg PO q8h; or 25-105 mg/kg/day PO when administered with phenobarbital
Vancomycin	Vancocin, Vancoled	Vials for injection (0.5 to 10 gm)	Dog: 15 mg/kg q6-8h IV infusion Cat: 12-15 mg/kg q8h IV infusion
Vasopressin (ADH)	Pitressin	20 U/ml (aqueous)	10 U per animal IV or IM
Verapamil	Calan, Isoptin	40-, 80-, and 120-mg tablet; 2.5-mg/ml injection	Dog: 0.05 mg/kg IV q10-30min (maximum cumulative dose is 0.15 mg/kg)
Vinblastine	Velban	1-mg/ml injection	2 mg/m^2 IV (slow infusion) once/wk
Vincristine	Oncovin, Vincasar, generic	1-mg/ml injection	Antitumor: 0.5-0.7 mg/m^2 IV (or 0.025-0.05 mg/kg) once/wk For thrombocytopenia: 0.02 mg/kg IV once/wk
Viokase	See Pancrelipase		
Vitamin A (retinoids)	Aquasol A	Oral solution: 5000 U (1500 RE) per 0.1 ml 10,000-, 25,000-, and 50,000-U tablets	625-800 U/kg PO q24h

Continued

Drug Name	Other Names	Formulations Available	Dosage
Vitamin B₁	See Thiamine		
Vitamin B₂ (riboflavin)	Riboflavin	Various-size tablets in increments from 10 to 250 mg	Dog: 10-20 mg/day PO Cat: 5-10 mg/day PO
Vitamin B₁₂ (cyanocobalamin)	Cyanocobalamin	Various-size tablets in increments from 25 to 100 μg and injections	Dog: 100-200 μg/day PO Cat: 50-100 μg/day PO
Vitamin C (ascorbic acid)	See Ascorbic acid	Tablets of various sizes and injection	100-500 mg/day
Vitamin D	See Dihydrotachysterol or Ergocalciferol		
Vitamin E (alpha-tocopherol)	Aquasol E, and generic	Wide variety of capsules, tablets, oral solution available (e.g., 1000 units per capsule)	100-400 U PO q12h (or 400-600 U PO q12h for immune-mediated skin disease)
Vitamin K₁ (phytonadione, phytomenadione)	AquaMEPHYTON (injection), Mephyton (tablets); Veta-K1 (capsules)	2- or 10-mg/ml injection; 5-mg tablet (Mephyton) 25-mg capsule (Veta-K1)	Short-acting rodenticides: 1 mg/kg/day IM, SC, PO for 10-14 days Long-acting rodenticides: 2.5-5 mg/kg/day and up to 6 wk IM, SC, PO for 3-4 wk Birds: 2.5-5 mg/kg q24h
Warfarin	Coumadin, generic	1-, 2-, 2.5-, 4-, 5-, 7.5-, and 10-mg tablets	Dog: 0.1-0.2 mg/kg PO q24h Cat: Thromboembolism: Start with 0.5 mg/cat/day and adjust dose based on clotting time assessment
Xylazine	Rompun and generic	20- and 100-mg/ml injection	Dog: 1.1 mg/kg IV, 2.2 mg/kg IM Cat: 5-10 mg/kg q12h, PO or SC
Yohimbine	Yobine	2-mg/ml injection	0.11 mg/kg IV or 0.25-0.5 mg/kg SC, IM
Zidovudine (AZT)	Retrovir	10-mg/ml syrup; 10-mg/ml Injection	Cat: 5-10 mg/kg q12h, PO or SC
Zolazepam	See Tiletamine-zolazepam combination		
Zonisamide	Zonegran	100-mg capsule	Dog: 3 mg/kg q8h PO; it has also been administered to dogs at 10 mg/kg q12h PO Cat: Dose not established

APPENDIX II

Treatment of Parasites

LORA R. BALLWEBER, *Fort Collins, Colorado*

Drug(s)	Species	Target Parasites	Route*	Veterinary Formulations
HELMINTHS				
Emodepside/ Praziquantel	Feline only	*Toxocara cati, Ancylostoma tubaeforme, Dipylidium caninum, Taenia taeniaeformis*	Topical	Profender
Epsiprantel	Canine and feline	*Dipylidium caninum, Taenia* spp.	Oral	Cestex
Febantel/ Praziquantel/ Pyrantel pamoate	Canine only	*Toxocara canis, Toxascaris leonina, Ancylostoma caninum, Uncinaria stenocephala, Trichuris vulpis, Dipylidium caninum, Echinococcus granulosus, Echinococcus multilocularis, Taenia pisiformis*	Oral	Drontal Plus
Fenbendazole	Canine	*Toxocara canis, Toxascaris leonina, Ancylostoma caninum, Uncinaria stenocephala, Trichuris vulpis, Taenia pisiformis*	Oral	Panacur C, Safe-Guard
Imidacloprid/ Moxidectin	Canine and feline	*Toxocara canis, Toxascaris leonina* (dog), *Toxocara cati* (cat), *Ancylostoma caninum, Uncinaria stenocephala* (dog), *Ancylostoma tubaeforme* (cat), *Trichuris vulpis* (dog); *Dirofilaria immitis* prevention (dog/cat)	Topical	Advantage Multi
Ivermectin	Canine and feline	*Ancylostoma tubaeforme, A. braziliense* (cat), *Dirofilaria immitis* prevention (dog/cat)	Oral	Heartgard
Ivermectin/ Praziquantel/ Pyrantel pamoate	Canine only	*Toxocara canis, Toxascaris leonina, Ancylostoma caninum, Ancylostoma braziliense, Uncinaria stenocephala, Dipylidium caninum, Taenia pisiformis, Dirofilaria immitis* prevention	Oral	Iverhart Max
Ivermectin/ Pyrantel pamoate	Canine only	*Toxocara canis, Toxascaris leonina, Ancylostoma caninum, Ancylostoma braziliense, Uncinaria stenocephala, Dirofilaria immitis* prevention	Oral	Heartgard Plus, Iverhart Plus, TriHeart Plus, PetTrust Plus
Milbemycin oxime	Canine and feline	Roundworms, *Ancylostoma* spp., *Trichuris vulpis* in dogs; *Dirofilaria immitis* prevention	Oral	Sentinel (with lufenuron), Trifexis (with spinosad)
Praziquantel	Canine and feline	*Dipylidium caninum* (cat/dog), *Echinococcus* spp. (dog), *Taenia* spp. (cat/dog)	Oral, injectable	Droncit
Moxidectin	Canine	*Dirofilaria immitis* prevention	Injectable	ProHeart6
Praziquantel/ Pyrantel pamoate	Canine and feline	*Toxocara canis, Toxascaris leonina* (dog), *Toxocara cati* (cat), *Ancylostoma caninum, Ancylostoma braziliense, Uncinaria stenocephala* (dog), *Ancylostoma tubaeforme* (cat), *Dipylidium caninum, Taenia* spp. (dog/cat)	Oral	Drontal and numerous generic formulations
Pyrantel pamoate	Canine	*Toxocara canis, Toxascaris leonina, Ancylostoma caninum, Uncinaria stenocephala*	Oral	Nemex 2
Selamectin	Canine and feline	*Toxocara cati, Ancylostoma tubaeforme* (cat); *Dirofilaria immitis* prevention (dog/cat)	Topical	Revolution

Continued

1335

Drug(s)	Species	Target Parasite(s)	Route(s) and Frequency of Administration	Veterinary Formulations
ECTOPARASITES				
Dinotefuran/ Pyriproxyfen	Canine and feline	Fleas	Topical, monthly	Vectra
Dinotefuran/ Pyriproxyfen/ Permethrin	Canine only	Fleas, ticks, mosquitoes, biting flies, mites (not mange), lice	Topical, monthly	Vectra 3D
Deltamethrin	Canine only	Fleas, ticks	Collar, 6 months	Scalibor Protector Band
Fipronil	Canine and feline	Fleas, ticks, chewing lice	Topical, monthly	Frontline Plus, Parastar, and numerous generic formulations
Fipronil/ Amitraz/S-Methoprene	Canine only	Fleas, ticks, sarcoptic mange mites, chewing lice	Topical, monthly	Certifect
Fipronil/ Cyphenothrin	Canine only	Fleas, ticks, chewing lice	Topical, monthly	Parastar Plus
Imidacloprid/ Flumethrin	Canine only	Fleas, ticks, sarcoptic mange mites, lice	Collar, 8 months	Seresto
Imidacloprid/ Pyriproxyfen	Canine and feline	Fleas (dog/cat), chewing lice (dog)	Topical, monthly	Advantage II
Imidacloprid/ Moxidectin	Canine and feline	Fleas (dog/cat), ear mites (cat)	Topical, monthly	Advantage Multi
Imidacloprid/ Permethrin	Canine only	Fleas, ticks, mosquitoes, biting flies, chewing lice	Topical, monthly	Advantix II
Indoxacarb	Canine only	Fleas	Topical, monthly	Activyl
Indoxacarb/ Permethrin	Canine only	Fleas, ticks	Topical, monthly	Activyl Tick Plus
Ivermectin	Feline only	Ear mites	Topical, in ear canal, repeat once as necessary	Acarexx
Nitenpyram	Canine and feline	Fleas	Oral, daily	Capstar
Spinosad	Canine and feline	Fleas	Oral, monthly	Comfortis
Spinosad/ Milbemycin oxime	Canine	Fleas	Oral, monthly	Trifexis

Drug(s)	Species	Target Parasite(s)	Route of Administration and Dosages	Veterinary Formulations
PROTOZOA				
Amprolium	Canine	*Cystoisospora* spp.	Oral, 100 mg/kg q24h, 7-10 days	Corid
Atovaquone + Azithromycin	Feline	*Cytauxzoon felis*	Oral, 15 mg/kg q8h + 10 mg/kg q24h, 10 days	Mepron + azithromycin suspension
Azithromycin	Canine and feline	*Cryptosporidium*	5-10 mg/kg (dog) or 7-15 mg/kg (cat) q12h, 5-7 days or until clinical signs resolve	Azithromycin suspension
Clindamycin	Canine and feline	*Toxoplasma gondii* (systemic infections); *Neospora caninum*	Oral, 10-15 mg/kg q12h, 14-28 days as needed *(T. gondii)*; 7.5-20 mg/kg q12h for 2 weeks beyond clinical resolution *(N. caninum)*	Antirobe
Doxycycline	Canine and feline	*Toxoplasma gondii* (systemic infections)	Oral 5-10 mg/kg q12h, 28 days	Vibramycin
Fenbendazole	Canine and feline	*Giardia intestinalis*	Oral, 50 mg/kg q24h, 3-5 days	Panacur
Furazolidone	Feline	*Giardia intestinalis*	Oral, 4 mg/kg q12h, 7-10 days	
Imidocarb diproprionate	Canine and feline	*Babesia* spp., *Cytauxzoon felis*	IM or SC, 6.6 mg/kg, repeat in 14 days *(Babesia)*; 3.5 mg/kg, repeat in 7 days *(C. felis)*	Imizol
Metronidazole	Canine and feline	*Giardia intestinalis*	Oral, 15-25 mg/kg q12-24h, 5-7 days	Flagyl
Nitazoxanide	Canine and feline	*Giardia intestinalis, Cryptosporidium* spp.	Oral, 100 mg/kg q12h, 3 days *(G. intestinalis)*; 25 mg/kg q12h, at least 5 days *(Cryptosporidium)*	Alinia (Human)
Ponazuril	Canine and feline	*Cystoisospora* spp., *Toxoplasma gondii*	Oral, 15 mg/kg q24h, 3 days; 30 mg/kg q24h, 1 day	Marquis (Horses)
Ronidazole	Canine and feline	*Giardia intestinalis* (dog); *Tritrichomonas foetus* (cat)	Oral, 30-50 mg/kg q12h, 7 days *(G. intestinalis)*; 30 mg/kg q12h, up to 14 days *(T. foetus)*	Ridzol
Sulfadiazine and trimethoprim	Canine and feline	*Cystoisospora* spp., *Toxoplasma gondii* (intestinal infections)	Oral, 30 mg/kg q12h, 14 days as needed	Tribrissen
Sulfadimethoxine	Canine and feline	*Cystoisospora* spp., *Toxoplasma gondii* (intestinal infections)	Oral, 50 mg/kg day 1, then 25 mg/kg q24h for 14-21 days as needed	Albon
Tinidazole	Canine and feline	*Giardia intestinalis*	Oral, 44 mg/kg q24h, 3 days (dog): 30 mg/kg q12h, 7-10 days (cat)	Tindamax, Fasigyn
Tylosin	Canine and feline	*Giardia intestinalis*	Oral, 10-15 mg/kg q8h-q12h for 21 days	Tylan

*Follow manufacturer's recommendations for indicated use; see Appendix I, Table of Common Drugs: Approximate Dosages, for extralabel use.

Index

A

A-V block. *See* Atrioventricular (heart) block
AAFCO profiles, during pregnancy and lactation, 964-965, 966f
Abamectin
    for dermatologic disorders, e178
    for lung worms, e274-e275
ABCB1 gene, for predicting adverse effects of drug therapy, 175, 330, 433
Abdomen, septic, drainage techniques for, e13-e20
Abdominal effusion(s). *See* Ascites; Peritoneal effusion
Abdominal palpation, for pregnancy diagnosis, 944
Abdominocentesis
    for ascites
        from liver disease, 591-592
        from refractory heart failure, 781
    for malignant effusions, 342
Ablation, for supraventricular tachyarrhythmias in dogs, 744
Abortion. *See also* Pregnancy, medical termination of
    from hypothyroidism, e85
    infectious causes of, 1218
    misoprostol causing, 507
Abscess, orbital, 1198-1199
Abyssinian cat
    amyloidosis in, 855
    arterial thromboembolism in, 812-813
    hepatic amyloidosis in, 571b
    progressive retinal atrophy in, 1195
Acanthomatous ameloblastoma, 363, 365
Acarbose, for diabetes mellitus, in cats, e136f, e136t, e137
Acemannan
    as cancer immunotherapy, 335, 336t
    for feline retrovirus infections, 1280t-1281t, 1282
    for infectious disease immune therapeutics, 1230, 1230t
Acepromazine
    causing adverse skin reactions, 488t
    for postpartum agalactia, 958t
    for tracheal collapse, 664
    to calm respiratory distress pets, 47t
    use of
        with cardiovascular dysfunction, 64-65
        with intracranial pathology, 69

Acetaminophen (Tylenol)
    associated hepatotoxicity, 570b, 576-577, 581b
    N-acetylcysteine for toxicity of, 576-577
    S-adenosylmethionine (SAMe) for toxicity of, 577
    toxicity from, 117-118
Acetazolamide
    for craniocervical junction abnormalities, 1102
    for glaucoma in dogs, 1173-1174, 1173b
    for hydrocephalus, 1036
Acetic acid
    as topical therapy, 441t
    for *Malassezia* dermatitis, 442
Acetylcholine receptor (AChR) antibody test, for myasthenia gravis, 1109, 1111-1112, e226
Acetylcholinesterase inhibitor(s)
    action and use of, for motility disorders, 516-518, 517t
    from insecticide toxicity, 135
Acetylcysteine (Mucomyst)
    for canine bronchial diseases, 672
    for respiratory diseases, 627
    for rhinitis in cats, 647
    for Tylenol toxicity, e61t-e66t
Acetylsalicylic acid. *See* Aspirin
Achondroplasia, 649
Achromatopsia, 1190
Acid-base disorders
    compensatory responses with, e2b, e2t
    diagnosis and treatment of, e1-e8
Acidosis, acid-base disorders and, e1-e8
Acitretin
    for ichthyosis, 476
    for sebaceous adenitis, e211
Acorus toxicity, 124t
Acral lick dermatitis, e172-e178
    allergy testing with, e175-e176
    causes of, e172, e173b
    diagnosis of, e174-e175
    drug therapy for, 482-485
    perpetuating factors for, e174
    predisposing factors for, e173, e173b
    treatment of, e175-e178
Acromegaly
    feline, 216-221, 217f, 217t
    hypertension from, 727t
    insulin resistance with, 206b, 207
    risk of, with progestin drugs, 985
Acrylonitrile, causing reproductive toxicity, 1027b
Actinic dermatoses, 480-482
Actinomycin D, as rescue therapy for canine lymphoma, 382t
Activated charcoal
    for flatulence, e249-e250
    for toxin ingestion, 105, 113

Activated clotting time (ACT)
    in disseminated intravascular coagulation, 294t
    with anticoagulant rodenticide toxicity, 133
Activated protein C, replacement therapy, for disseminated intravascular coagulation, 295
Acute kidney injury. *See* Renal failure, acute
Acute myeloid leukemia, 314, 318
Acute respiratory distress syndrome (ARDS), 48-51
    diagnosis and treatment of, 48-51
    differential diagnoses for, 49b
    rational use of glucocorticoids for, 1301
    risk factors for, 49b
    with feline pancreatitis, 567
Acyclovir, for feline ocular herpesvirus 1, 1158
Adenocarcinoma
    anal sac, e189-e190
    mammary
        canine, 376
        feline, 378-380
    nasal
        in dogs, 641-643, 642f
        radiation therapy for, 338-340
    of ciliary body, in cats, 1209
    of the exocrine pancreas, 557
    of third eyelid, in dogs, 1203
    perianal, 366-369
    uterine, 1025-1026
Adenosine triphosphate (ATP), as energy source for brain, 1047
Adenovirus 1, vaccine causing uveitis in dogs, 1164
Adipokines, role in obesity, 254
Adiponectin, role in obesity, 254
Adipose tissue, role in obesity, 254
Adnexal disease, e363-e369
Adrenal disease(s)
    hyperadrenocorticism
        imaging for diagnosis of, 171
        therapy of, 229
    interpretation of tests results for, e97-e102
Adrenal gland(s)
    imaging of, for diagnosis of endocrine disorder(s), 170-172
    incidental mass of, 172
    secretion of sex hormone causing hyperadrenocorticism, 221
    with feline hyperaldosteronism
        hyperplasia, 241
        neoplasia, 238-239, 241
Adrenal insufficiency
    illness-related, 78-79, 174-178
    with shock, 24-25

Page numbers followed by "f" indicate figure, "t" indicate tables, "b" indicate boxes, and "e" indicate web chapters.

Adrenalectomy, for adrenal-dependent hyperadrenocorticism, 229
Adrenocorticotropic hormone (ACTH)
    ectopic syndrome of, 230-232, 231f
    stimulation test
        for illness adrenal insufficiency, 175-176
        for occult hyperadrenocorticism, 221
        interpretation of, e97-e98
        with alopecia X, 478
        with hypoadrenocorticism, in dogs, 233-235
    with illness-related adrenal insufficiency, 79
Advanced life support, 28-31
Adverse drug experience
    definition of, e35-e36
    reporting of, e36
Adverse drug reactions, cutaneous, 487-490, 488t
Adverse events
    from vaccines, 1249-1256
    reporting of, e35-e43
Adverse food reactions
    causing blepharitis, e365
    food elimination diets for, 422-424
Aelurostrongylus abstrusus
    as bronchopulmonary parasite, e273-e274
    common symptoms and syndromes caused by, 1214t-1215t
AeroKat and AeroDawg spacers, 623-624, 671, 678-680, 679f, 690, 690f
Aerophagia, causing flatulence, e248-e249
Aerosol spray(s), as respiratory toxicants, e46
Afghan hound(s), testicular tumors in, 1022-1023
Aflatoxicosis
    associated hepatotoxicity, 570b, 581b
    in dogs, 159-161
African violet(s), 121b
Agalactia, 958t
    postpartum, 959
Agent orange, in pot scrubbing sponges, 98
Aglepristone, for pregnancy termination, 991
Air pollutant(s), e45-e46
Air quality
    improving indoor, e47-e48
    index, e47-e48
Air-purifiers, causing ozone toxicity, e45-e46
Airflow, with brachycephalic airway syndrome, 651
Airway obstruction
    and evaluation, 26
    causes of, 46t
    large, causing respiratory acidosis, e4b
    with brachycephalic airway syndrome, 649-653
Airway resistance, 44
Akita(s)
    hyperkalemia and hyponatremia in, e93
    sebaceous adenitis in, e209-e210

Alanine aminotransferase (ALT)
    elevations from methimazole, e104
    monitoring of, before lomustine, 332-333
    with feline hepatic lipidosis, 609-610
    with hepatobiliary disease, 569-573
    with idiopathic vacuolar hepatopathy, 607
Alaskan husky, mitochondrial encephalopathy in, 1048-1051, 1049t, 1051t
Alaskan malamute(s)
    alopecia X in, 477-479
    zinc-responsive dermatosis, causing blepharitis in, e365
Alaskan sled dog(s), thyroid hormone differences in, 180t
Albendazole
    for Giardia spp., 530t
    for lung worms, e276
Albumin, 11
    characteristics of, 10t
    fluid dynamics and, 9-11
Albuminuria, detection and management of, 849-852
Albuterol
    for bronchial diseases, 671
    for feline asthma, 677
    for respiratory diseases, 623
    inhaler
        for feline asthma, 675, 677, 680
        for respiratory diseases, 623-624
Alcohol
    for disinfection of methicillin-resistant Staphylococcal sp., 456-457
    in ear cleaners, 472t, 473
    toxicity, 147
Aldosterone
    concentrations
        with atypical hypoadrenocorticism, 233, 235
        with feline hyperaldosteronism, 239-240, 240t
    escape, 854
Aldosterone receptor antagonists, for glomerular disease, 854, 854f
Aldosterone-to-renin ratio, 235
Alendronate, for feline idiopathic hypercalcemia, 246-247, 246f
Alfentanil, with maintenance anesthetic, 66, 67t
Alkaline phosphatase (ALP)
    bone, e243
    corticosteroid, e243
    elevations, e242-e246, e245b-e246b
        algorithm for evaluation of, e244f
        from methimazole, e104
    liver, e243
    pathophysiology of, e242-e243
    with feline hepatic lipidosis, 609-610
    with hepatobiliary disease, 569-573
    with idiopathic vacuolar hepatopathy, 606
Alkalosis, acid-base disorders and, e1-e8
Alkylamine, toxicity of, 118-119
Allergen(s)
    causing flares in atopic dermatitis, 405
    exposure to respiratory, e43-e44

Allergen(s) (Continued)
    extracts, for immunotherapy, 411
    house dust mite, e197-e198
Allergen-specific immunotherapy, 411-414
    causing adverse skin reactions, 488t
    client education with, 412b
    for atopic dermatitis, 407
    injection vs. sublingual, 413b
    schedule adjustments for, 413b
    with acral lick dermatitis, e176
Allergic reaction
    anaphylaxis, epinephrine use for, 16
    from canine vaccines, 1250-1251
Allergic rhinitis, 636b, 637
Allergy shots, 411-414. See also Allergen-specific immunotherapy
Allergy(ies)
    allergen-specific immunotherapy for, 411-414
    associated with eosinophilic pulmonary diseases, 690
    causing otitis, and treatment of, 458
    conjunctivitis from, 1140
    flea dermatitis, 424-425
    role of respiratory allergens with, e43-e44
    testing of, for diagnosis of canine atopy, 404
Allium plant toxicity, 147-148
Alloantibodies, 311
    in cat blood, e145-e146, e145
Allogeneic blood administration, 312
Allopurinol
    drug interactions with, 677
    for American leishmaniasis, e397
    for dissolution of urate stones, 902-904, 902f
Alopecia
    association to obesity, 255b
    bilaterally symmetric, in dogs, 164-166, 165b
        adrenal sex hormones abnormalities causing, 221-222
    from adverse drug reactions, 268, 377, 488t
    from bacterial folliculitis, 437-438
    from cornification disorders, in dogs, 475
    from demodicosis, 432-433
    from ectoparasitoses, 428, 430-431
    from flea allergy dermatitis, 408-409
    from imidacloprid, 141
    from infection site reactions, 489, 1251
    from petroleum hydrocarbons, 155
    from topical pyrethrins/pyrethroids, 138
    in ferrets with hyperadrenocorticism, e94
    nonpruritic, 165b
    pruritic, 164
Alopecia areata, use of cyclosporine for, 410b
Alopecia X
    causing alopecia, in dogs, 165b, 222-224
    diagnosis and treatment of, 477-479, 478b
    synonyms for, 478b

Alpha-agonist(s)
  causing bradyarrhythmias, 731-732
  for feline glaucoma, 1179
Alpha-blocker agent(s), for urinary
  retention disorders, 918
Alpha-hydroxy acids, in ear cleaners,
  472t, 473
Alpha-linolenic acid, requirements
  during pregnancy and lactation,
  963
Alpha2-adrenergic agonist(s)
  adverse effects of, 60
  causing syncope, e328
  dosages for, 62t
  reversal agents for, 30
Alpha2-antagonists, to promote
  ureterolith passage, 894
AlphaTRAK, point-of-care analyzer,
  191-192, 196
Alprazolam
  for behavior-related dermatoses, 483t,
  484
  toxicity of, 113-114
Altrenogest, for low progesterone levels
  during pregnancy, 947-948
Aluminum hydroxide, as antacid
  therapy, 506b, 507
Aluminum toxicity, from sucralfate,
  507
Alveolar-arterial oxygen gradient,
  calculation of, with acid-base
  disorders, e3, e3b
Amanita mushroom hepatotoxicity,
  570b, 581b
Amantadine, 61
Amblyomma americanum
  transmitting cytauxzoonosis, e405
  transmitting *Ehrlichia ewingii*, 1228
Amblyomma maculatum, causing
  Hepatozoon americanum, 1283-1284
American bulldog(s)
  actinic dermatoses in, 480
  direct mutation tests for, 1018t-1020t
  nonepidermolytic ichthyosis in, 475
American canine hepatozoonosis
  diagnosis and treatment of, 1283-1286,
  1284f-1285f
  prognosis for, 1285
American eskimo(s), direct mutation
  tests for, 1018t-1020t
American leishmaniasis, e396-e397
Amikacin
  causing renal failure, e31-e32
  for *Bartonella* spp., 1266t
  for infective endocarditis, e294t
  for methicillin-resistant Staphylococcal
  skin infections, 444
  for nontuberculous cutaneous
  granulomas, 448t
  for otitis, 466t
  for pneumonia, 683t
  for superficial bacterial folliculitis, 438t
Amino acid therapy, for superficial
  necrolytic dermatitis, 486
Aminobisphosphonates, for
  osteosarcoma, 391-392
Aminocaproic acid, for treatment of von
  Willebrand disease, 290-291

Aminoglycoside antibiotics
  adverse effects of, 34t-35t
  causing fetal disorders, 1010
  causing renal failure, e31-e32
  drug incompatibility with, 33t
  for lower respiratory tract infection(s),
  1220t, 1222
  for musculoskeletal infections, 1220t,
  1222-1223
  for *Pseudomonas spp.* otitis, 466t, 467
  for septicemia, 1220t
  ototoxicity from, 468b, 469
Aminophylline. *See also* Theophylline
  for atrial arrhythmias, in cats,
  750f-751f
  for feline bronchitis and asthma,
  677
Amiodarone
  associated hepatotoxicity, 570b, 577,
  581b
  for arrhythmias
    with congestive heart failure,
    764t-765t, 771-772, 783-784
    with dilated cardiomyopathy, in
    dogs, 799
  for supraventricular tachyarrhythmias
  in dogs, 742t, 743-744
  for ventricular arrhythmias, 746-748,
  747f, 747t
  for ventricular fibrillation during CPR,
  30
Amitraz
  causing adverse skin reactions, 488t
  drug interactions with, 34t-35t
  for demodicosis, 433, 433t
  for tick control, 1274-1275, 1294
  toxicity, 138-139
Amitriptyline
  for urinary incontinence disorders,
  917
  to promote ureterolith passage, 894
Amlodipine
  for glaucoma in dogs, 1173b, 1174
  for heart failure in dogs, 764t-765t,
  768
  for hypertension, 728-729
    and kidney disease, 861-862
    from acute renal failure, 870
    with retinal detachment, 729
  for hyperthyroid cats, e103t, e105
  for myocarditis, e306
  for proteinuria and glomerular disease,
  855
  rectal use of, 870
  toxicity of, use of IV lipid emulsion
  therapy for, 106
Ammonia
  for evaluation of hepatobiliary disease,
  573
  reduction of, for
  hepatoencephalopathy, 582-583,
  593-594, 593b
Ammonium urate urolithiasis, 901
Amoxicillin
  for hepatoencephalopathy, 593-594
  for urinary tract infections, 1219-1220,
  1220t
  protocol for *helicobacter* spp., 511t

Amoxicillin-clavulanate
  for feline pancreatitis, 567t
  for infective endocarditis, e294t, e297
  for lower respiratory tract infection(s),
  1220t, 1222
  for musculoskeletal infections, 1220t,
  1222-1223
  for otitis, 466
  for pneumonia, 682t-683t, 683
  for pyoderma, 1220t, 1221-1222
  for superficial bacterial folliculitis, 438t
  for upper respiratory tract infections,
  1220t, 1222
  in cats, 631t
  for urinary tract infections, 881b,
  1219-1220
Amphetamine toxicity, 109-110
Amphotericin
  drug incompatibilities with, 33t
  for fungal rhinitis in cats, 647-648,
  647t
Amphotericin B
  adverse effects of, 1235
  use and protocols for, 1234-1238,
  1235t
Amphotericin B deoxycholate, use and
  protocols for, 1234-1238, 1235t
Amphotericin B lipid complex, use and
  protocols for, 1235-1236, 1235t
Ampicillin, for infective endocarditis,
  e294t
Amprolium, target parasites and dosage
  of, 1335-1337
Amputation
  for osteosarcoma, 389-390
  with open fractures, 85
Amylase
  changes with exocrine pancreatic
  insufficiency, 558-559
  changes with exocrine pancreatic
  neoplasia, 557
  elevations with insecticide toxicity,
  137
  for the diagnosis of pancreatitis,
  554-555
  with diabetes and pancreatitis, e77-e78
  with feline pancreatitis, 558-559
  with leptospirosis, 1287
Amylin, insulin resistance and, 205
Amyloidosis
  diagnosis and treatment of, 855
  hepatic, breeds predisposed to, 571b
  role of, in diabetic remission, 205
Anaerobes
  common symptoms and syndromes
  caused by, 1213t
  with open fractures, 84-85
Anagen or telogen defluxion, causing
  alopecia, in dogs, 165b
Anal furunculosis, e190
Anal sac(s)
  anatomy and function of the, e187,
  e187-e188
  apocrine glands tumors, 367-369
  impaction, e188-e190
  infection and abscess, e188-e189
  inflammation, e188-e189
  neoplasia, e189-e190

Analgesia
  constant rate infusions, 61
  epidural, 61
  in the critical care patient, 59-63
  local, 61
  transdermal, 61-63
Anaphylaxis, epinephrine use for, 16
Anaplasma phagocytophilum
  causing nonregenerative anemia, e161,
    e161b
  causing polyarthritis, 1225-1226
  common symptoms and syndromes
    caused by, 1214t
Anaplasma platys
  as cause of thrombocytopenia,
    281t-282t, 283
  common symptoms and syndromes
    caused by, 1214t
Ancyclostoma spp. infection
  as cause of thrombocytopenia,
    281t-282t
  drugs targeting, 1335-1337
Ancyclostoma tubaeforme, common
  symptoms and syndromes caused by,
  1214t-1215t
Ancylostoma caninum, common
  symptoms and syndromes caused by,
  1214t-1215t
Androgen receptor blockers, for
  hyperadrenocorticism in ferrets, e95
Androgen(s)
  excess, 996
  for estrus suppression in the bitch,
    985, 987
  synthesis or action disorders, 997
Androgenic anabolic steroid associated
  hepatotoxicity, 581b
Anemia
  causing syncope, e329
  diagnostic workup for, 315f
  feline
    causing arrhythmias, 750f-751f
    from cytauxzoonosis, e405-e409
    from *Mycoplasma haemofelis*, e398
    from *Bartonella* spp. infections, 1264
    from hypothyroidism, e86
    from inflammatory disease, e160
  hemolytic
    autoimmune
      bone marrow role in, 314-318
      immunosuppressive drugs for,
        268-274
      lymphocytosis associated with,
        305
      management of, 275-279
      nonregenerative, e162
      pulmonary thromboembolism
        with, 705, 708
      thromboembolic disease with, 812
      treatment of hypercoagulability,
        300
      triggers for, 275
      vaccine-induced, 1250-1251
    from cytauxzoonosis, e407
    from *Mycoplasma haemocanis*, e398
  infectious causes of, 1217
  nonregenerative, e160-e164
    diagnostic approach to, e161b

Anemia *(Continued)*
  refractory, 317
  with chronic kidney disease, 862-863
  with thrombocytopenia, 283-284
Anesthesia
  as cause for esophagitis, e237-e238
  causing gastroesophageal reflux, 501,
    503
  ear-flushing techniques under, 471-472
  for cesarean sections, 955t
  in critical care, 63-70
    induction of, 65-66
    maintenance of, 66, 67t
    with cardiovascular dysfunction, 64-68
    with intracranial pathology, 68-70, 1040
    with respiratory dysfunction, 68
Anesthetic agents, topical, as antipruritic
  agents, 419
Angioedema, from adverse drug
  reactions, 488t
Angiography
  with patent ductus arteriosus, e311
  with ventricular septal defect, e338
Angiostrongylus vasorum, as cause of
  thrombocytopenia, 281t-282t
Angiotensin II type 1 receptor blockers
  aldosterone escape with, 854
  antihypertensive effect of, 855
  for glomerular disease, 854-855, 854f
Angiotensin-converting enzyme (ACE)
  inhibitor(s)
  adverse effects of, 766-767, 779, 791
  aldosterone escape with, 854
  antihypertensive effect of, 855
  balancing renal function with, 779
  for asymptomatic heart disease,
    765-766, 775-777, 790
  for canine dilated cardiomyopathy,
    797-799
  for canine heart failure, 763b, 766-768,
    777-779
  for cardiogenic shock, 783
  for feline myocardial disease, 805-809
  for glomerular disease, 854-855
  for hypertension, 728-729
    and kidney disease, 729, 861-862
Aniline, causing reproductive toxicity,
  1027b
Animal cruelty, and pet poisonings, e51
Animal health diagnostic companies,
  role of, 306-307
Anion gap
  calculation of, with acid-base
    disorders, e2, e3b
  from ethylene glycol toxicity, 151-152
Anisocoria
  causes of, e392, e393t
  diagnosis and treatment of, e388-e395
  from optic chiasm lesions, 1137
  spastic pupil syndrome causing, e395
  types of, e388
Anorexia
  from chronic kidney disease, 863
  from feline hepatic lipidosis, 609
  from heart disease, 722
  from toxicity of chemotherapeutic
    drugs, 331
  palatability enhancers for, 723-724

Anovulvar cleft, 976-977
Antacid therapy, 505-508
  drug incompatibilities with, 33t
Anterior uveal melanoma, 1204
Anti-T_3 and Anti-T_4 antibodies, 184
Anti-Xa assay, for monitoring
  antithrombotic agents, 707
Antiandrogen(s), for alopecia X, 479
Antiangiogenesis, 354-355
Antiangiogenic therapy, for
  hemangiosarcoma, 396
Antiarrhythmic drugs
  during CPR, 30
  for arrhythmogenic right ventricular
    cardiomyopathy, 803, e280
  for bradyarrhythmias, 731-737
  for dogs, 763b, 764t-765t
    with congestive heart failure,
      771-772, 783
  for supraventricular tachyarrhythmias,
    741-744, 742t
  for ventricular tachycardia, 746-748,
    747f, 747t
Antibiotic therapy
  during pregnancy complications,
    947-948
  effect of, on urine cultures, 923-924
  for acral lick dermatitis, e175-e176,
    e175l
  for acute pancreatitis in dogs, 563
  for atopic dermatitis, 405
  for canine bronchial diseases,
    671-672
  for canine parvovirus, 535
  for canine respiratory tract infections,
    633-634
  for enteropathies, 518-522
  for feline asthma, 678
  for feline pancreatitis, 567t, 568
  for feline upper respiratory tract
    infections, 630, 631t
  for gall bladder diseases, 603
  for gastric dilation-volvulus, e17
  for hemotropic mycoplasmosis, e401
  for hepatoencephalopathy, 593-594
  for infective endocarditis, e294t,
    e296-e298
  for inflammatory bowel disease,
    538-539
  for methicillin-resistant Staphylococcal
    skin infections, 444
  for neutrophilic cholangitis, 616-618,
    617b
  for open fractures, 84
  for pneumonia, 682t, 683, 687
  for prostatitis, 1014
  for pyothorax, 696
  for respiratory diseases, 627-628
  for rhinosinusitis in cats, 646
  for septic metritis, 958
  for shock, 23-24
  for superficial bacterial folliculitis, 438,
    438t
  for urinary tract infections with
    urolithiasis, 881-882, 893-894
  ototoxicity from, 468b
  probiotic therapy with, 527
  rational empiric, 1219-1223, 1220t

Antibiotic therapy (Continued)
  topical
    for corneal ulcers, 1149-1151
    for keratoconjunctivitis sicca, 1147
    for otitis, 464t
  with heat-induced illness, 73
  with hematologic toxicity from
    chemotherapeutic drugs, 331
Antibiotic(s)
  aminoglycoside, causing renal failure,
    e31-e32
  causing adverse skin reactions, 488t
  formula for interval adjustment with
    renal failure, 34t-35t
  tylosin-responsive diarrhea, e262-e265
Antibodies, development of with
  autoimmune hemolytic anemia, 275
Antibody test(s)
  for Borrelia burgdorferi, 1272-1273
  for canine Bartonella spp., 1264-1265
  for canine heartworm disease, 832
  for ehrlichiosis, 1292-1293
  for feline Bartonella spp., 1269
  for feline heartworm disease, 827
  for masticatory muscle myositis, 1114
  for Toxoplasma gondii, 1296-1297
Anticancer drugs, new, e139-e142. See
  also under Chemotherapy
Anticholinergics, for CPR, 29
Anticoagulant rodenticide toxicity,
  133-134
Anticoagulant therapy
  for arterial thromboembolism, 815
  for autoimmune hemolytic anemia,
    276-278, 277t
  for disseminated intravascular
    coagulation, 296
  for hypercoagulable states, 295
  for protein-losing enteropathy, 544
  for thromboprophylaxis, 708-709
  with continuous renal replacement
    therapy, 873-875
Anticoagulation process, with
  disseminated intravascular
  coagulation, 294f
Anticollagenase therapy
  for keratoconjunctivitis sicca, 1147
  for keratomalacia, 1151
Anticonvulsant therapy
  emergent, 1059-1060
  for inflammatory central nervous
    system disorders, 1065
  new maintenance, 1054-1057
  with intracranial tumors, 1045
Antidepressants and anxiolytics, toxicity
  of, 112-114
Antidote(s)
  approved for animal toxicosis, e56t
  for rodenticide toxicities, 133-135
  IV lipid emulsion therapy as, 106-109,
    115-116
  used to treat toxicities, 101-105,
    102t-104t
Antiemetic(s)
  for acute renal failure, 870
  for canine parvovirus, 535
  for chronic renal disease, 863
  for feline cholangitis, 617, 617b

Antiemetic(s) (Continued)
  for feline pancreatitis, 567t
  for hepatic lipidosis, 612
Antierythrocyte antibodies, with
  autoimmune hemolytic anemia, 275
Antifibrotic drug(s)
  as hepatic support therapy, e257
  for chronic hepatitis, 587
Antifreeze. See Ethylene glycol toxicity
Antifungal drugs
  associated hepatotoxicity, 576
  augmentation with immunotherapy,
    1232
  causing fetal disorders, 1010
  for dermatophytosis, 449-451, 450t
  reactions from, 489
  shampoos, 450t
  systemic, 1234-1238
  topical
    for otitis, 465t
    for pyoderma, 440-441
Antigen receptor gene rearrangements,
  for feline gastrointestinal
  lymphoma, 546
Antigen test(s)
  for canine heartworm disease, 832
  for feline heartworm disease, 827
Antigens, causing hypersensitivity
  reactions to vaccines, 1250-1251
Antihistamine(s)
  for atopic dermatitis, 405-406
  for behavior-related dermatoses, 483,
    483t
  for rhinitis, 637
  topical use of, 419, 1031
  toxicity of, 118-119
  use of, during blood transfusions,
    312-313
Antihypertensive drug(s)
  for cats, 729
  for dogs, 729-730
  with NSAID causing risk of
    nephrotoxicity, 865-866, 865t
Antiinflammatory drug(s). See also
  Glucocorticoid(s); Nonsteroidal
  antiinflammatory drug(s) (NSAID's)
  doses of glucocorticoids, 1301t
  for bronchial diseases, in dogs,
    670-671
  for canine colitis, 551b
  for inflammatory bowel disease, 539
  for respiratory diseases, 625-627
  for rhinosinusitis in cats, 646
  potency of systemic glucocorticoids,
    461t
  topical, with acral lick dermatitis,
    e176-e177
Antileukotrienes, for feline asthma, 678
Antimicrobial susceptibility testing. See
  also under Culture(s)
  for superficial bacterial folliculitis,
    437-438
Antimicrobial therapy. See also Antibiotic
  therapy
  augmentation with immunotherapy,
    1232
  concentration-dependent, 1219, 1220f
  for atopic dermatitis, 405

Antimicrobial therapy (Continued)
  for feline caudal stomatitis, 494
  for otitis
    systemic, 466-467
    topical, 462-465, 464t
  for pyoderma, topical, 439-443, 441t
  for shock, 23-24
  for superficial bacterial folliculitis, 438,
    438t
    topical, 438-439
  prophylactic for urinary tract
    infection, 881-883
  rational empiric, 1219-1223, 1220t
  time-dependent, 1219, 1220f
  topical, 439-443
    for hot spots, e207-e208
Antimüllerian hormone, 1002
Antimuscarinic agents, for urinary
  incontinence disorders, 917
Antioxidants
  as hepatic support therapy, e255-e257
  for heart disease, 725, 763b, 770, 787
  for metabolic brain disorders, 1052
Antiplatelet antibodies, 280-281
Antiprotease therapy, for keratomalacia,
  1151
Antipruritic agents, topical, 420t
  with acral lick dermatitis, e176-e177
Antipyretic agents
  with heat-induced illness, 73
  with vaccine-associated reactions, 1251
Antiseptic(s)
  ear, 473-474
  for pyoderma, 440
  ototoxicity from, 468b
Antithrombin
  replacement therapy, for disseminated
    intravascular coagulation, 295
  with disseminated intravascular
    coagulation, 292, 294f, 294t
Antithrombotic agents
  for arterial thromboembolism, 814-815
  for pulmonary thromboembolism,
    705-707
  monitoring of, 706
Antithyroglobulin antibodies, 182-184
Antitplatelet drug(s)
  for arterial thromboembolism, 814-815
  for pulmonary thromboembolism,
    705, 709-710
Antitumor mechanisms, 354-355
Antitussive drugs
  for canine bronchial disease, 672
  for canine respiratory tract infections,
    633
  for respiratory diseases, 622-623
  for tracheal collapse, 664
Antiviral drugs
  for canine parvovirus, 535
  for feline ocular herpesvirus 1, 1158
  for feline retrovirus infections,
    1277-1280, 1279t
  for feline rhinosinusitis, 646-647
  for feline upper respiratory infections,
    630
  for papillomatosis, e186
  role of interferons in immunity, 1229
Antiyeast drugs. See Antifungal drugs

Anuria, from acute renal failure, 869-870
Anxiety, with behavior-related dermatoses, 484-485
Anxiolytics, toxicity of, 112-114
Aortic body tumor, e167-e168
    causing pericardial effusion, 817
Aortic stenosis, prevalence of, in cats, 757t
Aplastic anemia, 316, e162
Apocrine gland hidrocystoma, eyelid, 1207
Apocrine glands tumors of the anal sac, 366-369
Apomorphine, for emesis induction, 105
Apraclonidine, for feline glaucoma, 1179
Aqueous flare, 1130-1131, 1131f
    with canine uveitis, 1162, 1163t
    with feline uveitis, 1166-1167
Aqueous humor
    cytology, for canine neoplasia, 1201
    misdirection syndrome, 1178
    role of, in canine glaucoma, 1170-1171
Aqueous paracentesis, for identification of ocular neoplasia, 1209-1210
Araceae plant toxicity, 121b
Arachnoid cysts, intracranial, 1038-1039
Arginine production in cats, 592
Arnica toxicity, 124t
Aromatase inhibitors, for hyperadrenocorticism in ferrets, e95
Arrhythmia(s)
    anesthesia for patients with, 64-68
    brady
        cardiac pacing for, e281-e286
        diagnosis and treatment of, 731-737
    canine
        drug therapy for, 764t-765t
        supraventricular tachy, 737-744, 742t
        ventricular, 745-748
        with dilated cardiomyopathy, 799
    cardioversion for, e286-e291
    caused by infectious disease, 1212-1213
    causing syncope, e326-e329
    drugs that stimulate, 677
    feline
        diagnosis and treatment of, 748-755, 750f-751f
        with cardiomyopathy, 809
    from endocarditis, e292-e293
    from human drugs of abuse, 109-112
    from hypothyroidism, e85-e86
    induced right ventricular cardiomyopathy, 801-804, e277-e281
    pacemakers for (See Pacemaker)
    pacing in the ICU setting for, e21-e28, e23f
    ventricular
        causing syncope, e326
        from dilated cardiomyopathy, 799
        in dogs, 745-748
        magnesium chloride for, 250-251
        with feline cardiomyopathy, 809
        with gastric dilation-volvulus, e16-e17

Arrhythmogenic right ventricular cardiomyopathy
    in cats, e277-e281, e306-e307
    in dogs, 801-804, e308
Arsenic
    associated hepatotoxicity, 570b
    causing reproductive toxicity, 1027b
Artemisia, for canine babesiosis, 1259
Arterial blood gas analysis, use of, 52
Arterial thromboembolism. See under Thromboembolism
Arteriosclerosis
    causing Ischemic strokes, 1119-1120
    from hypothyroidism, e86
    pulmonary thromboembolism associated with, 705
Arthritis. See also Polyarthritis
    from borreliosis, 1271
    masitinib for, 361t
    septic
        common pathogens causing, 1222-1223
        empiric antimicrobial therapy for, 1220t
    with lumbosacral stenosis, 1106-1107
Arytenoid lateralization, 660-661
Asbestos fibers, as respiratory toxicant, e47
Asbestos-free sterilizing talc, for malignant effusions, 342
Ascensia Elite point-of-care analyzer, 196
Ascites
    from gall bladder disease, 603
    from hepatobiliary disease, 572, e257-e258
    from liver disease, 591-594, 592f
    from liver failure, 580-581
    with chronic hepatitis, 585f, 587
    with nephrotic syndrome, 856
    with refractory heart failure, 781
Ascorbic acid. See Vitamin C
Asparaginase associated hepatotoxicity, 570b
Aspartate aminotransferase (AST), with hepatobiliary disease, 569-573
ASPCA Animal Poison Control Center toxin exposures, 92-93, 92t
Aspergillosis
    antifungal therapy for, 1234-1238
    causing aflatoxicosis in dogs, 159-161
    causing epistaxis, 1216
    common symptoms and syndromes caused by, 1214t
    nasal
        in cats, 644-648, 645f
        in dogs, 636-640, 639f
Aspermia/oligospermia caused by retrograde ejaculation, e350-e353, e352f
Aspirin
    as anticoagulant therapy, for autoimmune hemolytic anemia, 277-278, 277t
    associated hepatotoxicity, 581b
    causing nephrotoxicity, e32-e33
    for arterial thromboembolism, 814
    for disseminated intravascular coagulation, 296

Aspirin (Continued)
    for feline cardiomyopathy, 806t
    for feline heartworm disease, 830
    for feline infectious peritonitis, 1305t
    for feline thromboembolism, 810, 814
    for feline uveitis, 1169t
    for hypercoagulable states, 299-300
    for prevention of cerebrovascular accidents (stroke), 1122
    for protein-losing enteropathy, 544
    for proteinuria with renal disease, 861
    for thromboprophylaxis, 709-710
    influence on thyroid function, 181t
    ototoxicity from, 468b, 471
    toxicity of, 116-117
Assault rodenticide toxicity, 134
Assisted ambulation/gait training, e358
Assisted devices, for rehabilitation, e359
Assisted feeding, for patients with cancer, 352-353
Asthma, feline, 673-680
    clinical findings with, 674-675
    crisis, catecholamine use for, 15t
    diagnosis and treatment of, 673-680
    masitinib for, 361t
    natural vs. experimentally induced, 673-674
    vs. lungworms, e273-e274
Asystole, 29f
Ataxia
    from vestibular disease, 1067
    infectious agents that cause, 1212
Atenolol
    adverse effects of, 34t-35t
    for asymptomatic heart disease, 766
    for feline arrhythmias, 750f-751f, 752
    for feline cardiomyopathy, 805-807, 806t
    for heart failure, in dogs, 764t-765t, 792
    for hypertension, 729
    for hyperthyroid cats, e103t, e105
    for sinus tachycardia, in cats, 749
    for supraventricular tachyarrhythmias in dogs, 742t
    for ventricular arrhythmias, 747-748, 747t
    in cats, 753-754
Atipamezole, 30
    as reversal agent, 60, e56t
    dosage for, 62t
Atlantoaxial subluxation, 1082-1090
    anatomy and pathophysiology of, 1082, 1083f-1084f
    diagnosis of, 1083-1085, 1085f-1086f
    prognosis for, 1088-1089
    treatment of, 1085-1088, 1086f
Atlantooccipital overlap in dogs, 1100, 1100f
Atopic dermatitis
    allergen-specific immunotherapy for, 411-414
    and food allergy, 403
    causing blepharitis, e365
    causing conjunctivitis, 1140
    causing hot spots, e206-e208

Atopic dermatitis (Continued)
  causing otitis, treatment of, 458
  causing perivulvar dermatitis, 971
  cyclosporine for, in dogs, 403
  diagnosis of, in dogs, 403-404, 404b
  house dust mites and, e197-e199
  treatment of, 405-407
    cyclosporine for, 269-271, 405
    glucocorticoids for, 415-417
    hypoallergenic dietary therapy,
      422-424
    interventions of no benefit, 406
    masitinib for, 361-362, 361t
    pentoxifylline for, e203-e204
    tacrolimus for, 271
    topical, 419-421
    topical immunomodulators for,
      e217-e218
    with bathing, 405
    with interferons, e200-e201, e201
  with acral lick dermatitis, e175-e176
Atopica. See Cyclosporine
Atovaquone
  for canine babesiosis, 1257-1260,
    1258t
  for cytauxzoonosis, e408
Atovaquone-azithromycin, target
  parasites and dosage of, 1335-1337
Atractylis gummifera associated
  hepatotoxicity, 581b
Atrial arrhythmias, in cats, 752-753
Atrial fibrillation, 738, 740f, 741, 742t
  cardioversion for, e288-e289, e288,
    e289f
  from hypothyroidism, e85-e86
  in cats, 749-753, 750f-751f
  with dilated cardiomyopathy, 799
  with heart failure, 783-784
    in dogs, 770-771
Atrial flutter, 738, 740f, 742t
  cardioversion for, e290, e290f
Atrial natriuretic peptide (ANP), with
  valvular heart disease, 790
Atrial septal defect, prevalence of
  in cats, 757, 757t
  in dogs, 756, 757t
Atrial standstill, 733-734
  causing syncope, e328, e328f
  in cats, 750f-751f, 755
Atrial tachycardia, 740f, 742t
  in cats, 749-753, 750f-751f
Atrioventricular (heart) block
  cardiac pacing for, e281-e286
  causing syncope, e328f
  from hypothyroidism, e85
  in cats, 750f-751f, 754-755
  second-degree, 734
  third-degree, 734-735
  temporary pacing for, e25f
Atrioventricular conduction
  abnormalities, 734-735
Atrioventricular node-blocking drugs, for
  supraventricular tachyarrhythmias,
  743
Atrioventricular reciprocating
  tachycardias, 738, 740f, 742t
Atrioventricular septal defect, prevalence
  of, in cats, 757t

Atropine
  adverse effects with α$_2$-adrenergic
    agonist, 60
  causing anisocoria or mydriasis, e392
  for atrioventricular block, in cats, 755
  for bradycardias, 736
  for canine uveitis, 1165
  for CPR, 29
  repeated use of, causing
    keratoconjunctivitis sicca, 1144
  topical
    for corneal ulcers, 1149, 1151
    for feline uveitis, 1169, 1169t
  use of prior to cesarean section, 955
Atropine response test, with sick sinus
  syndrome, e330
Audiometry, for evaluation of hearing,
  469
Auscultation. See also under Heart
    murmur(s)
  for tachyarrhythmias, 738-739
Australian cattle dog(s)
  direct mutation tests for, 1018t-1020t
  mitochondrial encephalopathy in,
    1048-1051, 1049t, 1051t
Australian shepherd(s)
  avermectin toxicity in, 145
  direct mutation tests for, 1018t-1020t
Autoagglutination, with blood typing,
  e144
Autoantibodies
  for myasthenia gravis, 1109
  vaccine-associated, 1255-1256
Autoimmune diseases
  atrophic lymphocytic pancreatitis,
    558
  causing inflammatory central nervous
    disease, 1063-1066
  immunosuppressive drugs for, 268-274
  of the skin, glucocorticoids for, 416t,
    417
Autoimmune hemolytic anemia. See
  Anemia, hemolytic
Automotive product toxins, 92t, 151-155
Autosomal factor deficiencies, 289
Autumn crocus toxicity, 121b
Avermectin(s)
  causing adverse skin reactions, 488t
  for dermatologic disorders, e178-e184
  toxicity, 145-146
Azaglynafarelin, for estrus suppression in
  the bitch, 988
Azathioprine (Imuran)
  associated hepatotoxicity, 581b
  for autoimmune hemolytic anemia,
    278-279
  for canine colitis, 551b, 552
  for canine uveitis, 1165
  for immunosuppression, 268
  for myasthenia gravis, 1110-1111,
    e228-e229
  for protein-losing enteropathy, 544
  for thrombocytopenia, 285t
  hepatotoxic effects of, 576
  use of, with glucocorticoids, 576
Azithromycin (Zithromax)
  for canine babesiosis, 1257-1260,
    1258t, 1265-1266, 1266t

Azithromycin (Zithromax) (Continued)
  for canine respiratory infection
    complex, 634
  for cytauxzoonosis, e408
  for feline babesiosis, 1270
  for feline upper respiratory infection,
    631t
  for Giardia spp., 531
  for lower respiratory tract infection,
    1220t, 1222
  for nontuberculous cutaneous
    granulomas, 448t
  for pneumonia, 682t
  for rhinosinusitis in cats, 646
  for upper respiratory tract infection,
    1220t, 1222
  target parasites and dosage of,
    1335-1337
Azole antifungals associated
  hepatotoxicity, 576
Azotemia. See also Renal Failure
  from amphotericin therapy, 1234-1235
  from diabetes mellitus, e76
  from heart failure therapy, 779, 791
  infectious agents that cause, 1212
  predicting, with renal failure, 187
  prognostic significance of, with renal
    failure, 187
  with heart disease, anorexia from, 722

B
B-cell leukemia, 303-304
B-cell lymphoma, 303-304
Babesia conradae
  common symptoms and syndromes
    caused by, 1214t-1215t
  treatment of, 1258t
Babesia gibsoni
  common symptoms and syndromes
    caused by, 1214t-1215t
  treatment of, 1258-1259, 1258t
Babesia vogeli
  common symptoms and syndromes
    caused by, 1214t-1215t
  treatment of, 1258t
Babesiosis
  as cause of thrombocytopenia,
    281t-282t
  dosage for and drugs targeting,
    1335-1337
  rational use of glucocorticoids for,
    1300-1301
  treatment of canine, 1257-1260, 1258t
Bacille Calmette-Guérin (BCG)
  as cancer immunotherapy, 335, 336t
  for feline retrovirus infections,
    1280t-1281t, 1282
Bacilli, appearance with nontuberculous
  cutaneous granulomas, 446, 447f
Baclofen toxicity, use of IV lipid
  emulsion therapy for, 108, 115-116
Bacteremia. See also Sepsis
  as cause of thrombocytopenia,
    281t-282t
  causing endocarditis, e291-e292
  common pathogens causing, 1223
  empiric antimicrobial therapy for,
    1220t

Bacteria. *See also* Methicillin-resistant
    Staphylococcal infections
  appearance with nontuberculous
      cutaneous granulomas, 446,
      447f
  associated with bronchitis and asthma
      in cats, 676
  causing blepharitis, e363
  causing food poisoning associated
      hepatotoxicity, 581b
  causing hospital-acquired urinary tract
      infections, 876-879
  causing infective endocarditis,
      e293-e294
  causing myocarditis, e304t
  causing pneumonia, 681-682, 686
  causing pregnancy loss, 1005t, 1006,
      1008-1009
  causing prostatitis, 1013
  causing pyothorax, 695
  causing vulvar discharge, 972-973
  Helicobacter spp., 508-513, 510f
  in anal sac fluids, e188
  in raw meat diets, 1240-1241
  list of, causing various clinical signs,
      1213t
  normal isolates
    in the female reproductive tract,
        970t
    in the trachea, 682b
  overgrowth of, in the intestine,
      518-522
Bacterial folliculitis, 437-439
Bacterial viruses, for persistent urinary
    tract infections, 883
Bacteriophages, for persistent urinary
    tract infections, 883
Bacteriuria
  from hospital-acquired urinary tract
      infections, 876-879
  with *Escherichia coli*, causing persistent
      infection, 880-883
  with urolithiasis, 881-882, 893-894
Balanoposthitis, 1030
Balloon valvuloplasty
  for congenital heart disease, 760-761
  for pulmonic stenosis, e317-e318
  for subaortic stenosis, e323
Bandage(s)
  with open peritoneal drainage, e16
  with vacuum-assisted wound closure,
      88, 89f
Barbiturate(s)
  causing adverse skin reactions, 488t
  for emergent seizures, 1059-1060
  toxicity of, 111
Barium-impregnated polyethylene
    spheres (BIPS), for evaluation of
    gastric emptying, 515
Baroreceptor reflex, 732f
Bartonella henselae
  causing infection in humans, 1212,
      1266
  common symptoms and syndromes
      caused by, 1213t, 1261-1262
Bartonella rochalimae, common
    symptoms and syndromes caused by,
    1261-1262

Bartonella spp. infection
  as cause of chronic hepatitis, 584t,
      586, 1263b
  as cause of thrombocytopenia,
      281t-282t, 1261-1262, 1263b
  causing endocarditis, e292, e292-e293,
      e294-e295, e294t, e296-e298
  causing gingivostomatitis, 1216
  causing infection in humans, 1266
  causing lameness, 1216-1217, 1263b
  causing myocarditis, e303-e304,
      e307-e308
  causing nervous system signs, 1212,
      1263b
  causing polyarthritis, 1225-1226, 1263b
  causing systemic disease, 1263b
  clinical signs of, 1263-1264, 1263b
  epidemiology of, 1262, 1267-1268
  in cats, 1267-1271
  in dogs, 1261-1262, 1262t
  reported diagnoses in dogs, 1263b
  transmission and risk factors for, 1262,
      1267-1268
  treatment of, 1265-1266, 1266t,
      1269-1270
Bartonella vinsonii
  causing infection in humans, 1266
  common symptoms and syndromes
      caused by, 1213t
Bartonellosis
  canine, 1261-1267
    causing uveitis, 1263b
  feline, 1267-1271
    causing uveitis, 1168
Basenji(s)
  direct mutation tests for, 1018t-1020t
  inflammatory bowel disease in, 536
  protein losing enteropathy in, 540-541
Basic life support, 26-28
Bassett hound(s)direct mutation tests for,
    1018t-1020t
Bath oils, for sebaceous adenitis,
    e210-e211
Bathing, for atopic dermatitis, 406
Baylisascaris procyonis, common
    symptoms and syndromes caused by,
    1214t-1215t
Beagle(s)
  actinic dermatoses in, 480
  coagulation factor deficiencies in, 289
  direct mutation tests for, 1018t-1020t
  glaucoma in, 1171b
  hyperlipidemia in, 261
  hypothyroidism in, 178-179
  intracranial arachnoid cysts in, 1038
  risk of bladder cancer in, 371t
  thyroid cancer in, 397-398
  vestibular disease in, 1068
Bearded collie(s), hypoadrenocorticism
    in, 233
Beclomethasone dipropionate, inhaled,
    for respiratory diseases, 626t
Bedlington terrier(s)
  acinar hypoplasia in, 1144
  copper-associated liver disease in,
      588-590, e231-e236
  genetic marker test for copper
      toxicosis, 1021t

Beef jerky, causing nephrotoxicity, e34
Behavior(s)
  abnormalities from hydrocephalus,
      1034
  aggression from hypothyroidism, e85
  assessment of, with neuro-ophthalmic
      exam, e390-e392
  concerns regarding, with early age
      neutering, 982
  feline
    chewing, 913
    elimination, 912
    environmental enrichment for
        domestic, 909-914
    making changes to minimize
        problems, 913, 913b
    observable positive and negative,
        911t
    prey-seeking for food, 911
    social interaction, 912-913
Behavior-related dermatoses, 482-485
Belching, e247
Belgian sheepdog(s), atypical pannus in,
    1141
Belladonna toxicity, 124t
Belt loop gastropexy, for gastric dilation-
    volvulus, e18
Benazepril
  adverse effects of, 766-768
  for asymptomatic heart disease,
      765-766
  for cough from bronchial compression,
      782
  for feline cardiomyopathy, 809
  for glomerular disease, 854-855
  for heart failure, in dogs, 764t-765t,
      766-768, 777-779
    balancing renal function and, 779
  for hypertension, 729
    from acute renal failure, 870
  for hyperthyroid cats, e103t, e105
  for occult dilated cardiomyopathy, in
      dogs, 797-798
Bence Jones proteinuria, 849
Benign prostatic hypertrophy, 1012-1015
Benzene, causing reproductive toxicity,
    1027b
Benzodiazepine(s)
  adverse effects of, 34t-35t
  dosing of, with liver disease, 32-33
  drug incompatibities with, 33t
  for behavior-related dermatoses, 483t,
      484
  for emergent seizures, 1059
  reversal agent for, 30
  toxicity of, 112-114
  use of
    with cardiovascular dysfunction,
        64-65
    with opioids for anesthetic
        induction in critical patients, 66
Benzoic acid associated hepatotoxicity,
    581b
Benzopyrene, causing reproductive
    toxicity, 1027b
Benzopyrones, for chylothorax, 699
Benzoyl peroxide, for pyoderma, 440,
    441t

Benzyl alcohol associated hepatotoxicity, 581b
Benzyl benzoate, for dust mite control, e198-e199
Bernese mountain dog(s)
  cervical spondylomyelopathy in, 1092
  direct mutation tests for, 1018t-1020t
Bernoulli equation, and pulmonary artery pressure, 713-714
Beryllium, causing reproductive toxicity, 1027b
Beta-adrenergic receptor agonists
  drug interactions with, 677
  for respiratory diseases, 623-624, 671
    adverse effects of, 624
Beta-blocker(s)
  causing syncope, e328, e328f
  for asymptomatic heart disease, 766, 790
  for atrial fibrillation, 743
    with dilated cardiomyopathy, 799
  for dilated cardiomyopathy, in dogs
    occult, 797-798
    with heart failure, 799
  for feline arrhythmias, 752
  for feline hyperthyroidism, e106
  for glaucoma
    in cats, 1179
    in dogs, 1173b, 1174
  for heart failure, in dogs, 763b, 770-771, 776, 792
  for supraventricular tachyarrhythmias, 742t
Beta-cell dysfunction, 205, 216
Beta-lactam antibiotic(s)
  drug incompatibilities with, 33t
  for Pseudomonas spp. otitis, 466t, 467
Betamethasone, for otitis
  systemic, 461t
  topical, 460t
Betaxolol
  for feline glaucoma, 1179
  for glaucoma in dogs, 1173b
Bethanechol
  for myasthenia gravis, e229-e230
  for urinary retention disorders, 917t, 918
Bevacizumab (Avastin)
  for hemangiosarcoma, 396
  for malignant effusions, 344
  metronomic chemotherapy of, 344
Bicalutamide, for hyperadrenocorticism in ferrets, e95
Bicarbonate. See Sodium bicarbonate
Bicarbonate concentration, and acid-base disorders, e1
Bichon Frise, risk of urolithiasis in, 897
Bifidobacterium animalis, as probiotic, 526
Bile acid testing
  evaluation with alkaline phosphatase elevations, e245-e246
  for evaluation of hepatobiliary disease, 572-573
  with portal vein hypoplasia, 599-600
Biliary mucoceles, e221-e224
Biliary tract disease
  diagnostic approach to, 569-575
  extrahepatic, management of, 602-605

Biliary tract disease (Continued)
  feline cholangitis and, 614-618
  surgery for, 605
Bilirubinemia, elevations from methimazole, e104
Bimatoprost, for glaucoma in dogs, 1173, 1173b
Bioactive enzyme(s), in ear cleaners, 474
Biochemical test(s), for hereditary disorders, 1016
Biologic respiratory contaminants, e43-e44
Biological safety cabinets, for hazardous drugs, 326-327
Biomarkers
  as outcome predictors for intervertebral disk disease, 1073-1074
  for cancer, 356-357
  for hemangiosarcoma, 395
  for valvular heart disease, 790
Biopsy
  bone, for osteosarcoma, 388
  conjunctival, e386, e386f
  esophageal, 502
  for mammary cancer, 376, 376t
  for ocular neoplasia, 1201-1202
  for protein-losing enteropathy, 540-544
  for soft tissue sarcomas, e149
  incisional vs. excisional, e170
  kidney, for glomerular disease, 849
  liver
    for evaluation of hepatobiliary disease, 574-575
    for feline cholangitis, 616
    with alkaline phosphatase elevations, e245
    with chronic hepatitis, 585f, 586
    with feline hepatic lipidosis, 610
    with liver failure, 581-582
    with portal vein hypoplasia, 600
  lung, for interstitial diseases, e268
  muscle
    for canine hepatozoonosis, 1285
    for evaluation of dysphagia, 498-499, e261
  nasal, 338, e157
    in cats, 646
    in dogs, 637
  nerve, for evaluation of dysphagia, 498-499, e261
  postreport conflicts, 325-326
  skin
    for actinic dermatoses, 480
    for dermatophytosis, 449
    for diagnosis of alopecia, 166
    for ichthyosis, 475-476
    of acral lick dermatitis lesions, e174
    with alopecia X, 478
    with superficial necrolytic dermatitis, 486
    with vaccine-associated sarcoma, in cats, 1254
  specimen collection principles, 322, 323b
  thyroid, 398

Biopsy and specimen submission, 322-326
Biphosphate(s), for cholecalciferol toxicity, e33-e34
Bipyridyl herbicide toxicity, 130-131
Birch, toxicity of, 125t
Bismuth salicylate toxicity, 117
Bismuth subsalicylate
  for flatulence, e250
  protocol for helicobacter spp., 511, 511t
Bisoprolol
  for asymptomatic heart disease, 766
  for heart failure, in dogs, 792
Bisphosphonates
  for feline idiopathic hypercalcemia, 246-247
  for multiple myeloma, 385
  to prevent postoperative hypocalcemia, e126
Bite wounds
  causing pyothorax, 695-697
  from pets to humans, 1244-1246, 1245t
Biting flies, drugs targeting, 1335-1337
Bittersweet toxicity, 124t
Black cohosh associated hepatotoxicity, 581b
Bladder
  cancer of the urinary, 370-374
  lithotripsy for stones in the, e340-e344, e342t-e343t
  stones (See Urolithiasis)
Blast cell, 314
Blastomyces dermatitidis, common symptoms and syndromes caused by, 1214t
Blastomycosis
  antifungal therapy for, 1234-1238
  causing nervous system signs, 1212
  causing uveitis
    in cats, 1168
    in dogs, 1163-1164, 1164b
  immunosuppressive therapy for, 1232-1233
Bleach ingestion, 98
Bleeding. See also Hemorrhage
  testing of, with thromboelastography, 74-77
Bleeding disorders
  and coagulation factor deficiencies, 286-291
  screening questions for, 287b
Bleomycin, for pleurodesis, 342
Blepharitis, e363-e365
  allergic, e365
  bacterial, e363
  fungal, e363-e364
  iatrogenic, e367
  immune-medicated, e366-e367
  metabolic-nutritional, e365-e366
  neoplastic, e368
  parasitic, e364
Blepharospasm, from anterior uveitis, 1163t
Blind immunotherapy, 412-413
Blindness
  assessment of, e390-e391
  causes of, 1136t

Blindness (Continued)
  congenital stationary night, direct
      mutation test for, 1018t-1020t
  differential diagnosis for, e382-e383
  evaluation of, 1134-1138
  from canine uveitis, 1163t
  from glaucoma, in dogs, 1170
    surgical options for, 1176b
  from hydrocephalus, 1034
  from optic tract lesions, 1137f-1138f
  in briard with congenital retinal
      dystrophy, 1190
  toxicities causing, e383
  visual pathway, 1135f, e382
Blisters, from adverse drug reactions,
    488t
Bloat. See Gastric dilatation-volvulus
    (GDV)
Blood
  characteristics of, 10t
  donors, e144-e145
  purification with renal replacement
      therapy, 871-875
Blood chemistry profile, and blood gas
    measurement, e1
Blood compatibility, 311-312
Blood crossmatching, 311-312
  and typing to ensure blood
      compatibility, e143-e148
  procedure, e146-e147
Blood dyscrasias
  drug induced, e160, e162
  from methimazole, e103
Blood film evaluation, in the clinic
    laboratory, 307
Blood flow
  during CPR, 27
  impairment, in hypercoagulable states,
      297, 298f
  improvement in collateral, 814
Blood gas interpretation, e1-e3
Blood glucose
  continuous monitoring systems for,
      198
  home monitoring, 196-197
  levels with insulinomas, e130
  monitoring of, with diabetes mellitus,
      194-195
    in cats, 214
    in dogs, 191
  point-of-care analyzer for, 191-192,
      196, 210
  values with diabetic ketoacidosis, e79,
      e80-e81t, e82
Blood groups, 311
Blood patching, for treatment of
    pneumothorax, 704
Blood pH, and acid-base disorders, e1
Blood pressure. See also Hypertension;
    Hypotension
  for staging of kidney disease, 859-860,
      860t
  indications for measurement of, 727b
  monitoring in dogs with murmurs,
      786
  monitoring with nitroprusside therapy,
      767-768
  tips for measurement of, 727-728

Blood products
  for treatment of von Willebrand
      disease, 290t
  types of, 310-311
Blood testing
  coagulation testing with
      thromboelastography, 74-77
  with hereditary coagulation factor
      deficiencies, 286-291
Blood transfusions
  best practices of, 309-313
  causing adverse skin reactions, 488t
  drug incompatibilities with, 33t
  effect of liver failure on, 580-581
  for disseminated intravascular
      coagulation, 295
  for therapy of shock, 21-22
  for treatment of von Willebrand
      disease, 290, 290t
  guidelines for, 309-313
  indications for, 309-310
  monitoring, 312-313
  pleural, for treatment of
      pneumothorax, 704
  reactions, 312-313
  typing and crossmatching to ensure
      compatibility of, e143-e148
Blood types
  in cats, e145-e146, e145t
  in dogs, e143-e144, e144t
Blood typing
  and crossmatching to ensure blood
      compatibility, e143-e148
  procedure, e144-e145
Blood vessel neoplasia, e167-e168
Bloodroot toxicity, 124t
Blue-green algae toxicity, 123, 570b, 581b
Body condition score, 38-39, 254-255,
    256f-258f
  with cancer cachexia, 351
Body fat index, 257f-258f
Body weight, estimating ideal, 255,
    256f-258f
Bone grafts, with open fractures, 86
Bone marrow
  aspirate
    cytologic evaluation of, 314-315
    prior to use of chemotherapeutic
        drugs, 330
    with thrombocytopenia, 284
  dyscrasias, 314-318
  neoplasia, causing nonregenerative
      anemia, e164
Bone tumor, from osteosarcoma, 388-392
Boneset toxicity, 124t
Boots, for feet protection, e359
Borates, for dust mite control, e199
Borborygmus, e247
Border terrier(s), sebaceous gland
    hyperplasia in, 476-477
Bordetella bronchiseptica
  canine
    bronchopneumonia from, 634, 681,
        682t, 687, 1218
    causing respiratory infection,
        632-633, 1217-1218
    causing rhinitis, 636-637, 636b,
        1217-1218

Bordetella bronchiseptica (Continued)
    nebulization of gentamicin for, 628,
        634, 671
    vaccination, 634-635
  causing infection in humans, 1246
  common symptoms and syndromes
      caused by, 1213t
  feline
    causing pneumonia, 681, 682t
    causing upper respiratory infections,
        629, 630t, 1217-1218
Boric acid
  as topical therapy, 441t
    for otitis, 465t
  causing reproductive toxicity, 1027b
  for Malassezia dermatitis, 442
Borreliosis. See Lyme disease
Borzoi(s), hypothyroidism in, 178-179
Boston ferns, 121b
Boston terrier(s), risk of vaccine
    hypersensitivity in, 1250-1251
Botanical insecticides, examples of, 136b
Botanical oil extract toxicity, 139-140
Botulinum toxin A, for treatment of
    cricopharyngeal dysphagia, 500
Bougienage, of esophageal structures,
    503-504, e240
Bouvier des Flandres, laryngeal paralysis
    in, 659-661
Bovine cross-linked collagen, for urinary
    incontinence, e348-e349, e348
Bowen's disease, topical
    immunomodulators for, e220
Boxer dog
  arrhythmogenic right ventricular
      cardiomyopathy in, 801-804
  canine leproid granuloma in, 446
  granulomatous colitis in, 519b, 520t,
      552-553
  indolent corneal ulcers in, 1151-1152
  neurocardiogenic syncope in,
      e326-e327
  risk of vaccine hypersensitivity in,
      1250-1251
  sick sinus syndrome in, 732-733
  subaortic stenosis in, e319
  testicular tumors in, 1022-1023
  ventricular arrhythmia in, 745
Brachycephalic airway obstruction
    syndrome, 649-653
  abnormalities associated with, 650t
  as risk for heat-induced illness, 71
  prognosis of, 652
  treatment of, 651-652
Bradyarrhythmias
  cardiac pacing for, e281-e286
  diagnosis and treatment of, 731-737
  feline, 750f-751f
  iatrogenic, 731-732
  pathologic, 732-737
  physiologic, 731
  temporary pacing for, e21-e22
  with heart failure, temporary pacing
      for, e22
Bradycardia(s). See also Bradyarrhythmias
  atropine response test with, e330
  causing syncope, e326-e328, e328, e328f
    drug induced, e328

Bradycardia(s) *(Continued)*
from calcium administration, e126
from hypothyroidism, e85
reflex-mediated, 736
sinus, with syncope, e330
Bradyzoites, from toxoplasmosis, 1295
Brain disorders
hydrocephalus, 1034-1037
intracranial arachnoid cysts causing, 1038-1039
intracranial tumors causing, 1039-1047
metabolic, 1047-1053
Brain energy metabolism, 1047-1048
Brainstem auditory evoked response (BAER), for evaluation of hearing, 469
Brake fluid toxicity, 154
Bravo capsule pH test, 502-503
Breathing
patterns with respiratory distress, 45-46
with ventilator therapy, 56
work of, 44
Breed(s)
affected with von Willebrand disease, 288t
predisposed to glaucoma, 1171b
predisposed to hepatobiliary disease, 571b
thyroid hormone differences in, 180t
with reported disorders of sexual development, 995b
Breeding
and pregnancy loss, 1003-1011
dystocia management from, 948-956
estrus suppression in the bitch and, 984-989
management of the bitch, 930-935
optimal time for breeding, 930-935, 931t
nutrition during pregnancy and lactation, 961-966
pregnancy diagnosis in companion animals, 944-948
screening of *brucella canis* before, 972, e404
soundness exam and normal ejaculation behavior, e353
toxins affecting, 1026-1028
use of endoscopy transcervical insemination, 940-944, 941f
Briard(s)
congenital night blindness of, 1190
hyperlipidemia in, 261
Brinzolamide
for canine glaucoma, 1173-1174, 1173b, e381
for feline glaucoma, 1179, e381
British anti-Lewisite (BAL), for lead toxicity, 158
Brodifacoum rodenticide toxicity, 133-134
Bromadiolone rodenticide toxicity, 133-134
Bromethalin rodenticide toxicity, 134
Bromocriptine, for pregnancy termination, 990-991

Bromovinyldeoxyuridine, for feline ocular herpesvirus 1, 1158
Bronchial
compression from heart enlargement, 782
deformities with brachycephalic airway obstruction syndrome, 650t
lavage, for feline asthma, 675-676
Bronchial collapse
and brachycephalic airway obstruction syndrome, 650t
stenting for, 668
Bronchial disease
antiinflammatory drugs for, 625-627
chronic, causing pulmonary hypertension, 711, 712t
diagnosis and treatment of
in cats, 673-680
in dogs, 669-672
Bronchiectasis, 671-672
Bronchitis. *See also Bordetella bronchiseptica*; Tracheobronchitis
chronic
in cats, 673-680
in dogs, 669-672
common infectious agents causing, 1218
Bronchoalveolar lavage
collection of cytology specimens from, e155
for diagnosis of parasites, e269-e276
for diagnosis of pneumocystosis, e410
for diagnosis of pneumonia, 686
Bronchoconstriction, 44
from feline asthma, 675
Bronchodilator(s)
for canine bronchial disease, 671
for feline asthma, 675-680
for pneumonia, 687
for respiratory diseases, 623-625
for tracheal collapse, 664
inhalers, 623-624, 678-680
Bronchogenic carcinoma, causing secondary ocular changes, 1210
Bronchomalacia in dogs, 669-672, 670f
Bronchopulmonary parasites, e271-e276
Bronchoscopy, 669, 670f
for bronchopulmonary parasites, e271-e276, e271f
for eosinophilic pulmonary diseases, 689, 689f
for feline asthma, 675-676
for interstitial lung diseases, e267
Broom plant toxicity, 124t
Brucella canis
aspermia from, e350
causing infection in humans, 1247
causing pregnancy loss, 1005t, 1008, 1218
common symptoms and syndromes caused by, 1213t
diagnosis of, 972
screening for, 972
treatment of, 972
Brucellosis, e402-e404
and pregnancy loss, 1004, 1008
causing uveitis in dogs, 1163-1164, 1164b

Brucellosis *(Continued)*
clinical signs of, e402-e403
diagnosis of, e403-e404, e403f
prevention of, e404
treatment of, e404
zoonosis of, e402
Buccal mucosa bleeding time, with bleeding abnormalities, 287
Budd-Chiari syndrome, stenting for, 347
Budesonide, for inflammatory bowel disease, 539
Buffer composition in fluid therapy, 3t
Bulking agents, injectable, for urinary incontinence disorders, e345-e350, e347-e348, e347f
Bull terrier(s), laryngeal paralysis in, 659-661
Bulldog(s), brachycephalic airway obstruction syndrome in, 650t
Bullmastiff(s), direct mutation tests for, 1018t-1020t
Buphthalmos, from canine glaucoma, 1171
Bupivacaine, 62t
toxicity of, use of IV lipid emulsion therapy for, 106
use of with cesarean section, 955
Buprenorphine
dosage for, 62t
for epidural analgesia, 61
for feline pancreatitis, 566-567, 567t
for the critical patient, 59
for thromboembolism pain, 814
oral transmucosal route for, 59-60
use of, with cardiovascular dysfunction, 65t
Buprenorphine SR, 59-60
dosage for, 62t
Bupropion toxicity, use of IV lipid emulsion therapy for, 106
Burning bush, Eastern, toxicity of, 124t
Burns, fluid movement with, 9t
Butorphanol
dosage for, 62t
for coughing, 622-623, 672
for feline pancreatitis, 567t
for heart failure
in cats, 808
in dogs, 764t-765t, 790-791
for thromboembolism pain, 814
to calm respiratory distress pets, 47t
use of, with cardiovascular dysfunction, 65t
Butterfly ingestion, 99

C

C-reactive protein, with inflammatory bowel disease, 538
Cabergoline
for postpartum puerperal tetany, 958t
for pregnancy termination, 990-991
for septic mastitis, 959
for termination of lactation, 960
Cachexia, from cancer, 349-354
Cadmium, causing reproductive toxicity, 1027b

Cairn terrier(s)
  direct mutation tests for, 1018t-1020t
  risk of urolithiasis in, 897
Calamus toxicity, 124t
Calcidiol, supplement for hypocalcemia,
    e127-e128, e128t
Calcimimetics, for feline idiopathic
    hypercalcemia, 247
Calcineurin inhibitor(s)
  as topical immunomodulators,
    e216-e220, e217f
  for immunosuppression, 269-271
  safety concerns of, e219-e220
Calcinosis cutis, corticosteroid-induced,
    489-490
Calcitriol
  for chronic kidney disease, 862
  for hyperparathyroidism, e70-e71
  for hypoparathyroidism, e124-e129
  measurement for evaluation of
    hypocalcemia, e125f
  supplement for hypocalcemia,
    e127-e128, e128-e129, e128t
Calcium. See also Hypercalcemia;
    Hypocalcemia
  composition in fluid therapy, 3t
  concentrations
    with feline idiopathic hypercalcemia,
      242-248, 245f
    with hyperparathyroidism, e70, e72
    with puerperal tetany, 959-960
  monitoring during IV injections of,
    e126
  oral formulations of, e127-e128, e127t
  pathophysiology and risk of oxalate
    urolithiasis, 897-898
  supplementation for tetany or seizures,
    e126, e126-e127, e126t
Calcium carbonate
  for hypocalcemia, e127-e128, e127t
  for postpartum puerperal tetany, 958t,
    960
Calcium channel blocker(s)
  causing syncope, e328, e328f
  drug incompatibilities with, 33t
  for atrial fibrillation with dilated
    cardiomyopathy, 799
  for dogs, 763b
  for feline arrhythmias, 752
  for hypertension, 728-729
    and kidney disease, 861-862
  for supraventricular tachyarrhythmias,
    742t, 743
  toxicity of, use of IV lipid emulsion
    therapy for, 106
Calcium chloride
  for hypocalcemia tetany or seizures,
    e126, e126t
  monitoring during injection with,
    e126
  oral, for hypocalcemia, e127-e128,
    e127t
Calcium citrate, for hypocalcemia, e127t
Calcium EDTA, for lead toxicity, 158
Calcium gluconate
  drug incompatibilities with, 33t
  for atrial standstill, 755
  for dystocia, 952f, 954

Calcium gluconate (Continued)
  for hypocalcemia tetany or seizures,
    e126, e126t
  for postpartum puerperal tetany, 958t,
    960
  monitoring during injection with,
    e126
  oral, for hypocalcemia, e127t
Calcium lactate, for hypocalcemia,
    e127t
Calcium oxalate crystalluria, 926
  from ethylene glycol toxicity, 152
Calcium oxalate urolithiasis, 897-901
  and nephroliths, 926
  laser lithotripsy for, e341f
  with hypercalcemia, 244
Calcium-related degenerative
    keratopathy, 1153
Calicivirus. See Feline calicivirus
Callilepis laureola toxicity, 581b
Calorie(s)
  composition in fluid therapy, 3t
  decreasing intake of, with obesity,
    255-260
  dietary requirements for, with diabetes
    mellitus, 202-203, 204t
  estimating desired intake of, 259
  in parenteral nutrition products, 40,
    41b-42b
  needs in patients with cancer, 352
  requirements during pregnancy and
    lactation, 961-963, 966f
Calprotectin, with inflammatory bowel
    disease, 538
Camellias, 121b
Camphor, as topical antipruritic agents,
    419
Campylobacteriosis, 520
  causing diarrhea, 519
  causing pregnancy loss, 1005t, 1006,
    1008
  common symptoms and syndromes
    caused by, 1213t
  in raw meat diets, 1240-1241, 1240b
  treatment for, 520t
Canaliculus
  imperforate, e375-e376
  laceration of, e376
  obstructed, e376
Cancer. See also Neoplasia
  adverse effects from therapy of,
    330-333
  cell targeting, 355
  nutrition for the patient with, 349-354
  talking to clients about, 318-321,
    e169-e170
Cancer cachexia, 349-354
Cancer immunotherapy, 334-337
Cancer vaccine, 335, 336t
Candida spp.
  causing hospital-acquired urinary tract
    infections, 876
  causing perivulvar dermatitis, 971
Candidatus mycoplasma haemominutum,
    e399
Candidatus mycoplasma turicensis, e399
Candidiasis, antifungal therapy for,
    1234-1238

Canine adenovirus 1, common
    symptoms and syndromes caused by,
    1215t
Canine adenovirus type 2 (CAV-2)
  causing canine respiratory infection,
    632, 1217-1218
  common symptoms and syndromes
    caused by, 1215t
Canine atopic dermatitis, 403-404
Canine bartonellosis, 1261-1267
Canine blood groups, 311
Canine breeding management of the
    female, 930-935
Canine colitis, 550-554
Canine conjunctivitis, 1138-1143
Canine coronavirus, common symptoms
    and syndromes caused by, 1215t
Canine demodicosis, 432-434
Canine distemper virus (CDV)
  as cause of thrombocytopenia,
    281t-282t
  causing canine respiratory infection,
    632, 1217-1218
  causing nervous system signs, 1212
  causing pregnancy loss, 1005t, 1009
  common symptoms and syndromes
    caused by, 1215t
Canine granulocytic anaplasmosis, as
    cause of thrombocytopenia,
    281t-282t
Canine hemotropic mycoplasmas,
    e398-e401
Canine herpesvirus (CHV)
  as cause of thrombocytopenia,
    281t-282t
  causing canine respiratory infection,
    632, 634, 1217-1218
  causing conjunctivitis, 634, 1141-1142,
    1142f
  causing pregnancy loss, 1005t, 1009
  causing vulvar discharge, 972
  common symptoms and syndromes
    caused by, 1215t
Canine hyperlipidemia, diagnosis and
    treatment of, 261-266
Canine infectious respiratory diseases,
    632-635
  diagnosis of, 633
  treatment and prognosis of, 633-634
Canine influenza virus (CIV)
  causing canine respiratory infection,
    632, 1217-1218
  common symptoms and syndromes
    caused by, 1215t
Canine inherited disorders, diagnostic
    tests for, 1015-1021
Canine leproid granuloma, 445-448,
    446f, 448t
Canine leukocyte adhesion deficiency,
    direct mutation test for, 1018t-1020t
Canine lymphoma, rescue therapy for,
    382t
Canine multifocal retinopathy, 1188
  direct mutation test for, 1018t-1020t
Canine ocular neoplasia, 1201-1206
Canine orthopedic trauma, 80-83
Canine papillomatosis. See
    Papillomavirus

Canine parainfluenza virus (CPiV)
    causing canine respiratory infection,
        632, 1217-1218
    common symptoms and syndromes
        caused by, 1215t
Canine parvoviral enteritis, 533-536
Canine parvovirus
    causing pregnancy loss, 1005t, 1009
    common symptoms and syndromes
        caused by, 1215t
    use of interferons for, e201
Canine pigmented plaques, e185
Canine respiratory coronavirus (CRCoV)
    causing canine respiratory infection,
        632, 1217-1218
    common symptoms and syndromes
        caused by, 1215t
Canine thyroid carcinoma, 397-400, 398f
Capillaria aerophilia, e275
Capillaria boehmi, causing nasal
        discharge, 636-637, 636b
Capsaicin, action and use of, for motility
        disorders, 517-518
Carbamate peroxide, in ear cleaners,
        472t
Carbamate toxicity, 135-137, 136b
Carbamazepine toxicity, use of IV lipid
        emulsion therapy for, 106
Carbapenem, for pneumonia, 683t
Carbimazole, for hyperthyroid cats,
        e103t, e105
    with kidney failure, 188
Carbohydrate(s)
    dietary, with weight loss diets, 255-259
    dietary requirements for, with diabetes
        mellitus, 200-201, 201t, 204t,
        210-215
Carbon dioxide
    and acid-base disorders, e1
    tension, disorders of, e3-e5
Carbon monoxide toxicity, 1027b, e45
Carbon tetrachloride toxicity, 570b
Carbonic anhydrase inhibitor(s)
    causing drug reaction conjunctivitis,
        1140
    for canine glaucoma, 1173-1174,
        1173b, e381
    for feline glaucoma, 1178-1179, e381
Carboplatin
    adverse effects of, 330-331
    for osteosarcoma, 391t
    for thyroid cancer, 400
    for urinary bladder cancer, 373
    ototoxicity from, 468b
Carcinogen, in second-hand smoke,
        e44-e45
Carcinomatosis, causing malignant
        effusions, 341
Cardiac
    effects of potassium supplementation,
        253
    toxicity from chemotherapeutic drugs,
        332
Cardiac atony, and brachycephalic
        airway obstruction syndrome, 650t
Cardiac biomarkers
    for congenital heart disease, 759
    for valvular heart disease, 790

Cardiac cachexia, 722-724
Cardiac hypertrophy, secondary to
        hypertension, 726
Cardiac neoplasia, e167
Cardiac pacemaker. See Pacemaker
Cardiac pump theory, 27
Cardiac tamponade, from pericardial
        effusion, 816-817
Cardiac troponin I
    for congenital heart disease, 759
    use in respiratory distress, 47
    with hemangiosarcoma, 395, 820
    with myocarditis, e305, e305f
Cardigan Welsh corgi(s), direct mutation
        tests for, 1018t-1020t
Cardiomyopathy
    arrhythmogenic right ventricular
        direct mutation test for, 1018t-1020t
        in cats, e277-e281, e306-e307
        in dogs, 801-804, e308
    canine
        classification and staging with,
            775-781
        dilated
            cardiogenic shock with, 783
            causing pulmonary hypertension,
                711
            classification and staging with,
                775-781
            diagnosis and treatment of,
                795-800
            direct mutation test for,
                1018t-1020t
            genetic marker test for, 1021t
            nutritional recommendations for,
                724
            prognosis, 800
            treatment of asymptomatic,
                775-777
            with arrhythmogenic right
                ventricular, 802
        feline, 804-810, 806t
            asymptomatic, 805-807
            dilated, 809
                nutritional recommendations for,
                    724-725
            hypertrophic, 807-809
                with arrhythmias, 809
                with congestive failure, 806t, 808
                recurrent, 806t, 809
                with thromboembolism, 809-815
            nutritional recommendations for,
                720-725
        pulmonary thromboembolism
            associated with, 705
Cardioprotective drugs, 762
Cardiopulmonary arrest
    diagnosis of, 26
    epinephrine use in, 15-17, 15t
    fluid therapy considerations with, 6
    temporary pacing for, e22
Cardiopulmonary resuscitation (CPR),
        26-31
    open chest, 31
    post arrest care, 31
    prognosis with, 31
Cardiovascular changes, from
        hypothyroidism, 179

Cardiovascular dysfunction
    anesthesia for patients with, 64-68
    premedication and sedation with,
        64-65, 65t
Cardiovascular effects, from plants,
        121b
Cardioversion, e286-e291, e288f
    for atrial fibrillation, e288-e289, e288,
        e289f
    for supraventricular tachyarrhythmias
        in dogs, 742t, 744
    indications and contraindications for,
        e286-e287
    procedure, e287-e288
Carminatives, for flatulence, e249-e250
Carmustine, for intracranial tumors,
        1041t, 1044
Carnitine. See L-Carnitine
Carotid body tumor, e167-e168
Carotid sinus massage, in cats, 753
Carotid sinus syncope, e328
Carpal hypertension, 80
Carpal trauma in dogs, 81
Carprofen
    adverse effects of, 60
        cutaneous, 489
    for canine uveitis, 1165t
    hepatotoxicity from, 570b, 578, 581b
    influence on thyroid function, 181t
Carts, for rehabilitation, e359
Carvedilol
    for asymptomatic heart disease, 776
    for dilated cardiomyopathy, in dogs
        occult, 797-798
        with heart failure, 799
    for heart failure, in dogs, 763b,
        764t-765t, 770-771, 792
    for myocarditis, e306
    for valvular heart disease, 790, 792
    toxicity of, use of IV lipid emulsion
        therapy for, 106
Caspofungin, use and protocols for,
        1235t
Castor beans toxicity, 121b
Castration
    early age, in dogs and cats, 982-984
    for benign prostatic hypertrophy,
        1013
    for perianal adenoma, 367
    risk of prostate cancer and, 1023-1024
Cat fur mite infestation, 431
Cat litter, hypokalemia from ingestion
        of, 252
Cat(s)
    population control for, 142-144
    temporary pacing in, e28
    use of cisplatin in, 333
Cataract(s)
    causing uveitis, 1184
    classification of, 1182t
    diabetic, 193, 1183, e78
    diagnosis and treatment of, 1181-1185,
        1182f
    direct mutation test for, 1018t-1020t
    hypermature, 1181-1183, 1183f
    immature, 1181-1183, 1182f
    mature, 1181-1183, 1182f
    surgery, 1184-1185

Catecholamine(s)
  commonly used, 15t
  for cardiogenic shock, 783
  for critical care patients, 14-17
  for heart failure, in dogs, 769
  for septic shock, 17
  hypokalemia from, 251b
  receptor activities of, 15t
Caterpillar ingestion, 99
Cathartic(s), for toxin ingestions, 105
Catheter(s)
  central venous, with acute respiratory
    distress syndrome, 50
  for parenteral nutrition products,
    40-41
  pulmonary artery, 19-20
  wound, lidocaine use with, 61
Catheterization
  heart, for diagnosis of pulmonary
    hypertension, 711
  of cervix
    for breeding, 942
    for pyometra treatment, 962-963
  urinary
    antegrade of bladder, 889-891
    as risk factor for hospital-acquired
      urinary tract infections, 877-879
Cationic liposomes, for infectious disease
  immune therapeutics, 1230t
Cattery(ies)
  multicat outbreaks with
    dermatophytosis in, 452-454
  upper respiratory infection in, 629
Caudal occipital malformation
  syndrome, 1098
Caval syndrome, 833
Cavalier King Charles spaniel(s)
  craniocervical junction abnormalities
    in, 1098-1102
  masticatory muscle myositis in,
    1113-1114
  nonepidermolytic ichthyosis in, 476
  otitis media with nasopharyngeal
    disorders in, 654
  strokes in, 812
  valvular heart disease in, 784
CCNU. See Lomustine
CD34+ cells, causing lymphocytosis, 303
Cefadroxil
  for pyoderma, 1220t, 1221-1222
  for septic mastitis, 959
  for superficial bacterial folliculitis,
    438t
  for upper respiratory tract infection(s),
    1220t, 1222
  for urinary tract infections, 1220-1221,
    1220t
Cefazolin
  adverse effects of, 34t-35t
  before musculoskeletal surgery, 1220t,
    1222
  for septicemia, 1220t, 1223
  for therapy with open fractures, 84-85
Cefovecin, for superficial bacterial
  folliculitis, 437-438, 438t
Cefoxitin, for septicemia, 1220t, 1223
Cefpodoxime, for superficial bacterial
  folliculitis, 438, 438t

Ceftazidime sodium (Fortaz), for otitis,
  466t, 467
Celecoxib toxicity, 116-117
Celinski v. State, e49-e50
Cellulitis, juvenile, use of cyclosporine
  for, 410b
Center of veterinary medicine, FDA,
  reporting adverse events to, e38,
  e39f
Centipede ingestion, 99
Central nervous system
  disease from Bartonella spp. infections,
    1263b
  disorder causing dysphagia, 496b
  disorder from hypothyroidism,
    e76-e77
  infections, use of glucocorticoids for,
    1300
  noninfectious and inflammatory
    diseases of, 1063-1066
  signs, infectious agents that cause,
    1212
  vascular disease of, 1119-1126
Central nervous system stimulant(s),
  toxicity of, 109-112
Centronuclear myopathy, direct
  mutation test for, 1018t-1020t
Cephalexin
  for feline upper respiratory infection,
    631t
  for methicillin-resistant Staphylococcal
    infections, 444
  for otitis, 466
  for pyoderma, 1220t, 1221-1222
  for superficial bacterial folliculitis, 438t
  for upper respiratory tract infection(s),
    1220t, 1222
  for urinary tract infections, 1220-1221,
    1220t
Cephalosporin(s)
  adverse effects of, 34t-35t
  causing adverse skin reactions, 488t
  for lower respiratory tract infection(s),
    1222
  for musculoskeletal infections, 1220t,
    1222-1223
  for therapy with open fractures, 84-85
Cephalothin
  adverse effects of, 34t-35t
  drug incompatibilities with, 33t
Ceramide(s), topical, 420t
Cerebral blood flow
  and energy metabolism, 1047-1048
  considerations of anesthesia with,
    68-70, 69f
Cerebral perfusion, with cerebrovascular
  accidents (stroke), 1120-1123
Cerebrospinal fluid (CSF)
  acidosis, 67
  analysis for inflammatory central
    nervous system disorders, 1064
  analysis with fibrocartilaginous
    embolism, 1124-1125
  biomarkers for intervertebral disk
    disease, 1073-1074
Cerebrovascular accident (stroke)
  diagnosis and treatment of, 1119-1126,
    1121f

Cerebrovascular accident (stroke)
  (Continued)
  hemorrhagic, 1120
  ischemic, 1119-1120
  thromboembolic disease with, 812
Ceroid lipofuscinosis, direct mutation
  test for, 1018t-1020t
Ceruminolytic(s), for the ear, 472-473,
  472t
Cervical pain
  from atlantoaxial subluxation,
    1082-1090
  from cervical spondylomyelopathy,
    1090-1097
  from Chiari-like malformation,
    1098-1105
Cervical spondylomyelopathy,
  1090-1097
  algorithm for diagnosis and treatment
    of, 1095f
  diagnosis of, 1092-1094
  hypothyroidism with, 1094
  pathophysiology of, 1090-1091,
    1091f-1092f
  prognosis of, 1096-1097
  surgery for, 1094-1096
  treatment of, 1094-1096
Cervical vertebral instability. See Cervical
  spondylomyelopathy
Cervix, catheterization of, 942
Cesarean section, anesthesia for, 955t
Cetirizine hydrochloride
  for atopic dermatitis, 406
  toxicity of, 118-119
Chagas' disease, causing myocarditis,
  e307
Chalazion, e363
Chaparral toxicity, 570b, 581b
Chelation therapy
  for copper-associated liver disease,
    588-590, e234-e236
  for lead toxicity, 157-158
  hypomagnesemia from, 249b
Chemical toxins
  associated with hepatotoxicity, 570b
  exposure to respiratory, e44-e47
Chemistry analyzers, quality control of,
  with in-clinic, 307-309
Chemodectoma
  major vessel, e167-e168
  pericardial, 817, 823
Chemoembolization, for malignant
  obstructions, 348
Chemosis, from conjunctivitis, in dogs,
  1139
Chemotherapy
  adverse effects of, 330
  and risk of hospital-acquired urinary
    infections, 877
  antiviral, for feline retrovirus
    infections, 1277-1280, 1279t
  associated hepatotoxicity, 575-579,
    581b
  causing adverse skin reactions, 488t
  client questions about, 318-321
  drug handling and safety, 326-329
  for feline gastrointestinal lymphoma,
    547-548

Chemotherapy (Continued)
for hemangiosarcoma, 395-396
for insulinoma, e132-e133
for intracranial tumors, 1043t, 1044-1045
for malignant effusions, 343-344
for mammary cancer, 377, 379-380
for multiple myeloma, 385-386
for oral tumors, 364
for osteosarcoma, 390-391, 391t
for perianal adenocarcinoma, 368-369
for soft tissue sarcomas, e151
for urinary bladder cancer, 373
intraarterial, 347-348
for lower urinary tract, 890, 891f
intracavitary, 343-344
metronomic, 354-357
new anticancer drugs, e139-e142
ototoxicity from, 468b, 469
rescue therapy for canine lymphoma, 381-383, 382t
update on masitinib as, 360-362
waste handling, 328-329
Cherry eye. See under Nictitating membrane
Chesapeake Bay retriever(s), direct mutation tests for, 1018t-1020t
Chest tube. See Thoracostomy tube(s)
Chewing behavior in cats, 913
Cheyletiellosis
diagnosis and treatment of, 430
treatment options for, 430t
use of avermectins for, e182
Chiari-like malformation in dogs, 1098-1105, 1099f
Chigger mite(s), diagnosis and treatment of, 431-432
Chihuahua(s), risk of vaccine hypersensitivity in, 1250-1251
Chinese crested(s), direct mutation tests for, 1018t-1020t
Chlamydia felis
causing feline upper respiratory infections, 629, 630t, 1217-1218
common symptoms and syndromes caused by, 1213t
Chlorambucil
for feline gastrointestinal lymphoma, 547-548, 548t
for feline infectious peritonitis, 1305t
for inflammatory bowel disease, 539
for multiple myeloma, 386
metronomic chemotherapy of, 344
Chloramphenicol
adverse effects of, 34t-35t
causing adverse skin reactions, 488t
dosing of, with liver disease, 32-33
drug interactions with, 35t
for ehrlichiosis, 1293
for lower respiratory tract infection(s), 1220t, 1222
for methicillin-resistant Staphylococcal skin infections, 444
for superficial bacterial folliculitis, 438t
ototoxicity from, 468b
topical, for feline ocular herpesvirus 1, 1158
Chlordecone toxicity, 1027b

Chlorhexidine
as topical therapy, 441t
for disinfection of methicillin-resistant Staphylococcal spp., 455-456
for Malassezia dermatitis, 442
for pyoderma, 440
Chloride composition in fluid therapy, 3t
Chloride gap, calculation of, with acid-base disorders, e2
Chlorinated compounds toxicity, 581b
Chlorinated hydrocarbon toxicity, 570b
Chloroform toxicity, 581b, 1027b
Chlorophacinone rodenticide toxicity, 133-134
Chloroprene toxicity, 1027b
Chlorothymol, in ear cleaners, 472t
Chloroxylenol, as topical therapy for skin infections, 441t
Chlorpheniramine
causing adverse skin reactions, 488t
toxicity of, 118-119
Chlorpromazine
for cocaine toxicity, 110
for feline pancreatitis, 567t
for vomiting with acute renal failure, 870
Chlortetracycline toxicity, 581b
Chocolate
enterohepatic recirculation of, 105
toxicity, 98, 148-149, 148t
Cholangiocystography, 603
Cholangiohepatitis
feline, 614-619
with diabetes mellitus, e77
Cholangioles, reactive, 581-582
Cholangitis
complex, 614-615
feline, 614-619, 617b
lymphocytic, 618
neutrophilic, 615-618
Cholecalciferol
causing nephrotoxicity, e33-e34
supplement for hypocalcemia, e127-e128
Cholecystectomy, 604f-605f
for biliary mucoceles, e223
Cholecystitis, 603
Cholecystography, 603
Choledochal stenting, for acute pancreatitis in cats, 568
Cholelithiasis, 603-604, 604f
Cholestasis
causing alkaline phosphatase elevations, e245b
effect on drug metabolism, 33
Cholinergic drug(s)
for feline glaucoma, 1179-1180
for keratoconjunctivitis sicca, 1145
Cholinesterase inhibitor(s), 136b
for myasthenia gravis, 1110
for urinary retention disorders, 918
Chondrosarcoma, nasal, radiation therapy for, 338-340
CHOP protocol, rescue therapy for canine lymphoma, 381
Chordae tendineae rupture, 790-791, 793

Chorionic gonadotrophin stimulation protocol, 1001, 1002t
Chorioretinitis
canine, 1162
causing blindness, 1136
causing retinal detachment, in dogs, e371, e371f
feline, 1166, 1195-1196
Choristoma, 1153
Choroiditis, canine, 1162
Chromium, for diabetes mellitus, 202, e136t, e137-e138
Chromosomal sex, 993, 995t
Chronic axonal degeneration, 1117
Chronic bronchial disorders in dogs, 669-672
Chronic bronchitis
in cats, 673-680
in dogs, 669-672, 670f
Chronic demyelinating polyradiculoneuritis, 1117
Chronic intestinal pseudo-obstruction, 516
Chronic kidney disease. See under Renal failure, chronic
Chronic lymphocytic leukemia, 314
Chronic myeloid leukemia, 314, 317-318
Chylothorax, 695
causes of, 697-698
cytology of fluid from, 698-699
medical treatment of, 699
surgical treatment of, 699-700
Cidofovir
for feline ocular herpesvirus 1, 1158
intraocular, with glaucoma eye, 1175-1176
Cigarette toxicity, 119
Cilia abnormalities, 1155
Ciliary body
adenoma, 1204-1205, 1205f
procedures on, for glaucoma, 1175
Cimetidine (Tagamet)
causing adverse skin reactions, 488t
drug interactions with, 35t, 37, 677
potency and use of, 505, 506b
toxicity of, 119
Ciprofloxacin, for otitis, systemic, 466t
Circulation, during CPR, 27, 30
Cirrhosis, 584-585, 585f. See also Liver failure
causing ascites, 591-592
Cisapride (Propulsid)
action and use of, for motility disorders, 517t
for esophagitis, e239-e240
for gastroesophageal reflux, 503
for hepatic lipidosis, 612
for urinary retention disorders, 917t
use of, for motility disorders, 516-518
Cisplatin
for intrathoracic chemotherapy, 343
for nasal neoplasia, in dogs, 641-643, e158
for osteosarcoma, 391t
for urinary bladder cancer, 372-373
intraarterial delivery of, 348
metronomic chemotherapy of, 343
toxicity from chemotherapeutic drugs, 332-333

Citalopram toxicity, 113
Citrate, use of, with continuous renal replacement therapy, 873-875
Citrus aurantium toxicity, 123
Citrus oil, 126
CL/mAb 231, as immunotherapy for lymphoma, 335
Clarithromycin, for nontuberculous cutaneous granulomas, 448t
Cleaning
  associated with hazardous drugs, 328
  environments contaminated with resistant Staphylococcal spp., 455-457
  for dust mite control, e198
  the ear
    flushing techniques and solutions for, 471-474, 472t
    with otitis, 458
Cleaning product(s), toxic exposures to, 92t, 95t
Client confidentiality, and reporting human drugs of abuse exposure, e52
Client information sheets, for drugs, e41
Client(s)
  communication of hazardous drug handling, 329
  education with allergen immunotherapy, 412b
  talking about cancer with, 318-321
Climbing structures, to enrich cats environments, 910-911
Clindamycin
  drug interactions with, 677
  for canine babesiosis, 1259
  for feline pancreatitis, 567t
  for feline upper respiratory infection, 631t
  for lower respiratory tract infection(s), 1220t, 1222
  for methicillin-resistant Staphylococcal skin infections, 444
  for musculoskeletal infections, 1220t, 1222-1223
  for pyoderma, 1220t, 1221-1222
  for superficial bacterial folliculitis, 438t
  for toxoplasmosis, 1167, 1297
  target parasites and dosage of, 1335-1337
Clitoral hypertrophy, 972, 978-979, 978f
Clofazimine, for nontuberculous cutaneous granulomas, 448t
Clomipramine
  for behavior-related dermatoses, 482-483, 483t
  influence on thyroid function, 181t
  toxicity of, 114
    use of IV lipid emulsion therapy for, 106
Clonal bone marrow dyscrasias, 316-318
Clonality testing, for evaluation of lymphocytosis, 302
Clonazepam
  for behavior-related dermatoses, 483t, 484
  toxicity of, 113-114

Clopidogrel (Plavix)
  as anticoagulant therapy, for autoimmune hemolytic anemia, 277-278, 277t
  causing adverse skin reactions, 488t
  drug interactions with, 34t-35t
  for feline cardiomyopathy, 806t
  for feline thromboembolism, 810
  for hypercoagulable states, 300
  for prevention of cerebrovascular accidents (stroke), 1122
  for protein-losing enteropathy, 544
  for thromboprophylaxis, 710, 814-815
  to improve collateral blood flow, 814
  use of proton pump inhibitors with, 506
Cloprostenol, for pregnancy termination, 990-991
Clorazepate, for behavior-related dermatoses, 483t, 484
Closed system drug transfer devices, 327
Closed-suction drainage, for peritoneal drainage, e12-e13, e12f
Clostridium difficile, in tube feeds, e19
Clostridium perfringens, common symptoms and syndromes caused by, 1213t
Clostridium spp., 520
  associated hepatotoxicity, 581b
  causing diarrhea, 519
  treatment for, 520t
Clot formation, with thromboelastography, 74-75
CLOtest, 510, 510f
Clotrimazole (Veltrim)
  for nasal aspergillosis
    in cats, 648
    in dogs, 638-639
  topical, for otitis, 465t
Clotting abnormalities. *See* Coagulopathy
Cloxacillin, for pyoderma, 1220t, 1221-1222
Coagulase-negative staphylococci, 436
Coagulation factor deficiencies, 286-291
Coagulation testing
  evaluation of, with thrombocytopenia, 284
  with disseminated intravascular disorders, 292-296, 293f, 294t
  with hereditary factor deficiencies, 287f, 288t
  with thromboelastography, 74-77
Coagulopathy
  causing hemothorax, 694
  from hydroxyethyl starch solutions, 12-13
  from liver failure, 580-582
  from methimazole, e104
  from rodenticide exposure, 133
  hepatic-disease associated, 572, 574, e257
  with autoimmune hemolytic anemia, 276
  with feline hepatic lipidosis, 610, 612
  with gastric dilation-volvulus, e19
Cobalamin
  absorption, 522-523, 523f

Cobalamin (*Continued*)
  factors affecting the concentration of, 523t
  malabsorption, direct mutation test for, 1018t-1020t
  measurement of, 523
Cobalamin deficiency
  for protein-losing enteropathy, 543
  in cats, 522-525
  with chronic pancreatitis, 564
  with exocrine pancreatic insufficiency (EPI), 556, 560
  with feline gastrointestinal lymphoma, 546-547
  with feline pancreatitis, 567t
  with hepatic lipidosis, 612
  with inflammatory bowel disease, 539
Cocaine toxicity, 110
Cocamidopropyl betaine, in ear cleaners, 472t
Coccidioides immitis
  causing feline uveitis, 1167b
  common symptoms and syndromes caused by, 1214t
Coccidioides spp., causing nervous system signs, 1212
Coccidioidomycosis
  antifungal therapy for, 1234-1238
  causing feline uveitis, 1168
Coccidiomycosis, causing uveitis in dogs, 1163-1164, 1164b
Cocker spaniel(s)
  cardiomyopathy in, 795-796
  direct mutation tests for, 1018t-1020t
  progressive retinal atrophy in, 1188-1190, 1189t
  sick sinus syndrome in, 732-733
  vitamin A-responsive dermatosis in, 476
Cocoa bean or hull toxicity, 98
Cocoa mulch toxicity, 132
Codeine (Methylmorphine), for coughing, 622
Codeine toxicity, 111
Coenzyme Q$_{10}$
  for asymptomatic heart disease, 766
  for feline caudal stomatitis, 494
  for heart disease, 725
  for metabolic brain disorders, 1051, 1051t
  for mitochondrial encephalopathy, 1051, 1051t
  for neuromuscular disease, 1118
Coffee toxicity, 98, 148t
Coin ingestion, 99-100
Cola toxicity, 98
Colchicine
  as hepatic support therapy, e257
  for amyloidosis, 855
  for hepatic fibrosis, 587
Colitis
  canine
    causes of, 551t
    diagnosis and treatment of, 550-554
    medical management of, 551b
  effect of, on gastric emptying, 516
  granulomatous, 552-553
    antibiotic responsive, 519b, 520t

Collagen XXVII, with hemangiosarcoma, 395
Collie(s)
    avermectin toxicity in, 145
    dermatomyositis in, 1115
    exocrine pancreatic insufficiency (EPI) in, 558
    eye anomaly, 1136-1137
        direct mutation test for, 1018t-1020t
    hyperlipidemia in, 261
    ivermectin sensitivity in, e179
    progressive retinal atrophy in, 1188-1190, 1189t
Colloid fluids
    characteristics of, 10t
    clinical use of, 12-13, 12t
    for acute pancreatitis in dogs, 562
    for canine parvovirus, 534
    for gastric dilation-volvulus therapy, e15-e16, e16t
    for protein-losing enteropathy, 543-544
    for shock, 21
    pharmacology of, 8-11
    with crystalloid fluid therapy, 13, e15-e16
    with hypertonic saline, 21
Colloid osmotic pressure, 8, 9f
    conditions that change, 9t
Colloidal oatmeal, 420t
Colonic stenting, of malignant obstructions, 347
Color dilution alopecia, 164
Coltsfoot toxicity, 124t
Combustion-derived toxicant(s), e44-e47
Comfrey toxicity, 570b, 581b
Companion animal parasite council, stand on raw meat diets, 1242
Compensation, with acid-base equilibrium, e1-e2, e2b, e2t
Complete blood count (CBC)
    finding with respiratory distress, 47
    monitoring, prior to chemotherapeutic drugs, 330-331
    with hepatobiliary disease, 569
Compounding
    drugs, e58
    parenteral nutrition products, 40, 41b
Computed tomography (CT)
    attenuation values of normal thyroid gland, 168t
    for atlantoaxial subluxation, 1084-1085, 1085f
    for canine ocular neoplasia, 1201-1206
    for cervical spondylomyelopathy, 1093
    for congenital hydrocephalus, 1035-1036
    for diagnosis of feline hypersomatotropism, 216, 217f, 219
    for evaluation of dysphagia, 499
    for evaluation of hepatobiliary disease, 574
    for evaluation of osteosarcoma, 388
    for hemangiosarcoma, 393-395, 394f
    for inflammatory central nervous system disorders, 1064
    for interstitial lung diseases, e266-e267

Computed tomography (CT) (Continued)
    for intervertebral disk disease, 1073
    for lumbosacral stenosis, 1106
    for nasal tumors, 338, e158f
    for nasopharyngeal disorders, 654
    for pituitary macroadenoma, e89-e90
    imaging for diagnosis of endocrine disorders, 167-174
    of adrenal gland(s), 170-172, 171f
        for hyperaldosteronism in cats, 240-241
    of pancreas, 172-174
    of pituitary gland, 171f
    of thyroid gland, 167-170
    with fibrocartilaginous embolism, 1124
    with nasal discharge
        in cats, 645-646, 645f
        in dogs, 636-638, 639f-640f, 640-641, 642f
    with pericardial effusion, 819, 819f
    with pneumothorax, 701f
    with portal vein hypoplasia, 600
Concentration alkalosis, e6-e7
Conditioner(s), for sebaceous adenitis, e210-e211, e211
Conductive hearing loss, 468, 468b
    treatment and prevention of, 470
Cone degeneration, direct mutation test for, 1018t-1020t
Cone-rod dystrophy, 1190
Congenital disease(s)
    genetic testing for, 1015-1021
    hydrocephalus, 1034-1037
    nonulcerative corneal, 1153
    of the lens, 1181
    of the reproductive tract, 993-999
    vulvar and vaginal anomalies, 976-980
Congenital heart disease, 756-761
    prevalence of, 756-757, 757t
    prophylaxis with, e297-e298
    screening for, 757-759
    therapy of, 759-760
Congenital hydrocephalus, 1034-1037
Conjunctiva
    anatomy and physiology of, 1138
    biopsy of, for episcleritis, 1141
    changes in, with glaucoma in dogs, 1171t
    tumors of
        in cats, 1207-1208
        in dogs, 1201, 1203-1204
    ulcers of, 1139
Conjunctivitis
    allergic, 1139f, 1140
    canine, diagnosis and treatment of, 1138-1143
    frictional irritant, 1140, 1140f
    from feline herpesvirus 1, 1156-1158
    from feline upper respiratory infection, 630t
    from keratoconjunctivitis sicca, 1143
    immune-mediated, 1140-1141
    infectious, 1141-1142
    traumatic, 1139f, 1142
Contact allergy, pentoxifylline for, e203
Contamination, with methicillin-resistant Staphylococcal infections, 455-457, 456t

Continuous glucose monitoring systems, 198
Continuous renal replacement therapy, 871-875, 872f-874f, 875b
Contraceptives, in the bitch, 984-989
Conval lily, toxicity of, 124t
Convection, 71
Cooling methods, for treatment of heat-induced illness, 72-73
Copper
    chelator therapy, 588-590
    concentrations, e234, e234t-e235t
    metabolism, e231, e232f
    restriction, e236
Copper-associated hepatopathy, e231-e236
    breeds predisposed to, 571b
    chelator therapy for, 588-590
    diagnosis of, e231, e234t
    genetic marker test for, 1021t
    liver biopsy for evaluation of, 575
    pathophysiology of, 588
    treatment of, e234
Cor triatriatum sinister, prevalence of, in cats, 757t
Corgi(s), progressive retinal atrophy in, 1188-1190, 1189t
Coring technique for cytology, e154
Cornea. See also under Keratitis; Keratopathy
    anatomy of, 1148, 1149f
    changes in, with glaucoma in dogs, 1171t
    diseases of the, feline, 1156-1161
        clinical signs of, 1157b
    foreign body in, e380
    healing of, 1148-1149
    laceration of, e380
    lipid deposits in, 1153
    neoplasia of, 1156
    nonulcerative disease of, in dogs, 1152-1156
    perforation of, e380
    physiology of, 1148
    plaque on, 1159f
    signs of disease in cats, 1157b
    tumors of
        in cats, 1207-1208
        in dogs, 1204
Corneal edema, with canine uveitis, 1163t
Corneal lipidosis, from hypothyroidism, e85
Corneal sequestrum, 1159-1160, 1160f
    from feline herpesvirus 1, 1157t
    indications for surgery with, 1161t
Corneal ulceration
    causing uveitis in dogs, 1164
    complicated, 1150-1151, e379
    diagnosis and treatment of, 1148-1152, e379-e380
    diamond burr débridement for, 1152
    fluorescein dye for diagnosis of, 1132
    from feline herpesvirus 1, 1157t
    from feline upper respiratory infection, 630t
    indications for surgery with, 1161t
    indolent, 1151-1152, e379
    keratotomy for, 1151-1152

Corneal ulceration *(Continued)*
  simple, 1149-1150, e379
  with canine uveitis, 1166
Cornification disorders in dogs, 475-477
Coronavirus
  enteric, 1303-1304
  feline, as cause of thrombocytopenia,
    281t-282t
Corticosteroid. *See* Glucocorticoid(s)
Corticosteroid alkaline phosphatase
    (cALP), e243
Corticosteroid insufficiency, illness-
    related, 78-79, 174-178
Cortisol, precursor secretion causing
    alopecia, 221-222
Cortisol levels
  with ectopic ACTH syndrome,
    230-231, 231f
  with feline hyperaldosteronism, 240t
  with hypoadrenocorticism, 233-235
  with illness-related adrenal
    insufficiency, 175-176
  with illness-related corticosteroid
    insufficiency, 175-176
Cortisol-to-ACTH ratio, 235
Corynebacterium parvum
    (ImmunoRegulin), as cancer
    immunotherapy, 336t
Cosyntropin
  for testing hypoadrenocorticism,
    233-235
  for testing illness-related adrenal
    insufficiency, 78-79, 175-176
Cotton ball vision test, e391
Cough
  from asthma in cats, 673-674
  from bronchial compression with
    heart disease, 782
  induced syncope, e327
  infectious causes of, 1217-1218
  suppressants (*See* Antitussive drugs)
  treatment of, from tracheal collapse,
    663-664
  with heart disease, 792-793
Coupage, for pneumonia, 687
COX inhibitor(s), for urinary bladder
    cancer, 372-373
Coxiella burnetii
  causing infection in humans, 1246
  causing pregnancy loss, 1005t, 1009,
    1218
  common symptoms and syndromes
    caused by, 1214t
Coxofemoral joint trauma in dogs, 82
Cranberry extract, for persistent *E. coli*
    urinary tract infections, 881b, 882
Cranial nerve(s)
  assessment of with neuro-ophthalmic
    exam, e389, e390-e392
  deficits, from vestibular disease, 1067t
Craniocervical junction abnormalities in
    dogs, 1098-1105
  diagnosis of, 1102
  medical therapy for, 1102-1103
  surgery for, 1103-1104, 1103f-1104f
Cranioplasty, for Chiari-like
    malformation in dogs, 1103-1104,
    1103f-1104f

Cream(s)
  as topical therapy for skin infections,
    441t
  for topical antimicrobials, for otitis,
    463
  potency of topical steroid, 460f
Creatine kinase (CK)
  activity with various myopathies,
    1113-1118
  in CSF as outcome predictors with
    intervertebral disk disease,
    1073-1074
  with heat induced illness, 72
  with leptospirosis, 1287
  with *Neospora caninum*, 1290
  with toxoplasmosis, 1296
Creatinine
  as indicator of predicting renal failure
    with hyperthyroidism, 187
  changes with hospital acquired kidney
    injury, 845-846
  for staging of kidney disease, 858,
    859t-860t
  formula for adjustment of drug
    dosage, 36
  formula for adjustment of drug
    intervals, 36
  monitoring of, with ACE inhibitors,
    854
Crenosoma vulpis, as bronchopulmonary
    parasite, e274-e275
Cricopharyngeal achalasia, 499
Cricopharyngeal dyssynchrony, 499
Critical care
  acid-base disorders, management of,
    e1-e8
  analgesia in, 59-63, 62t
  anesthesia in, 63-70
  catecholamines use in, 14-17
  drug Interactions in, 32-38
  fluid therapy and, 2-14
  hyperthermia and heat-induced illness,
    70-74
  hypomagnesemia in, 248-251
  nutrition in, 38-43
  orthopedic trauma in dogs in, 80-83
  oxygen therapy in, 52-54
  pacing in, e21-e28, e23f
  respiratory distress in, 44-51
  treatment of open fractures in, 83-86
  use of thromboelastography in, 74-77
  ventilator therapy in, 55-59
Critical-illness related corticosteroid
    insufficiency, 78-79, 174-178, 177f
  pathophysiology of, 175
Crossmatching. *See* Blood crossmatching
Cruciate ligament trauma in dogs, 81-82
  concerns regarding risk, with early age
    neutering, 983t
Crushing injuries, and wound care,
    87-88
Cryo-poor plasma, 310-311
Cryoprecipitate, 310-311
  for therapy of shock, 21-22
  for treatment of von Willebrand
    disease, 290, 290t
Cryosupernatant, for treatment of factor
    deficiencies, 290, 290t

Cryotherapy, for glaucoma, 1175
Cryptococcosis
  antifungal therapy for, 1234-1238
  causing epistaxis, 1216
  causing feline rhinitis, 644, 648
  causing nasopharyngeal disease,
    654-656
  causing nervous system signs, 1212
  causing uveitis
    in cats, 1168
    in dogs, 1163-1164, 1164b
  immunotherapy for, 1232
Cryptococcus neoformans, common
    symptoms and syndromes caused by,
    1214t
Cryptorchidism, 998-999
  risk of testicular tumors with, 1022
Cryptosporidium spp. infection
  common symptoms and syndromes
    caused by, 1214t-1215t
  dosage for and drugs targeting,
    1335-1337
  in raw meat diets, 1240b, 1241
Crystalloid(s). *See* Fluid therapy
Crystalluria, asymptomatic, 926
Culture(s)
  blood, for endocarditis, e293-e294
  ear, for diagnosis of otitis, 463
  fecal, bacterial, 519
  for *Bartonella* spp., 1265, e293
    feline, 1269
  for lagenidiosis, e415
  for methicillin-resistant Staphylococcal
    skin infections, 444
  for pythiosis, e413
  for septic mastitis, 959
  fungal, for dermatophytosis, 449,
    452-454
  lung, 681-682
    with pneumonia, 681-682, 684-686,
    684f
  of *brucella canis*, e404
  prostatic, 1013-1014
  respiratory
    for canine infectious diseases, 633,
      671-672
    for feline asthma, 676
  skin
    for superficial bacterial folliculitis,
      437-438
    of acral lick dermatitis lesions, e175
    of Staphylococcus spp., 435-436
  urine
    for surveillance of hospital-acquired
      urinary infections, 877-878
    why results are negative FAQ,
      923-924
  uterine, 938
  vaginal, 937, 972-973
  wound, 87-88
    with open fractures, 84
Cuprate, e56t
Curschmann's spirals, 669-670
Cushing's disease. *See*
    Hyperadrenocorticism
Cutaneous adverse drug reactions,
    487-490, 488t
Cutaneous inverted papilloma, e185

Cutaneous pythiosis, e412-e413

Cutaneous vasculitis, topical immunomodulators for, e218-e219

Cuterebra, nasal, 656, e270

Cyanocobalamin. See also Cobalamin; Cobalamin deficiency
for cobalamin deficiency, 524

Cyanosis, diagnosis of, 52

Cycad toxicity, 570b, 581b

Cyclical flank alopecia, 165b

Cyclizine toxicity, 118-119

Cyclocryotherapy, 1175
for feline glaucoma, 1180

Cyclooxygenase inhibitors, in NSAID's, 37, 60, 116-117

Cyclooxygenase isoenzymes, 863-864

Cyclophosphamide (Cytoxan)
causing hemorrhagic cystitis, 332
for feline gastrointestinal lymphoma, 547-548, 548t
for hemangiosarcoma, 395-396
for mammary cancer, 377, 379-380
for multiple myeloma, 386
for myasthenia gravis, 1111
metronomic chemotherapy of, 343-344
rescue chemotherapy for canine lymphoma, 381-383
use of, for immunosuppression, 268

Cyclophotocoagulation, 1175
for feline glaucoma, 1180

Cyclosporine
adverse effect of, in cats, 409
and risk of ocular squamous cell carcinoma, 1204
as topical immunomodulators, e216-e220, e217
blood level measurement of, 270
contraindications for use of, in cats, 409
drug interactions with, 35t
for anal furunculosis, e190
for atopic dermatitis, 406
for autoimmune hemolytic anemia, 278-279
for canine colitis, 551b, 552
for chronic pancreatitis and diabetes, 564
for chronic superficial keratitis (Pannus), 1154
for eosinophilic pulmonary diseases, 690-691
for episcleritis, 1141
for feline asthma, 678
for feline caudal stomatitis, 494
for feline tear film disorders, e387
for inflammatory bowel disease, 539
for inflammatory central nervous system disorders, 1065
for keratoconjunctivitis sicca, 1145, 1155, e387
for myasthenia gravis, 1111
for protein-losing enteropathy, 544
for sebaceous adenitis, e211
for thrombocytopenia, 285t
psoriasiform-lichenoid dermatosis from, 489
topical, for eosinophilic keratitis, 1159

Cyclosporine (Continued)
use in dermatology, 407-410, 410b
use of
for immunosuppression, 269-271
with fluconazole, 408

Cyproheptadine
for appetite stimulation, 352
for feline asthma, 678
for hepatic lipidosis, 611
for management with GI effects of chemotherapeutic drugs, 331
for selective serotonin reuptake inhibitors toxicity, 113

Cystadenoma, ovarian, 1024-1025

Cystic duct catheterization, 603, 605

Cystic endometrial hyperplasia, 967
causing pregnancy loss, 1005-1006, 1005t

Cystic orbital disease, 1199-1200

Cystine crystalluria, 926

Cystinuria, direct mutation test for, 1018t-1020t

Cystitis. See Urinary tract infections

Cystocentesis, use of ultrasound for, 841, 844

Cystoisospora spp. infection, dosage for and drugs targeting, 1335-1337

Cystolithotomy, percutaneous, 890

Cystometrogram (CMG), e346

Cystoscopy
biopsy using, 907-908
for bladder cancer, 371
for delivering injectable bulking agents, e347f
guided laser ablation for ectopic ureters, 890-891, 891f
interventional strategies for urinary diseases, 884
minilaparotomy-assisted, for urocystoliths, 905-909, 906f-907f

Cystourethroscope, for insemination, 940-944

Cytarabine, for inflammatory central nervous system disorders, 1065

Cytauxzoon felis, common symptoms and syndromes caused by, 1214t-1215t

Cytauxzoonosis, e405-e409
clinical signs of, e407
diagnosis of, e406f, e407, e407-e408
dosage for and drugs targeting, 1335-1337
pathogenesis of, e405-e407
treatment of, e408

Cytochrome p450, 33-36
and cimetidine, 505
associated with drug induced liver disease, 575, 580
drug interactions based on, 35t

Cytokine(s)
adverse effects of, 1231
for feline retrovirus infections, 1280t-1281t
for immune therapeutics, 335, 1230
inhibitors, for immunosuppression, 271-273
interferon, e200-e201

Cytology
airway, with pneumonia, 686

Cytology (Continued)
bronchial, 669-670
brush, for Helicobacter spp., 509-510, 510f
collection of specimens for, e153-e156
corneal, with complicated ulcers, 1150
ear, for diagnosis of otitis, 458, 463
fecal, for exocrine pancreatic insufficiency, 556
fixation and staining of specimens, e155-e156
for feline asthma, 675-676
for pneumocystosis, e410
for pythiosis, e413
joint, with polyarthritis, 1224-1228
liver, with feline hepatic lipidosis, 610
lung
for interstitial lung diseases, e268
for parasites, e269-e276
nasal
for parasites, e269-e271
in cats, 644, 645f
in dogs, 636-637
nasopharyngeal, 654
of malignant effusions, 342
of skin, for diagnosis of alopecia, 165
of the eye, 1133
pericardial effusion fluid, 817, 820
pleural effusion fluid, characterization of, 692t, 694-696
prostatic, 1013-1014
rectal, 550
uterine, 938
vaginal, 932-933, 933f, 970
for breeding management, 933f
for diagnosis of disease, 937
technique for, 937
to detect ovarian remnant syndrome, 1001
with pyometra, 967
with pyometra or mucometra, 947
with septic metritis, 958
with eosinophilic pulmonary diseases, 689
with Malassezia spp., e213-e214

Cytopenias
diagnostic workup for, 315f
multiple, diagnostic approach to, e161b

Cytoprotective agents, action and use of, 506-507

Cytosine arabinoside
as rescue therapy for canine lymphoma, 382t
for intracranial tumors, 1041t, 1044-1045

D

D-dimer level, in disseminated intravascular coagulation, 294t

D-limonene, causing adverse skin reactions, 488t

D-Penicillamine
adverse effects of, e234-e236
for copper-associated hepatitis, e234-e236

Dacarbazine, as rescue therapy for canine lymphoma, 382t

Dachshund(s)
  direct mutation tests for, 1018t-1020t
  intervertebral disk disease in, 1071-1072
  lymphoplasmacytic rhinitis in, 640
  pneumocystosis in, e410
  risk of vaccine hypersensitivity in, 1250-1251
  sick sinus syndrome in, 732-733
Dacryocystitis, e376
Dacryocystorhinography, e374
Dacryops, e376
Dactinomycin, extravasation and tissue sloughing from, 333
Daily energy requirements, 259
Dairy products, drug incompatibilities with, 33t
Dalmatian(s), missing canine red cell antigen(s), 311
Dalteparin (Fragmin), 707, 813
  as anticoagulant therapy, for autoimmune hemolytic anemia, 277t
  for arterial thromboembolism, 815
Dampness and mold, as respiratory allergens, e44
Danazol toxicity, 581b
Dantrolene, for urinary retention disorders, 917t, 918
Darbepoetin, for anemia, from chronic kidney disease, 862-863
Dark adaptation test, e391-e392
Dazzle reflex, e391
DEA 1.1 blood type, 311
Deadly nightshade toxicity, 124t
Deafness, 468-469
  age-related, 469
  causes of, 468b
  from ototoxicity, 468
Débridement
  for wound care, 83
  with open fractures, 85
Decongestants, for respiratory diseases, 627
Decontamination
  associated with hazardous drugs, 328
  from toxins, 104-105
Decoquinate, for canine hepatozoonosis, 1285
DEET mosquito repellent, use of, on pets, 100
Defecation induced syncope, e327
Defibrillation
  electrical, during CPR, 30
  types of units for, 30
Degenerative lumbosacral stenosis, 1105-1108
Degenerative myelopathy, 1075-1081
  differential diagnosis for, 1077
  direct mutation test for, 1018t-1020t
  disease progression of, 1076-1077, 1076t
  exercise with, 1078-1080
  rehabilitation considerations with, e360, e362b
Degreaser toxicity, 154-155
Dehydration
  during pregnancy and lactation, 964
  estimates of, 5t

Delayed gastric emptying, 514-515, 514b
Deltamethrin, 426t
  target parasites of, 1335-1337
Demecarium bromide
  causing anisocoria or mydriasis, e392
  for glaucoma
    in cats, 1179-1180
    in dogs, 1173b, 1174
Demodex cati, e192-e193
Demodex gatoi, e191-e192
Demodicosis
  canine, 432-434
    treatment options for, 433t, e364
  causing blepharitis, e364
  feline, e191-e193
  use of avermectins for, e182-e183
  with sebaceous gland hyperplasia, 476-477
Denaturing agents, for dust mite control, e199
Dental disease
  antibiotic prophylaxis with, e297-e298
  with diabetes mellitus, e77
Dental extractions, for feline caudal stomatitis, 493-494
Deoxyribonucleic acid-based test(s), for hereditary disorders, 1016-1020
Depot deslorelin, for urinary incontinence disorders, 916t
Depot leuprolide, for urinary incontinence disorders, 916t
Deracoxib
  adverse effects of, 60
  dosage for, 62t
  for canine uveitis, 1165t
  for urinary bladder cancer, 372
  influence on thyroid function, 181t
Dermacentor variabilis, causing cytauxzoonosis, e405
Dermatitis
  acral lick, e172-e178
  atopic (*See also* Atopic dermatitis)
    allergen-specific immunotherapy for, 411-414
  cyclosporine for, 403-404
  from nonsteroidal anti-inflammatory drugs, 489
  of the eyelid, e363-e369
  perivulvar, 971, 977f
    concerns regarding risk, with early age neutering, 983t
  pyotraumatic (*See* Pyotraumatic dermatitis)
  scrotal, 1031
  superficial necrolytic, 485-487
Dermatologic disorder(s)
  acral lick dermatitis causing, e172-e178
  actinic dermatoses, 480-482
  allergen-specific immunotherapy for, 411-414
  alopecia X, 477-479
  atopy, in dogs, 403-407
  bilaterally symmetric alopecia, in dogs, 164-166, 165b
  cornification disorders in dogs, 475-477
  cutaneous adverse drug reactions, 487-490

Dermatologic disorder(s) (*Continued*)
  disinfection of environments with staphylococcal sp., 455-457
  drugs for behavior-related dermatoses, 482-485
  ear-flushing techniques for, 471-474
  feline demodicosis causing, e191-e193
  feline viral skin, e194-e197
  food elimination diets for adverse reactions, 422-424
  from *Bartonella* spp. infections, 1263b
  from demodicosis, 432-434
  from dermatophytosis, 449-451
    in multicat environments, 452-454
  from ectoparasitoses, 428-432
  from hypothyroidism, 179
  from superficial bacterial folliculitis, 437-439
  from superficial necrolytic dermatitis, 485-487
  generalized sebaceous gland hyperplasia, 476-477
  glucocorticoids for, 414-418, 416t
  ichthyosis, 475-476
  malassezia causing, e212-e216
  nasal parakeratosis, 476
  of the anal sac, e187-e190
  otitis
    principles of therapy for, 458-459
    systemic antimicrobials for, 466-467
    topical antimicrobials for, 462-465
  papillomaviruses causing, e184-e187
  pentoxifylline for, e202-e205
  periocular, e363-e369
  pyotraumatic dermatitis causing, e206-e208
  sebaceous adenitis causing, e209-e212
  staphylococci causing pyoderma, 435-436
  topical and systemic glucocorticoid for, 459-462
  topical immunomodulators for, e216-e221
  topical therapy for, 439-443, 441t
    with pruritus, 419-421
  use of avermectins for, e178-e184
  use of cyclosporine for, 407-410
  vitamin A-responsive dermatosis, 476
  with canine leproid granuloma, 445-446
  with feline leprosy syndrome, 446-447
  with nontuberculous cutaneous granulomas, 445-448
Dermatomyositis, 1115
  pentoxifylline for, e203
Dermatophagoides farinae, e197
Dermatophagoides pteronyssinus, e197
Dermatophyte test medium (DTM), 449
Dermatophytosis
  as cause of alopecia, 165
  causing blepharitis, e363
  investigating a multicat outbreak, 452-454
  treatment of, 449-451, 450b, 450t-451t
Dermatoses
  actinic, 480-482
  behavior-related, 482-485

Dermatosis
  psoriasiform-lichenoid, cyclosporine-
    induced, 489
  sterile neutrophilic, 489
Dermoid, 1153
  causing frictional irritant
    conjunctivitis, 1140
Descemet's membrane
  anatomy of, 1148
  with descemetocele, 1149
Deslorelin
  for benign prostatic hypertrophy, 1013
  for prostatic abscesses, 1015
Desmopressin acetate (DDAVP)
  dose adjustments of, e75
  for diabetes insipidus, e73-e75
  for mammary cancer, 377
  for von Willebrand disease, 290
  injectable, e74
  nasal and ophthalmic, e73-e74
  oral, e74
  preparations of, e73-e74
Desoxycorticosterone pivalate (DOCP),
    for hypoadrenocorticism, 236-237
Detemir insulin, 211, 212b
  storage of, 214
Detrusor atony of urinary bladder, 918
Detrusor-urethral dyssynergia, 918
Dexamethasone
  adverse effects of, 461
  for otitis
    systemic, 461t
    topical, 460t
  for pregnancy termination, 991, 991t
  use of, with hypoadrenocorticism
    testing, 234-236
Dexamethasone suppression test
  for alopecia X, 478
  interpretation of, e98-e99
  low dose, 221
Dexlansoprazole, action and use of,
    505-506
Dexmedetomidine
  adverse effects of, 60
  CRI, 62t
  dosage for, 62t
  use of
    with cardiovascular dysfunction,
      64-65
    with intracranial pathology, 69
Dexrazoxane, use of, prior to
    doxorubicin, 332
Dextran 70, for canine parvovirus, 534
Dextroamphetamine and amphetamine
    (Adderall), toxicity of, 109-110
Dextroamphetamine toxicity, 109-110
Dextromethorphan, for coughing, 623
Dextrose
  for shock, 24
  hypokalemia from, 251b
  supplementation with diabetic
    ketoacidosis, e80t-e81t
Diabetes insipidus, desmopressin for
    diagnosis and treatment of, e73-e75
Diabetes mellitus
  and risk of urinary tract infections, 877
  and superficial necrolytic dermatitis,
    485

Diabetes mellitus (Continued)
  canine
    adjusting therapy with, 191-192
    diagnosis and treatment of, 189-193
    dietary management of, 199-202
  causing alkaline phosphatase
    elevations, e243-e244
  causing cataracts, 1183, 1183f
  complicated, e76-e83
  concurrent with hypothyroidism,
    e87-e88
  diet and, 199-204, 201t
  feline, 208-215
    alternatives to insulin therapy,
      e135-e138, e136f, e136t
    diagnosis and treatment of, 208-215
    dietary management of, 202-204
    pathogenesis of, 208-210
    remission, 204-205, 209-210, 213
    with acromegaly, 216
  hyperadrenocorticism with, 207
  hyperosmolar nonketotic, e83
  hypertension from, 727, 727t
  hypokalemia from, 251b
  hypomagnesemia with, 248
  imaging of pancreas for, 172-174
  insulin resistance in, 205-208, 206b
    from feline hypersomatotropism and
      acromegaly, 216-221
  monitoring of, 193-199
  nephropathy from, e76
  neuropathy from, 1116, e76-e77
  pulmonary thromboembolism
    associated with, 705
  retinopathy from, 1192
  risk of, with progestin drugs, 985
  toxicity of herbal supplements used
    for, 125
  with chronic pancreatitis, 564
Diabetic ketoacidosis (DKA)
  diagnosis and treatment of, e78-e83,
    e80t-e81t
  hypomagnesemia with, 248-250
  influence on fructosamine, 194
  potassium levels with, 253
  role of insulin resistance in, 205
  with acute pancreatitis in dogs, 563,
    e77-e78
Diagnostic test(s)
  biopsy and specimen submission for,
    322-326
  for causes of thrombocytopenia,
    281t-282t
  for hereditary disorders, 1015-1021,
    1016t
  interpretation of, for adrenal and
    thyroid disease, e97-e102
  of bone marrow, 314-318
  quality control for the in-clinic
    laboratory and, 306-309
Dialysis
  use of, with nephroliths and
    ureteroliths, 895
  vs. continuous renal replacement
    therapy, 871
Diamond burr débridement, 1152
Diaphragmatic rupture, causing pleural
    effusion, 694

Diarrhea. See also under Colitis
  antibiotic-responsive, 518-522, 519b
  chronic
    diagnostic approach to, e264-e265,
      e264f
    idiopathic large bowel, 516
  common infectious agents causing,
    1213-1215
  from Tritrichomonas foetus, 528-530
  large bowel, 550-554
    causes of, 551t
  probiotic therapy for, 525-528
  tylosin-responsive, e262-e265
Diazepam (Valium)
  associated hepatotoxicity, 570b, 581b
  for appetite stimulation, 352
  for behavior-related dermatoses, 483t,
    484
  for emergent seizures, 1059
  for urinary retention disorders, 917t,
    918
  rectal administration of, 1059
  toxicity of, 113-114
  use of, with cardiovascular
    dysfunction, 64-65
  with fentanyl, for anesthetic induction
    in critical patients, 66
Diazoxide(s), for insulinomas, e133
Dibromochloropropane toxicity, 1027b
Dichlorobenzene toxicity, 1027b
Dichloroethane toxicity, 1027b
Dichloromethane toxicity, 1027b
Dichlorphenamide, for glaucoma in
    dogs, 1173-1174, 1173b
Diclofenac
  for actinic dermatoses, 481
  for canine uveitis, 1165t
Dicloxacillin, for pyoderma, 1220t,
    1221-1222
Dicyclomine HCl (Bentyl), for canine
    colitis, 551b
Didanosine, for feline retrovirus
    infections, 1278, 1279t
Diesel toxicity, 154-155
Diestrus, drugs for pregnancy
    termination during, 991-992
Diet and diabetes, 199-204, 201t
Dietary supplements
  for heart disease, 725
  of calcium, e127-e128, e127t
  of potassium, 253
  toxicity from, 122-129
Dietary therapy
  copper-restricted, 590
  food elimination, for adverse reactions,
    422-424
  for acute pancreatitis in dogs,
    563-564
  for calcium oxalate urolithiasis,
    898-899, 899t
  for cancer, 351-352
  for canine colitis, 551b, 552
  for canine parvovirus, 535
  for chronic diarrhea, e265
  for chronic hepatitis, 587-588
  for control of hepatoencephalopathy,
    593
  for copper-associated hepatitis, e236

Dietary therapy (Continued)
  for exocrine pancreatic insufficiency
    (EPI), 559-560
  for feline diabetes mellitus, e136-e137,
    e136f
  for feline hyperthyroidism, e107-e112
  for feline idiopathic hypercalcemia,
    244-246
  for heart disease, 720-725, 777, 790,
    792
  for hepatic lipidosis, 611-612
  for hyperlipidemia, 264
  for hypertension and kidney disease,
    861-862
  for inflammatory bowel disease, 538
  for insulinomas, e133-e134
  for nephroliths and ureteroliths,
    895-896
  for obesity, 255-259
  for patients with flatulence, e248-e249,
    e249b
  for portosystemic shunt, 596
  for protein losing enteropathy,
    542-543, 543t
  for urate urolithiasis, 902, 902f, 904,
    905b
  hypoallergenic, 422-424, e176
  infectious diseases from raw meat
    diets, 1239-1243
  modification to facilitate gastric
    emptying, 515
  relative to environmental needs of
    cats, 911-912
  sodium restriction, for ascites, from
    liver disease, 592
Diethylcarbamazine
  causing adverse skin reactions, 488t
  for feline retrovirus infections,
    1280t-1281t, 1282
Diethylene glycol toxicity, 154, e30-e31
Diethylstilbestrol (DES), for benign
    prostatic hypertrophy, 1013
Difloxacin, for lower respiratory tract
    infection(s), 1220t
Digital papillomatosis, e185
Digitoxin toxicity, anorexia from, 722
Digoxin
  adverse effects of, 34t-35t, 791-792
  causing bradyarrhythmias, 732
  drug incompatibilities with, 33t
  drug interactions with, 35t
  for arrhythmia with congestive heart
    failure, 783
  for asymptomatic heart disease, 766
  for atrial fibrillation, 743
    with dilated cardiomyopathy, 799
  for dilated cardiomyopathy, in dogs
    occult, 797-798
    with heart failure, 799
  for feline arrhythmias, 752
  for heart failure, in dogs, 764t-765t,
    768-770, 791-792
  for refractory heart failure, 781
  for supraventricular tachyarrhythmias,
    742t, 743
  interaction with GI drugs, 37
  monitoring therapy of, 791-792, 799
  use of, with hypokalemia, 34t-35t

Dihydrostreptomycin, for brucellosis,
    e404
Dihydrotachysterol, supplement for
    hypocalcemia, e127-e128, e128t
Diltiazem
  causing bradyarrhythmias, 732
  causing syncope, e328
  for atrial fibrillation, 743
    with dilated cardiomyopathy, 799
  for feline arrhythmias, 752
  for feline cardiomyopathy, 805-807,
    806t
  for heart failure, in dogs, 764t-765t
    with arrhythmias, 772
  for supraventricular tachyarrhythmias,
    742t, 743
  toxicity of, use of IV lipid emulsion
    therapy for, 106
Dilutional acidosis, e6-e7, e7b
Dimenhydrinate
  for intracranial tumors, 1041t
  toxicity of, 118-119
Dimethyl sulfoxide (DMSO), for
    amyloidosis, 855
Dimethylnitrosamine toxicity, 570b
Diminazene aceturate, for canine
    babesiosis, 1258t, 1259
Dinotefuran, 426t
Dinotefuran/permethrin/pyriproxyfen,
    426t
  target parasites of, 1335-1337
Dinotefuran/pyriproxyfen, target
    parasites of, 1335-1337
Dioctyl sodium sulfosuccinate (DSS)
  ear cleaner, 472-473
  in ear cleaners, 472t
Dioxane toxicity, 1027b
Diphacenone rodenticide toxicity,
    133-134
Diphenhydramine (Benadryl)
  to reduce risk of vaccine
    hypersensitivity, 1250
  topical, 420t
    for hot spots, e207
  toxicity of, 118-119
Diphenoxylate, for canine colitis, 551b
Dipivefrin, for glaucoma in dogs, 1173b,
    1174
Dipylidium caninum
  causing infection in humans, 1247
  common symptoms and syndromes
    caused by, 1214t-1215t
  drugs targeting, 1335-1337
Direct megakaryocytic
    immunofluorescence assay,
    evaluation of, with
    thrombocytopenia, 284
Direct mutation test(s), 1017,
    1018t-1020t
Dirlotapide, for treatment of obesity,
    259-260
Dirofilaria immitis
  causing infection in humans, 1248
  common symptoms and syndromes
    caused by, 1214t-1215t
  drugs targeting prevention of,
    1335-1337
Dirofilariasis. See Heartworm disease

Discoid lupus erythematosus
  tacrolimus for, e218
  use of cyclosporine for, 410b
Discospondylitis, from brucellosis,
    e403f
Disinfection, from Staphylococcal spp.,
    455-457
Disseminated candidiasis, as cause of
    thrombocytopenia, 281t-282t
Disseminated intravascular coagulation
    (DIC)
  diagnosis and treatment of, 292-296
  diseases associated with, 294b
  from heat-induced illness, 71-72
  laboratory values supporting, 294t
  risk of, with pancreatitis in dogs, 562
  thrombocytopenia and, 280, 283
Distemper. See Canine distemper virus
    (CDV)
Distichiasis, e369, e377
  causing frictional irritant
    conjunctivitis, 1140
Diuresis
  for malignant effusions, 342
  to promote ureterolith passage, 894
Diuretic(s)
  for ascites, from liver disease, 591,
    592f
  for heart failure, in dogs, 762-766,
    763b
  loop, ototoxicity from, 469
DNA amplification assay, for Bartonella
    spp., 1264-1265, 1269
Doberman pinscher(s)
  cardiomyopathy in, 795, 797
  cervical spondylomyelopathy in,
    1090-1097
  copper-associated liver disease in,
    589-590
  direct mutation tests for, 1018t-1020t
  hyperlipidemia in, 261
  hypothyroidism in, 178-179
  neurocardiogenic syncope in, e327
  prostatic disease in, 1012
  risk of bladder cancer in, 371t
  ventricular arrhythmia in, 745
  with color dilution alopecia, 164
Dobutamine
  drug incompatibilities with, 33t
  for cardiogenic shock, 783
  for heart failure
    in cats, 808
    in dogs, 764t-765t, 768-770
  receptor activities of, 15t
  use and dosage of, 15t, 16-17
  use of with shock, 23
Docetaxel, e140t, e141
  for mammary cancer, 377
  hypersensitivity reactions to, 333
Docosahexaenoic acid(s)
  for heart disease, 722-723
  requirements during pregnancy and
    lactation, 963
Dog erythrocyte antigen, 311
Dolasetron (Anzemet)
  for acute pancreatitis in dogs, 562-563
  for feline cholangitis, 617, 617b
  for feline pancreatitis, 567t

Dolasetron (Anzemet) (Continued)
for hepatic lipidosis, 612
for vomiting with acute renal failure, 870
Domperidone, action and use of, for motility disorders, 516-518
Dopamine
adverse effects of, with metoclopramide, 34t-35t
drug incompatibilities with, 33t
for cardiogenic shock, 783
for heart failure, in dogs, 768-770
receptor activities of, 15t
use and dosage of, 15t, 16
use of with shock, 22-23
Doppler, fetal monitoring with, 950, 950f
Doramectin
for demodicosis, 434, e183
for dermatologic disorders, e178, e180
for sarcoptic mange, e182
toxicity of, 145-146
Dorsal laminectomy
for intervertebral disk disease, 1073-1074
for lumbosacral stenosis, 1107-1108
Dorzolamide
for canine glaucoma, 1173-1174, 1173b, e381
for feline glaucoma, 1179, e381
Dorzolamide/timolol
for canine glaucoma, 1173-1174
for feline glaucoma, 1179
Double-outlet right ventricle, prevalence of, in cats, 757t
Doxapram, use of, to evaluate laryngeal function, 660
Doxepin
for behavior-related dermatoses, 482-483, 483t
toxicity of, use of IV lipid emulsion therapy for, 106
Doxil, for hemangiosarcoma, 395-396
Doxorubicin
associated hepatotoxicity, 581b
cardiac toxicity from chemotherapeutic drugs, 332
causing adverse skin reactions, 488t
extravasation and tissue sloughing from, 333
for feline gastrointestinal lymphoma, 547-548, 548t
for hemangiosarcoma, 395-396
inhalational, 396
for insulinomas, e132-e133
for mammary cancer, 377, 379-380
for multiple myeloma, 386
for osteosarcoma, 391t
hypersensitivity reactions to, 333
induced cardiomyopathy, 795
pegylated liposomal, e139-e140, e140t
rescue chemotherapy for canine lymphoma, 381-383
Doxycycline
associated hepatotoxicity, 570b
for Bartonella spp., 1265-1266, 1266t
for Borrelia burgdorferi, 1273-1274
for brucellosis, 972, e404

Doxycycline (Continued)
for canine bronchial diseases, 670-672
for canine heartworm disease, 833, 834f, 835
for canine respiratory infection complex, 633-634
for causes of thrombocytopenia, 281t-282t
for ehrlichiosis, 1293-1294
for feline heartworm disease, 830
for feline tear film disorders, e387
for feline upper respiratory infection, 630, 631t
for hemotropic mycoplasmosis, e401
for infectious polyarthritis, 1225
for infective endocarditis, e294t, e297
for keratomalacia, 1151
for leptospirosis, 1289
for lower respiratory tract infection, 1220t, 1222
for lymphoplasmacytic rhinitis, in dogs, 641
for methicillin-resistant Staphylococcal skin infections, 444
for Mycoplasma spp., 973
for nontuberculous cutaneous granulomas, 448t
for pneumonia, 682t
for rhinosinusitis in cats, 646
for sebaceous adenitis, e211
for superficial bacterial folliculitis, 438t
for upper respiratory tract infection, 1220t, 1222
for urinary tract infections, 1220t, 1221
target parasites and dosage of, 1335-1337
Drainage, techniques for septic abdomen, e13-e20
Drawer motion, 82
Drug dosage(s)
formula for adjustment of, with renal failure, 36
table of common, 1307-1334
Drug extravasation, with chemotherapeutic drugs, 333
Drug incompatibilities, 32-38
intravenous administered, 33t
Drug interactions, 32-38, 34t-35t
Drug labeling, e40-e41
Drug preparation equipment, for hazardous drugs, 326-327
Drug reaction(s)
adverse, 32-38, 34t-35t
effects of glucocorticoid, 461-462
causing conjunctivitis, 1140
cutaneous, 487-490, 488t
Drug therapy(ies)
adverse effects of chemotherapy, 330
analgesia, 59-63, 62t
antibiotic for enteropathies, 518-522
antiinflammatory potency of systemic glucocorticoids, 461t
approved vs. unapproved, e37
associated liver disease, 570b, 575-579
causing alkaline phosphatase elevations, e243-e244, e245b
causing blood dyscrasias, e160, e162

Drug therapy(ies) (Continued)
causing hyperlipidemia, 262t
causing pregnancy loss, 1010
causing renal failure, e30b
during CPR, 28-30
effect of topical formulation on glucocorticoid potency, 460f
effect of vehicle/formulation on potency of topical glucocorticoids, 460f
effect on gastric emptying, 514, 516
effects on thyroid function, 181t
for behavior-related dermatoses, 482-485
for causes of thrombocytopenia, 281t-282t
for hypothyroidism, 182
for respiratory diseases, 622-628
for treatment of common parasites, 1335-1337
for treatment of obesity, 259-260
for treatment of toxicities, 101-105
hypertension from, 727t
immunosuppressive, 268-274
in nutritional support, 43
incompatibilities of, 32-38
lists of approved, extralabel and unapproved, e54-e68
mineralocorticoid activity of systemic glucocorticoids, 461t
new maintenance anticonvulsant, 1054-1057
premedication and sedation with cardiovascular dysfunction, 64-65, 65t
reporting adverse events from, e35-e43
systemic antimicrobial for otitis, 466-467
to treat animal toxicosis, e56t
topical antimicrobials for otitis, 462-465
toxic exposures to, 95t, 96
transdermal (See Transdermal medication(s))
update on masitinib, 360-362
update on toceranib (Palladia), 358-360
use of IV lipid emulsion therapy for toxicities, 106-109
with antacids, 505-508
with topical glucocorticoid for otitis, 460, 460f, 460t
Drug toxicity. See also Ototoxicity
from antidepressants and anxiolytics, 112-114
from human drugs of abuse, 109-112
over-the-counter, 115-120
Drug(s)
compatibility with parenteral nutrition products, 40
formulary of common, 1307-1334
storage, for hazardous drugs, 327
Drug-herb interactions, 127
Drugs of abuse, human, toxicity from, 109-112
and legal considerations, e51
Dry eye. See Keratoconjunctivitis sicca (KCS)

Drying agents, for ears, 472t, 473
Duloxetine, for urinary incontinence disorders, 916t, 917
Duodenal ulceration, associated with *Helicobacter* spp., 509
Duodenum, deformities with brachycephalic airway obstruction syndrome, 650t
Dust mite hypersensitivity and control, e197-e199
Dynamic left ventricular outflow tract obstruction, 805, 806t, 807-808
Dysautonomia
    causing megaesophagus, e227
    effect on gastric emptying, 514, 516
Dysbiosis
    associated inflammatory bowel disease, 521
    of colon, 551
    with protein-losing enteropathy, 544
Dyschezia, 550
Dyscrasias of bone marrow, 314-318
Dysfibrinogenemia, coagulation factor abnormalities with, 288t, 289
Dysgranulopoiesis, 314
Dysmyelopoiesis, e163-e164
Dysphagia
    from gastroesophageal reflux, 501
    oropharyngeal, 495-500, e259-e262
        causes of, 496b
        clinical signs of, 496b, e260t
        history associated with, 497b
        treatment of, e261-e262
    with feline caudal stomatitis, 492
Dyspnea, 45. *See also* Acute respiratory distress syndrome (ARDS)
    drugs used with, 47t
    from acute respiratory distress syndrome, 48-51
Dystocia
    fetal causes of, 953
    management of, 948-956
    obstetrical monitoring equipment for, 950f, 953f-954f

E

EACA. *See* Aminocaproic acid
Ear mites, diagnosis and treatment of, 430-431, 431t. *See also* Otodectes cynotis
Ear(s). *See also* Otitis
    antiseptics, 473-474
    cleaning solutions, 472-474, 472t
        ototoxicity of, 474
    debris removal agents for, 472-473, 472t
    flushing techniques for, 471-474
    normalizing agents for, 473
Easter lily toxicity, 99, e34
Ebstein's anomaly, e332
Ecchymosis
    from adverse drug reactions, 488t
    with thrombocytopenia, 283
Echinocandins, use and protocols for, 1238
Echinococcus granulosa, common symptoms and syndromes caused by, 1214t-1215t

Echinococcus multilocularis, common symptoms and syndromes caused by, 1214t-1215t
Echinococcus spp. infection
    causing infection in humans, 1247
    drugs targeting, 1335-1337
    in raw meat diets, 1240b, 1241
Echocardiography
    for staging heart disease in dogs, 776
    with arrhythmogenic right ventricular cardiomyopathy, in cats, e278-e279, e278f
    with dilated cardiomyopathy in dogs, 796-797
    with feline heartworm disease, 828-829, 828f
    with feline myocardial disease, 804-810
    with hemangiosarcoma, 393-394
    with infective endocarditis, e295
    with mitral valve dysplasia, e300-e302, e301f
    with patent ductus arteriosus, e309-e310, e312f
    with pericardial effusion, 818-819, 818f-819f
    with pulmonary hypertension, 711, 712f-713f, 713-714
    with pulmonic stenosis, e315-e317, e315f-e316f
    with subaortic stenosis, e321, e321f
    with tricuspid valve dysplasia, e333-e334, e334f
    with valvular heart disease, 788-790, 789f
    with ventricular septal defect, e337-e338
Eclampsia. *See* Puerperal tetany
Ecology Works Anti-Allergen Solution, for dust mite control, e199
Ectoparasites
    drugs used to treat common, 1335-1337
    treatment of, 428-432
Ectopic ACTH syndrome, 230-232, 231f
Ectopic cilia, causing frictional irritant conjunctivitis, 1140
Ectopic ureters
    cystoscopic-guided laser ablation for, 890-891, 891f
    ultrasound findings with, 841-842
Ectropion, 1155, e369
Edrophonium chloride challenge test, for myasthenia gravis, 1109
Effusions
    malignant, 341-344
    pleural, 691-700 (*See also* Pleural effusion)
Ehrlichia canis
    causing nervous system signs, 1212
    causing nonregenerative anemia, 1217, e161, e161b
    causing polyarthritis, 1227-1228
    causing renal infections, 1212
    common symptoms and syndromes caused by, 1214t
    immunosuppressive therapy for, 1232-1233

Ehrlichia ewingii
    causing polyarthritis, 1228
    common symptoms and syndromes caused by, 1214t
Ehrlichiosis
    as cause of thrombocytopenia, 281t-282t, 283
    canine monocytotropic, 1292-1294
    causing uveitis in dogs, 1164b
    feline monocytotropic, 1294
    post-treatment monitoring of, 1293-1294
    prevention of, 1294
Eicosapentaenoic acid(s)
    for heart disease, 722-723
    requirements during pregnancy and lactation, 963
Eisenmenger's physiology, e339
Ejaculation
    normal antegrade, e351
    retrograde
        aspermia/oligospermia caused by, e350-e353
        clinical examples of, e352-e353
        spinal reflexes occurring during, e351t
Elbow luxation, 80
Elbow trauma in dogs, 81
Electrical-mechanical dissociation, 29f
Electrocardiography
    common arrest rhythms, 29f
    during CPR, 28
    for evaluation of causes of pulmonary hypertension, 713
    with arrhythmias in cats, 749, 750f-751f
    with arrhythmogenic right ventricular cardiomyopathy
        in cats, e278
        in dogs, 801-802
    with atrioventricular block, third degree, 735f
    with baroreceptor reflex, 732f
    with cardiac pacemaker, e283f-e284f
    with congenital heart disease, 758-759
    with dilated cardiomyopathy in dogs, 797
    with mitral valve dysplasia, e300
    with myocarditis, e304
    with pericardial effusion, 818
    with pulmonic stenosis, e315
    with sick sinus syndrome, 733f
    with supraventricular tachyarrhythmias, 739-741, 740f
    with transvenous pacing, e23-e24, e24f-e25f
    with tricuspid valve dysplasia, e332-e333, e333f
    with valvular heart disease, 788
    with ventricular arrhythmias, 746f
Electrodiagnostic testing, for evaluation of dysphagia, 498, e260-e261
Electrolyte(s)
    approach to low magnesium, 248-253
    approach to low potassium, 248-253
    in parenteral nutrition products, 40
Electromyography (EMG), for degenerative myelopathy, 1077

Electroretinography, 1133
  with progressive retinal atrophy,
    1188-1190
Elimination diets, for adverse food
  reactions, 422-424
Elongated soft palate, and
  brachycephalic airway obstruction
  syndrome, 649-653, 650t, 652f
Embolism
  cardiogenic, 812-813
  from blood transfusion reaction, 313
Embolization, for malignant
  obstructions, 348
Embryonic structure, identification by
  ultrasonography for pregnancy
  diagnosis, 946t
Emergency care
  gastric dilation-volvulus in, e13-e20
  of hypertensive crisis, 730
  of open fractures, 83-86
  of ophthalmic disorders, e377-e384
  of pneumothorax, 700-704
  of the eye, e377-e384
  pacing in, e21-e28
  stabilization of patient with respiratory
    distress, 44-48
  with acute hypoadrenocorticism,
    235-236
  with laryngeal paralysis, 660
  with orthopedic trauma, 80-83
  wound care and vacuum-assisted
    wound closure, 87-90
Emetic drugs
  for toxin ingestions, 105, 113
  to avoid with anesthesia, 68
Emodepside, target parasites of,
  1335-1337
Emodepside-praziquantel, target parasites
  of, 1335-1337
Empiric antimicrobial therapy,
  1219-1223
Enalapril (Enacard, Vasotec)
  adverse effects of, 34t-35t, 766-768
  for asymptomatic heart disease,
    765-766, 790
  for cough from bronchial compression,
    782
  for feline cardiomyopathy, 809
  for glomerular disease, 854-855
  for heart failure, in dogs, 764t-765t,
    766-768, 777-779
    balancing renal function and, 779
  for hypertension, 729
  for hyperthyroid cats, e103t, e105
  for occult dilated cardiomyopathy, in
    dogs, 797-798
Encapsulated sodium nitrite, for
  population control, 142-144
Encephalomyelopathy, 1052-1053
End-tidal carbon dioxide (ETCO$_2$),
  during CPR, 28
Endocardial cushion defects. *See*
  Atrioventricular septal defect
Endocardial fibroelastosis, prevalence of,
  in cats, 757t
Endocarditis
  clinical signs of, e292-e293
  diagnosis of, e293-e296, e296b

Endocarditis *(Continued)*
  differential diagnosis for, e296
  infective, e291-e299
  pathophysiology of, e292
  prognosis for, e298
  pulmonary thromboembolism
    associated with, 705
  treatment of, e294t
  with heart failure, e292, e297-e298
Endocrine
  causes of hepatobiliary enzyme
    elevations, 570b
  disruption, from reproductive toxins,
    1028
Endocrine disease(s)
  acromegaly, feline, 216-221
  bilaterally symmetric alopecia, in dogs,
    164-166, 165b
  causing hyperlipidemia, 262t
  critical-illness related corticosteroid
    insufficiency, 174-178
  diabetes mellitus
    alternatives to insulin therapy, in
      cats, e135-e138, e136t
    and diet, 199-204
    complicated, e76-e83
    in dogs, 189-193
    monitoring of, 193-199
  ectopic ACTH syndrome, 230-232
  feline idiopathic hypercalcemia,
    242-248
  feline primary hyperaldosteronism,
    238-242
  food-dependent hypercortisolism,
    230-232
  hyperadrenocorticism
    occult, 221-224
    with large pituitary tumor, e88-e91
  hyperparathyroidism, e69-e73
  hypersomatotropism, feline, 216-221
  hyperthyroidism
    and renal failure, 185-189
    medical treatment of, e102-e106
    nutritional management of,
      e107-e112
    radioiodine therapy for, e112-e122
  hypoadrenocorticism, 233-237
  hypoparathyroidism, e122-e129
  hypothyroidism, 178-185
  imaging for diagnosis of, 167-174
  insulinoma, treatment of, in dogs cats
    and ferrets, e130-e134
  interpretation of results for adrenal
    and thyroid disease, e97-e102
  polyglandular, with hypothyroidism,
    e87-e88
Endocrine pancreatic insufficiency,
  insulin resistance with, 206b
Endometritis, use of renourethroscope
  for diagnosis of, 943
Endoscopy
  brush cytology with, 509-510, 510f
  cervical, 938
  for esophagitis and strictures, e238-
    e239, e239f, e240
  for feline gastrointestinal lymphoma,
    547
  for gastric ulcerations, e254

Endoscopy *(Continued)*
  for gastroesophageal reflux, 502
  for gastrointestinal disorder in
    brachycephalics, 649-651
  for *Helicobacter* spp., 508-511
  for nasopharyngeal disorders, 654
  for protein-losing enteropathy,
    541-542
  interventional strategies for urinary
    diseases, 884-892
  transcervical insemination, 940-944,
    941f, 941t
  uterine, 937-938
  vaginal, 934, 936-937
Endothelial dystrophy, 1153
Endotoxemia, as cause of
  thrombocytopenia, 281t-282t
Endotracheal wash, for diagnosis of
  pneumonia, 686
Energy requirement(s)
  calculators, 259
  during pregnancy and lactation,
    961-963, 962f
English setter(s), direct mutation tests
  for, 1018t-1020t
English springer spaniel(s)
  atrial standstill in, 734
  mitochondrial encephalopathy in,
    1048-1051, 1049t, 1051t
Enilconazole
  for nasal aspergillosis, 638
  topical rinse, for dermatophytosis,
    450t
Enophthalmos, from orbital diseases,
  1197, 1198b, 1200
Enoxaparin, 707, 813
  as anticoagulant therapy, for
    autoimmune hemolytic anemia,
    277t
  for arterial thromboembolism, 815
Enrofloxacin (Baytril)
  causing retinopathy, e383
  drug interactions with, 35t, 677
  for *Bartonella* spp., 1266t
  for brucellosis, 972, e404
  for canine bronchial diseases, 671
  for canine colitis, 551b, 553
  for feline upper respiratory infection,
    631t
  for hemotropic mycoplasmosis, e401
  for infective endocarditis, e294t, e297
  for lower respiratory tract infection(s),
    1220t
  for otitis
    systemic, 466t
    topical, 464t
  for pneumonia, 682t, 683
  for septicemia, 1220t, 1223
  for superficial bacterial folliculitis, 438,
    438t
  for therapy with open fractures, 84-85
  retinopathy, 1195
Enteral nutrition, 42-43
  for acute pancreatitis in cats, 567-568
  for acute pancreatitis in dogs,
    563-564
  for hepatic lipidosis, 611-612
  for patients with cancer, 353

Enteritis, effect on gastric emptying, 514, 516

Enterococcus faecium, as probiotic, 527

Enterococcus spp.
    in raw meat diets, 1240, 1240b
    in tube feeds, e19

Enterohepatic recirculation, of toxins, 105

Enteropathies, antibiotic-responsive, 518-522, 519b, 519f

Enteropathogenic bacterial infection, 520-521

Entropion, 1155, e369
    causing frictional irritant conjunctivitis, 1140

Enucleation
    for feline glaucoma, 1180
    of glaucoma eye, 1175-1176

Environment(al)
    agents associated with hepatotoxicity, 570b
    associated hepatotoxicity, 581b
    cleaner for dermatophytosis, 450b
    control of dermatophytosis, 452-454
    control of giardiasis, 532
    disinfection from Staphylococcal sp., 455-457, 456t
    enrichment for domestic cats, 909-914
    influences on health of cats, 910-913

Enzyme-linked immunosorbent assay (ELISA)
    for canine parvovirus, 533-534
    for lagenidiosis, e415
    for pythiosis, e413
    for sarcoptic mange, 428

Eosinophilia, with feline heartworm disease, 826

Eosinophilic granuloma complex, with flea allergies, 424-425

Eosinophilic keratitis, 1157t, 1158-1159, 1159f
    indications for surgery with, 1161t

Eosinophilic meningoencephalitis, 1063-1066

Eosinophilic pulmonary diseases, 688-691, 689f

Ephedra toxicity, 123

Ephedrine, for urinary incontinence disorders, 915, 916t

Epibulbar melanoma, in cats, 1207-1208

Epichlorohydrin toxicity, 1027b

Epidermal hyperplasia, use of interferons for, e200-e201

Epidermoloytic ichthyosis, 475

Epidural analgesia, 61

Epilepsy
    new anticonvulsants for, 1054-1057
    treatment of cluster seizures and status epilepticus, 1058-1063

Epinephrine
    drug incompatibilities with, 33t
    for CPR, 28-29
    for respiratory diseases, 623
    receptor activities of, 15t
    use and dosage of, 15-16, 15t

Epiphora, e374-e377
    causes of, e374-e376, e375b, e375f

Epirubicin, extravasation and tissue sloughing from, 333

Episcleritis, 1140-1141, 1141f

Episiotomy
    for surgical approach to the vagina, 974-976, 975f
    with dystocia, 951

Epistaxis
    from nasal neoplasia in dogs, 641
    from rhinitis in dogs, 636
    infectious causes of, 1216

Epithelial cell tumors, ovarian, 1024-1025

Epithelial inclusion cyst, 1153

Epithelioma, 1202

Eplerenone, 763-765

Eprinomectin
    for dermatologic disorders, e178
    toxicity of, 145-146

Epsiprantel, target parasites of, 1335-1337

Epulis, 363, 365

Erection. *See also* Paraphimosis; Priapism
    physiology of, e354, e355f

Ergocalciferol, supplement for hypocalcemia, e127-e128, e128, e128t

Erythema, from methimazole, e103-e104

Erythema multiforme
    causing blepharitis, e367
    from drug reactions, 488
    use of cyclosporine for, 410b

Erythromycin
    action and use of, for motility disorders, 517t
    associated hepatotoxicity, 581b
    for pyoderma, 1220t, 1221-1222
    for superficial bacterial folliculitis, 438t
    topical, for feline ocular herpesvirus 1, 1158

Erythropoietin
    for anemia, from chronic kidney disease, 862-863
    for feline retrovirus infections, 1280t-1281t

Escherichia coli
    causing diarrhea, 519
    causing endocarditis, e293-e294, e294t
    causing oligospermia, e350
    causing persistent urinary tract infection, 880-883
    causing pneumonia, 681, 682t
    causing pregnancy loss, 1005t, 1006, 1008
    causing prostatitis, 1013
    causing pyometra, 967-968
    causing septic mastitis, 959
    role of
        with canine colitis, 553
        with feline cholangitis, 615
        with feline pancreatitis, 568
    uropathogenic, 880

Escherichia spp., in raw meat diets, 1240, 1240b

Escitalopram, toxicity of, 113

Esmolol
    for heart failure with arrhythmias, in dogs, 771
    for supraventricular tachyarrhythmias in dogs, 742t

Esomeprazole
    action and use of, 505-506
    toxicity from, 118

Esophageal
    pH monitoring, 502-503
    phase of swallowing, 495-496

Esophageal dilation, with myasthenia gravis, 1109-1110

Esophageal perforation, 501-502

Esophageal stenting
    for malignant obstructions, 347
    for strictures, e240-e241, e241f

Esophageal strictures, e237-e242, e238, e238-e239, e239f
    dilation of, 503-504, e240
    prognosis with, e241
    with gastroesophageal reflux, 503-504

Esophagitis
    causes of, e237
    clinical signs of, e237-e238
    diagnosis and treatment of, e237-e242
    diagnosis of, e238-e239
    from gastroesophageal reflux, 501-504
    treatment of, e239-e241
    use of sucralfate for, 507
    with brachycephalic airway obstruction syndrome, 650t
    with megaesophagus, e229

Esophagostomy tube(s), for hepatic lipidosis, 611-612

Esophagram
    contrast, 501-502, e227
    for evaluation of esophagitis and strictures, e238-e239, e238f

Esophagus
    deformities with brachycephalic airway obstruction syndrome, 650t
    disorders of, e225b
    functional anatomy of, e224-e225
    motility of, e237

Essential fatty acids. *See* Fatty acids

Essential oils, toxicity from, 125-127, 126t

Essential renal hematuria, 885-886, 886f

Estradiol cypionate, for pregnancy termination, 992

Estriol, for urinary incontinence disorders, 915-916, 916t

Estrogen
    concentration
        to detect ovarian remnant syndrome, 1001-1002
        with pyometra, 967
        with reproductive neoplasia, 1024-1025
    myelotoxicity and and sertoli cell tumors, 1022-1023
    therapy and risk of pyometra, 967
    therapy for urinary incontinence disorders, 915-916, 916t
    therapy for vaginitis, 973

Estrogen-receptor-positive breast cancer, 377, 379t

Estrus, 931-932
    drugs for pregnancy termination during, 991-992
    role of, in mammary cancer, 375
    suppression, 984-989

Eszopiclone toxicity, 113-114
Ethanol
    for ethylene glycol toxicity, 153
    toxicity, 147
Ethanol ablation, ultrasound-guided, for
    treatment of hyperparathyroidism,
    e72
Ethanolamine toxicity, 118-119
Ethmoidal turbinate, deformities with
    brachycephalic airway obstruction
    syndrome, 650t
Ethyl lactate, for pyoderma, 441-442,
    441t
Ethylene dibromide toxicity, 1027b
Ethylene dichloride toxicity, 1027b
Ethylene glycol toxicity, 151-153, e30-e31
    hepatic metabolism of, 152f
    metabolism of, e30-e31
Ethylene oxide toxicity, 1027b
Ethylenediamine toxicity, 118-119
Ethylenediaminetetraacetic acid (EDTA),
    for keratomalacia, 1151
Etodolac toxicity, 116-117
Etomidate
    effect on shock, 25
    for anesthetic induction in critical
        patients, 65
Etoposide
    for hemangiosarcoma, 396
    hypersensitivity reactions to, 333
Etretinate, for sebaceous adenitis, e211
Euculeus aerophilus, e275
Euculeus boehmi, e269-e270
    causing nasal discharge, 636b
Eutrombicula alfreddugesi, 431-432
Evening primrose oil, for sebaceous
    adenitis, e210-e211
Everolimus, use of, for
    immunosuppression, 271-272
Everted laryngeal ventricles, and
    brachycephalic airway obstruction
    syndrome, 650t, 651-652
Excreta, handling associated with
    hazardous drugs, 328-329
Exenatide, for diabetes mellitus, in cats,
    e136t
Exercise
    causing syncope, e329
    for degenerative myelopathy, 1078-
        1080, 1079f
    recommendations postop disk
        herniation, e361b
    recommendations with degenerative
        myelopathy, e362b
    rehabilitation, and physical therapy
        for neurologic disorders,
        e357-e362
    role of, with obesity, 259
Exercise energy requirements, 259
Exercise induced collapse, direct
    mutation test for, 1018t-1020t
Exocrine pancreatic disorders, feline,
    565-568
Exocrine pancreatic insufficiency (EPI)
    diagnosis and treatment of, 558-560
    dietary modification for, 559-560
    enzyme replacement therapy for, 559
    laboratory testing for, 556-557

Exocrine pancreatic neoplasia, 557
Exophthalmos, from orbital diseases,
    1197-1200, 1198b
Expectorants, for respiratory diseases,
    627
External skeletal fixation, with open
    fractures, 86
Extracorporeal shockwave lithotripsy, 885
Extractions. See Dental extractions
Extrahepatic biliary tract disease,
    602-605
Extralabel drug(s)
    approved, e59t-e61t
    not approved for use in animals,
        e61t-e66t
    unapproved, e67t
    use of, e57
Extramedullary plasmacytoma, 386-387
Extranasal sinus disorders, causing
    rhinitis in dogs, 636b
Extraocular muscle myositis, 1114-1115
Extraocular polymyositis, 1199
Extravasation of chemotherapeutic
    drugs, 333
Exudate(s), from malignant effusions,
    341-344
Eye
    diseases of the periocular skin,
        e363-e369
    drops and tear substitutes for, 1146t
    emergencies, e377-e384
    orbital anatomy, 1197
Eyelid
    dermatitis of, e363-e369
    diseases of the, e363-e369
    diseases secondary to abnormalities of
        the, 1155
    ectropion of, e369
    entropion of, e369
    laceration, e378-e379, e379f
    pigment changes of, e367-e368
    tumors
        in cats, 1207
        in dogs, 1201-1206, e368

F
Facial excoriation, from methimazole,
    e103-e104
Facial symmetry, assessment of with
    neuro-ophthalmic exam, e390-e392
Factor II deficiency, coagulation factor
    abnormalities with, 288t, 289
Factor IX
    activity, in hypercoagulable states,
        298f
    deficiency, coagulation factor
        abnormalities with, 288t, 289
Factor V deficiency, coagulation factor
    abnormalities with, 288t
Factor VII deficiency
    coagulation factor abnormalities with,
        288t, 289
    direct mutation test for, 1018t-1020t
Factor VIII
    activity, in hypercoagulable states,
        298f
    deficiency, coagulation factor
        abnormalities with, 288t, 289

Factor X deficiency, coagulation factor
    abnormalities with, 288t
Factor XI
    activity, in hypercoagulable states, 298f
    deficiency
        coagulation factor abnormalities
            with, 288t, 289
        direct mutation test for, 1018t-1020t
Factor XII deficiency, coagulation factor
    abnormalities with, 288t, 289
Fading puppy, from ventricular septal
    defect, e336-e337
False pregnancy. See Pseudocyesis
Famciclovir, for feline tear film
    problems, e386
Familial nephropathy, direct mutation
    test for, 1018t-1020t
Famotidine (Pepcid)
    for feline pancreatitis, 567t
    for gastric ulceration, e254
    for hepatic lipidosis, 612
    for vomiting with acute renal failure,
        870
    potency and use of, 505, 506b
    protocol for helicobacter spp., 511t
    toxicity of, 119
Fanconi syndrome, e34
Fanconi's injury, 580-581
Fat, dietary
    for diabetes mellitus management,
        200-201, 201t, 203, 204t
    recommendations for, with heart
        disease, 722-723
Fat overload syndrome, 108
Fatty acids
    for atopic dermatitis, 406
    for sebaceous adenitis, e210-e211
    requirements during pregnancy and
        lactation, 963
    role of, in development of feline
        hepatic lipidosis, 609
    topical, 420t, 421
Febentel
    for Giardia spp., 530t
    target parasites of, 1335-1337
Febentel/praziquantel/pyrantel, target
    parasites of, 1335-1337
Febreze, toxic exposure to, 98
Febuxostat, for dissolution of urate
    stones, 902
Fecal
    chymotrypsin, 556
    contamination from pets to humans
        causing disease, 1245t, 1246-1247
    for detection of bronchopulmonary
        parasites, e271-e276
    oocysts from toxoplasmosis, 1296
    pancreatic elastase-1, 556, 559
    proteolytic activity (FPA), 556
    trypsin, 556
Fecal culture, 519
Feeding protocol
    during pregnancy and lactation,
        965-966
    for hepatic lipidosis, 612-613
Feeding tube(s), 42-43
    for acute pancreatitis in dogs, 563-564
    for patients with cancer, 353

Felbamate
  associated hepatotoxicity, 578
  for seizures, 1055-1056
Felicola subrostratus, 429t
Feline acromegaly, 216-221
Feline allergic dermatitis, cyclosporine
    for, 408-409
Feline asthma. *See* Asthma
Feline bartonellosis, 1267-1271. *See also*
    Bartonellosis
Feline calicivirus
  causing pregnancy loss, 1009-1010
  causing skin lesions, e194-e195
  common symptoms and syndromes
      caused by, 1215t
  immunotherapy for, 1232
  role in feline stomatitis, 493-494
  upper respiratory infection from, 629,
      1217-1218
    clinical signs of, 630t
  use of interferons for, e201
Feline cholangitis, 614-619
Feline corneal disease, 1156-1161
Feline coronavirus, common symptoms
    and syndromes caused by, 1215t
Feline cowpox virus, e196
Feline eosinophilic keratitis, cyclosporine
    for, 269-271
Feline exocrine pancreatic disorders,
    565-568
Feline facial pheromone, for behavior-
    related dermatoses, 485
Feline foamy virus (FeFV), management
    of, 1275-1283
Feline granulocytic anaplasmosis, as
    cause of thrombocytopenia,
    281t-282t
Feline hemotropic mycoplasmas,
    e398-e401
Feline herpesvirus 1
  causing blepharitis, e364-e365
  causing keratoconjunctivitis,
      1156-1158
  causing pregnancy loss, 1006,
      1009-1010
  causing rhinitis, 646-647
  causing skin lesions, e194, e364-e365
    topical immunomodulators for, e220
  causing upper respiratory infection,
      629, 630t, 1217-1218
  common symptoms and syndromes
      caused by, 1215t
  immunotherapy for, 1232
Feline hypersomatotropism, 216-221,
    217f
Feline immunodeficiency virus (FIV)
  causing nonregenerative anemia,
      e161b, e162
  causing pregnancy loss, 1005t, 1006,
      1009
  causing skin lesions, e195
  causing thrombocytopenia, 281t-282t
  causing uveitis, 1168, 1177
  common symptoms and syndromes
      caused by, 1215t
  immunotherapy for, 1232
  in multicat households, 1276
  lymphocytosis associated with, 305

Feline immunodeficiency virus (FIV)
    (Continued)
  management of, 1275-1283, 1277b,
      1279t-1281t
  vaccination for, 1276
  vaccination of, 1276-1277
Feline infectious peritonitis (FIP),
    1303-1306
  as cause of thrombocytopenia,
      281t-282t
  causing feline uveitis, 1167-1168
  causing pleural effusion, 695, 1216
  causing pregnancy loss, 1010
  diagnosis of, 1304
  rational use of glucocorticoids for, 1300
  treatment of, 1305t
Feline interferon. *See also under*
    Interferon
  for cancer immunotherapy, 336t
  for feline infectious peritonitis,
      1305-1306, 1305t
  for feline retrovirus infections,
      1280t-1281t, 1282
  for infectious disease immune
      therapeutics, 1230t
Feline interstitial cystitis (FIC). *See* Feline
    lower urinary tract disease (FLUTD)
Feline leprosy syndrome, 445-448, 447f,
    448t
Feline leukemia virus (FeLV)
  association with lymphoma, 545
  causing anemia, 1217
  causing feline uveitis, 1168
  causing lymphocytosis, 305
  causing nonregenerative anemia,
      e161b, e162
  causing pregnancy loss, 1006, 1009
  causing skin lesions, e195
  causing thrombocytopenia, 281-283,
      281t-282t
  causing uveitis, 1177
  common symptoms and syndromes
      caused by, 1215t
  immunotherapy for, 1232
  in multicat households, 1276
  management of, 1275-1283, 1278b,
      1279t-1281t
  vaccination for, 1276
  vaccination of, 1276-1277
  vaccine-associated sarcomas from, 1253
Feline lower urinary tract disease
    (FLUTD)
  environmental enrichment with,
      909-914
  indications for perineal urethrostomy
      with, 925
  new treatments for, 925
Feline mammary cancer, 378-380
Feline mononuclear ehrlichiosis, as cause
    of thrombocytopenia, 281t-282t
Feline myocardial disease, 804-810, 806t
Feline panleukopenia virus
  causing pregnancy loss, 1005t, 1006,
      1009
  common symptoms and syndromes
      caused by, 1215t
Feline papillomavirus, causing skin
    lesions, e195-e196

Feline posttraumatic sarcoma, 1209
Feline primary hyperaldosteronism,
    238-242, 240t
Feline retrovirus-infections, management
    of, 1275-1283
Feline sarcoid, e196
Feline scabies, diagnosis and treatment
    of, 429-430
Feline syncytium-forming virus. *See*
    Feline foamy virus (FeFV)
Feline triaditis syndrome, 615-616
Feline upper respiratory tract infection,
    629-632
  causes of, 629, 630t
  causing pregnancy loss, 1009-1010
  clinical signs of, 629
  diagnosis of, 630
  immunotherapy for, 1232
  risk factors for, 629
  treatment of, 630, 631t
Feline urinary bladder cancer, 374
Feline uveitis, diagnosis and treatment
    of, 1166-1170, 1169t
Feline viral skin disease, e194-e197
Feline(s)
  blood groups, 311
  breed blood types, e145t
  breed predispositions, with diabetes
      mellitus, 208-209
  environmental enrichment for
      domestic, 909-914
  outbreaks with dermatophytosis in
      multiple, 452-454
  use of glucocorticoids in, 416t
Femur trauma in dogs, 82
Fenbendazole
  for canine colitis, 551b, 552
  for *Giardia* spp., 530t
  for lung worms, e274-e275, e276
  for nasal nematodes, 637, e270
  target parasites and dosage of,
      1335-1337
Fenoldopam, for oliguria with acute
    renal failure, 869-870, 869t
Fentanyl
  CRI, 62t
  for feline thromboembolism, 810
  for the critical patient, 59, 62t
  for thromboembolism pain, 810, 814
  toxicity, 111
  transdermal, 61-63, 62t
  with diazepam, for anesthetic
      induction in critical patients, 66
  with maintenance anesthetic, 66, 67t
Ferguson reflex, 949
Ferret(s)
  hyperadrenocorticism in, e94-e97
  population control for, 142-144
  treatment of insulinoma in, e130-e134
Fertilization period, 930, 931f, 931t
Fertilizer toxicity, 96, 130
Fetal
  complications during pregnancy,
      947-948
  death, 1003-1011, e85
  disorders, 1011
  distress, 950
  monitoring, 949-951

Fetus, reproductive toxins targeting the, 1026-1028

Fever, *vs.* heat-induced illness, 71-72

Fexofenadine hydrochloride toxicity, 118-119

Fiber
  dietary requirements for, with diabetes mellitus, 200
  diets for feline idiopathic hypercalcemia, 244-246
  supplementation with *Giardia* spp. infections, 531

Fibers, as respiratory toxicants, e46-e47

Fibrates, for hyperlipidemia, 265

Fibrin, abnormalities with disseminated intravascular disorders, 292, 293f

Fibrin degradation products (FDP), in disseminated intravascular coagulation, 294t

Fibrinogen
  activity, in hypercoagulable states, 298, 298f
  in disseminated intravascular coagulation, 294t

Fibrinogen deficiency, coagulation factor abnormalities with, 288t

Fibrinolysis, with disseminated intravascular disorders, 292, 293f

Fibrocartilaginous embolism, 1123-1125, 1123f
  diagnosis of, 1124-1125
  prognosis with, 1125
  rehabilitation considerations with, e360
  treatment of, 1125
  vs. acute disk disease, 1124

Fibromatous epulides, 363

Fibropapilloma, e196

Fibrosarcoma
  eyelid, 1203f
  immunotherapy for, 336t
  nasal, radiation therapy for, 338-340
  oral, 365

Filaroides hirthi, as bronchopulmonary parasite, e272-e273

Filaroides milksi, e273

Filgrastim, for feline retrovirus infections, 1280t-1281t

Finasteride (Proscar)
  for alopecia X, 479
  for benign prostatic hypertrophy, 1013
  for prostatic abscess, 1014-1015

Fine-needle aspiration
  for cytology specimen collection, e153-e154, e154b
  of acral lick dermatitis lesions, e174
  of bladder tumors, 371
  of kidney, use of ultrasound for, 841, 844
  of liver, 574
  of mammary masses, 376, 378
  of masses, client questions about, 319
  of perianal mass, 367-368

Finnoff transilluminator, 1128-1129

Fipronil (Frontline), 426t
  for cheyletiellosis, 430t
  for *Otodectes* infestation, 431t
  for pediculosis, 429t

Fipronil (Frontline) *(Continued)*
  for sarcoptic and notoedric mange, 429t
  target parasites of, 1335-1337
  toxicity of, 140-141

Fipronil/amitraz/s-methoprene, target parasites of, 1335-1337

Fipronil/cyphenothrin, target parasites of, 1335-1337

Fipronil/methoprene/amitraz, 426t

Firocoxib
  adverse effects of, 60
  dosage for, 62t

Fish oils. *See also* Omega-3 fatty acids
  for asymptomatic heart disease, 766
  for heart disease, 722-723, 777, 781
  for hyperlipidemia, 265

Fistulagram, for wound tracts, 87-88

Flail chest, 703

Flatulence, e247-e251
  assessment of patients with, e248
  feeding plans for patients with, e248-e249, e249b
  normal production of, e247-e248, e248t

Flatus, e247

Flaxseed, for idiopathic vacuolar hepatopathy, 607-608

Flea
  biology, 424
  bite hypersensitivity, 403
  infestation, use of avermectins for, e182-e183
  transmission of disease by, from pets to humans, 1248

Flea allergy dermatitis, 424-425
  flea control for, 424-427
  with acral lick dermatitis, e176

Flea control
  products, 1335-1337
    and risk of urinary bladder cancer, 370
    drug reactions from, 489
    for cats, 426t
    for dogs, 426t
    formulations of, dosage for and target parasites of, 1335-1337
    toxicity of, 135-141
  protocols, 427
  strategies, 425-427
  with flea allergy dermatitis, 424-427, 426t

Flecainide
  for heart failure, in dogs, 764t-765t
    with arrhythmias, 771
  toxicity of, use of IV lipid emulsion therapy for, 106

Flies, transmission of disease by, from pets to humans, 1248

Florida spots, 1153-1154

Flow cytometry, for evaluation of lymphocytosis, 302

Fluconazole
  associated hepatotoxicity, 576
  for cryptococcosis, 656
  for dermatophytosis, 451
  for fungal rhinitis in cats, 647-648, 647t

Fluconazole *(Continued)*
  for *Malassezia* spp. infections, e215, e215t
  for systemic mycoses causing feline uveitis, 1168
  use of
    and protocols for, 1235t, 1236-1237
    with cyclosporine, 408

Flucytosine
  for fungal rhinitis in cats, 647-648, 647t
  use and protocols for, 1235t, 1238

Fludrocortisone acetate (Florinef), for hypoadrenocorticism, 236-237

Fluid dynamics, 8, 9f, 9t

Fluid therapy
  calculation of requirements for, 5
  choice of, 2
  colloid, 8-14
    for shock, 21
    with crystalloid, 13, e15-e16
  composition of common, 3t
  crystalloid, 2-7
  during CPR, 30
  for acute hypoadrenocorticism, 235
  for acute pancreatitis in dogs, 562
  for acute renal failure, 868-869
  for canine parvovirus, 534
  for diabetic ketoacidosis, e81-e82, e82
  for disseminated intravascular coagulation, 295
  for feline pancreatitis, 566-567, 567t
  for gastric dilation-volvulus, e15-e17, e16t
  for heat-induced illness, 73
  for hepatic lipidosis, 610-611
  for prevention of hospital acquired kidney injury, 847-848
  for seizure patients, 1061t
  for shock, 20-22
  resuscitation goals of, 13
  routes for, 7
  with acute respiratory distress syndrome, 51
  with cerebrovascular accidents (stroke), 1122
  with nephrotic syndrome, 856

Flumazenil, 30

Flunisolide (AeroBid), inhaled, for respiratory diseases, 626, 626t

Flunixin meglumine toxicity, e32-e33

Fluocinolone
  for otitis, 460
  potency of, for otitis, 460t

Fluorescein dye testing, 1132
  for corneal ulcers, 1149
  for mucin deficiency, 1155

Fluorocarbons toxicity, 1027b

Fluorocytosine
  causing adverse skin reactions, 488t
  for fungal diseases, 1238

Fluoroquinolone(s)
  adverse effects of, 34t-35t
  causing adverse skin reactions, 488t
  causing fetal disorders, 1010
  drug incompatibilities with, 33t
  drug interactions with, 35t
  for canine respiratory infection complex, 634

Fluoroquinolone(s) *(Continued)*
  for hemotropic mycoplasmosis, e401
  for infective endocarditis, e297
  for lower respiratory tract infection(s), 1220t, 1222
  for musculoskeletal infections, 1220t, 1222-1223
  for open fractures, 84-85
  for pneumonia, 682t
  for *Pseudomonas spp.* otitis, 466t
  interaction with GI drugs, 37
Fluoroscopy
  for evaluation of esophagitis and strictures, e238-e239
  for evaluation of esophagus, 496f, 497-498, 498f, e227-e228
  for interventional strategies for urinary disease, 884-892
  for placing temporary pacing, e23-e24, e25f
  for swallowing studies, 497-498, 501-502
Fluorouracil (5-FU)
  for mammary cancer, 377
  toxicity of, 94
  use in cats, 333
Fluoxetine HCl (Prozac)
  for behavior-related dermatoses, 483-484, 483t
  toxicity of, 113, 483-484
Flurbiprofen
  for canine uveitis, 1165t, 1184t
  for feline uveitis, 1169t, 1209-1210
  use of, with glaucoma, 1177
Flutamide
  for benign prostatic hypertrophy, 1013
  for hyperadrenocorticism in ferrets, e95
Fluticasone propionate (Flovent)
  for feline asthma, 679-680
  for respiratory diseases, 626, 626t, 671
Follicular dysplasia, causing alopecia, in dogs, 165b
Follicular neutrophilic dermatitis, from nonsteroidal anti-inflammatory drug(s), 489
Folliculitis
  canine bacterial, 165-166
  superficial bacterial, 437-439
Fomepizole (4-MP)
  as antidote, 102t-104t, 154-155, e56t
  for ethylene glycol toxicity, 153
Food. *See also* Pet food
  poisoning bacteria associated hepatotoxicity, 581b
  probiotic and prebiotic additives in, 525
  reporting adverse events of, e35-e43
  toxic exposures to, 92t, 93-95, 95t
  toxicities with human, 147-150
Food allergy. *See* Atopic dermatitis
Food and drug administration (FDA), reporting adverse events to, e35-e43
Food-dependent hypercortisolism, 230-232, 232f
Foreign body(s), toxic exposures to, 92t
Forelimb trauma in dogs, 80-81

Formaldehyde
  causing reproductive toxicity, 1027b
  respiratory irritant from, e46
Formalin, for tissue fixation, 322-324
Formamide toxicity, 1027b
Foscarnet, for feline retrovirus infections, 1279, 1279t
Fosfomycin, for persistent *E. coli* urinary tract infections, 881b, 883
Fracture(s)
  and orthopedic trauma in dogs, 80-83
  of the os penis, 1031
  open
    classification of, 83, 84t
    diagnosis and treatment of, 83-86
    in dogs, 82-83
    treatment protocol for, 84b, 85-86
  orbital, 1200
Francisella tularensis, as cause of thrombocytopenia, 281t-282t
French bulldog, granulomatous colitis in, 552-553
Fresh frozen plasma, 310
Fructosamine
  and insulin resistance, 205-206
  for monitoring diabetes mellitus, 194
  in dogs, 192
  with feline hypersomatotropism and acromegaly, 219f
FTY 720, use of, for immunosuppression, 273
Fucosidosis, direct mutation test for, 1018t-1020t
Functional residual capacity, 44, 45f
Fundic examination, 1131
Fungal culture, for dermatophytosis, 165
Fungal disease(s). *See also* Dermatophytosis
  as cause of thrombocytopenia, 281t-282t
  associated hepatotoxicity, 581b
  causing blepharitis, e363-e364
  causing blindness, 1136
  causing chorioretinitis, 1195-1196
  causing myocarditis, e304t
  causing pneumonia, 1218
  causing rhinitis
    in cats, 644, 647-648, 647t
    in dogs, 636b, 637-640, 639f
  causing uveitis, 1218
    in cats, 1168
    in dogs, 1164b
  common symptoms and syndromes caused by, 1214t
  immunotherapeutics for, 1230t
  with dermatophytosis, 449-451
Fur mite infestation
  in cats, 431
  use of avermectins for, e182-e183
Furazolidone, target parasites and dosage of, 1335-1337
Furosemide (Lasix)
  adverse effects of, 34t-35t, 36-37, 763
  for acute heart failure
    in cats, 808
    in dogs, 783, 787t, 790-792
  for acute respiratory distress syndrome, 51

Furosemide (Lasix) *(Continued)*
  for ascites, from liver disease, 591, 592f, e257-e258
  for cough from bronchial compression, 782
  for dilated cardiomyopathy, in dogs, 798-799
  for feline cardiomyopathy, 806t, 808-809
  for heart failure, in dogs, 762-763, 764t-765t, 777-779
  for hydrocephalus, 1036
  for oliguria with acute renal failure, 869, 869t
  for pulmonary hypertension, 714
  for refractory heart failure, 781
  interaction with potassium bromide, 34t-35t, 37
  to promote ureterolith passage, 894

G

Gabapentin
  dosage for, 62t
  for cervical spondylomyelopathy, 1095f
  for chronic neuropathic pain, 61
  for craniocervical junction abnormalities, 1102
  for priapism, e356-e357
  for seizures, 1054-1055
Gait, assessment of with neuro-ophthalmic exam, e390-e392
Galactomannan, levels with feline nasal cryptococcosis, 644-645
Galactorrhea, from hypothyroidism, e85
Galactosidase, for flatulence, e250
Galega officinalis, as diabetes supplement, toxicity of, 125
Gallbladder. *See also under* Biliary
  anatomy, 602-603
  cholecystitis, 603
  cholelithiasis, 603-604
  mucocele, 604-605, e221-e224, e222f
    hypertriglyceridemia-associated, 261
    risk with hypothyroidism, e86
  rupture, 603
  stents of, 605
  surgery, 604f-605f, 605
Gamma-glutamyl transferase (GGT), with hepatobiliary disease, 569-571
Ganciclovir, for feline ocular herpesvirus 1, 1158
Gapeworm, nasal, 656
Gaps and gradients, calculation of, with acid-base disorders, e2-e3, e3b
Garage and automotive product toxicity, 95t, 96, 151-155, e30b
Garden products toxicity, 130-132
Garlic toxicity, 98-99, 147-148
Gas(es), as respiratory toxicants, e46
Gasoline toxicity, 154-155
Gastric acid
  secretion, 505, e251-e252, e252f
  suppressants, 505-506
Gastric and intestinal motility disorders, diagnosis and treatment of, 513-518
Gastric brush cytology, 509-510, 510f

Gastric decompression, for gastric dilation-volvulus, e17-e18
Gastric dilatation-volvulus (GDV)
  diagnosis and treatment of, e13-e20
  effect on gastric emptying after, 514
  prognosis for, e14
Gastric *Helicobacter* spp., 508-513
Gastric stasis, with brachycephalic airway obstruction syndrome, 650t
Gastric ulceration, e251-e254
  antacid therapy for, 505-508
  associated with *Helicobacter* spp., 509
  causes of, e252-e253
  from NSAID toxicity, 116-117, e252-e253
  influence on gastric emptying, 514
  therapy of, e254
  use of sucralfate for, 507
Gastric-inhibitory polypeptide (GIP), role in food-dependent hypercortisolism, 231-232, 232f
Gastrinoma, imaging for diagnosis of, 174
Gastritis
  effect on gastric emptying, 514
  with *Helicobacter* spp., 508-513
Gastrocentesis, for gastric dilation-volvulus, e17
Gastroesophageal reflux, 501-504, e237-e242
  and brachycephalic airway obstruction syndrome, 649
Gastrointestinal
  regulation of magnesium, 249-250
  regulation of potassium, 251-252
Gastrointestinal disorder(s)
  antacid therapy for, 505-508
  antibiotic therapy for, 518-522
  canine colitis, 550-554
  canine parvoviral enteritis, 533-536
  causes of hepatobiliary enzyme elevations, 570b
  causing cobalamin deficiency in cats, 523-524
  causing hyperkalemia and hyponatremia, e92, e93b
  cobalamin deficiency in cats, 522-525
  drug incompatibilities and interactions with, 37
  dysphagia, 495-500
  effects from plants, 121b
  exocrine pancreatic disorders in cats, 565-568
  exocrine pancreatic insufficiency (EPI) as, 558-560
  feline lymphoma, 545-549
  feline stomatitis, 492-495
  flatulence as, e247-e251
  from cyclosporine, 405
  gastric ulceration causing, e251-e254
  gastroesophageal reflux, 501-504
  Helicobacter spp. causing, 508-513
  hypokalemia from, 251b
  hypomagnesemia from, 249b
  in dogs with brachycephalic airway obstruction syndrome, 649
  inflammatory bowel disease, 536-540

Gastrointestinal disorder(s) (Continued)
  laboratory testing for the pancreas with, 554-557
  motility disorders causing, 513-518
  oropharyngeal dysphagia as, e259-e262
  pancreatitis
    in cats, 565-568
    in dogs, 561-565
  probiotic therapy for, 525-528
  protein losing enteropathy, 540-544
  protozoal, 528-532
  stenting of malignant obstructions due to, 346-347
  toxicity from chemotherapeutic drugs, 331-332
  tylosin-responsive diarrhea, e262-e265
  upset from methimazole, e104
Gastrointestinal hemorrhage
  from heat-induced illness, 71
  from NSAID toxicity, 116
  from shock, 24
  use of antacid therapy with, 505-508
  with chronic hepatitis, 585f
Gastrointestinal microbial homeostasis, 519f
Gastrointestinal pythiosis, e412
Gastropexy, effect on gastric emptying, 514
Gastrostomy tube(s), for hepatic lipidosis, 611-612
Gel(s), potency of topical steroid, 460f
Gemcitabine, e140t, e141-e142
  for osteosarcoma, 391t
  for urinary bladder cancer, 372-373
Gemfibrozil, for hyperlipidemia, 265
Gene therapy, for retinal dystrophy, 1191
Genetic marker test(s), 1017-1020, 1021f, 1021t
Genetic test(s)
  ABCB1, for predicting adverse effects of drug therapy, 330
  for arrhythmogenic right ventricular cardiomyopathy, 802
  for canine dilated cardiomyopathy, 797
  for degenerative myelopathy, 1077
  for hereditary disorders, 1015-1021, 1016t, 1017f
Genital papillomatosis, e185
Gentamicin (Gentocin)
  causing adverse skin reactions, 488t
  causing renal failure, e31-e32
  for brucellosis, e404
  for otitis
    systemic, 466t
    topical, 464t
  intraocular
    for feline glaucoma, 1180
    fro canine glaucoma, 1175-1176
  nebulization of, for respiratory diseases, 628
Geraniums, 121b
Geriatric screening tests, 858b
Germ cell tumors, 1039-1047
German pinscher(s), direct mutation tests for, 1018t-1020t

German shepherd dog(s)
  avermectin toxicity in, 145
  diarrhea in, 519-520
  direct mutation tests for, 1018t-1020t
  Ehrlichia canis in, 1292
  exocrine pancreatic insufficiency (EPI) in, 558
  limbal melanomas in, 1204
  metatarsal fistulation in, e219
  pannus in, 1154
    atypical, 1141, 1141f
  prostatic disease in, 1012
  risk of bladder cancer in, 371t
  subaortic stenosis in, e319
  testicular tumors in, 1022-1023
  use of cyclosporine for pyoderma in, 410b
German shorthaired pointer(s), direct mutation tests for, 1018t-1020t
Germander toxicity, 570b, 581b
Gestation
  normal in the bitch, 948-949
  normal in the queen, 949
  prolonged, 949
Giardia spp.
  common symptoms and syndromes caused by, 1214t-1215t
  dosage for and drugs targeting, 1335-1337
  in raw meat diets, 1240b, 1241
Giardiasis
  diagnosis and treatment of, 530-532, 530t
  probiotics for infections with, 531
  with *Clostridium perfringens*, 530-531
  with nematode infection, 531
Gibbs-Donnan effect, 8
Gingival hyperplasia, from cyclosporine, 405
Gingivitis, with feline caudal stomatitis, 492
Gingivostomatitis, infectious causes of, 1216
Glanzmann's thrombasthenia, direct mutation test for, 1018t-1020t
Glargine insulin, 191, 210-211, 212b
  storage of, 214
Glaucoma
  canine
    breed predisposed to, 1171b
    causes and pathogenesis of, 1171
    clinical signs of, 1171t, 1172f
    diagnosis and treatment of, 1170-1176, 1173b, e381f, e382-e383
    surgery for, 1174-1176, 1176b
    with uveitis, 1166, 1173t
  causing blindness, 1136
  feline
    clinical signs of, 1178
    diagnosis and treatment of, 1177-1180, 1178f, e381f, e382-e383
    with uveitis, 1177
  from toxoplasmosis, 1297
  secondary from ocular neoplasia, 1206
Glial tumors, 1039-1047, 1042t-1043t
Glimepiride, for diabetes mellitus, in cats, e136t
Gliomas, ocular, 1205-1206

Glipizide (Glucotrol), for diabetes mellitus, in cats, 214-215, e135-e137, e136f, e136t
Glomerular disease
  causing proteinuria, 850-851
  diagnosis and treatment of, 853-857
  hypertension and, 727, 727t
  immune-mediated, immunosuppressive drugs for, 268
  prognosis with, 856
Glomerular filtration, effect of nonsteroidal anti-inflammatory drugs on, 865-866
Glomerular filtration rate (GFR), effect of hyperthyroidism on, 185
Gloves, for handling hazardous drugs, 327
Glucagon
  concentration, with diabetes mellitus in dogs, 189-190
  levels, with superficial necrolytic dermatitis, 486
  to promote ureterolith passage, 894
Glucagonoma
  and superficial necrolytic dermatitis, 485-487
  insulin resistance with, 206b
Glucocorticoid(s)
  adverse effects of, when given with infectious diseases, 1302
  as risk factor for hospital-acquired urinary tract infections, 876-877
  associated hepatotoxicity, 581b
  causing fetal disorders, 1010
  causing gastric ulcerations, e253
  causing hyperlipidemia, 262t
  contraindications for, 417-418
  deficiency of, with hypoadrenocorticism, 233-237
  dose tapering with, 1301-1302
  during CPR, 30
  effect of vehicle and formulation on topical potency, 460f
  effect on adrenocorticotropic hormone testing, e97-e98
  effect on hepatobiliary enzymes, 570-571
  effects on immune system, 414
  food-dependent excess, 230-232
  for actinic dermatoses, 481
  for atopic dermatitis, 405-406
  for autoimmune hemolytic anemia, 278
  for canine colitis, 551b, 552
  for canine uveitis, 1165, 1165t
  for cervical spondylomyelopathy, 1094
  for chronic hepatitis, 586
  for cough from tracheal collapse, 664
  for craniocervical junction abnormalities, 1102
  for dermatologic disorders, 414-418, 416t
  for ehrlichiosis, 1293
  for eosinophilic keratitis, 1159
  for eosinophilic pulmonary diseases, 690-691
  for esophagitis, e240
  for feline asthma, 676

Glucocorticoid(s) (Continued)
  for feline bronchitis, 676
  for feline caudal stomatitis, 494
  for feline cholangitis, 616, 617b, 618
  for feline idiopathic hypercalcemia, 246f, 247
  for feline infectious peritonitis, 1305-1306, 1305t
  for feline uveitis, 1168-1169, 1169t
  for gastric dilation-volvulus, e17
  for hemotropic mycoplasmosis, e401
  for hydrocephalus, 1036
  for hypoadrenocorticism therapy, 235-237
  for immunosuppression, 269
  for infections, 1232-1233, 1299-1303
  for inflammatory bowel disease, 539
  for inflammatory central nervous system disorders, 1064-1065
  for insulinomas, e133
  for masticatory muscle myositis, 1114
  for myasthenia gravis, 1110-1111
  for otitis, topical or systemic, 459-462, 460t-461t
  for palliative cancer care, client questions about, 321
  for prolonged seizures, 1062
  for protein-losing enteropathy, 544
  for respiratory diseases, 625-626
    inhaled, 626, 626t, 671, 678-680
  for retinal detachment, in dogs, e373
  for rhinosinusitis in cats, 646
  for shock, 24-25
  for thrombocytopenia, 285
  for toxoplasmosis, 1297
  hyperadrenocorticism and insulin resistance with, 207
  hypertension from, 727t
  idiopathic vacuolar hepatopathy associated with, 606
  induced calcinosis cutis, 489-490
  influence on thyroid function, 181t
  interaction with NSAID's, 34t-35t
  monitoring use of, 418
  potency and dosing of, 1301t
  prednisone vs. prednisolone, 415
  rational use of, for infectious diseases, 1299-1303
  structure of, 414-415
  systemic
    adverse effects of, 461
    potency of, 461t
  topical
    adverse effects of, 461-462
    for hot spots, e207
    for keratoconjunctivitis sicca, 1147
    potency of, 460f, 460t
    use of, 419-421, 420t
    causing alopecia, in dogs, 165
  use of, with hypoadrenocorticism testing, 234
  use of prednisone in cats, 415
  with feline pancreatitis, 568
Glucose. See also Blood glucose
  composition in fluid therapy, 3t
  drugs that impair intestinal absorption of, e137

Glucose (Continued)
  drugs that inhibit hepatic release of, e137
  energy metabolism in, 1047-1048
  supplementation with liver failure, 582
Glucose curve
  monitoring of and interpretation, 194-196
  vs. home monitoring curve, 197
  with diabetes mellitus management in dogs, 192
Glucose nadir
  interpretation of, 195
  with diabetes mellitus management in dogs, 190, 192
Glutaraldehyde cross-linked bovine collagen, for urinary incontinence, e347f-e348f, e348
Glycated hemoglobin, for monitoring diabetes mellitus, 194
Glycemic index, effect of diet on, with diabetes mellitus, 200
Glycerin, in ear cleaners, 472t, 473
Glycerol, for glaucoma in dogs, 1172-1174, 1173b
Glycogen storage disease, idiopathic vacuolar hepatopathy from, 606
Glycopyrrolate
  adverse effects with α2-adrenergic agonist, 60
  use of prior to cesarean section, 955
Golden period, of wound contamination, 85
Golden retriever(s)
  laryngeal paralysis in, 659-661
  Lyme disease in, 1271-1274
  nonepidermolytic ichthyosis in, 475-476
  pigmentary uveitis in, 1163-1164
  risk of bladder cancer in, 371t
  risk of pyometra with prior pregnancy, 967
  subaortic stenosis in, e319
Gonadal sex, 993, 995t
Gonadectomy, relationship to obesity, 254
Gonadotrophin(s)
  for estrus suppression in the bitch, 988
  for urinary incontinence disorders, 916-917
  levels to detect ovarian remnant syndrome, 1001
Gonadotropin-releasing hormone (GnRH)
  analogs, for hyperadrenocorticism in ferrets, e95-e96
  protocol, 1001, 1002t
  reproductive toxins affecting, 1027
Gonads, reproductive toxins targeting the, 1027-1028
Gonioimplant, with glaucoma therapy, 1175
Gonioscopy, 1133
Gordon Setter(s), vitamin A-responsive dermatosis in, 476
Gossypol toxicity, 581b
Gowns, for handling hazardous drugs, 327

Grain aflatoxins, 159-161
Granuloma(s), nontuberculous cutaneous, 445-448
Granulomatous colitis, 520t, 521, 552-553
Granulomatous meningoencephalitis
cyclosporine for, 269-270
diagnosis and treatment of, 1063-1066
vestibular signs from, 1069
Granulosa cell tumor, with ovarian remnant syndrome, 1001
Grape and raisin toxicity, 98, 121b, 149
Grass, 121b
Gravel root toxicity, 124t
Greasy scale, topical therapy for, 441t
Great Dane dog(s)
cardiomyopathy in, 795-796
cervical spondylomyelopathy in, 1090-1097
Great Pyrenees Mountain dog(s)
common mutation tests for, 1018t-1020t
hyperlipidemia in, 261
Greater celandine toxicity, 581b
Green tea extract toxicity, 581b
Greenies, danger of, 99
Greyhound(s)
atypical pannus in, 1141
canine influenza virus in, 632
pannus in, 1154
thyroid hormone differences in, 180t
Grid keratotomy, 1151-1152
Griseofulvin
associated hepatotoxicity, 570b, 581b
causing adverse skin reactions, 488t
causing fetal disorders, 1010
for dermatophytosis, 450
Growth abnormalities, from hypothyroidism, 179
Growth factor inhibitor(s), for immunosuppression, 271-273
Growth factors
for feline retrovirus infections, 1280t-1281t
for retinal dystrophy, 1191
Growth hormone
and feline hypersomatotropism, 216-221
measurement of, 218-219, 219f
insulin resistance and, 207
Guaifenesin, for respiratory diseases, 627
Guarana toxicity, 123-124
Gustilo, fractures classification system, 83
Gymnema sylvestre, as diabetes supplement, toxicity of, 125

H

H_1-antihistamine(s), toxicity of, 118-119
H_2-antihistamine(s), toxicity of, 119
H_2-receptor antagonists
for esophagitis, e240
for gastric ulceration, e254
for gastroesophageal reflux, 503
potency and use of, 505
use with nephroliths and ureteroliths, 894-895
Haemobartonella spp. *See under* Mycoplasmosis

Hageman trait, coagulation factor abnormalities with, 288t
Hair
examination for dermatophytosis, 453
photomicrogram of, 165f
Hair loss. *See* Alopecia
Halo effect, from ethylene glycol toxicity, 152
Haloperidol, toxicity of, use of IV lipid emulsion therapy for, 106
Halothane-associated hepatotoxicity, 570b, 581b
Hamamelis extract, topical, 420t
HARDIONS-G acronym, 243b
Hazardous drugs, chemotherapeutic, 326-329
Head tilt, from vestibular disease, 1067, 1067t
Head trauma
colloid use for, 12t
fluid therapy considerations with, 6
Hearing loss. *See* Deafness
Heart, Also *see* under
Cardiacmyocardial effects of hypocalcemia on, 252
myocardial effects of magnesium on, 250
Heart block. *See* Atrioventricular (heart) block
Heart disease
anesthesia for patients with, 64-68, 65t
canine
asymptomatic, 775-777, 797-798
at risk for, 775
classifications of, 773-775
stages of and treatment recommendations for, 775-781
valvular, diagnosis and treatment of, 784-794, 785f, 787t, 789f
cardioversion with, e286-e291
causing pleural effusion, 694
congenital, 756-761
causing pulmonary hypertension, 711, 712t
prevalence of, 756-757
drug incompatibilities and interactions with, 36-37
feline
myocardial, 804-810
tachyarrhythmias and, 750f-751f
from *Bartonella* spp. infections, 1263b
from heartworms (*See* Heartworm disease)
from infective endocarditis, e291-e299
from mitral valve dysplasia, e299-e302
from myocarditis, e303-e308
from patent ductus arteriosus, e309-e313
from pulmonic stenosis, e314-e319
from subaortic stenosis, e319-e324
from tricuspid valve dysplasia, e332-e335
from ventricular septal defect, e335-e340
insulin resistance with, 206b
nutritional management of, 720-725
pulmonary thromboembolism associated with, 705

Heart disease (*Continued*)
syncope from, e324-e331
tips for medication administration with, 721b
with hypothyroidism, 184
Heart failure
adverse drug effects on, 34t-35t
bradyarrhythmias and, temporary pacing for, e22
canine
cardiogenic shock from, 783
catecholamine use for, 15t
chronic right-sided, 781
classifications of, 773-775
colloid use with, 12t
congenital heart disease, 760
drug therapy for, 762-772, 764t-765t, 767f, 778b
follow-up examination for, 777-779, 778b
from chronic valvular disease, 786-792, 787t
from dilated cardiomyopathy, 798-799
from heartworm disease, 832-833
from hypothyroidism, e85
management of, 772-784, 778b
overview of, 772-773
persistent cough with, 782
prognosis, 781-782
refractory, 780-781, 780b, 791
treatment of acute, 782-783, 787t, 790-791
with atrial fibrillation, 741
causing hyperkalemia and hyponatremia, e93, e93b
feline, with cardiomyopathy, 807-809
from ventricular septal defect, e336-e337
nutritional recommendations for, 720-725
with endocarditis, e292, e297-e298
Heart function, effect of ventricular arrhythmia on, 745
Heart murmur(s)
caused by infectious disease, 1212-1213
from mitral valve dysplasia, e300
with congenital heart disease, 757-759
with dilated cardiomyopathy in dogs, 796
with endocarditis, e292-e293
with feline myocardial disease, 804-805
with patent ductus arteriosus, e309
with pulmonic stenosis, e314, e314-e315
with subaortic stenosis, e320-e321
with tricuspid valve dysplasia, e332
with valvular heart disease, 785-786
asymptomatic, 786
with ventricular septal defect, e337
Heartworm disease
canine
causing uveitis dogs, 1164b
classification and staging of, 832-833
diagnosis and treatment of, 831-838
eliminating microfilariae, 836

Heartworm disease *(Continued)*
  life cycle of, 831-832
    role of Wolbachia in, 826
  causing pulmonary hypertension, 711, 712t, 716
  causing pulmonary thromboembolism, 705
  causing thrombocytopenia, 281t-282t
  feline
    diagnosis and treatment of, 824-831, 826t, 828f
    prevalence of, 825f
    prevention of, 829, 829t
    prognosis of, 830
Heartworm prevention
  for cats, 829, 829t
  for dogs, 836-837
  formulations of, dosage for and target parasites of, 1335-1337
  product switching of, 836-837
  resistance of, 837
  with flea control, 426t
Heat ablation, ultrasound-guided, for treatment of hyperparathyroidism, e72
Heat-induced illness, 70-74
Heavy metals
  associated hepatotoxicity, 570b, 581b
  causing nephrotoxicity, e30b
  ototoxicity from, 468b, 469
Heimlich valves, with thoracostomy tubes, 702
Heinz body(ies)
  from acetaminophen toxicity, 118
  from onion/garlic toxicity, 147-148
Helicobacter spp.
  causing diarrhea, 1213-1215
  causing gastric ulcerations, e253
  chronic vomiting from, 508-513
  common symptoms and syndromes caused by, 1213t
  diagnostic tests for, 509-511
  pathogenesis of, 508-509, 510f
  treatment failure with, 512
  treatment protocols for, 511-513, 511t
Heliotropium europaeum toxicity, 124t
Helminths, drugs used to treat common, 1335-1337
Hemangiosarcoma
  clinical staging of, 393b
  conjunctival, in cats, 1208
  cyclophosphamide for, 355-356
  diagnosis and treatment of, in dogs, 392-397
  immunotherapy for, 334, 336t
  masitinib for, 361t
  pericardial, 816-823, e167
Hematocrit, relationship to mean corpuscular hemoglobin concentration (MCHC), 307-308
Hematologic, toxicity from chemotherapeutic drugs, 330-331
Hematology analyzers, quality control of, with in-clinic, 307-309
Hematuria, effect of, on urine protein and albumin, 850
Hemilaminectomy, for intervertebral disk disease, 1073-1074

Hemoabdomen, fluid therapy for, 4
Hemodialysis
  for ethylene glycol toxicity, e31
  slow continuous renal, 873, 874f
Hemoglobin, relationship to mean corpuscular hemoglobin concentration (MCHC), 307-308
Hemoglobin-based oxygen carrier solutions, 11
Hemophagocytic syndrome, 316, e163
Hemophilia A and B, 289
Hemophilia B, direct mutation test for, 1018t-1020t
Hemoplasmas, canine, e399
Hemorrhage
  associated with disseminated intravascular coagulation, 292
  chronic, anemia from, e160
  colloid use with, 12t
  conjunctival, 1139
  from anticoagulant rodenticide toxicity, 133
  induced-strokes, 1120
  intraocular, secondary to hypertension, 726
  postpartum, 957, 958t
  subconjunctival, 1139, 1139f
  with open fractures, 84
Hemorrhagic cystitis, from chemotherapeutic drugs, 332
Hemothorax, 694
Hemotropic mycoplasmosis, as cause of thrombocytopenia, 281t-282t
Henbane toxicity, 124t
Heparin
  drug incompatibilities with, 33t
  for arterial thromboembolism, 815
  for autoimmune hemolytic anemia, 276-278, 277t
  for disseminated intravascular coagulation, 296
  for hypercoagulable states, 299
  for thromboembolism, 813
    feline, 810
    pulmonary, 706-707, 707t
  for thromboprophylaxis, 708-709
  low-molecular weight *vs.* unfractionated, 813
  low-molecular-weight, 707, 813
  monitoring therapy of, 813
  unfractionated, 706, 813
  use of, with thromboelastography, 706
  use with gastric dilation-volvulus, e19
  use with IV lipid emulsion therapy, 108
Hepatic disease. *See under* Liver
Hepatic encephalopathy
  from chronic hepatitis, 587
  from feline hepatic lipidosis, 613
  from liver disease, 591-594
  precipitating factor for, 593b
Hepatic fibrosis, 587
Hepatic lipidosis, 608-614
  and liver failure, 582-583
  diagnosis and treatment of, 608-614
  pathogenesis of, 609
  prognosis for, 613
  with diabetes mellitus, e77

Hepatic necrosis, 580-581
  from glucocorticoid(s), 571
  from xylitol toxicity, 150
Hepatic nodular hyperplasia, *vs.* idiopathic vacuolar hepatopathy, 607
Hepatic support therapy, e255-e258
Hepatitis. *See also under* Liver
  canine, as cause of thrombocytopenia, 281t-282t
  chronic
    immunosuppressive drugs for, 268
    therapy for, 583-588, 585f
  copper-associated, e231-e236
Hepatitis X, 159-161
Hepatobiliary disease
  breeds predisposed to, 571b
  diagnostic approach to, 569-575
  extrahepatic diseases causing enzyme elevations, 571b
  function tests for, 572-573
  toxins and agents associated with, 570b
Hepatocellular carcinoma, associated hepatic injury, 581b
Hepatocellular necrosis, 580-583
  drug induced, 575-579
  therapy of, 583-588
Hepatocellular steatosis, hypertriglyceridemia-associated, 261
Hepatocutaneous syndrome, and superficial necrolytic dermatitis, 485
Hepatopathy, vacuolar, 606-608
Hepatotoxicity
  agents causing, 570b, 581b
  drugs causing, 570b, 575-579, 576f, 581b
    chemotherapeutic, 332-333
    mechanism of, 576f
    methimazole, e104
  idiosyncratic, 577-579
  mechanisms of injury, 581b
  pathogenesis of, 577f, 580
Hepatozoon americanum
  causing myositis, 1115
  common symptoms and syndromes caused by, 1214t-1215t
  diagnosis and treatment for, 1283-1286, 1284f
  prognosis for, 1285
Herbal supplement toxicity, 94-95, 99, 122-129, 124t
Herbalife toxicity, 581b
Herbicide(s)
  and risk of urinary bladder cancer, 370
  causing endocrine disruption, 1028
  causing reproductive toxicity, 1027b
  exposures to, 92t, 96
  toxicity, 130-131
Hereditary disorders
  coagulation factor deficiencies, 286-291, 288t
  diagnostic tests for, 1015-1021, 1016t
Hernia, scrotal, 1031
Herpesvirus. *See* Canine herpesvirus (CHV); Feline herpesvirus 1
Heska E.R.D. Health Screen urine test, for urine protein and albumin, 850

Hetastarch, 11-12
  characteristics of, 10t
  for acute pancreatitis in dogs, 562
  for canine parvovirus, 534
  for protein-losing enteropathy,
    543-544
Heterodoxus spiniger, 429t
Hexachlorophene toxicity, 581b
Hiatal hernia, 501-502, e238-e239
  and brachycephalic airway obstruction
    syndrome, 650t
Hibiscus, 121b
Hill's Science Diet c/d-oxl, for calcium
    oxalate urolithiasis, 898-899
Hill's Science Diet SO, for calcium
    oxalate urolithiasis, 898-899
Hill's Science Diet u/d, for calcium
    oxalate urolithiasis, 898-899
Hill's Science Diet Y/D
  for hyperthyroid cats with kidney
    failure, 187-188, e110
  transitioning from, to other
    treatments, e111
  transitioning from methimazole to,
    e111
Himalayan cat(s)
  corneal sequestrums in, 1159-1160
  risk of urolithiasis in, 897
Hip dysplasia, concerns regarding risk,
    with early age neutering, 983t
Histiocytic colitis
  in boxer dogs, 552-553
  in non-boxer dogs, 553
Histiocytic ulcerative colitis, 552-553
Histiocytosis
  canine reactive, causing eyelid
    problems, e368-e369
  use of cyclosporine for, 410b
Histcytocytic sarcoma, associated
    hepatic injury, 581b
Histopathology
  client questions about, 319-320
  for pythiosis, e413
  grading of soft tissue sarcomas, e149
  identification of *Helicobacter* spp.,
    510-511, 510f
  lesions associated with causes of
    pulmonary hypertension, 712t
  of canine colitis, 550-551
  of chronic hepatitis, 586
  of copper-associated liver disease,
    588-589, e233-e234, e235t
  of feline cholangitis, 614-615
  of feline gastrointestinal lymphoma,
    545-546
  of fibrocartilaginous embolism, 1125
  of idiopathic vacuolar hepatopathy,
    606
  of inflammatory bowel disease, 538
  of injection site sarcomas, 1254
  of liver, 574
  of nontuberculous cutaneous
    granuloma lesions, 447
  of ovarian remnant syndrome, 1002
  of portal vein hypoplasia, 600, 601f
  of skin, for diagnosis of alopecia,
    166
  staging of mammary cancer, 376t

Histoplasma capsulatum
  causing anemia, 1217
  common symptoms and syndromes
    caused by, 1214t
Histoplasmosis
  antifungal therapy for, 1234-1238
  as cause of thrombocytopenia,
    281t-282t
  causing feline uveitis, 1168
  causing nervous system signs, 1212
  causing uveitis in dogs, 1164, 1164b
  immunosuppressive therapy for,
    1232-1233
Holter monitoring
  for arrhythmogenic right ventricular
    cardiomyopathy, 802-803
  for diagnosis of syncope, e329
  for supraventricular tachyarrhythmias
    in dogs, 741-744
  for ventricular arrhythmias, 745, 747
  in cats, 753-754
  with dilated cardiomyopathy, 799
Holz-Celsus procedure, e375
Home-cooked diets, for adverse food
    reactions, 423
Hop toxicity, 148
Hordeolum, e363
Hormone receptor expression, with
    mammary cancer, 379t
Hormone(s)
  assays, to detect ovarian remnant
    syndrome, 1001-1002
  role of
    in mammary cancer, 375
    in urinary incontinence, e341
  therapy, for mammary cancer, 377
Horner's syndrome, e395
  after ventral bulla osteotomy, 657
Horse chestnut toxicity, 124t
Hospital
  acquired kidney injury, recognition
    and prevention of, 845-848, 846t
  acquired pneumonia, 682-683, 683b
  acquired urinary tract infections,
    876-879
  contamination with resistant
    Staphylococcal infections, 456t
  managing the recumbent patient in
    the, e360
Hospitalization, as risk factor for
    hospital-acquired urinary tract
    infections, 877
Hot spots. *See* Pyotraumatic dermatitis
House dust, as respiratory toxicants,
    e46-e47
House dust mite control, e197-e199
Household product toxicity, 92t, 95-100,
    95t, e30b
Human albumin
  characteristics of, 10t
  for therapy of shock, 22
  use of, 13
Human drugs of abuse
  legal considerations with, e51
  toxicity from, 109-112
Human food toxicities, 147-150
Human γ–globulin, for
    thrombocytopenia, 285, 285t

Human interferon. *See under* Interferon
Human medication, toxic exposures to,
    92t, 94-95
Human recombinant interferon alfa, for
    infectious disease immune
    therapeutics, 1230t
Humidifiers, for pneumonia, 687
Humidity
  and dust mite control, e198
  effect on heat-induced illness, 70
Hung far oil toxicity, 125t
Hyalohyphomycosis, antifungal therapy
    for, 1234-1238
Hycodan. *See* Hydrocodone (Hycodan)
Hydralazine
  dosage and formulations of, 764t-765t
  for chronic valvular heart disease, in
    dogs, 787t
  for heart failure, in dogs, 764t-765t,
    768, 778b, 783
  for hypertension, 730, 862
    from acute renal failure, 870
    refractory, 729-730
  for hypertensive emergencies, 870-871
Hydraulic fluid toxicity, 154
Hydrocephalus, congenital, 1034-1037
Hydrochlorothiazide
  for calcium oxalate urolithiasis, 900
  for dilated cardiomyopathy, in dogs,
    798-799
  for feline cardiomyopathy, 809
  for heart failure, in dogs, 764t-765t,
    765-766, 791
  for insulinomas, e133
Hydrocodone (Hycodan)
  for coughing, 622-623, 664, 672
  for heart failure, in dogs, 764t-765t
  for tracheal collapse, 664
  toxicity, 111
Hydrocortisone. *See also under*
    Glucocorticoid(s)
  for illness-related corticosteroid
    insufficiency, 79, 177, 177f
  potency of, for otitis, 460t
Hydrogen peroxide, for emesis
    induction, 105
Hydrolyzed protein diets, 422-423
Hydromorphone
  adverse effects of, 60
  CRI, 62t
  dosage for, 62t
  for the critical patient, 59
  for thromboembolism pain, 814
  toxicity, 111
  use of
    with cardiovascular dysfunction, 65t
    with intracranial pathology, 69
Hydromyelia, 1098
Hydronephrosis, ultrasound findings
    with, 842-843, 843f
Hydrostatic pressure, conditions that
    change, 9t
Hydrotherapy, for degenerative
    myelopathy, 1079-1080
Hydroxyamphetamine, for localization
    of anisocoria, e395
Hydroxychloroquine, toxicity of, use of
    IV lipid emulsion therapy for, 106

Hydroxycut associated hepatotoxicity, 581b

Hydroxyethyl starch. *See* Hetastarch; Pentastarch

Hydroxyurea, for intracranial tumors, 1041t, 1044

Hydroxyzine
    causing adverse skin reactions, 488t
    for atopic dermatitis, 406

Hyoscyamine
    for atrioventricular block, in cats, 754
    for bradycardias, 736
    for feline arrhythmias, 750f-751f

Hyperadrenocorticism
    adrenal-dependent
        gland imaging for diagnosis of, 170-172
        therapy of, 229
    adverse effects of topical and systemic glucocorticoids and, 461-462
    and risk of urinary tract infections, 876-877
    causing alkaline phosphatase elevations, e243-e244
    causing alopecia, in dogs, 165b
    clitoral hypertrophy with, 978-979
    diabetes mellitus and, 207
    hypertension from, 727, 727t
    idiopathic vacuolar hepatopathy with, 606
    in ferrets, e94-e97
    insulin resistance with, 206-207, 206b
    interpretation of tests results for, e97-e102
    lymphocytosis associated with, 305
    myopathy from, 1116
    occult, 221-224
    pituitary-dependent
        imaging for diagnosis of, 171, 173f
        radiotherapy for, 229
        therapy of, 225-228
        with large pituitary tumors, e88-e91
    pulmonary thromboembolism associated with, 705
    surgical treatment options for, 225, 229
    testing in cats, e99
    therapy of, 225-229
    thromboembolic disease with, 812

Hyperalbuminemia, causing nonvolatile ion buffer acid-base abnormalities, e5b

Hyperaldosteronism
    feline primary, 238-242
    hypertension from, 727t, 729
    with hypertensive retinopathy, in cats, 1194

Hyperbaric oxygen therapy, 54

Hyperbilirubinemia
    from feline hepatic lipidosis, 609-610, 613
    from liver failure, 580-581

Hypercalcemia
    diagnosis and treatment of, in dogs, e69-e73
    feline idiopathic, 242-248
        diagnostic plan for, 245f
        differential diagnosis for, 243b
        treatment of, 244-247, 244b
    from cholecalciferol toxicity, e33-e34

Hyperchloremic acidosis, e7, e7b

Hypercholesterolemia
    from hepatobiliary disease, 572
    from hypothyroidism, e86
    treatment of, 264
    with diabetes mellitus, 200-201

Hypercoagulable state(s)
    causing feline thromboembolism, 811
    causing pulmonary thromboembolism, 705, 708
    diagnosis and treatment of, 297-301, 298f
    testing of, with thromboelastography, 74-77

Hypercortisolism. *See also under* Cortisol
    ectopic syndrome of, 230-232
    food-dependent, 230-232

Hyperestrogenism
    and sertoli cell tumors, 1022-1023
    causing alopecia, in dogs, 165

Hyperglobulinemia, in cats caudal stomatitis, 493

Hyperglycemia. *See also* Diabetes Mellitus
    role of insulin resistance in, 205-206
    with acute pancreatitis in dogs, 563

Hyperinsulinism, from insulinoma, e130-e134

Hyperkalemia
    causes of, e93b
    causing feline arrhythmias, 750f-751f, 755
    causing syncope, e328
    from acute renal failure, 870
    from renin-angiotensin-aldosterone system inhibition, 854-855
    from reperfusion after thromboembolism, 810, 813
    with hypoadrenocorticism, 233, 234t, 236
    with hyponatremia, differential diagnosis for, e92-e93

Hyperlipidemia
    approach to canine, 261-266
    causes of, 261, 262t, 263
    causing uveitis in dogs, 1164, 1164b
    complications of, 263t
    from hypothyroidism, e85-e86
    insulin resistance with, 206b

Hypernatremia
    from activated charcoal use, 105, 137
    with feline hyperaldosteronism, 239-240
    with hyperthermia, 73

Hyperosmolality
    from diabetic ketoacidosis, e79
    from nonketotic diabetic mellitus, e83

Hyperosmotic(s)
    for glaucoma in cats, 1179
    for glaucoma in dogs, 1172-1174, 1173b

Hyperparathyroidism
    diagnosis and treatment of, in dogs, e69-e73
    direct mutation test for, 1018t-1020t
    hypercalcemia from, in cat, 243b

Hyperphosphatemia
    causing nonvolatile ion buffer acid-base abnormalities, e5, e5b

Hyperphosphatemia *(Continued)*
    from xylitol toxicity, 150
    with chronic kidney disease, 861-862
    with urolithiasis, 892-893

Hyperplastic dermatosis, use of interferons for, e200-e201

Hypersensitivity reactions
    from canine vaccines, 1250-1251
    to chemotherapeutic drugs, 333
    with polyarthritis, 1224

Hypersomatotropism, feline, 216-221

Hypertension
    acute intracranial, 1045
    fluid movement with, 9t
    from acute renal failure, 870
    from idiopathic vacuolar hepatopathy, 607
    in cats
        causing hyphema, 1178
        retinal detachment from, 1193-1194
        retinopathy from, 1193-1194
        with hyperaldosteronism, 239
        with hyperthyroidism, e105
    in dogs
        causing retinal detachment, e371
        causing uveitis, 1164, 1164b
        retinopathy from, 1192
    pulmonary (*See* Pulmonary hypertension)
    systemic
        conditions associated with development of, 727t
        diagnosis and treatment of, 726-730, 768
    with asymptomatic heart disease, 790
    with cerebrovascular accidents (stroke), 1121-1122
    with kidney disease
        effects of on staging of, 860t, 861-862
        management of, 861-862
    with refractory heart failure, 781

Hyperthermia
    and heat-induced illness, diagnosis and treatment of, 70-74
    from adverse effects of hydromorphone, 60, 65t
    from prolonged seizures, 959-960, 1060
    from serotonin syndrome, 34t-35t

Hyperthyroidism
    and renal function, 185-189, 188f, e118
    causing feline arrhythmias, 750f-751f
    causing myopathy, 1115
    cobalamin deficiency with, 524
    diagnosis of, 169-170, 170f, e101, e107
    hypertension from, 727t, 729-730, e105
    iatrogenic, 184
    insulin resistance with, 206, 206b
    lymphocytosis associated with, 305
    medical therapy for, e102-e106, e103t, e108-e111
    nutritional management of, e107-e112
    prognosis for, e111
    pros and cons of major therapies, e103t

Hyperthyroidism (Continued)
  radioiodine therapy for, e114f (See also
    under Radioiodine therapy)
  thyroid physiology of, e107, e108f
Hypertonic crystalloids, use of, 2
Hypertonic solutions
  for cerebral edema from prolonged
    seizures, 1062, 1062t
  for seizure patients, 1061t
  for shock, 21
  use of, 2
Hypertriglyceridemia
  approach to, 261
  risk of pancreatitis with, 39-40, 261
  treatment of, 264
  with diabetes mellitus, 190, 200-201
  with hypothyroidism, 179
Hypertrophic cardiomyopathy. See under
  Cardiomyopathy
Hypertrophic osteodystrophy, from
  adverse reactions to vaccines, 1251
Hyperuricosuria, direct mutation test for,
  1018t-1020t
Hyperventilation, causing respiratory
  alkalosis, e4b
Hyperviscosity
  causing retinal detachment, in dogs,
    e371
  causing uveitis in dogs, 1164, 1164b
Hypervolemia, fluid movement with, 9t
Hyphema
  causes of, 1178
  causing feline glaucoma, 1178
  from brucellosis, 1163-1164
  with blindness, 1134-1135
  with canine uveitis, 1135-1138,
    1163-1164
  with feline uveitis, 1166-1167
  with glaucoma, 1170-1171, 1178
  with hypertension, 1193
Hypoadrenocorticism. See also Critical-
  illness related corticosteroid
  insufficiency
  acute, 235-236
  adrenal gland imaging for diagnosis of,
    171-172
  causing nonregenerative anemia,
    e161b
  causing syncope, e328
  concurrent with hypothyroidism,
    e87-e88
  diagnosis and treatment of, in dogs,
    233-237
  differential diagnosis for,
    hyponatremia and hyperkalemia,
    e92-e93
  effect on gastric emptying, 514
  interpretation of tests results for,
    e97-e102
  lymphocytosis associated with,
    304-305
  megaesophagus with, e226, e229
  primary vs. secondary, 235
  steroid therapy during shock, 25
Hypoalbuminemia
  causing ascites, 591-592
  causing nonvolatile ion buffer
    acid-base abnormalities, e5, e5b

Hypoalbuminemia (Continued)
  effect on drug therapy, 36
  fluid movement with, 9t
  from hepatobiliary disease, 572
  from liver failure, 580-581
  from protein-losing enteropathy,
    540-544
  human albumin therapy for, 22
  interaction with NSAIDs, 34t-35t
  with acute respiratory distress
    syndrome, 50
  with inflammatory bowel disease, 539
  with renal disease, acetylsalicylic acid
    for, 861
Hypoallergenic dietary therapy, 422-424
Hypocalcemia
  clinical signs of, e124b
  conditions causing, e123b
  diagnostic approach to, e125f
  during pregnancy and lactation, 963
  from blood transfusion reaction, 313
  from hypoparathyroidism, e123b, e124
  postpartum, 958t, 959-960
  supplementation of, for tetany or
    seizures, e126, e126-e127, e126t
  with dystocia, 954
  with secondary hypercalcemia, e129
Hypocapnia, e3-e4
Hypochloremia, from diuretic therapy,
  779
Hypochloremic alkalosis, e6
Hypochlorous acid
  as topical therapy for skin infections,
    441t
  in ear cleaners, 474
Hypocholesterolemia
  from hepatobiliary disease, 572
  from liver failure, 580-581
Hypocoagulation, testing of, with
  thromboelastography, 74-77
Hypofibrinogenemia, coagulation factor
  abnormalities with, 288t
Hypoglycemia
  biochemical, 213-214
  during pregnancy and lactation,
    963-964
  emergency treatment of, e131
  from heat-induced illness, 71
  from insulinoma, e130-e134
  from liver failure, 581-582
  from xylitol toxicity, 150
  with diabetes mellitus, e78
    in dogs, 192-193
    remission, in cats, 213
Hypokalemia
  approach to, 248-253
  causes of, 251-252, 251b
  causing feline arrhythmias, 750f-751f
  causing myopathy, 1116
  from diuretic therapy, 779
  from ectopic ACTH syndrome, 230
  renal disfunction from, 252
  treatment of, 252-253, 253t
  use of digoxin with, 34t-35t
  with acute renal failure, 870
  with chronic kidney disease, 863
  with diabetic ketoacidosis, e79,
    e80t-e81t, e82

Hypokalemia (Continued)
  with feline hyperaldosteronism, 239
  with gastric dilation-volvulus, e18-e19
  with hepatic lipidosis, 611
Hypoluteoidism, 1006
Hypomagnesemia
  approach to, 248-253, 249b
  causes of, 249-250
  from diabetic ketoacidosis, e79,
    e80t-e81t
  treatment of, 250-251
Hyponatremia
  causes of, e93b
  from diabetic ketoacidosis, e79
  with hyperkalemia, differential
    diagnosis for, e92-e93
  with hypoadrenocorticism, 233, 234t
Hypoparathyroidism
  differential diagnosis for, e122-e123,
    e123b
  managing complications with,
    e128-e129
  prognosis for, e129
  treatment of, e122-e129
Hypophosphatemia
  from diabetic ketoacidosis, e79,
    e80t-e81t, e82
  from xylitol toxicity, 150
  with hepatic lipidosis, 611
Hypophysectomy
  for pituitary-dependent
    hyperadrenocorticism, 225
  for treatment of feline
    hypersomatotropism, 219
Hypoproteinemia
  from protein-losing enteropathy,
    540-544
  with open peritoneal drainage, e16-e17
Hypopyon
  canine, 1162, 1163t, 1164-1165
  with blindness, 1134-1135
  with uveitis, 1162, 1163t
Hyposensitization, for eosinophilic
  pulmonary diseases, 690
Hypospadias, 998
Hypotension
  causing gastric ulcerations, e253
  fluid therapy for, 2-4
    resuscitation in cats, 13
  from cardiogenic shock, 783
  from gastric dilation-volvulus, e16
  from prolonged seizures, 1060, 1061t
Hypotestosteronism, causing alopecia, in
  dogs, 165b
Hypothalamus
  as thermoregulatory center, 70-71
  reproductive toxins targeting the,
    1027-1028
Hypothermia
  and hypotension, in cats, fluid therapy
    for, 13
  during CPR, 31
Hypothyroidism
  causing alopecia, in dogs, 165b
  causing megaesophagus, e226-e227
  causing myopathy, 1115
  causing nonregenerative anemia,
    e161b

Hypothyroidism *(Continued)*
  causing vestibular signs, 1068-1069, e84, e86
  complications and concurrent conditions with, e84-e88
  concurrent illness and, 184
  congenital, 179
  diagnosis and treatment of, 178-185, 180t, 183f
  diagnosis of, in dogs, 169
  direct mutation test for, 1018t-1020t
  in cats
    from over-treatment, 187-189, e111, e119, e119-e121
    therapy of, e121
  insulin resistance with, 206-207, 206b
  interpretation of tests results for, e99-e101
  monitoring of, 184
  myxedema coma from, e86-e87
  neuropathy from, 1116
  with cervical spondylomyelopathy, 1094
  with laryngeal paralysis, 659
Hypotonic crystalloids, 2
Hypoventilation, causes of, 52
Hypovolemia
  anesthesia for patients with, 64-68
  causing gastric ulcerations, e253
Hypoxemia
  causing feline arrhythmias, 750f-751f
  clinical signs of, 52
  from acute respiratory distress syndrome, 49
  from V/Q mismatch, 52
  in respiratory acid-base disorders, e3-e5, e3b-e4b
  with pneumonia, 686
  with seizure patients, 1061
Hypoxia, causing respiratory acidosis, e5
Hysteroscopy, transcervical, 937-938

I

Ibuprofen. *See also* Nonsteroidal antiinflammatory drug(s) (NSAID's)
  causing nephrotoxicity, e32-e33
  toxicity of, 116-117
Ichthyosis, 475-476
Idiopathic vacuolar hepatopathy, diagnosis and treatment of, 606-608
Idoxuridine, for feline ocular herpesvirus 1, 1158
Ifosfamide, e139, e140t
  toxicity from chemotherapeutic drugs, 332
IgA deficiency, diarrhea with, 519-520
Ileus, post-surgical, effect of, on gastric emptying, 516-518
Illicit human drug toxicity, 109-112
Illness-related corticosteroid insufficiency, 78-79
Imaging, for diagnosis of endocrine disorders, 167-174, 168b
IMHA. *See* Anemia, hemolytic
Imidacloprid
  for lung worms, e274
  for pediculosis, 429t
  toxicity, 140-141

Imidacloprid-flumethrin, 426t
  target parasites of, 1335-1337
Imidacloprid-moxidectin, 426t
  target parasites of, 1335-1337
Imidacloprid-permethrin, target parasites of, 1335-1337
Imidacloprid-permethrin-pyriproxyfen (K9 Advantix II), 426t
Imidacloprid-pyriproxyfen (Advantage II), 426t
  target parasites of, 1335-1337
Imidapril, for heart failure, 763b, 766-767, 777-779
Imidocarb
  for canine babesiosis, 1258, 1258t
  for cytauxzoonosis, e408
  target parasites and dosage of, 1335-1337
Imipenem
  for infective endocarditis, e294t
  for otitis, 466t, 467
Imipramine, for urinary incontinence disorders, 916t, 917
Imiquimod
  as topical immunomodulators, 335, 336t, e220-e221
  for actinic dermatoses, 481
  for papillomatosis, e186
Immune-mediated disease(s)
  causing blepharitis, e366-e367
  causing endocarditis, e292
  causing myocarditis, e304t
  causing neuropathies, 1117
  causing nonregenerative anemia, e161b
  causing pregnancy loss, 1007
  causing retinal detachment, in dogs, e371
  causing uveitis in dogs, 1162-1165, 1164b
  topical immunomodulators for, e217-e218
  vaccines causing, 1250-1251
Immune-mediated hemolytic anemia. *See* Anemia, hemolytic
Immune-mediated thrombocytopenia
  diagnosis and treatment of, 280-281, 281t-282t, 285t
  secondary, 280-281
Immune-stimulatory therapy. *See* Immunotherapy
ImmuneFx, 335
Immunity
  and risk of hospital-acquired urinary tract infections, 876-879, 881b
  concerns regarding, with early age neutering, 982
  impairment from diabetes mellitus, e77
  impairment from hypothyroidism, e86
  role of interferons in, 1229
Immunodeficiency
  direct mutation test for, 1018t-1020t
  immunotherapy for, 1231-1232
Immunofluorescent antibody test
  for American leishmaniasis, e396-e397
  for *Borrelia burgdorferi*, 1272-1273
  for feline *Bartonella* spp., 1269

Immunoglobulin
  E causing hypersensitivity reactions, to vaccines, 1250-1251
  for autoimmune hemolytic anemia, 279
Immunohistopathology, for feline gastrointestinal lymphoma, 545-546
Immunologic transfusion reactions, 312-313
Immunomodulators. *See under* Immunotherapy
Immunosuppression
  contributing to pneumonia, 681
  from topical glucocorticoids, 461
Immunosuppressive drugs, 268-274
  doses of glucocorticoids, 1301t
  for infectious diseases, 1229, 1232-1233
  for inflammatory bowel disease, 539
  for inflammatory central nervous system disorders, 1065
  for myasthenia gravis, 1110-1111
  for thrombocytopenia, 285t
Immunotherapy
  adverse effects of, 1231
  allergen-specific, 411-414
  and risk of ocular squamous cell carcinoma, 1204
  for cancer, 334-337
  for canine parvovirus, 535
  for feline infectious peritonitis, 1304-1306, 1305t
  for feline retrovirus infections, 1280-1283, 1280t-1281t
  for hemangiosarcoma, 396
  for infectious diseases, 1229-1233, 1230t
  for intracranial tumors, 1045-1046
  for keratoconjunctivitis sicca, 1145
  for *Malassezia* spp. infections, e215-e216
  for oral tumors, 364
  for papillomatosis, e186
  for persistent infections
    in dogs, 1231-1232
    viral, in cats, 1232
  metronomic chemotherapy and, 355
  to augment antimicrobial and antifungal therapy, 1232
  topical, 421, e216-e221
Imperforate canaliculus, e375-e376
Imperforate punctum, e375
Imprint cytology, e153
Inactivated parapoxvirus, for infectious disease immune therapeutics, 1230t
Inappropriate elimination. *See also* Urinary incontinence disorders
  and litter box care with environmental enhancement for cats, 912
Incretins, for diabetes mellitus, in cats, e138
Indirect calorimetry, with cancer cachexia, 350
Indirect fluorescent antibody (IFA) test, for ehrlichiosis, 1292-1293
Indolent corneal ulcers, 1151-1152
Indomethacin
  causing nephrotoxicity, e32-e33
  toxicity of, 116-117

Indoxacarb, 426t
    target parasites of, 1335-1337
Indoxacarb/permethrin, 426t
    target parasites of, 1335-1337
Infections. *See also* Methicillin-resistant
    staphylococcal infections
    causing canine respiratory disease,
        632-635
    causing chronic hepatitis, 584t
    causing diarrhea, 519
    causing dysphagia, 496b
    causing feline respiratory disease,
        629-632
    causing hepatobiliary enzyme
        elevations, 570b
    causing myositis, 1115
    causing nasal discharge, 636b
    causing polyarthritis, 1224-1228
    causing renal failure, e30b
    differentials of, for medical problems,
        1212-1218
    disinfection of environments with
        staphylococcal sp., 455-457
    drug incompatibilities and interactions
        with, 37
    empiric antibiotic therapy for,
        1219-1223, 1220t
    risk of, with diabetes mellitus, e77
    septic abdomen causing, drainage
        techniques for, e13-e20
    skin
        from staphylococci causing
            pyoderma, 435-436
        glucocorticoids for, 415-417
        secondary to demodicosis, 433
        superficial bacterial folliculitis,
            437-439
        topical therapy for, 439-443, 441t
    use of glucocorticoids for, 1300-1301
    with cholangitis in cats, 615
    with complicated corneal ulcers,
        1150-1151
    with dermatophytosis, 449-451
    with nontuberculous cutaneous
        granulomas, 445-448
Infectious bronchitis in dogs, 669-672
Infectious disease(s)
    causing canine uveitis, 1164b
    causing feline uveitis, 1167-1168
    causing nonregenerative anemia,
        e161-e162, e161b
    from American leishmaniasis,
        e396-e397
    from babesia, 1257-1260
    from *Bartonella* spp., 1261-1271
    from canine brucellosis, e402-e404
    from feline cytauxzoonosis, e405-e409
    from feline retrovirus, 1275-1283
    from *Hepatozoon americanum*,
        1283-1286
    from leptospirosis, 1286-1289
    from monocytotropic ehrlichiosis,
        1292-1294
    from *Neospora caninum*, 1290-1291
    from pets to humans, 1244-1249 (*See
        also* Zoonosis)
    from raw meat diets, 1239-1243
    from toxoplasmosis, 1295-1298

Infectious disease(s) (*Continued*)
    hemotropic mycoplasmosis causing,
        e398-e401
    immunosuppressive therapy for,
        1232-1233
    immunotherapy for, 1229-1233, 1230t
    lagenidiosis causing, e412-e415
    pneumocystosis causing, e409-e411
    pythiosis causing, e412-e415
    rational use of glucocorticoids for,
        1299-1303
    zoonoses spread from animals to
        humans, 1245t
Infective endocarditis, e291-e299
Inflammation
    gastric, effect on gastric emptying,
        514
    intestinal, effect on gastric emptying,
        514
    role of, with glomerular disease, 849
    with feline caudal stomatitis, 493
Inflammatory bowel disease
    and canine colitis, 550-551
    antibiotic-responsive, 519b
    classification of, 536
    cyclosporine for, 269-270
    diagnosis and treatment of, 536-540
    prognosis for, 539
    with cholangitis, in cats, 615-616
    with dysbiosis, 521
Inflammatory diseases
    causing anemia, e160
    causing neuropathies, 1117
    causing pregnancy loss, 1005-1006,
        1005t, 1008-1010
    of the liver, in cats, 614-619
Inflammatory mammary carcinoma, 375,
    378
Inflammatory myopathies, 1113-1115
Inhaler(s)
    for eosinophilic pulmonary diseases,
        690, 690f
    for feline asthma, 675, 678-680, 679f
    for respiratory diseases, 623-624, 626,
        626t, 671
Inheritance pattern for coagulation
    factor deficiencies, 288t
Injection site
    reactions, 489
    sarcomas, 1252-1255
Inking, specimens for evaluation, 324b
Insane root toxicity, 124t
Insect bite(s)
    causing allergic conjunctivitis, 1140
    exposures to, 92t
Insect growth regulator toxicity, 140-141
Insecticide toxicoses, 135-141, 136b
    causing adverse skin reactions, 488t
    toxic exposures to, 92t
Insemination, use of endoscopy
    transcervical, 940-944, 941f, 941t
Insulin. *See also* Insulin resistance
    CRI for diabetic ketoacidosis, e80t-
        e81t, e82
    determining dose and frequency for,
        191-192
    drugs that enhance peripheral
        sensitivity of, e137-e138

Insulin (*Continued*)
    drugs that enhance secretion of,
        e135-e137
    for cats, 210, 212b
        alternatives to, e135-e138, e136t
    for dogs, 190-192
    for treatment of hyperkalemia, 236
    hypokalemia from, 252
    IV incompatibility, 33t
    long-term monitoring of, 192
    resistance, hypertriglyceridemia-
        associated, 261
    with oral hypoglycemics, e138
Insulin resistance, 205-209, 206b
    hypersomatotropism and acromegaly
        as causes, in cats, 216-221
Insulin-like growth factor-1, for feline
    retrovirus infections, 1280t-1281t
Insulinoma
    imaging for diagnosis of, 174
    prognosis with, e134
    treatment of, in dogs cats and ferrets,
        e130-e134
Intensity-modulated radiation therapy,
    for nasal tumors, 338-339, 340f
Interferon type 1, role of, in antiviral
    immunity, 1229
Interferon(s)
    applications in dermatology,
        e200-e201
    α, e200
    β, e200
    γ, e200-e201
    ω, e201
    balanced production of, with effective
        immune therapies, 1229-1230
    classification of, e200
    for cancer immunotherapy, 336t
    for feline caudal stomatitis, 494
    for feline infectious peritonitis,
        1305-1306, 1305t
    for feline retrovirus infections,
        1280t-1281t, 1281-1282
    for infectious disease immune
        therapeutics, 1230t
    for papillomatosis, e186
    γ, role of, in antibacterial and
        antifungal immunity, 1229
    importance of production of, 1230
    mode of action of, e200
Intermittent positive pressure
    ventilation, in critical care, 66-67
International renal interest society,
    857-863
Interstitial cell tumors, 1022-1023
Interstitial lung diseases, e266-e269,
    e267b
Interventional oncology, 345-349
Interventional radiology, 345-349
Interventional strategies for urinary
    disease(s), 884-892
Intervertebral disk disease, 1070-1075
    glucocorticoids for, 1074
    herniation causing, 1071
    neuroprotective agents for, 1074
    pathophysiology of, 1070-1071
    rehabilitation considerations with,
        e360, e361b

Intervertebral disk disease *(Continued)*
  risk of urinary tract infections with, 876-877
  spinal cord injury scale with, 1072, 1072t
  surgery for, 1073-1074
  vs. fibrocartilaginous embolism, 1124
Intestinal bacterial overgrowth, antibiotic-responsive, 518-522, 519b
Intestinal gas, e248t
Intestinal microbiota, 525-526
  with inflammatory bowel disease, 537
Intestinal motility
  disorders, diagnosis and treatment of, 513-518
  physiology, 516
Intestinal mucosal immune system, 537
Intraarterial chemotherapy
  for lower urinary tract, 890, 891f
  for malignant obstructions, 347-348
Intracranial arachnoid cysts in dogs, 1038-1039
Intracranial elastance curve, 68f
Intracranial hypertension, 1045
Intracranial pathology, anesthesia with, 68-70, 69f
Intracranial pressure
  elevations from prolonged seizures, 1061-1062, 1062t
  with cerebrovascular accidents (stroke), 1120, 1122
Intracranial tumors, 1039-1047, 1041t-1042t
Intracranial volume, 68
Intradermal testing, for *Malassezia* hypersensitivity, e214
Intralesional injection, with acral lick dermatitis, e177
Intranasal vaccinations
  accidental injection of, 635
  canine, 634-635
  feline, 631-632
Intraocular pressure (IOP)
  measurement of, 1130
  normal values, 1130
    in cats, 1166-1167
  with canine glaucoma, 1170, 1174
    and uveitis, 1173t
  with feline glaucoma, 1177
Intraperitoneal chemotherapy, 343-344
Intrathoracic chemotherapy, 343-344
Intravascular fluid therapy, 4, 8
Intravenous, drug incompatibilities, 33t
Intravenous fat embolism. *See* Intravenous lipid emulsion therapy
Intravenous lipid emulsion therapy, 106-109, 115-116
Intravesical therapy, for urinary bladder cancer, 373
Iodinated contrast agents, for hyperthyroid cats, e106
Iodine restriction, for feline hyperthyroidism, e109-e111
Ion gap, calculation of, with acid-base disorders, e2
Iopanoic acid, for hyperthyroid cats, e103t, e106

Ipilimumab, as cancer immunotherapy, 334
Ipronidazole, for *Giardia* spp., 530-531, 530t
Iridociliary adenoma, 1204-1205
  in cats, 1209
Iris melanoma, in cats, 1208-1209, 1208f
Iris nevus, 1208f
Iris swelling, with canine uveitis, 1163t
Irish setter(s)
  direct mutation tests for, 1018t-1020t
  progressive retinal atrophy in, 1188-1190, 1189t
Irish wolfhound(s), cardiomyopathy in, 795-796
Iron deficiency anemia, e160
Ischemic
  myelopathy, 1123-1125
  renal injury, causing renal failure, e30b
  strokes, 1119-1120
Isoflurane
  anesthesia in critical care, 66
  use of with cesarean section, 955
Isoproterenol, for bradycardias, 736-737
Isospora spp., common symptoms and syndromes caused by, 1214t-1215t
Isotretinoin, for sebaceous adenitis, e211
Itraconazole (Sporanox)
  adverse effects of, 1236
  associated hepatotoxicity, 576
  drug reactions from, 489
  for dermatophytosis, 451, 451t
  for fungal rhinitis in cats, 647t
  for lymphoplasmacytic rhinitis in dogs, 641
  for *Malassezia* spp. infections, e215, e215t
  for nasal aspergillosis, 639-640
  for nasopharyngeal cryptococcosis, 656
  for otitis, 467
  use and protocols for, 1235t, 1236
Ivermectin
  adverse reactions to microfilariae from, e180
  causing adverse skin reactions, 488t
  enterohepatic recirculation of, 105
  for cheyletiellosis, 430t, e182
  for demodicosis, 433-434, 433t, e182
  for dermatologic disorders, e178, e179-e180
  for feline demodicosis, e192-e193
  for fur mite infestation, e183
  for lung worms, e275
  for nasal mites, 637, 655-656
  for *Otodectes*, 431t, e182
  for pediculosis, 429t
  for sarcoptic and notoedric mange, 429t
  for sarcoptic mange, e181
  for tick infestation, e183
  target parasites of, 1335-1337
Ivermectin toxicity, e179
  causing blindness, 1136, e383
  direct mutation test for, 1018t-1020t
  drug interactions potentiating, e179
  use of IV lipid emulsion therapy for, 106, 108, 115-116

Ivermectin/praziquantel/pyrantel, target parasites of, 1335-1337
Ivermectin/pyrantel, target parasites of, 1335-1337
Ixodes spp. ticks
  transmitting *Anaplasma phagocytophilum*, 1225-1226
  transmitting *Borrelia burgdorferi*, 1227
  transmitting *Ehrlichia canis*, 1292-1294

J

Jack Russell terrier(s)
  mitochondrial encephalopathy in, 1048-1051, 1049t, 1051t
  nonepidermolytic ichthyosis in, 475-476
Jaundice
  and approach to hepatobiliary disease, 569
  from acute liver failure, 580-581
  from drug-associated liver disease, 576, 578-579, 647t
  from feline hepatic lipidosis, 609
  with chronic hepatitis, 585f, 587
  with feline pancreatitis, 566, 568
Jejunostomy feeding tubes
  for canine pancreatitis, 563-564
  for feline cholangitis, 617
  for feline pancreatitis, 568
  for nutrition in critical care, 24, 42-43
  for the cancer patient, 353
Jimsonweed
  causing anisocoria or mydriasis, e392
  toxicity, 124t
Jin Bu Huan toxicity, 570b
Joe Pye weed toxicity, 124t
Joint effusion
  collection of cytology specimens from, e155
  with infective endocarditis, e293
  with orthopedic trauma, 81
  with polyarthritis, 1224-1228
Joint function and rehabilitation, e357-e358
Jones test, 1132
Junctional tachycardia, 740f, 742t
Juvenile cellulitis
  causing eyelid dermatitis, e368
  rational use of glucocorticoids for, 1301

K

Kalanchoe toxicity, 121b
Kanamycin, causing renal failure, e31-e32
Kaopectate toxicity, 117
Kava toxicity, 570b, 581b
Keeshond
  direct mutation tests in, 1018t-1020t
  risk of urolithiasis in, 897
Kennel cough. *See* Tracheobronchitis
Keratectomy
  for corneal dermoid, 1153
  lamellar, for corneal sequestrum, 1159-1160
Keratinization disorders in dogs, 475-477

Keratitis
  in cats
    cyclosporine for, 269-271
    eosinophilic, 1158-1159, 1159f
    from herpesvirus 1, 1156-1158,
      1157t
    from upper respiratory infection,
      630t
    indications for surgery with, 1161t
  in dogs
    causing uveitis, 1164b
    chronic superficial (Pannus), 1154
    from keratoconjunctivitis sicca,
      1143
    pigmentary, in the pug, 1154
    superficial punctate, 1153
Keratoconjunctivitis
  feline herpesvirus 1, 1156-1158
  proliferative, 1158-1159
Keratoconjunctivitis sicca (KCS)
  cyclosporine for, 269-271
  diagnosis and treatment of, 1143-1147,
    1154-1155
  from feline herpesvirus 1, 1157t, 1158
  hypothyroidism with, e85
  indications for surgery with, 1161t
  Schirmer tear test for evaluation of,
    1132
  surgery for, 1147
  tear substitutes for, 1146t
  with corneal ulcers, 1150
Keratomalacia, 1151
Keratopathy
  calcium-related degenerative, 1153
  lipid, 1153
Keratotomy
  diamond burr, 1152
  grid, 1151-1152
  multiple punctate, 1152
Kerosene toxicity, 154-155
Kerry blue terrier(s), direct mutation tests
    for, 1018t-1020t
Ketamine
  CRI, 62t
  dosage for, 62t
  for feline pancreatitis, 567t
  use in critical care, 60
  use of, with intracranial pathology, 69
Ketamine/valium combination, for
    anesthetic induction in critical
    patients, 65
Ketoconazole
  adverse effects of, 1237-1238,
    1301-1302
  as topical therapy for skin infections,
    441t
  associated hepatotoxicity, 570b, 576,
    581b
  drug interactions with, 35t
  for anal furunculosis, e190
  for dermatophytosis, 450
  for ichthyosis, 476
  for Malassezia spp. infections, 442,
    e214-e215, e215t
  for nasopharyngeal cryptococcosis,
    656
  for otitis, 467
    topical, 465t

Ketoconazole (Continued)
  for pituitary-dependent
    hyperadrenocorticism, 228
  use and protocols for, 1235t,
    1237-1238
  use of, with cyclosporine, 270, 408
Ketone, measurement with diabetic
    ketoacidosis, e81
Ketoprofen
  adverse effects of, 60
  dosage for, 62t
  for feline uveitis, 1169t
  influence on thyroid function, 181t
  toxicity of, 116-117
Ketorolac
  for canine uveitis, 1165t
  toxicity of, 116-117
Kidney
  aspirate of, 841, 844
  biopsy, for glomerular disease, 849
  injury, hospital acquired, 845-848,
    846t
  interventional approach to
    nephrolithiasis, 884-889
  normal size of, 841-842
  ultrasound of, 840-845, 841f
Kidney disease. See Renal disease
Kidney failure. See Renal failure
Killed Propionibacterium
    (ImmunoRegulin), for infectious
    disease immune therapeutics, 1230,
    1230t
Klebsiella spp.
  causing pneumonia, 682t, 1216, 1222
  causing prostatitis, 1013
  causing thrombocytopenia, 281t-282t
  causing urinary infections, 1217,
    1219-1221
  isolates
    in feline airways, 676
    in trachea of healthy animals, 682b
    in vagina of healthy dogs, 970t
KOH prep, 164
Kratom toxicity, 124
Kwan loon medicinal oil toxicity, 125t

L

L-2-Hydrooxyglutaricaciduria, 1052
L-2-Hydroxyglutaricaciduria, direct
    mutation test for, 1018t-1020t
L-Asparaginase
  as rescue therapy for canine
    lymphoma, 382t
  associated hepatotoxicity, 581b
  for feline gastrointestinal lymphoma,
    548t
  hypersensitivity reactions to, 333
L-Carnitine
  for asymptomatic heart disease,
    721-722, 724
  for diabetes mellitus, 201
  for feline hepatic lipidosis, 609, 613
  for heart failure, 777
  for liver disease, 582-583
  for mitochondrial encephalopathy,
    1051, 1051t
  for neuromuscular disease, 1118
  requirements with heart disease, 724

L-Deprenyl, 228
L-Lysine. See Lysine
L-MTP-PE
  as cancer immunotherapy, 336t
  for hemangiosarcoma, 396
Labor and delivery
  dystocia, 948-956
  monitoring of, 951, 953f
  normal, in the bitch and queen,
    948-949
Laboratory
  quality control for the in-clinic,
    306-309
  techniques for biopsy and specimen
    submission, 322-326
  techniques for collection of cytology
    specimens, e153-e156
  tests for hereditary disorders,
    1015-1021
Laboratory test(s)
  for disseminated intravascular
    coagulation, 294t
  for evaluation of lymphocytosis, 302
  for heartworm disease in cats, 826-827,
    826t
  for hepatobiliary disease, 569-575
  for hypercoagulable states, 298
  for hypothyroidism, 179-182, 180t
  of the exocrine pancreas, 554-557
Labrador retriever(s)
  atrioventricular conduction
    abnormalities in, 734
  carprofen toxicity in, 578
  copper-associated liver disease in,
    589-590
  craniocervical junction abnormalities
    in, 1098-1100
  direct mutation tests for, 1017,
    1018t-1020t
  encephalomyelopathy in, 1052-1053
  hyperthermia in, 71-72
  laryngeal paralysis in, 659-661
  limbal melanomas in, 1204
  lumbosacral stenosis in, 1105, 1106f
  Lyme disease in, 1271-1274
  nasal parakeratosis in, 476
  obesity in, 254
  osteosarcoma in, 388
  pericardial effusion in, 817
  portosystemic vascular anomalies in,
    571b
  progressive retinal atrophy in,
    1188-1190, 1189t
  risk of pyometra with prior pregnancy
    in, 967
  testicular dysgenesis in, 997
  vitamin A-responsive dermatosis in, 476
  von Willebrand disease in, 288t
Lacrimomimetic(s), for
    keratoconjunctivitis sicca, 1145-
    1147, 1146t
Lacrimostimulant(s), e386-e387
  for keratoconjunctivitis sicca, 1145
Lactate
  as indicator for temporary pacing, e21
  effect of fluid therapy on, 2
  levels in shock, 19
  with gastric dilation-volvulus, e14, e18

Lactated Ringer's solution (LRS), drug incompatibilities with, 33t
Lactation
  antibiotics during, 958t
  hypomagnesemia from, 249b
  nutrition during, 961-966
  termination of, 960
Lactitol, for hepatoencephalopathy, 593
Lactobacillus probiotic(s)
  for persistent urinary tract infections, 882
  for treatment of vaginitis, 973
  therapy, 525, 527
Lactoferrin
  as topical therapy for skin infections, 441t
  for feline retrovirus infections, 1280t-1281t, 1282-1283
Lactoperoxidase, as topical therapy for skin infections, 441t
Lactulose
  enema with liver failure, 582-583
  for hepatoencephalopathy, 593, 596
  use of, with feline hepatic lipidosis, 613
Lagenidiosis, e412-e415, e414-e415
  clinical findings with, e414
  diagnosis of, e414-e415
  treatment of, e415
Lagerstroemia speciosa, as diabetes supplement, toxicity of, 125
Lagophthalmos, 1155
Lameness
  from bartonellosis, 1263-1264, 1263b
  from cervical spondylomyelopathy, 1092
  from craniocervical junction abnormalities, 1101
  from Cushing's myopathy, 1116
  from degenerative myelopathy, 1076-1077
  from *Hepatozoon americanum*, 1284
  from lumbosacral stenosis, 1105-1106
  from Lyme disease, 1213t, 1271
  from obesity, 255b
  from osteosarcoma, 388
  from polyarthritis, 1224-1228
  from trauma, 80-82
  from various infectious agents, 1213t-1215t, 1216-1217
Lamivudine, for feline retrovirus infections, 1278, 1279t
Lansoprazole (Prevacid)
  action and use of, 505-506
  for esophagitis, e240
  for gastric ulceration, e254
  toxicity from, 118
Lantus. *See* Glargine insulin
Laparoscopic surgery
  cholecystectomy, 605
  for gastric dilation-volvulus, e18
Laparotomy, to detect ovarian remnant syndrome, 1002, 1003f
Laryngeal collapse, with brachycephalic airway obstruction syndrome, 652, 661
Laryngeal diseases, diagnosis and treatment of, 659-662

Laryngeal masses, 661-662
Laryngeal paralysis
  causing megaesophagus, e227
  from hypothyroidism, e76
  in cats, 661
  in dogs, 659-661
    with heat-induced illness, 71, 73
Laryngoscopy
  for evaluation of dysphagia, 498
  for evaluation of laryngeal paralysis, 660
Larynx, deformities with brachycephalic airway obstruction syndrome, 650t, 652
Laser procedures
  ablation
    for actinic dermatoses, 481
    of ectopic ureters, 890-891, 891f
  for acral lick dermatitis, e176
  for glaucoma, 1174-1175
  lithotripsy for uroliths, e340-e344
Latanoprost
  causing anisocoria or mydriasis, 1163t, e392
  for glaucoma in cats, 1180
  for glaucoma in dogs, 1173, 1173b, 1173t
  for lens instability, 1186
Lavage
  for open fractures, 85
  for open wounds, 87-88
Lawn and garden product(s)
  risk of urinary bladder cancer from, 370
  toxic exposures to, 92t, 95-96
  toxicity of, 130-132
Lead toxicity, 156-159, 1027b
Leflunomide
  for autoimmune hemolytic anemia, 279
  for immunosuppression, 272-273
Left atrial tear or splitting, 793
Legal, considerations with pet poisoning, e49-e52
Leiomyoma, uterine, 1025-1026
Leiomyosarcoma, uterine, 1025-1026
Leishmaniasis
  American, diagnosis and treatment of, e396-e397
    diagnosis of, e396-e397
  associated hepatotoxicity, 581b
  causing myositis, 1115
  causing nonregenerative anemia, e161-e162
  causing thrombocytopenia, 281t-282t
  common symptoms and syndromes caused by, 1214t-1215t
Lens
  capsule rupture, 1183, 1183f
  changes in, with glaucoma in dogs, 1171t
  disorders, diagnosis and treatment of, 1181-1187
  implantation, 1185, 1185f
  induced uveitis, 1184, 1184t
  luxation, 1185-1187, 1186f
  normal structure and function of, 1181
  trauma, 1187

Lens-induced uveitis, 1164
Lenticular sclerosis, 1181, 1182f
Lentigo simplex, e367
Leonberger(s)
  chronic axonal degeneration in, 1117
  hypoadrenocorticism in, 233
Leopard's bane toxicity, 124t
Leptin, role in obesity, 254
Leptospirosis, 1286-1289
  associated hepatotoxicity, 581b
  causing infection in humans, 1247-1248
  causing pregnancy loss, 1005t, 1006, 1008
  causing renal infections, 1212
  causing thrombocytopenia, 281t-282t
  causing uveitis in dogs, 1164b
  common symptoms and syndromes caused by, 1213t
  diagnosis of, 1287-1289
    effect of vaccination on, 1288
  treatment of, 1289
  uncommon manifestations of, 1287
Leukemia, 317-318
  associated hepatotoxicity, 581b
  causing lymphocytosis, 302-305
  nonregenerative anemia from, e164
Leukopenia, from canine parvoviral enteritis, 533
Leukotriene inhibitors, for respiratory diseases, 626-627
Levamisole
  causing adverse skin reactions, 488, 488t
  for feline retrovirus infections, 1280t-1281t, 1282
Levetiracetam (Keppra)
  for emergent seizures, 1060
  for intracranial tumors, 1041t
  for seizures, 1056
Levey-Jennings control chart, 308
Levorphanol toxicity, 111
Levosimendan, for heart failure, in dogs, 768-770
Levothyroxine
  causing adverse skin reactions, 488t
  for hypothyroidism, 179, 183f, 184-185
    with complications or concurrent disease, e84-e88
  for myxedema coma, e87
  use of, with cardiac disease, 184
Lhasa apso
  hydrocephalus in, 1034-1035
  intracranial arachnoid cysts in, 1038
  risk of urolithiasis in, 892, 897
Lice infestation. *See* Pediculosis
Licorice associated hepatotoxicity, 581b
Lidocaine
  adverse effects of, 34t-35t
  CRI, 62t
  dosage for, 62t
  for feline arrhythmias, 750f-751f
  for feline pancreatitis, 567t
  for heart failure, in dogs, 764t-765t
    with arrhythmias, 771, 783
  for local analgesia, 61

Lidocaine (Continued)
  for supraventricular tachyarrhythmias, 742t, 743
  for ventricular arrhythmias, 746-747, 747f, 747t
  for ventricular fibrillation during CPR, 30
  toxicity of, use of IV lipid emulsion therapy for, 106-107
  transdermal patch, 62t, 63
  use, with gastric dilation-volvulus, e18
Lily of the valley toxicity, 124t
Lily toxicity, 121b
Limb salvage surgery, for osteosarcoma, 390
Limbal melanomas, in cats, 1207-1208
Limbus tumors, 1204
Lime sulfur dip
  for cheyletiellosis, 430t
  for dermatophytosis, 450t
  for feline demodicosis, e192-e193
  for pediculosis, 429t
  for sarcoptic and notoedric mange, 429t
Lincomycin
  drug interactions with, 677
  for pyoderma, 1220t, 1221-1222
  for superficial bacterial folliculitis, 438t
Linguatula serrata, nasal mite, e270-e271
Linognathus setosus, 429t
Lipase. See also Pancreatic lipase immunoreactivity (Spec cPL)
  for the diagnosis of pancreatitis, 554-555, 561
Lipemia, causing hyperkalemia and hyponatremia, e93
Lipid emulsion
  for parenteral nutrition, 39-40
  therapy, 106-109
Lipid keratopathy, 1153
Lipid metabolism, with diabetes mellitus, 200-201
Lipid(s)
  approach to canine hyperlipidemia, 261-266
  as emulsion therapy, 106-109
Lipogranulomas, for protein-losing enteropathy, 544
Lipoic acid, associated hepatotoxicity, 581b
Liposome based immunotherapy, 334, 336t
Lipstick ingestion, 99-100
Lithotripsy
  extracorporeal shockwave, 885
  for uroliths, e340-e344
    complications of, e344
    indications for, e342-e343
    limitations, e343-e344, e343t
    procedure for, e341-e342, e342t
Litter box, care and environmental enrichment for domestic cats, 912
Liver
  bile duct anatomy of, 602-603
  biopsy, 574-575
    for feline cholangitis, 616
    with chronic hepatitis, 585f, 586
    with feline hepatic lipidosis, 610

Liver (Continued)
    with liver failure, 581-582
    with portal vein hypoplasia, 600
  enzyme elevations, 569-573
    of the alkaline phosphatase, e242-e246
    with biliary mucocele, e221-e224
    with copper-associated hepatitis, e233
    with feline cholangitis, 614-619
    with feline hepatic lipidosis, 609-610
    with hepatobiliary disease, 569-573, 570b
    with hepatotoxicity, 575-579
    with idiopathic vacuolar hepatopathy associated, 606-607
    with liver failure, 580-581
  function tests, 572
    with portosystemic shunt, 595
Liver disease
  and superficial necrolytic dermatitis, 485-486
  associated with hypertriglyceridemia, 261, 262t
  causing nonregenerative anemia, e161b
  copper-associated, 588-590, e231-e236
  drug-associated, 575-580, 576f, 581b
  effect on drug therapy, 32-36
  extrahepatic biliary tract disease, 602-605
  feline cholangitis, 614-619, 617b
  from Bartonella spp. infections, 1263b
  from feline hepatic lipidosis, 608-614
  from heat-induced illness, 71
  from leptospirosis, 1287
  from plants, 121b
  hepatic support therapy for, e255-e258
  hepatitis (See Hepatitis)
  idiopathic vacuolar hepatopathy, 606-608
  insulin resistance with, 206b
  portal vein hypoplasia, 599-602
  portosystemic shunt (See Portosystemic shunts (PSS))
  toxin-associated, 581b
  treatment of ascites from, 591-594, e257-e258
  treatment of hepatoencephalopathy from, 591-594
  with concurrent feline pancreatitis, 566
  with diabetes mellitus, e77, e79
Liver failure
  acute, 580-583
  drug effects on, 34t-35t
  from aflatoxins, 159-161
  treatment of ascites with, 591-592
  treatment of hepatoencephalopathy with, 592-594
Lomustine
  as rescue therapy for canine lymphoma, 382t
  associated hepatotoxicity, 332-333, 570b, 577, 581b
  for hemangiosarcoma, 396
  for intracranial tumors, 1041t, 1044
  for multiple myeloma, 386
  metronomic chemotherapy of, 343-344

Loperamide
  for canine colitis, 551b
  toxicity, 111
Loratadine toxicity, 118-119
Lorazepam
  for behavior-related dermatoses, 483t, 484
  toxicity of, 113-114
Losartan, as hepatic support therapy, e257
Lotion(s)
  for Malassezia spp. infections, e215
  for topical antimicrobials, for otitis, 463
  potency of topical steroid, 460f
Low fat diets, for hyperlipidemia, 264
Lower motor neuron, signs with degenerative myelopathy, 1077
Lower respiratory tract infection(s). See also under Pneumonia; Respiratory tract infection(s)
  common pathogens causing, 1222
  empiric antimicrobial therapy for, 1220t
Lufenuron
  for dermatophytosis, 451
  for Malassezia spp. infections, e215
  toxicity, 136b, 140-141
Lumbosacral stenosis, 1105-1108
  diagnosis of, 1105-1106
  medical treatment for, 1106-1108
  surgery for, 1107-1108
Lung
  acute inflammatory disorder of, 48-51
  injury from ventilator therapy, 58
Lung diseases
  causing respiratory acidosis, e4b
  causing respiratory alkalosis, e4b
  from leptospirosis, 1287
  interstitial, e266-e269
    diagnosis of, e266-e268
Lung lobe torsion, causing pleural effusion, 694, 698
Lung neoplasia, e165
Lung volume, 44
Lungworms, e269-e276
Luteinizing hormone
  measurement of, 934-935
  surge, 930-931, 931f
    and ovulation timing, 931t
    and pregnancy complications relative to, 947-948
    and pregnancy diagnosis using abdominal palpation, 944
    and pregnancy diagnosis with relaxin concentrations, 947
  to detect ovarian remnant syndrome, 1001-1002
Lyell's syndrome, from drug reactions, 489
Lyme disease, 1271-1275
  causing infection in humans, 1216
  causing lameness, 1216-1217
  causing myocarditis, e307
  causing nephritis in dogs, 1272
  causing polyarthritis, 1227
  causing uveitis in dogs, 1164b

Lyme disease *(Continued)*
  common symptoms and syndromes
      caused by, 1213t, 1271
  diagnosis of, 1272-1273
  differential diagnosis for, 1273
  prevention of, 1274-1275
  renal infections with, 1212
  treatment of, 1227, 1273-1274
  vaccination, 1274-1275
Lymph node(s)
  involvement in mammary cancer, 375,
      380t
  involvement of, with of thyroid
      tumors, 398-399, 399t
  involvement with perianal tumors,
      368-369
  role in cancer surgery, e170-e171
Lymphatic
  abnormalities causing chylothorax,
      697-698
  involvement with mammary cancer,
      376, 376t
  obstruction, causing malignant
      effusions, 341
Lymphocytic cholangitis, 617b, 618
Lymphocytic plasmacytic colitis,
    551-552
Lymphocytic plasmacytic enteritis, 550
Lymphocytic portal hepatitis, 615
Lymphocytic-plasmacytic stomatitis, in
    cats, 492-495
Lymphocytosis
  diagnosis and treatment of, 301-305
  in cats, 305
  in dogs, 302-305
  nonneoplastic, 305
Lymphoma
  associated hepatic injury, 581b
  association with bipyridyl herbicide
      toxicity, 131
  causing eyelid changes, e368
  causing hyperlipidemia, 262t
  causing lymphocytosis, 302-305
  causing malignant effusions, 341-342
  causing retinal detachment, in dogs,
      e371
  causing secondary ocular neoplasia,
      1206, 1206f, 1209-1210
  causing uveitis, in cats, 1168
  gastrointestinal
      cobalamin deficiency with, 523-524
      feline, 545-549
        prognosis, 548-549, 548t
        protocols, 548t
  immunotherapy for, 334-335, 337
  mediastinal, e166-e167
  myocardial, feline, e167
  nasopharyngeal, 658
  nonregenerative anemia from, e164
  ocular, in cats, 1168
  of the exocrine pancreas, 557
  rescue therapy for canine, 381-383,
      382t
Lymphoplasmacytic rhinitis, in dogs,
    637, 640-641, 640f
Lymphoproliferative disorders, causing
    lymphocytosis, 302
Lynxacarus radovskyi, 431

Lysine
  for feline ocular herpesvirus 1, 1158
  for feline upper respiratory infections,
      630
  for rhinosinusitis in cats, 646-647
Lysozyme, as topical therapy for skin
    infections, 441t

M
Ma huang toxicity, 123
Maalox toxicity, 117
Macadamia nut toxicity, 98-99, 148
Macroadenoma(s), pituitary, e88
Macrolides, causing adverse skin
    reactions, 488t
Macropalpebral fissure, 1155
Macrophage depletion therapy, 335-337
Macules, from adverse drug reactions,
    488t
Magnesium
  approach to low levels of, 248-253,
      249b
  chloride supplementation, 250-251
  composition in fluid therapy, 3t
  dietary, recommendations for, with
      heart disease, 723
  ionized, 248, 250-251
  physiologic role and function of,
      248-249
  role in parathyroid hormone
      production, e123
Magnesium hydroxide, as antacid
    therapy, 506b, 507
Magnesium sulfate cathartic, for toxin
    ingestions, 105
Magnetic resonance imaging (MRI)
  for atlantoaxial subluxation, 1084-
      1085, 1086f
  for canine ocular neoplasia, 1201-1206
  for cerebrovascular accidents (stroke),
      1121f
  for cervical spondylomyelopathy, 1093
  for Chiari-like malformation in dogs,
      1098-1102, 1099f
  for congenital hydrocephalus,
      1035-1036, 1035f
  for degenerative myelopathy, 1077
  for diagnosis of feline
      hypersomatotropism, 216, 219
  for evaluation of dysphagia, 499
  for evaluation of hepatobiliary disease,
      574
  for evaluation of nasal discharge, in
      dogs, 636-637
  for evaluation of pericardial effusion,
      819
  for fibrocartilaginous embolism, 1124,
      1125f
  for inflammatory central nervous
      system disorders, 1064
  for intervertebral disk disease, 1073
      as outcome predictors, 1073-1074
  for intracranial arachnoid cysts in
      dogs, 1038, 1039f
  for lumbosacral stenosis, 1106, 1107f
  for myocarditis, e305
  for nasal tumors, 338
  for pituitary macroadenoma, e89-e90

Magnetic resonance imaging (MRI)
    (Continued)
  for portal vein hypoplasia, 600
  imaging for diagnosis of endocrine
      disorders, 167-174
  of adrenal gland(s), 170-172
      for hyperaldosteronism in cats, 240
  of pancreas, 172-174
  of pituitary gland, 172, 173f
  of thyroid gland, 167-170
  to evaluate for causes of dysphagia,
      e260, e261f
Maine coon cat
  blood type of, e145t
  diabetes mellitus in, 208
  myocardial disease in, 804
Major vessel neoplasia, e167-e168
Malassezia infection(s)
  causing blepharitis, e364
  dermatitis, e212-e216
      perivulvar, 971
      topical therapy for, 441t, 442-443
  otitis, e212-e216
      topical therapy for, 463-464
Malignancy. *See also* Neoplasia
  causing hypercalcemia, in cats, 243,
      243b
Malignant effusions, 341-344
Malignant glaucoma, 1178
Malignant histiocytosis
  cancer immunotherapy for, 336t
  nonregenerative anemia from, e164
Malignant obstruction(s)
  interventional oncology for, 345-347
  urethral stenting for, 889-890
Malnutrition, in critical care, 38
Malonic aciduria, 1052-1053
Maltese
  glaucoma in, 1171b, 1176f
  hepatobiliary disease in, 571b
  mammary tumors in, 375, 377-378
  portosystemic shunts in, 594
  protein-losing enteropathies in,
      540-541
  risk of urolithiasis in, 897
  von Willebrand disease in, 288t
Mammary neoplasia
  cancer immunotherapy for, 336t
  comparison between canine and
      feline, 379t
  diagnosis and treatment of, 375-380
  immunotherapy for, 336t
  in cats, 378-380, 380t
  risk of, with progestin drugs, 985
Mammomonogamus ierei, nasal, 656, e270
Manchester terrier(s), direct mutation
    tests for, 1018t-1020t
Mandibular tumors, 363-364
Mandrake toxicity, 124t
Manganese toxicity, 1027b
Mannitol
  for cerebral edema from prolonged
      seizures, 1061-1062, 1062t
  for cerebrovascular accidents (stroke),
      1122
  for glaucoma in cats, 1179, e381
  for glaucoma in dogs, 1172-1174,
      1173b, e381

Mannitol (Continued)
for intracranial tumors, 1041t
for oliguria with acute renal failure, 869, 869t
to promote ureterolith passage, 894
Manometry, for evaluation of the esophagus, e227-e228
Marbofloxacin
drug interactions with, 35t
for otitis
systemic, 466t
topical, 464t
for superficial bacterial folliculitis, 438, 438t
Marijuana
enterohepatic recirculation of, 105
toxicity, 110-111
Maropitant (Cerenia)
for canine pancreatitis, 562-563
for feline cholangitis, 617, 617b
for feline pancreatitis, 567t
for hepatic lipidosis, 612
for management with GI effects of chemotherapeutic drugs, 331
for vomiting
with acute renal failure, 870
with canine parvovirus, 535
Masitinib, 360-362
Mast cell tumor(s)
associated hepatic injury, 581b
causing eyelid changes, e368
immunotherapy for, 336t
masitinib for, 360-362, 361t
scrotal, 1023
Mastication, role in swallowing, 495-496
Masticatory muscle myositis, 1113-1114, 1199
Mastiff(s)
cervical spondylomyelopathy in, 1092
colitis in, 553
cystine crystalluria in, 926
hereditary tests for, 1018t-1020t
retinopathies in, 1188
Mastitis, septic, 959, 959f
Maternal causes of pregnancy loss, 1005-1010
Matrix metalloproteinase 9, with intervertebral disk disease, 1073-1074
Maxillary tumors, 363-364
Mayapple toxicity, 124t
Mayflower toxicity, 124t
MDR-1 gene, predicting adverse effects of drug therapy, 330
Meadowsweet toxicity, 125t
Mean arterial pressure, and intracranial dysfunction, 68-69, 69f
Mean corpuscular hemoglobin concentration (MCHC), and in-clinic laboratory quality, 307-308
Mebendazole associated hepatotoxicity, 570b, 581b
Mechanical occluder devices for urinary incontinence, 919-923, 920f
Mechlorethamine, as rescue therapy for canine lymphoma, 382t
Meclizine
for intracranial tumors, 1041t
for vestibular disease, 1045

Medetomidine, use of
with cardiovascular dysfunction, 64-65
with intracranial pathology, 69
Mediastinal mass
lymphocytosis associated with, 304
neoplasia, e166-e167
Medical records, considerations of, with legal claim with poisonings, e50-e52
Medication error(s), e37
Medications. See under Drug(s)
Medroxyprogesterone acetate
adverse effects of, 1013
for benign prostatic hypertrophy, 1013
for estrus suppression in the bitch, 986-987
Medulloepitheliomas, 1205
Megacolon, feline idiopathic, 516
Megaesophagus, e224-e230
acquired, e226-e227
causes of, e225b
congenital, e226
diagnosis of, e227-e228
from hypothyroidism, e76
functional anatomy of, e224-e225
idiopathic, e227
prognosis of, e230
treatment of, e228-e230
Megestrol acetate (Ovaban)
for benign prostatic hypertrophy, 1013
for eosinophilic keratitis, 1159
for estrus suppression in the bitch, 984-986
Meglumine antimoniate, for American leishmaniasis, e397
Meibomian gland
adenoma, e368
function of, 1143-1144
infection, e363-e365
tumors, 1202, 1202f-1203f
Melaleuca oil, 126-127, 140
Melanocytoma, uveal, 1204
Melanoma
limbal, 1204
masitinib for, 361t
ocular, in cats, 1207-1209, 1208f
oral, treatment of, 364-365
tumor vaccine for, 335
uveal, 1204
Melarsomine dihydrochloride (Immiticide)
adverse effects of, 835
for heartworm disease
in cats, 829-830
in dogs, 833-835, 834f
Melatonin
for alopecia X, 479
for hyperadrenocorticism in ferrets, e96
for idiopathic vacuolar hepatopathy, 607-608
Meloxicam
adverse effects of, 60
dosage for, 62t
for canine uveitis, 1165t
for feline uveitis, 1169t
for kidney disease, 865-866
influence on thyroid function, 181t
toxicity of, 116-117

Melphalan (Alkeran)
as rescue therapy for canine lymphoma, 382t
for multiple myeloma, 385-386
Memantine, for glaucoma in dogs, 1173b, 1174
Membranoproliferative glomerulonephritis, 855-856
Membranous glomerulopathy, 855
Menace test, 1134-1135, e390-e391
Meningioma, 1039-1047, 1042t-1043t
of the optic nerve, 1205
Meningitis, use of glucocorticoids for, 1232-1233
Menthol, as topical antipruritic agents, 419
Meperidine
toxicity, 111
use of, with cardiovascular dysfunction, 65t
Mepivacaine, toxicity of, use of IV lipid emulsion therapy for, 106
Mercury toxicity, 1027b
Meropenem, for otitis, 466t, 467
Mesalamine, for canine colitis, 551b
Mesenteric portography, with portal vein hypoplasia, 600
Mesna, given with ifosfamide, e139
Mesothelioma, e165-e166
causing malignant effusions, 341
causing pleural effusion, 694-695
pericardial, 817, 820
Metabolic
causes of dysphagia, 496b
complications of hypomagnesemia, 250
Metabolic acidosis
causing hyperkalemia and hyponatremia, e93, e93b
common causes of, e7b
compensatory response to, e2t
from diabetic ketoacidosis, e79, e80t-e81t, e82
management of acid-base disorders and, e5-e8
sodium bicarbonate for, 67-68
with acute kidney disease, 870
with chronic kidney disease, 862
with gastric dilation-volvulus, e16
with hypoadrenocorticism, treatment of, 236
with maintenance anesthetic, 67
Metabolic alkalosis
common causes of, e8b
compensatory response to, e2t
from diuretic therapy, 779
from hyperthermia, 70-71
hypokalemia and, 252
management of acid-base disorders and, e5-e8
Metabolic brain disorders, 1047-1053
Metabolic disorder(s)
causing pregnancy loss, 1007
causing seizures, 1058
Metabolism, and cancer cachexia, 350
Metaflumizone/amitraz (ProMeris), drug reactions from, 489
Metaldehyde toxicity, 96

Metatarsal fistulation, topical immunomodulators for, e219

Metatarsal sinus tracts, use of cyclosporine for, 410b

Metatarsal trauma in dogs, 81

Metergoline, for pregnancy termination, 990

Metformin, for diabetes mellitus, in cats, e136t, e137

Methadone
adverse effects of, 60
dosage for, 62t
for feline thromboembolism, 810
for the critical patient, 59
to calm respiratory distress pets, 47t
toxicity, 111
use of, with cardiovascular dysfunction, 65t

Methanol
in ear cleaners, 472t
toxicity, 151

Methazolamide, for glaucoma in dogs, 1173-1174, 1173b, e381

Methemoglobinemia
from acetaminophen toxicity, 118
from onion/garlic toxicity, 147-148

Methenamine hippurate, for persistent E. coli urinary tract infections, 881b, 882

Methicillin-resistant Staphylococcal infections
causing pyoderma, 435
diagnosis and treatment of, 443-445
disinfection of environments with, 455-457, 456t
from raw meat diets, 1240-1241
resistance, 435
topical therapy for, 440, 441t, 442
vaginal, 973

Methimazole (Tapazole)
adverse reactions from, 488t, 489, e103-e104
associated hepatotoxicity, 578, 581b
clinical monitoring of, e104
for hyperthyroid cats, e102-e106, e103t, e108-e111
with kidney failure, 188
transdermal, e104-e105
transitioning to limited-iodine diets from, e111

Methoprene toxicity, 140-141

Methotrexate
associated hepatotoxicity, 570b
for feline gastrointestinal lymphoma, 548t
use of, for immunosuppression, 268-269

Methoxyflurane toxicity, 581b

Methyl chloroform toxicity, 1027b

Methyl ethyl ketone toxicity, 1027b

Methyl n-butyl ketone toxicity, 1027b

Methylmalonic aciduria, 1052-1053

Methylphenidate toxicity, 109-110

Methylprazole (4-MP), for ethylene glycol toxicity, 153, e31

Methylprednisolone. See also under Glucocorticoid(s)
drug incompatibilities with, 33t

Methylprednisolone (Continued)
for feline asthma and chronic bronchitis, 676
for feline caudal stomatitis, 493-494
for feline gastrointestinal lymphoma, 547
for intracranial tumors, 1041t
for otitis, systemic, 461t
for respiratory diseases, 626
structure and use of in dermatology, 414-418

Methylxanthine(s)
for atrioventricular block, in cats, 754
for feline asthma, 677
for respiratory diseases, 624-625, 671
toxicity, 148-149, 148t

Metipranolol, for glaucoma in dogs, 1173b

Metoclopramide (Reglan)
action and use of, for motility disorders, 516-518, 517t
adverse effects of, 34t-35t
with dopamine, 34t-35t
drug incompatibilities with, 33t
for acute pancreatitis in dogs, 562-563
for esophagitis, e239-e240
for feline pancreatitis, 567t
for gastroesophageal reflux, 503
for hepatic lipidosis, 612
for vomiting with acute renal failure, 870
use of prior to cesarean section, 955

Metoprolol
for asymptomatic heart disease, 766
for heart failure, in dogs, 770-771, 792
for supraventricular tachyarrhythmias in dogs, 742t

Metritis
causing pregnancy loss, 1005-1006, 1005t
postpartum, 958, 958t

Metronidazole (Flagyl)
adverse effects of, 34t-35t
dosing of, with liver disease, 32-33
for antibiotic-responsive diarrhea, 519
for canine colitis, 551b, 552
for epiphora, e375
for Giardia spp., 530t
for hepatoencephalopathy, 593-594
for protein-losing enteropathy, 544
protocol for helicobacter spp., 511t
target parasites and dosage of, 1335-1337
toxicity, causing vestibular signs, 1068-1069

Metronomic chemotherapy, 354-357
for hemangiosarcoma, 396
with soft tissue sarcomas, e151

Mexiletine
for arrhythmia with congestive heart failure, 783
for arrhythmia with dilated cardiomyopathy, in dogs, 799
for heart failure, in dogs, 764t-765t
for ventricular arrhythmias, 747-748, 747t
with arrhythmogenic right ventricular cardiomyopathy, 803

Mibolerone (Cheque drops), for estrus suppression in the bitch, 984

Miconazole
for Malassezia spp. infections, 442, e215
for otitis, topical, 463-464, 465t
for pyoderma, 440-441
for skin infections, topical, 441t

Microalbuminuria, 850
from diabetes mellitus, e76

Microbial homeostasis, gastrointestinal, 519f

Microfilarial test
for canine heartworm disease, 832
for feline heartworm disease, 826-827

Micronutrient, supplementation of, with diabetes mellitus, 201-202

Microscopic agglutination test (MAT) titers, for leptospirosis, 1287-1289

Microscopy, for Bartonella spp., 1265

Microsomal triglyceride transfer protein inhibitors, 260

Microsporum spp.
causing blepharitis, e363-e364
causing dermatophytosis, 449-451
in multicat environments, 452-454

Microvascular dysplasia. See Portal vein hypoplasia

Midazolam
adverse effects of, 34t-35t
drug interactions with, 35t
for emergent seizures, 1059
toxicity of, 113-114
use of, with cardiovascular dysfunction, 64-65

Mifepristone, for pregnancy termination, 991

Milbemycin oxime
for cheyletiellosis, e182
for demodicosis, 433t, 434, e183
for dermatologic disorders, e178, e180-e181
for lung worms, e275
for nasal mites, 637, 655-656, e270
for Otodectes infestation, 431t
for sarcoptic and notoedric mange, 429t
for sarcoptic mange, e181
target parasites of, 1335-1337
toxicity of, 145-146

Miliary dermatitis, 424-425

Milk thistle. See Silymarin

Milrinone, for heart failure, in dogs, 763, 768-770

Mineralization, from high phosphorus and calcium, 244

Mineralocorticoid(s)
activity of systemic glucocorticoids, 461t
deficiency of, with hypoadrenocorticism, 233-237
excess, with feline hyperaldosteronism, 238
for hypoadrenocorticism therapy, 236-237

Miniature pinscher(s), direct mutation tests for, 1018t-1020t

Miniature schnauzer(s), vitamin A-responsive dermatosis in, 476
Minilaparotomy-assisted cystoscopy for urocystoliths, 905-909, 906f
Minimum inhibitory concentration, with antimicrobial therapy, 1219
Minocycline, for feline upper respiratory infection, 631t
Miosis
    causes of, e392
    from canine uveitis, 1163t
Miotic(s), for glaucoma in dogs, 1173b, 1174
Mirtazapine
    adverse effects of, 34t-35t
    dosage with renal failure, 34t-35t
    for hepatic lipidosis, 611
    for management of GI effects with chemotherapeutic drugs, 331
Misoprostol
    action and use of, 506-507
    for gastric ulceration, e254
    for pregnancy termination, 990
Mistletoe associated hepatotoxicity, 581b
Mite(s), drugs targeting, 1335-1337
Mithramycin associated hepatotoxicity, 581b
Mitochondrial encephalopathy, 1048-1051, 1049t, 1051t
Mitocidal therapies, for demodex, 433-434, 433t
Mitomycin C
    for esophageal strictures, e240-e241
    for urinary bladder cancer, 373
Mitotane (o,p'-DDD, Lysodren)
    associated hepatotoxicity, 581b
    for adrenal-dependent hyperadrenocorticism, 229
    for alopecia X, 479
    for hyperadrenocorticism in ferrets, e95
    for idiopathic vacuolar hepatopathy, 607-608
    for pituitary-dependent hyperadrenocorticism, 225-229
    monitoring therapy of, e98
Mitoxantrone
    as rescue therapy for canine lymphoma, 381-383, 382t
    for intrathoracic chemotherapy, 343
    for mammary cancer, 379-380
    for urinary bladder cancer, 373
Mitral regurgitation. See also Valvular heart disease
    asymptomatic, 765-766, 790
    atrial tear from, 793
    heart failure from, 766-768, 790-792
    neurocardiogenic syncope with, e326-e327
Mitral valve disease
    causing pulmonary hypertension, 711, 712t
    diagnosis and treatment of, chronic, 784-794, 785f
    staging of, 787t
Mitral valve dysplasia
    diagnosis and treatment of, e299-e302, e301f

Mitral valve dysplasia (Continued)
    prevalence of
        in cats, 757, 757t
        in dogs, 756, 757t
    prognosis for, e302
Mitratapide, for treatment of obesity, 259-260
Moisturizers, as antipruritic agents, 419, 420t
Mold(s)
    as respiratory allergens, e44
    immunotherapy for, 411
Mometasone furoate, potency of, for otitis, 460t
Momordica charantia, as diabetes supplement, toxicity of, 125
Monoclonal antibody therapy, for mammary cancer, 377-378
Montelukast, for feline asthma, 678
Morgagnian cataract, 1181-1183, 1183f
Morphine
    adverse effects of, 60
    CRI, 62t
    dosage for, 62t
    drug incompatibilities with, 33t
    for epidural analgesia, 61
    for the critical patient, 59
    to calm respiratory distress pets, 47t
    toxicity, 111
    use with cardiovascular dysfunction, 65t
    use with intracranial pathology, 69
Mosapride
    action and use of, for motility disorders, 516-518, 517t
    for esophagitis, e239-e240
Mosquito(s)
    drugs targeting, 1335-1337
    prevention products, pet exposure to, 100
    transmission of disease by, from pets to humans, 1248
Motilin agonists, action and use of, for motility disorders, 516-518, 517t
Motility disorders, gastric and intestinal, 513-518
Moxidectin
    causing adverse skin reactions, 488t
    for cheyletiellosis, 430t
    for demodicosis, 433t, 434, e183
    for dermatologic disorders, e178, e181
    for lung worms, e274-e275
    for Otodectes, 431t, e182
    for sarcoptic and notoedric mange, 429t
    for sarcoptic mange, e181-e182
    target parasites of, 1335-1337
    toxicity of, 145-146, e181
    use of IV lipid emulsion therapy for, 106, 108
Moxidectin/imidacloprid, target parasites of, 1335-1337
Mucin deficiency, 1155
Mucinolytic agent(s), for keratoconjunctivitis sicca, 1147
Mucoceles, of the gall bladder, 604-605, e221-e224

Mucolytic drug(s)
    for canine bronchial diseases, 672
    for pneumonia, 687
    for respiratory diseases, 627
Mucometra, 947
Mucopolysaccharidosis IIIB, direct mutation test for, 1018t-1020t
Mucopolysaccharidosis VI, direct mutation test for, 1018t-1020t
Mucopolysaccharidosis VII, direct mutation test for, 1018t-1020t
Mucosa-associated lymphoid tissue (MALT) lymphoma, Helicobacter spp associated, 509
Mulch toxicity, 131-132
Müllerian agenesis or hypoplasia, 996
Müllerian duct syndrome, persistent, 997-998, 998f
Multicat household(s)
    conflict in, 912-913
    environmental enrichment for, 909-914
    management of retrovirus infections in, 1276
    outbreaks with dermatophytosis in, 452-454
    upper respiratory infection in, 629
Multidrug resistance (MDR-1) gene, avermectin toxicity and, 145-146, e179
Multiple myeloma, 384-386
    causing secondary ocular neoplasia, 1206
    diagnosis and treatment of, 384-386, 385b
    nonregenerative anemia from, e164
Mupirocin
    for hot spots, e207-e208
    for lick granulomas, e178
    for skin infections, 441t, 442
Murmurs. See Heart murmur(s)
Muscle
    atrophy, with degenerative myelopathy, 1079
    disorder as cause of dysphagia, 496b
    injury as cause of hepatobiliary enzyme elevations, 570b
Musculoskeletal
    concerns regarding, with early age neutering, 983
    problems, empiric antimicrobial therapy for, 1220t
Musculoskeletal disorder(s)
    degenerative myelopathy, 1075-1081
    infectious causes of polyarthritis, 1224-1228
Musculoskeletal infection(s)
    common pathogens causing, 1222-1223
    infectious causes of polyarthritis, 1224-1228
    treatment of neuropathies and myopathies, 1113-1118
Mushroom toxicity, 94, 95t
Mustargen, extravasation and tissue sloughing from, 333
Myasthenia gravis
    acquired, from methimazole, e104
    causing megaesophagus, e226, e228

Myasthenia gravis *(Continued)*
diagnosis of, 1109, e226
immunosuppressive drugs for, 268
monitoring the course of, 1111-1112, e228-e229
therapy of acute fulminating, 1111
treatment of autoimmune, 1109-1112, e228-e229
Mycobacterium
causing nontuberculous cutaneous granulomas, 445-448
using immunotherapy for, 1232
Mycophenolate mofetil
for autoimmune hemolytic anemia, 279
for myasthenia gravis, 1111
for thrombocytopenia, 285t
use of, for immunosuppression, 272
Mycoplasma haemocanis, 1213t
Mycoplasma haemofelis, 1213t, e399
Mycoplasma haemominutum, 1213t
Mycoplasma hematoparvum, 1213t
Mycoplasma turicensis, 1213t
Mycoplasmosis
as cause of thrombocytopenia, 281t-282t
carrier status of, e399, e400f
causing canine respiratory infection, 632 633, 1217-1218
causing feline upper respiratory infections, 629, 1217-1218
causing pneumonia, 681, 683t, 687-688
causing pregnancy loss, 1005t, 1006, 1010, 1218
causing thrombocytopenia, 281t-282t
causing vaginitis, 972-973
common symptoms and syndromes caused by, 1213t
diagnosis of, e400-e401
features of, e399
hemotropic, e398-e401
in feline airways, 676
in the female reproductive tract, 938
normal isolates in healthy dogs, 973b
rational use of glucocorticoids for, 1300-1301
treatment of, e401
with feline asthma and bronchial disease, 678
Mycotoxin(s), exposures to, 95t
Mydriasis, causes of, e392
Mydriatic(s), for canine uveitis, 1165t
Myelin basic protein, with intervertebral disk disease, 1073-1074
Myelodysplastic syndrome, 314, 317, e163-e164
Myelofibrosis, secondary, e163
Myelography
for cervical spondylomyelopathy, 1093
for intervertebral disk disease, 1073
for lumbosacral stenosis, 1106, 1106f
with fibrocartilaginous embolism, 1124
Myeloid to erythroid ratio, 315f
Myelonecrosis, e162-e163
Myelopathy
degenerative, 1075-1081
ischemic, 1123-1125

Myelosuppression, from chemotherapeutic drugs, 330-331
Myelotoxic drug(s), for immunosuppression, 268-269
Myocardial disease, feline, 804-810
Myocardial infarction
as cause of sudden death, 782
causing hypokalemia, 251b, 252
with cardiogenic shock, 783
with corticosteroid insufficiency, 174
with feline myocardial disease, 804
Myocarditis, e303-e308
atrial, e308
causes of, e304t
diagnosis of, e304-e306
feline, e306-e307
pathophysiology of, e303-e304
treatment of, e306
Myopathy(ies)
from hyperadrenocorticism, 1116
from hyperthyroidism, 1115
from hypokalemia, 1116
from hypothyroidism, 179, 1115, e76
from steroids, 1116
rehabilitation considerations with, e360-e362
treatment of, 1113-1118
Myositis
dermato-, 1115
extraocular muscle, 1114-1115
masticatory muscle, 1114, 1199
poly-, 1114
Myotomy, for cricopharyngeal achalasia, 499-500
Myotonia
congenita, direct mutation test for, 1018t-1020t
from hyperadrenocorticism, 1116
Myxedema coma, e86-e87
Myxosarcoma, scrotal, 1023

N

N-acetylcysteine
for acetaminophen toxicity, 118, 576-577
for liver failure, 582
N-methyl-*D*-aspartate antagonist(s), use in critical care, 60-61
N-terminal pro-B-type natriuretic peptide (NT-proBNP)
in asymptomatic cats, 805
in dogs with murmurs, 786-787
with canine DCM, 797
with congenital heart disease, 759
with feline arrhythmias, 750f-751f
with feline myocardial disease, 804-805
with respiratory distress, 47, 793
with valvular heart disease, 790
Nabumetone toxicity, 116-117
Nail bed
epithelial inclusion cyst, e185
inverted squamous papillomas, e185
Naloxone, 30
as antidote, e56t
dosage for, 62t
for opioid toxicity, 111
Naproxen toxicity, 116-117, e32-e33

Narcolepsy, direct mutation test for, 1018t-1020t
Narcotic(s), use of prior to cesarean section, 955
Nasal
deformities with brachycephalic airway obstruction syndrome, 650t
disease from *Bartonella* spp. infections, 1263b
parasites, 636b, 655-656, e269-e271
Nasal arteritis, use of cyclosporine for, 410b
Nasal biopsy, 637
Nasal catheter, for oxygen administration, 53
Nasal discharge
in cats, 644-648
in dogs, 635-643, 636b
Nasal neoplasia, e157-e159
chemoembolization for, 348, 348f
in cats, 644, 648, e159
in dogs, 641-643, 642f
radiation therapy for, 338-340
staging of, e157
Nasal parakeratosis, 476
Nasal polyps, 656-657
in dogs, 641-643
Nasoesophageal tube(s), for hepatic lipidosis, 611
Nasogastric tube(s), and risk of aspiration pneumonia, 685
Nasolacrimal apparatus
cannulation of, 1132-1133
obstruction of, e376
testing of, 1132
Nasopharyngeal disorders, 653-658
cysts, 657-658
diagnosis of, 654-655
foreign bodies causing, 655
mucous, 655
neoplasia, 658
parasites causing, 655-656
turbinates, 657
Nasopharyngeal polyps, 656-657
causing vestibular signs, 1068
Nasopharyngoscopy, for evaluation of nasal neoplasia in dogs, 641
Nasopharynx
deformities with brachycephalic airway obstruction syndrome, 650t
surgical access to, 655
Nebulization
for pneumonia, 687
of gentamicin, 628, 634, 671
Nebulizers
for canine bronchial diseases, 672
for respiratory diseases, 623-624
Neck pain
from atlantoaxial subluxation, 1082-1090
from cervical spondylomyelopathy, 1092-1093
from Chiari-like malformation, 1098-1105
Necrolytic dermatitis, 485-487
Necrotizing leukoencephalitis, 1063-1066
Necrotizing meningoencephalitis, 1063-1066

Nemotodal, causes of thrombocytopenia, 281t-282t
Neomycin
    causing adverse skin reactions, 488t
    causing drug reaction conjunctivitis, 1140
    for hepatoencephalopathy, 593-594
    topical, for otitis, 464t
Neonatal corneal dystrophy, 1153
Neoplasia
    adrenal gland, with feline hyperaldosteronism, 241
    associated hepatic injury, 581b
    association of, with *Helicobacter* spp., 508
    association with herbicide toxicity, 131
    biopsy and specimen submission for, 322-326
    bladder
        diagnosis and treatment of, 370-374, 371t
        ultrasound findings with, 843, 844f
    blepharitis, e368
    bone marrow, anemia from, e164
    cardiac, e167
    causing neuropathies, 1117
    causing nonregenerative anemia, e161b
    causing pleural effusion, 694-695
    causing pregnancy loss, 1007
    causing pulmonary hypertension, 711, 712t
    causing retinal detachment, in dogs, e371, e372f
    collection of specimens for cytology with, e153-e156
    ectopic ACTH syndrome with, 230
    effusions from, 341-344
    exocrine pancreatic, 557
    hemangiosarcoma, 392-397
    immunotherapy for, 334-337
    incomplete resection and local recurrence, e172
    insulin resistance with, 206b
    interventional oncology and, 345-349
    intraarterial chemotherapy for, 347-348
        lower urinary tract, 890, 891f
    intracranial, 1039-1047, 1042t
    laryngeal, 661-662
    lung, e165
        ectopic ACTH syndrome with, 230
        from second-hand smoke, e44
    lymphoma (*See* Lymphoma)
    major vessel, e167-e168
    mammary, 375-380
        comparison between canine and feline, 379t
    mediastinal, e166-e167
    metronomic chemotherapy for, 354-357
    multiple myeloma, 384-386
    nasal, e157-e159
        from second-hand smoke, e44
        in cats, 644, 648
        in dogs, 641-643, 642f
        radiation therapy for, 338-340
    nasopharyngeal, 658

Neoplasia (*Continued*)
    new anticancer drugs for, e139-e142
    ocular
        corneal, 1156
        in cats, 1207-1210
            causing glaucoma, 1177-1178
        in dogs, 1201-1206
            causing uveitis, 1164, 1164b
        orbital, 1199
    oral, diagnosis and treatment of, 362-366
    osteosarcoma, 388-392
    palliative *vs.* curative surgery, e171
    perianal, 366-369
    perineal, 366-369
    plasma cell, 384-387
    plasmacytoma, 386-387
    pleural space, e165-e166
    pulmonary, e165-e168
    pulmonary thromboembolism associated with, 705
    renal, ultrasound findings with, 842, 843f
    reproductive, 1022-1026
    soft tissue sarcomas, e148-e152
    stenting for obstructions caused by, 345-347, 889-890
    talking to clients about, 318-321
    thromboembolic disease with, 812
    thyroid tumors, 397-400
    toceranib (Palladia) update for, 358-360
    urethral, ultrasound findings with, 844f
    vaccine-associated, in cats, 1252-1255
    vaginal, 972
    with diabetes mellitus, e77
Neoplastic obstruction(s), interventional oncology for, 345-347, 889-890
Neoral, 270
Neorickettsia helminthoeca, common symptoms and syndromes caused by, 1214t
Neorickettsia risticii, common symptoms and syndromes caused by, 1214t
Neorickettsial, causes of thrombocytopenia, 281t-282t
Neospora caninum, 1290-1291
    causing myositis, 1115
    causing nervous system signs, 1212
    causing pregnancy loss, 1218
    common symptoms and syndromes caused by, 1214t-1215t
    diagnosis of, 1290
    dosage for and drugs targeting, 1335-1337
    in raw meat diets, 1240b, 1241-1242
    treatment of, 1290-1291
Neotrombicula autumnalis, 431-432
Nepafenac, for canine uveitis, 1165, 1165t
Nephrolithiasis
    concurrent infections with, 893-894
    interventional approach to kidney and ureter, 884-889
    lithotripsy for, 884-889
    medical management of, 892-896
    percutaneous removal of, 885f
    when they should be treated, 925-926

Nephropathy. *See also* Protein-losing nephropathy
    familial, direct mutation test for, 1018t-1020t
    from diabetes mellitus, e76
Nephroscopy, interventional strategies for urinary diseases, 884
Nephrostomy
    percutaneous, for ureteral obstructions, 887, 888f
    tubes, use of, with nephroliths and ureteroliths, 895
Nephrotic syndrome
    causing hyperkalemia and hyponatremia, e93
    diagnosis and treatment of, 853-857
Nephrotic-range proteinuria, 853
Nephrotomy, effect on glomerular filtration, 884-885
Nephrotoxicity
    causes of, e29-e34, e30b
    from amphotericin, 1234-1235
    from nonsteroidal anti-inflammatory drugs, 864, 865t, 866-867
Nerve, lesions causing anisocoria or mydriasis, e390, e390f, e393t
Nerve conduction velocities, for degenerative myelopathy, 1077
Nerve injury, peripheral, rehabilitation considerations with, e360-e362
Nerve sheath tumor, eyelid, 1207
Netilmicin, causing renal failure, e31-e32
Neural tumors, 1039-1047
Neurally mediated syncope, e326-e327, e327f
Neuro-ophthalmic examination, e388-e395
Neurodiagnostic testing, for degenerative myelopathy, 1077
Neuroepithelial tumors, 1039-1047
Neurologic disorder(s)
    causing anisocoria or mydriasis, e392-e395
    causing dysphagia, 496b
    craniocervical junction abnormalities in dogs, 1098-1105, 1099f
    degenerative myelopathy, 1075-1081
    drug incompatibilities and interactions with, 37
    from atlantoaxial subluxation, 1082-1090
    from cerebrovascular accidents (stroke), 1119-1126
    from cervical spondylomyelopathy, 1090-1097
    from congenital hydrocephalus, 1034-1037
    from encephalomyelopathy, 1052-1053
    from intervertebral disk disease, 1070-1075
    from lumbosacral stenosis, 1105-1108
    from malonic aciduria, 1052-1053
    from methylmalonic aciduria, 1052-1053
    from mitochondrial encephalopathy, 1047-1053
    from myasthenia gravis, 1109-1112
    from organic acidopathies, 1052-1053

Neurologic disorder(s) (Continued)
  infectious agents that cause, 1212
  inflammatory diseases of the CNS, 1063-1066
  intracranial arachnoid cysts in dogs, 1038-1039
  intracranial tumors, 1039-1047
  new anticonvulsants for, 1054-1057
  physical therapy and rehabilitation for, e357-e362
  secondary to hypertension, 726
  treatment of cluster seizures and status epilepticus, 1058-1063
  treatment of neuropathies and myopathies, 1113-1118
  vestibular, 1066-1070
  with pituitary macroadenoma, e89
  with pituitary-dependent hyperadrenocorticism, 228
Neuromuscular disease
  adjunctive therapy for, 1117-1118
  causing respiratory acidosis, e4b
Neuronal ceroid lipofuscinosis, direct mutation test for, 1018t-1020t
Neuropathy(ies)
  from diabetes mellitus, e76-e77
  from hypothyroidism, e84-e85
  ototoxicity from, 468b
  treatment of, 1113-1118
Neuroprotective agent(s)
  for glaucoma in dogs, 1173b, 1174
  for intervertebral disk disease, 1074
Neutering
  early age, in dogs and cats, 982-984
    summary of risks, 983t
  for benign prostatic hypertrophy, 1013
  for treatment of alopecia X, 479
  risk of prostate cancer and, 1023-1024
Neutral protamine Hagedorn (NPH) insulin, 190-191, 210
Neutropenia
  diagnostic workup for, 315f
  from canine parvoviral enteritis, 533
  from chemotherapeutic drugs, 330-331
  from methimazole, e103
Neutrophilic cholangitis, 615-618, 617b
Newfoundland dog(s)
  cardiomyopathy in, 795-796
  dilated cardiomyopathy in, 724, 795-796
  direct mutation tests in, 1018t-1020t
  laryngeal paralysis in, 659
  polymyositis in, 1114
  subaortic stenosis in, e319
Niacin, for hyperlipidemia, 265
Niacinamide, causing adverse skin reactions, 488t
Nicotine toxicity, 119-120
Nictitating membrane
  neoplasia of
    in cats, 1207
    in dogs, 1203
  prolapsed gland of, 1203
Nightshade toxicity, 124t
Nitazoxanide
  for Giardia spp., 531
  target parasites and dosage of, 1335-1337

Nitenpyram, 426t
  target parasites of, 1335-1337
  toxicity of, 140-141
Nitrofurantoin
  causing toxic polyneuropathy, 1116-1117
  for urinary tract infections, 924, 1220-1221, 1220t
Nitrogen dioxide toxicity, 1027b, e45
Nitrogen mustard compounds, ototoxicity from, 468b
Nitroglycerine ointment, for heart failure, in dogs, 764t-765t, 767-768
Nitroprusside
  for cardiogenic shock, 783
  for heart failure, in dogs, 764t-765t, 767-768
  for hypertension, 870-871
    from acute renal failure, 870
  with chordae tendineae rupture, 793
Nitrous oxide
  anesthesia in critical care, 66
  use of with cesarean section, 955
Nitrovasodilators, for heart failure, in dogs, 767-768
Nizatidine
  for esophagitis, e240
  for motility disorders, 516-518
  potency and use of, 505, 506b
  toxicity of, 119
Noise, ototoxicity from, 468b, 469
Non-immunologic transfusion reactions, 313
Nonbenzodiazepine hypnotic agents, toxicity of, 112-114
Noncardiogenic pulmonary edema
  as cause of respiratory distress, 46-47, 46t
  from herbicide toxicity, 131
  from seizures, 1058, 1061
  vs. acute respiratory distress syndrome, 49-50
  with fluid therapy in critical care, 6
Nonepidermolytic ichthyosis, 475-476
Noni juice toxicity, 124-125
Nonsteroidal antiinflammatory drug(s) (NSAIDs)
  adverse effects of, 34t-35t, 60
    cutaneous, 489
    gastric ulcerations, e252-e253, e253f
  dosages for, 62t
  for canine uveitis, 1165, 1165t
  for feline caudal stomatitis, 494
  for feline uveitis, 1168-1169, 1169t
  for hemangiosarcoma, 396
  for kidney disease, 863-867
  for treatment of cancer, 359
  influence on thyroid function, 181t
  interaction of, with glucocorticoids, 34t-35t
  metabolism of, e33
  renal effects of, 864-866, 865t
  role of cyclooxygenase isoenzymes of, 863-864
  topical use of, 419-421
  toxicity of, 116-117, 864, e32-e33
    animals at risk for, 864-865, 865t
  use of

Nonsteroidal antiinflammatory drug(s) (NSAIDs) (Continued)
  with chronic kidney disease, 866-867, 866b
  with misoprostol, 506-507
Nonthermal irreversible electroporation, for intracranial tumors, 1046
Nontuberculous cutaneous granulomas, 445-448, 446f-447f, 448t
Nonulcerative corneal disease in dogs, 1152-1156
Nonvolatile buffer ion
  acid-base abnormalities, causes of, e5b
  acidosis, e5
  alkalosis, e5
Norepinephrine
  for seizure patients, 1061t
  receptor activities of, 15t
  use and dosage of, 15t, 16
Norepinephrine reuptake inhibitors toxicity, 112-114
Norfolk terrier(s)
  epidermolytic ichthyosis in, 475
  glaucoma in, 1171b
  ichthyosis in, 475
  portal vein hypoplasia in, 599
Nosodes, for feline retrovirus infections, 1280t-1281t, 1283
Notoedric mange
  diagnosis and treatment of, in cats, 429-430
  treatment options for, 429t
Nova Scotia duck tolling retriever(s)
  direct mutation tests for, 1018t-1020t
  hypoadrenocorticism in, 233
NPH insulin. See Neutral protamine Hagedorn (NPH) insulin
NT-proBNP. See N-terminal pro-B-type natriuretic peptide (NT-proBNP)
Nuclear scintigraphy
  for localizing parathyroid tissue, e71
  for portosystemic shunt, 595
Nutraceuticals
  causing pregnancy loss, 1007-1008
  for asymptomatic heart disease, 766
  for heart disease, 777, 778b
  for liver disease, 587, 596, 598f, 617-618, 617b
  probiotic, 527
  toxic exposures to, 94-96, 95t, 569
Nutrition
  after stabilization of shock, 24
  and feeding with hepatic lipidosis, 610-612
  and risk reduction of urinary bladder cancer, 370
  assessment of, 38-39
  association to cancer, 319
  causing polyneuropathy, 1116-1117
  during pregnancy and lactation, 961-966
  enteral support of, 42-43, 42b
  feeding tubes (See Feeding tube(s))
  food elimination diets for adverse reactions, 422-424
  for the cancer patient, 349-354
  for the heart patient, 720-725
  in critical care, 38-43

Nutrition (Continued)
  management of obesity, 254-260
  pharmacologic agents in support of, 43
  problems causing pregnancy loss, 1007
  with diabetes mellitus, 199-204, 201t
    in cats, 210
Nutritional requirements, calculation of, 39
Nutritional supplements, for neuromuscular disease, 1118
Nystagmus, from vestibular disease, 1067, 1067t
Nystatin, otic therapy, 465t

O

Obesity
  and risk of hospital-acquired urinary infections, 877
  and risk of urinary bladder cancer, 370
  as risk for heat-induced illness, 71
  causing hyperlipidemia, 262t
  diagnosis and treatment of, 254-260
  diseases associated with, 255b
  impact of, on canine bronchial diseases, 672
  in cats, management of, with diabetes mellitus, 203
  insulin resistance with, 206-207, 206b
  role of, in development of feline hepatic lipidosis, 609
Obsessive-compulsive disorder, with acral lick dermatitis, e177
Obstetrical monitoring equipment, 949-951, 950f
Obstructive uropathy, causing renal failure, e30b
Occult hyperadrenocorticism, 221-224
Octreotide
  for feline hypersomatotropism, 219
  for insulinomas, e134
  for superficial necrolytic dermatitis, 487
Ocular. See also under Ophthalmic disease(s)
  changes secondary to hypertension, 726
  changes with diabetes mellitus, e78
  complications of hypothyroidism, e85
  emergencies, e377-e384
Ocular neoplasia
  canine, 1201-1206
  feline, 1207-1210
Odontogenic fibroma, 363
Off-Gassing emissions, e46
Oils
  in ear cleaners, 472t, 473
  toxicity from
    botanical oil extract, 139-140
    citrus, 126
    essential, 125-127, 126t
    melaleuca, 126-127, 140
    pennyroyal, 127, 139-140
    salicylate-containing, 125t
Ointment(s)
  as topical therapy for skin infections, 441t
  for keratoconjunctivitis sicca, 1146t, 1147

Ointment(s) (Continued)
  for Malassezia spp. infections, e215
  potency of topical steroid, 460f
Old English mastiff(s), direct mutation tests for, 1018t-1020t
Old English sheepdog(s), avermectin toxicity in, 145
Oleander toxicity, 121b
Oligospermia, e350-e353
Oliguria
  associated with hospital acquired kidney injury, 845
  from acute renal failure, 869-870
Ollulanus tricuspis, common symptoms and syndromes caused by, 1214t-1215t
Oltipraz, for aflatoxicosis, 161
Omega-3 fatty acids
  for asymptomatic heart disease, 766
  for heart disease, 722-723
  for hyperlipidemia, 265
  requirements during pregnancy and lactation, 963
  supplementation of, with diabetes mellitus, 201
Omega-6 fatty acids, for heart disease, 722-723
Omentalization
  for chylothorax, 699
  for local peritonitis, e14-e15
Omeprazole (Prilosec)
  action and use of, 505-506, 506b
  drug interactions with, 34t-35t, 37
  for craniocervical junction abnormalities, 1102
  for esophagitis, e240
  for gastric ulceration, e254
  for gastroesophageal reflux, 503
  for hydrocephalus, 1036
  for vomiting with acute renal failure, 870
  toxicity from, 118
Oncept vaccine, 335, 336t
Onchocerca spp., causing conjunctivitis, 1142
Oncology. See also under Neoplasia
  interventional, 345-349
  reproductive, 1022-1026
  surgical principles for, e168-e172
Oncotic support
  for canine parvovirus, 534
  for protein-losing enteropathy, 543-544
Ondansetron
  for adverse effects from cancer therapy, 331
  for canine pancreatitis, 562-563
  for canine parvovirus, 535
  for feline cholangitis, 617, 617b
  for feline pancreatitis, 567t
  for hepatic lipidosis, 612
  for vomiting with acute renal failure, 870
Onion toxicity, 98-99, 147-148
Onychodystrophy, systemic lupoid, pentoxifylline for, e204
Open fractures, 83-86
Open peritoneal drainage, e10-e12, e15-e17

Ophthalmic disease(s)
  canine
    conjunctivitis, 1138-1143
    glaucoma, 1170-1176, 1171b, 1171t, 1173b
    nonulcerative corneal disease, 1152-1156
    ocular neoplasia, 1201-1206
    retinal detachment, e370-e374
    retinopathy, 1188-1192
    tear film disorders, 1143-1147
    uveitis, 1162-1166
  corneal ulcers, 1148-1152
  emergencies, e377-e384
  epiphora, e374-e377
  evaluation of blindness, 1134-1138
  feline
    corneal, 1156-1161
    glaucoma, 1177-1180
    herpesvirus 1, 1157t
    ocular neoplasia, 1207-1210
    retinopathy, 1189f, 1193-1196, 1194f
    uveitis, 1166-1170, 1169t
  from Bartonella spp. infections, 1263b
  hyperlipidemia and, 263t
  involving the eyelid, e363-e369
  involving the periocular skin, e363-e369
  keratoconjunctivitis sicca, 1143-1147
  lens disorders, 1181-1187
  orbital, 1197-1200
  pearls of the examination for, 1128-1133
Ophthalmic examination
  direct vs. indirect ophthalmoscopy, 1131
  evaluating anisocoria, e388-e395
  fluorescein dye, 1132
  fundic, 1131
  pearls of the, 1128-1133
  retroillumination, 1128-1129, 1129f
  Schirmer tear test, 1132
  slit lamp, 1130-1131
  tonometry, 1130
  transillumination, 1128-1129, 1129f
Ophthalmoscope, use of direct and indirect, 1131
Opiates, causing syncope, e328f
Opioid(s)
  adverse effects of, 34t-35t, 60
  causing bradyarrhythmias, 731-732
  for nephroliths and ureteroliths pain, 894-895
  for the critical patient, 59-60, 62t
  reversal agent for, 30
  toxicity of, 111
  use of
    prior to cesarean section, 955
    with cardiovascular dysfunction, 64-65, 65t
    with benzodiazepine, for anesthetic induction in critical patients, 66
Optic chiasm lesions, 1137, 1137f-1138f
  causing anisocoria or mydriasis, e390f, e393t, e394

Optic nerve disorders
  causing anisocoria or mydriasis, e390f,
    e393t, e394
  causing blindness, 1136-1137, 1136t
  coloboma, 1136
  hypoplasia, 1136
  neuritis, 1136-1137, e383
  tumors, 1205-1206
  with glaucoma in dogs, 1171t
Optic tract lesions, 1137, 1138f
  causing anisocoria or mydriasis, e394
OptiChamber spacers, 623-624
Oral
  evaluation
    with caudal stomatitis, in cats,
      492-493
    with oropharyngeal dysphagia,
      495-500
  irritation from plants, 121b
  phases of swallowing, 495-496
Oral neoplasia, 362-366
Orbifloxacin
  for lower respiratory tract infection(s),
    1220t
  for superficial bacterial folliculitis, 438t
  topical, for otitis, 464t
Orbital
  abscess, 1198-1199
  ccllulitis, 1198-1199
  disease, 1197-1200
    evaluation of, 1128-1133
  neoplasia, 1199
  tumors of, 1205-1206
Orchidectomy, early age, in dogs and
  cats, 982-984
Orchids, 121b
Orchitis, causing oligospermia, e350
Organic acidopathies, 1052-1053
Organic acidosis, e7-e8, e7b
Organic phosphorus/phosphonomethyl
  herbicide toxicity, 130
Organophosphate toxicity, 135-137,
  136b
Ormetoprim/sulfadimethoxine, for
  superficial bacterial folliculitis, 438t
Oropharyngeal dysphagia, 495-500,
  e259-e262
Oropharynx, deformities with
  brachycephalic airway obstruction
  syndrome, 650t
Orthopedic trauma in dogs, 80-83
Oseltamivir, for canine parvovirus, 535
Oslerus osleri
  as bronchopulmonary parasite,
    e271-e272, e271f-e272f
  common symptoms and syndromes
    caused by, 1214t-1215t
Oslerus rostratus, e272
Osmol gap, from ethylene glycol
  toxicity, 151-152
Osmolarity
  composition in fluid therapy, 3t
  of parenteral nutrition products, 40-41
Osteo-allograft mix, for open fracture
  repair, 86
Osteomyelitis
  common pathogens causing,
    1222-1223

Osteomyelitis (Continued)
  empiric antimicrobial therapy for,
    1220t, 1222-1223
  from bartonellosis, 1261
  from borreliosis, 1273
  infectious causes of, 1214t, 1216-1217
  with open fractures, 84
Osteosarcoma
  diagnosis and treatment of, 388-392,
    391t
  immunotherapy for, 334, 336t
  nasal, radiation therapy for, 338-340
Otitis
  causing deafness, 468-469, 468b
    treatment and prevention, 470
  contact, from adverse drug reactions,
    488t
  ear-flushing techniques for, 471-474
  from demodicosis, 432
  from Pseudomonas, 459, 463
    glucocorticoids for, 459
    systemic antimicrobials for, 466-467,
      466t
    topical antimicrobials for, 458
  from staphylococci causing pyoderma,
    435-436
  glucocorticoids for, 416t, 417
    systemic, 460-462, 461t
    topical, 460, 460t
  principles of therapy for, 458-459
  topical antimicrobials for, 462-465,
    464t
  treating severe fibrosis and stenosis,
    460-461
Otitis interna, causing vestibular disease,
  1068
Otitis media, 466
  causing vestibular disease, 1068
  causing xeromycteria, in dogs, 643
  primary secretory with Chiari-like
    malformation, 1101
  with nasopharyngeal disorders, 654
Otoacoustic emissions, 469-470
Otodectes cynotis
  causing otitis, and treatment of, 458
  diagnosis and treatment of, 430-431,
    431t
  use of avermectins for, e182
Ototoxicity, 468-471
  causing vestibular disease, 1068
  from ear cleaners, 474
  from topical therapy, 464
  treatment and prevention of, 468-471
Ovarian remnant syndrome, 1000-1003
Ovarian tumors, 1024-1025
Ovaries, reproductive toxins targeting
  the, 1027-1028
Ovariohysterectomy
  early age, in dogs and cats, 982-984
  for ovarian tumors, 1024-1025
  for uterine tumors, 1025-1026
  ovarian remnant syndrome from,
    1000-1003, 1001f
  urethral sphincter mechanism
    incompetence from, 919
  with cesarean section, 955-956
  with mammary tumor removal, 377
Over-the-counter drug toxicosis, 115-120

Overfeeding, 39
Overgrooming, drug therapy for
  behavior-related dermatoses e.g.,
  482-485
Ovotestes, 997
Ovulation, 930, 931f
  and luteinizing hormone surge, 931f,
    931t
  relationship to proestrus, 932f
  relationship to progesterone
    concentration, 933f, 935f
  relationship to vaginal cytology, 933f
Oxacillin, for pyoderma, 1220t,
  1221-1222
Oxazepam
  for behavior-related dermatoses, 483t,
    484
  toxicity of, 113-114
Oxibendazole, associated hepatotoxicity,
  581b
Oxibendazole-DEC associated
  hepatotoxicity, 570b
Oxybutynin, for urinary incontinence
  disorders, 916t
Oxycodone toxicity, 111
Oxygen
  consumption in the brain, 1047-1048
  delivery and oxygen consumption, 19f
  needs with seizure patients, 1061
  saturation, 20
Oxygen therapy, 52-54
  cage for, 53-54
  for heat-induced illness, 73
  for pneumonia, 687
  for pneumothorax, 701
  for respiratory acidosis, e5
  for shock, 18-20, 19f
  hyperbaric, 54
  techniques for administration of,
    52-54
  toxicity from, 54, 58
  weaning from, 54
  with anesthesia in critical care
    patients, 68-69
Oxyglobin, 11, 13
  characteristics of, 10t
Oxymorphone
  dosage for, 62t
  for the critical patient, 59, 64, 66
  for thromboembolism pain, 814
Oxytetracycline/polymyxin B ointment
  (Terramycin), for keratomalacia,
  1151-1152
Oxytocin
  for dystocia, 952f, 954-955
  for postpartum hemorrhage, 957, 958t
  levels with normal gestation, 949
Ozagrel hydrochloride, for feline
  infectious peritonitis, 1305t, 1306
Ozone, causing reproductive toxicity,
  1027b

P

P-glycoprotein, 33-36
Pacemaker
  advances in artificial, e283-e285
  biventricular, e284
  conventional, e282-e283

Pacemaker (Continued)
  dual-lead dual-chamber, e284, e284f
  for arrhythmias, in cats, 750f-751f
  for atrioventricular block, 735
    in cats, 754-755
  for bradyarrhythmias, e281-e286
  for persistent atrial standstill, 734
  programmable parameters for, e282t
  rate responsive ventricular, e283-e284,
    e284f
  single-lead atrial synchronous,
    e284-e285, e284f-e285f
  temporary, e285
  transvenous pacing prior to, e21-e28
Pacing in the ICU setting, e21-e28, e23f,
    e285
Paclitaxel, e140-e141, e140t
  for hemangiosarcoma, 396
  hypersensitivity reactions to, 333
  premedication and protocol for, e141b
Pad inverted papillomas, e185
Pain, causing feline arrhythmias,
    750f-751f
Pain management
  after cesarean section, 956
  for feline cholangitis, 617, 617b
  for feline pancreatitis, 567, 567t
  for nephroliths and ureteroliths,
    894-895
  for open fractures, 85
  for thromboembolism, 810, 814
  in the critical patient, 59-63, 62t
Paint thinner toxicity, 154-155
Pak far oil toxicity, 125t
Palatability enhancers, 723-724
Palatoplasty, for brachycephalic airway
    obstruction syndrome, 651
Palliative care, client questions about, 321
Palmar-plantar erythrodysesthesia
    syndrome, from doxorubicin,
    e139-e140
Palpation
  of canine orthopedic trauma, 80-82
  of pregnancy, 944
Pamidronate
  for cholecalciferol toxicity, e33-e34
  for feline idiopathic hypercalcemia,
    246-247
  for multiple myeloma, 385
  for osteosarcoma, 391-392
Pancreas. See also Exocrine pancreatic
    insufficiency (EPI)
  evaluation of, for insulinoma tumor,
    e131-e132
  imaging of, for diagnosis of endocrine
    disorder(s), 172-174, 173t
  islet amyloidosis of, insulin resistance
    and, 205
  laboratory testing of the exocrine,
    554-557
  measuring fecal elastase-1, 556, 559
  serum pancreatic lipase
    immunoreactivity (PLI) of,
    555-557
  serum trypsin-like immunoreactivity
    (TLI) of, 555, 559
Pancreatectomy, for insulinoma,
    e131-e132

Pancreatic abscess, treatment of local
    peritonitis with, e14-e15
Pancreatic endocrine neoplasia, imaging
    of, 174
Pancreatic enzyme(s)
  for flatulence, e250
  replacement therapy, 559
Pancreatic insufficiency
  laboratory testing for, 556-557
  with diabetes mellitus, e77-e78
Pancreatic lipase immunoreactivity (Spec
    cPL)
  for the diagnosis of pancreatitis, 554,
    561
  with chronic pancreatitis, 564
Pancreatic lipase immunoreactivity (Spec
    fPL), for the diagnosis of
    pancreatitis, 566
Pancreatitis
  after pancreatic surgery, e132
  canine
    acute vs. chronic, 561-565
    nutritional support with, 563-564
    treatment of, 561-565
  causing exocrine pancreatic
    insufficiency (EPI), 558
  causing hyperlipidemia, 262t
  effect of, on gastric emptying, 514,
    516
  feline, 565-568
    medical therapies for, 567t
    with cholangitis, 615-616
    with diabetes mellitus, 209
  from hypothyroidism, e86
  imaging for, 172-174
  insulin resistance with, 206, 206b
  laboratory testing for, 554-557
  pulmonary thromboembolism
    associated with, 705, 708
  risk of
    with diabetes mellitus, 200-201
    with hypertriglyceridemia, 261
  with diabetes mellitus, e77-e78, e77,
    e83
Panleukopenia, feline, as cause of
    thrombocytopenia, 281t-282t
Pannus. See also under Keratitis
  atypical, 1141, 1141f
Panting, to dissipate heat, 70-71
Pantoprazole
  action and use of, 505-506, 506b
  for vomiting with acute renal failure,
    870
  toxicity from, 118
Panuveitis, canine, 1162
Papillary adenomas, ovarian, 1024-1025
Papilloma, of the eyelid, e368
Papillomavirus
  canine
    diagnosis and treatment of,
      e184-e187
    exophytic, e185
    oral, e184
  cutaneous inverted, e185
  feline, causing skin lesions, e195-e196
  from cyclosporine, 405
  immunotherapy for, 1231-1232, 1231f,
    e220-e221

Papillon(s)
  direct mutation tests for, 1018t-1020t
  von Willebrand disease in, 288t
Papule(s)
  from adverse drug reactions, 488t
  from superficial bacterial folliculitis,
    437
Para-aminopropiophenone, for
    population control, 142-144
Parachlorometaxylenol, in ear cleaners,
    472t, 473
Paragonimus kellicotti
  as bronchopulmonary parasite,
    e275-e276
  common symptoms and syndromes
    caused by, 1214t-1215t
Paranasal sinus disorders, causing
    rhinitis in dogs, 636b
Paraneoplastic
  causes of hepatobiliary enzyme
    elevations, 570b
  syndrome, causing cachexia, 350
Paraparesis, from degenerative
    myelopathy, 1076-1077, 1076t
Paraphimosis, 1029-1030, 1030b
  concerns regarding risk, with early age
    neutering, 983t
  vs. priapism, e354
Paraquat herbicide toxicity, 130-131, e266
Parasite(s)
  causing blepharitis, e364
  causing conjunctivitis, 1142
  causing myocarditis, e304t
  causing pregnancy loss, 1010
  causing uveitis in dogs, 1164b
  common symptoms and syndromes
    caused by, 1214t-1215t
  flea and tick control products for, 426t
  in raw meat diets, 1240b
  nasal, 636b, 655-656, e269-e271
  respiratory, e269-e276
  skin, treatment of, 428-432
  target parasites of common drugs,
    1335-1337
  treatment of common, 1335-1337
Parasiticide toxicoses, avermectins,
    145-146
Parathyroid gland, imaging of, for
    diagnosis of endocrine disorder(s),
    170
Parathyroid hormone (PTH)
  injections for hypoparathyroidism,
    e124
  testing
    for diagnosis of
      hyperparathyroidism, e70-e71
    for diagnosis of hypoparathyroidism,
      e122-e123, e124, e125f
  values of, with hypercalcemia in cats,
    242-243
Parathyroid hormone-related protein
    (PTHrP), for diagnosis of
    hyperparathyroidism, e71
Parathyroidectomy, hypocalcemia from,
    e124-e125
Parenteral nutrition, 39-40, 42b
  administration of, 40-42
  complications of, 43

Parenteral nutrition (Continued)
  compounding, 40
  for acute pancreatitis
    in cats, 567-568
    in dogs, 563-564
  for patients with cancer, 353
  with gastric dilation-volvulus, e19-e20
  worksheet for calculating, 41b-42b
Paroxetine HCl (Paxil)
  for behavior-related dermatoses,
    483-484, 483t
  toxicity of, 113
Pars planitis, 1167
Partial thromboplastin time (PTT)
  for monitoring antithrombotic agents,
    706-707, 707t
  in disseminated intravascular
    coagulation, 294t
  with bleeding abnormalities, 287f
Parturition, use of ultrasound and
  radiology for predicting, 945t-946t
Parvovirus infection
  and risk of hospital-acquired urinary
    infections, 877
  canine
    causing thrombocytopenia,
      281t-282t
    diagnosis and treatment of, 533-536
    causing myocarditis, e307
    causing nonregenerative anemia, e161,
      e161b
    effect on gastric emptying, 514
  feline, causing thrombocytopenia,
    281t-282t
Pasturella spp.
  causing pneumonia, 682t
  human infection from pets, 1244-1246
  role of with feline caudal stomatitis,
    492
Patent ductus arteriosus (PDA),
  e309-e313
  classification scheme for, e311, e311f
  complications of ductal closure, e313
  device occlusion for, e310-e311,
    e310-e312, e310f, e311-e312
  diagnosis of, e309-e310
  prevalence of
    in cats, 757t
    in dogs, 756, 757t
  surgery ligation for, e312-e313
  treatment of, e310-e313
Pathologist, tips for tissue sample
  submission, 322-326, 325b
Paw pad, lesions with superficial
  necrolytic dermatitis, 485-486
PCR testing. See Polymerase chain
  reaction (PCR) testing
Pediculosis
  diagnosis and treatment of, 428
  drugs targeting, 1335-1337
  lice species affecting dogs and cats,
    429t
  use of avermectins for, e182-e183
Pelvic, abnormalities causing dystocia,
  951
Pelvic bladder, ultrasound findings with,
  842
Pelvic trauma in dogs, 81-82

Pembroke Welsh corgi(s)
  degenerative myelopathy in,
    1076-1077
  direct mutation tests for, 1018t-1020t
  glaucoma in, 1171b
  von Willebrand disease in, 288t
Pemoline toxicity, 109-110
Pemphigus erythematosus, causing
  blepharitis, e366-e367
Pemphigus foliaceus
  causing blepharitis, e366
  from metaflumizone/amitraz
    (ProMeris), 489
  glucocorticoids for, 417
  use of cyclosporine for, 409-410
Penciclovir, for feline ocular herpesvirus
  1, 1158
Penicillamine
  for copper-associated liver disease, 589
  for lead toxicity, 158
Penicillin G
  for leptospirosis, 1289
  legend of spinal cord damage with, 99
Penicillin(s)
  adverse effects of, 34t-35t
  drug incompatibility with, 33t
  for septicemia, 1220t, 1223
  skin reactions from, 488t
Penicillium mold toxicity, 149
Penicillium spp., causing epistaxis, 1216
Penis
  nonneoplastic disorders of the,
    1029-1031
  paraphimosis and the, 1029-1030
  physiology of the erection and, e354,
    e355f
  priapism and the, e354-e357
  tumors of, 1023
Penny toxicity, 99-100
Pennyroyal oil, 127, 139
  associated hepatotoxicity, 570b
Pennyroyal senna associated
  hepatotoxicity, 581b
Pentastarch, 11-12
  characteristics of, 10t
Pentobarbital
  drug incompatibilities with, 33t
  for central nervous system stimulant
    toxicity, 110
  for emergent seizures, 1045, 1059-1060
  for strychnine toxicity, 134
Pentosan polysulfate, for persistent
  urinary tract infections, 882-883
Pentoxifylline
  adverse effects of, e203
  for cutaneous drug reactions, 488-489
  for feline infectious peritonitis, 1305t,
    1306
  for vasculitis, from vaccines, 1251
  use of, e202-e205
Pepsinogen, e251
Peptic ulcers, 509
Pepto-Bismol, toxicity from, 117
Percorten-V. See Desoxycorticosterone
  pivalate (DOCP)
Percutaneous cystolithotomy, 890
Percutaneous nephrolithotomy, 885,
  885f

Percutaneous ultrasound-guided
  ablation, for treatment of
  hyperparathyroidism, e72
Perfusion
  fluid therapy and
    using colloids, 8
    using crystalloids, 4
  monitoring of, with shock, 18-20
  problems from prolonged seizures,
    1060
Perianal adenocarcinoma, 366-369
Perianal adenoma, 366-369
Perianal fistulas, e190, e219
  cyclosporine for, 269-271, 409
  topical immunomodulators for,
    e219
Perianal gland tumor, 366
Pericardectomy, 821-823, 822f
  for chylothorax, 699
  for hemangiosarcoma, 395
Pericardial disease
  causing chylothorax, 698
  causing effusion, 816-823, 822b
Pericardial effusion
  causes of, 817
  collection of cytology specimens from,
    e155
  diagnosis and treatment of, 816-823,
    821f, 822b
  fluid analysis from, 817
  malignant, 341-344
Pericardiocentesis, 820-821, 821f, 822b
Perineal tumors, 366-369
Perineal urethrostomy, indications for,
  925
Perinephric pseudocysts, ultrasound
  findings with, 843
Perinuclear antineutrophilic cytoplasmic
  antibodies, with inflammatory bowel
  disease, 538
Periocular skin diseases, e363-e369
Periodontitis, with feline caudal
  stomatitis, 492
Peripheral nerve dysfunction
  from hypothyroidism, 179, e84
  rehabilitation considerations with,
    e360-e362
  treatment of, 1116-1117
Peritoneal
  drainage
    comparison of techniques, e16t
    methods of, e10t
  lavage, for septic abdomen, e14
Peritoneal chemotherapy, 343-344
Peritoneal effusion. See also Ascites
  causing hyperkalemia and
    hyponatremia, e93, e93b
  collection of cytology specimens from,
    e155
  malignant, 341-344
Peritoneocentesis, with nephrotic
  syndrome, 856
Peritonitis
  determining the severity of, e11b
  effect of, on gastric emptying, 516
  from biliary mucoceles, e223
  septic, drainage techniques for,
    e13-e20

Perivulvar dermatitis, 971, 977f
    concerns regarding risk, with early age
        neutering, 983t
Periwinkle toxicity, 124t
Permethrin
    for flea control, 426t
    for pediculosis, 429t
    for tick prevention, 1274-1275, 1294
    toxic exposures to, 95-96, 115-116,
        136b, 427, 489
    toxicity of
        muscle relaxants for, 102t-104t
        use of IV lipid emulsion therapy for,
            115-116
Persian cat
    cholangitis in, 618
    corneal sequestrums in, 1159-1160
    glaucoma in, 1177
    portosystemic vascular anomalies in,
        571b
    retinal degeneration in, 1195
    risk of urolithiasis in, 897
Persistent atrial standstill, 733-734
Persistent Müllerian duct syndrome,
    997-998, 998f
Persistent right aortic arch, prevalence of
    in cats, 757t
    in dogs, 757t
Personal protective equipment, for
    hazardous drugs, 327
Pertechnetate, of thyroid gland, 167-168
Pesticide(s)
    causing nephrotoxicity, e30b
    for vertebrate pest species, 142-144
    reporting adverse events of, to FDA,
        e37-e38
Pet food
    aflatoxins in, 159
    nephrotoxins in, e29-e34
    reporting adverse effect of, e38
Pet Partners program, stand on raw meat
    diets, 1242
Pet Poison Helpline toxin exposures,
    93-96, 95t
Pet-associated illness, 1244-1249
Petechiae
    from adverse drug reactions, 488t
    with thrombocytopenia, 283
Petroleum compound toxicity, 154-155
pH
    changes, with acid-base disorders,
        e1-e8
    composition in fluid therapy, 3t
Phacoemulsification, 1184-1185
Phaeohyphomycosis, antifungal therapy
    for, 1234-1238
Phallopexy, 1029
Pharyngeal
    phase of swallowing, 495-496
    weakness, 499
Pharyngoscopy, for evaluation of
    dysphagia, 498
Phenazopyridine associated
    hepatotoxicity, 581b
Phenobarbital
    adverse effects of, 34t-35t
    associated hepatotoxicity, 570b, 576,
        581b

Phenobarbital (Continued)
    causing hyperlipidemia, 262t
    dosing of, with liver disease, 32-33
    drug interactions with, 35t, 677
    effect on hepatobiliary enzymes,
        570-571
    enterohepatic recirculation of, 105
    for emergent seizures, 1059-1060
    for intracranial tumors, 1041t, 1045
    influence on thyroid function, 181t,
        184
Phenolic chemicals associated
    hepatotoxicity, 581b
Phenols associated hepatotoxicity,
    581b
Phenothiazine(s)
    causing syncope, e328f
    toxicity of, 118-119, 581b
Phenotypic sex, 993, 995t
Phenoxy acid herbicide toxicity,
    130-131
Phenoxybenzamine
    for urinary retention disorders, 917t,
        918
    to promote ureterolith passage, 894
Phentermine, toxicity of, 109-110
Phenylbutazone
    associated hepatotoxicity, 581b
    causing nephrotoxicity, e32-e33
Phenylephrine
    causing anisocoria or mydriasis, e392
    for feline uveitis, 1169, 1169t
    for localization of anisocoria, e395
    for priapism, e356
    use of, with shock, 23
Phenylpropanolamine
    as decongestant, 627
    for urinary incontinence disorders,
        915, 916t, 925
    hypertension from, 727, 727t, 780b
Phenytoin (Dilantin)
    associated hepatotoxicity, 581b
    causing adverse skin reactions, 488t
    drug interactions with, 119, 507, 677
Pheochromocytoma
    hypertension from, 727t, 729
    imaging for diagnosis of, 171
    insulin resistance with, 206b
Pheromone, for behavior-related
    dermatoses, 485
Phimosis, 1029-1030, 1030b
    concerns regarding risk, with early age
        neutering, 983t
Phosphate binders, with chronic kidney
    disease, 862
Phosphate intake restriction, with
    chronic kidney disease, 862
Phosphofructokinase deficiency, direct
    mutation test for, 1018t-1020t
Phosphorus, and calcium, causing
    mineralization, 244
Physaloptera canis, common symptoms
    and syndromes caused by,
        1214t-1215t
Physical examination
    findings relative to dehydration, 5t
    of the eye, 1128-1133
    with respiratory distress, 45-46

Physical therapy
    and rehabilitation for neurologic
        disorders, e357-e362
    for degenerative myelopathy,
        1078-1080
    for neuromuscular disease, 1118
Phytosphingosine, 420t
    in ear cleaners, 474
    topical, 420t, 421, 441t
Pilocarpine
    causing anisocoria or mydriasis, e392
    for canine glaucoma, 1173b, 1174
    for feline glaucoma, 1179-1180
    for keratoconjunctivitis sicca, 1145,
        1155
Pimecrolimus
    as topical immunomodulators,
        e216-e220, e219
    safety concerns of, e219-e220
    topical, 420t, 421
Pimobendan (Vetmedin)
    for asymptomatic heart disease, 766
    for cardiogenic shock, 783
    for congenital heart disease, 760
    for dilated cardiomyopathy, in dogs
        occult, 797-798
        with heart failure, 799
    for feline cardiomyopathy, 806t,
        808-809
    for heart failure
        in cats, 808
        in dogs, 764t-765t, 768-770,
            777-779, 787t, 791
    for myocarditis, e306
    for pulmonary hypertension, 714, 716
    with valvular heart disease, 793-794
Pind-avi/Pind-orf, for feline retrovirus
    infections, 1280t-1281t, 1282
Pine oil associated hepatotoxicity, 570b
Pineal gland tumors, 1039-1047
Pinnal-pedal reflex, with sarcoptic
    mange, 428
Pioglitazone, for diabetes mellitus, in
    cats, e137-e138
Piperazine toxicity, 118-119
Piperidine toxicity, 118-119
Piroxicam
    as cancer therapy, 336t, 359
    for hemangiosarcoma, 396
    for inflammatory mammary
        carcinoma, 378
    for ocular neoplasia, 1207
    for oral tumors, 364
    for rhinosinusitis in cats, 646
    for urinary bladder cancer, 372-373
    metronomic chemotherapy of,
        343-344
    toxicity of, 116-117, 359, e32-e33
    use of, with toceranib, 359
Pituitary gland
    imaging of, for diagnosis of endocrine
        disorders, 172
    reproductive toxins targeting the, 1027
    tumors
        adenoma, 172
        causing acromegaly, in cats,
            216-217
        causing blindness, 1137

Pituitary gland (Continued)
  diagnosis and treatment of, 1039-1047, 1042t
  large, with pituitary-dependent hyperadrenocorticism, e88-e91
Placental site subinvolution, 957
Plant(s)
  and herbs of toxic concern, 124t
  causing nephrotoxicity, e34
  salicylate containing, 125t
  toxic and nontoxic, 121, 121b
  toxic exposures to, 92t, 94, 95t
Plaque
  as cause of thrombocytopenia, 281t-282t
  bacteria, role in feline caudal stomatitis, 494
Plasma
  characteristics of, 10t
  for treatment of von Willebrand disease, 290, 290t
Plasma cell neoplasms, 384-387
Plasma protein C
  with acute liver failure, 600
  with portal vein hypoplasia, 599-600
  with portosystemic shunt, 595-596
Plasma transfusions
  for canine pancreatitis, 562
  for disseminated intravascular coagulation, 295
  for feline pancreatitis, 567t
  for hypoalbuminemia, 543-544
  for therapy of shock, 21-22
Plasma von Willebrand factor, 287-288
Plasmacytic stomatitis, use of cyclosporine for, 410b
Plasmacytomas, diagnosis and treatment of, 386-387
Plasmapheresis, for multiple myeloma, 385
Plasminogen, with disseminated intravascular coagulation, 294f
Platelet function analyzer, use of, with bleeding abnormalities, 287
Platelet inhibition, for autoimmune hemolytic anemia, 277-278
Platelet transfusion(s), for thrombocytopenia, 284-285
Platelet(s). See also Thrombocytopenia
  activation, with autoimmune hemolytic anemia, 275-276
  activity, in hypercoagulable states, 298, 298f, 811-815
  assessment with thrombocytopenia, 283-284
  counts with hereditary factor deficiencies, 287f
  function, with disseminated intravascular coagulation, 292, 293f, 294t
Platelet-rich plasma, 311
Platinum toxicity, 1027b
Plerixafor, for feline retrovirus infections, 1279-1280, 1279t
Pleural chemotherapy, 343-344

Pleural effusion
  causes of, 692b
  causing hyperkalemia and hyponatremia, e93, e93b
  characterization of, 692-695, 692t
  chylous, 695
  clinical signs of, 692
  collection of cytology specimens from, e155
  diagnosis and treatment of, 691-700
  hemorrhagic, 694
  infectious causes of, 1216
  malignant, 341-344
  neoplastic, 694-695, e165-e166
  septic, 695-697
  transudates, 694
  types of, 694-695
  with cardiogenic shock, 783
  with feline pancreatitis, 567
  with refractory heart failure, 781
Pleural port placement, for chylothorax, 699-700
Pleural space disease
  anesthesia for patients with, 68
  causes of, 46t
Pleural space neoplasia, e165-e166
Pleurectomy, for malignant effusions, 343
Pleurodesis
  for malignant effusions, 342
  for treatment of pneumothorax, 704
Pleuroperitoneal shunt
  for chylothorax, 699
  for malignant effusions, 343
Pneumocystosis, e409-e411
  clinical findings with, e410
  diagnosis of, e410
  treatment of, e410-e411
Pneumonia
  anesthesia for patients with, 68
  aspiration, 681, 683-685, 683b
    post-op with laryngeal paralysis surgery, 661
    prevention of, 685
    with megaesophagus, e229
    with myasthenia gravis, 1109-1110
  common infectious agents causing, 1218
  community-acquired, 681-682, 682t
  diagnosis and treatment of, 681-688, 684f
  eosinophilic, e267b
  from canine infectious respiratory complex, 633-634
  hospital-acquired, 682-683, 682t-683t, 683b, 684f
  reasons for treatment failure with, 687-688
  risk factors for, 683b, 684-685
  with feline pancreatitis, 567
  with ventilator therapy, 58
Pneumonyssoides caninum
  common symptoms and syndromes caused by, 1214t-1215t
  nasal mite, 655-656, e270
Pneumonyssus caninum, causing nasal discharge, 636b, 637

Pneumothorax
  anesthesia for patients with, 68
  blood patching for, 704
  diagnosis and treatment of, 700-704
  iatrogenic, 693-694, 703, 703f
  spontaneous, 703
  traumatic, 702
Pododermatitis
  from cornification disorders in dogs, 475
  from Malassezia spp., e213
  use of cyclosporine for, 410b
Poinsettia toxicity, 99
Poison. See Toxicity(ies)
Poison hemlock toxicity, 124t
Poison tobacco toxicity, 124t
Pollakiuria, infectious causes of, 1217
Polyarthritis
  diagnosis of, 1225
  differential diagnosis for, 1224-1225
  from feline upper respiratory infection, 630t
  infectious causes of, 1216-1217, 1224-1228
  treatment of, 1225
Polybrominated biphenyls toxicity, 1027b
Polychlorinated biphenyls toxicity, 1027b
Polydimethylsiloxane, for urinary incontinence, e349, e349f
Polyglandular endocrinopathy, with hypothyroidism, e87-e88
Polyinosinic:poly-cytidylic acid, for feline retrovirus infections, 1280t-1281t, 1282
Polymerase chain reaction (PCR) testing
  for American leishmaniasis, e396-e397
  for bacteremia with endocarditis, e293-e294, e294-e295
  for canine hepatozoonosis, 1285
  for canine leproid granuloma, 446
  for canine parvovirus, 533-534
  for canine respiratory infection, 633
  for cytauxzoonosis, e407-e408
  for feline Bartonella spp., 1269
  for feline upper respiratory infection, 630
  for hemotropic mycoplasmosis, e400-e401
  for leptospirosis, 1287-1289
Polymyopathy
  causing laryngeal paralysis, 659
  from hypernatremia, 1116
  hypokalemic, with feline hyperaldosteronism, 239
Polymyositis, 1114
  causing dysphagia, 496b
  extraocular, 1199
  from ehrlichiosis, 1292
Polymyxin
  ototoxicity from, 468b
  topical, for otitis, 464t
Polyneuropathy, 1116-1117
Polyprenyl, for feline infectious peritonitis, 1306
Polyps
  nasal, 656-657

Polyps (Continued)
nasopharyngeal, 656-657
vestibular signs from, 1068
Polysaccharopeptide, for
hemangiosarcoma, 396
Polysulfated glycosaminoglycans, for
persistent urinary tract infections,
882-883
Polytetrafluoroethylene paste, for urinary
incontinence, e348
Polyuria, from acute renal failure, 870
Polyuria and polydipsia (PU/PD)
fluid therapy considerations with, 6
from glucocorticoids, 461
potassium supplementation and, 6-7
Pomeranian, risk of urolithiasis in, 897
Ponazuril
for canine hepatozoonosis, 1285
for toxoplasmosis, 1297
target parasites and dosage of,
1335-1337
Poodle(s)
alopecia X in, 166
atlantoaxial subluxation in, 1083
congenital hydrocephalus in, 1034
dilated cardiomyopathy in, 795-796
direct mutation tests for, 1018t-1020t
glaucoma in, 1171b
hypoadrenocorticism in, 233
mammary cancer in, 375
paraphimosis in, 1029
pericardial effusion in, 817
progressive retinal atrophy in,
1188-1190, 1189t
retinal atrophy in, 1189t
risk of bladder cancer in, 371t
sebaceous adenitis ion, e209,
e209-e210
testicular dysgenesis in, 997
thrombocytopenia in, 283
von Willebrand disease in, 288t
Population control, pesticides for
vertebrate pest species, 142-144
Porcine Lente insulin (Vetsulin),
190-191, 210
Portal circulation, 599
Portal hypertension
causing ascites, therapy of, 591-592
compared to portal vein hypoplasia,
601
from hepatobiliary disease, 572-574,
581-582, 584-585
postoperative PSS surgery, 597-598
Portal vein hypoplasia
as differential diagnosis for
portosystemic shunt, 595-596
compared to portal hypertension, 601
compared to portosystemic shunt,
599-600
diagnosis and treatment of, 599-602,
600b
with portosystemic shunt, 599
Portosystemic shunts (PSS), 594-598
breeds predisposed to, 594
compared to portal vein hypoplasia,
599-600
diagnosis of, 594-595
liver function tests for, 595

Portosystemic shunts (PSS) (Continued)
medical management of, 596
postoperative care with, 597-598, 598f
prognosis with, 596
surgery for, 596-597
treatment of hepatoencephalopathy
with, 592-594
with portal vein hypoplasia, 599
Portosystemic vascular anomalies
breeds predisposed to, 571b
ultrasound changes with, 573-574
Portuguese water dog(s)
direct mutation tests for, 1018t-1020t
genetic marker test for dilated
cardiomyopathy in, 1021t
Posaconazole
for fungal rhinitis in cats, 647t
topical, for otitis, 463-464
use and protocols for, 1235t, 1237
Positive end-expiratory pressure (PEEP),
with ventilator therapy, 56
Positive inotropic drugs
for heart failure, in dogs, 763b,
768-770
for therapy of shock, 22-23
Postobstructive hypokalemia, 251-252
Postpartum disorders, diagnosis and
treatment of, 957-960, 958t
Postprandial hyperlipidemia, 262t
Potassium. See also Hyperkalemia;
Hypokalemia
approach to low levels of, 248-253
composition in fluid therapy, 3t
diagnostics for, 252
dietary recommendations for, with
heart disease, 723, 763
role and function of, 251
supplementation
IV, 253t
with fluid therapy, 6-7, 7t, e80t-e81t,
e82
with gastric dilation-volvulus, e17,
e18-e19
Potassium blocker(s), causing syncope,
e328, e328f
Potassium bromide
influence on thyroid function, 181t
interaction of, with furosemide,
34t-35t, 37
with intracranial tumors, 1045
Potassium channel blockers
for dogs, 763b
for supraventricular tachyarrhythmias,
742t, 743-744
for ventricular arrhythmias, 746-748
Potassium chloride
for glaucoma in dogs, 1173b
supplementation, 253, 253t
Potassium citrate, for calcium oxalate
urolithiasis, 899-900
Potassium gluconate, supplementation,
252-253
Potassium penicillin G, before
musculoskeletal surgery, 1220t, 1222
Pradofloxacin
for Bartonella spp., 1265
for feline upper respiratory infection,
631t

Pradofloxacin (Continued)
for nontuberculous cutaneous
granulomas, 448t
Pralidoxime hydrochloride, as antidote,
e56t
Pramoxine, topical, 420t
Praziquantel
for Giardia spp., 530t
for lung worms, e276
target parasites of, 1335-1337
Praziquantel/pyrantel, target parasites of,
1335-1337
Prazosin
for urinary retention disorders, 917t,
918
to promote ureterolith passage, 894
Prebiotic therapy, 525
Precorneal tear film, e384, e385f
Prednisolone. See also Glucocorticoid(s)
for otitis, systemic, 461t
use of, for immunosuppression, 269
Prednisone. See also Glucocorticoid(s)
as rescue therapy for canine
lymphoma, 382t
for feline gastrointestinal lymphoma,
547-548, 548t
for multiple myeloma, 385-386
for otitis
systemic, 461t
topical, 460t
for rescue chemotherapy for canine
lymphoma, 381-383
Prednisone sodium succinate, use of,
with hypoadrenocorticism testing,
235-236
Pregabalin, for craniocervical junction
abnormalities, 1102
Pregnancy. See also Dystocia
and risk of pyometra, 967
antibiotic therapy during pregnancy,
947-948
breeding management of the bitch for
optimal, 930-935
complications of, 947-948
diagnosis, 944-948
with radiography, 938
with ultrasound, 939
differential diagnosis of, 947
false, 947
loss in the bitch and queen, 1003-
1011, 1005t
infectious agents causing, 1218
medical termination of, 989-992
nutrition during, 961-966
postpartum disorders after, 957-960
use of endoscopy transcervical
insemination, 940-944, 941t
Premature atrial complexes, in cats,
749-753, 750f-751f
Premedication, with cardiovascular
dysfunction, 64-65
Prepuce, nonneoplastic disorders of the,
1029-1031
Preputial hypoplasia, concerns
regarding risk, with early age
neutering, 983t
Preputial tumors, 1023
Presbycusis, causing deafness, 468b

Prescription diet(s), for diabetes mellitus, 201t, 204t

Priapism, e354-e357, e355f
    pathophysiology of, e354-e356

Primidone associated hepatotoxicity, 581b

Proanthocyanidin, for persistent *E. coli* urinary tract infections, 881b, 882

Probiotic therapy, 525-528
    for flatulence, e250
    for persistent *E. coli* urinary tract infections, 882
    mechanism of action of, 526

Procainamide
    causing adverse skin reactions, 488t
    for heart failure, in dogs, 764t-765t
        with arrhythmias, 771
    for supraventricular tachyarrhythmias, 743
    for ventricular arrhythmias, 746-747, 747f, 747t

ProcalAmine, 40

Procarbazine, as rescue therapy for canine lymphoma, 382t

Proestrus, 931
    relationship to ovulation, 932f

Progesterone
    changes with pyometra, 967
    concentrations
        and pregnancy complications, 947-948
        relationship to ovulation, 933f, 935, 935f
        to detect ovarian remnant syndrome, 1001-1002
        with normal gestation in the bitch, 949
    excess, insulin resistance with, 206b
    supplementation during pregnancy complications, 947-948
    to maintain pregnancy, 1006

Progesterone receptor blocker(s), for pregnancy termination, 991

Progestins, for estrus suppression in the bitch, 984-985

Progressive retinal atrophy
    direct mutation test for, 1018t-1020t
    in cats, 1195
    in dogs, 1188-1190, 1189f
    classifications of, 1189t

Progressive rod cone degeneration, direct mutation test for, 1018t-1020t

Prokinetic drug(s)
    for hepatic lipidosis, 612
    for motility disorders, 516-518
        action and use of, 517t
    for urinary retention disorders, 918

Prolactin, concentrations with false pregnancy, 947

Prolactin inhibitor(s), for pregnancy termination, 990-991
    used with prostaglandin F$_{2\alpha}$, 990-991

Proligestone, for estrus suppression in the bitch, 987

Propane toxicity, 154-155

Propantheline
    for bradycardias, 736
    for urinary incontinence disorders, 916t

Propentofylline, for feline infectious peritonitis, 1305t, 1306

Propionibacterium acnes
    for cancer immunotherapy, 335
    for feline retrovirus infections, 1280t-1281t, 1282

Propofol
    drug interactions with, 35t
    for cesarean section, 955
    for emergent seizures, 1060
    long term use of, in cats, 55
    to calm respiratory distress pets, 47t
    to evaluate laryngeal function, 660
    with intracranial pathology, 69
    with ventilator therapy, 55

Propranolol
    adverse effects of, 34t-35t
    causing adverse skin reactions, 488t
    drug interactions with, 35t
    for hyperthyroid cats, e103t
    influence on thyroid function, 181t
    toxicity of, use of IV lipid emulsion therapy for, 106

Proprioceptive deficits
    exercises to build strength with, e358, e358-e359
    from vestibular disease, 1067t

Proptosis, e377-e378, e378f

Propylene glycol
    causing adverse skin reactions, 488t
    in ear cleaners, 472-473, 472t
    toxicity, 153-154

Propylthiouracil
    causing adverse skin reactions, 488t
    for hyperthyroid cats, e103t, e105

Prostaglandin analog(s)
    for canine glaucoma, 1173, 1173b, e381
    for feline glaucoma, 1180, e381

Prostaglandin F$_{2\alpha}$
    for postpartum metritis, 958t
    for pregnancy termination, 990
        used with prolactin inhibitors, 990-991
    for pyometra, 963
    side effects of, 990

Prostaglandin(s), role of, with kidney disease, 863

Prostate
    cancer, 1023-1024
        immunotherapy for, 336t
        urethral stenting for, 346f
    disease, causing oligospermia, e350
    fluid collection from, 1013-1014

Prostatic abscess, treatment of, 1014-1015
    local peritonitis with, e14-e15

Prostatic hypertrophy, benign, 1012-1015

Prostatitis, diagnosis and treatment of, 1012-1015

Prosthesis, eye, with glaucoma, 1175-1176, 1176f

Prosthesis, for feline glaucoma, 1180

Protamine zinc insulin, 211, 212b

Protectant(s), as antipruritic agents, 419

Protein
    catabolism, with diabetes mellitus, 201
    dietary
        needs in patients with cancer, 352
        recommendations with diabetes mellitus, 200-201, 201t, 203, 204t
        recommendations with heart disease, 722
        requirements in parenteral nutrition products, 40, 41b
        with weight loss diets, 255-259

Protein C, role of, in hypercoagulable states, 297

Protein electrophoresis, for multiple myeloma, 384-385

Protein-losing enteropathy
    causes of, 540-541
    comparisons of diets for, 542-543, 543t
    diagnosis of, 540-544
    pulmonary thromboembolism associated with, 705
    treatment of, 539-544

Protein-losing nephropathy
    causing hyperlipidemia, 262t
    from *Borrelia burgdorferi*, 1272, 1274
    pulmonary thromboembolism associated with, 705, 812

Proteinuria
    asymptomatic, when to worry, 926-927
    causes of, 850-851
    detection and management of, 849-852
    for staging of kidney disease, 858-859, 860t
    from amyloidosis, 855
    from *Borrelia burgdorferi*, 1273
    from glomerular disease, 853-855
    from idiopathic vacuolar hepatopathy, 607
    localization of the source of, 850-851
    treating hypertension with, 729
    treatment of, with chronic kidney disease, 861

Prothrombin deficiency, coagulation factor abnormalities with, 288t

Prothrombin time (PT)
    in disseminated intravascular coagulation, 294t
    with anticoagulant rodenticide toxicity, 133
    with bleeding abnormalities, 287f

Proton pump inhibitor(s)
    action and use of, 505-506
    for esophagitis, e240
    for gastric ulceration, e254
    for gastroesophageal reflux, 503
    for vomiting with acute renal failure, 870
    intravenous formulations of, 506
    protocol for *helicobacter* spp., 511-513, 511t
    toxicity from, 118

Protozoa
    causes of thrombocytopenia, 281t-282t
    causing gastrointestinal disease, 528-532

Protozoa (Continued)
  causing myocarditis, e304t
  causing uveitis in dogs, 1164b
  drugs used to treat common, 1335-1337
Provera, for estrus suppression in the bitch, 987
Prucalopride, action and use of, for motility disorders, 516-518
Pruritic alopecia, in dogs, 164
Pruritus
  from adverse drug reactions, 488t
  from atopic dermatitis, 406
  from methimazole, e103-e104
  glucocorticoids for, 415-417, 416t
  topical therapy for, 419-421
Pseudocyesis, 947
  from hypothyroidism, e85
Pseudoephedrine
  for priapism, e356-e357
  for urinary incontinence disorders, 915, 916t
Pseudomonas infection
  causing aspermia, e350
  causing endocarditis, e293-e294, e294t
  causing prostatitis, 1013
  in feline airways, 676
  otitis, treatment of, 458-459, 463, 466-467, 466t
    ear-flushing techniques for, 472
    with glucocorticoids, 459
Pseudopelade, use of cyclosporine for, 410b
Pseudothrombocytopenia, 280
Psoriasiform-lichenoid dermatosis, cyclosporine-induced, 489
Psoriasis cream toxicity, e33-e34
Psychogenic alopecia, drug therapy for behavior-related dermatoses e.g., 482-485
Psychotropic drugs, behavior-related dermatoses, 482-484
Psyllium, for canine colitis, 551b, 552
Ptyalism, from feline hepatic lipidosis, 613
Puerperal tetany, 958t, 959-960
Pug(s)
  brachycephalic airway obstruction syndrome in, 650t
  encephalitis, 1064
  pigmentary keratitis in, 1154
  risk of vaccine hypersensitivity in, 1250-1251
Pulmonary artery catheter, for monitoring shock, 19
Pulmonary artery pressure, 711, 713-714
Pulmonary artery velocity profile, 714
Pulmonary capillary leak, from acute respiratory distress syndrome, 49-50, 50f
Pulmonary compliance, 45f
Pulmonary contusions, fluid therapy considerations with, 6
Pulmonary diseases. See also under Respiratory disease(s)
  eosinophilic, 688-691

Pulmonary edema
  as cause of respiratory distress, 45, 46t
  causing feline arrhythmias, 750f-751f
  from chronic valvular disease, 786-788, 787t
  from heart failure, 767-769, 767f
    in dogs, 773, 778b, 782
  from hemoglobin-based oxygen solutions, 11, 13
  morphine use with, 47t
  oxygen therapy for, 52
  post-arrest, 31
  reexpansion, after thoracocentesis, 693-694
  toxins causing, 125, 131, 152-153
  with acute respiratory distress syndrome, 48, 49b
  with brachycephalic airway obstruction, 649
  with cardiogenic shock, 783
  with dilated cardiomyopathy, 796-798
  with feline myocardial disease, 805, 807-809
  with feline pancreatitis, 567
  with pericardial effusion, 816
  with pneumonia, 687
  with pulmonary hypertension, 716
  with ruptured chordae tendineae, 793
  with status epilepticus, 1061
Pulmonary fibrosis, e267, e267b
  acetylcysteine for, 627
  causing pulmonary hypertension, 711, 712t
Pulmonary function tests, 690
Pulmonary hypertension
  arterial, 714-715, 715f
  associated with lung disease, 716
  associated with thrombosis, 716
  causes of, 712t
  classification and histologic lesion of, 712t
  clinical signs of, 711
  diagnosis and treatment of, 711-717, 715f, 768
  neurocardiogenic syncope with, e327, e329
  prognosis for, 716
  venous, with left-sided heart failure, 716
  with congenital heart disease, 760
  with interstitial lung disease, e268
  with refractory heart failure, 781
  with valvular heart disease, 793-794
  with ventricular septal defect, e336-e337
Pulmonary mineralization, e267b
Pulmonary neoplasia, e165-e168
Pulmonary parenchymal disease, causes of, 46t
Pulmonary thromboembolism
  diagnosis and treatment of, 705-710
  prevention of, 708-710
  with cardiogenic shock, 783
  with hemolytic anemia, 812
Pulmonary valve stenosis, e314-e319
  classification of disease severity, e317
  diagnosis of, e314-e317

Pulmonary valve stenosis (Continued)
  interventional therapy for, e317-e318, e318-e319
  prevalence of
    in cats, 757t
    in dogs, 756, 757t
  therapy of, 759-760
  treatment of, e317-e319
Pulse oximetry, use of, 52
Pulseless electrical activity, 29f
Pulsus paradoxus, 816
Punctum
  imperforate, e375
  obstructed, e376
Pupillary escape, e391
Pupillary light reflex
  abnormalities, e388-e395, e393t
  assessment of, e391
  defects of the, e390f
  direct vs. consensual, e391
  evaluation of, 1134, 1135f
  functional anatomy of the, e389
  grid to record, e389f
Puppy strangles, rational use of glucocorticoids for, 1301
Purina Glucotest, 197-198
Purine content of foods, 905b
Pustule, from superficial bacterial folliculitis, 437
Pyelocentesis, use of ultrasound for, 844
Pyelography
  for diagnosis of nephroliths and ureteroliths, 893
  use of ultrasound for, 844
Pyelonephritis
  infectious agents that cause, 1212
  ultrasound findings with, 842-843
  with urolithiasis, 893-894
Pyloric atony, with brachycephalic airway obstruction syndrome, 650t
Pyloric mucosal hyperplasia, with brachycephalic airway obstruction syndrome, 650t
Pyloric stenosis, with brachycephalic airway obstruction syndrome, 650t
Pyoderma
  common pathogens causing, 1221-1222
  empiric antimicrobial therapy for, 1220t
  from Staphylococcus spp. infection, 435-436
  immunotherapeutics for, 1230t
  topical therapy for, 440-442, 441t
  with methicillin-resistant Staphylococcal, 442, 444
  with superficial necrolytic dermatitis, 486
Pyogranulomatous dermatitis, from nontuberculous cutaneous granulomas, 446-447
Pyometra, 947
  causing pregnancy loss, 1005-1006, 1005f, 1005t
  diagnosis and treatment of, 967-969
  pathogenesis of, 967

Pyometra (Continued)
  risk
    with progestin drugs, 985
    with tamoxifen, 377
  use of renourethroscope for treating, 943-944
Pyothorax, 695-697
  blood patching for, 704
  causes of, 695-697, 1216
  medical treatment of, 696-697
  surgery treatment of, 697
Pyotraumatic dermatitis, e206-e208
  causes of, e207b
  treatment of, e207-e208
Pyrantel
  for Giardia spp., 530t
  target parasites of, 1335-1337
Pyrethrin
  for Otodectes infestation, 431t
  for pediculosis, 429t
  toxicity, 95-96, 136b, 137-138
Pyrethroid toxicity, 136b, 137-138
Pyridostigmine
  for myasthenia gravis, 1110-1111, e228-e229
  for urinary retention disorders, 917t
Pyrimethamine, for canine hepatozoonosis, 1285
Pyriproxyfen
  for dust mite control, e199
  toxicity, 140-141
Pyruvate dehydrogenase 4 gene mutation, testing for canine dilated cardiomyopathy, 797
Pyruvate kinase deficiency, direct mutation test for, 1018t-1020t
Pythiosis, e412-e415
  antifungal therapy for, 1234-1238
  diagnosis of, e413
  treatment of, e413-e414
Pyuria, effect of, on urine protein and albumin, 850
PZI. See Protamine zinc insulin

Q
Quadrigeminal cyst, 1038-1039
Quality control, for the in-clinic laboratory, 306-309
Quaternary ammonium compounds, for methicillin-resistant Staphylococcal sp., 455-456
Queen-of-the-meadow toxicity, 124t
Questions, to consultants, urinary, 923-927
Quetiapine, toxicity of, use of IV lipid emulsion therapy for, 106

R
Rabeprazole
  action and use of, 505-506
  toxicity from, 118
Rabies vaccine, injection site reactions from, 489
Rabies virus
  causing nervous system signs, 1212
  common symptoms and syndromes caused by, 1215t

Rabies virus (Continued)
  human infection from, 1244
  vaccine-associated sarcomas from, 1253
Radiation therapy
  client questions about, 320-321
  for acral lick dermatitis, e176
  for hemangiosarcoma, 396
  for intracranial tumors, 1043-1044
  for mammary cancer, 378
  for multiple myeloma, 385
  for nasal tumors, 338-340, e157-e159
    in cats, 648
    in dogs, 641-643
  for oral tumors, 364
  for osteosarcoma, 391
  for perianal adenocarcinoma, 367-369
  for pituitary macroadenoma, e90-e91
  for soft tissue sarcomas, e151
  for thyroid tumors, 399-400
  for treatment of feline hypersomatotropism, 219-220, 220f
  for urinary bladder cancer, 372
  for vaccine-associated sarcoma, 1254
  with interventional oncology, 348
Radioactive iodine therapy. See Radioiodine therapy
Radiography
  for diagnosis of nephroliths and ureteroliths, 893
  for diagnosis of osteosarcoma, 388
  for diagnosis of prostatic enlargement, 1012
  for evaluation of causes of pulmonary hypertension, 713
  for evaluation of dysphagia, 497
  for evaluation of hepatobiliary disease, 573
  for evaluation of hypercalcemia and hyperparathyroidism, in dogs, e69-e70
  for evaluation of kidney size, 841
  for evaluation of the eye, 1133
  of the ear, with otitis, 458
  of the female reproductive tract, 938
    for predicting parturition, 946t
    for pregnancy diagnosis, 945-947, 946f-947f
    to determine pregnancy loss, 1004
    with contrast, 939
  of the heart
    with congenital heart disease, 758
    with dilated cardiomyopathy in dogs, 797
    with mitral valve dysplasia, e300
    with myocarditis, e304-e305
    with pericardial effusion, 817-818
    with pulmonic stenosis, e315
    with tricuspid valve dysplasia, e333, e334f
    with valvular heart disease, 788, 789f, 792-793
    with ventricular septal defect, e337
  of the lungs
    for evaluation of respiratory distress, 46-47

Radiography (Continued)
  with acute respiratory distress syndrome, 50f
  with bronchopulmonary parasites, e269-e276
  with eosinophilic pulmonary diseases, 689
  with feline asthma, 675
  with feline heartworm disease, 827-829, 828f
  with interstitial lung diseases, e266-e267
  with pleural effusion, 691-700
  with pneumonia, 685-686
  with pneumothorax, 701f
  with atlantoaxial subluxation, 1083-1084, 1085f
  with barium, for evaluation of gastric emptying, 515
  with biliary tract disease, 603
  with cervical spondylomyelopathy, 1093
  with hemangiosarcoma, 393-394, 394f
  with intervertebral disk disease, 1072-1073
  with lumbosacral stenosis, 1106
  with nasal discharge
    in cats, 645-646
    in dogs, 636-637, 640-641
  with nasopharyngeal disorders, 654
  with pancreatitis in dogs, 561
  with portosystemic shunt, 595
  with thyroid gland neoplasia, 168-169
  with urinary bladder cancer, 371
  with urolithiasis, 906f
    calcium oxalate, 898
    urate
      double-contrast cystography, 902f
      monitoring of, 903
Radioiodine therapy, 399-400
  adverse effects of, e118, e119-e121, e119
  estimation of dose for, e117-e118
  failure to respond to, e119
  follow-up testing after, e118-e121
  for thyroid carcinoma, e118
  mechanism of action of, e107, e112-e122
  medical therapy before, e105
  prognosis after, e121
  pros and cons of, e103t
Radiology, interventional, 345-349
  strategies for urinary disease(s), 884-892
Radionuclide iodine imaging, of thyroid gland, 167-168
Radiosurgery, stereotactic, for osteosarcoma, 392
Radius trauma in dogs, 81
Radon, as respiratory toxicants, e47
Raison. See Grape and raison toxicity
Ranitidine (Zantac)
  action and use of, for motility disorders, 516-518, 517t
  for esophagitis, e240
  for feline pancreatitis, 567t
  for gastric ulceration, e254
  potency and use of, 505, 506b
  toxicity of, 119

Rapamycin, use of, for immunosuppression, 271-272
Rapid urease test, 510, 510f
Rauwolscine, for retrograde ejaculation, e351-e352
Raw meat diets
  causing disease transmission from pets to humans, 1245t, 1248
  causing pregnancy loss, 1007-1008
  during pregnancy and lactation, 965
  infectious diseases from, 1239-1243
  Neospora caninum from, 1290-1291
  toxoplasmosis from, 1297-1298
Receptors for cancer immunotherapy, 334-335
Recombinant cytokine therapy, 335
Recombinant human granulocyte colony-stimulating factor, for canine parvovirus, 535
Recombinant human NPH insulin, 190-191
Rectal neoplasms, immunotherapy for, 336t
Rectovaginal fistula, 977-978
Rectovestibular fistula, 977-978
Red blood cell transfusions, 309-313
Red cell aplasia, 316, e162
Red flower oil toxicity, 125t
Red puccoon toxicity, 124t
Red root toxicity, 124t
Reflux, gastroesophageal, 501-504
Rehabilitation
  and physical therapy for neurologic disorders, e357-e362
  recommendations postop disk herniation, e361b
Rehydration, fluid therapy for, 4-5
Relative adrenal insufficiency, 78-79, 174-178
  rational use of glucocorticoids for, 1301
Relaxin
  for pregnancy diagnosis, 947
  with pregnancy loss, 1004
Remifentanil, with maintenance anesthetic, 66, 67t
Renal
  regulation of magnesium, 249-250
  regulation of potassium, 251-252
Renal aplasia, ultrasound findings with, 841
Renal cell carcinoma, immunotherapy for, 335
Renal cysts, ultrasound findings with, 842
Renal disease
  and risk of urinary tract infections, 877
  anemia from, e160
  causing hyperkalemia and hyponatremia, e92, e93b
  drug incompatibilities and interactions with, 36
  from complications of hypoparathyroidism, e129
  from diabetes mellitus, e76
  from heat-induced illness, 72
  from hypothyroidism, e85

Renal disease (Continued)
  from plants, 121b
  glomerular disease and nephrotic syndrome, 853-857
  hypertension and, 726-727, 727t, 729-730
  hypokalemia from, 251b
  hypokalemia-induced, 252
  hypomagnesemia from, 249b
  insulin resistance with, 206, 206b
  use of H2 receptor antagonists with, 505
  use of nonsteroidal anti-inflammatory drugs for, 863-867
Renal dysplasia, ultrasound findings with, 841, 842f
Renal failure
  acute
    from leptospirosis, 1286-1287
    hospital acquired, 845-848
    management of, 868-871
    oliguria or anuria with, 869-870
    pathophysiologic stages of, 868
    polyuria with, 870
    prognosis with, 870-871
    treatment of toxin induced, e32b
    use of continuous renal replacement therapy with, 871-875, 875b
  and hypercalcemia, in cats, 242-243, 243b
  anemia from, e160
  causes of, e29, e30b
  chronic
    and risk of hospital acquired infections, 877
    diagnosis of, 857-863, 858b
    management of, 857-863
    staging of, 857-863
    substaging of, 858-860, 859t-860t
    treatment of, effect on staging, 860t
    use of NSAID's with, 866-867, 866b
  continuous renal replacement therapy for, 871-875
  drug effects on, 34t-35t
  formula for adjustment of antibiotic intervals, 34t-35t, 36
  formula for adjustment of drug dosage and intervals, 36
  from amphotericin, 1234-1235
  from ethylene glycol toxicity, 151
  from NSAID toxicity, 116
  hyperthyroidism and, 185-189, 188f, e104, e118
  nephrotoxins causing, e29-e34
    treatment of, e32b
  pancreatic lipase immunoreactivity (PLI) testing with, 556
  potassium supplementation with, 6-7
  subcutaneous fluid administration for, 7
  trypsin-like immunoreactivity (TLI) testing with, 557
  with proteinuria and albuminuria, 851-852
Renal function
  with drugs used to treat heart failure, 779
  with hyperthyroidism, 186-187

Renal infarct(s)
  from feline thromboembolism, 812
  ultrasound findings with, 842
Renal replacement therapy, 871-875
Renal threshold, for diabetes mellitus, in cats, 208
Renal transplantation
  immunosuppressive drugs for, 268-274
  with nephroliths and ureteroliths, 895
Renin-angiotensin-aldosterone system
  function of, 238, 766
  nutritional effects on, with heart disease, 720-722
  sites of action of inhibitors on, 854-855, 854f
  stock and, 18
Renourethroscope, 943-944. See also Vaginoscopy
  for pyometra treatment, 943-944
Repetitive licking behavior, drug therapy for, 482-485
Reporting
  adverse drug and product events to (FDA), e35-e43
  animal cruelty, e52
  human drugs of abuse, e52
Reproductive disorder(s)
  aspermia/oligospermia caused by retrograde ejaculation, e350-e353
  benign prostatic hypertrophy, 1012-1015
  controversy with early age neutering, 982-984
  effects of hypothyroidism, e85
  estrus suppression in the bitch and, 984-989
  inherited, 993-999
  medical termination of pregnancy, 989-992
  neoplasia, 1022-1026
  of the female reproductive tract, 936-939
  ovarian remnant syndrome, 1000-1003
  postpartum, 957-960
  pregnancy loss, 1003-1011, 1005t
  priapism as, e354-e357
  problems of the male external genitalia, 1029-1032
  prostatitis, 1012-1015
  pyometra, 967-969
  surgical repair of vaginal anomalies in the bitch, 974-981
  toxins and teratogens, 1026-1028
  vaginitis, 969-973
  vulvar discharge from, 969-973
Reproductive physiology
  breeding management in bitch and, 930-935
  exfoliative vaginal cytology, 932-933
  female, 930
  normal sexual development, 993, 994f
  onset of vulvar softening, 932
  optimal time for breeding, 930-935
  relationship of ovulation to luteinizing hormone surge, 931f, 931t
  proestrus, 932f

Reproductive physiology (Continued)
  progesterone concentration, 933f, 935f
  vaginal cytology, 933f
  reproductive toxins causing changes to, 1027-1028
Reproductive toxins and teratogens, 1026-1028, 1027b
Reproductive tract
  diagnosis of diseases of the female, 936-939
  examination of caudal, 932-934
  female, figure of, 970f
  inherited disorders of the, 993-999, 995t
Rescue chemotherapy, for canine lymphoma, 381-383, 382t
Resistance
  from methicillin, with Staphylococcal infections, 443-445
  multidrug, associated with pneumonia, 683b, 683t, 686
Resolve cleaner, toxic exposure to, 98
Respiratory acidosis
  causes of, e4b
  compensatory response to, e2t
  management of acid-base disorders and, e4-e5
Respiratory alkalosis
  causes of, e4b
  compensatory response to, e2t
  management of acid-base disorders and, e3-e4
Respiratory depression, intermittent positive pressure ventilation for, 66-67
Respiratory disease(s)
  anesthesia for patients with, 68
  as risk for heat-induced illness, 71
  brachycephalic airway obstruction syndrome, 649-653
  canine infectious, 632-635
  chronic bronchial, in dogs, 669-672
  chronic bronchitis and asthma in cats, 673-680
  drug therapy for, 622-628
  eosinophilic pulmonary, 688-691
  feline upper, 629-632
  heartworm-associated, in cats, 826t
  interstitial lung, e266-e269, e267b
  laryngeal, 659-662
  nasopharyngeal disorders causing, 653-658
  parasites causing, e269-e276
  pleural effusion with, 691-700
  pneumonia, 681-688
  pneumothorax, 700-704
  pulmonary hypertension and, 711-717
  pulmonary thromboembolism, 705-710
  rhinitis
    in cats, 644-648, 1232
    in dogs, 635-643
  tracheal collapse, 663-668
  with concurrent heart disease, 792-793
Respiratory distress
  acute syndrome of, 48-51, 49b
  causes of, 46t

Respiratory distress (Continued)
  from feline cardiomyopathy, 807-809
  from heart failure, 782-783
  from pleural effusion, 693-694
  from tracheal collapse, 664-665
  pathophysiology of, 44
  physical examination with, 45-46
  stabilization of patient with, 44-48
  syndrome, causing interstitial lung disease, e267b
  treatment plan for, 46t, 47-48
Respiratory failure, 44-45
Respiratory particle spread, from pets to humans causing disease, 1245t, 1246
Respiratory protection, for handling hazardous drugs, 327
Respiratory toxicant(s), e43-e48
Respiratory tract infection(s)
  canine infectious, 632-635
  common pathogens causing, 1222
  empiric antimicrobial therapy for, 1220t
  feline upper, 629-632, 1232
  use of glucocorticoids for, 1300
Resting energy requirements (RER), 39, 41b-42b, 259
Resuscitation. See also Cardiopulmonary resuscitation (CPR)
  end points for shock, 24
  fluid therapy for
    using colloids, 8, 12t
    using crystalloids, 2-4
  monitoring of, 19-20
Retina
  artificial, 1192
  changes in, with glaucoma in dogs, 1171t
  tumors of, 1205-1206
Retinal degeneration
  in cats, 1194-1195
  in dogs, 1192
Retinal detachment
  causing anisocoria, e392
  from chorioretinitis, 1162
  from hypertension, 726, 729, 1122, 1192
  gemcitabine causing, e141
  in cats, 1193-1194, 1194f
  in dogs
    causes of, e370-e372
    diagnosis of, e372-e373, e372f
    from hypothyroidism, e85
    pathogenesis of, e370
    prognosis for, e373-e374
    treatment of, e373
  in dogs and cats, e383
Retinal disease, causing anisocoria or mydriasis, e394
Retinal dysplasia, in dogs, 1188, 1189f
Retinal dystrophy, 1190-1192
Retinal pigment epithelial dystrophy, 1190
Retinochoroiditis, causing retinal detachment, in dogs, e371
Retinoids
  causing adverse skin reactions, 488t
  for actinic dermatoses, 481
  for sebaceous adenitis, e211

Retinopathies
  causing blindness, 1135-1136, 1136t
  direct mutation test for, 1018t-1020t
  in cats, 1193-1196, 1194f
    hypertensive, 1193-1194
    taurine, 1194-1195
  in dogs, 1188-1192
Retrobulbar pain, from orbital diseases, 1198
Retrograde ejaculation, aspermia/oligospermia caused by, e350-e353
Retroillumination, 1128-1129, 1129f
  with the neuro-ophthalmic exam, e391-e392
Retropulsion of the globe, 1132, 1197
Reverse sneezing, with nasopharyngeal disorders, 653
Rheumatoid arthritis, immunosuppressive drugs for, 268, 272
Rhinitis
  antibiotics for, 1220t, 1222
  in cats
    diagnosis of, 644-646
    from upper respiratory infection, 630t
    treatment of, 646-648
  in dogs, 635-643
    causes of, 636b
    treatment of, 637-643
Rhinoplasty, for brachycephalic airway obstruction syndrome, 651
Rhinoscopy
  for diagnosis of nasal disorders in dogs, 637
  of cats with nasal discharge, 645-646
Rhinosinusitis, chronic, in cats, 644-648
Rhinosporidium seeberi, causing rhinitis in dogs, 637-640
Rhipicephalus sanguineus tick, transmitting Ehrlichia canis, 1227-1228, 1292-1294
Rhodesian ridgeback(s)
  degenerative myelopathy in, 1075-1076
  epidermolytic ichthyosis in, 475
  papillomatosis in, 1231f
Rhododendron toxicity, 121b
Rhodotorula spp., causing perivulvar dermatitis, 971
Ribavirin, for feline retrovirus infections, 1279
Riboflavin, for mitochondrial encephalopathy, 1051, 1051t
Rickettsial infection(s)
  canine and feline monocytotropic ehrlichiosis, 1292-1294
  causing myocarditis, e304t
  causing nervous system signs, 1212
  causing polyarthritis, 1224-1228
  causing renal infections, 1212
  causing thrombocytopenia, 281t-282t
  common symptoms and syndromes caused by, 1214t
  immunosuppressive therapy for, 1232-1233

Rickettsial infection(s) (Continued)
  immunotherapy for, 1231-1233
  rational use of glucocorticoids for,
    1300-1301
Rifampicin
  for methicillin-resistant Staphylococcal
    skin infections, 444
  for nontuberculous cutaneous
    granulomas, 448t
Rifampin
  for Bartonella spp., 1266t
  for brucella canis, 972
  for superficial bacterial folliculitis, 438t
Right-to-left vascular shunt, with
    hypoxemia, 52
Riluzole, for degenerative myelopathy,
    1078
Rinse(s), for pyoderma, 441t
Rituximab, as cancer immunotherapy,
    334
Robenacoxib
  adverse effects of, 60
  dosage for, 62t
Rocky Mountain spotted fever
  causing thrombocytopenia, 281t-282t
  causing uveitis in dogs, 1164b
Rod cone dysplasia, direct mutation test
    for, 1018t-1020t
Rodenticide toxicity, 133-135
  exposures to, 92t, 96
Ronidazole
  for Tritrichomonas foetus, 528-530, 529f
  target parasites and dosage of,
    1335-1337
Ropivacaine, toxicity of, use of IV lipid
    emulsion therapy for, 106
Rose bengal stain, 1132
  with keratoconjunctivitis sicca, 1144
Roses, 121b
Rosiglitazone, for diabetes mellitus, in
    cats, e137-e138
Rottweiler(s)
  cervical spondylomyelopathy in, 1092
  colitis in, 553
  hyperlipidemia in, 261, 262t
  hypoadrenocorticism in, 233
  laryngeal paralysis in, 659
  osteosarcoma in, 388
  protein losing enteropathies in,
    540-541
  risk of pyometra in, 967
  subaortic stenosis in, e319, e320f
Royal Canin Veterinary diet Urinary SO,
    for calcium oxalate urolithiasis, 899t
Rubeosis iridis, with canine uveitis,
    1163t
Rush immunotherapy, 412
Rutin, for chylothorax, 699

S

S-adenosylmethionine (SAMe)
  as hepatic support therapy, e256-e257
  for toxicities, 139-140, 143, 150,
    161, 332-333, 577
  for acetaminophen toxicity, 577
  for chronic hepatitis, 585f, 587
  for extrahepatic biliary tract disease,
    604

S-adenosylmethionine (SAMe) (Continued)
  for feline hepatic lipidosis, 613
  for idiopathic vacuolar hepatopathy,
    608
  for liver failure, 582
  for portal vein hypoplasia, 600
  for portosystemic shunts, 596
Sachet fresh-packet exposure, 97-98
Safety, associated with hazardous drug
    handling, 329
Sago palms toxicity, 121b
Salicylate(s)
  containing oils, 125t
  containing plants, 125t
  containing preparations, 125
  ototoxicity from, 468b
  toxicity of, 117
Salicylic acid
  as topical therapy for skin issues, 441t
  ear cleaner, 472-473
  in ear cleaners, 472t
Salmon poisoning disease, as cause of
    thrombocytopenia, 281t-282t
Salmonella spp., 520
  causing diarrhea, 519
  causing pregnancy loss, 1005t, 1006,
    1008
  causing thrombocytopenia, 281t-282t
  common symptoms and syndromes
    caused by, 1213t
  in raw meat diets, 1240b, 1241
Salmonella typhimurium (Tapet), as
    cancer immunotherapy, 335, 336t
Saluki(s)
  glaucoma in, 1171b
  thyroid hormone differences in, 180t
Samoyed(s)
  alopecia X in, 477-479
  direct mutation tests for, 1018t-1020t
  glaucoma in, 1171b
  sebaceous adenitis in, e209-e210
  uveitis in, 1164
Sandimmune, 270
Sandostatin, for insulinomas, e134
Sarcoma(s)
  feline mammary, 378
  soft tissue, e148-e152
  vaccine-associated, in cats, 1252-1255
Sarcoptic mange, 403
  diagnosis and treatment of, 428-430
  treatment options for, 429t
  use of avermectins for, e181-e182
Sargramostin, for feline retrovirus
    infections, 1280t-1281t
Scaling, from adverse drug reactions,
    488t
Scapula trauma in dogs, 81
Schiff-Sherrington syndrome, from
    intervertebral disk disease, 1072
Schirmer tear test
  technique and use of, 1132
  with keratoconjunctivitis sicca, 1144,
    1155
Schnauzer(s)
  direct mutation tests for, 1018t-1020t
  fibrocartilaginous embolism in, 1123
  hyperlipidemia in, 261
  risk of pancreatitis in, 261

Schnauzer(s) (Continued)
  risk of urolithiasis in, 892, 897
  sick sinus syndrome in, 732-733, 733f
Scintigraphy
  for evaluation of esophagus, e227-e228
  for evaluation of hepatobiliary disease,
    573-574
  for portosystemic shunt, 595
  with portal vein hypoplasia, 600
Sclera tumors, 1204
Sclerosing agents, for malignant
    effusions, 342
Sclerotherapy, for essential renal
    hematuria, 886f
Scotch broom, toxicity of, 124t
Scott sliding potassium scale, 7t
Scottish terrier(s)
  breed related alkaline phosphatase
    elevations, e245b, e246
  direct mutation tests for, 1018t-1020t
  idiopathic vacuolar hepatopathy in,
    607
  prostatic hypertrophy in, 1012
  risk of bladder cancer in, 371t
Scraping, for cytology, e154
Scratch, from pets to humans causing
    disease, 1245t, 1246
Scratching behavior in cats, 913
Scrotum
  nonneoplastic disorders of the, 1031
  tumors of, 1023
Sebaceous adenitis
  diagnosis of, e210
  therapy of, e209-e212
  use of cyclosporine for, 409
Sebaceous gland hyperplasia, 476-477
Seborrhea, use of cyclosporine for, 410b
Seborrhea oleosa, with Malassezia spp.
    infections, e213
Seborrhea sicca, with Malassezia spp.
    infections, e213
Secnidazole, for Giardia spp., 530-531
Second-hand smoke, e44
Sedation
  for thoracocentesis, 693
  with cardiovascular dysfunction, 64-65
Sedums, 121b
Seidel's test, 1132
Seizure(s)
  causes of, 1058-1059, 1059t
  fluid resuscitation in, 1061t
  from hypoparathyroidism, e123-e124
  from insulinoma, e130
  infectious agents that cause, 1212
  new anticonvulsants for, 1054-1057
  pathophysiology of, 1058
  therapy for increased intracranial
    pressure from, 1061-1062, 1062t
  treatment of cluster, 1058-1063
  treatment of status epilepticus,
    1058-1063
  vs. syncope, e325
  with portosystemic shunt, 596
Selamectin (Revolution), 426t
  for cheyletiellosis, 430t, e182
  for dermatologic disorders, e178, e180
  for flea infestation, e183
  for lung worms, e274

Selamectin (Revolution) *(Continued)*
  for nasal mites, 637, 655-656, e270
  for *Otodectes* infestation, 431t, e182
  for pediculosis, 429t
  for sarcoptic and notoedric mange,
    429t
  target parasites of, 1335-1337
  toxicity of, 145-146
Selective serotonin reuptake inhibitors
    (SSRIs)
  for behavior-related dermatoses,
    483-484, 483t
  toxicity of, 112-114
Selenium associated hepatotoxicity,
    570b
Self-mutilating behavior(s)
  drug therapy for, 482-485
  with hot spots, e206
Semen
  and endoscopy transcervical
    insemination, 943
  frozen, fresh or chilled, 943
Seminomas, 1022-1023
Senile retinal degeneration, 1192
Sensorineural hearing loss, 468-469,
    468b
  treatment and prevention of, 470-471
Sepsis
  causing gastric ulcerations, e253
  causing uveitis in dogs, 1164b
  drainage techniques for the abdomen,
    e13-e20
  drug incompatibilities and interactions
    with, 37
  from heat-induced illness, 71
  pulmonary thromboembolism
    associated with, 705
  rational use of glucocorticoids for,
    1301
Septic abdomen, drainage techniques for,
    e13-e20
Septic arthritis, common pathogens
    causing, 1220t, 1222-1223
Septic shock, 18
  catecholamine use for, 15t
Septicemia
  as cause of thrombocytopenia,
    281t-282t
  common pathogens causing, 1223
  empiric antimicrobial therapy for,
    1220t
Serology
  for *Borrelia burgdorferi*, 1272-1273
  for feline *Bartonella* spp., 1269
Serotonin, and acral lick dermatitis,
    e177
Serotonin antagonist reuptake inhibitors
    (SARIs)
  for behavior-related dermatoses, 483t,
    484, e177
  toxicity of, 112-114
Serotonin syndrome, signs of, 34t-35t
Serotoninergic effects, of prokinetic
    drugs, 516-518, 517t
Serratia marcescens, for feline retrovirus
    infections, 1280t-1281t, 1282
Sertoli cell tumor, 1022-1023
  causing alopecia, in dogs, 165

Sertraline
  for behavior-related dermatoses,
    483-484, 483t
  toxicity of, 113
Serum pancreatic lipase
    immunoreactivity (PLI), with
    pancreatitis, 555-556
Serum proteomics, with myocarditis,
    e305
Serum therapy, for keratomalacia, 1151
Serum trypsin-like immunoreactivity
    (TLI)
  with exocrine pancreatic insufficiency,
    556-557, 559
  with feline pancreatitis, 566
  with pancreatitis, 555
Sevoflurane, anesthesia in critical care,
    66
Sex chromosome disorders of sexual
    development, 994, 995t
Sex hormone
  panel testing, 223
  role in alopecia X, 477
Sexual development
  disorders of, 993-999, 995t
  normal, 993, 994f
Shampoo therapy
  for atopic dermatitis, 405
  for dermatophytosis, 450t
  for ichthyosis, 476
  for *Malassezia* spp. infections, e215
  for methicillin-resistant Staphylococcal
    skin infections, 444
  for pyoderma, 439-443, 441t
  for sebaceous adenitis, e210-e211
Shar-pei dog, amyloidosis in, 855
Shelter(s)
  canine respiratory infection in, 632,
    634-635
  feline upper respiratory infection in,
    629, 631-632
  multicat outbreaks with
    dermatophytosis in, 452-454
Shetland sheepdog(s)
  avermectin toxicity in, 145
  dermatomyositis in, 1115
  direct mutation tests for, 1018t-1020t
  hyperlipidemia in, 261
  mitochondrial encephalopathy in,
    1048-1051, 1049t, 1051t
  risk of bladder cancer in, 371t
Shih tzu dog(s)
  Chiari-like malformation in, 1101
  cilia abnormalities in, 1155
  glaucoma in, 1171b
  hepatobiliary disease in, 571b
  intracranial arachnoid cysts in, 1038
  mammary cancer in, 377-378
  mitochondrial encephalopathy in,
    1048-1051, 1049t, 1051t
  risk of urolithiasis in, 892, 897
Shock, 18-25
  cardiogenic, 783
    dobutamine for treatment of, 16-17
    dopamine for treatment of, 16
    use of catecholamines for, 15t
  causing gastric ulcerations, e253
  classifications and examples of, 19b

Shock *(Continued)*
  dose of fluids, 2-4, 20-22
  hypovolemic
    fluid therapy for, 2, 12t
    physical findings with, 5t
  resuscitation end points for, 24
  septic (*See* Septic shock)
  therapy for, 20-25
  with illness-related corticosteroid
    insufficiency, 78, 174-178
Shoulder trauma in dogs, 81
Shunt reversal, 760
Siamese cat
  chylothorax in, 698
  glaucoma in, 1177
  hepatic amyloidosis in, 571b
  progressive retinal atrophy in, 1195
  resting nystagmus in, 1067
  retinal degeneration in, 1195
  risk of asthma in, 674
  risk of diabetes in, 208
  vestibular disease in, 1068
Siberian husky
  alopecia X in, 477-479
  breed related alkaline phosphatase
    elevations, e245b
  direct mutation tests for, 1018t-1020t
  laryngeal paralysis in, 659-661
  zinc-responsive dermatosis, causing
    blepharitis in, e365
Sick sinus syndrome, 732-733
  causing syncope, e328f, e330
  temporary pacing for, e21
Sildenafil (Viagra)
  for heart failure, in dogs, 764t-765t,
    768
  for pulmonary hypertension, 715-716
    with valvular heart disease,
    793-794
Silibin/phosphatidylcholine (PPC)
  for feline hepatic lipidosis, 613
  for liver failure, 582
Silver sulfadiazine, topical, for otitis,
    464t
Silymarin (milk thistle)
  as hepatic support therapy, e256
  for cholangitis, 617-618, 617b
  for hepatic lipidosis, 613
  for portosystemic shunts, 596-598
  for toxicities, 102t-104t, 161
Simethicone, for flatulence, e250
Sinoatrial node abnormalities, 732-733
Sinus arrest, temporary pacing in, e28f
Sinus tachycardia, with gastric dilation-
    volvulus, e17
Sinusitis, causing rhinitis in dogs,
    637-640
Sirolimus, use of, for
    immunosuppression, 271-272
Skin. *See also* under Dermatologic
    disorder(s)
  disease from *Bartonella* spp. infections,
    1263b
  lesions from adverse drug reactions,
    488t
Skin biopsy, for diagnosis of alopecia,
    166
Skin scale, 475-477

Skin scraping
  for demodex as cause of alopecia, 165
  for demodicosis, 432-433
  for sarcoptic mange, 428
Slide preparation for cytology, e154-
    e156, e155f
Slings, e359
Sloughi(s)
  direct mutation tests for, 1018t-1020t
  thyroid hormone differences in, 180t
Small intestinal bacterial overgrowth,
    520-521
  antibiotic-responsive, 519
  treatment for, 520t
Smears, for cytology, e155, e155f
Smog toxicity, e45-e46
Smoke, second-hand, e44
  and risk of asthma, 675
Sneezing
  and rhinitis in dogs, 635-648
  infectious causes of, 1217-1218
Snoring, with nasopharyngeal disorders,
    653
Sodium
  composition in fluid therapy, 3t
  requirements during pregnancy and
    lactation, 963
  restriction with heart disease, 721b,
    723, 777, 790, 792
  treats, 721t
Sodium bicarbonate
  drug incompatibilities with, 33t
  during CPR, 30
  for acid-base disturbances, e5-e8
  for acute renal failure acidosis, 870
  for diabetic ketoacidosis, 236, e80t-
    e81t, e82
  for gastric dilation-volvulus acidosis,
    e16
  formula for calculation of deficit,
    870
Sodium channel blockers
  for dogs, 763b, 771
  for supraventricular tachyarrhythmias,
    742t, 743
  for ventricular arrhythmias, 746-748,
    799
Sodium chloride, supplementation
    with calcium oxalate urolithiasis,
    898-899
Sodium hypochlorite
  as topical therapy for skin infections,
    441t
  for disinfection of methicillin-resistant
    Staphylococcal sp., 456
Sodium lauryl sulfate, in ear cleaners,
    472t
Sodium polyborate, for dust mite
    control, e199
Sodium stibogluconate, for American
    leishmaniasis, e397
Sodium tetraborate pentahydrate
    (Borax), in ear cleaners, 472t
Sodium-chloride difference, calculation
    of, with acid-base disorders, e2, e3b
Sodium/potassium ratio (Na/K ratio),
    with hypoadrenocorticism, 233,
    234t

Soft palate
  deformities with brachycephalic
    airway obstruction syndrome,
    650t, 651, 652f
  surgical access to, 655
Soft tissue sarcoma, e148-e152
  cancer immunotherapy for, 336t, 337
Solitary osseous plasmacytoma, 387
Somatostatin, for insulinomas, e134
Somogyi phenomenon, 195, 213
Sorbitol cathartic(s), for toxin ingestions,
    105
Sotalol
  causing bradyarrhythmias, 732
  causing syncope, e328
  for arrhythmia with congestive heart
    failure, 783-784
  for arrhythmia with dilated
    cardiomyopathy, in dogs, 799
  for feline arrhythmias, 750f-751f, 752
  for feline cardiomyopathy, 806t
  for heart failure, in dogs, 764t-765t
    with arrhythmias, 771
  for supraventricular tachyarrhythmias
    in dogs, 742t, 743-744
  for ventricular arrhythmias
    in cats, 753-754
    in dogs, 746-747, 747f, 747t
  with arrhythmogenic right ventricular
    cardiomyopathy, 803
Space, and environmental enrichment
    for domestic cats, 910-911
Spastic pupil syndrome, e395
Specialist referral, with legal claim
    regarding poisonings, e50-e51
Specimen(s), tissue handling and fixation
    of, 322-326, 323b
Spill management, associated with
    hazardous drugs, 328
Spinal cord
  injury from intervertebral disk disease,
    1071
  injury scores, 1072, 1072t
  reflexes occurring during ejaculation,
    e351t
Spindle cell tumor, ocular, 1205
Spindle tree, European toxicity, 124t
Spinosad, 426t
  potentiation of ivermectin toxicity
    with, e179
  target parasites of, 1335-1337
Spinosad/milbemycin, 426t
  target parasites of, 1335-1337
Spirochetes, causing myocarditis, e304t
Spironolactone
  causing adverse skin reactions, 488t
  for ascites, from liver disease, 591,
    e257-e258
  for asymptomatic heart disease, 766
  for dilated cardiomyopathy, in dogs,
    798-799
  for feline cardiomyopathy, 805-807,
    806t, 809
  for glomerular disease, 854
  for heart failure, in dogs, 763-765,
    764t-765t, 777-779, 791
  for hepatic fibrosis, 587
  for pulmonary hypertension, 714

Spitz(s), alopecia X in, 477-479
Splenectomy, for thrombocytopenia,
    285-286
Splenic
  disease from *Bartonella* spp. infections,
    1263b
  injury with gastric dilation-volvulus,
    e14, e18-e19
  masses with arrhythmogenic right
    ventricular cardiomyopathy, 802
Splenic hemangiosarcoma, 394
Splint(s), with open fractures, 84
Sponge(s), pot scrubbing, ingestion of,
    98
Sporothrix schenckii
  causing epistaxis, 1216
  common symptoms and syndromes
    caused by, 1214t
Sporotrichosis, antifungal therapy for,
    1234-1238
Sporozoites, from toxoplasmosis, 1295
Spray(s)
  for pyoderma, 441t
  potency of topical steroid, 460f
Springer spaniel(s
  atrial standstill in, 734
  direct mutation tests for, 1018t-1020t
  hepatobiliary disease in, 571b
  mammary cancer in, 375
  oropharyngeal dysphagia in, 497
Squalene, in ear cleaners, 472t
Squamous cell carcinoma
  anal sac, e189-e190
  eyelid, e368
  immunotherapy for, 336t
  mammary
    canine, 376
    feline, 378
  nasal, radiation therapy for, 338-340
  ocular
    in cats, 1207-1210
    in dogs, 1204
  oral, 365
  papillomaviruses causing, e185
  penis and preputial, 1023
  scrotal, 1023
  topical immunomodulators for, e220
Squamous papillomas, 1202
Staging
  of canine heartworm disease, 826-827
  of heart disease, 773-775, 787t
  of mammary cancer, 376t
  of nasal tumors, e157
  of renal failure, 857-863
  of thyroid tumors, 399t
  tumor, e170
Stanozolol, associated hepatotoxicity,
    570b
Staphage lysate (SPL)
  for infectious disease immune
    therapeutics, 1230t
  for superficial bacterial folliculitis, 439
Staphylococcus aureus
  causing endocarditis, e292-e293, e294t
  causing pyoderma, 435
  in raw meat diets, 1240-1241, 1240b
Staphylococcus intermedius, causing
    endocarditis, e293-e294, e294t

Staphylococcus protein A, for feline retrovirus infections, 1280t-1281t, 1282
Staphylococcus pseudintermedius
    causing pyoderma, 435
    common symptoms and syndromes caused by, 1213t
Staphylococcus schleiferi, causing pyoderma, 435-436
Staphylococcus spp. infection
    causing blepharitis, e363
    causing conjunctivitis, 1141-1142
    causing keratoconjunctivitis sicca, 1144
    causing otitis, 466
    causing pneumonia, 682t
    causing pregnancy loss, 1005t, 1006
    causing prostatitis, 1013
    causing pyoderma, 435-436
    causing septic mastitis, 959
    disinfection of environments with, 455-457
    methicillin-resistant infections, 443-445
    role of, in hot spots, e206
    topical therapy for, 440-442, 441t
    with open fractures, 84, 86
Starch, dietary requirements for, with diabetes mellitus, 200-201
Starling-Landis equation, 8, 9f
Statins, for hyperlipidemia, 265-266
Status epilepticus, 1058-1063
Stavudine, for feline retrovirus infections, 1278, 1279t
Stenosis, lumbosacral, 1105-1108
Stenotic nares, and brachycephalic airway obstruction syndrome, 649-653, 650t
Stenting
    bronchial, 668
    choledochal, in cats, 568
    of malignant obstructions, 345-347
    tracheal, 664-668, 666f-667f
    ureteral, 887-888
    urethral, 889-890, 889f-890f
Stereotactic radiation therapy, for nasal tumors, 338-339
Stereotactic radiosurgery, for osteosarcoma, 392
Sterile neutrophilic dermatosis, 489
Steroid contraceptives, 984-985, 987
Steroid myopathy, 1116
Steroid tachyphylaxis, 461
Steroid(s). *See* Glucocorticoid(s)
Stertor, with nasopharyngeal disorders, 653-654
Stevens-Johnson syndrome, from drug reactions, 488
Stevia rebaudiana, as diabetes supplement, toxicity of, 125
Stifle joint trauma in dogs, 81-82
Stillbirth. *See* Pregnancy
Stomach, deformities with brachycephalic airway obstruction syndrome, 650t
Stomatitis
    feline caudal, 492-495
    from feline upper respiratory infection, 630t
    infectious causes of, 1216

Stone basketing, 890
Strabismus
    from orbital diseases, 1197, 1198b
    from vestibular disease, 1067, 1067t
Straelensia cynotis, 431-432
Streptococcus canis
    causing endocarditis, e293-e294, e294t
    causing feline upper respiratory infections, 629
Streptococcus equi var. *zooepidemicus*
    causing respiratory infections, 1217-1218
    common symptoms and syndromes caused by, 1213t
Streptococcus spp. infection
    causing conjunctivitis, 1141-1142
    causing pneumonia, 681, 682t
    causing pregnancy loss, 1005t, 1006
    causing prostatitis, 1013
    causing septic mastitis, 959
Streptokinase, for pulmonary thromboembolism, 707-708
Streptozocin, toxicity from chemotherapeutic drugs, 332
Streptozotocin, for insulinomas, e132-e133
Stress
    causing pregnancy loss, 1010-1011
    effect of, with feline upper respiratory infection, 629, 631
Stress related mucosal disease (SRMD), from shock, 24
Stroke. *See* Cerebrovascular accident
Strong ion difference
    acidosis, causes of, e6-e8, e7b
    alkalosis, causes of, e6, e6b
    calculation of, with acid-base disorders, e2
    disorders of, e5-e8
    mechanisms for, e6t
Strong ion gap, calculation of, with acid-base disorders, e2, e3b
Strongyloides stercoralis, common symptoms and syndromes caused by, 1214t-1215t
Struve urolithiasis, and nephroliths, 926
Struvite crystalluria, 926
Strychnine toxicity, 134
Styrene toxicity, 1027b
Subaortic stenosis, e319-e324
    causes of, e319
    diagnosis of, e320-e323, e320f-e321f, e323f
    pathophysiology of, e320
    predisposing to endocarditis, e291-e292
    prevalence of, in dogs, 756, 757t
    prophylaxis with, e297-e298
    therapy of, 759-760, e323-e324
Subcutaneous fluid therapy, 7
Subinvolution of placental sites, 957
Sublingual immunotherapy, 413, 413b
Succimer, for lead toxicity, 158
Sucralfate (Carafate)
    action and use of, 507
    drug incompatibilities with, 33t
    for esophagitis, e240
    for gastric ulcerations, e254
    for gastroesophageal reflux, 503

Suction, with thoracostomy tubes, 702
Sudden acquired retinal degeneration, e383
Sudden death
    with arrhythmogenic right ventricular cardiomyopathy, 803
    with dilated cardiomyopathy, 798
Sulfadiazine/trimethoprim, target parasites and dosage of, 1335-1337
Sulfadimethoxine, target parasites and dosage of, 1335-1337
Sulfasalazine
    for canine colitis, 551b
    for inflammatory bowel disease, 539
Sulfonamide(s)
    adverse effects of, 34t-35t
    associated hepatotoxicity, 570b, 577-578
    causing adverse skin reactions, 488t
    causing keratoconjunctivitis sicca, 1144
Sulfosalicylic acid (SSA) precipitation test, 849
Sulfur, as topical therapy for skin issues, 441t
Sulfur dioxide toxicity, e45
Sulindac toxicity, 116-117, e32-e33
Sun exposure, as risk factor for ocular neoplasia, 1207
Sun protection
    for actinic dermatoses, 480-482
    with clothing, 481
    with sunscreens, 481
Superficial bacterial folliculitis, 437-439
Superficial necrolytic dermatitis, 485-487
    causing blepharitis, e365-e366
Superficial punctate keratitis, 1153
Superior vena cava syndrome, stenting for, 347
Superoxide dismutase 1 gene, in degenerative myelopathy, 1075-1076
Supraventricular tachyarrhythmias, in dogs, 737-744
    classification of, 738
    clinical signs of, 738-739
    treatment of, 741-744, 742t
Supraventricular tachycardia, in dogs, 739
Suprofen, for canine uveitis, 1165t
Suramin, for feline retrovirus infections, 1278-1279, 1279t
Surgery
    cesarean section, 951-956
    empiric antimicrobial therapy for musculoskeletal, 1220t
    for acral lick dermatitis, e176
    for atlantoaxial subluxation, 1086-1088, 1087f-1089f
    for canine glaucoma, 1174-1176
    for cataracts, 1184-1185
    for congenital heart disease, 760-761
    for correction of vaginal anomalies in the bitch, 974-981, 975f-976f
    for craniocervical junction abnormalities, 1103-1104, 1103f
    for feline cholangitis, 617
    for feline corneal disease, 1160, 1161t

Surgery *(Continued)*
    for feline gastrointestinal lymphoma, 547
    for feline glaucoma, 1180
    for gastric dilation-volvulus, e18
    for hemangiosarcoma, 395
    for hyperadrenocorticism in ferrets, e95
    for insulinoma, e131-e132
    for intervertebral disk disease, 1073-1074
    for intracranial tumors, 1039-1047
    for keratoconjunctivitis sicca, 1147
    for laryngeal paralysis, 660-661
    for ligation of patent ductus arteriosus, e312-e313
    for malignant effusions, 342-343
    for mammary cancer, 377
    for mechanical occluder devices, 921
    for nontuberculous cutaneous granulomas, 448
    for oral neoplasia, 363-364
    for osteosarcoma, 389-390
    for pituitary macroadenoma, e90
    for portosystemic shunt(s), 596-597, 598f
    for pyothorax, 697
    for soft tissue sarcomas, e150-e151, e151
    for thyroid tumors, 399, 399f
    for treatment of hyperparathyroidism, e72
    for urinary bladder cancer, 372
    for vaccine-associated sarcoma, 1254
    for valvular heart disease, 794
    for ventriculoperitoneal shunt, 1036-1037, 1037f
    indications for post-op peritoneal drainage with, e14
    margins, demarcating specimens for evaluation, 324, 324b
    minilaparotomy-assisted cystoscopy for urocystoliths, 905-909, 906f-907f
    of the gall bladder, 602-605
    of the nasopharynx, 655
    palliative *vs.* curative, e171
    pericardectomy, 821-823, 822f
    principles for oncology, e168-e172
    pulmonary thromboembolism associated with, 705
    technique for early age neutering, 983
    to detect ovarian remnant syndrome, 1002, 1003f
Susceptibility testing, for methicillin-resistant Staphylococcal skin infections, 444
Suture pattern
    for eyelid laceration, e379f
    temporary tarsorrhaphy, e378f
Swallowing
    phases of, 495-496, e224-e225, e259
    signs of dysfunction, e260t
    studies, 497-498
Sweet cane toxicity, 124t
Sweet cinnamon toxicity, 124t
Sweet flag toxicity, 124t
Sweet root toxicity, 124t
Swiffer WetJet ingestion, 97

Swinging flashlight test, e391
Swiss Mountain dog(s), cervical spondylomyelopathy in, 1092
Symblepharon, from feline herpesvirus 1, 1157t
Sympathomimetic agent(s)
    for glaucoma in dogs, 1173b, 1174
    for retrograde ejaculation, e352-e353
    for urinary incontinence disorders, 915, 916t
Symptoms, causing by common infectious agents, 1212-1218
Synbiotic(s), for flatulence, e250
Syncope, e324-e331
    and arrhythmia in cats, 748, 750f-751f
    causes of, e326-e329
    diagnosis of, e329
    pathophysiology of, e325
    reflex-mediated, 736
    temporary pacing for, e22
    treatment of, e329-e330
    vs. seizure, e325
    with congenital heart disease, 759-760
Syringomyelia, 1100-1101
Systemic illness, from adverse reactions to vaccines, 1251
Systemic inflammation
    and cancer cachexia, 350
    drug incompatibilities and interactions with, 37
    with disseminated intravascular coagulation, 292, 293f
Systemic inflammatory response syndrome (SIRS), 18
    fluid movement with, 9t
    from heat-induced illness, 71
    rational use of glucocorticoids for, 1301
    with feline pancreatitis, 567
Systemic lupoid onychodystrophy, pentoxifylline for, e204
Systemic lupus erythematosus, causing blepharitis, e367

T

T-cell leukemia, 303-304
T-cell lymphoma, 303-304
    masitinib for, 361t
Table of common drugs: approximate dosages, 1307-1334
Tachyarrhythmias
    feline, 750f-751f
    supraventricular, in dogs, 737-744
Tachycardia
    causing syncope, e326
    sinus, in cats, 749
    supraventricular tachyarrhythmias causing syncope, e326
    in dogs, 737-744
Tachycardiomyopathy, 738
Tachyzoites, from toxoplasmosis, 1295
Tacrolimus
    and risk of ocular squamous cell carcinoma, 1204
    as topical immunomodulators, e216-e220, e217
    for anal furunculosis, e190
    for atopic dermatitis, 406, e217-e218

Tacrolimus *(Continued)*
    for chronic superficial keratitis (Pannus), 1154
    for discoid lupus erythematosus, e218
    for episcleritis, 1141
    for immune-mediated diseases, e218
    for keratoconjunctivitis sicca, 1145, 1155
    monitoring blood levels of, 271
    safety concerns of, e219-e220
    topical, 420t, 421
    use of, for immunosuppression, 271
Tadalafil (Cialis), for pulmonary hypertension with valvular heart disease, 793-794
Taenia spp. infection
    common symptoms and syndromes caused by, 1214t-1215t
    drugs targeting, 1335-1337
Tamoxifen, for mammary cancer, 377
Tamsulosin
    for urinary retention disorders, 917t, 918
    to promote ureterolith passage, 894
Tannic acid
    associated hepatotoxicity, 570b
    for dust mite control, e199
Tape preparation, of skin, for diagnosis of alopecia, 165
Tapetal reflex, 1128-1129
Taurine
    deficiency cardiomyopathy, 795, 797, 800, 809
    for asymptomatic heart disease, 766
    for feline hepatic lipidosis, 613
    requirements with heart disease, 724
    retinopathy, 1194-1195
Tea
    as poisoning antidote, 98
    toxicity, 98, 148t
Tear film disorders
    in cats, e384-e388
        diagnosis of, e385-e386
        lipid layer abnormalities, e385
        mucin layer abnormalities, e385
        physiology and pathophysiology of, e384, e384-e385, e385f
        treatment of, e386-e387
    in dogs, 1143-1147
        causes of, 1144
        mucin deficiency causing, 1155
Tear substitutes, e386-e387
    for keratoconjunctivitis sicca, 1145-1147, 1146t
Tearing. *See* Epiphora
Tellurium, causing reproductive toxicity, 1027b
Temazepam toxicity, 113-114
Temozolomide, e140t, e142
Temporary tarsorrhaphy, e378f
Tenosynovitis
    common pathogens causing, 1222-1223
    empiric antimicrobial therapy for, 1220t
Tepoxalin, for canine uveitis, 1165t
Teratogens, 1026-1028

Terbinafine
  for dermatophytosis, 451, 451t
  for fungal rhinitis in cats, 647-648,
    647t
  for *Malassezia* spp. infections, e215,
    e215t
  for nasal aspergillosis, 639-640
  use and protocols for, 1235t, 1238
Terbutaline
  for atrioventricular block, in cats, 754
  for bradycardias, 736
  for bronchial diseases, 671
  for feline asthma, 675, 677
  for premature labor, 947-948
  for priapism, e356-e357
  for respiratory diseases, 623
  for tracheal collapse, 664
Terminator rodenticide toxicity, 134
Terrier(s), sebaceous gland hyperplasia
    in, 476-477
Testicle
  dysgenesis, partial, 997
  nonneoplastic disorders of the,
    1031-1032
  reproductive toxins targeting the,
    1027-1028
  tumors of the, 1022-1023
Testosterone, for estrus suppression in
    the bitch, 987
Tetrachloroethylene toxicity, 1027b
Tetracycline(s)
  adverse effects of, 34t-35t
  associated hepatotoxicity, 570b,
    581b
  causing adverse skin reactions, 488t
  causing pregnancy loss and fetal
    disorders, 1010
  drug incompatibilities with, 33t
  for brucellosis, e404
  for canine babesiosis, 1259
  for epiphora, e375
  for feline tear film disorders, e387
  for hemotropic mycoplasmosis, e401
  for keratomalacia, 1151
  for lower respiratory tract infection(s),
    1220t, 1222
  for pleurodesis, 342
  for sebaceous adenitis, e211
  for urinary tract infections, 1220t,
    1221
  interaction with GI drugs, 37
  topical, for feline ocular herpesvirus 1,
    1158
Tetralogy of Fallot, e339-e340
  prevalence of
    in cats, 757t
    in dogs, 757t
Tetramine, for copper-associated liver
    disease, 589, e236
Tetraplegia, from degenerative
    myelopathy, 1076-1077, 1076t
Tetrastarch, 11-12
  characteristics of, 10t
Thallium, causing reproductive toxicity,
    1027b
Thelazia spp., causing conjunctivitis,
    1142
Theobromine toxicity, 148-149

Theophylline
  adverse effects of, 625
  drug interactions with, 35t, 677
  enterohepatic recirculation of, 105
  for canine bronchial diseases, 671
  for feline bronchitis and asthma, 677
  for tracheal collapse, 664
  formulations of, 624
  pharmacokinetics and dosing of,
    624-625
Thermal injury, 71
Thermal tumor ablation, for malignant
    obstructions, 348
Thermoregulatory center, 70-71, 73
Thiabendazole
  causing adverse skin reactions, 488t
  topical, for otitis, 465t
Thiabendazole/neomycin/
    dexamethasone, for *Otodectes*
    infestation, 431t
Thiacetarsemide
  aplastic anemia from, e162
  associated hepatotoxicity, 570b, 581b
Thiamine deficiency
  causing vestibular signs, 1068-1069
  with liver failure, 582
Thiazide diuretic(s)
  for calcium oxalate urolithiasis, 900
  for congestive heart failure, 798
  for feline myocardial disease, 809
  for hypercalciuria, e128
  for hypoparathyroidism, e128
  for insulinomas, e133
  impact on potassium levels, 122-123,
    251-252, 251b, 723, e93
Thiazolidinedione, for diabetes mellitus,
    in cats, e135, e136f, e137-e138
Third eyelid. *See* Nictitating membrane
Thoracic pump theory, 27
Thoracocentesis
  complications of, 693-694
  for malignant effusions, 342
  for pleural effusion, 692-693
    with refractory heart failure, 781
  for pneumothorax, 701
  procedure for, 693
Thoracoscopic subtotal pericardectomy,
    822f, 823
Thoracostomy tube(s)
  "three strikes" rule for placement of,
    702-703
  for pneumothorax, 701-702
  for pyothorax, 696-697
Thoracotomy
  for pleural effusion, 697, 699-700
  for pneumothorax, 702
Thorn apple toxicity, 124t
Thoroughwort toxicity, 124t
Three-dimensional conformal radiation
    therapy, for nasal tumors, 339,
    339f-340f
Thrombi formation
  in hypercoagulable states, 297-301, 298f
  reduction of, 813
  risk of, 708
Thrombin, abnormalities with
    disseminated intravascular disorders,
    293f

Thrombocytopenia
  determining the cause of, 283-284
  diagnosis and treatment of, 280-286
  diagnostic workup for, 315f
  from canine parvoviral enteritis, 533
  from chemotherapeutic drugs, 331
  from heat-induced illness, 72
  from methimazole, e103
  immune-mediated,
    immunosuppressive drugs for, 268
  infectious causes of, 281-283,
    281t-282t
  prognosis for, 286
Thromboelastography, 74-77, 75t, 706,
    710
Thromboembolic disease, 812-813
  causing pulmonary hypertension,
    712t, 716
  from hypercoagulable states, 297-301
  risk of, with protein-losing
    enteropathy, 544
Thromboembolism
  causing Ischemic strokes, 1119-1120
  feline arterial, 809-815
    thromboprophylaxis for, 710
  from autoimmune hemolytic anemia,
    276
  from cytauxzoonosis, e408
  from endocarditis, e293
  from feline heartworm disease, 830
  from glomerular disease, 854-855
Thrombolysis, 813-814
  for pulmonary thromboembolism,
    707-708
Thrombophilia, causing pulmonary
    thromboembolism, 705
Thrombophlebitis, from parenteral
    nutrition products, 40-41
Thymectomy, for myasthenia gravis,
    1111
Thymidine kinase, with
    hemangiosarcoma, 395
Thymol, as topical antipruritic agents,
    419
Thymoma, lymphocytosis associated
    with, 304
Thyroid diseases, interpretation of tests
    results for, e97-e102
Thyroid gland
  CT images of, 168f
  imaging of, for diagnosis of endocrine
    disorder(s), 167-170, 168t
  influence of drugs on function of,
    181t
  physiology, in cats, e107, e108f
Thyroid scintigraphy, 167, e113-e117,
    e114f-e115f, e116f
Thyroid tumors
  diagnosis and treatment of
    in cats, 400
    in dogs, 397-400
  staging of, 399t
Thyroid-stimulating hormone
  levels in hypothyroidism, 181-182,
    182t
  suppression with radioiodine therapy,
    e119-e120
  test, 182, e100

Thyroidectomy, e109
  hypocalcemia post, e124-e125
  pros and cons, e103t
Thyroiditis
  diagnosis and treatment of, 182-184
  hypothyroidism with, 178-179
Thyroxine (T4)
  levels with hyperthyroidism, 169-170,
    e101, e107
  levels with hypothyroidism, 178-185,
    180t, e99-e101, e100
    age related differences, 180t
    autoantibodies with, e100
    effect of drugs on, 181t
    free, 180, e100
    total, 180
  levels, while on glucocorticoids, 461
  test sensitivity of, 181t
Tibetan terrier(s), direct mutation tests
    for, 1018t-1020t
Ticarcillin-clavulanate (Timentin)
  for feline pancreatitis, 567t
  for infective endocarditis, e294t,
    e297
  for otitis, 466t, 467
  for pneumonia, 683, 683t
Tick collar toxicity, 138-139
Tick prevention product(s)
  avermectins as, e182-e183
  drug reactions from, 489
  for cats, 426t
  for dogs, 426t, 1294
  formulations of, dosage for and target
    parasites of, 1335-1337
Tick(s)
  causing cytauxzoonosis, e405
  causing *Hepatozoon americanum*,
    1283-1284
  drugs targeting, 1335-1337
  transmission of disease by, from pets
    to humans, 1248
  transmitting polyarthritis, 1224-1228
  vectors for ehrlichiosis, 1292
Tiger balm liniment toxicity, 125t
Timolol
  for canine glaucoma, 1173b, 1174,
    e381
  for feline glaucoma, 1179, e381
Tinidazole
  for *Giardia* spp., 530-531, 530t
  target parasites and dosage of,
    1335-1337
Tissue factor
  with disseminated intravascular
    coagulation, 292, 293f-294f
  with hypercoagulable states, 297
Tissue factor pathway inhibitor(s), for
    disseminated intravascular
    coagulation, 296
Tissue handling and fixation, for biopsy
    and specimen submission, 322-323,
    323b
Tissue plasminogen activator (t-PA), 813
  for feline thromboembolism, 810
  for pulmonary thromboembolism,
    707-708
Tissue sloughing, from extravasation of
    chemotherapeutic drugs, 333

Tobramycin, causing renal failure,
    e31-e32
Toceranib (Palladia)
  for malignant effusions, 344
  for oral tumors, 364
  for osteosarcoma, 392
  for thyroid cancer, 400
  toxicity of, 359-360
Tocodynamometer, 950, 950f
Tolazoline hydrochloride, as antidote,
    e56t
Tolbutamide, associated hepatotoxicity,
    581b
Toll-like receptor agonists, for local
    immunotherapy, 335
Tolmetin toxicity, e32-e33
Toluene toxicity, 1027b
Toluidine toxicity, 1027b
Tongue tumors, 364-365
Tonka and tonka bean toxicity, 124t
Tono-pen, 1171-1172
Tonometry, 1130
  for canine glaucoma, 1171-1172, 1174
  in cats
    artificial elevations of, 1178-1179
    with glaucoma, 1178
Tonsillar tumor, 365
Tooth resorption, for feline caudal
    stomatitis, 493
Topical therapy
  for acral lick lesions, e176-e177
  for atopic dermatitis, 406
  for dermatophytosis, 450, 450t
  for hot spots, e207-e208
  for infectious skin diseases, 439-443,
    441t
  for *Malassezia* spp. infections, e215
  for otitis
    antimicrobials, 462-465
    with glucocorticoids, 460t
  for pruritus, 419-421
  ototoxicity from, 468b
Torsemide
  for heart failure, in dogs, 762-763,
    764t-765t
  for refractory heart failure, 781
Total parenteral nutrition, 39-40, 41b
Toxic epidermal necrolysis, from drug
    reactions, 489
Toxicity(ies)
  and risk of urinary bladder cancer, 370
  ASPCA Animal Poison Control Center
    exposures, 92-93
  causing blindness, e383
  causing hepatobiliary disease, 569,
    570b, 581b
  causing myocarditis, e304t
  causing polyneuropathy, 1116-1117
  causing pregnancy loss, 1010
  causing retinal detachment, in dogs,
    e371
  deaths from, 94, 94t
  drug-associated liver, 575-579
  drugs used to treat, 101-105, 102t-104t
  exposures to, 92-93
  from aflatoxins, 159-161
  from antidepressants and anxiolytics,
    112-114

Toxicity(ies) *(Continued)*
  from automotive and garage items,
    151-155
  from chemotherapeutic drugs, 330-333
  from cyclosporine, 270-271
  from essential oils, 125-127, 126t
  from herbal supplements, 122-129
  from human drugs of abuse, 109-112
  from human foods, 147-150
  from lawn and garden products,
    130-132
  from mycophenolate mofetil, 272
  from plants, 121, 121b
  insecticide, 135-141
  IV lipid emulsion therapy for, 106-109
  lead, 156-159
  legal claim considerations with,
    e49-e52
  nephrotoxins causing, e29-e34
  pesticides for vertebrate pest species,
    142-144
  Pet Poison Helpline exposures to,
    93-96
  regulatory points to consider with
    treatment of, e54-e68
  reporting adverse events from, e35-e43
  reproductive, 1026-1028, 1027b
  respiratory, e43-e48
  rodenticide, 133-135
  source of help for, e53
  urban legends of, 97-100
Toxocara canis, common symptoms and
    syndromes caused by, 1214t-1215t
Toxocara cati, common symptoms and
    syndromes caused by, 1214t-1215t
Toxocara leonina, common symptoms
    and syndromes caused by,
    1214t-1215t
Toxocara spp. infection
  causing infection in humans, 1247
  drugs targeting, 1335-1337
  in raw meat diets, 1240b, 1242
Toxoplasma gondii, 1295
  causing infection in humans, 1216,
    1246-1247
  causing myocarditis, e307
  causing myositis, 1115
  common symptoms and syndromes
    caused by, 1214t-1215t
  in raw meat diets, 1240b, 1242
Toxoplasmosis, 1295-1298
  associated hepatotoxicity, 581b
  causing blindness, 1136
  causing corneal sequestrums,
    1159-1160
  causing feline uveitis, 1167
  causing nervous system signs, 1212
  causing pregnancy loss, 1010, 1218
  causing thrombocytopenia, 281t-282t
  causing uveitis, 1218
  clinical features of
    in cats, 1295-1296
    in dogs, 1296
  cyclosporine use with, 403
  diagnosis of, 1296-1297
  dosage for and drugs targeting,
    1335-1337
  feline, 1295-1296

Toxoplasmosis (Continued)
  immunotherapy for, 1231-1232, 1232f
  lymphocytosis associated with, 305
  treatment of, 1297
  zoonosis from, 1297-1298, 1298b
Trachea
  deformities of, with brachycephalic
    airway obstruction syndrome,
    650t, 652
  normal bacterial isolates in, 682b
Tracheal carcinoma, stenting for, 346f
Tracheal catheter, for oxygen
    administration, 53
Tracheal collapse
  as risk for heat-induced illness, 71
  causing pulmonary hypertension, 711
  diagnosis and treatment of, 663-668
  stenting for, 664-668, 666f
  with concurrent bronchial disease,
    672
Tracheal stenting, of malignant
    obstructions, 346-347, 346f
Tracheobronchial culture, for feline
    asthma, 676
Tracheobronchial disease, with
    concurrent heart disease, 792-793
Tracheobronchitis
  canine infectious, 632-635
  from feline upper respiratory infection,
    630t
Tracheostomy tube care, 57b
Traction alopecia, in dogs, 165b
Tramadol
  after cesarean section, 956
  dosage for, 62t
  drug interactions with, 34t-35t
  for cervical junction abnormalities,
    1102-1103
  for cervical spondylomyelopathy,
    1095f
  for corneal ulcerations, 1149
  for degenerative lumbosacral stenosis,
    1106-1107
  for orbital cellulitis or abscess,
    1198-1199
  for the critical patient, 59
Tranexamic acid, for treatment of von
    Willebrand disease, 290-291
Transcervical hysteroscopy, 937-938
  for insemination, 940-944
Transcolonic pertechnetate scintigraphy
    (TCPS),for evaluation of
    hepatobiliary disease, 574
Transcutaneous external pacing, e21-e28
  technique for, e26-e28, e27f
Transdermal medication(s)
  amlodipine, 729
  analgesia, 61-63, 62t
  carbimazole, e103t
  methimazole, e104-e105, e104
    toxicity with, 579, e103t, e108
  nitroglycerine, 764t-765t
  toxicity of nicotine, 119-120
Transfusions. See Blood transfusions
Transillumination, 1128-1129, 1129f
Transitional cell carcinoma, bladder
  diagnosis and treatment of, 370-374
  immunotherapy for, 336t

Transitional cell carcinoma, bladder
    (Continued)
  intraarterial chemotherapy for, 890, 891f
  ultrasound findings with, 843, 844f
Transmissible venereal tumors, penis and
    preputial, 1023
Transsplenic portal scintigraphy, for
    evaluation of hepatobiliary disease,
    574
Transtracheal wash
  collection of cytology specimens from,
    e155
  for diagnosis of pneumonia, 686
Transurethral resection of bladder, for
    urinary bladder cancer, 372
Transvenous pacing, e21-e28
  technique for, e22-e26, e24f
  troubleshooting problems with,
    e24-e26
Tratruzumab, as cancer immunotherapy,
    334
Trauma
  associated sarcoma of the eye, in cats,
    1209
  causing pregnancy loss, 1010-1011
  causing retinal detachment, in dogs,
    e370
  causing uveitis in dogs, 1164, 1164b
  cellular, causing hyperkalemia and
    hyponatremia, e93, e93b
  colloid use for, 12t
  induced pneumothorax, 702
  open fractures from, 83-86
  orbital, 1200
  orthopedic, in dogs, 80-83
  pulmonary thromboembolism
    associated with, 705
  to the penis and prepuce, 1030-1031
  to the testes, 1031-1032
  wound care with, 87-90
Travoprost, for glaucoma in dogs, 1173,
    1173b
Trazodone, for behavior-related
    dermatoses, 483t, 484
Treats, sodium-restricted, 721t
Tree(s), toxicity of, 124t
Tremorgenic mycotoxins, 149
Trephination, for treatment of nasal
    aspergillosis, 638-639
Triaditis syndrome, in cats, 615-616
Triamcinolone
  causing adverse skin reactions, 488t
  for feline caudal stomatitis, 493-494
  for otitis
    systemic, 461t
    topical, 460t
  inhaled, for respiratory diseases, 626t
  subconjunctival, for eosinophilic
    keratitis, 1159
  submucosal esophageal injections of,
    503-504
  topical, for hot spots, e207
Triazapentadiene compounds, amitraz,
    136b
Triazole herbicide toxicity, 131
Trichiasis, e369, e377
  causing frictional irritant
    conjunctivitis, 1140

Trichloroethylene toxicity, 1027b
Trichodectes canis, 429t
Trichogram, 164
Trichophyton mentagrophytes, causing
    blepharitis, e363-e364
Trichophyton spp., causing
    dermatophytosis, 449-451
Trichuris vulpis
  common symptoms and syndromes
    caused by, 1214t-1215t
  drugs targeting, 1335-1337
Tricuspid valve disease. See also Valvular
    heart disease
  diagnosis and treatment of, 784-794
  staging of, 787t
Tricuspid valve dysplasia, e332-e335
  diagnosis of, e332-e334
  prevalence of
    in cats, 757, 757t
    in dogs, 756, 757t
  treatment of, e334-e335
Tricuspid valve stenosis, e332
Tricyclic antidepressant drugs
  for behavior-related dermatoses,
    482-483, e177
  for urinary incontinence disorders, 917
  influence on thyroid function, 181t
  toxicity of, 112-114
Trientine, for copper-associated liver
    disease, 589
Triethanolamine polypeptide oleate, ear
    cleaner, 472-473, 472t
Trifluridine, for feline ocular herpesvirus
    1, 1158
Triiodothyronine (T3), levels in
    hypothyroidism, 178-185
Trilostane
  for adrenal-dependent
    hyperadrenocorticism, 229
  for alopecia X, 479
  for idiopathic vacuolar hepatopathy,
    607-608
  for pituitary-dependent
    hyperadrenocorticism, 225-229,
    227f
  monitoring therapy, e98
Trimethoprim sulfonamide/
    sulfamethoxazole, induced
    thrombocytopenia, 280-281
Trimethoprim/sulfadiazine, for canine
    babesiosis, 1259
Trimethoprim/sulfonamide
  associated hepatotoxicity, 581b
  for superficial bacterial folliculitis, 438t
  for toxoplasmosis, 1297
  influence on thyroid function, 181t
Tritrichomonas foetus, 528-530
  causes and prevention of treatment
    failure of, 529-530
  common symptoms and syndromes
    caused by, 1214t-1215t
  treatment of, 529f
Tritrichomonas spp. infection, dosage for
    and drugs targeting, 1335-1337
Troglitazone, for diabetes mellitus, in
    cats, e137-e138
Trombiculiasis, diagnosis and treatment
    of, 431-432

Tromethamine/
ethylenediaminetetraacetic acid
(Tris-EDTA)
in ear cleaners, 472t, 473-474
topical, for otitis, 464t
Tropicamide
causing anisocoria or mydriasis, e392
for feline uveitis, 1169t
Troponin. See Cardiac troponin I
Tru-Cut biopsy, of liver, 574-575
Trypanosoma cruzi
causing myocarditis, e303-e304
causing myositis, 1115
common symptoms and syndromes
caused by, 1212-1213,
1214t-1215t
Trypsin-like immunoreactivity (TLI),
555-557
Trypsinogen-activation peptide (TAP), for
the diagnosis of pancreatitis, 554
Tubulopapillary carcinoma, mammary,
379t
Tularemia, as cause of
thrombocytopenia, 281t-282t
Tumor ablation, for malignant
obstructions, 348
Tumor biology, e169
Tumor biopsy, and specimen submission,
322-326
Tumor excision, surgical oncology
principles for, e168-e169
Tumor immunotherapy. See
Immunotherapy
Tumor-node-metastasis staging system,
for mammary cancer, 376, 376t,
380t
Tutin, for population control, 142-144
Tylenol. See Acetaminophen
Tylosin
for canine colitis, 551b, 552
for protein-losing enteropathy, 544
target parasites and dosage of,
1335-1337
Tylosin-responsive diarrhea, 519b, 520t,
521, e262-e265
Tympanic membrane, assessment of,
471-472, 474
Tyrosine kinase inhibitor(s)
induced cardiomyopathy, 795
masitinib, 360-362
toceranib, 358-360

U
Ulna trauma in dogs, 81
Ultrafiltration, slow continuous renal,
872, 872f
Ultrasonography
fetal monitoring with, 949-951
for endocrine disorders, 167-174
for evaluation of hypercalcemia and
hyperparathyroidism, in dogs,
e69-e70
for evaluation of respiratory distress,
47
for feline gastrointestinal lymphoma,
546-547
for hemangiosarcoma, 393-394, 394f
for localizing parathyroid tissue, e71

Ultrasonography (Continued)
for pancreatitis
in cats, 566
in dogs, 561
of adrenal gland(s), 170-172
for hyperaldosteronism in cats, 240
of the eye, 1133, 1197
of the female reproductive tract, 939
of ovaries for follicular dynamics,
934
to detect ovarian remnant
syndrome, 1002
with septic mastitis, 959, 959f
of the liver
and gall bladder, 603, 604f,
e222-e223
for biliary tract disease, 603
for biopsy acquisition, 574-575, 610
for feline hepatic lipidosis, 610
for hepatobiliary disease, 573-574
for idiopathic vacuolar hepatopathy,
607
for portal vein hypoplasia, 600
for portosystemic shunt, 595
with alkaline phosphatase
elevations, e245
with superficial necrolytic dermatitis,
485-486
of the prostate
for prostatic hypertrophy, 1012
for prostatitis, 1014
of the thyroid gland, 167, 169-170
of the urinary tract, 840-845
for nephroliths and ureteroliths,
893, 903
for urinary bladder cancer, 371-372
interventional strategies for urinary
disease, 884-892
ureter, 840-845
with urachal diverticulum, 842
of the uterus
for pregnancy diagnosis, 944-945,
945f, 945t-946t
for pyometra or mucometra, 947
to determine pregnancy loss, 1004,
1006
with priapism, e355-e356, e356f
Uncinaria spp. infection, drugs targeting,
1335-1337
Upper airway obstruction, as risk for
heat-induced illness, 71
Upper motor neuron, signs with
degenerative myelopathy,
1076-1077
Upper respiratory tract infection(s)
common pathogens causing, 1222
empiric antimicrobial therapy for,
1220t
feline, 629-632
Urachal diverticulum, ultrasound
findings with, 842
Urate crystalluria, 904, 926
Urban legends of toxicology, 97-100
Ureaplasma spp. infection, causing
pregnancy loss, 1010
Urease test, for Helicobacter spp., 510
Uremia, treatment of signs with acute
renal failure, 870

Ureter(s)
bypass device placement, 888-889,
889f
interventional approach to
nephrolithiasis, 884-889
stenting, 887-888, 889f
ultrasound of, 840-845
Ureteral, stenting of malignant
obstructions, 346
Ureterocele, ultrasound findings with,
841-842
Ureterolithiasis
concurrent infections with, 893-894
medical management of, 892-896
Ureteroscopy
for essential renal hematuria, 886
for laser lithotripsy, e341
Urethra
antegrade catheterization of,
889-891
indications for perineal urethrostomy
of, 925
interventional approach to stones in,
890
lithotripsy for stones in the, e340-
e344, e342t-e343t
stent placement, 890f
ultrasound of, 840-845
Urethral
hypertonicity causing urinary
retention, 917
pressure profile, e346
stenting of malignant obstructions,
345-346, 346f
Urethral sphincter
artificial, 919-922, 920f, 921t, 922f
mechanism incompetence, 919
Urethrospasms, treatment of, 918
Uric acid, metabolism causing
urolithiasis, 901
Urinalysis
changes with hepatobiliary disease,
572
crystals in
asymptomatic, 926
urate, 904, 926
for monitoring urate urolithiasis, 903
for surveillance of hospital-acquired
urinary infections, 878
leukocyte indicators on dipsticks, 923
pH
and risk of oxalate urolithiasis, 898
monitoring, 900
target, and risk of oxalate
urolithiasis, 899t
protein in (See Proteinuria)
Urinary bladder
antegrade urethral catheterization of,
889-891
atony, treatment of, 918
interventional approach to stones,
890
minilaparotomy-cystoscopy assisted,
surgery of, for urocystoliths,
907f-908f
ultrasound of, 840-845
Urinary bladder cancer, 370-374, 371t
staging of, 371b

Urinary diseases. *See also* Renal disease; Renal failure
  albuminuria and, 849-852
  as risk factors for urinary tract infections, 881b
    hospital-acquired, 877
  calcium oxalate urolithiasis, 897-901
  causing hyperkalemia and hyponatremia, e92, e93b
  glomerular disease, 853-857
  hospital-acquired urinary tract infections, 876-879
  incontinence disorders, 915-919
    mechanical occluder devices for, 919-923
  interventional strategies for, 884-892
  laser lithotripsy for uroliths, e340-e344
  medical management of nephroliths and ureteroliths, 892-896
  minilaparotomy-assisted cystoscopy for urocystoliths, 905-909
  nephrotic syndrome, 853-857
  persistent *Escherichia coli* infection, 880-883, 881b
  proteinuria and, 849-852
  retention disorders, 915-919
  risk of hospital acquired infections, 876-879
  top questions to consultants, 923-927
  urate urolithiasis, 901-905
  use of biomarkers for diagnosis of, 846-847
  use of ultrasound for diagnosis of, 840-845
Urinary incontinence disorders
  causes of, e341
  causing vestibulitis, 970-971
  concerns regarding risk, with early age neutering, 983
  diagnosis of, 915-919, e341-e342
  mechanical occluder devices for, 919-923
  not responsive to standard therapy, 925
  treatment of, 915-919, 916t, e346-e349
    with injectable bulking agents, e345-e350, e347f
Urinary retention disorders, 915-919
  therapeutic options for, 917t
Urinary retinol-binding protein, 846-847
Urinary tract
  diagnosis of disease with ultrasound of, 840-845
  toxicity from chemotherapeutic drugs, 332
Urinary tract infections
  asymptomatic, treatment of, 924-925
  common pathogens causing, 1217, 1219-1221
  concerns regarding risk, with early age neutering, 983
  concurrent urolithiasis with, 881-882, 893-894
  conditions that predispose to, 881b
  empiric antimicrobial therapy for, 1219-1221, 1220t
  from cyclosporine, 405
  from diabetes mellitus, e77, e81

Urinary tract infections (*Continued*)
  highly resistant, treatment of, 924
  hospital-acquired asymptomatic, 876-879
  multidrug resistance in, 881
  nonantimicrobial therapies for, 882-883
  persistent *Escherichia coli* causing, 880-883, 881b, 924
  prophylactic antimicrobial therapy for, 881-883
  reinfection, 880, 924
  relapse, 880-881, 924
  superinfection, 881
  ultrasound findings with, 843, 844f
Urinary tract obstruction
  from urinary bladder cancer, 370, 373
  in ferrets with hyperadrenocorticism, e96
  potassium levels from, 253
  with portosystemic shunt, 594
Urination-induced syncope, e327
Urine
  bile acids, 573
  ketone monitoring with diabetic ketoacidosis, e81, e83
  production with acute renal failure, 869-870
  protein and albumin, 849-852
  protein and enzyme markers, 846-847
  tests for human drugs of abuse, e51
Urine antigen tests, for urinary bladder cancer, 371
Urine biomarkers, 846-847
Urine cortisol:creatinine ratio
  use of test with hyperadrenocorticism, e99
  with alopecia X, 478
Urine culture
  for surveillance of hospital-acquired urinary infections, 877-878
  why results are negative FAQ, 923-924
  with highly resistant infections, 924
  with long-term use of glucocorticoids, 418
  with recurrent infections, 924
Urine glucose
  monitoring of
    with diabetes mellitus, 197-198
    with diabetic ketoacidosis, e81, e83
  threshold for, in cats, 208
Urine protein-creatinine (UPC) ratio
  elevations from diabetes mellitus, e76
  for staging of chronic kidney disease, 859t-860t
  with glomerular disease, 849-851
  with proteinuria and albuminuria, 849, 851, 926-927
  with pyometra, 967-968
Urine specific gravity, as indicator of predicting renal failure with hyperthyroidism, 187
Urogenital
  concerns regarding, with early age neutering, 983
  disease transmission from pets to humans, 1245t, 1247-1248

Urohydropropulsion, of urate urolithiasis, 902f, 903
Urokinase, 813
Urolithiasis
  calcium oxalate, 897-901
    monitoring for recurrence, 900
    target pH of diets for, 898-899, 899t
  concurrent infections with, 893-894
  interventional approach to, 890
  laser lithotripsy for, e340-e344
  medical management of nephroliths and ureteroliths, 892-896
  minilaparotomy-assisted cystoscopy for, 905-909, 906f-907f
  percutaneous cystolithotomy for, 890
  stone basketing for, 890
  ultrasound findings with, 843, 844f
  urate, canine, 901-905, 902f
    medical dissolution of, 902-903, 902f
    reoccurrence of, 904
Ursodeoxycholic acid
  for cholelithiasis, 603-604
  for chronic hepatitis, 582, 585f, 587
  for feline cholangitis, 617-618, 617b
  for portal vein hypoplasia, 600
Ursodiol, for biliary mucoceles, e223
Urticaria, from adverse drug reactions, 488t
Urticaria pigmentosa, use of cyclosporine for, 410b
Usnic acid, associated hepatotoxicity, 581b
Uterine
  causes of vaginal discharge, 970t
  culture, 938
  cytology, 938
  hypercontractility, 954-955, 954f
  inertia causing dystocia, 951, 954f
  prolapse, 957-958
  stump granuloma, 938
  tumors, 1025-1026
Uteroverdin, 949
Uterus. *See* Pyometra
Uvea
  anatomy and physiology of, 1162
  tumors of, 1204-1205, 1204f
Uveitis
  aqueous flare causing, 1130-1131, 1131f
  canine
    causes of, e382b
    diagnosis and treatment of, 1162-1166, 1163t, 1164b, e382
    differential diagnoses of, 1163t
    from leptospirosis, 1287
    with glaucoma, 1166, 1173t
  feline
    causes of, 1167b, 1177, e382b
    diagnosis and treatment of, 1166-1170, 1169t, e382
    with glaucoma, 1178
  infectious causes of, 1218
  lens induced, 1183-1184, 1184t
  with complicated/melting corneal ulcers, 1151
  with ocular neoplasia, 1206

V

Vaccination
accidental injection of intranasal, 635
for canine respiratory infection complex, 634-635
for feline immunodeficiency virus, 1276
for feline leukemia virus, 1276
for feline upper respiratory infections, 631-632
for lyme disease, 1274-1275
of retrovirus-infected cats, 1276
with leptospirosis, effect on titers, 1288
Vaccine(s)
adverse effects of
in cats, 1252-1256
associated sarcoma, 1252-1255
in dogs, 1249-1252
causing uveitis, 1164b
allergic reactions to, 1250-1251
autoimmune reactions to, 1250-1251
failure, 1251
induced thrombocytopenia, 280-281
influence on testing for feline herpesvirus 1, 1157-1158
reporting adverse events of, to FDA, 1251, e38
tumor, 335
Vacuolar hepatopathy, 606-608
Vacuum-assisted closure
for peritoneal drainage, e17-e18
of wound, 87-90, 88b, 89f
Vagal
maneuver in cats, 753
triggers causing syncope, e326-e327, e327f-e328f
Vaginal
anomalies in the bitch, surgical repair of, 974-981, 975f, 978f
band, septum and stenosis, 979-980
culture, 937
cytology
for breeding management, 932-933
for diagnosis of disease, 937
technique for, 937
to detect ovarian remnant syndrome, 1001
with pyometra, 967
with pyometra or mucometra, 947
with septic metritis, 958
discharge, diagnosis and treatment of, 969-973
postpartum, 957
with normal gestation, 949
with pyometra, 967-968
edema, 980
endoscopy, 934
fluid changes, 933-934
hyperplasia, 980, 981f
prolapse, 980-981
Vaginitis
adult-onset, 970
concerns regarding risk, with early age neutering, 983t
diagnosis and treatment of, 969-970
puppy, 970, 978f

Vaginoscopy
for breeding management, 934, 943
use and technique of, 936-937
with ovarian remnant syndrome, 1001, 1003f
Vaginourethrogram, 979f
Vaginourethrography, retrograde, 939
Valerian associated hepatotoxicity, 581b
Valsalva leak point pressure, e346
Valvular heart disease
asymptomatic, 775-777, 790
with murmur, 786
atrial tear with, 793
classification and staging of, 775-781, 786t-787t
congestive failure with, 790-792
refractory, 780-781, 791
diagnosis and treatment of, 775-781, 784-794, 785f, 787t, 789f
pulmonary hypertension with, 793-794
ruptured chordae tendineae with, 793
surgery for, 794
with concurrent respiratory disease, 792-793
Vanadium, for diabetes mellitus, in cats, e136f, e136t, e137-e138
Vapor(s), as respiratory toxicants, e46
Vaporizer(s), for pneumonia, 687
Vascular, causes of hepatobiliary enzyme elevations, 570b
Vascular access, for shock fluid therapy, 20
Vascular disease, of the central nervous system, 1119-1126
Vascular endothelial growth factor, causing malignant effusions, 341, 344
Vascular injury, in hypercoagulable states, 298f
Vascular permeability factor, causing malignant effusions, 341
Vascular ring anomaly, prevalence of
in cats, 757t
in dogs, 757t
Vascular stenting, of malignant obstructions, 347
Vasculitis
cutaneous,topical immunomodulators for, e218-e219
from adverse reactions to vaccines, 1251
from feline upper respiratory infection, 630t
from leptospirosis, 1287
infections causing, with nervous system signs, 1212
pentoxifylline for, e204
Vasodilation, from prolonged seizures, 1060
Vasodilator drugs
adverse effects of, 768
for heart failure, in dogs, 763b, 766-768
Vasopressin
during CPR, 28-29
for seizure patients, 1061t

Vasopressin (Continued)
for the diagnosis and treatment of diabetes insipidus, e73-e75
receptor activities of, 15t
use and dosage of, 15t, 17
use of with shock, 23
Vasopressor(s)
during CPR, 28-29
for therapy of shock, 22-23
therapy for seizure patients, 1061t
use of, with feline pancreatitis, 567-568, 567t
Vasovagal syncope, e324-e325
Vector, disease transmission from pets to humans, 1248
Vehicle
effect on potency of topical steroids, 460f
for topical antimicrobials, for otitis, 462-463
Venovenous hemofiltration, slow continuous renal, 872-873, 873f
Ventilation
during CPR, 27-28
for acute respiratory distress syndrome, 50-51
issues associated with prolonged seizures, 1060-1061
mechanical during CPR, 31
Ventilation/perfusion (V/Q)
fluid therapy considerations with, 6
with hypoxemia, 52
Ventilator therapy, 55-59
available studies of, 56t
causing respiratory acidosis, e4b
causing respiratory alkalosis, e4b
choosing settings for, 55-56
complications of, 58
patient care with, 56-58
sedation for, 55
tracheostomy tube care and, 57b
weaning from, 58-59
Ventral bulla osteotomy, in cats with polyps, 656-657
Ventricular arrhythmias
in cats, 753-754
in dogs
diagnosis and treatment of, 745-748, 747f, 747t
treatment of with heart failure, 771
with dilated cardiomyopathy, 797
with congestive heart failure, 783-784
Ventricular fibrillation, 29f
drug therapy for, 30
electrical defibrillation for, 30
Ventricular premature complexes
from arrhythmogenic right ventricular cardiomyopathy, 801-804
in cats, 753-754
in dogs, with dilated cardiomyopathy, 797
treatment of, with heart failure, 771, 783-784
Ventricular septal defect (VSD), e335-e340
diagnosis of, e337-e338
left-to-right shunting with, e338-e339

Ventricular septal defect (VSD) (Continued)
pathophysiologic features of, e336-e337
prevalence of
in cats, 757, 757t
in dogs, 756, 757t
right-to-left shunting with, e339-e340
surgery for, e339
Ventricular tachycardia, 746-748, 747f, 747t
cardioversion for, e290
causing syncope, e326
in cats, 750f-751f, 753-754
in dogs, with dilated cardiomyopathy, 797
treatment of with heart failure, 771, 783-784
Ventriculoperitoneal shunt, for hydrocephalus, 1036-1037, 1037f
Verapamil, toxicity of, use of IV lipid emulsion therapy for, 106
Vertebrate pest species pesticides, 142-144
Vesicles, from adverse drug reactions, 488t
Vestibular
anatomy, 1066-1067
central system, 1067
peripheral system, 1066
Vestibular disease
causes of, 1068-1069
congenital, 1068
from hypothyroidism, 1068, e84, e84-e85, e86
from neoplasia, 1068-1069
idiopathic, 1068
paradoxic, 1068-1069
peripheral and central, 1066-1070, 1067t
with nasopharyngeal disorders, 654
Vestibulitis, 970-971
Vestibulovaginal malformations, 971-972
Veterinary Perinatal Service, 950
Vetsulin. See Porcine Lente insulin
Vidarabine, for feline ocular herpesvirus 1, 1158
Vinblastine, extravasation and tissue sloughing from, 333
Vincristine
adverse effects of, 331
extravasation and tissue sloughing from, 333
for feline gastrointestinal lymphoma, 547-548, 548t
for hemangiosarcoma, 395-396
for multiple myeloma, 386
for thrombocytopenia, 285
rescue chemotherapy for canine lymphoma, 381-383
Vinorelbine, e140t, e141
extravasation and tissue sloughing from, 333
Vinyl chloride toxicity, 1027b
Vinylidene chloride toxicity, 1027b
Viral infection(s)
causing conjunctivitis, 1141-1142
causing myocarditis, e304t

Viral infection(s) (Continued)
causing pregnancy loss, 1005t, 1009-1010
causing skin disease, in cats, e194-e197
causing skin lesions in cats, e194-e197
causing thrombocytopenia, 281t-282t
causing uveitis in dogs, 1164b
causing vulvar discharge, 972
common symptoms and syndromes caused by, 1215t
immunotherapy for, 1229-1233, 1230t
Viral papilloma, ocular, 1204
Virchow's triad
factors causing thrombosis, 298f, 705
from heat-induced illness, 71
Virus isolation, for canine infectious respiratory diseases, 633
Vision
assessment of, e390-e391
evaluation of, 1134-1138
grid to record visual status and reflexes, e389f
loss of (See also Blindness)
from canine uveitis, 1163t
with canine glaucoma, and surgical options, 1174-1175, 1176b
Visual pathway
defects of the, e390f
lesions of the, e393f
signs of lesions in, e393f, e393t
Vitamin A
for actinic dermatoses, 481
for sebaceous adenitis, e210-e211
requirements during pregnancy and lactation, 963
responsive dermatosis, 476
toxicity of, 99
Vitamin B complex, drug incompatibilities with, 33t
Vitamin B_1, drug incompatibilities with, 33t
Vitamin B_{12}. See Cobalamin; Cobalamin deficiency
Vitamin B_3, for hyperlipidemia, 265
Vitamin C, drug incompatibilities with, 33t
Vitamin D
for evaluation of hypocalcemia, e125f
for postpartum puerperal tetany, 960
requirements during pregnancy and lactation, 963
role of, in idiopathic hypercalcemia in cats, 245-246
supplements for hypocalcemia, e127-e128, e128t, e129
toxicity of, 99
Vitamin E
as hepatic support therapy, e255-e256
for chronic hepatitis, 587
for liver failure, 582
for protein-losing enteropathy, 543
for retinal dystrophy, 1190-1191
Vitamin K_1
deficiency
from feline hepatic lipidosis, 610, 612
from hepatobiliary disease, 572
from liver failure, 582

Vitamin K_1 (Continued)
for hepatic-disease associated coagulopathy, e257
for protein-losing enteropathy, 543
for rodenticide toxicity, 133-134
supplementation with liver failure, 582
Vitiligo, of the eyelid, e367
Vitis fruit toxicity, 149
Vivonex, 542
Vizsla(s)
polymyositis in, 1114
sebaceous adenitis ion, e209-e210
VLA Quality Assurance System, 308-309
Vogt-Koyanagi-Harada-like syndrome
causing canine uveitis, 1164
of eyelid, e367-e368
Volvulus, gastric dilation and, e13-e20
Vomiting
chronic, from Helicobacter spp., 508-513
control of
with acute pancreatitis in dogs, 562-563
with canine parvovirus, 535
from intestinal motility disorders, 513-518
from uremia with acute renal failure, 870
induced syncope, e327
induction of, 105
von Willebrand disease, 286-291
blood products for, 290t
direct mutation test for, 1018t-1020t
subtype classification, 288t
Voriconazole
adverse effects of, 1237
for fungal rhinitis in cats, 647t
for nasal aspergillosis, 639-640
use and protocols for, 1235t, 1237
Vulva hooded, 971, 971f, 978f
Vulvar discharge
diagnosis and treatment of, 969-973, 971f
from pyometra or mucometra, 947
Vulvar hypoplasia, 977
Vulvar softening, 932

W

Wahoo, toxicity of, 124t
Walchia americana, 431-432
Warfarin (Coumadin)
for arterial thromboembolism, 815
for feline thromboembolism, 810
for hypercoagulable states, 299
for thromboprophylaxis, 708-709
Warfarin rodenticide toxicity, 133-134
Water, as antipruritic agent, 419
Wedge biopsy, of liver, 574-575
Weight gain
diagnosis and treatment of obesity, 254-260
during pregnancy, 961-963, 962f
Weight loss
diets, 255-259
from protein losing enteropathy, 541
with cancer cachexia, 349-354

Weimaraner(s)
  cervical spondylomyelopathy in, 1092
  hypertrophic osteodystrophy in, 1251
  masticatory muscle myositis in, 1199
  pruritic alopecia in, 164
  risk of vaccine hypersensitivity in,
    1250-1251
  vaccine reactions in, 1250
West Highland white terrier(s)
  atopic dermatitis in, 403
  copper-associated hepatopathy in,
    571b
  direct mutation tests for, 1018t-1020t
  glaucoma in, 1171b
  hyperplastic dermatosis in, e201
  hypoadrenocorticism in, 233
  intracranial arachnoid cysts in, 1038
  metabolic brain disorder in, 1052
  plasmacytomas in, 386
  pulmonary fibrosis in, 501, e267
  risk of urinary bladder cancer in,
    371t
  sick sinus syndrome in, 732-733
Wheals, from adverse drug reactions,
    488t
Wheelchairs, for rehabilitation, e359
WhelpWise veterinary orders, 952f
Whippet(s)
  actinic dermatoses in, 480
  avermectin toxicity in, 145
  direct mutation tests for, 1018t-1020t
  glaucoma in, 1171b
  thyroid hormone differences in, 180t
White flower oil toxicity, 125t
Willow, white toxicity, 125t
Windhound(s), avermectin toxicity in,
    145
Windshield washer fluid toxicity, 151
Wintergreen oil toxicity, 125t
Wipes, for pyoderma, 441t
Wirehaired terrier(s)
  risk of bladder cancer in, 371t
  sebaceous gland hyperplasia in,
    476-477
  von Willebrand disease in, 288-289,
    288t
Wireless motility capsule, for evaluation
    of gastric emptying, 514-515, 515f
Wobbler syndrome. See Cervical
    spondylomyelopathy
Wolbachia, role in heartworm disease,
    820, 826
Wolf's bane, toxicity of, 124t
Wood's lamp examination, for
    dermatophytosis, in multicat
    environments, 449, 453
Woody, toxicity of, 124t

Wound care
  and vacuum-assisted wound closure,
    87-90
  closure and, 88
  with open fractures, 84-86
Wound healing, 87

X
X-lined factor deficiencies, 289
Xanthine oxidase inhibitor(s), for
    dissolution of urate stones, 902
Xanthine urolithiasis, dose of allopurinol
    to dissolve urates and prevent,
    903-904
Xenobiotic(s), causing nephrotoxicity, e29
Xeromycteria, in dogs, 643
XX disorders of sexual development,
    994-996, 995t
XY disorders of sexual development,
    997-999
Xylazine
  for emesis induction, 105
  for retrograde ejaculation, e351-e352
  use of, with cardiovascular
    dysfunction, 64-65
Xylene toxicity, 1027b
Xylitol toxicity, 98, 149-150, 570b, 581b

Y
Yeast bread dough toxicity, 147
Yersinia pestis
  causing infection in humans, 1246
  causing thrombocytopenia, 281t-282t
  common symptoms and syndromes
    caused by, 1213t
Yew toxicity, 121b
Yohimbine, 30
  action and use of, for motility
    disorders, 517-518
  as antidote, e56t
  for retrograde ejaculation, e351-e352
Yorkshire terrier(s)
  acinar hypoplasia in, 1144
  alopecia in, 164
  atlantoaxial subluxation in, 1083
  Chiari-like malformation in, 1101
  encephalitis in, 1063
  hydrocephalus in, 1034
  intracranial arachnoid cysts in, 1038
  mammary tumors in, 375
  mitochondrial encephalopathy in,
    1048-1051, 1049t, 1051t
  ovarian tumors in, 1024
  portosystemic shunts in, 594
  protein-losing enteropathies in, 540-541
  risk of urolithiasis in, 892, 897
Yucca schidigera, for flatulence, e250

Z
Zafirlukast, for feline asthma, 678
Zalcitabine, for feline retrovirus
    infections, 1278, 1279t
Zaleplon, toxicity of, 113-114
Zidovudine (AZT), for feline retrovirus
    infections, 1277-1278, 1279t
Zileuton, for feline asthma, 678
Zinc
  role of, with diabetes mellitus, 202
  to restrict copper update, e236
  toxicity, from coin ingestion, 99-100
Zinc acetate, for flatulence, e250
Zinc chloride, in Febreze, 98
Zinc phosphide toxicity, 134-135
Zinc therapy
  for copper-associated liver disease,
    590
  for hepatoencephalopathy, 593
Zinc-responsive dermatosis, causing
    blepharitis, e365
Zolazepam, toxicity of, 113-114
Zoledronate, for osteosarcoma, 391-392
Zollinger-Ellison syndrome
  imaging for diagnosis of, 174
  proton pump inhibitors for, 118
Zolpidem toxicity, 113-114
Zonisamide
  associated hepatotoxicity, 570b, 578,
    581b
  for intracranial tumors, 1041t
  for seizures, 1056-1057
Zoonosis, 1244-1249, 1245t
  and disinfection of environments with
    staphylococcal spp., 455
  associated with raw meat diets, 1248,
    1291
  from dermatophytosis, 449, 450b
  from intranasal vaccination, 635
  from methicillin-resistant
    Staphylococcal infections, 444
  from toxoplasmosis, 1297-1298,
    1298b
  individuals at risk for, 1246b
  prevention of, 1248-1249
  route of transmission of, 1244-1248
  spread from animals to humans,
    1245t
  with American leishmaniasis, e396
  with Bartonella spp., 1266, 1270-1271
  with Brucella canis, 972
  with brucellosis, e402
  with Giardia spp., 531
  with Helicobacter spp., 509
  with Malassezia spp. infections, e213
Zygomycosis, antifungal therapy for,
    1234-1238